PHYSICAL MEDICINE AND REHABILITATION

SECOND EDITION

Associate Editors

Ralph M. Buschbacher, M.D.
Clinical Assistant Professor
Department of Physical Medicine and Rehabilitation
Indiana University Hospital
Indianapolis, Indiana

Daniel Dumitru, M.D., Ph.D.
Professor and Residency Program Director
Department of Rehabilitation Medicine
University of Texas Health Science Center at San Antonio
San Antonio, Texas

Ernest W. Johnson, M.D.
Professor, Department of Physical Medicine and Rehabilitation
Ohio State University College of Medicine
Dean of External Affairs
College of Medicine and Public Health
Columbus, Ohio

Dennis J. Matthews, M.D.
Associate Clinical Professor
Department of Rehabilitation Medicine
University of Colorado School of Medicine
Chairman and Medical Director
The Children's Hospital Rehabilitation Center
Denver, Colorado

Mehrsheed Sinaki, M.D., M.S.
Consultant, Department of Physical Medicine and Rehabilitation
Mayo Clinic and Mayo Foundation
Professor of Physical Medicine and Rehabilitation, Mayo Medical School
Rochester, Minnesota

PHYSICAL MEDICINE AND REHABILITATION

SECOND EDITION

Randall L. Braddom, M.D., M.S.

CEO and Medical Director
Wishard Health Services
Indianapolis, Indiana

W.B. SAUNDERS COMPANY

A Harcourt Health Sciences Company

Philadelphia London New York St. Louis Sydney Toronto

W.B. SAUNDERS COMPANY

A Harcourt Health Sciences Company

The Curtis Center
Independence Square West
Philadelphia, Pennsylvania 19106

Library of Congress Cataloging-in-Publication Data

Physical medicine and rehabilitation / editor, Randall L. Braddom ; associate editors, Ralph M. Buschbacher . . . [et al.].—2nd ed.
p. ; cm.
Includes bibliographical references and index.
ISBN 0-7216-8076-3
1. Physical therapy. 2. Medical rehabilitation. I. Braddom, Randall L. II. Buschbacher, Ralph M. III. Physical medicine & rehabilitation.
[DNLM: 1. Physical Medicine. 2. Rehabilitation. WB 460 P5774 2000]
RM700 .P465 2000
615.8′2—dc21
00-025389

PHYSICAL MEDICINE AND REHABILITATION ISBN 0-7216-8076-3

Printed in the United States of America.

Last digit is the print number: 9 8 7 6 5 4 3 2 1

This book is dedicated to
Carolyn Jean Lentz Braddom, Ed.D.,
the most remarkable person
I have ever known.

CONTRIBUTORS

JUDY ADKINS, O.T.R.
Department of Occupational Therapy
Indiana University Medical Center
Indianapolis, Indiana
Chapter 18, Prescription of Wheelchairs and Seating Systems

JAMES C. AGRE, M.D., Ph.D.
Physiatrist
Howard Young Medical Center
Woodruff, Wisconsin
Chapter 46, Rehabilitation Concepts in Motor Neuron Diseases

AUGUSTA S. ALBA, M.D.
Associate Professor
Clinical Rehabilitation Medicine
New York University Medical Center
Chief
Rehabilitation Medicine
Coler Goldwater Memorial Hospital
New York, New York
Chapter 33, Concepts in Pulmonary Rehabilitation

RENÉE J. ANDERSEN, O.T.
Occupational Therapist
Department of Physical Medicine and Rehabilitation
Mayo Clinic and Mayo Foundation
Rochester, Minnesota
Chapter 26, Rehabilitation of Patients with Swallowing Disorders

KAREN L. ANDREWS, M.D.
Assistant Professor
Mayo Medical School
Consultant
Department of Physical Medicine and Rehabilitation
Director
Amputee Services
Mayo Foundation for Educational Research
Rochester, Minnesota
Chapter 56, Vascular Disease: Evaluation and Management

JAMES W. ATCHINSON, D.O.
Associate Professor
Department of Orthopaedics and Rehabilitation
Division of Physical Medicine and Rehabilitation
University of Florida, College of Medicine
Gainesville, Florida
Chapter 20, Manipulation, Traction, and Massage

MATTHEW N. BARTELS, M.D., M.P.H.
Assistant Professor of Clinical Rehabilitation Medicine
College of Physicians and Surgeons
Columbia University
Director of Cardiac and Pulmonary Rehabilitation/ Director of Human Performance Laboratory
New York–Presbyterian Hospital
Columbia Presbyterian Campus
New York, New York
Chapter 32, Cardiac Rehabilitation

CLAIRE E. BENDER, M.D.
Consultant
Department of Diagnostic Radiology
Mayo Clinic and Mayo Foundation
Associate Professor of Radiology
Mayo Medical School
Rochester, Minnesota
Chapter 26, Rehabilitation of Patients with Swallowing Disorders

DONNA JO BLAKE, M.D.
Associate Professor
Department of Rehabilitation Medicine
University of Colorado Health Sciences Center
Staff Physician
Denver Veterans Affairs Medical Center
Denver, Colorado
Chapter 35, Employment of Persons with Disabilities

DONNA BLOODWORTH, M.D.
Assistant Professor
Department of Physical Medicine and Rehabilitation
Baylor College of Medicine
Houston, Texas
Chapter 42, Chronic Pain Syndromes: Evaluation and Treatment

CORWIN BOAKE, Ph.D.
Assistant Professor
Department of Physical Medicine and Rehabilitation
University of Texas–Houston Medical School
Neuropsychologist
The Institute for Rehabilitation and Research
Houston, Texas
Chapter 49, Brain Injury Rehabilitation

RANDALL L. BRADDOM, M.D., M.S.
CEO and Medical Director
Wishard Health Services
Indianapolis, Indiana
Chapter 18, Prescription of Wheelchairs and Seating Systems

SUSAN BRAUN, M.L.S., O.T.R.
Information Specialist
Uniform Data System for Medical Rehabilitation
State University of New York at Buffalo
Buffalo, New York
Chapter 8, Quality and Outcome Measures for Medical Rehabilitation

ANDREW D. BRONSTEIN, M.D.
Clinical Assistant Professor
Department of Radiology
University of Washington
Seattle, Washington
Radiology Consultants of Washington
Bellevue, Washington
Chapter 7, Neurological and Musculoskeletal Studies

ALLEN W. BROWN, M.D.
Assistant Professor
Department of Physical Medicine and Rehabilitation
Mayo Medical School
Medical Director
Brain Rehabilitation Services
Consultant
Department of Physical Medicine and Rehabilitation
Mayo Clinic
Rochester, Minnesota
Chapter 21, Physical Agent Modalities

LOIS BUSCHBACHER, M.D.
Clinical Assistant Professor
Department of Physical Medicine and Rehabilitation
Indiana University School of Medicine
Indianapolis, Indiana
Chapter 47, Rehabilitation of Patients with Peripheral Neuropathies

RALPH M. BUSCHBACHER, M.D.
Clinical Associate Professor and Interim Chair
Department of Physical Medicine and Rehabilitation
Indiana University School of Medicine
Indianapolis, Indiana
Chapter 18, Prescription of Wheelchairs and Seating Systems
Chapter 34, Deconditioning, Conditioning, and the Benefits of Exercise

OCTAVIO CALVILLO, M.D., Ph.D.
Associate Professor
Director, Center for Pain Medicine
Department of Anesthesiology
Baylor College of Medicine
Houston, Texas
Chapter 42, Chronic Pain Syndromes: Evaluation and Treatment

DENISE I. CAMPAGNOLO, M.D., Ph.D.
Associate Professor
Department of Physical Medicine and Rehabilitation
UMDNJ–New Jersey Medical School
Clinical Director
Spinal Cord Injury Program
University Hospital
Newark, New Jersey
Chapter 9, Research in Physical Medicine and Rehabilitation

DIANA D. CARDENAS, M.D.
Professor
Department of Rehabilitation Medicine
University of Washington
Project Director
Northwest Regional Spinal Cord Injury System
University of Washington Medical Center
Seattle, Washington
Chapter 27, Management of Bladder Dysfunction

STEPHANIE K. CARLSON, M.D.
Senior Associate Consultant
Department of Diagnostic Radiology
Mayo Clinic and Mayo Foundation
Rochester, Minnesota
Chapter 26, Rehabilitation of Patients with Swallowing Disorders

BRIAN A. CASAZZA, M.D.
Clinical Assistant Professor
Department of Physical Medicine and Rehabilitation
University of Virginia School of Medicine
Staff Physiatrist
Martha Jefferson Hospital
Charlottesville, Virginia
Chapter 39, Musculoskeletal Disorders of the Lower Limbs

KEVIN M. CAVES, B.S.M.E., A.T.P.
Director
RERC on Communication Enhancement
Clinical Associate
Department of Surgery
Duke University Medical Center
Durham, North Carolina
Chapter 23, Computer Assistive Devices and Environmental Controls

ANDREW J. COLE, M.D.
Clinical Assistant Professor
Department of Physical Medicine and Rehabilitation
University of Washington Medical Center
Seattle, Washington
Medical Director
The Spine Center at Overlake Hospital and Medical Center
Bellevue, Washington
Chapter 7, Neurological and Musculoskeletal Imaging Studies

ANN C. COTTER, M.D.
Clinical Assistant Professor
University of Medicine and Dentistry of New Jersey
Medical Director
Mind Body Center for Complementary Medicine
Morristown Memorial Hospital
Associates in Rehabilitation Medicine
Morristown, New Jersey
Chapter 20, Manipulation, Traction, and Massage

BARBARA J. deLATEUR M.D., M.S.
Professor and Director
Department of Physical Medicine and Rehabilitation
Johns Hopkins University School of Medicine
Baltimore, Maryland
Chapter 19, Therapeutic Exercise

ANNE DEUTSCH, M.S., R.N., C.R.R.N.
Adjunct Instructor
School of Nursing
Research Analyst
Uniform Data System for Medical Rehabilitation
State University of New York at Buffalo
Buffalo, New York
Chapter 8, Quality and Outcome Measures for Medical Rehabilitation

JULIUS P. A. DEWALD, P.T., Ph.D.
Assistant Professor
Departments of Physical Therapy and Human Movement Science, Physical Medicine and Rehabilitation, and Biomedical Engineering
Northwestern University
Senior Clinical Research Scientist
Rehabilitation Institute of Chicago
Chicago, Illinois
Chapter 29, Spasticity

MARY E. DILLON, M.D.
Medical Director of Physical Medicine and Rehabilitation
Clinton Memorial Hospital
Wilmington, Ohio
Chapter 60, Rehabilitation Management in Persons with AIDS and HIV Infection

MARY L. DOMBOVY, M.D.
Associate Professor of Neurology and Rehabilitation
University of Rochester
Vice President
Managed Care and Integrated Services
Chair
Department of Physical Medicine and Rehabilitation
Unity Health System
Rochester, New York
Chapter 51, Rehabilitation Concerns in Degenerative Movement Disorders of the Central Nervous System

DANIEL DUMITRU, M.D., Ph.D.
Professor and Residency Program Director
Department of Rehabilitation Medicine
University of Texas Health Science Center at San Antonio
University Hospital and Audie Murphy Veterans Hospital
San Antonio, Texas
Chapter 10, Electrodiagnostic Medicine I: Basic Aspects

ALBERTO ESQUENAZI, M.D.
Associate Professor
Temple University and Drexel University
Director
Gait and Motion Analysis Laboratory and the Regional Amputee Rehabilitation Center
Moss Rehabilitation
Philadelphia, Pennsylvania
Chapter 5, Gait Analysis: Technology and Clinical Applications
Chapter 13, Upper Limb Amputee Rehabilitation and Prosthetic Restoration

FRANK J. E. FALCO, M.D.
Clinical Assistant Professor
Department of Physical Medicine and Rehabilitation
Temple University School of Medicine
Philadelphia, Pennsylvania
Medical Director
Mid-Atlantic Pain Institute
Wilmington, Delaware
Elkton, Maryland
Chapter 37, Assessment and Treatment of Cervical Spine Disorders

VIRGIL W. FAULKNER, C.P.O.
Associate Professor
Hong Kong, Polytechnic University
Hong Kong, China
Chapter 14, Lower Limb Prostheses

GERALD FELSENTHAL, M.D.
Clinical Professor
University of Maryland School of Medicine
Chief
Department of Rehabilitation Medicine
Sinai Hospital of Baltimore
Baltimore, Maryland
Chapter 59, Principles of Geriatric Rehabilitation

ROGER C. FIEDLER, Ph.D.
Assistant Professor of Rehabilitation Medicine
University at Buffalo
Associate Professor of Occupational Therapy
D'Youville College
Buffalo, New York
Chapter 8, Quality and Outcome Measures for Medical Rehabilitation

STEVEN V. FISHER, M.D.
Associate Professor
University of Minnesota Medical School
Medical Director of Rehabilitation Services
Hennepin County Medical Center
Minneapolis, Minnesota
Chapter 17, Spinal Orthoses in Rehabilitation

DAVID J. FORDYCE, Ph.D.
Section of Physical Medicine and Rehabilitation
Neuropsychology and Rehabilitation Psychology
Virginia Mason Medical Center
Seattle, Washington
Chapter 4, Psychological Perspectives on Rehabilitation: Contemporary Assessment and Intervention Strategies

GERARD E. FRANCISCO, M.D.
Clinical Assistant Professor
Department of Physical Medicine and Rehabilitation
University of Texas Health Science Center
Baylor College of Medicine
Associate Director
Brain Injury Program
The Institute for Rehabilitation and Research
Houston, Texas
Chapter 49, Brain Injury Rehabilitation

FREDERICK S. FROST, M.D.
The Cleveland Clinic Foundation
Cleveland, Ohio
Chapter 55, Spinal Cord Injury Medicine

DEBORAH GAEBLER-SPIRA, M.D.
Associate Professor
Department of Physical Medicine and Rehabilitation
Assistant Professor
Department of Pediatrics
Norwestern University Medical School
Attending Physician
Pediatric and Adolescent Rehabilitation
Rehabilitation Institute of Chicago
Chicago, Illinois
Chapter 53, Rehabilitation of Children and Adults with Cerebral Palsy

JAN C. GALVIN, L.L.C.
The Galvin Group, Ltd.
Tucson, Arizona
Chapter 23, Computer Assistive Devices and Environmental Controls

LAURA M. GARBER, O.T.R., C.H.T.
Clinical Supervisor
Professional Rehabilitative Services, Inc., P.A.
Kansas City, Kansas
Chapter 15, Upper Limb Orthotic Devices

FAE H. GARDEN, M.D.
Associate Professor
Department of Physical Medicine and Rehabilitation
Baylor College of Medicine
Houston, Texas
Chapter 57, Principles of Cancer Rehabilitation

DIANE M.-L. GILBERT, M.D.
Clinical Faculty
University of Texas Health Science Center
San Antonio, Texas
Chapter 30, Sexuality Issues in Persons with Disabilities

THERESA A. GILLIS, M.D.
Associate Professor
Chief, Section of Physical Medicine and Rehabilitation
Medical Director, Rehabilitation Services
University of Texas M. D. Anderson Cancer Center
Houston, Texas
Chapter 57, Principles of Cancer Rehabilitation

ROBERT J. GOLDMAN, M.D.
Assistant Professor
Department of Rehabilitation Medicine
University of Pennsylvania School of Medicine
Director
Comprehensive Chronic Wound Program
Attending Physician Hospital of the University of Pennsylvania, Presbyterian Hospital
University of Pennsylvania Healthcare System
Philadelphia, Pennsylvania
Chapter 31, Prevention and Management of Pressure Ulcers and Other Chronic Wounds

MARTIN GRABOIS, M.D.
Professor and Chairman
Department of Physical Medicine and Rehabilitation
Baylor College of Medicine
Chief of Service
Department of Physical Medicine and Rehabilitation
The Methodist Hospital
Houston, Texas
Chapter 42, Chronic Pain Syndromes: Evaluation and Treatment

CARL V. GRANGER, M.D.
Professor and Chairman
Department of Rehabilitation Medicine
Director
Center for Functional Assessment Research
Uniform Data System for Medical Rehabilitation
University at Buffalo
Buffalo, New York
Chapter 8, Quality and Outcome Measures for Medical Rehabilitation

RICHARD L. HARVEY, M.D., M.P.H.
Assistant Professor
Department of Physical Medicine and Rehabilitation
Northwestern University Medical School
Wesley and Suzanne Dixon Stroke Chair
The Rehabilitation Institute of Chicago
Chicago, Illinois
Chapter 50, Rehabilitation of Stroke Syndromes

ROSS M. HAYS, M.D.
Associate Professor
Department of Rehabilitation Medicine and Pediatrics
University of Washington School of Medicine
Children's Hospital and Regional Medical Center
Seattle, Washington
Chapter 54, Rehabilitation Concepts in Myelomeningocele

PHALA A. HELM, M.D.
Professor
Department of Physical Medicine and Rehabilitation
University of Texas Southwestern Medical Center
Parkland Hospital
Zale Lipshy Hospital
Dallas, Texas
Chapter 56, Vascular Disease: Evaluation and Management

WILLIAM J. HENNESSEY, M.D.
Medical Director
Rehabilitation Services
Latrobe Area Hospital
Latrobe, Pennyslvania
President
Pennsylvania Physical Medicine
Greensburg, Pennsylvania
Chapter 16, Lower Limb Orthoses

CINDY B. IVANHOE, M.D.
Assistant Professor
Department of Physical Medicine and Rehabilitation
Baylor College of Medicine
Director
Brain Injury Program
The Institute for Rehabilitation and Research
Houston, Texas
Chapter 49, Brain Injury Rehabilitation

REBECCA D. JACKSON, M.D.
Associate Professor of Internal Medicine and Physical Medicine and Rehabilitation
Division of Endocrinology, Diabetes, and Metabolism
Ohio State University
Columbus, Ohio
Chapter 22, Electrical Stimulation

ERNEST W. JOHNSON, M.D.
Professor
Department of Physical Medicine and Rehabilitation
Ohio State University
Dean of External Affairs
College of Medicine and Public Health
Columbus, Ohio
Chapter 16, Lower Limb Orthoses
Chapter 38, Upper Limb Musculoskeletal Pain Syndromes

MARK V. JOHNSTON, Ph.D.
Associate Professor
Department of Physical Medicine and Rehabilitation
New Jersey Medical School
University of Medicine and Dentistry of New Jersey
Newark, New Jersey
Director of Outcomes Research
Kessler Medical Rehabilitation Research and Education Corporation
West Orange, New Jersey
Chapter 8, Quality and Outcome Measures for Medical Rehabilitation

RICHARD T. KATZ, M.D.
Associate Clinical Professor of Physical Medicine and Rehabilitation
University of Kansas
Kansas City, Kansas
Chapter 9, Research in Physical Medicine and Rehabilitation
Chapter 29, Spasticity

MARGARET KELLY-HAYES, Ed.D. R.N., C.R.R.N.
Clinical Professor
Department of Neurology
Boston University School of Medicine
Boston, Massachusetts
Investigator
Framingham Heart Study
Framingham, Massachusetts
Chapter 8, Quality and Outcome Measures for Medical Rehabilitation

JOHN C. KING, M.D., B.S.E.E.
Associate Professor
Department of Rehabilitation Medicine
University of Texas Health Science Center at San Antonio
Staff Physician
South Texas Veterans Health Care System
Audie L. Murphy Division
San Antonio, Texas
Chapter 28, Neurogenic Bowel: Dysfunction and Management

SUNIL KOTHARI, M.D.
Fellow, Brain Injury Rehabilitation
Department of Physical Medicine and Rehabilitation
Baylor College of Medicine
The Institute for Rehabilitation and Research
Houston, Texas
Chapter 49, Brain Injury Rehabilitation

FRANCIS P. LAGATTUTA, M.D.
Assistant Clinical Professor
Loyola University Stritch School of Medicine
Maywood, Illinois
Chapter 37, Assessment and Treatment of Cervical Spine Disorders

EDWARD R. LASKOWSKI, M.D.
Associate Professor
Department of Physical Medicine and Rehabilitation
Mayo Medical School
Consultant
Mayo Clinic and Mayo Foundation
Rochester, Minnesota
Chapter 44, Concepts in Sports Medicine

BRIAN LAY, B.S.
Rehabilitation Technology Specialist
Hamilton's ATS
Indianapolis, Indiana
Chapter 18, Prescription of Wheelchairs and Seating Systems

JEFFREY A. LEHMAN, M.D.
Attending Physiatrist
Sinai Hospital
Baltimore, Maryland
Chapter 59, Principles of Geriatric Rehabilitation

TED A. LENNARD, M.D.
Clinical Assistant Professor
Department of Physical Medicine and Rehabilitation
University of Arkansas for Medical Sciences
Little Rock, Arkansas
Springfield Physical Medicine and Rehabilitation
Springfield, Missouri
Chapter 24, Joint and Soft Tissue Injection Techniques

ELLEN I. LEONARD, M.D.
Clinical Associate Professor
University of Texas Health Science Center
Pediatric Medical Director
Warm Springs Rehabilitation Hospital
San Antonio, Texas
Chapter 14, Lower Limb Prostheses

MARIA LOMBA, M.D.
Assistant Professor
University of Texas Health Science Center
San Antonio, Texas
Medical Director
Rehabilitation Institute at McKenna Hospital
New Braunfels, Texas
Chapter 14, Lower Limb Prostheses

SHANE E. MACAULAY, M.D.
Clinical Assistant Professor
University of Washington
Seattle, Washington
Radiology Consultants of Washington
Bellevue, Washington
Chapter 7, Neurological and Musculoskeletal Imaging Studies

TERESA L. MASSAGLI, M.D.
Associate Professor
Department of Rehabilitation Medicine and Pediatrics
University of Washington School of Medicine
Attending Physician
Children's Hospital and Regional Medical Center
Seattle, Washington
Chapter 54, Rehabilitation Concepts in Myelomeningocele

DENNIS J. MATTHEWS, M.D.
Associate Clinical Professor
Department of Rehabilitation Medicine
University of Colorado School of Medicine
Chairman and Medical Director
The Children's Hospital Rehabilitation Center
Denver, Colorado
Chapter 2, Examination of the Pediatric Patient
Chapter 46, Rehabilitation Concepts in Motor Neuron Diseases

MICHAEL E. MAYO, M.B.B.S.
Professor
Director, Residency Program
Department of Urology
University of Washington School of Medicine
Seattle, Washington
Chapter 27, Management of Bladder Dysfunction

ROBERT D. McANELLY, M.D.
Associate
Mountain Rehabilitation Services
Las Vegas, Nevada
Chapter 14, Lower Limb Prostheses

LISA A. McPEAK, M.D.
Associate Professor
Department of Rehabilitation Medicine
University of Kansas Medical Center
Medical Director
Rehabilitation Unit
Baptist Medical Center
Kansas City, Missouri
Chapter 1, Physiatric History and Examination

CRISTINA M. MIX, O.T.R./L.
Occupational Therapist
Arlington Pediatric Therapy Management Services, Ltd.
Arlington Heights, Illinois
Chapter 25, Achieving Functional Independence

BAHRAM MOKRI, M.D.
Professor of Neurology
Mayo Medical School
Consultant
Department of Neurology
Mayo Clinic and Mayo Foundation
Rochester, Minnesota
Chapter 40, Low Back Pain and Disorders of the Lumbar Spine

JONATHAN R. MOLDOVER, M.D.
Chairman
Department of Physical Medicine and Rehabilitation
Beth Israel Medical Center
St. Luke's/Roosevelt Hospital
New York, New York
Chapter 32, Cardiac Rehabilitation

W. JERRY MYSIW, M.D.
Bert C. Wiley Professor
Department of Physical Medicine and Rehabilitation
The Ohio State University
Columbus, Ohio
Chapter 22, Electrical Stimulation

MARGE C. NELSON, O.T.
Occupational Therapist
Department of Physical Medicine and Rehabilitation
Mayo Clinic and Mayo Foundation
Rochester, Minnesota
Chapter 26, Rehabilitation of Patients with Swallowing Disorders

MAUREEN R. NELSON, M.D.
Associate Professor
Physical Medicine and Rehabilitation, Pediatrics
Baylor College of Medicine
Chief
Department of Physical Medicine and Rehabilitation
Texas Children's Hospital
Houston, Texas
Chapter 48, Rehabilitation Concerns in Myopathies

JOHN J. NICHOLAS, M.D.
Chairman and Professor
Department of Physical Medicine and Rehabilitation
Temple University School of Medicine
Philadelphia, Pennsylvania
Chapter 24, Joint and Soft Tissue Injection Techniques
Chapter 36, Rehabilitation of Patients with Rheumatological Disorders

STEPHEN F. NOLL, M.D.
Assistant Professor of Physical Medicine and Rehabilitation
Mayo Medical School
Consultant
Department of Physical Medicine and Rehabilitation
Mayo Clinic and Mayo Foundation
Rochester, Minnesota
Chapter 26, Rehabilitation of Patients with Swallowing Disorders

MICHAEL W. O'DELL, M.D.
Assistant Professor
Department of Physical Medicine and Rehabilitation
Albert Einstein College of Medicine
New York, New York
Medical Director
Regional Center for Brain Injury and Rehabilitation
Bay Shore, New York
Chapter 60, Rehabilitation Management in Persons with AIDS and HIV Infection

ANTHONY ORESTE, M.D.
Clinical Instructor
Department of Physical Medicine and Rehabilitation
Albert Einstein College of Medicine
New York, New York
Head
Section of Adult Physical Medicine and Rehabilitation
Long Island Jewish Medical Center
New Hyde Park, New York
Chapter 60, Rehabilitation Management in Persons with AIDS and HIV Infection

ATUL T. PATEL, M.D.
Associate Professor
Department of Rehabilitation Medicine
University of Kansas Medical Center
Medical Director of Rehabilitation Services
Research Medical Center
Kansas City, Missouri
Chapter 15, Upper Limb Orthotic Devices

BARBARA A. PIPPIN, M.D.
Resident Physician
Department of Physical Medicine and Rehabilitation
University of Rochester
Rochester, New York
Chapter 51, Rehabilitation Concerns in Degenerative Movement Disorders of the Central Nervous System

C. DOUGLAS PORTER, M.D.
Assistant Clinical Professor
Department of Rehabilitation and Restorative Care
Wright State University School of Medicine
Dayton, Ohio
Medical Director
Department of Physical Medicine and Rehabilitation
Greene Memorial Hospital
Xenia, Ohio
Chapter 34, Deconditioning, Conditioning, and the Benefits of Exercise

MICHAEL M. PRIEBE, M.D.
Associate Professor
Department of Physical Medicine and Rehabilitation
University of Texas–Southwestern Medical Center
Chief
Spinal Cord Injury Service
V.A. North Texas Health Care System
Dallas, Texas
Chapter 9, Research in Physical Medicine and Rehabilitation

PAUL R. RAO, Ph.D.
Visiting Professor
Loyola College
Baltimore, Maryland
Gallaudet University
Washington, D.C.
Vice President
Clinical Services, Quality Improvement, and Corporate Compliance
National Rehabilitation Hospital
Washington, DC
Chapter 3, Adult Communication Disorders

JOHN B. REDFORD, M.D.
Distinguished Professor
Department of Rehabilitation Medicine
University of Kansas Medical Center
Kansas City, Missouri
Chapter 15, Upper Limb Orthotic Devices

LAWRENCE R. ROBINSON, M.D.
Professor, Department of Rehabilitation Medicine
Adjunct Professor, Department of Otolaryngology, Head and Neck Surgery
University of Washington School of Medicine
Chief, Rehabilitation Medicine
Director, Electrodiagnostic Medicine
Harborview Medical Center
Seattle, Washington
Chapter 11, Electrodiagnostic Medicine II: Clinical Evaluation and Findings

ROBERT D. RONDINELLI, M.D., Ph.D.
Professor and Chairman
Department of Rehabilitation Medicine
University of Kansas Medical Center
Medical Director of Rehabilitation Services
Health Midwest
Kansas City, Missouri
Chapter 6, Practical Aspects of Impairment Rating and Disability Determination

THOM W. ROOKE, M.D.
Professor of Medicine
Director
Vascular Laboratory
Head, Section of Vascular Medicine
Mayo Clinic
Rochester, Minnesota
Chapter 56, Vascular Disease: Evaluation and Management

KIRSTEN K. ROSSNER, M.S., P.T., A.T.C.
Graduate Assistant (Ph.D. student)
University of Virginia
Charlottesville, Virginia
Chapter 39, Musculoskeletal Disorders of the Lower Limbs

ELLIOT J. ROTH, M.D.
The Dr. Paul B. Magnuson Professor and Chairman
Department of Physical Medicine and Rehabilitation
Northwestern University Medical School
The Donnelley Senior Vice President and Medical Director
Rehabilitation Institute of Chicago
Chicago, Illinois
Chapter 50, Rehabilitation of Stroke Syndromes

RICHARD SALCIDO, M.D.
Professor and Chair
Department of Rehabilitation Medicine
University of Pennsylvania School of Medicine
Director of Rehabilitation Services
University of Pennsylvania Healthcare System
Philadelphia, Pennsylvania
Chapter 31, Prevention and Management of Pressure Ulcers and Other Chronic Wounds

BRIAN D. SCHMIT, Ph.D.
Research Assistant Professor
Northwestern University
Associate Director
Sensory Motor Performance Program
Rehabilitation Institute of Chicago
Chicago, Illinois
Chapter 29, Spasticity

JOHN A. SCHUCHMANN, M.D.
Associate Professor
Department of Physical Medicine and Rehabilitation
Texas A & M University College of Medicine
Chairman
Department of Physical Medicine and Rehabilitation
Scott and White Clinic
Temple, Texas
Chapter 45, Occupational Rehabilitation

DAN D. SCOTT, M.D.
Assistant Professor
Department of Rehabilitation Medicine
University of Colorado Health Sciences Center
Staff Physician
Denver V. A. Medical Center
Denver, Colorado
Chapter 35, Employment of Persons with Disabilities

MEHRSHEED SINAKI, M.D., M.S.
Consultant
Department of Physical Medicine and Rehabilitation
Mayo Clinic and Mayo Foundation
Professor of Physical Medicine and Rehabilitation
Mayo Medical School
Rochester, Minnesota
Chapter 40, Low Back Pain and Disorders of the Lumbar Spine
Chapter 41, Prevention and Treatment of Osteoporosis

KEVIN SMITH, M.D.
Assistant Professor
Departments of Anesthesiology and Physical Medicine and Rehabilitation
Baylor College of Medicine
Houston, Texas
Chapter 42, Chronic Pain Syndromes: Evaluation and Treatment

DONNA PIEPER SPECHT, P.T.
Physical Therapist II
The Children's Hospital
Denver, Colorado
Chapter 25, Achieving Functional Independence

M. CATHERINE SPIRES, M.D., M.A.
Director, Residency Training
Associate Chair of Clinical Affairs
Assistant Clinical Professor
Department of Physical Medicine and Rehabilitation
University of Michigan
Ann Arbor, Michigan
Chapter 58, Rehabilitation of Patients with Burns

BARRY D. STEIN, M.D.
Northwest Hospital
Baltimore, Maryland
Chapter 59, Principles of Geriatric Rehabilitation

LYNNE M. STEMPIEN, M.D.
Associate Professor
Department of Rehabilitation Medicine
University of Colorado
Assistant Medical Director
Department of Rehabilitation Medicine
The Children's Hospital
Denver, Colorado
Chapter 53, Rehabilitation of Children and Adults with Cerebral Palsy

STEVEN A. STIENS, M.D., M.S.
Associate Professor
University of Washington School of Medicine
Department of Rehabilitation Medicine
Attending Physician
V.A. Puget Sound Health Care System
University Hospital
Harborview Medical Center
Seattle, Washington
Chapter 28, Neurogenic Bowel: Dysfunction and Management
Chapter 61, Rehabilitation Aspects of Organ Transplantation

SCOTT T. STOLL, D.O., Ph.D.
Assistant Professor and Interim Chairman
Department of Osteopathic Manipulative Medicine
University of North Texas Health Science Center
Medical Director, S.M.A.R.T. Institute
Medical Director, Rehab Center
Osteopathic Medical Center of Texas
Medical Director
Easter Seals Society of Tarrent County
Fort Worth, Texas
Chapter 20, Manipulation, Traction, and Massage

KATHRYN A. STOLP-SMITH, M.D., M.S.
Associate Professor
Department of Physical Medicine and Rehabilitation
Mayo Medical School
Associate Dean
Mayo Graduate School of Medicine
Rochester, Minnesota
Chapter 12, Electrodiagnostic Medicine III: Case Studies

JEFFREY A. STRAKOWSKI, M.D.
Clinical Assistant Professor
Department of Physical Medicine and Rehabilitation
The Ohio State University
Associate Director
Medical Education Department of Physical Medicine
Grant Riverside Methodist Hospital
Columbus, Ohio
Chapter 38, Upper Limb Musculoskeletal Pain Syndromes

MUKUL TALATY, M.S., Ph.D.
Research Engineer
Gait and Motion Analysis Laboratory
Moss Rehabilitation
Philadelphia, Pennsylvania
Chapter 5, Gait Analysis: Technology and Clinical Applications

RONALD S. TAYLOR, M.D.
Clinical Associate Professor
Wayne State University Medical School
Detroit, Michigan
Director
Rehabilitation Services
William Beaumont Hospital
Royal Oak, Michigan
Chapter 52, Rehabilitation of Persons with Multiple Sclerosis

JEFFREY M. THOMPSON, M.D.
Associate Professor
Department of Physical Medicine and Rehabilitation
Mayo Medical School
Consultant
Department of Physical Medicine and Rehabilitation
Mayo Clinic and Mayo Foundation
Rochester, Minnesota
Chapter 43, The Diagnosis and Treatment of Muscle Pain Syndromes

LANCE E. TREXLER, Ph.D.
Clinical Assistant Professor
Department of Physical Medicine and Rehabilitation
Indiana University School of Medicine
Clinical Director
Center for Neurological Rehabilitation
Community Hospitals Indianapolis
Indianapolis, Indiana
Chapter 4, Psychological Perspectives on Rehabilitation: Contemporary Assessment and Intervention Strategies

DAVID C. WEBER, M.D.
Assistant Professor
Mayo Medical School
Consultant
Department of Physical Medicine and Rehabilitation
Mayo Clinic
Rochester, Minnesota
Chapter 21, Physical Agent Modalities

J. WILLIAM WIAND, D.O.
Ohio University
Athens, Ohio
Medical Director
Department of Radiology
Riverside Methodist Hospital
Columbus, Ohio
Chapter 38, Upper Limb Musculoskeletal Pain Syndromes

PAMELA E. WILSON, M.D.
Assistant Professor
Department of Physical Medicine and Rehabilitation
University of Colorado School of Medicine
Assistant Professor
Department of Physical Medicine and Rehabilitation
The Children's Hospital
Denver, Colorado
Chapter 2, Examination of the Pediatric Patient

ROBERT B. WINTER, M.D.
Clinical Professor
Department of Orthopedic Surgery
University of Minnesota
Research Consultant
Twin Cities Spine Center
Minneapolis, Minnesota
Chapter 17, Spinal Orthoses in Rehabilitation

JEFFREY L. YOUNG, M.D., M.A.
Attending Physiatrist
Hospital for Special Surgery
New York, New York
Chapter 39, Musculoskeletal Disorders of the Lower Limbs

MARK A. YOUNG, M.D., F.A.C.P.
Faculty
The Sinai-Johns Hopkins University Residency Program
Co-chair
Department of Physical Medicine and Rehabilitation
The Maryland Rehabilitation Center
Baltimore, Maryland
Chapter 61, Rehabilitation Aspects of Organ Transplantation

PREFACE TO THE SECOND EDITION

This second edition is written and edited to expand the well-received traditions established in the first edition. In the first edition, our goals included coverage of the breadth of the field of physical medicine and rehabilitation and creation of a practical, clinically useful, and user-friendly work. In the second edition, additional emphasis has been placed on keeping "reader efficiency" in mind. The text, figures, and tables are designed to allow the reader to learn the "most per minute" of reading.

The editors are proud of the book's very high production values. A couple examples of these production values are the index and the new color figures. The index was created by hand, rather than relying on a computer program, to ensure its accuracy and usefulness to form an index. Color is used in some figures in this edition to add the most to the reader's comprehension.

It is literally true that one could write an entire book about the topic of each of the chapters in this text. One of the tasks of the authors and editors was to take the huge body of information that now comprises the field of Physical Medicine & Rehabilitation and condense it into a textbook of reasonable size. The length of each chapter in this edition again reflects the editors' feelings about the current importance of that topic relative to others. Since some details had to be left out, the authors have prepared an extensive reference list at the end of each chapter for readers wanting to explore a subject in greater depth. The advantage of each chapter's reference list is that it is prepared by an expert in the field, and is not just a cold computer search that results in a polyglot of references that might or might not be clinically useful. In this edition we have also listed some suggested internet web sites at the end of some chapters. These web sites also have been selected by the authors.

This edition incorporates many of the helpful comments and suggestions sent by readers from around the world. All suggestions were reviewed by the editors. This led to changes in chapter numbering, lengthening of some chapters, shortening of others, and adding a new chapter on the rehabilitation of patients with transplantations.

The book is again divided into four major sections. Section I deals with the evaluation of patients typically seen in the practice of physical medicine and rehabilitation (Chapters 1–12). Section II deals with treatment techniques and special equipment used in the field of physical medicine and rehabilitation (Chapters 13–24). Section III discusses the therapeutic issues and problems that are commonly seen in the practice of physical medicine and rehabilitation (Chapters 25–35). Section IV deals with specific diagnoses faced by the physiatrist, both in physical medicine and in rehabilitation (Chapters 36–61).

Considerable care was given to make sure that the chapters match in terms of syntax, readability, and quality. One problem in any edited textbook is the potential for unevenness in the various chapters written by different authors. The chapters in this work were contributed by more than 100 authors, all of whom had a different writing style. Some of the submitted chapters were rewritten by the Editor in Chief to accomplish a similarity in writing style. The redactors and grammarians at W.B. Saunders helped tremendously in this regard as well. Since a large portion of the book's reading audience includes residents in physical medicine and rehabilitation, each chapter was read and critiqued at the galley stage by a senior resident from the Indiana University School of Medicine Department of Physical Medicine and Rehabilitation.

Every chapter in this edition has been thoroughly updated. It is the policy of the editors to rotate the authors of some chapters in each edition to maintain the freshness of the material and its point of view. Consequently, five of the chapters in this edition are completely new.

Chapter 49, Brain Injury Rehabilitation, is dedicated to the memory of Catherine F. Bontke, M.D. Dr. Bontke was the author of this chapter in the first edition.

As with the first edition, we welcome comments, suggestions, and constructive criticism from members of the physical medicine and rehabilitation community and from all readers.

Randall Braddom, M.D.

ACKNOWLEDGMENT

Sincere appreciation is extended to all those who helped write, edit, and assemble the book, especially Cindy Poehler, Paul Hoffmann, David Stensland, James Crawford, Dolores Meloni, and Lisette Bralow. I would also like to thank Betty Dinius and Gordon King at Wishard Health Services for their help and encouragement.

NOTICE

CONTENTS

Color insert appears after page 648.

I

SECTION

EVALUATION

1 CHAPTER

Lisa A. McPeak, M.D.

Physiatric History and Examination

The physiatric history and physical examination are the basis for all therapeutic decision making. Although many physicians are familiar with the conventional history and physical examination, outlined in common medical reference texts such as DeGowin and DeGowin's *Bedside Diagnostic Examination* (New York, Macmillan, 1994) and Bates's *A Guide to Physical Examination* (Philadelphia, Lippincott–Raven, 1998), the physiatric history and physical examination are quite different and are in many respects unique. The purpose of this chapter is both to outline and to highlight these differences.

The conventional history and physical examination are the basis on which the physiatric history and examination are built. The physiatrist tailors the procedures of the conventional history and physical process to elucidate the problems of the physiatric patient population. Each section in this chapter focuses on the specific concerns that a physiatrist should emphasize during the history and examination.

The physiatric history and examination emphasize functional capacity in both the home and the community. The physiatrist determines not only physical deficits but also the functional impact of these deficits. The identification of functional problems allows the assignment of functional goals that become the basis for developing a therapeutic management plan.

The physiatric history and physical examination should identify an individual's impairments, disabilities, and handicaps as defined by the World Health Organization (Table 1–1). [30] Although an individual can have multiple impairments, the impairments might not cause a disability or handicap unless they affect function in the home or community. For example, an impairment such as a 20-degree flexion contracture of the right arm might cause no disability or handicap in an individual with the ability to walk. This same impairment can cause considerable disability in an individual with complete paraplegia who must fully extend the elbow to accomplish a wheelchair transfer. To define an impairment as a disability or handicap, the physiatrist must assess the patient's function based on the physiatric history and examination.

In 1997 the World Health Organization revised its definitions of disablement and functioning. In the future, the physiatrist may look for impairments, activities, and participation during the history and examination. These new definitions, also included in Table 1–1, are not commonly used clinically at present.[31]

Table 1–2 lists the major categories involved in the physiatric history and examination. Note that this table, if copied, will fit in a coat pocket and then can be used during each physiatric history and examination.

PHYSIATRIC HISTORY

Introduction

Most of a patient's problems can be identified with a thorough history. The physiatric history should be obtained in an organized manner so that no important items are missed.

Proper history taking involves listening carefully to the patient or caregiver, as he or she can best relate how the disease or injury results in functional problems. Try to use the patient's own words and avoid the temptation to reframe them in your own words. The patient is often unable to identify the problem directly, especially if a cognitive or psychosocial component of the problem exists. In these situations, the examiner must closely observe the patient during the interview for any implied indication of problems. This involves careful

TABLE 1–1 World Health Organization Definitions

1980: Definitions of Impairment, Disability, Handicap

Impairment: Any loss or abnormality of psychological, physiological, or anatomical structure or function.
Disability: Any restriction or lack resulting from an impairment of the ability to perform an activity in the manner or within the range considered normal for a human being.
Handicap: A disadvantage for a given individual, resulting from an impairment or a disability, that limits or prevents the fulfillment of a role that is normal for that individual.

1997: Definitions of Impairment, Activity, and Participation

Impairment: Any loss or abnormality of body structure or of a physiological or psychological function (essentially unchanged from 1980 definition).
Activity: The nature and extent of functioning at the level of the person.
Participation: The nature and extent of a person's involvement in life situations in relationship to impairments, activities, health conditions, and contextual factors.

From World Health Organization: International Classification of Impairments, Disabilities, and Handicaps, 1980, and International Classification of Impairments, Activities, and Participation, 1997. Geneva, World Health Organization.

scrutiny of body language, attitude, cooperativeness, and social awareness. A good physiatric history often includes identification of both implied and stated problems.

Obtaining a complete history requires the physiatrist to develop a rapport with the patient. Collect the history in a professional but caring and empathic manner. Shake hands with the patient (or use another greeting gesture if the patient is unable to shake hands), give an appropriate introduction, and address the patient by the last name. Introduction of the physician to any family or friends present is also important. Be aware of any signs of social or physical discomfort due to either the topic of discussion or pain. Both types of discomfort tend to decrease the patient's participation and accuracy during the interview process.

The physician should act as a facilitator, allowing the patient to speak freely, and should only occasionally ask a question to clarify the topic of discussion. The physician should ask specific questions to obtain all the necessary information, but the patient should answer these questions freely. Without development of verbal rapport, the patient can feel uncomfortable, and problems can be missed or inadequately discussed.

The sources of the information for the physiatric history are varied. The patient is the obvious source for most of the physiatric history, but if communication or cognitive difficulties are present, the history might also need to be taken or confirmed through interviews with family members and friends. Technical information about the patient's medical or physical problems can be obtained by questioning the patient's therapists, nurses, aides, and other physicians. It is not unusual for an examiner to find that individuals who provide care for a patient have different opinions as to the patient's problems and functional skills. If differences are noted, the physiatric examination should be tailored to help identify which opinions are the most factual.

TABLE 1–2 Outline of the Physiatric History and Examination

Physiatric history
- Chief complaint
- History of present problem
- Functional history
  - Mobility activities
  - Activities of daily living
  - Household activities
  - Community activities
  - Cognition
  - Communication
  - Vocation
  - Assistive devices
- Psychosocial history
  - Substance abuse
  - Family/friend support
  - Living situation
  - Vocational history
  - Avocational history
  - Psychiatric history
  - Sexual history
  - Finances
- Medications/allergies
- Diet
- Past medical/surgical history
- Family history
- Review of systems

Physiatric examination
- Functional examination
  - Mobility activities
  - Activities of daily living
  - Household activities
  - Driving
- Musculoskeletal examination
  - Inspection
  - Palpation
  - Joint stability
  - Range of motion
  - Contractures
  - Manual muscle testing
- Neurological examination
  - Level of consciousness
  - Mental status
  - Communication
  - Cranial nerves
  - Sensation
  - Motor control
  - Reflexes
- General medical examination

Summary
Problem list
Management plan
Goals

Chief Complaint

The chief complaint in a physiatric history, as in a conventional history, should be transcribed from the patient's own words, whenever possible, and is usually only one or two sentences in length. Unlike the conventional history, it should focus on the functional loss or the reason for the functional loss. For example, on transfer to an inpatient rehabilitation facility, a patient who has had a cerebrovascular accident often complains of inability to walk or to dress, due to stroke-caused weakness. The chief complaint of the outpatient with low back pain might be inability to perform a job because of decreased capability to stand and walk. Focusing on functional losses is a unique aspect of the physiatric history. Table 1–3 lists common presenting chief complaints of patients with physiatric problems and the corresponding discharge diagnoses.

History of Present Problem

In a physiatric setting, identifying the problem is not only discovering an illness but also uncovering the functional implications. For this reason, the "history of the present illness" might more appropriately be labeled "history of the present problem." The problem should be described in a clear, chronological narrative that lists all of the patient's functional, medical, surgical, physical, and cognitive deficits. The date of onset of the illness or injury, subsequent problems, treatment provided, and complications since the onset should be recorded. The history of the present problem should include the functional losses or restrictions that have occurred due to

TABLE 1–3 Common Chief Complaints with Corresponding Possible Diagnoses

Chief Complaint	Discharge Diagnosis
Pain in calves after walking several blocks	Peripheral vascular disease or lumbar stenosis
Weak left leg and arm	Stroke
Trouble with balance and clumsiness Recent falling Incoordination of right leg and arm	Multiple sclerosis
Stiffness Recent falling Inability to walk and talk well	Parkinsonism
Leg weakness	Transverse myelitis
Back pain spreading to left leg; pain increases with prolonged walking	Lumbosacral radiculopathy
Headaches and memory problems along with inability to organize self at work that began after a fall	Mild traumatic brain injury
Right wrist pain noted during computer use; pain wakes individual at night	Carpal tunnel syndrome
Low back pain for 3 months, does not go to either leg	Myofascial pain in the lumbosacral paraspinal muscles

the illness or injury. Table 1–4 lists common questions that are asked in developing the history of the present problem.[23]

Functional History

Functional losses and restrictions should be well documented, as they are key items in the physiatric history. Patients should be specifically questioned about their ability to perform all necessary activities to function at home and in the community. List both the functional skills prior to and since the recent illness or injury. Each functional activity should be described as accurately as possible and the specific assistance levels required from a caregiver should be included. The Functional Independence Measure (Table 1–5) is a scale that describes the assistive levels commonly used for documentation purposes.[13] Physicians and others reading the functional history should be able to develop a clear picture of the patient's lifestyle both before and after the injury or illness. Functional activities usually discussed in the functional history are listed in Table 1–6.

TABLE 1–4 Items Necessary to Develop the History of the Present Problem

1. Date of onset.
2. Character and severity (especially pain problems).
3. Location of problem (and referral area for pain problems).
4. Associated complaints.
5. Aggravating and alleviating factors (especially pain problems).
6. Previous medical and rehabilitation treatment plans and outcomes.

Adapted from Members of the Department of Neurology: Mayo Clinic Examinations in Neurology, ed 7. Philadelphia, Mosby, 1998.

TABLE 1–5 Description of the Levels of Function and Their Scores: Modified from the Functional Independence Measure (FIM)

Level of Function	Score	Definition
Independent		Another person is not required for the activity (NO HELPER).
	7	*Complete independence*—All of the tasks described as making up the activity are performed safely, without modification, assistive devices, or aids, and within a reasonable amount of time.
	6	*Modified independence*—One or more of the following may be true: The activity requires an assistive device, the activity takes more than reasonable time, or there are safety considerations.
Dependent		The patient requires another person for either supervision or physical assistance for the activity to be performed (REQUIRES HELPER).
	5	*Supervision or setup*—Patient requires no more help than standby or cueing without physical contact, or the helper sets up needed items.
	4	*Minimal contact assistance*—Patient requires no more help than touching and expends 75% or more of the effort.
	3	*Moderate assistance*—Patient requires more help than touching and expends 50% to 75% of the effort.
	2	*Maximal assistance*—Patient expends 25% to 50% of the effort.
	1	*Total assistance*—Patient expends less than 25% of the effort.

Adapted from the Guide for the Uniform Data Set for Medical Rehabilitation (Adult FIM), version 4.0. Buffalo, State University of New York, 1993.

Mobility Activities

Mobility is the capability of movement. Many times, an impairment resulting from an injury or an illness results in decreased independence in mobility. Each patient should be questioned about the ability to perform all the mobility activities, ranging from bed mobility to ambulation, both at home and in the community. Often an individual with an impairment requires assistive devices to improve function. Table 1–7 is a list of commonly used mobility assistive devices. Based on the functional history, the physiatrist should develop a good understanding of the patient's safety and independence in all mobility activities.

Bed mobility activities include rolling from one side of the bed to the other, and rolling from a supine to a prone position and back. Inability to do these activities places a patient at high risk for skin pressure ulcers. Patients with poor bed mobility skills require the help of a caregiver. Frequently, an individual with a new

TABLE 1–6 Functional Activities That Should Be Discussed in the Functional History

Mobility activities	Household activities
Bed mobility	Cooking
Transitional movements	Cleaning
Supine to sitting	Lawn work
Sitting to standing	Community activities
Sitting	Driving
Standing	Shopping
Ambulation	Social outings
Stair climbing	Cognition
Wheelchair activities	Communication
Propulsion	Vocational activities
Parts management	
Transfer activities	
Activities of daily living	
Feeding	
Grooming	
Dressing	
Bathing	
Toileting	

impairment is mobile in the hospital bed, with the use of side rails, but is unable to move in a regular bed. A bed with a soft mattress or a waterbed tends to make bed mobility skills more difficult. Individuals with leg weakness should be questioned about their ability to move their legs in bed.

Transitional movements allow the individual to change from one level of mobility to another. For example, transitional movements include going from a supine to a sitting position and from a sitting to a standing position and back again. Patients with an impairment might not have difficulty with either sitting or standing, but might be unable to perform the transitional movements required to move from one position to the other.

Sitting is an important functional skill. Sitting balance requires adequate trunk and neck stability or strength and appropriate midline orientation. Midline orientation enables the patient to recognize normal upright body position. Midline orientation in patients with sensory-perceptual or muscular impairments is often poor. An individual with a new impairment might be unable to sit without support from one or both arms or without back support.

Good standing skills are required prior to functional ambulation. Independent standing requires adequate midline orientation, trunk stability, strength, and balance. Standing also requires adequate bilateral leg stability and strength. Standing is often achieved only through arm support in an individual with impairments. Individuals with sitting difficulties are usually unable to stand without assistance. This support can be supplied by assistive devices (Table 1–7) such as a straight cane or walker.

Walking involves several physical skills such as balance, strength, coordination, and midline orientation. As in standing, support for walking activities is also often required. Table 1–7 lists the devices commonly used to improve ambulation activities. As walking is usually more difficult on carpeted or uneven surfaces, the individual should be questioned as to the ability to walk on different surfaces.

Climbing or descending stairs is often an essential activity for an individual whose home has a few entry steps, or if the bedroom is on the second floor. Stair mobility should also be investigated because many community buildings are still only accessible by stairs. The level of assistance and devices required for stair mobility activities should be noted. The number of stairs an individual can or might need to ascend or descend is valuable functional information.

Many patients with impairments can be functional within the home and the community using a wheelchair as the primary mode of mobility. Transfer activities, lower limb management in the wheelchair, wheelchair parts management, and wheelchair propulsion skills are important functional activities. The patient should be questioned specifically as to the ability to do all these activities. Transfers are performed in different ways to differing surfaces, with or without assistance. The most common types of transfers are the stand pivot or the half-stand pivot transfer, the sliding board transfer, and the lateral lift transfer. Both types of stand pivot transfers require that the patient stand either partially or fully and pivot around toward a new surface. The sliding board transfer utilizes a wooden or a plastic board between two surfaces. The patient uses the upper extremities to lift and move the body along the board with each lift, until the new surface is reached. The lateral lift transfer requires that the patient lift the body in a lateral direction from one surface to another. Floor to wheelchair transfer ability is also investigated, because any patient using a wheelchair for mobility is at risk for falling out of the wheelchair. A patient who is unable to assist in the transfer activities is considered dependent

TABLE 1–7 Commonly Used Mobility Assistive Devices

- Axillary crutches
- Canes
  - Straight cane
  - Wide-based or narrow-based quad cane
  - Hemiwalker or pyramid cane
- Forearm orthoses
  - Lofstrand
  - Platform
- Walkers
  - Standard or pickup walker
  - Wheeled walker
  - Platform walker
- Wheelchairs
  - Types
    - Manual
    - Motorized
  - Common modifications/specifications
    - Lightweight
    - Rigid or folding frame
    - Elevated or removable footrests
    - Removable armrests
    - Reclining
- Off-the-shelf ankle-foot orthoses
- Common custom orthoses
  - Plastic ankle-foot orthosis
  - Metal ankle-foot orthosis
  - Knee orthosis
  - Knee-ankle-foot orthosis

for this skill, and needs the assistance of one or more caregivers for transfers. Specifics as to the transfer style and assistive devices utilized by the caregivers should be documented in the history.

Lower limb management in the wheelchair is an important factor in transfer activities. Patients with severe lower limb weakness must be able to manipulate their legs so the transfer can proceed without injury. They should also be able to place the legs correctly on the wheelchair leg rest to prevent injuries during wheelchair propulsion. Wheelchair parts management includes the individual's ability to remove and replace armrests and leg rests, and appropriate use of the wheelchair brakes. Improper use of the parts can make wheelchair transfer and propulsion activities unsafe.

More difficult wheelchair activities are important for the patient who is active within the community. This patient is questioned about wheelchair propulsion activities on carpets, up and down inclined surfaces, on uneven surfaces, and over curbs. Information concerning driving and the assistive devices required for driving is useful. The patient should be able to relate how to maneuver the wheelchair in and out of the car. Also, knowing how an individual who uses the wheelchair for mobility is able to go up and down a few stairs, if necessary, is important. Although this type of activity is not often recommended, it is occasionally done if the patient must go into a building with entry steps.

Activities of Daily Living

The history should assess activities of daily living (ADL), including feeding, grooming, dressing, bathing, and toileting activities. All of these tasks can require the use of assistive devices. Table 1–8 lists the assistive devices commonly used to improve ADL functional skills (see Chapters 23 and 25 for a more detailed discussion of ADL and assistive devices).

TABLE 1–8 Common Activities of Daily Living and Household Assistive Devices

Arm orthoses	Devices for dressing
Utilized to hold equipment	Reacher
Adapted hand orthosis	Button aid
Adapted wrist-hand orthosis	Zipper pull
Universal cuff	Long-handled shoehorn
Utilized to assist movement	Stocking aid
Balanced forearm orthosis	Devices for bathing
Overhead sling suspension orthosis	Bath mitt
Devices for feeding	Long-handled sponge
Adapted utensils	Devices for cooking
Plate guard	Suction scrub brush
Rocker knife	Rocker knife
Adapted cup or cup holder	Adapted cooking utensils
Straw	Suction cutting board
Devices for grooming	Suction bowl holder
Adapted brush and comb	One-handed jar opener
Wash mitt	Reacher
Adapted manual razor	Devices for cleaning
Electric razor	Dust mitt
Adapted toothbrush	Adapted handles for cleaning equipment
Suction denture brush	Reacher

Feeding activities are often quite difficult for an impaired individual. Independent feeding requires the ability to open food packages before eating and the ability to use utensils correctly. The patient must also have the muscle strength, joint range, and coordination to bring the food or drink to the mouth. The patient also needs the endurance necessary to complete a full meal. A loss of the ability to do any of these activities prevents independence in feeding.

Grooming includes all of the hygiene activities done each morning, including face and body bathing at the sink, brushing of teeth or dentures, applying antiperspirant or cologne, shaving, and hair combing or brushing. These activities require strength, coordination, endurance, and adequate limb range of motion to complete.

Dressing skills require both fine and gross motor coordination, balance, strength, and adequate limb range of motion. Upper body dressing includes donning underwear and a shirt or a dress. Pullover items are easier to don if the patient has adequate over-head shoulder range of motion. Buttoned items do not require the over-head shoulder range of motion but require fine motor coordination to manipulate the buttons. Independence in lower body dressing requires enough range of motion to reach the feet to don shoes and socks. The patient must have adequate balance and strength to pull up underwear, pants, or skirt. Those items can be donned while the patient is in bed, but he or she must have the ability to lift the buttocks to allow items to be pulled to the waist. The history should include specific information concerning whether the patient dresses in bed, from a chair, or in a standing position.

Bathing requires the ability to get in and out of the bathtub or shower safely, to sit or stand for the activity, and to do the cleansing activity itself. Several assistive devices can help the patient to perform bathing mobility skills safely. Items such as a transfer tub bench, a bath chair, and a handheld shower head can improve the individual's independence for bathing activities. The actual cleansing activity during bathing requires strength, coordination, and range of motion to bathe every part of the body. Assistive devices, such as a long-handled sponge, can help the individual to reach all parts of the body.

Toileting skills include mobility activities such as transferring on and off the toilet, sitting on the toilet, and standing. Assistive devices such as grab bars, elevated toilet seats, and bedside commodes are often used by the individual with an impairment to make such mobility activities easier and safer. Clothing management and hygiene at the toilet are also important components in toileting activities. The individual requires good coordination, balance, and range of motion to complete these clothing and hygiene activities.

Household Activities

Many individuals consider household activities such as cooking, cleaning, and lawn work essential to their daily routine. For individuals who walk, these activities require good standing balance and endurance. Usually, these household activities require the use of both upper limbs. If an individual uses an assistive device such as a cane or a walker, household activities can be quite difficult. Household activities can also be performed from a wheelchair. Individuals who use the wheelchair as their primary mode of mobility are often able to perform fairly difficult household activities if the necessary household items are placed within reach. An individual who does not have the balance or endurance to do the household activities while standing can utilize either a stationary chair or a wheelchair to do the activities. Individuals often use assistive devices to help with household tasks; Table 1–8 lists some common household assistive devices.

Community Activities

Community activities such as driving, shopping, going to church, or participating in social outings are very important to many individuals. Assessing the community activities that patients consider important helps to delineate their lifestyle. It is important to know if new impairments are preventing individuals from performing their usual community activities. The individual should be specifically asked about desires to return to all or some of these activities.

Cognition

Cognition is the act or process of knowing. It includes adequate orientation to person, place, time, and situation, good memory skills, judgment, and capacity for abstract thought. Frequently, an individual with poor cognition is unable to recognize cognitive deficits and might not indicate cognition as a problem. When cognitive deficits are suspected, it is helpful to question family, friends, or health care workers who have come in contact with the patient. At other times, the patient can have some awareness of problems but might be unable to accurately describe the deficits. The history in this case should reflect the difficulties described by the caregivers or patient.

Communication

Communication is a process by which information is exchanged among individuals. Communication is primarily accomplished verbally, but nonverbal gestural and written communication are also important. It is important to learn whether the patient or family members have identified a new communication problem. The individual might report decreased speech quality or dysarthria. Aphasia is a deficit in communication resulting from a central nervous system problem. If the patient or family is aware of a problem in speech or in written or gestural communication, this might represent aphasia. Both nonverbal gestural and written communication can be impaired when a neuromuscular problem affecting limb movement is present. Good communication skills also rely on adequate hearing and sight. It is important to note whether the patient has a problem with hearing or sight, and whether hearing aids or glasses are required to correct the problem (see Chapters 3 and 50 for further information on communication and aphasia).

Vocational Activities

For many individuals, return to vocational activities is a reasonable goal. The history should assess the vocation of the individual just prior to the recent injury or illness, some specific information as to the physical and cognitive job requirements, and the individual's ability to perform the job since the injury or illness (see Chapters 35 and 45 for further information).

Patient's Own Functional Goals

It is tempting to set goals without inquiring about the patient's specific goals. Goal attainment depends on patient motivation and cooperation. The history should document the specific wishes or goals of the patient. If the physician fails to ask the patient about goals, it might not be noted that the patient has unrealistic goals. These problems can be avoided with careful assessment of the patient's personal goals or wishes.

List of Functional Devices

During the functional history, many patients report having or needing multiple assistive devices or equipment items. These devices are usually used to improve either mobility skills or ADL and homemaking skills. There are actually hundreds of such assistive devices, but the most common are listed in Tables 1–7 and 1–8 (see also Chapter 25).

Psychosocial History

The psychosocial history provides vital information. The individual with a new impairment often has psychosocial problems related to the impairment and decreased functional skills. If the patient can no longer work, the loss of income places stress on the whole family. If a previously independent individual requires physical assistance from family members, the role of both the patient and family member within the home can be changed, leading to a stressful situation. It is important to understand the psychosocial situation so that the treatment plan addresses the patient's lifestyle and expected discharge options (see Chapter 4 for further information).

Substance Abuse

Knowledge of past substance abuse helps the physiatrist understand possible future medical problems, recommend counseling for the patient to prevent future problems, and understand possible difficulties in the recovery process. The patient's history of smoking, alcohol abuse, and illegal drug abuse should be assessed. The patient must be made aware that truthfulness about past abuse of these items is important because continued abuse may slow recovery from the new injury or illness.

Chronic alcohol or illegal drug abuse typically decreases a patient's ability to participate in a rehabilitation program. Because of close patient supervision, abuse is rare during an inpatient rehabilitation program. The inpatient with a history of substance abuse should receive counseling to prevent a return to the abuse after discharge. Disabled individuals who are unable to return to their prior lifestyle are more likely to consider either alcohol or drug abuse after discharge, as a result of boredom and increased free time. The physiatrist should be able to recognize an individual at risk for such problems in the initial psychosocial history, so that counseling can begin early.

Smoking often leads to serious cardiopulmonary difficulties and interferes with a therapeutic exercise program. Smoking cessation should be aggressively encouraged and pursued.

Family/Friend Support

After an illness or injury, many individuals need assistance with functional skills. This assistance is usually obtained from family members and occasionally from friends. At the time of admission, a possible primary caregiver should be identified. The patient should also identify any other family members or friends who will be available to help periodically. The physical status of these potential caregivers should be known to identify possible problems with the patient's plan. If the patient has cognitive deficits that prevent safe decision making, the individual who is the primary decision maker should be identified.

Living Situation

It is important to document the patient's premorbid living situation. This entails asking such questions as whether the patient lived alone or with family members, the location of the bedroom, the number of steps into the home and into the bedroom, the size of the bathroom, and the type of floor covering. Early knowledge of restrictions to mobility within the home might prompt a home evaluation or the use of home modifications and special equipment items. Whether the home is owned or rented can be important if the patient cannot return to the previous home, or if extensive modifications are needed.

Vocational History

The patient's present job description was obtained in the functional history. Documentation of educational level and all previous job positions is necessary for the psychosocial history. The physiatrist must ensure that the rehabilitation program is appropriate to an individual's educational level. Information concerning prior job experience is also helpful if the patient will be unable to return to the previous job position.

Avocational History

Avocational activities are frequently as important to the individual as vocational activities. Restrictions in the ability to participate in previous hobbies and social activities can be very stressful for the patient. A short summary of previously enjoyed leisure activities will help all members of the rehabilitation team understand the patient's previous lifestyle and possible future goals.

Psychiatric History

Patient motivation and cooperation are imperative for a successful rehabilitation program. Psychiatric problems such as depression, anxiety, and suicidal or homicidal ideation can have a major influence on an individual's ability to cooperate. Depression is common immediately after a disabling injury, and patients should be questioned as to whether they have noted any feelings of sadness or depression since the new problem developed. The stress of a new illness or injury can trigger a recurrence of a previous psychiatric problem. Instituting preventive measures such as supportive psychotherapy or psychiatric medications can prevent problems that could interfere with accomplishing the patient's goals for the program.

Sexual History

Questions concerning sexuality are often avoided by health practitioners. Sexuality and sexual activity are very important aspects of an individual's lifestyle. Questions concerning sexuality should be presented in such a manner that the patient or caregiver remains sufficiently comfortable to provide accurate answers. Past sexuality problems can become worse after a new illness or injury. Some diagnoses treated by physiatrists are associated with hypersexuality, and any premorbid sexual problems can be compounded. Erectile dysfunction, ejaculation difficulties, and decreased libido are common in male patients after an injury or illness. Likewise, female patients may commonly have problems with irregular menses, dysmenorrhea, dyspareunia, or decreased libido. Identification of sexual problems and consideration of counseling or medical management in the initial physiatric management plan can be very helpful (see Chapter 30 for further information).

Finances

Loss of income due to a new illness or injury can cause stress-related problems in the patient and the family. Early recognition of this problem can help decrease stress by allowing family members to work with the social worker and other physiatric team members to solve some of the financial difficulties.

Medications and Allergies

A complete list of medications and allergies should be obtained during the history. Any prescription or over-the-counter medications or "home remedies" that the patient takes should be documented. Patients will omit mention of using over-the-counter medications and home remedies unless carefully questioned. The medication list should be reviewed for each medication's indication, side effects, and interactions. Many medications have unwanted cognitive and physical side effects, and reduction or avoidance of such medications is recommended.

Diet

Evaluation of the present diet is necessary to see if it is appropriate for the patient's current condition. The individual's medical problems should be reviewed to ensure that the diet will not present a risk of further complications. Bowel problems are very common in patients with new impairments. After a review of the patient's physical status and a gastrointestinal examination, a dietary change might be appropriate. If the patient complains of swallowing or chewing difficulties, a diet modification could be necessary.

Past Medical and Surgical History

Many medical and surgical problems can affect the patient's present function. Often individuals have learned to compensate effectively for a previous illness or injury, but when a new problem or impairment occurs, the ability to compensate for the previous problem might be lost. Many problems are progressive and are likely to cause further functional deficits as the patient ages.

Previous problems in any of the major body systems can affect the physiatric patient's performance in a therapeutic program. The physiatrist should follow the conventional history format to inquire about problems in all systems. The patient's cardiac, pulmonary, rheumatologic, neurological, and musculoskeletal system history is particularly pertinent information. As motivation to participate in the prescribed program is critical, the questions already outlined in the psychiatric history are of major importance as well.

Cardiovascular

Adequate cardiac function is necessary for improvement in a physiatric program. Many patients have histories of congestive heart failure, myocardial infarction, arrhythmias, and severe coronary artery disease. Previous surgical procedures, such as pacemaker placement and coronary artery bypass surgery, are common as well. These problems at times need to be discussed in detail with the patient's cardiologist or primary physician. Further cardiac testing might be necessary prior to exercise prescription. Only with accurate information can the exercise prescription include specific cardiac precautions and exercise intensity to allow the patient the maximal safe exercise level (see Chapter 32 for further information).

Notation of symptoms of intermittent claudication and peripheral vascular disease, as well as the history of old amputations or gangrenous areas, is important. Individuals with serious vascular problems might need exercise restrictions, which should be identified and followed strictly to prevent further vascular compromise. Periodic monitoring of vascular signs and symptoms during exercise is often warranted.

Pulmonary

Both obstructive and restrictive pulmonary problems can interfere with a patient's exercise tolerance. Investigation of previous pulmonary testing and discussion of the present physical status with the patient's primary medical physician can aid in exercise prescription. If there are questions concerning present pulmonary problems, pulmonary function tests might be necessary prior to any therapeutic activity. Attention should be paid to any airway problems, especially if an individual has a tracheostomy for airway protection. Oxygen requirements and stability on present oxygen level are important to assess (see Chapter 33 for further information).

Rheumatologic

Rheumatic disorders are common in the physiatric patient population. An exercise program can exacerbate rheumatologic symptoms. The history should include information concerning the rheumatologic disorder, previous sites of joint involvement, and the present level of disease activity. Information from the primary physician concerning the patient's course to date can be helpful (see Chapter 36 for further information).

Neurological

Chronic and progressive neurological problems can have a major effect on the patient's ability to improve or to tolerate the program. Specific history questions should elicit information about congenital neurological problems, seizure disorders, peripheral neuropathies, progressive neurological diseases, spinal cord and other central nervous system diseases, or trauma. Questions concentrating on such symptoms as muscular weakness, sensory loss, balance, and coordination are also helpful in assessing the patient's neurological status.

Specific questions concerning past cognitive and communication problems are important, as is information concerning previously effective communication techniques. Information about devices that improve communication, including hearing aids or eyeglasses, is valuable.

Musculoskeletal

Chronic or progressive musculoskeletal disorders can have a major impact on the physiatric therapeutic program. It is important to document disorders such as congenital muscular problems, progressive muscular diseases, amputations, joint contractures, traumatic injuries, osteoporosis, and previous bone fractures. Past musculoskeletal problems can medically restrict the patient from certain activities. The patient and, if necessary, the physicians who managed these problems previously should be questioned concerning any activity restrictions.

Individuals with previous neurological and musculoskeletal problems may progress slowly in a rehabilitation program. This should be considered when determining the goals and estimating the length of time needed to achieve the goals. Some of these patients return to their previous functional levels, but they need a longer period to do so. Others are not able to return to previous functional levels, and the program goals should reflect this. Also, the program goals should anticipate changing care and physical needs in patients with progressive neurological or musculoskeletal disorders.

Family History

The physiatrist should ask specific questions concerning family members known to have the same disease as the patient. This helps with overall disease prognostication for the patient. It is essential to learn whether any other family members have signs and symptoms similar to the patient's, as this can help identify family members with an as yet undiagnosed genetic problem.

Other questions concerning cardiac, pulmonary, rheumatologic, neurological, and psychiatric illnesses in family members may help to determine the patient's risk for such medical problems in the future.

Review of Systems

A comprehensive review of systems often uncovers problems not previously noted that can affect the patient's clinical course. The physician should follow a conventional history-taking format to inquire about problems in all systems of the body. The following discussion highlights common problems identified in the physiatric patient population. Table 1–9 provides sample review of systems questions that are specific to the physiatric history. Some systems, such as the pulmonary and cardiovascular systems, were discussed in other sections of this chapter and will not be addressed again.

Skin

Skin problems are common in patients with loss of mobility or sensation. Questions concerning rashes and skin pressure areas can help identify these problems (see Table 1–9). Notation of any open surgical wounds or drains is important, as these sites might need specific care and precautions during therapeutic activities.

Gastrointestinal Status

Trouble swallowing and complaints of coughing during eating activities or the sensation of food "getting stuck" while swallowing can indicate significant problems that need further investigation. Symptoms of gas, heartburn, mild stomach pain, poor digestion, nausea, occasional vomiting, hemoptysis, and darkened stools can indicate subacute gastric problems, including gastrointestinal bleeding that could lead to anemia. Diarrhea, constipation, and bowel incontinence not only interfere with an individual's ability to participate in a physiatric program, but can also indicate a neurogenic bowel that requires management. Many individuals require a specific bowel program, including dietary modification and oral and rectal medications. The individual with a colostomy should be questioned as to the frequency and consistency of bowel movements through the colostomy and necessary colostomy care (see Chapter 28 for further information).

Genitourinary Status

Complaints of urinary frequency, polyuria, nocturia, dysuria, hematuria, urgency, and hesitancy can all indicate significant problems such as urinary tract infection, bladder outlet obstruction, kidney stones, and neurogenic bladder. Past surgical urinary tract procedures, such as nephrostomy, ileostomy, or suprapubic catheter placement, should be documented. Inquire about nonsurgical bladder management programs, including indwelling catheter or intermittent catheter programs (see Chapter 27 for further information).

Nutritional Status

Without adequate nutrition it is often difficult for a patient to participate effectively in a physiatric program. Poor nutrition can be secondary to many different problems, ranging from swallowing dysfunction to decreased appetite. Individuals might be taking medication that decreases appetite or changes taste sensation. Depres-

TABLE 1–9 Review of Systems: Sample Questions Specific to the Physiatric History

System	Questions
Skin	1. Do you have any rashes?
	2. Can you tell me the size and location of open skin areas, if present?
	3. Do you have problems changing your position in bed?
	4. How long do you stay in one position in bed?
	5. How long do you sit up in the same chair?
	6. What are you using to treat your skin problem?
	7. Do you have any special cushions or a special mattress to prevent skin problems?
Gastrointestinal	1. Do you have any problems swallowing? Do you note the sensation of food "getting stuck," or do you cough while eating?
	2. Do you have problems with gas, heartburn, stomach pain, poor digestion, nausea, vomiting, diarrhea, constipation, or darkened stools?
	3. Are you on a bowel program? What is your bowel program?
Genitourinary	1. Do you have problems with frequency, burning with urination, dark or bloody-appearing urine, urgency, or hesitancy?
	2. Are you on a bladder program? What is your bladder program?
Nutritional	1. Do you have swallowing problems?
	2. Do you have appetite problems?
	3. Do you think you are eating and drinking enough?
	4. Do you eat or drink any nutritional supplements?
Neuromuscular	1. Do you have headaches often?
	2. Do you have any neurological problems such as weakness or sensory, visual, coordination, balance, or memory deficits that we have not yet discussed?
	3. Do you have any endurance problems?
	4. Do you have any musculoskeletal problems such as joint or muscle pain, abnormal joint motion, muscle atrophy, and muscle spasticity that we have not yet discussed?

sion also often leads to poor appetite and inadequate nutrition.

Questions concerning recent food and fluid intake help the physician determine whether the patient is at risk for an overall poor nutritional and hydration status. Documentation of the need for either caloric or protein supplementation is essential. Specifics concerning type of supplementation and the mode of supplementation (oral intake or nasogastric or gastrostomy tube) are important.

Neuromuscular Status

Specific neurological questions concerning headaches, weakness, numbness, tingling, visual problems, incoordination, disorientation, and memory problems should be asked if they have not been covered earlier in the history. Specific musculoskeletal questions about overall muscular endurance, joint and muscular pain or stiffness, abnormal joint motion, muscle atrophy, fasciculation, and spasticity are important.

Physiatric Examination

The main purpose of the physiatric examination is to confirm or disprove the diagnostic impression formed after obtaining the physiatric history and to identify other impairment or disabilities. The basis for the physiatric examination is the conventional physical examination, as outlined in such texts as DeGowin and DeGowin[8] and Bates.[3] The physiatrist uses all of the basic evaluation methods of inspection, palpation, percussion, and auscultation along with additional methods that assess impairment and disability.

As with the physiatric history, functional skills are emphasized in the physiatric examination. Special attention is paid to the ability to perform activities on request. This type of examination helps to assess the individual's physical impairments as well as cognitive and communication skills. If the individual is unable to follow commands, the physiatrist must use inventive techniques to increase the patient's ability to participate in the evaluation process. Basic knowledge of different cognitive and communicative deficits and utilization of techniques to decrease the deficits improve the physiatrist's ability to evaluate such patients.

The physiatrist must also use inventive means to evaluate an individual's functional skills. The physical examination should actually begin at the time of initial patient contact and continue throughout the physiatric history and examination. During this time the patient can demonstrate functional skills without the need for formal testing. At times the patient and the family have an inaccurate perception of functional capabilities and limitations. Careful observation might provide a more accurate estimate of the patient's skills.

The physiatric examination also includes a detailed evaluation of the musculoskeletal and neurological systems. The specific impairments that led to the patient's functional deficits should be identified. Since both physical impairments and disability are addressed in a physiatric therapeutic program, the physiatric examination must evaluate both types of problems. Specific attention is paid to impairments that might prevent the patient from safely participating in a physiatric program or that can slow the patient's progress in a prescribed program.

Functional Examination

The functional examination includes evaluation of mobility skills, ADL, household activities, and community activities. Evaluation of cognitive and communication skills is also performed; it is described later in the section on the neurological examination.

The examiner should determine the functional skills, the required level of assistance, and the need for assistive devices. Of the many methods for describing functional level, one that is becoming more commonly used is the Functional Independence Measure (see Table 1–5).[13]

For an accurate patient evaluation, it is helpful to have the appropriate assistive device available. This is not always possible, especially if the patient uses a unique or custom-fabricated device that was not brought to the examination. In these cases it might be necessary to provide the most appropriate replacement item or to re-examine the patient at a later date when the equipment is available.

A full patient assessment during the initial physiatric examination is not always possible due to safety issues and time limitations. The patient can have physical deficits that make it difficult for one person to perform safely the functional mobility examination of the patient. If there is no one available for assistance, it is better that the activity not be attempted, for the safety of both the patient and the examiner. With experience, most physiatrists develop an efficient examination technique that minimizes the time necessary for the formal functional examination.

Mobility Activities

The examination of mobility should proceed methodically, initially evaluating the most basic mobility skills and proceeding to increasingly difficult activities. Documentation of the assistance needed for each activity is important. Note whether the patient utilizes good body mechanics during mobility skills.

The most basic mobility activity is bed mobility. Examine whether the patient can roll from side to side, roll from supine to prone, and roll from prone to supine. This can be performed on an examination table or mat, but mobility is more difficult on a softer surface, such as a bed. Note whether the patient must use the side rails of the bed or examination table for assistance. If the patient has weakness in one or more limbs, his or her limb management ability in the bed should also be noted.

The ability to move from supine to sitting should be observed, since it is the most basic transitional movement. This movement is difficult if the individual is unable to roll onto one side or the other. Patients usually find it easier to first roll from the supine to the side-lying position, and then to push up with the upper limbs into a seated position while simultaneously swinging the legs down to the floor. This activity uses proper body mechanics to complete the task. To go directly from supine to sitting and then turn the body to swing the legs down to the floor not only requires a higher energy expenditure but significant abdominal and trunk muscle strength.

When examining an individual's ability to sit, it should be noted whether the individual is able to sit up straight in the midline (adequate midline orientation), and whether he or she can sit without back support. The patient might need to use one or both arms to maintain the seated position. If the patient is able to sit in the midline, with or without support, then the sitting balance should be physically challenged. This is commonly done by applying a mild or moderate pressure or push in all directions to see if the individual is able to maintain the seated position. The push is done such that the patient can be safely prevented from falling if loss of balance occurs.

The next transitional movement examined is the act of going from the seated to the standing position. Observe whether the patient can safely bend forward to bring the upper body weight anterior to and over the lower legs. The patient must then be able to lift the body into a standing position. Going from sitting to standing requires at least 100 degrees of knee flexion in one lower limb. The patient may or may not use the upper limbs initially to help push out of the seated position. Individuals with adequate lower limb strength should be able to go from sitting to standing without upper limb assistance.

With the patient in the standing position, evaluate midline orientation. The need for upper limb support and type of the assistive device utilized is documented. Standing balance is evaluated similarly to sitting balance, by providing the physical challenge of a pressure or push in all directions (within limits of safety).

Walking requires adequate standing skills, either with or without an assistive device, and should not be attempted unless the patient is able to demonstrate the required standing skills. Basic aspects of gait should be assessed, such as the individual's ability to maintain midline during walking, with or without an assistive device; the size of the base of stance; the fluidity of lower limb movements throughout all phases of the gait cycle; abnormal lower limb movements; appropriate use of an assistive device, if needed; and upper limb movements. Observe the patient's gait from the anterior, posterior, and both lateral positions if necessary. (For further information on gait analysis, see Chapter 5.)

If the patient can walk safely, the ability to descend and ascend stairs is tested. The number of stairs, the need for either one or two hand rails, the ability to use an assistive device if required, and the safety of ascending and descending stair technique is assessed. In an individual with an impairment in one leg, the stronger or normal leg should lead in ascending and the impaired leg should lead in descending.

Individuals using a wheelchair for mobility should be assessed for transfer and wheelchair propulsion skills. Patients should identify by name or description the type of transfer they intend to demonstrate. This knowledge helps in the event the examiner must provide assistance. It should be noted whether the patient uses the stand pivot transfer, the half-stand pivot transfer, the sliding board transfer, or the lateral lift transfer. Assess whether the patient can appropriately place and set up the wheelchair for the type of transfer performed. The transfer activity should be monitored for both safety and correct body mechanics. Observation of the patient's ability to transfer to different surface heights is also important, as most individuals are required to transfer to different surface levels during their daily routine. Some patients require either partial or total assistance for a transfer activity. If the caregiver who assists with the transfer is present, the caregiver and the patient should demonstrate the transfer technique.

Wheelchair propulsion activities on level surfaces can be observed on initial presentation to the clinic or hospital. If an individual is required to propel the wheelchair on different surfaces, try to test wheelchair skills on such surfaces. It is also helpful to examine the patient's ability to propel the wheelchair up and down ramps, onto and off curbs, and on uneven surfaces, if possible. In many cases, the examiner should assess the patient's ability to get back into the wheelchair from the floor or ground.

Activities of Daily Living

Observation of ADL might not be possible if the patient requires some assistive devices that are not present during the examination. Many different types of each assistive device are available, and each brand usually has a variation that might aid one patient but not another. Common items should be available for the patient to demonstrate functional abilities (see Table 1–8). If a patient's equipment requirements are very specific, the patient should provide the equipment.

Feeding skills include the ability to set up a meal, use utensils or hold finger foods, and use upper limb movement to bring food to the mouth. Grooming activities usually include toothbrushing or denture care, washing the face and body at the sink, shaving, and hairbrushing. Patients are observed to see if they can use the equipment appropriately and to see how they use upper limb movement to complete the activity.

A full bathing and toileting evaluation is difficult to observe during the functional examination process because of patient modesty issues. Observing the individual perform the movement activities required for the transfer and the upper limb and body motions required for the activities is helpful. Dressing skills should be assessed. Patients should demonstrate their ability to open and close different fasteners, such as buttons, zippers, and shoelaces. Observing patients as they don and doff a coat or shirt is helpful.

Household Activities

During the functional evaluation the physiatrist is unable to test household activities in an environment similar to the home. Asking patients to demonstrate as closely as possible some of these activities might be the best option available to the examiner. Patients can easily demonstrate the ability to reach overhead items or items at their feet. They can also demonstrate sweeping or vacuuming activities. Cooking skills are hard to demonstrate outside of a kitchen, but they can use eating utensils to demonstrate such simple activities as cutting food for meal preparation.

Driving

Although driving skills cannot be fully assessed without driving a vehicle, demonstration of how the skill is performed (including proper upper and lower limb use) can be done in the clinic or hospital. If a patient uses a wheelchair for mobility activities, an assessment can include observing the transfer technique into the car, and assessing the ability to place the wheelchair in the car.

Musculoskeletal Examination

The musculoskeletal examination is a major portion of the total physiatric examination. It requires inspection and palpation as well as unique tests, such as range of motion and manual muscle testing.[3, 5, 8, 15]

Inspection

All muscles, bones, and joints are closely inspected for any outward appearance of abnormality. Individual muscle shape, size, atrophy, and symmetry are inspected. If a difference is seen in side-to-side muscle symmetry or if an abnormality is noted in one muscle or muscle group, then objective measures such as limb circumference measurements are appropriate for documentation purposes. Joints and bones are inspected for deformities, swelling, redness, and abnormal positions. If present, note amputation levels, lengths, and shape.

Palpation

Patients often exhibit signs of muscle tenderness during this part of the examination. Note the activity that produces the tenderness and the site of the tenderness, and whether referred pain symptoms are present. The muscles are palpated to identify any abnormal swelling, warmth, and tight muscle bands. The exact position of a tight muscle band or area of tenderness within a muscle should be noted. Muscle tone is examined both during the range of motion and muscle palpation. The examiner should note whether the muscle palpated appears to have normal, increased, or decreased tone. During the bone and joint examination, each area should be palpated to identify the extent of any deformities, warmth, swelling, and pain with palpation.

Range of Motion

Adequate joint and limb range of motion (ROM) is essential for functional activities. Loss of joint ROM in the lower limbs can cause gait abnormalities or increased energy expenditure with walking, or it can prevent walking. Poor ROM in the upper limbs can prevent the performance of simple ADL.

The evaluation includes assessment of both active and passive ROM. Passive ROM is assessed by the examiner while the patient is relaxed. Each joint is moved through all planes of motion by the examiner and is measured for the extent of its range. Active ROM is assessed by having the patient perform the maneuvers without the assistance of the examiner. It should be noted whether the ROM activity produces pain.

Exact measurement of ROM activities is most often performed using a universal goniometer (Fig. 1–1). The universal goniometer consists of two movable arms that pivot around one point. Portable goniometers with arms 6 inches long are commonly used, but, depending on the joint measured, larger or smaller sizes are available. The measurement scale is in 1-degree intervals, 0 to 180 degrees in half-circle scales and 0 to 180 or 0 to 360 degrees in full-circle scales.

Goniometry is a relatively reliable method of ROM measurement.[14, 24] The clinician should utilize a systematic technique during each ROM examination to ensure reliability of the measurement. Accurate goniometry evaluation depends on standardized techniques that have been well described in reference texts.[2, 15, 24] The joint is initially placed in the anatomical position. The goniometer is placed lateral to the joint, except in the cases of a few joint motions (e.g., radioulnar supination and pronation). The examiner carefully instructs the patient in the motion required and the plane of movement necessary. Figure 1–2 depicts the three planes of movement. For measuring ROM, the patient moves the joint according to the instructions provided. The stationary arm of the goniometer remains in the anatomical joint position while the other goniometer arm is fixed carefully at the end of the patient's motion. The examiner reads the scale to obtain the active ROM measure-

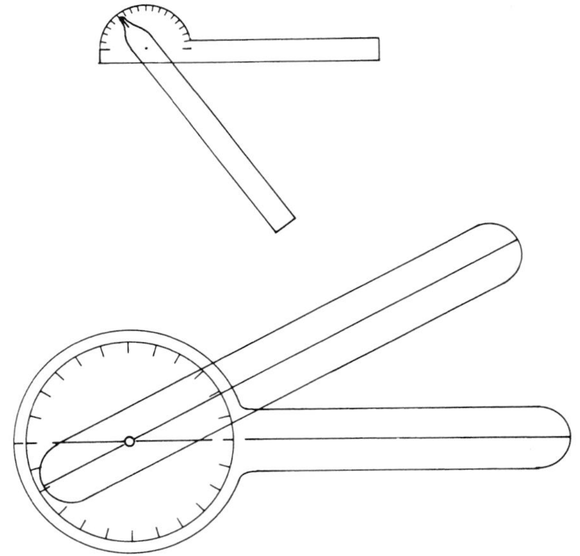

FIGURE 1–1. Two examples of universal goniometers commonly used by the clinician. (From Cole TM, Barry DT, Tobis JS: Measurement of musculoskeletal function. In Kottke FJ, Lehman JF (eds): Krusen's Handbook of Physical Medicine and Rehabilitation, ed 4. Philadelphia, WB Saunders, 1990, p 21.)

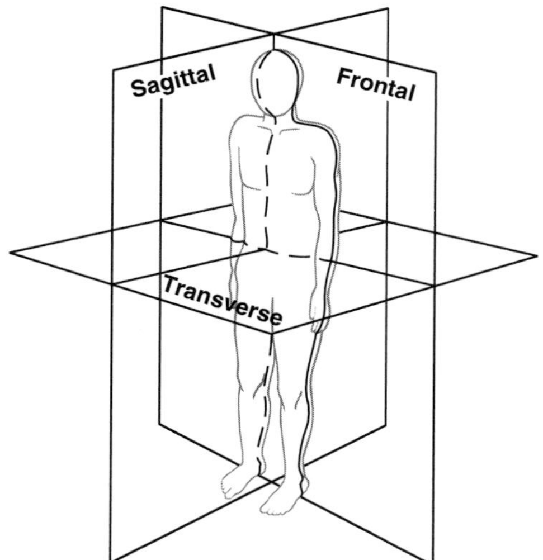

FIGURE 1–2. Three planes of motion.

ment. Passive ROM measurements require the same technique, except that the examiner moves the joints through the desired motions.

Several systems of measurement have been described in the past. The two most common include the 360-degree system proposed by Knapp and West[20, 21] and the 180-degree system proposed by Norkin and White.[26] In the 360-degree system, the patient is placed in anatomical position with the 0-degree point located over the patient's head and the 180-degree point below the patient's feet. In the sagittal plane, 0 to 180 degrees is anterior to the body and 180 to 360 degrees is posterior to the body. The 180-degree system identifies the anatomical position as 0 degrees and movement away from the anatomical position in any of the three planes of motion is described by a positive number between 0 and 180 degrees. For example, Figure 1–3 shows normal shoulder flexion and extension in both systems. The normal range from flexion to extension is 0 to 240 degrees in the 360-degree system. In the 180-degree system, flexion is from 0 to 180 degrees, and extension is measured separately as 0 to 60 degrees.[4, 24]

Most reference textbooks utilize the 180-degree system in an attempt to standardize measurement techniques.[2, 10, 19, 24, 26] Figures 1–4 through 1–19 describe the ROM examination on commonly evaluated joints utilizing the 180-degree system. Each figure outlines patient positioning, plane of motion, and goniometer placement. The shaded areas indicate normal ROM.

Spinal ROM is more difficult to measure, and techniques utilizing goniometers, plumb lines, and measuring tapes have been described. The reliability of these differing techniques is questionable.[10, 24] Inclinometers have also been suggested for accurate measuring of spinal ROM.[2, 11] The inclinometer is a fluid-filled instrument with either a 180- or 360-degree scale. It is placed on the patient's spine and utilizes gravity to determine a change in spinal position after movement. For example, the examiner places the inclinometer on a vertebral spinous process with the initial fluid level at 0 degrees and asks the patient to flex the spine. The examiner reads the measurement change produced when the instrument moves with the spine, but the fluid line remains stable due to the force of gravity. Cervical, thoracic, and lumbar spine movements in all planes can be measured utilizing inclinometers. Measurements are done with either one or two inclinometers.

The reader should refer to either the American Medical Association's *Guides to the Evaluation of Permanent Impairment*[2] or Gerhard's *Documentation of Joint Motion*[11] for specific inclinometer techniques to be used for each spinal segment range of motion. As examples,

Text continued on page 20

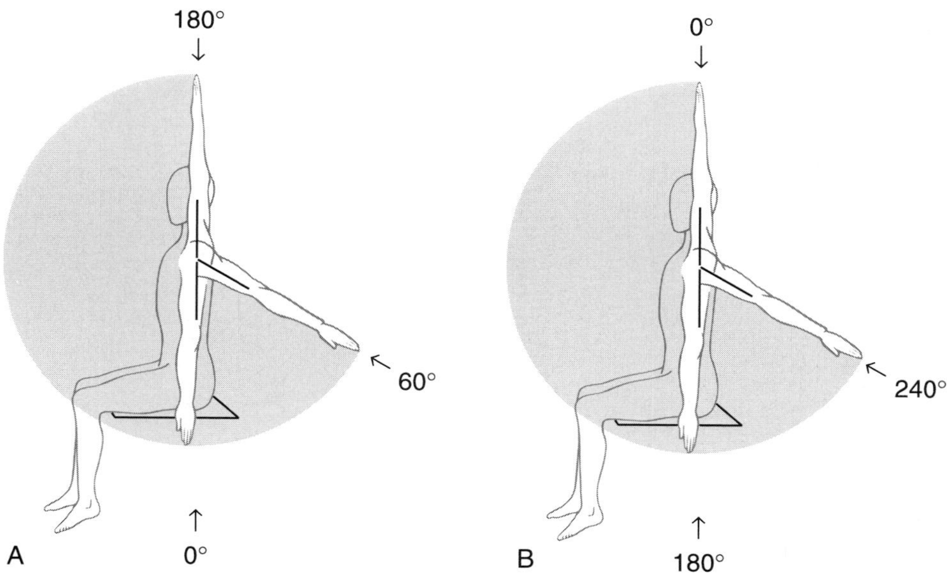

FIGURE 1–3. Shoulder flexion and extension. *A.* 180-degree system. *B.* 360-degree system.

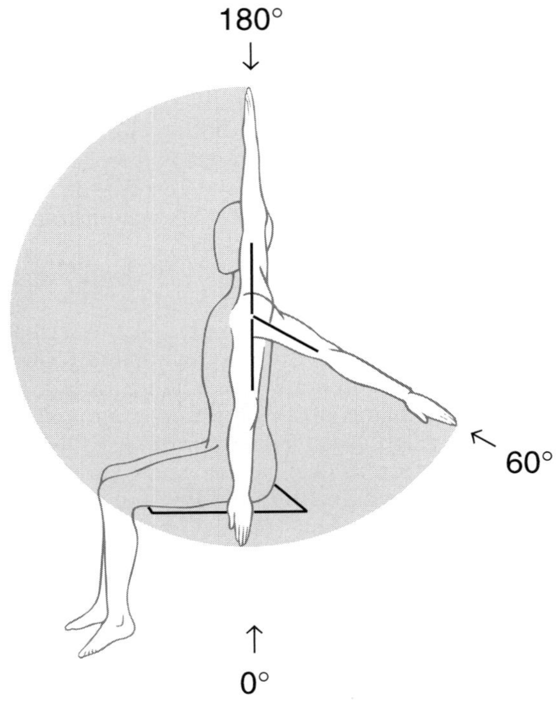

FIGURE 1–4. Shoulder flexion and extension.

Patient Position: Supine or sitting, arm at side, elbow extended.
Plane of Motion: Sagittal.
Normal ROM: Flexion, 0 to 180 degrees; extension, 0 to 60 degrees.
Movements Patient Should Avoid: Arching back, trunk rotation.
Goniometer Placement: Axis is centered on the lateral shoulder, stationary arm remains at 0 degrees, movement arm remains parallel to humerus.

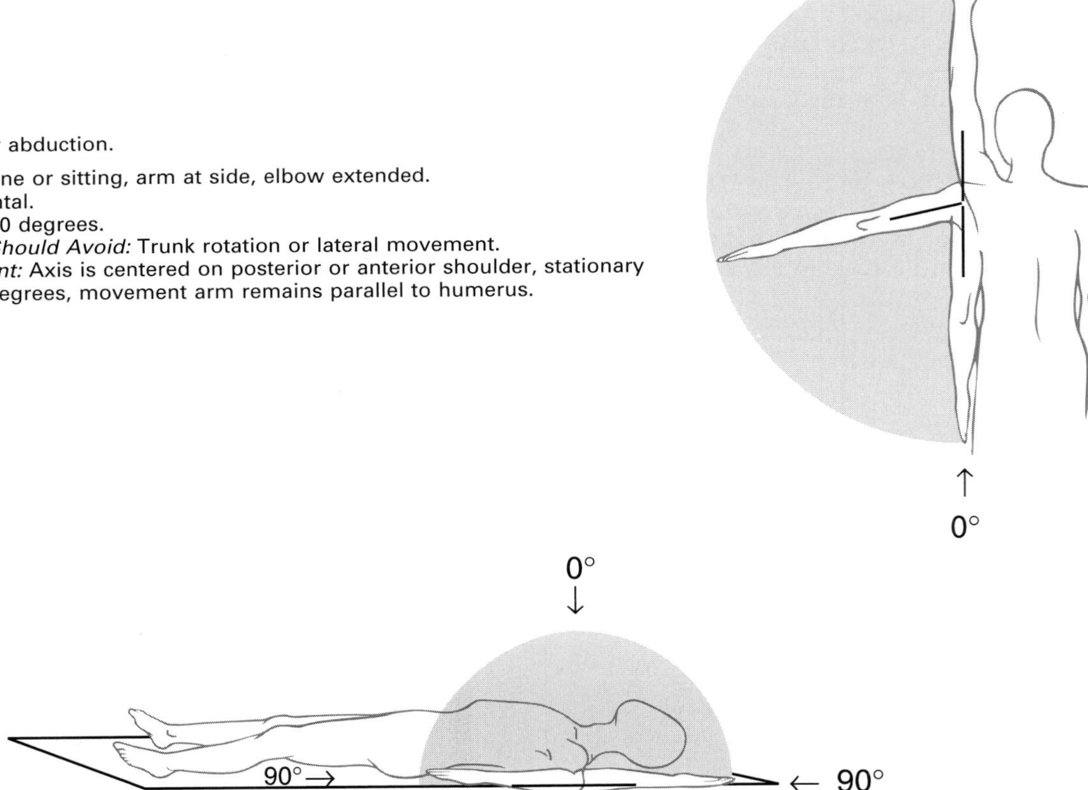

FIGURE 1–5. Shoulder abduction.

Patient Position: Supine or sitting, arm at side, elbow extended.
Plane of Motion: Frontal.
Normal ROM: 0 to 180 degrees.
Movements Patient Should Avoid: Trunk rotation or lateral movement.
Goniometer Placement: Axis is centered on posterior or anterior shoulder, stationary arm remains at 0 degrees, movement arm remains parallel to humerus.

FIGURE 1–6. Shoulder internal and external rotation.

Patient Position: Supine, shoulder at 90 degrees of abduction, elbow at 90 degrees of flexion, radioulnar joint pronated.
Plane of Motion: Transverse.
Normal ROM: Internal rotation, 0 to 90 degrees; external rotation, 0 to 90 degrees.
Movements Patient Should Avoid: Arching back, trunk rotation, elbow movement.
Goniometer Placement: Axis on elbow joint through longitudinal axis of humerus, stationary arm remains at 0 degrees, movement arm remains parallel to forearm.

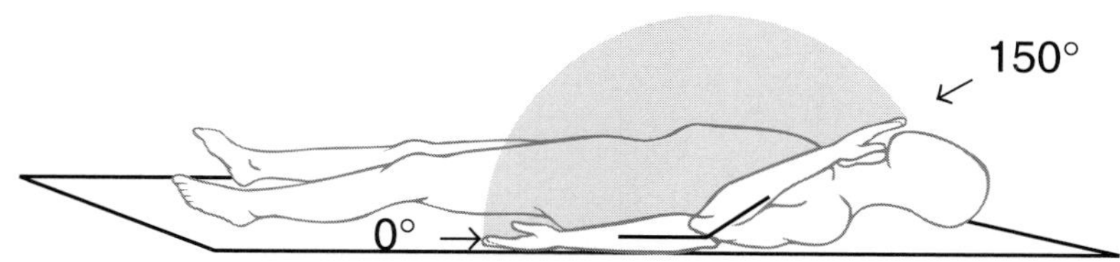

FIGURE 1–7. Elbow flexion.

Patient Position: Supine or sitting, radioulnar joint supinated.
Plane of Motion: Sagittal.
Normal ROM: 0 to 150 degrees.
Goniometer Placement: Axis is centered on lateral elbow, stationary arm remains at 0 degrees, movement arm remains parallel to forearm.

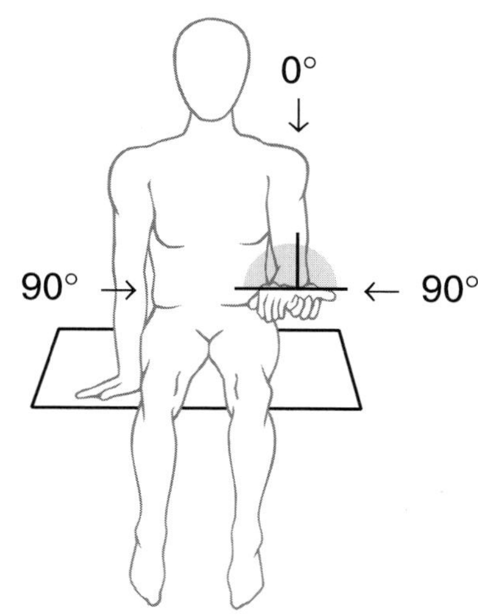

FIGURE 1–8. Radioulnar pronation and supination.

Patient Position: Sitting or standing, elbow at 90 degrees, wrist in neutral, pencil held in palm of hand.
Plane of Motion: Transverse.
Normal ROM: Pronation, 0 to 90 degrees; supination, 0 to 90 degrees.
Movements Patient Should Avoid: Arm, elbow, and wrist movements.
Goniometer Placement: Axis through longitudinal axis of forearm, stationary arm remains at 0 degrees, movement arm remains parallel to pencil held in patient's hand.

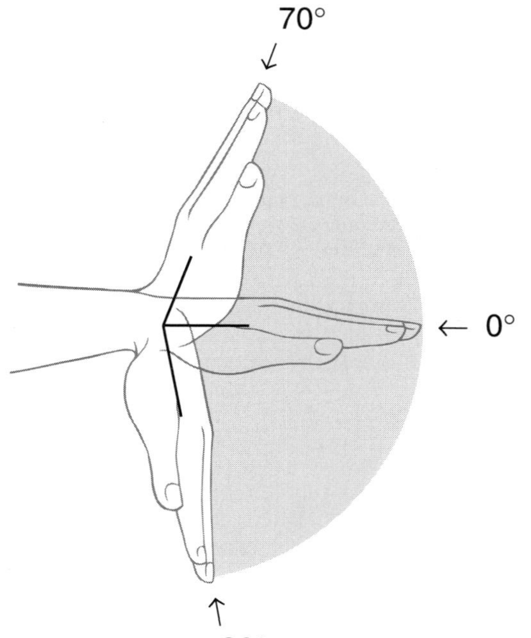

FIGURE 1–9. Wrist flexion and extension.

Patient Position: Elbow flexed, radioulnar pronated.
Plane of Motion: Sagittal.
Normal ROM: Flexion, 0 to 80 degrees; extension, 0 to 70 degrees.
Goniometer Placement: Axis is centered on lateral wrist over ulnar styloid, stationary arm remains at 0 degrees, movement arm remains parallel to fifth metacarpal.

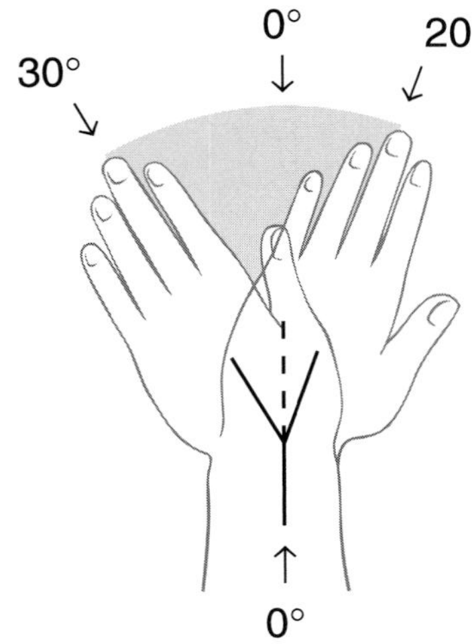

FIGURE 1–10. Wrist radial and ulnar deviation.

Patient Position: Elbow flexed, radioulnar joint pronated, wrist in neutral flexion and extension.
Plane of Motion: Frontal.
Normal ROM: Radial, 0 to 20 degrees; ulnar, 0 to 30 degrees.
Goniometer Placement: Axis is centered over dorsal wrist midway between distal radius and ulna, stationary arm remains at 0 degrees, movement arm remains parallel to third metacarpal.

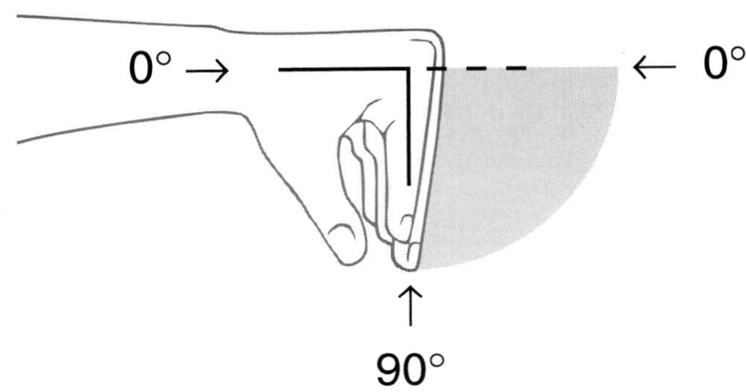

FIGURE 1–11. Second to fifth metacarpophalangeal flexion.

Patient Position: Elbow flexed, radioulnar joint pronated, wrist in neutral, fingers extended.
Plane of Motion: Sagittal.
Normal ROM: 0 to 90 degrees.
Goniometer Placement: Axis on dorsum of each metacarpophalangeal joint, stationary arm remains at 0 degrees, movement arm remains on dorsum of each proximal phalanx.

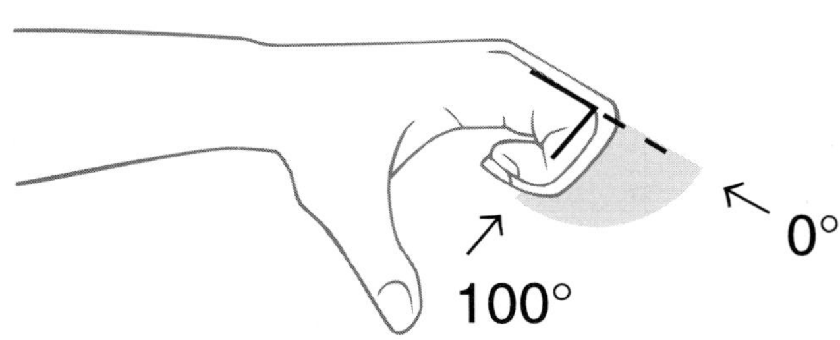

FIGURE 1–12. Second to fifth proximal interphalangeal flexion.

Patient Position: Elbow flexed, radioulnar pronated, wrist in neutral, metacarpophalangeal joints in slight flexion.
Plane of Motion: Sagittal.
Normal ROM: 0 to 100 degrees.
Goniometer Placement: Axis on dorsum of each interphalangeal joint, stationary arm remains at 0 degrees, movement arm remains on dorsum of each middle phalanx.

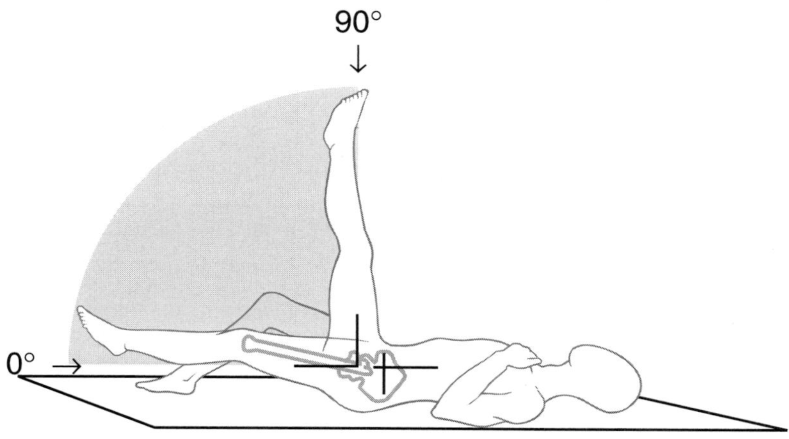

FIGURE 1–13. Hip flexion, knee extension.

Patient Position: Supine or lying on side, knee extended.
Plane of Motion: Sagittal.
Normal ROM: 0 to 90 degrees.
Movements Patient Should Avoid: Arching back.
Goniometer Placement: Axis is centered on lateral leg over greater trochanter, stationary arm remains at 0 degrees. (This is found by drawing a line from the anterior superior iliac spine to the posterior superior iliac spine, and then drawing another line, perpendicular to the first, that goes through the greater trochanter. The last line is 0 degrees.) Movement arm remains parallel to lateral femur.

FIGURE 1–14. Hip flexion, knee flexion.

Patient Position: Supine or lying on side, knee flexed.
Plane of Motion: Sagittal.
Normal ROM: 0 to 120 degrees.
Movements Patient Should Avoid: Arching back.
Goniometer Placement: Same as in Figure 1–13.

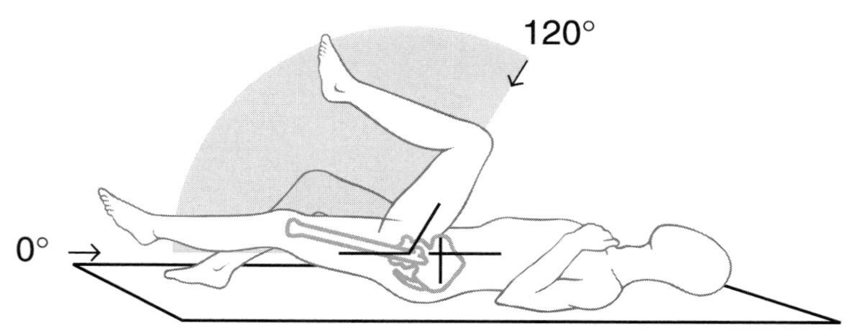

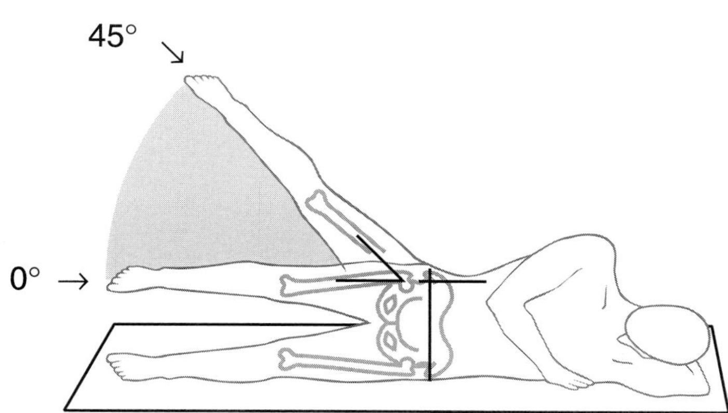

FIGURE 1–15. Hip abduction.

Patient Position: Supine or lying on side, knee extended.
Plane of Motion: Frontal.
Normal ROM: 0 to 45 degrees.
Movements Patient Should Avoid: Trunk rotation.
Goniometer Placement: Axis centered over greater trochanter, stationary arm is parallel to and below a line on patient drawn through both anterior superior iliac spines (this is perpendicular to 0 degrees), movement arm remains parallel to anterior femur.

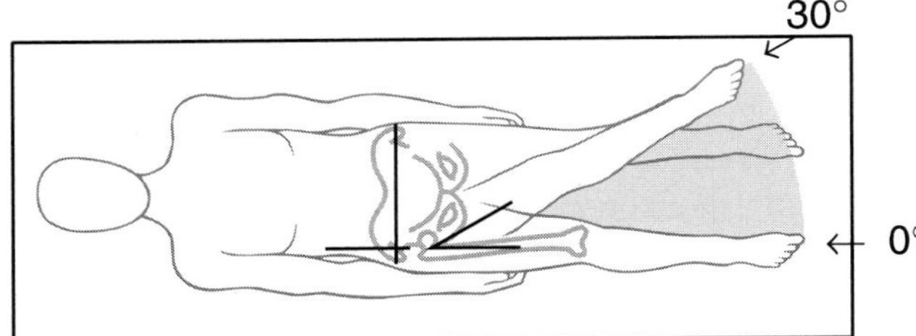

FIGURE 1–16. Hip adduction.

Patient Position: Supine, knee extended.
Plane of Motion: Frontal.
Normal ROM: 0 to 30 degrees.
Movements Patient Should Avoid: Trunk rotation.
Goniometer Placement: Same as in Figure 1–15.

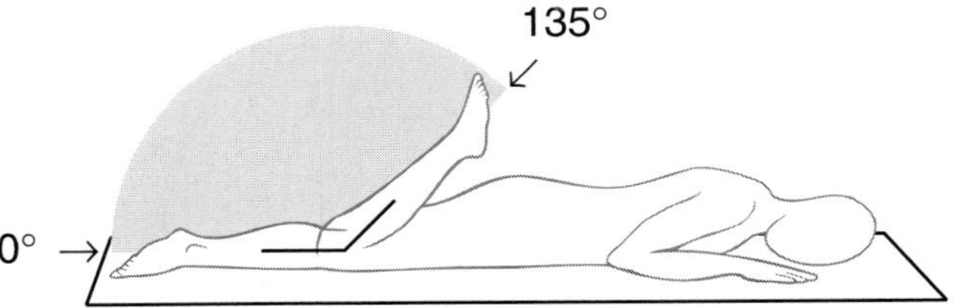

FIGURE 1–18. Knee flexion.

Patient Position: Prone or sitting, hip in neutral.
Plane of Motion: Sagittal.
Normal ROM: 0 to 135 degrees.
Goniometer Placement: Axis on lateral knee joint, stationary arm remains at 0 degrees, movement arm remains parallel to fibula laterally.

cervical flexion and extension are illustrated using a two-inclinometer technique (Fig. 1–20) and the one-inclinometer technique (Fig. 1–21).[2]

Joint Stability

The stability inherent in each joint depends on its bone integrity, ligamentous and joint capsule connections, and muscle activity. Each joint anatomically achieves stability differently. For example, shoulder joint stability depends mostly on muscle activity of the rotator cuff, whereas the hip joint depends on the ligamentous structures to provide much of the joint's stability. Basic knowledge of the joint anatomy is important for the clinician to be able to accurately diagnose joint instability problems.

Joint stability is evaluated by providing stress to all ranges of motion. If joint instability is noted, then a more specific examination of that joint using specialized tests is warranted, such as Lachman's test for ankle stability or McMurray's test for meniscus tear, which are well described in physical diagnosis texts.[3, 8, 15] (See also Chapters 39 and 44.)

Contracture

A contracture causes inability to perform full-joint ROM. It results from decreased tissue extensibility of soft tissues and muscle or from bony abnormalities.

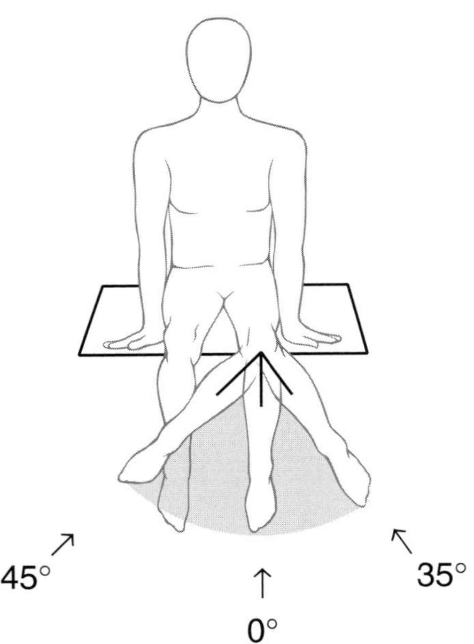

FIGURE 1–17. Hip internal and external rotation.

Patient Position: Supine or sitting, hip at 90 degrees flexion, knee at 90 degrees flexion.
Plane of Motion: Transverse.
Normal ROM: Internal, 0 to 35 degrees; external, 0 to 45 degrees.
Movements Patient Should Avoid: Hip flexion movement, knee movement.
Goniometer Placement: Axis over knee joint through longitudinal axis of femur, stationary arm remains at 0 degrees, movement arm remains parallel to anterior tibia.

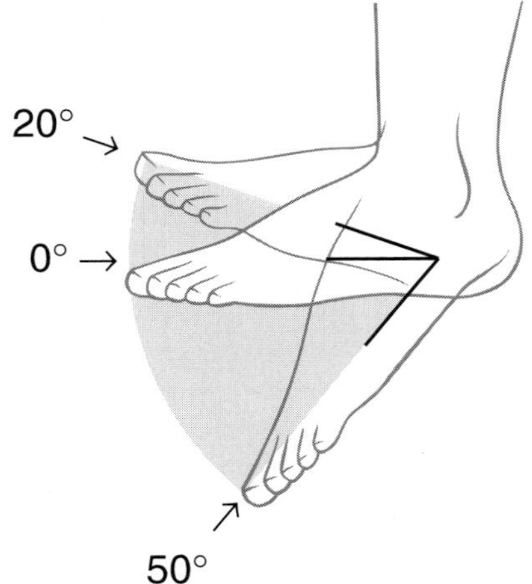

FIGURE 1–19. Ankle dorsiflexion and plantar flexion.

Patient Position: Sitting or supine with knee flexed to 90 degrees.
Plane of Motion: Sagittal.
Normal ROM: Dorsiflexion, 0 to 20 degrees; plantar flexion, 0 to 50 degrees.
Goniometer Placement: Axis is on sole of foot below lateral malleolus, stationary arm remains along shaft of fibula (this is perpendicular to 0 degrees), movement arm remains parallel to fifth metatarsal.

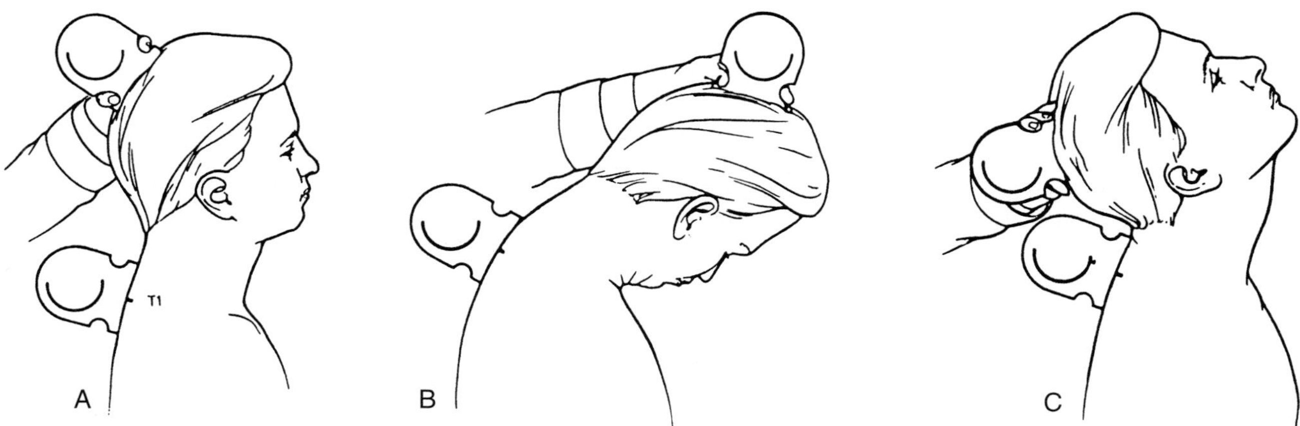

FIGURE 1–20. Two-inclinometer measurement technique for cervical flexion and extension.

1. With the patient seated, place the first inclinometer, aligned in the sagittal plane, over the T1 spinous process while holding the second inclinometer over the occiput. The head remains in neutral position while the inclinometers are set at 0 degrees (*A*).
2. Ask the patient to flex maximally and record both angles. Subtract the T1 angle from the occipital angle to obtain the cervical flexion angle. *B*. Ask the patient to return the head to the neutral position so that both inclinometers read 0 degrees again.
3. Ask the patient to extend the neck as far as possible, again recording both inclinometer angles. Subtract the T1 angle from the occipital angle to obtain the cervical extension angle (*C*).

(Adapted from Guides to the Evaluation of Permanent Impairment, ed 4. Chicago, American Medical Association, 1995, p 116.)

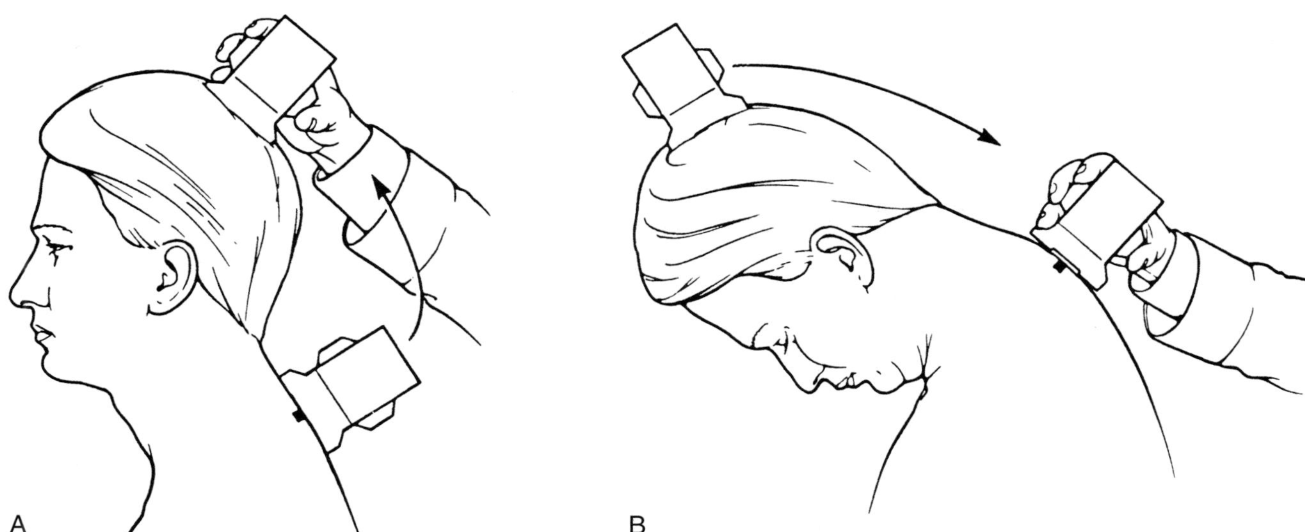

FIGURE 1–21. One-inclinometer measurement technique for cervical flexion and extension.

1. With the patient in the seated position, place the inclinometer, aligned in the sagittal plane, over the T1 spinous process and set the first 0-degree reading (*A*, position 1). Move the inclinometer to the occiput and set the second 0-degree reading (*A*, position 2).
2. Ask the patient to flex the head maximally and record the occipital flexion angle (*B*, position 3). Move the inclinometer to the T1 spinous process and record the angle while the subject maintains the head in flexion (*B*, position 4). Ask the patient to move the head back to the neutral position. Subtract the T1 reading from the occipital reading to obtain the cervical flexion angle.
3. After obtaining 0-degree readings, first from the T1 and then over the occiput, ask the patient to carry out full cervical extension. Record the angles first at the occiput and then over the T1 spinous process and subtract to obtain the cervical extension angles.

(From Guides to the Evaluation of Permanent Impairment, ed 4. Chicago, American Medical Association, 1995, p 117.)

Each contracture is evaluated for its possible cause. Significant joint contracture is often obvious just on visual inspection. Placing the joint, soft tissues, and muscles on gentle, prolonged, passive stretch can indicate whether the loss of motion is caused by abnormalities in bone, muscle, or soft tissue. Both soft tissue and muscle contractures often decrease after prolonged stretch is applied. Contractures due to bony abnormalities do not change with prolonged stretch.

Shortening of muscles that cross two or more joints is not a joint contracture, but is often noted during an examination for contractures, as shortening of these muscles can lead to ROM abnormalities. Muscles that cross two joints are normally at a length disadvantage, and even a mild loss of extensibility can lead to problems in gait and other movements.

An example of a joint motion that involves both one- and two-joint muscles is hip flexion, which involves the action of the iliopsoas, tensor fascia lata, rectus femoris, pectineus, and the adductor muscle group. This joint is specifically tested for shortness of both types of muscles using the Thomas test (Fig. 1–22). The patient is asked to lie supine with one leg dropped over the edge of the table so that the knee is free to flex. The other limb is lifted and pulled to the chest by the patient. The examiner notes whether the back flattens on the table. (The examiner should have one hand behind the patient's back to palpate for this.) Normal muscle length of both the one- and two-joint muscles allows the posterior thigh of the first leg to lie flat on the table with approximately 80 degrees of knee flexion (Fig. 1–22A). Shortened one-joint muscles (iliopsoas, pectineus, adductors) are noted when knee flexion ability is good, but the thigh rises up off the examination table (Fig. 1–22B). Shortened two-joint muscles (rectus femoris, tensor fascia lata) are diagnosed when the leg is able to maintain contact with the table but the knee cannot flex past 70 degrees (Fig. 1–22C). If both the one- and two-joint muscles are shortened, the thigh rises off the table and the knee is unable to flex past 70 degrees (Fig. 1–22D). Tensor fascia lata shortness can also cause abduction of the extended hip when this test is performed.[19]

Manual Muscle Testing

Manual muscle testing (MMT) is the technique physiatrists use to document muscle strength. MMT involves the actual test performance as well as muscle strength grading.

Prior to formal MMT, screening tests for muscle weakness can help identify areas needing specific evaluation. Upper limb strength is screened by having the patient grasp two of the examiner's fingers while the examiner attempts to free the fingers by pulling in all directions. A deep knee bend (squat and rise) screens proximal lower limb strength. Distal lower limb strength is evaluated by having the patient walk on the heels and then the toes, which tests ankle dorsiflexion and plantar

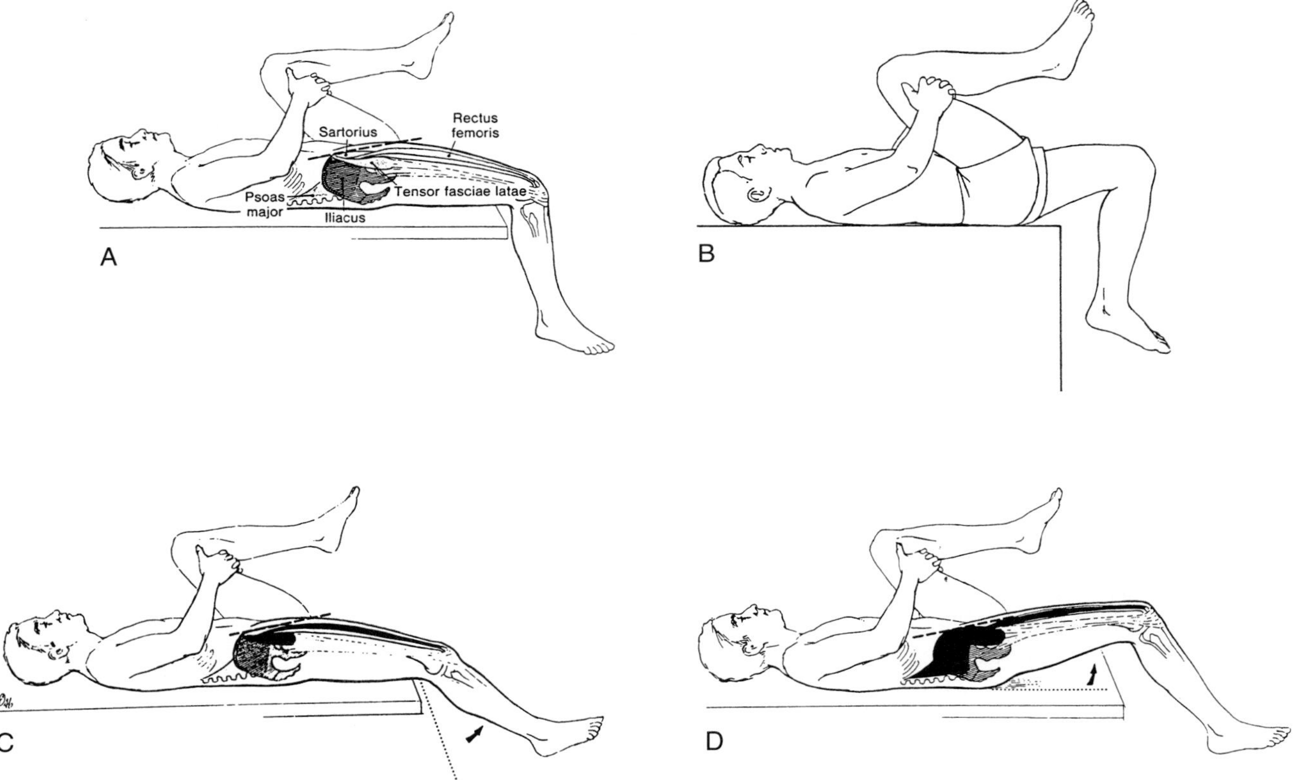

FIGURE 1–22. The Thomas test for hip flexor muscle tightness. *A.* Normal length of hip flexors. *B.* Shortness in one joint muscle only. *C.* Shortness in two joint muscles only. *D.* Shortness of both one and two joint muscles. (Adapted from Kendall FP, McCreary EK, Provance PG: Muscles Testing and Function, ed 4. Baltimore, Williams & Wilkins, 1993, pp 34–36.)

flexion strength, respectively. Increased walking cadence often increases gait abnormalities, causing them to be more evident. Abdominal strength is screened by observing a patient's ability to go from supine to sitting while the hips and knees are flexed. If the same activity is performed with the hips and knees extended, both abdominal and iliopsoas strength is evaluated.

Formal MMT requires that the examiner be proficient in the test procedures required to assess each muscle or muscle group. This proficiency requires a working knowledge of muscle function and of the techniques described in MMT reference texts such as Kendall and colleagues' *Muscles: Testing and Function*[19] or Daniels and Worthingham's *Muscle Testing: Techniques of Manual Examination.*[6] Proficiency also depends on developing expert manual skills, which typically come from practice in MMT.

The test procedure should generally be performed using the axiom "make and break." The patient is asked to "make" the muscle(s) being tested contract and to hold a specific position. The examiner then tries to "break" that muscle contraction by applying pressure at the distal end of the muscle or muscle tendon. The patient "makes" the muscle, contracting it into a set position, and the examiner attempts to "break" the muscle contraction.

MMT requires patient cooperation. Poor patient understanding of the test procedure or poor motivation to participate causes inaccuracies. Pain often prevents a full muscle contraction or causes the patient to release the contraction suddenly when resistance is provided. This is called *breakaway weakness,* and it should not be interpreted as true weakness. Documentation should reflect that pain prevented accurate MMT. A patient can also either consciously or subconsciously attempt to appear weak by a "ratchety" or inconsistent response to the resistance provided. Age, gender, pain, level of muscle conditioning, contractures, and joint stability are all factors that can lead to an inaccurate evaluation of normal muscle strength.

A few technique errors in MMT are important for the examiner to avoid. The examiner will generally want to place one hand above and one hand below the joint being affected by the muscle contraction. Avoid placing the hands so that pressure is applied across more than one joint (if possible). Often, patients try to use other muscles to assist a weak muscle or muscle group. This is called *substitution.* If it is observed, the patient should be counseled on how to avoid contaminating the MMT with substitution. At times it is necessary to intentionally place a muscle at a mechanical disadvantage to show a minor degree of weakness. For example, testing elbow extension with the elbow in 90 degrees of flexion rather than full extension can show minor weakness, especially when comparing the muscle on one side with the same muscle on the other side of the body.

MMT can also be quantified by the use of strain gauges, dynamometers, and other apparatus. Dynamometers record the force being resisted by the patient's muscles during testing. Inexpensive commercial versions are available and are commonly used, for example, to measure pinch or grip strength.

Muscle strength grading was developed to document the results of MMT. The two most common systems of muscle grading, which are listed and defined in Table 1–10, utilize numbers and words to document the results of the test. A third type of muscle strength grading, also listed in Table 1–10, uses percentages to describe muscle strength deficit and is used clinically for impairment rating.[2, 27] The examiner should do each test in a simple but standardized manner so that the results can be used for future comparisons.

When describing a muscle or muscle group that has weakness, the examiner should systematically proceed through the different grades. The patient is asked to contract the muscle while the examiner palpates it. If no movement is palpable in the muscle, it is graded 0 (zero). If muscle contraction is palpable but no joint movement is noted, the muscle is at least grade 1 (trace). Next, the examiner asks the patient to contract the muscle in a gravity-eliminated position. If the patient is able to move the body part through the full ROM then the muscle has at least grade 2 (poor) strength. The patient is asked to contract the muscle to move the body part against gravity. If the patient can move the body part through the full range of motion against gravity, there is at least grade 3 strength (fair). The examiner then provides resistance to the muscle activity, and if the patient is able to resist a moderate amount of pressure, the muscle strength is graded as 4 (good). If the patient is able to provide full resistance, the muscle strength is graded as 5 (normal). Grades 0 to 3 (zero to fair) are fairly objective, but both grades 4 and 5 (good to normal) depend on the examiner's subjective interpretation of the amount of resistance.[19, 27]

The actual MMT procedure is an evaluation of the individual's ability to perform a motion against resistance, not of the ability of one muscle to contract separately from all other muscles. Physiologically, cortical cells in the motor cortex of the brain represent the

TABLE 1–10 Systems of Muscle Strength Grading

Number	Work	Motor Deficit (%)	Definition
5	Normal	0	Complete joint range of motion against gravity with full resistance
4	Good	1–25	Complete joint range of motion against gravity with moderate resistance
3	Fair	26–50	Full joint range of motion against gravity
2	Poor	51–75	Full joint range of motion with gravity eliminated
1	Trace	76–99	Visible palpable or muscle contraction; no joint motion produced
0	Zero	100	No visible or palpable muscle contraction

Adapted from Stillwell GK, deLateur BJ, Fordyce WE, et al: Physiatric Therapeutics in Self-Directed Medical Knowledge Program in Physical Medicine and Rehabilitation, ed 2. Chicago, American Academy of Physical Medicine and Rehabilitation, 1986, p A1.

combined movements of multiple muscles, not individual muscles. When an individual is asked to do a specific movement to isolate the activity of one muscle, several other muscles also perform the movement and are actively assisting that muscle at the same time. Often the examiner positions the patient's joint so as to isolate one muscle as much as possible. For example, if the patient's radioulnar pronation is tested with the elbow in 90 degrees of flexion, this tends to isolate the pronator teres; but if pronation is tested with the elbow in full flexion (150 degrees), the pronator quadratus is preferentially isolated.

In the following sections, MMT of multiple muscles is described in a manner that emphasizes function. Functional muscle groups are discussed, with some muscles included in more than one category. The primary muscles involved in the movements are emphasized. Each muscle's peripheral and root level innervation are listed. The innervation listed is the most frequently described innervation, but anatomical variations are common. Functional anatomy reference texts such as *Hollingshead's Functional Anatomy of the Limbs and Back*[17] should be reviewed to learn the primary muscles involved in the movements. MMT references are recommended for learning the proper positioning and techniques for muscle testing.[6, 19]

SHOULDER MOVEMENTS

FLEXION (Fig. 1–23)

Deltoid, anterior portion (axillary nerve from posterior cord, C5, C6)

Pectoralis major, clavicular portion (medial and lateral pectoral nerve, C5 to T1)

Biceps brachii (musculocutaneous nerve from lateral cord, C5, C6)

Coracobrachialis (musculocutaneous nerve from lateral cord, C5, C6, C7)

TEST. The shoulder is placed in approximately 90 degrees of flexion with the elbow flexed. The examiner attempts to move the arm into extension by applying pressure over the distal humeral area. The anterior deltoid mainly produces this motion, although it is assisted by the other muscles.

EXTENSION (Fig. 1–24)

Deltoid, posterior portion (axillary nerve from posterior cord, C5, C6)

Latissimus dorsi (thoracodorsal nerve from posterior cord, C6, C7, C8)

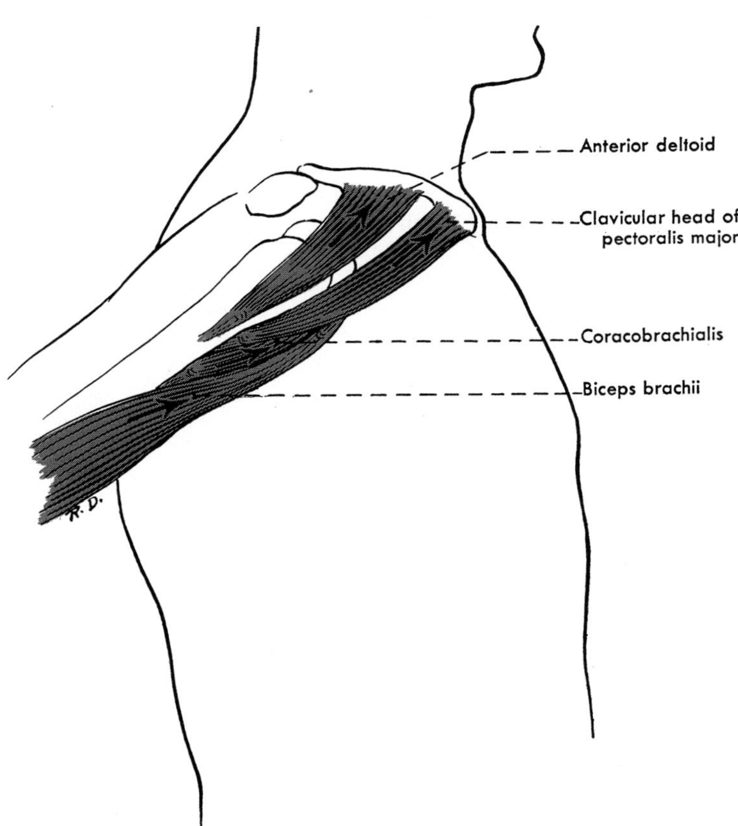

FIGURE 1–23. Shoulder flexors. (From Jenkins DB: Hollingshead's Functional Anatomy of the Limbs and Back, ed 6. Philadelphia, WB Saunders, 1998.)

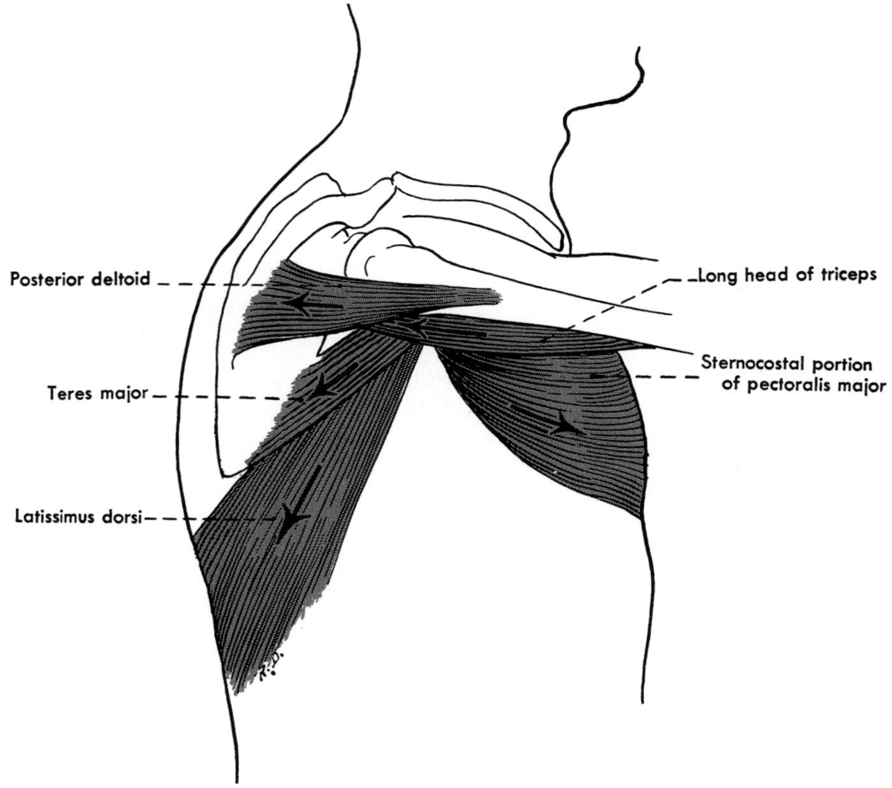

FIGURE 1–24. Shoulder extensors. (From Jenkins DB: Hollingshead's Functional Anatomy of the Limbs and Back, ed 6. Philadelphia, WB Saunders, 1998.)

Teres major (lower subscapular nerve from posterior cord, C5, C6)

TEST. The shoulder is placed in approximately 45 degrees of extension with the elbow extended. The examiner attempts to move the arm into flexion by applying pressure over the distal humeral area.

ABDUCTION (Fig. 1–25)

Deltoid, middle portion (axillary nerve from posterior cord, C5, C6)

Supraspinatus (suprascapular nerve from upper trunk, C5, C6)

TEST. The shoulder is placed in approximately 90 degrees of abduction. The examiner attempts to move the shoulder into adduction by applying pressure over the distal humeral area.

ADDUCTION (Fig. 1–26)

Pectoralis major (medial and lateral pectoral nerve, C5 to T1)

Latissimus dorsi (thoracodorsal nerve from posterior cord, C6, C7, C8)

Teres major (lower subscapular nerve from posterior cord, C5, C6)

TEST. The shoulder is placed at the side. The examiner attempts to pull the arm away from the side by applying pressure over the distal humeral area.

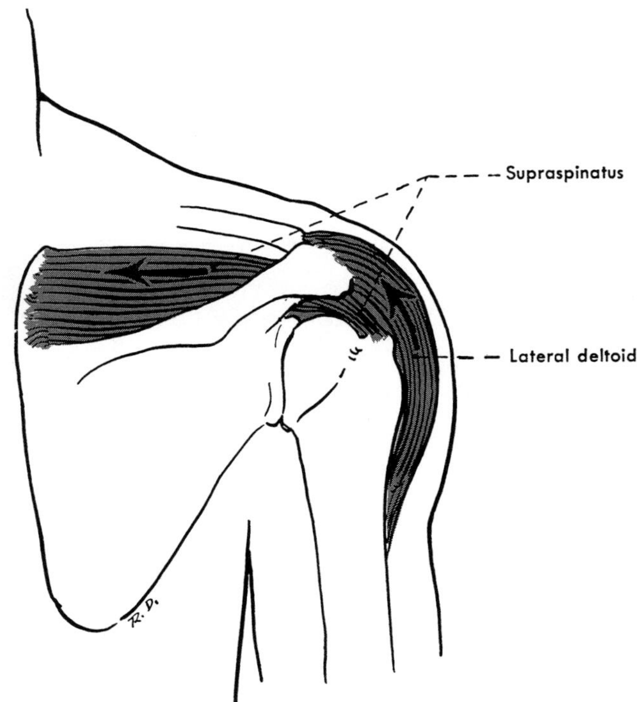

FIGURE 1–25. Shoulder abductors. (From Jenkins DB: Hollingshead's Functional Anatomy of the Limbs and Back, ed 6. Philadelphia, WB Saunders, 1998.)

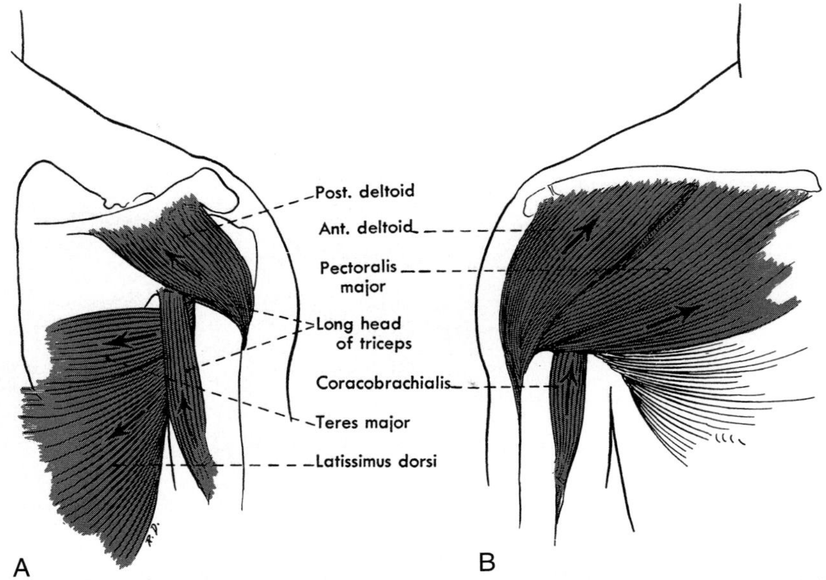

FIGURE 1–26. Shoulder adductors. *A.* Posterior view. *B.* Anterior view. (From Jenkins DB: Hollingshead's Functional Anatomy of the Limbs and Back, ed 6. Philadelphia, WB Saunders, 1998.)

INTERNAL ROTATION (Fig. 1–27)

Subscapularis (upper and lower subscapular nerve from posterior cord, C5, C6)

Pectoralis major (medial and lateral pectoral nerve, C5 to T1)

Latissimus dorsi (thoracodorsal nerve from posterior cord, C6, C7, C8)

Deltoid, anterior portion (axillary nerve from posterior cord, C5, C6)

Teres major (lower subscapular nerve from posterior cord, C5, C6)

TEST. The shoulder is placed in 90 degrees of abduction with full internal rotation and 90 degrees of elbow flexion. The examiner attempts to force the arm into

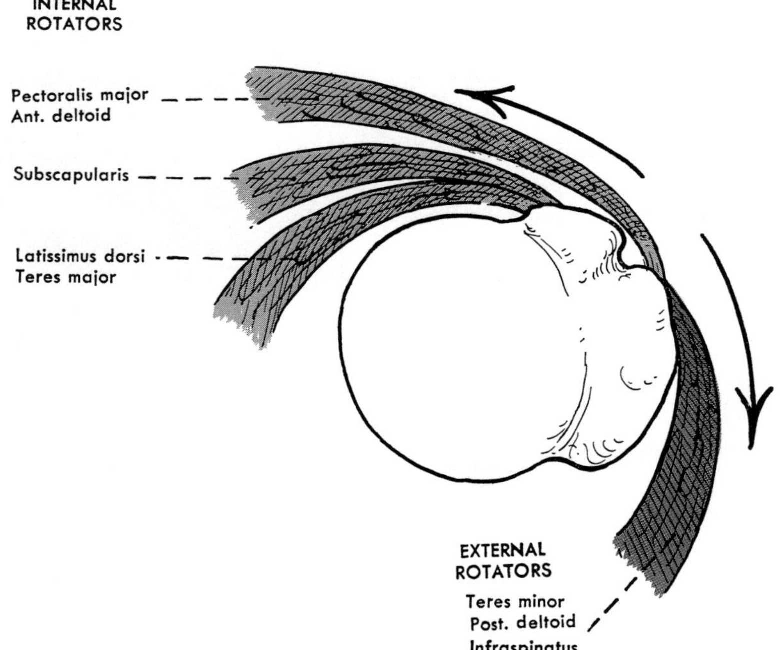

FIGURE 1–27. Shoulder internal and external rotators. (From Jenkins DB: Hollingshead's Functional Anatomy of the Limbs and Back, ed 6. Philadelphia, WB Saunders, 1998.)

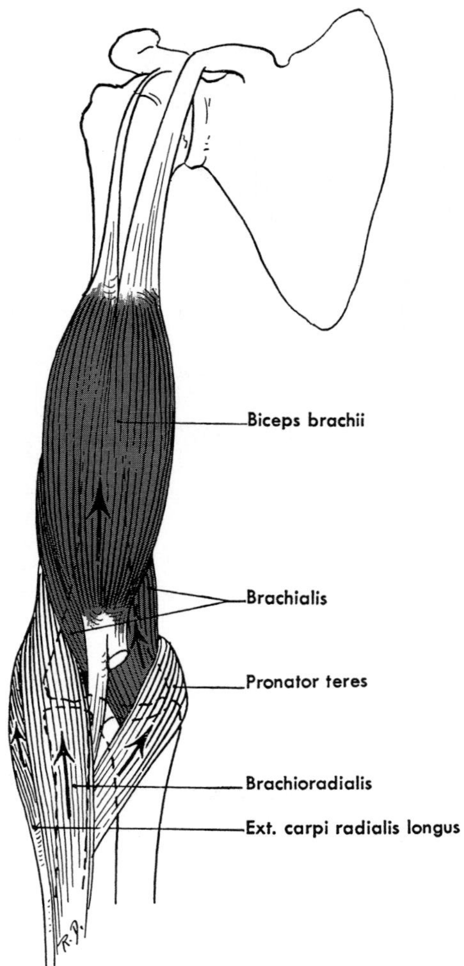

FIGURE 1–28. Elbow flexors. (From Jenkins DB: Hollingshead's Functional Anatomy of the Limbs and Back, ed 6. Philadelphia, WB Saunders, 1998.)

external rotation, applying pressure over the distal forearm.

EXTERNAL ROTATION (see Fig. 1–27)

Infraspinatus (suprascapular nerve from upper trunk, C5, C6)

Teres minor (axillary nerve from posterior cord, C5, C6)

Deltoid, posterior portion (axillary nerve from posterior cord, C5, C6)

TEST. The shoulder is placed in 90 degrees of abduction with full external rotation and 90 degrees of elbow flexion. The examiner attempts to force the arm into internal rotation, applying pressure over the distal forearm.

ELBOW MOVEMENTS

FLEXION (Fig. 1–28)

Biceps brachii (musculocutaneous nerve from lateral cord, C5, C6)

Brachialis (musculocutaneous nerve from lateral cord, C5, C6)

Brachioradialis (radial nerve from posterior cord, C5, C6)

TEST. The elbow is placed in approximately 90 degrees of flexion. The examiner attempts to force the elbow into extension, applying pressure over the distal forearm. Depending on the forearm position, the examiner is able to more specifically test each of the three muscles. In full radioulnar supination, the biceps muscle is the primary elbow flexor, whereas in full radioulnar pronation, the brachialis is the primary flexor. If the forearm is held in 0 degrees of flexion, or neutral position between pronation and supination ("thumbs-up" position), the main muscle of elbow flexion is the brachioradialis.

EXTENSION (Fig. 1–29)

Triceps (radial nerve from posterior cord, C6, C7, C8)

TEST. The elbow is placed in a few degrees of elbow flexion. (The number of degrees of elbow flexion can vary from 30 to almost full extension. The elbow is never in a fully extended position, because in that position the patient may be able to stabilize it, and a subtle elbow extension weakness might be missed.) The examiner

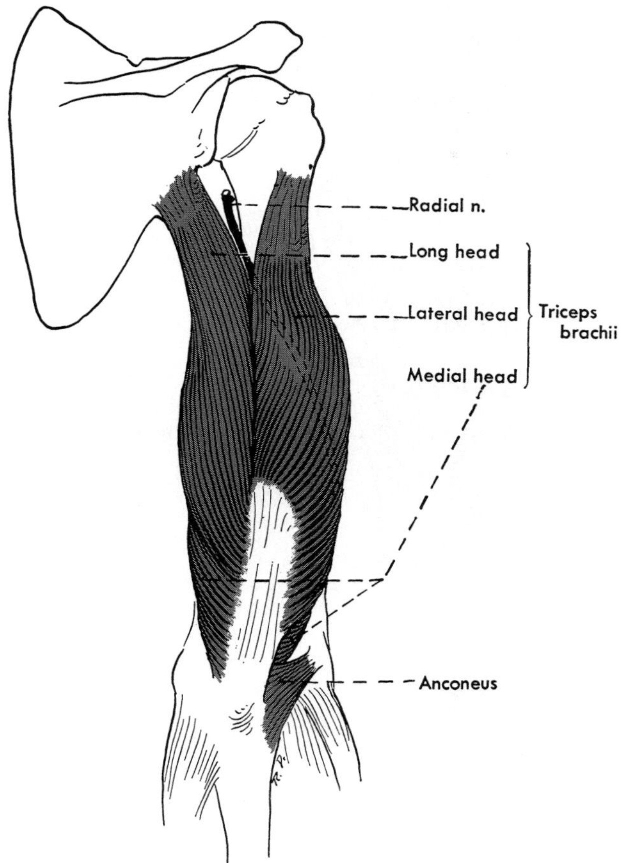

FIGURE 1–29. Elbow extensors. (From Jenkins DB: Hollingshead's Functional Anatomy of the Limbs and Back, ed 6. Philadelphia, WB Saunders, 1998.)

attempts to force the elbow into flexion, applying pressure over the distal forearm.

RADIOULNAR MOVEMENTS

PRONATION (Fig. 1–30)

Pronator quadratus (anterior interosseous branch of the median nerve, C7, C8, T1)

Pronator teres (median nerve from lateral cord, C6, C7)

TEST. The elbow is placed in a position of full pronation. The examiner attempts to force the radioulnar joint or forearm into supination, applying pressure at the distal forearm. If the elbow is partially flexed (90 degrees), the pronator teres is primarily tested. If the elbow is held in a position of full flexion, the pronator quadratus is the main pronator muscle.

SUPINATION (Fig. 1–31)

Supinator (radial nerve from posterior cord, C5, C6)

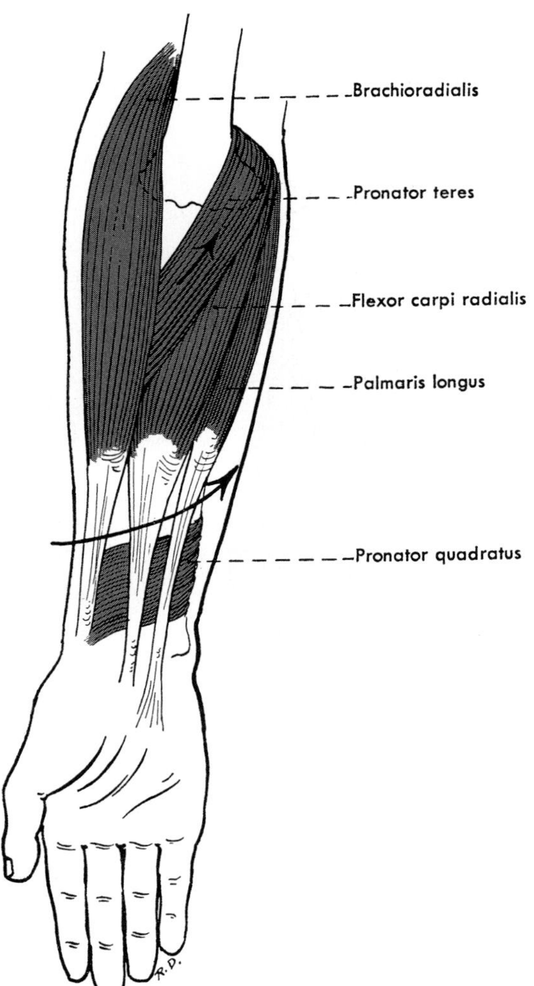

FIGURE 1–30. Radioulnar pronators. (From Jenkins DB: Hollingshead's Functional Anatomy of the Limbs and Back, ed 6. Philadelphia, WB Saunders, 1998.)

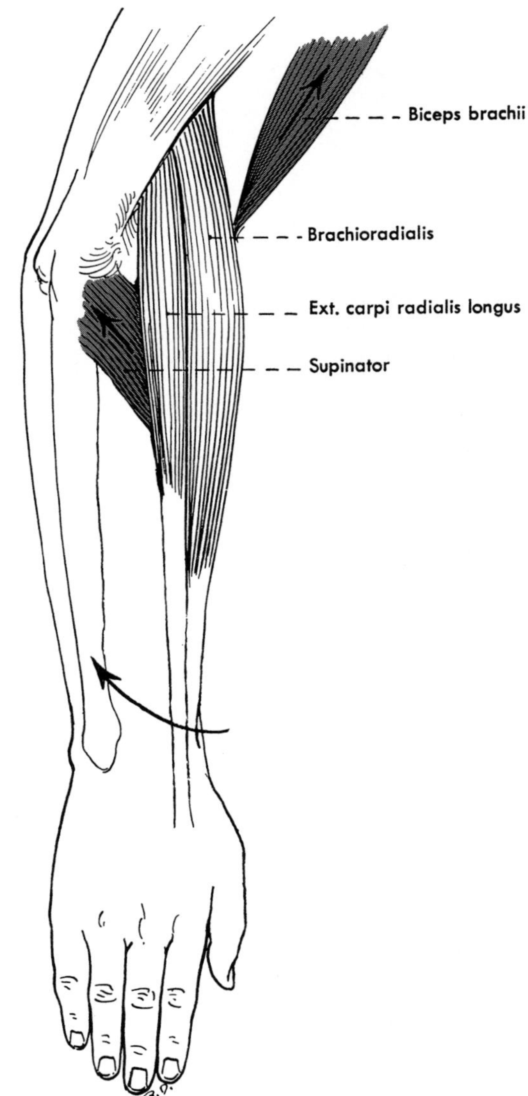

FIGURE 1–31. Radioulnar supinators. (From Jenkins DB: Hollingshead's Functional Anatomy of the Limbs and Back, ed 6. Philadelphia, WB Saunders, 1998.)

Biceps brachii (musculocutaneous nerve from lateral cord, C5, C6)

TEST. Because the biceps is tested by elbow flexion (see preceding section, Elbow Movements: Flexion), the arm should be placed in a position to favor the supinator muscle strength. To do this, the elbow is placed in full flexion with the radioulnar joint or forearm in full supination. In this position the biceps is unable to assist in the act of supination. The examiner attempts to force the radioulnar joint or forearm into pronation, applying pressure at the distal forearm.

WRIST MOVEMENTS

FLEXION (Fig. 1–32)

Flexor carpi radialis (median nerve from lateral cord, C6, C7)

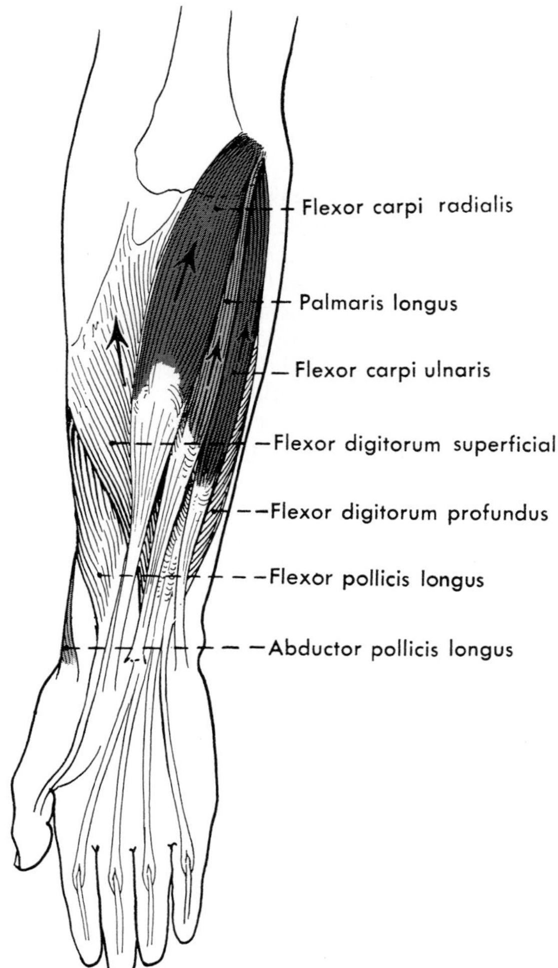

FIGURE 1–32. Wrist flexors. (From Jenkins DB: Hollingshead's Functional Anatomy of the Limbs and Back, ed 6. Philadelphia, WB Saunders, 1998.)

Flexor carpi ulnaris (ulnar nerve from medial cord, C8, T1)

TEST. The wrist is placed in a neutral position between radial and ulnar deviation and in full flexion, with the fingers extended. The examiner attempts to force the wrist into extension, applying pressure at the midpalm level. To more selectively test the flexor carpi radialis, the patient's wrist is placed in a position of radial deviation and full flexion. The examiner attempts to force the wrist into extension and ulnar deviation. To more selectively test the flexor carpi ulnaris, the patient's wrist is placed in a position of ulnar deviation and full flexion. The examiner attempts to force the wrist into extension and radial deviation.

EXTENSION (Fig. 1–33)

Extensor carpi radialis longus (radial nerve from posterior cord, C6, C7)

Extensor carpi radialis brevis (radial nerve from posterior cord, C6, C7)

Extensor carpi ulnaris (radial nerve from posterior cord, C6, C7, C8)

TEST. The wrist is placed in a neutral position between radial and ulnar deviation and in full extension, with the fingers extended. The examiner attempts to force the wrist into flexion, applying pressure over the dorsum of the hand. To more selectively test the extensor carpi radialis longus, the patient's wrist is placed in a position of radial deviation and full extension. The examiner attempts to force the wrist into flexion and ulnar deviation. To more selectively test the extensor carpi ulnaris, the patient's wrist is placed in a position of ulnar deviation and full extension. The examiner attempts to force the wrist into flexion and radial deviation. It is difficult to position the hand to isolate the extensor carpi radialis brevis because of the midline position of its tendon insertion in the wrist.

THUMB AND DIGIT MOVEMENTS

Only a few important strength testing movements are discussed; the reader should consult reference texts for additional thumb and digit tests.

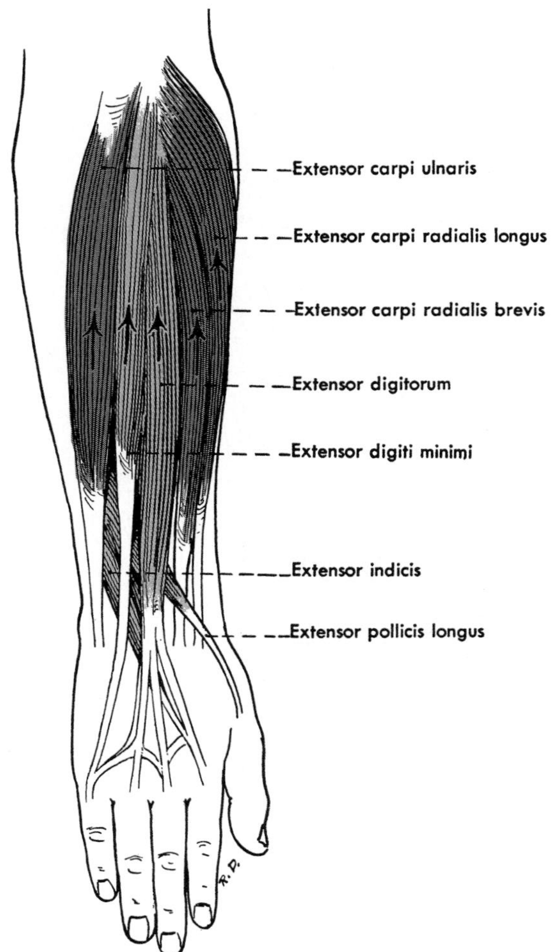

FIGURE 1–33. Wrist extensors. (From Jenkins DB: Hollingshead's Functional Anatomy of the Limbs and Back, ed 6. Philadelphia, WB Saunders, 1998.)

THUMB ABDUCTION (Fig. 1–34)

Abductor pollicis brevis (median nerve, C8, T1)

Abductor pollicis longus (radial nerve, C6, C7)

Extensor pollicis brevis (radial nerve, C6, C7)

TEST. The thumb is placed in abduction and perpendicular to the plane of the palm. The examiner attempts to force the thumb into adduction (toward the palm), applying pressure just above the first metacarpophalangeal joint.

THUMB OPPOSITION (see Fig. 1–34)

Opponens pollicis (median nerve, C8, T1)

Flexor pollicis brevis (superficial head: median nerve; deep head: ulnar nerve, C8, T1)

Abductor pollicis brevis (median nerve, C8, T1)

TEST. The thumb is placed in opposition. The examiner attempts to force the thumb back into anatomical position, applying pressure just above the first metacarpophalangeal joint.

SECOND TO FIFTH DIGIT FLEXION (see Fig. 1–34)

Flexor digitorum superficialis (median nerve, C7, C8, T1)

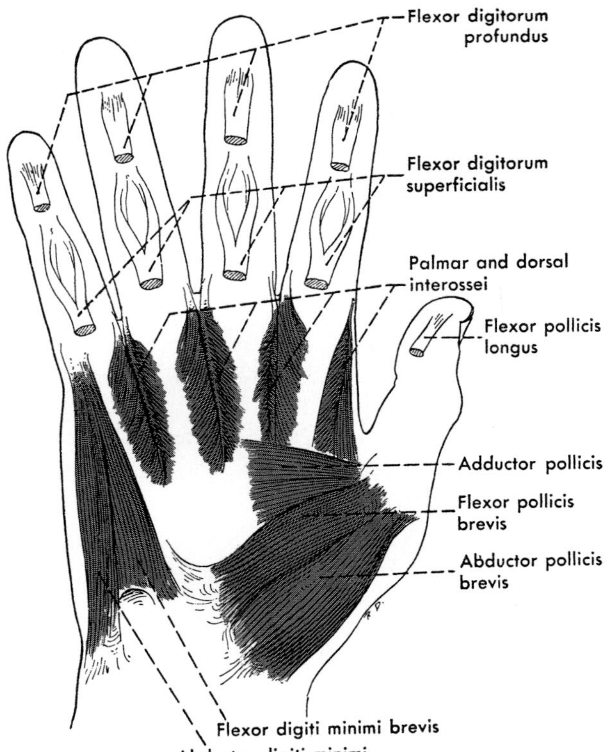

FIGURE 1–34. Muscles of the hand. (From Jenkins DB: Hollingshead's Functional Anatomy of the Limbs and Back, ed 6. Philadelphia, WB Saunders, 1998.)

Flexor digitorum profundus (lateral portion: median nerve, medial portion: ulnar nerve, C8, T1)

Lumbricals (lateral two: median nerve; medial two: ulnar nerve, C8, T1)

Interossei (ulnar nerve, C8, T1)

TEST. Because the tendons of the flexor digitorum profundus extend to the distal phalanges, the examiner tests the strength of this muscle by attempting to force each distal phalangeal joint into extension after it is placed in a position of flexion. The tendons of the flexor digitorum superficialis extend to the middle phalanx. The examiner tests both the superficialis and the profundus by attempting to force each middle phalangeal joint into extension after each is placed in a position of flexion. The primary flexors of the metacarpophalangeal joints of the second to fourth digits are the lumbricals and the interossei. The examiner tests these muscles by attempting to force each metacarpophalangeal joint into extension after each is placed in a position of flexion. The primary flexors of the fifth digit metacarpophalangeal joint are the flexors and abductor digiti minimi muscles, and MMT of flexion of this joint evaluates their strength.

SECOND TO FIFTH DIGIT EXTENSION (see Fig. 1–34)

Extensor digitorum (radial nerve, C6, C7, C8)

Extensor indicis (radial nerve, C7, C8)

Extensor digiti minimi (radial nerve, C6, C7, C8)

TEST. The second to fifth digits are placed in extension with the wrist in neutral position between flexion and extension (0 degrees). The examiner attempts to force each finger into flexion by applying a force over each proximal phalanx.

SECOND TO FOURTH DIGIT ABDUCTION, FIRST TO FIFTH DIGIT ADDUCTION (see Fig. 1–34)

Dorsal interossei (ulnar nerve, C8, T1)

Palmar interossei (ulnar nerve, C8, T1)

TEST. One method of testing adduction of these digits is to attempt to withdraw a piece of paper that has been placed between the patient's fingers while the patient attempts to retain the paper. Abduction is tested by placing each digit in abduction and attempting to force the digit into adduction. Note that the third digit cannot adduct, as movement of this digit to either side is abduction.

FIFTH DIGIT ABDUCTION (see Fig. 1–34)

Abductor digiti minimi (ulnar nerve, C8, T1)

Flexor digiti minimi (ulnar nerve, C8, T1)

TEST. The patient's fifth digit is placed in abduction. The examiner attempts to force the digit into adduction by applying pressure just above the metacarpophalangeal joint.

HIP MOVEMENTS

FLEXION (Fig. 1–35)

Iliacus (femoral nerve, L2, L3, L4)

Psoas (lumbar plexus, L2, L3, L4)

Tensor fascia latae (superior gluteal nerve, L4, L5, S1)

Rectus femoris (femoral nerve, L2, L3, L4)

Pectineus (femoral or obturator nerve, L2, L3)

Adductor longus, brevis, anterior portion of magnus (obturator nerve, L2, L3, L4)

TEST. Hip flexion is tested with the patient in both seated and supine positions. With the patient in a sitting position, the hip is placed in flexion by raising the knee. The examiner attempts to force the hip into extension, applying pressure over the distal anterior thigh. With the patient supine, the patient's hip is placed in flexion with the knee extended. The examiner attempts to force the hip into extension, applying pressure over the distal anterior thigh. The primary muscle of flexion is the iliopsoas, especially when resistance is applied.

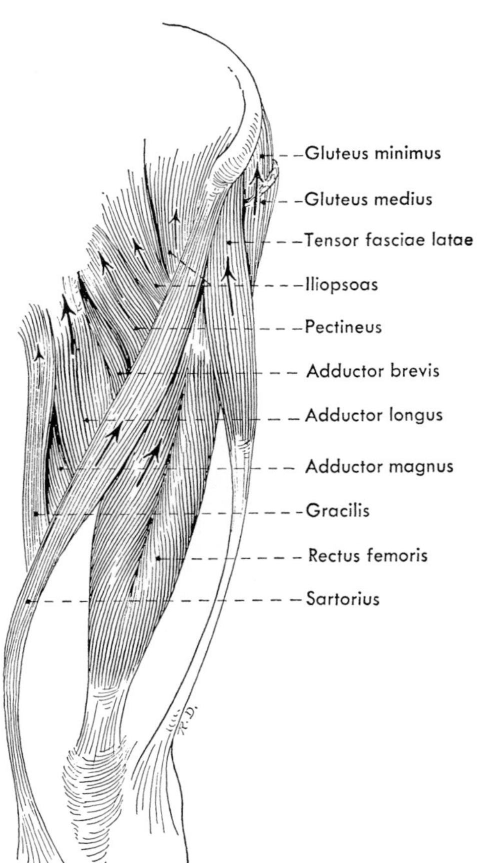

FIGURE 1–35. Hip flexors. (From Jenkins DB: Hollingshead's Functional Anatomy of the Limbs and Back, ed 6. Philadelphia, WB Saunders, 1998.)

EXTENSION (Fig. 1–36)

Gluteus maximus (inferior gluteal nerve, L5, S1, S2)

TEST. With the patient in a prone position, the hip is placed in extension with the knee flexed to 90 degrees. The examiner attempts to force the hip into flexion, applying pressure over the distal posterior thigh.

ABDUCTION (Fig. 1–37)

Gluteus medius (superior gluteal nerve, L4, L5, S1)

Gluteus minimus (superior gluteal nerve, L4, L5, S1)

Tensor fascia latae (superior gluteal nerve, L4, L5, S1)

TEST. With the patient in a side-lying position, the hip is placed in abduction. The examiner attempts to force the hip into adduction, applying pressure over the distal lateral thigh. An easier but less accurate test is performed with the patient seated. With the patient in a sitting position, the hips are placed in abduction (knees separated). The examiner attempts to force the hips into adduction, applying pressure over the distal lateral thighs.

ADDUCTION (Fig. 1–38)

Adductor brevis (obturator nerve, L2, L3, L4)

Adductor longus (obturator nerve, L2, L3)

Adductor magnus, anterior portion (obturator nerve, L3, L4)

Pectineus (femoral or obturator nerve, L2, L3)

TEST. The most accurate method requires the patient to assume a side-lying position. With the patient in a side-lying position, the examiner positions the top leg in abduction and the patient is asked to bring the bottom leg up into adduction to meet the top leg. The examiner attempts to force the bottom leg down into abduction, applying pressure over the distal medial thigh. An easier but less accurate test is performed with the patient in a sitting position. The hips are placed in adduction (knees together). The examiner attempts to force the hips into abduction, applying pressure over the distal medial thigh.

INTERNAL ROTATION (Fig. 1–39)

Tensor fasciae latae (superior gluteal nerve, L4, L5, S1)

Pectineus (femoral or obturator nerve, L2, L3)

Gluteus minimus, anterior portion (superior gluteal nerve, L4, L5, S1)

TEST. The patient is either seated with both knees bent at 90 degrees or prone with one knee bent at 90 degrees. In either position, the tested hip is placed in internal rotation. The examiner uses one hand to attempt to force the leg into external rotation, applying lateral pressure just above the ankle while stabilizing the knee with the other hand.

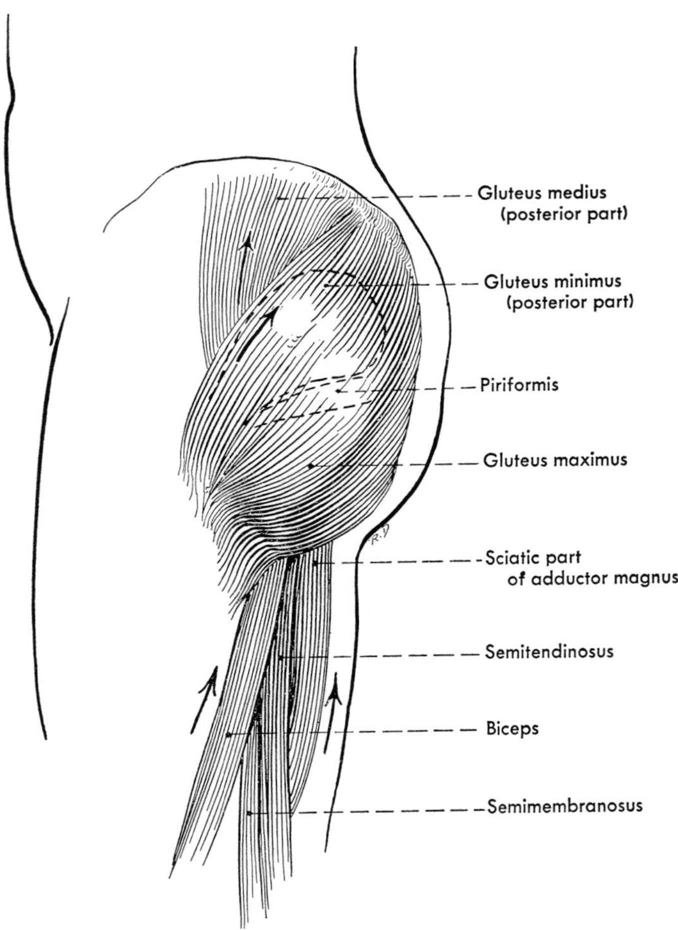

FIGURE 1–36. Hip extensors. Primary extensor is gluteus maximus. (From Jenkins DB: Hollingshead's Functional Anatomy of the Limbs and Back, ed 6. Philadelphia, WB Saunders, 1998.)

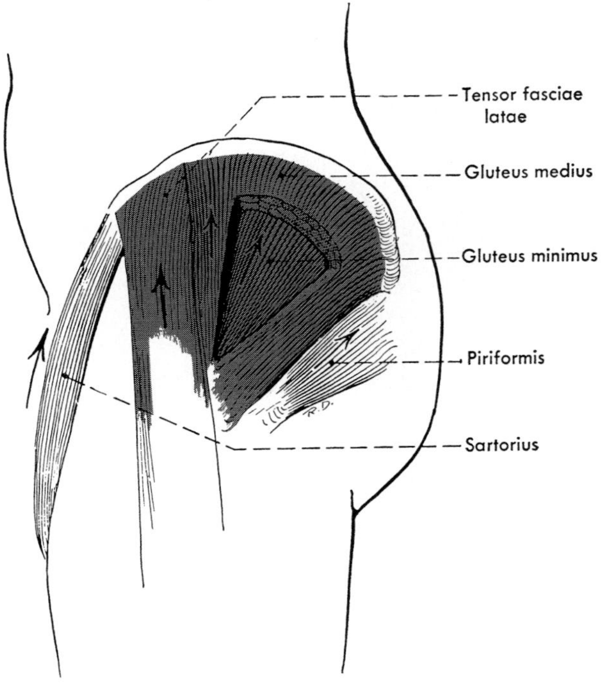

FIGURE 1–37. Hip abductors. (From Jenkins DB: Hollingshead's Functional Anatomy of the Limbs and Back, ed 6. Philadelphia, WB Saunders, 1998.)

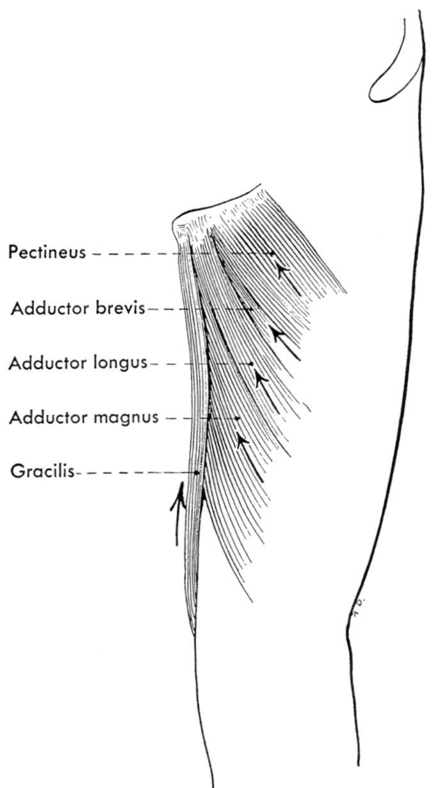

FIGURE 1–38. Hip adductors. (From Jenkins DB: Hollingshead's Functional Anatomy of the Limbs and Back, ed 6. Philadelphia, WB Saunders, 1998.)

EXTERNAL ROTATION (Fig. 1–40)

Gluteus maximus (inferior gluteal nerve, L5, S1, S2)

Piriformis (nerve to piriformis, S1, S2)

Superior gemelli and obturator internus (nerve to obturator internus, L5, S1, S2)

Inferior gemelli and quadratus femoris (nerve to quadratus femoris, L4, L5, S1)

TEST. The patient is either seated with both knees bent at 90 degrees or prone with one knee bent at 90 degrees. In either position, the tested hip is placed in external rotation. The examiner uses one hand to attempt to force the leg into internal rotation, applying pressure medially just above the ankle while stabilizing the knee with the other hand.

KNEE MOVEMENTS

FLEXION (Fig. 1–41)

Semitendinosus (tibial portion of sciatic nerve, L5, S1)

Semimembranosus (tibial portion of sciatic nerve, L5, S1)

Biceps femoris (tibial portion of sciatic nerve, L5, S1, S2)

TEST. The patient's knee is placed in 90 degrees of flexion while the patient is in a seated or prone position. The examiner attempts to force the leg into extension, applying pressure over the posterior tibial surface.

EXTENSION (Fig. 1–42)

Quadriceps femoris (femoral nerve, L2, L3, L4)

TEST. The knee is placed in approximately 30 degrees of flexion while the patient is in a seated or supine position. Full knee extension is avoided because the patient is able to stabilize the knee in that position, and minor quadriceps weakness might be missed. The examiner attempts to force the leg into flexion, applying pressure over the anterior tibial surface.

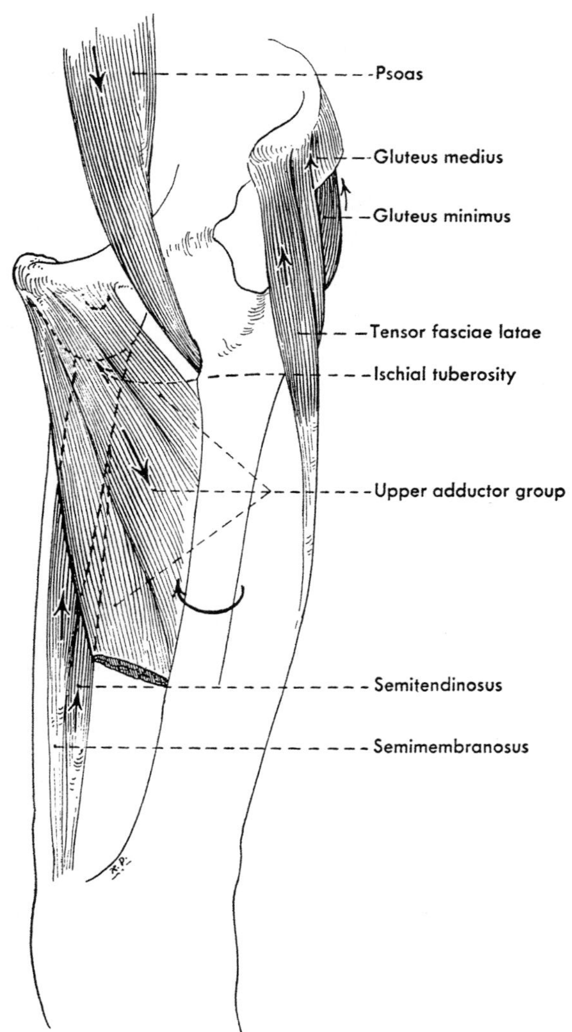

FIGURE 1–39. Hip internal rotators. Primary internal rotators are tensor fasciae latae, pectineus, and anterior portion of gluteus minimus. (From Jenkins DB: Hollingshead's Functional Anatomy of the Limbs and Back, ed 6. Philadelphia, WB Saunders, 1998.)

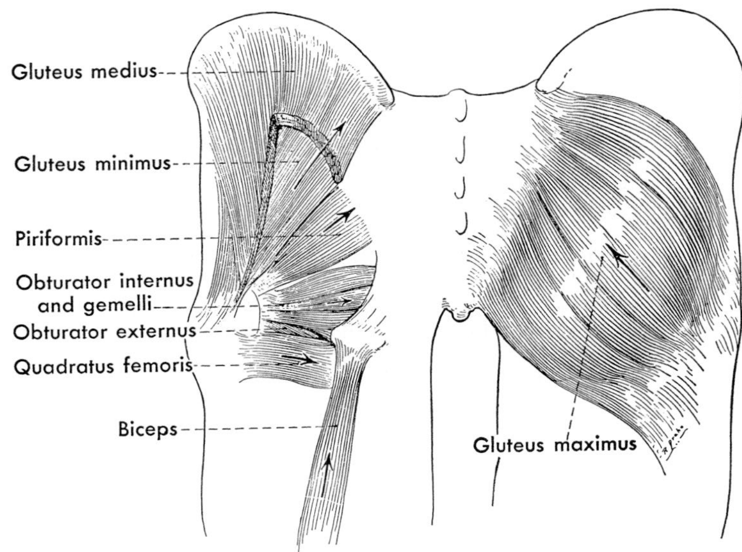

FIGURE 1–40. Hip external rotators. (From Jenkins DB: Hollingshead's Functional Anatomy of the Limbs and Back, ed 6. Philadelphia, WB Saunders, 1998.)

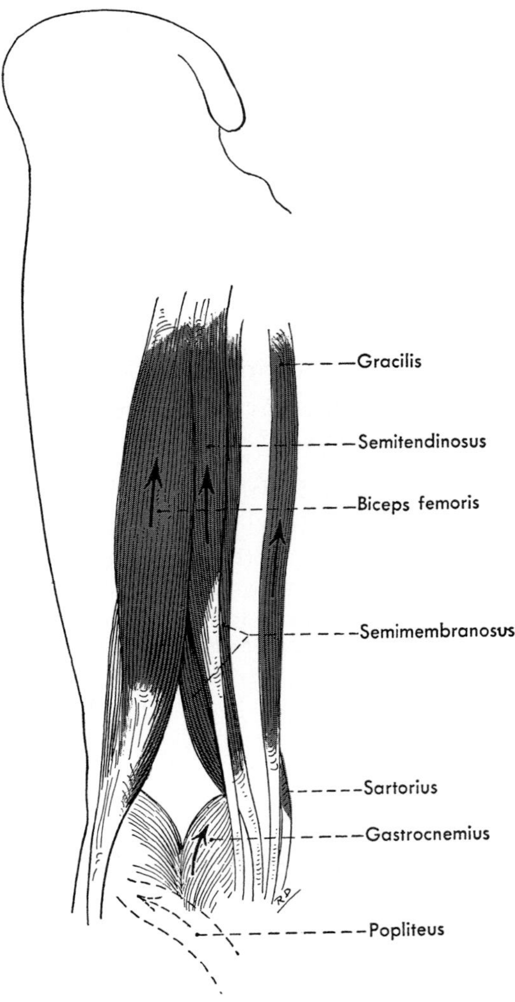

FIGURE 1–41. Knee flexors. (From Jenkins DB: Hollingshead's Functional Anatomy of the Limbs and Back, ed 6. Philadelphia, WB Saunders, 1998.)

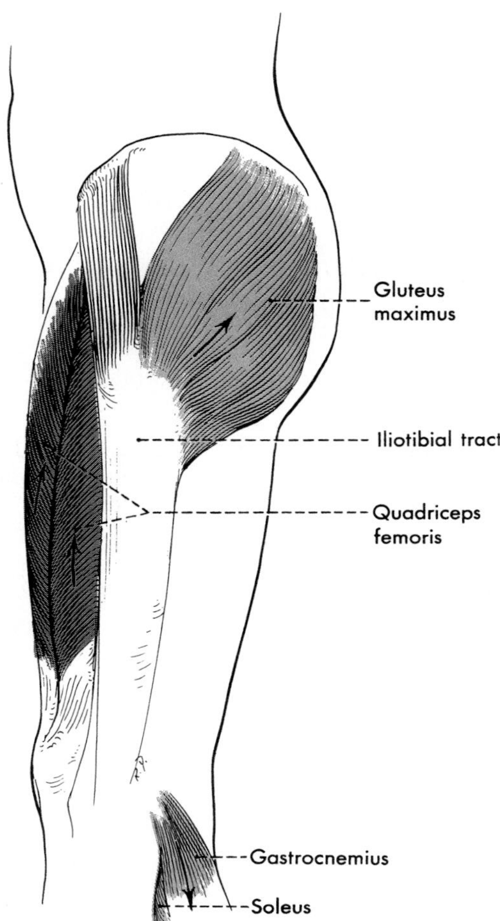

FIGURE 1–42. Knee extensors. Primary knee extensor is the quadriceps femoris. (From Jenkins DB: Hollingshead's Functional Anatomy of the Limbs and Back, ed 6. Philadelphia, WB Saunders, 1998.)

ANKLE MOVEMENTS

DORSIFLEXION (Fig. 1–43)

Tibialis anterior (deep peroneal nerve, L4, L5, S1)

Extensor digitorum longus (deep peroneal nerve, L4, L5, S1)

Extensor hallucis longus (deep peroneal nerve, L4, L5, S1)

TEST. All of these muscles work together to produce dorsiflexion when the foot is in a neutral position between inversion and eversion. The ankle is placed in dorsiflexion. The examiner attempts to force the ankle into plantar flexion, applying pressure over the dorsum of the foot. To more selectively test the tibialis anterior, the ankle is placed in a position of inversion and full dorsiflexion. The examiner attempts to force the ankle into plantar flexion and eversion. To more selectively test the extensor digitorum longus, the ankle is placed in a position of eversion and full dorsiflexion. The examiner attempts to force the ankle into plantar flexion and inversion.

PLANTAR FLEXION (Fig. 1–44)

Gastrocnemius (tibial nerve, S1, S2)

Soleus (tibial nerve, S1, S2)

TEST. The ankle is placed in plantar flexion. The examiner attempts to force the foot into dorsiflexion, applying pressure over the plantar surface of the foot. To selectively test the gastrocnemius, the knee is extended. To more selectively test the soleus, the knee is flexed to 90 degrees. These muscles are so strong that more functional tests such as standing or walking on toes might show weakness missed during MMT.

INVERSION (Fig. 1–45)

Tibialis anterior (deep peroneal nerve, L4, L5, S1)

Tibialis posterior (tibial nerve, L5, S1)

Flexor digitorum longus (tibial nerve, L5, S1)

Flexor hallucis longus (tibial nerve, L5, S1, S2)

TEST. The tibialis anterior is more selectively tested in a position of inversion and dorsiflexion. The examiner attempts to force the foot into eversion and plantar flexion, applying pressure on the medial surface of the

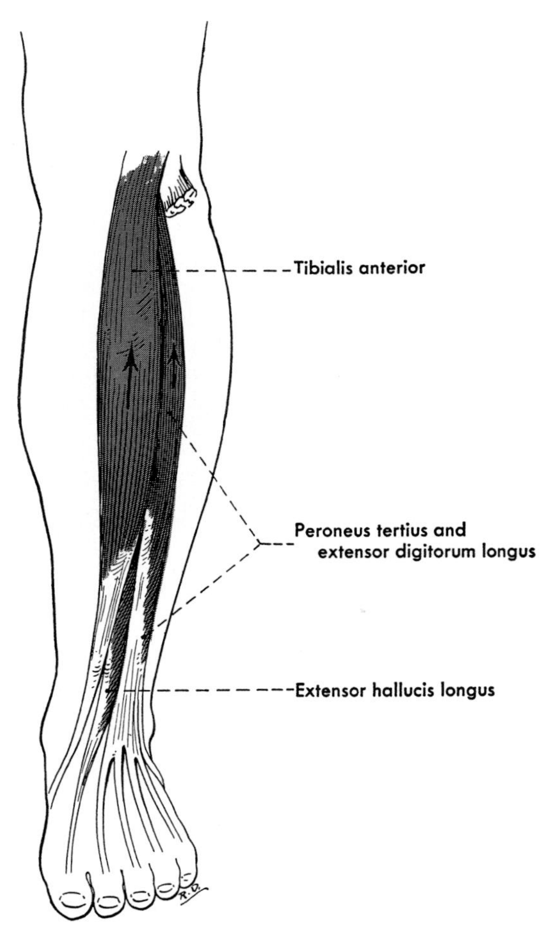

FIGURE 1–43. Ankle dorsiflexors. (From Jenkins DB: Hollingshead's Functional Anatomy of the Limbs and Back, ed 6. Philadelphia, WB Saunders, 1998.)

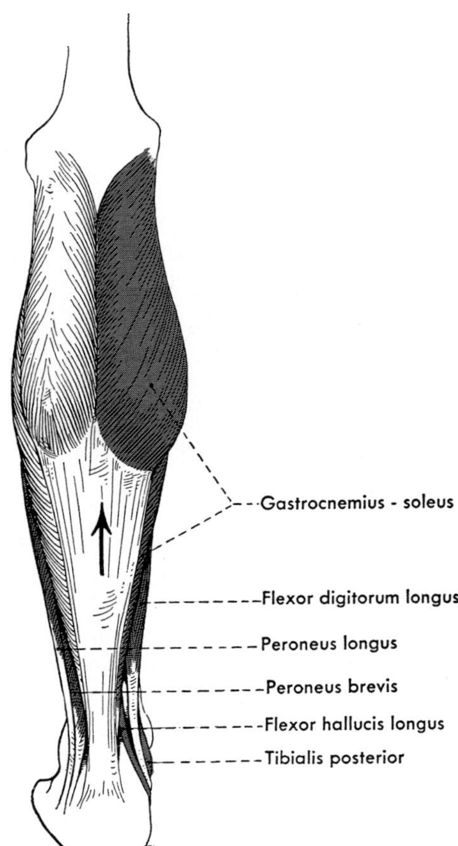

FIGURE 1–44. Ankle plantar flexors. (From Jenkins DB: Hollingshead's Functional Anatomy of the Limbs and Back, ed 6. Philadelphia, WB Saunders, 1998.)

foot. The other three muscles produce plantar flexion and inversion. They are more selectively tested with placement of the foot in inversion and plantar flexion. The examiner attempts to force the foot into eversion and dorsiflexion, applying pressure on the medial surface of the foot.

EVERSION (Fig. 1–46)

Extensor digitorum longus (deep peroneal nerve, L4, L5, S1)

Peroneus longus (superficial peroneal nerve, L4, L5, S1)

Peroneus brevis (superficial peroneal nerve, L4, L5, S1)

TEST. The extensor digitorum longus is more selectively tested in the position of eversion and dorsiflexion. The examiner attempts to force the foot into inversion and plantar flexion, applying pressure over the lateral surface of the foot. The peroneus longus and brevis produce plantar flexion and eversion. They are more selectively tested with placement of the foot in eversion and plantar flexion. The examiner attempts to force the foot into inversion and dorsiflexion, applying pressure over the lateral surface of the foot.

FOOT MOVEMENTS

FIRST DIGIT EXTENSION

Extensor hallucis longus (deep peroneal nerve, L4, L5, S1)

TEST. The first toe is placed in full extension. The examiner attempts to force it into flexion, applying pressure over the dorsum of the first toe.

SECOND TO FIFTH DIGIT EXTENSION

Extensor digitorum longus (deep peroneal nerve, L4, L5, S1)

Extensor digitorum brevis (deep peroneal nerve, L5, S1)

TEST. The second to fifth toes are placed in full extension. The examiner attempts to force them into flexion, applying pressure over the dorsum of the toes.

FIRST DIGIT FLEXION

Flexor hallucis longus (tibial nerve, L5, S1, S2)

Flexor hallucis brevis (medial plantar nerve, L5, S1)

TEST. The first toe is placed in full flexion. The examiner attempts to force it into extension, applying pressure over the plantar surface of the first toe.

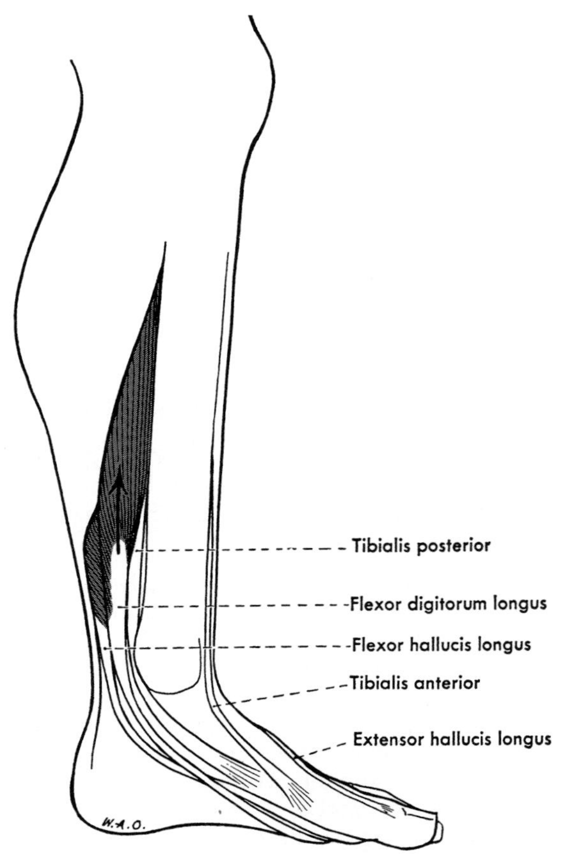

FIGURE 1–45. Ankle invertors. (From Jenkins DB: Hollingshead's Functional Anatomy of the Limbs and Back, ed 6. Philadelphia, WB Saunders, 1998.)

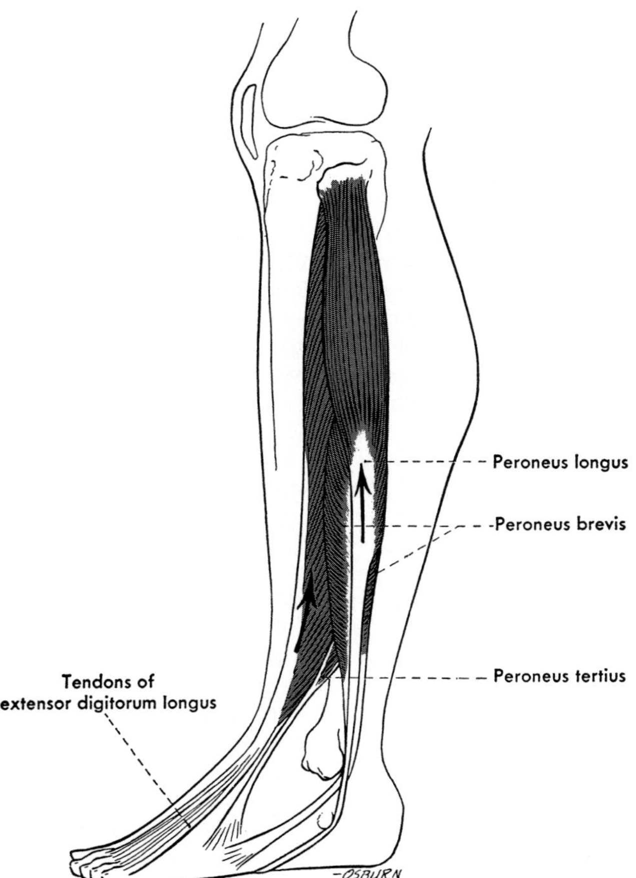

FIGURE 1–46. Ankle evertors. (From Jenkins DB: Hollingshead's Functional Anatomy of the Limbs and Back, ed 6. Philadelphia, WB Saunders, 1998.)

SECOND TO FIFTH DIGIT FLEXION

Flexor digitorum longus (tibial nerve, L5, S1)

Flexor digitorum brevis (medial plantar nerve, L5, S1)

TEST. The second to fifth toes are placed in full flexion. The examiner attempts to force them into extension, applying pressure over the plantar surface of the toes.

Neurological

Like the musculoskeletal examination, a complete neurological examination is essential to identify other impairments that help to clarify or confirm a diagnosis.

Level of Consciousness

A decreased level of consciousness can prevent or seriously limit a patient from participation in a physiatric therapeutic program. Descriptive statements, including such adjectives as *lethargic,* are helpful but are often misinterpreted by others due to the subjectivity of the information. Other subjective but sometimes helpful information includes the length of time and consistency with which an individual is able to attend to a task or to follow commands of the examiner before being unable to respond due to lethargy. This information is an indication not only of an individual's level of consciousness but also of endurance of attentiveness. A commonly used objective scale for an individual with impaired consciousness is the Glasgow Coma Scale (Table 1–11) which assigns a numerical value based on the best eye, motor, and verbal response. The scale ranges from 3 to 15, with 15 being the best score.[18] Patients with the diagnosis of a brain injury are initially evaluated by using a consciousness scale such as the Glasgow Coma Scale, and then periodically monitored for changes in their score. Note that the Glasgow Coma Scale does not include a measurement of functional capacity and should not be used by the practitioner to monitor function.

Mental Status

Many mental status examinations are commonly used to document cognitive ability. A simple, short evaluation is important to assess the patient's ability to participate in a therapeutic program. Usually this type of evaluation can be done in a few minutes. In-depth cognitive assessments and testing procedures often take several hours and should be completed under the direction of a practitioner who is familiar with the specific testing procedures. Referral to a specialist for such an in-depth evaluation is often helpful to assist the physiatrist in tailoring the treatment program.

The following tests can be performed in a short cognitive evaluation at the bedside or in a clinic. Table 1–12 lists items that can be included in such a short cognitive evaluation.[22, 23, 28] Adequate communication skills are necessary for participation in this type of evaluation. Patients with communication deficits might perform poorly or be unable to participate. If the patient is unable to answer the evaluation questions, it is appropriate to provide the patient with verbal cues to help with

TABLE 1–11 Glasgow Coma Scale

Eye opening	
Spontaneous	E 4
To speech	3
To pain	2
Nil	1
Best motor response	
Obeys	M 6
Localizes	5
Withdraws	4
Abnormal flexion	3
Extensor response	2
Nil	1
Verbal response	
Oriented	V 5
Confused conversation	4
Inappropriate words	3
Incomprehensible sounds	2
Nil	1
Coma score (E + M + V) = 3 to 15	

From Jennett B, Teasdale G: Assessment of impaired consciousness. Contemp Neurol 1981; 20:78.

TABLE 1–12 Brief Bedside Mental Status Evaluation

1. Orientation
   Person, place, time, situation
2. Attention span
   Digit retention
3. Memory
   Immediate recall
   Recall at 5- and 10-minute intervals
4. General information
   Remote memory
   Basic intellect
5. Calculation
   Serial 7s
   Simple mathematics
6. Abstract thinking
   Proverb explanation
7. Judgment
   Societal norms

Adapted from Mancall EL: Alpers and Mancall's Essentials of the Neurologic Examination, ed 2. Philadelphia, FA Davis, 1981.

better understanding of the questions. This evaluates the individual's ability to respond appropriately to cues.

Orientation is a basic cognitive skill, and severe disorientation often indicates severe cognitive impairments. Orientation is easily tested by asking patients their name, the place, the time and date, and the present situation or reason for the physiatric evaluation.

Attention span, as discussed previously, can be subjectively documented by noting whether the patient is able to attend to tasks consistently during the history and examination. Digit retention is a more objective test. The examiner asks the patient to recall a series of single-digit numbers immediately, both forward and backward. The patient with an adequate attention span is usually able to recall at least five or six numbers forward and four to five numbers backward.[22]

Memory depends on the ability of an individual both to store and to retrieve information provided. The examiner provides the patient with three items to remember and asks the patient to immediately recall the items. The patient without immediate recall ability has difficulty with information storage and is unable to remember all three items after a short period of time, with or without cues. The patient with adequate immediate recall is asked to recall the items at a later time, usually after 5 and 10 minutes. The patient with good storage and retrieval of information is able to recall the items without difficulty. The patient with good storage but poor retrieval of information might require cues to recall some or all of the items. A patient who is unable to recall the items with cues might have information storage difficulties. Documentation of memory ability should include the number of items recalled and whether cues were required.

Evaluation of general information helps assess the individual's remote memory and basic intellectual skills. The examiner should always take into account the patient's premorbid education and experience level and ask questions that the patient should be able to answer. Questions concerning common elected officials' names, such as that of the current U.S. President and those of recent past Presidents, state senators, and governors, are often appropriate. Well-known locations, such as state capitals and local tourist attractions, are common questions. Current events questions are appropriate for an individual who normally follows local or national news. Very simple questions concerning holidays are appropriate for the patient who is having difficulty with the preceding questions.

Calculation is tested by requesting that the patient serially subtract 7 from 100. Other simple addition, subtraction, multiplication, or division problems are appropriate. Problems with increasing difficulty can be presented if the patient is able to answer simple problems correctly. These questions are inappropriate for the patient who has not had formal mathematics education. If this patient normally purchases items without problems, then testing using monetary examples is appropriate.

Proverb explanation is commonly used to assess abstract thinking. A patient who has lost abstract thought ability will provide a concrete explanation, missing the basic principle of the proverb. Many individuals' educational backgrounds did not involve the use of proverbs, which can affect the patients' ability to answer correctly.

Judgment, like many of the other mental status activities, depends on the patient's background experience, but simple questions that reflect societal norms are often acceptable. Examples of such questions include what is done if a person smells smoke in a crowded theater, why it is inappropriate to yell "fire" in a theater, or what to do if a stamped and addressed envelope is found on the ground. (See Chapter 4 for further information.)

Communication

Communication deficits are often noted after an injury or illness. Specific in-depth evaluation of communication is necessary for any such individual, but a short examination at the hospital bedside or in the clinic can help guide the physiatrist in prescribing a more accurate treatment plan. Items often tested in a short communication examination are listed in Table 1–13.[7,16] It is inappropriate to make a specific communication diagnosis after completing only this short examination, but diffi-

TABLE 1–13 Brief Bedside Communication Evaluation

1. Comprehension
   Verbal, tactile, and gestural commands
   One- and two-step commands
2. Verbal communication
   Name items
   Repeat words or phrases
   Fluency
   Quality
3. Reading
   Written commands
   Matching item with written word
   Reading comprehension
4. Writing
   Personal items
   Write names of items
5. Gestural communication
   Observation

culties with the items identify impairments that need to be treated prior to or during the physiatric therapeutic program.

Comprehension is evaluated by asking the patient to follow commands. Initially, these commands should be presented only verbally, thus assessing only auditory comprehension. If no response is obtained, then other gestural or tactile cues are added and the patient is monitored for a response. For example, the examiner might ask the patient to raise an arm. If no response is elicited initially, then the examiner might repeat the command while touching the patient's arm, thus providing a tactile cue. If there is still no response, a gestural cue might be added by repeating the question and touching the patient's arm while the examiner also raises an arm. Document the cues required for the patient to perform the activity. This assessment allows the examiner to evaluate the patient's ability to comprehend by utilizing different types of stimulation. It also provides the examiner with insight concerning the most effective way to present information.

The patient is also examined as to the level of command comprehension. The initial commands presented should be simple one-step commands, such as "raise your arm," "open your mouth," "touch your nose." If the patient is able to do several of these commands without difficulty, then try two-step commands, such as "raise your arm, then open your mouth," which combine two activities that must be done in sequential order. If the patient is able to perform the two-step commands, the examiner might choose to evaluate the patient's ability to do more complex commands.

Verbal skills can be assessed by asking the patient to name simple, common items presented and to repeat simple words or phrases. The examiner should closely monitor the patient's verbal responses throughout the physiatric history and examination as to the appropriateness, the fluency of word utilization, and inappropriate speech repetition. Close monitoring often identifies common verbal problems such as anomias, inability to repeat, jargon, perseveration, and tangential speech. Documentation of decreased or absent verbalization is essential. If close monitoring of the individual with fluency problems is performed, the examiner can often identify the type of word (i.e., verb or noun) that the patient is having difficulty producing. The exact words that are spoken are documented in the individual with a very constricted vocabulary. Speech quality can be documented subjectively by a notation as to the articulation ability, phonation, pitch, tone, or prosody (see Chapter 3 for further information).

Reading and writing can be assessed in a patient with an adequate educational background. The patient's reading comprehension ability is assessed by writing a simple command and then asking the patient to read the command and perform it. The patient's ability to follow both one- and two-step written commands can be assessed in this way. Another common technique to help identify reading or communication problems is to ask the patient to match actual items with the written word. To assess both reading skills and comprehension, the patient is asked to read a sentence or paragraph and to verbally provide the examiner with a short synopsis. The examiner also can ask specific questions about either the same or another paragraph. Writing is evaluated by requesting that the individual write down simple personal data, such as name and address. If he or she is unable to do this, the patient should be asked to copy these items. Requesting that the patient write the names of specific items also helps to identify writing difficulties.

Patients who have difficulty with communication in both the verbal or the written form often use gestures to attempt to communicate. Documentation of appropriate use of gestures by an individual with otherwise poor communication skills helps other involved staff or family members improve communication. Gestural communication in the individual with adequate verbal skills is often utilized as a secondary form of communication. The observation of a patient's use of gestures and whether the gestures appropriately correspond to the verbal communication is important.

Cranial Nerve Examination

Evaluation of cranial nerve function is an essential part of the neurological evaluation. A good cranial nerve evaluation can help to identify the lesion site if an individual has a brainstem problem. Table 1–14 lists the cranial nerves, their function, and common evaluation procedures.[1, 22, 23]

Sensory Examination

Many clinicians believe that the sensory examination is the most difficult part of the neurological examination. The sensory evaluation can be extensive in the patient with a large number of sensory complaints. It also requires a significant degree of cooperation and subjective response from the patient. All of these facts can make the sensory examination difficult to interpret at times, but if the examination is performed in a systematic manner, valuable information is usually obtained.

The examiner should be aware of the normal dermatomal and peripheral nerve distribution to ensure completeness of the evaluation (Fig. 1–47). It is usually best to evaluate a normal area first, to ensure that the patient understands the sensory examination process. The sensory examination is organized to evaluate both superficial and deep somatic sensations along with discriminative sensory functions.[1, 22]

The three superficial somatic sensations are touch, superficial pain, and thermal sensations. Touch is easily tested with a wisp of cotton. Superficial pain is assessed by a careful pinprick evaluation, because harshly applied stimuli can draw blood. Usually, the patient is asked to tell the examiner where and when each type of stimulus (cotton wisp or pinprick) is applied. The patient can also be asked to compare each stimulus applied with the sensation felt when the same stimulus is applied to an area of known normal sensation. Thermal sensation is commonly evaluated by the use of test tubes, one with hot water and another with cold water or chipped ice. The patient is asked to relate which test tube is touching a specific skin area. Also, the examiner can test just one thermal sensation (either hot or cold) and

TABLE 1–14 Cranial Nerve Examination Techniques

Cranial Nerve	Test
I. Olfactory	Ask patient to smell common substances such as coffee, lemon, vinegar, peppermint, and rose water.
II. Optic	Perform funduscopic evaluation of optic nerve. Acuity testing can be done using standardized acuity charts if available. If charts are not available, then less accurate testing can be done by having the patient read different size newsprint. Visual field testing using the finger confrontation technique can reveal large visual field deficits. Small field deficits may require formal visual testing for diagnosis.
III. Oculomotor IV. Trochlear VI. Abducens	All three nerves are best tested together by checking ocular motility and pupillary reactions. The oculomotor nerve provides innervation to the superior rectus, the inferior rectus, the medial rectus, and the inferior oblique muscles of the eye. The trochlear nerve provides innervation to the superior oblique muscle, whereas the abducens provides innervation to the last eye muscle, the lateral rectus. The pupillary response is checked by flashing light in each eye and looking for an equal and contralateral pupillary contraction.
V. Trigeminal	This provides motor innervation to the masseter and temporal muscles, which are evaluated by asking the patient to clench his teeth; the examiner then palpates the cheek to feel the muscle contraction. The trigeminal nerve also supplies sensory innervation to the face and is easily evaluated using pinprick, thermal, or light touch sensations. The trigeminal nerve is also evaluated by the corneal reflex (see Table 1–17).
VII. Facial	This provides motor innervation to the muscles of facial expression and taste sensation of the anterior two-thirds of the tongue. The examiner evaluates facial muscle movement by forehead wrinkling, eye closure, lip pursing, smiling, or grimacing. Upper motor neuron lesions do not produce forehead weakness because this muscle is innervated by both sides of the cortex. A lower motor neuron lesion is manifest in weakness of all facial muscles. Taste on the anterior tongue can be tested using sugar or salt.
VIII. Auditory	The cochlear division is tested by using a tuning fork and performing the Rinne and Weber tests. Formal auditory testing is appropriate for the patient with auditory acuity problems. The vestibular portion is evaluated by observing for nystagmus. Caloric testing is appropriate in the patient with impaired consciousness.
IX. Glossopharyngeal	This supplies taste sensation to the posterior two-thirds of the tongue; it can be tested with either salt or sugar. It also supplies sensation to the pharynx and is tested along with the vagus nerve (next).
X. Vagus	This is the principal motor nerve to the pharynx and larynx. It is examined by watching the patient's soft palate and uvula move when saying "Ah." The gag reflex is tested by stimulating the back of the pharynx. The vagus nerve also provides motor innervation to the diaphragm muscle. Abnormal motion of the diaphragm indicates vagus nerve abnormality.
XI. Spinal accessory	This innervates the trapezius and sternocleidomastoid muscles. It is tested by resisting a shoulder shrug (trapezius) or by resisted head turning to one side (sternocleidomastoid).
XII. Hypoglossal	This innervates the tongue muscles. It is evaluated by tongue protrusion and observation for abnormal tongue movements.

request that the patient relate any abnormal sensation it produces in the different areas of the body.

Proprioception, vibration sense, and deep pain or pressure are all considered to be deep somatic sensations. Proprioception or joint position sensation is evaluated by testing the patient's perception of a distal joint position and motion. Often, the great toe in the lower limb and the small joints of the hand in the upper limb are used. If the patient has abnormal position sensation in the distal joints, then more proximal joints are tested to identify the level at which the patient's position sense is preserved. When moving the body part, it is important to grasp the sides of the body part rather than the top or the bottom, as the patient may be able to perceive pressure in those areas, which would make the test less accurate. Distal to proximal vibratory sensation is also tested in the limbs with a tuning fork with a low frequency and long duration of vibration (128 dv). Usually the patient is asked to state when the vibration of the fork touching a bony prominence has disappeared. The fork is then immediately placed over a normal bony sensory area and the examiner asks the patient if the vibration is still perceived. As an alternative, after the patient's sense of vibration has disappeared, the fork can be placed on the same area of the examiner's body to compare the patient's sense with the examiner's vibratory sense. Deep pain or pressure is evaluated in each limb by deep palpation of a muscle group or by a firm pinch applied to a muscle tendon.

Discriminative sensory functions are called *cortical* or *integrative sensations,* because an abnormality in these functions usually results from a lesion in the sensory cortex or thalamocortical pathways.[1] These functions include two-point discrimination, cutaneous tactile localization, graphesthesia, and stereognosis. All three of these sensory functions depend on adequate superficial and deep somatic sensations. Poor somatic sensation prevents accurate testing of the discriminative functions.

Two-point discrimination is accurately tested only with a calibrated compass, with both compass points applied simultaneously. A less accurate but often more practical technique uses a paper clip with the two ends separated and measured so the distance between them is known. The examiner asks the patient if one or two stimulation points are felt. The normal distance at which two separate points are distinguished varies depending on the body area being tested. Common areas for such evaluation include the fingertips (normal separation, 3

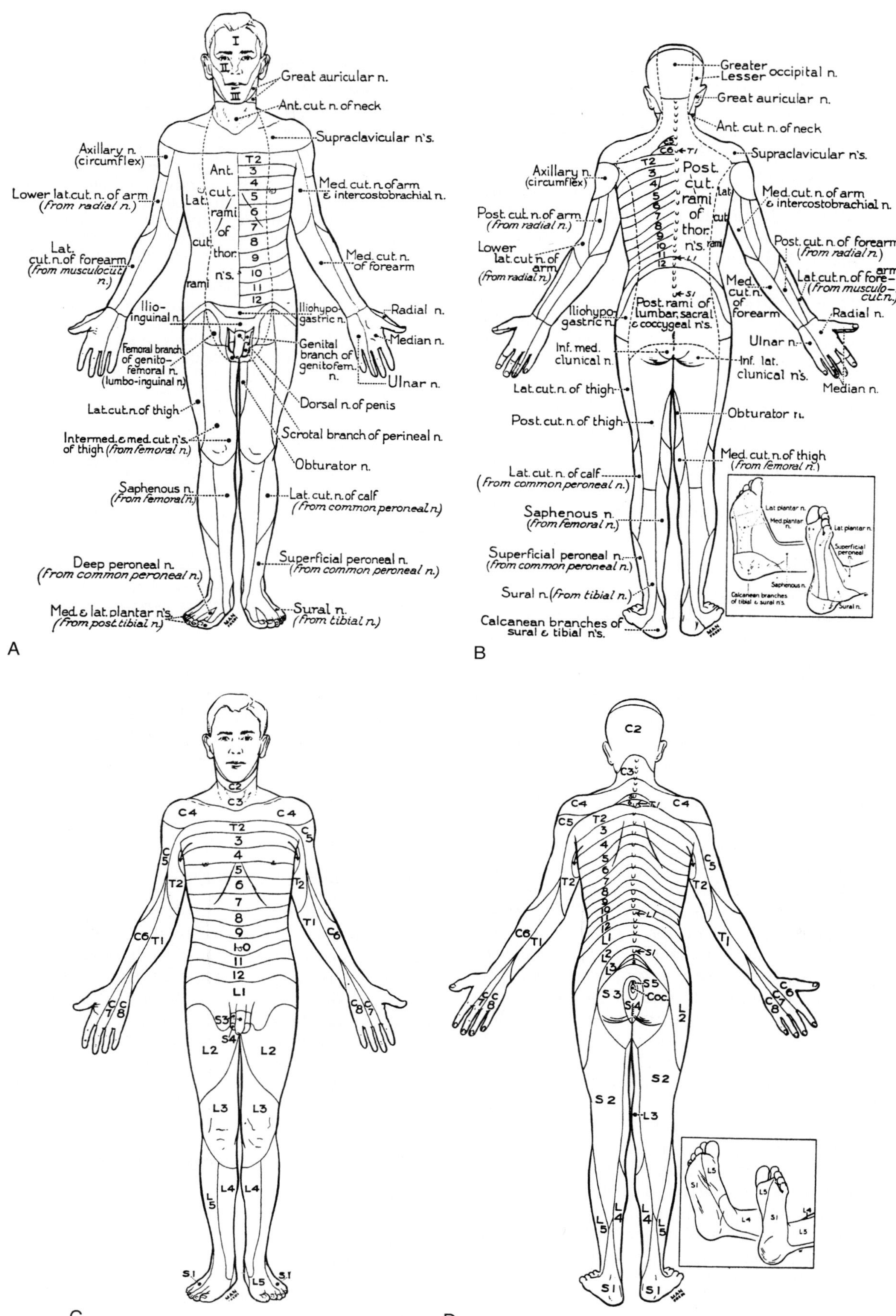

FIGURE 1–47. Distribution of peripheral nerves (*A, B*) and dermatomes (*C, D*). (From Haymaker W, Woodhall B: Peripheral Nerve Injuries, Philadelphia, WB Saunders, 1953.)

to 5 mm), the dorsal surface of the hands and feet (normal separation, 20 to 30 mm), and the trunk (normal separation, 4 to 7 cm).[22] Cutaneous tactile localization is evaluated by asking the patient to close the eyes and to indicate the area that is touched or stimulated with a pinprick by the examiner. The patient should be able to indicate the area accurately over the hands and fingers, and within a few millimeters over the rest of the body. Graphesthesia is the ability to recognize numbers or letters traced on the body, often on the palm of the hand. Stereognosis is the ability to recognize familiar objects, such as a coin or safety pin, that are placed in the hand. The patient should be able to indicate the type of coin (e.g., nickel or quarter) placed in the hand.[1]

The phenomenon of sensory extinction or inattention is a discriminative sensation abnormality. It is revealed by simultaneous bilateral presentation of cutaneous stimuli to one area of the body. Extinction is diagnosed if the stimulus on only one side of the body is perceived. This phenomenon is most often seen in patients with a right parietal cortical lesion, in which the stimulus to the left side is neglected or extinguished.[1]

Motor Control

Motor control depends on adequate muscle strength, balance, coordination, and adequate motor planning of an activity. The presence of involuntary muscle movements can also prevent functional abilities.

Manual muscle testing, already discussed, is performed to evaluate muscle strength. Sitting and standing balance is often tested by applying a mild to moderate pressure or push in all directions to a patient who is in one of those positions. This activity was discussed in the section on functional examination. Higher-level dynamic balance activities, such as tandem walking or braiding activities, can be tested in a patient who appears to have good standing balance.

Poor coordination can prevent independence in many functional skills. Gross motor coordination of the upper limb is evaluated by the finger-to-nose test. The patient should fully extend the limb to prevent inaccurate test results due to upper arm stabilization by the trunk muscles. Lower limb gross motor coordination is evaluated by the heel, knee-to-shin test. Fine motor coordination is best tested by rapid alternating movements. Hand movements such as hand tapping, rapid pronation and supination of the radioulnar joint or forearm along with hand tapping, and thumb to sequential finger movements evaluate upper extremity fine motor coordination. (The patient should be directed to touch the thumb to each fingertip in sequence, as quickly as possible.) Foot tapping evaluates fine motor movement in the lower limb. Asking the patient to rapidly repeat "ta" and "pa" evaluates tongue and mouth coordination.

The documentation of involuntary motor movements such as spasticity, tremors, chorea, athetosis, ballismus, and dystonia is important. Definitions of these involuntary movements are given in Table 1–15.

Apraxia is a loss or impairment in executing complex coordinated movements or in motor planning. An individual with apraxia can have difficulty with multiple functional skills, and the apraxia is often not noted until functional activities are evaluated. The examiner should observe the patient for motor planning problems during the functional examination. The patient is often unable to appropriately sequence the motor skills required to perform mobility activities but has adequate strength on formal MMT. Other patients might have difficulty with appropriate object use, such as inappropriate use of feeding utensils during meals and clothing management during dressing skills.

TABLE 1–15 Definitions of Involuntary Motor Movements

Type	Definition
Spasticity	A state of hypertonicity associated with involuntary quick muscle contraction, increased muscle tone, and increased muscle stretch reflexes.
Tremors	Involuntary repetitive movements of a body part or parts, most often in a distal limb. The activity may resemble quivering or trembling. May be seen at rest or in association with movement.
Chorea	Involuntary arrhythmic movements that are forcible, rapid, and jerky in quality. Most often the movements are seen in the proximal limbs. They are often incorporated into voluntary movements in an attempt to make them less noticeable.
Ballisimus	Unusually violent and flinging motions of the limbs.
Athetosis	A condition characterized by the inability to sustain a body part or parts in one position. Most often the distal limbs (fingers, hands, toes) are affected. The movements are relatively slow and fluid in nature.
Dystonia	A persistent posturing in one or more of the extremities, trunk, neck, or face.

From Adams RD, Victor M: Principles of Neurology, ed 5. New York, McGraw-Hill, 1993. Reproduced with permission of the McGraw-Hill Companies.

Motor Reflex Examination

Muscle stretch reflex (MSR) evaluation is essential. Each reflex is evaluated for symmetry as compared with the reflex on the opposite side, for hyporeflexic or hyperreflexic activity, and for spreading (reflex contraction noted not only in the muscle tested, but also in adjacent muscles). The MSRs should be observed to make certain that the appropriate response is obtained. Sometimes the opposite response occurs: the so-called *inverted reflex response.* Table 1–16 lists commonly evaluated MSRs.

TABLE 1–16 Muscle Stretch Reflexes

Reflex	Segmental Level
Biceps	C5, C6
Brachioradialis	C5, C6
Pronator teres	C6, C7
Triceps	C7, C8
Flexor digitorum profundus	C7, C8
Quadriceps (patella)	L2, L3, L4
Semitendinosus and semimembranosus (medial hamstrings)	L5, S1
Gastrocnemius and soleus (Achilles)	S1, S2

Superficial reflex abnormality is noted in many individuals with neurological impairments (Table 1–17). Corneal, pharyngeal, and palatal reflexes are important in the patient with a suspected brainstem lesion. The other listed reflexes are very important in diagnosing spinal cord dysfunction and the level at which it occurs.

Many abnormal reflexes can be observed after an illness or injury. The Babinski reflex, or abnormal plantar response, is common. The reflex is elicited by stroking along the base of the foot from the heel to the great toe. The normal plantar reflex is flexion of the toes. The Babinski reflex produces an abnormal extension and fanning of the toes. The Hoffmann reflex is noted in the hand. It is elicited by very quick flexion of the third digit distal interphalangeal joint. The abnormal motion observed is a quick flexion movement of the ipsilateral thumb. Both of these reflexes can be indicative of an upper motor neuron lesion. The Hoffmann reflex is normal in some individuals, especially in young women.

Primitive reflexes are abnormal adult reflexes that represent a return to a more infantile level of reflex activity. These abnormal reflexes often result from injury to the frontal cortex, but they are also seen in other disease processes. The *snout, rooting, palmomental,* and *reflex grasp reflexes* are all considered to be primitive reflexes.[22] The snout reflex is a lip-pursing response to a tap either just above or below the mouth. The rooting reflex is a quick contraction of the ipsilateral periorbital muscles toward a brushing tactile stimulus presented to the side of the mouth. A palmomental reflex is ipsilateral contraction of the chin facial muscles produced by a brisk tactile stimulation of the palm or brisk rotation motion of the thumb. Tactile stimulation of the palm can also produce a reflex grasp. The reflex grasp becomes stronger as the examiner attempts to remove his or her hand, which distinguishes the reflex from a voluntary grasp.

General Medical Examination

A general medical examination is completed for all patients to rule out problems that might have an impact on progress in a physiatric therapeutic program. The examiner should be familiar with the general medical examination techniques as described in such reference texts as those by DeGowin and DeGowin[8] and Bates.[3]

SUMMARY, PROBLEM LIST, PLAN, AND GOALS

After the physiatrist collects baseline patient data by history and examination, the information should be organized into a problem-oriented medical record.[9, 12, 29] This organization provides easy understanding of the data and allows other health care professionals quick access to information regarding the patient's status and treatment plans.

A summary of no more than a few sentences identifies the patient's major problems in a narrative form. The summary includes pertinent impairments, functional deficits, and medical and surgical problems. From the summary, the physician formulates a problem list. A recommended modification of the problem list separates the rehabilitation problems from the medical and surgical problems.[29] The separate problem lists help to further organize and simplify the problem list.

From this type of problem list the physiatrist develops a management plan, including treatment options for both the rehabilitation and medical or surgical problems. The management plan should be interdisciplinary and should address functional deficits, physical impairments, and psychosocial, medical, and surgical problems. The treatment plan addressing physical, occupational, or speech therapy options should identify specific recommendations for both exercise and treatment modalities. The physiatrist documents both therapeutic precautions and the treatment setting (either inpatient or outpatient).

In the rehabilitation setting, identification of treatment goals is necessary. The physiatrist identifies goals based on a realistic appraisal of rehabilitation and medical status, attainable after completion of the treatment plan. Obstacles to achieving the goals and the estimated time of goal attainment are recorded. A note as to the

TABLE 1–17 Important Normal Superficial Reflexes

Reflex	Elicited By	Response	Segmental Level
Corneal	Touching cornea with hair	Contraction of orbicularis oculi	Pons
Pharyngeal	Touching posterior wall of pharynx	Contraction of pharynx	Medulla
Palatal	Touching soft palate	Elevation of palate	Medulla
Scapular	Stroking skin between scapulae	Contraction of scapular muscles	C5–T1
Epigastric	Stroking downward from nipples	Dimpling of epigastrium ipsilaterally	T7–9
Abdominal	Stroking beneath costal margins and above inguinal ligament	Contraction of abdominal muscles in quadrant stimulated	T8–12
Cremasteric	Stroking medial surface of upper thigh	Ipsilateral elevation of testicle	L1, L2
Gluteal	Stroking skin of buttock	Contraction of glutei	L4, L5
Bulbocavernous (male)	Pinching dorsum of glans	Insert gloved finger to palpate anal contraction	S3, S4
Clitorocavernous (female)	Pinching clitoris	Insert gloved finger to palpate anal contraction	S3, S4
Superficial anal	Pricking perineum	Contraction of rectal sphincters	S5, coccygeal

Adapted from Mancall EL: Examination of the nervous system. In Alpers and Mancall's Essentials of the Neurologic Examination, ed 2. Philadelphia, FA Davis, 1993, p 25.

TABLE 1–18 Rehabilitation Plan

Summary Statement

L.R. is a 32-year-old right-handed African-American woman, previously an independent homemaker, with a history of sickle cell disease and left hip fracture treated with open reduction and internal fixation 1 year ago; she is presenting for rehabilitation for paraplegia due to an acute T12 spinal cord injury and compression fracture after a fall 1 week ago. The spine is stable if she wears a thoracic lumbar orthosis when out of bed and when the head of the bed is elevated more than 30 degrees. Physical impairments on examination include flaccid paralysis of the lower limbs, L1 sensory level, poor endurance with upper limb activities, left hip flexion and abduction contracture of 10 degrees each, no clitorocavernous reflex, and no rectal tone. Historically, the patient relates that she has had no bowel movement in 4 days; a Foley catheter is in place, and the only activity she is able to do without assistance is feed herself. Socially, she lives in a second-floor apartment (accessible only by stair climbing) with her husband, who works during the day.

Problem List

Rehabilitation problems

1. Functional deficits: Inability to perform any mobility activity, most activities of daily living, or household tasks, and to drive without assistance or assistive devices.
2. Flaccid paralysis of lower limbs bilaterally; poor lower limb management skills.
3. Poor endurance for upper limb activities.
4. Absent sensation below L1 level: High risk for skin pressure areas.
5. Left hip flexion and abduction contracture: Possible positioning problem, high risk for left lower limb skin areas due to positioning problems, possible difficulty with limb management.
6. Flaccid neurogenic bowel: Poor bowel regulation at present.
7. Neurogenic bladder: Needs evaluation for appropriate bladder management.
8. Patient and family adjustment to disability.
9. Sexuality concerns.
10. Discharge planning/living situation: Apartment not wheelchair accessible, equipment needs.

Medical/surgical problems

1. T12 compression fracture: Stable with appropriate wearing of thoracic lumbar orthosis.
2. Sickle cell disease: Stable at present, but will require monitoring.
3. Left hip fracture with surgical repair 1 year ago: Surgically healed, but patient has a residual flexion and abduction contracture.

Management Plan

1. Physical therapy (PT) to address mobility deficits, concentrating on wheelchair activities, transfer skills, upper extremity endurance for these activities, sitting balance, and tolerance. The physical therapist will instruct patient on lower limb range of motion and management, concentrating on decreasing the left lower limb contractures. All team members will reinforce the skills once patient has received basic instructions from the PT.
2. Occupational therapy (OT) will concentrate on upper limb strengthening and endurance, activities of daily living, and, when it is appropriate, have patient begin homemaking and driving with assistive devices. All team members will reinforce the skills once patient has received basic instructions from the OT.
3. Nursing (RN) to monitor skin and assist patient with bowel and bladder management.
4. The management team (physician, PT, OT, RN, recreational therapist, psychologist, social worker, etc.) presents a patient-specific rehabilitation education program concentrating on prevention of future problems related to accessibility, mobility, skin, bowel, bladder, sexuality, and psychosocial and medical/surgical problems.
5. Community issues such as accessibility, driving, social activities, and difficult psychosocial situations are addressed by the team.
6. Management team emphasis is placed on helping patient identify appropriate discharge placement, including accessible living arrangement, home modifications if needed, special equipment needs, and support systems for financial and psychosocial issues.
7. Management team continues to monitor for lower limb strength and sensory improvements.
8. Management team continues to monitor for emergence of muscle tone in rectal and lower limb muscles.
9. Spinal stability maintained by patient's wearing of the spinal orthosis. Periodic spinal radiographs taken when necessary.
10. Maintain stability of the sickle cell disease with close monitoring of blood count and symptoms. Provide blood transfusions or other treatments as necessary.

Therapeutic precautions: Patient to wear spinal orthosis when out of bed and when head of bed is elevated more than 30 degrees.

Therapeutic setting: Inpatient rehabilitation setting necessary because patient is not safe in or able to return to her previous living arrangement.

Goals

1. Independence with wheelchair mobility skills.
2. Independence with activities of daily living.
3. Independence with household tasks at a wheelchair level.
4. Independence with driving with assistive devices.
5. Supervision or independence for community reentry activities.
6. Independence with lower limb management and range of motion program.
7. Independence with the bladder management program.
8. Independence with the bowel management program, or if patient unable to provide own bowel care due to trunk range of motion limit from the spinal orthosis, then independence with ability to instruct another to perform the bowel management program.
9. Independence with skin management program.
10. Knowledge of sexuality related issues.
11. Independence in knowledge about future medical/surgical problems related to spinal cord injury.
12. Identify a safe, accessible living situation.
13. Obtain necessary equipment.

TABLE 1–18 Rehabilitation Plan *Continued*

14. Maintain stability of the sickle cell disease.
15. Maintain spinal stability.

Estimated time of goal attainment: 3 to 4 weeks.

Obstacles to goal attainment:

1. Decreased trunk range of motion due to spinal orthosis, which might prevent independence in some activities.
2. Left hip contractures might cause positioning and skin and limb management difficulties.
3. Poor upper limb endurance might prevent good progress in the rehabilitation program.

Time of reassessment of patient's status: 1 week.

time when the patient will be reassessed is important. Periodic re-evaluation of the patient's progress in the treatment program allows the physiatrist to identify problems that require a readjustment of the plan and goals.

Table 1–18 is an example of a problem-oriented medical record that includes summary, problem list, management plan, and treatment goals.

REFERENCES

1. Adams RD, Victor M: Principles of Neurology, ed 6. New York, McGraw-Hill, 1996.
2. American Medical Association: Guides to the Evaluation of Permanent Impairment, ed 4. Chicago, American Medical Association, 1995.
3. Bates B: A Guide to Physical Examination and History Taking, ed 7. Philadelphia, Lippincott-Raven, 1998.
4. Cole TM, Tobis JS: Measurement of musculoskeletal function. In Kottke FJ, Lehmann JF (eds): Krusen's Handbook of Physical Medicine and Rehabilitation, ed 4. Philadelphia, WB Saunders, 1990, pp 20–71.
5. D'Ambrosia RD: Musculoskeletal Disorders: Regional Examination and Differential Diagnosis, ed 2. Philadelphia, JB Lippincott, 1986.
6. Daniels L, Worthingham C: Muscle Testing: Techniques of Manual Examination, ed 6. Philadelphia, WB Saunders, 1995.
7. Darley FL: Treatment of acquired aphasia. Adv Neurol 1975; 7:111–145.
8. DeGowin EL, DeGowin RL: Bedside Diagnostic Examination, ed 6. New York, Macmillan, 1994.
9. Dinsdale SM, Massman PL, Gullickson G, et al: The problem-oriented medical record in rehabilitation. Arch Phys Med Rehabil 1970; 51:488–492.
10. Erickson RP, McPhee MC: Clinical evaluation. In Delisa JA, Gans BM (eds): Rehabilitation Medicine: Principles and Practice, ed 3. Philadelphia, Lippincott-Raven, 1998, pp 61–108.
11. Gerhard JJ: Documentation of Joint Motion—Revised, ed 3. Portland, Oregon Medical Association, 1992.
12. Grabois M: The problem-oriented medical record: Modification and simplification for rehabilitation medicine. South Med J 1977; 70:1383–1385.
13. Guide for the Uniform Data Set for Medical Rehabilitation (Adult FIM), version 4.0. Buffalo, NY, State University of New York, 1993.
14. Hellebrandt FA, Duvall EN, Moore ML: The measurement of joint motion: III. Reliability of goniometry. Phys Ther Rev 1949; 29:302–307.
15. Hoppenfeld S: Physical Examination of the Spine and Extremities. New York, Appleton-Century-Crofts, 1976.
16. Jayson MIV (ed): The Lumbar Spine and Back Pain, ed 4. London, Churchill Livingstone, 1992.
17. Jenkins DB: Hollingshead's Functional Anatomy of the Limbs and Back, ed 7. Philadelphia, WB Saunders, 1998.
18. Jennett B, Teasdale G: Assessment of impaired consciousness. Contemp Neurol 1981; 20:77–93.
19. Kendall FP, McCreary EK, Provance PG: Muscles: Testing and Function, ed 4. Baltimore, Williams & Wilkins, 1993.
20. Knapp ME: Measuring range of motion. Postgrad Med 1967; 42:A123–A127.
21. Knapp ME, West CC: Measurement of joint motion. Univ Minn Med Bull 1944; 15:405–412.
22. Mancall EL: Examination of the nervous system. In Mancall EL (ed): Alpers and Mancall's Essentials of the Neurologic Examination, ed 2. Philadelphia, FA Davis, 1981, pp 1–33.
23. Members of the Department of Neurology: Mayo Clinic Examinations in Neurology, ed 7. Philadelphia, WB Saunders, 1998.
24. Moore ML: Clinical assessment of joint motion. In Basmajian JV (ed): Therapeutic Exercise, ed 4. Baltimore, Williams & Wilkins, 1984, pp 192–224.
25. Moore ML: The measurement of joint motion: II. The technic of goniometry. Phys Ther Rev 1949; 29:256–264.
26. Norkin CC, White DJ: Measurement of Joint Motion: A Guide to Goniometry, ed 2. Philadelphia, FA Davis, 1995.
27. Stillwell GK, deLateur BJ, Fordyce WE, et al: Physiatric Therapeutics, ed 2. Chicago, American Academy of Physical Medicine and Rehabilitation, 1986.
28. Strub RL, Black FW: The Mental Status Examination in Neurology, ed 3. Philadelphia, FA Davis, 1993.
29. Weed LL: Medical Records, Medical Education, and Patient Care: The Problem-Oriented Record as a Basic Tool. Cleveland, The Press of Case Western Reserve University, 1971.
30. World Health Organization: International Classification of Impairments, Disabilities and Handicaps. Geneva, Switzerland, World Health Organization, 1980.
31. World Health Organization: International Classification of Impairments, Activities and Participation. Geneva, Switzerland, World Health Organization, 1997.

2 CHAPTER

Dennis J. Matthews, M.D., and Pam Wilson, M.D.

Examination of the Pediatric Patient

Examination of the child with suspected functional impairment requires understanding variations in normal childhood development as well as an assessment for dysfunction. The physiatrist must understand how organic pathological processes, normal development, and the child's psychosocial environment interact.

Establishing a diagnostic label is important, but determining the child's functional status is the first step in rehabilitation management. Although the evaluation of the child has many similarities to an adult's evaluation (see Chapter 1), it also has many unique features, as highlighted in this chapter.

DIAGNOSTIC EVALUATIONS

History

The clinical and developmental history is the basis of an accurate medical and rehabilitation diagnosis. The history is generally obtained from the parent or caretaker, but children are generally able to participate in the diagnostic interview by the time they reach school age. It is important to make both the child and the parents comfortable. With younger children, history taking can be facilitated and sped up by having the caregiver fill out a new patient questionnaire before the clinical examination is started.

Because cooperation is not assured and time is limited, it is important to identify the chief complaint quickly. The chief complaint focuses the history and the physical examination. It is important to develop a functional inventory with an emphasis on the child's development and the impact of the disability or impairment on the child's daily activities. It is equally important to note a child's abilities and compensatory functional solutions as it is to record limitations.

Many childhood disabilities reflect prenatal or perinatal problems. Maternal disease or acute illnesses, pregnancy and labor abnormalities, and the family history can help guide the diagnostic examination and investigational studies. The time and type of movements of the fetus should be noted in the record, as should the duration of the pregnancy, the ease or difficulty of labor, and whether any complications occurred during labor and delivery.

Events during the newborn period may retrospectively shed light on a current disorder. The examiner should record the infant's Apgar scores, any unusual cyanosis or respiratory distress, seizures, and other physical symptoms such as jaundice, anemia, and dysmorphic features. The parents' description of muscle tone and movement may suggest a picture of primary neuromuscular weakness.

The feeding history can suggest potential neurological abnormalities. The examiner should ask about and record any difficulties with sucking or swallowing, whether the baby is or was breast-fed or bottle-fed, and the volume and frequency of feedings. If feeding difficulties are present, determine the time of onset of the problems, the method of feeding, reasons for changes, the interval between feedings, the amount ingested at each feeding, associated crying, and weight changes.

The physical growth rate can be plotted on physical growth charts, which are readily available.[3, 4, 20, 27, 28, 32] The onset of organic or psychosocial illness is sometimes accompanied by a sudden acceleration in growth or cessation of growth. The child's growth rate should be considered in relation to what is normal for the child, the growth rates of immediate family members, and age-peer growth rates.

The examiner should determine the ages at which major developmental milestones were met, as this aids in assessing deviations from normal (Table 2–1). The achievement of major landmarks in gross motor, fine motor, and adaptive skills, in language, and in personal and social behavior should clarify whether the disability is confined primarily to the neuromuscular system or involves deficits in other areas as well. The coexistence of multiple problems influences the rehabilitation program, interventional methods, and ultimate outcome.

Familiarity with the normal landmarks of early childhood development helps in the assessment of the infant and toddler.[6, 10, 19, 21, 27, 31, 38] A more formal assessment of the child's development can be made with the use of standardized developmental evaluations (Table 2–2). Most of these tests are easy to administer, but they require some test familiarity and the cooperation of the child. Most important is the appropriate interpretation of the information obtained. Most infant evaluation measures rely heavily on motor responses to assess the child's interest in learning.[11] If a child has major physical disabilities, drawing correct inferences about the child's current or future intellectual abilities can be difficult.[11, 12, 29]

A psychosocial evaluation contributes to the understanding and management of the disabled child. It assesses the child's learning style, probable impediments to learning, and to what degree the child has built on previous learning experiences. It describes the behavioral and cognitive strengths and weaknesses so that specific programs can be implemented both at home and at school. A valuable strategy is to get a description of a typical day's schedule. This information provides insight into the functional impact of the impairment.

A family history of similar or related problems is helpful. A formal pedigree often helps delineate inherited or congenital problems. Formal genetic counseling and evaluation is mandatory whenever a familial disease is suspected or known to exist.

Physical Examination

There is no standardized approach to the physical examination of babies and children.[2, 6, 19, 20, 25] Each examination is tailored to the individual child. The examiner should be familiar with normal and abnormal patterns that may occur at different developmental stages. These developmental stages are key in evaluating both acute and chronic diseases. Young children should be examined with the parents present, but the parents' presence is optional for adolescents.

It is critical to develop rapport with the child before performing a hands-on examination. This can be achieved by playing with the child, talking with the child, or talking with the parents. During this time the examiner carefully observes the child's every movement and interaction. Observation is one of the primary tools used by a skilled practitioner. Even before touching the child the clinician has gained a wealth of information.

The actual hands-on approach varies from child to child. A flexible approach is recommended that capitalizes on opportunities to evaluate different systems as they present themselves. Young children often are best examined while sitting in a parent's lap, while the older child can be examined on the table. Since the child needs to be examined completely, the clothing should be removed. Removing clothing from very young children can be very stressful and should be done gradually. The modesty of older children must be respected.

General Inspection

This part of the examination is critical in planning the approach to the child. The general inspection can reveal abnormalities that need to be more closely evaluated. It begins with a general assessment of the child's appearance. This gives the examiner a sense of how the child interacts with the parents and information about the child's general movements, abnormal physical features, and overall general health (Fig. 2–1).

Evaluation of the skin includes an assessment of the nails and hair. The examiner looks for neurocutaneous lesions and other skin abnormalities. Café au lait spots

TABLE 2–1 Developmental Milestones

Age (mo)	Milestones
1	Lifts head (prone), vocalizes
3	Follows, laughs, smiles, has good head control
5	Plays with feet, reaches for and grasps objects
6	Sits with support
8	Sits without support; equilibrium reflexes present; looks for objects
9	Plays peekaboo, gets to sitting position; parachute reflex present; stranger anxiety
10	Pulls to stand, cruises, babbles
12–14	First words; walks
18	Multiple single words; uses spoon, removes clothes
24	Uses two-word phrases; throws overhand; "terrible twos"
30	Knows full name, puts on clothing
36	Jumps, pedals tricycle, learns nursery rhymes
48	Hops, plays with others

TABLE 2–2 Developmental Evaluation and Screening Tests

Test	Age Range	Scope and Value
Denver Developmental Screening Test[15]	Birth–6 yr	Quick screen for deviations from normal development of normal and near-normal children; pattern of functional deviations guides further evaluation
Bayley Scale of Infant Development[3]	Birth–30 mo	Separate mental and motor scales; well-standardized; heavily weighted with motor-based items, which limits predictive value in physically handicapped children
Gesell Developmental Schedule[17]	4 wk–6 yr	Indicator of current developmental level

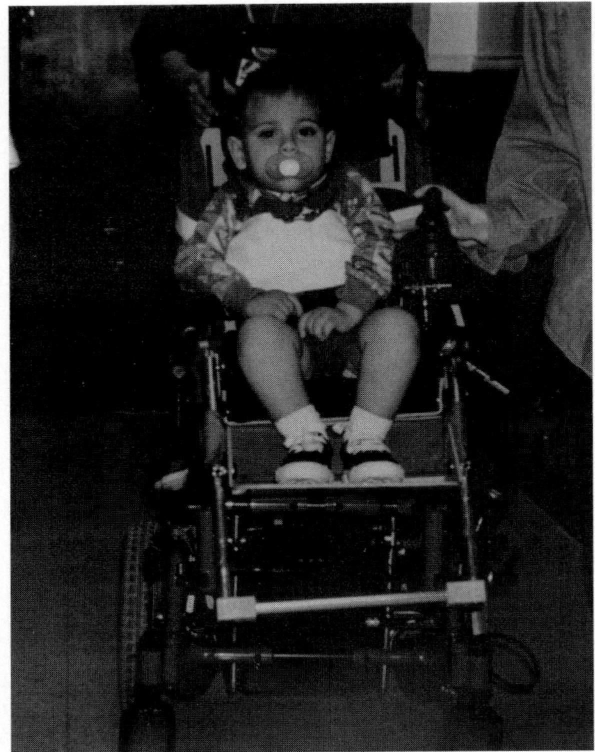

FIGURE 2–1. Young child with cervical level spinal cord injury. The examiner should evaluate general health, functional skills, development, and social interactions before performing the hands-on evaluation.

can indicate neurofibromatosis, while white ash leaf spots can point toward a diagnosis of tuberous sclerosis. Port wine stains, which are flat hemangiomas, that involve the first branch of the trigeminal nerve are associated with Sturge-Weber syndrome. Scars, calluses, and abrasions are often indicators of abnormal weight bearing.

The head, neck, and face are inspected for asymmetries and abnormalities. The size of the head should be measured and recorded. A small head can indicate microcephaly or craniosynostosis. A large head can be the result of hydrocephalus or intracranial mass. It is also important to record the parents' head sizes if familial patterns are suspected. The fontanels should be palpated. These close in a predictable sequence. The posterior fontanel closes at around 2 months of age and the anterior fontanel at around 12 to 18 months. The ears are evaluated for position and structure. Low-set ears or external anomalies can be associated with genetic diseases. Abnormalities of the neck such as torticollis can be caused by shortening of the sternocleidomastoid or by tumors. Klippel-Feil syndrome typically manifests with a short, broad neck with webbing and reduced range of motion.

Musculoskeletal Assessment

As with any other part of the pediatric examination, the musculoskeletal evaluation includes observation, palpation, range-of-motion assessment, and functional assessment. Observation focuses on posture, body symmetry, and movement. Palpation should include the skin, muscles, and joints. The muscle examination should evaluate size, bulk, and tone. The joints are palpated to detect tenderness, swelling, synovial thickening, and warmth. Range of motion should be assessed for all major joints and others in question.

Assessment of posture and position is part of the spinal evaluation. Evaluation includes having the child stand or sit and bend forward (Fig. 2–2). Any asymmetry most likely indicates a scoliosis, and further evaluation is needed. This generally is done by obtaining a spinal scoliosis series of x-rays. Children should also be evaluated for other spinal pathology (Table 2–3).

Examination of the lower extremities includes an evaluation of joint range of motion and torsional forces. Most torsional deformities tend to correct spontaneously with growth and development. Evaluation of the foot includes the toes and the three parts of the foot—forefoot, midfoot, and hindfoot. The shoes should be assessed for patterns of wear. A common problem of the forefoot is metatarsus adductus, which is medial deviation of the metatarsal bones (Figs. 2–3A and B). Pes planus, or flatfoot, is a common problem but does not cause functional limitations. It is characterized by ligamentous laxity and loss of the medial longitudinal arch. Pes cavus is seen in several neuromuscular disor-

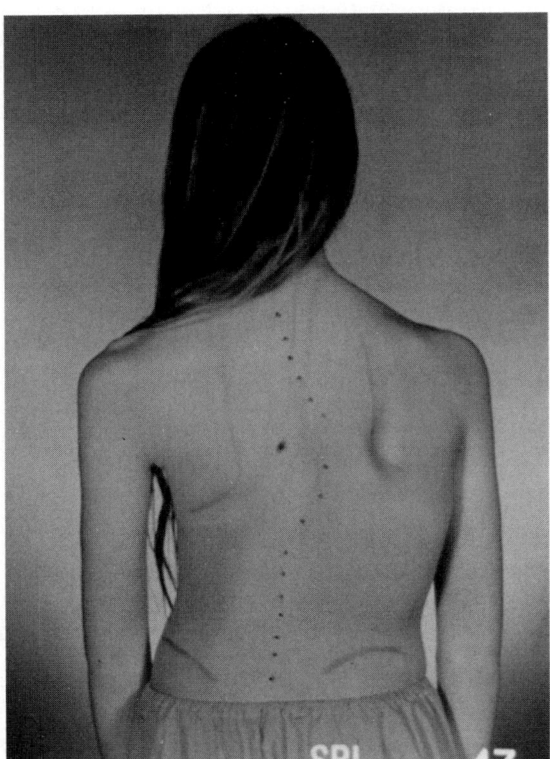

FIGURE 2–2. The evaluation of scoliosis includes an assessment of the spine with the child sitting or standing. This adolescent girl has an obvious curve in the standing position. She also has a rotational component.

TABLE 2–3 Spinal Abnormalities

Spine Abnormality	Clinical Findings
Scoliosis (idiopathic, congenital, neuromuscular)	Curvature of spine on forward bending Rib humping Shoulder asymmetry Pelvic obliquity
Kyphosis (congenital, Scheuermann's, neuromuscular)	Abnormal posture increases with flexion
Spondylolisthesis	Loss of lordosis, reduced range of motion Step-off back deformity Gait abnormalities Transverse abdominal creases

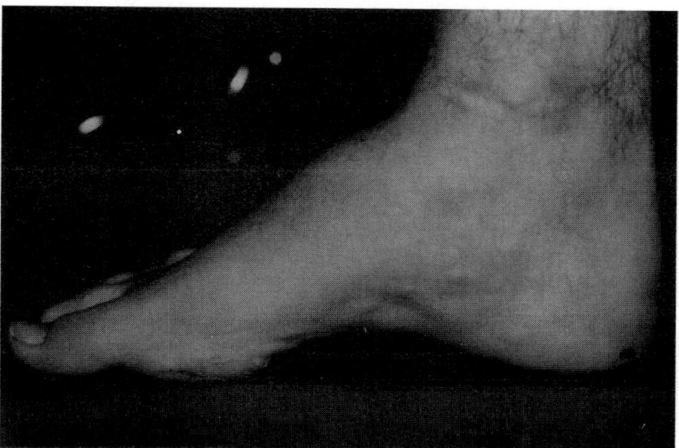

FIGURE 2–4. High-arched foot, or pes cavus, is seen in neuromuscular disorders.

ders, such as Charcot-Marie-Tooth disease (Fig. 2–4). Congenital vertical talus typically manifests with a rocker-bottom foot and can be seen in genetic disorders and myelodysplasia. Talipes equinovarus, or clubfoot deformity, can be seen in positional deformities or neuromuscular diseases. The foot classically presents as hindfoot equinus, or plantar flexion of the ankle, hindfoot varus, and forefoot adductus.

The knee should be evaluated for capsular tightness and joint stability. The child should be assessed for genu varum and genu valgum. A child normally progresses through these stages as the lower extremities mature. Genu varus is common in the 1- to 3-year-old age group and genu valgus in the 3- to 5-year-old range. Abnormal bowing of the legs is seen in Blount's disease. Tibial torsion can result in either internal or external rotation of the tibia and can be evaluated from the thigh-foot angle (Fig. 2–5).

The hip should be evaluated for torsional forces, including femoral anteversion and retroversion. These are best tested with the child prone (Fig. 2–5). Abduction of the hip should be assessed with the child supine (Fig. 2–6). Asymmetry can indicate hip subluxation, contracture, or spasticity. The hips of a newborn should be evaluated for developmental dysplasia. This can be done by using either the Ortolani or the Barlow test. Both tests are done with the infant supine and the hips flexed 90 degrees. In the Ortolani test the examiner attempts to relocate the hips. With the fingers placed over the greater trochanter, the examiner gently abducts the hips. A click or a clunk suggests a hip instability. In the Barlow method, the infant's hips are adducted with the examiner's fingers placed over the medial thigh. The examiner then applies pressure and feels for a posterior click or clunk.

The upper extremity is evaluated for range of motion and function. Common problems identified include brachial plexus injuries, Sprengel's deformity, congenital deformities, and functional limitations. The hand is critical in a child's ability to develop play skills. Hand movement progresses from a very primitive grasp-and-release pattern to a sophisticated ability to manipulate objects. Classically, many pathological processes are reflected in the position and appearance of the hand.

Gait should be carefully analyzed and evaluated. Evaluation includes both a stance and a swing phase

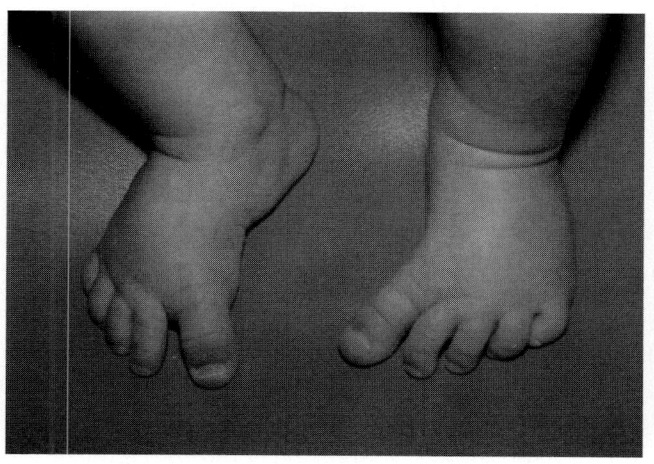

A

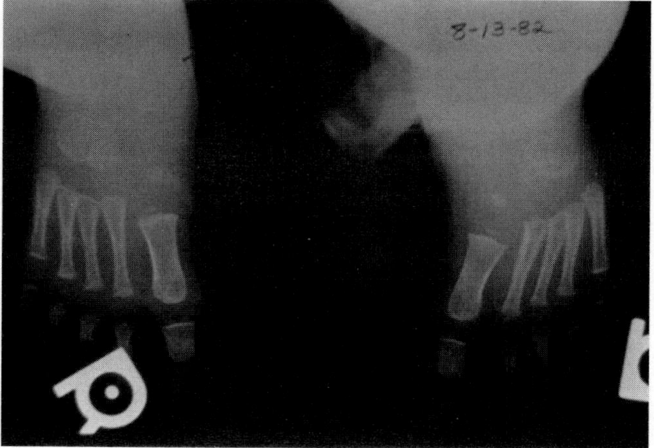

B

FIGURE 2–3. *A.* Child with bilateral metatarsus adductus. *B.* X-rays showing medial deviation of the metatarsal bones.

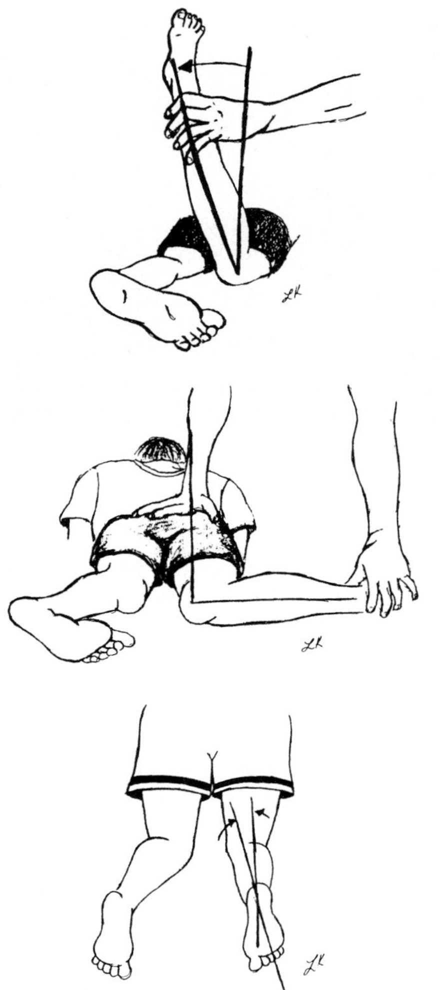

FIGURE 2–5. Evaluation of a child in the prone position allows assessment of the thigh-foot angle and internal and external rotation of the hip. The thigh-foot angle is demonstrated in the lower diagram and ranges from −3 degrees to +20 degrees.

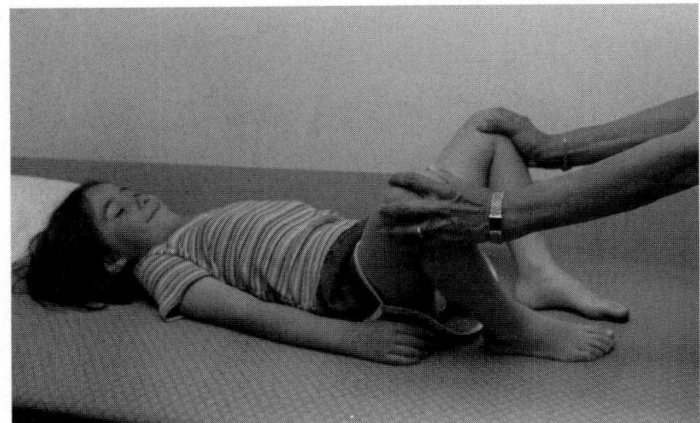

FIGURE 2–6. Examination of the hips should include passive range of motion, such as hip abduction, along with assessment of tone and spasticity.

TABLE 2–4 Gait Abnormalities

Gait	Characteristics	Clinical Association
Spastic	Adducted hips Internal rotation of hips Toe walking	Cerebral palsy
Crouched	Weak quadriceps Weak hip extensors Excessive dorsiflexion Hip or knee contractures	Neuromuscular disease Cerebral palsy
Hemiparetic	Posturing of upper extremity Circumduction of hip Inversion of foot	Cerebral palsy Cerebral vascular accident
Waddling (Trendelenburg)	Weakness of hip girdle	Neuromuscular disease
Ataxic	Wide-based gait Coordination problems Poor tandem walking	Cerebellar ataxia Friedreich's ataxia

analysis. Classic abnormal patterns are seen with certain diseases. Children move in the most efficient patterns and are masters of substitution. Movement patterns can indicate weaknesses or asymmetries. Gait generally matures by 7 years of age.[23] Milestones in gait maturation include walking by 15 months, running by 3 years, hopping and walking on the heels by 4 years, and skipping by 6 years. Understanding normal walking and gait facilitates an analysis of gait abnormalities (Table 2–4). In-toeing and out-toeing are common gait disturbances evaluated by clinical practitioners. These patterns are seen in torsional deformities of the femur and tibia. The most common cause of in-toeing is related to femoral anteversion and generally improves with maturation. Functional limitations, frequent tripping, or lack of hip rotation are reasons to consider surgical or nonsurgical interventions.

Neurologic Assessment

Examination of the neuromuscular system includes testing reflexes and evaluating tone, active motion, coordination, and strength. In children, most of these aspects are assessed simultaneously rather than sequentially.

Perhaps one of the most critical tools in evaluating neurological development is the evaluation and interpretation of developmental reflexes. The infantile developmental reflexes are related to various complex functions of the brainstem and spinal cord. Reflexive patterns appear and disappear predictably as the child passes through developmental stages (Table 2–5). This sequencing reflects cortical maturation, and persistence or reoccurrence of abnormal reflexes is a strong indicator of neurological dysfunction. Primitive reflexes are normally and eventually replaced by postural responses that allow the child to adapt to positional changes. The

TABLE 2–5 Developmental Reflexes

Reflex	Present At	Disappears By
Rooting	Birth	3 mo
Moro	Birth	4–6 mo
Asymmetrical tonic neck	Birth	6–7 mo
Symmetrical tonic neck	2 mo	6–7 mo
Protective reactions		
Forward	5–6 mo	Persists
Lateral	6–7 mo	Persists
Posterior	9–10 mo	Persists

presence of an obligatory tonic neck reflex is abnormal at any age and suggests a central nervous system disorder.

Muscle tone is the amount of resistance present in muscles through passive range of motion. Tone changes during development and can be affected by activity, alertness, and comfort. A newborn infant is more hypotonic than a toddler. Flexor tone predominates in the first several months of infancy. If true hypotonia persists, it generally indicates an abnormality in either the cerebrum, cerebellum, anterior horn cells, peripheral nerves, neuromuscular junction, or muscles. Hypertonicity can reflect damage to the cerebrum, brainstem, basal ganglia, or spinal cord. Hypertonicity manifests as either spasticity or rigidity. Severe spasticity and rigidity can present as opisthotonic posturing in the infant.

Muscle stretch reflexes are easily elicited in children of all ages. A reduction in or absence of reflexes can indicate an anterior horn cell disease, a peripheral neuropathy, or a myopathy. An increase in reflexes is often associated with an upper motor neuron process.

Strength testing or manual muscle testing can be formally applied in the school-age child. The scoring system is the same as in adults. Testing and scoring are more of a challenge in the younger child. In testing the strength of infants and very young children, reflexive patterns can be useful. Helpful techniques include holding the child under the arms and lifting the child into the air, ventral suspension, checking for age-appropriate head control, and observing the child sitting and standing. The older child can walk, get up off the floor, reach overhead, throw a ball, kick, or skip. Quantitative measurements are generally not required unless specific therapeutic interventions are contemplated.

Coordination is best assessed by evaluating gross motor and fine motor skills. Impaired coordination is a common sign of a central movement disorder. Specific tests can be done in the older child. Most children are able to walk a straight line, although unsteadily, by age 3 years. Tandem walking is a 5-year-old skill. School-age children can be more formally tested. Subtle symptoms can be seen by evaluating handwriting, drawing, and other higher-level physical skills. The avoidance of organized sports or physical activity can be a clue that coordination problems exist. Ataxia can be evaluated by having the child reach for an object, do the finger-to-nose test, sit or stand, and do tandem walking.

Sensory evaluation is difficult in young or uncooperative children. It has to be age adjusted to obtain information that is useful. A child of 4 to 5 years can interpret joint position, vibration, light touch, temperature, and pain. In the very young child, behavioral responses are the best indicator of sensory awareness. These responses include withdrawing, stopping the activity, and looking, crying, or squirming. A knowledge of infant movement patterns is helpful: for example, withdrawal with isolated spinal reflex activity can be confused with volitional responses.

The vision examination also must be adapted to the child's ability to cooperate. An infant is able to follow a stimulus with the eyes to midline by 1 month and through 180 degrees by 3 months. Central nervous system dysfunction frequently presents with ocular motor imbalance.

DEVELOPMENTAL ASSESSMENT

Familiarity with the normal landmarks of early child development is essential to the developmental assessment of the infant and toddler. The assessment includes observing and describing the child's gross motor and fine motor responses, verbal and nonverbal language, personal and social behavior, emotional characteristics, and adaptive skills. A formal assessment of the child's developmental status requires the use of a standardized examination. An interdisciplinary evaluation is particularly helpful when the initial diagnosis is being established or when interventions are being planned for a young child. It can also be used for periodic assessment of developmental progress throughout childhood and adolescence, especially for appropriate educational planning. It provides an assessment of overall development and its rate relative to other children. Diagnostic assessment relies on normed reference instruments that convey the child's developmental standing relative to a normal peer group. It provides valuable information on the assessment and formulation of the child's strengths and weaknesses for the purpose of individual program planning.

The results of infant tests are best interpreted as a measure of the infant's current developmental status relative to a normal peer group. Infant tests rely heavily on motor responses to assess the child's interest and learning. It can be difficult to draw inferences about the child's current or future intellectual ability in the presence of known physical limitations. Repeated studies have found low correlation between abilities measured on infant tests and later childhood intelligence quotients.[3, 10, 11] Infant test results must be considered provisional and followed by periodic re-evaluation for further diagnostic and prognostic clarification.

The assessment of preschool and school-age children includes assessment of both physical and intellectual abilities. The chief strength of intelligence tests lies in their correlation with school performance (Table 2–6). If the results are appropriately interpreted, the tests reflect the probability of standard academic achievement. It is important to note both the overall score and the subscores to assess whether a child's abilities are evenly developed, or whether there are patterns of

TABLE 2–6 Intellectual Evaluations

Test	Age Range	Scope and Value
Stanford-Binet Intelligence Scale[37]	2 yr–adult	Detailed diagnostic assessment (mental age and IQ); guidelines for hearing, visual, and motor handicaps
Wechsler Preschool and Primary Scale of Intelligence—Revised (WPPSI-R)[40]	3–6½ yr	Verbal, performance, and full-scale scores; delineates strengths and weaknesses; not appropriate for children with severe developmental delays
Wechsler Intelligence Scale for Children—Revised (WISC-R)[39]	6–16 yr	Verbal, performance, and full-scale scores; subtests point to specific areas of strength or dysfunction
Kaufman Assessment Battery for Children[24]	2½–12 yr	Measures mental processes independent of the content of acquired knowledge; useful for children from disadvantaged backgrounds

TABLE 2–7 Alternative Nonverbal and Motor-Eliminated Tests

Test	Age Range	Scope and Value
Peabody Picture Vocabulary Test (PPVT)[15]	2½–18 yr	Effective test of language, especially in children with speech and motor impairments
Leiter International Performance Scale[26]	2–18 yr	Measures nonverbal problem-solving abilities in deaf and speech- and motor-handicapped children
Pictorial Test of Intelligence[17]	3–8 yr	Measures intellectual ability of multiply handicapped children; requires receptive language
Raven's Progressive Matrices[35]	6 yr–adult	Measures nonverbal intelligence and concept formation

TABLE 2–8 Perceptual Evaluations

Test	Age Range	Scope and Value
Beery-Buktenica Development Test of Visual-Motor Integration[5]	2–16 yr	Assesses visual-motor performance; ability to copy geometric shapes; age equivalence
Bender Visual-Motor Gestalt Test[8]	5 yr–adult	Assesses visual-motor performance; easy to administer; nine geometric designs

TABLE 2–9 Academic Achievement Tests

Test	Grade Level/Age Range	Scope and Value
Wide-Range Achievement Test—Revised (WRAT)[21]	Kindergarten–12th grade	Yields academic achievement level in reading, spelling, arithmetic; can measure programs
Woodcock-Johnson Psychoeducational Battery: Test of Achievement[41]	3 yr–adult	Yields age and grade level, percentiles, and standard scores in reading, mathematics, written language, and general tasks
Peabody Individual Achievement Test[13]	Kindergarten–12th grade	Only pointing response for overview of achievement; useful for handicapped

strengths and weaknesses that are relevant to learning and general adaption.[11]

Most of the standardized intelligence tests rely heavily on language and motor performance. For some disabled children, such as those with central language impairments, significant motor difficulties, or sensory deficits, alternative nonverbal and motor-eliminated assessments might be needed (Table 2–7). Vocabulary tests typically show the strongest correlation with overall intellectual ability and school success.

The test composite scores, or full-scale scores (IQs), are used to designate a child's overall level of intellectual functioning.[11] This is derived by comparing an individual child's performance with the performance of hundreds of children in a representative age-stratified norm group. On most of these tests, the mean score is 100, which represents average or normal intelligence. Classifications as superior or subaverage typically refer to scores that fall 2 standard deviations above or below the mean. A definition of mental retardation includes three components: (1) subaverage general intelligence, (2) concurrent deficits in adaptive behavior, and (3) developmental delay. Generally, all three criteria must be present to make a formal diagnosis of mental retardation.

The classification of mild mental retardation (IQ of 55 to 69) encompasses the largest number of children with mental retardation. Generally they show delayed language development as toddlers and weaknesses in the acquisition of pre-academic writing skills. These children generally reach the third- to fifth-grade level academically. If the associated physical handicaps are mild, they can be independent in activities of daily living and achieve relative independence in adulthood.

Children with moderate mental retardation (IQ of 40 to 54) have a slower rate of developmental attainment. There is also a higher incidence of neurological and physical disabilities. These children are frequently in special classes and are taught primarily self-care and practical daily living skills. As adults, many are able to achieve some independence in self-care skills, but they usually continue to need supervision either at home or in group homes, and vocationally they function primarily in sheltered workshops or protected employment.

Children with severe mental retardation (IQ of 25 to 39) develop some functional language skills but no formal academic skills. They require intensive programming to master independence in activities of daily living. They need close supervision and supportive care as an adult. Profoundly retarded children (IQ less than 25) have limited language ability and limited potential for acquiring self-care skills. There is also a very high association with severe motor handicaps.

Several tests have been designed to evaluate visual-motor maturity in children, and to detect delays or impairment in visual-perceptual skills and eye-hand coordination (Table 2–8). Children with neurological and developmental disabilities sometimes exhibit difficulties in visual-perceptual, perceptual-motor, auditory, kinesthetic, and tactile functioning. A wide variety of instruments are available to test for these impairments. Achievement tests are designed specifically to evaluate the child's performance in school subject areas, such as reading and mathematics (Table 2–9). Scores are typically given in terms of school grade equivalence, which can provide an estimate of the child's level of academic skill, as well as standard scores based on age norms. Many are paper-and-pencil tests that penalize handicapped children for their slower pace, poor attention, or difficulty keeping track of their place on the page. It is important that a skilled observer administer the test since observation of task approach can be used to adjust quantitative results.

A complete assessment of the disabled child must include a description of social and adaptive abilities (Table 2–10). It is important to establish the level of achievement in locomotion, communication, and self-care activities such as feeding, dressing, and toileting. It is also important to assess the mode and methods of interaction with family members and peers, and the child's ability to assume increasing levels of responsibility. A number of social adaptive scales have been developed to look at the ages at which children usually achieve such competencies, along with emotional adjustment (Table 2–11).

Care must be taken when arriving at a specific diagnosis on the basis of developmental testing performed early in a child's life. In addition, central nervous system dysfunction is not incompatible with normal intelligence, and the degree to which a child may be intellectually impaired cannot be predicted solely from physical or motor deficits. Familiarity with the tests being utilized is essential when interpreting this information.

TABLE 2–10 Social and Adaptive Skills

Test	Age Range	Scope and Value
Vineland Adaptive Behavior Scale[36]	1 mo–adult	Questionnaire of social competence in communication, socialization, daily living skills, and motor skills; adjusted for handicapped
AAMD Adaptive Behavior Scale[33]	3 yr–adult	Activities of daily living; adaptive and maladaptive behaviors; assists in program planning

TABLE 2–11 Emotional Adjustment

Test	Age Range	Scope and Value
Manual Children's Apperception Test[7]	3–10 yr	Pictures of animals and humans in various situations; assesses adjustment patterns
Figure drawings[13]	4 yr–adult	Self-image and interpersonal relationships

SUMMARY

The pediatric examination shares a common purpose with all physiatric examinations: to ascertain the nature and cause of dysfunction. All the biological, environmental, and developmental factors should be identified. The physiatrist working with the child, family, and rehabilitation team seeks to foster an optimal developmental course so that each child can achieve maximal functional potential.[11]

REFERENCES

1. Alexander MA, Molnar GE: History and examination. In Molnar GE, Alexander MA (eds): Pediatric Rehabilitation. Philadelphia, Hanley & Belfus, 1999.
2. Barness CA: Manual of Pediatric Physical Diagnosis. St Louis, Mosby–Year Book, 1991.
3. Barness CA: Principles and Practice of Pediatrics. Philadelphia, JB Lippincott, 1994, pp 29–34.
4. Bayley N: Bayley Scale of Infant Development. New York, Psychological Corp, 1969.
5. Beery K, Buktenica N: Developmental Test of Visual-Motor Integration. Chicago, Follett, 1967.
6. Behrman RE, Vaughan VC (eds): Nelson's Textbook of Pediatrics. Philadelphia, WB Saunders, 1987.
7. Bellak L: Manual Children's Apperception Test. New York, Grune & Stratton, 1961.
8. Bender L: The Bender Visual-Motor Gestalt Test. New York, American Orthopsychiatric Association, 1946.
9. Bobath B: Abnormal Postural Reflex Activity Caused by Brain Lesions. London, Heinemann, 1971.
10. Capute AJ, Accardo PF, Vining EPG, et al: Primitive Reflex Profile. Baltimore, University Park Press, 1977.
11. Chinitz SP, Feder CZ: Psychological assessment. In Molnar GE (ed): Pediatric Rehabilitation. Baltimore, Williams & Wilkins, 1992.
12. DiBose R: Predictive value of infant intelligence scales with multiply handicapped children. Am J Ment Defic 1977; 81:388–390.
13. DiLeo J: Children's Drawings as Diagnostic Aides. New York, Brunner/Mazel, 1973.
14. Dunn L, Markwardt F: Manual: Peabody Individual Achievement Test. Circle Pines, MN, American Guidance Service, 1970.
15. Dunn LM: Peabody Picture Vocabulary Test—Revised. Circle Pines, MN, American Guidance Service, 1970.
16. Frakenburg WC, Dodds J, Archer P, et al: Denver II Technical Manual. Denver, Denver Developmental Materials, 1990.
17. French J: Manual: Pictorial Test of Intelligence. Boston, Houghton Mifflin, 1964.
18. Gesell A: Gesell Developmental Schedule. New York, Psychological Corp, 1940.
19. Green M: Pediatric Diagnosis: Interpretation of Symptoms and Signs in Different Age Periods. Philadelphia, WB Saunders, 1985.
20. Gundy JH: The pediatric physical examination. In Hoekelman RA (ed): Primary Pediatric Care. St Louis, Mosby–Year Book, 1992.
21. Illingworth RS: Development of the Infant and Young Child: Normal and Abnormal. New York, Churchill Livingstone, 1980.
22. Jastak S, Wilkinson GS: The Wide Range Achievement Test–Revised. Wilmington, DE, Jastak Associates, 1984.
23. Johnson EW: Examination for muscle weakness in infants and small children. JAMA 1958; 16:1306–1313.
24. Kaufman A, Kaufman N: Kaufman Assessment Battery for Children. Circle Pines, MN, American Guidance Service, 1983.
25. Kottke FJ, Lehman JF (eds): Krusen's Handbook of Physical Medicine and Rehabilitation. Philadelphia, WB Saunders, 1990.
26. Leiter R: The Leiter International Performance Scale. Chicago, Stoelting, 1969.
27. Lowery GH: Growth and Development of Children. St Louis, Mosby–Year Book, 1986.
28. Lustig JV: Growth and development. In Hathaway WE, Hay WW, Groothuis JR, et al (eds): Current Pediatric Diagnosis and Treatment. Norwalk, CT, Appleton & Lange, 1993.
29. Molnar GE: A developmental perspective for the rehabilitation of children with physical disabilities. Pediatr Ann 1988; 17:766–776.
30. Molnar GE, Alexander J, Gatfeld N: Reliability of quantitative strength measurements in children. Arch Phys Med Rehabil 1979; 60:218–221.
31. Molnar GE, Sobus KM: Growth and development. In Molnar GE, Alexander MA (eds): Pediatric Rehabilitation. Philadelphia, Hanley & Belfus, 1999, pp 2–20.
32. Nellhaus G: Head circumference from birth to eighteen years. Pediatrics 1968; 41:106–114.
33. Nihira K, Foster R, Shellhaas M, et al: AAMD Adaptive Behavior Scales. Washington, DC, American Association of Mental Deficiency, 1974.
34. Paine RS, Brazelton TB, Donovan DE, et al: Evolution of postural reflexes in normal infants and in the presence of chronic brain syndromes. Neurology 1964; 14:1036–1048.
35. Raven J: Raven's Progressive Matrices. Dumfries, Scotland, Crichton Royal, 1958.
36. Sparrow SS, Balla DA, Cicchetti DV: Vineland Adaptive Behavior Scale. Circle Pines, MN, American Guidance Service, 1984.
37. Thorndike RL, Hagen EP, Sattler JM: The Stanford-Binet Intelligence Scale, ed 4. Chicago, Riverside, 1986.
38. Twitchell TE: Normal motor development. Phys Ther 1965; 45:419–423.
39. Wechsler D: Wechsler Intelligence Scale for Children—Revised. New York, Psychological Corp, 1974.
40. Wechsler D: Wechsler Preschool and Primary Scales of Intelligence—Revised. San Antonio, Psychological Corp, 1989.
41. Woodcock R, Johnson MD: Woodcock-Johnson Psychoeducational Battery: Tests of Achievement. Allen, TX, DLM Teaching Resources, 1989.

3

CHAPTER

Paul R. Rao, Ph.D.

Adult Communication Disorders

> If all my possessions were taken from me with one exception, I would choose to keep the power of communication, for by it, I would soon regain the rest.
>
> *Daniel Webster*

OVERVIEW OF NORMAL COMMUNICATION PROCESSES

The ongoing, dynamic process of giving and getting information in our everyday lives is so routine that we often take for granted the gift of communication. Human communication is complex and multifaceted. Speech is just one component in the human repertoire of ways to get a message across. We use facial expression, gesture, tone of voice, writing, singing—many modes—to communicate a variety of intents. Besides strict information exchange, we communicate to describe events, converse, problem solve, play, persuade, punish, pray, or pun, and to participate in a host of other simple and sublime processes.

This chapter provides a brief overview of normal communication processes, followed by a discussion of adult communication disorders. What happens when you speak? Expression always begins with a thought. If it is to be spoken, it must first be organized by the language networks of the brain and according to certain linguistic rules. Only after the intended message has been arranged in a certain sequence is the brain ready to select the sequence of sounds to be spoken. Once the nervous system has encoded the message, the communication process commences with a symphony of synergy:

> [T]he *respiratory* muscles of the chest wall must be able to generate sufficient air pressure to drive the sound generator. The *phonatory* muscles of the larynx must generate enough vibrating energy for speech to be easily heard at a distance. The *articulatory* muscles of the vocal tract . . . must expand and contract this vibrating energy rapidly so that various sounds of speech that are shaped will fade quickly and not blur into each other. The *auditory* system of the ear must transform the acoustic waves of speech sounds into neural signals so that speakers can monitor their own performance and listeners can focus on the speaker of interest. Finally coming full circle, the auditory system, as it extends from the ear to the brain, must respond selectively to the special features of speech by which it is decoded so that the meaning of the message can be understood.[52]

As Figure 3–1 illustrates, speech is a circular process, whether one is attending to oneself or to another. The circularity of the speech process is illustrated in much greater detail in Figure 3–2, which shows that the process begins and ends with the brain.

HEARING

The human auditory mechanism analyzes sound according to changes in frequency (pitch) and intensity (loudness) over time. An audiologist uses an audiometer to measure hearing. Frequencies heard can be tested between 250 and 8000 hertz (Hz). Intensity is measured in decibels (dB) of sound pressure levels (SPLs), and can be tested from 0 to approximately 120 dB (the threshold for pain is around 125 dB). The most important part of the frequency spectrum is the range of frequencies critical for the understanding of speech. The human ear as a sensory receptor is remarkably responsive to the speech sounds that humans produce. The "speech range" extends roughly from 400 to 4000 Hz (4 kHz). Speech contains frequencies below 400 Hz and

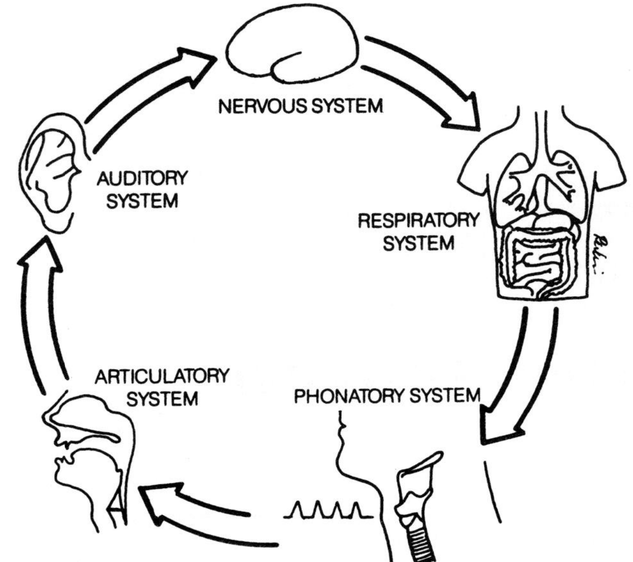

FIGURE 3–1. The circle of communication. (From Perkins WH, Kent RD: Functional Anatomy of Speech, Language, and Hearing: A Primer. Boston, Allyn and Bacon, 1986. Copyright 1986 by Allyn and Bacon. Reprinted by permission.)

above 4 kHz, but they are not necessary for nearly perfect intelligibility of routine conversational speech.

The mechanism of human hearing is simply one of transference of energy. The outer ear detects the sound pressure waves of speech in the air. These sound pressure waves are converted to mechanical vibrations, first by the tympanic membrane, and thereafter, in the middle ear, by a series of tiny bones (the ossicular chain) that leads to the cochlea of the inner ear. The cochlea is a fluid-filled, snail-shaped cavity within the temporal bone of the skull in which the mechanical vibrations are transformed into vibrations in fluid. The nerve endings in the cochlea act to transform the hydraulic vibration into nerve impulses, which are then sent to the brain via the eighth cranial nerve.[11]

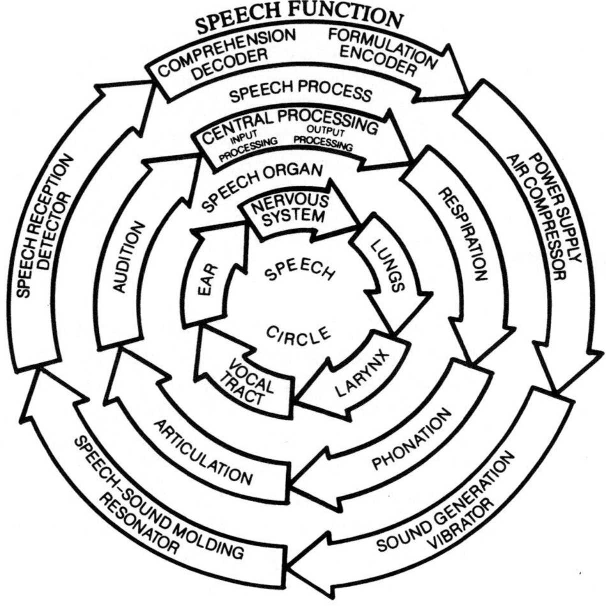

FIGURE 3–2. The processes of speech. (From Perkins WH, Kent RD: Functional Anatomy of Speech, Language, and Hearing: A Primer. Boston, Allyn and Bacon, 1986. Copyright 1986 by Allyn and Bacon. Reprinted by permission.)

VOICE

Voice is the audible sound produced by phonation, but is only one component of the total speech act. Phonation has been defined as "sound generated by rapid vocal fold movement excited by exhaled airstream."[6] The airstream refers to respiration, the power source for voice and speech. Normal voice and speech are produced during the exhalation phase of respiration wherein the vocal folds adduct to constrict the glottis. This momentary interruption of the flow of air from the trachea through the larynx is repeated hundreds of times per second, resulting in phonation. The terms most commonly used in the context of discussing phonation are found in Table 3–1. There are two types of phonation that occur during speech: voicing and whispering. In English there are approximately 40 phonemes (sounds), which are created by making exhaled air audible. Most speech sounds are voiced, but some are voiceless. Examples of voiced and voiceless sounds of American English are:

Voiced	**Voiceless**
All vowels	Aspirated *h*
b, d, g, z, v	*p, t, k, s, f*

The difference between voiced and voiceless speech can be easily heard and felt. For example, *b* and *p* are produced the same way, yet the larynx vibrates on *b* and is silent on *p*. If you feel your Adam's apple on "bay" and "pay," you will feel a vibration on *b* but not on *p*.

TABLE 3–1 Definitions of Terms Related to Phonation

Voice: Audible sound produced by phonation.
Vocal parameters: The elements of voice: pitch, loudness, quality, and flexibility.
  Pitch: The perceptual correlate of frequency.
  Loudness: The perceptual correlate of intensity.
  Quality: The perceptual correlate to complexity.
  Flexibility: The perceptual correlate of frequency, intensity, and complexity variations.
Dysphonia: Abnormal voice, as judged by the listener, involving either pitch, loudness, quality, flexibility, or combinations thereof.
Aphonia: Absence of a definable laryngeal tone. The voice is either severely breathy or whispered.
Mute: Unable to phonate and articulate.
Vocal folds: Synonymous with vocal cords—shelves of thyroarytenoid muscle covered with mucous membrane and fibroelastic tissue which project into the laryngeal airway.
Glottis: The space between and bordered by the vocal folds when the latter are partially or fully abducted.
Adduction (of vocal fold): Movement of the vocal folds medially, toward the midline of the laryngeal airway.
Abduction (of vocal fold): Movement of the vocal folds laterally, away from the midline of the laryngeal airway.

Adapted with permission from Aronson AE: Clinical Voice Disorders. New York, Thieme, 1985, p 5.

The outcome of speech has three phonological characteristics that are used to describe "voice"—pitch, quality, and loudness (Table 3–1). Fundamental frequency (pitch) and intensity (loudness) are two elements of voice and speech that are controlled primarily by the interaction of the respiratory and laryngeal systems. Vocal intensity increases as (1) subglottic air pressure increases and (2) the closed phase of the vocal folds increases. Essentially, we turn the volume up or down by manipulating both air pressure beneath the glottis and glottal resistance. Frequency increases as (1) subglottic pressure increases; (2) the larynx rises in the neck, shortening the pharyngeal dimensions; and (3) vocal fold length and tension increase.[6] The average fundamental frequency (pitch) for men is around 125 Hz; for women, it is around 200 Hz.

What is normal voice? Voices vary by age and sex, yet according to Moore,[48] they are judged as normal on the basis of cultural standards, education, environment, and other similar factors. Only general standards for normal voice can be stated[31]:

1. Quality must be pleasant.
2. Pitch level must be appropriate.
3. Loudness must be adequate.
4. Flexibility must be adequate.

Just as beauty is in the eye of the beholder, the "normal" voice is in the ear of the listener.

SPEECH

Speech is the motor activity by which the respiratory, laryngeal, and oral structures produce the sound patterns (phonemes) to communicate. Table 3–2 lists selected speech mechanisms and muscles and their motor innervations as they occur in the dynamically interactive systems of respiration, phonation, and articulation. The speech production mechanism can be likened to a peculiar instrument with a variable resonator, capable of producing sounds that are at one moment based on oscillation and at the next on turbulence. The entire system is powered by the air from the lungs.[11] The entire vocal tract is a dynamic series of cavities beginning at the vocal folds and ending at the lips. The primary articulatory structures along the vocal tract are the soft and hard palate, pharynx, tongue, teeth, lips, cheeks, and mandible. As air, voiced and voiceless, moves from the vocal folds along the vocal tract, the sequenced stream of sound evolves from the various modifications to the product that is finally heard. The vocal tract, with either voiced or voiceless sound, can function simultaneously as a sound filter (with various cavities such as the nares) and sound source (with various muscles and structures set in vibration by air, such as the "raspberry" made by vibrating the tongue and lips). For example, the resultant acoustic event for the speech sound /s/ begins as subglottal air puffs that are eventually expelled through the narrowed tongue, over the edges of the teeth and slightly parted lips, with an audible hissing sound.

Speech sounds are divided into vowels and consonants. Vowels are produced with a relatively open vocal tract, with the sound source beginning at the level of the larynx and the differentiation of one vowel from another determined primarily by tongue posture and degree of lip opening. During the classic throat examination, the tongue is down and the mouth is wide open to say "aah," the vowel sound produced in the word "caught." Consonants are produced at varying points along the vocal tract and at varying degrees of constriction, from completely closed for plosive sounds to closely constricted, as in the earlier example, for the /s/ sound. In this context the role of the velopharyngeal (V/P) port should be mentioned; when the V/P port is open and sound is being resonated through the nasal cavity, the nasal consonants /m/, /n/, and /ng/ are produced. This aspect of speech, termed *resonance,* relates to the degree of nasality in the speech, the amount of resonance.

In summary, the physiology of producing turbulence and pulse characteristics of consonants can be described under manner of articulation (e.g., plosive or fricative), place of articulation (e.g., lips-teeth or velum-tongue), and whether a voiced or voiceless airstream is being produced. Table 3–3 charts a selection of consonants according to manner, place, and voice.

TABLE 3–2 Selected Muscles of Speech Mechanism with Motor Innervation

Muscles	Motor Innervation
Respiration	
Diaphragm	Phrenic
Sternomastoid	Accessory (XI)
External intercostal	Intercostals T2–12
Internal intercostal	Intercostals T2–12
External and internal oblique	Intercostals T6–12
Transversus abdominis	Intercostals T7–12
Phonation	
Interarytenoid	Vagus (X), inferior
Lateral cricoarytenoid	Vagus (X), recurrent branch
Posterior cricoarytenoid	Vagus (X), recurrent branch
Thyroarytenoid	Vagus (X), recurrent branch
Cricothyroid	Vagus (X), recurrent branch
Articulation	
Tongue	
Superior longitudinal	Hypoglossal (XII)
Inferior longitudinal	Hypoglossal (XII)
Transversus	Hypoglossal (XII)
Styloglossus	Hypoglossal (XII)
Palatoglossus	Accessory (XI)
Hypoglossus	Hypoglossal (XII)
Genioglossus	Hypoglossal (XII)
Mandible	
Masseter	Trigeminal (V), anterior
Temporalis	Trunk of mandibular branch
Internal, external, and pterygoid	Trunk of mandibular branch
Velopharyngeal mechanism	
Levator palatini	Vagus (X)
Tensor palatini	Trigeminal (V)
Palatoglossus	Accessory (XI)
Pharyngeal constrictor	Vagus (X)

From Zemlin W: Speech and Hearing Sciences: Anatomy and Physiology, ed 3. Englewood Cliffs, NJ, Prentice-Hall, 1968, pp 403–405. Used by permission.

TABLE 3–3 Articulation of Consonants by Manner, Place, and Voice

Manner of Articulation	Place of Articulation							
	Both Lips		*Lips and Teeth*		*Tongue and Gum Ridge*		*Tongue and Velum*	
	−V	V	−V	V	−V	V	−V	V
Stops	*p*	*b*			*t*	*d*	*k*	*g*
Fricatives			*f*	*v*	*s*	*z*		
Nasals		*m*				*n*		*ng*

Abreviations: V, voiced; −V, voiceless.

FLUENCY AND PROSODY

Fluency is the smoothness with which sounds, syllables, words, and phrases are joined together during oral language with lack of hesitations or repetitions.[10] Rate of speech has a fairly broad range given the dialectical differences occurring throughout the country, such as the "Southern drawl." The average number of words per minute (wpm), or speaking rate, is 125; however, extremes of normal are seen in relation to a given person's educational, intellectual, and regional status. *Prosody* can also be discussed in the context of rate. Prosody encompasses the rate, rhythm, loudness, and pitch contours that signal stress and therefore carry additional meaning beyond individual speech sounds, words, or sequences of words.[81] Although we are unable to ascribe prosody to any given mechanism in the speech chain, prosody can have a dramatic impact on communication. Simply varying one's prosodics (e.g., vocal stress) can convey virtually any emotion or counter any verbal message. An example is the remark, "I am so happy my mother-in-law is visiting," which can be expressed in a number of different ways. Fluency and prosody are integral to getting a message across.

LANGUAGE

For the purposes of this chapter, the way one defines language directly influences who will be classified as language-disordered. In adults, language can be affected secondary to a host of neurological injuries, including stroke and brain injury. Current definitions of language are very broad and comprehensive. The definition developed by the American Speech-Language and Hearing Association's Committee on Language is:

> Language is a complex and dynamic system of conventional symbols that is used in various modes for thought and communication. Contemporary views of language hold that: a) language evolves within specific historical, social, and cultural contexts; b) language, as rule governed behavior, is described by at least 5 parameters—phonologic, morphologic, syntactic, semantic, and pragmatic; c) language learning and use are determined by the interaction of biological, cognitive, psychosocial, and environmental factors; and d) effective use of language for communication requires a broad understanding of human interaction including such associated factors as non-verbal cues, motivation and sociocultural roles.[5]

Table 3–4 includes definitions and examples of the five aspects of language included in the ASHA's definition.

To establish a context for discussing language disorders such as aphasia, I will introduce other terms and concepts not explicitly addressed by the ASHA's definition of language. The first concept is that language is *arbitrary* (e.g., the word "drink" is a sign that the community arbitrarily assigned meaning to) and that arbitrariness has implications for the rehabilitation of persons with a language impairment. Therapists might have to consider using *nonarbitrary* signals or tokens that have a direct relationship to the referent, such as pic-

TABLE 3–4 Definitions and Examples of the Five Dimensions of Language

Dimension	Definition	Example
Phonology	Rules governing the way the sounds of a language are organized	/ks/ sound in English can occur in the middle of a word (bo<u>x</u>er) or the end (boo<u>ks</u>), but never at the beginning.
Semantics	Rules governing the meaning of words and word combinations	Pen = an instrument consisting of ink and used for writing.
Morphology	Rules governing how words are formed	Grammatical morphemes may change the tense and aspect of sentences, e.g., play<u>s</u>, play<u>ing</u>, play<u>ed</u>.
Syntax	Rules governing how words are combined into larger meaningful units of phrases, clauses, and sentences	"Off the boat got" is *not* a well-formed grammatical sentence.
Pragmatics	Rules governing the use of language in context	A speaker must be appropriate in initiating a conversation or changing a topic.

TABLE 3–5 Scale of Hearing Impairment

Average Threshold Level (dB)	Suggested Description*
0–25	Normal hearing
26–40	Mild hearing loss
41–55	Moderate hearing loss
56–70	Moderately severe hearing loss
71–90	Severe hearing loss
≥91	Profound hearing loss

* Average threshold level per ANSI-1989 for 0.5, 1, and 2 kHz.
Modified with permission from Yantis P: Puretone Air-Conduction Threshold Testing. In Katz J (ed): Handbook of Clinical Audiology, ed 4. Baltimore, Williams & Wilkins, 1994, pp 97–108.

tures or gestures for drink that do not employ the arbitrary signs of language (i.e., the spoken or written word "drink"). The second concept is that there are *levels of language usage.* Adults possess automatic speech such as counting or reflexive language (e.g., profanity) that might not be used to convey a message and can be termed the *automatic* level of language usage. The next level of language usage is *imitation*—simply repeating what is heard. This level is also not typically at the level needed to get a need met. The highest level of language usage, and the one that gets at the functional nature of communication, is the *propositional* level of language. I may be able to recite the days of the week (automatic) or repeat what is said to me (imitative), but neither of these abilities will assist me in getting a need met. The core of communication is to *propositionalize*—to convey a message, a want or need, a joke, and so forth.

In summary, verbal language can be divided into phonology (sound), semantics (meaning), syntax (order), and pragmatics (use of language in context). Two underlying concepts that are emphasized for further reference are the arbitrariness of language and the levels of language usage, including automatic, imitative, and propositional. The essence of what humans must do is make propositions—to intend to give or get a message across to others.

ADULT COMMUNICATION DISORDERS

Hearing Impairment

Hearing impaired is a generic term that refers both to persons who are hard of hearing and those who are deaf. Hard of hearing refers to partial impairment of hearing sensitivity sufficient to cause difficulty with the comprehension of speech. Deafness refers to a degree of hearing loss in which hearing is nonfunctional for the ordinary purposes of daily life.[51] Hearing loss refers to the measured extent, or severity, of hearing impairment. As was mentioned earlier, hearing sensitivity is measured in decibels. The terms generally used to describe the extent of hearing loss are given in Table 3–5. Hearing impairment can also be categorized as unilateral or bilateral, and the impairment can be temporary, permanent, or progressive. Types of hearing impairment are related to the site of damage or dysfunction and are termed conductive, sensorineural, mixed, and central (Table 3–6).

Management of the person with hearing impairment begins with identification of the degree and type of hearing loss. When the hearing loss is conductive or mixed, consultation with an otolaryngologist should be sought. In many cases the hearing loss or disease process can be halted or reversed through proper treatment. When the hearing loss is sensorineural, otologic consultation should be pursued if there is an asymmetry in the degree of hearing loss, if the loss is sudden, or if the patient is experiencing concomitant vertigo or dizziness. In most cases of sensorineural hearing loss, hearing aids or other amplifying devices can be of help. Even persons with a mild hearing loss can experience significant difficulties in communication situations and benefit from the use of hearing aids. Technology in this field is evolving quickly, and hearing aids are best fit by a credentialed audiologist.

Voice Disorders

Normal voice falls within a wide range of acceptability, making it easier to define the disordered voice. A voice

TABLE 3–6 Definitions of Types of Hearing Loss and Various Causes

Type of Hearing Loss	Definition	Possible Causes
Conductive	Hearing loss resulting from dysfunction of the outer and/or middle ear systems	Occluding cerumen Perforated eardrum Otitis media Otosclerosis
Sensorineural	Hearing impairment resulting from damage/dysfunction of the inner ear (cochlea), or neural fibers of the eighth cranial nerve	Prebycusis Noise-induced Trauma Viral/bacterial illness Ménière's disorder Tumors Hereditary
Mixed	Hearing loss with both conductive and sensorineural components	See Conductive and Sensorineural
Central	Hearing impairment resulting from damage or dysfunction of the central auditory pathways; may influence ability to comprehend spoken language, especially in difficult listening situations.	Trauma Tumors Vascular damage Demyelinating disease

disorder is said to exist when the quality, pitch, or loudness of the voice, individually or severally, differs from that of other persons of similar age, sex, cultural background, and geographic location.[6,48,72] A common defining feature of a voice disorder is when a given voice draws attention to the speaker. The person who is usually the most critical of the voice is the owner of the voice.[72]

Laryngeal disorders have traditionally been classified as either functional or organic, depending on their specific causes. Disorders range from aphonia (no voice) to various dysphonias (disorders of sound quality). Four specific causes of voice problems will be discussed: (1) increased vocal fold or laryngeal mass, or both, (2) neurological, (3) psychosocial, and (4) surgical.

The person with a voice complaint should initially be seen by an otolaryngologist (ear, nose, and throat [ENT] specialist). The otolaryngologist typically examines the patient using indirect laryngoscopy, fiberoptic laryngoscopy, or video-stroboscopy to rule out life-threatening disease or to determine if further medical intervention is indicated (e.g., surgical removal of a vocal cord polyp). The voice evaluation should (1) attempt to determine the cause, (2) describe the current vocal status, and (3) arrive at a communication diagnosis, prognosis, and plan. The diagnostic workup typically includes an extensive interview, oral peripheral examination, voice analysis (including respiration, phonation, resonance, and prosody), and an objective voice analysis using instrumentation. This assessment is key to uncovering the factors contributing to the vocal problem, to determining the patient's stimulability to achieve an improved vocal cord approximation, to gauge the degree of the patient's understanding of the disorder, and finally to assess the patient's willingness to participate in a remediation program.

Adult dysphonias that are due to a mass effect are often caused by a faulty phonatory attack (voice misuse or abuse) or substance abuse (smoking and alcohol). The interruption of the smooth approximation of the vocal folds results in a dysphonia. Causes of dysphonias include vocal nodules (a callus formation at the anterior middle third of the vocal folds), laryngitis (an inflammation of the vocal fold mucosa), vocal polyps (fluid-filled sacs that can occur anywhere along the median edge of one or both vocal folds), and contact ulcers (which occur around the area of the arytenoid cartilages). Intervention for these dysphonias typically involves a systematic, step-by-step patient education and treatment implementation regimen that attempts to

1. Identify misuse or abuse
2. Describe the effects of the patterns of misuse or abuse
3. Define the specific instances or circumstances of abuse or misuse
4. Modify the behavior
5. Monitor vocal change

The regimen can include periods of voice rest and often includes counseling to reduce or eliminate substance abuse. Management of the vocal components basically involves re-establishing the proper coordination of respiration, phonation, resonance, and prosody and determining appropriate pitch, quality, and intensity.

Adult dysphonia of neurological origin (excluding dysarthria, which is discussed later) may be related to unilateral or bilateral vocal cord paralysis. The folds can be paralyzed in adduction (closed, a life-threatening condition) or in varying stages of abduction (opening). (For a discussion of the cause and treatment of vocal fold paralysis, see Aronson.[6]) Patients with cords fixed in an adducted position usually require a tracheostomy to maintain a functional airway. They phonate by occluding the stoma and exhaling for speech. In persistent closure due to abductor paralysis, surgical intervention might be indicated to reposition a cord laterally to provide sufficient opening for air. The surgical result, however, often leaves the patient with a breathy voice, as the cords are unable to fully approximate. In the case of adductor paralysis (folds in the open position), surgical intervention typically involves either injecting material into a fold to create a mass effect or surgically repositioning a cord to bring it closer to midline. The speech-language pathologist (SLP) typically is involved before and after surgery in an effort to optimize the patient's efforts at producing the most functional voice possible, given the physical condition of the laryngeal mechanism.[81]

Voice disorders of psychosocial origin may need psychological intervention in concert with the SLP voice regimen. As with all voice disorders, it is essential that a medical condition (especially a treatable one) be ruled out before therapy is initiated. The symptoms can range from a variety of dysphonias to complete aphonia.

A case of chronic hysterical aphonia (Case 1) was referred for SLP evaluation and treatment.

In another case (Case 2) the dysphonia resembled that due to an organic condition.

CASE STUDY 1

A 15-year-old boy presented who had not voiced in months. The ENT examination was unremarkable and the family rejected psychiatric consultation. By using vegetative, nonspeech approaches (e.g., lifting, sighing), voice was attained after several sessions. Normal phonation slowly evolved from aphonia to falsetto to functional voice as the patient progressed in his ability to talk about his dissatisfaction with his "strict parochial school" and "strict" parents. Once the family became involved in treatment and other school options and parenting strategies were explored, normal voice was regained and maintained at follow-up 1 year later.

CASE STUDY 2

A 26-year-old female schoolteacher was referred for chronic (1-year) severe dysphonia with normal ENT findings. The evaluation and treatment attempted to address the voice from an organic perspective (e.g., as would be employed to treat vocal nodules due to voice misuse), with training in the physiology and psychology of voice. No significant change was noted in the voice after a trial regimen of eight sessions in 1 month. At the conclusion of the trial regimen, the lack of results and the options remaining were discussed. It was at this point, when it appeared that the dysphonia was permanent, that the patient broke down and reported that she had been raped over a year ago and had been unable to report it, even to her doctor. She felt certain that her "stressed voice" condition was due to that trauma. She was referred to a rape crisis center for counseling and voice therapy was planned to continue. The patient's voice returned to normal in weeks and she enrolled in a course of psychotherapy to work through her trauma.

These cases illustrate the psychodynamics of voice, the potential for swift resolution, and the crucial role listening plays in the therapeutic process.

A voice disorder can also be one of the first symptoms of laryngeal cancer. Patients with laryngeal cancer may be candidates for a laryngectomy, the total or partial surgical removal of the larynx. A partial laryngectomy might or might not affect vocal quality, depending on whether vocal fold tissue has been excised. A total laryngectomy results in a sudden and complete loss of voice. The postlaryngectomy patient has at least three speaking and several nonspeaking options; these are described below.

Speaking Options

1. *Tracheoesophageal shunt:* A one-way valve prosthesis is inserted that permits air to pass from the trachea into the esophagus. "Esophageal sound" is produced by aerodynamics within the esophagus.
2. An *esophageal voice* is produced by oral injection of air into the esophagus followed by a rapid vibrating expulsion.
3. An *artificial larynx* is used by the speaker to generate sound for speech production purposes. The electrolarynx prosthesis can be a neck type or intraoral type and must be coordinated in placement and timing with articulated speech.

Nonspeaking Options

1. Writing
2. Complex and simple gestures
3. Communication board
4. Portable personal computer

Detailed information on laryngectomee rehabilitation can be found in Keith and Darley's *Laryngectomee Rehabilitation.*[33]

Speech Disorders

Apraxia of Speech

Two adult neurogenic communication disorders that fall under the generic term "speech" are apraxia of speech and dysarthria. *Apraxia of speech* (AOS) is a sensorimotor disorder of articulation and prosody that frequently accompanies Broca's aphasia and can also coexist with dysarthria. Just as the person with limb apraxia has difficulty programming the exact sequence of movements to complete a gesture, so the person with AOS presents with a volitional programming problem in "saying" what is meant. The four salient characteristics of AOS are

1. Effortful, trial-and-error, groping articulatory movements, and attempts at self-correction
2. Dysprosody unrelieved by extended periods of normal rhythm, stress, and intonation
3. Articulatory inconsistency on repeated productions of the same utterance
4. Obvious difficulty initiating an utterance[77]

AOS is believed by most experts to not be due to a language disorder, nor is it due to paralysis, weakness, or incoordination of the speech musculature.[19, 76] However, this "separate phenomenon" is a controversial issue since a number of experts are not convinced AOS exists in isolation.[3, 42] Patients with suspected AOS typically have left frontal lesions adjacent to Broca's area. The discriminating behaviors that differentiate AOS from aphasia and dysarthria are the following: relatively spared automatic speech; the absence of any significant motor control problems; and other language modalities that are superior to speech. The assessment of AOS should include a language screen and an extensive battery of speech production tests that elicit simple to complex volitional utterances under varying conditions (imitation, oral reading, spontaneous speech) (Case 3).[56, 57]

Treatment of AOS typically moves from automatic speech, such as counting and opposites (e.g., yes and no), to progressive meaningful speech sound sequencing. Rosenbek[65] suggests the use of an eight-step task continuum ranging from maximal cueing from the clinician to initiating responses in a role-playing situation. Dabul and Bollier[15] suggest a phonetic approach where the patient practices repetitive, volitional control of simple syllables (e.g., me, may, my, mow, moo). Finally, melodic intonation therapy (MIT)[71] has been suggested as a right hemisphere ("musical brain") facilitative approach to speech. MIT is a four-step program in which natural melody patterns are used to facilitate speech. Ideal candidates for MIT have good comprehension and

CASE STUDY 3

A 72-year-old woman presented with muteness with no hemiplegia. She had a history of unproductive home care for several months and was finally referred to a rehabilitation facility for a "more extensive speech work-up." Presenting symptoms were no speech, little or no speech initiation, no reported reading or writing skills, and no use of gestures or of her simple communication book. Evaluation of speech and language revealed a person who had nearly intact listening comprehension, functional reading and writing at the sentence level, and no useful speech.

The resultant revised communication diagnosis was severe apraxia of speech, since the other three language modalities (listening, reading, and writing) were relatively spared and speech initiation and oral motor control for speech were severely compromised. Treatment began with the elicitation of automatic speech and monosyllabic words relevant to her activities of daily living (ADL). Following 1 year of biweekly treatment, she was able to get her basic ADL messages across telegraphically and intelligibly. Her listening, reading, and writing skills were near normal at the time of discharge.

---

are verbally nonfluent. The treatment is painstaking and requires patience. In a Veterans Administration cooperative study in which 19 AOS patients received treatment, 14 patients (74%) improved with treatment.[65] Even the patient with severe AOS can generally establish some core functional verbal repertoire. Based on the cardinal signs of the disorder, therapy is designed to enhance the opportunity of speech being initiated to improve volitional control of the oral musculature for speech purposes, and to teach communication strategies that get the message across in the most efficient and effective manner possible.

Dysarthria

Dysarthria is a collective name for a group of motor speech disorders associated with disturbed neuromuscular control of speech due to central or peripheral nervous system damage.[19] Considering the systems involved in normal speech, neurological damage can affect respiration, phonation, articulation, resonance, and prosody.[49] It is important to point out that, unless a concomitant language disorder exists, language is *not* involved. Thus, the person with dysarthria is able to understand spoken language, read, write, and use a communication board, book, or device.

Differential Diagnosis

A Mayo Clinic study[16] demonstrated that six types of dysarthria can be distinguished on the basis of perceptual characteristics: (1) flaccid, (2) spastic, (3) ataxic, (4) hypokinetic, (5) hyperkinetic, and (6) mixed (Table 3–7). Each type of dysarthria has different auditory perceptual characteristics that can be distinguished clinically, and accurate identification has implications for localization (e.g., spastic dysarthria in upper motor neuron disease).

Assessment

Motor speech disorders can be assessed by both perceptual and physiological approaches. A basic clinical protocol for assessment of dysarthria begins with a detailed history. The clinician then screens hearing and vision and conducts an oral peripheral examination that includes testing alternating motion rates (e.g., rapid repetition of "puh, tuh, kuh") and sequential motor rates (e.g., rapid repetition of "puh, puh, puh"), and prolongation of "aah." The speech evaluation proper should involve contextual speech, stress testing (varying prosodic emphasis), and contrasting stress tasks (e.g., *I* am going home vs. I am going *home*). Finally an informal and formal speech intelligibility test should be considered as part of the evaluation, such as the Tikofsky word list (an unpublished list of 50 phonetically balanced words) or Assessing Intelligibility of Dysarthric Speech.[80] The latter test is used to assess speech intelligibility at the word and sentence level. It also provides an overall intelligibility quotient as well as a measure of speaking rate.

Treatment

The overall goal of dysarthria treatment is enhanced functional communication.[67] In the case of anarthria (no speech), a nonverbal communication system may be developed that permits the patient to reliably communicate basic daily living needs. In the case of a person with severe dysarthria who has the potential for verbal communication, treatment attempts to address three overriding goals, namely, maximization of speech intelligibility, speech efficiency, and functional independence. Clinicians may focus on the perceptual symptoms of the patient by attending to the most distinctive perceptual characteristics,[16] on the speech systems by employing a "physiological" approach,[49] or pragmatically and productively combine both approaches.[57] Figure 3–3 illustrates the vocal tract and the ten functional components that generate or valve speech airstreams, as well as the aerodynamic variables that allow diagnostic inferences. For example, malfunction of a given component could be due to variations in muscle strength and tone or to abnormalities in timing the onset, duration, and offset of muscle contractions.[49] The clinician must be judicious in selecting what variable to manipulate to obtain the greatest "speech" payoff. The general prioritized dysarthria hierarchy of treatment moves through three stages: (1) early, to establish functional verbal skills; (2) middle,

TABLE 3–7 Mayo Clinic Perceptual Classification of Dysarthrias

Type	Perceptual Characteristics	Localization	Causes	Neuromuscular Condition
Flaccid dysarthria	Breathy voice quality, hypernasality, consonant imprecision	Lower motor neuron	Viral infection (e.g., poliomyelitis), tumor, cerebrovascular accident (CVA), congenital conditions, disease (e.g., myasthenia gravis), palsies (e.g., bulbar, facial), trauma	Flaccid paralysis, weakness, hypotonia, muscle atrophy, fasciculation
Spastic dysarthria	Strained/strangled/harsh voice quality, hypernasality, slow rate, consonant imprecision	Upper motor neuron	CVA, tumor, infections (e.g., encephalitis), trauma, congenital conditions (e.g., spastic cerebral palsy)	Spastic paralysis, weakness, limited range of movement, slowness of movement
Ataxic dysarthria	Imprecise consonants, excess and equal stress, irregular articulatory breakdown	Cerebellar system	CVA, tumor, trauma, congenital condition (e.g., ataxic cerebral palsy, Friedreich's ataxia), infection, toxic effects (e.g., alcohol)	Inaccurate movement, slow movement, hypotonia
Hypokinetic dysarthria	Monopitch, monoloudness, reduced stress, imprecise consonants, inappropriate silences, short rushes	Extrapyramidal system	Parkinson's disease, drug-induced (e.g., reserpine or phenothiazine)	Slow movements, limited range of movement, immobility, paucity of movement, rigidity, loss of automatic aspects of movement, resting tremor
Hyperkinetic dysarthrias Predominantly quick	Imprecise consonants, prolonged intervals, variable rate, monopitch, harsh voice quality, inappropriate silences, distorted vowels, excess loudness variation	Extrapyramidal system	Chorea, infection, Gilles de la Tourette's syndrome, ballism	Quick involuntary movements (e.g., myoclonic jerks, tics, etc.), variable muscle tone
Predominantly slow	Imprecise consonants, strained/strangled/harsh voice quality, irregular articulatory breakdown, monopitch, monoloudness	Extrapyramidal system	Athetosis (e.g., acquired or congenital), infection, CVA, tumor, dystonia, drug-induced (e.g., tranquilizers), dyskinesia (e.g., torticollis, tardive dyskinesia)	Twisting and writhing movements, slow movements, involuntary movements, hypertonia
Mixed dysarthria Spastic-flaccid	Imprecise consonants, hypernasality, harsh voice quality, slow rate, monopitch, short phrases, distorted vowels, low pitch, monoloudness, excess and equal stress, prolonged intervals	Upper and lower motor neurons	Amyotrophic lateral sclerosis, trauma, CVA	Weakness, slow movement, limited range of movement
Spastic-ataxic-hypokinetic	Reduced stress, monopitch, monoloudness, imprecise consonants, slow rate, excess and equal stress, low pitch, irregular articulatory breakdown	Upper motor neuron, cerebellar, extrapyramidal	Wilson's disease	Intention tremor, rigidity, spasticity, slow movement
Variable (spastic-ataxic-flaccid)	Variable (e.g., slow rate, harsh voice quality, irregular articulatory breakdown)	Variable (e.g., upper motor neuron, cerebellar, lower motor neuron)	Multiple sclerosis	Variable (e.g., spasticity, weakness, slow movement, limited range of movement, inaccurate movement)
Others	Variable	Multiple CVAs, tumor, trauma, disease, etc.	Variable	

Data from Darley FL, Aronson AE, Brown JR: Motor Speech Disorders. Philadelphia, WB Saunders, 1975.

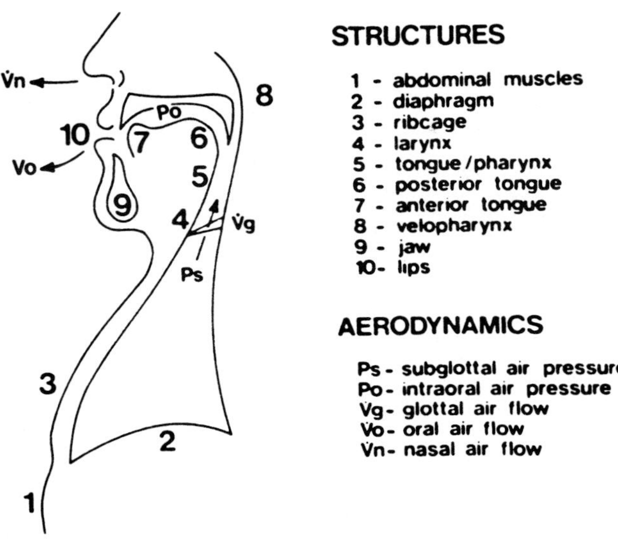

FIGURE 3–3. The vocal tract and designation of 10 functional components that generate or valve the speech airstream, and the aerodynamic variables that allow inferences as to malfunction of the various components. (From Netsell R, Daniel B: Dysarthria in adults: Physiologic approach to rehabilitation. Arch Phys Med Rehabil 1979; 60:502–508.)

to maximize speech intelligibility; and (3) final, to increase the naturalness of speech. The equipment that might be necessary at various stages of treatment includes an alphabet board to signal the first letter of each spoken word in the early stage, a palatal lift to reduce hypernasality and nasal emission in the middle stage, and a pacing board to control speech rate in the final stage.

A caveat to all of the above is that the approaches described are applicable only to the patient with dysarthria who is recovering from, for example, a stroke or traumatic brain injury. The treatment hierarchy for persons with dysarthria secondary to progressive diseases such as Parkinson's disease or multiple sclerosis is nearly the reverse. For example, in the latter stages of multiple sclerosis, the focus is on augmentative or alternative means of communication that can be used to get daily needs met.

Fluency Disorders

Stuttering is defined as gaps, prolongations, or involuntary repetitions of a sound or syllable that occur during speech production. The most common type of stuttering is developmental dysfluency. Acquired stuttering is fairly rare (only 2% of cases of stuttering begin after the age of 10 years[41]). Since acquired stuttering is primarily due to brain injury, it has been termed *cortical* or *neurogenic* stuttering. An additional variety of acquired stuttering that does not fit the above description except for its relative rarity is psychogenic stuttering of adult onset. Adult-onset dysfluency is consequently either neurogenic or psychogenic.

Differential Diagnosis

When conducting a differential diagnostic evaluation of a patient with a presumed adult-onset dysfluency disorder, it is critical that the clinician consider all possibilities in the clinical environment[68]:

1. Neurogenic stuttering vs. *Palilalia*—"repetitions of words or phrases in which each repetition gets faster and faster and it may or may not become more unintelligible."[62]
2. Neurogenic stuttering vs. *Multiple self-corrections*—primarily seen in persons with left hemisphere injury that affects language.[57]
3. Neurogenic stuttering vs. *Psychogenic stuttering*—"stuttering begun in adulthood as a result of emotional trauma."[41]
4. Neurogenic stuttering vs. *Malingering*—"stuttering that is feigned for some ulterior gain."[63]

At a minimum, the dysfluency assessment should include a detailed history relating to the onset of the dysfluency; an oral peripheral examination; a voice, speech, language, and cognitive screen; and an extensive speech sample that includes singing, imitation, oral reading, narrative discourse, and conversation.

Neurogenic Stuttering

Canter[13] classified neurogenic stuttering into three subgroups: dysarthric, dyspraxic, and dysnomic. Patients exhibit a fluency disorder that is predominantly either a disruption of motor speech, motor programming, or language, respectively. Rao[60] described Case 4.

This case illustrates an acquired dysfluency that appeared to be due to a combination of neurogenic dyspraxia (vocal control), dysarthria (motor control), and dysnomia (word finding). This dysfluency responded to treatment in all three subclasses of the disorder. The treatment approaches employed in acquired stuttering mirror the traditional approaches employed with developmental dysfluency[10]:

Bibliotherapy and patient education and counseling
Easy onset
Breathing exercises to control phonation
Use of masking noise to distract speakers from their own speech
Use of delayed auditory feedback, forcing the speaker to reduce speech rate
Use of pacing strategies such as finger tapping

Aphasia

Aphasia has been defined as an "acquired impairment of language processes underlying receptive and expressive modalities; caused by damage to areas of the brain that are primarily responsible for the language function."[17] The communication problems most common after a left hemisphere stroke are aphasia, AOS, and dysarthria.

CASE STUDY 4

A 52-year-old man developed severe neurogenic stuttering 1 hour after a motor vehicle accident in which he sustained no detectable trauma. He was referred for an SLP consultation to determine the nature of his fluency disorder, whether treatment would be beneficial, and whether resumption of his pretrauma vocational status was feasible. The differential diagnostic dilemma was whether his dysfluency was neurogenic, psychogenic, or malingering. Once the acquired stuttering was deemed to be due to a suspected small, focal hemisphere lesion, a 5-month treatment program was undertaken that used a novel prosthetic approach to restore fluency. Once fluency was restored with the use of an artificial larynx (an application of Netsell and Daniel's[43] physiological approach for dysarthria, in which a substitution is made for the phonatory component), with immediate and dramatic results, a residual dysnomic difficulty was discovered and treated.

The *volitional programming* aspects of AOS and the *motor speech* aspects of dysarthria, which were discussed earlier, can be easily contrasted with the devastating *language* disorder of aphasia.

Once related adult neurogenic communication disorders have been ruled out and aphasia has been diagnosed, the clinician should classify the type of aphasia. There are at least six existing classification systems in aphasiology, ranging from the simplistic severity system to the more complex syndrome approach (Table 3–8). Although syndromes seem to be the preferred approach in today's practice,[57] many experts contest the usefulness or even the existence of syndromes.[18] (See Rao[56] for a review of the controversies surrounding classification and localization in aphasia.) Kertesz[34] summarized the issue in favor of syndromes: "Most clinicians will agree that although aphasic disability is complex, many patients are clinically similar and will fall into recurring identifiable groups. . . . There are many classifications, indicating that none is altogether satisfactory, but also that this effort is useful and even necessary to diagnose and treat aphasics or to understand the phenomena."

Syndromes of aphasia are *not* hard neurological signs but simply suggestive of the presence of brain damage in a particular location of the brain. When a patient with a lesion in the third left frontal convolution is hemiplegic and has nonfluent speech with good comprehension, the patient is almost universally referred to as having a Broca's aphasia. Table 3–9 summarizes the various aphasia syndromes and suggested localization following a left cerebrovascular accident. Few cases are reported in the current literature using any grouping in aphasia other than syndromes.

Three particular discriminating binary language behaviors helpful in classifying aphasia by syndrome are (1) fluency, (2) comprehension, and (3) repetition. *Fluency* suggests a binary anteroposterior view of the left cortex, since nonfluent patients typically have anterior (frontal lobe) lesions whereas fluent patients typically have posterior (temporal, parietal, or occipital lobe) lesions. *Comprehension* is another binary dimension wherein patients who have suffered strokes in the distribution of the left middle cerebral artery (MCA) can exhibit some degree of deficit in listening comprehension, whereas patients who have suffered strokes in the left posterior cerebral artery (PCA) exhibit some degree of deficit in reading comprehension. *Repetition* distinguishes patients with MCA infarcts from those with lesions outside the MCA distribution. A left CVA patient who cannot repeat is thus suspected of having a Broca's, Wernicke's, conduction, or global aphasia. The aphasia syndromes listed in Table 3–9 are summarized briefly below.

Broca's Aphasia. Persons with Broca's aphasia are *nonfluent,* with telegraphic speech (like a telegram with the connecting words left out) and reduced verbal con-

TABLE 3–8 Classification Systems and Associated Tests for Aphasia

Criterion	Example(s)	Associated Tests	Proponent(s)
Severity	Mild, moderate, severe	Aphasia Language Performance Scales (ALPS)	Keenan & Brassell[32] (1975)
Modality	Receptive vs. expressive	Examining for Aphasia (EA)	Eisenson[21] (1954)
Behavioral	Simple aphasia, aphasia with visual involvement	Minnesota Test for the Differential Diagnosis of Aphasia (MTDDA)	Schuell[69] (1965)
Statistical	PICA 40%-ile PICA 75%-ile	Porch Index of Communicative Ability (PICA)	Porch[54] (1981)
Linguistic	Semantic aphasia Syntactic aphasia	Language Modalities Test (LMT)	Wepman & Jones[75] (1961)
Syndrome	Broca's aphasia Global aphasia	Boston Diagnostic Aphasia Examination (BDAE)	Goodglass & Kaplan[25] (1972)

Reprinted with permission from Rao P: The aphasia syndromes: localization and classification: In Topics in Stroke Rehabilitation. Rockville, MD, Aspen, 1994.

TABLE 3–9 Decision Tree for Classifying and Localizing Aphasia After a Left-Sided Cerebrovascular Accident

Impairment and Symptoms	Classification	Localization
Language impairment affecting linguistic components of semantics, syntax, phonology, or pragmatics, or any combination of these	Broca's	MCA, frontal lobe
	Wernicke's	MCA, temporal lobe
	Conduction	MCA, arcuate fasciculus
	Anomic	MCA, angular gyrus
	Global	MCA, multilobes
	Transcortical motor	ACA, prefrontal
	Transcortical sensory	PCA, parieto-occipital
	Isolation	ACA/PCA, watershed area
	Subcortical	Thalamus and basal ganglia
	Alexia with agraphia	PCA, angular gyrus
	Alexia without agraphia	PCA, medial-occipital and splenium of corpus callosum

Abbreviations: MCA, middle cerebral artery; ACA, anterior cerebral artery; PCA, posterior cerebral artery.

tent. Phrase length is generally less than four words, and the verbal repertoire is almost exclusively composed of content words (e.g., nouns and verbs), with a notable absence of function words (prepositions and conjunctions). Patients with Broca-type aphasia typically have functional comprehension but have trouble following complex grammatical statements.

Wernicke's Aphasia. Persons with Wernicke's aphasia are fluent with what is termed paragrammatism—speech running on with some semblance of grammatical structure. Phrase length is generally greater than five words and verbal productions are punctuated with paraphasic errors (word substitutions, e.g., pen for pencil) and poor repetition. Listening comprehension difficulty is a cardinal sign. In addition, the secondary language skills of reading and writing are typically also impaired.

Anomic Aphasia. Persons with anomic aphasia are most striking in their "loss of words" both orally and in writing. They tend to circumlocute (talk around a word) and generally have functional reading and listening skills. Their fluency and repetition skills are also unremarkable.

Global Aphasia. Persons with global aphasia are severely impaired in all language modalities, which results in an almost total inability to communicate orally. Fluency, repetition, and comprehension are all seriously compromised.

Conduction Aphasia. Persons with conduction aphasia have difficulty repeating a word or phrase back to the examiner. Spontaneous speech is relatively fluent with functional comprehension.

Transcortical Motor Aphasia. The patient with transcortical motor aphasia has fluency and comprehension resembling that of a person with Broca's aphasia, but the repetition skills are spared. A hallmark of this syndrome is adynamia (difficulty initiating speech).

Transcortical Sensory Aphasia. This relatively rare syndrome is similar to Wernicke's aphasia, save for the retained ability to repeat.

Isolation Syndrome. Persons with this rare syndrome are severely impaired in all language-processing abilities except for the oasis of being able to repeat.

Assessment

In the area of language assessment, the SLP is charged with conducting a differential diagnosis, establishing a prognosis, and determining whether or not treatment is indicated. Table 3–8 lists six tests for evaluation of a person with aphasia. Currently the two most frequently employed standardized aphasia examinations are the Boston Diagnostic Aphasia Examination (BDAE)[26] and the Western Aphasia Battery (WAB).[35] The tests are quite similar, employing the syndrome approach and systematically and comprehensively looking at spontaneous speech (content and fluency), auditory verbal comprehension, repetition, naming, reading, and writing.[36] An inventory of language input and output modalities is a general language assessment. Table 3–10 is a 4 × 4 matrix with 16 subtests that can easily serve as the basis for an inventory of language functions. Table 3–11 summarizes the components of a general language assessment.[53]

Functional communication assessment is an area that is increasingly coming under intense scrutiny. (See Rao[59] for a comprehensive review of functional communication assessment and outcomes in the elderly.) The rehabilitation clients (payers, patients, employers) are extremely interested in outcomes, and the optimal means to a functional outcome is a functional assessment. A useful definition for functional assessment of communication is as follows: "Assess the extent of the ability to communicate with others in a variety of contexts, considering environmental modifications, adaptive equipment, time required to communicate, and listener familiarity with the client. Special accommodations of the communicative partner to either receive or enhance reception must be considered."[23]

A functional communication assessment tool that is showing real promise in eliciting consumer input and measuring outcomes is the Communication Effectiveness Index (CETI).[38] The CETI focuses on communicative need and assesses communication for social need, life skill, basic need, and health threat. It is based on direct observation by the patient's significant other of the patient's ability to perform 16 communicative skills

TABLE 3–10 Stimulus Response Matrix in a Language Assessment

	Stimulus		Response	
	Point	*Say*	*Write*	*Do*
SEE OBJECT	Visual matching	Naming	Written naming	Pantomime (praxis)
HEAR WORDS (SENTENCES)	Word discrimination Sentence comprehension	Word repetition Sentence repetition or answering questions	Writing from dictation	Follow commands
SEE WORDS (SENTENCES)	Word-object matching	Oral reading	Copy	Follow written commands
FEEL OBJECTS	Visual-tactile matching (stereognosis)	Tactile naming	Tactile-written naming	

From Albert ML, Goodglass H, Helm N, et al: Clinical Aspects of Dysphagia, New York, Springer-Verlag, 1981. Used by permission.

relative to premorbid abilities in those skill areas. A sample of CETI items is (1) getting someone's attention, (2) communicating emotions, and (3) understanding writing.[38] The patient's performance is noted on a scale from "not at all able" to "as able as before stroke." When patients are at a high enough communication level, they can also be involved in rating their communication skills using the CETI. (See Rao[55] for a comprehensive case study utilizing CETI data for counseling the patient and spouse in coping with aphasia.)

Since the advent of managed care has prompted even greater scrutiny of the overall efficacy of medical rehabilitation in general and of speech-langauge pathology in particular, researchers and clinicians have been attempting to design tools that can be used to measure patients' functional status and the outcomes of service delivery. Two of the most current and comprehensive tools are the Functional Assessment of Communication Skills for Adults[23] and Communication Activities of Daily Living-2.[30]

TABLE 3–11 Components of the General Language Assessment

Auditory comprehension	Word identification/discrimination Yes/no reliability for personal/general questions Ability to follow commands, length and complexity Sentence/paragraph level retention and understanding
Visual comprehension	Ability to match symbols/letters Word identification skills Sentence/paragraph retention and comprehension Oral reading Functional reading skills
Speech	Social/automatic speech Word/sentence repetition Confrontation/responsive naming Verbal agility, mean length of utterance, fluency rating Analysis of form and content
Writing	Biographical information Letters, numbers: copyring/dictation Word/sentence level Spontaneous sample

From Porcelli J: Aphasia assessment and treatment. Phys Med Rehabil Clin North Am 1991; 2:487–500. Used by permission.

Prognosis

The prognostic variable approach is the most common one used to project ultimate communication status. Table 3–12 summarizes the research on prognostic variables important in aphasia and related neurogenic communication disorders following stroke. According to Rao,[57] the medical and speech and language variables are more potent than the subject or other variables. In formulating a prognosis, the team asks the following three questions:

1. Prognosis for what?
2. Which factors are positive?
3. Which factors are negative?

Although the correspondence is not one to one, the practitioner is able to make a best "guestimate" about the odds of recovery based on the answers to these questions. Once an overall prognosis is made for return of functional communication, the clinician must estimate the patient's response to treatment:

1. Will treatment help?
2. If so, what modalities should be treated and in what order?
3. What type of treatment should be used?

Four caveats that may rule out one's candidacy for aphasia treatment are found in Davis[18]:

1. Perseveration and severe auditory comprehension deficit
2. Inability to match objects
3. Unreliable yes/no responses
4. Jargon and empty speech without self-correction

Treatment

Today the focus of treatment is on function! One way to operationalize the "functional issues" with regard to aphasia treatment is to place the discussion in the context of the World Health Organization's model of consequences of pathology[39]: "Impairment (dysfunction at the organ level), activity (functional consequences of impairment that affect performance of daily tasks), and participation (social disadvantages resulting from an impairment or a disability)." With respect to aphasia, it is a result of a stroke that results in a disruption of language

TABLE 3–12 Prognostic Variables Important to Aphasia and Related Neurogenic Communication Disorders Following Stoke

Patient Variables	Medical Variables	Speech and Language Variables	Other Variables
Age at onset, education, intelligence, handedness, monolingual or multilingual	Etiologic factors, site of lesion; extent of lesion, coexisting medical problems	Severity of disorder, classification and type of disorder, coexisting communicative impairment, memory and attentional deficits, sensorimotor and perceptual deficits, history of earlier treatment	Months after onset, motivation, stimulability, environment

Modified with permission from LaPointe L: Aphasia therapy: Some principles and strategies for treatment. In Johns D (ed): Clinical Management of Neurogenic Communication Disorders, ed 2. Boston, Little, Brown, 1985, p 297.

activity and a consequent reduction in the ability to participate in communication activities.

A definition of *participation* is "the nature and extent of a person's involvement in life situations in relation to Impairments, Activities, Health Conditions, and Contextual Factors,"[39] representing a "limitation of choice." It is precisely in this area of "choice" that the aphasiologist must attempt to maximize communication options. The following three macro approaches to aphasia rehabilitation may be employed to meet this challenge[62]:

1. Enhance functional capacity by assisting the person with aphasia to change behavior through functional communication treatment.
2. Reduce demands of the environment by removing noise in the system (e.g., turning off the TV) and optimizing transmission of signals (e.g., having action pictures in a communication book available).
3. Provide assistive devices and alternative methods by determining the menu of core needs and abilities, then training the person with aphasia in the use of alternative communication options to convey wants and needs (the use of Amer-Ind Code is an example of this approach). (See Rao[62] for a comprehensive review of the use of Amer-Ind Code.)

Specific popular approaches to aphasia treatment that may be employed are the following:

Melodic intonation therapy.[71] This form of therapy utilizes the intact, "musical" right brain to "talk." Persons with good comprehension, poor fluency, and little available speech are thought to be ideal candidates.

Amer-Ind Code treatment.[62] A form of gestural communication that employs nearly 250 iconic gestural signals to get a message across.

Functional communication treatment.[7] Any therapeutic endeavor that seeks to improve the patient's reception, processing, and use of information germane to daily living.

Stimulation approach.[20] This approach, espoused by Hildred Schuell,[67] places primary emphasis on the stimulation presented to the person with aphasia; for example, the patient is asked to point to *X* and the patient responds.

Drawing.[58] Drawing brings unique visually based features to communication not present in speech, gesture, or writing.

An approach that is applicable to most functional methods is PACE therapy,[17] an acronym formed from *p*romoting *a*phasics' *c*ommunicative *e*ffectiveness. PACE is based on the following four principles: (1) the clinician and patient participate equally as senders and receivers of messages; (2) there is an exchange of new information between the clinician and patient; (3) the

CASE STUDY
5

A 35-year-old man suffered a left hemisphere stroke resulting in a markedly severe reduction in activity in all vital spheres. He could not walk, talk, bathe, or toilet. The prognosis was fairly grim for such a bright young man with a wife and two young children. He desperately wanted to get better and at the outset of treatment was assertively part of the team's planning and implementation process. He moved from yes-or-no questions and a simple communication book to an alphabet board, and finally to self-motivated internal coaching to arrive at his message and intent in a complete, coherent, and cogent manner. He progressed from severe apraxia of speech and Broca's aphasia to a mild residual anomia. His yearlong treatment program was totally vocationally focused because the patient demanded that the team assist him in returning to work as a customer service agent for a major U.S. airline. His daily regimen of SLP, vocational rehabilitation, and occupational therapy was designed to assist him to return to his work environment with several environmental adaptations. He returned to full-time employment 2 years after his devastating stroke and subsequently excelled at work (maintained for 7 years at the last report). (See Rao[61] for the individual's consumer testimony before the stroke panel of the Agency for Health Care Policy and Research.)

patient has a free choice as to which communication channels are used to convey new information; and (4) feedback is provided by the clinician, as a receiver, in response to the patient's success in conveying the message. This pragmatic approach to aphasia typifies the thrust of today's treatment, which involves getting a message across by any means possible, whether it be via language, drawing, gesture, tone of voice, or any of a variety of other expressive methods.

Efficacy

In an open letter to aphasiologists, Metter (a neurologist) charged that "A greater emphasis is needed on approaching each case with the most realistic long term expectations and being able to specify these clearly and how they will benefit the patient in his day to day life."[43] Medical rehabilitation care providers in this era of health system reform are increasingly called upon to present data proving that what they are doing works. Wertz et al.[77] reported on a tightly controlled Veterans Administration cooperative study on aphasia that indicated that individual and group treatment was effective: "If the traditional belief is correct, that significant spontaneous recovery is completed by three to six months post onset, significant improvement in both groups beyond 26 weeks post onset indicates both individual and group treatment are efficacious methods for managing aphasic patients." In a recent study, Nicholas et al[50] examined the evolution of severe aphasia in the first 2 years post onset and found that significant improvements in communicative functions were noted for up to 18 months, but the greatest improvement occurred in the first 6 months. Rao[50] reported on two patients who made dramatic progress in treatment: one patient returned home to enjoy a quality of life not experienced in 5 years post stroke and the other progressed from severe jargon aphasia to return to work in the customer service division of a major airline. Robey has produced the most current coverage of the critical issue of efficacy of aphasia therapy, and offers empirical support for aphasia treatment gleaned from 55 reports of clinical outcomes.[64]

Right Hemisphere Communication Disorder

Until 25 years ago, persons with right hemisphere damage were not typically enrolled in a communication treatment program unless they exhibited a severe motor speech impairment (dysarthria). In the mid-1970s, however, with aphasiology beginning to explore pragmatics, attention was also being directed to persons with right hemisphere damage. These "right CVAs"—cerebrovascular accidents—sounded alright—they could talk in complete sentences and did not appear to have any difficulty finding the right word. The physician, the family, and the patient did not refer them to the SLP because "speech wasn't the problem." The problem, as Myers[44] discovered, was with communication. The communication impairment secondary to right hemisphere stroke has been defined as "A breakdown in the expression and reception of complex, contextually based communicative events resulting from a disturbance of the attentional and perceptual mechanisms underlying nonsymbolic, experiential processing."[45] The key words in the definition are "context" and "attentional and perceptual mechanisms." In an isolated speech and language task, persons with right hemisphere stroke will typically exhibit no difficulty on language and speech tasks done in the laboratory. The patient will break down when the same task is done in a context, however, such as when the individual is required to appreciate the emotion in another's voice, the words on the left side of a newspaper, or the face of a friend or family member. These are the symptoms of a problem that has as its basis the visual-attentional processing mechanism of the right hemisphere. The assessment and treatment of persons with right hemisphere communication impairments (RHCIs) is still in its infancy compared to the 130 years of literature on aphasiology. Despite this, we now have a clearer picture of what the classic RHCI profile is (Case 6). The most current and comprehensive, standardized test that is commercially available for this population is the revised RIC evaluation in right hemisphere dysfunction.

According to Myers and Mackisack,[47] the communication deficits associated with RHCI can be divided into three broad categories:

Category	Examples of Problems
Linguistic	Confrontation naming and word fluency
Nonlinguistic	Left-sided neglect and visuospatial processing impairment
Extralinguistic	Facial recognition impairment and impulsivity of response

CASE STUDY 6

A 75-year-old man suffered a right hemisphere stroke with resultant left hemiparesis, left homonymous hemianopsia, left-sided neglect, and a moderate to severe RHCI. On admission and after 1 month of inpatient rehabilitation, the patient was rated as completely dependent in ADL. In team conference at 4 weeks' stay, the team recommended a daily regimen of SLP co-treatment of the patient, with occupational therapy and physical therapy to improve ADL skill development and carryover. At discharge, after 1 month of interdisciplinary co-treatment, he was rated as moderately independent in ambulation, dressing and hygiene, and leisure activity. At 1-month follow-up in a nursing home setting, he had maintained his level of independence in ADL and communication skills.

Although Myers and Mackisack use linguistic descriptions for the RHCI categories, it is important to restate that the problem is communication and the visual-attentional processing mechanism is the underlying basis for the disorder. It is certainly not surprising that a person with RHCI can have difficulty "getting the message in context" when left-sided neglect and impulsivity interfere with the reception and expression of a message.

Rao et al[63] presented an RHCI case that contrasted two approaches to SLP rehabilitation, favoring interdisciplinary co-treatment as a preferred approach. Table 3–13 compares a multidisciplinary and an interdisciplinary approach to RHCI.

In summary, according to Tonkovich,[74] right hemisphere lesions give rise to a number of communication disorders and associated deficits that can interfere with normal communicative interactions. The classification and treatment approaches employed with persons with RHCI continue to evolve. There is a clear need for efficacy and outcome data with respect to the types of interventions with RHCI in order for clinicians to make informed decisions on whether to treat or not treat, and what approaches to employ. At present, treatment tasks tend to focus on the "behaviors" that cause problems with communicating in context, and not typically on the underlying process. Some examples of compensation tasks are[46]

Story or scene interpretation: The goals of this task are to strengthen inferencing skills, to increase the amount of informative content and decrease the amount of extraneous content by improving macrostructure (outline of major topics) development.

Divergent questions: Patients can be asked open-ended or divergent questions that elicit an opinion. The goals of this task are to improve the patient's communication with respect to degree of completeness, integration, efficiency, and coherence.

Generating alternative meanings: The goal is to enhance the patient's flexibility and creativity in conversational contexts.

An exciting exception to the above-described compensation approach to RHCI is the approach of "edgeness," espoused by Myers and Mackisack.[47] This seven-stage technique appears to aid in the recovery of directed attention by presenting patients with a task that requires them to detect the boundaries of relevant space and perform tasks within that space. "Edgeness" readily translates into a reading technique called "bookness," wherein the patient must use the hand to outline the "edges" of the book, and then proceed to scan, then read edge to edge. We are really just on the edge of the literature that is exploring communication in RHCI.

Traumatic Brain Injury

Twenty years ago, few survived traumatic brain injury. With the advent of better emergency techniques and the proliferation of trauma centers, persons who sustain a traumatic brain injury are surviving in greater numbers than ever before. According to Ylvisaker and Szekeres,[66] the number of designated head injury rehabilitation programs in the United States increased from fewer than 50 in 1980 to nearly 1000 in 1994. Today, large numbers of rehabilitation professionals work exclusively with patients with traumatic brain injury in a variety of clinical settings. Patients who suffer traumatic brain injury can experience a variety of communication disorders that have been discussed: aphasia, anarthria, dysarthria, AOS, and cortical stuttering. The communication problem that is most commonly associated with traumatic brain injury, however, is not based on language, speech, or fluency but on cognition.

Cognitive-communication impairments[6] is the generic term used to refer to the cognitively based communication disorders resulting from deficits in both linguistic and nonlinguistic cognitive processes. This population differs from the language-impaired patients following stroke in that they are typically younger, have lesions that are more diffuse, have a longer recovery period, and frequently have academic and vocational reentry as significant functional goals. According to Adamovich,[1] specific cognitive skills that may be impaired in traumatic brain injury are attention, perception, discrimination, organization, recall, and reasoning/problem solving. Persons with traumatic brain injury can experience impairments in any or all stages of memory from attention and immediate recall to short- and long-term memory. Disturbances in executive functioning can occur even following a mild head injury with normal neuroradiological findings (see Chapter 49).

TABLE 3–13 Two Contrasting Approaches to Right-Sided Cerebrovascualr Accident Rehabilitation in Speech-Language Pathology

Traditional Multidisciplinary Treatment	Interdisciplinary Co-Treatment
Increase abstraction in all language modalities	Listing step by step the approach to accomplishing each ADL
Decrease impulsivity in treatment tasks via reminders, cues, etc.	Coaching with OT/nursing in shaving, brushing teeth, etc.
Increase left-sided awareness by introducing border concept, visual reminders, verbal cues	Coaching patient with PT stepwise in standing in parallel bars, transferring, wheelchair ambulation
Writing drills requiring print to remain within a highlighted border and cues and self-monitoring drills to decrease letter repetitions; reading from left to right with cues	Participating with therapeutic recreation in games—cueing patient in turn-taking, providing strategic and tactical advice, reminding of left-sided awareness
Reality orientation drills with log books	Log completion by each therapist after each activity, with patient reviewing same

Abbreviations: ADL, activities of daily living; OT, occupational therapy; PT, physical therapy.

Stages Of Recovery

The Rancho Los Amigos (RLA) Hospital Levels of Cognitive Recovery[27] is an eight-stage recovery scale that is widely used to rate the level of cognitive functioning. Ylvisaker and Szekeres[79] group RLA levels into three very broad stages: early, middle, and late.

Early Stages (RLA Levels 2 and 3). Functioning moves from generalized response to the environment to localized responses to specific stimuli, for example, pain, sound, visual tracking.

Middle Stages (RLA Levels 4 to 6). Functioning moves from the status where the patient is confused and agitated to the point where the patient is less confused, more appropriate in interaction, and, in a familiar environment, goal-directed.

Late Stage (RLA Levels 7 and 8). Functioning moves from the status where the patient is adequately oriented to the important aspects of life, is appropriate in interaction, and is goal-oriented, to the final stage, where the patient's ultimate neurological improvement may continue to include cognitive-communication impairments that may compromise community, academic, or vocational reentry.

Treatment

There is little efficacy data available to suggest what works and doesn't work in cognitive-communicative remediation. Ylvizaker and Szekeres[79] provide some general principles of treatment that they believe are critical in designing treatment programs that are germane to SLP. These principles are:

1. Success facilitates progress while building a positive self-concept.
2. Systematic gradation of activities carefully adjusted to meet individual needs facilitates improvement.
3. Generalization to real-world settings and activities must be a controlled component of intervention.
4. Sensitivity to executive system themes must be part of therapy sessions and the rehabilitation environment in general.
5. Integration of treatment among all staff and family members facilitates the individual's orientation, learning, and generalization of learned skills.
6. Whenever possible, personally meaningful activities and natural settings should be selected for cognitive-communicative treatment.
7. As much as possible, tasks should be designed that are consistent with the individual's pretraumatic personality, interests, and educational or vocational background as well as goals for the future. (See Case 7.)

Adamovich[1] summarizes the traumatic brain injury treatment issue of the 1990s:

> The treatment of patients with TBI extends from the intensive care and rehabilitation units to outpatient programs, including day treatment and transitional living. . . . If successful home, community, school, and work re-entry is to occur, clinicians must address executive or pragmatic skills in real life situations. Finally, our ultimate treatment goals should be to empower our patients to make as many decisions as they are capable of making throughout the process of rehabilitation.

Dementia

Dementia is an organic syndrome characterized by decline of memory and other intellectual functions in comparison with the patient's previous level of function. Conditions that can resemble dementia but are clearly distinguishable from it are delirium, psychiatric states, depression, and hearing loss. Dementia is a syndrome that can be due to numerous diseases, infections, toxins, and trauma.[8] Because many of the causes of dementia are treatable or reversible, a comprehensive case history and detailed diagnostic medical workup are crucial. Cummings and Benson[14] define dementia operationally as an "acquired persistent impairment of intellectual function with compromise in at least three of the following spheres of mental activity: language, memory, visuospatial skills, emotion or personality and cognition (abstraction, calculation, judgement, executive function and so forth)." According to Shekim,[70] the most common cause is Alzheimer's disease (AD), accounting for 50% to 60% of all patients with dementia. Vascular dementias (dementias caused by multiple infarcts or ischemia [MID]) are seen in 20% of demented patients. Alzheimer's dementia and multiple infarct disease cooccur in approximately 15% of the sample, and other conditions such as Pick's disease, Parkinson's disease, progressive supranuclear palsy, and Creutzfeld-Jakob disease, account for the remainder of the irreversible

CASE STUDY 7

A 20-year-old man suffered massive head injuries following a motor vehicle accident and was admitted to acute rehabilitation as a Rancho 2 (severe injury with only a generalized response to stimuli). He was quadraplegic and "locked-in." Following an aggressive 6-month interdisciplinary rehabilitation program that included his parents as co-therapists, he progressed from being unable to take anything by mouth, anarthric, and nonresponsive to managing a regular diet, being fully alert and responsive, and intelligible to familiar listeners 80% of the time at the phrase level. Today, 8 years later, he is attending junior college, living at home, and following professional sports with the acumen of a Vegas oddsmaker. He is cognitively intact, moderately intelligible, and uses an alphabet board for resolving any discrepancies in his communication.

CASE STUDY 8

A retired physician was originally seen and successfully treated for a severe Wernicke's aphasia secondary to a left-sided stroke. Following a 1-year course of in- and outpatient aphasia therapy, he recovered his language skills and resumed his retirement avocations of fishing and mentoring medical residents in dermatology. Five years later he was re-referred to SLP for an evaluation secondary to "another left CVA." His language skills had regressed markedly, and in addition, his spouse reported notable and frequent episodes of lability, irritability, and forgetfulness. He was found to have multi-infarct dementia. The patient was then enrolled in an adult day care program and his spouse joined an Alzheimer's disease support group. The second stroke, which appeared to result in a repeat episode of aphasia was, on a complete differential diagnostic evaluation, determined to have produced a dementia of vascular origin. (For additional elaboration of the various language profiles and the presumed sites of lesions for the various syndromes, see Albert et al.[3])

dementias. The rehabilitation team is charged with managing the patient and the family, with each discipline contributing a complementing component of care.

Differential Diagnosis

The communication problems commonly seen in dementia can be differentiated from those seen in single, left or right hemisphere strokes. According to Bayles,[8] there are at least six phenomena common to but distinguishable between aphasia and dementia:

1. Memory deficits
2. Anomia
3. Perseveration
4. Dysfluency
5. Jargon
6. Circumlocution

Dementia is differentiated from aphasia and the other adult communication disorders that have already been reviewed by their cause (AD or MID), course (decline), and constellation of symptoms (decrements in judgment, affect, memory, cognition, and orientation). (See Case 8.)

Assessment

Perhaps the most important portion of the assessment is the comprehensive case history obtained from the significant other to determine the type of onset, symptoms, and dysfunctional status of the person with dementia. The clinician should be sensitive to such reversible problems as drug use and depression, but also be eclectic in administering a battery of tests. A tool frequently used to screen for dementia is the Mini-Mental Status Examination (MMSE),[22] a 30-point screen that examines the patient's orientation, registration, calculation, memory, language, praxis, ability to follow commands, and level of consciousness. In addition, the SLP might administer the Arizona Battery for Communication Disorders in Dementia(ABCD),[9] the only commercially available standardized test designed to assess communication function in dementia. The results of the interview, the MMSE, and the ABCD should, in concert with the medical and laboratory findings, provide sufficient data for an examiner to determine whether an intellectual impairment exists, and if so, its current stage. Patients with dementia are often classified as being in the early, middle, or late stages of cognitive decline. Impairment is least in the *early stage.* In this stage, the person with dementia is just beginning to falter in the area of pragmatics, having difficulty with orientation and difficulty with words (e.g., semantic level of language). The syntax and phonology of language are generally unimpaired. In the *middle stage* there is further deterioration in pragmatic, orientation, and semantic functions, and gradual disruption of grammar (e.g., syntax) is now evident. In the *late stage,* function has deteriorated into global impairment, with no component of language being spared. Language sounds, words, grammar, and use all display severe levels of decrement. The patient at this level is oblivious to the environment and fairly nonresponsive. *The Thirty-Six Hour Day*[40] is a particularly useful book for family members as they cope with the staged, steady decline of dementia. Several recent articles on communication treatment for adults with dementia provide some degree of optimism in regard to slowing the intellectual decline.[12, 24]

ACKNOWLEDGMENT

Special thanks to Dr. Carmen Brewer, Director of Hearing and Speech at the Washington Hospital Center, for her input on the hearing impairment section of this chapter.

REFERENCES

1. Adamovich BB: Traumatic brain injury. In LaPointe LL (ed): Aphasia and Related Neurogenic Langauge Disorders, ed 2. New York, Thieme, 1997, pp 226–237.
2. Adamovich BB, Henderson JA, Auerbach S: Cognitive Rehabilitation of Closed Head Injury Patients. San Diego, College Hill Press, 1985.
3. Albert ML, Goodglass H, Helm N, et al: Clinical Aspects of Dysphasia. New York, Springer-Verlag, 1981.
4. American Speech-Language Hearing Association: The role of speech-language pathologists in the identification, diagnosis, and treatment of individuals with cognitive-communicative impairments. Rockville, MD, American Speech-Language Hearing Association, 1988.

5. American Speech-Language Hearing Association Committee on Language: Definition of language. ASHA 1983; 25:44.
6. Aronson AE: Clinical Voice Disorders. New York, Thieme, 1985.
7. Aten JL: Functional communication treatment. In Chapey R (ed): Language Intervention Strategies in Adult Aphasia, ed 3. Baltimore, Williams & Wilkins, 1994, pp 292–303.
8. Bayles KA: Management of neurogenic communication disorders associated with dementia. In Chapey R (ed): Language Intervention Strategies in Adult Aphasia, ed 3. Baltimore, Williams & Wilkins, 1994, pp 535–545.
9. Bayles KA, Tomoeda C: Arizona Battery for Communication Disorders of Dementia. Tucson, AZ, Canyonlands Publishing, 1991.
10. Bloodstein O: A Handbook of Stuttering. Chicago, National Easter Seal Society, 1981.
11. Borden GJ, Harris KS: Speech Science Primer. Baltimore, Williams & Wilkins, 1980.
12. Bourgeois MS: Communication treatment for adults with dementia. J Speech Hear Res 1991; 34:831–844.
13. Canter GJ: Observations on neurogenic stuttering: A contribution to differential diagnosis. Br J Disord Commun 1971; 6:139–143.
14. Cummings JL, Benson DF: Dementia: A Clinical Approach, ed 2. Boston, Butterworth-Heinemann, 1992.
15. Dabul B, Bollier B: Therapeutic approaches to apraxia. J Speech Hear Disord 1976; 41:268–276.
16. Darley FL, Aronson AE, Brown JR: Motor Speech Disorders. Philadelphia, WB Saunders, 1975, p 76.
17. Davis GA: A Survey of Adult Aphasia. Englewood Cliffs, NJ, Prentice-Hall, 1983, p 2.
18. Davis GA: A Survey of Adult Aphasia and Related Language Disorders, ed 2. Englewood Cliffs, NJ, Prentice-Hall, 1993.
19. Duffy JR: Differential diagnosis of acquired motor and psychogenic speech disorders. Course presented at the Riverside Rehabilitation Institute, Norfolk, VA, August 1991.
20. Duffy JR: Schuell's stimulation approach to rehabilitation. In Chapey R (ed): Language Intervention Strategies in Adult Aphasia, ed 3. Baltimore, Williams & Wilkins, 1994.
21. Eisenson J: Examining for Aphasia. New York, Psychological Corp, 1954.
22. Folstein MF, Folstein SE, McHugh PR: "Mini-mental state": a practical method for grading the mental state of patients for the clinician. J Psychiatr Res 1975; 12:189–198.
23. Frattali CM, Thompson CK, Holland AL, et al: Functional Assessment of Communication Skills for Adults: ASHA FACS. Rockville, MD, American Speech-Language Hearing Association, 1995.
24. Fromm D, Holland A: Functional communication in Alzheimer's disease. J Speech Hear Disord 1989; 54:535–540.
25. Goodglass H, Kaplan E: The Assessment of Aphasia and Related Disorders. Philadelphia, Lea & Febiger, 1972.
26. Goodglass H, Kaplan E: The Assessment of Aphasia and Related Disorders, ed 2. Philadelphia, Lea & Febiger, 1983.
27. Hagen C: Language disorders in head trauma. In Holland AL (ed): Language Disorders in Adults. San Diego, College-Hill Press, 1984.
28. Halper AS, Cherney LR, Burns MS, et al: The RIC Evaluation in Right Hemisphere Dysfunction—Revised (RICE-R). Gaithersburg, MD, Aspen, 1996.
29. Holland AL: Report from the consensus development conference on rehabilitation of persons with traumatic brain injury. Rockville, MD, ASHA Special Interest Division, 1999, vol 9, no 1, pp 2–4.
30. Holland AL, Frattali CM, Fromm D: Communication activities of daily living-2: CADL-2. Austin, TX, Pro-Ed, 1998.
31. Johnson W, Brown SF, Curtis JF, et al: Speech Handicapped School Children. New York, Harper, 1965.
32. Keenan JS, Brassell EG: Aphasia Language Performance Scales. Murfreesboro, TN, Pinnacle Press, 1975.
33. Keith RL, Darley FL: Laryngectomee Rehabilitation. Houston, College-Hill Press, 1986.
34. Kertesz A: Aphasia and Associated Disorders: Taxonomy, Localization, and Recovery. New York, Grune & Stratton, 1979.
35. Kertesz A: Western Aphasia Battery. New York, Grune & Stratton, 1982.
36. Kirk A, Kertesz A: Assessment of aphasia. In Hansen S, Tucker DM (eds): Neuropsychological Assessment. Physical Medicine and Rehabilitation: State of the Art Reviews. Philadelphia, Hanley & Belfus, 1992.
37. Knauf VH: Communication training. In Katz J (ed): Handbook of Clinical Audiology. Baltimore, Williams & Wilkins, 1978.
38. Lomas J, Pickard L, Bester SR, et al: The Communication Effectiveness Index: Development and psychometric evaluation of a functional communication measure for adult aphasia. J Speech Hear Disord 1989; 54:113.
39. Lux J: Towards a common language for functioning and disablement: ICIDH-2 (The International Classification of Impairments, Activities, and Participation). Rockville, MD, ASHA Special Interest Division, 1999, vol 9, no 1, pp 8–10.
40. Mace NL, Rabins PV: The Thirty-Six Hour Day, ed 2. Baltimore, Johns Hopkins University Press, 1991.
41. Mahr G, Leith W: Psychologenic stuttering of adult onset. J Speech Hear Res 1992; 35:283–286.
42. Martin AD: Some objections to the term "apraxia of speech." J Speech Hear Disord 1974; 39:53.
43. Metter J: An open letter to ASHA. ASHA 1985; 27:43.
44. Myers PS: Profiles of communication deficits in patients with right cerebral hemisphere damage. In Brookshire R (ed): Clinical Aphasiology: Conference Proceedings. Minneapolis, BRK, 1979.
45. Myers PS: Right hemisphere communication impairment. In Chapey R (ed): Language Intervention Strategies in Adult Aphasia. Baltimore, Williams & Wilkins, 1986.
46. Myers PS: Right hemisphere syndrome. In LaPointe LL (ed): Aphasia and Related Neurogenic Language Disorders, ed 2. New York, Thieme, 1997.
47. Myers PS, Mackisack EL: Right hemisphere syndrome. In LaPointe LL (ed): Aphasia and Related Neurogenic Language Disorders. New York, Thieme, 1990.
48. Moore GP: Organic Voice Disorders. Englewood Cliffs, NJ, Prentice-Hall, 1971.
49. Netsell R, Daniel B: Dysarthria in adults: Physiologic approach to rehabilitation. Arch Phys Med Rehabil 1979; 60:502–508.
50. Nicholas ML, Helm-Estabrooks N, Ward-Lonergan J, et al: Evolution of severe aphasia in the first two years post onset. Arch Phys Med Rehabil 1993; 74:830–836.
51. National Institute of Neurological Disease and Stroke: National Institutes of Health, US Department of Health, Education, and Welfare: Human Communication and Its Disorders: An Overview. Bethesda, MD, National Institute of Neurological Disease and Stroke Monograph, no 10, 1969.
52. Perkins WH, Kent RD: Functional Anatomy of Speech, Language, and Hearing: A Primer. San Diego, College Hill Press, 1986.
53. Porcelli J: Aphasia assessment and treatment. In Goldberg G (ed): Stroke Rehabilitation. Phys Med Rehabil Clin North Am 1991; 2:487–500.
54. Porch BE: Porch Index of Communicative Abilities, ed 3. Palo Alto, CA, Consulting Psychologists Press, 1981.
55. Rao P: Adult neurogenic communication disorders. In Crowe T (ed): Applications of Counseling in Speech-Language Pathology and Audiology. Baltimore, Williams & Wilkins, 1997.
56. Rao P: The aphasia syndromes: localization and classification. In Topics in Stroke Rehabilitation. Rockville, MD, Aspen, 1994.
57. Rao P: Communication disorders. In Ozer M, Materson RS, Caplan LR (eds): Management of Persons with Stroke. St Louis, Mosby–Year Book, 1994.
58. Rao P: Drawing and gesture as communication options in a person with severe aphasia. In Topics in Stroke Rehabilitation, vol 2. Rockville, MD, Aspen, 1995, pp 49–56.
59. Rao P: Functional communication assessment and outcomes. In Shadden B, Toner MA (ed): Aging and Communication. Austin, TX, Pro-Ed, 1997.
60. Rao P: Neurogenic stuttering as a manifestation of stroke and a mask of dysnomia. Clin Commun Disord 1991; 1:31–37.
61. Rao P: Testimony presented to the Agency for Health Care Policy and Research. In Topics in Stroke Rehabilitation, vol 2. Rockville, MD, Aspen, 1995, pp 80–81.
62. Rao P: Use of Amer-Ind Code by persons with aphasia. In Chapey R (ed): Language Intervention Strategies in Adult Aphasia, ed 3. Baltimore, Williams & Wilkins, 1994.
63. Rao P, Mackisack EL, Perr A, et al: An interdisciplinary approach to right CVA rehabilitation. Presented at the American Congress of Rehabilitation Medicine, Orlando, FL, October 12, 1987.

64. Robey R: A meta-analysis of clinical outcomes in the treatment of aphasia. J Speech Hear Res 1998; 41:172–187.
65. Rosenbek J: Treatment of apraxia of speech in adults. In Perkins WH (ed): Dysarthria and Apraxia. New York, Thieme, 1983.
66. Rosenbek J, Messert B, Collins M, et al: Stuttering following brain damage. Brain Language 1978; 6:82–96.
67. Rosenbek JC, LaPointe LL: The dysarthrias: Description, diagnosis, and treatment. In Johns DF (ed): Clinical Management of Neurogenic Communication Disorders. Boston, Little, Brown, 1985.
68. Roth CR, Aronson AE, Davis LJ: Clinical studies in psychogenic stuttering of adult onset. J Speech Hear Disord 1989; 54:634–646.
69. Schuell H: The Minnesota Test for Differential Diagnosis of Aphasia. Minneapolis, University of Minnesota Press, 1965.
70. Shekim L: Dementia. In LaPointe LL (ed): Aphasia and Related Neurogenic Language Disorders, ed 2. New York, Thieme, 1997.
71. Sparks RW, Deck JW: Melodic intonation therapy. In Chapey R (ed): Language Intervention Strategies in Adult Aphasia, ed 3. Baltimore, Williams & Wilkins, 1984.
72. Stemple J: Clinical Voice Pathology: Theory and Management. Columbus, OH, Charles E Merrill, 1984.
73. Stemple J: Voice disorders in adults. In Leahy MM (ed): Disorders of Communication: The Science of Intervention. New York, Taylor & Francis, 1989.
74. Tonkovich J: Communication disorders in the elderly. In Shadden B (ed): Communication Behavior and Aging: A Sourcebook. Baltimore, Williams & Wilkins, 1988.
75. Wepman J, Jones L: The Language Modalities Test for Aphasia. Chicago, University of Chicago Education Industry Service, 1961.
76. Wertz RT: Neuropathologies of speech and language: An introduction to patient management. In Johns DF (ed): Clinical Management of Neurogenic Communication Disorders. Boston, Little, Brown, 1985.
77. Wertz RT, LaPointe LL, Rosenbek JC: Apraxia of Speech in Adults. New York, Grune & Stratton, 1984.
78. Yantis P: Puretone air conduction threshold testing. In Katz R (ed): Handbook of Clinical Audiology, ed 4. Baltimore, Williams & Wilkins, 1994.
79. Ylvisaker M, Szekeres SF: Communication disorders associated with closed head injury. In Chapey R (ed): Language Intervention Strategies in Adult Aphasia, ed 3. Baltimore, Williams & Wilkins, 1994.
80. Yorkston KM, Beukelman DR: Assessment of Intelligibility of Dysarthric Speech. Austin, TX, Pro-Ed, 1981.
81. Yorkston KM, Beukelman DR: Speech and language disorders. In Kottke F, Stillwell G, Lehmann J (eds): Krusen's Handbook of Physical Medicine and Rehabilitation, ed 4. Philadelphia, WB Saunders, 1990.

4
CHAPTER

Lance E. Trexler, Ph.D., and David J. Fordyce, Ph.D.

Psychological Perspectives on Rehabilitation: Contemporary Assessment and Intervention Strategies

CONCEPTUALIZING PSYCHOLOGICAL ASPECTS OF REHABILITATION

Psychological variables significantly influence the rehabilitation process and outcome. Psychological variables often moderate the expression of a medical disability or determine the extent to which the disability has an impact on functional adaptation. Moreover, in the case of acquired brain damage, psychological disorders are often primary impairments toward which rehabilitation efforts are directed (e.g., disorders of mnestic functions or states of unawareness). For these reasons, rehabilitation psychologists and neuropsychologists often play a significant role in assessing and treating psychological and cognitive factors that not only affect outcome, but also determine the goals of rehabilitation. Psychologists in rehabilitation have become increasingly subspecialized since the mid-1970s. Subspecialities in rehabilitation include rehabilitation from chronic pain, inpatient medical rehabilitation, vocational and industrial rehabilitation, and brain injury rehabilitation. The theoretical and empirical literature in these areas has increased since the 1970s as well.

Overview of Psychological Approaches to Rehabilitation

Current formulations of human learning and emotional functioning provide a foundation for understanding the wide spectrum of recovery outcomes seen after injury, illness, or the onset of permanent impairment. This foundation also serves as a starting point for maximizing adjustment and rehabilitation effectiveness. The ultimate level of disability is influenced by a number of factors, including the individual's premorbid intellectual skills or endowments; premorbid personality (including coping, social, and emotional skills); and familial, social, and economic contingencies. It is clear that for virtually all medical conditions (diseases, injuries, or impairments), a one-to-one correspondence does not exist between the simple presence or magnitude of such a condition and associated functional disability. Similarly, the disease model of traditional medicine, consistent with Cartesian mind-body dualism, does not serve the rehabilitation enterprise well.[62] For example, different individuals report widely varying experiences of back pain or discomfort (or the lack thereof) despite having quite similar "objective" indices of tissue damage or pathological conditions. In this context, psychological assessment and intervention are not based on an illness model, and they are also not synonymous with, or a substitute for, psychiatric intervention. Rather, psychological services are best viewed as an integral component of medical rehabilitation. This is particularly true since psychological resources need to be incorporated into a rehabilitation intervention. Additionally, psychological factors often need to be treated so that the overall benefit of rehabilitation is not compromised.

Classification and Terminology in Rehabilitation: Implications for Psychological Assessment and Rehabilitation

The National Center for Medical Rehabilitation and Research (NCMRR)[124] has provided a new classification for terminology in rehabilitation that expands that provided by the World Health Organization.[193] The NCMRR model provides a much more usable model for conceptualizing psychological assessment and intervention in rehabilitation (Table 4–1).

Missing from the NCMRR model is a variety of preexisting individual variables, such as coping skills or level of intellectual functioning. These types of preexisting characteristics can have a significant impact on the reaction and adaptation to impairments, which often creates the form of, and the definition of, the disability. Moreover, these types of individual factors can have a significant influence on how pathophysiological limitations affect adaptation. Certainly psychological assessment seeks to provide insights into the individual characteristics of the patient. For example, the extent to which patients believe or perceive that they have some control over their behavior and that what happens to them is not merely the consequence of luck or fate (referred to as "locus of control" in the psychological literature) has been demonstrated to influence the length of hospitalization and/or outcome in many different medical conditions. This has been demonstrated in coronary bypass patients,[104] in the rate of recovery from stroke-induced hemiplegia,[126] and in significantly better levels of adaptation following traumatic head injury, even when severity of injury was controlled for.[101, 121, 122]

Psychological assessment and intervention can target different levels in the NCMRR model. Neuropsychological assessment has its historical antecedents in making inferences about the pathophysiology of brain lesions, with special reference to the following: (1) the presence or absence of brain damage, (2) the location of damage, if present, and (3) the type of brain injury (e.g., trauma, dementia, stroke).[38] A variety of psychological tests have been designed to assess emotional "impairments" and functional limitations that have directly resulted from pathophysiological sources or are a reaction to the resulting neurological impairments. Historically, psychological assessments have not emphasized the description of functional limitations or disability. Advances in brain injury rehabilitation have promulgated the development of tests designed to measure such outcomes as psychosocial adaptation[100] and community integration.[189] These instruments were developed to directly measure disability associated with acquired brain damage, because (1) the reasons for disability were unique to the type of pathophysiology (brain damage) and (2) the ability of neuropsychological tests to predict functional adaptation on a case-by-case basis is unclear.[2]

The impairments that result from a lesion and the attendant functional limitations and disabilities all interact dynamically in a manner that either facilitates or compromises adaptation. The quality of the interaction is largely determined by psychological and environmental variables. The model provided by the NCMRR provides a useful framework for determining the level at which, on a case-by-case basis, psychological assessment and interventions can be targeted.

TABLE 4–1 Terminology in Disability Classification: The National Center for Medical Rehabilitation and Research Model (1993)

Pathophysiology	Interruption or interference with normal physiological and developmental processes or structures
Impairment	Loss or abnormality of cognitive, emotional, physiological, or anatomical structure or function
Functional limitation	Restriction or lack of ability to perform an action in the manner or within the range consistent with the purpose of the organ or organ system
Disability	Inability or limitation in performing tasks, activities, and roles to levels expected within physical and social contexts
Societal limitation	Restriction, attributable to social policy or barriers (structural or attitudinal), which limits fulfillment of roles or denies access to services and opportunities that are associated with full participation in society

PSYCHOLOGICAL ASSESSMENT

The psychological evaluation provides for the following: (1) the study of individual differences, such as personality and intellectual and cognitive factors, that moderate the expression of physiological function; (2) some determination of how individual differences might influence rehabilitation processes; and (3) an evaluation of the presence and magnitude of certain "psychological impairments," such as depression, disinhibition, or short-term memory loss. Psychological assessment also strives to identify the factors that contribute to the propensity to report symptoms, and the factors that influence participation in rehabilitation and ultimate outcome levels in impairment and disability.

Purposes of Psychological Assessment

Psychological assessment is not just the administration of psychological tests and the reporting of psychometric test scores. Psychological assessment is a clinical endeavor directed toward theory-driven testing of hypotheses about human behavior. Psychological tests are generally constructed to provide objective, reliable, and valid observations about human behavior. However, the results of psychological tests must, by necessity, be integrated with clinical and subjective data, from which clinical interpretation can be provided. Psychological theories and constructs provide a framework that suggests which tests are administered. Some of the theories and constructs are discussed in the following section.

The Nature and Extent of Higher Cortical Impairment

Because individuals with brain dysfunction, either congenital or acquired, present with an altered capacity

TABLE 4–2 Determinants of Heterogeneity in Behavioral Effects of Brain Lesions

Premorbid factors	Intellect, psychosocial adjustment, coping skills
Age at onset	Children often "grow into" deficits; young adults recover better than older adults
Type of lesion	Diffuse lesions typically affect attention, memory, and metacognitive functions; focal lesions result in more specific syndromes; rapid-onset lesions result in more behavioral impairment than slow-onset lesions
Location of lesion	Cortical vs. subcortical, left vs. right hemisphere, anterior vs. posterior are relevant dimensions
Chronicity of lesion	Acute focal lesions present more immediate diffuse picture and resolve to more specific syndrome; diffuse lesions resolve in a more linear (severity) dimension

and style of learning, a distinctly unique approach to rehabilitation is required. Certain approaches to rehabilitation and certain environmental conditions can impede or enhance learning in persons with brain damage. Some patients are able to learn through certain sensory modalities but not others. Patients with brain damage also often have difficulty generalizing what they learn in one situation and applying it to the next. Therefore, despite learning a skill in a rehabilitation environment, the brain-damaged patient can mistakenly appear "unmotivated" simply because he or she is not able to generalize the strategy used. For example, a brain-injured patient might not complete a wheelchair transfer at home because the cues available in the clinic are not available in the home, or because the patient has a different type of wheelchair at home. Rehabilitation of the person with brain injury is also unique because reorganization or compensation for neuropsychological impairments is often the goal of the rehabilitation. As well, persons with brain damage often present with alterations in behavior and unique neurobehavioral syndromes that require medical and neuropsychological management. For these reasons, assessment of higher cortical functions has become an integral component of the medical rehabilitation of persons with brain damage.

Persons with brain damage are enormously heterogeneous in respect to the type of neuropsychological impairment. The reasons for this heterogeneity are summarized in Table 4–2.[84, 99, 167] Determining the location and evolution of the lesion, in both the acute and the chronic stages of brain injury, through neuroimaging and neuropsychological studies can be of assistance in choosing appropriate rehabilitation strategies.[14, 177, 191] For example, the size and location of a lesion on neuroimaging have been shown to predict recovery from aphasia.[123] Patients with left hemisphere occipital asymmetry (advantage), as demonstrated on computed tomography (CT), have better recoveries from aphasia.[23]

Langfitt and co-workers[90] suggested that the variety of neuroimaging strategies now available provides for the analysis of "morphology (metabolism and biochemistry), neural conduction and transmission (neurological and behavioral function)." This perspective provides for the study of recovery in persons with brain injury on a case-by-case basis and can be of some value in guiding both rehabilitative and pharmacological interventions.

It should also be noted, however, that contemporary research suggests that the best predictors of benefit from post-acute brain injury neuropsychological rehabilitation are measures of insight, awareness, and acceptance.[10, 134] This finding suggests that both pathophysiological factors (location, size, and type of lesion), as measured with neuroimaging techniques, and neuropsychological studies describe rehabilitation-relevant individual factors. The individual factors determine not only the prognosis for recovery, but also the type of brain injury rehabilitation strategies that should be employed.[169–171] Neuropsychological assessment is no longer solely a diagnostic endeavor but can be used to establish a framework for interventional[72] or ecological[173] neuropsychology.

It is important to note that any brain lesion can influence the patient's ability to learn from rehabilitation. The neuropsychological examination should provide information not only about what impairments might exist, but also as to how the rehabilitation staff should address or compensate for the impairments. Table 4–3 provides a gross classification of the types of disturbances of

TABLE 4–3 Disturbances of Higher Cortical Functions

Functions	Disturbances/Impairments
Motor and sensory	Hemiparesis Dyscoordination Dyspraxias Visual field defects Tactile, auditory, and visual sensitivity
Arousal and attention	Cognitive fatigue and poor endurance/sustained attention Distractability Modality-specific and global attention
Memory	Modality-specific (i.e., auditory, visual) memory Short-term working memory Prospective memory Autobiographical memory Episodic-semantic memory Procedural-declarative memory
Language and language-related	Dysphasias Dysgraphias Dyslexias Dyscalculias
Perceptual, visuospatial, and visuoconstructive	Agnosias Visual and auditory analysis and discrimination Hemispatial inattention and neglect Visuoconstructive disorders Dysprosodias
Executive and metacognitive	Problem-solving and abstraction Goal-directed behaviors Self-regulation Organization Monitoring

higher cortical functions that are evaluated in the neuropsychological assessment.

Brain injury can also result in organic changes in emotional behavior secondary to subtle alterations in the stability of temporolimbic functions.[154] Social interaction and integration are also often impaired secondary to neurobehavioral disorders (Table 4–4), that result from brain lesions.[16, 17, 99, 117, 154, 159] Patients are all different, and it is rare that a "pure" neurobehavioral syndrome is seen. Despite this, it is crucial in patient management that organic neurobehavioral changes following brain injury from posttraumatic emotional reactions be recognized and differentiated.

The cognitive, neurobehavioral, and emotional reactions to brain injury can, if not properly managed, interact and lead to a spiral of deterioration (Fig. 4–1). Goldstein[67] and Prigatano and co-workers[133] described a catastrophic reaction, usually precipitated by unexpected or unanticipated failure on tasks that had been easily accomplished before brain injury. Obviously, the patient's awareness of the failure or difficulty in performing the task is a requisite for the catastrophic reaction. The catastrophic reaction is characterized by angry outbursts, agitation, anxiety, and depression. Patients who are experiencing a catastrophic reaction often deteriorate in their approach to tasks and are unable to tolerate variability or a lack of rigid structure in the environment. Left undiagnosed and unmanaged, the overall adaptation of these patients typically deteriorates.

The spiral of deterioration often serves to sustain functional impairment of cognitive functions secondary to depression or anxiety following concussion or mild brain injury, despite the fact that neurologically based cognitive impairments might have resolved. The perpetuation of functional impairment following concussion or mild traumatic brain injury is therefore often mistakenly diagnosed as malingering.

Research has demonstrated that cognitive and neurobehavioral impairments following brain injury, and not physical impairments, create disabilities affecting long-term adjustment and social integration.[20, 21, 80, 164] The assessment, differential diagnosis, pharmacological management (the reader is referred to Gualtieri[73] for an excellent review), rehabilitation, and long-term case management of these disorders are essential.

TABLE 4–4 Partial Taxonomy of Neurobehavioral Disorders and Syndromes

Disorders of Awareness

Anosognosia: Unawareness or denial of illness or consequences of brain lesion

Anosodiaphoria: Lack of emotional reaction to a deficit caused by a brain lesion

Frontal Syndromes

Dorsolateral convexity: Indifference, cognitive slowness, inertia, "pseudo-depression"

Orbitofrontal: Euphoria, hyperkinesia, disinhibition, "pseudo-psychopathic" behavior

Temporolimbic Syndrome

Intensification of affect/ethical/religious feelings, spontaneous episodes of rage, hypergraphia, hypersexuality, and hyposexuality

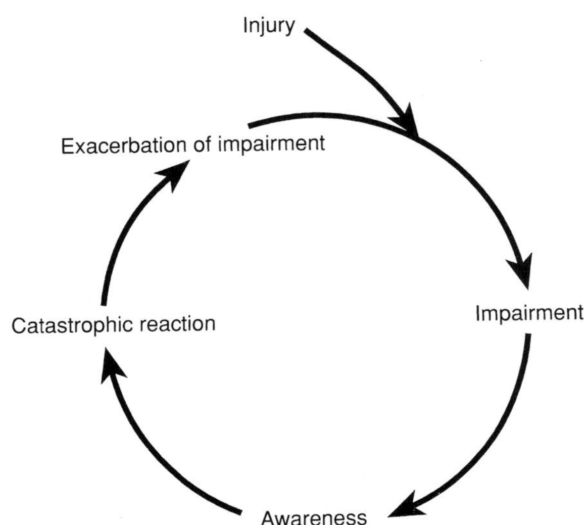

FIGURE 4–1. Spiral of deterioration.

Emotional Adjustment and Permanent Impairment

Developmental Stages

Emotional responses to acutely disabling conditions, such as spinal cord injury or stroke, or to the onset of a potentially disfiguring or fatal disease, such as cancer, have traditionally been thought to follow a natural course of evolution. The models essentially posit an initial state of significant distress or depression that, over time and as a result of some active process of "working through," resolves to a condition of acceptance and relative emotional harmony. It is now clear that such models reflect entrenched biases that are not well supported by empirical findings. Neither patients, nor victims of loss,[194] nor relatives[136] demonstrate consistent sequential trends in emotional adjustment. As reflected in group means, some general tendency for early distress to dissipate with time might exist,[52, 130, 148] although recent longitudinal data suggest some slight worsening of average ratings of life satisfaction over 20 years of adjustment to spinal cord injury.[87] Variability in emotional outcomes predominates, and there are some clinical conditions (e.g., amputation) that can produce fairly immediate psychological relief.[149] Most individuals never manifest a clinically significant depression, whereas in others such a state can develop and never resolve.[194]

Depression and Disability

Methodological problems or variations in experimental methods contribute to differing estimates of clinical depression in disabling conditions. Evaluating the presence of psychological distress in medical or disabled populations is not easy. Disturbances in sleep, appetite, arousal, motivation, communication, and affective modulation are common direct consequences of illness and medication. This can lead to either the overdiagnosis or the underdiagnosis of depression in medical populations.[150] Problems in evaluating the presence of depression are especially apparent in brain injury, in which alterations in language, arousal, attention, or emotional expressiveness can cloud the diagnostic picture.[146] Despite the complexities of diagnosing depression in medical populations, it is of serious concern. For example, the third leading cause of death among spinal cord-injured patients is suicide.[85]

In general, it appears that major psychological reactions occur in a minority of acutely impaired individuals. For example, in cross-sectional research, fewer than 30% of those who survive spinal cord injury evidence major emotional distress either in the acute stages of recovery[22, 41] or over longer periods of adaptation.[76] Rates of depression similar to those noted for spinal cord-injured patients have been reported for patients with rheumatoid arthritis,[63] multiple sclerosis,[45] type 1 diabetes mellitus,[157] burns,[130] and stroke.[69] Interestingly, these rates of depression are fairly typical of rates found in a variety of general outpatient and inpatient medical settings.[125, 142, 150] They exceed base rates for major depressive symptoms in the general population,[143] which confirms that illness and impairment are not emotionally benign events; the finding can also be demonstrated in surveys of individuals with disabilities who live in the community.[114, 175] Most individuals living with chronically disabling conditions, however, do not typically warrant a formal psychiatric diagnosis. Signs of distress during rehabilitation or in later adjustment might well reflect normal human emotional experience.[74, 130]

Human Resilience and Coping

Humans typically are fairly resilient in the face of difficult losses or the acquisition of permanent impairments, but significant depression is thought to be an understandable and natural response to loss. The fact that health care professionals frequently overestimate the degree of psychological distress in their patients might reflect this expectation.[39] More recent conceptualizations of normal human emotional functioning[28, 91] provide a framework for understanding responses to illness or impairment. Cassel's[28] formulation of emotional "suffering" is a useful example. It suggests that significant emotional distress is a common response to medical conditions that are perceived as threatening the future viability of the person. Such distress might last until the perceived threat has diminished. Within this context, it is not surprising that a variety of negative emotional states might occur during the course of adjusting to a chronic impairment. Their presence does not necessarily signify the presence of a pathological emotional process.

An examination of models of human emotional experience also helps to explain the frequent absence of clinically significant depression after injury or loss. For example, Lazarus and Folkman note that a particular emotional response arises out of a unique personal appraisal process.[91, 93] This process represents the product of assessments of personal meaningfulness, the level of possible control, the expectations for future change, and the potential to influence adjustment through coping. A particular emotional response flows from the appraisal of the event, not from the event itself. Appraisals are dependent on the personality, the experiences, the native endowment, the integrity of higher cortical functions, and the sociocultural context of the individual. Lazarus[92] has suggested that coping appraisals attempt to modulate emotional distress and that they can be roughly divided into problem-focused and emotion-focused domains (Table 4–5). Problem-focused coping typically refers to direct attempts to modify the stressor, avoid it, or develop some sense of control over its impact. Emotion-focused coping represents more avoidant-cognitive actions, such as denial or wishful thinking.

Recent research has attempted to understand the variability in emotional adjustment to impairment or loss through an analysis of individual differences in coping processes. While a thorough understanding of the relationships between personality, coping skills, and emotional adjustment remains elusive, the following points appear to be generally supported by the findings to date: (1) Various studies have defined very specific types of coping skills or strategies. Although these can eventually prove to have clinical utility in understanding emotional responses to impairment, this body of research remains to be fully developed. The general dichotomy between problem-focused and emotion-focused coping has been sufficiently validated to be of some help.[4] (2) Some evidence exists that the degree to which a particular illness or impairment interferes with daily function is positively related to resultant emotional distress.[45, 56] (3) Although it has been hypothesized that emotion-focused coping skills might be more likely to be employed in situations in which actual control of illness or impairment is impossible or limited,[91] the highly dynamic nature of coping processes has made it difficult to validate such a relationship. (4) Although there is some correlation between the types of coping skills an individual employs during two different periods,[76] it is clear that these processes are highly dynamic. The nature of appraisal, coping, and adjustment reflects the particular interaction of person, illness, and circumstance at a given point.[4, 76, 86] (5) Evidence exists that some avoidant emotion-focused coping strategies

TABLE 4–5 Some Examples of Coping Skills or Coping-Relevant Personality Traits

Problem-Focused	*Mixed*
Information seeking	Cognitive restructuring
Seeking social support	Selective ignoring
	Blame self
	Blame others
	Traits
Emotion-Focused	Locus of control
Avoidance	Learned resourcefulness
Denial	Monitoring
Threat minimization	Blunting

might be negatively correlated with emotional well-being.[139, 175] However, some avoidant strategies, such as denial, might be adaptive.

Denial

Those working in medical settings are familiar with the tendency for some disabled individuals and relatives to deny the existence (or ramifications) of acquired impairments. Denial is a highly dynamic, multifaceted coping process[26] that can be manifested through direct verbal report or inferred from behavior or from the absence of overt expressions of emotional distress. In the case of certain types of brain injury (e.g., nondominant stroke or traumatic head injury), apparent denial is likely to be reflective of impairments in information processing, emotional arousal, or emotional expression.[60, 109, 146, 187] Denial and related phenomena are clearly evident in a variety of other nonneurological situations of loss. In addition, in brain injury patients it is often very difficult to locate the boundary between psychological denial and neurological anosognosia.[60, 182]

Optimal mental health has historically been thought to depend on a generally realistic appraisal of self and the world. Denial was considered maladaptive and a target for psychotherapeutic intervention (see Taylor and Brown[162] for a discussion). Depression was similarly thought to be a natural response to loss, and its absence a matter of psychological concern. As previously noted, however, significant depression is not the modal response to impairment. In fact, it appears that emotion-focused coping is frequently employed after loss.[161, 194] Denial, in all of its forms, appears to be related phenomenologically to the generally positive illusory perceptual biases often found in cognitive psychological research of normal, nondepressed individuals. For example, we have a tendency to view ourselves more positively than others do, to accept more credit for positive personal outcomes (compared with more negative ones), to predict control over chance events, and to harbor a generally optimistic outlook about the future.[162] In contrast, mildly depressed individuals are more balanced in self-perceptions and evince more accurate predictions of control and future outcomes. More severe depression often yields quite negative appraisal tendencies.[9] If mental health is defined normatively, then the tendency to engage in positive illusory thinking might be reflective of optimal psychological function.[162]

Many avoidant strategies that disabled individuals employ for coping might be adaptive. As emotional distress in reaction to loss is not always resolved,[194] strong confrontations of denial might be counterproductive.[60] Seemingly unrealistic expressions of hope can actually reinforce progress through rehabilitation. If denial is determined to increase the probability of safety risk or psychosocial failure, then it should be sensitively confronted. At various times in adjusting to loss or chronic disability, however, avoidant emotion-focused coping strategies might well be quite adaptive and promote psychological well-being.

Psychological Forces That Have an Impact on Impairment and Disability

We often believe that we are aware of our actual internal physiological state, but the correlations between physiological activity and reported physical sensations are small. Physical and emotional symptom reporting is subject to a number of psychological processes. Major findings from recent research in the field of cognitive psychology (see Cioffi[33] or Pennebaker[131] for reviews) can be summarized as follows: (1) Whereas the encoding of information (stimuli) from both the internal and external environments occurs continuously, awareness of such stimulation is highly selective. (2) Attention and awareness are dependent on the relative strengths and numbers of competing stimuli. Awareness is also driven by perceptual biases, expectancies, and beliefs. (3) The subsequent interpretation and labeling of a physiological stimulus is an outcome of a complex psychological process. This process is dependent on prior experience, current circumstances, and associated cues, goals, and perceived or anticipated consequences. (4) The report of physical symptoms, or the manifestation of behaviors or actions reflective of an illness state, is a human behavior like all others. It is, as a result, subject to the laws of learning and, perhaps most important, to the effects of environmental consequences.[62]

Following a medical event, such psychological forces begin to play an increasingly important role in overall level of disability. They can parallel the effects of physiological healing and rehabilitation, and therefore promote a reduction in overall disability. Such forces can also impede recovery and contribute to more severe and prolonged disability. The more negative outcomes can be particularly prevalent in situations of less severe initial injury or in situations in which physiological healing is nearly always complete. Prototypical conditions are back injury and concussion, which result in chronic disability in a minority of individuals.[15, 62]

Sensations related to such secondary effects as depression, anxiety, and physical disuse can, over the course of time, become associated with sensations related to injury or impairment. After healing or recovery has progressed, the conditioned associations can lead to attributions of continued impairment that reinforce prolonged disability. Symptoms or sensations reflective of normal human function can, following injury, subsequently be attributed to the injury.[112] Base rates for sensations that comprise part of either the chronic pain or postconcussion syndromes (e.g., back pain, headache, inattention, word-finding problems, forgetfulness) are surprisingly frequent in the general population, particularly among non-neurologically impaired disability groups.[70, 94, 95, 131] Secondary conditions such as emotional distress, fatigue, and physiological changes associated with prolonged convalescence and disuse can generate internal sensations that become confused with the continuing effects of injury or tissue damage.[62, 176] Coincident and independent sources of distress from family or vocational settings can also become incorporated into the experience of suffering that accompanies the impairment. Note that these attributional phenomena often occur relatively unconsciously and automatically.

Social Factors and Rehabilitation

Alterations in social functioning following the onset of impairment can play a major role in concurrent and future adjustment. Social reinforcers can also exert a powerful influence on all aspects of recovery from injury. Illness and impairments are manifest in behaviors that are subject to influence by social consequences. Some symptoms such as pain are knowable only through behavioral expressions.[62] Although social support can ameliorate depression, perhaps by buffering the stresses associated with disability,[35] inappropriate social attention can accentuate suffering or enhance disability, pain, or dependency behaviors.[61, 174] Several studies of chronic pain patients have shown a positive relationship between a solicitous spouse responding to pain behavior and patient reports of pain and ratings of disability.[59, 144, 174] Entitlement systems such as worker's compensation insurance and Social Security disability insurance, and the compensatory forces associated with third-party lawsuits, can also influence symptom reporting and general levels of disability.[36, 71, 94, 110, 183,184] Intervention with patients and families must sort out and selectively guide attributions and interactions that serve to maintain disability.

The origins of social isolation associated with disability are multifactorial and complex. Isolation can naturally follow loss of mobility skills or of capacities for independent transportation. Brain injuries can alter communication skills through formal language impairments or through more subtle impairments of pragmatic communication. Nondisabled individuals experience a number of more negative psychosocial biases during their interactions with the disabled. These include heightened anxiety and devaluing beliefs that might well tend to decrease the likelihood of future contact.[47, 58] In disabled individuals, depression can also contribute to social isolation as well as be a consequence of reduced social contact. Depression and the quality and quantity of social relationships or interactions tend to covary in a negative fashion in nonmedical populations (see Barnett and Gotlib[5] for a review). Disability is often associated with a reduction in social contacts. Reduced socialization has been shown to correlate with an increased incidence of mortality in patients with spinal cord injuries[88, 89] and with depression in several disability groups.[52, 126, 140] Elliot, Frank, and others have shown that disabled individuals are viewed less favorably if they are depressed.[50, 51, 54]

The burden on families of the patient's altered social behavior can be substantial. This can be particularly true for the spouses or caregivers of brain-injured individuals,[20, 145, 156] for whom changes in the affected individuals' emotional and social behavior can have devastating consequences.

Types of Psychological Assessment

Psychological assessment is the integration of personal and medical history and behavioral observations with objectively derived test scores.[108] Psychological testing is therefore one component of a diagnostic process. The interpretation of objectively derived psychological test scores should, at a minimum, consider the following: (1) premorbid individual differences that might influence the patient's performance, (2) the circumstances in which the patient took the test and the medical condition, (3) the psychometric properties of the test (e.g., error of measurement, reliability, distribution of normative data), and (4) available research on ecological validity or predictive validity of the test. In this context, psychological tests are tools (albeit objective tools) that assist the psychologist with differential diagnosis and treatment planning.

The Clinical Interview and Behavioral Observations

Rehabilitation is intended to be a humanistically oriented enterprise. Meltzer,[116] a psychologist who suffered hypoxic encephalopathy, provided a particularly insightful series of recommendations to both patients and rehabilitation providers. After extensive inpatient and outpatient therapies, Meltzer concluded that no matter what particular intervention he received, it was the quality of the relationship between him and the therapist that determined the extent to which he benefited from therapy. The initial examiner, irrespective of his or her rehabilitation discipline, should consider these insights and their relevance for assessment in rehabilitation. Toward these ends, Strub and Black[158] have provided a very useful format for the mental status examination, which is a significant component of the initial clinical interview. Table 4–6 provides an overall format for the

TABLE 4–6 Major Components of the Initial Examination

History

1. Description of present illness: Nature of onset, duration of illness, behavioral changes
2. Other relevant organic behavioral symptoms: Social judgment, attention and concentration, memory, orientation, language, reading, writing, and calculations
3. Previous neurological, psychiatric, and psychological symptoms: Previous neurological disease or psychiatric illnesses, seizures, head injuries, or concussion, drug and alcohol use and misuse, toxic exposures, paranoia, hallucinations, delusions, depression or anxiety disorders, previous treatment, coping strategies
4. Birth and developmental history: Birth trauma, developmental delays in motor, language, intellectual, academic, and emotional/social domains
5. Educational and vocational history: Highest grade, level of performance, achievement scores, types of jobs, stability of jobs
6. Family history: Neurological or psychiatric illness, family predilection for disease process that might involve central nervous system (e.g., hypertension), family support, family coping strategies, family stability, family awareness, and goals

Behavioral Observations, Mood, and Neurobehavioral Status

1. General appearance: Age, height, weight, appearance for chronological age, posture, facial expression, eye contact
2. Personal cleanliness: Skin, hair, teeth
3. Habits of dress: Type of clothing, cleanliness and order of clothing, indications of neglect
4. Motor activity: Level of activity: placid-tense, hypokinetic-hyperkinetic, posturing
5. Mood: Appropriate to situation, sadness-euphoria, apathy-concern, stable or fluctuating
6. Emotional status: Anxiety, depression, agitation, anger, reality testing (delusions, hallucinations)
7. Neurobehavioral status: Orientation; awareness; motor, verbal, or affective impulsivity; other organic signs

initial examination, much of which comes from Strub and Black.[158] The initial interview provides an understanding of the individual patient as well as the framework or context in which a disability might exist. As previously discussed, the individual factors greatly influence the manifestation of the underlying impairment.

Based on the initial interview and review of the medical records, the psychologist determines which tests are clinically appropriate to administer, depending on the nature of the referral question and the needs of the individual. Following are general test categories that can be utilized in the rehabilitation setting.

Measures of Cognitive, Emotional, and Personality Functioning

Locus of Control Scales

As previously discussed, the extent to which the patient believes that he or she has some control over the impact of illness or disease can significantly influence outcome. Locus of control is easily measured with a brief questionnaire. The original scale was developed by Rotter,[147] but the version most applicable to rehabilitation is the Multidimensional Health Locus of Control Scale.[180] This Likert-type rating scale has three six-item subscales—Internal Health Locus of Control, Chance Health Locus of Control, and Powerful Others Externality. This scale has been well researched with respect to reliability and validity, and adequate normative data exist.

Sickness Impact Profile

The Sickness Impact Profile (SIP) is another behaviorally oriented measure of health status and is frequently used not only to measure the patient's perception of the effects of a given illness on everyday behavior, but also to measure the effectiveness of a specific health care program. The SIP consists of 136 items that load into three overall dimensions comprising 12 categories of behavior. The types of everyday activities measured by the SIP are summarized in Table 4–7.[12] The SIP has been modified to make it more specific to head injury-related issues, but the results did not support a significant advantage of the modified SIP over the standard SIP.[163] The SIP has also been used in a variety of illnesses, including myocardial infarction and cardiac arrest, chronic obstructive pulmonary disease, low back pain, cancer, and end-stage renal disease.[11, 46, 77, 111, 128, 160] Its reliability and validity have also been well documented.[13, 132]

TABLE 4–7 Behaviors Measured by the Sickness Impact Profile

Dimension	Category of Behavior
Independent categories	Sleep and rest
	Eating
	Work
	Home management
	Recreation and pastimes
Physical	Ambulation
	Mobility
	Body care and movement
Psychosocial	Social interaction
	Alertness behavior
	Emotional behavior
	Communication

Depression Inventories

There are a number of self-report screening measures of depression, including the Beck Depression Inventory,[6] the Zung Depression Scale,[195] and the Hamilton Rating Scale.[75] The Beck Depression Inventory is perhaps the best researched of these instruments. The primary disadvantage of these scales is that their intent is obvious, which makes dissimulation quite easy. Moreover, depression is not a unitary disorder and has physical or somatic symptoms, psychomotor retardation, mental slowness, and cognitive and affective components. The inventories are unfortunately deficient in assessing these in their entirety. Other approaches to the assessment of depression (e.g., the Minnesota Multiphasic Personality Inventory [MMPI]) allow for the psychometric separation of components of depression but are much longer than the Beck, Hamilton, and Zung scales.

Minnesota Multiphasic Personality Inventory

The MMPI is probably the most widely used objective test of personality functioning, although there are some advantages to the more recent Millon Clinical Multiaxial Inventory-II.[119] The latter instrument is designed around Millon's theory of personality,[120] which has certain heuristic value. The original MMPI was developed by Hathaway and McKinley in 1943 and is composed of 566 true/false questions that compose[14] clinical scales. The MMPI Handbook[40] described more than 550 possible scales that can be derived from the MMPI. More recently, the MMPI-2 has been developed,[24] with some clinically important differences from the MMPI. Administration of the MMPI-2 usually requires about 60 to 90 minutes. Patients must have a sixth grade reading level to comprehend the questions, and normative data begin at age 15 years. The 14 scales have descriptors, which have been summarized[44] and are provided in Table 4–8.

Taking the MMPI can be a trying experience for patients, and the rationale should be explained. It is very important that the psychologist explain the results to the patient, as failure to do so can lead to considerable anxiety and unfortunate misperceptions. The MMPI can be a very useful diagnostic tool, but the results should be interpreted only by a psychologist with specific training in the MMPI, and must be correlated with clinical observations. Elevations on certain scales can occur for a variety of reasons, and misinterpretations can obviously lead to misdiagnosis.

Intelligence and Achievement Tests

Intelligence tests are useful in rehabilitation for a variety of reasons, but are principally given either to assist with vocational or academic planning or as part of a neuro-

TABLE 4–8 Descriptors for High Scores on Validity and Clinical Scales of the Minnesota Multiphasic Personality Inventory

Scale	Name	Descriptor
Validity Scales		
L	L Scale	Conventional, rigid, self-controlled
F	F Scale	Restless, changeable, dissatisfied, opinionated
K	K Scale	Defensive, inhibited
Clinical Scales		
1	Hypochondriasis	Immature, self-centered, demanding, complaining
2	Depression	Pessimistic, withdrawn, slow, timid, shy
3	Hysteria	Immature, egotistical, suggestible, friendly
4	Psychopathic deviate	Rebellious, resentful, impulsive, energetic, irresponsible
5	Masculine/ feminine	Aggressive, dominant, masculine
6	Paranoia	Suspicious, hostile, rigid, distrustful
7	Psychasthenia	Worrying, anxious, dissatisfied, sensitive, rigid
8	Schizophrenia	Confused, imaginative, individualistic, impulsive
9	Hypomania	Energetic, enthusiastic, active, sociable, impulsive
0	Social introversion	Aloof, sensitive, inhibited, timid

Adapted from DeMendonca M, Elliot L, Goldstein M, et al: An MMPI-based behavior descriptor/personality trait list. J Personal Assess 1984; 48:483–485.

psychological examination for persons with known or suspected brain damage. The most commonly used test is the Wechsler Adult Intelligence Scale—Revised (WAIS-R).[181] The WAIS-R has also been revised by Kaplan and co-workers[82] to provide more useful information to neuropsychologists. The WAIS-R can be administered to persons 16 to 74 years of age. Administration of the WAIS-R typically takes 60 to 120 minutes. It is composed of 11 subtests, six of which statistically contribute to the Verbal Intelligence Quotient and five of which contribute to the Performance Intelligence Quotient. The scores are also combined in a way to yield a Full Scale Intelligence Quotient.

A great variety of cognitive and intellectual functions are measured by the WAIS-R, and each subtest can be multifactorial. For example, the Digit Span subtest is rather simple and requires the patient to repeat spoken numeric digits. The first part of the subtest requires the patient to repeat the digits. Then the patient is asked to repeat the digits backward. This task principally requires auditory attention, concentration, and mental control. The Picture Arrangement subtest, in comparison, requires that the patient put in order a series of pictures that tell a story, not unlike a cartoon sequence. This task requires a variety of cognitive functions, including visual scanning, identification of visual detail, sequencing, foresight, and planning. The patient also typically verbalizes, either overtly or covertly, through the task as a means to help solve the problem, adding a verbal and linguistic component to the task. As a consequence, patients can succeed or fail on these tasks for many reasons. A sizable body of literature exists about the WAIS-R (see Lezak[99] and Spreen and Strauss[155] for detailed reviews).

Measures of academic achievement are routinely given, such as intelligence tests, as part of neuropsychological testing or when questions regarding academic and vocational placement arise. The most comprehensive of the achievement tests is the Woodcock-Johnson Psychoeducational Battery—Revised.[192] This test provides a wide range of academic achievement information through nine subtests—Letter-Word Identification, Calculation, Applied Problems, Dictation, Writing Samples, Science, Social Studies, and Humanities. This test can be administered to persons as young as 2 years and requires approximately 60 minutes to administer. If clinically appropriate, portions of the battery can be administered. The Woodcock-Johnson has been well researched and has excellent psychometric properties.

Another commonly used achievement test is the Peabody Individual Achievement Test—Revised (PIAT-R).[106] This test is not as comprehensive as the Woodcock-Johnson battery but is better suited for patients with low verbal abilities.[155] The PIAT-R provides, in addition to a composite score, subtest scores for mathematics, reading recognition, reading comprehension, spelling, and general comprehension.

Neuropsychological Tests

Battery versus Individualized Approaches

The primary impetus for the development of neuropsychological assessment in the United States was to assist in neurological diagnosis. Prior to the development of CT, neuropsychological assessment was targeted at determining whether a brain lesion was present, and, if present, discerning its location and type. This diagnostic approach supported the development of the Halstead-Reitan Neuropsychological Test Battery (HRNTB).[137, 138] The Halstead-Reitan battery comprises five core tests, which were originally developed by Halstead, in addition to other tests that are referred to as "Allied Procedures." The Allied Procedures were developed by Reitan and associates.[18] The HRNTB typically requires an entire day to administer, particularly when done with other neuropsychological tests. All of the HRNTB tests are administered in a very standardized manner, irrespective of individual differences. The HRNTB provides an objective, statistical, and quantitative evaluation of neuropsychological functions. It was developed to detect the presence or absence of brain damage, but in a rehabilitation setting this is now of less obvious practical benefit.

As the HRNTB was being developed in the United States, a different approach to neuropsychological assessment was simultaneously being constructed in the former Soviet Union. Luria[102, 103] contributed the first organized neuropsychological theory of brain functions and developed examination procedures that emphasize individual differences. Luria's approach to the examination of patients with cerebral lesions was later organized and articulated by Christensen.[30] Although a core set of tests is administered in the Luria Neuropsychological Investigation, each evaluation proceeds differently and according to the patient's responses. In this approach to neuropsychological assessment, the examiner seeks to discover how the patient goes about performing the task, and whether or not the strategy the patient utilizes results in a successful outcome. When deficits in performance are noted, the examiner can manipulate the requirements of the test to determine the underlying (neuropsychological) reason for failure on the task. In this approach, the examiner can also manipulate the task to help determine what modifications are necessary to enable the patient to perform the task. This approach has obvious benefit from a rehabilitation perspective. The Luria Neuropsychological Investigation is wholly qualitative and yields no quantitative results, however.

Other approaches to neuropsychological assessment have been developing rapidly, including that of Kaplan, Milberg, and co-workers.[81, 118] Kaplan has developed a "process approach" to neuropsychological assessment that in many ways combines the advantages of the quantitative approach with those of the qualitative approach. The tests revised and developed by Kaplan emphasize (and quantify) the process (i.e., the strategies) that the patient uses while attempting to solve the problem. This approach still retains the achievement score, that is, the final score that reflects the extent to which the task was performed in a manner consistent with normative expectations. As previously mentioned, Kaplan and coworkers have revised the WAIS-R to enhance its utility in neuropsychological assessment, and other new tests have been developed that are of certain utility in a rehabilitation setting.[42] The interested reader is referred to Trexler and others[169] for further information on contemporary approaches to neuropsychological assessment in rehabilitation.

Purpose-Specific Neuropsychological Tests

In the case of brain injury, sequential monitoring of patients' overall orientation can be quite useful in determining the rate of progress and response to neuropharmacological treatment and in documenting evolution out of posttraumatic or anterograde amnesia. Too often patients are unknowingly discharged from the hospital in a state of posttraumatic or anterograde amnesia, often with disastrous results. The Galveston Orientation and Amnesia Scale[97] is a quick and objective measure that is invaluable. The Neurobehavioral Rating Scale[96] is also useful for rating the behavioral changes seen in brain injury. A variety of functions such as insight, emotional reactions, and disinhibition are rated on a seven-point scale. The Neurobehavioral Rating Scale is also helpful for tracking patient progress, and its reliability and validity have been studied in an inpatient rehabilitation setting.[37]

A variety of scales have been developed for measuring psychosocial and functional adaptation following brain injury and are sometimes used as part of neuropsychological assessment. The most useful include the Katz Adjustment Scale,[68, 83, 133] the Portland Adaptability Inventory[100] and a recent modification of this instrument,[105] and the Community Integration Questionnaire.[188, 189] These instruments provide valuable information about the patient's functional and psychosocial status, which is just as important as are neuropsychological data in the rehabilitation setting. When combined, the neuropsychological and functional-psychosocial data provide a more complete perspective from which to plan brain injury rehabilitation.

PSYCHOLOGICAL INTERVENTION

In rehabilitation settings, psychological interventions are typically divided into two broad areas: (1) maximizing general rehabilitation progress, and (2) teaching specific skills to facilitate ultimate psychosocial adjustment. Psychological goals and interventions are compatible with, and often support, the goals of other rehabilitation disciplines. Although traditional counseling sessions with rehabilitation clients or relatives might be employed, interventions are as likely to take the form of more frequent treatments of shorter duration. These can occur as "co-treatments" with other disciplines to reinforce general rehabilitation progress. Psychologists often also act in a consultation role with rehabilitation staff to assist in designing intervention strategies. Group interventions can be employed when issues of psychosocial adjustment or social skills are addressed. Psychologists are often also asked to assist with resistive patients, as well as to help staff manage their own reactions to the rehabilitation process.

Depressive Symptoms

Clinical depression or some subclinical depressive symptoms can have a negative impact on participation in rehabilitation and ultimate adjustment. Alterations in sleep or arousal secondary to significant depression can diminish the patient's energy available for rehabilitation. More important, the negative cognitive biases accompanying depression can have an impact on motivation, general activity level, socialization, and reactions to positive feedback.

Cognitive interventions for depression are based on the reasonably well validated finding[5, 74, 151] that depressed individuals tend to view themselves, their environments, and the future with a negative bias[7] and/or expect future negative or adverse occurrences to be largely uncontrollable.[1] These biases are fueled by such underlying information processing styles as the tendencies to overgeneralize, think dichotomously, abstract selectively, personalize, excessively employ "should" statements, catastrophize negative events, and minimize the importance of positive occurrences.[141] Although the onset of disability can precipitate depressive symptoms, these negative cognitive biases act to sustain them. From a behavioral perspective, prolonged hospitalization and permanent impairment with associated depression can lead to a decrease in the capacity to access pleasurable events[98] or reinforcers, effectively producing a condition of punishment.[62]

Cognitive therapy for depression strives to help the patient become aware of irrational negative perceptual biases and to modify associated information processing styles. In nonmedical populations, cognitive therapy for depression has been shown to be as effective as pharmacological interventions in the amelioration of depressive symptoms and to be possibly superior in preventing future depressive episodes.[79, 186] Cognitive therapy for depression can be an effective approach for treating the depressive symptoms of rehabilitation patients, although normal mood variations associated with loss should be distinguished from more psychologically serious conditions. "Supportive counseling" can have a role, but care must be taken not to generate or promote sadness for its own sake. A sense of progress or the reinforcement of effort or skill acquisition should be supported. Note also the importance of not necessarily confronting apparent illusory positive beliefs (or at least self-reports) if such beliefs appear unrelated or nondetrimental to rehabilitation outcome or ultimate psychosocial adjustment.

Various behavioral strategies can also be employed to intervene in depressive symptoms. In fact, most psychological interventions for depression employ a mixture of cognitive and behavioral strategies. Use of these can help alleviate the depressive forces normally stimulated by the rehabilitation process. During rehabilitation, patients can confront firsthand the magnitude of their disability. Both past reinforcing and current pleasurable experiences are typically lacking in inpatient settings. The rapid pace of delivery of rehabilitation services, especially now with shortened lengths of hospital stay, can produce fatigue and compound feelings of uncontrollability. Rehabilitation staffing, scheduling, and goal-setting decisions are often inappropriately made with little or no input from the patient. Individual therapies emphasize component or foundation skills in preparation for (or in lieu of) more functional and personally meaningful behaviors. Patients can have difficulty appreciating the relevance of these for their more important functional goals. Effective rehabilitation facilitates adjustment by actively including the patient in goal-setting and treatment-planning discussions. Documentation or charting of progress in therapies, allowing some personal control in the daily schedule or choice of therapists, and promoting access to pleasurable activities are all interventions that can help reduce suffering and increase participation in rehabilitation. Facilitating generalization from the rehabilitation environment to more personally meaningful settings and establishing a specific outpatient program prior to discharge can assist the transition home and help alleviate associated concerns.

Psychological Treatment of Anxiety

The onset of serious illness or injury can set the stage for the development of anxiety symptoms. Hemiplegia, amputation, or other impairments affecting physical stability or balance can generate notable fears of falling. Some conditions such as chronic obstructive pulmonary disease or certain cardiac impairments can create chronic anxiety related to doubts about future survival. These interact with the underlying medical state to further compromise function. Amputation, ostomy procedures, or other conditions altering physical appearance can induce a set of social avoidance behaviors that can compromise ultimate adjustment. Social anxiety and associated withdrawal can accompany awareness of alterations in interactional or communicative skill secondary to brain injury. A similar situation can arise over fear of incontinence from several conditions affecting bowel or bladder control.

Treatment of anxiety disorders is based on controlled exposure to the feared event or circumstance under conditions that optimize successful function. Anxiety nearly always leads to avoidance, perpetuating the emotional foundation and beliefs that continue to promote the anxiety. In addition to skill development during rehabilitation, several psychological interventions can promote easier exposure to the feared situation. Like depression, anxiety can be maintained by a set of irrational cognitive biases.[8, 29] Specific cognitive interventions designed to correct these beliefs facilitate recovery. Anxiety also generates a particular constellation of physiological responses, typically characterized by excessive sympathetic arousal. Teaching skills that modulate the magnitude of such arousal has served as a cornerstone for desensitization strategies. A variety of relaxation techniques are available (see Anderson[3] for a recent review) that, in combination with cognitive intervention and specific skill building, offer the anxious individual some sense of mastery and self-control.

Interventions with Excessive Chronic Disability

Specific interventions are required in cases in which excessive disability seems related to faulty attributions or psychosocial contingencies. For example, the foundation for effective intervention in chronic pain is physical reactivation and the eroding of reinforcement contingencies that serve to maintain pain and related disability behaviors.[57, 61] Supervised progressive physical activity occurs despite the presence of pain behaviors or reports of pain. Rest, analgesics, and social attention are programmed to occur at times that are not pain reinforcing. Attempts are made to intervene in family and vocational arenas to maximize the probability that social forces reinforce independence and function rather than disability (see Chapter 42).

To accomplish these goals, an attempt must be made to alter the attributions and beliefs of the patient. Cognitions about the meaning of pain must be altered or "reframed." Through teaching, patients learn about the complex, multifactorial nature of the perception of pain, and that chronic pain does not, in most cases, signify harm or danger.

Similar strategies can be effective for other conditions in which misattribution and social contingencies reinforce excessive disability. Individuals experiencing prolonged postconcussive symptoms can benefit from progressive cognitive rehabilitation activities designed to underline their skills and progress in problem areas.

Education about the natural course of recovery from concussion can facilitate the recasting of attributions of neuropsychological impairment into more reasonable directions that include the role of conditioning and the influence of emotional distress associated with early impairments. It is crucial to intervene in social or vocational domains that continue to promote disability.

Social Skills Training

Social skills training can assist ultimate psychosocial adjustment and minimize the relationship between disability and social isolation.[47] The nature of social interaction in traditional rehabilitation settings frequently offers little preparation for the disabled individual to deal with more natural social environments. In addition to the work on communication skills and social appropriateness that is typically included in brain injury rehabilitation activities, disabled individuals benefit from consideration of, and practice in, managing the more difficult social circumstances that they might have to confront. These can include the social ramifications of disability-specific issues (e.g., incontinence, wheelchair mobility, forgetfulness), but also present methods of minimizing uncomfortableness on the part of nondisabled interactional partners. Practice in statements that reduce disability-related uncertainty and anxiety in a communication partner can promote more successful social interactions.[127]

Resistive or "Unmotivated" Patients

Seemingly unmotivated, resistive, manipulative, or angry patients are not uncommon to the rehabilitation setting and can serve as a significant source of stress and frustration for staff. Not uncommonly, such behaviors are labeled as reflective of a personality flaw and lead to decisions to terminate services. They frequently reflect understandable responses to internal and external events (Table 4–9), however, and often offer opportunities for intervention.[19, 27] An analysis and discussion of which of these forces might be operating can lead to interventions that maximize participation, as well as to alleviation of negative staff reactions. The shorter hospitalizations that are secondary to the pressures of recent health care changes have unfortunately made it easier to inappropriately dismiss the "resistive" or "unmotivated" patient as an inappropriate candidate for rehabilitation.

TABLE 4–9 Common Sources of Resistance or Poor Motivation in Rehabilitation

Medical/Physical Factors	Psychological Factors
1. Effects of acute illness	1. Depression, anxiety, fear effects
2. Effects of acute pain	2. Lack of reinforcement/pleasure
3. Lack of sleep/fatigue	3. Denial
4. Medicine effects	4. Efforts at sustaining control
5. Brain injury/delirium effects	5. Limited input into established program/goals
a. Anosognosia	6. Poor understanding of rehabilitation rationale
b. Disorientation/confusion	7. Poor appreciation of progress/gains
c. Agitation	8. Personality conflict with therapist/physician
d. Memory impairment	9. Characterological traits of patient

Neuropsychological Rehabilitation

The literature on neuropsychological approaches to brain injury rehabilitation has flourished since the early 1980s. A variety of types of interventions have been developed. In general, neuropsychological treatment of cognitive impairments either employs a theoretical-clinical or a psychometric approach.[165] Interventions that are driven by a theoretical-clinical approach utilize principles of brain function and the effects of brain lesions on cognitive function for the individual patient. In contrast, the psychometric approach bases the intervention on the results of tests of cognitive function.

Trexler and Thomas[168] have provided a taxonomy of neuropsychological interventions that describes essentially two levels of intervention. The first type of intervention is targeted at specific cognitive deficits that occur secondary to acquired brain injury (e.g., memory impairment, hemispatial inattention). Interventions that aim for the amelioration of specific cognitive deficits can be categorized into cognitive remediation and compensatory strategies. Remediation strategies largely seek to restore human abilities, whereas compensatory strategies involve the performance of an integrated set of performances. Cognitive remediation strategies are targeted at either restoration of the lost ability or at reorganizing the lost ability through incorporating intact or spared functions. Compensatory strategies employ either a task reorganization or a task substitution approach. Task reorganization refers to adding to or modifying the inputs, stages, or outputs of a task in a manner that can be performed by the patient and incorporated into daily life with practice. Task substitution refers to the training of entirely new skills that replace the impaired function (e.g., memory notebook).

A great variety of studies have addressed the efficacy of interventions for specific cognitive disorders, and the available research provides support for neuropsychological interventions that seek to compensate for residual cognitive impairments. As an example, Sohlberg and Mateer[153] developed a systematic training procedure for utilizing a memory notebook. Some clinicians have naively attempted to encourage brain-damaged patients with memory deficits to compensate by using a notebook, but these investigators demonstrated that without rigorous and systematic training, patients did not learn to incorporate new behaviors into their daily life. The reader is encouraged to review the plethora of recent contributions for more specific information about specific neuropsychological interventions.[32, 55, 115, 152, 179]

Another neuropsychological intervention can be best described as an organized program of specialized rehabilitation, referred to as "holistic" neuropsychological rehabilitation.[10] The efficacy of postacute neuropsychological rehabilitation that employs a "holistic" approach has been demonstrated in a variety of studies.[10, 31, 105, 134, 135] A holistic approach to the rehabilitation of the person with acquired brain damage employs a therapeutic milieu with a variety of group therapies emphasizing awareness and emotional acceptance of residual deficits and compensation or remediation of cognitive impairments. Families must be quite involved, particularly from a psychotherapeutic standpoint, and these programs all emphasize a gradual and structured reentry into a target discharge environment, such as a vocational placement. The length of treatment is sometimes fixed; that is, all patients are admitted and discharged at the same time, or it is individually determined by time of referral, and patients are admitted and discharged continuously. These programs are typically provided within a day treatment framework for 4 to 5 days a week, and the average length of stay is typically 3 to 6 months, depending on the program and the patient. Two of the studies of outcome have been controlled,[134, 135] and the others have examined patients who were considerably past the period of spontaneous recovery with a pre-post methodology. When considered collectively, these studies demonstrated significant gains in psychosocial adaptation, independent living, employment status, reductions in health care utilization and costs, and cost savings[113] when individuals with acquired brain damage were provided with holistic neuropsychological rehabilitation.

PSYCHOLOGICAL ASPECTS OF REHABILITATION STAFF FUNCTIONING

Rehabilitation is unique among medical or allied health professions for the intensity and sometimes lengthy durations of typical interventions. The psychological reactions of both patients and staff can influence, as well as be stimulated by, the multiple rehabilitation interactions occurring throughout the course of treatment. Even seasoned rehabilitation professionals can be caught off guard by the emotional reactions generated around the care of a particular patient. Paradoxically, the rehabilitation environment is frequently staffed by relatively young professionals. Recent economic constraints, in addition to increasing general stress through shortened length of stays or managed care pressures, have also limited resources for staff development, support, and education. This state of affairs can further potentiate conflicts between staff members and between staff and patients. The highly stressful and emotionally laden rehabilitation environment offers a rich opportunity for a variety of transference forces to flow freely between patient and staff. In addition to the patient's own emotional responses, rehabilitation staff frequently develop strong emotional reactions to their work in general (burnout) or to particular patients (countertransference). These reactions are frequently based in differing staff and patient expectations, the repertoire of coping skills staff bring to the rehabilitation enterprise, and situational stresses present within the rehabilitation environment.

Staff members appear to carry to the rehabilitation setting expectations and biases about how patients should respond, as well as about their own roles in facilitating cooperation and recovery. It is of some interest that correlations between patient and staff ratings of mood[25] or behavioral competency[43, 60] have been found to be modest. Specific diagnoses can yield particular expectations of the degree of expected psychological reactions,[66, 185] with violations of these expectations being likely to color patient-staff interactions. For example, sometimes rehabilitation professionals underestimate the degree of emotional distress a patient has experienced.[65] Minimization of a patient's emotional distress might be based in the staff's struggle to accept a patient's disability and the staff's own general level of emotional exhaustion.[66] More often, professional helpers tend to overestimate the degree of psychopathology in their patients, particularly those who are more resistive.[190] It has been noted that professionals can overestimate both the presence of depression among spinal cord-injured patients relative to staff[172] and the degree of clinically significant depressive disorder in a general inpatient rehabilitation setting.[65] Similar tendencies have been noted in ratings of social impairment among brain-injured patients.[60] Caplan[25] has noted that different disciplines can systematically vary in tendencies to assign depressive symptoms to patients within a rehabilitation setting, and that to some extent members of a discipline selectively attend to different aspects of depressive phenomena.

Gans[66] perceptively described certain recurrent themes and offered possible methods of dealing with them. Patients can develop negative reactions to rehabilitation or to particular staff members because of their relative intactness, their constant scrutiny of the patients in difficult and sometimes embarrassing situations, their position of control, their self-confidence, or their perceived responsibility in any lack of progress that the patient experiences during rehabilitation. Trexler[166] suggested that the inherent stress in rehabilitation environments and the tendency to project blame on others often lead rehabilitation staff to be more territorial with respect to the roles of specific disciplines, to set unrealistic expectations for patients, or to blame the patient and family for either not making enough progress or not complying with therapy. Staff can also develop negative feelings as a consequence of dealing with the variety of resistive, splitting, manipulative, or blaming behaviors exhibited by some of their patients. All of these forces can act to increase conflict among rehabilitation staff. Interpersonal conflict has been reported to be the most frequent stressor among nurses in a rehabilitation setting.[53]

Dealing with staff reactions to the rehabilitation process is crucial, both with respect to the care of particular patients and with respect to preventing burnout and decreasing staff turnover. Recent theoretical accounts of rehabilitation staff burnout have focused on components of emotional exhaustion, depersonalization of the patient, and a reduced sense of personal accomplishment.[107] In addition to such personality variables as natural problem-solving style and stress tolerance, situational factors such as size of caseload, opportunities for job advancement, and general job satisfaction have been linked to rehabilitation job stress.[107] The tendency to employ certain classes of coping skills, particularly those focused on emotions, is also associated with increased feelings of burnout.[34, 53] Gans[66] notes that rehabilitation staff rarely have sufficient training in psychology to deal adequately with the emotions and conflicts they experience at work. He emphasizes active intervention in all cases in which conflicts arise, often involving a psychological evaluation with other rehabilitation team members present. The purpose of these meetings is to help staff understand the patient better so that they might be better able to modify their own behavior. He noted the importance of staff appreciating (1) that conflict in rehabilitation is inevitable (and sometimes desirable), (2) that premorbid emotional and personality problems are frequently the cause of conflictual patient behaviors in rehabilitation, and (3) that understanding these facts and basic themes of psychological defense can help staff not to personalize or tend to resist the more negative emotional and behavioral characteristics of their patients. Careful attention to issues of staff tension and burnout by supervisors and rehabilitation managers provides another tool for supporting staff. Helping staff develop new tools for coping with difficult patients can minimize burnout. Ensuring opportunities for advancement, promotion, continuing education, and wage increases can also offset the inherent strains of doing rehabilitation work. A book edited by Durgin and colleagues,[49] is a very useful text that addresses staff development and training in brain injury rehabilitation.

SUMMARY

Psychological assessment and treatment are increasingly valuable in all types of physical rehabilitation, from occupational rehabilitation to brain injury rehabilitation. Rehabilitation teams should include, or at least have access to, a psychologist. Rehabilitation clinicians also need to have at least a superficial understanding of the use and limitations of current psychological tests.

REFERENCES

1. Abramson LY, Seligman MEP, Teasdale J: Learned helplessness in humans: Critique and reformulation. J Abnorm Psychol 1978; 87:49–74.
2. Acker MB: A review of the ecological validity of neuropsychological tests. In Tupper DE, Cicerone KD (eds): The Neuropsychology of Everyday Life: Assessment and Basic Competencies. Boston, Kluwer Academic Publishers, 1990, pp 19–56.
3. Anderson JP: Relaxation training and relaxation-related procedures. In Doleys DM, Meredith RL, Ciminero AR (eds): Behavioral Medicine: Assessment and Treatment Strategies. New York, Plenum Press, 1982, pp 69–82.
4. Auerbach SM: Stress management and coping research in the health care setting: An overview and methodological commentary. J Consult Clin Psychol 1989; 57:388–395.
5. Barnett PA, Gotlib IH: Psychosocial functioning and depression: Distinguishing among antecedents, concomitants, and consequences. Psychol Bull 1988; 104:97–126.
6. Beck AT: Beck Depression Inventory: Manual. San Antonio, Psychological Corp, 1987.
7. Beck AT: Cognitive Therapy and Emotional Disorders. New York, International Universities Press, 1976.
8. Beck AT: Cognitive therapy: Past, present, and future. J Consult Clin Psychol 1993; 61:194–198.
9. Beck AT, Rush AJ, Shaw BF, et al: Cognitive Therapy of Depression. New York, Guilford Press, 1979.
10. Ben-Yishay Y, Silver SM, Piasetsky E, et al: Relationship between employability and vocational outcome after intensive holistic cognitive rehabilitation. J Head Trauma Rehabil 1987; 2:35–48.
11. Bergner L, Bergner M, Hallstrom AP, et al: Health status of survivors of out-of-hospital cardiac arrest six months later. Am J Public Health 1984; 74:508–510.
12. Bergner M, Bobbitt RA, Carter WB, et al: The Sickness Impact Profile: Development and final revision of a health status measure. Med Care 1981; 14:787–805.
13. Bergner M, Bobbitt RA, Pollard WE, et al: The Sickness Impact Profile: Validation of a health status measure. Med Care 1976; 14:57–67.
14. Bigler ED, Kurth S, Blatter D, et al: Day-of-injury CT as an index to pre-injury morphology: Degree of post-injury degenerative changes identified by CT and MR neuroimaging. Brain Injury 1993; 7:125–134.
15. Binder L: Persisting symptoms after mild head injury: A review of the postconcussive syndrome. J Clin Exp Neuropsychol 1986; 8:323–346.
16. Bisiach E, Geminiani G: Glossary. In Prigatano GP, Schacter DL (eds): Awareness of Deficit After Brain Injury: Clinical and Theoretical Issues. New York, Oxford University Press, 1991, pp 263–264.
17. Blumer D, Benson DF: Personality changes with frontal and temporal lobe lesions. In Benson DF, Blumer D (eds): Psychiatric Aspects of Neurologic Disease. New York, Grune & Stratton, 1975, pp 151–170.
18. Boll TJ: The Halstead-Reitan neuropsychology battery. In Filskov SB, Boll TJ (eds): Handbook of Clinical Neuropsychology. New York, John Wiley & Sons, 1981, pp 577–607.
19. Brockway JA, Fordyce WE: Psychological assessment and management. In Kottke FJ, Lehmann JF (eds): Krusen's Handbook of Physical Medicine and Rehabilitation. Philadelphia, WB Saunders, 1990, pp 153–170.
20. Brooks N, McKinlay W: Personality and behavior change after severe blunt head injury—a relative's view. J Neurol Neurosurg Psychiatry 1983; 46:336–344.
21. Brooks N, McKinlay W, Symington C, et al: Return to work within seven years of severe head injury. Brain Injury 1987; 1:5–19.
22. Buckelew SP, Baumstark KE, Frank RG, et al: Adjustment following spinal cord injury. Rehabil Psychol 1990; 35:101–110.
23. Burke HL, Yeo RA, Delaney HD, et al: CT scan cerebral hemispheric asymmetries: Predictors of recovery from aphasia. J Clin Exp Neuropsychol 1993; 15:191–204.
24. Butcher JN, Dahlstrom WG, Graham JR, et al: MMPI-2: Minnesota Personality Inventory–2: Manual for Administration and Scoring. Minneapolis, University of Minnesota Press, 1989.
25. Caplan B: Staff and patient perception of patient mood. Rehabil Psychol 1983; 28:67–78.
26. Caplan B, Shechter J: Denial and depression in disabling illness. In Caplan B (ed): Rehabilitation Psychology Desk Reference. Rockville, MD, Aspen, 1987, pp 345–364.
27. Caplan B, Shechter J: Reflections on the "depressed," "unrealistic," "inappropriate," "manipulative," "noncompliant," "denying," "maladjusted," "regressed," etc. patient. Arch Phys Med Rehabil 1993; 74:1123–1124.
28. Cassel EJ: The nature of suffering and the goals of medicine. N Engl J Med 1982; 306:639–645.
29. Chambless DL, Gillis MM: Cognitive therapy of anxiety disorders. J Consult Clin Psychol 1993; 61:248–260.
30. Christensen A-L: Luria's Neuropsychological Investigation Test. Copenhagen, Munksgaard, 1974.
31. Christensen A-L, Pinner EM, Moller Pedersen P, et al: Psychosocial outcome following individualized neuropsychological rehabilitation of brain damage. Acta Neurol Scand 1992; 85:32–38.
32. Christensen A-L, Uzzell BP (eds): Brain Injury and Neuropsychological Rehabilitation: International Perspectives. Hillsdale, NJ, Lawrence Erlbaum, 1994.

33. Cioffi D: Beyond attentional strategies: A cognitive-perceptual model of somatic interpretation. Psychol Bull 1991; 109:25–41.
34. Clanton LD, Rude SS, Taylor C: Learned resourcefulness as a moderator of burnout in a sample of rehabilitation providers. Rehabil Psychol 1992; 37:131–140.
35. Cohen S, Wills TA: Stress, social support, and the buffering hypothesis. Psychol Bull 1985; 2:310–357.
36. Cook JB: The post-concussional syndrome and factors influencing recovery after minor head injury admitted to hospital. Scand J Rehabil Med 1972; 4:27–30.
37. Corrigan JD, Dickerson J, Fisher E, et al: The Neurobehavioral Rating Scale: Replication in an acute, inpatient rehabilitation setting. Brain Injury 1990; 4:215–222.
38. Crockett D, Clark C, Klonoff H: Introduction—An overview of neuropsychology. In Filskov SB, Boll TJ (eds): Handbook of Clinical Neuropsychology. New York, John Wiley & Sons, 1981, pp 1–37.
39. Cushman LA, Dijkers MP: Depressed mood in spinal cord injured patients: Staff perceptions and patient realities. Arch Phys Med Rehabil 1990; 71:191–196.
40. Dahlstrom WG, Welsch GS: An MMPI Handbook: A Guide to Use in Clinical Practice and Research, vols 1 and 2. Minneapolis, University of Minnesota Press, 1960, 1975.
41. Davidoff G, Roth E, Thomas P, et al: Depression among acute spinal cord injury patients: A study utilizing the Zung self-rating depression scale. Rehabil Psychol 1990; 35:171–180.
42. Delis DC, Kramer JH, Friedlund AJ, et al: A cognitive science approach to neuropsychological assessment. In McReynolds P, Rosen JC, Chelune GJ (eds): Advances in Psychological Assessment. New York, Plenum Press, 1990, pp 101–132.
43. Dellario D, Anthony W, Rogers S: Client-practitioner agreement in the assessment of severely psychiatrically disabled persons' functional skills. Rehabil Psychol 1983; 28:243–248.
44. DeMendonca M, Elliott L, Goldstein M, et al: An MMPI-based behavior descriptor/personality trait list. J Personal Assess 1984; 48:483–485.
45. Devins GM, Seland TP, Klein G, et al: Stability and determinants of psychosocial well-being in multiple sclerosis. Rehabil Psychol 1993; 38:11–26.
46. Deyo RA, Diehl AK, Rosenthal M: How many days of bed rest for acute low back pain? A randomized clinical trial. N Engl J Med 1986; 315:1064–1070.
47. Dunn M: Social skills and rehabilitation. In Caplan B (ed): Rehabilitation Psychology Desk Reference. Rockville, MD, Aspen, 1987, pp 345–364.
48. Durgin CJ: Preparing staff to provide quality rehabilitation services: Problems and proposed solutions. In Durgin CJ, Schmidt ND, Fryer LJ (eds): Staff Development and Clinical Intervention in Brain Injury Rehabilitation. Gaithersburg, MD, Aspen, 1993, pp 3–22.
49. Durgin CJ, Schmidt ND, Fryer LJ (eds): Staff Development and Clinical Intervention in Brain Injury Rehabilitation. Gaithersburg, MD, Aspen, 1993.
50. Elliot TR, Frank RG: Social and interpersonal reactions to depression and disability. Rehabil Psychol 1990; 35:135–148.
51. Elliot TR, Frank RG, Corcoran J, et al: Previous personal experience and reactions to depression and physical disability. Rehabil Psychol 1990; 35:111–120.
52. Elliot TR, Herrick SM, Witty TE, et al: Social support and depression following spinal cord injury. Rehabil Psychol 1992; 37:37–48.
53. Elliot TR, Shewchuk R, Hagglund K, et al: Occupational burnout, tolerance for stress, and coping among nurses in rehabilitation units. Rehabil Psychol 1996; 41:267–284.
54. Elliot TR, Yoder B, Umlauf R: Nurse and patient reactions to social displays of depression. Rehabil Psychol 1990; 35:195–204.
55. Ellis DW, Christensen A-L (eds): Neuropsychological Treatment After Brain Injury. Boston, Kluwer Academic Publishers, 1989.
56. Felton BJ, Revenson TA: Coping with chronic illness: A study of controllability and the influence of coping strategies on psychological adjustment. J Consult Clin Psychol 1984; 52:343–353.
57. Fey SG, Williamson-Kirkland TE: Chronic pain: Psychology and rehabilitation. In Caplan B (ed): Rehabilitation Psychology Desk Reference. Rockville, MD, Aspen, 1987, pp 101–130.
58. Fichten CS, Robillard K, Judd D, et al: College students with physical disabilities: Myths and realities. Rehabil Psychol 1989; 34:243–258.
59. Flor H, Kerns RD, Turk DC: The role of spouse reinforcement, perceived pain, and activity levels of chronic pain patients. J Psychosom Res 1987; 31:251–259.
60. Fordyce DJ, Roueche JR: Changes in perspectives of disability among patients, staff, and relatives during rehabilitation of brain injury. Rehabil Psychol 1986; 31:217–229.
61. Fordyce WE: Behavioral Methods for Chronic Pain and Illness. St Louis, Mosby–Year Book, 1976.
62. Fordyce WE: Pain and suffering: A reappraisal. Am Psychol 1988; 43:276–283.
63. Frank RG, Chaney JM, Clay DL, et al: Depression in rheumatoid arthritis: A re-evaluation. Rehabil Psychol 1991; 36:219–230.
64. Fuhrer MJ, Rintala DH, Hart KA, et al: Depressive symptomatology in persons with spinal cord injury who reside in the community. Arch Phys Med Rehabil 1993; 74:255–260.
65. Gans JS: Depression diagnosis in a rehabilitation hospital. Arch Phys Med Rehabil 1981; 64:386–389.
66. Gans JS: Facilitating staff interaction in rehabilitation. In Caplan B (ed): Rehabilitation Psychology Desk Reference. Rockville, MD, Aspen, 1987, pp 185–218.
67. Goldstein K: The effects of brain damage on the personality. Psychiatry 1952; 15:245–260.
68. Goran DA, Fabiano RJ: The scaling of the Katz Adjustment Scale in a traumatic brain injury rehabilitation sample. Brain Injury 1993; 7:219–229.
69. Gordon WA, Hibbard MR, Egelko S, et al: Issues in the diagnosis of post-stroke depression. Rehabil Psychol 1991; 36:71–88.
70. Gouvier WD, Cubic B, Jones G, et al: Postconcussion symptoms and daily stress in normal and head-injured college populations. J Clin Exp Neuropsychol 1992; 7:193–211.
71. Greenough CG, Fraser RD: The effects of compensation on recovery from low-back injury. Spine 1998; 14:947–955.
72. Gross Y: A conceptual framework for interventive cognitive neuropsychology. In Trexler LE (ed): Cognitive Rehabilitation: Conceptualization and Intervention. New York, Plenum Press, 1982, pp 99–114.
73. Gualtieri CT: Neuropsychiatry and Behavioral Pharmacology. New York, Springer, 1991.
74. Haaga DAF, Dyck MJ, Ernst D: Empirical status of cognitive theory of depression. Psychol Bull 1991; 11:215–236.
75. Hamilton M: Development of a rating scale for primary depressive illness. Br J Soc Clin Psychol 1967; 6:278–296.
76. Hanson S, Buckelew SP, Hewett XX, et al: The relationship between coping and adjustment after spinal cord injury: 5-year follow-up study. Rehabil Psychol 1993; 38:41–52.
77. Hart LG, Evans RW: The functional status of ESRD patients as measured by the Sickness Impact Profile. J Chron Dis 1987; 40:1175–1305.
78. Hathaway SR, McKinley JC: Booklet for the Minnesota Multiphasic Personality Inventory. New York, Psychological Corp, 1943.
79. Hollon SD, Shelton RC, Davis DD: Cognitive therapy for depression: Conceptual issues and clinical efficacy. J Consult Clin Psychol 1993; 61:270–275.
80. Jacobs H: The Los Angeles Head Injury Survey: Procedures and initial findings. Arch Phys Med Rehabil 1988; 69:425–431.
81. Kaplan E: Process and achievement revisited. In Wapner S, Kaplan B (eds): Toward a Holistic Developmental Psychology. Hillsdale, NJ, Lawrence Erlbaum, 1983.
82. Kaplan E, Fine D, Morris R, Dellis D: WAIS-R as a Neuropsychological Instrument. San Antonio, Psychological Corp, 1991.
83. Katz MM, Lyerly SB: Methods for measuring adjustment and social behavior in the community: I. Rationale, description, discriminative validity and scale development. Psychol Rep 1963; 13:503–535.
84. Kertesz A (ed): Localization and Neuroimaging in Neuropsychology. San Diego, Academic Press, 1994.
85. Kewman DG, Tate DG: Suicide in SCI: A psychological autopsy. Rehabil Psychol 1998; 43:143–151.
86. Kleinke CL: How chronic pain patients cope with depression: Relation to treatment outcome in a multidisciplinary pain clinic. Rehabil Psychol 1991; 36:207–218.

87. Krause JK: Changes in adjustment after spinal cord injury: A 20-year longitudinal study. Rehabil Psychol 1998; 43:41–55.
88. Krause JS: Survival following spinal cord injury: A 15-year prospective study. Rehabil Psychol 1991; 36:89–98.
89. Krause JS, Crewe NM: Prediction of long-term survival of persons with spinal cord injury. Rehabil Psychol 1987; 32:205–214.
90. Langfitt TW, Obrist WD, Alavi A, et al: Regional structure and function in head-injured patients: Correlation of CT, MRI, PET, CBF, and neuropsychological assessment. In Levin HS, Grafman J, Eisenberg HM (eds): Neurobehavioral Recovery from Head Injury. New York, Oxford University Press, 1987, pp 30–42.
91. Lazarus RS: Cognition and motivation in emotion. Am Psychol 1991; 46:352–367.
92. Lazarus RS: Progress on a cognitive-motivational-relational theory of emotion. Am Psychol 1991; 46:819–834.
93. Lazarus RS, Folkman S: Stress, Appraisal, and Coping. New York, Springer, 1986.
94. Lees-Haley PR, Brown RS: Neuropsychological complaint base rates of 170 personal injury claimants. Arch Clin Neuropsychol 1993; 8:203–209.
95. Lees-Haley PR, Fox DD: Neuropsychological false positives in litigation: Trail Making Test findings. Percept Mot Skills 1990; 70:1379–1382.
96. Levin HS, High WM, Goethe KE, et al: The Neurobehavioral Rating Scale: Assessment of the behavioral sequelae of head injury by the clinician. J Neurol Neurosurg Psychiatry 1987; 50:183–193.
97. Levin HS, O'Donnell VM, Grossman RG: The Galveston orientation and amnesia test: A practical scale to assess cognition after head injury. J Nerv Ment Dis 1979; 167:675–684.
98. Lewinsohn PM, Graff M: Pleasant activities and depression. J Consult Clin Psychol 1978; 41:271–278.
99. Lezak MD: Neuropsychological Assessment, ed 2. New York, Oxford University Press, 1983.
100. Lezak MD: Relationships between personality disorders, social disturbances, and physical disability following traumatic brain injury. J Head Trauma Rehabil 1987; 2:57–69.
101. Lubuski AA, Moore AD, Stambrook M, Gill DD: Cognitive beliefs following severe traumatic brain injury: Association with post injury employment. Brain Injury 1994; 8:65–70.
102. Luria AR: Higher Cortical Functions in Man. New York, Basic Books, 1980.
103. Luria AR: The Working Brain. New York, Basic Books, 1973.
104. Mahler HI, Kulik JA: Preferences for health care involvement, perceived control and surgical recovery: A prospective study. Soc Sci Med 1990; 31:743–751.
105. Malec JF, Smigielski JS, DePompolo RW, Thompson JM: Outcome evaluation and prediction in a comprehensive-integrated post-acute outpatient brain injury rehabilitation programme. Brain Injury 1993; 7:15–29.
106. Markwardt FC: Peabody Individual Achievement Test—Revised. Circle Pines, MN, American Guidance Service, 1989.
107. Maslach C, Florian V: Burnout, job setting, and self-evaluation among rehabilitation counselors. Rehabil Psychol 1988; 33: 85–94.
108. Matarazzo JD: Psychological assessment versus psychological testing: Validation from Binet to the school, clinic, and courtroom. Am Psychol 1990; 45:999–1017.
109. McGlynn SM, Schacter DL: Unawareness of deficits in neuropsychological syndromes. J Clin Exp Neuropsychol 1989; 11: 143–205.
110. McKinlay WW, Brooks DN, Bond MR: Post-concussional symptoms, financial compensation, and outcome of severe blunt head injury. J Neurol Neurosurg Psychiatry 1983; 46:1084–1091.
111. McSweeney AJ, Grant I, Heaton RK, et al: Life quality of patients with chronic obstructive pulmonary disease. Arch Intern Med 1982; 142:473–478.
112. Mechanic D: Social psychologic factors affecting the presentation of bodily complaints. N Engl J Med 1972; 286:1132–1139.
113. Mehlbye J, Larsen A: Social and economic consequences of brain damage in Denmark: A case study. In Christensen A-L, Uzzell B (eds): Brain Injury and Neuropsychological Rehabilitation: International Perspectives. Hillsdale, NJ, Lawrence Erlbaum, 1994, pp 257–268.
114. Mehnert T, Krauss HH, Nadler R, Boyd M: Correlates of life satisfaction in those with disabling conditions. Rehabil Psychol 1990; 35:3–18.
115. Meier MJ, Benton AL, Diller L (eds): Neuropsychological Rehabilitation. London, Churchill Livingstone, 1987.
116. Meltzer ML: Poor memory: A case report. J Clin Psychol 1983; 39:3–10.
117. Mesulam, M-M (ed): Principles of Behavioral Neurology. Philadelphia, FA Davis, 1985.
118. Milberg WP, Hebben N, Kaplan E: The Boston process approach to neuropsychological assessment. In Grant I, Adams KM (eds): Neuropsychological Assessment in Neuropsychiatric Disorders. New York, Oxford University Press, 1986.
119. Millon T: Millon Clinical Multiaxial Inventory II Manual. Minneapolis, National Computer Systems, 1987.
120. Millon T: A theoretical derivation of pathological personalities. In Millon T, Klerman GL (eds): Contemporary Directions in Psychopathology: Toward the DSM-IV. New York, Guilford Press, 1986.
121. Moore AD, Stambrook M: Coping strategies and locus of control following traumatic brain injury: Relationship to long-term outcome. Brain Injury 1992; 6:89–94.
122. Moore AD, Stambrook M, Wilson KG: Cognitive moderators in adjustment to chronic illness: Locus of control beliefs following traumatic brain injury. Neuropsychol Rehabil 1991; 1:185–198.
123. Naeser MA: Neuroimaging and recovery of auditory comprehension and spontaneous speech in aphasia with some implications for treatment in severe aphasia. In Kertesz A (ed): Localization and Neuroimaging in Neuropsychology. New York, Academic Press, 1994, pp 245–296.
124. National Center for Medical Rehabilitation Research: Research Plan for the National Center for Medical Rehabilitation Research. NIH publication no. 93-3509. Washington, DC, US Department of Health and Human Services, National Institutes of Health, 1993.
125. Nielsen AC, Williams TA: Depression in ambulatory medical patients. Arch Gen Psychiatry 1980; 37:999–1004.
126. Oades-Souther D, Olbrisch ME: Psychological adjustment to ostomy surgery. Rehabil Psychol 1984; 29:221–238.
127. Orr E, Aronson E: Relationships between orthopedic disability and perceived social support: Four theoretical hypotheses. Rehabil Psychol 1990; 35:29–42.
128. Ott CR, Sivarajan ES, Newton KM, et al: A controlled randomized study of early cardiac rehabilitation: The Sickness Impact Profile as an assessment tool. Heart Lung 1983; 12:162–170.
129. Partridge C, Johnston M: Perceived control of recovery from physical disability: Measurement and prediction. Br J Clin Psychol 1989; 28:53–59.
130. Patterson DR, Everett JL, Bombardier CH, et al: Psychological effects of severe burn injuries. Psychol Bull 1993; 113:362–378.
131. Pennebaker JW: The Psychology of Physical Symptoms. New York, Springer-Verlag, 1982.
132. Pollard WE, Bobbitt RA, Bergner M, et al: The Sickness Impact Profile: Reliability of a health status measure. Med Care 1976; 14:146–155.
133. Prigatano GP, Fordyce DJ, Zeiner HK, et al: Neuropsychological Rehabilitation After Brain Injury. Baltimore, Johns Hopkins University Press, 1986, p 35.
134. Prigatano GP, Fordyce DJ, Zeiner HK, et al: Neuropsychological rehabilitation after closed head injury in young adults. J Neurol Neurosurg Psychiatry 1984; 47:505–513.
135. Prigatano GP, Klonoff PS, O'Brien KP, et al: Productivity after neuropsychologically oriented milieu rehabilitation. J Head Trauma Rehabil 1994; 9:91–102.
136. Rape RN, Bush JP, Slavin LA: Toward a conceptualization of the family's adaptation to a member's head injury: A critique of developmental stage models. Rehabil Psychol 1992; 37:3–22.
137. Reitan RM: Theoretical and methodological bases of the Halstead-Reitan neuropsychological test battery. In Grant I, Adams KM (eds): Neuropsychological Assessment of Neuropsychiatric Disorders. New York, Oxford University Press, 1986, pp 3–30.
138. Reitan RM, Wolfson D: The Halstead-Reitan Neuropsychological Test Battery: Theory and Clinical Interpretation. Tucson, Neuropsychology Press, 1985.

139. Revenson T, Felton BA: Disability and coping as predictors of psychological adjustment to rheumatoid arthritis. J Clin Consult Psychol 1989; 57:344–348.
140. Rintala DH, Young ME, Hart KA, et al: Social support and the well-being of persons with spinal cord injury living in the community. Rehabil Psychol 1992; 37:155–164.
141. Robins CJ, Hayes AM: An appraisal of cognitive therapy. J Consult Clin Psychol 1993; 61:205–214.
142. Rodin G, Voshart K: Depression in the medically ill: An overview. Am J Psychiatry 1986; 143:696–705.
143. Romano JM, Turner JA: Chronic pain and depression: Does the evidence support a relationship? Psychol Bull 1985; 97:18–34.
144. Romano JM, Turner JA, Friedman LS, et al: Observational assessment of chronic pain patient-spouse behavioral interactions. Behav Ther 1991; 22:549–567.
145. Rosenbaum M, Najenson T: Changes in life patterns and symptoms of low mood as reported by wives of severely brain-injured soldiers. J Consult Clin Psychol 1976; 44:881–888.
146. Ross ED, Rush AJ: Diagnosis and neuroanatomical correlates of depression in brain-damaged patients. Arch Gen Psychiatry 1981; 38:1344–1354.
147. Rotter JB: Generalized expectancies for internal versus external control of reinforcement. Psychol Monogr 1966; p 80.
148. Rubonis AV, Bickman L: Psychological impairment in the wake of disaster: The disaster-psychopathology relationship. Psychol Bull 1991; 109:384–399.
149. Rybarczyk B, Nicholas JJ, Nyenhuis DL: Coping with leg amputation: Integrating research and clinical practice. Rehabil Psychol 1997; 42:241–256.
150. Schulberg HC, Saul M, McClellan M, et al: Assessing depression in primary medical and psychiatric practices. Arch Gen Psychiatry 1985; 42:1164–1170.
151. Segal ZV: Appraisal of the self-schema construct in cognitive models of depression. Psychol Bull 1988; 103:147–162.
152. Sohlberg MM, Mateer CA: Introduction to Cognitive Rehabilitation: Theory and Practice. New York, Guilford Press, 1989.
153. Sohlberg MM, Mateer CA: Training use of compensatory memory books: A three-stage behavioral. J Clin Exp Neuropsychol 1989; 11:871–891.
154. Spiers PA, Schomer DL, Blume HW, et al: Temporolimbic epilepsy and behavior. In Mesulam M-M (ed): Principles of Behavioral Neurology. Philadelphia, FA Davis, 1985, pp 289–326.
155. Spreen O, Strauss E: A Compendium of Neuropsychological Tests: Administration, Norms, and Commentary. New York, Oxford University Press, 1991.
156. Stein PN, Gordon WA, Hibbard MR, et al: An examination of depression in the spouses of stroke patients. Rehabil Psychol 1992; 37:121–130.
157. Stone JB, Bluhm HP, White MI: Correlates of depression among long-term insulin-dependent diabetics. Rehabil Psychol 1984; 29:85–94.
158. Strub R, Black FW: The Mental Status Examination in Neurology, ed 2. Philadelphia, FA Davis, 1985.
159. Stuss DT, Gow CA, Hetherington CR: "No longer Gage": Frontal lobe dysfunction and emotional changes. J Consult Clin Psychol 1992; 60:349–359.
160. Sugarbaker PH, Barofsky I, Rosenberg SA, et al: Quality of life assessment of patients in extremity sarcoma clinical trials. Surgery 1982; 1:17–23.
161. Taylor SE: Adjustment to threatening events: A theory of cognitive adaptation. Am Psychol 1983; 38:1161–1173.
162. Taylor SE, Brown JD: Illusion and well-being: A social psychological perspective on mental health. Psychol Bull 1988; 103:193–210.
163. Temkin N, McLean A, Dikman S, et al: Development and evaluation of modifications to the Sickness Impact Profile for head injury. J Clin Epidemiol 1988; 41:47–57.
164. Thomsen IV: Late outcome of very severe blunt head trauma: A 10–15 year follow-up. J Neurol Neurosurg Psychiatry 1984; 47:260–268.
165. Trexler LE: Neuropsychological rehabilitation in the United States. In Meier MJ, Benton AL, Diller L (eds): Neuropsychological Rehabilitation. London, Churchill Livingstone, 1987, pp 473–480.
166. Trexler LE: Professional issues in neuropsychological rehabilitation. In Ellis DW, Christensen A-L (eds): Neuropsychological Treatment After Brain Injury. Boston, Kluwer Academic Publishers, 1989, pp 363–378.
167. Trexler LE, Thomas JD: Behavioral and cognitive deficits in cerebrovascular accident and closed head injury: Implications for cognitive rehabilitation. In Trexler LE (ed): Cognitive Rehabilitation: Conceptualization and Intervention. New York, Plenum Press, 1983, pp 27–62.
168. Trexler LE, Thomas JD: Research design in neuropsychological rehabilitation. In von Steinbuchel N, von Cramon DY, Poppel E (eds): Neuropsychological Rehabilitation. Berlin, Springer-Verlag, 1992, pp 79–87.
169. Trexler LE, Webb PM, Zappala G: Strategic aspects of neuropsychological rehabilitation. In Christensen A-L, Uzzell BP (eds): Brain Injury and Neuropsychological Rehabilitation: International Perspectives. Hillsdale, NJ, Lawrence Erlbaum, 1994, pp 99–123.
170. Trexler LE, Zappala G: Neuropathological determinants of acquired attention disorders in traumatic brain injury. Brain Cogn 1988; 8:291–302.
171. Trexler LE, Zappala G: Re-examining the determinants of recovery and rehabilitation of memory defects following traumatic brain injury. Brain Injury 1988; 2:187–203.
172. Trieschmann RB: Spinal Cord Injuries: Psychological, Social, and Vocational Adjustment. New York, Pergamon Press, 1980.
173. Tupper DE, Cicerone KD: Introduction to the neuropsychology of everyday life. In Tupper DE, Cicerone KD (eds): The Neuropsychology of Everyday Life: Assessment and Basic Competencies. Boston, Kluwer Academic Publishers, 1990, pp 3–18.
174. Turk DC, Kerns RD, Rosenberg R: Effects of marital interaction on chronic pain and disability: Examining the down side of social support. Rehabil Psychol 1992; 37:259–274.
175. Turner RJ, McLean PD: Physical disability and psychological distress. Rehabil Psychol 1989; 34:225–242.
176. Uomoto JM, Esselman PC: Traumatic brain injury and chronic pain: Differential types and rates by head injury severity. Arch Phys Med Rehabil 1993; 74:61–64.
177. Uzzell BP, Dolinskas CA, Wiser RF, et al: Influence of lesions detected by computed tomography on outcome and neuropsychological recovery after severe head injury. Neurosurgery 1987; 20:396–402.
178. Vitaliano PP, Katon W, Maiuro RD, et al: Coping in chest pain patients with and without psychiatric disorders. J Consult Clin Psychol 1989; 57:338–343.
179. von Steinbuchel N, von Cramon DY, Poppel E: Neuropsychological Rehabilitation. Berlin, Springer-Verlag, 1992.
180. Wallston KA, Wallston BS, Devellis R: Development of the Multidimensional Health Locus of Control (MHLC) scales. Health Educ Monogr 1978; 6:160.
181. Wechsler D: Wechsler Adult Intelligence Scale—Revised: Manual. San Antonio, Psychological Corp, 1981.
182. Weinstein EA, Kahn RL: Denial of Illness. Springfield, IL, Charles C Thomas, 1955.
183. Weissman HN: Distortions and deceptions in self presentation: Effects of protracted litigation in personal injury cases. Behav Sci Law 1990; 8:67–74.
184. Weissman HN: Forensic psychological assessment and the effects of protracted litigation on impairment in personal injury litigation. Forensic Rep 1991; 4:417–429.
185. Westbrook MT, Nordholm LA: Effects of diagnosis on reactions to patient optimism and depression. Rehabil Psychol 1986; 31:79–94.
186. Whisman MA: Mediators and moderators of change in cognitive therapy of depression. Psychol Bull 1993; 114:248–265.
187. Willanger R, Danielsen UT, Ankerhus J: Denial and neglect of hemiparesis in right-sided apoplectic lesions. Acta Neurol Scand 1981; 64:310–326.
188. Willer B, Ottenbacher KJ, Coad ML: The Community Integra-

tion Questionnaire: A comparative examination. Am J Phys Med Rehabil 1994; 73:103–111.
189. Willer B, Rosenthal M, Kreutzer JS, et al: Assessment of community integration following rehabilitation for traumatic brain injury. J Head Trauma Rehabil 1993; 8:75–87.
190. Wills TA: Perceptions of clients by professional helpers. Psychol Bull 1978; 85:968–1000.
191. Wilson JTL: Review: The relationship between neuropsychological function and brain damage detected by neuroimaging after closed head injury. Brain Injury 1990; 4:349–363.
192. Woodcock RW, Mather N: Woodcock-Johnson Tests of Achievement. Allen, TX, DLM Teaching Resources, 1989.
193. World Health Organization: International Classification of Impairments, Disabilities, and Handicaps: A Manual of Classification Relating to the Consequences of Disease. Geneva, World Health Organization, 1980.
194. Wortman CB, Silver RC: The myths of coping with loss. J Consult Clin Psychol 1989; 57:349–357.
195. Zung WWK: A self-rating depression scale. Arch Gen Psychiatry 1965; 12:63–770.

5 CHAPTER

Alberto Esquenazi, M.D., and Mukul Talaty, Ph.D.

Gait Analysis: Technology and Clinical Applications

For over 20 years gait analysis has been a useful clinical tool in the management of walking and movement problems. Technology and our understanding of its clinical application have improved greatly in recent years. Gait analysis was initially used as an investigational technique by the Weber brothers, working in the 1890s. Muybridge contributed to the understanding of movement with his famous sequential photographs of horses, and later of walking and running men.[12] (There are World Wide Web sites that have compiled some of Muybridge's original work into animated sequences; see *http://web.inter.NL.net/hcc/anima/muybridg/html-uk/muybr-01.htm* for a series of animations as well as additional links to Muybridge photo sequences.) Marey et al[10] used light-colored marking strips on dark-clad subjects for the analysis of body movements. Bernstein initiated the formal study of kinematics, using his detailed photographic studies of normal human locomotion movement.[2] In 1947, Schwartz and co-workers made the first quantitative studies of the forces generated at the floor-foot interface during walking.[15] Eventually electromyographic (EMG) recordings were possible, and Inman's group at the University of California Biomechanics Laboratory refined the simultaneous recording of the activity of multiple muscle groups during normal ambulation.[8]

Gait analysis has evolved into a recognized medical evaluation that is necessary for the appropriate planning of surgery or other therapeutic interventions in the management of spasticity, and for the prescription and optimization of orthotic and prosthetic devices. Other applications include sports analysis, the treatment of many musculoskeletal conditions, and clinical outcomes measurement. Perhaps the most important contribution of gait analysis is in the quantitative assessment of movement in general, and walking in particular. In some advanced centers, computer models of a patient walking are used to drive simulation models in which possible treatment interventions are entered to determine whether the proposed treatment can achieve the desired goal.

These advances have been possible in large part because of improvements in technology to record movement and forces, and because of the availability of dynamic EMG. The ease with which computers can be used to analyze large amounts of data obtained simultaneously from a variety of sources (such as force transducers, foot switches, EMG electrodes, motion analysis systems, and the like) has also been a major factor. Computers can be combined with data-gathering specialized transducers to record a physiological phenomenon, such as movements or muscle potentials, and then to transform the data into a digital signal that can be captured and analyzed with almost any standard computer. Data can be easily saved and retrieved for future reference. The data can then be analyzed to provide information on body segment velocities, accelerations, joint moments, powers, and mechanical energy. Under certain conditions, internal joint forces can also be estimated. The recent proliferation of gait analysis laboratories has been driven both by the clinical need to quantify neurophysiological function and by the rapid progress in computer technology.

Understanding gait analysis data and interpreting it in a clinically meaningful way, however, remains a challenge for many physicians. For gait analysis to be useful in the clinical evaluation of patients, certain criteria must be fulfilled. The measured parameters should

- Supply additional and more pertinent information than the clinical examination.

- Correlate with the functional capacity of the subject.
- Be accurate and repeatable.
- Result from a test that does not alter or alters very little the natural performance of the subject.
- Be interpreted by experienced clinicians familiar with the scope of the test protocol, instrumentation, and limitations of the equipment.

These criteria require that the clinician be familiar with the complex physiological interactions of normal gait biomechanics, know the normal and abnormal patterns of motor control, and be familiar with the technology used for its assessment. In addition, the clinician must be able to relate these features to any pathological motion that is observed during walking in order to effectively diagnose and address the problems of pathological gait. The clinician must be able to understand *what* the problem is, *where* and *when* it is present, and *why* it occurs. Knowledge of appropriate available interventions, a good medical history-taking ability, and good examination skills are requisite to determining the most appropriate treatment interventions.[6]

NORMAL HUMAN LOCOMOTION

Humans are the only animals that characteristically walk upright. The fundamental goal of ambulation is to move from one place to another safely and efficiently.[3] Because of the complex interaction of the lower limbs, head, trunk, and arms during gait, several time-based descriptors have evolved to describe normal and pathological gait. Gait is cyclic and can be characterized by the timing of foot contact with the ground. An entire sequence of functions by one limb is identified as a *gait cycle*.[3, 8] Each gait cycle has two basic components, *stance phase* and *swing phase*. Stance phase describes the duration of foot contact with the ground. Swing phase is the entire period during which the foot is in the air for the purpose of limb advancement. Swing phase can be further divided into three functional subphases: (1) *initial swing*, (2) *mid-swing*, and (3) *terminal swing*. The stance phase can be divided into five subphases: (1) *initial contact*, (2) *loading response*, (3) *mid-stance*, (4) *terminal stance*, and (5) *pre-swing*. (Fig. 5–1).[1, 5]

Alternatively, the stance phase can be divided into three periods according to foot-floor contact patterns. The beginning and the end of the walking stance phase mark the period of *double support*, during which both feet are in contact with the floor, allowing the weight of the body to be transferred from one limb to the other. Using this descriptor, one definition of running is locomotion in which double support is absent. *Single limb support* begins when the opposite foot is lifted from the ground for the swing phase. For normal subjects walking at self-selected comfortable speeds, the normal distribution of the floor contact period during the gait cycle is roughly 60% for stance phase and 40% for swing phase. Approximately 10% of the total cycle is overlap for each double support time. These ratios vary greatly with changes in walking speed (Fig. 5–2).

The *step period* is the time measured from an event in one foot to the next occurrence of the same event in the opposite foot. There are two steps in each stride or gait cycle. The step period is useful for identifying and measuring asymmetry between the two sides of the body in pathological conditions. *Step length* is the maximum distance between the feet in the direction of progression

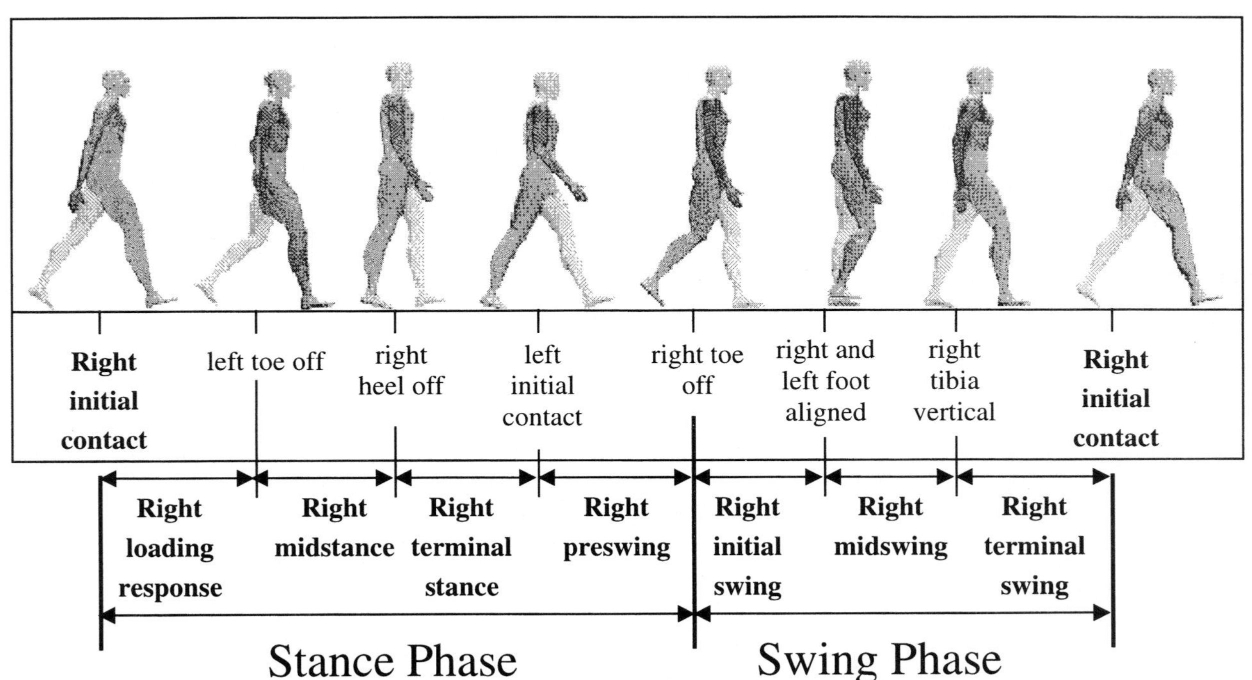

FIGURE 5–1. The gait cycle.

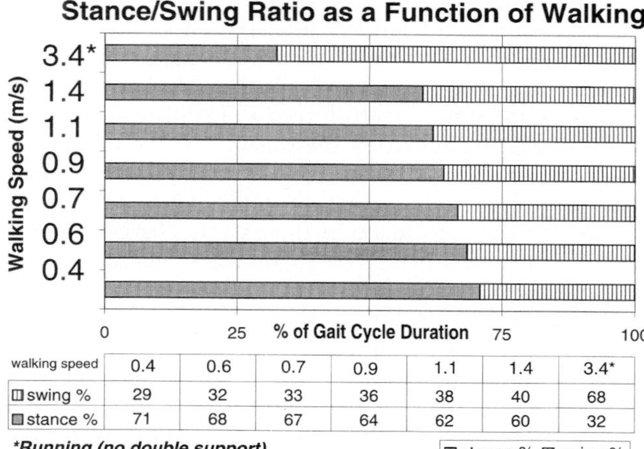

walking speed	0.4	0.6	0.7	0.9	1.1	1.4	3.4*
swing %	29	32	33	36	38	40	68
stance %	71	68	67	64	62	60	32

FIGURE 5–2. Effects of speed on the stance/swing ratio, from slow walking to running. As walking speed increases, the stance phase accounts for relatively less of the total gait cycle and the swing phase for proportionately more. In the example shown, the subject spends more time in swing phase than in stance phase when running at 3.4 m/sec.

during one step. The *stride period* is defined as the time from an event of one foot until the re-occurrence of the same event for the same foot. *Stride length* is the maximum distance traversed by the same foot in the direction of progression during one stride and is most often studied as the distance from the initial contact of one foot to the initial contact of the same foot. In most conditions for normal and pathological ambulators, left and right stride measures are equal. The stride period is often time-normalized for the purpose of averaging gait parameters over several strides, both between and within subjects (i.e., the absolute time is transformed to 100%). *Cadence* denotes the number of steps in a period of time (commonly expressed as steps per minute). Step length, step time, and cadence are fairly symmetrical between legs in normal individuals. These are all useful parameters for evaluating pathological gait. The base of support refers to the lateral distance between the feet. It is usually measured as the perpendicular distance between the medial borders or centerlines of the left and right feet.

GAIT DYSFUNCTION

Because of the complex relationship of multiple body segments, it is difficult to clearly identify the primary cause and compensation (substitution) in a gait deviation. One approach is to look at the different phases of locomotion and identify factors that affect the particular expected functional component. For this functional approach, the stance phase dysfunctions can be categorized into three groups: ankle-foot instability, knee instability, and hip instability (Table 5–1). A brief description of each follows.

Ankle-Foot Instability

The foot interaction with the ground is inadequate, interfering with the inherent weight-bearing function of the foot. An example as the abnormal posture of the foot present such conditions as equinus, equinovarus, ankle valgus with or without equinus, toe flexion, or hallux extension (hitchhiker's great toe).[11] Inadequate foot-ground interaction may also result from excessive ankle dorsiflexion, such as that seen with insufficient plantar flexor strength. This is commonly seen in the patient with neurological sequelae after central nervous system injury.

Knee Instability

Knee instability refers to flexed, hyperextended, varus or valgus knee posture. In the sagittal plane, it can be a compensatory response to avoid limb instability like that seen secondary to knee extensor or ankle plantar flexor weakness. Excessive knee hyperextension or valgus or varus knee can also be the result of an inherently unstable joint. An adducted hip or flexed hip can also affect knee stability.

Hip Instability

Hip instability typically involves hip abductor or extensor weakness or limited hip extension range of motion. Abnormal hip posture can also be a compensation for an abnormal base of support or limb instability. As an example, the patient with knee extensor weakness leans forward to improve knee stability by moving the center of mass anterior to the knee joint.

Swing Phase Deviations

Swing phase deviations can be divided into those of *impaired limb clearance* and those of *impaired limb advancement.* Impaired limb clearance can result from a drop foot, stiff knee, limited hip flexion, excessive or untimely hip adduction, and/or pelvic drop. Impaired limb advancement can be the result of a flexed knee, limited hip flexion, or contralateral hip extension, limitation, and adducted hips.

QUANTITATIVE GAIT ANALYSIS

Informal visual analysis of gait is routinely performed by clinicians and used as the basis to develop the initial

TABLE 5–1 Stance Limb Problems

Ankle-Foot Instability	*Hip Instability*
Equinus	Flexion
Varus	Extension
Equinovarus	Adduction
Valgus	Abduction
Equinovalgus	
Excessive dorsiflexion	
Toe curling	
Hallux hyperextension	
Knee Instability	
Excessive flexion (buckling)	
Hyperextension	
Varus	
Valgus	

questioning and examination of a patient. This sometimes casual observation can be more useful, although with many limitations, if performed in a careful and systematic manner. It can yield good descriptive information, especially when slow-motion video technology is used. The complexity and speed of the events that occur during walking, coupled with the deviations and possible compensations of a pathological gait, define the limitations of a visual-based qualitative analysis of locomotion.[3] Fortunately, many tools are available for quantifying gait as well.

In the laboratory, gait can be studied through the collection of a wide range of information. The four primary components of quantitative gait analysis that can be recorded are (1) kinetics (analysis of forces that produce motion), (2) poly-EMG or dynamic EMG (analysis of muscle activity), (3) kinematics (analysis of motion and resulting temporal and stride measures), and (4) energetics (analysis of metabolic or mechanical energy).

Kinetics

Kinetic analysis deals with the forces produced during walking. Sir Isaac Newton described basic but critical concepts that are useful in understanding the effect of gravity on gait. His third law of motion states that for every action there is an equal and opposite reaction. For our purposes, as long as gravity is present, there is a reaction force when the body interacts with the ground. The ground reaction force (GRF) is a reflection of body weight and acceleration. This force can be resolved into a convenient set of directions, such as vertical, anteroposterior (AP), and mediolateral. The AP shear forces are sometimes referred to as propulsion and braking forces. Friction is responsible for the generation of shear forces. The forces in all three directions measured by the force plates together make up the total force (Fig. 5–3).

A force plate is a sophisticated scale that can measure vertical (downward) force, similar to the body weight registered on a scale, as well as shear forces. Triaxial force plates measure the total force (a vector summation of all three components) acting on the center of pressure (a focal point under the foot at which the force is idealized to be concentrated). Preferably two platforms placed adjacent to each other are used so that the total force under each foot can be recorded independently and simultaneously. In most instances the force platforms are placed in the midpoint of the walkway and concealed in the floor so that steady-state, natural walking parameters are measured.

In our laboratory the components of the total force are measured using two triaxial force platforms. An innovation, however, is that the force is superimposed in real time as a visible line on an image of the walking subject at the location at which the force acts. This is accomplished using laser optics.[4] This force-line visualization system has significant clinical utility as it provides visual information regarding the effects of gravity on joint rotation without the need to instrument the patient.

A force is transmitted from the floor to the foot, then passed on up to all other body segments. The product of the magnitude of the GRF under each foot and its location with respect to a given joint center (ankle, knee, hip, etc.) are major factors that determine the torque or moments produced by the external force about that joint. This moment is a measure of the joint rotational tendency (flexion/extension, ab-/adduction, internal/external rotation) produced by the external force. Internal forces, generated primarily by muscles, ligaments, and the geometry of the joint articulation (bony contact), act to control the rotation of the joints caused by this external force. For example, the GRF when positioned anterior to the knee produces a moment that tends to drive the knee into extension and must be countered and controlled by muscle force (knee flexors/extensors, etc.).

Other components that contribute to the total joint moment are the products of the accelerations and masses of individual lower limb segments. It is important to note that the product of force and distance plus the product of mass and acceleration quantities constitute the total joint moment. The product of force and distance alone provides only an estimate of the total joint moment. The product of mass and acceleration (inertial effects) contributes a relatively small component to this total. Error caused by omitting inertial effects increases with increasing distance of a joint from the point of contact with the floor (1% at the ankle, 5% at the knee, and 8% at the hip).

The relative motion of body segments produces forces that affect the motion of the entire body. The inertial effects error just described is in part a reflection of the fact that all body segments are connected. This brings to light an important but not commonly considered concept that is currently an area of research in a few laboratories, namely, that the acceleration of each body segment affects the acceleration of all other segments in the body. A fairly sophisticated engineering analysis is necessary to quantify these interactions, but these effects should further our understanding of whole-body mechanics and interactions, and might ultimately reshape some of the traditional lines of thinking in gait biomechanics.

While force plates measure the sum or total force acting under the entire foot, it is sometimes useful to measure discrete components of that force acting over specific areas of the foot (the distribution of pressure). Pressure is defined as a force acting over a certain area: Pressure = Force/Area. A given force acting over an area of given size produces larger pressures than the same force acting over a large area. The pressure/time characteristics of the contact surface can have profound effects on the gait pattern. The forces generated at the point of contact with the floor can be measured with force platforms, as described above. Measuring the force distribution, for example, as it occurs inside the shoe necessitates using devices that can be placed inside the footwear and in direct contact with the foot without disturbing the foot-shoe interface. Ultrathin Mylar pressure-resistive sensors and specialized software permit the collection of multiple gait cycles. Analysis of this data is done by calibrated color pressure grids. Software allows evaluation of force and pressure as well as inte-

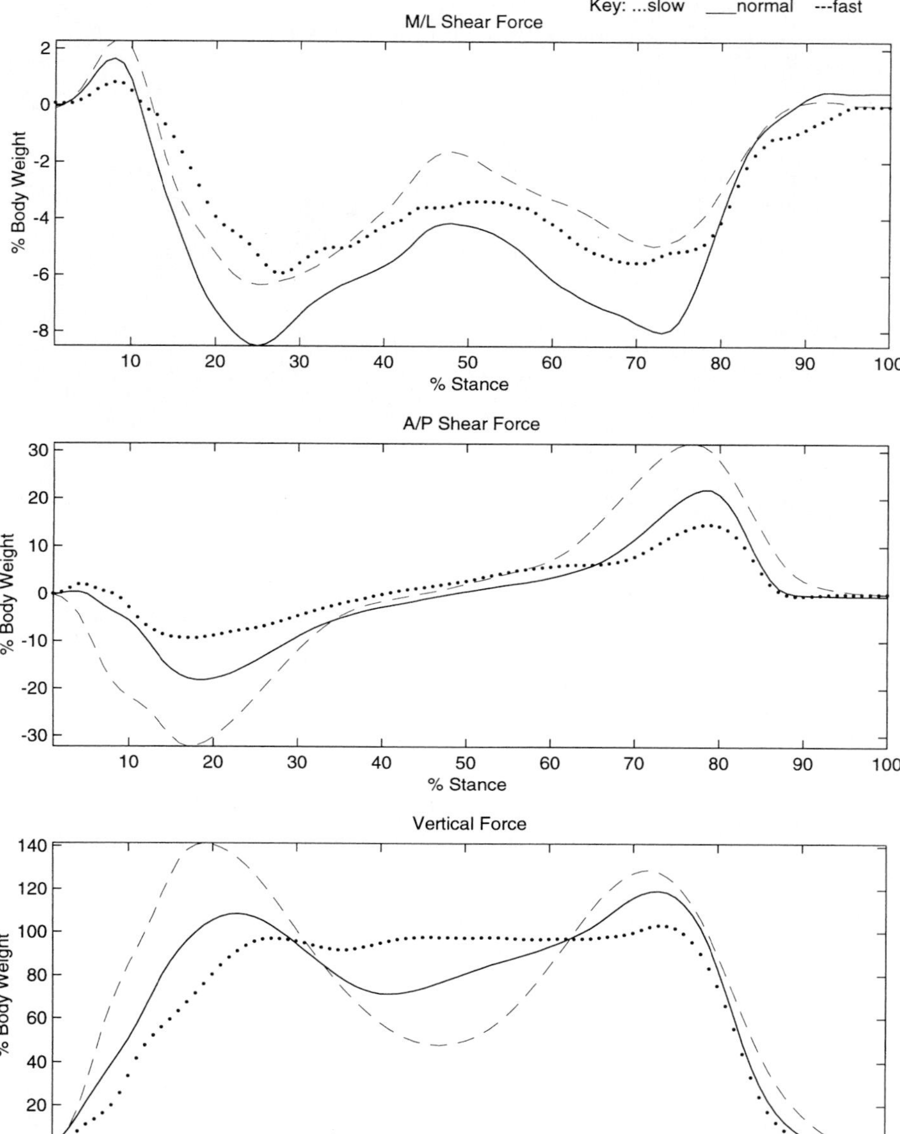

FIGURE 5–3. Effects of walking speed on force plate data (vertical, anteroposterior [A/P], and mediolateral [M/L] at slow, normal, and fast walking speeds). As walking speed increases, the peak forces of all components become more pronounced. At the fast speed, vertical force peaks at 140% of body weight.

grals of these measures. These systems are produced by TekScan in the United States and by others in Europe and Japan. Floor-embedded pressure sensor mats are also available to measure discrete pressures. One disadvantage of the floor mat is that only one step at a time can be captured, and frequent guidance to capture a complete step may be necessary because of the size of the mat sensor. Pressure measurement devices have clinical value particularly in the assessment of the deformed, insensate, or painful foot, and in the evaluation and fitting of customized foot or ankle-foot orthoses (Fig. 5–4).

Dynamic Polyelectromyography

In normal locomotion the body elicits forces from 28 muscles in each lower limb to carefully control the gravitational forces. The end result is a smooth, coordinated, energy-efficient movement pattern. Redundancy exists in the relationship between muscles and the joints upon which they act. This means that the association between a particular movement and the muscle forces producing the movement is not unique. The cause of a particular movement cannot be specifically assigned to a muscle based on the observed movement. Persons with spastic paraparesis secondary to brain or incomplete spinal cord injuries often present diagnostic challenges because muscle function is disrupted at many levels, and the overlay of spasticity often causes the muscle pattern expressed during clinical evaluation to differ significantly from the muscle pattern used during walking and standing.

The electrical activity of all of the muscles that are capable of producing the target movement needs to be evaluated, not just the electrical activity of a muscle

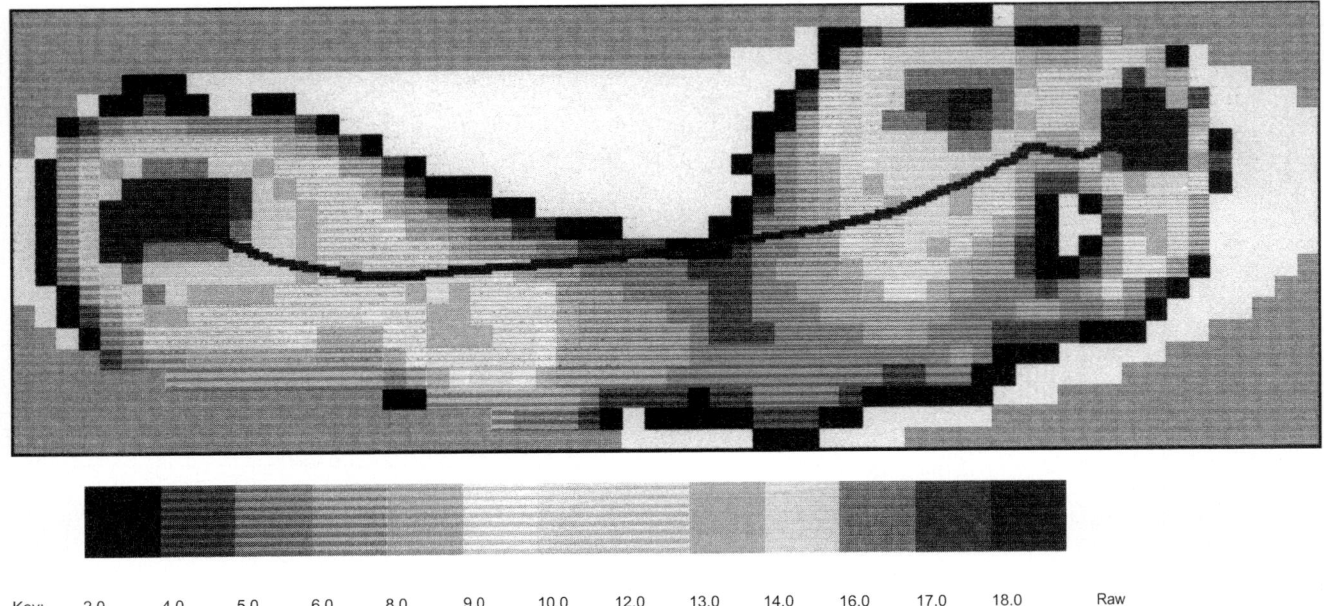

FIGURE 5–4. Graphic view of F-scan foot pressures. Top trace ishows a two-dimensional pressure map where shade (normally color) intensity indicates variations in pressure under the foot. Note the shade intensity (normally color coded) pressure key under the top trace. The horizontal line through middle of the foot is a trace of the center of pressure as the subject moves over the foot in the stance phase of gait cycle. The lower plot is a three-dimensional contour map showing the same pressure distribution as in the foot above. Peaks indicate high-pressure regions; valleys indicate lower-pressure regions. Outputs are normally provided in color; they are shown in gray scale for this text only.

directly spanning a particular segment or joint. EMG recordings provide information about the timing and duration of muscle activation (Fig. 5–5). Under certain conditions relative strength can also be determined. The EMG signal is an accurate indicator of muscle activation and can be used to infer neurological control information. Superficial muscles are preferentially studied using surface bipolar electrodes secured to the skin with double-sided tape after the skin has been prepared. For deep muscles or to differentiate between adjacent mus-

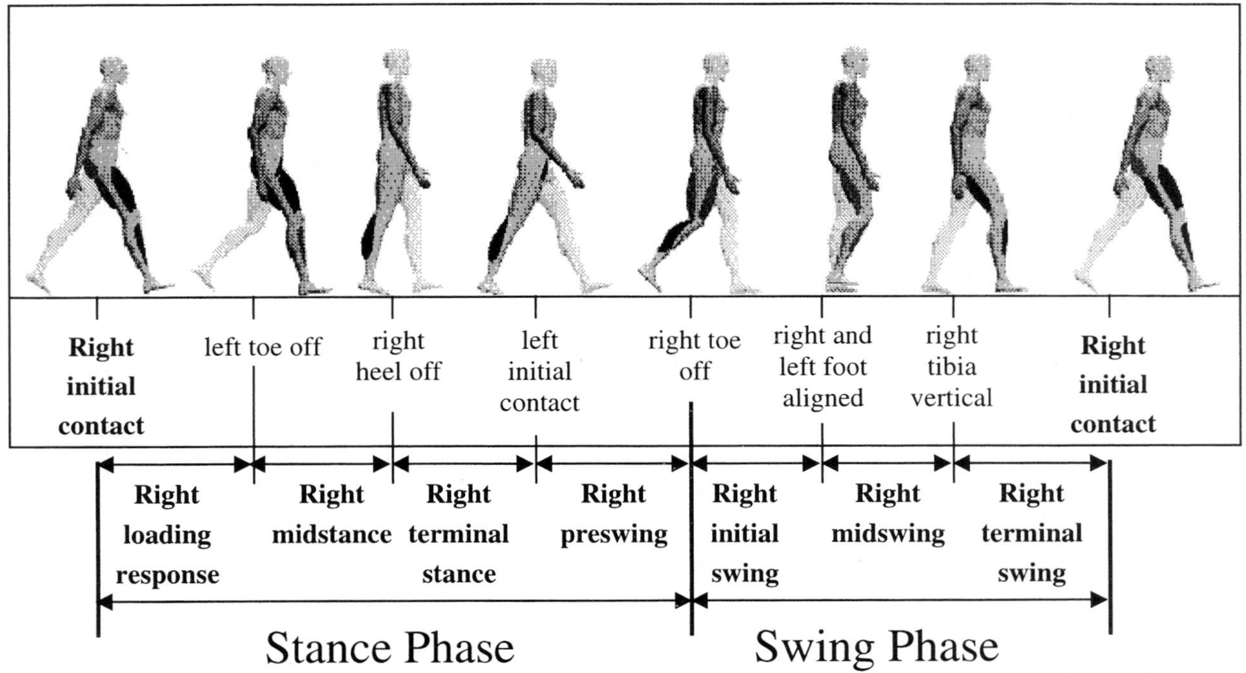

FIGURE 5–5. Normal walking gait cycle terminology with selected lower limb EMG representation. Human figures in the different phases of gait with superimposed primary gait muscles. Muscle shade intensity is roughly proportional to strength of muscle contraction.

cles when crosstalk might be of concern, a pair of indwelling fine wire electrodes is inserted through a 25-gauge hypodermic needle that is then immediately removed, leaving only the wires behind. The thin wires are 50 μ in diameter and are coated with Teflon or nylon except at their tips (Fig. 5–6).

EMG patterns are highly sensitive to walking speed. For this reason, it is incorrect and potentially misleading to compare the recording of a patient with a slow gait to that of an able-bodied control subject walking at a higher speed with a natural cadence. In addition to timing, amplitude of the EMG signal can provide valuable information for clinical decision making. A particular muscle can be over- or underactive during a given portion of the cycle. Such deviations should be carefully correlated with patient kinematics. When interpreting dynamic EMG data, it is important to distinguish cause from effect.

Patient EMG profiles can be compared to the mean and standard deviations of tabulated normative data, if speed matched, to identify how the patient's timing deviates from normative data. The timing classification scheme for EMG activity shown in Table 5–2 was devised in an attempt to standardize terminology.[9]

TABLE 5–2 Classification of Dynamic EMG Activity

I. Premature
II. Premature prolonged
III. Prolonged
IV. Out of phase
V. Normal

Kinematics

A kinematic analysis considers the patterns of motion, regardless of what forces (external or internal) are producing those motions, and the resulting temporal and spatial parameters.

Temporal and Spatial Descriptive Measures

Temporospatial measures afford a relatively simple and integrated method of quantifying some useful gait parameters. Temporospatial footfall patterns are the end product of the total integrated locomotor movement. Since gait is periodic, data from a single cycle or, better yet, an average of several cycles can be used to partially characterize a gait pattern. Measurement of basic temporal-spatial variables in stance and swing phases is often done. The data can be obtained by measuring the distances and timing that characterize the foot-floor contact patterns.

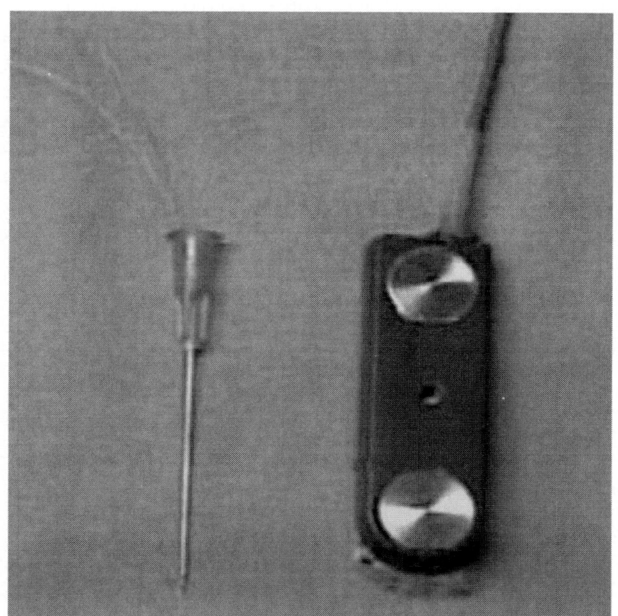

FIGURE 5–6. A wire EMG electrode. The needle shown is 24 gauge and 1.5 inches long. A standard surface electrode is shown for reference.

Available techniques range in sophistication from simpler systems using ink and paper, foot switches, and instrumented walkways to complex systems that require the patient to be instrumented. One example of a system that requires no patient instrumentation is the Electronic Gait Mat II. This instrumented walkway, 3.8 meters long, contains approximately 10,000 electronic switches, scanned at 100 Hz. Patients can use gait aids or shoes and braces, if necessary. They walk over the mat, which is mounted flush with the laboratory floor. A recording of foot contact generates a timed "electronic footprint." A printout provides calculated data about walking speed, cadence, and stance and swing times for each foot, as well as stride lengths, step lengths, and the width of the base of support.[6, 16] The data can be easily stored for future reference or analyzed in other ways.[7] Data from a subject's left and right sides can be compared to determine the extent of unilateral impairment. Comparisons can also be made to normative sex-, age-, and walking-speed-matched data. This allows an inference of the level of dysfunction.

Motion Analysis

Motion analysis produces a quantitative description of the motion of body segments without regard to the forces that are responsible for generating this motion. However, kinetic quantities such as joint reaction forces and moments are often combined with motion data to give a more complete picture of the coordinated total body movement pattern *and* the forces that are responsible for creating it. Measuring body segment motion in three dimensions is preferable, but it is sometimes done in two dimensions, due mainly to cost limitations. Early techniques included photographic and cinematographic analysis. Other techniques involve the use of accelerometers and electrogoniometers. Most modern systems use specialized optoelectronic apparatus. For the optoelectronic system, passive or active optical sources (e.g., infrared-reflecting markers or self-powered light-emitting diodes, respectively) are attached to the subject and serve as markers. Calibrated cameras or detectors track each marker as it moves with the subject. When two or more cameras or detectors identify the same marker, three-dimensional coordinates can be generated by mathematical triangulation, similar to the way in which we see an object with both eyes to gauge its depth (the third dimension).

Video and passive optoelectronic systems utilize retroreflective markers applied to the subject. The markers are illuminated by an external power source and are tracked by the detectors (camera). Near automatic marker identification and digitization is reliable if marker paths do not cross—as can usually be expected for standard marker placements in normal walking. However, conversion into quantitative data can require some manual intervention for marker identification in pathological gait, where increased limb rotation, sudden motions, or crossover of segment paths can occur. Manual digitization/tracking of the raw data can be error prone and in some instances time-consuming.[5, 13] With active optoelectronic systems, each marker is self-illuminated (hence the designation *active*). No postcollection marker identification is needed, because time sequencing between marker illumination and detector reception uniquely identifies each LED.[5] Each marker is activated at a slightly different (on the order of microseconds) instant in time. Telemetry (via infrared transmitters) in newer active systems such as the CODA MPX30 (Charnwood Dynamics Ltd., England) have eliminated the use of long wires or "umbilical cords" to power each marker. This has the advantage of ease of setup and cleanup, yet the subject is free from physically and psychologically restrictive cabling that was once the signature disadvantage of active systems.

Once the marker trajectories are available as three-dimensional data, they can be processed and displayed as a function of time or as a percentage of the gait cycle (normalized). Joint angles, linear and angular velocities, and accelerations are some of the commonly calculated measures that can be obtained once 3-D marker position is known. When these data are combined with anthropometric and kinetic (force) data, joint moments and powers as well as mechanical energy can be calculated. The physical meaning behind these quantities must be clearly understood if they are to provide any useful diagnostic information about the cause(s) of dysfunction.

ENERGETICS

Normal walking requires a relatively low level of metabolic energy consumption during steady state at comfortable walking speeds. Normal gait on level surfaces is most efficient at a walking speed of 1 to 1.3 m/sec, which is equivalent to 60 to 80 m/min or 3 miles/hr. Comfortable walking speed for an individual usually corresponds to minimum energy cost per unit distance. The center of mass is a point where all the mass of the body is idealized to be concentrated. In a homogeneous object, the center of mass is simply the geometric center of the object. For a symmetric object, like a sphere or cube, the center of mass is the center of the object. For the human body, the center of mass has been experimentally found to be located 2 cm in front of the second sacral vertebrae (in anatomic position). It has a dynamic nature (meaning that its location changes as the orientation of the body changes) and under certain conditions can even be located outside the body. The position of the center of mass is intimately related to the location of the GRF—simply put, they move in tandem. During walking the center of mass moves in a sinusoidal path with a mean of 5 cm of vertical and horizontal displacement. This displacement of the center of mass requires work, which in turn has an energy cost. The six determinants of gait described by Inman and colleagues (Table 5–3) were identified as the strategies necessary to produce forward progression with the least energy expenditure by minimizing the excursion of the center of mass.[14]

There is a link between motion of the center of mass and the energy expended during walking. Sudden acceleration or deceleration of the center of mass increases energy consumption. The three main events that consume energy during walking are controlled deceleration toward the end of swing phase, shock absorption at heel strike, and forward propulsion of the center of mass at push-off. Running is more efficient than walking, if walking speed is faster than 2 m/sec. Walking on a 10% to 12% incline doubles energy expenditure.

There are several methods of metabolic energy measurement, including indirect calorimetry, expired air collection, and heart rate monitoring. This last method can be used to calculate the energy expenditure index by subtracting the resting heart rate from the walking heart rate and dividing by the walking speed. This technique is subject to an error of 10% to 15% when compared with the other methods.

PATHOLOGICAL GAIT

At the beginning of this chapter, we used an anatomical approach to describe gait deviations. In this section we adopt a more functional approach in describing the various gait deviations likely to be seen and diagnosed clinically. Discussed are some common problems with base of support, limb and trunk instability, and limb clearance and advancement. We outline possible biomechanical implications and the manifestations of each disorder, and strategies to properly diagnose it. It should be noted

TABLE 5–3 Inman's Six Determinants of Gait

1. **Pelvic rotation in the horizontal plane:** The swinging hip moves forward faster than the stance hip.
2. **Pelvic tilt in the frontal plane:** The pelvis on the side of the swinging leg is lowered. This is controlled by activity in the hip abductors of the stance limb.
3. **Early knee flexion** (15 degrees) during the first part of stance.
4. **Weight transfer from the heel to flat foot** associated with controlled plantar flexion during the first part of stance.
5. **Late knee flexion** (30–40 degrees) during the last part of the stance phase.
6. **Lateral displacement of the pelvis toward the stance limb.** The aim of this determinant is to reduce the displacement of the CM.

that the biomechanics described are often similar, if not identical, for different base-of-support problems; the same can be said of other gait dysfunctions such as limb instability or impaired clearance. This suggests that biomechanics are not unique within a particular dysfunction or across dysfunction modalities. More important, this redundancy emphasizes the need to properly understand, diagnose, and treat the *primary* cause of the overall gait problem first. In some instances, after the primary cause has been treated, the additional abnormalities or deficiencies (compensations) in the gait pattern completely remedy themselves. Usually there is at least some change in gait character and severity once the patient has had a chance to come to a new plateau after treatment of the primary problem. Remaining deficiencies in the gait pattern can be addressed utilizing the same approach as indicated above.

Abnormal Base of Support

Base of support is presented first because it is literally the foundation upon which a stable gait pattern is built. An adequate base of support is critical to all aspects of gait. This is particularly true in regard to safety and comfort, since it is the foot-floor interaction that transmits the entire weight of the body to the ground and characterizes the GRF interaction with the body. The rate and magnitude of the loading (i.e., the gradual increasing of force under the stance leg) and unloading (the gradual decreasing of force as the leg prepares for swing phase) responses are shaped in large part by the interaction of the foot or feet with the ground. In addition, it is the location and magnitude of the GRF in relation to the joints that ultimately largely determine the joint moments that the muscles will have to stabilize and counteract.

Equinus Foot or Ankle

Equinus foot deformity is frequently seen after an upper or lower motor neuron injury. This deformity can also be the result of ankle immobilization, fractures, and surgery. The foot and ankle are in a toe-down and, frequently, turned-in (varus) position. Toe curling can coexist. In the resulting pathological gait, limb contact with the ground occurs first with the forefoot, and the weight is borne primarily on the anterior and lateral border of the foot and can be concentrated in the area of the fifth metatarsal, resulting in an antalgic gait. Toe flexion can be present, particularly in neurological injuries or cases where a plantar flexion contracture is present. Limited ankle dorsiflexion during mid-stance prevents forward progression of the tibia over the stationary foot, increasing pressure over the metatarsals, promoting ankle instability, and causing knee hyperextension. During the swing phase, sustained plantar flexion of the foot can result in a limb clearance problem unless proximal mechanisms of compensation such as increased hip and knee flexion are used.

A lower limb prosthesis set in excessive plantar flexion or set anterior to the trochanter-knee-ankle (TKA) line, or limited dorsiflexion of an articulated foot, can result in the same abnormal gait pattern. An ankle-foot orthosis that limits dorsiflexion beyond 8 degrees of equinus can also result in this same gait deviation (Fig. 5–7).

Ankle equinus posture during late stance and preswing interferes with rollover, push-off, and forward propulsion. This can be seen in the configuration of the vertical and AP GRFs. Clinical examination, combined with kinetics, kinematics, and dynamic EMG recordings, can elucidate the cause of the deformity. Overactivation of ankle plantar flexors during swing and/or stance phases or underactivation of ankle dorsiflexors during swing phase can lead to inadequate position of the foot during the stance phase. This can be seen on dynamic EMG studies, as well as manifesting as reduced or inadequate ankle range of motion. It also can be reflected in abnormal power generation or absorption. When it is difficult to differentiate between the muscular contribution of tibialis anterior and tibialis posterior to a varus deformity, a diagnostic tibial nerve block with lidocaine can be performed. If the deformity is corrected, then the tibialis posterior is most likely the offending muscle.

Case 1 is a clinical case presented to exemplify the use of the described methodology and technology for the evaluation of gait disorders and formulation of a treatment plan.

Equinovalgus Foot

The equinovalgus foot can be caused by a number of different problems, including limited ankle dorsiflexion, particularly in the child or young adult, in whom the subtalar joint can accommodate limited dorsiflexion with valgus posture. Upper or lower motor neuron injury, bony and ligamentous injuries, surgery, and prolonged immobilization with loss of ankle range of motion can all contribute to this deformity. During gait,

Text continued on page 106

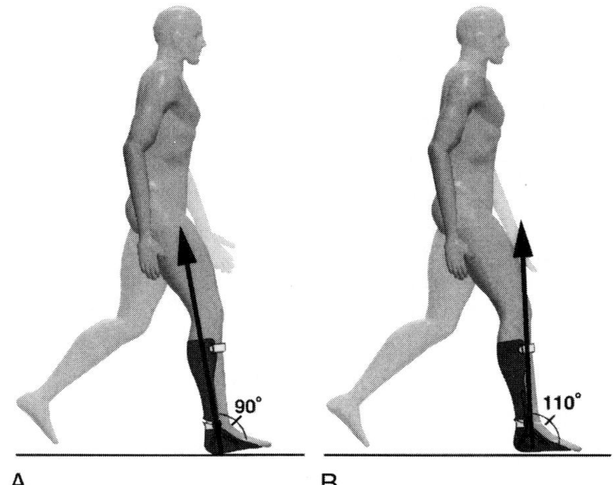

FIGURE 5–7. Effect of plantar flexed brace on position of force line. Note the position of the ground reaction force, indicated by an arrow from the floor through the leg. In the relatively dorsiflexed brace (*A*), the force vector passes slightly posterior to the knee joint center, thus producing a knee flexion moment. In *B*, the brace is more plantar flexed, and the force vector passes anterior to the knee joint, now producing a knee extension moment.

CASE STUDY 1

The patient is a 52-year-old man who was involved in an automobile collision with a truck 26 months prior to evaluation. He sustained severe craniocerebral trauma with residual spastic right hemiparesis. No pelvic or lower limb fractures were evident. He presented to the gait laboratory with difficulty ambulating and complaints of right ankle and knee pain aggravated by walking, as well as reduced balance. His right toes dragged against the ground if he did not pay attention to his walking. He used a right ankle-foot orthosis (plastic, moderate resistance, set in neutral ankle position) and a straight cane for walking outdoors. He walked without a cane at home. His past medical history was noncontributory.

Clinical Features of the Problem

Equinovarus of the right ankle-foot in terminal swing and stance phases. Right knee hyperextension in stance phase. Right stiff knee gait and occasional right toe drag. Poor balance with unstable gait.

Differential Diagnosis and Analysis

R/O ankle ligamentous instability or peripheral neuropathy.
R/O soft tissue contracture (static), dynamic deformity, or both.
Determine specific muscle(s) causing the ankle-foot deformity, i.e., gastrocnemius, soleus, tibialis anterior, tibialis posterior, extensor hallucis longus (EHL), flexor digitorum longus (FDL), peroneus longus.

Diagnostic Workup

On examination the patient was an alert, pleasant, cooperative, moderately obese man in no acute distress. His body weight was 105 kg. Passive range-of-motion and manual muscle testing yielded the following data:

	Right	*Left*	*Normal*
Ankle			
Dorsi./plantar	−15/50	0/50	0 to 20/0 to 50
Strength	0/3+	4+/5	5/5
Inv./eversion	30/20	30/20	0 to 30/0 to 20
Strength	3+/0	5/5	5/5
Knee			
Ext./flexion	−5/130	0/130	0/135
Strength	4+/4+	5/5	5/5
Hip			
Ext./flexion	−10/120	0/120	0/120
Strength	4+/4+	5/4+	5/5
Abd./Add.	25/30	25/30	0 to 50/0 to 30
Strength	4+/5	5/5	5/5
IR/ER	30/50	30/50	30/50
Scoliosis: none			
Flexibility			
Ely Test	+	−	
SLR	−	−	
LE Ashworth	2	1	
Ankle selective control	I	N	
Knee selective control	I	N	
Hip selective control	N	N	
Ankle joint instability/effusion	−	−	
Knee joint instability/effusion	+	−	
Clonus			
Ankle	+ sustained	+ unsustained	
Patellar	−	−	
Sensation			
Light touch	+	+	
Proprioception	+	+	
Leg length (cm)	95.5	96	

Key: Ashworth Scale: 0 = none, 1 = slight increase ½ ROM, 2 = increase all ROM, 3 = difficult PROM, 4 = rigid. MS = 0 to 5/5. Selective control: N = normal, I = impaired, U = unable.

Expected Functional Penalties

These included impaired right limb weight bearing, decreased balance, and decreased right leg weight acceptance. Also expected were increased right loading phase time and decreased unloading phase time, as well as increased pressure over the lateral portion of the right foot with decreased heel weight bearing and resulting ankle inversion instability. Right forefoot and ankle pain during the loading phase, prolonged right stance time, shortened right step length, right genu recurvatum with knee pain, and hip flexion during stance phase were also expected. Impaired smooth, forward progression of the center of gravity (CG), increased vertical displacement of CG, functional leg length discrepancy (ankle equinus), and increased energy consumption were predicted as well.

Instrumented Gait Analysis

Video with slow motion and superimposed force line visualization was done with temporospatial parameters of locomotion. Poly-EMG was done of the gastrocnemius, soleus, tibialis anterior, tibialis posterior, extensor hallucis longus, flexor digitorum longus, and peroneus longus. To simplify the analysis, hip and knee muscles were not evaluated at this time. Kinematic data were gathered to quantify ankle equinus and varus, as well as the effect of this deformity on other joints and temporospatial parameters of locomotion. Kinetic analysis to quantify joint moments and powers was included.

Findings (Fig. 5–8)

Video frame-by-frame analysis disclosed abnormal right ankle foot posture with equinus, varus, and toe flexion in swing phase. Ankle equinus and varus as well as toe curling were evident in stance phase. Abnormal force line location in front of the right knee was notes (Fig. 5–8). Kinematic data demonstrated limitation in right hip range of motion. The right hip was abducted and slightly externally rotated. The right knee exhibited reduced flexion with valgus in late stance phase. Increased internal rotation of the knee was evident. The right ankle exhibited markedly increased inversion and limited dorsiflexion. Slight limitation in left ankle dorsiflexion was also evident. Other parameters appeared to be within normal limits (Fig. 5–8). Kinetic data demonstrated a reduction in the right hip and knee extensor moment and reduced power generation. The right ankle also exhibited a reduction in power generation (Fig. 5–8). Poly-EMG demonstrated the gastrocnemius more than the soleus having abnormal activation (out of phase) in swing phase and premature activation in stance phase. The peroneus longus exhibited premature-prolonged activation in stance with abnormal activity in swing phase—a compensation attempting to control ankle posture. The tibialis posterior exhibited no significantly abnormal activation in swing phase, but appeared to activate prematurely in stance phase. The tibialis anterior activated prematurely in swing phase and abnormally in late stance phase. This muscle appeared to be the primary cause of the ankle inversion during swing phase. The FDL demonstrated increased activation in stance phase. The EHL demonstrated increased activation in swing phase and an abnormally low level of activation in the stance phase that was most likely to supplement the tibialis anterior and/or because of spastic response.

Impression

The right equinus posture appeared to be caused by overactivation of gastrocnemius more than of the soleus. The ankle varus resulted from out-of-phase activation of the tibialis anterior and EHL. No abnormal activation of the tibialis posterior was evident in the

Case study continued on following page

Gait Analysis Report MossRehab Hospital

JW061409.MDR JW061409.MDR

Patient Data:

Sex	Age	Date of Birth	Height (m)	Weight (kg)
Male	52	07/46	1.899	105

Gait Parameters	Left	Right	Normal
Speed (m/s)	1.10	1.03	1.66
Stride Length (m)	1.14	1.03	1.54
Stride Time (s)	1.04	1.00	0.92
Strides/Minute	57.69	60.30	64.86
Step Length (m)	0.68	0.46	0.77
Step Time (s)	0.52	0.52	0.46
Steps/Minute	114.94	115.16	129.73
Percent Stance	79.04	68.94	65.95
Single Support (s)	0.31	0.22	0.31
Double Support (s)	0.30	0.21	0.15

Joint Angles (deg)	Left	Right
Hip Range	41.30	22.00
Hip Max	35.20	23.60
Hip Min	−6.10	1.60
Knee Range	41.50	30.70
Knee Max	39.90	25.90
Knee Min	−1.60	−4.80
Ankle Range	24.10	17.20
Ankle Max	14.70	10.90
Ankle Min	−9.40	−6.30

FIGURE 5–8. Patient data generated by CODA mpx30. See Case 1 text.

Illustration continued on following page

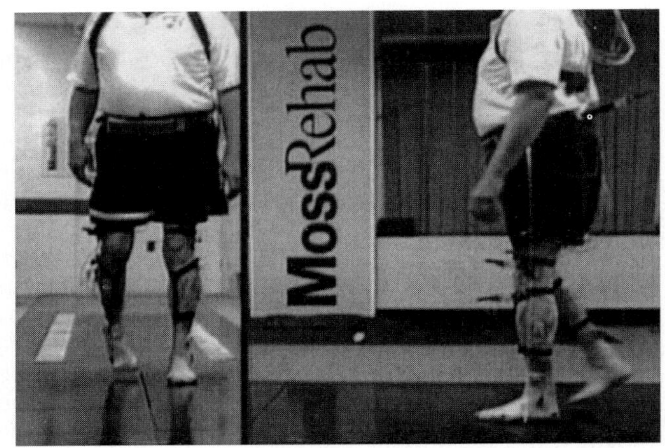

Kinematics: Single Cycle

MossRehab Gait Lab

Page 2

Left: JW061409.MDR

Right: JW061409.MDR

Normal:

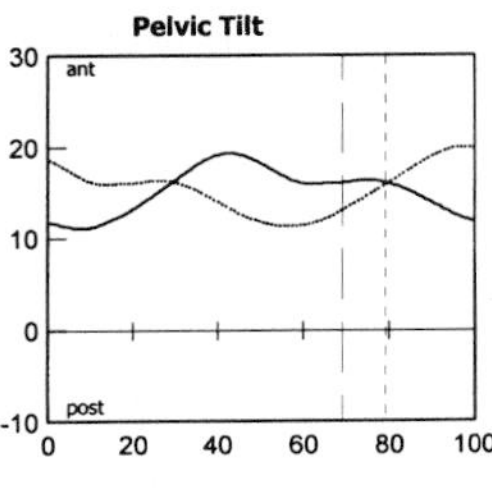

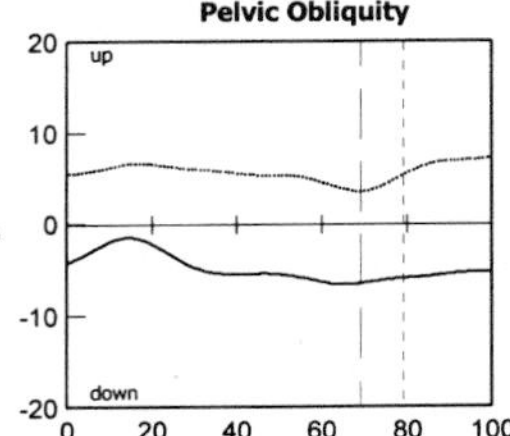

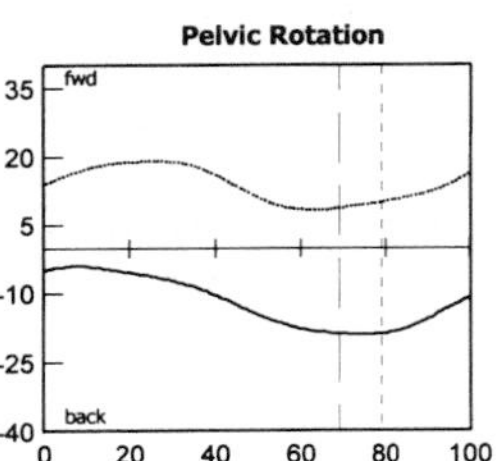

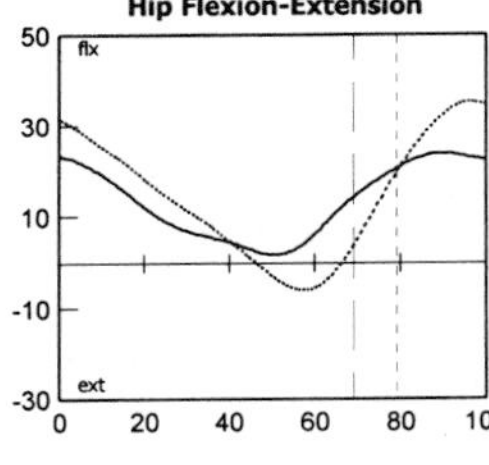

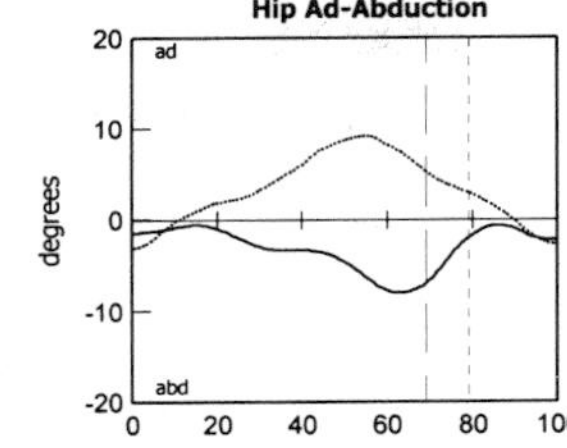

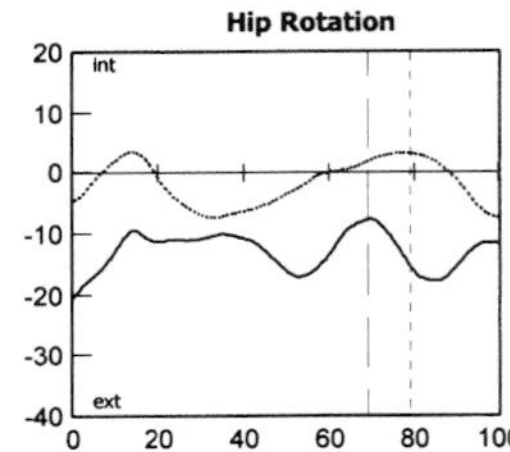

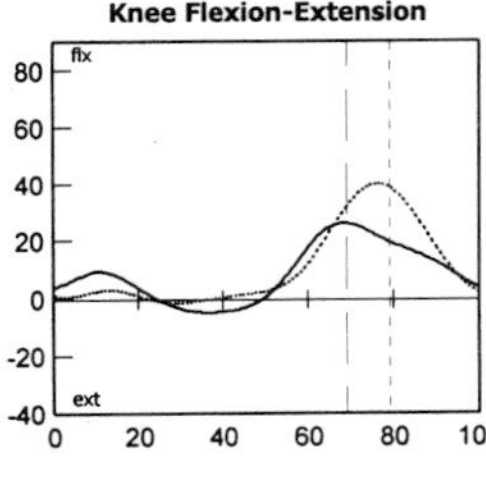

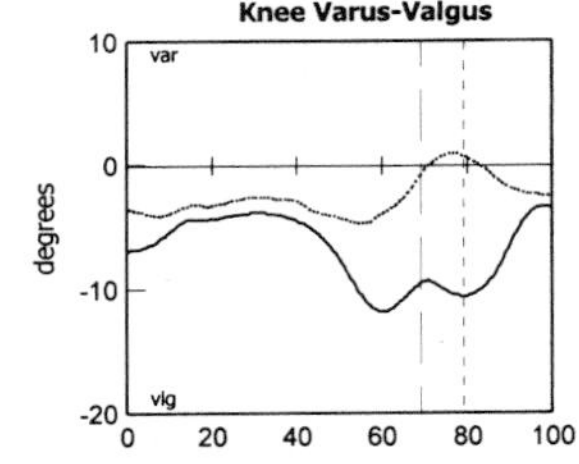

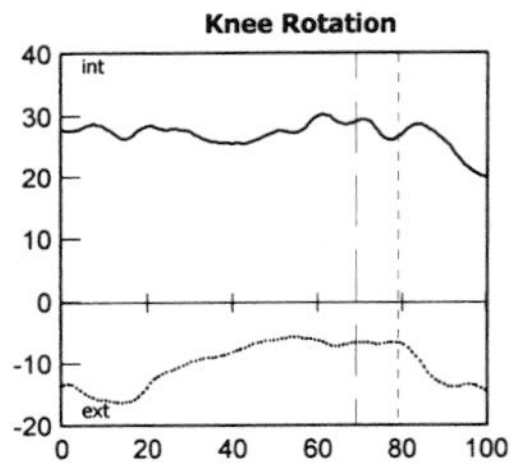

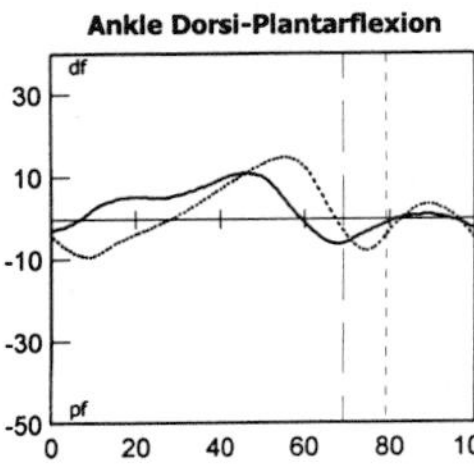

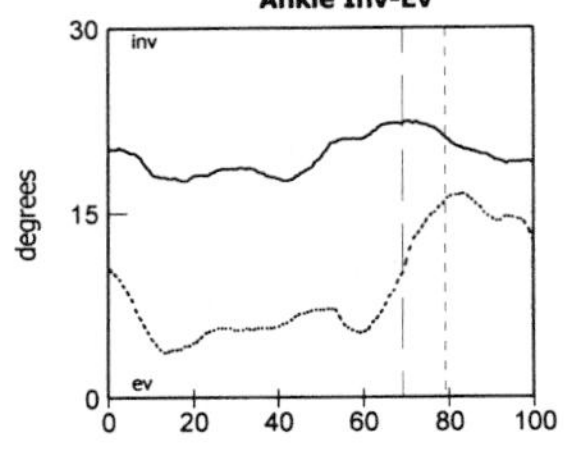

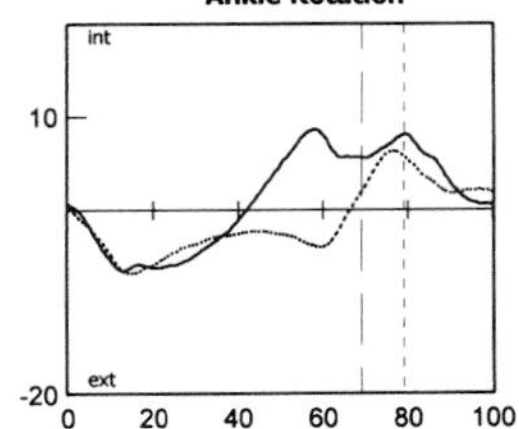

FIGURE 5–8 *Continued*

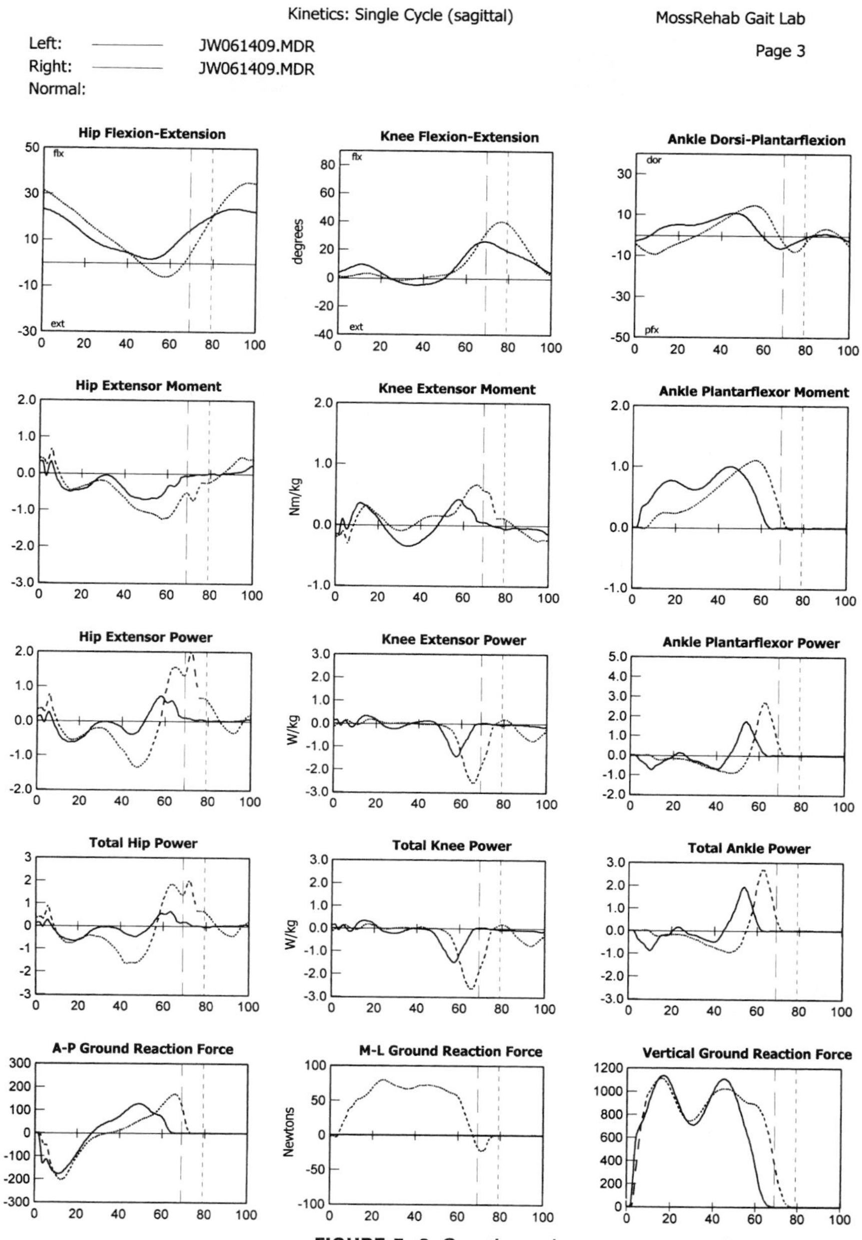

FIGURE 5–8 *Continued*

Illustration continued on following page

swing phase of this evaluation. The reduction in right hip, knee, and ankle power were felt to be related to the abnormal-ankle-foot posture. A spastic right "stiff knee" could not be ruled out. There was no evidence of right knee hyperextension on the kinematic data, but this could be related to the mechanical joint limitation in extension (see findings under Examination). Stretching of the hamstrings during stance phase was felt to be the cause of knee pain.

Possible Treatment Interventions

1. Imaging of the right knee to rule out bony block or a foreign intra-articular body.
2. Possible use of Botox or other focal antispasticity intervention applied to right ankle plantar flexors (gastrocnemius more than soleus) and tibialis anterior (avoid overdose for this muscle), followed by rehabilitation interventions to stretch the Achilles tendon and strengthen the ankle dorsiflexors; also, gait retraining is warranted.
3. Since Botox will most likely require repeated injections and the patient is more than 2 years post injury, surgical intervention in the form of Achilles tendon lengthening (TAL), split tibialis anterior tendon transfer (SPLATT), and myotendinous lengthening of the EHL can be considered. To supplement the weak ankle plantar

Case study continued on following page

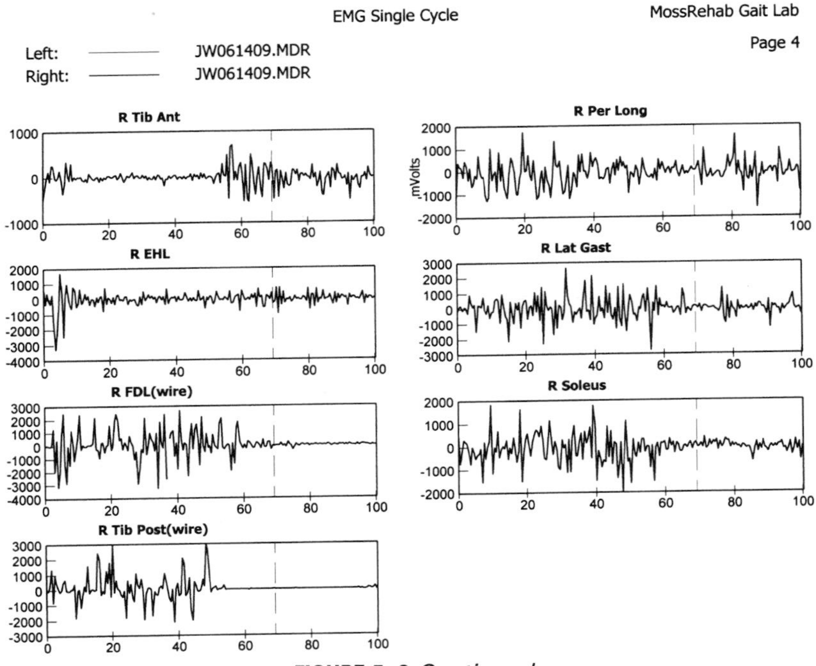

FIGURE 5–8 *Continued*

flexors and avoid toe curling when the ankle dorsiflexion ROM is increased, a release and transfer of the long toe flexors to the os calcis can be considered. Rehabilitation interventions to strengthen ankle plantar flexors and dorsiflexors are appropriate. Gait retraining followed by reevaluation for stiff knee is recommended if gait deviation continues.

contact with the ground occurs with the forefoot and weight is borne primarily on the medial aspect of the foot. This position is maintained or worsened during the stance phase and interferes with weight bearing. Antalgic gait can be present if the navicular is overloaded. During the swing phase, sustained plantar flexion of the foot can result in a limb clearance problem unless proximal mechanisms of compensation such as increased hip and knee flexion are used.

Combined with clinical and radiographic examinations, dynamic EMG recordings provide greater detail in delineating the cause of the deformity. If the deformity is muscular in type and due to an upper motor neuron injury, it can be difficult to differentiate between the valgus contribution of the peroneus longus and the peroneus brevis; for this a diagnostic lidocaine motor point block of one of them can be performed.

Flexion Deformity of the Toes

The toes might be held in flexion during the swing and stance phases of gait. When wearing shoes, the patient complains of pain at the tips of the toes and also over the dorsum of the phalangeal joints; the pain worsens with weight bearing. Callus formation in these areas is frequently seen. The gait pattern typically shows gradual loading of the affected limb and shortening of the step length and stance time. Likely causes include neurological injuries, a complex regional pain syndrome, prolonged immobilization, and contractures. Clinical examination combined with kinetics and dynamic EMG recordings can be helpful in sorting out the cause of the deformity. In patients with spasticity the recordings likely will demonstrate prolonged or out-of-phase activation of the flexor digitorum longus and flexor hallucis longus, and can demonstrate abnormal co-activation of the gastrocnemius and soleus or lack of activation of the toe extensors.

Hitchhiker's Great Toe

This deformity is seen in patients with upper motor neuron dysfunction. The great toe is held in extension during stance and frequently during the swing phase. Equinus and varus posture of the ankle might accompany this deformity. When wearing shoes, the patient frequently complains of pain at the dorsum and the tip of the big toe, as well as under the first metatarsal head during the weight-bearing phase of the gait cycle. During gait, big toe extension can interfere with the weight-bearing phase of locomotion. Overactivation of the extensor hallucis longus and reduction or lack of activation of the flexor hallucis longus frequently contribute to this deformity. The combination of clinical examination and dynamic EMG recordings is helpful in determining the source of the deformity and whether it is obligatory or compensatory in nature.

Joint Instability

Ankle Instability ("Drop-off" Gait)

This deviation is caused by excessive and untimely forward progression of the tibia in the mid- to late stance phase. This is usually the result of insufficient calf musculature, which is needed to control the forward progression of the tibia over the stationary foot. In the older literature this clinical picture is referred to as a "weak calf limp." Manual muscle testing of the ankle plantar flexors can be performed by having patients walk on their toes. Obtaining kinetic and kinematic data and dynamic EMG recordings may be necessary to elucidate the biomechanical causes of the problem.

Knee Instability

Knee instability refers to either knee buckling or hyperextension and typically occurs in early stance phase when knee flexion would normally occur; it is usually due to quadriceps weakness. This weakness can be seen in persons with a lower motor neuron syndrome, other types of knee extensor weakness, or quadriceps tendon rupture. It can also be seen in the early phase of recovery after upper motor neuron injury, when the involved limb is flaccid and weak. A knee flexion deformity further complicates this problem. If knee buckling occurs, the patient might need to use the upper extremities for support. The patient might not produce the normally expected full knee extension in either late swing phase or stance phase, further compromising limb stability. Bilateral knee and hip flexion may be present and can result in a crouched gait. This posture increases energy consumption markedly and results in muscle fatigue and joint pain. The lack of full knee extension in terminal swing limits limb advancement and reduces step length.

Knee hyperextension can be a compensation for knee extensor weakness during stance phase. Knee hyperextension can also be present in this phase of gait as a result of an ankle plantar flexion contracture or as a result of spastic ankle equinus produced by increased activity of the gastrocnemius-soleus group. Marked weakness of the ankle plantar flexor muscle group can produce a "drop-off" gait that the patient may compensate for with knee hyperextension in an attempt to prevent knee flexion. Spasticity of the knee extensors and forward trunk flexion can be another cause of knee hyperextension during the stance phase.

Hip Instability

Excessive hip flexion during stance phase is a less common gait deviation. This deformity is characterized by sustained hip flexion that interferes with limb positioning during gait. During the stance phase, excessive hip flexion interferes with contralateral limb advancement and results in a shortened step length. Possible causes include degenerative changes of the hip joint, bony deformities such as heterotopic ossification, knee extensor weakness and ankle plantar flexor posture, hip flexion contractures, and hip flexor spasticity.

Hip adduction that occurs during the swing phase interferes with limb clearance and advancement. During stance phase, hip adduction results in a narrow base of support with a potential balance impairment. Because many patients can compensate for hip flexion weakness by using the hip adductors to advance the limb during the swing phase, the clinician needs to be certain that reducing or eliminating hip adductor activity does not interfere with hip flexion. Dynamic poly-EMG of the hip flexors, adductors, and abductors can provide critical information on this issue. Some patients also benefit from a temporary diagnostic obturator nerve block so that the clinician can fully delineate the gait issues involved. In addition to causing a gait problem, severe hip adduction can interfere with hygiene, dressing, toileting, and sexual expression.

Trunk Instability

Trunk instability is an abnormal anterior or lateral lean of the trunk during walking, when the trunk normally is mostly upright. Trunk instability can result from hip extensor weakness, limited hip extension, compensation for knee extensor weakness and ankle plantar flexor posture, and hip flexor spasticity. Hip hiking and contralateral trunk lean can be used to compensate for decreased limb advancement and swing phase clearance problems.

Limb Clearance and Advancement

Limb clearance and advancement occur during the swing phase of gait and are vital precursors to proper limb positioning so that the leg can accept the body weight during the ensuing stance phase. When limb clearance is inadequate, limb advancement is usually compromised. Impaired limb clearance can cause a patient to trip and fall, particularly when walking on uneven, inclined or carpeted surface. Reduction of limb advancement produces shortening of step length and a reduction in walking speed.

Stiff Knee Gait

Stiff knee gait is most commonly seen in patients with spastic hemiplegia. The use of a locked knee prosthesis for the transfemoral amputee or a locked knee brace by a patient who really needs a knee-ankle-foot orthosis can also cause this gait deviation. In stiff knee gait, the knee and hip maintain an extended attitude in the swing phase instead of flexing up to the normal 60 degrees for the knee and 30 degrees for the hip. Even if the ankle-foot system has an appropriate dorsiflexed position, the lack of adequate limb clearance can result in a foot drag. At times only a mild reduction in range of motion of the knee and hip is present, but it can be delayed in relationship to the gait cycle. The patient's inability to flex the knee in an appropriate manner results in increased inertia, which requires more hip flexion activity to advance the leg during the swing phase. The patient will use compensatory mechanisms for limb clearance. These mechanisms may include trunk and ipsilateral hip mechanisms. Contralateral limb compensatory motions such as vaulting (early heel rise) can also be present.

Excessive Pelvic Obliquity (Pelvic Drop)

Increased hip adduction can interfere with limb advancement by contacting the contralateral stance leg. In contrast to ipsilateral swing phase hip adductor activity, stance phase hip abductor weakness can compromise both limb clearance and advancement. Normally, hip abductors help counter gravity's pull on the swing side pelvis by producing an abductor moment that helps keep the pelvis level. Weakness can allow the pelvis to sag (more obliquity). Imbalance in the abductor and adductor muscle groups is the main cause. Because many hemiplegic patients use the adductors to compensate for reduced hip flexion in limb advancement, the clinician needs to be certain that elimination or reduction of adductor activities does not result in the patient becoming nonambulatory.

Inadequate Hip Flexion

Inadequate hip flexion is another cause of abnormal limb clearance. This problem effectively prevents physiological "shortening" of the limb, producing a swing-phase toe drag or early foot contact. The use of compensatory techniques such as hip external rotation or circumduction to promote the use of the adductors to advance the limb should be attempted. The use of a shoe lift to cause functional lengthening of the contralateral limb can also be done.

Drop Foot

Drop foot refers to the lack of ankle dorsiflexion during the swing phase, which can result in impairment of limb clearance during swing phase. Compensation for this frequently includes increased knee and hip flexion (steppage gait), or vaulting up on the toes of the contralateral limb to make it functionally longer. A frequent cause of drop foot is lack of activation of the tibialis anterior. This can be secondary to a peroneal nerve injury, loss of strength such as that seen in residual polio, spastic imbalance between ankle plantar flexors and dorsiflexors, or out-of-phase activation of the tibialis anterior in the swing phase of locomotion.

SUMMARY

Gait analysis is a key adjunct to clinical examination and other diagnostic studies in the management of walking and mobility problems. When used appropriately by a clinician who can adequately interpret the data, these tools and methods can provide direct evidence of cause and effect in an otherwise redundant physiological system, a system that can produce a deformity or deviation based on many different muscle and joint interactions or adaptive mechanisms. Gait analysis can also help differentiate primary problems from those that are compensatory in nature. Gait analysis should be seen as a necessary diagnostic test to guide the development of a rational treatment intervention strategy in patients with moderate to severe gait dysfunction. This is particularly true if surgery or other nonreversible treatment is being considered. Computerized gait analysis also can be used as an outcome assessment tool to determine the effects of therapeutic interventions or to assess progression of conditions affecting gait. The results of gait analysis can be used to address gait dysfunction treatment, including the prescription of therapeutic exercises, the optimal design and alignment of orthoses, pharmacological treatment (local or intrathecal or systemic), prosthetic alignment optimization, and surgical planning. A clear understanding of the biomechanics of normal locomotion, pathological gait, and the potential pitfalls of gait analysis is necessary to use this technique appropriately for the benefit of patients.

REFERENCES

1. Bampton S: A Guide to the Visual Examination of Pathological Gait. Philadelphia, Temple University–Moss Rehabilitation Hospital, Rehabilitation Research and Training Center, no 8, 1979.
2. Bernstein N: The technique of the study of movements. In Conrady G, Farfel V, Slonim A (eds): Textbook of the Physiology of Work. Moscow, 1934.
3. Cappozzo A: Gait analysis methodology. Hum Movement Sci 1984; 3:27–50.
4. Cook TM, Cozzens BA, Kenosian H: A Technique for Force-Line Visualization. Rehabilitation Engineering Center, no 2, Moss Rehabilitation Hospital. Philadelphia, Temple University, March 1979.
5. Esquenazi A, Hirai B: Assessment of gait and orthotic prescription. Phys Med Rehab: Clin North Am 1991; 2(3):473–485.
6. Esquenazi A, Keenan MAE: Gait analysis. In Delisa J, Gans B (eds): DeLisa's Rehabilitation Medicine: Principles and Practice, ed 2. Philadelphia, JB Lippincott, 1993, pp 122–130.
7. Esquenazi A, Talaty M: Gait analysis. In Physical Medicine and Rehabilitation: "The Complete Approach." Cambridge, MA, Blackwell Science, in press.
8. Inman VT, Ralston HJ, Todd F: Human Walking. Baltimore, Williams & Wilkins, 1981.
9. Keenan MAE, Haider T, Stone LR: Dynamic electromyography to assess elbow spasticity. J Hand Surg 1990; 15A:607–614.
10. Marey EJ: La Methode graphique dans les sciences experimentales et particularierement en physiologie et en medicine. Deuxieme tirage augmente d'un supplement sur le development de le methode graphique par l'emploi de la photographie. Paris, Masson, 1885.
11. Mayer N, Keenan MA, Esquenazi A: Limbs with restricted or excessive motion after traumatic brain injury. In Rosenthal M, Griffith ER, Kreutzer JS, Pentland B (eds): Rehabilitation of the Adult and Child with Traumatic Brain Injury, ed 3. Philadelphia, FA Davis, 1999, pp. 503–535.
12. Muybridge E: Animal Locomotion: An Electro-Photographic Investigation of Consecutive Phases of Animal Movements. Philadelphia, Published under the auspices of the University of Pennsylvania, 1887.
13. Rowell D, Mann RW: Human movement analysis. Soma 1989; 3(2):13–20.
14. Saunders JB, Inman VT, Eberhart HD: The major determinants in normal and pathological gait. J Bone Joint Surg Am 1953; 35:543–558.
15. Schwartz RP, Health AL, Misiek W, et al: Kinetics of human gait: The making and interpretation of electrobasographic records of gait. J Bone Joint Surg Am 1934; 16:343–350.
16. Taylor DR: An instrumented gait mat. In Proceedings of the International Conference on Rehabilitation Engineering. Toronto, IEEE Society, 1980, pp 278–279.

6

CHAPTER

Robert D. Rondinelli, M.D., Ph.D.

Practical Aspects of Impairment Rating and Disability Determination

Within the field of physical medicine and rehabilitation, the topics of impairment rating and disability determination have generally been overlooked in the preparation of formal teaching materials, in establishing preceptorships within the major training programs, in key rehabilitation texts written by and for physiatrists, and in the attention given to the subject by the American Board of Physical Medicine and Rehabilitation. Physiatric representation and participation on the physician advisory panel to the American Medical Association's *Guides to the Evaluation of Permanent Impairment,*[2] which is the standard reference manual for rating worker compensation injuries in the United States, appears disproportionately low. Physiatrists represent only about 5% of physician contributors to this text, even though approximately 40% of the content is devoted to the musculoskeletal system. This is particularly problematic because impairment, disability, and handicap are the conceptual underpinnings of our specialty and the clinical focal point of virtually all rehabilitative problem solving.

This chapter attempts to provide the reader with a working vocabulary and conceptual understanding of the processes of impairment rating and disability determination. The discussion equally considers their inherent shortcomings and pitfalls at the present time. The chapter is also intended to provide an orientation to the AMA *Guides,* and to focus on key aspects of the examination and reporting requirements for the physician examiner in cases of compensable injury. All of this information should foster a heightened awareness of the importance of these topics to our field and the need for more formalized didactic treatment and research efforts by physiatrists.

DEFINITIONS AND TERMINOLOGY

Definitions

The World Health Organization (WHO) definitions are as follows[39]:

Impairment: "any loss or abnormality of psychological, physiological, or anatomic structure or function."

Disability: "any restriction or lack (resulting from an impairment) of ability to perform an activity in the manner or within the range considered normal for a human being."

Handicap: "a disadvantage for a given individual, resulting from an impairment or a disability, that limits or prevents the fulfillment of a role that is normal (depending on age, sex, and social and cultural factors) for that individual."

The fourth edition of the AMA *Guides*[2] provides the following working definitions for purposes of medical reporting:

Impairment: "the loss, the loss of use, or derangement of any body part, system or function" (p. 315).

Permanent impairment: "impairment that has become static or well stabilized with or without medical treatment, and is not likely to remit despite medical treatment" (p. 315).

Disability: "a decrease in, or the loss or absence of the capacity of an individual to meet personal, social, or occupational demands or to meet statutory or regulatory requirements" (p. 317).

Permanent disability: "occurs when the limiting loss or absence of capacity becomes static or well stabilized and is not likely to change in spite of continuing use of medical or rehabilitative measures" (p. 317).

Handicap: "refers to 'obstacles' to accomplishing life's basic activities that may be overcome only by . . . compensation or accommodation" (p. 2).

Impairment can be considered in absolute terms, but its relationship to disability and handicap tends to be a relative one. Disability and handicap are perhaps best viewed in the context of performing specific tasks or functions (Table 6–1). In terms of employment, for example, if the impaired individual can perform the task or function required of the job without specific accommodation, no disability or handicap exists relative to that function. If the impaired individual can successfully perform only in the presence of specific accommodation, and if that accommodation is provided, again no disability or handicap exists relative to that function. If the impaired individual can successfully perform only in the presence of accommodation, yet the accommodation is not provided, both disability and handicap exist. If the impaired individual cannot successfully perform even in the presence of "reasonable accommodation," a disability exists and a handicap might exist, depending upon the degree to which social barriers preclude full accommodation.

Although disability can arise out of impairment, it is not determined solely (or, for that matter, in large part) by the impairment. In fact, similar levels of impairment can give rise to substantially different disabilities. Handicap can be considered the degree to which social barriers (e.g., "undue hardship" or "direct threat") to accommodation exist and, consequently, bears an inverse relationship to accommodation.

Terminology

Following are some of the terms that frequently appear in the process and procedures of impairment evaluating and reporting.

Aggravation: A circumstance or event that (temporarily or permanently) worsens a preexisting or underlying and susceptible condition.[2]

Apportionment: A determination of percentage of impairment directly attributable to preexisting or resulting conditions and directly contributing to the total impairment rating derived.[2]

Causality: An association between a given cause (an event capable of producing an effect) and an effect (a condition that can result from a specific cause) within a reasonable degree of medical probability. Causality requires determination that:

An event took place.

The claimant experiencing the event has the condition (impairment).

The event could cause the condition (impairment).

It is medically probable that the event caused the condition (impairment).[2, 29]

Diagnosis-related estimates (DREs): Estimates of impairment assigned on the basis of a diagnosis rather than on the basis of findings on physical examination.[2, p. 84] The AMA *Guides* provide DREs for regional impairments affecting the spine and extremities. The rating physician must choose between the impairment estimate derived by diagnostic and that derived by examination criteria for a specific region. The physician is encouraged to use whichever approach yields the greater estimate.

Ergonomics: The science of matching the job to the worker and the product to the user. An effective match optimizes efficiency, safety, comfort, and ease of use.

Functional capacity assessment (FCA): A generic assessment of an individual's job-related functional abilities, including strength, flexibility, endurance, and overall capability to perform physical work. The FCA can be useful in case disposition in which no specific job is available to an impaired individual, and when general guidelines and restrictions are needed for purposes of job counseling and vocational rehabilitation.[18]

Functional capacity evaluation (FCE): A comprehensive assessment of an individual's strength, flexibility, endurance, and job-specific functional abilities. An FCE includes a feasibility assessment of the impaired individual's ability to perform the essential functions of a specific job and could be the most valid predictor of return-to-work potential and restrictions applicable in a given case.[1]

Independent medical evaluation (IME): In cases involving workers' compensation in which either party disputes maximum medical improvement (MMI; see below), an administrative law judge can refer to a separate physician examiner for a second opinion regarding MMI and impairment rating.[2, 29] Some regard an IME as any examination done for evaluation purposes by a physician other than the treating physician.

Job description: A formal listing of the essential functions that constitute a particular job in terms of their specific physical performance requirements.[18]

TABLE 6–1 Relationships of Impairment, Disability, and Handicap

Impairment Present	Individual Can Perform Essential Functions	Accommodation Necessary to Perform	Accommodation Provided	Disability	Handicap
Yes	Yes	No	No	No	No
Yes	No	Yes	No	Yes	Yes
Yes	No	Yes	Yes	No	No
Yes	No*	Yes*	Yes	Yes	Possibly

* May not be able to perform even in presence of accommodation.

Job site evaluation (JSE): An on-site analysis of the workplace to determine optimal ergonomic design and to validate specific physical performance requirements of the job. A JSE can be useful in concert with an FCE to determine applicable return-to-work restrictions and to help ensure employer/employee compliance when necessary.[18]

Maximum medical improvement (MMI): The point at which medically determined impairment resulting from injury becomes stable and no further treatment is reasonably expected to improve the condition. MMI is felt to occur when the following criteria have been satisfied:

- The healing period has ended (a minimum documented duration of 6 months since injury onset has been proposed in prior editions of the AMA *Guides*); or
- The medical condition has fully resolved; or
- No further reasonable progress occurs or is expected to occur toward resolution of the medical condition.

MMI does not preclude the deterioration of a condition that is expected to occur with the passage of time; neither does it preclude allowances for ongoing follow-up or maintenance care.[2, 29]

Medical possibility: Something could occur due to a particular cause (probability of 50% or less).[2]

Medical probability: Something is more likely to occur than not (probability exceeds 50%).[2]

Scheduled loss: Allocation of a specified value for purposes of indemnification to a regional anatomical or functional unit to which an impairment rating can be assigned. The specified value allowed for a given unit can be expressed in terms of weeks or months of lost wages.[2]

Unscheduled loss: Estimated functional loss to the "whole person" for purposes of indemnification and accorded to a physiological system rather than to a regional anatomical or functional unit.[2] The cardiopulmonary, gastrointestinal, and central nervous systems are examples of systems to which an unscheduled loss can apply.

"Waddell's signs": Findings on physical examination that are thought to reflect a "nonorganic" basis of physical complaints and collectively serve to invalidate the examination itself.[38] Five markers are described:

1. Tenderness that is provoked by superficial palpation and/or that is nonanatomical in distribution
2. Pain on simulated provocation by axial loading or sham rotation of the spine
3. Inconsistency of findings with patient distraction
4. Regional weakness or sensory loss
5. Overreaction to the examination

Work hardening: A work-oriented treatment program, delivered in a highly structured environment that simulates the workplace, designed to improve job productivity of an injured or deconditioned worker. Productivity goals can pertain to work tolerance, job proficiency, or job efficiency.[18]

Work simulation: An individually focused work-hardening exercise program that simulates specific components of a specific job for purposes of making a transition to work-ready status and documenting work-ready status.[18]

HISTORICAL DEVELOPMENT OF IMPAIRMENT RATINGS AND DISABILITY DETERMINATIONS

Workers' Compensation

Workers' compensation is the earliest known disability system,[25] with origins dating at least to Roman times. By the late 1600s, the buccaneers of the West Indies had written articles of agreement that stipulated compensable sums to which injured crew members would be entitled for injuries and losses suffered during the course of a particular voyage. For example, 600 pieces-of-eight would be awarded for loss of a right arm, 500 for loss of a left arm, 500 for loss of a right leg, and 100 for loss of an eye.[13]

Von Bismarck first introduced a comprehensive social insurance system in Europe that included provisions for workers' compensation in the 1880s. Contemporary developments in England included the Employers' Liability Act of 1880, followed by the Workers' Compensation Law in 1887. Prior to that time, injured employees were unlikely to receive help from their employer unless they filed suit and could demonstrate that the employer was at fault and the claimant was free from "contributory negligence." Unsuccessful claims went uncompensated, whereas successful litigants might receive large monetary rewards that could jeopardize the financial viability of a company and the jobs available to other constituent workers. A "no-fault" system was adopted to resolve this dilemma whereby eligibility for coverage was automatic if the claim could be shown to have arisen directly during the course of one's employment activity.[25]

In St. Petersburg, Russia, a disability indemnification schedule was developed in 1907 in which regional injuries and resulting physical impairments could be awarded a specified percentage of total "disability" according to the whole person concept.[25]

The United States' system of workers' compensation was created in 1908 under the Federal Employees Compensation Act. Subsequently, the California Industrial Accident Act of 1914 created a schedule of impairment indemnification according to claimant's age, specific occupation, and physical impairment rating. By 1949, workers' compensation was available to all states.[25]

Workers' compensation in the United States is a federally mandated system of health and disability insurance administered at the state level. Its purpose is to provide benefits to disabled workers for any and all claims of injury or illness arising directly out of employment. Under workers' compensation, a disability is defined as the "immediate inability, because of work-related injury, to perform gainful activity as defined by one's most recent occupation" or similar suitable occupation for the claimant's level of training and experience.[31] Recipients are eligible for three types of benefits, which include the following:

1. Benefits to an employee's survivor in cases of death
2. Coverage of expenses of hospitalization and medical and rehabilitative care
3. Wage-loss compensation

Wage-loss compensation benefits are of four types[2, 22] and include the following:

1. *Temporary total*—Benefits are typically equal to two thirds of the usual and customary wages up to a maximum allowable cap, which varies by state. For example, temporary benefits are payable monthly from onset of injury until maximum medical improvement is reached if the claimant is judged medically to be unable to continue working during the specified period of coverage.
2. *Temporary partial*—Benefits paid during the period of onset of injury through maximum medical improvement if the injured worker is returned to modified duty. Benefits are generally equal to two thirds of the difference between pre-injury versus modified duty wages up to the temporary total cap for each state.
3. *Permanent partial*—Benefits can be "scheduled" or "unscheduled." Scheduled benefits are awarded in specific amounts associated with specific impairments affecting particular body parts and in accordance with predetermined disability tables that specify the number of weeks for which benefits must be paid at an average weekly wage rate. Unscheduled benefits typically require the estimation of percentage of impairment to the "whole person," from which proportional compensation against total possible loss can be determined. Benefits are payable at MMI.
4. *Permanent total*—Benefits are awarded up to a state-recognized percentage of pre-injury wages if the employee is found to be permanently incapable of returning to work at a level suitable to his or her training and experience. Benefits are payable at maximum medical improvement.

Other Disability Systems

Social Security

The Social Security Disability Act of 1954, and subsequent establishment of Social Security Disability Income (SSDI) in 1956, provided for a federally administered disability insurance program within the Social Security Administration (SSA) with benefits for individuals who are unable to work because of a disability. The SSA defines disability as the "inability to engage in any substantial gainful activity by reason of any medically determinable physical or mental impairment which can be expected to result in death or has lasted or can be expected to last for a continuous period of not less than 12 months."[31, p. 38] SSDI is available to claimants who meet the definition of disability according to the SSA:

Can demonstrate a recent work history (actively working for at least 5 of the preceding 10 years)
Have remained unemployed for the previous 6-month period
Have a current income of less than $300 per month

Entitlement is based on the claimant's contributions from prior earnings to Old Age, Survivors and Disability Insurance (OASDI) or by meeting criteria of a "means test." Benefits include a monthly stipend, Medicare supplemental insurance, and coverage for vocational rehabilitation.[31]

Supplemental Security Income (SSI) provides SSA disability benefits to individuals who meet the SSA definition of disability but who lack evidence of a recent work history. Entitlement is based on financial need according to the means test, and benefits include a monthly stipend, Medicaid insurance supplement, and coverage for vocational rehabilitation.[31]

For both SSDI and SSI, a physician must render an impairment rating according to a List of Impairments Schedule (or estimate of equivalent rating) as provided by the SSA.

Department of Veterans Affairs

The Department of Veterans Affairs (VA) maintains a federally administered disability program available to veterans whose disability is recognized as any condition "which is sufficient to render it impossible for the average person to follow a substantially gainful occupation, but only if it is reasonably certain that such disability will continue throughout the life of the disabled."[31, p. 58] Service-connected entitlement requires determination that the disability be related to injury or disease incurred during the course of active military duty, whereas non-service-connected entitlement requires determination that the disability was not incurred during the course of active military duty. Benefits awarded to eligible service-connected veterans include a disability pension with monthly financial support, hospitalization and medical care at VA facilities, prosthetic and orthotic devices, durable medical equipment, and home and motor vehicle modifications as necessary and appropriate. The rating physician must estimate the nature and severity of impairment according to a VA schedule.

Americans With Disabilities Act

With the passage of the Americans With Disabilities Act (ADA) in 1990, disabled Americans were guaranteed equal rights to employment opportunities, transportation, and public access. The ADA defines disability as "a physical or mental impairment that substantially limits one or more of the major life activities of such individual, a record of such impairment or being regarded as such an impairment."[3] Although it is broad and somewhat imprecise, this definition is narrowed under Title 1 of ADA (Employment) to recognize employment as a major life activity, and views disability within the context of performance of the "essential functions" of an employment position with or without "reasonable accommodation." Reasonable accommodation can include structural modifications at the work site to improve accessibility, availability of modified duty options, and acquisition of adaptive equipment or devices to enable an otherwise qualified worker with a disability to perform the essential functions of the job. Accommodations exempted under ADA include those that would pose "undue hardship" to the employer in terms of cost or feasibility of implementation, or those that would pose a "direct threat" to the health and safety of the disabled individual and/or co-workers.[3]

Impairment Rating Systems

Early Systems

The earliest attempts at medical impairment rating systems were anatomically based and regional in scope, with emphasis on the musculoskeletal system. This regional approach lent itself well to the concept that a schedule of discrete disability values could be assigned to anatomical units or subunits of the spine and extremities. For example, Smith in 1959 provided a system for workers' compensation to evaluate industrial "disability" according to scheduled losses affecting the extremities (expressed as functional units or "radicals"), eyes, or ears, and according to unscheduled losses affecting other organ systems.[36] Structural criteria (amputation, ankylosis) and joint active range of motion (ROM) formed the basis for rating the extremities. In 1962 the American Academy of Orthopaedic Surgeons (AAOS) published a manual devoted entirely to scheduled impairments of the spine and extremities using structural criteria (amputation, ankylosis), ROM, and sensory loss as criteria for rating.[1] Subsequently Rice described an anatomical system of impairment rating for the spine and extremities whose sole criterion was loss of ROM.[33]

McBride in 1963 introduced additional functional criteria for impairment rating that included strength, coordination, speed of movement, dexterity, and endurance. However, he did not provide a precise method to follow when impairment determinations were made according to these additional criteria. Kessler[23] carried the notion of functionally based impairment ratings forward by considering losses in strength, sensation, and coordination as well as in ROM. Strength was assessed relative to the contralateral limb via strain gauge testing or manual muscle testing (MMT). Functional prehension and precision grip testing was also used. Losses due to coordination and sensation remained poorly defined.

The AMA *Guides*

In 1956, the AMA created an ad hoc committee to address medical impairment rating practices, and this resulted in 13 separate publications in the JAMA from 1958 to 1970. These publications were subsequently compiled into the AMA *Guides,* the first edition of which was published in 1971. By 1981, an advisory panel had been formed to update and revise the *Guides,* and four subsequent revisions appeared from 1984 through 1993. Although traditionally anatomically based, the most recent edition seeks to surmount many pitfalls inherent in that system through the introduction of the "diagnosis-related model," as described below.

APPLICATION OF THE AMA *GUIDES* (MUSCULOSKELETAL SYSTEM)

General Consideration

The fourth edition of the AMA *Guides* is a standard reference for evaluating and reporting medical impairment and is the preferred rating system where permitted by law. It has direct application to the majority of workers' compensation jurisdictions, being mandated or recommended in 29 (55%) of 53 jurisdictions and not mandated or recommended, but frequently used in an additional 11 (21%) of 53 jurisdictions.[2]

The following brief overview is intended to orient the reader conceptually to the musculoskeletal section of the AMA *Guides.* The reader is encouraged to consult the *Guides* directly for greater detail and discussion than space permits here.

Qualitative Impairments

Qualitative impairments are anatomically based and belong to discrete, mutually exclusive categories that can only be measured in descriptive terms. Nominal or ordinal scales of measurement can apply to such groupings to yield hierarchical assembly, but the actual magnitude of difference between groupings is nonuniform and lacks true proportionality to assigned numerical value. Examples of qualitative impairments pertaining to the extremities and recognized by the AMA *Guides* include amputation, joint ankylosis, sensory change (present versus absent), and cosmetic disfigurement (present versus absent).

Quantitative Impairments

Quantitative impairments are also anatomically based. They are measured according to continuous scales (interval or ratio) whose units represent fixed values, the ordering of which reflects a uniform and consistent increase in magnitude. The AMA *Guides* recognizes loss of motion (in degrees) in each cardinal plane of function for a given joint as representing quantitative impairment relative to the normally accepted range of motion for that joint.

Diagnosis-Based Impairments

The fourth edition of the AMA *Guides* has advanced a diagnosis-related estimates (DRE) as an alternative approach to impairment rating. It is categorical in nature, less dependent on findings during physical examination, and emphasizes the key elements of history of injury and corroborative, objective findings on diagnostic testing. Where applicable, the DRE model has advantages of simplicity and ease of determination, and it is perhaps less biased in terms of the concrete rating guidelines provided.

Shortcomings and Pitfalls

Any person who uses the AMA *Guides* should recognize the following key shortcomings.

First and foremost, the process whereby functional loss is inferred and extrapolated from anatomically determined impairment might not be valid. More specific and objective determinations concerning normal functioning of an organ system and the impact of impairments on an organ system are needed. The contributors to the AMA *Guides* have "estimated the extent of impairments on the basis of clinical experience, judgment, and consensus. The estimates of the well qualified persons contributing to . . . [the AMA *Guides*], most of them physicians . . . [are judged to be] more convincing than those of most others in estimating the severity of people's impairments."[2, p. 3] Such validation by consensus remains largely unsupported by rigorously collected, behaviorally based data,[34] and consequently lacks a sound scientific foundation at this time. This shortcoming applies both to anatomically based and diagnosis-based impairment ratings.

Second, concerns abound with regard to the validity and reliability of the impairment measures conventionally in use. For example, surface inclinometry is the adopted procedure of choice for determining spinal mobility, according to the AMA *Guides*. However, the degree to which surface inclinometry reflects underlying spinal mobility has been questioned.[27] Furthermore, loss of spinal flexibility might not predict back pain disability, and one study has even suggested an inverse relationship between pain-induced disability and lumbar flexibility.[24] High inter-rater and intrarater reliability have been reported using the two-inclinometer method to measure lumbar flexion and extension.[21] Other authors have shown, however, the presence of significant measurement error and unacceptably low reliability estimates for this technique (based on intraclass correlations). This was found to be true even when applied by experienced observers to healthy and fully compliant subjects.[35]

Subjectivity of the patient and examiner and performance effort put forth during any examination and testing can have a negative impact on the validity of impairment measures derived. Whereas true malingering/complaint fabrication is an exceptional occurrence, the examiner can expect to frequently encounter elements of symptom magnification.[26] This is particularly likely in compensable injury cases.[36] Such exaggeration and inconsistencies need to be recognized and appropriately discounted, hopefully without penalizing the patient who exhibits them. Waddell's signs[38] can aid the examiner in this regard, and meticulous record keeping of observations on successive visits, where possible, can serve as a further internal check on the consistency of findings during examination. Isokinetic ergometers have gained acceptance as an exercise and evaluation tool for assessment of the consistency of effort, based on coefficients of variability established for healthy subjects. However, a recent review[30] questions the applicability of these coefficients to subjects experiencing true nociception and those with symptom magnification.

Finally, the issue of pain as it pertains to impairment deserves further consideration. The role of pain in disability determinations has been dealt with extensively.[31] The logistical and conceptual issues surrounding the measurement of pain behavior are beyond our immediate scope, although they are well documented elsewhere.[14] Simply stated, pain as a phenomenon is entirely subjective and cannot be measured directly. Consequently, pain behavior or complaints should not serve as the only basis for ratable impairment determination in the absence of corroborative objective criteria.[2]

Extremities as Regional Units

The Hand and Upper Extremity

The AMA *Guides* has adopted a system for evaluating hand and upper extremity impairment that was originally developed and approved by the International Federation of Societies for Surgery of the Hand in association with the American Society for Surgery of the Hand. This regional unit is divided for purposes of separate evaluation into five regional units: thumb, finger, wrist, elbow, and shoulder.

Qualitative impairments are as follows: Total loss of motion or sensation within a regional unit or ankylosis/malposition that precludes functional use of same is equated to total functional loss, as would result from amputation of that unit. Ankylosis of a unit or subunit in optimal functional position is considered the least impairment of that unit. The impairments are assigned numerical values that are presented in tabular form for each regional unit.

Estimates of impairment resulting from peripheral nerve dysfunction involve losses attributable to sensory deficits, pain, or weakness. Sensory loss estimates are equated to 50% of comparable functional loss due to amputation. To be ratable, pain or sensory deficits must be shown to interfere with functional performance of the unit, to follow recognizable neuroanatomical pathways, and to be corroborated by other objective signs of peripheral nerve dysfunction. Similarly, objective and reproducible deficits in strength enable ratable estimates of functional loss attributable to motor weakness if the pattern of weakness is consistent with dysfunction along a peripheral nerve pathway.

Quantitative impairment in terms of restricted ROM for a given member is presented in tabular form as a percentage loss of the normative range for that member. Estimates of ROM are determined goniometrically, using procedures illustrated in the AMA *Guides*. The AMA *Guides* specifies that active ROM determination takes precedence over passive ROM whenever possible, and ROM estimates are rounded to the nearest 10 degrees. Although the AMA *Guides* fails to specify this, the unaffected contralateral extremity (if applicable) might serve as a more valid baseline reference for a given individual's expected ROM than the normative range estimated for that particular joint. Consequently, use of contralateral range loss estimates as the normative basis for comparison is recommended whenever possible.

In some cases, categorical (i.e., diagnosis-based) losses due to joint instability, implants, or other connective tissue disorders not covered in the preceding discussion are ratable according to the appropriate tables of the AMA *Guides*.

The Lower Extremity

The lower extremity is considered in terms of five regional units: hip, knee, ankle, foot, and toes. Qualitative impairments for amputation and ankylosis are recognized, and tabular references for these are provided. Losses due to peripheral nerve dysfunction affecting the lower extremities and attributable to sensory deficits, pain, or weakness are treated in similar fashion as those affecting the upper extremity. In addition, categorical impairment estimates according to limb-length discrepancies, gait "derangements," and muscle atrophy are separately recognized and tabulated. Quantitative impairments due to losses against expected arc of motion can be goniometrically determined and interpreted according to tables provided for each member, and in a manner similar to that for the upper extremity.

Diagnosis-Based Estimates

The AMA *Guides* separately recognizes diagnosis-based categories of impairment of the lower extremity, including fractures of the regional units, endoprosthetic replacement of the hip or knee, and major skin grafting procedures. Separate reference tables are provided. The examiner is encouraged to use diagnosis-based ratings as an alternative to (*never* in addition to) anatomically based ratings for each specific impairment and to select whichever option yields the greater impairment in any given case.

Spine as Regional Units

Qualitative Impairments and Diagnosis-Related Estimates

The AMA *Guides* has developed the DRE approach to the assessment of impairments of the spine in an attempt to recognize and differentiate clinical findings due to illness or injury from those that accompany the normal aging process. The DRE or *injury model* recognizes specific diagnostic categories for which diagnosis-based ratings can be derived (e.g., vertebral body compression graded according to severity; fracture of vertebral posterior elements or transverse processes; loss of motion segment integrity; cauda equina syndrome; paraplegia). The spine is treated as three regional units (cervicothoracic, thoracolumbar, and lumbosacral) for which maximal impairment estimates of 35%, 20%, and 75%, respectively, can be derived. Eight categories of gradation of severity are developed that are applicable to recognized disorders of each regional unit; categorical differentiators for each emphasize objective and reproducible evidence of neurological dysfunction or loss of structural integrity. For example, loss of reflexes or focal atrophy (≥2 cm), although recognized, is weighted less than electrodiagnostic findings of acute or chronic nerve root compromise (e.g., multiple positive sharp waves or fibrillation potentials, H-wave absence or delay, polyphasic waves). Similarly, cystometrogram findings outweigh those from physical examination. Loss of motion segment integrity is radiographically defined according to anteroposterior translations in flexion/extension views of at least 3.5 mm for cervical or at least 5 mm for thoracic or lumbar regions in the sagittal plane. Specific angular displacements identified radiographically between adjacent motion segments in the sagittal plane are also recognized. The DRE system enables the examiner to rate appropriate spinal diagnoses according to region and severity with all ratings rendered according to whole person estimates (see following discussion).

Quantitative Impairments and Inclinometry

The traditional, anatomically based approach to impairment rating of the spine is termed the *range of motion model,* and the AMA *Guides* currently recommends its use "only if the Injury Model is not applicable, or if more clinical data are needed."[2, p. 112] Under this model the three regions of the spine are cervical, thoracic, and lumbar, for which maximal ratings for loss of motion are 80%, 40%, and 90%, respectively. All impairment ratings are rendered to the whole person (see following discussion) and detailed procedural descriptions are provided for one- and two-inclinometer techniques to determine regional spinal motion in flexion/extension, lateral flexion, and rotation as applicable. Normative tables are provided by region to determine impairment according to degrees of motion loss. Procedural issues of concern with spinal inclinometry include the cumbersome need to provide at least three replicate measurements of each plane of motion to ensure accuracy, the need to average each set of three measurements, and the need to discard measurements that vary by more than 5 degrees or 10% (whichever is larger). Validation procedures for determining lumbosacral flexion and extension are potentially confusing and labor intensive. Application of the DRE approach obviates these concerns and is currently the favored method of the AMA *Guides.*

Impairments Due to Specific Spine Disorders

In situations where the range-of-motion model is being applied, four categories of diagnoses (separate from the DRE model) are recognized including fractures, intervertebral disk or soft tissue, spondylolysis/spondylolisthesis (unoperated), and spinal stenosis/segmental instability/spondylolisthesis (operated). In contrast to the DRE model, this option enables the examiner to take into account surgical interventions and multiple operative procedures in developing the final impairment rating. Such an approach is largely descriptive and does not take into account functional outcomes following surgery in determining the impairment weight assigned in any given case.

Combining Impairments and Whole Person Ratings

Impairment ratings derived independently for each regional unit or subunit of the spine and extremities are expressed in terms of scheduled values for each unit (exceptions being the unscheduled expressions of whole person ratings derived by the DRE model or other diagnosis-based ratings described earlier). It is possible for the examiner to combine these scheduled and unscheduled ratings to achieve a single cumulative impairment rating for the whole person according to a *combined values chart* provided by the AMA *Guides.* This chart is designed to ensure that cumulative scheduled ratings of regional subunits do not exceed the total value of the unit itself, and that a cumulative whole person impairment rating does not exceed 100%. In using the combined values chart, all scheduled impairments must first be converted to whole person equivalents using the appropriate conversion charts provided in each section of the *Guides.* Alternatively, regional impairments to the extremity can be converted to whole person equivalents by multiplying an upper extremity impairment value by 0.6 and a lower extremity impairment value by 0.4. When two whole person ratings from different regional units are combined (using the combined values chart), the larger value indicates the appropriate row and the smaller value the appropriate column from which to determine the appropriate combined value. The process is repeated until all unit values have been included into an overall rating.

IMPAIRMENT AND DISABILITY REPORT WRITING

The following illustrations of impairment rating and disability report writing are based on the workers' compensation systems for those jurisdictions accepting the AMA *Guides.* The disability examining physicians must be thoroughly familiar with the rules, jurisdictional requirements, and nuances applicable to the particular system and locale in which they are working.

Worksheet for History and Physical Examination

A sample worksheet is provided (Fig. 6–1) that is intended to aid the physician examiner and ensure that a consistent, systematic, and complete data base is gathered during the IME. If it is used as a teaching aid for preceptorships in industrial rehabilitation, the preceptor should validate key items of the history and physical examination and ensure that adequate and appropriate documentation takes place. The worksheet also serves as a reference to enable rapid, thorough, and accurate dictation of the IME report.

A number of risk factors for *delayed recovery* syndromes have been described[12, 16] and are important items to address in the IME patient history. These risk factors are:

Occupational
Time off work
Low job satisfaction
Patient perception of mismatch between physical capacity and job demands
Lack of modified duty options
Psychosocial
Poor English proficiency
Disabled spouse
Anger toward system
Ongoing or prior litigation/compensation
Disability convictions by patient or physician
Medical
Prior history of injury
History of substance abuse
Poor cardiovascular fitness

The history serves as an important screening tool to identify patients as high risk, and should address these items inclusively. It is well documented that the likelihood of return to work following injury decreases precipitously as time off work following injury increases, regardless of the illness or injury (see Chapter 45).[15] Specifically, probability decreases to 50% or less at 6 months and to 20% at 1 year post injury. Research has shown that 6 or more consecutive months out of work in the presence of amotivation, symptom magnification, and pain, unaccompanied by secondary medical conditions, presents a chronicity syndrome for which the prognosis for functional recovery is guarded (see Chapters 42 and 45).[37] The IME physician should be circumspect about recommending continued therapy in such cases and should judiciously monitor functional progress achieved if therapies are to continue. Justification for discontinuing therapy can be based, in part, on knowledge and documentation of the above.

Symptom magnification[26] refers to embellishment (conscious or otherwise) of the patient's subjective pain and suffering and displays of pain behavior that are out of proportion to what is supported by objective data in a particular case.

PHYSICIAN RESPONSIBILITIES/ REPORTING REQUIREMENTS

IME

In cases involving a dispute between the claimant and the insurer concerning MMI determination or impairment rating derived, a physician examiner unfamiliar with the case can accept a referral from an administrative law judge or other official. The physician should review the case records, examine the claimant independently, and render a second opinion concerning the findings. In some cases, additional testing and treatment is authorized to be undertaken by the examiner to satisfy an MMI determination.

MMI Determination

The physician examiner is typically required to complete a physician's initial report, supplemental interim reports, and a maximal medical improvement form at the time of case disposition.[29] Reporting requirements vary by state, but they are generally similar and must include an estimate of when MMI occurred or is expected to occur. The decision of MMI must be rendered before case closure can be achieved. The claimant is usually deemed not to be at MMI as long as expectations for further functional improvement continue to be met by demonstrable and ongoing performance gains. The distinction between functional versus pain-oriented goal setting must be maintained during treatment, so that progress toward goal achievement can be measured and monitored objectively. When functional progress is no longer evident or tenable and at least a 6-month healing period has been completed, MMI is felt to have occurred.

WORKSHEET FOR HISTORY AND PHYSICAL EXAMINATION		
Date:		
Patient Name:	**ID#**	
Referred by:		
Date of onset of injury/illness:		
Employer:		
Nature of injury/illness:		
Medical/diagnostic/therapeutic treatment rendered:		
Present symptoms/complaints:		
Pain:		
locality	quality	
severity (0 - 5 point scale)	duration (constant/intermittent)	
aggravating factors	palliating factors	
Weakness:		
distribution (regional vs focal)		
Sensory changes:		
numbness/paresthesias	distribution (regional vs focal)	
Bladder/Bowel dysfunction		
Present treatment strategies:		
Medications: type/frequency:		
Therapies: exercise/modalities:		
type/frequency		
Equipment: corset	TENS	other
Review of Systems:		
Sleep habits/changes since onset of injury/illness:		
Weight gain/loss/appetite changes		
Present disability:		
Basic mobility/self-care activity		
Work related: Duration of time out of work:		
modified duty/restrictions (if applicable):		
Avocational:		
Employment History:		
Nature of job		
Time on-the-job at onset of injury/illness:		
Job satisfaction/performance history		
Previous employers/duration of employment		
Educational level/English proficiency		
Major Life Stressors:		
Financial:		
Marital/familial:		

FIGURE 6–1. Worksheet for history and physical examination.

Illustration continued on following page

Past Medical History:			
Constitutional illness/symptoms			
Use of tobacco	alcohol	caffeine	illicit drugs
Allergies to foods or medications			
Peptic ulcer disease/aspirin intolerance			
Pregnancies			
Past Surgical History:			
Family History of Major Illness:			
Psychiatric/psychological treatment or medications:			
Prior history of injury:			
Work related:			
Non-Work Related:			
Previous compensation/impairment rating:			
Present litigation:			
Social History:			
Marital status:			
Active dependents:			
Child support?			
Other disabled family members?			
Patient's goals/expectations:			
PHYSICAL EXAM - General:			
Height:	**Weight:**	**Vital Signs:**	
HEENT:			
Cardiopulmonary:			
Abdominal:			
Extremities: Pulses:		Erythema/edema/trophic changes:	
Affect/cognitive:			
Neurological: Tone:		Coordination:	
Muscle stretch reflexes: upper extremity:		lower extremity:	sacral:
Sensory: touch:	pinprick:	proprioception:	vibration:
Musculoskeletal: Posture			
lordosis/kyphosis:	scoliosis:	abdominal tone:	
guarding/protective/splinting/spasm:			
tender points: location/distribution:			"jump sign":
Flexibility (Spine:)	**Cervical**	**Thoracic**	**Lumbar**
flexion/extension:			
lateral flexion:			
rotation:			

FIGURE 6–1 *Continued*

R.O.M. (Extremities)

Upper	L	R		Lower	L	R
Shoulder				Hip		
Elbow				Knee		
Wrist				Ankle		
Hand				Foot		

Muscle Bulk/Symmetry

Upper	L	R		Lower	L	R

Manual Muscle Testing

Upper	L	R		Lower	L	R
Scapulothoracic				Hip flex/ext		
Deltoid				Hip abd/add		
Bicep				Quad		
Tricep				Hamstring		
Wrist flex/ext				Ankle dorsiflex /evert		
Intrinsic				Ankle plantarflex /invert		

Special Tests	Pos	Neg		Functional Gait	Normal	Abnormal
Spurling's:				Heel / toe		
Adsen's:				Tandem		
Tinel's:						
Phalen's:				Trendelenburg/		
Yergason's:				stationary		
Straight leg raise:				dynamic		

Waddell's Signs	Positive	Negative
Superficial/non-anatomic tenderness		
Sham provocation of pain/discomfort		
Inconsistencies		
Regional weakness/sensory loss		
Overreaction		

FIGURE 6–1 *Continued*

Illustration continued on following page

The physician examiner is also required to determine the exact date of MMI and to address issues of medical stability from that point forward. Deterioration that might normally be expected with the passage of time (e.g., progression of an osteoarthritic condition) does not preclude MMI determination. The physician should also further address issues of future medical management and follow-up that are anticipated to be necessary to maintain MMI for a given condition.

Impairment Rating, Causality, and Apportionment

The physician examiner must determine the nature and degree of physical impairment, if any, according to the

Diagnostic Database
Labs:
Radiographic:
Other:
Assessment:
Rehabilitation diagnoses:
Functional prognosis/goals:
Recommendations:
Additional diagnostic/consultative procedures:
Additional therapeutic intervention:
MMI determination (if appropriate):
Final impairment rating:
Case Disposition:
Return-to-work restrictions:
Vocational rehabilitation referral:
Other recommendations:

FIGURE 6–1 *Continued*

guidelines outlined above. Impairments can be expressed in terms of functional loss to the unit or to the whole person.

The physician examiner might be asked to render a medical opinion "within reasonable certainty" as to causality of a specific impairment. A direct or "proximate" causal relationship is thought to exist if a medical probability exists that the impairment is a direct result of reported illness or injury.[2] Consequently, examiners must distinguish between medical probability and medical possibility in such cases, and do so to their best ability according to the guidelines stated above.

In cases involving preexisting conditions and/or recurrent injury, apportionment is necessary and involves the physician's best estimate of the relative contributions of preexisting or resulting conditions to the impairment rating that is ultimately derived. McBride[28] has recommended an impartial and objective solution to this problem that requires the development of three contingent "ratings" from which the apportioned percentage can be extracted:

A total impairment rating (A) is derived irrespective of preexisting/resulting conditions
A second "baseline" rating (B) is derived that accounts solely for preexisting conditions and progression over time without associated or aggravating re-injury
A third rating (C) is derived in which preexisting conditions are discounted

The physician might logically choose to award the greater of the two differences between the first minus the second rating (A − B) or the first minus the third rating (A − C) as the amount of total impairment apportioned to the resulting condition. To illustrate, consider Case Study 1.

In the above example, the "total impairment" (A) = 2% (ROM) combined with (10% + 1% + 3%) = 16%. The "baseline impairment" (B) = 2% combined with (10% + 1% + 2%) = 15%. The impairment without baseline (C) = 2% + 10% = 12%. You might logically render a 16% WP impairment rating and apportion 4% (the greater difference between 16% minus 15% or 16% minus 12%) for resulting re-injury and the third operation.

Disability Determination/ Return-to-Work Restrictions

The AMA *Guides* recognizes that disability benefits, in terms of wage-loss compensation for work-related impairment, are independent of the impaired individual's capacity to work and are formulated in terms of expected long-term negative financial impact of a given impairment category.[2] Indemnification schedules exist and vary by individual states with stipulations of the maximum number of weeks of average lost wages payable for loss of use of body parts. Consequently, the impairment rating and other medical information rendered by the physician ultimately assists a legal and administrative panel that is involved in making such determinations in any given case.

During the initial, interim, and MMI phases of reporting, the physician examiner is asked to complete a work status report, an example of which is provided in Figure 6–2. If treatment is ongoing and transitional work is available, the physician might recommend *modified duty* in terms of restrictions on the number of hours of work and permissible activities during the transitional healing period. If modified duty options are unavailable, the physician might be required to render a *temporary total disability* determination until MMI is reached. The probability of returning to work decreases precipitously as time out of work increases,[4] so the physician should make every effort to return the claimant safely to a transitional work setting as soon as possible. In cases in which transitional return to work options are unavailable, work hardening should be considered as a viable alternative to forced inactivity and should be implemented whenever feasible and medically necessary (see Chapter 45). At the point of MMI determination and case closure, the physician must render a final opinion on permanent restrictions applicable from that point forward.

A number of standardized assessment tools are available to assist the physician in determining valid and reliable physical performance expectations for an injured worker:

FCE is a comprehensive assessment of the individual's strength, flexibility, endurance, and safety in perform-

CASE STUDY 1

A 45-year-old man is diagnosed with recurrent low back strain with "failed back" syndrome. He had undergone an L4–5 laminectomy and discectomy 8 years previously, and a subsequent L5–S1 laminectomy and discectomy 2 years later. He suffered recurrent low back "strain" 2 years ago and ultimately had a recurrent L5–S1 laminectomy and excision of scar tissue 6 months later (18 months ago). He is at MMI and an impairment rating is requested. You elect to determine the whole person (WP) impairment to the spine according to the range-of-motion model. You calculate lumbosacral flexion limitation to 45 degrees for 2% whole person impairment. Lumbosacral extension and lateral flexion limitations are within normal limits, and there is no focal associated weakness or sensory change. According to Table 75 (p. 113) in the *Guides,* you note the following:

Surgical Rx for discectomy = 10% WP.
Multiple levels (add 1%/level) for 2nd level = 1% WP.
Multiple operations with residual (2nd operation) = 2% WP; "new" 3rd operation = 1% WP.

PATIENT STATUS:

PATIENT NAME: ______________________________ DATE OF INJURY: ______________

DIAGNOSIS: ______________________________ STATUS: ☐ Improved ☐ Same ☐ Worse ☐ Resolved

WORK STATUS:

☐ RETURN TO FULL DUTY

☐ RETURN TO LIMITED DUTY NUMBER OF HOURS/DAY: _______

☐ (OFF) UNABLE TO WORK UNTIL FOLLOW-UP PROJECTED RETURN TO WORK DATE: ______________

RESTRICTIONS:

CHECK THE FREQUENCY AND NUMBER OF HOURS/DAY THE WORKER IS ABLE TO DO THE FOLLOWING ACTIVITIES:

	FREQUENCY		NUMBER OF HOURS/DAY								
Activity	**Continuous**	**Intermittent (with rest)**	**0**	**1**	**2**	**3**	**4**	**5**	**6**	**7**	**8**
Sitting											
Standing											
Walking											

	Never	**Occasionally (up to 33%)**	**Frequently (34-66%)**	**Continuously (67-100%)**
Movements:				
Bend/Stoop				
Squat				
Kneel				
Crawl				
Climb				
Pushing/Pulling				
Reach above shoulder level				
Lift:				
Up to 10 lbs				
11 - 25 lbs				
26 - 50 lbs				
> 50 lbs				
Carry:				
Up to 10 lbs				
11 - 25 lbs				
26 - 50 lbs				
> 50 lbs				

RETURN APPOINTMENT:

RETURN APPOINTMENT (DATE): ______________ TIME: __________

IS PATIENT AT MMI? ☐ YES ☐ NO IF NOT, PROJECTED MMI DATE: ______________

______________________________ ______________________________

Provider signature/MD Date of Exam

FIGURE 6–2. Example of typical work status report.

ing job-specific activities, and it is perhaps the most valid predictor of appropriate restrictions to activity during various points of recovery and at MMI. In cases in which no specific job exists or is available, FCA provides suitable alternative information of a generic nature. The impaired individual's performance during an FCE or FCA can be assessed with respect to degree of effort, consistency, and reliability during testing.[18] In situations in which lack of consistency or incomplete effort results in questionable validity of performance measured, return-to-work restrictions must remain subjective.

A *job description* is frequently available from the employer and can provide a useful list of the essential functions of the job in question for purposes of assessing functional capacities and addressing specific restrictions that can apply.

Job site evaluation can be carried out by a specially trained therapist to validate the essential functions listed in the job description with respect to critical physical demands and relative amounts of time spent performing specific activities of each essential function. In some cases ergonomic analysis can be useful to quantify physical demands relative to observed physical capacities, and to enable specific recommendations for reasonable accommodation in terms of job redesign or workplace modification. Finally, employer and employee willingness to comply with recommended restrictions and accommodation can be addressed.

Physician examiners should avail themselves of these assessment tools in order to ensure that their prognostic inferences and sanctions are founded on valid, empirical, and functionally based data to the fullest extent possible.

LEGAL, ETHICAL, AND OTHER CONSIDERATIONS

Because of the medicolegal nature of many, if not most, workers' compensation referrals, the physician examiner can frequently expect to serve as an expert witness and to undergo deposition and courtroom testimony. The physician can be expected to testify with respect to even minute details of a specific case, often months or years after completion of the IME. A systematically collected, thorough, and well-organized database and record file can significantly reduce the need for additional testimony[6] and can facilitate preparation for testimony and enable rapid retrieval of key items of information by the physician deponent under questioning.

At time of deposition or courtroom testimony, the physician is required to submit evidence attesting to credibility as an expert witness. A curriculum vitae that adequately reflects relevant training and experience and highlights accomplishments pertaining to the area of claimed expertise is helpful. The physician examiner should be prepared to disclose information concerning customary fee schedules, percentage of practice devoted to workers' compensation claims and medicolegal testimony,[6] and percentage of referrals generated from plaintiff versus defendant camps.

W. Johnston[20] offers the following tips for physicians engaging in medical testimony:

Always know your file.

Listen to the question and answer only the question asked.

Answer yes/no whenever appropriate, and keep answers short and to the point.

Always elaborate on questions that go to the main issue of the case.

Always be ready to concede the weak points, but never concede points that are the foundation of your opinion.

In effect, good testimony is provided when an honest and well-prepared physician is willing to give honest answers to hard questions.[20]

The physician examiner must also confront the ethical challenge posed by the patient as a claimant. The traditional paternalistic view of the physician as the zealous advocate of the patient's best interests has given way to a contractual view encompassing patient autonomy, informed consent, and rights to privacy and self-determination. More recently, an *educational model* has been proposed for patients rehabilitated within a team framework.[9] It emphasizes shared responsibility and decision making, while recognizing team leadership and authority. Although such a model seeks to preserve patient autonomy it must be "carried out in an environment where financial considerations are playing an increasingly important role in determining access to and discharge from rehabilitation."[9 p. 317] The examiner who seeks to uphold the changing moral imperatives of the doctor-patient relationship must also be sensitive and responsive to the paradox of compensable injury, which is that financial compensation can discourage return to work and thereby promote disability.[5] Furthermore, the prolongation of an open claim (through inappropriate and excessive diagnostic and/or therapeutic endeavors, however well intended) might further serve to legitimize disability in the claimant's mind, and can also inhibit the likelihood of functional recovery and return to work. Decisions to terminate treatment of compensable injury and reach MMI might not always be mutually agreeable to claimant and examiner, and decisions in such cases are more likely to rest with the final authority of the physician rather than that of the patient. Perhaps the most useful beacon to guide decision making when treating compensable injuries is to promote functional recovery to the fullest extent, to terminate treatment when functional recovery is no longer tenable, and to render impairment ratings and return-to-work decisions that enable patients to use their residual abilities (through accommodation when necessary) as soon as possible and to the fullest extent possible.

The physician examiner is empowered to determine MMI, impairment rating, if any, and when and to what extent an injured worker can return to work or continue working. Physicians are becoming increasingly accountable for their medical opinions in this arena; this is hardly surprising, if one considers the disproportionately high health care costs of occupationally related temporary total and permanent partial disability compensation.[4] Physician impairment rating practices have been shown to vary widely with respect to acceptance of rating criteria, methods of application, and time of rating determination.[7, 11, 17] Lack of uniform standards of application and the resulting inconsistencies have been a source of embarrassing frustration to physicians themselves,[10] and the process of impairment rating often appears reduced to "educated guesswork."[8] Rating parameters should ideally meet the standards of objectivity, reliability, and content validity of measurements currently established in the field,[19] and should be widely accepted and employed by the rating community. The AMA *Guides* continues to reflect shortcomings in several of these areas, as discussed earlier in this chapter. These ideals can perhaps be realized if the body of qualified examiners continues to adopt uniform standards for acceptable rating criteria, reference materials, and methods of application, and continues to undergo specialized training and certification to promote quality and uniformity of the impairment rating process.[29]

REFERENCES

1. American Academy of Orthopaedic Surgeons: Manual for Orthopaedic Surgeons in Evaluating Permanent Physical Impairment. Chicago, American Academy of Orthopaedic Surgeons, 1975.
2. American Medical Association: Guides to the Evaluation of Permanent Impairment, ed 4. Chicago, American Medical Association, 1993.
3. Americans With Disabilities Act: Part 1: Employment (29CFR part 1630). Federal Register. July 26, 1991, pp 35726–35756.
4. Andersson GB, Pope MH, Frymoyer JW, et al: Epidemiology and cost. In Pope MH, Andersson GB, Frymoyer JW, et al (eds): Occupational Low Back Pain: Assessment, Treatment, and Prevention. St Louis, Mosby–Year Book, 1991, pp 95–113.
5. Beals RK: Compensation and recovery from injury. West J Med 1984; 140:233–237.
6. Bonfiglio RP, Bonfiglio RL: Medical testimony in Workers' Compensation matters. In Johnson EW (ed): Phys Med Rehabil Clin North Am 1992; 3:665–676.
7. Brand RA, Lehmann TR: Low-back impairment rating practices of orthopaedic surgeons. Spine 1983; 8:75–78.
8. Burd JG: The educated guess: Doctors and permanent partial disability percentage. J Tenn Med Assoc 1980; 73:441.
9. Caplan AL: Informed consent and provider-patient relationships in rehabilitation medicine. Arch Phys Med Rehabil 1988; 69:312–317.
10. Carey TS, Hadler NM: The role of the primary physician in disability determination for Social Security Insurance and Workers' Compensation. Ann Intern Med 1986; 104:706–710.
11. Clark WL, Haldeman S, Johnson P, et al: Back impairment and disability determination: Another attempt at objective, reliable rating. Spine 1988; 13:332–341.
12. Derebery VJ, Tullis WH: Delayed recovery in the patient with a work compensable injury. J Occup Med 1983; 25:829–835.
13. Esquemeling J: The Buccaneers of America, 1684–5. In Stallybrass W (ed): Broadway Translations. London, G. Routledge & Sons, 1924, p 60.
14. Fordyce WE: Behavioral Methods for Chronic Pain and Illness. St Louis, CV Mosby, 1976.
15. Frymoyer JW, Andersson GB: Clinical classification. In Pope MH, Andersson GB, Frymoyer JW, et al (eds): Occupational Low Back Pain: Assessment, Treatment, and Prevention. St Louis, Mosby–Year Book, 1991, pp 44–70.
16. Frymoyer JW, Cats-Baril W: Predictors of low back pain disability. Clin Orthop Rel Res 1987; 221:89–98.
17. Greenwood JG: Low-back impairment-rating practices of orthopaedic surgeons and neurosurgeons in West Virginia. Spine 1985; 10:773–776.
18. Isernhagen SJ: Work Injury Management and Prevention. Rockville, MD, Aspen, 1988.
19. Johnston MV, Keith RA, Hinderer SR: Measurement standards for interdisciplinary medical rehabilitation: Part I. General principles and technical standards. Arch Phys Med Rehabil 1992; 73(suppl):3–12.
20. Johnston W: Importance of communication between physician and attorney. Phys Med Rehabil Clin North Am 1992; 3:677–694.
21. Keely J, Mayer T, Cox R, et al: Quantification of lumbar function: Part 5. Reliability of range of motion measures in the sagittal plane and an in vivo torso rotation measurement technique. Spine 1986; 11:31–35.
22. Kemp JD, Pope MH: Workers' Compensation. In Kemp JD, Pope MH (eds): Occupational Low Back Pain: Assessment, Treatment and Prevention. St Louis, Mosby–Year Book, 1991, pp 296–304.
23. Kessler HH: Disability-Determination and Evaluation. Philadelphia, Lea & Febiger, 1970.
24. Lankhorst GJ, Van de Stadt RJ, Van der Korst JK: The natural history of idiopathic low back pain. Scand J Rehabil Med 1985; 17:1–4.
25. Luck J, Florence D: A brief history and comparative analysis of disability systems and impairment rating guides. Orthop Clin North Am 1988; 19:839–844.
26. Matheson LN: Symptom magnification syndrome structured interview: Rationale and procedure. J Occup Rehabil 1991; 1:43–56.
27. Mayer T, Tencer A, Kristoferson S, et al: Use of noninvasive techniques for quantification of spinal range-of-motion in normal subjects and chronic low back dysfunction patients. Spine 1984; 9:588–595.
28. McBride ED: Disability Evaluation and Principles of Treatment of Compensable Injuries, ed 6. Philadelphia, JB Lippincott, 1963.
29. Mueller KL, Goldman B (eds): Division of Workers' Compensation Level II Accreditation Course. Denver, State of Colorado Department of Labor and Employment, Division of Workers' Compensation, 1993.
30. Newton M, Waddell G: Trunk strength testing with isomachines: Part I. Review of a decade of scientific evidence. Spine 1993; 18:801–811.
31. Osterweis M, Kleinman A, Mechanic D (eds): Pain and Disability: Clinical, Behavioral, and Public Policy Perspectives. Washington, DC, National Academy Press, 1987.
32. Pheasant S: Ergonomics, Work and Health. Gaithersburg, MD, Aspen, 1991, p 4.
33. Rice CO: Calculation of Industrial Disability of the Extremities and the Back, ed 2. Springfield, IL, Charles C Thomas, 1968.
34. Rondinelli R, Dunn W, Hassanein K, et al: A simulation of hand impairments: Effects on upper extremity function and implications toward medical impairment rating and disability determination. Arch Phys Med Rehabil 1997; 78:1358–1363.
35. Rondinelli R, Murphy J, Esler A, et al: Estimation of normal lumbar flexion with surface inclinometry: A comparison of three methods. Am J Phys Med Rehabil 1992; 71:219–224.
36. Smith WC: Principles of Disability Evaluation. Philadelphia, JB Lippincott, 1959.
37. Strang JP: The chronic disability syndrome. In Aronoff GM (ed): Evaluation and Treatment of Chronic Pain. Baltimore, Urban & Schwartzenberg, 1985, pp 603–623.
38. Waddell G, McCulloch J, Kummel E, et al: Nonorganic physical signs in low-back pain. Spine 1980; 5:117–125.
39. World Health Organization: International Classification of Impairments, Disabilities and Handicaps. Geneva, World Health Organization, 1980.

7

CHAPTER

Andrew D. Bronstein, M.D., Shane E. Macaulay, M.D., and Andrew J. Cole, M.D.

Neurological and Musculoskeletal Imaging Studies

Multiple imaging modalities are available to help in making a neurological or musculoskeletal diagnosis. This chapter describes imaging methods, indications, contraindications, and artifacts specific to various types of imaging methods. The chapter also presents the preferred imaging methods for specific anatomical areas and tissues. The purpose of the discussion is to help the physiatrist, in concert with the consulting radiologist, choose the most appropriate imaging study or studies for a patient.

The American College of Radiology (ACR) has developed appropriateness criteria for various imaging modalities for specific clinical indications.[2] As of 1996, clinical indications pertinent to the physiatrist that have appropriateness criteria include suspected ankle injury in patients meeting Ottawa rules, cervical spine trauma, unilateral or bilateral hip pain, soft tissue mass, suspected primary bone tumors, stress/insufficiency fractures (excluding vertebral fractures), metastatic bone disease, painful hip or knee prostheses, acute shoulder trauma, nontraumatic knee pain, acute lower back pain with radiculopathy, and myelopathy. The appropriateness of a given imaging study on a scale of 1 to 9 is tallied for each clinical situation by expert panels. Ratings of the appropriateness criteria are presented under the specific anatomical discussions later in this chapter.

IMAGING MODALITIES

Plain Radiography and Its Variants (Stress Radiography, Arthrography, Myelography, Discography, Fluoroscopy, and Videofluoroscopy)

Plain radiographs are obtained when an x-ray beam is directed through the body part being imaged to a sensitized plate; part of the beam is absorbed by the body, producing a shadow image on the plate. Five different types of tissues can be imaged with plain radiography: gas, fat, soft tissue/water, bone, and metal (metals, barium, iodinated contrast material). The differentiation of tissue within each of these five groups is limited, however, which makes it difficult to differentiate entities such as edema from blood or muscle from tumor. Nevertheless, plain radiographs are a relatively inexpensive way to assess fractures or bony abnormalities.

It is crucial to have plain radiograph protocols for each body part. The protocols should specify the number of views, technique, and film-screen combination. To exclude a fracture, at least two orthogonal views perpendicular to each other are necessary, and often three or more are needed, depending on the body part. Patient history and skin markers placed on the region of interest can help identify abnormalities and might alter the patient positioning or imaging technique.

Stress radiography is a procedure in which stress is placed on a given joint to assess for any change in joint width or alignment caused by ligamentous laxity or disruption, usually in comparison to the asymptomatic normal side. Acromioclavicular joint views holding weights, telos stress examination of the ankles with varus or posterior stresses,[19] and valgus stress on the elbow[80] are examples of stress radiography. Flexion and extension views of the cervical spine can also be considered stress views, although the stress is achieved passively using the weight of the head and the tension of the cervical muscles.

Arthrography is a procedure in which iodinated contrast material or air (or both) is instilled into a joint before plain radiographs are obtained. This outlines the joint space as well as structures within or surrounding the joint. Arthrography can be performed on virtually any synovial joint, but at present it is used less often than in the past because of the development of newer, noninvasive modalities. The risks of arthrography are those of a needle puncture, including hemorrhage, infection, and drug reaction. Tenography involves injection of iodinated contrast material into a tendon sheath to assess for tendon pathology or rupture of a ligament and abnormal communication with an adjacent joint space.

Myelography is plain radiography performed after instillation of iodinated contrast material into the thecal sac. Nonionic iodinated contrast material can be injected via a lateral C1–2 approach or posterior upper lumbar approach. Although myelography has largely been supplanted by magnetic resonance imaging (MRI), there are some advantages of myelography over MRI. Myelography and postmyelography computed tomography (CT) better show bony detail and subtle impressions on the nerve roots. Myelography also allows imaging of the lumbar spine in the upright weight-bearing position as well as in flexion and extension. The risks of myelography include hemorrhage, infection/meningitis, drug reaction, nerve damage, and cerebrospinal fluid (CSF) leak/spinal headache, but these risks can be minimized with careful technique.

Discography is a procedure in which plain radiography is performed after instillation of iodinated contrast material into the intervertebral disk spaces. Suspected symptomatic disks are injected along with a "control" disk. The most important aspect of discography is whether pressurization of the disk space during injection reproduces the location and quality of the patient's symptoms.[50, 68] Unequivocal concordant symptoms during the injection correlate with that disk being the pain generator. The risks of discography are similar to those of myelography, except for a slightly higher risk of infection due to the low vascularity of the intervertebral disk space.

Fluoroscopy is the real time x-ray visualization of structures and is used during spinal diagnostic and therapeutic procedures and in the instillation of contrast medium for arthrography, myelography, and discography. Fluoroscopy might or might not involve obtaining plain radiographs.

Videofluoroscopy entails recording fluoroscopic images to study the motion of joints. It can demonstrate dynamic abnormalities during motion, such as in the cervical spine and especially in the atlanto-axial-occipital region. When there is a question of vertebral fusion in a postoperative patient, dynamic videofluoroscopy can sometimes be helpful.

Computed Tomography

Computed tomography is the production of cross-sectional images of the body by selective absorption of a traveling x-ray or electron beam. Multiple detectors measure the transmission of the beam at multiple angles, and computer algorithms are used to form images from the data. Contrast between different tissue types is significantly higher with CT than with plain radiography, and there is more precise localization of structures on the cross-sectional imaging. The imaging plane is usually axial or axial oblique, although coronal images of the foot and ankle and sagittal or coronal images of the wrist and elbow can be obtained with variations in patient positioning. CT has a definite advantage over MRI in the imaging of cortical bone. Additionally, CT can better image chondroid and osteoid matrices. The detection of fractures and delineation of positioning of fracture fragments are achieved well with CT, but a fracture tangential to the imaging plane can be missed, in part due to partial voluming artifact.

Axial images can be reformatted into sagittal, coronal, oblique, or complex planes,[78] but the resolution depends on the section thickness of the original images and is degraded if there is patient motion during the scan. Three-dimensional reformatted images can also be obtained and may occasionally be helpful for surgical reconstruction of complex fractures.[56]

CT with Contrast Agent Enhancement

CT with intravenous (IV) contrast agent enhancement is more commonly used for imaging the brain, neck, chest, abdomen, and pelvis. Intravenous contrast medium is rarely used to image the spine or extremities except in the detection of soft tissue tumors or in the evaluation of postoperative spine patients, especially when MRI cannot be performed because of contraindications or artifacts from metal internal fixation devices.

Postarthrography CT delineates well the joint space as well as surrounding bony structures. Postarthrography CT of the shoulder is good at delineating the glenoid labrum but is limited to the axial plane. Air and a low volume of contrast agent are injected into a joint if CT is to be performed.

CT-Myelography and Postdiscography CT

Postmyelography CT is a requisite adjunct to myelography. The bony intervertebral foramina and spondylosis are best seen on axial CT images. Furthermore, intraforaminal or far lateral disk abnormalities can be invisible on the plain film myelogram and are best shown on CT. Disk abnormalities at L5–S1 might be invisible on myelography (because of the ample ventral epidural fat at this level), but visible on CT. The postmyelography CT levels should include any levels with abnormality detected on myelography, as well as any levels of clinical abnormality. The L5–S1 level should be included on all lumbar CT-myelograms because of the insensitivity of myelography owing to the ventral epidural fat at this level.

Postdiscography CT is an adjunct to discography to better demonstrate the anatomy of an annular tear (Fig. 7–1).

Magnetic Resonance Imaging

Magnetic resonance imaging is the production of cross-sectional images of the body through placement of the imaged body part in a large static magnetic field with a

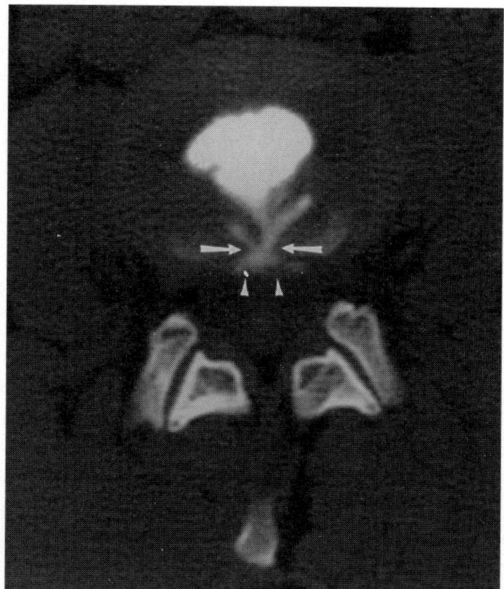

FIGURE 7–1. Postdiscography CT scan of a posterior central annular tear demonstrating iodinated contrast material extending from the nucleus through a midline tear (*arrows*) to a subannular location posteriorly (*arrowheads*). No focal convexity to the posterior disk margin is present; this abnormality would not be seen on plain CT or postmyelography CT.

TABLE 7–1 Relative Advantages and Disadvantages of MRI and CT

CT	MRI
Advantages	
Rapid acquisition time Less sensitive to motion than MRI Detection of calcification and ossification Less artifact from metallic foreign bodies or prostheses than MRI Good patient tolerance	Anatomical and pathological information (proton density, T1, T2, chemical shift) Better tissue contrast than CT Direct multiplanar imaging No ionizing radiation
Disadvantages	
Anatomical information predominantly; less pathological information than with MRI Ionizing radiation Limited imaging planes	More sensitive to motion than CT Longer acquisition time than CT, but getting faster Lower resolution for cortical bone or calcification than CT Considerable signal loss from metallic foreign bodies or prostheses Some problems with claustrophobia, although lessened with large-bore or open MRI scanners

varying magnetic gradient pulsed in such a way as to allow the resonance of hydrogen to be detected.[76] The data obtained are then converted by computer algorithms into cross-sectional images. These images depend on the number of mobile hydrogen atoms and specific tissue characteristics of the hydrogen. Pulse sequence parameters can be adjusted to accentuate certain inherent qualities of tissues, allowing for much higher contrast between different types of tissue (Table 7–1). For example, fat-containing tissues can be accentuated or suppressed; water-containing tissues can be accentuated or suppressed.

Since the patient is placed in proximity to a large magnetic field, there are contraindications to MRI. Patients with pacemakers, pacemaker wires, implanted electronic devices, ferromagnetic cerebral aneurysm clips, and metal around or within the orbits should not be scanned. Some other metallic devices are contraindications to MRI, and if there is a question of compatibility with the scanner, the consulting radiologist should be contacted prior to the examination.

MRI has multiple available imaging planes, including complex imaging planes. Multiple magnetic gradient pulse sequences are also available to accentuate different characteristics of tissues (Table 7–2). Standard pulse sequences include T1 weighting, proton density, T2 weighting, short inversion time/inversion recovery (STIR), and fat suppression imaging. Numerous pulse sequences are available on any given MR scanner, and different manufacturers may use different abbreviations for the sequences. The advent of fast spin-echo sequences has shortened imaging times. However, the natural fat signal suppression on T2-weighted spin-echo images is partially lost on fast spin-echo T2-weighted images unless additional fat suppression techniques are included.

The signal-to-noise ratio and image quality of an MR image depend on multiple factors, including magnetic field strength, surface coil design, field of view, matrix size, number of repetitions of the pulse sequences, other pulse sequence parameters, and patient size and body habitus.

STIR imaging shows additive T1 and T2 characteristics and has a high sensitivity for edema and many types of tumors. There is also suppression of the signal from fat, which causes the fat to appear dark, although some nonfat tissues can be suppressed if they have a short T1.[48]

TABLE 7–2 MR Signal Characteristics of Different Tissues

Tissue	T1-Weighted Images	T2-Weighted Images
Fat	High	Low*
Cortical bone	Low	Low
Fatty bone marrow	High	Low*
Red bone marrow	Intermediate	Intermediate
Muscle	Low–intermediate	Low–intermediate
Tendon	Low	Low
Ligament	Low	Low
Fluid	Low	High
Intervertebral disk	Low	High
Desiccated disk	Low	Low

* Low signal with routine spin-echo imaging. Fast spin-echo T2-weighted images do not show as much loss of fat signal.

Kinematic MR images are obtained as a joint is moved stepwise through a range of motion. This is useful to assess patellar tracking abnormalities.[93] Kinematic imaging of the temporomandibular joint and shoulder[88] can also be performed for specific clinical indications.

MRI with Contrast Agent Enhancement

Intravenous gadolinium contrast agents have several specific indications when used in conjunction with MRI. In spine imaging, IV contrast material is useful for assessing for postoperative scar versus recurrent or residual disk extrusion. Gadolinium contrast agents can show a breakdown of the blood-brain barrier with intramedullary or extramedullary intradural tumors. Musculoskeletal tumor detection can also be improved with IV contrast, although additional fat suppression techniques accentuate this enhancement.

Dilute gadolinium contrast material injected into joints significantly improves the delineation of many intra-articular and periarticular structures,[42] including the glenoid labrum and glenohumeral ligaments,[7, 71] the acetabular labrum,[24] a postoperative meniscus,[4] and the articular cartilage. Intra-articular gadolinium can also improve differentiation of partial-thickness from full-thickness tears of the rotator cuff. Nonenhanced bursal fluid has a different signal characteristic than intra-articular gadolinium. The risks of intra-articular injection of gadolinium are the same as for arthrography: hemorrhage, infection, and, rarely, anaphylactic reactions.

Nuclear Medicine Studies

Radionuclide bone scintigraphy is performed after IV injection of a bone-seeking isotope such as ^{99m}Tc-MDP to detect areas of increased bone turnover. Multiple lesions throughout the skeleton can be demonstrated in a single study, but radionuclide scintigraphy often has a low specificity. It can be useful for whole-body screening for bony metastases, but bony metastases in a given area can also be detected with MRI, which has a higher specificity and spatial resolution. A bone scan of the foot and ankle for chronic foot pain can help isolate the location of the abnormality, which might then be studied with MRI or CT. In the patient with mechanical back pain, a bone scan may help show the level of facet joint abnormality, although the facet joint with abnormal activity might not necessarily be the one that is painful. Often the contralateral facet is painful from abnormal stresses caused by the "hot" facet joint. Bone scanning is often used to detect stress or insufficiency fractures, but MRI might actually show these lesions earlier and provide better spatial resolution and specificity.

Single-photon emission computed tomography (SPECT) is an adjunct to the planar bone scan. It provides cross-sectional images of the body (axial, coronal, sagittal) using the same radioisotope emissions as a bone scan, but with a moving gamma camera. This is especially useful in the spine to show whether activity is greatest at the vertebrae anteriorly or around the facet joints or other posterior elements. The signal-to-background ratio is also improved with SPECT imaging. However, SPECT imaging takes additional time and adds expense, so it is used only for specific indications.

Radiolabeled white blood cell imaging is sometimes used to identify areas of osteomyelitis or infection. However, some noninfected areas such as around the tip of an orthopedic prosthesis or an amputated bone end can show increased activity.

Ultrasound

Shoulder ultrasound (US) for rotator cuff pathology was initially popular[55] but has become less utilized with the advent of improved shoulder MRI. US does not provide information about bone, the supraspinatus outlet anatomy, the glenoid labrum, or the glenohumeral ligaments. Shoulder US is very operator dependent, with the attendant variation in sensitivity and specificity.

High-resolution US allows targeted assessment of tendons and muscles for higher grade tears, hematomata, and calcification, and can be used to guide aspiration and injection of cysts or hematomas. However, US is operator dependent, and MRI is much more sensitive in the detection and grading of muscle and tendon pathology.

IMAGING ARTIFACTS

Imaging artifacts exist in great variety. Some of the most common artifacts are discussed here as they are routinely seen on image interpretation.

Plain Radiography Artifacts

On plain radiographs, a common artifact is the Mach line, which occurs when a bony edge overlaps another bone. A thin dark line appears just adjacent to the overlapping bone and can be mistaken for a fracture (Fig. 7–2).

CT Artifacts

The three artifacts seen most commonly with CT are those of partial voluming, streak, and beam hardening. A partial voluming artifact occurs because a CT section has a finite thickness (1, 3, 5, or 10 mm). If a structure extends only through a portion of the section, the attenuation is averaged with that of the structure beside it in the section. For this reason, partial voluming is more likely to occur with thicker sections. Partial voluming can result in missing a fracture in the axial plane, where it is averaged with the solid bone on either side of the fracture. Use of a thinner section thickness minimizes this artifact, which is why cervical spine CT images are obtained with a 1 or 1.5 mm section thickness. CT of ankle or foot fractures is performed with a relatively thin section thickness of 3 mm in both the coronal and axial planes, which minimizes the likelihood of missing a fracture from partial voluming.

Reconstruction of the CT data to form an image assumes a constant energy of the x-ray beam as it circles around the patient. An area of increased density, such as thick bone, can attenuate the lower-energy portion

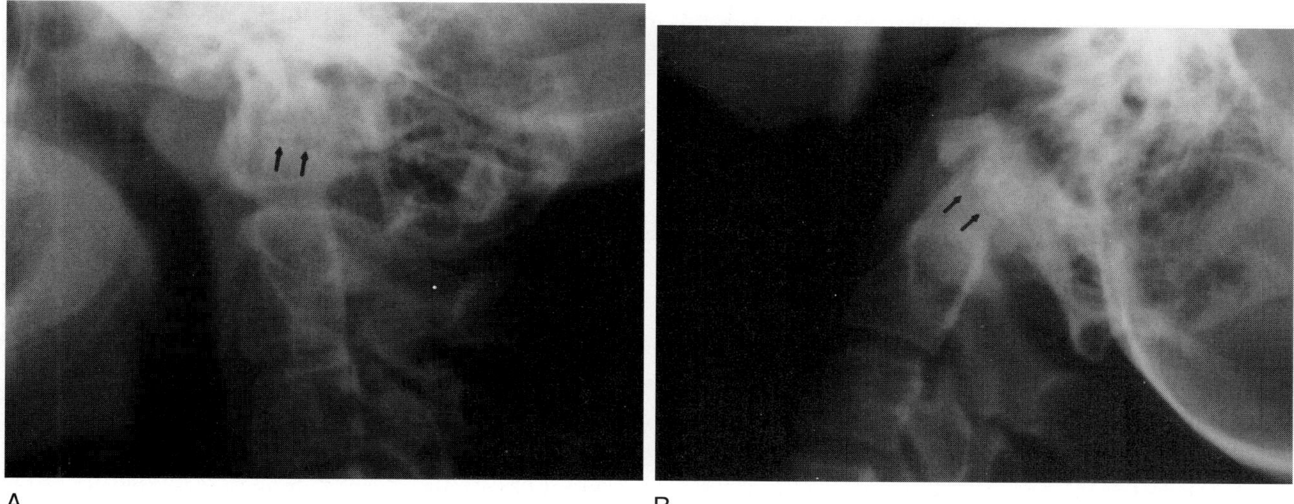

FIGURE 7–2. Mach line simulating a dens fracture. *A.* Lateral plain film of the cervical spine demonstrates a curvilinear lucency traversing the dens (*arrows*), but this parallels the undersurface of the C1 ring and mastoid bones as well as extending past the margins of the dens. *B.* Repeat extension lateral view of the same patient demonstrates no fracture line at the same site, and there is a fainter Mach line, now located more caudad (*arrows*).

of the x-ray spectrum and cause a relatively higher-energy beam to pass through. This difference in energy over a portion of the data stream can result in beam-hardening artifact, with variable attenuation central to the high-density bone (Fig. 7–3).

Streak artifact occurs where there is an interface between tissues of very different attenuation, such as bone and air, resulting in linear streaks extending along the plane of the interface. This can be seen at the bone-air interface of sinuses or at the interface of a metal prosthesis and bone. A metal prosthesis can result in both beam hardening and streak artifacts. Certain CT reconstruction algorithms can reduce these artifacts but not totally eliminate them.

MRI Artifacts

Partial voluming can occur with MRI in that there is a finite thickness of tissue sample to make an image and there can be averaging of signal from tissue components

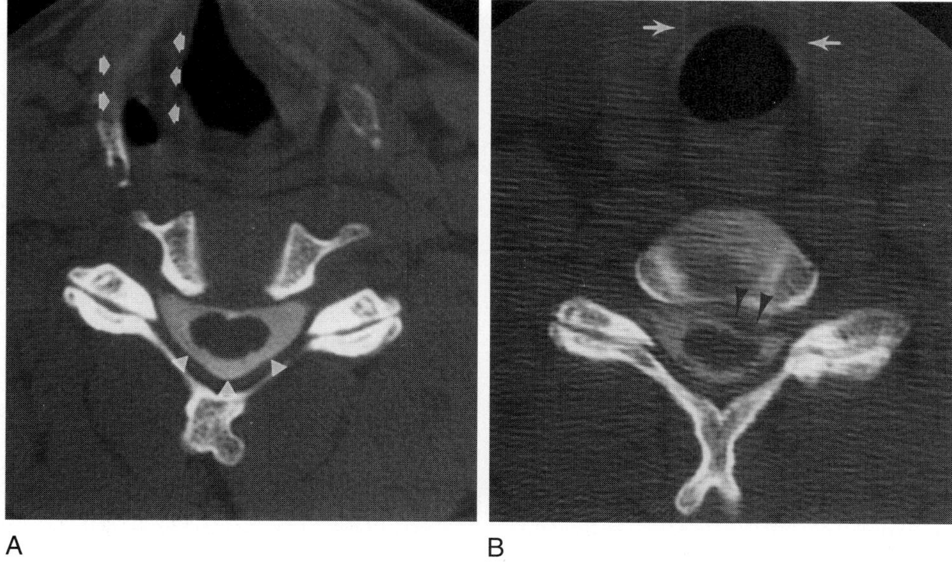

FIGURE 7–3. Streak and beam hardening artifact on CT. *A.* Postmyelography CT demonstrates low- and high-attenuation anteroposterior streaks at the air-soft tissue interfaces of the piriform sinuses (*arrows*). This image, obtained at the midcervical level, does not show beam hardening artifact from the shoulders, and the spinal cord cross section is well delineated, surrounded by intrathecal iodinated contrast material (*arrowheads*). *B.* A more caudal image in the same patient shows beam hardening artifact from the shoulders with multiple transverse lines degrading the image and making it more difficult to detect the left posterior extrusion tilting the cord (*arrowheads*). Streak artifact is seen at the air-soft tissue interface of the trachea (*arrows*).

within the thickness of the section. This effect can be reduced with thinner section thickness.[102] Partial voluming is routinely seen on sagittal images obtained through the spine at the lateral edge of the thecal sac, where there is partial voluming of the CSF with the epidural fat. Partial voluming of the edge of the spinal cord with the adjacent CSF on sagittal images can artifactually increase the signal intensity of the cord on the most lateral images of the cord.

Magic angle artifact is a phenomenon seen on imaging of anisotropic structures that course 55 degrees (the "magic angle") relative to the main magnetic field in the MR scanner.[30, 31] There is an artifactually increased signal within the structure at this angle. This artifact most commonly occurs during imaging of tendons that are anisotropic and course at a 55-degree angle to the main magnetic field, such as in the rotator cuff supraspinatus tendon[106] or the ankle tendons as they course around the malleoli. The artifact is especially problematic in the rotator cuff, where increased T1 and proton density signal in the critical zone (which may course 55 degrees relative to the main magnetic field) can represent tendinopathy. A partial-thickness or full-thickness tear of the supraspinatus should not be confused with the increased signal intensity arising from imaging at the magic angle, as T2-weighted images show more signal abnormality with tears and less magic angle effect.

Chemical shift artifact is seen because the resonance frequency of hydrogen varies with the structure that the hydrogen is within.[102] The resonance frequency of fat is slightly different from that of water because of the different hydrogen bonds. Consequently, the reconstruction algorithm can position fat slightly differently than water-containing structures, leading to artifacts in the frequency encoding direction. This can cause misregistration of fatty bone marrow in relation to soft tissues adjacent to the bone, giving an asymmetry and inaccuracy of cortical bone thickness in the extremities[27] or at the vertebral end-plate/cortex.

Motion artifact is usually visible on MR images as blurring or double images.[102] Flow artifact from vessels or CSF can cause artifacts, usually in a line in the phase encoding direction. These artifacts can often be minimized with flow compensation or saturation bands in the imaging protocol. However, if there is an unusual round focus of signal not expected within a structure, it is worth checking to see if it lies in a horizontal or vertical line with a blood vessel and if it is of the same caliber.

Metal artifact occurs when either microscopic or macroscopic metal fragments cause a localized change in the homogeneity of the magnetic field. This can result in a focus of signal void with an adjacent high-signal-intensity ring.[102] These artifacts are dramatically evident when a prosthesis or internal fixation device is present, and they appear as small foci in the postoperative patient if microscopic fragments of metal break off the drills or other instruments during surgery. The small high-signal ring or partial ring near the signal void will help differentiate this artifact from a calcification or hemosiderin. Artifact from metal can be reduced by using T2-weighted fast spin-echo techniques rather than conventional spin-echo techniques.[104]

IMAGING OF THE SPINE

Trauma

Plain radiography is the best initial screening procedure to use in assessing for fracture. In the cervical spine, a minimum three-view examination (lateral, AP, and open mouth odontoid) should be obtained. All of C7 and the C7–T1 interspace should be visualized. If a fracture is seen or suspected, thin-section CT with reformatting or helical CT can better delineate that fracture and can also disclose other associated vertebral fractures not seen on the plain radiographs.[1, 69] MRI can best show any traumatic disk extrusion or spinal cord abnormality if the patient has myelopathic symptoms.[29] Fast spin-echo T2-weighted images with fat suppression can show soft tissue edema or hemorrhage associated with ligamentous tearing in whiplash injuries in the acute setting, but this study is not routinely done in patients without myelopathy or neurological deficit.

For cervical spine trauma, the ACR Appropriateness Criteria unanimously give a Least Appropriate rating to plain radiographs in the asymptomatic and alert patient with normal physical examination findings, with or without a cervical collar. If the patient is symptomatic or has neurological signs or symptoms of cervical injury, then a minimal screening examination of three-view plain radiographs is given a Most Appropriate rating. If the patient has normal plain radiographs but neurological signs or symptoms are present, MRI is given a Most Appropriate rating, with CT-myelography as an alternative if MRI is not possible.

MRI performed before and after IV gadolinium instillation can help differentiate vertebral collapse due to osteoporosis from that due to malignancy.[23]

Intramedullary Abnormalities

MRI is the procedure of choice for assessing the intramedullary spinal cord. Six MRI patterns have been defined by their appearance on T1-weighted images, before and after contrast injection, and on T2-weighted images, with a short differential diagnosis for each.[12]

ACR Appropriateness Criteria are available for different types of myelopathy, including traumatic, painful, sudden-onset, stepwise progressive, slowly progressive, seen in an infectious disease patient, and seen in an oncology patient, with high ratings for MRI in all instances, and predominantly high ratings for plain radiography. The addition of post-contrast enhancement MRI is considered appropriate in several of the situations, such as the infectious disease patient or stepwise progressive condition, or if the non-contrast-enhanced MRI is negative or symptoms are not explained in an oncology patient. If the myelopathy is painful, of sudden onset, or of slow progression, contrast studies might be appropriate if MRI is negative, or to better characterize a known abnormality.

Intramedullary primary and metastatic neoplasms are well shown on MR T2-weighted images. Most intramedullary spinal tumors enhance with gadolinium contrast agents.[73] Contrast-enhanced MRI can help differentiate enhancing tumor from nonenhancing demyelination or a nonenhancing myelitis. Metastatic tumors can show a very focal enlargement of the cord as opposed to the more diffuse enlargement with primary gliomas.

The abnormalities of multiple sclerosis can be located entirely in the cervical spinal cord without brain involvement. Spinal cord multiple sclerosis plaques are characteristically peripherally located, are less than two vertebral segments in length, and occupy less than half the cross-sectional area of the cord.[105] If a cord lesion is suspicious for multiple sclerosis, either by imaging or by clinical criteria, MRI of the head should be performed to look for additional lesions and to strengthen the putative diagnosis.

MRI can well demonstrate enlargement of the cord from syringomyelia and may demonstrate an associated Chiari I malformation. If a syrinx involves the entire cervical region with no Chiari malformation to explain it, consideration can be given to imaging the rest of the cord, as cord tumors located more caudally can be associated with a holocord syrinx.

Increased T2 signal within the cord can be seen in areas of chronic compression from degenerative disk disease and from spondylosis. The likelihood of detecting increased cord signal is proportional to the severity of the clinical myelopathy and the degree of spinal canal compression.[103] The response to surgical or medical treatment is less favorable in patients with increased cord signal than in those without. Improvement in this imaging parameter after surgical treatment is a good prognostic indicator.

Intradural Extramedullary Abnormalities

MRI with IV gadolinium contrast is the most sensitive imaging study for assessing abnormalities within the dural sac, including drop metastases, hematogenous leptomeningeal metastases, meningitis, and arachnoiditis (Fig. 7–4).[36] T2-weighted axial images without contrast can well demonstrate the three different types of arachnoiditis seen on MRI. These include nerve clumping, tumefactive mass-like arachnoiditis, and the "empty sac" sign of the roots being attached to the thecal sac.[85] Residual Pantopaque, a possible cause for arachnoiditis, may be seen as fat signal on MRI due to its oily base.

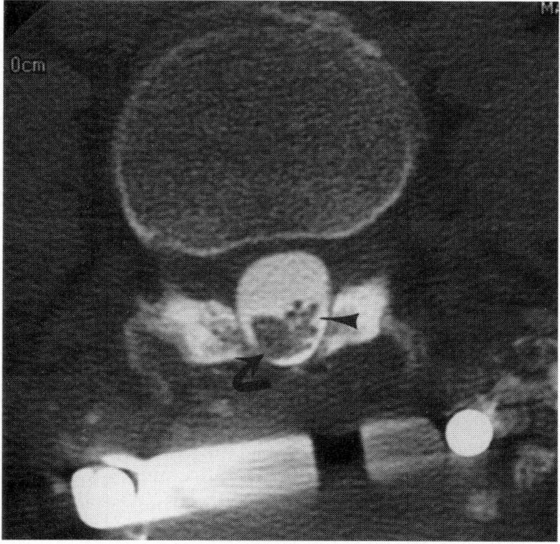

FIGURE 7–4. Postmyelography CT of arachnoiditis following laminectomy, fusion, and dural tear demonstrates clumping of the right-sided roots (*arrow*), with more evenly spaced left-sided roots (*arrowhead*). This clumping was seen just cephalad to the site of dural repair and dural surgical clips.

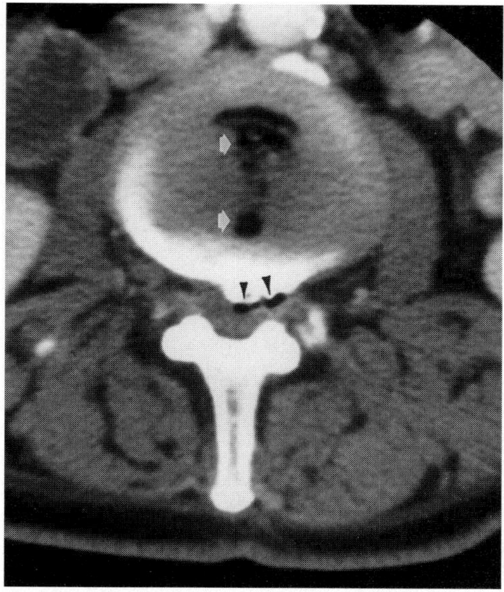

FIGURE 7–5. Non-contrast-enhanced CT of the spine demonstrating "vacuum" phenomenon with gas in the disk space (*arrows*) and extension of gas into the left ventral epidural space (*arrowheads*), indirect evidence of an annular tear. The ventral epidural gas is just posterior to the left paracentral endplate osteophyte contributing to acquired spinal stenosis.

Nerve root tumors such as schwannomas or neurofibromas can actually be well shown on myelography, as they may move with the roots with upright and prone positioning, indicating their origin. Nevertheless, MRI with contrast agent enhancement increases the conspicuity of intradural or intradural-extradural root sheath tumors and their relation to the nerve root.

Extradural Abnormalities

Degenerative Disk Disease and Spondylosis

MRI is probably the single best examination to assess the intervertebral disk and surrounding structures. However, plain CT and postmyelography CT can both demonstrate any morphological abnormalities of the disk contour as well. Plain CT or postmyelography CT can show gas within the epidural space from extension through a full-thickness annular tear when the degenerated disk space contains gas, the "vacuum phenomenon" (Fig. 7–5). There is little correlation between plain radiograph findings and the presence or absence of a disk extrusion.

The high incidence of asymptomatic imaging abnormalities in the general population makes it difficult to prove that an imaged abnormality is the pain generator. Discography with pressurization of the disk space may be the most accurate method of determining whether an abnormal-appearing disk is a generator of lower back pain[68] or a generator of pain radiating to the lower extremities in a patient with no MRI evidence of nerve root compression,[50, 61] if the patient has unequivocal concordant symptoms during pressurization different from a control disk level. Controversy remains regarding the utility of discography.[66, 68]

The ACR Appropriateness Criteria for lower back pain include ratings for variants of uncomplicated lower back pain with no red flags, acute lower back pain in the setting of trauma, steroid use, osteoporosis or age over 70, acute lower back pain with suspicion of cancer or infection, acute lower back pain with radiculopathy, acute lower back pain with prior lumbar surgery, and acute lower back pain with cauda equina syndrome. For uncomplicated lower back pain with no red flags, all imaging modalities are assigned a Low Appropriateness rating. MRI becomes more appropriate in the other clinical settings and is rated more appropriate than plain lumbar radiography in all of the different variants of lower back pain except for that seen with trauma, steroid use, osteoporosis, and age over 70.

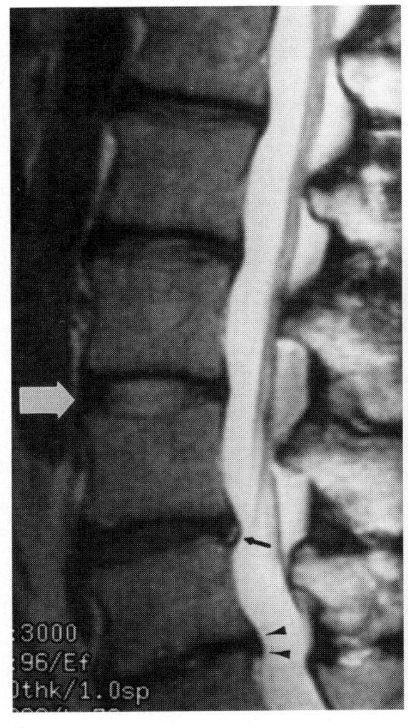

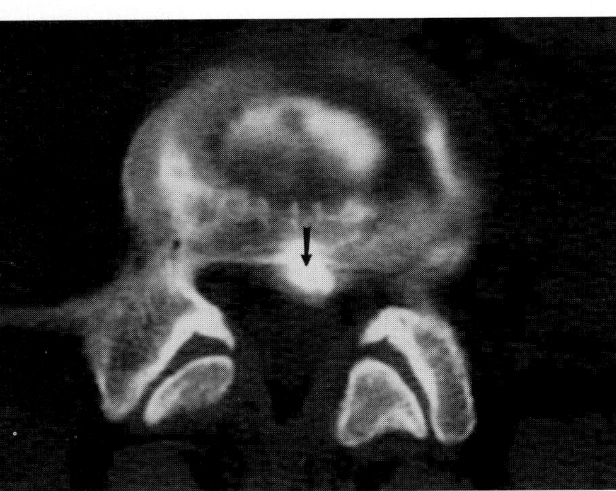

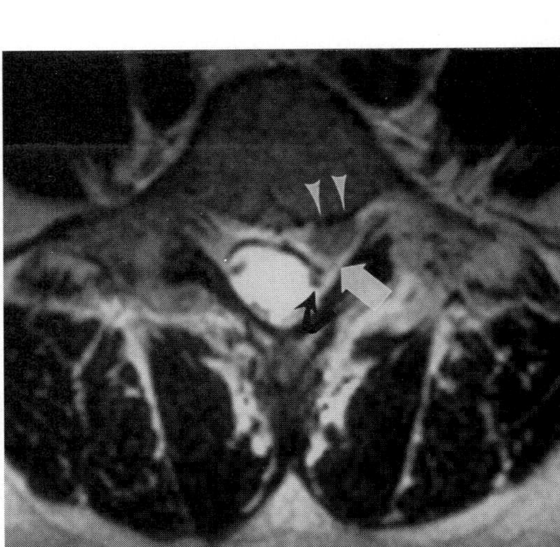

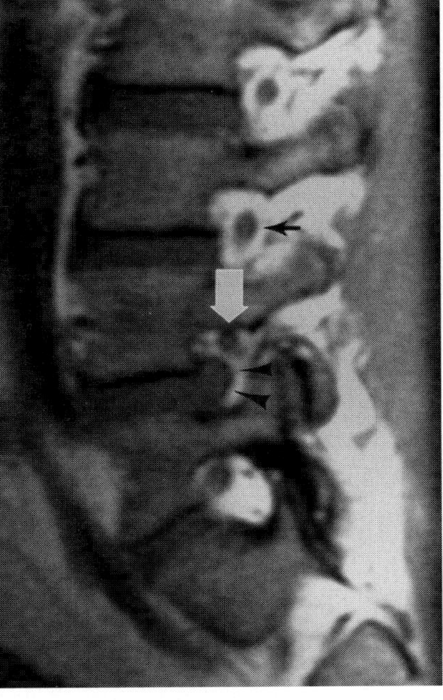

FIGURE 7–6. Various disk abnormalities. *A.* T2-weighted sagittal MRI of the lumbar spine demonstrates normal height and hydration of the L3–4 disk (*thick arrow*). The L5–S1 disk space is severely narrowed, with loss of hydration and low T2 signal intensity as well as a circumferential bulging of the disk (*arrowheads*). The L4–5 disk space shows moderate loss of height and hydration, with a focal convexity to the posterior disk having a focus of increased T2 signal intensity (*thin arrow*), consistent with annular tear and protrusion. *B.* Postdiscography CT demonstrates extension of contrast material into a left paracentral subannular region (*arrow*), consistent with an annular tear and protrusion. This disk lesion is similar to that seen at L4–5 in *A. C.* Axial T2-weighted MRI of the lumbar spine demonstrates a focal convexity to the disk extending caudad from the left posterior aspect of the disk, consistent with a focal extrusion, as the depth is greater than the width (*arrowheads*). This extrusion impinges on the exiting left root just posterior (*thick arrow*) and deviates the descending root within the thecal sac just adjacent (*arrow*). *D.* Sagittal T1-weighted MRI obtained more laterally at the intervertebral foramina shows a focal convexity to the L4–5 disk, which extends cephalad into the intervertebral foramen (*arrowheads*) and deviates the exiting L4 root superiorly (*thick white arrow*), representing an intraforaminal extrusion. The adjacent normal intervertebral foramen shows a low-signal exiting root (*black arrow*) surrounded by high T1 signal foraminal fat.

The normal intervertebral disk has a low T1 and high T2 signal, with a lower T2 signal cleft centrally and a surrounding low-signal annulus. With disk degeneration, the T2 signal of the nucleus begins to decrease as the nucleus dehydrates. Once the disk has lost T2 signal, the signal does not return. Loss of the T2 signal can be seen with either intravertebral disk space narrowing or normal disk height, but more commonly with the former.

Disk herniation is an ambiguous term denoting some form of disk pathology; the pathology can be more precisely described. Other than disk desiccation, there are four stages in the progress of disk herniation (Fig 7–6)[14]:

1. Circumferential bulging of the disk, consistent with weakening of the annulus fibrosis.
2. Protrusion of the disk, in which a focal convexity has a width wider than depth, consistent with a partial-thickness tear through the annulus fibrosis. These partial tears can also show a focus of increased T2 signal that represents fluid or granulation tissue extending through the annular tear. These annular lesions can sometimes appear more like a radial tear, and in some cases more like a partially circumferential tear, shaped like a bucket-handle tear.
3. Extrusion of the disk, in which a focal convexity has a depth greater than the width, consistent with the nucleus extending through a full-thickness tear of the annulus and extending extra-annularly. Other criteria for extrusion that can be used are extension of the nuclear material cephalad and caudad past the levels of the end-plates or visible extension through the annulus and posterior longitudinal ligament.
4. Sequestered or free fragment, in which the extruded disk material is not connected with the native nucleus pulposus. These fragments can be located well cephalad or caudad from the donor site and can extend into the intervertebral foramen. Often these sequestered fragments have different signal characteristics than the native disk.

Imaging findings of degenerative disk disease must be correlated with clinical history, physical examination findings, and possibly diagnostic injection results; many abnormal imaging findings can be asymptomatic. In 60 asymptomatic patients 20 to 50 years old, the patient prevalence of lumbar disk bulge was 20% to 28%. For protrusion it was 38% to 42%, for annular tears 32% to 33%, for extrusion 18%, and there were no disk sequestrations.[113] Disk extrusion, sequestration, nerve root compression, end-plate abnormalities, and moderate to severe facet joint osteoarthritis were rare in asymptomatic patients younger than 50 years when the prevalence among all 300 lumbar intervertebral disk levels in the study was considered.[113] In 36 patients (17 to 71 years old) without lower back pain or sciatica, the prevalence of disk bulge was 81%, protrusion 33%, and annular tears 56%, with no extrusions noted.[101] Annular tears showed contrast enhancement in 96%. However, assessment of T2 high-intensity zones in the disk (annular tears) by other authors in other studies showed a high correlation with pain at discography and a low prevalence in asymptomatic patients.[5, 89] A high prevalence

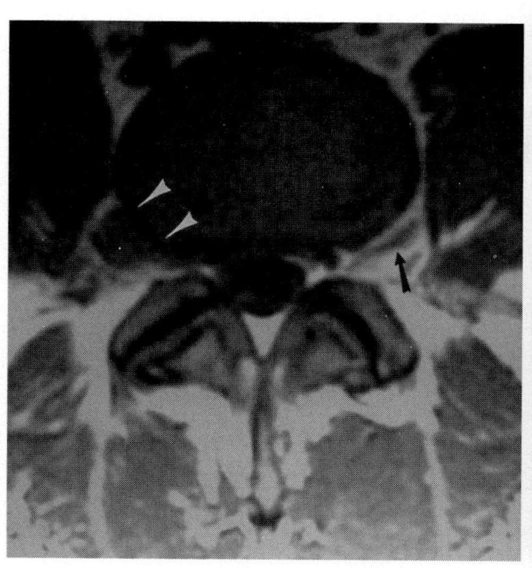
E

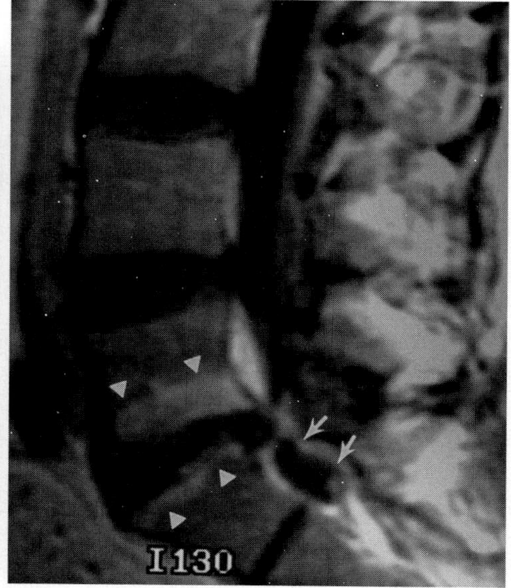

F

FIGURE 7–6 *Continued. E.* Axial T1-weighted image of the lumbar spine demonstrates a focal convexity to the right far lateral disk (*arrowheads*) deviating the exited nerve root in comparison to the normally exiting root on the contralateral side (*arrow*). The disk abnormality has a depth similar to width, best described as an extrusion. *F.* Sagittal T1-weighted image of the lumbar spine after intravenous injection of gadolinium contrast agent demonstrates narrowing of the L5–S1 disk space and degenerative changes of the adjacent end-plate (*arrowheads*). Just caudad to the posterior aspect of the disk space is a nonenhancing mass (*arrows*) that is separate from the native disk space and best described as a free fragment or sequestered disk.

of abnormal findings on cervical MRI of asymptomatic individuals, increasing with age, is also seen.[10]

Intervertebral disk contour abnormalities can occur anywhere along the circumference of the disk and are usually described by location as central, paracentral, posterior, posterolateral, and far lateral. Posterolateral disk abnormalities can be further described as occurring at the entrance zone, within the foramen, or at the exit zone of the foramen. MRI criteria to differentiate subligamentous from transligamentous disk extrusion, such as the presence of a continuous low-signal-intensity line posterior to the extrusion, disk extrusion size less than 50% of the size of the spinal canal, and absence of disk fragments, are unreliable.[94]

Small epidural hematomas can be associated with disk extrusions[38] and cause a larger mass effect than can be accounted for by the extrusion itself. If the extradural mass effect trails along a root sheath toward the foramen or has signal characteristics more like those of fluid or hemorrhage, then a small epidural hematoma should be considered.

End-plate degenerative changes associated with disk degeneration have been classified into type 1 (low T1 and high T2 signal), edema or fibrovascular signal; type 2 (high T1 and high T2 signal), fat signal[64]; and type 3, low T1 and low T2 signal, consistent with discogenic sclerosis.

Facet Joint Abnormalities

Facet and pars interarticularis abnormalities can often be seen with plain radiography. Oblique views are necessary to assess for a pars defect (spondylolysis). CT with bone detail is the most accurate means of assessing for a pars defect and can demonstrate any hypertrophic bone formation at the facet or pars contributing to foraminal narrowing (Fig. 7–7). MRI is relatively insensitive to cortical bone defects and so 30% of cases of lumbar spondylolysis may be undiagnosed if the physician relies on direct visualization of pars interarticularis defects.[109] However, 97% of levels of spondylolysis have been shown to yield one or more secondary MRI signs, including increased sagittal diameter of the spinal canal, wedging of the posterior aspect of the vertebral body, and reactive marrow changes in the pedicle distinct from normal adjacent levels.[109] Spondylolysis without spondylolisthesis can appear as widening of the sagittal dimension of the spinal canal because of dorsal subluxation of the posterior elements.[108] Fluoroscopy during facet joint injection below a pars defect shows flow of the contrast agent into the pars defect and often then to the facet joint above the pars defect.

Facet degenerative changes of sclerosis, joint space narrowing, and marginal osteophytosis can be shown on oblique plain radiographs but are optimally demonstrated with CT. MRI is relatively insensitive for demonstrating cortical bone or osteophyte, and shows foraminal narrowing indirectly by effacement of fat around the exiting root. Cartilage degeneration and sclerosis are related to age, lumbar spinal level, and overall facet joint angle, while tropism at the facet joints may result in slightly more sclerosis but not cartilage degeneration.[37]

Synovial cysts are best demonstrated on MRI, where the signal characteristics of the lateral extradural mass are usually those of fluid, with low T1 and high T2 signal (Fig. 7–8). This will also demonstrate the associated lateral recess stenosis. Postmyelography CT can also be diagnostic if the cyst is large enough to show water attenuation, and the adjacent bony facet joint abnormalities are also shown.

Spinal Stenosis

Spinal stenosis can be described as congenital/developmental or acquired. Acquired spinal stenosis can be

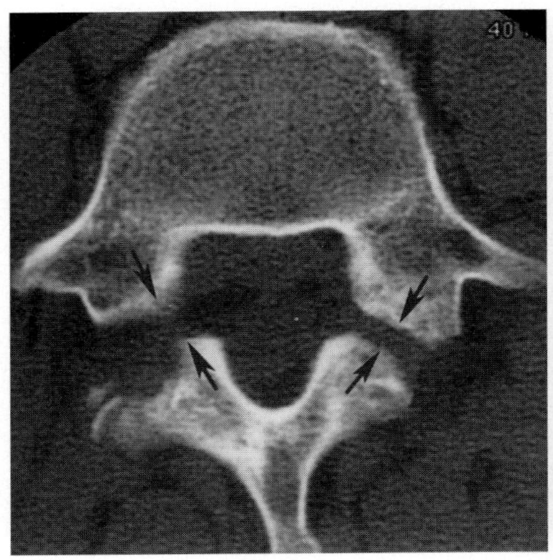

A

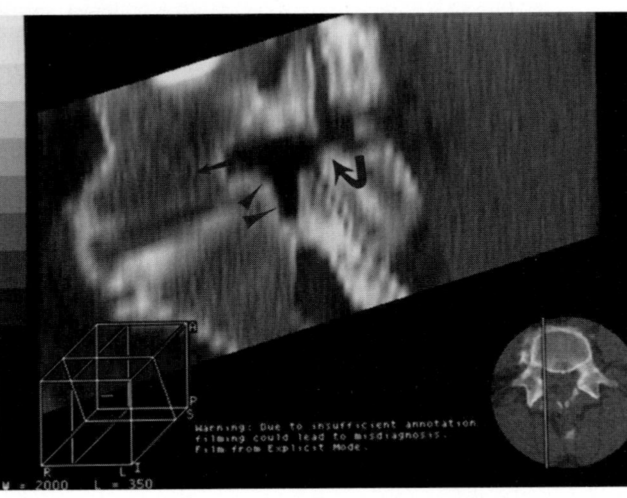

B

FIGURE 7–7. CT of pars interarticularis defects. *A*. Axial CT scan demonstrates discontinuity of the lumbar vertebral ring (*arrows*). *B*. Sagittal reformation of axial CT images obtained at a plane through the facet joints and pars interarticularis demonstrates the pars defects (*curved arrow*) as well as a grade 1 spondylolisthesis (*straight arrow*). The combination of disk space narrowing and anterolisthesis contributes to bony foraminal narrowing (*arrowheads*).

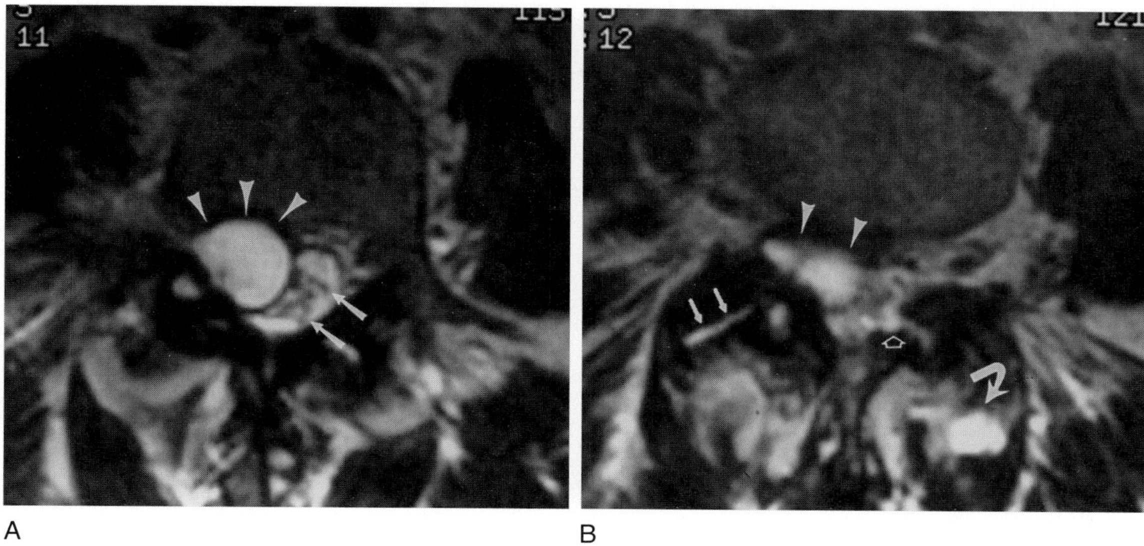

FIGURE 7–8. MRI of a large synovial cyst associated with facet degenerative joint disease (DJD). *A.* Axial T2-weighted image of the lumbar spine demonstrates a right lateral extradural mass with high T2 signal (*arrowheads*) impinging on the thecal sac containing the descending roots (*arrows*). *B.* An image obtained just inferior to that in *A* again shows the high T2 signal mass (*arrowheads*) as well as its association with a narrowed and sclerotic facet joint (*arrows*). On the left are two additional synovial cysts, with the smaller just medial to the facet joint (*open arrow*) and another just posterior to the facet joint (*curved arrow*).

further classified as central, lateral recess, and foraminal. Central and lateral recess stenosis are usually caused by a combination of disk degeneration, facet hypertrophic change, and ligamentum flavum enlargement. While MRI and CT-myelography can both demonstrate narrowing of the spinal canal, myelography and postmyelographic CT have the additional benefit of showing facet bony detail and end-plate osteophytosis, and allow upright weight-bearing views, which often accentuate the stenosis. Symptoms of spinal stenosis are usually worse with standing or walking, and there is often a discrepancy in the imaging appearance when the patient is imaged standing versus supine or prone. Foraminal narrowing is often well demonstrated on sagittal MRI images, where there is normally an exiting root surrounded by epiradicular fat. Disk space narrowing and consequent craniocaudal foraminal narrowing, any anterolisthesis, and facet hypertrophic change can be well shown on MRI.

Nerve Roots

Visualization of the nerve roots is excellent on MRI, especially on sagittal images of the lumbar region and thin-section axial images of the cervical region. However, cervical myelography can be better at showing subtle impressions on the root sleeves that are difficult to discern on MRI. Furthermore, postmyelography CT affords a more accurate measurement of the foraminal caliber than MRI, for cervical foraminal narrowing is often accentuated by the pulse sequences used with MRI. There has been preliminary work in MR-neurography using high-resolution surface coils, with some correlation between enhancement of the cervical root and associated radiculopathic symptoms.

Lumbar nerve root enhancement can correlate with root compression and radicular symptoms,[36, 44] but transient enhancement at the affected level can be seen in asymptomatic patients in the first 6 months following surgery.[28]

Postoperative Spine Imaging

Postoperative spine patients with residual or recurrent symptoms have special imaging considerations. Plain radiographs can often demonstrate any hardware positioning or failed fusion.[96] If hardware is present, both CT and MRI have some limitations,[104] as described previously. Flexion and extension plain radiographs can show motion at a failed fusion site. CT can show gas within the disk space (vacuum phenomenon), which is an indicator of movement. If the patient is asked to fully flex and then fully extend prior to CT, the vacuum phenomenon can develop and can be utilized as a sign of nonfusion. With posterior fusions, if the facet joint remains visible and there is resorption of fusion bone, this is an indicator of nonfusion. Persistent lucency above or below a bone plug or anterior fusion cage also suggests nonfusion if enough time has elapsed since the surgery.

Recurrent or residual disk extrusion is best assessed with MRI before and after IV contrast agent injection to differentiate extruded disk material from epidural scar or fibrosis (Fig. 7–9).[28] Extruded disk material does not show central enhancement during the first 15 minutes following IV gadolinium administration but may show some central enhancement later.[43] An extruded disk can exhibit superficial enhancement due to an inflammatory component or surrounding scar (the "wrapped disk"). It might be reasonable to perform both MRI and CT-myelography in problematic diagnoses, since some end-plate osteophytes, calcified disk fragments, or facet osteophytes can be relatively invisible on MRI. Spear-like osteophytes impinging on

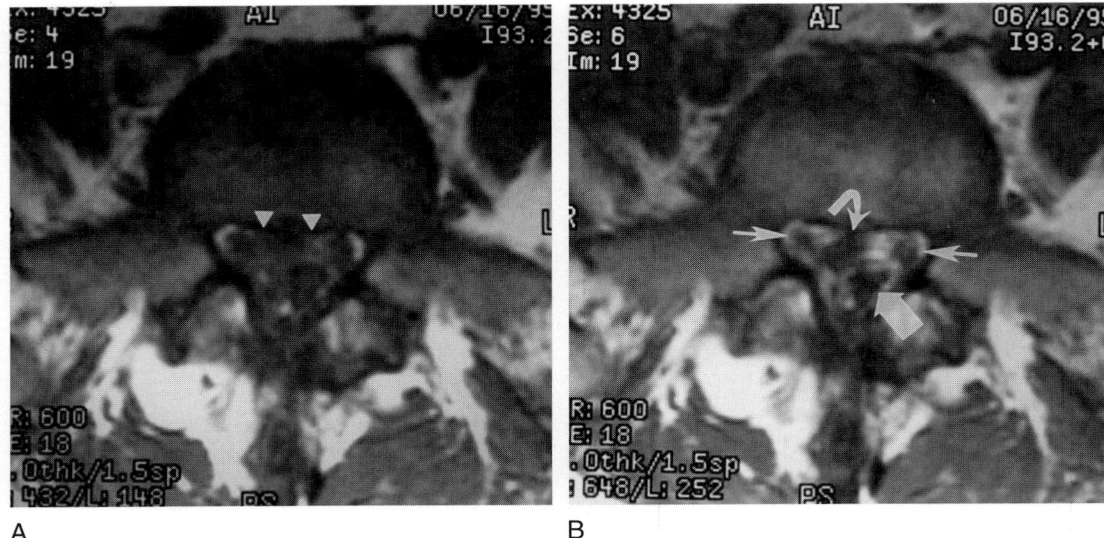

FIGURE 7–9. MRI of a recurrent disk extrusion after previous discectomy. *A.* Axial T1-weighted image obtained without contrast enhancement demonstrates low T1 signal material within the spinal canal and poor delineation of the thecal sac and nerve roots (*arrowheads*). *B.* Postcontrast axial T1-weighted image obtained at the same level as that in *A* shows enhancement of epidural fibrosis and better delineation of the thecal sac (*thick arrow*), descending nerve roots (*thin arrows*), and recurrent disk extrusion (*curved arrow*).

the spinal cord or nerve roots might also be invisible on MRI.

The postoperative disk can show linear enhancement—two thin bands paralleling the end-plates, sometimes with end-plate enhancement—as well as enhancement at the curettage site in asymptomatic patients.[86]

Non-contrast-enhanced MRI or myelography/postmyelography CT is usually sufficient for imaging the cervical postoperative patient. Contrast-enhanced MRI sequences are not usually indicated in a cervical postoperative patient, as most operations are performed by the anterior approach and there is rarely scar formation in the cervical epidural space. If the patient has had a foraminotomy or surgical complication, then cervical spine MRI with contrast agent enhancement might be a consideration.

Infection

Classic plain radiographic findings of discitis or osteomyelitis can clinch the diagnosis if disk space narrowing and end-plate loss are shown. However, MRI can demonstrate the disk space narrowing, abnormal disk space signal, end-plate loss, and adjacent changes in the vertebral marrow (Fig. 7–10).[63] There is a decrease in the normal high T1 signal from fatty marrow as well as

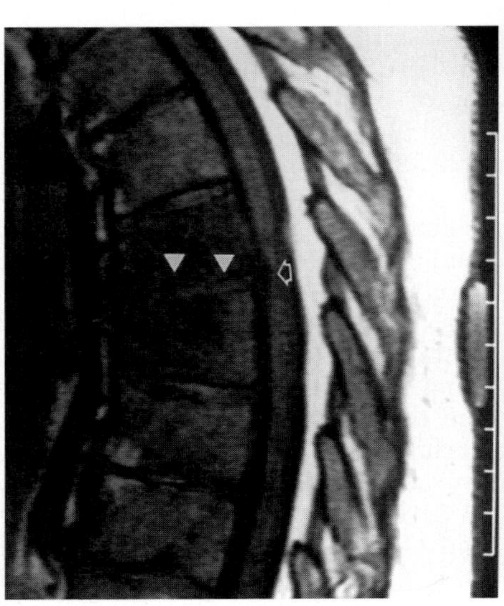

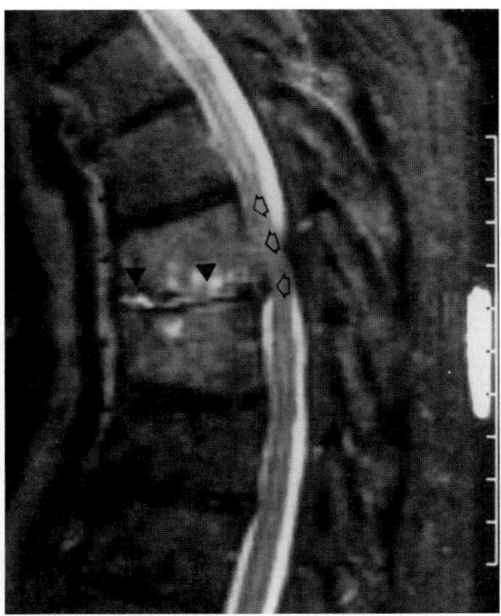

FIGURE 7–10. MRI of discitis and osteomyelitis. *A.* Sagittal T1-weighted image at the midline shows decreased signal within the thoracic vertebral bodies adjacent to a narrowed disk space with an irregular end-plate (*arrowheads*). The spinal cord is indented ventrally at the disk level (*open arrow*). *B.* Sagittal T2-weighted image obtained through the same area as *A* demonstrates increased T2 signal within the vertebral marrow and disk space with irregular end-plates (*arrowheads*). There is a ventral extradural mass effect on the cord at the disk level and posterior to the vertebral body (*open arrows*), consistent with epidural extension of the infection.

increased T2 signal in the marrow. Most narrowed disk spaces exhibit low T2 signal from desiccation, so if the T2 signal within the narrowed disk is increased, discitis is a consideration. Vertebral end-plate degenerative changes with low T1 and high T2 signal can mimic the marrow changes of osteomyelitis but are not associated with high disk T2 signal.

Postoperative discitis or osteomyelitis can sometimes be problematic in that a postoperative disk can exhibit increased T2 signal from scar, and there might be degenerative marrow changes showing low T1 and high T2 signal edema. However, the end-plates usually remain sharp and intact in the postoperative patient as opposed to patients with osteomyelitis or discitis. In the patient with infection, contrast-enhanced MRI is the best means of assessing for any epidural spread or paravertebral abscess.

Tumors and Extraspinal Abnormalities

Non-contrast-enhanced MRI is more sensitive in demonstrating vertebral metastatic disease than is radionuclide bone scan. MRI is especially sensitive (relative to radionuclide bone scan or plain radiography) in demonstrating myeloma involvement.[25] However, bone scintigraphy has the advantage of being able to survey the whole body for metastases. If the only area of interest is the vertebrae, then MRI can be both more sensitive and more specific. Additionally, MRI shows any extradural mass effect on the thecal sac, spinal cord, or nerve roots. STIR images are most sensitive for marrow-replacing tumors.[60] Intravenous gadolinium administration can actually make MRI less sensitive for vertebral metastases, as the usual appearance—low T1 signal metastases upon a bed of high T1 signal fatty marrow—becomes less conspicuous with enhancement and increased T1 signal of the metastases (Fig. 7–11).

In the setting of a primary vertebral tumor, it is imperative to obtain plain radiographs and possibly CT scans to assess for chondroid or osteoid matrix. Radionuclide bone scan can be helpful in determining whether the tumor is monostotic or polyostotic.

MRI, with its multiplanar capabilities, can demonstrate extraspinal abnormalities,[70] but the field of view might be limited, as the images are usually tailored (and filmed) to the spinal structures. Coronal images of the spine can show causative paraspinal abnormalities in patients with scoliosis.

MUSCLE IMAGING

Muscle is seen as a soft tissue attenuation on plain radiographs, demarcated by adjacent fat planes. Differentiation of the separate muscles and muscular abnormalities is usually not possible with plain radiography.

Imaging assessment of muscles includes assessment of position, size, and MR signal intensity. CT can be used to assess for position and often size of the muscles, but except for hemorrhage within a muscle, there is little CT attenuation difference between normal and abnormal muscle. MRI is best for assessing muscle position, size, and pathological changes.

Muscle position is assessed for evidence of retraction, as with a full-thickness muscle or tendon tear, such as with the supraspinatus tendon in rotator cuff injury. Anomalous muscles, such as an accessory soleus muscle

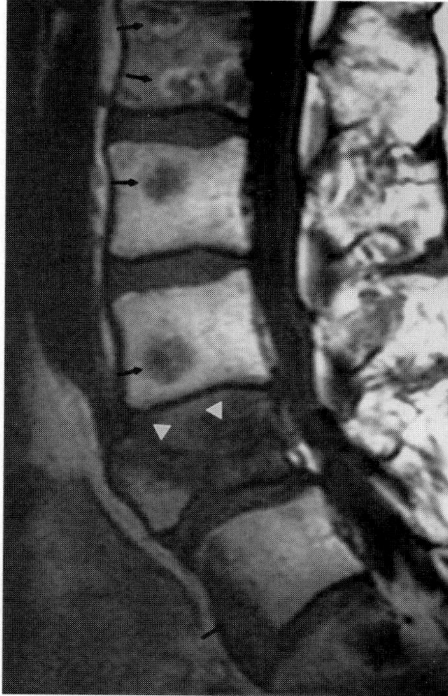
A

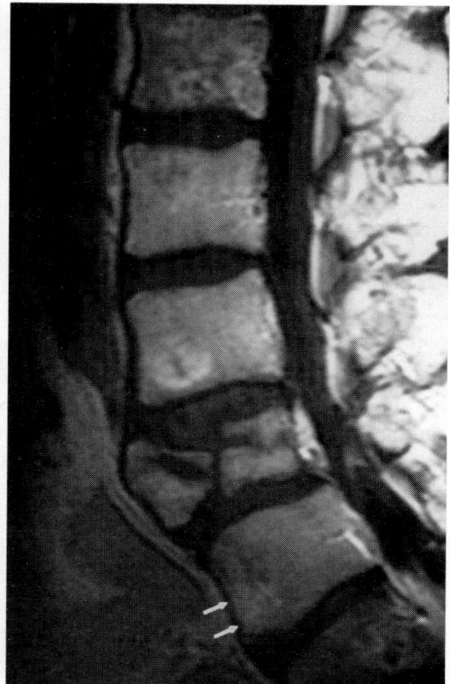
B

FIGURE 7–11. MRI of vertebral metastases before and after intravenous injection of gadolinium contrast. *A.* Sagittal T1-weighted image of the lumbar spine obtained without contrast enhancement in a patient with multiple vertebral metastases (*arrows*) and L4 pathological vertebral compression fracture (*arrowheads*) demonstrates predominantly low T1 signal of the lesions against the higher-signal fatty marrow. *B.* After intravenous injection of gadolinium contrast, the metastases enhance and become less conspicuous. The lesion involving the anterior aspect of the L5 vertebral body has become much less apparent (*arrows*). The tumor involving the L4 compressed vertebral body enhances to demonstrate the bony fragments.

causing an asymmetry between the calf muscles, should not be confused with a tumor.

Muscle size can vary over a wide range of normal, but a large asymmetry can be indicative of muscle atrophy if there is volume loss, such as can be seen in the paraspinal muscles with previous poliomyelitis. Increased muscle size can be seen with weight training, but the muscles retain their normal MR signal. Increased muscle size with abnormal signal intensity can be seen with muscle inflammation, edema, or contusion. Increased muscle size and abnormal signal can be seen with delayed-onset muscle soreness or rhabdomyolysis from exercise-induced injury.

Normal muscle has a low T1 and low to intermediate T2 signal. Increased T1 signal can be seen with old intramuscular hemorrhage or chronic fatty atrophy. On STIR sequences an increased T2 signal within the muscle can be seen with trauma, inflammation, and acute to subacute denervation.

Muscle trauma can be graded on a spectrum from strain (grade 1) to partial tear (grade 2) to full-thickness tear (grade 3). Muscle strain is characterized by a mild, poorly circumscribed, increased T2 signal and greater increased STIR signal, with an intact muscle and no discrete fluid collections within the muscle. There can be some fluid collection in the fascial planes between muscles or beneath the muscle capsule.[13] A partial tear is characterized by a more discrete focus of increased T2 signal intensity, with possibly some disrupted muscle fibers or fluid tracking longitudinally between muscle fibers. There should be no retraction of the muscle. A full-thickness tear is characterized by retraction of the muscle and free edges, usually with material of increased T2 signal intensity in the gap.

Muscle strains are an indirect injury to muscle caused by excessive stretch. The muscles most commonly involved are those that contain the highest proportion of fast twitch (type II) muscle fibers: the hamstrings, quadriceps, adductors of the hip, medial gastrocnemius, the triceps and biceps brachialis, and abdominal wall muscles. Muscles involved in eccentric action (lengthening) are those most likely to be strained. Clinical grading can be difficult owing to swelling and pain. MRI allows detection and grading of complications such as hematoma or muscle herniation.

Acute to subacute denervation of muscle results in a mildly increased T2 signal and more prominently increased STIR signal.[87, 114] Increased muscle signal in the acute to subacute stage changes to fatty atrophy with increased T1 signal and loss of muscle mass in the chronic stage. Idiopathic peroneal nerve palsy can result in early changes of abnormal increased T2/STIR signal within the extensor digitorum longus and tibialis anterior muscle (Fig. 7–12). Acute to subacute denervation changes can be seen in the infraspinatus and supraspinatus muscles with impingement on the suprascapular nerve by a paralabral ("ganglion") cyst.[33, 107] Transection of a muscle with proximal innervation can result in denervation changes distal to the transection or partial transection. Neurotoxic chemotherapy can result in a patchwork appearance of muscle signal changes.

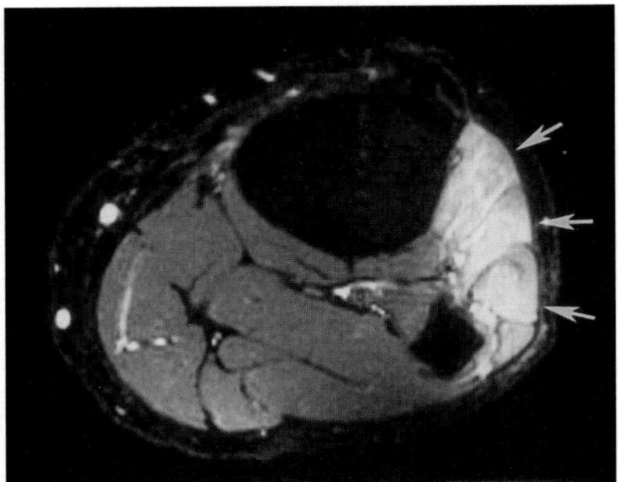

FIGURE 7–12. Axial STIR image of the proximal leg demonstrates markedly increased signal in the tibialis anterior, extensor digitorum longus, and peroneus longus muscles (*arrows*) in a patient with peroneal nerve palsy clinically. These signal abnormalities resolved over a time course similar to that of the clinical improvement.

NERVE IMAGING

The larger peripheral nerves can be imaged in cross section on CT when they are surrounded by fat. They are better imaged with MRI, where they have a low T1 signal surrounded by high-signal fat, or with STIR sequences, where they have an intermediate to high signal surrounded by low-signal fat. MRI is excellent for assessing an extrinsic mass effect on nerves, such as in the spinoglenoid notch from a suprascapular paralabral cyst or in the brachial plexus from a tumor. Intrinsic abnormalities of the nerves are more difficult to assess on routine MRI unless there is an enlargement of the nerve to indicate the level of abnormality. However, high-resolution experimental phased array surface coil imaging can show areas of intrinsic nerve abnormality.[57] The field of view can be relatively small with high-resolution scans, so the site of suspected abnormality needs to be established as accurately as possible prior to the scan.

TENDON IMAGING

The tendons can be assessed in imaging studies for position, size, and MR signal intensity.[32, 46, 91, 116] As with muscle, CT can demonstrate tendon position and (to an extent) size, but is unable to show intrinsic abnormalities. It is also sometimes limited by the fact that adjacent muscle, ligament, and tendon can have a similar CT attenuation. The multiplanar capabilities and tissue discrimination available with MRI make it the best imaging modality to assess tendons.

Tendon position is assessed both in the setting of a complete rupture, where there is retraction, as well as in subluxation or dislocation of an intact tendon, as can be seen with the biceps tendon in a subscapularis tendon tear or transverse ligament tear.

Tendon caliber is best assessed in a true cross section, which in some cases can require an oblique plane, as with curving of the peroneal tendons behind the lateral malleolus.[46] Imaging in planes tangential to the tendon can be compromised by partial voluming with adjacent fat. Assessment of tendons should include the musculotendinous junction, where many of the traumatic injuries occur.

Tendon size is easily comparable between extremities as well as between adjacent tendons (Fig. 7–13). Tibialis posterior tendon tears are graded as a grade 1, partial tear with enlargement of the tendon and longitudinal split; grade 2, partial tendon tear with attenuation of size and disruption of some of the tendon fibers; and grade 3, full-thickness tendon tear with retraction of the tendon.[84] Enlargement of a tendon can be seen with an acute partial tear and longitudinal split with fluid between the tendon fibers, with a chronic tendon tear and scar tissue increasing the girth of the tendon, as well as with acute or chronic tendinitis. The signal characteristics of the enlarged tendon help to differentiate these entities.[116]

The normal tendon is of very low, homogeneous T1 and T2 signal intensity. The magic angle phenomenon can artifactually increase signal intensity within the tendon when it is coursing at a 55-degree angle to the main magnetic field. The problem is greatest at the supraspinatus tendon in the rotator cuff[106] and at the ankle tendons as they course around the malleoli, for in these two cases, the region of artifactually increased signal is also that where pathology is most likely to be seen.

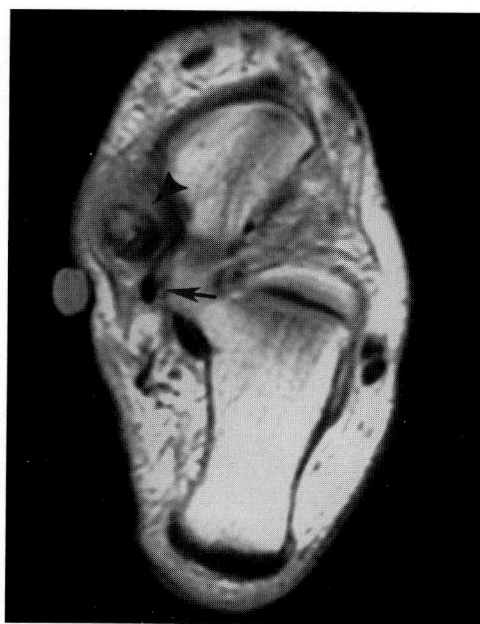

FIGURE 7–13. Axial T1-weighted image of the hindfoot demonstrates a grade 1 partial tear and longitudinal split with enlargement and increased signal in the tibialis posterior tendon (*arrowhead*) and lower signal surrounding the tendon, consistent with soft tissue edema. The tendon is markedly enlarged in comparison to the adjacent flexor digitorum longus tendon (*arrow*), which shows a uniform low signal intensity and normal caliber.

Increased T1 and proton density signal in the tendon can be seen with tendinosis (degeneration) or with tendinitis. Tendinosis usually becomes less evident with increasing T2 weighting, whereas tendinitis might or might not. Fluid or hemorrhage within the tendon becomes increasingly evident with increased T2 weighting. Chronic scarring of the tendon is usually of low signal intensity on all sequences, similar to the native tendon, and may appear as an enlargement of the tendon.

Fluid within the tendon sheath can be a normal finding in specific tendons, such as the biceps tendon or the flexor hallucis longus tendon, which communicate with the joint space. Fluid within other tendon sheaths, such as the peroneus longus tendon sheath, can be indicative of a calcaneofibular ligament tear with fluid extending from the mortise joint. Synovitis or tenosynovitis are also considerations when fluid is seen between the tendon sheath and a normal or enlarged tendon, respectively. Fluid surrounding a tendon that has no tendon sheath, such as the Achilles tendon, would be consistent with a peritenonitis, shown best on T2-weighted images with fat saturation.

LIGAMENT IMAGING

Ligaments can be indirectly assessed on plain radiographs by the presence of subluxation or dislocation, or movement with stress maneuvers. The telos stress examination is used to assess the ankle ligaments with posteriorly directed and varus stress.[19] Three-compartment arthrography is utilized to indirectly assess the carpal ligaments for rupture.[115]

Direct visualization of ligaments is best performed with MRI.[19, 47, 81, 92, 99, 110] Ligaments are assessed for continuity, size, and signal intensity.

A ligament should be continuous from insertion to insertion, with a smooth linear or curvilinear contour. Waviness of the ligament is consistent with a tear and partial retraction. Some ligaments will have a normal curvature in certain joint positions, and this should be taken into account during assessment; the posterior cruciate ligament takes a more curvilinear course with the knee in extension and a more linear course with the knee in flexion. The course of the ligament must also be assessed in that some complete ligament tears can heal in an abnormal position, such as a chronic anterior cruciate ligament tear that has healed in a more horizontal position.[110]

Knowledge of the range of normal ligament calibers is helpful during assessment. Many ligaments, such as the anterior talofibular ligament, are uniform in thickness along their lengths. Others, however, are comprised of multiple smaller fascicles and can assume a more fan-shaped appearance, such as the posterior-inferior tibiofibular ligament. Thickening or thinning of the ligament can occur with an acute or chronic partial tear.

Ligaments have homogeneous, low T1 and low T2 signal intensity on MRI. Increased T1 and T2/STIR signal intensity within or around the ligament is suggestive of a sprain or partial tear, whereas a complete tear disrupts the ligament, usually with intervening high T2 signal intensity in the acute stage (Fig. 7–14). A healing or healed full-thickness ligament tear might show low T2 signal material at the site of the tear, making it more difficult to delineate the location or even presence of a tear.[110]

CARTILAGE IMAGING

Cartilage thickness cannot be directly seen on plain radiographs, although secondary changes of severe chondromalacia such as joint space narrowing, subcortical sclerosis, and cyst formation can be seen.[41] Chondrocalcinosis is probably best detected on plain radiographs. Arthrography can demonstrate the thickness and surface contour of hyaline cartilage, as can postarthrography CT.[41] MRI and MR-arthrography best demonstrate cartilage thickness, contour, and any intrinsic signal abnormalities.[41, 82] Fat-suppressed proton-density images show excellent contrast between bone, cartilage, and intra-articular fluid (Fig. 7–15).[82]

There are four arthroscopic stages of chondromalacia. The earliest chondromalacia appears as a small focus of softening. This grade of chondromalacia may not be visible on MRI, but with probing it may be identified as a focal soft area on arthroscopy. Grade 2 chondromalacia is a focally increased thickness, with the cartilage showing some increased T2 signal, like a small blister or edema. Grade 3 chondromalacia is a thinning and focal irregularity of cartilage. Grade 4 chondromalacia is loss of cartilage to the bone, possibly with additional cortical sclerosis and/or cystic changes.

MR-arthrography is superior to CT-arthrography for demonstrating osseous and cartilaginous intra-articular bodies.[16] MRI and CT without intra-articular contrast

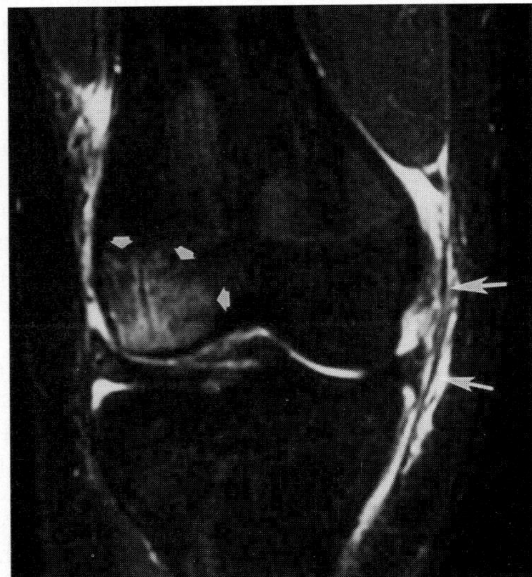

FIGURE 7–14. Coronal STIR image of the knee demonstrates high-signal fluid deep and superficial to the medial collateral ligament (*arrows*), which is avulsed from its femoral attachment, indicating grade 3 (complete) tear. Increased signal intensity within the lateral femoral condyle (*short arrows*) is consistent with a bone bruise, as may be seen with a varus injury at the knee.

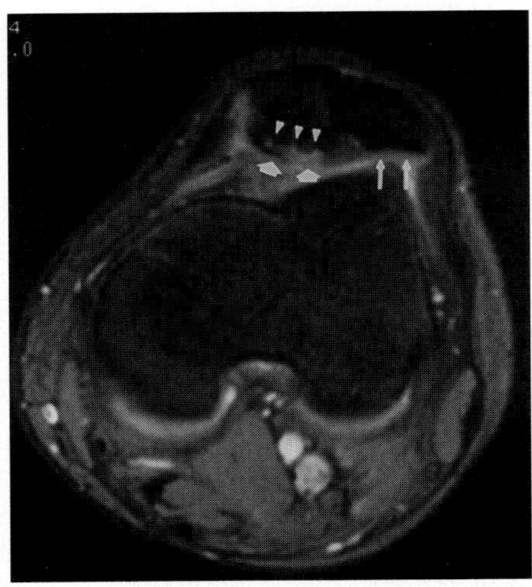

FIGURE 7–15. Axial proton-density fat-suppressed image of the knee demonstrates grade 3 and grade 4 chondromalacia of the patellar cartilage. Focal loss of cartilage to the bone (*short arrows*) is accompanied by abnormal signal within the adjacent marrow (*arrowheads*). A small area of normal cartilage shows intermediate signal intensity and normal underlying cortex (*thin arrows*).

are less accurate than either MR-arthrography or CT-arthrography.

BONE IMAGING

Plain radiography is the initial screening procedure for assessing fractures throughout the body except in the skull, where head CT is the initial procedure of choice. Orthogonal views of the body part of interest are mandatory to exclude a fracture. Some regions require a special view, such as a mortise view in the ankle, an oblique view in the hand, wrist, and foot, and an axillary or transscapular view in the shoulder.

Non-contrast-enhanced CT with or without multiplanar reformatting is utilized to assess the position of fracture fragments in more complex fractures, such as those involving the wrist or ankle-foot. Preoperative assessment of highly comminuted fractures can include CT.[56]

MRI is insensitive in assessing cortical bone. MRI images mobile hydrogen, and cortical bone has very little mobile hydrogen. MRI does well in assessing bone marrow, as well as bone marrow edema, making it quite sensitive to any fractures or processes that change the normal bone marrow signal. Fat within the bone marrow gives marrow a high T1 signal, depending on the degree of fatty versus red marrow, and a lower T2 signal. Consequently, any process that decreases the T1 signal and increases the T2 signal, such as edema or intratrabecular hemorrhage, might be quite conspicuous on MRI. The high sensitivity of MRI to bone marrow signal changes is best shown on non-contrast-enhanced T1-weighted and highly T2-weighted or STIR images. Intravenous contrast enhancement of marrow processes can decrease the conspicuity of the abnormality in relation to the high T1 signal intensity of marrow.

MRI is highly sensitive in the detection of reticular infractions (bone bruises), geographic infractions, stress or insufficiency fractures (Fig. 7–16), osteochondral fractures, and, indirectly, macrofractures.[15, 72, 111] Bone bruises can occur in typical locations for a given injury, such as lateral knee bone bruises with the "terrible triad of O'Donohue," the medial patellar facet and lateral femoral condyle with a patellar dislocation, and anteroinferior glenoid with an anteroinferior humeral dislocation. These bone bruises may be the only sign of a previous dislocation if there has been spontaneous reduction. Some authors have thought that osteochondral defects can be a sequela of certain geographic infractions.[111]

Palmer et al showed in 78 fractures of the knee and shoulder that MRI demonstrates prominent marrow edema with impaction fractures and minimal edema with distraction fractures.[72] Furthermore, impaction fractures are more often missed on plain radiographs, and distraction fractures (such as Segond fractures) are more often missed on MRI.

The ACR has Appropriateness Criteria for imaging of suspected stress/insufficiency fractures (excluding vertebral fractures). Eleven different clinical scenarios are presented, each with recommended imaging studies. The first imaging study should be plain radiography.

Assessment for avascular necrosis (AVN) should initially be performed with plain radiography. If the study is negative, then MRI imaging is highly sensitive and specific for AVN.[22] Bone scintigraphy might be able to demonstrate AVN in earlier stages, as "cold spots." However, there is a crossover period when AVN might not be detected by bone scan, between when the bone scan is "cold" and when it becomes "hot."[22] Even if a hip radiograph indicates AVN, MRI can be considered to assess for asymptomatic AVN in the contralateral hip. MRI is useful in assessing the percent involvement of the femoral head as well as in characterizing the marrow signal within the avascular region. The "double-line sign" of low and high T2 signal intensity at the margin of AVN is a relatively specific finding, seen in 80% of cases.[62]

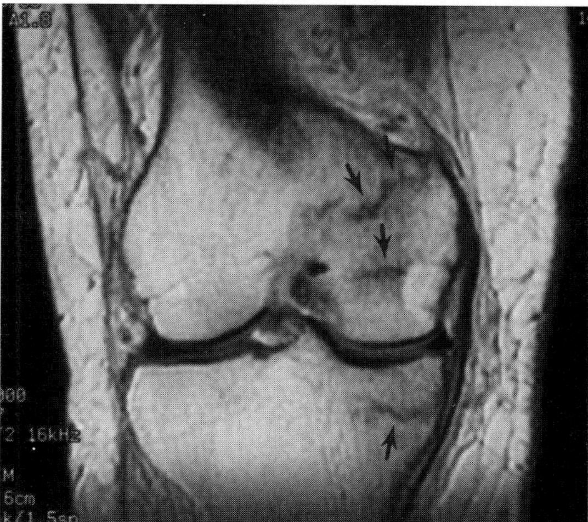

FIGURE 7–16. Coronal T1-weighted MRI of the knee demonstrates stress fractures of the medial femoral condyle and medial tibial plateau with serpentine linear low T1 signal (*arrows*) on a background of high T1 signal fatty marrow.

Osteochondritis dissecans in its intermediate to severe stages can be well shown on plain radiographs and non-contrast-enhanced CT scans. However, the earliest phase of geographic marrow edema is not visible on plain radiographs, but it is well shown on MR, especially STIR sequences (Fig. 7–17). MR further shows the condition of the cartilage overlying the bony defect and can show if there is loosening, indicated by high T2 signal fluid extending around the lesion or displacement of the osteochondral fragment.[41]

BONE AND SOFT TISSUE TUMORS

ACR Appropriateness Criteria for suspected primary bone tumors list routine radiography as an absolute requirement in a patient with a suspected bone lesion. If the radiograph is normal and there is focal pain, then MRI is the second imaging study. If the radiograph shows a lesion suspicious for malignancy, MRI is indicated, and if the lesion appears benign on radiographs, CT or MRI is indicated only for preoperative planning. If the lesion is a suspected osteoid osteoma, CT is recommended.

Non-contrast-enhanced CT can be considered for more accurate localization of bone lesions or assessment of any cartilaginous or osteoid matrix. A whole-body bone scan is useful to assess the entire skeleton to determine whether the lesion is single or multiple. Sometimes bone tumor MR signal can be pathognomonic, such as with an intraosseous lipoma with uniform high T1 fatty signal, or an aneurysmal bone cyst with blood product layering. However, a significant percentage of lesions might not be accurately categorized as benign or malignant with MRI, even with plain radiographic correlation.[53] MRI is effective at demonstrating origin, margins, and extension into bone marrow or adjacent soft tissue structures, as well as subperiosteal tracking and marrow "skip" lesions.

The ACR has Appropriateness Criteria ratings for imaging metastatic bone disease in 13 different clinical scenarios. In some scenarios no imaging is recommended, and in others a different combination of plain radiography, bone scan, MRI, and/or CT is considered most appropriate.

The ACR Appropriateness Criteria indicate routine radiography as the first imaging study for suspected soft tissue mass. MRI is usually the second imaging examination recommended, except that CT can be useful for characterizing types of calcification and assessing myositis ossificans, and can possibly be more useful than MRI in areas with motion artifact. MRI is thought to be the most useful study to assess extension into bone marrow and adjacent soft tissues, while also providing multiplanar delineation of the tumor.

Certain MR signal characteristics can be helpful in characterizing soft tissue masses, such as high T1 signal fat with a lipoma or liposarcoma, or low signal hemosiderin with pigmented villonodular synovitis (PVNS).

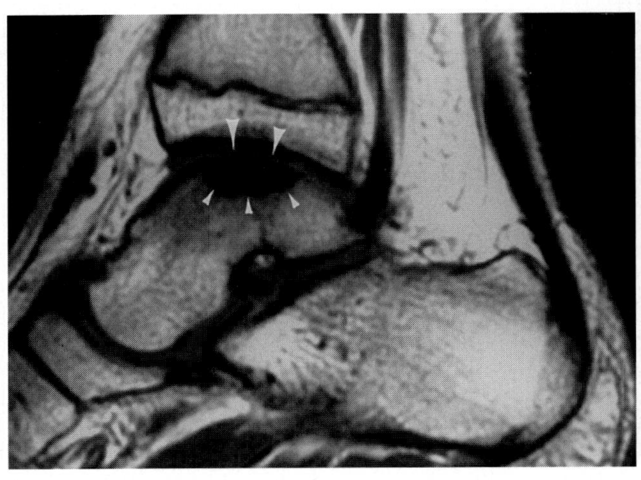

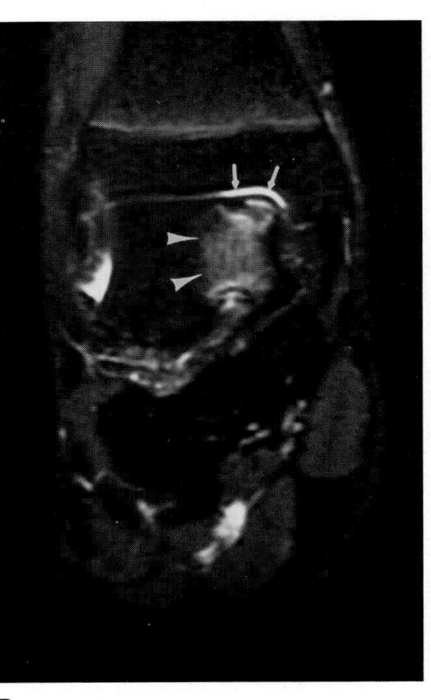

A B

FIGURE 7–17. MRI appearance of talar dome osteochondritis dissecans. *A.* Sagittal T1-weighted image of the hindfoot demonstrates a geographic focus of decreased T1 signal within the talar dome (*small arrowheads*). There is irregularity to the cortex overlying this lesion (*large arrowheads*). *B.* Coronal STIR image in the same patient demonstrates increased signal at the medial talar dome with at least a portion of the lesion having intact overlying cortex (*arrows*). The signal abnormality from bone marrow edema is more conspicuous on the STIR sequence (*arrowheads*) than on the T1-weighted sequence.

MRI is useful for primary subjective identification of some benign lesions (lipoma, superficial and deep skeletal muscle hemangiomas, arteriovenous malformations, periarticular cysts, hematomas), but for tumors with a nonspecific imaging appearance MRI is not reliable for distinguishing benign from malignant tumors.[53, 65]

To be considered benign, cystic lesions must meet three MRI criteria: (1) signal intensities that are homogeneous and lower than those of muscle on T1-weighted images, (2) T2 signal intensities homogeneously bright and similar to those of fluid, and (3) a uniformly thin rim, which may or may not enhance.[54] A thick rim, a multiseptated thick rim, or nodular components suggest that a simple cyst is not present.

IMAGING OF SPECIFIC BODY REGIONS

Shoulder Imaging

In the trauma setting, plain radiography is the initial imaging study of choice for the shoulder. Internal rotation and external rotation views, as well as an orthogonal view such as axillary or transscapular view, should be obtained. A posterior dislocation could theoretically be missed if only internal and external rotation views are obtained, unless one recognizes that there is limited rotation between the views because of the dislocation.

ACR Appropriateness Criteria for imaging in the setting of acute shoulder trauma to rule out fracture or dislocation recommend an AP view and an axillary lateral or scapular Y-view as most appropriate. If a patient has persistent shoulder pain and has had normal radiographs within the preceding 2 weeks, there is no consensus as to the most appropriate study; some experts say that MRI is indicated and some recommend repeating plain radiography. In the patient with subacute shoulder pain and a question of bursitis or calcific tendinitis of approximately 3 months' duration, the first study recommended is radiography with internal and external rotation views.

Impingement and Rotator Cuff Tears

The ACR Appropriateness Criteria indicate routine MRI for suspected rotator cuff tear or impingement in patients over the age of 40 with normal plain radiographs. Direct visualization of the tendons and muscles as well as detection of indirect evidence of rotator cuff tear is available with MRI (Fig. 7–18). MRI imaging of the shoulder has become more valuable as interpretation has improved and more attention has been paid to technique.[77, 95] Coronal oblique and sagittal oblique planes of imaging (perpendicular and tangential to the plane of the glenoid) are utilized to obtain images parallel or perpendicular to the muscles and tendons of the rotator cuff.

Assessment of rotator cuff tendon position, thickness, and signal intensity is optimal with MRI. Early impingement results in thickening of the tendon, usually of the supraspinatus. More advanced tendinopathy results in thinning of the tendon. When the rotator cuff abnormal-

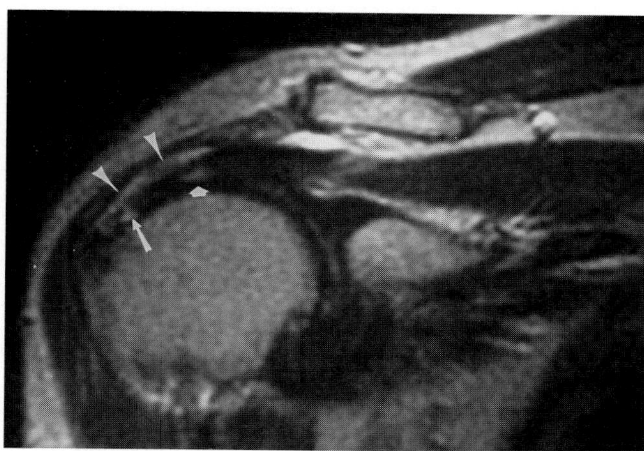

FIGURE 7–18. Coronal oblique T2-weighted image of the shoulder demonstrates a full-thickness tear of the distal supraspinatus tendon (*arrow*) with high T2 signal extending through the thickness of the tendon and increased T2 signal fluid within the subacromial-subdeltoid bursa (*arrowheads*). Increased T2 signal from a partial-thickness tear does not completely extend through the tendon (*short arrow*).

ity progresses to a partial-thickness tear, there is increased T1, proton-density, and T2 signal intensity within the tendon that reflects a morphological thinning. A full-thickness tear shows through-and-through increased signal; the position of the musculotendinous junction can be identified to determine whether there is any retraction from a full-thickness rotator cuff tear. The proximodistal and AP dimensions of a rotator cuff tear can be estimated. Unenhanced MRI is much less sensitive for partial tears than for full-thickness tears.[6]

Partial and complete rotator cuff tears can be seen on MRI in a significant percentage of asymptomatic individuals, the percentage increasing with age.[67] MRI-evident bone and peritendinous shoulder abnormalities are highly prevalent among asymptomatic individuals, but the prevalence of subacromial spurs, humeral head cysts, subacromial-subdeltoid bursal fluid, and disruption of the peribursal fat plane in each case is closely associated with an increasing severity of MRI-evident rotator cuff abnormalities.[67]

Contrast-enhanced arthrography with plain radiographs might demonstrate only articular side partial tears and not bursal side tears. Full-thickness tears can be shown with contrast-enhanced arthrography, but the size of the tear and the condition of the torn edges are poorly defined. Plain radiographs are useful for assessing for undersurface osteophytes at the acromion and acromioclavicular joint. They can also reveal the calcification of calcific tendinitis. Factors predisposing to impingement, such as undersurface osteophytes or a laterally downsloping acromion, can be detected using either arthrography or MRI. US is sometimes used to assess for rotator cuff tear, but it is highly operator dependent and provides less information than MRI.

In postoperative rotator cuff repair patients with a question of complication or recurrent tear, MRI is the best imaging technique, but sometimes scar in the rotator cuff can be associated with an abnormal signal intensity pattern mimicking that of a recurrent tear.[39] Arthrography or MRI with intra-articular contrast agent instillation can be helpful to assess for a recurrent tear and passage of fluid through the tendon and to differentiate the condition from the abnormal signal in the tendon from scar. Postarthrography CT is useful to assess for dislodgement of Mitek anchors used for rotator cuff repair.

Glenoid Labral Lesions and Instability

The ACR Appropriateness Criteria committee could not reach a consensus on a recommended imaging study when there is a suspicion of instability or labral tear, but listed CT-arthrography, MRI, or MR-arthrography as all being appropriate. CT can better show fractures of the bony glenoid. CT-arthrography yields high-definition images of the labrum, but the study is limited in its multiplanar capabilities and gives less information about any other possible causes of shoulder pain.[20] Unenhanced MRI[40] and MR-arthrography[7, 8] allow multiplanar imaging, which can be useful for assessing superior labral tears on coronal oblique images (Fig. 7–19), the inferior glenohumeral ligament on sagittal oblique and axial images, and the biceps tendon and rotator cuff. Nonenhanced MRI does not outline the labral structures as well as MR-arthrography if there is no significant effusion present, but some researchers have shown a high accuracy with unenhanced MRI.[40] The glenohumeral ligaments are best shown with postarthrography MRI.[8] The abduction–external rotation (ABER) position has been shown to best demonstrate the inferior glenohumeral ligaments,[49] but this position requires a longer imaging time and repositioning of the patient during the examination.

The labrum is evaluated for morphology, signal intensity, and position. There is variability in labral morphology, especially at the superior aspect of the anterior labrum.[52] Superior labral anterior to posterior (SLAP) lesions and involvement of the biceps–labral complex are ideally shown following intra-articular contrast agent injection where there is insinuation of the contrast agent between the cartilage and the superior labrum. The axial images can show a Hill-Sachs lesion or Bankhardt lesion of the bony glenoid or labrum if the patient has had a previous anteroinferior humeral dislocation.

Brachial Plexus

MRI of the brachial plexus can be used to screen for any extrinsic mass compressing or impinging on the brachial plexus.[9] It is also useful to assess for nerve root avulsion with enlargement and tearing of the root sleeve at the intervertebral foramen. However, intrinsic abnormalities of the brachial plexus are more difficult to assess unless there is enlargement of one of the components of the brachial plexus (Fig. 7–20). The components of the brachial plexus are best identified in their relationship to the subclavian artery on sagittal images, which show the nerves in cross section. The development of higher-resolution surface coils might allow better imaging of the intrinsic structure of the nerves of the brachial plexus.[57]

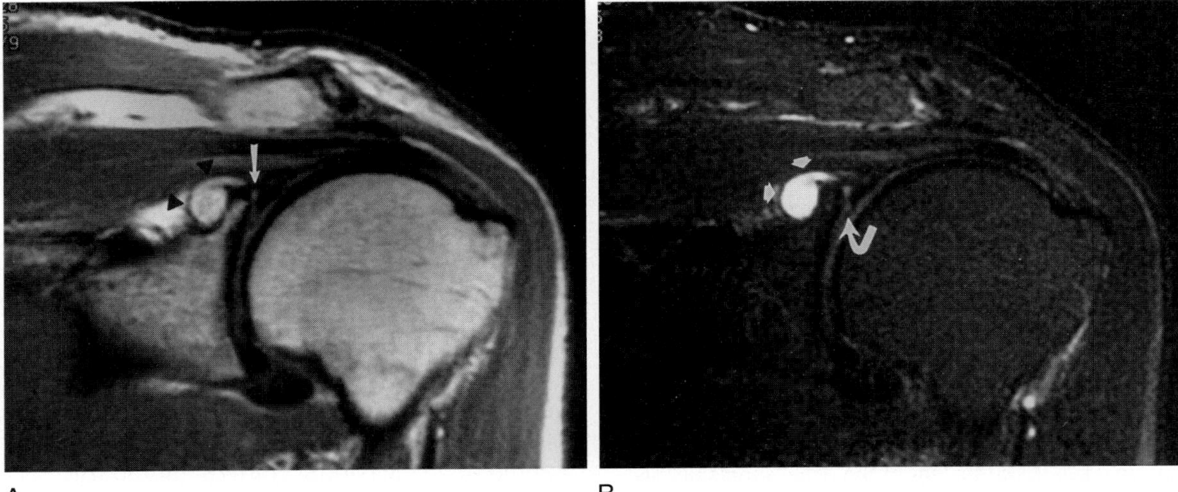

FIGURE 7–19. MRI appearance of a SLAP lesion and paralabral cyst. *A.* Proton-density coronal oblique image of the shoulder demonstrates a superior labral tear with increased signal intensity between the superior labrum and the bony glenoid (*arrow*). Just adjacent to this is a comma-shaped paralabral cyst (*arrowheads*). *B.* Coronal oblique T2-weighted fat-suppressed image demonstrates the labral tear (*curved arrow*) as well as the high-signal cyst (*short arrows*) more conspicuously. Denervation changes are not seen in the supraspinatus muscle, which is located just superior to the paralabral cyst and is innervated by the suprascapular nerve, which courses near the cyst.

Impingement on the suprascapular nerve, the first take-off of the brachial plexus, is relatively common and can cause denervation of the infraspinatus and possibly supraspinatus muscles.[33, 87] Suprascapular ganglion cysts (paralabral cysts) are well demonstrated on MRI, with high T2/STIR signal intensity. It is thought that most, if not all, suprascapular ganglion cysts are associated with labral tears,[107] but labral tears are often not demonstrated on MRI in these patients.

Elbow Imaging

Plain radiography in orthogonal planes is the first imaging study that should be obtained in the trauma setting. The posterior fat pad sign or anterior "sail" sign is indirect evidence of a fracture. Fractures in a child's elbow can be more difficult to assess on plain radiographs because of incomplete ossification; MRI can be helpful in these cases.

Because of its multiplanar capabilities and excellent contrast resolution, MRI is the best modality for assessing the elbow for muscular, ligamentous, or tendinous injuries, bone marrow edema, or osteochondral injury (Fig. 7–21).[34, 74, 100] Coronal imaging ideally assesses the collateral ligaments and extensor and flexor tendons; the annular ligament is best seen on axial imaging. The distal biceps tendon is best assessed on axial images.[32] Saline-enhanced MR-arthrography can better show partial tears of the ulnar collateral ligament than unenhanced MRI.[90]

Lateral epicondylitis ("tennis elbow") can manifest with increased T2 signal intensity and thickening of the common extensor tendon. Medial epicondylitis ("Little Leaguer's elbow" in children, medial tendinosis in adults) can manifest with bone marrow edema and medial epicondyle apophyseal separation in children and with increased T2/STIR signal intensity and thickening of the common flexor pronator tendons and muscles in adults. Valgus stress on the ulnar collateral ligament can result in traction osteophytes if chronic, while acute trauma can result in a sprain, a partial tear, or a full-thickness tear, with imaging characteristics similar to those of ligament injuries elsewhere in the body.

MRI can be useful for assessing ulnar nerve abnormalities at the elbow if there is an abnormality of size, signal, or position.[83, 100]

Wrist and Hand Imaging

In the setting of suspected wrist or hand fracture, preferably three views should be obtained: orthogonal AP and lateral views and an oblique view. If a scaphoid fracture is suspected, an additional scaphoid view can be obtained that lays out the length of the scaphoid. A carpal tunnel view can be useful in a suspected hook of hamate fracture. Knowledge of the clinical history and examination findings is helpful in determining which additional views are necessary to exclude a fracture. Some scaphoid fractures are occult and should be reimaged 7 to 10 days following the initial injury if there is a high suspicion of scaphoid fracture and snuffbox tenderness. The patient should be splinted until the follow-up radiograph. Alternatively, MRI is quite sensitive for occult fractures of the scaphoid and distal radius[15] where there is bone marrow edema and/or intratrabecular hemorrhage early after fracture.

Sacroiliac Joint Imaging

AP angled and bilateral oblique views of the sacroiliac joints are the standard initial workup. Limited sacroiliac joint CT has proved to be a cost-competitive screening

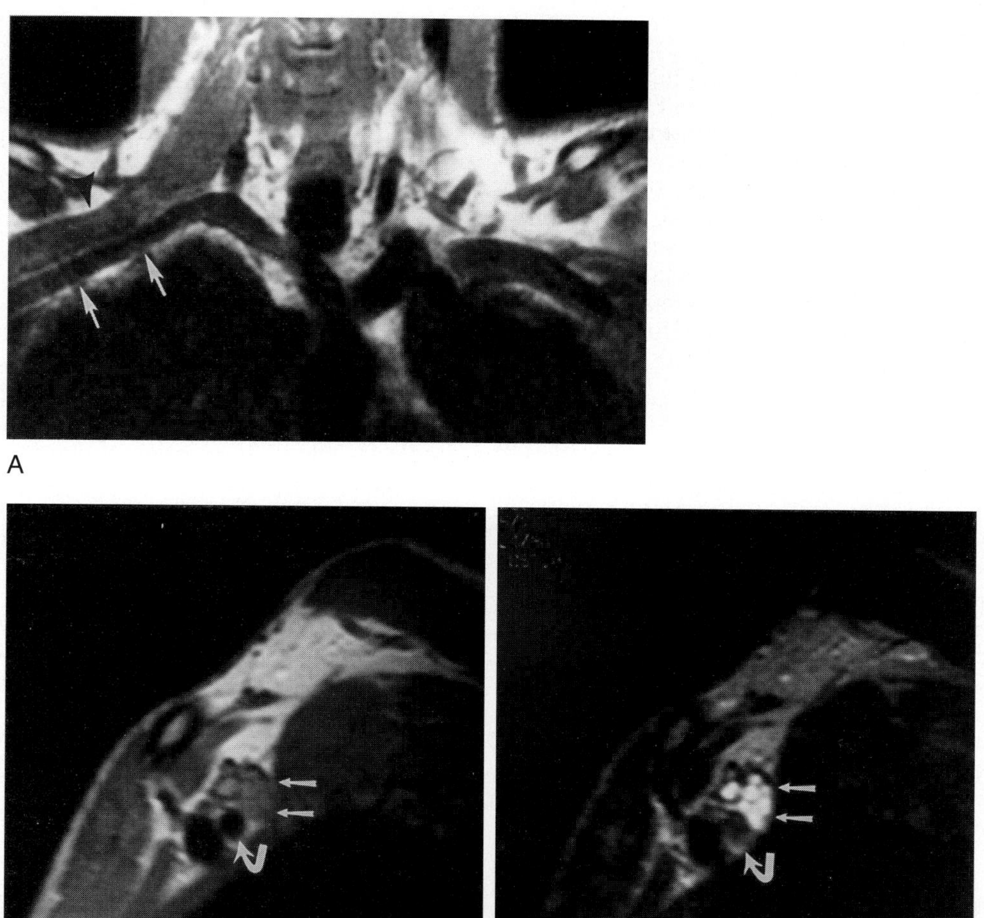

FIGURE 7–20. MRI appearance of brachial plexus neurofibroma. *A.* Coronal T1-weighted image including the right brachial plexus demonstrates diffuse thickening and enlargement of the brachial plexus components (*arrowheads*) coursing just above the right subclavian artery (*arrows*). *B* and *C.* Sagittal proton-density (*B*) and sagittal T2-weighted (*C*) images demonstrate the enlarged brachial plexus in cross section (*arrows*) located just above the subclavian artery (*curved arrow*).

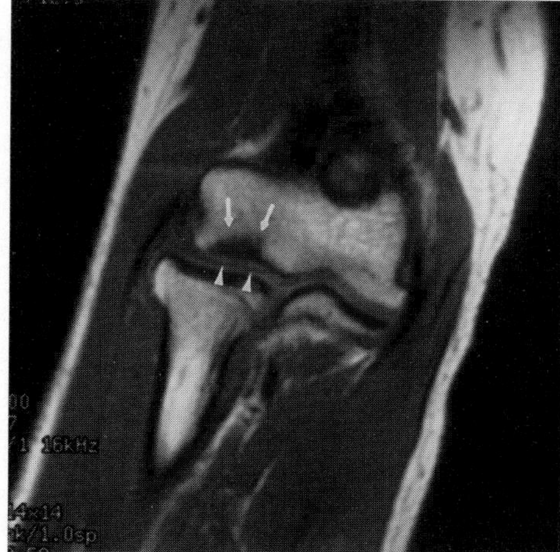

FIGURE 7–21. Coronal T1-weighted image of the elbow demonstrates osteochondritis dissecans of the capitellum (*arrows*) as a low T1 signal abnormality against normal fatty marrow. The overlying cartilage (*arrowheads*) appears intact.

examination that has higher sensitivity for subtle erosive changes of the sacroiliac joints and in the detection of subtle sclerosis.

Hip and Pelvis Imaging

In the trauma setting, orthogonal plain radiography is the initial imaging study. CT can be considered in the setting of more complex acetabular and pelvic fractures to aid in surgical planning.[22, 75] Fractures, muscle injuries, and soft tissue injuries can be detected with MRI of the pelvis in patients with nonrevealing radiographs after acute trauma.[11, 59] CT is the preferred modality for assessment of osseous-based abnormalities of the hip, and MRI is the preferred modality, following plain radiography, to image AVN, marrow replacement processes, musculoskeletal tumors, and osteomyelitis.[22] MR-arthrography has a much higher accuracy than nonenhanced MRI in the detection and staging of acetabular labral lesions when the labrum is being assessed for abnormalities of morphology, signal intensity, the presence or absence of a tear, and attachment to the acetabulum.[24]

Avascular Necrosis

In the setting of unilateral or bilateral hip pain when AVN is suspected clinically, AP pelvis and frog-leg lateral views of the hip or hips is the most appropriate imaging study, according to the ACR Appropriateness Criteria. If there is evidence of AVN on plain films, MRI can be considered to assess for occult AVN in the contralateral hip. If plain radiographs are suspicious but not definite for AVN or if there is a high clinical suspicion of AVN with normal plain radiographs, then MRI is the most sensitive and specific imaging study to assess for AVN.

Painful Prostheses

In the patient with a painful hip or knee prosthesis and a clinical suspicion of loosening or infection, the ACR Appropriateness Criteria give a Most Appropriate rating to plain radiography, with comparison with prior studies, as the first imaging study. If the initial plain radiographs are normal but there is clinical suspicion of loosening or infection, then joint aspiration with arthrography is considered the most appropriate study. If the plain radiographs are abnormal and consistent with loosening but infection is suspected, then aspiration, possibly with arthrography, is considered most appropriate. If aspiration is purulent, arthrography is contraindicated because increased pressure within the joint can lead to intravasation and hematogenous seeding of the infection.

Knee Imaging

In the setting of trauma, the minimum initial examination includes orthogonal AP and lateral views. If there is a high clinical suspicion of fracture or lipohemarthrosis, then further views, such as bilateral oblique, sunrise, and/or tunnel-notch, should be considered.[18] Bone bruise or occult stress fracture are best shown with MRI. MRI in a study of 84 patients with acute knee injury was shown to decrease the number of arthroscopic procedures, improve clinician diagnostic certainty, and change the management proposed prior to MRI.[58] MRI prior to arthroscopy in 50 patients who met clinical criteria for knee arthroscopy showed that 42% of the arthroscopies were unnecessary.[17]

The ACR Appropriateness Criteria recommend imaging studies for 12 variants of nontraumatic knee pain. The mandatory minimum initial study consists of AP and lateral plain radiographs, with an axial patellar view added if there are anterior patellofemoral symptoms. If the initial radiographs are normal or show joint effusion, then MRI is considered the next appropriate study. When the initial plain radiographs are abnormal, then other additional studies may or may not be considered appropriate.

Meniscal Injuries

MRI is the best method of assessing the meniscus in a patient who has not previously undergone surgery.[21, 45] MRI is noninvasive and multiplanar, allowing assessment of the meniscus. Radial imaging planes can be obtained that give similar views to that seen with knee arthrography.

Menisci are described according to the following scheme: (1) normal, with homogeneous low signal intensity on all sequences and normal morphology; (2) grade 1—degenerative change, manifesting as poorly circumscribed, increased T1/proton-density signal intensity within the meniscus not contacting an articular surface; (3) grade 2—degenerative change, manifesting as a horizontal line of increased T1 or proton-density signal intensity within the meniscus that does not contact an articular surface; or (4) grade 3—torn, manifesting as abnormal signal intensity extending from the meniscus to an articular surface, or when the morphology is definitely abnormal, possibly with a displaced bucket-handle fragment. In a series of 400 knee MRI studies with 333 meniscal tears, 6% of tears found on arthroscopy could not be identified on routine MRI, even in retrospect.[26] False positive diagnoses in the 400 patients occurred in 1.5% due to healed tears or tears missed at arthroscopy.

In the setting of an operated meniscus where the morphology can be abnormal and inherent degenerative change extends to the articular surface, knee arthrography or MRI with intra-articular contrast agent injection[4] can be considered to determine whether the fluid extends into a tear in the meniscus. Comparison with previous studies can be helpful in assessing for recurrent tear versus postoperative change. The two best signs of recurrent tear of the postoperative meniscus on routine MRI are (1) a line of abnormal meniscal signal intensity extending to an articular surface on proton-density-weighted images and (2) fluid extending into a linear area on T2-weighted images.[51]

Knee Ligament Injuries

The cruciate ligaments,[81, 99, 110] medial collateral ligament,[92] and lateral collateral ligament complex are best shown with multiplanar MRI. Again, the ligaments are assessed for continuity, caliber, and signal intensity. There is a continuum of sprain, partial tear, and full-thickness tear in the setting of ligamentous injury, similar to what is seen in ligaments elsewhere in the body.

Discontinuity of the anterior cruciate ligament (ACL) on sagittal and axial MRI planes and failure of the fascicles to parallel the Blumensaat line are the most accurate MRI signs of ACL tear (Fig. 7–22).[81] Multiple other indirect signs are good predictors of ACL tear, including disruption of the fascicles, a posterolateral tibial bruise, a buckled posterior cruciate ligament (PCL), a positive PCL line sign, a positive posterior femoral line sign, displacement of the lateral meniscus more than 3.5 mm posteriorly, displacement of the tibia more than 7 mm anteriorly, and a lateral femoral sulcus deeper than 1.5 mm.[35, 81] In 20 patients with two different sagittal MRI sequences of the ACL showing intact fibers on one sequence and disrupted or poorly seen fibers on the other sequence (discordant findings), the ACL fibers were found to be intact on arthroscopy.[97] A combination of plain radiography and MRI best assesses for complications after ACL repair.[79]

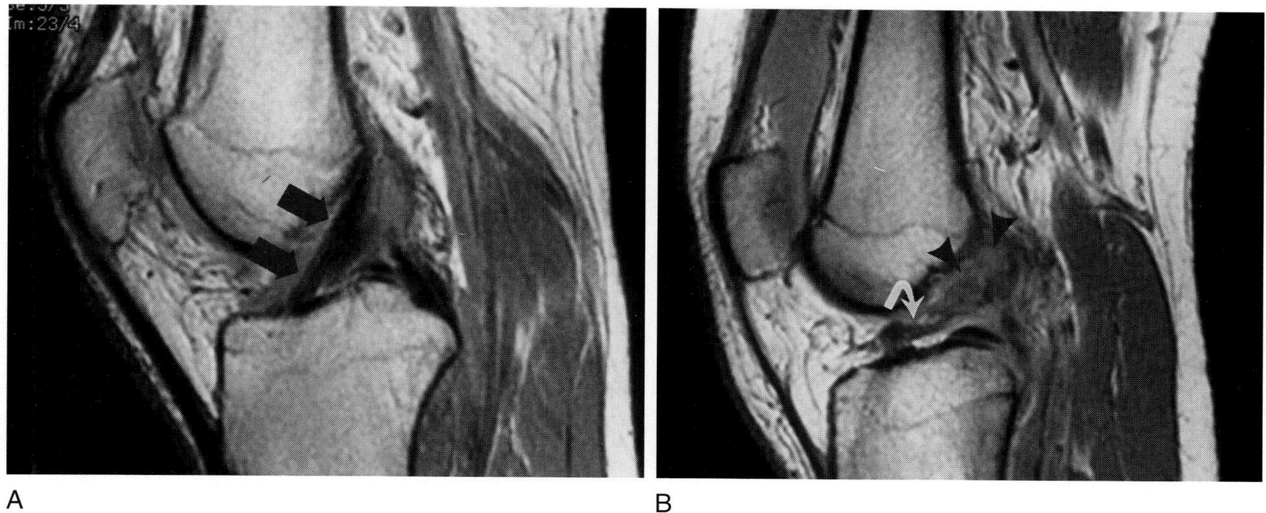

A B

FIGURE 7–22. MRI appearance of anterior cruciate ligament tear. *A.* Sagittal proton-density image of the knee demonstrates a normal intact anterior cruciate ligament (*arrows*) with uniform low signal, sharp linear contour anteriorly, and continuous extension from the femur to the tibia. *B.* Sagittal proton-density image demonstrates disruption of the anterior cruciate ligament with loss of the normal low-signal fascicles and intermediate-signal material in the expected location of the ligament (*arrowheads*). The distal stump of the ligament is folded downward (*curved arrow*).

Patellofemoral Abnormalities

Patellofemoral abnormalities are best assessed in the axial and sagittal planes on MRI.[98] Fat-suppressed proton-density MRI shows excellent contrast between the articular cartilage, bone, and any joint fluid.[82] Grading of chondromalacia is most accurate on axial MRI. Additionally, MRI can demonstrate patella baja/alta and the patellar position within the trochlear groove. Kinematic MRI studies are available to assess patellar tracking[93] and can show subluxation in certain positions. This can decrease or increase with knee flexion, depending on the cause of the tracking abnormality. Plain radiographs might or might not show patellar subluxation, depending on the degree of knee flexion utilized to obtain the axial patellar (sunrise) view.

Ankle and Foot Imaging

A three-view plain radiography that includes AP, lateral, and mortise views is considered the most appropriate by the ACR in patients with suspected ankle injury meeting Ottawa rules. Fluoroscopy with stress views may be necessary to assess for Lisfranc fracture dislocations. CT with reformations is often useful for preoperative planning in patients with complex comminuted fractures of the foot and ankle and can alter clinical management.[56]

Chronic ankle instability can be detected with a telos stress examination using posteriorly directed or varus stress, although MR-arthrography is more accurate and sensitive in the detection of anterior talofibular ligament tears.[19] In the patient with more diffuse foot pain of no definite cause, a radionuclide bone scan can localize the abnormality to a specific joint or joints.

MRI of the ankle or foot provides excellent delineation of ligaments,[19, 47] tendons,[46, 84, 91] and any abnormal bone marrow signal to indicate AVN or a bone bruise/stress fracture. In 81 patients referred for MRI of the foot and ankle by a group of four orthopedic surgeons and podiatrists, the post-MRI diagnosis differed from the pre-MRI diagnosis in 47%, and treatment plans were changed in 34%.[3]

The Achilles tendon is ideally shown with MRI in the sagittal and axial planes. MRI can be helpful in differentiating partial tears from tendinitis or peritenonitis. The tendon is assessed for continuity, caliber, and signal intensity as elsewhere in the body.

Tarsal coalition can be evident on plain radiographs and is clearly shown on CT if it is a bony coalition. Sometimes MRI will more effectively show a coalition that is fibrous.[112]

SUMMARY

Knowledge of the strengths and weaknesses of the multiple imaging modalities available can help the treating physician decide on the optimal imaging study in a given clinical situation for a specific anatomical site. Good communication between the referring physician and the consulting radiologist aids in selecting the most appropriate imaging study or studies and additionally helps in the interpretation of the study. Sometimes a single study is sufficient, but in other clinical situations more than one study might be necessary. Furthermore, treatment plans can dictate whether additional studies are required, in that some imaging is more for an interventional procedure or surgical planning than for simple diagnosis.

REFERENCES

1. Acheson MB, Livingston RR, Richardson ML, et al: High-resolution CT scanning in the evaluation of cervical spine fractures: Comparison with plain film examinations. Am J Radiol 1987; 148:1179–1185.
2. American College of Radiology: Appropriateness Criteria for Imaging and Treatment Decisions. Chicago, American College of Radiology, 1996.
3. Anzilotti, KJr, Schweitzer ME, Hecht P, et al: Effect of foot and ankle MR imaging on clinical decision making. Radiology 1996; 201:515–517.
4. Applegate GR, Flannigan BD, Tolin BS, et al: MR diagnosis of recurrent tears in the knee: Value of intraarticular contrast material. Am J Radiol 1993; 161:821–825.
5. Aprill C, Bogduk N: High intensity zone: A diagnostic sign of painful lumbar disc on magnetic resonance imaging. Br J Radiol 1992; 65:361–369.
6. Balich SM, Sheley RC, Brown TR, et al: MR imaging of the rotator cuff tendon: Interobserver agreement and analysis of interpretive errors. Radiology 1997; 204:191–194.
7. Beltran J, Bencardino J, Mellado J, et al: MR arthrography of the shoulder: Variants and pitfalls. Radiographics 1997; 17:1403–1412.
8. Beltran J, Rosenberg ZS, Chandnani VP, et al: Glenohumeral instability: Evaluation with MR arthrography. Radiographics 1997; 17:657–673.
9. Bilbey JH, Lamond RG, Mattrey RF: MR imaging of disorders of the brachial plexus. J Magn Reson Imaging 1994; 4:13–18.
10. Boden SD, McCowin PR, Davis DO, et al: Abnormal magnetic resonance scans of the cervical spine in asymptomatic subjects. J Bone Joint Surg 1990; 72:1178–1183.
11. Bogost GA, Lizerbram EK, Crues JV III: MR imaging in evaluation of suspected hip fracture: Frequency of unsuspected bone and soft-tissue injury. Radiology 1995; 197:263–267.
12. Bourgouin PM, Lesage J, Fontaine S, et al: Pattern approach to the differential diagnosis of intramedullary spinal cord lesions on MR imaging. Am J Radiol 1998; 170:1645–1649.
13. Brandser EA, El-Khoury GY, Kathol MH, et al: Hamstring injuries: Radiographic, conventional tomographic, CT, and MR imaging characteristics. Radiology 1995; 197:257–262.
14. Brant-Zawadski MN, Jensen MC, Obuchowski N, et al: Interobserver and intraobserver variability in interpretation of lumbar disc abnormalities: A comparison of two nomenclatures. Spine 1995; 20:1257–1264.
15. Breitenseher MJ, Metz VM, Gilula LA, et al: Radiographically occult scaphoid fractures: Value of MR imaging in detection. Radiology 1997; 203:245–250.
16. Brossman J, Preidler KW, Daenen B, et al: Imaging of osseous and cartilaginous intraarticular bodies in the knee: Comparison of MR imaging and MR arthrography with CT and CT arthrography in cadavers. Radiology 1996; 200:509–517.
17. Bui-Mansfield LT, Youngberg RA, Warme W, et al: Potential cost savings of MR imaging obtained before arthroscopy of the knee: Evaluation of 50 consecutive patients. Am J Radiol 1997; 168:913–918.
18. Capps GW, Hayes CW: Easily missed injuries around the knee. Radiographics 1994; 14:1191–1210.
19. Chandnani VP, Harper MT, Ficke JR, et al: Chronic ankle instability: Evaluation with MR arthrography, MR imaging, and stress radiography. Radiology 1994; 192:189–194.
20. Chandnani VP, Yeager TD, DeBerardino T, et al: Glenoid labral tears: Prospective evaluation with MR imaging, MR arthrography, and CT arthrography. Am J Radiol 1993; 161:1229–1235.
21. Cheung LP, Li KCP, Hollett MD, et al: Meniscal tears of the knee: Accuracy of detection with fast spin-echo MR imaging and arthroscopic correlation in 293 patients. Radiology 1997; 203:508–512.
22. Conway WF, Totty WG, McEnery KW: CT and MR imaging of the hip. Radiology 1996; 198:297–307.
23. Cuenod CA, Laredo JD, Chevret S, et al: Acute vertebral collapse due to osteoporosis or malignancy: Appearance on unenhanced and gadolinium-enhanced MR images. Radiology 1996; 199:541–549.
24. Czerny C, Hofmann S, Neuhold A, et al: Lesions of the acetabular labrum: Accuracy of MR imaging and MR arthrography in detection and staging. Radiology 1996; 200:225–230.
25. Daffner RH, Lupetin AR, Dash N, et al: MRI in the detection of malignant infiltration of bone marrow. Am J Radiol 1986; 146:353–358.
26. De Smet AA, Tuite MJ, Norris MA, et al: MR diagnosis of meniscal tears: Analysis of causes of errors. Am J Radiol 1994; 163:1419–1423.
27. Dick BW, Mitchell DG, Burk DL, et al: The effect of chemical shift misrepresentation on cortical bone thickness on MR imaging. Am J Radiol 1988; 15:537–538.
28. Dina TS, Boden SD, Davis DO: Lumbar spine after surgery for herniated disk: Imaging findings in the early postoperative period. Am J Radiol 1995; 164:665–671.
29. El-Khoury GY, Kathol MH, Daniel WW: Imaging of acute injuries of the cervical spine: Value of plain radiography, CT, and MR imaging. Am J Radiol 1995; 164:43–50.
30. Erickson SJ, Cox IH, Hyde JS, et al: Effect of tendon orientation on MR imaging signal intensity: A manifestation of the "magic angle" phenomenon. Radiology 1991; 181:389–392.
31. Erickson SJ, Prost RW, Timins ME: The "magic angle" effect: Background physics and clinical relevance. Radiology 1993; 188:23–25.
32. Fitzgerald SW, Curry DR, Erickson SJ, et al: Distal biceps tendon injury: MR imaging diagnosis. Radiology 1994; 191:203–206.
33. Fritz RC, Helms CA, Steinbach LS, et al: Suprascapular nerve entrapment: Evaluation with MR imaging. Radiology 1992; 182:437–444.
34. Fritz RC, Steinbach LS, Tirman PFJ, et al: MR imaging of the elbow. An update. Radiol Clin North Am 1997; 35:117–144.
35. Gentili A, Seeger LL, Yao L, et al: Anterior cruciate ligament tear: Indirect signs at MR imaging. Radiology 1994; 193:835–840.
36. Georgy BA, Snow RD, Hesselink JR: MR imaging of spinal nerve roots: Techniques, enhancement patterns, and imaging findings. Am J Radiol 1996; 166:173–179.
37. Grogan J, Nowicki BH, Schmidt TA, et al: Lumbar facet joint tropism does not accelerate degeneration of the facet joints. AJNR 1997; 18:1325–1329.
38. Gundry CR, Heithoff KB: Epidural hematoma of the lumbar spine: 18 surgically confirmed cases. Radiology 1993; 187: 427–431.
39. Gusmer PB, Potter HG, Donovan WD, et al: MR imaging of the shoulder after rotator cuff repair. Am J Radiol 1997; 168:559–563.
40. Gusmer PB, Potter HG, Schatz JA, et al: Labral injuries: Accuracy of detection with unenhanced MR imaging of the shoulder. Radiology 1996; 200:519–524.
41. Hayes CW, Conway WF: Evaluation of articular cartilage: Radiographic and cross-sectional imaging techniques. Radiographics 1992; 12:409–428.
42. Helgason JW, Chandnani VP, Yu JS: MR arthrography: A review of current technique and applications. Am J Radiol 1997; 168:1473–1480.
43. Hueftle MG, Modic MT, Ross JS, et al: Lumbar spine: Postoperative MR imaging with Gd-DTPA. Radiology 1988; 167:817–824.
44. Itoh R, Murata K, Kamata M, et al: Lumbosacral nerve root enhancement with disk herniation on contrast-enhanced MR. AJNR 1996; 17:1619–1625.
45. Justice WW, Quinn SF: Error patterns in the MR imaging evaluation of menisci of the knee. Radiology 1995; 196:617–621.
46. Khoury NJ, El-Khoury GY, Saltzman CL, et al: Peroneus longus and brevis tendon tears: MR imaging evaluation. Radiology 1996; 200:833–841.
47. Klein MA: MR imaging of the ankle: Normal and abnormal findings in the medial collateral ligament. Am J Radiol 1994; 162:377–383.
48. Krinsky G, Rofsky NM, Weinreb JC: Nonspecificity of short inversion time inversion recovery (STIR) as a technique of fat suppression: Pitfalls in image interpretation. Am J Radiol 1996; 166:523–526.

49. Kwak SM, Brown RR, Trudell D, et al: Glenohumeral joint: Comparison of shoulder positions at MR arthrography. Radiology 1998; 208:375–380.
50. Lebwohl NH: Diskography for the diagnosis of radiculopathy without nerve root compression. AJNR 1995; 16:1614–1615.
51. Lim PS, Schweitzer ME, Bhatia M, et al: Repeat tear of postoperative meniscus: Potential MR imaging signs. Radiology 1999; 210:183–188.
52. Liou JTS, Wilson AJ, Totty WG, et al: The normal shoulder: Common variations that simulate pathologic conditions at MR imaging. Radiology 1993; 186:435–441.
53. Ma LD, Frassica FJ, Scott WW Jr, et al: Differentiation of benign and malignant musculoskeletal tumors: Potential pitfalls with MR imaging. Radiographics 1995; 15:349–366.
54. Ma LD, McCarthy EF, Bluemke DA, et al: Differentiation of benign from malignant musculoskeletal lesions using MR imaging: Pitfalls in MR evaluation of lesions with a cystic appearance. Am J Radiol 1998; 170:1251–1258.
55. Mack LA, Nyberg DA, Matsen FA III: Sonographic evaluation of the rotator cuff. Radiol Clin North Am 1988; 26:161–177.
56. Magid D, Michelson JD, Ney DR, Fishman EK: Adult ankle fractures: Comparison of plain films and interactive two- and three-dimensional CT scans. Am J Radiol 1990; 154:1017–1023.
57. Maravilla KR, Bowen BC: Imaging of the peripheral nervous system: Evaluation of peripheral neuropathy and plexopathy. Am J Neuroradiol 1998; 19:1011–1023.
58. Maurer EJ, Kaplan PA, Dussault RG, et al: Acutely injured knee: Effect of MR imaging on diagnostic and therapeutic decisions. Radiology 1997; 204:799–805.
59. May DA, Purins JL, Smith DK: MR imaging of occult traumatic fractures and muscular injuries of the hip and pelvis in elderly patients. Am J Radiol 1996; 166:1075–1078.
60. Mehta RC, Marks MP, Hinks RS, et al: MR evaluation of vertebral metastases: T1-weighted, short-inversion-time inversion recovery, fast spin-echo, and inversion-recovery fast spin-echo sequences. AJNR 1995; 16:281–288.
61. Milette PC, Fontaine S, Lepanto L, et al: Radiating pain to the lower extremities caused by lumbar disk rupture without spinal nerve root involvement. Am J Neuroradiol 1995; 16:1605–1613.
62. Mitchell DG, Rao VM, Dalinka MK, et al: Femoral head avascular necrosis: Correlation of MR imaging, radiographic staging, radionuclide imaging, and clinical findings. Radiology 1987; 162:709–715.
63. Modic MT, Feiglin DH, Piraino DW, et al: Vertebral osteomyelitis: Assessment using MR. Radiology 1985; 157:157–166.
64. Modic MT, Steinberg PM, Ross JS, et al: Degenerative disk disease: Assessment of changes in vertebral body marrow with MR imaging. Radiology 1988; 166:193–199.
65. Moulton JS, Blebea JS, Dunco DM, et al: MR imaging of soft-tissue masses: Diagnostic efficacy and value of distinguishing between benign and malignant lesions. Am J Radiol 1995; 164:1191–1199.
66. Nachemson A: Lumbar discography: Where are we today? (editorial). Spine 1989; 14:555–557.
67. Needell SD, Zlatkin MB, Sher JS, et al: MR imaging of the rotator cuff: Peritendinous and bone abnormalities in an asymptomatic population. Am J Radiol 1996; 166:863–867.
68. North American Spine Society: Position statement on discography. Spine 1988; 13:1343.
69. Nunez DB, Zuluaga A, Fuentes-Bernardo DA, et al: Cervical spine trauma: How much more do we learn by routinely using helical CT? Radiographics 1996; 16:1307–1318.
70. Olson EM, Wong WHM, Hesselink JR: Extraspinal abnormalities detected on MR images of the spine. Am J Radiol 1994; 162:679–684.
71. Palmer WE, Caslowitz PL: Anterior shoulder instability: Diagnostic criteria determined from prospective analysis of 121 MR arthrograms. Radiology 1995; 197:819–825.
72. Palmer WE, Levine SM, Dupuy DE: Knee and shoulder fractures: Association of fracture detection and marrow edema on MR images with mechanism of injury. Radiology 1997; 204: 395–401.
73. Parizel PM, Baleriaux D, Rodesch G, et al: Gd-DTPA-enhanced MR imaging of spinal tumors. AJNR 1989; 10:249–258.
74. Patten RM: Overuse syndromes and injuries involving the elbow: MR imaging findings. Am J Radiol 1995; 164:1205–1211.
75. Potok PS, Hopper KD, Umlauf MJ: Fractures of the acetabulum: Imaging, classification, and understanding. Radiographics 1995; 15:7–23.
76. Prost R, Czervionke LF: How does an MR scanner operate? AJNR 1994; 15:1383–1386.
77. Quinn SF, Sheley RC, Demlow TA, et al: Rotator cuff tendon tears: Evaluation with fat-suppressed MR imaging with arthroscopic correlation in 100 patients. Radiology 1995; 195:497–501.
78. Rabassa AE, Guinto FC Jr, Crow WN, et al: CT of the spine: Value of reformatted images. Am J Radiol 1993; 161:1223–1227.
79. Recht MP, Piraino DW, Applegate G, et al: Complications after anterior cruciate ligament reconstruction: Radiographic and MR findings. Am J Radiol 1996; 167:705–710.
80. Rijke AM, Goitz HT, McCue FC, et al: Stress radiography of the medial elbow ligaments. Radiology 1994; 191:213–216.
81. Robertson PL, Schweitzer ME, Bartolozzi AR, et al: Anterior cruciate ligament tears: Evaluation of multiple signs with MR imaging. Radiology 1994; 193:829–834.
82. Rose PM, Demlow TA, Szumowski J, et al: Chondromalacia patellae: Fat-suppressed MR imaging. Radiology 1994; 193: 437–440.
83. Rosenberg ZS, Beltran J, Cheung YY, et al: The elbow: MR features of nerve disorders. Radiology 1993; 188:235–240.
84. Rosenberg ZS, Cheung Y, Jahss MH, et al: Rupture of the posterior tibial tendon: CT and MR imaging with surgical correlation. Radiology 1988; 169:229–235.
85. Ross JS, Masaryk TJ, Modic MT, et al: MR imaging of lumbar arachnoiditis. AJNR 1987; 8:885–892.
86. Ross JS, Zepp R, Modic MT: The postoperative lumbar spine: Enhanced MR evaluation of the intervertebral disk. AJNR 1996; 17:323–331.
87. Sallomi D, Janzen DL, Munk PL, et al: Muscle denervation patterns in upper limb nerve injuries: MR imaging findings and anatomic basis. Am J Radiol 1998; 171:779–784.
88. Sans N, Richardi G, Railhac JJ, et al: Kinematic MR imaging of the shoulder: Normal patterns. Am J Radiol 1996; 167:1517–1522.
89. Schelhaus KP, Pollei SR, Gundry CR, et al: Lumbar disc high-intensity zone: Correlation of magnetic resonance imaging and discography. Spine 1996; 21:79–86.
90. Schwartz ML, Al-Zahrani S, Morwessel RM, et al: Ulnar collateral ligament injury in the throwing athlete: Evaluation with saline-enhanced MR arthrography. Radiology 1995; 197:297–299.
91. Schweitzer ME, Caccese R, Karasick D, et al: Posterior tibial tendon tears: Utility of secondary signs for MR imaging diagnosis. Radiology 1993; 188:655–659.
92. Schweitzer ME, Tran D, Deely DM, et al: Medial collateral ligament injuries: Evaluation of multiple signs, prevalence and location of associated bone bruises and assessment with MR imaging. Radiology 1995; 194:825–829.
93. Shellock FG, Mink JH, Deutsch AL, et al: Patellofemoral joint: Identification of abnormalities with active-movement, "unloaded" versus "loaded" kinematic MR imaging techniques. Radiology 1993; 188:575–578.
94. Silverman CS, Lenchik L, Shimkin PM, et al: The value of MR in differentiating subligamentous from supraligamentous lumbar disk herniations. AJNR 1995; 16:571–579.
95. Singson RD, Hoang T, Dan S, et al: MR evaluation of rotator cuff pathology using T2-weighted fast spin-echo technique with and without fat suppression. Am J Radiol 1996; 166:1061–1065.
96. Slone RM, MacMillan M, Montgomery WJ: Spinal fixation: Part 3. Complications of spinal instrumentation. Radiographics 1993; 13:797–816.
97. Smith DK, May DA, Phillips P: MR imaging of the anterior cruciate ligament: Frequency of discordant findings on sagittal-oblique images and correlation with arthroscopic findings. Am J Radiol 1996; 166:411–413.
98. Sonin AH, Fitzgerald SW, Bresler ME, et al: MR imaging appearance of the extensor mechanism of the knee: Functional anatomy and injury patterns. Radiographics 1995: 15:367–382.
99. Sonin AH, Fitzgerald SW, Hoff FL, et al: MR imaging of the posterior cruciate ligament: Normal, abnormal, and associated injury patterns. Radiographics 1995; 15:551–561.

100. Sonin AH, Fitzgerald SW: MR imaging of sports injuries in the adult elbow: A tailored approach. Am J Radiol 1996; 167: 325–331.
101. Stadnik TW, Lee RR, Coen HL, et al: Annular tears and disk herniation: Prevalence and contrast enhancement on MR images in the absence of low back pain or sciatica. Radiology 1998; 206:49–55.
102. Taber KH, Herrick RC, Weathers SW, et al: Pitfalls and artifacts encountered in clinical MR imaging of the spine. Radiographics 1998; 18:1499–1521.
103. Takahashi M, Yamashita Y, Sakamoto Y, et al: Chronic cervical cord compression: Clinical significance of increased signal intensity on MR images. Radiology 1989; 173:219–224.
104. Tartaglino LM, Flanders AE, Vinitski S, et al: Metallic artifacts on MR images of the postoperative spine: Reduction with fast spin-echo techniques. Radiology 1994; 190:565–569.
105. Tartaglino LM, Friedman DP, Flanders AE, et al: Multiple sclerosis in the spinal cord: MR appearance and correlation with clinical parameters. Radiology 1995; 195:725–732.
106. Timins ME, Erickson SJ, Estkowski LD, et al: Increased signal in the normal supraspinatus tendon on MR imaging: Diagnostic pitfall caused by the magic-angle effect. Am J Radiol 1995; 164:109–114.
107. Tirman PFJ, Feller JF, Janzen DL, et al: Association of glenoid labral cysts with labral tears and glenohumeral instability: Radiologic findings and clinical significance. Radiology 1994; 190: 653–658.
108. Ulmer JL, Matthews VP, Elster AD, et al: Lumbar spondylolysis without spondylolisthesis: Recognition of isolated posterior element subluxation on sagittal MR. AJNR 1995; 16:1393–1398.
109. Ulmer JL, Matthews VP, Elster AD, et al: MR imaging of lumbar spondylolysis: The importance of ancillary observations. Am J Radiol 1997; 169:233–239.
110. Vahey TN, Broome DR, Kayes KJ, et al: Acute and chronic tears of the anterior cruciate ligament: Differential features at MR imaging. Radiology 1991; 181:251–253.
111. Vellet AD, Marks PH, Fowler PJ, et al: Occult posttraumatic osteochondral lesions of the knee: Prevalence, classification, and short-term sequelae evaluated with MR imaging. Radiology 1991; 178:271–276.
112. Wechsler RJ, Schweitzer ME, Deely DM, et al: Tarsal coalition: Depiction and characterization with CT and MR imaging. Radiology 1994; 193:447–452.
113. Weishaupt D, Zanetti M, Hodler J, et al: MR imaging of the lumbar spine: Prevalence of intervertebral disk extrusion and sequestration, nerve root compression, end plate abnormalities, and osteoarthritis of the facet joints in asymptomatic volunteers. Radiology 1998; 209:661–666.
114. West GA, Haynor DR, Goodkin R, et al: Magnetic resonance imaging signal changes in denervated muscles after peripheral nerve injury. Neurosurgery 1994; 35:1077–1085.
115. Yin Y, Evanoff BA, Gilula LA, et al: Surgeons' decision making in patients with chronic wrist pain: Role of bilateral three-compartment wrist arthrography. Prospective study. Radiology 1996; 200:829–832.
116. Zanetti M, Weishaupt D, Gerber C, et al: Tendinopathy and rupture of the tendon of the long head of the biceps brachii muscle: Evaluation with MR arthrography. Am J Radiol 1998; 170:1557–1561.

8
CHAPTER

Carl V. Granger, M.D., Margaret Kelly-Hayes, Ed.D., R.N., C.R.R.N., Mark Johnston, Ph.D., Anne Deutsch, M.S., R.N., C.R.R.N., Susan Braun, M.L.S., O.T.R., and Roger C. Fiedler, Ph.D.

Quality and Outcome Measures for Medical Rehabilitation

The quality of health care services has moved from being primarily an issue for regulating and accreditation agencies to a concern of clinicians, administrators, researchers, and consumers. The Institute of Medicine (IOM) has defined quality of care as the "degree to which health services for individuals and populations increase the likelihood of desired health outcomes and are consistent with current professional knowledge."[40] Since an important purpose of medical rehabilitation is to improve the functional status of patients, reliable and valid methods of functional assessment are necessary.

DEFINITION OF FUNCTIONAL ASSESSMENT

A *functional assessment* evaluates an individual's abilities and limitations. The essence of it is the measurement of an individual's use of the variety of skills included in performing tasks necessary to daily living, leisure activities, vocational pursuits, social interactions, and other required behaviors. For a comprehensive functional assessment, selected diagnostic descriptors, performance (skill or task) descriptors, and social role descriptors are used to assemble the information desired. The technique includes coding the component skills and tasks according to categories of activities required to support quality of daily living. The data help formulate judgments as to how well these essential skills are used, and to gauge the degree to which tasks are accomplished and social role expectations are met.

Figure 8–1 proposes that an individual's fulfillment and quality of daily living are a result of balancing functional opportunities and functional requirements or demands. We have chosen the term "quality of daily living" in preference to the more common term "quality of life" because it is less expansive, more subject to empirical investigation, and analogous to another commonly used term, activities of daily living (ADL). Functional opportunities are expressed as an individual's choices, options, and expectations. Functional requirements are expressed in physical, cognitive, and emotional terms. In order to achieve fulfillment and to maximize the quality of daily living, there must be a balance between improved opportunities through individual health and functioning and the reduction or removal of life's barriers causing constraints.

A clinician who is proficient in using functional assessment can obtain performance-oriented data that can be analyzed in conjunction with diagnostic descriptors of pathological conditions and impairment states. This integration of medical status with status in performance of tasks and fulfillment of social roles, together with knowledge of the individual's level of social supports, allows the construction of a set of data that profiles the whole person. Given this profile, problems and areas of

Except as otherwise indicated, all copyrights, service marks, and trademarks associated with UDSMR, FIM, WeeFIM, and LIFEware belong to Uniform Data System for Medical Rehabilitation, a division of UB Foundation Activities, Inc. ORYX is a trademark belonging to the Joint Commission on Accreditation of Healthcare Organizations. Penn Ability Systems is a registered trademark and PAS is a trademark belonging to the Trustees of the University of Pennsylvania.

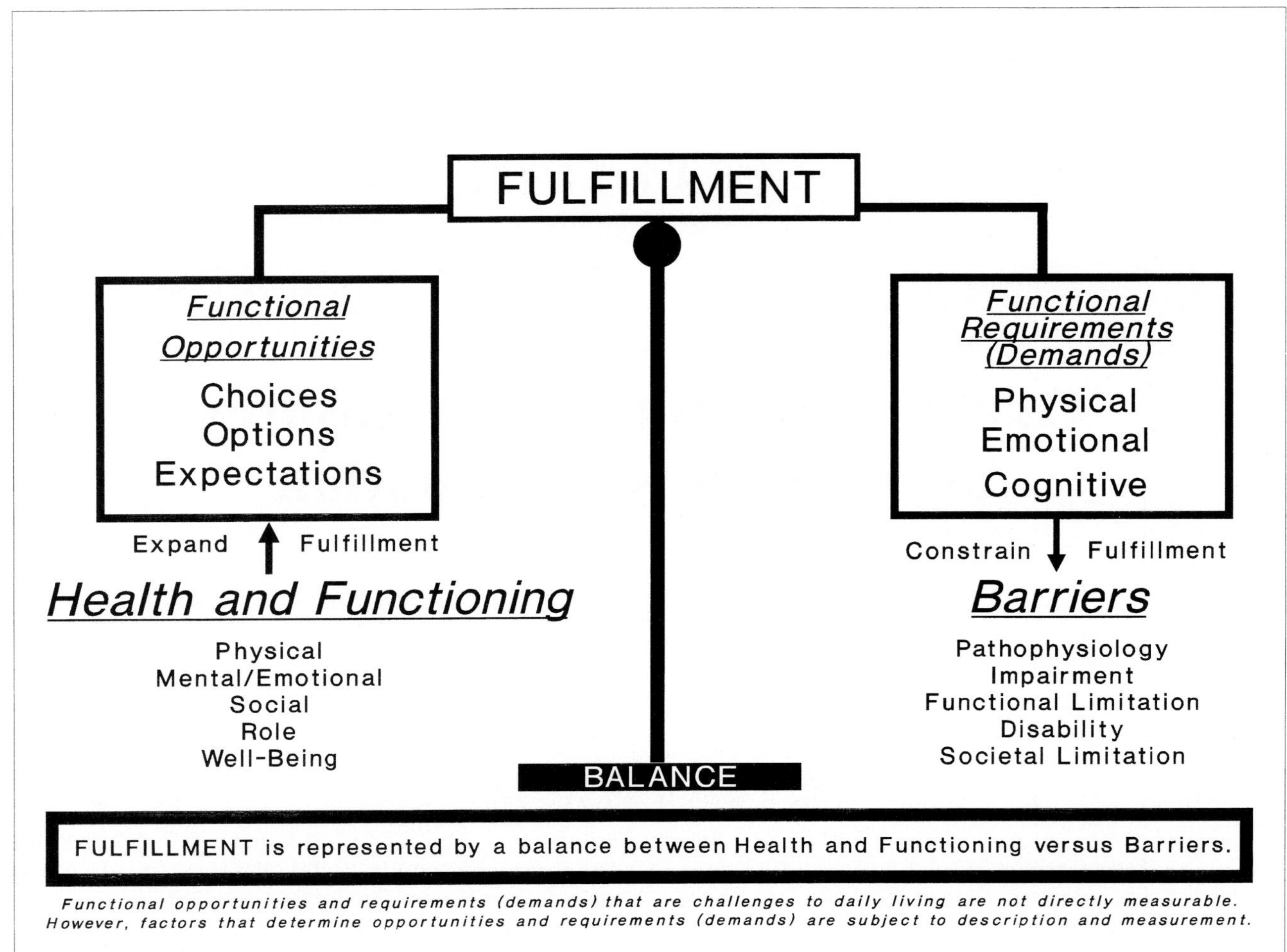

FIGURE 8–1. Challenges to quality of daily living.

need can be identified more accurately and reviewed in an orderly manner. Following analysis, interventions and coordination strategies (e.g., case management and critical pathways) can be developed that maximize personal independence and subjective well-being.

It is possible to compare the changes in status over periods of time for an individual or a group of individuals by assessing function at appropriate intervals. In this manner, outcomes of professional interventions of health care, rehabilitation, education, or psychological and social counseling may be described and monitored. Outcomes that are measurable are manageable.

The objectives of a functional assessment instrument that Donaldson and her co-workers summarized in 1973[11] still hold today. They are (1) objective description of functional status at a given point in time, (2) serial repetition allowing detection of changed functional status, (3) data collected through observation relevant to and useful in monitoring the treatment program, (4) enhancement of communication among treatment team members and between referral agencies, and (5) comparable clinical observations compatible with research questions.

The conceptual underpinnings for functional assessment are provided by disablement models proposed by Nagi,[48] Wood for the World Health Organization (WHO),[63] and the National Center for Medical Rehabilitation Research (NCMRR).[49] Although constructed slightly differently, the continuum from organ biology to the whole person and the social context is constant in each. The model of the NCMRR is the most recent and is intended to facilitate research efforts that probe how persons with a disability might interact with the rehabilitation process to achieve optimal accommodation with the environment. The terms specific to the NCMRR model are listed in Table 8–1. WHO is currently refining its disablement model.

Social norms are defined in the WHO document[63] within six key roles or dimensions of experiences in which competence is expected of the individual for survival: orientation, physical independence, mobility, occupation, social integration, and economic self-sufficiency. To satisfy these social roles, the individual employs a variety of functional skills that result in complex behaviors and in performance of tasks.

According to the WHO formulation, certain fundamental accomplishments or behaviors related to the existence and survival of people as social beings are expected in virtually every culture. The individual is expected to:

TABLE 8–1 Disablement Model Definitions

Term	Definition
Pathophysiology	Any interruption of, or interference with, normal physiological and developmental processes or structures
Impairment	Any loss or abnormality at the organ or organ system level of the body
Functional limitation	Any restriction or lack of ability to perform an action in the manner or within a range consistent with the purpose of an organ or organ system
Disability	Any limitation in performing tasks, activities, and roles to levels expected within physical and social contexts
Societal limitation	Any restriction attributable to social policy or barriers (structural or attitudinal) that limits fulfillment of roles or denies access to services and opportunities associated with full participation in society

Modified with permission from National Institutes of Health, National Institute of Child Health and Development: Research Plan for the National Center for Medical Rehabilitation Research. US Department of Health and Human Services, Public Health Service (NIH) publication no 93-3509. Rockville, MD, National Institutes of Health, March 1993.

1. Receive signals from surroundings (through seeing, listening, smelling, or touching), to assimilate these signals, and to express a response to what is assimilated.
2. Maintain a customarily effective independent existence with regard to the more immediate physical needs of the body, including eating, personal hygiene, and various other ADL.
3. Move around effectively in the environment.
4. Occupy time in a fashion appropriate to his or her gender, age, and culture, including following an occupation such as tilling the soil, laboring for others, running a household, bringing up children, and carrying out activities such as play or recreation.
5. Participate in and maintain social relationships with others.
6. Sustain socioeconomic activity and independence by virtue of labor or exploitation of material possessions, such as natural resources, livestock, or crops. This economic self-sufficiency customarily includes obligations to sustain others, such as members of the family.

MEASUREMENT STANDARDS AND PRINCIPLES OF SCALING

There have been many attempts to improve the quality of measurement in rehabilitation over the last 30 years.[16, 25, 34–36, 44] Experts have repeatedly warned that functional assessment scales and procedures now in common use have distinct failings. The empirical properties of scales—including basic validity, reliability, scaling characteristics, and standardization—have been insufficiently developed. Sometimes, the domains of functional assessment scaling have been stated in global, indistinct terms, such as "quality of life" or "function," without specification of the exact meaning of these terms. Rehabilitation facilities have commonly relied on locally developed scales and documentation procedures that lack formal study or development. Even simple clinical terms such as "mild," "moderate," and "severe," when applied without specific or objective reference, are used inconsistently.[60] All of the disciplines involved in medical rehabilitation face similar technical problems in the assessment of human function and performance.

Researchers and other leaders in rehabilitation had been communicating about problems in functional assessment for many years. Attempts to write specific measurement standards applicable to rehabilitation did not coalesce until the end of the 1980s, when the American Congress of Rehabilitation Medicine formed the Task Force on Measurement and Evaluation. This interdisciplinary task force included members of the American Congress of Rehabilitation Medicine and the American Academy of Physical Medicine and Rehabilitation. Disciplines represented in the task force included physiatry, psychology, physical therapy, occupational therapy, rehabilitation nursing, rehabilitation counseling, and others. After several years of work, "Measurement Standards for Interdisciplinary Medical Rehabilitation" was published in a special issue of the *Archives of Physical Medicine and Rehabilitation* in December 1992.[27]

The interdisciplinary standards document presents guidelines for the development and use of assessment procedures for measurement for the several disciplines involved in medical rehabilitation. Its purpose is to facilitate improved assessment in all of the disciplines. The interdisciplinary standards were designed to serve as a resource in courses and to guide the development, choice, use, and interpretation of assessments, both in research and in clinical practice.[26]

The relationship between pathophysiological processes and wider life issues is crucial to medical rehabilitation, both in research and in practice. Interdisciplinary measurement standards are intended to apply to the assessment of impairment (specific anatomical, physiological, and psychological functional limitations) as well as to the assessment of broader domains such as disability, societal limitations, and quality of daily living.

Similar measurement standards have been developed for psychology[2] and for physical therapy.[59] The interdisciplinary standards were designed to be consistent with the specific standards of these disciplines. Physical therapy standards are more stipulative than the interdisciplinary standards. The psychology standards are similar to the rehabilitation standards in that both are phrased primarily at the level of scientific principles; the two differ in the examples used to give content to the principles.

The documents addressing measurement standards differ fundamentally from systems that infer the impact on the "whole person" based on expert evaluation of severity of impairment alone. Some examples can be seen in the American Medical Association's Evaluation of Permanent Impairment, which is well established and periodically revised.[3] On the other hand, WHO's constructs of impairment, disability, and handicap have defined concepts that incorporate the whole person in a way that is understandable and scientifically defensible.[63] Current scientific understanding requires empirical testing of the reliability and validity of *disablement* and health-related scales.[1, 24, 26, 27, 37, 61, 64]

Validity and Related Guidelines

"Validity is the paramount criterion for choice and use of a measure. Validity is commonly regarded as the extent to which a test measures what it is intended to measure."[27] Validation involves linking a concept with specific operations involved in the assessment procedure and accumulating evidence that supports the logical inferences from the measurement procedure.

Scales of human function or performance may be quite broad or robust across diagnoses,[23, 39, 43] but they still cannot be assumed to have universal or unlimited validity. Validity is delimited by a particular construct, setting, and population or problem. Validity always relates to a specified use. Measurement standards are based on scientific validity principles. The initial standard (1.1) in the 1992 document states that a measure should have evidence of validity that is appropriate to its intended use.[27] Content validity, predictive validity, and construct validity are three types of validity that have stood the test of time.

Content validity is the extent to which a test contains items critical or appropriate to a domain. The content of a functional assessment domain must be examined to choose a scale that has items that are appropriate to the clinical problem. For example, an item addressing indoor mobility is appropriate to include in a basic functional assessment tool that measures independence in ADL. However, it is not an item that is sufficient to measure the abilities of persons who need speed and endurance in moving about in the community. A knowledge of pathophysiology is also helpful in analyzing functional assessment scales logically. Careful analysis of the sensibility of scales is essential in medical application.[14] Even though content validity is often established by a panel of experts representing experience and authority, only empirical evidence will resolve the many disputes about the validity and uses of functional assessment scales.

Predictive or criterion-referenced validity is the extent to which a scale is related to some outcome or external criterion. A truly useful assessment procedure should predict something outside of itself in the future. This is an acid test of the information provided by functional assessment scales. For example, a Barthel Index or FIM instrument rating can help to predict the likelihood of a patient's returning to the community versus going to a nursing home after discharge from a stroke rehabilitation program.[50] Occasionally, concurrent validity—the ability to predict something that occurs at the same point in time—is of interest. For instance, one may be interested in patient peformance at home, but it is impractical to leave the outpatient clinic to observe actual home performance. The outpatient clinic assessment should then be shown to correlate with home performance.

Construct validity is the extent to which a scale behaves as it should according to a theory. It involves study of the interactions of theoretically important constructs. A well-developed theory typically states that a construct should converge toward certain empirical criteria (convergent validity) on the one hand, but, on the other hand, the construct should be distinguishable by diverging from different criteria (divergent validity). Therefore, for a given scale there should be an accumulation of evidence of convergent and divergent relationships.[1, 24, 27] Construct validation involves study of the interactions of parameters that are theoretically important. For instance, one expects certain disease processes to affect related aspects of function, while unrelated aspects of function are not affected. This is an example of the dynamic logic by which rehabilitation is developing as a science. Tools that measure a physical quantity can often be validated against a single "gold standard" criterion. An inexpensive way to measure efficiency of ambulation can, for instance, be validated against an expensive and cumbersome laboratory measure of oxygen uptake. However, scales of complex concepts such as disability and societal limitation cannot be fully validated against a single ideal criterion. More complex construct validation analyses are required.

Guidelines for Reliability and Scaling

Functional assessment tools must have more than external validity characteristics such as predictive validity. They must also have internal validity characteristics such as reliability and internal homogeneity of the dimensional structure. Rehabilitation measurement standards require that adequate scales have numerical estimates of reliability (Standard 2.1).[27]

Reliability is usually defined as freedom from random error.[1, 37] It may be thought of as the extent to which the data contain relevant information with a high signal-to-noise ratio versus irrelevant static and confusion. Reliability is a necessary but not sufficient condition for validity. Although assessment tools of narrow physical quantities or impairments can attain high reliability coefficients, one cannot assume that such tools are more reliable or more valid than assessment tools of the wider and more complex behaviors, which often reveal much more about daily life and the priority needs of persons with disabilities.

Empirical testing of reliability begins with computation of the degree of agreement when a test is administered more than once under similar circumstances.[24] Agreement, however, is not precisely the same as reliability. Agreement means that the results of testing are similar despite variances in raters, time, or subjects tested. Percent of agreement is affected by population base rates, number of categories in the rating scale, and other factors that are not relevant to the balance between information and error in the measurement procedure. Several texts discuss the statistics that are used to estimate underlying reliability from surface-level agreement data.[13, 24, 37]

There are several ways of estimating reliability. Interrater reliability is crucial for rating scales that can be applied differently by various observers. Ratings of physical independence in basic ADL have shown high reliability coefficients in the range of .89 to .95.[43] (The coefficients are Pearson correlations, which are acceptable summaries of reliability only if there are no significant differences in rater means or variabilities, i.e., a normal distribution of the values.) Test-retest reliability is a critical form of reliability when results of the measurement procedure fluctuate over short periods of time, such that the ability to measure gain in basic status or ability is unlikely. When more than one form of a test is used, then parallel form reliability is needed.

A great deal hinges on the internal structure of tests involving multiple items. Internal consistency or unidimensionality is essential to a scale formed by adding up ratings from a series of items. If one adds up item ratings that are unrelated, the resulting sum is likely to fail to predict anything, even if some constituent items are in fact highly related to the criterion. Statistics such as split-half correlations and Cronbach's alpha have been used to estimate internal consistency.[1, 13, 24, 51] Factor analysis and Rasch analysis are used to identify latent factors or dimensions, that is, items that fit together.[1, 50]

The degree of ability or disability can be gauged by relating a person's performance to that of a wider age-gender-severity–adjusted comparison group. Explicit norms enhance the value of a test. Whenever possible, the characteristics of the comparison group used for evaluating patient performance should be explicitly stated (Standard 3.1).[27]

Guidelines for Clinical Application of Scales

Although measurement standards are based in science and apply most directly to researchers and developers of scales, they also have important implications for clinical practice. Simply stated, the idea is that scientific findings, when they exist and are relevant, should be applied to clinical assessment procedures. The first standard for use of measures is that "Users of measures should read the technical manual or relevant available documentation . . ." (Standard 6.1).[27] Users need to understand the scientific basis for the inferences they make from their clinical assessments (Standard 6.2) and the boundaries of this knowledge (Standards 6.3–6.6).

Scales used in rehabilitation often need to be altered to fit unusual impairments or problems, and these modifications ought to be made within bounds understood by the user (Standards 6.22–6.25). Additionally, it must be kept in mind that persons being assessed have rights that must be respected (Standards 7.1–7.4).

Guidelines for Program Evaluation, Quality Improvement, and Group Applications

Formal measures are frequently applied at a group or systems level rather than at the level of individual patients. Group applications include program evaluation, quality improvement, ongoing utilization review, and policymaking by government and managed-care organizations. Evidence of validity and reliability should be provided for measures used in all group applications, and the measures used should be shown to be relevant to the client populations involved (Standard 8.1).

The most respected scientific methodologies are based and validated on group rather than on single-subject studies. Usually individual outcomes are aggregated into some form of an average. When individual function varies greatly from the average, however, knowledge of the average may tell little about the individual. Standard 8.2 provides a caution, stating that comparisons of an individual with a group average need explicit justification.

Outcomes are affected by many factors other than the effectiveness of treatment. One can rarely infer effective treatment from outcomes alone. Rather, the effectiveness of rehabilitative interventions is based on a pattern of input, process, and outcome measures compared to some measured or assumed comparison.[29] One must adjust for case severity. Although severity adjustment is important everywhere in outcomes research, nowhere is it more critical than in rehabilitation, which specializes in treatment of persons with severe, permanent impairment. Standard 8.3 warns against evaluation of service providers on the basis of outcome scores alone in the absence of any other data.

The movement to improve and standardize measurement in rehabilitation should result in a smaller number of better-developed scales and measures. Quality and outcome monitoring will be facilitated by large sample sizes and valid comparisons.

CHARACTERISTICS OF EXISTING FUNCTIONAL ASSESSMENT INSTRUMENTS

Functional assessment methods have been influenced by changes in the concept of rehabilitation and technological advances. With the expanded scope of rehabilitation, there has been an increase in the number of domains routinely assessed as part of the rehabilitation process. It is currently common practice in rehabilitation services to utilize a large number of assessment instruments to document impairments, the ability to complete basic and more complex daily living skills, and perceptions of quality of daily living. The combination of these instruments provides the evaluation of the critical components that make up independent or interdependent active life. Although the assessment instruments can be either generic to rehabilitation patients or disease-specific, most documentation of functional abilities is determined using generic tools.

Comprehensive functional assessment is an essential clinical management component. It goes beyond disease categories and physical impairments to address the resultant disability that rehabilitation efforts target. The rationale or goal of treatment intervention guides the choice of instruments employed. Information from assessment instruments can be utilized for descriptive, evaluative, or predictive purposes. The use of functional assessment for descriptive purposes is a common screening method in rehabilitation and chronic illness, documenting the type and severity of disabilities at a given point in time. Assessment instruments are also used to set therapeutic goals and to monitor the clinical course of the disease, while measuring clinical changes over time. The predictive use of assessment instruments provides objective criteria to plan the treatment and evaluate the goals that have been set. Regardless of the instrument chosen, it should be practical, simple to administer, and yield meaningful results that can direct the rehabilitation process. The guiding principles in choosing a functional assessment scale are: that the scale be a valid measure of the function being tested, that previous studies document validity and adequate reliability, and that the measurement be sensitive enough to document clinically important change.[31]

The ability to distinguish between the concepts of functional capacity and functional performance is an important consideration for test administration. Methodological differences in obtaining the assessment measures and the type of populations being assessed are two sources of discrepancies. Often measures do not clearly differentiate between the presence of a functional impairment that makes an activity impossible to carry out and the actual performance of an activity. As a simple example, a low score in locomotion could mean either that the subject had severe paralysis of limbs or else lacked the will or ability to use limbs that were otherwise intact. Performance ADL was shown to have an integral cognitive component in the Framingham study of noninstitutionalized persons who had had strokes, and in patients after traumatic brain injury.[32, 35] This factor is a major consideration in rehabilitation. In addition, Nagi[48] has documented that disability, unlike functional limitation, has a major social component. Since disability reflects performance within a sociocultural context, one could expect that daily performance would be strongly influenced by social as well as physical factors. The goals of and rationale for choosing a specific functional assessment instrument need to take these considerations into account. One needs to be aware that performance-based functional assessment takes the social and physical contexts into account.

The functional assessment scale employed should be able to measure disability, monitor progress, enhance communications, measure the effectiveness of treatment, and document the benefits of rehabilitation interventions. Since assessment instruments are used repeatedly during the course of rehabilitation, the results should be reliable and valid measures for the disabilities being treated.

EXISTING ADULT FUNCTIONAL ASSESSMENT SCALES

Activities of Daily Living (ADL) Scales

Activities of daily living refer to those basic skills that one must possess in order to care for oneself independently. Instruments that assess ADL usually assess abilities in self-care (eating, bathing, grooming, dressing, etc.), transfers, continence, and, in most cases, locomotion. ADL scales are usually hierarchical in arrangement. They include easier activities such as eating, and more difficult tasks such as climbing stairs. The FIM and the Patient Evaluation and Conference System (PECS) are examples of scales that include the domains of functional communication and social cognition. Information is collected by observing actual performance rather than capacity as demonstrated in an artificial setting such as during therapy. There are a number of valid and reliable scales that document ADL. Most are administered by trained clinicians, although there are some that are based on subjective judgment. The utility of these instruments is that they provide a minimum number of items for describing physical functioning and can be used to track a clinical course of treatment.

Table 8–2 describes selected ADL scales that are currently in use in rehabilitation and that meet adequate validity and reliability standards.

Instrumental Activities of Daily Living (IADL) Scales

The ability to accomplish activities related to maintaining one's living environment is tested using IADL scales. These tasks can include using a telephone, shopping, preparing meals, and managing money. Developing and restoring these skills are often part of a rehabilitation program, but the skills are difficult to evaluate until the individual returns home. IADL scales can be rated either by an interviewer or by the individual, depending on the disability and circumstances. These scales might not be sensitive to change as not all activities are pertinent to everyone. Also, they do not take safety into account as a feature of performance.

Table 8–3 describes three IADL scales utilized in rehabilitation services.

Quality of Life Scales

Quality of life scales denote a wide range of capabilities, symptoms, and psychosocial characteristics that describe functional ability and satisfaction with life. Components of quality of life include social roles and interactions, functional performance, intellectual functioning, perceptions, and subjective health. Indicators can include standards of living and general satisfaction with life. Although there is controversy over the measurement of quality of life, it is a powerful indicator of successful rehabilitation. The relevance of these types of scales to populations with permanent disability has not yet been established. Rather than being criterion-referenced, these scales generally ask the subject to compare himself or herself with a prior healthy state.

Although several measures have been developed, only a few have been well tested in terms of reliability, validity, and sensitivity. Three that meet these criteria are described in Table 8–4.

PROGRAM EVALUATION AND CONTINUOUS QUALITY IMPROVEMENT

Definition

The Commission on Accreditation of Rehabilitation Facilities (CARF) defines *program evaluation* as a sys-

TABLE 8–2 Selected Measures of Activities of Daily Living (ADL)

Scale	Description and Type of Scale	Reliability, Validity, and Responsiveness	Time and Administration	Comments
Barthel Index (BI)[41]	Ordinal scale with total scores ranging from 0 (totally dependent) to 100 (independent); 10 weighted items: feeding, bathing, grooming, dressing, bladder control, bowel control, toileting, chair/bed transfer, mobility, and stair climbing	Well-documented reliability and validity; not sensitive to minor changes at higher levels of ADL functioning	Clinician observation: < 40 min; appropriate for screening, formal assessment, monitoring, maintenance	Widely accepted scale for disability; strong reliability and validity
Index of Independence in Activities of Daily Living[33]	Dichotomous rating in hierarchical order of dependency: bathing, dressing, toileting, transfer, continence, and feeding; cases ranked from A (independent in all 6 items) to G (dependent in all 6 items)	Documented reliability and validity; limited range of activities assessed; not as sensitive to change as BI or other instruments	Clinician observation: < 20 min; appropriate for screening, formal assessment, monitoring, maintenance	Widely accepted scale, especially in geriatrics; assesses some basic skills but not walking and climbing stairs
Kenny Self-Care Evaluation[57]	Ordinal scale with 17 specific activities under 6 major categories: bed activities, transfers, locomotion, personal hygiene, dressing, and feeding; measured on 5-point scale, 0 = dependence to 4 = independence; range of total scores: 0 to 24	Documented reliability and validity; reasonable sensitivity	Clinician observation or judgment: > 30 min; appropriate for formal assessment, monitoring, maintenance	Range of inclusive categories, geared to rehabilitation assessment; ratings can be subjective
FIM Instrument	Ordinal scale with 18 items, 7-level scale with scores running from 18 to 126; areas of evaluation include self-care, sphincter control, transfers, locomotion, communication, and social cognition	Well-documented reliability and validity; able to detect minor changes with 7 levels; physical and cognitive components able to detect increments of change; can be converted into two Rasch-derived measures	Clinician observation: < 20 min; appropriate for screening, formal assessment, monitoring, maintenance, and program evaluation	Widely accepted in medical rehabilitation, including international; proven measure of ADL and social cognition; standardized interobserver reliability by credentialing of clinicians; extensive training materials
Level of Rehabilitation Scale (LORS) and LORS American Data System (LADS) (LORS/LADS)[7]	Five interval subscales assessing ADL, mobility, communications, cognitive ability and memory, measured on 5-point scale from 0 = unable to perform activity to 4 = able to perform	Documented reliability and validity; specific to physical and cognitive measures in medical rehabilitation setting	Clinical observation: 10 min per subscale, > 60 min total; appropriate for screening, monitoring, maintenance, and program evaluation	Measures broad functional outcome categories; provides separate scores for subscales; does not measure bladder or bowel incontinence
Patient Evaluation and Conference System (PECS)[54]	Ordinal scale with 115 items in a 6-step scale ranging from total dependence to total independence; major headings include medicine, nursing, physical mobility, ADL, communication, medications, device utilization, pay, neuropsychology, social issues, therapeutic recreation, procedures, nutrition, pain, pulmonary	Documented reliability and validity; broad range of categories relating to medical rehabilitation services	Discipline-specific evaluations: < 60 min for most disciplines; appropriate for formal assessment, monitoring, maintenance, and program evaluation	Extensive number of items evaluated; focuses on long-term needs and program evaluation; an ADL subscale has been Rasch-analyzed

TABLE 8–3 Selected Measures of Instrumental Activities of Daily Living (IADL)

Scale	Description and Type of Scale	Reliability, Validity, and Responsiveness	Time and Administration	Comments
Functional Health Status[56]	Guttman scale containing 25 questions indicating ascending dependency; questions include out-of-home activities such as going to the movies, walking half a mile, and doing heavy work	Documented reliability and validity	Interviewer: < 30 min; appropriate for maintenance in community setting	Simple scale design with general functioning questions; limited utility with disabled population; difficult to validate in an institutional setting
Older Americans Resources and Services Multidimensional Functional Assessment Questionnaire (OARS MFAQ)[12]	Multidimensional assessment tool containing 105 questions in 5 domains: social resources, economic resources, mental health, physical health, and ADL	Documented reliability and validity	Interviewer: > 10 min; appropriate for maintenance in the community	Measures broad base of information necessary for independent living; complex domains assessed
Philadelphia Geriatric Center Instrumental Activities of Daily Living[13]	Guttman scale includes questions on use of telephone, walking, shopping, food preparation, housekeeping, laundry, public transportation, and medicine	Documented reliability and validity	Time: < 30 min	Strength: measures broad base of information necessary for independent living

tematic procedure for measuring the outcomes of care.[10] Quality assessment and quality improvement are "ongoing activities designed to objectively and systematically evaluate the quality of patient care and services, pursue opportunities to improve patient care and services, and resolve identified problems."[30] Gonnella[17] describes program evaluation as a branch of quality assessment and improvement. Other branches include utilization review, risk management, infection control, and documentation. The directives for achieving quality health care through program evaluation from CARF, the Joint Commission on Accreditation of Healthcare Organizations (Joint Commission), state health departments, and other agencies have been a major stimulus for documentation of outcomes in medical rehabilitation.

Program evaluation is one way to measure the effectiveness and efficiency of rehabilitation services. Structure, process, outcome, or a combination of these factors

TABLE 8–4 Selected Measures of Quality of Life

Scale	Description and Type of Scale	Reliability, Validity, and Responsiveness	Time and Administration	Comments
MOS 36-Item Short Form Survey (SF-36)[61]	Assesses 8 health domains including physical and social activities, mental health, general health perceptions, vitality, and discomfort	Documented reliability and validity	Interviewer in person or phone: < 30 min; appropriate for maintenance in community setting	Items well-standardized; widely used in community; utility for following persons with disability not known
Sickness Impact Profile (SIP)[8]	Subscales evaluate the following areas: ambulation, self-care, emotions, communications, alertness, habits, home and recreation, vocation, and social interactions	Adequate reliability and validity	Interviewer in person or phone: < 30 min; appropriate for maintenance in community setting	Comprehensive evaluation; behavioral rather than subjective health items; focus on community life; utility for following persons with disability not known
LIFEware System[4]	Subscales evaluate physical functioning, pain experience, affective well-being, and cognitive functioning	Initial reliability study showed overall high test-retest reliability; a validity study found adequate content, construct, and criterion validity using both raw scores and Rasch measures	Self-administered or conducted as an in-person interview: approximately 10 min	Items were selected through the use of Rasch analysis to assess the specific types of problems encountered with medical rehabilitation ambulatory care patients

can be addressed in the evaluation. Structural evaluation data include information about certification of professional health care providers. Process evaluation data include information about the provision of treatment in terms of number and type. Outcome evaluation data include information about the level of functional independence achieved or the level of patient satisfaction. Good patient outcomes are the culmination of the combined effects of structure and process. For practical purposes, then, program evaluation in medical rehabilitation has come to mean a comparison of the measurement of the functional performance of patients, as well as related variables, at the beginning of rehabilitation and after care has been completed.

Elements of Program Evaluation

The elements of program evaluation include a description of the purpose of the program (mission statement), program structure, program goals, program objectives, methods of applying measures, and utilization of outcome data in various reports and communications.[10]

The program mission statement is a broad summary of the rehabilitation program, the patients served, and the treatments provided. The program structure describes the organizational framework. This includes the type of facility, admission criteria, patients served, and services provided.[10] The program goals are derived from the mission statement and are written for each rehabilitation program (e.g., the stroke program). The goal statements are expressed in achievable terms.

Program objectives follow the program goals and are stated in terms that are measurable according to expected results. Achievement of objectives should relate to effectiveness and efficiency of the program and to satisfaction of the individuals served. Effectiveness objectives address the extent to which outcomes are attained. Efficiency objectives indicate the quantity of resources used to attain program goals.

For example, program objectives of a stroke program might be to (1) optimize self-care skills, (2) optimize sphincter management, (3) optimize transfer skills, (4) optimize locomotion skills, (5) optimize communication skills, (6) optimize social cognition skills, (7) return patients to the community, (8) optimize vocational independence, (9) ensure appropriate length of stay, and (10) optimize the average cost per unit of improvement (gain in function).

Functional assessment scales are used to determine whether these objectives have been achieved. They may reflect improvement from admission to discharge or else represent criterion levels to be matched or exceeded. Typically, this information is derived from using a functional assessment instrument that compares admission and discharge levels of independence. On the other hand, criterion measures indicate improvement to a predetermined level. An example of criterion measures might be a facility's objective to achieve a certain percentage of community discharges. From past performance, a facility might choose a level of 72% as minimally acceptable, with a goal of 80%, and an optimal level of 88%. A facility with less severely affected or younger patients might choose a percentage that is closer to 100% as optimal. Some facilities choose a criterion based on case-mix-adjusted (expected) data that are based on national data and the facility case mix.[10]

Additional data to be collected and analyzed for the program evaluation reports include demographic data and descriptors of the problems or barriers to individual success. Typically, demographic data include (1) average age and age distribution, (2) sex distribution, (3) average time from onset of impairment to admission to rehabilitation, (4) frequency of program interruptions, (5) vocational status prior to impairment, and (6) payment sources.

Having collected and aggregated the outcome data, feedback reports must be compiled to summarize the findings. The data are then used for management reports, quality improvement and research, and communications to the community and third-party payers.

Rationale and Usefulness

Forer[15] succinctly described the benefits of program evaluation:

1. Ensure that a program is functioning within predetermined standards.
2. Provide guidance for alignment of program goals and objectives with patient needs.
3. Facilitate collecting outcome data systematically for research purposes.
4. Make information available for evaluation of cost-effectiveness.
5. Plan for the future with the help of informed decision making.
6. Support marketing efforts with objective data.
7. Promote understanding and acceptance of the rehabilitation program by the community.

Program evaluation reports form the basis for monitoring the rehabilitation program. For example, they can be used to identify patients whose outcomes did not meet previously established goals and expectations. Identification of these patients can lead the quality improvement committee to suggest revision of existing programs, treatments, or interventions. By following certain indicators over time, administrators and clinicians may monitor the impact of those revisions and make further adjustments. It is important to establish a baseline of values with which results may be compared before and after a change of program is implemented.

Using outcome data to understand and improve the results of patient care is the most significant reason for doing program evaluation. Outcome data can identify those patients who fail to attain maximal benefits from the program as well as those patients who exceed expectations. Patients who may have had adjustment problems or medical complications or who have deteriorated in functional status may be identified and the program improved to serve them better.[15]

Outcome data from several facilities can be pooled to support research studies. For example, Granger et al[19] and Johnston et al[28] studied characteristics that predict outcomes for stroke patients in rehabilitation. The existence of a large and current data pool, such as the Uniform Data System for Medical Rehabilitation, allows investigators to study the interactions of many different factors in order to identify characteristics of patients with selected outcomes such as functional status, placement at discharge, and estimated length of stay.[58]

Outcome data can also be used to address a facility's operational issues such as the effectiveness and efficiency with which care is provided in relation to outcomes. The average charge per patient, the average length of stay, and the average cost per unit of improvement are important parameters for managing a facility. In these days of rapid changes in the manner of providing and paying for health care, planning for future program needs is another critical use of outcome data. Data should be used to monitor for changes in the following:[15]

1. Distribution of patient characteristics such as age and sex
2. Diagnostic mix
3. Case severity
4. Number of patients treated
5. Length of stay
6. Charges or costs per patient
7. Frequency of program interruptions
8. Discharge patterns
9. Intensity, modalities, and types of clinicians involved in treatment

Performance Measurement Systems

The medical rehabilitation industry has been interested in comparing facility data with national comparison data since the 1980s, and many programs subscribe to national performance measurement systems.

The largest measurement system is the Uniform Data System for Medical Rehabilitation, described below. Medirisk, now Care Data, offered the Formations Clinical Outcomes System, which maintained a database for inpatient medical rehabilitation programs. The Patient Evaluation Conference System (PECS), developed by Richard Harvey and Associates at Marianjoy Hospital, has been used by dozens of rehabilitation programs. The PECS provides a comprehensive assessment and is used to organize communication and set goals in the rehabilitation team conference, as well as to evaluate the rehabilitation program.

The Joint Commission on Accreditation of Healthcare Organizations' ORYX Initiative

The Joint Commission requires that facilities adhere to standards of patient care, staff education, and organizational performance. In 1987, the Joint Commission initiated its Agenda for Change, which emphasized the use of process and outcome measures to improve performance and quality of care.

In 1998, under the ORYX Initiative, hospitals and long-term care facilities accredited by the Joint Commission began working with performance measurement systems to collect and report performance measurement data in a standardized manner. The performance measurement systems then transmit a report summarizing the facility data as well as case-mix-adjusted comparison (e.g., national) data to the Joint Commission.

Beginning in 2000, the Joint Commission moved to the use of core measures so that data reported from different performance measurement systems can be compared.

Uniform Data System for Medical Rehabilitation

In 1983, a national task force was established to develop a uniform data set for medical rehabilitation that would document the outcomes and costs of medical rehabilitation. The task force recognized the need for the creation of a tool that could be used uniformly to measure the functional status of the person with long-term needs.[22] The work of the task force, supported by a grant from the National Institute of Handicapped Research (NIHR), resulted in the development of the FIM instrument (see Table 8–2) and the creation of the Uniform Data Set for Medical Rehabilitation. A nonprofit organization known as the Uniform Data System for Medical Rehabilitation (UDSMR) was established on the campus of the State University of New York at Buffalo to serve as a repository for information about medical rehabilitation. UDSMR, a division of U B Foundation Activities, Inc., owns all of the copyrights, trademarks, and service marks associated with the FIM instrument, the WeeFIM instrument, and the LIFEware System.[4] Subscribers to UDSMR sign license agreements in order to use the FIM System and the WeeFIM System, which consist of the adult and pediatric versions of the Uniform Data Set for Medical Rehabilitation; to use the data collection programs known as FIMware software and WeeFIMware software; and to receive UDSMR-produced reports. The data are downloaded to disk and returned to UDSMR on a quarterly basis for aggregation in large national databases. UDSMR uses the data to prepare standard and special reports that each subscriber can then use to examine the outcomes of their medical rehabilitation services, and for a variety of other purposes such as program evaluation, the ORYX Initiative, marketing, and so forth. This data set is now used on a regular basis in more than 70% of the medical rehabilitation facilities across the United States as well as in seven countries around the world.

The data set includes admission, discharge, and follow-up FIM scores (Fig. 8–2), as well as demographic, diagnostic, financial, and length-of-stay variables. Since 1987 more than 2.5 million complete data records have been collected on medical rehabilitation patients with a variety of diagnoses. The collection and analysis of comparable data from clinical sites around the country represented the next step in the development of an appropriate functional assessment scale for patients with disability.

The UDSMR Data Management Service provides subscribing facilities with quarterly reports on such variables as FIM items; subscale, domain, and total scores; demographics; charges; and length of stay. The report data are arranged in three columns, allowing direct comparisons of the clinical site with the region and nation.

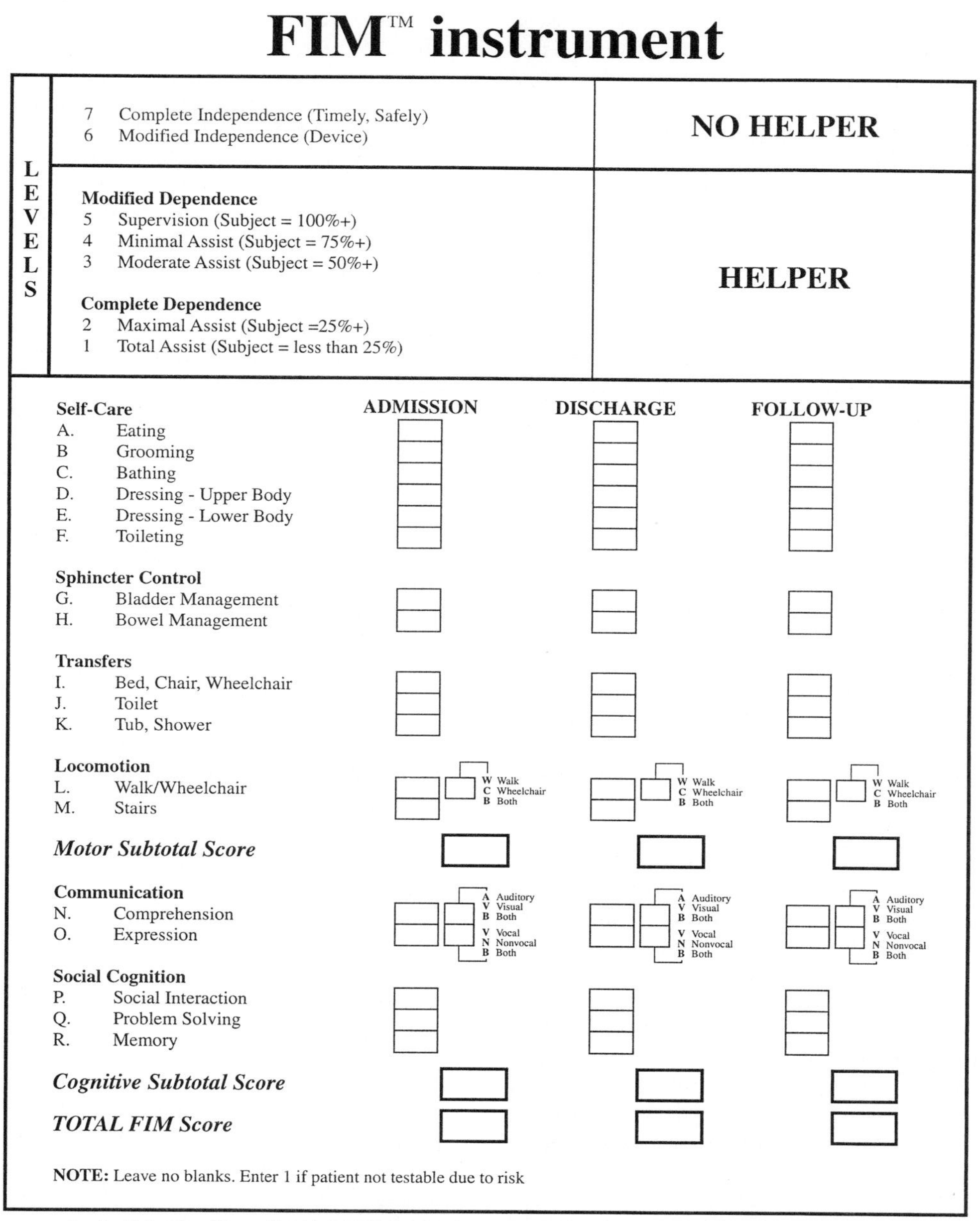

FIM™ instrument

LEVELS		
	7 Complete Independence (Timely, Safely) 6 Modified Independence (Device)	NO HELPER
	Modified Dependence 5 Supervision (Subject = 100%+) 4 Minimal Assist (Subject = 75%+) 3 Moderate Assist (Subject = 50%+) **Complete Dependence** 2 Maximal Assist (Subject =25%+) 1 Total Assist (Subject = less than 25%)	HELPER

	ADMISSION	DISCHARGE	FOLLOW-UP
Self-Care			
A. Eating	☐	☐	☐
B Grooming	☐	☐	☐
C. Bathing	☐	☐	☐
D. Dressing - Upper Body	☐	☐	☐
E. Dressing - Lower Body	☐	☐	☐
F. Toileting	☐	☐	☐
Sphincter Control			
G. Bladder Management	☐	☐	☐
H. Bowel Management	☐	☐	☐
Transfers			
I. Bed, Chair, Wheelchair	☐	☐	☐
J. Toilet	☐	☐	☐
K. Tub, Shower	☐	☐	☐
Locomotion			
L. Walk/Wheelchair	☐ ☐ W Walk C Wheelchair B Both	☐ ☐ W Walk C Wheelchair B Both	☐ ☐ W Walk C Wheelchair B Both
M. Stairs	☐	☐	☐
Motor Subtotal Score	☐	☐	☐
Communication			
N. Comprehension	☐ ☐ A Auditory V Visual B Both	☐ ☐ A Auditory V Visual B Both	☐ ☐ A Auditory V Visual B Both
O. Expression	☐ ☐ V Vocal N Nonvocal B Both	☐ ☐ V Vocal N Nonvocal B Both	☐ ☐ V Vocal N Nonvocal B Both
Social Cognition			
P. Social Interaction	☐	☐	☐
Q. Problem Solving	☐	☐	☐
R. Memory	☐	☐	☐
Cognitive Subtotal Score	☐	☐	☐
TOTAL FIM Score	☐	☐	☐

NOTE: Leave no blanks. Enter 1 if patient not testable due to risk

FIGURE 8–2. FIM instrument. (From Uniform Data System for Medical Rehabilitation: Guide for the Uniform Data Set for Medical Rehabilitation [including the FIM instrument], Version 5.1. Buffalo, State University of New York at Buffalo, 1997.)

Since the data set is uniform across clinical sites, these comparisons provide critical evaluation and planning data for any one site at any single point in time and across time from admission to discharge to follow-up. UDSMR also provides severity-adjusted data reports that use the national data and the facility case mix to calculate "expected" values.

The database can also be used as a tracking device by examining trends across reporting periods. Comparisons within sites allow clinicians and administrators to determine patterns of care within their facilities, while tracking of regional and national data across reports allows the same staff to be aware of changes in either regional or national medical rehabilitation policies and procedures. Because of the unique reporting by type of impairment across all diagnoses, the facilities can use the data to focus, with considerable detail, on their individual patient groups and to make comparisons within impairment types with regional and national trends.

A key advantage of a large national data repository or registry is that it allows for site-specific, multiple-site, regional, state, national, and international comparisons. Another advantage is the ability to study patterns of care and monitor trends over time. Statistical research often depends on the availability of large sample sizes to reach substantive conclusions about health care outcomes. A third advantage is that clinical sites can contribute to the national databases while at the same time keeping their own data in a readily accessible form for in-house data analysis and research efforts. This allows for improvements at both the local and national level and for comparisons of the trends at each clinical site with regional and national trends. These comparisons can be made on a quarterly basis or can be examined in trend form over periods of time.

Perhaps most important, large ongoing databases such as those maintained by UDSMR can provide national data of sufficient sample size that key indicators at admission can be incorporated into statistical models to predict more precisely the course of medical rehabilitation and the outcomes at discharge and follow-up. This predictive power of the FIM scores has been developed into models of Function Related Groups (Penn Ability Systems [PAS] FIM-FRGs) through the work of Stineman and colleagues.[58] The appearance of FIM-FRGs signals the next step in putting the national database to work for improving rehabilitative care. The database currently provides the data for prediction models with enough data left over for cross-validation studies of the predictive models to verify their accuracy and report their confidence limits.

In 1987, the FIM instrument was adapted for use in pediatrics by a multidisciplinary team of physicians, nurses, and therapists.[5, 6, 46] The resulting scale, known as the WeeFIM instrument,[22] is a measure of functional abilities and the need for assistance that is associated with levels of disability in children 6 months to 7 years of age. It can also be used with children well beyond the age of 7 when delays in functional performance are evident. The WeeFIM instrument measures functional status within a developmental framework. Function is measured by determining a child's ability to perform basic daily living skills at specific points in time. Development is measured by determining gross and fine motor, adaptive, personal/social, and cognitive skills over time. The WeeFIM instrument is associated with national inpatient and outpatient databases that are maintained by UDSMR. Approximately 105 pediatric service providers subscribe to the WeeFIM System.

The WeeFIM instrument utilizes the same items and rating scale as its parent. The 18 items have been reorganized into three subscales: self-care (eating, grooming, bathing, dressing upper and lower, toileting, bladder and bowel management), mobility (transfers, locomotion, stairs) and cognition (comprehension, expression, social interaction, problem solving, memory).[62] Each item is rated on a seven-level ordinal scale ranging from complete independence (Level 7) to total assistance (Level 1).

Pilot studies involving 111 children without documented disabilities were conducted in 1987 to 1988.[6, 47] The results revealed a strong association between WeeFIM ratings and chronological age. Items on the WeeFIM instrument appeared to progress in a developmental sequence. Less complex tasks, such as ambulation and eating, were performed independently at younger ages, while more complex tasks, such as dressing and problem solving, were completed at older ages.

In 1990, the first phase of a normalization study was completed when pediatric clinical nurse specialists and nurse practitioners who had been specially trained in the use of the WeeFIM instrument assessed 417 children without disabilities.[5, 46] The data were obtained by interviewing parents and primary caregivers at 11 pediatric primary care sites in the western New York area. Rasch analysis of the data led to the development of separate WeeFIM norms for the Motor and Cognitive subscales. Norms were also developed for the Total WeeFIM rating (the sum of the ratings for all 18 items) and for each of the individual items. The subscale and Total WeeFIM rating norms are included in the *WeeFIM System Clinical Guide, Version 5.0.*[62] Individual age-related item norms are in the UDSMR WeeFIMware software and are only available to subscribers. The calculations are based on the chronological age of the child at the time of the WeeFIM assessment.

In 1991, McCabe[42] concluded that the relationship between growth in functional independence and age in months, in children without disabilities, is logarithmic. She also determined that test-retest and inter-rater reliabilities were satisfactory, and that functional independence growth curves distinguish between children with disabilities and those without disabilities. The validity and reliability of the WeeFIM instrument have been well documented through numerous studies conducted by Ottenbacher and colleagues[52, 53] and by Msall and colleagues.[45, 47]

Although comparative follow-up assessments are available through UDSMR, more attention needs to be given to the follow-up of patients to study the impact of medical rehabilitation after discharge. Examination of both the short- and long-term impacts of medical rehabilitation on its patients becomes even more valuable when considering linkages of databases. When connections can be made between the UDSMR and other national data sets, as has been done with the ongoing study that is enhancing evaluation of the trauma system by incorporating the rehabilitation component,[20] then increasingly more detailed studies will become available. The development of UDSMR databases for skilled nursing facilities, outpatients, and children allows for a broad perspective on patients from birth through old age. The advantages of uniformity and matching measuring tools (FIM and WeeFIM instruments) allow for a unique opportunity to develop secondary prevention models by linking WeeFIM databases to adult databases to study lifetime outcomes.

The measurement of functional changes over time has received considerable attention in the statistical literature[9, 55] owing to the complicated nature of repeated measures statistics. The application of good measurement principles to both the FIM and WeeFIM instruments has resulted in tools that investigators can have confidence in using over time with little measurement error. UDSMR can be used with considerable statistical power and measurement confidence to provide unique insights into long-term care of patients in medical rehabilitation. The advantages of uniformity and large numbers of patients allow a broad range of clinical research to be applicable across the life span, from childhood to old age. This unique uniformity of measurement across time will provide an important key to understanding and meeting the needs of a diverse population with disabilities.

SUMMARY

Reviewing and assuring quality of health care delivery are daunting issues for all providers of health care. Almost two decades ago, medical rehabilitation adopted a model of program evaluation that is facility-based with certain common elements. Since an important purpose of medical rehabilitation is to improve the functional status of patients, reliable and valid methods of functional assessment are necessary.

Functional assessment is a method for describing a person's abilities and limitations. The essence of functional assessment is the measurement of a person's use of the variety of skills included in performing tasks necessary to daily living, leisure activities, vocational pursuits, social interactions, and other required behaviors. The data are used to help formulate judgments as to how well these essential skills are being used, and to gauge the degree to which tasks are accomplished and social role expectations are being met. Performance-based functional assessments take the social and physical contexts of the person into account.

It is possible to compare changes in status over periods of time for an individual or a group of individuals by assessing function at appropriate intervals. In this manner, outcomes of professional interventions of health care, rehabilitation, education, or psychological and social counseling may be described and monitored. Once outcomes become measurable they become manageable. However, care must be exercised in applying standards derived from group studies to the management of an individual. Factors that are unique to a particular case must be taken into account.

There have been many attempts to improve the quality of measurement in rehabilitation over the last 30 years. Validity is the paramount criterion for choice and use of a measure. Reliability is usually defined as freedom from random error and is necessary but not sufficient. The acid test of the utility of a functional assessment tool is that it predicts something in the future that is outside of itself.

Development of a sound functional assessment instrument involves having a good idea that is conceptually clear and feasible, operationalizing the idea in the form of a stable instrument with logical procedures, tedious testing, and, finally, dissemination, with opportunities to follow the consequences of use of the instrument.

The design of an effective program evaluation system involves many ingredients. Program evaluation data must be presented in a clear, concise, and timely manner. The information must be relevant and understandable to those reviewing the information. Some form of the information should be shared with managers, clinical staff, and others. Presentation may take a variety of formats including statistics, graphs, matrices, and narrative descriptions. This information should be used by providers to solve problems and improve the quality of care delivered to patients. The results of program evaluation could prove useful for evaluating alternative treatment modalities within a rehabilitation facility but will become crucial for evaluating outcomes among different types of rehabilitation settings.

In 1985, Granger[18] predicted that by the year 2000

> . . . all healthcare workers will be using standardized terminology to describe the problems consequent to chronic disease and we will be employing systematic computerized methods for tracking individuals' functional abilities and their unmet needs over time. Medical rehabilitation programs will be mandated into the healthcare plans of individuals disabled by accident or disease. However, authorization for payment by third parties will entail requirements for (a) an organized system of care with a comprehensive plan of management, (b) a functional prognosis in terms of probabilities for therapeutic gains in terms of quality of life, (c) efficient delivery of services, and (d) documentation of outcomes through periodic assessments of functional status in order to determine the most favorable benefit/cost ratios.[17]

As standardized functional assessment measures are developed that closely approximate the clinical situation, they will be used to predict the outcomes of care and they will be a part of the cost-benefit analysis that will be integral to decision making in the health and rehabilitative care systems. Functional assessment will allow comparison of the effectiveness and efficiency of alternative therapeutic interventions and settings. Finally, predictable relationships will emerge between the "dose" of rehabilitative services and the "response" of the patient.

REFERENCES

1. Allen MJ, Yen WM: Introduction to Measurement Theory. Monterey, CA, Brooks/Cole, 1979.
2. American Educational Research Association, American Psychological Association, National Council on Measurement in Education: Standards for Educational and Psychological Testing. Washington, DC, American Psychological Association, 1985.
3. American Medical Association: Guides to the Evaluation of Permanent Impairment, ed 4, rev. Chicago, American Medical Association, 1993.
4. Baker JG, Granger CV, Fiedler RC: A brief outpatient functional assessment measure: Validity using Rasch measures. Am J Phys Med Rehabil 1997; 76:8–13.
5. Braun S: The Functional Independence Measure for Children (WeeFIM instrument): Gateway to the WeeFIM System. J Rehabil Outcomes Meas 1998; 2:63–68.
6. Braun SL, Granger CV: A practical approach to functional assessment in pediatrics. Occup Ther Pract 1991; 2:46–51.
7. Carey RG, Posavac EJ: Program evaluation of a physical medicine and rehabilitation unit: A new approach. Arch Phys Med Rehabil 1978; 59:330–337.
8. Carter WB, Bobbitt RA, Bergner M, et al: Validation of an interval scaling: The Sickness Impact Profile. Health Serv Res 1976; 11:515–528.
9. Collins LM, Horn JL (eds): Best Methods for the Analysis of Change. Washington, DC, American Psychological Association, 1991.
10. Commission on Accreditation of Rehabilitation Facilities: Program Evaluation: A Guide to Utilization. Tucson, Commission on Accreditation of Rehabilitation Facilities, 1982.

11. Donaldson SW, Wagner CC, Gresham GE: A unified ADL form. Arch Phys Med Rehabil 1973; 54:175–179.
12. Duke University Center for the Study of Aging and Human Development: Multidimensional Functional Assessment: The OARS Methodology. Durham, NC, Duke University, 1978.
13. Dunn G: Design and Analysis of Reliability Studies. New York, Oxford University Press, 1989.
14. Feinstein AR: Clinimetrics. New Haven, Yale University Press, 1987.
15. Forer S: How to make program evaluation work for you. Neurorehabilitation 1992; 2:52–71.
16. Frey WD: Functional assessment in the '80s: A conceptual enigma, a technical challenge. In Halpern AS, Fuhrer MJ (eds): Functional Assessment in Rehabilitation. Baltimore, Paul H Brookes, 1984, pp 11–43.
17. Gonnella C: Program evaluation. In Fletcher GF, Banja JD, Jann BB, et al (eds): Rehabilitation Medicine: Contemporary Clinical Perspectives. Philadelphia, Lea & Febiger, 1992, pp 243–268.
18. Granger CV: Medical rehabilitation: Predicting needs and measuring outcomes for quality of life. In Gaitz CM, Niederehe G, Wilson NL (eds): Aging 2000: Our Health Care Destiny. Vol 2. Psychosocial and Policy Issues. New York, Springer-Verlag, 1985, p 255.
19. Granger CV, Hamilton BB, Fiedler RC: Discharge outcome after stroke rehabilitation. Stroke 1992; 23:978–982.
20. Grant no. R49-CCR 304550-03, Centers for Disease Control and Prevention. Enhancing Trauma System Evaluation: Incorporating the Rehabilitation Component (Wayne Copes, PI, ongoing).
21. Guide for the Uniform Data Set for Medical Rehabilitation (Including the FIM Instrument), Version 5.1. Buffalo, State University of New York at Buffalo, 1997.
22. Guide for the Uniform Data Set for Medical Rehabilitation for Children (WeeFIM). Version 4.0—Inpatient/Outpatient. Buffalo, State University of New York at Buffalo, 1993.
23. Heinemann AW, Linacre JM, Wright BD, et al: Relationships between impairment and physical disability as measured by the Functional Independence Measure. Arch Phys Med Rehabil 1993; 74:566–573.
24. Hinderer SR, Hinderer KA: Objective measurement in rehabilitation: Theory and application. In DeLisa J, Gans BM, Currie DM (eds): Rehabilitation Medicine: Principles and Practices, ed 2. Philadelphia, JB Lippincott, 1993.
25. Johnston MV, Findley TW, deLuca J, et al: Research in physical medicine and rehabilitation: XII. Measurement tools with application to brain injury. Am J Phys Med Rehabil 1991; 70:40–56.
26. Johnston MV, Keith RA: Measurement standards for medical rehabilitation and clinical applications. Phys Med Rehabil Clin North Am 1993; 4:425–449.
27. Johnston MV, Keith RA, Hinderer S: Measurement standards for interdisciplinary medical rehabilitation. Arch Phys Med Rehabil 1992; 73(suppl):S3–S23.
28. Johnston MV, Kirshblum S, Zorowitz R, et al: Prediction of outcomes following rehabilitation of stroke patients. Neurorehabilitation 1992; 2:72–97.
29. Johnston MV, Wilkerson DL, Maney M: Evaluation of the quality and outcomes of medical rehabilitation programs. In DeLisa J, Gans BM, Currie DM (eds): Rehabilitation Medicine: Principles and Practices. Philadelphia, JB Lippincott, 1993.
30. Joint Commission on Accreditation of Healthcare Organizations: 1993 Accreditation Manual for Hospitals. Oakbrook Terrace, IL, Joint Commission on Accreditation of Healthcare Organizations, 1992.
31. Kane RA, Kane RL: Assessing the Elderly: A Practical Guide to Measurement. Lexington, MA, Lexington Books, 1981.
32. Kaplan CP, Corrigan JD: The relationship between cognition and functional independence in adults with traumatic brain injury. Arch Phys Med Rehabil 1994; 75:643–647.
33. Katz S, Lord AB, Moskowitz RW, et al: Studies of illness in the aged: The index of ADL: A standardized measure of biological and psychological function. JAMA 1963; 185:914–919.
34. Keith RA: Functional assessment measures in medical rehabilitation: Current status. Arch Phys Med Rehabil 1984; 65:74–78.
35. Kelly-Hayes M, Jette A, Wolf PA, et al: Functional limitations and disability among elders in the Framingham Study. Am J Public Health 1992; 82:841–845.
36. Kelman HR, Willner A: Problems in measurement and evaluation of rehabilitation. Arch Phys Med Rehabil 1962; 63:172–181.
37. Kraemer HC: Evaluating Medical Tests: Qualitative and Objective Guidelines. Newbury Park, CA, Sage, 1992.
38. Lawton MP: Assessing the competence of older people. In Kent E, Kastenbaum R, Sherwood S (eds): Research Planning and Action for the Elderly. New York, Behavioral Publications, 1972.
39. Linacre JM, Heinemann AW, Wright BD, et al: The structure and stability of the Functional Independence Measure. Arch Phys Med Rehabil 1994; 75:127–132.
40. Lohr KN, Donaldson MS, Harris-Wehling J: Medicare: A strategy for quality assurance. Quality of care in a changing health care environment. Qual Rev Bull 1992; 18:120–126.
41. Mahoney FI, Barthel D: Functional evaluation: The Barthel Index. Md Med J 1965; 14:61–65.
42. McCabe MA: Evaluating the validity and reliability of the Pediatric Functional Independence Measure. Dissertation, Rush University, Chicago, 1991.
43. McDowell I, Newell C: Measuring Health: A Guide to Rating Scales and Questionnaires. New York, Oxford University Press, 1987.
44. Merbitz C, Morris J, Grip JC: Ordinal scales and foundations of misinference. Arch Phys Med Rehabil 1989; 70:308–312.
45. Msall ME, DiGaudio K, Duffy LC: Use of functional assessment in children with developmental disabilities. Phys Med Rehabil Clin North Am 1993; 4:517–527.
46. Msall ME, DiGaudio K, Duffy LC, et al: WeeFIM: Normative sample of an instrument for tracking functional independence in children. Clin Pediatr 1994; 33:431–438.
47. Msall ME, DiGaudio K, Rogers BT, et al: The Functional Independence Measure for Children (WeeFIM): Conceptual basis and pilot use in children with developmental disabilities. Clin Pediatr 1994; 33(7):421–430.
48. Nagi S: Disability concepts revisited. In Sussman MB (ed): Sociology and Rehabilitation. Washington, DC, American Sociological Association, 1965, pp 100–113.
49. National Institutes of Health, National Institute of Child Health and Human Development. Research Plan for the National Center for Medical Rehabilitation Research. US Department of Health and Human Services, Public Health Service (NIH) publication no 93-3509. Rockville, MD, National Institutes of Health, 1993.
50. Norusis MJ (ed): SPSS Guide to Data Analysis for SPSS-X. Chicago, SPSS, 1988.
51. Nunnally J: Psychometric Theory. New York, McGraw-Hill, 1978.
52. Ottenbacher KJ, Msall ME, Lyon NR, et al: Interrater agreement and stability of the Functional Independence Measure for Children (WeeFIM): Use in children with developmental disabilities. Arch Phys Med Rehabil 1997; 78:1309–1315.
53. Ottenbacher KJ, Taylor ET, Msall ME, et al: The stability and equivalence reliability of the Functional Independence Measure for Children (WeeFIM). Dev Med Child Neurol 1996; 38:907–916.
54. Patient Evaluation and Conference System (PECS). Available from Marianjoy Rehabilitation Hospital and Clinics, PO Box 795, Wheaton, IL 60189.
55. Rogosa DR, Willett JB: Understanding correlates of change by modelling individual differences in growth. Psychometrica 1985; 50:203–228.
56. Rosow I, Breslau N: A Guttman health scale for the aged. J Gerontol 1966; 21:556–559.
57. Schoening HA, Iversen IA: Numerical scoring of self-care status: A study of the Kenny self-care evaluation. Arch Phys Med Rehabil 1968; 49:221–229.
58. Stineman MG, Escarce JJ, Goin JE, et al: A case mix classification system for medical rehabilitation. Med Care 1994; 32:366–379.
59. Task Force on Standards for Measurement in Physical Therapy: Standards for tests and measurements in physical therapy practice. Phys Ther 1991; 71:589–622.
60. Wanlass RL, Reutter SL, Kline AE: Communication among rehabilitation staff: "Mild," "moderate," or "severe" deficits? Arch Phys Med Rehabil 1992; 73:477–481.
61. Ware JE, Sherbourne CD: The MOS 36-item short form survey (SF-36): Conceptual framework and item selection. Med Care 1992; 30:473–483.
62. WeeFIM System Clinical Guide. Buffalo, State University of New York at Buffalo; 1998.
63. World Health Organization: International Classification of Impairments, Disabilities, and Handicaps. Geneva, World Health Organization, 1980.
64. Wright BD, Masters GN: Rating scale analysis. Chicago, Mesa, 1982.

9 CHAPTER

Richard T. Katz, M.D., Michael M. Priebe, M.D., and Denise I. Campagnolo, M.D., Ph.D.

Research in Physical Medicine and Rehabilitation

There seems to be no study too fragmented, no hypothesis too trivial, no literature citation too biased or too egotistical, no design too warped, no methodology too bungled, no presentation of results too inaccurate, too obscure, and too contradictory, no analysis too self serving, no argument too circular, no conclusions too trifling or too unjustified, and no grammar and syntax too offensive for a patient to end up in print.

Drummond Rennie, M.D.

As recently delineated in the supplement on research published by the *American Journal of Physical Medicine and Rehabilitation*,[3] there are several key reasons why physiatrists must concentrate on research. We have enjoyed an unprecedented growth of specialists in physical medicine and rehabilitation, and this wealth of new physiatrists requires a solid research base on which to practice.

For physical medicine and rehabilitation to thrive as a specialty, we must develop a clear presence in medical schools, where academic physiatrists are carrying out research and education in contact with peers in other specialties. Physiatric research must demonstrate that the treatments we offer are clinically effective and cost-effective, so they will be covered in an age of unrelenting fiscal restraint.

Recent surveys demonstrate a need to increase the number of physiatrists who are engaged in research. A recent survey of physiatrists showed virtual unanimity for this sentiment.[11] Only 2% of physiatrists were spending more than one quarter of their time in research. The most common impediments were lack of funding and insufficient equipment.

Finally, research is critical for improving the day-to-day practice of medicine. The skills of clinical research are core knowledge for the improvement of clinical care and should be part of the repertoire for every physician, starting with the residency. Leaders in our field have argued strongly that a foundation of basic research skills should be included as part of residency training and incorporated into the lifelong learning of each physiatrist.[10]

This chapter serves as a primer to the broad knowledge base described in Table 9–1. The discussion is divided into six sections: (1) the research process, (2) experimental design, (3) an introduction to rudimentary statistics, (4) reading the medical literature, (5) grant application and funding, and (6) ethical issues.

THE RESEARCH PROCESS

Research is a process, not an outcome. Research at its core is nothing more than asking questions and answering them using the scientific method. Good research starts with a clinically important question that is refined into a focused, well-defined research question using the scientific literature and formulated as a hypothesis that can be tested (Table 9–2). A study is then designed so that when data are gathered and statistically analyzed, the question posed at the beginning can be answered. The process of asking and answering research questions typically raises more questions to be pursued, and the process starts anew. The key to doing good research, especially as a beginning researcher, is to follow the steps of the scientific process carefully and avoid the temptations to take shortcuts. The discussion in this

TABLE 9–1 Basic Research Skills

Defining a research question and formulating testable hypotheses
Critical review of the scientific literature in a selected area
Specifying subjects and sampling techniques
Precision and accuracy of measurements
Development and use of questionnaires
Using secondary data
Cohort study design
Cross-sectional and case-control design
Evaluation of diagnostic tests
Observational studies and inferences of causality
Experimental sample size
Ethical issues
Project management
Use of descriptive statistics
Use of analytic statistics
Use of statistical consultants
Organizing a pilot study—pretest, quality control
Technical skills in equipment, procedures, and questionnaires
Scientific writing
Oral presentation
Grant preparation
Computer use—word processing, database, statistics
Library reference search

From Findley TW, DeLisa JA: Research in physical medicine and rehabilitation: XI. Research training. Setting the stage for lifelong learning. American Journal of Physical Medicine and Rehabilitation 70(1):S107–S113, 1991.

section emphasizes the critical activities of asking the question and refining that question into a testable hypothesis.

Asking the Question

The significance of research is not found in the probability of the results being correct, but rather in the question asked. Finding the right research question is the most important factor in doing useful research.[17] If the research question is a good one, the outcome of research is more likely to be useful and important. Conversely, if one asks a bad question, no study design or statistical manipulation will make the outcome useful. The significance of a research study is not found in the *P*-value of the results, but rather in the question asked. How the question is asked determines what data are to be collected, what analysis is to be done, and what conclusions can be drawn. To avoid wasting time and energy collecting unnecessary data and, worse yet, drawing useless or incorrect conclusions from the data, it is critical to take the time to find the right research question.

What makes a good research question? The best research questions address problems that are *important and clinically relevant.* Start by asking yourself, Who cares about the answer? Is the answer important to my patients, their families, other physicians or researchers, administrators, or legislators? How will the answer affect the way I care for my patients? Is there currently debate or disagreement on this issue? How important is it to have the right answer? What are the implications of various possible answers? A good research question is *distinctive, yet grounded in the scientific literature.* What have others said about this problem? How is present opinion divided? Will the answer to the research question confirm or refute previous findings? Will it extend previous findings or provide new insights? Is there a theoretical model related to the question? By tying the question to a theoretical model, one can greatly boost the importance and the power of the research. A good research question is also *feasible.* Are subjects available? Are methods available to answer the question, or can they be developed? Are technical support and resources—time, money, facilities, and personnel—adequate to answer the question? Good research questions are *ethical.* What are the ethical implications of this question for the way the study needs to be conducted and the possible answers? Finally, a good research question must be *interesting to the investigator.* Research is a hard process. Important research takes time, a great deal of personal effort, and dedication to complete, and often has few rewards along the way. If the question posed is not of interest to the investigator it will rapidly become tedious and may never be completed.

When beginning the search for a good research question, the investigator must be wary of the risk for "perfection paralysis"—waiting to find the right question. It is better to begin with many questions that can be refined, restated, or rejected later than never to get started because the perfect question can't be found. There are important research questions surrounding us every day. They are most often found in day-to-day clinical situations. Questions raised on rounds by colleagues or by patients and their family members can lead to excellent research questions. Research questions can be found in team conferences, professional disagreements, or in problems that elicit in you a strong emotional response. Questions can be found by reading professional journals, by attending grand rounds, lectures, and journal club discussions, and by participating in scientific meetings. The key is to keep one's eyes and ears open for these potential questions every day. It often requires looking at problems from a different perspective, or listening to discussions with a different ear.

The first step in finding a good research question is to find as many potential questions as possible. When it is difficult to find the right question to begin, perform an exercise. Write down five questions every day for a month. At the end of the month review the questions. Likely, there will be patterns of repeated ideas on the list. These are the questions that may be of the greatest interest. Review the list for the qualities of a good re-

TABLE 9–2 The Research Process

Asking the question
Reviewing the literature
Refining the question into a testable hypothesis
Designing a project to answer the question
Writing the proposal
Obtaining institutional approval
Implementing the project and data collection
Managing the data
Analyzing the data
Reporting the results
Asking new questions

search question and select one to develop and refine into a testable hypothesis.

Reviewing the Scientific Literature

Place the question in the context of existing scientific literature by performing a literature search. It may be useful to locate two to four highly relevant articles as a starting point, then do a computerized literature search. This can be performed on CD-ROM in the medical library or through on-line computerized search services. The National Library of Medicine now provides free MEDLINE access through Internet Grateful Med and PubMed, available on the Internet. Integrate your literature review into a "conceptual review" in which the merits and value of various studies are weighed.

Refining the Question

Before a question can be answered it must be refined into a testable hypothesis. A hypothesis is simply a specific statement that will be deemed true or false as a result of the research. Most questions will be substantially transformed as they are refined into hypotheses because the original question usually contains many component questions, and therefore many hypotheses. Each hypothesis should correspond to one table, chart, or statistical analysis. Each revision of the question will narrow its scope, making the question easier to answer definitively.

To begin the process of refining the question, look for different ways to state the same question and for related questions that may address the question more directly. We can consider the following question: "How can one prevent deep venous thrombosis (DVT) and pulmonary embolism (PE) in persons with spinal cord injury (SCI)?" The question can be restated in many ways:

- Which method of prophylaxis for DVT and PE is most effective in SCI?
- What causes DVT and PE in SCI?
- What causes PE in persons with DVT and SCI?
- Who is at risk for PE after SCI?
- Which method of prophylaxis for PE is most effective in SCI?

The researcher can choose from the many possibilities to refine the question further based on the principles of relevance, distinctiveness, feasibility, ethical implications, and personal interest. Colleagues can be consulted to help advise which question is most to the point.

The next step is to define and expand each term. State the question in a simple, nontechnical, interrogative sentence. For example, "Which method of prophylaxis for DVT and PE is most effective in SCI?" Identify each major term and begin to define, clarify, and expand each one, adding terms to define the scope and focus of the question. A relatively simple question grows more complex. We can see this by examining each term or phase:

- *Which* This term implies a choice or a decision between at least two options.
- *method of prophylaxis* Based on the literature, you can select from numerous methods of prevention that have been studied and give the question a scientific context within which to work.
- *for DVT and PE* Should the clinical entity thromboembolism be defined as a single entity or as two unique but related problems? How will DVT and PE be detected? Will the study be restricted only to proximal lower extremity DVT? Again, the literature offers insights into the theoretical underpinnings of the pathophysiology of thromboembolic disease, contains data on the locations for DVT that are clinically most significant, and has information on which techniques are most sensitive and specific for the detection of DVT or PE.
- *is most effective* How will effectiveness be defined? Is the primary goal to prevent the disease itself, mortality due to the disease, complications such as missed therapy and loss of productivity as a result of the disease, or costs of treating the disease?
- *in SCI* What is the study population? Will it include individuals with acute or chronic SCI, traumatic or nontraumatic SCI, complete or incomplete SCI? What level of injury will be included? Will the study population include people of all ages, children to the elderly? Will persons with co-morbidities, such as multiple trauma, hemorrhage, or those on ventilators, be excluded?

At this point in the research process, consultation with a methodologist or statistician is vital. As the question is refined and each term defined, a large portion of the study design needed to answer the question will be determined, as well as the statistical analysis needed to test the hypotheses. Refining the question with the assistance of a statistician will ensure that the data collected will have meaning when they are analyzed. A common mistake of young researchers is to perform a study before consulting with a statistician. Once the data have been collected, no statistician can retrospectively fix a flawed study.

Once these and other related questions are answered and each term is defined or expanded, a very specific research question can be stated:

> Does early use (begun within 24 hours of injury) of low molecular weight heparin (enoxaparin, 30 mg given SC b.i.d.) result in a lower frequency of proximal (popliteal, femoral, or iliac vein) lower extremity DVT (obstructing intraluminal clot detected by duplex ultrasound performed daily for 2 weeks) than adjusted-dose heparin (8000–15,000 units given SC every 8 hours and adjusted to keep the aPTT between 29 and 34 seconds) in adults—16 years or older—with acute, traumatic, motor complete SCI at or above T_{12}?

A second question of equal importance could be asked specifically about PE by changing the key terms slightly. This carefully stated research question specifies the variables for data collection. It suggests the type of study to be done and the types of analysis to be performed. It defines the subjects to be included. By focusing the question, it becomes manageable and testable. If one were to make different choices concerning how to define each term, the research question and the study itself would be different.

Stating the question converts it into a hypothesis:

> Early use of low molecular weight heparin will result in a lower frequency of proximal lower extremity DVT than adjusted-dose heparin in adults with acute, traumatic, motor complete SCI.

This hypothesis can be tested after the data have been collected, and deemed to be either true or false, thereby answering the question. One can readily imagine a table listing the number of DVTs detected in each group. The statistician will help to determine which statistical analysis will be needed to test the hypothesis. These decisions should be made before proceeding further with the study. If the researcher wishes to study more than one of the possibilities raised by redefining the terms in the original question, separate hypotheses need to be created for each permutation. Once the hypotheses are clearly stated, the study can be designed.

EXPERIMENTAL DESIGN

Scientific studies may be divided into experimental and nonexperimental or observational studies. In an *experimental* study the investigator has control over the major variables, e.g., a drug or treatment. In *nonexperimental* studies researchers look for associations between variables, often in a search for causal relationships. As previously mentioned, once a possible causal relationship is suspected it must then be tested in an experimental design.

Clinical trials are experiments in which the subject is a human being. The prototype of clinical trials is the controlled clinical trial, in which the treatment group or groups are compared to a similar group of control *subjects.* Controlled trials are distinctly more advantageous than uncontrolled observations as causal inferences may be drawn and bias may be minimized through proper *randomization* (assignment of subjects to treatment and control groups purely by chance) and design methods. Randomized controlled trials can offer a persuasive argument that differences in treatment effect are not due to inherent differences between treatment and control groups or to differences in the handling of the groups during the course of an investigation (both of which would bias the study results).

Randomization is best carried out by using a random number list. An example of failure to adequately randomize treatment and control groups would be to compare treatment A on one hospital ward with treatment B on another. Are the same socioeconomic and diagnostic groups of patients admitted to both wards? Similarly, the assignment of alternate cases to the study or control group might be biased; did the referring doctors prefer one treatment method over the other and "load" one treatment group? With paired samples, randomization can be carried out using *crossover* design in which the patient serves as his or her own control. When drugs A and B are compared, one half of the subjects are randomized to receive the drugs ordered A–B, and the other half are randomized to receive drugs B–A.

Another method of randomization that is sometimes useful is *stratification,* also known as *randomized complete block design.* For example, if we were to design a study to assess the effect of GM-1 in minimizing neurotrauma in SCI, we might wish to stratify our treatment and control groups by level of injury and/or completeness of injury. Subjects would then be randomly assigned within each of these strata. Stratification is especially important with small samples, where straight randomization may still lead to unbalanced groups.

Matched controls are sometimes used as substitutes for true randomization. This strategy appears to be attractive at first, but should be used with caution. For example, we can place a subject with five "attributes" in one treatment group and a second individual with the same attributes in the control group. Unfortunately, we cannot always be informed enough to identify all of the important attributes. For example, suppose we identify two groups with the following attributes: (1) round, (2) found in a tree, (3) edible, (4) 3 to 5 inches in diameter, and (5) approximately one-half pound in weight. Although we might create a matched control group, we could still be comparing apples with oranges![6]

One type of control that is often used in drug trials is a *placebo* control. In this type of study a chemically inert sugar pill is formulated to look identical to the active drug to control for *placebo effect,* the positive psychological benefit derived from receiving a pill from a caregiver. In a *single-blind clinical trial* the subjects, but not the investigators, are blinded to the treatment identity for each subject. In a *double-blind clinical trial* both the investigators and the subjects are blinded.

Single-Subject Design

The randomized controlled study is often less suitable in the rehabilitation setting, where there are a large number of variables requiring substantial subject populations. One solution is to use a patient as his or her own control throughout the study, a strategy called *single-subject design.* A single-subject design is an example of *idiographic* or *within-subject designs,* which need not be limited to single subjects. Figure 9–1 shows an example of such a design. The effect of amitriptyline, 75 mg/day, versus placebo is being assessed in a traumatic brain injury patient for the control of agitation. A single patient is observed for several days to establish a baseline (days 0 to 5). A drug is started on the 5th day, and both patient and investigator might be blinded as to whether it is amitriptyline or placebo. The drug is stopped on day 10 and a 5-day "washout" period ensues. The second drug (in this case, amitriptyline) is started on day 15. This might similarly be followed by a subsequent washout period beginning on day 20 and a second baseline observation period from day 26 through 30. There are obviously many variations of baseline periods (A) and intervention periods (B) that could be constructed; some examples include AB, ABA, and ABAB.

The obvious advantage of single-subject design is that efficacy can be demonstrated without the benefit of large numbers of patients, or in settings in which a control group is difficult to define. The disadvantage is that the investigator must then prove that the results are generalizable to larger groups. Statistical methods for

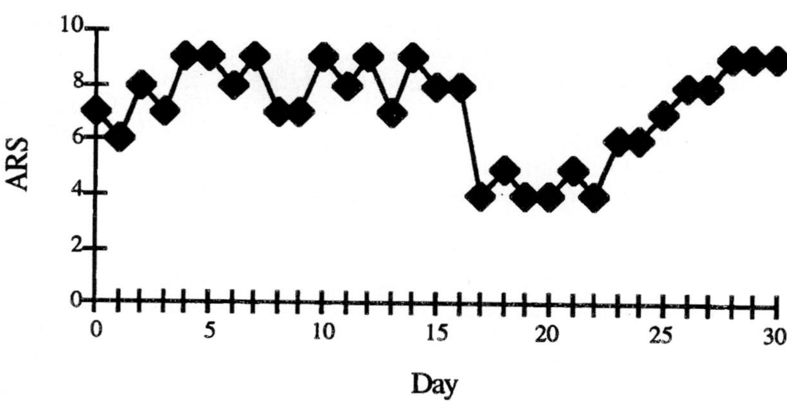

FIGURE 9–1. A data summary for a single-subject design or idiographic study. The *x*-axis represents a 30-day time period. The *y*-axis is a 10-point scale summarizing the patient's agitation for that day (Agitation Rating Scale). After a 5-day observation period, placebo is started on day 5. Placebo administration is stopped on day 10 and a 5-day washout period ensues. Amitriptyline is started on day 15. This is followed by a subsequent washout beginning on day 20 and a second baseline observation period from day 25 through 30.

manipulating data from single-subject designs are available but less well accepted and less robust than traditional statistics. These older views are changing, however, and single-subject design studies are becoming especially attractive in the rehabilitation research setting.[1, 19, 24]

Meta-Analysis

The number of *meta-analyses* in the medical literature is burgeoning. Meta-analysis combines the data from smaller studies into a larger sample size, which can then be statistically evaluated in a more robust fashion than the smaller samples. For example, suppose there are five studies of stroke outcome, each with a sample size of between 20 and 40. Perhaps there was no clinical benefit from speech therapy, and the investigator hypothesized this was because the sample size (N) was too small to demonstrate a statistically significant effect (this would be a Type I error). However, by grouping several studies together and reanalyzing the data, we might have the statistical power to demonstrate that the effect is statistically significant. Meta-analysis may be undermined when the original smaller studies were variable in quality, or when incongruous data are lumped together, or when negative studies fail to be published (*publication bias*).[4, 14, 20]

Epidemiologic Studies

Epidemiology is the study of the distribution of disease in a population and of the factors that influence that distribution. Epidemiologists often have the difficult task of making educated inferences about disease causation, even though they are making these inferences without the benefit of an experimental method.

Case-control studies are an example of *retrospective studies* in which the number of persons in a certain population suffering from a certain disease (that is, a known end point) are compared with another group not suffering from that disease. Both groups are then assessed for their exposure to a certain variable or variables—factors that are suspected of being causally related to that disease. For example, we wish to assess the contribution of excess alcohol consumption to the risk of sustaining traumatic brain injury (TBI). We could perform a retrospective analysis of 1000 TBI persons and 1000 normal controls to assess whether the incidence of excessive alcohol intake is higher or lower in the TBI group. We could then compare the treatment and control groups to determine whether the *relative risk* of suffering a TBI is higher in persons with higher alcohol consumption. There are four critical aspects of performing retrospective studies: (1) How did the investigator select the study subjects (TBI) and control subjects? (2) Are the study subjects and the control subjects comparable (e.g., are they from similar demographic backgrounds)? (3) How did the investigator define the factor under study (e.g., excess alcohol consumption)? (4) How accurate were the histories of exposure (e.g., to alcohol) in the study (TBI) and control groups.

Cohort studies are an example of *prospective studies.* Instead of "looking backward," as in a retrospective study, we "look forward" toward an unknown end point. We assess certain risk factors (e.g., risk factors for cardiovascular disease) in a certain population, and then follow this group of patients over time. We can then assess on long-term follow-up the relative risk of each of the potential risk factors (e.g., smoking, hypertension, obesity) in the development of a certain disease (e.g., angina, myocardial infarction, stroke—the unknown end point). The Framingham, Massachusetts, studies of cardiovascular disease are perhaps the most famous examples of this type of study. Prospective studies are less susceptible to historical bias than retrospective studies, but they often require very large populations in order to achieve an adequate sample size. One of the most difficult features of epidemiological studies is to minimize or eliminate bias in the control or comparison group (see the section titled Reading the Medical Literature, below).

INTRODUCTION TO RUDIMENTARY STATISTICS

Every physiatrist should have a working knowledge of statistics. As technology progresses, medicine is becoming increasingly quantitative. Medical research is reliant on statistical methodology, and statistics pervade the medical literature. The myriad of statistical methods may at first seem overwhelming, but studies have shown that the vast majority of studies in leading journals depend on a relatively small number of statistical concepts.[9, 28]

Descriptive statistics refers to the organization, presentation, and summarization of data. One type of descriptive statistics of interest to medicine is vital statistics, such as birth rates, mortality rates, and life expectancy. Another important concept is that of statistical inference, by which an investigator draws conclusions about a certain *target population* (e.g., all persons with SCI) by studying a *sample population* of that group (e.g., SCI patients drawn from model SCI centers). Obviously, there may be differences between the sample and target populations, which is generally referred to as *bias.* One method of minimizing sample bias is to obtain a *random sample,* where each member of the sample population has an equal and independent chance of being selected.

Data Collection

Data can be collected in several different ways:

- By using a *nominal scale.* A nominal scale (also called enumeration or attribute data) is one in which the data either fit the criteria (e.g., head-injured patients *with* heterotopic bone) or do not (head-injured patients *without* heterotopic bone).
- By using an *ordinal scale.* An ordinal scale is one in which there is a predetermined order among the response classifications. For example, a patient who undergoes a total joint replacement may be independent or may need minimal assistance, moderate assistance, maximal assistance, or be fully dependent for ambulation on postoperative day 7.
- By using a full *ranking scale.* A full ranking scale orders the members of a group from high to low. For example, there are 12 attending physicians in a physiatry group, and there is an administrative analysis to see which physicians are seeing the most outpatients. The physicians can be ranked from 1 through 12 according to their average monthly outpatient visits in the preceding 4 months.
- By using an *interval scale* or a *ratio scale.* An interval scale is one in which the distances between any two numbers are of equal size. For example, an increase in pinch strength from 5 to 10 pounds is equal to one of 10 to 15 pounds. Pinch strength is also an example or a ratio scale, because a pinch strength of 20 pounds is exactly double the force of 10 pounds.

Data may be numerically *discrete* (e.g., the number of irregular heartbeats per minute after acute quadriplegia) or *continuous* (e.g., the creatine kinase level in a patient with polymyositis).

The way in which we collect data is very important, but not without pitfalls. Functional assessment scales are commonly 7-point ordinal scales. Ordinal scales suffer from *nonlinearity,* that is, the distance from class to class is not known—an improvement from 3 to 4 on the scale may not be equivalent to an improvement from 4 to 5.[22] This has prompted a great deal of discussion in the rehabilitation literature because outcome measurement is extremely important. One solution has been to use a strategy called *Rasch analysis,* which transforms ordinal data into interval data.[5, 32]

When choosing a certain measure in data collection, one should have some idea as to its *validity.*[16] Validity refers to the *appropriateness,* meaningfulness, and usefulness of the specific inferences made from the test score. For example, the validity of IQ (intelligence quotient) scores has frequently been challenged as a predictor of school performance and achievement. *Reliability* refers to the *reproducibility* of the data. Suppose, for example, an electromyographer were to perform a new conduction test on a patient and record the results on the visual display. If the examiner manually moves the cursor to the take-off of the compound muscle action potential on two occasions, how close will the results of the first placement be in in comparison with those of the second (*intrarater reliability*)? If two electromyographers move the cursor to the takeoff of the same tracing, how close will the results be between examiners (*inter-rater reliability*)? If one electromyographer stimulates the patient on two occasions and measures the takeoff, how stable will the results be (*test-retest reliability*)?

Probability

Basic concepts of probability are an important element of statistical knowledge. Probability involves a random process—a repetitive process or operation that in any one trial may result in any one of a number of possible outcomes. These outcomes are determined by chance and are impossible to predict. For example, when a coin is tossed (assuming that it cannot land on its side) it will randomly land on heads or tails. The probability of a certain outcome (e.g., heads) occurring can be determined as a ratio of that outcome divided by all possible outcomes (for heads, 1/2). This is true only if the two outcomes are mutually exclusive—one outcome precludes the other (if the outcome is heads, the outcome cannot also be tails). If the probability of an SCI patient surviving 1 year is 0.9, there is a one out of ten or 10% chance that person will not survive 1 year.

One of the most important concepts of probability is that of *independent events.* Events are independent if the occurrence of one is totally independent (does not affect the probability of occurrence) of the other. For example, it is extremely common for SCI patients to also suffer a minor traumatic brain injury. Because these events are likely to occur in one person, they are *not* independent events. However, suffering an SCI as an adult and having strep throat as a child are almost certainly unrelated and thus can be considered independent events. Given two independent events A and B, the probability of *both* occurring is the product of the probability of A times the probability of B (multiplicative law of probability). Thus, if the probability of developing strep throat as a child is 0.4 and that of sustaining SCI is 0.01, the probability of one person being afflicted with both conditions in a lifetime would be the product $(0.4)(0.01) = 0.004$.

One has to be careful using the multiplicative law of probability. For example:

> If the possibility of surviving a cataract removal is 0.9 (or 90%), and the chance of surviving a tonsillectomy is 0.7 (or 70%), then (assuming the two procedures are independent events) a patient would have a (0.7) (0.9) = 0.63 or 63% chance of surviving both procedures.

However, examine a different example.

> The probability of contracting a urinary tract infection after catheterization is 0.1 (10%). The probability of contracting a urinary tract infection after two separate catheterizations is *not* (0.1)(0.1) = 0.01 (1%). The correct way of applying the multiplicative law (again assuming that these are independent events) is to recognize that the probability of *not* contracting a urinary tract infection is 0.9 (90%), and the probability of *not* contracting a urinary tract infection after two separate catheterizations would be (0.9)(0.9) = 0.81 (or 81%). The probability of contracting a urinary tract infection after two separate catheterizations would be 1 − 0.81 = 0.19 (or 19%).

Another possibility that often arises in probability analysis is when one or another of a group of mutually exclusive events may occur. The *additive law of probability* states that the probability of *A or B* occurring is the sum of the probability of *A* and the probability of *B*. For example, if we were to examine the relative frequency of 100% of confirmed lumbar radiculopathies in a series of patients, we might find that 1% occurred at L2, 2% at L3, 5% at L4, 42% at L5, and 50% at S1.

TABLE 9–3 Example of Frequency Distribution

Uric Acid Level (mg/dL)	Total (N = 100)
8.0–8.5	10
8.5–9.0	17
9.0–9.5	23
9.5–10.0	22
10.0–10.5	20
10.5–11.0	8

The additive law of probability allows us to state that the probability of suffering a radiculopathy at L5 *or* S1 is 0.42 + 0.50 = 0.92 (or 92%).

Displaying Data

Numerically discrete or numerically continuous data can be summarized in a *frequency distribution.* Table 9–3 shows uric acid levels for men with their first attack of gouty arthritis. After creating such a frequency distribution, the data can be charted on a bar-type graph (*histogram*) or *frequency polygon,* as in Figure 9–2.

Summarizing Data

Once data have been plotted, there are several useful parameters to help summarize the data. The mean, median, and mode are the most useful measures of central tendency or location. The *mean* or *arithmetic mean* (μ) is simply the total of the observations divided by the

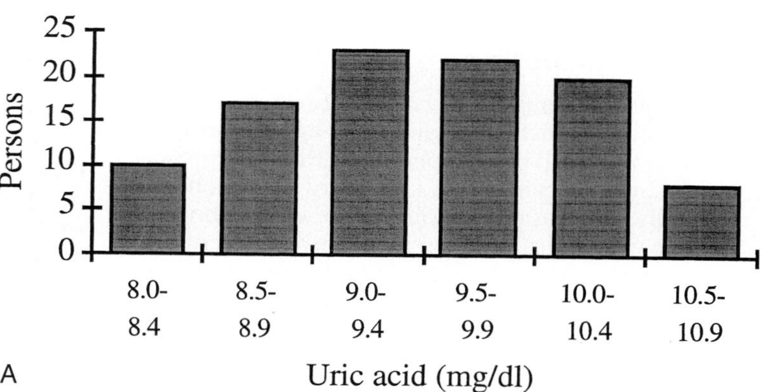

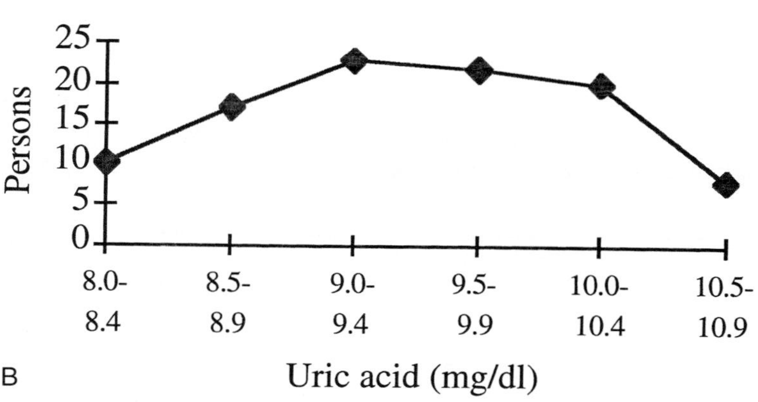

FIGURE 9–2. *A.* Histogram or bar-type graph demonstrating uric acid levels in 100 men and women with their first attack of gouty arthritis. *B.* Frequency polygram or line chart using the same data.

number of observations ($\Sigma x/n$, where Σ = summation sign, x = variable measured, and n = number of x values). The *median* is the observation "in the middle." The *mode* is the most frequently occurring value. For example, pinch strength is measured five times with measured values of 3, 4, 7, 8, and 3 pounds. The mean would be 5 (25 divided by 5), the median 4 (middlemost number), and the mode 3 (most commonly observed value). The mean is most often used in statistics but can be seriously affected by extreme values or *outliers*. The median is unaffected by outliers but is less amenable to statistical treatment.

The second important parameter in summarizing data is the spread or *variation*. The *range* of the data refers to the difference between the highest and lowest values (e.g., the pinch strengths ranged from 3 to 8 pounds, with a range of 5 pounds). Two other useful parameters are the *variance* (σ^2) and its square root, the *standard deviation* (σ). The mathematical formulas for these are

$$\sigma^2 = \frac{\Sigma x^2 - (\Sigma x)^2/n}{n - 1} \text{ and } \sigma = \sqrt{\frac{\Sigma x^2 - (\Sigma x)^2/n}{n - 1}}$$

The reader is referred to standard texts for their derivation and for further details of "sample" versus "population" standard deviations. An example of data needed to calculate variances and standard deviations of pinch strengths is shown in Table 9–4. It is easy to plug these numbers into our equations and determine the variance (σ^2) = 5.5, and the standard deviation (σ) = 2.34. The standard deviation is the most commonly used measure of variation in the medical literature.

Normal Distribution

The concept of a Gaussian or *normal distribution* is very important to statistical inference. The normal distribution is a symmetrical bell-shaped curve that can be characterized by its mean (μ) and standard deviation (σ). Empirically, the normal distribution is very important because many medical measurements in a given population approximate this curve (e.g., blood pressure, height, weight). Although the exact formulation of the normal distribution is beyond the scope of this discussion, several characteristics are worth mentioning. In Figure 9–3A, normal curves *A* and *B* have identical means but differing standard deviations. Curves *A* and *C* have identical standard deviations but different means. Many statistical tests are derived with the assumption that the variables being tested have a normal distribution; these are sometimes referred to as *parametric* tests.

In normal curves as well as other curves that are relatively bell-shaped, the $\mu \pm 1\sigma$ represents approximately 68% of observations that are charted (Fig. 9–3B). The mean $\mu \pm 2\sigma$ represents approximately 95%, and the $\mu \pm 3\sigma$ represents 99% of all observations. For example, if a sampling of body weights in 100 women with SCI were found to be in a normal distribution with $\mu = 120$ pounds and $\sigma = 10$ pounds, approximately 68% of all subjects would range in weight from 110 to 130 pounds, 95% from 100 to 140 pounds, and 99% from 90 to 150 pounds. These relationships do *not* hold true for curves that are asymmetrical (have a large degree of *skewness*). Such distributions are not well described by the mean and standard deviation. Remember that the term normal refers to a mathematical model, and has no biological or clinical connotation.

TABLE 9–4 Example of Data Needed to Calculate Variance and Standard Deviation

Trial	x (lb)	x^2
1	3	9
2	4	16
3	7	49
4	8	64
5	3	9
	$\Sigma x = 25$	$\Sigma x^2 = 147$

Normal Limits

In distributions that are normal, the mean + 2σ and the mean minus 2σ are frequently defined as the *upper and lower limits of normal*. In this context normal refers to *clinical normalcy*. Since $\mu \pm 2\sigma$ encompasses 95% of the subjects studied, this would represent the population between the 2.5 and 97.5 percentiles. Again, these concepts hold true only if the population studied falls into a normal distribution. Cholesterol values and motor nerve conduction velocities are examples of values that are *not* in a bell-shaped or normal distribution.[7]

Normal distributions can often be of use in studying differences between two populations. For example, suppose a new blood test (serum factor H) was being assessed for the detection of heterotopic bone (Fig. 9–4). Suppose that the normal distribution of serum factor H values obtained from 100 patients is represented by curve HO(−), and the normal distribution of serum factor H values from those with heterotopic ossification is represented by curve HO(+). Note that the curves overlap. Our goal for this new diagnostic test is to find an upper limit of normal for serum factor H. Clearly, anywhere we draw an arbitrary vertical line to signify the upper limit of normal serum factor H values is going to involve certain compromises. Our goal is to find a line where all patients without heterotopic bone will fall to the left of the line (*true negatives*) and all those with heterotopic bone will fall to the right (*true positives*). Because the HO(−) and HO(+) curves overlap, this is not possible. A small number of persons who do not have heterotopic bone will fall to the right of our upper limit discretionary value (*false positives*), and some with heterotopic bone will fall to the left of the line (*false negatives*).

With an ideal laboratory test the cutoff point distinguishes entirely between true negative and true positives. However, more often tests suffer from some degree of false positives and false negatives. The *sensitivity* of this test is the ratio of true positives divided by the sum of true positives and false negatives. The *specificity* of the test is a ratio of true negatives divided by the sum of true negatives and false positives. Suppose for

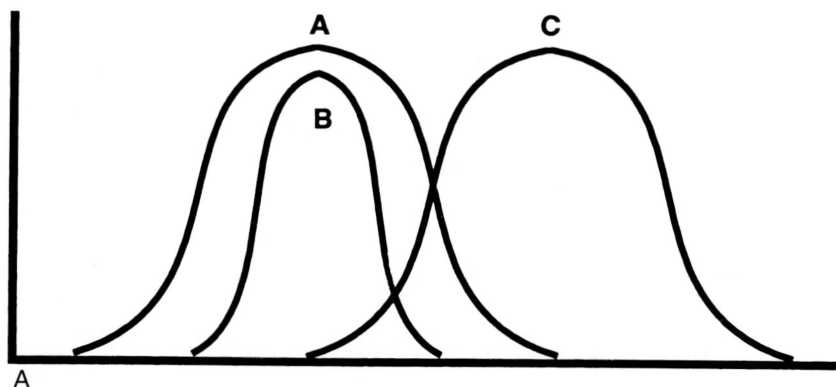

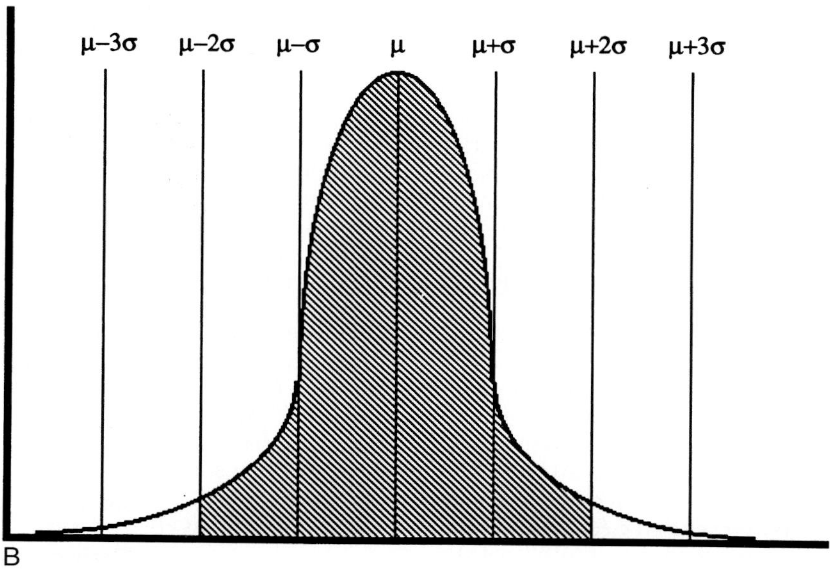

FIGURE 9–3. *A.* Three normal curves. Curves *A* and *B* have identical means (μ) but differing standard deviations (σ). Curves *A* and *C* have identical σ but different μ. *B.* Normal curve with vertical lines denoting the mean, μ, and standard deviations (σ) above or below the mean. *Cross-hatched area* represents 95% of the area under the curve.

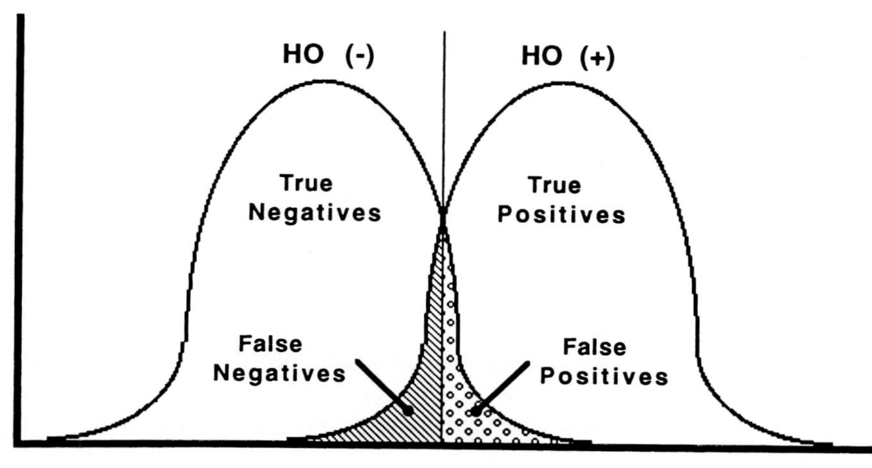

FIGURE 9–4. The distribution of serum factor H level is recorded for patients with heterotopic bone (HO(+)) and without heterotopic bone (HO(−)). The vertical line is arbitrarily placed to represent the upper limit of normal. As the two curves overlap, the upper limit of normal detemines the relative number of true negatives, true positives, false negatives, and false positives.

TABLE 9–5 Sample of Table Needed to Calculate Sensitivity and Specificity

Result of Serum Factor H Test	Persons With HO	Persons Without HO
Positive	80	10
Negative	20	190

our sample above we created the illustration shown in Table 9–5. The sensitivity of the test would be represented by 80 divided by (80 + 20) = 80%. The specificity would be 90 divided by (90 + 10) = 90%. Note that if we move our vertical line or cutoff to the right, we will increase our identification of true negatives and decrease our identification of false positives (specificity will improve, sensitivity will decrease). If we move it to the left, the opposite happens.

Sources of Variation

There are many sources of variation in a defined group of data. One type is true *biological variation,* which represents the actual differences that exist in different subjects. For example, if an investigator were studying weight fluctuation after SCI, actual weight loss in a group of patients may be found to vary from 0 to 20 pounds in the first 3 weeks post injury.

However, other types of variation can occur. *Temporal variation* is the natural variation that occurs over time. For example, due to physiological fluid changes, women may gain weight due to retained fluid during the menstrual cycle, and this may confound the observation of weight loss after SCI. Variation might result from *measurement error* on the part of the observer (e.g., one who reads the scale incorrectly) or the measurement instrument (e.g., a faulty scale).

Sampling variation is yet another important type of variation that can occur when we are studying large populations. Suppose we wished to study the level of a blood factor, serum factor K, in the American public. We could attempt to sample each and every one of the 250-plus million Americans. Obviously, this would be impossible; however, let us assume we could do it, and it was represented by a normal distribution with $\mu = 100$ and $\sigma = 10$. This would represent the *true* mean and standard deviation of factor K in the American public. The reality of the situation is that we would *not* be able to study all Americans but rather would have to select a random sample of Americans and sample their blood. We obtain samples from 100,000 Americans on five separate occasions and find the data shown in Table 9–6. As we can see from the table, none of the sample of the American public precisely represented the true mean and standard deviation, but they came quite close.

TABLE 9–6 Example of Data from Five Samples of a Large Population

Sample	$\mu \pm \sigma$
1	98.6 ± 10.3
2	100.1 ± 9.9
3	97.3 ± 9.8
4	103.1 ± 8.9
5	100.2 ± 11.0

The *central limit theorem* states that the *distribution* of the sample means in Table 9–6 (98.6, 100.1, 97.3, 103.1, and 100.2) will fall in a normal distribution around our true mean (100). Thus we can construct a normal curve (Fig. 9–5) not from the actual data, but from *the mean values for each of our samples.* This curve has its own mean (which hopefully is very close to the true mean of 100) and standard deviation (called the *standard error*).

The construction of such a normal curve of sample means allows us to define *confidence intervals.* From the previous discussion of normal distributions, we know that 95% of all observations fall within two standard deviations of the mean. Using the concept of the central limit theorem, we know that if we find the mean and standard deviation of our *curve of sample means,* we can state that there is a 95% chance that the *true* mean of serum factor K in the American public (100) would fall within the mean $\pm 2\sigma$ of our curve. This is the concept of defining a 95% confidence interval, and the values at each end of that interval are the *confidence limits.* It is a way of quantitating how "confident" we are that the true mean (of 100) falls within our sample estimate. From this discussion it is obvious that confidence limits provide a probability of specifying how successfully we have sampled the true mean value (in this case of serum factor K). Sample means based on a large sample have a better chance of truly estimating our mean value than smaller means. Thus a sample with a large number of observations has a *narrower* confidence interval.

Comparing Groups

Often in medicine we are asked to determine whether a new drug or treatment is superior to an older method, and we must design studies to assess the superiority of one of two (or more) methods. Suppose we had a new

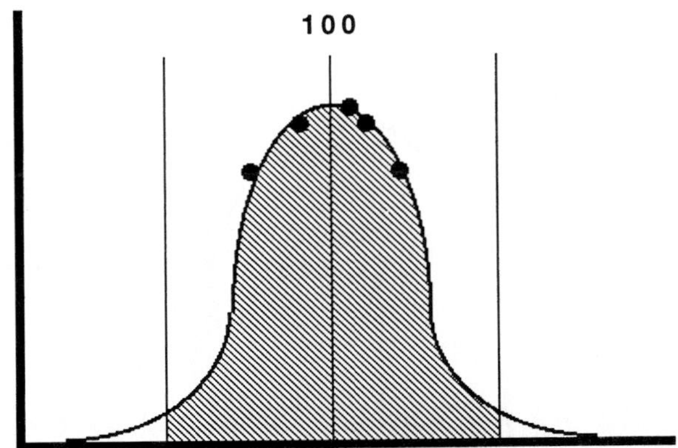

FIGURE 9–5. A normal curve of sample means derived from samples of serum factor K in the American population. The sample means are close to, but not exactly identical to, the true mean = 100. The central limit theorem states that the distribution of these sample means will fall in a normal distribution about the true mean.

antibiotic, genticillin, to treat urinary tract infections, and wished to compare it to a second antibiotic, ampicillin. If genticillin cured eight out of ten patients and ampicillin cured one out of ten, we would strongly suspect genticillin to be the superior drug. However, if genticillin cured six out of ten and ampicillin cured five out of ten, we would be less convinced of that superiority. Our question is, can we use statistical methods to determine whether there is a statistically significant superiority of genticillin as compared to ampicillin, or whether the difference is simply sampling variation (as discussed above).

One way of doing this is to construct a *null hypothesis* (abbreviated H_0) that there is *no* difference between our two treatments. If through statistical methods we can show there is an extremely low probability that the null hypothesis is correct (i.e., that there is no difference between genticillin and ampicillin), it would follow there is an extremely high probability that the converse is true (i.e., that there is a significant treatment difference between genticillin and ampicillin). This concept of *rejecting the null hypothesis* is the statistical hallmark of determining differences between various types of treatment.

Comparing Percentages

A *chi-squared test* is one such tool for determining statistical differences between two percentages (as compared to actual *measurement* data, see below). Suppose we were to compare our two antibiotics (Table 9–7). Let us set the following values for the variables in the table: $a = 8$, $b = 2$, $c = 1$, $d = 9$ and $n = a + b + c + d = 20$. The question is whether the success rate for genticillin (8/10) is superior to that of ampicillin (1/10). For any two-by-two table (two treatments—genticillin, ampicillin; two potential outcomes—success, failure), the chi-squared value (χ^2) may be computed by the formula

$$\chi^2 = \frac{(|ad - bc| - n/2)^2\, n}{(a + c)(b + d)(a + b)(c + d)}$$

(The chi-squared formula presented here uses the Yates correction. Readers are referred to statistical texts for details concerning use of the Yates correction.) The larger the treatment difference between the two drugs, the larger the χ^2 value will be. It can be determined from statistical tables of χ^2 values that only 5% of χ^2 values will exceed 3.84. Thus, if we compute from our example that $\chi^2 = 7.27$, there is a less than 5% chance that there is no treatment difference between genticillin and ampicillin. (In our example there is a less than 1% chance that there is no treatment difference between genticillin and ampicillin.) It is more reasonable, then, to *reject* our null hypothesis (no treatment difference) and accept the converse—that there *is* a treatment difference between genticillin and ampicillin. To put it another way, there is a less than 1 in 100 chance that the treatment difference between genticillin and ampicillin is due to sampling variation, and a greater than 99 out of 100 chance that it is due to a difference in drug efficacy. Using χ^2 values of 5% (or 0.05) or 1% (or 0.01) as the criterion for accepting or rejecting the null hypothesis is the basis of determining statistically significant differences between groups. This is commonly expressed as being statistically significant at the 0.05 ($P < 0.05$) or 0.01 ($P < 0.01$) level.

TABLE 9–7 Example of 2 × 2 Table to Compare the Results of Two Alternative Treatments

Antibiotic	Successes	Failures	Total
Genticillen	a	b	$a + b$
Ampicillen	c	d	$c + d$
Total	$a + c$	$b + d$	n

TABLE 9–8 Example of a Data Table for a Paired Measurement Study

Patient No.	Calcitonin (A)	Placebo (B)	Difference (A − B)
1	1.5	2.0	−0.5
2	3.0	2.0	1.0
3	1.0	4.0	0.6
4	2.5	2.0	0.5
5	1.2	1.0	0.2
	$\Sigma A/n = 1.84$	$\Sigma B/n = 2.2$	$\Sigma[A - B]/n = 0.36$

Comparing Measurements

There are many statistical significance tests for testing a null hypothesis when measurements are involved. The most commonly used method is the *Student's t-test.* There is a different *t*-test for *paired measurements* and for *unpaired measurements.*

Paired measurements involve an experimental design in which each subject in Group A has a correlate in Group B. This was discussed earlier in the section on study design, but examples of paired measurements are twin studies (one of each pair of identical twins in each treatment groups) and crossover design (where a patient may take either the active drug or placebo during phase one, and then the opposite during phase two). Suppose we examined the effect of calcitonin in treating immobilization hypercalcemia after SCI in five patients. Calcitonin and placebo treatment were each administered for 1 week to each patient; the order of treatment was randomized, and both patient and investigator were blinded to the identity of the drug. The reduction in serum calcium during calcitonin administration is shown in Table 9–8. If the null hypothesis states there is no difference between the active drug (calcitonin) and placebo in lowering serum calcium, we would expect the *mean difference* in calcium reduction to be zero. That is, if there are five paired comparisons, perhaps calcitonin would be better in two, placebo in two, and the same result in one. However, the arithmetic *mean* of those five ($\Sigma(A - B)/n$) would be zero. In our example the mean difference is 1.8/5 = 0.36.

The *paired t-test* helps us evaluate the question, "Is our mean difference in calcium reduction readily explainable by random chance, or is it due to a statistically significant treatment effect?" The derivation of the *t*-test is beyond the scope of this discussion (see references for further information), but suffice it to say that the *t*-test is a distribution curve that is shaped much like a Gaussian distribution and whose mean value is zero. Note that we can denote critical values that mark off the extreme 5% (2.5% in each tail) in the distribution with a sample size of *n*. The *t*-test will then tell us whether our calculated mean difference (0.36) is different enough from the mean difference of the perfect null hypothesis (zero) to justify rejecting the null hypothesis. If the disparity between our calculated mean difference and the "ideal" mean difference of the null hypothesis is significant at the 5% or 0.05 level, there is a less than 1 out of 20 chance that this difference can be explained on the basis of random chance alone. Thus we would usually reject the null hypothesis. (In our case the difference is not statistically significant.) Unlike χ^2 values, *t* values can be (+) or (−).

The *unpaired Student t-test* allows us to compare two groups or treatment effects when the individual members are not paired. Suppose we compare five patients taking calcitonin with five taking placebo (using the same data as in the previous example). The null hypothesis—that there is no difference between calcitonin and placebo—would argue that the average reduction in calcium in the treatment group would be equal to the reduction in the placebo group. Once again, the *t*-test could examine whether there is a statistically significant difference between the calcitonin group (mean reduction 1.84) and the placebo group (mean reduction 2.2). The *t*-test values are calculated using tables or a statistical computer program, and are dependent on the number of subjects in the group (referred to as *degrees of freedom*).

To be used appropriately, the *t*-test requires that the observations in treatment and control groups be normally distributed and that the variances be approximately the same. If these are not believed to be the case, other statistical tests are available.

Another feature to examine is the one-tailed versus the two-tailed *t*-test. For our example, we assume that calcitonin will lower the hypercalcemia more than placebo, and we are trying to prove that to be the case. We can use a *one-tailed t-test* to prove that the decline in calcium with calcitonin is greater. However, we may be making a critical error! Perhaps calcitonin were to have some sort of paradoxical effect and raise the calcium level. A *two-tailed t-test* would let us test the hypothesis that calcitonin is significantly more *or* less effective than placebo. The one-tailed test would only examine the statistical significance of calcitonin being *more* effective. The two-tailed *t*-test is the more conservative approach, and if there is any doubt about which *t*-test to use it should be the two-tailed.

Tests of comparison such as a *t*-test must be used judiciously. Suppose as investigators we were to collect a huge data set and then arbitrarily perform multiple *t*-tests looking for significant differences between measurements. As the number of *t*-tests increases, so does the likelihood that a "significant" difference may be found purely by random chance (when in actuality no significant difference really exists). When performing multiple simultaneous comparisons within a data set, it is more appropriate to use an analysis of variance.

Analysis of Variance

Yet another way of comparing differences is *analysis of variance,* abbreviated as ANOVA. ANOVA allows us to compare more than two groups at once, and it has become the most frequently encountered statistical test in the rehabilitation literature.[28] For example, suppose we were to measure the effect of four diets on post-SCI immobilization hypercalcemia. The four diets might be high calcium, low calcium, high sodium, and low sodium. Our null hypothesis would be that there would be *no difference in calcium levels in patients randomized to each of the four treatment groups.* A simple *one-way ANOVA* would be the statistical tool to compare each of the groups to each other and determine whether there is a significant likelihood that a *single* intervention (in this example, a type of diet) is effective an altering immobilization hypercalcemia.

In a simple one-way ANOVA, we compute a mean and variance for each dietary treatment group (high calcium, low calcium, high sodium, and low sodium). We then compare the means and the variance between the dietary treatment groups using the *F-statistic.* The F-statistic is a ratio of the variance *between the means* of each of the treatment groups, and the variance within each of the treatment groups. The F-statistic lets us answer the question, "Is the difference between the means among the four treatment groups due to chance, or is it most likely due to a treatment effect?" Similarly, we could investigate the role of two different treatments (e.g., diet and diuretics) simultaneously using a *two-way ANOVA.* More than two dependent variables can be assessed using a *multivariate ANOVA* (MANOVA).

Nonparametric Statistics

There are occasions when a body of data does not conform with the assumptions underlying traditional parametric statistical methods. Such a body of data does not fit in a normal distribution because it may be greatly skewed in one direction or it may have a large number of outliers. Such a body of data can be statistically analyzed using *nonparametric tests.* The *Wilcoxon signed rank test* is an example such a nonparametric method. It essentially compares the ranking in one group with the ranking in another. For example, assume 20 physicians are sitting for a board examination, 10 from Program A and 10 from Program B. Our question might be, "Do physicians in Group A perform in a superior manner?" In the signed rank test we would rank the scores from first place to 20th place and attempt to prove that Group A has significantly higher *rankings* than do the physicians from Group B. An alternative version of the Wilcoxon rank sum test is the *Mann-Whitney test.* The Wilcoxon signed rank test is the nonparametric equivalent of the paired *t*-test. Yet another nonparametric technique is *Spearman's rank correlation.*

Nonparametric statistics offer certain advantages and disadvantages. They are simpler to calculate for small groups, they make fewer assumptions of the data (remember, *t*-tests are used when one assumes there is approximately a normal distribution in the data), and they can be used when only rankings are available. For example if you knew from the test data that Program A had taken places 1, 3, 4, 5, 6, 7, 11, 12, 13, and 14, you could demonstrate this is significantly superior to Program B's placements of 2, 8, 9, 10, 15, 16, 17, 18, 19, and 20. When faced with large numbers of observations, nonparametric statistics are less practical, and the concept of confidence intervals is difficult to apply. In summary, nonparametric statistics may be viewed as valuable alternatives to *t*-tests.

Type I and Type II Error

In this entire section we have postulated a null hypothesis (e.g., calcitonin and placebo have no difference in therapeutic efficacy) that we have attempted to show with a statistical tool (e.g., *t*-test) to be an extremely unlikely possibility. As previously mentioned, we often choose that value of probability to be less than 1 out of 20 (abbreviated $P < 0.05$) or less than 1 out of 100 ($P < 0.01$). If we find our null hypothesis to be suitably unlikely, we feel comfortable rejecting our null hypothesis, and accepting the converse is most likely true (e.g., calcitonin is effective in lowering post-SCI hypercalcemia). Nonetheless, it is obvious that occasionally we may reject a null hypothesis that is actually true! At the 0.05 level of significance we have a 5% probability of rejecting a null hypothesis that is correct (e.g., accepting the therapeutic difference between calcitonin and placebo when in reality there is none). This first error of erroneously rejecting a true null hypothesis is called a *Type I error* or *α error*. Conversely, we can make a *Type II error* or *β error* by erroneously failing to reject a null hypothesis that is, in fact false (e.g., concluding there is no difference between calcitonin and placebo when indeed there is).

Type I and Type II errors are inherent in every study, and we attempt to minimize them by increasing the number of observations or subjects (N) in the experimental design. Also, the more powerful the treatment effect (e.g., the more dramatic the difference in efficacy between calcitonin and placebo), the less important Type I and Type II errors turn out to be. Beginning researchers often wonder how large an N must be used in any particular study. One can design a study with an appropriate N by determining the level of Type II error that is acceptable and estimating the difference in efficacy one can expect from the two treatment choices. This is called the *power* of a study, and it can be easily calculated for a variety of statistics. Lack of statistical power has been shown to be an important pitfall in the analysis of stroke rehabilitation clinical trials, in which the frequently small number of subjects limits the researcher's ability to detect small or medium treatment effects.[21, 25]

Clinical (Practical) versus Statistical Significance

Statistics can offer us a way of assessing the probable "truth" of a null hypothesis, but it cannot substitute for clinical judgment in assessing the practical value of that observation. Suppose we were to study the effect of a new drug, cognexin, in improving cognition after traumatic brain injury. We studied a huge number of patients (perhaps 100,000) and found those given cognexin had a 2-point greater score on the Wechsler Memory Scale at 1 year, and this was statistically significant at the 0.05 level. Nonetheless, as clinicians, we could state we are unsure what if any practical significance is found in this study unless other benefits are found from taking the drug. In this case we have discovered a statistically significant difference between the groups, which our common sense correctly identifies as having no clinical significance.

Linear Regression and Correlation

Sometimes while surveying certain groups, we may note certain factors or characteristics that seem to be "related." For example, if we study the incidence of diabetes mellitus and obesity, there appears to be a positive relationship between these two conditions. If we were to plot 8 a.m. blood glucose on the y-axis as a function of pounds in excess of ideal body weight for ten subjects, we might find a relationship such as that shown in Figure 9–6A. Eyeballing the *scattergram* would confirm our suspicion that the incidence of hyperglycemia increases with the degree of obesity. We can estimate a line that most closely fits the data according to the formula $y = ax + b$, the simple algebraic formula for a line where a = slope and b = y intercept. The formula for this line that most closely fits our data is called a *simple linear regression* and can be estimated statistically in several ways, one of which is called the *method of least squares.* The straight line that is selected is that which minimizes the sums of the squares of the vertical deviations between the points and the line (Fig. 9–6B).

Depending on the scattergram, certain linear regressions will fit the data very neatly, while others will fit it very poorly. The strength of a linear relation between y as a function of x is expressed as the *r value,* also called the *Pearson correlation coefficient.* Formulas for the calculation of r may be found in a statistics book, but the important thing to remember is that $-1 \leq r \leq 1$. An $r = 1$ implies a perfect correlation between two variables (e.g., the number of birthday parties one might have and one's age). An $r = -1$ implies a perfect inverse correlation. For example, if one has ten pieces of candy, how many pieces of candy are left after each piece is eaten? After eating one there would be nine left, after eating two there would be eight left, etc. An $r = 0$ implies absolutely no correlation between the x and y variables.

Another statistic useful in the study of linear relationships is the *coefficient of determination,* or r^2. The r^2 value provides a more useful measure of the predictability of y as a function of x than does the correlation coefficient alone. It follows that if $-1 \leq r \leq 1$, then $0 \leq r^2 \leq 1$.

We can use computer programs to calculate 95% confidence limits for a linear regression (95% confidence limits are commonly used), just as we can develop 95% confidence limits for our sample mean as discussed above. The 95% confidence interval for a linear regres-

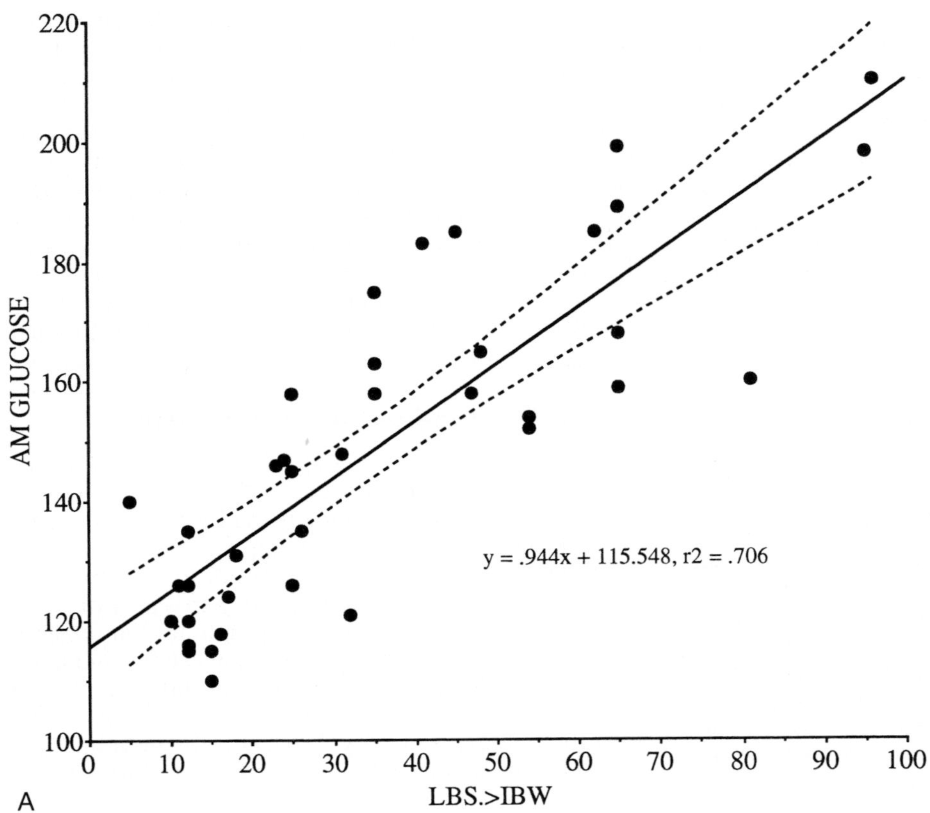

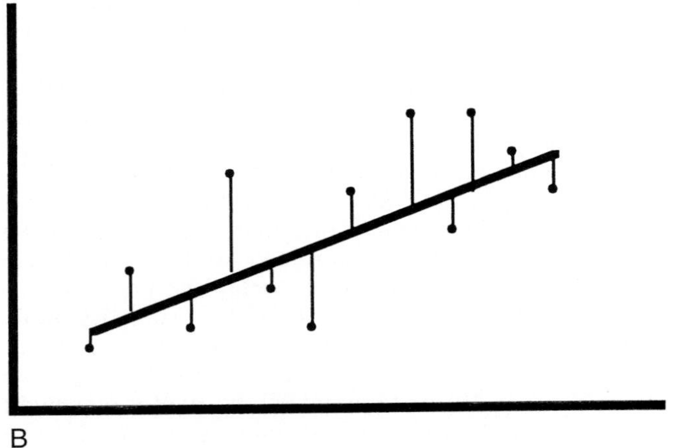

FIGURE 9–6. *A.* A scattergram plotting morning (AM) glucose values as a function of pounds above ideal body weight (IBW). The *solid line* is the regression line and is represented by the linear formula displayed on the figure. The *dotted curvilinear boundaries* represent the 95% confidence intervals for the regression line. *B.* A depiction of the method of least squares. The straight line used for the regression line is that which minimizes the sums of the squares of the vertical deviations between the points and the line.

sion implies that there is a less than 1 chance in 20 ($P < 0.05$) that the true algebraic formula for the linear regression ($y = ax + b$) *does not* fit within the curved lines denoting the confidence limits. We can also build more complex linear equations or models using more than one x variable. For example, if we measure nerve conduction velocity and collect a set of data about our subjects (e.g., age, sex, height, shoe size, arm span), we could perform a series of linear regressions to show how y (nerve conduction velocity) correlates to a series of x variables (age, sex, height, shoe size). We can perform such analysis one x at a time—*stepwise linear regression*—or for all of the x variables at once—*multiple linear regression.*

Linear regression models assume that a linear fit is the best fit for the data, but this may not be the case. For example, relationships between x and y may be better fit using quadratic or logarithmic instead of linear solutions. Second, as a general rule, *causal inferences* cannot be drawn without *experimentation.* That is, just because a strong correlation is found between x and y does not imply the x is the cause of y, or vice versa. To test causal relationships generally requires an experimental paradigm.

Vital Statistics

Vital statistics comprise another important area of descriptive statistics. *Mortality rates* can be estimated by the *crude annual death rate,* the ratio of total deaths for a given year divided by the population at risk in that year (usually measured at the midyear point). It is often helpful to stratify death rates by age group—*age-specific death rate*—because of the varying constitution of certain populations. Another special example of death rates is *cause-specific death rate;* for example, the number of deaths from motor vehicle accidents each year for the total population.

Morbidity rates are a ratio of the number of cases of a certain disease divided by the number of persons at risk for the disease. Morbidity rates can be reported as incidence and prevalence. The *incidence* is the number of new cases occurring during a given time period divided by the number at risk for the disease at that time. The *prevalence* of a disease represents the number of cases that exist at a specific instant divided by the number at risk for the disease. For example, in Table 9–9 two new patients suffered from the disease during the month of March, an incidence of 20%, with a prevalence of 50%.

READING THE MEDICAL LITERATURE

When reading the medical literature, the physiatrist must examine each research paper critically with the following principles in mind. These principles are similarly applicable for investigators preparing their own research paper.[3] (See also Additional References.)

- *There should be a clear statement of the objectives* (e.g., it is the hypothesis of this study to determine whether calcitonin is superior to placebo in the control of post-SCI immobilization hypercalcemia). The statement of objectives should include a brief review of the current medical literature demonstrating a synthesis of present medical knowledge.
- *The treatment and control groups should be clearly stated* (e.g., 100 male and 100 female persons with SCI between 10 and 50 years of age with no history of previous metabolic disorders). The demographic and socioeconomic features of the experimental subjects, as well as *inclusion* and *exclusion criteria,* should be clearly identified.
- *There should be random allocation of subjects to treatment and control groups* (e.g., the 200 subjects were randomized using a random number generator into treatment and control groups). The authors should demonstrate that there were no inherent differences between the treatment and control groups, and that the groups were similarly handled throughout the investigation. In criticizing a paper in a medical journal, it is not necessary to prove that there was bias in randomization of the treatment and control groups. It is enough to provide a cohesive argument that there *may* have been substantial bias in the way the treatment and control groups were compared.
- *There should be a rationale for choice of the particular experimental design* (e.g., a double-blind crossover study in which each patient serves as his/her own control). The methodology, including the variables studied and the method of quantitating these variables, should be sufficiently explained so that the work can be replicated by others. The type and range of values that can be obtained from each measurement instrument should be explained. This is especially important in rehabilitation research, where outcomes may be measured in quality of life or other idiosyncratic ways.[15, 16, 18]
- *The resulting data should be clearly and objectively presented and the methods of statistical analysis explained.* The methods of data collection and the strength and weakness of the data, figures, tables, and photographs should all be presented in a manner that facilitate understanding by the reader.
- *The conclusion should explain why the null hypothesis was accepted or rejected* (e.g., the data clearly demonstrated that daily subcutaneous calcitonin was effective in the control of immobilization hypercalcemia in persons suffering from acute SCI). There should be a justification of worthiness of the analysis, and a statement of conclusions that are justified by the data. The results should be discussed in light of previous research, and the implications of the work should be explained.

GRANT APPLICATION AND FUNDING ISSUES

The grant writer must approach grantsmanship as a business. Granting agencies are in the business of pro-

TABLE 9–9 Occurrence of a Disease by Month in Ten Patients

	Month											
Person	*Jan*	*Feb*	*Mar*	*Apr*	*May*	*Jun*	*Jul*	*Aug*	*Sep*	*Oct*	*Nov*	*Dec*
1	—	—	—									
2									—	—	—	
3												
4		—	—	—	—	—						
5												
6			—	—								
7	—	—	—	—	—							
8												
9			—									
10												

viding funding and support for projects that meet their needs and fulfill their mission. The grant applicant is in the business of pursuing his or her goals, and at the same time fulfilling the needs of the granting agency. Successful grant applicants not only must possess the research skills needed to complete the task, they must also convince the granting agency that the research idea is worth funding.

There are several key components to good grantsmanship: (1) understanding the mission of the potential funding agency, (2) understanding the grant review process, and (3) being able to write for the grant reviewer. Each of these factors is examined more closely with the goal of identifying the common deficiencies in grant writing.

Understanding the Mission

The potential researcher should stay informed and up to date as to the needs of the funding agencies from which he or she intends to seek support. For example, the mission of the National Institutes of Health (NIH) is to improve the health of the people of the United States; funding good science is simply a means to this end. Grant submissions should address the mission of the funding agency. This is especially important when applying for funds from a private foundation, whose mission might be very specific. Get as much information about the agency or foundation as possible. Most funding sources welcome questions from prospective applicants about their mission and focus or their funding. One excellent source of this type of information is the university or institutional office for grants and contracts (sponsored programs). The people and resources in this office can make the grant writing process smoother, and often have substantial experience to share.

The grant writer should be aware of the political overtones of grantsmanship. The major funding agencies are composed of federal employees within the executive branch of the federal government and are supported by federal monies. There are times when political priorities and pressures may have bearing on what types of research are funded. For example, women's health issues (e.g., cardiovascular disease in women, breast cancer) and AIDS are two areas in which national funding agencies have responded to strong political movements with increased funding support. This is most important when considering where to submit a proposal and how to tie research ideas to timely funding opportunities.

It is helpful to understand the structural hierarchy of the federal government agencies that fund rehabilitation research (Fig. 9–7). The NIH is an agency of the Public Health Service (PHS), which is within the U.S. Department of Health and Human Services. In 1990, legislation was signed that amended the NIH and created the National Center for Medical Rehabilitation Research (NCMRR) within the National Institute of Child Health and Human Development (NICHHD) at the NIH.[12] Also of interest to the researcher in rehabilitation interested in funding through the PHS is the Centers for Disease Control and Prevention (CDC), which fund research on injury prevention and rehabilitation through the National Center for Injury Prevention and Control.

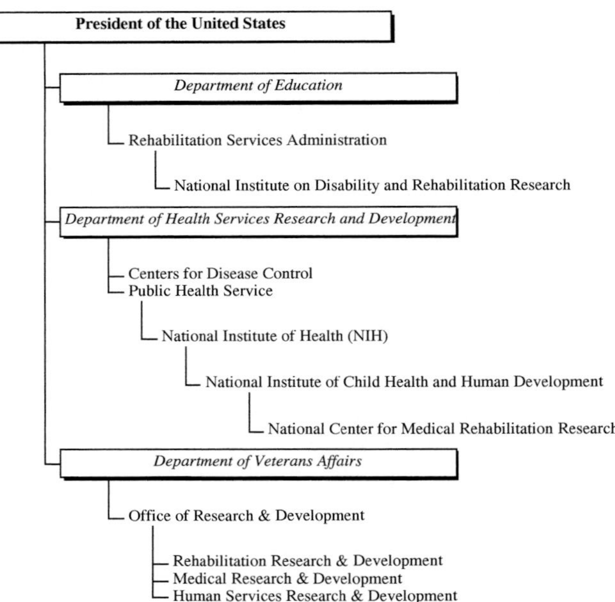

FIGURE 9–7. Federal agencies that primarily fund rehabilitation research.

The National Institute on Disability and Rehabilitation Research (NIDRR), an agency of the U.S. Department of Education, is currently the largest funding source for rehabilitation research. NIDRR was founded in 1978 as an outgrowth of the Rehabilitation Research and Demonstration Program administrated by the Rehabilitation Services Administration.[30] The mission of NIDRR is to generate, disseminate, and promote new knowledge that will substantially improve the capacities of people with disabilities to perform work and other activities in the community.[12] The annual priorities are published in the *Federal Register.* The Rehabilitation Services Administration (RSA) within the Department of Education funds training programs for rehabilitation professionals as well as persons with disabilities. The Department of Education also provides Vocational Rehabilitation state grants and Rehabilitation Engineering training grants.

The Department of Veterans Affairs (VA) funds research through its intramural programs, which are open to VA physicians and researchers and those who collaborate with them. Most of the rehabilitation research in the VA is funded through the Rehabilitation Research and Development Program, which funds numerous projects in the broad categories of spinal cord injury and neurological disorders, prosthetics, amputation and orthotics, and communications, cognition, and sensory aids.

Understanding the Grant Review Process

The NIH grant review process is typical of the steps used in a variety of federal granting agencies. A grant proposal is written and initiated by a principal investigator, then submitted to the NIH Division of Research Grants (DRG). The DRG is an advisory group responsible for setting up study sections to review grant proposals. The NIH has a two-tiered review process. The first part is the scientific merit review by the study section, also called the Initial Review Group. The second part is the priority and relevance review by the Advisory Council. When a grant proposal is received by the DRG, it is assigned a number that includes an abbreviation for the particular institute from which funding is sought (Table 9–10).

The DRG has approximately 12 referral officers who assign applications to the appropriate study section. Each study section has a scientific review administrator and approximately 14 to 20 basic and clinical scientist members, one of whom serves as a chairperson. The administrator of the study section, usually a scientist, is responsible for the administrative and technical review of the applications and for preparation of a summary statement with final recommendations.

Each grant application is assigned three primary reviewers. These individuals present a written report to the study section that encapsulates the scientific and technical merits of the proposal. Members serve as primary reviewers on several proposals, but additionally they may serve as secondary reviewers on scores of applications. Therefore it is extremely important to write a grant in a "reader-friendly" fashion. After the reports are read by the reviewers and their merit is evaluated, a vote is taken. Possible outcomes include (1) "not recommended for further consideration"; (2) deferred for additional information; and (3) assignment of a "priority score."

Occasionally, if the application involves a complex coordination of individuals or if inspection of the proposed site of research is needed to make a recommendation for funding, a site visit is arranged. Approximately 2 weeks after the study section meets, the priority scores are tabulated, percentile ranks are calculated, and results are forwarded to the applicant. Summary statements generally require 6 to 8 weeks to reach the principal investigator. Only the top 70% of grant applications assigned a priority score go on to the next stage of the review process. These are sent on to the Advisory Council meeting of the assigned institute/center/division to be considered for funding by a panel that includes both scientists and nonscientists.

The grant review process at NIDRR is somewhat different.[30] The NIDRR peer review process is based on policies contained in the Education Department Grant Administration Regulations (EDGAR), and detailed in the *Federal Register.* A short-term ad hoc review panel is established for each announced competition. Once applications are received in the application control center, they are inspected for completion and appropriateness by designated program staff. Selected reviewers read and score all assigned applications before the scheduled panel meeting in Washington, D.C. During this formal panel meeting discussion takes place and the applications are ranked for approval or disapproval. The panel manager checks all scores and evaluation materials. The panel's recommendations, as well as those of the program staff, are reviewed by the NIDRR director and other departmental officials in a prefunding conference. The final selections are then forwarded to the Department of Education's Grants and Contracts Services for negotiation and award.

TABLE 9–10 Abbreviations and Two-Letter Designations of the NIH Institutes/Funding Components

NEI (EY)	National Eye Institute
NIA (AG)	National Institute on Aging
NIDR (DE)	National Institute of Dental Research
NHLBI (HL)	National Heart, Lung and Blood Institute
NCI (CA)	National Cancer Institute
NIGMS (GM)	National Institute of General Medical Sciences
NIEHS (ES)	National Institute of Environmental Health Sciences
NIAID (AI)	National Institute of Allergy and Infectious Diseases
NINCDS (NS)	National Institute of Neurological and Communicative Disorders and Stroke
NIDDK (DK)	National Institute of Diabetes, Digestive and Kidney Diseases
NICHD (HD)	National Institute of Child Health and Human Development
NIAMS (AR)	National Institute of Arthritis, Musculoskeletal and Skin Diseases
NIDCD (DC)	National Institute of Deafness and Other Communication Disorders

Writing for the Grant Reviewer

Writing with the grant reviewer in mind is a necessary part of successful grantsmanship. Preparing a grant application is a scholarly endeavor that combines scientific skills with a clear, disciplined writing style.[8] Grant reviewers have a difficult, time-consuming job; it is essential to make the reviewer's job as easy as possible. The following suggestions seem timely for the potential grantee:

- Follow the instructions precisely on the grant application. Inability to follow directions will make a negative first impression.
- Keep to the page limits, and use the specific font and line spacing called for to make a neat and pleasing document. Carelessness in writing or presentation may suggest to the reviewer a potential carelessness in research.
- Begin to write the grant proposal early. Use an outline for each section of the proposal so that the logic of the discussion flows from section to section. It is much easier to detect logical errors when the manuscript is in skeletal form than when it is in full prose. It may help to prepare figures, tables, and photographs before writing the actual text of the proposal.
- Writing should be clear and concise, providing the reviewer with the maximum amount of information in the least number of words. Avoid redundancy and ambiguity while being consistent with terminology and abbreviations. Many individuals reading the grant application will not be physicians, so it is wise to avoid medical jargon. Ask more senior colleagues from the

basic and clinical science communities to read and critique your proposal—a "mock review" by a knowledgeable scientist in the field can be especially useful.

- It has been estimated that approximately 90% of applications submitted to the NIDRR are rejected for technical deficiencies each year.[30] Five types of errors account for 76.8% of all the deficiencies noted in these applications: (1) poor conceptualization of the problem or approach, (2) inadequate control of variables, (3) research design errors, (4) methodological errors, and (5) inappropriate statistical analysis.

Funding Sources

It is always difficult to decide where to apply for funding support. The university office of grants and contracts and the dean's office are good starting points to find what intramural funding is available. Small seed grants may be available to younger faculty and fellows to serve as startup funds for new research initiatives. Private foundations can serve as the source for startup funds when a new investigator works in a facility that is not part of a larger academic arena. Funding priorities in such organizations are often made by executive process rather than by peer review; final decisions are ratified by a board of directors. The *Foundation Directory,*[23] the standard reference work for information about private and community grant-making foundations in the United States, is available at most libraries.

Extramural funding is commonly solicited from the federal government through health research agencies such as NIH and NIDRR. There are two general methods of obtaining funding from these federal agencies. One can apply for *center-directed research,* in which the agency issues a request for grant applications or contract proposals (RFA or RFP respectively) and the investigator submits an application fitting the needs of this request. The other main type of application is for an *investigator-initiated research award* (R-01). This is the most common mechanism for funding research at the NIH. In addition to R-01 grants, the NCMRR offers a number of other funding avenues, which may be more appropriate for clinician-scientists and early career researchers. These include the small Business Innovation Research (SBIR), Mentored Clinical Scientist Development Award (K-08), and the Mentored Patient-Oriented Research Career Development Award (K-23). In addition, the National Center for Research Resources funds 74 General Clinical Research Centers (GCRC); the Clinical Associate Physician Award, which is similar to the K-08; and the Small Grants Award (R-03), which provides up to $50,000 per year for 2 years for preliminary and pilot studies. The Department of Health and Human Services publishes a web page called "GrantsNet." This web page provides links to all the major federal funding agencies (Table 9–11).

The private sector is also very interested in promoting research when it is related to the development of potential new drugs, products, services, or specific interests. Unfortunately, there is no central source of information for such funding sources and the potential grantee needs to seek these out on an individual basis. The National Science Foundation has partial listings of small businesses with research interests. An extensive list of resources is available in texts[19] as well as on the Internet (Table 9–11).

TABLE 9–11 URL Internet Addresses for Literature Searching and Grants Information

Internet Literature Search Sites

PubMed: http://www.ncbi.nlm.nih.gov/PubMed
Internet Grateful Med: http://igm.nlm.nih.gov/

Federal Agencies

Department of Education: http://ed.gov/
Federal Register: http://ocfo.ed.gov/fedreg.htm
NIDRR: http://ed.gov/offices/OSERS/NIDRR/
RSA: http://ed.gov/offices/OSERS/RSA/
Department of Health and Human Services: http://www.os.dhhs.gov/
CDC: http://www.cdc.gov/
NIH: http://www.nih.gov/
Department of Veterans Affairs
Office of Research and Development: http://www.va.gov/resdev/

Private and Federal Funding Agency Directories

National Center for Dissemination of Disability Research: http://ncddr.org/funding.html
Foundation Directory: http://fdncenter.org/
Government Grants: http://www.grantsnet.org

ETHICAL ISSUES

Ethics is perhaps the most important aspect of clinical research. Three general ethical principles serve as guidelines for clinical research: *respect for persons* (subjects), *beneficence,* and *justice.*

Respect for Persons

Patients who are enrolled in a clinical trial must be *volunteers* and are free to withdraw from the study at any time. *Informed consent* must be obtained before a human being may become part of a clinical experiment. In the case of persons who lack full autonomy because of brain injury, dehabilitated state, or immaturity, consent *by proxy* must be given by the legal guardian or his or her appointee. All information collected must be strictly confidential.

Beneficence

Investigators are obligated to design protocols that will produce valid and generalizable knowledge. Because *inherent risk* cannot be eliminated for volunteers in a clinical trial, the standard should be that the researcher has taken steps to preclude all *unnecessary* risks to the participants. For example, before a surgical technique or drug is tried in a clinical trial, it is usually assessed first in animal studies in mammals or other primates. Also, the benefits of the study to the patient, mankind, or science should clearly *outweigh* the risks to the subjects participating in the trial.

Federal law requires approval of any research project involving human subjects by an *institutional review board* (IRB). It is that board's responsibility to review the entire research proposal with consent form and to weigh the potential benefits and risks to patients who are participating in the study. Experimental devices or drugs additionally may require approval from the Food and Drug Administration.

Justice

The benefits and burdens of research should be distributed fairly among all members of society. Disadvantaged, disabled, or minority persons should not be asked to bear a disproportionate share. Scientific discoveries often have great societal impact; nowhere is this more visible than in the work done with AIDS patients. Science and technology are integral parts of society, and so investigators are often thrust into the public arena. They need to provide a successful interface so that the scientific value and merit of their work are not distorted in the public eye.

The question sometimes arises whether it is ethical to have a control group, or what type of control to use. This question is appropos in a rehabilitation research setting. Some examples are illustrative:

While it is easy to argue that the effect of a new antidepressant should be compared with an older antidepressant and/or a placebo, should speech therapy be compared to placebo speech therapy or to the absence of speech therapy?

Studies are presently under way investigating the use of a ganglioside, GM-1, as a method of minimizing SCI. As there is no present evidence that GM-1 is effective, a clinical trial is necessary to accept or reject the null hypothesis that GM-1 is *not* effective. Yet a prominent football player was able to obtain the drug outside of the experimental protocol.

How far can one go with placebos and dummy treatments? Should we perform sham back surgery as a control in comparison to a new surgical technique?

Conflicting and Proprietary Interests

Most journals and symposia require that the author or lecturer disclose whether he or she might have any financial or other type of interest that might bias results.[23] For example, a researcher who receives substantial research funding from a drug company might have difficulty reporting the uselessness of that company's product. Sometimes drug companies reserve the right to prohibit a clinical trial from being published if the results are adverse to their financial interest.

In other scenarios, investigators may be constrained to share data or other research tools because of proprietary interests. A new drug, reagent, or procedure might have significant financial potential, and a scientist or institution may reserve certain legal rights as to its future use. For example, a Wisconsin ophthalmologist was the innovator of botulinum toxin for the treatment of strabismus. The rights have since been acquired by a drug company because of its marketability not only to ophthalmologists, but for disorders such as torticollis, spasticity, and other movement disorders.

Communal Review of Scientific Results

The hallmark of scientific progress is the ability to communicate. Researchers communicate with others in their fields through informal dialogue and presentations at conferences, but most importantly through the submission of their work to peer-reviewed journals. This critical examination provides the only reliable method of self-correcting the progress of scientific progress. Information transmitted first through the mass media (e.g., trials of high-dose steroids in the treatment of acute SCI) may grossly prejudice the evaluation of these results and how the public perceives them. Many journals will not accept scientific papers without an agreement that they must be published before being presented to the lay press.

Error and Fraud

Error caused by the inherent limits on scientific theory can only be ascertained by the advancement of science. Despite the utilization of a scientific method, mistakes will inevitably occur. These errors should not be tolerated when they are the result of negligent work. There is a clear distinction between preventable error and outright fraud. *Fraud* can be defined as a conscious effort to publish inaccurate or misleading results. It is the gravest violation of the ethos of science.

Allocation of Credit in Collaborative Research

When scientific papers are published, credit is given in the list of authors, in the acknowledgments at the end of the text, and in the reference citations. As the number of authors in multidisciplinary or multicenter studies continues to increase, the issue of authorship ranking arises. In some fields the senior author is listed first, while in other fields the leader's name is last. Generally, these issues are handled most productively by discussing them early in the development of a research project and by ranking authors based on their contributions to the generation of the study idea, solicitation of funding, data collection and analysis, and finally the synthesis of results and manuscript(s).[13, 27, 29] Unfortunately, "authors" of scientific papers may be added for political reasons, and the ranking of non-first authors often is not based on their contribution to the research effort.[27] The most blatant misappropriation of credit in research is *plagiarism,* or intentionally seeking credit for another scientist's intellectual property.

REFERENCES

1. Backman CL, Harris SR, Chisholm JA, et al: Single-subject research in rehabilitation: Review of studies using AB, withdrawal, multiple baseline, and alternating treatment designs. Arch Phys Med Rehabil 1997; 78:1145–1153.
2. Braddom CL: Framework for writing and/or evaluating research papers. Am J Phys Med Rehabil 1991; 70(1):S169–S171.
3. Braddom RL: Why is physiatric research important? Am J Phys Med Rehabil 1991; 70(1):S2–S3.
4. Bulpitt CJ: Medical statistics: Meta-analysis. Lancet 1988; 2:93–94.

5. Chang WC, Chan C: Rasch analysis for outcomes measures: Some methodological considerations. Arch Phys Med Rehabil 1995; 76:934–939.
6. Deyo RA: Practice variations, treatment fads, rising disability. Spine 1993; 18:2153–2162.
7. Dorfman LJ, Robinson LR: Normative data in electrodiagnostic medicine. Muscle Nerve 1997; 20:4–14.
8. Eaves GN: Preview of research grant applications at the National Institutes of Health. Fed Proc 1972; 31:2–9.
9. Emerson JD, Colditz GA: Use of statistical analysis in the New England Journal of Medicine. N Engl J Med 1983; 309:709–713.
10. Findley TW, DeLisa JA: Research in physical medicine and rehabilitation: XI. Research training: Setting the stage for lifelong learning. Am J Phys Med Rehabil 1991; 70(1):S107–S113.
11. Grabois M, Fuhrer MJ: Physiatrists' views on research. Am J Phys Med Rehabil 1991; 70(1):S165–S168.
12. Gray DB, Graves WH, Cole TM: Federal funding of medical rehabilitation research: NCMRR and NIDRR. Phys Med Rehabil State Art Rev 1993; 70(2):381–392.
13. Huth EJ: Guidelines on authorship of medical papers. Ann Intern Med 1986; 104:269–274.
14. Ioannidis JPA, Cappelleri JC, Lau J: Issues in comparisons between meta-analyses and large trials. JAMA 1998; 279:1089–1093.
15. Johnston MV, Findley TW, DeLuca J, et al: Research in physical medicine and rehabilitation: XII. Measurement tools with application to brain injury. Am J Phys Med Rehabil 1991; 70(1):S114–S130.
16. Johnston MV, Keith RA, Hinderer SR: Measurement standards for interdisciplinary medical rehabilitation. Arch Phys Med Rehabil 1992; 73(suppl):S1–S23.
17. Kahn CR: Picking a research problem: The critical decision. N Engl J Med 1994; 330:1530–1533.
18. Keller RB, Rudicel SA, Liang MH: Outcomes research in orthopaedics. J Bone Joint Surg Am 1993; 75:1562–1574.
19. Larson EB, Ellsworth AJ, Oas J: Randomized clinical trials in single patients during a two-year period. JAMA 1993; 270:2708–2712.
20. LeLorier J, Genevieve G, Benhaddad A, et al: Discrepancies between meta-analyses and subsequent large randomized controlled trials. N Engl J Med 1997; 337:536–542.
21. Matyas TA, Ottenbacher KJ: Confounds of insensitivity and blind luck: Statistical conclusion validity in stroke rehabilitation clinical trials. Arch Phys Med Rehabil 1993; 74:559–565.
22. Merbitz C, Morris J, Grip JC: Ordinal scales and foundations of inference. Arch Phys Med Rehabil 1989; 70:308–312.
23. Olson S, Feczko MM (eds): Foundation Directory, ed 13. New York, Foundation Center, 1991.
24. Ottenbacher KJ: Clinically relevant designs for rehabilitation research: The idiographic model. Am J Phys Med Rehabil 1991; 70(1):S144–S150.
25. Ottenbacher KJ: Why rehabilitation research does not work (as well as we think it should). Arch Phys Med Rehabil 1995; 76:123–129.
26. Reif-Lehrer L: Writing a Successful Grant Application, ed 2. Boston, Jones and Bartlett, 1989.
27. Rennie D, Yank V, Emanuel L: When authorship fails: Proposal to make contributors accountable. JAMA 1997; 278:579–585.
28. Schwartz SJ, Sturr M, Goldberg G: Statistical methods in rehabilitation literature: Survey of recent publications. Arch Phys Med Rehabil 1996; 77:497–500.
29. Shapiro DW, Wenger NS, Shapiro MF: Contributions of authors to multi-authored biomedical research papers. JAMA 1994; 271:438–442.
30. Thomas JP, Lawrence TS: Common deficiencies of NIDRR research applications. Am J Phys Med Rehabil 1991; 70(1):S161–S164.
31. Witt MD, Gostin LO: Conflict of interest dilemmas in biomedical research. JAMA 1994; 271:547–551.
32. Wright BD, Linacre JM: Observations are always ordinals; measurements must be interval. Arch Phys Med Rehabil 1989; 70:857–867.

ADDITIONAL REFERENCES

Monographs

American Medical Association: Code of Medical Ethics: Current Opinions with Annotations. Chicago, American Medical Association, 1994.

Bailar JC III, Mosteller F: Medical Uses of Statistics, ed 2. Boston, New England Journal of Medicine Books, 1992.

Colton T: Statistics in Medicine. Boston, Little, Brown, 1974.

Committee on the Conduct of Science, National Academy of Sciences: On Being a Scientist. Washington, DC, National Academy Press, 1989.

Duncan RC, Knapp RG, Miller MC: Introductory Biostatistics for the Health Sciences, ed 2. New York, John Wiley & Sons, New York, 1983.

Edwards AL: Multiple Regression and the Analysis of Variance and Covariance, ed 2. New York, WH Freeman, 1985.

Haas JF (ed): Medical Ethics Series Supplement. Am J Phys Med Rehabil 1995; 74(1).

Hulley SB, Cummings SR: Designing Clinical Research: An Epidemiologic Approach. Baltimore, Williams & Wilkins, 1988.

Krauth J: Distribution-Free Statistics. An Application-Oriented Approach. Amsterdam, Elsevier, 1988.

Leaverton PE: A Review of Biostatistics: Program for Self-Instruction, ed 2. Boston, Little, Brown, 1978.

Sokal RR, Rohlf FJ: Biometry. The Principles and Practices of Statistics in Biological Research, ed 2. New York, WH Freeman, 1981.

Journal Series on Research and Critical Reading of the Medical Literature

Evidence-Based Medicine Working Group: Users Guides to the Medical Literature. JAMA 1993; 270:2093–2095, 2598–2601; 1994; 271:59–63, 389–391, 703–707, 1615–1619; 272:234–237, 1367–1371; 1995; 273:1292–1295, 1610–1613, 274:570–574, 1630–1632, 1800–1804; 1996; 275:554–558, 1435–1439; 1997; 277:1232–1237, 1552–1557, 1802–1806; 1998; 279:545–549 (series in progress).

O'Brien PC, Shampo MA: Statistics for Clinicians. Mayo Clin Proc 1981; 56:45–49, 126–128, 196–197, 274–276, 324–326, 393–394, 452–454, 513–515, 573–575, 639–640, 709–711, 753–756.

O'Brien PC, Shampo MA: Statistics Series. Mayo Clin Proc 1988; 63:813–820, 918–920, 1043–1045, 1140–1143, 1245–1249.

Physiatric Research: Hands-on Approach. Am J Phys Med Rehabil 1991; 70(1):S1–S171.

Sackett DL, Haynes RB, Tugwell PX, et al: How to Read Clinical Journals. Can Med Assoc J 1981; 124:555–558, 703–710, 869–872, 985–990, 1156–1162.

Victoria CG, Grisso JA, Carpenter LM, et al: Facts, Figures and Fallacies. Lancet 1993; 2:97–99, 157–160, 221–223, 286–288, 345–348, 418–421, 479–481, 530–532.

10
CHAPTER

Daniel Dumitru, M.D., Ph.D.

Electrodiagnostic Medicine. I. Basic Aspects

The electrodiagnostic medicine consultation is the practice of medicine and as such is predicated on a thorough understanding of the basic science and clinical aspects of nerve and muscle physiology. In addition to the normal physiological functioning of these two primary tissues, the physician must also comprehend the manner in which nerve and muscle tissues react to various diseases. The practitioner must be aware of how the instrument detects and displays the recorded physiological potentials. Once these basic principles are mastered, the practitioner has taken the first step toward being able to perform an electrodiagnostic medicine consultation.

ACTION POTENTIAL GENERATION

The two basic excitable tissues in the human body are nerve and muscle. For our purposes, the basic principles of action potential generation in nerve and skeletal muscle are relatively similar, with the primary difference being that the intracellular action potential in muscle has a longer duration compared to nerve. Additionally, the muscle's intracellular action potential is monophasic positive, whereas that for nerve is biphasic and initially positive. The reader is strongly encouraged to read basic physiology texts[23, 26] to gain a more complete appreciation of the intricate relationship between excitable cells and their associated action potentials.

Resting Membrane Potential

All living cells have a transmembrane potential across their cell membranes, with the intracellular region negative compared to the extracellular environment.[26] When an action potential is not present, the cell is said to be in the resting state and the potential difference across the cell membrane is referred to as the resting membrane potential. The development and maintenance of the resting membrane potential can be explained by a simple model.

Suppose that a beaker is divided into left and right halves by an impermeable membrane with two different concentrations of potassium chloride (KCl) solution, 10 millimolar and 100 millimolar (Fig. 10–1).[12] In solution, the KCl exists as positive potassium (K^+) ions (cations) and negative chloride (Cl^-) ions (anions). If a voltmeter (a device that measures potential differences) is placed across the two solutions, it will not measure a potential difference because there is a lack of physical continuity between the left and right halves of the beaker. There is no pathway for current to flow, and without current flow there can be no potential difference. If we can open only potassium channels in the membrane, then K^+ cations will flow down their concentration gradient from the high (100 millimolar) to low (10 millimolar) ion concentration side of the beaker (Fig. 10–1). The potassium ions will continue to flow into the low-concentration side of the container until there is a balance between (1) the forces of the physical concentration gradient difference driving potassium to the lower concentration region and (2) the electrical gradient opposing this directional ion flow. Recall that the negative chloride ions cannot pass through the membrane and remain on the high-concentration side of the beaker. As more and more positive potassium ions leave one side of the beaker, there begins to develop an unbalanced or "excess" amount of negative charges (Cl^-) on the high-concentration side of the beaker, with an equal buildup of excess positive charges (K^+) on the other side of the beaker. The increasing net negative charge of the beaker half with the remaining chloride ions begins to make it increasingly difficult for the positive potassium charges to leave the high-concentration side

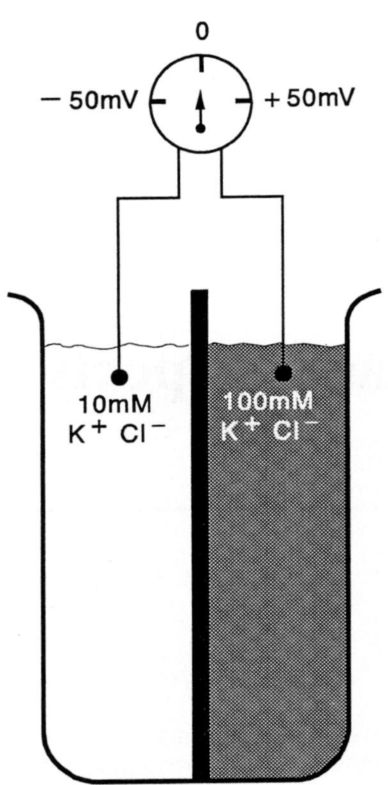

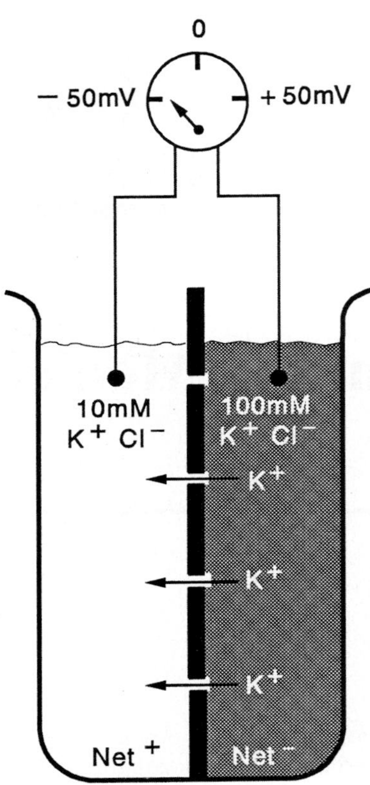

FIGURE 10–1. A beaker containing two different concentrations (10 millimolar and 100 millimolar) of a potassium chloride solution (KCl) existing as potassium (K^+) and chloride (Cl^-) ions. An impermeable partition separates the two different concentration solutions. A voltmeter placed across the partition fails to register any voltage difference. If the partition is now made selectively permeable to just the potassium ions, the concentration gradient difference will drive potassium ions into the lower-concentration side of the beaker until the electrical attraction from the accumulating negatively charged chloride ions prevents and further net K^+ ion movement, thus establishing a dynamic equilibrium. At this point, a potential difference exists across the partition and represents the equilibrium potential. (From Dumitru D: Electrodiagnostic Medicine. Philadelphia, Hanley & Belfus, 1995, p. 6.)

of the beaker, while at the same time an increasing amount of positive potassium ions on the low potassium concentration side of the beaker begins to repel additional potassium ions attempting to enter this side of the beaker.

At some point, the opposing electrical charges on the two sides of the beaker prevent any more potassium from leaving the high-concentration side of the beaker, even though there is still a higher potassium concentration on one side than on the other. A balance is now established between the concentration forces driving potassium ions from the high- to low-concentration regions and the electrical forces tending to keep potassium ions in the more concentrated portion of the beaker. Any potassium ions that randomly enter the lower-concentration side of the beaker are balanced by potassium ions similarly crossing in the opposite direction. The situation where a balance between electrical and concentration forces exists is said to be a dynamic equilibrium. Placing a voltmeter across the partition now measures a negative potential difference, as electrical continuity is now present between the two halves of the beaker through the open potassium ion channels.

This simple example can be applied to all cells in the body, and in particular to nerve and muscle cells. We will now use the nerve cell's axon as our example, although the same principles apply to muscle cells. The nerve cell is known to have a specialized cell membrane, or plasmalemma, permeable primarily to potassium and chloride ions in the resting state because of intramembranous ion channels. It is said to be selectively permeable, or semipermeable.[29] The potassium channels are passive because they are always open and permit the free flow of this ion. Contained within the axon but incapable of crossing the cell membrane are large negatively charged protein molecules. This negative charge attracts potassium ions from outside the cell to enter into the cell through the passive potassium channels, resulting in a buildup of potassium ions within the axon. This process continues until there is so much potassium within the axon that the continued entry of more potassium ions is prevented by the high intracellular potassium concentration, even though not all of the negative charges have been balanced. This is because the potassium concentration gradient force now attempting to drive potassium out of the cell is just large enough to balance the negative electrical attraction force of anions pulling potassium ions into the cell. Similar to the beaker example, a dynamic equilibrium develops between (1) the intracellular negative charges pulling potassium in and (2) the high intracellular potassium concentration attempting to push potassium out. This dynamic equilibrium occurs at a point when the large intracellular negative potential is reduced by the inflowing potassium ions to a value of a transmembrane potential difference approximating a negative 80–90 millivolts (mV) compared to the extracellular environment.

Nernst Equation

The above examples of beakers and cells can be expressed mathematically by simply saying that the net work of the electrical gradient (W_{elec}) and the concentration gradient (W_{con}) is zero in the resting state

($W_{elec} + W_{con} = 0$). This means that the work or energy of developing the concentration gradient (W_{con}) is balanced by, or equal but opposite to, that developed by the electrical gradient (W_{elec}) during the resting state: $W_{elec} = -W_{con}$. The negative sign is present to denote the "opposite" or balanced aspect of the work. The electrical work is expressed as $W_{elec} = Z_iFE_m$. The symbols designate specific aspects of defining electrical ion work: Z_i is the ion's charge; F is Faraday's constant, and E_m is the transmembrane potential. The work required to move ions across the membrane can be expressed as the natural logarithm of the ionic concentration differences between the intracellular ($[I]_i$) and extracellular ($[I]_e$) ions. Universal gas (R) and temperature (T) constants are conversion factors necessary to balance units between all of the variables. Substituting the above-noted variables into the balanced work equation results in:

$$W_{elec} = -W_{con}$$
$$Z_iFE_m = -RT\,\{\mathrm{Ln}\,[\,I\,]_i - \mathrm{Ln}\,[\,I\,]_e\}$$

This formula can be rearranged to find the potential at which the electrical work just balances the concentration work—i.e., the dynamic equilibrium or resting membrane potential—by solving the above equation for E_m.

$$E_m = \frac{-RT}{Z_iF}\,\mathrm{Ln}\,\frac{[I]_i}{[I]_e}$$

The above equation is more commonly known as the Nernst equation and is a mathematical statement of the potential at which all of the electrical and concentration forces are balanced in the resting state, which is the resting membrane potential.[26, 29] By substituting the actual values for the different variables and using the more familiar base 10 logarithm, the equation converts to the more recognizable form. Also, the approximate concentration ratio of intracellular to extracellular potassium is 20:1 (Table 10–1). The Nernst equation then becomes:

$$E_m = -(26\text{ mV})\ 2.3\ \log_{10}\,[20 \div 1]$$
$$E_m = -75\text{ mV}$$

Sodium Pump

Experimentation has shown that the Nernst equation predicts the resting membrane potential quite well with different extracellular potassium concentrations as long as the potassium concentration is relatively high. At low extracellular potassium concentrations there is a deviation of the resting membrane potential from that predicted, with a less negative potential achieved. This finding suggests that at low potassium ion concentrations another ion (sodium: Na^+) has some influence on the resting membrane potential. It turns out that sodium has a very high extracellular compared to intracellular ion concentration, which results in small quantities of sodium ions leaking into the membrane through a few passive sodium channels in the cell's membrane. This relative impermeability of positive sodium ions, combined with a high extracellular but low intracellular concentration, and the resulting electrical drive to enter the cell (negative inside), would tend to "run down" the cell's resting membrane potential over time. Fortunately, the cell has developed a mechanism whereby this "rundown" is prevented. Located within the cell membrane is an energy-dependent sodium-potassium pump, which pumps in potassium ions and pumps out sodium ions in just the right ratio of the sodium ions entering and the compensatory potassium exiting the cell. This ratio is two sodium ions extruded for every three potassium ions taken into the cell. This pump maintains the exact ionic balance necessary to maintain the resting membrane potential.

TABLE 10–1 Cellular Ionic Concentrations

Ion	Squid Axon		Mammalian Muscle	
	Intracellular	*Extracellular*	*Intracellular*	*Extracellular*
Na^+	50	440	10	145
K^+	400	20	160	4
Cl^-	52	560	3	114
A^-	385	—	163	34

The ionic concentrations are in millimoles/liter. A^- refers to the intracellular organic anions.[23, 26, 28, 29]

Goldman-Hodgkin-Katz Equation

An important modification of the Nernst equation is the inclusion of ion permeability as the primary influence on the cell's transmembrane voltage. Specifically, the greater an ion's permeability, the more likely it is to influence the transmembrane potential, because the equilibrium potential of the most permeable ion in effect becomes the cell's membrane potential. The equation accounting for the different permeability (designated as p in the equation below) factors is known as the Goldman-Hodgkin-Katz equation[26, 28, 29]:

$$E_m = \frac{-RT\ 2.3\ \log_{10}\{pK[K^+]_i + pNa[Na^+]_i + pCl[Cl^-]_e\}}{F\,\{pK[K^+]_e + pNa[Na^+]_e + pCl[Cl^-]_i\}}$$

In this equation it can be seen that the cell's transmembrane voltage (E_m) is primarily dependent on which ion has the greatest permeability. For example, in the resting state, we know that the permeability of potassium is relatively high due to nonvoltage-gated passive leak potassium channels, while that of sodium is very low. Chloride ions are distributed through chloride channels, and thus the chloride ion adjusts to whichever ion's permeability predominates between potassium and sodium as dictated by the net transmembrane potential. With a high potassium and low sodium permeability, the above equation simplifies to the Nernst equation, i.e., potassium is the predominant ionic species and E_m becomes −75 mV. If sodium permeability were to increase dramatically, then E_m would approach the sodium ion equilibrium potential of +55 mV. It would not quite reach this value because potassium continues to have some influence and would hold the maximum potential to a less positive (more negative) value of about +40 mV.

Action Potential Generation

In addition to the passive (always open) potassium channels and relatively few passive sodium channels, there is a second set of sodium and potassium channels within nerve and muscle cell membrane that are modulated by transmembrane voltage differences. They are voltage gated because they open and close depending on the voltage across the membrane.[23] Muscle and unmyelinated nerve contain both sodium and potassium voltage-gated channels. The voltage-gated sodium and potassium ion channels are closed at the resting membrane potential. If the transmembrane voltage changes in the depolarization direction (less negative) and reaches about 15 to 20 mV less negative than the resting membrane potential, the voltage-gated sodium channels open. This results in an increased permeability of the sodium ion, a process known as sodium activation. As noted above, the Goldman-Hodgkin-Katz equation predicts that the transmembrane potential shifts toward the sodium ion equilibrium potential. This massive shift in transmembrane potential is referred to as depolarization. After staying open for a short period of time, the sodium gates automatically close (sodium inactivation), with a return of the resting membrane potential again dictated by the resting state ion permeabilities (repolarization). In muscle and unmyelinated nerve membranes, a delayed opening of potassium voltage-gated channels occurs secondary to the depolarization during sodium inactivation and serves to repolarize the cell.

It should be recognized that very few ions have to physically cross the membrane either for sodium-induced depolarization or for potassium-mediated repolarization to occur. The important factor is the increase in permeability that drives the transmembrane shifts in both the depolarization and repolarization direction. The region of membrane where there are large numbers of voltage-gated sodium channels in the open position acts as a current sink for sodium ions to "sink" into the cell's interior. This implies that a nearby source for the sodium ions must be present. The surrounding membrane acts as the current source, thus permitting a current flow from the region about the current sink. Sodium ions are thereby removed from the outside of the membrane surrounding the sink (making this region relatively more negative) and deposited on the inside of the cell (Fig. 10–2). The ions within the cell migrate within it to help neutralize some of the interior's negative charge. This flow of current, or charge transfer from extracellular to intracellular, is referred to as a *local circuit current*. The net effect of this charge transfer is to make the cell's interior less negative and exterior more negative, thus acting to shift the transmembrane voltage in the depolarized direction about the current sink. If the charge transfer is sufficient to depolarize the cell by 15 to 20 mV, the membrane surrounding the sink is induced to permit sodium activation and hence undergo depolarization. This process can then continue along the length of the cell.

The above process creates an action potential spike at the original site of sodium activation. A mechanical, chemical, or electrical stimulus that causes the membrane potential to reach threshold over a localized region is all that is required to initiate action potential generation. Once the process begins, it is self-sustaining as long as there are sufficient ion channels to repeat the process of depolarization. The intracellular action potential is essentially a monophasic positive spike: −75 mV resting potential; +40 mV spike; return to resting −75 mV with sodium inactivation and potassium activation (Fig. 10–2). The membrane's threshold value must be reached in order to generate the self-sustaining action potential that is the same at all regions of the membrane. This concept is referred to as an all-or-none phenomenon. Since in a good volume conductor like the body there are many ions to sustain passive current flows, the local circuit currents spread out in all directions.[12] It is the voltage generated by the depolarization-induced current flows that generates all of the potentials we observe on the instrument's cathode ray tube (CRT) screen.

Of note, in myelinated nerve, the nodes of Ranvier lack voltage-gated potassium channels and contain voltage-gated sodium channels.[43, 44] The action potential, therefore, "jumps" from one node to the next, creating an efficient means of action potential propagation that is referred to as saltatory conduction. Repolarization in myelinated nerve, therefore, does not require a delayed potassium current for repolarization. As noted above, the resting membrane potential is restored once the permeability of sodium is reduced. Passive "back-leak" sodium and potassium currents are believed to mediate the discharge of the membrane's capacitance which accumulates over time with multiple action potential discharges.

PHYSIOLOGICAL FACTORS AFFECTING ACTION POTENTIAL PROPAGATION

A number of physiological factors have a direct effect on action potential propagation. These factors can be divided into those that can be altered by the practitioner and those that are intrinsic to the subject and beyond control. The most important factor readily amenable to change is a limb's surface temperature. Physiological variables beyond the control of the clinician include the subject's sex, age, height, and digit circumference.

Sex

Only a few studies have attempted to investigate the difference in nerve conduction between males and females.[3] A slight increase in the antidromic sensory nerve action potential amplitudes for both the median and ulnar nerves recorded from the digits has been noted in women. Also, women demonstrate a greater nerve conduction velocity for upper and lower limb nerves than men. Both of these differences, however, are eliminated when limb length and digit circumference are considered (see below).[36]

Age

Several generalizations can be made regarding peripheral evoked sensory nerve action potentials (SNAPs)

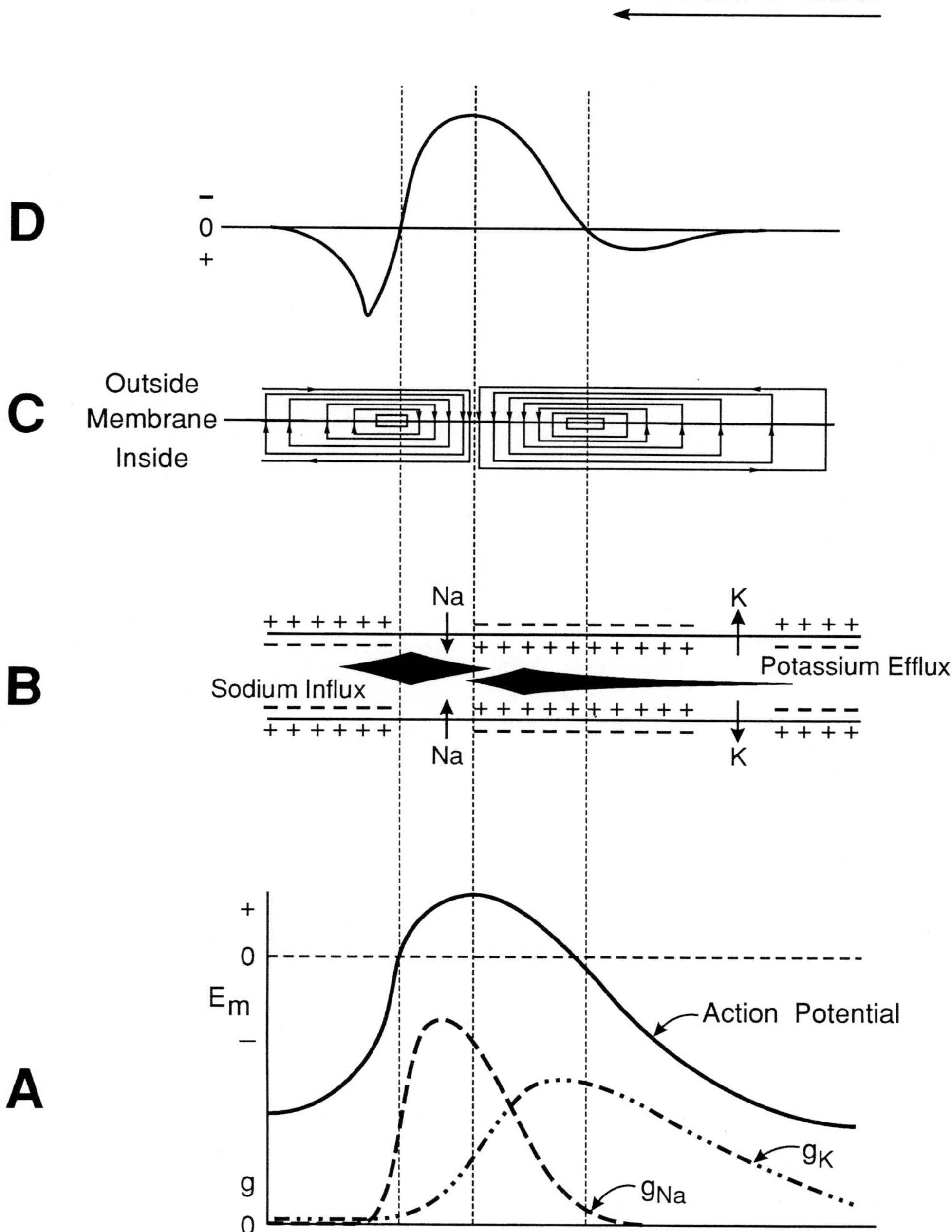

FIGURE 10–2. *A.* Sodium (g_{Na}) and potassium (g_K) ion conductances over time result in an alteration of the transmembrane potential, creating an action potential. *B.* Spatial relationship of the sodium and potassium ion influx during an action potential. Note alteration of the transmembrane ionic potential differences corresponding to depolarization and repolarization. *C.* Local circuit currents describe the pathways of extracellular sodium ions entering the cell and then migrating longitudinally within the cell. *D.* Triphasic extracellular waveform associated with the intracellular monophasic action potential. (From Dumitru D: Electrodiagnostic Medicine. Philadelphia, Hanley & Belfus, 1995, p. 32.)

and aging. The conduction velocity demonstrates a consistent decline approximating 1 to 2 m/sec per decade.[33] The SNAP's duration is about 10% to 15% longer in 40- to 60-year-olds and 20% longer in 70- to 88-year-olds than in persons 18 to 25 years old.[8] Compared to the 18- to 25-year-old group, the SNAP's amplitude is one-half and one-third, respectively, for the age groups 40 to 60 years and 70 to 88 years old. The distal sensory latencies reveal a similar prolongation with age. There is a suggestion that the median and radial nerves do not demonstrate considerable alteration with age.[17] At present there is disagreement as to the magnitude of change in SNAP parameters induced by the aging process.

The results of aging on conduction velocity have been examined in a number of upper and lower limb nerves.

Motor nerve conduction velocities reveal changes similar to those of sensory nerves. The newborn's motor nerve conduction velocities are about half of adult values, which are reached by 3 to 5 years of age.[2] After age 50, there is a progressive decline in the conduction velocity of the fastest motor fibers approximating 1 to 2 m/sec per decade. There is a concurrent increase in the distal motor latency and a decrease in the motor response's amplitude with advancing age. H-reflex latency demonstrates little alteration with aging in the healthy elderly.[18] The decrease in amplitude is difficult to ascertain clinically as there is such a wide range of normal H-reflex amplitudes.

Digit Circumference

Females consistently demonstrate significantly higher antidromic SNAP amplitudes for the median and ulnar nerves recorded from the second and fifth digits.[3] A negative linear correlation exists between finger circumference and amplitude for these two nerves. It is known that as the distance between the recording electrode and neural generator increases, the amplitude precipitously declines. Increasing the circumference of the finger displaces the electrode further from the nerve. Since men have significantly larger finger circumferences than women, this appears to explain the difference in SNAP amplitudes. There is no evidence that this difference is due to an intrinsic neural difference between male and female nerves.

Height

Several investigations have documented slower nerve conduction velocities in taller compared to shorter individuals with respect to lower limb nerve conductions.[9, 30] This difference is found to be independent of the limb's temperature or subject's age. The cause of the difference is unknown, but distal nerve tapering or an abrupt change in axon diameter has been speculated to account for this finding.[12]

Temperature

Temperature is one of the most profound factors influencing nerve conduction studies. As the temperature of the nerve is lowered, the amount of current required to generate an action potential increases. Neural excitability is lowered with a reduction in temperature. This decreased excitability is a direct temperature effect on the nerve's action potential-generating mechanism at the nodes of Ranvier, and not a result of membrane resistance changes, i.e., the transmembrane resistance is not increased by a drop in temperature.[24, 25] In addition to excitability, the morphology of an action potential is profoundly affected by a drop in temperature.

The action potential's amplitude, rise time, and fall time all increase as the nerve's temperature declines. The time required for the action potential of a cold nerve to reach its peak depolarization from the resting membrane level increases approximately 33%.[34] The time necessary for the action potential to return to its resting level is also increased, but much more so than the rise time (69%). Because both the duration and spike height increase, the area of the action potential increases dramatically at lower temperatures.

The compound muscle action potential (CMAP) arising from cooled muscle tissue demonstrates similar changes as those noted for SNAPs. The CMAP's amplitude, duration, rise time, and area all increase as the muscle's temperature is reduced. Intramuscular recordings also reveal that those motor units in close proximity to the recording electrode are also increased in the same parameters noted above.

Temperature also has an impact on nerve conduction velocities (NCV). Based on the prolongation of the rise and fall time noted above, we should be able to infer the nerve's response to cooling with respect to NCV. Since propagation is saltatory in myelinated nerves, decreasing the temperature results in an increase in the amount of time necessary to reach the action potential's peak at each node of Ranvier. As cooling increases the time required at each node, a slower conduction velocity results.

The first detailed investigation of temperature effects on NCV in human nerves revealed an NCV-to-temperature correlation of 2.4 m/sec/°C for median and ulnar motor conduction.[22] With every 1°C drop in temperature, there was a 2.4 m/sec decrease in the conduction velocity. Reductions in conduction velocity for upper extremity motor nerve fibers have also been found to approximate a decrease of 4% or 5% per degree Celsius.[10, 27] Correction factors utilizing subcutaneous and intramuscular readings are equally correct, but it is more convenient and less painful to use surface measurements.[20]

In the upper limb, the relationship between temperature and NCV has been investigated for the surface temperature range of 26 to 33°C, measured at the midline of the distal wrist crease. Calculations reveal that for median motor and sensory nerves, NCV is altered 1.5 and 1.4 m/sec/°C, respectively, while the distal latency for both changes 0.2 msec/°C.[19–21] The ulnar nerve demonstrated motor and sensory temperature relationships of 2.1 and 1.6 m/sec/°C, respectively, and a distal motor and sensory latency correlation of 0.2 msec/°C.[19–21]

Because of the profound effects of temperature on NCV, it is clear that reliable nerve studies require temperature control. A cool limb, irrespective of the ambient room temperature, can result in latencies, NCVs, and amplitudes that are not in the "normal" range. A normal limb study can yield results that are spuriously thought to be abnormal but that are only due to the low temperature. This is an especially important issue when an abnormal nerve is being studied. Correction factors are well known for normal nerve, but serious questions remain about how abnormal nerves respond to temperature variations. Although applying a correction factor is less time-consuming than heating the patient, it is questionable how accurately correction factors for temperature in normal nerves can be applied to abnormal nerves. Until more data are available regarding the best correction factor for diseased nerves, warming of the limb should be considered to be superior to using correction factors. It is recommended that the practitioner use at least a surface temperature between the stimulating and recording electrodes of 32°C for upper limbs and 30°C for lower limbs. In persons with ischemic limbs or those with altered sensation, great care must be exercised with respect to increasing the tissue's metabolic demand and injuring the patient when attempting to warm the limb.

WAVEFORM MORPHOLOGY GENERATION

As noted earlier, the current flow created by a depolarization sink is associated with a specific pattern of voltages known as isopotential lines (Figs. 10–2 and 10–3).[12] Recording a voltage at any point in space along this line results in the same voltage being recorded. As one moves further from the current sink, the corresponding voltages decline as the current density also decreases. The pattern of isopotential lines in space create three distinct regions of voltage. The current sink is associated with a negative voltage while the two surrounding (leading and trailing) current sources are considered zones of positive voltage. Separating the current sink zone from the current sources are zero isopotential lines. These lines correspond to regions of zero voltage, demarcated by that portion of the potential crossing the baseline on the CRT (Fig. 10–3).

An action potential with its local circuit current and associated isopotential lines propagating past an electrode can be considered essentially equivalent to a stationary action potential sequentially sampled with a recording electrode moving through its electrical field (Fig. 10–3). We shall use the latter situation as an example for discussion purposes because it is easier to visualize the ensuing action potential waveform. Suppose a propagating nerve or muscle action potential is frozen for an instant in time. A characteristic pattern of isopotential voltage lines is described in the region of the body surrounding the nerve or muscle. We can then move a recording electrode through the activated tissue's electrical field to simulate a propagating action potential (Fig. 10–3). The final waveform morphology associated with an action potential propagating along a straight portion of nerve or muscle is a triphasic waveform with a large negative spike flanked by an initial large and subsequent terminal small positive phase. For our discussion purposes, positive is denoted by a downward CRT deflection, while an upward CRT deflection designates a net negative potential difference between the two recording electrodes. This example implies that for both nerve and muscle, when an action potential approaches, reaches, and then travels past a recording electrode, the fundamental waveform morphology is a triphasic potential. These same simple principles can be applied to understand the morphological generation of essentially all potentials likely to be observed during the electrodiagnostic medicine examination.

NERVE AND MUSCLE WAVEFORM MORPHOLOGIES AND CHARACTERISTICS

Nerve Potentials

Sensory Nerve Action Potentials

Clinical Recordings. SNAPs can be obtained with either antidromic or orthodromic techniques.[8] The term

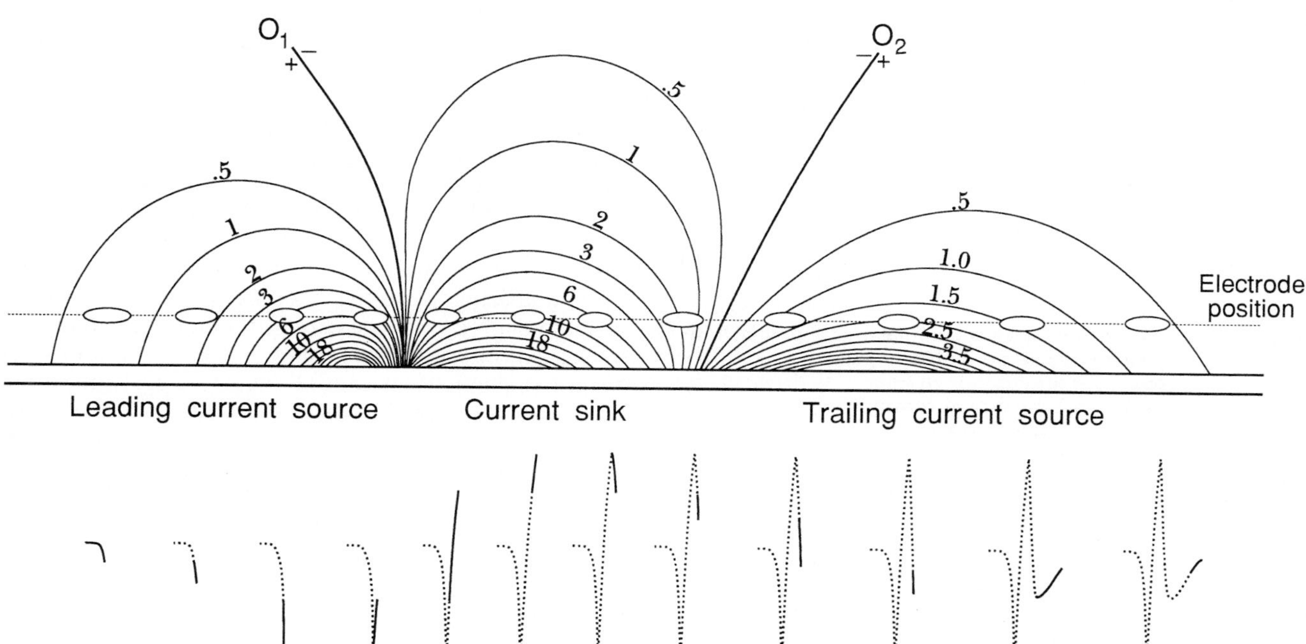

FIGURE 10–3. A propagating nerve or muscle action potential generates a characteristic pattern of voltages associated with the corresponding current flows. Passing an electrode through a hypothetically stationary action potential (open ovals) results in the recording of a triphasic extracellular waveform. This basic conceptualization of extracellular waveforms applies equally to nerve and muscle tissue. (From Dumitru D: Electrodiagnostic Medicine. Philadelphia, Hanley & Belfus, 1995, p. 35.)

antidromic implies that the induced neural impulse propagates along the nerve in a direction opposite to its physiological direction. Remember that the nerve will conduct an impulse proximally and distally when stimulated by a depolarizing current. On the other hand, stimulating the median sensory fibers on the second digit and recording from the wrist is an example of an orthodromic technique. In orthodromic recordings, the sensory fiber impulses are detected at a proximal location to the stimulus as they travel physiologically from the finger, through the wrist region, on their way to the central nervous system.

SNAP Morphology. Antidromic and orthodromic bipolar SNAP waveform recordings will typically be biphasic rather than triphasic. The biphasic, negative-positive potential is a result of the bipolar recording technique and not a violation of volume conductor theory. Biphasic SNAP waveforms can best be understood by use of bipolar and referential recording montages for median nerve stimulation at the wrist (Fig. 10–4).[13] The median SNAP is indeed a triphasic waveform and conforms to the principles of volume conduction but appears biphasic because of the recording montage used.

It is also possible to predict the optimal interelectrode separation to maximize the biphasic potential's amplitude in the bipolar recording.[16] The critical factor in this instance is the rise time, baseline to negative peak, of the biphasic potential. The recording electrodes must be located at a distance greater than the spatial extent represented by the rise time duration. The rise time of most SNAPs approaches 0.8 msec, which represents a longitudinal extent of 40 mm for an action potential conducting at 50 m/sec (50,000 mm/1000 msec = D/0.8 msec; D = 40 mm). If the two recording electrodes are separated by a distance of less than 40 mm, some similar information regarding the main peaks of the two potentials will be recorded by both electrodes and result in mutual cancellation of data, producing a potential with a smaller amplitude. A portion of the nerve will be depolarizing under the reference electrode while still in some degree of depolarization under the active electrode. At interelectrode separations of greater than 40 mm, the biphasic potential's negative peak amplitude will no longer grow, but the terminal positive phase will enlarge slightly and may change its morphology. These findings can be demonstrated by varying the distance between recording electrodes and observing the ensuing results (Fig. 10–5). In effect, as the recording distance decreases below 40 mm, the amplitude of the potential declines, and the peak latency shortens.

Activating the median nerve at the wrist will yield the expected biphasic SNAP of a particular duration and amplitude. Relocating the neural stimulator sequentially at more proximal activation sites results in a series of SNAPs with a progressively declining ampli-

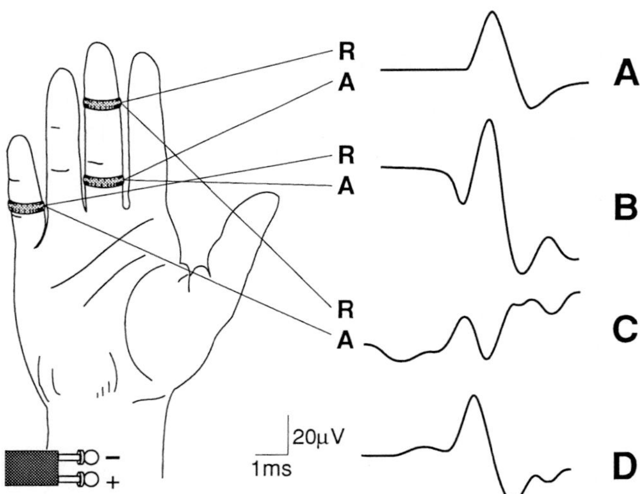

FIGURE 10–4. The median nerve is stimulated at the wrist with an antidromic sensory recording montage. Active (*A*) and reference (*R*) electrodes are located on fingers as designated above. *A.* Bipolar recording with the commonly observed biphasic median nerve sensory nerve action potential (SNAP). *B.* The same active electrode location as in *A* is referenced to the fifth digit, resulting in a triphasic SNAP. *C.* An active electrode placed on the fifth digit but referenced to the third digit permits one to observe what this electrode records when the median nerve is stimulated. An inverted triphasic potential of small magnitude is detected. It is inverted because of its connection to the inverting amplifier port. *D.* Electronically summating the potential recorded in *B* and *C* yields that recorded with a bipolar montage in *A.* (From Dumitru D: Volume conduction: Theory and application. In Dumitru D [ed]: Physical Medicine and Rehabilitation State of the Art Reviews: Clinical Electrophysiology. Philadelphia, Hanley & Belfus, 1989, pp. 665–681.)

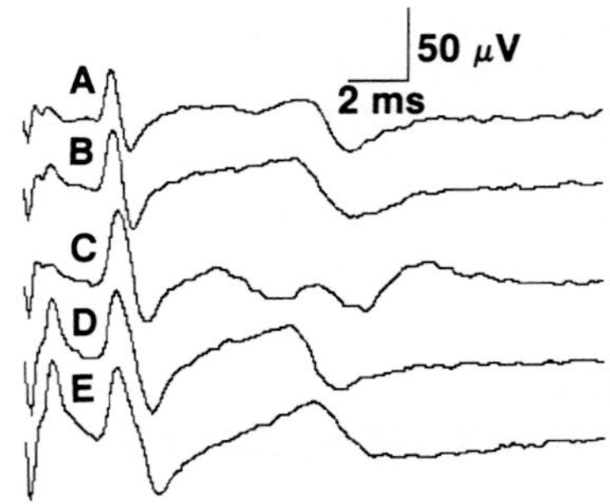

Trace	Interelectrode distance	Latency		Amplitude
		Onset	Peak	
	cm	*ms*		*μV*
A	1.0	2.7	3.0	56
B	2.0	2.7	3.1	72
C	3.0	2.7	3.3	77
D	4.0	2.7	3.3	86
E	5.0	2.7	3.3	86

FIGURE 10–5. The effect of interelectrode separation can be easily demonstrated by evoking an antidromic median sensory nerve action potential (SNAP) and progressively increasing the interelectrode separation between the active and the reference electrode. The active electrode remains in the same location while the reference electrode is sequentially displaced more distally on the digit. As can be seen, the SNAP amplitude increases, peak latency increases, and the onset latency remains the same. (From Dumitru D, Walsh NE: Practical instrumentation and common sources of error. Am J Phys Med Rehabil 1988; 67:55–65.)

tude and an area of the negative phase. This effect occurs because of increasing phase cancellation between the individual SNAPs contained within the peripheral nerve secondary to temporal dispersion manifesting over large distances. The significant reduction in SNAP amplitude with progressive increases in distance between the stimulating and recording electrodes precludes the use of SNAP amplitudes as accurate predictors of conduction block or axonal loss from widely separated stimulation sites within the same arm. Corresponding left/right amplitude comparisons for the same stimulus site, however, can be utilized to assess possible axonal loss.

Muscle Potentials

Needle Insertional Activity

Normal Insertional Activity. Placing a needle (monopolar or standard concentric) recording electrode into healthy muscle tissue and advancing it in quick but short intervals results in brief bursts of electrical potentials referred to as insertional activity (Fig. 10–6).[12] The observed electrical activity is believed to result from the needle electrode mechanically depolarizing the muscle fibers surrounding its leading edge as it pierces and pushes aside the tissue. Minimal and localized muscle tissue damage may occur from direct needle trauma and is the basis for the synonymous term, "injury potentials." The purpose of including insertional activity analysis as part of the electromyographic examination is that the probing needle may provoke transient or sustained membrane instability before this abnormal activity is present with the muscle at rest.

Decreased Insertional Activity. Muscle that has been replaced by fibrous tissue, or that is otherwise electrically inexcitable, is no longer capable of electrical activity. Consequently, the needle electrode is incapable of mechanically depolarizing this tissue. The result is that few if any electrical potentials will be detected following needle movement (Fig. 10–6).

Increased Insertional Activity. Practitioners have noted that insertional activity may appear to persist following needle movement cessation. This finding has led to the term "increased insertional activity." In disease states where the muscle is no longer connected to its nerve or the muscle membrane is inherently unstable from primary muscle pathology, the increased insertional activity completes a temporal continuum from the previously normal insertional activity to the development of sustained membrane instability potentials (Fig. 10–6).

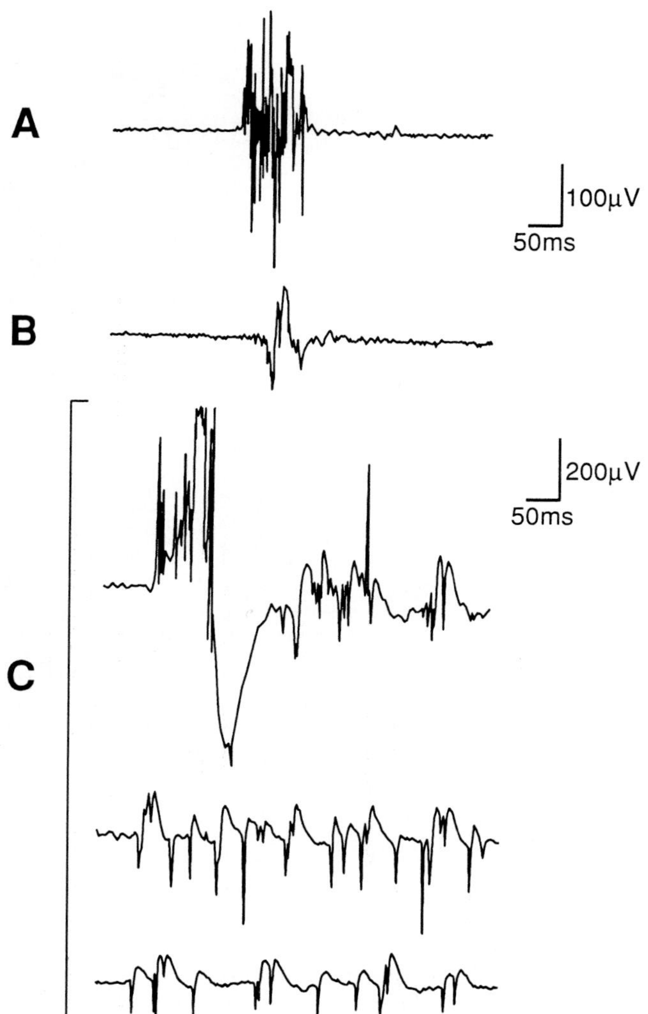

FIGURE 10–6. *A.* Inserting a monopolar needle in healthy muscle tissue results in mechanical depolarization of muscle tissue, which generates a brief burst of electrical activity designated as insertional activity. *B.* Inserting the same needle in fibrotic muscle or subcutaneous fatty tissue results in decreased insertional activity. *C.* Inserting a monopolar needle in denervated muscle tissue produces not only the initial burst of electrical activity, but associated positive sharp waves and fibrillation potentials that abate over several hundred milliseconds. (From Dumitru D: Electrodiagnostic Medicine. Philadelphia, Hanley & Belfus, 1995, p. 219.)

End-Plate Potentials

Miniature End-Plate Potentials (MEPPs). An active electrode located in the end-plate region can record two distinct potentials. One of the potentials that can be observed is a short duration (0.5 to 2 msec), small (10 to 50 μV), irregularly occurring (once every 5 sec per axon terminal) monophasic negative waveform.[12] These potentials represent the random release of acetylcholine vesicles. Volume conduction theory would suggest that for a potential to be monophasic and negative, the current sink would have to start and finish within the active electrode's recording area (Fig. 10–7A).

Clinically, multiple MEPPs are usually observed with an intramuscular recording electrode, and the sound is referred to as end-plate noise or "seashell murmur" (Fig. 10–7B).

End-Plate Spikes. A second potential that can be detected with an active electrode placed in the end-plate region is relatively short in duration (3 to 4 msec), of moderate amplitude (100 to 200 μV), irregularly firing, and biphasic with an initial negative deflection.[16] The biphasic potential has an initial negative phase,

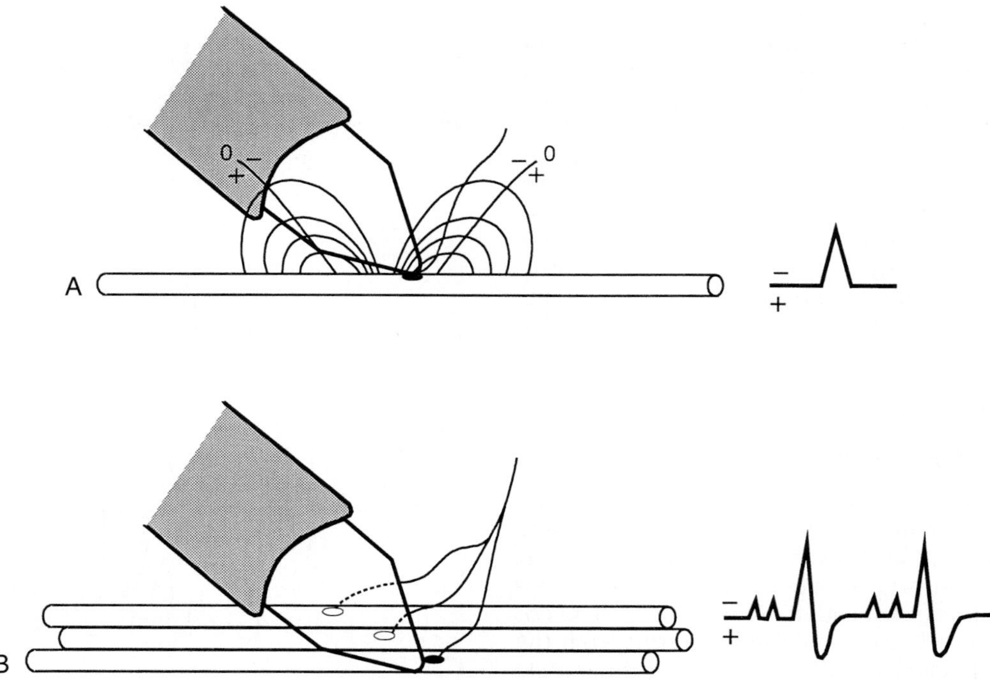

FIGURE 10–7. *A.* Monopolar needle electrode located over a muscle's end-plate records the spontaneous depolarization of a miniature end-plate potential. As the electrode is located over this potential's subthreshold central current sink and hence does not propagate, a monophasic negative potential is recorded. *B.* The large recording electrode is usually positioned over several end-plates, thus recording multiple miniature end-plate potentials and end-plate spikes. (From Dumitru D: Electrodiagnostic Medicine. Philadelphia, Hanley & Belfus, 1995, p. 49.)

produced when a current sink originates in the vicinity of the active electrode and then propagates away (Fig. 10–8). Triphasic end-plate spikes may also occur if the active electrode induces an action potential in the terminal axon but the electrode's recording surface is some distance from the end-plate. End-plate spikes and MEPPs are frequently observed together as they arise from the same region (Fig. 10–9).

Single Muscle Fiber

The single muscle fiber's extracellular waveform morphology, like nerve tissue, depends on the characteristics of the muscle's intracellular action potential. A muscle's action potential is approximately 4 to 20 times longer than a nerve's, due in particular to the prolonged repolarization process.[12] Aside from the longer duration of local circuit currents compared to that in neural tissue, the concept of a current sink surrounded by two source currents (source-sink-source) remains unchanged. A triphasic waveform with a small terminal phase should then be recorded from an extracellular active electrode placed adjacent to a propagating single muscle fiber action potential at some distance from the end-plate region (Fig. 10–10).

Motor Unit Potential Morphology

Anatomy. One anterior horn cell gives rise to a peripheral axon that splits into multiple terminal axons, each of which innervate a single muscle fiber. The anterior horn cell, its axon, and all the single muscle fibers supplied by that nerve are referred to as a motor unit. When the anterior horn cell fires, or the nerve that arises from it is stimulated, all of the muscle fibers that belong to that motor unit depolarize. The electrical activity from all of these muscle fibers summates to produce a motor unit action potential (MUAP). The anatomical distribution of the terminal axons with respect to the muscle fibers they innervate is particularly relevant to the morphological characteristics of the MUAP.

Let us consider one motor unit belonging to a human biceps muscle (Fig. 10–11A).[6,7] Upon reaching the muscle tissue, the peripheral nerve divides into a large number of terminal axons. Each terminal axon will form an end-plate region with a single muscle fiber. The length of an individual terminal axon from the point it divides to the end-plate is quite variable for each muscle fiber innervated (Fig. 10–11B). As a result, the spatial extent of the end-plate region from one motor unit may reach 30 mm longitudinally along the muscle. Additionally, the muscle fibers of a single motor unit are randomly distributed in an oval territory 4 to 6 mm in circumference (Fig. 10–11A). The random distribution implies that the single muscle fibers may be in groups of different numbers or singly arranged within the 4 to 6 mm. Five to ten or more different motor units may share this area.

Amplitude/Rise Time. The morphology of a MUAP can be described in terms of its *amplitude* (maximum peak-to-peak CRT trace displacement), *rise time* (temporal aspect of a potential's peak), *duration* (departure from and return to baseline), and number of *phases*

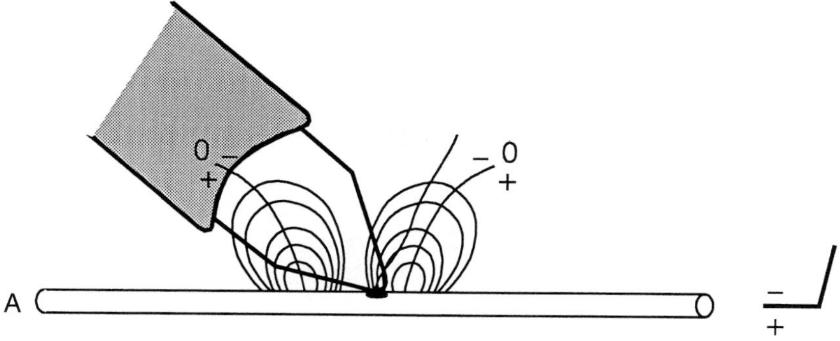

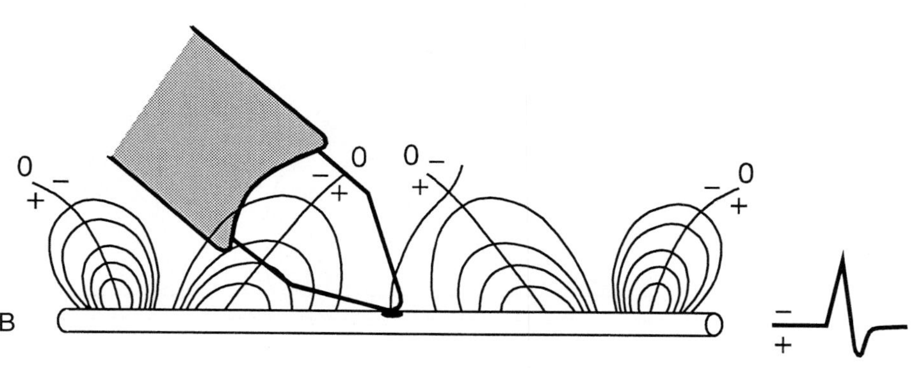

FIGURE 10–8. *A.* Irritation of the terminal axon results in a suprathreshold end-plate depolarization, thus generating a single muscle fiber potential. Because the electrode is located over the end-plate zone, an initial negative deflection is recorded. *B.* The terminal positive current sources are then recorded with action potential propagation, thereby generating a biphasic initially negative potential referred to as an end-plate spike. (From Dumitru D: Electrodiagnostic Medicine. Philadelphia, Hanley & Belfus, 1995, p. 49.)

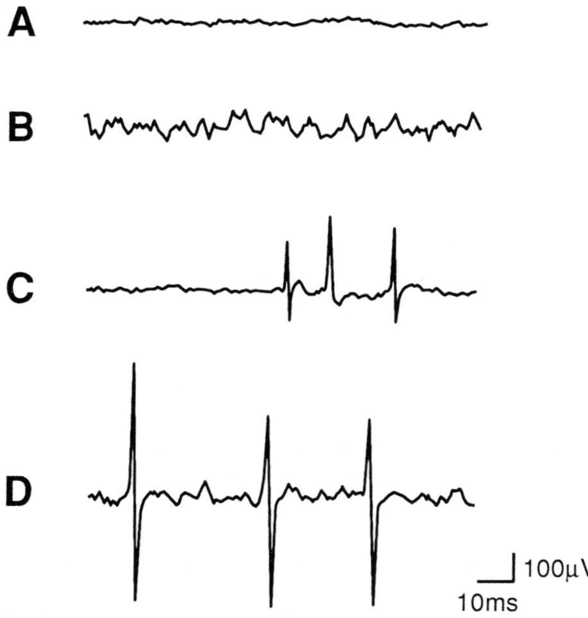

FIGURE 10–9. *A.* Monopolar needle located in a healthy muscle at rest. *B.* Slight needle movement positions the electrode in an end-plate region with the recording of multiple miniature end-plate potentials of a negative spike configuration. *C.* Repositioning the needle electrode to a slightly different region primarily records biphasic, initially negative end-plate spikes. *D.* Advancing the needle electrode slightly permits the simultaneous recording of both potentials noted individually in *B* and *C.* (From Dumitru D: Electrodiagnostic Medicine. Philadelphia, Hanley & Belfus, 1995, p. 220.)

(baseline crossings plus one) (Fig. 10–12). In the volume conductor of muscle tissue, the amplitude of potentials declines exponentially with increases in distance from the current generator. This occurs because the surrounding muscle and its supportive tissues impede potentials that change rapidly over a short period of time. The tissue acts as a high-frequency filter. As a result, the peak-to-peak MUAP's amplitude is believed to arise from fewer than 12 and possibly just one or two single muscle fibers located within 0.5 mm of the electrode's recording surface.

Duration. The MUAP's duration depends on (1) the shortest and longest lengths of terminal axons from the point they separate from the parent nerve to the end-plate, and (2) the conduction velocities of the terminal axons and muscle fibers, with respect to the recording electrode, and the muscle fiber length (Figs. 10–11 and 10–12).[6, 7] A MUAP's duration is the most sensitive clinical parameter in diagnosing disease.

Phases. As previously stated, the single muscle fiber usually has a triphasic appearance when recorded outside of the end-plate zone and away from the tendinous insertion. The voltages from all of the single muscle fibers belonging to one motor unit summate to yield a MUAP that is also usually triphasic: positive-negative-positive. This voltage summation does not always produce a smooth result, and small serrations or *turns* can occasionally be seen as part of a MUAP's major phase (Fig. 10–12). The number of *phases* is defined as the number of CRT trace baseline crossings plus one. Normal MUAPs are considered to have four or fewer phases. MUAPs with five or more phases are called

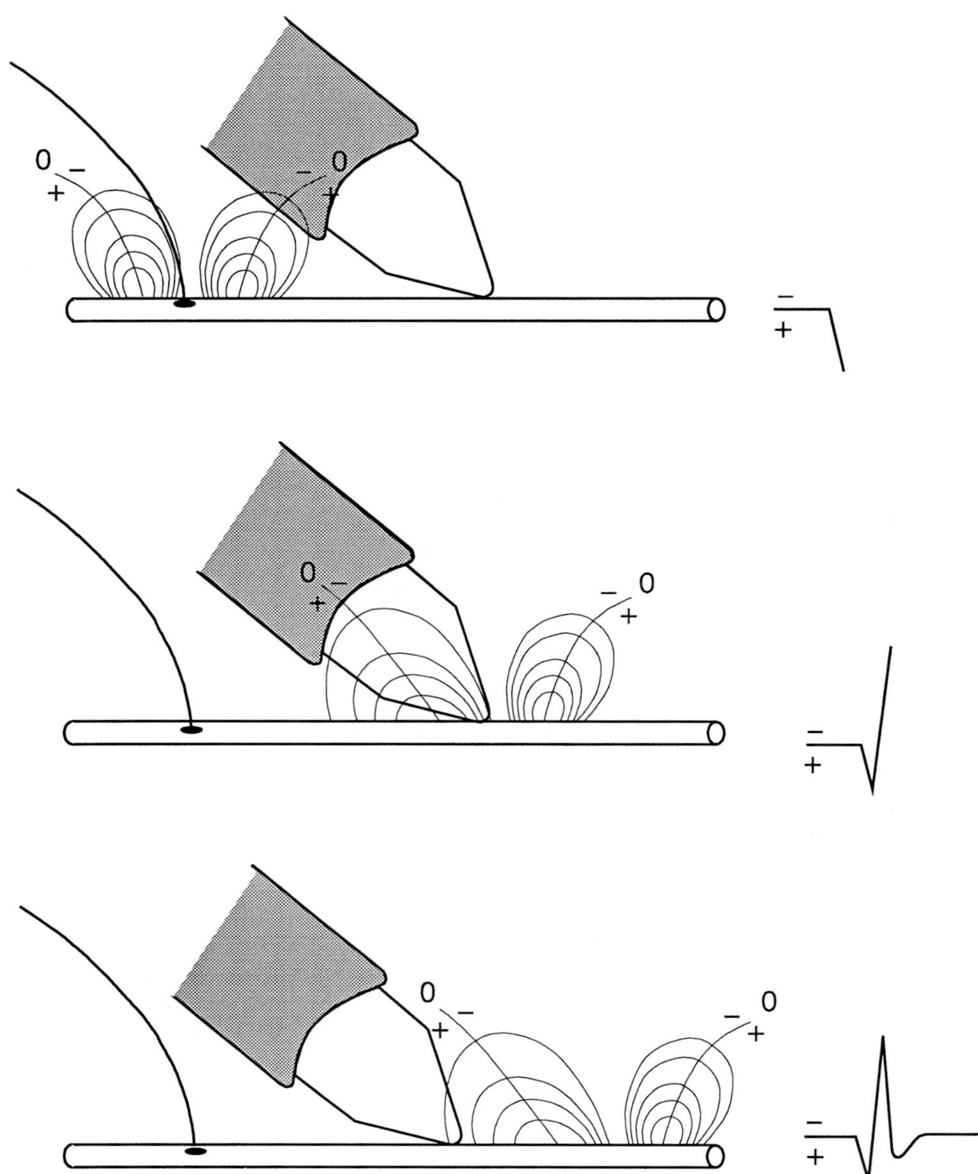

FIGURE 10–10. A single muscle fiber action potential propagating past a needle recording electrode results in a triphasic waveform. This is because the voltage distribution creates an initial and terminal positive voltage source surrounding a negative current sink zone. (From Dumitru D: Electrodiagnostic Medicine. Philadelphia, Hanley & Belfus, 1995, p. 218.)

polyphasic potentials. Recordings of multiple MUAPs from normal muscle tissue can have between 12% (concentric needle) to 35% (monopolar needle) polyphasic potentials, depending on the type of recording electrode used.[12] Slightly different MUAP morphologies can be expected, depending on the exact location of the recording electrode with respect to different single muscle fibers within the motor unit territory.

Pathology can also alter the number of phases a MUAP waveform can have. The motor unit can be affected in two general ways following injury or disease. A pathological condition may affect either the anterior horn cell or peripheral nerve, or the muscle fibers composing the motor unit. If the neural component of a motor unit is compromised severely enough to experience degeneration, all of the muscle fibers innervated by the parent nerve will become denervated. These denervated muscle fibers somehow induce nearby terminal axons of intact nerves to send out neural projections to reinnervate the orphaned muscle fibers. Through peripheral sprouting, the total number of muscle fibers belonging to a specific motor unit may increase dramatically (Fig. 10–13). Neurogenic diseases can lead over time to larger amplitude, longer duration, and highly polyphasic MUAPs.

If the muscle fibers comprising a motor unit undergo a random degeneration such as occurs in some myopathies, the total number of fibers belonging to that motor

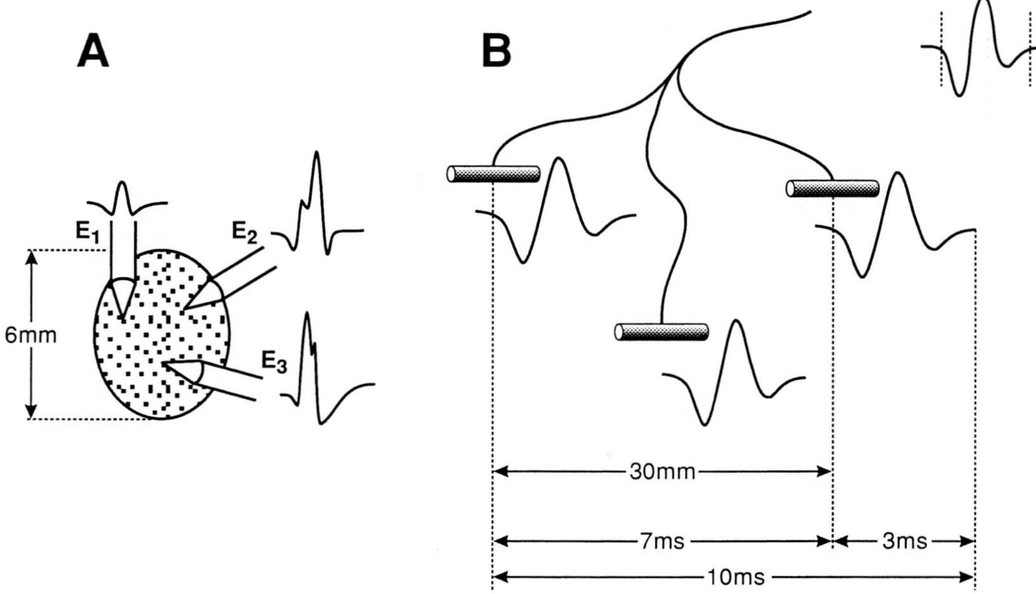

FIGURE 10–11. *A.* The single muscle fibers (*small dots*) composing a single motor unit in the biceps brachii muscle are depicted. Three needle recording positions are shown, each with a slightly different motor unit action potential (MUAP) morphology for the same motor unit. *B.* The total duration of a MUAP depends on the spatial expanse of the end-plate zone, terminal axon conduction velocity, and single muscle fiber conduction velocity. (From Dumitru D, DeLisa JA: Volume conduction. Muscle Nerve 1991; 14:605–624.)

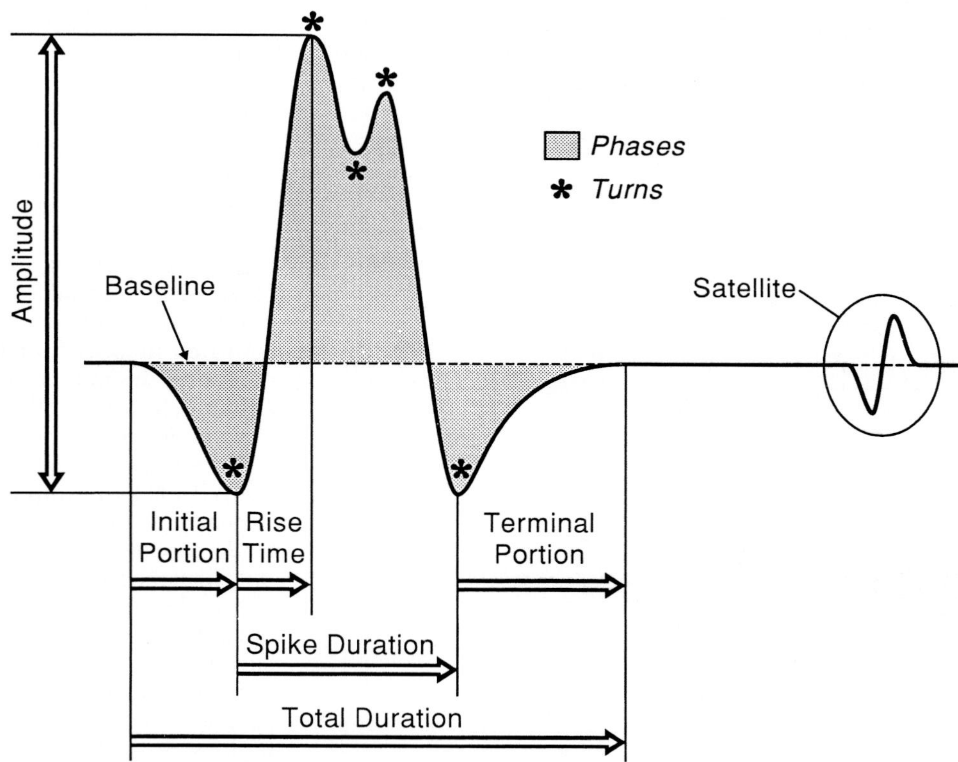

FIGURE 10–12. A motor unit action potential is depicted with various morphological aspects measured. (From Dumitru D: Electrodiagnostic Medicine. Philadelphia, Hanley & Belfus, 1995, p. 53.)

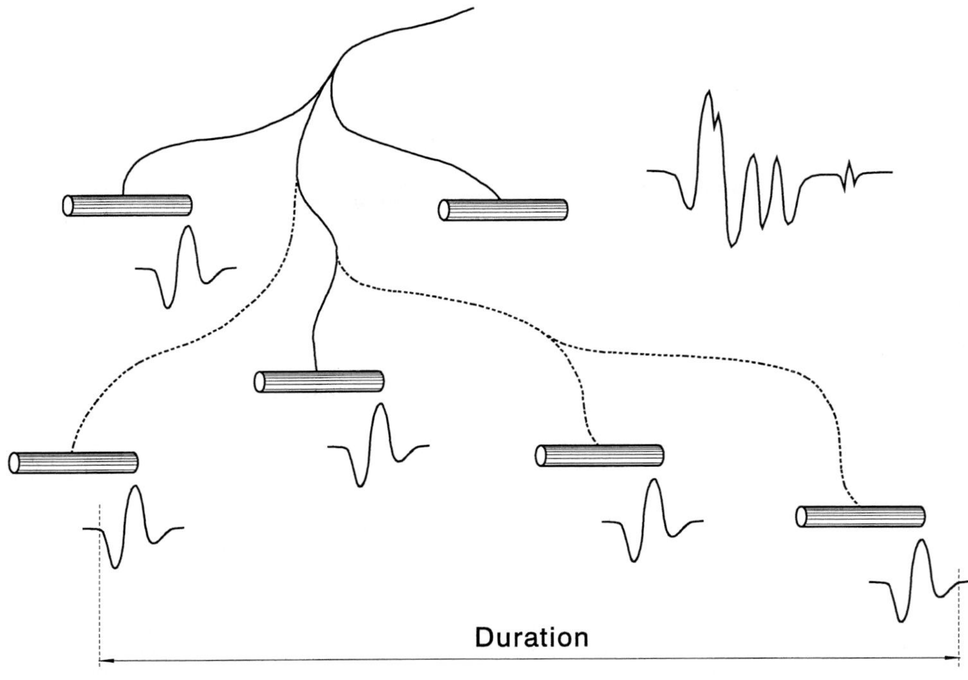

FIGURE 10–13. Several muscle fibers are denervated in this example. Collateral terminal nerve sprouts from an intact motor unit (*dotted lines*) grow to reinnervate those denervated muscle fibers. The end result is a large-amplitude, long duration potential with more phases. (From Dumitru D: Electrodiagnostic Medicine. Philadelphia, Hanley & Belfus, 1995, p. 54.)

unit decreases (Fig. 10–14). A decrease in muscle fibers would most likely result in a reduction of the MUAP's maximum amplitude. It is also conceivable that fibers at the extremes of the end-plate region may be involved. The result of these fibers' degenerating would cause a shortening of the MUAP duration. Finally, the dropout of single muscle fiber waveforms would produce less voltage with respect to the spatial summation of single fiber potentials. Fewer muscle fibers could lead to "gaps" in the MUAP waveform, causing an increase in the number of phases. A primary myopathic process tends to yield a shorter duration, highly polyphasic, low-amplitude MUAP.

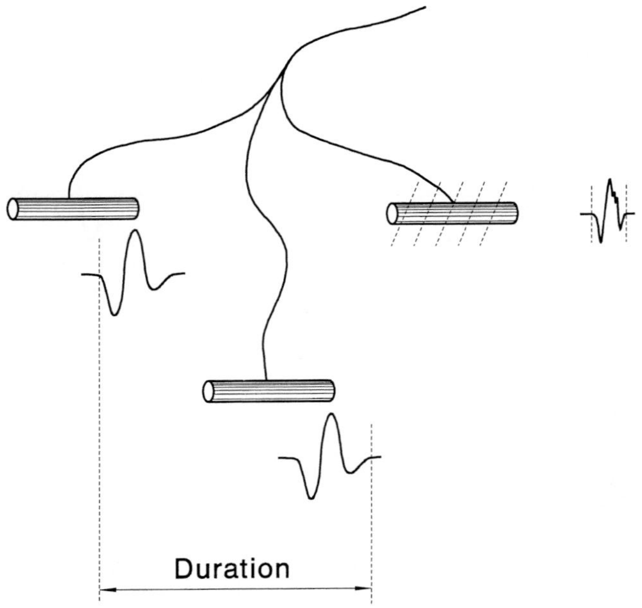

FIGURE 10–14. Loss of single muscle fibers from a motor unit results in the generation of motor unit action potentials with smaller amplitude, shorter durations, and possibly more phases. (From Dumitru D: Electrodiagnostic Medicine. Philadelphia, Hanley & Belfus, 1995, p. 54.)

Compound Muscle Action Potential

To elicit a CMAP from a particular muscle, the active electrode is located on the skin's surface directly over the muscle's motor point (end-plate region).[12] The end-plate region typically lies midway between the muscle's origin and insertion. The reference electrode is usually placed on or distal to the tendinous insertion of the muscle so as not to record electrical activity from the activated muscle. Stimulating the peripheral nerve innervating the muscle under investigation will result in a relatively large, biphasic waveform with an initial negative deflection (Fig. 10–15).

Occasionally a positive deflection can precede the CMAP's negative phase. Volume conductor theory can explain this observation (Fig. 10–16). The active electrode may not be located directly over the motor point but displaced longitudinally away from it. The region of muscle surrounding the end-plate zone serves as that portion of the volume conductor from which the source currents initially arise to complete the local circuit currents into the current sink. An active electrode located off the motor point will first record some portion of one of the source currents "feeding" the current sink. Recall that the leading portion of the source current will result in a positive deflection of the CRT trace. As propagation ensues in the muscle, the current sink will eventually reach the active electrode, resulting in a negative deflection. Finally, the terminal source current is detected

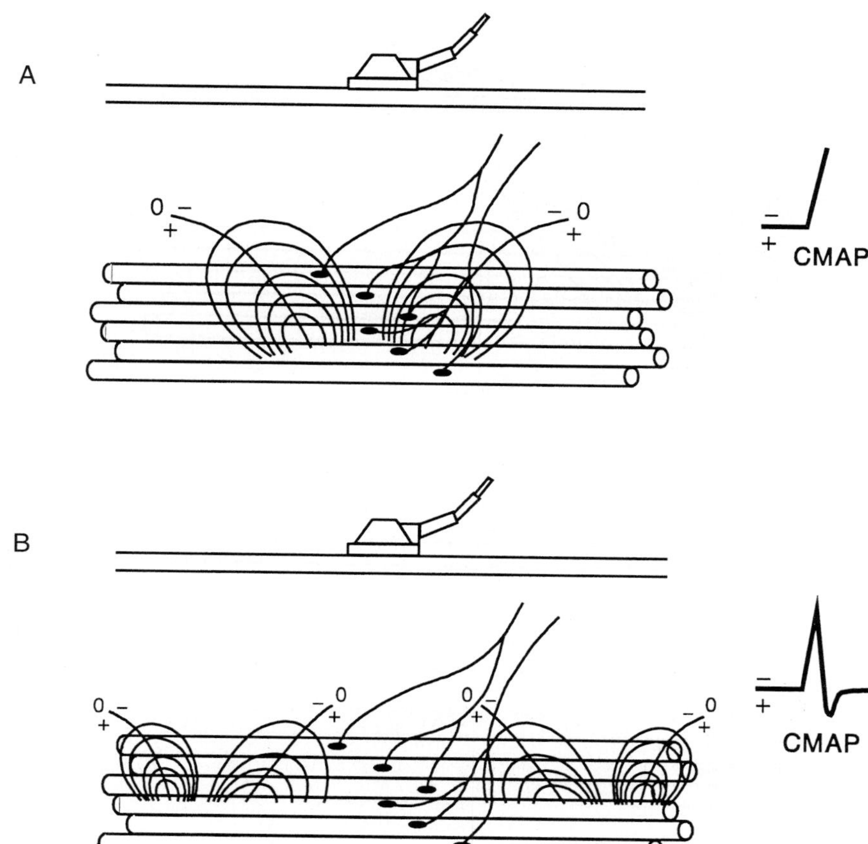

FIGURE 10–15. *A.* Locating an active recording electrode over the motor point of a muscle places this electrode over the central region of the negative current sink generating all of the muscle's action potentials. An initial negative deflection is recorded because of this location, thereby producing the compound muscle action potential's characteristic morphology. *B.* A terminal positive phase is then recorded as the action potential propagate away from the electrode. (From Dumitru D: Electrodiagnostic Medicine. Philadelphia, Hanley & Belfus, 1995, p. 55.)

producing a positive deflection. Instead of the anticipated biphasic potential, a triphasic positive-negative-positive waveform is recorded. Relocating the active electrode over the anticipated motor point region will usually remedy the situation.

MUSCLE GENERATORS OF ABNORMAL SPONTANEOUS POTENTIALS

Fibrillation Potentials

In vitro observations have shown that about 6 days or so after denervation, the muscle fiber's resting membrane potential decreases to a less negative level of −60 mV, compared to the normal value of −80 mV.[41] Additionally, the resting membrane potential begins to oscillate. Since the threshold level for starting the all-or-none self-sustaining action potential is now closer to the new resting membrane potential, the oscillating membrane potential will eventually reach the threshold level. Once threshold is achieved, a propagating action potential is induced in the muscle fiber which is referred to as a fibrillation potential. The repolarization phase of denervated muscle results in a temporarily more hyperpolarized (−75 mV or more) level than the previous resting membrane potential of −60 mV. Additionally, the muscle's repolarization actually hyperpolarizes the threshold level to that of −60 mV or slightly more negative. As the hyperpolarized membrane level (−75 mV or more) begins to return toward its resting membrane level of −60 mV (the new threshold level), an action potential is again produced. This process regularly repeats at a time interval dependent on the repolarization-to-threshold turnaround time. Fibrillation potentials may be reduced in number following a decrease in temperature, muscle ischemia, or *d*-tubocurarine administration.

The difference between the resting membrane potential and threshold level is less in the former end-plate region than along the muscle fiber. This may explain why fibrillation potentials appear to arise more commonly from the previous end-plate than at other portions of the muscle. Irregularly firing fibrillation potentials occur at times and are less well understood, but are thought to arise from spontaneous depolarizations within the transverse tubule system.

Fibrillation potentials are simply spontaneous depolarizations of a single muscle fiber and demonstrate waveform morphologies similar to those of single muscle fibers that are voluntarily activated (Fig. 10–17). Fibrillation potentials occur not only spontaneously, but also can be provoked by electrode movement in pathological tissue. Fibrillation potentials are typically short in duration (less than 5 msec), less than 1 mV in amplitude, and fire at rates between 1 and 50 Hz. They have a typical sound likened to a high-pitched tick or "rain on a tin roof" when amplified through a loudspeaker.

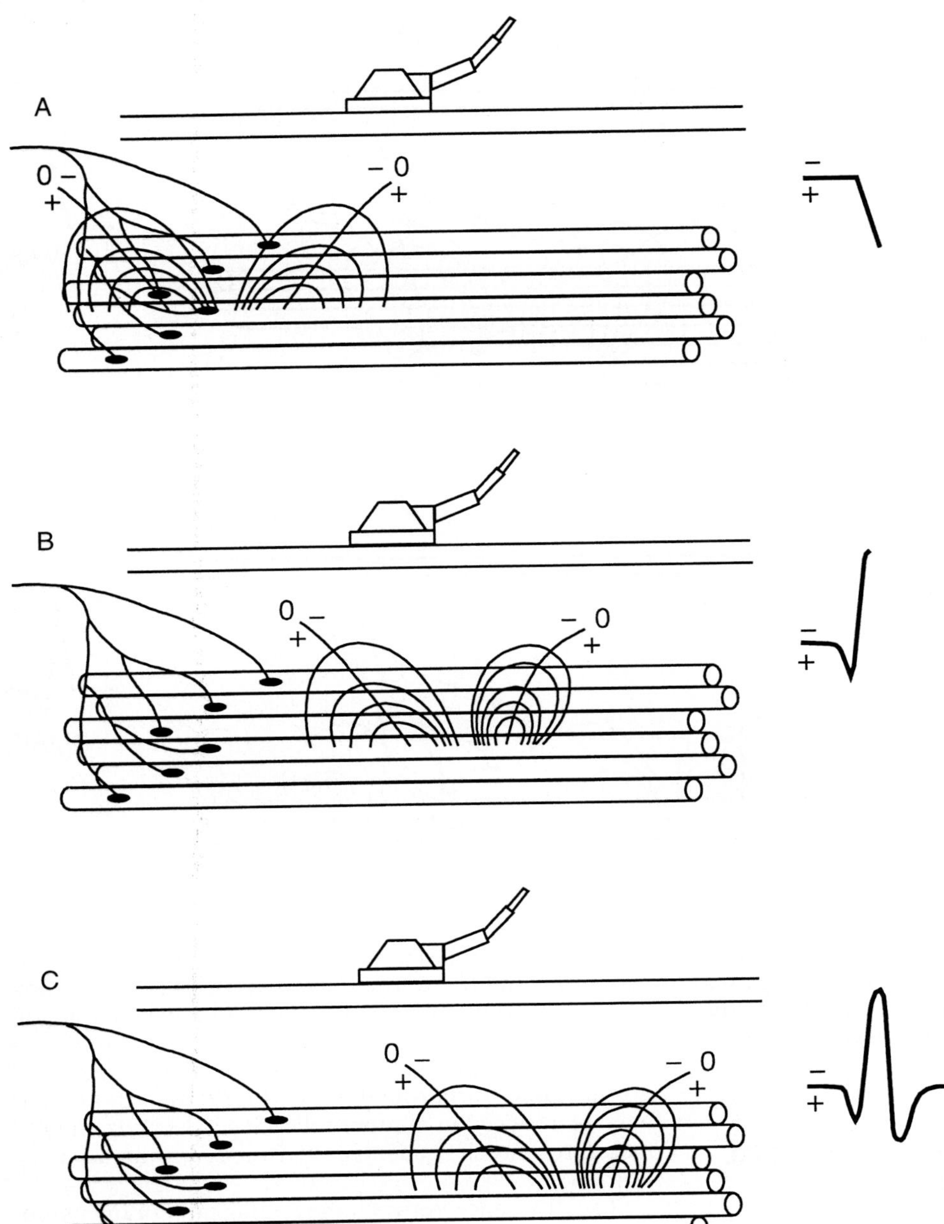

FIGURE 10–16. *A.* Relocating the active electrode in Figure 10–15 off the motor point results in a compound muscle action potential with an initial positive deflection, as some of the muscle's action potentials no longer originate under the electrode but propagate toward it. *B.* When the main negative sink reaches the electrode, the potential's main negative spike is detected. *C.* Finally, the terminal positive source currents are recorded generating the potential's terminal positive phase. (From Dumitru D: Electrodiagnostic Medicine. Philadelphia, Hanley & Belfus, 1995, p. 56.)

When the recording electrode is located in the previous end-plate zone of a denervated muscle, fibrillation potentials can be biphasic with an initial positive deflection. A recording electrode outside of the end-plate zone but far from the tendinous region will detect fibrillation potentials that are either biphasic (positive-negative) or triphasic (positive-negative-positive).

Positive Sharp Waves

A potential that can be recorded from a single muscle fiber having an unstable muscle membrane potential secondary to denervation or intrinsic disease typically has a large primary sharp positive deflection followed by a small or absent negative potential. These potentials are called positive sharp waves (PSWs) (Fig. 10–17). This waveform is believed to have the same clinical significance as a fibrillation potential in that it is a single muscle fiber discharge. Amplified through a loudspeaker, positive sharp waves have a regularly firing rate (1 to 50 Hz) and a dull thud sound. Their durations are from several milliseconds to 100 msec. Although observed to fire spontaneously, PSWs are more often provoked by electrode movement.

A number of other potentials can be observed that have the morphology of a PSW. As we have already described, a MUAP recorded from the tendinous region can also have an initial positive deflection followed by a negative potential because the current sink cannot pass beyond the recording electrode.[12] It is also possible

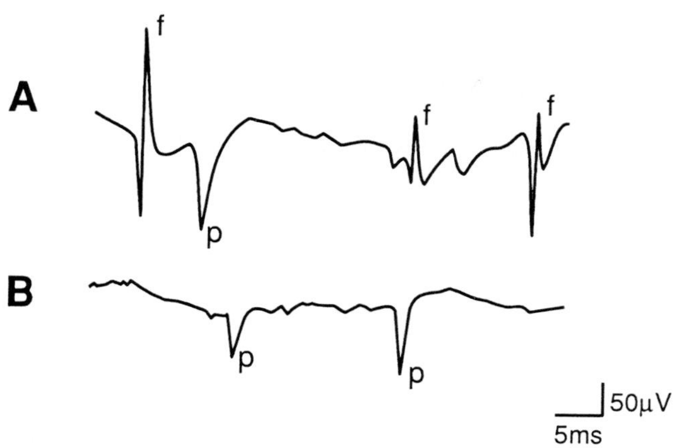

FIGURE 10–17. *A.* Monopolar needle recording of positive sharp waves (*p*) and fibrillation potentials (*f*). *B.* Only positive sharp waves are depicted. (From Dumitru D: Electrodiagnostic Medicine. Philadelphia, Hanley & Belfus, 1995, p. 230.)

for the recording electrode to damage a number of muscle fibers in close proximity to the recording surface, again preventing an action potential from passing its recording surface. This results in a primarily positive potential. An additional possibility is for the cannula of a concentric needle recording electrode to preferentially be located in the motor unit territory and invert the negative spike (cannula = reference electrode), making it appear positive and simulating a PSW. These three potentials can be distinguished from a PSW in that they are MUAPs and subject to voluntary control, whereas a PSW is not. Asking the individual to contract and relax the muscle under investigation should demonstrate that the potential has a variable firing rate. A PSW typically fires at a regular rate. If any doubt remains, the electrode should be repositioned until successful recordings are obtained. Transient runs of "PSW-appearing potentials" may be seen in healthy skeletal muscle, particularly in the paraspinal muscles. The "nonpathological" PSWs are believed to arise because the needle electrode is oriented in such a manner as to irritate a terminal axon, but extend the needle along the muscle fiber while injuring the tissue and preventing action potential conduction. The induced end-plate spike resembles a PSW.

Complex Repetitive Discharge

A complex repetitive discharge (CRD) is a spontaneously firing group of action potentials (formerly called a bizarre high-frequency discharge or pseudomyotonic discharge).[12] These potentials cannot be observed visually and require a needle recording electrode to be detected. Morphologically, these potentials are continuous runs of simple or complex spike patterns that regularly repeat at 0.3 to 150 Hz. The repetitive pattern of spike potentials has the same appearance with each firing and bears the same relationship with its neighboring spikes (Fig. 10–18). A distinct sound likened to heavy machinery or an idling motorcycle is produced by the firing of CRDs. In addition to the sound and repetitive pattern, a hallmark of these waveforms is that they start and stop abruptly. Complex repetitive discharges may begin spontaneously or may be induced by needle movement,

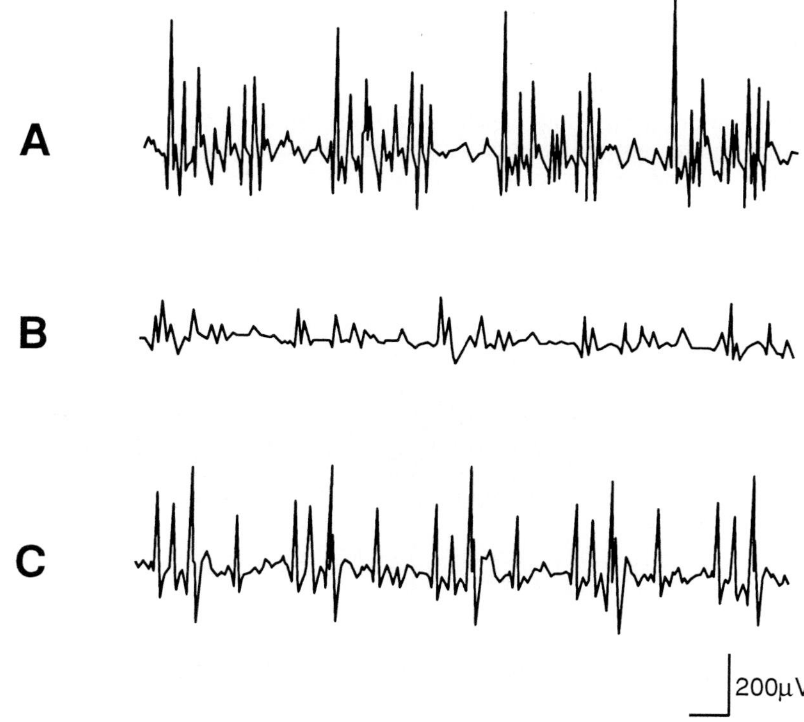

FIGURE 10–18. *A–C.* Several examples of complex repetitive discharges. Note how the same pattern of potentials repeats. The sound is like that of heavy machinery, and they start and stop abruptly. (From Dumitru D: Electrodiagnostic Medicine. Philadelphia, Hanley & Belfus, 1995, p. 232.)

muscle percussion, or muscle contraction. Nerve block and curare do not abolish CRDs, suggesting that the origin of these potentials is in muscle tissue.

Myotonic Discharges

The phenomenon of delayed muscle relaxation following muscle contraction is referred to as myotonia or action myotonia.[12] The finding of delayed muscle relaxation after reflex activation or induced by striking the muscle belly with a reflex hammer is called percussion myotonia. Clinical myotonia is usually accentuated by energetic muscle activity following a period of rest. Continued muscle contraction lessens the myotonia and is known as the "warmup." It is believed that cooling the muscle accentuates myotonia, but this finding has been objectively documented only in paramyotonia congenita.

Myotonic discharges may present in one of two waveform types (Fig. 10–19). The myotonic potential induced by needle electrode insertion usually assumes a morphology similar to that of a PSW. It is believed that the needle movement induces a repetitive firing of the unstable membranes of multiple single muscle fibers. This is because the recording needle is thought to have damaged that portion of the muscle fiber with which it is in contact. Myotonic potentials may also appear as a series of rapidly firing triphasic single muscle fiber potentials following muscle contraction. Regardless of the waveform type, the hallmark of myotonia is the waxing and waning in both frequency and amplitude. The myotonic discharge has a characteristic sound likened to a dive bomber and easily recognized. Amplitudes range from 10 μV to 1 mV and firing rates from 20 Hz to 100 Hz.

Myotonic discharges can occur with or without clinical myotonia. The observation of these potentials requires needle movement or muscle contraction. These potentials persist after nerve block, neuromuscular block, or frank denervation. This suggests that their site of origin is the muscle membrane itself. Although the exact mechanism of myotonic discharge production remains unclear, it is proposed that decreased chloride conductance is responsible at least in part for the findings in myotonia congenita. In addition to the syndromes noted above, myotonic discharges can also be detected at times in acid maltase deficiency and polymyositis.

NEURAL GENERATORS OF ABNORMAL SPONTANEOUS POTENTIALS

Fasciculation Potentials

The visible spontaneous contraction of a portion of muscle is referred to as a fasciculation. When these contractions are observed with an intramuscular needle recording electrode they are called fasciculation potentials.[12] A fasciculation potential is the electrically summated voltage of depolarizing muscle fibers belonging to all or part of one motor unit. Occasionally fasciculation potentials may only be documented with needle electromyography because they lie too deep in muscle to be seen.

Fasciculation waveforms can be characterized with respect to polyphasicity, amplitude, and duration (Fig. 10–20). Their discharge rate (1 Hz to many per minute) is irregular. They are not under voluntary control, nor are they influenced by mild contraction of the agonist or antagonist muscles. The site of origin of fasciculation potentials remains unclear, although it appears that the spontaneous discharge may arise from the anterior horn cell, or along the entire peripheral nerve (particularly the terminal portion), and at times within the muscle itself.

Fasciculation potentials occur in normal subjects and in patients with a variety of diseases. Typical diseases in which fasciculation potentials may be found include motor neuron disorders, radiculopathies, entrapment neuropathies, and cervical spondylotic myelopathy. Fasciculation potentials have also been described in metabolic disturbances, including tetany, thyrotoxicosis, and anticholinesterase overdose. Studies have unsuccessfully attempted to distinguish between benign (normal) and pathological fasciculation potentials. There is no reliable way to categorize whether fasciculation potentials indicate a disease state just by considering their inherent characteristics based on routine needle electromyography. Fasciculations with increased jitter and/or blocking on single-fiber electromyography may, how-

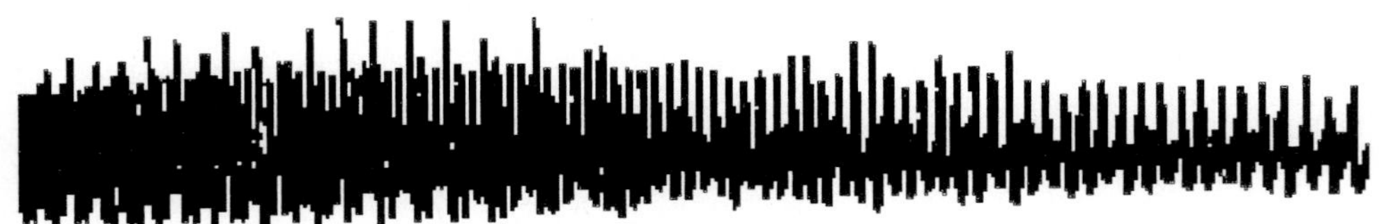

FIGURE 10–19. A run of myotonic potentials demonstrating both the positive sharp waves and negative spike form of the potentials. (From Streib EW: Differential diagnosis of myotonic syndromes. Muscle Nerve 1987; 10:603–615.)

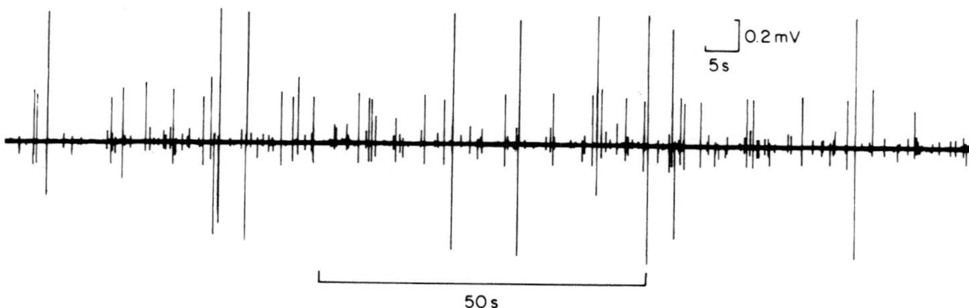

FIGURE 10–20. Multiple fasciculation potentials are depicted from a patient with amyotrophic lateral sclerosis. Note the random firing pattern of individual potentials. (From Brown WF: The Physiological and Technical Basis of Electromyography. Boston, Butterworth, 1984, pp. 317–368.)

ever, be considered abnormal. Perhaps the best way to evaluate fasciculation potentials is to analyze the company they keep. That is, a careful analysis of voluntary MUAP morphology combined with a search for abnormal spontaneous potentials is required prior to concluding that fasciculation potentials are either a normal or an abnormal finding.

Myokymic Discharge

Myokymia is a readily observable vermicular ("bag of live worms") or rippling movement of the skin. It is usually associated with myokymic discharges.[12] The myokymic discharge consists of bursts of normal-appearing motor units with interburst silent intervals. Typically the firing rate is 0.1 to 10 Hz in a semirhythmic pattern. Two to ten potentials within a single burst may fire at 20 to 150 Hz. These potentials are not affected by voluntary contraction (Fig. 10–21). The sound associated with these potentials is a type of sputtering often heard with a low-power motorboat engine. The actual discharge may be distinguished from CRDs in that myokymic discharges do not display a regular pattern of spikes from one burst to the next, nor do they typically start and stop abruptly. Myokymic discharges are groups of motor units, while CRDs represent groups of single muscle fibers. The groups of motor units within a burst may fire only once or possibly several times. The sputtering bursts of myokymic discharges sound quite different from the continuous drone of a CRD.

Myokymic potentials can be observed in the face (facial myokymia) as a result of multiple sclerosis or a brainstem neoplasm. Segmental myokymic discharges can be noted in syringomyelia or radiculopathies. Generalized myokymic discharges have been detected in uremia, thyrotoxicosis, and inflammatory polyradiculoneuropathy. Limb myokymic discharges have also been described, associated primarily with radiation plexopathy.

Continuous Muscle Fiber Activity

A number of relatively rare syndromes producing continuous muscle fiber activity associated with muscle stiffness have been reported.[12] Portions of both the central and peripheral nervous system have been implicated in generating the sustained firing of motor units. One syndrome with continuous muscle fiber activity is known as "stiff-man syndrome." The motor unit discharges in this condition are believed to have a central origin, as

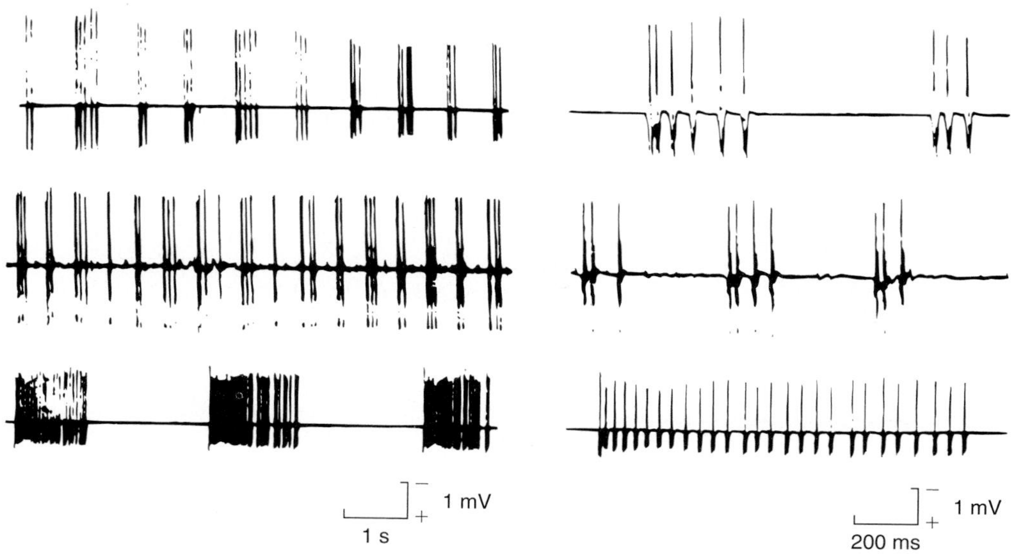

FIGURE 10–21. Multiple examples of myokymic discharges as recorded in patients with radiation plexopathy. Each burst of motor unit activity is relatively regular; however, the motor unit action potential content of each burst is somewhat variable. (From Albers JW, Allen AA, Bostron JD, et al: Limb myokymia. Muscle Nerve 1981; 4:494–504.) Copyright © 1981. Reprinted by permission of John Wiley & Sons, Inc.

they are abolished or attenuated by peripheral nerve block, neuromuscular block, spinal block, general anesthesia, and sleep. The continuous motor unit firing is diminished by diazepam but not by phenytoin or carbamazepine. The patient can voluntarily control motor unit activity, but when the patient relaxes the overriding involuntary firing returns. Progressive muscle stiffness involving all muscles (including the chest wall and pharynx) eventually occurs, resulting in contractures and profound impairment. A needle electrode recording reveals normal MUAPs producing a sustained interference pattern in both the agonists and the antagonists.

A "peripheral" form originating in the peripheral motor axon is referred to as Isaac's syndrome or neuromyotonia (Fig. 10–22). The continuous motor unit activity is eliminated by a neuromuscular block but not by a peripheral nerve block, spinal or general anesthesia, or sleep. The motor unit activity usually begins in the lower extremities in the late teens and progresses to all skeletal muscles.

Cramps

A sustained and possibly painful muscle contraction of multiple motor units lasting seconds or minutes may appear in normal individuals or specific disease states.[31] In healthy subjects a cramp usually occurs in the calf muscles or other lower extremity muscles following exercise, abnormal positioning, or maintaining a fixed position for a prolonged period of time. Cramps may also be induced by hyponatremia, hypocalcemia, vitamin deficiency, or ischemia. They also occur in early motor neuron disease and peripheral neuropathies. Familial syndromes have been reported that involve fasciculations and cramps; alopecia, diarrhea, and cramps; and simply autosomal dominantly inherited cramps.

A needle recording electrode placed into a cramping muscle shows multiple motor units firing synchronously at between 40 and 60 Hz and occasionally reaching 200 to 300 Hz (Fig. 10–23). A large portion of the muscle is simultaneously involved in a cramp, as opposed to the asynchronous excitation of motor units during voluntary activation. Cramps are believed to arise from a peripheral portion of the motor unit. A cramp that results in a taut muscle with electrical silence is the physiological contracture seen in McArdle's disease.

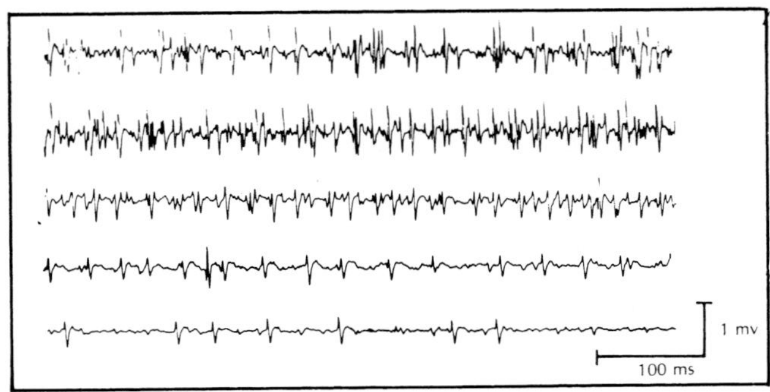

FIGURE 10–23. A characteristic muscle cramp as recorded with an intramuscular needle electrode. There is an initial burst of motor unit activity that eventually subsides as the cramp dissipates. (From Daube JA: Needle Examination in Electromyography. AAEM Minimonograph no. 11. Rochester, MN, American Association of Electrodiagnostic Medicine, 1979, pp. 1–8.)

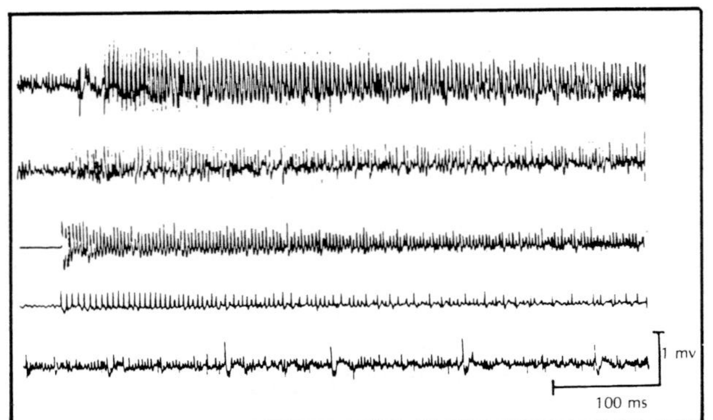

FIGURE 10–22. An example of neuromyotonia as recorded from a patient with Isaac's syndrome. The number of motor unit action potentials declines with time as the muscle's metabolic processes become exhausted. (From Daube JA: Needle Examination in Electromyography. AAEM Minimonograph no. 11. Rochester, MN, American Association of Electrodiagnostic Medicine, 1979, pp. 1–8.)

Multiplet Discharges

A clinical syndrome manifested by spontaneous muscle twitching, cramps, and carpopedal spasm is known as tetany.[12] This entity usually results from peripheral and/or central nervous system irritability associated with systemic alkalosis, hypocalcemia, hyperkalemia, hypomagnesemia, or local ischemia. Clinically one may induce tetany by tapping the facial nerve (Chvostek's sign), the peroneal nerve at the fibular head (peroneal sign), or inducing limb ischemia (Trousseau's sign).

In the above conditions, characteristic MUAPs may be observed. A single MUAP may fire rather rapidly with an interdischarge interval of 2 to 20 msec. If the motor unit fires twice, it is referred to as a doublet; if three times, it is called a triplet; and if more than three times, it is called a multiplet (Fig. 10–24). These potentials can be seen following voluntary contraction or can be observed to result spontaneously from the induction maneuvers noted above (Chvostek's sign or Trousseau's sign), in which MUAPs may fire in long trains or short bursts of 5 to 30 Hz (tetany). MUAPs with an interdischarge interval of 20 to 80 msec are called paired discharges but can arise in similar states as previously described.

NERVE INJURY CLASSIFICATION

Peripheral nerve injury is one of the most common types of pathology likely to be encountered during an electrodiagnostic medicine classification. It is necessary to be familiar with the various classification systems available to categorize an insult to neural tissue.

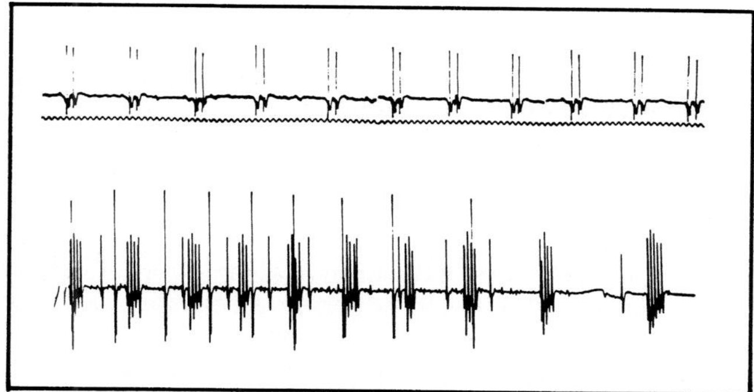

FIGURE 10–24. Examples of doublets (*upper trace*) and multiplets (*lower trace*), motor unit action potentials resulting from voluntary contraction. (From Daube JA: Needle Examination in Electromyography. AAEM Minimonograph no. 11. Rochester, MN, American Association of Electrodiagnostic Medicine, 1979, pp. 1–8.)

Seddon's Classification

The degree to which a nerve is damaged has obvious implications with respect to its present function and potential for recovery. There are essentially two general classification systems.[35, 39] One classification is that of Seddon, which considers neural injury from the perspective of a combination of functional status and histological appearance. In Seddon's scheme there are three degrees or stages of injury to consider: *neurapraxia, axonotmesis,* and *neurotmesis* (Table 10–2).

Neurapraxia

The term *neurapraxia* is used to designate a mild degree of neural insult that results in blockage of impulse conduction across the affected segment. It is also acceptable to designate this type of neural insult simply as *conduction block.* The most important aspect of conduction block is its reversibility. Muscle wasting usually does not occur in conduction block because muscle innervation is maintained and recovery is typically rapid enough to avoid disuse atrophy. Fibrillation potentials should not be observed in conduction block because the axon is not disrupted. Many nerve injuries, however, are mixed lesions in which some fibers have conduction block and some have axonal loss. In such cases it is certainly possible to observe fibrillation potentials.

TABLE 10–2 Nerve Injury Classification

Type	Function	Pathological Basis	Prognosis
LUNDBORG			
Physiological conduction block			
Type a	Focal conduction block	Intraneural ischemia; metabolic (ionic) block; no nerve fiber changes	Excellent; immediately reversible
Type b	Focal conduction block	Intraneural edema; increased endoneurial fluid pressure; metabolic block; little or no fiber changes	Recovery in days or weeks
SEDDON/SUNDERLAND			
Neurapraxia			
Type 1	Focal conduction block; primarily motor function and proprioception affected; some sensation and sympathetic function may be present	Local myelin injury, primarily larger fibers; axonal continuity; no wallerian degeneration	Recovery in weeks to months
Axonotmesis			
Type 2	Loss of nerve conduction at injury site and distally	Disruption of axonal continuity with wallerian degeneration; endoneurial tubes, perineurium, and epineurium intact	Axonal regeneration required for recovery; good prognosis since original end-organs reached
Type 3	Loss of nerve conduction at injury site and distally	Loss of axonal continuity and endoneurial tubes; perineurium and epineurium preserved	Disruption of endoneurial tubes, hemorrhage, and edema produce scarring; axonal misdirection; poor prognosis; surgery may be required
Type 4	Loss of nerve conduction at injury site and distally	Loss of axonal continuity, endoneurial tubes, and perineurium; epineurium intact	Total disorganization of guiding elements; intraneural scarring and axonal misdirection; poor prognosis; surgery necessary
Neurotmesis			
Type 5	Loss of nerve conduction at injury site and distally	Severance of entire nerve	Surgical modification of nerve ends required; prognosis guarded and dependent on nature of injury and local factors

Modified with permission from Lundborg G: Nerve Injury and Repair. Edinburgh, Churchill Livingstone, 1988.

Axonotmesis

The second degree of neural insult in Seddon's classification is *axonotmesis,* a specific type of nerve injury in which only the axon is physically disrupted, with preservation of the enveloping endoneurial and other supporting connective tissue structures (perineurium and epineurium). Compression of a profound nature or traction on the nerve are typical lesion etiologies. Once the axon has been disrupted, the characteristic changes of Wallerian degeneration occur. The fact that the endoneurium remains intact is a very important aspect of this type of injury. A preserved endoneurium means that once the remnants of the degenerated nerve have been removed, the regenerating axon simply has to follow its original course directly back to the appropriate end-organ. A good prognosis can be expected when neural damage results only in axonotmesis.

Neurotmesis

The greatest degree of nerve disruption is designated in Seddon's system as *neurotmesis.* This is complete disruption of the axon and all supporting connective tissue structures, including the endoneurium, perineurium, and epineurium, which are no longer in continuity. A neurotmetic lesion has a poor prognosis for complete functional recovery. Surgical reapproximation of the nerve ends will likely be required. Surgery does not guarantee proper endoneurial tube alignment, but at least it improves the chances that axonal growth will occur across the injury site.

Sunderland's Classification

A second popular and somewhat more detailed classification is that proposed and subsequently modified by Sunderland. This classification of nerve injury is based on the results of trauma with respect to the axon and its supporting connective tissue structures. Basically, Sunderland's classification is divided into five types of injury, based exclusively on which connective tissue components are disrupted (Fig. 10–25). Type 1 injury corresponds to Seddon's designation of neurapraxia. Seddon's axonotmesis is subdivided by Sunderland into three forms of neural insult (types 2 to 4). A type 2 injury involves loss of axonal continuity with preservation of all supporting neural structures, including the endoneurium (closely corresponding to Seddon's axonotmesis). Type 3 and 4 injuries result in progressively more neural disruption. Sunderland's type 5 injury corresponds to Seddon's neurotmesis (complete neural disruption).

INSTRUMENTATION

An electrodiagnostic instrument comprises many separate components. The most important of these are the electrodes, amplifier, filters, speaker, analog-to-digital (A/D) converter, CRT, and stimulator (Fig. 10–26).[15, 16, 37]

Electrodes

The two basic types of electrodes are surface and needle. Surface electrodes are manufactured in various sizes and shapes for conformity to the body part under investigation. The electrode is secured to the patient with sufficient tape to ensure a movement-free placement. Well-secured electrodes minimize movement artifact that could contaminate the desired signal. Commercially available disposable self-adhering electrodes are now available and eliminate the need for tape.

Two basic types of needle recording electrodes are commonly used, monopolar and concentric (Fig. 10–27). The monopolar needle is a solid stainless steel shaft coated completely with Teflon except for the bare metal tip. It is this bare metal tip that acts at the recording surface. The needle is typically 12 to 75 mm long and 0.3 to 0.5 mm in diameter, with a recording surface of 0.15 to 0.6 mm^2. Separate reference and ground electrodes are required. The concentric needle electrode is a hollow stainless steel hypodermic needle with a central platinum or nichrome-silver wire about 0.1 mm in diameter, surrounded by epoxy resin acting as an insulating material from the surrounding cannula. The cannula has a similar length and diameter as the monopolar needle. A separate ground is required, but the cannula serves as the reference electrode.

There has been considerable discussion about the merits of each of these electrodes compared to the other. Both electrodes have advantages and disadvantages, depending on the clinical circumstances. Monopolar needle electrodes have a wider recording territory and a distant reference, thereby making the recording "noisier" with respect to distant activity and interference. On the other hand, the Teflon coating reduces patient discomfort. The concentric needle electrode has the active and reference electrodes close together, making them quieter than monopolar needles. Concentric electrodes typically cause more patient discomfort. Concentric needle electrodes give the following as compared to monopolar needle electrodes: smaller potential amplitudes, possibly fewer phases, comparable durations, and less distant activity. The durations of potentials recorded with monopolar and concentric needle electrodes are the same. The introduction of commercially available disposable monopolar and concentric needle electrodes has eliminated such worries as Teflon peeling back on the monopolar needles and hook formation on the tip of the concentric needle electrodes. The quality of disposable needle electrodes has improved, eliminating the need to use nondisposable needle electrodes. If electrodes are reused, they should be properly sterilized, with presoaking in sodium hypochlorite and steam autoclaving.[12]

Single-fiber electrodes are essentially modified concentric needle electrodes. A small, 25-μm recording port is placed opposite the electrode's bevel and several millimeters from the tip. This makes this special electrode capable of recording the electrical activity from a single muscle fiber. The uptake area for this electrode is approximately 300 μm (Fig. 10–27). Occasionally subdermal electroencephalographic needle electrodes may be

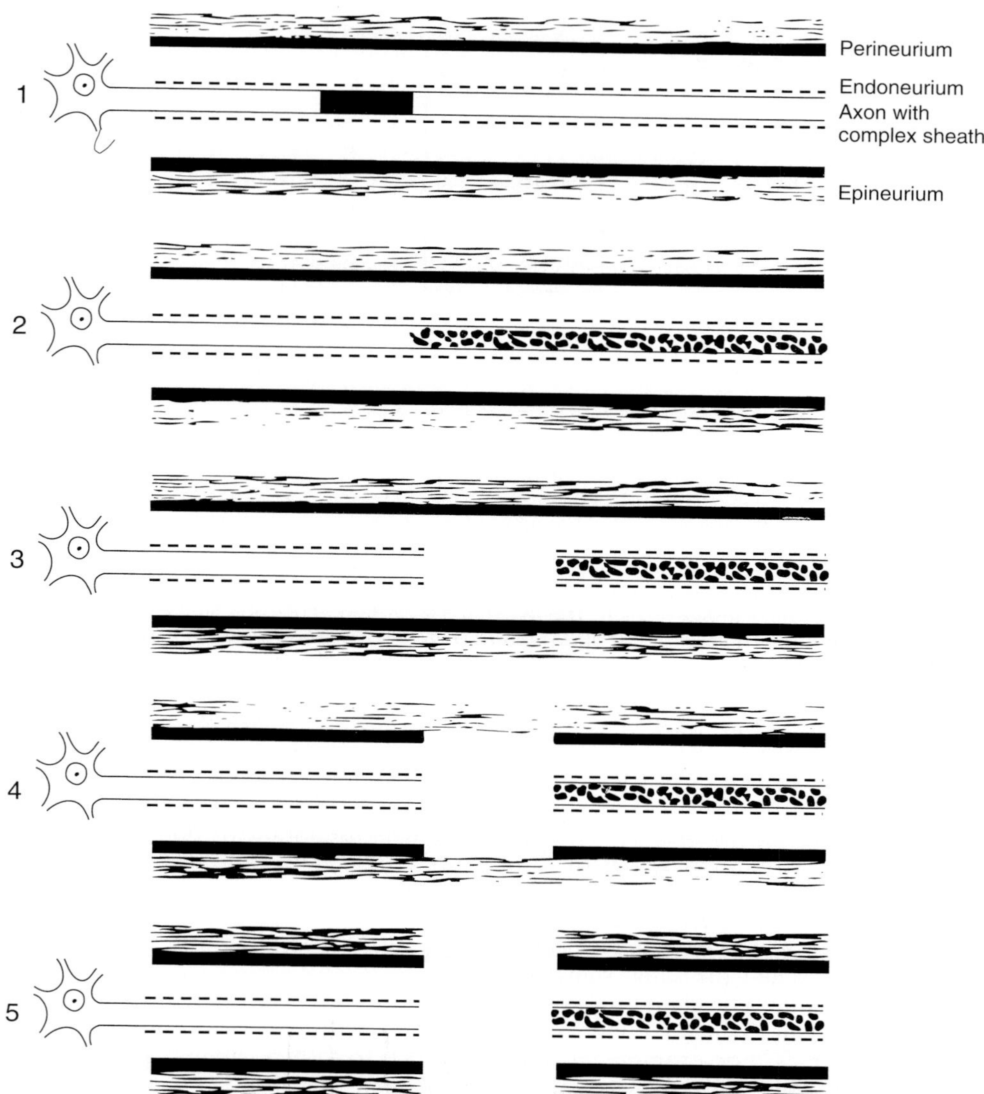

FIGURE 10–25. Shown are the five degrees of neural injury in Sunderland's classification. *1.* Conduction block. *2.* Wallerian degeneration occurring secondary to a lesion confined to the axon, with preservation of the endoneurial sheath. *3.* Disruption of the axon and endoneurial tube within an intact perineurium. *4.* Disruption of all neural elements except the epineurium. *5.* Complete discontinuity of the entire nerve trunk. (From Sunderland S: Nerve Injuries and Their Repair: A Critical Appraisal. Edinburgh, Churchill Livingstone, 1991, p. 222.)

used to record somatosensory-evoked potentials. The potentials detected with these electrodes are identical to those recorded with surface electrodes.[12] In the case of somatosensory-evoked potentials, all reusable electrodes (both surface and needle) must be sterilized. Surface electrodes are exposed to patients' serum if proper techniques are used to abrade the skin so as to reduce the skin's impedance.

Amplifier

The size of biological signals is on the order of microvolts or millivolts and thus must be amplified prior to being analyzed. An amplifier is simply a device with the ability to magnify the detected signal so that it can be displayed on the CRT.

Amplification is expressed as gain or sensitivity. Gain is a ratio of the signal's output divided by the input. For example, an output of 1 V for an input of 10 mV implies that the amplifier has a gain factor of 100,000 (output/input = 1 V ÷ 0.00001 V = 100,000). Sensitivity is the ratio of the input voltage to the size of deflection on the CRT and is usually measured in centimeters. For example, an amplifier that produces a 1 cm deflection for an input of 10 mV has a sensitivity of 10 mV/cm or 10 mV/division. The sensitivity or gain setting used is important because it can influence the onset latency. Increasing the sensitivity for a given waveform results in the instrument's detecting the potential's initial departure from baseline as occurring earlier in time.

The standard electromyograph has two amplifiers. The amplifier connected to the active electrode is known

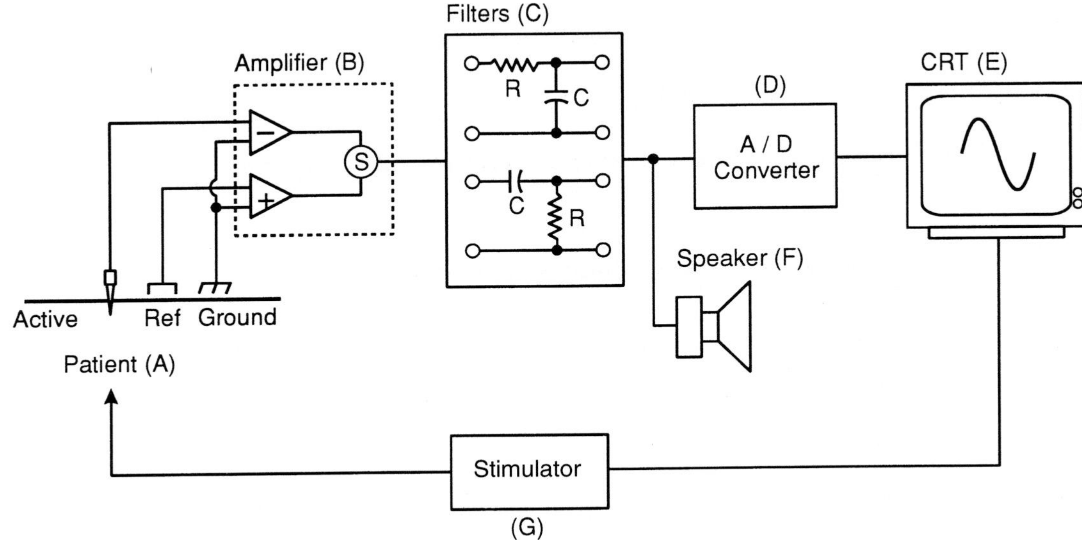

FIGURE 10–26. The subcomponents of the electrophysiologic instrument are depicted. Electrodes (*A*) on or in the patient detect bioelectrical changes, which are transmitted to a differential amplifier (*B*). This signal is filtered (*C*), undergoes analog-to-digital conversion (*D*), and is displayed on the cathode ray tube (*E*); the sound is presented through a loudspeaker (*F*). Time-locked evoked potentials can be generated with the stimulator (*G*). (From Dumitru D, Walsh NE: Electrophysiologic instrumentation. In Dumitru D [ed]: Physical Medicine and Rehabilitation State of the Art Reviews: Clinical Electrophysiology. Philadelphia, Hanley & Belfus, 1989, pp. 684–699.)

as the noninverting amplifier, while the reference electrode is connected to the inverting amplifier. The inverting amplifier magnifies the signal presented to it in the same manner as the noninverting amplifier with the exception of inverting the signal. Both amplified signals (inverted and noninverted) are then electronically summated, and like signals are canceled. This is the concept of differential amplification. When the same signal is presented to both amplifiers, theoretically there should be no output from the instrument as there is elimination of the same or common signals. For example, 60 Hz interference recorded by the active and reference electrodes is eliminated as a common mode signal. It is impossible to build two amplifiers with identical properties, so common mode rejection can never be perfect. The ratio of the instrument's output when the same signal is presented to both amplifiers is the common mode rejection ratio. This number should exceed 10,000:1.

Filters

Perhaps the least understood and most ignored aspect of the instrument is the filters. The main purpose of filters is to form a window or bandwidth of frequencies contained within the desired waveform, but excluding those frequencies not comprising the signal of interest ("noise"). Low- and high-frequency filters are used to

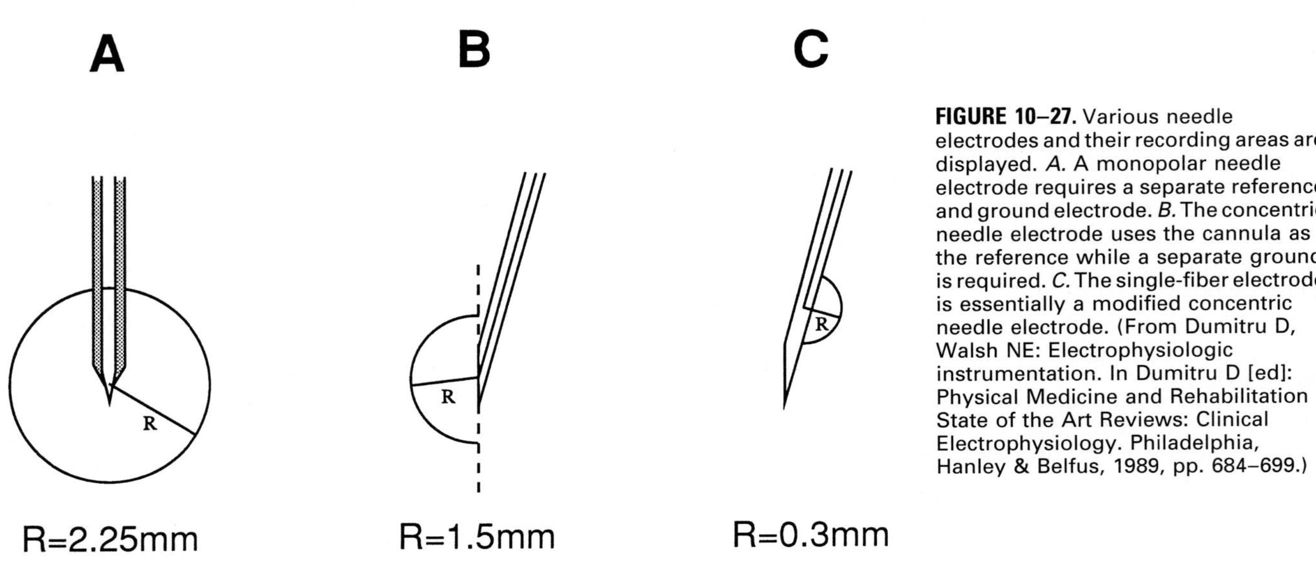

FIGURE 10–27. Various needle electrodes and their recording areas are displayed. *A.* A monopolar needle electrode requires a separate reference and ground electrode. *B.* The concentric needle electrode uses the cannula as the reference while a separate ground is required. *C.* The single-fiber electrode is essentially a modified concentric needle electrode. (From Dumitru D, Walsh NE: Electrophysiologic instrumentation. In Dumitru D [ed]: Physical Medicine and Rehabilitation State of the Art Reviews: Clinical Electrophysiology. Philadelphia, Hanley & Belfus, 1989, pp. 684–699.)

prevent those frequencies below and above the respective filter settings from being amplified and subsequently presented for display.

Any biological signal can be conceptualized as a series of sine waves of various frequencies and amplitudes. The combination of "appropriate" sine wave amplitudes and frequencies can result in the formation of essentially any waveform. In this way the biological signal recorded by the instrument consists of multiple subcomponent waveforms with specific frequency and amplitude characteristics. Eliminating any of these subcomponent waveforms results in a distortion of the waveform's appearance. This is exactly what can happen if the high or low frequency filters is set such that the desired biological waveform has various subcomponent frequencies eliminated. The examples provided below apply equally well to nerve and muscle potentials.

In our example a recorded median SNAP and CMAP are sequentially distorted by altering the low- and high-frequency filter settings. Let us begin with an arbitrary low-frequency filter setting of 1 Hz and a high filter cutoff of 10,000 Hz. Sequentially elevating the low-frequency filter from 1 Hz to 10 Hz, 100 Hz, and finally 300 Hz while maintaining a high-frequency filter of 10,000 Hz results in characteristic waveform distortions (Fig. 10–28). The onset latency does not change, the peak latency decreases, amplitude is serially reduced, and the total potential duration decreases. Also, an additional phase is created. The use of higher low-frequency filters removes low frequencies from the SNAP. In other words, the remaining potential now has a predominance of high frequencies contained in it as compared to the original potential. The onset of the potential is a quick departure from baseline and is not influenced by an alteration in the low-frequency content of the waveform. The remainder of the potential, however, is influenced by low-frequency subcomponent waveforms. By taking out the low frequencies, the amplitude is reduced as subcomponent waveforms are removed. The entire waveform is shifted to an earlier time of occurrence because of the high frequencies left in the SNAP. A third phase is created as the potential begins to appear more like a sine wave as the higher frequencies begin to emerge. A similar occurrence is noted for the CMAP.

Eliminating high frequencies results in a somewhat different set of alterations. Because we are removing waveforms from the total potential, a reduction in amplitude can be anticipated. The SNAP is thus biased toward a potential with more low frequencies and hence takes longer to occur in time. This results in a delay of both the onset and peak latencies (Fig. 10–29). Lowering the high-frequency filter while maintaining a constant low-frequency filter results in a waveform with a comparatively smaller amplitude, longer onset latency, and longer peak latency. Similar findings can be observed for a CMAP.

There are no universally agreed-upon filter settings for any electrodiagnostic medicine procedure. Arriving at optimal filter settings is highly empirical. The high- and low-frequency filters are respectively lowered and raised until waveform distortions are observed. The fil-

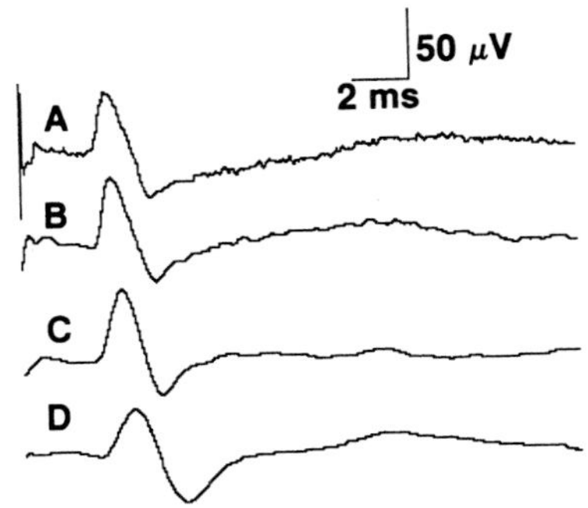

Trace	High frequency filter	Latency Onset	Latency Peak	Amplitude
	Hz	*ms*		*μV*
A	10,000	2.7	3.3	76
B	2,000	2.8	3.4	76
C	1,000	2.8	3.8	75
D	500	3.0	4.2	64

FIGURE 10–29. An antidromic median sensory nerve action potential is recorded from the third digit while a constant low-frequency filter of 10 Hz but different high-frequency filters are employed. Note how the onset and peak latencies are sequentially delayed with decreasing high-frequency filter settings. The potential's amplitude also decreases. (From Dumitru D, Walsh NE: Practical instrumentation and common sources of error. Am J Phys Med Rehabil 1988; 67:55–65.)

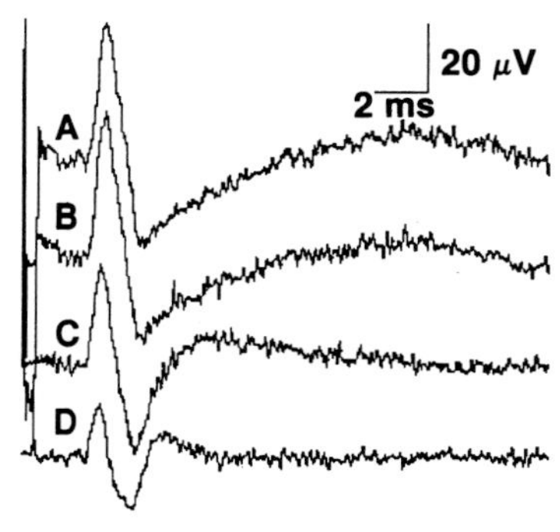

Trace	Low frequency	Latency Onset	Latency Peak	Duration negative spike	Amplitude
	Hz	*ms*		*ms*	*μv*
A	1	2.6	3.3	1.4	65
B	10	2.6	3.3	1.4	65
C	100	2.6	3.1	1.0	54
D	300	2.6	3.0	0.8	30

FIGURE 10–28. An antidromic median sensory nerve action potential is evoked from the third digit while the low frequency filter is sequentially elevated with a constant high frequency filter of 10,000 Hz. Note how the onset latency does not change, however, the peak latency decreases as does the potential's amplitude. A third phase is also produced at the low frequency filter setting of 300 Hz. (From Dumitru D, Walsh NE: Practical instrumentation and common sources of error. Am J Phys Med Rehabil 1988; 67:55–65.)

ters are then expanded until no waveform changes are noted. The goal is to include the major components of the waveforms while eliminating undesired signals or noise. The most important factor is to reproduce all filter settings originally described by those investigators whose normative data are being used (Table 10–3).

Sound

After the biological signal is filtered it is fed to a loudspeaker. The acoustic analysis of both normal and abnormal potentials is extremely important. It is not uncommon for practitioners to "hear" an abnormality prior to viewing it on the CRT. The instrument must have a relatively good speaker to accurately present the sounds associated with the biological signals.

Analog-to-Digital Conversion

All of today's commercially available instruments employ the conversion of a real-time analog signal to a digital representation of the recorded waveform. This is accomplished by sampling the potential at a given rate or frequency and assigning a digital representation of the waveform in the computer's memory. Complex signals with many changes over time and high frequencies must be sampled very fast in order to accurately reproduce them. If the sampling frequency is below that of the recorded waveform, considerable distortion can occur. The sampling frequency of the instrument must be at least twice as fast as the highest frequency contained in the waveform and is referred to as the Nyqvist frequency. For example, suppose the rise time, fast subcomponent, of a MUAP is 500 μs (0.5 msec). This rise time converts to a frequency of 2000 Hz:

$$\frac{1 \text{ time}}{0.5 \text{ msec}} \times \frac{1000 \text{ msec}}{1 \text{ sec}} = 200 \text{ Hz}$$

The Nyqvist frequency for this potential is 4000 Hz. The sampling frequency of the amplifier, therefore, must be at least 4000 Hz. This means that the instrument has to have a sweep speed capable of sampling the potential at the given frequency. For example, suppose our instrument has 1000 points (pts) of resolution across the screen for a sweep speed of 10 msec/div for a total screen of 10 division (100 msec). Our sampling frequency in this case is 10,000 Hz, which is more than enough to adequately resolve the waveform (1000 pts/100 msec × 1000 msec/1 sec = 10,000 pts/1 sec or 10,000 Hz). As noted above, the most useful conversion factor is 1000 msec/1 sec, as this converts how many times something happens per second into the appropriate number of Hz (Hz = Hertz = cycles per second).

TABLE 10–3 Recommended Filter Settings

Procedure	Low Frequency (Hz)	High Frequency (Hz)
NCV (Motor)	2–10	10,000
NCV (Sensory)	2–10	2,000
EMG (Routine)	20–30	10,000
EMG (Quantitative)	2–5	10,000
SFEMG	500–1,000	10,000–20,000
SEP	1–10	500–3,000

Abbreviations: NCV, nerve conduction velocity; EMG, needle electromyography; SFEMG, single-fiber electromyography; SEP, somatosensory-evoked potential.

From Dumitru D, Walsh NE: Practical instrumentation and common sources of error. Am J Phys Med Rehabil 1988; 67:55–65.

Averager

Most modern instruments typically have the capacity for averaging multiple responses. The goal of averaging a number of responses is to improve the size of the signal compared to the background noise, i.e., improve the signal-to-noise ratio. Responses can be averaged by taking advantage of the fact that the desired signal can be time-locked to appear in constant time referenced to a delivered electrical stimulus or internal instrument marker. The responses can thus be added while the randomly occurring noise phase cancels, thus improving the signal compared to the surrounding noise. This can be expressed mathematically as deriving the signal (S) to noise (N) ratio, which is directly proportional to the square root of the number of averages (n):

$$S/N = \frac{\text{Signal amplitude (S)} \times \sqrt{\text{Number of sweeps (n)}}}{\text{Noise amplitude}}$$

For example, if a signal has an amplitude of 2 mV while that of the noise is 4 mV, a single stimulus results in a signal-to-noise ratio (S/N) of 1/2 (S/N = [2 mV $\sqrt{1}$] ÷ 4 mV = 1/2). If four averages are performed, the S/N becomes 1/1. The S/N improved by the square root of the number of averages, or 2. Similarly, averaging 64 times results in an improvement by a factor of 8.

Stimulator

Two different types of stimulators are commercially available, constant current and constant voltage. For both types of devices, neural tissue is activated under the cathode (negative pole) while the anode (positive pole) completes the stimulating circuit. A constant current stimulator effectively delivers the desired current output for each stimulus irrespective of the resistance between the skin and cathode/anode. This is accomplished by varying the voltage or current driving force as is necessitated by any alterations in the skin/stimulator interface's resistance. Similarly, a constant voltage stimulator is designed to deliver the same voltage with each stimulus even if the resistance between the skin and stimulator changes. A compensatory increase or decrease in current is provided so as to maintain the same voltage level. In short, a constant current stimulator is effectively a variable voltage stimulator, while a constant voltage stimulator is also a variable current stimulator. Both stimulators are acceptable for most purposes. The constant current stimulator is preferred when the same current must be delivered for each stimulus in clinical situations requiring quantification of current delivery, e.g., somatosensory-evoked potentials, research, or evaluating side-to-side stimulation thresholds during facial nerve excitability testing.

An important problem associated with stimulators is the stimulus artifact. There is commonly a large potential recorded during the delivery of the stimulus, referred to as the shock or stimulus artifact. At times the magnitude of the potential is large enough to compromise the desired neural or muscular response. In such situations, it is necessary to minimize the shock artifact. An effective method of reducing the shock artifact is to employ fast recovery amplifiers that act to suppress this artifact by quickly recovering from the overwhelming voltage delivered. These amplifiers are not available on all instruments, and so other means must be found to deal with the artifact. The skin surface must be dry and any perspiration, body lotion, makeup, or other surface conductors should be removed. Wiping a large portion of the body segment under investigation with alcohol usually removes all surface conducting films. A ground electrode is best placed between the stimulus site and the active recording electrode. Wire leads between the patient and stimulator should be separated to avoid any type of capacitive interaction. The stimulator circuit should be isolated from the instrument's ground circuit, which is true of virtually all commercially manufactured instruments. Perhaps the most effective method of reducing stimulus artifact, once all of the above have been addressed, is to rotate the anode about the cathode. This optimizes the stimulator's voltage output as recorded by the active and reference electrode to take advantage of differential amplification and the elimination of the shock artifact as a common mode signal. An attempt is made to have both the active and reference electrodes record similar voltages, thereby minimizing the stimulator's signal from being amplified and displayed along with the signal.

Anodal block is an interesting concept that has been widely discussed but has little supporting experimental data. Theoretically the anode hyperpolarizes the neural tissue in its immediate vicinity and should result in an action potential failing to conduct past the anode. In humans, investigations employing bipolar and monopolar anodal current stimulation at the highest current outputs failed to document any type of anodal block. Since the anode is capable of stimulating neural tissue and not blocking it, at this time it appears that anodal block does not occur during the routine electrodiagnostic medicine consultation.

SUMMARY

Mastering the information provided in this chapter gives the practitioner a firm grasp of the fundamental principles that underpin the electrodiagnostic medicine consultation. Appreciating the formation and generation of an action potential is not a trivial matter. Of equal importance is the manner in which the electrophysiological instrument processes the biological signal of interest. An insufficient functional understanding of how the instrument can potentially distort the biological signal predisposes the practitioner to errors in diagnosis.

REFERENCES

1. Albers JW, Allen AA, Bastron JD, et al: Limb myokymia. Muscle Nerve 1981; 4:494–504.
2. Baer RD, Johnson EW: Motor nerve conduction velocities in normal children. Arch Phys Med Rehabil 1965; 46:698–704.
3. Bolton CF, Carter KM: Human sensory nerve compound action potential amplitude: Variation with sex and finger circumference. J Neurol Neurosurg Psychiatry 1980; 43:925–928.
4. Brown WF: The Physiological and Technical Basis of Electromyography. Boston, Butterworth, 1984, pp 317–368.
5. Buchthal F: Fibrillations: Clinical electrophysiology. In Culp WJ, Ochoa J (eds): Abnormal Nerves and Muscle Generators. New York, Oxford University Press, 1982, pp 632–662.
6. Buchthal F, Guld C, Rosenfalck P: Multielectrode study of the territory of a motor unit. Acta Physiol Scand 1957; 39:83–104.
7. Buchthal F, Guld C, Rosenfalck P: Volume conduction of the spike of the motor unit potential investigated with a new type of multielectrode. Acta Physiol Scand 1957; 38:331–354.
8. Buchthal F, Rosenfalck A: Evoked action potentials and conduction velocity in human sensory nerves. Brain Res 1966; 3:1–122.
9. Campbell WW, Ward LC, Swift TR: Nerve conduction velocity varies inversely with height. Muscle Nerve 1981; 4:520–523.
10. Cummins KL, Dorfman LJ: Nerve fiber conduction velocity distributions: Studies of normal and diabetic human nerves. Ann Neurol 1981; 9:67–74.
11. Daube JA: Needle Examination in Electromyography. AAEM Minimonograph no 11. Rochester, MN, American Association of Electrodiagnostic Medicine, 1979.
12. Dumitru D: Electrodiagnostic Medicine. Philadelphia, Hanley & Belfus, 1994.
13. Dumitru D: Volume conduction: Theory and application. In Dumitru D (ed): Physical Medicine and Rehabilitation State of the Art Reviews: Clinical Electrophysiology. Philadelphia, Hanley & Belfus, 1989, pp 665–682.
14. Dumitru D, DeLisa JA: Volume conduction. Muscle Nerve 1991; 14:605–624.
15. Dumitru D, Walsh NE: Electrophysiologic instrumentation. In Dumitru D (ed): Physical Medicine and Rehabilitation State of the Art Reviews: Clinical Electrophysiology. Philadelphia, Hanley & Belfus, 1989, pp 684–699.
16. Dumitru D, Walsh NE: Practical instrumentation and common source of error. Am J Phys Med Rehabil 1988; 67:55–65.
17. Falco FJE, Hennessey WJ, Braddom RL, et al: Standardized nerve conduction studies in the upper limb of the healthy elderly. Am J Phys Med Rehabil 1992; 71:263–271.
18. Falco FJE, Hennessey WJ, Goldberg G, et al: H reflex latency in the healthy elderly. Muscle Nerve 1994; 17:161–167.
19. Halar EM, DeLisa JA: Peroneal nerve conduction velocity: The importance of temperature control. Arch Phys Med Rehabil 1981; 62:439–443.
20. Halar EM, DeLisa JA, Brozovich FV: Nerve conduction velocity: Relationship of skin, subcutaneous and intramuscular temperatures. Arch Phys Med Rehabil 1980; 61:199–203.
21. Halar EM, DeLisa JA, Soine TL: Nerve conduction studies in upper extremities: Skin temperature corrections. Arch Phys Med Rehabil 1983; 64:412–416.
22. Henrikson JD: Conduction velocity of motor nerves in normal subjects and patients with neuromuscular disorders. Thesis, University of Minnesota, Minneapolis, 1956.
23. Hille B: Introduction to physiology of excitable cells. In Patton HD, Fuchs AF, Hille B, et al (eds): Textbook of Physiology, ed 21. Philadelphia, WB Saunders, 1989, pp 1–80.
24. Hodgkin AL, Huxley AF: A quantitative description of membrane current and its application to conduction and excitation in nerve. J Physiol 1952; 117:500–544.
25. Hodgkin AL, Katz B: The effect of temperature on the electrical activity of the giant axon of the squid. J Physiol 1949; 109:240–249.
26. Jewett DL, Rayner MD: Basic Concepts of Neuronal Function. Boston, Little, Brown, 1984.
27. Johnson EW, Olsen KJ: Clinical value of motor nerve conduction velocity determination. JAMA 1960; 172:2030–2035.
28. Katz B: Nerve, Muscle, and Synapse. New York, McGraw-Hill, 1966.

29. Koester J: Resting membrane potential and action potential. In Kandel ER, Schwartz JH (ed): Principles of Neural Science, ed 2. New York, Elsevier, 1985, pp 49–57.
30. Lang AH, Forsstrom J, Bjorkqvist SE, et al: Statistical variation of nerve conduction velocity: An analysis in normal subjects and uraemic patients. J Neurol Sci 1977; 33:229–241.
31. Layzer RB, Rowland LP: Cramps. N Engl J Med 1971; 285:30–31.
32. Lundborg G: Nerve Injury and Repair. Edinburgh, Churchill Livingstone, 1988.
33. Oh SJ: Clinical Electromyography: Nerve Conduction Studies, ed 2. Baltimore, Williams & Wilkins, 1993.
34. Schoepfle GM, Erlanger J: The action of temperature on the excitability, spike height and configuration, and the refractory period observed in the responses of single medullated nerve fibers. Am J Physiol 1941; 134:694–704.
35. Seddon H: Three types of nerve injury. Brain 1943; 66:237–288.
36. Soudmand R, Ward LC, Swift TR: Effect of height on nerve conduction velocity. Neurology 1982; 32:407–410.
37. Stolov W: Instrumentation and Measurement in Electrodiagnosis. AAEM Minimonograph no 16. Rochester, MN, American Association of Electrodiagnostic Medicine, 1981.
38. Streib EW: Differential diagnosis of myotonic syndromes (AAEM Minimonograph no 2). Muscle Nerve 1987; 10:603–615.
39. Sunderland S: A classification of peripheral nerve injuries producing loss of function. Brain 1951; 74:491–516.
40. Sunderland S: Nerve Injuries and Their Repair: A Critical Appraisal. Edinburgh, Churchill Livingstone, 1991.
41. Thesleff S: Fibrillation in denervated mammalian muscle. In Culp WJ, Ochoa J (eds): Abnormal Nerve and Muscle as Impulse Generators. New York, Oxford University Press, 1982, pp 678–694.
42. Trojaborg W: Motor nerve conduction velocities in normal subjects with particular reference to the conduction in proximal and distal segments of median and ulnar nerve. Electroencephalogr Clin Neurophysiol 1964; 17:314–321.
43. Waxman SG, Foster RE: Ionic channel distribution and heterogeneity of the axon membrane in myelinated fibers. Brain Res Rev 1980; 2:205–234.
44. Waxman SG: Action potential propagation and conduction velocity: New perspectives and questions. Trends Neurosci 1983; 6:157–161.

11
CHAPTER

Lawrence R. Robinson, M.D.

Electrodiagnostic Medicine II: Clinical Evaluation and Findings

CLINICAL ASSESSMENT

Among medical consultations and laboratory testing, the electrodiagnostic medical consultation is unique. Conceptually, it is a history and physical examination extended by the singular capabilities of electrophysiological testing, which can include nerve conduction studies, needle electromyography (EMG), somatosensory evoked potentials (SEPs), single-fiber EMG, and other studies. The consultation starts with a directed history and physical examination and uses electrophysiological testing to help distinguish among the possible differential diagnoses in a more sensitive fashion than is possible with clinical examination alone.

The electrodiagnostic consultation has important distinctions from laboratory tests. It relies greatly on the consultant's history and physical examination; moreover, it is a dynamic process. Specific methods employed depend on the clinical assessment and are contingent upon the outcomes of some of the initial tests. These can change dynamically throughout the consultation. In contrast, other types of laboratory testing (such as serum chemistries or electroencephalography [EEG]) are usually performed in a standard fashion and findings are interpreted after the patient leaves the office or hospital.

As with any other type of testing, the electrodiagnostic medical consultant must try to find electrophysiological abnormalities, preferably multiple ones, that are consistent with the patient's clinical presentation. Diagnoses should not be made solely on electrophysiological "abnormalities," but must always be made in the context of the patient's clinical presentation.

History

A directed history serves to generate a list of differential diagnoses and allows the examiner to plan the electrophysiological examination. The history should be initially directed toward the presenting chief complaint. A number of components of the history are especially pertinent to the electrodiagnostic medical consultation. Among these components are the time since onset of symptoms, the quality of those symptoms, and their distribution. The time since onset of symptoms is extremely important because the electrophysiological findings evolve over time. For instance, a radiculopathy studied five days after onset of symptoms is unlikely to show as much electrophysiological evidence of denervation as one studied 21 days after onset of symptoms. Finding out whether symptoms are intermittent or constant is also important, as the likelihood of finding abnormalities on the electrophysiological examination is higher in the case of constant symptoms. The distribution of symptoms is also relevant. Although symptoms are usually reported initially in one or two limbs, one should also ask about other limbs. The patient with hand numbness, for example, could have entrapment neuropathy in the upper limbs. However, if the lower limbs are also involved, the examiner should do a wider search for a peripheral polyneuropathy. For the examiner, then, it is critical to have information about the quality and distribution of symptoms, as well as an intimate knowledge of peripheral nervous system anatomy.

Although an extensive search of the past medical history is not always productive for the electrodiagnostic medical consultation, several points should always be raised. The examiner should routinely ask about patient medications, thereby eliciting other pertinent diagnoses and uncovering possible toxic exposures. Such questions may also reveal the possibility of anticoagulation (which is critical to know before starting a needle examination). It is also necessary to obtain a history of systemic disease that might contribute to the chief complaint, such as a history of diabetes mellitus, extensive alcohol intake, or rheumatologic disease. In addition, it is important to know whether or not the presenting symptoms have occurred in the past, so that finding old electrophysiological changes is not confusing.

Finally, the examiner should always inquire about the family history of similar or congenital diseases. Some peripheral polyneuropathies and myopathies are inherited disorders. Thus, it is occasionally necessary to examine or test potentially affected family members.

Physical Examination

Whereas the history contributes most significantly to establishing a differential diagnosis, physical examination offers more objective evidence of peripheral nervous system dysfunction. In most cases, the four most important examinations are muscle strength, sensation, muscle stretch reflexes, and provocative signs. The strength examination (manual muscle testing) should be directed to all four limbs, to look for widespread abnormalities and to assess any underlying poor effort. While weakness can be severe, in most cases it is mild or subtle. Accordingly, muscles should be tested near their "break" points, rather than in positions in which resistance cannot be overcome. The examiner must be sure to obtain a maximum mechanical advantage in performing the muscle strength testing, obtaining the maximal lever arm by applying force as far as possible from the joint. The examiner should also put particularly strong muscles at added stretch to put them at a mechanical disadvantage, using gravity and body weight as an aid to stress antigravity muscles maximally. Simply testing dorsiflexion or plantar flexion at the ankle against manual resistance, for example, is insufficient. The examiner should also have the patient walk on the heels and the toes or do a sequence of ten raises up on the toes.

Sensory testing should be directed at eliciting subtle deficits in sensation. Unlike patients with spinal cord injury, patients with entrapment neuropathies or radiculopathies often have mild or difficult-to-assess sensory losses. Finding out whether the patient can distinguish pinprick from dull touch is usually of insufficient sensitivity, except when severe deficits are present. Pinprick and light touch sensation in a questionable area should be compared with that of an asymptomatic area (such as the cheek or forehead) or with the same location on the other side if it is not symptomatic. A useful technique is to touch the asymptomatic area first, then the symptomatic area, asking the patient, "If this [asymptomatic] area is 100%, how much is this [symptomatic] area?" Two-point discrimination has been shown to pick up milder deficits in sensation than simple pinprick testing. Testing vibration is useful if particular involvement of large fibers (as in peripheral polyneuropathy) is expected or if the dorsal column pathways are expected to be spared (as in syringomyelia).

Muscle stretch reflexes (MSRs) are probably the most objective finding in the examination of the peripheral nervous system, as they are not easily influenced by patient cooperation or reporting. In addition to the commonly elicited reflexes in the upper limb (biceps, brachioradialis, and triceps) and lower limb (knee and ankle), other MSRs should be considered. In the lower limbs, the most common level for radiculopathy is L5. Because the knee jerk largely represents L4 input and the ankle jerk largely S1 input, it is quite easy to miss reflex changes in an L5 radiculopathy unless the medial hamstring or tibialis posterior reflexes are checked routinely. In the upper limb, C7 is the most common level for radiculopathy. Although the triceps reflex is useful in this regard, the pronator teres reflex (elicited by tapping the neutrally positioned forearm into supination and palpating over the pronator teres) can be useful for detecting C6 or C7 changes. Other reflexes, such as Hoffmann's or Babinski's reflexes, are useful to distinguish upper motor neuron from lower motor neuron changes (see Chapter 1 for additional information).

Several useful provocative tests can be employed in the physical examination prior to electrophysiological studies. When considering entrapment neuropathies, Phalen's test is a moderately sensitive and specific test for detecting median nerve compression at the wrist. This is performed by keeping the wrist in sustained flexion for 60 seconds and monitoring for paresthesias. Tinel's sign (which was originally developed for detecting the most distal site of peripheral nerve regeneration) is sensitive but not very specific. It can be elicited over the median nerve at the wrist or ulnar nerve at the elbow in the case of entrapment; however, many asymptomatic control subjects also have a positive test over many peripheral nerves. When considering the possibility of cervical radiculopathy, one should look for Spurling's sign by bringing the neck into extension and lateral flexion toward the side being tested. If one applies pressure to the top of the head and elicits pain extending out to the shoulder or beyond, this is a positive test and might indicate the presence of cervical radiculopathy. In the lower limb, straight leg raising tests or other sciatic stretch maneuvers can provide additional useful information about the presence of a lumbosacral radiculopathy.

Depending on the clinical presentation, other parts of the physical examination can be employed. For example, when looking for neuromuscular junction disease or motor neuron disease, a thorough cranial nerve examination should be performed. In suspected myopathies, one should look for muscle tenderness.

Differential Diagnosis

After reviewing the referring physician's request and performing a history and physical examination, the consultant should generate a credible list of differential diagnoses. Even if the referring physician's diagnosis is unlikely, the consultant should perform testing to address it specifically, as the referring physician is expecting a response about this specific diagnosis.

Initial Plan

Based on the list of differential diagnoses, an electrophysiological examination plan should be developed to look for and distinguish between the possibilities listed. This plan could start off with either electromyographic (EMG) or nerve conduction studies (NCS), depending on the differential diagnoses. The initial goal is to get as much pertinent information as possible in the shortest amount of time (and, consequently, at the lowest cost for the patient). For focal or distal problems where it is possible to stimulate proximal and distal to the suspected problem, it is usually best to begin with nerve conduction studies. Examples of such problems include carpal tunnel syndrome and ulnar neuropathy. For predominantly proximal lesions, such as radiculopathies, it is often best to start with needle EMG. For potentially diffuse or multifocal processes, needle EMG is usually a more rapid way of determining how widespread the problem is. There is a great variation among examiners as to whether they start with NCS or EMG. The underlying goal is to obtain the most useful information with the smallest number of tests. The goal also includes maximizing the marginal gain of each additional test and avoiding unnecessary tests.

The initial plan should not be rigid. Often, it has to be changed or modified as information is obtained. It is also inappropriate to use a single standardized protocol for all patients. Because the electrodiagnostic medical consultation is a dynamic process, the testing strategy should be changed quickly as new information is obtained and items on the differential diagnosis are either added or deleted.

NEEDLE ELECTROMYOGRAPHY

Preparing the Patient

Preparing the patient is a critical first step in performing a needle EMG. The patient should get a clear explanation of what is to happen and what the experience is like. Explanatory pamphlets (the American Association of Electrodiagnostic Medicine offers some good ones) are helpful; however, most patients require an additional verbal explanation—one that establishes an appropriate level of rapport with the examiner. Examiners vary widely in the wording they use to explain the procedure, but many find it useful to avoid words with strong negative connotations. It is often reassuring, for example, to say "pin" electrode rather than "needle," electrical "pulse" or "stimulus" as opposed to "shock," and "uncomfortable" instead of "painful." It is also helpful to give the patient some measure of control, saying, for instance, "Let me know if I get into an especially uncomfortable area." It is usually not helpful to show the patient the needle electrode, as most patients erroneously associate needle length with level of discomfort. While it is not standard practice to have the patient sign a consent form for the procedure, it is advisable to inform the patient of any risks that might be involved as well as the potential benefits. If one is performing a high-risk procedure (e.g., intercostal muscle EMG), then informed consent should be obtained.

Patient position is important for comfort as well as for ease and accuracy of the examination. The patient should be in a relaxed position, with the muscles to be examined easily accessible. Patients should be gowned and appropriately covered with a blanket or sheet. The room should be reasonably warm, both to keep the patient comfortable and to prevent distortion of the electrophysiological findings by cooling.

Deciding on an Electrode to Use

Assuming that the electrodiagnostic instrument is ready and the patient is prepared and adequately positioned, the next step is to choose an electrode for needle EMG. The two common types are monopolar and concentric electrodes. Each has advantages, with differences predominantly in recording surface area, price, and, possibly, level of discomfort.

The monopolar needle EMG electrode is composed of a single solid-core pin, which is Teflon-coated except for an exposed tip. Electrical potentials are usually measured with reference to a nearby surface electrode. The monopolar electrode has a larger recording area than the concentric electrode, is less expensive, and may (as many maintain) be less painful. The larger recording area is advantageous when recording potentials that might be distant, such as fibrillations or positive sharp waves. In performing quantitative motor unit potential analysis, however, the larger recording surface area is a disadvantage because extraneous noise from distant potentials is incorporated into the signal. Quantitative EMG reference data have generally been obtained with concentric electrodes, although motor unit action potential durations might not be very different when the two needles are compared. When reusable needle EMG electrodes are used, price can be a factor, as disposable monopolar electrodes are currently about one-fourth the cost of disposable concentric electrodes.

The concentric EMG needle electrode has a more standardized, smaller recording surface area. It does not use a surface reference electrode. The wire running through the center of the insulated shaft is electrically referenced to the exposed outside shaft of the needle. The concentric needle electrode is most useful in performing quantitative motor unit potential analysis. It is particularly useful if a recording is desired from a restricted area near the tip of the needle. Electrodiagnostic consultants should feel comfortable using either type of needle electrode for EMG and should be able to switch between the two types, depending on the clinical circumstances. Disposable needle electrodes have gained widespread acceptance due to fear of spreading infectious disease through reusable needles. The risk of spreading infection through properly sterilized reusable electrodes, however, is probably no greater than that for reusable surgical instruments. A review of proper sterilization techniques can be found in the *Guidelines in Electrodiagnostic Medicine,* published by the American

Association of Electrodiagnostic Medicine (421 First Avenue SW, Rochester, Minnesota).

When performing the needle examination, it is advisable to use appropriate safety precautions for exposure to bodily fluids. Both of the examiner's hands should be gloved during the examination, and needles should not be recapped using a two-handed technique. Needle electrodes that facilitate one-handed recapping are available. Another technique is to tape the cap onto the side of the electrodiagnostic instrument and to insert the needle using a one-handed technique. When the examination is finished, the needle should be disposed of in an appropriate container without recapping.

Steps of the Needle EMG Examination

The needle EMG examination for each muscle can usually be divided into four distinct steps: (1) insertional activity; (2) spontaneous activity; (3) examination of motor unit potentials; and (4) assessment of recruitment. An excellent summary of the findings on needle EMG examination can be found in a recently published review article.[6]

Insertional Activity

Insertional activity is examined by moving the needle through the muscle briefly and observing the amount and duration of the electrical potentials produced. These potentials are mechanically evoked due to the advancement of the needle. Usually, insertional activity and spontaneous activity should be examined using three to four insertions for each of the four different muscle quadrants. The duration of insertional activity varies from one examiner to another. After a brief, small movement of the needle, insertional activity usually persists for no more than 300 msec. The electrodiagnostic consultant can practice assessing the duration of insertional activity by using a slow sweep speed (such as 100 msec/division).

Insertional activity can be decreased or prolonged in duration. *Decreased insertional activity* means that the usual degree of injury potentials is not elicited. Decreased insertional activity can result from not being in muscle, or from being in a muscle that has fewer viable fibers than normal. Muscles that have become atrophied, been replaced by fat, or become fibrotic have reduced insertional activity. Muscles that have become necrotic due to compartment syndrome or other causes of ischemia also have reduced insertional activity, which is a poor prognostic sign for recovery. Muscles that have become electrically silent, such as during attacks of periodic paralysis, also have reduced insertional activity.

Increased insertional activity is usually considered to be prolonged muscle membrane activity lasting more than 300 msec after the needle movement stops. Prolonged or increased insertional activity, as an isolated finding, is a "soft" finding. No diagnosis can be made solely on the basis of this "abnormality." One exception is the *syndrome of diffusely abnormal increased insertional activity,* an autosomally dominant inherited syndrome without any clear associated symptomatology.[40] Increased insertional activity can also be seen in association with fibrillations or positive sharp waves, in which cases it supports the impression of either denervation or primary muscle pathological lesions. Some authors argue that increased insertional activity is an early finding after denervation, before sustained positive sharp waves or fibrillations become apparent.

Spontaneous Activity

Spontaneous activity consists of electrical discharges that are seen without needle movement or voluntary contraction. These are usually looked for after each needle placement or movement, when the needle is stationary. Some spontaneous activity, recorded near the endplate zone (endplate noise and endplate spikes), is normal.

Endplate noise (reflecting miniature endplate potentials, or MEPPs) and endplate spikes (reflecting endplate potentials, or EPPs) are normal findings. It is critical to recognize these for several reasons. First, the endplate zone is a painful area, and staying in this region increases the discomfort of the examination. Second, endplate spikes have short-duration biphasic morphological characteristics that can be mistaken for fibrillation potentials by the inexperienced examiner. In contrast to fibrillation potentials, however, endplate spikes are almost always initially negative (whereas fibrillations are initially positive) and they discharge in an irregular, sputtering rhythm. Third, if the needle electrode is put into the endplate zone and then pushed through it, the endplate spikes recorded from a distance can assume the morphological characteristics of fibrillation potentials with an initial positivity. It is important to recognize endplate noise and endplate spikes and to withdraw the needle from that area of the muscle quickly and proceed to another area.

Fibrillation potentials represent abnormal spontaneous single muscle fiber discharges. They are short in duration (usually less than 5 msec) and biphasic, with an initial positivity in almost all instances. Although fibrillation potentials are essentially always abnormal, they are a nonspecific finding. They represent abnormal muscle membrane irritability, which can occur in many disorders. Fibrillation potentials are often seen in denervated muscles. Myopathies can be associated with fibrillation potentials. This is especially common in inflammatory myopathies. They are the least likely to occur in chronic steroid or thyroid myopathies. Direct muscle trauma, intramuscular injections, or intramuscular bleeding have been noted to produce both immediate and chronic fibrillations. Neuromuscular junction disorders, particularly presynaptic disorders (e.g., botulism) or occasionally severe postsynaptic defects (e.g., myasthenia gravis), can produce fibrillation potentials. Upper motor neuron lesions, such as stroke and spinal cord injury, have also been shown to produce fibrillation potentials. These are usually seen early after onset of the lesion and can be confusing when trying to diagnose a peripheral nerve lesion superimposed on an upper motor neuron disorder.

Fibrillation potentials, as well as positive sharp waves, are usually graded on a subjective, qualitative scheme.

Usually this ranges from 1+ to 4+, with 1+ representing a reproducibly observed fibrillation in an isolated area and 4+ representing sustained fibrillation potentials, often obscuring the baseline, throughout the muscle. Grading schemes vary somewhat from one laboratory to another. It should be remembered, however, that this is an ordinal, nonquantitative, noninterval scale. A finding of 2+ fibrillation potentials does not necessarily represent twice as much denervation as a 1+. Because each axon supplies many muscle fibers, the loss of only a few axons can produce many fibrillation potentials. It takes relatively little axon loss to produce 4+ fibrillation potentials. In clinical studies comparing functional outcome with the grading of fibrillation potentials, there has not been very good correlation, because density of fibrillations does not reliably estimate the degree of axon loss. The size of the compound muscle action potential (CMAP) elicited distal to the lesion is a better reflection of the viable axon population than the grading of the number of fibrillation potentials.

Fibrillation potentials decrease in size over time.[21] Large-amplitude fibrillation potentials (greater than 100 μV) are seen within the first year after onset of denervation, and smaller amplitudes (less than 100 μV) are seen later. It has been postulated that this relationship reflects muscle fiber atrophy over time, with smaller diameter fibers producing smaller amplitude fibrillations. Consequently, large-amplitude fibrillations in the presence of a neuropathic lesion suggest recent denervation.

Fibrillation potentials after denervation are probably related to acetylcholine hypersensitivity. After denervation, extrajunctional receptors appear on muscle fibers and the muscle fiber membrane comes closer to its firing threshold. The time course for the appearance of fibrillation potentials is similar to that for the development of acetylcholine hypersensitivity. However, some debate exists as to whether this represents the true mechanism.[28] In the case of myopathies, segmental necrosis is thought to account for fibrillation potentials. A myopathic fiber can become necrotic over only a focal portion of its length, leaving a portion of viable muscle fiber (distal to the necrotic area and separated from the motor end-plate by the necrotic area) functionally denervated. Experimental evidence in human and animal models supports this hypothesis.[8, 30] For patients with upper motor neuron lesions, the etiology of fibrillations is less well delineated. Some authors have proposed that fibrillations are due to transsynaptic degeneration, whereby the lower motor neuron receives less trophic influence from the upper motor neuron.[38]

Positive sharp waves can be thought of in much the same way as fibrillation potentials. They also represent abnormal single muscle fiber discharges, although they are often evoked by needle movement and may be recorded in a different way (see Chapter 10). Positive sharp waves can be seen in essentially all of the same disorders in which fibrillation potentials are seen. In addition, positive sharp waves can be seen in some cases in which fibrillations are not typically seen.[22] In the autosomally dominant inherited syndrome of diffusely abnormal insertional activity, positive sharp waves are abundant, but fibrillations are not.[40] Early after denervation, particularly when recording with a monopolar electrode, positive sharp waves are much more prominent than fibrillation potentials (fibrillations become more prominent later). In some cases of muscle trauma, positive sharp waves can be seen in isolation, without associated fibrillations. Positive sharp waves are thought to have the same pathophysiology as fibrillation potentials and can be graded using the same scheme.

Complex repetitive discharges (CRDs), formerly known as bizarre high-frequency discharges, probably represent groups of muscle fibers firing in near synchrony. Single fiber electromyography has suggested that complex repetitive discharges are produced by a fibrillating muscle fiber that acts as a "pacer" and ephaptically (membrane to membrane, without any neurotransmitter-modulated synapse) activates adjacent muscle fibers. This has been likened to the reentry phenomenon associated with some cardiac arrhythmias. These groups of muscle fibers then discharge in near synchrony with constant interspike intervals. A hallmark of CRDs is that they start and stop abruptly, unlike positive sharp waves or myotonia. CRDs can have any wave shape, with rates varying from 0.3 to 150 Hz. Complex repetitive discharges are a nonspecific finding. They are usually seen in chronic neuropathic or myopathic conditions, but are occasionally seen acutely in inflammatory myopathies. When seen in isolation, CRDs are a nonspecific but usually abnormal finding, similar in diagnostic meaning to positive sharp waves and fibrillations. Some have reported observing CRDs in the iliopsoas muscle of normal individuals,[20] and this author has observed CRDs in the levator scapulae in several individuals without lower motor neuron lesions (personal observation).

Myotonia is a rarely seen discharge that waxes and wanes in both amplitude and frequency. Its sound, when heard on the electrodiagnostic instrument, has been likened to that of a dive bomber or a revving motorcycle. Myotonia can be seen in a variety of myotonic disorders, such as myotonic dystrophy, paramyotonia, or congenital myotonia,[35] but it can also be seen rarely in inflammatory myopathies.[6] Acid maltase deficiency has also been reported to produce myotonic discharges, particularly in the paraspinal or other proximal muscles.

Myotonia can be accentuated by tapping the muscle or by needle movement. In cases of clinically or electrophysiologically mild myotonia, cooling the limb often produces myotonic bursts of increased amplitude that persist longer. In many myotonic conditions the intrinsic hand muscles (e.g., thenar muscles) show the highest incidence of myotonia. Myotonia exists in many mammals, but its pathophysiology is not well understood. There is some evidence that abnormal chloride conductance at the muscle fiber membrane might be involved.[20]

Fasciculation potentials represent spontaneous discharges of all or of part of a single motor unit. As opposed to a fibrillation potential (in which just a single muscle fiber fires), a fasciculation potential involves multiple muscle fibers of the motor unit. Fasciculations produce enough muscle contraction that they are often visible through the skin on clinical examination. Because a fasciculation potential often involves the discharge of an entire motor unit, a *single* fasciculation potential cannot be distinguished from a *single* voluntary motor unit action potential. It is only by their firing patterns that the two can be distinguished. While voluntary motor unit potentials fire in a regular, semirhythmic pattern, typically at rates from 5 to 15 Hz during early recruitment, fasciculation potentials fire in a *random* pattern that is not under voluntary control. Fasciculation potentials are often generated at the anterior horn cell, as in motor neuron diseases, but they can also be generated ectopically distally along the axon, possibly even in intramuscular axons.

Fasciculation potentials can be seen in a variety of neuromuscular disorders. "Benign" fasciculations occur in otherwise healthy individuals in whom there are no other associated signs, symptoms, or electrophysiological abnormalities. They are often seen in healthy people who are stressed, tired, lack sleep, or who are sensitive to chemicals in the diet (e.g., caffeine). Benign fasciculation potentials tend to fire more rapidly than those in patients with motor neuron disease, but the difference in rate of firing is not sufficient to permit unequivocal distinction between the two syndromes. A more reliable judge of the clinical significance of fasciculations is the presence or absence of associated electrodiagnostic findings. Motor neuron disease is typically expected to show fibrillation potentials, positive sharp waves, and abnormal motor unit potentials in association with fasciculations. Benign fasciculations are seen in individuals who have no other electrophysiological findings. Complex fasciculation (polyphasic, long duration) potentials can be a reason for concern, because these indicate that the motor units that are discharging spontaneously have undergone some axonal sprouting and reinnervation. These are more likely to be seen in a lower motor neuron disorder than in benign fasciculation syndromes. Fasciculation potentials can also be seen in chronic radiculopathies, peripheral polyneuropathies, thyrotoxicosis, and overdosage of anticholinesterase medications.

Myokymia results from groups of motor units firing synchronously in a regular bursting pattern. This can often be seen through the skin surface as a wormlike (or vermicular) movement. When heard over the loudspeaker of the electrodiagnostic instrument, myokymia sounds like a platoon of marching soldiers. The pathophysiology of myokymia is poorly understood, but it probably arises in the lower motor neuron cell body (in the anterior horn of the spinal cord or the brainstem nucleus) or axon.

Myokymia is a rare finding, but it can be seen in a variety of neurological disorders. It is classified into two distinct groups: facial myokymia and limb myokymia. Facial myokymia has been reported with multiple sclerosis, brainstem neoplasia (pontine gliomas), facial palsy, and hemifacial spasm. Limb myokymia has been reported in radiation plexopathy/neuropathy and some chronic compression neuropathies, as well as in gold polyneuropathy (patients with rheumatologic disorders treated with gold agents). Knowledge of the association with radiation treatment becomes especially important when trying to identify whether a new brachial plexopathy after radiation treatment for malignancy (e.g., breast cancer) represents a recurrence of tumor or radiation plexopathy. Patients with radiation plexopathy usually have myokymia, upper trunk lesions, and paresthesias, whereas those with recurrent tumor typically have painful lower trunk lesions without myokymia but with Horner's syndrome.[24]

Motor Unit Analysis

A great deal of information can be obtained from analysis of voluntarily activated motor unit action potentials (MUAPs). This information is more diagnostically specific for neuropathic or myopathic changes than is the assessment of spontaneous activity at rest.

Theoretically, in neuropathic conditions in which partial denervation and reinnervation has occurred, changes representative of the underlying process of axonal sprouting can be seen (Fig. 11–1). Within days after partial denervation,[28] intramuscular axons that remain unaffected send out sprouts, usually emanating from distal nodes of Ranvier or axon terminals, to reinnervate nearby denervated muscle fibers. These sprouts are initially poorly myelinated and conduct slowly. Consequently, in the early phases of reinnervation, motor unit action potentials have increased polyphasicity and duration. This is the direct result of temporal dispersion in these newly formed sprouts and poor synchronization of muscle fiber discharges. The neuromuscular junctions at the terminals of these new sprouts are not yet mature and are unreliable with respect to consistently transmitting across the myoneural junction. Unstable MUAPs can be seen with morphological characteristics and size that vary with repetitive firing. As these sprouts mature, synchronization of muscle fiber discharges improves, and the polyphasicity is somewhat reduced. The final status of reinnervated MUAPs is that they are typically large in amplitude, long in duration, and sometimes polyphasic. The increase in amplitude is a result of the increased density of muscle fibers belonging to the same motor unit within the recording area of the tip of the EMG needle.

Myopathic changes in the MUAP result from loss of individual muscle fibers, impairment to muscle fibers, or temporal dispersion of conduction along muscle fibers. In myopathic conditions, the MUAPs are typically small in amplitude and short in duration. There are fewer muscle fibers from the same motor unit firing within the recording area of the needle electrode. Polyphasicity is increased, although the reasons behind this are not completely understood. In part, polyphasicity might result from dropout of muscle fibers, causing loss of the normally smooth synchronous discharge of all the muscle fibers firing together. Additionally, the affected muscle fibers might conduct more slowly than usual, increasing temporal dispersion and, consequently, polyphasicity within the MUAP.

Neuromuscular junction (NMJ) diseases tend in many ways to mimic the changes seen with myopathy. Because some of the individual muscle fibers in the motor unit cannot fire with the rest of the motor unit, the duration can be shortened and the amplitude reduced. Consequently, NMJ disease should also be considered whenever short-duration, low-amplitude MUAPs are

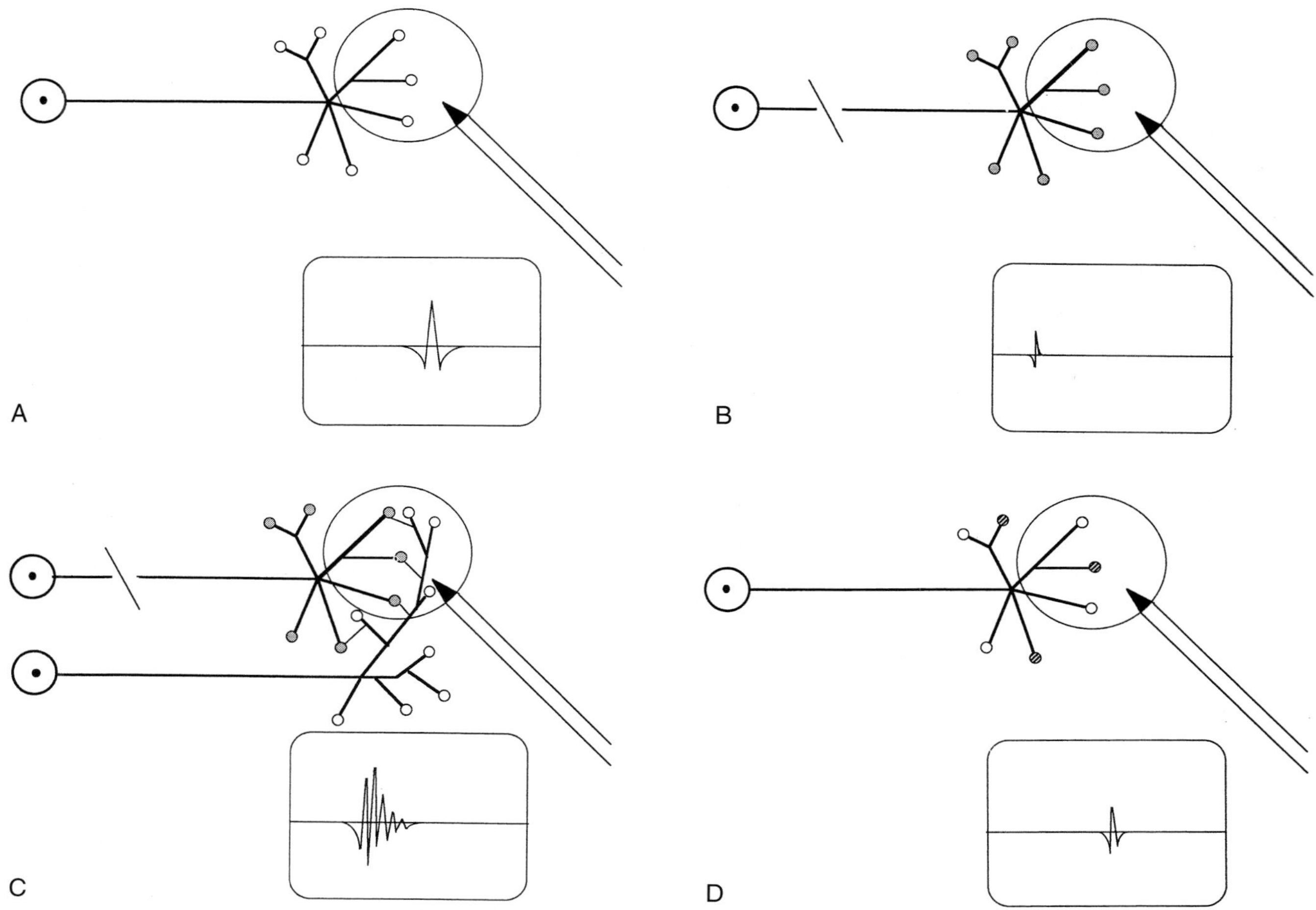

FIGURE 11–1. *A.* The normal motor unit action potential (MUAP). A needle electrode records from muscle fibers within the recording area of the needle. *B.* After denervation, single muscle fibers spontaneously discharge, producing fibrillations (or positive sharp waves). *C.* When reinnervation by axon sprouting has occurred, the newly formed sprouts conduct slowly, producing temporal dispersion (i.e., prolonged motor unit potential duration) and polyphasicity in the MUAP. The higher density of muscle fibers within the recording area of the needle that belong to the enlarging second motor unit results in an increased-amplitude MUAP. *D.* In myopathies, some muscle fibers in the motor unit become necrotic or dysfunctional and no longer contribute to the MUAP, producing shorter durations and smaller amplitudes.

observed. Motor unit variability or instability also increases in NMJ defects as a result of intermittent blocking of NMJ transmission.

The three most commonly used parameters of MUAPs are amplitude (peak to peak), duration, and number of phases. Amplitude is the easiest parameter to measure, but is largely a reflection only of those muscle fibers closest to the tip of the needle. In fact, the high-frequency components of more distant muscle fiber discharges are filtered out during passage through the volume conductor of the body—that is, the intervening tissue acts like a low-pass filter. An analogy can be made with sound waves transmitted through the air. (Consider your neighbor's stereo system for instance. The low rumble of drums is more bothersome than the high-voiced piccolos, because the high-frequency components are filtered out in transmission through the air.) Likewise, the high-frequency spike component of the MUAP where the amplitude is measured is representative of the few muscle fibers very close to the recording surface. Muscle fibers that are distant are recorded with much lower amplitudes and predominantly low-frequency components.

Electromyographers note empirically that amplitude is very dependent on distance from the electrode. A MUAP can be recorded as having a relatively small amplitude or large amplitude, depending on how much effort is put into "focusing" the needle close to the discharging muscle fibers. Typically the needle is moved to obtain the largest amplitude possible for a MUAP, which usually occurs when the potential sound is sharp rather than dull on the electrodiagnostic instrument. This sharp sound comes from the higher amplitude and rapid rise time of the chief spike of the MUAP. Although amplitude is to some extent a reflection of the density of muscle fibers within the MUAP, it is relatively unreliable as compared with other measures, because it depends on how much effort is put into "focusing" on the potential.

Duration from the onset to the end of the motor unit action potential is a better reflection of the number of active muscle fibers within the motor unit, i.e., the motor unit territory. Measurement of mean motor unit duration is the most reliable routine electrophysiological feature to use in distinguishing between "neuropathic" and "myopathic" conditions. It is less dependent on distance from the motor unit, because duration is being measured from both the initial and terminal low-frequency components of the potential conducted from distant muscle fibers. A problem with duration, however, is the technical difficulty inherent in its measurement. It is difficult to measure MUAP duration when watching voluntary motor units fly by on a regular sweep speed, except for detecting gross changes. One cannot easily tell where one motor unit starts and another stops when multiple potentials are present, and often baseline noise obscures the start or finish of the motor unit (Fig. 11–2). For an accurate representation of MUAP duration, a trigger and delay line should be used. To reduce random baseline noise, multiple discharges of a motor unit should be combined by averaging. It has been shown repeatedly that mean values for at least 20 different MUAPs must be taken to develop reliable MUAP measures.

Polyphasicity as an isolated finding is nonspecific and is often overreported and overinterpreted. The phases of a motor unit can be counted as the baseline crossings plus one. When MUAPs have more than five phases, they are termed *polyphasic potentials.* Most normal muscles have at least 10% polyphasic MUAPs, depending on the muscle examined and the type of needle electrode used. Increased polyphasicity can be seen in both neuropathic and myopathic conditions, but it is not specific for either. The electrodiagnostician should be reluctant to make a diagnostic statement solely on the basis of an isolated finding of increased polyphasicity.

Motor unit variability or instability is manifested as a change in amplitude or morphological characteristics of MUAPs during repetitive firing. This is usually due to instability or unreliability in neuromuscular junction (NMJ) transmission, either as a result of a primary defecte in the NMJ or as a result of recent reinnervation.

Several different methods are available to assess voluntary MUAPs during performance of an EMG. The optimal method can vary and depends on the clinical question being asked, the equipment and software available, the experience of the examiner with various techniques, and the probable subtlety of the findings expected.

The most commonly used method, usually when assessing for possible radiculopathy or entrapment neuropathy, is "semiquantitative." Several MUAPs are examined as they fire during low effort, without a trigger and delay line or any actual quantitative measurement (except possibly for peak-to-peak amplitude of a few of the larger MUAPs). The experienced examiner can notice marked changes in MUAPs, but this method is not sufficient to find more subtle changes. These semiquantitative methods are often acceptable when looking for neuropathic conditions in which other indications of neuropathy are typically present (such as positive sharp waves and fibrillations or changes on nerve conduction studies), or if the MUAP changes are marked.

An incremental improvement to this method is the employment of a trigger and delay line and a visual examination of several motor units (Fig. 11–3). The trigger feature allows the instrument to store selected MUAPs (exceeding a designated amplitude) for later analysis. If a trigger were used only for storage, a problem would occur with visualizing the entire MUAP, because only the part of the MUAP occurring after the trigger would be displayed. A delay line permits the instrument to "remember" what happened for several milliseconds before the trigger and to display the entire MUAP. While this still does not provide reliable quantitative information when just a few potentials are analyzed, it does permit closer examination of the motor units and better examination of the duration and morphological characteristics of the potentials.

Traditional quantitative methods were developed in the 1950s by Buchthal and colleagues.[3, 4] These methods involve recording at least 20 different MUAPs and taking mean values of their measurements. Motor unit potentials are recorded with concentric needle electrodes with wide filter settings (Fig. 11–4). The low-frequency filter is set at 2 Hz, rather than 20 Hz, to include the low-frequency initial and terminal phases of the potential (although this makes the baseline less stable). Display sensitivity is set at a consistent level of 100 μV per division. Since duration measurements are dependent on sensitivity of the display, increasing the sensitivity

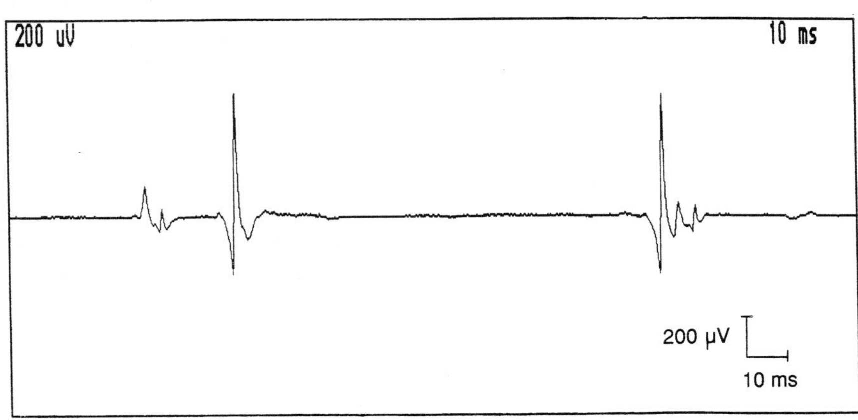

FIGURE 11–2. Two motor unit action potentials (MUAPs) examined during free sweep of the electromyograph. Note that the two potentials superimpose on the right, making it possible to erroneously identify the last potential as a long-duration, polyphasic MUAP.

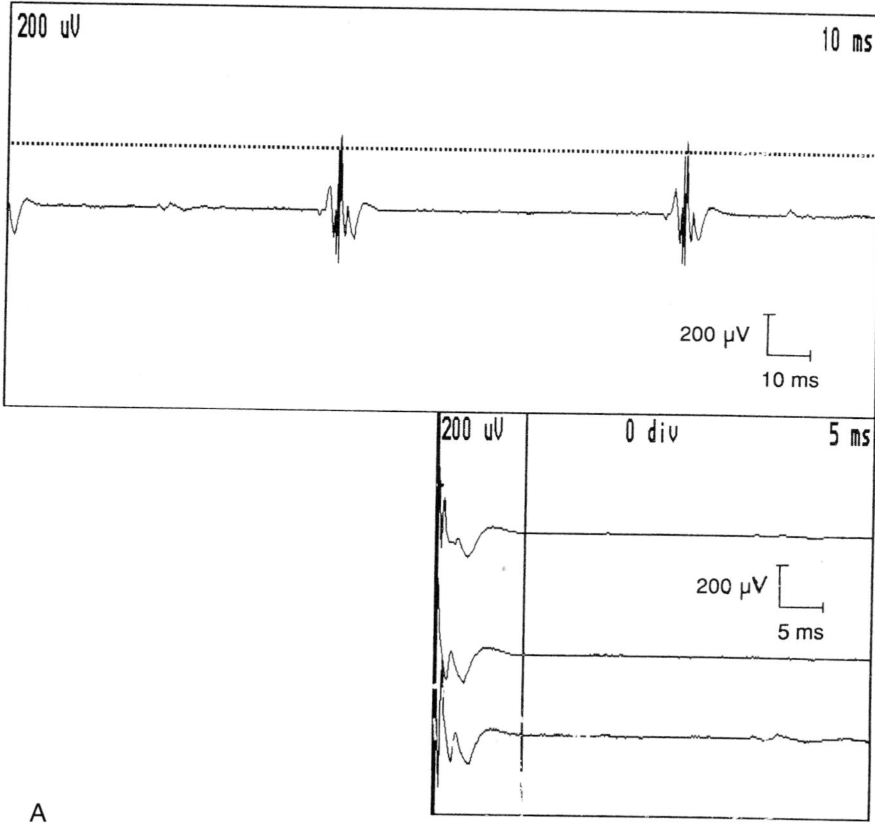

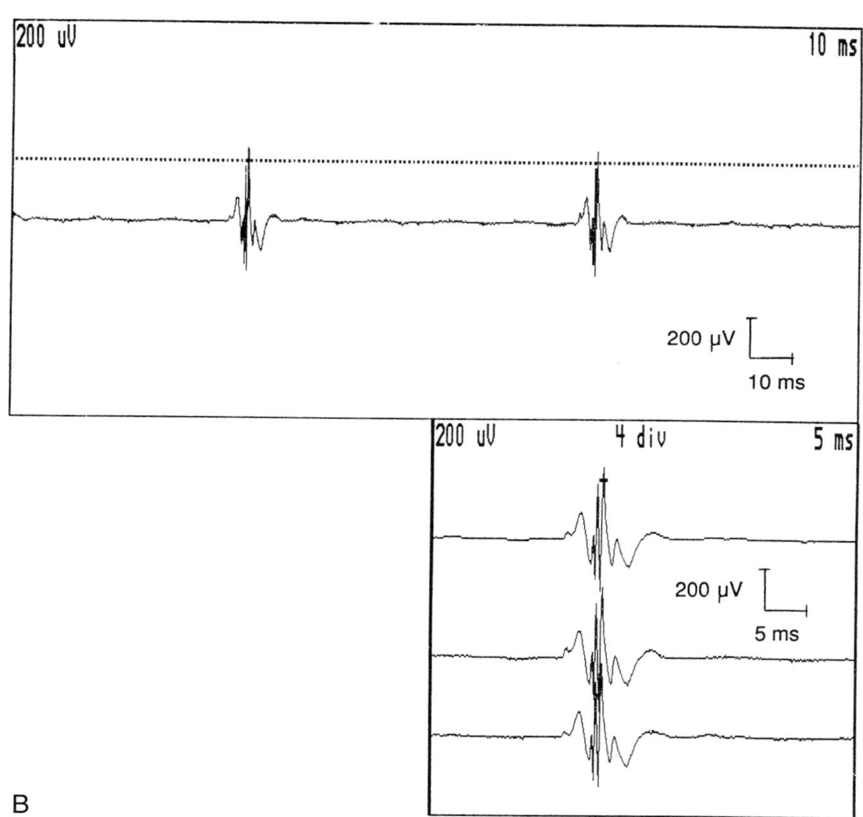

FIGURE 11–3. Examination of motor unit action potentials (MUAPs) with a free sweep (*top, A* and *B*), trigger only (*bottom, A*), and trigger and 40-msec delay line (*bottom, B*). When the trigger is used alone (*A*), only the part of the MUAP that occurs after the trigger is displayed. However, with both the trigger and the delay line (*B*), the whole MUAP can be clearly seen for measurement of duration, amplitude, and number of phases.

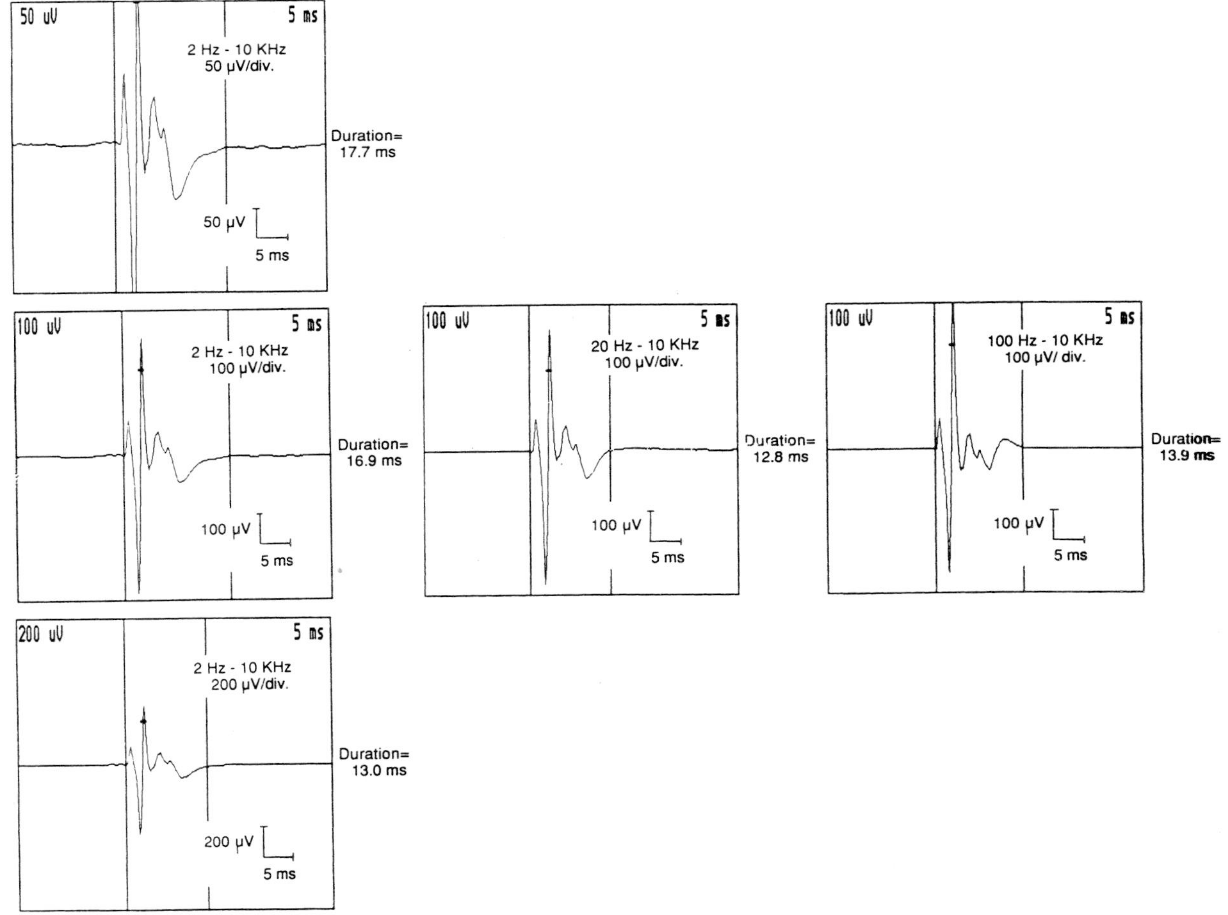

FIGURE 11–4. A single motor unit action potential (MUAP) recorded at various display sensitivities and filter settings. The standard fashion for recording is at 100 μV/division, 2 Hz to 10 kHz filters (*left, center*). As display sensitivity is increased (*top*) or decreased (*bottom*), duration changes markedly. As the low-frequency filter is increased to 20 Hz (*center*), the slow terminal phase is reduced in amplitude and duration is shortened. Further increase of the low-frequency filter to 100 Hz (*right*) adds an extra terminal phase as well.

(say, to 50 μV/division) produces longer durations, and lower sensitivity (say, 200 μV/division) produces shorter durations. During MUAP collection one should not select only the largest MUAPs, but should attempt to collect a representative sampling of all MUAPs near the tip of the needle.

Reference values have been studied extensively using these methods, and they are available for many different muscles and vary according to age.[32] Mean values are usually given. If a patient's mean value for MUAP duration in a muscle varies by more than 20% from the mean, it is determined to be outside the reference range. The primary role of this type of quantitative analysis is in the evaluation of myopathy.

Newer, automated techniques allow extraction of single MUAPs from contractions during which several motor units are firing simultaneously.[9] These allow for collection of more MUAPs in a rapid fashion. Often, five or more motor units can be recorded from a 10-second epoch (time period) during a moderate muscle contraction. The MUAPs that are selected with this technique, however, as well as the subsequent computational methodology employed, might differ from those of Buchthal and colleagues. The normal values to be used with each methodology of MUAP analysis have to be those that are standardized for that technique.

It is traditional to study at least 20 different MUAPs, but methods developed by Stålberg suggest that measurement of the number of outlier potentials with automated sampling can provide similar information using a lower number of analyzed potentials.[34] Those choosing to use this relatively new method should use the same motor unit sampling algorithm as that used by the original authors. The sensitivity of this technique versus that of more traditional methods is unknown.

Some automated methods for motor unit analysis do not depend on analysis of individual MUAPs. Stålberg and others[33] have studied computerized methods of looking at *turns,* defined as a change in direction of more than 100 μV, during minimal to moderate contractions (Fig. 11–5). Turns usually represent MUAPs or phases of MUAPs, but they are not resolved as MUAPs by the instrument and could represent noise or other types of discharges. Computationally, the mean ampli-

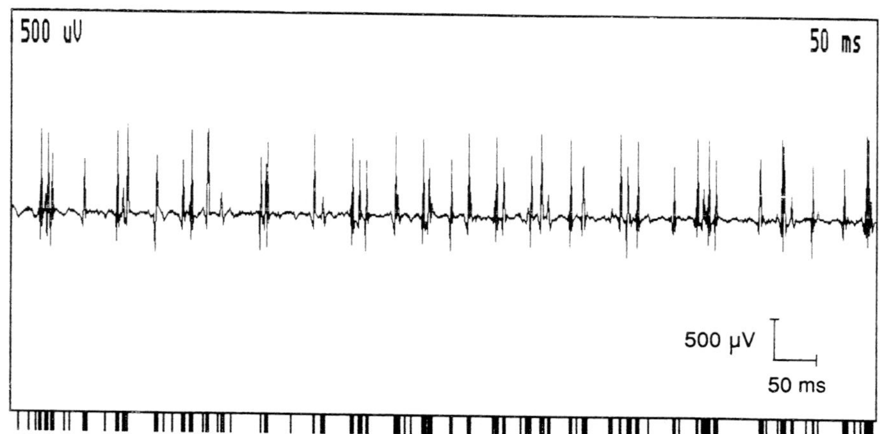

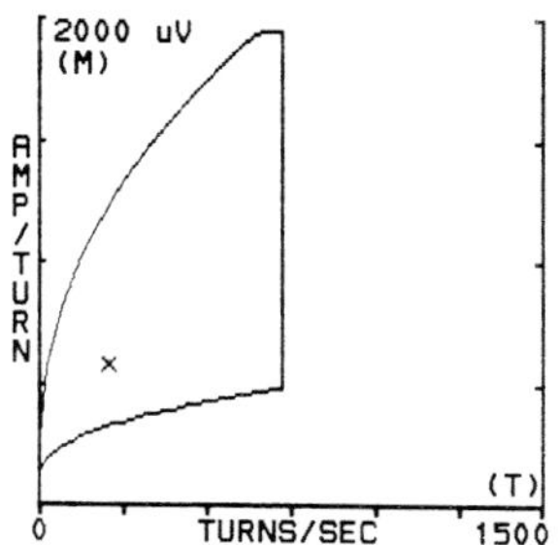

FIGURE 11–5. Turns amplitude (interference pattern) analysis during a minimal to moderate contraction. On the top screen, a 1-sec epoch of firing of motor unit action potentials is displayed. The instrument notes each turn (change in direction exceeding 100 μV) with a vertical line at the bottom of the screen. In the plot at *bottom,* the mean amplitude for each turn is plotted (on the *y*-axis) against the turns per second (on the *x*-axis). If more than 2 of 20 samples fall outside the normal "cloud," then the study is "abnormal."

tude for each turn (theoretically an index of MUAP amplitude) is plotted (on the *y*-axis) against the number of turns measured per second (theoretically an index of the strength of contraction or number of motor units recruited on the *x*-axis). This is done for 20 different 1-sec epochs. If more than two of the 20 samples fall outside the reference distribution ("normal cloud"), the test result is probably abnormal. If the reference data supplied by Stålberg and colleagues are being used, care must be taken to use the same methods and the same type of needle (concentric) as was used in collection of reference values. Myopathic conditions produce small-amplitude potentials and are below the normal cloud, whereas neuropathic conditions produce large-amplitude potentials above the cloud. This type of analysis might be somewhat better than simple "semiquantitative" analysis of amplitude, depending on the experience of the examiner. In effect, by plotting the amplitude per turn versus turns per second, one is controlling MUAP amplitude for the strength of voluntary contraction (larger-amplitude MUAPs are recruited with stronger contractions). Interference pattern analysis has been shown to be about as sensitive as conventional needle EMG, but it is probably not much more sensitive. It is likely not as sensitive or reliable as using the quantitative analysis methods as applied by Buchthal and colleagues.

Recruitment

Assessment of motor unit recruitment has a number of important purposes.[29] The most important of these is that it can assess whether reduced strength is due to a reduction in the lower motor neuron pool or to poor central effort. In myopathies, recruitment analysis also allows some qualitative assessment regarding how much force is being provided by each motor unit.

In distinguishing between reductions in the lower motor neuron pool versus poor central drive, the primary feature that should be measured is the rate of motor unit firing. This can be measured in several different ways, but the electromyographer should be facile at rapidly measuring the rate of motor unit firing. For measuring the firing rate of a motor unit, divide 1000 msec by the interpeak interval of two consecutive discharges of a MUAP. For instance, a motor unit whose potentials have an interpeak interval of 100 msec would be firing at 10 Hz (1000/100 = 10). If the sweep speed of the instrument is set at 10 msec/division, a quick way of estimating this is to count the number of divisions between the two motor units and divide the number into 100. If there are 10 divisions between the potentials, the rate would be 10 Hz, 9 divisions would be about 11 Hz, 8 divisions would be 12 Hz, and so on. A second way to estimate firing rates is to count the number of discharges of a given potential on the screen and multiply this number appropriately to arrive at the number that would be expected in 1 sec (1000 msec). If an MUAP fires twice during a 100-msec analysis time, the firing rate is about 20 Hz. The second method is less precise, because it does not take into account the possible variable position of the motor units across the screen.

There are several ways to use the measurement of firing rates to obtain a quantitative estimate of firing patterns. One method is to measure the firing rate of the first recruited motor unit just before the second MUAP starts to fire. This *recruitment frequency* is faster than normal in diseases that reduce the size of the available motor neuron pool. The upper limit of normal for recruitment frequency varies from one muscle to another. In most limb muscles, it is in the range of 12 to 15 Hz; but in the facial muscles, it can be as high as 30 Hz. Consequently, if one MUAP is firing at 20 Hz in a limb muscle, it is likely that the motor neuron pool is reduced (i.e., some axons are not able to fire and others are driven to fire faster to try to provide the requested force).

There are other alternative methods for measuring recruitment. The recruitment ratio compares the number of motor units firing during a minimal to moderate contraction with their frequencies. A rule of thumb is that (for moderate contraction) the rate of motor units firing divided by the number of motor units firing should be less than 5. A number higher than 10 is fairly clear evidence of a loss of motor units. Assessment of the interference pattern looks at how many motor units are firing at maximum voluntary contraction, but it is a more subjective measure. After assessing the firing rate, one should classify the recruitment as normal or full, central, reduced or discrete, or early (Fig. 11–6). Normal or full recruitment implies that the patient can give a full effort, with many MUAPs firing at normal rates. Central recruitment implies that reduced numbers of motor units are firing but are firing at a normal or slow speed. This is by far the most common "abnormality" in recruitment, but in isolation the finding is completely nondiagnostic. The central pattern of recruitment can be seen in patients with upper motor neuron lesions, pain, or poor voluntary effort. Reduced and discrete recruitment patterns are pathologically significant and imply reduced numbers of rapidly firing motor units. "Reduced" recruitment is less severe than "discrete" recruitment (in which just a few clearly identifiable motor units are firing rapidly, with baseline between them).

Assessment of recruitment is particularly useful in myopathies. In a myopathy each motor unit is "weak," and it takes more of them firing faster to accomplish a task. Consequently, in a myopathy, many MUAPs are activated to provide minimal levels of force. In a severe myopathy, it can be difficult for the patient to fire only a single motor unit as others are recruited quickly at low levels of force.

False-Positive and False-Negative Findings on Needle EMG

False-positive or false-negative needle EMG findings are common and have many potential causes. False-positive findings are usually related to overreading of "soft" or subtle changes. The most common examples include overreading increased insertional activity, mistaking end-plate potentials for fibrillation potentials, overestimating the percentage of polyphasic motor units or overinterpreting the finding of a few polyphasic potentials, and overreading central or reduced recruitment. False-negative findings are often related to timing. Needle EMG performed too early after the onset of symptoms can produce false-negative results, as it often takes two to three weeks for obvious findings such as positive sharp waves and fibrillations to develop. False-negative findings can also be produced if subtle MUAP changes are missed in a semiquantitative examination. Obviously, false-negative results could also come from insufficient breadth of the examination (e.g., too few muscles examined or each muscle insufficiently examined) or from not examining areas that are clinically involved.

Referring physicians usually prefer that the electrodiagnostic medical consultant "underread" findings. They tend to be understanding if a patient is subsequently

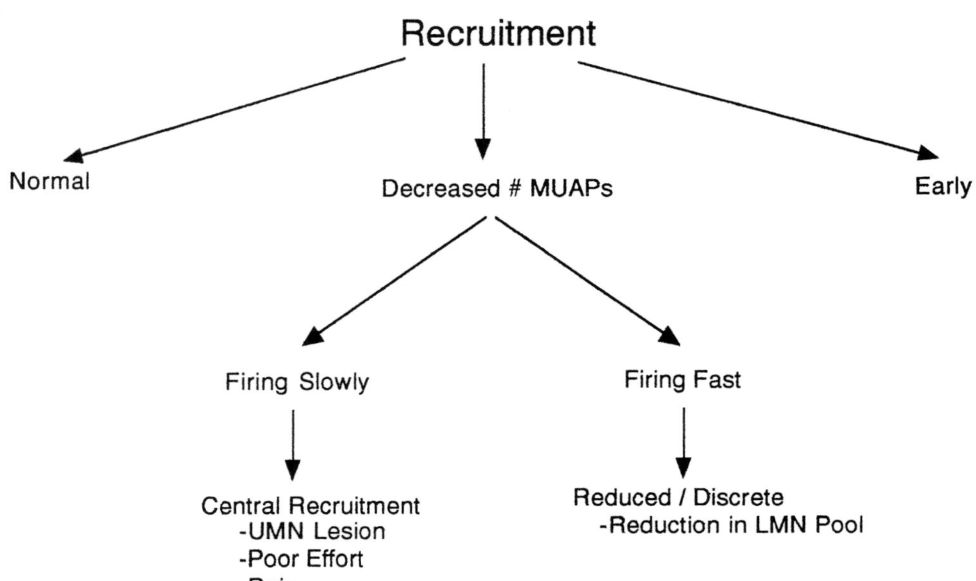

FIGURE 11–6. Assessment of recruitment. By examining firing rates, number of motor units firing, and level of force produced, recruitment should be classified as normal, central (nondiagnostic), reduced or discrete (suggesting reduction in the motor neuron pool), or early (reduced levels of force produced by each motor unit action potential, as seen in myopathy).

found to have a condition that could not be initially confirmed electrodiagnostically (false-negative findings). They are not as forgiving of a specific diagnosis that is later proved not to be present (false-positive findings).

NERVE CONDUCTION STUDIES

Nerve conduction studies are a very valuable part of the electrodiagnostic consultation. The instrumentation for these is discussed in Chapter 10. Specific case examples of the uses of nerve conduction studies are presented in Chapter 12.

Measurement of Compound or Sensory Nerve Action Potentials

There are usually two measures of nerve action potentials (NAPs): (1) speed of conduction (latency or velocity) and (2) size of the evoked response (amplitude). The speed of conduction for compound nerve action potentials (CNAPs) or sensory nerve action potentials (SNAPs) has traditionally been measured using peak latencies—i.e., the time between onset of stimulation and the peak of the potential. This is technically the easiest latency measurement to make because it is independent of display sensitivity; and on older instruments, it was often the only measurement that could be clearly discerned. The peak latency, however, is not always optimal in that it does not represent the arrival of the fastest conducting fibers, and it is affected by interelectrode separation (overly short active-to-reference separation produces shortened peak latencies; see Chapter 10). Onset latency, although more difficult to measure (particularly for small potentials or those with noisy baselines), does have the physiological advantage of representing arrival of the fastest conducting fibers and being less influenced by electrode separation.

Assuming that distance is held constant (e.g., 14 cm), CNAP latency can be used as an index of speed of conduction, or it can be used to calculate conduction velocity directly. Conduction velocity for CNAPs (in meters per second) can be derived in two ways. One method is to provide a single stimulus then divide the distance between the stimulation site (cathode) and the active electrode by the onset latency:

$$CV = d/t$$

where CV = conduction velocity in meters per second; d = distance between cathode and active electrode in millimeters; and t = onset latency in milliseconds. Onset latency should usually be used for these calculations because it is well understood physiologically and it is thought to represent the fastest fibers.

There is some controversy as to whether the time for activation of the nerve (activation time) should be introduced into the calculation. Some advocate subtracting a 0.1-msec activation time from the onset latency, although it is not clear whether this number is constant or if it can actually be longer than 0.1 msec.[23] Accounting for activation time, one would alter the equation to

$$CV = d/(t - AT)$$

where AT = activation time.

Another method for obtaining conduction velocity involves using two points of stimulation and dividing the distance between the two points by the difference in onset latencies. This method simply looks at the *difference* in latencies, so it cancels out any activation time inherent in both points of stimulation. Because it measures velocity between two points of stimulation rather than one, it is more difficult to measure conduction velocities over distal segments. Whatever method is used for measuring latency or conduction velocity, it should be well standardized and as close as possible to the methods that were used in developing reference (normal) values.

Latency and conduction velocity can be affected by a number of physiological and pathological factors, as discussed in Chapter 10. In healthy control subjects, slower conduction can be a result of cold limbs, aging, or increased height. Pathologically, demyelination produces slowing, as does loss of the faster conducting axons.

Amplitude of the CNAP can be measured (1) from baseline to peak, (2) from initial positive peak to subsequent negative peak if an initial positive peak is present, or (3) from initial negative peak to subsequent positive peak. In the setting of unstable or poorly defined baselines, the peak-to-peak measures are often easier to make, although any subsequent motor volume conducted response makes the later positive phase difficult to measure.

Amplitude can also be affected by a number of physiological and pathological factors. Cold increases the amplitude of the SNAP when the nerve at the active electrode is cooled. This is thought to result from an effect on Na^+ channel inactivation, which produces longer duration action potentials from each axon and a larger summed compound nerve action potential.[7] Whenever a prolonged latency or slowed conduction velocity is encountered in the face of a clearly normal or larger than usual amplitude, a cold limb is the probable cause. *Pathological* causes for slowed velocities or prolonged latencies usually produce small amplitudes. Amplitude is also influenced by the distance between the nerve and the recording electrode—i.e., the volume of tissue lying between nerve and electrode. Amplitude declines exponentially with distance from the generator. This explains why subjects with smaller finger circumferences have larger amplitude SNAPs.[1] Aging produces smaller amplitude SNAPs, probably as a result of loss of large myelinated axons.

The size of the CNAP is roughly proportional to the number of axons depolarizing under the active electrode. Loss of axons reduces the size of the CNAP accordingly. Distal lesions, occurring between the sites of stimulation and recording, drop the amplitude of the CNAP immediately. Proximal lesions (e.g., brachial plexus lesions) that separate the sensory axons from their cell bodies (in the dorsal root ganglion) produce distal axon loss due to axonal degeneration.[28] A reduced amplitude SNAP can be the result of an axonal lesion anywhere distal to the dorsal root ganglion.

Measurement of Compound Muscle Action Potentials

Principles of stimulation and recording for motor nerve conduction studies are similar to those used for sensory nerve conduction studies, with several exceptions. The primary difference is that motor nerve conduction studies involve recording a CMAP over muscle rather than recording directly from nerve. Consequently, the distal latency involves not only conduction along the nerve from the point of stimulation, but also neuromuscular junction transmission time (which takes ~1 msec) and conduction along muscle fibers (~3–5 m/sec). Although the onset latency from a distal stimulation site can easily be measured, it cannot be converted into a nerve conduction velocity as it can with the SNAP. To obtain conduction velocities, motor nerves are typically stimulated twice, and the distance between the two stimulation sites is divided by the difference in latency. The neuromuscular junction transmission time and the time for muscle fiber conduction are canceled out in this process.

Because each axon supplies many muscle fibers (usually hundreds or more) the compound muscle action potential is usually several hundred times the size of the corresponding nerve action potential. As a consequence, the onset latency of the CMAP is easy to delineate and it, rather than the peak, is usually used for measurement. Amplitudes of the response can be measured either from baseline to peak or from peak to peak, although the baseline-to-peak measurement is more commonly used.

Although many of the factors that affect sensory nerve conduction studies also affect motor nerve conduction studies, some important differences exist. First, because motor neuron cell bodies reside in the anterior horn of the spinal cord rather than in the dorsal root ganglion, the amplitude of the response is diminished by axon loss at the anterior horn cell or distally (not at the dorsal root ganglion). Second, because the recording is from muscle, neuromuscular junction transmission defects or primary myopathies can reduce the amplitude of the CMAP.

Occasionally, one may encounter the unusual finding of intact sensory nerve amplitudes with decreased motor amplitudes. It is helpful conceptually to think about areas in the spinal cord or along the peripheral nervous system that could account for these findings. Motor neuron disease or other intraspinal processes (such as tumor, syrinx, or carcinomatous meningitis) can reduce CMAP amplitudes; but because these are preganglionic lesions, they do not affect SNAPs. If sufficiently severe, radiculopathies (which almost always occur preganglionically) can result in small motor amplitudes with intact sensory responses. More peripherally, selective motor axonopathies produce a similar discrepancy, although these are relatively rare (e.g., heavy-metal neuropathies, porphyria, and some of demyelinating neuropathies). Neuromuscular junction defects (usually presynaptic) or primary myopathies can also selectively reduce motor amplitudes, because the CMAP is recorded over muscle and the SNAP over sensory axons.

The CMAP and SNAP amplitudes are useful in estimating the degree of axon loss. The degree of axon loss is roughly proportional to the drop in CMAP or SNAP amplitude that is elicited with distal stimulation (assuming that enough time has passed for wallerian degeneration).

Late Responses

There are several "late" responses (i.e., those that occur late after the CMAP or M wave) that sometimes provide useful information. These include the F wave, the H wave, and the A wave.[13] The F wave (so named because it was first recorded in foot muscles) is a late response usually recorded from distal muscles. When a motor nerve is stimulated distally, axons are depolarized in both directions: distally (orthodromically) and proximally (antidromically). Whereas the orthodromic volley activates the muscle distally, the antidromic volley proceeds proximally to the anterior horn cell. It is thought that the F wave occurs when a small percentage (3 to 5%) of antidromically activated motor cell bodies discharge and produce orthodromic activation of their motor axons. This is noted as a small-amplitude (~100 to 200 μV) late (~30 msec in the distal upper limb) potential.

The technique for obtaining F waves is similar to that for motor nerve conduction, with several important differences. First, because the F wave involves such a small percentage of the motor neuron pool, the sensitivity of the recording instrument needs to be greater (e.g., 200 μV/division versus a customary 2–5 mV/division for conventional motor studies). Second, since the F wave is a late response, having gone from the distal stimulation site to the spinal cord and back, the sweep speed needs to be slower so that a total of 50 msec (in the upper limbs) or 100 msec (in the lower limbs) can be measured in each sweep. Nerve stimulation for the F wave is typically at the same point in the limb as for distal motor latencies. It is customary practice, however, to turn the stimulating electrode around, with the anode facing distally rather than proximally. Although anodal block is probably not a common phenomenon in clinical nerve conduction studies, the concern for this possibility has led to the standard practice of reversing the stimulating electrodes. The small percentage of axons in the motor neuron pool that are activated for the F wave are not always the same with every stimulation. Consequently, to avoid sampling error, multiple stimulations need to be performed and multiple F waves measured. Some debate exists as to the number of F waves that need to be recorded,[13] but standard practice usually involves 10 to 20 recordings.

Multiple parameters can be measured in the 10 to 20 or more F waves that are collected. The most widely measured parameter is the minimal latency, as the shortest latency out of 10 or 20 stimulations. Some authors[13] advocate using the mean onset latency rather than the minimal latency, which may be more reliable. Other parameters that can be measured include penetrance or persistence (percentage of responses obtained), chronodispersion (the range between the shortest and longest latencies), and number of repeater F waves (frequency of obtaining the same F wave over time). Amplitude of the F wave is probably not very useful; but when it is measured, it is usually expressed as a ratio of the corresponding supramaximal CMAP amplitude.

F-wave measurements usually find their greatest applicability in the assessment of multifocal or diffuse processes, especially those affecting proximal areas of the peripheral nervous system. F waves are particularly helpful in assessing acquired or inherited demyelinating polyneuropathies, which produce multifocal or diffuse slowing of conduction velocity. In Guillain-Barré syndrome (acute inflammatory demyelinating polyradiculoneuropathy), abnormalities in F-wave measures can be the only electrophysiological abnormality early in the disease course. F waves are also useful in the assessment of syringomyelia, in which prolongation or absence of F waves can result from impaired turnaround time (central delay) at the anterior horn cell.[26]

Although it would seem appealing to use F-wave measurements for the diagnosis of brachial plexopathy or some entrapment neuropathies, they typically are not of significant help in these applications, nor do they offer unique information that cannot be obtained by conventional nerve conduction studies. There are two basic reasons for this. First, because the F wave is produced by just a small percentage of the motor axons, the presence of just a few normally conducting fibers can mask slowing of other fibers, resulting in a normal F-wave latency. Second, the F-wave volley traverses such a long distance of peripheral nerve that a focal lesion, unless it has severe demyelination, cannot be expected to produce marked abnormalities in F-wave latencies. Another limitation of F-wave measurements is that they usually can be recorded reliably only from distal muscles. When attempting to record F waves from proximal muscles, the latency becomes so short that the response is buried within the CMAP.

The H wave, unlike the F wave, does involve synaptic transmission at the spinal cord level. The H wave (also known as the H reflex) is in many ways analogous to the muscle stretch reflex. In the case of the muscle stretch reflex, the stretch receptors within the muscle are activated mechanically. But in the case of the H wave, the large-diameter afferent nerve fibers are directly activated electrically (many other fibers are probably activated as well). After the afferent volley reaches the spinal cord, a monosynaptic reflex excites alpha motor neurons and a late response is produced in the muscle. The H wave in adults is most easily elicited in the soleus muscle. In some subjects it can also be recorded from the flexor carpi radialis, foot intrinsic muscles, and the quadriceps. The H wave can be seen in many more muscles in children, especially those under three years old, possibly because the descending inhibitory pathways are not yet fully myelinated.

The H wave is recorded using somewhat different techniques than those for F-wave recording. For recording from the soleus muscle, stimulation is performed of the tibial nerve in the popliteal fossa. Although many authors report using a handheld stimulator, we have found it preferable to use a disk electrode taped over the middle of the popliteal fossa with an anode placed anteriorly over the knee, driving the current through the knee.[25] Recording is at a standardized site that is half the distance between the popliteal fossa and the proximal flare of the medial malleolus.[2] As opposed to the F wave, the H wave is largest in amplitude with stimulation levels that are submaximal for the corresponding M wave. The H wave should usually be higher in amplitude than the corresponding M response. Increasing the intensity of stimulation further causes the H wave amplitude to fall. The reason for this decrease in H-wave amplitude with higher levels of stimulation is not clearly known, but probably involves activation of inhibitory phenomena at the spinal cord level.

Because the H wave depends on a reflex at the spinal cord level, some unique concerns are applicable to obtaining these responses. The patient should be relaxed, since even minimal contractions, particularly of the ankle dorsiflexors, markedly reduce the amplitude of the response. Some authors utilize a minimal contraction of the ankle plantar flexors to facilitate the response. Also, there must be ample time between stimuli for the response to recover. Stimulating at rates more than about 0.2 Hz (one every 5 sec) alters the morphological characteristics of the H wave (except for the first one). Stimulation usually involves long-duration pulses, optimally between 0.5 and 1.0 msec, to preferentially activate the type Ia afferent fibers.

When performing the H-wave studies, a late response is sometimes seen after the M wave, and it might be unclear whether this is an H wave or an F wave. To differentiate the two, one should consider the size, the consistency of the response in latency and shape, and the current required to obtain the response. H waves tend to be large and are usually (but not always) greater in amplitude than the corresponding M wave seen when the H wave is elicited. They tend to be stable with little variability from one stimulation to the next, and they are best elicited at submaximal stimulation intensities and attenuate with higher intensities of stimulation. In contrast, the F wave is small (usually only about 3 to 5% of the M-wave amplitude), variable in morphological characteristics, and best seen with supramaximal stimulation intensities.

The H-wave latency is dependent on the age of the subject as well as on leg length; hence, reference values have been developed that account for these variables[2] and produce the mean expected latency. It is unusual, however, for a subject to have an H-wave latency that exceeds the mean plus 2 standard deviations (2 SD; 5.5 msec) generated by this calculation, except in severe neuropathies. More commonly, side-to-side differences exceed the reference range. Side-to-side latency differences exceeding 1.2 msec are probably abnormal.[2] H-wave amplitude is dependent on the intensity of stimulation as well as on the level of relaxation. This makes it difficult to compare an H-wave amplitude to absolute reference (normal) values, but side-to-side amplitude comparison has been found useful.[17] When comparing sides, the smaller response should not be less than 40% of the amplitude of the larger response.

The H wave can be abnormal in a variety of peripheral nervous system lesions. Tibial neuropathy, sciatic neuropathies, and lumbosacral plexopathies can all create abnormalities in the H-wave latency, amplitude, and shape. The most useful application of the H wave is in the detection of S1 radiculopathy. It has been shown that the H wave is more sensitive than needle EMG in the assessment of S1 radiculopathy,[2] probably related to the fact that the H wave can detect conduction block and demyelination, whereas needle EMG can detect only motor axon loss.

The A wave, formerly termed the *axon reflex,* is a rarely seen late response, usually observed in the setting of a peripheral nervous system lesion.[14] In most cases the A wave is thought to represent aberrant innervation after peripheral nerve injury such that single axons branch to innervate two different groups of muscle fibers. Stimulation distal to the site of the regenerated area of nerve causes depolarization antidromically to the other axon branch. This type of A wave is typically seen only at submaximal stimulation, because supramaximal stimulation simultaneously activates both branches and eliminates the A wave. The A wave usually represents an abnormality, since it reflects axon branching, although Sunderland has demonstrated axon branching in some normal subjects.[37] The A wave is easily missed in routine clinical nerve conduction studies if the sweep speed is too fast or the sensitivity too low to permit the observation of these small, late responses.

Another proposed etiology for the A wave is ephaptic transmission. It has been proposed that the A wave might result from the distal activation of an axon in a partially demyelinated nerve. When the volley reaches a demyelinated segment, slower conducting myelinated fibers could ephaptically activate nearby large-diameter faster conducting fibers (Fig. 11–7). This could be seen even in the case of supramaximal stimulation, in which both branches are activated (the refractory period in the faster fiber can already be over by the time the slow fiber is activated at the site of ephaptic transmission). Ephaptically generated A waves have been reported in early cases of Guillain-Barré syndrome.[39]

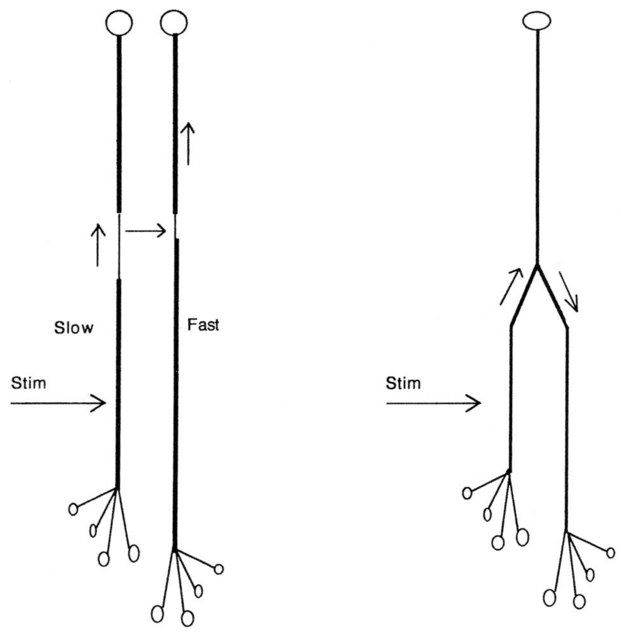

FIGURE 11–7. Axon waves can result from two different mechanisms. When demyelination is present, slowly conducting fibers can ephaptically activate nearby faster conducting fibers. In other cases, in which there is axon branching, selective stimulation of one branch activates the other branch; stimulation of both branches, however, causes collision and the A wave will be absent.

REPETITIVE STIMULATION STUDIES

Physiological Basis

Repetitive stimulation studies are most commonly used to search for abnormalities in neuromuscular junction transmission. To understand repetitive stimulation studies, it is first necessary to review the basic synaptic physiology at the neuromuscular junction (see Chapter 10 and reviews[19, 27]).

When a motor axon is activated, the depolarization proceeds down the axon to the presynaptic terminal. This depolarization produces a large influx of calcium into the presynaptic terminal, which in turn facilitates the release of acetylcholine-containing vesicles. A key point to remember when considering rates of stimulation is how long the calcium stays in the presynaptic terminal: usually about 100 to 200 msec. Given this timing, stimulation rates in excess of 5 to 10 Hz (interstimulus intervals of less than 100 to 200 msec) result in a buildup of calcium intra-axonally and a facilitation of release of acetylcholine to a greater degree than would otherwise occur. However, with stimulation at slow rates (below 5 Hz), calcium egresses from the presynaptic terminal between each stimulation and no accumulation occurs.

At the time of synaptic transmission, acetylcholine is released to travel across the neuromuscular junction and reaches receptors at the postsynaptic end-plate. Normally, about 3 to 5 times as much acetylcholine is released than is needed to fully activate the postsynaptic membrane. This margin of safety ensures that even though the amount of acetylcholine released during repetitive depolarizations normally progressively decreases, the muscle fiber is still fully activated.

Stimulation at slow rates (less than 5 Hz) is usually done to detect postsynaptic neuromuscular junction defects. With slow rates of stimulation in normal individuals, a successive decrease occurs in the amount of acetylcholine released. When the safety factor of release is normal, muscle fibers are still fully activated. When the safety margin is less than normal, progressively fewer and fewer muscle fibers are activated during repetitive stimulations at slow rates.

Fast rates of stimulation (e.g., 20 to 50 Hz) are primarily used to detect presynaptic defects in neuromuscular junction transmission. At these fast rates of stimulation, Ca^{2+} concentrations are progressively increased in the presynaptic terminal and more acetylcholine is released. Presynaptic defects, such as Lambert-Eaton myasthenic syndrome (LEMS) or botulism, produce marked increments (at least twofold) in the amplitude of the CMAP with high rates of stimulation.

Technical Considerations

There are a number of important technical variables to keep in mind when performing repetitive stimulation studies. First, because acetylcholinesterase is sensitive to temperature changes, the limb should be adequately warmed before studies are performed. When the limb is too cold (usually under 34°C), defects in neuromuscular junction transmission can be hidden. There is no correction factor for an overly cold limb, so the problem must be corrected by warming the limb to 34°C or greater. Movement artifact is probably the most common technical difficulty in repetitive stimulation studies. This can be reduced by securely taping down all electrodes. Stimulation should be via a block electrode taped to the limb rather than a handheld electrode whenever possible. When performing stimulation distally, such as in the hand, it is also advisable to use an arm board to stabilize the limb. Submaximal stimulation can be a potential problem. Using stimuli around the maximal level (rather than supramaximal) can result in intermittent submaximal stimuli and "pseudodecrements" with limb movement during stimulation. To avoid this problem, stimulation intensities should be at least 30% above the maximal level.

Although distal muscles are usually the least difficult technically to study, they are also usually the least diagnostically sensitive. It is often necessary to perform a progression of studies, starting with the ulnar nerve, which is technically easy to study, then moving proximally to the shoulder (e.g., Erb's point to deltoid or spinal accessory nerve to trapezius), and finally to the facial muscles (nasalis). Facial muscles are the most sensitive for detecting postsynaptic defects of neuromuscular transmission, but technical problems may arise owing to difficulty with stabilization and movement. If abnormal results are clearly seen in distal muscles, it is often not necessary to move to more proximal studies.

Exercise has a marked effect on repetitive stimulation studies. Immediately after exercise (usually defined as 30 seconds of isometric exercise), a brief period of postexercise potentiation occurs, acetylcholine release is facilitated, the margin of safety is improved, and initial decrements can be reduced. About 2 to 4 minutes after exercise, there is a period of postexercise exhaustion. During this period, release of acetylcholine from the presynaptic terminal is reduced and any defects in neuromuscular transmission become more apparent. Consequently, it is customary to perform slow (2 to 3 Hz) repetitive stimulations pre-exercise, immediately postexercise (during postexercise facilitation), and then at 1-minute intervals for four minutes to look for postexercise exhaustion.

Changes in Disease States

Presynaptic disorders of neuromuscular junction transmission are rare. Lambert-Eaton myasthenic syndrome is an autoimmune disorder that is often, but not always, associated with malignancy or autoimmune disease. Botulism results from exposure to the toxin from the bacterium *Clostridium botulinum.* These disorders have in common a reduced release of acetylcholine from the presynaptic terminal. Myasthenia gravis is an example of a postsynaptic neuromuscular junction disorder. In this disorder not only are the postsynaptic receptors blocked by specific antibodies, but the cleft between the presynaptic and postsynaptic terminals is also widened and an increased breakdown of acetylcholine occurs as it crosses the synaptic cleft.

Presynaptic disorders such as LEMS or botulism are usually characterized by their potentiation with high-frequency stimulation and exercise (Table 11–1). When studied either immediately after exercise or during high-frequency stimulation, the CMAP potential increases at least twofold, and often several fold, in affected muscles. Presynaptic disorders also display a decrement with slow rates of stimulation, but this is usually less marked than in postsynaptic disorders.

Postsynaptic disorders such as myasthenia gravis usually have a progressive decrement on slow repetitive stimulation studies, which is exacerbated during postexercise exhaustion. In some cases a decrement can become apparent only during postexercise exhaustion 2 to

TABLE 11–1 Expected Findings on Single and Repetitive Nerve Stimulation*

	CMAP Amplitude	CMAP After 10 sec Exercise	CMAP After 10 sec Exercise		
			Pre-Exercise	*Immediate Postexercise*	*2–4 min Postexercise*
Normal	Normal	No change	No change	No change	No change
Presynaptic defect	Very small	Markedly increased	Decrement, 1st to 4th stimulation	Markedly increased initial CMAP amplitude	Decrement similar to pre-exercise
Postsynaptic defect	Normal	No change	Decrement, 1st to 4th stimulation	Less decrement than pre-exercise	Decrement more than pre-exercise

* Recording the CMAP in normal subjects, patients with presynaptic lesions, and patients with postsynaptic lesions.
Abbreviation: CMAP, compound motor action potential.

4 minutes after exercise. Postsynaptic disorders also manifest postexercise facilitation, but this is far less marked than in presynaptic disorders. Repetitive stimulation studies are moderately sensitive for the diagnosis of myasthenia gravis, and most studies suggest that the sensitivity ranges from 60% to 70%. Single fiber EMG studies are probably more than 90% sensitive.

Abnormalities on repetitive stimulation studies are not entirely specific to neuromuscular junction (NMJ) disorders. After reinnervation, newly developed axon sprouts have immature and unstable NMJs, and can produce a decrement during repetitive stimulation at slow rates. Patients with motor neuron disease, peripheral polyneuropathy, or entrapment neuropathies can have decrements unrelated to any specific neuromuscular junction defect. Similar decrements have also been reported in myopathies.

INTERPRETATION

Normal versus Abnormal

As with any other type of testing, nerve conduction studies and quantitative measurements on EMG are not always conclusively normal or abnormal. Reference values have been derived for most quantitative measurements, but these do not unequivocally differentiate a healthy subject from one with disease.[5] Reference values provide only the *probability* of a result coming from a healthy subject versus from a patient with disease. When one uses a 2-SD level from mean for a reference value to determine abnormality, 97.5% of the subjects will fall on the normal side of that reference value. Since no diagnoses should be made due to too short a latency, too large an amplitude, or too fast a conduction velocity, a one-sided probability is used. However, 2.5% of the time, someone from the healthy control subject group will have a result outside of the reference values, and be considered "abnormal." It is the finding of multiple "abnormalities" consistent with the clinical presentation that helps to establish a diagnosis.

The use of 2 SDs to produce reference values at the 97.5 percentile level assumes a normal (gaussian) distribution to the data. It has been shown, however, that nerve conduction study data (and probably EMG data) do not follow a gaussian distribution.[31] Consequently, using a mean and 2 SDs to determine reference values is inappropriate and can lead to an increased number of false positives or false negatives. Appropriate adjustments to the data can be made to obtain more reliable reference values; however, these adjustments typically have not been performed in most literature studies.

Given these considerations, when deciding whether or not a study is "normal," one must view all reference values with a degree of healthy skepticism and avoid making a diagnosis based on a single unusual finding. Diagnoses based on the electrophysiological examination are best made when multiple "abnormalities" are demonstrated in a pattern consistent with the clinical presentation.

Principles of Localization

A number of principles are useful for localizing peripheral nerve lesions based on the electrophysiological examination. Nerve lesions that are very proximal cannot be studied with stimulation both proximal and distal to an entrapment site, making needle EMG the most helpful in their diagnosis and localization. Localization is based on the distribution of the abnormalities determined after examination of the muscles supplied by multiple peripheral nerves, roots, or areas of the plexus. Sciatic neuropathy can be distinguished from peroneal neuropathy, for example, if evidence is found of denervation in muscles supplied by both the peroneal and tibial nerves, with normal findings in the gluteal muscles. Localization is based on finding abnormalities distal to a branch point, with normal findings proximal to that point.

Although this approach often results in correct localization, there are many instances in which it leads to choosing an erroneous lesion site. Sunderland[36, 37] has shown that fascicles within peripheral nerves intertwine considerably as they move proximally through the limbs. Fascicles supplying the flexor carpi ulnaris muscle, for example, are not uniquely placed proximally within the ulnar nerve as it joins the medial cord of the brachial plexus. However, fascicles do become organized within peripheral nerves several centimeters prior to branch points. In this example, fascicles destined to supply the flexor carpi ulnaris become organized within the ulnar nerve several centimeters prior to supplying the muscle. Consequently, even though ulnar nerve entrapment at the elbow usually occurs proximal to the branch to flexor carpi ulnaris, this muscle is usually spared in ulnar neuropathy at the elbow. The fascicles for this muscle are isolated in a relatively protected area of the nerve at the entrapment site. If localization were based only on EMG using the known branch points, these lesions would be erroneously placed distal to the branch point and in the forearm (Fig. 11–8).

The ulnar nerve is not unique with regard to its specific intraneural topography causing potential problems in localization. Cases have been reported of neuropathy of the common peroneal nerve occurring proximal to the popliteal fossa but resulting only in deep peroneal deficits clinically.[10] Sciatic neuropathies, even when they occur near the hip joint, can result in a clinical picture of predominantly peroneal nerve lesions. The fascicular structure within the peroneal division of the sciatic nerve can make it more predisposed to injury than is the tibial division.[36] Although conventional EMG does make use of known anatomical branch points to arrive at localization, the electromyographer should be aware of the intraneural topography within the nerve and recognize that a partial lesion might be more proximal than predicted by the electrophysiological data.

Nerve conduction studies are best at localizing the site of the pathological lesion when demyelination is present. Demyelination causes focal slowing and conduction block. When present, these findings allow precise localization of a focal entrapment. A problem with localizing lesions based on nerve conduction studies

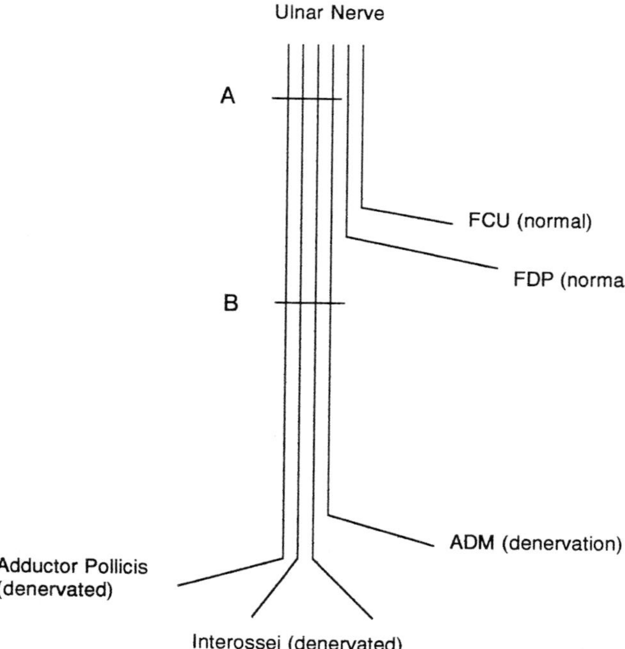

FIGURE 11–8. Predominantly axonal ulnar neuropathies with denervation in hand muscles and normal forearm muscles can be difficult to localize. Lesions in the forearm distal to the branches to flexor carpi ulnaris (FCU) and flexor digitorum profundus (FDP) can produce these findings (site *B*). More commonly, the lesion is at a higher location (site *A*), which spares the fascicles supplying the two forearm muscles.

arises when there is predominantly axon loss and little demyelination. In such cases, conduction velocity throughout the nerve is mildly slowed due to loss of the faster conducting fibers, but is not focally or markedly slowed. Although a diffuse reduction is seen in CMAP or SNAP amplitude at all sites of stimulation (due to axon loss and subsequent Wallerian degeneration), there is no focal drop in amplitude across the lesion site. Conduction block (in which a drop in amplitude of the CMAP is seen in moving from distal to proximal stimulation) is related only to demyelination and neurapraxia, and is not present in axon loss lesions after Wallerian degeneration has occurred (about seven days after onset).

This difficulty is exemplified when an attempt is made to localize an ulnar neuropathy at the elbow that is predominantly due to axon loss (e.g., post-traumatic lesions). Because there is no focal demyelination across the elbow, all segments of the ulnar nerve tested demonstrate mild slowing and have reduced-amplitude CMAPs. Because there are but two ulnar innervated muscles in the forearm and none in the arm, and because complications are introduced by the complex intraneural topography (see preceding discussion), localization by EMG is also difficult.

Localization of proximal lesions such as radiculopathies or plexopathies is usually best done utilizing needle EMG results and SNAPs. Study of motor nerve conduction studies and recording of CMAPs is less useful in localization because it is usually difficult to stimulate proximal to the site of the lesion. CMAP amplitude, however, is useful for assessing the degree of motor axon loss, and for making a prognosis.

A common problem in proximal localization is in distinguishing between plexus and root lesions. In most cases, only two findings distinguish between these two possibilities. One is the paraspinal needle EMG, which, if abnormal, speaks strongly for a lesion at or proximal to the posterior primary ramus (such as a root lesion). However, there are patients with root lesions in whom paraspinal muscles are reportedly normal on EMG. The second is the study of the sensory nerve action potential, assuming that there has been enough time for axonal degeneration after injury. This helps to distinguish between preganglionic and postganglionic (dorsal root ganglion) lesions. Plexopathies are usually expected to have small SNAPs, while radiculopathies usually have normal SNAPs. Some cervical radiculopathies occur laterally enough to involve the dorsal root ganglion, however, and result in small-amplitude SNAPs. Moreover, postganglionic lesions, such as brachial plexopathies, must have marked axon loss if axonal degeneration is to produce reduction of distal SNAPs. Because there is a wide range of "normal" SNAP amplitudes, a drop in amplitude from 60 to 30 μV, for example, might still leave the SNAP within "normal" limits.

Deducing the Pathophysiology from the Electrophysiological Results

Whenever possible, it is helpful to provide to the referring physician some indication of the pathophysiology within the peripheral nervous system (e.g., neurapraxia, demyelination, or axon loss) (Fig. 11–9).

Neurapraxia or focal conduction block is seen on nerve conduction studies when a larger amplitude CMAP or SNAP is elicited with stimulation distal to the site of the lesion, as compared to proximally. Purely neurapraxic injuries show no electrophysiological evidence for axon loss (fibrillation potentials or positive sharp waves) or reinnervation.

Demyelination is best demonstrated by slowing of conduction, often with conduction block. Slowing of conduction can take the form of slowed conduction velocities, prolonged distal latencies, increased temporal dispersion, or prolonged late responses. Slowing of conduction does not always mean that demyelination has occurred, since axon loss, particularly of the faster conducting fibers, similarly produces mild slowing of conduction as well.

Axon loss lesions are usually demonstrated by evidence of denervation on needle EMG examination as well as by small-amplitude CMAP and SNAP responses with stimulation and recording distal to the site of the lesion. Although needle EMG is a more sensitive indicator for motor axon loss, measurement of CMAP and SNAP amplitude is a better way to quantify the *degree* of axon loss and prognosis.

Timing of Electrophysiological Changes

The time course of electrodiagnostic changes after onset of a neuropathic lesion should always be kept in mind

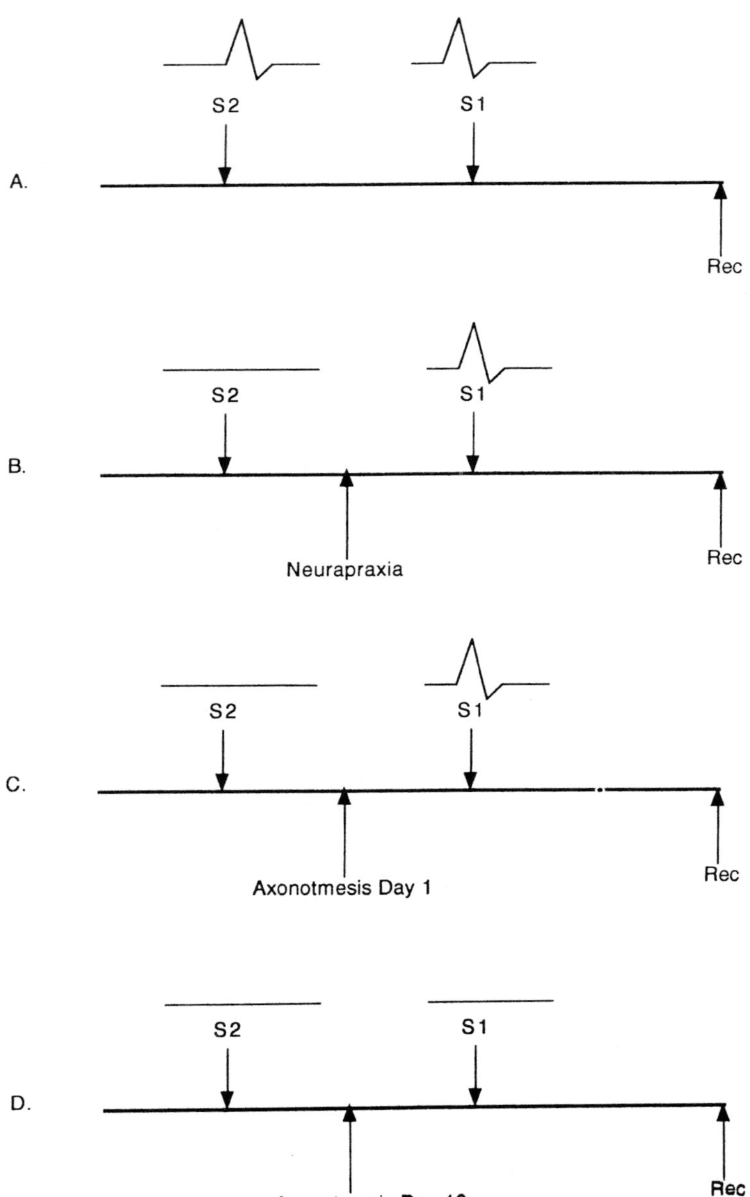

FIGURE 11–9. Normally, stimulation at two different points along a peripheral nerve produces similar-sized responses when recording distally from muscle (*A*). After a neurapraxic lesion (*B*), the distal nerve segment remains excitable, but a small-amplitude or absent response is elicited from proximal stimulation until recovery occurs. Similar findings are seen immediately after the occurrence of a lesion producing axonotmesis or neurotmesis (*C*). After sufficient time for axonal degeneration has elapsed, usually 7 to 10 days (*D*), the distal segment is inexcitable and no response is produced with distal stimulation.

when planning the electrophysiological examination. Neurapraxia, demyelination, and severe axon loss produce electrophysiological changes immediately if one can perform stimulation both proximal and distal to the lesion. Very proximal lesions, in which it is not possible to access a site both proximal and distal to the lesion, do not immediately produce changes on distal nerve conduction studies or EMG. Distinction between neurapraxia and axonotmesis cannot be made until after wallerian degeneration has occurred in cases of axonotmesis.

Day 1 After an Axon Loss Lesion. Immediately after onset of an axon loss lesion, some electrophysiological changes can be noted. On needle EMG the only potential abnormality is a change in recruitment, with reduced or discrete recruitment if enough axon loss has occurred. Mild lesions do not produce noticeable changes in recruitment. Nerve conduction studies distal to the site of the lesion are unchanged, but stimulation proximal to a lesion with recording distally might produce a small-amplitude response. Otherwise, nerve conduction studies and EMG are usually unremarkable.

Days 7 to 10. Seven days after a complete nerve lesion, wallerian degeneration will have progressed to a point at which stimulation of motor axons elicits no motor responses. Ten days after onset of a complete lesion, SNAPs will be absent as well. Incomplete lesions produce less marked changes, but with similar timing. Seven to ten days after onset, a neurapraxic injury can be distinguished by nerve conduction studies (in which case the distal amplitudes are normal) from an axonotmetic lesion (in which case the distal amplitudes are reduced).

Days 14 to 21. Two to three weeks after onset of injury the needle EMG starts to show fibrillation potentials and positive sharp waves. Proximal muscles typically demonstrate these abnormalities before distal ones. Radiculopathies, for example, can show paraspinal abnormalities at days 10 to 14 after onset, but distal limb muscle changes might not be apparent until three to four weeks after onset. In studies of peripheral nerve lesions in animal models, it has been documented that the longer the segment of nerve left attached to a muscle after section, the longer the interval before the appearance of fibrillation potentials. This has raised the question of the existence of some type of "antifibrillation" trophic factor stored in peripheral nerves, with fibrillations occurring only after it is depleted.

Fibrillations and positive sharp waves can persist for several months or even many years after a single injury, depending on the extent of reinnervation. Although the presence of positive sharp waves or fibrillations indicates that there has been some denervation, it does not necessarily indicate that there is "active" or "ongoing" loss of axons over time. Fibrillation amplitudes are sometimes helpful in determining the chronology of the lesion. This is due to the fact that the amplitude of fibrillation potentials decreases over the course of time. The presence of fibrillation potentials larger than 100 μV indicate an onset less than 1 year ago.[21]

Reinnervation. The timing and type of electrophysiological changes consequent to reinnervation depend in part on the mechanism of reinnervation. When reinnervation is a result of axonal regrowth from the site of the lesion, as in complete lesions, the appearance of new MUAPs does not occur until motor axons have had sufficient time to grow the distance between the lesion site and the muscle. Nerve regrowth usually occurs at 1 mm/day or 1 inch/month. When these new axons first reach the muscle, they innervate only a few muscle fibers, producing short-duration, small-amplitude potentials, sometimes referred to as *nascent potentials.* With time, as more muscle fibers are innervated and join the motor unit, the MUAPs become larger, more polyphasic, and longer in duration.

Motor unit potential changes also develop when reinnervation occurs by axonal sprouting. Polyphasicity and increased duration develop first as newly formed, poorly demyelinated sprouts supply the recently denervated muscle fibers. As the sprouts mature, large-amplitude, long-duration MUAPs develop and persist indefinitely.

Estimating Prognosis

Prognosis of a peripheral nerve lesion is related to the pathophysiological problem that has occurred, the time since onset, and the distance between the lesion and the target muscles. Those lesions that have had extensive axon loss are less likely to have recovery of function. Estimation of the extent of axon loss, however, should not be based solely or predominantly on findings during needle EMG, as it takes very little axon loss to produce profuse fibrillation potentials and positive sharp waves. The extent of axon loss should be determined chiefly by the distal CMAP amplitude.

Electrophysiological measures cannot, unfortunately, assess the integrity of supporting structures around the nerve and cannot distinguish axonotmesis from neurotmesis. Neurotmesis (which has complete or nearly complete disruption of supporting structures) carries a much worse prognosis for regeneration than axonotmesis, in which the supporting structures are largely intact. In these cases, careful periodic reexamination of proximal muscles (those expected to be reinnervated first) gives the best information as to ultimate prognosis for full reinnervation.

Lesions that are predominantly neurapraxic have a much better prognosis, because conduction block in these lesions rarely lasts more than a few months. Demyelinating lesions also have a better prognosis than axon loss, but the specific prognosis depends on what intervention is taken (e.g., release of entrapment sites).

When axon loss is present, it is important to remember that a critical window of time exists for peripheral nerve regeneration, after which the target muscles cannot be reinnervated. This "window" is usually in the range of 18 to 24 months. Because peripheral nerves regenerate roughly at a rate of 1 inch/month, proximal lesions with a great deal of axon loss have a poor chance of reinnervating distal hand or foot muscles. Complete brachial plexus injuries, for example, have very little chance of reinnervating ulnar innervated hand muscles. As a consequence, most neurosurgical interventions in brachial plexus lesions are directed at reinnervating proximal upper limb muscles. When looking for any electrophysiological evidence of reinnervation, keep in mind both the distance between the lesion and the time since injury, to know whether reinnervation should be expected at the time of the examination.

PEDIATRIC EMG

There are some special points to be considered when performing EMG on pediatric patients.[18] First, the indications for performing EMG in children are substantially different from those for adults, and the indications are changing over time. In the past, pediatric EMG was used to detect changes consistent with such diseases as Duchenne muscular dystrophy or Wernig-Hoffman disease. Now, however, there are well established gene probes that are more accurate than EMG for making these diagnoses. In the evaluation of possible infantile botulism, EMG plays less of a role than it used to, since the toxin can now be easily detected in the stool.

Nevertheless, pediatric EMG is still useful for a number of indications. It is particularly useful for evaluation of possible acute inflammatory demyelinating polyradiculoneuropathy (AIDP or Guillain-Barré syndrome) or the Fisher variant (Fisher syndrome or Miller Fisher syndrome). EMG is often helpful in the assessment of children for myopathies. It should be remembered, however, that many congenital myopathies look about the same on EMG and that more specific diagnosis requires consideration of the clinical picture and usually muscle biopsy.

Another significant difference between pediatric EMG and that in adults is the reference or "normal" value range. At birth, nerve conduction velocity is about half that of adults, since nerves are not yet fully myelinated. As children mature, nerve conduction velocity increases until it essentially reaches the adult range at about three years of age. Electromyographers should use age specific reference values, particularly when assessing for demyelinating neuropathies.

Perhaps one of the most significant differences between adult and pediatric EMG is the technique. Children simply don't tolerate the procedure as well as adults. Children less than six years of age generally don't tolerate the procedure, particularly if they have had bad experiences with prior medical procedures or if the parental anxiety level is high.[16] There are different schools of thought about whether or not sedation should be used for the procedure. Some electromyographers feel they can get through the procedure quickly without sedating the child and with minimal trauma. Others prefer to use sedation with midazolam or other short-acting sedatives to avoid unnecessary trauma to the child and to preserve the child's tolerance of future medical procedures. If sedation is used, personnel with appropriate training should be present. This often includes the presence of a pediatric anesthesiologist.

Finally, another important consideration in performing pediatric electromyography is the difference in the amount of data that can be obtained. While many muscles can be sampled in the adult, looking at both spontaneous activity and voluntary motor unit potentials, the same cannot be said for children. Generally, only a few nerves or muscles can be examined, and muscles can be examined primarily for either spontaneous activity (during sedation) or motor unit action potentials (when awake), but not both.

ELECTRODIAGNOSIS IN THE ELDERLY

The electrodiagnostic medical consultant needs to be aware of several important changes that occur with aging. These primarily need to be considered when deciding what is normal or abnormal. Most nerve conduction measures change with age. Latencies become longer, velocities slower, and amplitudes smaller with age. This is not necessarily a linear change with age and some data suggest that nerve conduction remains relatively constant until about age 60, and then declines in the 7th and 8th decades. As a consequence, it is preferable to use age-specific data[11, 12] rather than making linear adjustments for age. These data do not, however, take into account any interactions that can occur between age, temperature, and height.

Voluntary motor unit action potentials also change with age. Buchthal[4] and others[32] have shown that motor units become longer in duration and larger in amplitude as people age. This presumably reflects slow motor neuron loss over time, with consequent reinnervation by distal sprouting. While this change does not usually present problems when performing semiquantitative motor unit analysis, it can make a difference when performing quantitative motor unit analysis. Age-specific normative data[32] should be used when doing quantitative motor unit analysis.

WRITING THE ELECTRODIAGNOSTIC MEDICAL CONSULTATION REPORT

Guidelines for writing the electrodiagnostic medical consultation report can be found in the American Association for Electrodiagnostic Medicine guidelines for electrodiagnostic laboratories.[15] The report should identify the patient, state the referring problem and indication for the study, and list the findings from the electrophysiological examination. The conclusion should specify whether the study results are normal or abnormal, answer the referring physician's question (e.g., whether or not a specific diagnosis is present), and report any other diagnoses that can have come to light during the clinical or electrophysiological examination. Whenever possible, the pathophysiological basis of the lesion and the prognosis for recovery should be included.

REFERENCES

1. Bolton CF, Carter KM: Human sensory nerve compound action potential amplitude: Variation with sex and finger circumference. J Neurol Neurosurg Psychiatry 1980; 43:925–928.
2. Braddom RL, Johnson EW: Standardization of H wave and diagnostic use in S1 radiculopathy. Arch Phys Med Rehabil 1974; 55:161–166.
3. Buchthal F, Guld C, Rosenfalk P: Action potential parameters in normal human muscle and their dependence on physical variables. Acta Physiol Scand 1954; 32:200–218.
4. Buchthal F, Pinelli P, Rosenfalk P: Action potential parameters in normal human muscle and their physiological determinants. Acta Physiol Scand 1954; 32:219–229.
5. Campbell WW, Robinson LR: Issues and opinions: Deriving reference values in electrodiagnostic medicine. Muscle Nerve 1993; 16:424–428.
6. Daube JR: AAEM minimonograph no. 11: Needle examination in clinical electromyography. Muscle Nerve 1991; 14:685–700.
7. Denys EH: AAEM minimonograph no. 14: The influence of temperature in clinical neurophysiology. Muscle Nerve 1991; 14:795–811.
8. Desmedt JE, Borenstein S: Relationship of spontaneous fibrillation potentials to muscle fibre segmentation in human muscular dystrophy. Nature 1975; 258:531–534.
9. Dorfman LJ, McGill KC: AAEE minimonograph no. 29: Automatic quantitative electromyography. Muscle Nerve 1988; 11: 804–818.
10. Esselman PC, Tomski MA, Robinson LR, et al: Selective deep peroneal nerve injury associated with arthroscopic knee surgery. Muscle Nerve 1993; 16:1188–1192.
11. Falco FJ, Hennessey WJ, Braddom RL, et al: Standardized nerve conduction studies in the upper limb of the healthy elderly. Am J Phys Med Rehabil 1992; 71:263–271.
12. Falco FJ, Hennessey WJ, Braddom RL, et al: Standardized nerve conduction studies in the lower limb of the healthy elderly. Am J Phys Med Rehabil 1994; 73:168–174.
13. Fisher MA: AAEM minimonograph no. 13: H waves and F waves: Physiology and clinical applications. Muscle Nerve 1992; 15:1223–1233.
14. Fullerton PM, Gilliat RW: Axon reflexes in human motor nerve fibers. J Neurol Neurosurg Psychiatry 1965; 28:1–11.
15. Guidelines in Electrodiagnostic Medicine. Rochester, MN, American Association of Electrodiagnostic Medicine, 1994.

16. Hays RM, Hackworth SR, Speltz ML, et al: Physicians' practice patterns in pediatric electrodiagnosis. Arch Phys Med Rehabil 1993; 74:494–496.
17. Jankus WR, Robinson LR, Little JW: Normal limits of side-to-side H-reflex amplitude variability. Arch Phys Med Rehabil 1994; 75:3–7.
18. Jones HR, Bolton CF, Harper CM: Pediatric Clinical Electromyography. Philadelphia, Lippincott-Raven, 1996.
19. Keesey JC: AAEM minimonograph no. 33: Electrodiagnostic approach to defects of neuromuscular transmission. Muscle Nerve 1989; 12:613–626.
20. Kimura J: Electrodiagnosis in Diseases of Nerve and Muscle: Principles and Practice, ed 2. Philadelphia, FA Davis, 1989.
21. Kraft GH: Fibrillation potential amplitude and muscle atrophy following peripheral nerve injury. Muscle Nerve 1990; 13:814–821.
22. Kraft GH: Fibrillation potentials and positive sharp waves: Are they the same? Electroencephalogr Clin Neurophysiol 1991; 81:163–166.
23. Krarup C, Horowitz SH, Dahl K: The influence of the stimulus on normal sural nerve conduction velocity: A study of the latency of activation. Muscle Nerve 1992; 15:813–821.
24. Lederman RJ, Wilbourn AJ: Brachial plexopathy: Recurrent cancer or radiation? Neurology 1984; 34:1331–1335.
25. Little JW, Hayward LF, Halar E: Monopolar recording of H waves at various sites. Electromyogr Clin Neurophysiol 1989; 29:213–219.
26. Little JW, Robinson LR: Electrodiagnosis in post-traumatic syringomyelia: Case report and review of the literature. Muscle Nerve 1992; 15:755–760.
27. MacLean IC: Neuromuscular junction. In EW Johnson (ed): Practical Electromyography. Baltimore, Williams & Wilkins, 1980.
28. Miller RG: AAEM minimonograph no. 28: Injury to peripheral motor nerves. Muscle Nerve 1987; 10:698–710.
29. Petejan JH: AAEM minimonograph no. 3: Motor unit recruitment. Muscle Nerve 1991; 14:489–502.
30. Robinson LR: AAEM case report no. 22: Polymyositis. Muscle Nerve 1991; 14:310–315.
31. Robinson LR, Temkin NR, Fujimoto WY, et al: Effect of statistical methodology on normal limits in nerve conduction studies. Muscle Nerve 1991; 14:1084–1090.
32. Rosenfalk P: Electromyography in normal subjects of different age. Methods Clin Neurophysiol 1991; 2:47–52.
33. Stålberg E, Chu J, Bril V, et al: Automatic analysis of the EMG interference pattern. Electroencephalogr Clin Neurophysiol 1983; 56:672–681.
34. Stålberg E: Outliers, a way to detect abnormality in quantitative EMG. Muscle Nerve 1994; 17:392–399.
35. Streib EW: AAEE minimonograph no. 27: Differential diagnosis of myotonic syndromes. Muscle Nerve 1987; 10:603–615.
36. Sunderland S: The relative susceptibility to injury of the medial and lateral popliteal divisions of the sciatic nerve. Br J Surg 1953; 41:300–302.
37. Sunderland S: Nerves and Nerve Injuries, ed 2. Edinburgh, Churchill-Livingstone, 1968.
38. Taylor RG, Kewalramani LS, Fowler WJ: Electromyographic findings in lower extremities of patients with high spinal cord injury. Arch Phys Med Rehabil 1972; 53:558–562.
39. Wang L, Robinson LR: Axon reflexes resulting from ephaptic transmission in acute demyelinating polyneuropathy. Arch Phys Med Rehabil 1993; 74:1250.
40. Wright KC, Ramsey-Goldman R, Nielsen VK, et al: Syndrome of diffusely abnormal insertional activity: Case report and family study. Arch Phys Med Rehabil 1988; 69:534–536.

12

CHAPTER

Kathryn A. Stolp-Smith, M.D.

Electrodiagnostic Medicine III: Case Studies

The ability to perform nerve conduction studies (NCS) and needle electromyography (EMG) in a clinical setting significantly enhances our role as clinicians. Knowledge and skill in clinical neurophysiology allow the clinician a physiological extension and confirmation of the clinical examination. An analytical and sequential thought process, application of medical knowledge of anatomy, physiology, and pathophysiology, and familiarity with electrodiagnostic equipment are necessary to properly perform and interpret NCS and EMG. Clinical neurophysiological studies allow us immediate physiological feedback and confirmation of clinically suspected problems. The decision to perform electrophysiological studies is based on many factors. Confirming a clinical impression, exploring and excluding disorders in a differential diagnosis, highlighting findings that will alter clinical management, and, in some cases, providing objective evidence of a disorder for medicolegal reasons are all ways in which NCS and EMG can facilitate the practice of medicine.

The principal goal of the electrodiagnostic medicine consultation is to reach a diagnostic conclusion efficiently and reliably. Selection of NCS and muscles for EMG should be based not only on the anatomy and suspected pathophysiology but also on the patient's ability to tolerate the study, the ease and reliability with which the study can be performed, and the time allotted by the patient and clinician for the study.

Patient tolerance is to a large extent a function of the examiner's bedside manner. If the examiner shows patience, good technique, and a thoughtful approach to the study, all procedures are usually well tolerated. As a rule, when no disorder of the neuromuscular system is suspected based on the history and clinical examination, clinical neurophysiological studies are unnecessary. The precise NCS chosen and the muscles examined by EMG are determined by the clinical findings, knowledge of pathophysiology, and factors of patient compliance, positioning, and tolerance. The procedure performed can change depending on the data obtained as each step is completed. A "cookbook" approach to electrodiagnosis is flawed by lack of the necessary customization for each case, and is rarely if ever satisfactory for accurate results or for patient tolerance. Standard techniques may have to be varied in some situations, depending on the type of information sought. Studies performed can be limited by patient compliance, tolerance, coagulopathies, the presence of central vascular catheters or pacemakers, lymphedema, and other factors. Clinical judgment and knowledge of the risk of electrodiagnostic studies apply in all cases. In some cases, other types of studies may prove more useful and appropriate in reaching a diagnosis and determining a management plan.

The cases presented and discussed in this chapter are meant to highlight these principles. Each patient is unique, and the approach differs from patient to patient and from clinician to clinician. The approaches used are examples and not protocols. The purpose of the case studies is to show the logic of performing electrodiagnostic medicine studies and how the sequence of steps is recursive, as each step reflects findings from the preceding step. The cases described represent problems commonly encountered in the clinical neurophysiological laboratory. Some examples are classic cases, others are focal presentations of generalized problems. The problem of coexisting disorders is also described. Problems of the neuromuscular system are highlighted. Disorders of other organ systems, in particular the musculoskeletal system, are not discussed but often must be considered in the differential diagnosis.

Disorders most readily assessed by NCS and EMG include diseases of the neuron—the anterior horn cell or dorsal root ganglion; the nerve roots; the plexus; and the peripheral nerves. The disorders include entrapments, discrete proximal conduction block, distal nerve disorders, and neuromuscular junction and muscle disorders. The cases reported here demonstrate how to apply the basic science and techniques described in Chapters 10 and 11 to a clinical situation.

UPPER LIMB PROBLEMS

Many disorders affecting the upper extremity can be diagnosed during the electrodiagnostic medicine consultation. Common problems involving one or both upper limbs include cervical radiculopathy or root avulsion, brachial plexopathy, and radial, ulnar, and median nerve entrapments or compression. Entrapments or compression of other upper limb nerves can be determined, including the spinal accessory, long thoracic, dorsal scapular, suprascapular, axillary, musculocutaneous, thoracodorsal, and pectoral nerves. Cutaneous neuropathies of the lateral and medial antebrachial cutaneous, superficial radial, and dorsal ulnar sensory cutaneous nerves can also be seen. Disorders that may present in, but are not limited to, the upper limbs include motor neuron disease, multifocal motor neuropathy with conduction block, polyradiculoneuropathies, multiple multifocal mononeuropathies of acquired or hereditary cause, neuromuscular junction disease such as myasthenia gravis, and congenital, acquired, metabolic, or structural disorders of muscle. Clinical symptoms and signs can be acute or chronic, constant or intermittent, and focal or generalized, and include numbness, paresthesias, weakness, pain, fatigue, cramps, fasciculations, and position- and posture-related symptoms. Sensory loss, weakness, atrophy, depressed reflexes, fasciculations, myokymia, myotonia, and tremor can result from these disorders.

Neck and Arm Pain (Case 1)

Thought Process

The principal consideration in the differential diagnosis for this case is a right cervical radiculopathy at the C7 level. However, other root level involvement cannot be excluded by the history and examination alone because of overlap of myotomes and dermatomes and individual anatomical variation. An idiopathic or traumatic brachial plexopathy affecting primarily the posterior cord should also be considered. Radial nerve entrapment is a possibility. Median nerve entrapment at the wrist can cause shoulder symptoms, but there is little to suggest this disorder in our current evaluation. The history and physical examination do not support a diagnosis of root avulsion. A central nervous system (CNS) disorder with spinal cord injury at a cervical level or a discrete lesion rostral to the spinal cord could potentially explain these findings, and although these diagnostic possibilities should not be ignored, they would be unlikely, given the time course of the history and the focal findings, and would only rarely produce pain.

Selection of appropriate electrodiagnostic studies is based on the differential diagnosis. Needle EMG is an essential component of the evaluation to specifically define involved myotomes. Sensory NCS are important to exclude plexopathy and mononeuropathy. Motor NCS denote the severity of axonal loss and assist with myotome definition. F-wave studies, if included, can be useful in highlighting proximal slowing or conduction block in unsuspected areas of involvement. Given the sensory symptoms and findings, tests such as repetitive stimulation to study neuromuscular junction transmission are not indicated. The studies performed in this patient are listed in Table 12–1.

Discussion

As is typical for all but the most severe radiculopathies, the NCS results were normal.[61] Median and ulnar motor NCS were performed to study nerves commonly entrapped in the upper extremity, which can lead to pain, weakness, and numbness. The compound muscle action potentials from these muscles allow assessment of axonal integrity of the C8 and T1 nerve roots. F-wave studies assess slowing in proximal nerve segments as may be seen in radiculopathy, plexopathy, or multifocal motor neuropathy with conduction block. The me-

CASE STUDY 1

A 45-year-old male carpenter developed gnawing right-sided neck pain 1 day following a day of repetitive lifting and stacking of lumber. The pain began as a dull ache and gradually became more severe, with radiation down the right arm to the dorsum of the hand. Discomfort was exacerbated by turning the head to the right and was associated with transient tingling and numbness along the extensor forearm and dorsum of the hand. He had not found any measures that reduced the pain. Occasionally the arm felt heavy though not particularly weak. The pain became more severe, and 6 weeks after onset he sought a medical evaluation.

Clinical examination showed decreased cervical lordosis and decreased active neck range of motion. Passive range of motion was limited, and Spurling's maneuver significantly increased his neck pain, with paresthesias and pain radiating down the arm to the dorsum of the right hand. Shoulder range of motion was normal. Muscle stretch reflexes were normal except for an absent right triceps reflex. Sensory examination revealed decreased pain and touch sensation of the extensor forearm and dorsum of the hand, including the third digit. Manual muscle testing showed mild right triceps weakness.

TABLE 12–1 Case 1: Neck and Arm Pain

NERVE CONDUCTION STUDIES

Nerve Stimulation (Record)	Amplitude (μV)	Conduction Velocity (msec)	Latencies (msec)	
			Distal	*F-Wave*
Motor				
Median (thenar)	6800	52	3.5	29.0
Ulnar (hypothenar)	8300	54	3.0	29.5
Sensory				
Radial (hand dorsum)	28	—	3.3	—
Median (index)	42	63	3.0	—
Ulnar (fifth)	20	63	2.8	—

ELECTROMYOGRAPHY*

Muscle	Insertional Activity	Spontaneous Activity		Motor Unit Potentials		Phases/ Turns
		Fibrillation Potentials	*Fasciculation Potentials*	*Recruitment*	*Duration/Amplitude*	
First dorsal interosseous (manus)	Normal	0	0	Normal	Normal	—
Pronator teres	Increased	0	0	Normal	Slightly increased	—
Triceps	Increased	++	0	Reduced	Increased	Increased
Biceps	Normal	0	0	Normal	Normal	—
Extensor digitorum communis	Increased	+	0	Reduced	Increased	Increased
Deltoid	Normal	0	0	Normal	Normal	—
Midcervical paraspinal muscles	Increased	++	0	Not evaluated	Normal	—

*All needle examinations were performed with a concentric needle.

dian and ulnar antidromic sensory NCS were performed to evaluate the upper and lower trunks of the brachial plexus as well as to exclude common focal entrapments. The specific distribution of numbness by history and physical examination for this patient led to consideration of a radial neuropathy and the radial antidromic sensory NCS was performed. These studies are well tolerated and are technically reliable.

Needle examination should be as focused as possible, yet help to appropriately include or exclude disorders noted in the differential diagnosis. Performing a needle examination in at least two muscles of the suspected involved myotome increases the chances of finding an abnormality and better defines the root level involved. Needle examination of muscles that are clinically involved should always yield some abnormal finding. Severely involved muscles that are fibrotic provide abnormal but limited findings.

EMG can include the first dorsal interosseous of the hand, pronator teres, triceps, biceps brachii, deltoid or infraspinatus, cervical paraspinal muscles, and possibly a finger extensor muscle. Increased insertional activity in the pronator teres resulted in suspicion that a C6 or C7 radiculopathy was present and was evidence against a radial neuropathy. The myotome involved was further defined by the triceps abnormalities. Abnormal findings in the paraspinal muscles, taken together with the abnormalities in anterior myotomes limited principally to a single myotome, directed us away from the diagnosis of plexopathy and provided good evidence for a radiculopathy. Since the most severe findings were in the triceps with only mild pronator teres abnormalities and a normal biceps, and since both fibrillation potentials and motor unit potential (MUP) changes were present, the best explanation was an active or chronic and incompletely reinnervated radiculopathy at the right C7 root level.

Arm Numbness and Weakness (Case 2)

Thought Process

The most likely diagnosis for this patient is posttraumatic brachial plexopathy with primarily lower trunk involvement. Elbow flexor weakness with normal strength noted in other upper trunk–innervated muscles could indicate more extensive plexus involvement. The most important disorder to exclude in the differential diagnosis is the root avulsion, since prognosis and further treatment would be significantly altered by this possibility. Given the humerus fracture, multiple mononeuropathies at the level of the fracture could also explain these findings. The history of trauma and the physical examination findings suggest plexopathy or root avulsion coupled with a musculocutaneous neuropathy.

When considering a less clear-cut brachial plexopathy, other causes should be considered based on the clinical history, course, and portion of the plexus involved. Traction plexopathies typically involve the upper trunk of the brachial plexus.[37] Gunshot wounds more commonly affect the cords.[30] Nontraumatic onset of upper extremity pain with weakness and numbness, occasionally following a viral illness, leads to consideration of an idiopathic plexopathy or a neurological amyotrophy, as described by Turner and Parsonage.[57] This disorder can also involve the long thoracic nerve and phrenic nerve or cervical roots, resulting in findings that could be attributed to root involvement. Idiopathic brachial plexopathies often present bilaterally,[60, p. 924] and

CASE STUDY 2

A 60-year-old farmer developed left upper extremity weakness and numbness after falling from his tractor. His sleeve caught in the tractor doorframe and caused him to dangle freely before falling to the ground. He landed on his shoulder, fracturing the clavicle and humerus. The fractures required surgical fixation. He presented for an evaluation when the surgical wounds had healed.

Clinical examination revealed deformity of the shoulder with limited range of motion. Muscle stretch reflexes were absent in the affected upper limb. Manual muscle testing demonstrated normal strength with shoulder abduction, rotation, and no scapular winging. Moderate weakness of elbow flexion, forearm pronation, supination, elbow and wrist extension, and severe weakness of wrist flexion, finger extension and flexion, and hand intrinsics were noted. Atrophy of weak muscles and swelling and clawing of the hand were present. Sensory examination showed reduced pain and touch sensation in the forearm and hand, with relative sparing of the thumb, and completely absent sensation in the lateral forearm, medial hand, and fourth and fifth digits. Proximal to the elbow, the medial aspect of the arm exhibited significant sensory loss.

---

subclinical involvement of the contralateral extremity can be demonstrated on NCS and EMG.[57]

Lower trunk plexopathies that develop insidiously can be due to an apical lung tumor or metastatic breast carcinoma or to primary plexus tumors such as a neurofibroma or schwannoma.[60, p. 93] Often, differentiating recurrent tumor infiltration from postradiation plexopathy is challenging, but postradiation plexopathy is more likely to be associated with myokymic discharges on EMG and can occur up to 34 years after the radiation exposure.[22, 36] Healthy persons with droopy shoulders can develop symptoms of intermittent lower trunk compromise that can be due to vascular or lower trunk encroachment in the shoulder girdle by a rudimentary cervical rib or fibrous band.[19] Electrophysiological hallmarks of this disorder, known as thoracic outlet syndrome, are a low median compound muscle action potential (CMAP) and a markedly reduced or absent ulnar sensory nerve action potential (SNAP) with needle examination abnormalities in muscles that receive innervation from the lower trunk.[18] The NCS and EMG performed in this case are outlined in Table 12–2.

TABLE 12–2 Case 2: Arm Numbness and Weakness

NERVE CONDUCTION STUDIES

Nerve Stimulation (Record)	Amplitude (μV)	Conduction Velocity (msec)	Latencies (msec) Distal	Latencies (msec) F-Wave
Motor				
Median (thenar)	**1500**	**45**	**4.0**	**NR**
Ulnar (hypothenar)	**NR**	**NR**	**NR**	—
Musculocutaneous (biceps)	**1300**	**45**	**4.2**	
Axillary (deltoid)	5200	—	—	
Sensory				
Ulnar (fifth)	**NR**	**NR**	**NR**	
Lateral antecubital (forearm)	**NR**	—		
Median (index)	18	57	3.2	

ELECTROMYOGRAPHY

Muscle	Insertional Activity	Spontaneous Activity: *Fibrillation Potentials*	Spontaneous Activity: *Fasciculation Potentials*	Motor Unit Potentials: *Recruitment*	Motor Unit Potentials: *Duration/ Amplitude*	*Phases/ Turns*
Deltoid	Normal	0	0	Normal	Normal	—
Biceps brachii	Increased	++	0	Reduced	Increased/low	Increased
Pronator teres	Increased	+	0	Reduced	Increased	Increased
First dorsal interosseous (manus)	Increased	+++	0	None activated		—
Flexor pollicis longus	Increased	++	0	Reduced	Normal	Increased
Triceps	Increased	+	0	Reduced	Increased	Increased
Brachioradialis	Increased	+	0	Reduced	Increased	Increased
Infraspinatus	Normal	0	0	Normal		—
Midcervical paraspinals	Normal	0	0	—		—
Low cervical paraspinals	Increased	+++	0	—		—
High thoracic paraspinal muscles	Normal	0	0	—		—

Abbreviation: NR, no response.

Discussion

One of the electrodiagnostic challenges posed by this case is to completely assess the degree of the lesion without performing excessive NCS and to limit the needle examination. Both median and ulnar motor NCS were performed because (1) both median motor and ulnar motor and sensory nerve fibers course through the lower trunk of the brachial plexus; (2) the median CMAP reflects the integrity of primarily C8 axons and the ulnar CMAP represents primarily T1 axons; (3) F waves are readily obtainable with both; (4) both types of NCS are technically reliable; and (5) the ulnar nerve is ideally suited for stimulation at multiple points along its course, including the plexus and root level. Because of the suspected musculocutaneous neuropathy, this nerve and the lateral antebrachial cutaneous nerves were specifically studied.

The abnormalities on these studies alone do not exclude an upper trunk brachial plexopathy. This could be further defined using the needle examination. The normal results on axillary NCS pointed to a musculocutaneous neuropathy, although upper trunk plexopathy could not be completely excluded. The abnormal results on sensory NCS indicated a lesion distal to the dorsal root ganglion. In root avulsion without plexopathy, SNAPs should be preserved.[59]

Nerve root stimulation may be indicated to better define the level of involvement in some cases of brachial plexopathy. Nerve root stimulation can be technically difficult and uncomfortable for the patient and generally should not be performed unless the examiner is comfortable with the technique and familiar with the technical pitfalls that could affect the results. Root stimulation was not performed in this case.

The needle examination provided evidence of extensive denervation in the upper limb with sparing of upper trunk–innervated muscles except for those innervated by the musculocutaneous nerve. Muscles representing all plexus levels were examined. Relatively normal MUPs with reduced recruitment in the flexor pollicis longus indicated a lack of reinnervation.[29, p. 633] The presence of MUPs in this muscle was evidence against a complete C8 root avulsion. Long-duration, low-amplitude, highly polyphasic MUPs in the biceps are characteristic of nascent MUPs indicating early reinnervation. Low cervical paraspinal fibrillation potentials indicated root involvement and indeed likely avulsion at this level.

The conclusion from these studies was that of a middle and lower trunk brachial plexopathy with probable root avulsion of the C8 or T1 nerve root.

Arm Weakness (Case 3)

Thought Process

The patient's age, history, and examination findings are most characteristic of acquired myasthenia gravis.[20] Lambert-Eaton myasthenic syndrome (LEMS) could also produce these symptoms but usually manifests with dysautonomia and less pronounced bulbar symptoms. Weakening, rather than facilitation, of muscle strength and muscle stretch reflexes with repetitive testing was noted on clinical examination.[16, 34] The time of weakness onset was most consistent with an acquired disorder of muscle, although a congenital myopathy or dystrophy can present in later years.[6, 58] Myotonic dystrophy or other myotonic disorder of muscle can present in this way, but the examination findings and lack of cramping were not suggestive of this family of disorders.[24] Inflammatory myopathy, motor neuron disease, and motor neuropathy or inflammatory polyradiculoneuropathy must also be included in the differential diagnosis. Facial weakness is not characteristic of early motor neuron disease or inflammatory myopathy. Motor neuropathy or polyradiculoneuropathy usually present with depressed reflexes,[15, 45] and polyradiculoneuropathy is rarely only motor. Multifocal motor neuropathy with conduction block can present with normal or slightly increased reflexes.[35] The NCS and EMG performed in this case are presented in Table 12–3.

Discussion

Myasthenia gravis is the most likely diagnosis, given the clinical presentation. It is important to consider disorders of the neuromuscular junction when evaluating a patient for vague or more pronounced complaints of

CASE STUDY

3

A 42-year-old woman complained of fatigue and upper limb weakness that had developed over the preceding 6 months. She occasionally noted double vision, particularly later in the day, and had difficulty with overhead activities. Although she denied difficulty walking, she said her legs felt heavy, and she described some difficulty climbing stairs. There was no family history of a similar disorder.

Clinical examination revealed a healthy-appearing woman with a transverse smile. Muscle stretch reflexes, gag reflexes, and sensory examination results were normal. Manual muscle testing of facial muscles showed mild orbicularis oculi and oris weakness. With prolonged upward gaze the patient developed ptosis bilaterally. Prolonged phonation and repetitive lingual motions resulted in palatal weakness and dysarthria. Extraocular motions were full and conjugate. Upper extremity strength was normal distally. There was mild weakness of the shoulder rotators and abductors, and repeated contraction of these muscles resulted in moderate weakness. Lower extremity manual muscle testing was normal, but repeated squatting and rising from the floor became progressively more difficult.

TABLE 12–3 Case 3: Arm Weakness

NERVE CONDUCTION STUDIES

Nerve Stimulation (Record)	Amplitude (μV)	Conduction Velocity (msec)	Latencies (msec)	
			Distal	*F-Wave*
Motor				
Ulnar (hypothenar)*	8800	60	3.0	27.0
Facial (nasalis)*	2800	—	3.0	
Accessory (trapezius)	6000	—	4.2	
Peroneal (EDB)*	4000	46	5.1	55.5
Sensory				
Medial (index)	32	58	3.2	
Medial-plantar (ankle)	10	—	4.4	

Repetitive Stimulation	Ulnar	Facial	Accessory	Peroneal
Rest (% decrement)	10	18	20	3
Exercise duration (sec)	60	15	15	60
Postexercise (% decrement)				
Immediate	0	3	4	3
30 sec	0	6	8	2
1 min	2	10	12	1
2 min	8	18	19	3
3 min	10	22†	27†	3

ELECTROMYOGRAPHY

Muscle	Insertional Activity	Spontaneous Activity		Motor Unit Potentials	
		Fibrillation Potentials	*Fasciculation Potentials*	*Recruitment*	*Duration/Amplitude*
Anterior tibial	Normal	0	0	Normal	Normal
Vastus medialis	Normal	0	0	Normal	Normal
First dorsal interosseous (manus)	Normal	0	0	Normal	Normal
Biceps brachii	Normal	0	0	Normal but slight variation in MUP amplitude	
Upper trapezius	Normal	0	0	Slight short-duration MUP with amplitude varying	
Cervical paraspinals	Normal	0	0	—	

Abbreviations: EDB, extensor digitorum brevis; MUP, motor unit potential.
*Repetitive stimulation—2 Hz, % decrement (no increment).
†Ten-second exercise repeated and repair of decrement reproduced.

upper limb weakness. Myasthenia gravis can present initially with weakness in the upper extremity.[20] The patient described here has the more classic presentation, with facial and some lower extremity involvement as well.

The key to the electromyographer's approach is to determine whether the neuromuscular junction is involved. Whether the pathology is confined to the face or upper or lower limbs, and to prove that motor neuropathy, polyradiculoneuropathy, motor neuropathy, or myopathy is not present. The examiner must also demonstrate the characteristic pattern of decrement on repetitive nerve stimulation in at least two nerves to avoid false positive results. A decrement of greater than 10% is generally used, as technical limitations of repetitive stimulation can produce a small decrement, and a small decrement can be seen in some other disorders. The decremental response must be demonstrated to repair with exercise and to follow a pattern in which the greatest incremental percentage of decrement occurs between the first and second CMAP.[43] Decrement is calculated by comparing the amplitude or area of the first CMAP with the fourth or fifth CMAP resulting from a train of four or more stimuli.[50]

The nerves selected were chosen because (1) the ulnar nerve is technically the most reliable for repetitive stimulation (because of distal recording it may not show an abnormality); (2) the accessory nerve is a reliable and well-tolerated proximal NCS and is relatively sensitive (the axillary NCS may be more sensitive but is technically more difficult); (3) facial NCS evaluate facial symptoms and signs; (4) peroneal NCS can demonstrate lower limb involvement; (5) a median antidromic sensory study could be involved early in a polyradiculoneuropathy[1]; and (6) medial plantar NCS can exclude a subtle sensory neuropathy. Ideally, a proximal lower limb NCS should be performed, but it is technically difficult and more uncomfortable for the patient. The femoral NCS may show significant findings as one of the first abnormal nerve studies in LEMS. LEMS usually displays an initial low CMAP at rest and a more profound decremental response than is seen in myasthenia gravis, with a marked incremental response following brief periods of exercise.[25, 42]

The needle examination should include the proximal and distal muscles of the upper and lower limbs, to exclude myopathy, motor neuron disease, and define the extent of involvement. Myasthenia gravis is essentially an inflammatory myopathy and can present with EMG findings of occasional fibrillation potentials and short-duration, polyphasic, low-amplitude MUPs, leading to confusion with inflammatory myopathy.[53] Repetitive stimulation is necessary to differentiate these disorders. Looking for variation of amplitude with repetitive firing of a single MUP is a sensitive but nonspecific finding of neuromuscular junction involvement.[29, p. 265]

The diagnosis in this case is a postsynaptic disorder of neuromuscular junction transmission characteristic of the type seen in myasthenia gravis.

Arm Weakness (Case 4)

Thought Process

The primary concern in the differential diagnosis is motor neuron disease, specifically amyotrophic lateral sclerosis (ALS). Multifocal motor neuropathy with conduction block could present in this manner and warrants exclusion, given the prognostic implications, but is unlikely to be associated with brisk reflexes.[35] Other causes of motor neuropathy, polyradiculoneuropathy, neuromuscular junction disorders, and myopathies or dystrophies should be considered. Inclusion body myositis[38] could present in this manner, but the brisk reflexes and distribution of weakness would be somewhat unusual. Cervical spondylosis may also present with lower motor neuron findings in the upper limbs and upper motor neuron findings in the lower limbs.[47] The electrophysiological evaluation results are in Table 12–4.

Discussion

Nerve conduction studies were selected to assess motor nerves for degree of axon integrity and to exclude conduction block. The ulnar nerve was stimulated at the wrist, elbow, upper arm, and supraclavicular fossa to look for proximal conduction block. A search for proximal conduction block was also the purpose of the F-wave studies. Repetitive stimulation can be helpful to determine whether the disorder is more rapidly progressive. A decremental response and motor unit variability indicate immaturity and instability of neuromuscular junctions, a situation that occurs with rapid denervation and reinnervation.[13]

The diagnosis of ALS is a clinical diagnosis and cannot be made based solely on NCS and EMG data. The findings on these studies are sensitive and often uncover evidence of denervation in clinically unaffected muscles. In early motor neuron disease, MUP morphology often changes without fibrillation or fasciculation potentials being present. Given the prognosis of this disorder, fulfilling Lambert's EMG criteria of fibrillation potentials in at least two muscles innervated by different nerves and root levels in at least three limbs is recommended.[33] When bulbar symptoms are present, findings in cranial muscles, usually the tongue, can substitute for one of the three limbs. This finding is more specific for ALS. Fasciculation potentials in and of themselves are nonspecific and can be present normally and in many other disorders affecting the motor unit (see Chapter 11).[48, 49]

Unilateral hand weakness can be a presenting sign of ALS.[11] Occasionally, shoulder girdle weakness is the principal early finding, and shoulder girdle neuropathies such as long thoracic, spinal accessory, or suprascapular neuropathies should be considered and excluded if the clinical examination warrants. The NCS and muscles for needle examination should be selected based on the clinical findings.

Inclusion body myositis (IBM) is sometimes confused with motor neuron disease. The history of slowly progressive weakness and EMG findings of diffuse fibrillation and fasciculation potentials can cause confusion. The fasciculation potentials seen in IBM are typically fewer in number than in ALS. IBM can show long-duration, high-amplitude MUPs that distract the electromyographer from the simultaneous presence of short-duration, low-amplitude MUPs. The clinical examination in IBM generally demonstrates more severe involvement of the iliopsoas, quadriceps, biceps brachii, and triceps, and does not show hyperreflexia or other upper motor neuron signs.[38]

The findings in this case are classic for a diffuse disorder of motor neurons and, given the clinical history and examination, a diagnosis of ALS is most appropriate.

CASE STUDY

4

A 50-year-old dentist presented with weakness of the nondominant left hand and heaviness of the right arm, which he felt had progressed over the past 6 months. He denied sensory symptoms. He jogged regularly and noticed that jogging seemed to be more difficult, although his running distance remained the same. He had no difficulty chewing or swallowing and denied bowel or bladder difficulties. He complained of left-hand muscle loss and occasional cramps and muscle twitches.

Clinical examination showed normal sensory findings, brisk upper and lower extremity muscle stretch reflexes, positive Babinski signs in both feet, and a normal cranial nerve examination. Manual muscle testing demonstrated moderate weakness of the median- and ulnar-innervated left-hand intrinsics and forearm pronators, and mild right ulnar-innervated hand weakness, although the wrist and long finger flexors remained normal. Fasciculations were present in the calves and both upper extremities.

TABLE 12–4 Case 4: Arm Weakness

NERVE CONDUCTION STUDIES

Nerve Stimulation (Record)	Amplitude (μV)	Conduction Velocity (msec)	Latencies (msec)	
			Distal	*F-Wave*
Motor				
Peroneal (EDB)	4400	42	4.9	52.5
L ulnar* (hypothenar)	**4700**	54	3.0	28.0
L median (thenar)	**4300**	52	3.8	27.5
Sensory				
Sural (ankle)	10	45	4.0	27.5
L ulnar (fifth)	25	63	2.8	

ELECTROMYOGRAPHY

Muscle	Insertional Activity	Spontaneous Activity		Motor Unit Potentials		
		Fibrillation Potentials	*Fasciculation Potentials*	*Recruitment*	*Duration/ Amplitude*	*Phases/ Turns*
L anterior tibial	Increased	0	+	Reduced	Increased	—
L vastus medialis	Increased	0		Reduced	Increased	—
L gluteus medius	Increased	+	+	Reduced	Increased	Increased
L medial gastrocnemius	Increased	+	++	Reduced	Increased	—
L first dorsal interosseous (manus)	Increased	+++	++	Reduced	Increased	Increased
L flexor pollicis longus	Increased	+	+	Reduced	Increased	—
L pronator teres	Increased	++	++	Reduced	Increased	—
L biceps brachii	Increased	+	+	Reduced	Increased	—
R first dorsal interosseous (manus)	Increased	++	++	Reduced	Increased	—
R triceps	Increased	+	++	Reduced	Increased	—
R deltoid	Increased	+	+	Reduced	Increased	—
R cervical paraspinals	Increased	+	+			—
R midthoracic paraspinals	Increased	++	++			—

Abbreviations: EDB, extensor digitorum brevis; L, left; R, right.
*Includes four-point stimulation to Erb's point and 2-Hz repetitive stimulation at rest—15% decrement noted.

Hand Numbness and Weakness (Case 5)

Nerve conduction studies and EMG are very useful in determining the cause of hand numbness and weakness. Often the patient's report of symptoms is definite, yet vague in terms of distribution. Anatomical variation may also lead to confusion in the clinical evaluation and diagnosis of hand symptoms. The following cases illustrate the benefit of an electrophysiological evaluation.

Thought Process

The differential diagnosis in this case is complicated by many symptoms that could be attributed to a musculoskeletal etiology. The sensory loss in the entire hand can be characteristic of median neuropathy but is not clearly median only. The symptoms are common for carpal tunnel syndrome,[46] but a median neuropathy in the forearm or plexopathy or concomitant ulnar neuropathy should also be considered. The history and exami-

CASE STUDY

A 38-year-old woman working in a meatpacking plant described a 6-month history of forearm, wrist, and hand pain that began in the right hand and more recently occurred in the left. She had burning pain in the palms of both hands and frequently awoke at night with numbness of the entire hand and fingers. The numbness was often relieved by changing positions or shaking her hands. The pain was usually worse at the end of a day of work, after she performed repetitive manual activities. She also complained of neck pain and headaches. Her symptoms had become progressively worse.

Clinical examination revealed normal upper limb muscle stretch reflex and motor findings. Sensory examination revealed decreased pain and touch sensation along the palmar surface of the index and middle fingers of the right hand and positive Tinel's and Phalen's signs at the right wrist. A Tinel sign was also present at both elbows, although less pronounced. The neck and shoulder examination, including foraminal compression and thoracic outlet maneuvers, was normal except for soft tissue tenderness and some limited active range of motion of the neck.

TABLE 12–5 Case 5: Hand Numbness and Weakness

NERVE CONDUCTION STUDIES

Nerve Stimulation (Record)	Amplitude (μV)	Conduction Velocity (msec)	Latencies (msec) Distal	Latencies (msec) F-Wave
Motor				
R median (thenar)	6200	52	**7.8**	32.5
R ulnar (hypothenar)	7400	54	2.8	29.5
L median (thenar)	8000	54	4.0	29.5
L ulnar (hypothenar)	8000	54	3.0	29.5
Sensory				
R median (index)	**NR**			
R ulnar (fifth)	20	65	3.0	
L median (palm)	80	60	**2.5**	
L ulnar (palm)	50	63	1.8	

ELECTROMYOGRAPHY

Muscle	Insertional Activity	Spontaneous Activity: Fibrillation Potentials	Spontaneous Activity: Fasciculation Potentials	Motor Unit Potentials: Recruitment	Motor Unit Potentials: Duration/ Amplitude	Motor Unit Potentials: Phases/ Turns
R first dorsal interosseous (manus)	Normal	0	0	Normal	Normal	—
R abductor pollicis brevis	Increased	+	0	Decreased	Increased	Increased
R pronator teres	Normal	0	0	Normal	Normal	—
R flexor pollicis longus	Normal	0	0	Normal	Normal	—
L abductor pollicis brevis	Normal	0	0	Normal	Normal	—

nation do not support a diagnosis of radiculopathy. Burning pain in the hands could be due to a small-fiber neuropathy or other peripheral neuropathy, but this is highly unusual without simultaneous lower extremity symptoms. The results of the electrophysiological evaluation are presented in Table 12–5.

Discussion

Starting the evaluation with a median motor NCS guides the examiner to select the most appropriate sensory NCS. Stevens[54] has demonstrated that when comparing median and ulnar motor distal latencies in the same hand, values should be within 1.8 msec of each other. In this case, the distal latencies obtained in the right hand show a clear median-to-ulnar discrepancy. However, this does not necessarily mean the lesion is at the wrist. Because of the severity of the median nerve involvement, we no longer need a sensitive test to assess median nerve function. We need an accurate and reliable method to assess the sensory axons remaining in the median nerve. Therefore, a median antidromic sensory study was performed. Findings in the left hand showed no significant discrepancy in motor distal latencies. A very sensitive test that assesses conduction across the carpal tunnel was selected—palmar sensory studies.[26]

The purpose of doing ulnar motor and sensory conduction studies is to exclude ulnar neuropathy, plexopathy, and peripheral neuropathy, to assist in excluding a C8 radiculopathy, and to serve as a means of comparison of conduction at the wrist. When these NCS fail to reveal a clinically suspected abnormality, other conduction studies comparing median-to-radial sensory distal latencies at the thumb, ulnar-to-median latencies to the fourth finger, wrist-to-palm latency and amplitude to the middle finger, and antidromic digital nerve studies to the involved digits can be useful.[26]

The needle examination was initiated in the first dorsal interosseous nerve of the hand, as this is relatively well tolerated by the patient and helps exclude ulnar neuropathy or C8 radiculopathy. Examination of the abductor pollicis brevis (APB) is important to measure motor axon integrity and further define the severity of the neuropathy. If this is abnormal, a median neuropathy in the arm or forearm cannot be excluded. Therefore, the pronator teres was also studied. Pronator teres examination also allows assessment for a C6 or C7 radiculopathy, which can also present with index and middle finger numbness. To completely study all components of the median nerve, examination of the flexor pollicis longus can be performed to assess anterior interosseous function. Given the clear-cut median neuropathy at the right wrist and a much milder median neuropathy at the left wrist on NCS, only the left APB was examined. Because of the normal findings, further studies were not performed. Other coexisting problems could be present, and clinical judgment should be used to determine whether further studies are needed. In the case of hand numbness with normal nerve conduction studies and APB needle examination, a more thorough study of the upper limb is indicated to exclude radiculopathy.

The results of this evaluation demonstrate a focal median neuropathy at each wrist, more pronounced on the right, typical of carpal tunnel syndrome.

CASE STUDY

A 60-year-old diabetic man complained of left-hand numbness and weakness in the postoperative period following lumbar spinal fusion. He described neck pain that was worse when sitting and noted paresthesias along the medial aspect of the hand and fifth digit.

Clinical examination revealed focal findings in the left upper extremity with moderate weakness of the dorsal interossei, mild weakness of wrist flexors and lumbricals, and normal thumb opposition and flexion. Pain and touch sensation were diminished in the fifth digit and the medial aspect of the fourth digit and hand. Tinel's sign was not present at the wrist or elbow. Shoulder and neck examinations were remarkable only for some soft tissue tenderness in the posterior cervical musculature.

Hand Numbness and Weakness (Case 6)

Thought Process

The differential diagnosis in this case includes ulnar neuropathy, most likely due to compression at the elbow as a result of positioning during back surgery. Though the nerve is most vulnerable at the elbow, the patient could have compression at other sites along the course of the ulnar nerve. This patient may have had intravenous or intra-arterial catheters placed in the arm at the time of surgery and, depending on the location, could have a more distal ulnar nerve lesion. However, weakness of the wrist flexors indicates a lesion at the elbow or proximal to the elbow. Other considerations include a low cervical radiculopathy or lower trunk or medial cord plexopathy. The electrophysiological examination is described in Table 12–6.

Discussion

The findings are most consistent with a focal ulnar neuropathy with conduction block proximal to the below-elbow stimulation site. To further define the location of the conduction block, "short-segment stimulation" was performed as demonstrated in Figure 12–1. Conduction block was found at the level of the medial epicondyle.

TABLE 12–6 Case 6: Hand Numbness and Weakness

NERVE CONDUCTION STUDIES

Nerve Stimulation (Record)	Amplitude (μV)	Conduction Velocity (msec)	Latencies (msec)	
			Distal	*F-Wave*
Motor				
L median (thenar)	5600	55	3.8	29.5
L ulnar (hypothenar)			3.5	32.0
Wrist	8700	45		
Below elbow	8400	**48**		
Elbow	**5800**	**46**		
Upper arm	**5600**	**48**		
Supraclavicular	**5300**	**50**		
R ulnar (hypothenar)				
Wrist	8700		3.5	29.0
Elbow	8400	53		
Sensory				
L ulnar (fifth)	10	52	3.8	
L median (index)	12	52	3.8	

ELECTROMYOGRAPHY

Muscle	Insertional Activity	Spontaneous Activity		Motor Unit Potentials	
		Fibrillation Potentials	*Fasciculation Potentials*	*Recruitment*	*Duration/Amplitude*
R first dorsal interosseous (manus)	Increased	+	0	Reduced	Increased
R abductor pollicis brevis	Increased	+	0	Normal	Mildly increased
R flexor pollicis longus	Normal	0	0	Normal	Normal
R flexor carpi ulnaris	Normal	0	0	Reduced	Normal
R pronator teres	Normal	0	0	Normal	Normal
R triceps	Normal	0	0	Normal	Normal
L first dorsal interosseous (manus)	Increased	+	0	Reduced	Increased
R lower cervical paraspinals	Normal	0	0		

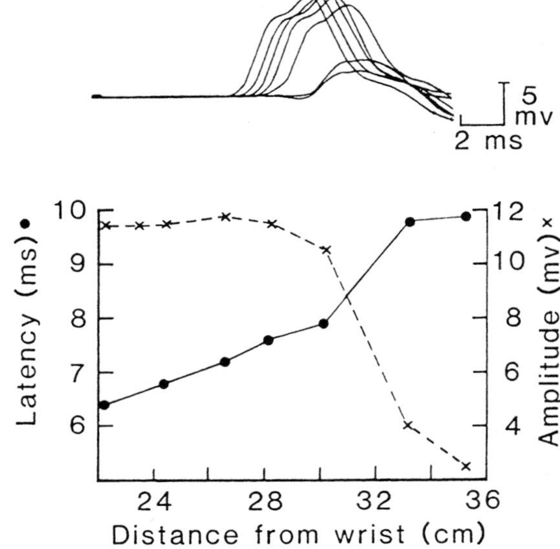

FIGURE 12–1. Ulnar neuropathy at the elbow. Localization with short-segment stimulation.

The borderline ulnar and median SNAP amplitudes, with slight slowing of conduction velocities and mild changes found in distal muscles of both upper limbs, could represent a peripheral neuropathy. If this finding does not clearly correlate with the clinical history and examination, further studies in the lower extremity are indicated to demonstrate electrophysiologically whether a neuropathy is present. To assess the presence of generalized neuropathy, one may begin NCS in the lower limb at the risk of performing multiple additional studies. This was not necessary in this case. The other possibility explaining these findings is median neuropathy at the wrist, but given a lack of discrepancy in median and ulnar sensory distal latencies, knowing that these were determined over the same distance, and with slowing of conduction velocities and first dorsal interosseous involvement, it is unlikely that a median neuropathy at the wrist explains these findings.

The needle examination was extended to additional upper extremity muscles to ensure that a more proximal process was not influencing the findings, particularly given the history of diabetes. The flexor digitorum profundus was examined because the flexor carpi ulnaris may be spared in ulnar neuropathy at the elbow.[10] The opposite extremity was studied, since the manner of positioning for spine surgery puts both ulnar nerves at risk and because many patients have bilateral ulnar neuropathies at the elbows given an anatomical and, in this case, a diabetic predisposition.[39]

The conclusion of these studies is that the patient has an ulnar neuropathy at the level of the left medial epicondyle. Reduced MUP recruitment in the flexor carpi ulnaris and flexor digitorum profoundus muscles indicates that this is most likely an acute conduction block lesion that will likely resolve. The severity and distribution of EMG findings in the hand muscles suggest an underlying peripheral neuropathy.

Hand Numbness and Weakness (Case 7)

Thought Process

The most likely diagnosis in this case is a radial nerve injury due to improper use of axillary crutches, since compression in the axilla by axillary crutches can result in radial nerve injury at this level. However, in this case, the sparing of the triceps and brachioradialis indicates that the radial nerve lesion is distal to the axilla, possibly at the humeral groove, where the radial nerve courses laterally and anterior to the humerus.[14] A classic cause of wristdrop is lead neuropathy, which, despite being a systemic illness, tends to have a predilection for asymmetrical involvement of the radial nerves.[51] Cervical radiculopathy, incomplete posterior cord plexopathy, inflammatory neuropathy, and a hereditary tendency to pressure palsies arc other considerations. The NCS and EMG results are presented in Table 12–7.

Discussion

The median antidromic sensory study was performed first. Since the radial SNAP may be technically more difficult to obtain, proving that the upper extremity sensory nerves are generally normal can make radial nerve findings easier to interpret later. In addition, because these findings could be explained by a plexopathy, early demonstration that nonradial sensory nerve fibers are normal contributes to the exclusion of plexopathy and peripheral neuropathy. With focal neurological examination findings, directing studies to the radial nerve is the next most logical step. Generally, in performing radial sensory and motor conduction studies, stimulating at the elbow is sufficient unless one specifically suspects a conduction block. In this case, more proximal stimula-

CASE STUDY

7

A 27-year-old skier fractured his right tibia, requiring ambulation with axillary crutches. One month after the fracture, he noticed tingling over the dorsum of his left hand. He ignored this and 2 weeks later awoke with a left wristdrop. He was otherwise symptom-free.

Clinical examination showed impaired pain sensation over the dorsum of the hand, thumb, index, and middle fingers. Motor examination revealed moderate weakness of the wrist and finger extensors with normal elbow flexion and extension, pronation, supination, and wrist and finger flexion. Upper extremity reflexes were normal except for a decreased left brachioradialis reflex.

TABLE 12–7 Case 7: Hand Numbness and Weakness

NERVE CONDUCTION STUDIES

Nerve Stimulation (Record)	Amplitude (μV)	Conduction Velocity (msec)	Latencies (msec)	
			Distal	*F-Wave*
Motor				
Radial (extensor indicis proprius)				
Elbow	4000	52	4.2	
Humeral groove*	NR			
Ulnar (hypothenar)	12000	53	3.2	29.0
Sensory				
Median (index)	57	68	3.0	
Radial (dorsum of thenar)	NR			

ELECTROMYOGRAPHY

Muscle	Insertional Activity	Spontaneous Activity		Motor Unit Potentials	
		Fibrillation Potentials	*Fasciculation Potentials*	*Recruitment*	*Duration/Amplitude*
Deltoid	Normal	0	0	Normal	Normal
Biceps brachii	Normal	0	0	Normal	Normal
Triceps	Normal	0	0	Normal	Normal
Brachioradialis	Increased	+	0	Decreased	Increased
Pronator teres	Normal	0	0	Normal	Normal
Extensor indicis proprius	Increased	+++	0	Decreased	Increased
Anconeus	Increased	+	0	Decreased	Increased

Abbreviation: NR, no response.
*Inching shows conduction block between the humeral groove and elbow stimulation sites.

tion disclosed a site of conduction block at an anatomically vulnerable site. The ulnar motor conduction study was performed to complete the study of brachial plexus levels and to exclude plexopathy.

The EMG was initiated by deltoid examination because this muscle is innervated by the axillary nerve, the other branch of the posterior cord of the brachial plexus. Normal findings here indicated that a plexopathy involving the posterior cord was unlikely. The biceps was examined to further assess the midcervical roots. Radial-innervated muscles were examined, starting with the most proximally innervated, the triceps. The triceps is innervated proximal to the humeral groove and was normal. The brachioradialis was then examined and found to be abnormal. The normal biceps brachii study supports a diagnosis of radial neuropathy rather than a C5 or C6 radiculopathy. The pronator teres was examined to study a median-innervated muscle that could be involved in a C6 or C7 radiculopathy or plexopathy. It was normal. A distal radial-innervated muscle was then examined and showed severe involvement. Finally, the anconeus, saved for last since it is a relatively difficult muscle to examine, was studied to determine at which level the axonal loss affecting the radial nerve occurred, because it is the next radial muscle innervated after the triceps branches.

The NCS findings indicated a radial neuropathy with conduction block at the humeral groove. The EMG showed evidence of axonal loss sparing the triceps but involving those muscles innervated distal to the radial nerve as it courses through the groove. These findings are also commonly seen in "Saturday night palsy," a compression neuropathy of the radial nerve at the humeral groove.

LOWER LIMB PROBLEMS

As in the upper extremities, disorders that affect the lower extremities may be localized or may represent generalized processes. Lumbar and sacral radiculopathies are more often bilateral than are cervical radiculopathies, but lumbar or sacral plexopathies are less often bilateral than are brachial plexopathies. Entrapment neuropathies in the lower limbs and mononeuropathies are also less common than in the upper limbs. Peroneal nerve compression at the fibular head is the most common lower extremity mononeuropathy. Less common lower extremity mononeuropathies include involvement of the femoral, tibial, sciatic, plantar, saphenous, and lateral femoral cutaneous nerves.

Generalized disorders that can begin or manifest with lower limb weakness or numbness include inflammatory myopathies, most peripheral neuropathies and polyradiculoneuropathies, inclusion body myositis, motor neuron disease, and neuromuscular junction disorders, particularly LEMS. The following cases illustrate the more common lower limb problems.

Low Back and Leg Pain (Case 8)

Thought Process

The differential diagnosis includes chronic lumbosacral radiculopathy or polyradiculopathy from spinal ste-

CASE STUDY 8

A 77-year-old woman with a 2-year history of non-insulin-dependent diabetes but who was otherwise healthy presented with a 10-year history of low back pain that had increased in the past year. She also noted leg pain in the past 6 months. When walking more than one block, she experienced aching in the posterior thighs and calves. If she stopped, leaned forward over a fence, or sat on a park bench, the pain resolved over 10 to 15 minutes. She noted less difficulty with leg pain while pushing a grocery cart while shopping. She noted some transient tingling in the legs and was not certain of the distribution or of exacerbating factors. She also experienced occasional stress incontinence but this had not changed in 15 years. Coughing or sneezing did not exacerbate the pain. Sitting was more comfortable than standing, but any static position for prolonged periods irritated her back. She denied weight loss, fatigue, or night pain.

Clinical examination showed normal lower extremity pulses and temperature. Spine examination showed limited lumbar range of motion and mild scoliosis with the major curve in the lumbar spine. There was no spine percussion pain. Straight leg raising was negative bilaterally. Muscle stretch reflexes were normal in the upper extremities and knees, but internal hamstring and Achilles reflexes were depressed bilaterally. Mild calf and foot intrinsic atrophy was present. Sensory examination was remarkable only for decreased vibratory sensation in the toes.

nosis or perhaps diabetes. A diabetic peripheral neuropathy could be present, but the examination and history are not suggestive. Peripheral neuropathies of other types should be considered. Other causes of polyradiculopathy such as conus ependymoma, other intraspinal tumors, or infectious disorders, including meningeal sarcoidosis, could present in this fashion but would usually have other features not present in this case. An inflammatory polyradiculopathy or vasculitis could cause these examination findings, but they usually also involve the upper extremities and follow a more stuttering course with acute or subacute worsening.[9, 44] These disorders are unlikely to cause the neurogenic claudication of which this patient appears to be complaining. A lumbosacral plexopathy could be present but is unlikely to be bilateral, and in diabetes it usually presents with acute and severe pain affecting a single lower extremity.[56, pp. 1228–1229] Cauda equina tumors or perhaps even conus medullaris tumors could present with some of these features, but usually more severe neurological findings and bladder and bowel symptoms would result. Spinal cord arteriovenous malformation is an important consideration. Of course, vascular disease as a cause of leg pain must also be considered. The NCS and EMG findings are presented in Table 12–8.

Discussion

NCS were performed to assess the degree of axonal loss from the suspected polyradiculopathy and to help exclude peripheral neuropathy, lumbosacral plexopathy, and nonstructural causes of polyradiculopathy. The peroneal motor study recording from the extensor digitorum brevis provided an assessment of the L5 root and sciatic and peroneal nerves. The tibial study provided information about the S1 root and sciatic and tibial nerves. A femoral NCS could have been done, but it is technically more difficult, more uncomfortable for the patient, and does not help exclude problems affecting distal peripheral nerves. The sural sensory NCS was performed because it is the most reliable lower extremity sensory conduction study, and it helped exclude lumbosacral plexopathy or peripheral neuropathy. Even though the sural SNAP was normal, a mild distal neuropathy could still be present as the sural SNAP is recorded along the nerve trunk at the ankle and not along its most terminal fibers. A medial-plantar SNAP could be attempted, particularly in a younger person, to exclude peripheral neuropathy, although is not likely to be present in normal persons at this age.[40] Further NCS were not performed, given the symmetry of the symptoms and signs. However, when findings include generally low CMAPs, LEMS should be considered. If weakness had been the predominant feature of this case, further motor conduction studies and repetitive stimulation would have been performed. An H-reflex can be performed if the needle examination is negative.

The needle examination strategy is to study muscles innervated by the principal nerve roots and nerves to the legs. The anterior tibial provides peroneal and L4–5 root assessment; the medial gastrocnemius. L5–S1 root and tibial nerve. Other L5-innervated muscles, such as the peroneus longus, posterior tibial, or extensor hallucis longus, could be examined. Given abnormalities in the L5–S1 distribution, the next level to assess is L4, so the vastus medialis was studied. With further abnormality here, we have not yet defined the level of the lesion. A severe peripheral neuropathy can explain these findings, so the proximal muscles were examined. The adductor longus provides information about the L2–3 roots and obturator nerve. Assessment of more proximal muscles innervated by L5, the tensor fascia lata, and S1, the gluteus maximus, also disclosed abnormal findings. Based on the information obtained so far, this appeared likely to be due to a root level disorder, but a plexopathy could not be completely excluded. Of concern in a diabetic patient is that multiple neurological problems can coexist.[56, pp. 1219–1230] To place the level of the disorder at the root, paraspinal muscles were examined. Because of the concern regarding a more widespread diabetic polyradiculopathy, paraspinous muscle examination was extended into the the thoracic level to exclude generalized spinal level involvement.[29, pp. 449–450]

TABLE 12–8 Case 8: Low Back and Leg Pain

NERVE CONDUCTION STUDIES

Nerve Stimulation (Record)	Amplitude (μV)	Conduction Velocity (msec)	Latencies (msec)	
			Distal	*F-Wave*
Motor				
Peroneal (EDB)	**1700**	42	5.3	58.0
Tibial (AH)	2300	42	4.9	60.0
Sensory				
Sural (ankle)	8		4.0	

ELECTROMYOGRAPHY

Muscle	Insertional Activity	Spontaneous Activity		Motor Unit Potentials		
		Fibrillation Potentials	*Fasciculation Potentials*	*Recruitment*	*Duration/Amplitude*	*Phases/Turns*
R anterior tibial	Normal	0	0	Reduced	Increased	—
R medial gastrocnemius	Increased	0	+	Reduced	Increased	—
R peroneus longus	Increased	+	+	Reduced	Increased	Increased
R vastus medialis	Normal	0	0	Reduced	Increased	—
R adductor longus	Normal	0	0	Normal	Normal	—
R tensor fascia lata	Decreased	0	0	Reduced	Increased	—
R gluteus maximus	Normal	0	+	Reduced	Increased	—
R lower lumbar paraspinals	Increased	+	0			—
R high lumbar paraspinals	Increased	+	0			—
R lower thoracic paraspinals	Normal	0	0			—
L peroneal longus	Increased	0	0	Reduced	Increased	—
L medial gastrocnemius	Increased	0	0			—
L vastus medialis	Normal	0	0			
L adductor longus	Normal	0	0	Normal	Normal	

Abbreviations: EDB, extensor digitorum brevis; AH, abductor hallucis.
*No conduction block or temporal dispersion noted.

The conclusion from the electrophysiological studies is that this patient has multiple chronic lumbosacral radiculopathies, more severe on the right. Given the clinical symptoms and signs, this is most likely structural, related to spinal stenosis. Further studies, including imaging of the lumbar spine, are warranted to exclude an intraspinal lesion, including arteriovenous malformation.[4]

Lower Extremity Weakness (Case 9)

Thought Process

The differential diagnosis includes polyradiculopathy or polyradiculoneuropathy. A primarily motor polyradiculopathy, such as an inflammatory polyradiculopathy, could present in this manner. Motor neuron disease is certainly a consideration, although, without hyperactive reflexes, this is not classic for ALS.[11] A myopathy or late-onset dystrophy or early LEMS could present in this way. Of particular note is the pattern of weakness, which is typical in IBM.[38] A disorder of the spinal cord, particularly involving anterior horn cells, could produce this picture. A combination of a motor disorder and a peripheral neuropathy must be considered, given the abnormal sensory examination. The electrophysiological findings are presented in Table 12–9.

CASE STUDY

9

A 60-year-old man with a 50-pack-year history of smoking complained of leg weakness that had begun approximately 6 months earlier. He denied pain and sensory or bowel or bladder changes, and primarily noted that his legs felt heavy and fatigued. Ascending or descending stairs was more difficult. The right leg seemed worse to him than the left leg. He denied difficulty chewing, swallowing, breathing, or double vision.

Clinical examination revealed normal mental status and cranial nerves. Muscle stretch reflexes were slightly depressed from normal in the lower limbs. Vibratory and touch sensations were mildly diminished distally. Motor examination revealed mild weakness of the triceps and most lower extremity muscle groups. The quadriceps was weaker than any other muscle group and the anterior thighs demonstrated significant atrophy.

TABLE 12–9 Case 9: Lower Extremity Weakness

NERVE CONDUCTION STUDIES

Nerve Stimulation (Record)	Amplitude (μV)	Conduction Velocity (msec)	Latencies (msec) Distal	F-Wave
Motor				
R peroneal (EDB)*	2300	42	4.8	55.0
R tibial (AH)	3600	41	5.2	56.0
R ulnar (hypothenar)	7200	52	3.2	
Sensory				
L sural (ankle)	**NR**			
R median (index)	**10**	**53**	3.4	
R ulnar (fifth)	**5**		3.0	

ELECTROMYOGRAPHY

Muscle	Insertional Activity	Spontaneous Activity: *Fibrillation Potentials*	*Fasciculation Potentials*	Motor Unit Potentials: *Recruitment*	*Duration/Amplitude*	*Phases/Turns*
R anterior tibial	Increased	+	0	Reduced	Increased and decreased	—
R medial gastrocnemius	Increased	+	0	Reduced	Increased and decreased	—
R abductor hallucis	Increased	++	0	Reduced	Increased	—
R rectus femoris	Increased	+++	+	Reduced	Increased and decreased	Increased
R tensor fascia lata	Increased	+	0		Increased and decreased	—
R first dorsal interosseous (manus)	Normal	0	0	Reduced	Increased	—
R triceps	Increased	+	+	Reduced	Increased and decreased	—
R biceps	Normal	0	+	Normal	Normal	—
R midthoracic paraspinals	Increased	0	+			—

Abbreviations: EDB, extensor digitorum brevis; AH, abductor hallucis; NR, no response.
*2-Hz repetitive stimulation at rest and following brief exercise is normal.

Discussion

NCS were initiated with the peroneal motor study to assess distal motor axons (proximal L5 root, peroneal nerve) and because this study lends itself to easy repetitive stimulation testing. The borderline amplitude could represent any of the above disorders or could be normal. Repetitive stimulation performed at rest to screen primarily for a presynaptic neuromuscular junction disorder was normal. The absent sural SNAP is likely due to a neuropathy. To further examine the sensory nerves, a median antidromic study was done. Low amplitude and slow conduction velocity correlate with a peripheral neuropathy, but a median neuropathy could also produce these findings. An ulnar SNAP study was performed that demonstrated an abnormality and supported the conclusion that a peripheral neuropathy was likely. An ulnar motor study was conducted to determine the extent of upper limb neuropathy.

On needle examination, the mixture of MUPs of both increased and decreased amplitude and duration in the anterior tibial muscle could represent a combined myopathy and neuropathy, chronic myopathy, or IBM. The medial gastrocnemius was examined to explore findings in a muscle at a comparable distal anatomical level, and similar findings were noted. Because of the question of a coexisting peripheral neuropathy, a foot muscle was studied and was found to be more severely involved, with only large MUPs present. This favored a coexisting neuropathy. Proximal lower limb muscles showed that the quadriceps was most severely involved. Moving to the upper limb becomes important, since subclinical findings of neuropathy and myopathy may be present. Here, more subtle changes were noted, again including a mixture of large and small MUPs in some muscles, with the most severe involvement in the triceps.

Based on the electrophysiological studies alone, a coexisting myopathy and peripheral neuropathy is the most likely diagnosis. However, taken together with the clinical pattern of weakness and the more severe involvement of the quadriceps and triceps confirmed by needle examination, IBM must be considered. This can be confirmed only on muscle biopsy.

IBM is often associated with some neuropathic findings and fasciculation potentials, which can be confusing. Sensory studies are often not as significantly affected as in the case presented here. A not uncommon mistake is to ignore or not recognize the presence of short-duration, low-amplitude MUPs in the presence of others of long duration and high amplitude, resulting in an incorrect conclusion of motor neuron disease. There is no cure for either condition, but the prognosis for IBM is more positive than for motor neuron disease.[38]

CASE STUDY 10

A 20-year-old college student awakened with right leg and ankle weakness and numbness. She had attended a party, where she used alcohol heavily, and had fallen asleep on her bedroom floor. She sought evaluation 3 days after onset of these symptoms.

Clinical examination was normal except for a patch of sensory loss on the dorsum of the right foot and weakness of the ankle dorsiflexors, evertors, and toe extensors.

Foot Numbness and Pain (Case 10)

Thought Process

The diagnosis here is almost certainly a peroneal neuropathy, most likely due to compression at the fibular head. Included in the differential diagnosis is a more proximal peroneal or sciatic neuropathy or an L5 radiculopathy. With a radiculopathy, the ankle invertors should also be weak. A lumbosacral plexopathy is unlikely to present with such isolated findings. Hereditary tendency to pressure palsies should also be considered, but in this patient there was no history of prior nerve palsies or family history of nerve problems. Table 12–10 outlines the electrophysiological findings.

Discussion

Starting with the peroneal motor NCS was the most logical first step, given the high clinical suspicion that a peroneal neuropathy was present. The large discrepancy between the ankle and knee CMAP amplitudes requires stimulation distal to the site most common for compression. Stimulation at or just below the fibular head showed an amplitude similar to the ankle amplitude, indicating a conduction block proximal to this point of stimulation. Short-segment stimulation was performed to specifically localize the lesion. The superficial peroneal nerve was studied to evaluate which divisions of the peroneal nerve were involved and to help exclude peripheral neuropathy or plexopathy. The tibial NCS was performed strictly to help exclude plexopathy, radiculopathy, or sciatic neuropathy.

The needle examination was performed in muscles that would (1) assess both deep and superficial divisions of the peroneal nerve; (2) explore the tibial division of the sciatic nerve; (3) differentiate an L5 radiculopathy from a peroneal neuropathy; and (4) demonstrate the level of the peroneal neuropathy. The relative acuity of the symptoms did not allow the examiner to define the degree of axonal loss, as the duration of the problem was not sufficient to significantly alter distal axon excitability or cause wallerian degeneration.[29, pp. 64–69] The conduction block signifies at least a neurapraxic lesion at the fibular head. If recovery does not ensue, a repeat study to assess for level of axonal loss and axonotmesis would be useful. The problem was diagnosed as a focal

TABLE 12–10 Case 10: Foot Numbness and Pain

NERVE CONDUCTION STUDIES

Nerve Stimulation (Record)	Amplitude (μV)	Conduction Velocity (msec)	Latencies (msec)	
			Distal	*F-Wave*
Motor				
R peroneal (EDB)				
Ankle	6000		5.2	53.0
Knee	**2500**	**40**		
Fibular head*	5800	51		
R tibial	8800	50	5.2	53.0
Sensory				
R Superficial peroneal (ankle)	20		4.5	

ELECTROMYOGRAPHY

Muscle	Insertional Activity	Spontaneous Activity		Motor Unit Potentials	
		Fibrillation Potentials	*Fasciculation Potentials*	*Recruitment*	*Duration/Amplitude*
Anterior tibial	Normal	0	0	Reduced	Normal
Medial gastrocnemius	Normal	0	0	Normal	Normal
Peroneal longus	Normal	0	0	Reduced	Normal
Posterior tibial	Normal	0	0	Normal	Normal
Biceps femoris, short head	Normal	0	0	Normal	Normal

Abbreviation: EDB, extensor digitorum brevis.
*Inching demonstrates focal conduction block 1 cm proximal to the fibular head.

CASE STUDY 11

A 55-year-old woman presented with a 3-month history of steadily increasing difficulty performing overhead activities such as washing her hair and reaching cupboards. She also noted difficulty arising from low chairs and climbing stairs. She had a history of goiter but was currently euthyroid and otherwise in good health. She denied sensory symptoms or difficulty with speech or swallowing, although on occasion she felt solids "sticking" in her esophagus. Her weakness did not fluctuate and was not exercise-related. She denied cramps and had no family history of similar problems.

The clinical examination was remarkable for normal facial strength, muscle stretch reflexes, and sensory examination. Motor examination showed moderate weakness of neck flexors, shoulder girdle, biceps brachii, and triceps muscles, hip girdle, quadriceps, and hamstring muscles. These muscles were not fatigable. Proximal muscle bulk appeared somewhat reduced. Myotonia was not present.

---

common peroneal neuropathy with conduction block 1 cm proximal to the fibular head.

Generalized Weakness (Case 11)

Thought Process

The most likely diagnosis was thought to be a proximal myopathy or dystrophy. Given the history of an autoimmune thyroid disease, the most likely possibility is another autoimmune disorder such as inflammatory myopathy or myasthenia gravis. The degree of limb involvement without facial involvement is more characteristic of polymyositis than of myasthenia gravis (as described in Case 3).

Other considerations in the differential diagnosis include late-onset dystrophy, motor neuron disease, motor neuropathy or polyradiculoneuropathy, thyroid-related myopathy, or a neuromuscular junction defect such as LEMS. The NCS and EMG findings are presented in Table 12–11.

Discussion

The approach used (1) demonstrated the degree of involvement of both the upper and lower limbs; (2) excluded motor neuropathy or a neuromuscular junction defect; and (3) proved the sensory system was not involved. The peroneal CMAP amplitude was at the lower limits of normal. The sural SNAP was normal. The ulnar motor conduction study was performed because of the ease of performing repetitive stimulation and was normal. Patchy involvement may be present in myasthenia gravis, so it is necessary to perform repetitive stimulation in an area that is clinically involved. The accessory NCS was chosen because the trapezius was clinically involved, and because of the relative technical ease of performing this study.

The needle examination was performed in proximal and distal muscles of the upper and lower limbs to define the distribution of involvement. In performing a needle examination in inflammatory myopathy, it is important to recognize that within a muscle, findings may be fairly

TABLE 12–11 Case 11: Generalized Weakness

NERVE CONDUCTION STUDIES

Nerve Stimulation (Record)	Amplitude (μV)	Conduction Velocity (msec)	Latencies (msec)	
			Distal	*F-Wave*
Motor				
Peroneal (EDB)	2500	44	5.2	56.0
Ulnar (hypothenar)*	10500	53	3.2	32.0
Accessory (trapezius)*	3600		4.0	
Sensory				
Sural (ankle)	18		4.0	

ELECTROMYOGRAPHY

Muscle	Insertional Activity	Spontaneous Activity		Motor Unit Potentials		Phases/ Turns
		Fibrillation Potentials	*Fasciculation Potentials*	*Recruitment*	*Duration/Amplitude*	
Anterior tibial	Increased	+	0		Decreased	—
Vastus medialis	Increased	++	0	Rapid	Decreased	Increased
Gluteus medius	Increased	++	0	Rapid	Decreased	Increased
First dorsal interosseous (manus)	Normal	0	0	Normal	Normal	—
Biceps	Increased	+	0	Rapid	Decreased	Increased

Abbreviation: EDB, extensor digitorum brevis.
*2-Hz repetitive stimulation at rest and following 1 minute of exercise did not produce a decrement or increment.

CASE STUDY 12

A 33-year-old female assembly line worker presented with forearm pain and hand cramps and noted that fine motor tasks were becoming increasingly more difficult. She denied sensory symptoms or symptoms characteristic of carpal tunnel syndrome. She denied cramps and weakness. She denied a family history of any nerve or muscle problems.

Clinical examination was normal except for weakness of the finger flexors. Obesity impeded the ability to assess for percussion myotonia in the limbs, though tongue myotonia was not present. She did exhibit a delayed relaxation of grip.

Further review determined that the patient had become amenorrheic in her late teens. She also noted increased hand cramping in the cold. She did not have a family history of muscle disease to her knowledge, but did have a family history of diabetes and fertility problems. On examination, the patient had long hair covering the forehead, but when the hair was lifted from her forehead, significant frontal balding was noted. The obese face did not display the atrophy that can be characteristic of myotonic dystrophy, but a lid lag was present after tightly closing the eyes.

localized, with some areas severely involved and other areas that are normal. A careful search in each muscle is important. In subtle cases, the only abnormality found may be in the paraspinous muscles.[2,55] Paraspinous muscles were not examined in this case owing to the obvious abnormalities in other proximal muscle groups. It is also important to remember that in more chronic myopathies, some long-duration, high-amplitude MUPs can be seen, and should not dissuade the examiner from a diagnosis of myopathy.[8] Myasthenia gravis can rarely present with needle examination findings similar to those seen in this case, highlighting the importance of performing repetitive stimulation to ensure that this disorder is not overlooked. The most likely diagnosis in this case is a myopathy that results in fiber splitting, vacuolization, and fiber necrosis, as is seen in polymyositis.[7]

Generalized Weakness (Case 12)

Thought Process

This was a puzzling case, given the limited features in a patient who was predisposed to have an overuse syndrome. If finger flexor weakness is not effort-related, a selective distal myopathy or perhaps incomplete nerve entrapment syndrome can produce these findings. The delayed grip relaxation could be a sign of a metabolic disturbance of muscle such as a myotonic disorder or tetany. A peripheral neuropathy could produce these findings, but the lack of sensory features and lower extremity involvement would be highly atypical. As the electrophysiological studies (Table 12–12) are initiated, the most likely diagnosis is not clear.

TABLE 12–12 Case 12: Generalized Weakness

NERVE CONDUCTION STUDIES

Nerve Stimulation (Record)	Amplitude (μV)	Conduction Velocity (msec)	Latencies (msec) Distal	Latencies (msec) F-Wave
Motor				
Median (thenar)	6800	56	3.2	31.5
Ulnar (hypothenar)	10300	55	2.8	31.0
Sensory				
Median (palm-wrist)	160	65	1.8	
Ulnar (palm-wrist)	90	67	1.8	

ELECTROMYOGRAPHY

Muscle	Insertional Activity	Spontaneous Activity: Fibrillation Potentials	Spontaneous Activity: Fasciculation Potentials	Motor Unit Potentials: Recruitment	Motor Unit Potentials: Duration/Amplitude	Motor Unit Potentials: Comment
First dorsal interosseous (manus)	Increased			Difficult to assess	Difficult to assess	Marked myotonic discharges
Pronator teres	Increased	+	0	Rapid	Decreased	Myotonic discharges
Biceps	Increased	0	0	Normal	Normal	Occasional myotonic discharges
Anterior tibial	Increased	+	0	Rapid	Decreased	Myotonic discharges
Gluteus medius	Increased	0	0	Normal	Normal	Occasional myotonic discharges
L cervical paraspinals	Increased	0	0			Myotonic discharges

Discussion

NCS were performed on the median and ulnar nerves looking for a nerve entrapment that would explain the finger flexor weakness. These studies were normal. The needle examination was somewhat surprising and clearly demonstrated myotonic discharges and myopathic MUP changes affecting the distal muscles most severely. Given these findings, a return to the clinical history and examination was necessary.

These findings are all characteristic of myotonic dystrophy. Myotonic dystrophy is a primarily distal myopathy and may have many associated features, including endocrine, dermatologic, and cardiac complications. The condition is dominantly inherited with incomplete penetrance, and some of these features may present in some family members and not others.[23, 24] This case demonstrates that at times the EMG shows unexpected findings, forcing the electrodiagnostician to go back to the drawing board by returning to the history and physical examination. This instant feedback on the veracity of one's history and physical examination makes the electrodiagnostician a better clinician over the course of time.

Generalized Numbness (Case 13)

Thought Process

The primary diagnostic consideration in this case was acute inflammatory demyelinating polyradiculoneuropathy (AIDP) or Guillain-Barré syndrome. An idiopathic or inflammatory etiology could be presumed, but other possibilities had to be considered, including arsenic toxicity, axonal neuropathy from a vasculitis, other toxins, including other heavy metals, or porphyria. A dysproteinemia or paraneoplastic syndrome can also present in this manner.[5] The history was strongly in favor of an acquired rather than a hereditary process. The pattern of electrophysiological findings was imperative in guiding the differential diagnosis, because the findings allowed differentiation of axonal from demyelinating and sensory from motor involvement (Table 12–13).

Discussion

This patient was far enough into the course (10 days) that fairly obvious electrophysiological features would be present and identifiable. These findings often lag behind the clinical course. As a rule, starting the NCS and EMG in the lower extremities and then moving to the upper extremities is fairly typical for a peripheral neuropathy assessment. However, if the severity of findings predicted in the legs is so severe that the examiner anticipates lack of evoked action potentials, beginning in the arms is often more feasible. It is also advisable in cases of suspected AIDP to perform studies on multiple motor nerves to define the presence of conduction block and to avoid common sites for conduction block due to compression.[1]

In this case, we were able to obtain reasonable CMAPs from the lower extremities. All studies showed significant temporal dispersion, and a focal conduction block was identified in the peroneal nerve just distal to the fibular head. The normal amplitude discrepancy between proximal and distal stimulation of the tibial nerve makes this nerve difficult to assess for conduction block and temporal dispersion unless they are pronounced. The sural SNAP was present and the median SNAP was absent, a finding not uncommon in AIDP. Sensory and motor nerves showed significant slowing. Motor nerves also showed temporal dispersion and conduction block in the upper limbs. Prolonged F-wave latencies were also noted. These were prolonged when corrected for conduction velocity using F-wave estimation, and demonstrated slowing in proximal nerve segments. A musculocutaneous conduction study was performed to demonstrate that proximal slowing was present. Given the severe limb involvement, blink reflexes were recorded and were found to be prolonged, indicating a very proximal peripheral nerve lesion.

The needle examination showed primarily recruitment abnormalities related to conduction block. Given some of the low CMAPs recorded distally over the next few weeks, one could expect fibrillation potentials to occur distally and in paraspinal muscles. Studying paraspinal muscles is important to place part of the lesion

CASE STUDY

13

A 29-year-old man noted tingling of the toes when he woke up one morning. While walking to work, he noted a tendency to catch his toes on sidewalk cracks. By midday his feet felt numb and walking was generally uncoordinated. Some hand tingling was also noted, and by that evening hand clumsiness was present. The patient decided to wait until morning to seek a medical evaluation when he awoke the next morning he was unable to get out of bed unassisted and could not walk. He was emergently admitted to a local hospital and over the next week continued to get weaker. Eventually he was electively placed on mechanical ventilation. He was in general good health but 3 weeks prior to the onset of these symptoms had experienced a flulike illness.

An EMG was requested 10 days into the course. Clinical examination showed generalized areflexia, sensory loss to all modalities that was worse in the distal upper and lower limbs, and flaccid quadriparesis.

TABLE 12–13 Case 13: Generalized Numbness

NERVE CONDUCTION STUDIES

Nerve Stimulation (Record)	Amplitude (μV)	Conduction Velocity (msec)	Latencies (msec)	
			Distal	*F-Wave*
Motor				
Peroneal (EDB)	1800	**28**	**6.5**	NR
Tibial (AH)	2700	**32**	**6.5**	77.5
Ulnar (hypothenar)	6600	**44**	**3.8**	51.0
Median (thenar)	4900	**42**	4.4	55.0
Musculocutaneous (biceps)	4500	58	5.2	
Sensory				
Sural (ankle)	**8**			
Median (index)	**NR**			
Ulnar (fifth)	15	**52**	3.5	
Blink Reflex				
R trigeminal (R orbicularis oculi)			R_1 = **18.0** R_2 = 42.5	

ELECTROMYOGRAPHY

Muscle	Insertional Activity	Spontaneous Activity		Motor Unit Potentials	
		Fibrillation Potentials	*Fasciculation Potentials*	*Recruitment*	*Duration/Amplitude*
Anterior tibial	Normal	0	0	None	
Tensor fasciae latae	Normal	0	0	Reduced	Normal
First dorsal interosseous (manus)	Normal	0	0	Reduced	Normal
Biceps	Normal	0	0	Reduced	Normal
L lumbar paraspinals	Normal	0	0		

Abbreviations: EDB, extensor digitorum brevis; AH, abductor hallucis; NR, no response.

proximally to confirm the diagnosis of polyradiculoneuropathy. The findings in this case were characteristic of AIDP.

CRANIOFACIAL PROBLEMS

Case 14

Disorders of the head and face are seen less commonly in the clinical neurophysiological laboratory but are important to recognize. Disorders that cause facial numbness, pain, twitching, or weakness are the most likely referrals for electrophysiological evaluation. Disorders that result in dysphagia, dysarthria, or vocal cord paralysis can also be evaluated less routinely. The case presented here is of Bell's palsy, since NCS and EMG may be useful in the diagnosis and prognosis of this disorder. Other disorders that lend themselves to evaluation include trigeminal and facial neuropathies from idiopathic, inflammatory, or compressive causes such as posterior fossa tumors, most commonly acoustic neuromas. Hemifacial spasm can be well-defined and differentiated from blepharospasm and synkinesis using NCS and EMG, and is usually the result of vascular compression of the facial nerve. As previously discussed, facial weakness can be due to myasthenia gravis or myasthenic syndrome as well as myopathies or dystrophies involving the face. Techniques that can be used for evaluating these problems include facial NCS; EMG of facial, ocu-

CASE STUDY

14

A 50-year-old woman awoke one morning and on looking in the mirror noticed a right facial droop that was especially pronounced when she smiled. She did not experience numbness but noted that it was difficult to completely close the right eye. Pursing her lips while eating was also difficult. She decided she had "slept wrong" and did not seek medical attention until 3 days later.

Clinical examination at that time revealed intact extraocular motions and visual fields, facial sensation, hearing, taste, and palatal and tongue motions. The right nasolabial fold was flattened and there was little movement of the right side of the face with smiling. The orbicularis oculi and oris were weak and she could not raise the right eyebrow.

TABLE 12–14 Case 14: Craniofacial Problems

NERVE CONDUCTION STUDIES

Nerve Stimulation (Record)	Amplitude (μV)	Distal Latency (msec)
R facial orbicularis oculi	**1500**	3.4
L facial orbicularis oculi	2900	3.2

Blink Reflex Latency (msec)	R_1	Ipsilateral R_2	Contralateral R_2
L trigeminal	10.7	36.0	**47.0**
R trigeminal	**23.1**	**48.1**	39.1

ELECTROMYOGRAPHY

Muscle	Insertional Activity	Spontaneous Activity: *Fibrillation Potentials*	Spontaneous Activity: *Fasciculation Potentials*	Motor Unit Potentials: *Recruitment*	Motor Unit Potentials: *Duration/Amplitude*
R orbicularis oculi	Normal	0	0	Reduced	Normal
R orbicularis oris	Normal	0	0	Reduced	Normal
R frontalis	Normal	0	0	Reduced	Normal
R mentalis	Normal	0	0	Reduced	Normal
L orbicularis oculi	Normal	0	0	Normal	Normal

lar, laryngeal, pharyngeal, and palatal muscles; reflex responses, including the blink reflex, masseter reflex, masseteric inhibitory reflex, and lateral spread response; as well as electrophysiological demonstration of synkinesis. Visual, brainstem, and trigeminal-evoked potentials may also be used in assessing these disorders.

Thought Process

The history, signs, and symptoms are classic for an idiopathic facial neuropathy, or Bell's palsy. Other possibilities include a posterior fossa tumor, multiple sclerosis, brainstem stroke, and, less likely, an infection-related facial neuropathy such as herpes zoster or Lyme disease.[28] Nerve conduction studies to evaluate the facial nerve and exclude other cranial neuropathies were performed (Table 12–14).

Discussion

Bilateral facial nerve conduction studies should be performed first. A low facial amplitude CMAP was recorded over the right orbicularis oculi. Blink reflexes (Fig. 12–2) are also important to define the site of the lesion relative to the facial nucleus. The right efferent limb of this reflex—that is, the facial nerve—was impaired. The fact that there was a normal facial nerve distal latency yet prolonged ipsilateral blink reflex latency is important. These findings suggest a lesion proximal to the stylomastoid foramen. Further studies to evaluate the bony segment and intracranial portion of the nerve are important. Depending on the clinical situation, brainstem auditory-evoked potentials, the masseter reflex, and accessory NCS can be performed to show that other cranial nerves are not involved.

Needle examination showed only reduced MUP recruitment, given the relatively early course of the problem. Because of future prognostic considerations, needle examination of muscles innervated by multiple branches of the facial nerve was performed to assess the extent of involvement, since routine facial NCS allows us to look only at a single branch.

NCS can be used prognostically in some cases. This is related to whether the lesion is merely demyelinating or includes axon loss. The facial CMAP amplitude measured after adequate time for wallerian degeneration to occur is probably the most useful prognostic measure. A facial CMAP amplitude that is less than 10% of that on the healthy side denotes delayed recovery for at least 6 to 12 months, with significantly limited function. An amplitude of 10% to 30% that of the unaffected side heralds mild to moderate dysfunction at 2 to 8 months. Facial CMAP amplitude greater than 30% of normal usually predicts full recovery within 2 months.[41] The electrophysiological findings are consistent with a right facial neuropathy.

L. Supraorbital nerve

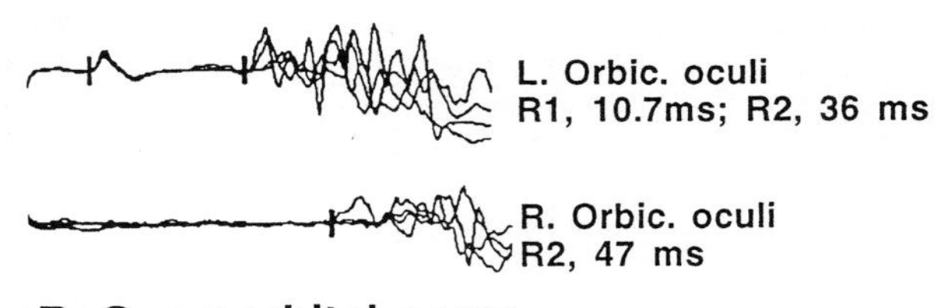

R. Supraorbital nerve

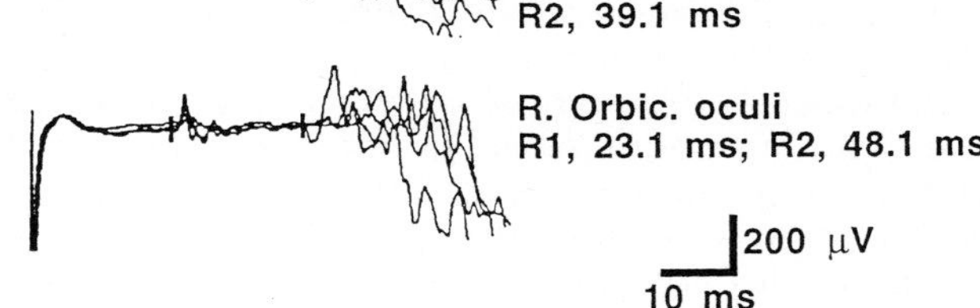

R. Facial nerve lesion

FIGURE 12–2. Blink reflexes.

PEDIATRIC ELECTROMYOGRAPHY

Case 15

Clinical neurophysiological testing in children is in many respects a specialty unto itself. The basic techniques of NCS and needle EMG are similar but require smaller electrodes and use of shorter distances, depending on the age and size of the patient. The basic physiological principles are similar to those in adults, but the clinician must understand age-related changes in the anatomy and physiology of nerve, neuromuscular junction, and muscle. Patient tolerance is a critical issue, and it requires a skilled examiner to glean crucial electrophysiological data in the most efficient manner possible. Each age group displays behavioral characteristics that must be recognized and managed skillfully to achieve the greatest level of cooperation possible for a complete study. Understanding and cooperation of the parents should not be overlooked.

The range of disorders that can exist in children is extensive, and normal electrophysiological parameters differ with age. Those in the 12- to 18-year-old age range will generally have amplitudes, conduction velocities, distal latencies, MUP morphology, and neuromuscular junction characteristics that are similar to normal adult values because nerves, muscles, and neuromuscular junctions have matured.[56, pp. 1219–1230] This age does not necessarily guarantee adult levels of cooperation, however.

Prior to age 12, development of the motor unit is not complete and CMAP amplitudes and MUP morphology differ from those of adults. Myelination begins in utero at 15 weeks' gestation. By age 3 to 5 years, peripheral nerve myelination is complete and conduction velocities and distal latencies approach normal adult values.[17] It is important to recognize that distal latencies are generally shorter than in adults because of shorter distances. Infants and toddlers have conduction velocities that are approximately 50% of normal adult values, but this varies in different nerves and with motor vs. sensory nerves. SNAP amplitudes generally approach adult values by age 7 months.[27]

Results of repetitive stimulation vary with age. Low rates of stimulation should not produce a decrement in normal persons of any age. Premature and full-term infants normally exhibit post-tetanic facilitation and exhaustion to repetitive stimulation at rates of 50 Hz. This is related to a reduced safety factor for neuromuscular transmission resulting from an immature neuromuscular junction and possibly poorly myelinated nerves. At 20 Hz, only premature infants demonstrate these findings. This becomes an issue when studying a floppy infant, especially when coupled with the technical problems of performing these studies in the neonatal intensive care unit.[31]

Disorders having onset at birth generally present with hypotonia, weakness, poor respiration, feeding problems, and often skeletal deformities. Disorders occurring in the neonate include hereditary disorders of nerve, muscle, and the neuromuscular junction most commonly, but acquired disorders such as acute or chronic inflammatory demyelinating polyradiculoneuropathy, infantile botulism, and neonatal myasthenia gravis can also occur.[3] Developmental and dystrophic disorders such as hypomyelinating neuropathy, motor neuron disease and spinal muscular atrophy, myotonic dystrophy, and other congenital myopathies, both metabolic and structural, can present in neonates. Mononeuropathies, although most often traumatic in this age group, can also occur, and the clinician should be alert for evidence of nerve or muscle hypoplasia.

Children ages 1 to 5 years can exhibit problems with delayed developmental milestones or begin to show deterioration in gait, coordination, and ability to keep up with peers. The classic disorder of this age group is Duchenne's muscular dystrophy. Other disorders, both acquired and hereditary, may manifest in this age range, as may essentially any acquired disorder that adults develop.

A complete discussion of the multitude of disorders affecting children is beyond the scope of this chapter. Case 15 illustrates a typical situation that may be encountered.

Thought Process

In a child of this age, the diagnosis usually depends on the clinical and family history, examination, electrophysiological studies, and nerve or muscle biopsy. The electrophysiological studies can be very helpful in the decision to pursue a biopsy and to order various bio-

CASE STUDY

15

A 1-month-old infant was referred for an electrophysiological evaluation because of ongoing problems with weakness. The infant was the product of a normal, full-term pregnancy, but had respiratory problems at birth requiring 1 week of intensive care. The mother reported relative lack of fetal movements in utero as compared to her previous pregnancies. Since birth, the infant had fatigued quickly when sucking, often drooling and coughing while swallowing. The mother denied a family history of neuromuscular disorders.

The infant was bright and alert. The infant showed little volitional movement of the extremities and was supine with legs abducted in a froglike position. There was little recoil of the limbs when stretched and released, and no effort to align the head with the torso when pulled from supine to sitting position. Muscle bulk was decreased. The infant withdrew the limbs from noxious stimuli, although not vigorously, and had a weak cry.

chemical studies. Because the study may be limited by cooperation, the first consideration is to determine whether the disorder is neuropathic, myopathic, or a neuromuscular junction disorder. The second consideration is to determine the extent and severity of involvement.

In the case of a truly floppy infant, the ability to conduct a complete study is facilitated by the child's inability to resist. However, the examiner must respect the fact that fear on the part of both patient and parents and discomfort remain factors, and should select the minimum number of studies necessary. The NCS and EMG data are listed in Table 12–15.

Discussion

The first step was to confirm the clinical impression that the disorder involved motor units with sparing of the sensory system. The medial plantar sensory NCS was selected because it is often easily performed in a child and reduces the problems with positioning required to perform a sural nerve study. The normal plantar study probably confirmed that this was primarily a motor disorder, although it did not totally rule out a multifocal neuropathy. A median antidromic sensory study was performed that was also normal. The peroneal motor conduction study is also easily performed in most children and in this case showed only a low CMAP amplitude and was otherwise normal.

Repetitive stimulation could have been performed here but, depending on the child, foot and leg movement may preclude adequate repetitive stimulation recordings at this site. The ulnar motor study was used for repetitive stimulation, as it was technically more feasible. A low ulnar CMAP was noted with normal repetitive stimulation at slow rates. A decrement could indicate immaturity of neuromuscular junctions in reinnervating nerve.[32] The findings of low CMAPs with normal sensory studies indicated a disorder of muscle, motor nerve, or motor neurons that affects both the upper and lower extremities. Normal repetitive stimulation with low-amplitude CMAPs excludes most disorders of neuromuscular junction transmission in this age group. Other rates of stimulation could be performed at this point, but in this case, the decision was made to return to this only if the needle examination was unrevealing.

The goal of the needle examination was to demonstrate the severity and extent of involvement and to define whether the disorder was primarily one of muscle, motor axons, or neurons. The findings of generalized fibrillation potentials, reduced recruitment, and large MUPs were most consistent with a disorder of motor axons or neurons. Given the clinical history and examination, the findings were typical of those seen in infantile spinal muscular atrophy as described by Werdnig and Hoffmann.[21]

Infantile neuronal degeneration and genetic or acquired neuropathies also produce similar clinical and electrophysiological findings but generally present with much slower conduction velocities owing to dysmyelination or demyelination.[52] Other disorders to consider that could show similar electrophysiological features include some congenital myopathies such as central core disease, although this generally lacks spontaneous activity, or acid maltase deficiency, although generally myotonic discharges would be seen. Poliomyelitis must also be included in the differential diagnosis. Had fibrillation potentials been less prominent and had low-amplitude, short-duration MUPs been the predominant finding, repetitive stimulation at high rates to exclude infantile botulism would have been performed.[12]

TABLE 12–15 Case 15: Pediatric Electromyography

NERVE CONDUCTION STUDIES

Nerve Stimulation (Record)	Amplitude (μV)	Conduction Velocity (msec)	Latencies (msec) Distal	Latencies (msec) F-Wave
Motor				
Peroneal (EDB)	**1100**	25	2.0	**NR**
Ulnar (hypothenar)*	**3200**	28	1.6	18.5
Sensory				
Median plantar (ankle)	10		1.8	
Median (index)	22	35	1.4	

ELECTROMYOGRAPHY

Muscle	Insertional Activity	Spontaneous Activity: Fibrillation Potentials	Spontaneous Activity: Fasciculation Potentials	Motor Unit Potentials: Recruitment	Motor Unit Potentials: Duration/ Amplitude	Motor Unit Potentials: Phases/ Turns
R anterior tibial	Increased	++	0	Reduced	Increased	—
R quadriceps	Increased	+++	+	Reduced	Increased	Increased
R first dorsal interosseous (manus)	Increased	++	0	Reduced	Increased	Increased
R biceps	Increased	++	0	Reduced	Increased	—

Abbreviations: EDB, extensor digitorum brevis; NR, no response.
*2-Hz repetitive stimulation at rest was normal.

OTHER USES OF ELECTRODIAGNOSTIC STUDIES

Routine electrodiagnostic medicine techniques can be used to evaluate many other types of conditions affecting the peripheral and central nervous systems. Combining information from NCS and EMG with data obtained using other electrodiagnostic techniques may be necessary. Basic techniques of NCS and EMG, evoked potentials, and surface EMG can be useful for diagnosis in many situations.

Surface EMG is useful in the assessment of movement disorders. Patterns of EMG activity can characterize tremor patterns and distinguish organic from functional tremor. This technique assists in determining patterns of muscle activation in dystonia, which significantly enhances the choice of muscles for denervation with botulinum toxin or via surgery. A combination of NCS techniques to elicit various types of reflexes and surface EMG recording may be useful in defining disorders causing spasticity and rigidity.

Some patients experience episodic weakness. Routine NCS techniques are applied in exercise testing for periodic paralysis.

Patients with incontinence may benefit from electrodiagnostic assessment to determine the neurological process responsible for incontinence or to characterize and sphincter coordination. Pudendal NCS and evoked potentials, coupled with sphincter EMG to determine appropriate levels of sphincter activation and relaxation with voluntary activation and Valsalva maneuvers, can be performed. Anal sphincter EMG is probably most useful for determining whether sphincter denervation is present.

Cranial nerves can also be assessed using these techniques. EMG of muscles innervated by cranial nerves, including cranial nerves V, VII, XI, and XII, is easily performed. Less readily accessible muscles include those innervated by cranial nerves IX and X. Fine-wire EMG of palatal muscles is useful in palatal myoclonus and for intraoperative monitoring during posterior fossa or other head and neck surgery. The extraocular muscles can be examined as well. Reflex studies, including tests of the blink reflex, masseter reflex, and masseter inhibitory reflex, can be performed, although the masseter reflexes require a reflex hammer that triggers the oscilloscope. The two-channel recording available on most standard EMG equipment is useful for demonstrating synkinesis and the lateral spread response, the latter characteristic of hemifacial spasm. Trigeminal somatosensory-evoked potentials and visual and brainstem auditory-evoked potentials are additional techniques that can assist in cranial nerve assessment.

The phrenic nerve can be assessed with NCS of each phrenic nerve in addition to needle EMG of the diaphragm. Intercostal EMG is also possible, but caution should be used because of the risk of pneumothorax. These techniques are useful in patients with respiratory symptoms, particularly if diaphragm dysfunction is suspected (as in patients with failure to wean from mechanical ventilation). Excluding more generalized nerve or muscle disease in these patients is critical.

Patients with thoracic pain or paresthesia may have radiculopathy or polyradiculopathy at this level. The most frequent cause of thoracic radiculopathy is diabetes mellitus, which is often associated with a neuropathy that can be subclinical. NCS and EMG are useful in defining both problems. Thoracic paraspinal EMG and EMG of abdominal muscles, when appropriate, should be performed.

Various techniques are useful for assessing CNS involvement. High-voltage or high-frequency stimulation of small myelinated fibers can elicit a withdrawal reflex in flexor muscles and assist in characterizing disorders of the CNS and the "stiff man" syndrome. Stimulation of a nerve during a muscle contraction in the upper limb results in suppression of activity for 90 to 130 msec (the silent period), which may be altered in some central disorders. In some subjects, a variable C-response occurs during the silent period at 40 to 70 msec. This so-called long loop reflex has also been reported to be abnormal in some central disorders. The H-reflex is useful for assessing proximal conduction, and comparing the amplitude of the maximum H-reflex with the maximum M-wave amplitude provides a ratio that may reflect central excitability, which may be useful in quantification of spasticity. Evoked potential techniques are also used for CNS study.

Intraoperative monitoring during peripheral nerve surgery, spine, and the aforementioned posterior fossa surgeries can be performed using relatively routine NCS, EMG, and evoked potential techniques.

SUMMARY

Electrodiagnostic medicine plays an important role in patient diagnosis and management. Training in neuromuscular disease and electrophysiological techniques is critical for useful diagnostic results from NCS and EMG. The ability to customize each study and alter the course of the study based on results obtained at each step is critical to a well-conducted evaluation. Electrodiagnosis plays a significant role in the practice of physical medicine and rehabilitation.

REFERENCES

1. Albers JW, Donofrio PD, McGonagle TK: Sequential electrodiagnostic abnormalities in acute inflammatory demyelinating polyradiculoneuropathy. Muscle Nerve 1985; 8:528–539.
2. Albers JW, Mitz M, Sulaiman AR, et al: Spontaneous electrical activity and muscle biopsy abnormalities in polymyositis and dermatomyositis. Muscle Nerve 1979; 2:503.
3. Al-Quadah AA, Shahar E, Logan WJ, et al: Neonatal Guillain-Barré syndrome. Pediatr Neurol 1988; 4:255–256.
4. Armon C, Daube JR: Electrophysiologic signs of arteriovenous malformations of the spinal cord. J Neurol Neurosurg Psychiatry 1989; 52:1176–1181.
5. Asbury AK, Arnason BGW, Karp HR, et al: Criteria for diagnosis of Guillain-Barré syndrome. Ann Neurol 1978; 3:565.
6. Banker BQ: The congenital myopathies. In Engel AG, Banker BQ (eds): Myology. New York, McGraw-Hill, 1986, pp 1527–1581.
7. Bohan A, Peter JB: Polymyositis and dermatomyositis. N Engl J Med 1975; 292:403–407.

8. Bradley WG: The limb girdle syndromes. In Unken PJ, Broyn GW (eds): Handbook of Clinical Neurology. Diseases of Muscle. Amsterdam, North-Holland, 1979, pp 433–469.
9. Bradley WG: Low back and lower limb pain. In Bradley WG (ed): Neurology in Clinical Practice. Boston, Butterworth-Heinemann, 1991, p 412.
10. Campbell WW, Pridgeon RM, Riaz G, et al: Sparing of the flexor carpi ulnaris in ulnar neuropathy at the elbow. Muscle Nerve 1989; 12:965–967.
11. Caroscio JT, Mulvihill MN, Sterling R, et al: Amyotrophic lateral sclerosis: Its natural history. Neurol Clin 1977; 5:3.
12. Cornblath DR: Disorders of neuromuscular transmission in infants and children. Muscle Nerve 1986; 9:606–611.
13. Daube JR, Mulder DW: Clinical electrophysiologic factors in prognosis in amyotrophic lateral sclerosis. Muscle Nerve 1982; 5:S107.
14. Dawson DM, Hallett M, Millender LH: Entrapment Neuropathies. Boston, Little, Brown, 1990, pp 199–203.
15. Dyck PJ, et al: Chronic inflammatory polyradiculoneuropathy. Mayo Clin Proc 1975; 50:621–627.
16. Eaton LM, Lambert EH: Electromyography and electric stimulation of nerve in diseases of motor units: Observations on myasthenic syndrome associated with malignant tumors. JAMA 1957; 163:1117.
17. Gamble HJ, Breathnach AS: An electron-microscopic study of human foetal peripheral nerves. J Anat 1965; 99:573–584.
18. Gilliatt RW: Thoracic outlet compression syndrome. Br Med J 1976; 1:1274–1275.
19. Gilliatt RW, Willison RG, Dietz V, et al: Peripheral nerve conduction in patients with a cervical rib and band. Ann Neurol 1978; 4:124–129.
20. Groh D, Brunner NG, Namba T: The natural course of myasthenia gravis and effect of therapeutic measures. Ann NY Acad Sci 1981; 377:652.
21. Harding AE: Inherited neuronal atrophy and degeneration predominantly of lower motor neurons. In Dyck PJ, et al (eds): Peripheral Neuropathy, Philadelphia, WB Saunders, 1993, pp 1053–1054.
22. Harper CM, Thomas JE, Cascino TL, et al: Distinction between neoplastic and radiation-induced brachial plexopathy with emphasis on the role of EMG. Neurology 1989; 39:502–506.
23. Harper PS: The Myotonic Disorders. In Walton JN (ed): Disorders of Voluntary Muscle. New York, Churchill-Livingstone, 1988, pp 569–587.
24. Harper PS: Myotonic Dystrophy. In Walton HN (ed): Major Problems in Neurology. Philadelphia, WB Saunders, 1979, pp 14–36.
25. Jablecki C: Lambert Eaton myasthenia syndrome. Muscle Nerve 1984; 7:250–257.
26. Jablecki CK, Andary MT, So YT, et al: AAEM Quality Assurance Committee: Literature review of the usefulness of nerve conduction studies and electromyography for the evaluation of patients with carpal tunnel syndrome. Muscle Nerve 1993; 16:1392–1414.
27. Jones HR: Pediatric electromyography. In Brown WF, Bolton CF (eds): Clinical Electromyography, ed 2. Boston, Butterworth-Heinemann, 1993, pp 698–704.
28. Karnes WE: Diseases of the seventh cranial nerve. In Dyck PJ, et al (eds): Peripheral Neuropathy, ed 3. Philadelphia, WB Saunders, 1993, pp 826–830.
29. Kimura J (ed): Electrodiagnosis in Diseases of Nerve and Muscle, ed 2. Philadelphia, FA Davis, 1989.
30. Kline D: Civilian gunshot wounds to the brachial plexus. J Neurosurg 1989; 70:166.
31. Koenigsberger MR, Patten B, Lovelace RE: Studies of neuromuscular function in the newborn: A comparison of myoneural function in the fullterm and premature infant. Neuropediatrics 1973; 4:350–361.
32. Kuntz NL, Gomez MR, Daube JR: Prognosis in childhood proximal spinal muscular atrophy. Neurology 1980; 30:378.
33. Lambert EH: Electromyography in amyotrophic lateral sclerosis. In Norris FH, Kurland LT (eds): Motor Neuron Diseases: Research on Amyotrophic Lateral Sclerosis and Related Disorders. New York, Grune & Stratton, 1969, pp 135–153.
34. Lambert EH, Eaton LM, Rooke ED: Defect of neuromuscular transmission associated with malignant neoplasms (abstract). Am J Physiol 1956; 187:612.
35. Lange DJ: Multifocal motor neuropathy with conduction block: Is it a distinct clinical entity? Neurology 1992; 42:497–505.
36. Lederman RJ, Wilbourn AJ: Brachial plexopathy: Recurrent cancer or radiation? Neurology 1984; 34:1331.
37. Leffert RD: Brachial plexus injuries. N Engl J Med 1974; 291:1059.
38. Lotz BP, et al: Inclusion body myositis: Observations in 40 patients. Brain 1989; 112:727–747.
39. Odesate K, Eisen A: An electrophysiological quantitation of the cubital tunnel syndrome. J Can Sci Neurol 1979; 6:403–410.
40. Oh SJ: Clinical Electromyography: Nerve Conduction Studies. Baltimore, University Park Press, 1984, p 231.
41. Olsen PZ: Prediction of recovery in Bell's palsy. Acta Neurol Scand Suppl 1975; 61:90.
42. O'Neill JH, Murray NMF, Newsom-Davis J: The Lambert-Eaton myasthenic syndrome: A review of 50 cases. Brain 1988; 111:577–596.
43. Ozdemir C, Young RR: The results to be expected from electrical testing in the diagnosis of myasthenia gravis. Ann NY Acad Sci 1976; 274:203.
44. Parry GJ: Diseases of spinal roots. In Dyck PJ, et al (eds): Peripheral Neuropathy, ed 3. Philadelphia, WB Saunders, 1993, pp 899–907.
45. Parry GJ, Clarke S: Multifocal demyelinating neuropathy masquerading as motor neuron disease. Muscle Nerve 1988; 11: 103–107.
46. Phalen GS: Reflections on 21 years experience with the carpal tunnel syndrome. JAMA 1970; 212:1365.
47. Preston DC, Kelly JJ: Atypical motor neuron disease. In Dyck PJ, et al (eds): Peripheral Neuropathy, ed 3. Philadelphia, WB Saunders. 1993, p 458.
48. Reed DM, Kurland LT: Muscle fasciculations in a healthy population. Arch Neurol 1963; 9:363–367.
49. Richardson AT: Muscle fasciculation. Arch Phys Med Rehabil 1954; 35:281–286.
50. Rivner MH, Swift TR: Electrical testing in disorders of neuromuscular transmission. In Brown WF (ed): Clinical Electromyography, ed 2. Boston, Butterworth-Heinemann, 1993, pp 630–631.
51. Seto DSY, Freeman JM: Lead neuropathy in childhood. Am J Dis Child 1964; 107:337.
52. Sladley JT: Chronic sensory-motor polyneuropathies in children. American Association of Electrodiagnostic Medicine Course A: Pediatric Electromyography. New Orleans: American Association of Electrodiagnostic Medicine, 1993, pp 7–12.
53. Stalberg E: Clinical electrophysiology in myasthenia gravis. J Neurol Neurosurg Psychiatry 1980; 43:622–633.
54. Stevens JC: AAEE minimonograph #26: The electrodiagnosis of carpal tunnel syndrome. Muscle Nerve 1987; 10:99–113.
55. Streib EW, Wilbourn AJ, Mitsumoto H: Spontaneous electrical muscle fiber activity in polymyositis and dermatomyositis. Muscle Nerve 1979; 2:14–18.
56. Thomas PK, Tomlinson DR: Diabetic and hypoglycemic neuropathy. In Dyck PJ, et al (eds): Peripheral Neuropathy, ed 3. Philadelphia WB Saunders, 1993.
57. Turner AJW, Parsonage MJ: Neurologic amyotrophy (paralytic brachial neuritis) with special reference to prognosis. Lancet 1957; 1:209.
58. Walton JN, Gardner-Medivin D: Muscular dystrophies. In Walton JN (ed): Disorders of Voluntary Muscle, ed 5. New York, Churchill-Livingstone, 1988, pp 519–569.
59. Warren J, Guttmann L, Figueroa AF Jr, et al: Electromyographic changes of brachial plexus root avulsions. J Neurosurg 1969; 31:137–140.
60. Wilbourn AJ: Brachial plexus disorders. In Dyck PJ, et al (eds): Peripheral Neuropathy, ed 3. Philadelphia, WB Saunders, 1993.
61. Wilbourn AJ, Aminoff MJ: AAEE minimonograph #32. The electro-physiologic examination in patients with radiculopathy. Muscle Nerve 1988; 11:1099–1114.

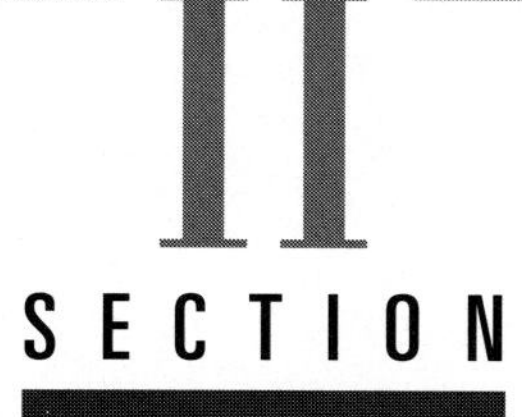

TREATMENT TECHNIQUES AND SPECIAL EQUIPMENT

13

CHAPTER

Alberto Esquenazi, M.D.

Upper Limb Amputee Rehabilitation and Prosthetic Restoration

INCIDENCE AND DEMOGRAPHICS

Based on the most recent information available from the National Center for Health Statistics, approximately 1,230,000 amputees are living in the United States (all levels of amputation), with approximately 50,000 new amputations performed annually.[33] The ratio of upper limb to lower limb amputation estimated from this information is 1:4.9. The most frequent causes of upper limb amputation are trauma and cancer, followed by vascular complications of disease. The most common major upper limb amputation is at the transradial level, which accounts for 57% of all arm amputations. Transhumeral amputation accounts for 23% of all amputations. The right arm is more frequently involved in work-related injuries. Sixty percent of arm amputees are between the ages of 21 and 64 years, and 10% are younger than 21 years.[11, 21]

Congenital upper limb deficiency has an incidence of approximately 4.1 per 10,000 live births.[33] The congenital limb deficiencies are best classified according to the International Organization of Standards and the International Society of Prosthetics and Orthotics classifications as modified from Frantz-O'Reilly. The limb deficiencies can be transverse or longitudinal. The term *terminal* is used to describe the fact that the limb has developed normally to a particular level, beyond which no skeletal element exists. In intercalary limb deficiency, a reduction or absence of one or more elements occurs within the long axis of the limb, and in this case normal skeletal elements may be found distal to the affected segments.[20] The most common congenital limb deficiency is the left terminal transverse radial limb deficiency (Table 13–1).

LIMB SALVAGE VERSUS AMPUTATION SURGERY

Severe hand injuries frequently challenge the skills of the surgeon to the point of having to consider amputation. The absolute surgical indication for amputation in trauma is ischemia in a limb with unreconstructible vascular injury. As reconstruction techniques have improved, more attempts at limb salvage have been made, although amputation is often ultimately required after multiple surgical procedures. Such surgical procedures also represent a substantial investment of time, money, and emotional energy. Massively crushed or burned muscle[10] and ischemic tissue release myoglobin and cell toxins, which can lead to renal failure, adult respiratory distress syndrome, and death. In addition, the risk of infection, contractures, and nerve injuries that interfere with function needs to be considered. Recent studies show the value of early amputation not only in saving lives, but also in preventing the emotional, marital, and financial disasters and narcotic analgesic addictions that can follow desperate attempts at limb salvage.

In establishing guidelines for immediate or early amputation of mangled limbs the surgeon must bear in mind that for the upper limb, salvage should be based on providing an extremity that has sufficient sensation to provide protective feedback, has a durable soft tissue cover, and can be used to interact with the environment. An upper limb with limited motion, multiple scars, or lack of sensation functions poorly because of the constant risk of tissue injury. This type of limb often functions worse than a modern prosthetic replacement. Recently, grading scales for mangled lower limbs have been

TABLE 13–1 International Terminology for the Classification of Congenital Limb Deficiencies, Derived from International Organization of Standards and the International Society of Prosthetics and Orthotics Classifications

Terminal: The limb has developed normally to a particular level, beyond which no skeletal elements exist.
Intercalary: There is a reduction or absence of one or more elements within the long axis of the limb, and normal skeletal elements may be present distal to affected segment.

developed and should serve as guidelines to help the surgeon assess the gravity of the injury and the subsequent risk of salvage.[13]

Amputation should never be viewed as surgical failure but rather as the means to return the patient to a more functional status. The value of approaching amputation with a positive and reconstructive approach cannot be over-emphasized. The decision to amputate is an emotional process for all involved, and the rehabilitation team should stand ready to respond and assist early in the process.

The selection of the surgical level of amputation is probably one of the most important decisions that must be made for the amputee. The viability of soft tissue and the amount of skin coverage with adequate sensation usually determine the most distal possible functional level for amputation. After surgery, the patient with an upper limb amputation should ideally be able to use a prosthesis (either body or externally powered) during most of the day. Bony prominences, skin scars, soft tissue traction, shear, and perspiration can complicate prosthesis use. For these reasons the residual limb must be surgically constructed with care to optimize the intimacy of fit, maintain muscle balance, and allow assumption of stresses necessary to meet the limb's new function. New surgical techniques that permit myocutaneous transfers, skin expansion methods, and bony lengthening procedures are available to optimize the residual limb shape, size, and function.[16] This optimization should preferably be done at the time of the amputation, but it can be done in a second stage. Using a staged approach delays prosthetic fitting and can decrease the success of prosthetic restoration. Early prosthetic fitting after arm amputation (1 to 4 months) is imperative if successful prosthetic restoration is to be expected.[30] Once healing has occurred, prevention of scar tissue adhesion formation is critical.

Levels of Amputation

Finger amputation can occur at the distal interphalangeal, proximal interphalangeal, and metacarpophalangeal levels (Fig. 13–1). Transcarpal amputation and wrist amputation are seen less frequently because of their limited functional outcome. Multiple finger amputations, including thumb and partial hand amputations and those through the wrist, need to be considered carefully in view of the possible functional and cosmetic implications of prosthesis fitting and restoration. Inappropriate choice of amputation site can result in a prosthesis with disproportional length or width. It can also preclude the use of externally powered devices.

The transradial amputation is preferred in most cases; it can be performed at three levels (resulting in long, medium, and short residual limbs). The long forearm residual limb is preferred when optimal body-powered prosthetic restoration is the goal. It is the ideal level for the patient who is expected to perform physically demanding work. The medium forearm residual limb is preferred when optimal externally powered prosthetic restoration is the goal. This length typically permits good function and cosmesis. The short transradial amputation level can complicate suspension and limit elbow flexion strength and elbow range of motion. Transradial amputation is the most common level and allows the highest level of functional recovery in the majority of cases. These three amputation levels require the same type of rehabilitation interventions and make use of similar prosthetic components. The suspension system for each one of them can be different.

The elbow disarticulation has some surgical and prosthetic advantages and disadvantages. The surgical technique permits reduction in surgery time and blood loss, provides improved prosthetic self-suspension while per-

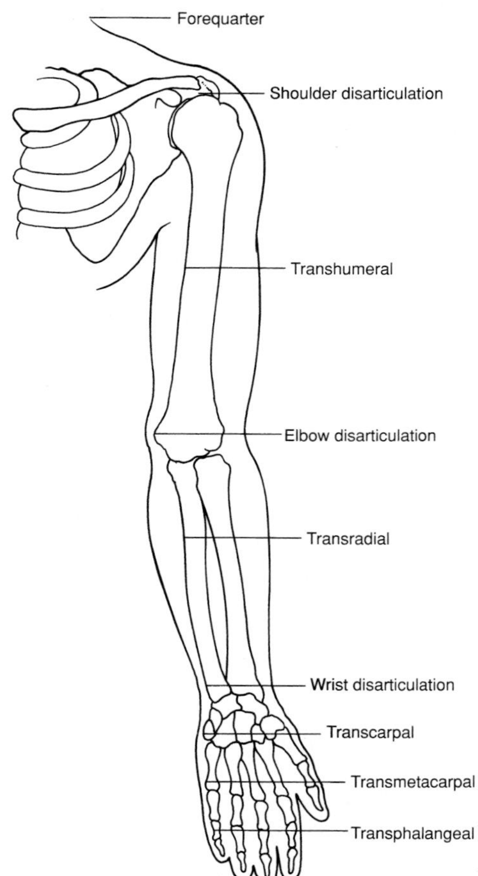

FIGURE 13–1. Upper limb levels of amputation and anatomical terminology.

mitting the use of a less encumbering socket, and reduces the rotation of the socket on the residual limb, as compared with the transhumeral level of amputation.[44] Major disadvantages are the marginal cosmetic appearance caused by the necessary external elbow mechanism, and current limitations in technology, which impede the use of externally powered elbow mechanisms at this level of amputation. These drawbacks often outweigh the advantages in the long run. In the patient for whom bilateral transhumeral amputation is the alternative, the elbow disarticulation is a more desirable level when feasible, despite the possible cosmetic problems.

The transhumeral amputation can be performed at three levels (long, medium, and short residual limbs). The long arm residual limb (7 to 10 cm from the distal humeral condyle) is preferred for optimal prosthetic restoration. These three amputation levels require the same type of rehabilitation interventions and, in most cases, require similar prosthetic components, which can be externally powered, body powered, passive, or a combination of these.

The shoulder disarticulation and forequarter amputations fortunately are seen less frequently than amputations at other levels. In most cases they are made necessary as part of the surgical intervention to remove a malignant lesion. Patients with these levels of amputation are the most difficult to fit with a functional prosthesis, owing to the number of joints to be replaced and the problems related to maintaining secure suspension of the prosthesis.

In regard to surgical techniques, soft tissue handling is especially critical to wound healing and functional outcome in amputation surgery. When tissues are excessively traumatized, the risk of wound failure and infection is high. Flaps should be kept thick, and unnecessary dissection between the skin, subcutaneous, fascial, and muscle planes should be avoided. All bone edges should be rounded, and prominences should be beveled for optimal force transmission during prosthetic use. Split-thickness skin grafts are generally discouraged except as a means to save essential residual limb length and with the understanding that future surgical revision might be necessary. Skin grafts do best with adequate soft tissue support and are most durable when not adherent to bone. Muscle loses its contractile function when the skeletal attachments are divided during amputation. Stabilizing the distal insertion of muscle can improve residual limb function and comfort. *Myodesis* is the direct suturing of muscle or tendon to bone. This technique is most effective in stabilizing muscles that are needed to counteract strong antagonistic muscular forces. *Myoplasty* involves suturing of muscles to periosteum. Myoplasty does not provide as secure a distal stabilization of the muscle as does myodesis. Care must be taken to prevent having a mobile sling of muscle over the distal end of the bone, which can result in formation of a painful bursa that could interfere with prosthetic fitting and use.

All transected nerves form a neuroma. Nerves should be transected cleanly, allowing the cut end to retract into the soft tissues away from the scar and prosthetic pressure points. The integrity of the peripheral nervous system should be assessed as early as feasible after traumatic amputation, because traction injuries frequently result in temporary or permanent nerve injury that has direct implications for arm function as well as for rehabilitation and prosthetic restoration programs.

The Amputee Rehabilitation Program

The amputee rehabilitation program should ideally be designed to cover the wide spectrum of care from preamputation to reintegration into the community. The proposed stages are outlined in Table 13–2.[31]

Preamputation Counseling

During this stage it is essential to develop direct communication involving the patient, the family, and the surgeon regarding the need for amputation and the expected surgical outcome. Communication with the physiatrist, therapists, and other members of the treatment team should be facilitated. At this point, it is appropriate for the clinician to have introductory discussions about phantom limb sensation, prosthetic devices, prosthesis fitting and training, and the timing of these events. When possible, a demonstration of a prosthesis by a trained volunteer with a similar level of amputation and discussion of realistic expected functional outcomes should be arranged. Family involvement throughout this process should be encouraged. For all levels of amputation a "prehabilitation" program should include strengthening exercises for the trunk and remaining upper limb musculature and range-of-motion exercises for the involved glenohumeral, scapulothoracic, and elbow joints (if present).

Amputation Surgery

Partial hand amputations should be carefully planned to ensure adequate residual sensation and movement. There is little point in salvaging a partial hand if no metacarpals are present to provide pinch. Prosthetic restoration of the thumb should be attempted before any pollicization procedures or toe transfers are attempted. Many patients find that a thumb prosthesis provides adequate functional restoration, and they choose to forgo further surgical reconstruction.[31] In addition, toe transfers can result in the partial loss of the normal foot function during walking.

Selecting a transhumeral level amputation over a transradial amputation presents a number of important dilemmas in rehabilitation. The lack of an anatomical

TABLE 13–2 Stages of Upper Limb Amputee Rehabilitation Program

1. Pre-amputation counseling
2. Amputation surgery
3. Acute postamputation period
4. Preprosthesis training
5. Preparatory prosthesis fitting
6. Prosthesis fitting and training
7. Reintegration into the community
8. Long-term follow-up

elbow joint requires increased effort and cost for prosthetic restoration and results in greater impairment. The selection of the level of amputation should take into consideration the amount of space necessary for the appropriate prosthetic components with adequate cosmesis. The transradial amputation has to be a minimum of 5 cm proximal to the distal radius to accommodate an externally powered terminal device. Transhumeral amputations should be performed 7 to 10 cm proximal to the distal humeral condyles to accommodate most of the prosthetic elbows. Longer residual limbs affect the location of the artificial elbow joint center of rotation, which can compromise cosmesis.

Transradial and Transhumeral Amputations

In the traumatic transradial and transhumeral amputation, it is not uncommon to find a more proximal fracture, a dislocation, or, occasionally, a peripheral nerve injury that can temporarily or permanently interfere with optimal prosthesis fitting and arm motion. Early diagnosis of these problems is needed to ensure inclusion of the necessary appropriate prosthetic modifications and alterations to the rehabilitation program.

Shoulder Disarticulation and Forequarter Amputation

Shoulder disarticulation is performed in severe electrical injuries, in trauma cases, and in tumor surgery. Prosthetic replacement in these cases is more successful in those who are healthy, young, and male. In the majority of cases, the loss of the anatomical shoulder necessitates the use of an external prosthetic shoulder joint. This joint requires control mechanisms in addition to the body-powered or externally powered control mechanisms needed for the elbow, wrist, and hand.

Forequarter amputation is rarely performed, but it may be required in some cases of severe trauma or malignant lesion involving the shoulder. Functional prosthetic use is uncommon after this procedure, as suspension is difficult to maintain. Special considerations should be made for providing a shoulder cap to allow the patient to wear clothing more easily and to improve cosmesis. An ultralight passive prosthesis is usually well accepted by the patient.

Acute Postamputation Period

Pain control, maintenance of range of motion and strength, and promotion of wound healing (Table 13–3) are the goals of this stage, which begins with the surgical closure of the wound and culminates in wound healing.

TABLE 13–3 Frequently Utilized Postoperative Wound Dressing Systems

Immediate postoperative rigid dressing
Immediate postoperative prosthesis
Elastic bandage dressing
Unna bandage
Soft dressing

Pain control and residual limb maturation should be pursued aggressively. Immediate application of postoperative plaster of Paris rigid dressing (IPORD) or soft elastic bandage and subsequent pneumatic compression are indicated for edema control. An increasingly popular method of wound protection, swelling control, early shaping and soft tissue shrinking, and return to function is the immediate postoperative prosthesis, as reported by Malone and others.[29] Soft compressive dressings or Unna bandages are used in many centers.[9] The dressing should be extended to the proximal joint to better control swelling and to improve the dressing suspension. Proper postoperative positioning and rehabilitation are essential to prevent elbow flexion and shoulder adduction contractures when wounds are present over or close to the joints. This is most important if the wounds are caused by burn injuries, open reduction, or internal fixation or if skin grafts were applied.

Acute Pain Management

Pain control can be best achieved initially with a patient-controlled analgesia (PCA) system, followed by the use of scheduled parenteral and oral analgesia. A skin desensitization program that includes gentle tapping, massage, soft tissue and scar mobilization, and lubrication is recommended for the patient with a soft or elastic dressing.

When the patient's condition is medically stable, early mobilization, general endurance, and strengthening exercise are started. Special attention is paid to the shoulder and scapulae and to the prevention of joint contractures. It is also important to carefully observe the remaining limbs, especially their strength and function, with attention to switching hand dominance if necessary. At this time, emotional counseling for the patient and the family should begin, with special focus on the significant other and children. Psychosocial evaluation of the patient and family should be initiated to assess and manage depression and anxiety. It is important during this phase to promote patient participation in the decision-making process to encourage independence and a sense of control.

Postoperative Care

Postoperative edema is common following amputation. If soft dressings are used they should be combined with elastic wrapping to control edema, especially if the patient is a candidate for a prosthesis. The ideal shape of the upper extremity residual limb is cylindrical, not conical. The major complication from elastic wrapping is applying the bandage too tightly at the proximal end in an attempt to improve bandage suspension. This causes congestion, worsens edema, and results in a dumbbell-shaped residual limb. The recommended elastic dressing involves the use of a figure-of-8 wrapping technique that extends over the proximal joint and that is reapplied every 4 to 6 hours.

The use of an IPORD to control postoperative edema, promote healing, protect the limb from trauma, decrease postoperative pain, desensitize the limb, and allow early mobilization and rehabilitation is the preferred treatment approach for the transradial level (Table 13–4). In some centers, the rigid dressing is applied and managed by a team of specialists that includes the surgeon, the physiatrist, and the prosthetist. In other facilities where the team approach to amputee management has not been implemented, the dressing can be applied by a trained clinician. The dressing is made out of plaster of Paris bandages that extend beyond the proximal joint for suspension. An IPORD should be replaced at 1-week intervals. By the time the second dressing is replaced, the prosthesis can be casted and a few days later it can be fitted. If the patient has a fever for which no other apparent cause can be determined, the IPORD should be removed and the wound inspected. The IPORD should be reapplied if the wound shows no signs of infection.

Phantom Limb, Phantom Pain, and Painful Residual Limb

Phantom limb sensation is the feeling that all or a part of the amputated limb is still present. This sensation is felt by nearly all "acquired" amputees, but is not always bothersome.[32] Phantom sensation usually diminishes over time, and telescoping (the sensation that the phantom hand has moved proximally) commonly occurs. Phantom sensation is not necessarily painful. As many as 70% of amputees perceive phantom pain in the first few months after amputation. However, such pain usually disappears or decreases sufficiently so that it does not interfere with prosthesis fitting and day-to-day activities.[5] A smaller percentage of patients experience long-term pain, whereas others have recurrent pain later in life. When pain persists for more than 6 months, the prognosis for spontaneous improvement is poor, and it can be extremely difficult to treat successfully. Perceived pain intensity is closely related to anxiety level, depression, prosthesis fitting problems, and other personal factors.[43]

The traditional explanation for phantom sensation and pain is that the remaining nerves in the amputated limb continue to generate impulses that flow through the spinal cord and the thalamus to the somatosensory areas of the cerebral cortex. Another theory suggests that the phantom arises from excessive, spontaneous firing of spinal cord neurons that have lost their normal sensory input from the missing body part. Another suggests that the phantom sensation is caused by changes in the flow of signals through the somatosensory circuit in the brain.[32]

Appropriate management of phantom limb begins by preventing prolonged periods of pain before the amputation, because preamputation pain often ends in postoperative phantom pain. Treatment includes prosthetic socket revisions, desensitization techniques, transcutaneous nerve stimulation, neuropharmacological intervention, and the voluntary control of the phantom limb (mental imaging).[41] For severe cases, nerve blocks, steroid injections, and epidural blocks can be useful. Nonsurgical interventions are far more successful than surgical ones.[19] Clearly, the etiology of the phantom limb phenomenon is more complex than any of the theories here presented would suggest, and treatment can be complex. An important issue to discuss with the patient is normal phantom sensation, phantom pain, and the relationship between phantom pain and tension, anxiety, stress, and pain perception.

TABLE 13–4 Indications for IPORD (Immediate Postoperative Rigid Dressing)

Pain control
Promote wound healing
Protection from trauma
Edema control
Desensitization
Prevent contractures

Joint Contractures

Joint contractures can occur between the time of amputation and prosthesis fitting. Efforts should be directed at preventing contractures with aggressive rehabilitation efforts, beginning soon after surgery. If burns, degloving injury, or severe trauma with proximal fractures are the cause of amputation, special attention should be given to the prevention of frozen shoulder and contractures induced by scar tissue formation. In the case of peripheral nerve or brachial plexus injury, appropriate positioning, splinting, and passive and assisted range of motion should be implemented to preserve joint mobility.

Preprosthetic Rehabilitation

It is not unusual for patients with amputations to be provided with artificial limbs without much attention being paid to prosthetic training or other special needs. With the advent of specialized treatment teams, regional centers, and new prosthetic devices, the outlook for the upper limb amputee has improved. A preprosthetic rehabilitation program must be initiated as soon as possible.[8] Pain control and residual limb maturation should be promoted during this phase. An IPORD or soft elastic bandages are indicated for edema control. This is also a time for the patient to initiate emotional adaptation to a body image without the artificial limb, and to learn basic skills without a prosthesis, which is essential for the times when the device is not worn. Soft tissue desensitization, early mobilization, improving general endurance, strengthening, avoidance of joint contractures, and emotional counseling are the key goals of this phase.

Often, limb loss is interpreted in our society as punishment for a misdeed. An amputation typically causes patients to initiate a process of introspection and reassessment of goals. This process can result in an individual taking a more mature approach toward life goals and actively pursuing plans. Occasionally, however, a patient can become so emotionally disturbed by the limb loss that the result can be a chronic failure to cope. This can have a very negative effect on the rehabilitation outcome.[6]

The use of the first prosthesis should be implemented as soon as possible in this stage. The early fitting of the prosthetic device is intended to promote prosthesis use for bimanual activities. As reported by Malone and others,[29, 30] there is a direct relationship between the time of fitting and long-term prosthetic use. There is a 3- to 6-month window of opportunity for the unilateral upper limb amputee. If a prosthesis is fitted during this period, there is a much greater rate of acceptance and integration of the artificial arm.

The first prosthesis is intended to promote residual limb maturation and desensitization, to build up wearing tolerance, and to allow the patient to become a functional user. Commonly, this is done with a body-powered or a switch-controlled externally powered prosthesis. Suction suspension or myoelectric control is not practical at this stage because of limb volume fluctuation, which results in the loss of the necessary intimate contact of the socket and electrodes with the soft tissues. When no significant volume fluctuation is noted in the residual limb over a period of 2 months, consideration should be given to proceeding with fitting of the first permanent prosthesis. Serial circumferential measurements of the limb at pre-established locations is the simplest method of determining residual limb size stability. Volumetric measurements in a water displacement chamber or with a computer-aided design system are more precise, although more time-consuming, techniques.

Prosthesis Fitting and Training

Prosthesis prescription options for the amputee have changed greatly since the mid-1980s. Selecting the most appropriate componentry for prosthetic restoration of the upper limb is an extremely challenging task in view of the variety and complexity of available prosthetic components (prosthetic terminal devices, wrists, elbows, and shoulders), socket fabrication techniques, suspension systems, and sources of power and control. This task should be accomplished by an expert team of professionals in close communication with the patient. Members of the team ideally should include the surgeon, a physiatrist who devotes time in practice to amputee rehabilitation and prosthetics, a certified prosthetist, an occupational therapist, a physical therapist, a recreational therapist, a psychologist, a social worker, and the patient and family. Other specialists can be added to the team as needed. The team members can best serve the needs of the patient if they have significant experience in the specialized rehabilitation techniques for the upper limb amputee and prosthetic fabrication and training. This typically occurs most commonly in large, specialized regional rehabilitation centers.

Terminal Devices

The functional capacity of the upper limb is determined by the development of multiple integrated spheres of action by the shoulder complex, elbow, wrist, and hand. Given the normal proportions of limb segments, this capacity is limited in relation to the surrounding space. The functional activities of the hand are extensive, but they can be grouped into nonprehensile and prehensile activities. The former include touching, feeling, pressing down with the fingers, tapping, vibrating the cord of a musical instrument, and lifting or pushing with the hand. Prehensile activities are grouped into precision and power grips. Three-jaw chuck involves grip with the thumb and index and middle fingers. A lateral or key grip involves contact of the pulp of the thumb with the lateral aspect of the corresponding finger. These two patterns provide precision prehension. Power grip predominantly involves the ulnar aspect of the hand, with less involvement of the ring and little fingers. The hook power grip involves flexion of both interphalangeal joints and minimal participation of the metacarpophalangeal (MCP) joint. This grip pattern is used in carrying a briefcase. The spherical grip is very much like the power grip but with minimal flexion of the fingers, which are abducted and rotated; the thumb is used to stabilize the object and to provide counter-pressure.

Most patients who have had an upper limb amputation and undergo prosthetic restoration require a terminal device for their prosthesis. The human hand is a very complex anatomical and physiological structure whose functions cannot be replaced by the current level of prosthetic technology. A variety of prosthetic terminal devices are available and include passive, body-powered, and externally powered hooks and hands (Fig. 13–2). They all lack sensory feedback and have limited mobility and dexterity. Prosthetic hands provide a three-jaw chuck pinch and hooks provide the equivalent of lateral or tip pinch. Body-powered terminal devices can be voluntary-opening (most common and practical) or voluntary-closing (most physiological). The voluntary-opening device is maintained in the closed position by rubber bands or tension springs. The patient can open the device by "pulling" with the cable on the harness system in preparation to grasp. To grasp, the patient releases the opened terminal device on an object; the rubber bands or spring provide the prehensile force. The maximum prehensile force possible is predetermined by the number of springs or rubber bands. To control the amount of prehensile force, the patient must generate an

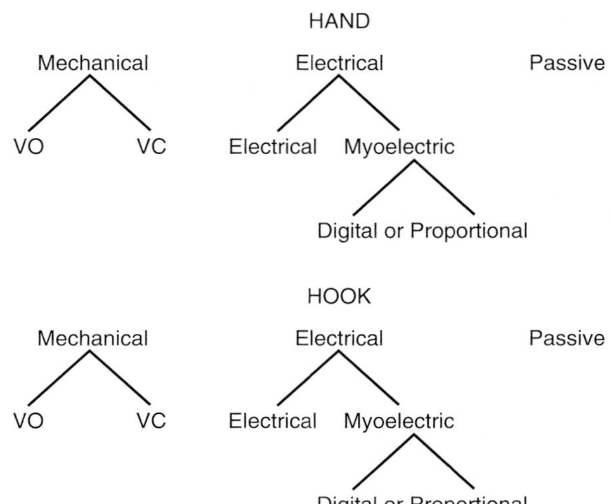

FIGURE 13–2. Classification and availability of terminal devices. VO, voluntary opening; VC, voluntary closing.

opening force all the time. Voluntary-closing terminal devices require that the patient close the device by "pulling" with the cable on the harness system to grasp an object. To release, the patient releases the pull on the harness, and a spring in the terminal device opens it. The maximum prehensile force possible is determined by the strength of the individual. One major disadvantage of this system is that prolonged prehension requires constant pull on the harness. The human hand normally does not reach out to grasp an object in the closed position, but rather uses the semi-open position to facilitate the interaction with the environment.

Externally powered devices can have digital (on/off) or proportional (stronger signal = faster action) control systems. More recently, a slip control system was introduced by the Otto Bock Company to improve hand grip. The device has a sensor that maintains a constant pressure on an object to prevent slippage. If the sensor perceives that the object is slipping, it automatically slightly increases the pressure on the object.

Prosthetic Wrists

The type of prosthetic wrist (Table 13–5) most commonly used allows passive pronation and supination. Spring-assisted rotation is available for the bilateral amputee. Quick-disconnect wrists are also available. The friction control permits ease of positioning, but it can rotate when lifting heavy objects. This is particularly problematic when the wearer is carrying a plate or tray. Quick-disconnect wrists permit rapid interchange of different terminal devices. In addition, when it is locked, the quick-disconnect wrist provides a secure control for wrist rotation. An externally powered switch or myoelectric control wrist pronosupination system exists, but it is prescribed primarily for bilateral transhumeral or higher level of amputation. A mechanical spring-assisted wrist flexion unit is indispensable for the bilateral upper limb amputee. This device permits the patient to reach the body's midline for grooming, feeding, hygiene activities, and buttoning of clothing.

Prosthetic Elbows

The prosthetic elbows available in the treatment of transhumeral amputation have either external or internal joints. These joints can be passive, body-powered, or externally powered (Figs. 13–3 and 13–4). These devices are controlled via mechanical cables, electrical switches, or myoelectric signals (Table 13–6). The externally powered systems have digital or proportional control mechanisms. The mechanical elbows have a locking mechanism that is manually applied using the contralateral hand, the chin, or the ipsilateral shoulder via a cable system. Electric elbows have an electromechanical brake or a switch-controlled lock mechanism to maintain the selected position. The rotation function of the arm (internal/external rotation) is provided through the use of a turntable. This device is useful to provide reach to the body midline. Electric elbows have limited active flexion force. The flexion force across a mechanical elbow is dependent on the wearer's strength, the comfort of the socket fit, and the ability to efficiently transfer the power from the residual limb to the prosthesis.

For elbow disarticulation, the external elbow joint is indicated in an attempt to maintain the optimal length of the arm. This joint is larger and protrudes in the medial aspect. Limited flexion strength and increased maintenance are some of the problems with this type of joint.

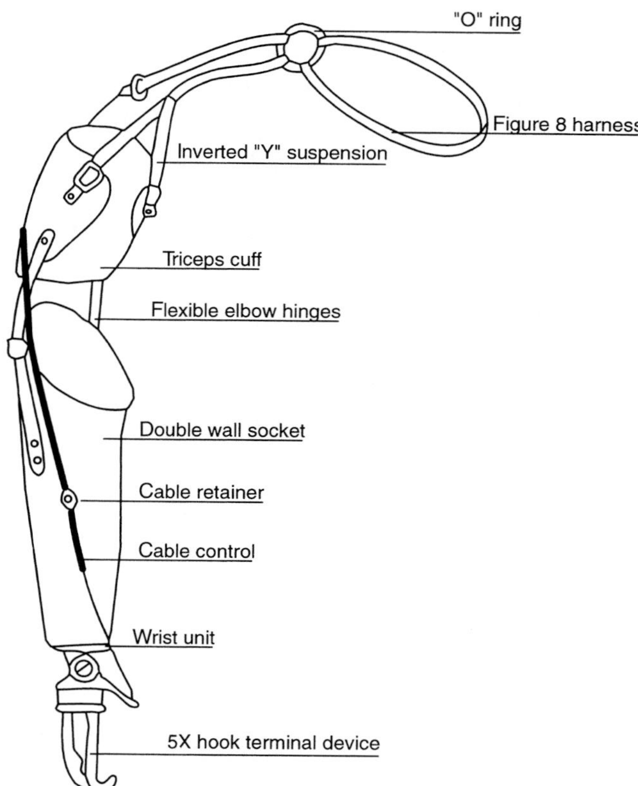

FIGURE 13–3. A body-powered transhumeral prosthesis with components identified.

TABLE 13–5 Types of Prosthetic Wrists

Mechanical
Pronosupination
Friction
Quick-disconnect
Spring-assisted
Flexion
Spring-assisted internal or external
Electric
Pronosupination
Myoelectric
Switch control

Prosthetic Sockets

Socket configuration and materials have improved greatly since the mid-1980s. The key functions of a prosthetic socket include comfortable total contact interface with the residual limb, efficient energy transfer from the

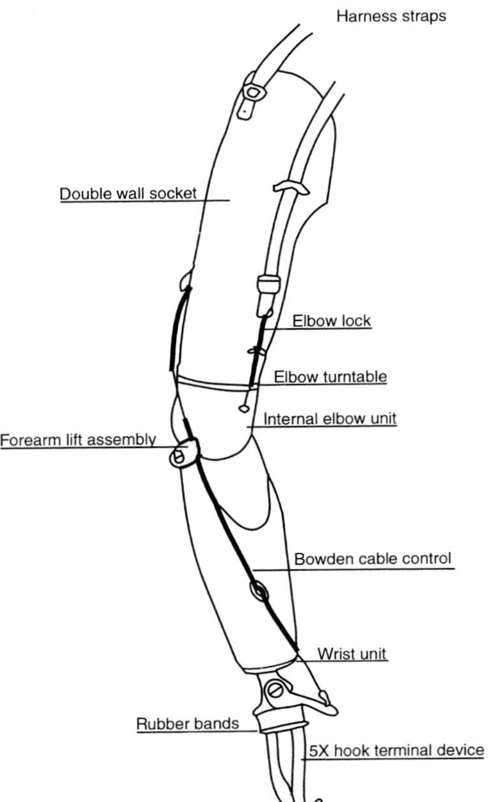

FIGURE 13–4. A body-powered transradial prosthesis with components identified.

residual limb to the prosthetic device, secure suspension, and cosmetic appearance (Table 13–7). A patient often fails to accept the prosthesis if the socket does not provide most of these characteristics.

Sockets used in the past were carved out of wood. These sockets had the disadvantage of being open-ended, which promoted distal residual limb swelling with potential development of chronic edema and trophic skin changes. With the development of high-temperature rigid plastic materials such as polyester resin, sockets with decreased weight and increased durability could be molded to have total contact. More recently, acrylic lamination, the use of carbon graphite, and the introduction of flexible thermoplastics have permitted the design of sockets with windows that are lined with flexible materials and are more comfortable, lighter, and durable.[17] Most upper limb prosthetic sockets have two layers. The first one is closely contoured to the residual limb and the external layer gives the necessary length and shape to the socket. It is to this external layer that the necessary prosthetic components (e.g., elbow, wrist) are attached.

Sockets are custom made by obtaining a negative impression of the residual limb by plaster of Paris wrap. This is then converted to a positive mold that can be modified by the prosthetist to appropriately distribute pressure throughout the entire surface of the residual limb. Routinely, a transparent plastic socket is first manufactured to permit direct visualization of the soft tissues. The transparent socket can be modified to ensure comfortable total contact. Eventually a final socket is fabricated. The concepts of computer-assisted design (CAD) and computer-assisted manufacturing (CAM) have been adapted to prosthesis fabrication. Direct surface video imaging of the residual limb, ultrasound and/or magnetic resonance imaging, and direct digitization from a plaster of Paris mold are being used in some centers as sources of digital data to be manipulated in a computer environment. From that point, a computer-controlled carver can create a positive mold of wax or plaster from which a socket can be manufactured from vacuum-formed thermoplastics.[2]

New flexible plastic materials have made sockets lighter and more comfortable.[11] The use of these new materials in prosthetics has resulted in the development of improved socket construction techniques.[23, 36, 40] The inner socket provides total contact with the residual limb and is the interface that provides suction suspension if desired. The outer socket or frame is made of a more rigid material, thermoplastic or resin, and provides the structural integrity of the socket. When double sockets are used, windows can be cut in the exterior frame to allow muscles to expand during contraction and to improve comfort and sensory feedback. The elasticity of the thermoplastic material results in a more comfortable fit. Although more costly and time-consuming to fabricate initially, the frame socket design has the added advantage of allowing replacement of the inner socket to accommodate small residual limb changes without changing the external frame to which the other prosthetic components are attached. It is a fairly simple process to pull out the old liner and slip in a new one. The inner socket is usually held in place by Velcro or another removable fastener. The frame socket design is particularly appealing for externally powered prosthe-

TABLE 13–6 Classification of Prosthetic Elbows

Body-Powered Elbow
External, with or without spring-assisted flexion
Internal, with or without spring-assisted flexion
Internal, with rotating turntable
Externally Powered Elbow
Digital switch control
Proportional switch control
Digital myoelectric control
Proportional myoelectric control
Passive Elbow
Manual lock

TABLE 13–7 Key Functions of the Prosthetic Socket

Comfortable residual limb–prosthesis interface
Efficient energy transference to the prosthesis
Secure suspension of the prosthesis
Adequate cosmesis

ses and self-suspended ones (wrist and elbow disarticulation and Muenster sockets). One disadvantage of these materials is their poor temperature insulation characteristics, which make them uncomfortable during cold weather. This can be partially corrected by using clothing layers to cover the arm.

Suspension Systems

The suspension and control system of a body-powered prosthesis needs to provide two distinct important functions to make the prosthetic device work. One of these is suspension, which is the means of securing the prosthetic device to the body. The other is to permit control of the prosthesis, including the terminal device. The more secure the suspension system, the more prosthetic control and comfort can be expected by the patient. The upper limb amputee has traditionally been provided with suspension systems that are uncomfortable and that limit mobility. They consist mostly of straps with metal and plastic attachments. The traditional suspension mechanisms (Table 13–8) for the upper limb sockets include a strap that suspends the prosthesis over the shoulder (figure-of-8 harness). The harness is used as a control mechanism to transmit body power to the terminal device and elbow. For the more proximal level amputation, a chest strap or shoulder saddle can be used to further improve suspension. Patients with wrist or elbow disarticulation or transradial amputations can use bony prominences for suspension. The Muenster[15] or condylar suspension is perhaps the best of these. When this type of suspension is used, a figure-of-9 harness can be used for control purposes only.

The transradial Muenster socket design was developed in Germany in the early 1950s[15] and was later modified at Northwestern University. This socket configuration provides excellent suspension by encasing the elbow condyles. The main disadvantage is the limitation in elbow range of motion for terminal extension and flexion. This can prevent its use as the preferred type of suspension for the patient with bilateral transradial amputations. This type of suspension works extremely well with externally powered, myoelectric control prostheses, as the patient can be completely free of straps.

In most cases, a sock is used as an interface between the residual limb and the socket. Using different numbers of sock layers can adjust for the physiological volume changes that occur from day to day. Socks also protect the skin and improve hygiene. The only exceptions are suction sockets, for which direct skin-to-socket contact is required, and socks cannot be used.

TABLE 13–8 Prosthetic Suspension Systems

Harness	Semisuction
Figure-of-8	Hypobaric
Chest strap	Semisuction
Shoulder saddle	Suction
Self-suspension	Full suction
Condylar	Silicone sock
Muenster	
Northwestern	

Hypobaric and semisuction suspension is best thought of as a transition between nonsuction and full-suction suspension. This suspension system utilizes socks that have a special silicone band in them, and the socket is provided with a one-way valve that permits the expulsion of air during donning. The band creates a seal between the socket and the skin of the residual limb and permits the development of suction that can be used for suspension. The advantage of this suspension system is that the changes in residual limb volume that typically occur early in the rehabilitation process can be accommodated simply by altering the number of plies (thicknesses) of socks used.

Silicone Suction Suspension Application to Upper Limb Body and External Powered Prostheses

Since 1986 the Icelandic roll on silicone sleeve (ICEROSS), invented by Kristinsson,[24] has been in use as a suspension system for the transtibial amputee, with consistent improvement in the suspension of the prosthesis. More recently its use has been extended to suspend the upper limb prosthesis while protecting the skin. It has also been applied more recently for upper extremity myoelectric prosthetics.[37]

The silicone liner provides improved suspension function by creating a negative atmospheric pressure and an adhesive bond to the skin.[28] The silicone sleeve also improves the socket-residual limb interface by protecting the skin through significant reduction of shear forces and added cushioning. The silicone sleeve provides improved suspension by reducing pistoning and shear, protects the skin, allows for volume adjustment with residual limb girth changes, and improves cosmesis, as it reduces or eliminates the need for harness suspension.[14]

Donning of the prosthesis is simplified and can be done with one hand. Silicone sleeve systems do not interfere with elbow range of motion, unlike other types of self-suspension systems such as supracondylar sockets. Patients perceive the prosthesis to be lighter and more comfortable when silicone suspension is used, owing to the improved suspension.

The system consists of a silicone sleeve with a distal attachment pin that interfaces with a shuttle lock mechanism built into the prosthetic socket (Figs. 13–5 through 13–7). The patient rolls on the silicone liner directly over the skin after spraying the external surface of the liner with alcohol (or, in the case of a prelined liner, just pulling it on). This results in a suspension system that makes use of negative pressure on the distal third of the residual limb and of friction and pressure between the sleeve and the skin in the upper two-thirds portion of the limb. Once in place, one or more socks can be applied over the silicone liner to improve fit, adjust for changes in the limb girth, and reduce friction between the silicone material and the prosthesis. Some systems rely on this friction to suspend the prosthesis if no pin mechanism is used. If a high degree of cushioning and pressure distribution is desirable, a thicker liner system can be used. Liner thickness ranges from 3 to 9 mm to provide optimal suspension and cushioning. More

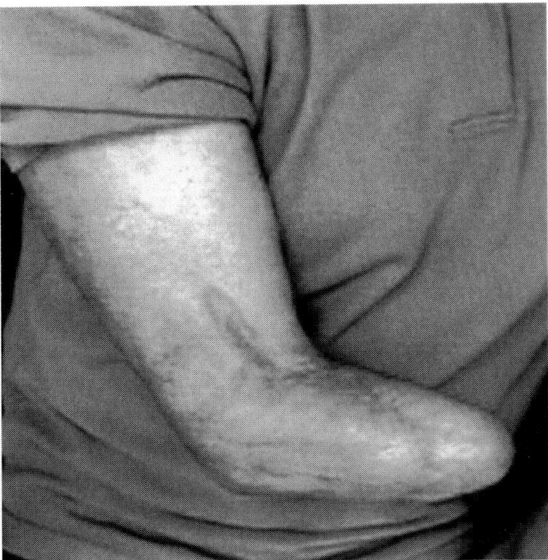

FIGURE 13–5. Transradial amputation with significant scar tissue that would benefit from silicone sleeve suspension.

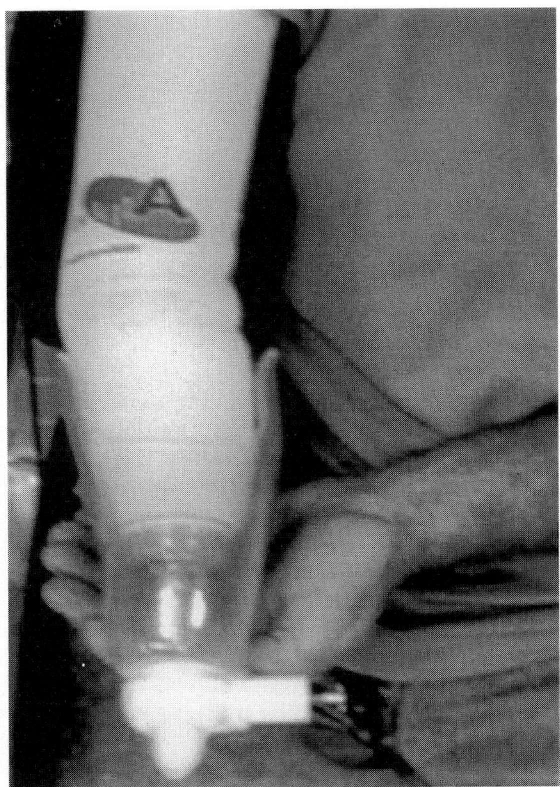

FIGURE 13–7. Patient demonstrating application of transradial check socket prosthesis over silicone sleeve suspension. Note the suspension pin, which will connect with the shuttle lock system.

recently available are silicone liners that have a variable thickness, and a distal silicone pad can be added to protect sensitive areas.

Excessive perspiration and irritation can occur with roll-on silicone sleeve use. Excessive perspiration can be controlled with antiperspirant lotions or Botox injections of the affected skin area to control the focal hyperhidrosis.[34] A contact dermatitis-like reaction can occur, even though silicone is a hypoallergenic material. Commonly this problem occurs only in the first weeks of use and when the weather is very warm. It affects primarily the edge of the sleeve where the transition of pressure gradients and the free edge of the silicone can trigger this dermatological reaction. A period of increased skin and sleeve hygiene and protecting the skin from direct contact by using a partial sock are recommended. A bland skin protectant agent such as zinc oxide or petrolatum paste (Desitin) can make for rapid resolution of the problem.[25]

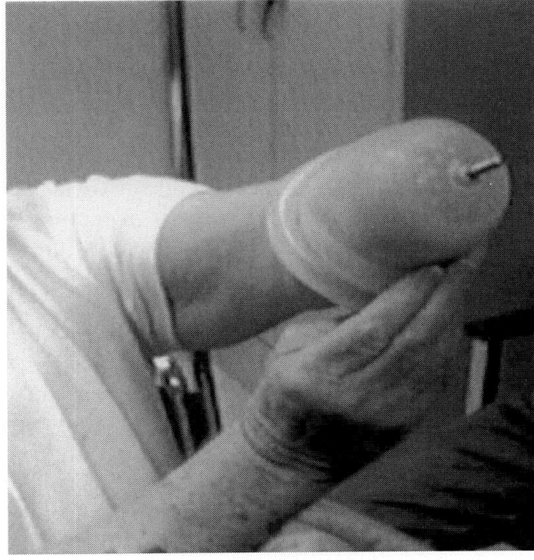

FIGURE 13–6. Patient demonstrating one-handed application of silicone sleeve suspension system.

Silicone sleeves are best used by patients who are likely to have problems with skin integrity, such as patients who have undergone skin grafting for burns or degloving injuries, those with delicate, insensate skin (such as patients with diabetes and scleroderma), or those with adhesive scar tissue. We have applied this type of suspension to the upper limb amputee (transradial and transhumeral) and expanded its use to externally powered prosthesis (myoelectric control), with excellent results.

Silicone sleeves afford excellent skin protection and are a good prosthetic suspension system for patients who are very active users, play sports, or have short, very sensitive or delicate residual limbs. Patients with skin grafts after burns, trauma or degloving injuries or those with areas of reduced sensitivity are also prime candidates for this type of suspension system.

In the upper limb externally powered socket design, silicone suspension can be implemented and can permit the use of myoelectric controls if the residual limb is not extremely short and other selection characteristics are met.

Individuals who live in areas of the world with warm and humid weather are more likely to develop dermatological problems. These can be minimized by strict hygienic care of the skin and the insert.

Control Mechanisms

When a body harness is used as a control mechanism for a body-powered prosthesis, the patient needs to be able to produce movements that generate the power requirements to activate the terminal device or elbow. These movements include scapular abduction; chest expansion; shoulder depression, extension, and abduction and humeral flexion; and elbow flexion and extension (see Fig. 13–5). These movements can be difficult to perform if the residual limb is short, painful, or has limited motion, or if the prosthetic socket does not fit well. A poorly adjusted harness decreases the power transmission of the movements.[7]

Electric switch control mechanisms can be activated with residual limb movements that depress a switch inside the socket. For other cases, a chest strap, waist belt, or figure-of-9 harness can be used. Servo controls that sense tension have been introduced into clinical use.

Myoelectric controls use the electrical activity generated during a muscle contraction to control the flow of energy from a battery to a motor in the prosthetic device. The control signals come from muscle sites in the amputated limb that still have normal innervation and voluntary control.[38] Ideally, muscles in the more distal portion of the residual limb should be used. Antagonistic muscles are best for this function (i.e., wrist or elbow flexor/extensor). This ensures that the control is easy to use, physiological, consistent, and precise. At times, more proximal muscles or muscles in the trunk or other limb can be used. Systems that use single-channel control mechanisms use two electrode sites, one to trigger hand closure or elbow flexion and the other to trigger hand opening or elbow extension. Multi-channel systems permit the use of one muscle to control two different functions. This requires that the patient be able to produce a slow, gentle muscle contraction for one function and a strong, faster one for the other function. Myoelectronic prosthetic components, such as the Boston or Utah arms, use an "electronic switch" to alternate between the hand and the elbow function. Some systems also include proportional controls, which respond to the speed and strength of the muscle contraction by correspondingly producing a faster or slower movement of the hand or elbow. A very snug fit of the socket is required to avoid shift of the muscles in reference to the electrodes for proper function. Hybrid systems combine two or more of the available control mechanisms, either electric or body-powered (Fig. 13–8).

Suction Suspension

For the transhumeral amputee, suction suspension (negative pressure) without the use of straps is the preferred type of suspension. For this system to work well, and to be able to don the prosthesis independently, the patient should have good contralateral upper limb strength, endurance, and coordination. The socket is made small enough and provided with a one-way valve that permits the expulsion of air during donning. The amputee dons the socket using a pull sock or Ace bandage or with a wet fit (using a lubricant liquid or powder). The intimate fit between the socket and the skin of the residual limb, especially distally, results in a tight seal between the socket and skin. Doffing requires breaking the vacuum seal. To maintain proper suspension over time, the residual limb must be mature and volume stable.[9]

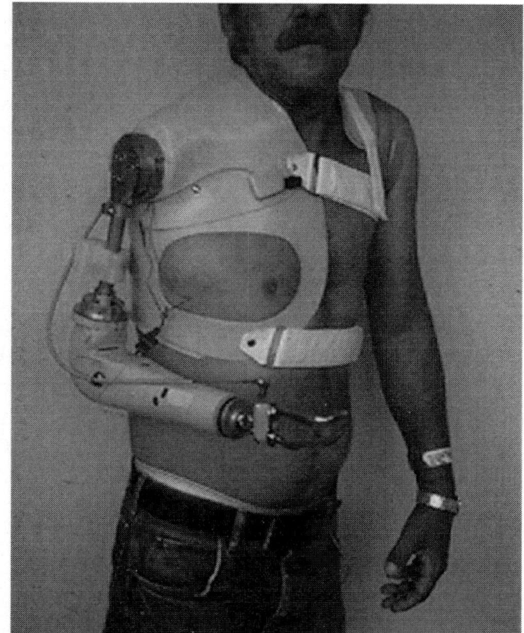

FIGURE 13–8. Hybrid forequarter amputation prosthesis. The device uses a MICA shoulder with chin control locks, Utah myoelectronic elbow, and interchangeable 5X voluntary opening hook or myoelectric hand.

Shoulder Disarticulation and Forequarter Amputation

There has been little change in the basic socket design for shoulder disarticulation or forequarter amputation since it was designed. The main changes have been modification of the socket trim lines and suspension and use of lighter materials to construct the socket. As in sockets for other levels of amputation, thermoplastic and silicone materials are being used to provide lighter, more secure, and more comfortable sockets at these proximal levels of amputation. Most of the advances in prosthetic design for these levels have occurred with externally powered components, which are described elsewhere in this chapter. A shoulder joint with a manual lock that provides improvement in the arm control and position is now available.

Cosmetic Covers

Cosmetic covers can be manufactured for a single digit, for the hand, or to extend to the elbow. They should be considered an integral part of the prosthesis, because for many patients the cover is the factor that determines success or failure of prosthetic restoration.

Custom-made silicone cosmetic covers can provide excellent cosmetic results, but they can be very expensive and difficult to maintain, and they deteriorate over time. Intrinsic coloration is a newer technique that provides a more realistic look. The colors are integrated at the time of fabrication instead of coloring the cover after it has been applied to the arm.

Activity-Specific Devices

To optimally perform at work, sports, or recreational activities, it might be necessary to provide the patient with a specially designed terminal device. Many devices are commercially available that are designed for participation in sports (e.g., golf, fishing, skiing). Many more have been designed by the users for activities such as construction, cooking, archery, and photography.

Prosthetic Prescription

The prosthetic prescription should be carefully prepared to satisfy the needs and desires of the patient. A team approach to prescription writing should be used. The prescription should clearly spell out the components, control system, suspension, materials, and any special features that might be required. The prescription should serve to clearly communicate with the prosthetist and the insurance company. A clear, well-thought-out, organized prescription should achieve this (Fig. 13–9).

Prosthetic Training

Training is integral to the rehabilitation process. A new amputee or an experienced one who receives a prosthetic device that has different components should participate in such training. In most cases, this program

MossRehab Upper Limb Prosthetic Prescription

Name:________________ Age:________ Date:__________

Diagnosis:________________ Patient ready: yes no Room#________

Prosthetist:________________ Third Party Coverage:____________

Preparatory Prosthesis Permanent Prosthesis

Circle and complete as necessary

Side: Right Left Bilateral

Site: Partial Hand Wrist Transradial Transhumeral Shoulder or Forequarter Disarticulation

Socket configuration: Frame Single wall Double wall Pre-flexed Silicone sleeve

Socket construction: Hard Flexible Suction Expandible Shuttle

Suspension: Biceps cuff Triceps cuff Muenster Suction Chest strap

Structure: Endoskeletal Exoskeletal Hybrid

Control: Myoelectric Procontrol Body powered External powered

Harness: Figure 8 Double "O" ring Figure 9 Chest strap Shoulder saddle None

Shoulder: Manual lock Friction Heavy duty

Elbow: Internal External Spring flexion assist Balanced forearm Electric Myoelectric

Lock: Manual Friction Cable control Electronic Switch control (rocker / pull / push)

Wrist: Oval Round Friction Quick disconnect Flexion unit

Spring prono/supination Electric prono/supination

Terminal device: Hand Hook VO VC Passive Myoelectric Electric (rocker / pull / push)

Cover: Cosmetic glove Semicustom glove Intrinsic coloration Custom

Power supply: Batteries#________ Chargers#________ 110 or 220 V

Socks: Nylon #______ 1Ply #______ 3Ply #______ Silipos#______ Pull socks#______

Special Instructions:______________________________

____

____

Signature ____________________ **M.D./D.O.**

FIGURE 13–9. Sample of an upper limb prosthetic prescription developed at the MossRehab Regional Amputee Center.

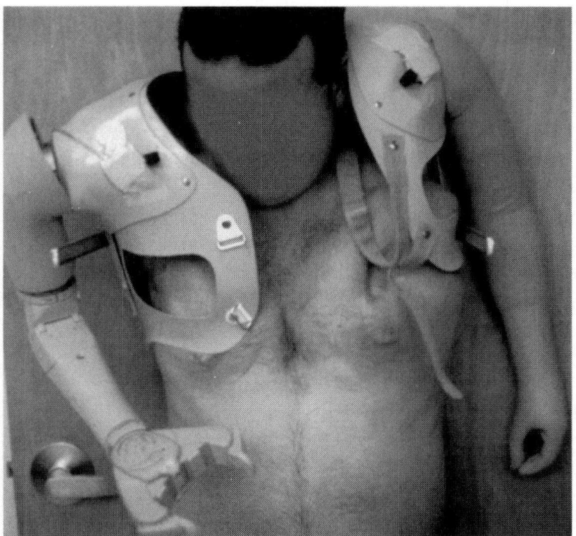

FIGURE 13–10. Patient demonstrating donning of bilateral shoulder disarticulation myoelectric prosthesis. Note right-sided Greifer terminal device, left-sided hand.

should be a coordinated effort among the occupational, physical, and recreational therapists and the prosthetist, with frequent physiatric input (kinesiotherapists are also used at some centers). Each of the team members uses different techniques to teach what needs to be learned by the amputee. Before initiating a program of upper limb prosthetic training, one must realistically orient the patient to what the prosthesis can and cannot do.[1] The patient should learn prosthetic management, including the basic principles behind the function, care, and maintenance of each of the components in the prosthesis. The patient should practice independently putting on and taking off the prosthesis. Skin care and inspection techniques are also reviewed. For the body-powered devices, dismounting the harness for washing and replacing it should be practiced. Written instructions are useful for explaining the care and maintenance of the batteries used in externally powered devices. A review and practice of the use of the prosthesis for bimanual activities, such as grooming, dressing, feeding, driving, sports, work, and recreation activities, should always be included in the training process.

Special Considerations for the Bilateral Upper Limb Amputee

For the bilateral upper limb amputee, training should promote the development of a dominant prosthesis and skills for independent donning. Alternative techniques for putting on the prosthesis are frequently required. This might include using the bed for setup and suspending the prosthetic devices from special wall hooks or frames. The prosthesis should have a wrist rotation and flexion device that permits access to the body midline.

For bathing activities, the patient with bilateral upper limb amputations ideally should have a modified shower with wall brushes and liquid soap dispensers. In some cases, simplified shower prostheses (devices that are waterproof) are a medical necessity, because they allow the patient to perform this activity independently (Fig. 13–10).

Brachial Plexus and Other Nerve Injuries

Brachial plexus injuries can be the result of many different causes, which can be divided into two main categories: closed injuries and open penetrating trauma. The majority of cases are caused by closed injuries. Traction on the upper plexus and the C5 and C6 roots occurs when the head and neck are stretched away from the shoulder. When the arm is stretched overhead, traction to the lower plexus and C8 and T1 roots occurs most frequently. The injuries can be preganglionic (indicating injury or avulsion of the nerve root proximal to the spinal ganglion) with resulting severe or even complete motor and sensory loss. This can also be accompanied by Horner's syndrome. Postganglionic injuries occur distal to the spinal ganglion and tend to have a more favorable prognosis (Table 13–9).

Reintegration into the Community

Reintegration into the community is best done gradually over a few weeks or months. This process can be initiated early in the rehabilitation program with the supervision of the team members during organized trips for shopping, recreation, and part-time work or school. When possible, the use of "day" rehabilitation programs, in which the patient participates in rehabilitation 6 hours a day, 5 days a week (with return to home every evening and weekend), is a good system to foster community reintegration.

The patient can return to work when safety concerns are met.[22] Initially, modified or restricted work should be provided, but the patient should not be discouraged from returning to the premorbid work level if it is safe to do so. Work simulation or supervised work are good techniques to reintroduce patients to their work environment. The use of a partial "day program" rehabilitation program in which the patient participates in rehabilitation for 3 hours a day, 5 days a week or 6 hours a day, 2 to 3 days a week also encourages and allows time for the return to part-time work in the community. The availability of psychological counseling or assistance from the team members during each of these steps is important for the smooth transition of patients and their families to independent functioning.

Functional Outcomes

Realistic goals for the majority of unilateral transradial or transhumeral amputees include independence in

TABLE 13–9 Types and Common Causes of Brachial Plexus Injuries

Closed Injuries	*Penetrating Injuries*
Traction	Gunshot
Compression	Fracture
Combined	Knife
Radiation	

all activities of daily living, most household activities, driving, and work (Table 13–10). Some restrictions should be imposed in relationship to handling delicate, heavy, or voluminous objects. The typical patient with a transradial amputation can be expected to lift 20 to 30 lb, unless the residual limb is very short or sensitive. The typical patient with a transhumeral amputation can be expected to lift 10 to 15 lb, unless the residual limb is very short or sensitive. This is also affected by the type of elbow used.

For the bilateral transhumeral amputee, realistic goals include independence in most activities of daily living after assisted donning, some household activities, driving with a spin ring, and most types of sedentary work with environmental modifications. Restrictions should be imposed in relationship to handling delicate, heavy objects (up to 20 lbs.), unless the residual limb is very short or sensitive, or voluminous objects.

If work is to take place where magnetic fields or large electrical currents are present, myoelectric prostheses may not work well unless special shielding materials are used during fabrication, to prevent interference.

Long-Term Follow-up

The patient who has successfully completed a rehabilitation program should be seen for follow-up by a minimum of two of the team members at least every 3 months for the first 18 months. These visits might need to be more frequent and include other members of the team if the patient is having difficulties with prosthesis fitting, the residual limb, specific activities, or psychosocial adjustment. After this critical period, the patient should be seen at least every 6 months to ensure adequate prosthetic fit and function and to assess the need for maintenance and the overall medical condition and functional level of the patient. When the patient's condition is stable it may be necessary to replace a prosthesis or parts of it every 18 months to 3 years for body-powered devices and every 2 to 4 years for myoelectric prostheses.

Neuromas

Neuroma is the formation of scar tissue around the distal end of the severed nerve. As previously mentioned, every time a nerve is cut it forms a neuroma. Good surgical technique results in the neuroma being buried under large soft tissue masses that serve to protect it from irritation. At times, because of limited soft tissue coverage or very large neuroma formation with compression of the nerve, adhesion of the tissues, or complications from the surgical technique, a neuroma may become symptomatic. This results in pain that can be perceived at the site of the neuroma and that radiates distally to the end of the residual limb (or, at times, into the phantom limb). A painful neuroma is palpable most of the time, and pressure over it reproduces the symptoms. Desensitization techniques, prosthetic modifications, and, at times, use of flexible materials with windowed frame construction to decrease pressure over the neuroma may help. Injection of the neuroma with a mixture of long- and short-acting local anesthetics and a corticosteroid should reduce the scar tissue pressure on the nerve and produce symptomatic improvement. When correctly performed, this technique reproduces the presenting symptoms with increasing severity as the needle is advanced. The injection can be repeated several times at 6- to 8-week intervals. Surgical removal of the neuroma with careful retraction of the nerve prior to cutting it should be reserved for those cases in which all other interventions have failed and in which the tissues allow repositioning of the neuroma to a less pressure exposed location.

TABLE 13–10 Typical Functional Outcomes for Upper Limb Amputation with Prosthesis

Unilateral transradial or transhumeral amputation
Independent ADLs, household activities, driving, and work, with some limitations
Bilateral amputation
After assisted donning of prosthesis, independent ADLs, household activities, driving, and work, with many limitations

Support Groups

Support groups are a source of information, peer counseling, and motivation for many patients. These groups ideally should constitute one more component of the comprehensive rehabilitation approach to the patient with an amputation. Patients who have recently sustained an amputation benefit from contact with experienced amputees; at the same time, the veteran amputee enjoys serving as a resource. This forum can also be used effectively as a resource for the family of the patient with an amputation.

Dermatological Problems

The skin of a patient who wears a prosthesis is subject to much abuse. Most prosthetic sockets prevent appropriate air circulation, thereby trapping perspiration moisture. This can result in a variety of problems such as hyperhidrosis, folliculitis, allergic dermatitis, and even skin breakdown where adherent scars are present. Poor hygiene is frequently the cause of some of these problems, and for this reason the patient should be trained in the proper washing technique for the residual limb, silicone liners, socks, and the socket and its interfaces. A daily routine of washing the skin and the internal wall of the socket with a mild soap might suffice. It can be necessary at times to use concentrated antiperspirants, bacteriostatic or bactericidal soaps, and, in some cases, antibiotics. Topical antibiotics or steroids should not generally be used if the prosthesis has silicone components as part of the socket materials that are in direct contact with the skin. Contact dermatitis can frequently occur because of this.[27]

Care of the Nonamputated Upper Limb

Jones and Davidson recently reported the first study of problems in the remaining arm of the unilateral upper limb amputee.[18] There is a high incidence of overuse injuries to the soft tissues, tendon-muscle complex, and the joint itself. In order of frequency, elbow, shoulder, and wrist injuries were reported. The more proximal the amputation, the more prevalent were the problems. A program of education to avoid overuse and promote habilitation, aggressive early management of injuries, and preventative care of the limb with avoidance of potentially injurious activities should be implemented.

PEDIATRIC LIMB DEFICIENCY AND AMPUTATION REHABILITATION

The pediatric patient can have an acquired or congenital limb deficiency. The child with a congenital limb deficiency has no sense of loss and does not have to go through the psychological adjustment process. The prosthesis is perceived as an aid rather than as a replacement. If the device cannot serve in this role it will be discarded. These children try to engage in the same types of activities as other children. Their only limitations are usually those imposed by adults. In contrast, the child with an acquired limb deficiency goes through the natural readjustment process of limb loss. How well they are able to adjust has a direct impact on their acceptance of an artificial limb.[43]

Some special considerations should be made for the pediatric patient with upper limb deficiency or amputation.[12] Three specific points to consider in this population are (1) normal growth and development, which will necessitate frequent prosthetic adjustments or replacements; (2) bony overgrowth; and (3) the more rigorous use that the device will be subjected to.[39] It can be expected that a prosthesis (socket only, or all of it) will need to be replaced yearly in the first 5 years of life, every 18 months from 5 to 12 years of age, and every 2 years until age 21 years.[3] To address growth problems, multilayered sockets (onion sockets) for body-powered devices can be used. These allow removal of one layer at a time to accommodate growth. This results in gradual enlargement of the socket to coincide with periods of growth. The socket made in this fashion increases the life span of the prosthesis from 6 months to as much as 18 months. Length adjustment is also important, although it is not as critical as with lower limb prostheses. This can be adjusted by adding material at the wrist or elbow sites when necessary. Harnesses and cables need to be adjusted for length and replaced more frequently.[4] For bony overgrowth, surgery with bony capping may be necessary.[26] For myoelectric devices, two problems are noted: (1) the limitation imposed by weight and size of the components[35] and (2) the necessary frequent alterations to the socket to maintain optimal electrode contact as the residual limb size changes.[42] Frequently required socket replacements can make myoelectric devices less practical for this population due to their cost. Terminal devices and elbows might need to be replaced frequently. Prosthetic component banks are available in some countries, which make myoelectric prosthetic component replacement less expensive.

Parental counseling and support are integral components in the rehabilitation of the pediatric amputee. The prosthetic fitting for the pediatric patient with upper limb deficiency or the pediatric amputee should be initiated at 3 to 9 months of age. This should coincide with sitting and the initiation of bimanual activities. The use of a passive mitten, hand, or inactive hook or California Amputee Pediatric Project (CAPP) terminal device and a preflexed fixed elbow is indicated at this stage. The terminal device can be activated at ages 18 to 24 months and the elbow at ages 36 to 48 months.[39] Myoelectric devices have been used at these young ages, with good results.[41] For very proximal upper limb deficiency, use of the feet should be encouraged.

SUMMARY

The rehabilitation process for the patient with an upper limb amputation is a complex one, and it is best accomplished by the patient who is able to work in a close cooperative relationship with a comprehensive, multidisciplinary, specialized treatment team. The team members should be ready and able to assist the patient throughout the rehabilitation program, from preamputation to community reintegration. The availability of psychological counseling and/or assistance from the team members during each one of these steps is very important for the smooth transition of the patient back into the community.

REFERENCES

1. Atkins D: Adult upper-limb prosthetic training. In Atkins DJ, Meier RH III (eds): Comprehensive Management of the Upper-Limb Amputee. New York, Springer-Verlag, 1989, pp 39–59.
2. CAD-CAM special issue. J Prosthet Orthot 1989; 1:116–190.
3. Challenor Y: Limb deficiencies in children. In Molnar G (ed): Pediatric Rehabilitation. Baltimore, Williams & Wilkins, 1992, pp 400–424.
4. Curran B, Hambrey R: The prosthetic treatment of upper limb deficiency. Prosthet Orthot Int 1991; 15:82–87.
5. Davis RW: Phantom sensation, phantom pain and stump pain. Arch Phys Med Rehabil 1993; 74:79–91.
6. Dise-Lewis J: Psychological adaptation to limb loss. In Atkins JD, Meier RH III (eds): Comprehensive Management of the Upper-Limb Amputee. New York, Springer-Verlag, 1989; pp 165–172.
7. Dobner DL: A prosthetic harness adaptation. Arch Phys Med Rehabil 1990; 71:436–438.
8. Edelstein JE: Preprosthetic management of patients with lower or upper limb amputation. Phys Med Rehabil Clin North Am 1991; 2:285–297.
9. Esquenazi A: Geriatric amputee rehabilitation. Geriatr Clin North Am 1993; 9:731–743.
10. Fletchall S, Hickerson WL: Early upper-extremity prosthetic fit in patients with burns. J Burn Care Rehabil 1991; 12:234–236.
11. Glatly HW: A statistical study of 12,000 new amputees. South Med J 1964; 57:1373–1378.
12. Gover AM, McIvor J: Upper limb deficiencies in infants and young. Infant Young Child 1992; 5:58–72.
13. Gregory RT, Gould RJ, Peclet M, et al: The mangled extremity syndrome (MES): A severity grading system for multisystem injury of the extremity. J Trauma 1985; 25:1147–1150.
14. Heim M, et al: Silicone suspension of external prostheses: A new era in artificial limb usage. J Bone Joint Surg Br 1997; 79:638–640.

15. Hepp O: Prothesen der oberen Extremitat. In Hohmann G, Hoackenbrock K, Lindemann L (eds): Handbuck der Orthopadie, vol 1. Stuttgart, Georg Thieme Verlag, 1957.
16. Illizarov GA: Possibilities offered by our method for lengthening various segments in upper and lower limbs. Basic Life Sci 1988; 48:323.
17. Jendrzejczyk D: Flexible socket systems. Clin Prosthet Orthot 1985; 9:27–31.
18. Jones LE, Davidson JH: Save that arm: A study of problems in the remaining arm of unilateral upper limb amputees. Prosthet Orthot Int 1999; 23:55–58.
19. Kamen LB, Chapis GJ: Phantom limb sensation and phantom pain. Phys Med Rehabil State Art Rev 1994; 8:73–88.
20. Kay H, Working Group, ISPO: A proposed international terminology for the classification of congenital limb deficiencies. Orthot Prosthet 1974; 28:33–48.
21. Kay HW, Newman JD: Relative incidence of new amputations: Statistical comparisons of 6,000 new amputees. Orthot Prosthet 1975; 29:3–16.
22. Kejlaa GH: The social and economic outcome after upper limb amputation. Prosthet Orthot Int 1992; 16:25–31.
23. Kristinsson O: Flexible above-knee socket made from low density polyethylene suspended by a weight-transmitting frame. Orthot Prosthet 1983; 37:25–27.
24. Kristinsson O: The ICEROSS concept: A discussion of philosophy. Prosthet Orthot Int 1993; 17:49–55.
25. Lake C, Sopan T: The incidence of dermatological problems in the silicone suspension sleeve user. J Prosthet Orthot 1997; 9:97–104.
26. Lambert C: Amputation surgery in the child. Orthop Clin North Am 1972; 3:473–482.
27. Levy WS: Skin problems of the amputee. In Bowker JH, Michael JW (eds): Atlas of Limb Prosthetics, ed 2. St Louis, Mosby–Year Book, 1992, pp 681–688.
28. Madigan RR, Fillaver KD: 3-S prosthesis: A preliminary report. J Pediatr Orthop 1991; 11:112–117.
29. Malone JM, Childers SJ, Underwood J, et al: Immediate postsurgical management of upper extremity amputation: Conventional, electric and myoelectric prosthesis. Orthot Prosthet 1981; 35:1.
30. Malone JM, Fleming LL, Roberson J, et al: Immediate, early and late postsurgical management of upper limb amputation. J Rehabil Res Dev 1984; 21:33.
31. Meier RH: Upper limb amputee rehabilitation. Phys Med Rehabil State Art Rev 1994; 8:165–185.
32. Melzack R: Phantom limbs. Sci Am, April 1992, pp 120–126.
33. National Center for Health Statistics: Current Estimates from the National Health Interview Survey. Washington, DC, US Department of Health and Human Services, 1990.
34. Neumann M, Bergmann I, Hoffmann U, et al: Botulinum toxin for focal hyperhydrosis: Technical considerations and improvements in application. Br J Dermatol 1998; 139:1123–1124.
35. Patton J, Shida-Tokeshi J, Setoguchi Y: Prosthetic components for children. Phys Med Rehabil 1991; 5:2.
36. Pritham CH, Fillauer, C, Fillauer K: Experience with the Scandinavian flexible socket. Orthot Prosthet 1985; 39:17–32.
37. Salem Y: The use of silicone suspension sleeves with myoelectric fittings. J Prosthet Orthot 1994; 6(4):119–120.
38. Scott RN: Biomedical engineering in upper-extremity prosthetics. In Atkins DJ, Meier RH III (eds): Comprehensive Management of the Upper-Limb Amputee. New York, Springer-Verlag, 1989, pp 173–189.
39. Setoguchi Y, LeBlanc M: Upper limb strength of young limb deficient children as a factor in using body powered terminal devices: A pilot study. J Assoc Child Prosthet Orthot Clin 1992; 27:89–96.
40. Setoguchi Y, Rosenfelder R (eds): The Limb Deficient Child. Springfield, IL, Charles C Thomas, 1982.
41. Sherman AR, Sherman JC, Gall GN: A survey of current phantom limb pain treatment in the United States. Pain 1980; 8:85–99.
42. Sorbye R: Myoelectric prosthetic fitting in young children. Clin Orthop 1980; 148:34–40.
43. Varni JW, Setoguchi Y: Effects of parental adjustment on the adaptation of children with congenital or acquired limb deficiencies. J Dev Behav Pediatr 1993; 14:13–20.
44. Wilson AB Jr: Limb Prosthetics, ed 6. New York, Demos, 1989, pp 69–90.

14 CHAPTER

Ellen I. Leonard, M.D., Robert D. McAnelly, M.D., Maria Lomba, M.D., and Virgil W. Faulkner, C.P.O.

Lower Limb Prostheses

The types of amputation by level are partial foot, Syme, transtibial (below-knee), knee disarticulation (through-knee), transcondylar/supracondylar, transfemoral (above-knee), hip disarticulation, transpelvic (hemipelvectomy), and translumbar (hemicorporectomy). The 1977 National Health Survey found 358,000 persons with major amputations living in the United States, yielding a rate of 1.7 major amputations per 1000 persons.[103] Of the major amputations, 91,000 were upper limb, 92,000 were transfemoral, 113,000 were transtibial, 22,000 were partial foot, 36,000 were bilateral lower limb, and 4000 were combined lower- and upper-limb amputations. An estimated 205,000 persons used an artificial leg or foot.[104] The subsequent 1990 National Health Survey unfortunately failed to differentiate finger amputations from major limb amputations.[101] Nonfederal hospitals in the year 1989, however, discharged patients with 30,000 transfemoral amputations, 24,000 transtibial amputations, and 11,000 partial foot amputations.[102]

Kaye and Newman surveyed 5830 new amputees for the causes of amputation.[47] They found that vascular disease and infection accounted for 70% of all amputations; trauma, 22%; tumor, 5%; and congenital deformity, 3%. The largest number of amputations for disease occurred in the 61- to 70-year age group; for trauma, the 21- to 30-year age group; and for tumor, the 11- to 20-year age group. Male amputees outnumbered female amputees in the disease group 2.1 : 1; in trauma, 7.2 : 1; in tumor, 1.3 : 1; and in congenital deformity, 1.5 : 1. The ratio of lower- to upper-limb amputations was 11 : 1. The distribution of lower-limb amputations by level was Syme, 3%; transtibial, 59%; knee disarticulation, 1%; transfemoral, 35%; and hip disarticulation, 2%.

Vascular diseases requiring amputation include diabetes mellitus, arteriosclerosis, and Buerger's disease. Diabetic patients not only experience vascular compromise, but also suffer motor, sensory, and autonomic neuropathy, all of which lead to ulceration.[6] Antibiotic drugs have greatly improved the control of infection in vascular cases, allowing amputation to be performed at a lower level. (See Chapter 56.)

In the past, it was common to amputate well proximal to the neoplastic lesion in malignancy cases. Advances in chemotherapy and radiation therapy with better tumor staging now make it possible, in many cases, to perform segmental limb resection with wide local excision of the tumor. Segmental limb resection in the region of the knee can allow options such as total knee arthroplasty or van Ness tibial rotationplasty (Fig. 14–1), in which the anatomical ankle joint is rotated 180 degrees to become a functional knee joint. Post-tumor amputee patients who have received doxorubicin (Adriamycin) require cardiac screening prior to prosthesis fitting.[54] Amputees on chemotherapy have residual limb volume fluctuation, and it is important to coordinate prosthetic and chemotherapy programs. Transfemoral socket fit and gait training should be done when the patient is feeling well, usually prior to chemotherapy.[14] For the transtibial amputee, after alignment and initial gait training, chemotherapy if indicated, can begin on the same day.[14] Almost every post-tumor amputee deserves a prosthesis trial, regardless of prognosis.[44, 49] The permanent prosthesis should not be prescribed until 6 weeks after termination of chemotherapy (with resolution of transient edema). (See Chapter 57.)

All combinations of congenital limb deficiency occur, including missing intermediate parts. For example, the thigh or upper arm can be missing, whereas the other parts of the limb can be present but malformed. If a malformed part is nonfunctional, surgical options might have to be considered for amputation or reconstruction.

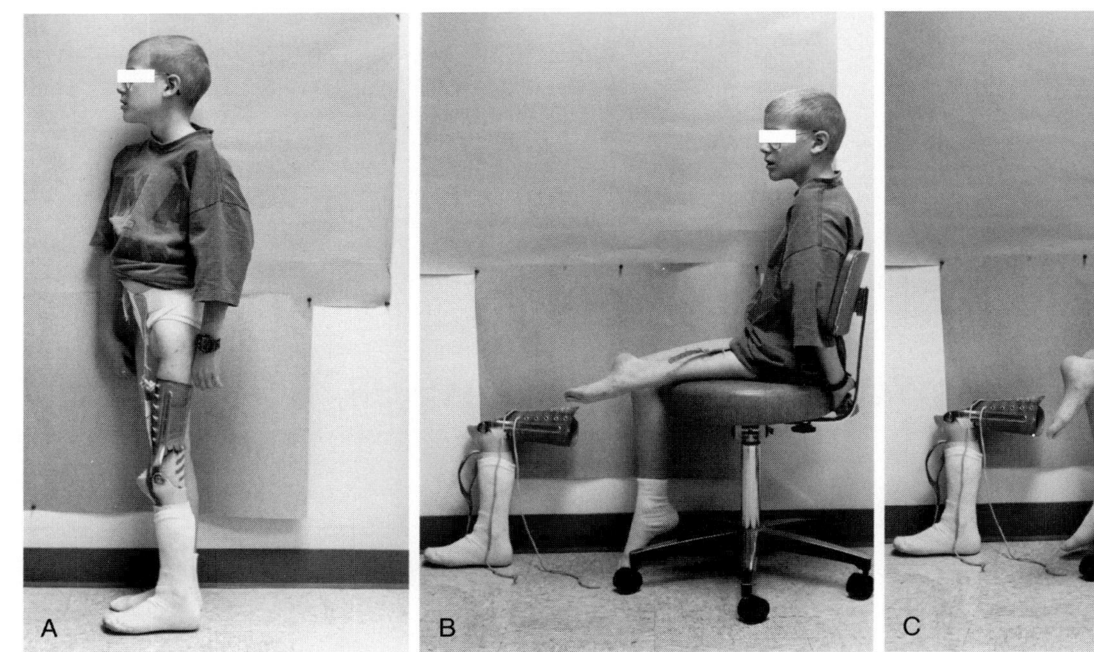

FIGURE 14–1. *A–C.* van Ness rotationplasty after tumor resection. (Courtesy of R. P. Williams, M.D.)

Trauma to a limb often involves vascular or nerve injury, burn injury, cold injury, and nonhealing fracture. These can render the limb permanently less functional than an artificial limb. In such cases, early amputation, rather than attempts at limb salvage, is often the best option.

PREOPERATIVE MANAGEMENT

Psychological Aspects

Preoperative counseling by the rehabilitation team and peer counseling by other amputees facilitates recovery. Preoperative therapy includes range-of-motion exercise, strengthening, and ambulation with an assistive device. Keep in mind that a new amputee typically experiences depression, especially if unaware of the prosthetic options for future function and ambulation.

Surgical Decisions and Level of Amputation

The rule of amputation is to save as much of the limb as possible, consistent with satisfactory healing and function. This rule demands a thoughtful accounting of advantages and disadvantages. The cost of limb salvage can be high: increased morbidity may occasion multiple operations, which can be financially and psychosocially ruinous. It is often better to choose early amputation and prosthetic fitting over limb salvage of questionable functional benefit.[5, 6, 33, 35, 36, 38, 56, 57] It is difficult to select the optimum level of amputation based on clinical assessment of tissue viability. Criteria such as poor skin edge bleeding during surgery and absence of pulses do not always correlate with failure to heal.[11] Many noninvasive vascular studies are available to determine level of amputation.[67, 77] Adequate nutrition and immunocompetence, as measured by albumin and total lymphocyte counts, also contribute to healing.

Preamputation arteriography in peripheral vascular disease is done chiefly to guide possible arterial reconstruction. It is of limited value for amputation level selection, however, because distal vessels are commonly not detected.[3] Despite angiography's limited prognostic value,[76] occlusion of both the deep and superficial femoral vessels indicates a poor prognosis for healing in transtibial amputation.[84]

Doppler-determined ankle blood pressure measurements are of little value in assessing partial foot amputation viability,[41, 70, 109] probably due to arteriovenous shunting that results in artificially elevated ankle blood pressures. Thigh blood pressure measurements above 70 mm Hg and possibly between 50 and 70 mm Hg, however, are predictive of success in transtibial amputation surgery.[88]

Intradermally injected radioisotope traces (^{133}Xe, ^{131}I, or ^{125}I-iodoantipyrine) provide a direct measure of skin blood flow, though the measurement is difficult to perform. Skin blood flow greater than 2.5 mL/100 g/min is correlated with healing at multiple amputation levels.[67, 71] Skin blood flow technique can be the most accurate measurement to assess skin viability, particularly around the knee joint.[65] But it is not as reliable in assessing regional blood flow.[64] Absolute skin perfusion pressure is also valuable.[34, 42, 100] Healing occurs in 90% of patients with skin perfusion calf pressure greater than 30 mm Hg, and in 67% with skin perfusion pressure from 20 to 30 mm Hg.[43]

Transcutaneous oxygen pressure ($TcPO_2$) is easy to measure but difficult to interpret. $TcPO_2$ levels greater

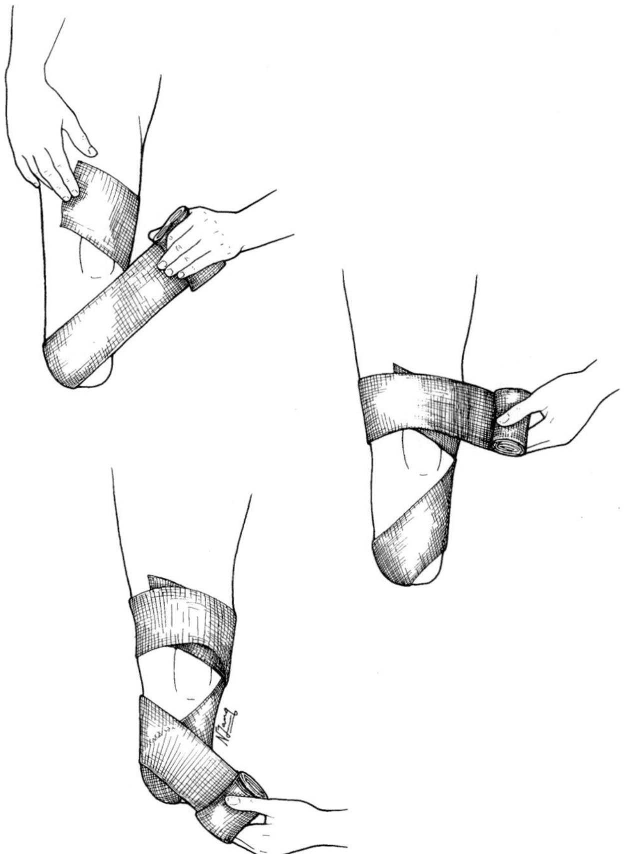

FIGURE 14–2. Wrapping a transtibial residual limb with elastic bandage in a figure-of-8 pattern to reduce edema. (Courtesy of the University of Texas Health Science Center at San Antonio.)

than 35 mm Hg at the calf predict that a transtibial amputation will heal, but values below this are not predictive.[11, 12, 23, 82, 110] Adding 100% oxygen inhalation to the test improves test reliability dramatically: Successful healing is predicted with a rate of change of 9 mm Hg/min on switching to 100% oxygen from room air, or with a rise in $TcPO_2$ of at least 10 mm Hg after 10 minutes of 100% oxygen inhalation compared with room air values.[37, 66]

Infrared thermography, intravenous fluorescein dye, and laser Doppler are less commonly utilized vascular studies. Infrared thermography is less valuable because much of the heat derives from deeper structures,[113] but it is a good indicator of skin flap viability.[65] Fluorescein dye can be injected intravenously to provide quantitative fluorometry criteria for skin flap viability,[68, 96] but this is rarely used because interpretation is difficult. Laser Doppler studies also provide some information about the microcirculation in a noninvasive mode.[40]

Preoperative noninvasive vascular studies are crucial in preserving limb length, so that the level selected is at the edge of tissue viability. If limb infection is present, then the limb blood flow should be evaluated to assess whether healing will occur.

Proper surgical technique requires suturing of cut muscles to each other and to the periosteum at the end of the cut bone (myoplasty) or to the bone itself (myodesis). In the most functional residual limbs, the muscles and their fascia are sutured directly to the bone through drill holes. In myoplasty, the muscles are joined to each other with minimal tension, which takes less operating time. The surgeon should taper the muscle mass to reduce distal bulk.

Residual Limb Management

A postoperative plaster of paris or fiberglass rigid dressing prevents edema, protects from trauma, and decreases postoperative pain. Postoperative edema occurs within a few minutes, so immediate replacement of the dressing is necessary. Once they are removed for inspection or suture removal, rigid dressings must be replaced within minutes to prevent recurrence of edema.

The removable rigid dressing (RRD) for the transtibial amputee consists of a plaster of paris or fiberglass cast suspended by a stockinet and supracondylar cuff, and is adjusted by adding or removing socks to maintain compression.[115, 116] The RRD provides good edema control with the advantage of allowing daily inspection.

When a rigid dressing is not being used, one can wrap cotton-elastic bandages around the residual limb if the patient is physically and mentally able to learn the wrapping technique (Figs. 14–2 and 14–3). Elastic bandages

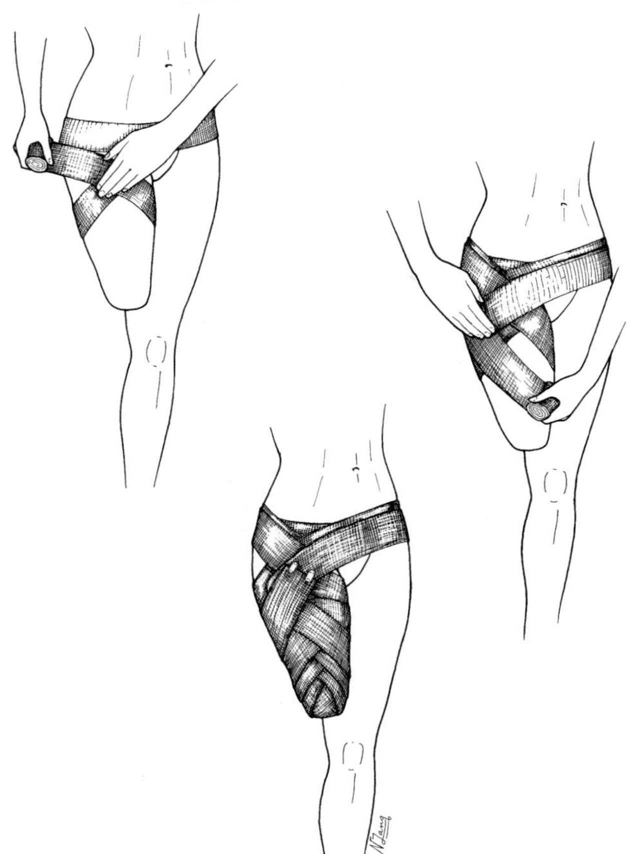

FIGURE 14–3. Wrapping a transfemoral residual limb with elastic bandage in a figure-of-8 pattern to reduce edema. (Courtesy of the University of Texas Health Science Center at San Antonio.)

are typically the least effective shrinkage device, because many patients fail to master the wrapping technique, which requires reapplication many times a day. Poorly applied elastic bandages also can cause circumferential constriction with distal edema. Double-length 4-inch bandages should be used for the transtibial limb, and double-length 6-inch bandages for the transfemoral limb.

Elastic shrinker socks are easy to apply and provide uniform compression, but are more expensive than elastic bandages (Fig. 14–4). They should fit snugly, and should reach the groin in the transfemoral amputee. They can also cause skin damage with constriction if not properly fitted and maintained.

The amputee should wear a shrinkage device 24 hours/day except for bathing or for ventilating an open sore for short periods during the day. A shrinkage device for the non-prosthesis candidate helps control pain and edema and facilitates healing. The shrinkage device can be discontinued after fitting the definitive prosthesis if the amputee wears the prosthesis regularly. The shrinkage device can be used overnight if edema is an ongoing problem.

A contracture is easy to prevent but difficult to correct. The amputee should not lie on an overly soft mattress or use a pillow under the back or thigh; nor should the head of the bed be elevated. Patients should also avoid standing with a transfemoral residual limb resting on a crutch. All of these practices lead to hip flexion contractures. The amputee should not place a pillow between the legs because this creates a hip abduction contracture. A transtibial amputee should not lie with the residual limb hanging over the edge of the bed, with a pillow placed under the knee, or with the knees flexed, and must not sit in a wheelchair with the knee flexed, because these positions lead to knee flexion contractures. The transtibial amputee should sit with the knee extended on a board under the wheelchair cushion, with a towel wrapped over the board. Crutch walking with or without a prosthesis promotes good range of motion and, when feasible, is preferred over wheelchair mobility. Amputees should lie prone for 15 minutes three times a day to help prevent hip flexion contractures. The amputee who cannot lie prone should lie supine and actively extend the residual limb while flexing the contralateral hip (this is essentially a Thomas test maneuver).

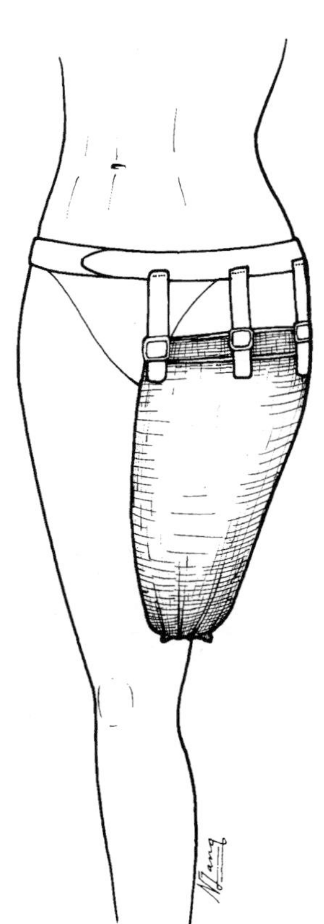

FIGURE 14–4. Elastic shrinker for the transfemoral residual limb. (Courtesy of the University of Texas Health Science Center at San Antonio.)

After suture removal, the residual limb should be cleansed daily with bland soap and tepid water (an antiseptic cleanser can be used if needed). The limb should be patted completely dry before application of any shrinkage device. Gentle massage decreases sensitivity to pressure, and deep friction massage perpendicular to the scar helps prevent scar adhesions. Be sure that the residual limb scar has mobility in all directions, because adherent scars can cause pain. One can use a thin layer of emollient to decrease the friction from massage, but should avoid the use of thick creams. For very dry skin, a thin emollient can be applied in the evening for absorption overnight. Shaving of the residual limb should be discouraged.

Preprosthetic Training

Preprosthetic training includes active range-of-motion exercises, positioning, muscle strengthening, skin care, wheelchair mobility, transfers, ambulation with assistive devices, self-care, and patient and family education. Goals should be realistic and individualized to challenge each amputee to his or her maximum potential based on functional considerations of age and health.

Immediate Postoperative and Early Prosthetic Training

In 1963, Weiss reported success in fitting amputees with prostheses immediately after surgery and beginning ambulation training the next day.[112, 117] The immediate postoperative weight bearing required by this technique has lost popularity owing to concerns over wound healing, but it is still common practice for pediatric and clean post-traumatic amputees. The usual technique is to apply a rigid plaster of paris or fiberglass dressing postoperatively to prevent edema and promote healing. A pylon and foot are attached to the rigid dressing for immediate postoperative weight bearing. It should be noted that patients should never be fully weight bearing on this type of socket. At 10 to 14 days after surgery, a preparatory prosthesis is provided if the wound has closed. If the wound has not closed, a new rigid dressing should be applied for 10 additional days. Others recommend waiting at least 21 days postoperatively before fitting or using a temporary prosthesis.

The amputee must learn to adjust the number of plies of prosthetic socks, to use a nylon sheath against the skin to prevent friction, and to don and doff the prosthesis and inserts. The amputee dons the nylon sheath before the prosthetic socks. The socks should not have wrinkles, and seams should not lie over bony areas or scars. The amputee should wash socks and sheaths daily, wipe the socket and insert daily with a damp cloth, and air non-gel inserts overnight. Gel inserts left out of the socket overnight can deform from their preferred shape.

Gait Training

Training for an efficient, cosmetically acceptable gait begins with the parallel bars and includes training in sit-to-stand transfers, balance, knee control, lateral weight shifting, and forward progression. Balancing techniques are taught first, with progression to limited weight bearing. The amputee should use open hands to avoid pulling up on the bars.

Advanced gait training progresses through gait aids (e.g., walker, crutches, canes) to ramps, curbs, stairs, clearing obstacles, and, if indicated, falling safety and floor-to-standing transfers. In stair climbing and ramp walking, the amputee ascends by leading with the sound foot and descends by leading with the prosthesis. ("Up with the good, down with the bad.") If skin pressure problems occur, the prosthesis wearing time should be temporarily decreased and the problem identified and corrected if skin pressure problems occur. Patients fitted immediately postoperatively should ideally wear the prosthesis at least 3 hours/day before discharge.

THE PROSTHESIS

All limb prostheses consist of a suspension device, a socket, rigid components, and a terminal device (foot). Some also include artificial joints. Most amputees require a prosthetic sheath and socks over the residual limb. The prosthesis-patient interface is the *fit,* and the geometry of the components is the *alignment.*

Preparatory/Temporary Prosthesis

Even when a patient's potential success at using a prosthesis is uncertain, a preparatory prosthesis should be provided as a trial. The preparatory or temporary prosthesis is usually uncosmetic, but is used during the period of residual limb shrinkage. The amputee uses the preparatory prosthesis until maximal shrinkage has been attained, usually 3 to 6 months post-surgery. Outpatient followup is best done with a prosthetic clinic team, including a physician, prosthetist, therapist, and social worker. When the ply of socks reaches 10 to 15 because of residual limb shrinkage, the amputee should be given a new socket—this many plies of difference in the size of the residual limb and the socket tends to result in pistoning.

Definitive/Permanent Prosthesis

The definitive or permanent prosthesis is cosmetically finished. Its fit, alignment, and components are chosen based on the amputee's experience with the preparatory prosthesis. A test or check socket is usually made to test fit just prior to fabricating the definitive socket. If the definitive prosthesis is fitted too early, the limb continues to shrink and the prosthetic socket becomes too large, necessitating replacement. Weight loss or gain of 5 lb can alter the fit. Diuretics, hemodialysis, chemotherapy, and alcohol consumption can also cause fluctuations in residual limb size. The definitive prosthesis typically requires replacement about every 3 years.[61]

PARTIAL FOOT AMPUTATIONS

Surgical Procedures

The most common types of foot amputation are (1) transmetatarsal, (2) Lisfranc, and (3) Chopart (Fig. 14–5). In transmetatarsal amputation, the surgeon sections the metatarsals transversely, usually just proximal to the metatarsal heads, and bevels them inferiorly.

The Lisfranc amputation is a tarsometatarsal disarticulation. The Chopart amputation is a disarticulation at the midtarsal joint through the talonavicular and calcaneocuboid joints (see Fig. 14–5). In both of these procedures, the remaining foot often develops a significant equinovarus deformity resulting in excessive anterior weight bearing with breakdown. Adequate extensor tendon implantation with Achilles tendon lengthening has been advocated to prevent this deformity. Such patients frequently require a postoperative rigid dressing for several weeks to try to prevent the equinus deformity.

The Boyd amputation consists of excision of all tarsals except the calcaneus. The Boyd amputation is rarely performed in the adult due to residual limb length problems, but is more commonly performed in the pediatric congenital amputee.

Prosthetic and Orthotic Prescription

For patients with toe amputation, wool, sponge rubber, or foam should be inserted in the shoe to serve as a

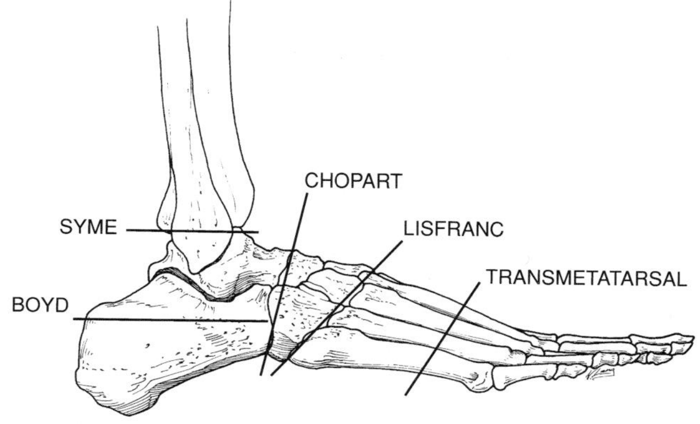

FIGURE 14–5. Syme and partial foot amputations: Boyd, Chopart, Lisfranc, and transmetatarsal. (Courtesy of the University of Texas Health Science Center at San Antonio.)

spacer and to prevent toe deformity. For an amputated great toe, a long steel spring shank, a metatarsal pad, and a rocker sole improve function. The transmetatarsal amputation requires a custom-molded insole and toe filler. The stiff insole should prevent shoe hyperextension proximal to the natural toe break. A thin, lightweight carbon fiber shank can be incorporated directly in the insert. The slipper-type prosthesis contains flexible and semi-flexible materials, and provides a plantar lever arm and cosmesis.

For the Lisfranc or Chopart amputee, a modified shoe or molded plastic socket, or a combination of the two, should be provided. Modern slipper-type prostheses terminate at the ankle joint, whereas the older devices, such as the prosthetic boot and ankle-foot orthosis (AFO), can extend up the ankle and inhibit subtalar and tibiotalar motion. The ground reaction force AFO with anterior and posterior plastic shells gives maximal control with minimal ankle motion and some limited proximal weight bearing, and is indicated for the muscularly imbalanced, active, or pressure-sensitive amputee.[2]

The Boyd amputation is fitted as a Syme amputation (see below), but it requires a contralateral shoe lift in adults because of leg length discrepancy.

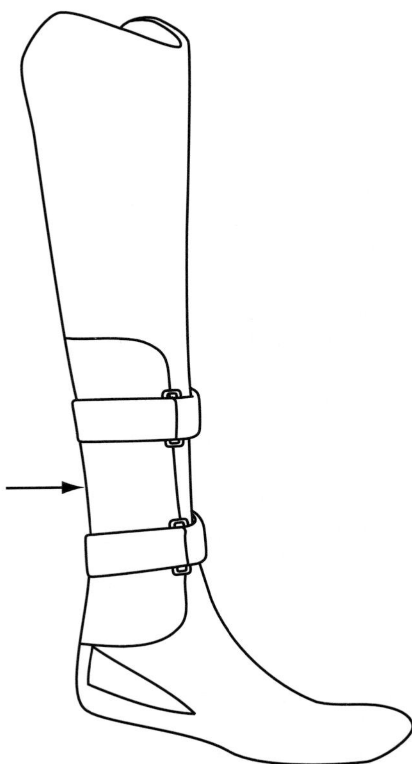

FIGURE 14–6. Syme-type prosthesis with medial opening socket. (From Cestaro JM: The Illustrated Guide to Orthotics and Prosthetics. Alexandria, VA, National Office of Orthotics and Prosthetics, 1992, p 234.)

SYME AMPUTATION

Surgical Procedures

Syme amputation is an ankle disarticulation for destructive and infective lesions of the foot that cannot be treated with a transmetatarsal amputation. The original Syme procedure is the best for this level. The main advantage is that if successful, the patient can walk on the Syme residual limb without a prosthesis, at least for short distances. One difficulty with Syme amputation is that the heel pad can migrate posteriorly or mediolaterally if it is not adequately anchored to the cut end of the tibia. Syme amputation prostheses are uncosmetic, because of the inability to match the shape of the contralateral leg. This amputation level compromises cosmesis in favor of function, and might not be cosmetically suitable for some persons.

Prosthetic Prescription

The Syme prosthesis usually has a removable medial window that allows the patient to push the residual limb into the socket (Fig. 14–6). The window, when replaced, provides suspension over the malleoli. The prosthesis gives excellent function. The prosthetic heel should be soft to accommodate lack of ankle motion. Feet for the Syme amputee include all of the SACH-type [solid ankle cushion heel] feet as well as some energy-storing feet; they are similar to the feet of the same name described under Transtibial Amputation (see below), but have a lower profile.

Gait speed is typically decreased 32% and oxygen consumption increased 13% per distance walked in the vascular Syme amputee with a prosthesis, compared with normal subjects without vascular disease.[108]

TRANSTIBIAL (BELOW-KNEE) AMPUTATION

Surgical Procedures

Transtibial amputation is usually performed at the junction of the upper and middle third of the tibia (Fig. 14–7). Some advocate a longer residual limb to provide a longer lever arm and more efficient gait, but this is harder to fit. A long posterior flap meets a shorter anterior flap to allow the gastrocnemius-soleus muscles to form the distal soft tissue.

Nearly full use of the knee allows the transtibial amputee to have a more efficient gait. In debilitated elderly persons with no walking or transfer potential, knee disarticulation is preferable to transtibial amputation to prevent knee flexion contracture and distal residual limb breakdown.[73] Unlike Syme amputation, the end of the transtibial residual limb cannot bear total body weight. Transtibial residual limbs as short as 2.5 inches can be successfully fitted with a prosthesis. Ertl recommended a distal tibiofibular synostosis to prevent fibular hypermobility and to improve weight bearing in the traumatic amputee.[19]

Prosthetic Prescription

Foot-Ankle Assemblies

Prosthetic feet are classified into five types: (1) the SACH foot, (2) the single-axis foot, (3) the multi-axis

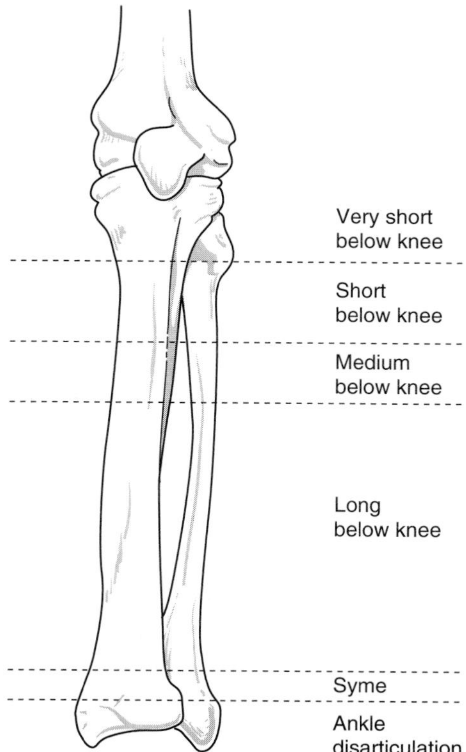

FIGURE 14–7. Categories of transtibial residual limb based on length. (From Epps CH: Surgery of the Musculoskeletal System, ed 2. New York, Churchill Livingstone, 1990, p 5124.)

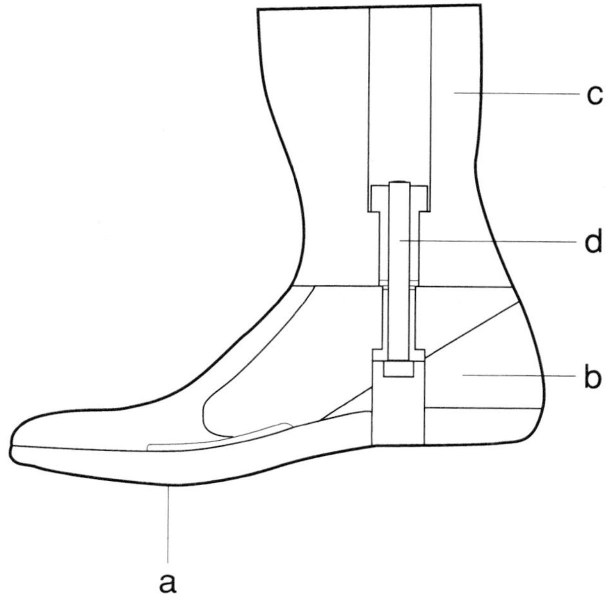

FIGURE 14–8. SACH (*s*olid *a*nkle *c*ushion *h*eel) foot. The plastic cover (*a*) is over a wooden core. The heel wedge (*b*) is elastic. The foot is attached to the wooden ankle block (*c*) by a bolt (*d*). (Courtesy of Otto Bock Orthopadische Industrie GmbH and Co.)

foot, (4) the solid ankle flexible keel foot, and (5) the energy-storing foot.[72] SACH is an acronym for solid ankle cushion heel. The SACH foot has a cushioned heel that compresses during heel-strike, simulating plantar flexion, and has a rigid anterior keel to roll over during late stance (Fig. 14–8). It is light, durable, inexpensive, and is most often prescribed for juvenile and geriatric amputees.

The single-axis foot has a single mechanical axis for plantar flexion and dorsiflexion motion limited by anterior and posterior bumpers, allowing quicker foot flat, which results in a more stable knee (Fig. 14–9). The single-axis foot is heavier and less durable than the SACH foot. The single-axis foot has some biomechanical advantages in gait over the SACH. It is most often used in transfemoral prostheses, but seldom in transtibial prostheses.

Multi-axis feet, such as the Greissinger, Endolite Multiflex, and stationary attachment flexible endoskeleton (SAFE) II, allow dorsiflexion, plantar flexion, inversion, eversion, and transverse rotation (Fig. 14–10). Multi-axis feet are good for walking on uneven ground or for an excessively scarred and sensitive residual limb, because of better shock absorption. They are heavier, less durable, and more costly than SACH feet.

Feet such as the Kingsley stored-energy (STEN) and Otto Bock 1D10 Dynamic foot are similar to the SACH foot but have a flexible anterior keel (Fig. 14–11). Solid ankle flexible keel feet are lighter than multi-axis feet, and provide limited inversion, eversion, and transverse rotation. They offer shock absorption in late stance and benefit the moderately active or obese amputee.

Energy-storing feet (dynamic response feet) store and release energy as the limb is weighted and unweighted,

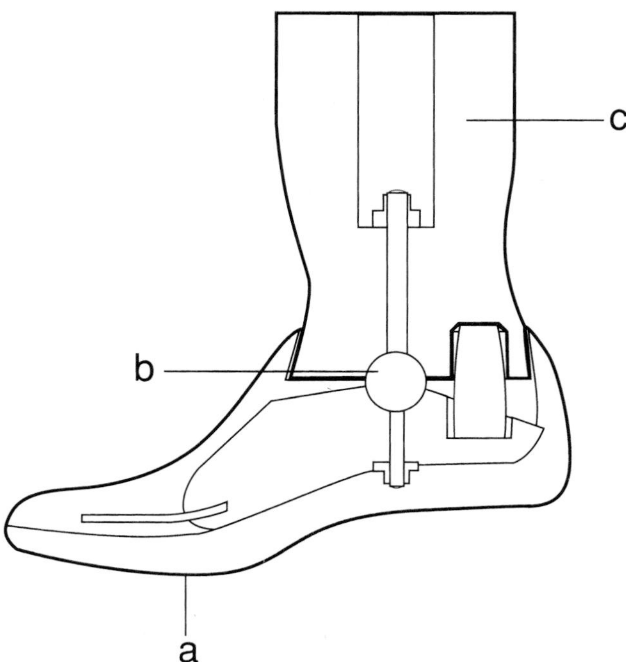

FIGURE 14–9. Single-axis foot allowing plantar and dorsiflexion. The foam cover (*a*) is over a wooden core. The single-axis joint (*b*) connects the foot to the ankle block (*c*). A rubber bumper limits plantar flexion, and a rigid stop limits dorsiflexion. (Courtesy of Otto Bock Orthopadische Industrie GmbH and Co.)

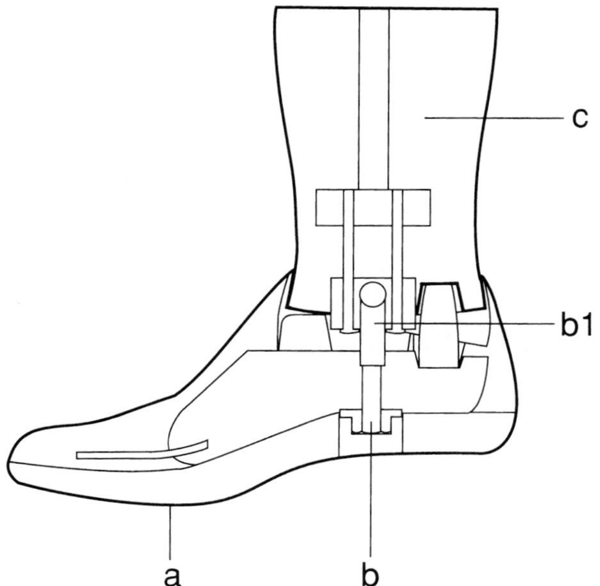

FIGURE 14–10. Multi-axis Greissinger foot. The foam cover (*a*) is over a wooden core. The Greissinger foot joint (*b*) connects the foot to the ankle block (*c*). Movement in all directions is permitted by the U-joint (*b1*). Rubber bumpers limit plantar flexion and dorsiflexion. (Courtesy of Otto Bock Orthopadische Industrie GmbH and Co.)

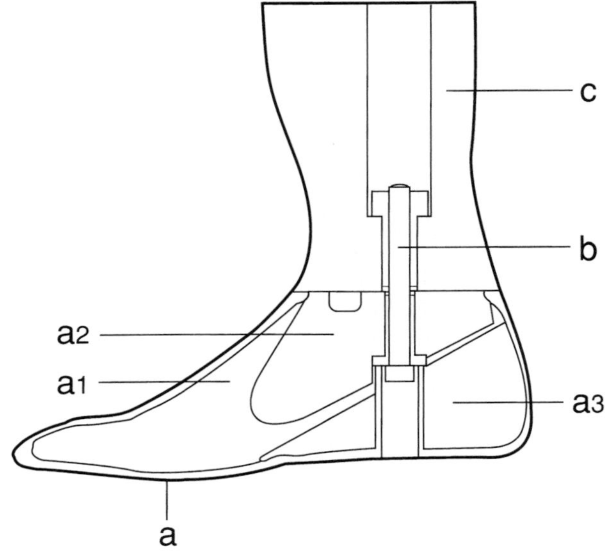

FIGURE 14–11. The Otto Bock 1D10 Dynamic foot is an example of a foot with a flexible keel. The foot (*a*) consists of a plastic inner foot (*a1*) with a wooden core (*a2*), and is coated by an exterior plastic material. The heel wedge (*a3*) is elastic. The foot is attached to the ankle block by a steel and titanium bolt (*b*). (Courtesy of Otto Bock Orthopadische Industrie GmbH and Co.)

giving a "springy" feeling (Fig. 14–12).[114] Examples include the Seattle foot, Seattle Light, Carbon Copy II, Carbon Copy II Light, Carbon Copy III, Quantum Foot, Flex Walk, Flex Foot (Fig. 14–13), and Springlite. Energy-storing feet result in a higher self-selected walking speed and are indicated for the more active amputee. They can be slightly more energy-efficient than SACH feet at normal speeds, with increased relative efficiency at higher speeds, although not all studies concur in this regard.[13, 75]

Shanks: Exoskeletal ("Crustacean") versus Endoskeletal (Modular)

The two basic designs for the shank are (1) the exoskeletal ("crustacean") and (2) the endoskeletal (modular). The exoskeletal "crustacean" system has a hard outer plastic shell. It is very durable, but does not allow alignment changes in the finished prosthesis. The endoskeletal system has a pylon covered by contoured, soft foam. The endoskeletal system is generally lighter and more cosmetic, and can be more easily accessed for adjustment and component change-out.

Socket Construction

"Patellar Tendon-Bearing Socket" Total Surface Weight-Bearing Socket

The conventional total-contact "patellar tendon-bearing" (PTB) socket is characterized by a bar in the anterior wall designed to apply pressure to the patellar tendon. The trimline extends anteriorly to the midpa-

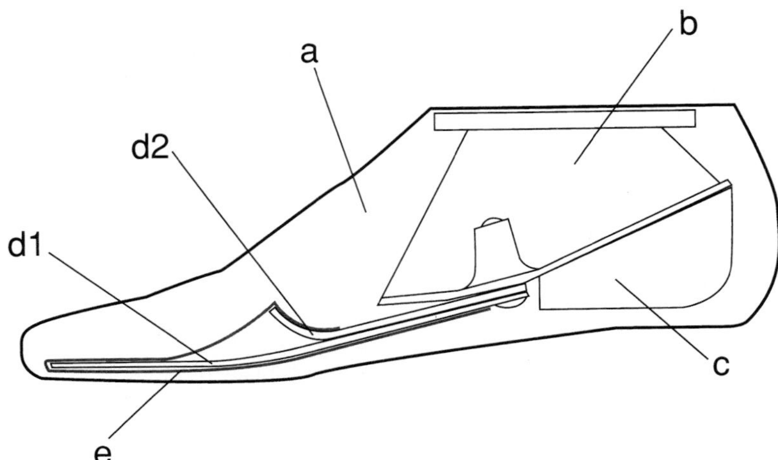

FIGURE 14–12. The Carbon Copy II is an example of an energy-storing foot. The flexible foam urethane foot (*a*) is over a rigid composite keel (*b*). The heel wedge (*c*) is elastic. Primary (*d1*) and secondary (*d2*) deflection plates store and release energy as the forefoot is weighted and unweighted. A Kevlar sock (*e*) prevents the plates from punching through the urethane. (Courtesy of Ohio Willow Wood Co.)

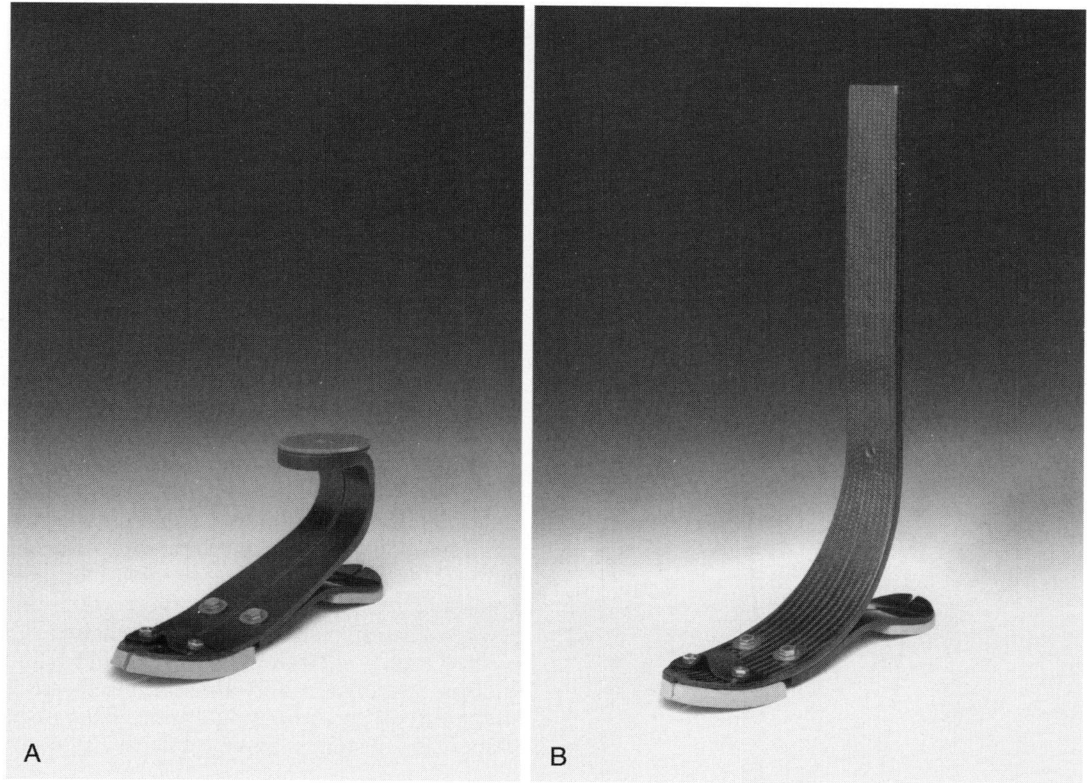

FIGURE 14–13. Flex-Walk II (*A*) and Flex-Foot Modular III (*B*) energy-storing feet store and release energy by way of graphite composite springs. There is also a cosmetic foam cover. (Courtesy of Flex-Foot, Inc.)

tella level, can extend mediolaterally to the femoral condyles, and extends posteriorly to below the level of the PTB bar. Pressure-sensitive areas include the tibial crest, tubercle and condyles, the fibular head, the distal tibia and fibula, and the hamstring tendons. Pressure-tolerant areas include the patellar tendon, the pretibial muscles, the gastrocnemius-soleus muscles, the popliteal fossa, the lateral flat aspect of the fibula, and the medial tibial flare (Fig. 14–14). Despite the name *patellar tendon-bearing,* pressure should be equally distributed over the pressure-tolerant areas and relieved over the pressure-sensitive areas. The PTB socket is a total-contact socket, because the distal part of the residual limb is in contact with the socket with minimal end-weight bearing.

Bent Knee or Kneeling Prosthesis and Bypass Prosthesis

The bypass prosthesis receives all pressure from the thigh, ischium, and gluteus, and bypasses the tibia. If the bypass is due to severe knee flexion contracture, it

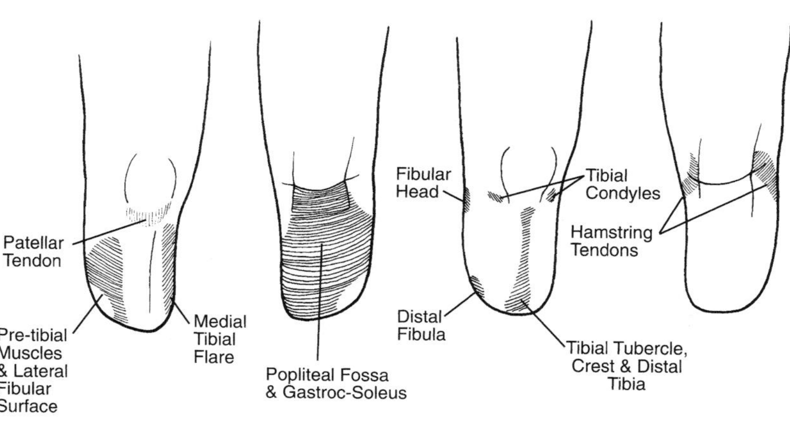

FIGURE 14–14. Pressure-tolerant and pressure-sensitive areas of the PTB socket. (Courtesy of the University of Texas Health Science Center at San Antonio.)

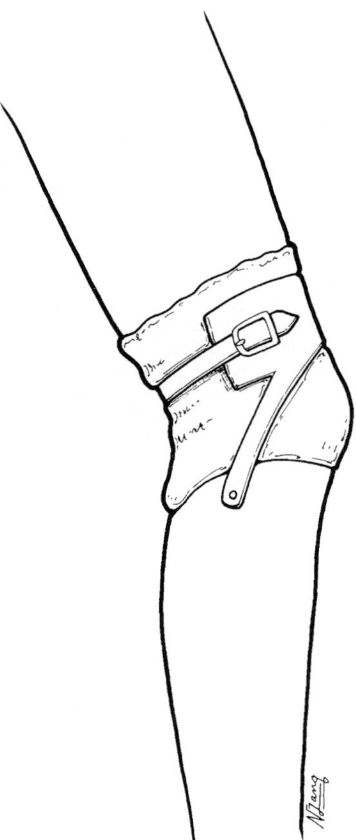

FIGURE 14–15. Supracondylar cuff for the transtibial amputee. (Courtesy of the University of Texas Health Science Center at San Antonio.)

is called a *bent knee* or *kneeling prosthesis.* Protruding external knee hinges are necessary. The biomechanics are the same as for the transfemoral prosthesis, with poorer cosmesis.

Soft and Hard Sockets

A plastic socket without an insert is a *hard socket,* and when fitted with an insert it is a *soft socket.* An insert provides extra protection for the residual limb, but reduces the intimate contact between limb and prosthesis. It is often fabricated from polyethylene foam, although a silicone gel insert protects the sensitive residual limb better. Inserts should be prescribed when peripheral vascular disease, extensive scarring, or reduced subcutaneous tissue is present. Inserts are almost always prescribed for transtibial prostheses.

Flexible Socket

Flexible sockets provide a softer, thermoplastic material for weight transmission. The flexible socket sits in a rigid frame and is described in greater detail in the section below on transfemoral amputation. Note that the term *flexible* refers to the socket material and not to the socket shape.

Suspension

Flexible Attachment

The supracondylar cuff is a simple cuff or strap fitted just above the femoral condyles to suspend the prosthesis during swing phase (Fig. 14–15). It can have a Velcro or buckle closure. A waist belt and elastic strap can be added for extra security.

Neoprene or rubber suspension sleeves provide excellent suspension, fitting snugly over the proximal prosthesis and several inches up on the thigh (Fig. 14–16). Sleeves should not be used for very short residual limbs or for amputees who need added knee stability with proximal trim lines. Perspiration and hygiene problems can occur, especially in hot, humid climates, and kneeling shortens the life of the sleeve.

The silicone suction suspension system (3S, ICEROSS, ALPS) is a thin-walled, highly compliant, closed-end insert or liner of silicone (Fig. 14–17).[28] The amputee rolls the silicone liner onto the bare residual limb, then attaches it to the socket by a shuttle lock system. The amputee pushes the residual limb into the prosthesis until a click (or clicks) is heard. The amputee pushes a button to doff the socket. The liner provides friction suspension and absorbs moderate impact and shear forces on the residual limb. The silicone suction suspension system is more expensive than most suspen-

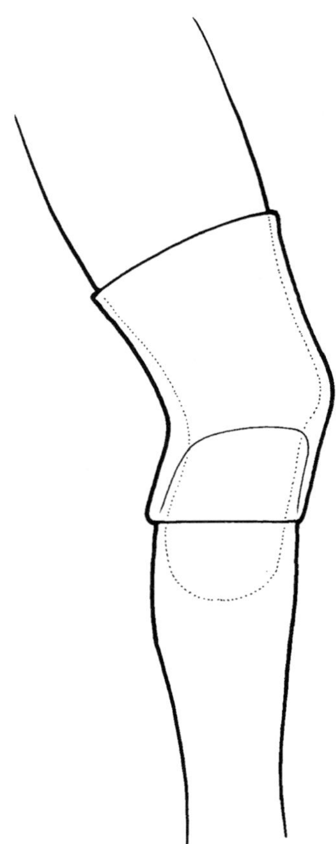

FIGURE 14–16. Elastic sleeve suspension for the transtibial amputee. (Courtesy of the University of Texas Health Science Center at San Antonio.)

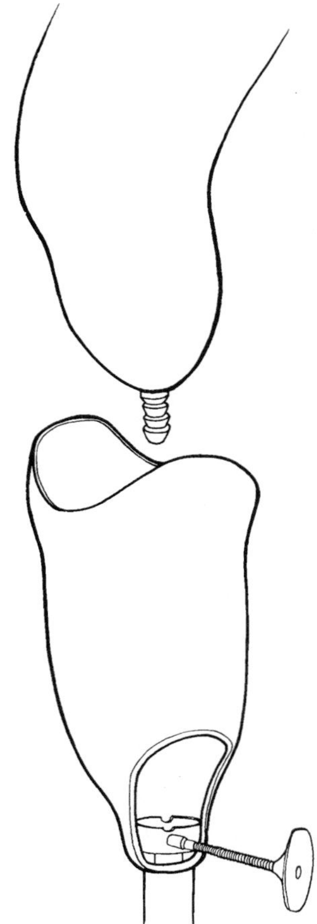

FIGURE 14–17. The 3S is an example of a silicone suction suspension system for the transtibial amputee. It attaches to the socket by a shuttle lock system. Silicone suction suspension systems are also available for the transfemoral amputee. (Courtesy of Durr-Fillauer Orthopedic Inc.)

sion systems, but it provides excellent suspension for the athlete and excellent skin protection for the scarred residual limb.

Suction suspension is very difficult to achieve in the transtibial amputee due to the presence of many bony channels, but has been achieved by using a flexible socket.

Brim Contour

Supracondylar. The patellar tendon-bearing socket with supracondylar wedge (PTB-SC) extends its mediolateral trimlines above the femoral condyles for suspension (Fig. 14–18). A wedge is either built into the liner or is completely separate, and is positioned above and over the medial femoral condyle. The PTB-SC provides extra mediolateral support and is helpful for short residual limbs and in overweight amputees.

Supracondylar/Suprapatellar. The patellar tendon-bearing socket with supracondylar/suprapatellar trimline (PTB-SC/SP) is a PTB-SC socket with suprapatellar trimlines (see Fig. 14–18). The alternative name, from France, is *prothèse tibiale supracondylien* (PTS). The suprapatellar trimline helps suspend the prosthesis and increases socket wall support of the expected stance phase varus moment; it is helpful for short residual limbs and for controlling genu recurvatum.

Thigh Corset

The patellar tendon-bearing socket with joints and corset (PTB w/J&C) adds a femoral corset to decrease residual limb weight bearing by 40% to 60%. It gives less knee control and worsens gait and is therefore the socket suspension of last resort (see Fig. 14–18). It provides control of significantly lax collateral knee ligaments and protects the knee from varus stresses during stance. It also provides additional mediolateral support for the patient with a short residual limb. The PTB w/J&C relieves weight on a residual limb with poor pressure tolerance, and it is often used for amputees involved in heavy manual labor.

Transtibial Prosthetic Care

The amputee should be taught to adjust the prosthetic socks so that the patellar tendon bar is over the midpoint of the patellar tendon. The insert should be donned before the prosthesis is donned. Inserting a clay ball the size of a pea, wrapped in plastic, at the bottom of the socket during weight bearing is a way to test fit. If the ball is partly but not totally flattened, then distal contact is adequate.

Gait Deviations: Static and Dynamic Analysis

Fit and Alignment

The weight-bearing surface is increased by aligning the PTB socket to hold the knee in 5 to 10 degrees of flexion. During mid-stance there should be a slight varus moment at the knee, pushing the knee laterally. The socket applies a counterposing force to the medial femoral condyle and the lateral fibular shaft. The foot is set medial to the socket center. Moving the foot medially

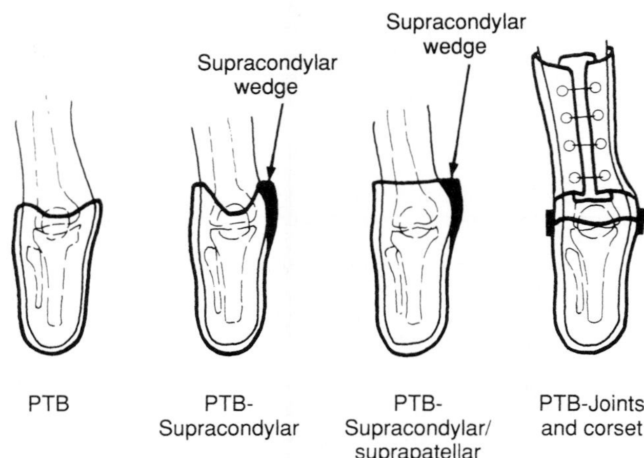

FIGURE 14–18. Examples of the variations of the PTB socket design. (From Karacoloff LA, Hammersley CS, Schneider FJ: Lower Extremity Amputation. Gaithersburg, MD, Aspen Publishers, 1986, p 27.)

increases the varus moment. Moving the foot laterally decreases the moment but can create a valgus moment, resulting in pressure over sensitive areas. Sagittal plane forces within the socket progress from anteroproximal and posterodistal in early stance, to anterodistal and posteroproximal in late stance.

Pistoning should be checked by marking the posterior brim of the socket against the sock while the amputee is standing. Pistoning of more than one-fourth of an inch indicates inadequate suspension or loose socket. If suspension is by elastic sleeve, then a portion of the proximal sleeve should be in direct contact with the amputee's skin.

Gait Analysis

Table 14–1 lists gait problems, causes, and solutions in the transtibial amputee.

Energy Expenditure

The average measured gait velocity of the vascular transtibial amputee is decreased 44%, with oxygen consumption increased 33% per distance walked. The gait velocity of the traumatic transtibial amputee is decreased only 11%, with oxygen consumption increased 7% per distance walked, as compared with normal subjects without vascular disease.[108] Longer residual limbs have lower oxygen requirements than short residual limbs, ranging from 10% to 40% increased oxygen requirement per distance walked.[30]

KNEE DISARTICULATION (THROUGH-KNEE AMPUTATION)

Surgical Procedures

Knee disarticulation is removal of the tibia and fibula at the knee. As in the Syme procedure, knee disarticulation provides the capacity for partial end-weight bearing.

Prosthetic Prescription

The socket is usually a modified quadrilateral socket with some ischial weight bearing, and a soft socket liner with supracondylar buildups to provide suspension. Proximal socket trimlines prevent socket rotation on the limb, though ischial weight bearing is not an absolute requirement, if the femoral condyles provide suspension. The problem in prosthetic fitting of a knee disarticulation is that the prosthetic knee's center of rotation needs to go through the distal residual limb. Fitting a knee unit distal to the residual limb has caused problems in the past, but the four-bar polycentric knee has helped to solve the problem (Fig. 14–19). The polycentric knee, unlike the single-axis knee, has an instantaneous center of rotation that changes, and is proximal and posterior

TABLE 14–1 Gait Analysis of the Transtibial Amputee

Problem	Cause	Solution
Delayed, abrupt, and limited knee flexion after heel-strike	Heel wedge is too soft; foot is too far anterior	Stiffen heel wedge; move foot posterior
Extended knee throughout stance phase	Too much plantar flexion	Dorsiflex foot
Toe stays off floor after heel-strike	Heel wedge too stiff; foot too anterior, too much dorsiflexion	Soften heel wedge; move foot posterior; plantar flex foot
"Hill-climbing" sensation toward end of stance phase	Foot too anterior, too much plantar flexion	Move foot posterior, dorsiflex foot
High pressure against patella throughout most of stance phase; heel is off floor when patient stands	Foot too plantar flexed	Dorsiflex foot
Knee too forcefully and rapidly flexed after heel strike; high pressure against anterodistal tibia at heel-strike and/or prolonged discomfort at this point	Heel wedge too stiff; foot too far posterior; foot too dorsiflexed	Soften heel; move foot anterior; plantar flex foot
Hips level, but prosthesis seems short	Foot too far posterior, foot too dorsiflexed	Move foot anterior; plantar flex foot
Drop-off at end of stance phase	Foot too far posterior	Move foot anterior
Toe off of floor as patient stands or knee flexed too much	Foot too dorsiflexed	Plantar flex foot
Valgus moment at knee (knockkneed) during stance phase; excessive pressure on distomedial limb and proximolateral surface of knee	Foot too outset	Inset foot
Excessive varus moment at knee (bowlegged) during stance phase (a varus moment at the knee should occur in stance phase but should never be excessive); the distolateral residual limb is painful	Mediolateral dimension of socket too large; foot too inset	Fit of socket should be checked; outset foot

Courtesy of Northwestern University Prosthetic-Orthotic Center, Chicago.

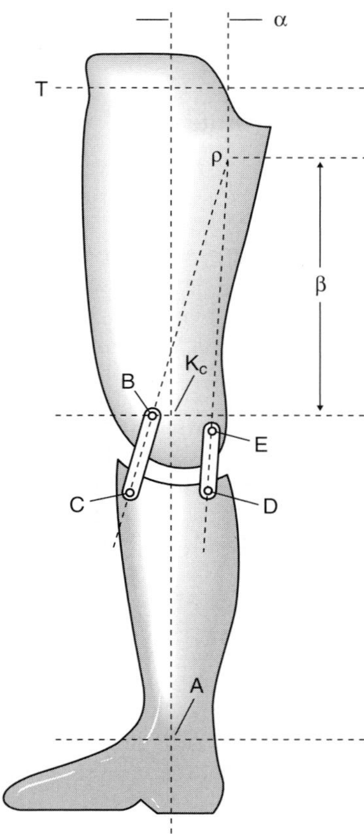

FIGURE 14–19. Four-bar polycentric knee with superiorly and posteriorly displaced instantaneous center of rotation. (From Greene MP: Four bar linkage knee analysis. Orthot Prosthet 1983; 37:17.)

to the knee unit itself. This allows greater knee stability, a more symmetrical gait, and equal knee length when sitting. Fluid control can be added for the active amputee.

Waters and colleagues found the average measured gait velocity for the traumatic through-knee amputee to be decreased 24%, with oxygen consumption increased 53% per distance walked, compared with normal subjects without vascular disease.[108]

TRANSCONDYLAR/SUPRACONDYLAR AMPUTATION

Surgical Procedures and Prosthetic Prescription

The Gritti-Stokes procedure provides partial but not total end-weight bearing, and eliminates the bulbous prosthetic profile seen in knee disarticulation. The amputation is done through the femoral condyles, and the patella is attached directly over the cut end of the femur. Gritti-Stokes amputation is a very difficult procedure and is now seldom used.[87]

In the transcondylar and supracondylar amputation, a conventional single-axis knee unit almost fits distal to the residual limb, although the prosthetic thigh is still slightly longer than the normal thigh. Suspension is also more difficult than in knee disarticulation.

TRANSFEMORAL (ABOVE-KNEE) AMPUTATION

Surgical Procedures

Transfemoral amputation is usually performed with equal anterior and posterior length flaps. This amputation does not tolerate total end-weight bearing. The surgeon typically transects the quadriceps just proximal to the patella, transects the adductor magnus from the adductor tubercle, and transects the smaller muscles 1 to 2 inches longer than the bone cut. If severed muscles are not sutured, they retract. An abduction contracture is likely to develop if most of the adductor muscles have been severed and have not been reattached. Flexion-abduction contracture can be minimized by reattaching the adductor magnus to the lateral aspect of the femur.[32]

With myoplasty or myodesis, the hamstrings are able to assist in hip extension and thereby stabilize the prosthetic knee. Myoplasty produces a smoother, more rounded cylindrical residual limb, though best results appear to be with myodesis or bony attachment. Muscle strength is proportional to its cross section and its length, and shortened muscle in a shortened residual limb is weaker (Fig. 14–20).

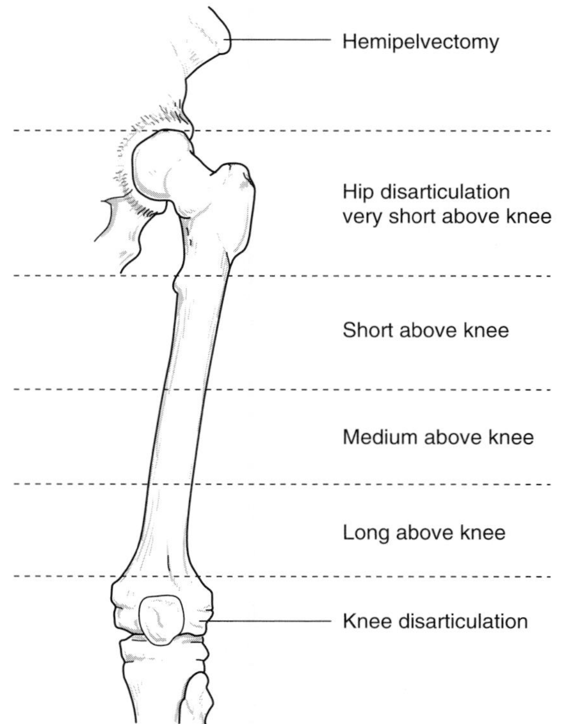

FIGURE 14–20. Categories of transfemoral residual limb based on length. (From Epps CH: Surgery of the Musculoskeletal System, ed 2. New York, Churchill Livingstone, 1990, p 5124.)

Prosthetic Prescription

The residual limb should be at least 8.5 to 13.6 cm in length, measured from the groin, to fit a transfemoral prosthesis; but no absolute measurement is prescriptive, because success is dependent on soft tissue volume.[87]

Foot-Ankle Assemblies

Compared with a transtibial amputee, a transfemoral amputee needs softer plantar flexion to enhance knee stability. The single-axis foot offers more knee stability than the SACH foot, but is also heavier. If a SACH foot is used, a softer heel is necessary. Energy-storing feet should also be considered. An ankle unit torque-absorber can be used to reduce transverse friction forces for the short residual limb.

Shanks

The choice between an endoskeletal (modular) and an exoskeletal (crustacean) shank is similar to that for the transtibial amputee. The hard shell of the exoskeletal system is more durable, whereas the endoskeletal system is lighter, more cosmetic, and allows easier prosthetic adjustment. The endoskeletal shank has gradually gained popularity over the exoskeletal shank. There are now more commercial components available for endoskeletal prostheses. Lightweight or ultralight prostheses are generally prescribed for geriatric amputees.

Knee Units

Knee units are either single-axis or polycentric. They are also either mechanical or fluid-controlled. All knee units, except for the hydraulic stance control units such as the Mauch S-N-S, attempt to keep the knee flexion-extension fixed at one angle (without relative motion) throughout the stance phase.

Mechanical Knee Units

Conventional constant-friction single-axis knees are light, durable, and inexpensive. Single-axis knees rely on alignment for stability, and work best at one speed. Excessive heel rise in early swing phase, as well as terminal swing impact in late swing phase, can occur at faster cadences. These problems can be corrected by manually adjusting the constant friction unit, which can only be set for one optimum cadence. The amputee must prevent knee buckling by activating the hip extensors. The debilitated amputee or amputee with a short residual limb cannot adequately contract the hip extensors, and requires a knee that is set posterior to the trochanter-knee-ankle (TKA) line (Fig. 14–21). This alignment has the disadvantage of causing difficulty in flexion of the knee for swing phase, which causes increased energy expenditure compared to other knee units.

A manual-locking knee provides maximum stability for the debilitated or elderly amputee, but this is accompanied by the worst gait efficiency and increased energy consumption. The knee can be manually unlocked for sitting. This knee is typically reserved for those with weakness and for those who are likely to sustain severe injuries if they fall.

The weight-activated stance control knee (*limited slip* or, formerly, *SAFETY knee*) can provide stable stance for up to 20 degrees of knee flexion by producing friction when weight increases during stance (Fig. 14–22). This knee design is for amputees with weak hip extensors or for geriatric amputees. The stance control is not auto-

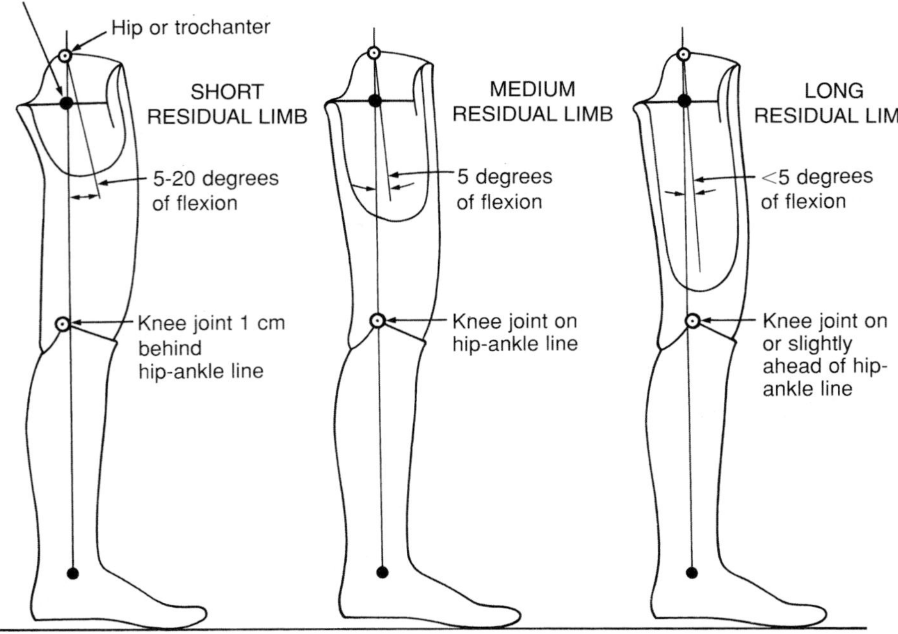

FIGURE 14–21. Trochanter-knee-ankle (TKA) alignment for the short, medium, and long transfemoral residual limb. (From Radcliffe CW: Biomechanics of above-knee prostheses. In Murdoch G (ed): Prosthetic and Orthotic Practice. London, Edward Arnold, 1970, p 191.)

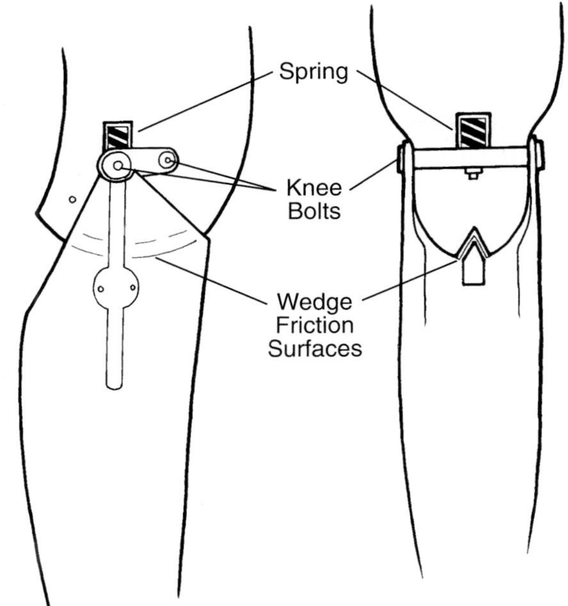

FIGURE 14–22. One type of weight-activated stance control knee (limited slip or, formerly, SAFETY knee).

matic, and the amputee must be able to initiate and maintain control of the knee.

The four-bar polycentric knee, previously mentioned in the section on knee disarticulation (see Fig. 14–22), works well for patients with very long residual limbs as well as for those with poor stability due to short residual limbs, poor balance, or weak hip extensors. Fluid control can be added, and some polycentric knees can be manually locked.

Extension aids are sometimes used with single-axis knees and polycentric knees, and are usually located within the shank. The extension aid is usually a compressible spring with screw adjustments that give constant resistance to knee flexion until flexion reaches 90 degrees, then it assists flexion. Extension aids improve knee stability at the expense of gait efficiency.

Hydraulic- and Pneumatic-Control (Fluid-Control) Knee Units

Both hydraulic and pneumatic control (fluid-control) knee units are cadence-responsive through cadence-dependent resistance. Pneumatic units are air-filled and are lighter in weight, but they cannot support the heavier or more athletic amputee as well as the hydraulic units can. Fluid-control knees are helpful for the active amputee who varies cadence and who can tolerate the extra weight and expense. Most fluid-control knees control the knee velocity during swing phase only, although hydraulic stance control knees (such as the Mauch S-N-S hydraulic knee; Fig. 14–23) give gradually yielding resistance to knee flexion during late stance phase as well. The Endolite pneumatic intelligent prosthesis has a computer-controlled valve that adjusts knee swing phase speed based on cadence. The Hydracadence knee is unique in that it also hydraulically controls ankle dorsiflexion and plantar flexion.

Sockets

An adjustable hinged socket for the temporary prosthesis is an option that allows adjustment for edema reduction. The quadrilateral socket is the usual choice. The choice for socket shape in the definitive prosthesis is between the traditional quadrilateral socket and the newer ischial containment socket. Both the quadrilateral and ischial containment sockets are total-contact sockets with ischiogluteal weight bearing.

Socket Shape

Quadrilateral Socket. The traditional quadrilateral socket has a flat, horizontal posterior shelf on which the ischial tuberosity and gluteal muscles rest. There is an inward bulge over the femoral triangle, and a channel for the rectus femoris. The femoral triangle bulge keeps the ischial tuberosity on the posterior shelf. Medially, there is an anterior channel for the adductor longus tendon. If an "adductor roll" of soft tissue is present over the medial brim, the medial wall needs higher extension or the roll needs to be pulled inside the socket. The quadrilateral socket has a wide mediolateral and a narrow anteroposterior dimension at the proximal socket edge.

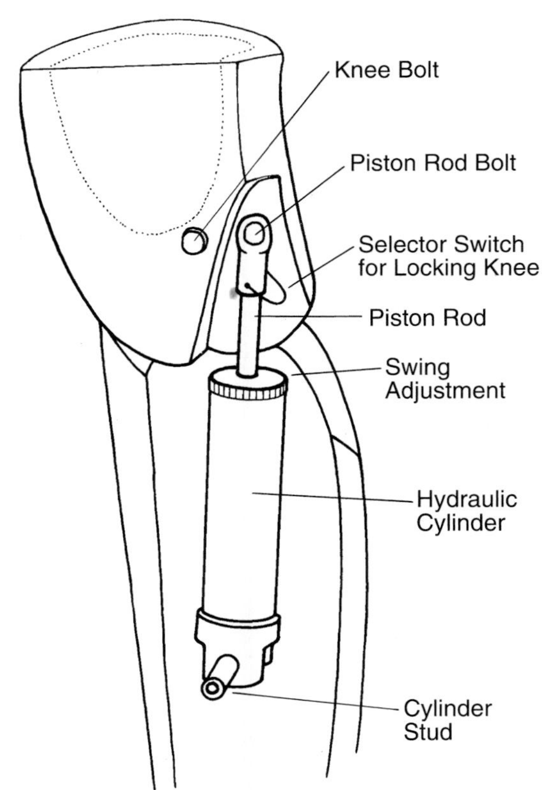

FIGURE 14–23. S-N-S Mauch hydraulic stance and swing-phase control knee unit. (Courtesy of the University of Texas Health Science Center at San Antonio.)

Ischial Containment Socket. The ischial containment socket (Narrow M-L socket) was developed as the normal-shape normal-alignment (NSNA) socket by Long, and as the contoured adducted trochanteric-controlled alignment method (CAT-CAM) by Sabolich (see Fig. 14–24).[59, 60, 86] The posterior wall is 0.75 to 1.25 inches proximal to the ischial level and is contoured to support the ischium and gluteal muscles. Compared with the quadrilateral socket, the ischial containment socket gives mediolateral control, or "bony lock," at the minor expense of increased anteroposterior movement, and has a narrow mediolateral dimension and wide anteroposterior dimension at the level of the ischial ramus. It does not, however, alter femoral adduction angle within the socket as compared to the quadrilateral socket.[29] The ischial containment socket gives more energy-efficient ambulation at high speeds[29] for the active amputee, and is helpful for the short residual limb or weak gluteus medius.

Bypass Prosthesis. For transfemoral amputees with a non-weight bearing lesion in the femur or insufficient pressure tolerance of the residual limb, a complete bypass of weight bearing allows fitting of a hip disarticulation-type prosthesis.

Socket Materials: Laminated versus Flexible

The choice in materials is between the traditional rigid plastic-laminate socket and a flexible thermoplastic socket. The flexible socket originated with the ISNY (Icelandic-Swedish-New York) transfemoral socket consisting of two separate structures: a thin, pliable, vacuum-formed thermoplastic socket to interface with tissues, and a rigid, outer supporting frame for weight transmission (Fig. 14–25).[46, 52] The soft, flexible socket is often translucent or transparent and is more comfortable. It gives better total contact, enables one to better sense external objects through the socket, and feels cooler, with better heat dissipation. Flexible sockets can be more rapidly fabricated and modified, but they are also more expensive. They are especially beneficial for the patient with scarring of the residual limb; and because of better adherence, they provide better suction suspension. The frames usually do not permit a hip joint and pelvic band to be attached.

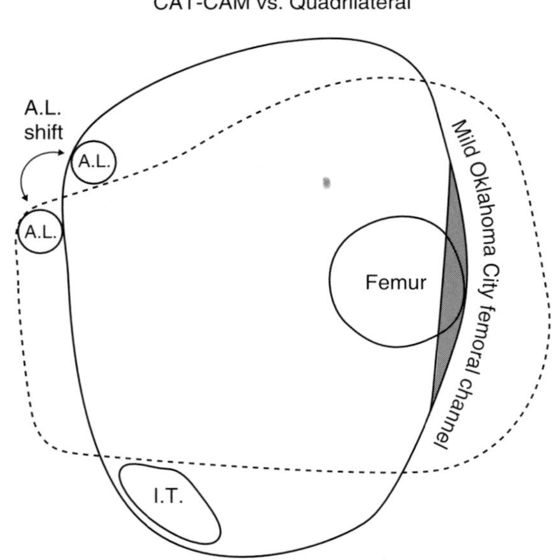

FIGURE 14–24. Comparison of CAT-CAM and quadrilateral sockets in a transverse view. The CAT-CAM is a type of ischial containment socket. In the CAT-CAM socket, the femur and ischial tuberosity are fixed, whereas the adductor longus tendon shifts a small amount compared with the quadrilateral socket. Note the Oklahoma City channel about the femur. (From Sabolich J: Contoured adducted trochanteric-controlled alignment method (CAT-CAM): Introduction and basic principles. Clin Prosthet Orthot 1985; 9:17.)

Suspension

Suspension systems for the transfemoral amputee include suction or partial suction, total elastic suspension (TES) belt, Silesian band, hip joint with pelvic band and waist belt, silicone suction suspension system, and hypobaric silicone suction system (Fig. 14–26).

Suction

The amputee usually dons a total suction prosthesis while standing. It requires that a pull sock or elastic bandage cover the residual limb. The sock or bandage is passed through the valve hole and is used to pull the limb into the socket. Alternatively, a wet fit can be used. The wet fit procedure uses a gel that turns into a liquid or powder after the prosthesis is donned. A one-way valve placed in the valve hole seals the socket by allowing air to escape but not to enter. Total suction is the best suspension biomechanically, but it requires minimal volume fluctuation of the residual limb, good hand strength and dexterity, good balance, and good skin tissue integrity.

Any socket that has a suction valve but requires the user to wear prosthetic socks is called "partial suction." Such a socket provides minimal suspension (except for the hypobaric silicone system described later), so auxiliary suspension is needed.

The hypobaric silicone suction system consists of a prosthetic sock impregnated with a proximal ring of silicone to provide an air seal for suction suspension. The amputee dons it while either sitting or standing. Once the residual limb is all the way in the socket, the amputee replaces the air valve. The hypobaric system allows suction in a looser-fitting socket.

The silicone suction suspension system, previously described for transtibial suspension, is a roll-on silicone sock attached to the distal socket, and is only occasionally used for transfemoral amputees.

No Suction

The TES belt is a neoprene belt attached to the prosthesis and pulled around the waist, providing a relatively cosmetic auxiliary suspension. The Silesian belt is a soft belt that encircles the pelvis and is attached proximally to the posterolateral aspect of the socket wall, and to the proximal anterior wall at the midline. The hip joint with pelvic band and waist belt gives excellent mediolat-

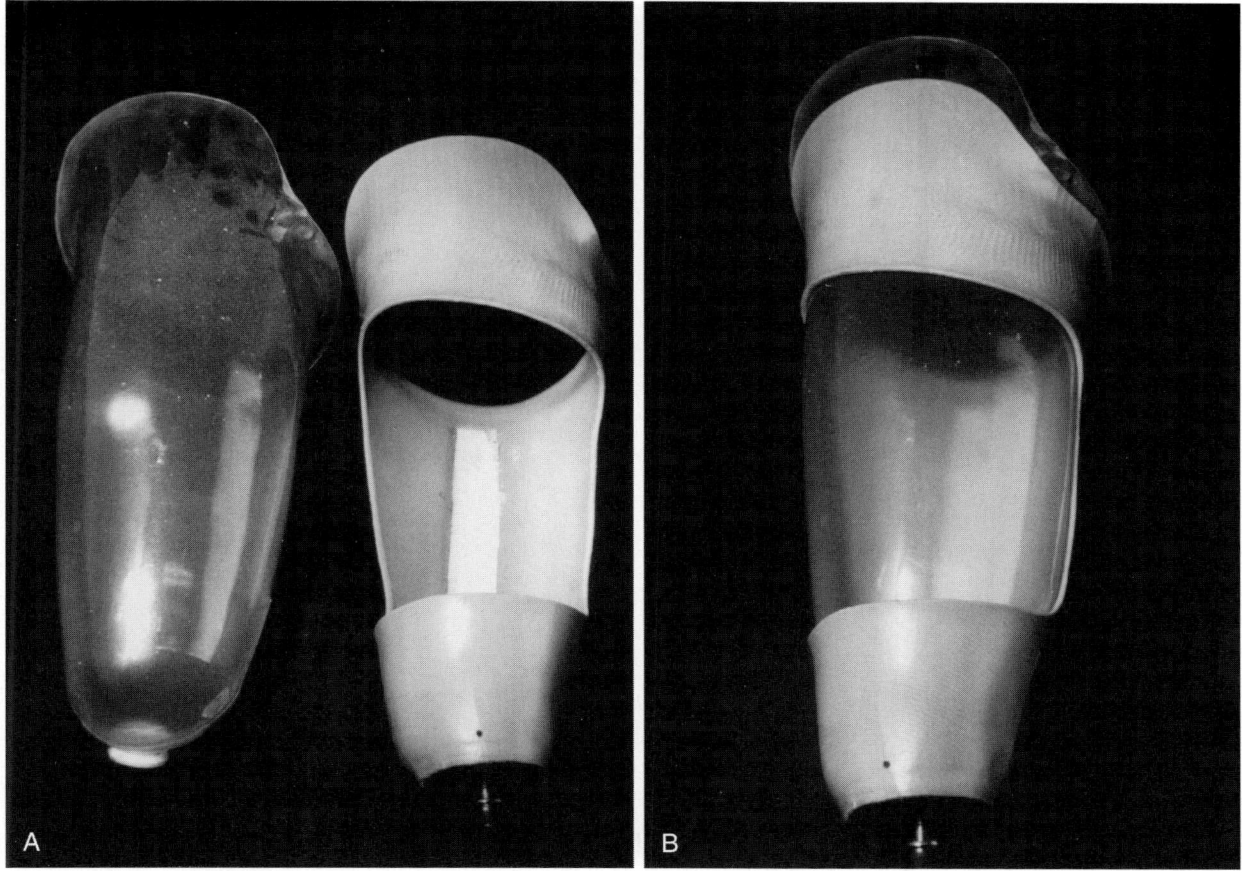

FIGURE 14–25. *A* and *B*. Flexible socket in a rigid frame for the transfemoral amputee. (Copyright Robert D. McAnelly, M.D.)

eral stability for the frail amputee or for the amputee with a short residual limb, but it is bulky, heavy, constricting, and cumbersome. Placement of these suspension mechanisms over bypass graft surgery sites and use in pregnant women are contraindicated.

Gait Deviations: Static and Dynamic Analysis

Fit and Alignment

For the quadrilateral socket, the ischium should rest on the posterior shelf, with firm but not excessive pressure between the tuberosity and socket. Insufficient pressure indicates the use of too many plies of socks or a palpable adductor roll, whereas excessive pressure indicates insufficient ply. The adductor longus tendon should be rotated to lie in the anteromedial corner.

For the ischial containment socket, the pubic ramus should be identified where it exits the medial wall. As the patient takes the weight off of the residual limb, he or she should check to see that the ischial tuberosity rests inside the ischial pocket or flare.

If a valve is present, the valve should be removed to see that the residual limb is in contact with the bottom of the socket. If there is no valve, the clay ball procedure, as described previously for the transtibial amputee, should be performed. The pelvis can be 1.4 inches lower on the prosthesis side to allow toe clearance during swing phase.

To allow the amputee to walk with an erect trunk and with a normal stride length, the initial socket flexion is set at 5 degrees of socket flexion plus the amputee's angle of hip flexion contracture. This puts the hamstrings on stretch, giving the amputee greater stance control. Sagittal plane forces within the socket progress from anteroproximal and posterodistal in early stance, to anterodistal and posteroproximal in late stance.

The TKA line is a line drawn in the sagittal plane through the greater trochanter and mid-ankle (see Fig. 14–21). If the knee joint is on this line, the knee is in *intermediate alignment.* If it is anterior to this line, it is said to be in *voluntary alignment,* because the amputee must actively extend the hip during stance to prevent knee buckling. If the knee is posterior to this line, the knee is in maximum stability and is said to be in *involuntary alignment.*

In the coronal plane, the center of rotation of the transfemoral amputee within the socket is about the ischium. A varus moment about the hip joint occurs naturally and must be stabilized by the lateral socket wall. Lack of intimate contact between the lateral femur and the socket wall makes the hip abductors inefficient and weak. The farther the foot is inset, or the heavier the amputee, the greater the varus moment. In the trans-

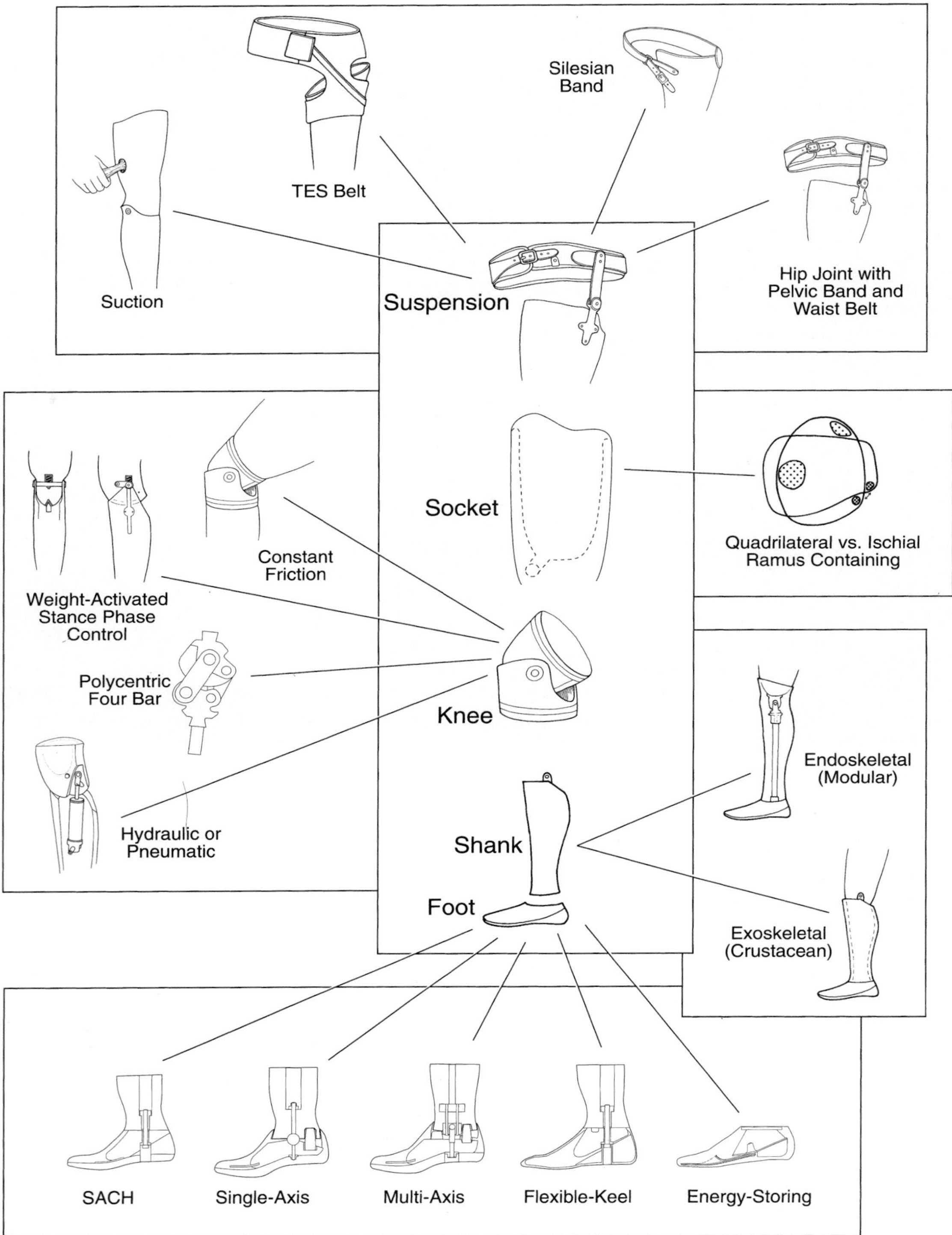

FIGURE 14–26. Prosthetic options for the transfemoral amputee. (Courtesy of the University of Texas Health Science Center at San Antonio.)

verse plane, foot toe-out should match that of the sound limb.

Gait Analysis

Table 14–2 lists gait problems and causes in the transfemoral amputee.

Energy Expenditure

The average measured gait velocity for the vascular transfemoral amputee is decreased by 55%, with oxygen consumption increased by 87%. The average measured gait velocity for the traumatic transfemoral amputee is decreased by 35%, with oxygen consumption increased

TABLE 14–2 Gait Analysis of the Transfemoral Amputee

Problem and Characteristics	Prosthetic Causes	Amputee Causes
Lateral bending of trunk: excessive bending occurs laterally from midline, generally to prosthetic side	• Prosthesis can be too short • Improperly shaped lateral wall may fail to provide adequate support for femur • High medial wall may cause amputee to lean away to minimize discomfort • Prosthesis aligned in abduction may cause wide-based gait, resulting in this defect	• Amputee may not have adequate balance • Amputee may have abduction contracture • Residual limb may be oversensitive and painful • Very short residual limb may fail to provide a sufficient lever arm for pelvis • Defect may be due to habit pattern
Abducted gait: very wide-based gait with prosthesis held away from midline at all times	• Prosthesis may be too long • Too much adduction may have been built into prosthesis • High medial wall may cause amputee to hold prosthesis away to avoid ramus pressure • Improperly shaped lateral wall can fail to provide adequate support for femur • Pelvic band may be positioned too far away from patient's body	• Patient may have abduction contracture • Defect may be due to habit pattern
Circumducted gait: prosthesis swings laterally in wide area during swing phase	• Prosthesis may be too long • Prosthesis may have too much alignment stability or friction in knee, making it difficult to bend knee in swing-through	• Amputee may have abduction contracture of residual limb • Patient may lack confidence for flexing prosthetic knee because of muscle weakness or fear of stubbing toe • Defect may be due to habit pattern
Vaulting: rising on toe of sound foot permits amputee to swing prosthesis through with little knee flexion	• Prosthesis may be too long • Socket suspension may be inadequate • Excessive stability in alignment or some limitation of knee flexion, such as knee lock or strong extension aid, may cause this deficit	• Vaulting is fairly frequent habit pattern • Fear of stubbing toe may cause this defect • Residual limb discomfort may be a factor
Uneven heel rise: prosthetic heel rises quite markedly and rapidly when knee is flexed at beginning of swing phase	• Knee joint may have insufficient friction • Extension aid may be inadequate	• Amputee may be using more power than necessary to force knee into flexion
Terminal swing impact: rapid forward movement of shin piece allows knee to reach maximum extension with too much force before heel-strike	• Knee friction is insufficient • Knee extension aid may be too strong	• Amputee may try to assure himself or herself that knee is in full extension by deliberately and forcibly extending the residual limb
Instability of the prosthetic knee creating a danger of falling	• Knee joint may be too far ahead of trochanter-knee-ankle (TKA) line • Insufficient initial flexion may have been built into socket • Plantar flexion resistance may be too great, causing knee to buckle at heel-strike • Failure to limit dorsiflexion can lead to incomplete knee control	• Amputee may have hip extensor weakness • Severe hip flexion contracture may cause instability
Medial or lateral whips: whips best observed when patient walks away from observer; a medial whip is present when heel travels medially on initial flexion at beginning of swing phase; a lateral whip exists when heel moves laterally	• Lateral whips may result from excessive internal rotation of prosthetic knee • Medial whips may result from excessive external rotation of knee • Socket may fit too tightly, thus reflecting residual limb rotation • Excessive valgus or "knock" in prosthetic knee may contribute to this defect • Badly aligned toe break in a conventional foot may cause twisting on toe-off	None
Drop-off at end of stance phase; downward movement of trunk as body moves forward over prosthesis	• Limitation of dorsiflexion of prosthetic foot is inadequate • Heel of SACH-type foot may be too short, or toe break of a conventional foot may be too far posterior • Socket may have been placed too far anterior in relation to foot	None

Table continued on following page

TABLE 14–2 *Continued*

Problem and Characteristics	Prosthetic Causes	Amputee Causes
Extensive trunk extension: amputee creates an active lumbar lordosis during stance phase	• Improperly shaped posterior wall may cause forward rotation of pelvis to avoid full weight bearing on ischium • Insufficient initial flexion may have been built into socket	• Amputee may have hip flexor tightness • Amputee may have weak hip extensors and may be substituting with lumbar erector spinae muscle; abdominal muscles may be weak • Defect may be due to habit pattern • Amputee may be moving shoulders backward in an effort to obtain better balance • Weak abdominal muscles may contribute to this defect

Courtesy of Northwestern University Prosthetic-Orthotic Center, Chicago.

by 33%, as compared with those of normal subjects without vascular disease.[108] Individual energy expenditure per distance walked increases with a shorter residual limb or with age. The energy expended in walking with a prosthesis is usually less than that in walking with crutches and without a prosthesis.[108] As a rule of thumb, if a patient can ambulate without the prosthesis and with crutches, he or she has the strength and endurance to ambulate with a prosthesis. Geriatric amputees are best fitted with lightweight "modular" prostheses using titanium or carbon fiber components. Stress testing is indicated for the patient with serious cardiac compromise to see if the energy level needed for ambulation can be tolerated.[16]

HIP DISARTICULATION AND TRANSPELVIC AMPUTATION (HEMIPELVECTOMY)

Surgical Procedures

A true hip disarticulation involves removal of the entire femur; in practice, however, the proximal femur is usually left to provide prosthetic stabilization and to avoid an uncosmetic cavity. Transpelvic amputation is the surgical removal of the lower limb and part or all of the ileum. These surgical procedures are usually done for malignant tumor, major trauma, or uncontrolled infection.

Prosthetic Prescription

The hip disarticulation amputee bears weight in the socket through the ischial tuberosity and gluteal muscles, whereas the transpelvic amputee bears weight on the soft tissue and lower rib cage. The hip disarticulation socket usually has good contact just above the iliac crest inside the socket rim, though reduced-trimline socket designs are available for young, active amputees (Fig. 14–27). Velcro socket closures secure the socket to the torso to prevent pistoning.

The transpelvic socket requires careful contouring, with gluteal bearing on the contralateral side (Fig. 14–28). The proximal border of the socket can be trimmed below the traditional second rib margin if distal contours provide precise fit.

The older Canadian-type exoskeletal hip disarticulation prosthesis has been replaced by the lightweight and ultralight endoskeletal prosthesis. Hip joint mechanisms for the hip disarticulation and transpelvic amputee are similar. The free hip joint has a posterior bumper extension stop and an anterior flexion stop, but allows no

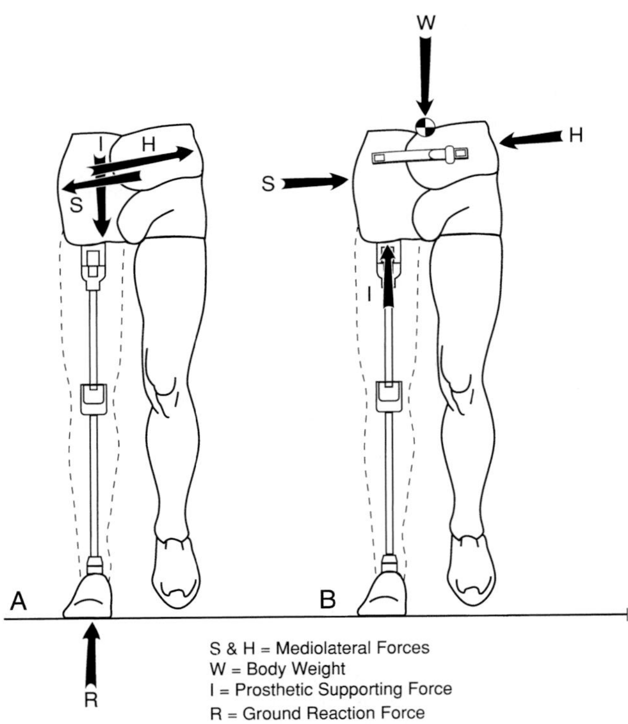

FIGURE 14–27. Mediolateral forces in the hip-disarticulation prosthesis during stance. *A.* Forces acting on the prosthesis. *B.* Forces acting on the amputee. (From Radcliffe CW: The biomechanics of the Canadian-type hip-disarticulation prosthesis. Artificial Limbs 1957; 4:34.)

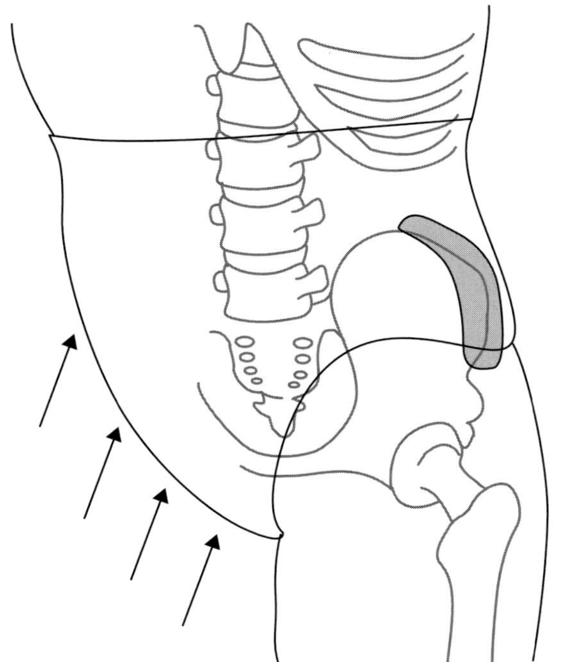

FIGURE 14–28. Transpelvic (hemipelvectomy) socket pressures. (From Lower Limb Prosthetics, New York, New York University, 1975, p 246.)

abduction or rotation. The hip joint is made to be stable by placing it anteriorly. A hip extension assist and lockable or four-bar polycentric hip joint are options.

Most of the knee units used with the transfemoral prosthesis can also be used with the hip disarticulation or transpelvic prosthesis, as can most prosthetic feet.[71] The active amputee might need a hydraulic knee, but otherwise the four-bar polycentric knee is an excellent choice. Adding a transverse rotation unit above the knee allows rotation of the distal prosthesis to assist in donning and doffing shoes and to allow cross-legged sitting. A torque-absorber can be added to prevent transverse shear forces at the socket-limb interface.

Successful gait training depends on mastering a posterior pelvic tilt to advance the prosthesis, then mastering prosthetic swing-through and weight-shift (Fig. 14–29). *Vaulting,* or intentionally rising up on the toes of the sound foot during prosthetic swing to clear the prosthesis, should be avoided.

The average measured gait velocity for the surgical hip disarticulation amputee is decreased by 41%, with oxygen consumption increased by 60% per distance walked. The average measured gait velocity for the surgical transpelvic amputee is decreased by 50%, with oxygen consumption increased by 93% per distance walked, as compared with normal subjects without vascular disease.[108] Due to the high energy requirements of hip disarticulation and transpelvic amputation ambulation, motivation and cardiopulmonary status are extremely important for prosthetic use. Most young men abandon these prostheses in favor of crutch-walking, whereas 50% of women retain their prosthesis for cosmesis.

TRANSLUMBAR AMPUTATION (HEMICORPORECTOMY)

Surgical Procedures

Translumbar amputation, or hemicorporectomy, is usually performed for pelvic malignancy, intractable decubitus ulcers, infection, or trauma. It is unique, involving the loss of the rectum and bladder as well as of most of the body mass. A segment of distal sigmoid colon can be used to create a continent urinary diversion.[107] A colostomy is also formed. The amputation is usually closed by approximating the anterior abdominal wall fascia to the lumbodorsal fascia. The need for considerable advanced psychological preparation for this procedure is obvious.

Prosthetic Prescription

Prosthetic training begins with a sitting device to increase sitting tolerance. The socket must accommodate and allow free access to the ostomy stomas. The amputee should learn stoma care and transfers in and out of the socket. Regular weight reliefs within the socket prevent skin breakdown. Attaching legs to the socket for limited ambulation impairs transfers, and so a second socket is needed if ambulation training is attempted. Successful ambulation is difficult, but cases of household

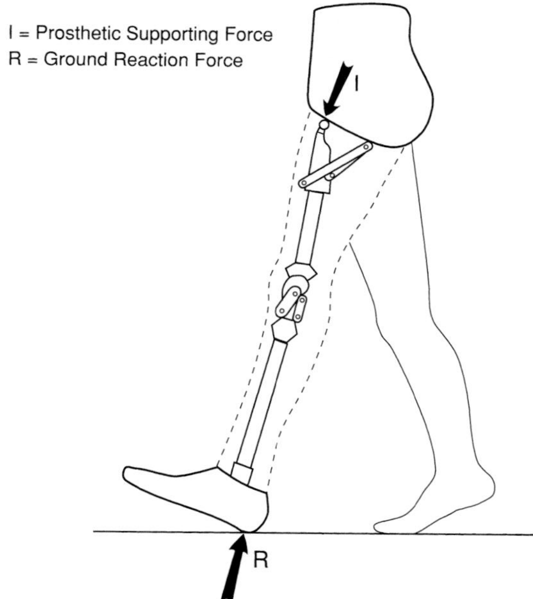

FIGURE 14–29. Hip disarticulation prosthesis at heel-strike. The ground reaction force R creates no flexion moments at the knee or hip, allowing the amputee to remain stable. (From Murdoch G (ed): Prosthetic and Orthotic Practice. London, Edward Arnold, 1970, p 287.)

and limited community ambulation are reported.[20] Prosthetic components should be lightweight and adjustable, and are similar to hip disarticulation components.

BILATERAL TRANSTIBIAL, TRANSFEMORAL, OR TRANSTIBIAL AND TRANSFEMORAL AMPUTATION

Prosthetic Prescription

For the bilateral amputee, as for the unilateral amputee, as much of the limb should be saved as will satisfactorily heal and be functional. For the bilateral hip disarticulation amputee, a molded jacket or bucket socket might be necessary to maintain sitting. If the bilateral hip disarticulation is from pressure ulcers related to spinal cord injury, the socket should be open-ended to relieve pressure over insensate areas, and should distribute weight over the chest wall without compromising respiration. A walking prosthesis is rarely indicated for the bilateral hip disarticulation amputee owing to excessive energy costs.

Bilateral transfemoral amputees are sometimes limited functional ambulators, but those in the geriatric population rarely ambulate. Lightweight or ultralight componentry should be used. The Mauch S-N-S knee and four-bar polycentric knee provide more stability than does the weight-activated stance control knee. Most dysvascular bilateral transfemoral amputees lack the cardiopulmonary reserve to ambulate. "Stubbies" are short, basic transfemoral prostheses without knee joints and with rocker-bottom feet. They require less energy to ambulate than standard transfemoral prostheses; however, stubbies leave the amputee at an uncosmetic and less functional height and result in energy-inefficient gait. Wheelchairs for bilateral transfemoral amputees and other proximal amputees require anti-tip devices and/or offset rear axles to maintain rolling stability.

Healthy bilateral transtibial amputees rarely require assistive devices, although the dysvascular amputee can require a cane. Bilateral transtibial amputees are generally better ambulators than unilateral transfemoral amputees, though limited data in the literature make direct metabolic comparisons difficult.[106, 108]

The combination transfemoral-transtibial amputee obviously has less function than a bilateral transtibial amputee or a unilateral transfemoral amputee, but has more function than a bilateral transfemoral amputee. The transfemoral-transtibial amputee usually ambulates with at least the help of a cane. Ambulation with this combination is usually done only by younger or post-traumatic amputees.

Hemiparesis on either side can prevent prosthetic ambulation in the unilateral amputee, depending on the predictive factors of severity of hemiparesis, level of amputation, and bowel and bladder continence.[1, 76, 105] In the unilateral amputee, amputation of the contralateral arm limits use of assistive devices, and so limits ambulation.

PROBLEMS OF AMPUTEES AND THEIR TREATMENT

Skin Problems

Skin lesions of the residual limb can expand rapidly, so early intervention is required, particularly for diabetic patients. Daily residual limb and socket washing is mandatory. In adults, split-thickness skin grafts cannot tolerate pressure, particularly over bony prominences, and require socket modifications. Painful bursae are common and are best managed by socket modifications, but surgical excision of a troublesome bony prominence might be necessary.

Choke Syndrome

Lack of total contact with proximal restriction results in distal edema called *choke syndrome.* The distal, strangulated residual limb becomes darkened with hemosiderin. Treatment might involve adding a distal pad, improving suspension, or changing sockets.

Verrucous hyperplasia is a wart-like skin overgrowth, usually of the distal residual limb, resulting from inadequate external compression and edema; it can be reversed with total contact within the socket.

Skin Infection

Folliculitis is a hair-root infection resulting from poor hygiene, sweating, poor socket fit, or pistoning. It is important to clean the area with antiseptic cleanser, to keep it dry, and to consider administration of oral antibiotics. Treat boils and abscesses with limited prosthetic use. Epidermoid cysts occur when sebaceous glands are plugged by keratin, and usually do not appear until months or years after a prosthesis is worn. They grow up to 5 cm in diameter and can break to discharge purulent fluid. They should be treated with topical or oral antibiotics, and in some cases with incision and drainage.

Tinea corporis and tinea cruris mainly result from sweating. They can be confirmed through culture or microscopy and are treated by topical or oral fungicides as well as by good residual limb and socket hygiene.

Excessive residual limb sweating can be controlled with cornstarch or unscented talc, but astringents and rubbing alcohol should be avoided. Antiperspirants or iontophoresis with copper sulfate or formalin might also be helpful.

Contact Dermatitis

Allergic contact dermatitis can arise from topical medications or from agents used in prosthetic manufacture. Eczema can appear acutely, with small blisters and, later, with scaling and erythema. Topical corticosteroids should be applied, and the offending agent should be identified and removed.

Bone Problems

Symptomatic bone spurs can arise from bone from which the periosteum was incorrectly stripped during surgery or trauma. Bone pain can also result from a hypermobile fibula that is left longer than the tibia. If a balanced myodesis was not performed in the transfemoral amputation, the femur can extrude through the muscle and present subcutaneously. If prosthetic adjustments, such as a flexible socket, are inadequate for the extruded femur, surgical intervention might be needed. If the amputee has severe hip joint arthritis, total hip arthroplasty is an option. If the sound limb and the prosthetic limb are of unequal length, a functional scoliosis occurs on standing, and requires shortening or lengthening of the prosthesis.

Pain

Incisional pain should subside with healing, although shear forces on an adherent scar can be painful. Deep massage helps prevent scar adhesions. Intermittent claudication pain in parts of the residual limb can be experienced by the amputee. After tumor amputation, local recurrence of tumor might also be an explanation for a painful residual limb. Remember that not all residual limb pain is the result of a poorly fitting prosthesis.

Neuromas

Every severed nerve develops a pressure-sensitive neuroma. The surgeon should sever nerves proximally to avoid socket pressure. Palpating directly over the neuroma typically elicits lancinating pain. The treatment for neuromas is socket adjustment. Direct injection of local anesthetic, with or without steroids, is helpful and aids in making the diagnosis. Neurolysis with phenol can be tried after multiple anesthetic injections have failed. If conservative measures fail, surgery to move the neuroma to a deeper or more proximal site should be considered.

Phantom Pain and Phantom Sensation

Patients with acquired amputation typically have the sensation of the amputated part, or "phantom sensation," which usually diminishes with time. Occasionally, new amputees have such a dramatic phantom sensation that they transfer out of bed in a darkened room at night and fall when the phantom limb fails to support them. A night light can help prevent such a fall.

Phantom pain can accompany the phantom sensation, localizing in the phantom limb rather than in the residual limb. Often described as cramping, aching, burning, and, occasionally, lancinating, this pain may be caused by neuron deafferentation hyperexcitability. The longer a person has pain in a limb before it is amputated, the more likely he or she is to have phantom pain. Phantom pain usually diminishes with time, and chronic phantom pain is rare. Occasionally, medical intervention is required, although tricyclic antidepressants, mexiletine, anticonvulsants, capsaicin, propranolol, and chlorpromazine offer some limited benefit.[17] Because the etiology is not precisely known, phantom pain is difficult to treat.[45, 58, 91–95] Vigorous desensitization techniques of the residual limb are usually of great benefit. If the patient can move the perceived phantom limb, "isometric exercise" of the phantom ankle in all planes might be helpful.[73] Psychological support with relaxation therapy and biofeedback might be indicated in severe cases, although phantom pain is not considered a psychosomatic complaint. Ambulation on a temporary prosthesis can help alleviate phantom pain. Transcutaneous electrical stimulation over the tibial nerve in the popliteal fossa and lumbar paravertebral sympathetic block at the L2 level should be considered if the phantom pain is burning and of a character similar to that of "reflex sympathetic dystrophy" (complex regional pain syndrome).[79] Intravenous regional guanethidine or reserpine blocks have been tried with little success.

Contractures

Maintaining the residual limb in extension is necessary to prevent flexion contractures. For severe knee flexion contractures beyond 25 degrees in an amputation without vascular disease, hamstring lengthening with posterior knee capsule release or a bent-knee prosthesis should be considered. Less severe contractures can be treated with stretching, with or without simultaneous ultrasound. When a contracture is less than 10 degrees, the patient should be encouraged to walk as much as is tolerated, as this might further reduce the contracture. More than 15 degrees of hip flexion contracture in the transfemoral amputee requires marked compensatory lumbar lordosis. Hip flexion contractures up to 25 degrees can be accommodated in the short transfemoral amputee with resulting loss of hip extensor power, but contractures are more difficult to accommodate for longer residual limbs. Hip flexion contractures result in knee instability and poor cosmesis, and often require that the prosthesis have a lockable knee. Contractures in children can lead to scoliosis.

Psychosocial Adjustments

Amputees can develop a sense of inferiority, inadequacy, or repulsiveness. They should be encouraged to discuss problems openly. Their sexual identity and body image are altered, and phantom pain can occur with orgasm. Some amputees need psychological counseling. Attention to cosmesis, such as the cosmetic "New Skin" prosthetic skin covering, can facilitate psychological adjustment.[98] The clinician should also remember never to refer to the residual limb as a "stump." New amputees often benefit from positive visits from "peer" amputees.

Activities of Daily Living and Vocational Adjustments

In dressing, the patient dons underwear first. Trousers are then put on the prosthesis before the prosthesis itself is donned. Shoe heel height cannot be changed unless foot wedges are used or unless an adjustable foot or second foot is available for the prosthesis. Driving a car can require moving the gas or brake pedal for the unilateral amputee, or installing hand controls for the bilateral amputee. Velcro closures are often needed for patients with poor hand dexterity.

The team should be aware of how much lifting, bending, climbing, and carrying of heavy objects is necessary in the patient's job, both for prosthetic training and for prosthetic prescription. Fine balance while standing can also be a job requirement to be addressed. Cosmesis can also be a significant part of the requirement. Retraining manual laborers for more sedentary work is often necessary (see Chapter 35).

Recreational Activities

Determining the capacity for sports activities requires a careful evaluation of the amputee by the physician and prosthetist. The transfemoral amputee with a mechanical knee must run with a hop-skip pattern, but with a hydraulic knee the person can run with a more normal motion. Recreational opportunities for the amputee are endless. The National Handicapped Sports (NHS) is the main U.S. organization for amputee sports, while the National Wheelchair Athletic Association offers wheelchair competition and the International Sports Organization for the Disabled (ISOD) organizes international competitions. The Paralympics began as an official competitive event sponsored by the International Olympics Committee in 1988.

PEDIATRIC AMPUTEE

Kaye and Newman's national survey of 5830 new amputees found that 3% of new amputees were in the first decade of life and 7% were in the second decade.[47] In the first decade, 68% of new amputations were from congenital deformity, 27% from trauma, 3% from tumor, and 2% from disease. In the second decade, 63% of new amputations were from trauma, 22% from tumor, 9% from disease, and 6% from late surgery for congenital deformity.

Differences Between Adult and Pediatric Amputees

Major pediatric amputee concerns include skill development, growth, and psychosocial issues. Just as for adults, all possible functional residual limb length should be preserved. A contraindication to lower limb amputation is severe upper limb deformities that make lower limb prehension necessary.

Pediatric bony overgrowth refers to pressure-related periosteal appositional growth, not epiphyseal growth. Bony overgrowth is a problem of the skeletally immature, particularly after mid-shaft amputation of the fibula or tibia. It occurs frequently enough in acquired amputations to require residual limb revision about 10% of the time, and it also can occur in congenital amputation. Bony overgrowth can cause the skin to become thin and shiny and be accompanied by pain, making prosthetic fitting difficult. The bone can even break through the skin. This overgrowth might require excision or reamputation. Capping or transplanting an amputated epiphysis over the bone end can limit the problem of recurrence.[81] To preserve the epiphysis, amputations should be done through a joint rather than through a bone. Unlike those in adults, the residual condyles in children tend to atrophy, resulting in a more cosmetic fitting prosthesis.

Leg length discrepancy from epiphyseal growth asymmetries can be substantial in the pediatric amputee. The epiphyseal plates about the knee give the greatest contribution to growth, with the distal femoral plate contributing 70% to femoral growth lengthening and the proximal tibial plate contributing 56% of tibial growth lengthening. Some residual limbs, such as a short transtibial limb, can be improved by skeletal lengthening. This procedure often requires a muscle flap for adequate skin coverage.

Unlike the case in adults, pediatric split-thickness skin grafts provide good residual limb coverage, even on end-bearing surfaces, and surgical incisions tolerate more tension. Symptomatic neuromas are rarely a problem in children, and socket modifications can usually relieve neuroma pain. Phantom limb pain is less frequent and of shorter duration in children. Knee and hip flexion contractures in children can largely be ignored and the affected limb fitted for conventional alignment, as those contractures usually stretch out with walking and growth.

Classification of Congenital Deformity

The new International Standard, ISO 8548-1:1989, "Method of Describing Limb Deficiencies at Birth," is a classification system to describe every level and type of congenital deficiency in simple terms.[18] This system categorizes congenital deformities as transverse and longitudinal (Figs. 14–30 and 14–31). A transverse deficiency has no distal skeletal elements; all others are longitudinal deficiencies. The transverse level is named after the segment beyond which no bony elements exist. Digital buds do not count. Longitudinal level names the bones affected, and indicates whether the bones are partly or totally affected.

Congenital limb deformities can be genetic or environmental. Embryologically, the limbs appear at about day 26 and are completely formed during the first 8 weeks of gestation. An estimated 1 of every 2000 human births has limb malformations,[25] primarily from unknown etiologies.[89]

When Krebs and Fishman surveyed 679 new amputees referred to specialized pediatric amputee clinics, they found that 48% of the patients were age 0 to 3 years and 11% were 4 to 6 years.[51] In these specialized clinics, congenital limb deficiencies outnumbered acquired amputations 1.6 : 1. They reported that 41% were unilateral upper limb amputees, 40% were unilateral lower limb amputees, and 19% were multiple limb amputees. Boys outnumbered girls 2.1 : 1 for acquired amputations and 1.5 : 1 for both congenital unilateral lower limb and multiple limb deficiencies. Girls outnumbered boys 1.1 : 1 for congenital unilateral upper limb deficiencies. Because previous attempts at surveying congenital anomalies by scientific classification had failed due to the sheer number of different anomalies, Krebs and Fishman instead asked in their survey for the prosthetic fitting of congenital amputees. They reported that 2% of congenital unilateral lower limb amputees were fitted as hip disarticulation, 21% as transfemoral, 6% as knee disarticulation, 37% as transtibial, 26% as Syme, and 8% as partial foot amputations.

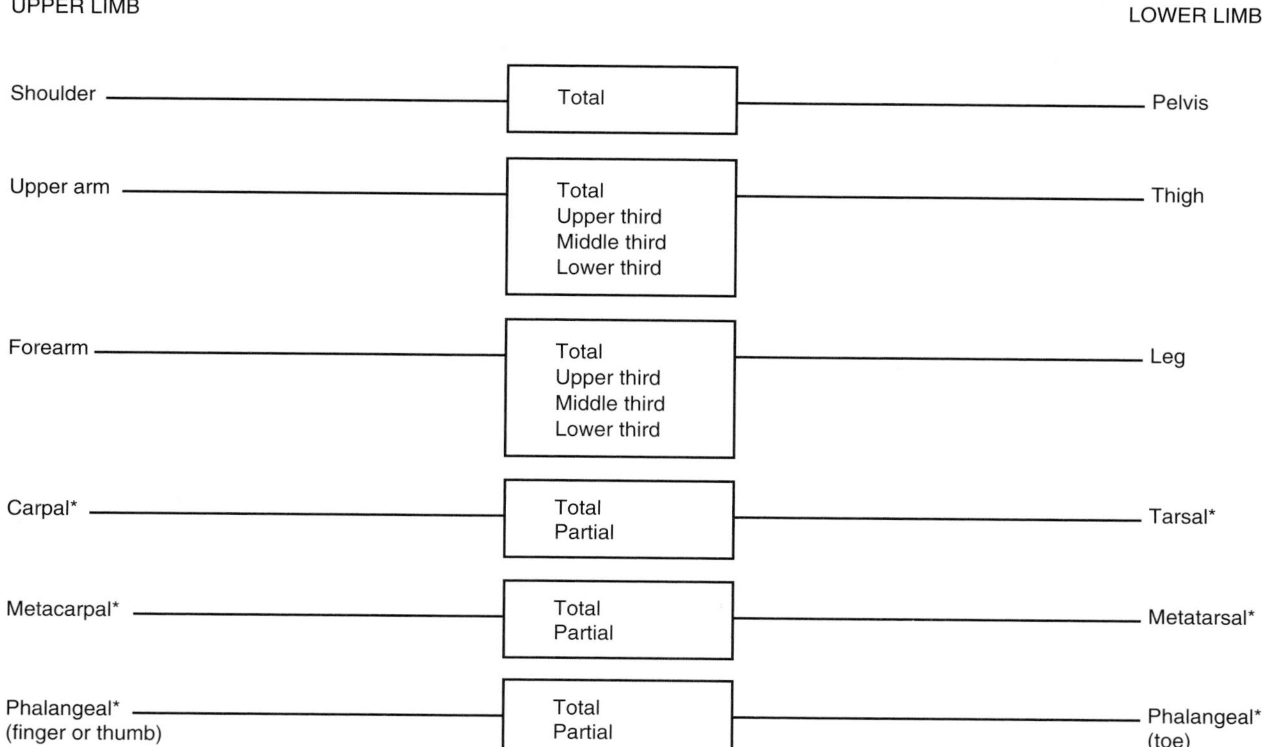

FIGURE 14–30. Designation of levels of congenital transverse deficiencies of the upper and lower limbs. Note that skeletal elements marked with an *asterisk* are used as adjectives in describing transverse deficiencies (e.g., tarsal transverse deficiency, total). A total absence of the shoulder or hemipelvis (and all distal elements) is a transverse deficiency. If only a portion of the shoulder or hemipelvis is absent, the deficiency is of the longitudinal type. (From Day HJB: The ISO/ISPO classification. In Bowker JH, Michael JW (eds): Atlas of Limb Prosthetics: Surgical, Prosthetic, and Rehabilitation Principles, ed 2. St Louis, Mosby–Year Book, 1992, p 744.)

Corrective Surgery: Surgical Possibilities

The goal of surgery is to improve the function of the child. Reasons for corrective surgery include bony overgrowth, better prosthetic fit, leg-length discrepancy, severe contracture, unstable joints, feet in a non-weight-bearing position, limb malrotation, severe neurological anesthesia, polydactyly, and cosmesis.[90] Surgery can be indicated to change a congenital anomaly to an amputation. The family can offer valuable insight into the potential effects of surgery. Surgery for congenital deformity should be planned, if possible, so that all surgical procedures can be carried out in one stage. Surgery for limb lengthening should be preceded by calculating the mature predicted discrepancy. Surgery done as early as 1 year of age provides early fitting and adaptation. Joint disarticulation is preferred over the long shaft of bones to preserve normal bone growth, to prevent bony overgrowth, and for distal end-bearing. The Ilizarov device increases length, epiphysiodesis stunts bone growth, osteotomy corrects malalignment, and joint fusion improves stability. Acetabuloplasties, shelf procedures, and femoral osteotomies can be used to stabilize the hip.

Prostheses

Several specialists—physicians, prosthetists, therapists, and social workers—are necessary to fully meet the needs of the pediatric amputee.

Timing of Prosthetic Fitting

Children generally do not need a lower limb prosthesis until they are ready to stand. Most children sit at about 6 months, crawl on all fours at about 8 to 9 months, and walk at about 1 year. Children are ready for a lower limb prosthesis between 9 and 12 months for standing. Some, however, fit pediatric transfemoral amputees at 6 months of age to promote a symmetrical sitting posture. A child with a high-level amputation is often fitted with a locked knee joint once he or she appears to be ready to ambulate. At age 3 years, the child can usually handle a constant friction knee joint with an extension strap. Children tolerate immediate postoperative fitting well, owing to good vascularity and sensation. Crutches can be tried at about 4.5 years of age.

Pediatric Prosthetic Components

Flexible thermoplastic transfemoral sockets within a rigid frame allow for some growth. Children are active and have prominent fat, and often require auxiliary suspension such as waist belts, bilateral shoulder suspension, elastic sleeves, or the silicone suction suspension system. Suction is more difficult to achieve due to growth. Alignment must be age-specific, because toddlers ambulate with legs externally rotated, abducted, and flexed. The prosthesis must adjust to the child's rapidly changing needs and challenges, such as to the prosthetically destructive teenager. Most prefer the

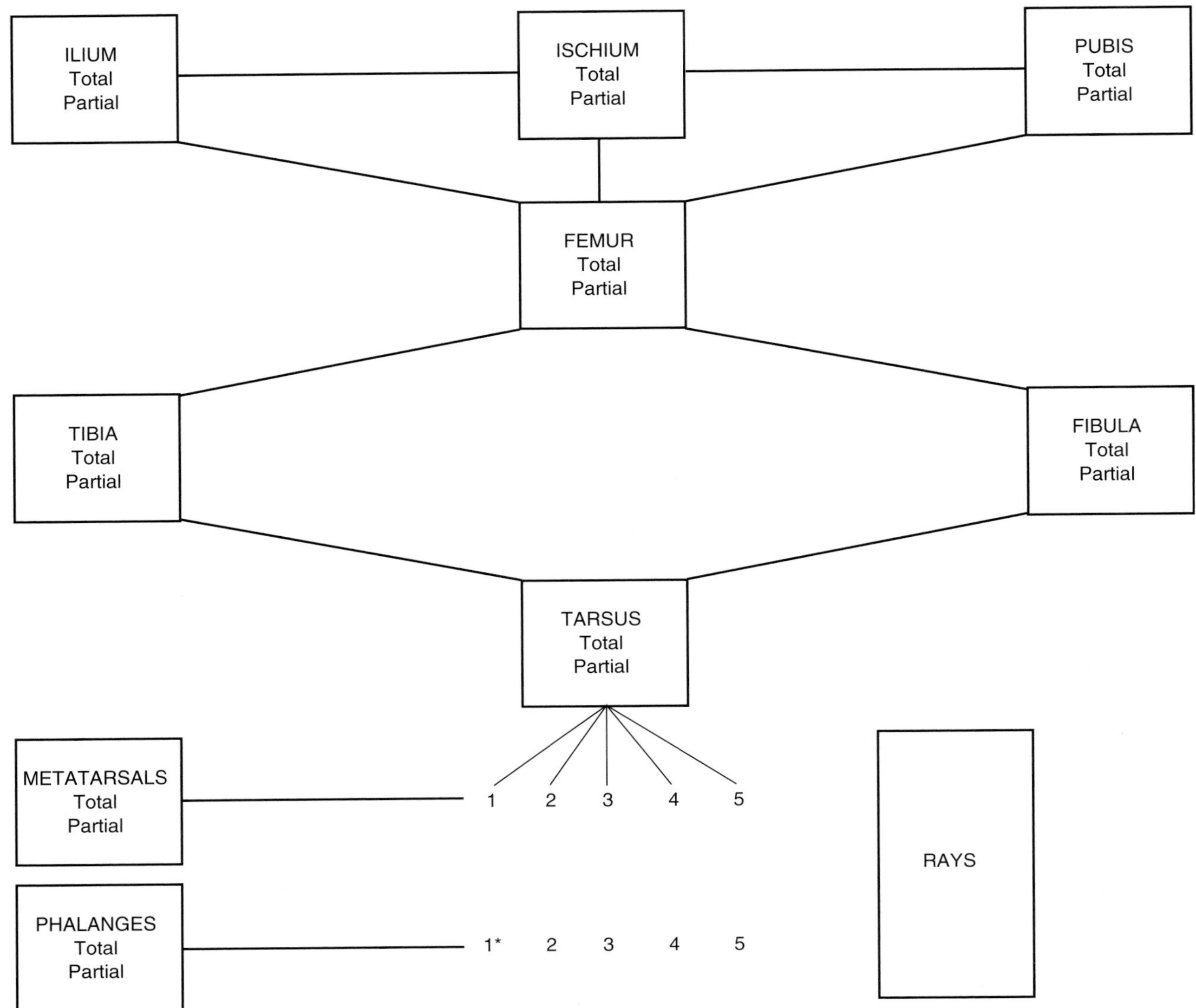

FIGURE 14–31. Description of congenital longitudinal deficiencies of the lower limb. The *asterisk* indicates the great toe, or hallux. (From Day HJB: The ISO/ISPO classification. In Bowker JH, Michael JW (eds): Atlas of Limb Prosthetics: Surgical, Prosthetic, and Rehabilitation Principles, ed 2. St Louis, Mosby–Year Book, 1992, p 746.)

greater durability of exoskeletal construction, unless the patient feels that cosmesis is a high priority. The ideal prosthesis for a young child should be lightweight and easily modified with growth.

Many common adult components, such as feet and mechanical knee joints, are also available in pediatric sizes. A good first non-locking knee unit around age 3 years is a constant friction hinge using an elastic extension aid to help prevent buckling. The active child and teenager are likely to want a hydraulic knee for activities, and will test prosthetic durability to the maximum. Hip disarticulation in children is accompanied by problems similar to those encountered in the adult.

Growth Considerations

Children require a new lower limb prosthesis at least annually up to age 5 years, biannually until age 12 years, and every 3 or 4 years until age 21 years.[53] Pediatric prostheses must be altered or replaced depending on the growth rate (or when the prosthesis has become more than 1 cm shorter than the sound limb). Pediatric limbs grow faster longitudinally than circumferentially. Growth can be accommodated by removing distal end pads or liners, extending an endoskeletal pylon, or adding wedges between the foot and exoskeletal shank. Scoliosis on standing that is not present on sitting might indicate unequal leg length.

Common Longitudinal Deficiencies

Fibular Longitudinal Deficiency, Total/Partial (Fibular Hemimelia)

Fibular longitudinal deficiency (formerly known as fibular hemimelia) is the most common congenital deficiency, and is bilateral in 25% of cases (Fig. 14–32). It consists of complete or partial absence of the fibula.

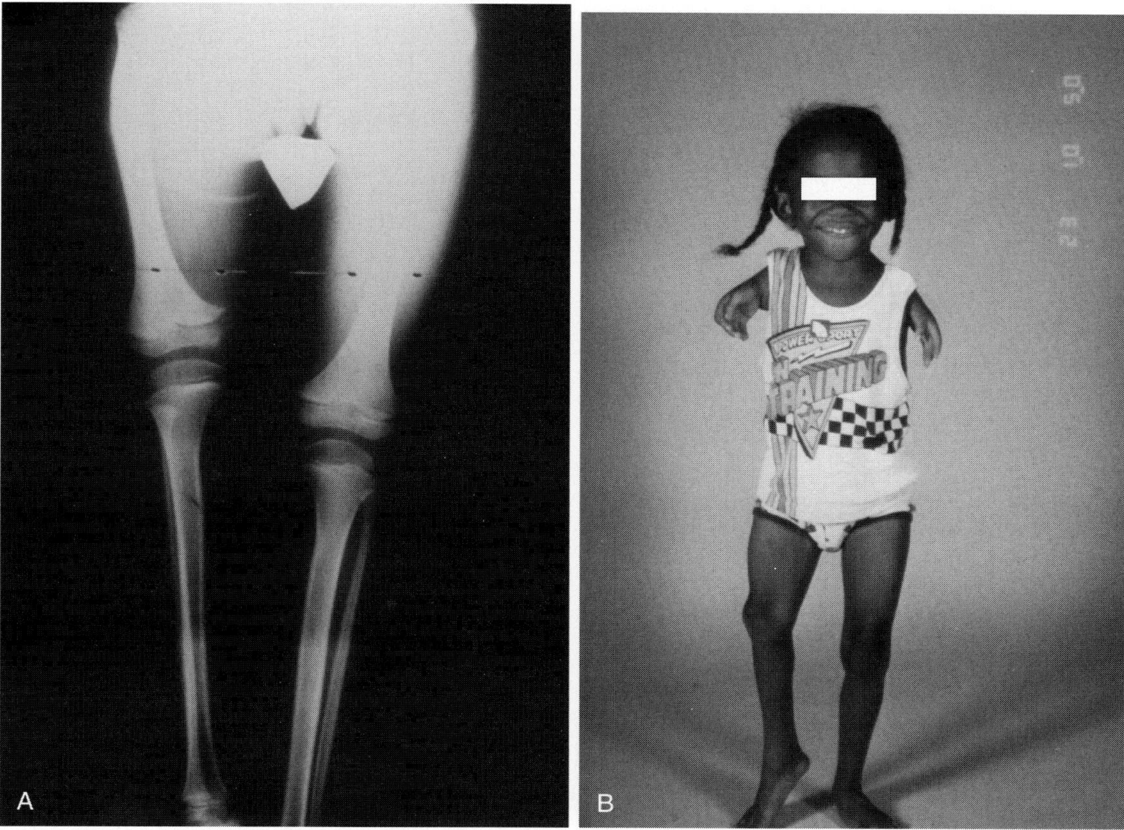

FIGURE 14–32. *A* and *B*. A patient with a longitudinal fibular deficiency and upper limb deficiency. (Courtesy of J. Sanders, M.D.)

The clinical picture is that of a shortened tibia with an anteromedial bow, foot equinovalgus deformity, occasionally a shortened femur, and leg length discrepancy. There can be a ball-and-socket ankle joint, fusion of tarsal bones, absent lateral rays, ankle instability, genu valgum, and abnormal distal tibial epiphysis. Anatomically, there is often a cartilaginous or a fibrous rudimentary fibula. The muscles originating on the fibula, such as the peroneals and flexor hallucis longus, can be deficient. Care is needed not to confuse this deformity with delayed ossification of the fibula.

The leg length inequality can be severe. The amount of inequality is roughly correlated with the percent of the fibular aplasia. There can also be some correlation with the severity of foot deformity, particularly the number of absent lateral rays. Conservative treatment is indicated if the final shortening is not expected to be greater than 7.5 cm.[99] Most of the treatment is to correct the limb length inequality with considerations of a shoe lift, bracing, contralateral epiphysiodesis (to stunt growth), ipsilateral limb lengthening, or Syme or Boyd amputation. The bow tends to straighten with growth after Syme or Boyd amputation. If the foot is retained intact, the surgeon can correct the bow with a tibial osteotomy. The Gruca procedure reinforces an unstable ankle with an osteotomy through the distal tibia and epiphysis, but can worsen leg length discrepancy. In most unilateral cases, the Gruca procedure is an interim procedure that does not compromise the result of subsequent Syme or Boyd amputation, but it can be considered definitive in cases of bilateral deformity.[99]

Proximal Femoral Focal Deficiency or Femoral Longitudinal Deficiency, Partial

Proximal femoral focal deficiency (PFFD) is characterized by partial deficiency of the proximal femur and involves the hip joint (Fig. 14–33). It comprises a spectrum of deformities, ranging from mild hypoplasia to complete absence of the proximal femur, classified as Aitken class A (mild) through D (severe).[10] The femur is typically short and held in flexion, abduction, and external rotation. Partial fibular absence and foot deformity are often present, with possible tibial shortening, hip and knee flexion contractures, and an unstable knee joint.[50] The incidence is about 1 in 50,000 births. About 10% to 15% are bilateral. Embryologically, this deformity is a failure of the proximal femoral growth plate and the chondrocytes to migrate proximally. Treatment depends on whether PFFD is unilateral or bilateral, if a hip joint is present, the amount of coxa vara, the presence of pseudarthrosis, and the estimated ultimate leg length inequality.[85]

Bilateral deformities should usually not be treated by amputation unless there is great likelihood the patient can walk with prostheses after bilateral amputations. For bilateral PFFD, the child with symmetrical shortening often is able to ambulate without a prosthesis. If the

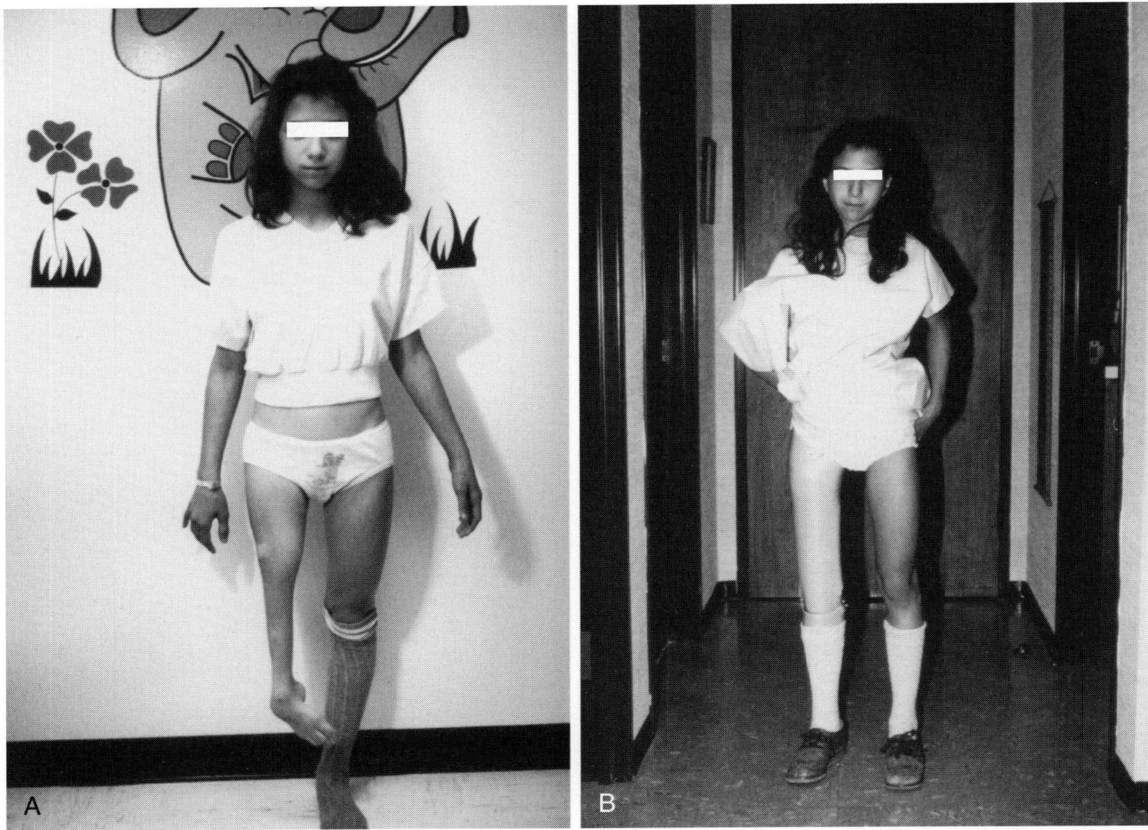

FIGURE 14–33. A patient with proximal femoral focal deficiency (PFFD) before (*A*) and after (*B*) Syme amputation with knee fusion. The patient was fitted as a knee disarticulation amputee. (Courtesy of K. Wilkins, M.D.)

upper limbs are either absent or severely deformed, both feet must be saved for self-care activities.

Options for PFFD include special prostheses to lengthen the leg, surgical limb lengthening, surgical correction of the coxa vara and the pseudarthrosis, hip stabilization with an iliofemoral fusion, Syme or Boyd amputation, knee disarticulation and prosthetic fitting, and knee fusion with a van Ness rotationplasty. The length of the shortened femur grows as a constant proportion to the length of the contralateral normal femur. If the predicted foot position at maturity is below the level of the opposite knee and the ankle is normal, a knee arthrodesis and van Ness tibial rotationplasty (see Fig. 14–1) allow fitting as a transfemoral amputee. One can try fitting a child with an unstable hip joint with an ischial containment socket to prevent the femur from pistoning.

Tibial Longitudinal Deficiency, Total/Partial (Tibial Hemimelia)

Tibial longitudinal deficiency occurs in approximately 1 in 1 million births and is characterized by complete or partial absence of the tibia (Fig. 14–34). Clinically, the foot is in severe varus, the leg is shortened, and there can be instability of the knee, ankle, or both. It can occur with PFFD and coxa valga. Associated upper limb deformities include supernumerary digits, partial adactyly (floating thumb), and central aphalangia of the hands ("lobster-claw" hands). Longitudinal tibial deficiency can be part of an inherited autosomal dominant syndrome, and 30% of cases are bilateral. Treatment depends on the anatomical abnormalities.

Treatment depends on the presence of any proximal tibia, the presence of a quadriceps mechanism, whether the foot and ankle are salvageable, and what the anticipated leg length discrepancy will be. The foot and ankle are usually not salvageable, and therefore require a Syme or Boyd amputation. If a proximal tibia and quadriceps mechanism are present, fusing the fibula to the remaining tibia allows the patient to function as a transtibial amputee. With no proximal tibia and no quadriceps mechanism, a knee disarticulation provides a functional amputation.

Training and Treatment Goals

Most children require minimal training because they adapt quickly and easily to new devices. Play is a primary motivation; thus, games with the prosthesis can be useful. Games keep the child's attention while increasing proficiency.

Toddlers should be encouraged, but not forced, to wear a prosthesis; they will wear a prosthesis if it truly helps them. Remember the milestones of the normal child: heel-to-toe gait at age 2 years, standing on one

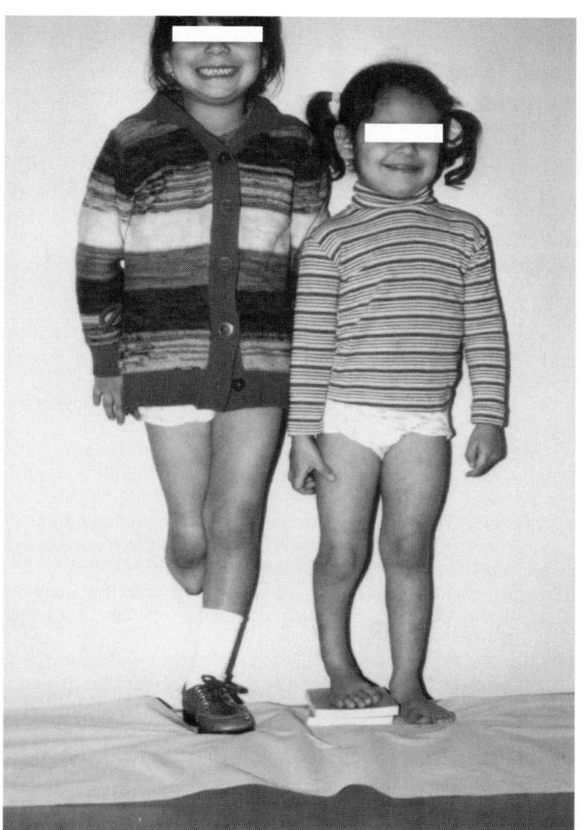

FIGURE 14–34. Sisters with the familial form of tibial longitudinal deficiency. The older sister has a short transtibial amputation; the younger sister, whose deformity was less severe, later had a Syme amputation. (Courtesy of K. Wilkins, M.D.)

foot with help at 20 months, and standing on one foot momentarily at 3 years.

Children should be encouraged to participate in as many activities as possible. Transtibial or more distal pediatric amputees can excel at athletics. Although they can develop valgus knee deformities and patellar instability, these rarely need surgical treatment.

When prostheses are contraindicated in severely impaired multiple amputees, alternative mobility should be provided at approximately 16 months of age. The alternative can be a caster cart, swivel-rocker, or electrically powered cart.[26]

Psychosocial Issues

Peer counselors make a significant difference in acceptance of the prosthesis. Congenitally limb-deficient children accept their deficiency more readily than do acquired amputees. Children deal with limb loss better if they are adequately prepared. Adolescents, of course, place a high priority on cosmesis. Parents should encourage the child to engage in as much normal physical activity as possible. Although most limb deficiencies occur sporadically, cases of tibial deficiency with a known heritable defect require genetic counseling.

RESEARCH AND DEVELOPMENT: WHAT'S ON THE HORIZON

Computer-aided design/computer-aided manufacturing (CAD-CAM) of prostheses has been in the making for 20 years (Fig. 14–35).[27, 69] The first step in CAD-CAM is for the computer to gather information about the residual limb. In the second step, the computer manipulates this information to generate specifications for fabricating a socket. In the third step, a model is produced on an automated carver for immediate socket manufacture. A fourth step is modification of a socket design, if needed, after checking it on the residual limb. The biggest advantage in CAD-CAM is the data bank of information about each patient's previous limbs and fittings, which constantly updates and improves the technique. Current shortcomings of CAD-CAM include the continued dependence on input from the prosthetist (with the associated expense and possibility of human error), software and hardware that is currently limited to transtibial or transfemoral sockets, and the inability of most CAD-CAM data input sensors to detect the location of bones and the density of deep tissues. When these problems are overcome, the amputee will reap

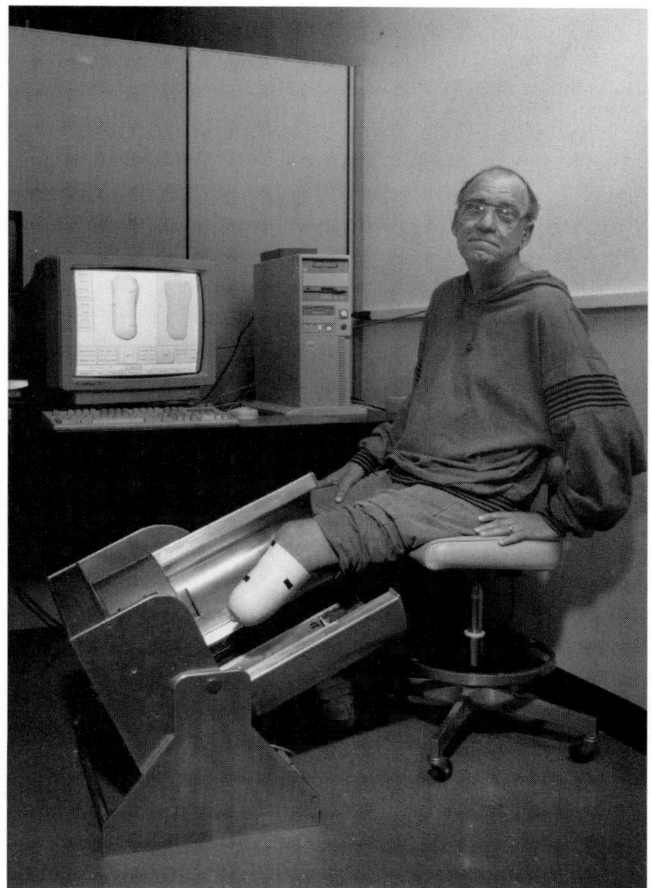

FIGURE 14–35. San Antonio computer-aided design/computer-aided manufacture (CAD-CAM) video laser imager and SOCKETS software. (Copyright Robert D. McAnelly, M.D.)

the rewards of continued improvement in the understanding of the socket-residual limb interface, and the payer will reap the rewards of time, labor, and cost savings.

REFERENCES

1. Altner PC, Rockley P, Kirby K: Hemiplegia and lower extremity amputation: Double disability. Arch Phys Med Rehabil 1987; 68:378.
2. Ayyappa E: Prosthetic Desk Reference–Revised, ed 5. Long Beach, CA, West Virginia Regional Medical Education Center, 1995.
3. Beard J, Scott DJA, Evans JM, et al: Pulse-generated runoff: A new method of determining calf vessel patency. Br J Surg 1988; 75:361.
4. Bodily KC, Burgess EM: Contralateral limb and patient survival after leg amputation. Am J Surg 1983; 146:280.
5. Bondurant FJ, Cotler HB, Buckle R, et al: The medical and economic impact of severely injured lower extremities. J Trauma 1988; 28:1270–1272.
6. Border J, Allgower M, Hanse ST, et al: Blunt Multiple Trauma: Comprehensive Pathophysiology and Care. New York, Marcel Dekker, 1990.
7. Boulton AJM, Kubrusly DB, Bowker JH, et al: Impaired vibratory perception and diabetic foot ulceration. Diabetic Med 1986; 3:335–337.
8. Bowker JH, Keagy RD, Pooneker PD: Musculoskeletal complications in amputees: Their prevention and management. In Bowker JH, Michael JW (eds): Atlas of Limb Prosthetics: Surgical, Prosthetic, and Rehabilitation Principles, ed 2. St Louis, Mosby–Year Book, 1992.
9. Boyd HB: Anatomic disarticulation of the hip. Surg Gynecol Obstet 1947; 84:364.
10. Bryant DD, Epps CH: Proximal femoral focal deficiency: Evaluation and management. Orthopedics 1991; 14:775.
11. Burgess EM, Matsen FA, Wyss CR, et al: Segmental transcutaneous measurements of pO_2 in patients requiring below-the-knee amputation for peripheral vascular insufficiency. J Bone Joint Surg Am 1982; 64:378.
12. Cina C, Katsamouris A, Megerman J, et al: Utility of transcutaneous oxygen tension measurements in peripheral arterial occlusive disease. J Vasc Surg 1984; 1:362.
13. Colborne GR, Naurmann S, Longmuir PE, et al: Analysis of mechanical and metabolic factors in the gait of congenital below knee amputees. Am J Phys Med Rehabil 1992; 71:272.
14. Cole WG, Klein RW, ValLith M, Jarvis R: Prosthetic program after above-knee amputation in children with sarcomata. J Bone Joint Surg Br 1982; 64:586–589.
15. Couch NP, David JK, Tilney NL, et al: Natural history of the leg amputee. Am J Surg 1977; 133:469.
16. Currie DM, Gilbert DML: Aerobic capacity with two leg work vs. one leg plus both arms work in peripheral vascular disease. Arch Phys Med Rehabil 1992; 73:1081–1084.
17. Davis RW: Phantom sensation, phantom pain, and stump pain. Arch Phys Med Rehabil 1993; 74:79–89.
18. Day HJB: The ISO/ISPO classification of congenital limb deficiency. Prosthet Orthot Int 1991; 15:67–69.
19. Deffer PA: More on the Ertl osteoplasty. Amputee Clin 1970; 2:7–8.
20. DeLateur BJ, Lehman JF, Winterscheid LC: Rehabilitation of the patient after hemicorporectomy. Arch Phys Med Rehabil 1989; 50:14.
21. Dormandy J: Natural history of intermittent claudication. Hosp Update, April 1991, pp 313–315.
22. Dormandy J, Mahir M, Ascady G, et al: Fate of the patient with chronic leg ischemia. J Cardiovasc Surg 1989; 30:50.
23. Dowd GSE, Linge K, Bentley G, et al: Measurement of transcutaneous oxygen pressure in normal and ischaemic skin. J Bone Joint Surg Br 1983; 65:79.
24. Eilber FR, Eckhardt J, Morton DL: Advances in the treatment of sarcomas of the extremity: Current status of limb salvage. Cancer 1984; 54:2695.
25. Evans DGR, Thakker Y, Donnai D: Heredity and dysmorphic syndromes in congenital limb deficiencies. Prosthet Orthot Int 1990; 15:70–77.
26. Faulkner V, Walsh N, Currie D: Early mobility aid for nonwalking children. Clin Prosthet Orthot 1987; 11:106–108.
27. Faulkner V, Walsh NE, Gall NG: A computerized ultrasound shape-sensing mechanism. Orthot Prosthet 1988; 41:57–65.
28. Fillauer CE, Pritham CH, Fillauer KD: Evolution and development of the silicone suction socket (3S) for below-knee prostheses. J Prosthet Orthot 1989; 1:92–103.
29. Gailey RS, Lawrence D, Burditt C, et al: The CAT-CAM socket and quadrilateral socket: A comparison of energy cost during ambulation. Prosthet Orthot Int 1993; 17:95–100.
30. Gonzalez EG, Corcoran PJ, Reyes RL: Energy expenditure in below knee amputees: Correlation with stump length. Arch Phys Med Rehabil 1974; 55:111–119.
31. Goorin A, Abelson H, Frei E: Osteosarcoma—15 years later. N Engl J Med 1985; 313:1637.
32. Gottschalk FA, Kourosh S, Stills M: Does socket configuration influence the position of the femur in above-knee amputation? J Prosthet Orthot 1989; 2:94–102.
33. Gregory RT, Gould RJ, Peclet M, et al: The mangled extremity syndrome (M.E.S.): A severity grading system for multi-system injury of the extremity. J Trauma 1985; 25:1147–1150.
34. Hammersgaard E, Baadsgaard K: Healing of below knee amputations in relation to perfusion pressure of skin. Acta Orthop Scand 1977; 48:335.
35. Hansen ST: Overview of the severely traumatized lower limb. Clin Orthop 1989; 243:17–19.
36. Hansen ST: The type IIIC tibial fracture. J Bone Joint Surg Am 1987; 69:799–780.
37. Harward TRS, Volny J, Golbranson F, et al: Oxygen inhalation-induced transcutaneous pO_2 changes as a predictor of amputation level. J Vasc Surg 1985; 2:220.
38. Helfet DL, Howey T, Sanders R, et al: Limb salvage versus amputation: Preliminary results of the mangled extremity severity score. Clin Orthop 1990; 256:80–86.
39. Hicks JH: Amputation in fractures of the tibia. J Bone Joint Surg Br 1964; 46:388–392.
40. Holloway GA, Burgess EM: Preliminary experience with laser Doppler velocimetry for the determination of amputation levels. Prosthet Orthot Int 1983; 7:63.
41. Holstein P: Distal blood pressure as guidance in choice of amputation level. Scand J Clin Lab Invest 1973; 31:245.
42. Holstein P, Lund P, Larsen B, et al: Skin perfusion pressure measured as the external pressure required to stop isotope washout. Scand J Clin Lab Invest 1977; 37:649.
43. Holstein P, Sager P, Lassen NA: Wound healing in below-knee amputations in relation to skin perfusion pressure. Acta Orthop Scand 1979; 50:49.
44. Jain AS, Stewart CPU: Tumor related lower limb amputation: A 23 year experience. Prosthet Orthot Int 1989; 13:82–85.
45. Jensen TS, Krebs B, Nielsen J, Rasmussen P: Immediate and long term phantom limb pain in amputees—incidence, clinical characteristics, and relationship to pre-amputation limb pain. Pain 1985; 21:267–278.
46. Kawamura I, Kawamura J: Some biomechanical evaluations of the ISNY flexible above-knee system with quadrilateral socket. Orthot Prosthet 1986; 40:17–23.
47. Kaye HW, Newman JD: Relative incidences of new amputations: Statistical comparisons of 6,000 new amputees. Orthot Prosthet 1975; 29:3–16.
48. Kihn RB, Warren R, Beebe GW: The "geriatric" amputee. Ann Surg 1972; 176:305.
49. King JC, Williams RP, McAnelly RD, Leonard EI: Rehabilitation of tumor amputees and limb salvage patients. In Garden FH, Grabois M (eds): Physical Medicine and Rehabilitation: State of the Art Reviews, vol 8, no 2, Cancer Rehabilitation. Philadelphia, Hanley & Belfus, 1994.
50. Krajbich I: Proximal femoral focal deficiency. In Kalamachi A (ed): Congenital Lower Limb Deficiencies. New York, Springer-Verlag, 1989.
51. Krebs DE, Fishman S: Characteristics of the child amputee population. J Pediatr Orthop 1984; 4:89–95.

52. Kristinsson O: Flexible above-knee socket made from low-density polyethylene suspended by a weight-transmitting frame. Orthot Prosthet 1983; 37:25–27.
53. Lambert C: Amputation surgery in the child. Orthop Clin North Am 1972; 3:473–482.
54. Lane JM, Kroll MA, Rossbach PG: New advances and concepts in amputee management after treatment for bone and soft-tissue sarcomas. Clin Orthop 1990; 256:22–28.
55. Lane RH, Harsh B, Boland P, et al: Osteogenic sarcoma. Clin Orthop 1986; 204:93.
56. Lange RH: Limb reconstruction versus amputation decision making in massive lower extremity trauma. Clin Orthop 1989; 243:92–99.
57. Lange RH, Bach AW, Hansen ST, et al: Open tibial fractures with associated vascular injuries: Prognosis for limb salvage. J Trauma 1985; 25:203–208.
58. Loeser JD: Pain after amputation: Phantom limb and stump pain. In Bonica JJ (ed): The Management of Pain, ed 2. Philadelphia, Lea & Febiger, 1990, p 244.
59. Long IA: Allowing normal adduction of the femur in above-knee amputations. Orthot Prosthet 1975; 29:53.
60. Long IA: Normal shape normal alignment (NSNA) above-knee prosthesis. Clin Prosthet Orthot 1985; 9:9.
61. Lowry R: Durability of lower extremity prostheses. Arch Phys Med Rehabil 1966; 47:742–743.
62. Malone JM: Complications of lower extremity amputation. In Moore WS, Malone JM (eds): Lower Extremity Amputation. Philadelphia, WB Saunders, 1989, pp 208–214.
63. Marcove R, Rosen G: En bloc resection for osteogenic sarcoma. Cancer 1980; 3040.
64. McCollum PT, Spence VA, Walker WF, et al: Amputation for peripheral vascular disease: The case for level selection. Br J Surg 1988; 75:1193.
65. McCollum PT, Spence VA, Walker WF, et al: Circumferential skin blood flow measurements in the ischaemic lower limb. Br J Surg 1985; 72:310.
66. McCollum PT, Spence VA, Walker WF, et al: Oxygen induced changes in the skin as measured by transcutaneous oxymetry. Br J Surg 1986; 73:882.
67. McCollum PT, Walker WF: Major limb amputation for end-stage peripheral vascular disease: Level selection and alternative options. In Bowker JH, Michael JW (eds): Atlas of Limb Prosthetics, ed 2. St Louis, Mosby–Year Book, 1992, pp 29–30.
68. McFarland DC, Lawrence PF: Skin fluorescence: A method to predict amputation site healing. J Surg Res 1982; 32:410.
69. Medhat MA, McAnelly RD: What's new in lower extremity amputation and prosthetics: IV. CAD-CAM. Surg Rounds Orthop, July 1990, pp 37–39.
70. Mehta K, Hobson RW, Jamil Z, et al: Fallibility of Doppler ankle pressure in predicting healing of transmetatarsal amputation. J Surg Res 1980; 28:466.
71. Michael J: Component selection criteria: Lower limb disarticulations. Clin Prosthet Orthot 1988; 12:99–108.
72. Michael J: Energy storing feet: A clinical comparison. Clin Prosthet Orthot 1987; 11:154–168.
73. Mooney V, Wagner FW, Waddell J, et al: The below-the-knee amputation for vascular disease. J Bone Joint Surg Am 1976; 58:365.
74. Moore WS, Henry RE, Malone JM, et al: Prospective use of xenon[133] clearance for amputation level selection. Arch Surg 1981; 116:86–88.
75. Nielson DH, Schurr DG, Golden JC, et al: Comparison of energy cost and gait efficiency during ambulation in below-knee amputees using different prosthetic feet: A preliminary report. J Prosthet Orthot 1989; 1:24–31.
76. O'Connell PG, Gnatz S: Hemiplegia and amputation: Rehabilitation in the dual disability. Arch Phys Med Rehabil 1989; 70:451.
77. Oishi CS, Fronek A, Golbranson FL: The role of non-invasive vascular studies in determining levels of amputation. J Bone Joint Surg Am 1988; 70:1520.
78. Otteman MG, Stahlgrew LH: Evaluation of factors which influence mortality and morbidity following major lower extremity amputation for atherosclerosis. Surg Gynecol Obstet 1965; 120:1217.
79. Personal oral communication, N. Gall, M.D., 1995.
80. Personal oral communication, R. Heimbach, M.D., 1995.
81. Pfeil J, Marquardt E, Holtz T, et al: The stump capping procedure to prevent or treat terminal osseous overgrowth. Prosthet Orthot Int 1991; 15:96–99.
82. Ratcliff DA, Clyne CAC, Chant ADB, et al: Prediction of amputation wound healing: The role of transcutaneous pO_2 assessment. Br J Surg 1984; 71:219.
83. Robbs JV, Ray R: Clinical predictors of below knee stump healing following amputation for ischaemia. S Afr J Surg 1982; 20:305.
84. Roon AJ, Moore WS, Goldstone J, et al: Below-knee amputation: A modern approach. Am J Surg 1977; 134:153.
85. Rossi TV, Kruger L: Proximal femoral focal deficiency and its treatment. Orthot Prosthet 1975; 29:37–57.
86. Sabolich J: Contoured adducted trochanteric-controlled alignment method (CAT-CAM): Introduction and basic principles. Clin Prosthet Orthot 1985; 9:15.
87. Sanders GT: Lower Limb Amputations: A Guide to Rehabilitation. Philadelphia, FA Davis, 1986.
88. Schwartz JA, Schuler JJ, O'Connor BJA, et al: Predictive value of distal perfusion pressure in the healing of amputation of the digits and forefoot. Surg Gynecol Obstet 1982; 154:865.
89. Scott CI: Genetic and familial aspects of limb defects with emphasis on the lower extremities. In Kalamachi A (ed): Congenital Lower Limb Deficiencies. New York, Springer-Verlag, 1989.
90. Setoguchi Y, Rosenfelder R: The Limb-Deficient Child. Springfield, IL, Charles C Thomas, 1982.
91. Sherman RA: Phantom limb pain mechanism-based management. Clin Podiatr Med Surg 1994; 11:85–106.
92. Sherman RA, Sherman CJ, Gall NG: A survey of current phantom limb treatment in the United States. Pain 1980; 8:85–99.
93. Sherman RA, Sherman CJ: A comparison of phantom sensations among amputees whose amputations were of civilian and military origins. Pain 1985; 21:91–97.
94. Sherman RA, Sherman CJ: Prevalence and characteristics of chronic phantom limb pain among American veterans. Am J Phys Med Rehabil 1983; 62:227–238.
95. Sherman R, Sherman CJ, Parker L: Chronic phantom and stump pain among American veterans: Result of a survey. Pain 1984; 18:83–95.
96. Silverman DG, Roberts A, Reilly CA, et al: Fluorometric quantification of low-dose fluorescein delivery to predict amputation site healing. Surgery 1987; 101:335.
97. Simon MA: Limb salvage for osteosarcoma in the 1980s. Clin Orthop 1991; 270:264–270.
98. Staats TB: Advanced prosthetic techniques for below knee amputations. Orthopedics 1985; 8:249–258.
99. Thomas IH, Williams PF: The Gruca operation for congenital absence of the fibula. J Bone Joint Surg Br 1987; 69:587.
100. Thyregod HC, Holstein P, Steen Jensen J, et al: The healing of through-knee amputations in relation to skin perfusion pressure. Prosthet Orthot Int 1983; 7:61.
101. US Department of Health and Human Services: Current Estimates from the National Health Interview Survey, 1990, series 10, 181. Washington, DC, Vital and Health Statistics, 1991, p 94.
102. US Department of Health and Human Services: Detailed Diagnoses and Procedures: National Hospital Discharge Survey, 1989, series 13, 108. Washington, DC, Vital and Health Statistics, 1989, p 119.
103. US Department of Health and Human Services: Prevalence of Selected Impairments: United States—1977, series 10, 134. Washington, DC, Vital and Health Statistics, 1981, pp 14–17, 28–29.
104. US Department of Health and Human Services: Use of Special Aids: United States—1977, series 10, 135. Washington, DC, Vital and Health Statistics, 1980, pp 12–13, 15–16, 23–25.
105. Varghese G, Hinterbuchner C, Mondall P, et al: Rehabilitation outcome of patients with dual disability of hemiplegia and amputation. Arch Phys Med Rehabil 1978; 59:121.
106. Volpicelli L, Chambers R, Wagner F: Ambulation levels of bilateral lower extremity amputees. J Bone Joint Surg Am 1983; 65:599.
107. Wagman LD, Terz JJ: Hemipelvectomy and translumbar amputation. In Moore WS, Malone JM (eds): Lower Extremity Amputation. Philadelphia, WB Saunders, 1989, pp 157–176.

108. Waters RL, Perry J, Chambers R: Energy expenditure of amputee gait. In Moore WS, Malone JM (eds): Lower Extremity Amputation. Philadelphia, WB Saunders, 1989, pp 250–260.
109. Welch GH, Leiberman DP, Pollock JG, et al: Failure of Doppler ankle pressure to predict healing of conservative forefoot amputations. Br J Surg 1985; 72:888.
110. White RA, Nolan L, Harley D, et al: Noninvasive evaluation of peripheral vascular disease using transcutaneous oxygen tension. Am J Surg 1982; 144:68.
111. Williard WC, Hajdu SI, Casper ES, et al: Comparison of amputation with limb-sparing operations for adult soft tissue sarcoma of the extremity. Am Surg 1992; 215:269–275.
112. Wilson AB: Limb Prosthetics, ed 6. New York, Demos Publications, 1989.
113. Wilson SB, Spence VA: Dynamic thermographic imaging method for quantifying dermal perfusion: Potential and limitations. Med Biol Eng Comput 1989; 27:496.
114. Wing DC, Hittenberger DA: Energy-storing prosthetic feet. Arch Phys Med Rehabil 1989; 70:330–335.
115. Wu Y, Keagy RD, Krick HJ, et al: An innovative removable rigid dressing technique for below-knee amputation. J Bone Joint Surg Am 1979; 61:724–729.
116. Wu Y, Krick H: Removable rigid dressing for below-knee amputees. Clin Prosthet Orthot 1987; 11:33–44.
117. Zettl JH: Immediate postoperative prostheses and temporary prosthetics. In Moore WS, Malone JM (eds): Lower Extremity Amputation. Philadelphia, WB Saunders, 1989, pp 177–207.

15 CHAPTER

Atul T. Patel, M.D., Laura M. Garber, O.T.R, C.H.T., and John B. Redford, M.D.

Upper Limb Orthotic Devices

This chapter provides a guide for indications and basic principles for using upper limb orthotic devices, commonly known as splints or braces. The word "orthosis" (derived from the Greek *orthos,* meaning to correct or make straight) encompasses the full spectrum of devices currently fabricated by therapists and orthotists. As defined by the International Standards Organization of the International Society for Prosthetics and Orthotics, *orthosis* is any externally applied device used to modify structural and functional characteristics of the neuromuscular skeletal system.[10] Thus, "orthosis"—or, alternatively, "orthotic device"[7]—is the preferred term. The terms "splint" and "brace" are less preferred because they imply mere immobilization and do not suggest either improved function or restoration of mobility. But these terms remain common. (Note: In this chapter, we use the terms "orthotic device" and "splint" interchangeably.)

PRINCIPLES AND INDICATIONS

Upper limb orthotic devices can be used in a number of different circumstances and clinical situations. The objectives of orthotic applications can be classified into three major areas: protection, correction, and assistance with function:

1. Protection: Orthotic devices can provide compressive forces and traction in a controlled manner, thus protecting the impaired joint or body part. Restricting or preventing joint motion allows for corrective alignment and serves to prevent deformity. Protective orthoses can also stabilize unstable bony components and promote healing of soft tissues and bones. Traction forces can permit joint motion with decreased compressive forces applied to the joint cartilage.
2. Correction: Orthoses help in correcting joint contractures and subluxation of joints or tendons, thus preventing or reducing joint deformities.
3. Assistance with function: Orthoses can assist function by compensating for deformity, muscle weakness, or increased muscle tone.

Physicians prescribe orthotic devices based on their knowledge of diagnosis and preferred treatment; other health professionals, including occupational therapists and orthotists, are involved in design and application of these devices.

CLASSIFICATION

We use many different terms to describe upper limb orthotic devices. We call them by the joint they cover, the function they provide (e.g., immobilization), or the condition they treat. Some are named by their appearance (e.g., banjo or sugar tong), and still others bear the name of the person who designed them (e.g., Kleinert).[6]

Most splints are known by their common names (see Table 15–1)—names that have evolved over time. But such names are not fully informative; moreover, they are not systematic, or even universally accepted. And this lack of a universally accepted terminology often presents a communication barrier between the physician and other health professionals. Consequently, more systematic naming systems have been developed—naming systems that classify orthotic devices according to anatomic region or to purpose and function. Table 15–1 compares the common names of several orthotic devices with those in three other naming systems.

TABLE 15–1 Nomenclature Systems in Current Use

Common Name	ASHT SCS[1]	ISO[12]	McKee and Morgan[6]
Humeral fracture brace	Nonarticular splint-humerus	N/A	Circumferential nonarticular humerus-stabilizing
Tennis elbow splint/brace	Nonarticular splint-proximal forearm	Elbow orthosis (EO)	Circumferential nonarticular proximal forearm strap
Long arm splint	45° elbow flexion immobilization; type 1[1]	Shoulder-elbow-wrist-hand orthosis (SEWHO)	Posterior static elbow/wrist orthosis
Resting hand splint	Index through small finger PIP extension, thumb CMC palmar abduction mobilization; type 3[16]	Wrist-hand orthosis (WHO)	Volar forearm-based static (or serial static) wrist-hand orthosis
Ulnar deviation splint	Index through small finger MP extension/radial deviation mobilization; type 0[4]	Hand orthosis (HO)	Circumferential hand-based dynamic traction D2-5 MCP corrective radial deviation orthosis
Kleinert splint Modified Kleinert splint Postop flexor tendon splint	Wrist, MP, PIP, DIP flexion immobilization/extension restriction; type 0[13]	Wrist-hand orthosis (WHO)	Dorsal forearm-based dynamic MCP-IP protective-flexion and MCP extension-blocking orthosis
Duran splint Postop flexor tendon splint	Wrist and finger flexion immobilization; type 0[4]	Wrist-hand orthosis (WHO)	Dorsal forearm-based static MCP-IP protective-flexion and MCP extension blocking orthosis
Postop dynamic extensor tendon splint	Wrist, MP, PIP, DIP extension immobilization/flexion restriction; type 0[13]	Wrist-hand orthosis (WHO)	Volar/dorsal forearm-based dynamic MCP-IP protective-extension and flexion-blocking orthosis
Swan neck splint	Index finger PIP extension restriction; Type 0[1]	Finger orthosis (FO)	Finger-based static PIP extension-blocking orthosis
Postop MCP arthroplasty splint Swanson splint	Index through small finger MP extension/radial deviation mobilization; type 1[5]	Wrist-hand-finger orthosis (WHFO)	Dorsal forearm-based dynamic D2-5 MCP assisted extension/radial deviation orthosis
Radial nerve palsy splint	Wrist extension, MP flexion mobilization/MP flexion, wrist extension mobilization; type 0[5]	Wrist-hand-finger orthosis (WHFO)	Dorsal forearm-based dynamic low-profile wrist and D1-5 MCP assistive-extension orthosis
Ulnar nerve palsy splint	Ring though small finger MP extension restriction; type 0[2]	Hand-finger orthosis (HFO)	Circumferential hand-based dynamic joint-aligned coil-spring D4-5 MCP assistive-flexion orthosis
Median nerve palsy splint	Index through small finger MCP flexion mobilization and thumb CMC opposition mobilization; type 0[5]	Hand-finger orthosis (HFO)	Circumferential hand-based dynamic joint-aligned coil-spring D2-5 MCP assistive-flexion and thumb assistive-oppositon orthosis

Flail arm splint	Not classified	Shoulder-elbow-wrist-hand orthosis (SEWHO)	Not classified
Dynamic finger flexion splint, forearm-based	Index through small finger MP flexion mobilization; type 3[7]	Wrist-hand-finger orthosis (WHFO)	Volar hand-based dynamic MCP corrective-flexion orthosis
Dynamic finger final flexion splint, hand-based	Index through small finger flexion mobilization; type 0[12]	Wrist-hand-finger othosis (WHFO)	Volar forearm-based dynamic MCP, PIP, DIP corrective-flexion orthosis
Dynamic finger extension splint, forearm-based	Index through small PIP & DIP extension mobilization; type 2[13]	Wrist-hand-finger orthosis (WHFO)	Volar forearm-based dynamic MP, PIP, DIP corrective-extension orthosis
Dynamic finger extension splint, hand-based	Index through small finger extension mobilization; type 0[12]	Wrist-hand-finger orthosis (WHFO)	Circumferential hand-based dynamic D4-5 MCP, PIP, DIP assistive-flexion orthosis
Static progressive splint	Index finger MP flexion mobilization; type 1[4]	Wrist-hand-finger orthosis (WHFO)	Volar forearm-based static progressive MERiT-screw MCP-flexion orthosis
Dynamic wrist flexion splint	Wrist flexion mobilization; type 0[1]	Wrist-hand orthosis (WHO)	Dorsal forearm-based dynamic-joint-aligned wrist assistive flexion orthosis
Dynamic wrist extension splint	Wrist extension mobilization; type 0[1]	Wrist-hand orthosis (WHO)	Dorsal forearm-based dynamic-joint-aligned wrist assistive extension orthosis
RIC tenodesis splint	Not classified	Functional orthosis (FO)	Volar forearm-based tenodesis wrist-hand orthosis
Elbow flexion splint	Elbow flexion mobilization; type 0[1]	Elbow-wrist orthosis (EWO)	Posterior dynamic elbow corrective-flexion orthosis
Elbow extension splint	Elbow extension mobilization; type 0[1]	Elbow-wrist orthosis (EWO)	Anterior serial static elbow corrective-extension orthosis
Dynamic pronation/supination splint	Forearm pronation/supination mobilization; type 2[3]	Elbow-wrist-hand orthosis (EWHO)	Posterior forearm-based dynamic radius/ulna corrective pronation/supination orthosis
Wrist splint, Carpal tunnel splint	Wrist extension immobilization; type 0[1]	Wrist orthosis (WO)	Volar forearm-based static wrist orthosis
Thumb spica splint	Thumb MP extension immobilization; type 2[3]	Wrist-thumb orthosis (WHFO)	Volar forearm-based static wrist-thumb orthosis
Mallet finger splint, DIP extension splint, Stax splint	Index finger DIP extension immobilization; type 0[3]	Finger orthosis (FO)	Volar finger-based static DIP-flexion-blocking orthosis
Capener splint	PIP extension mobilization; type 0[1]	Finger orthosis (FO)	Three-point finger-based dynamic joint-aligned coil-spring PIP corrective-extension orthosis
Figure-eight harness	Nonarticular splint-axilla	Shoulder orthosis (SO)	Figure-eight nonarticular axilla orthosis
Airplane splint	Shoulder abduction immobilization; type 3[4]	Shoulder-elbow-wrist-hand orthosis (SEWHO)	Lateral trunk-based static shoulder-elbow-wrist orthosis
Gunslinger splint			
Mobile arm support	Not classified	Shoulder-elbow-wrist-hand orthosis (SEWHO)	Not classified
Orthosis sugar tong splint	Elbow extension immobilization; type 3[4]	Shoulder-elbow-wrist-hand orthosis (SEWHO)	Bivalved static elbow orthosis

The simplest naming system is that developed by the International Standards Organization (ISO). It reports the anatomic region the orthotic device encompasses. A wrist-hand orthosis, for example, is called a WHO.[11] This system, however, fails to define the purpose or function of the orthosis.

In 1991, the American Society of Hand Therapists (ASHT) published the ASHT *Splint Classification System* (SCS).[1] This system provides standard nomenclature for splints based on function. It classifies splints by characteristics (e.g., articular or nonarticular) and location of body part covered. A humeral fracture brace, for example, is identified as a nonarticular splint-humerus (see Table 15–1). It also identifies the direction of the force applied, and whether the splint is for mobilization, immobilization, or restriction. Thus, a long arm splint is characterized as a 45° elbow flexion immobilization. In addition, this system provides a way to indicate the number of primary and secondary joints. A primary joint is the anatomic joint affected by a splint, while a secondary joint is a joint included in a splint to provide counterforce control, position, or stabilization of joint(s) immediately adjacent to primary articular structures. The numbering system is indicated by the word "type." The number that follows the word "type" indicates the number of secondary joints involved, while the number in brackets is the total number of joints included in the splint—the sum of the primary joints plus the secondary joints. Consider, for example, a thumb spica splint, forearm-based (Fig. 15–1), which is commonly used for deQuervain's stenosing tenosynovitis. In the ASHT SCS system, this splint is known as a thumb metacarpophalangeal (MCP) extension immobilization; type 2[3]. Type 2 refers to the two secondary joints covered (i.e., the wrist and thumb carpometacarpal [CMC] joint). The number in brackets, [3], refers to the total number of joints covered: the thumb MCP joint plus the wrist plus the thumb CMC joint).

DESIGN CATEGORIES

Orthotic devices can be classified by the support or forces provided to improve motion or function. Categories of splint design are as follows[6]:

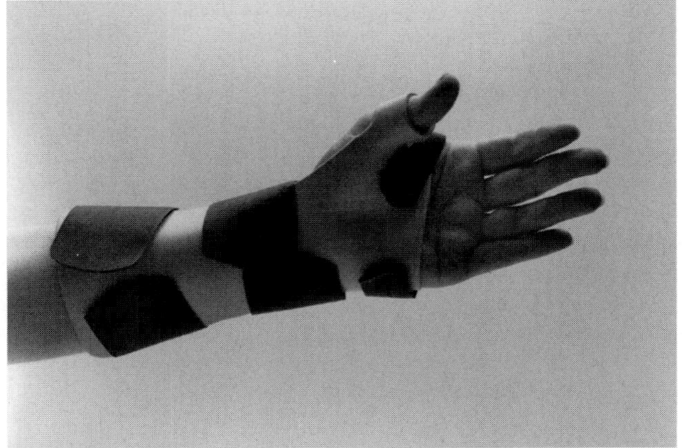

FIGURE 15–1. Forearm-based thumb spica splint used for deQuervain's stenosing tenosynovitis.

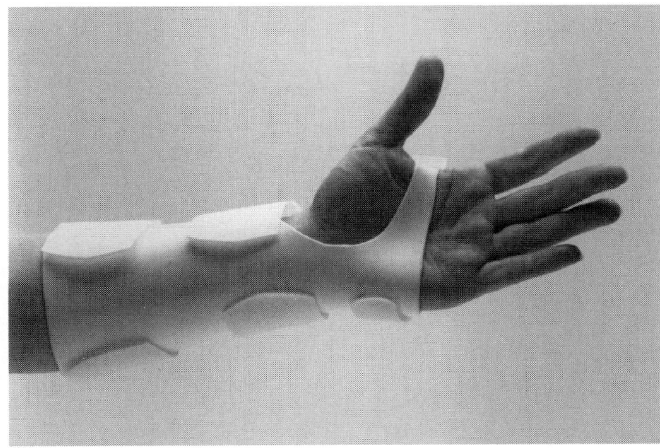

FIGURE 15–2. Wrist splint for carpal tunnel syndrome with the wrist in a position of 0 to 5 degrees of extension; distal palmar crease left free to allow for MCP motion.

Nonarticular: This type of splint provides support to a body part without crossing any joint and protects a bone or body part. For example, a humeral fracture splint provides circumferential support to the upper arm during fracture healing. Other examples are a sugar tong splint to immobilize a proximal radius fracture, or a shell splint to exert pressure over a healing scar to prevent hypertrophic scarring.

Static: This type of splint provides static support to hold a joint or joints stationary. For example, a volar wrist splint for acute carpal tunnel syndrome reduces motions and rests injured tissues (Fig. 15–2). Static splints can be used to protect healing structures, to decrease or prevent deformity, and to reduce tone in spastic muscles.

Serial static: This splint is also static but is periodically changed to alter the joint angle at which the splint is positioned. For example, a wrist splint is changed periodically to increase extension in a wrist with a flexion contracture after a wrist fracture. This serial repositioning provides a prolonged gentle stretch to involved structures, permitting a stiff joint to regain motion.

Static motion blocking: This type of splint permits motion in one direction but blocks motion in another. For example, a swan neck splint is designed to allow flexion but to block hyperextension of the proximal interphalangeal (PIP) joint. (See the section on Rheumatoid Arthritis.)

Static progressive: This type of splinting is the one most commonly used for regaining joint motion. Unlike the serial static splint, the orthosis is not remolded to increase joint motion; rather, it uses a static (nonelastic) line of pull that is tightened periodically to increase tissue length. One such device is similar in principle to a tuning screw on a guitar. The MERiT static progressive component[8] (available commercially) decreases the static line length as it is turned, thereby increasing the range of joint motion (Fig. 15–3). This type of splinting uses the principle advocated by Kenneth Flowers and Paul LaStayo,[3] placing the joint in a position of stretch to regain motion. As

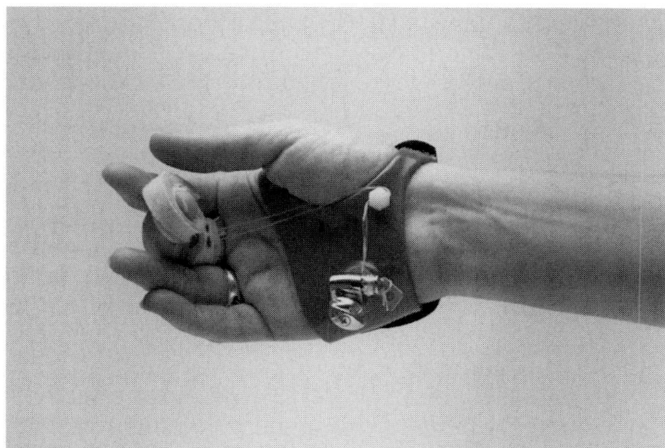

FIGURE 15–3. Static progressive flexion splint using a MERiT component. The MERiT component resembles a tuning screw on a guitar; tension increases on the static line as the MERiT is turned, thereby increasing the motion in the digit.

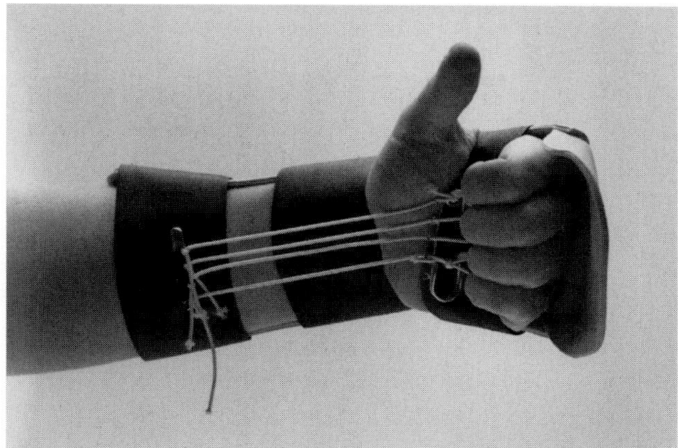

FIGURE 15–5. Kleinert splint used for postoperative care for patients with flexor tendon injuries. Allows for passive flexion, holding digits flexed at rest.

the joint begins to regain motion, the wearer can then increase the tension on the line. The joint is then statically held in this position using the principle of total end-range time (TERT), the length of time the joint is held at the end of its range: The longer the TERT, the more quickly a contracture will resolve.[7] This type of pull has been extremely effective in regaining joint motion, particularly in very stiff joints.

Dynamic: This type of splint provides an elastic force to regain motion. An example of such an orthosis is a Capener splint, which uses a spring coil assist to increase extension in a PIP joint with a mild contracture (Fig. 15–4).

Dynamic motion blocking: This type of splint allows certain motions but blocks others. It utilizes a passive, elastic line of pull in the desired direction but permits active motion in the opposite direction. An example is a Kleinert postoperative splint for flexor tendon repairs (Figs. 15–5 and 15–6). It passively pulls the finger into flexion with an elastic thread or rubber band, but allows active digital extension while parts of the splint block full extension of the MCP joint and the wrist.

Dynamic traction splints: This type of splint offers traction to a joint while allowing controlled motion. An example is a splint for an intra-articular fracture, which gives constant longitudinal traction while the joint is gently flexed and extended.

Tenodesis: This type of splint facilitates function in a hand that has lost motion due to nervous system injury. An example is a Rehabilitation Institute of Chicago (RIC) tenodesis splint (Fig. 15–7), which assists the patient with a C6 spinal cord injury to achieve a functional pinch. Active extension of the wrist produces, through tenodesis action, controlled passive flexion of the fingers against a static thumb post.

Continuous passive motion (CPM) orthoses: These are electrically powered devices that mechanically move joints through a desired range of motion. This keeps the joints supple and maintains articular, ligamentous, and tendinous structure mobility during the healing phases following injury or surgery.

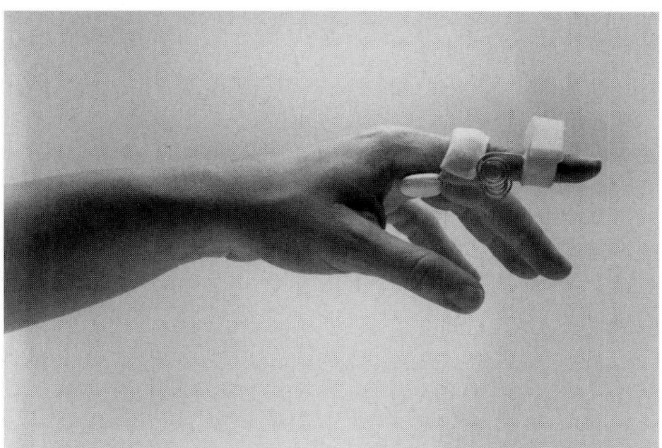

FIGURE 15–4. Capener splint for increasing extension in the PIP joint of the finger.

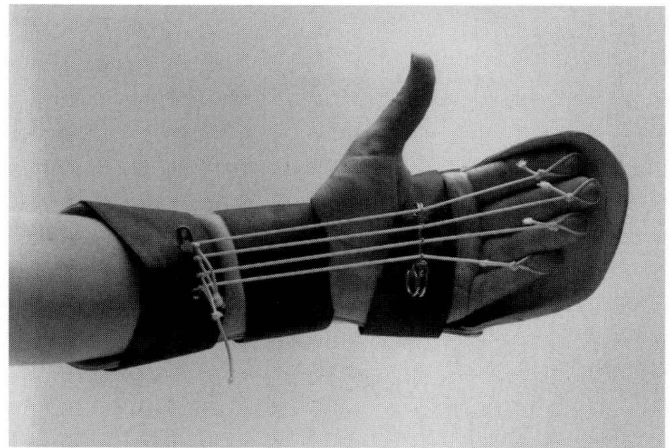

FIGURE 15–6. Kleinert splint used for postoperative care for patients with flexor tendon injuries. Allows for active extension within the constraints of the splint.

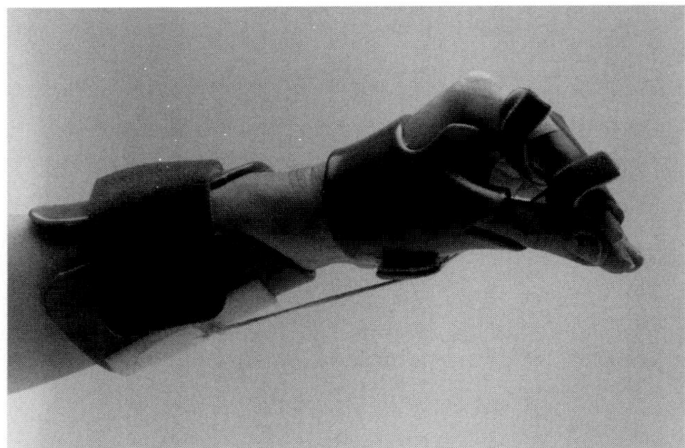

FIGURE 15–7. Rehabilitation Institute of Chicago (RIC) tenodesis splint, used for functional pinch during activities of daily living (ADL).

Adaptive/functional usage: These devices promote functional use of the upper limb with impairment due to weakness, paralysis, or loss of a body part. An example is the universal cuff, which encompasses the hand and holds various small items such as a fork, a pen, or a toothbrush (Fig. 15–8). This cuff allows patients to manipulate these items, known as activities-of-daily-living (ADL) tools, and gives them some degree of independence.

BIOMECHANICAL CONSIDERATIONS

Health care personnel involved in the fabrication and application of an orthotic device need a good understanding of biomechanics and anatomy as well as the physiological response to tissue healing. They also need technical and creative skills—skills that allow them to design and fabricate orthotic devices that win patient acceptance and meet treatment goals. Most upper limb splinting is performed by occupational therapists (OTR) and certified hand therapists (CHT), but is also done by physical therapists (RPT) and orthotists (CO). The physician ordering these devices needs to comprehend the technical factors involved in fabrication and fitting. Some of these are listed here.

1. When increasing joint range of motion with splinting, the angle of pull needs to be perpendicular to the bony axis that is being mobilized. If this is not taken into account, forces on the skin and underlying structures can be sufficient to cause injury through excessive pressure on the skin and deforming stresses on the underlying healing structures.
2. Wrist position is an important consideration in the design of a splint.[6] Power grasp is most effectively achieved when the wrist is extended slightly. When writing, most right-handed individuals extend the wrist; however, many left-handed individuals place their wrists in slight flexion. All of these examples indicate that individual considerations of wrist position can be paramount in fabricating a wrist orthosis.
3. To maintain tissue length through static positioning, one needs to consider the ligamentous structures involved, the anatomic angle of pull on structures, and the positions that may produce deformity. For example, when the hand is made nonfunctional after a dorsal burn, the metacarpophalangeal (MCP) joints tend toward hyperextension. This position alters the tension on the collateral ligaments of the MCP joints and puts them at risk of shortening, with subsequent loss of full flexion. In such a case, it is imperative to place the MCP joints in full flexion and the IP joints in extension. The wrist should also be placed in slight extension to maintain flexor tendon length and to improve hand function (Fig. 15–9).
4. A study by Flowers and LaStayo[2] demonstrated the TERT principle: that is, the improvement in range of motion is directly proportional to the length of time a joint is held at its end range. This principle is used with static progressive splinting, as noted previously. They also emphasize that the

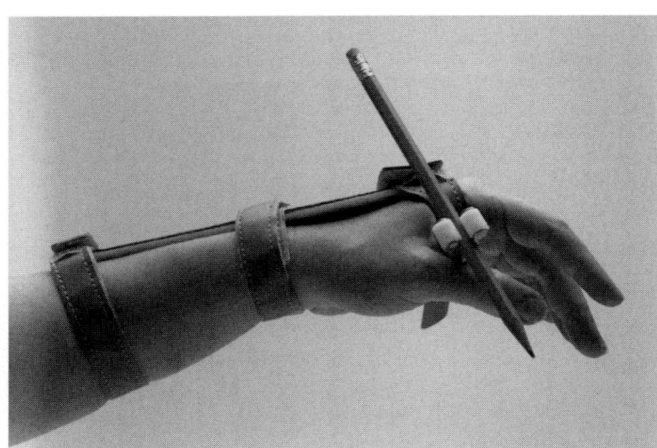

FIGURE 15–8. Universal cuff/splint used to assist in using ADL tools.

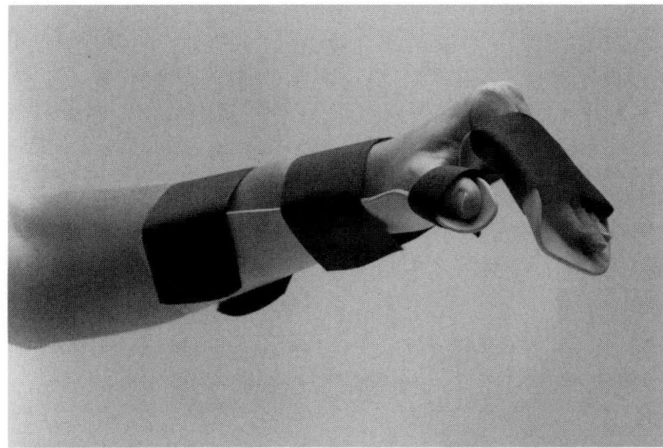

FIGURE 15–9. Splint used to position the hand and wrist, keeping the MCP joints flexed and the IP joints extended with the wrist in slight extension. Often used with burn patients.

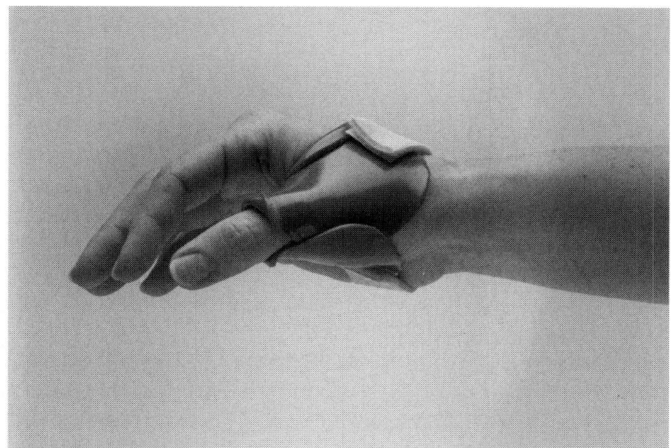

FIGURE 15–10. Hand-based thumb spica splint used to limit motion in the MCP and CMC joints of the thumb.

clinically safe amount of force covers a very narrow range.

5. When making a splint, the therapist should be sure to fabricate it in a position that enhances prehension and does not force the thumb into a position of extension and radial abduction. This position causes the rest of the arm to compensate for poor thumb positioning. To decrease the stresses on the hand and thumb, built-up pens and pencils can be used for improved function, especially with a thumb spica splint (Fig. 15–10). Thumb position is most often compromised in low median and ulnar nerve injuries, which leave the patient with no or weakened ability to place the thumb in opposition and palmar abduction.
6. Splints designed to encompass the hand must preserve both longitudinal and transverse arches. The distal palmar crease must not be blocked if full MCP flexion is desired (see Fig. 15–2).
7. In designing dynamic or static progressive hand splints to improve digital flexion, the direction of pull should be toward the scaphoid bone on the palmar surface to mimic the angle noted in the healthy hand.[8] The angle of pull across the palm is oblique, not straight down toward the wrist. This is most apparent when the fingers are flexed individually and less pronounced when flexed all at once.
8. The mobility of the ulnar two digits is critical to the power grasp of the hand. The radial three digits are used for pinch and prehension. Persons designing splints should keep both these principles in mind during splint fabrication.
9. Active and passive range of motion measurements need to be assessed to determine the mechanics of the joint. Joint torque angle measurements can be used to determine whether or not (1) a splint is needed, (2) conservative treatment would be beneficial, or (3) surgery is indicated. Torque angle measurement assesses what occurs at the joint as the force is applied at a given distance from the joint axis. This measurement gives the examiner an understanding of whether the joint has a "soft end feel" (more motion with a given force), or a "hard end feel" (little or no motion with the same force).

DIAGNOSTIC CATEGORIES AND SPLINT EXAMPLES

We have seen that orthotic devices are applied primarily to protect tissue, to correct deformity, or to enhance function. In this section, we discuss common conditions for which orthotic intervention is appropriate. We give a brief overview of the features of specific diagnoses, followed by the type of splint(s) commonly indicated for each diagnosis. This is not, however, an all-inclusive list. For a more comprehensive overview of upper limb orthotic devices, see texts that are devoted entirely to splinting or other references at the end of this chapter.[1, 3, 4, 6, 7, 10]

Musculoskeletal Conditions

Tendinitis, Tenosynovitis, and Enthesopathy

Tendinitis (inflammation of the tendon), tenosynovitis (inflammation of the tendon sheaths), and enthesopathy (inflammation at a muscle or tendon origin or insertion) can all result from excessive repetitive movement or unphysiological stress. In the upper limb the tendons most commonly involved are the wrist extensors or the abductor pollicus longus (APL) and extensor pollicus brevis (EPB) muscles of the thumb, commonly called deQuervain's stenosing tenosynovitis. The goal of splints for these conditions is to immobilize the affected structures in order to facilitate healing and decrease inflammation. The thumb spica splint, forearm-based, immobilizes the wrist, the carpometacarpal (CMC) joint, and the MCP joint of the thumb; the interphalangeal (IP) joint of the thumb does not need fixation because the affected tendons do not move this joint (see Fig. 15–1).

Lateral epicondylitis is the most common enthesopathy of the upper limb. It can be treated by a tennis elbow orthosis (Fig. 15–11). This is a forearm band that

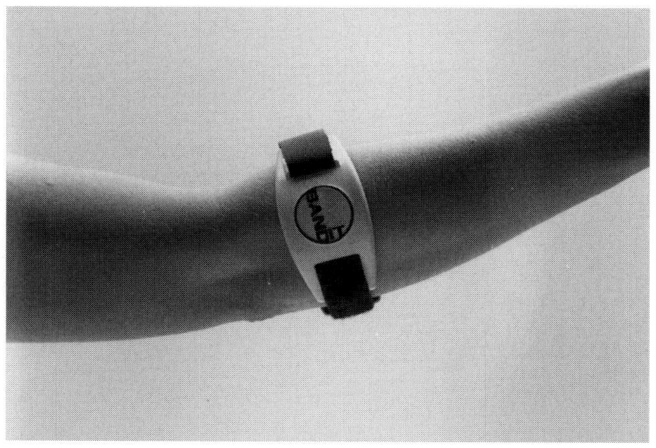

FIGURE 15–11. BAND-IT brace by Pro Band Sports Industries, Inc. Used for lateral epicondylitis.

changes the lever arm against which the wrist extensors pull; in essence, it puts the origin of the extensor muscles at rest and decreases the microtrauma from overuse. This orthotic device, placed approximately two fingerbreadths below the lateral epicondyle, is a firm strap against which the extensors press against when contracting. A similar brace is used for medial epicondylitis (also known as golfer's elbow; see Chapter 38).

Trigger finger describes a snapping sensation in the volar surface of the digits on release of grasp. It is usually a result of trauma to the flexor tendon sheath of the fingers or thumb, producing thickened tendinous sheaths and restriction of motion. In advanced trigger finger the digit can become "locked" in flexion. This can be due to an intense acute episode or repetitive trauma. The goal in this condition is to halt the repetitive motion temporarily to allow for healing. This is usually achieved by immobilization, but patients should have functional use of the hand while the affected digit is immobilized (Fig. 15–12). The splint for trigger finger covers the proximal phalanx and the MCP joint of the involved digit. This splint decreases the tendinous excursion through the first annular pulley, at the base of the MCP joint, and allows the inflamed structures to rest.

Sprains

Sprains are defined as momentary subluxations with spontaneous reduction that result in torn ligamentous structures. Patients experience pain, swelling, and decreased function. This situation requires joint immobilization in a position of function to allow for healing as well as functional use. Common sprains include dislocation of the IP and MCP joints caused by hyperextension injuries—often seen in sports injuries (see Chapter 44). For a first- or second-degree ligamentous tear, the goal is to protect and rest the area by applying functional splinting. The goal for a third-degree tear is to fully immobilize and approximate the ligaments.

Common splints used for digital sprains are finger extension splints that hold the PIP joint in extension but allow flexion of the distal interphalangeal (DIP) joint. This action keeps the oblique retinacular ligament and the terminal extensor tendon lengthened, preventing boutonnière deformities during healing. Ulnar collateral ligamentous injuries at the MCP joint of the thumb are treated with a hand-based thumb spica splint, producing immobilization during the healing phase (see Fig. 15–10). Wrist splints that place the wrist in slight extension are used for wrist sprains. For mild sprains, splints with no spline (metal bar insert) permit some motion, but avoid creating significant stiffness. They also keep available range to about 40 degrees of total motion (Fig. 15–13). Elbow neoprene sleeves are helpful for mild sprains at the elbow because they limit the extremes of range, but permit limited function.

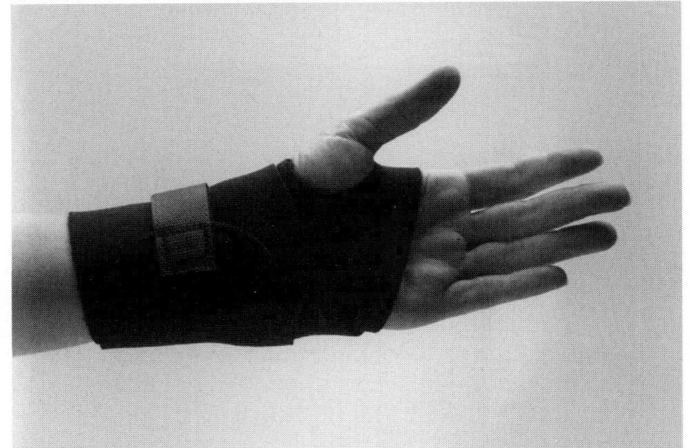

FIGURE 15–13. Neoprene splint used for wrist sprains or arthritis.

Fractures

Most major fractures need total immobilization, requiring casting and/or surgical intervention. Some fractures, however, do not need total immobilization and can be treated with orthotic devices (Fig. 15–14). These devices should immobilize the body part or the joint sufficient to promote healing, while also optimizing function. An example of such an orthotic device is the humeral fracture brace, which has a circumferential design to hold healing bony parts in alignment. This ortho-

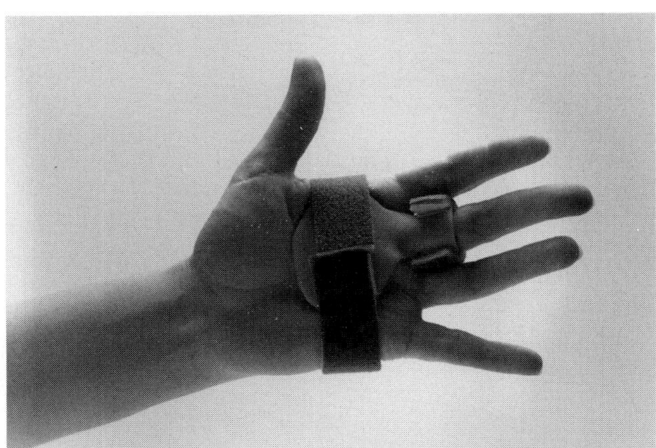

FIGURE 15–12. Trigger finger splint used for conservative treatment.

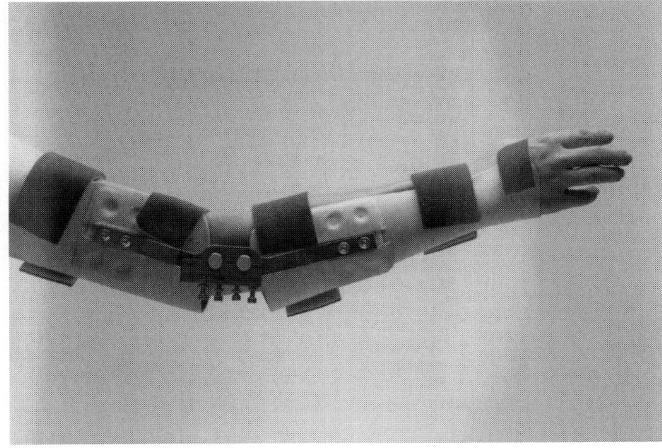

FIGURE 15–14. Hinged elbow splint with stops to limit extremes of motion during the rehabilitation phase after a fracture.

sis permits motion of the elbow, forearm, and hand, which is desirable because rigid arm immobilization can lead to the development of edema and resultant joint stiffness. Other examples are the traction-type splints that allow for very controlled motion during the healing phase of intra-articular finger fractures treated with pinning. Joint movement has been credited with enhancing cartilage nutrition and preventing intra-articular adhesions.[6]

Arthritis

Osteoarthritis is the most common disease affecting the joints in the upper limb. Joint diseases of the hand and wrist have the most significant impact upon function. Chronic inflammation often exposes these digital joints to further risk of deformity and injury. Orthotic devices can provide functional positioning to prevent further deformity and loss of use in arthritic diseases as well as protecting the joints from further injury.

Rheumatoid Arthritis

Rheumatoid arthritis is a chronic inflammatory disease that primarily affects synovial joints. The joints most frequently affected in the upper limb are the wrist, MCP, and PIP joints. Deformities include subluxation and ulnar deviation at the MCP joints, subluxation and radial deviation at the wrist, and swan-neck deformity and boutonnière deformity of the fingers. These deformities usually progress, especially if no attempt is made to rest and protect the affected joints from overuse.

Several options are available for splinting the rheumatoid hand. Ulnar deviation splints that pull the MCP joints toward radial deviation and increase the functional use of the hand are now lightweight and permit full MCP joint motion in flexion and extension. Wrist splints that provide light support for the wrist are usually tolerated very well (see Fig. 15–13). Swan neck and boutonnière splints can be made from thermoplastics, but are often bulky and cosmetically unpleasing. Very thin Siris Silver Ring Splints[12] are now available for digital deformities (Figs. 15–15 and 15–16). Made of sterling silver, these splints are cosmetically similar to jewelry; they provide excellent improvement in function and are well tolerated. The Silver Ring Splint Company[13] makes a wide variety of splints for the finger and thumb joints; each is individually tailored to exact specifications and reasonably priced. The swan neck splint allows for flexion of the digit but blocks hyperextension. The boutonnière splint holds the DIP or PIP joint in extension.

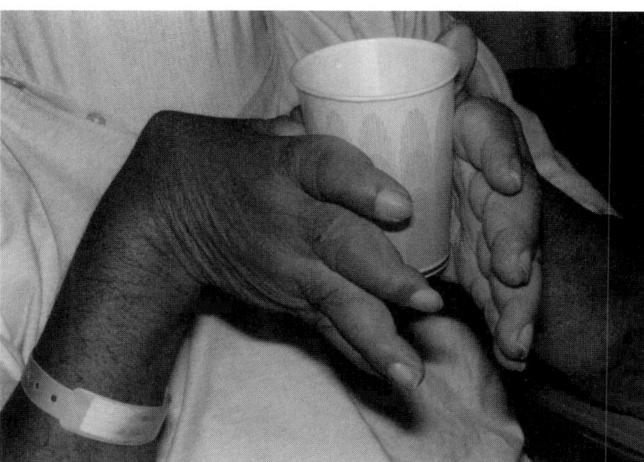

FIGURE 15–15. Swan neck deformities at the PIP joints. The patient is holding a cup without the aid of splints. (Courtesy of Silver Ring Splint Company.)

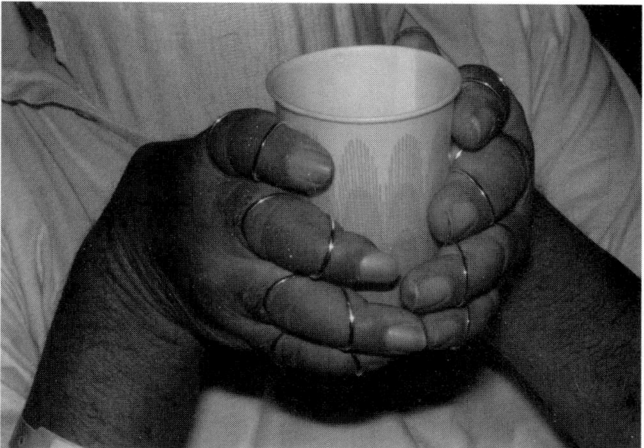

FIGURE 15–16. Siris Swan Neck Splints, which greatly enhance function of the digits for activities of daily living. The patient is holding a cup with the aid of these splints. (Courtesy of Silver Ring Splint Company.)

Osteoarthritis

Osteoarthritis, the most common form of arthritis, is primarily a disease of cartilage, not of the synovium. In the upper limb, it most commonly involves the carpometacarpal (CMC) joint of the thumb. A thumb spica hand-based (Fig. 15–10) or forearm-based (Fig. 15–1) splint can be prescribed for CMC joint osteoarthritis. By limiting motion at the base of the thumb, the splint decreases pain, especially with pinching-type activities.

Neuromuscular Conditions

Nerve Injuries

In a peripheral nerve injury, which can affect a nerve anywhere along its course, the level of injury determines the extent of deficit incurred. For example, in a distal median nerve injury, the type of deformity incurred is usually described as a simian hand and the function most affected is thumb abduction and opposition (Fig. 15–17). The goal of an orthotic device is to try to restore this function. The splint usually has a spring coil design holding the MCP joints in slight flexion but permitting MCP extension (Fig. 15–18). This splint also has a portion to position the thumb in palmar abduction. Distal median nerve palsy splints assist in flexion of all the MCP joints and thumb palmar abduction.

With radial nerve injuries distal to the humeral spiral groove, the most common presenting condition is wrist drop and finger drop. The goal of an orthotic device is to enhance wrist and finger extension. A radial nerve

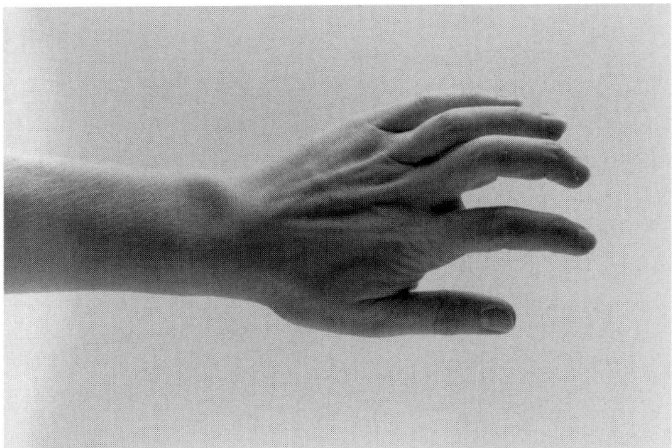

FIGURE 15–17. Simian hand, as seen in low combined median and ulnar nerve injuries.

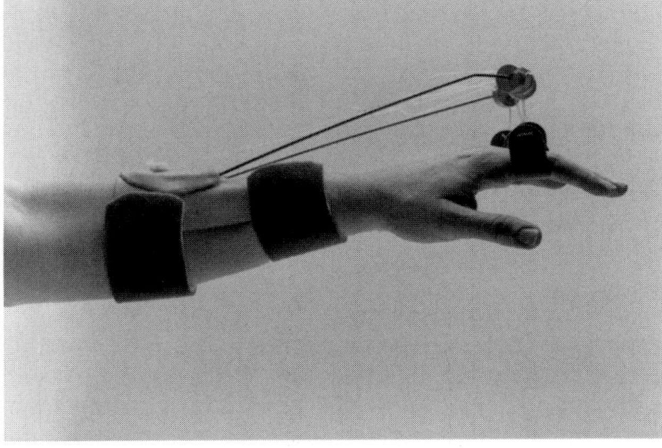

FIGURE 15–19. Radial nerve palsy splint. Assists with wrist and digit extension to improve functional use of the hand.

palsy splint is forearm-based with an outrigger that holds the wrist, fingers, and thumb in extension and allows for flexion of the digits (Fig. 15–19).

With a proximal ulnar nerve injury, the patient has what is called a "benediction hand," featuring hyperextension of the fourth and fifth MCP joints and flexion of the PIP joints due to the loss of balance between the extrinsic and intrinsic hand muscles. The goal with orthotic devices is to prevent fixed deformity of the fourth and fifth MP joints and improve function. An ulnar nerve palsy splint holds the MCP joints of the fourth and fifth fingers in slight flexion by a spring coil or figure of eight splint design. The spring coil design assists MCP flexion and permits extension of the MCP joints but blocks hyperextension (Fig. 15–20). This can also be accomplished by using a static splint that prevents hyperextension of the MCP joints of the fourth and fifth digits with the use of a "lumbrical bar."

Incomplete nerve injuries can be caused by compression without producing complete paralysis as, for example, median nerve injury from carpal tunnel syndrome. This can be due to an overuse syndrome producing an inflammatory response in the synovium surrounding the flexor tendons at the wrist causing decreased blood supply to the median nerve. The purpose of the splint is to immobilize the wrist to minimize swelling from overuse of the tendons. Complete resolution of this syndrome can occur if wrist orthoses are applied early when symptoms first appear. The splint is molded to the patient from a thermoplastic that offers excellent conformity to hold the wrist in 0 to 5 degrees of extension. Its common name, wrist cock-up splint, is misleading and should be avoided because this name implies that the wrist should be placed in extension (see Fig. 15–2). The patient should be instructed to reduce stresses at the wrist, and to wear the splint all night. Often the patient is instructed to wear it as much as possible during the day as well. The wearing schedule is controversial, however; most agree that it should be worn at night, but encouragement of daytime wear varies from source to source.[4]

A word of caution is in order for many prefabricated wrist splints. Many of these splints have a metal spline formed to hold the wrist at a 45-degree angle of exten-

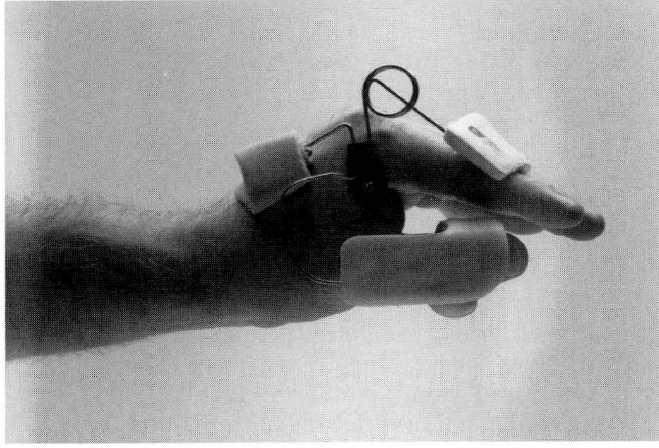

FIGURE 15–18. LMB MP Flexion Spring with Dynamic Thumb Abduction Spring Splint. Used for median nerve palsy to provide opposition of the thumb and flexion of the MCP joints.

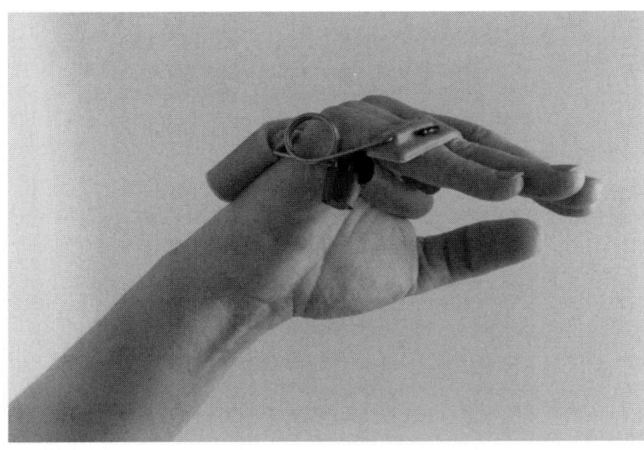

FIGURE 15–20. Ulnar nerve splint. Allows extension but blocks hyperextension of the MCP joints of the ring and small fingers.

sion (Fig. 15–21). This angle far exceeds the recommended 0 to 5 degrees of extension needed to decrease pressure in the carpal tunnel. Patients need to be instructed to remove the metal spline, flatten it, and then replace it in the fabric covering. Usually this splint should be worn for 4 to 6 weeks, with a gradual weaning from the splint, as well as a gradual return to activity with workstation modifications.

Long arm splints hold the elbow in 45 degrees of flexion, the forearm in neutral, and the wrist in 0 to 5 degrees of extension with thumb and fingers free; these splints are helpful with cubital tunnel syndrome (compression of the ulnar nerve at the elbow).

In patients with multiple nerve injuries or brachial plexopathy with essentially a flail arm, the goal with orthotic devices is to provide some functional use. One type of orthosis is in the form of an exoskeleton on the arm, similar to a prosthesis; this device uses a shoulder harness with scapular activation to produce elbow function, similar to scapular action in an above-elbow prosthesis.[3]

Brain Injury and Stroke

Depending on the area of brain injury and ensuing deficits, particularly an increase or decrease in muscle tone, orthotic devices should be designed to prevent deformities and to help adjust muscle tone. Resting and positioning orthotic devices are also necessary to prevent such complications as distal edema, joint subluxation, and contracture formation. In upper limb paralysis, a resting hand splint is commonly used to position the wrist in slight extension, the MCP joints in slight flexion, and the IP joints in extension. The thumb is supported in a position between palmar and radial abduction. Full support of the first CMC joint prevents ligamentous stresses on the thumb, especially in the insensate hand. This thumb position also utilizes the reflex inhibiting posture, which decreases tone in the hand (Fig. 15–22).

A mobile arm support can be used to enhance function for patients with proximal upper limb weakness, especially when the weakness is profound and the outlook for recovery is guarded. A mobile arm support is particularly helpful when performing such ADL (activities of daily living) tasks as eating and grooming.

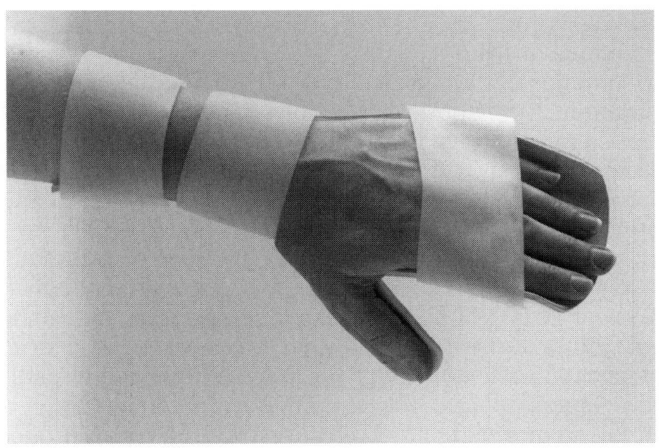

FIGURE 15–22. Resting hand splint.

Many types of slings are available for patients with decreased tone of the upper limb (Fig. 15–23). Decreased tone can result in shoulder subluxation, and these slings can help reduce the degree of this deformity. Unfortunately, nothing—no sling, no arm tray attached to a wheelchair—has been found to correct shoulder subluxation completely. But an overhead sling device can help increase the function of weakened shoulder and scapular musculature.

Spinal Cord Injury

In patients with spinal cord injury (SCI), orthotic devices are needed to enhance function and/or help with positioning. The type of such devices depends on the level of injury and the extent of neurological compromise. With spinal cord injury at C_1-C_3 level, the goal is to prevent contractures and hold the wrist and digits in a position of function with a resting hand splint (see Fig. 15–22). In a C_4 level injury, the goal is to use the available shoulder strength, providing a mobile arm support to enhance function as previously described. In a

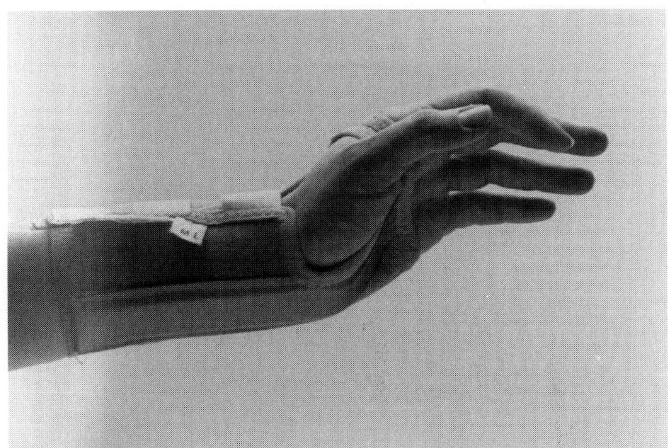

FIGURE 15–21. Commercially available wrist splint. The preset angle, which may be appropriate in some patients with wrist sprains, far exceeds that recommended for the treatment of acute carpal tunnel syndrome.

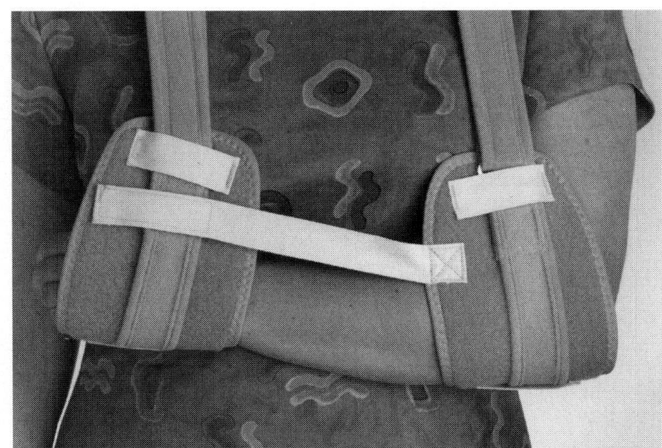

FIGURE 15–23. Rolyan Figure-of-8 sling used for reducing subluxation of the shoulder joint in a patient with hemiplegia.

C_5 level injury, the goal is to statically position the wrist in extension with a ratchet-type hinged orthotic device to hold devices and utilize the shoulder musculature for function. An orthotic device for a C_6 tetraplegic patient can enhance finger flexion using a tenodesis flexion effect from wrist extension. For example, a RIC tenodesis splint molded from thermoplastic materials has several positioning components (see Fig. 15–7). A thumb post component positions the thumb in palmar abduction. A dorsal finger piece component, which is attached with a static line to a volar forearm component, holds the PIP joints of the index and long fingers in slight flexion. When the patient extends the wrist, the static line pulls the fingers toward the thumb post. This produces a three-point pinch, allowing the patient to grasp on object. When the patient flexes the wrist, the fingers extend passively, releasing the object. The degree of pinch varies, depending on the strength of the wrist extensors and the degree of finger flexion, extension, and opposition. This custom-made thermoplastic tenodesis device is mainly used in training and practice. If a patient finds the device useful, a light metal custom-made tenodesis orthosis achieves better functional restoration.

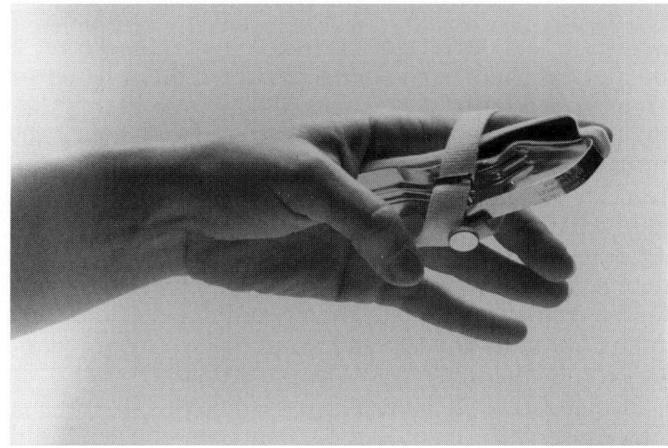

FIGURE 15–25. Joint Jack is a static progressive splint used to increase extension in the PIP joint.

Other Injuries

Post-Surgical and Post-Injury Orthosis

Many types of splints have been developed to regain motion in stiff joints. Examples of such splints include: (1) dynamic elbow flexion and extension splints during rehabilitation after upper arm or elbow fracture (see Fig. 15–14); (2) dynamic wrist flexion and extension after a Colles fracture; and (3) dynamic finger flexion (Fig. 15–24) and extension splints for stiffness after crush injuries to the hand. Similar splints can be fabricated using a static progressive approach. Joints that have "soft end feel" do well with dynamic splints; but for those with a "hard end feel," a static progressive approach is typically better. Examples of static progressive splints are the Joint Jack (Fig. 15–25) or cinch straps, and splints for PIP and DIP joint contractures using the MERiT components (see Fig. 15–3). Selection of forearm- or hand-based splints is determined by the need for stabilization. In general, the goal is to immobilize as few joints as feasible. Forearm pronation/supination splints using both dynamic and static features such as the Collelo splint are very helpful in regaining motion after fractures of the radius and ulna[3] (Fig. 15–26).

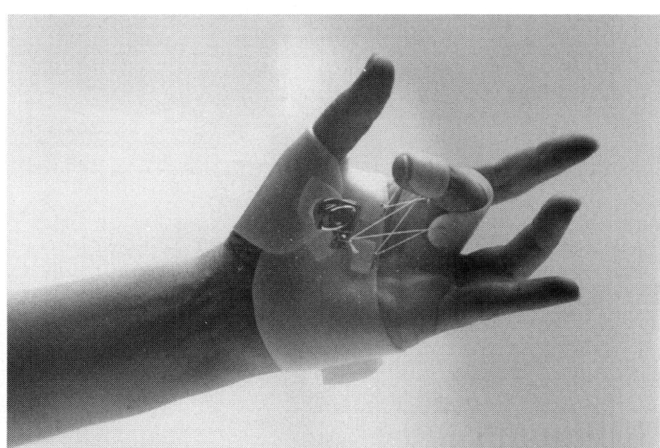

FIGURE 15–24. Finger flexion splint used to increase range of motion in the digit, and can be static or dynamic.

Following repair of tendon injuries, several splint designs are currently employed. Often the type of surgical procedure or injury level dictates the type of splint used, so that the splints cannot be used interchangeably. For flexor tendon repair, the Kleinert and Duran are common. The Kleinert splint (see Figs. 15–5 and 15–6) features dynamic traction into flexion but allows active digit extension within the constraints of the splint; the Duran splint statically positions the wrist and MCP joints in flexion and the IP joints in extension (Fig.

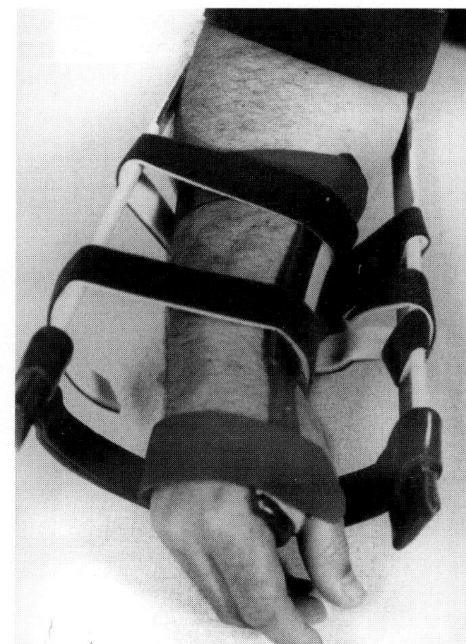

FIGURE 15–26. Dynamic Pronation/Supination splint, Collelo design, used to increase motion in the forearm.

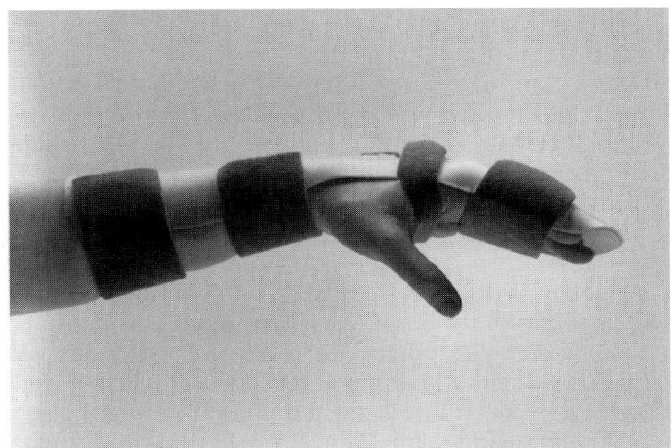

FIGURE 15–27. Duran flexor tendon repair splint used for postoperative care.

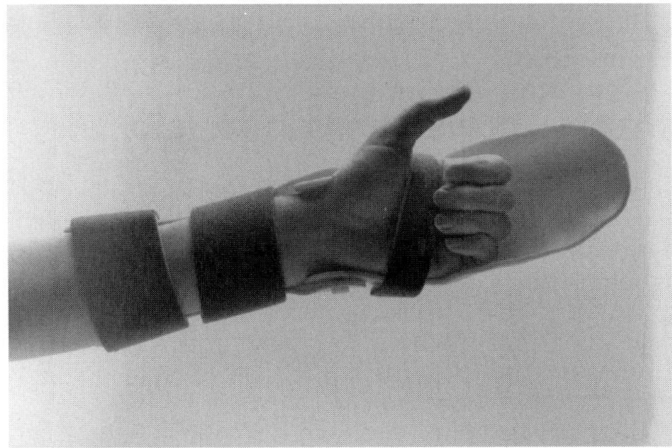

FIGURE 15–29. Indiana protocol postoperative flexor tendon splint; demonstration of passive flexion exercises.

15–27). The Indiana protocol splint can also be used (Figs. 15–28 and 15–29). This splint, which adds to the above components a tenodesis-type action splint for a specific, active assisted range of motion exercises, can be used only if a specific surgical suture technique has been utilized.

The form of extensor tendon repair splints depends on the level of injury. A mallet finger injury can require only a Stax splint—a static splint holding the DIP joint in full extension. A more proximal injury, however, needs a splint that holds the wrist statically in extension with dynamic extension of MCP and IP joints. Such a splint permits active flexion of the MCP joints within the constraints of the splint to an angle of approximately 30 degrees. Injuries to the thumb flexor or extensor tendons require more specific splinting, again dependent upon the level of the injury.

Postoperative joint replacements for the PIP, DIP, or the MCP joints of the hand require very specific splints that promote healing or encapsulation of the joints while preserving ROM during the healing phases (Fig. 15–30).

Burns

Burn patients typically prefer an adducted and flexed position of the upper limbs to maintain comfort, but this preference can lead to loss of functional range of motion. In this case, the splint acts as a preventative—it prevents contractures and deformities from developing. This is especially important when the patient cannot voluntarily maintain the range or when soft tissues underlying the skin are exposed. With tendon exposure, the splint plays a more protective role. It is important to monitor these patients frequently and reassess the needs for splinting.

After burn injuries, body parts should be positioned to prevent the tendency toward known deformities. For example, in burns of the dorsal surface of the hand, the wrist is kept in slight extension, the MCP joints in 60 to 70 degrees of flexion, the PIP and DIP joints in full extension, and the thumb between radial abduction and extension (see Fig. 15–9). To combat a tendency for shoulder adduction deformity after axillary burns, the shoulder should be held in abduction with an airplane splint. The tendency toward hypertrophic scarring after a burn is addressed with a selection of compression

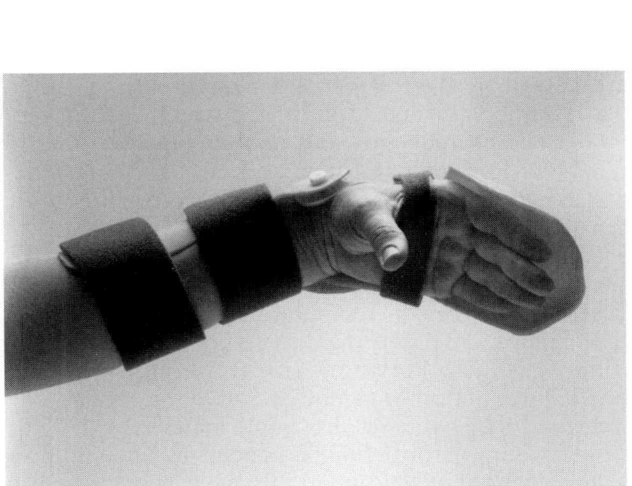

FIGURE 15–28. Indiana protocol postoperative flexor tendon splint; tenodesis exercises.

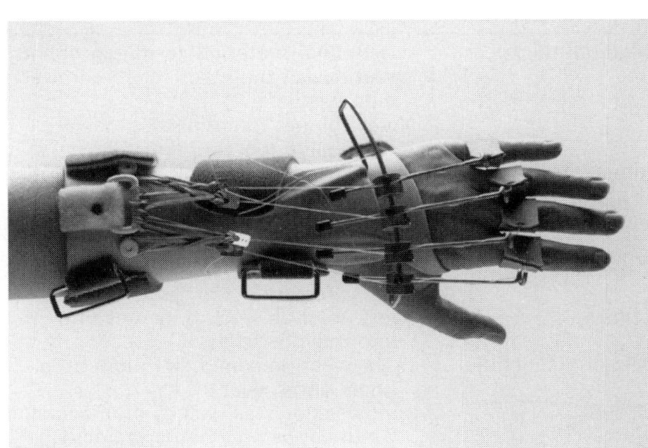

FIGURE 15–30. MCP arthroplasty postoperative splint; positions fingers in extension with a slight radial pull.

garments, elastomer molds, facial splints, shell splints, and silicone gel sheeting.

SPECIAL CONSIDERATIONS

Splints can be perfectly designed and skillfully fabricated. But an unworn splint, however ingenious, is a useless splint. The more choices and input patients have in splint design, the more compliant they will be with splint wear. It is important, then, to ask about the patient's goals for splinting and function before choosing a splint design. (See Table 15–2 for a list of points to consider for optimization of splint use.)

Cosmesis is often a problem for patients—they care about the way a splint will look. To assure splint wear, the splint has to be as cosmetically acceptable as possible. Patients should have every opportunity to assist in choosing design and appearance. Patients often have very good ideas about the design of a splint and suggest good ways to strap it into place. They may also have color preferences. Low-temperature thermoplastic materials are now available in a wide range of colors. The person's age or occupation may be factors. For example, a youthful patient who works in an amusement park might like a hot pink splint, while an older autoworker might prefer a black one. Adolescents should be given as much freedom as possible, encouraged to "decorate" their splints if they so desire, as long as the splint mechanics are not altered.

Comfort is also important. The thinner the materials used and the more care the therapist takes in making a close, comfortable fit, the better the acceptance of the splint. For example, areas around bony prominences need to be "popped" out to prevent pressure, while edges and joints might need to be padded to reduce skin irritation. Arthritic patients who have been taking corticosteroids for long periods of time often have fragile skin, so their splints should be padded throughout. Stockinette worn under splints also helps, particularly with perspiration in warmer weather.

TABLE 15–2 Points to Consider for Optimization of Splint Use

Material thickness	Use thinner materials for finger splints and thicker materials for forearm and elbow splints *Note:* Thinner materials cool faster, decreasing working time
Function	Consider patient's goals and functional needs
Patient input	Elicit patient's ideas, preferences, and goals
Cosmesis	Consider patient's age, occupation, and other factors
Color	Allow color choices to increase to improve cosmesis
Wearing schedule	Tailor wearing schedule to meet the goals of the splint
Design	Consider goals as well as biomechanics when choosing whether a splint should be static, static progressive, dynamic, etc.

The wearing schedule depends upon the goals you have for the splint and the patient's tolerance for wear. Suppose, for instance, you have a head-injured patient who is "storming"—sweating excessively and combative. In that case, a resting hand splint for positioning might be worn just 30 minutes on and 3 hours off. In contrast, a stroke patient with mild spasticity could wear a resting hand splint 2 hours on and 2 hours off during the day and keep it on all night. Static progressive splint wear depends upon tissue response to gentle stretching. The stretch should be perceived as mild, and it should never awaken the patient at night. In a patient with both flexion and extension splinting needs, the flexion splint can be worn 1 hour on, 2 hours off during the day, and the extension splint can be worn at night. Patients tolerate the splint better and spend more daytime with the splint off so they can do hand exercises.

A resting hand splint for positioning is often indicated when edema is present. But a splint can also induce edema—the result of an inflammatory response due to an overly aggressive stretch—particularly in a patient with increased tone. Splint design needs to address this possibility; often, special strapping techniques can lessen the response. Other tissue responses are also possible. Blueness or redness of the digits when wearing a splint tells the observer that an overly aggressive stretch is being applied to the shortened neurovascular bundles. These structures sometimes change in length due to the joint contracture, in which case splint tension must be decreased and the contracture stretch should be less aggressive.

Splint prescriptions should explain the diagnosis or problem to be addressed. A description of the function or motion desired helps to alleviate confusion. It can also open up discussion with the therapist, physician, and patient regarding the best design to meet agreed-upon goals. Finally, a good description can clarify misunderstandings arising from conflicting naming systems (see Table 15–1).

ORTHOTIC MATERIALS

Most splinting materials are low-temperature thermoplastics, some of which are listed in Table 15–3. Many are known by their trademark names, such as Orthoplast, Aquaplast, and Orfit.[9, 13] Low-temperature thermoplastics become soft and pliable when exposed to relatively low temperatures, and can be shaped in a water bath at 180°F. High-temperature thermoplastics are more durable, but require oven heating (up to 350°F) and placement over a mold to achieve the desired shape. All splinting materials have certain characteristics determined by the temperature and material properties. Some, like Ezeform,[13] are very rigid when cool while some, like Polyform,[13] are very drapeable when warm. Firm materials can be desirable for patients with increased tone, whereas drapeable materials can be desirable when conformability is needed, as when splinting a finger. Some plastic materials have a great deal of "memory." This means they return to their original shape when reheated. This characteristic can help con-

TABLE 15–3 Commonly Used Low-Temperature Thermoplastic Materials for Splint Fabrication

Material Name	Resistance to Stretch	Memory	Rigidity	Surface Finish	Typical Splint Uses
Aquaplast	Minimal	100%	Moderate	Marks with firm pressure	Wrist splint, thumb spica splint, finger splints
Ezeform	Maximum	Moderate	Maximal	Resists fingerprints	Resting hand splint, pronation/supination splint
Orfit	Moderate	100%	Moderate	Resists fingerprints	Thumb spica splints
Prism	Minimal	100%	Moderate; withstands application of dynamic components	Resists fingerprints	Wrist splint, thumb spica splint, flexor tendon splints (e.g., Duran and Kleinert)
Orthoplast	Moderate	Poor	Maximal	Resists fingerprints	Resting hand splint, humeral fracture brace
Polyform	Minimal	Maximal	Poor	Marks easily	Mallet finger splints, dynamic finger splints

trol costs, especially those incurred when providing serial static splinting.

Therapists use heat guns and water baths to heat thermoplastic materials to mold for splint fabrication. Velcro[9] straps are almost universally used to hold orthotic devices in place. There are multiple attachments available to add to the splint base to achieve particular goals; these include outriggers from wire, line guides to position the line of pull, and loops or slings to pull a digit into the desired position. Most often, the choices of attachments are based upon the therapist's experience with the materials, training, or continuing education.

SUMMARY

This chapter has provided guidelines concerning the principles and indications for upper limb orthotic devices as well as various classification systems and descriptions of design categories. To fabricate an orthosis, a sound understanding of the anatomy, biomechanics, and tissue physiology of the upper limb is required. Persons prescribing upper limb orthotic devices should have a thorough knowledge of the musculoskeletal and neurological conditions amenable to treatment by orthoses; they must also understand additional measures of treatment such as exercise therapy and be alert to surgical indications.

The most important principle in prescription of orthotic devices is gaining cooperation of the patient. Through attention and concern by the physician and therapist, the patient must see the benefit of the orthosis. It also must fit comfortably and be cosmetically appealing. All involved must have the same goals and purpose for the device, or it will end up in a closet soon after it has been fitted.

As we continue to learn more about the biomechanics of the hand, we better understand how to redress externally the internal imbalance caused by disease and injury. Keeping the internal dynamics of the hand in mind, we find that splinting is the most efficient and effective way to effect this mechanical rebalance.[4]

REFERENCES

1. American Society of Hand Therapists (ASHT), Splint Nomenclature Task Force: Splint Classification System. Garner, NC, ASHT, 1991.
2. Flowers KR, LaStayo P: Effect of total end range time. J Hand Ther 1989; 2:71.
3. Hunter JM, Mackin EJ, Callahan AD: Rehabilitation of the Hand: Surgery and Therapy, ed 3. St Louis, Mosby, 1990.
4. Hunter JM, Mackin EJ, Callahan AD: Rehabilitation of the Hand: Surgery and Therapy, ed 4. St Louis, Mosby, 1995.
5. Joint-Jack Company. Joint Jack is a trademark of the Joint-Jack Company.
6. McKee P, Morgan L: Orthotics in Rehabilitation, Splinting the Hand and Body. Philadelphia, FA Davis, 1998.
7. Malick MH: Manual on Dynamic Hand Splinting with Thermoplastic Materials, ed 2. Pittsburg, Harmarville Rehabilitation Center, 1982.
8. MERiT Static Progressive Component Product Catalog, 1998. MERiT is a trademark of UE Tech, Upper Extremity Technology.
9. North Coast Medical Company Hand Therapy Catalog, 1998. Prism, Orthoplast, Velcro, and Orfit are trademarks of the North Coast Medical Company.
10. Redford JB, Basmajian JV, Trautman P: Orthotics: Clinical Practice and Rehabilitation Technology. New York, Churchill Livingstone, Inc, 1995.
11. Schuch CM, Pritham CH: International Standards Organization Terminology: Application to prosthetics and orthotics. J Prosthetics Orthotics 1994; 6(1):29–48.
12. Silver Ring Splint Company Catalog, 1994. Siris and Silver Ring Splint are trademarks of the Silver Ring Splint Company.
13. Smith & Nephew Inc. Rehabilitation Division Catalog, 1997. Ezeform, Aquaplast, and Polyform are trademarks of Smith & Nephew, Inc.

16

CHAPTER

William J. Hennessey, M.D., and Ernest W. Johnson, M.D.

Lower Limb Orthoses

An orthosis is defined as a device attached or applied to the external surface of the body to improve function, restrict or enforce motion, or support a body segment.[28] Lower limb orthoses are indicated to assist gait, reduce pain, decrease weight bearing, control movement, and minimize progression of a deformity. Lower limb orthoses assist nonambulatory patients with transfer and mobility skills and assist ambulatory patients in becoming safe walkers. Ambulation aids can be used in combination with lower limb orthoses to help patients ambulate more safely. Ambulation aids represent extensions of the upper limb but are discussed in this chapter because of their importance in gait.

PRINCIPLES OF LOWER LIMB ORTHOSES

Orthoses should be used for the specific management of selected disorders. As in all fields of medicine, specific treatment should be based on a specific medical diagnosis, with an established goal of treatment.[39] Placement of orthotic joints should approximate anatomic joints. Table 16–1 outlines this principle as well as other common lower limb orthotic principles. Most orthoses utilize a three-point system to ensure proper positioning of the limb within the orthosis. For example, a knee that has a tendency to hyperextend, or "back knee," can be treated with a knee orthosis that applies force posterior to the knee but also applies forces anteriorly along the leg and the thigh. Such an orthosis ensures adequate control of the knee by exerting these forces proximal to, distal to, and at the knee joint.

TERMINOLOGY FOR LOWER LIMB ORTHOSES

Orthoses are frequently and incorrectly referred to as orthotics. Words ending in -ic are typically adjectives. *Orthotic* is the adjective derived from the noun *orthosis*. An orthosis can be referred to as an orthotic device. An orthosis is also made in an orthotic laboratory.

Terminology pertinent to the anatomy of the lower limb is also frequently used incorrectly. The term extremity specifically refers to the foot. The term leg should be used to refer to the portion of the lower limb between the knee and ankle joints. The thigh is located between the hip and knee joints. Lower limb refers to the thigh, leg, and foot.

Pathological abnormalities regarding angulation have also been referred to incorrectly as varus and valgus deformities at the knee and hip. Correct use of the Latin-derived terminology for these deformities requires the suffix of -us at the ankle, -um at the knee, and -a at the hip. Varus and valgus deformities of the foot are described for both the hindfoot and forefoot (i.e., hindfoot valgus or forefoot varus). A bow-legged condition is correctly referred to as genu varum. Deformity at the hip is referred to as coxa valga and coxa vara.

Lower limb orthoses are frequently referred to with abbreviations. Standard orthotic nomenclature uses the first letter of each joint the orthosis crosses from proximal to distal. It then lists the first letter of the limb to which it is affixed (i.e., "f" for foot). Lastly, the letter "o" is used to signify it is an orthosis. Thus, AFO designates an ankle-foot orthosis. KAFO means knee-ankle-foot orthosis. HKAFO means hip-knee-ankle-foot orthosis.

The orthotic literature uses variable medical terminology, which can make it difficult to understand the literature. The calcaneus is frequently referred to as the os calcis. A plantar flexion deformity is referred to as an equinus deformity. Torsion and rotation have incorrectly been used interchangeably. Torsion refers to twisting of a portion of a limb. Rotation of a limb occurs only at a joint. Pronation has been referred to as inroll-

TABLE 16–1 Principles of Lower Limb Orthoses

1. Use only as indicated and for as long as necessary.
2. Allow joint movement wherever possible and appropriate.
3. Orthoses should be functional throughout all phases of gait.
4. Orthotic ankle joint should be centered over tip of medial malleolus.
5. Orthotic knee joint should be centered over prominence of medial femoral condyle.
6. Orthotic hip joint should be in a position that allows patient to sit upright at 90 degrees.
7. Patient compliance will be enhanced if orthosis is comfortable, cosmetic, and functional.

ing, whereas supination has been referred to as outrolling. An orthosis is not put on and taken off but rather is donned and doffed. Checkout means an examination of the patient after the orthosis is fitted.

SHOES

The purpose of wearing shoes is to protect the feet. The normal foot does not require support from shoes. The sole should be pliable so as not to interfere with the normal biomechanics of the foot. A practical way of ensuring that a shoe is of adequate length is to determine whether the index finger can be placed between the tip of the great toe and the toe box.[42] The presence of calluses indicates areas of friction from poorly fitting (loose) shoes. The presence of corns indicates areas of friction over bony prominences, most often due to tight-fitting shoes. Leather shoes are good choices for all types of activity. They are durable, allow ventilation, and mold to the feet with time. A good pair of shoes can eliminate the need for foot orthoses and should be considered before orthotic prescription.

Shoe Parts

Two types of dress shoes are commonly worn, the Blucher and the Bal (Fig. 16–1). The tongue is part of the vamp in the Blucher shoe. The quarters overlap the vamp. A Blucher shoe is recommended for patients requiring an orthosis because there is more room to don and doff the shoe and the orthosis, owing to the open throat. In the Bal shoe style the quarters meet at the throat. The vamp is stitched over the quarters at the throat, thereby limiting the ability of the shoe to open and accommodate an orthosis.

A shoe with a welt should be recommended to patients. A welt is a narrow strip of leather used to unite the upper part of the shoe, the inner sole, and the outer sole of a shoe by means of stitching.[44] The welt design allows the orthotist to disassemble the shoe for modifications more easily than with other types of shoes. The presence of a welt can be easily noted by the horizontal stitching just above the sole. It is also present in most athletic shoes, at least along the anterior half of the shoe, to provide reinforcement for activities requiring frequent "cutbacks."

FOOT ORTHOSES

Foot orthoses (FOs) range from arch supports found at a local pharmacy or athletic store to customized orthoses fabricated by an orthotist. The effectiveness of an orthosis depends on proper diagnosis of the foot condition, the appropriate selection of orthotic material, and proper molding. FOs affect the ground reactive forces acting on the joints of the lower limb. They also have an effect on rotational components of gait (Fig. 16–2).

Mild conditions can be treated with over-the-counter orthoses. More severe problems require customized orthoses. These are available in three types. A soft type is most commonly used in over-the-counter orthoses. Orthotists usually provide semirigid orthoses, which provide more support than the soft type but are still shock absorbing. A rigid orthosis is indicated only for

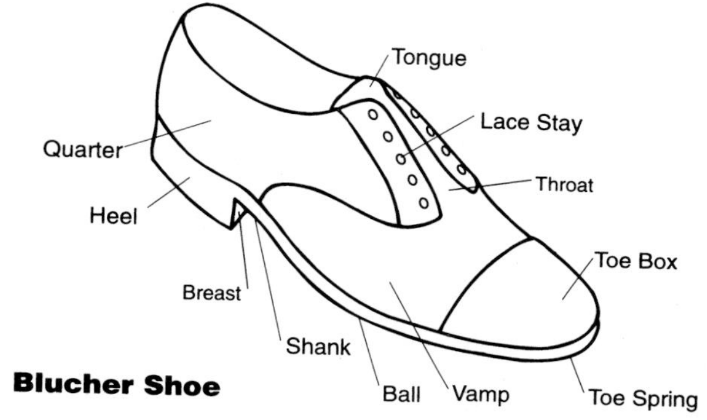

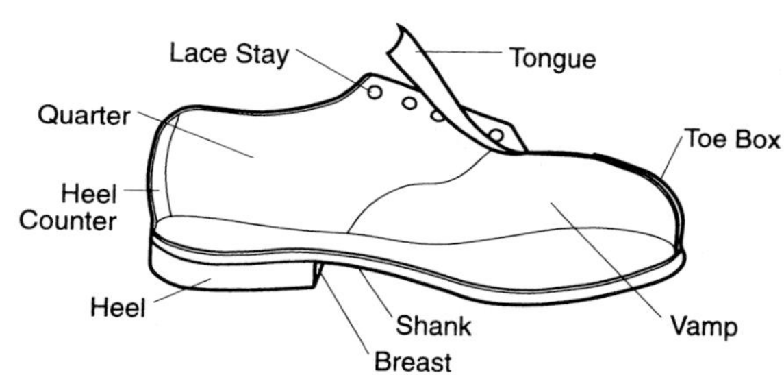

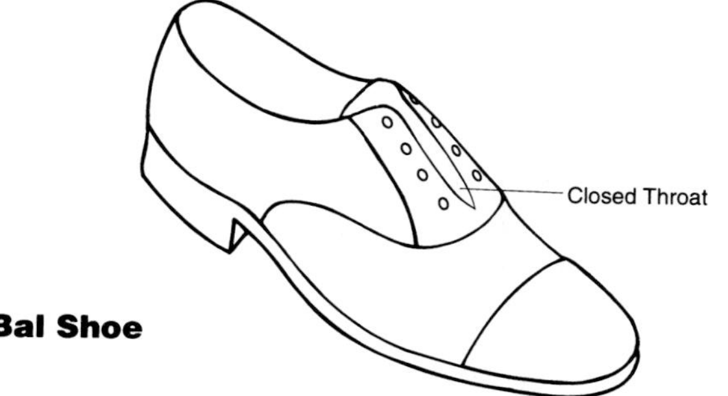

FIGURE 16–1. Shoe types and components. The open throat of the Blucher shoe accommodates an orthosis better than the Bal shoe.

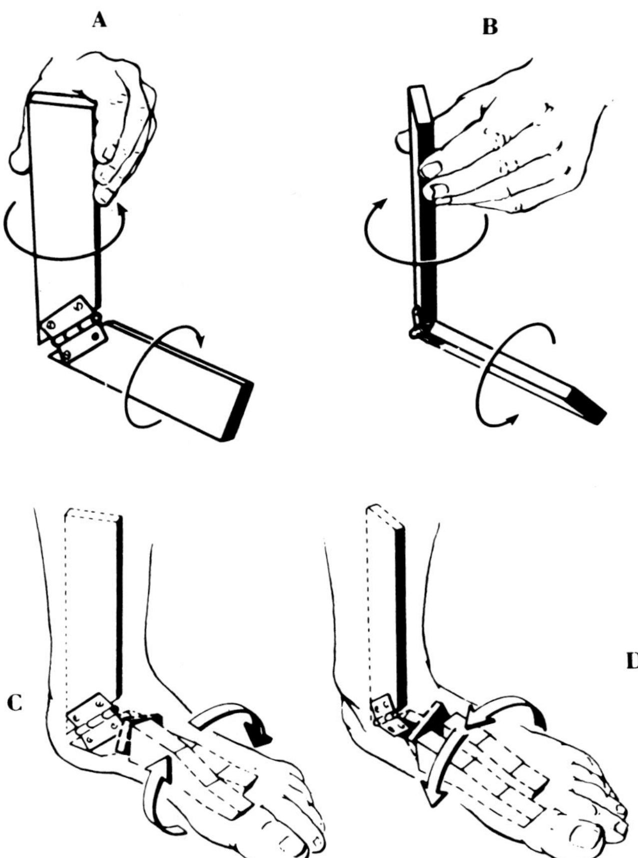

FIGURE 16–2. Analogy of subtalar axes to an oblique hinge. *A* and *C.* Outward rotation of the upper stick (tibia) results in inward rotation of the lower stick (calcaneus). This results in elevation of the medial border of the foot and depression of the lateral border. *B* and *D.* Inward rotation of the upper stick (tibia) results in outward rotation of the lower stick (calcaneus). This results in depression of the medial side of the foot with elevation of the lateral side. (Modified from Mann RA: Biomechanics of the foot. In American Academy of Orthopaedic Surgeons (eds): Atlas of Orthotics. St Louis, Mosby–Year Book, 1985, p 118.)

a problem that requires aggressive bracing to control the deformity.

To make a custom foot orthosis, the subtalar joint should be placed in a neutral position prior to casting. This position minimizes abnormalities related to foot and ankle rotation, such as hyperpronation, and it is also the position in which the foot functions best.[30] The foot is then covered with a parting agent, such as stockinet or a clear plastic wrap. The foot is then wrapped in either plaster of Paris strips or fiberglass tape and allowed to harden. Fiberglass casting is also used for difficult orthotic cases where the fiberglass casting itself can be used as a temporary orthosis to determine whether the mold properly controls the deformity. This negative mold is then removed to allow a positive mold to be made from the negative mold. The positive mold can be modified to increase the effectiveness of the orthosis. The custom orthosis is obtained by heating and forming (often by use of a vacuum) the plastic to the positive mold.

It should be noted that research has not determined the length of time an orthosis remains effective. The orthosis should be examined at each follow-up visit to determine when a new one is necessary.

COMMON FOOT CONDITIONS

Pes Planus (Flat Foot)

Symptomatic relief of pain is obtained by controlling excess pronation of the foot. Pronation of the foot can be defined as a rotation of the foot in the longitudinal axis resulting in a lowering of the medial aspect of the foot. Pronation is also referred to as inrolling. Pronation and abduction of the foot occur at the subtalar joint. Foot pronation is a component of eversion. Eversion involves pronation and abduction (at the subtalar joint) and dorsiflexion (at the ankle joint). The key to controlling excess pronation is controlling the calcaneus to keep the subtalar joint in a neutral position.

Pes planus can be due to abnormalities such as excessive internal torsion of the tibia (which results in pronation of the foot) or malalignment of the calcaneus. It is the interaction between the tibia and the foot at the subtalar joint that allows pathology outside the foot to cause inrolling of the foot (Fig. 16–2).

The reduction of pronation is accomplished by maintaining the calcaneus and the subtalar joint in correct alignment. The subtalar joint should be in a neutral position during the custom molding process. The subtalar joint neutral position prevents rotational deformities associated with excessive pronation or supination from occurring (parts C and D of Fig. 16–2). Elevation of the anteromedial calcaneus exerts an upward thrust against the sustentaculum tali to help prevent inrolling.[5] The orthosis should extend beyond the metatarsal heads to provide better leverage for control of the deformity. A custom-made foot orthosis designed to prevent hyperpronation is also referred to as a UCBL orthosis (or UCB), denoting the University of California Biomechanics Laboratory, where original work regarding this type of orthosis was performed in the 1940s.

Some cases of pes planus are due to ligamentous laxity within the foot. For these cases, a medial longitudinal arch support can be helpful for alleviating pain. Initial use of an arch that is too high can cause discomfort. The height of the arch can be increased as necessary as the foot develops a tolerance for the inlay. A Thomas heel extension (Fig. 16–3) can also offer medial support, particularly for heavier individuals. A most practical piece of advice for runners who have hyperpronation/pes planus is to purchase a pair of running shoes with a firm medial heel counter as well as shoes with a wide last at the shank (see Fig. 16–1). Each of these applications helps prevent pronation at the subtalar joint.

Pes Cavus (High-Arched Foot)

A typical complication of pes cavus is excess pressure along the heel and metatarsal head areas, which can

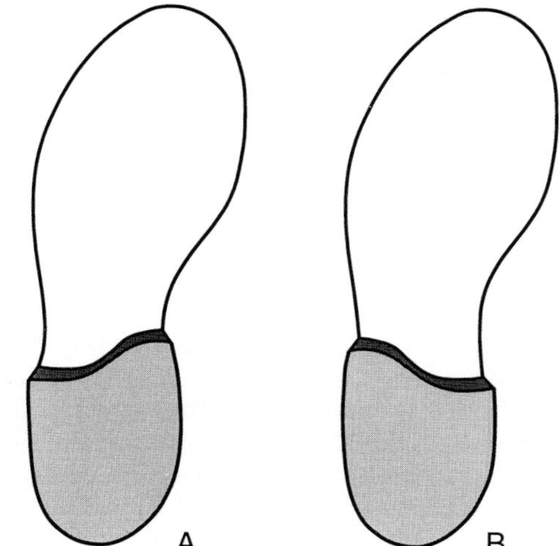

FIGURE 16–3. *A.* Thomas heel. *B.* Reverse Thomas heel.

lead to pain. This can be prevented by making the height of the longitudinal support just high enough to fill in the space between the shank of the shoe and the arch of the foot to distribute weight more effectively (Fig. 16–4). Weight should also be evenly distributed over the metatarsal heads. The lift is extended just to the metatarsal head area to help distribute and alleviate pressure over the metatarsal weight-bearing area. Since there is no tendency to pronate as in pes planus, the high point of the arch is located at the talonavicular joint. If the tibia is externally rotated (Fig. 16–2), this can give the appearance of an elevated arch as the foot supinates and the lateral aspect of the foot assumes additional weight-bearing responsibility. In these cases, a foot orthosis is custom molded with the subtalar joint in a neutral position to prevent excess supination from occurring.

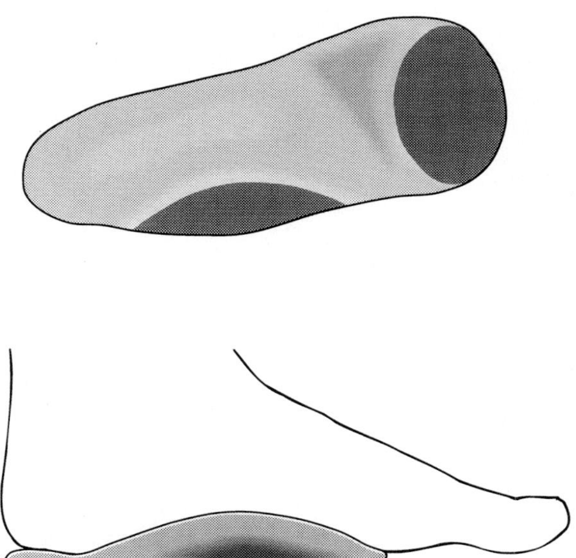

FIGURE 16–4. Pes cavus orthosis. (Modified from Diveley RL: Foot Appliances and Shoe Alterations: Orthopaedic Appliances Atlas. Ann Arbor, MI, Edward Brothers, 1952, p 464.)

Forefoot Pain (Metatarsalgia)

Relief of pain in the forefoot is accomplished by distributing the weight-bearing forces to an area proximal to the metatarsal heads. This can be done by either internal or external modification. A metatarsal pad (also referred to as a "cookie") can be placed inside the shoe just posterior to the second, third, and fourth metatarsal heads. It should also be just posterior to the lateral aspect of the first metatarsal head and medial to the fifth metatarsal head (Fig. 16–5). A metatarsal bar (Fig. 16–6) is recommended for cases in which the foot is too sensitive to tolerate a pad inside the shoe. The metatarsal bar is typically ¼ inch thick and tapers distally. The distal edge should be proximal to the metatarsal heads. It is often applied to a leather or neoprene sole.[26] The metatarsal bar can also be used for forefoot pain associated with pes cavus (Fig. 16–6).

Prevention of forefoot pain should also be emphasized to patients. Patients should avoid shoes with high heels or pointed toes, which place excess stress on the metatarsal heads.[3]

Heel Pain

The painful area can be alleviated by using an orthosis to help distribute weight. Rubber heel pads can be applied

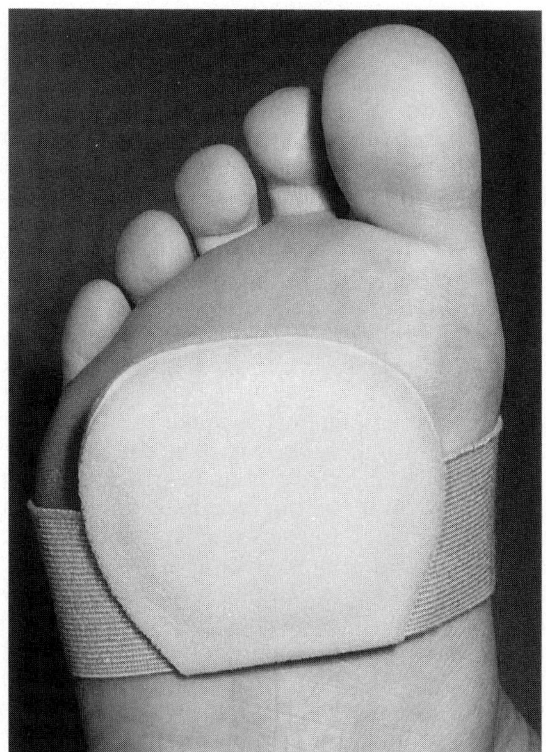

FIGURE 16–5. Metatarsal pad for forefoot pain. This should be placed proximal to the metatarsal heads in order to reduce weight distribution on the metatarsal heads. (Courtesy of Apex Foot Health Industries, South Hackensack, NJ.)

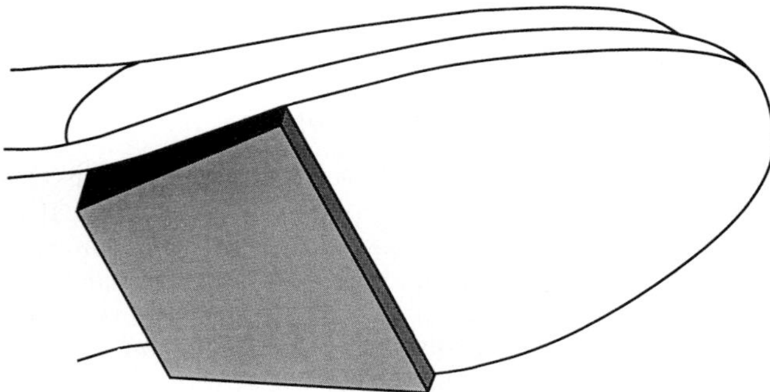

FIGURE 16–6. Metatarsal bar. (Modified from Pfeffinger LL: Foot orthoses. In American Academy of Orthopaedic Surgeons (eds): Atlas of Orthotics. St Louis, Mosby–Year Book, 1985, p 350.)

inside the shoe to offer relief in cases of minor discomfort. A calcaneal bar is recommended for cases in which the foot is too sensitive to tolerate a pad inside the shoe and the heel pain is associated with a chronic condition. The calcaneal bar is placed distal to the painful area to prevent the calcaneus from assuming full weight-bearing status.

A common cause of heel pain along the anteromedial calcaneus is plantar fasciitis. Pain occurs at the attachment site of the fascia along the medial aspect of the heel. Point tenderness is located over the anteromedial calcaneus. It is common in people who hyperpronate their feet, thereby placing excess stress on the medial longitudinal arch. A custom-made orthosis with the subtalar joint in a neutral position (such as that described for pes planus) helps prevent excessive inrolling from occurring and reduces the stress placed along the proximal arch. A custom-made orthosis is indicated for cases in which conservative treatment has failed. From an orthotic standpoint, conservative treatment should include the use of a pair of shoes with a firm medial heel counter and a wide shank.

Plantar fasciitis is also common in patients with high arches. For these patients, the medial longitudinal arch undergoes marked stress during weight bearing. This can be treated with either an elevated arch support or a heel well that helps distribute pressure along the medial longitudinal arch.

Heel spurs are frequently mistaken as the source of heel pain. Heel spurs related to plantar fasciitis are the result of mechanical stress acting through the plantar fascia onto its origin at the calcaneus and are not the source of the pain.[29] Inferior heel spurs are related to advancing age and are not painful in nature.

Heel lifts help some causes of Achilles pain by decreasing the amount of stretch placed on the Achilles tendon (by keeping the ankle joint plantar flexed). A heel lift can be used to treat Achilles enthesitis, an inflammatory reaction at the insertion of the tendon into the periosteum of the calcaneus. A heel lift can also be helpful for treating plantar flexion spasticity or contracture by increasing the total heel height to help ensure that the patient has a heel strike prior to toe touch during gait.

Toe Pain

The goal of orthotic intervention in toe pain is to decrease pain by immobilization. This is done by extending the steel shank forward to reduce the mobility of the distal joints. A metatarsal bar can also be used for partial immobilization. Common conditions associated with toe pain include hallux rigidus, gout, and arthritis.

Leg Length Discrepancy

A symptomatic leg length discrepancy should first be evaluated with proper measurement. True leg length is measured from the distal tip of the anterior superior iliac spine to the distal tip of the medial malleolus. Apparent leg length is measured from a midline point such as the pubic symphysis or umbilicus to the distal tip of each malleolus. This can be abnormal in cases in which the true leg length is normal but pelvic obliquity is present secondary to conditions such as scoliosis, pelvic fracture, or muscle imbalance. There is no support in the medical literature for treating low back pain associated with an alleged leg length discrepancy and it is not advised unless there is a traumatic event, such as a femur fracture, resulting in a significant acute onset "leg" (lower limb) length discrepancy.

Leg length discrepancies less than $\frac{1}{2}$ inch do not need correction. The total discrepancy is never corrected. At most, 75% of the leg length discrepancy should be corrected. The first ½ inch of the discrepancy can be managed with a heel pad. Additional correction requires the heel to be built up externally. The sole should also be built up proportionally when the heel is built up externally in order to provide a comfortable, stable gait. A taller sole should have a rocker bottom to help normalize the gait pattern at toe-off (Fig. 16–7).

Osteoarthritis of the Knee

Although osteoarthritis of the knee is not a foot condition, it is mentioned here since pain related to it can be alleviated with foot orthoses. Foot orthoses alter the ground reaction forces affecting the more proximal

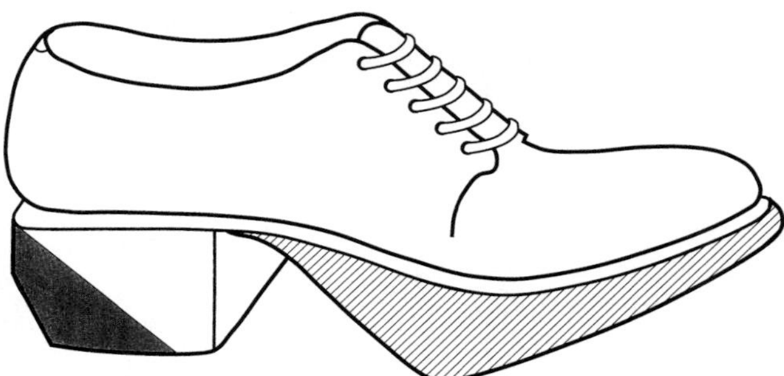

FIGURE 16–7. SACH heel and rocker bottom. Note that the elevated heel requires an elevated sole with rocker bottom to facilitate gait. The heel must also slant inward to prevent an excessive flexion moment at the knee at heel strike. (Modified from Pfeffinger LL: Foot orthoses. In American Academy of Orthopaedic Surgeons (eds): Atlas of Orthotics. St Louis, Mosby–Year Book, 1985, p 350.)

joints, such as the knee, and this relationship should be considered when prescribing a foot orthosis. Lateral heel wedges can be used for conservative treatment of osteoarthritis when medial compartment narrowing results in genu varum. The heel wedges used are ¼ inch thick along the lateral border and taper medially. Relief was obtained with heel wedges in 74 of 121 knees from 85 patients in one study.[11] Relief of pain was most frequently obtained in patients with mild osteoarthritis, but it was also documented in some patients with complete obliteration of the medial joint space. Wedge use widened the gait pattern.

Pediatric Shoes

Children's shoes should have a simple design. To facilitate gait, a heel should not be present. Soft soles are recommended to permit the natural development of feet. Tennis shoes are adequate for most children. A high quarter or three-quarter shoe will stay on a child's foot better than a low-cut shoe and is recommended during the first few years of life.

It is a common misconception that all flat feet need to be treated in children. Flat feet are usual in infants, common in children, and occur occasionally in adults.[36] Flat feet improve over time, in part because of the loss of subcutaneous fat and the reduction of laxity of the joints that occur with growth[36] and the maturation of the gait pattern. Intensive treatment with corrective shoes or inserts for a 3-year period did not alter the natural history of flat feet in 129 children who were 1 to 6 years of age.[41] One cannot make the asymptomatic person feel any better. Frequent shoe size change is necessary in the first few years of life.[42]

ANKLE-FOOT ORTHOSES

Ankle-foot orthoses (AFOs) are the most commonly prescribed lower limb orthoses. They were formerly known as short leg braces. Metal or plastic AFOs can be used effectively to control ankle motion. Metal AFOs are relatively contraindicated in children because the weight of the brace can cause external tibial rotation. Plastic AFOs are now more common in all age groups.

AFOs should provide mediolateral stability as a safety feature.[12] Although much emphasis with AFOs is placed on controlling the amount of dorsiflexion and plantar flexion, movements at the subtalar joint also significantly influence the biomechanics of gait. Supination and adduction occur at the subtalar joint, which results in the foot being in a varus position. Pronation and abduction occur at the subtalar joint, resulting in the foot being in a valgus position. Rotation at the subtalar joint is also accompanied by rotation of the tibia (Fig. 16–2).

AFOs can also stabilize the knee during gait.[18] They are prescribed for conditions affecting knee stability, such as genu recurvatum. An AFO should be considered for conditions affecting the knee, particularly when a concurrent problem exists at the ankle or subtalar joints. A proper AFO prescription considers the biomechanical influence of the orthosis at the foot, ankle, and knee in all planes of movement. *It should be remembered that plantar flexion creates a knee extension moment and dorsiflexion creates a knee flexion moment.*

Metal AFOs

Metal AFOs are now used much less commonly than the plastic type. They will be discussed for the following three reasons: (1) Much of the research regarding the biomechanical influence of AFOs on gait was performed with metal AFOs. These principles also apply to plastic orthoses. (2) Metal components (especially joints) are frequently used in combination with plastic orthoses. (3) Some older patients wish to continue to use the metal orthoses to which they have become accustomed.

The metal AFO consists of a proximal calf band, two uprights, ankle joints, and an attachment to the shoe to anchor the AFO (Fig. 16–8). The posterior metal portion of the calf band should be 1.5 to 3 inches wide in order to adequately distribute pressure.[7] The calf band should be 1 inch below the fibular neck to prevent a compressive common peroneal palsy. A leather strap with Velcro is used to close the calf band, since it pro-

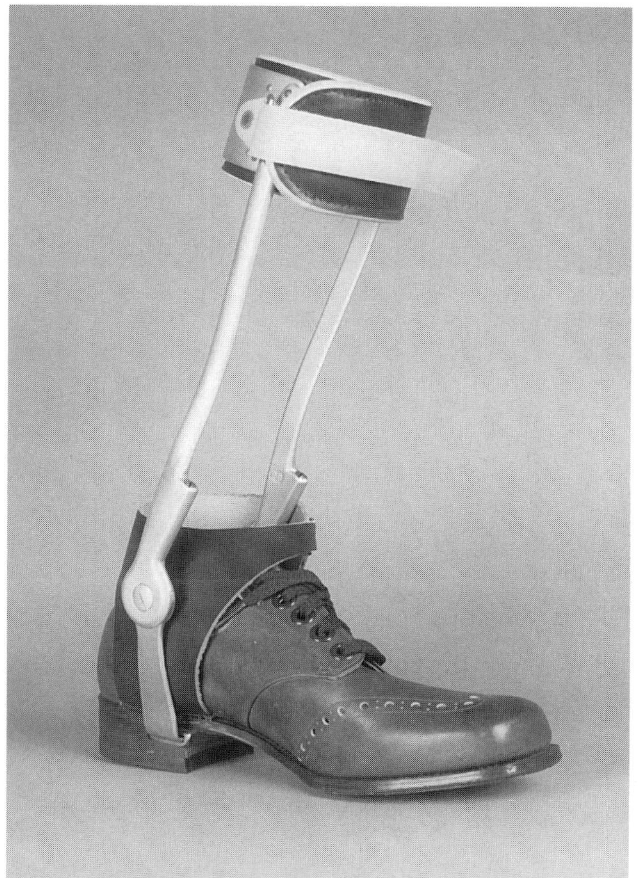

FIGURE 16–8. Metal double upright dorsiflexion assist AFO on left shoe with medial T strap for control of valgus deformity. The metal dorsiflexion assist ankle joint is also referred to as a *Klenzak ankle joint.* Note the split stirrup in the heel that allows the wearing of the orthosis with other shoes.

vides ease of closure for patients with only one functional upper limb.

Ankle joint motion is controlled by pins or springs inserted into channels (Figs. 16–9 through 16–11). The pins are adjusted with a screwdriver to set the desired amount of plantar flexion and dorsiflexion. The spring is also adjusted with a screwdriver to provide the proper amount of tension necessary to aid motion at the ankle joint (used to assist dorsiflexion). Longer channels help prevent the spring mechanism from "bottoming out" and provide for more precise control of ankle motion.

A solid stirrup is a U-shaped metal piece permanently attached to the shoe. Its two ends are bent upward to articulate with the medial and lateral ankle joints (Fig. 16–9). The proximal stirrup attachment sites are shaped to enforce the desired movements at the ankle joint (Fig. 16–11). The sole plate can be extended beyond the metatarsal head area for conditions requiring a longer lever arm for better control of plantar flexion (such as plantar spasticity).

A split stirrup can be used instead of a solid stirrup (Figs. 16–8 and 16–12). The split stirrup has a sole plate with two flat channels for insertion of the uprights. The two uprights are now called calipers, as they can open and close distally to allow donning and doffing of the AFO. A split stirrup allows removal of the uprights from the shoes so that the AFO can be worn with other shoes (Fig. 16–8). Other pairs of shoes should also have the sole plate with channels for calipers incorporated into the heel area. The split stirrup is not as stable as the solid stirrup.

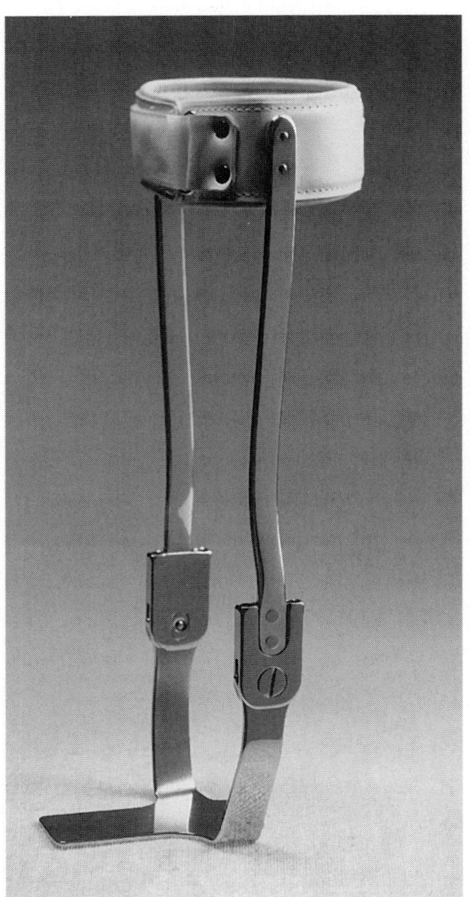

FIGURE 16–9. Double-action metal ankle joint with solid stirrup. (Courtesy of Becker Orthopedic Co., Troy, MI.)

Ankle Stops and Assists

The ankle joint can be positioned so that it is in a neutral, dorsiflexed, or plantar-flexed position, depending on the gait disturbance. It can be set to permit a partial range of motion or to eliminate a certain motion. An understanding of the effect on the placement of pins and screws into the two channels of an ankle joint (Fig. 16–10) facilitates the proper orthotic prescription for the patient. This section reviews the common uses of the posterior stop, anterior stop, and the posterior dorsiflexion assist. A spring in the anterior channel has not been demonstrated to be of clinical value.

Plantar Stop (Posterior Stop)

The plantar stop is used to control plantar spasticity or help incrementally stretch plantar contractures. The plantar stop is most commonly set at 90 degrees. A pin is inserted into the posterior channel of an ankle joint, such as that in Figure 16–10, to limit plantar flexion. An AFO with a plantar stop at 90 degrees produces a flexion moment at the knee during heel strike. Since the dorsiflexors cannot eccentrically activate to permit the foot to make contact with the ground, the ground reactive force remains posterior to the knee after heel strike, which creates a flexion moment at the knee (and possibly an unstable gait). The proximal portion of the AFO also has an effect on knee stability. The posterior portion of the proximal AFO exerts a forward push on the proximal leg to increase the knee flexion moment after heel strike (Fig. 16–13). The opposite occurs at toe-off, with an extension moment created at the knee. This concept has been used to develop what has been referred to as a plastic ground reaction AFO, with a solid proximal anterior tibial closing that provides a greater influence on the knee. This device will be discussed in more detail later. The greater the plantar flexion resistance, the greater the flexion moment at the knee at heel strike, and the greater the need for active hip extensors to prevent the body from collapsing forward on a buckling knee.

A solid ankle cushioned heel (SACH) heel wedge (see Fig. 16–7) can be used to reduce the flexion moment at the knee. The term SACH is a misnomer borrowed from the prosthetic literature. The "SA" (solid ankle) refers to the type of prosthetic ankle joint. The SACH heel wedge in this case should be referred to only as a cushioned heel. A cushioned heel serves as a shock absorber at heel strike, and is able to partially substitute for the dorsiflexors, which cannot be activated when an AFO's ankle plantar stops are set at 90 degrees. A cushioned heel also helps move the ground reactive force more anteriorly. In essence, a soft heel helps stabilize the knee. It helps keep the ground reaction force anterior to the knee joint. A firm heel decreases knee

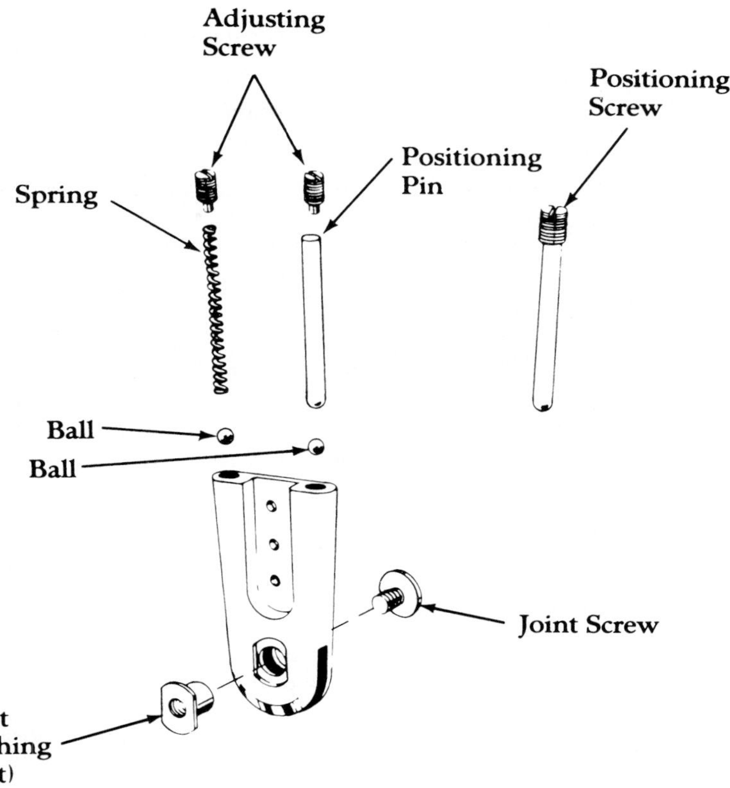

FIGURE 16–10. Schematic drawing of metal ankle joint components. This type of ankle joint has also been referred to as a *double-action ankle joint,* a *double Klenzak ankle joint,* and a *BiCAAL* (bichannel adjustable ankle locking) joint. (Courtesy of USMC, Pasadena.)

stability via a knee flexion moment while moving the ground reaction force posterior to the knee joint. A cushioned heel can also be used with an AFO to minimize the amount of plantar flexion spasticity present after heel strike.

The posterior stop should be set at the minimal amount of plantar flexion required to clear the foot during swing-through.[13] Remember, plantar flexion creates a knee extension moment at the knee after heel strike. This provides a more stable knee during gait than when the ankle plantar stops are set in any degree of dorsiflexion.

A balanced decision should be made between providing resistance to plantar flexion to clear the foot during the swing phase of gait and the amount of instability at the knee during the stance phase of gait. No AFO is effective in reducing the amount of knee flexion to "normal" levels during the stance phase of gait.[15]

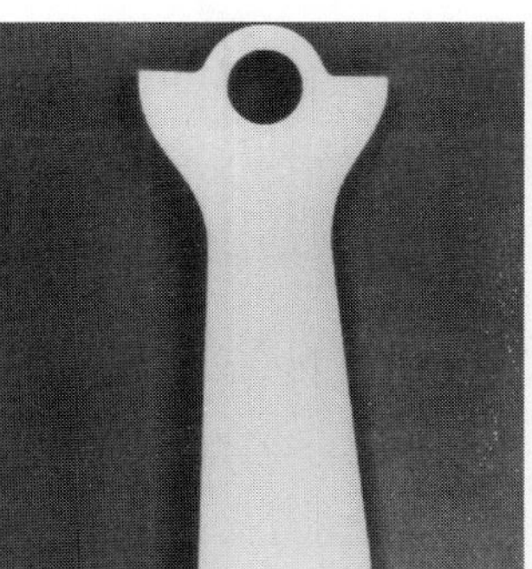

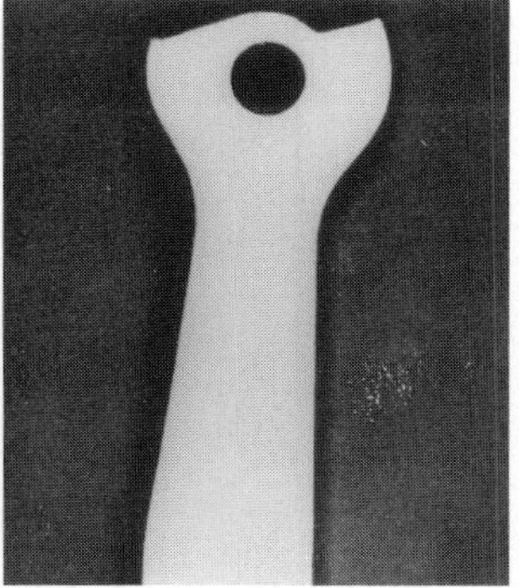

FIGURE 16–11. Dorsiflexion assist and double-action stirrups, used with the ankle joints shown in Figures 16–9 and 16–8, respectively. (Courtesy of USMC, Pasadena.)

Dorsiflexion Stop (Anterior Stop)

An anterior stop is used to substitute for the function of the gastrocnemius/soleus complex. It is used in conditions with weak calf muscles or weak quadriceps (because of its effect on the knee). Weak calf musculature allows the ankle to enter dorsiflexion. The anterior stop set at 5 degrees of dorsiflexion best substitutes for gastrocnemius/soleus function.[13, 15]

The anterior stop assists with push-off and assists the knee joint into extension. It should be used in combination with a stirrup with a sole extension to the metatarsal heads, to simulate the action of the calf muscles. The dorsiflexion stop simulates the gastrocnemius/soleus function by causing the heel to rise during the latter part of stance rather than remaining flat on the ground. The shoe pivots over the metatarsal heads, creating an extension moment at the knee that helps stabilize the knee from midstance to toe-off.

The earlier the dorsiflexion stop occurs during the stance phase, the greater the extension moment at the knee. This is useful in clinical situations where quadri-

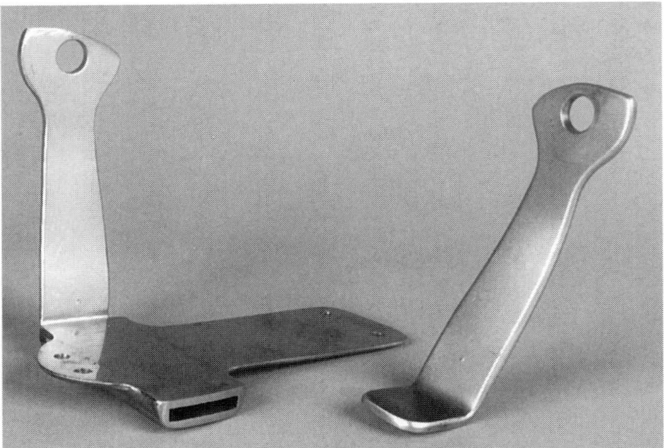

FIGURE 16–12. Split stirrup. The stirrup extends anteriorly to attach at the shank area of a shoe for stability.

ceps weakness is also present. If the extension moment at the knee is too great for too long, then genu recurvatum ("back knee") can occur. A balance should be obtained such that the extension at the knee is sufficient to stabilize the knee in extension yet prevent genu recurvatum. If too much dorsiflexion is permitted by the anterior stop, there will be too much knee flexion during gait from midstance to toe-off.

Dorsiflexion Assist (Posterior Spring)

The posterior spring serves two purposes. It substitutes for concentric contraction of dorsiflexors to prevent flaccid foot drop after toe-off. It also substitutes (inadequately) for the eccentric activation of the dorsiflexors after heel strike. The metal dorsiflexion assist ankle joint is also known as a Klenzak ankle joint (see Fig. 16–8).

The posterior spring prevents rapid plantar flexion at heel strike during its compression in the posterior channel. The posterior spring is again compressed during plantar flexion during late stance prior to toe-off. The posterior spring assists with toe clearance during the swing phase of gait by providing a downward thrust posterior to the ankle joint at toe-off, which results in dorsiflexion anterior to the ankle joint. The longer the channel, the greater the ability to control dorsiflexion.

A summary of some of the common indications for the various channel components is found in Table 16–2.

Metal AFO Varus/Valgus Control

Varus and valgus deformities are associated with rotation at the subtalar joint. A T strap is attached along the side of the shoe distal to the subtalar joint to help minimize the deformity (Fig. 16–8). T straps are also used to help prevent worsening of the deformity. T straps also help distribute pressure properly along the foot during weight bearing.

T straps are referred to as being either medial or lateral. A medial T strap is sown to the medial aspect of the shoe and the belt is cinched around the lateral upright of the AFO (Fig. 16–8). A medial T strap is used to control a valgus deformity. The belt is secured with a buckle around the lateral upright. This helps create a force directing the subtalar joint inward which counteracts the pronation and abduction tendency that would result in excess valgus. The opposite is true for a varus deformity with the T strap being laterally located. A pressure ulcer can develop over the malleolus if the T strap is buckled too tightly.

The T strap inadequately substitutes for the foot pronators, supinators, abductors, and adductors because it

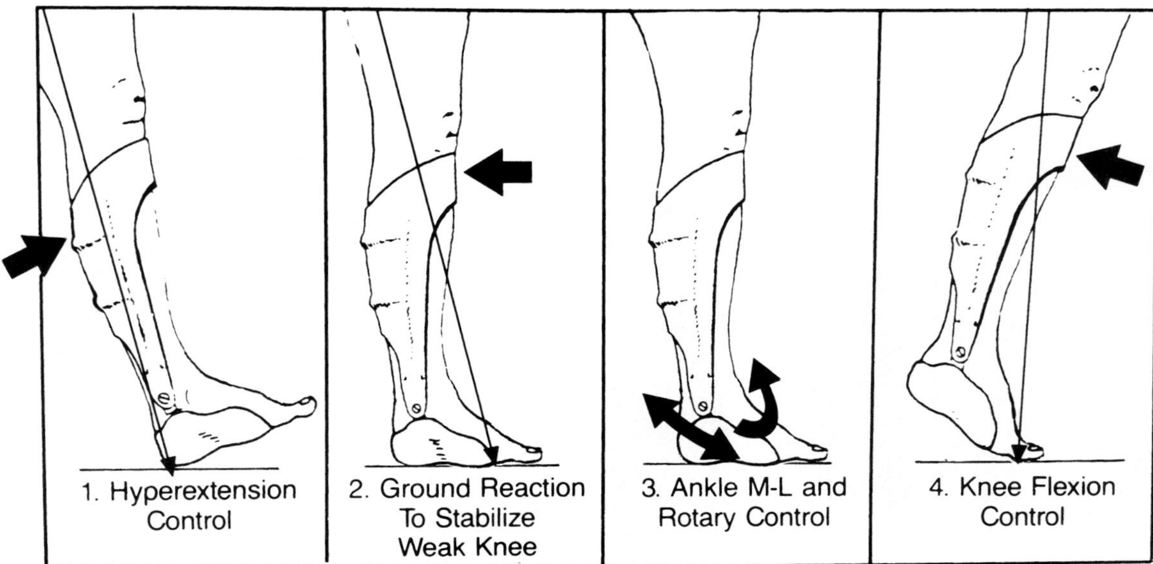

FIGURE 16–13. Ground reaction AFO dynamic illustration. Note the effect of the proximal portion of the AFO on the knee throughout gait. (Courtesy of Oregon Orthotic System, Albany, OR.)

TABLE 16–2 Clinical Indications for Various Metal Ankle Channel Components

Channel	Rod or Spring	Function	Clinical Indications
Posterior	Rod	Limits plantar flexion	Plantar spasticity, toe drag, pain with ankle motion
Posterior	Spring	Assists dorsiflexion	Flaccid footdrop, knee hyperextension
Anterior*	Rod	Limits dorsiflexion	Weak plantar flexors, weak knee extensors, pain with ankle motion
Anterior	Spring	Assists plantar flexion	None

*Used in combination with an extended sole plate to metatarsal head area to help compensate for weak plantar flexors.

does not have an attachment on the plantar surface of the foot to create the mechanical advantage offered by the plantar-attached muscles and tendons.

Plastic AFOs

Plastic AFOs are the most commonly used AFOs because of their cost, cosmesis, light weight, interchangeability with shoes, ability to control varus and valgus deformities, provision of better foot support with the customized foot portion, and ability to achieve what is offered by the metal AFO (Fig. 16–14). Energy consumption is equal with a plastic solid AFO or a metal double upright AFO.[2] Although a plastic orthosis weighs less than its metal counterpart, the weight of the orthosis is not as important as the influence of the ground reactive force created by the presence of the orthosis. The same orthotic principles apply to orthoses made of plastic or metal. The plastic AFO's effect on knee stability should be recognized. The plastic AFO prescribed for toe clearance should be just rigid enough to provide resistance for toe clearance. Excessive resistance to plantar flexion can make the knee unstable (create a flexion moment) after heel strike.[16]

Plastic AFOs can be prefabricated or custom made. The reasons for prescribing a custom-molded orthosis include long-term need, conformed molding for comfort or insensate feet, placement of the orthosis in a fixed amount of plantar or dorsiflexion, better control of rotational deformities, and further reduction of weight bearing for a tibial fracture or diabetic plantar ulcer. The custom process is similar to that previously described in this chapter for foot orthoses, with the positive mold serving as the model for the orthosis.

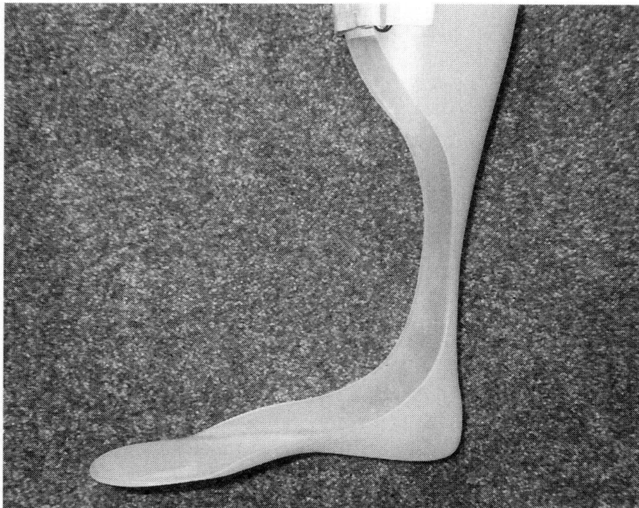

FIGURE 16–14. Custom plastic solid (means no ankle joint although still flexible) AFO with posterior trimline to allow some flexibility with plantar flexion. This is the most commonly prescribed AFO for foot drop.

Some practical advice should be offered to the patient regarding the use of a plastic AFO. If changing shoes, it is best to have another pair with a similar heel height, to prevent altering the biomechanical effects at the foot, ankle, and knee. Tennis shoes are most accommodating for donning and doffing of the AFO. However, if dress shoes are to be worn, patients should also be told that their shoe size might need to be one-half size greater and the next width larger to accommodate the orthosis. A Blucher-style dress shoe helps accommodate the orthosis (see Fig. 16–1).

Plastic AFO Components

The foot component of the AFO should extend beyond the metatarsal heads. The footplate can be extended beyond the toes to reduce the spasticity aggravated by toe flexion. The shape and molding of the foot portion influence the biomechanics of more proximal joints.

The ankle and subtalar joints can be made more stable under four circumstances: (1) the trim line extends more anteriorly at the ankle level (a trim line is the anterior border of the plastic AFO), (2) the plastic material is thicker, (3) carbon inserts are placed along the medial and lateral aspects of the ankle joint, and (4) corrugations are made within the posterior leaf of the AFO. The strength of the AFO should be matched to the patient's weight and activity level.

Plastic AFOs can also be hinged at the ankle. Ankle hinges allow full or partial ankle motion, which can permit a more natural gait. They should be considered when complete restriction of ankle motion is not required. Plastic ankle joints are light and are a good choice for children. Metal ankle joints are preferred for adults, particularly heavy adults. Newer designs have a single midline posterior rod/spring mechanism (Fig. 16–15). This midline spring functions like the more traditional medial and lateral dual posterior spring assist mechanism (see Figs. 16–8 and 16–9). This makes the AFO narrower in the mediolateral direction and slightly longer in the anteroposterior direction, which better conforms to the design of most pants.

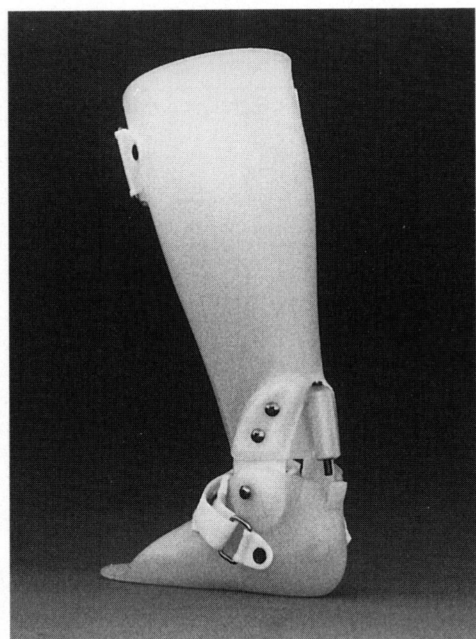

FIGURE 16–15. Elite midline posterior stop articulated AFO. Note the use of a plastic ankle joint to further decrease weight. Plastic ankle joints are more common in children (lightweight individuals). The use of a plantar stop with ankle joints is recommended for an active lightweight patient with plantar spasticity (e.g., a child with cerebral palsy).

The leg component should encompass three quarters of the leg and should be padded along its internal surface.[7] The proximal extent should end 1 inch below the fibular neck to prevent a compressive common peroneal nerve palsy.

To Hinge or Not to Hinge

There is often great controversy among the various health care providers (physiatrists, orthotists, and physical therapists) as to whether or not an AFO should be hinged. This controversy also exists frequently within the aformentioned health care provider categories. Unfortunately, there is no medical research available on this topic to provide general guidelines. We recommend that a plastic AFO for foot drop not be hinged. This keeps the orthosis more narrow to accommodate shoe wear, and needs less maintenance. Some movement at the ankle can still be achieved by making the AFO flexible with a posterior trim line. We recommend a hinged AFO for an active patient with plantar spasticity, who would take advantage of some of the range of motion permitted at the ankle (e.g., a child with cerebral palsy or a young adult with a traumatic brain injury).

The Solid Plastic AFO

The solid plastic AFO is the most commonly prescribed plastic AFO (Fig. 16–14). It can be made to serve several purposes. The term solid refers to an AFO that is made of a single piece of plastic. It does not have ankle joints. A solid AFO can still be flexible enough to allow some ankle motion, and it should be flexible with a posterior trim line for the treatment of a foot drop. A solid AFO should be truly solid (not flexible) for the treatment of plantar spasticity.

Solid AFOs set at 90 degrees are commonly used for foot drop. Less obvious but equally important is the solid AFO's ability to treat conditions affecting the knee. Again, it should be remembered that plantar flexion creates knee extension and dorsiflexion creates knee flexion at heel strike. The AFO can be fixed in a few degrees of plantar flexion to provide stability at the knee during the stance phase of gait. Genu recurvatum can also be treated with a solid AFO. The more rigid the AFO, the greater the flexion moment at the knee at heel strike, which helps reverse the extension moment at the knee associated with genu recurvatum. The flexion moment at the knee also becomes greater during midstance if the ankle is placed in a few degrees of dorsiflexion.

Plastic AFO Varus/Valgus Control

The goal of orthotic intervention is to alter the ground reactive forces with custom molding to help maintain proper alignment of the lower limb by "building up" selected portions of the AFO. A three-point system is used to provide the counter forces necessary to oppose the forces of the deformity (Fig. 16–16).[23] Some orthotists believe that an orthosis should be firm ("not conforming") in order to control a deformity. Pressure points should be present in expected areas at follow-up visits if the orthosis is serving its purpose. A custom ground reaction orthosis provides appropriate foot support that influences the rotation of more proximal joints (Fig. 16–17). The anterior tibial shell closing helps stabilize the knee during gait (see Fig. 16–13).

An equinovarus (or inversion) deformity is controlled by applying forces medially at the metatarsal head area and calcaneus. The next force is applied more proximally along the lateral aspect of the fibula. This helps prevent inversion at the subtalar and ankle joints. A more proximal medial tibial force is applied to provide stabilization of the leg portion of the plastic AFO by providing an opposing force to the fibular area (Fig. 16–16). A three-point system also exists at the foot level to help prevent supination of the foot related to the equinovarus deformity (Fig. 16–16). A three-point system is again applied to control the plantar flexion deformity associated with equinovarus (Fig. 16–16).

The reverse of the above described three-point system to control varus can be used to control valgus at the foot. Movements in all joints should be considered when prescribing an orthosis.

Patellar Tendon-Bearing AFOs

A patellar tendon-bearing (PTB) AFO uses the patellar tendon and the tibial condyles to partially relieve weight-bearing stress on skeletal structures distally with more weight bearing distributed along the medial tibial condyle.[20] PTB is a misnomer for this orthosis because only about 10% of the weight is distributed along the patellar tendon and the medial tibial condyle. Most of

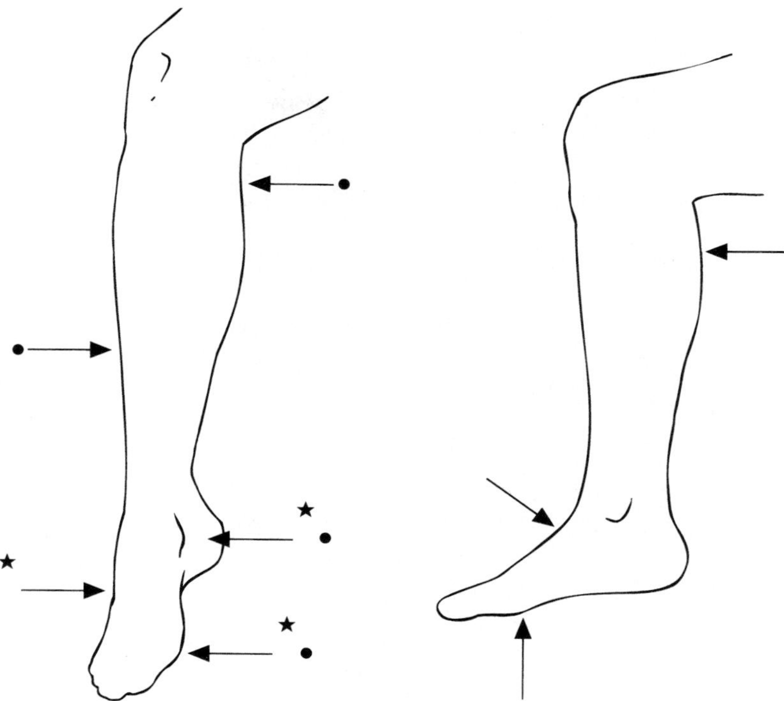

FIGURE 16–16. Three-point system control of equinovarus deformity. *Left:* Control of varus rotational component at the foot (*) and subtalar joint (●). *Right:* Control of equinus deformity. (Modified from Marx HW: Lower limb orthotic designs for the spastic hemiplegic patient. Orthot Prosthet 1974; 28:14.)

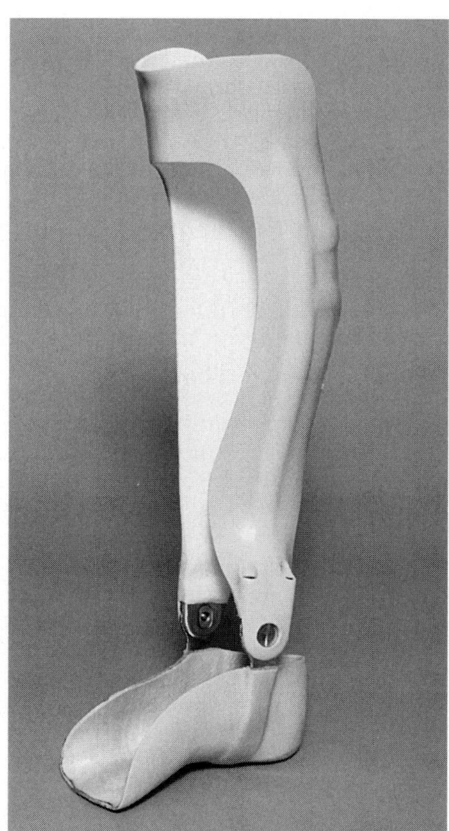

FIGURE 16–17. OOS rotational control AFO. Note the corrugations that add strength to the orthosis. Also note the metal ankle joint that is similar to those in Figure 16–9 and 16–10. (Courtesy of Oregon Orthotic System, Albany, OR.)

the weight bearing is distributed throughout the soft tissues of the leg that are compressed by an appropriately fitted orthosis. Compression of the soft tissues of the leg is also responsible for maintaining alignment and length of the tibia after a fracture.[33, 34]

PTB AFOs are often prescribed for diabetic ulcerations of the foot, tibial fractures, relief of the weight-bearing surface in painful heel conditions such as calcaneal fractures, postoperative ankle fusions, and avascular necrosis of the foot or ankle. The orthoses are made of plastic and so are of light weight and high durability. They are bivalved and fit snugly with the use of Velcro straps or buckles similar to those of ski boots (Fig. 16–18). A custom-molded PTB AFO can reduce weight bearing in the affected foot by up to 50%.

Custom-made PTB AFOs are indicated when maximum weight-bearing reduction is necessary to ensure proper healing (such as in a debrided diabetic heel ulcer) and reduction of pain. It should first be determined that the painful condition is associated with weight bearing rather than with range of motion. If pain occurs with range of motion, then the pain-producing range of motion should be eliminated.

The solid plastic orthosis makes contact with the ground before the reactive force is absorbed significantly by the foot and then distributes this force more proximally along the leg. Compared to a prefabricated AFO, a custom-made PTB AFO more effectively distributes pressure over a greater surface contact area for maximal weight-bearing reduction. Additional weight-bearing reduction is obtained by eliminating ankle movement (carbon graphite inserts can be used, as in Fig. 16–18) and the use of a rocker bottom (see Fig. 16–7), which eliminates active push off.[21] A rocker bottom is directly incorporated into the plastic orthosis.

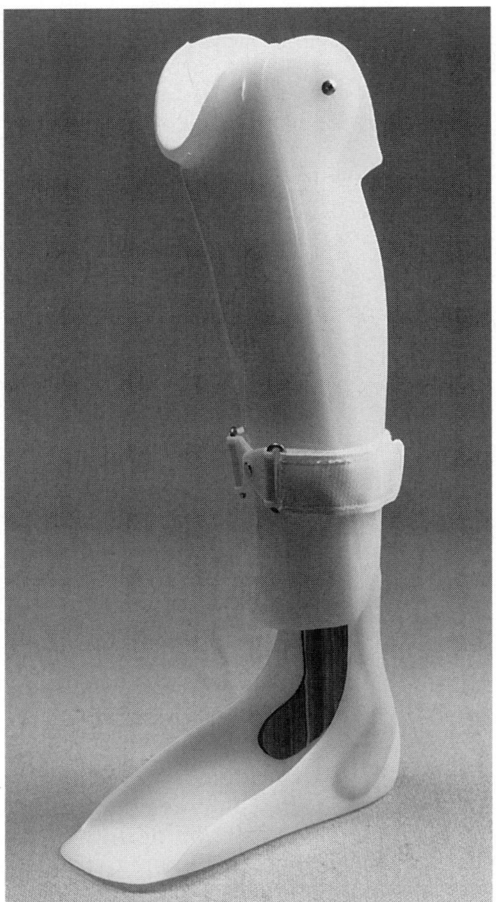

FIGURE 16–18. Prefabricated bivalved PTB AFO. Note the carbon inserts, which help eliminate ankle motion and therefore help eliminate active push-off. (Courtesy of Becker Orthopedic Co., Troy, MI.)

Checkout

The patient should be examined after fitting and use of the orthosis. The first and most obvious form of a checkout is to verify that the gait pattern is improved with the orthosis in comparison to without the orthosis. The orthotic ankle joint should coincide with the tip of the medial malleolus. The patient is to be checked for ease of donning and doffing the orthosis, and while it is off, observed for areas of skin breakdown. If the AFO was prescribed to control spasticity, the orthotic evaluation should include determining its effectiveness in a dynamic setting, since spasticity can worsen with ambulation. In cases where significant deformity is being addressed with orthotic intervention, some redness can and should be present if the orthosis is doing its job. Some redness is acceptable as long as it is dispersed in as large an area as possible and as long as there is no skin breakdown.

KNEE-ANKLE-FOOT ORTHOSES

Knee-ankle-foot orthoses (KAFOs) were formerly referred to as long leg braces. The components are the same as those of an AFO but also include knee joints, thigh uprights, and a proximal thigh band. Various knee joints and knee locks are available for a variety of conditions. KAFOs are used in patients with severe knee extensor and hamstring weakness, structural knee instability, and knee flexion spasticity. The purpose of the KAFO is to provide stability at the knee, ankle, and subtalar joints during ambulation. They are most commonly prescribed bilaterally for patients with spinal cord injuries and unilaterally for patients with polio. There is a common misconception that patients with a complete femoral neuropathy (i.e., no quadriceps function) should have their knees braced. From a functional anatomical standpoint, it should be kept in mind that there are three stabilizers to the knee: the quadriceps, the hamstrings (via eccentric activation at heel strike), and the plantar flexors (plantar flexion creates a knee extension moment). These stabilizers should all be evaluated carefully by physical examination before a KAFO is prescribed.

KAFOs can be prescribed for functional ambulation or exercise (or both). The benefits of exercise to the patient requiring bilateral KAFOs include preventing lower limb contractures, enhancing cardiovascular fitness, maintaining upper body strength for activities of daily living, delaying the development of osteoporosis, and fewer medical complications such as deep venous thromboses.

The use of KAFOs often complements the use of a wheelchair for ambulation. The proprioceptive level is a reliable indicator of which spinal cord-injured patients can achieve ambulation status.[40] It is helpful to have sensation and proprioception in the lower limbs in order to ambulate safely with KAFOs. The level of the spinal cord injury is also important in predicting the ability to ambulate. Adult spinal cord-injured patients with lesions at or above T12 generally are not functional ambulators because of the metabolic cost involved.[25] Children have a higher center of gravity and can have a functional gait with a higher spinal cord lesion. Muscle function is a predictor of the quality of ambulation. Good trunk control and upper body strength are needed in order to ambulate with KAFOs because these devices are used in combination with ambulation aids, such as walkers and Lofstrand forearm orthoses.

Some paraplegic patients, such as those with lower lumbar lesions with some knee extensor strength, are able to ambulate without KAFOs. Ambulation in these patients can often be accomplished with the use of bilateral plastic ground reaction AFOs (Figs. 16–13 and 16–17) with the ankles fixed in 10 to 15 degrees of plantar flexion. The plantar flexion provides an extension moment at the knee during gait for stability with ambulation. The proximal anterior tibial shell closing provides further stability at the knee from mid-stance to toe-off (see part 4 of Fig. 16–13). A walker or two Lofstrand forearm orthoses can be used for additional support and balance.

Knee Joints

There are three basic types of knee joints. The straight set knee joint provides rotation about a single axis (Fig.

16–19). It allows free flexion but prevents hyperextension. It is often used in combination with a drop lock, which keeps the knee in extension throughout all phases of gait for further stability.

The polycentric knee joint uses a double-axis system to simulate the flexion-extension movements of the femur and tibia at the knee joint (Fig. 16–20). Although this concept is theoretically sound, the polycentric knee joint has not proved to be advantageous over the straight set knee joint and it is less commonly used. It also adds bulk to the orthosis. It is most frequently used in sport knee orthoses.

The third type of knee joint is the posterior offset knee joint (Fig. 16–21). It is prescribed for patients with weak knee extensors and some hip extensor strength. It allows free flexion and extension of the knee during the swing phase of gait and helps keep the *orthotic* ground reactive force in front of the knee axis for stability during stance. The center of gravity is normally posterior to the knee at heel strike, creating a flexion moment at the knee, which requires knee extensor muscle contraction to counteract this force. The offset knee joint component of the KAFO helps place the ground reactive force anterior to the orthotic knee joint, creating an extension moment at the knee during stance to compensate for the weak knee extensors. The offset knee

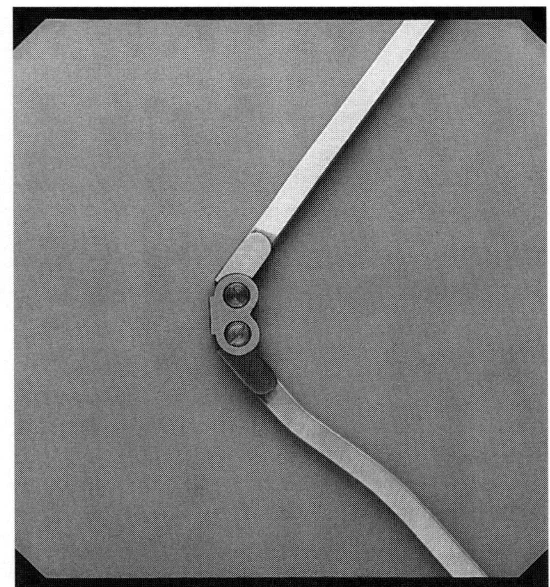

FIGURE 16–20. Polycentric knee joint. (Courtesy of Becker Orthopedic Co., Troy, MI.)

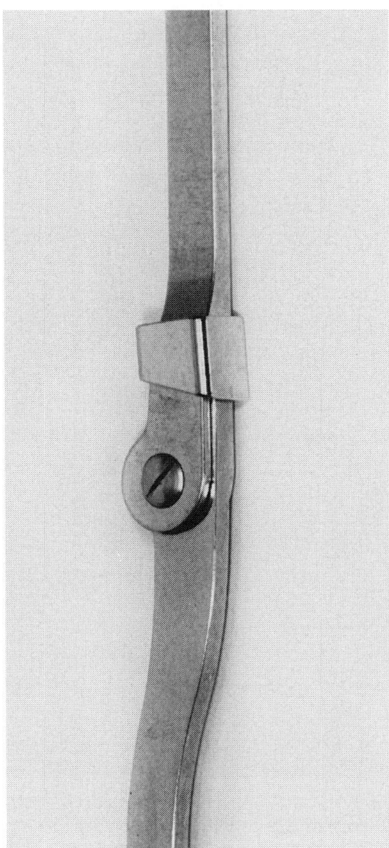

FIGURE 16–19. Straight-set knee with drop lock. (Courtesy of USMC, Pasadena.)

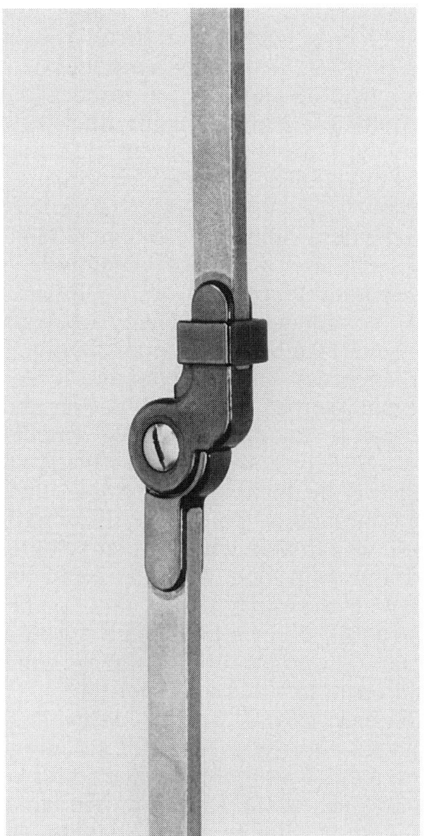

FIGURE 16–21. Offset knee joint with drop lock. (Courtesy of USMC, Pasadena.)

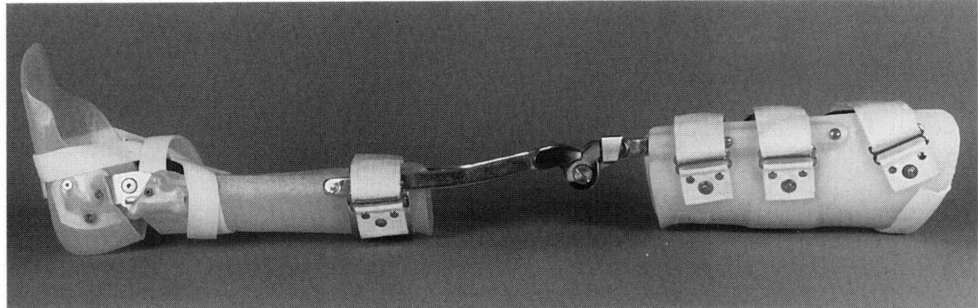

FIGURE 16–22. Plastic-metal KAFO. The 10 degrees of plantar flexion and the posterior offset knee joint initially provided stability at the knee for the patient. A drop lock had to be added because of advancing knee extensor weakness.

joint should have a hyperextension stop to help prevent genu recurvatum.

Occasionally, the offset knee joint does not provide adequate stability at the knee. The ankle component of the KAFO can then be set in 10 to 15 degrees of plantar flexion to further help create an extension moment at the knee for stability (Fig. 16–22).

Knee Locks

Knee locks are used to provide complete stability at the knee. There are four common types of knee locks; these are discussed in order of their frequency of use, beginning with the most commonly used.

The ratchet lock has recently become the most commonly prescribed knee lock (Fig. 16–23). The ratchet lock has a catching mechanism that operates in 12-degree increments. As the user rises from a seated to a standing position, if there is a tendency for the knee to become unstable and flex, the ratchet lock prevents that movement and keeps the gains made toward extension. Once the patient is standing with the knees extended, knee flexion is achieved by pressing down on a release lever.

Prior to the development of the ratchet lock, the drop lock (ring lock) was used most commonly in both the medial and lateral uprights of the KAFO (see Fig. 16–19). Its advantage is simplicity of design without bulk. However, fine motor coordination skills are needed to lock the knee in complete extension. The drop lock can "settle" after ambulation and might be difficult to pull up to unlock the knee. The disadvantage of the drop lock in comparison with the ratchet lock is that there is no locking mechanism until full knee extension is obtained. Consequently, a patient's knee can collapse into flexion when not sufficiently extended to activate the drop lock. A collapse into flexion does not occur with the ratchet lock, and so the patient is less likely to fall. A drop lock can be used unilaterally along the lateral upright if the patient is relatively lightweight and has a low activity level.

The bail lock (Swiss, French, Schweitzer, or pawl lock) provides an easy method of simultaneously unlocking the medial and lateral knee joints of a KAFO (Figs. 16–24 and 16–25). Lifting up the bail posteriorly releases the knee joint to permit flexion, allowing the patient to sit down. The patient can also catch the bail on the edge of a chair to release the lock mechanism

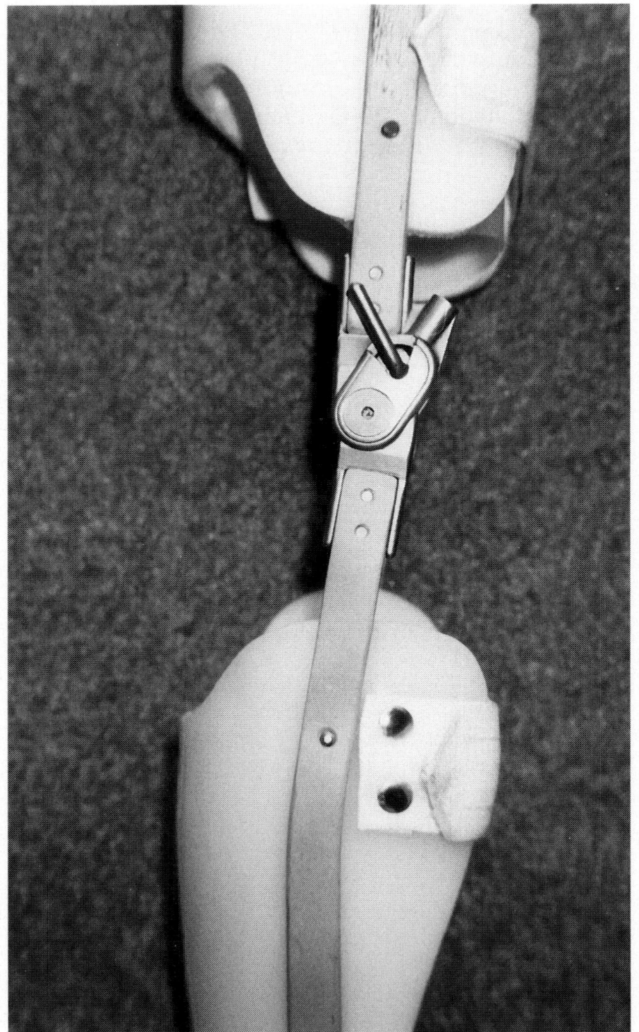

FIGURE 16–23. Ratchet lock. The 12 degree increments gained with knee extension prevent the knee from going into flexion and thereby adding stability and a safety factor as one rises from a seated to a standing position. The mechanism is released to allow one to resume a seated position by using the lever arm.

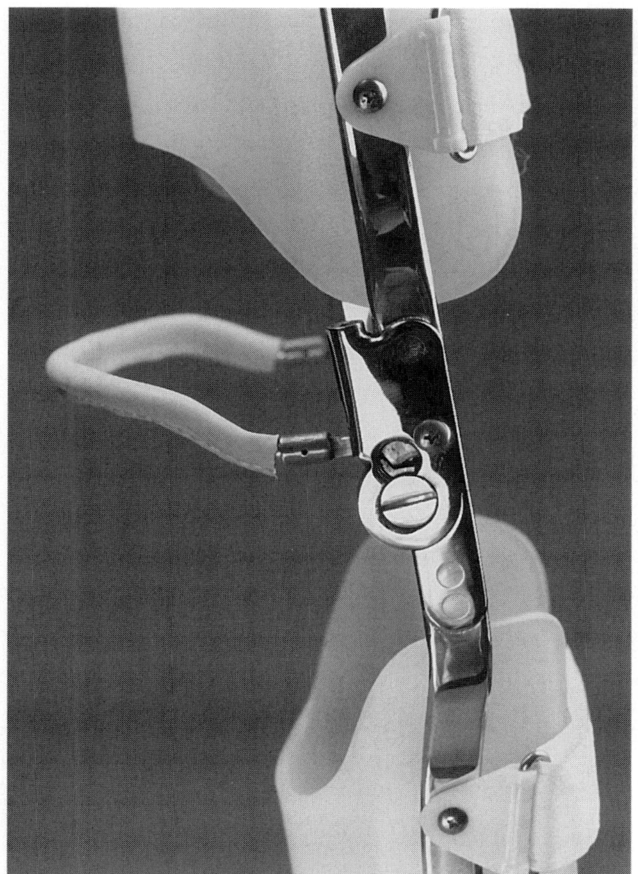

FIGURE 16–24. Spring-loaded bail lock. (Courtesy of Becker Orthopedic Co., Troy, MI.)

to permit sitting. The locking mechanism is often spring-loaded to assist locking the knee into extension (Fig. 16–25). The bail is often padded with rubber to protect the clothing from being torn or soiled. The KAFO with a bail lock can be worn over or under clothes, depending on the size of the bail lock and the size of the clothing.

The dial lock (formerly known as a turn buckle) is used to stabilize the knee in varying amounts of flexion (Fig. 16–26). It can be adjusted in 6-degree increments and is more precise for the management of a knee with a flexion contracture than a KAFO with ratchet locks. Its uses include helping prevent progression of a flexion contracture or assisting with the gradual reduction of a flexion contracture.

The Thigh Component of a KAFO

The thigh band needs to be wide enough to adequately distribute the pressure of the ground reactive force transmitted through the knee axis. A partial plastic thigh shell can provide a greater contact area and decrease high-pressure areas if properly fitted. Plastic-metal combination KAFOs also decrease the weight of the KAFO, which can increase patient comfort and usage. A low thigh band is used to prevent genu recurvatum.

Scott Craig Orthosis

The Scott Craig orthosis (Fig. 16–27) was designed to provide the paraplegic patient having a complete lesion at L1 or higher with a more functional and comfortable gait.[35] It was also designed to reduce unnecessary hardware, to be a KAFO of lighter weight, and to be easy to don and doff.

The orthotic design consists of an ankle joint with anterior and posterior pin stops, a sole plate extending to the metatarsal heads, a crossbar added to the metatarsal head area for mediolateral stabilization, and an offset knee joint with a bail lock.[35] A rigid anterior tibial band is positioned directly below the tibial tubercle. A rigid proximal thigh band is positioned posteriorly and is closed anteriorly with a soft strap secured with Velcro. These two bands should be shallow enough to hold the knee in extension. A three-point system helps keep the knee in extension by applying pressure at the proximal thigh posteriorly, the proximal tibia anteriorly, and at the calcaneus posteriorly.[17] The ankle joint functions with a dorsiflexion stop used to simulate the triceps surae function as previously described and with a posterior stop set at 90 degrees to prevent toe drag.

A group headed by Lehmann analyzed the Scott Craig orthosis and found that it was the easiest of the KAFOs

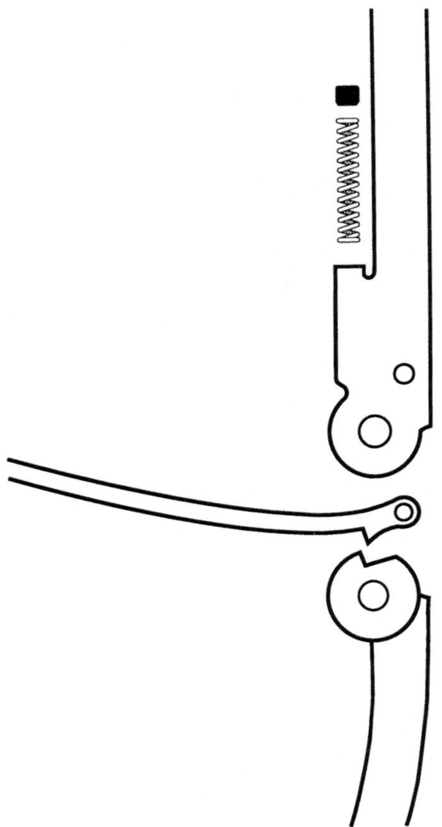

FIGURE 16–25. Spring-loaded bail lock mechanism. Lifting the bail permits free flexion for sitting and the spring mechanism helps lock the knee joint into extension.

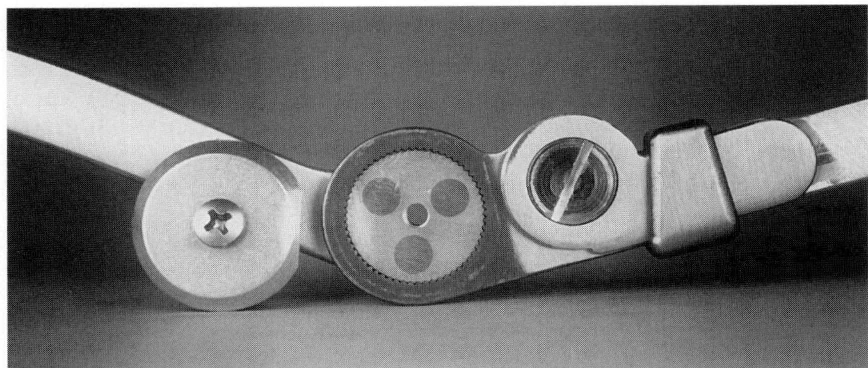

FIGURE 16–26. The dial lock may be adjusted every 6 degrees for precise control of knee flexion.

tested to don and doff.[19] The original design of this orthosis is still being prescribed for paraplegic patients.

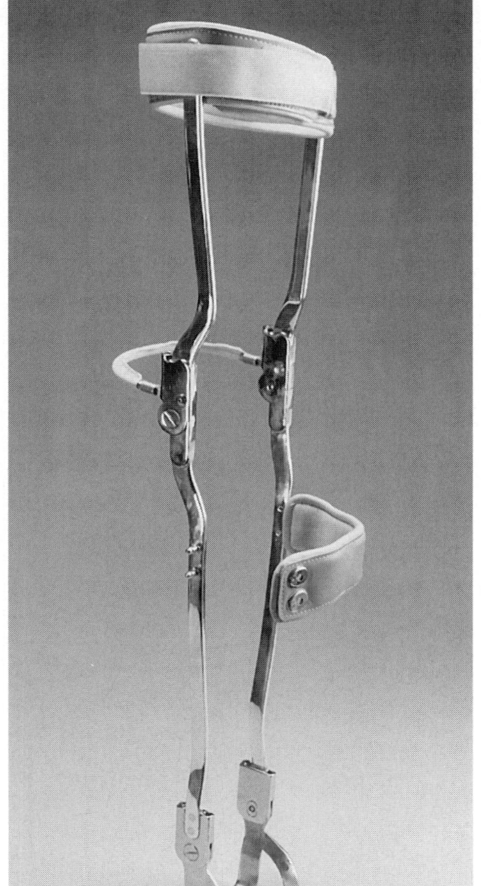

FIGURE 16–27. Scott Craig KAFO. (Courtesy of Becker Orthopedic Co., Troy, MI.)

KNEE ORTHOSES

Swedish Knee Cage

The knee orthosis (KO) known as a Swedish knee cage (Fig. 16–28) is used to control minor to moderate genu recurvatum due to ligamentous or capsular laxity. It was previously available in a nonarticulated form but should be prescribed only in an articulated form. The nonarticulated version does not allow any knee flexion or extension and therefore is no longer the recommended version of the Swedish knee cage for genu recurvatum. The articulated version allows full knee flexion and prevents hyperextension. The articulated version is recommended for the treatment of genu recurvatum. It uses a three-point system with two bands placed anterior to the knee axis (one above and one below the knee) and a third band posterior to the knee joint in the popliteal area. It also has an additional thigh band with longer uprights to obtain better leverage at the knee joint. Severe genu recurvatum might need to be controlled with longer lever arms, such as that offered by a KAFO.

Genu recurvatum can also be controlled with a solid plastic AFO that resists plantar flexion. This can be used in cases where pathology also affects the ankle or subtalar joints. The more rigid the AFO, the greater the flexion moment at the knee during heel strike (which counters the extension moment of the recurvatum). An additional flexion moment at the knee during midstance can be obtained by fixing the AFO in a few degrees of dorsiflexion.

Osteoarthritis Knee Orthoses

The same orthotic three-point principle that has been applied for years in the Swedish knee cage for genu recurvatum has recently also been applied to osteoarthritis of the knee, more commonly with medial compartment narrowing (Fig. 16–29). The three-point system distribution is achieved by a strap that is applied across the knee joint. In a recent study, 19 of 20 patients

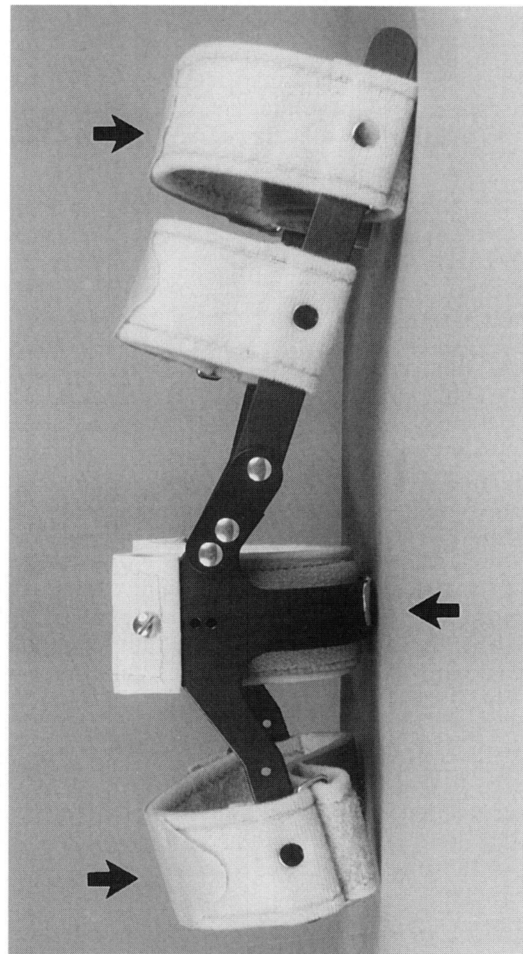

FIGURE 16–28. The articulated Swedish knee cage, which uses a three-point system to control genu recurvatum.

with varying degrees of osteoarthritis experienced significant relief of knee pain.[24] Radiographic improvement in joint alignment was also noted. The limiting factor regarding this knee orthotic prescription is the patient's weight. A morbidly obese patient with an abundance of fatty tissue around the knee will not support the knee orthosis adequately. In such cases where this KO and surgery are precluded, the foot orthoses with lateral buildup as described earlier in this chapter should be considered.

Sport Knee Orthoses

There is an increasing abundance of sport orthoses on the market. There is also a lack of definitive research regarding their role in sports. This can lead to much confusion regarding their prescription, unless the KO is reviewed systematically. Sport KOs can be divided into prophylactic, rehabilitative, and functional categories.[27]

Prophylactic knee bracing attempts to prevent or reduce the severity of knee injuries. There is currently no evidence to support the use or cost benefit of these orthoses. Some studies have found that the use of these orthoses actually increased the number of athletes with knee injuries.[32, 37] It is theorized that knee-braced players can put themselves in compromising positions because of overreliance on the orthosis and that this can contribute directly to the increasing injury rates observed. The use of prophylactic knee bracing has also been associated with increased energy consumption, which can impair athletic performance.[9]

Rehabilitative knee bracing is used to allow protected motion within defined limits.[27] It is useful for postoperative and conservative management of knee injuries.

Functional knee bracing is designed to assist or provide stability for the unstable knee. Functional knee bracing does not replace the need for rehabilitation of the knee. Knee braces are used most commonly to stabilize a laterally subluxing patella or an anterior cruciate ligament–deficient knee (Fig. 16–30). Their use

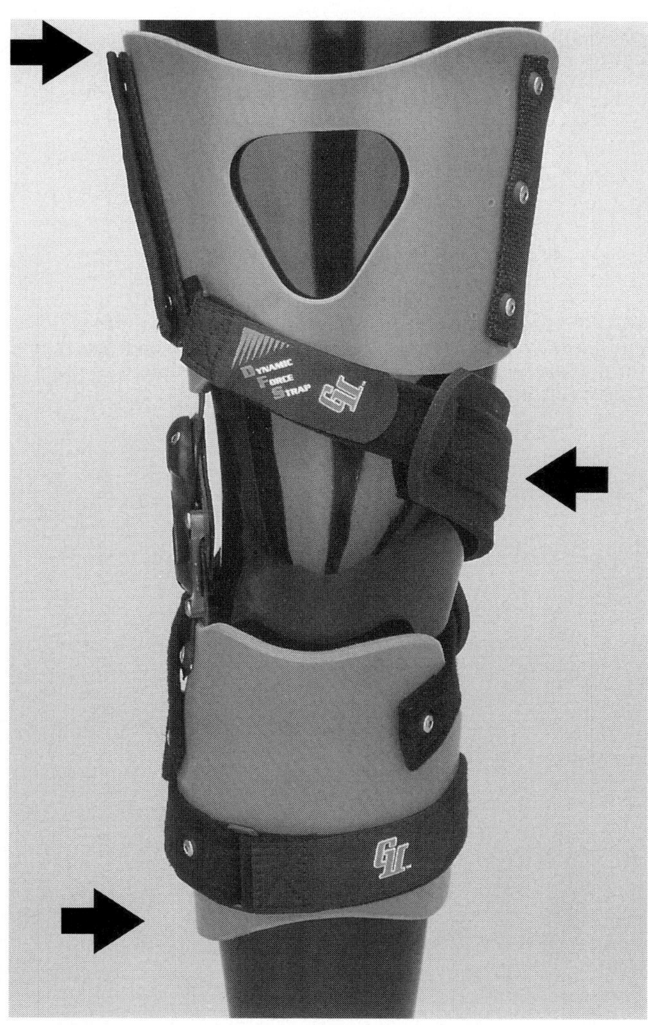

FIGURE 16–29. The Generation II knee orthosis for tricompartmental osteoarthritis of the knee. This utilizes the standard orthotic three-point distribution system in a medial-lateral distribution rather than in an anterior-posterior distribution as was noted with the Swedish knee cage (Fig. 16–28).

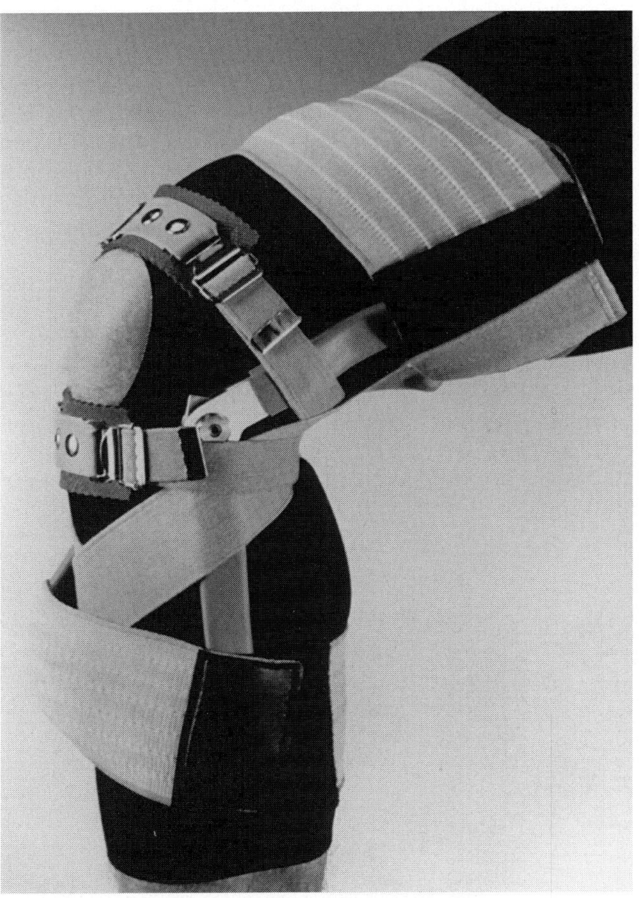

FIGURE 16–30. Lenox Hill Spectralite knee orthosis, which is commonly prescribed for anterior cruciate-deficient knees and for patellas with a tendency to lateral subluxation. (Courtesy of Lenox Hill Brace Co., Bethesda, MD.)

has been shown to be effective only at loads much lower than those placed on the knee during athletic participation. In summary, functional knee bracing can possibly play a role in the treatment of pathological laxity by possibly decreasing the frequency of unstable episodes.[27]

PEDIATRIC ORTHOSES

Caster Cart

The disabled child should identify early with motion so that ambulatory skills can progress naturally.[1] Without familiarity with motion, disabled children lack the desire to ambulate once placed in a parapodium or reciprocating gait orthosis.

The caster cart (Fig. 16–31) is used for children with a developmental delay in ambulatory skills, and it serves as an initial mobility aid. It is most often prescribed for children with spina bifida. Most children are upright and cruising by 10 months.[10] Children with paraplegia should be fitted for a caster cart once they have obtained enough upper limb strength and trunk balance to propel themselves. If balance is a problem for the child, a deep seat bucket can be prescribed to help provide balance so that the child can use the upper limbs for propulsion.

The caster wheel at the back of the cart facilitates multidirectional movement. Initially, the child can be pushed around in the cart with a handle attached posteriorly so that the cart serves as a stroller.

Standing Frame

The use of a standing frame (Fig. 16–32) typically follows successful use of a caster cart. The age range for initial use is usually 8 to 15 months. Children can continue to use their caster carts during this time. Children who are pulling themselves up along furniture are typi-

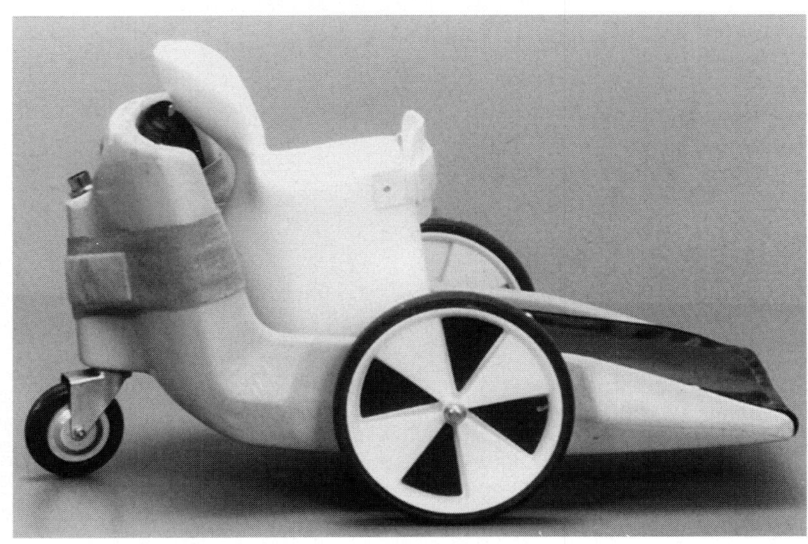

FIGURE 16–31. Caster cart. This is an initial mobility aid for the disabled child. The child uses it as a "prewheelchair device." The deep seat bucket stabilizes the seated ataxic child while permitting free use of the upper limbs for ambulation. (Courtesy of the Hugh MacMillan Rehabilitation Center, Toronto.)

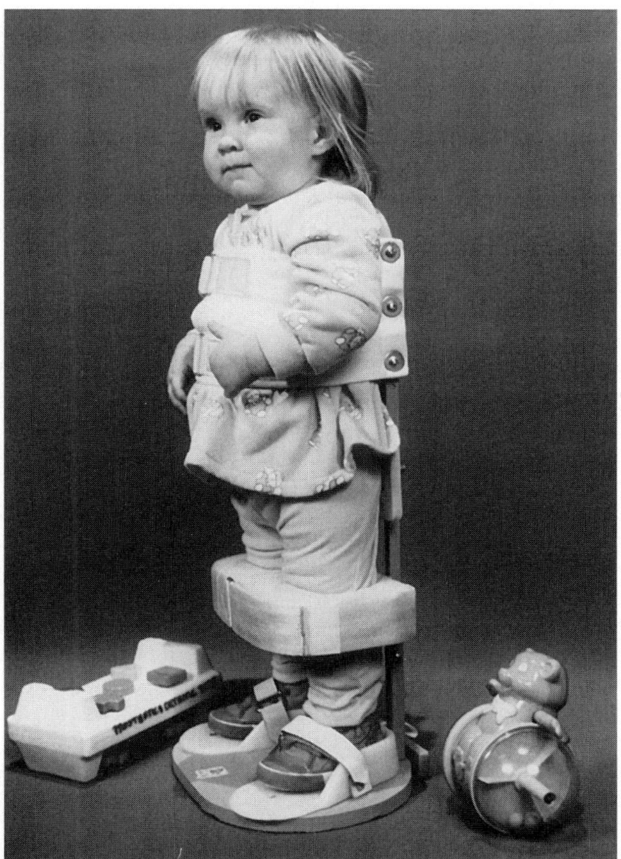

FIGURE 16–32. A standing frame being used by a spina bifida toddler with a T12 neurosegmental level lesion. (Courtesy of the Hugh MacMillan Rehabilitation Center, Toronto.)

cally ready for a standing frame. This is the first sign that they are interested in standing and moving.[10]

The standing frame helps balance the body in space and allows free use of the upper limbs for participation in activities. Children with thoracic level lesions need AFOs to provide good ankle and foot support in the standing frame or parapodium. Initial gait training can occur with the use of the standing frame via a swing-through gait with the assistance of parallel bars.

Parapodium

The parapodium was also referred to in the past as a swivel orthosis (Fig. 16–33). Before children are given a parapodium, they should first demonstrate adequate use of a standing frame and exhibit a desire to ambulate. A child's standing frame can be evaluated for wear and tear to determine whether it has been used sufficiently so that the child can advance to a parapodium. A frequently used standing frame (or any orthosis) will look dirty and scratched up, and have lint in the Velcro straps. It is important to note this, since parents frequently set expectations too high for the disabled child. A child who has not used a standing frame will likely be unable or unwilling to ambulate with a parapodium.

A parapodium is an appropriate prescription for children who are unlikely to become functional walkers owing to the severity of their impairment. It often complements wheelchair use.[21] It is most commonly prescribed for children between 2½ and 5 years of age.

A parapodium allows crutchless gait. Ambulation occurs by the child pivoting the hips and using "body English" to swivel one side of the oval-based stand forward and then repeating the same event for the other side. Its design is similar to the standing frame, but it has hip and knee joints. The hip and knee joints remain locked in extension to permit ambulation in the upright position but can be unlocked (simultaneously in some models) to permit sitting. The difficulties experienced with the use of this orthosis include donning and doffing and rising from a seated position to a standing position.

Reciprocating Gait Orthosis

The reciprocating gait orthosis (RGO) was formerly known as a hip-guided orthosis (HGO) (Fig. 16–34). It can also be referred to as a bilateral hip-knee-ankle-foot orthosis (HKAFO). The purpose of the RGO is to provide contralateral hip extension with ipsilateral hip flexion. The RGO is appropriate for children who have

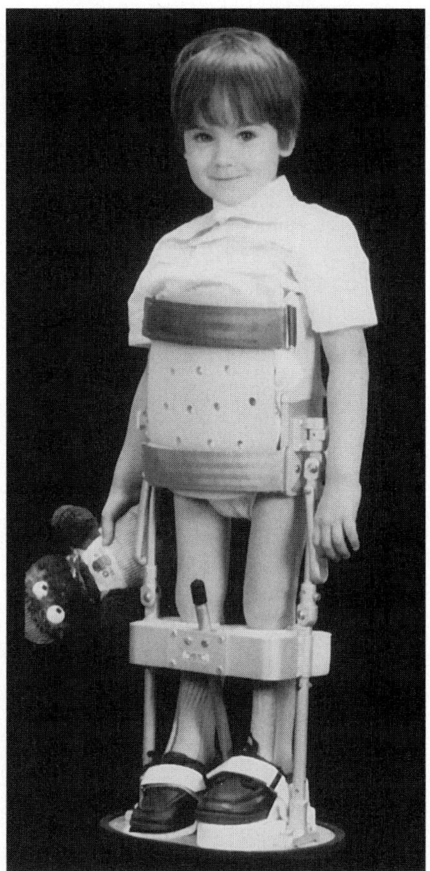

FIGURE 16–33. Parapodium. Note the lift on the left leg to compensate for a leg length discrepancy and the wide abdominal support pad to assist in upright posture. (Courtesy of the Hugh MacMillan Rehabilitation Center, Toronto.)

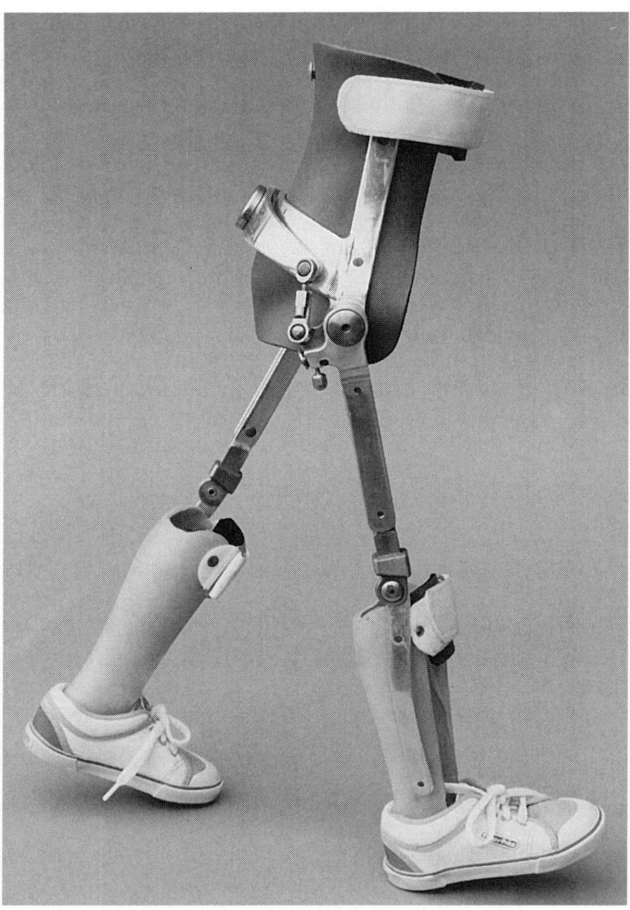

FIGURE 16–34. Isocentric reciprocating gait orthosis (RGO): dynamic view. (Courtesy of Center for Orthotic Design, Redwood City, CA.)

used the standing frame, developed good trunk control and coordination, can safely stand, and are mentally prepared for ambulation. Good upper limb strength, trunk balance, and active hip flexion are important positive variables for ambulation.[6] Obesity, advanced age, lack of patient or family motivation, scoliosis, spasticity,[6] and contractures are significant negative factors in the long-term use of the RGO. This type of orthosis clearly only complements the use of a wheelchair for mobility purposes.

Spinal cord injury level of spinal cord level injury is not a very reliable predictor of ambulation capability for children. As children with spinal cord injuries grow taller, they might experience more difficulty walking as their center of gravity becomes lower.

The RGO is prescribed most commonly for children ages 3 to 6 years. The concept of the RGO was developed by researchers working with a patient who had active hip flexion and no hip extension. Gait is initiated with unilateral hip flexion and can be assisted by swaying the trunk when hip flexion is inadequate. This type of gait pattern can also be considered to be a form of physical therapy, since hip extension occurs passively with each step, helping to reduce flexion contractures. Cables were initially used to provide the necessary hip motion, but newer mechanical methods of reciprocal gait employ a "teeter-totter" concept (Fig. 16–34). This type of RGO has been reported to be more energy efficient than an RGO with cables.[43]

Crutches are used with the RGO to provide a control mechanism, taking advantage of the forward momentum to produce small propulsive forces when needed.[22] This also is a disadvantage of this orthosis (compared to the parapodium) because the upper limbs are not free for other activities. The patient with an RGO is able to negotiate a greater variety of surfaces than would be possible with the parapodium.[31]

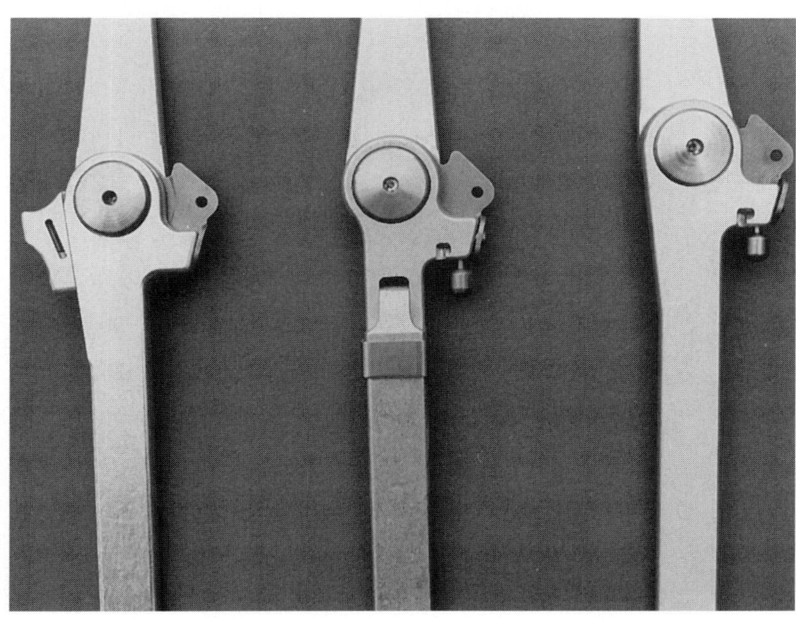

FIGURE 16–35. Unique hip joints for use with the isocentric RGO. *Left:* "Pre-selected" with easy-to-lock and -unlock lever. *Middle:* "Abduction hinge" hip joint for easy catheterization without removal of the brace. *Right:* Conventional hip joint as used on cable braces. (Courtesy of Center for Orthotic Design, Redwood City, CA.)

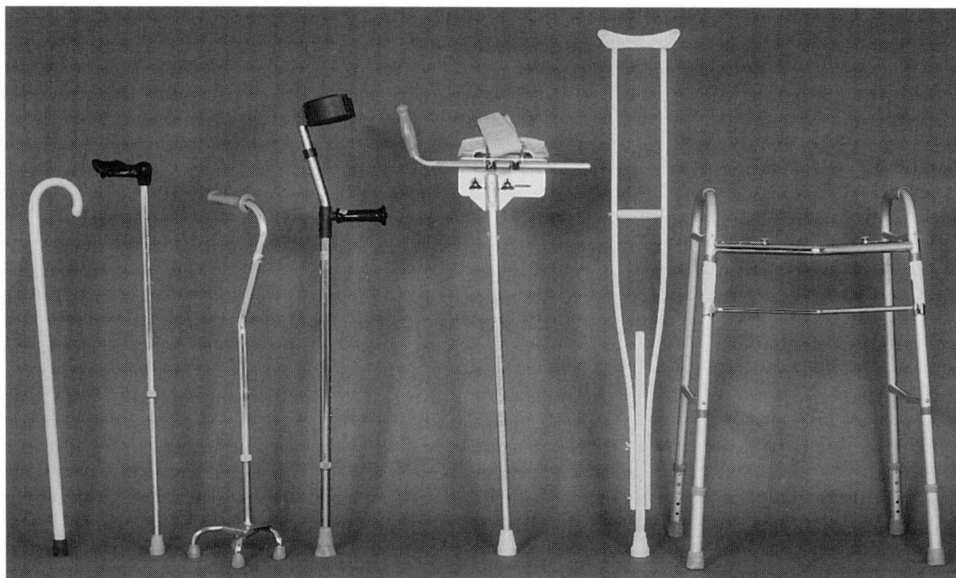

FIGURE 16–36. Ambulation aids. *Left to right:* C cane, functional grip cane, quad cane, Lofstrand forearm orthosis, platform forearm orthosis, crutch, and walker.

The hip joints of the RGO have hip flexion and abduction capabilities upon release of the locking mechanisms (Fig. 16–35). It is recommended that one hip joint have abduction capability to permit catheterization and to allow sitting in a hip-flexed and abducted position.

AMBULATION AIDS

The purpose of using ambulation aids (Figs. 16–36 and 16-37) is to increase the area of support for patients who have difficulty maintaining their center of gravity safely over their own support area. A variety of aids are available for the individual needs of patients. Ambulation aids improve balance, redistribute and extend the weight-bearing area, reduce lower limb pain, provide small propulsive forces, and provide sensory feedback. They should be considered an extension of the upper limb. Their proper use requires adequate upper limb strength and coordination. An exercise program for the upper limbs is useful and can complement ambulation with the aid by increasing endurance and stability. A supervised period of training is recommended after prescription of an aid.

The type of aid needed depends on how much balance and weight-bearing assistance is needed. The body weight transmission for a unilateral cane opposite the affected side is 20% to 25%.[4] It is 40% to 50% with the use of a forearm or arm cane.[4] Body weight transmission with bilateral crutches is estimated at up to 80%.[4]

Canes

Prescription: Measure the tip of the cane to the level of the greater trochanter with the patient in an upright position to determine the proper cane length.[38]

The elbow should be flexed approximately 20 degrees, which is a desirable elbow position for all ambulation

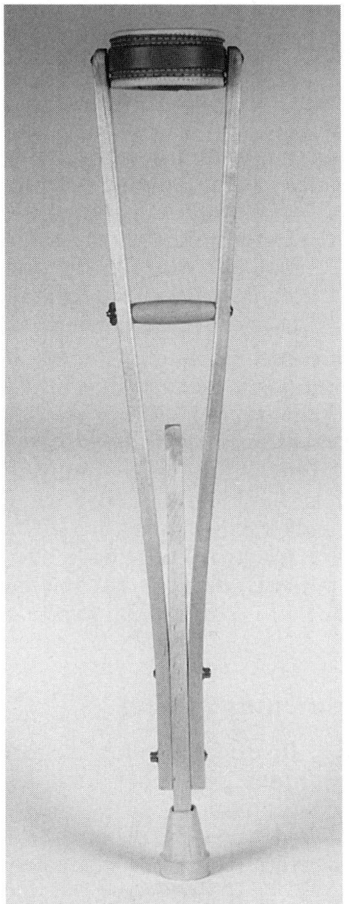

FIGURE 16–37. Wooden forearm orthosis (Kenny stick). The leather band encloses the proximal forearm.

aids. Canes are made of wood or aluminum, with the aluminum alloy cane having adjustable notches so that "one cane fits all."

There are three common types of canes (see Fig. 16–36). The C cane is most commonly used. It is also known as a crook top cane or a J cane. A functional grip cane offers the patient a grip that can be more comfortable than with the C cane. A quad cane provides an increased area of support compared to the other canes. Quad canes also come in narrow- and wide-based forms for different degrees of support. The lateral two legs are directed away from the body.

A cane is used on the side opposite the supporting lower limb. It is advanced with the opposite lower limb. It is usually held on the patient's unaffected side. This can be done to lessen the force exerted on a hip with pathology. The load is increased by four times the body weight on the stance side during gait due to the gravitational forces and the gluteus medius-minimus force exerted across the weight-bearing hip.[4] The cane helps decrease the force generated across the affected hip joint by decreasing the work of the gluteus medius-minimus complex. This occurs when the upper limb exerts force on the cane to help minimize pelvic drop on the side opposite the weight-bearing lower limb.

Patients should be instructed on how to ascend and descend stairs. The pneumonic "up with the good and down with the bad" serves as an easy reminder. The patient should always have the "good" lower limb assume the first full weight-bearing step on level surfaces.

Walker

Prescription:
1. Place the front of the walker 12 inches in front of the patient (the walker should partially surround the patient).
2. Determine the proper height of the walker by having the patient stand upright with the shoulders relaxed and the elbows flexed 20 degrees.[38]

A walker provides maximum support for the patient but also necessitates a slow gait. It is useful for hemiplegic and ataxic patients. Wheels can be added to the front legs to facilitate movement of the walker for those who lack coordination in the upper limbs. Patients using wheeled models should be supervised initially to ensure safety. Some walkers also have a front U-shaped extension with extra supports to provide stability for stair climbing. A patient needs to be motivated and have good strength and coordination to use this model of walker.

Visual Impairment Cane

Prescription:
1. Instruct the patient to flex the shoulder until the upper limb is parallel with the floor.
2. Measure the distance from the hand to the floor. That is the proper length.

A visual impairment cane should be lightweight, flexible, and easily collapsible. The distal inches of the cane are red.

Crutches

Prescription:
1. Crutch length: Measure the distance from the anterior axillary fold to a point 6 inches lateral to the fifth toe with the patient standing with the shoulders relaxed.
2. Handpiece: Measure with the patient's elbow flexed 30 degrees, the wrist in maximal extension, and the fingers forming a fist. This is measured *after* the total crutch height is determined with the crutch 3 inches lateral to the foot.[38]

A crutch is defined as a device that provides support from the axilla to the floor. Although there are different types of crutches and canes, they can all be referred to as orthoses because they are applied to the external surface of the body to improve function.

The patient should be able to raise the body 1 to 2 inches by complete elbow extension. Despite the popularity of padding the axillary area of the crutch, this should not be done. It needs to be emphasized to the patient that crutches are not designed to be rests for body support. This point should be made to the patient in order to reduce the incidence of compressive radial neuropathies.

Nonaxillary Crutches

Nonaxillary crutches are more appropriately called forearm or arm canes, or forearm or arm orthoses. The Loftstrand forearm orthosis, Kenny sticks, the Everett or Warm Spring orthosis, the Canadian crutch, and the platform forearm orthosis will be discussed (Figs. 16–36 and 16–37).

FOREARM ORTHOSES

Lofstrand Forearm Orthosis

Prescription: Measure the handpiece as described above for crutches, with the patient standing upright and the elbow in 20 degrees of flexion.

The proximal portion of the orthosis is also angled at 20 degrees to provide for a comfortable, stable fit. It is often made of tubular aluminum. It provides less support than crutches for ambulation, but is sufficient for many patients. Lofstrand forearm orthoses are most often used bilaterally. The open end of the cuff is placed on the lateral aspect of the forearm to permit elbow flexion and grasping without dropping the orthoses. The advantages of this orthosis are that it is shorter than an axillary crutch, and the forearm cuff pivots to allow the patient to lean on the crutch for hand activities.

Wooden Forearm Orthosis (Kenny Stick)

Another forearm orthosis option is the Kenny stick (Fig. 16–37). It was named after Sister Kenny, who sawed off the top half of wooden crutches and placed a leather band around the proximal portion of the forearm. It was designed for polio patients who had satisfactory proximal upper limb musculature but were weak distally and unable to effectively hold and control the orthosis. Its advantage over the Loftstrand orthosis is the presence of a closed leather band. This assures the patient (more so than the Lofstrand forearm orthosis does) that he or she will not drop the ambulation aid.

Platform Forearm Orthosis

Prescription: Have the patient stand upright with the shoulders relaxed and the elbows flexed 90 degrees. The distance from the ground to the forearm rest is the proper length.

This orthosis is helpful for patients with painful wrist and hand conditions as well as for those with elbow contractures. Velcro straps are applied around the forearm, especially for patients with weak hand grips.

Triceps Weakness Orthoses (Arm Orthoses)

These orthoses, also known as triceps weakness crutches, were originally developed for poliomyelitis patients. The metal version is known as a Warm Spring crutch or Everett crutch. The wooden version is known as a Canadian crutch. These crutches resemble the "axillary" crutches in style, but end proximally with a cuff at the mid-arm level. These ambulation aids help prevent flexion (buckling) of the elbow during gait.

Crutch Tips and Hand Grips

The purpose of crutch tips is to absorb shock and prevent slippage. Crutches are only as safe as the quality of their crutch tips. Special crutch tips are available for rainy and icy conditions (Fig. 16–38). At each checkup, the physician should make sure that the crutch tips are not worn out. Hand grips are used to reduce pressure on the hands and are also safety features because they help prevent slippage.

Crutch Gaits

Strength, balance, coordination, and walking surface all have an effect on which crutch gait should be used under different circumstances. Each patient should be comfortable with more than one type of crutch gait. There are two-point, three-point, and four-point crutch gaits. The swing-through, swing-to, and drag-to gaits will also be discussed. Although these gaits have traditionally been referred to as crutch gaits, their use applies to the other ambulation aids as well.

The four-point crutch gait follows the sequence: left crutch → right foot → right crutch → left foot → repeat. Its advantage is stability. At least three points are always in contact with the ground. This gait is useful ataxic patients and those with marked lower limb weakness. It is more difficult to learn than the other gait patterns and is a relatively slow form of ambulation.

The three-point crutch gait follows the sequence: both crutches and the weaker lower limb → "good" lower limb → repeat. The advantage of the three-point gait is that all weight bearing on the affected lower limb is eliminated. This gait is commonly used by patients with lower limb fractures or amputations. It is also known as the non-weight-bearing gait. The patient should have good balance to perform this gait.

The alternate two-point crutch gait follows the sequence: left crutch and right foot → right crutch and left foot → repeat. This gait pattern provides stability and is useful for ataxic patients and with decreased lower limb weight-bearing capabilities. It is faster than the four-point gait and provides some weight-bearing relief to both lower limbs.

Gait can also be classified as swing-through, swing-to, and drag-to. The swing-through pattern sequence is: both crutches → advancement of both lower limbs past the crutches. It is very energy-consuming and its use requires functional abdominal muscles. The swing-through gait is the fastest gait (even faster than abled body walking). The swing-to gait sequence is: both crutches → advancement of both lower limbs almost to the crutch level. There are alternate and simultaneous forms of drag to gait. The alternate sequence is: left crutch → right crutch → drag to crutch level. The simultaneous sequence is: both crutches → drag to crutch level. These are useful as initial gait patterns for paraplegic patients. They can advance to another gait pattern. These patterns provide stability during gait but are slow and laborious methods of ambulation.

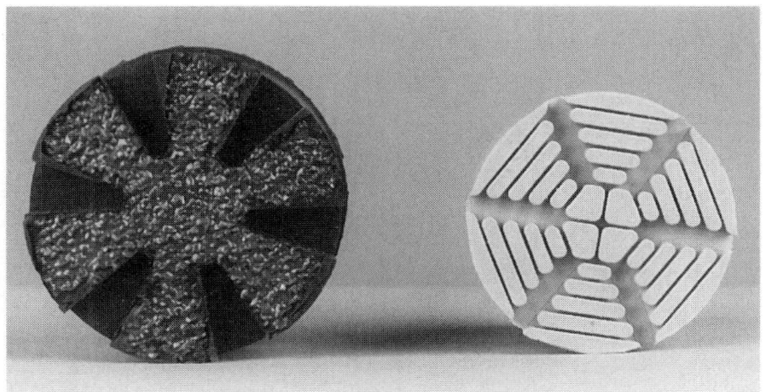

FIGURE 16–38. *Left,* Snow Boot crutch tip for use in snowy and icy conditions. *Right,* Rain Guard crutch tip for use in wet conditions. (Courtesy of Hi-Trac Industris, Holley, MI.)

Prescription

A medical diagnosis with delineation of the impairment and any resulting disability should be made before an orthotic prescription is written. The orthotic goals should be documented for the orthotist. An AFO prescription should include the type of ankle (rigid, flexible, or jointed) and the position of the ankle (neutral, dorsiflexed, or plantar-flexed). If the ankle is jointed, the range of motion should be specified. In the case of a compressive peroneal nerve palsy, for example, the physical impairment would be a flaccid foot drop. The ankle should be flexible and held in a neutral position with a plastic AFO set at 90 degrees. The goals include toe clearance during swing-through and prevention of foot slap during early stance.[14]

LOWER LIMB ORTHOTIC PRESCRIPTION

NAME: ______________________ AGE: _______

DIAGNOSIS: ______________________

ORTHOTIC GOALS: ______________________

JUSTIFICATION: ______________________

ORTHOTIC COMPANY: ______________________

REFERRING PHYSICIAN: ______________________

❑ FO ❑ AFO ❑ KAFO ❑ HKAFO ❑ KO

❑ Right ❑ Left ❑ Bilateral

❑ Custom

❑ Plastic ❑ Metal ❑ Combination

ANKLE TYPE: ❑ Solid (flexible) ❑ Solid (rigid) ❑ Hinged: ___ dorsi-assist
___ dorsi-stop
___ plantar stop

ANKLE ROM: ❑ Plantar flexion ______ degrees
❑ Dorsiflexion ______ degrees
❑ Neutral (90°)

KNEE TYPE: ❑ Straight set ❑ Posterior offset ❑ Polycentric

KNEE LOCKS: ❑ Two per knee joint ❑ One per knee joint

KNEE LOCK TYPE: ❑ Drop lock ❑ Bail lock ❑ Dial lock ❑ Ratchet lock ❑ Fan lock

HIP JOINTS with drop locks: ❑ Standard ❑ Abduction

MISCELLANEOUS: ______________________

______________________ ______________________
Physician Name Date

FIGURE 16–39. Lower limb orthotic prescription sheet.

TABLE 16–3 Summary Reference for Prescription Pad

FO:

UCBL (University of Ca. Biomechanics Laboratory)—hyperpronating "flat" foot
metatarsal pad—temporary mild to moderate metatarsalgia
metatarsal bar to shoe—severe metatarsalgia (can't stand something in shoe) or permanent metatarsalgia (e.g. arthritis)
heel lift—temporary use for achilles tendinitis or plantar fasciitis
heel cup—fat pad syndrome (heel bruise)
lateral heel wedge—OA with medial compartment narrowing

AFO:

over-the-counter—for a trial basis only
custom—for long term use
plastic—for almost everyone
metal—for the patient >250# with a hinged AFO

Common types:

custom solid (flexible) AFO set at 90°—foot drop
custom solid (rigid) AFO set at 90°—plantar spasticity

Hinge indications:

1) significant mediolateral instability at subtalar joint but patient with ankle dorsi & plantar flexion (rare)
2) tight plantar flexors in a spastic patient with improving lower limb function (they can take advantage of a more "normal" gait via dorsiflexion from midstance to toe off and plantar stretching is therapeutic over this part of the gait cycle)
3) an active patient with foot drop or plantar flexor spasticity can take advantage of the hinged feature during stair climbing, rising from sit to stand, frequent walking, etc.

KAFO:

knee type:
straight set—most common; always used unless posterior offset is indicated
posterior offset—patient with weak knee extensor triad (quads, plantar flexors, and hamstrings)
polycentric—a two joint system that theoretically simulates femur—tibia translation
—standard on most sport orthoses for the above marketing purpose
—no clear cut indications
knee locks:
drop lock—most common; can be difficult to pull up after "settling in" from walking
bail lock—bulkier and less desirable then the drop locks for most patients but necessary for those without fine hand control
dial/fan lock—used to lock an unstable knee in extension but they are adjusted to account for knee flexion contractures

Hip joints (common to prescribe one of each of the below):

standard—allows flexion & extension
abduction—permits flexion and extension but also permits abduction to allow self urinary bladder straight catheterization and seating in a hip-flexed & abducted position

From an orthotic prescription standpoint, most of this chapter is concisely summarized in Figure 16–39, a full-size prescription pad with convenient check boxes and room at the top of the page to copy this onto letterhead for clinical use. Adjacent to this sheet is a quick summary reference that can be copied onto the back of the prescription sheets (Table 16–3).

SUMMARY

An appropriate lower limb orthotic prescription requires a thorough biomechanical analysis of gait and knowledge of the available orthotic components available to treat specific conditions. The prescribing physician should maintain a close working relationship with the certified orthotist to make certain that the patient is receiving the best orthotic options available.

Patient complaints about orthoses usually are related to cosmesis, comfort, clothing soiling or damage, weight, and difficulty with donning and doffing. All practitioners should work toward the goal of achieving the ideal orthosis for the patient that enhances comfort, cosmesis, and function. Accomplishing this will in turn enhance compliance. The ideal orthosis would be weightless, invisible, without cost, maintenance free, comfortable, and strong, and would normalize the gait pattern while simultaneously reducing energy consumption to within normal limits.

ACKNOWLEDGMENTS

A special thanks to Bradd L. Rosenquist, C.P.O., of Columbus Orthopaedic Prosthetic and Orthotic Center, Inc., Mike Russell, C.P.O., and colleagues of Hanger Orthopedics, Rosalind Batley, M.D., and Kurt Kuhlman, D.O., and Richard Kozakiewicz, M.D., for reviewing this chapter. Our gratitude also goes to Steve Brady, medical illustrator, and to Jenny Torbett, photographer, for their contributions to several figures in this chapter. We also thank Pearl Liss of Apex Health Industries, R. Douglas Turner of Becker Orthopedic, Wally Motloch, C.O., of the Center for Orthotic Design, Inc., Robert Evans of High-Trac Industries, Greg Belbin, C.O., of the Hugh MacMillan Rehabilitation Center, Carol Hiemstra-Paez of Hanger Orthopedic

Group, Inc., Deanna Fish, C.P.O., of O.O.S., Inc., Stacey Whiteside, C.O., of Precision O & P Components, Inc., and Wayne Janke, of USMC, for providing photographs of their products for this chapter.

Thanks for the assistance provided by the following product suppliers: Apex Foot Health Industries, Inc., South Hackensack, NJ; Becker Orthopedic, Troy, MI; Center for Orthotic Design, Inc., Redwood City, CA; High-Trac Industries, Holley, MI; the Hugh MacMillan Rehabilitation Center, Toronto, Canada; Lenox Brace Company, Long Island City, NY; the JA Preston Corportion, Jackson, MI; Oregon Orthotic System, Inc., Albany, OR; Precision O & P Components, Inc., Tempe, AZ; and United States Manufacturing Company, Pasadena, CA.

REFERENCES

1. Bleck EE: Developmental orthopaedics: III. Toddlers. Dev Med Child Neurol 1982; 24:533–555.
2. Corcoran PJ, Jebsen RH, Brengelmann GL, et al: Effects of plastic and metal leg braces on speed and energy cost of hemiparetic ambulation. Arch Phys Med Rehabil 1970; 51:69–77.
3. D'Ambrosia RD: Conservative management of metatarsal and heel pain in the adult foot. Orthopedics 1987; 10:137–142.
4. Deathe AB, Hayes KC, Winter DA: The biomechanics of canes, crutches, and walkers. Crit Rev Phys Rehab Med 1993; 5:15–29.
5. Diveley RL: Foot appliances and alterations. In American Academy of Orthopaedic Surgeons (eds): Orthopaedic Appliances Atlas. Ann Arbor, JW Edwards, 1952, vol 1, pp 463–464.
6. Guidera KJ, Smith S, Raney E, et al: Use of the reciprocating gait orthosis in myelodysplasia. J Pediatr Orthop 1993; 13:341–348.
7. Halar E, Cardenas D: Ankle-foot orthoses: Clinical implications. Phys Med Rehabil State Art Rev 1987; 1:45–66.
8. Harvey LA, et al: Functional outcomes attained by T9–12 paraplegic patients with the Walkabout and the Isocentric reciprocal gait orthoses. Arch Phys Med Rehabil 1997; 78:706–711.
9. Houston ME, Goemans PH: Leg muscle performance of athletes with and without knee support braces. Arch Phys Med Rehabil 1982; 63:431–432.
10. Johnson EW, Spiegel MH: Ambulation problems in very young children. JAMA 1961; 175:858–863.
11. Keating EM, Faris PM, Ritter MA, et al: Use of lateral heel and sole wedges in the treatment of medial osteoarthritis of the knee. Orthop Rev 1993; 22:921–924.
12. Lehmann JF: The biomechanics of ankle foot orthoses: Prescription and design. Arch Phys Med Rehabil 1979; 60:200–207.
13. Lehmann JF, Condon SM, de Lateur BJ, et al: Ankle-foot orthoses: Effect on gait abnormalities in tibial nerve paralysis. Arch Phys Med Rehabil 1985; 66:212–218.
14. Lehmann JF, Condon SM, de Lateur BJ, et al: Gait abnormalities in peroneal nerve paralysis and their correlation by orthoses: A biomechanical study. Arch Phys Med Rehabil 1986; 67:380–386.
15. Lehmann JF, de Lateur BJ, Warren CG, et al: Biomechanical evaluation of braces for paraplegics. Arch Phys Med Rehabil 1969; 50:179–188.
16. Lehmann JF, Esselman P, Ko MJ, et al: Plastic ankle foot orthoses: evaluation of function. Arch Phys Med Rehabil 1983; 64:402–407.
17. Lehmann JF, Warren CG: Restraining forces in various designs of knee ankle orthoses: Their placement and effect on anatomical knee joint. Arch Phys Med Rehabil 1976; 57:430–437.
18. Lehmann JF, Warren CG, de Lateur BJ: A biomechanical evaluation of knee stability in below knee braces. Arch Phys Med Rehabil 1970; 51:687–695.
19. Lehmann JF, Warren CG, Hertling D, et al: Craig Scott orthosis: A biomechanical and functional evaluation. Arch Phys Med Rehabil 1976; 57:438–442.
20. Lehmann JF, Warren CG, Pemberton DR, et al: Load bearing function of patellar tendon bearing braces of various designs. Arch Phys Med Rehabil 1971; 52:367–370.
21. Liptak GS, Shurtleff DB, Bloss JW, et al: Mobility aids for children with high-level myelomeningocele: Parapodium versus wheelchair. Dev Med Child Neurol 1992; 34:787–796.
22. Major RE, Stallard J, Rose GK: The dynamics of walking using the hip guidance orthosis (hgo) with crutches. Prosthet Orthot Int 1981; 5:19–22.
23. Marx HW: Lower limb orthotic designs for the spastic hemiplegic patient. Orthot Prosthet 1974; 28:14–20.
24. Matsuno H, Kadowaki, Tsjui H: Generation II knee bracing for severe medial compartment osteoarthritis of the knee. Arch Phys Med Rehabil 1997; 78:745–749.
25. Merritt JL: Knee-ankle-foot orthotics: Long leg braces and their practical applications. Phys Med Rehabil State Art Rev 1987; 1:67–82.
26. Milgram JE, Jacobson MA: Footgear: Therapeutic modifications of sole and heel. Orthop Rev 1978; 7:57–61.
27. Millet C, Drez D Jr: Knee braces. Orthopedics 1987; 10:1777–1780.
28. Redford JB: Orthoses. In Basmajian JV, Kirby RL (eds): Medical rehabilitation. Baltimore, Williams & Wilkins, 1984, p 101.
29. Reid DC: Heel pain and problems of the hindfoot. In Reid DC (ed): Sports Injury Assessment and Rehabilitation, ed 1. New York, Churchill Livingstone, 1992, pp 196–212.
30. Riegler HF: Orthotic devices for the foot. Orthop Rev 1987; 16:293–303.
31. Rose GK, Stallard J, Sankarankutty M: Clinical evaluation of spina bifida patients using hip guidance orthoses. Dev Med Child Neurol 1981; 23:30–40.
32. Rovere GD, Haupt HA, Yates CS: Prophylactic knee bracing in college football. Am J Sports Med 1987; 15:111–116.
33. Sarmiento A: A functional below the knee brace for tibial fractures: A report of its use in 135 cases. J Bone Joint Surg Am 1970; 52:295–311.
34. Sarmiento A, Gersten LM, Sobol JA, et al: Tibial shaft fractures treated with functional braces: Experience with 780 fractures. J Bone Joint Surg Br 1989; 71:602–609.
35. Scott BA: Engineering principles and fabrication techniques for Scott-Craig: Long leg brace for paraplegics. Orthop Prosthet 1974; 28:14–19.
36. Staheli LT, Chew DE, Corbett M: The longitudinal arch. J Bone Joint Surg Am 1987; 69:426–428.
37. Teitz CC, Hermanson B, Kronmal RA, et al: Evaluation of the use of braces to prevent injury to the knee in collegiate football players. J Bone Joint Surg Am 1987; 69:2–9.
38. Varghese G: Crutches, canes, and walkers. In Redford JB (eds): Orthotics Etcetera, ed 2. Baltimore, Williams & Wilkins, 1980, pp 453–463.
39. Von Werssowetz OF: Basic principles of lower extremity bracing. Orthot Prosthet Appl J 1962; 323–350.
40. Waters RL, Miller L: A physiologic rationale for orthotic prescription in paraplegia. Clin Prosthet Orthot 1987; 11:66–73.
41. Wenger DR, Mauldin D, Morgan D, et al: Foot growth rate in children age one to six years. Foot Ankle 1983; 3:207–210.
42. Wenger DR, Mauldin D, Speck G, et al: Corrective shoes and inserts as treatment for flexible flatfoot in infants and children. J Bone Joint Surg Am 1989; 71:800–810.
43. Winchester PK, Carollo JJ, Parekh RN, et al: A comparison of paraplegic gait performance using two types of reiprocating gait orthoses. Prosthet Orthot Int 1993; 17:101–106.
44. Zamosky I, Redford JB: Shoes and their modifications. In Redford JB (eds): Orthotics Etcetera, ed 2. Baltimore, Williams & Wilkins, 1980; 388–452.

17 CHAPTER

Steven V. Fisher, M.D., and Robert B. Winter, M.D.

Spinal Orthoses in Rehabilitation

CLINICAL USE OF SPINAL ORTHOSES

Descriptions of splints date back to 2700 BCE in ancient Egypt, where healers used splints to protect a damaged body part from further outside injury. The Egyptians did not, however, use splints to hold bone fragments rigid, either to allow healing or to prevent further damage from movement of the body parts.[52] In the Middle Ages, the armorer's skill lent itself to brace making.[62] Later, in the 16th century, French surgeon Ambroise Paré (c.1510–1590) pioneered the modern art of brace making. His inventions included metal corsets. Lorenz Heister (1638–1731) is credited with developing the first spinal brace. Heister's brace shared some of the basic components of today's cervical orthoses, including a halo-like structure for the head, with an axillary sling, shoulder straps, and a waist or pelvic belt for thoracic stabilization. Since that time, neither the basic concept nor the mechanisms of bracing have undergone significant change.[60] In the 19th century, Hugh Owen Thomas, an orthopedic physician, developed a cervical orthosis that still bears his name, despite later modifications. New materials and research have contributed to more effective bracing. Coupled with the tremendous explosion in spinal surgery, new materials, have brought about a significant change in the actual orthoses used for the spine.[60] Relatively few external appliances merit application for the treatment of most spinal deformities. However, many devices have been fabricated, some bearing the inventor's name, some named for the locality where they were designed, and some carrying a descriptive name.[62]

There are four primary objectives for the application of an orthosis: (1) controlling the position of the spine by the use of external forces; (2) applying corrective forces to abnormal curvatures; (3) aiding spinal stability when soft tissues cannot adequately perform their stabilizer role; and (4) restricting spinal segment movement after acute trauma or surgery to protect against further injury.[5, 28] In the case of traumatic spinal injury, the most important objective is the protection of the spinal cord and nerve roots. In other words, the goal of an orthosis is to control the position of the spine by the application of an external force for protection, immobilization, support, or correction of a deformity.[62]

These objectives are achieved through the biomechanical effects of trunk and head support, motion control, and spinal realignment.[62] When dealing with the cervical spine, an additional biomechanical effect is partial weight transfer of the head to the trunk when the patient is upright.[26, 62]

Spinal orthoses can also have negative effects, including axial muscle atrophy secondary to reduced muscle activity. The control of motion by the orthosis also promotes contractures of the immobilized part. Moreover, psychological dependency can occur, thereby increasing physical dependence on the orthosis. Psychosocial and economic elements may also play a negative role in a patient's continued use of an orthosis.

Cervical Orthoses

Proper prescription of a cervical orthosis requires knowledge of the general principles of bracing and the biomechanics of the cervical spine (see Chapter 37), as well as an understanding of the indications and limitations of specific cervical orthoses. All spinal orthoses utilize the principle of a three-point pressure system. The corrective component of force is ideally located midway between the opposing forces. As in a first-class lever system, any corrective force applied depends on its point and force of application and the distance from the axis of rotation. The effectiveness of a cervical orthosis is determined by its ability to resist not only gross motion, but intersegmental motion as well. As discussed later, it is the control of intersegmental motion that is difficult, especially in the cervical spine, due to its extreme flexibility at multiple levels.

The occipito-atlanto-axial complex (C1 and C2) is a distinct anatomical and functional unit. The occiput-C1 articulation is capable of very significant flexion and extension, with minor degrees of lateral bending and very little axial rotation. The atlanto-axial joint (C1-C2) is more complex and is also more frequently involved in pathological processes. The primary motion is rotation, with a much smaller component being flexion-extension. The rotation at this joint accounts for nearly 50% of the rotation of the entire cervical spine in the adult. The combined movement of the occipito-atlanto-axial complex allows total flexion of approximately 23 degrees and a total axial rotation of 47 degrees. Lateral bending at this complex is approximately 8 degrees of motion. In the lower cervical spine, C3-C7, each unit functions similarly. The vertebral bodies are wider anteriorly than posteriorly, and the facet joints are aligned at an angle to the body that causes lordosis and allows flexion-extension, lateral bending, and axial rotation movement. The greatest flexion-extension takes place at C5-C6, followed closely by C6-C7. Lateral bending and axial rotation are greatest in the upper part of the cervical spine (C2-C3 and C3-C4) and decrease in the lower cervical spine.[26, 60]

The biomechanical consequences of the spinal orthosis are therefore dependent on the points of application, the direction and magnitude of the force applied by the device, the tightness with which the device is worn, and the amount of force the patient exerts against it. The patient's body habitus also plays a significant role in the effectiveness of the orthosis. Spinal trauma produces unpredictable instability at times; hence a given orthosis must be "tested" to assure its effectiveness. In order to judge the effectiveness of an orthosis on a particular patient, a clinician must take radiographs in different positions while the patient is wearing the orthosis.

In applying a cervical orthosis, the clinician's objective is to control the position of the spine by the use of external force. The cervical spine, however, is the most mobile part of the entire spine, and has multiple planes of motion. Moreover, little body surface area is available for adequate contact of the orthosis. The amount of external force applied over the small surface area of the chin and occiput needs to be limited to prevent local ischemic pressure problems. Adequate contact of the orthosis on the bony structures of the skull and thorax is anatomically difficult. The occiput is rounded and the chin can easily be lifted away from the mandibular support by extending the upper cervical spine. Additionally, the shoulders and clavicle are mobile. Any strong force that acts on the head or over the clavicles is unpleasant for the patient. The chin becomes tender rather easily with undue pressure, especially in males who need to shave, and complications such as skin breakdown and local pain may develop.

Currently, there is significant interest in new cervical collars for prehospitalization/extrication use. (In 1999, there were more than 30 manufacturers of cervical extrication collars, collectively projecting a $40-million market for the year 2000.) In the acute prehospitalization arena, immediate decisions are made, and rigid immobilization of the cervical spine is of paramount importance to prevent further injury. Some of these orthoses seem to have use in the rehabilitation arena.

Cervical orthoses can be categorized in several different ways. Some arrange cervical appliances into four basic designs: (1) cervical collars; (2) poster appliances; (3) cervicothoracic orthoses; and (4) halo devices. Probably the most widely used orthoses are (1) the soft and hard collars; (2) Philadelphia orthosis; (3) SOMI (*s*ternal-*o*ccipital-*m*andibular *i*mmobilizer) orthosis; (4) poster orthosis (two or four); (5) Yale-type cervicothoracic orthosis; (6) thermoplastic Minerva body jacket (TMBJ); and (7) halo jacket or vest.

There are several basic types of cervical collars. The first is a soft cervical collar (Fig. 17–1). Made of foam rubber covered by stockinet, this device is low in cost, easy to fabricate, and well tolerated by most patients. It does not restrict cervical motion in any plane (Table 17–1). It provides warmth and psychological comfort but no support. It probably serves only as a reminder to hold the neck relatively still.

The second type of collar is a hard collar made of a rigid polyethylene. It can have an optional occipital and mandibular support. The hard collar without the mandibular and cervical support does not significantly immobilize the cervical spine. With the two supports, it gives more restriction in flexion and extension, but it is not truly effective. It does not limit lateral bending or

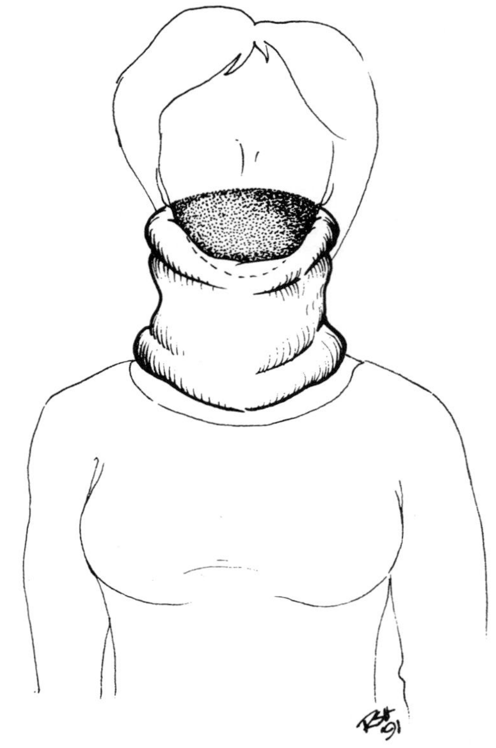

FIGURE 17–1. Soft collar.

TABLE 17–1 Normal Cervical Motion from Occiput to First Thoracic Vertebra and the Effects of Cervical Orthoses

	Mean of Normal Motion (%)		
	Flexion/ Extension	**Lateral Bending**	**Rotation**
Normal*	100.0	100.0	100.0
Soft collar*	74.2	92.3	82.6
Philadelphia collar	28.9	66.4	43.7
SOMI brace	27.7	65.6	33.6
Four-poster brace	20.6	45.9	27.1
Yale cervicothoracic brace	12.8	50.5	18.2
Halo device*	4.0	4.0	1.0
Halo device†	11.7	8.4	2.4
Minerva body jacket‡	14.0	15.5	0

* Data from Johnson RM, Hart DL, Simmons EF, et al: Cervical orthoses: A study comparing their effectiveness in restricting cervical motion in normal subjects. J Bone Joint Surg [Am] 1977; 59:332.

† Data from Lysell E: Motion in the cervical spine, thesis. Acta Orthop Scand Suppl 1969; 123.

‡ Data from Maiman D, Millington P, Novak S, et al: The effects of the thermoplastic Minerva body jacket on cervical spine motion. Neurosurgery 1989; 25:363–368.

rotation. It does not contact onto the thorax. It can press on the clavicles, creating areas of high pressure with subsequent discomfort.

The Philadelphia ("collar") orthosis (Fig. 17–2) is made of plastazote reinforced with anterior and posterior plastic struts. The front and rear halves fasten with Velcro closures. This orthosis has a molded mandibular and occipital support. The anterior and posterior caudal aspects of the brace extend onto the upper thorax. The Philadelphia orthosis does restrict cervical spine motion, particularly in flexion and extension (see Table 17–1). This is probably due to the better fit at the occiput and chin, as well as the improved contact on the upper thorax. However, the Philadelphia orthosis is relatively ineffective in controlling rotation and lateral bending (see Table 17–1). Depending on the prominence of the clavicles of the individual wearer, the Philadelphia orthosis may be quite uncomfortable.

Another brace in this category is a Jobst Vertebrace constructed from a high-density polyethylene sheet with its periphery cushioned with soft, closed-cell polyethylene foam. It provides full contact along its costal end to the sternum and it closely cups the mandible. A radiological study[53] of 10 normal volunteers showed that this orthosis functioned as well as, or better than, the Yale (see below) and Philadelphia orthoses. The investigators concluded that it was a good orthotic choice for use in emergency transport situations. It does not, however, appear to be comfortable enough for long-term rehabilitation use. The Miami J, NecLoc, and Newport/Aspen are other, newer orthoses, which were initially designed for emergency extrication purposes. However, the Miami J, the Aspen (formerly known as the Newport), and the NecLoc are probably comfortable enough to be used in the rehabilitation phase of management.[14] Askins and colleagues[2] found the Aspen orthosis to be at least as good as the Philadelphia collar, and perhaps superior to it at some cervical levels. They also found that in 20 healthy volunteers the NecLoc was most effective in immobilization in flexion and extension, with the Miami J superior to the Aspen or Philadelphia.

The four-poster brace (Fig. 17–3) represents the first true cervical thoracic orthosis discussed here. It has a molded mandibular and occipital support with adjustable struts attaching to anterior and posterior padded thoracic plates. The mandibular and occipital supports can be held together with straps running below the ears. The anterior and posterior thoracic pads are connected by leather shoulder straps. There are no straps under the axilla. The Guilford brace (Fig. 17–4) is a two-poster brace with a front and back strut connecting the anterior and posterior thoracic plates to the chin and occipital piece. The strapping runs over the shoulder as well as under the axilla. These orthoses are relatively effective in limiting range of motion in flexion and extension (see Table 17–1).

Another true cervical thoracic brace is the Yale orthosis (Fig. 17–5). This cervicothoracic orthosis was originally a modified Philadelphia collar with molded plastazote reinforced with plastic struts. It extends down onto the anterior and posterior thorax, with strapping beneath the axilla. The occipital piece can extend higher on the skull than does the original Philadelphia orthosis. The increased contact on the body surface at the occiput and onto the thorax improves the stability that this brace offers (see Table 17–1).

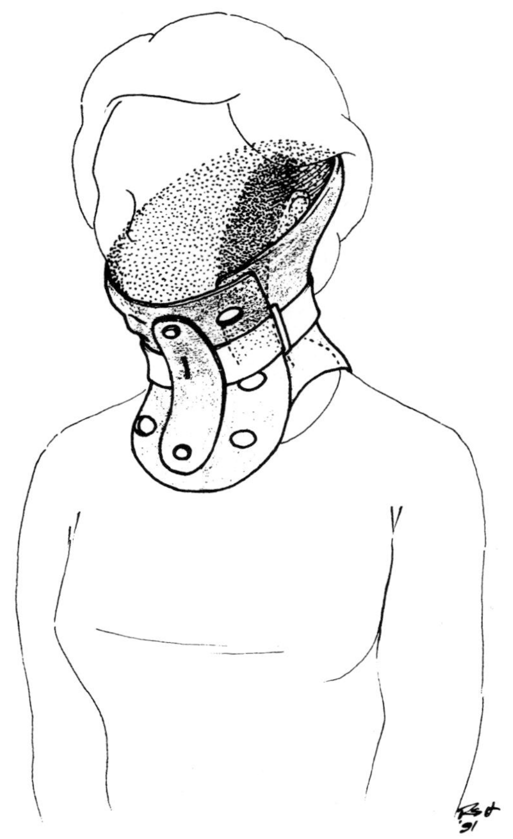

FIGURE 17–2. Philadelphia collar.

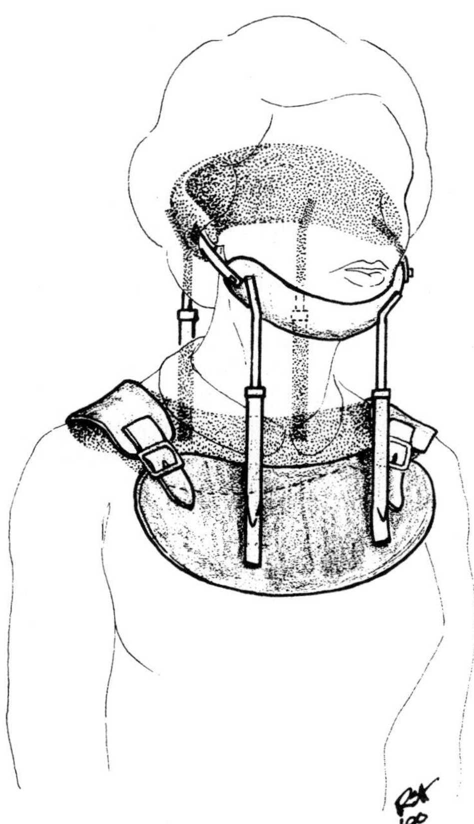

FIGURE 17–3. Four-poster collar.

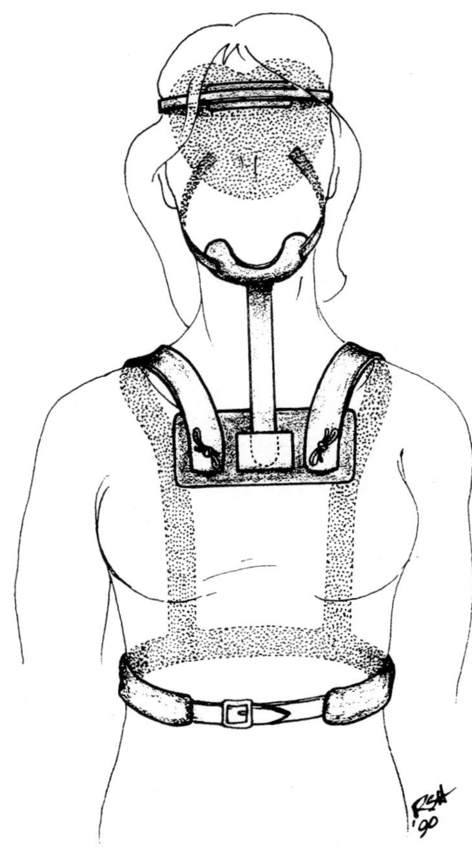

FIGURE 17–4. Two-poster orthosis (Guilford).

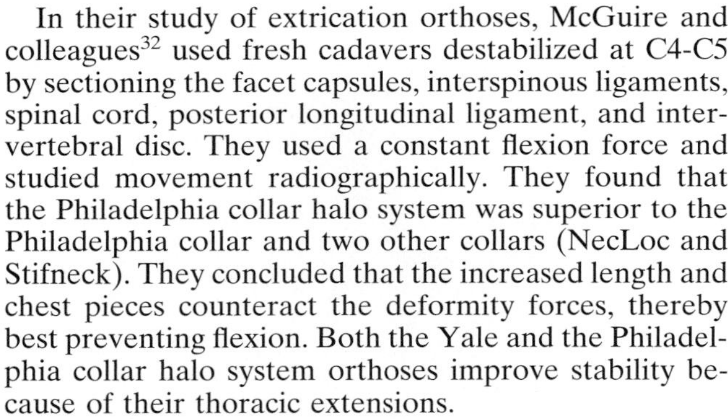

In their study of extrication orthoses, McGuire and colleagues[32] used fresh cadavers destabilized at C4-C5 by sectioning the facet capsules, interspinous ligaments, spinal cord, posterior longitudinal ligament, and intervertebral disc. They used a constant flexion force and studied movement radiographically. They found that the Philadelphia collar halo system was superior to the Philadelphia collar and two other collars (NecLoc and Stifneck). They concluded that the increased length and chest pieces counteract the deformity forces, thereby best preventing flexion. Both the Yale and the Philadelphia collar halo system orthoses improve stability because of their thoracic extensions.

The SOMI orthosis (Fig. 17–6) is also a cervicothoracic orthosis. It has a rigid anterior plastic chest piece and shoulder straps. The occipital piece is attached with two posters, which run anteriorly. The mandibular piece has a single poster, which also attaches anteriorly. These posts are made of rigid aluminum. The strapping crosses under the arms to the base of the chest piece. The SOMI brace is well tolerated. This brace can be applied without moving the patient from the supine position—an advantage in the spinal cord–injured patient in skeletal tong traction. It is supplied with an optional headpiece that snaps onto the occipital rest and passes around the forehead. This allows removal of the mandibular support while eating. It is relatively effective in restricting flexion-extension (see Table 17–1).

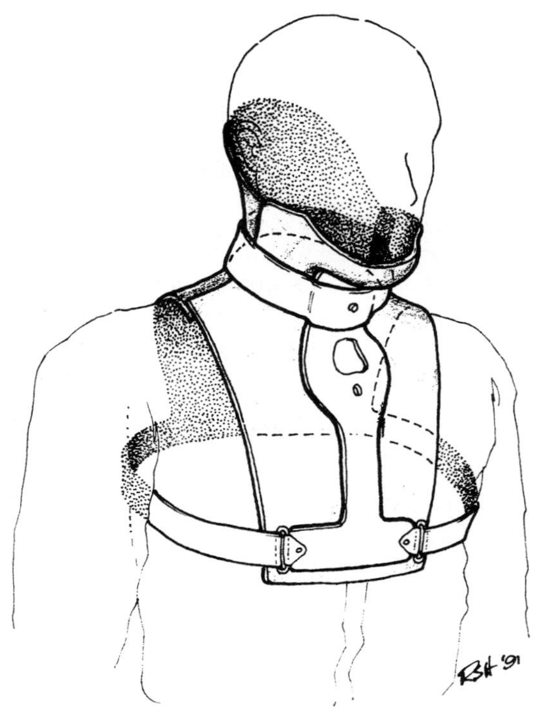

FIGURE 17–5. Yale cervicothoracic orthosis.

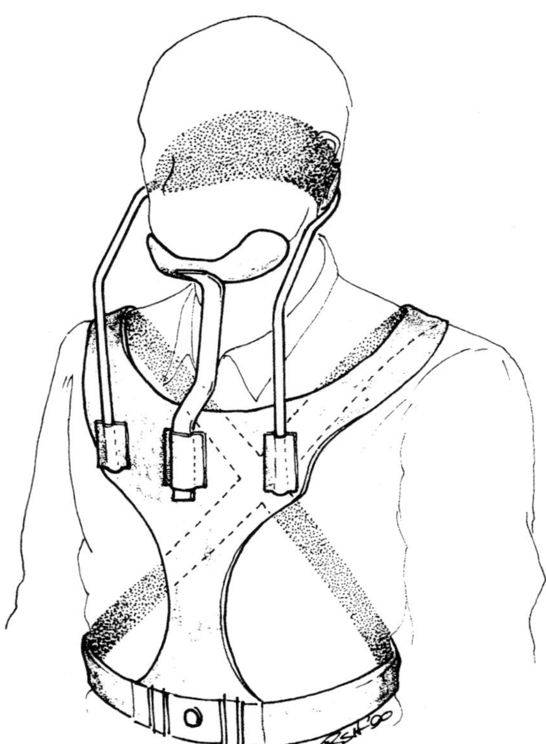

FIGURE 17–6. Sterno-occipital mandibular immobilization orthosis (SOMI).

There have been several studies in the last 15 years documenting the effectiveness of cervical orthoses. The most widely referenced study was performed by Johnson and associates[15] (see Table 17–1). Normal subjects were fitted with a soft collar, Philadelphia collar, SOMI brace, four-poster brace, cervicothoracic brace, and a halo with plastic body vest. Flexion-extension and lateral bending were measured radiographically and rotation was measured using overhead photography. Fisher and colleagues[11] studied normal subjects radiographically using the polyethylene hard collar, plastazote Philadelphia orthosis, a four-poster, and a SOMI orthosis. This study measured only flexion and extension. Although there were some differences in the range of motion at specific cervical levels, the results of the two separate studies generally agree and trends can be recognized. It is known that no cervical orthosis totally immobilizes the cervical spine. There is a recognized "snaking" of the cervical spine, with some segments moving into flexion and others into extension, especially when forced flexion-extension is attempted against the orthosis. The differences noted in these studies at specific cervical levels are probably due to the variable degree of snaking of the spine with forced movements against the orthosis.

Soft collars allow 75% to 100% of normal unrestricted flexion and extension motion, while plastic collars allow 25% to 30%. Four-posters, two-posters, and the SOMI allow 10% to 28%. The Yale orthosis and the Minerva body jacket (TMBJ), discussed later, provide more restriction in this plane (see Table 17–1).

In the United States, the halo brace (Fig. 17–7) has become the most frequently used method of treating cervical fractures or dislocations. It was first described by Perry and Nickel[44] in 1959 and reviewed by them again in 1968.[43]

There are basically two types of halo orthotic devices currently used to control neck motion. They are the halo cast and halo vest. The halo component is the same on each type and consists of a rigid metal or graphite ring attached to the skull with four fixation pins, two anteriorly, usually in the frontal region, and two posteriorly in the parieto-occipital area. The ring is bolted to four posters which run down onto either a rigid polyethylene vest or a plaster cast, both of which extend to about the umbilicus. If further intimate contact on the thorax is needed, a body cast is fabricated distally with contact onto the pelvis.

Johnson and colleagues[15] and Lysell[29] studied the restriction of motion provided by the halo. Their results are summarized in Table 17–1. Koch and Nickel[10] first studied forces within the halo vest device coupled with range-of-motion measurements. There was a strikingly wide variety of values in different patients and a wide range of values for each individual in different positions. The variability was partially related to the fit of the vest. The forces could be either compressive or distractive. They also found that the absolute motion in the halo vest had been underestimated in previous studies using normal subjects, and that an average of 31% of normal spine motion was observed in their patient population.

Walker and co-workers[57] found the same magnitude of vertical forces noted by Koch,[19] but observed that

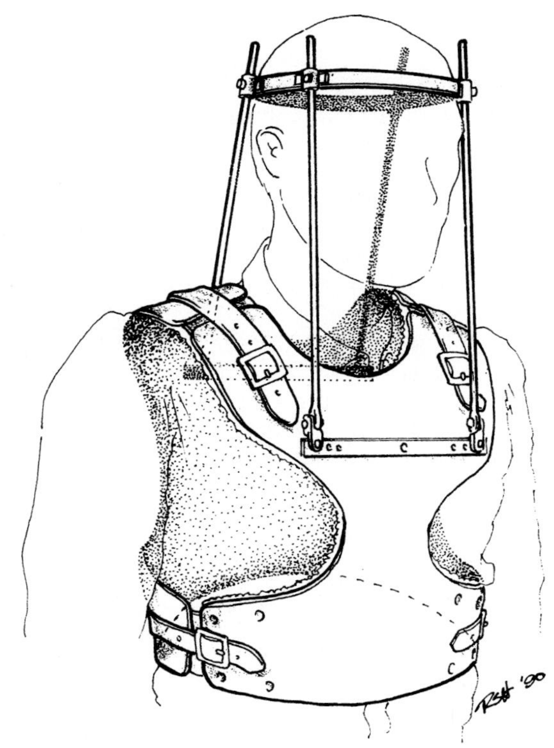

FIGURE 17–7. Halo device/vest.

these forces would be applied infrequently over a typical day. The vest was again thought to be the weak link in terms of movement and distortion. The forces on the pins in the skull are primarily shear forces acting in multiple directions, which explains why pinholes enlarge in a crater-like fashion.

Lind and others[24] found the same snakelike motion described by Johnson[15] and great individual variability, as noted above. They found that the maximal cervical motion in the halo apparatus was 70% of the normal motion and that most of this motion occurred in the upper cervical spine area. Rehabilitation exercises did not cause any greater movement to the spine than did daily motion and activity.

Wolf and Jones[63] studied 21 patients: 7 patients in a halo cast and 14 in a plastic body jacket. They found no significant difference in the amount of motion in flexion-extension and lateral bending as determined radiographically. Patient acceptance and comfort were greater in the plastic jackets. The frequency of pin loosening was twice as high in the heavier halo cast.

Wang and associates[58] studied the relationship of vest length to the stability of the cervical spine. A half-vest to the level of the nipples was compared with a short extended vest to the twelfth rib and a full vest extended to the iliac crests in 12 normal subjects. There was no rotation of the cervical spine, regardless of vest length. There was a variable amount of flexion and extension of the upper cervical spine regardless of vest length. More motion was seen in the lower cervical spine than in the upper. The authors concluded that a lesion of the upper cervical spine could be treated with a half-vest, which improves comfort and ease of patient care. However, they recommended a full vest.[58]

Given the overestimation of restriction in motion and the level of variability noted, it is not surprising that the literature on treatment of cervical fractures is unclear on the indications for halo alone, or for surgical intervention coupled with halo immobilization. Sears and Fazi[49] studied 173 acute cervical injuries. They found that those patients with facet joint dislocation formed a distinct subgroup in which only 44% achieved stability with halo alone, but half of these had a poor anatomical result. Of the patients without facet joint dislocation, 70% achieved stability and 75% had good results anatomically.

Clark and White[7] studied patients with fractures of the dens, which is another area of management controversy. Their results support the surgical approach of type II (fractures of the junction of the dens and central body of the axis) with either angulation or displacement. Unstable type III (fractures that go deep into the body of the axis) are also believed to require surgery. When one realizes that the halo device does not immobilize as well as was first thought, and that most motion occurs in the upper cervical spine, it is unsurprising that upper cervical spine injuries require frequent surgical intervention as well as halo immobilization.

Glaser and others[13] reviewed 245 cases treated with halo vests. They concluded that halo vests protect cervical fracture patients from neurological injury, but do not absolutely immobilize or even prevent deformity. After 3 months of halo immobilization, surgery might be required in some cases involving ligamentous and osseous injuries to achieve stability. The United Kingdom has been very cautious in adopting the halo device, but a relatively recent publication suggests acceptance of this device versus the more traditional skull caliper-bed immobilization treatment.[42]

The original Minerva molded-type orthosis (Fig. 17–8) contacts the head or thorax, but not any better than the more traditional Philadelphia or four-poster. The newer design of the Minerva body jacket (TMBJ), shown in Figure 17–9, runs down the thorax to a level similar to that of the halo vest and provides significant contact on the head with its circumferential forehead adaptation. It is obviously much lighter in weight than its forerunner, the plastic Minerva jacket. And it is noninvasive—an advantage over the halo device whose pins inherently present the risk of infection and slippage.

Millington and colleagues[34] introduced the TMBJ in 1987; and later Maiman, Millington, and colleagues[30] studied the effectiveness of this device in 21 normal subjects. That study is summarized in Table 17–1. The investigators doubted the accuracy of their rotation measurements secondary to inadequate stabilization of the trunk. They concluded, however, that flexion-extension compared favorably with that found for halo devices in studies by other researchers. The authors caution that this study was on normal subjects—a fact that must be considered when applying their results to actual patients.

Benzel and co-workers[3] compared the TMBJ and halo devices in 10 ambulatory patients with an unstable cervical spine. The patients initially underwent 6 to 8 weeks of immobilization with a halo device followed by the

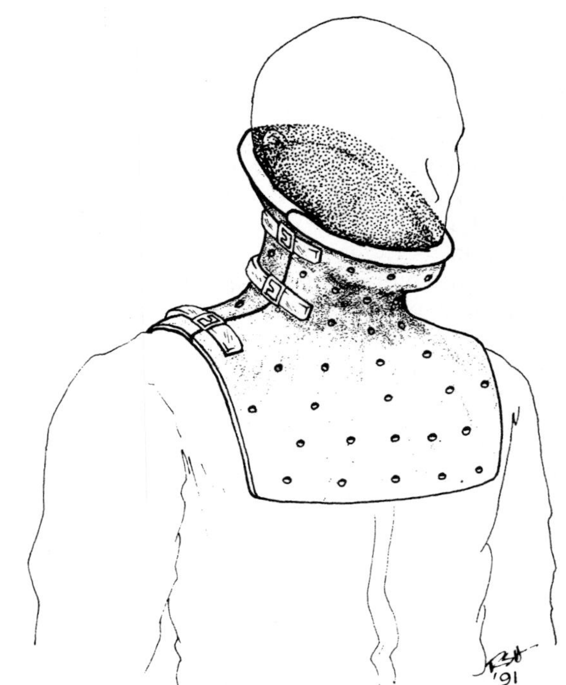

FIGURE 17–8. Custom-molded cuirass orthosis (original Minerva design).

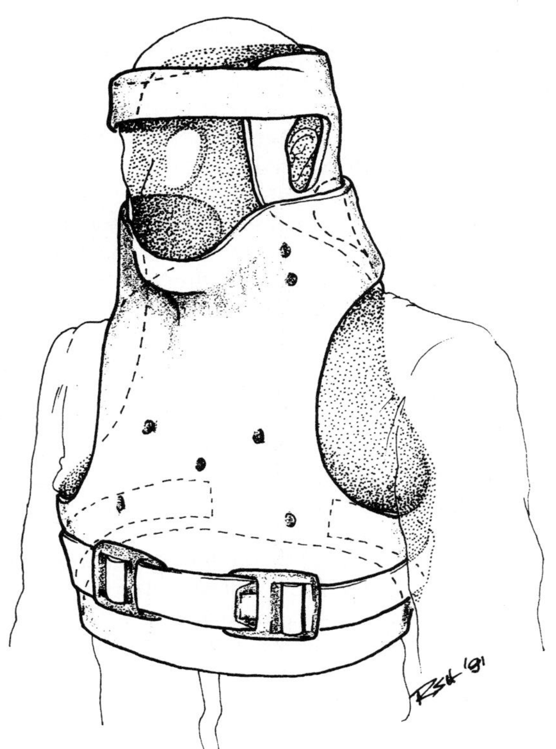

FIGURE 17–9. Thermoplastic Minerva body jacket (TMBJ).

TMBJ. Prior to removal of the halo, flexion-extension radiographs were taken. Two to three weeks later, similar films were taken while the subjects were wearing the TMBJ. The average spine movement in the TMBJ was less than that in the halo. The authors attributed the difference to the snaking of the cervical spine noted in the halo device.

In his review article, Pringle[46] stated that both the Minerva and the halo vest are far superior to other cervical thoracic orthoses, and are the treatment of choice in the ambulatory management of the unstable cervical spine. Additionally, there is literature that supports the use of the Minerva vest in preference to the halo vest in children of preschool age. The Minerva vest provided necessary stabilization and yet was lighter and more comfortable, thereby allowing mobilization of the patient for rehabilitation with satisfactory stabilization of the cervical spine.

It appears that the TMBJ can be an alternative to the halo in selected patients. Further clinical studies certainly are required, but the TMBJ seems to be a promising addition to cervical orthotic management.

There is very little published on the management of upper thoracic fractures. The typical thoracic orthoses, such as the Jewett hyperextension device or the chair-back brace with sternal pad, provide immobilization up to the level of T6 at the maximum and are therefore of no value in the upper thoracic spine. The ribs act as support struts in the thorax, but many times there are associated rib fractures which reduce the desired stability. If neurological compromise is a risk in a given upper thoracic fracture with instability, a halo device is needed. Surgical stabilization can also be required.[8] Other orthoses can be utilized for attempted posture control if the spinal cord is not in jeopardy of compromise. Upper thoracic fractures require either a halo cast to the pelvis or a Milwaukee-type orthosis (cervicothoracolumbosacral orthosis, CTLSO) if surgery is not selected.[61]

Thoracolumbosacral Orthoses

Lumbosacral (LSO) and thoracolumbosacral (TLSO) orthoses are prescribed more frequently than cervical orthoses. There are more variations of design for each type and hence more eponyms. The following discussion focuses on the most commonly prescribed devices and the representative types of design and material.

As with cervical orthoses, proper prescription of a thoracolumbar orthosis (TLO) requires knowledge of the general principles of bracing and the biomechanics of the thoracic and lumbar spine, as well as an understanding of the indications and limitations of specific thoracic and lumbar orthoses. It is outside the scope of this chapter to deal in detail with these subjects, but a few general considerations are necessary.

The sacrum can be considered the "foundation" of the spinal column. The sacrum is rigidly attached to the ilium to form the pelvis, which rotates freely on the femoral heads. In the upright standing posture, flexion of the pelvis on the femur causes a compensatory extension of the lumbar spine (increased lumbar lordosis with an increase in the lumbosacral angle). Likewise, if there is an increase in lumbosacral lordosis, there can be an increased thoracic flexion or kyphosis.

As in the cervical spine, the range of motion of each spinal segment is directly related to the anatomy of the region. In the thoracic spinal column, the facets are primarily oriented in the horizontal plane. Each vertebra is bilaterally attached to a rib, with the upper 10 ribs attaching directly to the sternum, and the spinous processes are overlapping. These factors severely limit thoracic spine mobility in flexion and extension. The rib cage plays a great role in enhancing the stiffness of the thoracic spine. It has been demonstrated that the spine is 27%, 45%, 31%, and 132% stiffer in flexion, lateral bending, axial rotation, and extension, respectively, due to the rib cage.[1] Rotation and lateral bending are the predominant movements possible: about 6 degrees of lateral bending at each segment, and 8 to 9 degrees of axial rotation. There is an average of 4 degrees of flexion and extension in the upper portion and 6 degrees in the middle segments of the thoracic spine. The transitional segments from thoracic to lumbar spine (T10-T12) have much greater flexion-extension (average 12 degrees). There is also increased lateral bending (average 8 degrees) and less rotation (2 degrees). This is in part because the ribs do not articulate with the sternum in the last segments and the facet joints are in transition from the alignment in the thoracic spine to that of the lumbar spine.

The lumbar spine has five large vertebrae, large intervertebral discs, and nearly sagittally placed articular processes with posteriorly directed spinous processes. Because of the anatomical alignment of the facets, there is between 12 degrees of flexion and 17 degrees of extension, 3 to 6 degrees of lateral bending, and only 1 to 2 degrees of axial rotation at any given level. The greatest flexion-extension, and the least lateral bending and axial rotation, occurs at L5 to S1.[60]

The objectives of thoracolumbar orthosis usage are similar to those of the cervical region: controlling the position of the spine by the use of external forces, applying corrective forces to abnormal curvatures, aiding spinal stability when soft tissues cannot adequately perform their stabilizing role, and restricting spinal segment movement. Currently, a different objective has aroused much interest—the use of lumbar supports to prevent injury or to increase the individual's actual lifting capacity. In the case of trauma, however, the most important objective is the protection of the spinal cord, cauda equina, and nerve roots.

The work of Norton and Brown[41] on the effectiveness of back braces was the first and remains one of the most important. There is very significant variability in the effectiveness of back braces. This relates to an individual's lumbar flexion pattern. Orthotic devices that are well fixed to the chest but inadequately so to the pelvis leave the lumbosacral segments unsupported. Braces such as the chairback brace, which has shorter supports, tend to pull away from the pelvis less, thereby giving more support to the lumbosacral (LS) area.[41] While no brace can totally immobilize, bracing can limit, interspinous motion. If an orthosis is to be effective, it must supply sufficient pressure over bony prominences to remind the wearer to change position or maintain posture.[27] All braces employ a three-point pressure system. The more contact the brace has with the wearer, the more evenly the pressure is distributed and the better the control achieved. The total-contact custom-molded thermoplastic orthosis is an example of an orthosis in which the three-point pressure principle is diffused by the total contact against the patient.

Morris and associates[35] demonstrated that increasing the abdominal pressure by using an orthosis decreases the net force applied to the spine when lifting a weight from the floor. However, when extra loading of the spine occurs, the amount of compression necessary is not well tolerated. They argued that since the spinal column is attached to the sides of the abdominal and thoracic cavities, the action of the trunk muscles converts the thoracic and abdominal chambers into nearly rigid containers. These containers transmit part of the forces (generated in loading the spine when lifting), thereby relieving the load directly on the spine.[35] Other investigators have studied the effect of lumbosacral belts on intra-abdominal pressure. Lander and colleagues[21, 31] found an increase in intra-abdominal pressure, but others have not reported consistent results.

Nachemson and co-workers,[39] however, noted that no LSO significantly raised intragastric pressure. Intra-abdominal pressure increases only with closure of the glottis during muscular activity. The LS support, when tightened within patient tolerance, decreases the intradiscal pressure at the lumbar spine by approximately 30%.[37] Nachemson[39] demonstrated that wearing a lumbosacral orthosis reduces disc pressure values during about two-thirds of a set of exercises and increases pressure during the remaining third.[39] The biomechanical models to predict compressive and shear forces in these studies[1] have, however, been criticized.[40]

Morris and associates[35] found that the chairback brace and the LS corset decreased or had no effect on the electrical activity of back muscles. Nachemson and colleagues[39] also found no consistent trends when studying four normal volunteers performing six tasks while using an orthosis. The erector spinal myoelectrical activity was at times increased and at other times reduced by a like amount.

Later studies of lumbosacral corsets and EMG activity while lifting have not diminished the controversy regarding the correlation of EMG activity and intra-abdominal pressure.[20, 21, 31] In his review, Calmels[6] noted the scarcity of good evidence for the actual immobilization ability of an orthosis, and argued in favor of their proprioceptive efficacy.

A 1994 NIOSH report[40] concluded that there is no scientific evidence that lumbosacral belt wearing is protective to an industrial population on the basis of changes in intra-abdominal pressure and trunk muscle EMG. The report states further that there is no conclusive evidence that spinal compressive forces or shear forces are significantly reduced with lumbosacral supports.

Lantz and Shultz[22] also found inconsistent changes in the myoelectrical activity with normal volunteers, and some of the increased activity was thought to be due to antagonistic muscle activity. It was considered, but not verified experimentally, that low back pain patients wearing an orthosis daily "relax into the brace" and perhaps reduce antagonistic muscle activity. Segmental motion can be increased at each end of the immobilized spine as the spine moves, possibly exacerbating a condition the orthosis is attempting to treat.[26]

The studies mentioned earlier of thoracic-lumbar orthoses were in large part carried out on normal volunteers. The authors did not take into consideration important complicating factors such as pain, decreased muscular strength, insensate skin, altered biomechanics secondary to trauma and instability, or surgical changes.[54] Since there is significant variability of fit and effectiveness, radiographic analysis of spinal motion is necessary for a given patient to determine the effectiveness of the device in limiting unwanted motion.

These appliances can be classified as corsets, rigid braces, hyperextension braces, hyperflexion braces, and jackets. All spinal orthoses, with the exception of hyperextension braces, give abdominal support. The ability of these devices to restrict motion has not been measured in as great detail as with the cervical orthoses. The evaluation of effectiveness is therefore more subjective.

The most commonly prescribed lumbosacral support is the LS corset.[45] In general, a corset is made of canvas with rigid back stays often made of steel. There is adjustable side or back lacing. A corset is a stock item and can usually be fitted by a corsetier without difficulty. The corset can be lumbosacral (LS) or thoracolumbosacral (TLS). The stays can be either rigid or semirigid. Fidler[9] and Lantz[22] found that a corset significantly reduced spinal motion by as much as two-thirds. The stays actually give only a small amount of support, but they supply painful stimuli if the patient leans against them, especially the lateral ones. The corset gives minimal actual support and its effectiveness might be more related to the discomfort it can produce for patients[41] because it reminds them to maintain adequate posture.

Despite the possible potential biomechanical effects of lumbar supports, Van Poppei and colleagues[56] found that in a large study of airline cargo workers, neither lumbar supports nor education reduced the incidence of low back pain or the incidence of sick leave.

Lumbosacral Orthoses. The chairback brace is the most popular of the rigid braces. It consists of an anterior corset or apron front with midaxillary metal uprights (Fig. 17–10). It can also have two paraspinal uprights and two uprights in the midaxillary line (Fig. 17–11). It is designed to control flexion-extension and lateral motion.

Another commonly prescribed lumbosacral orthosis is the William's back brace, which is used primarily to control extension and lordosis and to give some lateral control (Fig. 17–12). It is a specialized orthosis in that it allows free flexion but limits extension and uses a lever action and abdominal support to reduce lumbar lordosis.

Thoracolumbosacral Orthoses. There are two major types of thoracolumbosacral orthoses (TLSOs). The more common is the Taylor orthosis, which is con-

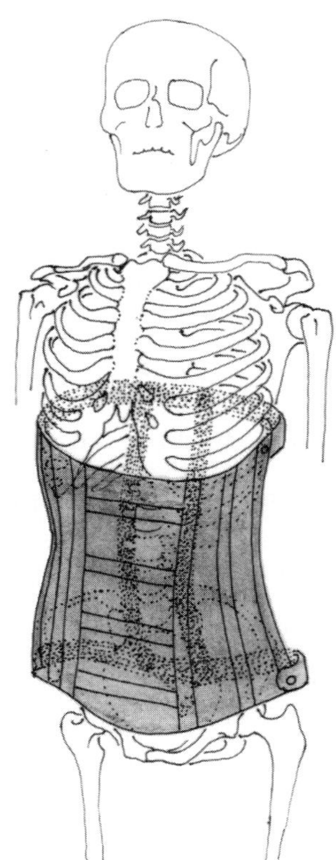

FIGURE 17–11. Chairback lumbosacral orthosis with paraspinal uprights in addition to the midaxillary line supports.

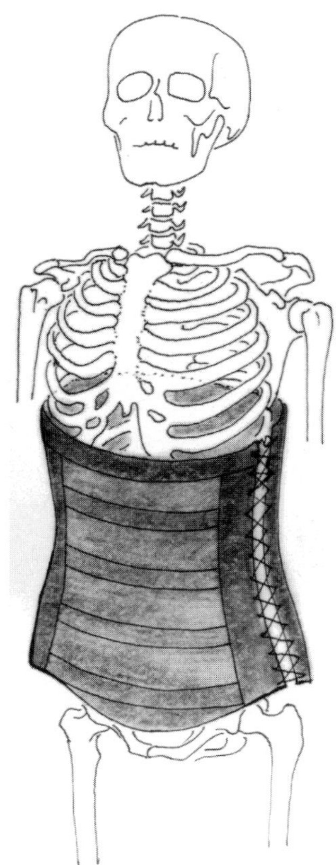

FIGURE 17–10. Chairback lumbosacral orthosis with side lacing attachment to an abdominal apron.

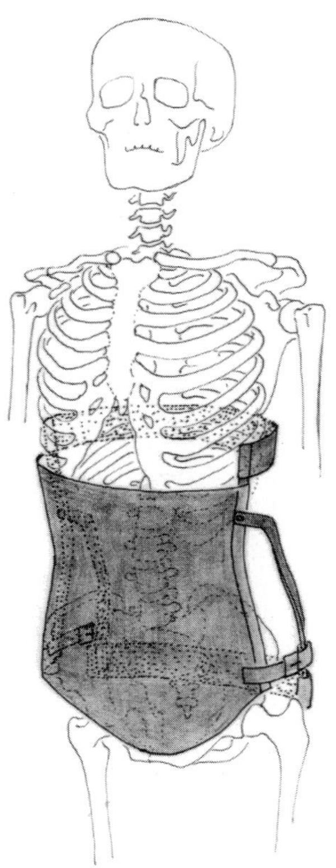

FIGURE 17–12. William's hyperextension lumbosacral orthosis.

structed to restrict flexion and extension (Fig. 17–13). This type of orthosis is relatively ineffective for limiting lumbar spine motion.[41] The Taylor orthosis limits thoracic motion only if the axillary straps are tightened to the point of discomfort. This orthosis appears to be a poor choice for thoracolumbosacral immobilization. The chairback brace has cowhorn or sternal pad attachments (Fig. 17–14), which transmit pressure through the sternum and ribs directly to the spine. This provides better lumbosacral and thoracic immobilization than a brace that transmits force through the pectoral girdle and is attached to the spinal axis only by muscles and the sternoclavicular joints.

Molded jackets are made either of plaster of paris or a thermoplastic material to conform to the contours of the body (Fig. 17–15). If made properly, they become a nearly total contact type of orthotic device. The pressure distribution is more uniform and more support is provided. Fidler and Plasmans[9] and Lantz and Schultz[22] verified that the molded TLSO restricts spinal movement better than a corset or chairback brace. A spica attachment to the molded TLSO was best at restricting movement, presumably by partially immobilizing the pelvis. These jackets are used frequently for patients with spinal fractures or low back fusions to allow early mobilization and rehabilitation. They also may be of value when there are metastases in vertebrae, to provide support and control pain. Donning and doffing the molded jacket is more difficult than with other orthoses.

The hyperextension orthosis differs from other devices because it does not have an abdominal apron and

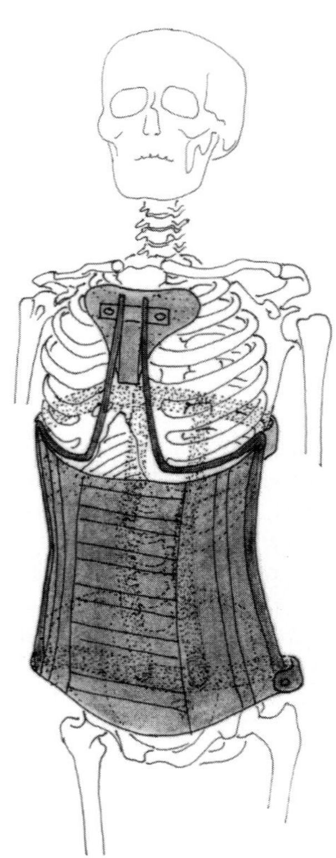

FIGURE 17–14. Chairback brace with sternal pad transmitting bony support to the lower thoracic spine.

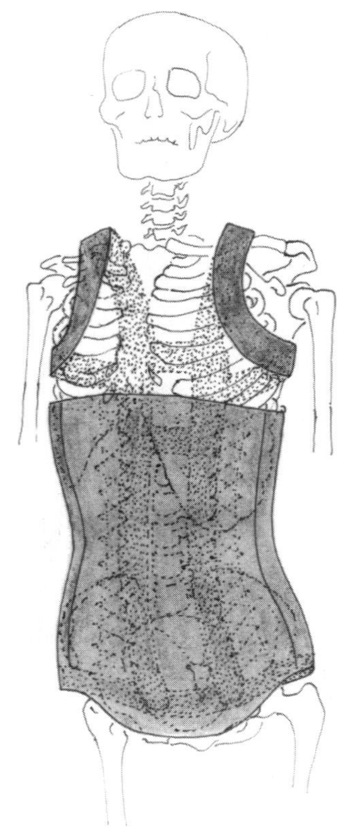

FIGURE 17–13. The Taylor thoracolumbosacral brace.

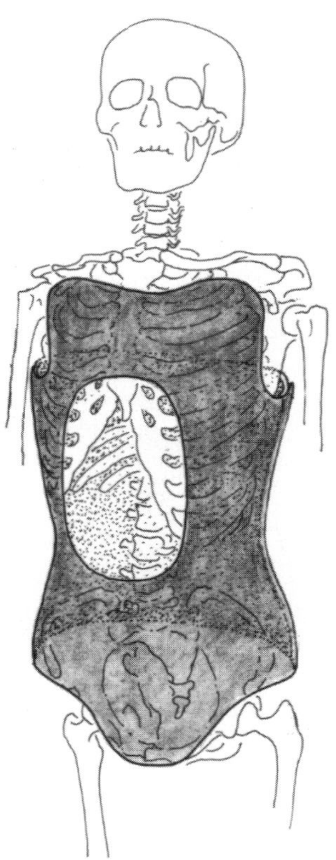

FIGURE 17–15. The custom-molded thermoplastic jacket-type thoracic lumbosacral orthosis.

does not give abdominal support. It functions to give a hyperextension moment (Fig. 17–16). This hyperextension brace applies three-point pressure over the sternum and the pubis anteriorly and over the upper lumbar spine posteriorly. This hyperextension orthosis is used to permit the upright position, while preventing flexion after a compression fracture of a vertebral body. It is not recommended in the management of compression fractures in osteoporotic elderly patients because it can place excessive hyperextension forces on lower lumbar vertebrae, possibly inducing posterior element fractures or exacerbating a degenerative arthritis condition.

It should be stressed that orthoses only partially limit rather than immobilize the spine. Spinal orthoses should be considered to be temporary devices. At the same time that the orthotic device is prescribed, a rehabilitation treatment plan should be outlined to attempt to rid the patient of the need for the device in the future.

SPINAL ORTHOSES FOR SPINAL DEFORMITY

In this section we describe the orthoses used for the management of spinal deformities, discussing the goals of these devices, the indications and contraindications for their use, and attendant problems. Thirty years ago, bracing was purely empirical. But since the 1960s, clinical research from around the world has made the orthotic management of spinal deformities a well-established, proven technique.

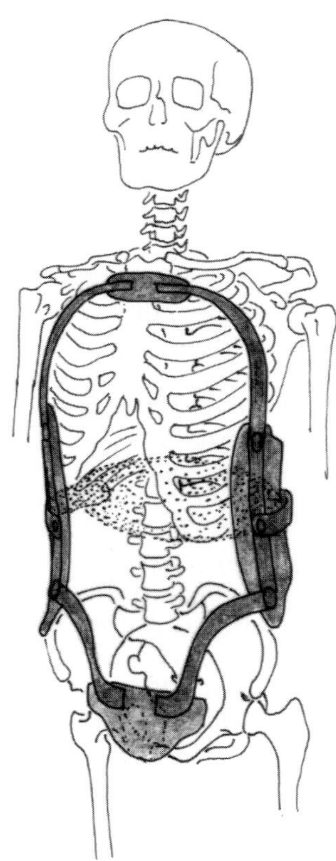

FIGURE 17–16. Jewett hyperextension orthosis restricts spinal flexion by anterior pressure over the sternum and pubic symphysis, and posterior pressure across the lower thoracic/upper lumbar region.

History

Bracing for spinal deformity has gone through many historical stages. Prior to the first spinal fusion for scoliosis by Hibbs in 1915, bracing was the only treatment method available. At that time, highly sophisticated orthoses were available, especially in Germany. In the next decades, surgery was refined, becoming increasingly safe and effective; these improvements prompted an understandable diminution in enthusiasm for bracing. But surgery still presented significant risks; moreover, patients, who had to spend many months in bed in a heavy plaster cast, found the postoperative experience very unpleasant.

The late 1940s saw a major milestone when Blount and Schmidt, of Milwaukee, collaborated on a new brace design. This Milwaukee brace was first used for postsurgical correction and stabilization, then was modified for nonoperative treatment. A tremendous surge of enthusiasm for brace management followed on the heels of accumulating evidence that braces could not only halt the progression of curvatures but could sometimes effect lasting improvement. This was actually an overzealous swing of the pendulum away from surgery toward bracing.

By the late 1970s, however, pessimistic voices began to rise, reaching maximum levels in the late 1980s and early 1990s. The disenchantment was so severe that many orthopedic surgeons pronounced braces to be "of no use at all" and insisted that "bracing really did not affect the natural history of scoliosis." But this, too, was an overzealous swing. Thanks to diligent work over many years in several centers, it has been amply demonstrated that orthotic management can have a very positive effect on many spinal deformities.

Biomechanics

Scoliosis is a three-dimensional problem. Rotation of vertebrae is an integral component of all structural scolioses. The frontal plane radiograph—both anteroposterior (AP) and posteroanterior (PA)—must be studied, as well as lateral films. However, the physical examination of the patient typically reveals the rotational aspects far better than radiographs. Bracing affects the spinal column itself; but it also affects the physiology of internal organs, playing a role, for example, in pulmonary function.[17, 18]

The biomechanics of the spine are quite dynamic. A common error is to think only in terms of *passive* forces. Many orthoses, especially the Milwaukee brace (CTLSO), are designed to stimulate *active* corrective forces on the part of the patient. In a well-fitted Milwaukee brace for a right thoracic idiopathic scoliosis, for example, there is a constant force only in the pelvic section. It is a circumferential force, but so mild that pressure sores do not develop and the patient experiences no pressure-related discomfort. The design is such that the patient's neck "floats" within the neck ring;

that is, there are usually zero forces anywhere on the neck. The main corrective force pad—the right thoracic pad—is broad, thus distributing the force over a wide area of skin. The patient can, at any time, shift the thorax to the left so that there are zero forces under the pad.

While ensuring that no skin sores will form, the ability to "get away from the pad" guarantees that the patient is actively using trunk muscles only in a way that corrects the curvature. The neck ring also acts in an active manner. If the patient slumps in the brace, the throat will come down onto the occipital pads and throat mold. The ensuing discomfort prompts the patient to elongate the spine again, using trunk muscles in a curve-correcting way. In a well-fitting Milwaukee brace, trunk muscles are constantly being used, but always in a positive mode relative to the curve. These muscles are quiet only at night. Bracing therefore does not produce severe muscle atrophy.

These concepts of dynamic muscle activity can be carried over into underarm orthoses (TLSOs) if they are carefully designed. The great virtue of the Milwaukee brace is its open design and its lack of circumferential torso constriction. The torso is allowed to shift to the left (in a typical right thoracic curve pattern) since there is no "wall" of plastic on the left to block the shift.

Thus a TLSO can be designed which incorporates a "space" into which the torso can shift. The counterforce opposing the right thoracic pad must therefore be a high axillary padded margin of the TLSO above the space area. Because this high axillary contact point can be an irritant if the patient sags down, the patient will tend to "elongate" and lean the upper thorax to the right, adding to the effectiveness of the right thoracic pad.

Lumbar pads, whether in a TLSO or a Milwaukee brace, tend to be much more passive than thoracic pads. However, the brace should provide a space into which the patient can actively shift the spinal segments.

These dynamic concepts apply only to those patients with active muscle power and a good sense of muscle control. The orthoses used in patients with neuromuscular problems are passive.

Types of Orthoses for Spinal Deformities

Milwaukee Brace. The Milwaukee brace (CTLSO) was the first to have statistically proven positive results in spinal deformity; it is thus a "gold standard" against which other orthoses can be compared. It consists of a well-molded pelvic section (originally made of leather, but now almost universally made of plastic), two posterior uprights, a single anterior upright, and a neck ring. These components are always made in straight alignment; that is, the pelvic section is level, the uprights are all perfectly vertical, and the neck ring is centered over midpelvis.

Curve correction is achieved by one or more pads attached to the basic frame. Ideally, the deformed spine is brought to the perfect vertical alignment. A patient with a leg-length difference should have a shoe lift such that the pelvis is leveled. The two most common corrective pads for scoliosis are the thoracic pad and the lumbar pad. Other pads less often used are the oval pad, the trapezius pad, and the shoulder ring. The axillary sling is not a corrective pad; rather, it is a device against which the patient pushes in order to center the neck within the neck ring. For kyphosis, two thoracic kyphosis pads are used, one on each posterior upright (Fig. 17–17*A* and *B*).

Thoracolumbosacral Orthosis. The thoracolumbosacral orthosis (TLSO) reaches only to the axillary level and exerts no corrective action on the upper thoracic spine. It is typically used for scolioses having their apex at T9 or lower, and for kyphoses having their apex at the thoracolumbar junction. Many different styles exist, under many different names (often derived from the city or institution in which they were developed). But whatever the name, it is the design concepts that are important. Any orthosis worth its salt must have a positive effect on the curve to be treated, and it must do no harm.

There are corrective types designed primarily for adolescents with idiopathic scoliosis and passive TLSOs made with the patient held in a corrected alignment (Fig. 17–18*A* and *B*). These latter types are most commonly used for neuromuscular deformities.

Lumbosacral Orthosis. The lumbosacral orthosis (LSO) is a specific design only for lumbar scolioses. It is firmly locked to the pelvis, has a strong force pad against the apex of the lumbar curve, and no thoracic extension on the opposite side. The correction is done by the patient's own active righting reflexes and muscle power. It is intended only for idiopathic scoliosis patients (Fig. 17–19*A* and *B*).

Bracing for Infantile Idiopathic Scoliosis

Idiopathic infantile scoliosis is an idiopathic curvature occurring in a child less than 3 years old. There must be no anomalous vertebrae, and magnetic resonance imaging (MRI) or myelogram must demonstrate the absence of a syrinx, tumor, or any other neurological abnormality. Since 80% to 85% of infants with this type of scoliosis have spontaneous resolution of their curvature, it is important to avoid bracing a mild curve that will disappear on its own. Similarly, it is important to aggressively treat those children with progressive curves. One useful measure of prognosis is Mehta's rib-vertebral angle difference (RVAD). If the curve exceeds 20 degrees, the prognosis is poor and treatment is indicated. Curves progressing past 30 degrees should also be treated. Although Mehta prefers serial plaster casts, the author favors the use of the classic Milwaukee brace. It takes a skilled orthotist to create such a brace for children as young as 6 months.

The brace is worn on a full-time schedule (23½ hours per day), being removed only for the daily bath. Under these conditions, children readily adapt to the brace. Normal developmental activities are encouraged, and the children soon largely forget that life existed without it.

In many cases, these children will have a cure of their problem with a vigorous brace program. The spine is

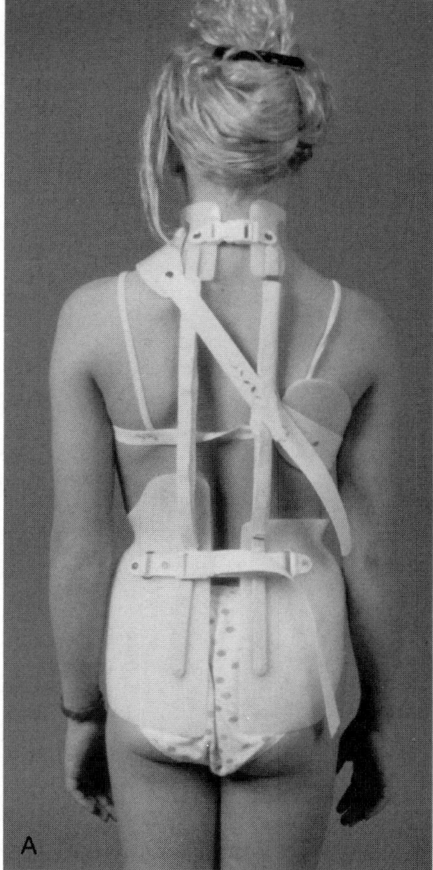

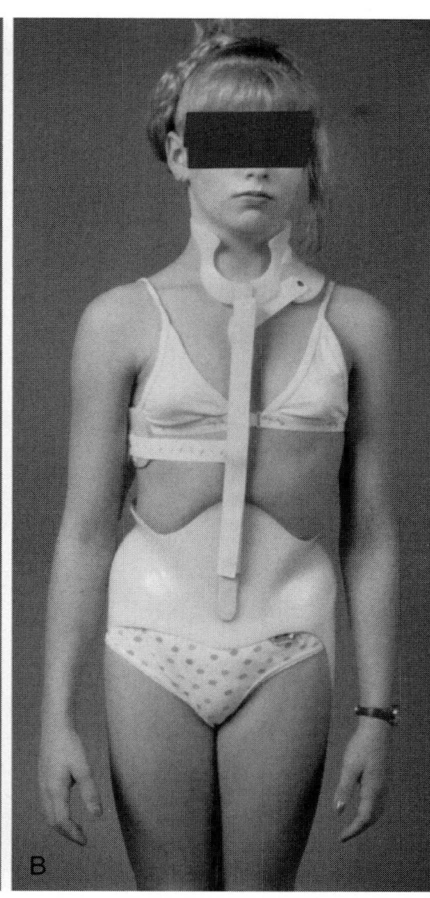

FIGURE 17–17. *A.* Posterior view of a modern Milwaukee brace showing the pelvic section, a lumbar pad, a right thoracic pad, a left trapezius pad, and the new style plastic neck-ring. *B.* Frontal view of the same patient, again showing the pelvic section, the anterior upright, the trapezius pad, and the modern plastic neck-ring, which avoids all dental problems and is much more aesthetically acceptable to the patient.

held straight in the brace for a few months; then the brace is gradually removed (the "weaning" process). At times, however, the spine does well as long as the brace is on, but deforms with attempts at weaning. In this case, long-term bracing is necessary until the pubertal growth spurt, at which point the curve usually gets worse despite the brace so surgical fusion typically becomes necessary. Brace failure can also occur; that is, the curve may fail to respond to the brace from the beginning. In that case, serial Risser casts should be used, followed by another brace trial. When all such nonoperative attempts fail, epiphysiodesis and rodding without fusion may be required.

Bracing for Juvenile Idiopathic Scoliosis

Juvenile idiopathic scoliosis is far more common in North America than is infantile idiopathic scoliosis, and it is more likely to affect females than males. Curves developing after age 3 years, but before puberty onset, are in this category.

Unlike infantile idiopathic scoliosis, the juvenile type almost never spontaneously resolves. Moreover, because there are several years of growth during which progression can take place, extremely severe curves can develop.[10, 15] In North America, this is the type of idiopathic scoliosis most likely to cause adult cor pulmonale and early death. Because of the very poor prognosis of this scoliosis, and the great desire to avoid fusion at a young age, bracing becomes an extremely important method of management.

Thoracic curves predominate, although a compensatory lumbar curve can become quite significant. Because of the thoracic curve, and because the rib cage is soft and pliable, it is critical to use a Milwaukee brace rather than any type of TLSO. Early bracing with the correct orthosis is imperative for success.

Brace treatment should begin when the curve reaches approximately 25 degrees; but curves as high as 60 degrees can still respond to a brace.

The outcomes in juvenile idiopathic scoliosis are similar to those of infantile idiopathic scoliosis: total success with brace management only; successful bracing until the pubertal growth spurt, then surgery; complete brace failure, with surgery needed before the onset of puberty.

Brace wearing always begins with a full-time (23 hours per day) schedule with subsequent adjustments according to the curve's response. It is not unusual for a child to require 5 to 8 years of full-time brace wearing. This may seem unduly harsh; however, children this age adapt readily, and the alternative of curve progression is unacceptable.

Bracing for Adolescent Idiopathic Scoliosis

This is the most common diagnosis for which scoliosis bracing is used. The indications for bracing are a grow-

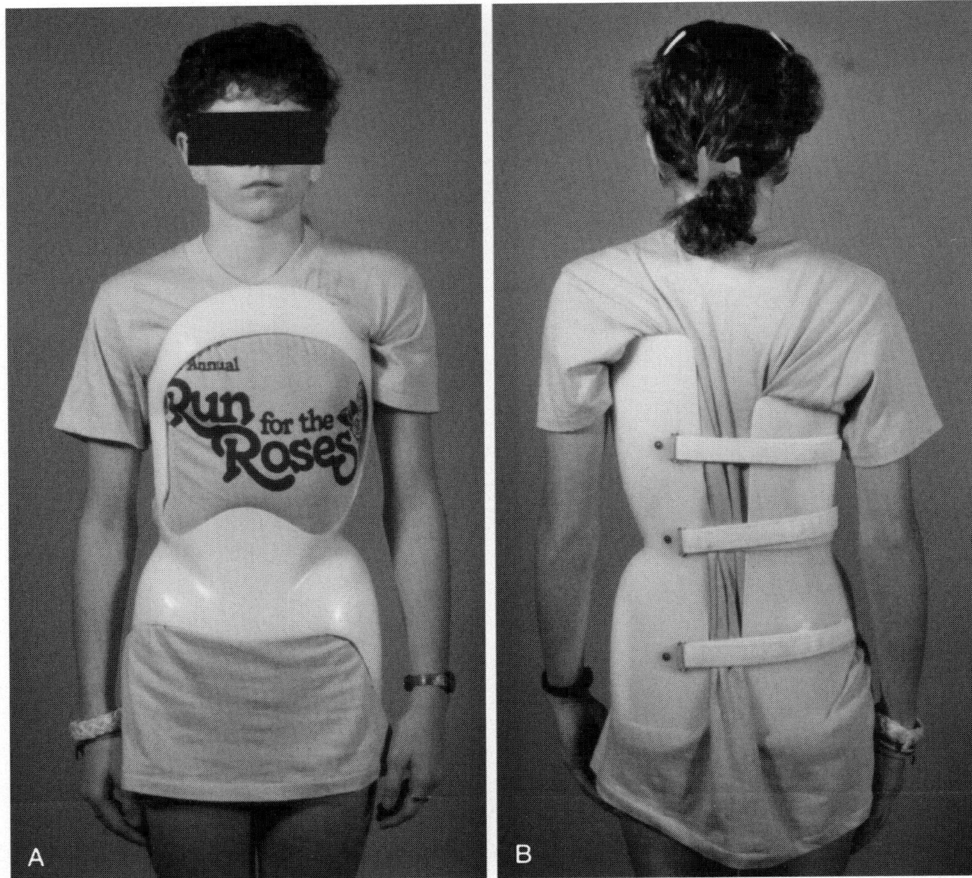

FIGURE 17–18. *A.* Anterior view of a TLSO with a large anterior window for good pulmonary function. Note the excess room on the left side, allowing truncal shift. The patient also has a trochanteric extension on the left. *B.* Posterior view of the same patient shows the posterior opening brace (with three Velcro straps) and the asymmetrical upper end of the brace, which provides right lower thoracic support and high left axillary support.

ing child with a curve of between 25 and 45 degrees. Below 25 degrees there are too many curves that are nonprogressive to justify treatment, and above 45 degrees bracing is ineffective. The highest-risk child for progression is the premenstrual girl with a thoracic curve.

These adolescent scolioses are associated with a variety of highly standardized curve patterns: single thoracic (almost always to the right), single lumbar (almost always to the left); single thoracolumbar (apex at the thoracolumbar junction); double thoracic (high left thoracic T1-T5 and low right thoracic T5-T12); and double major right thoracic and left lumbar.

As mentioned earlier, curves with an apex at T9 or lower can be managed with a TLSO, but curves with an apex higher than that require a Milwaukee brace. The high left curve T1-T5 of the double thoracic pattern requires a trapezius pad mounted on a Milwaukee brace. Single lumbar curves do best with the dynamic LSO; low thoracic and thoracolumbar curves, with the TLSO; and higher thoracic curves, with the Milwaukee brace.

In most cases, bracing should begin with a 22-hour schedule; then, after a year, some modification can sometimes be done. Some children require the full 22-hour schedule until growth has stopped.[33] Although nighttime-only bracing has some advocates, comparative studies have shown it to be much less effective.[16, 47] Electrical stimulators are ineffective, yielding results no different from the natural history of the disease.[25] Comparisons of the Milwaukee brace with the natural history of the disease have clearly demonstrated its effectiveness, even in the highest risk premenarchal female with a right thoracic curve of 20 to 39 degrees.[25, 37]

Bracing for Scheuermann's Disease

Scheuermann's disease is a developmental disorder of the discs and vertebral end-plates occurring in adolescents. The etiology is unknown, but there is a strong genetic tendency. Males and females are affected equally. Second only to adolescent idiopathic scoliosis, Scheuermann's disease is the most frequent diagnosis for which bracing is prescribed. There are two locations of the condition: the classic midthoracic with apex at T7, T8, T9, and the less common thoracolumbar apex. The latter is more likely to present with pain, the former with deformity.

The indications for bracing are a growing child with an increasing deformity, pain, or both. The upper limit of normal thoracic kyphosis is 50 degrees. For midthora-

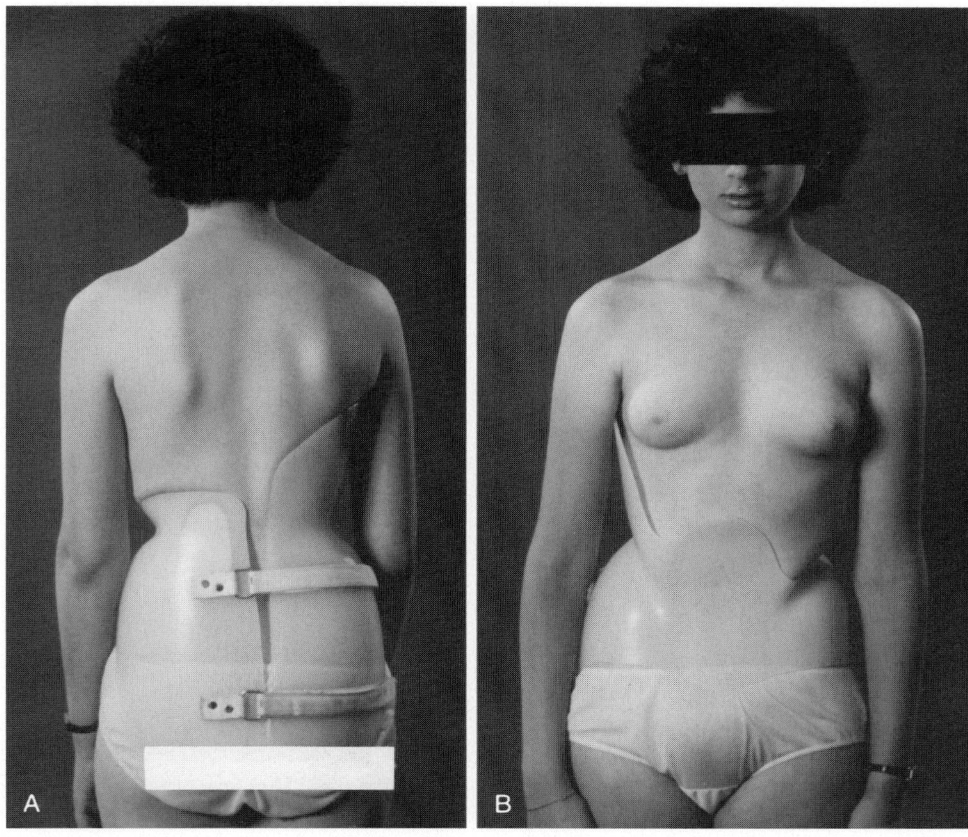

FIGURE 17–19. *A.* Posterior view of a lumbosacral orthosis fitted for a left lumbar curve. Note the pad in the region of the left lumbar prominence, the pelvic section, and the counterpoint on the right thoracic area. *B.* Anterior view of the same brace showing the total lack of any constriction of the thorax.

cic disease, a brace candidate is one in whom there is a deformity with radiological evidence of disc space narrowing, end-plate irregularity, vertebral body wedging, and lack of normal extension flexibility.

For lesions at the thoracolumbar junction, the degree of kyphosis is not relevant, since any kyphosis at this level is pathological. The old definition of "three consecutive vertebrae wedged 5 degrees or more" is no longer considered valid, since this represents end-stage disease and is not amenable to bracing.

For the classic midthoracic disease, the only brace of proven value is the Milwaukee brace. All underarm braces (TLSOs) have failed for deformity at this level, but are the braces of choice for lesions at the thoracolumbar junction. The duration of bracing depends greatly on the time of onset of the problem, since bracing to the end of growth is usually necessary.[61] Short-duration programs (i.e., 18 months) have failed. The intensity and duration of bracing are also related to the severity of the disease process, since there is a wide spectrum within the diagnosis (Fig. 17–20).

Bracing for Neuromuscular Scoliosis

Neuromuscular spine deformities include a very large number of different diagnoses, not all having the same natural history or the same response to bracing. Flaccid deformities are different from spastic, and children with absent skin sensation present a different problem for bracing than those with intact sensation.

The original experience with neuromuscular curves was largely with poliomyelitis, a flaccid paralysis with intact skin sensation. Given an early curve diagnosis, a responsive curve pattern, a good orthosis, and a good wearing schedule, most of these children responded well to a brace until the pubertal growth spurt, at which time the curve would increase and surgery was necessary. This pattern of adequate curve control until the pubertal growth spurt with subsequent surgery has proved to be quite consistent in the neuromuscular diagnoses. Rarely, if ever, is bracing done to prevent surgery entirely.

Good brace results are seen in patients with cerebral palsy, myelomeningocele, traumatic paraplegia, and spinal muscular atrophy. Bracing has *not* proved to be of value in patients with Duchenne muscular dystrophy, Friedreich's ataxia, or syringomyelia.

Virtually all bracing in neuromuscular diseases is achieved with TLSOs. These can be back-opening, front-opening, or bivalved.

Bracing for Congenital Spine Deformity

Bracing is of no value in congenital kyphosis or congenital lordosis, but does have limited value in some congenital scolioses. The curvatures most likely to benefit from bracing are the long curve (10 vertebrae or more) which

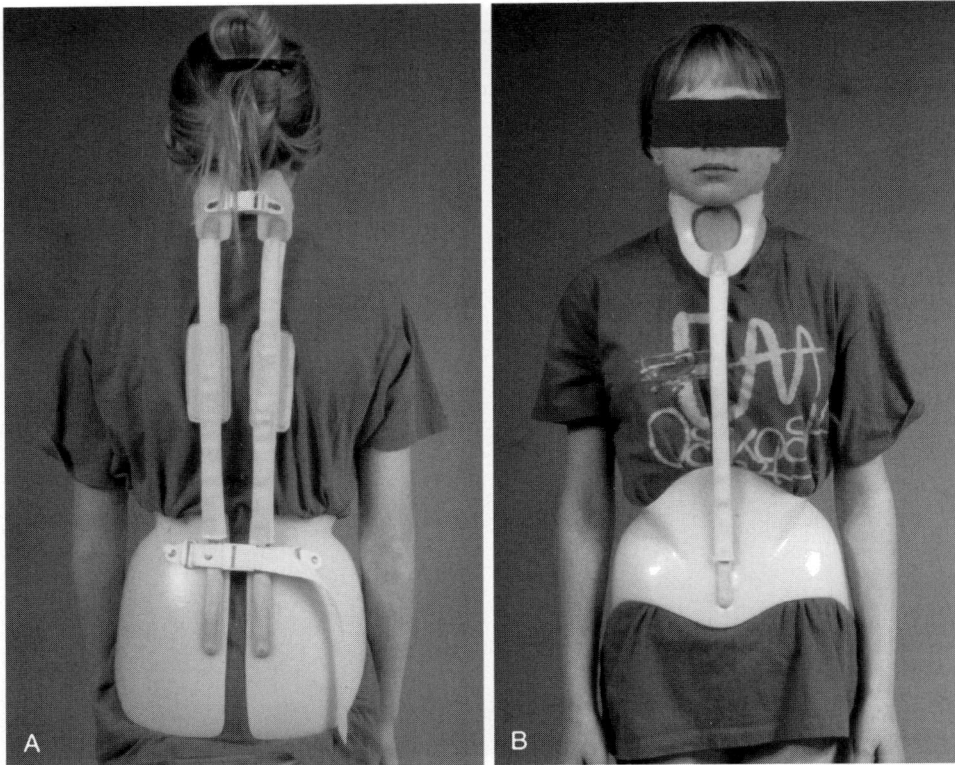

FIGURE 17–20. *A.* This patient is wearing a Milwaukee brace for a typical midthoracic kyphosis of Scheuermann's disease. Note the plastic pelvic section, the single strap, the two kyphosis pads (one mounted on each upright), and the modern plastic neck-ring. *B.* A frontal view of the same patient shows the pelvic section, the single, narrow upright, and the modern plastic neck-ring.

demonstrates considerable flexibility (at least 50% on a supine bending radiograph as compared to an upright radiograph). As with neuromuscular scolioses, the goal of bracing in congenital scoliosis is to control the curve until the adolescent growth spurt, at which time fusion is done. Bracing is also used to control compensatory curves after fusion of the primary congenital scoliosis.

Bracing for Other Scolioses

The previous material has covered the more common diagnoses, but other diagnoses remain. In less common scoliotic conditions, a child with a progressive curvature is a candidate for bracing if he or she is at an age when fusion is undesirable or when there is hope that surgery can be prevented. The exceptions are those conditions for which bracing is generally useless: Duchenne muscular dystrophy, congenital kyphosis, and congenital lordosis, as well as dystrophic neurofibromatosis and Marfan's syndrome. These patients typically require surgical fusion. In progressive problems involving loss of respiratory function, the fusion should be done early while there is adequate vital capacity to prevent surgical morbidity and mortality.

REFERENCES

1. Andriacchi TP, Schultz AB, Belytschko TB, et al: A model for studies of mechanical interactions between the human spine and rib cage. J Biomech 1974; 7:487.
2. Askins V, Eismont FJ: Efficacy of five cervical orthoses in restricting cervical motion: A comparison study. Spine 1997; 22:1193–1198.
3. Benzel EC, Hadden TA, Saulsberry CM: A comparison of the Minerva and halo jackets for stabilization of the cervical spine. J Neurosurg 1989; 70:411–414.
4. Berg U, Aaro S: Long term effect of Boston brace treatment on renal function in patients with idiopathic scoliosis. Clin Orthop 1983; 180:169–172.
5. Berger N, Lusskin R: Orthotic components and systems. In Atlas of Orthotics: Biomechanical Principles and Applications. St Louis, Mosby–Year Book, 1975.
6. Calmels P: An update on orthotic devices for the lumbar spine based on a review of the literature. Rev Rhum (Engl Ed) 1996; 63:285–291.
7. Clark CR, White AA III: Fractures of the dens. J Bone Joint Surg [Am] 1985; 67:1340–1348.
8. Denis F: Personal communication, Minnesota Spine Center, Minneapolis, May 1991.
9. Fidler MW, Plasmans CMT: The effects of four types of supports on the segmental mobility of the lumbosacral spine. J Bone Joint Surg [Am] 1983; 65:943–947.
10. Figueredo UM, James JIP: Juvenile idiopathic scoliosis. J Bone Joint Surg [Br] 1981; 63:61–72.
11. Fisher SV, Bowar JF, Awad EA, et al: Cervical orthoses effect on cervical spine motion: Roentgenography and goniometric method of study. Arch Phys Med Rehabil 1977; 58:109–115.
12. Gaskill SJ, Marlin AE: Custom fitted thermoplastic Minerva jacket in the treatment of cervical spine instability in preschool age children. Pediatr Neurosurg 1990; 91:35–39.
13. Glaser JA, Whitehill R, Stamp WG, et al: Complications associated with the halo-vest, a review of 245 cases. J Neurosurg 1986; 65:762–769.
14. Hughes SJ: How effective is the Newport/Aspen collar? A prospective radiological evaluation in healthy adult volunteers. J Trauma 1998; 45:374–378.

15. Johnson RM, Hart PL, Owen JR, et al: The Yale cervical orthosis: A study comparing their effectiveness in restricting cervical motion in normal subjects. J Bone Joint Surg [Am] 1977; 59:332–339.
16. Katz DE, Richards S, Browne RH, et al: A comparison between the Boston brace and the Charleston brace in adolescent idiopathic scoliosis. Spine 1997; 22:1302–1312.
17. Kennedy JD, Robertson CF, Hudson I, et al: Effect of bracing on respiratory mechanics in mild idiopathic scoliosis. Thorax 1989; 44:548–553.
18. Kennedy JD, Robertson CF, Olinsky A, et al: Pulmonary restrictive effect of bracing in mild idiopathic scoliosis. Thorax 1987; 42:959–961.
19. Koch RA, Nickel UL: The halo vest, an evaluation of motion and forces across the neck. Spine 1978; 3:103–107.
20. Kumar S: The effect of sustained spinal load on intra-abdominal pressure and EMG characteristics of trunk muscles. Ergonomics 1997; 40:1324–1334.
21. Lander JE, Simonton RL, Giacobbe J: The effectiveness of weight belts during the squat exercise. Med Sci Sports Exer 1992; 22:117–124.
22. Lantz SA, Schultz AB: Lumbar spine orthosis wearing. Restriction of gross body motion. Spine 1986; 11:834–837.
23. Lantz SA, Schultz AB: Lumbar spine orthosis wearing. II. Effect on trunk muscle myoelectric activity. Spine 1986; 11:838–842.
24. Lind B, Shlbom H, Nordwall A: Forces and motions across the neck in patients treated with the halo vest. Spine 1988; 13:162–167.
25. Lonstein JE, Winter RB: Milwaukee brace treatment of adolescent idiopathic scoliosis: A review of 1020 patients. J Bone Joint Surg [Am] 1994; 76:1207–1221.
26. Lucas BD: Spinal bracing. In Licht S (ed): Orthotics, Etcetera. New Haven, CT, Waverly Press, 1966, pp 275–305.
27. Lumsden RM, Morris JM: An in vitro study of axial rotation and immobilization at the lumbosacral joint. J Bone Joint Surg [Am] 1968; 50:1591–1602.
28. Lusskin R, Berger N: Prescription Principles. In Atlas of Orthotics: Biomechanical Principles and Applications. St Louis, Mosby–Year Book, 1975.
29. Lysell E: Motion of the cervical spine: Thesis. Acta Orthop Scand Suppl 1969; 123.
30. Maiman D, Millington P, Novak S, et al: The effects of the thermoplastic Minerva body jacket on cervical spine motion. Neurosurgery 1989; 25:363–368.
31. McGill SM, Norman RW, Sharratt MT: The effect of an abdominal belt on trunk muscle activity and intra-abdominal pressure during squat lifts. Ergonomics 1990; 32:147–160.
32. McGuire RA, Degnan G, Amundson GM: Evaluation of current extrication orthoses in immobilization of the unstable cervical spine. Spine 1990; 15:1064–1067.
33. Miller JAA, Nachemson A, Schultz AB: Effectiveness of braces in mild idiopathic scoliosis. Presented to the Scoliosis Research Society, New Orleans, 1983.
34. Millington P, Ellingsen J, Hauswirth B, et al: Thermoplastic Minerva body jacket—A practical alternative to current methods of cervical spine stabilization. Phys Ther 1987; 67:223–225.
35. Morris JM, Lucas DB, Bresler B: Role of the trunk in stability of the spine. J Bone Joint Surg [Am] 1961; 43:327–351.
36. Morris JM: Low back bracing. Clin Orthop 1974; 102:126–132.
37. Nachemson A, Morris JM: In vivo measurement of intradiskal pressure: Discometry, a method for the determination of pressure in the lower lumbar discs. J Bone Joint Surg [Am] 1964; 46:1077–1092.
38. Nachemson A, Peterson L: Effectiveness of treatment with a brace in girls who have adolescent idiopathic scoliosis. J Bone Joint Surg [Am] 1995; 77:815–822.
39. Nachemson A, Schultz A, Andersson G: Mechanical effectiveness studies of lumbar spine orthoses. Scand J Rehabil Med Suppl 1983; 9:139–149.
40. National Institute for Occupational Safety and Health (NIOSH): Workplace Use of Back Belts: Review and Recommendations. DHHS no 94-122. Washington D.C., U.S. Department of Health and Human Services, 1994.
41. Norton PL, Brown T: The immobilization efficiency of back braces, their effect on the posture and motion of the lumbosacral spine. J Bone Joint Surg [Am] 1957; 39:111–139.
42. Parry H, DeLargy M, Burt A: Early mobilization of patients with cervical cord injury using the halo brace device. Paraplegia 1988; 26:226–232.
43. Perry J, Nickel UL, Garrett A, et al: The halo—A spinal skeletal traction fixation device. J Bone Joint Surg [Am] 1968; 50:1400–1409.
44. Perry J, Nickel UL: Total cervical spine fusion for neck paralysis. J Bone Joint Surg [Am] 1959; 41:37–60.
45. Perry J: The use of external support in the treatment of low back pain. J Bone Joint Surg [Am] 1970; 52:1440–1442.
46. Pringle RG: Review article: Halo versus Minerva—Which orthosis? Paraplegia 1990; 28:281–283.
47. Rowe DE, et al: A meta-analysis of the efficacy of non-operative treatment for idiopathic scoliosis. J Bone Joint Surg [Am] 1997; 79:664–674.
48. Sachs B, Bradford DS, Winter RB, et al: Scheuermann's kyphosis: Long-term results of Milwaukee brace treatment. J Bone Joint Surg [Am] 1987; 69:50–57.
49. Sears W, Fazi M: Prediction of stability of cervical spine fracture managed in the halo vest and indications for surgical intervention. J Neurosurg 1990; 72:426–432.
50. Sharpe KP, Rao S, Ziogas A: Evaluation of the effectiveness of the Minerva cervicothoracic orthosis. Spine 1995; 20:1457–1479.
51. Sinaki M: A new back support in rehabilitation of osteoporosis program exercise: Posture training support. Osteoporosis 1990; 3:1355–1357.
52. Smith GE, Cantab MA: The most ancient splints. Br Med J 1908; 1:732–734.
53. Solot JA, Winzelberg GG: Clinical and radiologic evaluation of Vertebrace extrication collar. J Emerg Med 1990; 8:79–83.
54. Stillo JV, Stein AB, Ragnarsson KT: Low back orthoses. In Lehmann JF (ed): Orthotics. Phys Med Rehabil Clin North Am 1992; 3:57–94.
55. Tolo VT, Gillespie R: The characteristics of juvenile idiopathic scoliosis and results of its management. J Bone Joint Surg [Br] 1978; 60:181–188.
56. Van Poppei MNM, Koes BW, van der Ploeg T, et al: Lumbar supports and education for the prevention of low back pain in industry. J Am Med Assoc 1998; 279:1789–1794.
57. Walker PS, Lamser D, Hussey RW, et al: Forces in the halo vest. Spine 1984; 9:773–777.
58. Wang GJ, Moskal JT, Albert T, et al: The effect of halo-vest length on stability of the cervical spine. J Bone Joint Surg [Am] 1988; 70:357–361.
59. White AA III, Panjabi MM: The basis of kinematics of the human spine. Spine 1984; 9:12–20.
60. White AA III, Panjabi MM: Clinical Biomechanics of the Spine. Philadelphia, JB Lippincott, 1990.
61. Winter RB: Personal communication, Minnesota Spine Center, Minneapolis, April 1994.
62. Wolf JW, Johnson RM: Cervical orthoses. In The Cervical Spine. Philadelphia, JB Lippincott, 1983, pp 54–61.
63. Wolf JW, Jones HC: Comparison of cervical immobilization in halo-cast and halo-plastic jackets. Orthop Trans 1981; 5:118.

18 CHAPTER

Ralph M. Buschbacher, M.D., Judy Atkins, O.T.R., Brian Lay, and Randall L. Braddom, M.D., M.S.

Prescription of Wheelchairs and Seating Systems

Having the optimal wheelchair and seating system is critical to the habilitation or rehabilitation and ongoing well-being of patients with mobility impairment and many other types of disorders. Because a wheelchair is often used during all waking hours and during all activities, having the right one can make the difference between independence and dependence. A patient of one author once confided that "having the wrong wheelchair is worse than having the wrong spouse." Due to the myriad brands and types that are now available, the wheelchair user has never had more choices. For the same reason, it has never been more difficult for the practitioner to prescribe a wheelchair.

Although the types, brands, and choices of components are numerous, constantly changing, and can seem overwhelming to the practitioner, the basic principles of prescribing wheelchairs have not changed. This chapter discusses the types of wheelchairs and seating systems that are available and the principles of prescription.

PURPOSES OF WHEELCHAIRS AND SEATING SYSTEMS

Britell[1] cites the five following major goals of wheelchair prescription (Table 18–1):

- Maximization of efficient independent mobility
  The wheelchair should provide mobility in the environment with as little energy consumption as possible and with minimal assistance from others.
- Prevention/minimization of deformity or injury
  The wheelchair and seating system should help to prevent pressure ulcers, contractures, joint deformities, and other injuries.
- Maximization of independent functioning
  The wheelchair should allow the user to meet the environment in the most functional manner. Because use of the head and upper extremities is essential for function, the wheelchair should maximize stable positioning and limit abnormal tone or dysfunctional movements.
- Projection of a healthy, vital, attractive body image
  Because able-bodied individuals often view the wheelchair user and the wheelchair as a unit, the wheelchair and seating system should have as aesthetically appealing an appearance as possible.
- Minimization of short-term and long-term equipment cost
  With the current emphasis on containing health care costs, the practitioner should prescribe wheelchairs that are the most cost-effective, not necessarily the least expensive. The overall expense of a wheelchair includes not only the purchase price, but also the costs of maintenance and repair.[1]

Practitioners have to be assertive in explaining to third-party payers that it is "pennywise and pound foolish" to prescribe an inappropriate, stripped-down, or nondurable wheelchair because of its lower purchase cost. Teenagers and young adults in particular can test the physical limits of a wheelchair. Prescribing a nondurable wheelchair will likely result in such patients frequently having a "broken" chair, which adds considerable repair costs. However, patients getting a wheelchair for the first time often pressure the practitioner to prescribe every avail-

TABLE 18–1 Purposes of Wheelchair and Seating Prescription

1. Maximizatiion of efficient independent mobility
2. Prevention/minimization of deformity or injury
3. Maximization of independent functioning
4. Projection of a healthy, vital, attractive "body image"
5. Minimization of short-term and long-term equipment cost

able option. Patients rapidly learn that a wheelchair that has too many options is not always better, as it is heavier, more prone to break down, often more difficult to propel, and more difficult to place in vehicles.

HISTORY OF WHEELCHAIRS

Perry[12] has provided a summary of the likely history of wheelchairs. The development of the wheelchair first required the invention of the chair (documented as early as 2900 BCE) and the wheel/axle (documented as early as 3500 BCE). The wheelbarrow was the most-used vehicle for mobility-impaired persons in the Middle Ages and the Renaissance (it was probably invented in China in the third century CE and used in Europe by the 12th century CE). Putting wheels on chairs probably occurred in the 15th century CE, with the addition of a hand-crank mechanism in the 17th century, to permit propulsion by the user.

By the 18th century, a manually powered wheelchair with two large front wheels and a small rear wheel was developed. The 19th century saw the introduction of smaller and lighter wheelchairs made of wood, with bicycle-type wheels that had hand rims. During the American Civil War, the wheelchair was typically a manually powered nonfolding wooden type with large front wheels and two small rear wheels (Fig. 18–1). The first folding wheelchair is believed to have been developed in the United States by the father of a mobility-impaired daughter, in collaboration with the superintendent of a wheelchair manufacturing company who also had a mobility-impaired daughter. The wheelchair was made of steel, and, when folded, it was 20 inches wide.[12]

The next major advance in wheelchair design occurred in 1933 when Herbert A. Everest (a paraplegic individual) and Harry C. Jennings (a mechanical engineer) invented the modern folding metal wheelchair.[12] Although the wheelchair has been developed over thousands of years, modern advances in materials and design are causing improvements to occur at a dizzying and accelerating pace.

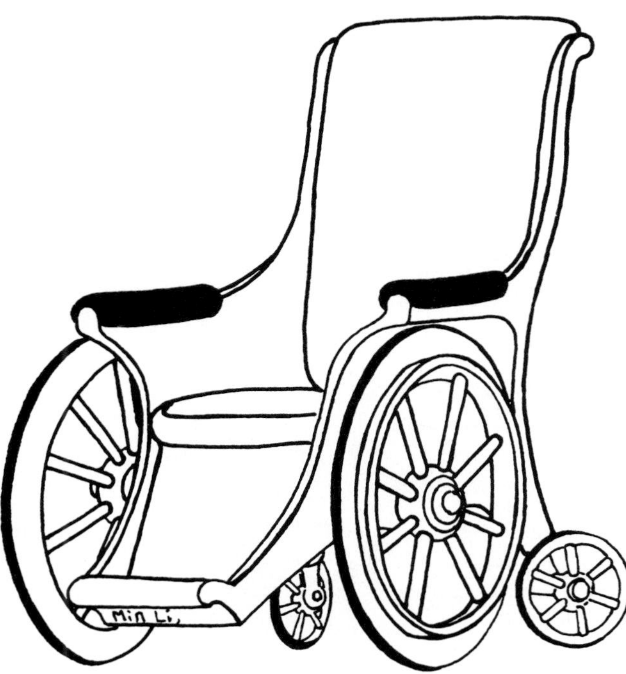

FIGURE 18–1. Civil War era wheelchair.

COMMONLY USED WHEELCHAIR TYPES

The types of wheelchairs now available can be variously categorized in the following ways: adult/pediatric, heavy/moderate/lightweight/ultralight, manually propelled/powered, folding/nonfolding/standup frame, reclining/nonreclining, tilting/nontilting, and metal/composite. Table 18–2 lists the major types of wheelchairs on the market that are prescribed commonly. These wheelchairs are described in more detail later in the chapter.

TABLE 18–2 Basic Types of Wheelchairs and Their Characteristics

Wheelchair Type	Characteristics
Rigid frame	Nonfolding; commonly used in institutions; used in sports chairs
X-frame	Common folding wheelchair
User-propelled	User propels chair
Assistant-propelled	Assistant pushes chair; usually large wheels are placed forward (or has four small wheels); commonly used in institutions
Motorized	Various types of battery-powered scooters or chairs available
Standard weight	Usual configuration
Ultra-lightweight	For especially active individuals
Sports chairs	For specific events
Adult chairs	Usual configuration
Pediatric chairs	Various sizes available
Standing frame	Allows user to gain height; motorized and nonmotorized units available
Nonreclining	Usual configuration
Reclining	Useful in patient with hypotension and for pressure relief, though some units increase shear force on sacrum
Nontilting	Usual configuration
Tilting	Useful in high-tone patients, for pressure relief, for pulmonary posture changes

TABLE 18–3 Types of Frames and Their Common Uses, Advantages, and Disadvantages

	Uses	Common Advantages	Disadvantages
Rigid	Institutions	More stable, energy efficient	Difficult to transport
Folding	Community mobility	Compact transport	Heavier, more energy use

MANUAL WHEELCHAIR COMPONENTS

Frames

The most common type of wheelchair frame in use is the folding type (Table 18–3). Rigid wheelchairs are more energy-efficient because they have less wasted internal motion during movement; however, they are not as easy to transport as a folding frame type. The rigid chair (Fig. 18–2) can have quick-release wheels and a fold-down back to make it more compact and transportable, but it is still more cumbersome than the folding type. Folding chairs (Fig. 18–3) utilize a cross-linkage (X-shaped) bar frame assembly. The chair is folded by lifting the center of the seat, which to some extent limits the seating support and cushions that can be fitted to the chair. Because the folding chair has more parts, it is typically heavier than the rigid type, and usually weighs around 27 lb.

In the past, most wheelchairs were made of steel and wood. They were strong, inexpensive, and easy to construct, but were too heavy for ordinary use. The wooden and steel wheelchair is still used by many hospitals and other institutions for internal patient transport, primarily because this wheelchair is very durable and tends to be stolen much less frequently than the more modern styles.

Most wheelchairs are now constructed of aluminum. This makes the chair durable enough for ordinary use and lighter than the steel chair, and it can be purchased at a reasonable cost. Even lighter chairs, made of titanium, are available. They are very durable but also very expensive. The lightest chairs are made of composite materials, although these are currently prohibitively expensive and are not very durable. In developing nations, ease of construction and the ready availability of replacement parts are of greatest importance. Wheelchairs in these countries are often constructed of various bicycle parts.

Wheels and Tires

Two basic types of wheels are available: "mag" wheels and spoked wheels (Table 18–4). The most commonly

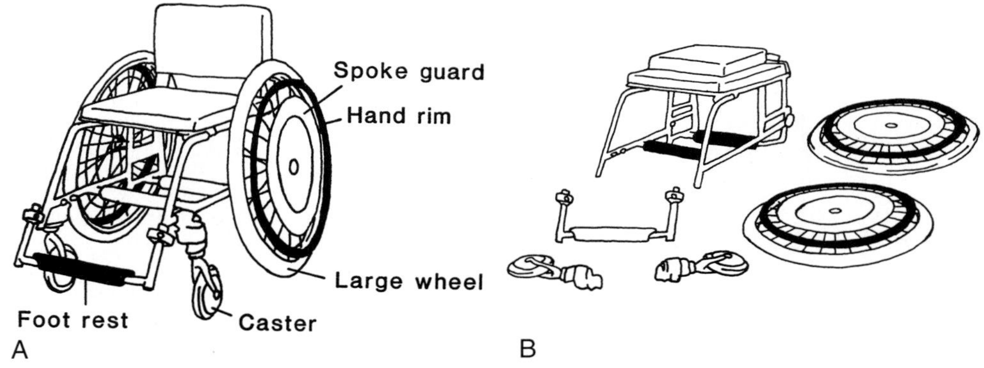

FIGURE 18–2. Rigid chair. *A.* Assembled. *B.* Disassembled with casters, wheels, and footrest removed and seat back folded.

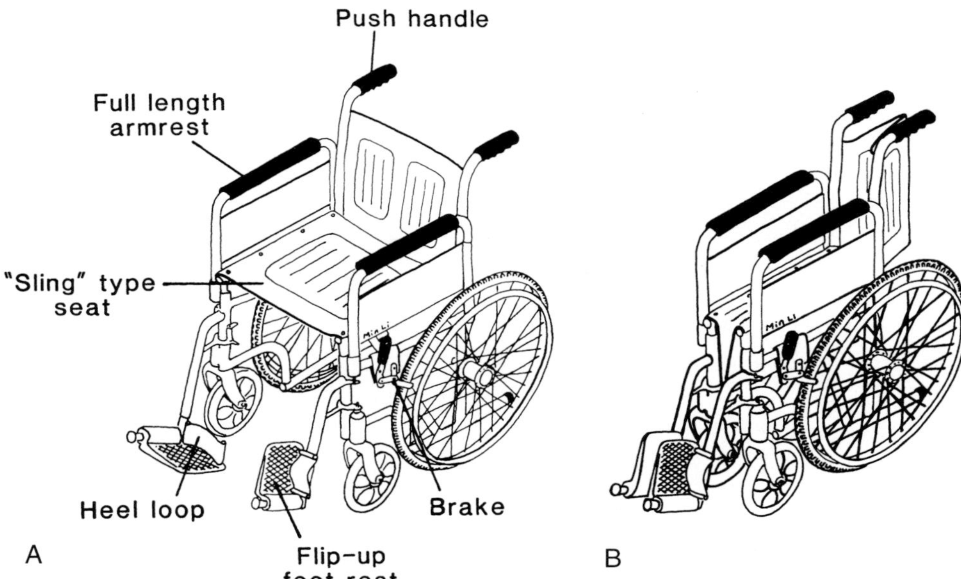

FIGURE 18–3. Folding chair: *A.* open; *B.* folded.

used is the mag wheel. The mag wheel was first made out of magnesium, which is how it got its name. It was also first used in bicycles. Now most mag wheels are actually made out of plastic. Although these wheels are typically heavier than their spoked counterparts, they require virtually no maintenance. Spoked wheels are lighter, but the spokes tend to loosen and must be retightened periodically. Mag wheels are very durable and, unlike spoked wheels, are unlikely to bend with heavy use.

Three types of tires can be fitted to the wheels (Table 18–5): hard rubber, pneumatic, and pneumatic with flat-free inserts. Hard rubber tires are very durable and have a low rolling resistance, especially on flat, smooth surfaces. On rough terrain they create a harsh ride. They are also relatively heavy.

Pneumatic tires utilize an outer tire casing with an inner tube. They are lightweight and give the best ride on most surfaces, although on flat, smooth surfaces they have a higher rolling resistance than hard rubber tires. Unfortunately, they can have "flats." To solve this problem, the flat-free insert has been developed, which is basically a piece of soft rubber or latex gel that takes the place of the inner tube. It provides nearly as good a ride as the pneumatic tire, without the risk of flats. Because it is heavier than the inner tube, it also carries added weight, however.

Wheels and tires come in several size options, the most common being 24 inches in diameter; 22- and 20-inch wheels are also commonly used to vary the height of the chair.

Wheel placement is an important consideration in chair construction. Many chairs allow for adjustment of the wheel up and down as well as forward and backward (Fig. 18–4). Up and down adjustments are used to vary the height of the chair. This can improve positioning and, in the case of chairs for patients with hemiplegia, allow a user to reach the floor with the "good" foot. Forward and back wheel adjustments alter the stability of the chair. The further forward the wheel is placed, the more easily the chair will tip backward. This can be desirable for a patient with paraplegia who does "wheelies" to negotiate curbs. It is undesirable in the bilateral lower extremity amputee,

TABLE 18–4 Types of Wheels and Their Common Uses, Advantages, and Disadvantages

	Common Uses	Advantages	Disadvantages
Mag	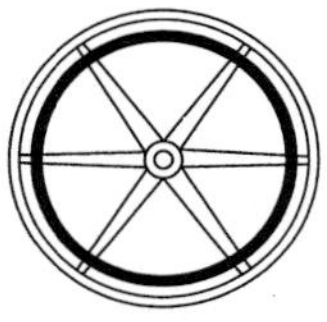 Community mobility	Durable, low maintenance	Heavier
Spokes	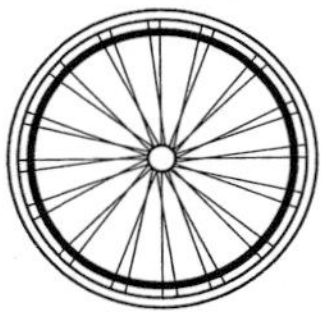 Community, institutions, sports	Lighter	Greater maintenance, less durable

TABLE 18–5 Types of Tires and Their Common Uses, Advantages, and Disadvantages

	Common Uses	Advantages	Disadvantages
Hard rubber	Institutions	Low rolling resistance	Harsh ride on rough terrain, heavy
Pneumatic	Community mobility	Best all-around ride, lightweight	Tendency to develop flats
Pneumatic with flat free inserts	Community mobility	Good ride with no flats	Moderately heavy

as the lack of forward-placed (leg) weight makes it even easier to tip the chair backward. The wheels also need to be placed posteriorly for some types of reclining or posterior-tilting wheelchairs. Unfortunately, the further posterior the rear wheels are placed, the greater are the rolling resistance and the turning radius. The tradeoff of stability versus rolling ease must be factored into the wheel-placement decision.

Camber is the angle the wheel makes from the vertical axis. A wheelchair demonstrating increased camber is shown in Figure 18–2A. The more the bottom of the wheel is moved outward, the greater its camber and stability. Increasing the camber makes it easier to manually propel the chair and is especially useful in sports chairs. A greater camber also improves the user's ability to propel the wheelchair at higher speeds, and tightens the turning radius. The tradeoff is a wider chair and greater wear and tear (mainly on the tires, but also on doorways and furniture).

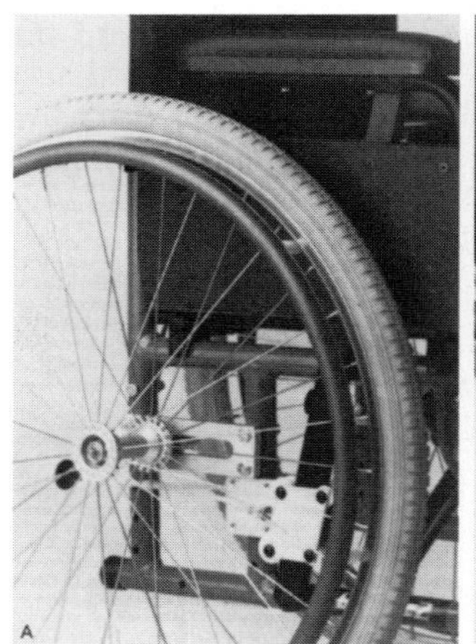

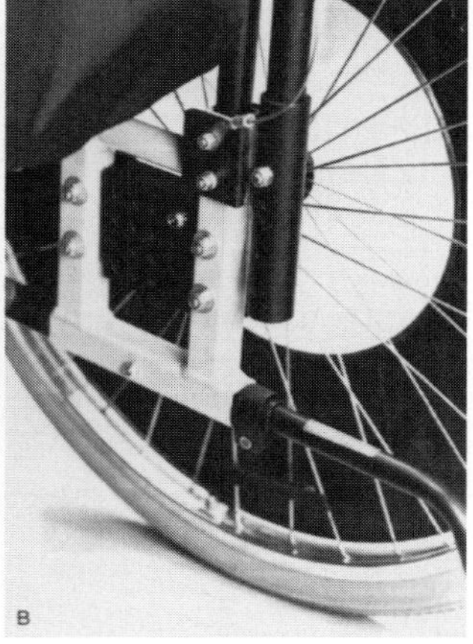

FIGURE 18–4. Wheel adjustment devices. *A.* Axle lies in a plate with a groove for forward/backward adjustment. The plate can be moved up or down. *B.* Plate with multiple holes. Axle can be fitted into any of the holes. (From Britell CW: Wheelchair prescription. In Kottke FJ, Lehmann JF (eds): Krusen's Handbook of Physical Medicine and Rehabilitation, ed 4. Philadelphia, WB Saunders, 1990, pp 548–563.)

Hand Rims

Hand rims are placed slightly lateral to the wheel and are smaller in diameter than the wheel (Table 18–6). The larger the hand rim's diameter, the easier it is to propel the chair, but more arm strokes are required to cover a given distance. Larger hand rim diameters are the most practical for general use, but wheelchair athletes often opt for smaller-diameter rims to maximize the distance covered with each stroke.

Hand rims can be varied in thickness, and different coatings can be used to foster optimal grip. The thicker the rim the easier it is to grip, but weight and width are added to the chair. Some patients with very poor grip, such as those with quadriplegia, benefit from the attachment of knobby projections to the rim.

Casters

Casters are the small wheels typically found on the front of the chair (Table 18–7). They come in different diameters, widths, and materials. In general, the smaller casters are suited for rapid maneuverability; these are often used on sport chairs. Narrow, hard casters are good on smooth, level surfaces but perform poorly on rough terrain or on outside surfaces. They also tend to shimmy (wobble) when moving longitudinally along a grade, as is often the case on slightly tilted sidewalks. Larger and wider casters are easier to use on rough terrain, although

TABLE 18–6 Types of Hand Rims and Their Common Uses, Advantages, and Disadvantages

	Common Uses	Advantages	Disadvantages
Large diameter	Community, institutions	Easy to propel	Less distance per stroke
Small diameter	Active individual, sports	Greater distance per stroke	More force required
Thick	Poor hand grip	Easier to grip	More weight and width
Knobby	Poor hand grip	Easier to push	More weight and width

on smooth, level surfaces they increase rolling resistance. For most purposes an 8 inch diameter caster of relatively wide configuration is optimal.

Seats and Backs

The seats and backs that are standard on most wheelchairs are referred to as *sling upholstery* or *hammock* style (see Fig. 18–3A). They consist of a piece of material that is suspended between the frame posts of the chair and are lightweight and easy to fold. The most common material used for such slings is vinyl, which is inexpensive, durable, and easy to clean, and comes in a number of colors. Vinyl tends to become quite warm with use and promotes perspiration. Because of this problem, materials such as Dacron and nylon are often used instead, as they are lighter in weight and more breathable. They are not as easy to clean, however, and tend to accumulate dirt and stains.

Since sling-type chairs provide little support, a solid seat is often placed on top of them. This solid support can be removed when the chair is folded. Other styles utilize a solid folding seat; however, this adds weight to the chair and cannot easily be modified.

The seat plane angle is the angle the seat makes with the horizontal. The most common seat plane angles range from 0 to 5 degrees, although in sports applications angles up to 20 degrees may be used. The greater angle creates greater stability but can also cause pressure problems.[3]

Seat Cushions

A number of more specialized seating surfaces are available (Table 18–8). They include air-cell cushions, which can help prevent local pressure-induced skin breakdown. The pressure in each cell can be individually adjusted to provide proper pressure distribution.

TABLE 18–7 Types of Casters and Their Common Uses, Advantages, and Disadvantages

	Common Uses	Advantages	Disadvantages
Large	Community, institutions	Rough terrain	Increased rolling resistance
Small	Sports	Maneuverability	Poor outdoor performance

TABLE 18–8 Types of Cushions and Their Common Uses, Advantages, and Disadvantages

	Common Uses	Advantages	Disadvantages
Foam	General use	Good stability, low cost	Pressure relief not optimal
Coated, contoured foam	General use	Excellent stability, cleanability, durability	Heat buildup, expensive
Gel-filled	General use	Good pressure relief, cleanability, heat dissipation	Expensive
Contoured foam with gel insert	When improved pressure distribution needed	Good pressure relief, stability, cleanability, durability	Expensive, heat buildup
Air-filled villous	Optimal pressure relief needed	Excellent pressure relief, cleanability, heat dissipation	Expensive, suboptimal seating stability

From Britell CW: Wheelchair prescription. In Kottke FJ, Lehmann JF (eds): Krusen's Handbook of Physical Medicine and Rehabilitation, ed 4. Philadelphia, WB Saunders, 1990, pp 548–563.

Another seat cushion that provides improved pressure distribution is the gel-filled type, which can be fitted with modular components to optimize the configuration. Custom-molded seats and seat backs can also provide optimal pressure distribution while helping to control posture. Wheelchairs can also be customized with lateral supports and headrests (Fig. 18–5). Pelvic and leg position can be maintained with abductor wedges and a proper cushion.

For some persons it is important when creating a custom seat to allow rotation of the pelvis when the person bends forward. If such rotation is not allowed, the lumbar spine will compensate with an extreme kyphosis. The seat should help maintain the lumbar spine in slight lordosis.[3]

Seat backs vary in height, depending on the level of control and mobility that is desired. The higher the back, the more support, and the less freedom of mobility. If the back is too low, it leads to a slumped "sacral seating" posture with a tendency toward development of thoracic kyphosis. If the back is too high, it pushes the scapulae forward. Most wheelchair users require seat backs that come to mid-back or to a level a few inches below the inferior poles of the scapulae. Quadriplegic persons require higher back heights, and paraplegic persons sometimes do well with a lower height. Seat backs are usually fitted with push handles to allow an aide to maneuver the chair. Most seat backs are placed at a 0- to 5-degree tilt from the vertical plane.[3]

Reclining Backs

Persons prone to the development of pressure ulcers or orthostatic hypotension often benefit from the reclining or semireclining posture. Semireclining and reclining chairs are available (Fig. 18–5A) and come with a variety of release mechanisms, including cable releases and hydraulic units that help hold the weight of the patient. Not all chairs recline equally, and this must be considered when ordering a chair. Reclining chairs also add weight, width, and bulk, and can make transport more difficult. Simple reclining chairs may create shear stress over the back and sacrum during position changes. In the person at risk for pressure ulcers, special nonshear recliners are indicated. They allow the seat or back to slide during movement, instead of having only a simple hinge.

Tilt-in-Space Seats

An alternative to the reclining seat back is the tilt or tilt-in-space chair (Fig. 18–5B), which utilizes a system whereby the entire seat and back are tilted posteriorly as a single unit. Such systems generally utilize a hydraulic cylinder to aid in movement. The advantage of tilt systems is that they do not create shear stress during movement. Like reclining units, they also help with pressure release and orthostasis and are sometimes used for patients in need of help with pulmonary secretions. They may offer an advantage over the reclining units in patients with tone or spasticity problems, in whom reclining can trigger spasticity. Tilt models tend to be unstable if used for large persons. They also require a higher seating position and do not allow the patient's body to straighten toward the supine position.

Footrests/Leg Rests

Fixed and Swing-away Footrests

Footrests and leg rests help provide balance and positioning and afford protection to the wheelchair user. They also decrease the load on the buttocks and thigh.[3] Swing-away footrests (Fig. 18–6A) are used most commonly. They allow the footrest to be moved out of the way, which makes transfers easier, as the user can position the chair closer to chairs, beds, or toilets. Removable footrests can also improve the portability of the wheelchair.

Fixed, or nonremovable, footrests are available as well. They generally make the chair lighter and more rigid but interfere with transfers and portability.

Elevating Footrests

Elevating footrests (Fig. 18–6B) are available for situations in which the knee cannot or should not be flexed. They can also be used to help minimize dependent edema. Elevating leg rests are of two types: one is level with the seating surface, called the *low pivot-point* style; the other projects higher than the seat, called the *goose*

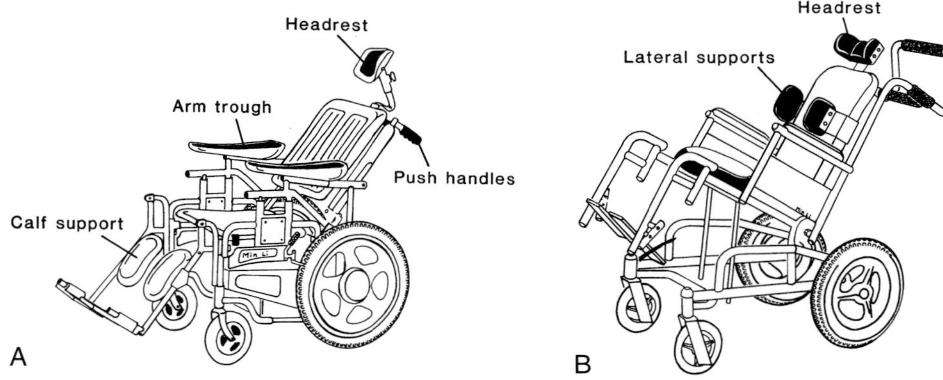

FIGURE 18–5. *A.* Reclining chair with modular supports added. Unit shows headrest and arm troughs. *B.* Tilt chair with modular headrest and lateral trunk supports.

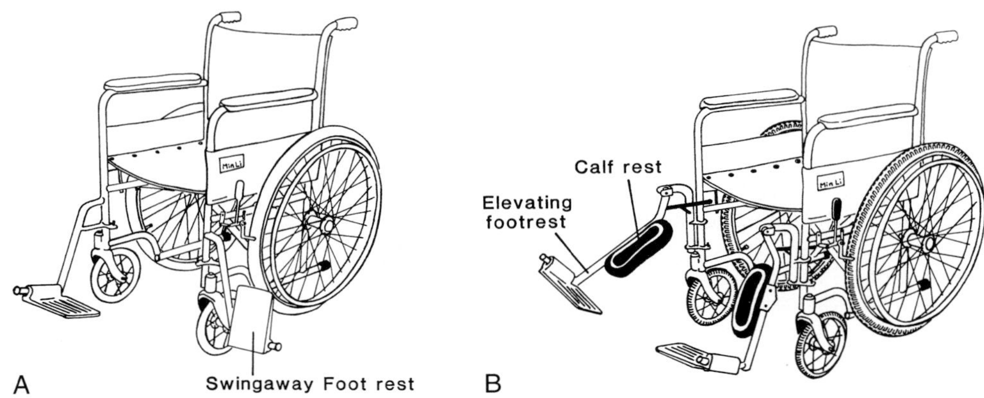

FIGURE 18–6. Footrests/leg rests. *A.* Standard swing-away. *B.* Elevating.

neck style. The goose neck is less desirable as it can interfere with transfers and provides a point of pressure contact with the leg. Elevating footrests usually come with calf supports to hold the lower leg, and for this reason they are often referred to as "leg rests."

Other Footrests

Specialized footrests are available for many clinical situations. In a chair for paraplegics, the footrest is generally a single bar that connects the two sides of the chair (see Fig. 18–2A). This improves structural rigidity but eliminates the folding option. When more leg and foot control is necessary, the footrest can be ordered with special loops or pads. Heel loops (see Fig. 18–3A) are often used instead of the leg rest portion of the unit, as they reduce weight. Most footrests can also be flipped up to aid in transfers (see Fig. 18–3A).

Armrests/Lap Trays

Armrests are added to wheelchairs for a number of reasons (Fig. 18–7). They help provide balance and stability by allowing the user to rest the elbows. They also help provide a point of pushoff for weight shifting and pressure release. In addition, they decrease intradiskal pressures.[3] Many types and styles of armrests are available. The choice of armrest style can affect the patient's independence level, function, and the ability to use certain seating systems.

Fixed Armrests

The main advantages to fixed armrests are that they are inexpensive and cannot be lost. Their chief disadvantages are that they can make fitting of a seating system more difficult and can also hinder transfers.

Removable Armrests

Removable armrests make transfers easier. They can generally be adjusted in height or replaced to accommodate growth. Their disadvantage is that they increase the width and weight of the chair.

Wraparound Armrests

The wraparound armrest design reduces the width of the wheelchair. This is accomplished by attaching the armrest behind the seat back rather than next to the seat. These armrests can generally be moved or detached for transfers.

Desk-Length Armrests

Both fixed and removable armrests are available in full or desk lengths. Full-length armrests extend from the seat back to the front of the chair. They provide more area for resting the arm or for pushing the body forward in a transfer. However, full-length armrests interfere with the ability to maneuver the chair close to tables and desks. Desk-length armrests extend forward only partially, and allow the user to slide the knees under a desk. Because elbow and shoulder positioning is important, adjustable-height armrests are available to accommodate individuals of different sizes.

Other Armrests

In addition to the styles described previously, there are swing-away or flip-up armrests. Young persons with paraplegia often prefer chairs with no armrests at all. Persons who need more control of their limbs often require trough-style armrests (see Fig. 18–5A) to hold the forearms in place. In power chairs, one armrest generally has an attached joystick control unit. Hemiplegic individuals often do well with a lap tray instead of regular armrests. The tray provides a larger surface on which to rest the arm and may help prevent the pain of shoulder subluxation. It can also be used to hold a communication board or a daily schedule. If a lap tray is to be used, proper armrests that can accommodate such a tray are needed.

Brakes/Grade Aids

All wheelchairs are available with wheel locks, commonly known as *brakes* (Fig. 18–8). This mechanism is a very important safety feature. Wheel locks are devices that put pressure on the larger wheels or tires to lock them into position. They are installed to prevent unintended rolling of the chair, either on a grade or during transfers. They are not, however, foolproof, and they should not be used as a substitute for good wheelchair technique.

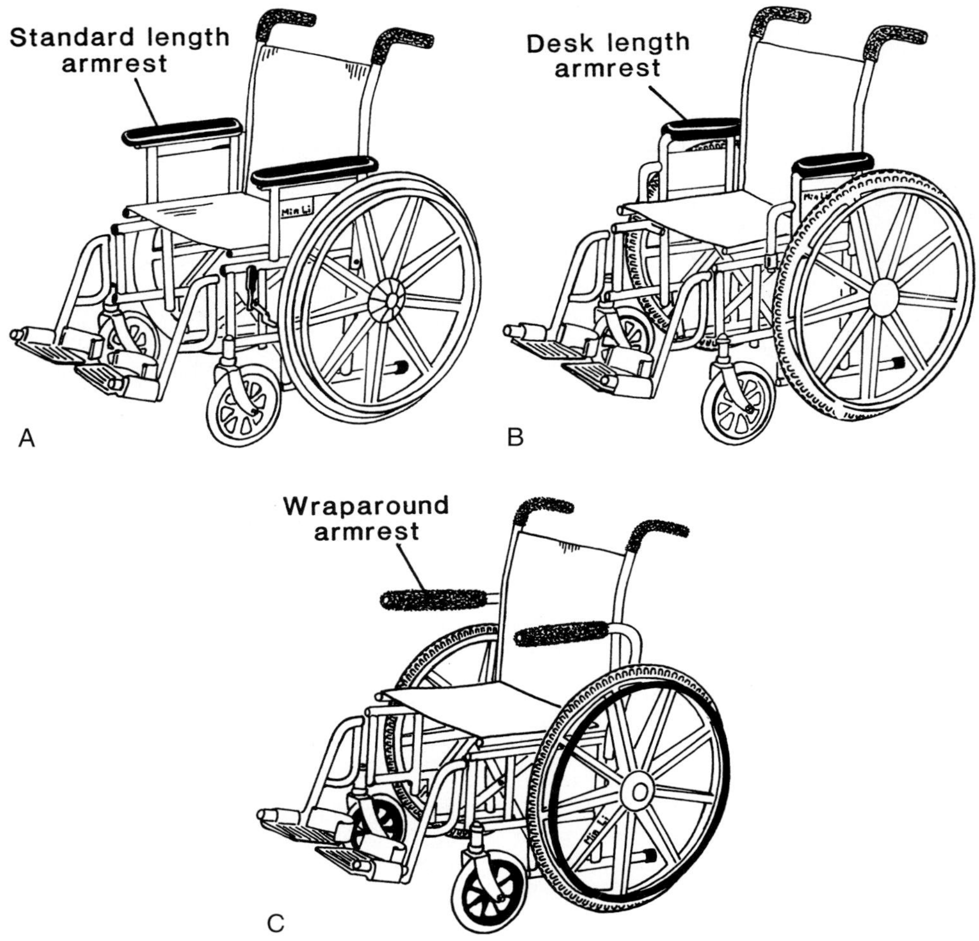

FIGURE 18–7. Armrests. *A.* Standard. *B.* Desk length. *C.* Wraparound.

Wheel locks attach to the sideframe of the chair and are available in either a "push-to-lock" or a "pull-to-lock" mechanism. They are also available in a low mounting style, which places them out of the way so they do not interfere with transfers. Persons who do not have the cognitive ability to decide when to lock and unlock the chairs can have the brakes placed in the rear of the chair where the brakes can be activated only by an attendant or caregiver. Persons with hemiplegia who are not able to activate or release the brake on one side often benefit from an extended handle so that their "good" arm can reach both brakes. In cases in which greater stability is required, the casters can be locked as well.

Wheel locks are available in both a lever style and a toggle style. The lever can be set in different notches to provide varying degrees of holding power. This can be an advantage on a steep grade, but its use requires greater control and strength. Toggle-style brakes are used more commonly. The "power" of the lock is preset, but can be adjusted.

Grade aids, or "hill holders," are devices that prevent the chair from rolling backward but do not interfere with forward motion. They are useful for persons with poor strength or endurance on inclines, where the chair might roll backward between forward thrusts (Fig. 18–9).

Anti-tippers

Patients at risk of falling backward in the chair often benefit from the addition of anti-tippers (Fig. 18–10). These devices can be fixed or removable, and they are capable of being turned. Turning the anti-tipper to the "up" position can help during such maneuvers as negotiating curbs, when the device might interfere. Anti-tippers are useful for above-knee amputees, who have a more posterior center of gravity. They are generally not used for paraplegic patients who practice "wheelies" to help in climbing curbs. In rare cases, forward facing anti-tippers are necessary.

One-Arm Drive

Patients who have the ability to propel a wheelchair with one arm only are sometimes given one-arm drive chairs (Fig. 18–11). On these chairs, both propelling rims are on one side. When both are turned, the chair moves straight ahead. Turning one or the other steers the chair. One-arm drive chairs are wider and heavier than standard chairs, and they often require a longer

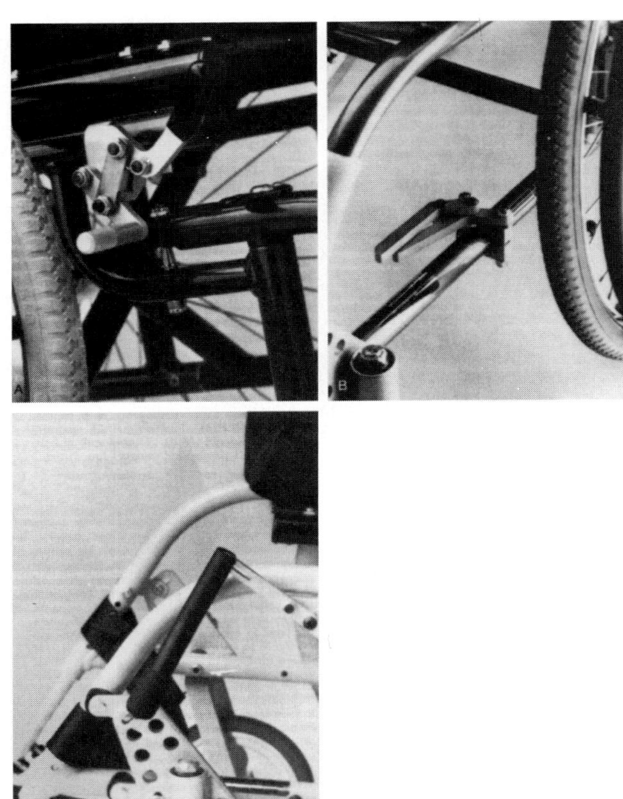

FIGURE 18–8. Several designs of wheelchair brakes. (From Britell CW: Wheelchair prescription. In Kottke FJ, Lehmann JF (eds): Krusen's Handbook of Physical Medicine and Rehabilitation, ed 4. Philadelphia, WB Saunders, 1990, pp 548–563.)

wheel base. They are rarely used successfully, as propelling them requires a fairly high degree of strength and coordination. A practical alternative in most hemiplegic patients is to use one hand rim and one foot to properly guide the chair. A motorized chair is also sometimes a more practical solution than the one-arm drive wheelchair.

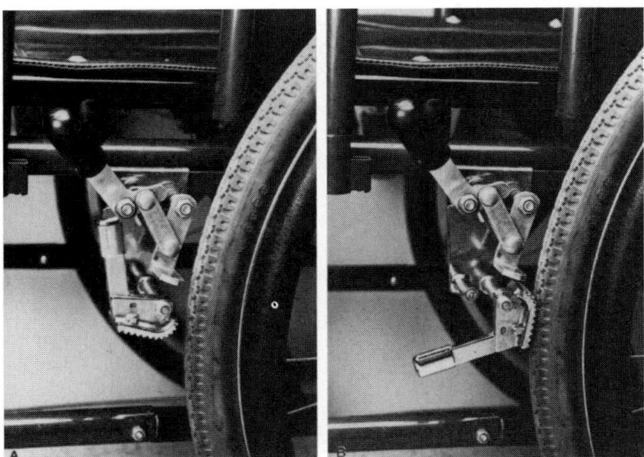

FIGURE 18–9. Grade aid connected to a wheel lock (upper mechanism). *A.* Disengaged. *B.* Engaged. (From Britell CW: Wheelchair prescription. In Kottke FJ, Lehmann JF (eds): Krusen's Handbook of Physical Medicine and Rehabilitation, ed 4. Philadelphia, WB Saunders, 1990, pp 548–563.)

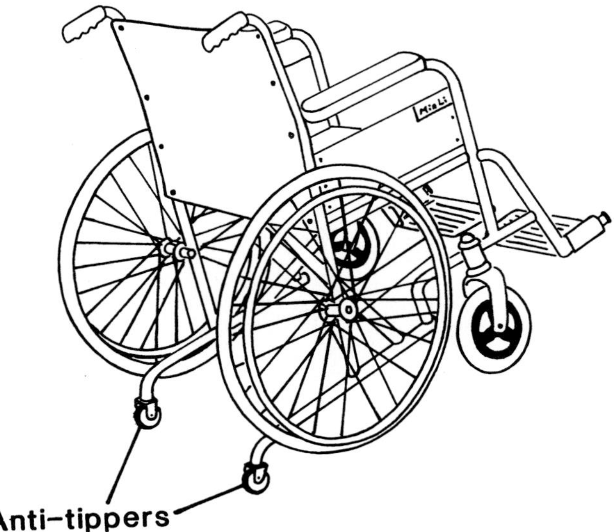

FIGURE 18–10. Anti-tipper device.

Hemichair

Hemiplegic patients are often able to utilize the "good" leg to help propel the chair, but the seat height in a regular chair is too high for their legs to reach the floor effectively. Hemichairs are made lower to the ground and allow the user to propel the chair with the "good" arm and ipsilateral leg.

Stand-up Chairs

The stand-up design allows the patient to stand within the frame of the chair (Fig. 18–12). Patients can benefit from being able to stand for a number of reasons, including having access to more jobs and experiencing an improved psychological outlook. Standing chairs also provide weight-bearing benefits on bone and improved pressure release. They are available in both motorized

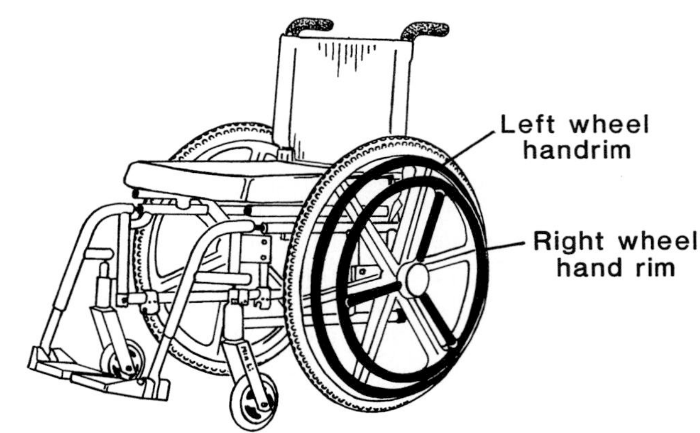

FIGURE 18–11. One-arm-drive chair.

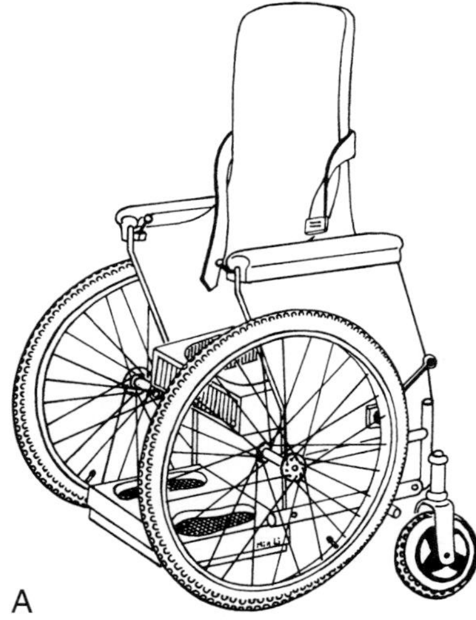

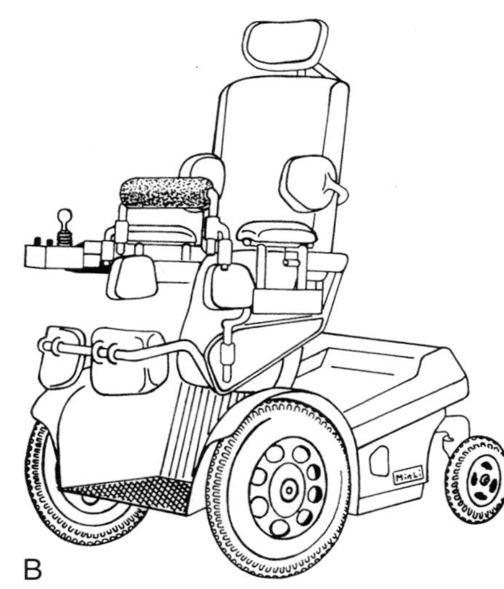

FIGURE 18–12. Stand-up chairs. *A.* Manual. *B.* Power.

and manual versions, but have drawbacks of increased weight, width, cost, and complexity.

MOTORIZED WHEELCHAIRS AND SCOOTERS

Individuals who do not have the strength or dexterity to efficiently propel a manual wheelchair usually need a motorized wheelchair. Such chairs can provide a high degree of independence, and with modern reclining and tilting models, even severely impaired persons can perform pressure release maneuvers.

Although manual wheelchairs permit much needed exercise, many users are better served in the long run with a motorized model. Although they may be able to operate a manual chair for short distances, they might not have the endurance for long distance travel. Manual wheelchair use can also hasten the deterioration of the shoulders, so that in the long term the patient may lose function for such critical activities as transfers and activities of daily living.[11, 13] This is becoming an ever more prevalent problem in active paraplegic patients, who typically have a high incidence of shoulder problems and compressive neuropathies.

Three types of motorized wheelchairs are available: (1) direct drive, (2) belt driven, and (3) add-on units. Scooters constitute a separate category.

Direct-Drive Motorized Wheelchairs

Direct-drive wheelchairs (Fig. 18–13A) are commonly referred to as *power base chairs.* They have a rigid main frame that contains the drive components and provides the base for the required seating system. Direct-drive chairs commonly have four small balloon tires, but some newer models offer larger wheels in the rear. They are durable and suited for rough terrain.

Belt-Driven Motorized Wheelchairs

Belt-driven wheelchairs (see Fig. 18–13B) usually have large rear tires and small front casters. They are more stable than direct-drive units and are generally capable of reaching greater speeds, but they tend to be less durable. Belt-driven chairs are more versatile than direct-drive versions, because the frames are better suited to modification and the addition of different components.

Add-on Power Packs

For individuals requiring a motorized chair that is easily transported, a few add-on power packs are available (see Fig. 18–13C) that convert a manual chair to a motorized chair. These units give the user an advantage in transportability. They are mainly helpful for individuals who use a manual chair most of the time but who occasionally need power assistance for long distance travel or rough terrain. They can be mounted on folding or rigid frames and are less expensive than conventional power chairs. They are also not as durable, have less power and smaller batteries, and are less adaptable than standard power chairs.

Motorized Scooters

Three- and four-wheeled scooters (see Fig. 18–13D) are a good choice of powered mobility for individuals who have the upper body dexterity and strength to manually steer the unit. They are not available with as much "custom fitting" as other wheelchairs and generally do not have as good a seating position. They are more difficult to transfer into and out of than most other motorized chairs. They are optimally used by the person who can ambulate, transfer, and perform most activities of daily living but who lacks the endurance to ambulate for long distances or to use a manual wheelchair. They are also useful in persons who must avoid overuse of their limbs. They are well suited to many patients with rheumatoid arthritis or severe cardiac or degenerative joint disease, and to some patients with multiple sclerosis or motor neuron or neuromuscular junction disease.

Three-wheeled scooters are available with both front- and rear-wheel drive. Front-wheel drive is less powerful and limits the user to smooth, flat terrain. Front-wheel

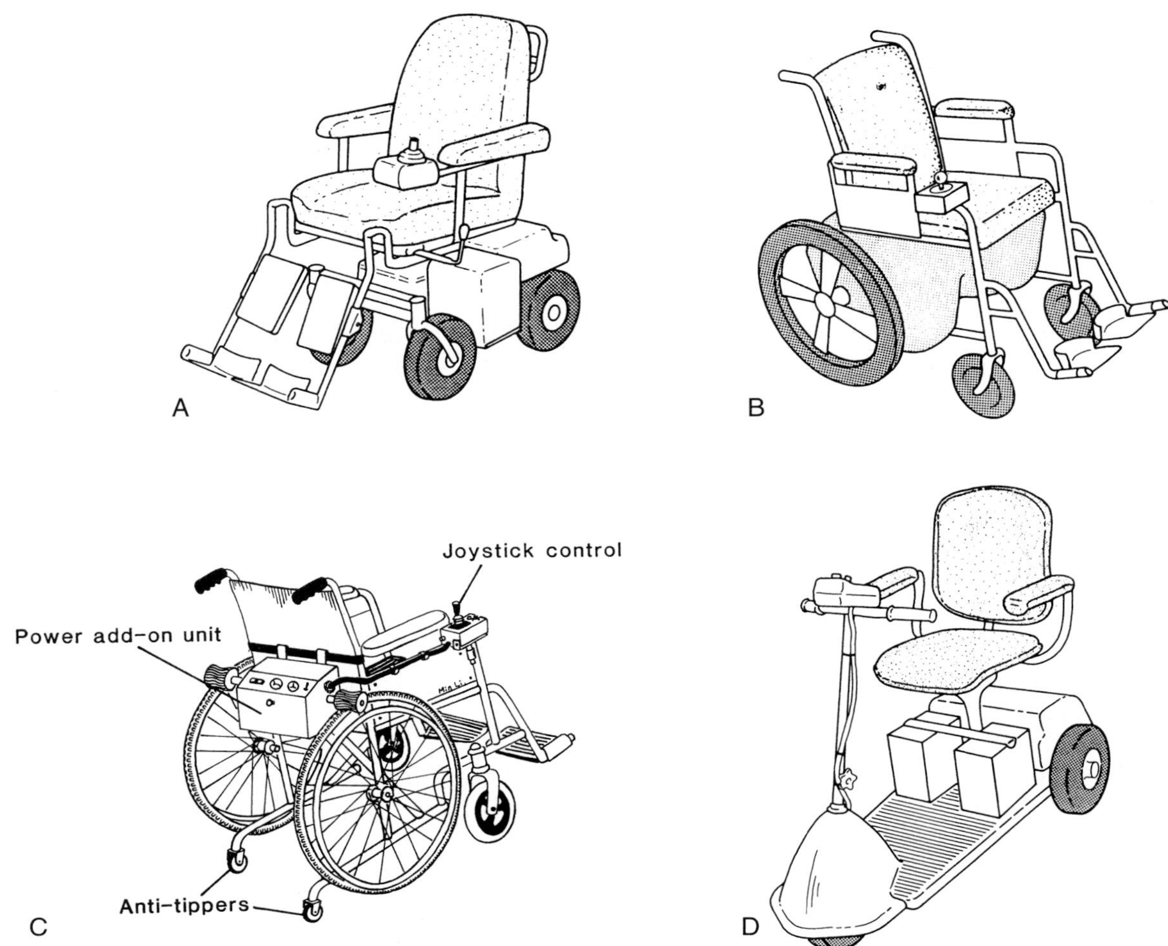

FIGURE 18–13. Power chairs: direct-drive (*A*), belt-drive (*B*), add-on power unit (*C*), and three-wheeled scotter (*D*). (*A, B,* and *D* from Britell CW: Wheelchair prescription. In Kottke FJ, Lehmann JF (eds): Krusen's Handbook of Physical Medicine and Rehabilitation, ed 4. Philadelphia, WB Saunders, 1990, pp 548–563.)

drive units can be built with smaller dimensions and are best suited to indoor or light use.

Four-wheeled scooters are available in both rear- and four-wheel drive models. These units are more stable than three-wheeled models, but they are not as compact and are harder to transport. Although they are more stable than three-wheeled scooters, caution is still advised. All scooters have a tendency to be top-heavy and can tip easily, especially when operating at high speed.

Control Systems for Motorized Chairs

Control systems for motorized wheelchairs can be classified as either proportional (graded response) or nonproportional (on/off). Proportional systems are used most commonly. They require the ability to incrementally control the push or pull of a joystick (see Fig. 18–13C) by the hand, head, or foot. Pushing the joystick further increases the speed of the wheelchair or the angle of a turn. Proportionally operated power chairs are generally fitted with what is known as a *high brake bias.* When there is no input to propel the chair, it brakes automatically.

Nonproportional systems are used when an individual cannot operate a joystick. They basically have an "on-or-off" type of control. As little as one switch can be used, along with a scanning system. Several switches are usually used, each for a different command or direction. Switches can be placed at any point of the body at which the person can generate enough movement to activate them. Switch sensitivity can be controlled, and in patients with severe spasticity (for safety reasons), the unit can be programmed to ignore excessively rapid movements. Air-controlled "sip-and-puff" drive controls are nonproportional controls used for individuals with high-level quadriplegia who have the capacity to control their breathing. They are sometimes used even in conjunction with ventilator use.

Voice-controlled wheelchairs are only experimental at this time, but practical voice-controlled units will probably be available in the future.

SPORT WHEELCHAIRS

Sport wheelchairs have a rigid frame and are usually made of lightweight material, such as titanium. They are usually not the primary chair of the user. These chairs are generally expensive, cannot easily be modified, and are of limited use outside their intended sport. Basketball chairs have thin indoor-type wheels with little tread and small casters. Camber is large, and depending on the type of impairment (usually level of paraplegia), these chairs allow fairly unrestricted upper body mobility.

Racing chairs (Fig. 18–14) are highly specialized. They compress the athlete's body into a compact shape, have a large camber, and have small-diameter hand rims to help get maximum distance from each arm stroke. Due to body position, wheelchair racers tend to have problems with skin irritation and breakdown. Incidentally, because wheelchairs propel the body mass with little or no vertical or side-to-side displacement of the center of gravity, they are more efficient than running, and in long-distance events, such as marathons, the wheelchair athletes routinely have shorter finishing times than the runners.

Wheelchair exercise provides both physical and psychological benefits to the participant, and if it is properly structured, such exercise can provide training comparable to standard aerobic exercise.[2]

ENERGY CONSIDERATIONS IN WHEELCHAIR USE

As described in previous sections, certain wheelchair modifications and styles affect rolling resistance and energy consumption. The most important of these is probably tire and caster width. Narrower tires have less rolling resistance and are ideal for use on hard, flat surfaces, such as within institutions. They require much more force to propel over uneven surfaces (such as gravel) and are not suited for outdoor use. The same holds true for small casters, which are mainly used for maneuverability in sports such as basketball. Weight obviously is another consideration in calculating energy consumption, and for sports applications, very lightweight chairs are available. In one study,[8] sports chairs were found to require 17% less energy to propel than standard chairs.

The energy consumption of wheelchair use is lowest on a flat, hard surface. Carpeting, rough terrain, and even small inclines or slopes greatly increase the energy cost of mobility.[6, 7, 17] This increase can be prohibitive in elderly or debilitated patients. Powered mobility may be a more realistic option in these patient populations.

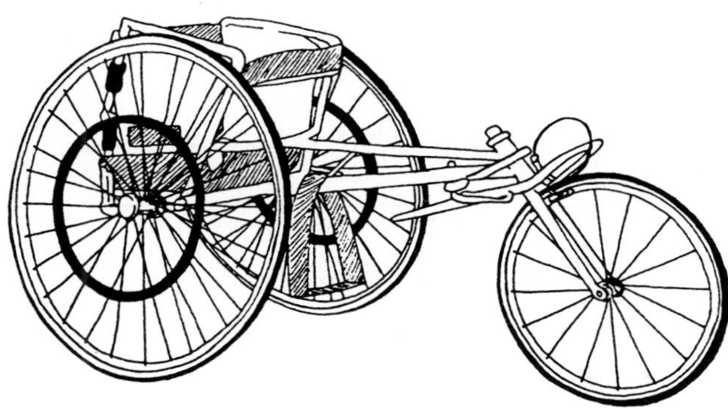

FIGURE 18–14. Racing chair.

TABLE 18–9 Indications for Manual Mobility

1. Physical limitation not compatible with ambulation
2. Need for increased independence at work or school
3. Poor endurance/distance walking

To optimize energy consumption, careful selection of all components of the wheelchair is important.[10] Alternative wheelchair propulsion designs have been investigated. Although some of these have been shown to be more energy efficient than those currently in use,[9, 14, 16] none have yet gained wide popularity.

GENERAL CONSIDERATIONS IN WHEELCHAIR SELECTION

When prescribing wheelchairs for adults it is important to note whether the mobility impairment is of adult onset or has existed since birth or childhood. Developmentally disabled adults present with problems of abnormal muscle tone deformity, and contractures. Some require custom-molded seating to correct or accommodate these abnormalities.

Adults with traumatic paraplegia are typically best fitted with high-strength lightweight wheelchairs. High-level quadriplegic persons usually need powered mobility with sophisticated control systems such as chin controls or sip-and-puff systems. Adults with multiple sclerosis often do well with powered scooters, and adults with stroke typically use a hemi-height manual wheelchair, which they propel with the "good" arm and leg.

Traumatic brain injury patients often initially require a complex wheelchair system, but frequently progress to needing a less sophisticated system or no wheelchair over the course of time.

The most important prescribing considerations in all cases include the diagnosis, clinical picture, living situation, family involvement, funding, and previous experience of the patient/caregiver with wheelchairs. Tables 18–9 and 18–10 list some of the indications for choosing either a manual or power chair. Table 18–11 lists some of the issues important in prescribing a power chair, whereas Table 18–12 lists some of the disadvantages of powered chairs.

PEDIATRIC CONSIDERATIONS IN WHEELCHAIR PRESCRIPTION

Pediatric patients present with all of the challenges in wheelchair selection seen in adults, but with specific

TABLE 18–10 Indications for Powered Mobility

1. Physical limitations not compatible with manual wheelchair mobility
2. Need for increased independence level at school and work
3. To improve self-esteem
4. To increase efficiency of mobility
5. To spare the upper limb joints from premature deterioration

TABLE 18–11 Evaluation Factors for Powered Mobility

1. Physical ability
2. Intelligence level
3. Age
4. Judgment
5. Perception
6. Transportability of device
7. Reimbursement
8. Follow-up availability/maintenance
9. Family acceptance

additional concerns. These include accommodating the patient's growth, fostering development of self-esteem, and enabling proper interaction with peers and the environment. Children have different needs based on their developmental level and age. They need physical contact and handling (as do adults), and the equipment they use should not limit that physical contact. For example, wheelchair lap trays used in classrooms can sometimes cause peers to keep their distance, and they do not permit the same interaction as occurs at a desk or a table or in a circle on the floor.

Cosmetic Concerns

Children are very conscious of their appearance and like brightly colored equipment. Most adults are more concerned about the reliable operation of equipment, with appearance being a somewhat secondary concern. Children, however, have very definite ideas about the appearance and color of their equipment. They frequently reject the traditional chrome frame wheelchair "look." Manufacturers have responded to this concern with brightly colored choices. Some vendors monogram the name of the child at no extra charge.

Growth Concerns

Manufacturers offer both manual and power-drive wheelchairs with "growth potential," and decisions should be made on the basis of whether the child can self-propel the chair or will be able to in the future. Some chairs can be expanded in width and depth with modular and expanding frames. Growth of the legs can be accommodated with longer footrest hangers. Prescribers of wheelchairs for children should be familiar with which products "grow," how they grow, and their growth ranges. In general, one should strive to obtain a chair that meets the child's needs for a 5-year period. However, prescribing a chair that is initially too large can be counterproductive, as it decreases the child's independence and makes propelling the chair more difficult.

Family Concerns

Dealing with children requires carefully listening to the parents or primary caregivers regarding function, appearance, and utility of the end product. It is often psychologically difficult for a parent with a very young child to use a device that looks like a wheelchair. The parents are usually still hopeful that the child will learn to sit, have head control, and walk. Although they realize the need for good positioning and proper body alignment to help prevent contractures and added deformity, they often want the seating components fitted into a device that looks more like a stroller. They might also want the capacity to use the seating system as a car seat. Some manufacturers make FDA-approved car seats that interface with a mobility base for transport, which may or may not be the best choice for the child. Most parents want to be intimately involved in the wheelchair decision-making process.

Ventilators and Wheelchairs

Growing numbers of children are ventilator dependent. For these children not only must one choose the best seating system to support function, growth, and positioning needs, but the system must also house and transport the ventilator and other support equipment. If respiratory status improves, one should be able to modify the system for increased independence and function.

Progressive Disorders

Functional independence is always a goal in working with children, but for children who have degenerative or progressive disorders, future loss of control has to be considered. Sometimes it is not possible to predict how quickly changes will be required, but the system of choice should be adaptable to those changes when they occur.

Power Chairs

Power chairs should be considered for children who have adequate intelligence and judgment but lack the necessary muscle control to propel a manual wheelchair. Varying opinions exist about how early a child has the judgment and control to use a power chair. Many 3-year-olds can safely use power chairs, and power has even been successfully used with some 2-year-olds. It is obviously important that the wheelchair should not be allowed to pose a safety threat to the child or others.

Powered mobility should be considered in children with a number of diagnoses, including cerebral palsy, muscular dystrophy, hemiplegia, severe arthrogryposis, traumatic quadriplegia, or bronchopulmonary dysplasia. Children with severe juvenile arthritis or cardiac dysfunction often need powered mobility for more freedom of movement. A scooter often meets their needs, as a special seating system is typically not needed. How-

TABLE 18–12 Potential Disadvantages of Powered Mobility

1. Relatively high cost
2. Weight
3. Transportation difficulty
4. Maintenance
5. Technological dependence
6. Limited environmental accessibility
7. Lack of physical exercise

ever, most children who require powered mobility also require a special seating system for support and control. The optimal type of system is determined by considering the diagnosis, degree of deformity, functional ability, and overall clinical picture.

TRANSPORTING THE WHEELCHAIR

Manual Wheelchairs

Manual wheelchairs are easily transported in motor vehicles. Most manual wheelchairs have folding frames and can be lifted into a trunk or back seat. The lifting weight can be lessened by removing the footrests, the armrests, and, on some models, the rear wheels. Trunk lifts are also available for those who lack the strength to put the chair in the trunk by themselves.

Although rigid frame wheelchairs do not fold, they are usually fitted with quick-release axles for easy removal of the rear wheels. Their backs can also be folded down. If necessary, the push handles can be made to turn down, and casters can be made with quick-release mechanisms.

Transporting tilt wheelchairs is very similar to transporting rigid frame wheelchairs. Tilt wheelchairs can be made with a seating system that snaps out, armrests and backs that fold down, and rear wheels that can be removed. This generally leaves a manageable size for storage in the trunk or on the back seat of a car.

Power Wheelchairs

Power wheelchairs present complex transport problems. Although some can be disassembled, this is not practical or recommended on a daily basis. Transport of power wheelchairs generally is best done with a van, van lift, and an approved tie-down system. A ramp system can be used instead of a lift, but for safety reasons, the wheelchair has to be pushed or driven up the ramp by someone other than the user. The width of the van door and roof clearance are critical measurements to consider when a power wheelchair is purchased. Roof clearance can be increased with an extra top on the vehicle, but because the resultant seating and transfer position is usually too high, the van must often be modified by lowering the floor.

Adolescents and adults who operate their own vans generally remove the driver's seat so that they can substitute their wheelchair. They use a lift and tie-down so that they can drive while seated in the restrained wheelchair. The tie-down system in these cases is usually an automatic system that can be operated by a driver-controlled button. This system promotes maximum independence for individuals who can drive.

Power Add-on Units

Power add-on systems do not decrease portability, because the unit is easily removed. These systems have worked well with many patients and have become popular when used with high-strength lightweight wheelchairs.

Scooters

Scooters can usually be disassembled for relatively easy transport in a car. They are often too heavy for the user to lift, so trunk lifts are often prescribed. However, lifts of any variety are rarely funded by third-party payers, making them difficult for many patients to procure. Vocational rehabilitation programs can sometimes help in the purchasing of a lift, especially if it is necessary to provide work access.

TRANSPORTING THE WHEELCHAIR USER

Adults or children who use wheelchairs and seating systems can usually be transferred to the car seat (or child safety seat) and wear a regular seat belt. Sometimes, large children or adults with cognitive problems must be restrained with a vest in combination with the auto seat belt. Persons who must be transported in their wheelchairs require vans with an FDA-approved tie-down system. Although manufacturers do not recommend that individuals be in their wheelchairs for transport, it is often the most acceptable or the only practical method.

Airline Travel

For air travel, the wheelchair user is advised to call ahead to let the airline know that specific accommodations might be necessary. Most major carriers have aids to assist the traveler in this regard. When power chairs are to be transported, they must have approved batteries, because airlines will not allow some batteries to be transported on board.

Bus Travel

When traveling by bus, the same general considerations apply as for air travel. The user should call ahead to learn about any specific requirements. Most municipal bus systems now offer wheelchair-accessible facilities. Cities also often provide alternative transport with a van, if necessary, although this usually has to be arranged in advance.

For school bus transportation, the parents should contact their local school district for any specific recommendations or requirements. In some states, safety standards recommend using forward-facing four-point tie-downs. Weight restrictions might apply as well. Upper extremity supports, such as lap trays, might be prohibited due to their potential for causing injury in the case of an accident. The child should be safely secured in the seating system, and the wheelchair and seat should be secured to the bus. Special accommodations might be necessary for ventilator-dependent children.

SIZING THE WHEELCHAIR

Determining the size of the mobility base and seating system components requires careful measurement of the patient. The measurements that should be taken are depicted in Figure 18–15. The thickness of cushions and padding should be taken into consideration and added to the chair's dimensions.

MAINTENANCE AND SAFETY CONSIDERATIONS

Wheelchairs have many moving parts that must regularly be lubricated, cleaned, and maintained. The user (or caregiver) must make sure that the chair is in proper working order, to maximize both durability and safety. Wheelchairs should not be immersed in water, as some parts can rust. Bearings should be periodically replaced. Power chairs should be taken out of gear when not in use.

SEATING SYSTEMS

A proper seating system is important for the patient, both in and out of the wheelchair. Proper seating is necessary in the young child who does not yet need a wheelchair for mobility (Fig. 18–16). In the elderly, seating is important for general care and to prevent deformity. This section addresses the seating prescription, both as a subset of the wheelchair selection process and as an independent need.

Goals of Seating Systems

Selection of a seating system is a complex process that requires input from the patient, family, primary caregiver, physician, therapists, vendor, and educator. The team approach can help to ensure a more positive outcome. Goals of seating include the following.

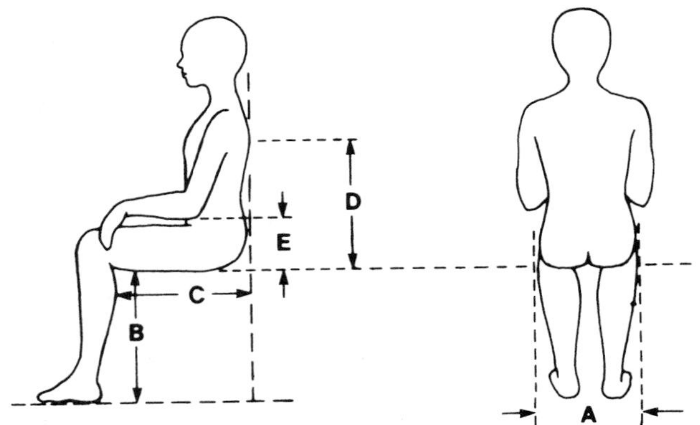

FIGURE 18–15. Standard measurements required for wheelchair dimensions. Seat width: 1 inch wider than the width of the widest part of the buttocks (*A*). Seat height: 2 inches higher than the distance from the bottom of the heel to the popliteal area (*B*). Seat depth: 1 to 2 inches shorter than the distance from the popliteal area to the back of the buttocks (*C*). Back height: 2 inches less (may vary) than the distance from the bottom of the scapulae to the sitting surface (*D*) Armrest height: Distance from bottom of buttocks to elbow (*E*). (From Britell CW: Wheelchair prescription. In Kottke FJ, Lehmann JF (eds): Krussen's Handbook of Physical Medicine and Rehabilitation, ed 4. Philadelphia, WB Saunders, 1990, pp 548–563.)

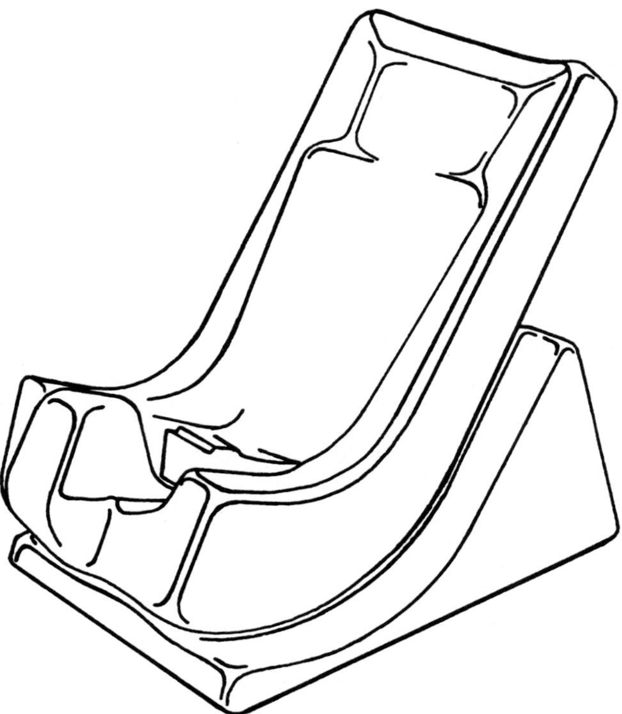

FIGURE 18–16. Tumbleform pediatric seating device.

Control Abnormal Tone and Reflexes. Proper support can help normalize tone and inhibit abnormal reflexes. Abnormal tone and reflexes produce abnormal movement patterns and poor posture, which in turn contribute to the development of muscle contractures and skeletal deformities. Maintaining proper alignment can help prevent these deformities.

Correct or Accommodate Deformities. The seating position should help correct or prevent deformities, such as hip adduction contractures and ankle plantar flexion contractures. When a deformity cannot be prevented or corrected, it has to be accommodated to prevent its worsening or the development of new compensatory deformities.

Above all, the seating system should not cause new deformity. One of the problems with the commonly used "hammock" or "sling" wheelchair seat is that it can promote poor posture (Fig. 18–17), and it should be avoided in patients at risk for such deformity.

Enhance Function and Improve Control. Function is enhanced by optimum posture and position. For example, proper support to the head and neck can improve swallowing and decrease the risk of aspiration during eating. Proper alignment and support can also free the upper extremities for self-care activities or for self-propulsion.

Improve Comfort and Improve Sitting Tolerance. A seating system should provide the necessary support with the least possible restriction of movement. Proper support should provide a secure, stable base and enhance the patient's sitting tolerance.

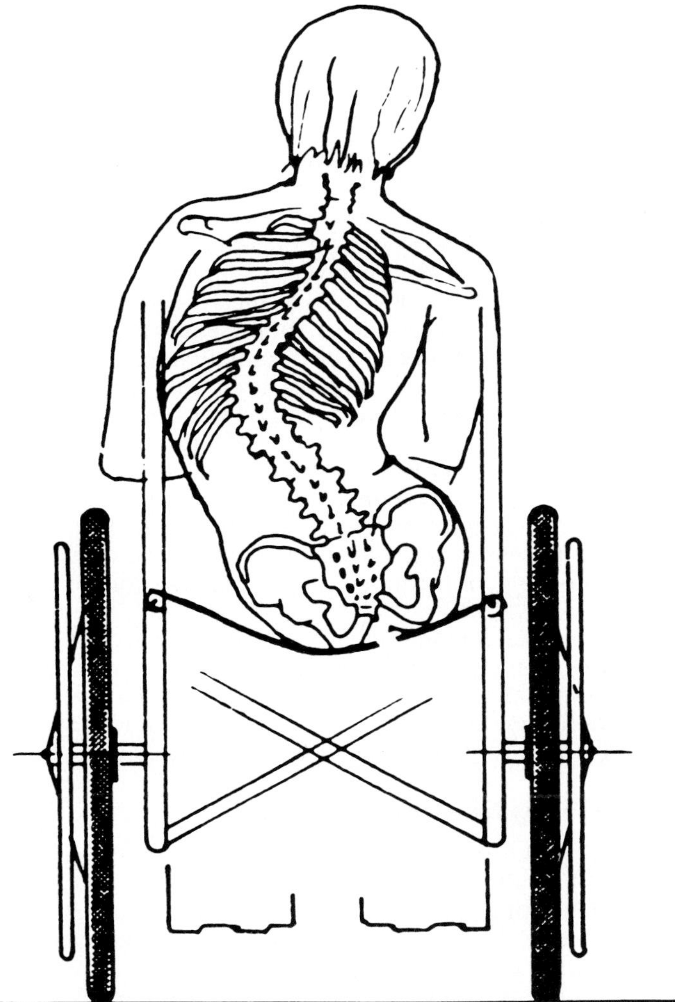

FIGURE 18–17. Sling effect of standard chairs, which can promote deformity. (From Letts RM (ed): Principles of Seating Prescription. Boca Raton, FL, CRC Press, 1991.)

Provide Pressure Relief and Skin Protection. The able-bodied child or adult shifts position frequently to redistribute pressure and prevent skin breakdown. Individuals with a lack of sensation or with physical or cognitive limitations are not always capable of such weight shifts, nor do they always understand the need for them. A seating system that equalizes pressure distribution, prevents shear force, and provides proper support decreases the incidence of pressure ulcers.

Facilitate Management and Care. Seating cannot improve function or control in some patients with very severe neurological impairments. A proper seating system can, however, allow them to be placed in an upright position to improve respiration, digestion, and urinary function. It also allows them to be transported more easily and helps others to do their care and hygiene.

Principles of Seating

Sitting should provide the necessary support to the body while fostering a comfortable, symmetrical midline posture. Proper sitting position is generally considered to be with the head in midline, trunk erect, hips flexed to 90 degrees, knees at 90 to 100 degrees, and feet in neutral position, with the spine stable and the pelvis level. Seating systems are traditionally grouped into three categories: (1) planar systems (see Fig. 18–5B for an example), (2) contoured systems (see Fig. 18–16 for an example), and (3) custom-molded systems.

Planar, also known as *linear seating systems,* are constructed of a support covered with upholstery to provide a relatively flat surface. Possible planar components include seats, seat backs, lateral/head/sternal supports, abductor supports, lap trays, footrests, and cushions. The planar components are generally inexpensive and can readily be modified, repaired, or replaced.

Contoured seating systems are used when patients require a more customized shape to accommodate their bodies. They can be simple or complex. Simple contours can be constructed by using varying densities of foam in the seat cushions to accommodate the body (see Table 18–8). More commonly, however, a more complex design is required. Preformed bases can be obtained with curves to better fit the body. These are then covered with foam or gel to which special add-on pads can be applied, such as lateral supports and thigh abductors. Contoured systems are useful for patients who require mild to moderate support and who are free of severe deformity.

If more support is necessary, or if the patient's deformity is such that standard seating systems will not fit, a custom-molded seat is needed. Custom-molded systems tend to be used with patients who have more severe deformities and a history of skin breakdown. They are not usually advisable for use in very young children due to their cost and the inability to change the system to accommodate growth. Most of these systems cannot be modified and require replacement if they do not fit properly.

The covering of the seating system is important. Some patients are allergic to and do not tolerate materials such as latex or neoprene. Incontinence is a problem for some patients, and the material used must be either easily cleaned or impervious to urine. Some coverings can cause increased shear pressure in transfers, which presents a problem in the patient at risk for pressure ulcers.

Assessing patients for wheelchairs typically requires removal of their clothing. Clothing can hide gastrostomy tubes, bony deformities, and pressure ulcers. Patients or families often fail to mention these factors, and they are essential for making a good seating choice.

Prescribing Seating Systems

The availability of numerous wheelchair bases combined with multiple seating options requires that the seating team thoroughly assess the patient to successfully prescribe the best system. Prescription of the system is further compounded by funding limitations and family resources. Modern technology can enhance the user's potential for independence, but it is not always affordable or practical based on funding restrictions and the environment in which such equipment is to be operated. Clinical assessment should include the following items (also summarized in Table 18–13).

Tone/Spasticity. Patients presenting with tone or spasticity problems often require special seating considerations, such as rolled seats (thinner over the ischial tuberosities to properly position the pelvis), anti-thrust seats, abduction devices, and special back-to-seat angles. They also require parts that are reinforced or made of stronger and more durable materials. Patients with low tone often require lumbar supports to promote spinal extension, tilt mechanisms to improve head and trunk control, or custom headrests. Patients with athetosis may require stabilization of an upper and lower extremity to effectively use the remaining upper extremity functionally. Other patients have fluctuating tone, and the seating system should support this flexibility. Tone can also change over time as the patient's medical condition changes.

TABLE 18–13 Items to Consider in the Clinical Assessment for Wheelchair or Seating Systems

1. Muscle tone	6. Visual impairments
2. Contractures	7. Hearing impairments
3. Abnormal reflexes	8. External orthotics
4. Sensory deficits	9. Bony deformities
5. Tissue integrity	10. Behavioral problems

Contracture. Contractures create a number of problems for the patient and for the clinician prescribing or recommending equipment. Knee flexion contractures can affect caster size and the type of footrest that can be used. Hip extension contractures require a more open hip angle and might necessitate a reclining back feature. Assessment of contractures should include whether the patient has a fixed deformity or abnormal posturing.

Pathological Reflexes. The presence of abnormal or pathological reflexes, such as an asymmetrical tonic neck reflex, directly affects posture and control. Many cognitively aware patients can utilize these reflexes to enhance function, whereas others are hindered by them. The type of headrest used can position the head to allow the patient to effectively "break through" these abnormal reflexes for added postural control.

Impaired Sensation/Body Awareness. Sensation has a direct impact on positioning, and sensory deficits can impair balance as well as predispose to pressure ulceration. A proper sense of body awareness is important. Patients with perceptual problems, such as hemineglect, often injure themselves in their wheelchairs. They might drag a foot on the floor without realizing that it has fallen from the footrest. Sometimes they injure a hand or arm as it dangles and gets caught in the wheel. Special seating and wheelchair restrictions are needed to prevent these problems.

Skin Integrity. Tissue integrity should also be assessed. Children and adults with no history of breakdown usually tolerate regular planar seating systems. Clients with current ulcers or a history of previous pressure ulcers require more creative seating and the use of foam, air-cell, or pressure pads.

Other Seating Considerations. A number of other items should be noted, as they can necessitate special seating or wheelchair arrangements. These items include the status of vision and hearing, need for orthoses, presence of deformities, and behavior problems. Table 18–14 lists some of the more common problems in seating along with their causes and possible solutions.

WHEELCHAIR SAFETY

Wheelchairs can, of course, be involved in accidents. Falls and tips are the most common of these.[3] Therefore, it is important to match a person's cognitive capabilities to the type of device being prescribed. Anti-tippers, proper brakes, grade aids, proper axle position, proper seating position, and wheel camber, among others, can all be modified to enhance stability. Special care must be taken when prescribing reclining, tilting, standing, or power chairs.

Wheelchairs require regular maintenance and inspection. Metal fatigue fractures or other deterioration is expected, especially in the more active user.[3]

TABLE 18–14 Troubleshooting in Postural Seating and Wheelchair Prescription

	Problem	Possible Causes	Possible Solutions
Pelvis	Posterior tilt (sacral sitting or sliding out of chair)	Hypotonia Tonic labyrinth prone (TLP) reflex (producing flexed posture) Limited active hip flexion (causing compensatory loss of low lumbar curve) Tight hamstrings with seat too long or with too high a wedge in seat, footrests preventing knee flexion Improper positioning in seat Lap belt located too high	Decrease seat length Reduce seat wedge/roll height Lumbar or sacral pad Change position of head in space and thereby influence TLP Raise height of tray Adjust position of footrests to allow more knee flexion Reposition pelvis (flex pelvis) Lower lap belt attachment point
	Lateral tilt (weight on one buttock)	Asymmetrical muscle tone Scoliosis with pelvic obliquity Dislocated or subluxated hip "Hammock" of wheelchair seat	Solid base to seat Midline orientation by using lateral pelvic blocks Three-point pressure support of trunk and pelvis Contour seat to facilitate equal weight distribution
Trunk	Scoliosis	Postural Position of pelvis not midline Hypotonia-hypertonia asymmetrical muscle tone (asymmetrical tonic neck reflex, asymmetrical distribution of tone, hemiplegia, etc.) Environmental or functional demands Structural Persistent asymmetrical posture (fixed deformity)	Midline pelvic orientation Three-point support Midline trunk or chest harnesses Recessed back or midline orientation Tray to help with midline orientation Reduce abnormal tone Hip angle Neck collar Change orientation of functional work Recline back to reduce effects of gravity
	Kyphosis	Postural Posterior pelvic tilt Structural Fixed deformity	Surgery or othotic management See previous solutions, pelvic tilt Add chest panel or bandolier harnesses Lumbosacral pad Surgery or orthotic management
Shoulder girdle	Retraction	Thoracolumbar scoliosis Extensor thrust Asymmetrical tonic neck reflex Instability of upper trunk	Reduce extensor tone Roll or wedge seat Decrease hip angle Neck collar Alter head position in space (gravity) Protract shoulders Tray extensions or rounded seat back with wings Lower tray Stabilize upper trunk with straps
	Protraction	TLP Kyphosis	Lumbosacral pad Raise tray height Chest panel Change attitude of body in space (gravity)
Head and neck	Hyperextension	Extensor hypertonicity Poor flexor control Headrest or neck collar positioned too low Improper neck or head support (i.e., headrest placed on occipital) Thoracolumbar scoliosis	Neck collar positioned just below occipital region Reduce total extensor hypertonicity at pelvis (see above) Position neckrest slightly anterior Alter position of head in space (gravity)
	Protraction	Hypotonia Neckrest too high or too far forward TLP Tray work too low Kyphosis	Lower neckrest and align in neutral position Raise and/or tilt tray Low lumbosacral pad Alter position of head in space (gravity)

Table continued on following page

TABLE 18–14 Troubleshooting in Postural Seating and Wheelchair Prescription *Continued*

	Problem	Possible Causes	Possible Solutions

	Rotation	Atonic neck reflex
		
		Sensory deficit
		  Visual
		  Auditory
		Unstable spine
		Generalized domination of primitive pathosis
			Inhibit atonic neck reflex
			Midline orientation of pelvis and trunk
			Protraction of shoulders
			Thoughtful positioning for function
			Reduce general hypertonicity

	Side flexion	Hypertonicity Hydrocephalus Severe retardation Sensory deficits	Reposition of neck or headrest Larger neck or headrest More stable chest support Recline body in space (gravity)
Hips	Extension-adduction	Thoracolumbar scoliosis Positive supporting reaction	Roll seat, with roll one finger width behind knee

	Internal rotation	Extensor thrust
		Dislocated hip
		Seat too short
		Seat belt too long or poorly positioned
			Increase hip flexion by
			  Higher roll
			  Wedge
			  Flexing seat back anterior of vertical
			Pommel (as a last resort); keep it short enough so it is nowhere near groin area
			Platform shoes to reduce positive supporting reaction (PSR)
			Seat belt at 45 degrees to thigh
			Alter attitude of body in space to affect tonic labyrinth supine reaction (gravity)
			Have removable footrests for initial fittings
			Caution: watch pelvis as you increase hip flexion if hamstrings are tight

	Flexion-abduction	Hypotonia Adductor releases	Adduction blocks with good foot position (footpads or straps)
Knees	Flexion	Primitive patterns Flexion contractures	Inhibit flexor tone by adjusting (roll or wedge) Position feet in neutral (if tight hamstrings, watch effect on pelvis) Surgery
	Extension	Extension patterns (usually dynamic response to abnormal tone)	Inhibit extensor tone with roll or wedge Decrease hip angle Neutral strapping of feet Shorten seat
Feet	Plantar flexion	Extension pattern Positive supporting reaction Heel cord contractures Footrest too low	Check footrest height and place foot in slight dorsiflexion to inhibit PSR Surgery Inhibit tone with roll/wedge Platform shoes
	Inversion-eversion	Same as above	Footrest height Platform shoes Footpads or straps Ankle-foot orthosis

From Letts RM (ed): Principles of Seating Prescription. Boca Raton, FL, CRC Press, 1991.

Falls can also occur when braking a power chair. Seat belts and leg rests can minimize such mishaps.[4]

SUMMARY

The wheelchair and seating options currently available are numerous and increasing rapidly. It is nearly impossible for one person to keep abreast of all the latest developments, but by adhering to the basic principles outlined in this chapter and by listening to the patient and family, it is possible to achieve better outcomes than ever before. This is most efficient and effective with the use of a wheelchair team approach that includes the patient, family, physician, therapist, and vendor, all working toward the common goal of prescribing the best wheelchair and seating system available for each patient.

REFERENCES

1. Britell CW: Wheelchair prescription. In Kottke FJ, Lehmann JF (eds): Krusen's Handbook of Physical Medicine and Rehabilitation. Philadelphia, WB Saunders, 1990, pp 548–563.
2. Cardus D, McTaggart WG, Ribas-Cardus F, et al: Energy requirements of gamefield exercises designed for wheelchair-bound persons. Arch Phys Med Rehabil 1989; 70:124–127.
3. Cooper RA: Wheelchair Selection and Configuration. New York, Demos, 1998.
4. Cooper RA, Dvorznak MJ, O'Connor TJ, et al: Braking electric powered wheelchairs: Effect of braking method, seatbelt, and legrests. Arch Phys Med Rehabil 1998; 79:1244–1249.
5. DuBow LL, Witt PL, Kadaba MP, et al: Oxygen consumption of elderly persons with bilateral below knee amputations: Ambulation vs wheelchair propulsion. Arch Phys Med Rehabil 1983; 64:255–259.
6. Glaser RM, Barr SA, Lauback CC, et al: Relative stresses of wheelchair activity. Hum Factors 1980; 22:177–181.
7. Glaser RM, Sawka MN, Wilde SW, et al: Energy cost and cardiopulmonary responses for wheelchair locomotion and walking on tile and on carpet. Paraplegia 1981; 19:220–226.
8. Hilbers PA, White TP: Effects of wheelchair design on metabolic and heart rate responses during propulsion by persons with paraplegia. Phys Ther 1987; 67:1355–1358.
9. Linden AL, Holland GJ, Loy SF, et al: A physiological comparison of forward vs reverse wheelchair ergometry. Med Sci Sports Exerc 1993; 25:1265–1268.
10. McLaurin CA, Brubaker CE: Biomechanics and the wheelchair. Prosthet Orthot Int 1991; 15:24–37.
11. Nichols PJR, Norman PA, Ennis JR: Wheelchair user's shoulder. Scand J Rehabil Med 1979; 11:29–32.
12. Perry RAF: The history of wheelchairs. In Letts RM (ed): Principles of Seating the Disabled. Boca Raton, FL, CRC Press, 1991, pp 331–337.
13. Rodgers MM, Gayle GW, Figoni SF, et al: Biomechanics of wheelchair propulsion during fatigue. Arch Phys Med Rehabil 1994; 75:85–93.
14. Sawka MN, Glaser RM, Wilde SW, et al: Metabolic and circulatory responses to wheelchair and arm crank exercise. J Appl Physiol 1980; 49:784–788.
15. Smith PA, Glaser RM, Petrofsky JS, et al: Arm crank vs handrim wheelchair propulsion: Metabolic and cardiopulmonary responses. Arch Phys Med Rehabil 1983; 64:249–254.
16. Van Der Woude LHV, DeGroot G, Hollander AP, et al: Wheelchair ergonomics and physiological testing of prototypes. Ergonomics 1986; 29:1561–1573.
17. Waters RL, Lunsford BR: Energy cost of paraplegic locomotion. J Bone Joint Surg Am 1985; 67:1245–1250.

19 CHAPTER

Barbara J. deLateur, M.D., M.S.

Therapeutic Exercise

THEORETICAL CONSIDERATIONS

It is common knowledge that strength is somehow related to the ability to lift objects in a gravitational field. It is intuitive that this strength is greater with larger muscles and is also related to the technique of lifting. Scientific research and research-based practice, however, require greater precision of definition.

One- and Ten-Repetition Maxima

A useful definition is the one-repetition maximum (1 RM), that is, the largest weight that can be lifted once and only once through the full range of motion of a given joint. The 1 RM lends itself to use with highly technical isokinetic equipment, an example of which would be the peak torque developed at any point in the range of a given joint at a given contraction velocity. It could also be given as an angle-specific torque, for example, the torque developed by the quadriceps at 60 degrees/sec at an angle of 60 degrees of flexion. Another useful definition is the 10 RM, that is, the highest weight that can be lifted through the full range of motion 10 times only. The 10 RM is useful if a set of weights is available but not an isokinetic apparatus or other dynamometer.

Determinants of Strength

Absolute Muscle Strength

It has been known from antiquity that larger muscles are stronger. It has been known since the late 19th century that strength or the ability to develop force is related to the cross-sectional area of the muscle. This has been further refined to relate muscle strength to the physiological cross-sectional area, which is the cross section at the bulkiest part of the muscle for long parallel muscles such as the sartorius (Fig. 19–1). For pennate muscles, multiple cross sections must be taken at right angles to the fibers until all fibers have been included (Fig. 19–2). Because many more (necessarily shorter) muscle fibers can be packed into a pennate muscle of the same volume as a parallel muscle, such muscles are said to be adapted to force rather than speed. Although figures in the literature vary, a generally accepted value for the absolute muscle strength is 3.6 kg/cm^2 of physiological cross-sectional area.[1, 48] This should be listed technically as 3.6 kp/cm^2 (a kilopond, abbreviated as kp, is the force exerted by the mass of 1 kg in Earth's gravitational field). This is generally implied rather than stated, and the convention is simply to give the force in kilograms.

Neural or Learning Factors in Strength

In 1967 Gordon and co-workers reported that in rats, high-force or high-intensity performance could be enhanced without a substantial overall increase in muscle bulk.[30] This work has been confirmed in humans by Moritani and deVries[40] and by Milner-Brown et al[39] Moritani and deVries make use of the fact that if one assesses integrated surface electromyographic (IEMG) activity over the same spot of the same muscle with the same angle of the joint, and if the contraction is kept purely isometric, there will be a linear relationship between force and IEMG activity. Figure 19–3 shows theoretically possible outcomes of training. In Figure 19–3A there is, as a result of training, an increase in the amount of EMG activity that can be produced at maximal effort. There is no change in the amount of force achieved for any given amount of effort. The line is simply extended upward. Figure 19–3B shows another theoretically possible outcome in which the amount of force generated for any given amount of EMG activity is greater. This

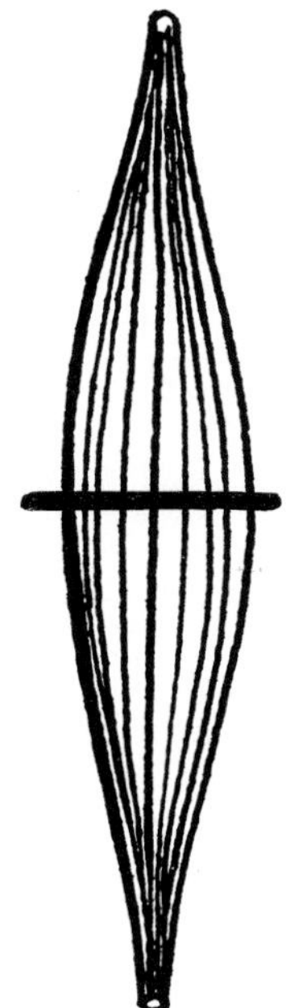

FIGURE 19–1. Parallel arrangement of muscle fibers. "Physiological" cross section is equal to cross-section of muscle belly. (From Brunnstrom S: Clinical Kinesiology, ed 2. Philadelphia, FA Davis, 1966.)

electrical efficiency, as Moritani and deVries term it, presumably reflects hypertrophy. Figure 19–3C shows how one can determine the relative contributions of (1) increased EMG activity reflecting neural or learning factors, and (2) increased efficiency, reflecting hypertrophy.

Figure 19–4A shows IEMG: force data from trained and untrained arms of a female subject over the course of 8 weeks of training. In the figure, the IEMG-force relationships measured at baseline (week 0) and at the end of 2 weeks of training virtually superimpose, but the line of week 2 extends beyond that of week 0. This suggests that there was no hypertrophy in the first 2 weeks of training, but something happened with learning or the ability to recruit or rapidly fire motor units or a combination of these. By week 4 the IEMG-force line has moved to the right, indicating that hypertrophy has taken place, and for any given level of effort (IEMG), greater force results. The same happens for subsequent weeks. There is little or no further upward extension of the line beyond week 4 in this subject.

Cross-Training. The question of whether strengthening one limb results in strength increases in the opposite, untrained limb is of practical as well as theoretical interest. As currently used, the term *cross-training* means training in one sport to benefit performance in another sport. In the older literature, cross-training meant the extent to which training one limb benefited the opposite limb. This might be of interest, for example, if the untrained side is in a cast. The series of measurements shown in Figure 19–4B show that there is a learning effect but no hypertrophy. This finding is reasonable because it is the same brain that is being utilized and trained, and one would not expect hypertrophy when muscles are not subjected to tension-producing activity.

Endurance, Fatigue, and the Relationship of Endurance to Intensity of Activity

Endurance is the ability to continue a prescribed task in the desired manner. Virtually all definitions of endurance are variations on this theme. In contrast, *fatigue* can be defined in more than one way. For example, fatigue could be defined as the time elapsed (measured in seconds) in an attempted sustained contraction (or the number of contractions in a dynamic task) until the peak force or torque reaches a specified percentage of the initial force or torque, for example, the time at which 60% of the initial value is reached. This definition is useful in assessing the response to training or to various therapeutic interventions. A broader definition of fatigue, useful to coaches and others concerned with athletic competition, is any decrement in performance resulting from previous performance.[43]

Figure 19–5 shows the results in a subject attempting to sustain a maximal isometric contraction for 5 seconds. In the figure, it takes (this muscle group) approximately 1 second to reach peak force, and this true peak can be held for only 1 second despite sustained effort. The decrement in force over the next 4 seconds reflects fatigue in the broadest sense. Thus defined, fatigue need

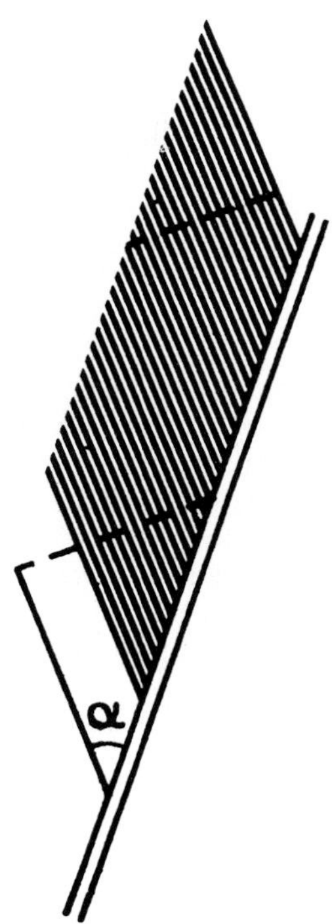

FIGURE 19–2. In pennate muscle, the physiological cross section is determined by multiple sections taken at right angles to the fibers until all are included (From Brunnstrom S: Clinical Kinesiology, ed 2. Philadelphia, FA Davis, 1966.)

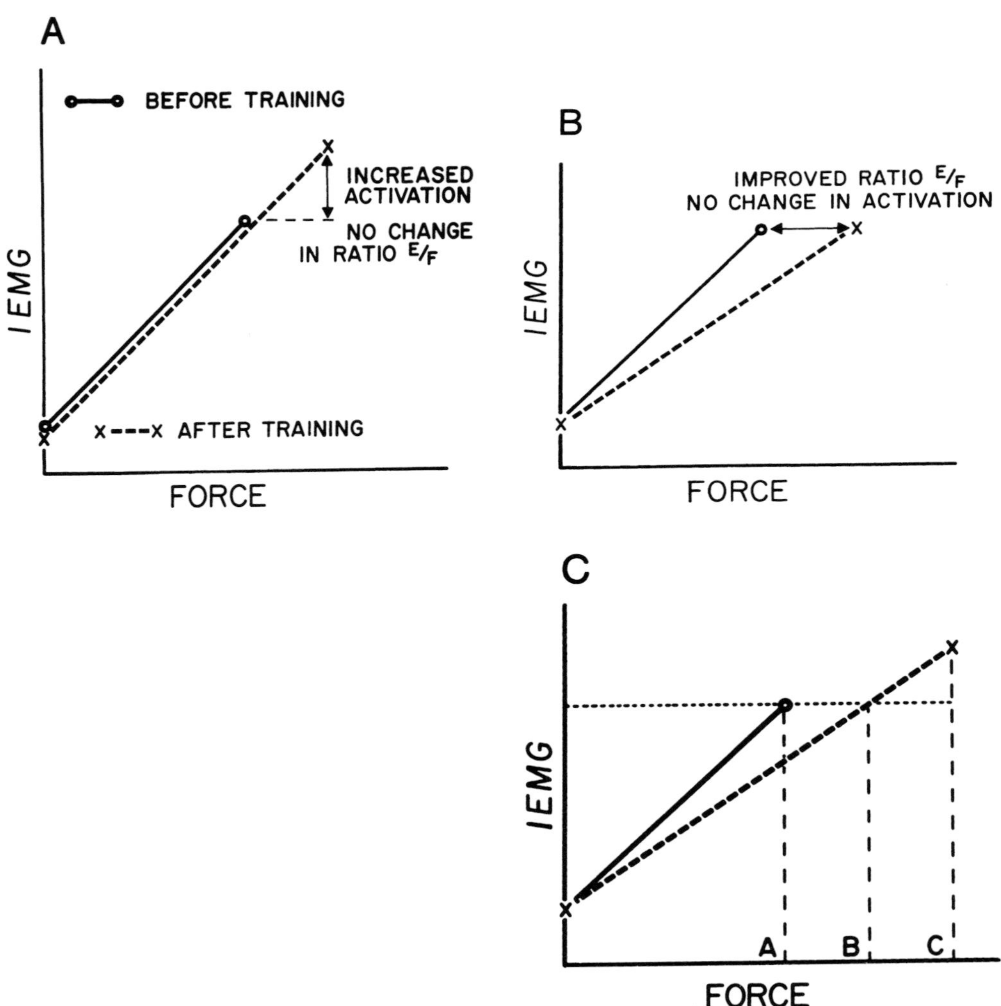

FIGURE 19–3. *A.* Increasing integrated electromyographic activity (IEMG) plotted against force of contraction as an index of strength due to neural factors gained during training. *B.* Strength gained due to hypertrophy when neural activity is maintained constant. *C.* Schema for evaluation of relative contributions of neural factors (N.F.) and muscular hypertrophy (M.H.) to the gain of strength through progressive resistance exercise based on efficiency of electrical activity (EEA). Strength increase percent (M.H.) = (B − A)/(C − A) × 100. Strength increase percent (N.F.) = (C − B)/(C − A) × 100. (Redrawn from Moritani T, deVries HK: Neural factors versus hypertrophy in the time course of muscle strength gain. Am J Phys Med 1979; 58:115–130.)

not imply total exhaustion. The latter would be a very narrow definition and also a rare occurrence. In the figure, fatigue is also reflected in the fact that after 10 minutes of 1 second on, 1 second off contractions at only 5% of maximal effort, a lower peak force is generated on attempted maximal contraction. It should be observed that the general configuration of the curve remains the same as the pre-exercise attempted maximal curve.

Absolute Endurance versus Relative Endurance

Absolute endurance is the time that a subject can sustain a given workload; or, the number of seconds a given force can be held; or, the number of repetitions of a given load. Some examples are the number of seconds that a given bicycle ergometer can be pedaled by a subject at 100 W, the number of seconds a force of 50 N can be held, or the number of times a subject can lift with the right biceps a loaded barbell weighing 10 lb. Note that these activities all have units, such as watts, newtons, and pounds.

Figures 19–6 and 19–7 show the relationship of endurance to intensity of activity. In Figure 19–6, absolute units are recorded on the abscissa. In Figure 19–7 the abscissa reflects relative force from 20% to 100% of the maximal voluntary contraction (MVC). In relative endurance, strength and endurance are not related because no matter how strong or weak one is, 100% is still 100% and the true maximal isometric contraction can be held only for 1 second, as seen in Figure 19–5. On the other hand, if one looks at absolute endurance, for example, how long one can hold a given weight, strength and endurance are very much related. If the MVC of my right biceps is 20 lb and I go on a strength-training program and double the strength of my MVC to 40 lb, then I will be able to hold the force of 20 lb for more than 1 minute. My new MVC of 40 lb, which is now

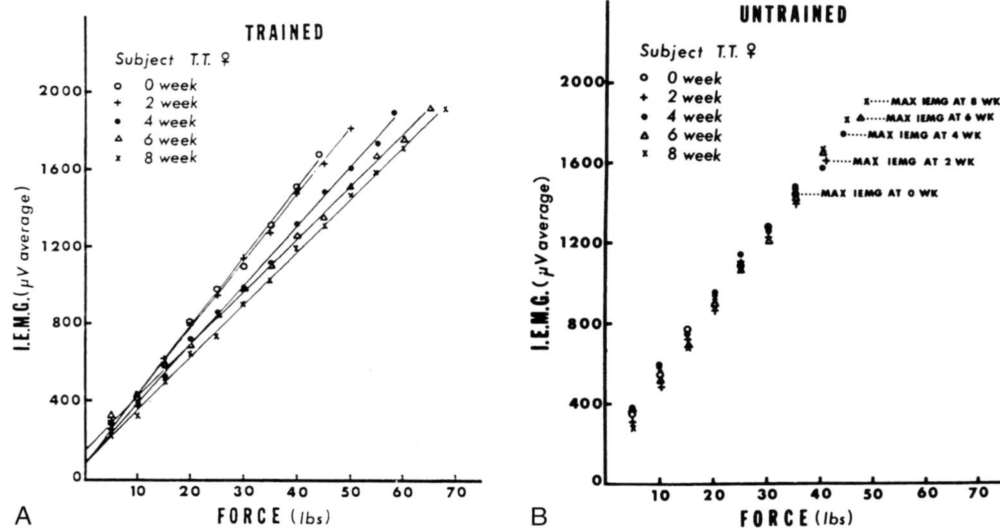

FIGURE 19–4. Data plotted to show typical changes in the trained arm (*A*) as compared with the untrained (*B*) arm. Both arms gained in strength, but only the trained arm showed significant changes in the E/F ratio, which is the amount of electrical activity required per unit of force generated (hypertrophy). (From Moritani T, deVries HK: Neural factors versus hypertrophy in the time course of muscle strength gain. Am J Phys Med 1979; 58:115–130.)

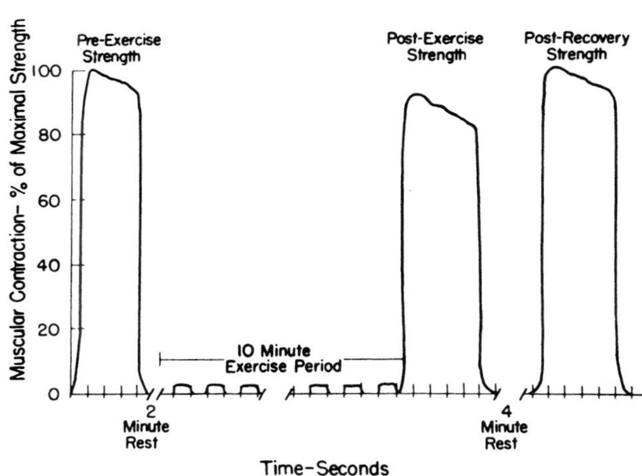

FIGURE 19–5. Maximal tension can be maintained during a voluntary maximal contraction of hand grip for less than 1 second before evidence of fatigue appears as the available supply of adenosine triphosphate (ATP) is exhausted. Fatigue (unavailability of ATP) increases in proportion to the intensity of activity but can be demonstrated following 10 minutes of intermittent contractions at 5% of maximal. (From Mundale MO: The relationship of intermittent isometric exercise to fatigue of hand grip. Arch Phys Med Rehabil 1970; 51:532–539.)

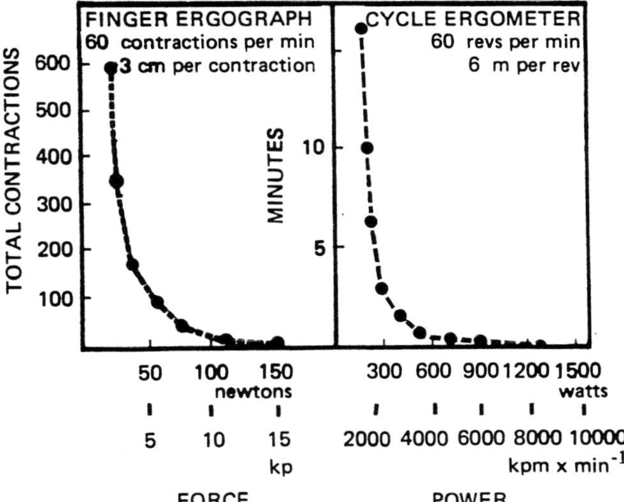

FIGURE 19–6. *A.* Relationship of endurance (as total contractions) of repeated flexion of third digit to effective force of contraction. *B.* Relationship of endurance (as minutes to fatigue) of cycle ergometer exercise to external power production. In both panels, the intercept with the abscissa represents the exercise intensity for which the maneuver could be performed only once (and, therefore, the strength of the concentric movement). In both panels, endurance could be presented as either total contractions or minutes to fatigue and, as the contraction rate and velocity are designated, either abscissa could be designated as force (per individual repetition) or power (work per unit time). (From Knuttgen HG: Development of muscular strength and endurance. In Knuttgen HG (ed): Neuromuscular Mechanisms for Therapeutic and Conditioning Exercises. Baltimore, University Park Press, 1976, pp 97–118.)

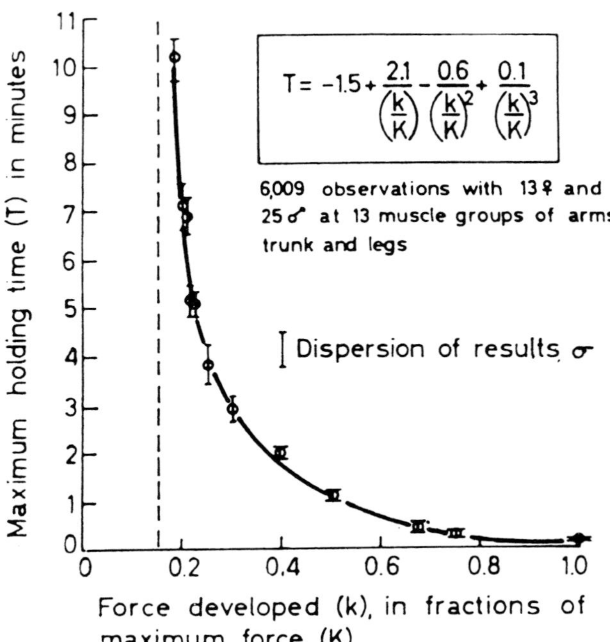

FIGURE 19–7. Endurance and intensity of work. Static work: tension at fractions of maximum strength. (From Simonson E: Recovery and Fatigue. Springfield, IL, Charles C Thomas, 1971, pp 440–458.)

100% of the MVC, can be held for only 1 second. This distinction between absolute muscle endurance and relative muscle endurance should resolve much of the apparent conflict in the literature about the relationships of strength and endurance.

Length-Tension Relationships

Figure 19–8 shows the classic force-velocity relationships, also known as a Blix diagram. Attention is directed to curve *C*. In this relationship the tendon of insertion of the relaxed muscle of the anesthetized animal is removed from the insertion and connected to a tension-measuring device. At very short lengths no tension registers in the muscle-tendon relationship. That length at which tension just begins to exceed zero is known as the resting length. As the muscle is drawn out (stretched) further and further, tension increases exponentially. If the muscle then is returned to a much shorter length (in the figure to 88% of the resting length) and a tetanizing volley of electrical stimuli is delivered to the motor nerve, tension is developed in the muscle. This is known as active tension. At all points below 100% of the resting length, the active and total tension are the same. At a point beyond 100% of the resting length, the active tension (curve *B*) is obtained by subtracting the passive tension (*C*) from the total tension (*A*). It can be seen that the tension (total) that can be developed in the muscle is greatest at this theoretical resting length, and it is inferred that the active tension drops off markedly at greater than 100% of the resting length. It is difficult to determine this theoretical resting length in living subjects, and the term resting length can be misleading, since the muscle can be at rest (relaxed) at many lengths. As a practical matter, the resting length, sometimes called the neutral length, of the intact subject could be considered to be at about the midpoint of the joint range or slightly longer.

Leverage Effect

Leverage curves that were determined by looking at the angle of application of the tendon of insertion at various joint angles are shown in Figure 19–9. Any muscle force can be broken down into two forces normal (perpendicular) to each other: a rotatory force and a stabilizing force, as can be seen in Figure 19–10. The rotatory force is equal to the product of the total muscle force times the sine of the angle of application. Since the sine of 90 degrees is 1, the full muscle force is converted to rotatory force only if the angle of insertion is 90 degrees. Leverage is a function of the site of application of the tendon of insertion, that is, the perpendicular distance of the site of application from the joint.

Before isokinetic devices became available, torque-angle curves had to be determined by measurement of isometric force at each angle and computation of torque according to one of the methods shown in Figure 19–10. Examples of such curves are shown in Figures 19–11, 19–12, and 19–13. Leverage is determined by this site of application as well as the angle of application. If the leverage so defined were the only determinant of torque, it would be inferred from Figure 19–9 that the brachioradialis was the strongest of the elbow flexors. However, the force or tension developed by the muscle is, as we

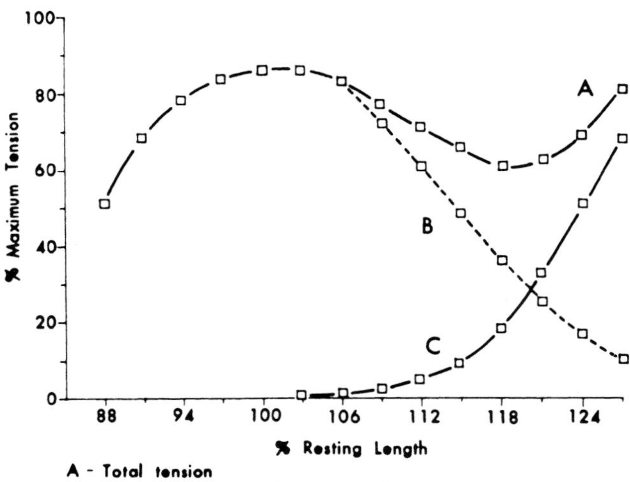

FIGURE 19–8. Length-tension diagram for passive stretch of an unsimulated muscle is shown in lower curve *C*. Curve *A*, showing total isometric tension when the muscle was stimulated at various lengths from maximal stretch through moderate shortening, represents the summation of active contraction plus passive tension due to the stretch. Active tension due solely to muscular contraction is obtained by subtracting passive tension (*C*) from total tension (*A*) and is represented by curve *B*. Normal resting length is 100, represented by curve *B*. Normal resting length is 100%. (Redrawn from Schottelius BA, Senay LC: Effect of stimulation-length sequence on shape of length-tension diagram. Am J Physiol 1956; 186:127–130.)

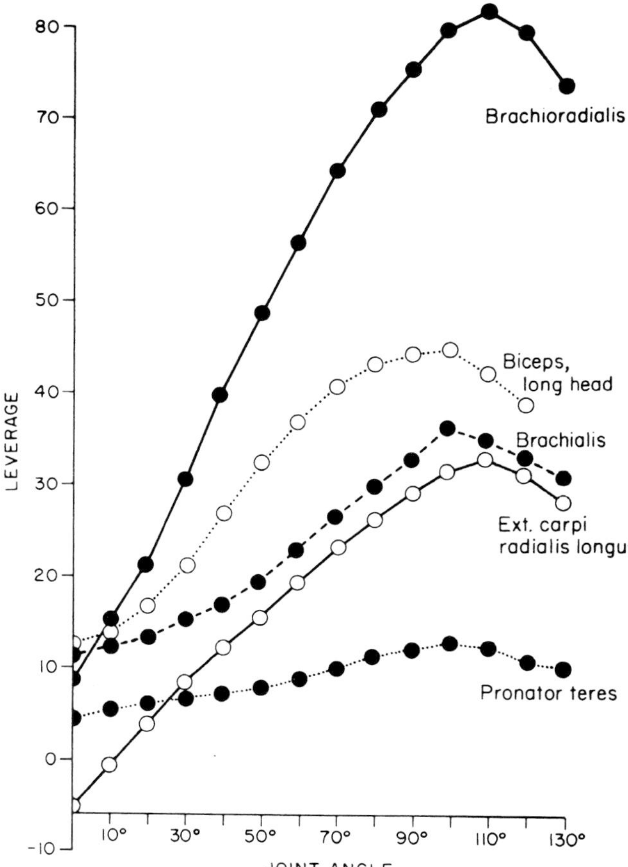

FIGURE 19–9. Leverage curves of elbow flexors; 0 degrees: elbow extended. Leverage is effective lever arm length: *lf* × sine α, where *lf* is the distance from joint axis to site of application of tendon of insertion and α is the angle of insertion of the tendon at that joint angle. (From Brunnstrom S: Clinical Kinesiology, ed 2. Philadelphia, FA Davis, 1966.)

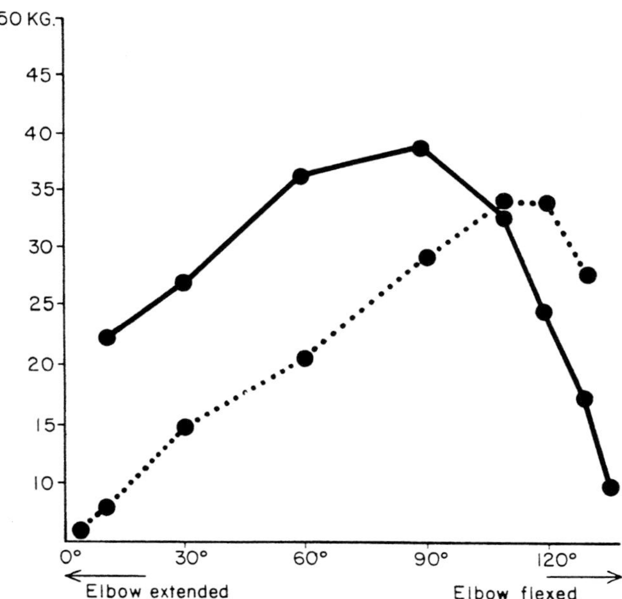

FIGURE 19–11. Torque curves for flexion and extension of right elbow, from determinations in four male subjects. *Solid curve,* elbow flexion curve; *dotted curve,* elbow extension. (From Brunnstrom S: Clinical Kinesiology, ed 2. Philadelphia, FA Davis, 1966.)

have seen, a function of the physiological cross-sectional area of the muscle. The torque developed (the effectiveness of the muscle for producing rotation about the joint) is the net result of muscle size (physiological cross-sectional area) and leverage.

Torque-Velocity Relationships

Modern isokinetic devices allow easy measurement of torque as it varies throughout the range of motion. They also permit the measurement of such torque-angle curves at varying velocities of contraction. Consequently, there are whole families of torque-angle-velocity curves. The point of maximum torque even shifts with the velocity of contraction. It is as though, at higher velocities, especially when the muscle is working

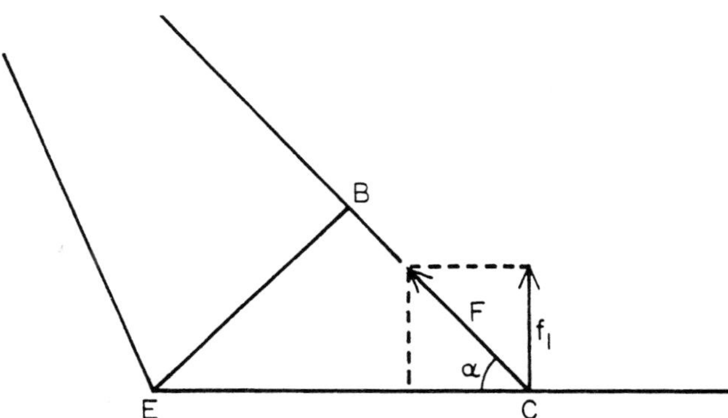

FIGURE 19–10. Two methods of computing torque. Torque equals f_1 × EC or F × EB. (From Brunnstrom S: Clinical Kinesiology, ed 2. Philadelphia, FA Davis, 1966.)

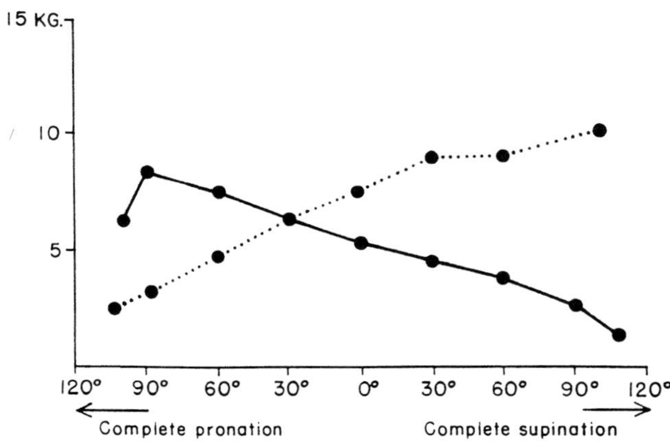

FIGURE 19–12. Torque curves for pronation and supination of right elbow, derived from determinations in four male subjects. Elbow is 90 degrees of flexion. *Solid curve,* supination; *dotted curve,* pronation; 0, thumb upward. (From Brunnstrom S: Clinical Kinesiology, ed 2. Philadelphia, FA Davis, 1966.)

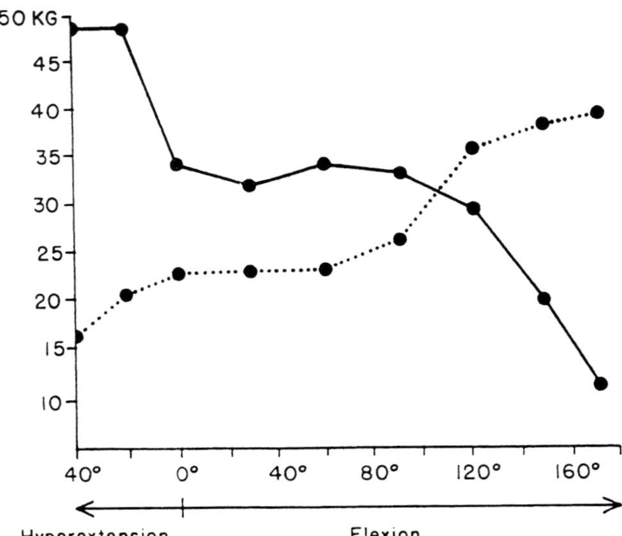

FIGURE 19–13. Torque curves for flexion and extension of right shoulder, derived from determinations in four male subjects. *Solid curve,* flexion; *dotted curve,* extension. (From Brunnstrom S: Clinical Kinesiology, ed 2. Philadelphia, FA Davis, 1966.)

against gravity (as when the seated subject uses the quadriceps to extend the knee), the muscle has to "catch up" with the resistance lever of the isokinetic device. Examples are shown in Figures 19–14 through 19–16. Figure 19–15 shows the torque-angle curve for the quadriceps and hamstrings of a seated subject at 3 rpm (18 degrees/sec), 10 rpm (60 degrees/sec), and 30 rpm (180 degrees/sec). The displacement or position angle in degrees is shown in the lower set of curves. With these synchronized curves one can see the point of maximal torque for the quadriceps and the hamstrings. Of greater importance, however, is the fact that despite exerting full effort the subject can produce less torque at 10 rpm than at 3 rpm, and less torque at 30 rpm than at 10 rpm. This illustrates the well-known torque-velocity relationships, which are plotted out in Figure 19–16. This plot shows that one can develop less torque with a fast shortening (concentric) contraction than with a slow shortening contraction, less torque with a slow shortening contraction than with an isometric contraction, less torque with an isometric contraction than with a slow lengthening (eccentric) contraction, and less torque with a slow lengthening contraction than with a rapid lengthening contraction. This relationship has important implications for therapeutic exercise for development of strength and for hypertrophy (see discussion of the overload principle, below).

Muscle Fiber and Motor Unit Types

In the human there appear to be two muscle fiber types, generally designated type I (slow oxidative or SO) and type II (fast-twitch or FT). There is at least one subdivision of fibers into fast glycolytic (FG) and fast oxidative-glycolytic (FOG). The categorization into types I and II is made on the basis of the twitch characteristics, that is, fast or slow (Fig. 19–17). The characteristics of the muscle fibers are determined by the type of motor unit (Table 19–1). These characteristics include such things as their metabolic processes and sources of fuel, along with the enzymatic activity, speed of contraction, and rate of fatigue. Descriptions of differences in muscle color and muscle fiber diameter relate more consistently or at least more obviously to animals than to humans, in whom the differences are more subtle. The distinction between light and dark meat in the Thanksgiving turkey is well known. The FOG motor unit, including the muscle fiber, can be thought of as a sort of hybrid that is defined as type II by its FT characteristics but retains some of the fatigue resistance associated with the oxidative phosphorylation seen in the type I or SO motor unit types.

Twitch characteristics of muscle are not easily determined in the intact subject and one generally uses histochemical markers to determine whether units in a given micrograph are type I or type II. Figure 19–18 shows type I (light-staining fibers) and type II (dark-staining fibers). Serial sections can be stained for other enzymatic features; the right panel in Figure 19–18 shows that the type I fibers have greater NADH diaphorase. The fuel utilized by the various motor units has important implications for therapeutic exercise, particularly fat reduction (see Exercise for Fat Reduction, below).

The Motor Unit Size Principle

Henneman[33] first enunciated the size principle, which has been supported by subsequent investigators. The smaller motor units have fewer muscle fibers, smaller motor unit action potentials, somewhat smaller cross-sectional areas, and a lower threshold of recruitment. In needle EMG, as motor units are recruited in succession, the smaller motor units come in first and the larger motor units later. Some later motor units appear smaller because of their distance from the exploring electrode. With the needle adjusted to focus on the motor unit, it becomes much larger. Another way of stating this is that smaller units can be recruited without the larger

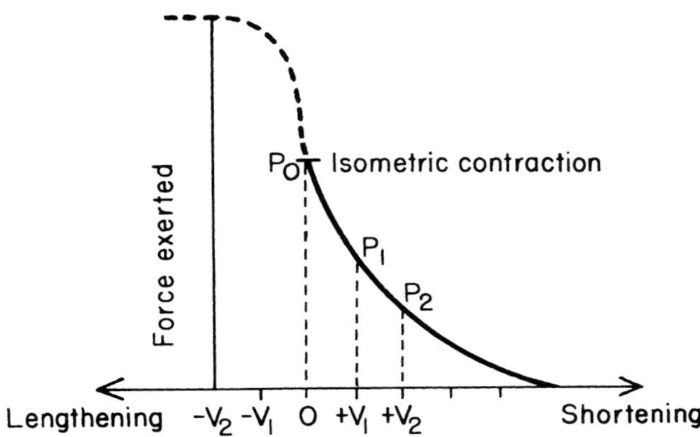

FIGURE 19–14. Force-velocity curve of human muscle. *Solid line,* data obtained from elbow flexors of human subjects. At the time this curve was drawn, the *dotted line* was made by extrapolation. This portion of the curve has subsequently been confirmed experimentally (see Fig. 19–16). (From Brunnstrom S: Clinical Kinesiology, ed 2. Philadelphia, FA Davis, 1966.)

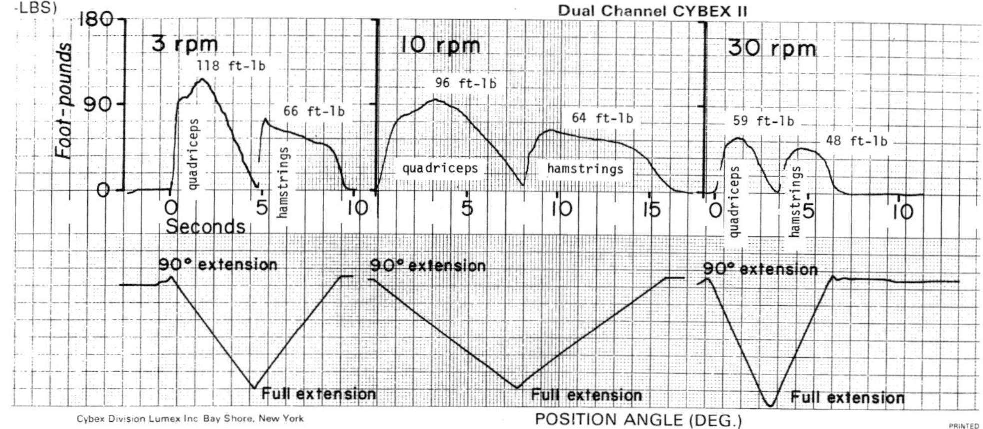

FIGURE 19–15. Torque curves of quadriceps and hamstrings throughout 90-degree range of motion and at various speeds. Note the greater strength of the quadriceps versus the hamstrings. With the subject seated, gravity hinders the quadriceps and helps the hamstrings progressively more at higher speeds. (From de Lateur BJ, Lehmann JF: Therapeutic exercise to develop strength and endurance. In Kottke FJ, Lehmann JF (eds): Krusen's Handbook of Physical Medicine and Rehabilitation, ed 4. Philadelphia, WB Saunders, 1990.)

units, but larger units cannot be recruited without the smaller units. Some variation of the size principle can be seen even among motor units of similar size.

Metabolic Aspects of Exercise

Gollnick et al have shown that the point of recruitment of the larger type II fibers depends on the type of exercise.[28] With sustained isometric contractions, type II motor units are brought in at 20% of the MVC. However, if the isometric effort is sustained long enough, type II fibers can be brought in at thresholds somewhat below 20% of MVC. With aerobic exercise, as on a bicycle ergometer, the reliance is on type I motor units below 100% of the maximal aerobic capacity ($\dot{V}O_{2max}$; see Fig. 19–19). Beyond this aerobic capacity, both type I and type II are relied upon, and the subject will rapidly go into oxygen debt secondary to anaerobic metabolism. However, the threshold for bringing in anaerobic pathways is generally about 70%, although it may be higher in endurance-trained (aerobic-trained) athletes.

Application of Principles to Therapeutic Exercise for Strength, Local Muscle Endurance, and Hypertrophy

Strength

Muscle performance, including performance on tests of strength, can be enhanced in various ways. These include increases in the amount of weight lifted (progressive resistance exercise, or PRE); increases in the

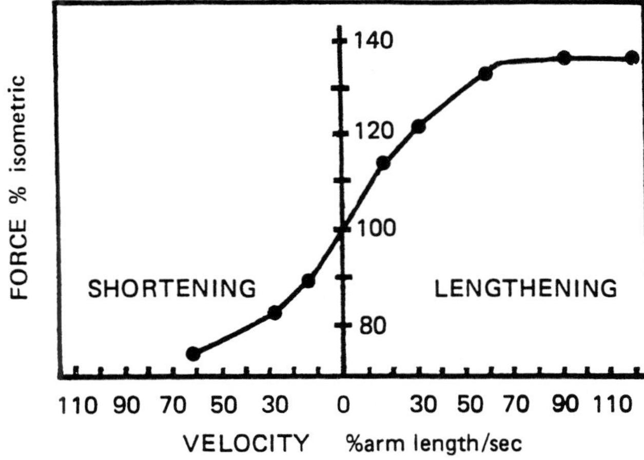

FIGURE 19–16. Relationship of maximal force of human elbow flexor muscles to velocity of contraction. Velocity on abscissa is designated as a percentage of arm length per second. (From Knuttgen HG: Development of muscular strength and endurance. In Knuttgen HG (ed): Neuromuscular Mechanisms for Therapeutic and Conditioning Exercises. Baltimore, University Park Press, 1976, pp 97–118.)

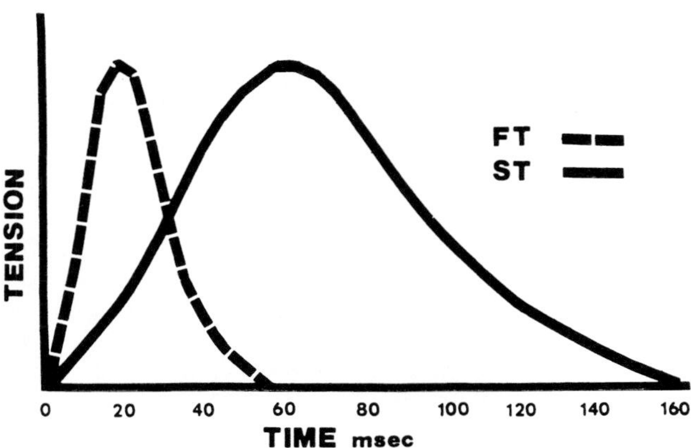

FIGURE 19–17. Twitch characteristics (contraction relaxation curves) of slow twitch (type I) and fast twitch (type II) muscles. (From Ianuzzo CD: The cellular composition of human skeletal muscle. In Knuttgen HG (ed): Neuromuscular Mechanisms for Therapeutic and Conditioning Exercise. Baltimore, University Park Press, 1976, pp 31–53.)

TABLE 19–1 A Characterization of Skeletal Muscle Fibers Based Upon Their Metabolic and Mechanical Properties

	Muscle Fiber Characteristics		
	Slow Oxidative (SO)	*Fast Glycolytic (FG)*	*Fast Oxidative-Glycolytic (FOG)*
Major source of ATP	Oxidative phosphorylation	Glycolysis	Oxidative phosphorylation
Mitochondria	Numerous	Few	Numerous
Myoglobin content	High	Low	High
Capillarity	Dense	Sparse	Dense
Muscle color	Red	White	Red
Glycogen content	Low	High	Intermediate
Glycolytic enzyme activity	Low	High	Intermediate
Myosin ATPase activity	Low	High	High
Speed of contraction	Slow	Fast	Fast
Rate of fatigue	Slow	Fast	Intermediate
Muscle fiber diameter	Small	Large	Intermediate

Abbreviations: ATP, adenosine triphosphate; ATPase, adenosine triphosphatase. From Kidd G, Brodie P: The motor unit: A review. Physiotherapy 1980; 66:146–152.

number of repetitions or sets, or both; and increases in the contraction velocity (while keeping the resistance and number of repetitions the same).

Progressive Resistance Exercise

This type of exercise was described and popularized by T. L. DeLorme, who at the time was a captain in the U.S. Army. It requires the determination, usually once a week, of the 10 RM. At each session, held 3 to 5 days per week, the subject performs 10 repetitions at each of a series of fractions of the 10 RM. In the early stages this was 10 repetitions each at 10%, 20%, 30%, . . . , up to 100% of the 10 RM.[19, 20] Because of the enormous amount of time necessary to train multiple muscles with this technique, a number of modifications of this program were devised and the final form was 10 repetitions each at 50%, 75%, and 100% of the 10 RM. This program has much to recommend it, including the fact that there is a built-in warmup at a lower intensity and the likelihood of fatigue limiting the number of contractions in the final set at 100%. Nevertheless, some workers were concerned about the inability to carry out the full prescribed 10 RM at 100%, and thus the "Oxford technique"[49] was developed. It begins with 10 repetitions at 100% and progresses down in weight to 10 repetitions at 75% and 50% of the 10 RM. Esselman et al[23] showed that as many as 40 extra repetitions at a lower resistance had virtually no effect on the results of 12 weeks of training. This observation strongly suggests

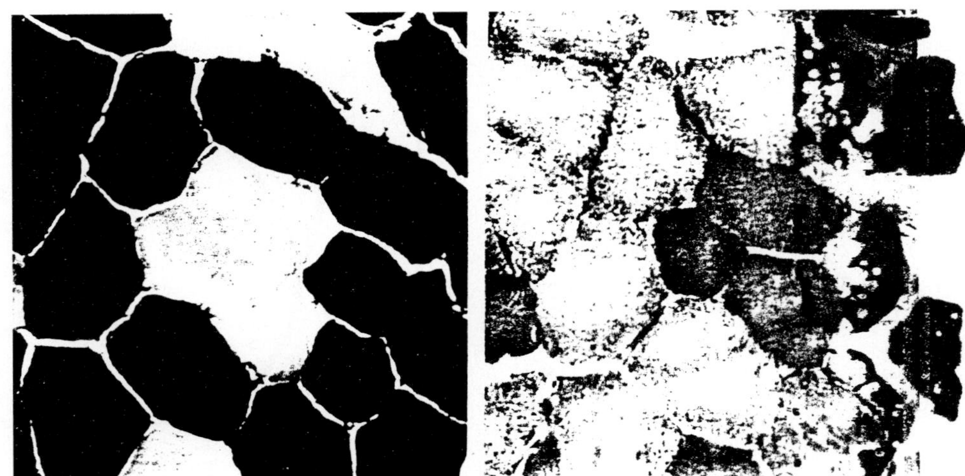

FIGURE 19–18. Histochemical micrograph illustrating the fast twitch (FT) and slow twitch (ST) muscle fibers in human skeletal muscle. The micrograph on the left has been stained for myofibrillar ATPase. The light- and dark-stained cells are ST and FT fibers, respectively. The micrograph at the right is from a serial section of the muscle and has been stained for DPNH-diaphorase, which indicates the aerobic potential of the fibers. These micrographs illustrate that in human skeletal muscle, ST fibers have a relatively high aerobic capacity, whereas FT fibers have a low capacity. (From Ianuzzo CD: The cellular composition of human skeletal muscle. In Knuttgen HG (ed): Neuromuscular Mechanisms for Therapeutic Conditioning Exercise. Baltimore, University Park Press, 1976, pp 31–53.)

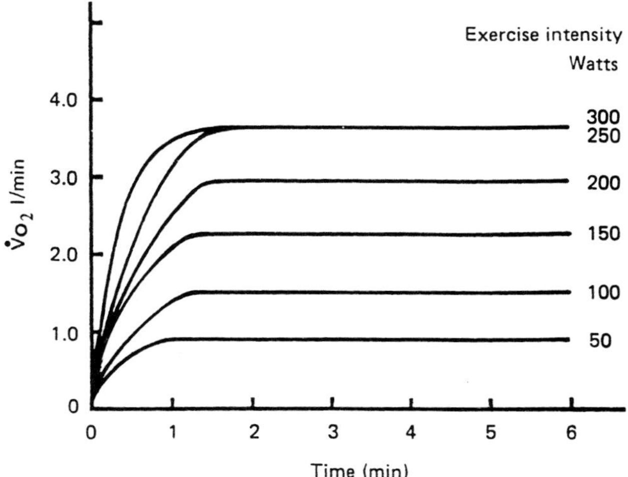

FIGURE 19–19. Relationship of oxygen uptake to various exercise intensities utilizing several muscle groups in reciprocal concentric contractions. There is no additional increase in oxygen uptake with a further increase in exercise intensity (external work) once maximal oxygen uptake is reached. (From Soule RG: Physiological response to physical exercise. In Knuttgen HG (ed): Neuromuscular Mechanisms for Therapeutic and Conditioning Exercise. Baltimore, University Park Press, 1976, pp 79–96.)

that the DeLorme technique is more effective than the Oxford technique, although the critical study in this regard has not yet been done. The reader is advised to determine what type of exercise training is actually performed when progressive resistive exercise is requested.

Increasing the Number of Repetitions

There is essentially 100% transfer-of-training when exercise with relatively high weights and few repetitions is compared with exercise with relatively low weights and more repetitions, as long as the exercise is continued to the point of fatigue.[17] However, two points should be noted. The first is that far more repetitions must be carried out with lower weights than with higher weights to reach the point of fatigue. It is likely that the subject will stop low-weight exercise for reasons other than true muscle fatigue. The amount of mechanical work done will be much greater with the lower weight. Mechanical work is far less relevant to muscle training than is the stimulus of muscle failure, that is, a short-lasting inability to carry out the task. There may be some circumstances in which the subject should avoid the risk of training that might occur with the higher weights. In general, however, exercising with higher weights to failure is both more effective and more efficient than exercising with lower weights to failure. One can also do multiple sets, continuing to fatigue with each set, with the higher weights. This might be necessary once a plateau has been reached in training.

Progressive Rate Training of Hellebrandt

Hellebrandt and Houtz showed that muscle performance can be improved by selecting a relatively high weight and using a metronome to control the contraction velocity.[23] A fixed number of repetitions can be used, such as 10 or, at most, 20. The metronome is set initially at the lowest rate and the weight is lifted on "tick" and lowered on "tock." Each day the metronome rate is set one notch higher. Almost imperceptibly the contraction velocity is thereby increased and the entire torque-velocity curve is shifted upward. This technique has the additional advantage that the exercise time required is shorter every day. It is also unnecessary to keep redetermining the 10 RM. With these advantages it is somewhat surprising that this technique is rarely used, but that is apparently the case.

A variation on this type of training is to use an isokinetic device with the initial velocity limit set very low. One might therefore start out at an 18 degrees/sec velocity limit and gradually increase it to as much as 360 degrees/sec, or the upper limit of some isokinetic machines.

Other Approaches

A simple but highly effective technique[16] is to find a relatively high weight, one that can be lifted three to five times prior to failure (temporary inability to lift the weight further), and record the number of repetitions. The exercise should be carried to the point of muscle fatigue or failure each session. The number of repetitions to fatigue is graphed on a daily basis. When the subject can perform some 15 to 20 repetitions, the weight is increased approximately 10% and the process is repeated. A variation on this process, useful when strength begins to reach a plateau, is to do multiple sets during a session, going to fatigue with each set.

CLINICAL AND SPORTS APPLICATIONS

The practice of sports medicine is characterized by a number of maxims, perhaps one of the most important and useful of which is "Get in shape to play. Do not play to get in shape." This maxim applies equally to clinical rehabilitation practice. Following this single maxim would do more to prevent injury than virtually any other practice. By doing so, one builds up a reserve in the mechanical, metabolic, and neuromuscular aspects of performance, and this reserve goes a long way toward preventing overuse injuries, strains, sprains, and so forth.

Are Athletes Born or Made?

Marked differences between athletes participating in different types of sports can be detected by the casual observer or the devotee of sport and in greater detail by the scientist in the human performance laboratory. The weightlifter is heavy and extremely strong. The distance runner is slight of build with very little body fat and relatively low strength but has the ability to continue running, literally for hours. Definite but more subtle changes are observed between the sprinter and the distance runner. Differences in local metabolic capacity of the muscle as well as fiber type differences have been determined by large-needle biopsy.[3] Gollnick et al sampled the upper and lower extremity muscles of athletes participating in various sports.[27] A total of 74 trained and untrained men were studied. The quantitative chemical studies that were carried out included succinate dehydrogenase (SDH) and phosphofructokinase (PFK), representing respectively the oxidative and glycolytic capabilities of the muscle sample as a whole, without distinction between fiber types. Histochemical studies included myosin adenosine triphosphatase (ATPase) for fiber typing, as well as NADH diaphorase and α-glycerophosphate dehydrogenase for estimating (semiquantitatively only) relative (type I versus type II) oxidative and glycolytic capabilities. The distribution of glycogen was estimated (in serial sections) from the periodic acid–Schiff (PAS) reaction. Standard photographs were made so that planimetry could be used for fiber areas. In addition, each subject's $\dot{V}O_{2max}$ was determined while he was either running on a treadmill or pedaling a bicycle. Whereas only minor differences existed for PFK (glycolytic capacity), remarkable differences were found in local muscle oxidative capacity (SDH) and in $\dot{V}O_{2max}$. The SDH and $\dot{V}O_{2max}$ of the weight lifters were no greater than those of the untrained men; in fact, the values were slightly less. The endurance-trained athletes had much higher $\dot{V}O_{2max}$ and local muscle SDH activity than the untrained men or the weight lifters.

Of particular interest is the selective effect on the muscles used predominantly in the sport. For instance, in the bicyclists, the SDH activity of the vastus lateralis (11.0 ± 1.0 μmol/g/min) was much greater than that of the deltoid (6.1 ± 0.2), whereas in canoeists, the SDH activity of the deltoid (7.9 ± 0.6) was much higher than that of the vastus lateralis (5.8 ± 0.9). Table 19–2 shows the fiber sizes, populations, and contributions to muscle area of several individual subjects. Note that in the untrained men, the weight lifters, and the sprinter, the slow-twitch (ST) fibers (type I) occupied a relatively small percentage of the muscle fiber area (21.9% to 30%), whereas in the endurance-trained athletes the ST fibers occupied as much as 84% of the area.

This study examined the athletes as they were and did not constitute a before-and-after experiment. It might be argued that very early in their athletic careers these athletes found they were able to compete much more effectively in one type of sport than in another and therefore, because of positive reinforcement, selected the sport at which they were successful. However, there is some suggestion that the changes seen in their muscles were at least to some extent the result of training, because one would anticipate genetically a more or less constant ratio of ST to FT fibers in the upper and lower extremities. This is not to say that the same ratio of ST to FT fibers in the deltoid and in the vastus lateralis would be expected. However, if the ST/FT ratio is X in the deltoid and Y in the vastus lateralis in one subject, and if the ST/FT ratio is A in the deltoid and B in the vastus in another subject, then, if differential usage (training) has no effect, one might expect X/Y to equal A/B. However, those athletes who used the upper or the lower extremity more in a specific sport had enhanced the metabolic capability and a larger percent area of ST fibers in the muscles used.

Gollnick et al also carried out a 5-month training program with biopsy studies before and after training.[26] The training program was 1 hour per day for 4 days a week at a load requiring 75% to 90% of maximal aerobic power. The subsequent biopsies showed an increase in the ratio of the areas of ST to FT fibers from 0.82 to 1.11 ($P < 0.01$). Oxidative capacity increased in both fiber types; anaerobic capacity increased only in the FT fibers. This study indicates the possibility of great enhancement of local muscle metabolic capability, particularly oxidative capacity, with endurance training and strongly supports the notion of some degree of specificity of training. In human subjects, fiber number does not appear to increase. However, in an animal study, Gonyea et al were able to excise and tease apart the fibers of an entire muscle using nitric acid digestion, and they found a small but significant increase in fiber number in response to unilateral exercise.[29] The fact that they found significance means either that a rare thing had happened (the animals had been born with more fibers on one side than on the other) or that there was an actual increase in fiber number in response to exercise.

Regarding the question of whether athletes are born or made, it appears that the genotype sets the rather wide limits, with the actual performance capability determined by the extent and type of training.

Studies on the Specificity of Training

The exercise literature and clinical experience both strongly support the observation that the poorer the initial condition of the subject (provided that no specific neuromuscular disorder is present), the greater the percentage response to training and the greater the generalizability of the training. Conversely, the more elite the athlete or performer, the greater the requirement for specific training (see also Coordination, below). With very deconditioned subjects, aerobic training leads to increases in strength, and strength training leads to improved aerobic performance as well as enhanced local muscle endurance.[10, 14, 47]

High Weights versus Low Weights: The DeLorme Axiom

One study illustrates the transferability of training on relatively high weights to performance under low-weight conditions (and vice versa) utilizing a study design known as double-shift transfer-of-training design.[17] This type of design, long utilized by investigators in the realm of motor skills learning, requires the best performance a subject can produce during each training session. In this way each session yields a score and no other assessment is required. This type of design was utilized during World War II to see, for example, the extent to which training in flight simulators transferred to performance in airplanes (which were in relatively short supply). A similar design was used to determine whether gunnery training should be performed on small targets, which were thought to make the shooters sharp,

TABLE 19–2 Relationship of Exercise Training of Upper and Lower Extremity Muscles to Fiber Diameters, Total Cross-Sectional Areas, and Percentage of Slow Twitch and Fast Twitch Muscle Fibers

Subject	Sample Site	Group	Fiber Diameter (μm) ST	Fiber Diameter (μm) FT	Area (μ^2) ST	Area (μ^2) FT	ST Fibers (%)	Area of ST Fibers (%)
PG	L	Untrained	75.2 ± 2.9 (47.1 − 96.1)	85.8 ± 2.0 (69.3 − 101.7)	4567.5 ± 343.2 (1740 − 7250)	5843.0 ± 273.9 (3770−8120)	34.0	28.7
CS	L	Untrained	80.3 ± 3.3 (54.4 − 112.2)	93.2 ± 2.2 (71.9 − 110.4)	5234.5 ± 440.3 (2320 − 9860)	6902.0 ± 329.9 (4060 − 9570)	30.0	24.5
MKS	L	Untrained	63.4 ± 2.4 (47.1 − 79.4)	67.7 ± 2.4 (47.1 − 86.0)	3057.5 ± 273.6 (1740 − 4930)	3683.0 ± 250.0 (1740 − 800)	34.0	30.0
GK	A	Untrained	63.6 ± 2.0 (38.0 − 76.0)	67.3 ± 1.7 (53.8 − 79.2)	3234.0 ± 181.2 (1135 − 4540)	3594.0 ± 177.8 (2270 − 4918)	48.3	45.7
	L		72.2 ± 3.5 (43.9 − 98.2)	75.0 ± 1.4 (65.9 − 87.8)	4275.0 ± 382.1 (1513 − 7566)	4445.0 ± 169.1 (3405 − 6053)	48.6	47.6
NP	L	Sprinter	79.5 ± 2.6 (54.4 − 98.0)	89.4 ± 2.1 (74.4 − 101.7)	5060.5 ± 314.0 (2320 − 7540)	6336.5 ± 284.2 (4350 − 8120)	26.0	21.9
DM	L	Distance runner	67.1 ± 1.7 (54.4 − 83.3)	58.0 ± 1.3 (47.1 − 69.3)	3581.1 ± 186.2 (2320 − 5510)	2668.0 ± 1220 (1740 − 3770)	75.0	80.1
DS	L	Distance runner	85.1 ± 3.5 (57.7 − 105.3)	105.2 ± 2.5 (81.5 − 124.6)	5858.0 ± 445.8 (2610 − 8700)	8776.1 ± 403.2 (5220 − 12,179)	70.0	60.9
DF	L	Middle-distance runner	95.5 ± 3.2 (74.4 − 121.6)	87.9 ± 3.4 (47.1 − 115.3)	7307.8 ± 499.6 (4350 − 11,599)	6235.0 ± 448.2 (1740 − 10,439)	55.0	58.9
RP	L	Middle-distance runner	59.2 ± 2.7 (27.2 − 79.2)	71.6 ± 2.5 (50.9 − 98.0)	2856.5 ± 231.8 (580 − 4830)	4118.0 ± 295.9 (2030 − 540)	47.0	38.1
BA	L	Former weight lifter	107.1 ± 3.8 (83.8 − 135.9)	108.9 ± 3.4 (92.2 − 160.8)	9199.1 ± 656.7 (5510 − 14,499)	9482.9 ± 666.9 (6670 − 20,299)	24.0	23.5
MH	L	Weight lifter	85.6 ± 4.9 (47.1 − 113.7)	110.8 ± 3.0 (86.0 − 135.9)	6035.6 ± 629.4 (1740 − 10,149)	9758.1 ± 516.6 (5800 − 14,499)	25.3	23.5
	A		83.5 ± 2.4 (60.8 − 98.0)	105.0 ± 3.3 (74.4 − 135.9)	5553.5 ± 303.8 (2900 − 7540)	8917.2 ± 543.1 (4350 − 14,499)	48.4	36.9
JR	A	Bicyclist	83.1 ± 1.4 (71.9 − 96.1)	96.2 ± 1.9 (76.9 − 108.7)	5467.0 ± 187.9 (4060 − 7250)	7337.0 ± 273.7 (4640 − 9280)	52.1	48.6
	L		104.6 ± 2.3 (86.0 − 127.5)	112.2 ± 2.2 (98.0 − 137.2)	8651.5 ± 763.9 (5800 − 12,759)	9946.6 ± 401.5 (7540 − 14,789)	51.3	44.0
BL	A	Canoeist	101.9 ± 2.6 (86.3 − 129.5)	102.9 ± 2.3 (88.6 − 118.2)	8244.0 ± 570.3 (5850 − 13,162)	8391.0 ± 361.9 (5484 − 10,968)	57.9	74.6
	L		90.5 ± 2.7 (68.2 − 107.9)	80.3 ± 1.5 (68.2 − 91.6)	6544.0 ± 387.5 (3656 − 9140)	5100.0 ± 190.1 (3656 − 6581)	69.9	57.5
SH	A	Swimmer	88.0 ± 1.7 (71.6 − 101.2)	91.0 ± 2.4 (77.8 − 105.7)	6124.0 ± 233.9 (4022 − 8043)	6552.0 ± 263.2 (4753 − 8774)	85.3	84.4
	L		79.0 ± 2.0 (61.9 − 91.6)	93.6 ± 1.9 (74.8 − 105.7)	4954.0 ± 237.6 (2925 − 6581)	6928.0 ± 266.9 (4387 − 8774)	79.7	73.7

Note: Values are means ± SE. Values in parentheses are highest and lowest observations.
Abbreviations: ST, slow twitch; FT, fast twitch; L, leg; A, arm.
Modified from Gollnick PD, Armstrong RB, Sanbert CW IV, et al. Enzyme activity and fiber composition in skeletal muscle of untrained and trained men. J Appl Physiol 1972; 33:312–319.

or on large targets, which were reinforcing because of the higher time spent on target. Such transfer-of-training designs are ideally suited to test the DeLorme axiom, which states: "High weight (intensity), low repetition programs build strength; low weight (low intensity) high repetition exercises build endurance. Each of these types of exercise is wholly distinct and wholly incapable of producing the results obtained by the other."[19] In the extreme, this axiom must be true. However, there is a large middle ground in which this axiom is untrue, that is, in which there is a high degree of transferability from relatively low-weight conditions to relatively high-weight conditions as long as the subject goes to the point of fatigue. It should be noted that 50 lb lifted 10 times will have a different training effect from 10 lb lifted 50 times, even though the mechanical work performed by the muscle is the same. What counts is the relative intensity or tax on the muscle (see discussion of intensity-endurance relationships, above).

In a study, "A Test of the DeLorme Axiom," the authors randomly assigned a relatively homogeneous group of young, sedentary men to four training groups: two groups that trained on 55-lb weights and two groups that trained on the relatively low weight of 26 lb (26 lb was selected as the low weight because much below this level, even these sedentary subjects would have been able to repeat the exercise indefinitely without muscle failure).[17] Paced by a metronome, seated subjects raised the weighted limb to full extension of the knee on the count of 1, held it through the count of 6, lowered the weight on 7, and repeated the process at the next beat. To encourage maximal performance, subjects were paid per repetition and received more pay per high-weight repetition. At the end of the series of training sessions, one low-weight group switched to the high-weight condition and one high-weight group switched to the low-weight condition, and all groups continued performing their best for several more (test) sessions. There was a 100% transfer from one condition to another (Fig. 19–20). It could be said that the strength-trained group gained as much endurance as the endurance-trained group, and the endurance-trained group gained as much strength as the strength-trained group. Although one training condition was as *effective* as the other, the high-intensity (and therefore necessarily low-repetition) group took far less time and was therefore much more efficient.

Isometric versus Isotonic

A double-shift, transfer-of-training design is also well suited to sort out the controversy between the proponents of isometric exercise and the proponents of isotonic exercise. During the height of this controversy, one could find studies that purported to show the superiority of isometric over isotonic exercise and other studies that purported to show the reverse. It was stated that "one 6-second maximal isometric contraction was worth more than hours and hours in a weight room." The issue of test bias or training-to-task was generally not considered. In a 1972 study, the authors randomly assigned healthy sedentary young adult men to one of four groups, two of which trained on a 50-lb isometric task and two of which trained on a 50-lb isotonic task.[18] The weight was kept the same to avoid confounding by low versus high weights. For those training on the isometric condition, the experimenters lifted the weighted limb to the point of full extension of the knee and by the count of 3 the subject had to hold the weight himself. The extended limb lifted a light bar that triggered the stopclock, and the subject was paid per second held. This constituted the training task and yielded the score for each day. For those training on the isotonic task, the knee was fully extended and lowered to the count of a metronome. When the bar was lifted, however briefly, the repetition was counted and the subject was paid per repetition. There was no "hold" for the isotonic group. Each task was kept pure (no lift for the isometric group and no hold for the isotonic group). At the end of the series of training sessions, two of the four groups shifted to the opposite condition and all groups continued to perform their best for several more sessions.

The result, shown in Figure 19–21, was very interesting in that subjects always did better on the task on which they had trained. Figures 19–22 and 19–23 break out the results as though they had been performed as two single-shift, transfer-of-training studies. If one saw only Figure 19–22, one would conclude that isometric exercise was superior. If one saw only Figure 19–23, one would conclude that isotonic exercise was superior. This clearly illustrates the effect of training-to-task. From these results it can be concluded that for qualitatively identical tasks, as in the DeLorme axiom study, there are comparable results, as long as subjects go to the point of fatigue in training (remember that it will take much longer to go to true muscle fatigue for lower weights). For qualitatively different tasks (or for extreme quantitative differences), the best training for a task is that task itself. This is a good illustration of Aristotle's maxim, "Men become builders by building, lyre players by playing the lyre, and virtuous by doing virtuous acts."

Isokinetic Programs: Strength, and Hypertrophy; Specificity of Velocity of Training

Isokinetic programs require special isokinetic equipment. The type of training and testing involved is not reflective of everyday, nontechnical experience. This is in contrast to isotonic and isometric tasks, in which

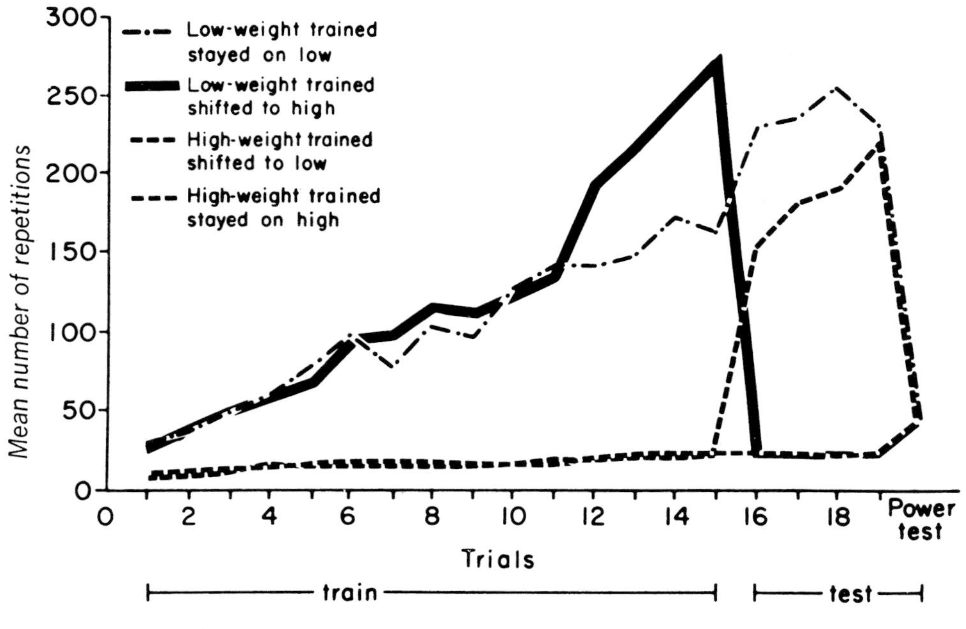

FIGURE 19–20. Mean scores for each of four groups on each of 15 training trials and each of four test trials. The mean score for each of the four groups on the power test is also shown. See text for details. (From de Lateur BJ, Lehmann JF, Fordyce WE: A test of the DeLorme axiom. Arch Phys Med Rehabil 1968; 49:245–248.)

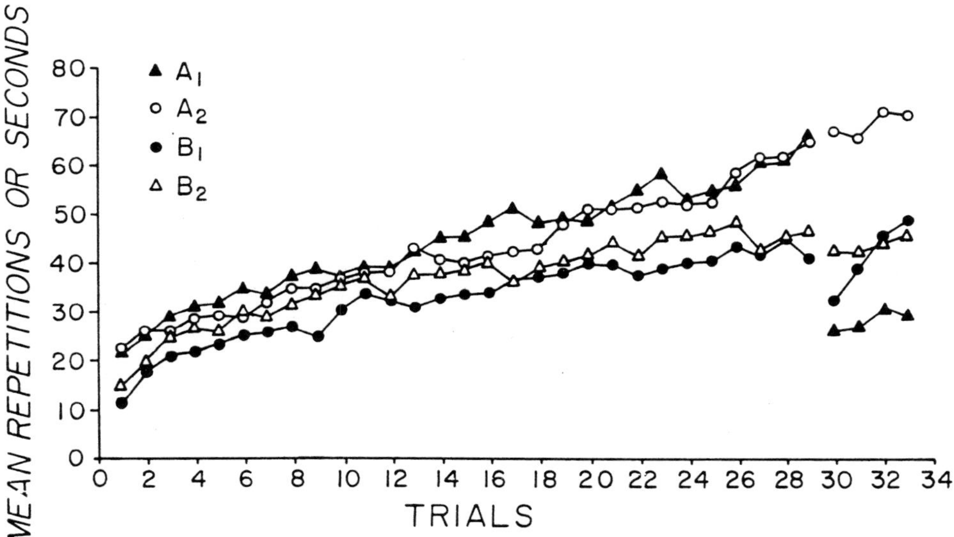

FIGURE 19–21. Results of the isotonic-isometric comparison. Groups A_1 and A_2 were isotonically trained. Groups B_1 and B_2 were isometrically trained. Group A_1 shifted to the isometric task on day 30. Group B_1 shifted to the isotonic task on day 30. (From de Lateur BJ, Lehmann J, Stonebridge J, et al: Isotonic vs. isometric exercises: A double-shift, transfer-of-training study. Arch Phys Med Rehabil 1972; 53:212–217.)

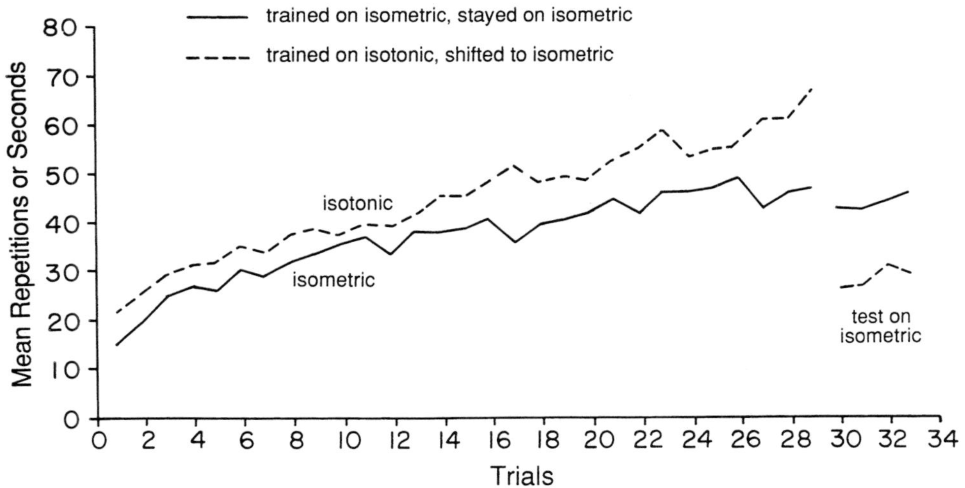

FIGURE 19–22. Comparison of isotonic versus isometric training-to-task. The group trained on isometric tasks (*solid line*) performed better on isometric tasks than did the group trained on isotonic tasks (*dashed line*). (From de Lateur BJ, Lehmann J, Stonebridge J, et al: Isotonic vs. isometric exercises: A double-shift, transfer-of-training study. Arch Phys Med Rehabil 1972; 53:212–217.)

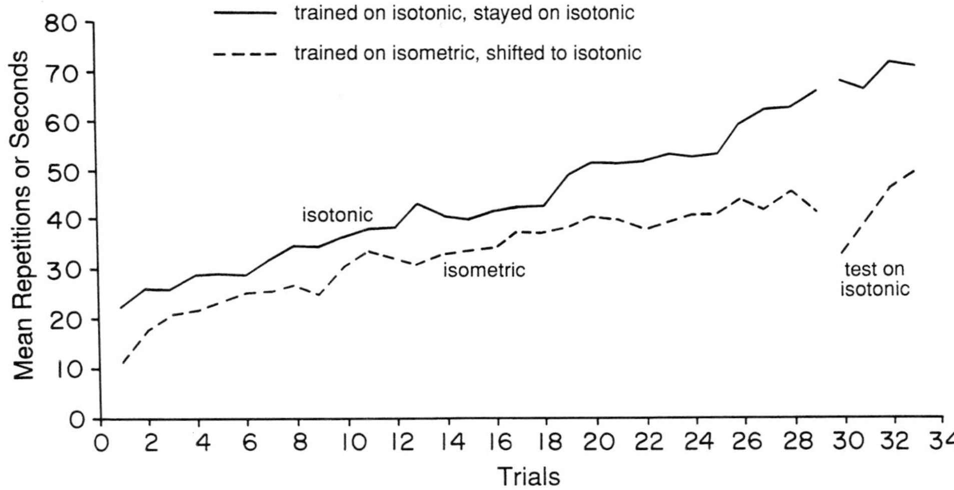

FIGURE 19–23. Comparison of isotonic versus isometric training-to-task. The group trained on isotonic tasks (*solid line*) performed better on isotonic tasks than did the group trained on isometric tasks (*dashed line*). (From de Lateur BJ, Lehmann J, Stonebridge J, et al: Isotonic vs. isometric exercises: A double-shift, transfer-of-training study. Arch Phys Med Rehabil 1972; 53:212–217.)

testing involves the ordinary activity of lifting or holding objects against gravity. Training to task and learning to perform on the isokinetic devices are heavily involved in isokinetic programs. Consequently, it is theoretically possible, and seems to be the case,[13, 23] that isokinetic performance can be greatly enhanced without significant hypertrophy. This is especially true if there is no eccentric component. Early isokinetic devices involved purely concentric exercise, since knee extension was carried out by the quadriceps (concentric) and knee flexion by the hamstrings (also concentric). In contrast, raising and lowering a weight has both a concentric and an eccentric component. More recent equipment, such as the Kin-Com, Lido (Loredan), and Biodex, as well as updated versions of the Cybex, allow either a mixed mode or a purely concentric mode. Although studies are conflicting,[37, 38] the preponderance of evidence suggests that if hypertrophy is desired, there should be at least a component of eccentric exercise in the training.

Specificity of Velocity of Training

If the best training for a task is that task itself, and if the task requires exerting force at high velocities, it would seem advantageous to train at high contraction velocities. The intrinsic shape of the torque-velocity curve (see Figs. 19–14, 19–15, and 19–16) implies that, regardless of effort, training at high contraction velocities will be less forceful, although the force exerted will gradually, with training, become higher. Esselman et al randomly assigned healthy sedentary young men to training at 6 rpm (18 degrees/sec) and 18 rpm (108 degrees/sec).[23] Because effort is all-important on isokinetic performance, subjects were paid a small amount per foot-pound of torque for every training or testing contraction. Torque-velocity curves were carried out at baseline and after 12 weeks of training. Subjects who trained at the slower contraction velocity limit (and therefore more forcefully) gained more than those who trained at a faster velocity limit, not only at the velocity at which they trained but throughout the entire torque-velocity curve, even at velocities far greater than those at which either group trained. Is this a violation of the specificity principle? Probably not, since what one was attempting to increase was the ability to produce torque (proportionate to force). It therefore appears that the more important variable in developing strength (forceful contractions) is the tension (force) produced in the muscle during training. To the extent that a skill is involved, however, such as throwing a baseball, it is extremely important to practice on the task itself.

Coordination

The maxim "Practice makes perfect" would be more accurate if restated as "*Perfect* practice makes perfect." Inaccurate practice leads to inaccurate performance, and wrong notes or skills are learned as readily as correct ones. Some extremely complex tasks involving more than one limb should be broken down into simpler tasks and performed slowly enough that the practice is essentially error-free. The simpler tasks should then be brought up to a faster speed, after which combined practice is undertaken at a slow speed. This speed is gradually increased until the combined performance can be carried out at a much faster speed than will be required in recital or concert (in the case of musical performance). This would be appropriate in the case of pipe organ performance for the training of the lower limbs for a pedal task, since the task of the hands is separated from the pedals. Care must be taken, however, not to develop some techniques that work at slow speeds or a separation of the limbs that would not be sustainable in faster or combined tasks. Accurate repetitions must

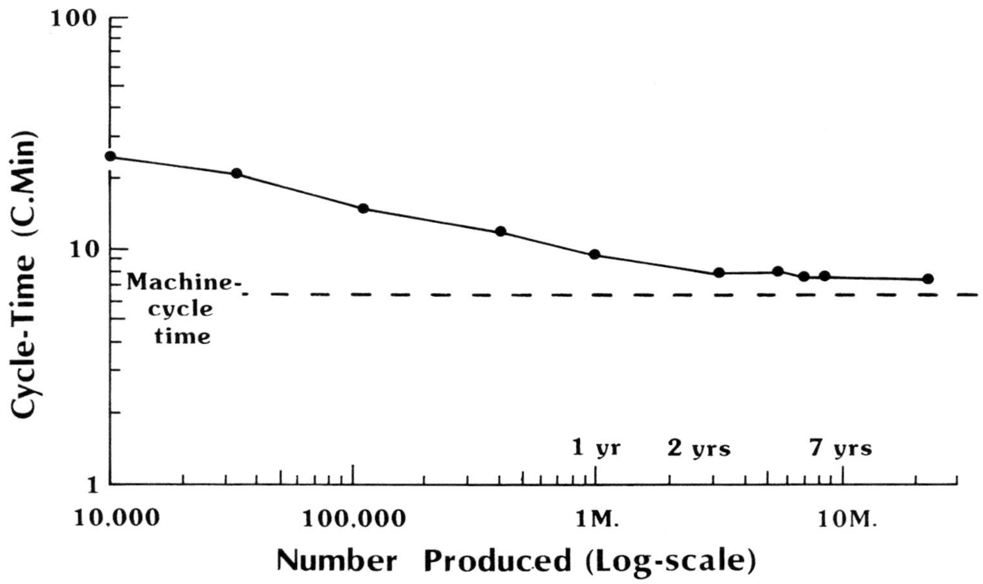

FIGURE 19–24. Practice and speed in cigar making. Each point is the average cycle time over 1 week's production for one operator. The ordinate is the total production by the operator since beginning work. (From Crossman ERFW: A theory of the acquisition of speed skill. Ergonomics 1959; 2:163–166.)

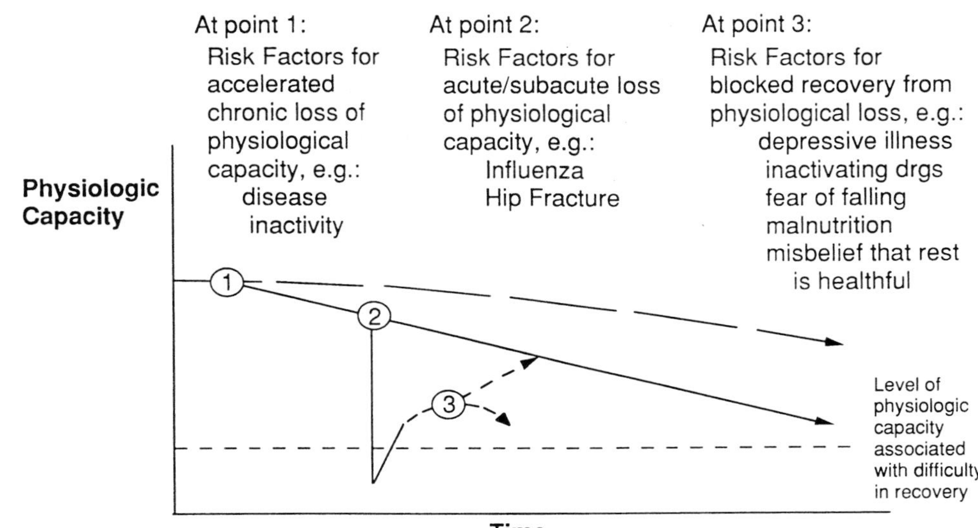

FIGURE 19–25. Conceptual model of how risk factors cause frailty. (From Buchner DM, Wagner EH: Preventing frail health. Clin Geriatr Med 1992; 8:1–17.)

be carried out until an engram is generated. A useful definition of an *engram* is a precise automatic performance implying a preprogrammed pattern.[36]

The number of repetitions required to generate an engram varies with the complexity of the task but is probably much higher than ordinarily thought. Figure 19–24 shows the gradually increasing performance of human cigar makers compared with the cigar-making machine.[15] Only with millions of repetitions does the human subject approach the machine's time as a limit. Specificity of training or practice is extremely important with highly coordinated tasks. This is the experience of musicians who go from one woodwind instrument to another or from one type of keyboard to another, such as piano to harpsichord, or mechanical action pipe organs to electropneumatic pipe organs. It is very clear that with this level of required skill, the best training for a given task is that task itself.

APPLICATIONS TO AGING

Strength Training

Evidence is accumulating that older people respond favorably to strength training.[4–8, 14, 24, 25, 41, 42] There were some data from the inferential technique of Moritani and deVries[41] that the improved performance on strength tasks of older subjects was due entirely to learning or neural factors, not to hypertrophy. However, the direct imaging used by Frontera et al showed that the muscles of older people can in fact improve their performance by hypertrophy as well as by learning.[25]

Frailty

Buchner and Wagner have defined *frailty* as "the state of reduced physiologic reserve associated with increased susceptibility to disability."[9] This is a more inclusive concept and more useful than the popular notion of frailty as thin and weak. Although those who are thin and weak are most often frail, many obese people are frail in that they have poor relative strength or strength-to-weight ratio. In either case, because of the loss of reserves, some disruption of their equilibrium by injuries or intercurrent illness might well lead to disability.

Conceptual Model of Frailty

Figure 19–25 illustrates this conceptual model. When subjects drop below a certain level they have difficulty getting back to the minimal strength or aerobic capacity required to carry out their ordinary functions or activities of daily living (ADL). Likewise, relative strength, or strength-to-weight ratio, is much more important than the absolute strength in the matter of self-perceived impairment. Figure 19–26 shows that there is a threshold of relative strength below which subjects are likely to see themselves as impaired and that this threshold is lower in older subjects (the old old) than in younger

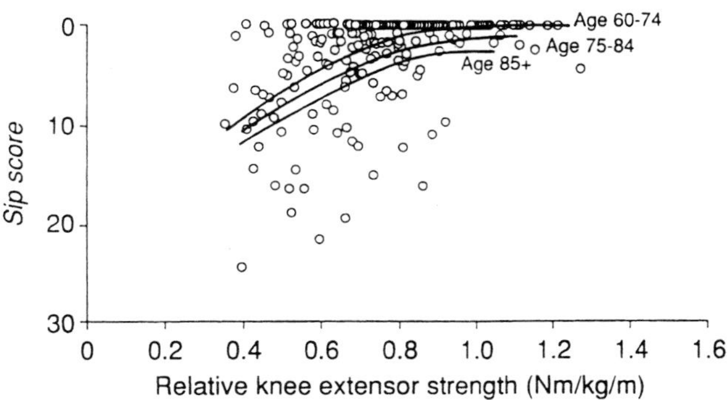

FIGURE 19–26. Relative knee extensor strength vs. Sickness Impact Profile (SIP) physical dimension score. Data are from 434 adults aged 60 years or older with only every other point plotted. The SIP scale is oriented so that higher scores, which reflect poorer function, are at the bottom. Curves were derived from polynomial regression. (From Buchner DM, de Lateur BJ: The importance of skeletal muscle strength to physical function in older adults. Ann Behav Med 1991; 13:91–98.)

geriatric subjects.[8] Strengthening muscles beyond this threshold does not yield any less perceived impairment but would lead to a greater reserve so that the individuals do not as easily slip below that threshold. There are two basic ways to improve relative strength. One is by strength training and the other is by weight reduction, especially fat reduction in the obese.

Exercise for Fat Reduction

Evidence is accumulating that the size of the fat cells is regulated in the same way that many things in the body, such as oxygen tension, carbon dioxide tension, calcium levels, blood sugar, and temperature, are regulated,[2] and that this "lipostat"[34] is high in some persons and low in others, with all gradations in between. Efforts to reduce fat by restricting caloric intake severely have only a temporary result because the body interprets this restriction as a famine, and mechanisms to defend the fat cell size over the long term are brought into play. The first line of defense is hunger. If this does not succeed in restoring the caloric intake, the next line of defense is energy conservation by decreased production of heat and a strong disinclination to exercise. People who attempt to control their weight without exercise generally have poor long-term results and tend to put on as much or more weight than they took off. In addition, when weight is lost by caloric restriction without exercise, there is some loss of muscle mass as well as fat. When the weight is put back on without exercise, it is mostly fat that is restored. The subject can wind up being more obese, in terms of percentage body fat, than at the start of the program.

Muscles are the furnaces in which fat is burned. Progressive loss of muscle makes it more and more difficult to burn off even an ordinary intake of calories. The only way to successfully live below a high set-point, that is, to reduce body fat in the face of a high set-point, is by prolonged aerobic exercise.

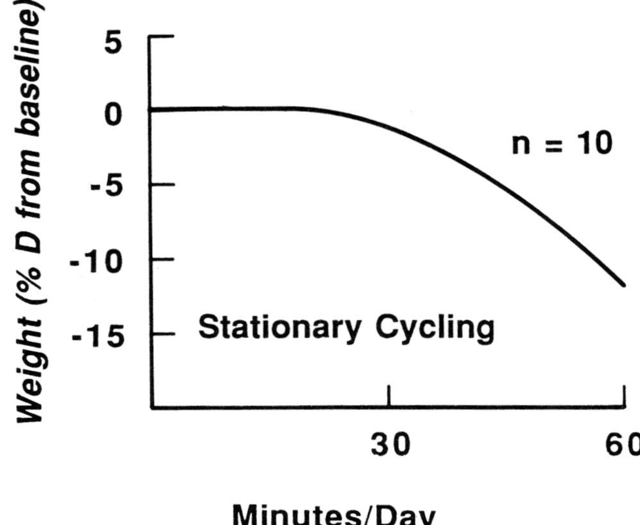

FIGURE 19–28. The relationship between percent change from baseline weight and the time spent each day in stationary cycling. (From Gwinup G: Weight loss without dietary restriction: Efficacy of different forms of aerobic exercise. Am J Sports Med 1987; 15:275–279.)

Gwinup recruited moderately obese subjects who were all long-term failures at repeated dieting, and randomly assigned them to one of three groups: (1) walking or jogging, (2) stationary bicycling, and (3) lap swimming.[31] They were exercised 7 days a week for 6 months. They were told to pay as little attention to dietary intake as they could, and no records were kept of their intake. Figures 19–27 through 19–29 show the results. The

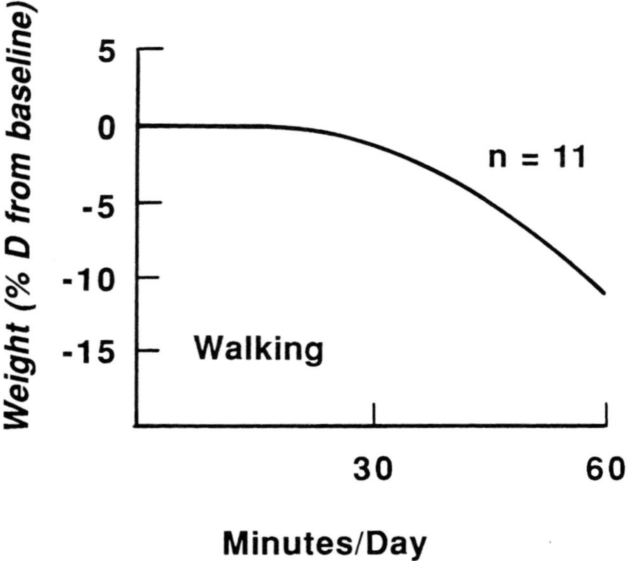

FIGURE 19–27. The relationship between percent change from baseline weight and time spent walking each day. (From Gwinup G: Weight loss without dietary restriction: Efficacy of different forms of aerobic exercise. Am J Sports Med 1987; 15:275–279.)

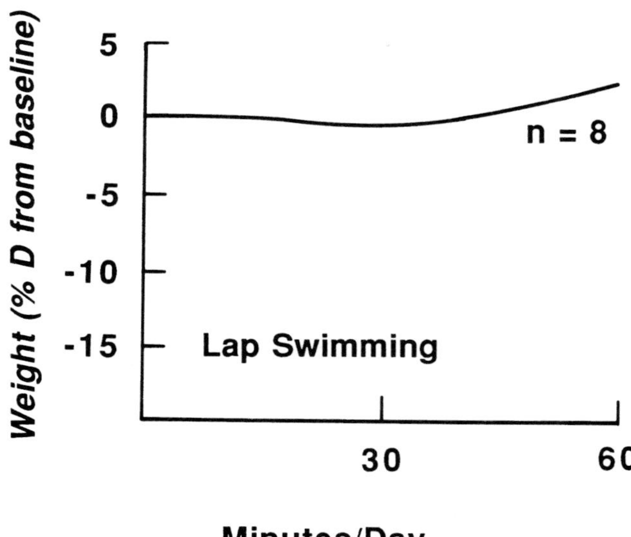

FIGURE 19–29. The relationship between percent change from baseline weight and time spent lap swimming each day. (From Gwinup G: Weight loss without dietary restriction: Efficacy of different forms of aerobic exercise. Am J Sports Med 1987; 15:275–279.)

threshold for change in body weight was 30 minutes of exercise per day. Much more marked changes were observed with 60 min/day. The stationary cyclists and walkers lost 10% to 12% of their body weight, all fat. The swimmers, who exercised 60 min/day, showed no change in their body fat, but put on approximately 10% body weight, which was all muscle. This no doubt related to their initial condition of fitness (or lack thereof). The exact numbers varied depending on greater or lesser extent of initial physical fitness. The figures do not imply that swimming cannot be useful as an adjunct to moderate caloric restriction, and in fact swimming may be the only type of exercise tolerable by those with certain disorders such as arthritis. They do imply that swimming alone is not a useful means of fat reduction.

Reaction Time

Cross-sectional studies clearly indicate that fitter is faster.[11, 12, 21, 22] Spirduso has shown for such things as simple reaction time or movement time that, although young active subjects are fastest and old sedentary subjects are slowest, old active subjects may be as fast as or slightly faster than young sedentary subjects.[44–46] This does not, however, establish cause and effect. Perhaps the quickness of some subjects makes their motor activity more pleasurable and reinforcing, and actually promotes their participation in activity, rather than the activity promoting the quickness. More research needs to be done to determine whether putting older subjects on a progressive activity or exercise program will, in fact, improve their reaction time and general quickness. This is important to determine, since quick reaction time can be important in the prevention of falls.

EQUIPMENT CONSIDERATIONS

Equipment ranges from simple resistance devices to complex electronic and compression devices available for both resistance and metabolic exercise.

Simple Resistance Training Devices

These devices fall into two basic categories: elastic resistance devices and free weights. *Elastic resistance* devices, whether they involve tension or compression, have resistance that varies with displacement. Surgical tubing is a commonly used example of an elastic resistance device. It is available in bulk and can be cut to the length needed. It has the advantage of portability, ease of use, low cost, and adaptability to a rather wide range of muscles. Such a device can even be used in the weightless environment of space. A disadvantage is the lack of feedback regarding what is done in precise terms or of the progress being made. With *free weights,* there is a similar advantage of simplicity and versatility for upper extremity use. For the lower limb, adaptations must be made such as the quadriceps boot or DeLorme boot, which is a short bar with circular weights and collar attachments with a metal plate and straps for attaching to the foot. The disadvantage is that numerous weights must be used to adapt to muscles of different strength or to the increasing strength of a given muscle. This greatly restricts the portability of such a device. Progress can be noted by counting repetitions or recording the change in the amount of weight lifted.

Complex Resistance Training Devices

The past decade has seen the development of a number of complex devices with computerized feedback systems attached. Such devices can be programmed to compare left and right sides, the quadriceps-to-hamstrings strength ratio, and other information considered of interest. Some form of feedback is of great importance, both for its cue value and for its reinforcement or reward value. One need only look at the response to the daily stock market report to see the effect of information feedback about performance.

Relatively simple mechanical devices can be very useful in strengthening some muscles that are ordinarily awkward to subject to resistance training or to give relatively uniform stress and training throughout the range of motion. An example of the former is the Elgin table, shown in Figures 19–30 and 19–31. In Figure 19–30 the subject is strengthening his hip extensors in

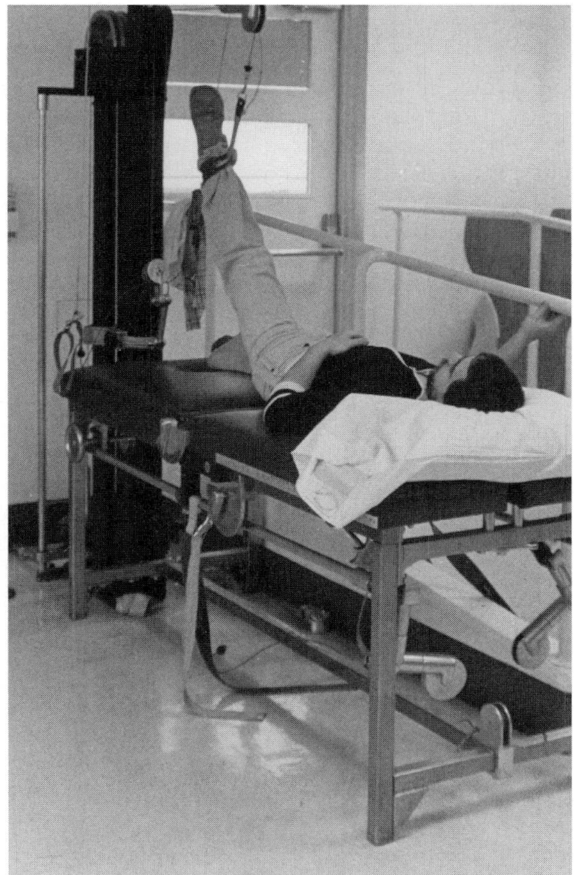

FIGURE 19–30. The Elgin table used to strengthen hip extensors in the supine position. (From de Lateur BJ, Lehmann JF: Therapeutic exercise to develop strength and endurance. In Kottke FJ, Lehmann JF (eds): Krusen's Handbook of Physical Medicine and Rehabilitation, ed 4. Philadelphia, WB Saunders, 1990.)

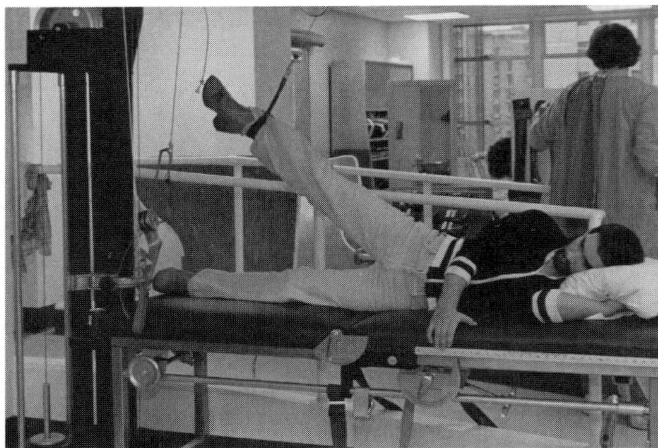

FIGURE 19–31. The Elgin table used for adductor strengthening. (From de Lateur BJ, Lehmann JF: Therapeutic exercise to develop strength and endurance. In Kottke FJ, Lehmann JF (eds): Krusen's Handbook of Physical Medicine and Rehabilitation, ed 4. Philadelphia, WB Saunders, 1990.)

the supine position. The weight-and-pulley system allows exercise throughout at least a 60 degree range, with gradations from a very mild, gravity-assisted exercise to severe progressive loading. These muscles, the hip extensors, cannot be satisfactorily trained with the subject in the prone (face down) position, since the excursion of the muscles and the joint has been used up in the extended position and the subject winds up forcibly hyperextending the lumbar spine. Likewise, the adductors are difficult to strengthen without special equipment. Figure 19–31 shows the Elgin table being used for adductor strengthening. This allows excursion of at least 45 degrees and perhaps as much as 70 degrees, again with a resistance ranging from gravity-assisted exercise (the weight does not fully counterbalance the weight of the limb) to heavy resistance.

Another simple device is the N-K table, shown in Figures 19–32 and 19–33. This has at least two advantages, namely, relative safety and ease of attaching weights. A third advantage is the ability to change the point in the range at which the muscle begins to exert substantial force. In Figure 19–32, the force arm and weight arm are parallel and not much force is required in the early part of the range. In Figure 19–33, the relative positions of the force and weight arm have been changed such that a substantial force is required even before the 90-degree flexed position is reached.

Recent years have seen the development of accommodating resistance devices that allow concentric and also allow eccentric exercise. With accommodating resistance devices, exemplified by the Cybex, Lido, Kin-Com, and Biodex, the operator presets a maximum contraction velocity. Accommodating resistance is developed when the subject attempts to accelerate the resistance arm beyond the preset limit. Passive devices such as the original Cybex and Cybex II permit only concentric training. For example, with training of the muscles about the knee, extension of the knee is produced by concentric contraction of the quadriceps and flexion is produced by concentric contraction of the hamstrings. Robotic devices allow eccentric training as well. For example, the subject attempts to accelerate the (robotically moving) resistance arm as it moves toward extension of the knee, and to decelerate (eccentrically) the resistance arm as it moves toward flexion of the knee. This allows development of different levels of force with concentric and eccentric exercise. The latter appears to be very important for hypertrophy as well as for maximum strength training. In the early phases of strength training, however, it would be safer to use an all-concentric mode.

Newer devices involving electronic programming and compressors permit the partial counterbalancing of the subject's weight to permit upper body chin-and-dip exercise for subjects whose upper body strength would not otherwise be great enough to permit these rather severe exercises. Such a device is the Gravitron, made by Stairmaster. The subject steps on the platform, turns on the device, and enters his or her accurate body weight, including the weight of the training clothes and shoes. The subject then selects a level of intensity from 1 to 17. With the lowest level, the machine counterbalances all but a small fraction of the weight. As the subject's strength increases, he or she can increase either the amount of training weight (by decreasing the amount of the body weight counterbalanced), the number of repetitions, or both, with each chin-and-dip rou-

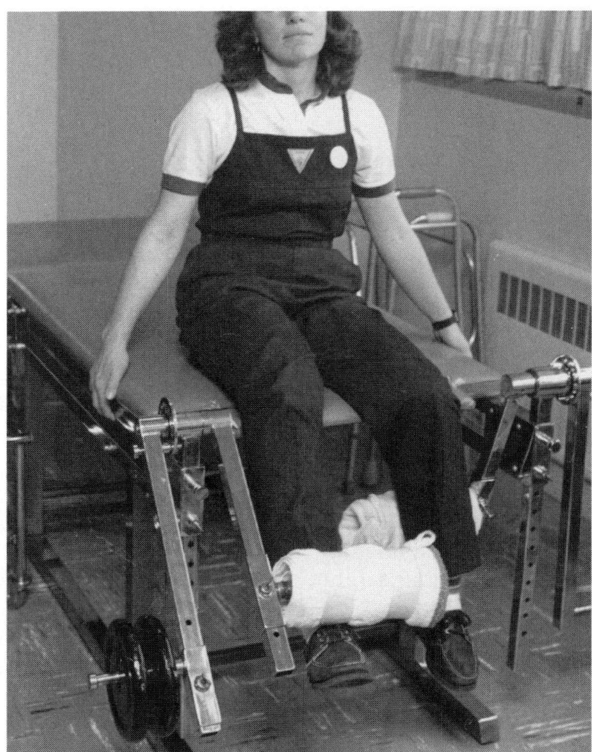

FIGURE 19–32. Little force is required when the N-K table is used with the force arm and weight arm parallel. (From de Lateur BJ, Lehmann JF: Therapeutic exercise to develop strength and endurance. In Kottke FJ, Lehmann JF (eds): Krusen's Handbook of Physical Medicine and Rehabilitation, ed 4. Philadelphia, WB Saunders, 1990.)

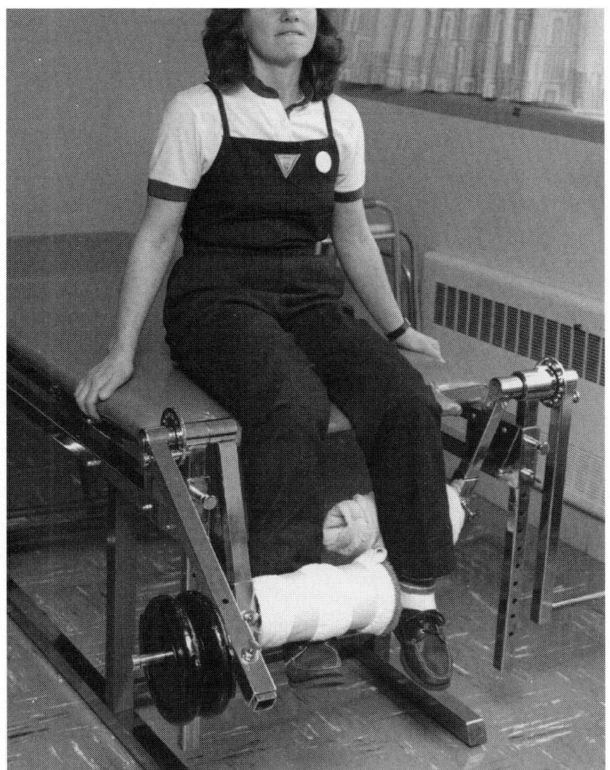

FIGURE 19–33. A substantial force is required even before the 90-degree flexed position is reached, simply by changing the positions of the force and weight arms on the N-K table. (From de Lateur BJ, Lehmann JF: Therapeutic exercise to develop strength and endurance. In Kottke FJ, Lehmann JF (eds): Krusen's Handbook of Physical Medicine and Rehabilitation, ed 4. Philadelphia, WB Saunders, 1990.)

tine. It will be valuable when such devices as these are adapted for persons who use wheelchairs.

Equipment for Metabolic Exercise

A wide range of equipment is available for metabolic exercise. Some devices are equipped with computers that estimate the number of calories expended based on body weight or typical efficiencies. Arm ergometers range from simple mechanical devices such as the Monark to the more complex electromechanical devices with attached computer software which not only give caloric readouts but also allow competition with built-in pacers. Depending on the initial state of training of the subject and the intensity of the activity, strength may be increased as well as aerobic capacity.[10] Similarly, for the lower body, one can use a simple bicycle-type attachment to a chair, or one may go to the much more complex devices made by Cybex, Lifecycle, or other devices such as the Wind Trainer. These devices may be upright or recumbent. A device that allows simultaneous or separate use of the upper and lower limbs is the Schwinn Airdyne. The lower limbs move in a circular fashion, as with any bicycle, and the upper limbs move in a forward-and-back motion as they move long levers. Resistance is provided by calibrated air-resisting paddles attached to the wheel. As with any wind resistance, the resistance is in proportion to the square of the speed. This type of device allows a very smooth aerobic employment of large numbers of muscles in a reciprocal fashion. As such, it is virtually ideal for burning fat (see Exercise for Fat Reduction).

Treadmills allow weight-bearing aerobic activity at precise speeds and grades. The subject can clip an infrared-based pulse meter to the earlobe and monitor the pulse. Speed and grade are varied to bring the heart rate into the desired range.

Finally, nonambulatory hemiparetic patients may be able to walk on the treadmill with partial body-weight support. Hesse and co-workers[34] examined the effect of just such treadmill training with partial body-weight support in nine nonambulatory hemiparetic patients who were, on the average, 129 days post stroke. Standard physical therapy carried out at least 3 weeks prior to the treadmill training did not lead to marked improvement in their gait. After 25 additional treadmill training sessions, the functional ambulation category (ranked 0 to 5) improved by an average of 2.2 points and the Rivermeade motor assessment score improved 3.9 points for gross function and 3.2 points for leg and trunk section and cycle gait parameters (significant at $P < 0.01$). During this time no significant changes were noted in strength or muscle tone of the paretic lower limb.

REFERENCES

1. Arkin AM: Absolute Muscle Power: The Internal Kinesiology of Muscle. Thesis, Department of Orthopedic Surgery, State University of Iowa, 1939.
2. Bennett W, Gurin J: The Dieter's Dilemma. New York, Basic Books, 1982.
3. Bergstom J: Muscle electrolytes in man. Scand J Clin Lab Invest 1962; 68(suppl 14):11–13.
4. Buchner DM, Cress ME, de Lateur BJ, et al: Variability in the effect of strength training on skeletal muscle strength in older adults. Facts Res Gerontol 1993; 7:143–153.
5. Buchner DM, Cress ME, de Lateur BJ, et al: The effect of strength and endurance training on gait, balance, fall risk and health services use in community living older adults. J Gerontol: Medical Sciences 1997; 52A(4):M218–M224.
6. Buchner DM, Cress ME, Wagner EH, et al: The role of exercise in fall prevention: Developing targeting criteria for exercise programs. In Vellas B, Troupet M, Rubenstein L, et al (eds): Falls, Balance and Gait Disorders in the Elderly. Amsterdam, Elsevier, 1992.
7. Buchner DM, Cress ME, Wagner EH, et al: The Seattle FICSIT/MoveIt Study: The effect of exercise on gait and balance in older adults. J Am Geriatr Soc 1993; 41:321–325.
8. Buchner DM, de Lateur BJ: The importance of skeletal muscle strength to physical function in older adults. Ann Behav Med 1991; 13:91–98.
9. Buchner DM, Wagner EH: Preventing frail health. Health Promotion Dis Prev 1992; 8:17.
10. Clarke DH, Stull GA: Endurance training as a determinant of strength and fatigability. Res Q 1970; 41:19–26.
11. Clarkson PM, Kroll W: Practice effects on fractionated response time related to age and activity level. J Motor Behav 1978; 10:275–286.
12. Clarkson-Smith L, Hartley AA: Relationships between physical exercise and cognitive abilities in older adults. Psychol Aging 1989; 4:183–189.
13. Côté C, Simoneau J-A, Lagassé P, et al: Isokinetic strength training protocols: Do they induce skeletal muscle fiber hypertrophy? Arch Phys Med Rehabil 1988; 69:281–285.

14. Cress ME, Essleman PC, de Lateur BJ, et al: Lower limb strength predicts $\dot{V}O_{2max}$ in frail elderly. Med Sci Sports Exerc 1992; 24(suppl 5):S15.
15. Crossman ERFW: A theory of the acquisition of speed-skill. Ergonomics 1959; 2:153–166.
16. de Lateur BJ, Lehmann JF: Therapeutic exercise to develop strength and endurance. In Kottke FJ, Lehmann JF (eds): Krusen's Handbook of Physical Medicine and Rehabilitation, ed 4. Philadelphia, WB Saunders, 1990, p 512.
17. de Lateur BJ, Lehmann JF, Fordyce WE: A test of the DeLorme axiom. Arch Phys Med Rehabil 1968; 49:245–248.
18. de Lateur BJ, Lehmann JF, Stonebridge JB, et al: Isotonic versus isometric exercise: A double-shift, transfer-of-training study. Arch Phys Med Rehabil 1972; 53:212–217.
19. DeLorme TL: Restoration of muscle power by heavy-resistance exercises. J Bone Joint Surg Am 1945; 27:645–667.
20. DeLorme TL, Watkins AL: Progressive Resistance Exercise. East Norwalk, CT, Appleton-Century-Crofts, 1951.
21. Dustman RE, Emmerson RY, Ruhling RO, et al: Age and fitness effects on EEG, ERPs, visual sensitivity, and cognition. Neurobiol Aging 1990; 11:193–200.
22. Engle VF: The relationship of movement and time to older adults' functional health. Res Nurs Health 1986; 9:123–129.
23. Esselman PC, de Lateur BJ, Alquist AD, et al: Torque development in isokinetic training. Arch Phys Med Rehabil 1991; 72:723–728 [erratum, p 970].
24. Fiatarone MA, O'Neill EF, Ryan ND, et al: Exercise training and nutritional supplementation for physical frailty in very elderly people. N Engl J Med 1994; 330:1819–1820.
25. Frontera WR, Meredith CN, O'Reilly KP, et al: Strength conditioning in older men: Skeletal muscle hypertrophy and improved function. J Appl Physiol 1988; 64:1038–1044.
26. Gollnick PD, Armstrong RB, Saltin B, et al: Effect of training on enzyme activity and fiber composition of human skeletal muscle. J Appl Physiol 1973; 34:107–111.
27. Gollnick PD, Armstrong RB, Saubert CW IV, et al: Enzyme activity and fiber composition in skeletal muscle of untrained and trained men. J Appl Physiol 1972; 33:312–319.
28. Gollnick PD, Karlsson J, Piehl K, et al: Selective glycogen depletion in skeletal muscle fibres of man following sustained contractions. J Physiol 1974; 241:59–67.
29. Gonyea WJ, Sale DG, Gonyea FB, et al: Exercise induced increased in muscle fiber number. Eur J Appl Physiol 1986; 55:137–141.
30. Gordon EE, Kowalski K, Fritts M: Protein changes in quadriceps muscle of rat with repetitive exercises. Arch Phys Med Rehabil 1967; 48:296–303.
31. Gwinup G: Weight loss without dietary restriction: Efficacy of different forms of aerobic exercise. Am J Sports Med 1987; 15:275–279.
32. Hellebrandt FA, Houtz SJ: Methods of muscle training: The influence of pacing. Phys Ther Rev 1958; 38:319–322.
33. Henneman E: Peripheral mechanisms involved in the control of muscle. In Mountcastle VB (ed): Medical Physiology, ed 13. St Louis, Mosby–Year Book, 1974.
34. Hesse S, Bertelt C, Schaffrin A, et al: Restoration of gait in nonambulatory hemiparetic patients by treadmill training with partial body-weight support. Arch Phys Med Rehabil 1994; 75:1087–1093.
35. Kennedy GC: The role of depot fat in the hypothalamic control of food intake in the rat. Proc R Soc Lond Biol 1953; 14:579–592.
36. Kottke FJ, Halpern D, Easton JKM, et al: The training of coordination. Arch Phys Med Rehabil 1978; 59:567–572.
37. Lacerte M: Effects of Concentric versus Combined Concentric-Eccentric Isokinetic Training Programs on Peak Torque and Hypertrophy of Human Quadriceps Femoris Muscle. Thesis, University of Washington, Seattle, 1989.
38. Lacerte M, de Lateur BJ, Alquist AD, et al: Effects of concentric versus combined concentric-eccentric isokinetic training programs on peak torque of human quadriceps femoris muscle. Arch Phys Med Rehabil 1992; 73:1059–1062.
39. Milner-Brown HS, Stein RB, Lee RG: Synchronization of human motor units: Possible role of exercise and supraspinal reflexes. EEG Clin Neurophysiol 1975; 38:245–254.
40. Moritani T, deVries HA: Neural factors versus hypertrophy in the time course of muscle strength gain. Am J Phys Med 1979; 58:115–130.
41. Moritani T, deVries HA: Potential for gross muscle hypertrophy in older men. J Gerontol 1980; 35:672–682.
42. Morris-Chatta R, Buchner DM, de Lateur BJ, et al: Isokinetic testing of ankle strength in older adults: Assessment of inter-rater reliability and of stability of strength over six months. Arch Phys Med Rehabil 1994; 75:1213–1216.
43. Mundale MO: The relationship of intermittent isometric exercise to fatigue of hand grip. Arch Phys Med Rehabil 1970; 51:532–539.
44. Spirduso WW: Physical fitness, aging and psychomotor speed: A review. J Gerontol 1980; 35:850–865.
45. Spirduso WW: Reaction and movement time as a function of age and physical activity level. J Gerontol 1975; 30:435–440.
46. Spirduso WW, Clifford P: Replication of age and physical activity effects on reaction and movement time. J Gerontol 1978; 33:26–30.
47. Stull GA, Clarke DH: High-resistance, low-repetition training as a determiner of strength and fatigability. Res Q 1970; 41:189–193.
48. Von Recklinghausen H: Gliedermechanik und Lähmungsprothesen. Berlin, Springer-Verlag, 1920.
49. Zinovieff AN: Heavy-resistance exercises: The "Oxford" technique. Br J Phys Med 1951; 14:129–132.

20 CHAPTER

James W. Atchison, D.O., Scott T. Stoll, D.O., Ph.D., and Ann Cotter, M.D.

Manipulation, Traction, and Massage

In recent years, spinal care for back and neck disorders has moved toward an "aggressive" conservative (nonoperative) approach. There has been growth in comprehensive treatment programs utilizing multidisciplinary teams and many treatment modalities. This nonoperative trend in spinal care has increasingly emphasized the traditional physical therapeutic interventions (heat, cold, exercise, traction, and massage). "Complementary or alternative" interventions such as manipulation, acupuncture, and mind-body have also gained popularity. Also emerging within our present medical system is the trend of identifying cost-effective treatment options. Physiatrists should be well versed in the medical indications and contraindications for all nonoperative spine treatment options, whether or not they perform them themselves.

Well trained in the "functional approach" to a patient, the physiatrist typically has the added advantage of working as part of a team of health professionals, each assisting in therapeutic interventions. Physiatrists are ideally suited to provide efficient and cost-effective musculoskeletal care with conservative treatment such as heat/cold modalities, exercise, manipulation, traction, massage, acupuncture, or mind-body.

MANUAL MEDICINE

Manipulation: Definition and Goal

The International Federation of Manual Medicine[161] defines *manipulation* as "the use of the hands in the patient management process using instructions and maneuvers to maintain maximal, painless movement of the musculoskeletal system in postural balance." The goal of manipulation or manual medicine is to help maintain optimal body mechanics and to improve motion in restricted areas, thus enhancing maximal, pain-free movement in postural balance and optimizing function.[42, 69, 138] This is accomplished by treatments that attempt to restore the mechanical function of a joint and normalize altered reflex patterns,[105, 111, 138] as evidenced by optimum range of motion, body symmetry, and tissue texture. The indications for and success of manual medicine techniques are determined by structural evaluation before and after treatment.[69, 105, 138]

Manual medicine can involve manipulation of both spinal and peripheral joints, although lately spinal manipulation has received the most attention. The indications for the use of manual medicine are based, in part, on the theories of how manual medicine works, and include: (1) restoration of normality and symmetry at either the disc or facet level[36, 84, 92]; (2) mechanically restoring optimal muscular and myofascial range and ease of motion, thereby restoring function[110]; (3) therapy-induced reduction of afferent signal transmission to the cord, thereby diminishing pain awareness through a gate theory effect[105, 110, 111]; (4) endorphin release, which increases the pain threshold or reduces pain severity[68, 92, 111]; or (5) placebo effect.[55] Selection of a particular manipulative treatment is based on the pathology encountered and the theoretical mechanism of action of each treatment model.

The effectiveness and risks of manual medicine have been and continue to be controversial. As with most other forms of conservative treatment for spinal pain syndromes, randomized controlled studies to determine long-term benefit are not available. Studies that are available have been limited by the variability of the clinical source and duration of the pain, the variety of manual medicine techniques utilized, the difficulty of blinding treatments, and the lack of widely accepted or validated outcome measures.[12, 13, 54, 64, 75, 77, 87, 123, 129, 169, 180, 196, 197]

There have been several recent reviews[1, 4, 6, 93, 107, 164] of manual medicine studies indicating effectiveness in certain subpopulations, especially in persons with low back pain of 2 to 4 weeks' duration.[77, 123] These reports contributed to the support for their use in *Guidelines for Acute Low Back Problems* by the Agency for Health Care Policy and Research (AHCPR).[3] There are no current guidelines for treatment regimens regarding the cervical or thoracic spine, but several studies support the use of manipulation in these areas.[23, 75, 93] Manual medicine continues to be widely practiced and is in high demand by patients,[46] as evidenced by the estimated 12 to 17.6 million Americans[148, 152] receiving manipulations each year with a high degree of patient satisfaction.[24]

History

Manual medicine has regained popularity over the past 30 to 40 years, but it dates back to the time of Hippocrates (*fl.* 460–377 BCE), Galen (*fl.* 131–202 CE), and Ambroise Pare (1510–1590 CE).[78, 83] Many other physicians (e.g., Sydenham, Hahnemann, Boerhaave, Shultes) deviated from the traditional disease-oriented form of medicine during the 16th and 17th centuries,[83] but manual medicine fell out of favor until the 19th century. The pioneers of manual medicine at that time included the "bonesetters" of England (Richard Hutton, Wharton Hood, Sir Herbert Baker),[20, 83] Andrew Taylor Still, the founder of osteopathic medicine in 1874,[69] and Daniel David Palmer, the founder of chiropractic in 1895.[69, 83]

Still's philosophy stressed wellness and wholeness of the body and included: (1) the unity of the body—all systems depend upon and influence all other systems; (2) the body's natural ability for self-healing; (3) the somatic component of disease; (4) the interrelationship of structure and function; and (5) the use of manipulative therapy.[69, 83] His use of manual medicine was based not only on restoration and maintenance of the structural-functional relationship within the musculoskeletal system, but also the neural-hormonal relationship with all other systems.

"Traditional" medical professionals have also shown interest in manual medicine. James Mennell[130] and his son John McM. Mennell,[131] as well as Edgar and James Cyriax,[36] have espoused the use of joint manipulation within the British medical community. Beginning in the 1940s, James Cyriax, a British orthopedic surgeon, published several works related to manipulation, incorporating massage, traction, and injections[36] in the treatment programs. His books are still used today as reference texts for injections, but his use of manual medicine has not been as widely accepted. Travell's[179] use of manual techniques for examination purposes has been well accepted. This section on manual medicine is intended as a brief introduction to these techniques and others, which are widely used throughout the world.

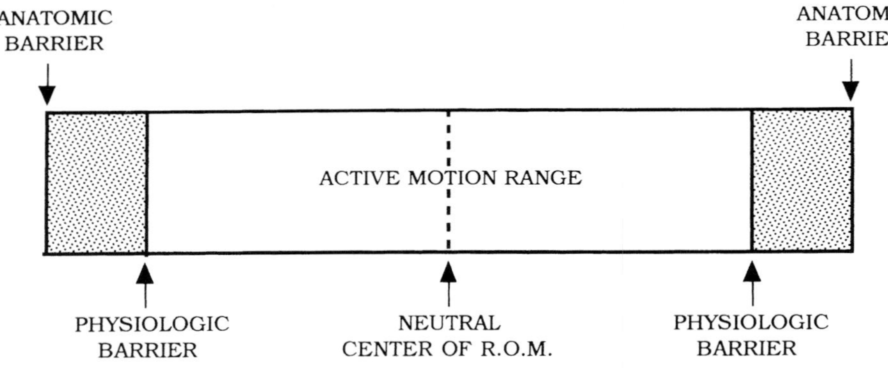

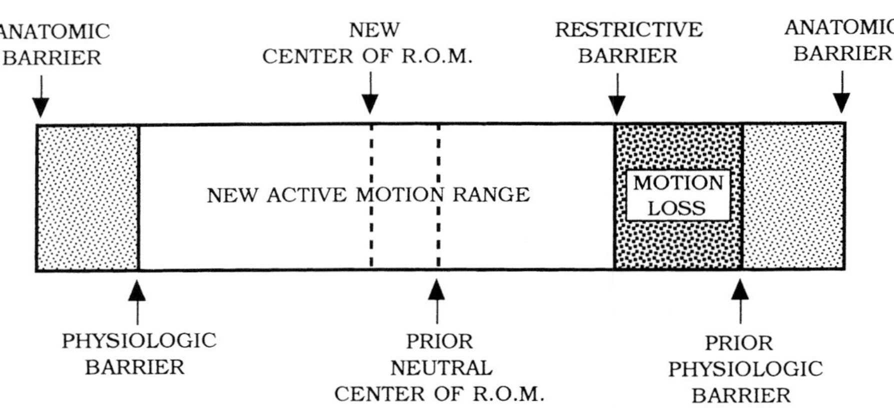

FIGURE 20–1. The barrier concept for normal joint motion (*top*) and with somatic dysfunction (*bottom*). All joints have an optimal range of motion with a physiological and an anatomical barrier at each end. A restrictive barrier causes motion loss and establishes a new center to the active range of motion. This shift in neutral positioning aids in the diagnosis of somatic dysfunction. (From Kimberly PE: Formulating a prescription for osteopathic manipulative treatment. J Am Osteopath Assoc 1980; 79:508.)

Nomenclature

One of the problems in learning and teaching manual medicine lies in understanding exactly what is being manipulated. Over the years, the nomenclature for the musculoskeletal pathology or "manipulable lesion" has repeatedly changed. At present, it is labeled "somatic dysfunction," while previous terms include osteopathic lesion, subluxation, joint blockage, loss of joint play, and joint dysfunction.[110, 111, 138]

Somatic dysfunction is defined as impaired or altered function of related components of the somatic (body framework) system; skeletal, arthrodial, and myofascial structures; and related vascular, lymphatic, and neural elements.[69, 138] Somatic dysfunction is manifested as *t*enderness, structural *a*symmetry, altered *r*ange of motion, and *t*issue texture changes (TART). There can be decreased mobility at any point along the physiological range of motion of any joint[15, 69, 105] (Fig. 20–1). Joint play[69, 78] is usually decreased and there is muscle contraction or tissue texture changes associated with the restricted joint. Early findings can include vasodilation, edema, pain, and tenderness; and, chronically, fibrosis, paresthesia, itching, and persistent tenderness are often present. These findings are generally asymmetrical. Moreover, there can be other reflex effects on the function of tissues that are innervated from the same spinal segmental level as the somatic dysfunction.[68, 105, 110, 111]

Manipulation has traditionally been equated with the high-velocity/thrusting techniques; currently, however, manipulative methods encompass a broad range of techniques. They have historically ranged from the "barbaric" stretching techniques of Hippocrates[83] to Cyriax's combinations,[36] Mitchell's use of muscle forces[133, 134] (see Figs. 20–2, 20–3), and Jones's passive positioning techniques.[17, 26, 98] In the European literature the term *mobilization* means only thrusting procedures. In the U.S. literature, however, manipulation encompasses mobilization techniques—techniques that utilize thrusting (high-velocity, low-amplitude, or mobilization with impulse) forces (see Figs. 20–2, 20–4, 20–5, 20–6)—together with many other nonthrusting procedures, as listed in Table 20–1.

Indications and Goals of Treatment

Manual medicine techniques are potentially useful for treatment of any musculoskeletal problem demonstrating somatic dysfunction. This can include many specific conditions, including acute and chronic cervical pain,[10, 23, 68, 75, 93, 108, 157] thoracic pain,[55, 68, 125, 126] rib pain,[68, 125] functional and mechanical low back pain,[13, 47, 55, 77, 87, 107, 123, 124, 126, 129] chronic low back pain,[1, 13, 87, 108, 129, 180] bulging intervertebral disc,[35, 36, 125, 142] facet syndrome,[39, 98] piriformis syndrome,[22, 69, 98] sciatica,[45, 124, 142, 151] headaches,[55, 124, 125, 160, 172, 183, 189] and sacroiliac syndromes.[55, 69, 71, 76, 78, 98, 126, 196]

The assessment for somatic dysfunction starts with a history and physical examination that includes a careful neuromusculoskeletal examination. This is followed by a detailed structural evaluation, which incorporates observation, palpation, and segmental motion testing (see Fig. 20–7). The structural examination requires sophisticated palpatory skills to assess for tenderness, body asymmetry, altered range of motion, and tissue texture changes (see Greenman's 12-step screen[69]; Table 20–2). Tissue texture changes are assessed by observation and palpation of the tissues, from the most superficial tissues down to bony prominences. Muscle, tendon, and fascia can show signs of vasodilation, edema, flaccidity, contraction, and or contracture. Musculoskeletal asymmetry can appear as structural or functional asymmetry or both. The examiner should observe for asymmetrical joint range of motion, tenderness, strength, posture, positioning, or muscle tone. This complex evaluation is designed to distinguish multilevel versus segmental abnormalities and to determine whether dysfunction is due to hypomobility or hypermobility.

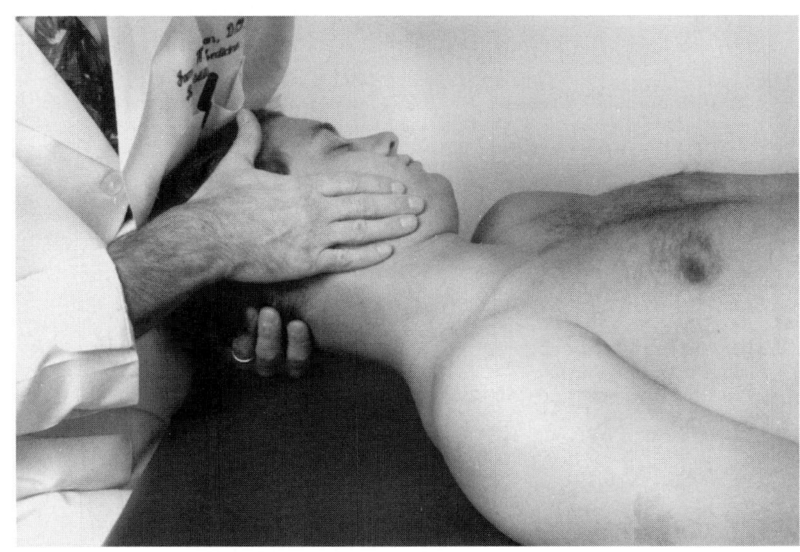

FIGURE 20–2. Hand placement for high-velocity/low-amplitude (HVLA) or muscle energy (ME) treatment for the cervical spine with left rotation dysfunction. For muscle energy, the right thumb is resisting the patients' attempts to rotate the head toward the right (midline). The more cephalad the dysfunction, the more the cervical spine is concomitantly flexed. For HVLA, the thrust is provided by the thumb and the metacarpophalangeal area of the index finger (right hand) through the transverse process being contacted to induce rotation and sidebending. With high cervical dysfunction the opposite (left) hand provides distraction prior to the thrust.

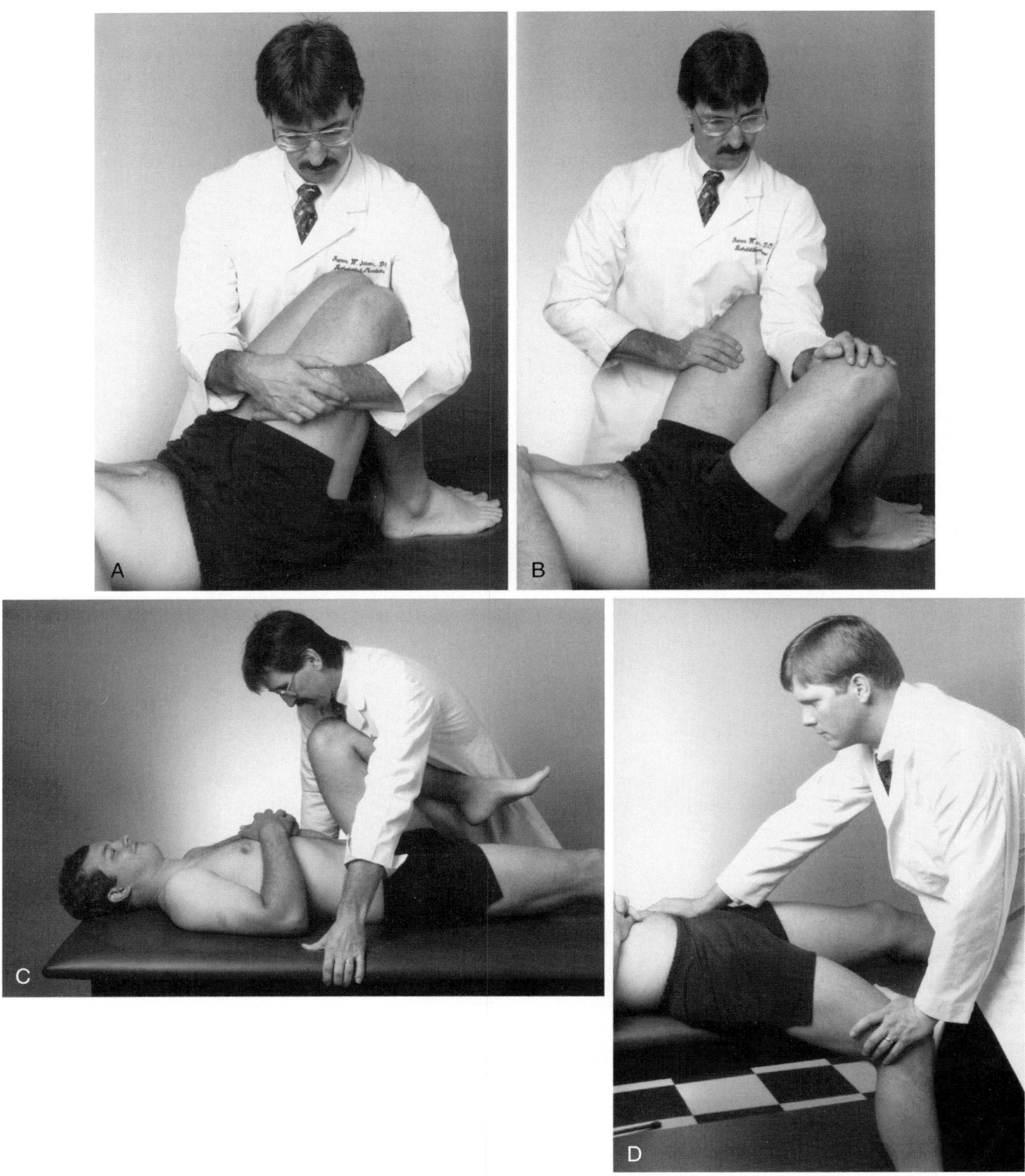

FIGURE 20–3. Muscle energy treatment for the sacroiliac joint may include: (*A*) supine, resisted abduction (both hips): (*B*) supine, resisted adduction (both hips); (*C*) supine, resisted extension (left hip); (*D*) supine, resisted flexion (right hip). These maneuvers are use in varying combinations, depending on the patients structural examination findings.

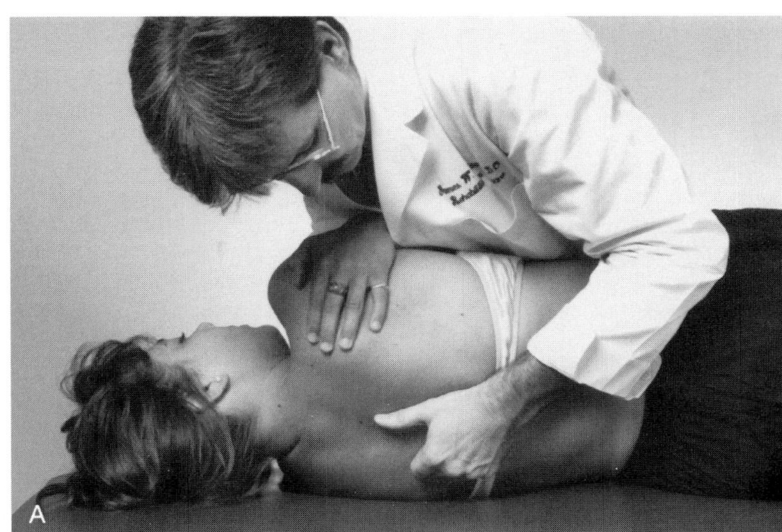

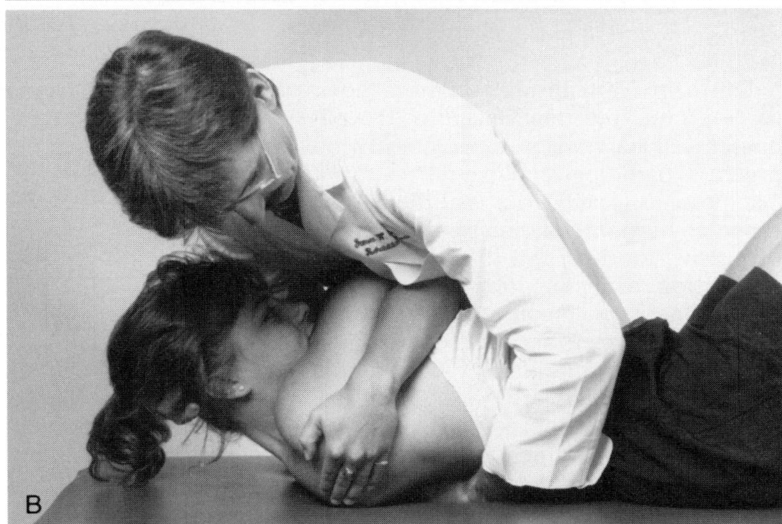

FIGURE 20–4. High-velocity/low-amplitude treatment (crossed-arm technique) for the thoracic spine in a supine position. *A.* The hand is placed with the thenar eminence contacting the transverse process of the dysfunctional vertebrae. *B.* The force is then directed to the hand by thrusting through the patient ipsilateral (right) arm.

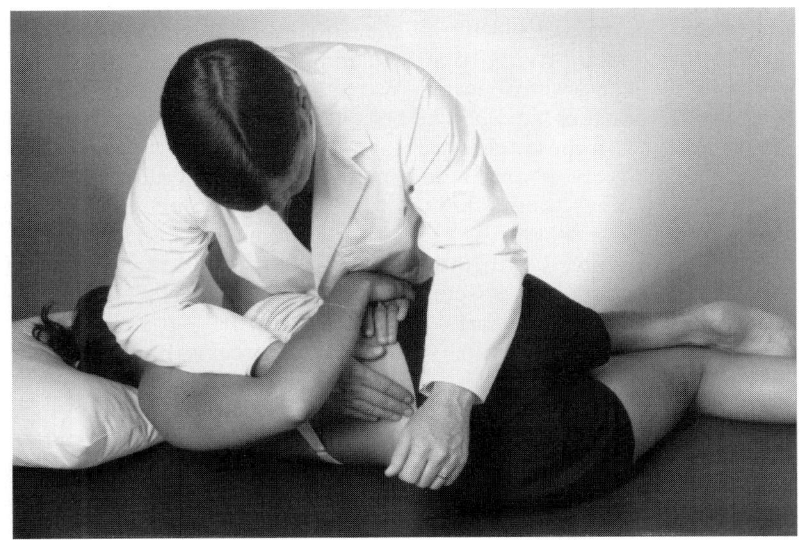

FIGURE 20–5. High-velocity/low-amplitude treatment for the lumbar spine with rotatory thrusting. The patient is positioned below the level of dysfunction in flexion, left rotation, and right sidebending, and above the level in extension, right rotation, and left sidebending. The practitioner thrusts by dropping his shoulders and forcing the patient's shoulder toward the table and the hip toward himself.

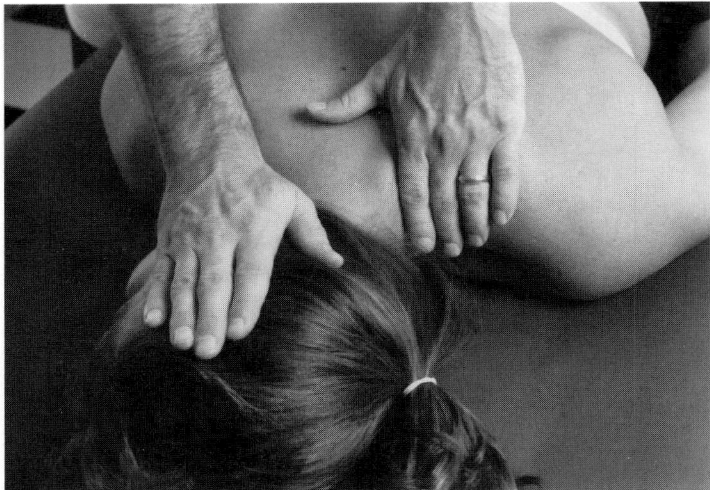

FIGURE 20–6. High-velocity/low-amplitude treatment for elevated first rib on the left. In the supine position, the head is rotated right to allow the right hand thrust to induce distraction, while the left hand thrusts caudally and toward the midline.

During the structural evaluation, the practitioner tries to determine the relationship of the physiological and anatomical barriers to movement, while assessing for potential pathological barriers[15, 69, 105, 138](see Fig. 20–1). The physiological barrier is at the end of normal, active range of motion. The anatomical barrier is at the end of passive motion, and if exceeded, leads to fracture, dislocation, or ligamentous damage. There is a normal feel of increasing resistance as the physiological and anatomical barriers are approached. A pathological barrier limits the usual range of motion or alters the ability of the tissues to perform throughout the usual range of motion, and is evidence of dysfunction.[68, 105]

Because it is possible to find some evidence of somatic dysfunction in asymptomatic persons[38] and multiple areas in acutely ill patients,[68] the practitioner must determine the clinical significance of each area of dysfunction and decide which areas require treatment.[105] A complete structural evaluation of all areas of the body (see Table 20–2) is necessary to establish a diagnosis, to differentiate primary from secondary areas of dysfunction, and to determine the appropriate treatment technique(s) that can be applied[15, 69, 105, 138, 144] (see Fig. 20–7). There is no indication for manipulation if there is no structural evidence of somatic dysfunction.[105, 138]

TABLE 20–1 Manual Medicine Techniques

Thrusting
Mobilization with impulse/high-velocity, low-amplitude
Nonthrusting
Mobilization without impulse/articulatory technique
Muscle energy
Counterstrain
Functional technique
Myofascial release
Soft tissue
Craniosacral

Classification of Manual Medicine Techniques

Manual medicine encompasses many different types of treatment techniques. Classification regimens include (1) the type of procedure (thrusting or non-thrusting); (2) the type of force utilized (intrinsic or extrinsic); (3) the patient contribution to the force (active or passive); and (4) the type of movement approach to the pathological barrier (direct or indirect).[54, 68, 97] The effects of these different techniques are classified by five basic theoretical models of interaction with the body: (1) postural-structural or biomechanical,[68, 69] (2) neurological,[68, 92, 111] (3) respiratory-circulatory,[68, 92, 132, 138] (4) bioenergy,[92, 113, 172, 183, 198] and (5) behavioral-psychosocial.[25, 68, 92, 167] Each of the various treatment techniques involves combinations of the models to explain the benefits and effects of the procedure.

When considering manipulative treatment options in a patient, the type of activating treatment force involved can be extrinsic or intrinsic. *Extrinsic forces*[15, 68, 105] are applied from the outside of the body and can be provided by gravity, straps, and pads or by another person. The practitioner can use a thrusting, springing, or guiding technique.[69] The patient is usually passively involved with these techniques. *Intrinsic forces*[68, 105] occur within a person's body and include muscle forces, respiratory forces, and inherent forces, such as fluctuating body fluid pressures.[69] Patients are considered to be actively involved with these treatments if they are consciously contracting specific muscle groups or performing respiratory sequences.

The direction of treatment force is related to the barrier concept (see Fig. 20–1). *Direct methods*[68, 69, 105, 138] involve moving the patient toward the pathological barrier or in the direction of increasing resistance. Once the barrier has been engaged, a force is applied to move through the pathological barrier toward the normal physiological or anatomical barrier (see Figs.

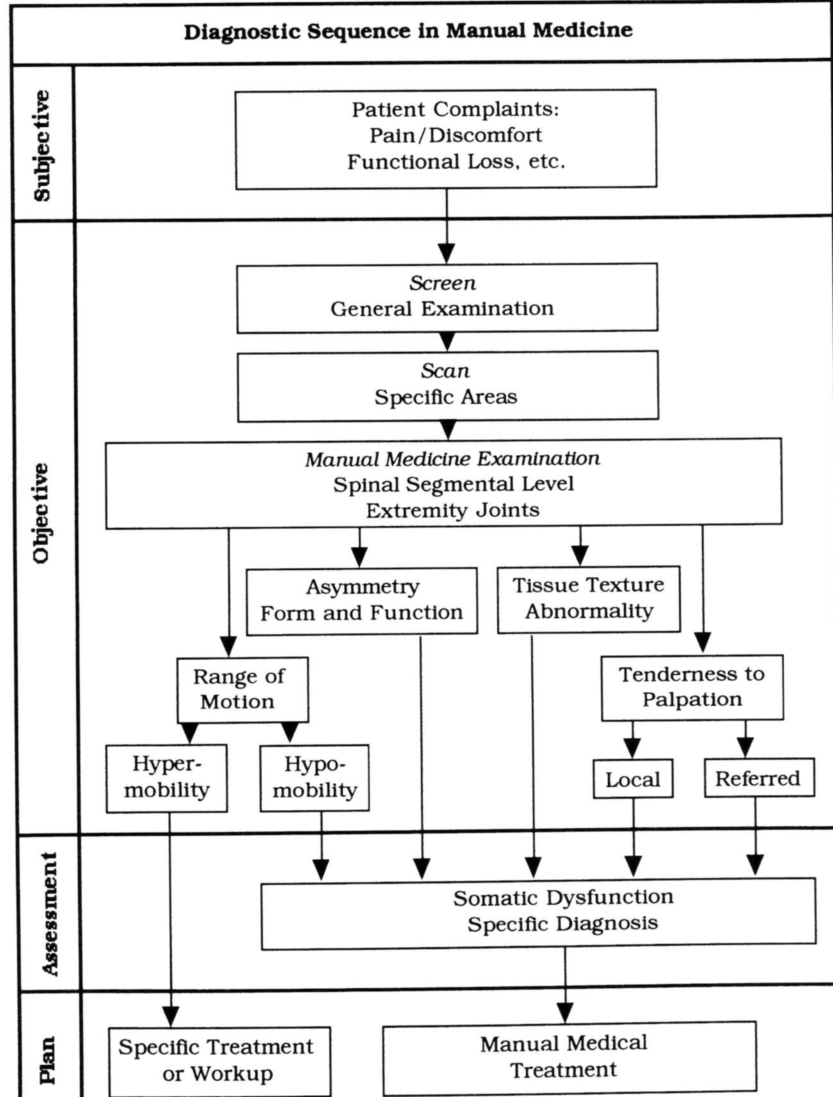

FIGURE 20–7. The diagnostic sequence in manual medicine. The general and/or specific examinations reveal objective changes that help to establish the diagnosis of a specific somatic dysfunction and plan the appropriate treatment. (Modified from Neumann H-D: Introduction to Manual Medicine. Berlin, Springer-Verlag, 1989, p 14.)

TABLE 20–2 Twelve Step Screening Examination

Step	
Step 1.	Gait analysis in multiple directions
Step 2.	Observation of static posture and palpable assessment of paired anatomical landmarks
Step 3.	Dynamic trunk sidebending
Step 4.	Standing flexion test
Step 5.	Stork test
Step 6.	Seated flexion test
Step 7.	Screening test of upper extremities
Step 8.	Trunk rotation
Step 9.	Trunk sidebending
Step 10.	Head and neck mobility
Step 11.	Respiration of thoracic cage
Step 12.	Lower extremity screening

From Greenman PE: Principles of Manual Medicine, ed 2. Baltimore, Williams & Wilkins, 1996, p 18.

20–2, 20–3, 20–4, 20–5, 20–6). All mobilization techniques (with or without impulse) use direct methods, as do some types of soft tissue, muscle energy, and myofascial release treatments. *Indirect methods*[68, 69, 105, 138] involve movement of the patient or segment in the direction of least resistance, away from the pathological barrier. This allows the body's inherent and muscle energy forces to enhance mobility, permitting changes in the relationship between the position of the pathological barrier and the normal physiological barrier. Counterstrain, functional indirect, myofascial release, and craniosacral techniques are most often utilized. Often, *combined methods*[68, 69] are used. *Physiological response methods,*[68, 69, 92, 105, 138] such as respiratory assistance or exaggerated movements, can also be involved with both direct and indirect techniques. These are activities performed by the patient which increase the effect of the simultaneous practitioner-directed techniques.

Specific Types of Manual Medicine Techniques

Mobilization with Impulse. Mobilization with impulse is more commonly known as the thrust maneuver[84] or the high-velocity/low-amplitude (HVLA) form of manual medicine. This is a direct form of treatment, and is commonly prescribed for cervical[15, 19, 23, 36, 59, 93, 108, 149] (see Fig. 20–2), thoracic[36, 59, 69] (see Fig. 20–4), lumbar[13, 15, 36, 54, 59, 64, 69, 77, 87, 107, 109, 123, 129, 152, 164, 169] (Fig. 20–5), rib[15, 59, 69, 124] (Fig. 20–6), sacroiliac,[15, 36, 55, 59, 69, 76, 124] (see Fig. 20–3), and extremity[15, 36, 69, 124] dysfunctions. These are the techniques most commonly associated with the term manipulation. They are frequently performed because they offer the quickest mode of releasing a dysfunctional segment or region. Often, a "crack" or "pop" occurs when a restricted joint is released.[18] In itself, this noise has no effect on the treatment outcome; rather, the treatment benefit lies in the reintroduction of movement into the restricted or dysfunctional area.[84]

The preparation of the patient for HVLA is as important as the thrust itself.[69, 84, 138] The more precise the localization by positioning, the more directed the treatment and the less thrusting force necessary. High thrusting forces should be avoided to prevent possible injury to the neighboring soft tissue or joints. After localizing and engaging the barrier, there is a momentary waiting period to allow the patient to relax the muscles in the area. During this time, the practitioner monitors the patient's respiratory cycle, then delivers the treatment thrust at the point of deepest exhalation. This allows maximal relaxation of the surrounding muscles. The force of the thrust varies with the location of the treatment, with cervical requiring the least and thoracic the greatest force.[85] The duration of the thrust is very short, less than 0.5 sec.[178] Immediate relief of pain symptoms might not occur, but an improvement in the range of motion of the treated joint should occur.

The patient has to be relaxed to get maximal effectiveness. Tightening of the muscles or "guarding" can limit the amount of movement resulting from the thrust and increase the amount of thrusting force required. Treatment should always be provided in a pain-free direction, enhancing relaxation and avoiding guarding. Somatic dysfunction rarely restricts movement along all planes simultaneously.[138] If a patient cannot be positioned without exacerbating pain in any of the three planes (flexion-extension, sidebending, rotation), it is likely that the pain or restriction arises from a source other than somatic dysfunction[78] (e.g., inflammatory or destructive process; see Table 20–3), in which case thrusting should not be performed.

The following techniques have fewer contraindications and require less training to perform safely, but are more time-consuming than HVLA techniques.

Articulatory Technique. Articulatory technique,[69, 138] or mobilization without impulse, is a direct segmental technique popularized by Maitland.[126, 127] In this technique, a combination of leverage, patient ventilatory movement, and a fulcrum is used to achieve mobilization of the dysfunctional segment. This is most often done by repeatedly applying a low-velocity/high-amplitude force to engage the barrier directly, then move away from it.[143] This repeated "tapping" on the barrier is designed to move the pathological barrier gently toward the physiological barrier (see Fig. 20–1), improving the range of motion. This is the graded oscillation form of the technique. Less commonly, a progressive or sustained-loading technique is used.[144] These procedures can be used as an extension of the diagnostic evaluation for range of motion, and can be combined with soft tissue or thrust techniques.[69]

TABLE 20–3 Contraindications for High-Velocity Manipulation Techniques

Unstable fractures
Severe osteoporosis
Multiple myeloma
Osteomyelitis
Primary bone tumors
Paget's disease
Any progressive neurological deficit
Spinal cord tumors
Cauda equina compression
Central cervical intervertebral disc herniation
Hypermobile joints
Rheumatoid arthritis
Inflammatory phase of ankylosing spondylitis
Psoriatic arthritis
Reiter's syndrome
Anticoagulant therapy
Congenital bleeding disorder
Acquired bleeding disorder
Inadequate physical and spinal examination
Poor manipulative skills

From Haldeman S: Spinal manipulative therapy in the management of low back pain. *In* Finneson BE (ed): Low Back Pain. Philadelphia, JB Lippincott, 1980, p 250.

Muscle Energy Technique. Introduced by F. L. Mitchell Sr.,[134] muscle energy (ME) technique[65, 133] involves the patient's voluntary contraction of muscles (isometric, concentric, or eccentric) against resistance supplied by the practitioner (see Figs. 20–2, 20–3). An active manual medicine treatment, ME can be applied to most muscle groups in the body as either a direct or indirect technique. The goal is to increase the mobility of hypomobile segments, increase functional range of motion, allow the return of symmetrical motion to affected segments, strengthen weakened muscles, and lengthen contracted or spastic muscles.[65, 69] ME is also believed to have an effect on the nervous system.[65, 69, 111, 149] It is a relatively safe technique, with few contraindications, since the patient controls the degree of force applied to the dysfunctional area.

Most practitioners perform the direct form of ME manipulation. First, the patient is passively moved to the pathological barrier or restriction; then he or she actively contracts the muscles in an attempt to move away from the barrier while the practitioner resists the movement (isometric contraction). The patient tries to maintain a mild-to-moderate degree of sustained contraction for 3 to 7 seconds. With instruction by the practitioner, the patient chooses the degree of active contraction, avoiding contracting hard enough to induce pain or actual movement. The practitioner provides only static resistance of a distal attachment of the muscle, thus allowing the contraction to move the proximal segment.

Following the contraction, the patient completely relaxes the muscles, which usually takes 1 or 2 seconds. The patient should not be moved during this time. Then the practitioner passively moves the patient directly to the new pathological barrier. This step-by-step procedure is repeated three to five times in an attempt to increase muscle length and advance motion toward the physiological barrier. Dubbed "contract-relax" by physical therapists, this technique can often be learned by patients as part of a home exercise program. The cervical spine[15, 69, 133] (see Fig. 20–2) and sacroiliac/pelvic regions[15, 69, 133, 196] (see Fig. 20–3) are more easily and safely treated with ME than with HVLA.

Strain-Counterstrain. Strain-counterstrain (CS) is a manual medicine technique that attempts to passively place a spinal segment or other joint into its position of greatest comfort or ease. This is an indirect, functional technique[16, 69] developed by Jones[98] aimed at relieving painful dysfunction through a reduction in inappropriate afferent proprioceptor activity.[68, 111, 149] Prior to using CS treatment, structural evaluation is required to determine the areas of dysfunction and specify the location of Jones's "tender points."[17, 26, 98] These Jones points are palpably tense and tender areas located deep in the tissue, and can involve muscle, fascia, tendon, or ligament. The tender points can be widely distributed throughout the body and are not limited to the area of dysfunction. They are different from the "myofascial trigger points" described by Travell.[179] For each Jones point, there is a position that will relieve the pain. Identification and treatment of anterior tender points (chest wall, abdomen, and anterior pelvis) associated with spinal complaints can enhance a practitioner's therapeutic armamentarium.

Following localization of a tender point, the practitioner uses one hand on the point as a "monitoring hand" while the other hand moves the patient into various positions trying to relax the muscle. The monitoring hand discerns tissue relaxation versus tightening, and verbal interaction with the patient is used to localize the exact position that provides the greatest relief of pain. Once the position of relief (ease) is determined, it should be maintained for 90 to 120 seconds. During this time, the monitoring hand can continue to provide palpatory pressure on the tender point. This is somewhat controversial, as some practitioners feel it might be associated with a form of acupressure. Continual fine-tuning can occur during the 120 seconds of positioning; and often, as the tender point releases, the monitoring hand will feel a pulsatile sensation. It is essential to return the person to the neutral position very slowly in order to let the muscle spindles reset themselves.[65, 111] Often it is best to treat and to move in one plane at a time (rotation, then sidebending, etc.). The patient must remain relaxed and should not assist by firing any of the involved muscles.

CS has widespread indications for symptomatic relief, and few contraindications are associated with this passive, indirect technique. Limiting factors to CS treatment are the time required to release tender points (1.5 to 2 minutes each) and the varying length of time for which the treatment can provide symptomatic relief. These techniques must also be dosed appropriately: Some patients become "addicted" to this form of passive release, surrendering active responsibility for their own recovery. But if used correctly, CS often allows a patient to begin an active back treatment program earlier than would otherwise be possible, and can even be effectively incorporated into a patient's home treatment program.

Other Functional Techniques. Other functional techniques[16, 69] also involve the evaluation and treatment of the quality of motion instead of the range of motion. A palpating hand is placed over the dysfunctional segment to "listen" while motion is introduced into the area either actively by the patient or passively by the practitioner. The "listening hand" is trying to determine which direction allows easy and free movement (*ease*) and which direction is difficult (*bind*). Motion is introduced in every direction in a sequential pattern while monitoring for ease in each direction. Functional techniques are theoretically a part of the neurological model and can be used in both acute and chronic problems because they are not painful and depend on a release of soft tissue rather than a structural change.[69]

Myofascial Release. Myofascial release[20, 69, 186] treats the neuromuscular-somatic unit as a whole, combining soft tissue, ME, and craniosacral principles. It involves the release of somatic dysfunction or related imbalances, whether affecting a discrete region, a vertebral segment level, an entire limb, or the whole body. This can be accomplished by using intrinsic and extrinsic forces with direct or indirect methods. Direct treatment engages the restrictive barrier and pushes against it with a constant force until tissue release occurs. With the indirect technique, dysfunctional tissues are guided along the path of least resistance until free movement is achieved. Each of the techniques uses a combination of manual traction and twisting maneuvers to achieve tension on the soft tissues, aiming to effect biomechanical and reflex changes.[69, 186] Initial treatment is directed at the short, tight muscle groups. The stretch should always follow the long axis of the fascia; then a twisting force can be added to localize the traction. Palpation throughout the treatment process is important to monitor tissue response, following the concept that tightness creates asymmetry while weakness permits it.[69] The release is a dynamic process; thus, it cannot be predetermined by the practitioner but must be continually adjusted according to the response of the patient's tissues. General principles have been established by Ward[186] and others, but experience and expert palpatory skills are essential for treatment success. This form of manual medicine is becoming widely used by physical therapists in both acute and chronic musculoskeletal pain syndromes. It is, however, passive and therefore needs to be combined with parts of an active treatment program (see Chapters 40 and 42).

Craniosacral Therapy. Craniosacral therapy[69, 73, 172, 183] is a manual medicine technique for diagnosis and treatment of the body by way of the primary respiratory mechanism. It was pioneered by Sutherland,[172] who perceived that the cranial bones undergo subtle cyclical motion about the cranial sutures at a rate of 8 to 12 Hz. This motion is felt most easily at the cranium and the sacrum, but is palpable everywhere in the body. He termed this inherent motion the *primary respiratory mechanism* and claimed that it comprises five body components: (1) the articular mechanism of the cranial bones, (2) involuntary motion of the sacrum between the ilia, (3) fluctuation of the CSF, (4) reciprocal tension of the dural membranes, and (5) inherent motion of the central nervous system.

Craniosacral therapy consists of assessing the amplitude, rate, symmetry, and quality of the primary respiratory mechanism. Gentle pressure applied to the body in rhythm with the palpated inherent motion can be used to passively move toward optimal mobility.[172, 183] A variety of practitioners have evinced growing interest in the applicability and appropriateness of craniosacral therapy in patients suffering head trauma and postconcussive syndrome.[70, 72] There is some basic anatomical and physiological research on the movement of the cranial sutures and CSF dynamics[2, 141]; overall, however, craniosacral therapy enjoys more hypothetical than hard scientific support.

Soft Tissue Techniques. Soft tissue techniques can involve lateral stretching (Fig. 20–8), linear stretching (Fig. 20–9), deep pressure (Fig. 20–10), or traction, or any combination of these, directed at separating the origin and insertion of a muscle.[69] It incorporates procedures similar to traditional massage, but can also include acupressure, Travell's trigger point release,[179] diaphragmatic release,[69] mesenteric release,[69] and lymphatic drainage techniques.[69, 113, 198] Soft tissue techniques can be used for generalized treatment programs in people with chronic illnesses such as multiple sclerosis, hemiplegia, or any immobility syndrome. They are also used preceding other forms of more active treatment programs or manipulation.

Lymphatic Pump. The lymphatic pump[69] is a soft tissue technique that utilizes the muscle forces and intrathoracic pressure changes to enhance lymphatic flow.

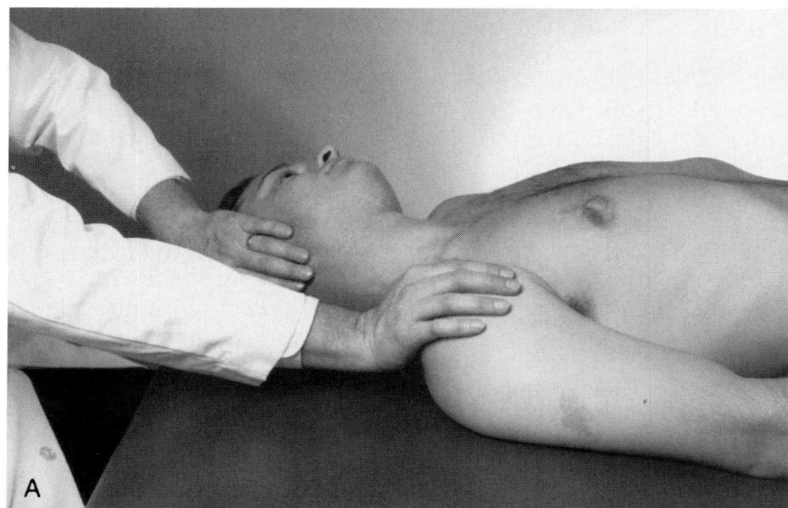

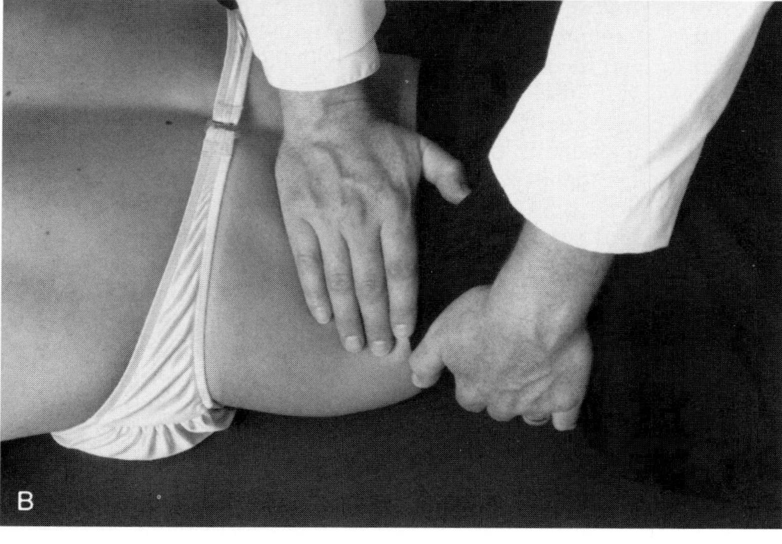

FIGURE 20–8. Soft tissue release by elongated lateral stretch. *A.* Sidebending: the patient's right shoulder is stabilized by the practitioner's right hand, while the left hand provides passive left sidebending. *B.* Rotation: the practitioner's left hand is hooked under the ASIS and is pulled back toward the practitioner, while the base of the right hand is placed firmly against the medial border of the paraspinal muscles; the hand is then pushed toward the table and away from the midline.

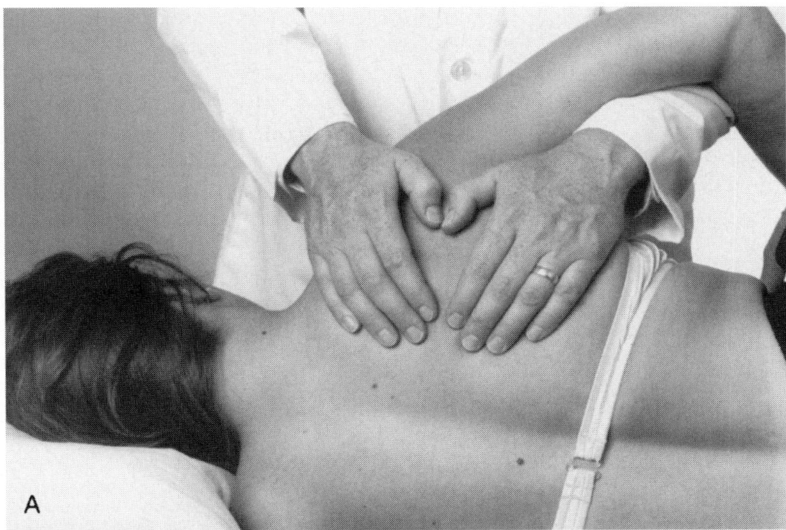

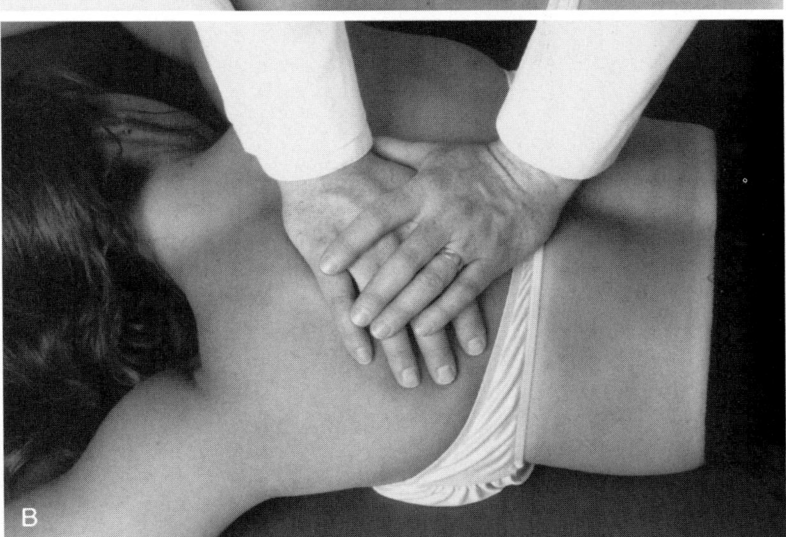

FIGURE 20–9. Linear soft tissue release by scapular mobilization. *A.* Side-lying: the practitioner's finger pads are hooked under the medial border of the scapula and lifted upward. *B.* Prone: the thenar eminences of both hands are placed in contact with the medial border of the scapula and a gentle force is directed toward the table and laterally.

Intermittent compression of the thoracic cage in a rhythmic fashion enhances the return of lymph through the thoracic inlet, which relieves vascular engorgement to allow resumption of normal tissue motion.[170] Other lymphatic techniques can be similarly performed with repetitive movements of the arms or legs. These techniques are often performed distal-to-proximal, similar to the centripetal massage techniques[88, 194] used to relieve edema in the extremities.

Contraindications and Risks

Each of the manual medicine techniques has its own set of contraindications. Mobilization with impulse (HVLA) has the greatest number of absolute contraindications[78] (see Table 20–3). Soft tissue, muscle energy, counterstrain, and myofascial release techniques have few contraindications, since they have a much lower inherent risk to the patient than HVLA thrusting techniques. Once the contraindications and specific treatment procedures have been appropriately established for a particular clinical situation, the incidence of "complications" decreases.[43]

There are a few general precautions to be followed for all manual medicine techniques for safety and effectiveness. Neck positioning is important, especially in elderly patients. Prolonged neck extension should be avoided, due to the risk of potential vertebral artery abnormalities and the possibility of irritating arthritic facet joints or compromising cervical nerve roots. Prolonged, extreme neck rotation can be dangerous in patients with carotid artery disease. Many practitioners use an extension-rotation test of the neck to try to determine clinical safety prior to treatment, but this test has not been validated as a useful screening tool.[32] All levels of the spine should be carefully positioned in persons with significant osteoporosis, as marked or prolonged flexion can lead to compression fractures (see Chapter 41). Extension should be limited in patients with lumbar stenosis (see Chapter 40). With all techniques, the patient must be kept relaxed and breathing freely to avoid ex-

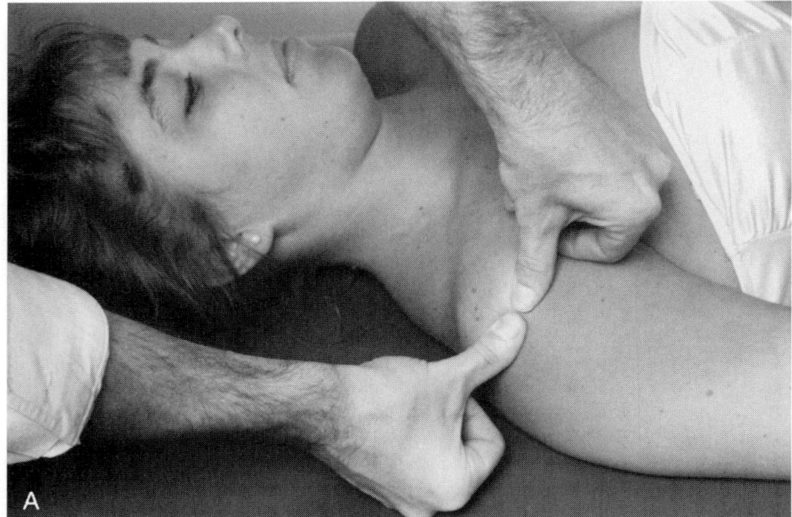

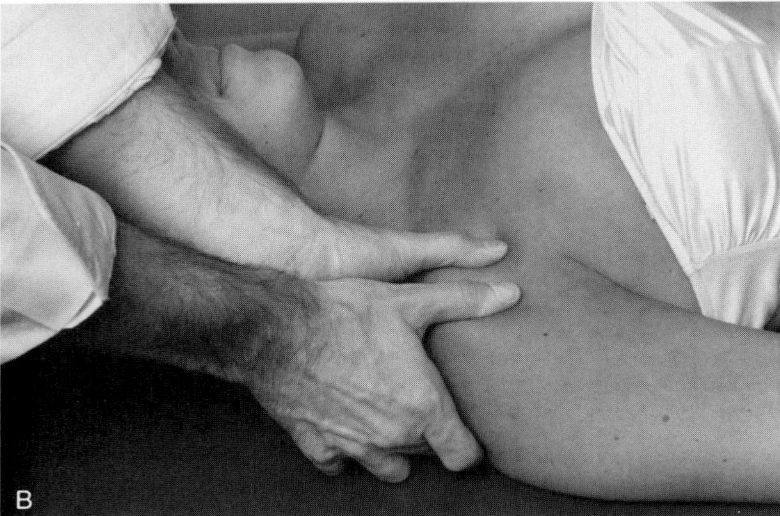

FIGURE 20–10. Soft tissue release by deep friction message. *A.* Supraspinatus tendon: the thumb pads are placed between the acromion and the humeral head, with deep pressure used to roll the fingers back and forth without losing contact with the skin. *B.* Biceps tendon: the entire thumb is placed on either side of the tendon as it progresses cephalad. Deep pressure is applied by rhythmically bringing the thumbs together without losing contact with the skin.

cessive changes in blood pressure, as well as increased intra-abdominal or spinal canal pressure.

There are potential side effects that can occur even when manual medicine treatment is successful, including increased autonomic effects (hypotension, increased menses, perspiration, etc.) and a transient increase in discomfort.[82, 118] Other side effects are mostly related to inadequate skill of a practitioner, improper diagnosis, or the use of an inappropriate technique for a particular dysfunction. Catastrophic outcomes have been reported—stroke,[5, 112, 119, 154, 166] myelopathy,[5, 119, 147] quadriplegia,[93, 152] cauda equina syndrome,[5, 80, 152] cardiac arrest,[66] even death[164]—mostly the result of manipulation of the cervical spine with improper technique or misdiagnosis or both. These cases provide the basis for most arguments against the use of manual medicine; however, their frequency is low, at just one case per 1 to 1.5 million manipulations.[152]

There have been reports of manual medicine causing progressive neurological changes in a radicular pattern,[119, 152] vertebral osteomyelitis,[121] compression fractures,[81] and worsening of herniated disks.[5, 91, 156] But these syndromes have a highly variable course, making it difficult to determine whether the manipulation or the natural course of the disease process worsened the conditions in these cases. Although some practitioners advocate manipulative procedures in the presence of an acute spondylolisthesis or a disk herniation with radiculopathy, the general guideline is to not use thrusting techniques at that particular level (unless in the hands of a highly trained practitioner). Nonthrusting techniques are typically preferred in these cases and are safely performed at nearby levels with dysfunction.

Using Manual Medicine in Practice

The structural examination necessary to determine somatic dysfunction is a "hands-on" approach that can easily be incorporated into the routine physiatric physical examination. Greenman[69] has proposed a 12-step examination to screen for structural abnormalities, many of which are already done in a routine physiatric examination (see Table 20–2). Asymmetry of the shoulders, scoliosis, asymmetry at the lumbosacral junction, joint dysfunction in the legs, and leg length differences influence the overall motion, loading, and forces of the spine and the lower extremities. This can lead to impaired functional activities or pain complaints.

A physiatrist's goal during a musculoskeletal examination is to determine whether there is a structural or pathophysiological abnormality present that is treatable. Somatic dysfunction is just one of many things that must be assessed; but if present, it can easily be treated during the same office visit. If the examining physician cannot provide the treatment, a patient can be referred to another practitioner who is trained in manual medicine (i.e., a D.O., D.C., P.T., or M.D. with additional training). It is recommended that physiatrists doing musculoskeletal medicine establish these relationships prior to treatment, so that no confusion arises as to who will be primarily managing the patient and what specific treatments are being requested.

Some general guidelines for the duration and frequency of manipulative treatment have been proposed.[3, 79, 164, 165] To date, however, most of this has been by consensus of expert panels and debate continues regarding parameters.[7] Treatment plans for all types of manual medicine must be developed on an individual basis in relation to the patient's structural diagnosis, the type and location of the somatic dysfunction, the type of manual medicine techniques being performed, and the patient's response to treatment. With each patient visit, the practitioner must reevaluate these parameters to determine the need for continued manipulative treatment. Clearly, if the patient receives no measurable benefit after 2 to 4 weeks of treatment (6 to 8 visits), the underlying diagnosis must be reconsidered. The indiscriminate use of manual medicine for weeks or months without the proper indications is inappropriate.

The philosophies of the use of manual medicine and the practice of physical medicine and rehabilitation (PM&R) are consistent in their goals to increase function. In manual medicine, this increase in function is gauged by increased motion and body symmetry, as well as functional activities. The two most widely quoted studies supporting the use of manual medicine in patients with acute low back pain (Hadler[77] and MacDonald[123]) demonstrated improvement in functional outcome measurements at a faster rate than nontreated subjects. A review of current manipulation trials revealed that the highest rated studies for methodological quality generally demonstrated positive patient response with manual medicine.[6] Manual medicine contributes only one part of a comprehensive musculoskeletal treatment program, and should be incorporated into an active exercise program[15, 104, 155, 173, 182] to enhance the long-term outcome. Manipulation techniques can be combined with specific spinal injections to reduce pain and permit the active treatment program.[8, 39, 137] Some forms of manual medicine, such as muscle energy and counterstrain, are more easily incorporated into the home exercise program.

TRACTION

Traction: Definition and Goals

Traction is the technique in which a pulling force is used to stretch soft tissues and to separate joint surfaces or bone fragments.[86] The goal of spinal traction is to obtain pain relief and functional improvement. Traction involves applying a force of sufficient magnitude and duration in the proper direction, while simultaneously resisting movement of the body by an equal and opposite force. With proper positioning of the patient and the correct angle of pull, traction can be localized to a specific spinal area. The force is generally applied through a mechanical pulley system with weights, and stabilization by either a chin strap for the cervical spine (Figs. 20–11, 20–12) or a pelvic belt for the lumbar spine[158]

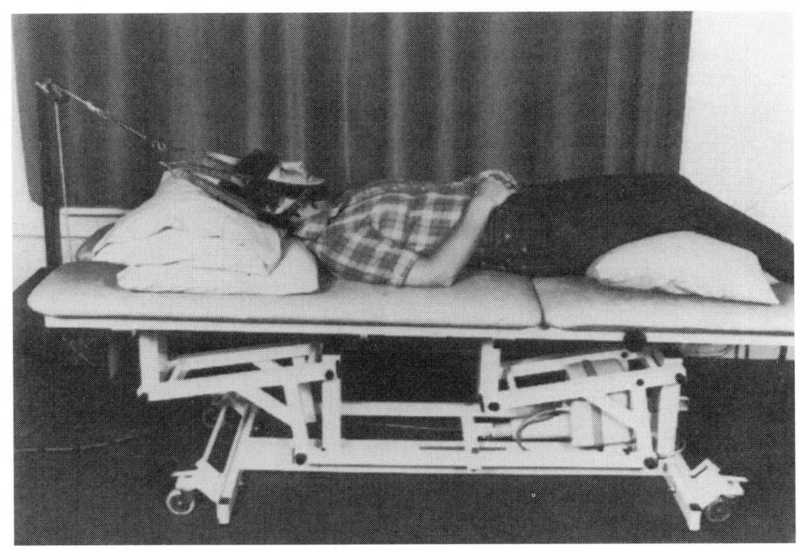

FIGURE 20–11. Mechanical cervical traction. Patient in a supine position with the neck slightly flexed. (Note spring balance in series to monitor the amount of force applied.) (From Grieve GP: Mobilisation of the Spine, ed 5. New York, Churchill Livingstone, 1991, pp 270–271.)

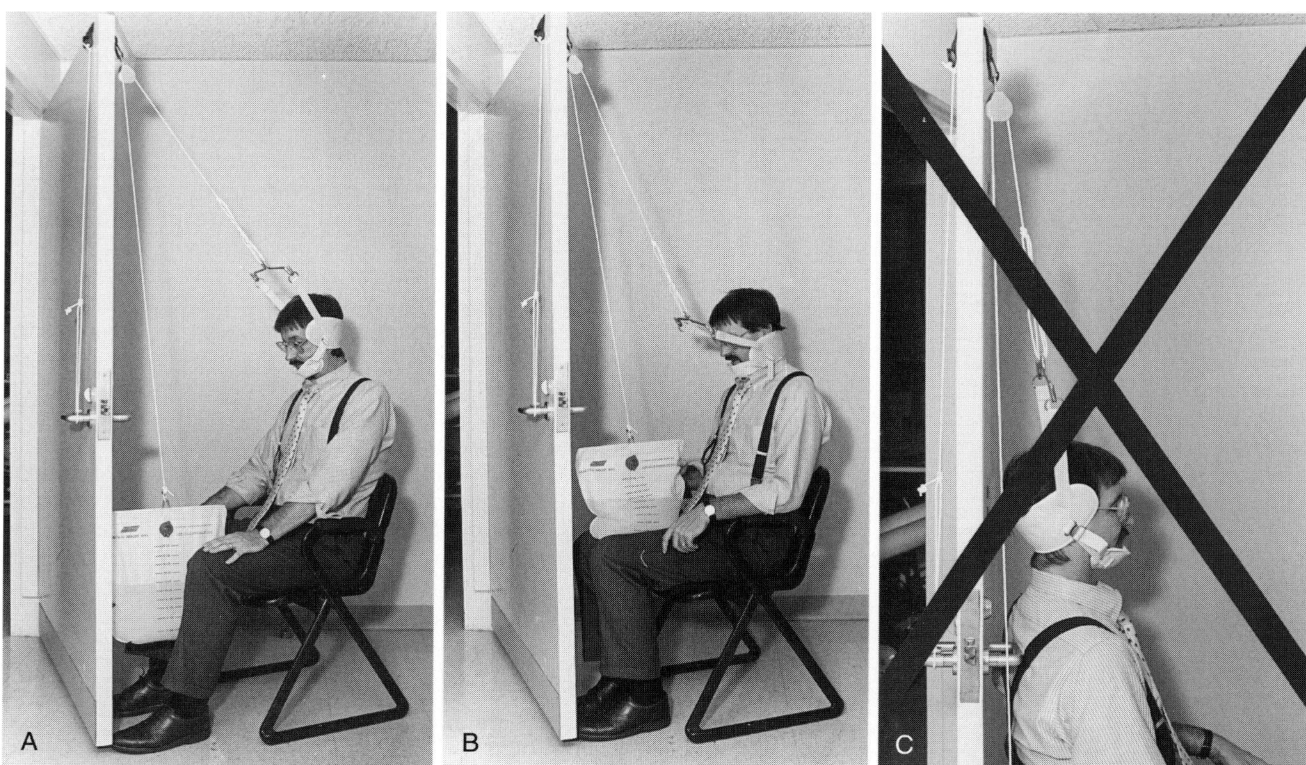

FIGURE 20–12. Home cervical traction. *A.* Properly performed distraction, with the patient facing the door (pulley) to allow the force to be applied through a slightly flexed cervical spine. *B.* To perform intermittent traction, the position of the patient is maintained while the weight (water bag) is placed to allow the rope to be relaxed *C.* Improper positioning with the neck in extension is not appropriate and may lead to further cervical injury. Make sure the door is not accidentally moved during the treatment.

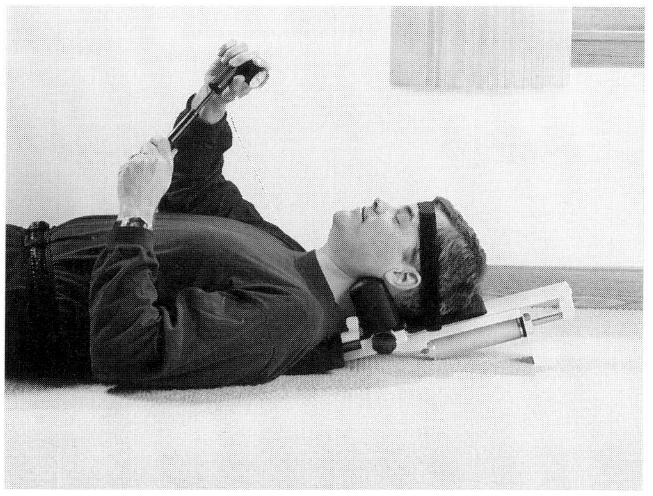

FIGURE 20–13. Alternative home cervical traction. The patient is supine (with gravity eliminated) with the neck slightly flexed by the device. The neck fits into a groove in the pad, which pushes caudally against the base of the occiput. The patient controls the amount of distractive pressure by using the hand pump. (Courtesy of The Saunders Group, 5250 Norex Drive, Chaska, MN 55318-3047.)

(Figs. 20–14, 20–15). The various techniques can be performed in standing, sitting, or lying positions (see Figs. 20–11 to 20–15).

History

Traction was originally utilized in the treatment of fractures and dislocations. Hippocrates recommended traction for spinal disorders such as scoliosis and excessive kyphosis.[86, 90] The early use of traction was limited by soft tissue or skin interfacing with the traction apparatus, so that any pull on the bone had to be transferred through the soft tissue. This type of traction is effective for conditions such as burn contractures,[116] but it remains a limitation today for most forms of spinal traction. Skeletal traction with the use of hooks (Malgaigne), pins (Steinmann), and wires (Kirshner) has improved in the limbs,[86] but these devices are not useful for spinal traction except with surgical stabilization or "Halo" bracing.

Cyriax,[35, 36] in the 1950s, popularized the use of traction for lumbar disc lesions. Since then, Judovich,[99, 101, 102,] Colachis and Strohm,[27, 29] and others[11, 34, 57, 58, 61, 90, 120, 135, 146, 153, 159, 162, 176, 184, 192, 193, 195] have extensively studied the parameters and effects of traction in both the neck and low back. No consensus with regard to maximal clinical benefit has emerged. Traction can be used in conjunction with other forms of conservative

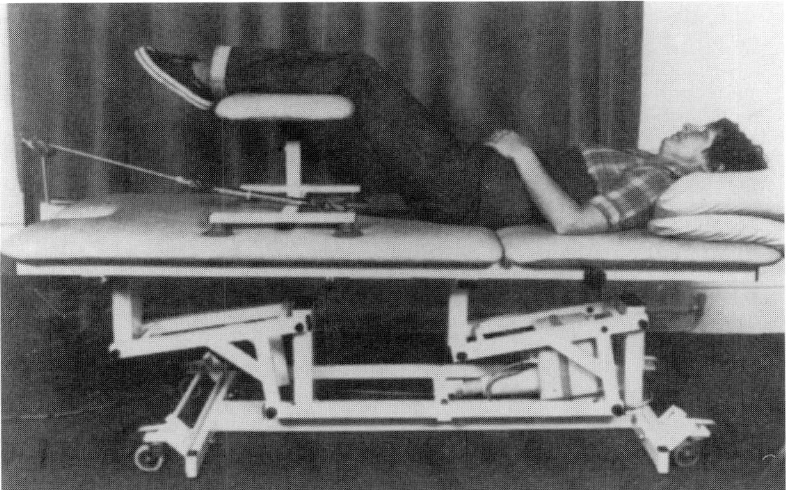

FIGURE 20–14. Motorized lumbar traction with patient in a supine position with hips and knees flexed. The distractive force is directed through the pelvic belt, while the upper belt stabilizes the patient. (From Grieve GP: Mobilisation of the Spine, ed 5. New York, Churchill Livingstone, 1991, p 261.)

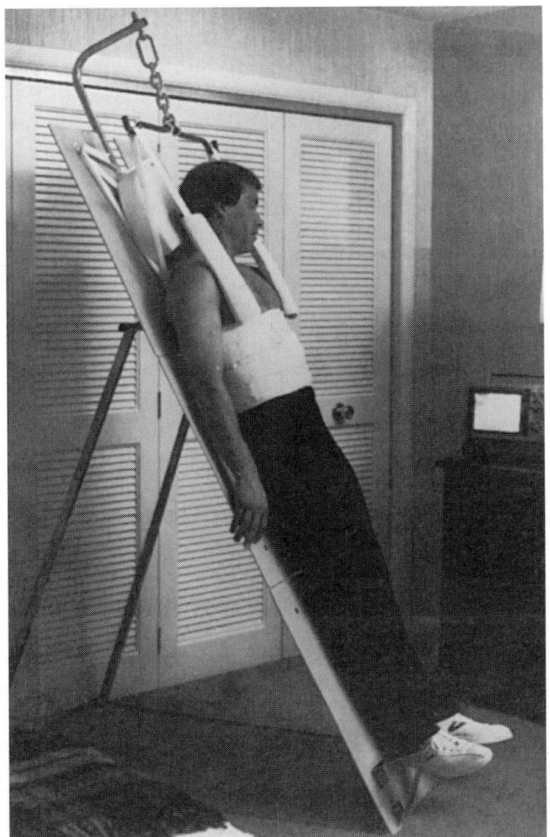

FIGURE 20–15. Gravitational lumbar traction. The patient's weight provides the force of distraction, while the thoracolumbar belt must be able to stabilize the upper body. In this position, the lumbar spine is in neutral or slight extension, which may assist or hinder the treatment process. (From Grieve, GP: Mobilisation of the Spine, ed 5. New York, Churchill Livingstone, 1991, p 264.)

treatment of low back and neck pain to improve symptomatic outcome,[35, 61, 90, 159, 162] but evidence of long-term benefit remains scanty. Most recent changes in the techniques have been related to positioning,[158, 162, 193] the development of stabilizing tables,[60, 153, 162, 176] motorized delivery systems,[153, 158, 162, 193] and inversion techniques.[58]

Indications and Goals of Treatment

It is generally held that any condition involving irritation or compression of nerve roots—whether related to trauma, a degenerative process, or compression from the disc—can benefit from a trial of traction. It is most often used for neck or arm pain secondary to cervical nerve root compromise or radiculopathy[99, 124, 136, 159] (see Figs. 20–11 to 20–13) and low back pain from lumbar radiculopathy[35, 60, 90, 162] (see Figs. 20–14, 20–15). Some practitioners also prescribe traction for patients with nonspecific low back pain, acute cervical or lumbar strain, and other soft tissue abnormalities.[11, 57, 74, 124, 146, 162] However, few data indicate that traction is any more effective than placebo in these conditions, and some practitioners assert that the only benefit can be due to the temporary immobilization while undergoing treatment.[158] The effects of traction in the thoracic area and sacrum or pelvis are minimal, and use in these areas is limited to stabilization for fractures, dislocations, or correction of congenital deformity or scoliosis.

Although specific clinical indications for traction are controversial, the anatomical basis for the use of traction is well established. Traction has been shown to (1) enlarge intervertebral foramina,[27, 28, 30, 31, 193] (2) separate apophyseal joints,[27, 28, 30, 31, 193] (3) stretch muscles and ligaments,[31] (4) tighten the posterior longitudinal ligament to exert a centripetal force on the adjacent annulus fibrosus,[86] and (5) enlarge the intervertebral space[27, 31] (possibly producing a suction effect on the disc[95]). Traction is theoretically indicated for any condition that could benefit from these anatomical changes (see Table 20–4). The magnitude, duration, position, and direction of pull vary with the treatment goals.

TABLE 20–4 Theoretical and Observed Changes with Axial Spine Traction

Diminution of disc protrusion
Reduction of cervical disc space pressure
Enlargement of intervertebral foramen
Opening up of the intervertebral disc space
Separation of intervertebral joints
Stretching a tight or painful capsule
Release of entrapped synovial membrane
Freeing of adherent nerve roots
Production of central vacuum to reduce herniated disc
Production of posterior longitudinal ligament tension to reduce herniated disc
Relaxation of muscle spasm

From White AA, Panjabi MM: Clinical Biomechanics of the Spine, ed. 2. Philadelphia, JB Lippincott, 1990, p 432.

Types of Traction

There are several different methods of delivering traction to a patient. These include manual,[36, 69, 74, 124] mechanized,[86, 158] (see Fig. 20–11), motorized or hydraulic,[153, 158, 162, 193] (see Fig. 20–14), special tables[60, 86, 153, 158, 162, 176] (see Figs. 20–14, 20–15), and inversion[58] methods. The pull can be continuous, sustained, intermittent, or intermittently pulsed, and can vary based on the magnitude, duration, and direction of pull.[86] All types of treatment, though, must overcome the body's surface resistance to traction, which is equal to about one-half of the weight of the body segment[99, 101] plus the resistance of the involved soft tissues. This resistance is also a function of the patient's position and changes depending on whether the patient is supine, inclined or tilted, or sitting. Gravity can be used either to assist or resist the pulling force. The force required is obviously greater for lumbar traction than for cervical traction, but in either type the force necessary for vertebral separation can be more than a patient can safely tolerate.

Continuous traction uses a low force over a long period of time, say, 20 to 40 hours.[86] This is hard for many patients to tolerate, and any change in the patient's position can change the direction of the pull. It is often used in spinal traction for the low back, mostly to assure that a person remains at rest, or for orthopedic uses other than for the spine.

Sustained traction uses force greater than that used in continuous traction, but less than that in intermittent. The pull is maintained for 20 to 60 minutes.[86] This is still difficult to tolerate if too much force is used. Sustained traction is more practical time-wise for therapy departments. Split traction tables or autotraction tables are typically used. Sustained traction treatments can be given at varying frequencies, although it is common practice to treat inpatients daily and outpatients three times per week.

Intermittent traction techniques allow for the use of greater forces, but for a shorter period of time. The force is gradually increased and decreased during each treatment cycle, and can be administered by pulley or motorized system. The duration can be adjusted, and can be on a timed, rhythmic schedule or controlled manually by the patient. For a preprogrammed treatment protocol, the time sequences can vary from as little as 7 to 10 seconds of tractive force with a 5-second rest, up to 30 to 60 seconds of tractive force followed by 10 to 15 seconds of rest.[28, 31] The on-off cycle is repeated for 15 to 25 minutes.[30, 31] The patient-controlled protocol is based more on tolerance; and the amount of time with a tractive force and resting is variable for each sequence, depending on that patient's tolerance. Intermittent traction is used in the cervical region to allow the use of progressively higher forces (up to 50 lbs.), which increases vertebral separation.[28, 99, 117]

Cervical Traction. Cervical traction is most commonly administered by a manual force[36, 74] (often with manipulation) or with the use of a head or chin sling by a mechanized or motorized force (see Fig. 20–11). The sling (Sayre[86, 124] is the most common), which should fit so that it does not compress any vascular structures in the neck or the ears, is designed to provide more pull on the occipital region than the mandible. Colachis and Strom[27] have demonstrated that posterior vertebral separation is related to the angle of the pull, with maximum separation occurring at 24 degrees of flexion. The best clinical relief reportedly occurs between 20 and 30 degrees of cervical flexion.[33, 34] The most common reason clinically for cervical traction to fail or to exacerbate symptoms is applying the force in extension rather than flexion (see Fig. 20–12). There is no effective way to deliver cervical traction with an inversion system.

The optimal force for cervical traction varies depending on the method of delivery. At least 10 lbs. of force is necessary to counter the effects of gravity on the head,[95] while 25 lbs. of force is necessary to provide straightening of the cervical lordotic curve and the earliest separation of posterior vertebral segments.[99] Several studies have shown that larger forces definitely cause more separation,[28, 99] but higher forces cannot always be tolerated by patients. When tolerated, the longer a constant force can be applied, the greater the separation.[28] The maximum separation occurs anteriorly at C4 to C5 after 25 minutes and posteriorly at C6 to C7 after 20 minutes.[30] The distraction effect is short-lived, since 20 minutes after traction there is no evidence of posterior separation.[30]

Cervical traction in the inclined position[86] uses the effect of gravity on the body to pull against a stable chin strap. In the supine position,[193] the weight of the head is reduced, but there is increased frictional resistance between the head and the table. This position gives the patient better control of the neck and allows for better relaxation. In many cases, however, the patient has difficulty staying flat on the table if the angle of pull remains at 24 degrees of flexion. This can cause the patient to actively fire the neck muscles, causing pain and limiting the effect of the traction.

Many clinicians prescribe traction in the seated position because it is easier to position the patient for the correct angle of pull and the patient's body weight counters the force of the pull. In this position, however, the neck is more uncontrollable than in the supine position, and some patients have difficulty relaxing the muscles in this position. The pulley systems and motorized instruments can be used in either the sitting or the supine position (see Fig. 20–11). Each patient should be assessed for the position of best individual tolerance.

When a patient is noted to be benefiting from cervical traction, it can be performed with a home over-the-door unit as long as the correct angle for pull is maintained[174] (see Fig. 20–12). The patient should always be facing the door to which the pulley is attached (see Fig. 20–12). This keeps the cervical spine in flexion and allows the patient to manipulate the weight with both hands. There are newer inflatable collar units and supine posterior distraction units that are more expensive than the standard over-the-door units (see Fig. 20–13). These alternative devices are indicated primarily when the head sling cannot be tolerated due to temperomandibular joint syndrome or headaches. Patients using traction at home should never be alone, as someone might need to assist them if any untoward effects arise. The optimal frequency of treatments has not yet been established for any of the methods of delivery.

Lumbar Traction. Lumbar traction that provides vertebral separation requires significantly larger forces than cervical traction to overcome the body's resistance.[57, 101, 120, 153, 162] Pelvic belts (see Fig. 20–14) or the use of gravity by tilting[162, 163] (see Fig. 20–15) or inversion[58] are necessary to deliver sufficient tractive force to the lumbar spine. Due to the large amount of weight necessary to overcome the body's resistance in this area, either a thoracic or chest belt or corset is necessary to hold the upper body in place during distraction of the lower body. These chest harnesses are often uncomfortable and can limit breathing and venous return,[86] affecting a patient's cardiovascular status.

Lumbar traction can be delivered by continuous, sustained, intermittent or pulsed intermittent methods. Several studies have shown that the larger the force, the greater the vertebral separation; but these high forces (300 to 400 lbs.) have to be delivered intermittently for patients to tolerate them.[120] The use of sustained delivery methods with less weight (40, 50, 80, 100, and 132 lbs.)[31, 195] becomes more effective when surface resistance is reduced by increasing lumbar flexion,[31, 100, 162] using a Scott traction frame[117] or a standing technique.[120] Split-traction and autotraction tables also reduce the body's surface resistance so that less force is required to provide the same degree of vertebral separation.

Split-traction tables[86, 90, 101, 153, 162] have a mobile and a stationary half. The lower body rests on the mobile half, which separates from the stationary portion. This arrangement stabilizes the upper body and allows vertebral separation with less force at the level where the table is separating. Because the force necessary to overcome surface resistance is reduced, treatment can be provided with as little as 80 to 150 lbs.[86, 101, 162] rather than 300 to 400 lbs.[57, 120] Optimal treatment frequency and duration have not yet been established. Newer computerized versions of these tables can be more effective than traditional tables when utilized as part of a comprehensive treatment program[162]; however, reports of systems' "pulling" a herniated disc back into the disc space are unsubstantiated.

The autotraction table allows both sections of the table to move, which induces rotational and sidebending forces into the spine. The patient is assisted by a therapist to assume the most pain-free position, similar to the beginning of a neutral spine exercise program. The patient performs this active traction by pulling on an overhead bar for 3 to 6 seconds. This controls the amount of tractive force. The patient then uses the feet to push or pull on a bar at the foot of the bed, which alternates compressive and distracting forces. The patient rests about 60 seconds between each tractive sequence, and repeats the treatment for 30 to 60 minutes. Optimal frequency or length of treatment has not been established, but the studies showing symptomatic benefit have provided treatment every 2 to 3 days for 6 to 10 treatments.[176]

There has been no definitive study of lumbar traction to determine optimal magnitude, duration, frequency, or angle of pull for clinical use. It has been shown that pain relief is quicker with the lumbar spine in flexion[86, 162]; and Colachis and Strohm[31] found that, with the hips flexed to 70 degrees, an angle of pull of 18 degrees provided the greatest vertebral separation. The duration of beneficial treatment varies with the amount of force used; but even in studies showing a strong clinical benefit, there is no evidence of residual effect following removal of the tractive force.[181] A home treatment table has been proposed,[181] but has not been as widely accepted as home cervical traction. Due to the large forces necessary for lumbar vertebral separation, manual traction is not an option.

Contraindications and Risks

Absolute contraindications to traction (see Table 20–5) include malignancy,[86, 114] infectious diseases such as tuberculosis, osteomyelitis or discitis, osteoporosis, rheumatoid arthritis, cord compression, pregnancy, previous fusion, and hypertension or cardiovascular disease. In the cervical region, midline disc herniation[35, 99] is also a contraindication, since traction could pull the cord into contact with the disc. Traction should be used with caution in all elderly patients, and should not be used in those with evidence of significant carotid or vertebral artery disease. Most clinicians recommend that no one

TABLE 20–5 Contraindications to Traction

- General
  - Osteomyelitis or discitis
  - Primary bone tumor or spinal cord tumor
  - Unstable fracture
  - Severe osteoporosis
  - Hypertension
  - Cardiovascular disease
  - Inadequate expertise
- Cervical
  - Central intervertebral disc herniation
  - Hypermobile joints
  - Rheumatoid arthritis
  - Carotid or vertebral artery disease
- Lumbar
  - Pregnancy
  - Cauda equina compression

should have a trial of traction unless x-rays have ruled out instability, infection, and other contraindications. Lumbar traction should be performed with caution in persons with abdominal problems, such as peptic ulcer and hiatal or other hernias; aortic aneurysm; or hemorrhoids.[86] Patients with neurogenic bladder related to nerve root entrapment should not receive lumbar traction.

Inversion traction[58] involves more risk than standard traction, as it can increase systolic and diastolic blood pressure, decrease heart rate, and cause persistent blurred vision, persistent headaches, and periorbital/pharyngeal petechiae. Since the center of gravity in adults is at the vertebral level of S2, there is a greater force across the lumbar disks if the patient is hanging upright.

Traction of any type should be discontinued in those who experience nausea, dizziness, exacerbation of temporomandibular joint dysfunction, or increased pain in the soft tissues of the neck. In the lumbar region, pain can be worsened by the traction itself, at the contact points of the pelvic belt, or at the upper body-belt or -corset interface. Frazer[57] reports an "untoward sequelae" rate of just 6 per 25,000 with lumbar traction, and reports of problems associated with cervical traction are rare.[168]

Using Traction in Practice

In clinical practice, traction is used most often for patients who present with signs and symptoms of cervical radiculopathy.[159] It can be used as both a diagnostic and treatment tool, since patients with nerve root compression often receive benefit, while patients with soft tissue or myofascial pain frequently have an exacerbation of symptoms. The limiting factor for successful cervical traction treatment is often the amount of weight the patient can tolerate. Manual traction during the examination can give an initial indication whether a patient can tolerate cervical traction. Another benefit of cervical traction is that it can potentially be used at home, but initial instruction and testing of a home unit should always be done under the supervision of a physician or physical therapist.

The use of lumbar traction has become less frequent in recent years.[37] This is due to patient intolerance and the difficulty with stabilizing a patient and delivering the amount of force necessary for traction to be effective.[184] Regulations limiting hospital admissions for low back pain have further decreased its use. Aggressive nonoperative low back programs for either soft tissue or radicular symptoms have not typically found lumbar traction necessary, although it can be effective within the framework of a comprehensive treatment program. It should be considered in some patients as an adjunct modality so as to enhance their ability to initiate or maintain an active treatment program. It has been combined empirically with other modalities, such as heat, cold, massage, and electrical treatments; but there are, as yet, no studies proving that such combinations improve clinical outcomes.

MASSAGE

Massage: Definition

In 1884, Graham[67] defined massage as "a group of procedures which are usually done with the hands, such as friction, kneading, rolling and percussion of the external tissues of the body in a variety of ways, either with a curative, palliative or hygienic object in view." Massage and manipulation have common ancient roots. In modern times these modalities have become separated, but they continue to share considerable overlap in terminology, philosophy, and technique.

History

Massage has been celebrated in the writings of poets, philosophers, historians, and physicians from ancient to modern times. From its beginnings, massage has waxed and waned as a respected form of health promotion and healing. The philosophy, technical practice, and goals of massage have evolved through the millennia and continue to change today. There is considerable debate as to the etymology of the term *massage.*[103] Most likely origins include the Arabic verb *mass,* to touch; the Greek word *massein,* to knead; or possibly the Sanskrit term *makch,* to strike, press or condense.[67, 103]

The most ancient references to the use of massage come from Babylonia, China, and India followed later by Greek and Roman literature. Around 900 BCE, Babylonian-Assyrian medical writings prescribed massage to expel demons[103] and to aid in healing. Documented use of massage in China dates back to a text written on kung-fu in 2700 BCE.[103] The Nei Ching, written around 1000 BCE,[185] and Taoism, originated by Lao-tzu in the 6th century BCE[103] embraced massage. The Ayur-Veda, the oldest medical writing known in India (1500–1200 BCE), also makes reference to the use of massage.[103]

References to massage are common in ancient Greek and Roman literature. Hippocrates (460–375 BCE), Plato (427–347 BCE), and Socrates (470–399 BCE) refer to the benefits of anointing with oils,[67] and Galen, a Greek physician who settled in Rome, wrote extensively about exercise and massage.[103] The Greek physician Asclepiades, considered by some the father of physical medicine, referred to hydrotherapy, exercise, and massage as the three most important treatments that he recommended.[103]

The most common terminology employed today can be traced to Per Henrik Ling (1776–1839), who was a Swedish teacher of physical education. Ling adopted the French terms for various massage strokes translated from ancient writings. He classified and systematized a series of movements of the soft tissues and then the joints. He used terms such as *rolling, slapping, pinching, shaking,* and *vibration;* and he promoted the use of the French terms *effleurage, petrissage, friction massage,* and *tapotement*[63] (see Fig. 20–16). Ling emphasized strictly defined massage techniques, employed rationally on a foundation of mechanical and anatomical principles. A royal institute for the practice, promotion, and teaching of what came to be known as Swedish massage was established in Stockholm in 1813 under Ling's direction.[103] Ling's students later opened similar institutes in

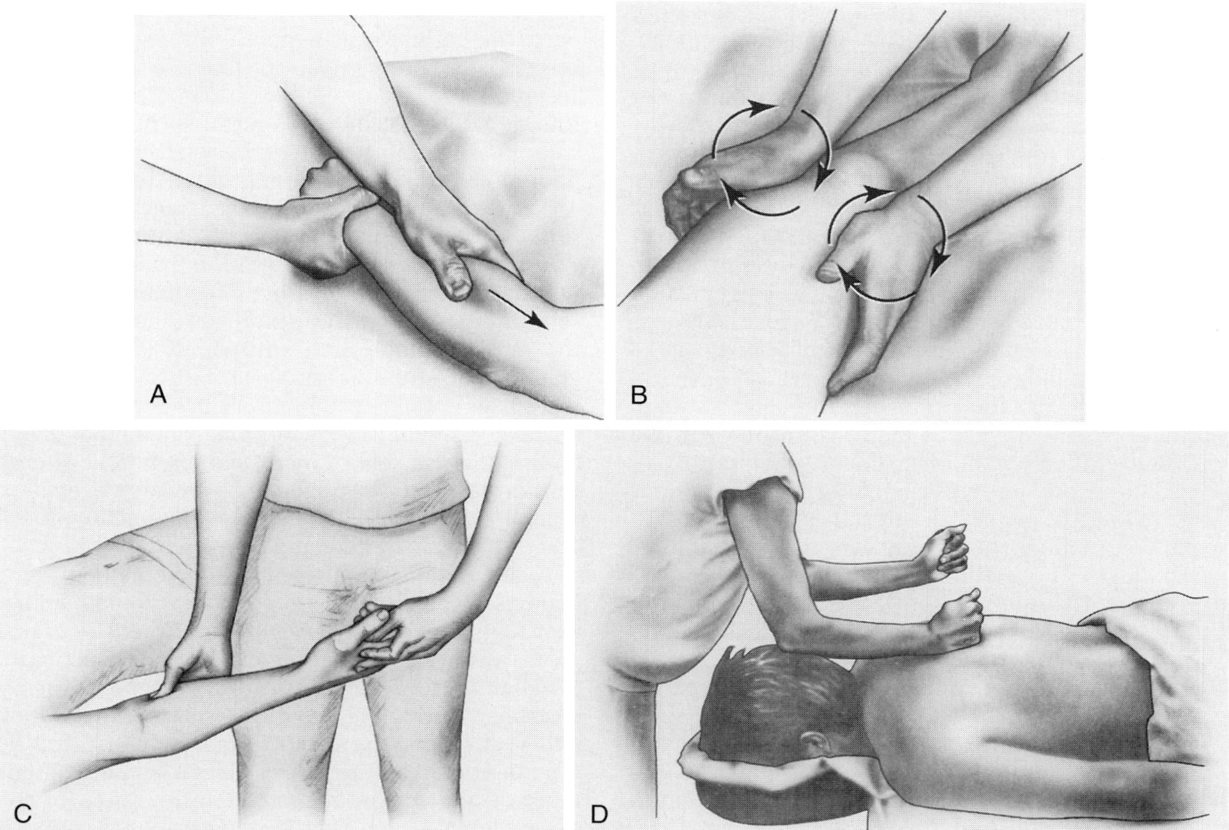

FIGURE 20–16. The common Swedish massage techniques. *A.* Effleurage or gliding strokes cover large area, and generally go from distal to proximal with light strokes. *B.* Pettrissage or compression involves movement of deeper tissues in a nonlocalized area. *C.* Friction involves the practitioner using the thumb or fingers in a small area to go from superficial tissue to deeper layers. *D.* Tapotement or percussion involves rhythmic alternating movements of the hands and may be used as superficial or deep tissue. (From Loving, JE: Massage Therapy: Theory and Practice. Stamford, CT, McGraw-Hill, 1999, pp. 83, 86, 89, 90. Reproduced with permission of The McGraw-Hill Companies.)

the capitals of Europe, and in 1916 an institute was established in New York.[103]

Many systems of massage have evolved in the 20th century and are currently popular. Today, massage holds neither the prominent place nor the level of prestige it enjoyed during the Roman Empire, or even the 19th-century British Empire. The decline is attributable to several modern trends, including scientific advances, the medical profession's emphasis on medications, and a greater faith in advanced technologies than in the hands. Nevertheless, in recent years an increasing number of people are seeking the benefits of manipulation and massage therapy,[46, 148, 152] and traditional medical education is beginning discussions of "alternative medicine" or complementary therapies, of which massage is considered a mainstay.[115, 188]

Indications and Goals of Treatment

There are mechanical, reflex, neurological, and psychological effects of massage.[20, 36, 194] Any massage elicits a combination of these effects. The magnitude of these effects and their exact characteristics depend on the technique employed and the manner of its application. The goals of treatment can include sedation, adhesion reduction (see Figs. 20–9, 20–10), fluid mobilization, muscular relaxation (see Fig. 20–8), and vascular changes. Massage can be useful with any diagnoses in which mobilization of tissues, relief of muscle hypertonicity, relief of discomfort, or reduction of swelling would benefit the patient.

The mechanical effects of massage are the most evident and easily understood; they are also the most studied and quantified. They are based on mobilizing individual muscle fibers and constricting the blood vessels to mechanically squeeze blood and lymph centrally. Deep continuous stroking of an extremity from distal to proximal compresses the low-pressure vasculature and augments venous return.[21, 150, 191] As blood is expressed from the periphery into the central venous system, arterial blood flow is augmented and flows more freely into the vacated tissue capillary beds.[21, 191] Edema is alleviated by massage-induced increase in tissue hydrostatic pressure. Vascular stasis is a risk factor for thrombosis, edema, ischemia, and their consequent morbidities. Massage can be used effectively to help alleviate vascular stasis via the mechanisms described above.

Massage clearly has temporary effects on cutaneous blood flow.[62] This can be readily observed by the hyperemia of the skin after vigorous cutaneous stimulation or the increased prominence of superficial veins. The specific mechanisms responsible for changes in cutaneous blood flow are multiple and not well delineated. Mechanical stimulation of mast cells in the skin causes release of histamine. Local histamine release causes the triple response of redness, flare, and then wheal formation at the site of cutaneous stimulation. Autonomic neurological reflex changes are also probably involved.

The lymphatic system returns fluids and macromolecules from the interstitium to the vascular system. Stroking techniques performed slowly with deep, constant pressure can mobilize lymphatic flow.[194] There is smooth muscle in the walls of venous and lymphatic vessels to assist in moving fluid centrally. However, the cyclical contraction and relaxation of skeletal muscle through which these vessels travel is a major contributor to the flow of fluid. Many conditions, such as pain, paralysis, or debilitation, prevent sufficient muscle contractions to mobilize fluid. Massage can be used as a substitute for muscular contractions to augment venous and lymphatic flow in patients who are immobile.[194] Retrograde massage is frequently used to control the edema seen with hemiparesis after stroke or reflex sympathetic dystrophy or following axillary node dissection.

Deep massage also has mechanical effects on fascia and connective tissue.[20, 194] The fascia surrounds, infiltrates, and supports the musculoskeletal system as well as most of the visceral organs. Restrictions, microadhesions, and scarring in the fascial system lead to diminished musculoskeletal mobility, contracture, and consequent stasis. Fascia is believed to have colloidal properties, which enable it to be molded and stretched by sustained pressure. Deep friction massage can, for example, be used to treat shoulder hypomobility secondary to myofascial and tendinous restrictions (see Fig. 20–10). Deep friction massage can result in an immediate increase in shoulder mobility and decrease in pain by easing fascial restrictions.

In the past, massage was believed to increase muscle strength—a notion no longer considered valid.[177] Massage has been shown to facilitate the recovery of muscle ability to perform exercise after being fatigued by work or electrical stimulation.[21] Massage has also been shown to improve myofascial flexibility.[140, 194] Although it does not increase strength, massage can aid in developing strength by enabling more exercise with decreased probability of injury. Massage does not, however, stimulate the metabolism of fat, as health spas once maintained.

Musculoskeletal hypomobility, intra- and extravascular fluid stasis, and subsequent pain are hypothesized to form a self-perpetuating/feedback loop. Pain and splinting of a joint occur after musculoskeletal injury. Decreased movement in the injured muscles around the joint can cause fluid stasis, which allows for the accumulation of metabolic byproducts. The increasing local concentration of these metabolites is thought to cause irritation and pain, resulting in more involuntary splinting. By mechanically deforming and lengthening connective tissue, massage can alleviate the hypomobility. Massage could also augment the dispersion of the metabolites by its direct effects on venous and lymphatic flow. Pain is relieved as muscle splinting is diminished and noxious metabolites are mobilized. Once the self-perpetuating cycle of hypomobility, stasis, and pain is broken, the body's own restorative mechanisms can complete the healing process. Daily massage has been found to decrease anxiety and stress hormone levels, as well as self-reported and physician-assisted levels of pain in children with rheumatoid arthritis.[51]

Neural reflex reactions to massage have also been proposed to explain some of the its widespread effects. Afferent nerves carry information from the somatic system to the spinal cord. This information includes pain sensation and proprioception as well as feedback from the muscle spindle and autonomic afferents. When a given part of the somatic system is dysfunctional, there is a sustained increase in afferent neural input into the spinal column at that given spinal segmental level. This continuous barrage of increased segmental afferent information is hypothesized to have an effect on other neural elements at that same spinal segmental level, creating a "facilitated spinal segment."[110, 111, 149]

A facilitated spinal segmental level is one that has a decreased threshold for depolarization of all neurons in that segment owing to excessive afferent neural input. At the facilitated spinal segment, any given stimulus for efferent neuronal depolarization causes an exaggerated efferent outflow. This hypothesis implies that all somatic and visceral tissues can be negatively affected if they are innervated by the nerves from a spinal segment that receives afferent information from an area of somatic dysfunction. If this is true, alleviation of somatic dysfunction via massage could result in improved function of somatic and visceral systems that are innervated by the same spinal segment.

Many massage strokes do not necessarily mobilize fluids, release myofascial restrictions, or initiate reflex neurological effects. These strokes are comforting and relaxing and have their greatest effect on the psychological health of the patient. A positive impact on the psychological state of a patient appears to have widespread benefits. The emerging field of psychoneuroimmunology documents the favorable impact of a positive mental attitude on the immune system.[25, 167] Massage in a group of HIV-positive men shows a significant improvement in measures in immune function,[94] and massage in an otherwise healthy population under significant stress increases levels of immune modulators.[199] Alternatively, pain, depression, and anxiety exert a negative effect on the body's immune system. The uplifting and relaxing experience of an expertly given, painless massage could have more than just a psychological benefit, but further documentation of this is needed in future studies.

Massage functions via a variety of mechanisms to benefit a wide variety of conditions. Patients with low back pain, neck pain, fibromyalgia, arthritis, bursitis, tendinitis, fascitis, and even neuromas can benefit from massage techniques. Complications associated with multiple sclerosis, cerebral palsy, hemiplegia, or spinal cord injury such as spasticity, reflex sympathetic dystrophy, edema, and contracture can also be significantly improved. Specific techniques for respiratory problems can help persons with respiratory muscle paralysis. Limited use with varicose ulcers, localized draining infections, and following skin grafting has been reported. Light massage with a lubricant can be useful on a recent skin graft. Deeper massage techniques can be beneficial later after skin grafting to prevent or model scar tissue. Massage can also release deep scar adhesions and contracture following amputations to improve prosthetic fit and comfort.

Types of Massage

The most commonly accepted types of hand movements used in therapeutic massage are from the Swedish system. The four basic stroke types are called (1) effleurage, (2) petrissage, (3) friction and (4) tapotement[89, 194] (see Fig. 20–16). These manipulations are described below.

Effleurage. Effleurage, or stroking massage,[36, 88, 194] involves lightly running the hand over the skin. This can be performed with either superficial or deep pressure and provides different effects depending on the depth of treatment. Deep stroking involves mechanical effects and should be performed with continuous contact of the hands from distal to proximal on the extremities, the back, or the neck. Once the proximal extent is reached, the hands can be drawn back to the distal position applying light contact or no contact at all. Effleurage is especially effective in assisting return of venous or lymphatic drainage, such as following joint sprains, peripheral muscle strains or bruising, and vascular congestion related to surgery, peripheral vascular disease, or reflex sympathetic dystrophy.

Superficial stroking can be performed in any direction and involves mostly reflex and psychological effects to enhance relaxation, especially with muscle hypertonicity or spasticity. One or two hands can be used with varying rate and pressure, depending on the desired effect. A slow rate is used for relaxation, a rapid rate for stimulation. Stroking can also include a rapid hand-over-hand series of short strokes progressing from proximal to distal along a portion of the body.

Petrissage. Petrissage, or compression massage,[36, 69, 88, 194] includes *kneading, picking up, wringing, rolling* and *shaking.* The common characteristic is the compression of the body's soft tissues between two hands or between the hand and the underlying skeletal tissue (see Fig. 20–8). These techniques are designed to mobilize fluid and tissue deposits, as well as to break up tissue and muscle adhesions (see Fig. 20–9). *Kneading* indicates circular movements of one hand superimposed on the other, a single hand, the knuckles, the finger pads, or the thumb compressing superficial soft tissues against deeper ones. *Picking up* includes four basic steps: (1) compression of soft tissue against underlying structures, (2) grasping of the soft tissue, (3) release of the soft tissue, and (4) moving the hands to a new position. *Wringing* resembles picking up, except once the tissue is grasped using two hands side-by-side, one hand pulls while the other pushes. This generates a shear force in the tissue planes. *Rolling* is the motion of gathering skin alone or muscle and skin between fingers and thumb and allowing the tissue to "roll" between these digits before releasing and taking another nearby grasp. In *shaking,* once the soft tissue is firmly grasped between thumb and fingers, the hands are shaken vigorously side to side as they move down the length of the muscle.

Friction Massage. Friction massage,[36, 69, 88, 194] is performed by applying circular or transverse motions through the fingers, thumb, or the heel of the palm of the hand to a small area of tissue (see Fig. 20–10). Treatment progresses from superficial to deep by increasing the pressure through the hand to the level of tissue problem (i.e., muscle, tendon, ligament, or myofascial junction). When applied correctly, no motion should occur between the fingertips and the skin, as the movement should occur deeper in the tissues. Deep friction can be uncomfortable and even cause mild bruising, but it is especially effective for soft tissue problems such as tendinitis or fascitis (e.g., lateral epicondylitis, supraspinatus tendinitis, subacromial bursitis, and plantar fascitis) and trigger points as described by Travell.[179]

Tapotement. Tapotement, or percussion massage,[36, 88, 194] produces stimulation by rhythmic, alternating movements of the hands on the soft tissue of the patient. *Clapping, hacking, vibrations, beating, pounding,* and *tapping* are all types of tapotement massage. *Clapping,* or cupping, is the technique wherein the open palms are cupped and repetitively strike the surface of the body. Often a sheet or towel is placed between the striking hands and the skin. The cupped hand produces a dull noise and affects deeper tissues. A flat hand makes a sharper, high-pitched noise, and stimulates predominantly the skin. *Hacking* consists of repetitively striking the body with the medial border of the hands, with the plane of the open hand perpendicular to the surface of the body. The hands alternate as they strike the body at a rate of 2 to 6 Hz, providing superficial stimulation. *Vibrations* should be distinguished from shakings. Vibrations require a rapid up-and-down motion of pressure and release within the soft tissue without losing contact with the skin. Shaking is a side-to-side, rapid oscillating motion and is not a form of tapotement. *Beating* and *pounding* are rarely used techniques wherein the loosely clenched fists are used to repetitively strike the body in an alternating manner. Beating strikes the body palm down and pounding strikes the body with the medial border of the fist. *Tapping* uses the finger pads to percuss. The second through fourth fingers of each hand in rapid succession alternately rise and fall in small, sensitive areas such as the face.

There are many different styles of massage other than the commonly employed Swedish forms described above. Alternative techniques include acupressure, shiatsu, reflexology, Rolfing and its offshoots, Trager therapy, and lymphatic massage.

Acupressure. Acupressure[175] is a technique of applying constant, circular friction pressure to specific points for treatment purposes. It uses the principles and points of acupuncture defined more than 3000 years ago in China. Acupuncture specialists contend that there are hundreds of points energetically aligned within 12 energy meridians which interconnect and course longitudinally throughout the human body. Disease is believed to result from imbalances in the body's energy systems, or chi (*ki*); therefore, the goal of treatment is to balance the flow of energy through the meridians to allow the body to regain homeostasis and heal itself. In traditional acupuncture, these points are accessed by fine needles, which can be further stimulated by the use of heat, manual manipulation, or electricity. In acupressure, practitioners use their fingers, thumbs, or hands to stimulate these points by circular friction. The art as practiced in China is now taught in some U.S. medical schools. While it is often offered as a distinct treatment, the more widespread use is by massage therapists integrating the technique into their practice. Acupressure can be used as a nonpharmacologic technique to (1) control nausea and vomiting related to morning sickness,[41] chemotherapy,[40] spinal anesthesia,[171] or postoperatively[9, 48]; (2) decrease postoperative pain[49]; (3) treat headache and temporomandibular joint pain[139]; or (4) assist with pulmonary rehabilitation.[122] As a noninvasive approach to a number of problems, acupressure can be safely taught to patients for self-administration at home as one part of a comprehensive rehabilitation program.

Shiatsu. Shiatsu (which means "finger pressure" in Japanese) massage[175] is based on the Japanese interpretation of the acupuncture theory and flow of chi. In shiatsu massage, heavy pressure is applied perpendicularly to the body over a given meridian with the palm of the hand or heel of the foot. The mental attitude of the practitioner is felt to be critical to successful balancing of the energy meridians, and some believe the use of upper body musculature to apply the necessary force requires the practitioner to be too tense to adequately sense patient responses and appropriately guide therapy. Different forms of shiatsu have evolved. Some of them incorporate Western anatomy and physiology as well as diet, breathing, exercise, and lifestyle guidance. In the U.S. and Japan, Shiatsu is taught and practiced as a distinct entity, rather than in combination with Swedish massage. Some practitioners use it for episodic treatment of headache, back pain, menopausal symptoms, constipation, or stress-related conditions, while other practitioners use it on a regular basis as a preventative. Shiatsu as a noninvasive treatment option is beginning to be discussed in traditional medical settings.[187]

Reflexology. Reflexology[175] embraces the philosophic tenet that there is a homuncular representation of the entire human body mapped out on the ear, hand, and sole of the foot. The practice of foot reflexology probably dates back to ancient Egypt, but the notion that discrete ear, hand, foot, and other areas influence the condition of more proximal body structures and functions also has roots in Chinese acupuncture. By palpating the entire surface of these distal regions, one will find areas of point tenderness which correspond to organs or tissues in the body which are dysfunctional. Once these areas are identified, the tender points are treated by circular deep friction massage. Reflexology massage must be firm and can be uncomfortable, but the practitioner should not induce extreme discomfort. Foot reflexology is taught and practiced as a separate discipline in the U.S. Some hand and foot reflexology is often part of Swedish massage training and can be included into a total body massage session. It is often used in patients who cannot tolerate massage to sensitive body areas, or who do not wish to expose their body to the extent required for the total body massage. Practitioners most commonly treat conditions such as back pain, headache, hypertension, stress, fatigue, and digestive complaints, but reflexology can be attempted as a preventive measure. Medical conditions such as hypertension should be monitored closely in order to prevent patient injury if reflexology is to be attempted without more traditional medical treatments. A group of patients experiencing premenstrual symptoms has demonstrated significant improvement with reflexology as compared to placebo.[145] Proposed mechanisms of action include an influence on adrenocortical stress reactivity[145] and centrally mediated effects through the stimulation of peripheral sensory fibers.[56] Although gaining more recognition in medical and lay circles within the U.S., reflexology has not been incorporated into the medical setting to the same extent as other massage techniques such as Swedish massage and acupressure.

Rolfing. Rolfing[20](structural integration) is a method of restructuring and realigning the deep fascial planes in the body through a variety of deep friction massage techniques. Ida Rolf (1896–1979), a chemist, developed and promoted this type of deep fascial massage. The goal is to balance and align the human body in the gravitational field. Rolfing treatment traditionally consists of a series of massages that concentrate on specific body areas, each session building on the previous one, followed by more integrative work. Rolfing theory adheres to the concept of mind-body integration and attempts to favorably influence the psychological state as it corrects physical problems. In the past this type of deep friction was often described as uncomfortable but effective. More recent Rolfers have refined the approach into gentler, less painful techniques more tolerable to patients. There are offshoots of Ida Rolf's original work; two of the best known are Hellerwork and Aston-patterning. Hellerwork combines connective tissue manipulation, movement re-education, and verbal dialogue to assist in release of chronic tension patterns. Aston-patterning practitioners work with the body's spirally directed patterns and include fitness and environmental considerations in their treatment plans. The three styles are gaining popularity in the U.S. and are most frequently performed by independent practitioners outside the medical setting. In the medical rehabilitation setting, physical therapists with specific training are able to integrate the techniques into traditional musculoskeletal and neurological rehabilitation programs.

Trager Psychophysical Integration. Trager psychophysical integration is a combination of gentle, hands-on tissue work, movement re-education, and relaxation exercises. Developed by Milton Trager, M.D., in the 1940s, it attempts to teach patients to move with ease and efficiency. The hands-on work consists of gentle rocking and stretching movements to relax and enliven tense areas of the body. The movement work emphasizes ease and pleasure in movement. Tragerwork has been used mostly outside the medical community, although it has been shown to increase vital capacity in COPD patients.[190] It is currently being investigated for relief of chronic shoulder pain in spinal cord–injured persons.[44]

Lymphatic Massage. First developed in Europe by the Danish physiotherapists Estrid and Emil Vodder in the 1930s, lymphatic massage was later refined by Foldis in Germany and the Casley-Smiths in Australia. The approach uses gentle manual pressure to encourage lymph flow from obstructed to unobstructed lymph nodal areas. Using specialized hand motions such as "stationary circles" and "pumping movements," lymph is directed toward "watershed" areas, or areas drained by a single lymphotome (group of nodes).[14] The focus is more superficial than with deep muscle massage. A typical session lasts approximately 45 minutes, and is used in combination with other modalities. Usually, treatment consists of skin care followed by manual treatment, bandaging, use of compression garments, and exercises aimed at maintaining range of motion and muscle strength and tone. Clinical literature stresses the importance of long-term maintenance for continued volume reduction in the limb, which can range from 25%[96] to 63%.[14] This end reduction in limb volume compares favorably with sequential pneumatic compression, and its popularity in the U.S. is increasing for post-mastectomy arm lymphedema and post-inguinal node resection leg lymphedema.

Contraindications and Risks

There are numerous contraindications to Swedish massage, but the absolute and relative contraindications for acupressure, shiatsu, and reflexology have not been determined. Massage should not be performed over areas of malignancy, cellulitis, or lymphangitis.[106] The effects of massage on mobilizing vascular and lymphatic fluid may only serve to disseminate tumor cells or spread infection.

Areas of recent trauma or bleeding can re-bleed if massage is applied too soon after injury or surgery. Massage is commonly used to increase elasticity and mobility in scar tissues, but caution should be taken not to disrupt the incision by beginning massage before healing is complete. When performing massage after joint replacement, the therapist should be familiar with the allowable range of motion of the replaced joint. Massage should not be performed over any open area where the therapist can be exposed to bloodborne pathogens.

Massage should not be applied over an area of known deep venous thrombosis or over a known atherosclerotic plaque. Deep massage might dislodge venous or arterial thrombi, which can potentially cause pulmonary, cerebral, or peripheral embolic infarcts.

Massage should be done only when the reason for the massage, the cause of the condition being treated, and the goals of therapy are known. For example, if massage is prescribed as a treatment for edema, the cause of the edema should be known (renal failure, heart failure, reflex sympathetic dystrophy, deep venous insufficiency, lymphatic obstruction, immobility, infection, postoperative, etc.).

Using Massage in Practice

The ability to perform structural diagnosis is not essential for prescribing massage techniques, but it can be beneficial in determining the type of treatment that is indicated. There are many similarities between massage techniques and manual medicine techniques such as myofascial release, the lymphatic pump, and other soft tissue release techniques. Knowledge of the indications and contraindications for each treatment approach is essential for safe and effective treatment. There is a risk of psychological patient dependence with these physical modalities, just as there is with medications or manipulation. Contrarily, massage can be used to help treat the anxiety and depression associated with some disorders.[50, 52, 53]

Massage can be very effective within the context of a comprehensive rehabilitation program, and is increasingly being integrated into inpatient and outpatient treatment plans. Since massage is a passive modality, any massage technique must be supplemented with an active treatment program at the proper time. During the initial stages after a fracture or dislocation, tissue mobilization and soft tissue stretching without joint or bone movement is beneficial; but eventually, the patient needs to begin an active movement program to resume normal function. Other diagnoses for which massage is commonly prescribed, such as lumbar sprain or strain, cervical sprain or strain, fibrositis or fibromyalgia, supraspinatus tendinitis, and lateral epicondylitis should have some form of active range-of-motion program started at the time of initial treatment, and should eventually be progressed into a strengthening program when appropriate. For a few disorders such as post-mastectomy lymphedema,[14, 96] rheumatoid joints,[51] COPD,[122, 190] and headaches,[128] massage can be considered for isolated use. Since there are no studies to date that indicate the optimal treatment frequency or duration for any of the massage techniques, repeated clinician evaluations are necessary to follow the progress of a patient. Prescription for treatment should include the diagnosis, area of concentration, goals, precautions, and number of visits necessary for a particular patient complaint.

The basic principles of massage treatment are as follows: (1) the patient must be comfortable, relaxed and not too cold; (2) the therapist must be comfortable and able to complete the technique without shifting position; (3) the therapist should have clean hands, short nails, and no areas of broken skin; (4) the use of lubricants can facilitate ease of techniques; and (5) the skill of the practitioner lies more in the ability to distribute even pressures throughout the hands rather than in strength.

Mastering the art of massage is time-consuming. Practice is essential, as is a natural ability to "listen" with the hands; and incorporating oriental philosophies and principles can require extensive continuing medical education. Some techniques can be difficult to master; hence some practitioners argue against instructing patients or families in home programs. However, for a patient who has demonstrated therapeutic response and benefit, it can become part of a complete home program so that patients can receive ongoing benefit.

REFERENCES

1. Abenhaim L, Bergeron AM: Twenty years of randomized clinical trials of manipulative therapy for back pain: A review. Clin Invest Med 1992; 15:527–535.
2. Adams T, Heisey RS, Smith MC, et al: Parietal bone mobility in the anesthetized cat. J Am Osteopath Assoc 1992; 92:599–622.
3. Agency for Health Care Policy and Research: Acute low back problems in adults: Assessment and treatment. Clin Pract Guide Quick Ref Guide Clin 1994; 14:1–25.
4. Anderson R, Meeker WC, Wirick BE, et al: A meta-analysis of clinical trials of spinal manipulation [see comments]. J Manipulative Physiol Ther 1992; 15:181–194.
5. Assendelft WJ, Bouter SM, Knipschild PG: Complications of spinal manipulation: A comprehensive review of the literature. J Fam Pract 1996; 42:475–480.
6. Assendelft WJ, Koes BW, Knipschild PG, et al: The relationship between methodological quality and conclusions in reviews of spinal manipulation [see comments]. JAMA 1995; 274:1942–1948.
7. Atchison JW: Manipulation. In Gonzalez EG, Matheson RS (eds): The Nonsurgical Management of Acute Low Back Pain. New York, Demos Vermande, 1997, pp 187–198.
8. Atchison JW, Stoll ST, McDowell S: Manipulation under local anesthesia: Lumbar sympathetic blocks followed by high velocity–low amplitude treatment. Arch Phys Med Rehabil 1996; 77:956 (Abstract).
9. Barsoum G, Perry E, Fraser R: Postoperative nausea is relieved by acupressure. J Royal Soc Med 1990; 83:86–89.
10. Beal MC, Vorro J, Johnston WL: Chronic cervical dysfunction: Correlation of myoelectric findings with clinical progress. J Am Osteopath Assoc 1989; 89:891–900.
11. Beurskens AJ, de Vet HC, Koke AJ, et al: Efficacy of traction for nonspecific low back pain: 12-week and 6-month results of a randomized clinical trial. Spine 1997; 22:2756–2762.
12. Blomberg S, Hallin G, Grann K, et al: Manual therapy with steroid injections—A new approach to treatment of low back pain. Spine 1994; 19:569–577.
13. Blomberg S, Svardsudd K, Mildenberger F: A controlled, multicentre trial of manual therapy in low-back pain. Initial status, sick-leave and pain score during follow-up. Scand J Prim Health Care 1992; 10:170–178.
14. Boris M, Weindorf S, Lasinski B: Persistence of lymphedema reduction after noninvasive complex lymphedema therapy. Oncology 1997; 11:99–114.
15. Bourdillon JF, Day EA, Bookout MR: Spinal Manipulation. Oxford, Butterworth-Heinemann Ltd, 1992.
16. Bowles CH: Functional technique: A modern perspective. J Am Osteopath Assoc 1981; 80:326–331.
17. Brandt B Jr, Jones LH: Some methods of applying counterstrain. J Am Osteopath Assoc 1976; 75:786–789.
18. Brodeur R: The audible release associated with joint manipulation. J Manipulative Physiol Ther 1995; 18:155–164.
19. Brodin H: Cervical pain and mobilization. Med Phys 1983; 6:67–72.
20. Cantu RL, Grodin AJ: Myofascial Manipulation: Theory and Clinical Application. Gaithersburg, MD, Aspen Publishers, Inc., 1992.
21. Carrier EB: Studies on physiology of capillaries; reaction of human skin capillaries to drugs and other stimuli. Am J Physiol 1922; 61:528–547.
22. Cassidy JD, Kirkaldy-Willis WH: Manipulation. In Kirkaldy-Willis WH (ed): Managing Low Back Pain. New York, Churchill Livingstone, 1988, pp 287–296.
23. Cassidy JD, Lopes AA, Yong-Hing K: The immediate effect of manipulation versus mobilization on pain and range of motion in the cervical spine: A randomized controlled trial. J Manipulative Physiol Ther 1992; 15:570–575.
24. Cherkin DC, MacCornack FA: Patient evaluations of low back pain care from family physicians and chiropractors [see comments]. West J Med 1989; 150:351–355.
25. Chrousos GP, Gold PW: The concepts of stress and stress system disorders. JAMA 1992; 267:1244–1252.
26. Cislo S, Ramirez MA, Schwartz HR: Low back pain: Treatment of forward and backward sacral torsions using counterstrain. J Am Osteopath Assoc 1991; 91:255–259.
27. Colachis SC Jr, Strohm BR: A study of tractive forces and angle of pull on vertebral interspaces in the cervical spine. Arch Phys Med Rehabil 1965; 46:820–830.
28. Colachis SC Jr, Strohm BR: Cervical traction: Relationship of traction time to varied tractive force with constant angle of pull. Arch Phys Med Rehabil 1965; 46:815–819.
29. Colachis SC Jr, Strohm BR: Radiographic studies of cervical spine motion in normal subjects: Flexion and hyperextension. Arch Phys Med Rehabil 1965; 46:753–760.
30. Colachis SC Jr, Strohm BR: Effect of duration of intermittent cervical traction on vertebral separation. Arch Phys Med Rehabil 1966; 47:353–359.
31. Colachis SC Jr, Strohm BR: Effects of intermittent traction on separation of lumbar vertebrae. Arch Phys Med Rehabil 1990; 50:251–258.
32. Cote P, Kreitz BG, Cassidy JD, et al: The validity of the extension-rotation test as a clinical screening procedure before neck manipulation: A secondary analysis [see comments]. J Manipulative Physiol Ther 1996; 19:59–164.
33. Crue BL: The importance of flexion in cervical traction for radiculitis. U.S. Air Force Med J 1957; 8:374–380.
34. Crue BL, Todd EM: The importance of flexion in cervical halter traction. Bull Los Angeles Neurol Soc 1965; 30:95–98.
35. Cyriax J: Conservative treatment of lumbar disc lesions. Physiotherapy 1964; 50:300–303.
36. Cyriax J, Russell G: Textbook of Orthopaedic Medicine, vol 2: Treatment by Manipulation, Massage and Injection. London, Bailliere Tindall, 1980.
37. Deyo RA, Tsui Wu YJ: Descriptive epidemiology of low-back pain and its related medical care in the United States. Spine 1987; 12:264–268.
38. Dreyfuss P, Dreyer S, Griffin J, et al: Positive sacroiliac screening tests in asymptomatic individuals. Spine 1994; 19:1138–1143.
39. Dreyfuss P, Michaelsen M, Horne M: MUJA: Manipulation under joint anesthesia/analgesia: A treatment approach for recalcitrant low back pain of synovial joint origin. J Manipulative Physiol Ther 1995; 18:537–546.
40. Dundee JW, Ghaly RG, Fitzpatrick KTJ: Optimizing aniemesia in cancer chemotherapy. Br Med J 1987; 294:179.
41. Dundee JW, Sourial F, Ghaly RG, et al: P6 acupressure reduces morning sickness. J Royal Soc Med 1988; 81:439–441.
42. Dvorak J, Dvorak V: Manual Medicine: Diagnostics. Stuttgart, Thieme, 1990.
43. Dvorak J, Dvorak V, Schneider W: Manual Medicine. Berlin, Springer-Verlag, 1984.
44. Dyson-Hudson T: Personal communication, 1998.
45. Edwards BC: Low back pain and pain resulting from lumbar spine conditions. Aust J Physiother 1969; 15:104–110.
46. Eisenberg DM, Kessler RC, Foster C, et al: Unconventional medicine in the United States: Prevalence, costs, and patterns of use. N Engl J Med 1993; 328:246–252.
47. Erhard RE, Delitto A, Cibulka MT: Relative effectiveness of an extension program and a combined program of manipulation and flexion and extension exercises in patients with acute low back syndrome. Phys Ther 1994; 74:1093–1100.
48. Fan C-F, Tanhui E, Joshi S, et al: Acupressure treatment for prevention of postoperative nausea and vomiting. Anesth Analg 1997; 84:821–825.
49. Felhendler D, Lisander B: Pressure on acupoints decreases postoperative pain. Clin J Pain 1996; 12:326–329.
50. Field T, Grizzle N, Scafidi F, et al: Massage and relaxation therapies' effects on depressed adolescent mothers. Adolescence 1996; 31:903–911.
51. Field T, Hernandez-Reif M, Seligman S, et al: Juvenile rheumatoid arthritis: Benefits from massage therapy. J Pediatr Psychol 1997; 22:607–617.
52. Field T, Ironson G, Scafidi F, et al: Massage therapy reduces anxiety and enhances EEG pattern of alertness and math computations. Int J Neurosci 1996; 86:197–205.
53. Field T, Quintino O, Henteleff T, et al: Job stress reduction therapies. Altern Ther Health Med 1997; 3:54–56.

54. Fisk JW: A controlled trial of manipulation in a selected group of patients with low-back pain favouring one side. NZ Med J 1979; 10:288–291.
55. Fisk JW: Medical Treatment of Neck and Back Pain. Springfield, IL, Charles C Thomas, 1987.
56. Frankel B: The effect of reflexology on baroreceptor reflex sensitivity, blood pressure and sinus arthythmia. Complement Ther Med 1997; 5:80–84.
57. Frazer EH: The use of traction in backache. Med J Aust 1954; 41:694–697.
58. Gianakopoulos G, Waylonis GW, Grant PA, et al: Inversion devices: Their role in producing lumbar distraction. Arch Phys Med Rehabil 1985; 66:100–102.
59. Gibbons RW: The evolution of chiropractic: Medical and social protest in America. In Haldeman S (ed): Modern Developments in the Principles and Practice of Chiropractic. New York, Appleton-Century-Crofts, 1980, pp 3–24.
60. Gillstrom P, Ehrnberg A: Long-term results of autotraction in the treatment of lumbago and sciatica. Arch Orthop Trauma Surg 1985; 4:294–298.
61. Gillstrom P, Ericson K, Hindmarsh T: Computed tomography examination of the influence of autotraction on herniation of the lumbar disc. Arch Orthop Trauma Surg 1985; 104:289–293.
62. Goats GC: Massage—the scientific basis of an ancient art: Part 1. The techniques. Br J Sports Med 1994; 28:149–152.
63. Goats GC: Massage—The scientific basis of an ancient art: Part 2. Physiological and therapeutic effects. Br J Sports Med 1994; 28:153–156.
64. Godfrey CM, Morgan PP, Schatzker J: A randomized trial of manipulation for low-back pain in a medical setting. Spine 1984; 9:301–304.
65. Goodridge JP: Muscle energy technique: Definition, explanation, methods of procedure. J Am Osteopath Assoc 1981; 81:249–254.
66. Gorman RF: Cardiac arrest after cervical spine mobilization. Med J Aust 1978; 2:169–170.
67. Graham D: Practical Treatise on Massage. New York, Wm. Wood, 1884.
68. Greenman PE: Models and mechanisms of osteopathic manipulative medicine. Osteopathic Med News 1987; 4:1–20.
69. Greenman PE: Principles of Manual Medicine, ed 2. Baltimore, Williams & Wilkins, 1996.
70. Greenman PE: Craniosacral manipulation in persons with traumatic brain injury. Symposium on Rehabilitation of Traumatic Brain Injury patients. East Lansing, MI, Kellogg Center, Feb 1991.
71. Greenman PE: Syndromes of the lumbar spine, pelvis, and sacrum. In Kraft GH, Stanton DF, Mein EA (eds): Physical Medicine and Rehabilitation Clinics of North America: Manual Medicine 1996; 7(4):773–785.
72. Greenman PE, McPartland JM: Cranial findings and iatrogenesis from craniosacral manipulation in patients with traumatic brain syndrome. J Am Osteopath Assoc 1995; 95:182–188.
73. Greenman PE, Mein EA, Andary M: Craniosacral manipulation. In Kraft GH, Stanton DF, Mein EA (eds): Physical Medicine and Rehabilitation Clinics of North American: Manual Medicine 1996; 7(4):877–896.
74. Grieve GP: Mobilisation of the Spine. New York, Churchill Livingstone, 1991.
75. Gross AR, Aker PD, Quartly C: Manual therapy in the treatment of neck pain. Rheum Dis Clin North Am 1996; 22:579–598.
76. Guo X, Zhao Y: Treating subluxation of sacroiliac joint by manipulation—A report of 100 cases. J Tradit Chin Med 1994; 14:192–194.
77. Hadler NM, Curtis P, Gillings DB, et al: A benefit of spinal manipulation as adjunctive therapy for acute low-back pain: A stratified controlled trial. Spine 1987; 12:702–706.
78. Haldeman S: Spinal manipulative therapy in the management of low back pain. In Finneson BE (ed): Low Back Pain. Philadelphia, J.B. Lippincott Company, 1980, pp 245–275.
79. Haldeman S, Chapman-Smith D, Petersen DM: Guidelines for chiropractic quality assurance and practice parameters. Proceedings of the Mercy Center Consensus Conference. Gaithersburg, MD, Aspen Publishers, 1993.
80. Haldeman S, Rubinstein SM: Cauda equina syndrome in patients undergoing manipulation of the lumbar spine. Spine 1992; 17:1469–1473.
81. Haldeman S, Rubinstein SM: Compression fractures in patients undergoing spinal manipulative therapy. J Manipulative Physiol Ther 1992; 15:450–454.
82. Haldeman S, Rubinstein SM: The precipitation or aggravation of musculoskeletal pain in patients receiving spinal manipulative therapy. J Manipulative Physiol Ther 1993; 16:47–50.
83. Harris JD: History and development of manipulation and mobilization. In Basmajian JV (ed): Manipulation, Traction and Massage. Baltimore, Williams & Wilkins, 1985, pp 3–21.
84. Heilig D: The thrust technique. J Am Osteopath Assoc 1981; 81:244–248.
85. Herzog W, Conway PJ, Kawchuk GN, et al: Forces exerted during spinal manipulative therapy. Spine 1993; 18:1206–1212.
86. Hinterbuchner C: Traction. In Basmajian JV (ed): Manipulation, Traction and Massage. Baltimore, Williams & Wilkins, 1985, pp 172–201.
87. Hoehler FK, Tobis JS, Buerger AA: Spinal manipulation for low back pain. JAMA 1981; 245:1835–1838.
88. Hofkosh JM: Classical massage. In Basmajian JV (ed): Manipulation, Traction and Massage. Baltimore, Williams & Wilkins, 1985, pp 263–269.
89. Hollis M: Massage for Therapists. Oxford, Blackwell Scientific Publications, 1987.
90. Hood LB, Chrisman D: Intermittent pelvic traction in the treatment of the ruptured intervertebral disk. Phys Ther 1968; 48:21–30.
91. Hooper J: Low back pain and manipulation: Paraparesis after treatment of low back pain by physical methods. Med J Aust 1973; 1:549–551.
92. Hruby RJ: Pathophysiologic models and the selection of osteopathic manipulative techniques. J Osteopathic Med 1992; 6:25–30.
93. Hurwitz EL, Aker PD, Adams AH, et al: Manipulation and mobilization of the cervical spine. A systematic review of the literature. Spine 1996; 21:1746–1759.
94. Ironson G, Field T, Scafidi F, et al: Massage therapy is associated with enhancement of the immune system's cytotoxic capacity. Int J Neurosci 1996; 84:205–217.
95. Jackson R: The Cervical Syndrome. Springfield, IL, Charles C Thomas, 1958.
96. Johannson K, Lie A, Ekdah C, et al: A randomized study comparing manual lymph drainage with sequential pneumatic compression for treatment of postoperative arm lymphedema. Lymphology 1998; 31:56–64.
97. Johnston WL: Passive gross motion testing: Part I. Its role in physical examination. J Am Osteopath Assoc 1982; 81:298–303.
98. Jones LH: Strain and Counterstrain. Newark, OH, American Academy of Osteopathy, 1992.
99. Judovich BD: Herniated cervical disc: A new form of traction therapy. Am J Surg 1952; 84:646–656.
100. Judovich BD: Lumbar traction therapy and dissipated force factors. Lancet 1954; 74:411.
101. Judovich BD: Lumbar traction therapy—Elimination of physical factors that prevent lumbar stretch. JAMA 1955; 159:549–550.
102. Judovich BD, Nobel GR: Traction therapy: A study of resistance forces. Am J Surg 1957; 93:108.
103. Kanemetz HL: History of Massage. In Basmajian JV (ed): Manipulation, Traction and Massage. Baltimore, Williams & Wilkins, 1985, pp 211–255.
104. Khalil TM, Asfour SS, Martinez LM, et al: Stretching in the rehabilitation of low-back pain patients. Spine 1992; 17:311–317.
105. Kimberly PE: Formulating a prescription for osteopathic manipulative treatment. J Am Osteopath Assoc 1980; 79:506–513.
106. Knapp ME: Massage. In Kottke FJ, Lahman JF (eds): Krusen's Handbook of Physical Medicine and Rehabilitation. Philadelphia, WB Saunders Company, 1990, pp 433–435.
107. Koes BW, Assendelft WJ, van der Heijden GJMG, et al: Spinal manipulation for low back pain. An updated systematic review of randomized clinical trials. Spine 1996; 21:2860–2871.
108. Koes BW, Bouter LM, van Mameren H, et al: A randomized clinical trial of manual therapy and physiotherapy for persistent back and neck complaints: Subgroup analysis and relationship between outcome measures [see comments]. J Manipulative Physiol Ther 1993; 16:211–219.

109. Koes BW, Bouter LM, van Mameren H, et al: Randomised clinical trial of manipulative therapy and physiotherapy for persistent back and neck complaints: Results of one year follow up [see comments]. Br Med J 1992; 304:601–605.
110. Korr IM: Proprioceptors and somatic dysfunction. J Am Osteopath Assoc 1975; 74:638–650.
111. Korr IM: Somatic dysfunction, osteopathic manipulative treatment, and the nervous system: A few facts, some theories, many questions. J Am Osteopath Assoc 1986; 86:109–114.
112. Krueger BR, Okazaki H: Vertebral-basilar distribution infarction following chiropractic cervical manipulation. Mayo Clin Proc 1980; 55:322–332.
113. Kurz W, Litmanovitch YI, Romanoff H, et al: Effect of manual lymph drainage massage on blood components and urinary neurohormones in chronic lymphedema. Angiol 1981; 32:119–127.
114. LaBan MM, Meerschaert JR: Quadriplegia following cervical traction in patients with occult epidural prostatic metastasis. Arch Phys Med Rehabil 1975; 56:455.
115. Laken MP, Cosovic S: Introducing alternative/complementary healing to allopathic medical students. J Altern Complement Med 1995; 1:93–98.
116. Larson DL, Evans EB: Skeletal suspension and traction in the treatment of burns. Ann Surg 1968; 168:981.
117. Lawson GA, Godfrey CM: A report on studies of spinal-traction. Med Services J Can 1958; 14:762.
118. Leboeuf YC, Hennius B, Rudberg E, et al: Side effects of chiropractic treatment: A prospective study. J Manipulative Physiol Ther 1997; 20:511–515.
119. Lee KP, Carlini WG, McCormick GF, et al: Neurologic complications following chiropractic manipulation: A survey of California neurologists [see comments]. Neurology 1995; 45:1213–1215.
120. Lehmann JF, Brunner GD: A device for the application of heavy lumbar traction: Its mechanical effects. Arch Phys Med Rehabil 1958; 39:696–700.
121. Lewis M, Grundy D: Vertebral osteomyelitis following manipulation of spondylitic necks—A possible risk. Paraplegia 1992; 30:788–790.
122. Maa S, Gauthier D, Turner M: Acupressure as an adjunct to a pulmonary rehabilitation program. J Cardiopulm Rehabil 1997; 17:268–276.
123. MacDonald RS, Bell CM: An open controlled assessment of osteopathic manipulation in nonspecific low-back pain [published erratum in Spine 1991; 16(1):104]. Spine 1990; 15:364–370.
124. Maigne R: Orthopedic Medicine: A New Approach to Vertebral Manipulations. Springfield, IL, Charles C Thomas, 1972.
125. Maigne R: Manipulation of the spine. In Basmajian JV (ed): Manipulation, Traction and Massage. Baltimore, Williams & Wilkins, 1985, pp 71–134.
126. Maitland GD: Vertebral Manipulation. London, Butterworths, 1986.
127. Maitland GD: Peripheral Manipulation. London, Butterworth-Heinemann, 1991.
128. Matsumura WM: Use of acupressure techniques and concepts for nonsurgical management of TMJ disorders. J Gen Orthod 1993; 4:5–16.
129. Meade TW, Dyer S, Browne W, et al: Low back pain of mechanical origin: Randomised comparison of chiropractic and hospital outpatient treatment. Br Med J 1990; 300:1431–1437.
130. Mennel J: The Science and Art of Joint Manipulation. Vol. II: The Spinal Column. London, J. & A. Churchill Ltd, 1952.
131. Mennel JM: Joint Pain: Diagnosis and Treatment Using Manipulative Techniques. London, J. & A. Churchill Ltd, 1964.
132. Mitchell FL Jr: The respiratory-circulatory model: Concepts and applications. In Greenman PE (ed): Concepts and Mechanisms of Neuromuscular Functions. Berlin, Springer-Verlag, 1984.
133. Mitchell FL Jr, Moran PS, Pruzzo NA: An Evaluation and Treatment Manual of Osteopathic Muscle Energy Procedures. Valley Park, MO, Mitchell, Moran, and Pruzzo Associates, 1979.
134. Mitchell FL: Structural pelvic function. AAO Yearbook 1958; 71–89.
135. Nanno M: Effects of intermittent cervical traction on muscle pain. Flowmetric and electromyographic studies of the cervical paraspinal muscles. Nippon Ika Daigaku Zasshi 1994; 61:37–147.
136. Nayak NN: Cervical traction: Prescription patterns. Arch Phys Med Rehabil 1993; 74:1268 (Abstract).
137. Nelson L, Aspegren D, Bova C: The use of epidural steroid injection and manipulation on patients with chronic low back pain. J Manipulative Physiol Ther 1997; 20:263–266.
138. Neumann H-D: Introduction to Manual Medicine. Berlin, Springer-Verlag, 1989.
139. Nixon M, Teschendorff J, Finney J, et al: Expanding the nursing repertoire: The effect of massage on post-operative pain. Aust J Adv Nurs 1997;14:21–26.
140. Nordschow M: Influence of manual massage on muscle relaxation: Effect on trunk flexion. J Am Phys Ther Assoc 1962; 42:653.
141. Norton JM: A tissue pressure model for palpatory perception of the cranial rhythmic impulse. J Am Osteopath Assoc 1991; 91:975–994.
142. Nwuga G, Nwuga V: Relative therapeutic efficacy of the Williams and McKenzie protocols in back pain management. Physiother Practice 1985; 1:99–105.
143. Nwuga VCB: Manipulation of the Spine. Baltimore, Williams & Wilkins, 1976.
144. Nyberg R: Manipulation: Definition, types, application. In Basmajian JV, Nyberg R (eds): Rational Manual Therapies. Baltimore, Williams & Wilkins, 1993, pp 21–47.
145. Oleson T, Flocco W: Randomized controlled study of premenstrual symptoms treated with ear, hand, and foot reflexology. Obstet Gynecol 1993; 82:906–911.
146. Olson VL: Whiplash-associated chronic headache treated with home cervical traction. Phys Ther 1997; 77:417–424.
147. Padua L, Padua R, LoMonaco M, et al: Radiculomedullary complications of cervical spinal manipulation. Spinal Cord 1996; 34:488–492.
148. Paramore LC: Use of alternative therapies: Estimates from the 1994 Robert Wood Johnson Foundation National Access to Care Survey. J Pain Symptom Manage 1997; 13:83–89.
149. Patterson MM: Louisa Burns Memorial Lecture 1980: The spinal cord—Active processor not passive transmitter. J Am Osteopath Assoc 1980; 80:210–215.
150. Pemberton R: The physiologic influence of massage and the clinical application of heat and massage in internal medicine. In Principles and Practices of Physical Medicine, vol I. Hagerstown, MD, W.F. Prior Co., 1932.
151. Postacchini F, Facchini M, Palieri P: Efficacy of various forms of conservative treatment in low back pain. A comparative study. Neuro-orthopedics 1988; 6:28–35.
152. Powell FC, Hanigan WC, Olivero WC: A risk/benefit analysis of spinal manipulation therapy for relief of lumbar or cervical pain. Neurosurgery 1992; 33:73–78.
153. Ramos G, Martin W: Effects of vertebral axial decompression on intradiscal pressure [see comments]. J Neurosurg 1994; 81:350–353.
154. Raskind R, North CM: Vertebral artery injuries following chiropractic cervical spine manipulation—Case reports. Angiol 1990; 41:445–452.
155. Reitman C, Esses SI: Conservative options in the management of spinal disorders, Part II. Exercise, education, and manual therapies. Am J Orthop 1995; 24:241–250.
156. Richard J: Disk rupture with cauda equina syndrome after chiropractic adjustment. NY State J Med 1967; 67:2496–2498.
157. Rogers RG: The effects of spinal manipulation on cervical kinesthesia in patients with chronic neck pain: A pilot study. J Manipulative Physiol Ther 1997; 20:80–85.
158. Rogoff JB: Motorized intermittent traction. In Basmajian JV (ed): Manipulation, Traction and Massage. Baltimore, Williams & Wilkins, 1985, pp 201–207.
159. Saal JS, Saal JA, Yurth EF: Nonoperative management of herniated cervical intervertebral disc with radiculopathy. Spine 1996; 21:877–883.
160. Saghafi D, Curl DD: Chiropractic manipulation of anteriorly displaced temporomandibular disc with adhesion. J Manipulative Physiol Ther 1995; 18:98–104.
161. Scientific Advisory Committee, International Federation of Manual Medicine: Workshop. Fischingen, Switzerland, 1983.
162. Shealy CN, Borgmeyer V: Emerging technologies: Preliminary findings. Decompression, reduction, and stabilization of the lumbar spine: A cost-effective treatment for lumbosacral pain. AJPM 1997; 7:63–65.

163. Sheffield FJ: Adaptation of tilt table for lumbar traction. Arch Phys Med Rehabil 1964; 45:469.
164. Shekelle PG, Adams AH, Chassin MR, et al: Spinal manipulation for low-back pain [see comments]. Ann Intern Med 1992; 117:590–598.
165. Shekelle PG, Adams AH, Chassin MR, et al: The Appropriateness of Spinal Manipulation for Low Back Pain: Indications and Ratings by an All-Chiropractic Expert Panel. Santa Monica, CA, RAND, 1992.
166. Sherman DG, Hart RG, Easton JD: Abrupt change in head position and cerebral infarction. Stroke 1981; 12:2–6.
167. Shors TJ, Weiss C, Thompson RF: Stress induced facilitation of classical conditioning. Science 1992; 257:537–539.
168. Simmers TA, Bekkenk MW, Vidakovic VM: Internal jugular vein thrombosis after cervical traction. J Intern Med 1997; 241:333–335.
169. Sims-Williams H, Jayson MIV, Young SMS, et al: Controlled trial of mobilisation and manipulation for low back pain: Hospital patients. Br Med J 1979; 2:1318–1320.
170. Sleszynski SL, Kelso AF: Comparison of thoracic manipulation with incentive spirometry in preventing postoperative atelectasis. J Am Osteopath Assoc 1993; 93:834–835.
171. Stein D, Birnback D, Danzier B, et al: Acupressure vs. intravenous metclorpramide to prevent nausea and vomiting during spinal anesthesia for cesarean section. Anesth Analg 1997; 84:342–345.
172. Sutherland Cranial Teaching Foundation of the Cranial Academy: Osteopathy in the Cranial Field. Kirksville, MO, The Journal Printing Company, 1976.
173. Sweeney T: Neck school: Cervicothoracic stabilization training. Occupational Medicine: State of the Art Reviews 1992; 7:43–54.
174. Swezey RL, Swezey AM, Warner K: Efficacy of home cervical traction therapy. Am J Phys Med Rehabil 1999; 78(1):30–33.
175. Tappan F: Healing Massage Techniques: Holistic, Classic, and Emerging Methods. Norwalk, CT, Appleton & Lange, 1988.
176. Tesio L, Merlo A: Autotraction versus passive traction: An open controlled study in lumbar disc herniation. Arch Phys Med Rehabil 1993; 74:871–876.
177. Tiidus PM: Manual massage and recovery of muscle function following exercise: A literature review. J Orthop Sports Phys Ther 1997; 25:107–112.
178. Tobis JS, Hoehler F: Musculoskeletal Manipulation: Evaluation of the Scientific Evidence. Springfield, IL, Charles C Thomas, 1986.
179. Travell J, Simonsen M: Myofascial Pain and Dysfunction: The Trigger Point Manual. Baltimore, Williams & Wilkins, 1983.
180. Triano JJ, McGregor M, Hondras MA, et al: Manipulative therapy versus education programs in chronic low back pain. Spine 1995; 20:948–955.
181. Turner D: New apparatus: A spinal traction treatment table. Br J Phys Med 1957; 20:259.
182. Twomey L, Taylor J: Exercise and spinal manipulation in the treatment of low back pain. Spine 1995; 20:615–619.
183. Upledger JE, Vredevoogd JD: Craniosacral Therapy. Seattle, WA, Eastland Press, 1983.
184. van der Heijden GJMG, Beurskens AJ, Koes BW, et al: The efficacy of traction for back and neck pain: A systematic, blinded review of randomized clinical trial methods. Phys Ther 1995; 75:93–104.
185. Veith I: The Yellow Emperor's Classic of Internal Medicine. Baltimore, Williams & Wilkins, 1949.
186. Ward RC: Myofascial release concepts. In Basmajian JV, Nyberg R (eds): Rational Manual Therapies. Baltimore, Williams & Wilkins, 1993, pp 223–241.
187. Weintraub M: Shiatsu massage therapy: A remarkable healing technique in spine pain. J Back Musculoskeletal Rehab 1996; 195–197.
188. Wetzel M, Eisenberg D, Kaptchuk T: Courses involving complementary and alternative medicine at U.S. medical schools. JAMA 1998; 280:787–787.
189. Whittingham W, Ellis WB, Molyneux TP: The effect of manipulation (toggle recoil technique) for headaches with upper cervical joint dysfunction: A pilot study. J Manipulative Physiol Ther 1994; 17:369–375.
190. Witt P, MacKinnon J: Trager psychophysical integration: A method of improving chest mobility of patients with chronic lung disease. Phys Ther 1998; 66:214–217.
191. Wolfson H: Studies on effect of physical therapeutic procedures on function and structure. JAMA 1931; 96:2020–2021.
192. Wong AM, Lee MY, Chang WH, et al: Clinical trial of a cervical traction modality with electromyographic biofeedback. Am J Phys Med Rehabil 1997; 76:19–25.
193. Wong AMK, Leong CP, Chen C-M: The traction angle and cervical intervertebral separation. Spine 1992; 17:136–138.
194. Wood EC: Beard's Massage: Principles and Techniques. Philadelphia, WB Saunders, 1974.
195. Worden RE, Humphrey TL: Effect of spinal traction on the length of the body. Arch Phys Med Rehabil 1964; 45:318–320.
196. Wreje U, Nordgren B, Aberg H: Treatment of pelvic joint dysfunction in primary care—A controlled study [published erratum appears in Scand J Prim Health Care 1993 Mar;11(1):25]. Scand J Prim Health Care 1992; 10:310–315.
197. Yong HK: Sacro-iliac joint pain: Etiology and conservative treatment. Chir Organ Mov 1994; 79:35–45.
198. Zanolla R, Monzeglio C, Balzarini A, et al: Evaluation of the results of three different methods of postmastectomy lymphedema treatment. J Surg Onc 1984; 26:210–213.
199. Zeitlin, D: Unpublished data, 1998.

21 CHAPTER

David C. Weber, M.D., and Allen W. Brown, M.D.

Physical Agent Modalities

Modalities are physical agents that are utilized to produce a therapeutic response in tissue. They include heat, cold, water, sound, electricity, and electromagnetic waves (including infrared, visible, or ultraviolet [UV] light; shortwaves; and microwaves) (Fig. 21–1). This chapter focuses on these physical agent modalities, except for most of the therapeutic uses of electrical stimulation (which are covered in Chapter 22). These modalities are generally considered adjunctive treatments, rather than primary curative interventions. This chapter reviews the physiological effects, common uses, techniques of application, and precautions for the therapeutic use of modalities.

MODALITY PRESCRIPTION

The elements of a prescription for heat or cold are listed in Table 21–1. The condition for which the modality is being used should be clearly indicated. The location to be treated influences modality selection in that large areas can preclude the use of modalities such as ultrasound (US) or ice massage. The surface to be treated can also influence selection. If using US over an irregular surface, degassed water may be preferred over a gel coupling agent. If using superficial heat over an irregular surface, hot packs or heating pads can result in focal heating over prominences, so radiant heat might be preferred. Intensity should be indicated where appropriate (e.g., US power output, hydrotherapy, Fluidotherapy, paraffin bath temperature). Most modalities allow only qualitative dosimetry as currently used in physical medicine, and therefore rely on patient perception of thermal intensity for safety. Duration for most modalities is 20 to 30 minutes, except for US, which is typically 5 to 10 minutes per site. Frequency is based on the severity of the condition being treated and on clinical judgment. Although information about duration and intensity of treatment is noted in this chapter, it is intended only as a guideline, and should be modified by clinical experience and the clinical condition.

Modality selection is influenced by multiple factors (Table 21–2). In selecting a modality, one should recognize that there are few well-designed clinical trials demonstrating the efficacy of *specific* modalities in *specific* conditions. However, there are numerous studies that review the physiological effects of modalities. Having a firm understanding of the physiological effects of a particular modality allows one to make an educated selection. One must understand the heating or cooling capabilities of the various modalities to ensure the selection of the proper modality for the target tissue. Body habitus influences modality selection in that subcutaneous adipose affects the depth of penetration of many modalities. Co-morbid conditions should also be considered. For example, both cold and heat can have adverse effects in the patient with significant arterial insufficiency. Cold can have harmful effects via the production of arterial vasoconstriction, and heat can cause complications via the production of increased metabolic activity, which may exceed the potential increase in blood supply and produce ischemia. Age is also a factor in modality selection. In the pediatric population, US should generally be avoided near open epiphyses.[117] In the elderly population, there can be co-morbidities that will affect modality choice. Gender may also play a role in modality use, since fetal malformations have been reported following US near a gravid uterus.[85]

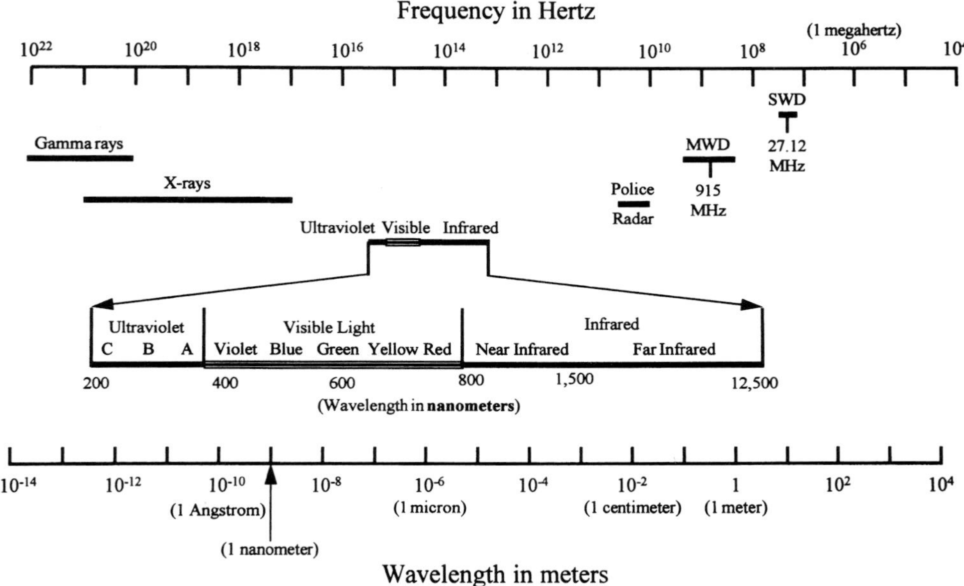

FIGURE 21–1. Electromagnetic spectrum.

HEAT

Forms of heat can be broadly classified by depth of penetration and form of heat transfer (Table 21–3). Depth of penetration is arbitrarily divided into superficial and deep. Superficial heat includes hot packs, heating pads, paraffin baths, Fluidotherapy, whirlpool baths, and radiant heat. Deep heating agents (or diathermies) include US, shortwave, and microwave. Mechanisms of heat transfer include conduction, convection, radiation, evaporation, and conversion (Fig. 21–2). *Conduction* is the transfer of thermal energy between two bodies in direct contact. *Convection* uses movement of a medium (e.g., water, air, blood) to transport thermal energy, although the actual transfer of thermal energy is ultimately by conduction. *Radiation* refers to the thermal radiation emitted from any body whose surface temperature is above absolute zero (−273.15°C or −459.67°F). *Evaporation* involves the transformation of a liquid into a gas, a process that requires thermal energy. Evaporation is actually a process of heat dissipation, and plays a role in cooling modalities such as vapocoolant sprays. For each gram of water that evaporates from the body surface, approximately 0.6 calorie (kilocalorie) of heat is lost.[51] *Conversion* refers to the transformation of energy (e.g., sound, electromagnetic) to heat. Likewise, the human body converts protein, carbohydrates, and fats to thermal energy via numerous metabolic processes. The next section reviews the physiological effects (Table 21–4) of the therapeutic use of heat, followed by discussions of the general uses of heat (see Table 21–5), some general precautions (see Table 21–6), and descriptions of the agents currently used in physical medicine.

Physiological Effects of Heat

Hemodynamic

Localized heating produces a variety of hemodynamic effects. A two- to threefold increase in forearm blood flow has been demonstrated following hydrotherapy at 44 to 45°C (111.2 to 113°F) or shortwave diathermy.[1] This vasodilation results in increased ingress of nutrients, leukocytes, and antibodies, and increased egress

TABLE 21–1 Elements of a Prescription for Heat or Cold

Indication/diagnosis
Modality
Location
Intensity
Duration
Frequency

TABLE 21–2 Factors to Consider in Modality Selection

Target tissue
Depth of heating or cooling desired
Intensity of heating or cooling desired
Body habitus (i.e., amount of subcutaneous adipose)
Co-morbid conditions (e.g., cancer, vascular disease, neuropathy, etc.)
Specific patient features (e.g., metal implants, pacemaker, cold allergy, etc.)
Age (e.g., open epiphyses)
Sex (e.g., pregnant female)

TABLE 21–3 Classification of Various Types of Heating

	Depth	Main Mechanism of Energy Transfer
Hot packs/heating pads	Superficial	Conduction
Paraffin baths	Superficial	Conduction
Fluidotherapy	Superficial	Convection
Whirlpool baths	Superficial	Convection
Radiant heat	Superficial	Radiation
Ultrasound	Deep	Conversion
Shortwave diathermy	Deep	Conversion
Microwave	Deep	Conversion

TABLE 21–4 Physiological Effects of Heat

Hemodynamic
- Increased blood flow
- Decreased chronic inflammation
- Increased acute inflammation
- Increased edema
- Increased bleeding

Neuromuscular
- ?Increased group Ia fiber firing rates (muscle spindle)
- ?Decreased group II fiber firing rates (muscle spindle)
- ?Increased group Ib fiber firing rates (Golgi tendon organ)
- Increased nerve conduction velocity

Joint and connective tissue
- Increased tendon extensibility
- Increased collagenase activity
- Decreased joint stiffness

Miscellaneous
- Decreased pain
- General relaxation

of metabolic byproducts and tissue debris, and may facilitate resolution of inflammatory conditions.[50, 107] Unfortunately, vasodilation with heating may also contribute to increased bleeding and increased edema formation, and can exacerbate acute inflammatory conditions.[107] There are a number of experimental animal models of acute and chronic inflammation which support the general clinical impression that acute inflammatory conditions tend to react unfavorably to heat, whereas chronic inflammatory conditions tend to benefit from heat.[107]

Neuromuscular

Animal experiments of localized heating have demonstrated increased firing rates in all group Ia fibers (muscle spindle) and many group Ib (Golgi tendon organ) fibers, and decreased firing rates in the majority of group II fibers (muscle spindle).[88] It should be noted that all experiments on muscle spindle and Golgi tendon organ firing rates are significantly influenced by the length and tension at which they are performed. This factor likely accounts for many of the differences among investigators.[39, 88] In contrast, the effects of temperature change on nerve conduction velocity are much more consistent. Heating produces modest increases in conduction velocity, whereas cooling is capable of producing dramatic decreases in conduction velocity. Abramson et al[1] noted increases in conduction velocity of up to 7.5 m/sec following hydrotherapy at 44 to 45°C (111.2 to 113°F) or shortwave diathermy, whereas cooling produced conduction velocity decreases of up to 35.8 m/sec. The effects of temperature in clinical neurophysiology are succinctly summarized elsewhere.[32]

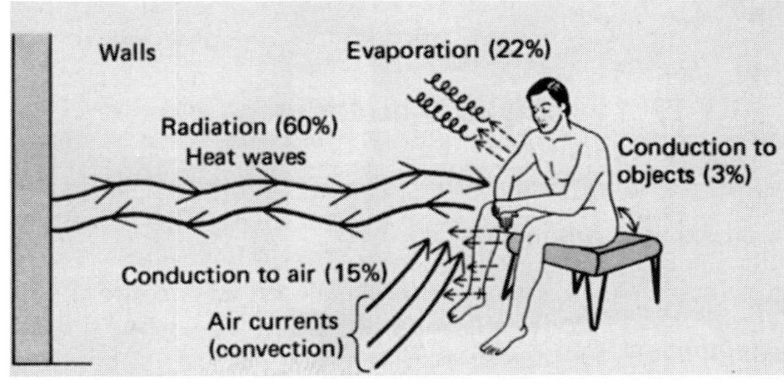

FIGURE 21–2. Mechanisms of heat transfer. (From Guyton AC: Body temperature, temperature regulation, and fever. In Guyton AC (ed): Textbook of Medical Physiology, ed 8. Philadelphia, WB Saunders, 1991, pp 797–808.)

Joint and Connective Tissue

In vitro experiments demonstrate the importance of combined heating and stretching to maximize tendon extensibility. Lehmann et al[73] measured tendon extensibility under a variety of temperature and loading conditions. Tendon extensibility was greater at 45°C (113°F) than at 25°C (77°F). Furthermore, simultaneous use of heating and stretching produced significantly increased tendon extensibility when compared to the isolated use of either agent. Sustaining stretching during the cool-down period also facilitated tendon elongation. Other investigators[130] have demonstrated metacarpophalangeal joint stiffness to decrease by as much as 20% at 45°C (113°F) compared to 33°C (91.4°F). Temperature also affects enzymatic activity. In vitro experiments have shown a fourfold increase in collagenase activity with a temperature increase from 33 to 36°C (91.4 to 96.8°F).[52]

Miscellaneous Effects of Heat

It is generally accepted that heat produces an analgesic effect. A variety of mechanisms for the analgesic effect of heat have been postulated.[40, 66] These include (1) cutaneous counterirritant effect, (2) vasodilation resulting in decreased ischemic pain, (3) vasodilation resulting in washout of pain mediators, (4) endorphin-mediated response, (5) alteration of nerve conduction, and (6) alteration of cell membrane permeability. Elevation of pain threshold has been demonstrated following therapeutic application of US, microwave, and infrared radiation.[67] Many patients also find heat to have a general relaxation effect, although the specific mechanisms are not well defined.

General Uses of Heat in Physical Medicine

The general uses of heat are summarized in Table 21–5. These uses are based on the physiological effects previously described. Heat is used in a variety of musculoskeletal conditions because of its potential to produce analgesia and muscle relaxation, and to facilitate resolution of inflammation. Increased soft tissue extensibility and decreased joint stiffness make heat useful in contractures and a variety of arthritides.

General Precautions for the Use of Heat

The general precautions for the use of heat are listed in Table 21–6. As noted earlier, heat can exacerbate acute inflammation, and should generally be avoided in the acute management stage.[107] In the patient with impaired circulation, increased metabolic activity with heating may exceed the capacity of arterial supply, so heat should be used with caution in this patient population. Vasodilation from heat can result in increased bleeding in persons with bleeding diatheses. Likewise, it can produce increased edema. Since scars can be relatively avascular and have reduced ability for heat dissipation, they can be selectively heated. Heat should generally be avoided in areas of impaired sensation because of obvious potential for thermal injury due to the lack of precise dosimetry in modality use. This same reason justifies caution in using heat in patients with impaired cognition or communication, which precludes reporting of pain. Lehmann[66] cautions against the use of heat over malignancies because of the potential for increased rate of tumor growth or hyperemia increasing hematogenous spread. However, this should be distinguished from the use of specific local hyperthermia in the adjunctive treatment of malignancies.[100] It also does not preclude the use of heat for adjunctive analgesia in the terminally ill cancer patient.

SUPERFICIAL HEAT

Superficial heating agents achieve their maximum tissue temperatures in skin and subcutaneous fat. Deeper tissue heating is limited by vasodilation (which dissipates heat), and the insulating properties of fat. Superficial heating agents can heat via conduction (hot packs, heating pads, and paraffin baths), radiation (heat lamps), or convection (Fluidotherapy and whirlpool baths). Superficial heat is used in osteoarthritis, rheumatoid arthritis, neck pain, low back pain, muscle pain syndromes, and a variety of musculoskeletal conditions.[66]

TABLE 21–5 General Uses of Heat in Physical Medicine

Musculoskeletal conditions (tendinitis, tenosynovitis, bursitis, capsulitis, etc.)
Pain (neck, low back, myofascial, neuromas, postherpetic neuralgia, etc.)
Arthritis
Contracture
Muscle relaxation
Chronic inflammation

TABLE 21–6 General Precautions for the Use of Heat

Acute trauma, inflammation
Impaired circulation
Bleeding diatheses
Edema
Large scars
Impaired sensation
Malignancy
Cognitive or communication deficits that preclude reporting of pain

Hot Packs

Commercially available hot packs, such as Hydrocollator packs, typically contain silicon dioxide encased in a canvas pack. They come in a variety of sizes and styles for use over different areas. Hot packs are immersed in tanks at 74.5°C (166°F) and applied over several layers of insulating towels.[76] After several minutes, the skin should be inspected briefly to ensure that the heating is not excessive. Total treatment time is usually 30 minutes. Lehmann et al[76] showed that 30-minute application of a Hydrocollator pack to the posterior thigh produced approximately 3.3 and 1.3°C tissue temperature elevations at 1- and 2-cm depths, respectively. Other investigators observed a 1.1°C temperature rise 4 cm deep in the brachioradialis muscle following a 30-minute application of a Hydrocollator pack.[2] A 1.2°C increase in intra-articular temperature (knee) has also been demonstrated following hot pack application.[127] General heat precautions should be observed. The patient should not lie on the pack. This can squeeze water from the pack, wetting the insulating towels, thereby raising their thermal conductivity and increasing the risk of burns. Similarly, the focal pressure from lying on a hot pack can produce increased heating over bony prominences. Hot packs are among the more common causes of burns in physical therapy. This is because heat has sedative effects and the patient is typically not directly supervised when this modality is used.

Heating Pads

Two main types of heating pads are available—electric heating pads and circulating-fluid pads. Electric heating pads usually control heat output by regulating current flow. Circulating fluid (e.g., water) heating pads usually control heat output thermostatically. Peak temperatures of nearly 52°C (125°F) were achieved with an electric heating pad set on the *lowest* setting.[33] Periodic temperature oscillations of up to 5°C were also noted.[33] General heat precautions should be observed with heating pads. There is an obvious potential for electric shock, particularly when used in conjunction with moist toweling.

Many commercially available heating pads are designed to be used in conjunction with moist toweling, but caution should be taken to inspect them regularly to ensure that all insulating materials are intact. The patient should not lie on a heating pad, as this can result in focal temperature increases, leading to burns. This is of particular concern in the slender or cachectic patient with minimal subcutaneous adipose over bony prominences. Figure 21–3 shows a typical heating pad burn. The patient was an elderly woman who had not received adequate instruction in home use of her modalities, and had been repeatedly lying supine on an electric heating pad. Repeated and prolonged skin exposure to heat can result in erythema ab igne, a skin condition characterized by reticular pigmentation, and telangiectasia, which has been noted following the use of a variety of superficial heating modalities.[34]

Radiant Heat

Radiant energy, including infrared (IR) radiation, is emitted from any substance with a temperature above absolute zero. IR is the portion of the electromagnetic spectrum adjacent to the long-wavelength, low-frequency (red) end of the visible spectrum. Luminous IR heat lamps emit radiation in the near-infrared spectrum (wavelength 770 to 1500 nm), and nonluminous IR heat lamps emit radiation in the far-infrared spectrum (wavelength 1500 to 12,500 nm).[66] IR produces heating by inducing molecular vibration.[34] A 1.3°C temperature rise has been noted at a depth of 2 cm following heat lamp application.[76]

The main determinants of intensity of radiant heating are distance and angle of delivery. The inverse square law states that the intensity of radiation varies inversely with the square of the distance from the source (Fig. 21–4). This means that doubling the distance from a heat lamp reduces the heating intensity by a factor of 4. Conversely, decreasing the distance from the heat lamp by half would increase the intensity fourfold. Typical distances are 30 to 60 cm from the patient's body, depending on heat lamp wattage.[66] Angle of delivery also affects the intensity of thermal radiation. Maximal radiation is applied when the source of radiation is perpendicular to the surface. As the angle away from perpendicular increases, the intensity of radiation decreases in proportion to the cosine of the angle.

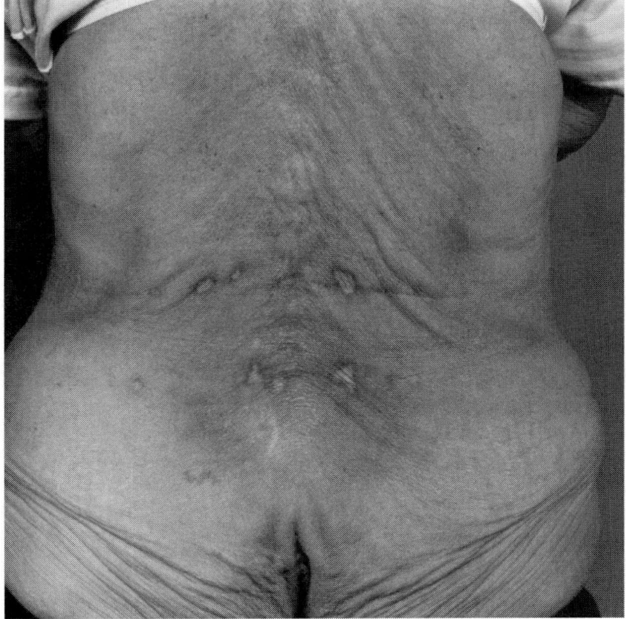

FIGURE 21–3. Typical heating pad burn. Note the focal hypopigmentation from burns at areas of increased pressure. Also note the more diffuse hyperpigmentation changes (erythema ab igne).

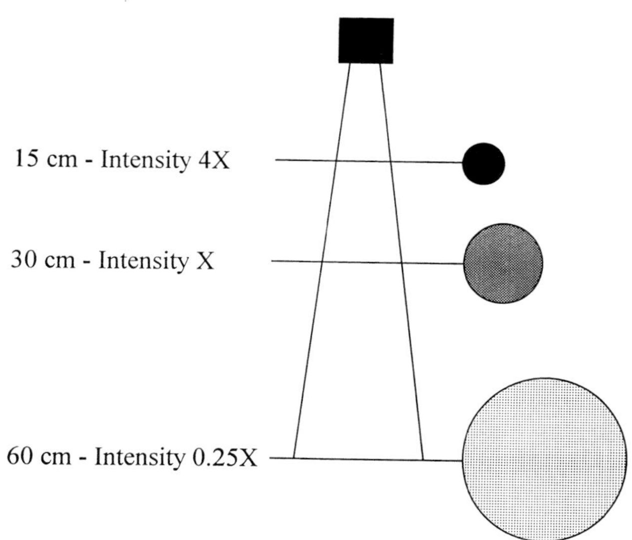

FIGURE 21–4. Example of inverse square law with the intensity arbitrarily defined as *x* at a distance of 30 cm. With a change in distance from the heat source, the area of heating changes and, therefore, the heat intensity per unit of area changes.

Radiant heat is often preferable in patients who cannot tolerate the weight of hot packs. Caveats for the use of radiant heat include (1) general heat precautions, (2) light sensitivity, (3) skin drying, and (4) dermal photoaging.[34, 66] Some laboratory data suggest a potential for IR acting synergistically with UV radiation in cutaneous photocarcinogenesis, but the clinical significance of this, if any, remains to be determined.[34]

Fluidotherapy

Fluidotherapy is a superficial, dry heating modality that uses convective heating with forced hot air and a bed of finely divided solid particles.[14] This solid–gas system reportedly behaves like a heterogeneous fluid of low viscosity, a phenomenon labeled fluidization.[13] Reputed advantages include the massaging action of the highly turbulent solid–gas mixture, and the freedom to perform range-of-motion exercises.[13] Peak hand muscle and joint capsule temperatures of nearly 42°C (107.6°F) and peak foot muscle and joint capsule temperatures of approximately 39.5°C (103.1°F) have been achieved following 20 minutes of Fluidotherapy at 47.8°C (118°F).[14] Both the temperature and the amount of agitation can be controlled. The typical temperature range is 46.1 to 48.9°C (115 to 120°F). Decreased degrees of agitation can be utilized for sensitive areas. General heat precautions should be observed, and infected wounds should probably be avoided because of the risk of cross-contamination.

Paraffin Baths

A paraffin bath is a superficial heating agent that uses conduction as the primary form of heat transfer. Paraffin wax and mineral oil are mixed in a ratio of 6:1 or 7:1.[66] Treatment temperatures are 52.2 to 54.4°C (126 to 130°F). These are tolerated because of the low heat conductivity of the paraffin mixture.[66] A thermometer should be used to ensure proper temperature. A thin film of unmelted paraffin on the tank walls generally indicates a safe temperature. Methods of application include dipping, immersion, and brushing. After removing all jewelry, thoroughly wash and dry the area to be treated. The dipping method involves 7 to 12 dips followed by wrapping in plastic and towels or insulated mitts to retain heat.[2] The immersion method involves several dips to form a thin glove of paraffin, followed by immersion for 30 minutes.[2] The brushing method involves brushing on several coats of paraffin, followed by covering with towels. The brushing method is more cumbersome and infrequently used in the adult population. However, children may find paraffin brushing to be fun, thereby improving their treatment compliance. Paraffin brushing can also be useful for areas difficult to immerse. For home treatment, patients can use a double boiler, although commercial paraffin tanks are reasonably inexpensive and probably safer. The equipment safety precautions should be carefully reviewed. General heat precautions apply to paraffin use. Open wounds and infected areas should be avoided.

The immersion method produces the greatest quantity and duration of temperature increase, with peak forearm subcutaneous tissue temperatures of 5.5°C over baseline and brachioradialis temperatures of 2.4°C over baseline.[2] The dip method produces a 4.4°C peak forearm subcutaneous tissue temperature rise and a 1.0°C brachioradialis temperature rise, but these temperature rises decrease significantly by 15 to 20 minutes post-dipping.[2] In a study of scleroderma patients, paraffin baths in conjunction with friction massage and active range-of-motion exercise resulted in statistically significant improvement in skin compliance and overall hand function.[4] In a study of rheumatoid arthritis patients, statistically significant improvements in range of motion and grip function were noted following paraffin treatment in conjunction with active range-of-motion exercises, whereas paraffin baths alone had no statistically significant effect.[31] This again emphasizes the importance of using exercise in combination with the modality.

DEEP HEAT

Diathermy is derived from *dia* (through) and *therme* (heat), and refers to several forms of deep heating, namely shortwave, microwave, and US. Since the target tissue in physical medicine is generally muscle, tendon, ligament, or bone (rather than skin or subcutaneous fat), the goal of early investigators was to discover a mode of heating that minimized skin and subcutaneous tissue heating, but maximized heating of deeper tissues.[50] The challenge of diathermy developers was to discover a modality that could penetrate the skin and subcutaneous fat to produce a maximum temperature rise in underlying soft tissues. Conversely, the modality should not produce excessive temperatures in more superficial tissues (subcutaneous fat, being relatively avascular compared to muscle, is unable to adequately dissipate heat via vasodilation). The therapeutic target temperature is generally considered to be 40 to 45°C (104 to 113°F).[50] Lower temperatures may not produce adequate vasodilation and increased metabolism, whereas higher temperatures can result in tissue damage. Since the thermal pain threshold is approximately 45°C (113°F), pain perception may be used to monitor intensity of heating.[50] One gradually increases modality intensity to the earliest pain perception, then slightly decreases intensity. However, there is a fine line between the therapeutic temperature range and potential thermal injury.

Ultrasound

Ultrasound is defined as acoustic vibration with frequencies above the audible range (i.e., greater than 20,000 Hz). Medical uses of US can be diagnostic or therapeutic. Diagnostic US is used for a variety of obstetric, urological, cardiovascular, and other imaging studies, and is outside the scope of this chapter. Therapeutic US involves the use of high-frequency acoustic energy to produce thermal and nonthermal effects in tissue. Ultrasonic signals are typically generated using the reverse piezoelectric effect. Certain quartz crystals and synthetic ceramics have piezoelectric characteristics, such that when they vibrate they produce an electric current.[119] Conversely, by passing an electric current across such crystals, vibration at a specific frequency is produced.

As ultrasonic waves travel through tissue, they lose a proportion of their energy, a process called attenuation.[131] *Attenuation* in tissue is produced by several mechanisms: absorption, beam divergence, and deflection.[131] *Absorption* is the major cause of US attenuation.[131] Ultrasonic energy is absorbed by the tissue, and is ultimately converted into heat.[131] For most tissues, attenuation increases as frequency increases, so a 1.0-MHz signal would penetrate deeper than a 3.0-MHz signal because of its lower attenuation by the tissue.[131] *Beam divergence* is the amount that the beam spreads out from the transducer. Beam divergence decreases as frequency increases, so a higher frequency signal has a more focused beam.

Deflection includes the processes of *reflection, refraction,* and *scattering.*[131] The *angle* of the reflected wave is equal to the angle of the incident wave (Fig. 21–5). The *magnitude* of the reflected wave depends on the difference in acoustic impedance between the tissues

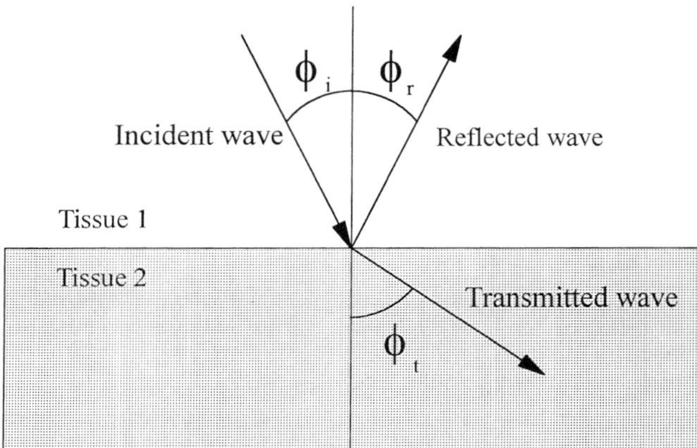

FIGURE 21–5. Example of reflection and refraction at a tissue interface. ϕ_i = Angle of incident wave; ϕ_r = angle of reflected wave; and ϕ_t = angle of transmitted wave.

TABLE 21–7 Ultrasound Parameters

Frequency—millions of cycles per second (MHz)
Power—total energy per unit time (W)
Effective radiating area—the area of the transducer that actually radiates ultrasonic waves (cm^2)
Intensity—may be expressed in terms of peak or average and spatial or temporal (W/cm^2)
  Spatial average intensity—total power output divided by effective radiating area
  Spatial peak intensity—maximal intensity anywhere within the beam
  Temporal average intensity—average intensity of "on" and "off" periods of a pulsed signal
  Temporal peak intensity—maximal intensity of "on" period of a pulsed signal
Duration—generally 5–10 min per site
Additional parameters for pulsed ultrasound
  Pulse duration—time of actual ultrasound pulse ("time on")
  Pulse repetition period—time interval from one pulse to the next ("time on" and "time off")
  Pulse repetition frequency—number of pulses per second
  Duty factor—fraction of total time during which ultrasound is emitted (calculated by dividing pulse duration by pulse repetition period)

on each side of the reflecting surface.[131] Acoustic impedance is a measure of the resistance to the transmission of a sound wave and is the product of the velocity of sound and density of the medium.[119, 131] The magnitude of the reflected wave is proportional to the following formula[119]:

$$A_2 - A_1/A_2 + A_1$$

where A_2 is the acoustic impedance of tissue 2 and A_1 is the acoustic impedance of tissue 1. Therefore, the greater the mismatch of acoustic impedance of the two tissues, the greater the magnitude of the reflected wave. Since the impedance mismatch between skin and air is extremely high, essentially all of the acoustic signal is reflected if a coupling agent is not used (see below).[131] *Refraction* is a deviation of beam direction as it is transmitted between two media (see Fig. 21–5). The angle of the transmitted (refracted) wave is determined by the velocity of sound in the two media, and is given by Snell's law[131]:

$$\text{sine } 1/\text{sine } 2 = \text{velocity } 1/\text{velocity } 2$$

where sine 1 is the sine of the incident wave, sine 2 is the sine of the transmitted wave, velocity 1 is the velocity of sound in the first tissue, and velocity 2 is the velocity of sound in the second tissue. *Scattering* is the last mechanism of beam deflection. It occurs when surface irregularities scatter the signal. Scattering is minimized when surface irregularities are small with respect to the wavelength.

Parameters for therapeutic US are noted in Table 21–7. Frequency is generally in the range of millions of cycles per second (or megahertz, MHz). In the United States, the most commonly used frequencies are in the range of 0.8 to 1.1 MHz, although frequencies around 3.0 MHz are also fairly common. Power is total energy per unit time, whereas intensity is power per unit area. Intensity can be expressed in terms of peak or average intensity, and spatial or temporal intensity, and is indicated in units of watts per square centimeter. These different measures of intensity are defined in Table 21–7. The World Health Organization and the International Electrical Commission both recommend limiting spatial average intensity to 3 W/cm^2.[56] Most clinically used intensities of therapeutic US are in the 0.5 to 2.0 W/cm^2 range. Temperatures of up to 46°C (114.8°F) in deep tissues (e.g., bone–muscle interface) are easily achieved with US.[69–71] If very deep heating (e.g., hip joint) is the goal, US appears to be superior to microwave or shortwave diathermy.[75]

Ultrasound delivery can be continuous or pulsed. Pulsed delivery involves the emission of brief bursts or pulses of US, interspersed with periods of silence (Fig. 21–6). For pulsed US delivery, additional parameters should be indicated.[119] These include pulse duration, pulse repetition period, pulse repetition frequency, and duty factor, and are defined in Table 21–7. In most US units, selecting a duty factor automatically determines the other parameters. Duty factor commonly ranges from 10% to 50%. For example, a 2-ms pulse duration might be interspersed with 8 ms of silence. The pulse repetition period would be 10 ms, the pulse repetition frequency would be 100 Hz, and the duty factor would be 20%. Pulsed delivery, especially at low duty factors, results in less heating than continuous-wave US, and thereby presumably emphasizes nonthermal effects.

The physiological effects of US can be divided into thermal and nonthermal effects. Thermal effects are produced when acoustic energy is absorbed, producing

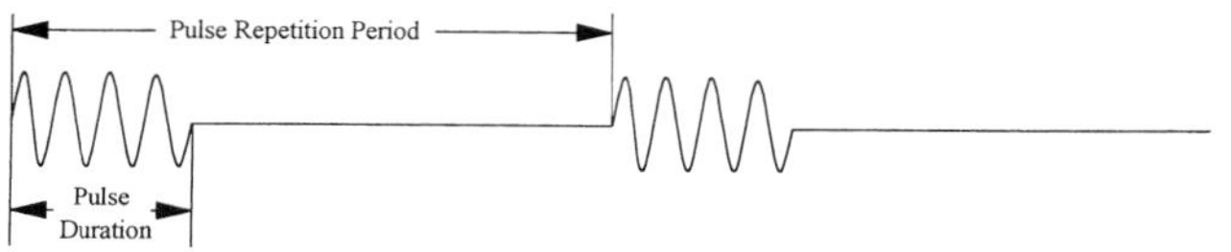

FIGURE 21–6. Example of pulsed ultrasound signal.

molecular vibration, which results in heat production.[22] Nonthermal effects include cavitation, media motion (acoustic streaming, microstreaming), and standing waves. *Cavitation* is the production of gas bubbles in a sound field.[22] These bubbles can expand and contract with alternating compressions and rarefactions of a sound wave.[22] Stable cavitation refers to bubbles that oscillate in size within the sound field.[36] Unstable cavitation refers to bubbles that continue to grow in size and then collapse. The high temperatures and pressures generated by this can produce platelet aggregation, localized tissue damage, and cell death.[36] Both forms of cavitation are capable of mechanical distortion, movement of material, and alteration of cellular function, but their clinical significance is not yet clearly defined.[22, 90]

Media motion includes acoustic streaming and microstreaming. Acoustic *streaming* is defined as unidirectional movement in an ultrasonic pressure field, and results from an ultrasonic wave traveling through a compressible medium.[36] Acoustic *microstreaming* is produced by stable cavitation. As the stable cavitation bubbles oscillate in size, the surrounding fluid is set in motion, with nearby particles being attracted to the oscillating bubble.[36] In addition to movement of material, acoustic streaming and microstreaming can result in cell membrane damage and accelerate metabolic processes.[36]

Standing waves are produced by the superimposition of incident and reflected sound waves and can result in focal heating at tissue interfaces of different densities.[36] Stasis of red blood cells at one-half wavelength intervals in a sound field has also been demonstrated in the laboratory.[37] Although numerous subcellular, cellular, and tissue nonthermal US effects have been reported, their clinical significance remains to be elucidated.[22, 28, 36, 37, 90] Certain measures can minimize the nonthermal effects of US. Higher frequency, lower intensity, and pulsed delivery mode minimizes acoustic cavitation.[28] Stroking technique of application minimizes standing wave formation.[36]

As noted previously, the amount of US reflected at an interface between two media depends on the difference in acoustic impedance, so the ideal coupling medium is one with an acoustic impedance similar to tissue. Three factors have an impact on the effectiveness of a coupling medium: (1) absorption by the medium, which attenuates the ultrasound power; (2) impedance match between the coupling media and the transmitter sound head, which determines the amount of power reflected into the US source; and (3) impedance match between the coupling medium and the body tissue, which determines the amount of power reflected into the medium.[5] Degassed water is a commonly used coupling medium and is used to prevent bubble formation on the skin surface. Allowing tap water to stand overnight should allow for adequate gas evaporation. In tests of acoustic transmissivity, mineral oil and several commercially available coupling gels had similar transmissivities to the reference standard of distilled degassed water.[122] However, the hydrocortisone phonophoresis coupling agents tested had a significantly lower transmissivity, presumably related to microscopic air bubbles introduced into the media. Variation in transducer pressure produced dramatic differences in transmissivity, which outweighed the differences between the various coupling media. These investigators concluded that coupling media can be chosen primarily on the basis of cost and convenience, without compromising function.[122] Encased silicon gel shows promise for use as a coupling agent over irregular body surfaces, sensitive skin areas, and open wounds, if the issue of impedance mismatch with the sound head can be rectified.[5] In addition to accommodating for impedance mismatches, coupling media also lubricate to permit smooth movement of the transducer over the skin.

The most common technique of US application is the stroking technique. It allows a more even energy distribution over the site being treated. The applicator is moved slowly over an area of approximately 25 cm^2 (4 sq inches) in a circular or longitudinal manner.[66] The applicator size (usually 5 to 10 cm^2) limits the size of the area that can be treated, so multiple fields of treatment may be needed for larger areas (i.e., shoulder and hip anterior, lateral, and posterior ports). The stationary technique generally should be avoided because of the potential for standing waves and the production of hot spots.[95] Intensity is indicated by specifying the particular watts per square centimeter or by titrating to just below pain threshold. In surveys of performance of ultrasonic therapy equipment, variations in frequency and power output were common.[56, 114] Although the frequency of commercially available US applicators was typically within 5% of manufacturer's specifications, the overwhelming majority (85%) of applicators tested had power output variations of over 20%.[114] Therefore, US applicators should be recalibrated regularly.

More than 35 clinical uses of US have been described, but many of these are not well supported by experimental evidence.[117] Falconer et al[40] summarized the literature addressing the effectiveness of US in a variety of musculoskeletal conditions, including periarticular inflammatory conditions (bursitis, capsulitis, epicondylitis, tendinitis), other "chronic inflammatory conditions" (rheumatoid arthritis, ankylosing spondylitis, nonspecific musculoskeletal pain, low back pain, frozen shoulder), and osteoarthritis. Study differences precluded meta-analysis, so a quantitative synthesis was performed instead. The overall quality of many of the studies was questionable. Only 5 of 35 studies were blinded and placebo-controlled. As one would expect, uncontrolled or unblinded studies were more likely to produce positive outcomes. The authors concluded that pain and range of motion appear to improve following US treatment in acute periarticular inflammatory conditions and osteoarthritis, but not in chronic periarticular inflammatory conditions.[40] Pain relief was theorized to be related to alterations in nerve conduction, washout of pain mediators by increased blood flow, or alterations in cell membrane permeability that result in decreased inflammation.[40] The authors emphasized a significant placebo effect and experimenter expectancy bias and noted that well-designed clinical trials (e.g., randomized, controlled, blinded studies) are necessary to resolve the issue of ultrasound efficacy.[40]

TABLE 21–8 Ultrasound Precautions

General heat precautions
Near brain, eyes, reproductive organs
Gravid or menstruating uterus
Near pacemaker
Near spine, laminectomy sites
Malignancy
Skeletal immaturity
Arthroplasties?
Methyl methacrylate or high-density polyethylene?

Ultrasound precautions are summarized in Table 21–8.[85, 95, 117] Concern about the use of heat near malignancies was discussed previously. Deep heating over an open epiphysis could result in either increased growth (from hyperemia) or decreased growth (from thermal injury). Avoiding US near pacemakers is reasonable because of potential thermal or mechanical injury to the pacemaker. US over laminectomy sites could theoretically result in spinal cord heating. US at therapeutic dosage over the peroneal nerve has been shown to produce a reversible conduction block in some patients with polyneuropathy.[58] There are also case reports of increased radicular pain with US.[44] There are even case reports of patient abuse of US.[79] The concern with US use over arthroplasties and other metallic implants is the potential for focal heating. Gersten[43] reported that temperature rises near metal were actually lower than temperature rises near bone, so metal per se should not be a contraindication to US. However, Lehmann[66] cautions against the use of US near methyl methacrylate or high-density polyethylene because of their high coefficient of absorption. The effect of US on bony ingrowth arthroplasties is not yet well defined. Since the effects of US on arthroplasties are not yet completely delineated, the most prudent course would be to avoid US over these areas whenever possible.

Shortwave Diathermy

Shortwave diathermy (SWD) is a modality that produces deep heating via conversion of electromagnetic energy to thermal energy. Oscillation of high-frequency electrical and magnetic fields produces movement of ions, rotation of polar molecules, and distortion of nonpolar molecules, with resultant heat generation.[45, 60] The Federal Communications Commission (FCC) limits industrial, scientific, and medical (ISM) use to 13.56 MHz (22-m wavelength), 27.12 MHz (11-m wavelength), and 40.68 MHz (7.5-m wavelength).[62] The 27.12-MHz frequency is most commonly used. The heating pattern produced depends on the type of shortwave unit and on the water content and electrical properties of the tissue. Tissues can be grossly divided into those with high water content (muscle, skin, blood, etc.) and those with low water content (bone, fat, etc.).[60]

Shortwave diathermy units can be inductive or capacitive. Inductive applicators use induction coils which apply a magnetic field to induce circular electrical fields in the tissue.[50] They achieve higher temperatures in water-rich tissues with higher conductivity.[62] These applicators may have a cable or drum configuration.[62] Cables are semiflexible induction coils which can be formed to the contour of the area to be treated. Drum applicators consist of induction coils enclosed in a rigid housing or drum. For a capacitive applicator, the patient is placed between two metal condenser plates (Fig. 21–7). The plates and the patient's intervening tissue act as a capacitor (an object that stores electrical charge), and heat is generated by rapid oscillations in the electric field from one plate to the other.[45] Capacitive applicators may achieve higher temperatures in water-poor tissues such as subcutaneous adipose.[50, 62]

Currently available shortwave applicators do not allow precise dosimetry, so initial pain perception is used to monitor intensity. Terrycloth towels are used for spacing and to absorb sweat, which is highly conductive and could result in potentially severe focal heating.[66] Typical treatment time is 20 to 30 minutes. Specific applicator configuration can greatly affect the distribution of heating.[62, 74] In a review of several different induction applicators, the ratio of muscle heating versus fat heating ranged from 0.39 to 2.67 for the various applicators tested.[74]

Lehmann et al[68] evaluated the effect of subcutaneous fat thickness and technique of SWD application. In comparing distance from the applicator, 2 cm of air space between patient and applicator produced a more desirable heating pattern than did 3 mm of terrycloth between patient and applicator. Depth of subcutaneous fat also had a significant effect on temperature distribution. Muscle temperature rise in subjects with less than 1 cm of subcutaneous fat was 9.5°C, compared with 5.6°C in subjects with more than 2 cm of subcutaneous fat.[68] SWD has been purported to be useful in a variety of musculoskeletal conditions.[45] The precautions are listed in Table 21–9. Metal can result in focal heating and should be strictly avoided. All jewelry should be removed, and the treatment table ideally should not contain metal. Likewise, electromagnetic energy can seriously interfere with pacemaker function, so a pacemaker is an absolute contraindication. Contact lenses are a concern because of the potential for focal heating.[108] The other precautions listed are self-explanatory.

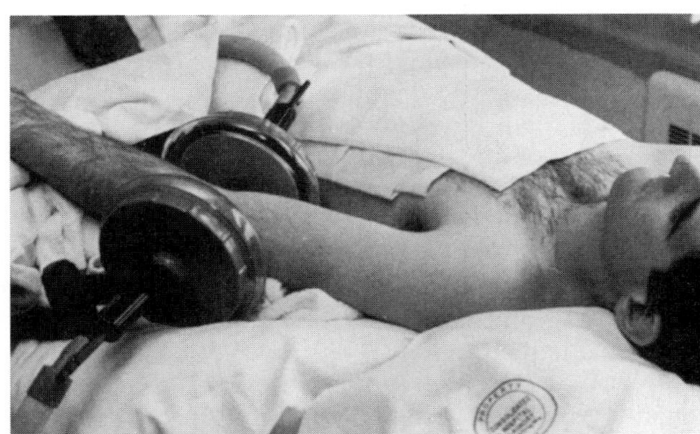

FIGURE 21–7. Example of shortwave diathermy application with capacitive applicator (condenser plates). (From Kotke FJ, Lehmann JF (eds): Krusen's Handbook of Physical Medicine and Rehabilitation, ed 4. Philadelphia, WB Saunders, 1990, p 293.)

TABLE 21–9 Shortwave Precautions

General heat precautions
Metal (jewelry, pacemakers, intrauterine devices, surgical implants, etc.)
Contact lenses
Gravid or menstruating uterus
Skeletal immaturity

Microwave Diathermy

Microwave diathermy is another form of electromagnetic energy which uses conversion as its primary form of heat production. Thermal energy is produced by increased kinetic energy of molecules within the microwave field.[99] FCC-approved frequencies for therapeutic microwave are 915 MHz (wavelength 33 cm) and 2456 MHz (wavelength 12 cm).[66] The lower frequency has the advantage of increased depth of penetration, but disadvantages of greater beam dispersion and the requirement of larger applicators.[99]

Temperature distribution in a particular tissue is affected largely by its water content. The fraction of power absorbed in a particular tissue depends on several factors, including the frequency of the electromagnetic wave, the dielectric constant, and the electrical conductivity of the tissue.[99] In general, tissues with high water content absorb greater amounts of energy, and are selectively heated.[66] If muscle heating is a primary objective, 915-MHz applicators are preferable to 2456-MHz applicators.[72] Nonthermal effects of microwave diathermy have been documented, but Lehmann points out that there is no evidence that these are of any therapeutic significance.[66] Average temperatures of approximately 41°C (105.8°F) at a depth of 1 to 3 cm have been demonstrated.[30] Microwave, although once quite popular, has been largely replaced by other modalities such as US and hot packs.[115] However, a study by Weinberger did demonstrate some potential benefit in rheumatoid arthritis. In this study, treatment with 915-MHz microwave to the rheumatoid knee resulted in statistically significant improvements in pain score index and walking speed.[126]

General heat precautions should be observed with microwave. Metal implants, pacemakers, sites of skeletal immaturity, reproductive organs and brain, and fluid–filled cavities (eye, bullae, effusions, etc.) should be avoided.[61, 66]

CRYOTHERAPY

All forms of cryotherapy (therapeutic use of cold) are considered superficial cooling agents, usually transferring thermal energy by conduction. Exceptions include convective cooling in the whirlpool, and evaporative cooling with vapocoolant sprays (Table 21–10). This section reviews the physiological effects (Table 21–11), general uses (Table 21–12), and general precautions (Table 21–13) for cryotherapy, followed by a discussion of the agents currently used in physical medicine.

TABLE 21–10 Classification of Various Types of Cooling

	Depth	Main Form of Energy Transfer
Cold packs	Superficial	Conduction
Ice massage	Superficial	Conduction
Cold water immersion	Superficial	Conduction
Cryotherapy-compression units	Superficial	Conduction
Vapocoolant spray	Superficial	Evaporation
Whirlpool baths	Superficial	Convection

Physiological Effects of Cold

Hemodynamic

Application of cold to the skin results in immediate cutaneous vasoconstriction through sympathetically mediated reflex mechanisms and by directly stimulating smooth muscle contraction.[51, 101] Lewis[81] observed phasic oscillations of temperature in the fingers after initial vasoconstriction during cold water immersion. The initial vasoconstriction is thought to be due to a cold-induced increase in the affinity of the postjunctional alpha-adrenergic receptors for existing norepinephrine in vascular smooth muscle.[111] Reactive vasodilation occurs as further cooling interrupts norepinephrine release. Vasodilation warms the tissues, again releasing norepinephrine to sensitized receptors, and the cycle repeats. This "hunting" of temperature is believed to be a mechanism by which peripheral exposed parts of the body are protected from cold injury. Others have demonstrated vasodilation after cooling of the hand and forearm, without the phasic oscillations observed by Lewis.[21, 41] The effects of localized cooling on heart rate and blood pressure are variable, and have been summarized elsewhere.[86] Cryotherapy has also been

TABLE 21–11 Physiological Effects of Cold

Hemodynamic
- Immediate cutaneous vasoconstriction
- Delayed reactive vasodilation
- Decreased acute inflammation

Neuromuscular
- Slowing of conduction velocity
- Conduction block and axonal degeneration with prolonged exposure
- Decreased group Ia fiber firing rates (muscle spindle)
- Decreased group II fiber firing rates (muscle spindle)
- Decreased group Ib fiber firing rates (Golgi tendon organ)
- Decreased muscle stretch reflex amplitudes
- Increased maximal isometric strength
- Decreased muscle fatigue
- Temporarily reduced spasticity

Joint and connective tissue
- Increased joint stiffness
- Decreased tendon extensibility
- Decreased collagenase activity

Miscellaneous
- Decreased pain
- General relaxation

shown to moderate inflammation, more effectively in the acute phase than in the chronic phase.[107]

Neuromuscular

The initial response of peripheral nerve to cold application is a marked slowing of conduction velocity.[1, 32] With more prolonged exposure there is conduction block, cessation of axoplasmic transport, and eventual axonal degeneration.[94] Decreased muscle spindle (both group Ia and II fibers) and Golgi tendon organ (group Ib fibers) firing rates have been demonstrated after local cooling in animals.[39] The clinical neuromuscular effects of cooling include a decrease in gastrocnemius muscle stretch reflex amplitude,[11, 65] an increase in maximal isometric strength,[20, 84] and slowing in the rate of muscle fatigue.[20] Cold has also been shown to temporarily reduce spasticity in patients with hemiplegia and multiple sclerosis, improving exercise tolerance and enhancing function.[55, 89] However, other investigators have noted increased spasticity after cold application in some subjects.[17, 103]

Joint and Connective Tissue

Topical cold application (approximately 4°C) to the knee in dogs induced significant and sustained depression of intra-articular temperature without significant effect on core temperature.[12] Synovial collagenase activity also decreases with temperature. In vitro experiments demonstrate negligible synovial collagenase activity after cooling to 30°C (86°F), suggesting that therapy that decreases intra-articular temperature in inflammatory arthropathies may slow the rate of collagenolysis.[52] However, it should be noted that in one study of the use of cryotherapy after cruciate ligament surgery, skin temperature had to be lowered to 20°C in order to produce significant intra-articular temperature declines.[26] Potentially negative effects such as decreased tendon extensibility and increased joint stiffness have also been demonstrated following cooling.[73, 130]

Miscellaneous Effects of Cold

The analgesic effect of cold may be related to reflex muscle relaxation, cutaneous counterirritation, or its effects on nerve conduction.[86] As with heat, some patients note cold to produce a general relaxation, although the mechanisms are not well defined.

General Uses of Cryotherapy in Physical Medicine

The general uses for therapeutic cold are summarized in Table 21–12. Cryotherapy is most commonly used acutely after musculoskeletal injury to minimize formation of edema, and for symptomatic relief in painful soft tissue and articular inflammatory states.[47, 57, 86, 87, 120] Two recent reviews nicely summarize the use of modalities in arthritis.[53, 98] Studies of the use of cryotherapy following orthopedic procedures have produced mixed results: some investigators report favorable effects on factors such as range of motion, pain, analgesic use, swelling, postoperative blood loss, and hospital length of stay, while others demonstrate no significant effect from cryotherapy.[6, 23, 27, 38, 54, 59, 78, 80, 105, 125, 128] Likewise, there have been mixed results with the use of cryotherapy in spasticity management.[17, 55, 89, 103, 123] Cryotherapy in the form of immediate ice water immersion is advocated as emergent primary treatment for minor burns.[113]

TABLE 21–12 General Uses of Cryotherapy in Physical Medicine

Musculoskeletal conditions (sprains, strains, tendinitis, tenosynovitis, bursitis, capsulitis, etc.)
Myofascial pain
Following certain orthopedic surgeries
Component of spasticity management
Emergent treatment of minor burns

TABLE 21–13 General Precautions for the Use of Cold

Cold intolerance
Cryotherapy-induced neurapraxia/axonotmesis
Arterial insufficiency
Impaired sensation
Cognitive or communication deficits that preclude reporting of pain
Cryopathies
Cryoglobulinemia
Paroxysmal cold hemoglobinuria
Cold hypersensitivity
Raynaud's disease/phenomenon

General Precautions for the Use of Cold

The general precautions for the use of cold are outlined in Table 21–13. The most common relative contraindication to the use of cold is simple cold intolerance. A patient who does not tolerate cold application will tend to increase muscle guarding and co-contraction, which is directly counterproductive to the therapeutic goals. Simple cold intolerance should be distinguished from true cold hypersensitivity discussed below. Caution should also be used when applying cold over the course of superficial nerves, as peroneal and ulnar palsies have been reported following cryotherapy.[35] Application of cold over areas of compromised arterial vascularity can theoretically produce further ischemia from local vasoconstriction and should be avoided. Likewise, because of the potential for cold injury, cryotherapy should be used with caution in areas of impaired sensation, or in patients who have cognitive or communication deficits that preclude reporting of pain.

The cryopathies are also contraindications to the use of cold.[104] Cryoglobulinemia is a condition that results in the precipitation of immune complexes at low temperatures. Paroxysmal cold hemoglobinuria is a rare disorder resulting from an antibody directed against a red blood cell surface antigen, with hemolysis precipitated by cold exposure. Cold hypersensitivity is a mast cell–mediated process producing urticaria and angioedema on exposure to cold. Raynaud's *disease* is an idiopathic condition characterized by arteriolar spasm precipitated by cold exposure or stress. Raynaud's *phenomenon* is secondary to other rheumatologic conditions (rheumatoid arthritis, scleroderma, systemic lupus erythematosus, etc.) and is classically manifested by digital pallor, followed by cyanosis and eventual reactive hyperemia.

Cryotherapy Agents

Cold Packs

Cold packs include Hydrocollator packs, endothermic chemical gel packs, and ice packs. Hydrocollator packs are cooled in a freezer to −12°C (10°F) and applied over a moist towel.[65] Endothermic chemical gel packs have separate compartments with compounds such as ammonium nitrate and water that, when mixed, undergo a heat-absorbing reaction. They are portable, pliable, and easily used in the field. Although many endothermic chemical gel packs are designed for one-time use, some have the advantage that they can be refrozen and reused as a simple cryogel pack. Ice packs are easily used at home and may be best applied by elastic bandage or tape, as external compression appears to increase their cooling effectiveness.[7] The duration of application is typically 20 to 30 minutes. With application of a cooled Hydrocollator pack, the skin is cooled immediately, subcutaneous tissues are cooled within minutes, and muscle at a depth of 2 cm is cooled by approximately 5°C after 20 minutes.[65] Precautions for cold packs are as listed in Table 21–13.

Ice Massage

Ice massage is the direct application of ice to the skin using gentle stroking motions. It combines the therapeutic effects of cooling with the mechanical effects of massage. Water is frozen in a paper cup, with the ice being exposed by tearing the top rim of paper off as the ice melts (Fig. 21–8). Alternatively, a wooden tongue depressor can be placed in the water, to be used as a handle after the water is frozen. Ice massage is generally used for localized symptoms and applied for 5 to 10 minutes per site, depending on the amount of subcutaneous adipose tissue.[83] Typically, there is a phasic response to ice massage, beginning with an initial perception of coolness, followed by a burning or aching, then hypesthesia and analgesia.[47] Intramuscular temperatures at a depth of 2 cm after 5 minutes of ice massage have been reported to be reduced by 4.1°C in the posterior thigh[124] to as much as 15.9°C in the biceps brachii muscle.[83] In his initial description of ice massage, Grant[47] reported a "satisfactory treatment result" in over 80% of a series of over 7000 patients with a variety of painful musculoskeletal conditions treated with ice massage and mobilization exercises, although no statistical analysis was reported. Precautions for ice massage are as listed under general cold precautions.

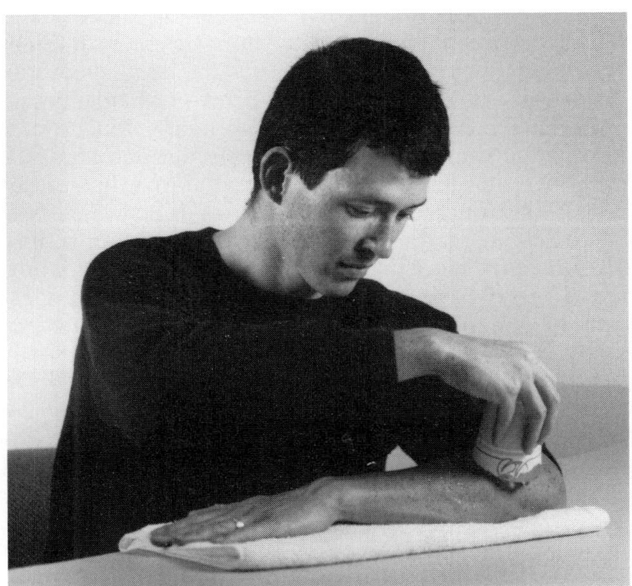

FIGURE 21–8. Example of ice massage.

Cold Water Immersion

Immersion in cold water is best suited for circumferential cooling of the limbs, usually at temperatures of 5 to 13°C (41 to 55.4°F).[113] It is often uncomfortable and poorly tolerated, though reportedly effective with localized burns, as skin temperature rapidly approaches water temperature.[113] Gastrocnemius muscle temperature decreases to approximately 6°C below baseline after 30 minutes of cold water immersion.[89, 102] Precautions for cold water immersion are listed in Table 21–13.

Cryotherapy-Compression Units

Cryotherapy-compression units consist of a cuff or boot through which cold water is circulated and can be pneumatically compressed statically or in a serial, distal-to-proximal pumping action. They are designed to combine the beneficial effects of cryotherapy with the advantages of pneumatic compression. They are used primarily after acute musculoskeletal injury with soft tissue swelling and after some surgical procedures.[106] Typical temperatures of 45°F (7.2°C) and pressures up to 60 mm Hg are used.

Vapocoolant Spray

Vapocoolant spray-and-stretch methods are used by some practitioners to treat myofascial and musculoskeletal pain syndromes. The technique consists of a series of unidirectional applications of Fluori-Methane spray, which has replaced the highly flammable ethyl chloride spray in clinical usage.[120] Treatment begins in the "trigger area" (area of deep myofascial hypersensitivity) and extends over the "reference zone" (area of referred pain) while passively stretching the muscle.[120] The spray and stretch is performed parallel to the muscle fibers, at an approximate rate of 4 inches/sec. Waiting briefly between applications helps prevent skin freezing. The therapeutic effect of spray and stretch is postulated to result from a counterirritant phenomenon.[120] Precautions include general cold precautions and avoidance of cutaneous freezing.

HYDROTHERAPY

Hydrotherapy is defined as the external application of hot or cold water, in any form, for the treatment of disease.[42] The main forms of hydrotherapy are whirlpool baths, the Hubbard tank, the shower cart, and contrast baths. Their primary uses are in arthritis and a variety of musculoskeletal conditions, and in the cleansing and debridement of burns and other dermal injuries.

Whirlpool Baths and Hubbard Tanks

Whirlpool baths and Hubbard tanks control water temperature and agitate it by aeration, dispersing thermal energy by convection (although, as noted previously, the actual transfer of heat to or from the body is by conduction). Whirlpool baths come in a variety of sizes and are typically used for treatment of a limb or localized lesion. Because only a portion of the body is immersed, greater extremes of temperature can be tolerated without significant core body temperature change.[42, 102] As more body surface area is immersed and the extremes of temperature increase, there is increasing potential for alteration of core body temperature. Hubbard tanks are larger tanks generally used for whole-body immersion, so neutral temperatures (34 to 36°C/93 to 97°F) should be used to prevent core temperature fluctuations.

An immersed body experiences a vertical antigravity force equal to that of the volume of the displaced water, decreasing stress on bones and joints.[42] This property, along with the therapeutic effects of the water temperature, make hydrotherapy appropriate for adjunctive treatment of degenerative arthritis, acute musculoskeletal injuries, burns, and skin ulceration and infection.[42] Antiseptic conditions can be used for hydrotherapy of burns or infected areas, but truly sterile conditions are not easily achieved. Sodium hypochlorite is the most commonly used antibacterial solution used in burn programs.[118] Likewise, for Hubbard tank treatment of large wounds, salt may be added to minimize fluid shifts. Isotonic saline is 0.9% sodium chloride (0.9 g NaCl/100 mL H_2O), so 900 g (approximately 2 lbs.) of salt should be added per 100 L (approximately 25 gallons) of water.

Shower Cart

Hydrotherapy has several features that are desirable for treatment of burns or other wounds. It loosens adherent dressings to facilitate removal, allows for removal of antimicrobial cream prior to reapplication, and softens eschar to facilitate debridement.[121] However, there is a risk of autocontamination and cross-contamination with conventional whirlpool baths or Hubbard tanks.[121] The shower cart was developed in response to this risk.[121] It allows for gentle spray or shower hydrotherapy during mechanical debridement of large surface area burns and other wounds under relatively sterile conditions.[121] Typical units have overhead retractable shower heads (Fig. 21–9), with independently adjustable water temperature and pressure. A shower cart also uses significantly less water, less space, and requires less maintenance than a Hubbard tank.

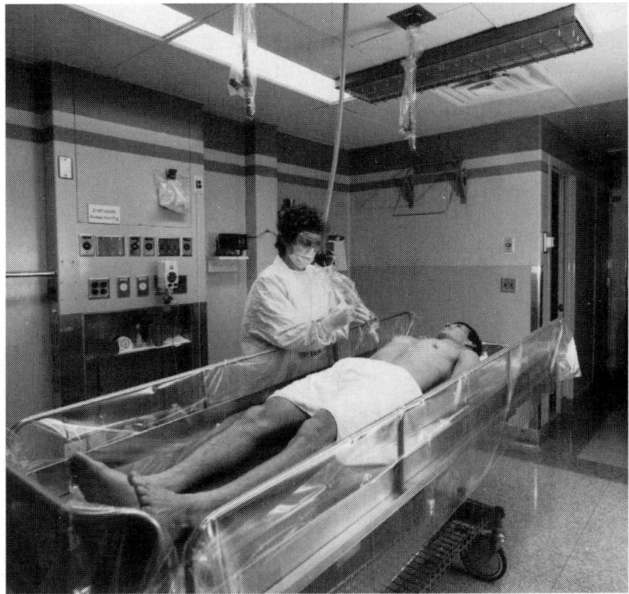

FIGURE 21–9. Shower cart.

Contrast Baths

Contrast baths consist of alternating immersion of the distal limbs in hot (42 to 45°C/108 to 113°F), then cold (8.5 to 12.5°C/47 to 55°F) water.[129] The effect is believed to be related to the cyclic vasoconstriction and vasodilation produced by the temperature extremes. Thirty-minute treatment sessions are typical, beginning with a 10-minute immersion in hot, followed by alternating immersions of 1 minute cold and 4 minutes hot, ending the session with cold immersion to theoretically limit swelling. The technique may be beneficial in the treatment of rheumatological disease, neuropathic pain, or other chronic pain syndromes such as complex regional pain syndrome.

OTHER MODALITIES

Ultraviolet

Ultraviolet radiation is that part of the electromagnetic spectrum adjacent to the short-wavelength, high-frequency (violet) end of the visible light spectrum. Historically, UV radiation has been used in physical medicine for the treatment of skin ulcers, but now its therapeutic use is almost exclusively dermatological.[92] Most current treatments with UV radiation utilize either UVA (wavelength 320 to 400 nm) or UVB (wavelength 290 to 320 nm) radiation.[92] The minimal erythema dose (MED) may be used to titrate intensity, and is determined by exposing small areas of skin to different durations of UV radiation. The MED is that duration of exposure which produces erythema. Although originally used mainly in the treatment of psoriasis, there are now more than 30 dermatological disorders for which UV radiation may be efficacious.[92] Potential adverse effects include premature aging of the skin, non-melanoma skin cancer, and cataracts.[92]

Iontophoresis

Iontophoresis is the migration of charged particles across biological membranes under an imposed electrical field.[77] Its primary use has been in transcutaneous systemic or local delivery of medicines. For systemic drug delivery it avoids the problems associated with oral or intravenous routes such as gastric irritation, first-pass hepatic metabolism, and variable serum concentrations.[18, 19] Iontophoresis in physical medicine is used to deliver medicines directly to soft tissues, limiting systemic absorption.[16, 24, 82] Ionic medications (local anesthetics, corticosteroids, analgesics, antibiotics) or plain tap water have been used with this technique. The ionic solution to be iontophoresed is placed on the electrode of the same polarity, and then the negative, positive, and ground electrodes are applied to the skin. A direct current, typically between 10 and 30 mA, is applied to drive the solution away from the electrode and into the surrounding tissues.[112] The quantity of solution transported appears to be dependent on the local current density, duration of treatment, and the solution concentration.[97] Though the mechanisms by which it causes transdermal delivery of drugs to the soft tissues have yet to be indisputably determined, and treatment efficacy remains incompletely supported by rigorous clinical research, iontophoresis is a modality commonly used by practitioners to treat numerous musculoskeletal conditions.[16, 24, 82, 112] Iontophoresis is generally well tolerated, although miliarisis has been reported when treating hyperhydrosis.[112]

Phonophoresis

Phonophoresis involves the use of US to facilitate transdermal migration of topically administered medications. Corticosteroids are the most frequently used phonophoresis agents. The anti-inflammatory effects of US and corticosteroids are thought to be synergistic.[93] The actual mechanism of transdermal migration has not been well defined, but may involve increased cell permeability from the thermal effects of US.[93] Standard ultrasonic coupling gel is mixed with 1% or 10% hydrocortisone solution or with 1% lidocaine to produce the phonophoresis coupling agent.[93] Typical phonophoresis treatment parameters are similar to those of standard US-pulsed mode, 1-MHz transducer frequency, stroking technique, at 1.0 to 1.5 W/cm^2, for approximately 5 minutes per site.[93] Proposed indications for phonophoresis include osteoarthritis, bursitis, capsulitis, tendinitis, strains, fasciitis, epicondylitis, tenosynovitis, contracture, scar tissue, neuromas, and adhesions.[49, 93] Like iontophoresis, phonophoresis is a commonly used modality with some measure of clinical effectiveness; but its basic mechanism of action and efficacy in treating specific clinical conditions remain to be established by ongoing research.[15] Precautions for and contraindications to phonophoresis are listed in Table 21–8.

Low-Energy Laser

Laser is the acronym for *l*ight *a*mplification by *s*timulated *e*mission of *r*adiation. It consists of a coherent (in-phase), collimated (restricted in area) beam of photons of identical frequency. Low-energy lasers typically deliver less than 90 mW, and should be distinguished from the higher-power (10 to 100+ W) lasers utilized in surgery, dermatology, and ophthalmology. Low-energy lasers deliver minimal energies (between 1 and 4 J) and can be considered a form of intense, focal light therapy.[8] They have been shown to affect many subcellular and cellular processes, although the mechanisms have not been well defined.[8] However, it is important to note that low-energy laser does not produce significant tissue temperature changes, so any potential physiological effects appear to be nonthermal. Low-intensity laser therapy has been used experimentally to treat a wide variety of clinical conditions, but no consensus regarding indication or effectiveness has been established.[9, 10, 25, 91] The equipment, experimental designs, and techniques used in the low-energy laser literature are highly variable, and close attention should be paid to treatment parameters when reviewing and comparing these studies.[8] Low-energy laser is not currently approved by the Food and Drug Administration for any therapeutic indication. Protective goggles should be worn by both the patient and treating therapist to protect against potential retinal injury.

Interferential Current Therapy

Interferential current therapy (IFC) is a modality that utilizes two alternating current signals of slightly different frequency. To understand the mechanism of IFC, one must have an understanding of how waves interact. Figure 21–10 illustrates that interaction. At the intersec-

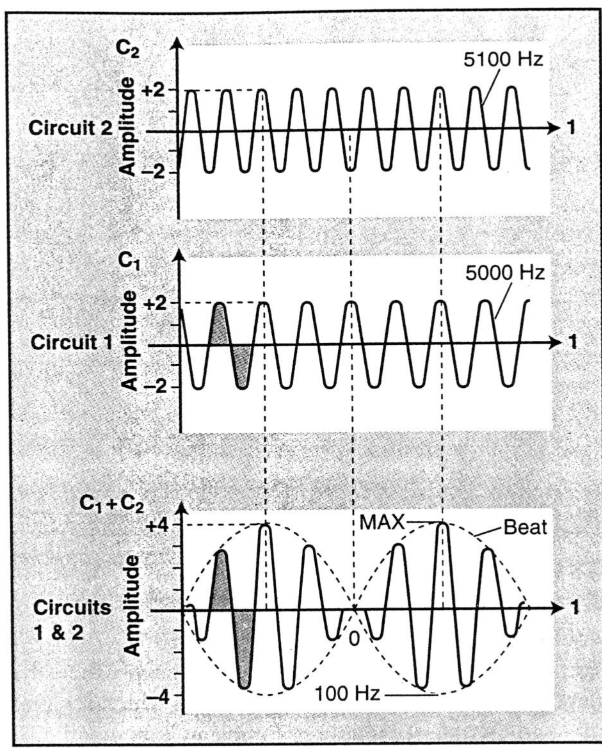

FIGURE 21–10. Interaction of two sinusoidal waves of slightly different frequency, demonstrating cyclical constructive and destructive interference. (From Nemectrodyn Model 7 Manual of Nemectron GmbH, Daimlerstr. 15, Karlsruche/Germany, 1984, with permission.)

tion of two sinusoidal waveforms, the "interference" of the two waves produces a summated wave. When the two waves are in phase, there is *constructive interference:* the summated wave has an amplitude equal to the sum of the individual wave amplitudes.[46] When the two waves are out of phase, there is *destructive interference:* the summated wave has a lower amplitude because the opposite polarities of the waves partially cancel each other.[46] When two waves of equal amplitude and frequency are exactly in phase, the amplitude of the summated wave is exactly twice that of the individual waves. When two waves of equal amplitude and frequency are out of phase by exactly one-half wavelength (i.e., the peak of one wave intersects with the trough of the other wave), the amplitude of the summated wave is zero. As noted, IFC utilizes two alternating current signals of slightly different frequencies. As these two waveforms intersect, they are periodically in phase (constructive interference) and periodically out of phase (destructive interference). This periodic interference results in a new wave with cyclical modulation of amplitude, owing to the cyclical constructive and destructive interference. The amplitude of the summated wave will modulate at a "beat frequency," equal to the difference in frequency between the two signals.[46] For example, if one applicator channel frequency is 5100 Hz and the other is 5000 Hz, the beat frequency would be 100 Hz (5100 − 5000 = 100).

IFC machines typically use medium-frequency currents of approximately 4000 to 5000 Hz. Alternating currents of medium frequency (1000 to 10,000 Hz) have lower skin resistance than low-frequency currents (<1000 Hz); it is therefore postulated that they penetrate tissue more easily.[46, 110] However, many factors other than signal frequency also affect skin resistance and depth of penetration.[3, 63, 64] Most IFC machines use two, four, or six applicators. These can be arranged in the same plane (*planar*), as in the lumbar area, or in different planes (*coplanar*), as in the shoulder. Figure 21–11 demonstrates a typical quadripolar IFC application. The classic "clover leaf" pattern of interference produced between two circuits in a perfectly homogeneous medium is diagrammed. However, due to the marked heterogeneity of electrical conductance of human tissues, the actual summation is unlikely to occur as precisely as this diagrammatic representation.[3]

IFC parameters that can be manipulated include signal frequency, beat frequency, amplitude, and cycle time. IFC machines allow for either a fixed frequency difference (most machines are capable of producing beat frequencies from 1 to 120 Hz) or for a modulated frequency difference where the beat frequency varies over time.[64] Frequency modulation is sometimes referred to as "sweep."[109] In theory, the use of frequency modulation limits neural adaptation.[63] Amplitude may also be fixed or modulated. By manipulating the ampli-

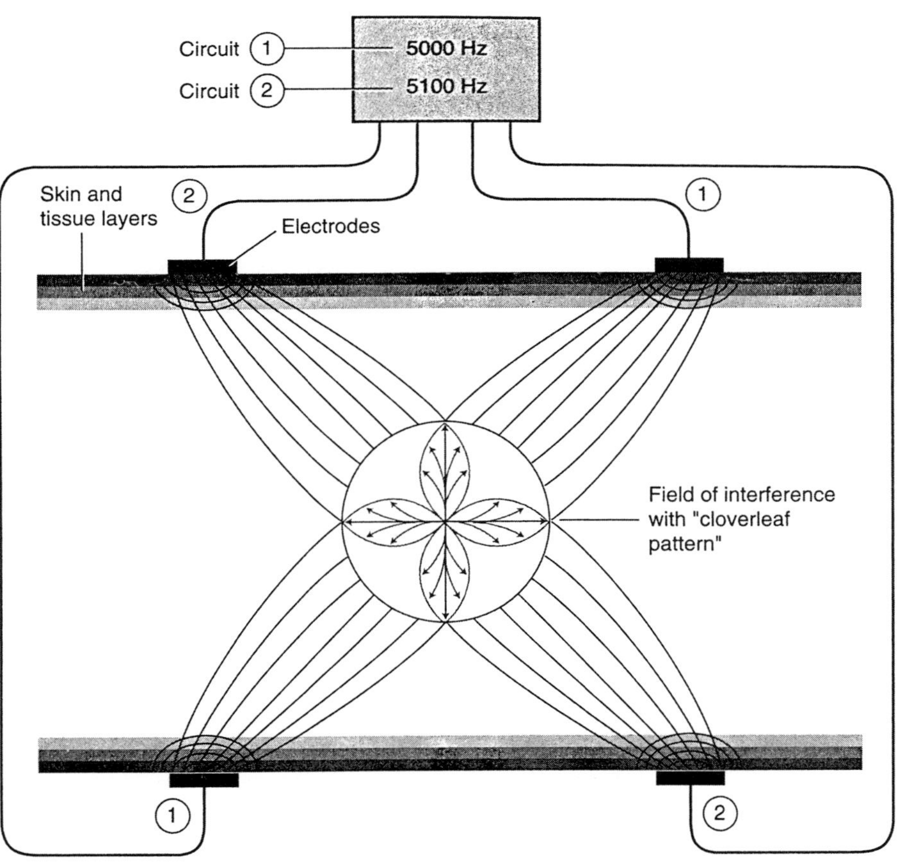

FIGURE 21–11. Quadripolar IFC application demonstrating classic "clover leaf" pattern of interference. (From Nemectrodyn Model 7 Manual of Nemectron GmbH, Daimlerstr. 15, Karlsruche/Germany, 1984, with permission.)

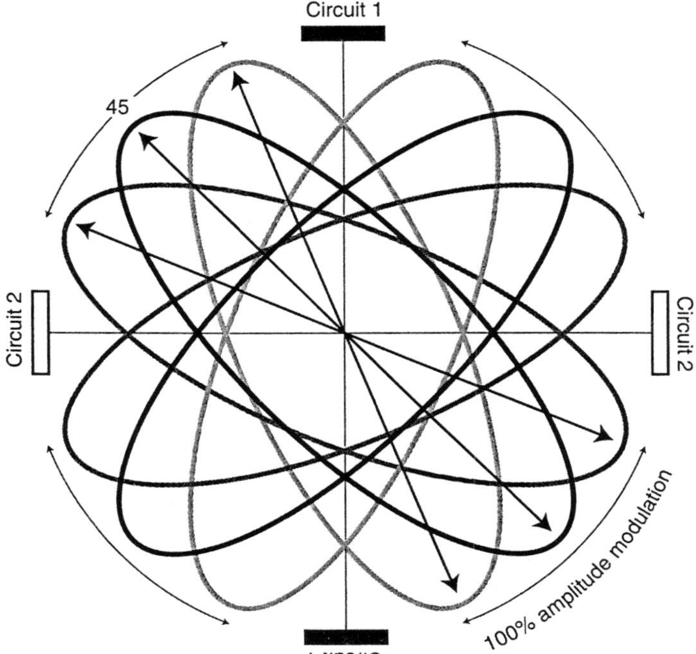

FIGURE 21–12. IFC amplitude modulation or "scanning." If the amplitude is increased or decreased in a circuit, the zone of maximum interference rotates toward or away from that circuit, respectively. (From Kloth LC: Interference current. In Nelson RM, Currier DP (eds): Clinical Electrotherapy, ed 2, Norwalk, Appleton & Lange, 1991, with permission.)

tude, the point of maximal amplitude interference changes. As Figure 21–12 shows, with equal amplitude in each circuit, the field of interference is at a 45-degree angle to the circuits. If the amplitude of circuit 1 is increased, the field will rotate toward circuit 1. Conversely, if the amplitude in circuit 1 is decreased, the field will rotate away from circuit 1. Amplitude modulation is sometimes referred to as "scan."[109] IFC scan mode may be preferable when the treatment area is large or poorly localized; theoretically, the area of tissue stimulation is larger with modulated amplitude than with fixed amplitude IFC.[109] Some IFC machines also allow for on/off cycling. IFC treatment parameters may be manipulated to produce stimulation parameters similar to the different categories of TENS delivery—conventional, acupuncture-like, hyperstimulation, or burst modes.[63, 64] But Kloth[63] notes that a major difference between IFC and TENS may be the ability of IFC to deliver higher currents than TENS.

Some have reported that IFC is useful in a variety of musculoskeletal conditions, neurological conditions, and in the management of urinary incontinence,[29, 48, 64, 110] although other literature fails to demonstrate its superiority over other interventions[96] or placebo.[116] As with some other modalities, there is a dearth of randomized, placebo-controlled trials documenting the clinical efficacy or optimal treatment parameters for the many clinical entities for which it is commonly used.

Precautions and contraindications for IFC are the same as those for other forms of transcutaneous electrical stimulation.[46, 64] IFC should not be used near implanted stimulators (pacemakers, intrathecal pumps, spinal cord stimulators, etc.) because of the potential for interference with the function of these devices.[46, 64] One should be aware of the potential for vascular responses when IFC is used near sympathetic ganglia or the carotid sinus.[64] IFC should not be used near open incisions or abrasions because of the potential for concentration of electrical current.[64] It should not be used near the gravid uterus, because of concern about potential adverse effects on fetal development or potential for stimulating uterine contractions.[46, 64] In the presence of venous thrombosis, IFC could result in mechanical stimulation of vascular smooth muscle, with the theoretical potential of precipitating emboli.[46, 64] It should not be used in an insensate area or in a patient cognitively incapable of accurately reporting pain.[64] Additionally, IFC should not be used near short-wave diathermy because of the potential for interference, with resultant excessive electrical stimulation.[64]

CONCLUSION

This chapter has reviewed the physiological effects, common uses, techniques of application, and precautions for the therapeutic use of modalities. It is important to remember that these modalities are adjunctive treatments, to be used in conjunction with appropriate therapeutic exercise and medications. Because of the potential for deleterious effects, their use should generally be preceded by appropriate professional evaluation. Having a firm understanding of the physiological basis of modality selection is crucial to their proper use.

REFERENCES

1. Abramson DI, Chu LSW, Tuck S, et al: Effect of tissue temperatures and blood flow on motor nerve conduction velocity. JAMA 1966; 198:1082–1088.

2. Abramson DI, Tuck S, Chu SW, et al: Effect of paraffin bath and hot fomentations on local tissue temperatures. Arch Phys Med Rehabil 1964; 45:87–94.
3. Alon G: Interferential current news (letter). Phys Ther 1986; 66:280–281.
4. Askew LJ, Beckett VL, An K, et al: Objective evaluation of hand function in scleroderma patients to assess effectiveness of physical therapy. Br J Rheumatol 1983; 22:224–232.
5. Balmaseda MT, Fatehi MT, Koozekanani SH, et al: Ultrasound therapy: A comparative study of different coupling media. Arch Phys Med Rehabil 1986; 67:147–150.
6. Barber FA, McGuire DA, Click S: Continuous-flow cold therapy for outpatient anterior cruciate ligament reconstruction. Arthroscopy 1998; 14(2):130–135.
7. Barlas D, Homan CS, Thode HC: In vivo tissue temperature comparison of cryotherapy with and without external compression. Ann Emerg Med 1996; 28:436–439.
8. Basford JR: The clinical and experimental status of low energy laser therapy. Crit Rev Phys Rehabil Med 1989; 1:1–9.
9. Basford JR: Low intensity laser therapy: Still not an established clinical tool. Lasers Surg Med 1995; 16:331–342.
10. Basford JR, Malanga GA, Krause DA, et al: A randomized controlled evaluation of low-intensity laser therapy: Plantar fasciitis. Arch Phys Med Rehabil 1998; 79:249–54.
11. Bell KR, Lehmann JF: Effect of cooling on H- and T–reflexes in normal subjects. Arch Phys Med Rehabil 1987; 68:490–493.
12. Bocobo C, Fast A, Kingery W, et al: The effect of ice on intra-articular temperature in the knee of the dog. Am J Phys Med 1991; 70:181–185.
13. Borell RM, Henley EJ, Ho P, et al: Fluidotherapy: Evaluation of a new heat modality. Arch Phys Med Rehabil 1977; 58:69–71.
14. Borell RM, Parker R, Henley EJ, et al: Comparison of in vivo temperatures produced by hydrotherapy, paraffin wax treatment, and Fluidotherapy. Phys Ther 1980; 60:1273–1276.
15. Byl NN: The use of ultrasound as an enhancer for transcutaneous drug delivery: Phonophoresis. Phys Ther 1995; 75(6):539–553.
16. Chantraine A, Ludy JP, Berger D: Is cortisone iontophoresis possible? Arch Phys Med Rehabil 1986; 67:38–40.
17. Chiara T, Carlos J, Martin D, et al: Cold effect on oxygen uptake, perceived exertion, and spasticity in patients with multiple sclerosis. Arch Phys Med Rehabil 1998; 79:523–528.
18. Chien YW, Banga AK: Iontophoretic (transdermal) delivery of drugs: Overview of historical development. J Pharm Sci 1989; 78:353–354.
19. Chien YW, Siddiqui O, Shi WM, et al: Direct current iontophoretic transdermal delivery of peptide and protein drugs. J Pharm Sci 1989; 78:376–383.
20. Clarke DH, Stelmach GE: Muscular fatigue and recovery curve parameters at various temperatures. Res Q 1966; 37:468–479.
21. Clarke RS, Hellon RF, Lind AR: Vascular reactions of the human forearm to cold. Clin Sci 1958; 17:165–179.
22. Coakley WT: Biophysical effects of ultrasound at therapeutic intensities. Physiotherapy 1978; 64:166–169.
23. Cohn BT, Draeger RI, Jackson DW: The effects of cold therapy in the postoperative management of pain in patients undergoing anterior cruciate ligament reconstruction. Am J Sports Med 1989; 17:344–349.
24. Costello CT, Jeske AH: Iontophoresis: Application in transdermal medication delivery. Phys Ther 1995; 75(6):554–563.
25. Craig JA, Barlas P, Baxter GD, et al: Delayed-onset muscle soreness: Lack of effect of combined phototherapy/low-intensity laser therapy at low pulse repetition rates. J Clin Laser Med Surg 1996; 14(6):375–380.
26. Dahlstedt L, Samuelson P, Dalen N: Cryotherapy after cruciate knee surgery. Acta Orthop Scand 1996; 67(3):255–257.
27. Daniel DM, Stone ML, Arendt DL: The effect of cold therapy on pain, swelling, and range of motion after anterior cruciate ligament reconstructive surgery. Arthroscopy 1994; 10(5):530–533.
28. Daniels S, Blondel D, Crum LA, et al: Ultrasonically induced gas bubble production in agar based gels. Part I: Experimental investigation. Ultrasound Med Biol 1987; 13:527–539.
29. Dumoulin C, Seaborne DE, Quirion-DeGirardi C, et al: Pelvic-floor rehabilitation, part 1: Comparison of two surface electrode placements during stimulation of the pelvic-floor musculature in women who are continent using bipolar interferential currents. Phys Ther 1995; 75:1067–1074.
30. DeLateur BJ, Lehmann JF, Stonebridge JB, et al: Muscle heating in human subjects with 915 MHz microwave contact applicator. Arch Phys Med Rehabil 1970; 51:147–151.
31. Dellhag B, Wollersjo I, Bjelle A: Effect of active hand exercise and wax bath treatments in rheumatoid arthritis patients. Arthritis Care Res 1992; 5:87–92.
32. Denys EH: AAEM minimonograph no. 14: The influence of temperature in clinical neurophysiology. Muscle Nerve 1991; 14:795–811.
33. Diller KR: Analysis of burns caused by long-term exposure to a heating pad. J Burn Care Rehabil 1991; 12:214–217.
34. Dover JS, Phillips TJ, Arndt KA: Cutaneous effects and therapeutic uses of heat with emphasis on infrared radiation. J Am Acad Dermatol 1989; 20:278–286.
35. Drez D, Faust DC, Evans JP: Cryotherapy and nerve palsy. Am J Sports Med 1981; 9:256–257.
36. Dyson M: Non-thermal cellular effects of ultrasound. Br J Cancer 1982; 45(suppl):165–171.
37. Dyson M, Woodward B, Pond JB: Flow of red blood cells stopped by ultrasound. Nature 1971; 232:572–573.
38. Edwards DJ, Rimmer M, Keene GCR: The use of cold therapy in the postoperative management of patients undergoing arthroscopic anterior cruciate ligament reconstruction. Am J Sports Med 1996; 24(2):193–195.
39. Eldred E, Lindsley DF, Buchwald JS: The effect of cooling on mammalian muscle spindles. Exp Neurol 1960; 2:144–157.
40. Falconer J, Hayes KW, Chang RW: Therapeutic ultrasound in the treatment of musculoskeletal conditions. Arthritis Care Res 1990; 3:85–91.
41. Folkow B, Fox RH, Krog J, et al: Studies on the reactions of the cutaneous vessels to cold exposure. Acta Physiol Scand 1963; 58:342–354.
42. Franchimont P, Juchmes J, Lecomte J: Hydrotherapy—mechanisms and indications. Pharmacol Ther 1983; 20:79–93.
43. Gersten JW: Effect of metallic objects on temperature rises produced in tissue by ultrasound. Am J Phys Med 1958; 37:75–82.
44. Gnatz SM: Increased radicular pain due to therapeutic ultrasound applied to the back. Arch Phys Med Rehabil 1989; 70:493–494.
45. Goats GC: Continuous shortwave (radiofrequency) diathermy. Br J Sports Med 1989; 23:123–127.
46. Goats GC: Interferential current therapy. Br J Sports Med 1990; 24:87–91.
47. Grant AE: Massage with ice (cryokinetics) in the treatment of painful conditions of the musculoskeletal system. Arch Phys Med Rehabil 1964; 45:233–238.
48. Green RJ, Laycock J: Objective methods for evaluation of interferential therapy in the treatment of incontinence. IEEE Trans Biomed Eng 1990; 37:615–623.
49. Griffin JE, Echternach JL, Price RE, et al: Patients treated with ultrasonic driven hydrocortisone and with ultrasound alone. Phys Ther 1967; 47:594–601.
50. Guy AW, Lehmann JF, Stonebridge JB: Therapeutic applications of electromagnetic power. Proc IEEE 1974; 62:55–75.
51. Guyton AC: Body temperature, temperature regulation, and fever. In Guyton AC (ed): Textbook of Medical Physiology, ed 8. Philadelphia, WB Saunders, 1991, pp 797–808.
52. Harris ED, McCroskery PA: The influence of temperature and fibril stability on degradation of cartilage collagen by rheumatoid synovial collagenase. N Engl J Med 1974; 290:1–6.
53. Hayes KW: Heat and cold in the management of rheumatoid arthritis. Arth Care Res 1993; 6(3):156–166.
54. Hecht PJ, Bachmann S, Booth RE, et al: Effects of thermal therapy on rehabilitation after total knee arthroplasty. Clin Orthop 1983; 178:198–201.
55. Hedenberg L: Functional improvement of the spastic hemiplegic arm after cooling. Scand J Rehabil Med 1970; 2:154–158.
56. Hekkenberg RT, Oosterbaan WA, vanBeekum WT: Evaluation of ultrasound therapy devices. Physiotherapy 1986; 72:390–394.
57. Hocutt JE, Jaffe R, Rylander CR, et al: Cryotherapy in ankle sprains. Am J Sports Med 1982; 10:316–319.
58. Hong C-Z: Reversible conduction block in patients with polyneuropathy after ultrasound thermotherapy at therapeutic dosage. Arch Phys Med Rehabil 1991; 72:132–137.

59. Ivey M, Johnston RV, Uchida T: Cryotherapy for postoperative pain relief following knee arthroplasty. J Arthroplasty 1994; 9(3):285–290.
60. Johnson CC, Guy AW: Nonionizing electromagnetic wave effects in biological materials and systems. Proc IEEE 1972; 60:692–718.
61. Jones SL: Electromagnetic field interference and cardiac pacemakers. Phys Ther 1976; 56:1013–1018.
62. Kantor G: Evaluation and survey of microwave and radiofrequency applicators. J Microwave Power 1981; 16:135–150.
63. Kloth LC: Electrotherapeutic alternatives for the treatment of pain. In Gersh MR (ed): Electrotherapy in Rehabilitation. Philadelphia, FA Davis Company, 1992.
64. Kloth LC: Interference current. In Nelson RM, Currier DP (eds): Clinical Electrotherapy, ed 2, Norwalk, CT, Appleton & Lange, 1991.
65. Knutsson E, Mattsson E: Effects of local cooling on monosynaptic reflexes in man. Scand J Rehabil Med 1969; 1:126–132.
66. Lehmann JF: Therapeutic Heat and Cold, ed 4. Baltimore, Williams & Wilkins, 1990.
67. Lehmann JF, Brunner GD, Stow RW: Pain threshold measurements after therapeutic application of ultrasound, microwaves and infrared. Arch Phys Med Rehabil 1958; 39:560–565.
68. Lehmann JF, DeLateur BJ, Stonebridge JB: Selective muscle heating by shortwave diathermy with a helical coil. Arch Phys Med Rehabil 1969; 50:117–123.
69. Lehmann JF, DeLateur BJ, Warren CG, et al: Heating produced by ultrasound in bone and soft tissue. Arch Phys Med Rehabil 1967; 48:397–401.
70. Lehmann JF, DeLateur BJ, Warren CG, et al: Therapeutic temperature distribution produced by ultrasound as modified by dosage and volume of tissue exposed. Arch Phys Med Rehabil 1967; 48:662–666.
71. Lehmann JF, DeLateur BJ, Warren CG, et al: Heating of joint structures by ultrasound. Arch Phys Med Rehabil 1968; 49:28–30.
72. Lehmann JF, Johnston VC, McMillan JA, et al: Comparison of deep heating by microwaves at frequencies 2456 and 900 megacycles. Arch Phys Med Rehabil 1965; 46:307–314.
73. Lehmann JF, Masock AJ, Warren CG, et al: Effect of therapeutic temperatures on tendon extensibility. Arch Phys Med Rehabil 1970; 51:481–487.
74. Lehmann JF, McDougall JA, Guy AW, et al: Heating patterns produced by shortwave diathermy applicators in tissue substitute models. Arch Phys Med Rehabil 1983; 64:575–577.
75. Lehmann JF, McMillan JA, Brunner GD, et al: Comparative study of the efficiency of short-wave, microwave and ultrasonic diathermy in heating the hip joint. Arch Phys Med Rehabil 1959; 40:510–512.
76. Lehmann JF, Silverman DR, Baum BA, et al: Temperature distributions in the human thigh, produced by infrared, hot pack and microwave applications. Arch Phys Med Rehabil 1966; 47: 291–299.
77. Lekas MD: Iontophoresis treatment. Otolaryngol Head Neck Surg 1979; 87:292–298.
78. Leutz DW, Harris H: Continuous cold therapy in total knee arthroplasty. Am J Knee Surg 1995; 8:121–123.
79. Levenson JL, Weissberg MP: Ultrasound abuse: Case report. Arch Phys Med Rehabil 1983; 64:90–91.
80. Levy AS, Marmar E: The role of cold compressive dressings in the postoperative treatment of total knee arthroplasty. Clin Orthop Rel Res 1993; 297:174–178.
81. Lewis T: Observations upon the reactions of the vessels of the human skin to cold. Heart 1930; 15:177–208.
82. Li LC, Scudds RA: Iontophoresis: An overview of the mechanisms and clinical application. Arthr Care Res 1995; 8(1):51–61.
83. Lowdon BJ, Moore RJ: Determinants and nature of intramuscular temperature changes during cold therapy. Am J Phys Med 1975; 54:223–233.
84. McGown HL: Effects of cold application on maximal isometric contraction. Phys Ther 1967; 47:185–192.
85. McLeod DR, Fowlow SB: Multiple malformations and exposure to therapeutic ultrasound during organogenesis. Am J Med Genet 1989; 34:317–319.
86. Meeusen R, Lievens P: The use of cryotherapy in sports injuries. Sports Med 1986; 3:398–414.
87. Melzack R, Jeans ME, Stratford JG, et al: Ice massage and transcutaneous electrical stimulation: Comparison of treatment for low-back pain. Pain 1980; 9:209–217.
88. Mense S: Effects of temperature on the discharge of muscle spindles and tendon organs. Pflugers Arch 1978; 374:159–166.
89. Miglietta O: Action of cold on spasticity. Am J Phys Med 1973; 52:198–205.
90. Miller DL: A review of the ultrasonic bioeffects of microsonation, gas-body activation, and related cavitation-like phenomena. Ultrasound Med Biol 1987; 13:443–470.
91. Mokhtar B, Baxter GD, Walsh DM, et al: Double-blind, placebo-controlled investigation of the effect of combined phototherapy/low intensity laser therapy upon experimental ischaemic pain in humans. Lasers Surg Med 1995; 17(1):74–81.
92. Morison WL: Phototherapy and photochemotherapy. Adv Dermatol 1992; 7:255–271.
93. Newman JT, Nellermoe MD, Carnett JL: Hydrocortisone phonophoresis. J Am Podiatr Med Assoc 1992; 82:432–435.
94. Nukada H, Pollock M, Allpress S: Experimental cold injury to peripheral nerve. Brain 1981; 104:779–811.
95. Oakley EM: Dangers and contraindications of therapeutic ultrasound. Physiotherapy 1978; 64:173–174.
96. Olah KS, Bridges N, Denning J, et al: The conservative management of patients with symptoms of stress incontinence: A randomized, prospective study comparing weighted vaginal cones and interferential therapy. Am J Obstet Gynecol 1990; 162: 87–92.
97. O'Malley EP, Oester YT: Influence of some physical chemical factors on iontophoresis using radio-isotopes. Arch Phys Med Rehabil 1955; 36:310–316.
98. Oosterveld FGJ, Rasker JJ: Treating arthritis with locally applied heat or cold. Sem Arthr Rheum 1994; 24(2):82–90.
99. Paliwal BR, Shrivastava PN: Microwave hyperthermia: Principles and quality assurance. Radiol Clin North Am 1989; 27:489–497.
100. Perez CA, Emami B: Clinical trials with local (external and interstitial) irradiation and hyperthermia—current and future perspectives. Radiol Clin North Am 1989; 27:525–542.
101. Perkins JF, Li M, Nicholas CH, et al: Cooling as a stimulus to smooth muscles. Am J Physiol 1950; 163:14–26.
102. Petajan JH, Watts N: Effects of cooling on the triceps surae reflex. Am J Phys Med 1962; 41:240–251.
103. Price R, Lehmann JF, Boswell-Bessette S, et al: Influence of cryotherapy on spasticity at the human ankle. Arch Phys Med Rehabil 1993; 74:300–304.
104. Ritzmann SE, Levin WC: Cryopathies: A review. Arch Intern Med 1961; 107:186–204.
105. Scarcella JB, Cohn BT: The effect of cold therapy on the postoperative course of total hip and knee arthroplasty patients. Am J Orthop 1995; 24(11):847–852.
106. Scheffler N, Sheitel P, Lipton M: Use of Cryo/Cuff for the control of postoperative pain and edema. J Foot Surg 1992; 31:141–146.
107. Schmidt KL, Ott VR, Rocher G, et al: Heat, cold and inflammation (a review). Z Rheumatol 1979; 38:391–404.
108. Scott BO: Effects of contact lenses on short-wave field distribution. Br J Ophthalmol 1956; 40:696–697.
109. Selkowitz DM: Electrical currents. In Cameron MH (ed): Physical Agents in Rehabilitation: From Research to Practice. Philadelphia, WB Saunders, 1999.
110. Shafshak TS, El-Sheshai AM, Soltan HE: Personality traits in the mechanisms of interferential therapy for osteoarthritic knee pain. Arch Phys Med Rehabil 1991; 72:579–581.
111. Shepherd JT, Rusch NJ, Vanhoutte PM: Effect of cold on the blood vessel wall. Gen Pharmacol 1983; 14:61–64.
112. Shrivastava SN, Singh G: Tap water iontophoresis in palmoplantar hyperhidrosis. Br J Dermatol 1977; 96:189–195.
113. Shulman AG: Ice water as primary treatment of burns. JAMA 1960; 173:96–99.
114. Stewart HF, Harris GR, Herman BA, et al: Survey of use and performance of ultrasonic therapy equipment in Pinellas County, Florida. Phys Ther 1974; 54:707–714.
115. Stuchly MA, Repacholi MH, Lecuyer DW, et al: Exposure to the operator and patient during short wave diathermy treatments. Health Phys 1982; 42:341–366.

116. Taylor K, Newton RA, Personius WJ, et al: Effects of interferential current stimulation for treatment of subjects with recurrent jaw pain. Phys Ther 1987; 67:346–350.
117. Ter Haar G, Dyson M, Oakley EM: The use of ultrasound by physiotherapists in Britain, 1985. Ultrasound Med Biol 1987; 13:659–663.
118. Thomson PD, Bowden ML, McDonald K, et al: A survey of burn hydrotherapy in the United States. J Burn Care Rehabil 1990; 11:151–155.
119. Thornton KL: Principles of ultrasound. J Reprod Med 1992; 37:27–32.
120. Travell J: Ethyl chloride spray for painful muscle spasm. Arch Phys Med 1952; 33:291–298.
121. Walk EE, Himel HN, Batra EK, et al: Aquatic access for the disabled. J Burn Care Rehabil 1992; 13:356–363.
122. Warren CG, Koblanski JN, Sigelmann RA: Ultrasound coupling media: Their relative transmissivity. Arch Phys Med Rehabil 1976; 57:218–222.
123. Watson CW: Effect of lowering of body temperature on the symptoms and signs of multiple sclerosis. N Engl J Med 1959; 261:1253–1259.
124. Waylonis GW: The physiologic effects of ice massage. Arch Phys Med Rehabil 1967; 48:37–42.
125. Webb JM, Williams D, Ivory JP, et al: The use of cold compression dressing after total knee replacement: A randomized controlled trial. Orthopedics 1998; 21(1):59–61.
126. Weinberger A, Fadilah R, Lev A, et al: Treatment of articular effusions with local deep microwave hyperthermia. Clin Rheumatol 1989; 8:461–466.
127. Weinberger A, Fadilah R, Lev A, et al: Intra-articular temperature measurements after superficial heating. Scand J Rehabil Med 1989; 21:55–57.
128. Whitelaw GP, DeMuth KA, Demos HA, et al: The use of the Cryo/Cuff versus ice and elastic wrap in the postoperative care of knee arthroscopy patients. Am J Knee Surg 1995; 8(1):28–31.
129. Woodmansey A, Collins DH, Ernst MM: Vascular reactions to the contrast bath in health and in rheumatoid arthritis. Lancet 1938; 2:1350–1353.
130. Wright V, Johns RJ: Quantitative and qualitative analysis of joint stiffness in normal subjects and in patients with connective tissue diseases. Ann Rheum Dis 1961; 20:36–45.
131. Ziskin MC: Fundamental physics of ultrasound and its propagation in tissue. Radiographics 1993; 13:705–709.

22

CHAPTER

W. Jerry Mysiw, M.D., and Rebecca D. Jackson, M.D.

Electrical Stimulation

The history of electrical stimulation as an adjunct to traditional medicine has its roots in Greek philosophy. Although early applications with a variety of electricity-generating devices were advocated for use in the treatment of many different medical conditions, its initial association with quackery limited its general acceptance. Acceptance has gradually grown as the systematic collection and analysis of scientific and clinical data have helped to define its beneficial impact. Current clinical applications of electrical stimulation therapy have crossed the lines of many specialties, including rehabilitation medicine, neurology, urology, gynecology, orthopedics, dermatology, and pain management.

The first significant application of electrical stimulation to improve muscle function dates back to 1950, with the invention of the cardiac pacemaker.[171] Effective application of functional electrical stimulation (FES) in a rehabilitation system is generally credited to Liberson, who applied electrical stimulation to the peroneal nerve to produce ankle dorsiflexion in hemiplegic patients during the swing phase of gait.[150] This was followed by reports of the use of electrical stimulation of the quadriceps to aid in static standing following spinal cord injury (SCI).[126] Together, these are the first reports of functional electrical stimulation utilizing electrical stimulation to serve as a neuro-orthosis or external control of motor function.

Since the 1960s, advances have come rapidly. The gate theory of pain by Melzack and Wall, described in 1965,[162] provided the rationale for the development of such stimulation techniques as transcutaneous electrical nerve stimulation (TENS) and the use of both implanted dorsal column and conus medullaris root stimulators for neuropathic pain or neurogenic bladder control. Most recently, electrical stimulation has returned to its functional roots in cardiology and has been applied to the development of latissimus dorsi cardiomyoplasty assist devices for the treatment of cardiomyopathy.

Over the past several decades, improvements in electronic technology and a better understanding of neuromuscular physiology have worked together to improve the use of electrical stimulation for functional and therapeutic purposes. Today, there is a substantial body of experimental data supporting its application in the treatment of a variety of medical conditions, based on its unique properties in modifying certain biological and chemical aspects of biological tissues in vivo and increasing the contractile properties of muscle.

PHYSIOLOGICAL EFFECTS OF NEUROMUSCULAR ELECTRICAL STIMULATION

Normal Muscle Physiology

The motor unit involved in contraction consists of an alpha motor neuron, its axon, the myoneural junction, and the muscle fibers that it innervates. The alpha motor neurons differ in size and function, with the small motor neurons, which have the lowest activation frequency, innervating slow muscle fibers and the large motor neurons innervating fast fibers. Muscle fibers within the motor unit can be classified into three main categories[161] based on specific functional, metabolic, and histochemical features of the individual muscle fibers (Table 22–1). Within each motor unit, all muscle fibers are histologically identical,[29] although with any muscle, all fiber types can be present in varying amounts, resulting in unique contractile characteristics.

During normal muscle contraction, a motor unit with a low axonal conduction velocity (or activation frequency) is recruited before a unit with a higher conduc-

TABLE 22–1 Properties of Muscle Fiber Types

	I	IIa	IIb
Morphology			
Name	Red	Intermediate	White
Capillary density	↑	Intermediate	↓↓
Histochemical			
Myosin ATPase	↓	↑	↑
Mitochondria	↑	↑	↓
Glycogen	Low	Intermediate	High
Myosin HC	HC_s	HCfa	HCfb
Myosin LC	$LC_{1a, 1b, 2}$	$Lcf_{1, 2, 3}$	$Lcf_{1, 2, 3}$
Metabolism			
Type	Oxidative	Oxidative/ glycolytic	Glycolytic
	Aerobic	Mixed	Anaerobic
Contractile properties			
Twitch	Slow	Fast	Fast
Fatigability	Slow	Intermediate	Rapid

tion velocity.[103, 104] This size principle suggests that axonal conduction of a motor unit is related to the muscle fiber parameters such that a unit with low conduction velocity has a slow twitch force, long contraction time, and higher resistance to fatigue. This theory explains the orderly progression of fiber activation with the onset of isometric voluntary contraction. Weak, slowly conducting, fatigue-resistant motor units containing type I fibers are recruited first to allow for slow increases in firing rate and increasing tension in the muscle.[165, 166] This is followed sequentially by the recruitment of the high conduction velocity, type IIb fibers, which can increase gain.[168]

When the motor unit is stimulated by artificial rather than voluntary action, this orderly progression of fiber activation does not always occur.[132] With functional neuromuscular stimulation, the order of recruitment is reversed because activation of motor units is dependent on the excitation current threshold, which varies inversely with the diameter of the nerve fiber.[247] This results in initial stimulation of type II fibers, followed by activation of the slow type I fibers with continued stimulation.

Response of Muscle Fibers to Electrical Stimulation

Following chronic, continuous, low-frequency (10-Hz) electrical stimulation of normal, fast-twitch skeletal muscles, a stereotypical series of events occurs, resulting in transformation of the muscle fiber from a fast-twitch type IIb fiber to a composition with slow-twitch type I characteristics (Table 22–2). Although most of the data come from studies in mammalian models in which different low-frequency, continuous stimulation regimens were used, the consistency of changes reported supports generalization of the results to many animals, including humans.

Within 2 to 4 days of the onset of stimulation, initial changes are noted in the sarcoplasmic reticulum. First, there is a decrease in the rate and capacity of ionized calcium uptake that is associated with a decrease in the activity of calcium-dependent adenosine triphosphatase (ATPase) and its phosphorylated intermediate.[102, 156, 219, 235] There also occur an associated decrease in calsequestrine, the major calcium-binding protein in the sarcoplasmic reticulum,[101] an increase in the specific membrane proteins that are typical of the slow-twitch type I sarcoplasmic reticulum,[270] and a rearrangement of the membrane phospholipid matrix.[237] The transformation of the sarcoplasmic reticulum is associated with a decline in parvalbumin, the calcium-binding cytosolic protein, which almost completely disappears within 3 weeks of stimulation.[131] These histochemical changes result in both a decrease in calcium sequestration in the sarcoplasmic reticulum and a reduction in calcium-buffering capacity, which functionally affects contractile properties by increasing the time to peak velocity within the first week.[101, 206] The isotonic twitch characteristics, a function of myosin heavy and light chains and other contractile proteins, are unaltered during this early stage of transformation.[2]

Ultrastructurally, there is an early decrease in T-tubuli, terminal cisternae, and sarcoplasmic reticulum,[65] as well as a decrease in calcium-transporting membranes. In addition, there is a decrease in high-density intermembranous particles of the sarcoplasmic reticulum. These particles are thought to be oligomers of calcium-pumping ATPase, and their decline is associated with a reduction in the rate and capacity of calcium uptake in the sarcoplasmic reticulum.[62]

TABLE 22–2 Chronic Low-Frequency Stimulation of Fast-Twitch Muscle: Sequence of Events in Transformation

	Acute (0–3 wk)	Subacute (4–8 wk)
Contractile	↑ resistance to fatigue ↑ time to peak twitch ↑ time to half relaxation ↑ tetanus-to-twitch	↓ maximal velocity of shortening
Ultrastructural	Swelling SR ↑ T system ↓ particle in SR bilayer ↑ mitochondrial fraction ↑ Z band width	Broad Z band Declining mitochondria
Histochemical	↑ Type IIA, ↓ type IIB HC	↓ Type IIA → type I HC ↓ LC_2 → ↑ LC_{2s} ↓ LC_3 then ↓ LC_1 ↓ NCH_3-histidine
Metabolic	↑ oxidative enzyme mRNA Δ α-, β-tropomysin ↓ Ca transport + Ca-active ATPase ↓ glycolytic enzymes mRNA	↑ oxidative enzyme activity ↓ glycolytic activity
Morphological	↑ capillary density ↑ blood flow	↓ muscle fiber area ↓ muscle fiber wet weight

Although the most rapid transformation responses to electrical stimulation are centered on the sarcoplasmic reticulum, continued low-frequency stimulation can eventually affect the myosin contractile proteins to result in the ultimate transformation to a slow fiber type. Calcium-activated myosin ATPase activity begins to decline by 3 weeks, eventually reaching the low levels typical of slow type I muscle fibers. Concomitantly, there is an increase in the alkali lability of the myosin ATPase corresponding to changes in myosin light chain (LC) patterns.[248] Changes in LC patterns occur at both the level of transcription and translation during the transformation from fast to slow fiber type. In an orderly sequence, the fast DTNB-LC chain (LC-f2) is replaced by its slow counterpart (LC-S2), followed by declines in LC-f3, then LC-f1, with replacement by the corresponding slow LC.[23, 230, 242] The changes in the DTNB-LC occur simultaneously with the initial changes in myosin heavy chain (MHC). MHC messenger RNA (mRNA) expressed in each muscle fiber encodes a unique myosin cross-bridge for types I, IIa, and IIb fibers that is responsible for the characteristic intrinsic velocity of contraction and economy of force for each muscle fiber type. Within 4 days of the onset of electrical stimulation, there is a decline in the mRNA of the MHC characteristics of type IIb fibers (MHC-fb), with eventual suppression of these mRNA levels by 90% after 21 days (Fig. 22–1).[26] This is followed by a decline in MHC-fb protein within 12 days.[100] The decreasing MHC-fb is initially replaced by an MHC reflecting the type IIa fiber (MHC-fa), and only after prolonged stimulation is the phenotypic transformation completed with replacement of MHC-fa by MHC-s.[23] However, if electrical stimulation is combined with stretch, there is a synergistic effect of mechanical and electrical forces leading to a rapid (within 4 days) stimulation of MHC-s mRNA (Fig. 22–2).[84] This asynchronous transformation from fast to slow type within the different myosin subunits can lead to the coexistence of both slow and fast isoforms of myosin within a single muscle fiber (type IIc fibers).[156, 204, 232]

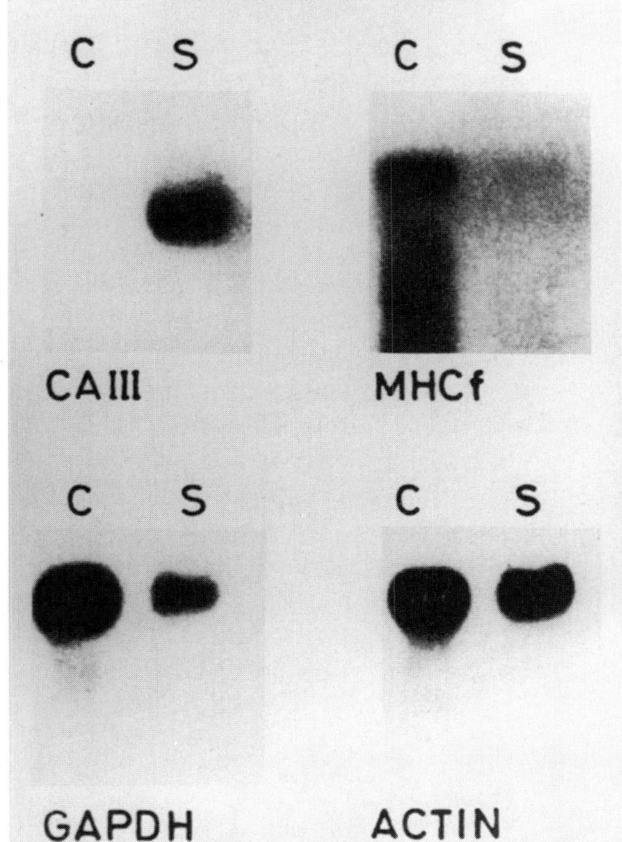

FIGURE 22–1. Northern blot analysis of changes in messenger RNA expression of four different muscle genes in response to 21 days of electrical stimulation of the tibialis anterior muscle. There is a stimulation of carbonic anhydrase III (CAIII) expression and suppression of both glyceraldehyde-3-phosphate dehydrogenase (GAPDH) and the fast myosin heavy chain (MHCf) with electrical stimulation-induced fast-to-slow transition. (From Brownson C, Isenberg H, Brown W, et al: Changes in skeletal muscle gene transcription induced by chronic stimulation. Muscle Nerve 1988; 11:1183–1189. Reprinted by permission of John Wiley & Sons, Inc.)

By 3 weeks after the onset of stimulation, alpha and beta tropomyosin changes from fast to slow type,[231] and Z lines become evident, with a corresponding development of the M-band structure. Conversion of fiber type is completed within 8 weeks of initiation of chronic, low-frequency stimulation.[202] This new type I muscle fiber composition is functionally associated with both an increase in resistance to fatigue and a decrease in the maximum velocity of shortening.

The changes in ultrastructural and contractile properties from a fast- to a slow-twitch muscle fiber are also associated with important changes in metabolic activity from use of an anaerobic, glycolytic pathway in the type IIb fiber to the aerobic Krebs cycle–associated pathway of type I fibers. With the onset of continuous low-frequency electrical stimulation, there is an enhancement of the enzymes responsible for phosphorylation and oxidation of glucose. Within 10 days of initiation of electrical stimulation, there is a rapid rise in Glut-4, a facilitative glucose transporter isoform present in skeletal muscle.[68] The stimulatory effect of both insulin and exercise on glucose transport is higher in the more oxidative type I and IIa fibers than in glycolytic type IIb fibers. However, electrical stimulation increases glucose uptake similarly in both oxidative type I and IIa fibers and glycolyte type IIb fibers, presumably due to the fact that electrical stimulation similarly increased plasma membrane content of Glut-4 in both types of fibers.[230] In contrast, the activity of citrate synthase (an enzyme of the Krebs cycle) increases more slowly after the onset of electrical stimulation, with rises in protein levels over 30 to 40 days and a plateauing of the peak effect by day 60 to 90, reflecting the metabolic change to an aerobic oxidative enzyme system. The mRNA of carbonic anhydrase II, an enzyme that facilitates carbon dioxide movement in muscle, is also rapidly stimulated with electrical stimulation to reach levels seen in type I fibers over 10 to 20 days (Fig. 22–1).[26] Finally, there is a pronounced increase in many other enzymes involved in terminal subtrate oxidation and fatty acid and ketone body oxidation.[28, 115, 131, 203, 205, 221] These metabolic changes are

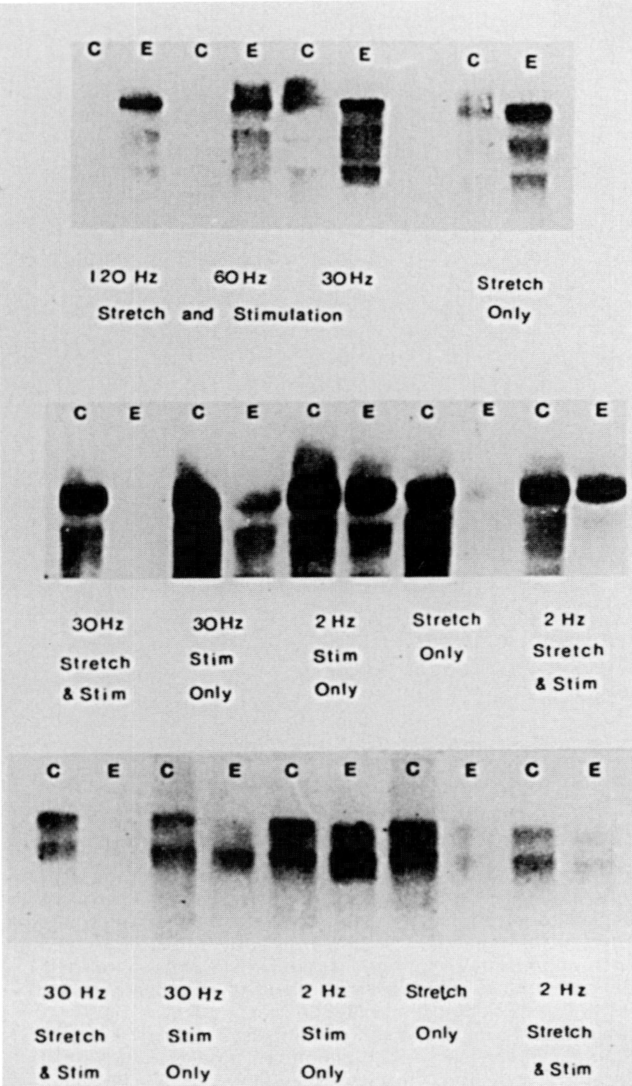

FIGURE 22–2. Northern blot analysis of RNA from normal (*C*) and electrically stimulated and stretched (*E*) rabbit tibialis anterior muscle after 4 days. There is activation of slow myosin heavy chain (*panel A*) with repression of both fast type IIb myosin heavy chain (*panel B*) and myosin heavy chain genes detected with a myosin light chain 1 and 3 probe (*panel C*). Note that the two bands in panel C represent the two light chains encoded by the same gene. (From Goldspink G, Scutt A, Martindale J, et al: Stretch and force generation induce rapid hypertrophy and isoform gene switching in adult skeletal muscle. Biochem Trans 1991; 19:368–373.)

also associated with pronounced increases in capillary density[24, 117, 221] and oxygen consumption, which in combination might be responsible for the development of increased resistance to fatigue.[116]

In addition to the increase in oxidative capacity, there is a suppression of enzymes involved in anaerobic glycogenolysis. There are progressive declines in the level of phosphorylase kinase (PK),[145] a regulator of glycogen metabolism that promotes glycogenolysis by phosphorylating and activating phosphorylase enzyme. These changes might reflect the very early changes in metabolic activity in the sarcoplasma reticulum in response to electrical stimulation, as this enzyme is allosterically activated by calcium through its delta subunit, calmodulin, thus providing a potential link between electrically stimulated calcium changes and glycogenolysis. There are also dramatic changes in mRNA levels of glyceraldehyde-3-phosphate dehydrogenase (GAPDH), a glycolytic enzyme abundant in fast twitch fibers (see Fig. 22–2).[26] There are steady declines in GAPDH mRNA to the levels seen in slow-twitch fibers after 21 days of electrical stimulation, suggesting that part of the regulation of fast- to slow-twitch fiber transformation is occurring at the level of gene transcription. When temporal data of GAPDH enzyme activity are compared with the temporal data of its mRNA, it appears that the declines in mRNA concentration precede the observed protein changes.[131, 201] This is similar to a pattern of events described for aldolase,[273] an enzyme adjacent to GAPDH in the glycolytic pathway. These data suggest that there is a relative delay in the turnover of the glycolytic proteins that potentially delays the rate of change observed in metabolic activity in response to electrical stimulation.

Several studies have helped to confirm the applicability of some aspects of these data derived from animal models to the effects of electrical stimulation on human muscle in vivo. After 21 days of electrical stimulation (50 Hz, alternating current) in normal muscle, there is a significant increase in total capillary length per tissue volume, a decrease in intercapillary distance, and a decrease in Krogh cylinders, leading to an improvement in capillary supply to muscle[34]; these findings are similar to those changes noted in animal models. Using intermittent electrical stimulation (square wave, 20 to 30 Hz, 0.003-sec pulse, 33% duty cycle) with surface electrodes for 30 minutes twice a day for 90 days in individuals with chronic SCI, electrical stimulation of the lower extremity has resulted in an increase in the number of type IIa muscle fibers (Fig. 22–3).[86] Munsat and associates have shown more dramatic changes in fiber type in response to electrical stimulation, with type I muscle fibers increasing from 4% to 48% after FES of the quadriceps in patients with disuse atrophy.[172] Studies using electrical stimulation of triceps surae muscle for 20 days at medium (50 Hz) and high (2500 Hz) frequencies have also shown an increase in fiber size, mitochondrial fraction, and DNA fiber content.[32, 33] Finally, similar changes have also been noted in normal muscle from subjects with scoliosis, in whom chronic, low-intensity electrical stimulation resulted in increases in type I and IIc muscle fiber percentages after 6 months of continuous stimulation. In addition to changes in muscle fiber types, an increase was also noted in citrate synthase activity, suggesting a move toward an oxidative metabolism[90] and a more fatigue-resistant muscle.

After discontinuation of electrical stimulation, the muscle fiber type begins to transform to its prestimulation characteristics in a time course that reflects a "first in, last out" relationship. Within 6 weeks, the former fast-twitch muscle fiber regains its previous contractile behavior with a change in maximum velocity of contraction. This is associated with changes in N-methyl-

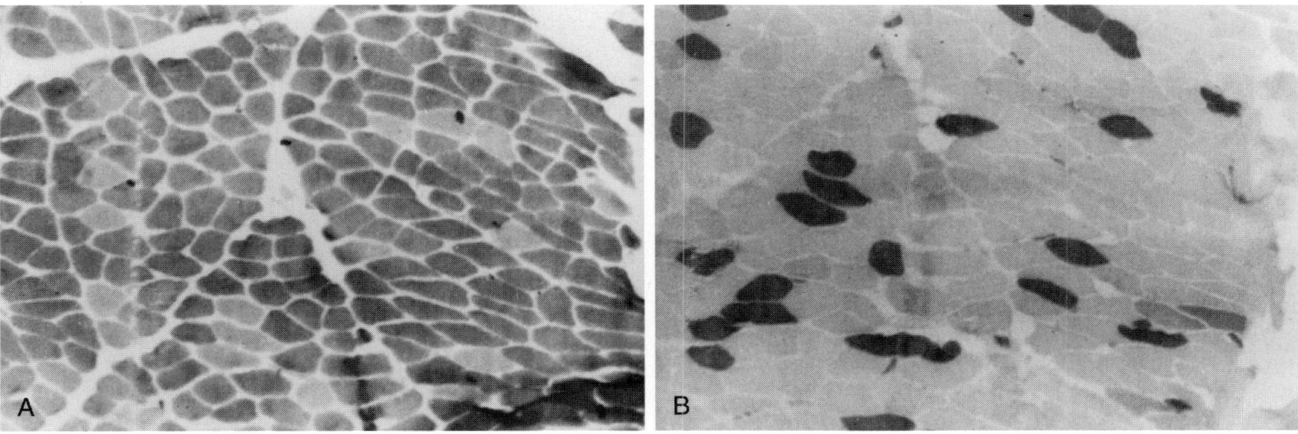

FIGURE 22–3. Biopsy of vastus lateralis of the quadriceps femoris muscle from a subject with a spinal cord injury before (*A*) and after (*B*) undergoing functional electrical stimulation for 90 days. The muscle biopsy was stained with a dye for ATPase myofibrillar activity. Note the increase in type IIa fibers after electrical stimulation. (From Greve JMD, Muszkat R, Schmidt B, et al: Functional electrical stimulation (FES): Muscle histochemical analysis. Paraplegia 1993; 31:764–770.)

histidine content, myosin ATPase, and LC. Changes in oxidative and glycolytic enzymes lag behind the contractile protein changes, with a return to an anaerobic metabolic pathway by 12 weeks. Capillary density changes are one of the last features to be modified and may be present for up to several months.[234] If electrical stimulation therapy is discontinued, a series of changes occurs in the muscle fiber that depends on the length of discontinuation of therapy. This can affect the muscle response to resumption of electrical stimulation (detraining effect).

The importance of stimulation frequency for fiber transformation has also been a subject of intense investigation.[235] Application of low-frequency (10 Hz) stimulation for 8 hours per day results in a delay of the acquisition of the transformation from fast- to slow-twitch muscle fiber composition when compared with a continuous (24 hours per day), low-frequency (10 Hz) stimulation protocol.[203] Despite this delay, similar changes in contractile properties eventually occur with both stimulation regimens. If an equal number of stimuli is given per minute as a short burst of high-frequency (40 Hz) stimuli, versus continuous low-frequency (10 Hz) stimulation, similar histochemical changes reflecting a transition from fast- to slow-twitch muscle fiber type are noted in both groups.[118] Increases in succinate dehydrogenase activity are also seen in response to each of these stimulation patterns, although the increase in succinate dehydrogenase occurs at a slower rate when the stimulation frequency is 40 Hz.[207] Using even higher frequencies (2.5-sec trains at 60 Hz delivered every 10 sec) with the number of stimuli equivalent to continuous low-frequency (10 Hz) stimulation over a 5-week period produced nearly identical changes in ATPase, fiber type, calcium uptake, and contractile properties with each regimen.[249]

The impact of a change in frequency, however, is dramatically different if there is an increase in *both* frequency and number of stimuli. In the denervated rat soleus model, intermittent high-frequency (100 Hz) electrical stimulation resulted in conversion of the muscle from a slow- to fast-twitch fiber type.[152, 153] In contrast, continuous low-frequency (10 Hz) stimulation of this muscle maintained the slow-twitch characteristics of the denervated soleus muscle.[153] It appears that both the specific frequency and the number of stimuli per minute with electrical stimulation can dramatically affect the phenotypic expression of the muscle fiber in response to treatment. This switch from slow- to fast-twitch fiber type, at this point, is unique to denervated muscle and has never been reported in innervated muscle.

To exclude the influence of the release of local neurotropic factor(s) on the transformation of muscle fiber type in response to electrical stimulation, investigations have focused on the response of denervated muscle to electrical stimulation. Using a 1-sec train of low-frequency (10 Hz) pulses every 2 sec, electrical stimulation started within 24 hours of denervation resulted in a decrease in atrophy and maintenance of oxidative enzyme levels at or above normal levels in 95% of samples.[176] Somewhat surprising, however, were findings that the late-onset initiation of electrical stimulation (28 days post denervation) using an intermediate frequency (25 Hz) stimulus with a long bidirectional impulse duration (200 μsec) markedly retarded atrophy and induced a hybrid fiber type with mitochondrial changes suggestive of a type I fiber and type IIb myofibrillar ATPase expression.[167] These studies and other histological and biochemical data suggest that denervated muscles exhibit some properties of plasticity independent of neurological input.

WAVES

Therapeutic electricity is characterized according to its waveform, amplitude, duration, and frequency. Three basic types of waveforms exist: direct current, alternating current, and pulsed current. Direct current involves the unidirectional flow of a charge with no change in waveform characteristics over time. This type of uninterrupted direct current waveform is not applicable to FES systems. *Alternating current* refers to an uninterrupted bidirectional flow of charged particles that can be symmetrical or asymmetrical (Fig. 22–4).[139, 173] The pulsed waveforms are the most common waveforms applied for therapeutic purposes.[139] Pulsed waves can be further classified as *monophasic* or *biphasic.* The biphasic waveforms can be symmetrical or asymmetrical with respect to the baseline. The reference to symmetry applies to any combination of parameters, such as current intensity, duration, rise time, or decay of the waveform.[173]

Pulsed or alternating currents can be varied, or modulated, with respect to amplitude, duration, or frequency.[139, 173] These modulations can be sequential, intermittent, or variable. *Ramping* refers to a form of modulation in which either the pulse amplitude or the duration is increased (ramped up) or decreased (ramped down) over time. A *burst* refers to a type of modulation in which a finite series of pulses, or an envelope of alternating current, is delivered at a specific frequency (carrier frequency) over a specified time interval (burst duration). The interval between bursts is referred to as the *interburst interval* (Fig. 22–4). The *duty cycle* is defined as the ratio between burst duration and the total cycle time, where the total cycle time equals the duration of the burst duration plus the interburst interval. The duty cycle is often expressed as a percentage; therefore, a duty cycle ratio of 1:4 corresponds to a duty cycle of 20%.

A number of studies have been done to explore the impact of different waveforms and stimulation parameters on patient comfort, force of contraction, strengthen-

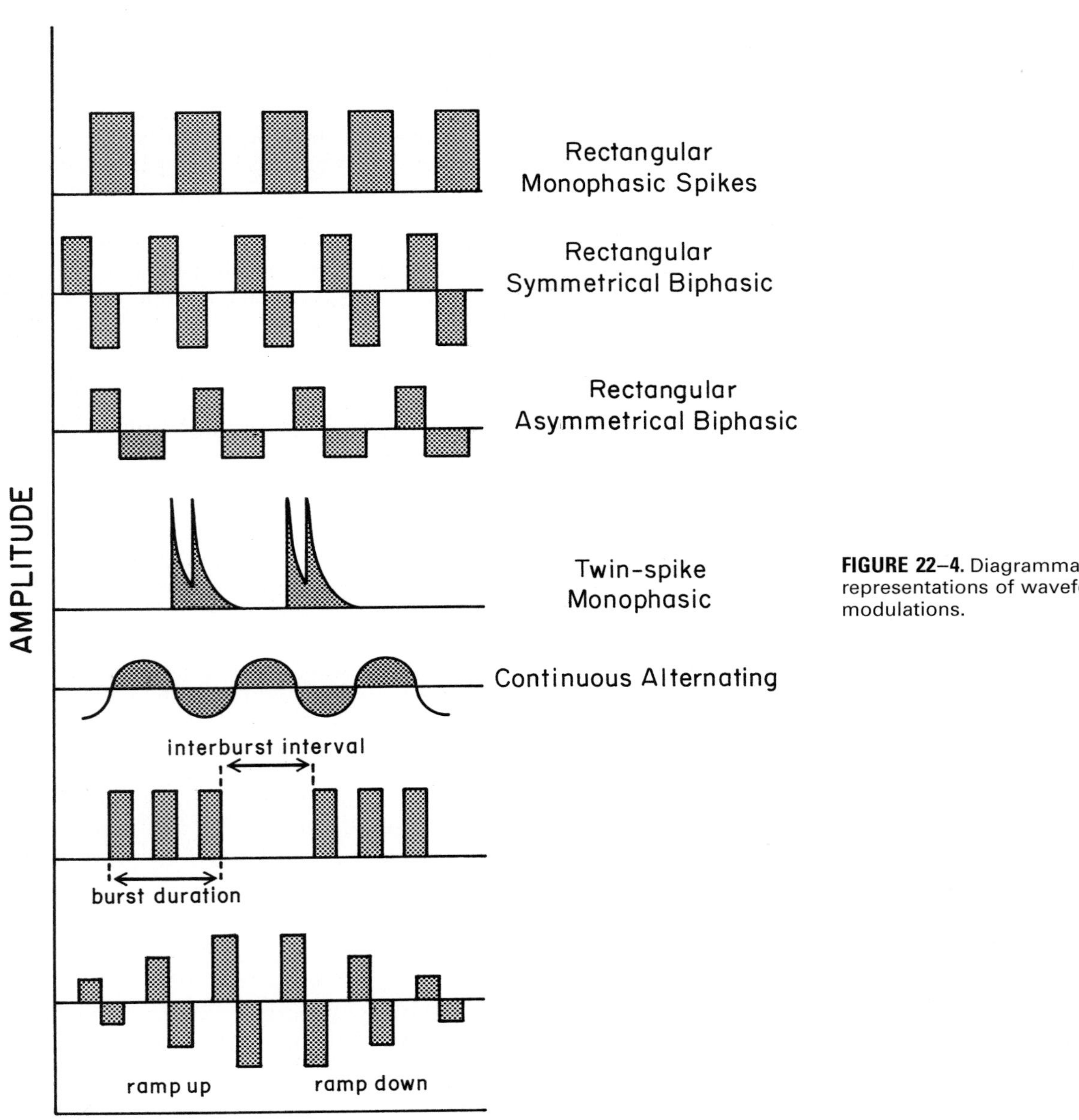

FIGURE 22–4. Diagrammatic representations of waveforms and modulations.

ing effect, and fatigue. The majority of these studies have been done in normal muscle, and these data are presumably transferable to upper motor neuron and myopathic conditions.

Both burst-modulated alternating current and asymmetrical biphasic pulsed current appear to induce the most forceful contractions.[136, 265] No consensus exists as to which waveform provides the greatest patient comfort. Various studies have advocated the burst-modulated alternating current, asymmetrical biphasic pulsed current, symmetrical biphasic pulsed current, and twin spiked monophasic pulsed currents.[8, 90, 277]

The relationship between current amplitude (milliamperes [mA]) and the force of muscle contraction is linear.[139] A stimulus duration in excess of 200 μsec is likely to produce a more forceful muscle contraction, but waveforms with durations in excess of 60 μsec are also associated with greater pain.[20, 113] Stimulation frequencies of 60 to 100 Hz are necessary to produce the most forceful muscle contraction, but stimulation at these rates rapidly results in muscle fatigue.[16] Muscle fatigue is significantly diminished by utilizing stimulation rates of approximately 20 Hz, but this results in approximately a 35% drop in the force generated at higher stimulation frequencies.[124] Current studies are attempting to maximize the effectiveness of stimulation parameters through the manipulation of duty cycles and the development of biophysically based mathematical models of how muscle responds to electrical stimulation, in the hope that these models will optimize FES-generated movement.[57, 58] In summary, data demonstrate that waveform amplitude, duration, and frequency can all be manipulated to control both the force and endurance of muscle contraction, but the optimal combinations of stimulation parameters for therapeutic or functional purposes are not identical. This area is an area of active research.

ELECTRODES

The development of neuromuscular stimulation electrodes remains problematic. A number of different types of electrodes are available, including surface, epimysial, intramuscular, juxtaneural, nerve cuff, epineural, intraneural/intrafascicular, and intraspinal.[253] The choice of an electrode type is based on the goal of the electrical stimulation program and its ease of use for the patient. In addition, selection criteria for the choice of an electrode type should include general biocompatibility of the electrode and leads, electrochemistry at the electrode-tissue interface, the possibility of actively or passively induced tissue damage by the electrodes or leads, electrode invasiveness, ease of surgical placement, ease of electrode retrieval and/or replacement, electrode reliability and failure rate, selectivity of the desired elicited muscle contractions, potential for side effects, repeatability and reproducibility of the muscle responses over time, dependence of contractile responses over time, dependence of contractile responses on muscle length and joint angle, and electrode system economics.[253]

Surface electrodes remain the most commonly utilized electrode type for most FES therapeutic and functional interventions. The force of muscle contractions induced with surface electrodes is influenced by electrode size and alignment. Longitudinal placement of electrodes produces as much as a 64% increase in the maximal tolerable torque when compared with a transverse placement.[139] Larger surface electrodes result in a more forceful muscle contraction and cause less discomfort than smaller surface electrodes.[139]

Electrical stimulation protocols that require multiple surface electrodes are often impractical if long-term FES utilization is anticipated. In an effort to improve the practicality of surface stimulation, a number of electrode garments have been developed (Fig. 22–5). These garments are particularly useful for FES cycle ergometry and standing and gait protocols in that they decrease preparation time for FES, increase patient independence, and provide more consistent electrode placement.

Patient discomfort associated with surface stimulation and the lack of precision achieved with surface stimulation are, at least in part, overcome with implanted electrode systems. Epimysial, intramuscular, and nerve cuff electrodes are the most common examples of implanted electrodes presently utilized. A number of material science issues need to be resolved to be able to design neuromuscular stimulation electrodes that minimize tissue injury while maintaining electrode reliability. For example, failure rates of percutaneously inserted intramuscular electrodes have apparently been reduced from an early failure rate of 20% to a subsequent failure rate of approximately 1% per year.[267] However, percutaneous intramuscular electrodes resulted in local tissue injury when the voltage output that created the maximum contraction was utilized. This problem can be somewhat circumvented by inserting electrodes into multiple motor points of a muscle, with subsequent sequential or simultaneous stimulation at a lower voltage. This decreases the problems with fatigue and presumably tissue injury.[143]

Cuff electrodes, which are placed around peripheral nerves that innervate several muscles, offer the opportunity to activate numerous muscles through a single electrode, thereby diminishing the extent of required hardware. Snug-fitting cuff electrodes are available that can improve selectivity by stimulating portions of a peripheral nerve.[195] Endoscopic implantation techniques have been explored for cuff electrodes that overcome the lack of precision of surface and percutaneous electrodes while avoiding the need for surgical exposure of target nerves.[185] Problems with electrode movement continue to cause variability of the input-output properties of nerve cuff stimulating electrodes.[88] Implanting nerve cuff electrodes also results in the loss of axons during the first several weeks, but follow-up studies document considerable regeneration.[140] Stimulation techniques such as decreasing the duration of stimulation, stimulating at lower rates (20 Hz vs. 50 Hz), and using a shorter duty cycle require ongoing development to minimize neural damage from cuff electrodes.[1]

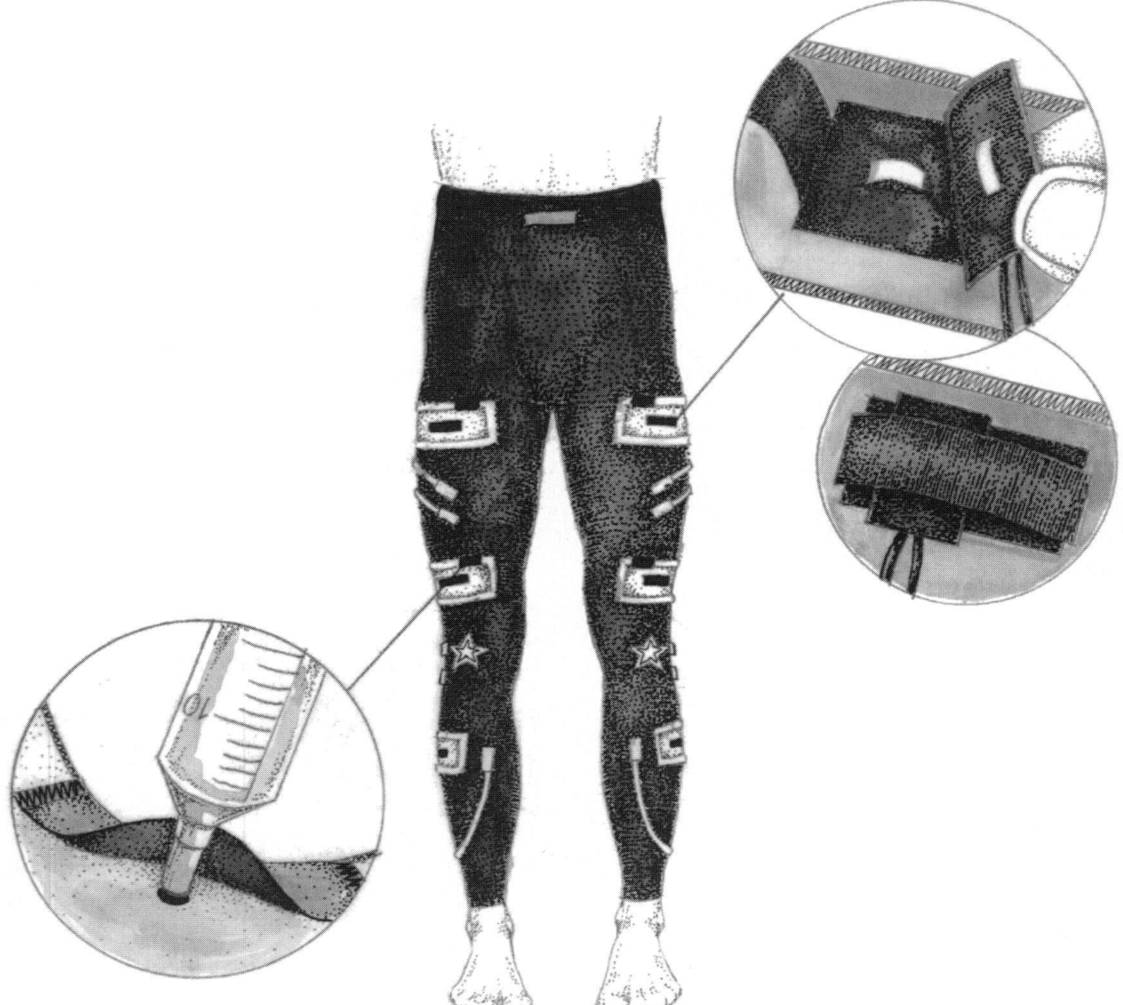

FIGURE 22–5. Example of a custom-made electrode garment manufactured by Bioflex, Inc. Electrodes are made of stretch materials and conductive gel is inserted into the pocket on the side of the electrode. Velcro connectors are arranged to allow connection of all anteriorly and posteriorly placed electrodes to stimulators while the patient is seated.

THERAPEUTIC NEUROMUSCULAR ELECTRICAL STIMULATION FOR MUSCLE STRENGTHENING

Stimulation of Normal Muscle

Although electrical stimulation therapy has been shown to be effective in improving muscle force,[31] there are no data to suggest that the use of neuromuscular electrical stimulation (NMES) in a normal healthy human results in substantial improvement in muscle strength compared with that achieved by voluntary isometric exercise. Multiple studies comparing the efficacy of NMES with isometric voluntary contraction of the quadriceps have shown that similar gains in isometric muscle strength occur with both exercise regimens.[51, 52, 93, 136, 138, 144] When a combination of neuromuscular stimulation and voluntary exercise was compared with either program alone, no significant augmentation of quadriceps strength was seen after combined training. Similarly, NMES can improve the endurance of muscle in sedentary humans trained with stimulation rates of 8 Hz, but the benefit did not exceed the endurance noted in normal active adults.[256] The lack of additional benefit from NMES in combination with voluntary contraction for strengthening probably reflects the fact that with maximal voluntary contraction, nearly 100% of the recruitable motor units are activated. Consequently, the additional stimulation provided by NMES is unable to recruit additional motor units to result in further increments in force.

Despite the fact that NMES and voluntary exercise result in comparable increases in isometric strength, these two training regimens differ. With voluntary training, type I fibers are activated first, followed by the progressive recruitment of type II fibers with increasing force. In contrast, the NMES protocols lead to an activation of type II fibers to a greater extent than type I fibers. As maximal force depends on type II fiber activation, selected augmentation of the type II muscle fibers by

NMES might lead to greater increases in the overall strength of the muscle at submaximal training intensity. This hypothesis has been supported by data showing that voluntary exercise groups train at higher muscle contraction intensity (78% to 119% of initial maximal voluntary isometric contraction [MVIT]) than NMES groups (33% to 68% MVIT) to achieve an equivalent degree of strengthening.[52] In one study of isometric strength training in elderly men, these higher workloads resulted in increases in heart rate during the training sessions. Subjects randomized to NMES, in contrast, had similar gains in strength without a change in cardiovascular work.[35] NMES strengthening might offer specific advantages in training over voluntary contraction in certain populations of individuals who have cardiovascular disease or other limitations that preclude training at higher workloads.

Studies of NMES or voluntary isometric contraction of the adductor pollicis of the nondominant hand have shown the importance of understanding the unique contractile properties of the specific muscle involved in the training regimen. Both NMES and voluntary training result in increases in muscle force, although the observed increase in response to NMES was significantly smaller. With voluntary training, a greater increase was seen in tetanic force of contraction, speed of contraction, and speed of relaxation in comparison to NMES. Training with NMES, however, had no effect on mechanical twitch tension and resulted in no reduction in fatigue. Finally, voluntary training resulted in faster kinetics of contraction, whereas no improvements were noted with NMES. The authors concluded that in small muscles, such as the adductor pollicis,[59] all or nearly all motor units were recruited during voluntary contractions, but not during electrical stimulation. Thus, the number of trained motor units was different with the two training regimens. In this specific muscle group, voluntary contraction using activation of synaptic ionic current with excitation-contraction coupling was more efficient in stimulating the smaller motor neurons with the higher-input resistance that were present in the hand. In contrast, electrical stimulation affected changes in peripheral processes beyond the membrane ionic mechanisms of the muscle excitation-contraction coupling, recruiting larger cells with lower external input, which reflected a smaller population of the motor units within the hand muscle. Based on these data, it is clearly important to understand the motor unit composition of the muscle in order to determine the most appropriate therapeutic intervention and response.

NMES might also have a therapeutic application in augmenting strengthening at skeletal regions in which attainment of maximal volitional contraction is difficult to achieve. NMES at both high (2000 Hz) and moderate (50 Hz) frequencies has been shown to increase maximal isometric force of the triceps surae.[31] NMES with voluntary contraction can also result in significantly higher gains in abdominal strength and endurance when compared with NMES or voluntary exercise alone.[6] Finally, biphasic NMES of the back muscles has been shown to improve isokinetic strength to a degree that is equal to voluntary exercise, with the added benefit of enhanced endurance.[125]

Not only has NMES been shown to increase muscle strength, it has also been shown to improve functional performance. NMES applied to the quadriceps femoris muscle bilaterally has been shown to improve performance on force measurements from a squat machine, the 25-yard dash time, and vertical jump.[276] Another benefit of NMES in normal muscle is in the prevention of the muscle atrophy associated with prolonged immobilization. Individuals undergoing knee immobilization following ligament reconstruction surgery experience significant muscle atrophy, as demonstrated by decreases in strength, endurance, muscle mass, and oxidative capacity.[139] Early intervention with NMES of the quadriceps femoris (Fig. 22–6) results in improved preservation of quadriceps muscle strength, muscle mass,[169] and succinate dehydrogenase activity[139] as well as in higher isokinetic peak torque values.[99, 271] In a study using NMES protocols (30 Hz, 300 μsec) for isometric quadriceps contraction for a 10-minute session repeated four times per day, three times per week, together with voluntary quadriceps contraction, versus exercise alone, the combination of NMES plus voluntary exercise resulted in a significant reduction in muscle wasting, a reduction in the loss of isometric torque, and preserva-

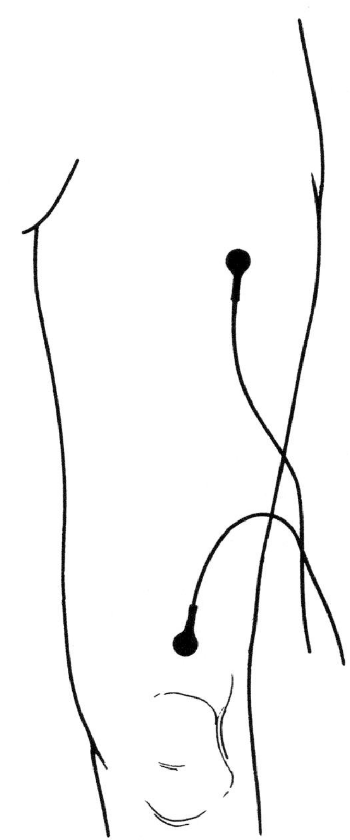

FIGURE 22–6. Electrode placement for isometric quadriceps fermoris strengthening. The active electrode is placed proximally and the indifferent electrode is placed both laterally and distally to stimulate the vastus lateralis muscle. The lateral position is used to avoid stimulation of the rectus femoris, which if stimulated would cause knee extension and hip flexion.

TABLE 22–3 Effects of Neuromuscular Electrical Stimulation on the Quadriceps Femoris During Immobilization (% Change)

	Isometric Torque	Cross-sectional Area	Citrate Synthesis Activity	TPDH Activity
Electrical stimulation	−39.2	−22.9	−5.8*	−10.1*
Control	−57.8	−25.9	−29.4	−16.8

* $P < 0.05$, electrical stimulation vs. control.

tion of oxidative enzyme activity as defined by the levels of citrate synthase and triphosphate dehydrogenase (TPDH) during the period of immobilization (Table 22–3).[271]

The benefit of NMES appears to be limited to the period of immobilization. In one prospective study of NMES after knee immobilization, although losses of thigh girth and maximal voluntary contraction during immobilization were significantly smaller with the use of NMES, by 12 weeks post surgery (6 weeks after discontinuation of immobilization), no significant differences were seen in maximal voluntary isokinetic torque or thigh girth between patients randomized to the nonexercise control or NMES group.[55] This suggests that NMES could be of greatest benefit in the treatment of elite athletes or other individuals who desire a rapid return to maximal performance levels. It might be of little or no benefit in individuals who can afford the delay in return to peak physical activity until after the period of immobilization and reconditioning is complete.

NMES (30 Hz per 18% duty cycle for 1 hour per day), using surface electrodes on the quadriceps femoris, prevents the development of disuse muscle atrophy in individuals immobilized with a long-leg cast for a tibial fracture. This preservation of muscle mass was associated with maintenance of muscle protein synthesis and rate of muscle protein synthesis per unit of muscle RNA (Fig. 22–7).[79] NMES of the calf muscles (7 Hz for 30 minutes twice a day) in patients hospitalized in the intensive care unit for postoperative ventilatory failure or cerebral infarctions, decreased urinary 3-methylhistidine and creatinine excretion, reflecting a slowing of negative nitrogen balance and improved preservation of muscle mass, in contrast to nonstimulated controls.[19] These studies taken together suggest a potential role for NMES in preserving muscle mass in individuals undergoing prolonged periods of immobilization for a variety of reasons.

One final application of NMES in normal muscle is to help in evaluating the etiology of weakness in a patient. Under conditions of normal volitional central control, a decrease occurs in electrical stimulation-induced contraction response with increasing voluntary muscle contraction at different levels (Fig. 22–8A).[226] Thus, if a subject is volitionally attempting to maximally contract muscle, leading to an optimal pattern of recruitment of all the motor units, direct electrical stimulation of the muscle will not lead to a further increment in muscle

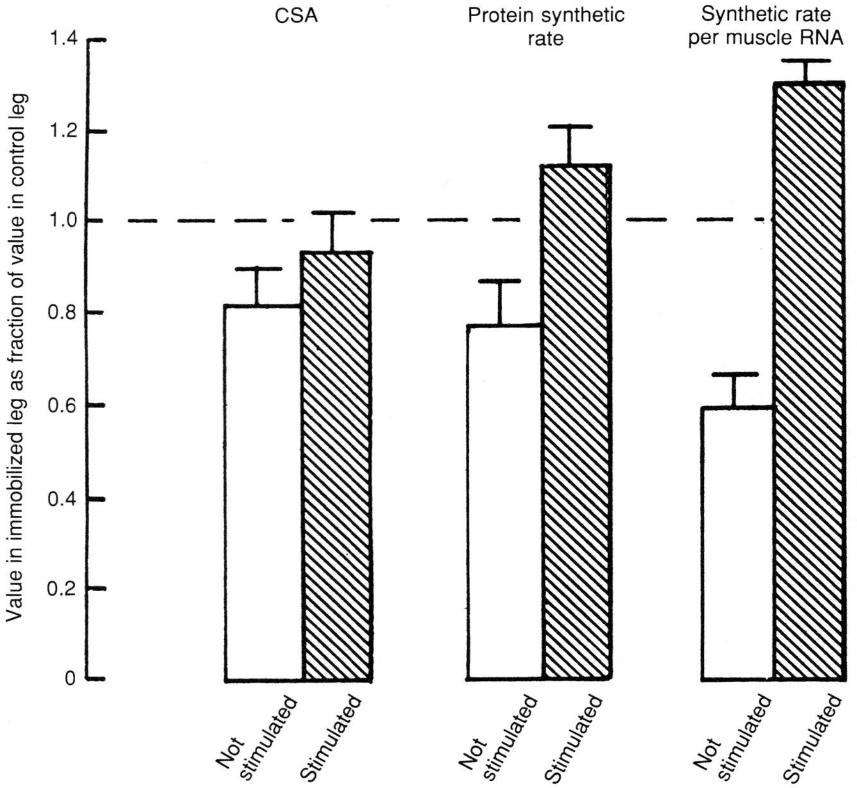

FIGURE 22–7. Effect of 6 weeks of electrical stimulation of the cast-immobilized quadriceps femoris muscle on muscle protein synthesis and quadriceps cross-sectional area in comparison to the same parameters in immobilized controls. (From Gibson JNA, Smith K, Rennie MJ: Prevention of disuse muscle atrophy by means of electrical stimulation: Maintenance of protein synthesis. Lancet 1988; 2(8614):767–769.)

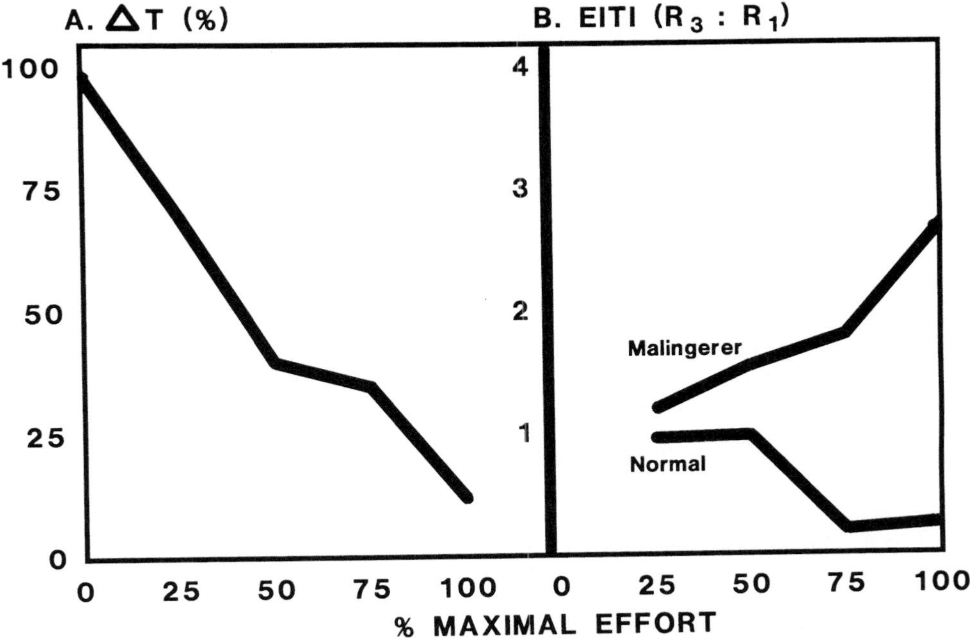

FIGURE 22–8. Effect of central and peripheral factors in fatigue elicted by electrical stimulation with voluntary contraction of the quadriceps femoris. *Panel A* reflects the dependence of the amplitude of electrically stimulated torque increments (T) on the percent of maximal voluntary contraction (% MVC). *Panel B* shows the utility of measuring the ratio of the electrically induced torque increments (EITI) in the third to the first trial (R3 : R1), to detect malingerers. The amplitude of force at 100% maximal voluntary force drops on successive trials in normal control subjects due to fatigue, but the target torque is dramatically different in the malingerer. (Data from Latash ML, Yee MJ, Orpett C, et al: Combining electrical muscle stimulation with voluntary contraction for studying muscle fatigue. Arch Phys Med Rehabil 1994; 75:29–35.)

force. If, however, the subject is not maximally trying (or if other forces contribute to a drop in volitional muscle force), electrical stimulation will lead to an increase in muscle force. This is best seen as a striking difference in the ratio of the electrically induced torque increment (EITI) in the fourth to first stimulation in response to increases in voluntary contraction in normal controls versus malingerers (Fig. 22–8B). The decrease in the fourth to first EITI ratio in normal subjects at 75% and 100% voluntary contraction reflects the effect of the development of peripheral fatigue at near-maximal contractions, which subsequently results in a reduced responsiveness of the motor unit to electrical stimulation.[52]

Stimulation of Myopathic Muscle

There remains considerable controversy regarding the benefit of electrical stimulation in preservation of motor function in individuals with neuromuscular disease. Previous studies have suggested that aggressive physical exercise might result in overwork weakness and a loss of physical function.[121, 262] In dystrophic animal models, low-frequency electrical stimulation has been shown to improve muscle function, delay degeneration of muscle fibers, and increase the quantity of oxidative enzymes.[54, 155, 222, 264] In the genetically dystrophic chicken, NMES applied early after hatching delayed the onset of righting disability, gradually increased muscle mass, increased dystrophic protein by 29%, and increased circulating creatine phosphokinase (CPK) levels. Surprisingly, however, electrical stimulation in this model resulted in a discernible shift toward a glycolytic metabolism, which is the opposite of the effect seen with NMES in normal muscle.[114]

When low-frequency electrical stimulation is applied to dystrophic muscle in children with muscular dystrophy, improvements occur in maximal voluntary contraction of the stimulated muscle[164, 238, 239, 280] and in torque, with no increase in fatigue.[280] If, however, electrical stimulation is initiated after significant strength has already been lost, there appears to be no benefit from electrical stimulation treatment. After discontinuation of NMES, strength gains are lost rapidly.[164] It appears that if NMES is to be used for strengthening in neuromuscular disease, it is only of benefit in individuals who have retained more than 15% of normal strength, and that the benefit is likely to be short-lived, resulting in only a delay of the inevitable outcome.

Stimulation of Denervated Muscle

The therapeutic relevance of NMES in a denervated muscle model is predicated on the ability of the technique to prevent or reduce atrophy and the ability of the technique to enhance reinnervation. Denervated muscle appears to have some plasticity, as NMES has been shown to facilitate the transformation from fast- to slow-twitch (or slow- to fast-twitch) fiber. This result has been associated with improved maintenance of muscle fiber area[81, 187] and muscle girth[92, 179] for a short time interval until reinnervation sets in. NMES, however, has no benefit in maintaining certain isometric contractile properties that are associated with prolongation of the action potential, including the twitch to peak time and twitch half-relaxation time.[45]

The data are mixed on the effect of initiating NMES late after denervation injury. If the electrical stimulation is initiated immediately at the time of injury, the acceleration of the half-life of the slow-degrading acetylcholine receptor can be prevented.[7] If started after the acetylcholine receptor has begun to destabilize, NMES cannot reverse the switch to a faster-degrading receptor nor can it slow the degradation of the rapid acetylcholine receptor. These data suggest that maximal maintenance of normal motor unit characteristics in a short-term stimulation program depends on very early initiation of stimulation.

In contrast, NMES using an unusually long duration (200 μsec), bidirectional, rectangular impulse at a frequency of 25 Hz, begun 28 days after denervation, has been shown to preserve muscle fiber diameter and to induce a hybrid fiber type having properties of both slow- and fast-twitch muscle.[167] The authors of the study postulated that the relatively dramatic results of this late application of NMES might be due in part to the long impulse duration used in the stimulation protocol. This is consistent with data from a previous study comparing 8 Hz/1 msec with 1 Hz/7 msec stimulation regimens in the denervated rabbit fast-twitch muscle, which found that only the lower-frequency stimulation pattern reduced atrophy.[178] The overall consensus of several studies on the dose-response of tetanic stimulation in prevention of muscle atrophy is that stimulation durations ranging from 5 to 45 μsec are beneficial, with no utility of shorter-duration impulses.[268] Although the application of NMES for muscle denervated for 4 to 10 months did cause some improvement in muscle tension, the resultant upper end of tension noted in the studies was only 10% of normal values.[3]

The data supporting the efficacy of NMES in human studies are less clear than noted in an animal model. For example, in man, low-frequency NMES started within 7 weeks of injury and continued for more than 35 weeks resulted in no benefit over the long term as measured by clinical muscle force testing, dynamometry, muscle mass measurement (by CT or ultrasound), or maximal amplitude or frequency of denervation activity.[18] In contrast, galvanic stimulation (30 stimulations three times per day) has been reported to maintain hand muscle bulk.[121] The discrepancies among these studies, other data in the literature, and the animal models could reflect differences in stimulation parameters and muscle characteristics. Additional research is needed to resolve the conflicting recommendations as to the optimal stimulation parameters. Parameters that have been shown to be most effective to date for NMES in denervation are high voltage and short duration or long duration and low voltage, both of which can be clinically impractical due to discomfort.[105]

There are no data to support that NMES of denervated muscle speeds the process of reinnervation.[229] In fact, a number of studies have suggested that stimulation inhibits terminal sprouting and reinnervation.[61] The mechanism for this is unclear and appears to contradict experiments that show an increase in the trophic factor, neurotrophin-4, after electrical stimulation.[74] That is, neurotrophin-4 promotes axonal sprouting, and its levels have been shown to increase in response to NMES in a denervation model. Despite this observed increase in neurotrophin-4, other studies have consistently shown that reinnervation is at least partially suppressed by NMES.[61]

Ultimately, the decision to use any therapeutic intervention should depend on evidence of an improved outcome. Such a benefit has been shown in an animal study comparing outcomes after nerve repair in a group receiving NMES and a second group that did not receive NMES. Both the morphology and the functional capacity of the muscle were improved in the NMES-treated group.[272] Hence, in a denervated muscle, long-term NMES might be effective in improving functional outcome by preventing atrophy when reinnervation is expected over a long period of time, such as after a surgical nerve repair.

Stimulation of Decentralized Muscle

Electrical stimulation of muscle following CNS injury or SCI can result in reversal of the muscular atrophy seen in association with the relative immobilization associated with these disorders. Although applications of NMES after cerebral vascular accident have, in general, been limited to use of NMES as an orthotic assist rather than as a therapeutic adjunct to strengthening, NMES has been used successfully in the small superficial muscles of the hand and wrist to improve strength and decrease atrophy.[188] Recommendations for electrical stimulation in the hand muscles suggest that strength is maintained at greater than 80% of initial value over an 8-month period at a 1:5 duty cycle, with decreases in dorsiflexion force output as duty cycle is equalized to 50%. Modification of electrical stimulation parameters to meet the fatigability of the muscles undergoing training is necessary, especially in situations in which spasticity and severe weakness can limit therapeutic gain.

Much more attention has been paid to the use of NMES as a modality for rehabilitation of paralyzed muscle following SCI. Following SCI, type I and type IIa fibers, myofibrillar ATPase, succinate dehydrogenase activity, and the capillary-to-fiber ratio are reduced in comparison to what is seen in normal control muscles.[38] In addition, loss of muscle bulk, a decrease in fiber cross-sectional area, a reduction in torque, a significant slowing of contractile speed, and increased fatigability have been noted.[244] Electrical stimulation (20 Hz for 15% of a duty cycle) of the tibialis anterior in individuals with chronic SCI resulted in an increase in the proportion of type I fibers from 14% ± 8% to 25% ± 10% (although the final level was well below that of control muscles), but had no effect on the distribution of fiber sizes or mean fiber area.[160] In addition, NMES enhanced the oxidative capacity of the muscle, as defined by an increase in succinate dehydrogenase activity. These results are similar to those seen with the application of low-frequency electrical stimulation to normal muscle.

Muscle strength and contractile properties also showed a positive response to NMES. Daily NMES increased endurance of the muscle to levels found in able-bodied control subjects, with a slowing of the time course of contraction and half-relaxation.[229a, 252] These data suggest substantial increases in fatigue resistance from characteristics of a fast-twitch, fatigable muscle (type IIb) to a fast-twitch fatigue-resistant type (type IIa). Despite these improvements in fatigue, there was no marked change in muscle force with a stimulation pattern. This is consistent with the reciprocal relationship between strength and endurance in normal motor units.[85] Other studies of NMES in SCI have shown that increases in force are achieved with stimulation when the stimulated muscle contracts against resistance.[85]

Although NMES-induced muscle contraction has been shown to increase certain contractile and histochemical properties of decentralized muscle, actual increases in muscle strength and endurance are most dramatically seen when NMES is combined with resistance training or functional activities. Since the mid-1980s, isometric quadriceps strengthening using NMES to move the knee through a 45-degree arc with increasing resistance has resulted in increases in quadriceps endurance and mass. The development of a functional electrical stimulation hybrid cycle ergometry system (FES-CE) (Fig. 22–9) has resulted in further therapeutic benefits. The system uses a rectangular, monophasic waveform of 30 Hz, 0 to 130 mA at 375 μsec duration, to sequentially stimulate the quadriceps, hamstrings, and gluteal muscles to produce a smooth pedaling motion of a Monark lower extremity cycle ergometer. This closed-loop system is set to maintain a cycling rate of 35 to 50 rpm, with automatic shutoff if the impedance is greater than 16,000 Ω, if the voltage exceeds 220, or if the pedaling rate is less than 35 rpm (suggesting fatigue). Using FES cycle ergometry, several investigators have shown increases in thigh circumference,[196, 197, 217] muscle strength and endurance,[212] quadriceps muscle area (by CT),[189] and quadriceps muscle protein synthesis rates (from 0.071% to 0.0985% per hour) with no change in whole body protein turnover.[189] Changes in contractile properties include a decrease in the initial slope of quadriceps twitch, which is assumed to be compatible with a disproportionate increase in the function of slow-twitch fibers.[212]

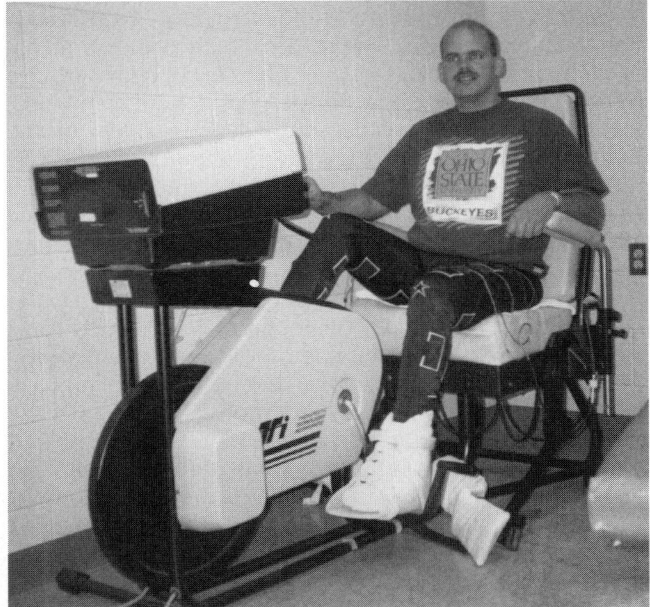

FIGURE 22–9. Functional electrical stimulation (FES) cycle ergometer by Therapeutic Technologies, Inc. Cycling is produced with sequential stimulation of the quadriceps femoris, hamstring, and gluteal muscles, using surface electrodes.

Not only can FES result in changes in localized muscle mass, it can also affect overall body composition. Following SCI, lean body mass decreases and fat mass increases. Data from our laboratory have shown, however, that individuals with chronic SCI who were randomized to an FES-CE protocol showed gains in total body lean body mass of 7.9% with a decrease in percent body fat of 12.1%. These gains in lean body mass were primarily attributed to gains in the lower extremity lean body mass, which increased 9.7% over baseline. FES-CE is also a promising intervention to prevent the losses in lean body mass associated with acute SCI. Initiation of FES-CE within 3 months of acute SCI has been shown to prevent lower limb muscle atrophy after 3 months of training and to cause muscle hypertrophy after 6 months of training.

Finally, the use of NMES to stimulate muscle contraction and maintain muscle mass might be applicable to the prevention of pressure sores. In an animal model, chronic stimulation at 10 Hz for 8 hours per day resulted in an increase in capillarization in as little as 7 days.[64, 96] NMES (50 Hz for 33% of the duty cycle) resulted in an increase in blood flow under the ischial tuberosity of humans. During electrical stimulation in untrained SCI subjects, this change was not statistically significant. Because significant benefits were noted in able-bodied subjects, the authors postulated that fatigue might have contributed to a reduction in the increment of blood flow in the SCI subjects, and that training might improve the hemodynamic benefit. In addition, NMES (50 Hz) of the gluteus maximus (Fig. 22–10) in able-bodied subjects can produce appreciable changes in seating interface pressure distribution and result in substantial shape changes of the buttocks at stimulation levels producing only a small fraction of maximum voluntary contraction.[149] The buttock shape obtained during stimulation more nearly resembles the shape of the suspended buttocks, implying a reduction in tissue distortion. If similar results could be obtained in an SCI population, NMES could have a potential application as a form of "pressure release" to decrease the incidence of pressure sores.

ELECTRICAL STIMULATION TO PREVENT COMPLICATIONS OF DISUSE

Following a neurological insult, a person is predisposed to a number of complications that arise over the long term due to the resultant decrease in physical activity. This is especially true in patients with SCI. With the

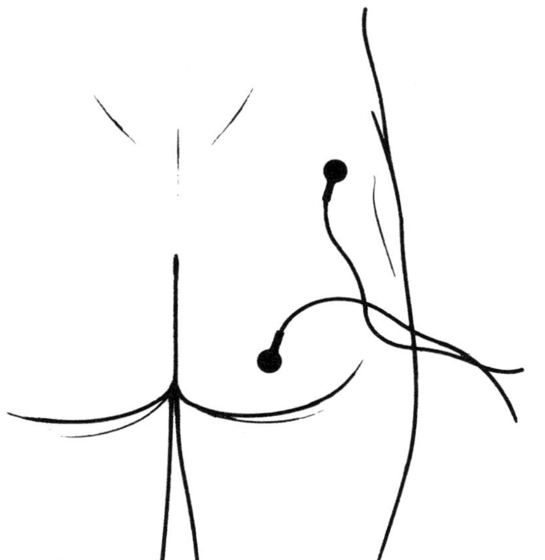

FIGURE 22–10. Hip extension is produced with placement of the active electrode on the gluteus maximus below the posterior superior iliac crest, and the indifferent electrode is placed inferiorly on the muscle.

loss of voluntary bipedal locomotion, individuals with SCI are at greater risk for cardiovascular disease, osteoporosis, pressure ulcers, and thromboembolic disease. In addition, changes in self-image can have a major influence on well-being. In an attempt to reduce these disuse-associated medical conditions, physicians have turned to NMES techniques.

Cardiovascular Deconditioning

During the past few decades, with improvement in bladder and skin management, cardiovascular disease has become the primary cause of death in individuals with SCI. A body of evidence shows that SCI is associated with a decrease in cardiopulmonary performance.[210] Within the first 3 months of SCI, a significant decline occurs in aerobic capacity, with declines in maximal oxygen consumption (Vo_{2max}) of more than 40%.[66] After discharge from rehabilitation, the workload of a paraplegic individual performing independent activities of daily living (ADL) is only 24% of the maximal work capacity, which is insufficient to maintain cardiovascular fitness.[110] This cardiovascular deconditioning is even more pronounced in quadriplegic persons, for whom data show a decrease in maximum heart rate, stroke volume, and cardiac output[186] and the development of left ventricular atrophy.[175] Studies of Vo_{2max} in persons with chronic SCI reveal an inverse relationship to the level of SCI.[111]

Cardiovascular deconditioning, however, is not an inevitable consequence of SCI. Wheelchair athletes have been shown to have significantly higher Vo_{2max}, cardiac output, and stroke volume than sedentary SCI individuals.[183, 281] In addition, their lipid levels are nearly the same as those of able-bodied individuals, with the exception of a lower HDL_3 level.[22] Arm crank ergometry has been proposed as a means to improve cardiovascular training, but it is inefficient, because recruitment of small muscle mass during exercise results in a Vo_2 level that is 15% to 35% lower than that which can be obtained with lower extremity exercises.[49, 67, 216] For quadriplegic individuals, arm crank ergometry can be impractical because of upper limb weakness. Attention has therefore turned toward the therapeutic use of NEMS as an intervention to improve cardiovascular fitness. Chronic use of arm crank ergometry might also accelerate the deterioration of the shoulder joints seen in chronic SCI.

A consensus has existed since the initial studies in the late 1980s that short-term training with FES-CE can produce an increase in both endurance and Vo_{2max} when stress testing is performed with the lower limb cycle ergometer.[175, 208] FES-CE can also result in an improvement in the left ventricular mass of quadriplegic persons.[175] This lower limb training, however, has not been shown to translate to a cardiovascular improvement when exercise testing is done via arm crank ergometry stress testing.[111] This is consistent with data in able-bodied individuals that indicate that a training effect is specific to the muscle groups that are trained.[42]

During an acute bout of FES-CE, a relative increase occurs in Vo_2, pulmonary ventilation, heart rate, and stroke volume, with greater increases noted in paraplegic versus quadriplegic persons. The increase in Vo_2 is thought to be due to augmented blood flow to the exercised muscles. Work by Petrofsky and Stacy[200] has shown that the respiratory efficiency of FES cycling is only 3.6% (3.6% of the energy of cycling is converted to energy to move the pedals), which is substantially lower than the value of 20% to 30% for lower limb ergometry in able-bodied individuals. Despite the low respiratory efficiency, however, prolonged training with FES-CE does result in increases in blood pressure, heart rate, cardiac output, and Vo_{2max} that are linear with the metabolic demand on the muscle.

In an attempt to increase the efficiency of cardiovascular training, studies have combined arm crank ergometry with lower extremity FES. Training with these hybrid systems has shown improved increments in Vo_2, minute ventilation, cardiac output, and stroke volume in comparison with arm crank ergometers or FES-CE alone.[141, 209] New approaches include the combination of FES quadriceps extension against 20 lb of resistance with arm crank ergometry at 50 rpm,[63] FES-CE with voluntary arm crank ergometry,[137] or FES-rowing.[141]

In summary, advances in functional electrical stimulation have resulted in the development of several systems that can increase muscle mass, reduce venous pooling, increase stroke volume and cardiac output, and improve cardiorespiratory fitness.[91] Additional long-term data analyzing the efficacy of various FES techniques and treatment protocols are necessary to determine whether the short-term improvements in cardiorespiratory fitness can be maintained over long periods of time and whether they will have a substantial influence on cardiovascular morbidity and mortality.[91]

Osteoporosis

One prominent metabolic consequence of SCI is an acute disruption of normal calcium balance, which contributes to a rapidly evolving osteopenia that is a permanent consequence of the injury. The severe osteopenia results in an increased risk of fractures, and as many as 9% of all SCI patients present with one or more fractures within the first 10 years after injury.[218] Cross-sectional studies of regional bone mass changes have documented that bone mass loss is not uniform below the level of neurological injury, but that the magnitude of loss is determined, at least in part, by the degree of reduction in biomechanical loading.[15] One of the mechanisms thought to contribute to this profound bone loss is the loss of muscle contraction and mechanical loading in the SCI patient. Based on Wolff's law, which states that the form and structure of bone are organized to optimally resist perceived loads from functional demands, attention has been focused on the therapeutic use of NMES to reduce immobilization, increase biomechanical strain, and potentially improve bone mass at localized skeletal regions.

Initial studies by Leeds and associates[147] and Pacy and colleagues[189] showed no benefit of FES-CE on bone mass at the proximal femur or lumbar spine in individuals with SCI of long duration. More recent work has supported a positive effect of FES on bone mass. One group demonstrated a 0.2% to 3.3% reduction in tibial bone loss in a group of chronic SCI subjects training with FES-CE.[95] Data from our laboratory suggest FES-CE can produce small increments in bone mass in patients with chronic SCI, but these benefits are localized to the two skeletal regions (proximal tibia and distal femur) receiving the greatest mechanical strain with the exercise regimen.[17] In addition, as seen in able-bodied individuals, these increments in bone mass are dependent on achieving a sufficient workload, with gains limited to individuals who were able to cycle at workloads of 18 W or greater. Additional studies in our laboratory suggest that FES-CE could be of greater benefit for the prevention of neurogenic osteopenia. This is consistent with all other forms of osteoporosis, for which there are no known strategies to date for reversing significant osteopenia. Early intervention with FES-CE following acute SCI has been reported to significantly slow rates of bone loss and to decrease hypercalciuria.[174] Longer duration studies with continued use of FES-CE will help to define whether NMES is a practical and an effective means of preventing osteopenia and of reducing the incidence of fractures.

Deep Venous Thrombosis

Another complication associated with the relative immobilization seen after a neurological insult is an increase in the risk of thromboembolic disease. Following a cerebrovascular accident, there is a 23% to 75% incidence of deep venous thrombosis (DVT) and a 10% incidence of pulmonary emboli during the first 6 months. The role of reduced muscle activity is suggested by data that show that the DVT is most commonly localized to the paretic limb (5- to 10-fold increase). The incidence of DVT is even greater following SCI, with a reported incidence between 47% and 100% in the first year post SCI. Thromboembolic disease accounts for 37.5% of acute deaths in this population. Because some individuals have contraindications to subcutaneous heparin prophylaxis (e.g., blood in CNS), there has been some exploration of the use of NMES to reduce the incidence of thromboembolic disease. NMES (10 Hz, 50-μsec pulse for a 33% duty cycle) of the tibialis anterior and gastrocnemius-soleus muscle groups for 23 hours per day over a 28-day period in combination with low-dose heparin in patients with acute SCI showed a significant decrease in the incidence of DVT in comparison with a group receiving low-dose heparin alone.[163] This result might be due in part to the effects of NMES in increasing plasma fibrinolytic activity.[127] Promising results from FES were also seen in a stroke population, in which FES compared favorably with adjusted dose heparin and intermittent pneumatic compression in preventing DVT.[190]

Psychological Effects

A number of psychosocial problems have been reported in patients following SCI, including mood disorders and diminished social and vocational functioning. It has been proposed that exercise might result in some psychological benefits, such as improved self-esteem. Utilizing FES-CE, 62% of paraplegic and 56% of quadriplegic patients reported improved self-image with participation.[246] Other benefits included increased self-esteem,[92, 246] well-being,[12] and independence[98] and diminished depression.[4] Not all changes, however, are positive: some subjects also report decreased motivation and increased anger and tension. Expectations played an important role in resultant negativity, with individuals with unrealistic expectations (e.g., anticipation of improved neurological function) showing the fewest psychological benefits.[21] The positive feelings noted with FES-CE can have a physiological explanation, as regular exercise with FES-CE has been shown to significantly increase beta-endorphin levels.[260]

THERAPEUTIC FUNCTIONAL ELECTRICAL STIMULATION

Urinary Incontinence

Urinary incontinence is a significant public health problem that carries an economic burden estimated at $10 billion per year.[37] Although Kegel introduced exercises for the management of urinary incontinence in the late 1940s and early 1950s, the primary method of intervention has remained surgical intervention.[27] The conservative management of urinary incontinence is, however, considered to be the wave of the future.[27]

Caldwell was the first to report positive results after implantation of an electrical stimulation system for the correction of urinary incontinence in 1963 (reviewed in Jonasson et al[123]). A subsequent study treated women with both stress- and motor-urge incontinence with intravaginal electrodes. After 12 weeks of stimulation, 20 minutes daily, a markedly diminished leakage of urine was noted in 35% of women with stress incontinence and in 65% of women with motor-urge urinary incontinence.[123] Another study combined pelvic floor exercises with intravaginal maximal electrical stimulation. After 6 weeks of stimulation for 15 minutes daily, 89% of women with stress-urge incontinence, 73% with motor instability, and 70% with mixed incontinence demonstrated improvement. Long-term follow-up demonstrated that 80% of women maintained the improvement.[37] Subsequent studies suggested cure rates of 30% to 50% and improvement rates of 67% to 90% for stress incontinence with FES.[279]

The mechanism for this therapeutic response is believed to be secondary to the fact that incontinence might represent a denervation injury; that is, the observed improvements could be due to the muscle strengthening properties of electrical stimulation.[27] The validity of this hypothesis is questioned in view of the fact that many humans do not tolerate stimulation intensities sufficiently high to directly stimulate motor nerves. Therefore, it is suggested that pelvic floor afferents with reflex connections to the muscle are stimulated.[72]

The stimulation systems for the management of bladder incontinence include electrodes implanted into pelvic floor muscles and external electrodes that are primarily intra-anal or intravaginal.[279] The intravaginal electrodes appear to be the most commonly utilized technique. Both anal and vaginal external electrodes are recommended because of safety and ease of use. Stimulation programs typically utilize biphasic pulsed waveforms. Less than 10 Hz stimulation is optimal for bladder inhibition, whereas stimulation rates approaching 50 Hz are recommended for optimal urethral closure. Mixed stress and urge incontinence protocols utilize stimulation rates of 20 Hz.[72] Pulse duration and amplitude are adjusted to the maximal tolerable level. However, controversy continues as to the relative benefit of chronic (long-term, continuous) stimulation versus short-term stimulation.[279]

In summary, data clearly suggest that the electrical stimulation of pelvic floor muscles is an important adjunct to the conservative management of stress and motor-urge urinary continence. It has been suggested that this technique is primarily suited as an adjunct to therapy for individuals who are not able to voluntarily stop urine flow and who cannot contract the pelvic floor muscles.[27]

Electrical stimulation has also been utilized extensively for the restoration of bladder function after SCI. Sphincter stimulation with an anal plug stimulator for 30 minutes twice daily did not improve cystometric findings in one study, and most patients in this study did not wish to continue utilizing this technique.[120] Similarly, pudendal nerve stimulation via the penis or clitoris for 20 minutes, five times per week for 4 weeks, did not improve bladder capacity or incontinence.[214] However, stimulation of the pudendal nerve at twice the bulbocavernosus threshold has been shown to increase bladder capacity.[215]

Implanted electrodes have been applied to the bladder wall, pelvic splanchnic nerves, conus medullaris, mixed sacral nerves, and sacral anterior roots. The greatest attention has been directed toward stimulation of the sacral anterior roots. The procedure is, however, complicated by the reflex activation of sphincters. A number of techniques have been explored to reduce the subsequent outflow obstruction, such as pudendal neurectomy, external sphincterotomy, and the development of stimulation parameters that sufficiently maintain the peak contraction of the sphincter and bladder out of phase to produce micturation between bursts.[48] In an animal model, a new FES system was successfully tested on the sacral roots that could generate one signal composed of two independent waveforms delivered by a single bipolar electrode. This permitted selective blockade of the external urethral sphincter during simultaneous detrusor stimulation, with subsequent more physiological voiding.[243] Somewhat similar results were noted in humans using a tripolar electrode to stimulate the sacral root.[244]

Posterior root rhizotomy has been advocated in conjunction with sacral anterior root stimulation as a means of abolishing uninhibited reflex bladder contractions, thereby increasing bladder capacity, restoring bladder compliance to normal, and abolishing reflex contraction of the sphincter.[48, 126] The disadvantages of the posterior root rhizotomy include the loss of reflex erection and reflex ejaculation. The combination of these techniques is useful in that they decrease residual urine volume, improve bladder compliance, improve urinary incontinence, and decrease reflux and hydronephrosis. Additional benefits of these two interventions are restoration of full erections sufficient for coitus in 60% of patients and production of defecation with the stimulator alone in 50% of patients.[48]

Numerous other techniques have been explored to improve bladder continence using electrical stimulation technology, with results that are intriguing. These techniques include stimulation of the thigh muscles 20 minutes daily for 14 days, with a resulting improvement in the bladder capacity of patients with detrusor hyperreflexia or instability.[182] Additionally, neurovascularly intact gracilis muscle transposition to the proximal urethra, with subsequent stimulation of the transposed muscle using intramuscular electrodes and a subcutaneously placed pulse generator, has resulted in a decrease in urinary incontinence.[40]

Ejaculatory Failure

Ejaculatory failure is noted in approximately 95% of SCI survivors. Semen retrieval, however, is possible with subcutaneous physostigmine, vas aspiration, vibratory stimulation, and electrostimulation by rectal probe.[118] Ejaculation via rectal probe stimulation is apparently accomplished with either sinusoidal or pulsed waveforms utilizing a variety of stimulation parameters.[194, 240] This technique does not adversely affect sperm motility.[233] One other study documented that in a group of 25 SCI survivors, electro-ejaculation resulted in bidirectional emission in 12 patients, antegrade in 9, retrograde in 1, and failure in 3.[266] Sperm quality or quantity did not correlate with SCI level, age at injury, or patient age. Ejaculation via electrostimulation appears to be well tolerated and safe, with minimal autonomic dysreflexia and mild rectal mucosal changes.[266]

Management of Spasticity

Electrical stimulation has been used therapeutically for the management of spasticity since Duchenne's first use of it in 1871. Since then, electrical stimulation for the management of spasticity has been administered by epidural, implanted, subcutaneous, and surface stimulation. Most of the available information regarding the efficacy of this modality is based on observations noted during the application of electrical stimulation for functional purposes. Few studies have attempted to systematically evaluate the therapeutic efficacy of this modality in spasticity. Short-term effects of surface electrical stimulation utilizing an intensity of 100 mA, a duration of 0.5 msec, a stimulation frequency of 20 Hz, and a compensated monophasic waveform, with a duty cycle ratio of 1:1 for 20 minutes in 12 SCI survivors, resulted in a significant improvement in the pendulum drop test. This improvement did not persist past 24 hours.[226]

In contrast, application of an 8-week electrical stimulation protocol in which SCI subjects received 20 minutes of electrical stimulation twice a day, 6 days per week, demonstrated a tendency toward increasing spasticity with long-term surface electrical stimulation.[228] However, a 3-month program of FES decreased spasticity and improved both gait patterns and velocity (determined by gait analysis) in a subject with familial spastic paraplegia.[191]

Observations noted in hemiplegic individuals have been more consistently favorable for the benefits of FES in the management of spasticity. One study, for example, followed up a group of hemiplegic patients receiving surface stimulation and via an implanted peroneal stimulator for 12 months. The stimulation parameters were described as a pulse width of 0.5 msec and a stimulation frequency of 30 to 33 Hz. This group noted a significant decrease in passive resistance and tonic reflex activity. These changes were thought to result in improved voluntary control in agonist and antagonist muscle groups.[250] A second study applied electrical stimulation to wrist extensors of hemiplegic individuals with flexor spasticity. Their stimulation program involved training individuals for three 30-minute periods per day, 7 days per week, with stimulation parameters described as square wave pulses at 33 Hz, a pulse width of 200 μsec, and a pulse amplitude of 100 mA. The stimulation cycle was described as 7 sec on, followed by a 10-sec rest interval. This group also demonstrated a decrease in flexor spasticity, a decrease in the contractures noted in persons with chronic hemiplegia, and a prevention of flexion contractures noted in "subacute" hemiplegic individuals.[11]

More recent applications of FES in the management of spasticity have documented benefit when FES is used in conjunction with botulinum toxin.[106, 107] One randomized, double-blind, placebo-controlled trial used FES three times, one-half hour each, for 3 days after injection, in a group of stroke survivors. Follow-up at 2, 6, and 12 weeks evaluated tone and arm function. The use of FES appeared to enhance the response to the botulinum toxin injections.[106]

In summary, these data clearly indicate that electrical stimulation results in a short-term decrease in spasticity that can persist for several hours after a treatment session. There also appears to be evidence to suggest that both short-term treatment in conjunction with botulinum toxin and long-term treatment decreases spasticity in hemiplegic individuals. However, the data are less clear regarding the impact of long-term stimulation on SCI survivors. More information is needed to determine whether the type and completeness of the lesion affect the observed responses from long-term functional electrical stimulation intervention.

Upper Limb in Hemiplegia

The most common application of electrical stimulation in the upper limb of hemiplegia is in the treatment and prevention of shoulder subluxation. Electrical stimulation is thought to be a superior option because it does not restrict the use of the limb as physical supports do. One study demonstrated that electrical stimulation could reduce existing subluxation. The study protocol involved stimulating the supraspinatus and posterior deltoid muscles (Fig. 22–11) with an asymmetrical biphasic waveform over a 6-week period.[10] The results indicated that electrical stimulation was superior to slings and wheelchair arm supports in reducing subluxation, but this apparently had no impact on reduction of shoulder pain. A subsequent controlled study evaluated the efficacy of electrical stimulation in a group of recent

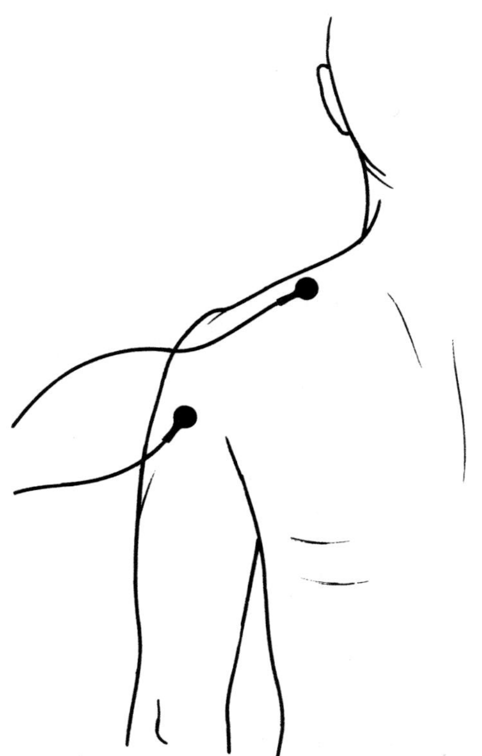

FIGURE 22–11. Use of electrical stimulation for treatment of shoulder subluxation involves placement of electrodes over the supraspinatus and posterior deltoid muscles.

hemiplegic stroke patients. The goal was to evaluate the efficacy of electrical stimulation in the prevention of glenohumeral joint stretching and subsequent subluxation, and to facilitate recovery of the flaccid shoulder. The protocol also involved placing the active electrode over the posterior deltoid and the passive electrode over the supraspinatus muscles. Stimulation frequency was set at 33 Hz and the intensity was adjusted to elicit the desired response. The duty cycle varied throughout the duration of the study. Patients were treated for 1.5 to 6 hours per day over a 6-week period. The results suggested that FES resulted in improvement in arm muscle tone and function, decreased shoulder subluxation, and a more rapid recovery of arm function.[69] This observation was supported by a meta-analysis of randomized controlled trials of FES in stroke. These pooled data supported FES as promoting recovery of muscle strength after stroke.[82]

It has also been demonstrated that electrical stimulation can improve functional use of a chronically hemiplegic upper limb (more than 6 months after cerebrovascular accident) by combining electrical stimulation techniques with voluntary effort. One particular study assigned subjects to four groups that received electromyographically (EMG) induced electrical stimulation of wrist extensors, low-intensity electrical stimulation of wrist extensors combined with voluntary contractions, proprioceptive neuromuscular facilitation exercises, or no treatment. The EMG-initiated electrical stimulation protocol (0.2-msec biphasic square wave, pulse at 30 to 90 Hz and a constant current of 20 to 60 μV) utilized low-level voluntary EMG activity in target muscles to trigger electrical stimulation of forearm wrist extensor muscles to produce a joint movement. The group with low-intensity electrical stimulation of wrist extensors with combined voluntary contractions received 30 minutes of stimulation to the wrist extensors with a 0.3-msec square wave pulse at 30 to 90 Hz. The stimulation intensity was adjusted to increase voluntary range of wrist extension. The subjects were told to perform voluntary wrist extension exercises during the stimulations. The results of this study are compelling in that the electrical stimulation appeared to improve the function of chronically hemiparetic upper limbs, with subjects who received the EMG-induced electrical stimulation of wrist extensors demonstrating the greatest improvement. In addition, these gains were retained for 9 months.[133]

Phrenic Nerve Stimulation

Modern phrenic nerve stimulation dates to 1948.[180] Since that time, the technique has proved to be a valuable adjunct in the care of the patient with chronic ventilatory insufficiency who has a normal phrenic nerve, diaphragm, and lungs. Specifically, this technique is useful in persons with high-level quadriplegia accompanied by respiratory paralysis and central hypoventilation syndromes.[180] It has been estimated that, nationally, 100 SCI survivors would annually meet the criteria for use of a phrenic nerve pacer.[180] The goal of this technique is to circumvent the need for mechanical ventilation. One series demonstrated that 40% of all quadriplegic patients who received the device were supported full-time by the phrenic nerve pacers.

Initial protocols involved pacing a single phrenic nerve with high-frequency stimulation (25 to 30 Hz) at a respiratory rate of 12 to 17 per minute. Problems with this approach included loss of efficiency secondary to paradoxical motion of the contralateral unpaced side and myopathic changes noted in animal diaphragms subjected to the same stimulation program.[83] In 1981, protocols evolved that utilized uninterrupted simultaneous pacing of both hemidiaphragms using low-frequency stimulation (7 to 8 Hz) and a respiratory rate of 5 to 9 per minute. This approach improved minute volumes and resulted in better air mixing.[83] In addition, it is speculated that the low-frequency stimulation converts the normal mixture of fast-twitch and slow-twitch fibers to a preponderance of fatigue-resistant type I fibers.[83] This speculation is supported in part by the fact that endurance and respiratory function improve slowly after initiation of phrenic nerve pacing.

Several battery-powered implanted systems exist, which differ in electrode systems and waveforms.[47] Benefits from phrenic pacing include decreased infections, the ability to speak and smell more normally, and reduced cost and time for ventilation care.[47]

THERAPEUTIC FUNCTIONAL ELECTRICAL STIMULATION AS AN ORTHOTIC DEVICE

Scoliosis

The importance of bracing in the prevention of scoliosis curve progression was documented in the 1970s and 1980s. During the same period, studies were initiated that examined the efficacy of FES in the management of scoliosis. The technique involved placement of electrodes along the convex portion of the curve above and below the apex. Stimulation parameters typically approximate a stimulation rate of 35 Hz, a pulse width of 200 μsec, and a pulse amplitude of 0 to 100 mA. In addition, the stimulation was modulated to deliver 5 sec of stimulation followed by 25 sec of rest. The advantage of this technique is that the electrical stimulation was performed only for 8 to 10 hours per night.[73]

Although the technique was typically well tolerated with few complications, the efficacy of the technique remains unclear. Some studies have documented that electrostimulation was equal in efficacy to a Milwaukee brace in the treatment of adolescents with mild curves (20 to 40 degrees).[73] However, other studies documented failure rates with electrostimulation that approximated the rates of progression noted in studies examining the natural history of this disorder.[61] Moreover, patients whose curves progressed with electrostimulation then underwent bracing, with a subsequent halting of the progression of the scoliosis.[60, 73]

Therefore, the data examining the efficacy of electrical stimulation in the management of idiopathic scoliosis are inconclusive. Although some data indicate that electrostimulation is as effective as a Milwaukee brace in halting the progression of the disease, other data imply that electrical stimulation does not alter the natural course of the disorder.[61, 73] A meta-analysis of the efficacy of nonoperative treatments for idiopathic scoliosis suggested that lateral electrical surface stimulation is equal in outcome to observation only.[229] Therefore, the role for electrical stimulation in the management of idiopathic scoliosis is at best limited to use in a patient who is unable to tolerate appropriate bracing.

Hemiplegic Gait

Electrical stimulation has been utilized as a neural orthosis since 1961.[150] Since that time, NMES has been an important adjunct in the rehabilitation of patients with hemiplegia. Primarily this has involved utilizing NMES to improve the gait pattern of hemiplegics by increasing the torque output of the ankle dorsiflexors and reciprocally decreasing spastic reflexes in the plantar flexors (Fig. 22–12).[56] Additionally, NMES can be applied to gluteal muscles and/or to the quadriceps muscles in an effort to enhance the stance phase of gait. Finally, NMES can be utilized to facilitate the swing phase of gait in hemiplegia with stimulation of the sole, dorsum of the foot, or lower posterior thigh in an effort to induce the flexion reflex.[56] The greatest role for NMES in hemiplegic gait appears to be early during the acute rehabilitation phase of recovery.

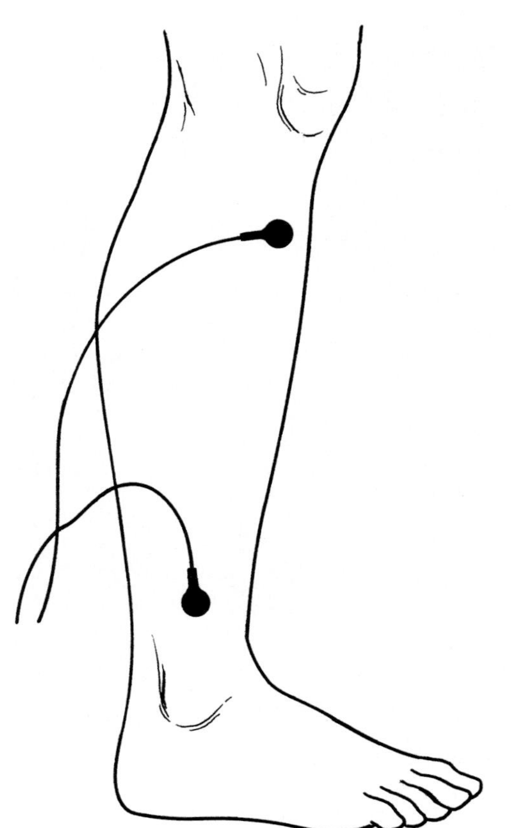

FIGURE 22–12. Ankle dorsiflexion is produced with placement of the active electrode proximally over the anterior tibialis and peroneal muscle groups and placement of the indifferent electrode distally over the tendons of the peroneal muscle.

More recent studies attempting to enhance hemiplegic gait patterns with FES have begun to address the inherent disadvantages of foot switches, which require wires or telemetry, the use of shoes that are insensitive, and are cosmetically unappearing. Tilt sensors have been successfully applied in NMES as a neural orthosis to control FES stimulation to the peroneal nerve through a device attached below the knee.[53]

FUNCTIONAL NEUROMUSCULAR STIMULATION: CLINICAL APPLICATIONS

Standing and Gait

Since the 1970s, FES for gait restoration after SCI has progressed from feasibility studies to the development of a commercially available, FDA-approved ambulation system.[135, 245] Despite the considerable progress, a number of barriers remain that continue to render this a cumbersome clinical application of technology. In addition to requiring a user-friendly system, the ideal FES gait system should be safe (in that it does not cause additional injury, such as degenerative joint changes), reliable, sufficiently functional to provide community ambulation, and both inexpensive and cosmetically acceptable. Many of these goals have not yet been realized.

The typical components of the FES system include a power source plus cables, a control mechanism, display and ground, stimulator with cables, and electrodes.[211] Additionally, FES systems require a feedback mechanism. In open-loop systems, the feedback is controlled by the patient or therapist in response to observations. More sophisticated, closed-loop systems automatically incorporate feedback into the FES system. This permits the FES system to adjust to changes in muscle spasticity and fatigue. In addition, closed-loop systems likely improve endurance by keeping the stimulation intensity to the minimum necessary to accomplish a given functional task. Finally, closed-loop systems require less concentration on the part of the ambulator. Types of FES feedback systems include input from (1) external sensors, (2) EMG of muscle, (3) sensory nerve, or (4) motor areas of the brain.[159] The most common and practical sensors are externally mounted devices that feed back information regarding limb position and movement.

The number of channels in FES ambulation systems varies according to the sophistication of the system. Two-channel systems typically stimulate the knee extensors, while four-channel systems typically activate knee extensors and hip flexors.[108, 245] FES ambulation systems employing more than eight channels often require implanted electrodes to provide more precise stimulation and to avoid the stimulation of adjacent muscles. Finally, the FES ambulation systems available today range from totally external devices (Fig. 22–13) to more experimental systems that are virtually completely implanted.

A survivor of a thoracic-level SCI presently has three options for pursuing the ability to walk. These include

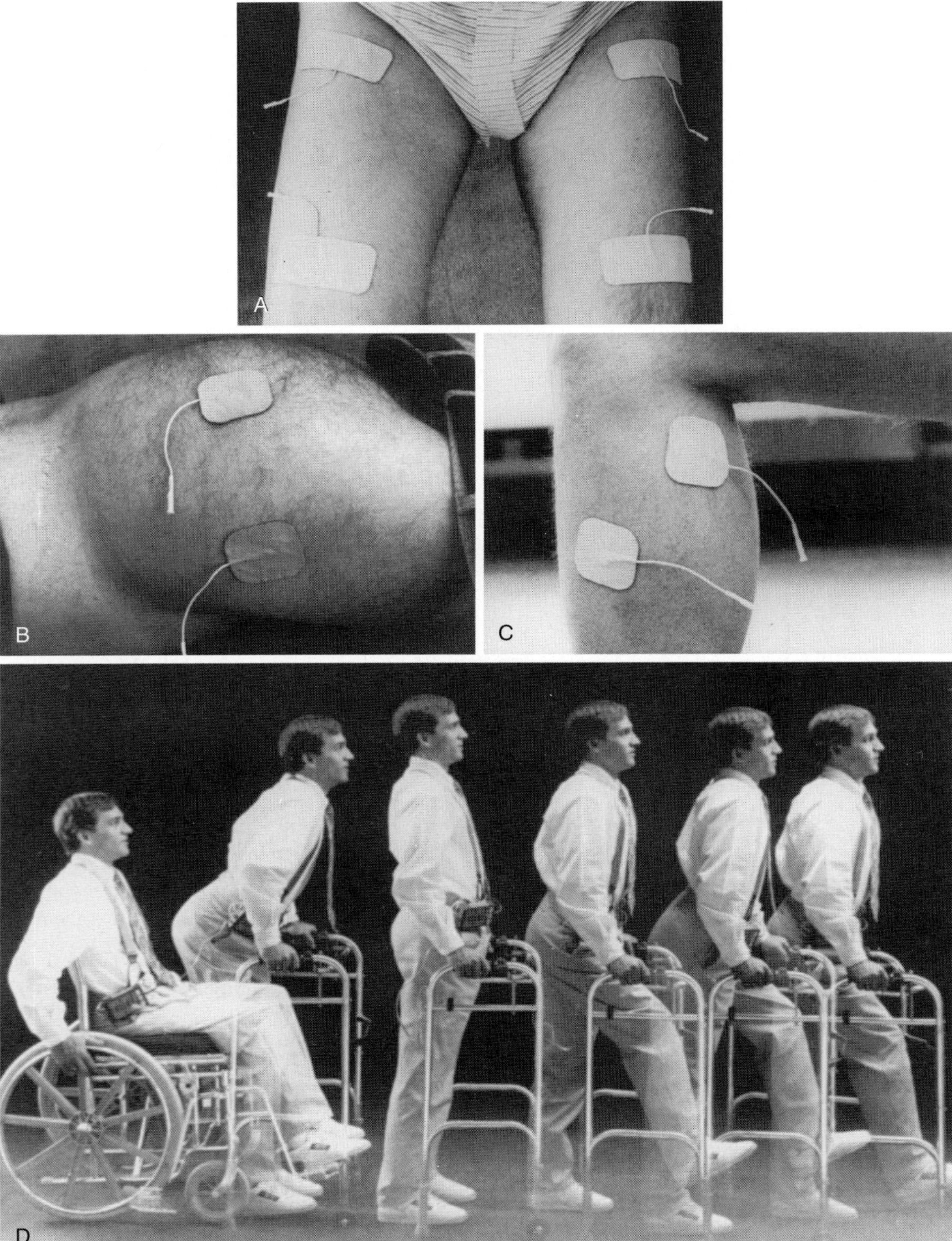

FIGURE 22–13. Parastep system developed by Sigmedics, Inc. These systems use surface electrodes. Both four- and six-channel systems exist that assist spinal cord injury individuals to stand and ambulate with use of a walker. Electrodes are placed over the quadriceps (*panel A*), peroneal nerve behind the fibula head and tibialis anterior (*panel C*), and gluteus medius and maximus (*panel B*; six-channel system only) to allow for standing and walking (*panel D*).

utilizing a mechanical orthosis (reciprocal gait orthosis, long-leg brace, etc.), an FES gait system, or a hybrid system that utilizes a mechanical orthosis with the assistance of FES. Ambulation with a mechanical orthosis alone is impractical, in part because the energy consumption is three to nine times that needed in normal controls.[44] However, FES gait systems also consume considerable energy, as it has been estimated that these patients utilize 59% to 75% of their maximum aerobic power.[158] It appears that the energy consumption of some FES systems rival, if not exceed, that required for walking with a mechanical orthosis.

FES ambulation systems are also somewhat impractical because they permit only a limited range of activity. The typical standing time for these systems ranges from minutes to hours.[135] The speed of ambulation is slow, typically in the range of 0.1 to 0.4 m/sec.[130] Finally, the walking distance with these devices is limited to approximately 20 meters although distances of more than 1000 meters have been reported.[135, 157]

The fatigue associated with FES ambulation is attributed to several factors. First, considerable energy is expended in stimulating the muscles necessary to maintain a standing position.[158] The rapid onset of FES-induced muscle fatigue is also in part caused by the preferential recruitment of rapidly fatiguing, type II muscle fibers.[154] In an effort to minimize this fatigue, several stimulation techniques have been developed. First, stimulation intensities are limited to the minimum necessary to achieve a desired functional response. Second, stimulation rates are kept within the physiological ranges of 15 to 50 Hz.[158] Specifically, lower stimulation rates are desirable, presumably because of the greater likelihood of stimulating slow-twitch fatigue-resistant muscle fibers.[36] The third approach to diminishing muscle fatigue involves an electrode distribution that permits the stimulation of portions of muscles or muscle groups. In this electrode distribution muscle fatigue is diminished by sequentially activating portions of an individual muscle or muscle group, thereby producing the minimum necessary force to accomplish a functional task.[109, 195]

Because the technology does not yet exist for FES to produce truly functional community ambulation, most FES systems are hybrid systems that concomitantly utilize FES with a mechanical orthosis. This combination of devices offers several advantages. First, the mechanical orthosis permits standing without considerable energy expenditure.[135] Hybrid systems also appear to use less energy than either mechanical orthoses or FES ambulation systems. One study specifically compared the energy consumption during ambulation with a reciprocating gait orthosis (RGO), RGO and FES, FES alone, long-leg braces, and a hip-guided orthosis. The order of energy expenditure (from lowest to highest) was (1) RGO with FES to the thigh muscles, (2) hip-guided orthosis, (3) long-leg brace, and (4) FES systems. The addition of FES to the RGO decreased energy consumption by approximately 16% in one study but increased energy consumption in another study.[108, 254] Finally, hybrid systems increase the speed of ambulation.[170, 177] The addition of FES to an RGO increases the optimum speed of ambulation from 1.2 km/hr with the RGO to 2.4 km/hr with the hybrid system.[177] However, studies have also shown that RGO use at home is low and that the addition of electrical stimulation does not increase RGO use.[255]

Advances in FES gait systems have extended to the commercial availability of an FDA-approved ambulation system.[245] However, the technology is still not capable of resolving or compensating for issues such as FES-induced muscle fatigue, excessive energy expenditure associated with FES ambulation, reduced FES-induced joint torques, autonomic hyperreflexia, osteoporosis, modified reflex activity, and spasticity.[157] Because FES ambulation systems to date are unable to meet many of the criteria for a truly functional system, the patients who might benefit from existing FES ambulation systems are relatively few. One study estimated that approximately 10% of patients admitted to an SCI service are candidates for an FES gait restoration program. Only half of those, or 5% of survivors in the cohort, eventually learned to walk, but fewer than 3% of those patients ultimately utilized the FES ambulation system functionally within their home.

The therapeutic benefit of FES in gait might extend beyond simply functioning as an orthotic device. The combination of FES with locomotion training in motor-incomplete SCI subjects has been shown to increase walking speed. This gain in speed is retained when the FES is temporarily not utilized. This observed therapeutic benefit suggests a potential role for FES in facilitating neural plasticity.[13]

Restoration of Upper Limb Function

The traditional option for survivors of a high cervical SCI with loss of hand function has included functional restoration via orthotic devices or surgical procedures, such as arthrodesis and tendon transfers. The goal of FES in this population is to provide palmar and lateral prehension grasp and to develop a means to easily change from one type of grasp to the other.[192]

To accomplish this goal, intramuscular or epimysial electrodes have been utilized to stimulate the flexor digitorum superficialis and profundus, flexor pollicis longus, abductor pollicis, flexor pollicis brevis, abductor pollicis brevis, extensor digitorum, and extensor pollicis longus.[192] The stimulation parameters typically involve amplitudes of approximately 20 mA and pulse widths of approximately 200 μsec. Variations in stimulation frequency between 15 and 50 Hz permit smooth transitions in force of muscle contraction.[192]

Implanted FES hand systems to provide grasp and release for individuals with tetraplegia can be controlled through three systems. These include shoulder position, wrist position, and myoelectric activity from wrist extensors. Each system offers advantages based on function, cosmesis, neurological status, and preference that warrant consideration prior to commitment.[97]

Functional ADL skills achieved through this technology have included handling eating utensils, cups, writing instruments, books, and the telephone. More complex tasks, such as pouring, washing, brushing teeth, and handling computer diskettes have also been demonstrated.[192] Operative procedures such as arthrodesis, tenodesis, and tendon transfers are also available to minimize joint movement and to improve upper limb stability for FES utilization.[192]

A prerequisite for increasing hand functioning in the future is the development of a sensory feedback system for joint position, contact, force, slippage, pressure, and temperature.[120] To date, a single-element subcutaneous electrode in the C5 dermatome has been utilized.[120] A more intriguing feedback mechanism that has been explored involved an implanted cuff electrode that permits recording from peripheral sensory nerves.[225]

The results from the upper limb neuroprostheses have been favorable. A recent survey of 34 individuals with a hand neuroprosthesis were surveyed, with high satisfaction and improved function noted in over 80% of patients.[278] However, the applicability is limited to patients who have primarily C6-spared SCIs. In addition, problems with peripheral nerve injuries involving the upper limb further limit the utility of this technique.

ELECTRICAL STIMULATION FOR THE TREATMENT OF SOFT AND HARD TISSUE INJURY

Wound Healing

A body of scientific evidence has been accumulating to suggest that electrical stimulation can be used to promote the healing of wounds. Investigators have previously demonstrated that the surface of human skin is electronegative with respect to the inner layers. Wounded skin demonstrates the existence of a natural bioelectric current, with the ionic body fluids allowing for transmission of electricity between outer and inner layers. When electrical stimulation is applied to a wound, a number of biological processes in the wound are modified that might lead to enhanced healing. Electrical stimulation increases the number and function of fibroblasts,[50, 77] collagen, protein, and DNA synthesis,[14] and causes changes in expression of cellular receptors for transforming growth factor beta,[71] enhancing calcium uptake and neurite growth. The fibroblasts and epithelial cells move along the path of the voltage gradient (the galvanotaxic effect)[46, 274] toward the cathode. Electrical stimulation has also been shown to increase the relative number of neutrophilic granulocytes while suppressing the number of mast cells.[269] This suppression of mast cells has been postulated to result in improved wound healing with a decrease in fibrotic scarring and, thus, better cosmetic results. It appears that electrical stimulation can augment the endogenous chemical factors that initiate the inflammatory stage of healing. Evidence also indicates that electrical stimulation has bacteriostatic and bactericidal properties.[119] The duration of exposure and voltage shows a linear relationship with inhibition of growth of several common wound pathogens when negative polarity is used.[129]

Electrical stimulation can also improve blood flow.[119] The improved vascularity has been associated with decreased lipid peroxidation and prevention of damage to oxygen-derived free radicals. High-voltage pulsed current, however, has also been shown to have a bimodal effect on foot blood flow in humans at risk for diabetic ulcers. One study found that 27% of subjects increased transcutaneous oxygen, whereas 73% of subjects showed a decrease in transcutaneous oxygen. The mechanism for this bimodal response is not understood.[80]

Several studies published since the mid-1960s[263] have demonstrated the effectiveness of electrical stimulation to promote the healing of dermal ulcers (Table 22–4). The initial studies were nonrandomized, prospective trials undertaken to determine the safety and efficacy of electrical stimulation in the treatment of chronic dermal ulcers. The use of electrical stimulation to treat pressure ulcers or ischemic ulcers in a variety of patient populations showed a significant increase in ulcer healing. When patients entered into a study were found to have more than one ulcer, several trials utilized those patients to randomize one ulcer to treatment with electrical stimulation and the other to a nonelectrical stimulation control group. In these substudies, significant improvements were noted in the rate of ulcer size reduction and number of healed ulcers in the ulcers receiving electrical stimulation in comparison to control ulcers. Recognizing the need for randomized trials, several studies have subsequently been published comparing electrical stimulation to sham-treated ulcers. In general, these studies have shown increased rates and percentages of healing with electrical stimulation in comparison to control populations (see Table 22–4), with no significant complications. Recent studies have focused on the use of pulsed galvanic electrical stimulation, with demonstration of similar benefits.[78] In summary, the data suggest that electrical stimulation can augment wound healing, and the efficacy appears to be generalizable to ischemic ulcers and pressure ulcers as well as to other types of deep wounds.

The more effective stimulation pattern is pulsed electrical stimulation, because it allows for higher current density without tissue irritation or burning. Asymmetrical biphasic waveforms have been shown to be more effective in healing diabetic ulcers than symmetrical biphasic or square wave pulses.[9] Recent studies have used alternating polarities, beginning with a negative polarity; the alternating-polarity protocol is thought to have antibacterial effects and is associated with increased vascular support. When no further improvements in wound healing are noted (*plateauing*), polarity is changed. The absolute charge density needed to cause successful wound healing is on the order of 0.1 to 2.0 coulombs/cm^2,[220] and the duration of treatment sessions can vary from 1 to 24 hours per day.

SUMMARY

Electrical stimulation is a historical physiatric modality, but an explosion of new interest in this subject has occurred since the mid-1970s. In addition to rehabilitation medicine, a renewed interest in electrical stimulation has been demonstrated in various fields such as physiology, molecular biology, engineering, neurosur-

TABLE 22–4 Effect of Electrical Stimulation on Wound Healing

NONRANDOMIZED TRIALS

	Unilateral Ulcer		Bilateral Ulcers (% Healed)	
Type of Ulcer	*No. Participating*	*% Healing*	*Electrical Stimulation*	*Control*
Chronic[257]	75	13.4	27	5
Ischemic	150	20.0	28.3	8.3
Ischemic[75]	106	28.4	30	14.7
Elderly[244]	223	89.7	—	—

RANDOMIZED TRIALS

		Electrical Stimulation			Control		
Type	**No.**	*% Δ Ulcer Size*	*% Healed*	*Time to Heal (Days)*	*% Δ Ulcer Size*	*% Healed*	*Time to Heal (Days)*
Pressure	8	—	100	50.1	+13.8	—	74
Pressure[126]	16	−38*	100	50	+28.9	—	52
Mixed[245]	17	—	88.9	51.2	—	37.5	77
Pressure[85]	17	−80			−52		
Diabetic[150]	64	−61	42	84	−41	15	84

* Improvement in ulcer size after cross-over of ulcers from sham treatment to electrical stimulation.

gery, neurology, orthopedics, urology, and plastic surgery. The result has been a significant improvement in the technology available for functional applications. A far greater understanding has also developed of the physiological basis for the improvements noted with therapeutic applications of electrical stimulation.

Electrical stimulation appears to have growing importance as a modality in rehabilitation medicine. This is apparent in the increasing number of FDA-approved FES systems available to treat paralysis-related conditions.[184] Continued research is, however, needed to ensure that this technology is maximally utilized. Toward this end, continued advancements in technology, a better understanding of optimal stimulation parameters, and a better understanding of the physiological changes induced by this technology are required.

REFERENCES

1. Agnew WF, McCreery BB, Yuen TGH, et al: Histologic and physiologic evaluation of electrically stimulated peripheral nerve: Considerations for the selection of parameters. Ann Biomed Eng 1993; 17:39–60.
2. al-Amood WS, Buller AJ, Pope R: Long-term stimulation of cat fast-twitch skeletal muscle. Nature 1973; 244:225–227.
3. al-Amood WS, Lewis DN, Schmalbruch H: Effects of chronic electrical stimulation on contractile properties of long-term denervated rat skeletal muscle. J Physiol 1991; 441:243–256.
4. Alexander CJ, Sipski ML: Electrical stimulation bicycle ergometry with spinal cord injured patients: Potential medical and physiological benefits. SCI Psychosoc Proc 1990; 3:18–20.
5. Almay BG, Johansson F, von Knorring L, et al: Long-term high frequency transcutaneous electrical nerve stimulation (hi-TENS) in chronic pain: Clinical response and effects on CSF-endorphins, monoamine metabolites, substance P-like immunoreactivity (SPLI) and pain measures. J Psychosom Res 1985; 29:247–257.
6. Alon G, McCombe SA, Koutsantonis S, et al: Comparison of the effects of electrical stimulation and exercise on abdominal musculature. J Orthop Sports Phys Ther 1987; 8:567–573.
7. Andreose JS, Xu R, Lomo T, et al: Degradation of two AchR populations at rat neuromuscular junctions: Regulation in vivo by electrical stimulation. J Neurosci 1993; 13(8):3433–3438.
8. Baker LL, Bowman BR, McNeal DR: Effects of waveform on comfort during neuromuscular electrical stimulation. Clin Orthop Rel Res 1988; 233:75–85.
9. Baker LL, Chambers R, DeMuth SK, et al: Effect of electrical stimulation on wound healing in patients with diabetic ulcers. Diabetes Care 1997; 20:405–412.
10. Baker LL, Parker K: Neuromuscular electrical stimulation of the muscles surrounding the shoulder. Phys Ther 1986; 66:1930–1937.
11. Baker LL, Yeh C, Wilson D, et al: Electrical stimulation of wrist and fingers for hemiplegic patients. Phys Ther 1979; 59:1495–1499.
12. Baker RC, Heinemann AW, Yarkony GM, et al: Functional neuromuscular stimulation for standing and ambulation: Six month evaluation of psychological effects. In Proceedings of the RESNA 12th Annual Conference. New Orleans, 1989, pp 401–402.
13. Barbeau H, Ladoucer M, Norman KE, et al: Walking after spinal cord injury: Evaluation, treatment and function. Arch Phys Med Rehabil 1999; 80:225–235.
14. Bassett CA, Hermann I: The effect of electrostatic fields on macro-molecular synthesis by fibroblast in vitro. J Cell Biol 1968; 39:9A.
15. Biering-Sorensen F, Bohr H, Schaadt O: Bone mineral content of the lumbar spine and lower extremities years after spinal cord lesion. Paraplegia 1988; 26:293–301.
16. Binder-MacLeod SA, Guerin T: Preservation of force output through progressive reduction of stimulation frequency in human quadriceps femoris muscle. Phys Ther 1990; 70(10):619–625.
17. Bloomfield SA, Mysiw WJ, Jackson RD: Bone mass and endocrine adaptations to training in spinal cord injured individuals. Bone 1996; 19:61–68.
18. Boonstra AM, van Weerden TW, Eisma WH, et al: The effect of low-frequency electrical stimulation on denervation atrophy in man. Scand J Rehabil Med 1987; 19:127–134.
19. Bouletreau P, Patricot MC, Saudin F, et al: Effects of intermittent electrical stimulation on muscle metabolism in intensive care patients. J Parenter Enteral Nutr 1987; 11:552–555.
20. Bowman BR, Baker LL: Effects of waveform parameters on comfort during transcutaneous neuromuscular electrical stimulation. Ann Biomed Eng 1985; 13:59–74.
21. Bradley MB: The effect of participating in a functional electrical stimulation exercise program on affect in people with spinal cord injuries. Arch Phys Med Rehabil 1994; 75:676–679.
22. Brenes G, Dearwater S, Shapera R, et al: High density lipoprotein cholesterol concentration in physically active and sedentary spinal cord injured patients. Arch Phys Med Rehabil 1986; 67:445–450.

23. Brown MC, Holland RL: A central role for denervated tissues in causing nerve sprouting. Nature 1979; 282:724–726.
24. Brown MD, Cotter MA, Hudlicka O, et al: The effects of different patterns of muscle activity on capillary density, mechanical properties and structure of slow and fast rabbit muscles. Pflugers Arch 1976; 361:241–250.
25. Brown WE, Salmons S, Whalen RG: The sequential replacement of myosin subunit isoforms during muscle type transformation induced by long-term electrical stimulation. J Biol Chem 1983; 258:14686–14692.
26. Brownson C, Isenberg H, Brown W, et al: Changes in skeletal muscle gene transcription induced by chronic stimulation. Muscle Nerve 1988; 11:1183–1189.
27. Brubaker L, Kotarinos R: Kegel or cut? Variations on his theme (review). J Reprod Med 1993; 38:672–678.
28. Buchegger A, Nemeth PM, Pette D, et al: Effects of chronic stimulation on the metabolic heterogeneity of the fibre population in rabbit tibialis anterior muscle. J Physiol 1984; 350:109–119.
29. Burke RE, Levine DN, Tsairis P, et al: Physiological types and histochemical profiles of motor units of the cat gastrocnemius. J Physiol 1973; 234:723–748.
30. Bushnell MC, Marchand F, Tremblay N, et al: Electrical stimulation of peripheral and central pathways for the relief of musculoskeletal pain. Can J Physiol Pharmacol 1991; 69:697–703.
31. Cabric M, Appell HJ: Effect of electrical stimulation of high and low frequency on maximum isometric force and some morphological characteristics in man. Int J Sports Med 1987; 8:256–260.
32. Cabric M, Appell HJ, Resic A: Effects of electrical stimulation of different frequencies on the myonuclei and fiber size in human muscle. Int J Sports Med 1987; 8:323–326.
33. Cabric M, Appell HJ, Resic A: Fine structural changes in electrostimulated human skeletal muscle: Evidence for predominant effects on fast muscle fibers. Eur J Appl Physiol 1988; 57:1–5.
34. Cabric M, Appell HJ, Resic A: Stereological analysis of capillaries in electrostimulated human muscles. Int J Sports Med 1987; 8:327–330.
35. Caggiano E, Emrey T, Shirley S, et al: Effects of electrical stimulation or voluntary contraction for strengthening quadriceps femoris muscles in an aged male population. J Orthop Sports Phys Ther 1994; 20:22–28.
36. Campbell J: Efficacy of volitional versus electrically evoked knee extension exercise. In Proceedings of the RESNA 10th Annual Conference. San Jose, CA, June 19–23, 1987, pp 648–650.
37. Caputo RM, Benson JT, McClellan E: Intravaginal maximal electrical stimulation in the treatment of urinary incontinence. J Reprod Med 1993; 38:667–671.
38. Castro MJ, Apple DF, Staron RS, et al: Influence of complete spinal cord injury on skeletal muscle within 6 months of injury. J Appl Physiol 1999; 86:350–358.
39. Chae J, Hart R: Comparison of discomfort associated with surface and percutaneous intramuscular electrical stimulation for persons with chronic hemiplegia. Am J Phys Med Rehabil 1998; 77:516–522.
40. Chancellor MB, Heesakkers JP, Janknegt RA: Gracilis muscle transposition with electrical stimulation for sphincteric incontinence: A new approach. World J Urol 1997; 15:320–328.
41. Cheng RSF, Pomeranz B: Electroacupuncture analgesia could be mediated by at least two pain relieving mechanisms: Endorphin and non-endorphin systems. Life Sci 1979; 25:1957–1962.
42. Clausen JP: Circulatory adjustments to dynamic exercise and effect of physical training in normal subjects and in patients with coronary artery disease. Prog Cardiovasc Dis 1976; 18:459–495.
43. Clement-Jones V, McLoughlin L, Tomlin S, et al: Increased beta-endorphin but not met-enkephalin levels in human cerebrospinal fluid after acupuncture for recurrent pain. Lancet 1980; 2:946–948.
44. Clinkingbeard JR, Gersten JW, Hoehn D: Energy cost of ambulation in traumatic paraplegia. Am J Phys Med Rehabil 1964; 43:157–165.
45. Cole BG, Gardiner PF: Does electrical stimulation of denervated muscle, continued after reinnervation, influence recovery of contractile function? Exp Neurol 1984; 85:52–62.
46. Cooper MS, Schliwa M: Electrical and ionic controls of tissue cell locomotion in DC electric fields. J Neurosci Res 1985; 13:223–244.
47. Creasey G, Elefteriades J, DiMarco A, et al: Electrical stimulation to restore respiration. J Rehabil Res Dev 1996; 33:123–132.
48. Cresey GH: Electrical stimulation of sacral roots for micturition after spinal cord injury. Urol Clin North Am 1993; 20:505–515.
49. Crowell LL, Squires WG, Raven PB: Benefits of aerobic exercise for paraplegics: A brief review. Med Sci Sports Exerc 1982; 18:501–508.
50. Cruz NI, Bayron FE, Suarez AJ: Accelerated healing of full thickness burns by the use of high-voltage pulsed galvanic stimulation in the pig. Ann Plast Surg 1989; 23:49–55.
51. Currier DP, Lehman J, Lightfoot P: Electrical stimulation in exercise of the quadriceps femoris muscle. Phys Ther 1979; 59: 1508–1512.
52. Currier DP, Mann R: Muscular strength development by electrical stimulation in normal individuals. Phys Ther 1983; 63: 915–921.
53. Dai R, Stein RB, Andrews BJ, et al: Application of tilt sensors in functional electrical stimulation. IEEE Trans Rehabil Eng 1996; 4:63–71.
54. Dangain J, Vrbova G: Effect of chronic electrical stimulation at low frequency on the passive membrane properties of muscle fiber from dystrophic mice. Exp Neurol 1983; 79:630–640.
55. Delitto A, Rose SJ, McKowen JM, et al: Electrical stimulation versus voluntary exercise in strengthening thigh musculature after anterior cruciate ligament surgery. Phys Ther 1988; 68: 660–663.
56. DeVahl J: NMES and rehabilitation. In Gersh M (ed): Electrotherapy in Rehabilitation. Philadelphia, FA Davis, 1992, pp 244–245.
57. Ding J, Binder-Macleod SA, Wexler AS: Two-step, predictive, isometric force model tested on data from human and rat muscles. J Appl Physiol 1998; 85:2176–2189.
58. Dorgan JJ, O'Malley MJ: A nonlinear mathematical model of electrically stimulated skeletal muscle. IEEE Trans Rehabil Eng 1997; 5:179–194.
59. Duchateau J, Hainaut K: Training effects of sub-maximal electrostimulation in a human muscle. Med Sci Sports Exerc 1988; 20:99–104.
60. Durham JW, Moskowitz A, Whitney J: Surface electrical stimulation versus brace in treatment of idiopathic scoliosis. Spine 1990; 15:888–892.
61. Eberstein A, Eberstein S: Electrical stimulation of denervated muscle: Is it worth it? Med Sci Sports Exerc 1996; 28:1463–1469.
62. Edstrom L, Grimby L: Effect of exercise on the motor unit. Muscle Nerve 1986; 9:104–126.
63. Edwards BG, Marsolais EB: Metabolic responses to arm ergometry and functional neuromuscular stimulation. J Rehabil Res Dev 1990; 27:107–113.
64. Egginton S, Hudlicka O: Early changes in performance, blood flow and capillary fine structure in rat fast muscles induced by electrical stimulation. J Physiol 1999; 515(Pt):265–275.
65. Eisenberg BR, Salmons S: The reorganization of subcellular structure in muscle undergoing fast-to-slow type transformation: A stereological study. Cell Tissue Res 1981; 220:449–471.
66. Ellenberg M, MacRitchie M, Franklin B, et al: Aerobic capacity in early paraplegia: Implications for rehabilitation. Paraplegia 1989; 27:261–268.
67. Emes CG: Fitness and the physically disabled. A review. Can J Appl Sport Sci 1981; 6:176–178.
68. Etgen GJ Jr, Farrar RP, Ivy JL: Effect of chronic electrical stimulation on GLUT-4 protein content in fast-twitch muscle. Am J Physiol 1993; 264:r816–819.
69. Faghri PD, Rodgers MN, Glaser RM, et al: The effects of functional electrical stimulation on shoulder subluxation, arm function recovery, and shoulder pain in hemiplegic stroke patients. Arch Phys Med Rehabil 1994; 75:73–79.
70. Fakhri O, Amin M: The effect of low-voltage electric therapy on the healing of resistant skin burns. J Burn Care Rehabil 1987; 8:15–18.
71. Falanga V, Bourguignon GJ, Bourguignon LY: Electrical stimulation increases the expression of fibroblast receptors for transforming growth factor-beta. J Invest Dermatol 1987; 88:488.
72. Fall M, Lindstrom S: Electrical stimulation: A physiologic approach to the treatment of urinary incontinence. Urol Clin North Am 1991; 18:393–407.

73. Fisher DA, Rapp GF, Emkes M: Idiopathic scoliosis: Transcutaneous muscle stimulation versus the Milwaukee brace. Spine 1987; 12:987–991.
74. Funakoshi H, Bellvardo N, Arenas E, et al: Muscle-derived neurotrophin-4 as an activity-dependent trophic signed for adult motor neurons. Science 1995; 268:1495–1499.
75. Gault WR, Gatens PF: Use of low intensity direct current in management of ischemic skin ulcers. Phys Ther 1976; 56:265–269.
76. Gentzkow GD: Electrical stimulation to heal dermal wounds. J Dermatol Surg Oncol 1993; 19:753–758.
77. Gentzkow GD, Miller KH: Electrical stimulation for dermal wound healing. Clin Podiatr Med Surg 1991; 8:827–841.
78. Gentzkow GD, Pollick SV, Kloth LC, et al: Improved healing of pressure ulcers using dermapulse, a new electrical stimulation device. Wound 1991; 3:158–170.
79. Gibson JN, Smith K, Rennie MJ: Prevention of disuse muscle atrophy by means of electrical stimulation: Maintenance of protein synthesis. Lancet 1988; 2(8614):767–769.
80. Gilcreast DM, Stotts NA, Froelicher ES, et al: Effect of electrical stimulation on foot skin perfusion in persons with or at risk for diabetic foot ulcers. Wound Repair Regen 1998; 6:434–441.
81. Girlanda PR, Dattola R, Vita G, et al: Effect of electrotherapy on denervated muscles in rabbits: An electrophysiological and morphological study. Exp Neurol 1982; 77:483–491.
82. Glanz M, Klawansky S, Stason W, et al: Functional electrical stimulation in poststroke rehabilitation: A meta-analysis of the randomized controlled trials. Arch Phys Med Rehabil 1996; 77:549–553.
83. Glenn WW, Hogan JF, Loke JS, et al: Ventilatory support by pacing of the conditioned diaphragm in quadriplegia. N Engl J Med 1984; 310:1150–1155.
84. Goldspink G, Scutt A, Loughna PT, et al: Gene expression in skeletal muscle in response stretch and force generation. Am J Physiol 1992; 262:r356–363.
85. Gordon T, Mao J: Muscle atrophy and procedures for training after spinal cord injury. Phys Ther 1994; 74:50–60.
86. Greve JMD, Muszkat PT, Schmidt B, et al: Functional electrical stimulation (FES): Muscle histochemical analysis. Paraplegia 1993; 31:764–770.
87. Griffin JW, Tooms RE, Mendius RA, et al: Efficacy of high voltage pulsed current for healing of pressure ulcers in patients with spinal cord injury. Phys Ther 1991; 71:433–442.
88. Grill WM, Mortimer JT: Stability of the input-output properties of chronically implanted multiple contact nerve cuff electrodes. IEEE Trans Rehabil Eng 1998; 6:364–373.
89. Grimby G, Nordwell A, Hulten B, et al: Changes in histochemical profile of muscle after long-term electrical stimulation in patients with idiopathic scoliosis. Scand J Rehab Med 1985; 17:191–196.
90. Grimby G, Wigerstad-Lossing I: Comparison of high- and low-frequency muscle stimulators. Arch Phys Med Rehabil 1989; 70:835–838.
91. Gurney AB, Robergs RA, Aisenbray J, et al: Detraining from total body exercise ergometry in individuals with spinal cord injury. Spinal Cord 1998; 36:782–789.
92. Gutmann E, Gutmann L: Effects of electrotherapy on denervated and reinnervated muscles in rabbit. Lancet 1942; 1:169–170.
93. Halbach JW, Straus D: Comparison of electro-myostimulation to isokinetic power of the knee extensor mechanism. J Orthop Sports Phys Ther 1980; 2:20–24.
94. Han JS, Chen XY, Sun SL, et al: The effect of low- and high-frequency TENS on metenkephalin-Arg-Phe and dynorphin A immunoreactivity in human lumbar CSF. Pain 1991; 47:295–298.
95. Hangartner TN, Rodgers MM, Glaser RM, et al: Tibial bone density loss in spinal cord injured patients: Effects of FES exercise. J Rehabil Res Dev 1994; 31:50–61.
96. Hansen-Smith F, Egginton S, Hudlicka O: Growth of arterioles in chronically stimulated rat muscle. Microcirculation 1998; 5:49–59.
97. Hart RL, Kilgore KL, Peckham PH. A comparison between control methods for implanted FES hand-grasp systems. IEEE Trans Rehabil Eng 1998; 6:208–218.
98. Harvey JR, Bradley MB: Staff perceptions of the psychological benefits of FES training: A grounded therapy approach. SCI Psychosoc Proc 1992; 5:8.
99. Haug J, Wood LT: Efficacy of neuromuscular stimulation of the quadriceps femoris during continuous passive motion following total knee arthroplasty. Arch Phys Med Rehabil 1988; 69(6):423–424.
100. Heilig A, Pette D: Changes induced in the enzyme activity pattern by electrical stimulation of fast twitch muscle. In Pette D (ed): Plasticity of Muscle. Berlin, Walter de Gruyter, 1980, pp 409–420.
101. Heilmann C, Pette D: Molecular transformation in sarcoplasmic reticulum of fast-twitch muscle by electro-stimulation. Eur J Biochem 1979; 93:437–446.
102. Heilmann C, Muller W, Pette D: Correlation between ultrastructural and functional changes in sarcoplasmic reticulum during chronic stimulation of fast muscle. J Membr Biol 1981; 59: 143–149.
103. Henneman E, Somjen G, Carpenter DO: Excitability and inhibitability of motoneurons of different sizes. J Neurophysiol 1965; 28:599–620.
104. Henneman E, Somjen G, Carpenter DO: Functional significance of cell size in spinal motoneurons. J Neurophysiol 1965; 28:560–580.
105. Herbison GJ, Jaweed MM, Ditunno JF Jr: Exercise therapies in peripheral neuropathies. Arch Phys Med Rehabil 1983; 64: 201–205.
106. Hesse S, Mauritz KH: Management of spasticity. Curr Opin Neurol 1997; 10:498–501.
107. Hesse S, Reiter F, Konrad M, et al: Botulinum toxin type A and short-term electrical stimulation in the treatment of upper limb flexor spasticity after stroke: A randomized, double-blind, placebo-controlled trial. Clin Rehabil 1998; 12:381–388.
108. Hirokawa S, Grimm M, Le T, et al: Energy consumptions in paraplegic ambulation using the reciprocating gait orthosis and electric stimulation of the thigh muscles. Arch Phys Med Rehabil 1990; 71:687–694.
109. Hjeltnes N, Lannem A: Functional neuromuscular stimulation in four patients with complete paraplegia. Paraplegia 1990; 28:235–243.
110. Hjeltnes N, Vokac Z: Circulatory strain in everyday life of paraplegics. Scand J Rehabil Med 1979; 11:67–73.
111. Hoffman MD: Cardiorespiratory fitness and training in quadriplegics and paraplegics. Sports Med 1986; 3:312–330.
112. Hooker SP, Figoni SF, Glaser RM, et al: Physiologic responses to prolonged electrically stimulated leg-cycle exercise in the spinal cord injured. Arch Phys Med Rehabil 1990; 71:863–869.
113. Howson DC: Peripheral neural excitability: Implications for transcutaneous electrical nerve stimulation. Phys Ther 1978; 58:1467–1473.
114. Hudecki MS, Caffiero AT, Gregorio CC, et al: Effects of percutaneous electrical stimulation on functional ability, plasma creatine kinase, and pectoralis musculature of normal and genetically dystrophic chickens. Exp Neurol 1985; 90:53–72.
115. Hudlicka O, Aitman T, Heilig A, et al: Effects of different patterns of long-term stimulation on blood flow, fuel uptake and enzyme activities in rabbit fast skeletal muscles. Pflugers Arch 1984; 402:306–311.
116. Hudlicka O, Brown M, Cotter M, et al: The effect of long-term stimulation of fast-muscles on their blood flow, metabolism and ability to withstand fatigue. Pflugers Arch 1977; 369:141–149.
117. Hudlicka O, Dodd L, Renkin EM, et al: Early changes in fibre profile and capillary density in long-term stimulated muscles. Am J Physiol 1982; 243:h528–535.
118. Hudlicka O, Tyler KR, Srihari T, et al: The effect of different patterns of long-term stimulation on contractile properties and myosin light chains in rabbit fast muscles. Pflugers Arch 1982; 393:164–170.
119. Im MJ, Lee WP, Hoopes JE: Effect of electrical stimulation on survival of skin flaps in pigs. Phys Ther 1990; 70:37–40.
120. Ishigooka M, Hashimoto T, Hayami S, et al: Electrical pelvic floor stimulation: A possible alternative treatment for reflex urinary incontinence in patients with spinal cord injury. Spinal Cord 1996; 34:411–415.
121. Johnson EW, Braddom R: Over-work weakness in fascioscapulohumeral muscular dystrophy. Arch Phys Med Rehabil 1971; 52:333–336.

122. Johnson MI, Ashton CH, Thompson JW: The consistency of pulsed frequencies and pulse patterns of transcutaneous nerve stimulation (TENS) used by chronic pain patients. Pain 1991; 44:231–234.
123. Jonasson I, Larsson B, Pschera H, et al: Short-term maximal electrical stimulation: A conservative treatment of urinary incontinence. Gynecol Obstet Invest 1990; 30:120–123.
124. Jones DA, Bigland-Ritchie B, Edwards RH: Excitation frequency and muscle fatigue: Mechanical responses during voluntary and stimulated contractions. Exp Neurol 1979; 64(2): 401–413.
125. Kahanovitz N, Nordin M, Verderame R, et al: Normal trunk muscle strength and endurance in women and the effect of exercises and electrical stimulation: 2. Comparative analysis of electrical stimulation and exercises to increase trunk muscle strength and endurance. Spine 1987; 12:112–118.
126. Kantrowitz A: Electronic Physiologic Aids. Brooklyn, NY, Maimonides Hospital, 1960, pp 4–5.
127. Katz RT, Green D, Sullivan T, et al: Functional electrical stimulation to enhance systemic fibrinolytic activity in spinal cord injury patients. Arch Phys Med Rehabil 1987; 68:423–426.
128. Keith MW, Peckham CH, Thrope GB, et al: Functional neuromuscular stimulation neuroprostheses for the tetraplegic hand. Clin Orthop Rel Res 1988; 233:25–33.
129. Kincaid CB, Lavoie KH: Inhibition of bacterial growth in vitro following stimulation with high voltage, monophasic, pulsed current. Phys Ther 1989; 69:651–655.
130. Kloth LC, Feedar JA: Acceleration of wound healing with high voltage, monophasic, pulsed current. Phys Ther 1988; 68:503–508.
131. Klug G, Wiehrer W, Reichmann H, et al: Relationships between early alterations in parvalbumins, sarcoplasmic reticulum and metabolic enzymes in chronically stimulated fast twitch muscle. Pflugers Arch 1983; 399:280–284.
132. Knaflitz M, Merletti R, Deluca CJ: Inference of motor unit recruitment order in voluntary and electrically elicited contraction. J Appl Physiol 1990; 68:1657–1667.
133. Kraft GH, Fitts SS, Hammond MC: Techniques to improve function of the arm and hand in chronic hemiplegia. Arch Phys Med Rehabil 1992; 73:220–227.
134. Kralj A, Bajd T, Turk R: Enhancement of gait restoration in spinal injured patients by functional electrical stimulation. Clin Orthop Rel Res 1988; 233:34–43.
135. Kralj AR, Bajd P, Munih M, et al: FES gait restoration and balance control in spinal cord injured patients. Prog Brain Res 1993; 97:387–396.
136. Kramer JF, Semple JE: Comparison of selected strengthening techniques for normal quadriceps. Physiol Ther Can 1983; 35:300–304.
137. Krauss JC, Robergs RA, Depaepe JL, et al: Effects of electrical stimulation and upper body training after spinal cord injury. Med Sci Sports Exerc 1993; 25:1054–1061.
138. Kubiak RJ, Whitman KM, Johnston RM: Changes in quadriceps femoris muscle strength using isometric exercise versus electrical stimulation. J Orthop Sports Phys Ther 1987; 8:537–541.
139. Lake DA: Neuromuscular electrical stimulation: An overview and its application in the treatment of sports injuries. Sports Med 1992; 13:320–336.
140. Larsen JO, Thomsen M, Haugland M, et al: Degeneration and regeneration in rabbit peripheral nerve with long-term nerve cuff electrode implant: A stereological study of myelinated and unmyelinated axons. Acta Neuropathol 1998; 96:365–378.
141. Laskin JJ, Ashley EA, Olenik LM, et al: Electrical stimulation-assisted rowing exercise in spinal cord injured people: A pilot study. Paraplegia 1993; 31:534–541.
142. Latash ML, Yee MJ, Orpett C, et al: Combining electrical muscle stimulation with voluntary contraction for studying muscle fatigue. Arch Phys Med Rehabil 1994; 75:29–35.
143. Lau HK, Liu J, Pereira BP, et al: Fatigue reduction by sequential stimulation of multiple motor points in a muscle. Clin Orthop Rel Res 1995; 321:251–258.
144. Laughman RK, Youdas JW, Garrett TR, et al: Strength changes in the normal quadriceps femoris muscle as the result of electrical stimulation. Phys Ther 1983; 63:494–499.
145. Lawrence JC Jr, Krsek JA, Salsgiver WJ, et al: Phosphorylase kinase isozymes in normal and electrically stimulated skeletal muscles. Am J Physiol 1986; 250:c84–89.
146. Leandri M, Parodi CI, Corrieri N, et al: Comparison of TENS treatments in hemiplegic shoulder pain. Scand J Rehabil Med 1990; 22:69–71.
147. Leeds EM, Klose KJ, Ganez W, et al: Bone mineral density after bicycle ergometry training. Arch Phys Med Rehabil 1990; 71:207–209.
148. Levin MF, Hui-Chan CWY: Relief of hemiparetic spasticity by TENS is associated with improvement in reflex and voluntary motor functions. Electroencephalogr Clin Neurophysiol 1992; 85:131–142.
149. Levine SP, Kett RL, Cederna PS, et al: Electric muscle stimulation for pressure sore prevention: Tissue shape variation. Arch Phys Med Rehabil 1990; 67:108–116.
150. Liberson WT, Holmquest HJ, Scot D, et al: Functional electrotherapy: Stimulation of the personeal nerve synchronized with the swing phase of gait of hemiplegic patients. Arch Phys Med Rehabil 1961; 42:101–105.
151. Lewis SM, Clelland JA, Knowles CJ, et al: Effects of auricular acupuncture-like transcutaneous electrical nerve stimulation on pain levels following wound care in patients with burns: A pilot study. J Burn Care Rehabil 1990; 11:322–329.
152. Lomo T, Westgaard RH, Dahl HA: Contractile properties of muscle: Control by pattern of muscle activity in the rat. Proc R Soc Lond Biol 1974; 187:99–103.
153. Lomo T, Westgaard RH, Engebretsen L: Different stimulation patterns affect contractile properties of denervated rat saveus muscle. In Pette D (ed): Plasticity of Muscle. Berlin, Walter de Gruyter, 1980, pp 297–309.
154. Lundeberg TCM, Eriksson SV, Malm M: Electrical nerve stimulation improves healing of diabetic ulcers. Ann Plast Surg 1992; 29:328–331.
155. Luthert P, Vrbovà G, Ward KM: Effects of slow frequency electrical stimulation on muscles of dystrophic mice. J Neurol Neurosurg Psychiatry 1980; 43:803–809.
156. Mabuchi K, Szvetko D, Pinter K, et al: Type IIB to IIA fiber transformation in intermittently stimulated rabbit muscles. Am J Physiol 1982; 242:c373–381.
157. Marsolais EB: FES ambulatory assist. In Neural Prosthesis: Motor Systems IV. Engineering Foundation Conferences. New York, July 23–28, 1994.
158. Marsolais EB, Edwards BG: Energy costs of walking and standing with functional neuromuscular stimulation and long leg braces. Arch Phys Med Rehabil 1988; 69:243–249.
159. Marsolais EB, Kobetic R, Barnicle K, et al: FNS application for restoring function in stroke and head injury patients. J Clin Eng 1990; 15:489–496.
160. Martin TP, Stein RB, Hoeppner PH, et al: Influence of electrical stimulation or the morphological and metabolic properties of paralyzed muscle. J Appl Physiology 1992; 72:1401–1406.
161. McDonagh JC, Binder MD, Reinking RM, et al: Tetrapartite classification of motor units of cat tibialis posterior. J Neurophysiol 1980; 44:696–712.
162. Melzack R, Wall PD: Pain mechanism: A new theory. Science 1965; 150:171–179.
163. Merli GJ, Herbison GJ, Ditunno JF, et al: Deep vein thrombosis: Prophylaxis in acute spinal cord injured patients. Arch Phys Med Rehabil 1988; 69:661–664.
164. Milner-Brown HS, Miller RG: Muscle strengthening through electrical stimulation combined with low-resistance weights in patients with neuromuscular disorders. Arch Phys Med Rehabil 1988; 69:20–24.
165. Milner-Brown HS, Stein RB, Yemm R: The contractile properties of human motor units during voluntary isometric contractions. J Physiol 1973; 228:285–306.
166. Milner-Brown HS, Stein RB, Yemm R: The orderly recruitment of human motor units during voluntary isometric contraction. J Physiol 1973; 230:359–370.
167. Mokrusch T, Engelhardt A, Eichorn KF, et al: Effects of long-impulse electrical stimulation on atrophy and fibre type composition of chronically denervated fast rabbit muscle. J Neurol 1990; 237:29–34.

168. Monster AW, Chan H: Isometric force production by motor units of extensor digitorum communis muscle in man. J Neurophysiol 1977; 40:1432–1443.
169. Morrissey MC, Brewster CE, Shields CL Jr, et al: The effects of electrical stimulation on the quadriceps during postoperative knee immobilization. Am J Sports Med 1985; 13:40–45.
170. Mortiemer JT: Extra neural neuromuscular stimulating electrodes. In Neuroprosthesis: Motor Systems IV. Engineering Foundation Conferences, New York, July 23–28, 1994.
171. Mullett K: State-of-the-art in neurostimulation. PACE 1987; 10:162–175.
172. Munsat TL, McNeal D, Waters R: Effects of nerve stimulation on human muscle. Arch Neurol 1976; 33:608–617.
173. Myklebust BM, Kloth L: Electrodiagnostic and electrotherapeutic instrumentation: Characteristics of recording and stimulation systems and principles of safety. In Gersh MR (ed): Electrotherapy in Rehabilitation. Philadelphia, FA Davis, 1992, pp 51–100.
174. Mysiw WJ, Jackson RD: Hypercalciuria permitted by functional electrical stimulation (abstract). Arch Phys Med Rehabil 1990; 71:795.
175. Nash MS, Bilsker S, Marcillo AE, et al: Reversal of adaptive left ventricular atrophy following electrically-stimulated exercise training in human tetraplegics. Paraplegia 1991; 29:590–599.
176. Nemeth PM: Electical stimulation of denervated muscle prevents decreases in oxidative enzymes. Muscle Nerve 1982; 5:134–139.
177. Nene AV, Patrick JH: Energy cost of paraplegic locomotion using the ParaWalker electrical stimulation "hybrid" orthosis. Arch Phys Med Rehabil 1990; 71:116–120.
178. Nix W: Effect of electrical stimulation on denervated muscle. In Nix WA, Vrbovà G (eds): Electrical Stimulation and Neurodisorders. Berlin, Springer-Verlag, 1986, pp 115–124.
179. Nix WA: The effect of low-frequency electrical stimulation on the denervated extensor digitorum longus muscle of the rabbit. Acta Neurol Scand 1982; 66:521–528.
180. Nochomovitz ML, Peterson BK, Stellato TA: Electrical activation of the diaphragm. Clin Chest Med 1988; 9:349–358.
181. Noland MF: Selected problems in the use of transcutaneous nerve stimulation for pain control: An appraisal with proposed solutions. Phys Ther 1988; 68:1694–1698.
182. Okada N, Igawa Y, Ogawa A, Nichizawa O: Transcutaneous electrical stimulation of thigh muscles in the treatment of detrusor overactivity. Br J Urol 1998; 81:560–564.
183. Okuma H, Ogata H, Hatada K: Transition of physical fitness in wheelchair marathon competitors over several years. Paraplegia 1989; 27:237–243.
184. O'Malley-Teeter J, Brown-Triolo DL: Exploring today's FES options. FES Update 1999; 9:1–2.
185. Osman SG, Marsolais EB: Endoscopic implantation of cuff electrodes on the hamstring branches of the sciatic nerve in paralyzed subjects. In Neuroprosthesis: Motor Systems IV. Engineering Foundation Conferences, New York, July 23–28, 1994.
186. Osterman AL, Bora FW Jr: Electrical stimulation applied to bone and nerve injuries in the upper extremity. Orthop Clin North Am 1986; 17:353–364.
187. Pachter B, Eberstein A, Goodgold J: Electrical stimulation effect on denervated skeletal myofibers in rats: A light and electron microscopic study. Arch Phys Med Rehabil 1982; 63:427–430.
188. Packman-Braun R: Relationship between functional electrical stimulation duty cycle and fatigue in wrist extensor muscles of patients with hemiparesis. Phys Ther 1988; 68:51–56.
189. Pacy PJ, Hesp R, Halliday DA, et al: Muscle and bone in paraplegic patients, and the effect of functional electrical stimulation. Clin Sci 1988; 75:481–487.
190. Pambianco G, Orchard T, Landan P: Deep vein thrombosis prevention in stroke patients during rehabilitation. Arch Phys Med Rehabil 1995; 76:324–330.
191. Pease WS: Therapeutic electrical stimulation for spasticity: Quantitative gait analysis. Am J Phys Med Rehabil 1998; 77: 351–355.
192. Peckham PH, Keith MW, Freehafer AA: Restoration of functional control by electrical stimulation in the upper extremity of the quadriplegic patient. J Bone Joint Surg Am 1988; 70:144–148.
193. Pentland B: Quadriplegia and cardiorespiratory fitness. Lancet 1993; 341:413–414.
194. Perkash I, Martin DE, Warner H, et al: Electroejaculation in spinal cord injury patients: Simplified new equipment and technique. J Urol 1990; 143:305–307.
195. Petrofsky JS: Sequential motor unit stimulation through peripheral motor nerves in the cat. Med Biol Eng Comput 1979; 17:87–93.
196. Petrofsky JS, Phillips CA: The use of functional electrical stimulation for rehabilitation of spinal cord injured patients. Central Nerv Syst Trauma 1984; 1:57–74.
197. Petrofsky JS, Phillips CA, Heaton HH, et al: Bicycle ergometer for paralyzed muscle. J Clin Eng 1984; 9:13–19.
198. Petrofsky JS, Phillips CA, Stafford DE: Closed loop control for restoration of movement in paralyzed muscle. Orthopedics 1984; 7:1289–1302.
199. Petrofsky JS, Smith JB: Physiologic costs of computer-controlled walking in persons with paraplegia using a reciprocating gait orthosis. Arch Phys Med Rehabil 1991; 72:890–896.
200. Petrofsky JS, Stacy R: The effect of training on endurance and the cardiovascular responses of individuals with paraplegia during dynamic exercise induced by functional electrical stimulation. Eur J Appl Physiol 1992; 64:487–492.
201. Pette D: Activity-induced fast- to slow-transition in mammalian muscle. Med Sci Sports Exerc 1984; 16:517–528.
202. Pette D, Müller W, Leisner E, et al: Time dependent effects on contractile properties, fibre population, myosin light chains and enzymes of energy metabolism in intermittently and continuously stimulated fast twitch muscle of the rabbit. Pflugers Arch 1976; 364:103–112.
203. Pette D, Ramirez BU, Müller W, et al: Influence of intermittent long-term stimulation on contractile, histochemical and metabolic properties of fibre populations in fast and slow rabbit muscles. Pflugers Arch 1975; 361:1–7.
204. Pette D, Schnez U: Coexistence of fast and slow type myosin light chains in single muscle fibres during transformation as induced by long-term stimulation. FEBS Lett 1977; 83:128–130.
205. Pette D, Smith ME, Staudte HW, et al: Effects of long-term electrical stimulation on some contractile and metabolic characteristics of fast rabbit muscles. Pflugers Arch 1973; 338:257–272.
206. Pette D, Staudte HW, Vrbovà G: Physiological and biochemical changes induced by long-term stimulation of fast muscle. Naturwissenschaften 1972; 59:469–470.
207. Pette D, Tyler KR: Response of succinate dehydrogenase activity in fibres of rabbit tibialis anterior muscle to chronic nerve stimulation. J Physiol 1983; 338:1–9.
208. Phillips CA, Petrosky JS, Hendershot DM, et al: Functional electrical exercise: Comprehensive approach for physical conditioning of spinal cord injured patients. Orthopedics 1984; 7:1112–1123.
209. Phillips WT, Burkett LN: Augmented upper body contribution to oxygen uptake during upper body exercise with concurrent leg functional electrical stimulation in persons with spinal cord injury. Spinal Cord 1998; 36:750–755.
210. Phillips WT, Kiratli BJ, Sarkarati M, et al: Effect of spinal cord injury on the heart and cardiovascular fitness. Curr Probl Cardiol 1998; 23:641–716.
211. Polando G, Schiner A, Marsolais EB: Reliability of lower extremity FES systems: Analysis of a current laboratory system. In Neuroprosthesis: Motor Systems IV. Engineering Foundation Conferences, New York, July 23–28, 1994.
212. Pollack SF, Axen K, Spielholtz N, et al: Aerobic training effects of electrically-induced lower extremity exercises in spinal cord injured people. Arch Phys Med Rehabil 1989; 70:214–219.
213. Popovic DB: Finite state model of locomotion for functional electrical stimulation systems. Prog Brain Res 1993; 97:397–407.
214. Previnaire JG, Soler JM, Perrigot M: Is there a place for pudendal nerve maximal electrical stimulation for the treatment of detrusor hyperreflexia in spinal cord injury patients? Spinal Cord 1998; 36:100–103.
215. Previnaire JG, Soler JM, Perrigot M, et al: Short-term effect of pudendal nerve electrical stimulation on detrusor hyperreflexia in spinal cord injury patients: Importance of current strength. Paraplegia 1996; 34:95–99.
216. Ragnarsson KT: Physiologic effects of functional electrical stimulation-induced exercises in spinal cord injured individuals. Clin Orthop Rel Res 1988; 233:53–63.

217. Ragnarsson KT, Pollack SF, O'Daniel W, et al: Clinical evaluation of computerized functional electrical stimulation after spinal cord injury: A multicenter pilot study. Arch Phys Med Rehabil 1988; 69:672–677.
218. Ragnarsson KT, Sell G: Lower extremity fractures after spinal cord injury: A retrospective study. Arch Phys Med Rehabil 1981; 62:418–423.
219. Ramirez BU, Pette D: Effect of long-term electrical stimulation on sarcoplasmic reticulum of fast rabbit muscle. FEBS Lett 1974; 49:188–198.
220. Reich JD, Tarjan PP: Electrical stimulation of skin. Int J Dermatol 1990; 29:395–400.
221. Reichmann H, Hoppeler H, Mathieu-Costello O, et al: Biochemical and ultrastructural changes of skeletal muscle mitochondria after chronic electrical stimulation in rabbits. Pflugers Arch 1985; 404:1–9.
222. Reichmann H, Pette D, Vrbovà G: Effects of low frequency electrical stimulation on enzyme and isozyme patterns of dystrophic mouse muscle. FEBS Lett 1981; 128:55–58.
223. Rieb L, Pomeranz B: Alterations in electrical pain thresholds by use of acupuncture-like transcutaneous electrical nerve stimulation in pain free subject. Phys Ther 1992; 72:658–667.
224. Rijkhoft NJ, Hendrickx LB, van Verrebroeck PE, et al: Selective detrusor activation by electrical stimulation of the human sacral nerve roots. Artific Organs 1997; 21:223–226.
225. Riso RR, Gorman PH: Viability of the cutaneous innervation of the fingers in C5 and C6 level quadriplegic subjects studied using evoked sensory nerve action potentials. In Neuroprosthesis: Motor Systems IV. Engineering Foundation Conferences, New York, July 23–28, 1994.
226. Robinson CJ, Kett NA, Bolam JM: Spasticity in spinal cord injured patients: 1. Short-term effects of surface electrical stimulation. Arch Phys Med Rehabil 1988; 69:598–604.
227. Robinson CJ, Kett NA, Bolam JM: Spasticity in spinal cord injured patients: 2. Initial measures and long-term effects of basic electrical stimulation. Arch Phys Med Rehabil 1988; 69:862–888.
228. Robinson LR, Mustovic EH, Lieber PS, et al: A technique for quantifying and determining the site of isometric muscle fatigue in the clinical setting. Arch Phys Med Rehabil 1990; 71:901–904.
229. Rowe DE, Bernstein SM, Riddick MF, et al: A meta-analysis of the efficacy of non-operative treatments for idiopathic scoliosis. J Bone Joint Surg Am 1997; 79:664–674.
229a. Roy D, Johannsson E, Bonen A, et al: Electrical stimulation induces fiber type-specific translocation of GLUT-4 to T tubules in skeletal muscle. Am J Physiol 1997; 273:E688–E694.
230. Roy RK, Mabuchi K, Sarkar S, et al: Changes in tropomyosin subunit pattern in chronic electrically stimulated rabbit fast muscles. Biochem Biophys Res Commun 1979; 89:181–187.
231. Rubinstein N, Mabuchi K, Pepe F, et al: Use of type-specific antimyosins to demonstrate the transformation of individual fibers in chronically stimulated rabbit fast muscles. J Cell Biol 1978; 79:252–261.
232. Saito K, Kinoshita Y, Hosaka M: Direct and indirect effects of electrical stimulation on the motility of human sperm. Int J Urol 1999; 6:196–199.
233. Salmons S, Henriksson J: The adaptive response of skeletal muscle to increased use. Muscle Nerve 1981; 4:94–105.
234. Salmons S, Sreter FA: Significance of impulse activity in the transformation of skeletal muscle type. Nature 1976; 263:30–34.
235. Salmons S, Vrbovà G: The influence of activity on some contractile characteristics of mammalian fast and slow muscles. J Physiol 1969; 210:535–549.
237. Sarzala MG, Szymanska G, Wiehrer W, et al: Effects of chronic stimulation at low frequency on the lipid phase of sarcoplasmic reticulum in rabbit fast-twitch muscle. Eur J Biochem 1982; 123:241–245.
238. Scott OM, Hyde SA, Vrbovà G, et al: Therapeutic possibilities of chronic long-frequency electrical stimulation in children with Duchenne muscular dystrophy. J Neurol Sci 1990; 95:171–182.
239. Scott OM, Vrbovà G, Hyde SA, et al: Responses of muscles of patients with Duchenne muscular dystrophy to chronic electrical stimulation. J Neurol Neurosurg Psychiatry 1986; 49:1427–1434.
240. Seager SW, Halstead LS: Fertility options and success after spinal cord injury. Urol Clin North Am 1993; 20:543–548.
241. Sebrille A, Boudoux-Jahan M: Effects of electrical stimulation in previous nerve injury on motor function recovery in rats. Brain Res 1980; 193:560–565.
242. Seedorf K, Seedorf U, Pette D: Coordinate expression of alkali and DTNB myosin light chains during transformation of rabbit fast muscle by chronic stimulation. FEBS Lett 1983; 158:321–324.
243. Shaker HS, Tu LM, Robin S, et al: Reduction of bladder outlet resistance by selective sacral root stimulation using high-frequency blockade in dogs: An acute study. J Urol 1998; 160:901–907.
244. Shields RK, Law LF, Reiling B, et al: Effects of electrically induced fatigue on the twitch and tetanus of paralyzed soleus muscle in humans. J Appl Physiol 1997; 82:1499–1507.
245. Sigmedics: Parastep Update. Northfield, IL, Sigmedics, 1994.
246. Sipski ML, Delisa JA, Schweer S: Functional electrical stimulation bicycle ergometry: Patient perceptions. Am J Phys Med Rehabil 1989; 68:147–149.
247. Solomonow M: External control of the neuromuscular system. IEEE Trans Biomed Eng 1984; 31:752–763.
248. Sréter FA, Gergely J, Salmon S, et al: Synthesis by fast muscle of myosin light chain characteristic of slow muscle in response to long-term stimulation. Nature 1973; 241:17–19.
249. Sréter FA, Pinter K, Jolesz F, Mabuchi K: Fast to slow transformation of fast muscles in response to long-term phasic stimulation. Exp Neurol 1982; 75:95–102.
250. Stefanoviska A, Gros N, Vodovnik L, et al: Chronic electrical stimulation for the modification of spasticity in hemiplegic patients. Scand J Rehabil Med 1988; 17(suppl):115–121.
251. Stein RB: Methods for using feedback to control functional electrical stimulation. In Neuroprosthesis: Motor Systems IV. Engineering Foundation Conferences, New York, July 23–28, 1994.
252. Stein RB, Gordon T, Jefferson J, et al: Optimal stimulation of paralyzed muscle after human spinal cord injury. J Appl Physiol 1992; 72:1393–1400.
253. Sweeney JD: Selection criteria for neuromuscular stimulation electrodes. In Neuroprosthesis: Motor Systems IV. Engineering Foundation Conferences, New York, July 23–28, 1994.
254. Sykes L, Campbell IG, Powell ES, et al: Energy expenditure of walking for adults with spinal cord lesions using the reciprocating gait orthosis and functional electrical stimulation. Spinal Cord 1996; 34:659–665.
255. Sykes L, Ross ER, Powell ES, et al: Objective measurement of use of the reciprocating gait orthosis (RGO) and the electrically augmented RGO in adult patients with spinal cord lesions. Prosthet Orthot Int 1996; 20:182–190.
256. Theriault R, Boulay MR, Theriault G, et al: Electrical stimulation-induced changes in performance and fiber type proportion of human knee extensor muscles. Eur J App Physiol Occup Physiol 1996; 74:311–317.
257. Tulgar M, McGlone F, Bowsher D, et al: Comparative effectiveness of different stimulation modes in relieving pain: II. A double blind controlled long-term clinical trial. Pain 1991; 47:157–162.
258. Twist DJ, Culpepper-Morgan JA, Ragnarsson KT, et al: Neuroendocrine changes during functional electrical stimulation. Am J Phys Med Rehabil 1992; 71:156–163.
259. Unger PG: A randomized clinical trial of the effect of HVPC on wound healing. Phys Ther 1991; 71:S118.
260. Unger PG, Rainastry S: A controlled study of the effect of high voltage pulse current (HVPC) on wound healing. Phys Ther 1991; 71:S119.
261. Van Kerrebroeck PE: The role of electrical stimulation in voiding dysfunction. Eur Urol 1998; 34(suppl 1):27–30.
262. Vignos PJ, Watkins MP: The effect of exercise in muscular dystrophy. JAMA 1966; 197:843–848.
263. Vodovnik L, Karba R: Treatment of chronic wounds by means of electrical and electromagnetic fields: I. Literature review. Med Biol Eng Comput 1992; 30:257–266.
264. Vrbovà G, Ward K: Observations on the effects of low frequency electrical stimulation on fast muscles of dystrophic mice. J Neurol Neurosurg Psychiatry 1981; 44:1002–1006.
265. Walsfley RP, Letts G, Booyf J: A comparison of torque generated by knee extension with a maximal voluntary muscle contraction: Vis-a-vis electrical stimulation. J Orthop Sports Phys Ther 1984; 6:10–17.

266. Wang YH, Chiang HS, Wu CH, et al: Electroejaculation in spinal cord injured males. J Formosa Med Assoc 1992; 91:413–418.
267. Weber RJ: Functional neuromuscular stimulation. In DeLisa JA, Gans BM (eds): Rehabilitation Medicine: Principles and Practice. Philadelphia, JB Lippincott, 1993, pp 463–476.
268. Wehrmacher WH, Thomson JD, Hines HM: Effects of electrical stimulation on denervated skeletal muscle. Arch Phys Med Rehabil 1945; 26:261–266.
269. Weiss DS, Eaglstein WH, Falanga V: Pulsed electrical stimulation decreases scar thickness at split thickness graft donor sites (abstract). J Invest Dermatol 1989; 92:3.
270. Wiehrer W, Pette D: The ratio between intrinsic 115 kDa and 30 kDa peptides as a marker of fibre type-specific sarcoplasmic reticulum in mammalian muscles. FEBS Lett 1983; 158:317–320.
271. Wigerstad-Lossing I, Grimby G, Jonnson T, et al: Effects of electrical stimulation combined with voluntary contractions after knee ligament surgery. Med Sci Sports Exerc 1988; 20: 93–98.
272. William HB: The value of continuous electrical muscle stimulation using a completely implantable system in the preservation of muscle function following motor nerve injury and repair: An experimental study. Microsurgery 1996; 17:589–596.
273. Williams RS, Salmons S, Newsholme EA, et al: Regulation of nuclear and mitochondrial gene expression by contractile activity in skeletal muscle. J Biol Chem 1986; 261:376–380.
274. Winter GD: Movement of epidermal cells over the wound surface. Adv Biol Skin 1964; 5:113.
275. Wolcott LE, Wheeler PC, Hardwicke HM, et al: Accelerated healing of skin ulcers by electrotherapy: Preliminary clinical results. South Med J 1969; 62:795–801.
276. Wolf SL, Ariel GB, Saar D, et al: The effect of muscle stimulation during resistive training on performance parameters. Am J Sports Med 1986; 14:18–23.
277. Wong RA: High voltage versus low voltage electrical stimulation: Force of induced muscle contraction and perceived discomfort in healthy subjects. Phys Ther 1986; 66:1209–1214.
278. Wuolle KS, VanDoren CL, Bryden AM, et al: Satisfaction with and usage of a hand prosthesis. Arch Phys Med Rehabil 1999; 80:206–213.
279. Yamanish T, Yasuda K: Electrical stimulation for stress incontinence. Int Urogyn J Pelvic Floor Dysfunction 1998; 9:281–290.
280. Zupan A, Gregoric M, Valencic V, et al: Effects of electrical stimulation on muscles of children with Duchenne and Becker muscular dystrophy. Neuropediatrics 1993; 24:189–192.
281. Zwiren LD, Bar-Or O: Responses to exercise of paraplegics who differ in conditioning level. Med Sci Sports 1975; 7:94–98.

23 CHAPTER

Keven Caves, B.S.M.E., A.T.P., and Jan C. Galvin, L.L.C.

Computer Assistive Devices and Environmental Controls

Computers have changed the way Americans think, work, and play. They have become a part of our everyday life. The microchip is embedded in virtually everything we use, from toys and games to cell phones, televisions, remote controls, microwave ovens, and ATM machines. Even the mundane iron now contains a microchip that tells it when to switch off.

Computers are now helping change the world for individuals with disabilities, opening up opportunities for independence, community integration, education, and employment. Children with disabilities are using computers in the classroom, from pre-school to postsecondary school, to play, communicate, and learn. Adults with disabilities are using computers in the workplace to access and disseminate information, design buildings, and teach. Older Americans are taking advantage of computerized environmental control systems in the home for both safety and security, using them to switch lights on and off, to open and close doors, and to call for help if needed. A vast array of computer-related equipment is available to assist individuals with disabilities. Ten years ago an individual with quadriplegia and a law degree could not hope to work independently, let alone live independently. Now through the use of an adapted computer, such an individual can research documents from every law library in the United States, write briefs, and if the courtroom is wheelchair-accessible, vigorously defend his or her client. After winning the case, the lawyer can go home in an adapted van to a barrier-free, automated environment. An attendant might still be required to assist with bathing, grooming, and eating, but the individual is able to be a productive member of society through the assistance of computers and computer adaptations.

How can you find out what types of computer-related equipment are available? How can you determine the consumer's needs? How do you know if the different components interface with each other? Finally, who pays for computer-related technology? This chapter focuses on the different types of adapted computer technologies that are available and ways of evaluating a patient's need for such equipment. It also identifies the motor and cognitive factors that affect assistive technology interventions.

BACKGROUND

The Internet has revolutionized the way we access information. We can purchase airline tickets and books, obtain the latest news, join chat rooms, book a hotel in Europe, play interactive games, and invest in stocks and bonds 24 hours a day. Just a decade ago, e-mail was the province of a select group of university researchers; now, more than 100 million users from around the world access mail via the computer.

Computer technology is one of the most rapidly changing fields in the world. As telephone and cable companies merge their fiberoptic lines over the next five years, the television will become an interactive tool for the whole family—a necessity for school, work, and leisure. But because computers are now so pervasive, it is easy to forget that many individuals find their use difficult. Many are unable to access computers via such "usual" methods as the standard QWERTY keyboard.

By its very nature, the computer is an extremely flexible tool, one that can be used in many different ways. It can be used as a diagnostic or learning tool, for example, or as a method of providing equal access to an education. In the workplace, it can be used as a tool for achieving successful employment; and in the home, it can help procure safety, security, and a means of independent living. Each of these uses can involve different computers, different types of components, and different constraints. But the success of the technology has more to do with people than machines. The key to success lies in making the right parts and pieces work together so that even the most severely incapacitated individual has access to information.

EDUCATION

In a school environment, children with disabilities generally use computers with special software programs. These programs are designed to evaluate or develop skills, such as reading, spelling, and language. Computers provide a flexible learning and play environment, and they can serve as a tool for discovery-oriented activities. Development of a child can be hampered by the inability to participate in typical play behaviors because of physical, sensory communication, or cognitive barriers. It has been shown that the early use of switches and computers can help forestall the development of learned helplessness and learning deficits in these children,[2, 3] and may lay the foundation for transition to more sophisticated computer and augmentative communication devices.[9, 16]

In many colleges and universities, homework, examinations, and grades are all communicated via e-mail. Therefore, all students must be familiar with computer use. For a high school or college student with a disability, assistive technology labs provide access to computer technology. These labs provide the support, technology, and training that can create equal access and integration by students into the world of technology. Students with visual impairments might not be able to see the computer screen well enough to use the computer productively. Programs that produce raised line drawings, enlarge hard copies of materials, magnify the screen, or convert text into speech or Braille enable the student to access class materials. Large-print keyboards, alternative lighting, and text scanners also can assist the student in a learning environment.

Conventional techniques used to input to the computer can present a barrier to a student with mobility impairments. Support is available through a voice recognition system, an on-screen keyboard, word predictor, joystick, or an ergonomic keyboard and arm supports. For the student with learning disabilities, using all the standard support functions of the word processing programs, such as spell and grammar checkers and thesaurus, provides a good foundation for writing. Also available are word predictors, customized screen colors, and academic support software in math, speed reading, and grammar.

DISTANCE LEARNING

Distance learning is defined as "the linking of a teacher and students in several geographic locations via technology that allows interaction. Distance learning is simply a form of telecommuting."[5] This emerging method of teaching via computer networking and distance learning is spawning a revolution in education. Educators are beginning to realize that students learn differently. Computers allow students to work at their own pace and revisit courses as often as necessary. For the first time in history, extremely large databases, encyclopedias, popular books (both fiction and nonfiction), dictionaries, thesauruses, library catalogs, and the like are available through the Internet. People who cannot be physically present because of a disability need only sit at a computer to enjoy the benefits of an education.[15]

EMPLOYMENT

The Americans with Disabilities Act of 1990 prohibits discrimination in the workplace and provides for reasonable accommodations to ensure that persons with a disability, if qualified for the job, have an equal opportunity to enter employment. Computers are now so integrated into all educational levels and most employment situations that people with disabilities must be able to use them along with everyone else in order to participate and compete effectively in these environments. The person with a disability must be able to access not just a computer, but the specific computer and software that is found in the school or job.[10, 14] The growth in computer technology, in conjunction with the changing nature of commerce and industry, continues to provide opportunities for individuals with disabilities to be productive.

Industry is discovering that telecommuting has many benefits; employees are less stressed, use less sick-time, and are often more productive and creative. The growing attraction of telecommuting has many benefits for the disabled worker. Transportation (the bane of many a disabled person's life) ceases to be an issue, freeing these employees to spend many productive hours in familiar surroundings accessing their work on computers at home.

Sophisticated applications are now in use for most occupations. Architects no longer stand long hours at a drawing board, but design and build virtual 3-D buildings on the computer. A severely disabled architect is able to operate, via a single input device, a powered wheelchair, an augmentative communication device, and a computer to design houses. The tetraplegic lawyer can use a personal computer with a voice-recognition system to control such programs as word processors, databases, spreadsheets, telecommunications, and other applications. Its extensive vocabulary and ability to learn new words enables the lawyer to speak to the computer as one would type words. Verbal commands are also recognized, including "delete," "print," and "merge." The workstation consists of a raised-height desk so that the employee in a wheelchair can roll right up to the desk.

Workstations are often altered to meet the needs of a worker with a disability (Fig. 23–1). These alterations are simple and inexpensive, and provide access for workers who may have sensory, cognitive, or physical

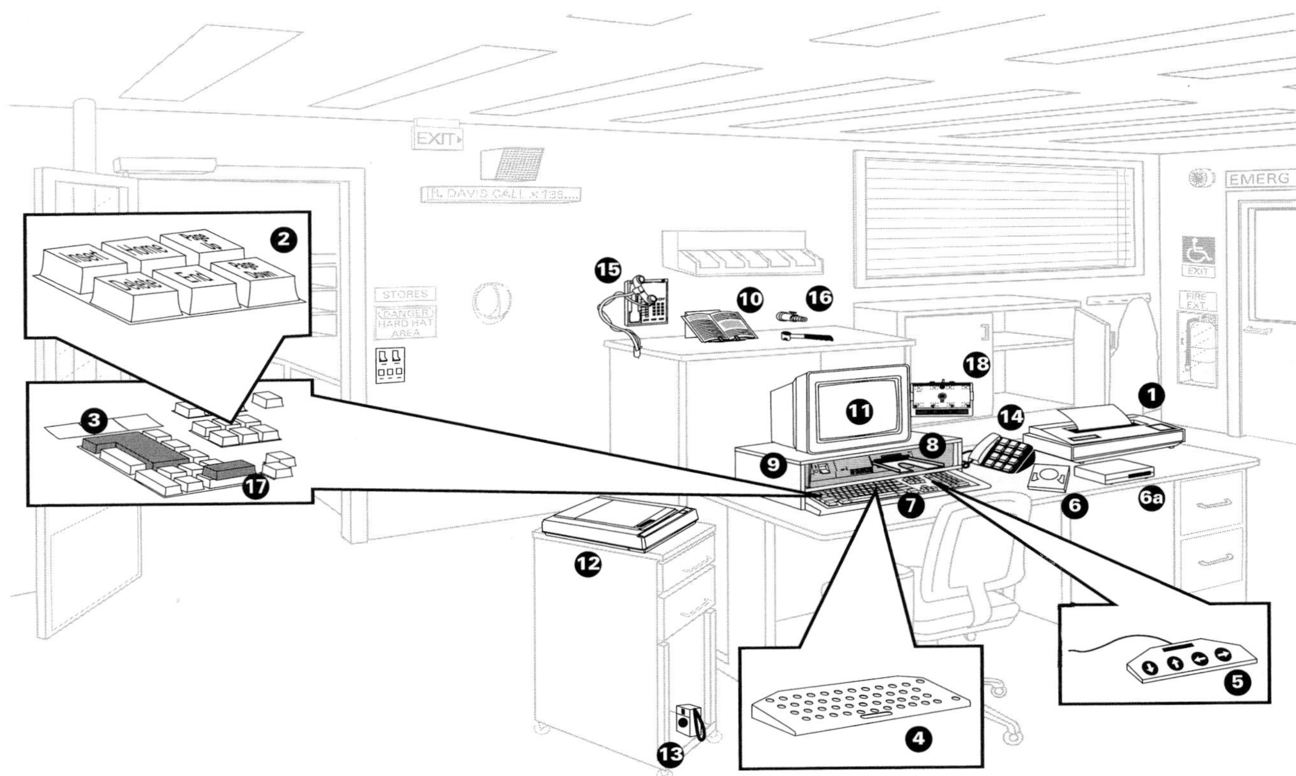

FIGURE 23–1. Computers, information displays, communication devices, and controls: assistive modifications for workers with incoordination. *A,* Graphic illustration of a typical workstation setup for an individual with coordination problems. *B,* Key to features in *A.* (From Mueller J: The Workplace Workbook 2.0: An Illustrated Guide to Workplace Accommodation and Technology. McLean, VA, HRD Press, 1992.)

disabilities. The growing emphasis on ergonomically designed workstations also benefits all workers, providing improved positioning, lighting, and comfort.

HOME AND COMMUNITY

Safety and security in the home are major considerations for all, but particularly for the individual who is disabled and/or frail and elderly. An environmental control unit (ECU) can be used to manipulate and interact with the environment to alert police or medical personnel to emergency issues or danger. Accessing one or more electrical devices via switches, voice activation, remote control, computer interface, and other technological adaptations activates the ECU. For a hearing-impaired elderly person who is alone most of the day and needs to take medication at a designated time, the ECU is programmed to turn on the lights as a reminder. A tetraplegic individual can use an ECU to open doors, turn on the coffeepot, dial the telephone, and control the television and radio.[1] Access to the Internet also brings companionship, albeit virtual, with 24-hour access to the whole world. Banking and shopping online obviates the need to travel. The advent of telemedicine and telerehabilitation is providing a mechanism whereby interdisciplinary providers can deliver or support delivery of healthcare long distance.

TRENDS IN PREVALENCE OF ASSISTIVE TECHNOLOGY DEVICES

According to findings from the 1990 National Health Interview Survey (NHIS) on Assistive Devices, which was cosponsored by the National Center for Health Statistics (NCHS) and the National Institute on Disability and Rehabilitation Research (NIDRR), more than 13.1 million Americans (about 5.3% of the population) use assistive technology devices to accommodate physical impairments.[8] It is also estimated that 37.3 million noninstitutionalized persons aged 15 years and older living in the United States have a chronic health disability that limits their ability to participate fully in life. More than 70 chronic conditions are listed in the NHIS report, and each of these has the potential to cause one or more functional limitations that could be ameliorated by the use of appropriate assistive technology. In addition, a significant number of individuals are surviving catastrophic trauma and living with severe functional losses. More children are being born with learning disabilities resulting from in utero drug addiction or lack of prenatal care. These individuals can also potentially benefit from the use of adaptive computer technologies.

The potential of technology to help individuals with disabilities to achieve maximum independent functioning is well recognized in rehabilitation. Several pieces of legislation—notably the Rehabilitation Act of 1973 (as amended), the Americans with Disabilities Act of 1990, the Individuals with Disabilities Education Act of 1990, and the Technology Related Assistance for Individuals with Disabilities Act of 1988—have particularly emphasized the use of assistive technology as part of the continuum of services.[6] It is important to remember, however, that as technology is used to increase opportunities for individuals with disabilities, the needs of the whole person must be taken into account to ensure maximum benefit from the technology. All professionals in assistive technology service delivery must be technology-literate so that appropriate referrals and selections can be made.[11]

EVALUATING FOR APPROPRIATE PERSON/DEVICE MATCH

An evaluation is performed to gather the information necessary to identify the appropriate technology for a given person. The purpose of the evaluation is to ensure that the equipment will meet the user's needs. The evaluation can involve persons from several different backgrounds with different areas of expertise. A team of individuals, including occupational, physical, and speech therapists, as well as engineers, assistive technologists, rehabilitation counselors, nurses, and physicians, often performs these evaluations. This technology team should include the person for whom the evaluation is being performed, who must be an equal partner in the process.

There are as many different styles of evaluation as there are rehabilitation professionals. However, an evaluation should provide enough information to allow the team to identify the appropriate technology.[4, 7] An outline for a typical evaluation follows.

Identify Consumer Goals and Tasks. The first portion of the assessment is used to gather information about the goals of the individual and the need for equipment. This may be the most important step of the process. The needs assessment is used to identify why the individual is seeking technology. Different people use equipment in different ways and for different purposes. The needs assessment provides the technology team with information about what the user wants to be able to do, and about the "type" of user the person will be. For example, a computer programming student's computer technology requirements will likely be greater than those of the home computer user, and hence the level of control and access may be more complex. It is also important to conduct a task analysis of activities (i.e., to look at the components of the activity and determine what actions are required to do it).

Get Comprehensive Information. Get information about the person, the environment, and the devices. Assess the consumer's functional abilities, personal preferences, environmental barriers, and resources, and ascertain product availability (Table 23–1). The information-gathering step is typically ongoing until the final decision is made. In most cases, the evaluation of functional capabilities rests with the physicians and clinical professionals involved. A comprehensive evaluation of the consumer's environment is also essential. Clinicians conducting functional evaluations need to consider environmental issues. The counselor might have special expertise in the work and community settings. Consumers returning to previously held jobs have the best understanding of the work environment and are a crucial source of information.

TABLE 23–1 User's Functional Abilities

User's Functional Abilities	
Disability	Type, severity, age at onset, prognosis
Motor	Strength, endurance, range of motion, fine and gross motor coordination, positioning to use device, type of control that can be operated
Cognitive	Intelligence, judgment, attention span, problem-solving, memory
Communication	Voice quality, pronunciation, speed
Sensory	Vision, hearing, tactile perception
User's Personal Characteristics	
Psychosocial	Interests/activities, personal values, adjustment to disability, coping style, motivation/desire, attitude toward devices, concept of independence
Family and social support	Family, friends, co-workers, neighbors, etc.
Environment	
Environmental compatibility	Usable in home, work, play, community; architectural barriers, getting into and out of rooms, access to lighting, kitchen, phones, bath
Resources available	Space, electronics, wiring compatible
Impact on others in environment	Family, housemates, co-workers
Service delivery system	Training provided, follow-up provided, user support services available, installation, timely delivery

From Galvin J, Barnicle K, Perr A: Evaluating and Choosing Assistive Technology. Proceedings of the Technology and People with Disabilities Conference. Northridge, Calif, California State University, 1992.

Establish Criteria for a Successful Choice. Based on the consumer's goals, abilities, and preferences, identify the specific, objective criteria that can be used to judge potential solutions. To make the best match, you must consider multiple issues: the tasks to be accomplished, the consumer's functional abilities and personal characteristics, the environment, and the device. The interaction of these issues must then be considered, because they all affect the use of the device. The major areas of concern are summarized in Table 23–2.

Make a Final Selection. Apply the criteria to possible solutions to narrow down the options. Determine which of these solutions best meets the criteria. Equipment trials utilizing loaner or rental equipment are extremely useful, especially in the area of augmentative and alternative communication (AAC). In lieu of equipment trials, recommendations are made and equipment is procured, set up, and configured. Training and appropriate

TABLE 23–2 Device Selection Evaluation Criteria

Performance	Effectiveness, reliability, durability, safety, comfort
Ease of use	Easy to set up, learn to use, operate, maintain, repair
Aesthetics	Attractive, quiet, well-designed
Cost	Purchase, maintenance, repairs
Convenience	Easy to store, transport, etc.
Flexibility	Compatible with other devices, expandable

From Galvin J, Barnicle K, Perr A: Evaluating and Choosing Assistive Technology. Proceedings of the Technology and People with Disabilities Conference. Northridge, Calif, California State University, 1992.

follow-up are integral parts of the evaluation process, to ensure the success of the technology solution.

Although these steps are presented as a linear process, the operation is really cyclical. Information gathered at each step might necessitate adjustment of decisions made in earlier steps. A device selected for one activity might also have an effect on another activity. For example, in a work setting, hand-held typing sticks might be the best method for typing. However, if the user must also answer the telephone, the typing stick might interfere and make overall activity more difficult. All of the benefits and drawbacks should be weighed within the larger context. When evaluating for computer-related technologies, it is important to ensure that the technologies interface with each other. The hardware, the software, and the user must successfully interact to achieve the optimal result. It is also important to be aware of other related factors, such as an employer's using only a specific type of computer. Cognitive factors, as well as sensory and motor skills, should also be taken into account. Tables 23–3 and 23–4 illustrate some of the factors affecting computer use.

It is important to realize that any piece of equipment works best when used as designed. When an assistive technology intervention is necessary, the simpler the intervention the better. The same rule applies when looking at computer adaptations. First, try the device as designed. If this is not workable, try to identify the simplest appropriate intervention, using more complicated interventions only if needed. Avoid the temptation to use a "high-tech" solution when a "low-tech" solution might be best.

TABLE 23–3 Cognitive Factors That Affect Assistive Technology Interventions

Cognitive Factors	Impact on Use of Technology
Attention deficits	Failure to follow screen prompts and directions Inability to consistently perform multi-step procedures Inability to filter information on busy screens Difficulty with large amounts of computer speech
Sensory deficits	Inability to separate command menus from other screen data Inability to track user information on rapidly changing screens Slow visual-motor dexterity Difficulty understanding computer speech
Memory deficits	Unable to complete multi-step operations or device commands Unable to follow set-up directions Unable to locate and recall disk files Difficulty recalling knowledge of computer symbols and commands
Abstract reasoning and thinking deficits	Unable to analyze equipment procedures and generalize operations Unable to understand scanning methods Unable to build abstract symbol sets to infer selections or choices Unable to reproduce a sequence of operational tasks
Problem-solving deficits	Unable to operate device because of a hardware or software procedure problem Unable to use software or hardware rules to back out of an operation Unable to use device prompts or cues to accomplish task Unable to sequence steps to complete computer commands

From Church G, Glennen S: The Handbook of Assistive Technology. San Diego, Singular Publishing, 1992.

TABLE 23–4 Motor Factors That Affect Assistive Technology Interventions

Motor Factors	Impact on Use of Technology
Voluntary motor deficits	Inability to make deliberate switch and keyboard selections Limited control of trunk and extremities during movement Eye twitching resulting in overshooting the mark when reaching for objects Limited ability to produce speech communication
Fixed-posture and positioning deficits	Limited hand positioning and stabilization for access to assistive and peripheral devices
Recurring purposeless motion	Accidental triggering of switches and keys Limited fine motor control in isolating symbol, key, and button selections
Motor paralysis	Changes in muscle tone interfere with motor movements Spastic movements result in poor control and accidental selections Limited movement of arm, face, or leg that limits access to keyboard or mouse
Low muscle tone	Loss of balanced muscle control in extremity for selection and stability
Rigidity	Inhibits arm and leg movements and good positioning
Spasticity	Limits full range of motion Reduces accurate and consistent motor movements for switch, key, and button selection
Tremors	Inhibits the precision of fine and gross motor precision selection tasks

From Church G, Glennen S: The Handbook of Assistive Technology. San Diego, Singular Publishing, 1992.

COMPUTER ADAPTATIONS

Computer systems consist of hardware (the actual computer plus the monitor, printer, and other peripherals) and software (programs such as the operating system, or applications such as word processors or Web browsers). A large range of adaptations is now available for individuals with disabilities who have difficulty using a computer. It is possible to get information in and out of a computer in a number of ways. Many different types of computers are available, from personal computers to minicomputers and mainframe computers. Most personal computers now use graphical user interfaces (such as the Macintosh or Microsoft Windows user interfaces). All of these factors contribute to the decision to use a given solution over another. This section focuses on personal computer solutions and adaptations for input and output (Table 23–5).

Positioning

One of the first areas to evaluate is positioning of the individual and the computer equipment. Ergonomically designed office chairs, footrests, arm supports, and wrist rests can help positioning so that equipment is more easily accessed. Devices such as keyboard trays, copy holders, monitor arms, and printer stands can all help to make access easier. Many of these devices are available from computer and stationery stores; and when used properly, this type of equipment can help to prevent computer-related disabilities, such as repetitive stress syndromes. Proper prescription and use is crucial to ensuring that the equipment is appropriate. An ergonomist or occupational therapist can be helpful in selecting the proper equipment and assisting with its appropriate setup and use.

Keyboard Accommodations

It is preferable to access equipment in the standard way, as it was designed to be accessed, but traditional input devices and methods can be difficult or impossible for persons with disabilities to use. The QWERTY keyboard (named for the letter arrangement of the top left-hand row of keys) works very well for people with ten working fingers, but can severely slow down a person who types using a single hand, or even a single finger. Fortunately, a number of strategies and devices have been developed to accommodate persons with disabilities.

TABLE 23–5 Common Adapted Computer Input and Output Hardware and Software

Alternative computer keyboard	Braille input devices
Braille translation	Braille printers/embossers
Computer keyboard enhancers	CD-ROM
Digitizers	Environmental control unit (ECU)
Expanded keyboards	Facsimile machines
Graphical user interface (GUI)	Keyguards
Keyboard emulators	Large-print software
Magnified CRT displays	Morse code input
Mouse/trackball input	Optical character recognition (OCR)
Refreshable Braille displays	Screen reader software
Signaling systems	Speech synthesizers
Speech recognition	Speech amplification
Telephone amplifiers	Telephone device for the deaf (TDD)
Touch screens	Word prediction software

Free software packages have been built into both the Macintosh and Windows operating systems that modify the way the keyboard responds (e.g., delaying the automatic repeat, or permitting one-finger typists to press the shift key sequentially rather than simultaneously when capitalizing). It is now fairly simple to change the keyboard layout from QWERTY to one that is designed to facilitate typing by one-hand typists.

Keyboards come in a variety of sizes and shapes, key type, and layout. Many different keyboards are available for individuals who cannot use the standard keyboard. Mini-keyboards are available for individuals whose range or strength is limited. Expanded keyboards can be obtained for individuals who lack fine motor control. Membrane keyboards (similar to those found on microwave ovens and ATM machines) enable the typist to slide the hand across other keys without causing unwanted keystrokes. Keyboards with different layouts can facilitate typing for one-hand or one-finger typists. Keyboards that take advantage of an individual's present keyboarding skills, such as a Braille keyboard, are also available. When access cannot be accomplished through a keyboard, an alternative form of access may be successful (see Fig. 23–1).

Alternative Access

Alternative access methods range from selection of characters from scanning arrays or inputting dots and dashes in Morse code via switches to using actual voice input. But these alternative methods are more complex to set up and harder to learn because they usually require additional hardware and software.

Switches have been designed to capture virtually any movement that a person can make. Developers have created hardware and software able to translate switch closures into keystrokes or mouse movements that can be used to operate the computer. Switches can be activated by the head, hands, feet, or even eye movements. Switches are used to provide input to a computer in one of two ways. The first involves scanning, in which the person uses a switch to make selections from an array of characters. Scanning can allow severely physically disabled persons to use computers, even if only able to access a single switch. Switches can also be used to send coded input to the computer. For example, switches can be used to send Morse code, which the computer translates into letters and numbers.

Technology such as optical character recognition (OCR), voice input systems, and handwriting recognition can also be used to provide input to computers. With OCR, the computer is programmed to recognize printed material and to convert the printed text into information the computer can understand. OCR involves using a scanner to "take a picture" of the printed page, then using software that recognizes the picture as letters and numbers. OCR is often limited to certain typefaces and font sizes. Computer systems that can be trained to recognize an individual's handwriting are becoming more common, with handwriting recognition being built into hand-held computers called personal digital assistants (PDAs). Voice input systems allow persons to dictate into the computer. The computer is "trained" to recognize a sound and to provide a word or computer action in response. These systems can be trained to understand tens of thousands of words. But the computer is not nearly as good at "recognition" as the human brain. Computers can only match to a pattern, and typically have difficulties if the pattern is varied (e.g., if a word is spoken more softly, or loudly, or at a different rate). People are able to understand spoken and written information even if a substantial portion is missing because they can "fill in the blanks" by using content or emotion cues. While voice recognition technology is rapidly improving, these solutions are inherently complex, and can require significantly more training, setup, and support time.

Word prediction software can assist a user in recognizing and predicting keystrokes, building on a dictionary of words and phrases. This can speed up the entry process and enable the user to communicate more rapidly. Abbreviation expansion or macro capability allows the user to retrieve a sentence or phrase with only a few representative keystrokes.

Mouse Substitution and Emulation

A mouse is the standard way to access a graphical user interface (GUI). Programs, commands, and document files are represented on the screen by pictures, or icons. The user opens documents and runs programs by using the mouse to move the cursor around the screen. The point-and-click, icon-based Windows and Macintosh OS interfaces are examples of GUIs. The GUI makes learning to use a computer easier for most people. If an individual has difficulty using a mouse, access to the computer might be limited were it not for the availability of mouse substitution or emulation.

A wide variety of commercially available mouse "pointing" devices have been designed as alternatives to the traditional mouse. For example, a trackball is like an upside-down mouse. Instead of moving the mouse around the desktop, the user moves just the ball, which rotates in a stationary holder. The trackball can be set in different positions to improve access, allowing the foot or even the chin to operate it. Trackballs are inexpensive adaptations that are 100% compatible and are available in local computer stores. Another such device is a track pad. There are also inductive or pressure-sensitive tablets that detect movements without any moving parts. Other solutions include digitizers, touch screens, and head pointers. *Digitizers* are position-sensitive tablets on which the user provides input by using a stylus or puck. *Touch screens* are see-through, pressure-sensitive mats that fit over the monitor and allow direct pressure to activate the desired area of the screen. *Head pointing* is an emulation; it employs sensors to track the user's head position and translates the head movements to pointer positions. Digitizers, touch screens, and head pointers are more technologically complex and expensive and require additional training and support.

Keyboard Equivalents

Many programs (especially those written for the Windows operating environment) have equivalent keystrokes for every mouse command. For example, one way to print a document might be to select "print" from the "file" menu of a GUI. The user points to and clicks on "file," causing a menu to drop down. Pointing to and clicking on "print" then initiates the print process. Alternatively, there is often a keyboard equivalent to using the mouse to point and click, such as pressing the "shift" and "F10" keys simultaneously. The Windows operating system has an extensive set of keyboard equivalents for actions commonly completed using the mouse. Built into both the Macintosh and Windows operating systems is MouseKeys, a feature that allows the user to directly control the movement and clicking of the mouse through the keyboard, eliminating the need for a separate mouse altogether.

Output Accommodations

Just as the keyboard and the mouse are the traditional input devices for the computer, the cathode ray tube (CRT), or monitor, and the printer are the traditional output devices. Although a variety of printers and monitors are on the market, they are visual devices, rendering them largely unusable by individuals with visual deficits. As the software industry has moved to the GUI as the industry standard, the need to comprehend visual information has become more important.

Visual limitations can sometimes be accommodated by the use of a larger monitor. Most off-the-shelf monitor screens measure 13 to 15 inches diagonally. Computer monitors as large as 21 to 25 inches can be purchased, but they can be more expensive. Monitor prices appear to be dropping, a trend that could make the use of a larger monitor a more realistic possibility for more people. Flat screen computer display technology is also becoming more affordable, and many people find these, large, clear displays easier to read. Built into the latest versions of the Macintosh and Windows operating systems is the ability to custom-tailor the default text size and the default background and text colors. There are even several "standard" high- and reversed-contrast setups for people to use.

Magnifying lenses can be attached to the front of screens to enlarge the output, but the amount of magnification that they provide is usually limited. Programs that enlarge a portion of the screen to full screen size can be utilized. These programs can enlarge portions of the screen 12 to 15 times normal, but display just one section at a time. This is akin to looking at the monitor through a drinking straw: to see the whole screen, the user must move the straw across the screen, then put the pieces together. Screen readers can be used to supplement visual information. A screen reader consists of a speech synthesizer and software that converts text on the screen into audible speech. Many individuals with visual deficits use screen readers as their sole source of feedback from the computer.

When a screen reader is to be used with a GUI, the graphical information must be converted into text that the speech synthesizer will recognize. For example, when an individual using a screen reader encounters an icon on the screen, several pieces of information are needed—information that a seeing person would get visually, including the type of icon (e.g., program, document, or system file) and the file name. Screen reader packages are designed to speak this "visual" information.

Printers

The main differences among printers are speed and print quality, and the ability to print in color. Individuals using printers often have problems in seeing the printed page or in managing the paper. The most common problem is difficulty loading the paper into the printer or unloading the finished pages. Paper-loading problems can be minimized with a printer that uses continuous-feed paper. Pullout trays and top-feed printers might be considered. Regular paper printouts can be difficult or impossible to read for individuals with visual limitations. Printing in a larger font can be a simple adaptation. For those who read Braille, there are Braille printer embossers. Some Braille printers have the capability to produce tactile graphics. If printer noise (especially from dot matrix or Braille printers) is an issue, dome covers or insulated tiles can be used to provide a sound barrier.

COMMUNICATION TECHNOLOGIES

Augmentative Communication

Many individuals have difficulty communicating verbally. For example, persons with cerebral palsy, neuromuscular disease, traumatic brain injury, or stroke can have difficulty producing speech. Communication boards that have words, letters, or pictures are a common method for communicating basic needs. For many speech-impaired individuals, however, these manual communication boards are insufficient. The advent of computer technology has made possible the creation of electronic augmentative or alternative communication systems (AACs). These systems which have the ability to produce spoken output and are available in a wide variety of configurations. Augmentative communication devices have developed rapidly. Since the late 1980s, more than 250 augmentative communication hardware and software items have become available. Sophisticated AAC systems can offer speech synthesis in up to ten age- and gender-appropriate voices and foreign languages. These offer access by touch, pointer, switch, and scanning, or even by ocular eyegaze monitors that electronically measure eye movements.[13]

Systems can be further customized to ensure they meet the unique needs and abilities of the user. For example, AAC systems for children can teach communication through play. Games, bedtime stories, prayers, descriptive concepts, basic math, and core vocabulary programs make learning and communicating fun. A developmentally delayed individual who doesn't read or write can have a picture-based system—one that generates unique phrases and sentences, even though the individual can't read them. Stephen Hawking, who has a form of amyotrophic lateral sclerosis, dictated his best-selling book *A Brief History of Time* through a personal computer adapted for single-switch scanning access with speech output through a speech synthesizer.

AAC technology is complex, and evaluating a nonverbal individual for a communication system has become equally complex. The individual's expressive language skills, receptive language skills, symbol recognition skills, sequencing, and functional abilities to access the technology, all must be evaluated to ensure an appropriate match between the person and the device. These evaluations are generally performed by speech and language pathologists with expertise in AAC.

Telecommunications

Telephone devices for the deaf (TDD) enable individuals who are hearing-impaired, deaf, or speech-impaired to communicate by telephone. The TDD utilizes a QWERTY keyboard. The message is typed in and displayed on an LED screen while being transmitted over the telephone lines. A Braille version is available for individuals who have both severe hearing and visual impairment. Computers with PC/TDD modems are also used as a means of communication. Conversations are typed in and responses are received on the computer screen.

Environmental Controls

An environmental control system allows an individual with functional or sensory disabilities to independently control the immediate surroundings. These systems typically utilize a set of modules that plug into standard electrical outlets and can be used to operate lights or television, initiate or answer telephone calls, and unlock doors. Even for the able-bodied, environmental control units (ECUs) are becoming familiar as tools for enhancing security (e.g., light-activated daylight sensors, movement and noise sensors). For an individual with a disability, an ECU can confer a sense of freedom, independence, and security. They can activate radios and televisions, electric beds, thermostats, and telephones, and they offer a lifeline to emergency response teams. ECUs can be activated through a range of access strategies, from voice input to touch. ECU technology ranges from the simple, commercially available remote control for switching lights on and off to a fully functional "smart house." The computerized house is controlled by a central processing unit that monitors the complete environment. It regulates the thermostats in each room for energy saving and monitors the children at play outside or visitors at the door. By means of strategically placed sensors, the system alerts home owners to such hazards as stove burners that have been left on, and continuously monitors the exterior to ensure security.

FUNDING FOR COMPUTER ASSISTIVE DEVICES

Despite the federal mandates for comprehensive consumer-responsive assistive technology and technology-related services, obtaining such devices and services remains an arduous task both for the individual user and for the professional. The physician can facilitate the funding process by providing sufficient clinical information to support the written justification for financing computer-related technologies. The rehabilitation team should begin gathering funding information during the evaluation process, and should determine how much funding is required. It is critical to include adequate funds to cover any necessary installation costs, training fees, and service contracts.

The team should ensure that appropriate language is utilized in writing the justification. For example, if educational funding sources are requested, the justification should reflect that the equipment will assist the individual in scholastic endeavors. Medicaid requires that the equipment be deemed "medically necessary." If a vocational rehabilitation agency is to be approached for funding, the justification should clearly express that the equipment is work-related. If an employer is to be approached, the justification should describe how the recommended equipment relates to the essential functions of the job. Under the Americans with Disabilities Act, reasonable accommodations are required in the workplace for qualified individuals with disabilities. Although no direct funding is available under the Act, companies have various tax relief options available for the purchase of equipment and other barrier removal activities. Table 23–6 lists some of the funding sources that might be appropriate for your patient. Private funding sources should also be investigated. The family may need to consider its own resources, since a mix-and-match approach is often necessary to obtain all of the required funding. Private medical insurance can be approached, as can advocacy agencies (such as the National Easter Seal Society or the Muscular Dystrophy Association) and community groups (such as the Lions Club or Rotary Club). Corporations and private foundations may help, but should usually be considered only as a last resort.

SUMMARY/FUTURE TECHNOLOGIES

The field of computers and computing is evolving rapidly, and the next five years should see dramatic changes. One trend is patently obvious: computers will continue to get faster, smaller, and cheaper. New computers will offer built-in features, such as speech recognition, and will have increased storage capacity that allows them to handle sophisticated software more easily. Described briefly below are some of the technological advances that are emerging.

Computers and information appliances will be connected to each other in a wireless fashion. The new Java ring from Sun Microsystems, a piece of jewelry with a powerful built-in minicomputer, can be used as a digital key to open a door or log on to a computer with the appropriate software and current encryption technology. Credit card-sized disks that slip into one's pocket will allow access to information anywhere in the world. The development of knowledge-based systems reflecting a general trend in information management is gaining momentum. These expert systems "jog" one along the decision-making path, whether it is in diagnostic medicine or computing tax returns.

Virtual technologies are becoming commonplace for training and recreation and will be a routine part of simulation for all kinds of planning and product design. Libraries are gradually becoming virtual. Digital books can be downloaded to a small flat tablet with a touch pad for page turning.

Everything will be "smart," that is, responsive to its external or internal environment, by virtue of embedding microprocessors and sensors in devices or by creating materials that respond to such physical variables as heat light, noise, odors, and the like. Future fabrics will have built-in microprocessors that can cool or heat the body. A shift from mass marketing to one-on-one marketing of technology-driven advances will cause a paradigm shift in the design, production, development, and

TABLE 23–6 Funding Sources for Assistive Technology

Public Programs	Alternative Financing	U.S. Tax Code
Medicare	Private insurance	Medical care expense deduction
Medicaid	Private foundations	Business deductions
Individuals with Disabilities Education Act (IDEA)	Employee accommodation programs	ADA credit for small business
State grants—vocational rehabilitation	Corporate-sponsored loans	Targeted jobs tax credit
The Developmental Disabilities State grants	Community groups	Charitable contributions deduction
CHAMPUS	Religious organizations	
Workers' Compensation programs	Service clubs	
The Technology Related Assistance programs	Advocacy organizations	
Social Security Administration—PASS Program	Family/friends	
Veterans benefits		

delivery of programs, products, and services. In the design of many commercial products such as homes, furnishings, and vehicles, the customer will participate directly with the specialist in the design. Customized products will dominate large parts of the manufacturing market. Manufacturers will offer customers unlimited variety in their products.

By 2015 there will be an Electronic Global Village based on a worldwide, broadband network utilizing high-speed fiberoptics. Face-to-face, voice-to-voice, and data-to-data communication will be available to any place at any time. Voting and more frequent referenda will be on-line in all advanced nations. Networked schools will emerge. As schools around the world get "wired," we will see increased cooperation among schools around the globe. For example, native speakers will teach language classes via videophone.

As these new technologies and information systems evolve, the needs of all people with all types, degrees, and combinations of disabilities must be kept in mind. As wonderful as these new technologies can potentially be, their use may create new barriers. Computers are rarely, if ever, a solution in and of themselves. We must remember that the computer is a tool; and if that tool is applied appropriately, it can enhance all our lives.

REFERENCES

1. Bain B, Ledger D (eds): Assistive technology: An interdisciplinary approach. New York, Churchill Livingstone, 1997.
2. Behrman M, Lahm E: Babies and robots: Technology to assist learning. Rehabilitation literature 1984; 45(7):194–201.
3. Bradley M: Computers for the very young: From the ridiculous to the sublime. Closing the Gap 1991; 13(2):15.
4. Church G, Glennen S: The Handbook of Assistive Technology. San Diego, Singular Publishing Group, 1992.
5. Coombs N: Using distance education technologies to overcome physical disabilities. In Mason R, Kaye A (eds): Mindweave: Communication, computers and distance education. New York, Pergamon Press, 1988.
6. Galvin J, Scherer M: Evaluating, selecting and using appropriate assistive technology. Gaithersburg, MD, Aspen Publishers, 1996.
7. Galvin J, Barnicle K, Perr A: Evaluating and choosing assistive technology. Proceedings of the Technology and People with Disabilities Conference. Northridge, California State University, 1992.
8. LaPlante M, Rendershot G, Moss A: Assistive technology devices and home accessibility features: Prevalence, payment, needs and trends. Advance data from Vital and Health Statistics, no. 217. Hyattsville, MD, National Center for Health Statistics, 1992.
9. Mann W, Lane J: Assistive technology for persons with disabilities, ed 2. Bethesda, MD, American Occupational Therapy Association, 1995.
10. Mueller J: The Workplace Workbook 2.0: An Illustrated Guide to Workplace Accommodation and Technology. McLean, VA, HRD Press, 1992.
11. Scadden L: Technology: Training awareness and needs. In Penman LG, Hansen CE (eds): Technology and Employment of Persons with Disabilities: A Report of the Mary E. Switzer Memorial Seminar. Alexandria, VA, National Rehabilitation Association, 1989.
12. Scherer MJ: Living in a State of Stuck: How Assistive Technologies Affect the Lives of People with Disabilities. Cambridge, MA, Brook-line Books, 1996.
13. Vanderheiden G, Lloyd LL: Communication systems and their components. In Blackstone S, Ruskin D (eds): Augmentative Communication: An Introduction. Rockville, MD, ASHA Press, 1986.
14. Vanderheiden G: Computer access and use by people with disabilities. In Galvin J, Scherer M (eds): Evaluating, selecting and using appropriate assistive technology. Gaithersburg, MD, Aspen Publishers, 1996.
15. Vitali A: Interactive technologies. In Galvin J, Scherer M (eds): Evaluating, selecting and using appropriate assistive technology. Gaithersburg, MD, Aspen Publishers, 1996.
16. Wilds ML: Effective use of technology with young children. NICHY News Digest 1989; 13:6–7.

PRINT RESOURCES

American Medical Association: Primary Care for Persons with Disabilities: Guidelines for the Use of Assistive Technology. Evaluation, Referral, Prescription. Chicago, AMA, 1994. (AMA Department of Geriatric Health (312) 464-5085.)

Bower K, Vanderheiden G, Sheikh N: Trace Resource Book: Assistive Technologies for Communication, Control and Computer Access, 1998/9 ed. Madison, WI, Trace R&D Center, 1998.

Church G, Glennen S: The Handbook of Assistive Technology. San Diego, Singular Publishing Group, 1992.

Galvin J, Scherer M: Evaluating, selecting and using appropriate assistive technology. Gaithersburg, MD, Aspen Publishers, 1996.

Lazzaro J: Adaptive Technologies for Learning and Work Environments. Chicago, American Library Association, 1993.

Mueller J: The Workplace Workbook 2.0: An Illustrated Guide to Workplace Accommodation and Technology. McLean, VA, HRD Press, 1992.

The Alliance for Technology Access: Computer Resources for People with Disabilities. Alameda, CA, Hunter House, 1997.

WEB SITES

Trace Research and Development Center. One of the most comprehensive resources on computer access.
http://trace.wisc.edu/

Apple—the disability connection. Apple computer's worldwide disabilities solutions group web site.
http://www2.apple.com/disability/message.html

Home page of DO-IT program at the University of Washington. One of the best and most complete disability and technology-related web sites.
http://www.disability.com

The Job Accommodation Network (JAN). Exceptional resource for reasonable accommodations in the workplace.
http://janweb.icdi.wvu.edu/kinder/

Computer Access Center. Good resource for computer access.
http://www.cac.org/

ABLEDATA. This site lists more than 22,000 assistive technology devices.
http://www.abledata.com/index.htm

University of Kansas. Excellent resources on assistive technology for the computer user with disabilities, and other links.
http://www.sped.ukans.edu/speddisabilitiesstuff/univs.html

Microsoft
http://www.microsoft.com/enable/microsoft.htm

Augmentative and Alternative Communication Journal.
http://aac.unl.edu/AACtabcon.html

American Foundation for the Blind. Good resource for a wide range of assistive technologies for children and adults who are blind or visually impaired.
http://www.afb.org/afb

RESNA (Rehabilitation Engineering and Assistive Technology Society of North America). Excellent resource for identifying assistive technology practitioners and rehabilitation engineers.
http://www.resna.org

Project EASI: Equal access to Software and Information. Excellent resource for individuals who are blind or visually impaired.
http://www.rit.edu/~easi

Spinal Cord Injury Association. Excellent Web page on disability related issues with many links.
http://www.spinalcord.org

24 CHAPTER

John J. Nicholas, M.D., and Ted A. Lennard, M.D.

Joint and Soft Tissue Injection Techniques

The modern era of therapeutic joint injections began with Joseph Lee Hollander in the 1940s. Hollander, however, credited George Thorn with first injecting hydroxycorticosterone (17-hydroxycorticosterone) into the inflamed knee joints of patients with rheumatoid arthritis (RA), osteoarthritis, sprained knee, acute gouty arthritis, disseminated lupus erythematosus, Sjögren's syndrome, subdeltoid bursitis, and olecranon and prepatellar bursitis. Hollander and colleagues[42] subsequently reported injecting hydrocortisone acetate, 25 to 37.5 mg, into the joints of 69 patients. In six of seven cases in which measurements were made, the total synovial cell count fell by 50%, and the temperature within the joint fell in all seven cases. In a subsequent report, Hollander described postinjection flare, aseptic necrosis of weight-bearing joints, and a frequency of infection of 1 in 15,000 injections.[41] Overall, he reported on a total of 250,000 injections in 8000 patients.

INTRA-ARTICULAR INJECTIONS

Benefits

Many authors have described the effectiveness of intra-articular (IA) steroid injections for patients with inflammatory arthritis. For example, in 1962 Stolzer et al[81] described 2360 injections in 589 patients. Pain relief occurred in 97%, and there were no infections. Flanagan et al[27] in 1988 described injections of triamcinolone under fluoroscopic control into the hip joints of British patients awaiting total hip replacement. Those injected with triamcinolone obtained greater relief than those injected with bupivacaine or saline. At 1 month, nine patients had improved, one was unchanged, and two were worse. In addition to pain relief, it was asserted that function and strength were improved in muscles surrounding the injected joints. Geborek et al[29] in 1990 reported the results of IA injection into 11 knee joints in seven patients. They noted that extensor muscle torque had increased, range of motion had improved, and knee circumference had diminished when measured 7 and 14 days after injection. They also noted that removal of synovial fluid alone increased extensor muscle torque.

It has even been suggested that the benefits of the longer-acting steroid preparations have been so successful that the frequency of surgical synovectomy has decreased.[10] Stefanich[78] in 1986 reviewed the effects and complications of IA steroid injections.

Indications

The reason for injecting joints is that IA steroids decrease inflammation. Any inflamed joint is a candidate for injection, provided there is no joint infection or other contraindication. The use of IA steroids in osteoarthritis (minimally inflamed joints) has been debated.[67] The current consensus is that patients with osteoarthritis should undergo a trial of IA steroid injections. IA injections should be utilized along with all other appropriate treatments. Only rarely do they constitute the only treatment method.

Precautions

IA injection precautions include avoiding joint infections.[4] It has been asserted, however, that little additional damage occurs when an infected joint is injected with steroids, although the discovery of the infection can be delayed for 24 to 48 hours.[85] The infection might be accelerated in some cases. Proper technique diminishes the small likelihood of infecting the joint at the time of IA injection.

Many authors suggest an injection of a mixture of anesthetic and steroid. Using the steroid only has the advantage of the physician's knowing the exact site of the needle tip and being able to ascertain the location of the injection. The diffusion of a local anesthetic agent into the surrounding tissue can obscure the exact site of the needle tip. There seems to be relatively little advantage to the inclusion of anesthesia for joint or soft tissue injection as it provides at most only temporary relief of symptoms.

It is not clear whether injecting the joint is beneficial to patients with a hemarthrosis. The injection of a joint in a patient taking an anticoagulant or who has a bleeding disease must be done very carefully and only after a discussion of the potential harm or benefit with the hematologist or other physician managing the anticoagulation.[83] Adjacent skin infections can be a hazard and should be avoided at sites of IA injection. IA injection in immunocompromised patients should be performed only after consultation with the attending physician.

It is generally held that no more than three or four injections should be made in the same joint in any 12-month period, in order to avoid cartilage damage or infection.[68, 69]

Chatham has described an interesting study in which 30 patients with RA were divided into those rested for 48 hours after joint injection and those who were not rested.[16] The results suggest that there is no symptom difference at 48 hours between those rested and those not rested after the injection. However, Chakravarty et al[13] recently demonstrated that 1 day of complete bed rest following knee injection resulted in better walking time, improved CRP, less perceived pain and perceived stiffness, and a greater reduction in knee circumference than in those who did not rest.

Preparations

Many steroid preparations are available for joint injections. The choice in a particular case depends on associated complications and the intent of the treating physician. The preparation chosen must be designated "for intra-articular use." The preparations vary in strength, concentration, and duration of effect (Table 24–1).[6] Currently available preparations include the following:

Methylprednisolone acetate (Depo-Medrol, Pharmacia-Upjohn), IA, 40 and 80 mg/mL
Triamcinolone acetonide (Kenalog, Bristol-Myers Squibb), IA, 40 mg/mL
Triamcinolone hexacetonide (Aristospan, Fuzisawa), IA, 20 mg/mL
Betamethasone sodium phosphate and acetate (Celestone Soluspan, Schering), IA, 6 mg/mL

Blyth et al[7] recently demonstrated that triamcinolone hexacetonide provides greater pain relief than triamcinolone acetonide in RA patients.

Strength

The contents of a 1.0-mL vial of any of the above preparations can be injected into a joint cavity. Larger doses have been suggested for larger joints and smaller doses for smaller joints, but there are no data to substantiate the efficacy of this practice. It is important that a new and never previously used, single vial be used, to eliminate the possibility of contamination from previous withdrawal of steroid or anesthetic from the vial. It has not been shown that there are harmful side effects directly from any dose contained in a single 1.0-mL dose vial.

TABLE 24–1 Relative Strengths of Steroids

Duration of Action	Equivalent Glucocorticoid Dose (mg)	Glucocorticoid Potency
Short-acting		
Cortisone	25.0	0.8
Hydrocortisone	20.0	1.0
Prednisone	5.0	4.0
Prednisolone	5.0	4.0
Methylprednisolone	4.0	5.0
Intermediate-acting		
Triamcinolone	4.0	5.0
Long-acting		
Dexamethasone	0.75	30.0
Betamethasone	0.6	25.0

New Preparations

The results of current trials with IA preparations of hyaluronic acid have suggested some efficacy for use in human arthritis. Hyalgan (sodium hyaluronate) and Synvisc (hylan G-F 20) have been approved by the Food and Drug Administration (FDA) for use in patients with osteoarthritis of the knee.[59] The drugs have been studied mainly in animals[11, 28, 60, 70, 75] and in patients outside the United States.[2, 45, 53, 55, 89]

Technique

The "no-touch" technique described by Hasselbacher[38] is strongly recommended. With this technique, no drapes or sterile room are required, but universal precautions require wearing gloves to prevent contact with bloodborne pathogens.

The first step is for the operator to select the site of injection through the skin. The injection site is chosen based on available bony landmarks. Bony landmarks are usually quite stable, while soft tissue landmarks can vary from patient to patient and from time to time. Once the site has been chosen, it is carefully outlined with a marker, usually with a circle (as a target) at least 3 cm in diameter. A larger field is not required. After the site has been outlined with a marker, a common technique is to clean the area with three swipes of Betadine (povidone-iodine) and one swipe of alcohol, taking care not to remove the landmarks.[76] Hasselbacher[38] recommends that "the patient's skin should not be touched with the bare finger after preparation. Identification of landmarks with ink, or impressions made on the skin with a pointed object before cleaning, will facilitate recognition of the aspiration site." There are other techniques of skin preparation, but this one is well accepted.[26] A 25-gauge needle is used to inject an anesthetic into the epidermis, producing a skin wheal. After waiting 30 to 60 seconds to allow for the anesthetic effect, the operator places a 1.5-inch (3.8-cm), 21-gauge needle on the syringe filled with anesthetic and enters the skin through the wheal. The patient should not feel pain at needle entry. The operator should stop and aspirate every 0.5 cm, and inject another small bolus of anesthetic agent. The patient should not perceive undue pain and should remain relaxed during the procedure. When the joint capsule is entered, the patient will experience some discomfort, but injection of additional anesthetic should eliminate this. When the joint has been entered, the hub of the needle should be clasped with a hemostat, the syringe with anesthetic removed, and an aspirating syringe, or series of aspirating and injecting syringes, applied. If the hub of the needle is grasped for syringe exchange with the fingers, inevitably the needle shaft will be touched by the operator and contaminated and then thrust back under the skin. The hemostat is cleaner and more secure. If these precautions and equipment are used, the only likely source of contamination would be the vials of anesthetic agent or steroid.

Once the joint is entered, the color and consistency of the synovial fluid are observed and a sample is removed for laboratory analysis. Examination should be performed promptly,[48] and the sample should be sent to the laboratory for white blood cell (WBC) count and polarized light microscopic examination. Evaluation for the presence or absence of crystals and Gram's stain and culture for the presence of bacteria should be performed if indicated. The operator should determine, by letting a drop of fluid drip from the end of the syringe or by palpating a sample between the fingertips, whether there is a normal consistency and viscosity to the fluid. Normal synovial fluid will stretch approximately 2.5 cm between the fingertips. The WBC count of the fluid can be estimated by attempting to read 0.25-inch print through a standard test tube of the fluid. If the print can be read, the fluid is probably noninflammatory. If the print cannot be read, it likely indicates inflammation or infection. Additional tests, including tests for rheumatoid factor, complement, and albumin, protein electrophoresis, and glucose level determination, have not been shown to help in the diagnosis of the patient's condition or to determine whether or not the sample is infected.[73]

There are few articles describing infections following joint injections. The senior author's experience is limited to a knowledge of only three joint infections in many years of practice. Each of these joints was injected with multiple punctures through the skin in an effort to obtain specimens of joint fluid. Multiple skin punctures are to be avoided. If joint fluid is not readily obtained at the first attempt, the needle should be redirected but not removed or pulled out of the skin. The tip of the needle should be pulled out to within a short distance of the skin and then redirected while still under the skin surface.

CHOICE OF SITE

Many articles have described joint injection techniques. Readers are referred to Hendrix et al[39] for a description of injection of the sacroiliac joint. The hip joint is usually injected under fluoroscopic guidance to ensure entrance into the site, especially when no synovial fluid is obtained. The temporomandibular joints are not routinely injected because of their proximity to the facial nerve, artery, and parotid gland. Spinal facet joint injections also require fluoroscopic guidance. Pertinent review articles have been published by Gray and Gottlieb,[34] Samuelson et al,[72] Leversee,[52] and Zuckerman et al.[90] Eustace et al[26] demonstrated, not surprisingly, that shoulder injections are more effective if the steroid is deposited accurately into the shoulder joint and not into the surrounding tissue.

Sternoclavicular Joint

The sternoclavicular joint cannot ordinarily be entered by a needle. The site of the injection is actually on the top or superior aspect of the joint where the clavicle attaches to the sternum. The deposit is made in the subcutaneous tissues adjacent to the joint. The bony surfaces of the sternum and clavicle can be readily palpated (Fig. 24–1A).

Acromioclavicular Joint

The approach is similar to that for the sternoclavicular joint. The injected steroid is deposited superior to the joint, where the clavicle joins the acromion, approximately 12.5 mm (0.5 inch) medial to the tip of the acromion (Fig. 24–1A). The site is readily palpable.

Long Head of the Biceps Tendons

The injection is made at the point of maximum palpable tenderness in the bicipital groove (bony landmark) in the head of the humerus (Fig. 24–1B). No attempt is made to inject the tendon sheath, but the steroid is deposited in immediate proximity to the point of tenderness.

Short Head of the Biceps Tendon

The steroid is injected at the point of greatest tenderness, which is usually right on top of the coracoid process (Fig. 24–1B). The tendon arises from the coracoid process, and clinical inflammation seems maximal at this site (bony landmark).

Shoulder

The bony landmarks are the coracoid process and the head of the humerus (Fig. 24–1A). A site is chosen just lateral to the coracoid process. The joint is entered either between the head of the humerus and the coracoid process or 0.5 cm superior to this site. An injection medial to the coracoid process might result in harm to the brachial plexus, subclavian artery, vein, or lung. The steroid preparation is deposited approximately 1.5 inches (3.8 cm) below the skin surface, after entering directly perpendicular to the skin at the described site. Entrance into the shoulder joint from a posterior approach is less reliable because there are no good bony landmarks.

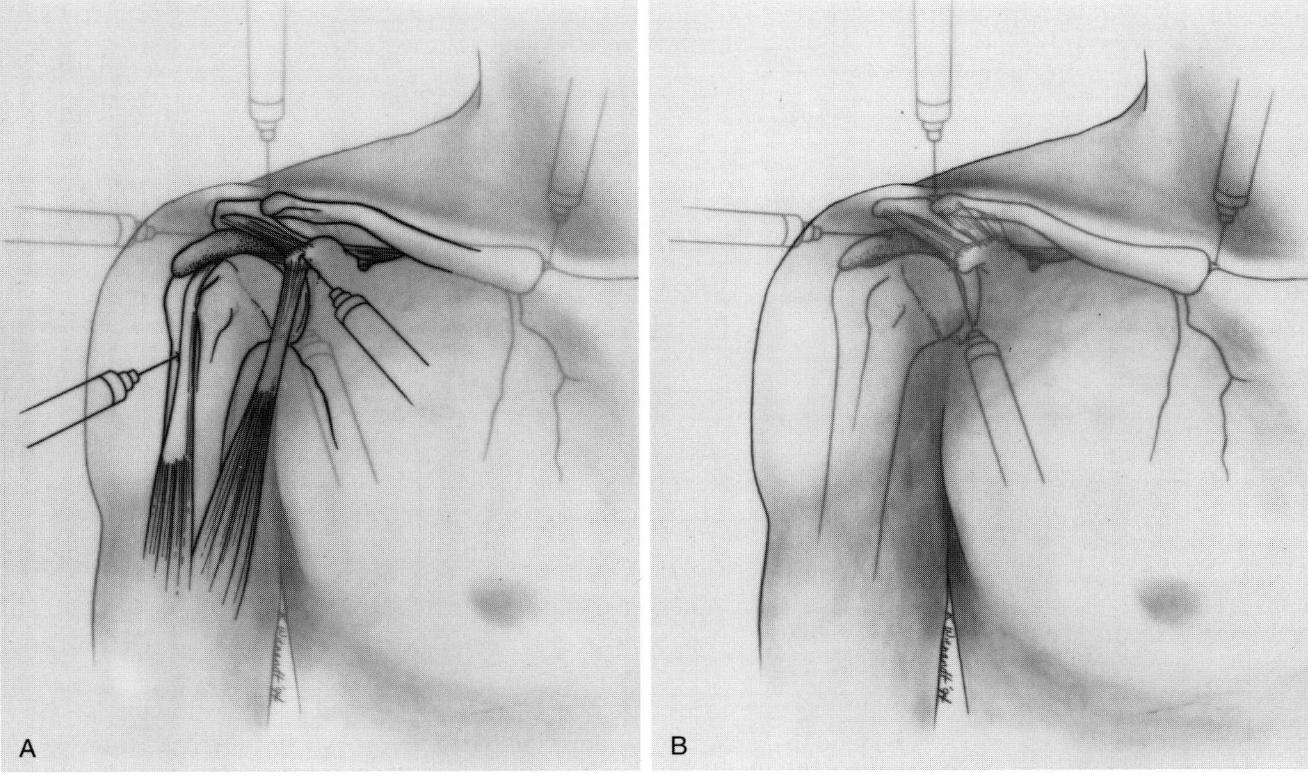

FIGURE 24–1. *A.* It is important to identify the acromioclavicular joint, the acromion, and the coracoid process as bony landmarks to aid joint injection around the shoulder. *B.* The bony bicipital groove can be palpated at the anterior aspect of the humerus.

Subacromial Bursa

The subacromial bursa lies beneath the tip of the acromion (bony landmark), and the steroid is deposited approximately 1.5 cm under the skin beneath the tip of the acromion process and superior to the head of the humerus (Fig. 24–1A).

Supraspinatus Tendon (Impingement Syndrome)

The tendon is approached posteriorly and just beneath the acromio-clavicular joint (bony landmark). There should be no resistance to needle insertion. A tender area will be "discovered" by the point of the injecting needle.

Elbow

The elbow joint can be entered anteriorly, but this approach can present a hazard to the biceps tendon, brachioradialis tendon, median nerve, radial nerve, and branches of the radial artery. A medial approach is to be avoided because of potential ulnar nerve injury, so a lateral site is generally best. The bony landmarks are the olecranon process, the head of the radius, and the lateral epicondyle. These landmarks form a triangle. The joint can be entered just anterior to the center of this triangle and posterior to the head of the radius (Fig. 24–2). If there is considerable synovial fluid, there will be a slight bulge. The needle must be moved toward where the operator estimates the center of the joint to be (much as when performing a spinal tap). There is not much room to maneuver through a bony tunnel at this site, but if bony landmarks are chosen carefully and consistently, good results are obtained.

Olecranon Bursitis

The olecranon bursa overlies the olecranon process of the ulna. The needle is directed into the most fluctuant part of the enlarged bursal sac.

Carpal Joints

The ulnar and radial styloids are the bony landmarks for carpal joint injection. A line connecting these two bony landmarks defines the proximal row of carpal bones. Injections should not be made too far proximally. There are many carpal joints, each with its own synovial cavity. Injections of each should be done at the point of maximal tenderness.

De Quervain's Disease

The tendons of the extensor pollicis brevis and abductor pollicis longus can be located by palpation (Fig. 24–3). The point of injection should be at the site of maximal tenderness. The operator should not attempt to enter

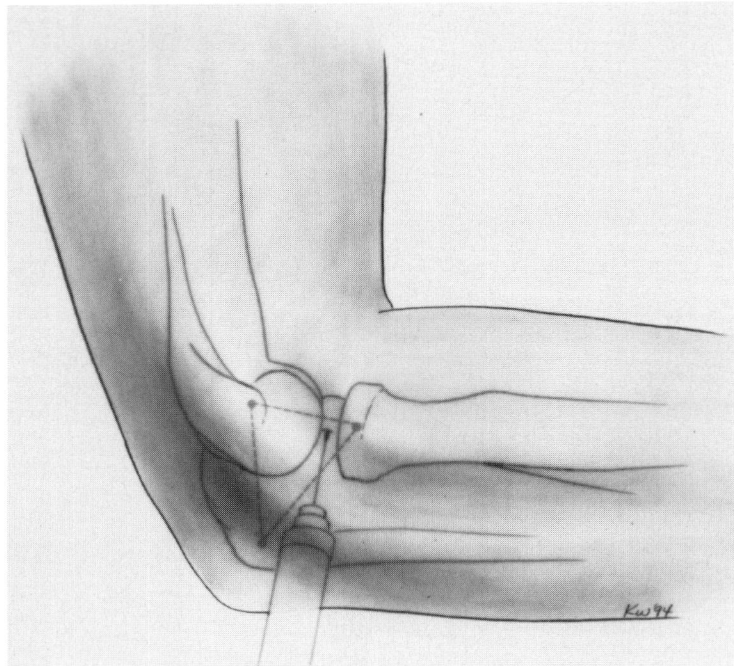

FIGURE 24–2. The site of injection at the elbow lies just inferior and posterior to the head of the radius.

the tendon sheath because of potential tendon damage. The steroid should be deposited subcutaneously in the area of maximal tenderness.

Carpometacarpal Joint of the Thumb

The anatomical snuffbox lies between the abductor pollicis longus and extensor pollicis longus, and the extensor brevis pollicis tendons of the thumb. Osteoarthritis at this site usually results in tenderness on palpation. The operator should inject the steroid at the point of tenderness, approximately 12.5 mm (0.5 inch) below the skin.

Metacarpophalangeal Joint of the Thumb and Fingers

This joint is one of the more difficult joints to inject. When the fist is clenched and the knuckles protrude (bony landmark), the joint can be palpated just *distal* to the apex of the knuckle (Fig. 24–4). It can be readily palpated just beyond the bulge of the knuckle. The joint should be entered with a 25-gauge needle at an angle, not directly laterally or directly superiorly, in order to avoid the digital nerve, artery, vein, and the extensor tendon apparatus on the superior aspect of each digit.

Distal Interphalangeal and Proximal Interphalangeal Joints

These joints cannot readily be entered by a needle, and any effort to do so can result in joint damage. The operator should palpate the bony landmarks in a fashion similar to palpating the bony landmarks of the metacarpophalangeal joints, and then deposit the steroid subcutaneously in the area just beyond the apex of the knuckle

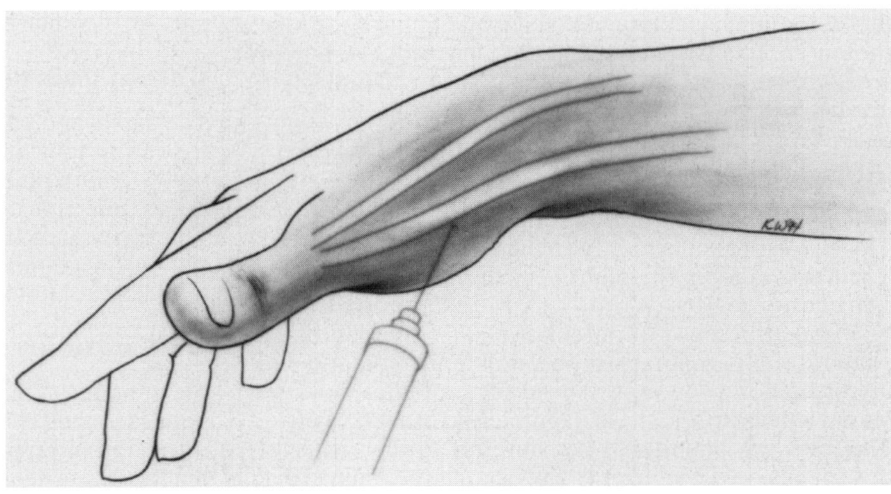

FIGURE 24–3. The tendon of the extensor pollicis brevis can be readily palpated and identified beneath the skin without the aid of a bony landmark.

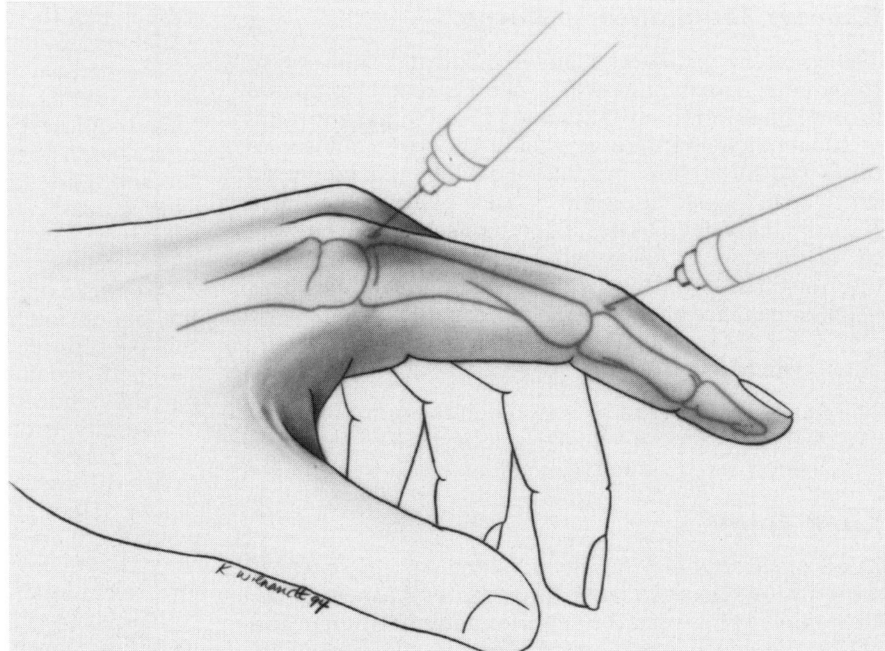

FIGURE 24–4. The metacarpophalangeal joint is more distal than usually thought, just beyond the bony prominence of the distal end of the metacarpal bone (the knuckle).

of the proximal or distal interphalangeal joints. This is where the joint will most likely be, and the medication will get into the joint space.

Carpal Tunnel

The boundaries of the carpal tunnel can be readily determined if the pisiform and trapezoid bones are palpated on the palmar aspect of the proximal hand (bony landmark) (Fig. 24–5). A line connecting these bony landmarks shows the position of the transverse carpal ligament. The median nerve enters the palm just medial (ulnarward) to the trapezoid. The injection is made through the transverse carpal ligament in this area, approximately 6 mm below the surface of the skin. If paresthesias occur due to the needle being on or near the median nerve, the operator should maneuver the needle more laterally and less deep.

An alternative injection technique is to determine the site of the palmaris longus tendon and enter the skin at a point on the radial side of the tendon. The needle should be directed toward the palm of the hand in the hope of entering the carpal tunnel near the site of the median nerve entrapment.

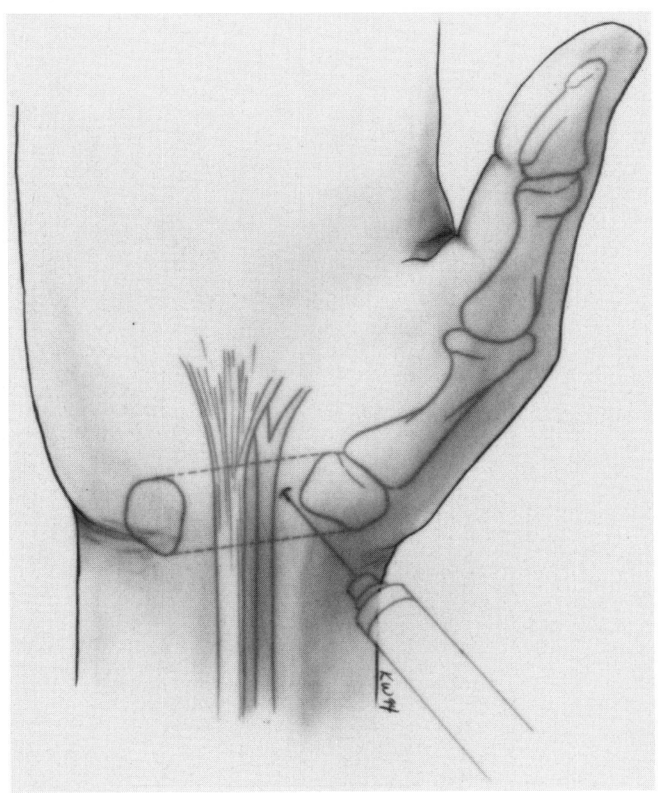

FIGURE 24–5. The boundaries of the carpal tunnel are defined by the pisiform and the trapezoid bones.

Hip Joint

The hip joint is routinely injected only under fluoroscopic control and is beyond the scope of this chapter.

Ischial Bursitis

Inflammation of a bursa inferior to the ischial tuberosity can occur from persistent sitting ("weaver's bottom"). Injection of this bursa is rarely required, but the ischial tuberosity should be palpated and injection made directly into the point of maximum tenderness.

Greater Trochanteric Bursa

The greater trochanteric bursa is located superior to the greater trochanter, which can be readily palpated through the skin (bony landmark) (Fig. 24–6). The point of maximal tenderness is usually superior, but sometimes inferior, to this bony landmark. The skin is entered using a spinal needle in most cases, because the bursa is surprisingly deep. After a depth of several inches, the tip of the needle will touch a tender area superior to but not directly on top of the greater trochanter. This is the site where the steroid should be deposited.

Sacroiliac Joint

The sacroiliac joint can be injected at the point of maximal tenderness, or it can be injected more certainly under fluoroscopic guidance.[39]

Knee Joint

Knee injections are generally performed poorly because most authors describe entering the lateral aspect of the knee midway between the superior and inferior margins of the patella and beneath the patella. There is very little room at this site for the operator to insert a needle between the femur and patella. Commonly the joint surfaces are engaged by the needle, causing the patient to contract the quadriceps muscle in pain and narrow the joint space even further. The recommended procedure is that the operator outline the patella with a pen, and then select a site just superior to the superior margin of the patella on the medial aspect of the knee. This site should be low enough on the medial aspect of the knee to allow direction of the needle below the quadriceps *tendon* (Fig. 24–7). This puts the medication into the suprapatellar pouch, which is contiguous with the synovial cavity. Since it lies below the quadriceps tendon, it can be readily entered without causing undue pain or contraction of the quadriceps muscle.

An alternative method is to inject the knee joint with the patient supine or sitting and the knee flexed. In this procedure, the tibial tubercle and the patella are outlined and are connected with lines to outline the patellar tendon. The needle can be directed medially or laterally just below the superior margin of the patella toward the operator's sense of where the knee joint cavity is located. The joint can be entered without any bony contact. This is an especially advantageous site when there are osteophytes around the patella or when the patient is very obese. The disadvantage of the flexed knee technique is that only rarely can fluid be obtained from this position, apparently because the fluid migrates to a posterior position in the knee during flexion.

"Housemaid's Knee"

Housemaid's knee is an inflammation of the prepatellar bursa. No bony landmarks are needed. The prepatellar bursa can be injected at the site of maximal fullness.

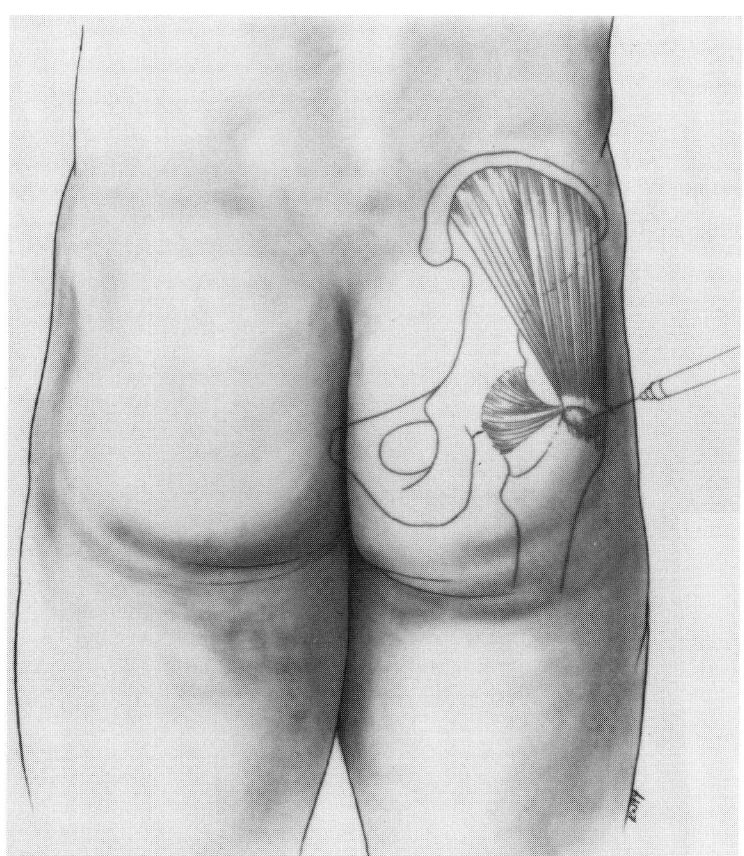

FIGURE 24–6. The bony prominence of the greater trochanter is best palpated with the patient lying on the uninvolved side.

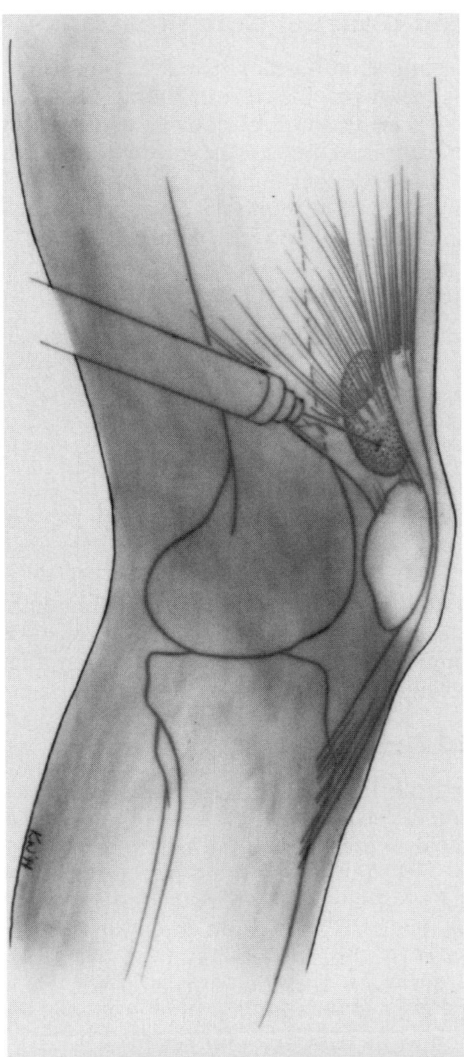

FIGURE 24–7. Palpation of the superior margin of the patella allows the operator to avoid inserting the needle between the patella and the femur.

Anserine Bursa

The anserine bursa is located approximately 5 cm distal to the tibial joint line on the medial aspect of the tibia and somewhat posterior (bony landmark). The site for injection should be determined by palpation. The bursa is often surprisingly deep below the skin, but tenderness to the tip of the needle will indicate the location of the inflamed bursa (Fig. 24–8).

Ankle Joint

The bony landmarks are the medial and lateral malleoli. A line is drawn 1 cm superior to these two structures, joining them. This line outlines the distal end of the tibia (Fig. 24–9). The patient is asked to dorsiflex the foot, and the anterior tibial and extensor communis tendons can be readily identified. The dorsalis pedis artery is beneath these structures. The operator then should select a site on either the medial or lateral aspect of the joint, so that the needle will enter beneath the landmark line at the end of the tibia, but avoiding the tarsal bones and tendinous structures.

Metatarsophalangeal Joints

The metatarsophalangeal joints are injected from the dorsal aspect. Bony landmarks are difficult to find because of the overlying soft tissue. The patient should flex the foot, and the operator should recall that the joint is probably distal to the largest palpable part of the joint. To avoid important structures, the site chosen should not be lateral or superior but between these two planes.

Morton's Neuroma

Morton's neuroma commonly occurs between the distal metatarsal bones of the second and third or third and fourth digits of the foot. The exact site can be determined by palpating the point of maximal tenderness. The preparation is deposited through the skin of the dorsum of the foot into the tender area.

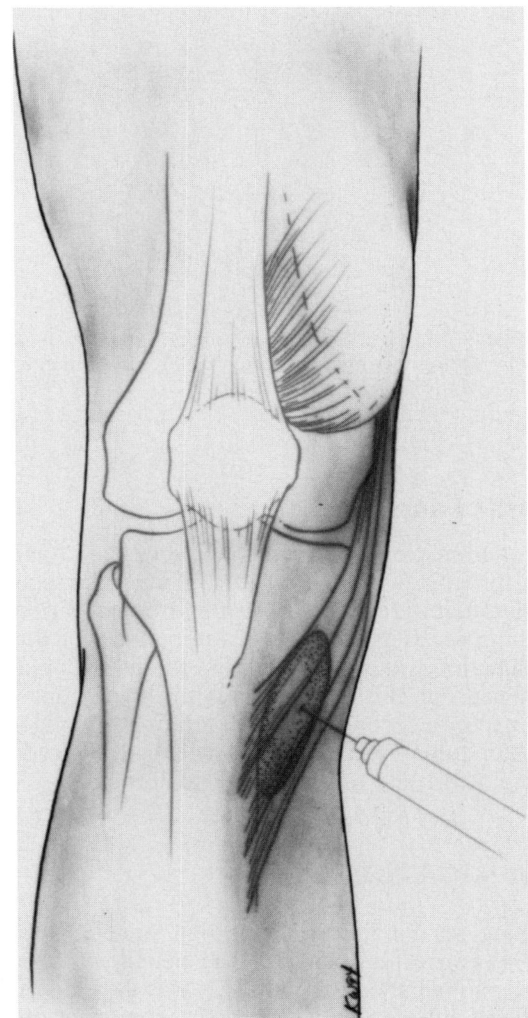

FIGURE 24–8. The anserine bursa lies medial and distal to the knee joint. An inflamed anserine bursa can often be palpated.

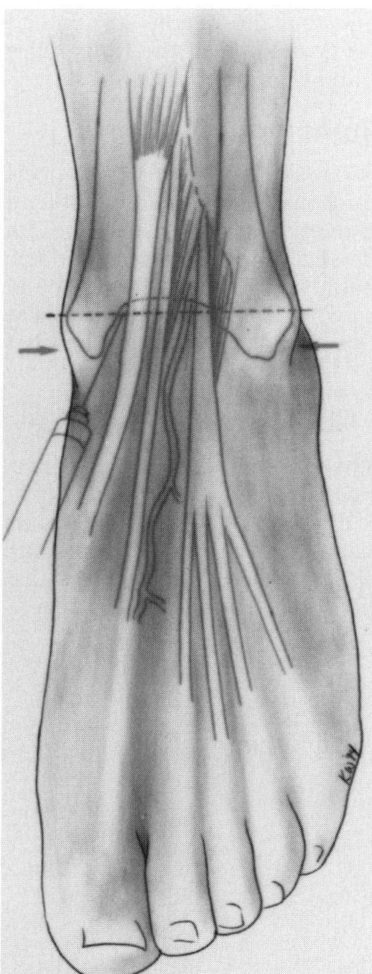

FIGURE 24–9. The medial and lateral malleoli are bony landmarks that help outline the inferior margin of the tibia or superior boundary of the tibiotalar joint.

Plantar Fasciitis

The inflammation occurs at the site of the attachment of the plantar fascia to the calcaneum. The exact site of inflammation can be determined by palpation. The site is approached from the plantar aspect of the foot. The injection is quite painful, and the use of epidermal anesthesia can also be quite painful. Rarely does a patient ask for a second injection, although the injections are often quite effective. The steroid is deposited in the midline at the site of maximum tenderness.

COMPLICATIONS

A debate was held at the Heberden Society (published in 1984) concerning whether the benefits of using IA steroids outweighed the risks.[43] It was decided that the benefit of steroids outweighed the complications, but there are many complications which the operator should be aware of and attempt to avoid.

Rare and Unusual Complications

Gladman and Bombardier[32] in 1987 reported a sickle cell crisis following IA steroid therapy for RA in two patients. Facial flushing after IA steroid injection has also been reported, but has never been observed in the senior author's experience. Gray and Gottlieb[34] reported an estimated frequency of complications following IA injections of steroids (Table 24–2).

Postinjection Flare

The postinjection flare has been clearly described by McCarty and Hogan,[58] who reproduced it by injecting mongrel dogs with various steroid preparations. The authors attributed it to the microcrystalline structure of the steroids. They and others found that prednisolone acetate and hydrocortisone acetate, but not triamcinolone acetonide, produced such flares.

Periarticular Calcifications

Sparling et al,[77] Gilsanz and Bernstein,[31] Dalinka et al,[19] Gerster and Fallet,[30] and McCarty[57] have all reported asymptomatic periarticular calcifications in finger joints following injections.

Steroid Arthropathy

Following the introduction and widespread use of IA steroid injections, authors began to describe radiological and clinical evidence of progressive joint destruction occurring after multiple steroid injections.[33] The senior author (J.J.N.) has seen patients who seemingly benefited greatly from IA steroid injections, with marked suppression of clinical inflammation, only to have the radiographs show continued progression of joint destruction. Chandler and Wright[14] also described this phenomenon in patients who received four injections over approximately 1 year. Sweetnam et al[82] reported that aseptic necrosis of the hip can follow oral and IA steroid administration. Steinberg et al[80] reported that a patient who received 22 injections into the shoulder in 24 months' time developed a Charcot-like joint. Bentley and Goodfellow[5] reported that 12 weekly injections into the left knee and 26 more weekly injections into the right knee were followed by Charcot-like disorganization of

TABLE 24–2 Prevalence of Complications Following Intra-Articular Steroid Injection

Complication	Prevalence (%)
Postinjection flare	2–5
Steroid arthropathy of weight-bearing joints	0.8
Tendon rupture	<1
Facial flushing	<1
Skin changes	<1
Infection	<0.1000006
Transient paresis of injected extremity	Rare
Hypersensitivity	Rare
Asymptomatic periarticular calcification	Rare

Adapted from Gray RG, Gottlieb NL: Intra-articular corticosteroids: An updated assessment. Clin Orthop 1983; 177:235–236.

the knee joints. Further credence to the assertion of joint destruction was supplied in 1970 by Moskowitz and colleagues,[63] who showed that triamcinolone acetonide injected into rabbit joints caused destructive changes. More recently, Parikh and colleagues[66] in 1993 reported that 18 injections over a 4-month period caused a Charcot-like arthropathy of the shoulder joint.

Miller and Restifo[61] in 1966 reviewed the literature and reported that there was evidence to suggest that joint destruction was related to the injections only in cases in which there had been an unusual frequency of injections. Stefanich[78] in 1986 further reviewed this topic and agreed there was little evidence to support the concept of steroid arthropathy, other than in exceptional cases of multiple injections.

Skin Changes

Skin changes can appear following intradermal, subcutaneous, or intramuscular injection of steroid preparations. Local depigmentation, scarring, and depression of the skin have been described. The hardened scar resembles a lupus skin plaque. There can be destruction of underlying hair follicles and sebaceous and sweat glands. These scars are not harmful but can be unsightly. Atrophy of the underlying subcutaneous tissues causes the scar to becomes depressed. Atrophy of underlying muscle has also been reported. Some patients feel that such atrophy on the back, shoulder areas, or hands is unsightly and highly undesirable. These complications can be avoided by using less concentrated preparations. Triamcinolone preparations can cause these complications with increased frequency.

Cassidy and Bole[12] reported skin changes in eight patients following injection of methylprednisolone acetate, triamcinolone diacetate, triamcinolone acetonide T.B.A., and hydrocortisone T.B.A. They reproduced these findings in rabbits. Dymant[25] reported skin atrophy in a 3-year-old girl following triamcinolone acetonide injection. McCarty[57] reported skin atrophy over 13 proximal interphalangeal and five metacarpophalangeal joints after triamcinolone hexacetonide injection. Morris[62] reported hypopigmentation and atrophy of the subcutaneous tissues following the use of triamcinolone acetonide, triamcinolone hexacetonide, and betamethasone sodium phosphate and acetate for interlesional injections of keloids. Steffey[79] reported subcutaneous gluteal atrophy following intramuscular injection of triamcinolone in six of 45 asthma patients, and no skin changes in 45 patients injected with methylprednisolone acetate. Abdel-Fattah[1] reported subcutaneous atrophy in eight of 144 patients after triamcinolone acetonide injection of keloids. Rowe[71] published a photograph of the subcutaneous atrophy that occurs with injections around the shoulder. Lemont and Hetman[50] reported linear depigmentation of the foot of a patient after IA injection of triamcinolone acetonide.

These unsightly skin lesions are said to remit after a number of years. Lund et al[54] reported that the skin lesions improved over a period of 5 years. Their occurrence can be avoided by the selection of steroid preparation, but they are probably unavoidable in a small percentage of patients.

Systemic Effects

IA steroids do not remain solely within the joint cavity. Serum levels can be detected shortly after injection, and suppression of the pituitary-adrenal axis occurs if injections are frequently repeated. Triamcinolone hexacetonide and betamethasone sodium phosphate seem to remain within the joint cavity longer than methylprednisolone acetate, and their systemic effect is limited because of their low serum levels and prolonged release time. Aseptic necrosis and Cushing's syndrome occur concurrently with suppression of the pituitary-adrenal axis if IA steroids are given frequently enough and for a prolonged period of time.[6, 23, 46, 65, 86]

Tendon Rupture

Ismail et al[44] reported a patellar ligament rupture in a high jumper following injection of either hydrocortisone or triamcinolone into the area of the patellar ligament on four occasions in a 12-month period. Karpman et al[47] reported ruptures of the extensor communis tendon of the hand, the extensor tendon of the ring finger, and the extensor tendons of the thumb and little finger, and of the long head of the biceps, in four patients with RA following IA injections with prednisolone tebutate, triamcinolone hexacetonide, and prednisolone tebutate. Although spontaneous tendon rupture can occur following trauma and RA, these rare examples illustrate a complication of IA steroids.

PHONOPHORESIS AND IONTOPHORESIS

Phonophoresis or iontophoresis has been suggested as a substitute technique for delivering adrenocorticosteroid preparations to inflamed soft tissue areas. Chantraine and colleagues[15] studied the transmission of adrenocorticosteroids by iontophoresis through cadaver skins and in the urine of rabbits after administration through shaved thighs. They found no evidence of the passage of adrenocorticosteroids through the skin. They also described 188 patients, 56% of whom said they felt better after iontophoresis of triamcinolone acetonide. They concluded that there was no evidence that iontophoresis provided transmission of adrenocorticosteroids through the skin.

Agostinucci and Powers[3] studied the effect of lidocaine hydrochloride on motor neuron excitability through the skin by iontophoresis and found that both lidocaine and placebo were effective in changing motor nerve excitability. These authors and Chantraine and co-workers concluded that electrical current might affect soft tissue inflammation and motor neuron excitability without involving the passage of any substances through the skin.

Kleinkort and Wood[49] described 285 patients with soft tissue pain and inflammation and reported a very small difference in the beneficial effect of between 1% and 10% hydrocortisone ointment with phonophoresis.

They quoted Griffin and Touchstone,[35, 36] who claimed hydrocortisone could penetrate 7 cm into porcine soft tissue through the skin with iontophoresis.

The actual penetration of adrenocorticosteroid beneath the skin of human subjects through the use of phonophoresis has not been substantiated. It may well be that electrical current and ultrasound waves provide some analgesic or anti-inflammatory effects, however. A review by Singh and Roberts[74] is consistent with this view.

LUMBAR INJECTIONS FOR PAIN MANAGEMENT

Spinal injections are a useful tool in alleviating pain or identifying pain generators that originate within the neuroaxial and posterior compartments of the spinal column. These injections can be used as an extension of the physical examination, as outcome predictors of decompressive surgeries,[20, 24, 40] or to provide pain relief to facilitate a higher level of function.[56]

This section reviews the procedural techniques used with lumbar epidural and facet joint injections. It is beyond the scope of the present discussion to review discography, radiofrequency techniques, sacroiliac joint injections, sympathetic blocks, and injections into the thoracic and cervical spine. Other sources are available on these subjects.[18, 51] The discussion also assumes the reader is knowledgeable in the vascular, bony, ligamentous, neurological, and radiographic anatomy of the lumbar spine.

Lumbosacral Epidural Injections

Midline and Paramedian Approach

Midline and paramedian epidural steroid injections are the most commonly used approaches for spinal analgesia. They can be used effectively for pain management when placed at the level of pathology in cases of disk herniations, degenerative disk disease, central stenosis, or compression fractures. The techniques are performed quickly and easily by the skilled injectionist. They have classically been performed with the patient in the lateral decubitus or upright sitting slumped position. However, under fluoroscopy the patient is placed in the prone position. Studies show that fluoroscopy facilitate proper needle placement.[9, 87]

With the patient prone, the desired injection interval is marked on the skin under fluoroscopic guidance. This includes the inferior border of the lamina of the upper injection interval and the superior border of the lamina of the lower injection interval. The patient's skin is cleaned with Betadine or Hibiclens, draped with sterile towels, and anesthetized with approximately 5 mL of 1% anesthetic solution. The operator places a large-bore, blunt spinal needle (18-gauge or 20-gauge Tuoy) directly in the lower portion of the injection interval in the midline. Using a sharp-tipped, 18-gauge needle to initially penetrate the skin and supraspinous ligaments can be helpful. With the Tuoy needle in place and attached to a small-volume glass syringe, the needle is slowly advanced anteriorly through the supraspinous and interspinous ligaments to the ligamentum flavum. As the needle is advanced, slight pressure is applied to the syringe. Once the needle tip has been advanced through the ligamentum flavum, immediate loss of resistance will be noted with the syringe (Fig. 24–10). Using a glass syringe lubricated with sterile water or lidocaine affords greater sensitivity to this loss of resistance. Once the epidural space has been located, careful aspiration is necessary to avoid intrathecal or intravascular injection. Many practitioners inject a test dose of anesthetic solution and observe the patient for a few minutes for signs of intrathecal or intravascular injections. Two to four mL of contrast dye can then be injected and observed under fluoroscopy for typical epidural dye patterns (Fig. 24–11). Once these patterns are confirmed and the needle is thought to be properly placed, a solution of Celestone Soluspan (2 mL) and lidocaine (usually 2 to 3 mL of 1% methylparaben free) is slowly injected. The needle is removed and the patient is cleaned and transferred to a recovery room.

As an alternative to the midline approach, a paramedian approach can be used. This approach is usually more comfortable for the patient and easier for the physician. It differs from the midline approach in needle placement. The Tuoy needle is placed adjacent to the supraspinous and interspinous ligaments rather than directly in these ligaments. The needle tip is advanced down to the superior edge of the lamina and slowly "walked off" this edge through the ligamentum flavum. As with the midline approach, a loss of resistance to syringe pressure will be noted by the operator.

Transforaminal Technique

As an alternative to midline or paramedian blocks, the transforaminal or selective nerve root block can be performed for disk herniations with or without radiculopathies, foraminal stenosis, or discogenic disease. A greater concentration of medication can be placed at the site of pathology because of the proximity of the foramina to most spine pathology (i.e., nerve root and

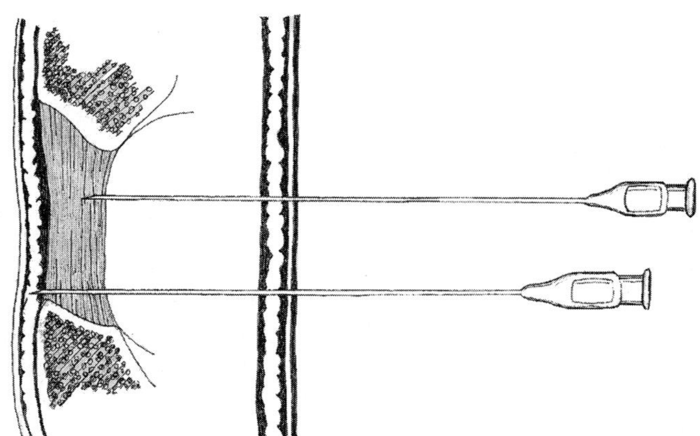

FIGURE 24–10. Illustration of tissue layers through which the needle advances during a paramedian epidural injection. *Top:* needle is located in the ligamentum flavum. *Bottom:* needle is located in the epidural space.

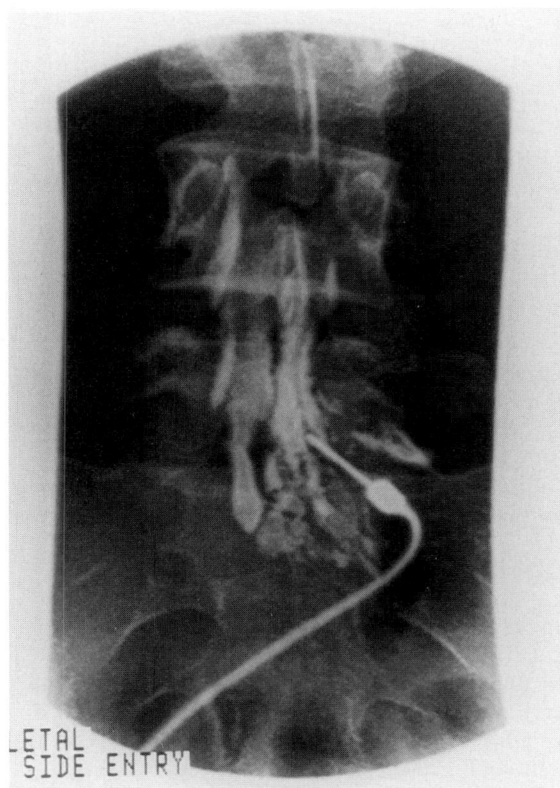

FIGURE 24–11. Midline epidural approach to lumbar injection. An AP lumbar x-ray shows contrast material in the epidural space following injection.

disk).[22] It is usually the procedure of choice in postoperative patients because of the scar tissue typically found in the midline.

The transforaminal injection is performed with the patient prone. There are unique aspects of the technique when the S1 foramen is injected as compared to the L1–L5 foramina.

If the S1 nerve root is the desired target, the S1 foramen is initially located under fluoroscopy and marked on the skin. This landmark radiographically is often difficult to locate, especially in older individuals. In patients with excessive lumbar lordosis, a pillow can be placed under the hips to change the angle of the S1 foramen as it relates to the x-ray beam. The S1 foramen is usually equidistant between the S2 foramen and the L5–S1 facet joint. Once the operator is confident of the landmark, the skin is scrubbed with Betadine or Hibiclens and a fenestrated drape is applied. Three to five mL of 1% lidocaine can then be injected into the skin and subcutaneous tissue. Once proper anesthesia is obtained, a 22-gauge, 3½-inch spinal needle is slowly inserted into the S1 foramen. Usually the initial puncture is made at the inferior aspect of the foramen and the needle is advanced cephalad under fluoroscopic guidance at a 10-degree angle. Lateral views can be helpful to confirm needle depth. Once the operator becomes experienced in this technique, the needle depth can usually be judged from the location of the needle on the AP views. When the needle is thought to be in the proper location, the inner trocar of the 22-gauge needle is removed and a syringe with nonionic contrast material is attached. After careful aspiration, the contrast material is slowly injected. Correct dye flow patterns are evaluated under fluoroscopy. The characteristic pattern is of dye flowing along the S1 nerve root (Fig. 24–12). The patient might experience radiating pain or numbness in an S1 nerve distribution during infusion of the medication, but this quickly resolves when syringe pressure stops. If a dense, well-localized pattern is noted directly over the S1 foramen, the needle is likely to be too superficial or in the soft tissue lying over the foramen. Syringes are then changed and 4 to 6 mL of a mixture of steroid and lidocaine is injected. The syringes and needles are removed, the skin is cleaned, and a bandage is applied. The patient is then monitored in a recovery room.

For injections around the lumbar nerve roots, slight modifications from the S1 injection technique are necessary. With the patient prone, a sterile preparation with Betadine or Hibiclens is performed. Either a posterior or an oblique approach can be used. For an L5 SNRB, landmarks include the L5 transverse process, L5 lamina, and the upper portion of the sacrum. Once proper anesthesia is obtained, a 22-gauge spinal needle can be advanced at the inferomedial portion of the transverse process. The tip of the needle is directed toward the inferior aspect of the pedicle superior to the exiting nerve root, or in the 6 o'clock position, with the round pedicle read as a clock face. A "safe triangle" in this region has been described that includes the base of the pedicle, the outer vertical border of the intervertebral foramen, and the diagonal nerve root and dorsal ganglion.[22] Once the needle is deemed to be in proper position, 2 to 4 mL of contrast agent is injected (Fig.

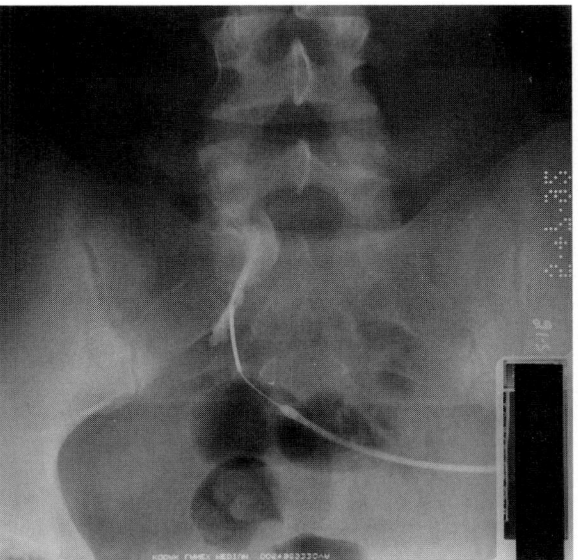

FIGURE 24–12. S1 selective epidural nerve root block. An AP radiograph shows contrast material that has been injected into the epidural space through the S1 foramen. The dye flows superiorly along the S1 nerve root.

24–13), followed by injection of a solution of steroid and anesthetic.

A double-needle technique is often used in place of the 22-gauge needle technique. An 18-gauge 3½-inch needle replaces the 22-gauge needle. The inner trocar is removed and a 23-gauge, 6-inch needle is placed within the 18-gauge needle that is already implanted in the skin and soft tissue. The 23-gauge needle is then slowly advanced under fluoroscopic guidance while the 18-gauge needle remains stable between the physician's fingertips. When this technique is used the advancing needle never touches the skin, therefore reducing the risk of infection. In addition, the distal tip of the 23-gauge needle can be intentionally bent by the physician and reinserted into the 18-gauge needle. When the 23-gauge needle is advanced through the distal portion of the 18-gauge needle, the 23-gauge needle will curve into areas that may normally be difficult to reach.

Caudal Technique

Caudal or transsacral epidural injections are usually indicated in discogenic disease, disk herniations, or central stenosis involving the lower lumbar disk. That is, they are mainly performed for disk abnormalities at the L4–5 and L5–S1 levels, and usually at the latter.

A caudal injection begins with the patient prone. With the index finger of the nondominant hand, the operator palpates the sacral cornu and hiatus. In obese patients these landmarks may be obscured; in this case, the operator locates the coccyx and slowly moves the palpating finger cephalad on the posterior aspect of the coccyx while applying pressure. Usually the sacral cornu can be located. The skin is then cleaned with Betadine or Hibiclens and a fenestrated drape is applied. The surrounding skin is anesthetized with 1% lidocaine solution, usually 2 to 3 mL. During infusion of the anesthetic, the operator's index finger should be maintained directly over the hiatus. This avoids loss of the palpable surface anatomy, which often occurs in this specific location. Once proper anesthesia is obtained, a 3½-inch, 22-gauge spinal needle is directed cephalad through the hiatus at a 30- to 45-degree angle. As the needle advances the bevel should be rotated ventrally until slight contact with bone is made. The needle is then withdrawn several millimeters and readvanced at a 5- to 10-degree angle approximately 2 to 3 cm or superiorly to the S3 vertebrae (Fig. 24–14). The inner trocar of the 22-gauge needle is removed and a syringe containing nonionic contrast material is applied to the existing needle. After careful aspiration reveals no blood or CSF return, the contrast dye is injected and the dye flow pattern is analyzed under fluoroscopy. If the needle is properly placed, a typical epidural pattern (Fig. 24–15) will be observed. Minimal resistance is noted as the contrast dye is injected. A dense, well-localized pattern indicates improper needle placement into the soft tissue. Improper placement is usually associated with increased resistance. Once the correct dye pattern is confirmed, 10 to

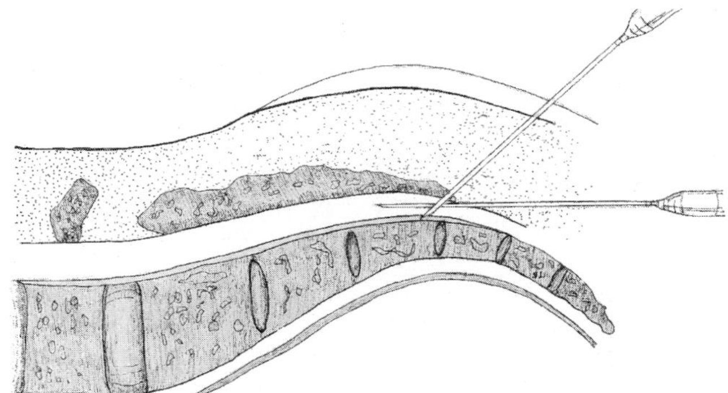

FIGURE 24–14. Needle angles and advancement during a caudal approach to lumbar injection.

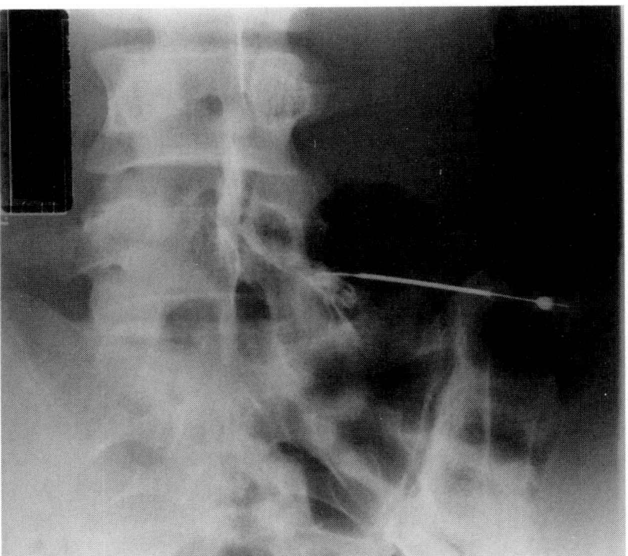

FIGURE 24–13. L5 selective epidural nerve root block. An AP radiograph shows contrast material that has been injected into the epidural space through the L5 foramen. The dye flows inferior to the pedicle.

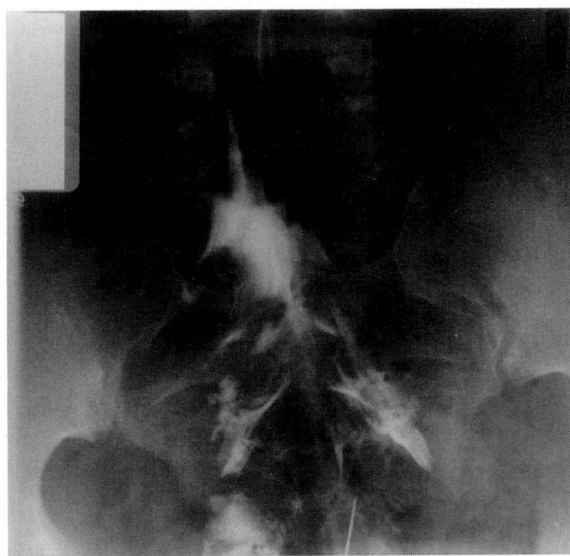

FIGURE 24–15. Caudal epidural injection. Note the superior dye flow pattern with several sacral nerve roots outlined.

15 mL of a steroid-anesthetic solution is slowly injected in fractions. The needles are withdrawn, the skin is cleaned, and a bandage is applied. The patient can be monitored in the recovery room.

Lumbar Facet Injections

Lumbar facet injections are indicated when posterior element pain is suspected as the pain generator.[21] This may occur when these joints are suspected as the primary source of pathology or in conjunction with discogenic disease. IA injections typically precede medial branch blocks when determining whether the facet joint is the putative source of pain. Medial branch blocks are commonly done to predict the response to denervation procedures.

Intra-Articular Injections

IA facet or zygoapophyseal joint injections of the lumbar spine are performed with the patient prone and the table tilted obliquely. The zygoapophyseal joints are marked on the skin under fluoroscopic guidance. The patient is cleaned with Betadine or Hibiclens, anesthetized with 3 to 4 mL of 1% lidocaine, and dressed with sterile drapes. A 22-gauge spinal needle is slowly advanced directly into the joint under fluoroscopic guidance. Several needle adjustments may be required before the needle is felt to enter the joint contents. Usually the joint edge is noted initially and the needle tip can be "walked" into the joint space (Fig. 24–16). If an arthrogram is desired for further needle confirmation, 1 mL of contrast agent can be injected and later aspirated. Dye injection can be followed by injection of a steroid-anesthetic solution, usually 1 mL of Celestone Soluspan and 1 mL of 1% or 2% lidocaine. Other, longer-acting anesthetics such as marcaine may be desired.

Often, injection of the L5–S1 joint from an oblique approach is not possible owing to the location of the iliac crest, in which case a direct posterior approach is used. The patient is placed prone and the lower edge of the L5–S1 joint is noted under fluoroscopy. The needle is advanced and the injection is made using the same technique described above.

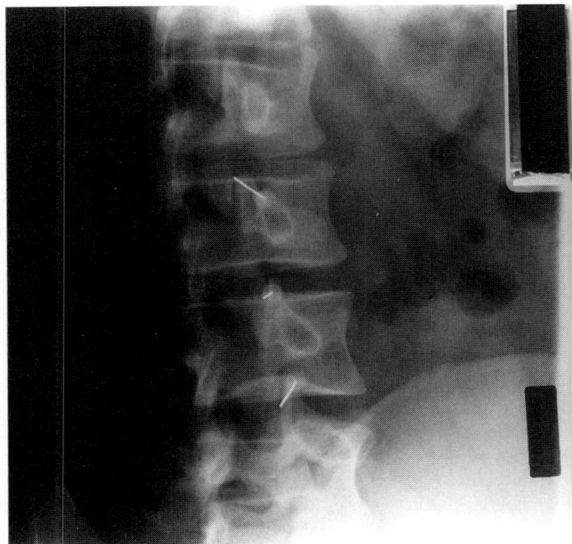

FIGURE 24–16. Lumbar intra-articular facet injection. An oblique-view radiograph shows needle placement within the lumbar facet joints prior to contrast enhancement.

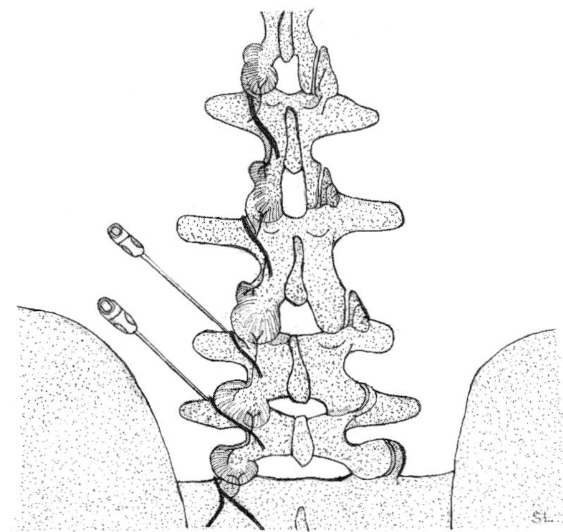

FIGURE 24–17. Needle placement for medial branch blocks. Each needle shown is located adjacent to the medial branch.

Medial Branch Blocks

Anesthetic injections of the medial branch of the posterior ramus, or medial branch blocks, can be helpful in diagnosing the painful zygoapophyseal joint or in preparation for a denervation procedure. Because a zygoapophyseal joint has dual innervation, two medial branch blocks are necessary to anesthetize a single joint (Fig. 24–17). For example, to anesthetize the nerve supply to the L4–5 zygoapophyseal joint, the L3 medial branch (located at the L4 transverse process) and the L4 medial branch (located at the L5 transverse process) are injected.

The block technique is simple and is performed under fluoroscopic guidance with the patient prone. Target sites for each block are marked on the skin, and the patient is cleaned and draped in sterile fashion and anesthetized with 2 to 4 mL of 1% lidocaine at each proposed injection site. A small-gauge spinal needle, either 22 gauge or 25 gauge, is commonly used. The needle is advanced in a superior to inferior approach[21] to the target site. For the L1–4 medial branches this site is on the posterior surface of the transverse process at the mamilloaccessory ligament and notch. The target location for the L5 nerve is the interval between the sacral ala and the S1 superior articular process. Contrast material can be injected to rule out vascular uptake. Small volumes of either 1% or 2% lidocaine or marcaine, usually 0.5 mL, are then injected at each target site.

Complications

Potential complications during lumbar injections range from the insignificant to the serious. These injections fortunately have a very low rate of serious complications and are quite safe when performed by experienced physicians and when proper precautions are observed.

Inherent to most needle procedures are transient postinjection soreness, minor swelling, and local tissue bleeding. These symptoms are usually alleviated with ice, limitation of activity, and analgesics. Bleeding complications can be reduced by taking a good medical history, including a history of recent medication intake. Aspirin should be discontinued 7 to 10 days prior to epidural procedures.[56] Anticoagulant's and other antiplatelet drugs are also contraindications to epidural procedures. Vasovagal syncope or fainting is a relatively common complication with lumbar injections. Venodilator drugs, recent exhaustive exercise, relative dehydration, hypoglycemia, and aortic stenosis are predisposing factors.[17, 37, 84] Infection is rare.

Allergic reactions to injected drugs are always a possibility. These reactions can range from skin lesions, which include urticaria, pruritus, and angioedema, to gastrointestinal symptoms. Bronchospasm, wheezing, respiratory distress, and cardiopulmonary arrest represent the most severe form of reactions.

Dural puncture and associated headaches occur after 0.5% to 5% of spinal epidural injections.[8, 64] They are primarily associated with midline or paramedian approaches.

Other complications are usually related to anesthetic toxicity and include CNS or cardiovascular problems. CNS complications vary considerably, based on plasma levels. They range from anxiety, visual and auditory disturbances, nausea, twitching, and drowsiness to seizures and coma. Medications that lower the seizure threshold should be noted; they include CNS stimulants, antipsychotic agents, tricyclic antidepressants, phenothiazine derivatives, and monoamine oxidase inhibitors. Cardiovascular complications usually parallel CNS side effects with toxic anesthetic doses. These symptoms range from hypotension, arrhythmias, peripheral dilation, and myocardial depression to cardiac arrest.

Benefits

Lumbar injections provide considerable pain relief to patients when used in the appropriate clinical setting. They also provide valuable diagnostic information for the spine physician. These injections are generally safe, easy to perform, and carry a low side effect profile. The technical performance of these injections requires proper training, a good knowledge of lumbar gross and radiological anatomy, and the ability to manage any complications resulting from the procedure.

REFERENCES

1. Abdel-Fattah AM: Unusual complications of triamcinolone injected keloids: Tissue necrosis and systemic corticosteroid effects. Br J Plast Surg 1976; 29:283.
2. Adams ME, Atkinson MH, Lussier AJ, et al: The role of viscosupplementation with hylan G-F 20 (Synvisc) in the treatment of osteoarthritis of the knee: A Canadian multicenter trial comparing hylan G-F alone, hylan G-F 20 with nonsteroidal anti-inflammatory drugs (NSAIDs) and NSAIDs alone. Osteoarthr Cartilage 1995; 3:213–225.
3. Agostinucci J, Powers WR: Motoneuron excitability modulation after desensitization of the skin by iontophoresis of lidocaine hydrochloride. Arch Phys Med Rehabil 1992; 73:190–194.
4. Axelrod L: Glucocorticoids. In Kelly WN, Harris ED, Ruddy S, et al (eds): Textbook of Rheumatology. Philadelphia, WB Saunders, 1993, pp 779–796.
5. Bentley G, Goodfellow JW: Disorganisation of the knees following intraarticular hydrocortisone injections. J Bone Joint Surg Br 1969; 51:498–502.
6. Bertouch JV, Meffin PJ, Sallustio BC, et al: A comparison of plasma methylprednisolone concentrations following intra-articular injection in patients with rheumatoid arthritis and osteoarthritis. Aust NZ J Med 1983; 13:583–586.
7. Blyth T, Hunter JA, Stirling A: Pain relief in the rheumatoid knee after steroid injection: A single-blind comparison of hydrocortisone succinate, and triamcinolone acetonide or hexacetonide. Br J Rheumatol 1994; 33:461–463.
8. Bogduk N, Cherry D: Epidural corticosteroid agents for sciatica. Med J Aust 143:402–406, 1985.
9. Bush K, Hillier S: A controlled study of caudal epidural injections of triamcinolone plus procaine for the management of intractable sciatica. Spine 16:572–575, 1991.
10. Carlsson A, Lindmark B, Marsal L: Intra-articular steroids: An alternative to knee synovectomy in rheumatoid arthritis? Scand J Rheumatol 1984; 13:375–377.
11. Caron JP, Kaneene JB, Miller R: Results of a survey of equine practitioners on the use and perceived efficacy of polysulfated glycosaminoglycan. JAMA 1996; 209:1564–1668.
12. Cassidy JJ, Bole GG: Cutaneous atrophy secondary to intra-articular corticosteroid administration. Ann Intern Med 1966; 65:1008–1018.
13. Chakravarty K, Pharoah PD, Scott DG: A randomized controlled study of post-injection rest following intra-articular steroid therapy for knee synovitis. Br J Rheumatol 1994; 33:464–468.
14. Chandler GN, Wright V: Deleterious effect of intra-articular hydrocortisone. Lancet 1958; 27:661–663.
15. Chantraine A, Ludy JP, Berger D: Is cortisone iontophoresis possible? Arch Phys Med Rehabil 1986; 67:38–40.
16. Chatham W, Williams G, Moreland L, et al: Intraarticular corticosteroid injections: Should we rest the joints? Arthritis Care Res 1989; 2:70–74.
17. Come PC, Bertram P: Nitroglycerin-induced severe hypotension and bradycardia in patients with acute myocardial infarction. Circulation 1976; 54:624–628.
18. Cousins MJ, Bridenbaugh PO (eds): Neural Blockade, ed 2. Philadelphia, JB Lippincott, 1988.
19. Dalinka MK, Stewart V, Bomalaski JS, et al: Periarticular calcifications in association with intra-articular corticosteroid injections. Radiology 1984; 153:615–618.
20. Derby R, Kine G, Saal J, et al: Response to steroid and duration of radicular pain as predictors of surgical outcome. Spine 1992; 17:5176–5183.
21. Derby R, Bogduk N, Schwarzer A: Precision percutaneous blocking procedures for localizing spinal pain: Part 1. The posterior lumbar compartment. Pain Digest 1993; 3:89–100.
22. Derby R, Bogduk N, Kine G: Precision percutaneus blocking procedures for localizing spinal pain: Part 2. The lumbar neuroaxial compartment. Pain Digest 1993; 3:175–188.
23. Derendorf H, Möllmann H, Grüner A, et al: Pharmacokinetics and pharmacodynamics of glucocorticoid suspensions after intra-articular administration. Clin Pharmacol Ther 1986; 19:313–317.
24. Dooley JF, McBroom RJ, Taguchi T, et al: Nerve root infiltration in the diagnosis of radicular pain. Spine 1988; 13:79–83.
25. Dyment PG: Local atrophy following triamcinolone injection. Pediatrics 1970; 46:136–137.
26. Eustace JA, Brophy DP, Gibney RP, et al: Comparison of the accuracy of steroid placement with clinical outcome in patients with shoulder symptoms. Ann Rheum Dis 1997; 56:59–63.
27. Flanagan J, Casale FF, Thomas TL, et al: Intra-articular injection for pain relief in patients awaiting hip replacement. Ann R Coll Surg Engl 1988; 70:156–157.
28. Gaustad G, Larsen S: Comparison of polysulphated glycosaminoglycan and sodium hyaluronate with placebo in treatment of traumatic arthritis in horses. Equine Vet J 1995; 27:356–362.

29. Geborek P, Mansson B, Wollheim FA, et al: Intraarticular corticosteroid injection into rheumatoid arthritis knees improves extensor muscles strength. Rheumatol Int 1990; 9:265–270.
30. Gerster JC, Fallet GH: Periarticular hand hydrozyapatite deposition after corticosteroid injections. J Rheumatol 1987; 14:1156–1159.
31. Gilsanz V, Bernstein BH: Joint calcification following intraarticular corticosteroid therapy. Radiology 1984; 151:647–649.
32. Gladman DD, Bombardier C: Sickle cell crisis following intraarticular steroid therapy for rheumatoid arthritis. Arthritis Rheum 1987; 30:1065–1068.
33. Gogia PP, Brown M, al-Obaidi S: Hydrocortisone and exercise effects on articular cartilage in rats. Arch Phys Med Rehabil 1993; 74:463–467.
34. Gray RG, Gottlieb NL: Intra-articular corticosteroids: An updated assessment. Clin Orthop 1983; 177:235–263.
35. Griffin JE, Touchstone JC: Ultrasonic movement of cortisol into pig tissue: I. Movement into skeletal muscle. Am J Phys Med 1963; 42:77–85.
36. Griffin JE, Touchstone JC: Ultrasonic movement of cortisol into pig tissue: II. Movement into paravertebral nerve. Am J Phys Med 1965; 44:20–25.
37. Hargreaves AD, Muir AL: Lack of variation in venous tone potentiates vasovagal syncope. Br Heart J 1992; 67:486–490.
38. Hasselbacker P: Synovial fluid analysis. In Utsinger PD, Zvaifler NJ, Ehrlich GE (eds): Rheumatoid Arthritis. Philadelphia, JB Lippincott, 1985, pp 194–196.
39. Hendrix RW, Lin PJ, Kane WJ: Simplified aspiration or injection technique for the sacroiliac joint. J Bone Joint Surg 1982; 64:1249–1252.
40. Herron LD: Selective nerve root block in patient selection for lumbar surgery: Surgical results. J Spin Disord 2:75–79, 1989.
41. Hollander JL: Intrasynovial corticosteroid therapy in arthritis. Md State Med J 1970; 19:62–66.
42. Hollander JL, Brown EM Jr, Jessar RA, et al: Hydrocortisone and cortisone injected into arthritic joints. JAMA 1951; 147:1629–1635.
43. Intra-articular steroids (letter, Heberden Society). Lancet 1984; 18:385.
44. Ismail AM, Balakrishnan R, Rajakumar MK, et al: Rupture of patellar ligament after steroid infiltration: Report of a case. J Bone Joint Surg Br 1969; 51:503–505.
45. Itokazu M, Matsunaga T: Clinical evaluation of high-molecular-weight sodium hyaluronate for the treatment of patients with periarthritis of the shoulder. Clin Ther 1995; 17:946–955.
46. Jarratt MT, Spark RF, Arndt KA: The effects of intradermal steroids on the pituitary-adrenal axis and the skin. J Invest Dermatol 1974; 62:463–466.
47. Karpman RR, McComb JE, Volz RG: Tendon rupture following local steroid injection. Postgrad Med 1980; 68:169–174.
48. Kerolus G, Clayburne G, Schumacher HR Jr: Is it mandatory to examine synovial fluids promptly after arthrocentesis? Arthritis Rheum 1989; 32:271–278.
49. Kleinkort JA, Wood F: Phonophoresis with 1 percent versus 10 percent hydrocortisone. Phys Ther 1975; 55:1320–1324.
50. Lemont H, Hetman J: Cutaneous foot depigmentation following an intra-articular steroid injection. J Podiatr Med Assoc 1991; 81:606–607.
51. Lennard TA (ed): Physiatric Procedures in Clinical Practice. Philadelphia, Hanley & Belfus, 1995.
52. Leversee JH: Aspiration of joints and soft tissue injections. Primary Care 1986; 13:579–599.
53. Listrat V, Ayral X, Patarnello F, et al: Arthroscopic evaluation of potential structure modifying activity of hyaluronan (Hyalgan) in osteoarthritis of the knee. Osteoarthr Cartilage 1997; 5: 153–160.
54. Lund IM, Donde R, Knudsen EA: Persistent local cutaneous atrophy following corticosteroid injection for tendonitis. Rheumatol Rehabil 1979; 18:91–93.
55. Lussier A, Cividino AA, McFarlane CA, et al: Viscosupplementation with hylan for the treatment of osteoarthritis: Findings from clinical practice in Canada. J Rheumatol 1996; 23:1579–1585.
56. Macdonald R: Aspirin and extradural blocks (editorial). Br J Anaesth 1991; 66:1–3.
57. McCarty DJ: Treatment of rheumatoid joint inflammation with triamcinolone hexacetonide. Arthritis Rheum 1972; 15: 157–173.
58. McCarty DJ Jr, Hogan JM: Inflammatory reaction after intrasynovial injection of microcrystalline adrenocorticosteroid esters. Arthritis Rheum 1964; 7:359–367.
59. Med Lett 1998; 40:69–70.
60. Miller JA, Ferguson RL, Powers DL, et al: Efficacy of hyaluronic acid/nonsteroidal anti-inflammatory drug systems in preventing postsurgical tendon adhesions. J Biomed Mater Res (Appl Biomater) 1997; 38:25–33.
61. Miller WT, Restifo RA: Steroid arthropathy. Radiology 1966; 86:652–657.
62. Morris WJ: Undesirable side effects following intralesional corticosteroid therapy. Calif Med 1972; 116:55.
63. Moskowitz RW, Davis W, Sammarco J, et al: Experimentally induced corticosteroid arthropathy. Arthritis Rheum 1970; 13:236–243.
64. Okell RW, Sprigge JS: Unintentional dural puncture: A survey of recognition and management. Anaesthesia 1987; 42:1110–1113.
65. O'Sullivan MM, Rumfeld WR, Jones MK, et al: Cushing's syndrome with suppression of the hypothalamic-pituitary-adrenal axis after intra-articular steroid injections. Ann Rheum Dis 1985; 44:561–563.
66. Parikh JR, Houpt JB, Jacobs S, et al: Charcot's arthropathy of the shoulder following intraarticular corticosteroid injections. J Rheumatol 1993; 20:885–887.
67. Pelletier JP, Martel-Pelletier J: The therapeutic effects of NSAID and corticosteroids in osteoarthritis: To be or not to be. J Rheumatol 1989; 16:266–269.
68. Pfenninger JL: Injections of joints and soft tissue: Part I. General guidelines. Am Fam Physician 1991; 44:1196–1202.
69. Pffenninger JL: Injections of joints and soft tissue: Part II. Guidelines for specific joints. Am Fam Physician 1991; 44:1690–1701.
70. Pozo MA, Balazs EA, Belmonte C: Reduction of sensory responses to passive movements of inflamed knee joints by hylan, a hyaluronan derivative. Exp Brain Res 1997; 116:3–9.
71. Rowe CR: Injection technique for the shoulder and elbow. Orthop Clin North Am 1988; 19:773–777.
72. Samuelson CO Jr, Cannon GW, Ward JR: Arthrocentesis. J Fam Pract 1985; 20:179–184.
73. Shmerling RH, Delbanco TL, Tosteson AN, et al: Synovial fluid tests. What should be ordered? JAMA 1990; 264:1009–1104.
74. Singh J, Roberts MS: Transdermal delivery of drugs by iontophoresis: A review. Drug Design Deliv 1989; 4:1–12.
75. Smith GN Jr, Myers SL, Brandt KD, et al: Effect of intraarticular hyaluronan injection in experimental canine osteoarthritis. Arthritis Rheum 1998; 41:976–985.
76. Smith RW, Campbell MJ, O'Connell S, et al: Methods of skin preparation prior to intra-articular injection. Br J Rheumatol 1993; 32:648.
77. Sparling M, Malleson P, Wood B, et al: Radiographic follow-up of joints injected with triamcinolone hexacetonide for the management of childhood arthritis. Arthritis Rheum 1990; 33:821–826.
78. Stefanich RJ: Intraarticular corticosteroid in treatment of osteoarthritis. Orthop Rev 1986; 15:65–71.
79. Steffey JM: Subcutaneous atrophy following intramuscular administration of triamcinolone acetonide. Am J Dis Child 1973; 126:561–562.
80. Steinberg CL, Duthie RB, Piva AE: Charcot-like arthropathy following intra-articular hydrocortisone. JAMA 1962; 181: 145–148.
81. Stolzer BL, Eisenbeis CH Jr, Barr JH Jr, et al: Intra-articular injections of adrenocorticosteroids in patients with arthritis. Pa Med J August 1962; pp 911–914.
82. Sweetnam DR, Mason RM, Murray RO: Steroid arthropathy of the hip. Br Med J 1960; 1:1392–1394.
83. Thumbo J, O'Duffy JD: A prospective study of the safety of joint and soft tissue aspirations and injections in patients taking warfarin sodium. Arthritis Rheum 1998; 41:736–739.
84. van Lieshout JJ, Wieling W, Karemaker JM, et al: The vasovagal response. Clin Sci 1991; 81:575–586.

85. Weiss MM: Corticosteroids in rheumatoid arthritis. Semin Arthritis Rheum 1989; 19:9–21.
86. Weiss S, Kisch ES, Fischel B: Systemic effects of intraarticular administration of triamcinolone hexacetonide. Isr J Med Sci 1983; 19:83–84.
87. White AH, Derby R, Wynne G: Epidural injections for the diagnosis and treatment of low back pain. Spine 1980; 5:78–82.
88. Woodward JL, et al: Epidural procedures in spine pain management. In Lennard (ed): Physiatric Procedures in Clinical Practice. Philadelphia, Hanley & Belfus, 1995, pp 260–291.
89. Wu JJ, Shih LY, Hsu HC, et al: The double-blind test of sodium hyaluronate (ARTZ) on osteoarthritis knee. Chin Med J (Taipei) 1997; 59:99–106.
90. Zuckerman JD, Meislin RJ, Rothberg M: Injections for joint and soft tissue disorders: When and how to use them. Geriatrics 1990; 45:45–52.

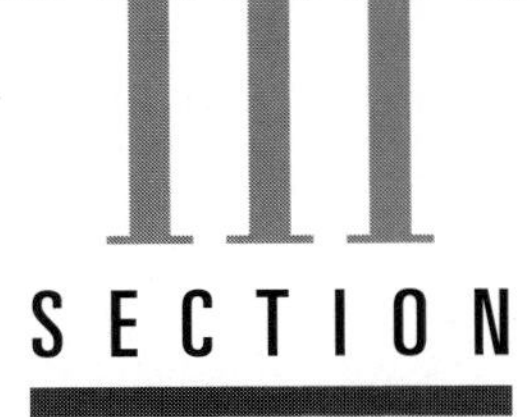

SECTION III

COMMON CLINICAL PROBLEMS IN PHYSICAL MEDICINE AND REHABILITATION

25 CHAPTER

Cristina M. Mix, O.T.R., and Donna Pieper Specht, P.T.

Achieving Functional Independence

Functional independence is the ability to perform daily living skills without help. Independence has been described as freedom from the influence, control, or determination of one or more others. Being independent includes performance of living tasks in a manner customary to that person's sex, age, and culture.[25] Disabled or not, everyone must regularly carry out certain tasks or activities to live and participate in society.[4] These activities include tasks of self-maintenance, mobility, communication, home management, and leisure skills, as well as school work and play skills.[19] If a person fails to achieve functional independence in any one of these activities, he or she cannot be self-sufficient and will need another person's assistance to meet daily living needs. Such dependence can affect the person's ability to work, live in his or her own home, and travel.[4]

Minimizing a person's dependence on assistance is one of rehabilitation's most cherished goals.[11] Dependence can have a major impact on a person's quality of life. Quality of life includes those activities that a person enjoys and values. The foundations of independent living skills begin in infancy and are refined—with nurturing, time, and opportunity—through various stages of development and mastery until functional independence is achieved. Attainment of independent living skills is generally believed to be critical to the development of a positive self-image,[20] which is enhanced by the person's participation in productive and enjoyable activities.

Health professionals need to be sensitive to what persons consider to be meaningful in their lives. Everyone has goals and aspirations to fulfill during life. As health professionals, we are instrumental in assisting people whose physical or mental challenges interfere with achieving their goals. Such assistance includes restoration of the components of function, education of the patient and family in compensatory techniques, and instruction in the use of adaptive equipment.[12]

Families are important to everyone. In the process of assisting people, we need to include families and significant others who play significant roles in the person's life. *Family-centered care* is a set of philosophies, attitudes, and approaches to care for persons with special needs and their families.[10] It refers to a relationship between the person, family, and health care professional that builds on the person's and family's priorities and responds to their mutual goals.[5] Family-centered care supports families by building on the strength of the family as a whole, as well as the unique strengths of individual family members. Families differ in the strategies they use to reach for their dreams; there is no single approach that is right for all families. Health professionals should respect this diversity.[10]

Some key elements in family-centered care include recognizing family strengths, respecting different methods of coping, facilitating family and professional collaboration at all levels of health care, and sharing complete and unbiased information with families on a continuing basis and in a supportive manner. These elements also include designing accessible health-care systems that are flexible, culturally competent, and responsive to family-identified needs.[10] A family- or person-centered philosophy encourages and respects family involvement in decisions made for individual family members. Family members play an important role in the evaluation process, treatment program, and advocacy for the person in need of rehabilitation services.

EVALUATION

Evaluation of performance skills identifies impairments that interfere with a person's achieving the goals of functional independence. Evaluation includes assessment of patients' abilities and limitations in school, work, play, leisure activities, mobility, self-care, and home maintenance.[19] Multiple evaluation tools and assessments exist which assist in identifying a person's abilities and limitations.

The evaluation begins with an interview with patient and family to identify the person's interests, premorbid status, and current perception of impairment. Within the evaluation, component areas of involvement that can interfere with function are assessed. These component areas include assessment of range of motion (ROM), strength, tone, sensation, balance and coordination, visual perception, and cognition. Direct observation of functional activities ensures accuracy and shows which areas of limitations are problematic.[4] Throughout the treatment phase of rehabilitation, it is important to measure patient progress according to functional outcome, which provides information about rehabilitation effectiveness, rehabilitation progress, and program efficacy. Many outcome-oriented scales exist. One scale is the Children's Hospital Rehabilitation Independence Scale (CHRIS),[7] which is specific to pediatrics and is used at The Children's Hospital in Denver, Colorado. Other scales are the Rehabilitation Institute of Chicago Functional Assessment Scale (RICFAS)[13] and the Functional Independence Measure (FIM).[22] Centers choose the scale appropriate to their needs.

This chapter reviews the general principles involved in developing functional independent living skills underlying self-maintenance, mobility, communication, home management, leisure skills, and occupational activities. Suggested uses of adaptations and modifications to allow functional independence are included.

SELF-MAINTENANCE

Basic self-maintenance activities include feeding, upper- and lower-extremity dressing, and grooming and hygiene.

Feeding

The process of self-feeding involves adequate range of motion (ROM), as well as coordination and strength sufficient to scoop and bring the hand to the mouth from a surface while grasping a utensil or cup. When coordination is difficult, stabilization of dishes may be needed. Mats made of nonskid materials such as Dycem are uesful for this purpose. For persons with functional use of just one hand, commercially available scoop dishes or plate guards (Fig. 25–1) allow food to be stabilized against the raised side. Weighted utensils and cups and swivel utensils may help when hand control is limited. A rocker knife is useful when bilateral upper extremity motor skills are impaired, as with involvement such as hemiplegia. A rocker knife is used by pushing the knife down into food and rocking the knife until the food is cut. This avoids the traditional sliding method while stabilizing the food with a fork in the opposite hand (Fig. 25–2).

A variety of adapted and built-up utensils are available for use when grasp is weak or absent. These include utensil cuffs and splints with utensil slots, as well as lightweight cups or cups with special handles that make grasping easier. A common way to build up handles is to place built-up foam over the utensil. The foam is cylindrical with a hole in the center, and comes in various widths to conform to the palm and grip (Fig. 25–3). Utensils such as knives can also be adapted with the use of orthotic material by fabricating a custom-made palmar cuff. The knife is attached to the cuffs facing down near the ulnar border of the hand with orthotic material. A sheath for the knife is often fabricated for safety when storing. Many kinds of adapted knives are also commercially available.

If ROM is limited for hand-to-mouth activity, long straws for drinking, long-handled and curved utensils, and sandwich holders can help, as can mobile arm supports or suspension slings (Fig. 25–4). A mobile arm support is a system that supports the forearm while assisting and maximizing such motions as shoulder flexion and extension, horizontal abduction and adduction, external and internal rotation, and elbow flexion and extension. For the mobile arm support to be used successfully, a person should exhibit some functional upper-extremity movement in the these gravity-eliminated planes, with strength in upper extremities of at least trace (1+) to poor (3−). Electrical and mechanical feeders and elevated spoon and plate setups are also available for persons with moderate to severe physical limitations.

Adequate oral motor skills such as sucking, lip closure to utensil, and tongue mobility are necessary for eating. Oral motor skills can be facilitated by a variety of feeding tools, such as various nipples for children when bottle-drinking, spoons made of sturdy plastic with a shallow bowl, and cups with nose cutouts or spouts (Fig. 25–5). It is important to have an optimal functional position for self-feeding and oral intake.

Dressing

Dressing involves donning and doffing clothing, which includes managing fasteners (buttons, zippers, snaps) and handling accessories such as belts and shoes. The person's usual clothing should be used when evaluating and performing dress training. Dressing requires adequate active ROM, coordination, strength, and gross mobility skills (rolling, trunk control, and sitting balance).

Some modifications that permit independent dressing are very simple. One can, for example, avoid clothes with many fasteners or choose loose clothing (pullover shirts and dresses, pants and shorts with elastic waistbands, no elastic at cuffs). For those with limited dexterity, choosing clothes with larger buttons can help. And when fine motor skills are weak, button aids, zipper

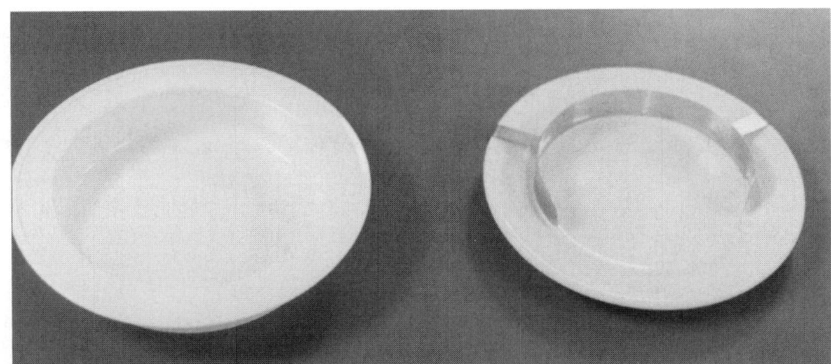

FIGURE 25–1. Scoop dish and plate with plate guard are used by pushing food against rim to scoop; it also aids as a guide.

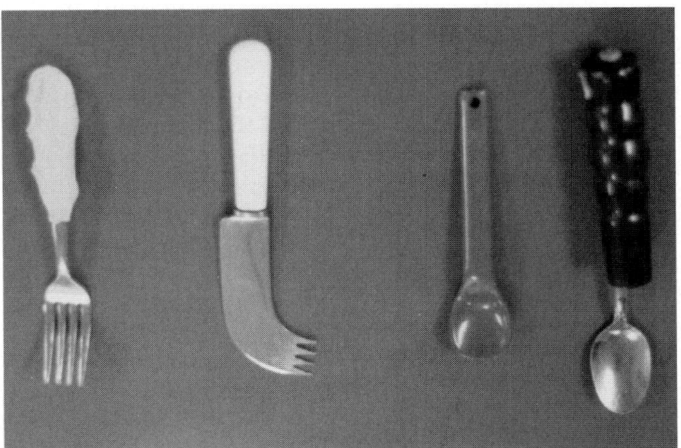

FIGURE 25–2. Adapted utensils from *left* to *right:* weighted utensils used by a person with decreased stability. Rocker knife used by an individual with functional use of one hand; spoon with plastic shallow bowl; custom-made handle made of putty.

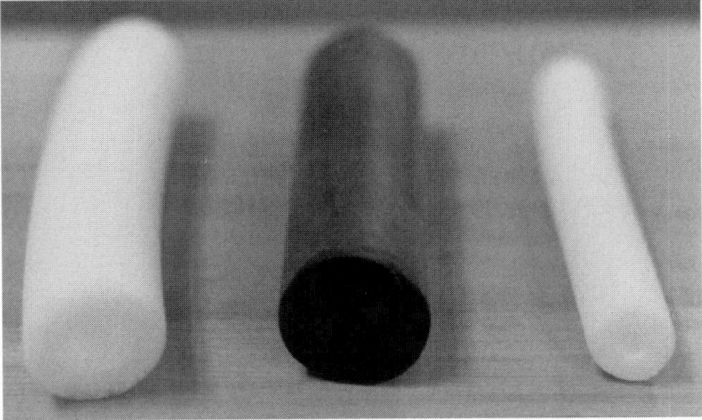

FIGURE 25–3. Built-up foam used to build up various handles (e.g., utensils, writing tools) when grasp is limited.

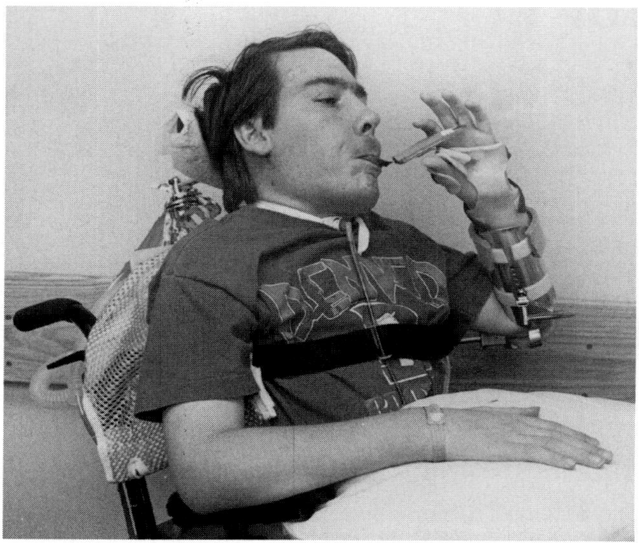

FIGURE 25–4. Mobile arm support used with a long opponens splint and vertical holder to aid in feeding: mobile arm supports and upper extremity function when shoulder or forearm strength is weak. The subject also has a long opponens splint with a utensil and a vertical holder for a spoon for feeding.

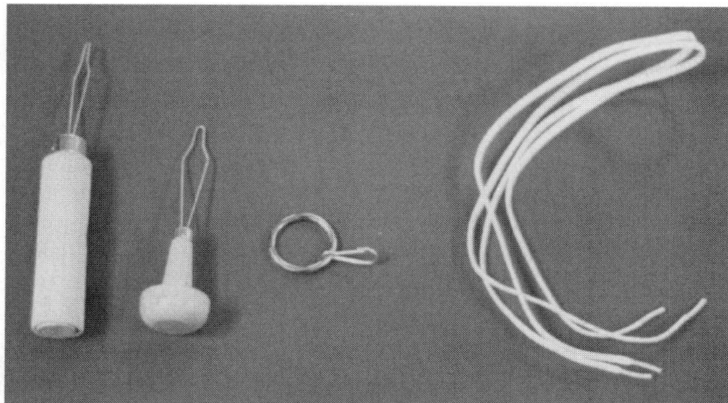

FIGURE 25–6. Fastener adaptions, *left* to *right:* button aid, knob handle button aid, zipper pull, and elastic laces.

pulls, elastic shoelaces, and Velcro are available to help manage fasteners. A button aid consists of a wire loop that hooks around the button and is then pulled through the hole. It works especially well for those with reduced manipulation and bilateral motor skills. Zipper pulls can be as simple as a loop tied to the zipper or a wire hook used to pull the zipper up. It is used primarily by those with limited prehension. Elastic shoelaces are similar to regular cloth laces, except that the elastic laces do not need to be untied or retied each time. They stretch when the foot enters the shoe, adapting to the shoe (Fig. 25–6). Modified clothing is now commercially available; but simple, "home-made" modifications can be effective, too. For example, when hand strength is limited, it's useful to put loops on socks to assist in pulling up. Velcro openings on pants can facilitate toileting. Finally, in the case of perceptual or cognitive problems, it can help to label clothes so the person can distinguish front from back.

When a person has limited reach and mobility, he or she may find a commercially available reacher useful for retrieving items of clothing. A reacher is an extended stick, usually made of lightweight aluminum, with a grasping unit at the end. It is operated by squeezing the handle, which activates the gripper position to open and close. Reachers come in many lengths and handle types to adapt to a person's ability to grasp (Fig. 25–7). A variety of dressing sticks, which are long sticks with a hook at the end, aid in pulling up pants and socks. Stocking aids have a sock holder and an attached rope; the person puts a stocking over the sock holder, places the holder in front of the foot, then uses the rope to pull up (Fig. 25–8). The rope is long enough to reach the person's lap, which reduces the need to bend at the hips.

When providing recommendations for adapted dressing modifications or equipment, it is important to consider developmental age, cognitive abilities, motivation to use the equipment, and its potential to enhance or impede independence (Fig. 25–9).

Grooming and Hygiene

To perform hygiene and grooming skills, a person must have a grasp that permits holding appropriate tools and

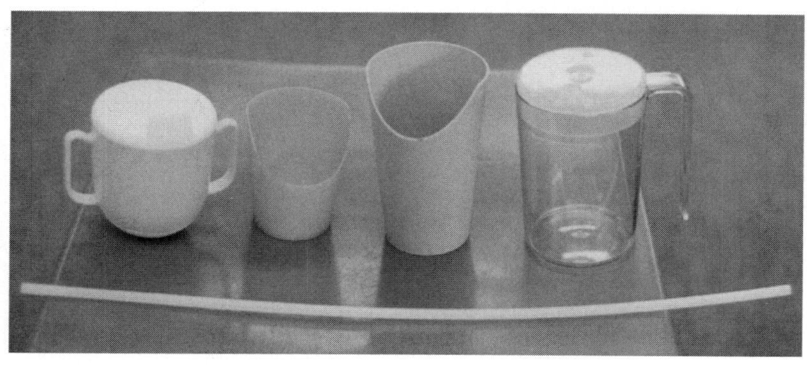

FIGURE 25–5. Various cups to assist with oral control. *Left* to *right:* tippy cup, small and large nose cut-out cup, and cup with handle and spout.

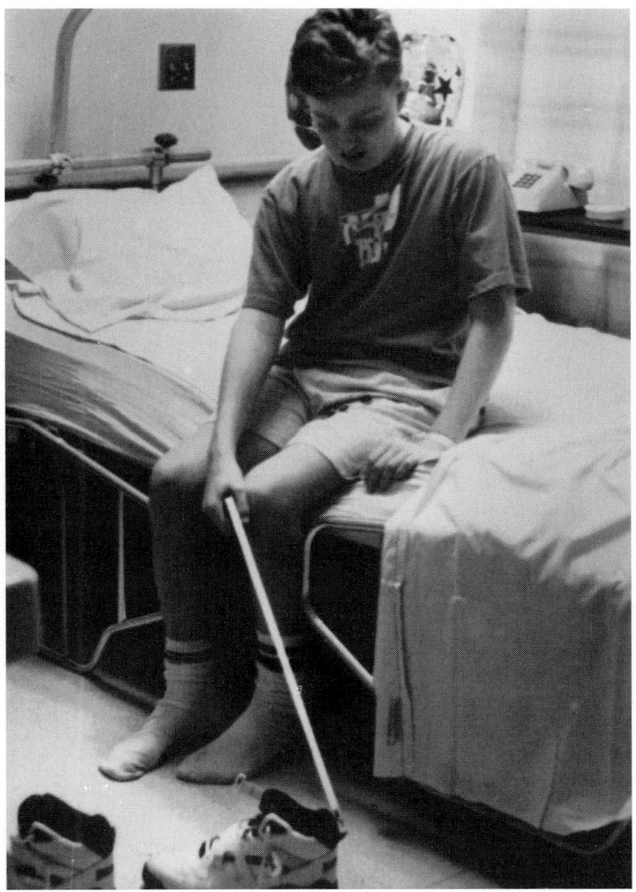

FIGURE 25–7. Reacher used to assist in picking up objects from floor. A reacher aids persons with limited lower extremity and upper extremity mobility. It is operated by squeezing the handle, which opens the tongs. The handle is released to maintain grasp.

enough ROM to reach all areas of the head and body, as well as bilateral hand function, fine and gross motor coordination, strength, trunk control, and sitting balance (Fig. 25–10).

When hand function is limited due to decreased strength or diminished ROM, several adaptations can be used to enhance that function. A utensil cuff is a palmar strap with a slot into which small items, such as a toothbrush, can be inserted and stabilized. The cuffs are commercially available, but they can also be fabricated from orthotic material or webbing. Built-up foam and Velcro straps can be used in conjunction with a toothbrush. A razor or electric shaver, electric toothbrushes, and Water Piks can greatly assist those whose strength and endurance are limited. Soap-on-a-rope and wash mitts (which hold the soap inside the mitt) assist with face washing. Attaching a suction brush to the sink facilitates nail and denture care when bilateral hand function is limited. One can also attach a nail clipper and emery board to a board backed with Dycem or suction cups to compensate for the strength necessary to pinch or hold a clipper.[8]

The adaptations discussed consider weak hand strength and incoordination. When shoulder strength is weak, long handles added to such grooming tools as brushes or combs can enhance reach. A mobile arm support or balanced forearm orthosis can also allow one to work in reduced antigravity planes, maximizing motion.

Bowel and Bladder

An important factor in hygiene is bowel and bladder care. Such care requires adequate upper-extremity ROM, hand function, mobility, endurance, and ability to manage clothes. Therapists work closely with the patient, family, and nurses to discuss possible adaptations and positioning to allow the patient to perform this care. Reaching aids that hold toilet tissue are available. Various commode chairs, raised toilet seats, and potty chairs can be used when standard toilets make toileting difficult. To facilitate catheterization, dynamic splints or catheter inserters are helpful, as are labia spreaders for females. For those using leg bags, there are various adapted leg bag emptiers and catheter clamps, as well as modified strapping for urinary drainage bags. Adapted condom catheter holders can help to secure condom catheters. Bowel care might require use of adapted suppository inserters or digital stimulators to aid those with weak hand strength or incoordination.[14] Bowel and bladder care is discussed in detail in Chapters 27 and 28.

Skin Management

Another aspect of care is skin management, especially for those with absent or reduced sensation. A long-handled mirror allows one to personally perform skin inspection. Specialized timers provide an auditory reminder to perform weight shifts to assist in preventing pressure sores. The timer, which is placed beneath the wheelchair, beeps every 15 minutes to remind a person to perform a pressure relief. (See also Chapter 31.)

Menstrual Care

Menstrual care can also require the use of a dynamic splint to allow handling and adequate placement of hygiene products when prehension is weak.

Bathing

Bathing is a complex activity, involving gross motor mobility skills performed in a potentially dangerous (i.e., slippery) environment. In addition, one must have adequate active ROM, fine motor coordination, and sitting balance.

Various environmental adaptations can assist with bathing and safety. These include grab bars placed outside and inside the bathing area, nonskid strips inside the tub, handheld shower heads, and automatic water temperature controls. A variety of bath chairs are available for those whose mobility and balance are impaired. The bath chairs vary, depending on the person's size and motor abilities (e.g., a bath ring is appropriate for a small child). A wheelchair commode or shower chair is recommended for those who have a roll-in shower.

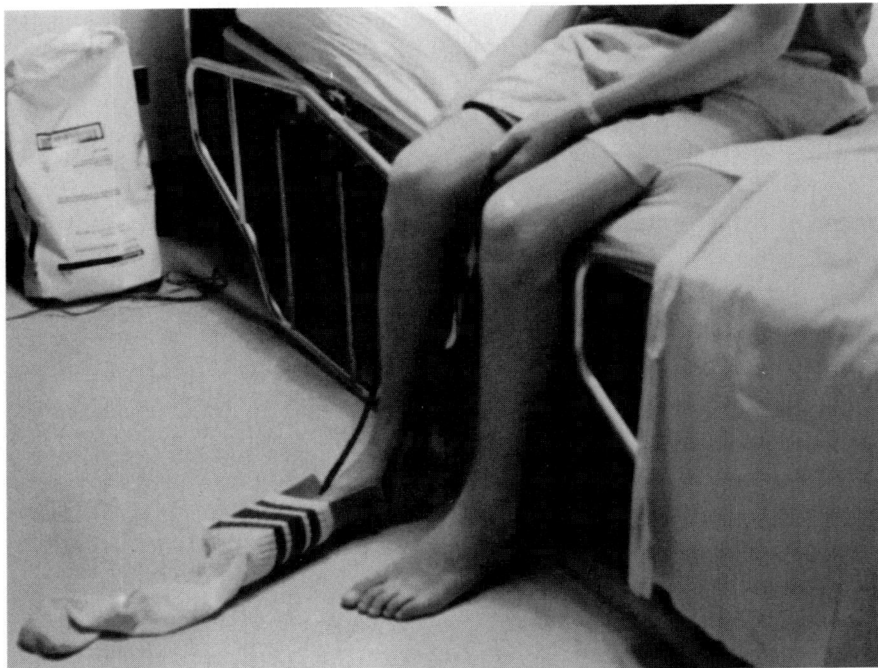

FIGURE 25–8. Stocking aid used when a person is limited in reaching down to the feet or when lower extremity mobility limits bringing the foot near to the hands. A person places stocking over sock holder, places the holder in front of foot, and pulls at rope to pull up.

Other equipment or modifications to assist those with limited reach or grasp include bath mitts, long-handled brushes with soap holders (including a loop or built-up handle if grasp is impaired), soap-on-a-rope, pump dispensers for shampoo, and finger ring brushes for scrubbing the hair. For those who have severe physical difficulties, inflatable bed baths and shampoo trays are available.

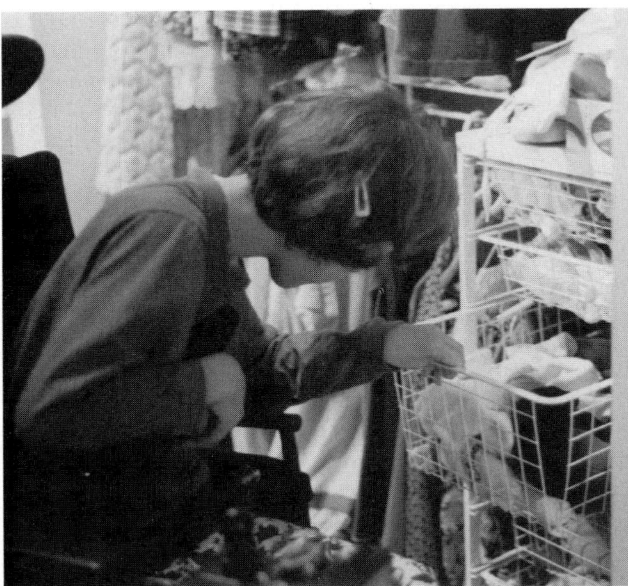

FIGURE 25–9. Commercially available closet organizer with mesh basket drawers allows a person with limited hand function to easily open and close drawers.

MOBILITY

Functional mobility is defined as the ability to move from one position in space (sitting, lying down, standing, etc.) to another position regardless of distance between starting and ending point.[4] Functional mobility includes bed mobility, transfers, ambulation, wheelchair mobility, and driving.

Bed Mobility

Bed mobility includes rolling in bed; scooting up, down, or toward either edge of the bed; and coming to a sitting position at the edge of the bed. Independence in bed mobility means being able to get into bed, position or reposition oneself to sleep, and get out of bed without the assistance of another person. Good head control, as well as upper-extremity strength and endurance, is needed to achieve bed mobility. Motor planning skills are also important for efficient and timely mobility.

Bed mobility can be challenging and exhausting, depending on the person's physical or mental limitations. Loops attached along the edge of the bed or onto the bed railing can decrease the amount of time needed for bed mobility and conserve one's energy. When trunk strength is inadequate, loops allow a person to roll to either side by pulling with the upper extremities. An overhead trapeze bar can help a person to sit at the edge of the bed or scoot up or down in bed. A step stool placed on the floor at the edge of the bed makes it easier to get into and out of bed. An electric bed is also helpful. When the head of the bed can be raised or lowered, it is easier for a person to come to a sitting position in or at the edge of the bed.

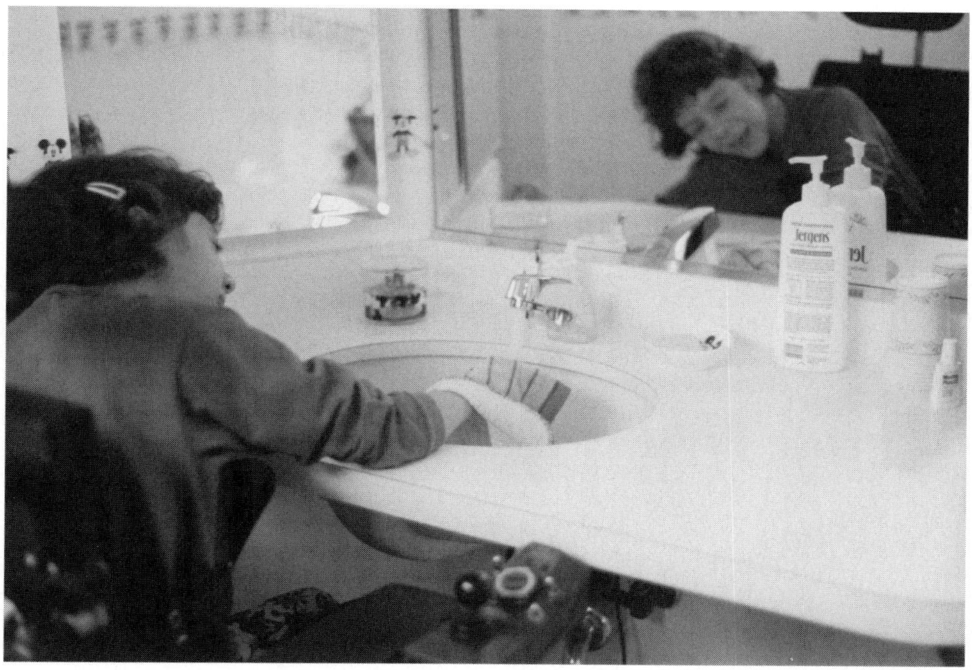

FIGURE 25–10. Sink with infrared sensor for easily turning water on and off when performing grooming and hygiene activities at the sink.

Transfers

A transfer is the act of moving a short distance from one position in space to another. The ability to transfer is necessary for anyone who uses a wheelchair for mobility. For a person to be independent in daily living tasks, independent transfers must be performed to wheelchair, bed, commode, tub, and car (if a van is not adapted for the wheelchair). Children must learn to transfer from the wheelchair to the floor so they can participate in activities with other children. It is desirable that all wheelchair users be adept at wheelchair-to-floor and floor-to-wheelchair transfers in case of a fall. (Sometimes, a small bench can be used as an intermediate step to go halfway between the floor and the wheelchair seat.) There are many different ways in which a person can perform a transfer. Depending on the functional limitations, certain transfers are faster and more efficient than others and might change as the person's abilities change. Some of the common methods of performing transfers are described below.

Stand-Pivot Transfer. For persons who can attain and maintain standing for short periods of time, the stand-pivot transfer is the most efficient method. Adequate hip and knee extension and good sitting balance are required. In this transfer, the person rises from a seated to a standing position and pivots to the adjacent chair to sit down. A modification of the stand-pivot transfer is the sit-pivot transfer, in which good sitting balance and upper-extremity strength are used to lift the hips up and across to another chair without standing. The feet are usually positioned on the floor; but if, as in children, the legs are too short to reach the floor, the feet can remain positioned on the footrests of the wheelchair or on a step stool.

Sliding Board Transfer. Sliding boards bridge the gap between transferring surfaces.[18] One end of the sliding board must be positioned securely under the individual's buttocks and the opposite end placed solidly on the other surface. Once the board is positioned securely between the surfaces, the person scoots his hips across the board to the new surface (Fig. 25–11). As with the sit-pivot transfer, the feet can be positioned on the floor or remain on the footrests of the wheelchair. Sliding boards are available in many shapes and sizes, and adaptations can be added according to a person's individual situation.

Wheelchair-to-Floor Transfers. There are a variety of ways to transfer from the wheelchair to the floor. Using the forward method, the footrests are rotated to the side and the feet placed on the floor. Then, flexing far forward in the wheelchair, the person places his hands on the floor and lowers himself to the floor.

Pivoting to the floor is another method. With the footrests removed or rotated to the side, the person scoots to the edge of the wheelchair and pivots the hips so that he or she is sitting on one buttock. Hands are placed on the seat of the wheelchair. Using strong upper extremities, the body is pivoted out of the wheelchair and the knees are lowered to the floor. From the kneeling position facing the wheelchair, the person can then lower the hips to the floor into a side-sitting position.

Yet another method is used when long leg braces are worn. In this case, the footrests must be removed or rotated to the side, hips are moved to the edge of the

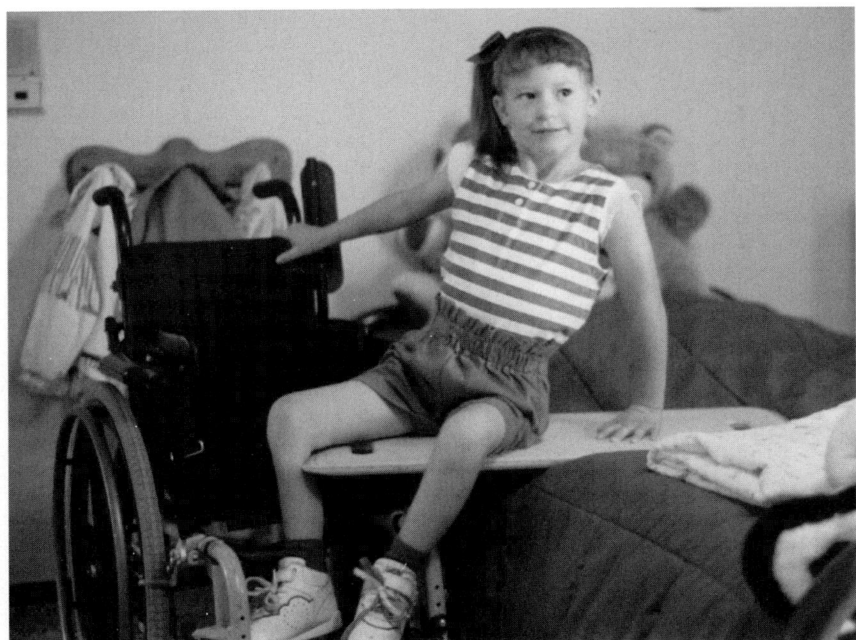

FIGURE 25–11. Sliding board transfer: the sliding board bridges the gap between the wheelchair and bed. The person uses upper extremities to scoot across the surface from the wheelchair to the bed.

wheelchair, and the knees are extended with the heels placed on the floor. Then, placing the hands on the forward-most frame of the wheelchair, the person lowers the hips to the floor. This method requires good upper-extremity strength and long arms for leverage to control the lowering movement for the entire distance to the floor. Children's wheelchairs, with a lower floor-to-seat height, can help some children perform this type of transfer; however, the wheelchair might still be too high for a child to perform this method of transfer.

The last two methods can be reversed to transfer from the floor back into the wheelchair. The last method is more difficult, since very good upper-extremity strength and leverage are important for success.

Ambulation

A person's level of functional independence can be significantly affected by the ability to ambulate. In order to ambulate, one must have sufficient lower-extremity and trunk strength, as well as balance, coordination, and cognitive skills for safety and timing. (See Chapter 5 for a discussion of gait analysis.) If limitations exist in these areas, physical compensations, orthoses, and other assistive ambulation devices can be used singly or in combination to help a person be independent with ambulation.

Many physical compensations (e.g., locking the knee during the stance phase of gait, abducting the leg during the swing-through phase, or placing the foot flat instead of heel-strike at initial contact) are neither energy- nor time-efficient. Through therapy programs and the use of orthoses and assistive ambulation devices, these compensations can be minimized. Many orthoses that support various joints of the lower extremity can help one to compensate for physical limitations. Chapter 16 describes the variety of lower-limb orthoses that are available. It is important to remember that in order to be independent, a person must also be able to don and doff orthotic devices without help.

There are a variety of assistive gait devices. In general, walkers provide the most stability and are prescribed for persons with more significantly decreased balance, coordination, or strength. Crutches provide moderate stability, and canes provide the least stability. Careful assessment of a person's function allows the recommendation of the device that maximizes function and best meets the person's needs.

Figures 25–12 to 25–15 show some examples of assistive ambulation devices.

Wheelchair Mobility

For people who are unable to ambulate or are able to ambulate only short distances, use of a wheelchair for mobility can still allow functional independence in the community. Proper positioning in the wheelchair, good sitting tolerance, strength, endurance, and cognitive skills are necessary for efficient and safe mobility in a wheelchair.

Proper positioning in the wheelchair (described in Chapter 18) is necessary to maintain alertness, increase comfort in and tolerance of the wheelchair, and allow for efficient use of the upper extremities—either to propel a manual wheelchair or to activate a switch for a power wheelchair. In order to propel a manual wheelchair, a person must have sufficient strength in at least one upper extremity (e.g., a person with hemiplegia operating a one-arm-drive wheelchair) or in bilateral upper extremities (e.g., a person with paraplegia) (Fig. 25–16). Lighter-weight wheelchairs, such as sports models, are easier to propel and maneuver over a variety of surfaces

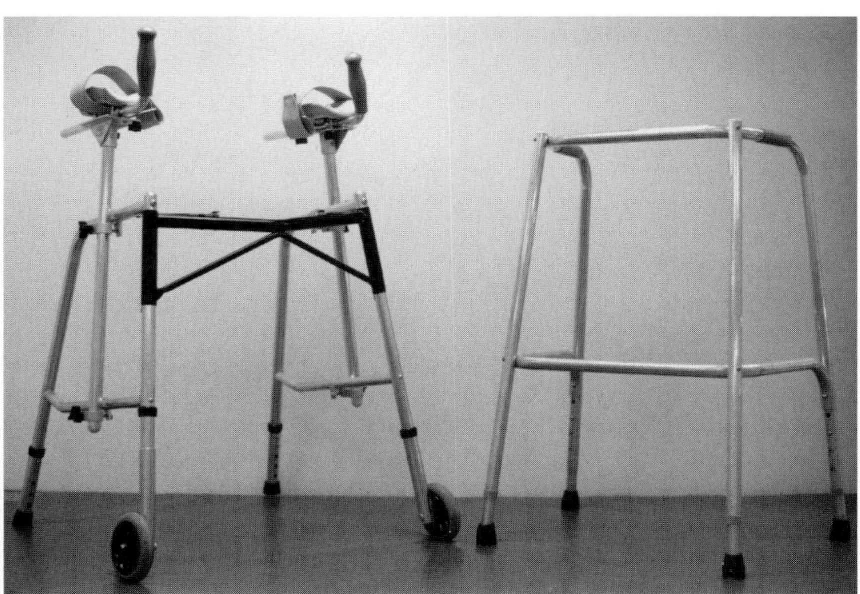

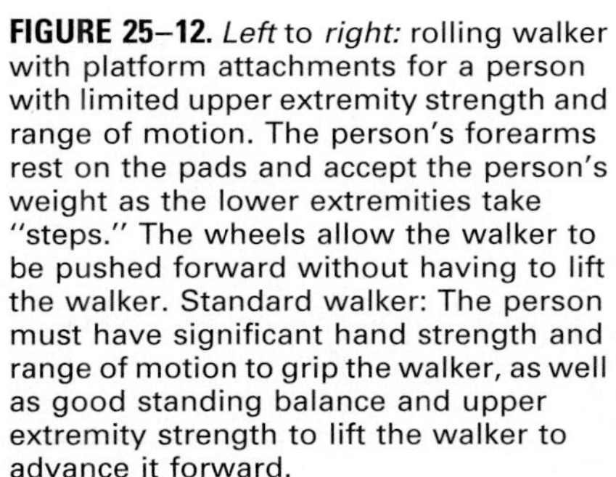

FIGURE 25–12. *Left* to *right:* rolling walker with platform attachments for a person with limited upper extremity strength and range of motion. The person's forearms rest on the pads and accept the person's weight as the lower extremities take "steps." The wheels allow the walker to be pushed forward without having to lift the walker. Standard walker: The person must have significant hand strength and range of motion to grip the walker, as well as good standing balance and upper extremity strength to lift the walker to advance it forward.

such as grass, curbs, and thick carpeting (Fig. 25–17). Adaptations, such as lateral trunk supports for balance or quad pegs to the rims of wheels for a person with decreased hand function, increase the weight of the wheelchair, but are sometimes necessary to enhance a person's independence with wheelchair mobility.

As a result of advances in technology, even persons with significant limitations in upper- and lower-extremity function can still be independent in wheelchair mobility. There are many ways to control a power wheelchair. Some examples include using a straw

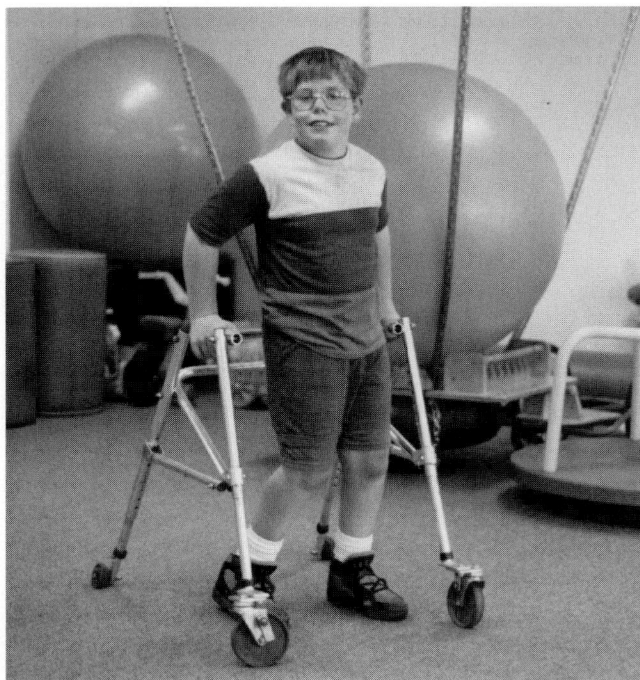

FIGURE 25–13. Reverse walker is used to facilitate extension posture with a person who tends to maintain a flexed posture while standing.

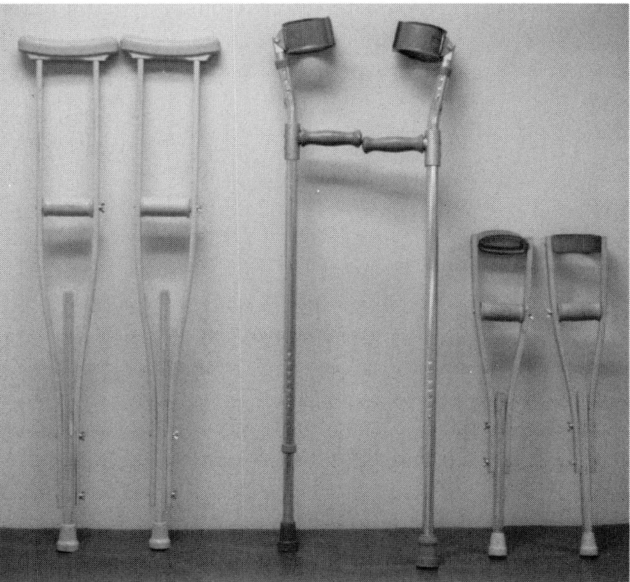

FIGURE 25–14. *Left* to *right:* axillary crutches used by individuals with good balance and coordination: length of time crutches are required is usually short. Forearm crutches have a cuff around the forearm that is open at the front or side, and are used mostly by individuals needing crutches on a long-term basis (e.g., individual with paraplegia who may require bracing with ambulation). Kenney crutches are used mostly by children who need total contact around their forearm.

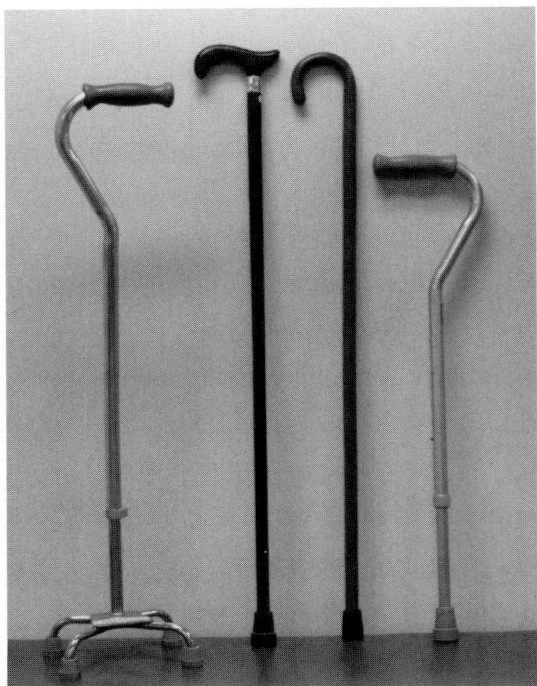

FIGURE 25–15. *Left* to *right:* quad cane and various standard canes used by individuals who need minimal assistance for balance during ambulation and who may or may not have limited use of one upper extremity. The quad cane provides more stability due to the four prongs at the base.

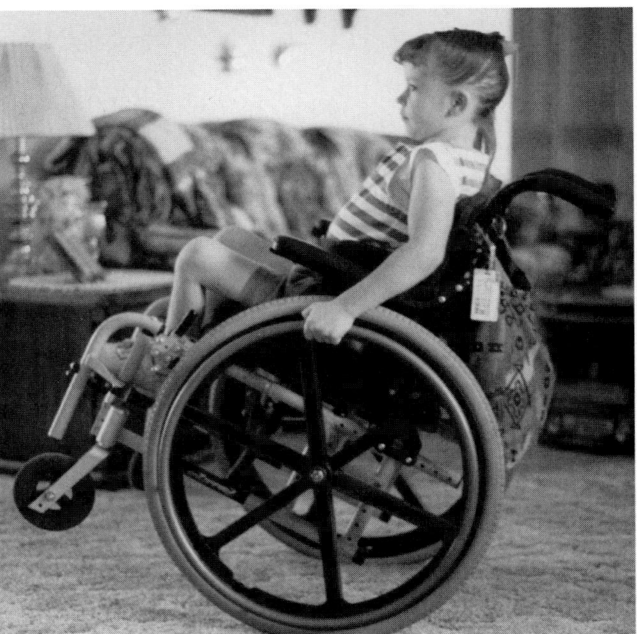

FIGURE 25–17. Demonstration of "wheelie" for ease in wheelchair mobility over obstacles or through rough terrain, such as grass or thick carpeting.

(sip-and-puff), proportional head controller, separate switches for directions, and joysticks. A person must understand the concepts of mobility in order to safely and efficiently drive a power wheelchair. Children as young as 2½ to 3 years old can be taught to operate a power wheelchair safely.[9] Physical and occupational therapists are an integral part of the team in helping a person decide which type of wheelchair best meets his or her positioning and mobility needs.

Driving

Transportation is an important aspect of a person's functional independence. Those who are unable to drive

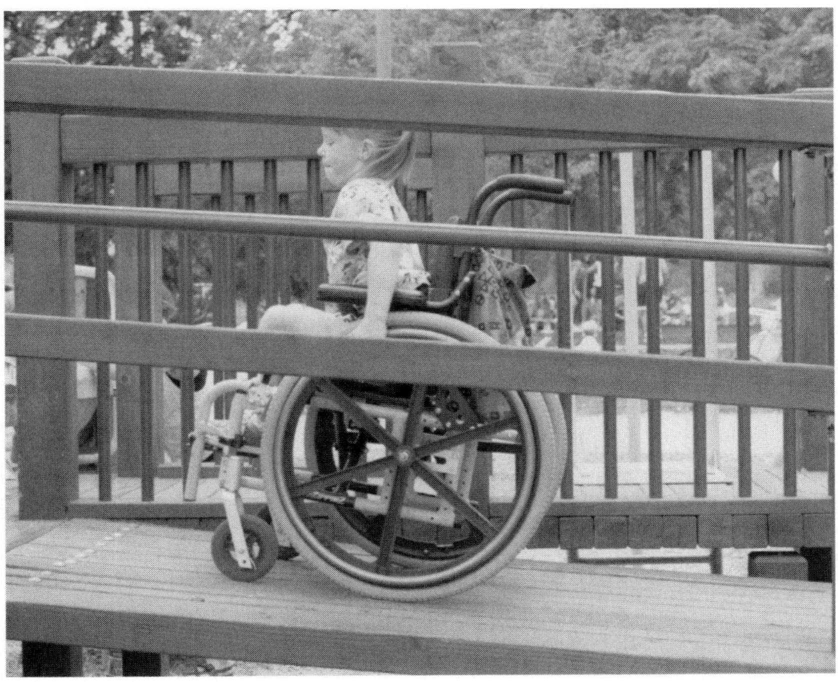

FIGURE 25–16. Good upper extremity strength is needed for self-propelling a wheelchair up a ramp.

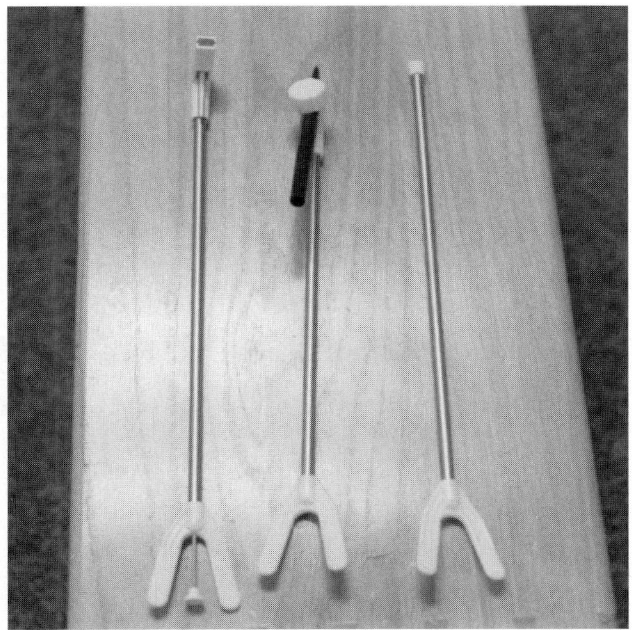

FIGURE 25–18. Various mouthsticks are used to perform different functions. *Left* to *right:* pincer mouthstick used by pushing tongue forward onto center piece, which then opens up the distal end to pick up light objects. Middle mouthstick holds writing tools from pencil to crayon. Pointer mouthstick used for turning pages and pushing forward.

must rely on others or on public transport. All people must be properly restrained in the seat of a car or wheelchair, and children must be restrained in a car seat. Harness systems can be used for people who need added trunk support.

Many people with physical limitations can drive with adaptations to the vehicle. Hand controls for driving and braking accommodate diminished upper extremity strength. Levers and knobs can be attached to the controls for optimal function. Adaptations vary, depending on whether the person will be driving from the wheelchair or from a captain's chair in a van. Electric lifts and wheelchair tie-down systems are available for vans. Portable ramps can be used when there is a large step to enter the vehicle. Assistance may be required to set up the ramp, supervise the stability of the ramp, and for maneuvering up the ramp if strength is inadequate. If a person is able to transfer from the wheelchair to the seat of the car, the wheelchair can be loaded into the back seat or onto an electric car top carrier.

Companies that specialize in custom van modifications for disabled persons and some car dealerships can provide information regarding the latest modifications available.

COMMUNICATION

Patients are often limited in their choice of nonverbal communication tools (writing, typing, computer, phone use, and book). The use of communication tools requires adequate fine motor strength, coordination, reach, and grasp to use the device.

Adaptations for writing tools can vary. They include built-up foam, cuffs, or mouthsticks with pens or pencils, hand splints and writing devices that support and compensate for weak hand musculature while positioning and holding writing tools, and weighted pens for controlling coordination of movement for writing. Figures 25–18, 25–19, and 25–20 show some adaptations for writing tools. Bookholders, page-turners, mouthsticks, or head sticks can help in handling books.

Typing, either on a typewriter or computer, can be performed by the use of typing sticks with adapted handles and splints with a slot for a typing stick (e.g., a vertical holder, pointer mouthstick, or head pointer). If coordination is impaired, keyguards and a key latch can facilitate accuracy. Alternative keyboards are also

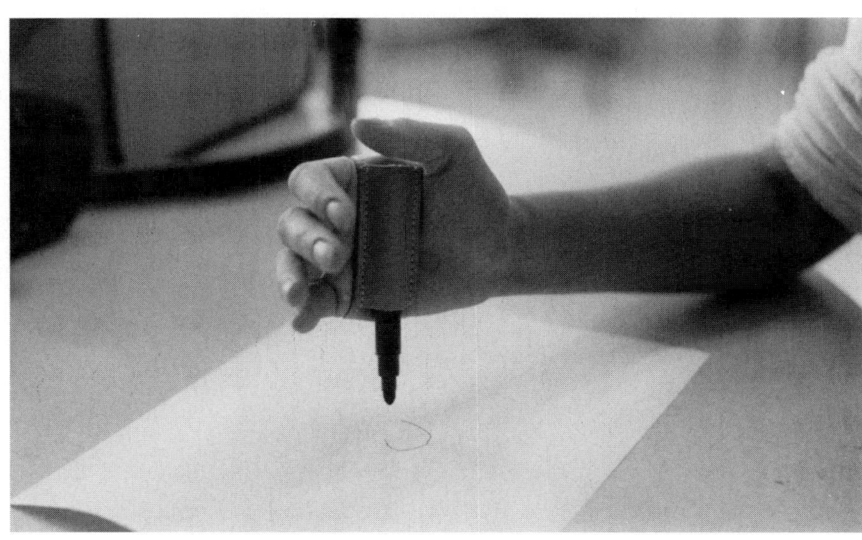

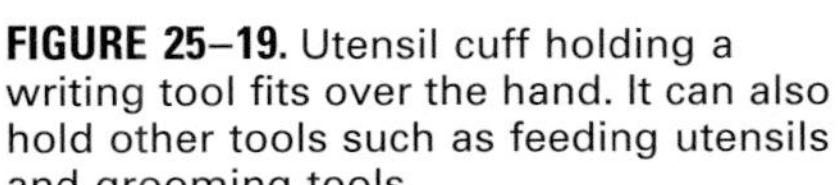

FIGURE 25–19. Utensil cuff holding a writing tool fits over the hand. It can also hold other tools such as feeding utensils and grooming tools.

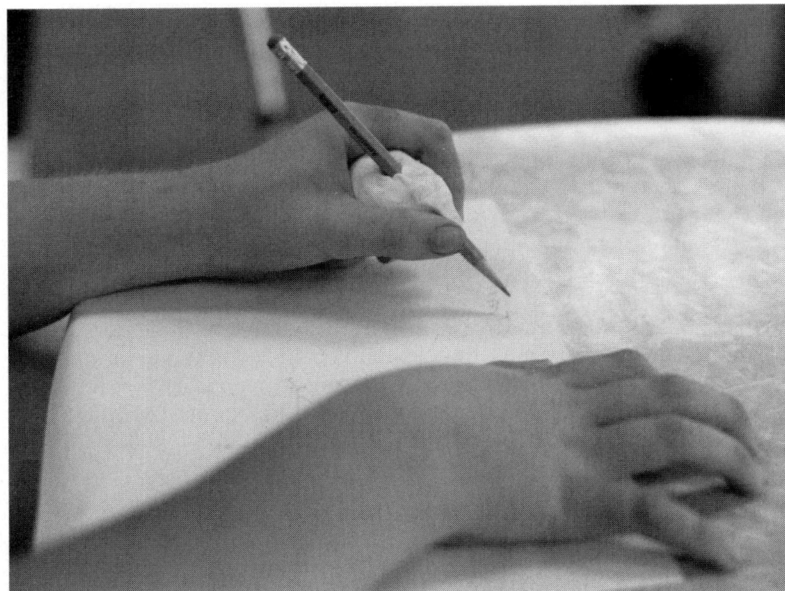

FIGURE 25–20. Built-up handle made out of setting putty was conformed to person's grasp to facilitate functional tripod grasp for writing. Modifications can vary from application of foam to commercially available plastic grips.

available, such as the expanded keyboard or a small keyboard. Adapted switches (i.e., single-switch or sip-and-puff) can also be added for the use of a computer. Armrests, mobile arm supports, or overhead slings can be used for typing if arm strength and endurance are limited. For phone use, telephone clip holders, dialing sticks, speakerphones with quick-dial features, and goosenecks to hold the receiver are available. Environmental control units and technology aids are discussed in Chapter 23.

HOME MANAGEMENT

Home management involves cooking, cleaning, and safely and appropriately using tools and appliances. Before providing recommendations, it is important that the therapist assess the individual while performing homemaking activities to determine which activities can be done safely with or without adaptations (Fig. 25–21). It is also important to educate and train the individual in energy conservation and work simplifica-

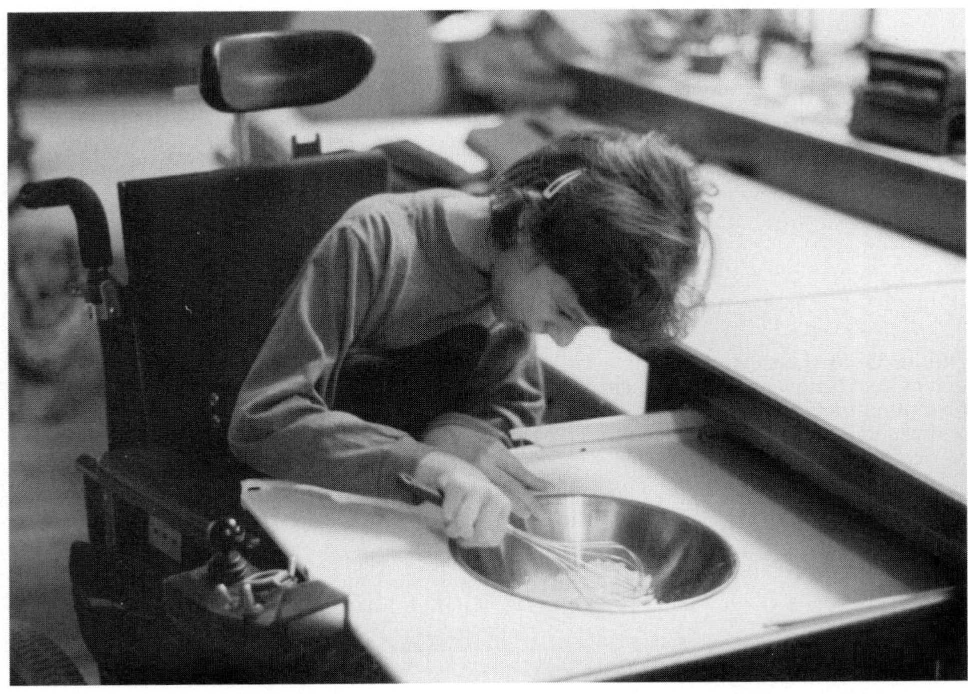

FIGURE 25–21. House with wheelchair-accessible cooking area so child with physical limitations can participate in cooking activities, such as mixing ingredients for a cake.

tion techniques for incorporation into home management activities.

These tasks require gross motor mobility skills and upper-extremity fine and gross motor coordination and strength. When limitations exist, environmental adaptations and assistive devices can be used in conjunction with work simplification and energy conservation techniques. Examples include reachers to retrieve items; lever-type handles to faucets, doorknobs, and appliances; adapted cooking utensils with loop Velcro handles; stabilizers such as Dycem; cutting boards with suction cups on the bottom and prongs to hold vegetables (Fig. 25–22); commercially available power appliances (e.g., can opener); and extended handles for reach (e.g., dustpan, broom).

Home Accessibility

Many adaptations exist for performance of home management skills. Home modifications are also important to allow persons to live efficiently and successfully in their homes. Examples of modifications range from very simple ones, such as rearranging the furniture and placing commonly used items within reach, to complex ones such as widening doorways, adding a ramp (Figs. 25–23 and 25–24), and construction of a roll-in shower. A thorough home assessment by a therapist is recommended for persons who have or may have difficulty functioning within their home environment.

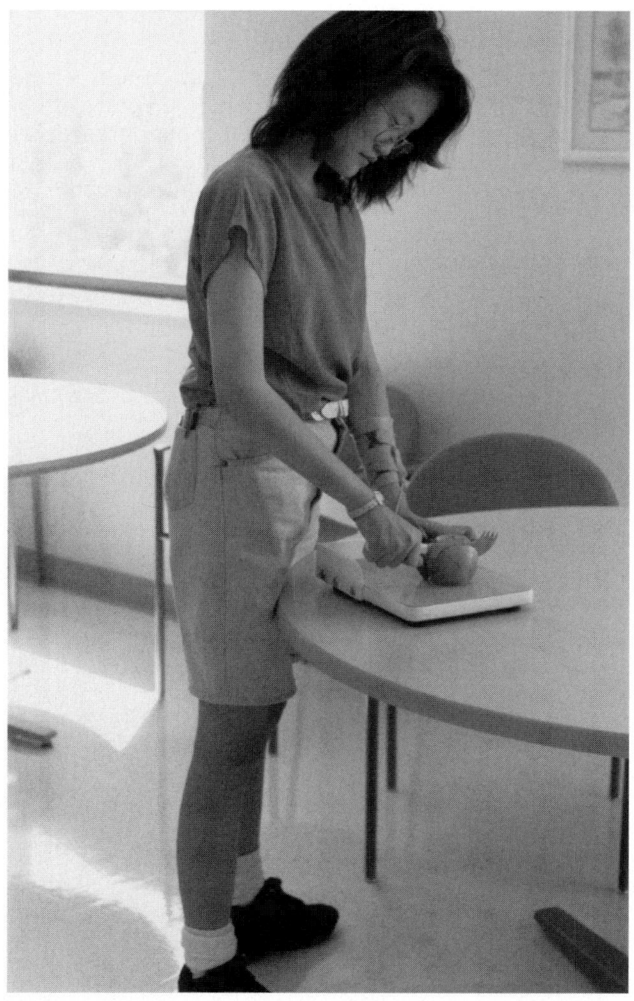

FIGURE 25–22. A rocker knife and an adapted cutting board with rubber feet, to avoid slippage of board, and prongs and edges, to hold the food, assists the person with functional use of one upper extremity. A rocker knife with fork edges cuts food by rocking down on food: the traditional sliding motion often receives stabilization from the opposite upper extremity. The fork edges are used in place of a fork, avoiding the need for two utensils.

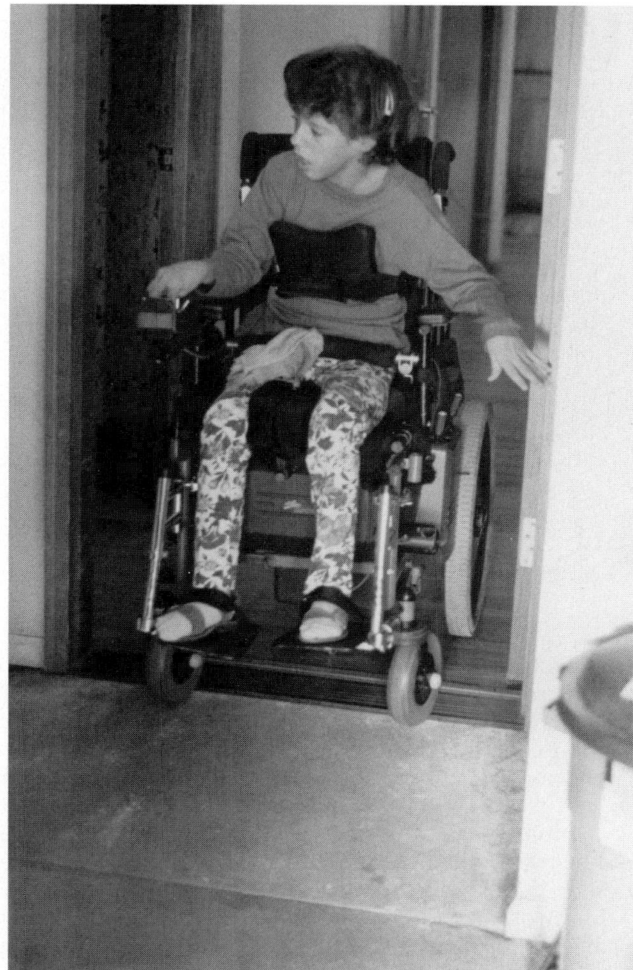

FIGURE 25–23. Ramp in residential setting: this small ramp provides accessibility over one step. Longer ramps are necessary to provide accessibility over several steps: the recommended slope of the ramp is 12 in. run for every 1 in. of rise.

LEISURE SKILLS

Leisure is "free" time, during which a person indulges in rest and recreation, etc.[24] Recreational activities benefit people both physically and emotionally through enjoyment, exercise, competition, and meeting other people.[6, 30] If the person is in a rehabilitation setting, therapists can facilitate independence in leisure activities through a community reintegration program, either individually or in groups. Goals of community reintegration include performing self-maintenance, mobility

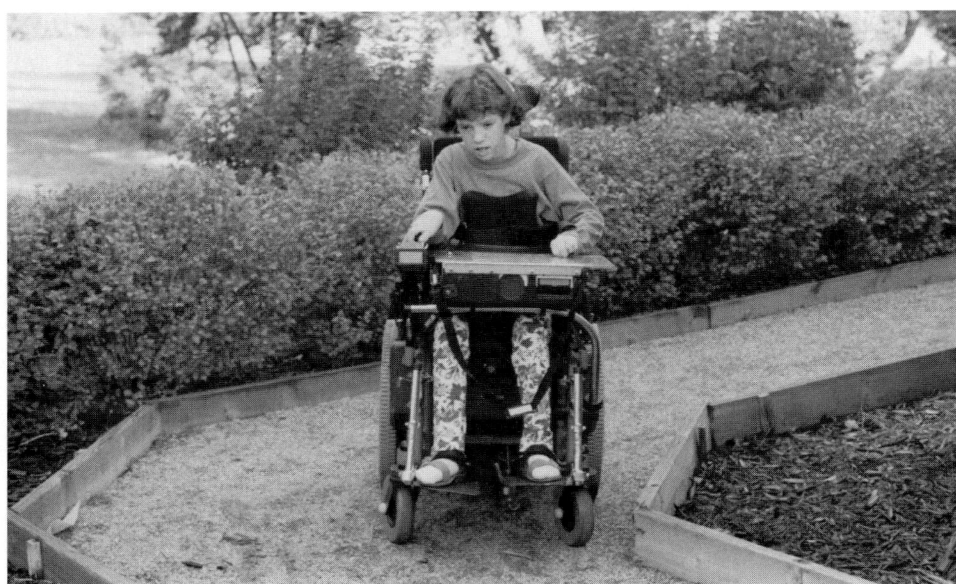

FIGURE 25–24. Specially designed walkway through yard provides accessibility outdoors when grass is an obstacle.

skills, and problem solving in a community setting so the person can perform comfortably in school, work, and leisure activities in the community (Fig. 25–25). Some examples of activities that can be practiced include popping a wheelchair over a curb, reaching for items on a high or low shelf, negotiating a wheelchair at a counter to pay, and practicing toileting skills in a public restroom. Exposure to various community activities facilitates comfortable functioning in social settings.

Many organizations exist throughout the country that provide programs especially designed for people with special needs. Information about these programs can be obtained from local parks and recreation departments, churches, and national organizations, which may be disability-specific (e.g., the National Head Injury Foundation). An example of an outdoor sports organization is the National Sports Center for the Disabled (NSCD) in Winter Park, Colorado. Activities at this center include alpine skiing, biking, hiking, white-water rafting, fishing, rock-climbing, and camping. Camps can be sports-specific[2] or include a variety of activities such as a tennis camp or a week filled with canoeing, rock-climbing, and camping.

Many adaptations exist to compensate for a person's mental limitations and physical disability. These include equipment as well as environmental modifications. Occupational and physical therapists are instrumental in helping individuals access resources, and perform task analysis and identify adaptations for participation in leisure activities.

Figures 25–26 to 25–30 illustrate some examples of adapted activities that serve as therapeutic modalities and, more importantly, offer enjoyment.

OCCUPATIONAL ENVIRONMENTS

Work has been described as "a behavior which is motivated by an intrinsic urge to be effective in the environment . . . influenced by cultural tradition and learned through the process of socialization."[16] Work can be a mere source of livelihood.[17, 23] Occupations are age-specific. A preschool child's occupation may be play and learning, whereas a school-age child's occupation

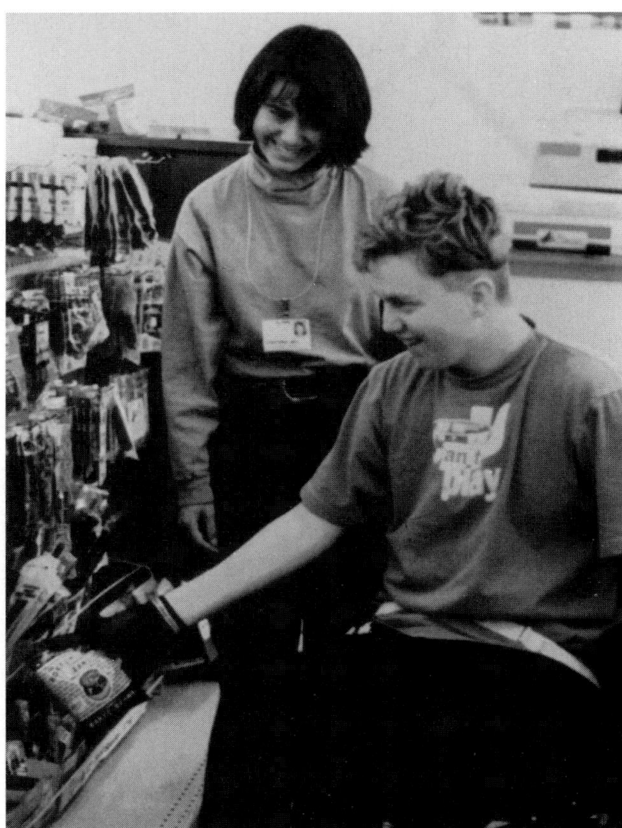

FIGURE 25–25. Problem-solving in the community: therapist facilitating independence in the community. Person is solving problem of how to reach items off the shelf in a grocery store.

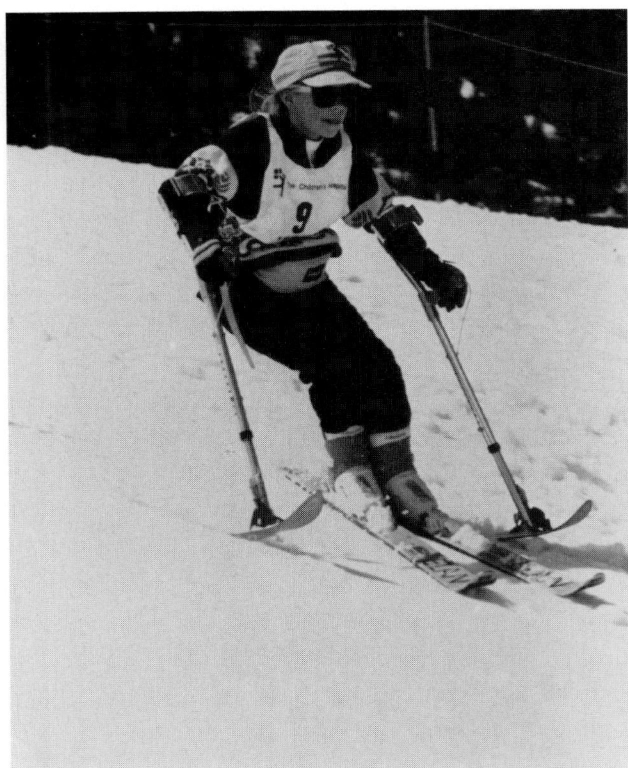

FIGURE 25–26. Outrigger skis used while skiing by a person who has difficulty shifting weight, maintaining upright stance, and maintaining balance. A person must be able to stand independently but may have difficulty with coordination.

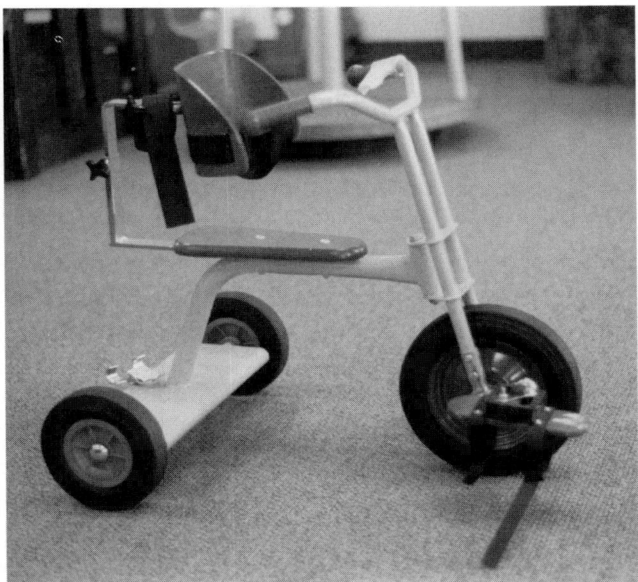

FIGURE 25–28. Tricycle adapted with footplates and straps, trunk support, and an extended seat, for children with limited balance, coordination, and strength.

is school activities and play, and an adult's occupation is work and leisure activity (Fig. 25–31).

Limitations can interfere with a person's ability to perform a job. Public laws exist that have provisions that allow a person with disabilities to enter work more easily. The Americans with Disabilities Act of 1990 (ADA)[1] supports people with disabilities in competing in the workforce.[15, 21] The ADA provides persons with disabilities with civil rights protection in areas of employment, public services, transportation, public accommodation, and telecommunication. Therapists play a vital role in providing information regarding the ADA as well as in task analysis of the person's job, providing input for environmental and tool adaptations, and information on changing and problem-solving architectural barriers.

Some examples of how therapists can assist include assessment of work environments. Considerations to be

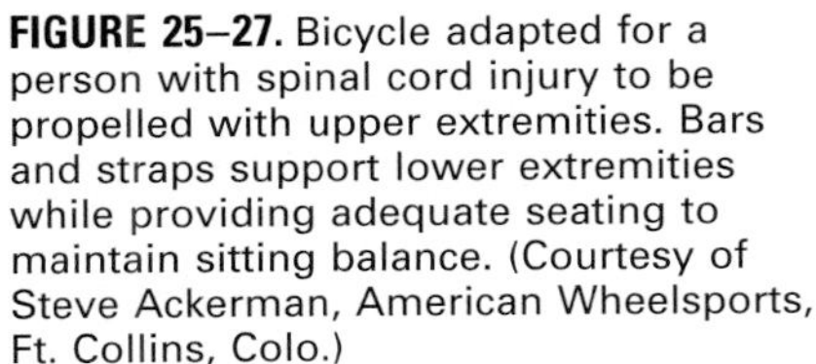

FIGURE 25–27. Bicycle adapted for a person with spinal cord injury to be propelled with upper extremities. Bars and straps support lower extremities while providing adequate seating to maintain sitting balance. (Courtesy of Steve Ackerman, American Wheelsports, Ft. Collins, Colo.)

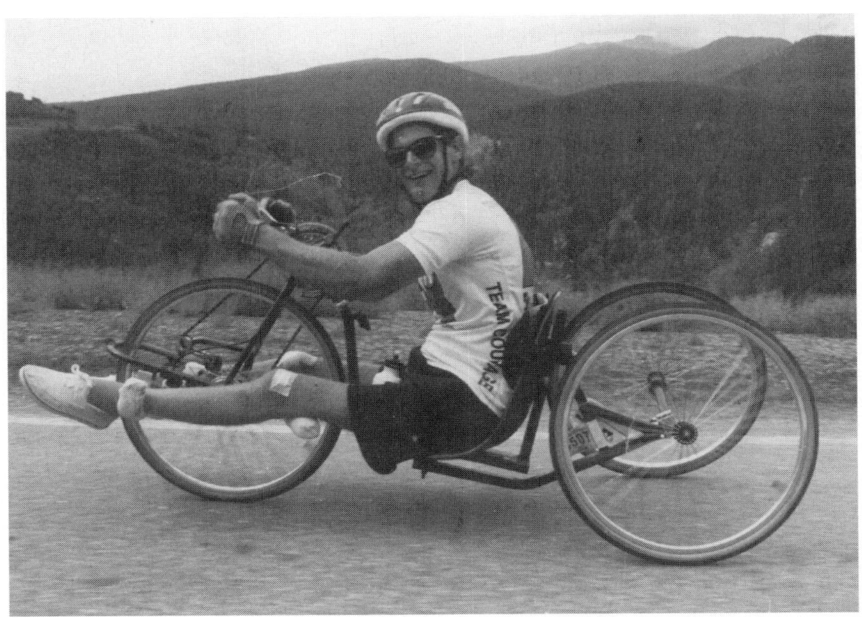

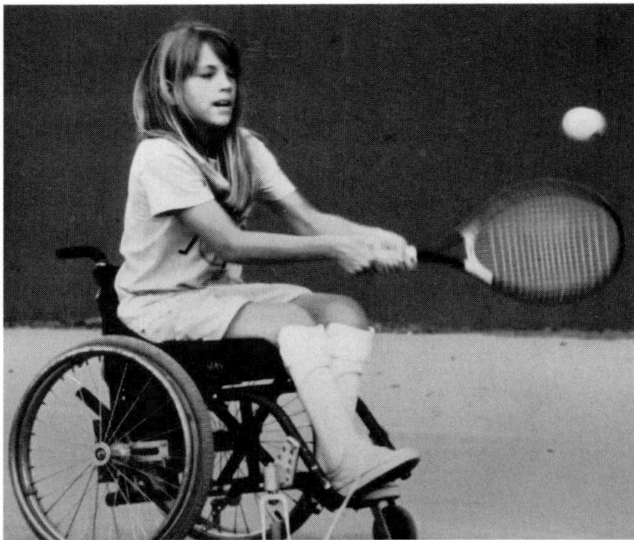

FIGURE 25–29. Many sports, such as tennis, basketball, and rugby, can be adapted for participation by a person in a wheelchair.

taken into account for the work environment include the following:

1. Is the person able to enter and exit the work (school, play) environment?
2. Is the person able to be mobile inside the environment (i.e., access all necessary rooms)?
3. Can the person efficiently use all necessary equipment (e.g., computer, water fountain, restroom, swings) (Fig. 25–32)?
4. Can the person communicate effectively with coworkers and peers?

A variety of modifications are available that can facilitate work (school, play) access and function. The modifications vary according to the person's physical or mental limitations. Some examples of modifications that facilitate entering and exiting an environment include[1,3]:

1. Ramps built at a ratio of 12 inches of length to 1 inch of rise.
2. Wide landings at the top of ramps (5 ft. × 5 ft.).
3. Platforms built from sidewalks to playground equipment (Fig. 25–33).

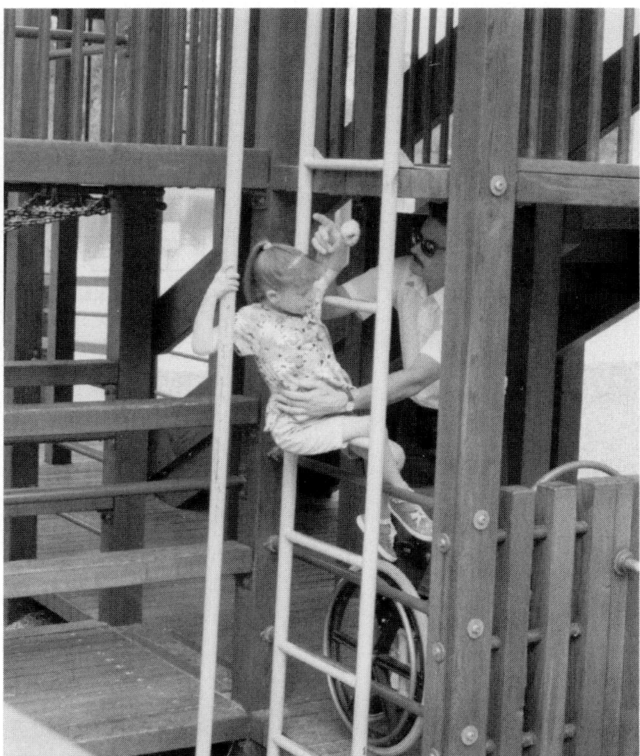

FIGURE 25–31. Parent helping child adapt to playground environment.

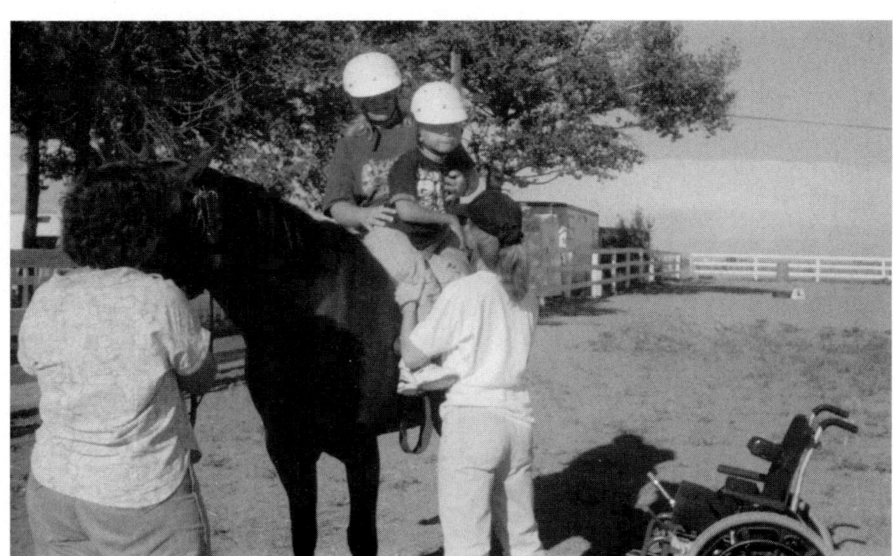

FIGURE 25–30. Therapeutic horseback riding can be used as an alternative to traditional therapy programs and as a recreational activity. Saddles can be adapted for those with decreased strength in lower extremities and trunk.

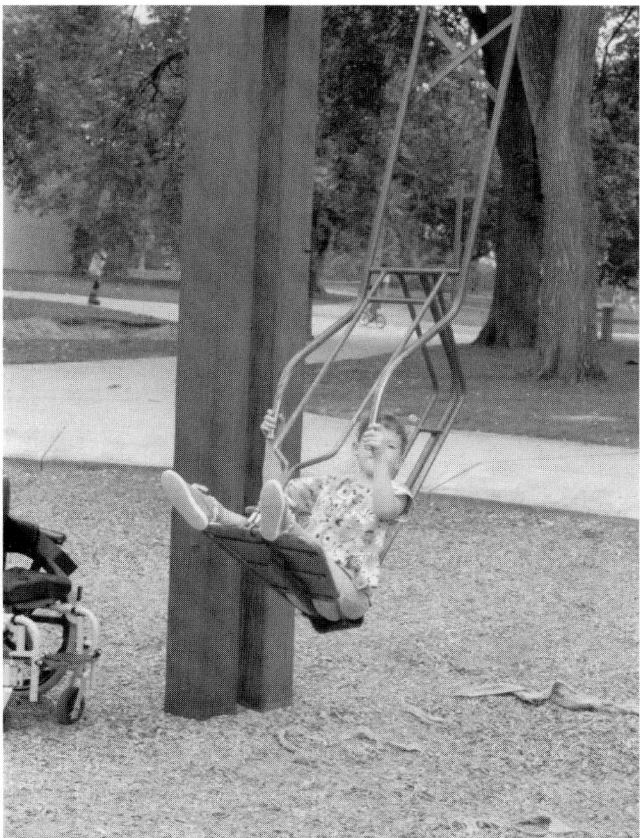

FIGURE 25–32. Adapted swing. Movement of the swing is achieved by pushing and pulling on the handles, using the arms.

Some examples of modifications that allow a person to be mobile inside environments include:

1. Wide doorways (36 inches)
2. Elevators
3. Ramps
4. Rearrangement of furniture or equipment (especially the restroom area)
5. Avoid thick carpeting and throw rugs.

Some examples of modifications to equipment include:

1. Computers with appropriate access (e.g., Headmaster, switches, scanning devices, etc.)
2. Lowering water fountains and providing a variety of buttons and levers to activate them
3. Handicapped-accessible swings
4. Modifications to toys (e.g., switch-activated, adapted handles, stabilizing surface)
5. Appropriate work surface (e.g., a desk or table at an appropriate height, width, length, and with space underneath)
6. Wheelchair needs to allow optimal positioning for maximum performance and interaction with the environment as well as minimizing skin and postural problems
7. Restrooms facility accessible to provide functional use (e.g., grab bars and levers to flush toilet)

Some examples to foster effective communication:

1. Augmentative communication devices and telephone with adaptations
2. Proximity of student to chalkboard
3. Effective use of all communication tools (i.e., computer and all necessary software and writing tools)

Therapists are helpful in providing suggestions to teachers or employers regarding ways to allow a person to function in his or her environment.

CONCLUSION

There are many adaptations and modifications available to help a person with physical and mental limitations to achieve functional independence in the home and community. It is essential that the person's developmental and cognitive level, motivation, physical abilities, and goals be considered in collaboration with patient and family before recommending any adaptations. The adaptations should enhance function without interfering with independence.

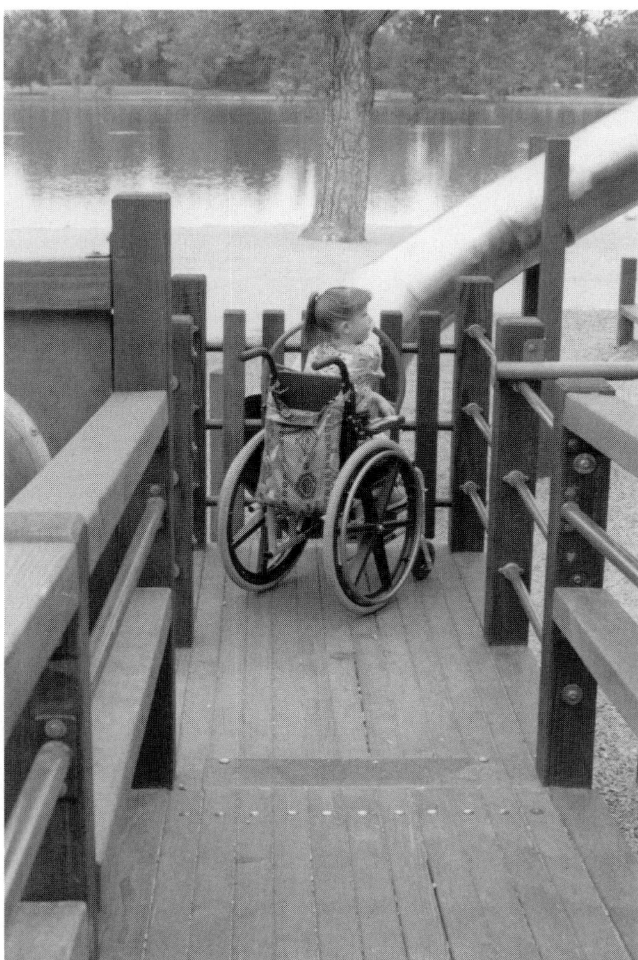

FIGURE 25–33. Playground equipment accessible by wheelchair, with platforms and ramps.

REFERENCES

1. Americans with Disabilities Act of 1990. Public Law 101–336, US Code, vol 42, sec 1210.
2. American Wheelsports. 721 N. Taft Hill Road, Ft. Collins, CO 80521.
3. Architectural and Transportation Barriers Compliance Board: Americans with Disabilities Act, accessibility guidelines for buildings and facilities. Federal Register 1991; 56(July 26):35408–35453.
4. Brandstater ME: Disability: Activities of daily living. In Basmajian JV, Kirby RL (eds): Medical Rehabilitation: A Student's Textbook. Baltimore, Williams & Wilkins, 1984, pp 246–259.
5. Breske S: When it comes to rehabilitation, family matters. Adv Phys Ther 1992; 23:4.
6. Bundy AC: Assessment of play and leisure: Delineation of the problem. Am J Occup Ther 1993; 47:217–222.
7. The Children's Hospital Rehabilitation Independence Scale (CHRIS). The Children's Hospital, Denver, Department of Rehabilitation.
8. Coley IL, Procter SA: Self-maintenance activities. In Pratt PN, Allen AS (eds): Occupational Therapy for Children. St Louis, Mosby–Year Book, 1989, pp 260–294.
9. Dietz JC: Functional evaluation of pediatric powered mobility devices. Arch Phys Med Rehabil 1989; 70:A–20.
10. Edleman L: Getting on Board: Training Activities to Promote the Practice of Family-Centered Care. Bethesda, MD, Association for the Care of Children's Health, 1991.
11. Fisher AG: Functional measures: Part 1. What is function, what should we measure, and how should we measure it? Am J Occup Ther 1992; 46:183–185.
12. Haley S, Baryza MJ, Webster HC: Pediatric rehabilitation and recovery of children with traumatic injuries. Pediatr Phys Ther 1992; 4:24–30.
13. Intagliata S, Sullivan B: Development and implementation of the Rehabilitation Institute of Chicago Functional Assessment Scale. Occup Ther Pract 1991; 2:26–37.
14. Jones R: Bladder and bowel management. In Hill JD, Intagliata S (eds): Spinal Cord Injury: A Guide to Functional Outcomes in Occupational Therapy. Rockville, CO, Aspen Press, 1986, pp 145–168.
15. Kalscsheur JA: Benefits of the Americans with Disabilities Act of 1990 for children and adolescents with disabilities. Am J Occup Ther 1992; 46:419–426.
16. Kielhofner G: Health Through Occupation: Therapy and Practice in Occupational Therapy. Philadelphia, FA Davis, 1983, p 136.
17. Mills CW: The meanings of work throughout history. In Best F (ed): The Future of Work. Englewood Cliffs, NJ: Prentice-Hall, 1973, pp 6–13.
18. Nawoczenski DA, Rinehart ME, Duncanson P, Brown BE: Physical management. In Buchanan LE, Nawoczenski DA (eds): Spinal Cord Injury Concepts and Management Approaches. Baltimore, Williams & Wilkins, 1987, pp 123–184.
19. Pedretti LW: Activities of daily living. In Pedretti LW, Zoltan B (eds): Occupational Therapy: Practice for Physical Dysfunction, St Louis, Mosby–Year Book, 1989, pp 230–271.
20. Procter SA: Adaptations for independent living. In Pratt PN, Allen AS (eds): Occupational Therapy for children. St Louis, Mosby–Year Book, 1989, pp 335–357.
21. Reed KL: History of federal legislation for persons with disabilities. Am J Occup Ther 1992; 46:397–408.
22. Uniform Data System (UDS): Functional Independence Measures (FIM). University of Newark at Buffalo. Department of Rehabilitation Medicine. Buffalo General Hospital, Buffalo.
23. Velazo CA: Work evaluations: Critique of the state of the art of functional assessment of work. Am J Occup Ther 1993; 47: 203–209.
24. Webster's New World Dictionary. New York, William, Collins, & World, 1976, p 807.
25. Whitneck G: Quantifying handicap: A new measure of long-term rehab outcomes. Arch Phys Med Rehabil 1992; 73:519–526.

26 CHAPTER

Stephen F. Noll, M.D., Claire E. Bender, M.D., Marge C. Nelson, O.T., Stephanie K. Carlson, M.D., and Renée J. Andersen, O.T.

Rehabilitation of Patients with Swallowing Disorders

Dysphagia can represent yet another barrier and another loss to a person already limited in mobility or self-care. The inability to swallow without drooling, coughing, or choking robs a person of enjoyment in eating and of the socialization that often accompanies eating. But more than a loss of pleasure, dysphagia also is a serious threat to a person's health from the risk of aspiration pneumonia and malnutrition. *Dysphagia,* a Greek word that means disordered eating, is difficulty in eating as a result of disruption of the swallowing process.

THE SWALLOWING PROCESS

Normal deglutition is a smooth, coordinated process that has been divided into three phases: oral, pharyngeal, and esophageal.[36, 80] Each phase is associated with a specific function, and if the functions are impaired by disease, specific symptoms result (Fig. 26–1 and Table 26–1).

The oral preparatory phase is the early component of the oral phase. In the oral preparatory phase the bolus is prepared and placed on the tongue. Intact lip closure, a mobile tongue, and functional muscles of mastication are needed for successful execution of this phase. Mastication not only modifies the bolus but also stimulates salivation, without which swallowing is difficult and delayed.[66] Once it is properly positioned, the bolus is propelled into the pharynx by a syringe-like action.[14] An important event that occurs simultaneously with the initiation of swallowing is the inhibition of breathing. Before the onset of swallowing, however, the airway is open. If a portion of the bolus slips into the pharynx early because of poor oral control or coordination, aspiration can occur before swallowing.[80]

The pharyngeal phase is of particular importance, because without intact laryngeal protective mechanisms, aspiration is most likely to occur during this phase (Fig. 26–2). Protection from laryngeal penetration and aspiration is afforded in several ways: by folding of the epiglottis over the laryngeal opening, by closure of the vocal cords, and by elevation and anterior displacement of the larynx.[80] Elevation and anterior displacement positions the larynx under the base of the tongue while opening the upper esophageal sphincter by traction, increasing the diameter of the pharynx, and engulfing the bolus.[36] Bolus propulsion by the tongue and pharyngeal constrictors is also an important factor[62]; propulsion through the pharynx lasts only about 0.6 seconds. If this function is slow or ineffective, there is greater laryngeal exposure to the bolus. In the normal state, the tongue, the pharyngeal palate, and a portion of the superior pharyngeal constrictors (the Passavant cushion) also close the oral and nasal cavities to prevent regurgitation.[60]

The pharynx is used in both deglutition and respiration. Of concern are potential food traps within this structure that are located near the laryngeal opening: the valleculae and pyriform sinuses (Figs. 26–2 and 26–3A). Ordinarily, food is cleared from these spaces with repeated swallowing. Retention of food in these

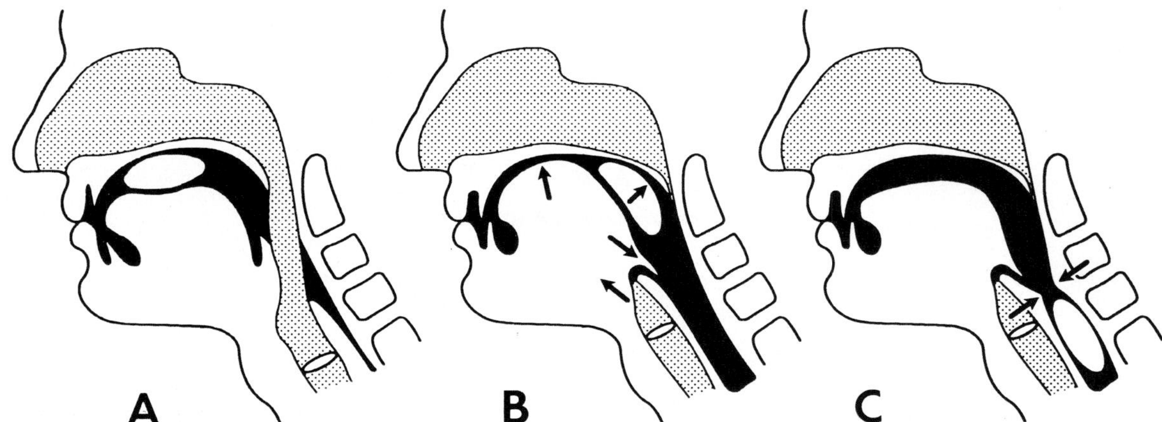

FIGURE 26–1. Three phases of normal deglutition. *A.* Oral preparatory/oral. *B.* Pharyngeal. *C.* Esophageal.

recesses, however, allows for spillage (penetration) into the larynx after swallowing and for possible aspiration into the tracheobronchial tree.[60, 80]

The cricopharyngeus muscle and pharyngoesophageal sphincter (PES) mechanism, called the *upper esophageal sphincter,* can also serve as a pharyngeal trap. The cricopharyngeus is unique among the pharyngeal constrictors[15] (Fig. 26–3B) and tonically contracts while other pharyngeal constrictors are at rest. The cricopharyngeus muscle, however, is only a portion of the physiological mechanism that serves as a closed portal to prevent esophageal reflux into the pharynx.[32, 45] With pharyngeal weakness, the propulsive force generated in the pharynx might not be great enough to transport the bolus past the upper esophageal sphincter. With pharyngeal incoordination, a form of dyssynergia can occur if the PES remains uninhibited and fails to relax during the swallowing process. In either of these instances, a portion of the bolus is retained in the pharynx and can result in aspiration after swallowing.[60, 80]

The esophageal phase, the last phase, is notable for being the longest phase, lasting approximately 6 to 10 seconds. Peristalsis is responsible for the bolus transport through the esophagus.[36] The lower esophageal sphincter is a high-pressure zone that, like the PES, relaxes to allow peristaltic movement of the bolus distally.[66] Disorders of the esophageal phase are diagnostically problematic, because symptoms of this phase can be referred to the pharyngeal region.[60]

The organization of deglutition is neurologically highly complex, much like the process it controls. Simply stated, however, the swallowing process requires the following elements: sensory input from the peripheral and central nervous systems, a coordinating center or centers, and a subsequent motor response sent back through these systems.[36] Sensory input from the peripheral system is primarily through cranial nerves V, VII, IX, and X. Sensory receptors take on several forms, including taste, fluid, or pressure sensors.[66] The fauces, pharynx, and posterior larynx appear to be key areas from which the most effective swallowing stimuli originate.[36] Centrally, cortical and subcortical pathways modulate the swallowing threshold,[90] although the exact role of the cerebral cortex is un-

TABLE 26–1 Stages of Deglutition

	Stage		
	Oral Preparatory/Oral	*Pharyngeal*	*Esophageal*
Purpose	Bolus preparation and transport	Bolus transport without aspiration	Bolus transport with limited reflux
Requirements	Mastication and salivation for bolus modification Lip closure for bolus containment Lingual control for bolus manipulation, positioning, and transport	Tongue elevation to prevent oral regurgitation Palatal elevation to prevent nasal regurgitation Laryngeal elevation, folding of epiglottis, and vocal cord adduction to prevent aspiration Coordinated pharyngeal motility and cricopharyngeal relaxation for bolus transport	Coordinated peristalsis and lower esophageal sphincter relaxation for bolus transport Cricopharyngeal tonic contraction to prevent pharyngeal regurgitation Relaxation of lower esophageal sphincter
Symptoms	Drooling Pocketing (squirreling) Repeated swallowing attempts Head tilt	Oral/nasal regurgitation Food sticking Cough or choke Wet, gurgling voice	Food sticking Heartburn

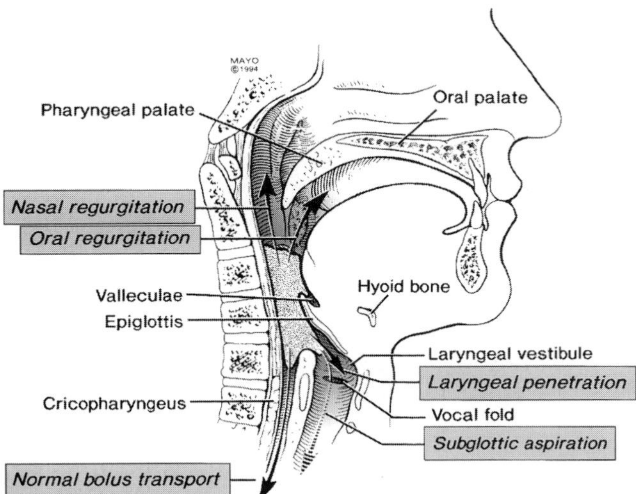

FIGURE 26–2. Pharyngeal phase of swallowing. Without laryngeal protective mechanisms, aspiration can occur. (Reproduced by permission of Mayo Foundation.)

clear.[88] The brainstem swallowing centers receive the input, organize it into a programmed response, and transmit the response.[36, 66, 115] Swallowing is only one of the possible programmed responses from these centers; the gag is another.[36] Output from the swallowing centers is passed to nuclei of cranial nerves V, VII, IX, X, and XII, and subsequently to the muscles they innervate. In response to the output, there is also a sensory feedback system that varies depending on the swallowing phase.[90]

CLINICAL ASSESSMENT

A thorough clinical assessment, or the "bedside" evaluation, is one method to determine how the swallowing process is impaired and which stage or stages are involved (Fig. 26–4).

History

Documentation of the course of the disease and specific symptoms of dysphagia is imperative, but other information is also important.[50, 71, 100] For example, dental disorders or the presence of dentures can affect the oral phase of swallowing. A history of recurrent pneumonia raises the question of aspiration. The presence of significant cardiopulmonary disease, such as chronic obstructive lung disease or congestive heart failure, can increase morbidity from aspiration. Previous neck surgery or radiation and cervical spondylosis or ankylosis can also alter the mechanics of swallowing or limit compensatory options for treatment. A dietary history provides clues to the problem based on the types and textures of food that a person has chosen.

Examination

Cranial nerve testing (nerves V, VII, IX, X, and XII) is done to elicit physical evidence of oral or pharyngeal dysfunction and allows direct observation of lip closure, jaw closure, tongue mobility and strength, palatal elevation, and oral sensitivity. However, additional observations are necessary to unveil other impairments that can affect swallowing.[71, 89, 100] For example, the level of alertness and cognitive status can significantly affect the safety of swallowing and also a person's ability to learn compensatory measures. Foamy oral secretions or an altered voice quality points to pharyngeal dysfunction and possible aspiration. Testing for the gag reflex is helpful, but an absent gag does not imply the inability to swallow safely.[80]

Assessing respiratory function is essential during the evaluation for many reasons. If the breathing rate is rapid because of respiratory distress, the timing and energy of swallowing can be difficult. If there is inadequate respiratory force with a cough or with clearing the throat, the risk of aspiration is increased. Chest auscultation can uncover an unsuspected pneumonitis or evidence of obstructive lung disease. Palpating for laryngeal excursion while a patient swallows helps identify the presence or absence of a key laryngeal protective mechanism (Fig. 26–5).

One final step in evaluation (if clinically appropriate and safe) is a diagnostic feeding assessment with various food textures. This assessment allows the opportunity to observe swallowing behavior directly. The "3-oz water swallow test" has compared favorably with the video swallow in identifying aspiration.[35] The result of this test is positive if the patient's voice develops a wet, hoarse quality or if the patient coughs within 1 minute after swallowing 3 oz of water.

The bedside evaluation has some predictive capabilities for determining the risk of aspiration. For example, the presence or absence of the gag reflex or a cough has been used to identify patients with bilateral infarctions who are at greatest risk for aspiration.[53] But the bedside evaluation tends to underestimate the occurrence of aspiration, particularly in older patients, in patients with expressive aphasia, and when more than 30 days has elapsed after onset of injury.[79, 128]

Laboratory Data

Chest radiography is a simple assessment for aspiration pneumonia. No pathognomonic sign of aspiration is seen on the chest radiograph, but the presence of infiltrates in a patient at risk raises suspicion. Pulse oximetry can be an adjunct to the identification of aspiration when performed before, during, and after a swallow.[31] Other routine laboratory tests are also useful. For example, the serum albumin value can be a marker of nutritional status. A low value suggests chronic nutritional insufficiency or chronic illness.[30]

TECHNICAL ASSESSMENT OF DYSPHAGIA

Radiographic Imaging

Videofluoroscopy. Most swallowing disorders are best evaluated with the dynamic recorded videofluoroscopy technique. Although many of the newer imaging methods (ultrasonography, computed tomography [CT],

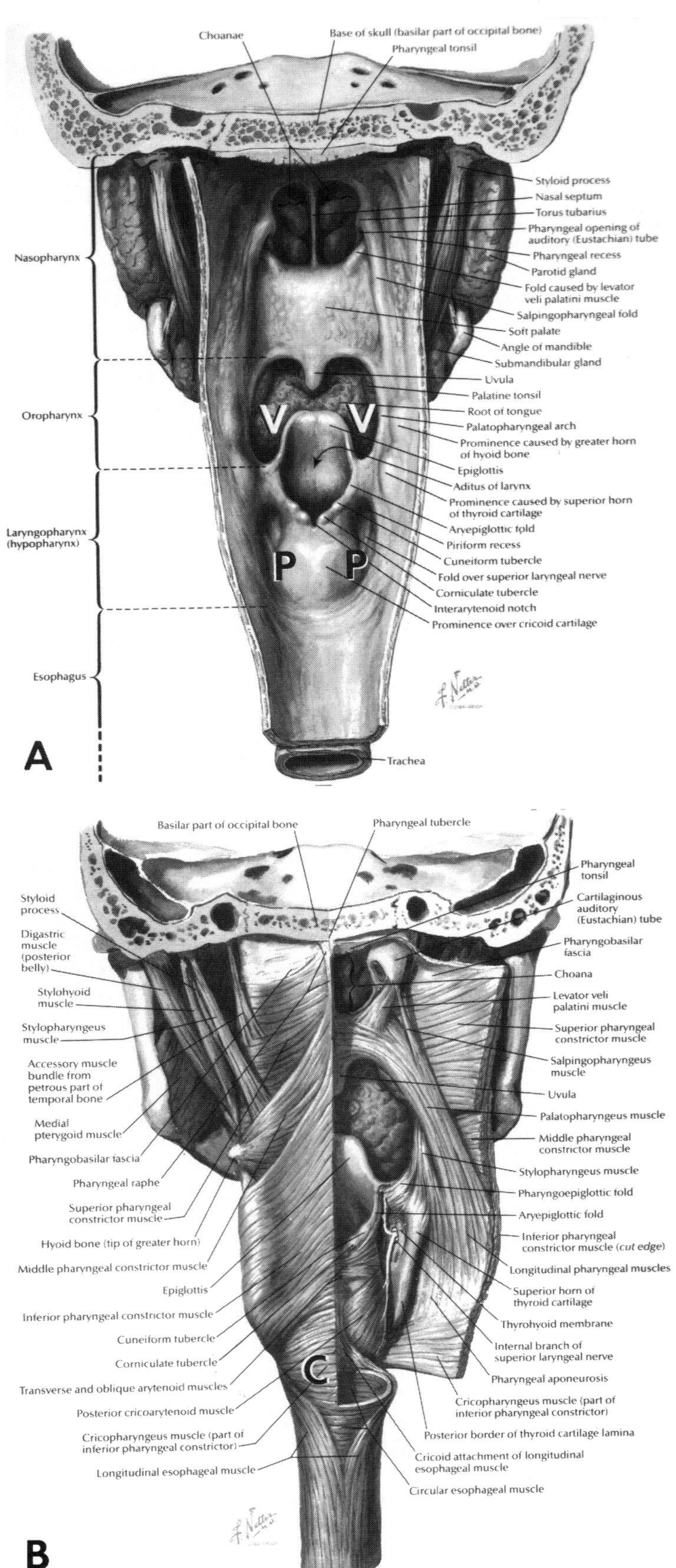

FIGURE 26–3. *A.* Pharynx: opened posterior view. P, pyriform sinuses; V, vallecula, which sits between base of tongue and epiglottis. *B.* Muscles of pharynx: partially opened posterior view. *C.* Cricopharyngeus muscle. (From Netter FH: Atlas of Human Anatomy, plates 60 and 61. Summit, NJ, Pharmaceuticals Division, CIBA-GEIGY Corp, 1989. Reproduced by permission of Novartis.)

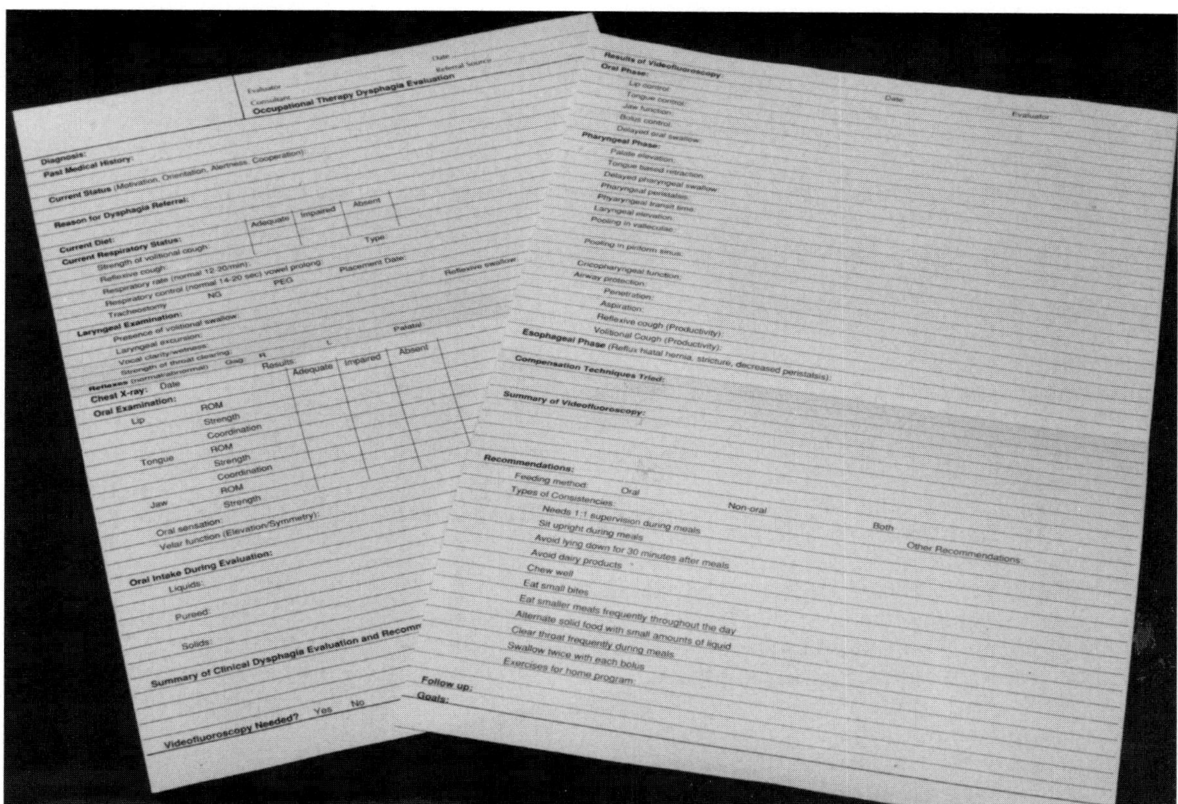

Occupational Therapy Dysphagia Evaluation

Evaluator
Consultant
Date
Referral Source

Diagnosis:
Past Medical History:
Current Status (Motivation, Orientation, Alertness, Cooperation):
Reason for Dysphagia Referral:
Current Diet: Type:
Current Respiratory Status: Adequate Impaired Absent
Strength of volitional cough:
Reflexive cough:
Respiratory rate (normal 12-20/min):
Respiratory control (normal 14-20 sec) vowel prolong:
Tracheostomy NG PEG Placement Date:
Laryngeal Examination:
Presence of volitional swallow Reflexive swallow
Laryngeal excursion:
Vocal clarity/wetness:
Strength of throat clearing:
Reflexes (normal/abnormal): Gag R L Palatal
Chest X-ray: Date Results:
Oral Examination: Adequate Impaired Absent
Lip ROM Strength Coordination
Tongue ROM Strength Coordination
Jaw ROM Strength
Oral sensation:
Velar function (Elevation/Symmetry):
Oral Intake During Evaluation:
Liquids:
Pureed:
Solids:
Summary of Clinical Dysphagia Evaluation and Recomm
Videofluoroscopy Needed? Yes No

Results of Videofluoroscopy Date: Evaluator:
Oral Phase:
Lip control
Tongue control
Jaw function
Bolus control
Delayed oral swallow
Pharyngeal Phase:
Palate elevation
Tongue based retraction
Delayed pharyngeal swallow
Pharyngeal peristalsis
Pharyngeal transit time
Laryngeal elevation
Pooling in valleculae
Pooling in piriform sinus
Cricopharyngeal function
Airway protection:
Penetration
Aspiration
Reflexive cough (Productivity):
Volitional Cough (Productivity):
Esophageal Phase (Reflux hiatal hernia, stricture, decreased peristalsis):
Compensation Techniques Tried:
Summary of Videofluoroscopy:
Recommendations:
Feeding method: Oral Non-oral Both
Types of Consistencies:
Other Recommendations:
Needs 1:1 supervision during meals
Sit upright during meals
Avoid lying down for 30 minutes after meals
Avoid dairy products
Chew well
Eat small bites
Eat smaller meals frequently throughout the day
Alternate solid food with small amounts of liquid
Clear throat frequently during meals
Swallow twice with each bolus
Exercises for home program
Follow up:
Goals:

FIGURE 26–4. Sample assessment form used in the evaluation of patients with dysphagia.

magnetic resonance imaging [MRI], scintigraphy, and endoscopy) have been used for workup, videofluoroscopic technique with the use of existing fluoroscopy systems, which are easily connected to inexpensive videotape recorders, continues to be the standard

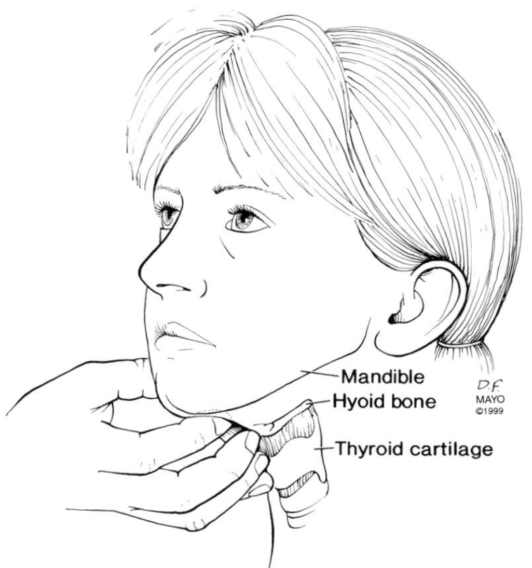

FIGURE 26–5. Palpating for laryngeal excursion to detect protective mechanisms active during swallowing. (Reproduced by permission of Mayo Foundation.)

Although this system has some loss of quality when compared with the more expensive, specialized cinefluorography systems, it is easier to use. However, radiation is still being used, and radiation exposure to the patient, fluoroscopist, and swallowing therapist exists and carries attendant risks.

Radiation Risk. Imaging with x-rays (as in videofluorscopy and plain radiography) delivers low-dose ionizing radiation that has been associated with tissue damage, genetic injury, and cancer. The risks associated with low-dose exposures have been extrapolated downward from high-dose data; consequently, the precise risks cannot be determined. It is important to note that low levels of radiation exist in our natural environment (air, ground, and water). During any x-ray study, it is the responsibility of the clinician to keep the amount of radiation at a minimum for the patient and for all personnel in the examining room.

Radiation effects depend on the amount of radiation energy absorbed. One gray (Gy) results from the absorption of 1 joule of radiation energy in a kilogram of tissue (1 Gy = 100 rad). Levels of x-ray doses are more commonly described in millirad or rad. Another measurement is the dose equivalent (1 sievert [Sv] = 100 rem). For general purposes, 1 Sv = 1 Gy; 1 rem = 1 rad.

Radiation effects can be (1) nonstochastic (i.e., with a threshold dose that must be exceeded for effects to occur) or (2) stochastic (i.e., the biological effect is all or nothing, the probability of the effect increases with dose [but *not* its severity], and there is no threshold dose level below which the effect cannot occur).[10] An example of nonstochastic effect is lens cataract induction with a single-exposure dose-equivalent of 200 rem. Stochastic effects include the principal health risks of diagnostic levels of radiation, such as the potential induction of cancer and genetic mutation.

The embryo and fetus, like all rapidly growing tissues, are particularly sensitive to the effects of radiation. Caution must be exercised when the patient, fluoroscopist, or therapist is pregnant. Videofluoroscopy for a swallowing evaluation does not directly irradiate the pelvic region of the patient, so fetal exposure is very minimal. It is during the first trimester of pregnancy that the most severe effects can be induced (e.g., spontaneous abortion, gross organ malfunction).

Currently, the National Council on Radiation Protection and Measurements recommends that a pregnant radiation worker (therapist, fluoroscopist) not exceed 500 mrem (0.5 cSv) exposure during the entire gestation period, and not exceed 50 mrem exposure in any 1 month. With proper shielding, the pregnant female operator can safely remain within these limits.

Exposure dose to the patient during videofluoroscopy is dependent on exposure times, the technique of the fluoroscopist, the equipment, and patient characteristics (cooperativeness, size). Exposure to the patient is determined by multiplying the number of minutes (seconds) of fluoroscopy by the dose (to a particular body part) per minute. Generally, the exposure to the patient is small.

The following key steps protect both the patient and the operators:

- Minimize the duration of exposure to x-rays.
- Think before you perform fluoroscopy (check the position of the patient and the equipment maintenance and handling).
- Ensure x-ray beam collimation (image only the area or areas of interest).
- Locate personnel at appropriate positions (Fig. 26–6).
- Use lead shielding (e.g., aprons, glasses, thyroid shields).
- Screen for pregnancy.
- Ensure that radiation monitor badges are worn by all radiation workers, including therapists, who assist in videofluoroscopy.

The image document (the videotape) becomes part of the patient's medical record. If additional documentation is warranted, image transfer to film can be achieved, but the image is of lesser quality than traditional spot filming or overhead filming for a permanent record. These techniques add to the overall exposure dose to the patient during the evaluation.

Equipment. Fluoroscopy is performed with standard radiographic and fluoroscopic units with image intensification. The x-ray tube is located beneath the tabletop. A videotape recorder (½-in.) with audio recording capability is adapted to the fluoroscopy unit for audiovisual examination. To facilitate the investigation of swallowing disorders in patients who are difficult to image, we have utilized a special lightweight mobile

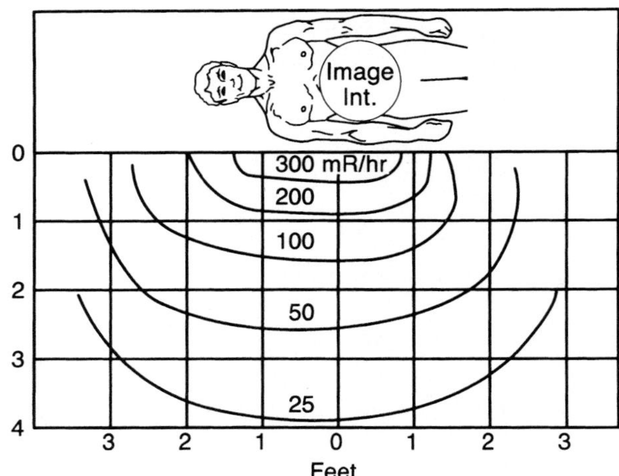

FIGURE 26–6. Radiation exposure to personnel depends on the inverse square law: intensity of beam is inversely proportional to the inverse square of the distance from the x-ray beam ($I \alpha 1/d^2$). Int, intensifier.

chair (Fig. 26–7). This equipment has the following benefits[24]:

- Narrow dimensions, which permit use with standard fluoroscopic units.
- Rugged yet lightweight construction for ease in mobility.
- Easy rotation of chair for posteroanterior and lateral viewing.
- Safety features, including seat belts, head restraints, locking wheels, and footrests.
- Can be modified to transportable chair for ease of patient transportation.

Procedural Guidelines. The examination is facilitated by coordinated consultation between the swallowing therapist and the radiologist (fluoroscopist). The videofluoroscopic swallowing evaluation team includes the therapist, the fluoroscopist, the radiology nurse or technologist, and the patient. A standardized examination protocol is often followed to make studies consistent and reproducible. A standard videofluorographic examination is described in Table 26–2.[101]

The standard procedure is performed with the patient in the upright (sitting) position; posteroanterior and lateral views are obtained. Swallowing is evaluated (and documented) by simultaneous video and audio recording, and the following methods or agents are used: dry swallow, thin liquid barium, thick liquid barium, pudding-thick barium, or solid barium cookie.

Individual patient needs might require that the examination be modified (such as by use of a semi-upright or a supine position instead of a sitting position).[35] The dry swallow is a screening tool to evaluate how the patient handles secretions. This can be further adapted by having the patient swallow sips of water.[46] Aspirated barium is usually well tolerated, but complications have occasionally occurred.[48] Water-soluble agents with high osmolality (such as diatrizoate meglumine [Gastro-

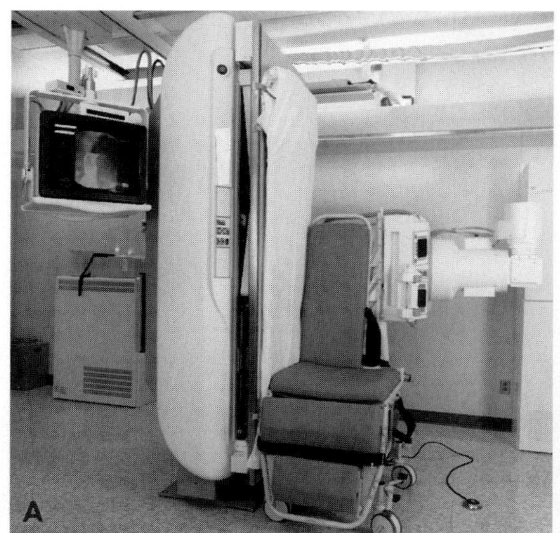

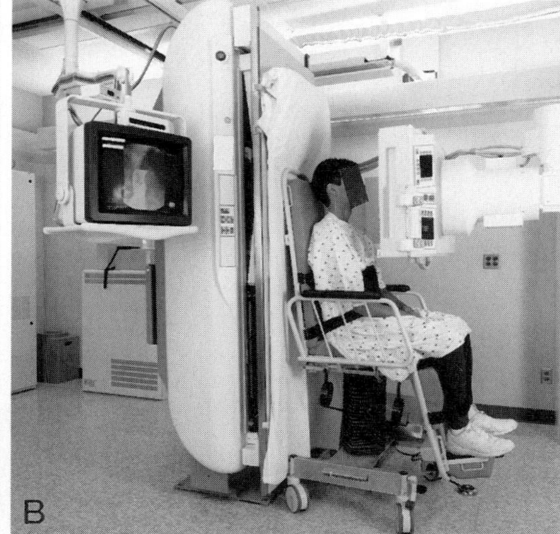

FIGURE 26–7. Lightweight chair mounted on special transporter. (Videoimaging Chair is manufactured by Hausted, Medina, OH.) *A.* Chair positioned for lateral fluoroscopy. *B.* Chair rotated for posteroanterior fluoroscopy. Note belts for head and body restraints.

grafin]) should not be used because of the risk of aspiration-induced pulmonary edema. The newer, more expensive, low-osmolar, iodinated contrast materials can be used with less risk of pulmonary or allergic reaction.

Interpretation. Diagnosis by fluoroscopy is a skill achieved through dedicated training and experience. The fluoroscopy diagnosis is recorded by the radiologist in the patient's permanent record. The entire upper gastrointestinal tract (from the mouth to the ligament of Treitz of the jejunum) should be evaluated to avoid missing an underlying disease (such as obstructing gastric carcinoma with aspiration).

There is a distinct clinical difference between the video-fluoroscopic examination and the routine upper gastrointestinal series. Both examinations evaluate the gastrointestinal tract from the mouth to the small intestine. The videofluoroscopic evaluation of swallowing has *both* diagnostic and potentially therapeutic capabilities. After aspiration is diagnosed, changes in the texture of the barium meal or variations in head positioning can provide immediate feedback for treatment of a swallowing problem.[105]

Quantitative evaluation of the pharyngeal transit time (measured during fluoroscopy) can be useful for following the progress of patients with dysphagia and for evaluating the effects of remedial therapy.[57]

Plain Film Analysis. Plain radiographic documentation is obtained if any abnormality is observed. Spot film analysis can be performed at the time of videofluo-

TABLE 26–2 Standard Sequence for Videofluorography

Lateral projection, patient sitting in usual position of comfort
Speech sample
Swallow 5 mL of thick liquid from a spoon
Drink thick liquid from a cup (1 swallow)
Swallow 5 mL of thin liquid from a spoon
Drink thin liquid from a cup (1 swallow)
Modifications and other liquids as appropriate
Masticate and swallow 1 tsp (or ¼ cookie) of formable solid food (category A)—patient seated in usual position of comfort with head in neutral position
Masticate and swallow 1 tsp of particulate solid food (category B)
Modifications and other foods as appropriate
Posteroanterior projection, patient sitting upright with neck slightly extended if possible
Take thin liquid from a cup, hold it in the mouth, and then swallow
Modifications or other foods as appropriate
Additional swallows of thin liquid as needed for imaging the esophagus

From Palmer JB, Kuhlemeier KV, Tippett DC, et al: A protocol for the videofluorographic swallowing study. Dysphagia 1993; 8:209. Reprinted by permission of Springer-Verlag, New York.

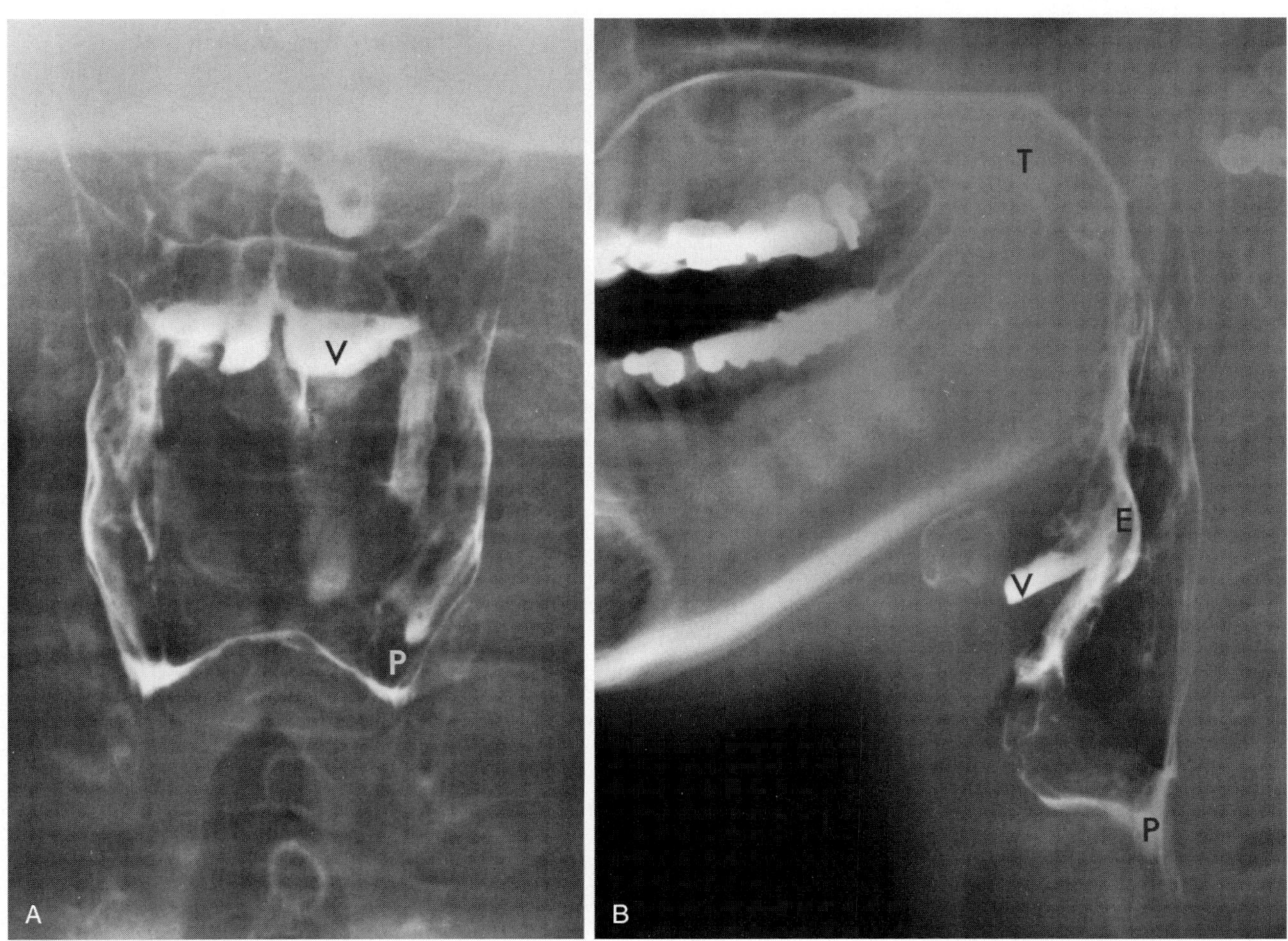

FIGURE 26–8. *A.* Normal posteroanterior view of pharynx. *B.* Normal lateral view of pharynx. E, epiglottis; P, pyriform sinus; T, tongue; V, valleculae.

roscopy, or overhead films can be taken after fluoroscopy. Any variety of views (anteroposterior, posterolateral, lateral, oblique) can be obtained to document the diagnosis (Figs. 26–8 through 26–12).

Ultrasonography. Dynamic US examination during swallowing is helpful in the evaluation of tongue and pharyngeal muscle function.[51, 57] As with any US technique, it has advantages and disadvantages (Table 26–3). When the swallowing mechanism is evaluated, only the region of the tongue posterior to the hyoid level can be studied.[85] The major advantage is the delineation of soft tissues within this region (Fig. 26–13).

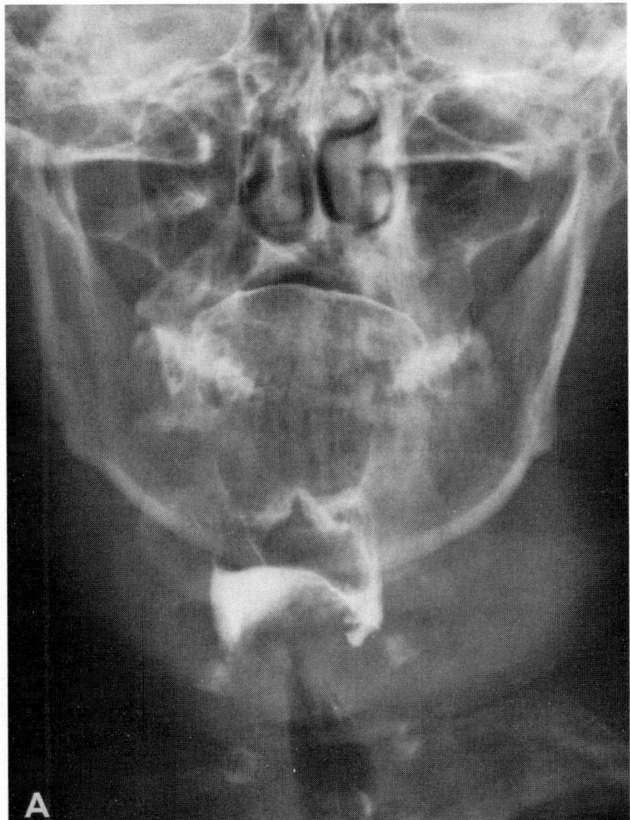

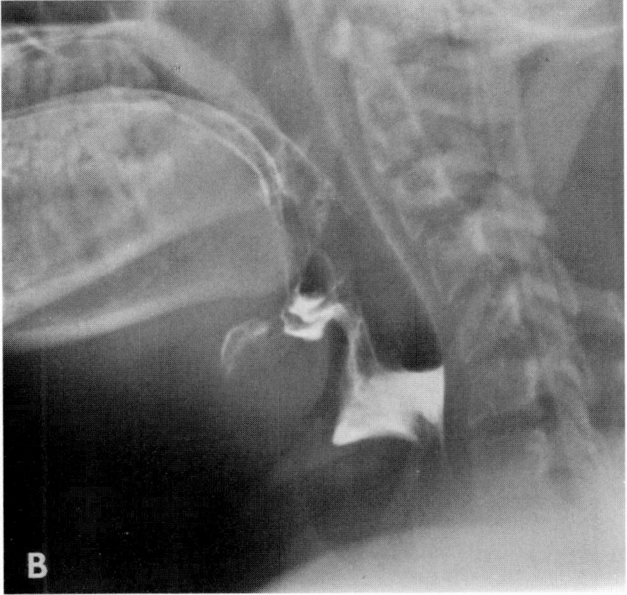

FIGURE 26–9. Pooling of barium in asymmetrically enlarged right pyriform sinus in patient who had had a stroke. No aspiration. *A.* Posteroanterior view. *B.* Lateral view.

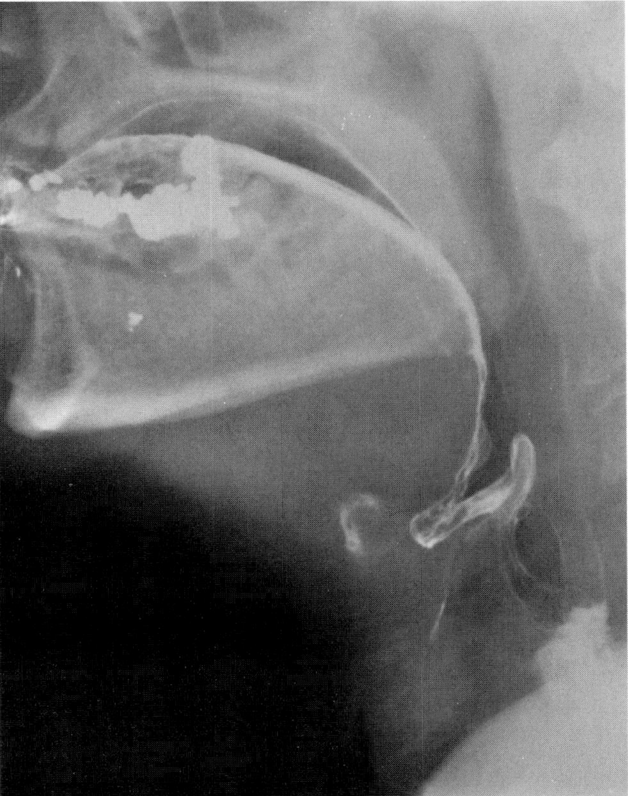

FIGURE 26–10. Lateral view, showing laryngeal penetration of barium due to poor covering of epiglottis. Calcified hyoid bone is just anterior to valleculae.

Most real-time US systems can be used to evaluate swallowing. For viewing the oropharynx, a real-time sector scanner should be used; for evaluating the larynx, a linear array system should be used. A 5-MHz transducer provides the best focal depth for both areas. US may be used with baseline videofluoroscopy to document aspiration and to further evaluate esophageal activity.[126]

The recent development of 2.7-mm endoluminal US probes now allows evaluation of the esophageal wall. This can be very helpful in the evaluation of dysphagia due to such common diseases as benign and malignant esophageal strictures, esophagitis, achalasia, cricopharyngeal dysfunction, and motility disorders (Fig. 26–14). Endoluminal US may also be helpful in following patients with benign strictures after esophageal dilation procedures.[124]

CT and MRI. The major indications for cross-sectional imaging in the evaluation of patients with a swallowing disorder include the following: (1) identification

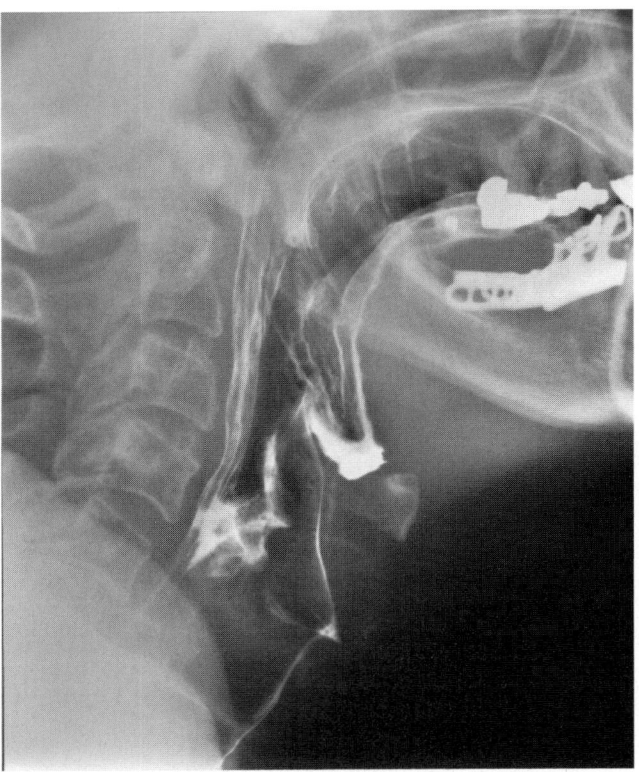

FIGURE 26–11. Tracheal aspiration of barium due to overflow of barium pooled in valleculae in patient who had had a stroke.

and staging of a mass in the upper digestive tract and (2) diagnosis of a central or peripheral nervous system mass to explain the pathophysiology of the swallowing disorder.

Fast CT scanning techniques now allow dynamic imaging of swallowing at a preselected level in the axial plane. This can be useful in assessing the degree of soft palate closure during swallowing, in evaluating the hypopharyngeal wall and detecting lateral hypopharyngeal pouches, and in detecting vertebral osteophytes that may encroach on the upper esophageal sphincter in the cervical esophagus and mimic primary upper esophageal sphincter dysfunction.[77] Because this technique evaluates only a single level at a time, it is only complementary to the standard videofluorographic examination. With the rapid development of MRI technology, CT has taken a lesser role. MRI is noninvasive, whereas CT utilizes ionizing radiation. Speech, tongue movements, and the swallowing motion can now be studied in motion series using the fast low-angle shot MRI (FLASH-MRI) tomography technique.[48] Studies using high-speed MRI (turbo-FLASH technique) and an oral contrast agent can even more accurately delineate the swallowing motion.[130]

Scintigraphy. Nuclear medicine techniques are becoming more widely used in the analysis of swallowing disorders. Procedures have been developed to assess gastric emptying, gastroesophageal reflux, esophageal motility disorders, and airway penetration and aspiration (Fig. 26–15).[119] Patients can be imaged both dynamically during swallowing and after they have swallowed a cupful of thin liquid containing 1 to 2 mCi of technetium-99m sulfur colloid. Compared with videofluoroscopy, computer-assisted scintigraphy, according to recent literature, provides more accurate data concerning the severity of airway penetration and the degree of airway clearing after penetration or aspiration. Identifying persons with airway penetration that is limited or vigorously cleared can assist in the decision whether to restrict liquid ingestion.[118]

Manometry. Although the barium swallow examination remains the screening procedure of choice, manometry can be a useful adjunct, particularly in patients with normal results on barium swallow examinations, patients with motility disorders, and patients with dysfunction of the cricopharyngeus muscle. Pharyngeal manometry provides an objective method of assessing swallowing dysfunction by measurement of intraluminal pressures during swallowing. Simultaneous videofluorography (videomanometry) confirms accurate placement of the manometric sensors (Figs. 26–16 and

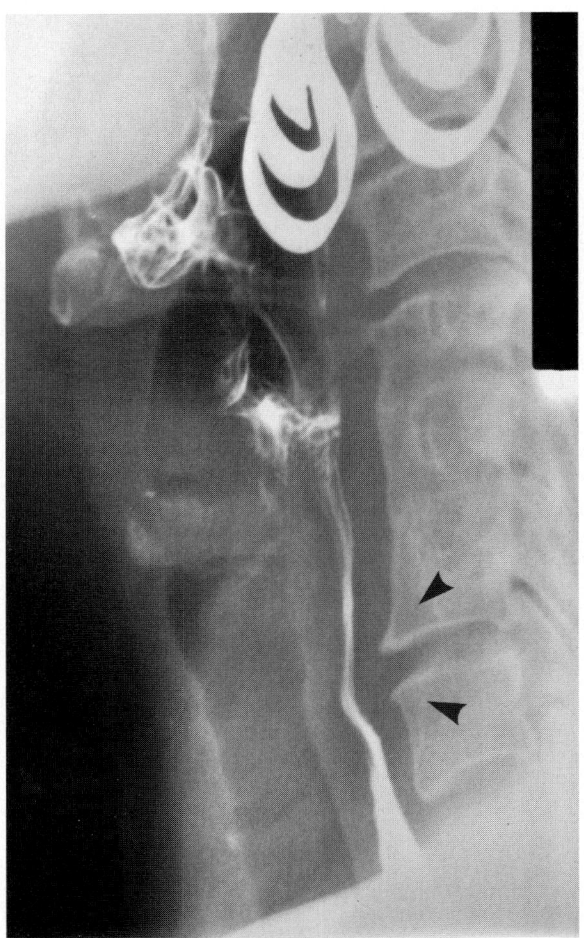

FIGURE 26–12. Prominent osteophytes (*arrowheads*) can result in dysphagia. Extrinsic compression of upper posterior esophagus is noted on lateral view.

TABLE 26–3 Advantages and Disadvantages of Ultrasonography for Evaluation of Swallowing

Advantages	Disadvantages
Noninvasive	Limited scanning region
Soft tissue delineation	Air, bone artifacts
Multiplanar imaging: sagittal, parasagittal, coronal, transverse	Missed aspirations
No contrast agent given	
Video recording	
Hard copy prints	

26–17). This helps to eliminate sensory displacement during laryngeal elevation and allows for more accurate measurements, particularly when assessing upper esophageal sphincter relaxation.[97, 99, 112] Manometry is time-consuming, however, and may be uncomfortable to the patient because of the placement of a peroral multilumen catheter system (Fig. 26–16).

Endoscopy. Fiberoptic endoscopic examination of swallowing (FEES), also referred to as videoendoscopic examination of swallowing (VEES), is a relatively new technique for evaluating the pharyngeal phase of swallowing (Fig. 26–18).[9, 74] This procedure is a sensitive technique for detecting premature spillage, laryngeal penetration, tracheal aspiration, and pharyngeal residue. The endoscope is passed transnasally to view the larynx and pharynx. Swallowing is directly evaluated using measured quantities of liquid dye with blue food coloring for contrast and food (such as applesauce or bread). Although the videofluoroscopic examination remains the standard for evaluation of swallowing disorders, certain patients are more amenable to endoscopy, such as critically ill patients who are unable to tolerate any risk of aspiration, patients in intensive care units who cannot be transferred to the fluoroscopy suite, and patients who require immediate evaluation. FEES is also valuable in patients with anatomical or neurological impairment of the laryngopharynx, such as those who have had a stroke or those recovering from head and neck operation. Some authors now advocate using FEES as the primary screening tool for dysphagia and for follow-up of patients postoperatively or during treatment, and using videofluoroscopy on a more selective basis.[9] The biggest drawback of FEES is its inability to assess the esophagus (Tables 26–4 and 26–5).

DYSPHAGIA IN SPECIFIC DISORDERS

Dysphagia has been reported in multiple types of disorders, and for purposes of categorization, it can be classified as neurological or nonneurological (Table 26–6). In rehabilitation medicine, the neurological swallowing disorders are more frequently encountered, and a few deserve further discussion.

Stroke

The frequency of dysphagia after stroke has been reported to be as high as 30% to 45%[53, 132] and has been associated with increased mortality, increased length of hospital stay, and decreased level of functional outcome,[123] although not in all studies.[96] Dysphagia is not limited to brainstem or bilateral infarctions. Unilateral lesions also result in dysphagia.[6, 82, 107] The most common swallowing impairments associated with stroke are reduced lingual control, reduced pharyngeal peristalsis, and a delayed swallowing reflex.[135] Aspiration is frequently associated with dysphagia in stroke, but it cannot be predicted by the imaged location of the stroke.[1] The presence of a cough after swallow, an absent or

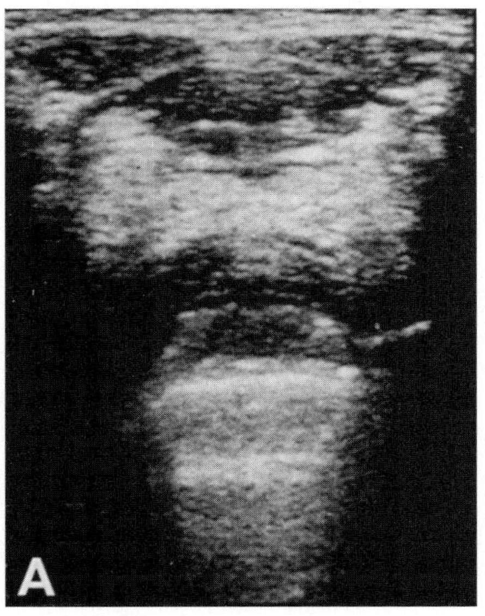

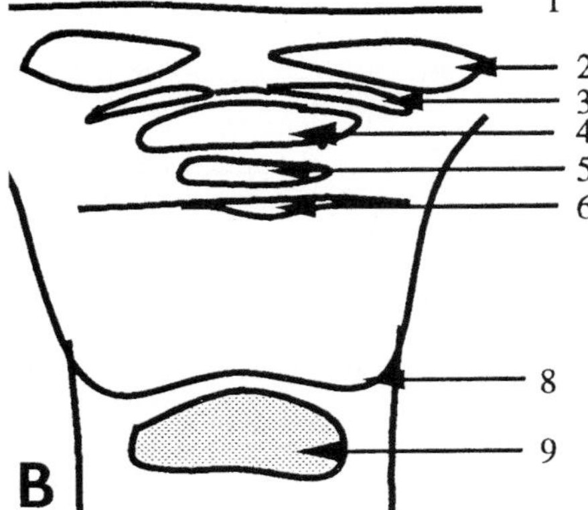

FIGURE 26–13. *A.* Ultrasound scan of coronal section of tongue during swallowing. Lateral borders of tongue are elevated to form a hollow, which contains the bolus. *B.* 1, superficial plane; 2, anterior belly of digastric muscle; 3, mylohyoid muscle; 4, geniohyoid muscle; 5, genioglossus muscle; 6, alveololingual groove; 8, superior or dorsal surface of tongue; 9, bolus. (From Maniere-Ezvan A, Duval J-M, Darnault P: Ultrasonic assessment of the anatomy and function of the tongue. Surg Radiol Anat 1993; 15(1):55. Reproduced by permission of Springer-Verlag France.)

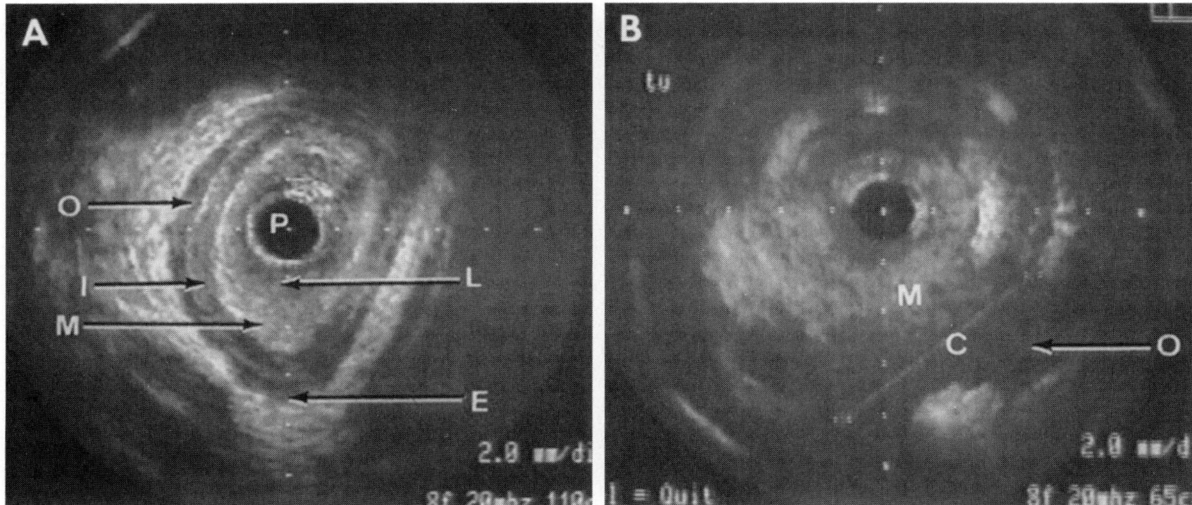

FIGURE 26–14. *A.* Normal ultrasonic image of the esophagus. P, probe; L, lumen; M, mucosa and submucosa; I, inner circular part of muscularis propria; O, outer longitudinal part of muscularis propria; E, outer limit of esophagus. Scale = 2.0 mm/division. *B.* Esophageal carcinoma. The carcinoma (C) infiltrates all layers of the esophagus. Note the dissolved mucosa-submucosa (M) and the absence of the outer limit (O) of the esophagus. Scale = 2.0 mm/division. (From Sobin J, Nathanson A, Engstrom CF: Endoluminal ultrasonography: A new method to evaluate dysphagia. ORL J Otorhinolaryngol Relat Spec 1996; 58:107. Reprinted by permission of S. Karger AG, Medical and Scientific Publishers.)

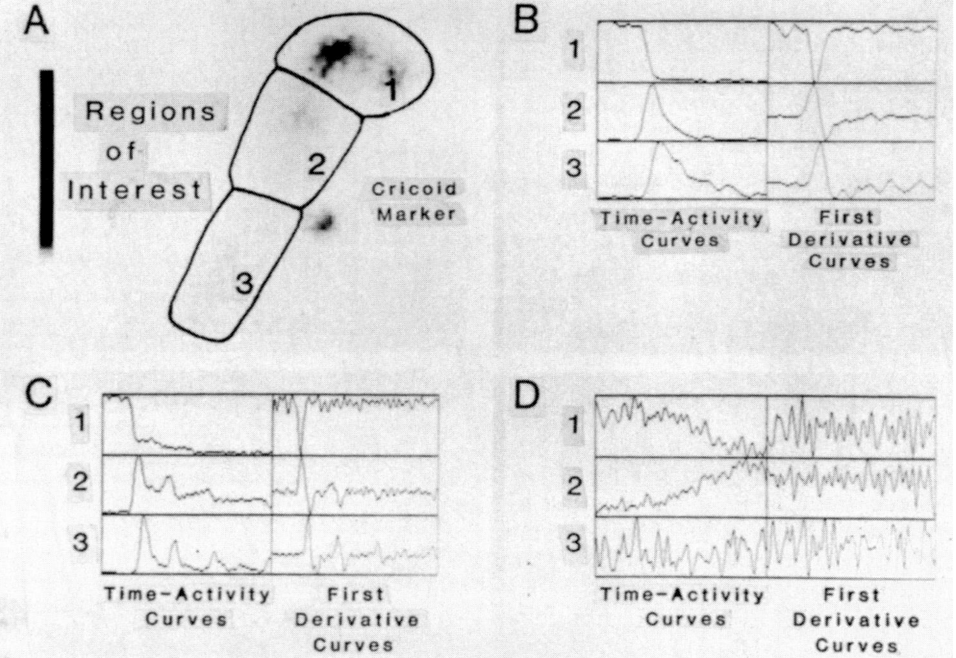

FIGURE 26–15. *A.* Scintiscan of oropharynx in which selected regions of interest have been drawn to represent the mouth (1), pharynx (2), and esophagus (3). The time-activity curves (time on horizontal axis, counts on vertical axis) that are constructed from the area of the mouth (1), pharynx (2), and esophagus (3) together with corresponding first-derivative curves are shown in *B*, *C*, and *D*. The peaks and nadirs correspond to peak emptying or filling rates of the respective compartments. *B.* Transit data recorded during swallowing in the control subject. *C* and *D.* Abnormal bolus transit in two patients (one with bulbar palsy and one with myasthenia gravis) manifested by major change in pattern of the time-activity and first-derivative curves. (From Holt S, Miron SD, Diaz MC, et al: Scintigraphic measurement of oropharyngeal transit in man. Dig Dis Sci 1990; 35(10):1198. Reproduced by permission of Plenum Publishing Corporation.)

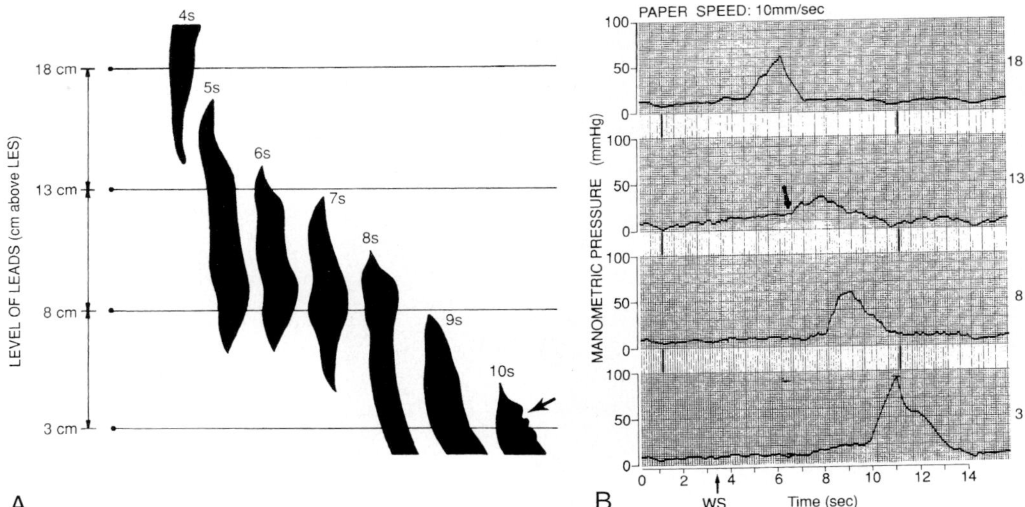

FIGURE 26–16. *A.* Temporal tracings of a 5-mL barium bolus at 1-second intervals show normal primary peristalsis at fluoroscopy. Tapered tops of the barium column correspond to the peristaltic contraction wave seen at manometry. Mild tertiary activity (*arrow*) affects tracing at 10 seconds. Numbers on vertical axis represent positions of the catheter ports. *B.* Manometric tracing of bolus in *A.* Wet swallow (WS) occurred at 3.4 seconds. Time scale is synchronous with the temporally labeled barium tracings. On the lead 13 cm above the lower esophageal sphincter (LES), peristaltic onset is at about 6.6 seconds (*arrows*), corresponding precisely to the fluoroscopic level of primary peristalsis. (From Ott DJ, Chen YM, Hewson EG, et al: Esophageal motility: Assessment with synchronous video tape fluoroscopy and manometry. Radiology 1989; 173(2);419. Reproduced by permission of the Radiological Society of North America.)

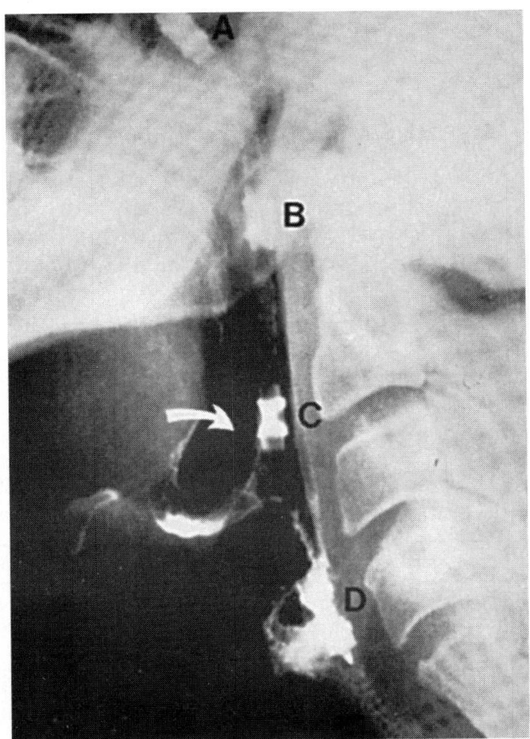

FIGURE 26–17. Lateral radiograph of neck with correct positioning of the manometric sensors (A, B, C, D). The second sensor (B) is located at the tongue base level. The third sensor (C) is close to epiglottis (*white arrow*). D is the region of the upper esophageal sphincter. (From Olsson R, Nilsson H, Ekberg O: Simultaneous videoradiography and pharyngeal solid state manometry (videomanometry) in 25 nondysphagic volunteers. Dysphagia 1995; 10:36. Reprinted by permission of Springer-Verlag, New York.)

abnormal gag,[33, 54] and findings such as dysphonia, dysarthria, abnormal volitional cough, and voice change after swallow indicate a risk for aspiration in acute stroke.[33] But aspiration is "silent" (without symptoms or signs) in many persons with stroke.

When aspiration is detected on videofluoroscopy, the chances of pneumonia developing are significantly greater than if aspiration is not present.[113] A prolonged pharyngeal transit time also helps predict patients in whom pneumonia will develop.[58] In general, the prognosis for oral feeding after stroke is good, and the risk for aspiration pneumonia decreases over time.[52, 54, 131] Nonetheless, monitoring oral feedings over time after stroke is warranted because dysphagia persists for some patients, and in other patients dysphagia seemingly does not develop until later in the course of their illness.[122]

Traumatic Brain Injury

Dysphagia in the head-injured population is not uncommon. Cognitive impairment is often the most significant factor, followed by motor control difficulties.[140] The motor deficits often impair both the oral and the pharyngeal phases of swallowing and increase the risk of aspiration.[28] Behavioral difficulties also can interfere, necessitating various behavioral strategies, such as systematic desensitization of oral hypersensitivity.[18] Drooling may be a significant problem in this population. Several treatment options exist, usually beginning with oral motor exercises to control oral secretions, followed by administration of drugs, such as atropine sulfate, to dry oral secretions, and, finally, surgical intervention to block oral secretions.[37]

Motor Neuron Disease

Upper and lower motor neuron dysfunction occurs commonly in a significant number of patients with motor

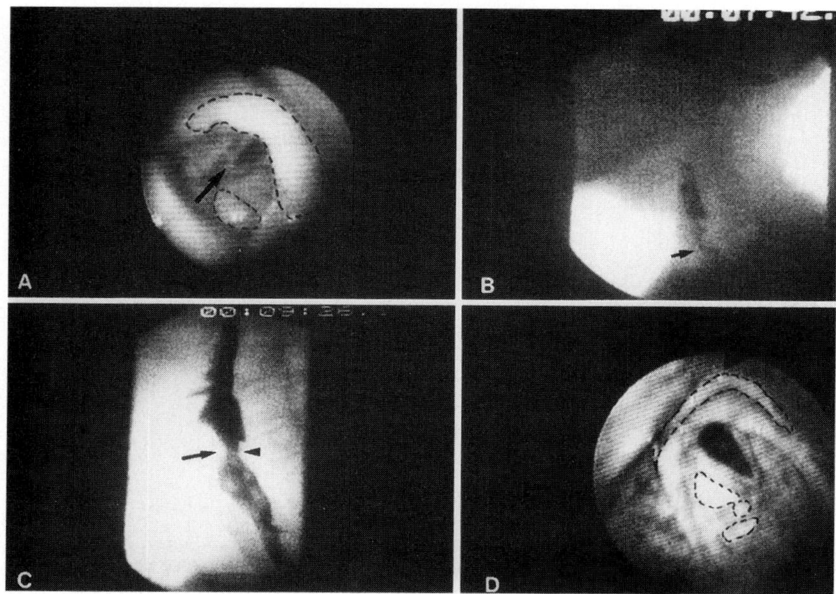

FIGURE 26–18. *A. Arrow,* anterior commissure. *Dotted lines* outline pudding pooled in pyriforms and postcricoid area, about to spill over into laryngeal vestibule. *Small dotted circle* denotes small amount of laryngeal vestibule soiling. *B.* Videophotograph of VFSS, showing marked cricopharyngeus hypertrophy and very "narrow" bolus through this area (*arrow*). *C.* Magnified postmyotomy view showing altered cricopharyngeus impression (at *arrowhead*) and widened bolus passing through this area. *D.* VESS postmyotomy view. *Dotted line* outlines smaller amount of pyriform postcricoid pooling of pudding, which is also pooled to a much lower level. A small amount of laryngeal vestibule soiling is still in evidence. (From Bastian RW. The videoendoscopic swallowing study: An alternative and partner to the videofluoroscopic swallowing study. Dysphagia 1993; 8:364. Reprinted by permission of Springer-Verlag.)

neuron disease and results in oral and pharyngeal dysphagia.[16, 20] Because of the progressive nature of this disorder, difficult emotional and ethical issues often arise. Various treatment measures can be used in this disorder, including surgical options such as laryngeal diversion.[25]

Parkinson's Disease

Patients with Parkinson's disease can present with dysphagia and nutritional deficits, in part due to oropharyngeal motility problems.[137] On videofluoroscopic examination, oral phase dysfunction is very common, occurring in up to 92% of patients complaining of dysphagia. Aspiration is also common[129] and can be silent. Swallowing function usually improves with administration of levodopa, but improvement in parkinsonian signs does not always signify improvement in swallowing.[23, 55]

Poliomyelitis

With careful examination, oropharyngeal function is found to be disturbed to some degree in many patients with post-polio syndrome.[127] Videofluoroscopy reveals not only neurogenic dysfunction, such as weakness of the pharyngeal constrictors, poor laryngeal elevation, and aspiration without a cough, but also structural le-

TABLE 26–4 VESS versus VFSS: A Preliminary Comparison of Capabilities by Findings

Item	VESS	VFSS
Palate mobility and closure	Excellent	Good
Pharynx squeeze	Excellent	Good
Vocal fold mobility and closure	Excellent	Fair
Sensation	Excellent	Fair
Anatomical detail	Excellent	Fair
Pooling	Excellent	Excellent
Aspiration	Good	Excellent
Latency	Good	Excellent
Duration	Good	Excellent
Laryngeal elevation	Good (include neck palpation)	Excellent
Oral cavity behavior	Fair (use direct inspection)	Excellent
Esophagus	Poor	Excellent

Abbreviations: VESS, videoendoscopic swallowing study; VFSS, videofluoroscopic swallowing study.
From Bastian RW: Videoendoscopic evaluation of patients with dysphagia: An adjunct to the modified barium swallow. Otolaryngol Head Neck Surg 1991; 104:339. Reprinted by permission of CV Mosby.

TABLE 26–5 VESS versus VFSS: A Comparison of Clinical Usefulness

Clinical Circumstance or Disorder	VESS	VFSS
Initial workup	Good	Excellent
Esophageal disease	Poor	Excellent
Cranial neuropathies	Excellent	Fair
Postsurgical anatomy	Excellent	Good
Rapidly evolving swallowing disorder	Excellent	Fair
Bedfast patient	Excellent	—
Biofeedback, as to teach pharyngeal squeeze	Excellent	Poor

Abbreviations: VESS, videoendoscopic swallowing study; VFSS, videofluoroscopic swallowing study.
From Bastian RW: Videoendoscopic evaluation of patients with dysphagia: An adjunct to the modified barium swallow. Otolaryngol Head Neck Surg 1991; 104:339. Reprinted by permission of CV Mosby.

TABLE 26–6 Disorders Associated with Dysphagia

Neurological

- Central nervous system
  - Vascular
    - Stroke
    - Intracranial hemorrhage
  - Motor neuron disorders
    - Progressive spinal muscular atrophy
    - Progressive bulbar palsy
    - Amyotrophic lateral sclerosis
    - Infantile spinal muscular atrophy
    - Poliomyelitis
  - Degenerative/extrapyramidal
    - Parkinsonism
    - Spinocerebellar degeneration
    - Olivopontocerebellar atrophy
    - Progressive supranuclear palsy
    - Huntington's disease
    - Alzheimer's disease
    - Adrenoleukodystrophy
    - Dystonia
    - Tardive dyskinesia
  - Immune-mediated
    - Multiple sclerosis
  - Infectious
    - Encephalitis/meningitis
  - Structural
    - Neoplasm
    - Arnold-Chiari malformation
    - Syringomyelia, syringobulbia
  - Exogenous
    - Traumatic brain injury
    - Drug-induced
- Peripheral nervous system
  - Guillain-Barré syndrome
  - Sarcoidosis
  - Porphyria
- Myopathy/dystrophy
  - Inflammatory myopathy (polymyositis, dermatomyositis)
  - Metabolic myopathy (mitochondrial myopathy, dysthyroid myopathy)
  - Myotonic dystrophy
  - Oculopharyngeal dystrophy
- Neuromuscular junction
  - Myasthenia gravis
  - Eaton-Lambert syndrome
  - Botulism

Nonneurological

- Structural
  - Cervical osteophytes
  - Goiter
  - Neoplasm
  - Foreign body
  - Congenital anomalies
  - Vascular aneurysm or anomaly
  - Schatzki's ring
  - Zenker's diverticulum
  - Esophageal webs
- Esophageal dysmotility
  - Gastroesophageal reflux
  - Achalasia
  - Diffuse esophageal spasm
  - "Nutcracker" esophagus
- Other gastrointestinal disorders
  - Crohn's disease
  - Ulcerative colitis
  - Amyloid
  - Plummer-Vinson syndrome
- Rheumatologic
  - Scleroderma
  - Sjögren's syndrome
  - Systemic lupus erythematosus
  - Mixed connective tissue disease
  - Rheumatoid arthritis
- Infectious
  - *Candida*
  - Herpesvirus
  - Cytomegalovirus
  - Tuberculosis
  - Acute pharyngitis
  - Retropharyngeal abscess
  - Epiglottitis
  - Human immunodeficiency virus (HIV)
- Psychiatric
  - Globus
- Skin diseases
  - Mucous membrane pemphigoid
  - Epidermolysis bullosa dystrophica
  - Lichen planus
  - Psoriasis
  - Stevens-Johnson syndrome
  - Chronic graft-vs.-host disease
- Metabolic
  - Hypercalcemia
  - Diabetes mellitus
- Treatment-related
  - Postoperative head and neck radiation
  - Foreign device (tracheostomy tube, nasogastric tube)
  - Medication-induced injury

Data from Brin and Younger,[17] Buchholz,[20] Buchin,[22] Jones et al.,[61] Kosko,[72] and Schechter.[111]

sions, including pharyngeal pouches, Zenker's diverticulum, and focal stenosis.[21, 59]

Multiple Sclerosis

Management of dysphagia can vary significantly over time in the patient with multiple sclerosis because of the disease course. If it is relapsing and remitting, interventions might be intermittent. If the course is progressive, more permanent compensatory measures could be necessary.[20]

Myasthenia Gravis

Swallowing difficulties in myasthenia gravis are sometimes greater than expected from the symptoms and are not necessarily amenable to pharmacological intervention.[70]

Myotonic Dystrophy

Although dysphagia is not common in Duchenne muscular dystrophy, the facial and pharyngeal muscular weakness in myotonic dystrophy often results in significant dysphagia.

Nonneurological Disorders

In addition to the neurological causes, nonneurological causes for dysphagia are important to consider in the rehabilitation setting. The patient with primarily neurological dysphagia might also have a concurrent, nonneurological cause that is aggravating the swallowing process, such as cervical osteophytes (see Fig. 26–12) or Zenker's diverticulum (Fig. 26–19). The presence of pain or difficulties in swallowing solids early in the course of dysphagia raises a strong suspicion of a nonneurological cause.[71]

AGE CONSIDERATIONS IN DYSPHAGIA

Elderly Patients

Aging is not a cause of dysphagia. However, motor and sensory changes and changes in central and peripheral processes that are associated with aging can result in a predisposition to dysphagia or can aggravate dysphagia in an older person.[4, 44, 106] Some of those changes affect the oral stage, such as poor dentition, atrophy of the tongue and alveolar ridge, and diminished taste and smell sensitivity. Others can affect the pharyngeal stage, such as decreased muscle tone and increased ligamentous laxity, which impair pharyngeal clearing capabilities and limit laryngeal elevation. In addition to these changes, certain illnesses, such as stroke, parkinsonism, and hiatal hernia with gastroesophageal reflux, occur more commonly with age.[38, 41, 116, 125]

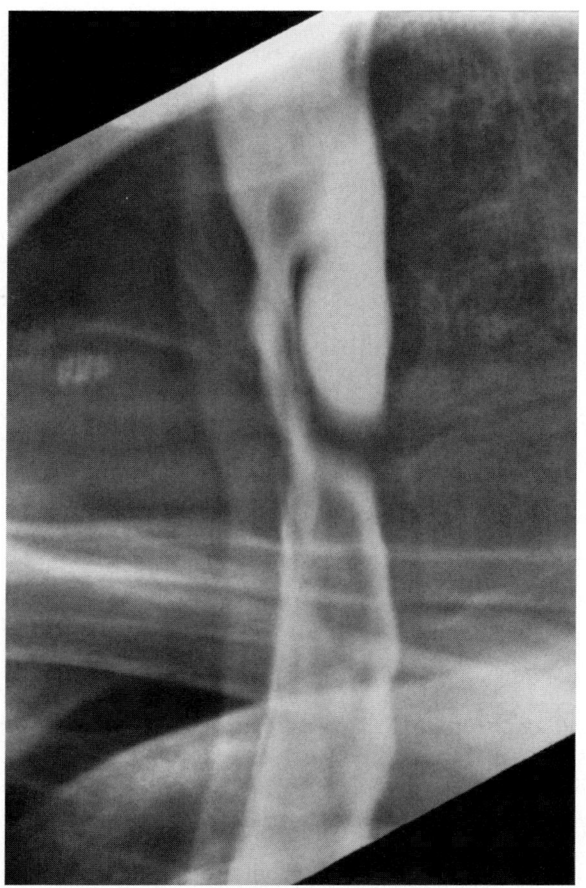

FIGURE 26–19. Lateral projection of video swallow test demonstrates large Zenker's diverticulum arising posteriorly from upper esophagus.

Aspiration during the swallowing process results from oral phase or combined oropharyngeal phase dysfunction in the elderly as commonly as, if not more commonly than, pharyngeal stage problems alone. Abnormalities identified on videofluoroscopy during the oral stage include difficulties with bolus containment and poor coordination of bolus movement orally with the initiation of a swallow. Retention of the bolus in the pharynx and inadequate laryngeal protection are common defects visualized during the pharyngeal stage.[40]

Management of the elderly patient with dysphagia can involve special considerations. From a dietary standpoint, the older patient might routinely take in fewer calories and have secondary deficiencies in vitamins and minerals, particularly vitamin D, calcium, zinc, copper, and chromium.[67] From a standpoint of nutrition delivery, ethical issues may arise. For example, a mentally competent patient might not choose to accept enteral feeding despite a risk of aspiration. Such choices are often difficult for the swallowing team. More difficult are decisions about the management of an elderly patient with end-stage dementia or severe brain injury. Specific goals for treatment, clearly understood by family and team members, help alleviate ethical concerns.[114]

Young Patients

Swallowing difficulties in children result in the same medical concerns as in adults: poor nutrition and aspiration. Certain factors make dysphagia in children unique, however. For example, in infants, the tongue fills the oral cavity, the space between the soft palate and epiglottis is contracted, and the larynx is positioned closer to the base of the tongue. These anatomical differences enhance airway protection. Evolution toward the adult configuration begins by age 3 to 4 months and continues until bone growth is complete.[2, 79]

Just as the child normally grows and develops, so too does the swallowing process. Differences between the infant and adult are most apparent in the oral phase of swallowing. *Suckling* is an early feeding behavior that consists of a rhythmic compression of the nipple by the tongue and lower jaw against the palate and upper jaw. Suckling activity is important for infants, even if it is with a nonfeeding nipple (*nonnutritive suck*).[134] With development, this behavior evolves through a series of chewing functions until about age 3 years, and becomes further coordinated by about age 6 years, when the oral phase approximates that of the adult. The pharyngeal phase in the infant is similar to that of the adult from early on, although the swallow typically occurs with greater frequency and speed in an infant.[73]

Dysphagia in infants and children can be assessed with videofluoroscopy. Studying the very young, however, requires modification in positioning and in supplies. Typically, infants age 0 to 6 months are optimally positioned semi-upright with the head in midline. After 6 months, children are positioned increasingly more upright as postural control and tone allow, so that by age 3 years they are ideally studied fully upright. Barium textures and feeding utensils vary with the age of the child. For example, infants younger than 6 months are studied with liquid barium from a bottle or syringe, whereas pureed or chewable textures of barium are added as developmental readiness allows.[3]

Difficulties in feeding and swallowing arise from several sources. For example, prematurity by itself can result in poor coordination of sucking and breathing, often manifested by apnea and bradycardia.[83] Neurological impairment, as occurs in cerebral palsy, is a common cause of dysphagia in the young. Affected children can exhibit findings such as the bite reflex, tongue thrust, poor trunk control, and slowness in eating.[136] The degree of swallowing difficulty typically parallels the degree of impairment in cerebral palsy, but aspiration can remain clinically hidden, even with severe disability. Videofluoroscopy documents that silent aspiration is very common in this population.[108] Coordination of deglutition and ventilation is frequently impaired and is associated with a prolonged, exhausting feeding time. Because hypoxemia can occur while a child with swallowing difficulties eats, pulse oximetry during mealtime can be useful in these situations to help direct treatment.[109]

As with the adult, gastroesophageal reflux is a common problem in very young children, and contributes to both feeding and respiratory difficulties.[83] Gastric pH changes with age, and the lowest mean pH (1.99) occurs in the pediatric age group.[84] This low pH places the child at particular risk for aspiration-induced chemical pneumonitis.

Congenital structural lesions can interfere with the normal anatomical transport of a bolus. Multiple disorders can occur, ranging from choanal atresia, cleft lip and palate, and craniofacial syndromes to vascular anomalies, such as a double aortic arch or an aberrant right subclavian artery.[72, 138] With certain structural lesions, prosthetic devices or adapted feeding equipment, including modified nipples, might be necessary. A Chiari malformation is another type of structural lesion that can result in neurogenic dysphagia.[104]

Management of the pediatric patient requires a special approach.[2, 3] Cognitive, developmental, and behavioral issues can affect treatment options. If a child has acquired dysphagia after having learned feeding skills, treatment can be drawn from the child's prior experience. If dysphagia is congenitally acquired, feeding skills must be learned for the first time, often in the face of neurological or structural impairments.[29]

Treatment does not necessarily imply the use of feeding therapy.[91] Addressing such problems as tonal abnormalities, postural control, adverse behavior, and primitive reflexes might precede any attempt at oral feeding. When feeding does begin, it is clear from both clinical experience and videofluoroscopy that positioning and dietary makeup are important for the neurologically impaired child. Isolated oral phase dysfunction is usually best managed with feeding in a reclining position, whereas an erect position, if possible, is most effective for pharyngeal phase problems.[92] In addition, children with cerebral palsy typically manage solid boluses more easily than liquid boluses, and small liquid boluses more easily than large liquid boluses.[26]

COMPLICATIONS OF DYSPHAGIA

Aspiration Pneumonia

Dysphagia is a major risk factor for aspiration pneumonia,[87] but it usually results in pneumonia only when present with other risk factors such as dependency for feeding, medical comorbidities, poor oral hygiene, and decreased functional status.[75] Aspiration typically occurs at the time of eating, but it can also occur at other times. Some persons without dysphagia even aspirate during sleep.[56] Not every episode of aspiration results in pneumonia. Aspiration results in pneumonia primarily by three mechanisms: chemical injury, bacterial infection, and obstruction (Table 26–7).[8, 68, 69]

Chemical pneumonitis typically presents with acute dyspnea and hypoxemia. It develops from the burn of gastric acid present in the aspirate and implies gastric reflux. The pH and volume of the aspirate seem to be the most important determinants of whether pulmonary injury will occur. When the pH is less than approximately 2.5, there is particular concern for chemical pneumonia.[8, 133] The natural course of pneumonia is variable. Rapid improvement typically occurs over about 5 days. In other instances, improvement occurs initially, followed by a superimposed infection. Least commonly, but most worrisome, the course is fulminant, and death occurs. Treatment is supportive, with fluids and ventilation provided as needed. The role of steroids and antibiotics is not clearly defined in this type of aspiration pneumonia.[8]

Bacterial pneumonia typically presents with fever and sputum production in the course of a more insidious onset. Anaerobes present in oral flora are common pathogens in community-acquired pneumonia, whereas gram-negative bacilli and *Staphylococcus aureus* become more prominent in hospital-acquired disease.[8, 42, 68, 69] This information can guide antibiotic selection in the absence of culture identification.

Aspiration of particles of food can result in airway obstruction. The right mainstem bronchus territory is typically involved, and symptoms include wheezing, coughing, choking, and respiratory distress.[68] The severity of this condition partially depends on the size of the particle aspirated. The potential for aspiration of particulate matter mandates that persons caring for any patient with dysphagia know the Heimlich maneuver. A superimposed bacterial infection can also occur in this type of aspiration as a result of obstruction of normal pulmonary drainage.[8]

In addition to specific treatment for dysphagia, measures to prevent aspiration pneumonia include elevation of the head of the bed, use of H_2-blocking agents or antacids to increase gastric pH above 2.5, and decrease in food intake before sleep.[8]

TABLE 26–7 Classification of Aspiration Pneumonia

Inoculum	Pulmonary Sequelae	Clinical Features	Therapy
Acid	Chemical pneumonitis	Acute dyspnea, tachypnea, tachycardia with or without cyanosis, bronchospasm, fever Sputum: pink, frothy X-ray: infiltrates in one or both lower lobes Hypoxemia	Positive-pressure breathing Intravenous fluids Tracheal suction Corticosteroids
Oropharyngeal bacteria	Bacterial infection	Usually insidious onset Cough, fever, purulent sputum X-ray: infiltrate involving dependent pulmonary segment or lobe, with or without cavitation	Antibiotics
Inert fluids	Mechanical obstruction Reflex airway closure	Acute dyspnea, cyanosis with or without apnea Pulmonary edema	Tracheal suction Intermittent positive pressure breathing with oxygen and isoproterenol
Particulate matter	Mechanical obstruction	Dependent on level of obstruction, ranging from acute apnea and rapid death to irritating chronic cough with or without recurrent infections	Extraction of particulate matter

From Bartlett JG: Aspiration pneumonia. In Baum GL, Wolinsky E (eds.): Textbook of Pulmonary Diseases, ed 5, vol 1. Boston, Little, Brown, 1994, p. 593. Reprinted by permission of the publisher.

Malnutrition

Poor nutritional status is a common problem in the general hospital patient[12] as well as in patients admitted for rehabilitation[95] and may affect the length of stay in the rehabilitation unit and the functional improvement rate.[43] Presumably, the patient with dysphagia is in a particularly high-risk category for undernutrition.[120]

As part of the dysphagia evaluation, some measure of nutritional status is useful as a baseline. Multiple measures are available, but all have limitations.[117] A simple practical screen is to determine weight, albumin value, and total lymphocyte count.[7] A recent weight loss of more than 10% to 15% and weight below 90% of ideal body weight represent significant malnutrition.[63, 65, 120] The body mass index (BMI), the quotient of weight in kilograms divided by height in meters squared, is useful for identifying someone who is underweight. The BMI is typically between 22 and 27.[7] The visceral protein compartment can be measured from serum albumin and transferrin levels. Because of albumin's long half-life (20 days), the albumin value does not reflect acute nutritional deficiencies, but a level less than 3.5 g/dL raises nutritional concerns.[30] The total lymphocyte count (the product of the total leukocyte count and the percentage lymphocytes) correlates with the albumin value and is decreased in malnutrition. A count less than 1400 may indicate nutrition problems.[7]

In cases of malnutrition, the daily caloric needs are traditionally determined with the Harris Benedict formula for basal energy expenditure (BEE), which takes into account weight, height, and age:

$$\text{BEE for women} = 655 + (9.6 \times \text{weight [kg]}) + (1.8 \times \text{height [cm]}) - (4.7 \times \text{age [yr]})$$

$$\text{BEE for men} = 66 + (13.7 \times \text{weight [kg]}) + (5 \times \text{height [cm]}) - (6.8 \times \text{age [yr]})$$

This formula was derived from healthy individuals at rest. Adjustment factors have been defined for activity and injury. General hospital patients require 120% of BEE, whereas medically stressed patients can require 150% to 200%.[30] An estimate of caloric need is typically 25 to 30 calories/kg of ideal body weight. Protein requirements are typically estimated at 1.0 to 1.5 g/kg/day, but are increased in catabolic states and decreased in significant renal or liver disease.[65] Daily caloric counts, serial weight determinations, and monitoring of nutritional measures, such as nitrogen balance, help direct further refinement of dietary needs.

When nutritional needs can be met orally only partially or not at all, enteral feeding is the usual route of choice unless there is a need to eliminate the risk of aspiration completely.[121] An initial feeding route is easily accomplished with a soft nasogastric feeding tube. If enteral feeding is prolonged, the use of a gastrostomy tube, typically placed percutaneously, is better tolerated by the patient, provides the prescribed nutrition more reliably, and results in more weight gain than the long-term use of a nasogastric feeding tube.[102] The absence of a nasogastric tube also facilitates swallowing interventions, although a nasogastric tube is not a contraindication to therapeutic feeding.[100] The absence of a nasogastric tube does not eliminate the risk of aspiration. Whether a tube placed in the jejunum affords greater protection from aspiration than a gastric tube is unclear.[76] Data from patients hospitalized for acute conditions who were enterally fed by various routes suggest that the incidence of aspiration is only 2.4 per 1000 tube-feeding days, and there is no excess mortality and only minimal morbidity. Continuous feedings by infusion pump result in the least gastric distention and might be preferable in patients at high risk for reflux aspiration.[93] Continuous feedings are also useful in patients with poor enteral motility or in persons who require hypertonic formulas. Intermittent or bolus feeding, however, is less disruptive to rehabilitation activities and to general daily living.[132]

TREATMENT MENU FOR DYSPHAGIA

Dietary Modification

Modification of the diet for the patient with dysphagia is a critical step in establishing a therapeutic feeding program. If oral feedings, in some form, are determined to be appropriate, the type of food to be administered needs careful consideration. Although thin liquids can result in less pharyngeal residue, they are often difficult for the patient with a neurological disorder to manage. Liquids can be thickened with various thickening agents. These agents typically are added to, for example, hot or cold beverages or soups. A thicker consistency can be beneficial to patients who have a delayed swallow reflex because there is less tendency for the material to fall over the base of the tongue before the swallow is triggered. The patient or a family member can be instructed in the amount of thickening agent to be added to obtain an optimal consistency.

Food can be modified to have a pureed, semisolid, or solid consistency, depending on the results of the patient's clinical or videofluoroscopic evaluation. Pureed consistencies can be used for patients who demonstrate difficulty chewing or an inability to form a cohesive bolus because of decreased tongue function. As tongue function, chewing ability, and pharyngeal function improve, patients may tolerate advancing their food types to soft, semisolid, and regular consistencies. Many centers have adapted the "dysphagia diet" concept as a means for organizing and administering appropriate foods. The benefit of the dysphagia diet is that it links similar foods. Examples of a dysphagia diet are in the first column of Table 26–8.

As the patient demonstrates clinical or radiographic improvement, the dysphagia diet can be advanced to the next level (Table 26–8). Careful monitoring of the patient with the introduction of each new food type is important to ensure safety and to avoid the risk of aspiration. Because many patients are instructed in various compensatory techniques to be used during mealtimes, monitoring the patient during mealtime is essential. This can be done by nurses or family members after instruction by the swallowing therapist.

Oral hygiene needs careful consideration. Dried secretions can accumulate on the tongue and palate, reducing oral sensitivity and promoting growth of bacteria in the mouth.[47] Lemon-glycerin, plain swabs, or a damp wash-cloth can be used to remove the secretions. This step should be done before treatment or administration of food substances.

Exercise and Facilitation Techniques

Numerous exercises and methods of facilitation have been described for the patient with dysphagia. Clinical experience and anecdotes indicate the effectiveness of these techniques despite the lack of research to scientifically support their benefits. The techniques and exercises require that the patient be able to follow directions and participate in a therapy program. The indications for use of the exercises are outlined in Table 26–9.

Exercises designed to facilitate oral motor strength, range of motion, and coordination are best done frequently (five to ten times per day).[79] Patients and family members can be instructed by the swallowing therapist to perform the exercises between therapy sessions. The variety of exercises is limited only by the clinician's creativity.

Examples of exercises for the lips to facilitate the ability to prevent food or liquid from leaking out of the oral cavity, are as follows:

- Smile or grin
- Purse lips together, gradually increasing the time they are held together
- Close lips around a tongue blade, swab stick, or spoon
- Blow through a straw, party favor, or windmill, or blow bubbles

TABLE 26–8 Dysphagia Diet

Group: Date:	Initial Evaluation	Re-evaluation	Re-evaluation
1. Thin liquids (fruit juice, coffee, tea)			
2. Nectar-thick liquids (tomato juice, sherbet, cream soup)			
3. Honey-thick liquids (liquids thickened to a honey consistency)			
4. Pudding-thick liquids/foods (mashed bananas, purees, cooked cereal)			
5. Mechanical soft foods (baked beans, casseroles, meatloaf)			
6. Chewy foods (cheese, bagels, pizza)			
7. Foods that fall apart (breads, muffins, rice)			
8. Mixed textures			

TABLE 26–9 Indications for Exercises in Patients with Dysphagia

Clinical Diagnosis	Clinical Observation	Exercise/ Technique
Decreased lip range of motion, strength, or coordination	Drooling, facial droop	Lip exercises
Decreased tongue range of motion, strength, or coordination	Inability to propel food from front to back of mouth Food pooling in sulci	Tongue exercises
Decreased jaw range of motion, strength, or coordination	Inability to chew food adequately	Jaw exercises
Weak or absent cough	Nonproductive cough	Respiratory exercises
Increased respiratory rate	Rapid or shallow breathing	Respiratory exercises
Decreased airway protection	Wet or "gurgly" voice Hoarse voice Coughing during the swallow	Vocal cord adduction exercises
Delayed/absent swallow reflex	Decreased laryngeal elevation during swallow Coughing before the swallow	Thermal stimulation
Incomplete contact between tongue base and posterior pharyngeal wall	Pooling in the valleculae	Tongue base retraction exercises

Examples of exercises for the tongue to facilitate manipulation of the bolus and its propulsion through the oral cavity[49] include:

Protrude tongue
Push tongue into side of cheek
Push tongue against a tongue blade in front and to the side
Move tongue from side to side

Residue in the valleculae and along the posterior pharyngeal wall can occur after the swallow if the range of tongue base movement is restricted.[27] To assist the pharyngeal swallow by improving tongue base retraction, exercises are as follows:

Pull tongue toward the back of the throat and hold
Hold tongue between the teeth and swallow
Yawn[79]
Pretend to gargle[79]

An exercise to enhance elevation of the larynx involves having the patient sing in a falsetto manner.[79] The patient is asked to do the following:

Take a deep breath, and say "ah" with a deep-pitched voice
Hold the "ah" and slowly raise the voice to the highest pitch possible, returning to the deepest pitch

Examples of exercises for the jaw to facilitate the rotary movements required for mastication are as follows:

Open mouth as wide as possible, relax, repeat
Move jaw from side to side

Increasing the length of time the exercises are held and the amount of resistance applied advances the difficulty of these exercises.

Patients with impaired respiratory status are at increased risk for aspiration because of their inability to successfully cease respiration in order to swallow. Their inability to successfully clear penetrated or aspirated material from the airway also compromises safe swallowing. Several exercises can improve respiratory strength, as follows:

Take in a big breath, inhale deeply, and exhale slowly
Take in a big breath. Repeat "ah" as long as possible
Blow through a straw, a windmill, or party favor
Read poems or sing a song

Vocal cord adduction exercises are performed as an attempt to strengthen weak cords and approximate them to prevent aspiration. Examples of these exercises include the following:

Repeat "ah, ah, ah," while pushing down on a chair or pushing hands together
Say "ah" for 5 seconds while pushing down on a chair

Because these vocal cord adduction exercises create a Valsalva effect, caution is necessary when they are being performed by a patient with a cardiac disorder.

Strap muscles are important contributors to laryngeal elevation during the swallow. Strengthening of these muscles can be accomplished by lifting one's head slowly off the mat when supine and holding this position for 3 to 5 seconds.

Thermal-tactile stimulation is a facilitative technique designed to increase the speed at which the swallow occurs. It can be performed with a laryngeal mirror (size 00) or a metal rod of similar size. The mirror is placed in ice until cold and then placed along the area of the anterior facial arch (bilaterally) and rubbed five times. After this icing procedure, the patient is asked to swallow.[79] This technique can be performed frequently throughout the day as well as before or during mealtimes. If oral feedings are not recommended, the therapist can use this technique without food to facilitate the swallow reflex. This technique has been found to be of clinical benefit in some patients,[34] although long-term results are inconclusive.[110] Patients might report an easier time initiating a swallow when the technique is done immediately before mealtime.

If abnormal oral reflexes (such as tongue thrust or bite reflex) are found during the clinical evaluation, attempts should be made to inhibit them.[47] Inhibitory techniques[39] for the bite reflex include:

Sustained pressure applied to the tongue using a padded tongue blade

TABLE 26–10 Indications for Compensatory Techniques in Patients with Dysphagia

Clinical Diagnosis	Clinical Observations	Compensatory Technique
Delayed swallow reflex	Coughing before the swallow Aspiration	Chin tuck Supraglottic swallow
Decreased pharyngeal peristalsis (unilaterally)	Unilateral pooling in the pharyngeal region Coughing after the swallow	Turning of head to weaker side Tilting of head to stronger side
Decreased pharyngeal peristalsis	Coughing after the swallow	Effortful swallow Double swallow Alternating liquids and swallows
Decreased laryngeal closure	Coughing during or after the swallow	Chin tuck Supraglottic swallow
Decreased opening of cricopharyngeal region	Coughing after the swallow Pooling in the pyriform sinus	Mendelsohn's maneuver Turning of head to weaker side

Positioning of the head in an upright position with the chin tucked

Techniques to inhibit tongue thrust include, sequentially:

Applying pressure under the chin to the tongue retraction musculature
Manually vibrating under the tongue
Applying a quick stretch of the tongue into protrusion to facilitate retrusion

The gag reflex can be either hypoactive or hyperactive. Although a normal gag reflex is not required for safe swallowing, attempts to normalize it are recommended. Facilitation of a hypoactive gag can be achieved by applying a tongue depressor, cotton-tipped swab, or a quick tap or a stretch to the arch of the soft palate in an upward and outward direction. A hyperactive gag can be desensitized by slowly "walking" back on the tongue while applying firm pressure with a tongue depressor.[98] As the gag reflex becomes less sensitive, the tongue depressor can be advanced farther back in the mouth.

Compensatory Techniques

Positioning the patient's head and trunk can compensate for swallowing dysfunction (Table 26–10). The ideal position for most patients with a neurological disorder is seated upright in a chair with the head in the midline, the trunk erect, and the neck slightly flexed forward. Pillows and other supports can be used to maintain trunk support and to support the limbs.

Common postural techniques used to decrease or eliminate aspiration include tilting the chin down, turning the head, or tilting the head to the right or left. As described by Logemann,[79] the chin tuck can be beneficial in that it narrows the opening of the airway and may widen the vallecular space (Fig. 26–20). This technique is particularly useful for patients who have a delayed pharyngeal swallow, reduced tongue base retraction, or reduced airway entrance closure. In the case of aspiration due to a delayed swallow reflex, the chin tuck provides greater airway protection by allowing food substances to sit in the valleculae until the reflex is triggered. Recent research shows that the chin tuck may be beneficial in that it decreases the space between the base of the tongue and the posterior pharyngeal wall, creating increased pharyngeal pressure to move the bolus through the pharyngeal region.[139]

Turning the head to the affected side may be beneficial when decreased pharyngeal peristalsis is noted unilaterally (Fig. 26–21). This maneuver helps direct food down the stronger or more normal side of the pharynx. Upper esophageal sphincter function also improves with head turning.[81]

Tilting the head to the right or left toward the stronger side can be of similar assistance in that it keeps food on the stronger side of the pharynx.[79] It also is effective for patients who have unilateral tongue weakness because it directs food toward the stronger side of the tongue. From clinical experience, these techniques can be effective for decreasing or eliminating aspiration in some, but certainly not in all, cases. Therefore, videofluoroscopy is useful to determine the effectiveness of these techniques.

Other compensatory techniques include effortful swallows and double swallows. For the effortful swallow, the patient swallows "hard" while eating in an attempt to help propel food through the pharyngeal cavity in a forceful and timely manner. For double swallowing, the

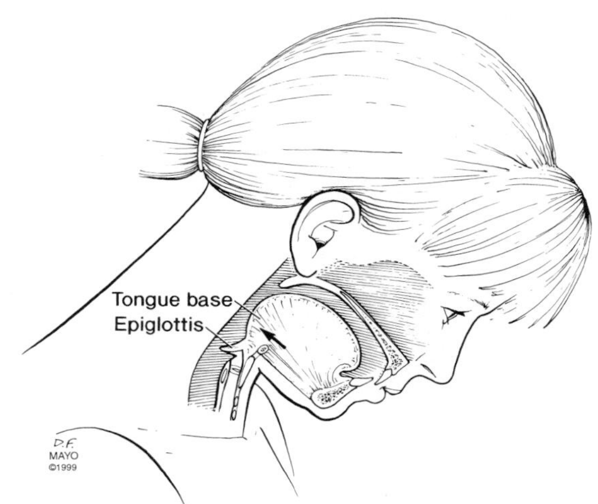

FIGURE 26–20. Chin tuck to protect the airway and prevent aspiration. (Reproduced by permission of Mayo Foundation.)

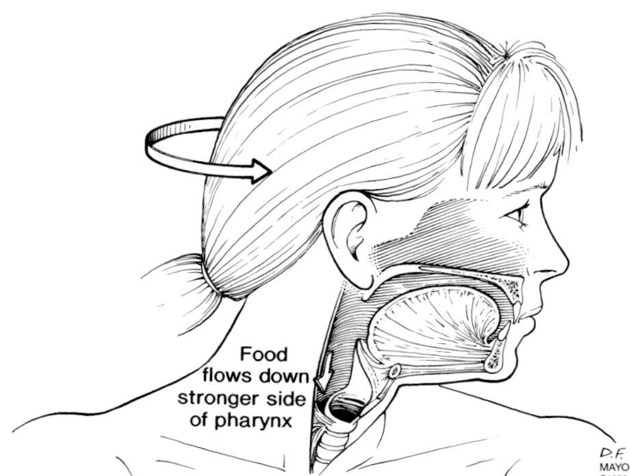

FIGURE 26–21. Turning head to the side directs food down stronger side of the pharynx. (Reproduced by permission of Mayo Foundation.)

patient swallows once again (or repeatedly, if needed) after the initial swallow. One or both of these techniques can be beneficial for cases in which decreased pharyngeal peristalsis is noted on videofluoroscopy.

Alternating liquids and solids can be another effective technique in some cases in which decreased pharyngeal peristalsis is present. The liquid swallows help to clear any material remaining in the pharyngeal recesses.

The supraglottic swallow is a technique designed to close the airway voluntarily.[79] It incorporates closure of the vocal folds along with clearing the airway of any aspirated material after the swallow. This technique can be useful for patients who have reduced laryngeal closure. The steps of the supraglottic swallow are as follows:

1. Take a bite of food or a sip of liquid.
2. Chew well.
3. Take a deep breath and hold it.
4. Swallow while holding the breath.
5. Cough immediately after the swallow.
6. Relax and breathe normally.

This technique may be used with just one or with all consistencies of food. Because numerous steps are required, the patient must demonstrate the ability to follow and sequence the instructions.

The super supraglottic swallow incorporates the supraglottic swallow while the patient bears down on a table or presses the hands together to create a Valsalva effect.[79] This technique may assist in creating additional laryngeal closure.

The Mendelsohn maneuver is a technique designed to prolong the opening of the cricopharyngeal region.[103] The technique may be indicated for cases in which decreased laryngeal elevation and subsequent decreased cricopharyngeal opening exist. To perform this maneuver, patients are asked to concentrate on the feeling of the Adam's apple rising while they swallow. Next, they are instructed to hold the swallow for 2 to 3 seconds when the pharynx is at its uppermost point. Finally, they are asked to complete the swallow and relax.[49] It is one of the few techniques that may be of assistance in working with a disorder of the cricopharyngeal region.

Biofeedback techniques also may be of assistance in swallowing retraining. They can be useful for oral motor and facial exercises and for giving the patient feedback on the actual swallow.[19]

Adaptive Equipment

Numerous devices are available to assist patients who have difficulty with the motor or perceptual components of feeding. Examples include rocker knives, swivel utensils, built-up handles on utensils, scoop dishes, nonskid mats, and large-handled cups (Fig. 26–22). These devices compensate for decreased upper extremity function, including limited grasp, incoordination, decreased

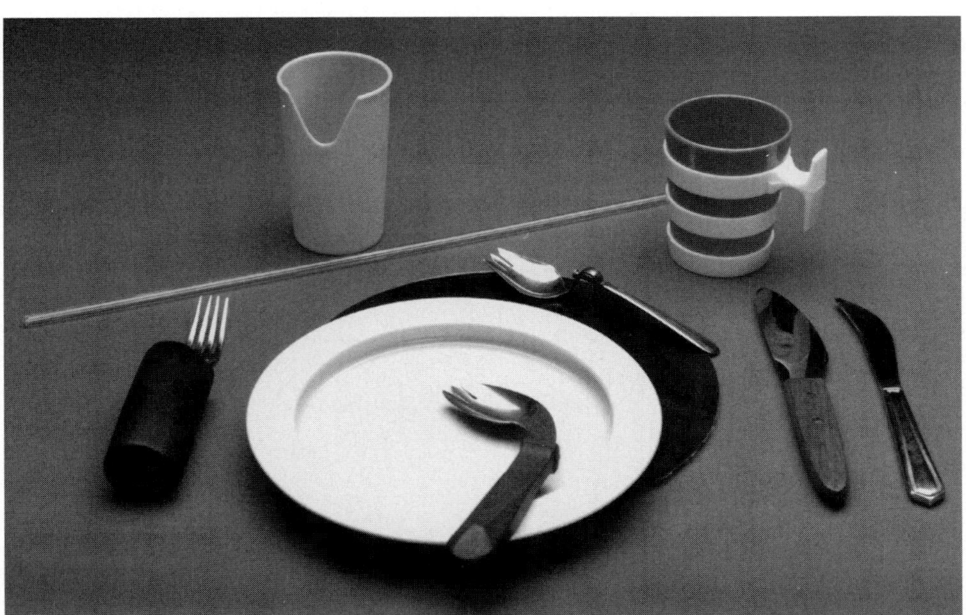

FIGURE 26–22. Adaptive equipment used to compensate for limited upper extremity function. *Left to right:* built-up fork, nose cutout cup, long straw, inner lip plate, nonskid mat, offset spoon and fork, large-handled mug, and rocker knives.

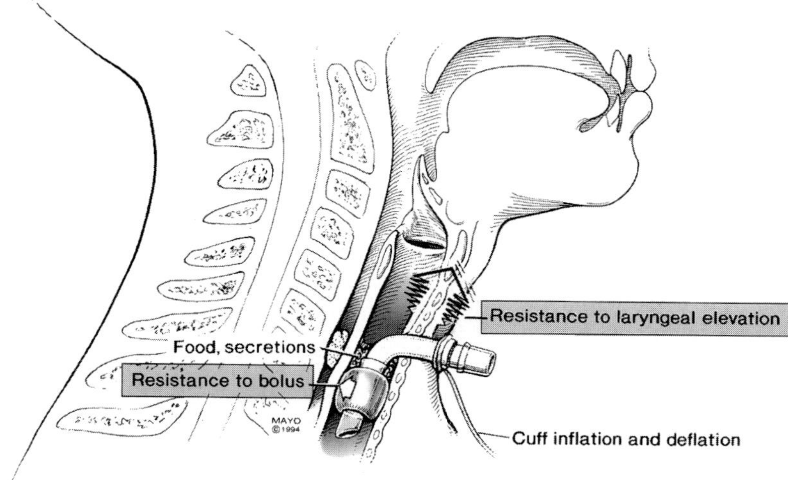

FIGURE 26–23. The swallowing impairments from a tracheostomy. (Redrawn from Nash M: Swallowing problems in the tracheotomized patient. Otolaryngol Clin North Am 1988; 21:701. Reproduced by permission of Mayo Foundation.)

range of motion, hemiparesis, and hemiplegia (see Chapter 25).

Surgical Procedures

Operative intervention is another option in the treatment of dysphagia. It is particularly helpful when conservative measures have failed and swallowing difficulties arise from a focal neuromuscular disorder or obstruction.

A tracheostomy is commonly used to provide optimal pulmonary ventilation and hygiene, and it also serves as a short-term solution for airway protection from aspiration.[13] Ironically, it can also be a risk factor for aspiration. After tracheostomy, laryngeal elevation is impaired, which increases the risk of aspiration. Aspiration can also be associated with cuff inflation or deflation. The inflated cuff applies a compressive force to the esophagus and may increase resistance to the passage of a food bolus. The deflated cuff allows food or secretions that have been retained above the cuff to pass into the trachea,[94] and careful suctioning after cuff deflation is necessary (Fig. 26–23).

Cricopharyngeal myotomy is often done in patients with Zenker's diverticulum and is effective in the treatment of cricopharyngeal achalasia.[5, 11] Myotomy is not generally recommended for conditions in which a generalized failure of the swallowing process is present,[13] although it has been used successfully in neuromuscular disease.[78] Videofluoroscopy has limitations in the assessment of cricopharyngeal function, and manometry or newer study tools can be helpful in making decisions regarding myotomy.[32] Moreover, botulinum toxin (Botox) injections have been used to identify patients who will benefit from myotomy.[141]

Several procedures have been devised for protection of the larynx, including vocal cord augmentation in mild aspiration and laryngeal diversion for more severe and chronic cases. Microsurgical techniques and progress with microprocessors in the application of electrical stimulation give hope that a more functional solution to severe aspiration will evolve with time.[7, 13]

OUTCOMES OF THE TEAM APPROACH

Dysphagia is a complex symptom that can be evoked by a myriad of disorders. The assessment and treatment of this symptom and its cause often transcend one specialty or discipline. Consequently, utilization of a multidisciplinary treatment team, functioning in an interdisciplinary manner, has become common. In the rehabilitation setting, a team frequently consists of a speech pathologist, an occupational therapist, a physiatrist, a radiologist, a dietitian, and a rehabilitation nurse with consultation from a gastroenterologist, an otolaryngologist, and other subspecialists as needed. Use of this team approach for evaluation and treatment seems to result in improved outcomes. The risk of aspiration cannot be completely eliminated, but patients managed with this approach aspirate less often than their control group counterparts,[64] and they also have greater caloric intake and weight gain.[86]

REFERENCES

1. Alberts MJ, Horner J, Gray L, et al: Aspiration after stroke: Lesion analysis by brain MRI. Dysphagia 1992; 7:170.
2. Arvedson JC: Dysphagia in pediatric patients with neurologic damage. Semin Neurol 1996; 16:371.
3. Arvedson JC, Lefton-Greif MA: Pediatric Videofluoroscopic Swallow Studies: A Professional Manual with Caregiver Guidelines. San Antonio, Communication Skill Builders, 1998.
4. Aviv JE: Effects of aging on sensitivity of the pharyngeal and supraglottic areas. Am J Med 1997; 103:74S.
5. Baredes S: Surgical management of swallowing disorders. Otolaryngol Clin North Am 1988; 21:711.
6. Barer DH: The natural history and functional consequences of dysphagia after hemispheric stroke. J Neurol Neurosurg Psychiatry 1989; 52:236.
7. Barrocas A, Belcher D, Champagne C, et al: Nutrition assessment: Practical approaches. Clin Geriatr Med 1995; 11:675.
8. Bartlett JG: Aspiration pneumonia. In Baum GL, Wolinsky E (eds): Textbook of Pulmonary Diseases, ed 5, vol 1. Boston, Little, Brown, 1994, p 593.
9. Bastian RW: The videoendoscopic swallowing study: An alternative and partner to the videofluoroscopic swallowing study. Dysphagia 1993; 8:359.

10. Beck TJ, Gayler BW: Image quality and radiation levels in videofluoroscopy for swallowing studies: A review. Dysphagia 1990; 5:118.
11. Berg HM, Jacobs JB, Persky MS, et al: Cricopharyngeal myotomy: A review of surgical results in patients with cricopharyngeal achalasia of neurogenic origin. Laryngoscope 1985; 95:1337.
12. Bistrian BR, Blackburn GL, Vitale J, et al: Prevalence of malnutrition in general medical patients. JAMA 1976; 235:1567.
13. Blitzer A: Approaches to the patient with aspiration and swallowing disabilities. Dysphagia 1990; 5:129.
14. Bosma JF: Deglutition: Pharyngeal stage. Physiol Rev 1957; 37:275.
15. Bosma JF, Donner MW, Tanaka E, et al: Anatomy of the pharynx, pertinent to swallowing. Dysphagia 1986; 1:23.
16. Briani C, Marcon M, Ermani M, et al: Radiological evidence of subclinical dysphagia in motor neuron disease. J Neurol 1998; 245:211.
17. Brin MF, Younger D: Neurologic disorders and aspiration. Otolaryngol Clin North Am 1988; 21:691.
18. Brown GE, Nordloh S, Donowitz AJ: Systematic desensitization of oral hypersensitivity in a patient with a closed head injury. Dysphagia 1992; 7:138.
19. Bryant M: Biofeedback in the treatment of a selected dysphagic patient. Dysphagia 1991; 6:140.
20. Buchholz D: Neurologic causes of dysphagia. Dysphagia 1987; 1:152.
21. Buchholz D, Jones B: Dysphagia occurring after polio. Dysphagia 1991; 6:165.
22. Buchin PJ: Swallowing disorders: Diagnosis and medical treatment. Otolaryngol Clin North Am 1988; 21:663.
23. Busmann M, Dobmeyer SM, Leeker L, et al: Swallowing abnormalities and their response to treatment in Parkinson's disease. Neurology 1989; 39:1309.
24. Cameron DC, Guy D: The design of a lightweight mobile chair for use with video fluoroscopy in the investigation of swallow disorders. Australas Radiol 1990; 34:274.
25. Carter GT, Johnson ER, Bonekat HW, et al: Laryngeal diversion in the treatment of intractable aspiration in motor neuron disease. Arch Phys Med Rehabil 1992; 73:680.
26. Casas MJ, Kenny DJ, McPherson KA: Swallowing/ventilation interactions during oral swallow in normal children and children with cerebral palsy. Dysphagia 1994; 9:40.
27. Cherney LR: Clinical Management of Dysphagia in Adults and Children, ed 2. Gaithersburg, MD, Aspen, 1994.
28. Cherney LR, Halper AS: Swallowing problems in adults with traumatic brain injury. Semin Neurol 1996; 16:349.
29. Christensen JR: Developmental approach to pediatric neurogenic dysphagia. Dysphagia 1989; 3:131.
30. Ciocon JO: Indications for tube feedings in elderly patients. Dysphagia 1990; 5:1.
31. Collins MJ, Bakheit AM: Does pulse oximetry reliably detect aspiration in dysphagic stroke patients? Stroke 1997; 28:1773.
32. Cook IJ: Cricopharyngeal function and dysfunction. Dysphagia 1993; 8:244.
33. Daniels SK, Brailey K, Priestly DH, et al: Aspiration in patients with acute stroke. Arch Phys Med Rehabil 1998; 79:14.
34. de Lama Lazzara G, Lazarus C, Logemann JA: Impact of thermal stimulation on the triggering of the swallowing reflex. Dysphagia 1986; 1:73.
35. DePippo KL, Holas MA, Reding MJ: Validation of the 3-oz water swallow test for aspiration following stroke. Arch Neurol 1992; 49:1259.
36. Dodds WJ: Physiology of swallowing. Dysphagia 1989; 3:171.
37. Dworkin JP, Nadal JC: Nonsurgical treatment of drooling in a patient with closed head injury and severe dysarthria. Dysphagia 1991; 6:40.
38. Ergun GA, Miskovitz PF: Aging and the esophagus: Common pathologic conditions and their effect upon swallowing in the geriatric population. Dysphagia 1992; 7:58.
39. Farber SD: Neurorehabilitation: A Multisensory Approach. Philadelphia, WB Saunders, 1982, p 115.
40. Feinberg MJ, Ekberg O: Videofluoroscopy in elderly patients with aspiration: Importance of evaluating both oral and pharyngeal stages of deglutition. AJR 1991; 156:293.
41. Feinberg MJ, Knebl J, Tully J, et al: Aspiration and the elderly. Dysphagia 1990; 5:61.
42. Finegold SM: Aspiration pneumonia. Rev Infect Dis 1991; 13(suppl 9):S737.
43. Finestone HM, Greene-Finestone LS, Wilson ES, et al: Prolonged length of stay and reduced functional improvement rate in malnourished stroke rehabilitation patients. Arch Phys Med Rehabil 1996; 77:340.
44. Frederick MG, Ott DJ, Grishaw EK, et al: Functional abnormalities of the pharynx: A prospective analysis of radiographic abnormalities relative to age and symptoms. AJR 1996; 166:353.
45. Goyal RK, Martin SB, Shapiro J, et al: The role of cricopharyngeus muscle in pharyngoesophageal disorders. Dysphagia 1993; 8:252.
46. Gray C, Sivaloganathan S, Simpkins KC: Aspiration of high-density barium contrast medium causing acute pulmonary inflammation: Report of two fatal cases in elderly women with disordered swallowing. Clin Radiol 1989; 40:397.
47. Groher ME: Dysphagia: Diagnosis and Management. Boston, Butterworth, 1984.
48. Hagen R, Haase A, Matthaei D, et al: Oropharyngeale Funktionsdiagnostik mit der FLASH-MR-Tomographie. HNO 1990; 38:421.
49. Hardy E, Robinson NM: Swallowing Disorders: Treatment Manual. Bisbee, AZ, Imaginart Communication Products, 1993.
50. Hendrix TR: Art and science of history taking in the patient with difficulty swallowing. Dysphagia 1993; 8:69.
51. Holt S, Miron SD, Diaz MC, et al: Scintigraphic measurement of oropharyngeal transit in man. Dig Dis Sci 1990; 35:1198.
52. Horner J, Buoyer FG, Alberts MJ, et al: Dysphagia following brain-stem stroke: Clinical correlates and outcome. Arch Neurol 1991; 48:1170.
53. Horner J, Massey EW, Brazer SR: Aspiration in bilateral stroke patients. Neurology 1990; 40:1686.
54. Horner J, Massey EW, Riski JE, et al: Aspiration following stroke: Clinical correlates and outcome. Neurology 1988; 38:1359.
55. Hunter PC, Crameri J, Austin S, et al: Response of parkinsonian swallowing dysfunction to dopaminergic stimulation. J Neurol Neurosurg Psychiatry 1997; 63:579.
56. Huxley EJ, Viroslav J, Gray WR, et al: Pharyngeal aspiration in normal adults and patients with depressed consciousness. Am J Med 1978; 64:564.
57. Johnson ER, McKenzie SW, Rosenquist CJ, et al: Dysphagia following stroke: Quantitative evaluation of pharyngeal transit times. Arch Phys Med Rehabil 1992; 73:419.
58. Johnson ER, McKenzie SW, Sievers A: Aspiration pneumonia in stroke. Arch Phys Med Rehabil 1993; 74:973.
59. Jones B, Buchholz DW, Ravich WJ, et al: Swallowing dysfunction in the postpolio syndrome: A cinefluorographic study. AJR 1992; 158:283.
60. Jones B, Donner MW: How I do it: Examination of the patient with dysphagia. Dysphagia 1989; 4:162.
61. Jones B, Ravich WJ, Donner MW: Dysphagia in systemic disease. Dysphagia 1993; 8:368.
62. Kahrilas PJ: Pharyngeal structure and function. Dysphagia 1993; 8:303.
63. Kamel PL: Nutritional assessment and requirements. Dysphagia 1990; 4:189.
64. Kasprisin AT, Clumeck H, Nino-Murcia M: Efficacy of rehabilitative management of dysphagia. Dysphagia 1989; 4:48.
65. Kelly KG: Advances in perioperative nutritional support. Med Clin North Am 1993; 77:465.
66. Kennedy JG III, Kent RD: Physiological substrates of normal deglutition. Dysphagia 1988; 3:24.
67. Kerstetter JE, Holthausen BA, Fitz PA: Nutrition and nutritional requirements for the older adult. Dysphagia 1993; 8:51.
68. Khawaja IT, Buffa SD, Brandstetter RD: Aspiration pneumonia: A threat when deglutition is compromised. Postgrad Med 1992; 92:165, 173, 181.
69. Kirsch CM, Sanders A: Aspiration pneumonia: Medical management. Otolaryngol Clin North Am 1988; 21:677.
70. Kluin KJ, Bromberg MB, Feldman EL, et al: Dysphagia in elderly men with myasthenia gravis. J Neurol Sci 1996; 138:49.
71. Koch WM: Swallowing disorders: Diagnosis and therapy. Med Clin North Am 1993; 77:571.

72. Kosko JR, Moser JD, Erhart N, et al: Differential diagnosis of dysphagia in children. Otolaryngol Clin North Am 1998; 31:435.
73. Kramer SS, Eicher PM: The evaluation of pediatric feeding abnormalities. Dysphagia 1993; 8:215.
74. Langmore SE, Schatz K, Olson N: Endoscopic and videofluoroscopic evaluations of swallowing and aspiration. Ann Otol Rhinol Laryngol 1991; 100:678.
75. Langmore SE, Terpenning MS, Schork A, et al: Predictors of aspiration pneumonia: How important is dysphagia? Dysphagia 1998; 13:69.
76. Lazarus BA, Murphy JB, Culpepper L: Aspiration associated with long-term gastric versus jejunal feeding: A critical analysis of the literature. Arch Phys Med Rehabil 1990; 71:46.
77. Lindbichler F, Raith J, Uggowitzer M, et al: Functional imaging of the pharynx using electron beam tomography. Dysphagia 1998; 13:101.
78. Lindgren S, Ekberg O: Cricopharyngeal myotomy in the treatment of dysphagia. Clin Otolaryngol 1990; 15:221.
79. Logemann JA: Evaluation and Treatment of Swallowing Disorders, ed 2. Austin, TX, Pro-Ed, 1998.
80. Logemann JA: Swallowing physiology and pathophysiology. Otolaryngol Clin North Am 1988; 21:613.
81. Logemann JA, Kahrilas PJ, Kobara M, et al: The benefit of head rotation on pharyngoesophageal dysphagia. Arch Phys Med Rehabil 1989; 70:767.
82. Logemann JA, Shanahan T, Rademaker AW, et al: Oropharyngeal swallowing after stroke in the left basal ganglion/internal capsule. Dysphagia 1993; 8:230.
83. Loughlin GM: Respiratory consequences of dysfunctional swallowing and aspiration. Dysphagia 1989; 3:126.
84. Manchikanti L, Colliver JA, Marrero TC, et al: Assessment of age-related acid aspiration risk factors in pediatric adult and geriatric patients. Anesth Analg 1985; 64:11.
85. Maniere-Ezvan A, Duval JM, Darnault P: Ultrasonic assessment of the anatomy and function of the tongue. Surg Radiol Anat 1993; 15:55.
86. Martens L, Cameron T, Simonsen M: Effects of a multidisciplinary management program on neurologically impaired patients with dysphagia. Dysphagia 1990; 5:147.
87. Martin BJ, Corlew MM, Wood H, et al: The association of swallowing dysfunction and aspiration pneumonia. Dysphagia 1994; 9:1.
88. Martin RE, Sessle BJ: The role of the cerebral cortex in swallowing. Dysphagia 1993; 8:195.
89. Milazzo LS, Bouchard J, Lund DA: The swallowing process: Effects of aging and stroke. Phys Med Rehabil 1989; 3:489.
90. Miller AJ: Neurophysiological basis of swallowing. Dysphagia 1986; 1:91.
91. Morris SE: Development of oral-motor skills in the neurologically impaired child receiving non-oral feedings. Dysphagia 1989; 3:135.
92. Morton RE, Bonas R, Fourie B, et al: Videofluoroscopy in the assessment of feeding disorders of children with neurological problems. Dev Med Child Neurol 1993; 35:388.
93. Mullan H, Roubenoff RA, Roubenoff R: Risk of pulmonary aspiration among patients receiving enteral nutrition support. J Parenteral Enteral Nutr 1992; 16:160.
94. Nash M: Swallowing problems in the tracheotomized patient. Otolaryngol Clin North Am 1988; 21:701.
95. Newmark SR, Sublett D, Black J, et al: Nutritional assessment in a rehabilitation unit. Arch Phys Med Rehabil 1981; 62:279.
96. Nilsson H, Ekberg O, Olsson R, et al: Dysphagia in stroke: A prospective study of quantitative aspects of swallowing in dysphagic patients. Dysphagia 1998; 13:32.
97. Olsson R, Nilsson H, Ekberg O: Simultaneous videoradiography and pharyngeal solid state manometry (videomanometry) in 25 nondysphagic volunteers. Dysphagia 1995; 10:36.
98. O'Sullivan N: Dysphagia Care: Team Approach With Acute and Long-Term Patients. Los Angeles, Cottage Square, 1990.
99. Ott DJ, Chen YM, Hewson EG, et al: Esophageal motility: Assessment with synchronous video tape fluoroscopy and manometry. Radiology 1989; 173:419.
100. Palmer JB, DuChane AS: Rehabilitation of swallowing disorders due to stroke. Phys Med Rehabil Clin North Am 1991; 2:529.
101. Palmer JB, Kuhlemeier KV, Tippett DC, et al: A protocol for the videofluorographic swallowing study. Dysphagia 1993; 8:209.
102. Park RH, Allison MC, Lang J, et al: Randomized comparison of percutaneous endoscopic gastrostomy and nasogastric tube feeding in patients with persisting neurological dysphagia. Br Med J 1992; 304:1406.
103. Penington GR, Krutsch JA: Swallowing disorders: Assessment and rehabilitation. Br J Hosp Med 1990; 44:17, 20, 22.
104. Pollack IF, Pang D, Kocoshis S, et al: Neurogenic dysphagia resulting from Chiari malformations. Neurosurgery 1992; 30:709.
105. Rasley A, Logemann JA, Kahrilas PJ, et al: Prevention of barium aspiration during videofluoroscopic swallowing studies: Value of change in posture. AJR 1993; 160:1005.
106. Robbins J: Normal swallowing and aging. Semin Neurol 1996; 16:309.
107. Robbins J, Levine RL, Maser A, et al: Swallowing after unilateral stroke of the cerebral cortex. Arch Phys Med Rehabil 1993; 74:1295.
108. Rogers B, Arvedson J, Buck G, et al: Characteristics of dysphagia in children with cerebral palsy. Dysphagia 1994; 9:69.
109. Rogers BT, Arvedson J, Msall M, et al: Hypoxemia during oral feeding of children with severe cerebral palsy. Dev Med Child Neurol 1993; 35:3.
110. Rosenbek JC, Robbins J, Fishback B, et al: Effects of thermal application on dysphagia after stroke. J Speech Hearing Res 1991; 34:1257.
111. Schechter GL: Systemic causes of dysphagia in adults. Otolaryngol Clin North Am 1998; 31:525.
112. Schima W, Stacher G, Pokieser P, et al: Esophageal motor disorders: Videofluoroscopic and manometric evaluation: Prospective study in 88 symptomatic patients. Radiology 1992; 185:487.
113. Schmidt J, Holas M, Halvorson K, et al: Videofluoroscopic evidence of aspiration predicts pneumonia and death but not dehydration following stroke. Dysphagia 1994; 9:7.
114. Serradura-Russell A: Ethical dilemmas in dysphagia management and the right to a natural death. Dysphagia 1992; 7:102.
115. Sessle BJ, Henry JL: Neural mechanisms of swallowing: Neurophysiological and neurochemical studies on brain stem neurons in the solitary tract region. Dysphagia 1989; 4:61.
116. Sheth N, Diner WC: Swallowing problems in the elderly. Dysphagia 1988; 2:209.
117. Signore J, Erickson RV: Nutritional assessment of the stroke patient. Phys Med Rehabil 1989; 3:501.
118. Silver KH, Van Nostrand D: The use of scintigraphy in the management of patients with pulmonary aspiration. Dysphagia 1994; 9:107.
119. Silver KH, Van Nostrand D, Kuhlemeier KV, et al: Scintigraphy for the detection and quantification of subglottic aspiration: Preliminary observations. Arch Phys Med Rehabil 1991; 72:902.
120. Sitzmann JV: Nutritional support of the dysphagic patient: Methods, risks, and complications of therapy. J Parenteral Enteral Nutr 1990; 14:60.
121. Sitzmann JV, Mueller R: Enteral and parenteral feeding in the dysphagic patient. Dysphagia 1988; 3:38.
122. Smithard DG, O'Neill PA, England RE, et al: The natural history of dysphagia following a stroke. Dysphagia 1997; 12:188.
123. Smithard DG, O'Neill PA, Parks C, et al: Complications and outcome after acute stroke. Does dysphagia matter? Stroke 1996; 27:1200.
124. Sobin J, Nathanson A, Engstrom CF: Endoluminal ultrasonography: A new method to evaluate dysphagia. ORL J Otorhinolaryngol Relat Spec 1996; 58:105.
125. Sonies BC: Oropharyngeal dysphagia in the elderly. Clin Geriatr Med 1992; 8:569.
126. Sonies BC: Ultrasound imaging and swallowing. In Jones B, Donner MW (eds): Normal and Abnormal Swallowing: Imaging in Diagnosis and Therapy. New York, Springer-Verlag, 1991, p 109.
127. Sonies BC, Dalakas MC: Dysphagia in patients with the post-polio syndrome. N Engl J Med 1991; 324:1162.
128. Splaingard ML, Hutchins B, Sulton LD, et al: Aspiration in rehabilitation patients: Videofluoroscopy vs bedside clinical assessment. Arch Phys Med Rehabil 1988; 69:637.
129. Stroudley J, Walsh M: Radiological assessment of dysphagia in Parkinson's disease. Br J Radiol 1991; 64:890.

130. Suto Y, Kamba M, Kato T: Technical note: Dynamic analysis of the pharynx during swallowing using Turbo-FLASH magnetic resonance imaging combined with an oral positive contrast agent: A preliminary study. Br J Radiol 1995; 68:1099.
131. Teasell RW, Bach D, McRae M: Prevalence and recovery of aspiration poststroke: A retrospective analysis. Dysphagia 1994; 9:35.
132. Teasell RW, Finestone HM, Greene-Finestone L: Dysphagia and nutrition following stroke. Phys Med Rehabil 1993; 7:89.
133. Terry PB, Fuller SD: Pulmonary consequences of aspiration. Dysphagia 1989; 3:179.
134. Tuchman DN: Cough, Choke, sputter: The evaluation of the child with dysfunctional swallowing. Dysphagia 1989; 3:111.
135. Veis SL, Logemann JA: Swallowing disorders in persons with cerebrovascular accident. Arch Phys Med Rehabil 1985; 66:372.
136. Waterman ET, Koltai PJ, Downey JC, et al: Swallowing disorders in a population of children with cerebral palsy. Int J Pediatr Otorhinolaryngol 1992; 24:63.
137. Waxman MJ, Durfee D, Moore M, et al: Nutritional aspects and swallowing function of patients with Parkinson's disease. Nutr Clin Pract 1990; 5:196.
138. Weiss MH: Dysphagia in infants and children. Otolaryngol Clin North Am 1988; 21:727.
139. Welch MV, Logemann JA, Rademaker AW, et al: Changes in pharyngeal dimensions effected by chin tuck. Arch Phys Med Rehabil 1993; 74:178.
140. Winstein CJ: Neurogenic dysphagia: Frequency, progression, and outcome in adults following head injury. Phys Ther 1983; 63:1992.
141. Wisdom G, Blitzer A: Surgical therapy for swallowing disorders. Otolaryngol Clin North Am 1998; 31:537.

27 CHAPTER

Diana D. Cardenas, M.D., and Michael E. Mayo, M.B.B.S.

Management of Bladder Dysfunction

The first section of this chapter describes the neuroanatomy and classification of the neurogenic bladder. The discussion then addresses methods of clinical evaluation, management, surgical techniques, and common complications. Bladder dysfunction is commonly found in patients cared for by physiatrists, and basic knowledge of these areas is essential.

NEUROANATOMY

Structure and Function

The detrusor muscle in humans is said to have no gap junctions, which suggests a one-on-one nerve-to-muscle-cell innervation. In the striated muscle of the distal sphincter the majority of fibers are slow twitch, while those in the pelvic floor are a mixture of fast- and slow-twitch fibers. Contraction of the detrusor muscle is started by phosphorylation of the light myosin chain and relaxed by dephosphorylation. Contraction is initiated by a rise in intracellular calcium concentration from release of calcium from intracellular sources and, more important, from an influx of calcium into the cell. This influx is controlled by as many as four calcium channels (three voltage sensitive and one receptor sensitive). This probably explains why calcium channel blockers are not effective inhibitors of detrusor activity in the clinical setting. Relaxation of the detrusor is associated with the efflux of potassium into the cell. In addition to smooth muscle, collagen forms nearly 50% of the bladder wall in healthy subjects, and this proportion increases considerably in disease states.

Receptors

The receptors active during bladder contraction are cholinergic muscarinic (M_2 and M_3) receptors and are widely distributed in the body of the bladder, trigone, bladder neck, and urethra. Adrenergic receptors are concentrated in the trigone, bladder neck, and urethra and are predominantly α_1. These have recently been subdivided into α_{1a}, α_{1b}, and α_{1d}. Identification of the subgroups should allow increased specificity with regard to future therapeutic agents. Norepinephrine-containing nerve cells are also found in the paravesical and intramural ganglia, and a few authors describe norepinephrine terminals in the striated muscle of the distal sphincter, although most would dispute this. When these cells are active, they have excitatory effects and maintain continence by contraction of the bladder neck and urethral smooth muscle. α_2-adrenergic receptors are found in the bladder neck and also in the body of the bladder. These receptors are inhibitory when activated and can produce relaxation at the bladder neck on initiation of voiding and relax the bladder body to enhance storage (Fig. 27–1). In humans, however, the storage role seems to be a minor one. The striated sphincter muscle contains cholinergic nicotinic receptors.

Other lower tract transmitters have been considered, but much of the evidence for their presence and activity is from animal preparations. The role of these other transmitters in normal and disease states in humans is uncertain. Many lower tract transmitters have opposing effects on lower tract function, depending on their site of action. Purine receptors (P_1, stimulated by adenosine, and P_2, stimulated by adenosine triphosphate) have their effects at the pelvic ganglia and the neuroeffector junction, and have inhibitory and facilitative effects respectively on the detrusor muscle. Vasointestinal polypeptide, on the other hand, enhances transmission of acetylcholine in pelvic ganglia and inhibits acetylcholine-mediated contraction in the detrusor. Neuropeptide Y has excitatory functions on detrusor

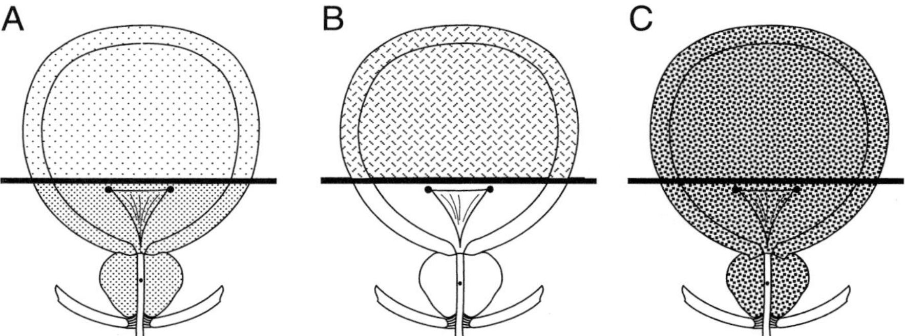

FIGURE 27–1. *A.* Distribution of the α-adrenergic receptors, with few in the dome of the bladder and more in the base of the bladder and prostate. *B.* Distribution of the β-receptors, which are largely in the dome. *C.* Distribution of the cholinergic receptors, which are widely distributed throughout the dome and the base of the bladder and the urethra.

muscle and indirect facilitative effects by inhibiting norephinephrine release. This transmitter also has inhibitory effects by blocking acetylcholine release and blocks the atropine-resistant bladder contraction. Tachykinins are found mostly in afferent nerves, where their effects are to augment the micturation reflex and also transmit pain sensation. Thus tachykinins augment the contractile and vascular response in inflammatory states. Prostaglandin causes the slow onset of contractions of the detrusor, while parathyroid hormone–related peptide causes a relaxation.

The main effector transmitter for contraction of the urethra is norepinephrine, via the α_1 receptors. Smooth muscle relaxation is mediated by acetylcholine and probably by nitric oxide. Prostaglandins, in contrast to their effects on the detrusor, cause a relaxation of the urethral muscle. Prostaglandins have been tried in various clinical states of retention but without consistent results. Serotonin appears to be an antagonist that causes urethral muscle contraction; it might be important in the production of irritable urethral symptoms. The role of estrogens on the lower urinary tract in women is confined to the modification of tissues and receptors. Apparently they have no direct transmitter effects.

In the brainstem and spinal cord the various transmitters described above can have a variety of inhibitory and facilitative actions, depending on their site of action. Serotonin might have inhibitory detrusor effects at the midbrain level, and uptake of serotonin might be blocked by tricyclics (which are used in treating nocturnal enuresis). Activation of opiate receptors in the brainstem and sacral spinal cord inhibits voiding. This might partly explain the retention of urine seen with the use of these agents.[31] A complete discussion of the pharmacology of the lower urinary tract can be found in Steers.[31]

Innervation

The afferent and efferent peripheral pathways include the autonomic through the pelvic (parasympathetic) and hypogastric (sympathetic) nerves, and the somatic through the pudendal nerves (Fig. 27–2 and Table 27–1). Recently a subpopulation of the C-afferent fibers has been identified that is sensitive to the neurotoxin capsaicin. In health these fibers might modulate the normal micturition reflex via their effects on the afferent Aδ fibers. In pathological states they might mediate inflammatory reactions. In suprasacral neurogenic bladder disease these capsaicin-sensitive primary afferents have a major role in the pathogenesis of hyperreflexia. Intravesical capsaicin has been used experimentally to treat hyperreflexia when it does not respond to the usual pharmacological agents.

Central Connections and Control

The reflex center for the bladder lies in the pons along with the other autonomic centers (Fig. 27–3). Not shown in Figure 27–3 is a reflex with afferent axons originating from the bladder and synapsing on the pudendal nerve nucleus at S2, S3, and S4. This allows inhibition of pelvic floor activity during voiding. Another important reflex is the local segmental innervation of the external sphincter with afferents from the urethra, sphincter, and pelvic floor and efferents in the pudendal nerve. Higher (voluntary) control over the pelvic floor is achieved through afferents that ascend to the sensory cortex. Descending fibers from the motor cortex synapse with the pudendal motor nucleus.[5]

BLADDER FUNCTION

Urodynamic studies in both intact patients and those with neurological disease have yielded clinical insights into the normal and abnormal function of the lower urinary tract over the course of life.

Infant and Young Child

Neonates and infants have truly reflex bladders that empty at approximately 50- to 100-mL volumes. Sometime after the first year of life, the child begins to show some awareness of bladder evacuation and can begin to delay urination for a brief period by contracting the voluntary sphincter. For normal control, the detrusor reflex has to be inhibited by the higher centers at the level of the pontine nucleus. By 5 years of age, approximately 90% of children have normal control. The remaining 10% have a more infantile or immature pattern, with detrusor activity between voluntary voidings that produces frequency, urgency, and occasionally urge incontinence and nocturnal enuresis. Most of these children gradually develop inhibition of the detrusor reflex by the onset of puberty.

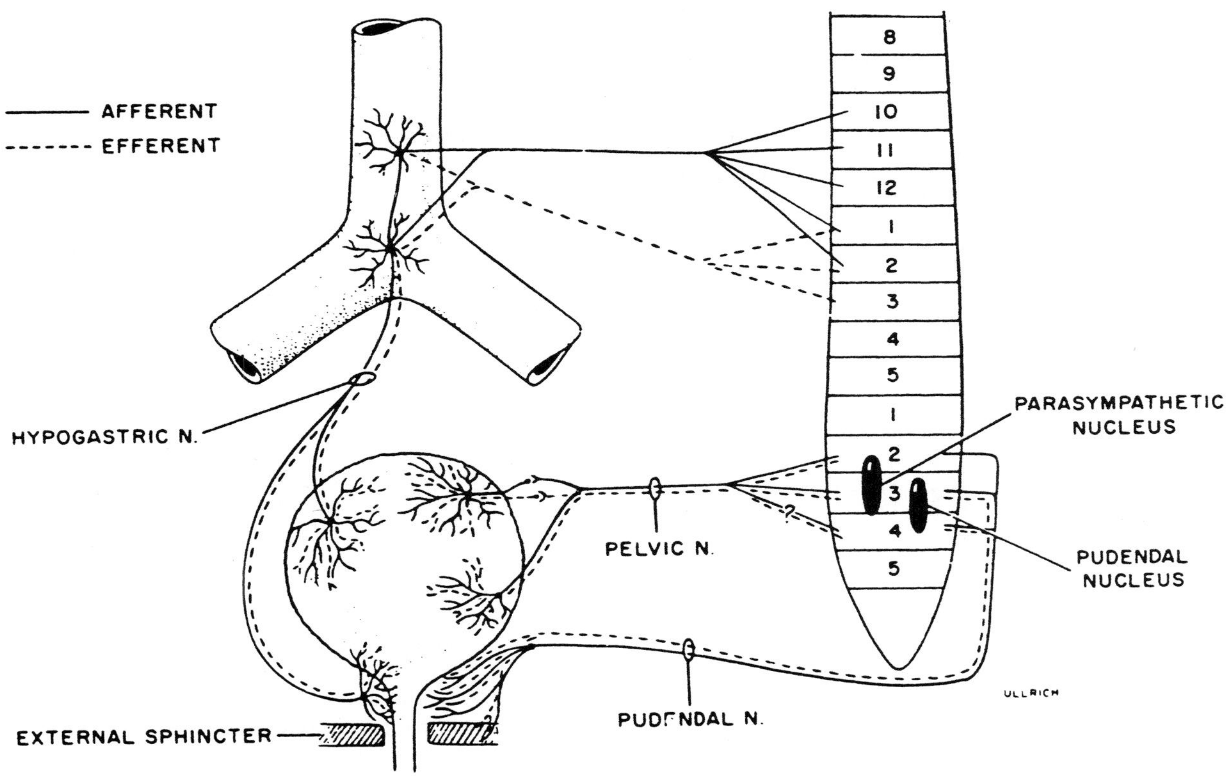

FIGURE 27–2. The parasympathetic, sympathetic, and somatic nerve supply to the bladder, urethra, and pelvic floor. (From Blaivas JG: Management of bladder dysfunction in multiple sclerosis. Neurology 1980; 30(2):12–18.)

Adult

With bladder filling, there is only a minimal rise in intravesical pressure (accommodation) together with an increase in recruitment of activity in the pelvic floor and voluntary sphincter. Normal voiding is initiated by voluntary relaxation of the pelvic floor with subsequent release of inhibition of the detrusor reflex at the pontine level. The detrusor contraction is maintained steadily throughout voiding, and the pelvic floor remains quiescent.

Elderly

Frequency, urgency, and incontinence with incomplete emptying are common in the elderly. Urodynamic studies show that many elderly persons have bladder contractions during filling, producing frequency, urgency, and incontinence. These contractions are poorly sustained during voiding and result in incomplete evacuation. Elderly men can have prostatic obstruction, and women can have incontinence related to impaired sphincter activity or stress incontinence. In the absence of these mechanical factors, changes in bladder function in the elderly have been ascribed to loss of cerebral control due to minor strokes, and to changes in the bladder wall due to collagen deposition. Changes in bladder function can also result from polyuria secondary to reduced renal concentrating ability, diuretic use, lack of normal increase in antidiuretic hormone secretion at night, and lower extremity edema during sleep.

CLASSIFICATION

The neurogenic bladder has been classified in a variety of ways, beginning with the anatomical classification of Bors and Comarr.[4] The first functional classification was based on cystometric findings, and five basic groups were described: (1) reflex, (2) uninhibited, (3) autonomous, (4) motor paralytic, and (5) sensory neurogenic bladders.[26] This system does not take into account the function of the sphincter mechanisms, however, and

TABLE 27–1 Bladder Afferent Pathways

Receptor	Pelvic (Parasympathetic)	Hypogastric (Sympathetic)	Pudendal (Somatic)
Bladder wall tension	+	−	−
Bladder mucosal nociception (pain, temperature, chemical irritation)	+	+	−
Urethral mucosal sensation (pain, temperature, passage of urine)	−	−	+

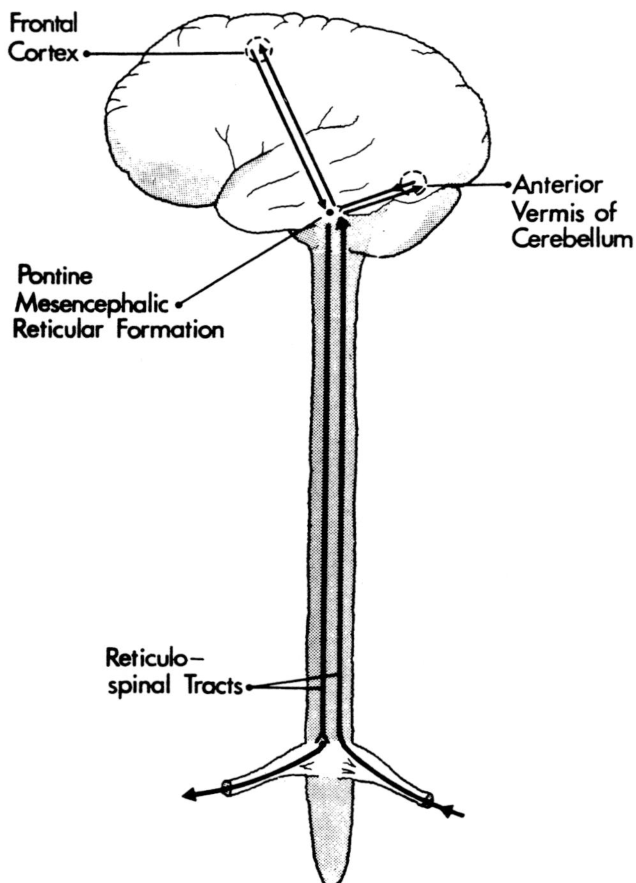

FIGURE 27–3. The central connections of the bladder reflex are shown, with the afferents ascending possibly in the reticulospinal tracts or the posterior columns to the pontine mesencephalic reticular formation and the efferents running down to the sacral outflow in the reticulospinal tracts. The pontine center is largely influenced by the cortex but also by other areas of the brain, particularly the cerebellum and basal ganglia. (From Bradley WE, Brantley SF: Physiology of the urinary bladder. In Campbell's Urology, ed 4. Philadelphia, WB Saunders, 1978, p 106.)

there are a few patients in whom the detrusor reflex does not return after spinal cord injury above the sacral outflow. Later a more anatomical classification system was proposed in which the neurogenic bladder was subdivided into types such as supraspinal, suprasacral spinal, infrasacral, peripheral autonomic, and muscular lesions (Fig. 27–4). At the same time others developed functional classifications, all of which were based on conventional urodynamic evaluations. This was an attempt to categorize the lower urinary tract according to the passive storage ability of the bladder and the activities and coordination of the detrusor and sphincter mechanisms (Table 27–2). In practice it is common to use a combination of both anatomical and functional classifications, with any known neurological lesion described in anatomical terms (e.g., supraspinal, suprasacral). Management is based on functional changes as demonstrated by conventional urodynamic testing.

HISTORY AND PHYSICAL EXAMINATION

Although the symptoms associated with neuropathological bladder processes are often misleading and correlate poorly with objective findings, relief of symptoms is one of the patient's main concerns. It is often helpful to have the patient or attendant record fluid intake, output, and incontinence episodes over several 24-hour periods. Such record keeping can show whether there is excessive intake or reversed diurnal rhythm of urine production. The history should help determine whether there were voiding symptoms prior to the putative neurological event, any premorbid conditions such as diabetes or cerebrovascular accidents, or prior urological or pelvic surgery. The neurological diagnosis, especially the level of the lesion and its completeness, is important in predicting the type of lower urinary tract dysfunction that might be expected.

The physical examination should assess mental status and confirm the neurological level (if present). The perineal sensation and pelvic floor muscle tone are particularly important in lower spinal cord and peripheral lesions. Reflexes are also important, but the bulbocavernous, cremasteric, and anal reflexes are sometimes difficult to elicit, even in intact persons. The skin of the perineum, state of bladder supports, and, in women, degree of vaginal support and estrogenization should be assessed. The prostate in males should be evaluated, but size or consistency alone is not a good indicator of obstruction. Lastly, an assessment should be made of the patient's motivation, lifestyle, body habitus, and other physical impairments.

DIAGNOSTIC TESTS

Indications

The extent of upper and lower urinary tract testing has to be individualized for each patient and the neurologi-

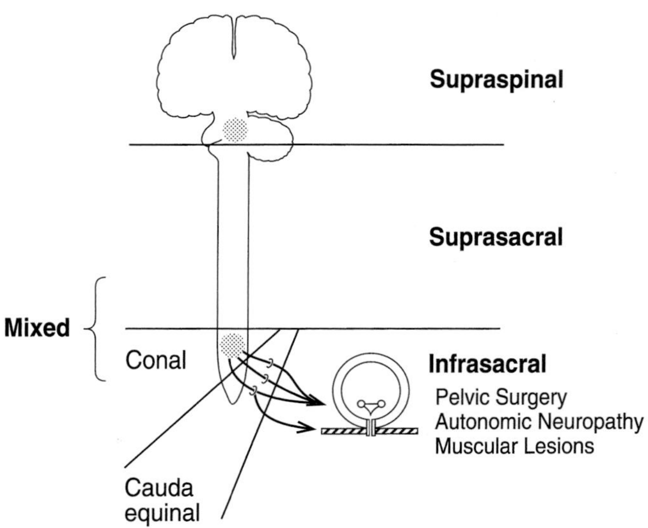

FIGURE 27–4. Anatomical classification of the neurogenic bladder.

TABLE 27–2 Functional Classification of the Neurogenic Bladder

Type of Failure	Bladder Factors	Outlet Factors
Failure to store	Hyperreflexia Decreased compliance	Denervated pelvic floor Bladder neck descent Intrinsic bladder neck sphincter failure
Failure to empty	Areflexia Hypocontractility	Detrusor-sphincter dyssynergia (striated sphincter and bladder neck) Nonrelaxing voluntary sphincter Mechanical obstruction (benign prostatic hypertrophy or stricture)

cal condition. The upper tracts need evaluation if there are symptoms suggestive of pyelonephritis or prior history of renal disease. Some neurological conditions such as strokes, Parkinson's disease, and multiple sclerosis rarely or only occasionally cause upper tract involvement. For these conditions, a simple baseline screening test such as renal ultrasonography (US) is sufficient. Conditions such as those involving a complete spinal cord lesion and myelodysplasia need more extensive and regular upper tract surveillance with both structural and functional tests. The lower urinary tract evaluation can be quite simple, from urinalysis to urine culture to measurement of postvoid residual. A full urodynamic evaluation might be necessary, however, especially if incomplete bladder emptying, incontinence, recurrent bacteriuria, or upper tract changes are present.

The bladder findings on urodynamic studies cannot be used to determine the level of neurological lesion. For example, a suprasacral neurogenic bladder from a complete spinal cord injury can remain areflexic, and a conal or cauda equinal bladder can exhibit high pressures from poor compliance. The anatomical level of the neurological lesion can suggest to the clinician the commonest pattern of bladder dysfunction, but urodynamic testing should always be performed to confirm this.

Upper Tract Tests

Ultrasonography

Ultrasonography is a low-risk and relatively low-cost test for routine evaluation of the upper urinary tract. It is not sensitive enough for evaluating acute ureteral obstruction, and in this clinical setting non-contrast-enhanced computed tomography (CT) should be performed. US is adequate for imaging chronic obstruction and dilation, scarring, renal masses (both cystic and solid), and renal stones. The ureter is seen only if dilated. The bladder, if partially filled, can be evaluated for wall thickness, irregularity, and the presence of bladder stones.

Plain Radiography of the Urinary Tract—Kidneys, Ureter, and Bladder (KUB)

A KUB study is often combined with US to identify any possible radiopaque calculi in the ureter or bladder stones not seen on US.

Computed Tomography

CT is often performed without contrast agent enhancement and has replaced KUB, US, and excretory urography in the evaluation of the upper tracts when acute obstruction from stones is a possibility.

Excretory Urography or Intravenous Pyelography

The term excretory urography has replaced intravenous pyelography, as modern techniques show much more than the collecting system. Renal tomograms obtained 1 to 3 minutes after contrast agent injection should show a clear nephrogram. If the serum creatinine concentration is more than 1.5 mg/dL or if the patient has insulin-dependent diabetes, intravenous contrast agent administration increases the risk of contrast-related nephropathy. In these cases, alternative studies include US, radioisotope renography, and possibly cystoscopy with retrograde pyelography.

Creatinine Clearance Time

This has been the gold standard for assessing renal function and is said to approximate the glomerular filtration rate, but its accuracy depends on meticulous urine collection. In quadriplegic patients with low muscle mass and a 24-hour creatinine excretion of less than 1000 mg, the calculated creatinine clearance time can be too inaccurate to be clinically useful.

Isotope Studies

The technetium 99m DMSA (dimercaptosuccinic acid) scan is still the best study for both differential function and evaluation of the functioning areas of the renal cortex. The renogram obtained with ^{99m}Tc-MAG 3 (mertiatide) also gives information on urinary tract drainage, as well as a good assessment of differential function. In patients who might have ureteral reflux, these studies should be done with the bladder drained with an indwelling catheter.

Lower Tract Tests

Urinalysis, Culture and Sensitivity Testing

These tests are done routinely for all patients with neurogenic bladder disease and should be repeated as often as necessary. Bacteriuria should be treated before any invasive test is performed.

Postvoid Residual

By itself, a low postvoid residual (PVR) of less than 20% of capacity is not indicative of a "balanced" bladder as it was once defined. High intravesical pressures can be present in spite of low PVR values. The PVR is simple to determine and clinically useful, when compared with prior recordings and taken in conjunction with the bladder pressure, clinical symptoms, and the appearance of the bladder wall. A catheter insertion has been used for PVR in the past, but there are now simple US machines that can noninvasively obtain the PVR.[8]

Cystography

This study is usually performed to test for the presence or absence of ureteral reflux, and it also shows the bladder shape and outline. The procedure is usually performed in the radiology department, often with no control over the rate of bladder filling and without any monitoring of intravesical pressure. It is often helpful in planning management to know the level of intravesical pressure at which ureteral reflux occurred. Significant bacteriuria should be treated before the test is performed. Blood pressure should be monitored throughout the test in all patients with spinal cord lesions above T-6 who are at risk for autonomic dysreflexia. In many cases a full videourodynamic study, which includes fluoroscopy of the bladder and monitoring of the intravesical pressure, is more clinically useful. This study is described later.

Cystometrography

Cystometrography (CMG) is a filling study and gives little information about the voiding phase of bladder function. Although carbon dioxide as a filling medium is convenient with the commercially available apparatus, this type of testing has shown considerable variability, poor reproducibility, and the presence of artifacts due to leakage of CO_2 gas around the catheter. Hyperemia of the bladder mucosa has also been noted at cystoscopy immediately after CO_2 use. An advantage of the CO_2 CMG is that any size of catheter can be employed, as there is little resistance to flow and therefore no pressure artifact from the pump.

Water CMGs are best obtained with a two-channel catheter, with one channel used for filling and the other for pressure recording. A rectal pressure trace is also helpful in many patients to help distinguish intravesical pressure variations (due to intra-abdominal transmission) from contractions of the detrusor itself. Reported filling rates vary but are usually in the range of 25 to 60 mL/min. During filling, patients are asked to suppress voiding. Normal values include a capacity of 300 to 600 mL, with an initial sensation of filling at approximately 50% of capacity. The sensation of normal fullness is said to be appreciated in the lower abdomen with a sense of urgency in the perineum. The change in volume divided by the rise in baseline pressure during filling (i.e., in the absence of a detrusor contraction) describes the bladder's compliance. This value should be greater than 10 mL/cm H_2O, and 10 to 20 mL/cm is borderline if the bladder capacity is reduced. Normal persons are able to suppress detrusor contractions during this test. Any detrusor contraction during the test, usually defined as a phasic pressure change of more than 15 cm H_2O, is abnormal. If the patient is neurologically intact, these contractions are referred to as uninhibited. If the patient has a suprasacral or supraspinal lesion, these contractions are called hyperreflexic.[1]

Although patients can be instructed to try to void at capacity, many are unable to generate a detrusor contraction. The presence of an easily obtainable involuntary detrusor contraction confirms the presence of hyperreflexia in a patient with a suprasacral or supraspinal lesion. The absence of a contraction, however, does not necessarily imply true areflexia in a patient with an infrasacral lesion. The CO_2 CMG is a useful bedside test to monitor the return of a detrusor reflex in the spinal shock phase of spinal cord injury, and to confirm the presence of detrusor hyperreflexia in patients with supraspinal or cerebral insult before pharmacotherapy is started.

Sphincter Electromyography

Sphincter electromyography (EMG) can be combined with the CMG or preferably with a full multichannel videourodynamic study.[23] Recordings have been made with a variety of electrodes (monopolar, coaxial needle, and surface electrodes) from the levator, perianal, or periurethral muscles. Because some authors claim there is a functional dissociation between these muscle groups, periurethral recordings are preferred. The integrated EMG is displayed on the same trace as the bladder pressure. EMG activity gradually increases as bladder capacity is reached during bladder filling, and then becomes silent just prior to voiding. In complete spinal cord injury, low levels of EMG activity with no recruitment during filling are a common pattern. In these patients, however, as a reflex detrusor contraction occurs, EMG activity in the sphincter can increase rather than decrease. With this detrusor-sphincter dyssynergia, voiding often occurs toward the end of the detrusor contraction, as the striated sphincter relaxes more quickly than the smooth muscle of the bladder. This type of sphincter EMG does not display individual motor units and cannot be used for the evaluation of infrasacral denervation of the pelvic floor musculature (for which standard needle EMG is needed).

Videourodynamics

This study is designed to give the maximum information about the filling and voiding phases of lower urinary tract function, and every effort is made to make it as physiological as possible.[3] A videourodynamic study is indicated in the following patients: those with incomplete spinal cord lesions with incontinence who have some ability to void and inhibit voiding voluntarily but empty incompletely; persons with mechanical obstruction (e.g., benign prostatic hyperplasia) with neuropathy; candidates for sphincterotomy, to assess detrusor contraction and the presence or absence of bladder neck obstruction in addition to striated sphincter dyssynergia; those who fail to respond to pharmacotherapy; those who will undergo any surgical procedures such as augmentation, continent diversion, or placement of an artificial sphincter or a suprapubic catheter; patients who have deterioration of the upper tracts; and finally, patients who relapse frequently with symptomatic bacteriuria.

The procedure requires placement of a 7-F two-channel catheter in the bladder and an 8-F balloon catheter in the rectum. EMG of the sphincter is recorded along with bladder, rectal, and detrusor (bladder minus rectal) pressures. A contrast solution delivered at 50 mL/min is used to fill the bladder, with the patient sitting or lying as appropriate. The blood pressure is recorded in patients with spinal cord lesions above T6 to determine if there is any autonomic dysreflexia. The bladder image is monitored intermittently with fluoroscopy, and the combined radiographic and urodynamic image is mixed on the same screen and recorded on videotape (Fig. 27–5). If the patient can sit and void during the study, a flow rate can also be recorded. A videourodynamic study in children with myelodysplasia or spinal cord injury might have to be modified, and adequate clinical information can often be obtained by recording bladder pressure combined with fluoroscopy. Table 27–3 lists urodynamic terms used to categorize bladder and outlet abnormalities.

Cystoscopy

The only routine indication for cystoscopy is the presence of a long-term indwelling suprapubic or urethral catheter, as there can be a risk of bladder tumor development.[19] Cystoscopy is recommended after 5 years in high-risk patients, such as smokers, or after 10 years in those with no risk factors. Cystoscopy should also be

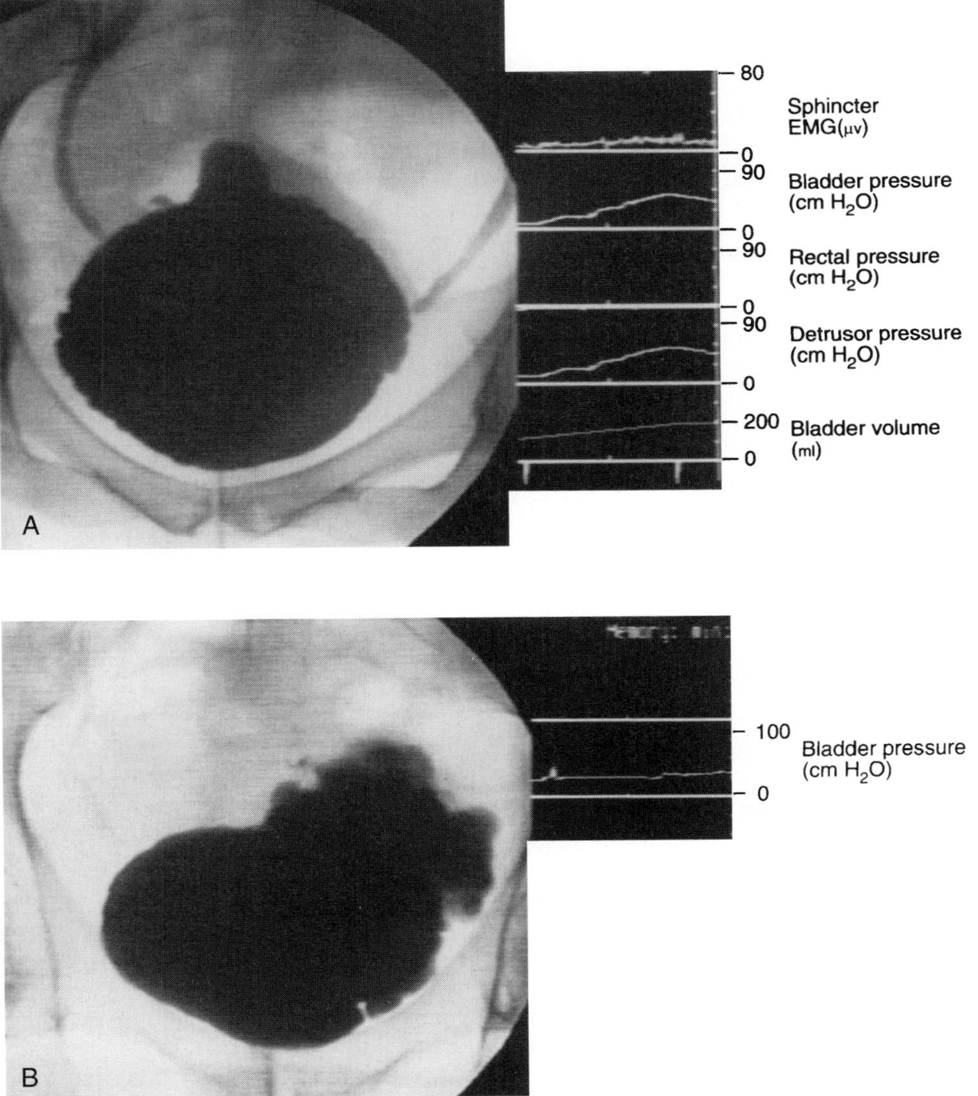

FIGURE 27–5. *A.* A videourodynamic study showing a hyperreflexic bladder in a woman with bilateral ureteral reflux. The detrusor pressure maximum is about 60 cm H_2O, and the rise in detrusor pressure is associated with a rise in sphincter EMG; the bladder neck stays closed. There are moderate bladder wall changes, with trabeculation and a small diverticulum. *B.* A videourodynamic study showing a very irregular, asymmetrical bladder that is very noncompliant. The baseline pressure has risen to just over 30 cm H_2O and the volume of contrast material in the bladder at that time is 150 mL. This gives a compliance of 5 mL per cm H_2O.

TABLE 27–3 Urodynamic Definitions

Bladder	
Hyperreflexia	Uninhibited contractions of the detrusor during filling due to neurological disease
Hypocontractility	Unsustained contractions causing failure to empty
Areflexia	Absent contractions with attempt to void
Compliance	Change in volume divided by change in baseline pressure with filling (<10 mL/cm H_2O abnormal; 10–20 mL/cm H_2O borderline if capacity reduced)
Outlet	
Detrusor-sphincter dyssynergia	
1. At bladder neck	Usually in high quadriplegic patients with autonomic hyperactivity
2. At striated sphincter	Uncoordinated pelvic floor and striated sphincter contraction with detrusor contraction during attempts to void
Nonrelaxing sphincter	Poor voluntary relaxation of voluntary sphincter in patients with areflexia attempting to void by Valsalva's maneuver
Decreased outlet resistance	Incontinence due to damage to the bladder neck or striated sphincter, pelvic floor descent, or denervation

performed after excretory urography in patients who have gross or microscopic hematuria that cannot be clearly associated with urinary tract infection (UTI), stones, or trauma. Bladder stones can usually be detected on plain radiographs or US, but persistent infection can be associated with gravel too small to be detected on imaging studies. Consequently, repeated lower tract infections can be an indication for cystoscopy.

Other Tests

Long-Term Monitoring

Monitoring over 12 to 24 hours of bladder and rectal pressures with sphincter EMG is now possible with solid-state microtip transducers and miniaturized digital recorders. The patients can go about their normal daily activities and cue in any symptoms, incontinence, or voiding episodes. Studies to date indicate that reduced compliance might not be as important in upper tract decompensation as is currently believed.[35]

Transrectal or Transvaginal Ultrasound

This imaging study can demonstrate the bladder base and posterior urethra continuously during urodynamic studies, without exposing the patient to ionizing radiation. However, the bladder wall and ureteral reflux cannot be evaluated, and the rectal transducer is large and uncomfortable for patients with perianal sensation.[29]

Urethral Pressure Profiles

Urethral pressure profiles are obtained by withdrawing a measuring device (microtip transducer or perfused side-hole catheter) gradually down the urethra and measuring the centrally oriented forces. It has limited value except in determining whether a sphincter-active area is still present after a sphincterotomy.

Urecholine (Bethanechol) Stimulation Test

The urecholine stimulation test is based on Cannon's law of denervation, which says that an end-organ becomes supersensitive to its neurotransmitter when denervated. In practice, the test is performed in patients with possible infrasacral lesions when the detrusor appears to be areflexic. A rise in baseline pressure of more than 20 cm H_2O on CMG at a volume of 100 mL is considered a positive result. Unfortunately, false positives and false negatives do occur, and the test is positive only in complete decentralization.

MANAGEMENT

General Principles

Bladder management must be undertaken in the context of the whole person. Patient goals are to empty the bladder not more than every 3 to 4 hours, remain continent, sleep without interference from the urinary drainage system, and avoid recurrent UTI or other complications. Less than optimal bladder management decreases the person's social, vocational, and avocational potential. The following discussion describes specific management approaches (Table 27–4).

Approaches and Rationale

Behavioral Management

Timed Voiding

For patients with hyperreflexia producing urgency or reflex incontinence, a timed voiding program can help by having the patient urinate before the anticipated detrusor contraction. The limitation to this program is that persons with dementia need continual reminding. It is also useful in patients with sphincter weakness, as the incontinence is worse when the bladder is full, and timed voiding reduces the amount of urine leakage.

Bladder Stimulation

Various maneuvers have been tried to stimulate the bladder. Stroking or pinching the perineal skin, which is intended to cause reflex stimulation, is rarely effective. Suprapubic tapping or jabbing over the bladder causes a mechanical stretch of the bladder wall and subsequent contraction. Controlled studies have shown that deeper indentation of the bladder with a jabbing technique is the most effective maneuver.[9] This can be used by spinal cord–injured patients with condom catheters. It is most effective in patients with paraplegia who have good upper extremity function.

TABLE 27–4 Bladder Management Options

Failure to Store	
Bladder factors	
Behavioral	Timed voids
Collecting devices	Diaper, condom catheter, indwelling catheter
CIC	With drugs to lower bladder pressure
Drugs	Anticholinergics, musculotropics, intrathecal baclofen,* calcium channel blockers,* intravesical capsaicin*
Surgery	Augmentation, continent diversion, denervation procedures*
Outlet factors	
Behavioral	Timed voids, pelvic floor exercises
Collecting devices	Diaper, condom catheter, indwelling catheter
Drugs	α-Agonists, imipramine, estrogens
Surgery	Collagen injection, fascial sling, artificial sphincter, Teflon injection*
Failure to Empty	
Bladder factors	
Behavioral	Timed voids, bladder stimulation, Valsalva's and Credé's maneuvers
Collecting devices	Indwelling catheter
CIC	
Drugs	Bethanechol
Surgery	Neurostimulation*
Outlet factors	
Behavioral	Anal stretch void
Collecting devices	Indwelling catheters
CIC	
Drugs	α-Blockers, oral striated muscle relaxant, intrathecal baclofen*
Surgery	Sphincterotomy incision, bladder neck incision, prostate resection, pudendal neurectomy,* stent sphincterotomy*
Failure of Storage and Emptying with Nonusable Urethra	
Surgery	Suprapubic catheter ± bladder neck closure, ileal conduit, continent diversion

Abbreviation: CIC, clean intermittent catheterization.
* Experimental or nonstandard management.

Valsalva's and Credé's Maneuvers

Patients with areflexia and some denervation of the pelvic floor (infrasacral lesions) are able to void by effecting a Valsalva maneuver or straining. This is most effective in women because the paralyzed pelvic floor descends with straining and the bladder neck opens. Over time, however, the pelvic floor descent increases as the paralyzed muscles atrophy and stretch, and the patient complains of worsening stress incontinence. Credé's maneuver, usually performed by an attendant, mechanically pushes urine out of the bladder in patients with quadriplegia. The abdominal wall must be relaxed to allow Credé's maneuver to be effective, and there is a theoretical risk of producing ureteral reflux by the long-term use of this method.

Anal Stretch Voiding

In patients with paraplegia who have a spastic pelvic floor, effective voiding has been achieved by an anal stretch technique. This technique involves relaxing the pelvic floor by first stretching the anal sphincter and then evacuating by Valsalva's maneuver.[20] It requires transfer onto a toilet for bladder emptying, absence of anal sensation, and the ability to generate adequate intra-abdominal pressure. For these reasons it is not widely used, even though the technique was well described more than 20 years ago.

Pelvic Floor Exercises

Pelvic floor exercises are effective only in female patients with stress incontinence due to pelvic floor descent. Most patients with infrasacral neuropathy need surgery to achieve continence.

Urine Collection Devices

External Condom Catheters

External condom catheters are convenient and often the best management for men with tetraplegia who are unable to perform self-catheterization, provided that any outflow obstruction is adequately treated. Although attendants and family members can perform intermittent catheterization, the program often breaks down if the patient is at school or work. Bacteriuria with fever is more common in those who have intermittent catheterization done by an attendant than in those on any other bladder management program, including indwelling catheterization.[10] Problems with skin breakdown and urethral damage can occur if the condom is applied too tightly. There is also an increased risk of UTI because of poor hygiene. The risk is increased in patients who have to do intermittent catheterization because of inadequate emptying and who also need a condom catheter for incontinence.

Indwelling Catheters

Indwelling catheters can be either urethral or suprapubic, and are typically used because other programs have failed or for patient convenience. The combination of sphincterotomy and condom drainage, although ideal for men with tetraplegia, often fails because of inadequate detrusor contractions or penile skin problems. In the past, indwelling catheters had a justifiably bad reputation, but there are recent reports that some patients with indwelling catheters do no worse than those on other methods of management.[12] This change is due to a number of factors, including improved catheter materials. Good catheter care is still very important. Some of the important aspects of care include monthly catheter changes, copious fluid intake, control of hyperreflexia with medication, sterilization of the collecting bags with bleach, and avoidance of traction on the catheter. The prevalence of squamous cell carcinoma of the bladder associated with an indwelling catheter might be lower than reported.[19] Most centers continue to recommend yearly cystoscopy, cytology, and biopsy, if indicated, when the patient has had an indwelling catheter in place for 10 years or more, and possibly after only 5 years if there are increased risk factors such as smoking.

Adult Diapers and Other Protective Garments

Protective garments have improved considerably over the past few years, and a high-absorbency gel-impregnated material is now used that allows the lining against the patient's perineal skin to stay dry. Protective garments are commonly used in incontinent demented patients who have adequate bladder emptying.

Clean Intermittent Catheterization

Intermittent catheterization using a sterile technique was introduced by Guttmann and Frankel in the 1950s for the management of patients with acute spinal cord injury. Lapides et al in 1972 proposed a nonsterile but "clean" technique for the management of chronic retention and infection.[21] The technique has since been employed extensively for neurogenic bladder disease. An intermittent catheter program requires a low-pressure bladder of adequate capacity (>300 mL) and enough outflow resistance to maintain continence with normal daily activities. If the bladder is not sufficiently areflexic and compliant, anticholinergics or musculotropics can be used. If these fail, some form of surgery, such as augmentation, can be done to achieve a low-pressure reservoir. Men with lesions at C6 and below and women with lesions at C7 and below can manage self-catheterization. Patients should restrict fluid intake to maintain an output of not more than 600 mL in the time period chosen. Some patients have enough sensation to be able to catheterize on demand, but most have to do so on a timed schedule. A minimum of three catheterizations per 24 hours is recommended, since longer intervals between catheterizations theoretically increases the risk of symptomatic bacteriuria. Most patients wash their catheters with soap and water. If recurrent bacteriuria becomes a problem, sterilization by soaking in Cidex (a glutaral preparation) or boiling the catheters is recommended. Rarely, a completely sterile technique is used.

The most common problems with self-catheterization are symptomatic bacteriuria, urethral trauma, and incontinence. Occasionally a bladder stone formed on a nidus of hair or lint is found, and patients should be warned to avoid introducing foreign material into the bladder with the catheter. Urethral trauma and catheterization difficulties are usually due to sphincter spasm. This can be managed by using extra lubrication and local anesthetic urethral gel (lidocaine 2%). Sometimes a curved-tip (coudé) catheter is helpful. Repeated urethral bleeding suggests the presence of a break in the urethral mucosa or a false passage, and using an indwelling urethral catheter for a period of time might be necessary for this to resolve. Urethroscopy and unroofing of a false passage is occasionally necessary.

Drugs

Many drugs for lower urinary tract management have been tried, with the rationale for their use often based on animal and organ bath experiments. Bladder management drugs in humans have generally been disappointing. The most effective group are those that inhibit detrusor activity.

Cholinergic Agents

The detrusor is innervated by cholinergic muscularinic (M_2 and M_3) receptors. Bethanechol, a cholinergic agonist, can be helpful in detrusor areflexia by increasing detrusor activity. Although a pharmacological effect can be seen with a parenteral dose when the bladder is partially innervated, oral doses are not effective at levels that can be tolerated by patients. Double-blind, controlled clinical trials have not been performed, and the use of this drug has declined.[14]

Anticholinergic Agents

Anticholinergic agents have been used for many years for suppression of detrusor activity. Propantheline bromide (15 to 30 mg three times a day) is the prototype, and hyoscyamine (0.125 to 0.25 mg three or four times a day) is regaining popularity. Oxybutynin hydrochloride, a more recent preparation, when taken at 5 to 10 mg three times a day has similar actions, but it is effective mostly on the muscle cell membrane (musculotropic) rather than on anticholinergic endings. Oxybutynin in solution can be administered as an intravesical instillation in patients on intermittent catheterization. It appears to be effective, although somewhat delayed serum levels result that are almost as high as with the oral route. Side effects appear to be less than when the drug is given by the oral route.[22] A problem with this technique is that, at present, there is no sterile liquid form, and the 5-mg tablet has to be dissolved in sterile water. Imipramine is recommended by several authors for its presumed anticholinergic actions. It is said to be additive in its effectiveness, but not in its side effects, when combined with other agents such as oxybutynin and propantheline. A new agent, tolterodine, in a dose of 2 mgs twice daily has anticholinergic activity and fewer troublesome side effects from dry mouth and constipation.

Calcium Channel Blockers

Pure calcium channel blockers, although promising in experimental preparations, do not seem to be effective inhibitors of detrusor activity in humans. Terodiline was effective and was available in Europe until recently, but it was withdrawn from the market because of its association with cardiac arrhythmias.

Adrenergic Antagonists

The α-adrenergic receptor antagonist phenoxybenzamine (10 to 30 mg/day) has α_1- and α_2-blocking actions and has been used for inhibiting smooth muscle activity at the bladder neck and in the prostate. Newer agents with more specific α_1-blocking actions are available, such as prazosin, terazosin, and doxazosin. These are typically given in doses of 1 to 20 mg/day as tolerated. These agents have a number of effects: they appear to reduce the irritative symptoms in men with obstruction due to benign prostatic hyperplasia and to increase emptying in patients with neurogenic voiding dysfunction. Beneficial effects have also been reported, including increasing compliance secondary to decentralization. A new, more specific agent, tamsulosin, has been introduced for the treatment of benign prostatic hyperplasia. This agent has fewer vascular effects and rarely causes hypotension. Its effects on the neurogenic bladder have not yet been reported. These agents are effective in control of the vascular manifestations of autonomic dysreflexia, and phenoxybenzamine, with its α_1- and α_2-blocking action, might be better in this regard than the pure α_1-blocking agents.

Adrenergic Agonists

Adrenergic agonists have been used to increase urethral resistance in patients with mild stress incontinence. Anecdotally, ephedrine (25 to 75 mg/day) has been effective in children with myelodysplasia, but controlled studies are lacking, and adrenergic agonists are rarely used in adults with bladder neuropathy. The α-agonists and antagonists seem to have little effect on normal or neuropathic bladder function in humans.

Estrogens

Postmenopausal women often have atrophy of the urethral submucosa, which can lead to stress incontinence. Estrogen administration often restores or maintains this tissue and can be helpful in women with a partially denervated pelvic floor and stress incontinence.

Muscle Relaxants

Diazepam, dantrolene sodium, and baclofen are frequently used for skeletal muscle spasticity (see Chapter 29) but have never been shown to be effective in controlled studies in patients with detrusor striated sphincter dyssynergia. Baclofen given intrathecally by infusion pump for severe lower extremity spasticity depresses pelvic floor reflexes but also depresses the detrusor reflex.[32] This net result is a lower-pressure bladder that might empty less effectively. Insofar as intrathecal baclofen is indicated in some patients with tetraplegia, this overall decrease in bladder emptying might not be desirable.

Surgery on the Bladder or Bladder Nerves

To Increase Bladder Capacity

Bowel Procedures

Augmentation. Bladder augmentation is often recommended for patients who have detrusor hyperreflexia or reduced compliance that fails to respond to anticholinergic or musculotropic drugs.[30] The patient must be motivated to continue indefinitely with clean intermittent catheterization and must have adequate outflow resistance. The patient must be fully informed of the immediate surgical risks and the possible long-term sequelae of this procedure. Immediate surgical risks include prolonged intestinal ileus or obstruction, anastomotic leak with peritonitis, wound infection, and pulmonary complications such as pneumonia, deep venous thrombosis, and pulmonary emboli. All the long-term sequelae are unknown, because bladder augmentation procedures have been performed for only about 20 years. The known sequelae include chronic bacteriuria, a theoretical risk of neoplastic change, possible diarrhea or malabsorption from a shortened gut or decreased intestinal transit time, and hyperchloremic acidosis due to absorption of urine with secondary mobilization of skeletal calcium (acting as a buffer).

The bladder is opened widely in this procedure, and an opened and reconfigured segment of bowel is sewn in. A 20- to 30-cm segment of distal ileum is usually used, but an ileocecal segment, sigmoid, or even a wedge of stomach can be employed (Fig. 27–6). The procedure is intended to result in a 600-mL-capacity, low-pressure reservoir without the use of any drugs. Mucus production is the main day-to-day problem initially, especially in those with active urinary infection. With good intermittent catheterization technique and the use of bladder irrigations as necessary, this is rarely a problem after the first 3 months. Because the risk of neoplastic change is unknown with this procedure, yearly cystoscopy should probably begin 10 to 15 years after the augmentation.

Continent Diversion. In this procedure, bowel is used not just to increase effective bladder capacity but also to form a continent catheterizable channel that opens onto the abdominal wall. It is particularly useful in women for whom intermittent self-catheterization via the urethra is difficult or impossible because of leg spasticity, body habitus, severe urethral incontinence, or the need to transfer from a wheelchair. Men who are unable to perform intermittent catheterization because of strictures, false passages, or fistulas are also potential candidates. However, severe urethral disease in men is typically due to poor personal care, and it is inappropriate to perform these procedures on patients who cannot or will not follow through with appropriate techniques. If the patient fails to catheterize after augmentation and continent diversion, the bowel segment can rupture internally before overflow incontinence occurs through the urethra or catheterizable channel.

The procedure involves enlarging the bladder and constructing some form of continent catheterizable channel. The terminal ileum and the ileocecal valve work well, but intussuscepted small bowel, the appendix, and a defunctioned segment of ureter have all been used. The bladder neck might require closure if there is sphincter-related incontinence.

Denervation Procedures. The denervation technique for bladder hyperreflexia, although theoretically attractive, is not widely used. Operative approaches include sectioning of the sacral nerve roots or interrupting the peripheral nerve supply near the bladder. Selective sacral rhizotomies have been attempted. The technique involves identifying the nerve root (usually S3 on one side) that carries the detrusor reflex by doing differential sacral local anesthetic blocks while monitoring the detrusor reflex by CMG. Surgical or chemical destruction of S3 usually results in temporary areflexia. Over time

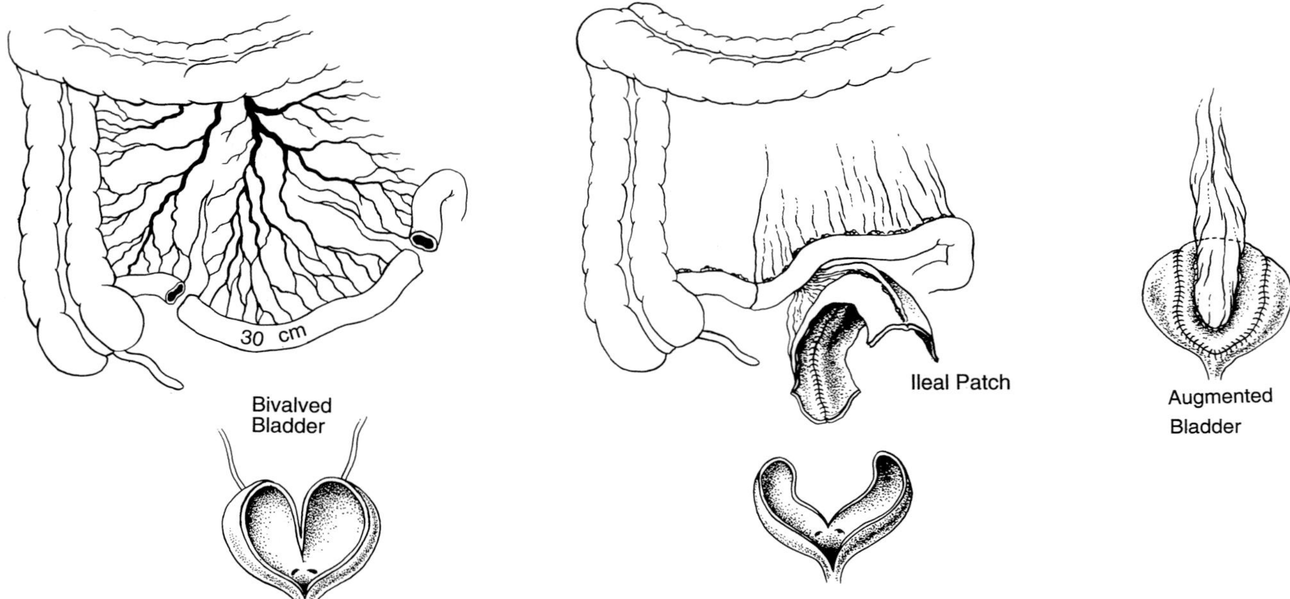

FIGURE 27–6. Augmentation cystoplasty. A 30-cm segment of small bowel is opened and reconstructed as a U-shaped patch and then sewn into the bivalved bladder.

the detrusor reflex typically reroutes through the intact sacral nerves. Bilateral S2, S3, and S4 rhizotomies permanently abolish the reflex, but at the expense of loss of reflex erections and worsening of the bowel evacuation problem.[15]

Peripheral denervation of the detrusor has been attempted by transecting the detrusor above the trigone and resuturing it, or by removing the paravesical ganglia via a vaginal approach, or by overdistending the bladder with the intent of damaging the intramural nerves and muscle fibers. In fact, in one clinical study, in patients with complete paraplegia, the bladder was intentionally distended in the spinal shock phase with the intent of preventing the return of the bladder reflex. The prevalence of areflexia in the short term following distention was 63%, compared with an expected 15%.[18] None of these peripheral denervation procedures have become commonly accepted, and long-term results of intentional overdistention of the bladder in spinal shock have not yet been reported. The neurotoxic agent capsaicin is being tried experimentally in hyperreflexia for its effects on the C-afferent fibers, which are implicated in its pathogenesis. Encouraging short-term results are reported with intravesical instillation in selected patients.

To Increase Bladder Contraction

Electrical Stimulation. Attempts have been made to stimulate detrusor contraction using electrodes driven by an implanted receiver conveying a stimulus generated by an external transmitter. The electrodes have been implanted on the bladder wall, pelvic nerves, sacral roots, and conus. At present, the only site being used clinically is the sacral roots, and most of the reported series come from Europe.[6] The electrodes are placed on the anterior roots either intradurally or extradurally. To prevent spontaneous hyperreflexic contractions and antidromic reflex contractions, bilateral S2, S3, and S4 dorsal rhizotomies are usually performed. Pelvic floor contraction with anterior root stimulation will still obstruct voiding, and European centers have elected to stimulate intermittently. This leads to intermittent voiding, as the striated pelvic floor muscle relaxes more quickly than the smooth muscle detrusor. In the center developing this device in the United States, pudendal neurectomies are performed to decrease outflow resistance.[34] Adequate bladder emptying at acceptable intravesical pressures with preservation of the bladder wall as well as upper tract morphology and function has been reported.[6] One important disadvantage of bilateral S2, S3, and S4 rhizotomies is that reflex erections are abolished; usable erections occurring as a result of sacral root stimulation occur in less than 30% of patients. Bowel evacuation, however, is improved in many patients. Further refinements such as supraselective rhizotomies, with modification of stimulus parameters and electrode design, are future possibilities. This technique has just been approved for routine clinical use in the United States.

Surgery on the Bladder Outlet

To Increase Outlet Resistance

Incontinence due to decreased outlet resistance is relatively uncommon in bladder dysfunction secondary to neurological disease. It is seen in children with myelodysplasia and in women with infrasacral lesions and a denervated pelvic floor. It can occur in active men with complete denervation, but this is rare. Although α-adrenergic agonists might help minor incontinence, more severe leakage typically requires some form of urethral compressive procedure. The options include injection therapy into the bladder neck and urethra to increase the bulk of tissue under and around the bladder neck muscle, a fascial sling, or an artificial sphincter. Electrical stimulation of pelvic floor muscles or nerves, or muscles and nerves, via rectal, vaginal, or implanted electrodes has been tried but has not been effective enough to achieve widespread popularity.

Injection Therapy. Teflon has been used for years in the urethra for certain types of stress incontinence, but its use has recently declined because of the danger of particle migration. Autologous fat and bovine collagen have been tried recently, and one to three injections seem to help some proportion of patients. The procedure has few potential side effects and is especially suitable for elderly and poor-risk patients.

External Compressive Procedures. In the fascial sling procedure, a 2-cm strip of fascia is taken from the anterior rectus abdominis fascia or tensor fascia lata. It is wrapped around the bladder neck and fixed anteriorly to the abdominal fascia or pubic tubercle. Patients who are candidates for this procedure must have compliant low-pressure bladders. They will be unable to void by Valsalva's maneuver after a successful sling procedure and must be willing to perform self-catheterization indefinitely in exchange for being continent.

The artificial urinary sphincter consists of a cuff, a pressure-regulating balloon, and a control pump. The cuff is usually implanted around the bladder neck in both sexes and less commonly around the bulbar urethra in men. The pump in the labia or scrotum allows the patient to open the cuff for voiding. Reinflation of the cuff is automatic and takes about 3 to 5 minutes. Mechanical failure, cuff erosion, and infection can occur with this device. Patients can use Valsalva's maneuver to void and do not have to be on self-catheterization. In patients with myelodysplasia, although the detrusor is naturally areflexic or can be rendered so by drugs, uncontrolled hyperreflexia occurs in 10% in the first year after implantation of an artificial sphincter. This probably results from activation of dormant urethrovesical reflexes. Careful follow-up is essential, and if hyperreflexia occurs, an augmentation procedure can be done secondarily.

To Decrease Outlet Resistance

Sphincterotomy. In male spinal cord–injured patients unable or unwilling to do self-catheterization, the use of a condom catheter is a practical alternative. As it is unusual to find a lower urinary tract that has adequate detrusor contraction and a coordinated pelvic floor in these patients, some procedure to decrease outflow resistance is usually indicated. The results are poor in patients without adequate detrusor contractions. Preoperative parameters suggested for a good outcome are low volume (<200 mL), spontaneous contraction with a quick rise time (<20 seconds), adequate amplitude (>50 cm H_2O), and an adequate duration of approximately 2 minutes or more. Ablation of the striated sphincter, usually by incision, is the standard procedure. It is now performed anteriorly to avoid the cavernous artery and nerve, which lie lateral to the membranous urethra (which, if damaged, can lead to impotence). Some patients also have bladder neck obstruction either because of primary hyperactivity (e.g., high quadriplegic patients) or because of total bladder wall hypertrophy (which follows striated sphincter dyssynergia). They need bladder neck ablation either by resection or by incision. In older men, prostatic obstruction from benign disease can also contribute to increased outflow resistance and might require prostatic resection. The immediate morbidity from sphincterotomy—bleeding, clot retention, and infection—is relatively high. The long-term results are compromised because of recurrent obstruction from stricture or recurrent dyssynergia. An implantable stainless steel stent is undergoing trial currently and should reduce morbidity and improve long-term results. This stent material is inert, and the epithelium grows through the spaces between the wires of the stent, completely covering them.[25]

Other Methods of Decreasing Outflow Resistance. Intrathecal baclofen given for severe spasticity decreases the pudendal reflexes, but the detrusor reflex and contractions are reduced as well. Consequently it cannot be used as a chemical sphincterotomy. Botulinum toxin injected into the striated sphincter has also been used experimentally, but its effects last only a few months.[13]

Urinary Diversion

The use of any urinary diversion procedure should be restricted to patients with severe urethral problems such as stricture, fistula, periurethral abscess, and intractable incontinence with perineal skin breakdown. The simplest method is to insert a suprapubic catheter and close the bladder neck. If the bladder cannot be preserved because of malignant disease, contracture, or ureteral reflux, a standard bowel conduit is recommended with removal of the bladder in most cases. Usually a 10- to 15-cm segment of small bowel is used. Because a nonrefluxing ureterointestinal anastomosis is desired, the ileocecal segment or sigmoid colon is preferred.

MANAGEMENT OF SPECIFIC DISEASES

Diseases of the Brain

Stroke

After an initial period of areflexia, stroke patients typically have hyperreflexia with frequency and urge incontinence but coordinated voiding and complete emptying (see Chapter 50). Anticholinergics and musculotropics frequently help ameliorate symptoms without adversely affecting emptying. Persistent areflexia and retention can occur with bilateral lesions. Retention in the elderly can occur due to prostatic obstruction. Videourodynamic studies are helpful in differentiating these conditions.

Parkinson's Disease

The prevalence of bladder symptoms in this disease is high (70%) (see Chapter 51). Most have frequency, urgency, and urge incontinence, and 50% complain of difficulty voiding. Evaluation shows hyperreflexia, but the contractions are poorly sustained and result in incomplete emptying. Failure to empty can also be due to bradykinesia secondary to failure of pelvic floor relaxation, the adrenergic effects of levodopa, or the anticholinergic effects of other antiparkinsonian drugs.[2] Treatment is difficult because there is frequently a combination of incontinence and retention. Detrusor inhibition with drugs makes emptying worse, and α-adrenergic blockers have a marginal effect in decreasing outflow resistance.[33] Intermittent catheterization and detrusor inhibition is often the best choice, but many patients do not have sufficient upper extremity dexterity to do this independently.

Dementia, Brain Tumors, and Trauma

Dementia, brain tumors, and trauma can all cause hyperreflexia with reflex or urge incontinence with complete emptying. If cognitive impairment is severe, incontinence often persists in spite of detrusor inhibition. Some type of collecting device is appropriate for many of these patients (see Chapter 49).

Diseases of the Brain and Spinal Cord

Multiple sclerosis is the commonest disease in this category, with 90% of patients developing urinary manifestations in the course of the disease (see Chapter 52). The bladder symptoms usually present because of an incomplete spinal cord lesion with hyperreflexia and hypocontractility. In this situation, detrusor inhibition with drugs worsens emptying. In the rare, predominantly encephalopathic variety, these agents might be useful. Patients with multiple sclerosis and with a predominantly conal lesion have bladder areflexia. Intermittent catheterization is eventually indicated in most patients with multiple sclerosis, but few are able to undertake it because of poor upper extremity strength and coordination. High-pressure bladders due to hyperreflexia and detrusor-sphincter dyssynergia are rare, but sphincterotomy in men is sometimes indicated.[24]

Diseases of the Spinal Cord

Injury, tumors, and vascular lesions of the spinal cord cause the majority of suprasacral neurogenic bladder problems (see Chapter 55). After a varying period of spinal shock, the detrusor reflex typically returns. With complete lesions, the center for this reflex develops in the sacral cord. Inhibitory control by the higher center is impaired, and because the long-routed detrusor reflex is interrupted, the detrusor contraction might not be completely sustained. Coordination and control of the pelvic floor are also impaired, leading to lack of voluntary contraction and relaxation. In complete lesions, this often causes discoordinated activity during voiding. This discoordination or detrusor-sphincter dyssynergia affects the striated voluntary sphincter, but in high complete quadriplegic patients excessive sympathetic activity can lead to detrusor-bladder neck dyssynergia as well. Incomplete lesions can produce the supraspinal pattern with urgency and adequate emptying, while patients with complete lesions have reflex incontinence and incomplete emptying due to detrusor-sphincter dyssynergia (in most cases). Some patients have hypocontractility or areflexia and retention. A truly balanced bladder with sustained detrusor contraction and coordinated pelvic floor is uncommon.

The onset and severity of the symptoms vary with the cause of spinal cord dysfunction, but the management discussed here is in relation to spinal cord injury. An indwelling catheter is typically maintained until the patient's medical state is stable and fluid intake can be regulated to achieve a urine output of 1500 to 2000 mL/day. Intermittent sterile catheterization is then started, if possible, by a dedicated catheterization team. The patient should learn self-catheterization when able to do so. A sterile technique is ideal in the hospital, but a clean technique can be used when the patient is discharged home. Maximum allowable bladder volume is 600 mL. In some of these patients, however, retention of interstitial fluid in the lower limbs when the patient is upright, with subsequent mobilization and dumping at night, is frequently a problem. The use of antiembolism stockings such as TED hose, recumbency early in the evening, and an extra catheterization in the middle of the night might all be necessary to manage this.

In the majority of spinal cord–injured patients, the detrusor reflex returns usually within the first 6 months. Its return is often indicated by episodes of incontinence, but the presence of the detrusor reflex should be confirmed by CMG. Anticholinergics and musculotropics can be given to suppress the reflex and allow intermittent catheterization to continue. Patients with lesions at the level of C7 and below, who are able to do self-catheterization, can continue this in the long term. If the detrusor reflex cannot be suppressed, the patient should consider augmentation, which remains the standard method today for achieving a low-pressure reservoir if medications fail.

In male patients unable or unwilling to do self-catheterization, and for those who refuse augmentation, sphincterotomy followed by use of an external catheter is probably the best alternative. Other options include intermittent catheterization by an attendant, although this has a greater risk of febrile UTIs.[10] Wearing an external collector can be done also, but only 15% of men with spinal cord injury have a suitable, truly "balanced" bladder with coordinated voiding at low pressure. Some men with quadriplegia end up with an indwelling catheter because of sphincterotomy failure, or inadequate detrusor contractions, or skin breakdown on the penile shaft. Women using intermittent catheterization might be unable to control urinary incontinence with medications and can choose to use an indwelling catheter. A regular long-term urinary tract surveillance program (Table 27–5) should be set up for spinal cord–injured patients who might, with good care, have a near normal life expectancy.

TABLE 27–5 Routine Urinary Tract Surveillance After Spinal Cord Injury

I. Initial rehabilitation admission.
   Urinalysis, initial and as needed.
   Urine culture and sensitivity, weekly.
   Renal and bladder ultrasound if on IC or condom catheter. Add KUB in patients with a Foley catheter.
   IVP only if US is abnormal.
   PVR.
   CMG or urodynamics (usually no cystogram at this point).
   CrCl, 24-hr urine.
II. Routine evaluations (yearly for the first 5 years and, if stable, every other year thereafter).
   Renal US and KUB for all annual evaluations.
   IVP or CT only if indicated by clinical status or US findings.
   Urodynamics determined on individual basis (often needed annually for the first few years).
   CrCl, 24-hr urine, annually.
   PVR (by portable US or catheter) annually unless indwelling catheter is in place.
   Other tests of renal function as needed.
III. Cystoscopy.
   Generally performed in patients after 10 years of chronic, continuous indwelling catheterizations (urethral or suprapubic), or earlier (at 5 years) if at high risk (heavy smoker, age > 40 years, or history of complicated UTIs) or in any patient with symptoms that warrant such a procedure.

Abbreviations: IVP, intravenous pyelography; SCI, spinal cord injury; CMG, cystometrography; PVR, postvoid residuals; US, ultrasound; CrCl, creatine clearance; KUB, kidneys, ureters, and bladder, plain film study; CUG, cystourethrogram; UTIs, urinary tract infections; IC, intermittent catheterization.

Diseases of the Conus, Cauda Equina, and Peripheral Nerves

Trauma, disk disease, lumbar stenosis, arachnoiditis, and tumors are some of the mechanical lesions that can affect this region of the spinal canal. The resulting bladder is typically areflexic or noncontractile and insensate. Pelvic floor innervation is frequently affected in conal lesions, which can lead to incontinence, especially in females. In cauda equinal lesions, the nonmyelinated pelvic nerve roots are more easily damaged and pelvic floor innervation is usually relatively more intact than the detrusor nerve supply. Autonomic neuropathy is most common secondary to diabetes, although at times it is the result of alcohol abuse. The detrusor afferents are affected first, with reduction of bladder sensation. Detrusor efferents are involved later. Because of lack of sensation, overstretching contributes to the end result, which is a noncontractile and insensate bladder.

Intermittent catheterization is the initial treatment in all cases. If the pelvic floor is severely paralyzed, patients might be able to void by straining. Men can be helped by α-adrenergic blocking agents to decrease outflow resistance. Women can often empty by straining, but tend to develop severe stress incontinence. These patients' can be candidates for a fascial sling or artificial sphincter. Reduced bladder compliance, usually found in patients after radical pelvic surgery, does not respond well to medications. In these cases an augmentation might be indicated, particularly if the outflow resistance is high and the upper tracts begin to dilate. Patients with diabetes can often maintain bladder function and contractility and avoid overdistention by timed voidings.

Diseases of the Spinal Cord and Conus

Myelodysplasia is the most common disease producing a mixed pattern of bladder dysfunction. Any combination of detrusor and sphincter activity can be found, but it is most common to have a hyperreflexic or noncompliant bladder, or both, with dyssynergia or a nonrelaxing sphincter.

Intermittent catheterization is used initially along with medication in infancy and childhood. In many cases, reconstructive surgery is necessary early if more conservative measures fail.

MANAGEMENT OF COMPLICATIONS

Bacteriuria

About one half of all hospital-acquired infections originate in the urinary tract in association with urinary catheters and other drainage devices. In patients with neurogenic bladders, UTIs are a common source of morbidity. Frequent exposure to antibiotics increases the risk of infection with antibiotic-resistant organisms, which further complicates the treatment of UTI. The diagnosis of UTI can be delayed or missed in patients with neurological disorders affecting bladder sensation. In patients with spinal cord disorders, signs and symptoms suggestive of UTI include fever, onset of urinary incontinence, increased spasticity, autonomic dysreflexia, increased sweating, cloudy and odorous urine, malaise, lethargy, or sense of unease.[27] Unexplained signs and symptoms suggestive of UTI in the presence of pyuria warrant empirical therapy for UTI. Absence of pyuria makes the diagnosis of UTI unlikely but does not exclude it.

Asymptomatic bacteriuria is very common in patients with neurogenic bladder, especially those using intermittent or indwelling catheterization. Most authorities recommend against routine treatment of asymptomatic bacteriuria. However, the presence of significant bacteriuria with urease-producing organisms that are associated with stone formation might warrant treatment.[28]

The spectrum of uropathogens causing catheter-associated UTI is much broader than that causing uncomplicated UTI. *Escherichia coli* causes the majority of uncomplicated UTIs. *E. coli* and organisms such as species of *Proteus, Klebsiella, Pseudomonas, Serratia, Providencia,* enterococci, and staphylococci are relatively more common in patients with catheter-associated UTI.[27] Polymicrobic bacteriuria is the rule in patients with indwelling catheters.

Patients with mild to moderate illness can be treated with an oral fluoroquinolone such as ciprofloxacin, norfloxacin, or ofloxacin. This group of antibiotics provides coverage for most expected pathogens, including *Pseudomonas aeruginosa.* Trimethoprim-sulfamethoxazole is another commonly used antibiotic for less ill patients, but it does not provide coverage against *P. aeruginosa.* It is less expensive than the fluoroquinolones and can be used empirically and continued according to the results of susceptibility testing. Amoxicillin, nitrofurantoin, and sulfa drugs are poor choices for empirical therapy because of the high prevalence of resistance to these agents among uropathogens typically involved in complicated UTIs.

In more seriously ill, hospitalized patients, ampicillin plus gentamicin or imipenem plus cilastatin provides coverage against most expected pathogens, including *P. aeruginosa* and most enterococci.[7] A number of other parenteral antimicrobial agents can also be used. Patients can be switched to oral treatment after clinical improvement. At least 7 to 14 days of therapy is generally recommended, depending on the severity of the infection.[28] There is no convincing evidence that regimens longer than this are beneficial. Patients undergoing effective treatment for UTI with an antibiotic to which the infecting pathogen is susceptible, should have definite improvement within 24 to 48 hours. If not, a repeat urine culture and imaging studies (US or CT) are indicated.

In a patient who has had UTI with high fever or hemodynamic changes suggestive of sepsis, or who is having recurrent symptomatic UTIs, an excretory urogram, cystogram, or urodynamic evaluation might be indicated after successful treatment to look for correctable anatomical or functional abnormalities.

Autonomic Dysreflexia

Paroxysmal hypertension, sweating, piloerection, headache, and reflex bradycardia are brought on by increased stimulation into and sympathetic output from the isolated spinal cord below a complete lesion. Injuries below T6 are rarely associated with this problem. Afferent stimulation frequently arises in the bladder, and the best treatment is prevention by avoiding overdistention. If symptoms persist when the bladder has been emptied or if the blood pressure is at a dangerously high level, 10 mg of sublingual nifedipine, a calcium channel blocking agent, can be given and repeated if necessary for a total of three doses. Long-term management with phenoxybenzamine (10 to 30 mg/day) has been used to prevent autonomic dysreflexia when all findable causes have been eliminated (see Chapter 55 for further explanation of the treatment of autonomic dysreflexia).

Hypercalciuria and Stones

Loss of calcium from the bones occurs in all spinal cord–injured patients and is worse in young males. Increased urinary calcium (>200 mg/24 hours) begins about 4 weeks after injury, reaches a maximum at 16 weeks, and can persist for 12 to 18 months. Renal stone incidence in the first 9 months is approximately 1.0% to 1.5% and is due mainly to hypercalciuria. Over the next 10 years upper tract stones are found in 8%, with many of these secondary to infection. The incidence of bladder stones in the first 9 months in patients on intermittent catheterization is 2.3%. In the presence of an indwelling catheter, and in spite of greater urine output, the prevalence is much higher, at 8.8%.[11]

Bladder stones are effectively treated with electrohydraulic lithotripsy. Small stones and particles can be dissolved by daily bladder irrigations with 30 mL of 10% of hemiacidrin (Renacidin) solution, which is left in the bladder for 30 minutes. Some patients with recurrent stones use this once or twice a week for prophylaxis. In patients who have ureteral reflux, it should be used with caution because of potential nephrotoxicity and absorption of magnesium. Caliceal calculi that are small (<1 cm) and asymptomatic can be followed expectantly, but 50% of these patients become symptomatic over 5 years and half of these will need some sort of invasive procedure.[16] Calculi that are growing or that are located in the renal pelvis should probably be treated before they pass into the ureter and cause obstruction (Fig. 27–7). Extracorporeal shock wave lithotripsy (ESWL) is the standard treatment. For large stones (>3 cm diameter), a percutaneous approach is preferred, as clearance of fragments is poor if patients are inactive.

Ureteral stones are potentially dangerous in patients with no renal sensation. These can be managed expectantly if they pass down within 2 to 3 weeks. There is

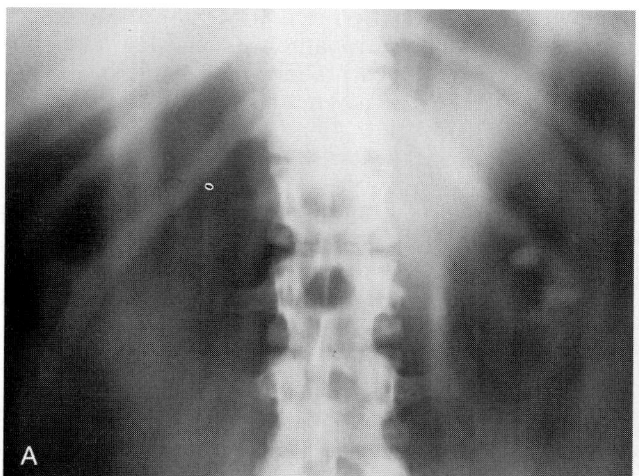

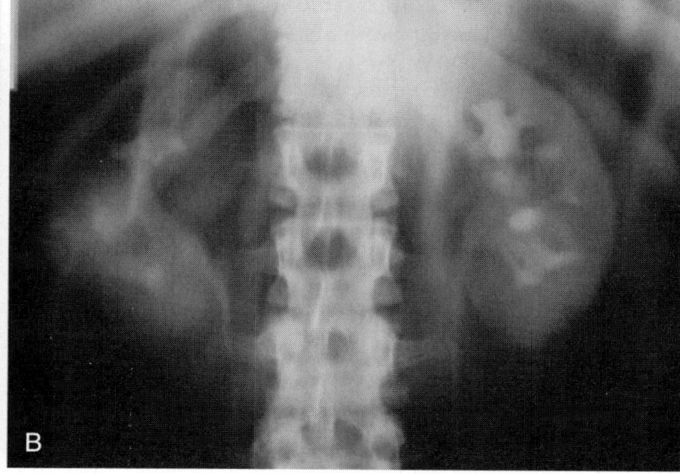

FIGURE 27–7. *A.* Tomograms of the kidneys showing partial staghorn calculi in the lower pole of the left kidney, with two smaller stones in the middle calices. *B.* The excretory urogram shows well-preserved morphology with minimal caliectasis.

an increased risk of renal damage, as these patients with reduced sensation will not perceive continuous pain, which would normally suggest severe continuing obstruction. Obstruction and infection together will require a drainage procedure as an emergency with a percutaneous nephrostomy or a retrograde stent, and this can be followed by an endoscopic removal or ESWL later.

Lower Urinary Tract Changes

Trabeculation occurs in the majority of patients after spinal cord injury and in many cases it happens despite appropriate management strategies. Sacculation and diverticula can occur when obstruction and high pressure are severe. If a diverticulum occurs at the ureteral hiatus, ureteral reflux is almost inevitable. Chronic infection of dilated prostatic ducts may be an important source for relapsing UTIs in men.

Ureteral Reflux and Upper Tract Dilation

Ureteral reflux or high bladder pressure in the absence of reflux can cause upper tract dilation (Fig. 27–8). Dilation without reflux is said to be due to decreased compliance, but recent data from long-term monitoring suggest that baseline pressure elevations are minimal with natural rates of filling, and that increased phasic activity may be more important.[35] With reflux, or ureteral dilation without reflux, the bladder pressure should be lowered with intermittent catheterization and anticholinergics. If reflux fails to improve but the bladder pressure responds, a surgical procedure to repair the reflux can be considered. If bladder pressures do not improve, the options are to augment the bladder or, in men, to perform a sphincterotomy and rely on free drainage.

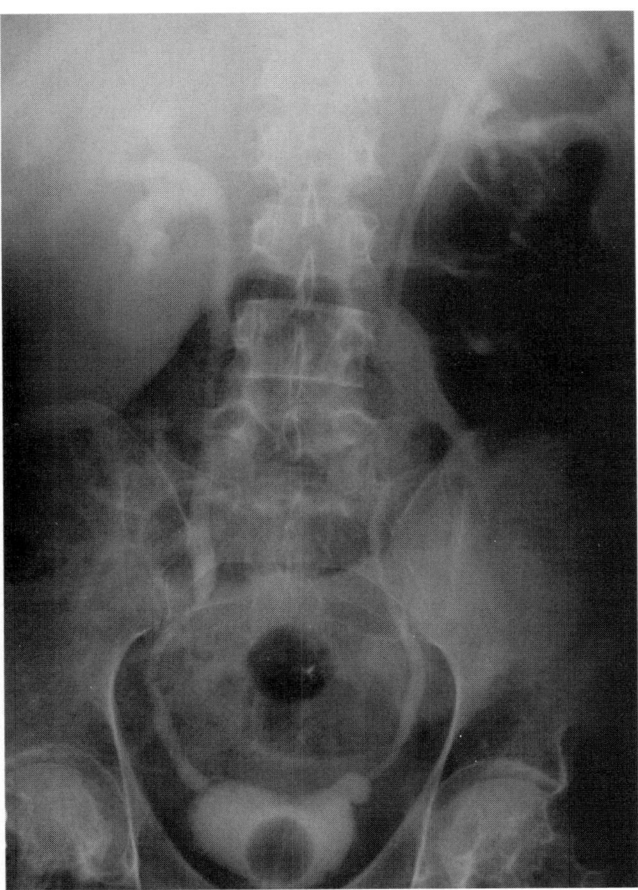

FIGURE 27–8. The 45-minute film from an excretory urogram of the patient whose urodynamic study is shown in Figure 28–5B. The Foley catheter draining the bladder is clamped, and at the low bladder volume shown an obvious holdup is noted at the ureterovesical junctions on both sides, particularly the right.

SUMMARY

The ultimate goal of bladder management is to prevent renal deterioration and reduce morbidity such as UTIs. The current demands of the health care market, however, are to reduce costs and length of hospital stays. These market demands are no doubt affecting daily decisions made by patients and providers regarding bladder management. Time will tell whether these market forces are changing outcomes (morbidity and mortality) related to the neurogenic bladder.

REFERENCES

1. Abrams P, Blaivas JG, Stanton SL, et al: Standardization of terminology of lower urinary tract function. In Krane RJ, Siroky MB (eds): Clinical Neurourology, ed 2. Boston, Little, Brown, 1991, pp 651–669.
2. Berger Y, Blaivas JG, DeLa Rocha ER, et al: Urodynamic findings in Parkinson's disease. J Urol 1987; 138:836–838.
3. Blaivas JG: Videourodynamics. In Krane RJ, Siroky MB (eds): Clinical Neurology, ed 2. Boston, Little, Brown, 1991, pp 265–274.
4. Bors E, Comarr AE: Neurological Urology. Baltimore, University Park Press, 1971.
5. Bradley WE: Physiology of the urinary bladder. In Walsh PC, Gittes RF, Perlmutter AD, et al: (eds): Campbell's Urology. Philadelphia, WB Saunders, 1986, pp 129–185.
6. Brindley GS, Rushton DN: Long-term follow-up of patients with sacral anterior root stimulator implants. Paraplegia 1990; 28:469–475.
7. Cardenas DD, Hooton TM: Urinary tract infection in persons with spinal cord injury. Arch Phys Med Rehabil 1995; 76:272–280.
8. Cardenas DD, Kelly E, Krieger JN, et al: Residual urine volumes in patients with spinal cord injury: Measurement with a portable ultrasound instrument. Arch Phys Med Rehabil 1988; 69:514–516.
9. Cardenas DD, Kelly E, Mayo ME: Manual stimulation of reflex voiding after spinal cord injury. Arch Phys Med Rehabil 1985; 66:459–462.
10. Cardenas DD, Mayo ME: Bacteriuria with fever after spinal cord injury. Arch Phys Med Rehabil 1987; 68:291–293.
11. DeVivo MJ, Fine PR, Cutter GR, et al: The risk of renal calculi in spinal cord injury patients. J Urol 1984; 131:857–860.
12. Dewire DM, Owens RS, Anderson GA, et al: A comparison of the urological complications associated with long-term management of quadriplegics with and without chronic indwelling urinary catheters. J Urol 1992; 147:1069–1072.
13. Dykstra DD, Sidi AA: Treatment of detrusor-sphincter dyssynergia with botulinum A toxin: A double-blind study. Arch Phys Med Rehabil 1990; 71:24–26.
14. Finkbeiner AE: Is bethanechol chloride clinically effective in promoting bladder emptying? A literature review. J Urol 1985; 134:443–449.
15. Gasparini ME, Schmidt RA, Tanagho EA: Selective sacral rhizotomy in the management of the reflex neuropathic bladder: A report on 17 patients with long-term follow-up. J Urol 1992; 148:1207–1210.
16. Glowacki LS, Beecroft ML, Cook RJ, et al: The natural history of asymptomatic urolithiasis. J Urol 1992; 147:319–321.

17. Guttmann L, Frankel H: The value of intermittent catheterization in the early management of traumatic paraplegia and tetraplegia. Paraplegia 1966; 4:63–84.
18. Iwatsubo E, Komine S, Yamashita H, et al: Over-distension therapy of the bladder in paraplegic patients using self-catheterization: A preliminary study. Paraplegia 1984; 22:210–215.
19. Kaufman JM, Fam B, Jacobs SC, et al: Bladder cancer and squamous metaplasia in spinal cord injury patients. J Urol 1977; 118:967–971.
20. Kiviat MD, Zimmerman TA, Donovan WH: Sphincter stretch: A new technique resulting in continence and complete voiding in paraplegics. J Urol 1975; 114:895–897.
21. Lapides J, Diokno AC, Silber SJ, et al: Clean intermittent self-catheterization in the treatment of urinary tract disease. J Urol 1972; 107:458–461.
22. Madersbacher H, Jilg G: Control of detrusor hyperreflexia by the intravesical instillation of oxybutynine hydrochloride. Paraplegia 1991; 29:84–90.
23. Mayo ME: The value of sphincter electromyography in urodynamics. J Urol 1979; 122:357–360.
24. Mayo ME, Chetner MP: Lower urinary tract dysfunction in multiple sclerosis. Urology 1992; 34:67–70.
25. McInerney PD, Vanner TF, Harris SAB, et al: Permanent urethral stents for detrusor sphincter dyssynergia. Br J Urol 1991; 61:291–294.
26. McLellan FC: The Neurogenic Bladder. Springfield, IL, Charles C Thomas, 1939, pp 57–70, 116–185.
27. Montgomerie JZ, Chan E, Gilmore DS, et al: Low mortality among patients with spinal cord injury and bacteremia. Rev Infect Dis 1991; 13:871–876.
28. National Institute on Disability and Rehabilitation Research Consensus Statement: The prevention and management of urinary tract infections among people with spinal cord injuries. J Am Paraplegia Soc 1992; 15:194–204.
29. Perkash I, Friedland GW: Transrectal ultrasonography of the lower urinary tract: Evaluation of bladder neck problems. Neurourol Urodynamics 1986; 5:299.
30. Sidi AA, Becher EF, Reddy PK, et al: Augmentation enterocystoplasty for the management of voiding dysfunction in spinal cord injury patients. J Urol 1990; 143:83–85.
31. Steers WD: Physiology and pharmacology of the bladder and urethra. In Walsh PC, Retch AB, Dawocott Vahnghan E, et al. (eds): Campbell's Urology, ed 7. Philadelphia, WB Saunders, 1998, chap 26, pp 870–915.
32. Steers WD, Meythaler JM, Haworth C, et al: Effects of acute bolus and chronic continuous intrathecal baclofen on genitourinary dysfunction due to spinal cord pathology. J Urol 1992; 148:1849–1855.
33. Swierzewski SJ III, Gormley EA, Belville WD, et al: The effect of terazosin on bladder function in the spinal cord injured patient. J Urol 1994; 151:951–954.
34. Tanagho EA, Schmidt RA, Orvis BR: Neural stimulation for control of voiding dysfunction: A preliminary report in 22 patients with serious neuropathic voiding disorders. J Urol 1989; 142:340–345.
35. Webb RJ, Styles RA, Griffiths CJ, et al: Ambulatory monitoring of bladder pressure in low compliance neurogenic bladder dysfunction. J Urol 1992; 48:1477–1488.

28

CHAPTER

John C. King, M.D., and Steven A. Stiens, M.D., M.S.

Neurogenic Bowel: Dysfunction and Management

Neurogenic bowel dysfunction may be relatively hidden from public view. It is often accompanied by other, more noticeable associated motor deficits. However, neurogenic bowel dysfunction alone can be particularly life-limiting if it is not thoroughly assessed and treated using rehabilitation principles. Interdisciplinary rehabilitative interventions focus on establishing a total management plan for bowel function, termed a bowel program, and for assisted defecation, known as bowel care.[48] Sensation and mobility might be limited, affecting a person's ability to anticipate the need for and to physically perform independent bowel care and hygiene. In spite of many abilities regained during the rehabilitation process, bowel care capabilities at the time of discharge are not always comparable to other skills that would be expected for a given level of function. Bowel management has been found to be one of the areas of least competence among rehabilitated spinal cord–injured (SCI) persons.[5] In spite of immobility, more than one-third of surveyed persons with SCI rated bowel and bladder dysfunction as having the most significant effect on their lives after SCI.[23] In a recent Swedish review of medical problems after SCI, 41% of subjects rated bowel dysfunction as a moderately to severely life-limiting problem.[29] Bowel programs and techniques for bowel care training should be more effectively pursued during inpatient rehabilitation. Some patients need attendants to help with bowel care, and they must be well trained as well.[49, 50] The burden of care for persons with neurogenic bowel is much higher if continence is not achieved or if bowel care evacuation times are excessive.[48, 56] Careful training of the patient and attendant care is necessary if satisfactory bowel management results are to be achieved.

EPIDEMIOLOGY

Neurogenic bowel dysfunction results from autonomic and somatic denervation, and produces fecal incontinence (FI), constipation and difficulty with evacuation (DWE). These symptoms are common. The prevalence of FI and fecal impaction ranges from 0.3% to 5.0% in the general population. The prevalence of DWE ranges from 10% to 50% among the hospitalized or institutionalized elderly.[44, 56] Although many gastrointestinal (GI) disorders can contribute to FI or DWE, disorders that impair the extrinsic (sympathetic, parasympathetic, or somatic) nervous control of the bowel and anorectal mechanisms are more common among the patient populations seen by physiatrists. Neurogenic bowel difficulties can be a primary disabling and handicapping feature for patients with SCI, stroke, amyotrophic lateral sclerosis, multiple sclerosis, diabetes mellitus, myelomeningocele, and muscular dystrophy.[8, 48]

IMPACT

Satisfactory functional outcomes depend on an individually designed, patient-centered and patient-managed bowel program.[49] The three primary objectives of the bowel program that apply to all cases are (1) to prevent unplanned bowel movements, (2) to promote efficient and effective bowel care, and (3) to prevent complications. FI decreases the return-to-home rates for stroke patients.[20] Almost one-third of persons with SCI report or exhibit worsening of bowel function 5 years beyond their injury, suggesting inadequate long-term management.[51] Recent evidence has shown some improvement in this area of management.[27] Nursing home costs are higher for patients with FI,[56] although restoring normal defecation might not be possible, *social continence,* defined as predictable, scheduled, adequate defections without incontinence at other times, is often achievable by persons with neurogenic bowel dysfunction. Embarrassment and humiliation from FI frequently result in extreme vocational and social disability. Vocational disability and excessive institutionalization add substantial costs to the care of neurogenic bowel dysfunction. A 1983 report estimated that $8 billion per year is spent in the United States for the care of fecally incontinent institutionalized patients.[44]

BOWEL ANATOMY AND FUNCTION

Anatomy: Structure and Innervation

The colon is the terminal segment of intestine that has been differentiated for fecal formation, storage, and defecation. The colon and anorectal mechanisms receive parasympathetic, sympathetic, and somatic innervation and contain the intrinsic enteric nervous system (ENS) between muscular layers and under the mucosa (Figs. 28–1 and 28–2). The neurogenic bowel is defined as the loss of direct somatic sensory or motor control functions, with or without impaired sympathetic and parasympathetic innervation.[48] However, the intrinsic ENS remains intact with most presenting injuries and illnesses. The most common exceptions are the developmental disorder of Hirschsprung's disease or cases of acquired autonomic neuropathy from diabetes mellitus, which can involve the ENS as well. Such diabetic ENS damage, however, does not necessarily correlate with the severity of the peripheral diabetic polyneuropathy. When intact, the intrinsic ENS continues to integrate and modulate bowel function, even without autonomic and somatic nervous system input, and can be the neurological substrate for bowel habit training.

Physiology: Normal Function

The colon is a reservoir for food waste until it is convenient for elimination. It also acts as a storage device as long as the colonic pressure is less than that of the anal sphincter mechanism. Fecal elimination occurs when colonic pressure exceeds that of the anal sphincter mechanism. Other functions of the colon are to reabsorb fluids (up to 30 L/day can be reabsorbed from the large and small bowel walls, with typically only 100 mL of water loss in feces) and gases (90% of the 7 to 10 L of gases produced by intracolonic fermentation is absorbed rather than expelled). The colon also provides an environment for the growth of bacteria needed to assist in digestion, and serves to absorb certain bacterial breakdown products as well.[21] The layers of the colon wall are depicted in Figure 28–2.

The ENS is the key to proper functioning of the entire GI tract. This collection of highly organized neurons is situated in two primary layers, the submucosal (Meissner's) plexus and the intramuscular myenteric

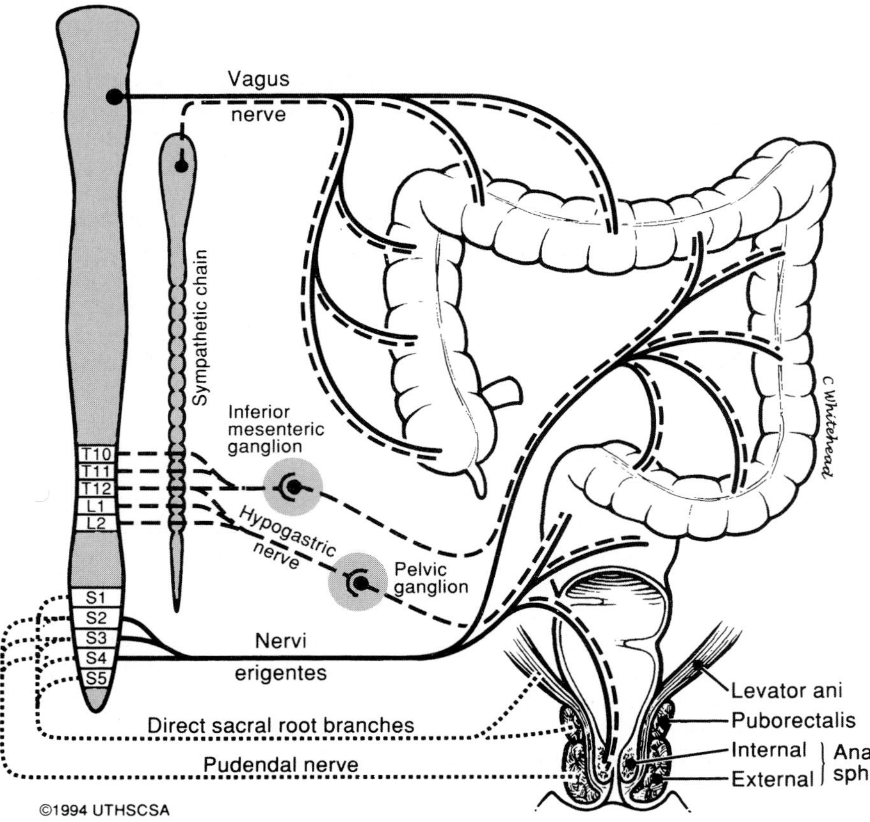

FIGURE 28–1. Neurological levels and pathways for the sympathetic, parasympathetic, and somatic nervous system innervation of the colon and anorectum. Not shown is the enteric nervous system, which travels along the bowel wall from esophagus to internal anal sphincter and forms the final common pathway to control the bowel wall smooth muscle.

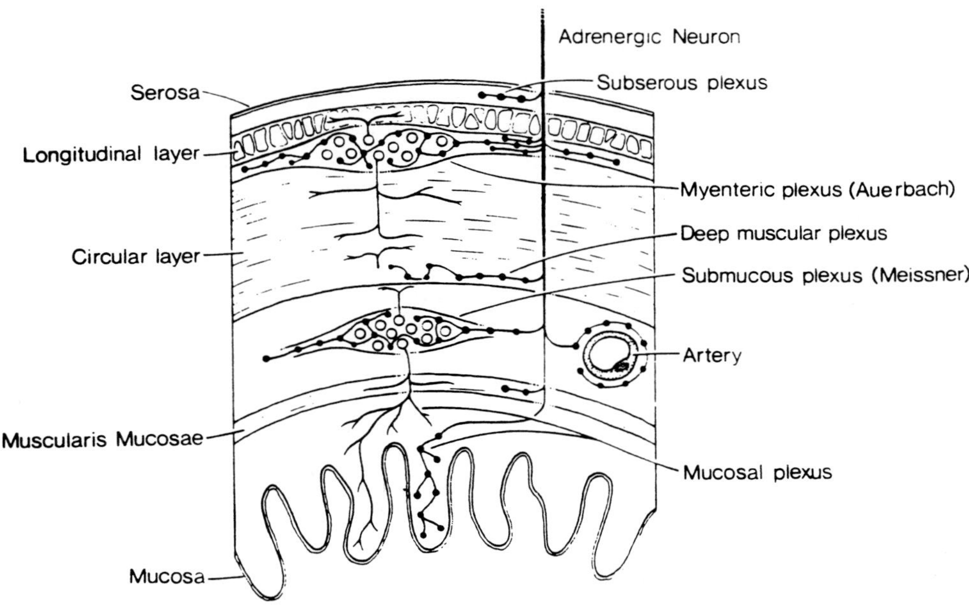

FIGURE 28–2. Diagram of a transverse section of the gut showing enteric plexus and the distribution of adrenergic neurons. Note the ganglionic plexuses of Auerbach and Meissner. The deep muscular plexus contains a few ganglia, the subserosal contains an occasional ganglion, and the mucosal plexus shows none. The adrenergic fibers are all extrinsic and arise from the prevertebral sympathetic ganglia. The adrenergic fibers are distributed largely to the mesenteric, submucous, and mucosal plexus and to blood vessels. (From Goyal RK, Crist JR: Neurology of the Gut. In Sleisenger MH, Fordtran JS (eds): Gastrointestinal Disease: Pathophysiology, Diagnosis, Management, ed 4. Philadelphia, WB Saunders, 1989, p 34.)

(Auerbach's) plexus. These plexi have an estimated 10 to 100 million neurons, plus two to three glial cells per neuron. That is more nerve cells than are contained in the spinal cord. The ENS glial cells, which resemble central nervous system (CNS) astrocytes, are much less abundant than the 20 to 50 glial cells per neuron in the CNS.[19] The coordination of segment-to-segment function is largely regulated by the ENS and considered by some as a third part of the autonomic nervous system.[59] The ENS also has its own nerve-blood barrier, similar to the CNS.[10]

The sympathetic and parasympathetic nervous systems seem to modulate the ENS, rather than directly controlling the smooth muscles of the bowel.[59] The smooth muscles of the bowel also have their own electromechanical automaticity, which is directly modulated by the inhibitory control of the ENS.[10, 19] Sympathetic nervous system stimulation tends to promote the storage function by enhancing anal tone and inhibiting colonic contractions, although little clinical deficit occurs from bilateral sympathectomy.[14] Parasympathetic activity enhances colonic motility, and its loss is often associated with DWE, including impactions and functional obstructions, such as Ogilvie's pseudo-obstructive syndrome.[14]

The normal intact colon wall has a 3 to 6 Hz pattern of slow electrical potential waves with irregularly occurring bursts of spike activity typically on the apex of these waves every 10 to 12 seconds. This spike activity is associated with development of bowel wall tension and with slow peristaltic waves of ring contractions. These ring contractions are several centimeters apart and travel at 1 to 2 mm/sec. These peristaltic waves seem to be paced from the transverse colon and travel both caudad to the rectum and cephalad to the cecum.[10]

The function of the transverse and ascending colon is largely storage, with propulsion generally retrograde toward the one-way ileocecal valve. This allows the haustral and colonic motility waves to mix and stir contents and also exposes contents to the colon wall for additional fecal liquid absorption.[10] Occasionally these proximal traveling colonic waves reverse, especially during a giant migratory contraction (GMC) of the colon. The GMC is associated with mass movement of feces as far as one-third the length of the colon.[59] In the fasting emptied colon, GMCs occur approximately four times per day, but twice or less per day in the normal colon.[59] The origin of the GMCs is poorly understood, but they commonly occur after meals with the gastrocolic response, or due to increased physical activity. The GMC does not seem to be under volitional control.[10]

The rectum is usually empty until just prior to defecation. The resting anal canal pressure is largely determined by the angulation and pressure at the anorectal junction by the puborectalis sling and smooth muscle internal sphincter tone. Continence is maintained by the anal sphincter mechanism,[34, 48] which consists of the internal anal sphincter (IAS), external anal sphincter (EAS), and the puborectalis muscle.[34] Only about 20% of the anal canal pressure is due to the static contraction of the somatically innervated striated EAS.[3] The EAS and puborectalis muscle are the only striated skeletal muscles whose normal resting state is tonic contraction, and these muscles consist mainly of slow-twitch fatigue-resistant type I fibers (unlike the situation in nonupright animals such as the cat or dog, in which it consists of predominately type II fibers).[3] Anal pressure can be increased volitionally by contracting the EAS and puborectalis muscles. Maximum volitional squeeze pressures, however, are not as high as can be generated reflexively against Valsalva pressure. The EAS is physically larger than the internal sphincter, and its contraction is under both reflex and volitional control. The volitional control is learned during the course of normal maturation. Normal baseline reflex action of the anorectal mechanism allows spontaneous stool elimination. The EAS is innervated by the S2 through S4 nerve roots via the pudendal nerve, and the puborectalis muscle is innervated by direct branches from the S1 to S5 roots (see Fig. 28–1).[41] The remarkable degree of learned EAS coordination allows the selective discrete passage of gas while balancing a variable mixture of solids, liquids, and gases.

Normal defecation begins with reflexes triggered by rectosigmoid distention (Fig. 28–3). A rectorectal reflex occurs in which the bowel proximal to the distending bolus contracts and the bowel wall distally relaxes, serving to propel the bolus further caudad. Reflex relaxation of the internal sphincter also occurs, which is enhanced by, but does not require, an extrinsic nerve supply. This relaxation, called the rectoanal inhibitory reflex, correlates with the urge labeled "the call to stool."[59] One can then volitionally contract the levator ani to open the proximal anal canal and relax the external sphincter and puborectalis muscles. This allows a straighter, shorter, and open anorectal passage (see Fig. 28–3), which permits the bolus to pass. Increasing the intra-abdominal pressure by squatting and by a Valsalva maneuver assists bolus elimination. For 90% of normal individuals only the contents of the rectum are expulsed, whereas 10% will clear the entire contents of the left colon from the splenic flexure distally.[13] One can elect to defer defecation, however, by volitionally contracting the puborectalis muscle and EAS. The reflexive IAS relaxation subsequently fades, usually within 15 seconds, and the urge resolves until the IAS relaxation is again triggered. The rectal wall accommodates to the bolus by decreasing its wall tension with time, resulting in less sensory input and less reflex triggering from that particular accommodated bolus. This continence and reflex process is somewhat analogous to the function of the striated external urethral sphincter in volitional control of urinary voiding.

The external sphincter generally tenses in response to small rectal distentions via a spinal reflex, although reflexive relaxation of the external sphincter occurs in the presence of greater distentions. These spinal cord reflexes are centered in the conus medullaris and are augmented and modulated by higher cortical influences. When cortical control is disrupted, as by SCI, the external sphincter reflexes usually persist and allow spontaneous defecation. During sleep, colonic activity, anal tone, and protective responses to abdominal pressure elevations are all decreased, while rectal tone increases.[10, 59]

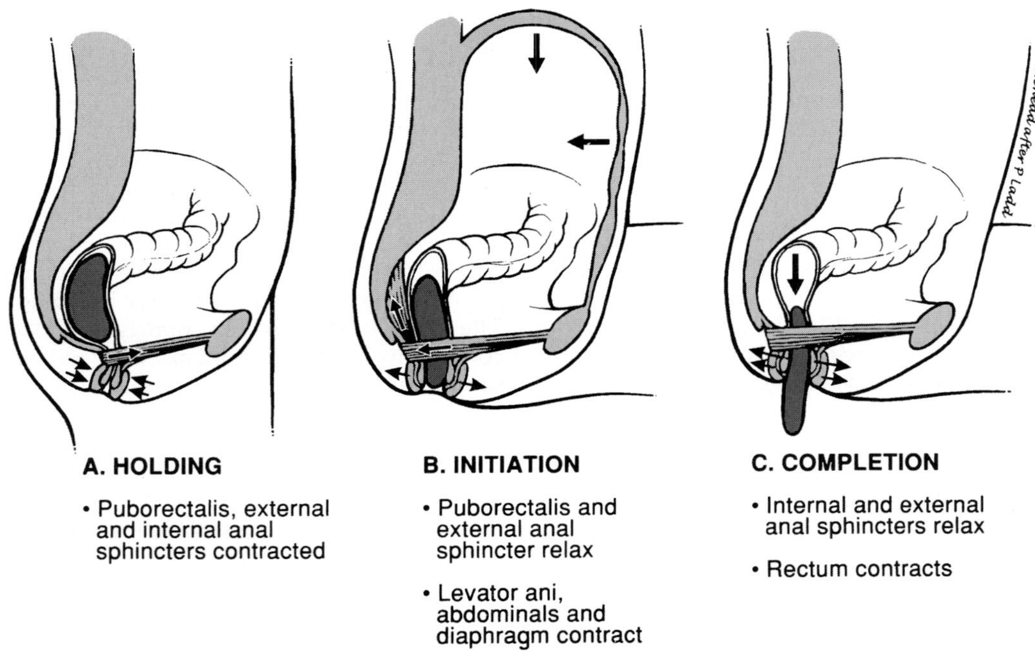

FIGURE 28–3. *A.* Defecation is prevented by a statically increased tone of the internal anal sphincter and puborectalis, as well as by the mechanical effects of the acute anorectal angle. Dynamic responses of the external anal sphincter and puborectalis to rectal distention reflexes or increased intra-abdominal pressures further impede defecation. *B.* To initiate defecation, the puborectalis muscle and external anal sphincter relax while intra-abdominal pressure is increased by Valsalva's maneuver, which is facilitated by squatting. The levator ani helps reduce the acute anorectal angle to open the distal anal canal to receive the stool bolus. *C.* Intrarectal reflexes result in continued internal anal sphincter relaxation and rectal propulsive contractions, which help expel the bolus through the open canal. (Modified from Shiller LR: Fecal incontinence. In Sleisenger MH, Fordtran JS (eds): Gastrointestinal Disease: Pathophysiology, Diagnosis, Management, ed 4. Philadelphia, WB Saunders, 1989, p 322.)

The "gastrocolonic response" or "gastrocolic reflex" refers to the increased colonic activity (GMCs and mass movements) that occurs in the first 30 to 60 minutes after a meal. This increased colonic activity appears to be modulated both by hormonal effects, from release of peptides from the upper GI tract (gastrin, motilin, cholecystokinin), which increase contractility of colonic smooth musculature, and by a reduction in the threshold for spinal cord–mediated vescicovescical reflexes.[10] Upper GI receptor stimulation also results in increased activity in the colon, possibly due to reflexively increased parasympathetic efferent activity to the colon. The possibility of a purely ENS-mediated activation exists, although the small bowel and colon motor activities do not seem to be synchronized. In SCI the measured increase in colonic activity after a meal is blunted as compared to normals.[10] The gastrocolonic response is often used therapeutically, even in SCI patients, to enhance bowel evacuation during this 30- to 60-minute postprandial time frame.[1, 16] Occasionally, certain foods can serve as trigger foods that are especially likely to induce bowel evacuation shortly after consumption.

PATHOPHYSIOLOGY: NEUROGENIC BOWEL DYSFUNCTION

Upper Motor Neurogenic Bowel (UMNB)

Any destructive CNS process above the conus, from SCI to dementia, can lead to the UMNB pattern of dysfunction. Spinal cortical sensory pathway deficits lead to decreased ability to sense the urge to defecate. Most persons with SCI, however, sense a vague discomfort when excessive rectal or colonic distention occurs, and 43% have chronic complaints of vague abdominal distention discomfort that eases with bowel evacuation.[33, 51] These sensations might be mediated by autonomic nervous system afferent fibers bypassing the zone of SCI via the paraspinal sympathetic chain or by means of vagal parasympathetic afferents.

Colonic compliance and sphincter tone have been experimentally evaluated in SCI subjects. Studies of colonic compliance in response to a continuous infusion of saline initially suggested rapid pressure rises and a hyperreflexic response.[39, 58] More recent studies have demonstrated normal colonic compliances in SCI subjects with UMNB.[32, 40] Passive filling of the rectum leads to increases in the resting sphincter tone. These increases are associated with increased external sphincter pressure development due to sacral reflexes that can be abolished by pudendal block.[3] This form of rectal sphincter dyssynergia has unfortunately been labeled decreased colonic compliance, even though intermittent or slow filling in the rectum appears to be associated with normal bolus accommodation and pressure relaxation.[32, 40] This contrasts with the true decreased compliance found in ischemic or postinflammatory rectal bowel wall due to fibrosis, which cannot accommodate and relax regardless of flow rates.

Internal sphincter relaxation upon rectal distention occurs in persons with SCI as well as in neurologically intact persons. After sufficient rectal distention the external sphincter might completely relax, resulting in expulsion of the fecal bolus. Rectal sphincter dyssynergia does not necessarily correlate with bladder sphincter dyssynergia, but it often results in DWE.[41] The protective vesicorenal reflex, whereby the external sphincter pressure increases in response to increased intra-abdominal pressure, is usually intact (Table 28–1).[3] Patients with UMNB also have normal or increased anal sphincter tone, intact anocutaneous (or anal wink) and bulbocavernosus reflexes,[48] a palpable puborectalis muscle sling, and normal anal verge appearance (Fig. 28–4).

Lower Motor Neurogenic Bowel (LMNB)

Polyneuropathy, conus medullaris or cauda equina lesions, pelvic surgery, vaginal delivery, or even chronic straining during defecation can impair the somatic innervation of the anal sphincter mechanism. These conditions can also produce sympathetic and parasympathetic innervation deficits. If an isolated pudendal insult has occurred, colonic transit times are normal and FI predominates. Colonic sluggishness can occur as a result of loss of parasympathetic supply, adding constipation and DWE to FI difficulties. This is an especially bad combination because the accumulation of a large amount of hard stool that can result from such colonic inertia can overstretch the weakened anal mechanism, resulting in a gaping, patulous, incompetent anal orifice. The denervation and atrophy of the EAS leads to loss of the protective vesicorectal reflex, which can result in stool soilage from the increased abdominal pressures associated with everyday activities. Rectal distention leads to the expected internal sphincter relaxation, but attenuated or absent external sphincter protective contractions result in FI or fecal smearing whenever boluses present at the rectum. The presence of a large bolus in the rectal vault can further compromise the rectoanal angulation at the pelvic floor and contribute to paradoxical liquid incontinence around a low (ball-valve effect) impaction.[3, 53, 60]

Patients with LMNB dysfunction have decreased anal tone due to the smooth muscle internal sphincter. If no tone is found initially upon inserting the examining finger, the examiner should wait up to 15 seconds to allow IAS reflex relaxation to recover and restore tone. Chronic overstretching has probably occurred if tone does not return. The anal-to-buttock contour typically appears flattened and "scalloped" (see Fig. 28–4) due to atrophy of the pudendal-innervated pelvic floor muscles and EAS.[3] The anocutaneous reflex is absent or decreased (depending on the completeness of the lesion). Likewise, the bulbocavernosus reflex is weak if present (see Table 28–1). The anal canal is shortened (as compared to the normal 2.5 to 4.5 cm length) and the puborectalis muscle ridge may not be palpable. Excessive perineal descent and even rectal prolapse may occur with Valsalva's maneuver.

Evaluation

The GI history should not only review for cardinal symptoms, but should also address the patient's general neu-

TABLE 28–1 Features of Colorectal Function in Normal Subjects and in Those with Upper Motor Neurogenic Bowel (UMNB), UMNB with Posterior Rhizotomy, and Lower Motor Neurogenic Bowel (LMNB)

	Normals	UMNB	UMNB and Posterior Rhizotomy	LMNB
Bowel dysfunction	Normal colon activity and defecation	Chronic intractable constipation, fecal impaction, reflex defecation ± incontinence	Chronic constipation; no reflex defecation	Chronic constipation; fecal impaction maximal in the rectum
Transit time (cecum to anus)	12–48 hr	Prolonged >72 hr	Very prolonged unless sacral nerve stimulator used	Prolonged >6 days, especially left colon
Colonic motility at rest	GMC approx. 4 per 24 hr	GMC may be reduced in frequency	Reduced GMC	Reduced GMC
In response to stimuli	GMC facilitated by defecation, exercise, and food ingestion	Less GMC facilitation by defecation, exercise, or food ingestion	Less GMC facilitation by defecation, exercise, or food ingestion	Less GMC facilitation by defecation, exercise, or food ingestion
Anal Sphincter Pressure (mm Hg)				
Resting tone	>30	>30	Normal	Reduced
Volitional squeeze	>30 (up to 1800)	Absent	Absent	Absent
Rectal compliance	Normal	Normal but sigmoid compliance decreased	Normal or increased	Rectum dilated; increased distention volume; increased compliance
Rectal Balloon Distention				
Effect on IAS	Normal RA inhibitory reflex	Normal RA inhibitory reflex	Normal RA inhibitory reflex	Normal RA inhibitory reflex
Effect on EAS	Causes contraction	Causes contraction	No contraction	No contraction
Sensory perception threshold	<20 mL volume	None	None	None
Stimulation of rectal contraction	Induced by balloon distention	Giant rectal contractions stimulated readily	Rectal contraction stimulation	Rectal contraction stimulation
Vesicoanal reflex	Present (>50 mm Hg)	Present	Absent	Absent
Valsalva protective reflex				
Reflex defecation	Yes	Yes	Impaired	Impaired
Perianal sensation (Cutaneous sensation—touch, pinprick)	Normal	No sensory perception	No sensory perception	Loss of perianal and buttock sensation due to injury to sacral nerves
Anocutaneous reflex ("anal wink")	Present	Present; may be increased	Absent	Absent due to injury to afferent/efferent sacral pathways
Bulbocavernosus reflex	Present	Present; may be increased	Absent	Absent
Anal appearance	Normal	Normal	Normal	Flattened, "scalloped," due to loss of EAS bulk

Abbreviations: GMC, giant migratory contractions; IAS, internal anal sphincter; EAS, external anal sphincter; RA, rectoanal.

Modified from Banwell JG, Creaswey GH, Aggarwal AM, et al: Management of the neurogenic bowel in patients with spinal cord injury. Urol Clin North Am 1993; 20:523; and Schiller LR: Fecal incontinence. In Sleisenger MH, Fordtran JS (eds): Gastrointestinal Disease. Philadelphia, WB Saunders, 1989, pp 317–330.

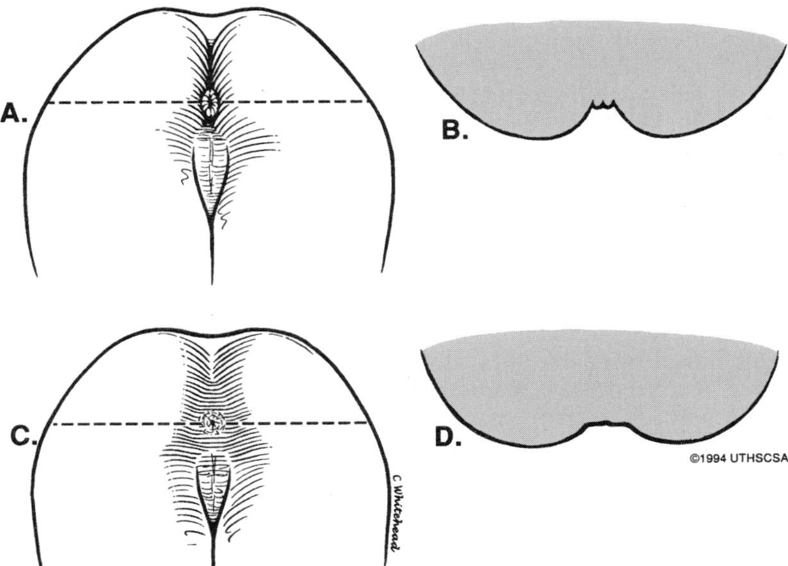

FIGURE 28–4. Upper motor neurogenic bowel presents an appearance similar to normal (*A*, rear view; *B*, profile from above). Anal contour of the lower motor neurogenic bowel (*C*, rear view; *D*, profile from above), with its atrophic external anal sphincter, shows a flattened, scalloped-appearing anal area.

romuscular and GI function. A detailed review of the patient's bowel program includes an assessment of fluids, diet, activity, medications, and aspects of bowel care.[26] A review of the technique and outcome of bowel care should include a description of schedule, initiation method (chemical or mechanical stimulation), facilitative techniques, time requirements, and characteristics of stool results.[48] The history should include premorbid bowel pattern information such as defecation frequency, typical time(s) of the day, associated predefecatory activities, bowel medications and techniques or trigger foods, and stool consistency. It is important to elicit any history of premorbid GI disease or dysfunction. The presence of GI sensations or pain, warning sensations for defecation, sense of urgency, and ability to prevent stool loss during Valsalva activities such as laughing, sneezing, coughing, or transfers should be noted. Excessively large-caliber hard stool can be ascertained by a history of toilet plugging.[37] The patient's goals and willingness to alter prior bowel patterns or management need to be established.[24]

The physical examination should include the GI system and the associated parts of the musculoskeletal and nervous systems required for independent management of the bowel program. The examination should be completed at the onset and then annually for SCI.[26] The purpose of the examination is to detect functional changes, screen for complications, and identify any new masses or lesions.

The abdomen should be inspected for distention, hernias, and other abnormalities. Percussion and auscultation should precede palpation for masses and tenderness. With the abdomen releaxed, the examiner transabdominally palpates the colon for hard stool. Palpable hard stool should not be present on the right side of the abdomen (ascending colon).

Physical examination continues with inspection of the anus. A patulous gaping orifice suggests a history of overdistention and trauma by a previous regimen. A normal anal-buttock contour (Fig. 28–4) suggests an intact EAS muscle mass, whereas its loss results in a flattened, fanned-out "scalloped"-appearing anal region. The patient should perform a Valsalva maneuver while the examiner observes the anus and perineum for excessive descent.[54] Perianal cutaneous sharp stimulation normally results in an externally visible anal sphincter reflexive contraction. This is the anocutaneous reflex, mediated by the inferior hemorrhoidal branch of the pudendal nerve (S2 to S5). This can be checked by tugging perianal hairs or by the application of the sharp edge of a broken cotton swab stick to the perianal skin. The anocutaneous reflex should be checked in all four quadrants, as selective (especially side-to-side) deficits can occur. Sensation to pinprick is tested at the same time. A gloved lubricated finger should then be inserted through the anus until no pressure is appreciated at the fingertip. The tone and voluntary squeeze strength of the EAS and tone of the IAS should be assessed. The length of the anus, where pressure is sensed, is normally 2.5 to 4.5 cm. The point where the pressure decreases marks the anorectal junction. Along the posterior wall, 1.5 to 2.5 cm from the anal verge, the puborectalis muscular sling can be palpated as a ridge that will push the finger forward as the subject resists defecation. No palpable ridge or push suggests puborectalis atrophy or dysfunction. A shortened length of anal pressure zone suggests EAS muscle atrophy. With the examiner's finger in place, the bulbocavernosus reflex can be elicited by rapidly tapping or squeezing the clitoris or glans penis. Multiple random trials are needed to be certain the vesicorectal Valsalva protective reflexes are not occurring at the same time by random chance. The response can be delayed up to a few seconds in pathological conditions. A consistent response to the stimulus indicates an intact bulbocavernosus reflex. Insertion of the finger in the anal canal occasionally triggers IAS relaxation, but more often triggers a tightening squeeze that is efferently equivalent to the bulbocavernosus reflex. If IAS and EAS relaxation occur, the examiner should wait several seconds for tone to be restored before testing the bulbocavernosus reflex. Ask the patient to volitionally squeeze the anus before removing the finger ("resist defecation") to check for volitional EAS and puborectalis tone and control.

Diagnostic Testing

The history and physical examination provide most of the necesary information. The clinical cause of neurogenic bowel dysfunction in most patients who are referred to physiatrists is readily apparent. Additional objective laboratory testing can be helpful when the cause of FI or DWE is obscure, the history appears doubtful, conservative interventions fail, or surgical interventions are contemplated. Table 28–2 lists some of the many tests available.

Basic laboratory tests complement the physical examination. A stool guaiac test is helpful to rule out the presence of blood in the stool. False positives are common after SCI because of hemorrhoids, as well as from anal trauma secondary to bowel care.[48] A flat plate radiograph of the abdomen can be helpful to rule out impaction,[60] megacolon, obstruction and a perforated viscus.

MANAGEMENT

General Principles

A bowel program is a comprehensive individualized patient-centered treatment plan focused on preventing incontinence, achieving effective and efficient colonic evacuation, and preventing the complications of neurogenic bowel dysfunction.[48] The subcomponents of a bowel program address diet, fluids, exercise, medications, and scheduled bowel care. Bowel care is the individually developed and prescribed procedure for defecation that is carried out by the patient or the attendant.[48]

The approach to the problems associated with neurogenic bowel is the same as for all issues that confront the patient in the rehabilitation process. All aspects of impairment and disability that limit a person's ability to maintain continence and volitionally defecate must be assessed within the perspective of the entire person. All aspects of personal performance should be addressed in person-centered rehabilitation, with the overall goal of maximizing independence in bowel management or direction of a bowel program.[48]

Neurogenic bowel dysfunction results in problems with fecal storage and elimination. Inability to volitionally inhibit spontaneous defecations leads to incontinence, while the inability to adequately empty leads to constipation and impactions. Paradoxically, impactions can result in diarrhea and incontinence. Providing adequate emptying must be combined with the inhibition of spontaneous defecations except at desired times in order to achieve social continence.

Disablement and Rehabilitation Models: Methods for Coordinating Efforts of the Interdisciplinary Team

The method of assessment and intervention for problems caused by neurogenic bowel is the same as for all issues that confront the patient in the rehabilitation

TABLE 28–2 Laboratory Tests of Colonic and Rectoanal Function

Test	Purpose
Colonoscopy, rectosigmoidoscopy, anoscopy	Visualize anatomy to identify lesions Limited benefit to assess function
Anal endosonography	Evaluate structure and continuity of pelvic muscles
Radiography	
Defecography	Visualize kinesiology of defecation
Barium enema	Identify structural defects; fluoroscopy time too limited to assess function in any detail
Serial radiographs of tiny radiopaque plastic beads ingested with food	Evaluate colonic transit time; useful to confirm constipation history and to identify dysfunctional segments that help plan colostomy level
Manometry	Assess giant migratory contractions and anal pressures; with intrarectal balloon inflation, to evaluate rectoanal inhibitory reflex
Kymography	Measure pressure and volume change by intraluminal balloons
Catheter	Measure pressures by catheter in various compartments of the bowel
Solid-sphere retention test	Measure maximal anal resistance force to extraction of spheres of standard sizes
Rectally infused saline continence test	Quantitative reproducible assessment of liquid continence ability
Electromyography	
Traditional	Assess motor nerve supply to puborectalis, anococcygeus, levator ani, and external anal sphincter; assess sensory pelvic afferents by nerve conduction studies, bulbocavernosus reflex testing, or somatosensory-evoked potentials
Mucosal electrosensitivity	Assess degree of mucosal wall sensibility
Intraluminal catheter	Research tool to assess colonic smooth muscle electrical potential activity

Information compiled from Christensen J: The motor function of the colon. In Yamada T (ed): Textbook of Gastroenterology. Philadelphia, JB Lippincott, 1991, pp 180–196; Schiller LR: Fecal incontinence. In Sleisinger MH, Fordtran JS (eds): Gastrointestinal Disease. Philadelphia, WB Saunders, 1993, pp 934–953; and Stone JM, Wolfe VA, Niro-Murcia M, et al: Colostomy as treatment for complications of spinal cord injury. Arch Phys Med Rehabil 1990; 71:514–518.

process.[48] The rehabilitation evaluation should be interdisciplinary in approach and include assessment not only of colon and pelvic floor dysfunction, but also of impairments of other organs or systems that could affect rehabilitative strategies to make bowel care independent or prevent unplanned bowel movements. The rehabilitation database should specifically note the level and degree of associated co-morbid motor and sensory deficits. The examination should assess reflex function to determine the impairment pattern (UMNB or LMNB) of colonic and pelvic floor dysfunction that is present. Next, the problem is succinctly described and included on the rehabilitation problem list as a UMNB or LMNB pattern of impairment. Disabilities that limit a person's ability to maintain continence and volitionally defecate must be assessed within the perspective of the entire person. Limitations of functional mobility as well as retained capabilities need to be considered. For example, any residual colonic reflex function can be exploited in bowel care. Task modifications, digital stimulation, or pharmacological interventions can be utilized to trigger and sustain defecation.[48] The rehabilitation process for bowel care requires knowledge of the individual person and derivation of person-centered goals.[25, 47] A single member of the rehabilitation team should coordinate this interdisciplinary intervention effort. Typically, this person is the primary nurse, acting in close association with the physiatrist and occupational therapist.

The role performance of the individual that will occur after the acute rehabilitation process is complete determines the timing and content of the new bowel care schedule. The demands of life activities, the duration of bowel care, and the needs of other members of the household should all be considered in scheduling. During inpatient rehabilitation, scheduling can be especially difficult because of the time-consuming nature of bowel care.[3] Evening bowel care often allows for more predictable attendance at daily therapies.

It is crucial to remember that the patient must take a decisive leadership role in designing a bowel program that includes a convenient bowel care schedule. Educating patients about their altered neurogenic bowel physiology and empowering them with options and techniques to construct a bowel care regimen compatible with their life interests are important aspects of the overall rehabilitation process.

Dietary Considerations

Food choices are important when colonic transit time is prolonged, as in SCI (96 hours vs. the 30 hours typically found in normal subjects).[3, 4, 38] Excessive fluid resorption can result in stool hardening and subsequent constipation. Gases and liquids are propelled 30 to 100 times faster than solids by the colon. Stools that have lost their plasticity might not be kneaded and folded by the haustra, and instead their transit can be impeded. To maintain a more fluid content, stool softeners, both docusate and food fiber, have been used. No increase in stool bulk, as would be expected with fluid retention, occurs from docusate in normal subjects, which brings its efficacy into question.[3] Fiber does increase stool bulk and plasticity, especially in the more physically coarse forms, which also tends to decrease colonic pressures.[3] Control of excessive stool hardness requires higher-fiber foods in preference to lower-residual foods.

The American norm has been found to be 100 g (though highly variable, with a range of 35 to 450 g in males and 5 to 335 g in females) of solid feces expelled daily or less frequently.[13, 44] However, the high pressures involved in moving solid feces probably contribute to the 90% incidence of hemorrhoids in Americans and to premature diverticula formation and hemorrhoidal complications in more than 70% of SCI patients.[51] Constant straining at stool can also contribute to peripheral neuropathic deficits in the anal sphincteric musculature.[13] Acceptance of softer stools, from a higher-fiber diet, might help reduce these complications and is often recommended for their treatment. A diet that contains at least 15 g of fiber daily is recommended.[26] Increases in the fiber content of the diets of persons with SCI do not decrease colonic transit time[7] but enhances the rectonal inhibitory reflex.[13] The effects of fiber intake on stool consistency and frequency and efficacy of evacuation should be evaluated in each individual patient. The longer perineal hygiene time required for softer stools might be a deterrent for some and should be discussed with patients. Increases in dietary fiber typically result in increased stool bulk, which can require more frequent bowel care.

A wide range of "normal" bowel patterns exists. Defecation frequencies in nonimpaired persons vary dramatically from several times per day to less than once per week. Ninety-five percent have a frequency of between three times per day and three times per week.[13, 42] Stool consistencies vary, from liquid to pudding, pasty, semisolid, soft-formed, medium-formed, and hard-formed. Patients rarely have an adequate vocabulary to describe this socially taboo subject.[50] Fully appreciating an individual's premorbid "normal" bowel function is important in the planning and goal setting for a new neurogenic bowel program.

Approaches and Rationale

Colonic transit time and fecal elimination are enhanced by softer stool. However, if the stool becomes too liquid, the protective angle provided by the puborectalis becomes less effective, and greater EAS pressures are required to maintain continence. Neurogenic bowel resting anal pressures are usually normal to slightly decreased, but are unable to develop the protective increases in EAS tone needed to control more liquid stool.[3] Some degree of stool firmness must be tolerated to prevent incontinence. To avoid incontinence upon straining, more firmness (medium-formed) is required for the weaker anal sphincter mechanism of LMNB than for UMNB (semiformed to soft-formed). Docusate is often used to try to increase fluid content and plasticity of the stool, although its clinical efficacy should be individually monitored. Fiber more consistently softens stool but also adds bulk. Bulkier stools can help stimulate the defecatory response more easily in LMNB, although less stimulus is needed in UMNB.[15, 31] The presentation of stool to the rectum, triggering defecation, can be associated with GMC and mass movements more than with the slow accumulation of sufficient rectal stool to trigger reflex defecation, and the GMC might be what is actually habituated.[44]

The frequency and specific timing of bowel care to induce adequate colonic emptying can be chosen, based on previous elimination patterns. Regular bowel emptying is recommended as the primary means for enhancing both elimination and decreasing incontinence between stooling. Incontinence is reduced by less stool accumulation, since stool is not presented to the rectum between desired defecation times. Adequate emptying is accomplished by (1) making stools easier to move by means of softening, (2) adding bowel stimulant medication if needed, and (3) triggering the defecatory reflex at consistent desired times to promote habituation.

Choosing long intervals between elimination allows more fluid reabsorption, resulting in harder stools, which can worsen DWE. Since 95% of unimpaired persons defecate three or more times per week, choosing a frequency of at least as often as every other day would seem more physiological and less likely to contribute to constipation.[13, 26, 42] One study of well-managed SCI patients found frequencies of bowel care to be chosen as daily by 24%, every other day by 46%, and more often than three times a week by 85%.[27] The desire to avoid the unpleasant task of stool elimination leads some to elect longer time intervals between bowel care sessions, but this carries the attendant risk for impaction or sphincter damage caused by rectal distention by larger-caliber, harder stools.

Chronic oral bowel stimulant medication use has been questioned because of concerns of developing the atonic "cathartic bowel" syndrome. Certain stimulants, especially in the anthraquinone family (senna, cascara, aloes), have been shown to damage myenteric neurons with chronic use.[11, 46] It has not been established whether late complications from chronic oral bowel stimulant medications occur in those with neurogenic bowel dysfunction. Approaches that appear effective initially need longer-term studies to verify their continued benefits, especially since there is a high incidence of late GI problems reported in an initially successfully managed SCI population.[51]

Triggering of defecation can be accomplished by digital stimulation, rectal stimulant medications, enemas, or electrical stimulation. All of these cause reflex relaxation of the IAS, and if strong enough can reflexly relax the EAS as well. This initiates the rectorectal reflex that helps to eliminate any stool that is present. The GMC and mass movement associated with the call to stool for many intact persons often occurs at consistent times, which can be trainable. If a bowel habit (consistent time or times of day when defecation typically occurs for that individual) existed premorbidly, its consistency should be encouraged by inducing defecation at similar times. Such bowel habits might be a trainable event that also enhance adequate emptying if consistent training is used. A change from the patient's usual pattern can be habituated, but can take several weeks of inducing defecations at the new desired time before incontinence at the prior time subsides.[24]

Theoretically, fewer long-term complications will occur if the following are minimized: anorectal overdistention (as with enemas), anal trauma (as by manual disimpaction), and oral stimulant medication use. An accelerating enema volume required for efficacy should be a warning that chronic rectal overdistention might be leading to less responsiveness.[24] Digital stimulation to induce defecatory reflexes should be favored over manual disimpaction because the latter can easily result in inadvertent overstretching of the insensate and more delicate anal mechanisms of the neurogenic bowel. Local rectal stimulant suppositories and mini-enemas with bisacodyl or glycerin do not carry the same risk as oral stimulant medications and do not appear to lead to chronic inflammatory changes of the rectal mucosa.

One approach to initiating neurogenic bowel training is outlined in Table 28–3. Each step is added only after 2 weeks' consistent trial of the previous step has been ineffective. In this approach, obtaining elimination at the desired time is emphasized as the first step and usually precedes development of complete continence by several weeks. This regimen is designed to enhance responsiveness and emptying at the habituated time with apparently less responsiveness, or less rectal or stool presentation, during periods between bowel care sessions.

Bowel function is a very private matter, and patients might be reluctant to seek advice or information despite its major importance to their overall well-being and self-concept.[44, 48, 49] Information should be freely disseminated in order to enhance the development of healthy

TABLE 28–3 Protocol for Progressive Steps in Bowel Habituation Program

1. Perform bowel clean-out if stool is present in the rectal vault or palpable proximal to the descending colon, by multiple enemas or oral cathartic.
2. Titrate to soft stool consistency with diet and bulking agents (fiber) and stool softeners (docusate).
3. Trigger defecation with a glycerin suppository or by digital stimulation 20–30 minutes after a meal; 10 minutes later have the patient attempt defecation on toilet, limited to less than 40 minutes, and relieving skin pressure every 10 minutes.
4. If defecation is not initiated, a trial of a bisacodyl suppository PR is initiated.
5. Digital stimulation. Start 20 minutes after suppository placement and repeat every 5 minutes.
6. Timed oral medications. Administer casanthranol–docusate sodium (Peri-Colace), senna (Senokot), or bisacodyl (Dulcolax) tablets timed so that bowel movement would otherwise result 30 minutes to 1 hour after anticipated triggered bowel timing.
7. If defecation occurs in less than 10 minutes after suppository insertion, transition to digital stimulation technique only. Once the patient is well habituated, straining alone may rarely trigger defecations at a desired time.

Note: Steps 1 to 3 are initial interventions and are always followed, with steps 4 to 6 incorporated only as needed. At least 2 weeks' trial with proper technique is pursued before advancing to the next step.

habits and minimize bowel complications. Basic education in GI function can be presented by lectures, review of SCI care manual chapters,[22] booklets,[49] and videos.[50] Bowel habituation training is more difficult to accept among those with long-established patterns of managing stool hygiene, even if their current methods are ineffective in eliminating incontinence or constipation and are identified by the patient as unsatisfactory.[24] The advantages to a bowel program need to be explicitly communicated and illustrated using the patient's bowel record as evidence for effectiveness.[49]

Intrinsic loss of the ENS, or any segment, including by surgical reanastomosis, can result in loss of the rectoanal inhibitory reflex, causing DWE. Oral laxative abuse can cause dysfunction of the ENS.[11, 46] If bowel training is not accomplishing defecation at the desired times or if repeated involuntary incontinence occurs, further diagnostic evaluation might be indicated (see Table 28–2).

When neurogenic bowel deficits are incomplete and some degree of control and sensation is present, biofeedback might offer a means of enhancing the patient's residual sensory and motor abilities. Improved sensory awareness after biofeedback training is an indicator of success. This typically requires only a few sessions, and most patients improve after just one session.[44] Among more severely impaired nonselected myelomeningocele children, biofeedback and behavioral training are equally effective in restoring continence.[44] For selected individuals with some degree of volitional EAS activation and some degree of anorectal sensation, biofeedback can be a tool to help restore not just social continence, but also normal defecatory control.

Surgical Options

Sacral nerve deficits interfere with the action of the puborectalis, levator ani, and EAS (see Fig. 28–1). The resulting pelvic floor descent impairs the protective puborectalis sling angle and decreases the efficacy of protective EAS contractions. Some patients have benefited from transposition of innervated gracilis, adductor longus, gluteus maximus, or free muscle graft palmaris longus to replace puborectalis function and restore the acute anorectal junction angle that this sling provides. Chronic electrical stimulation to enhance development of fatigue resistance is used with these transplants. Sensory deficits are not improved, but continence is somewhat restored with the ability to inhibit defecation if some degree of sensation remains.[34, 44]

Incomplete EAS relaxation during defecation (dyssynergia) results in a functional outlet obstruction and DWE. A prolonged descending colon transit time occurs, which does improve with an IAS and partial EAS myotomy.[14] This procedure relieves constipation in 62% of patients but results in FI in 16% and therefore has not become a popular option.[36]

Stimulation of anterior sacral roots S2, S3, and S4 by transrectal electric stimulation or via a stimulator surgically placed for micturition has been performed.[6, 9, 17, 32] Stimulation of S2 tends to promote nonperistaltic, low-pressure colorectal motor activity. Stimulation of S3 causes occasional high-pressure peristaltic waves, especially with repetitive stimulation. Stimulation of S4 increases both rectal and anal tone.[32, 57] Electrodefecation has been obtainable by sacral root stimulation in up to 50% of patients, but remains unpredictable.[2, 6, 9, 10] A reliable electroprosthesis for defecation remains an elusive goal.[2, 17] Artificial anal sphincters with a subcutaneous pump reservoir similar to urinary artificial sphincters suffer from high complication rates and poor outcomes, and their use remains investigative.[34]

In clinical scenarios of prolonged bowel care time, recurrent fecal impactions, or poor or intermittent response to rectal medications to initiate bowel care, the options of the antegrade continence enema should be considered.[28, 35, 55] This is an alternative method of orthograde enema delivery that requires the surgical construction of a catheterizable appendicocecostomy stoma. Through a horizontal right lower quadrant incision the appendix and right colon are mobilized and brought against the abdominal wall. The tip of the appendix is then amputated and the opening into the appendix lumen is modified into a catheterizable stoma on the abdominal wall. This stoma can be catheterized and infused with 200 to 600 mL of tap water to trigger a propulsive colonic peristalsis and defecation within 10 to 20 minutes.[61] Bowel care can then be additionally facilitated with digital stimulation in the usual fashion.

Colostomy has been shown to reduce bowel care time, especially when offered to those with chronic DWE.[43, 52] It may be indicated in three general scenarios: (1) when conservative medical measures and training have failed,[26, 48] (2) when intrinsic bowel deficits exist such as in Hirschsprung's disease, Chagas' disease, "cathartic colon," and when pressure ulcers or other skin lesions occur that cannot be effectively healed because of frequent soiling, or (3) when recurrent urinary tract seeding by repetitive bowel impactions occurs.[12, 43, 52] Although diversion for pressure ulcer healing is usually anticipated to be reversed, those with neurogenic bowel often elect to maintain the colostomy even after the pressure ulcer has healed.[43, 52] Colostomy carries a surgical risk, is cosmetically disfiguring, and is seldom necessary to achieve adequate social continence, but it remains a procedure of last resort for the treatment of FI or DWE.[2, 12, 26, 48, 51]

Complications

Significant bowel complications requiring medical treatment or lifestyle alterations are reported by 27% of SCI persons by 5 years or greater beyond their injury, even though bowel management was satisfactory during the first 5 years. Over 80% of persons with SCI had bowel impactions, and 20% had chronic bowel impaction and DWE problems.[51] Impactions have been reported to be complicated by perforation or even death.[60] Impactions have a morbidity ranging between 0% and 6% in the normal population, being higher in the cognitively impaired elderly.[60] Other late GI complications reported by SCI patients include gastroesophageal reflux, premature diverticulosis, and autonomic dysreflexia.[18, 51] Morbidity from colonic perforation by enema use has also been reported.[30]

Hemorrhoids are more symptomatic when patients have intact sensation, but in one study rectal bleeding due to hemorrhoids was reported by 74% of SCI patients.[51] Hemorrhoids develop as a result of frequent high pressures in the anorectal marginal veins and are associated with constipated hard stool passage. Stool softening is the best preventive and chronic treatment measure, but it should be balanced with the requirement to modulate stool consistency to maintain continence.

An overstretched patulous noncompetent sphincter associated with rectal prolapse often is the end result of chronic passage of very large hard stools through a weakened anorectal mechanism in LMNB. Overdistention of the weakened neurogenic anal mechanism should be avoided by use of stool softening and gentle care to dilate the sphincter whenever manual disimpaction is required, to minimize trauma to these denervated structures. Although the anus can be significantly dilated to accommodate two fingers for breaking up low impactions, anorectal overdistention has been hypothesized to lead to atonic segments similar to bladder overdistention. The bowel, however, cannot be as easily decompressed and rested to allow recovery as can the bladder. The IAS is smooth muscle that will shorten and remodel to eventually regain competent closure if the overstretching can be eliminated. Unfortunately, this might require months of incontinent, liquid to soft pasty stools, which is seldom tolerated. Should the patient require temporary colostomy for some other disease process, it might be possible, after many months, to then train toward social continence with the decompressed and restored IAS. However, such patients have usually had long courses of constant soiling and often prefer to keep their colostomy and continence rather than pursue surgical reversal and training.

Autonomic dysreflexia occurs in SCI patients with lesions at or above the midthoracic region. FI is a common and potentially dangerous cause of autonomic dysreflexia because of the substantial time that may be required for its clearance (see Chapter 55). If manual disimpaction is required, lubrication with lidocaine gel is recommended to decrease additional nociceptive sensory input from the richly innervated anal region.

Bloating and abdominal distention are common complaints of patients with neurogenic bowel dysfunction. These complaints can be reduced in SCI patients by increasing the frequency of bowel care. This complaint can be especially severe in those with hyperactive EAS protective responses to rectal distention, which can preclude the passing of flatus. Digital release of flatus might be required, in addition to diet modification to eliminate foods that produce excessive gases. The workup should also include assessment for any contributing aerophagia (air swallowing).

Treatment Outcomes

Bowel habituation training in children with myelomeningocele by means of suppositories, digital stimulation, or both resulted in 83% of compliant patients having less than one incontinent stool per month.[24] The continence catheter enema, which has a distal rectal balloon to avoid immediate enema expulsion, when used daily or every other day, reduced fecal incontinence to fewer than three episodes per month in children with myelomeningocele.[45]

FI nursing home residents with dementia evaluated to have UMNB were treated by medically constipating them (with codeine) and giving biweekly enemas. Those diagnosed to have LMNB had their stools softened with lactulose and received weekly enemas. Fecal continence was restored in 80% of those consistently treated by these protocols.[56]

Although all complete SCI patients have episodic FI,[33] this is a chronic problem for only 2%.[49] DWE appears to be a progressive problem that develops 5 years or more after SCI. This is rarely reported after training in the first 4 years but occurs in 20% by a mean of 17 years after injury.[49] GI problems in SCI are not merely nuisances; they also account for 10% of SCI late mortality.[18]

Patients with multiple sclerosis, parkinsonism, or muscular dystrophy have also been helped by methods to enhance bowel storage or elimination in the setting of deteriorating neuromuscular and anorectal function.[2, 8] Colostomy can also provide a means of achieving social continence in these patients. Colostomy complications include embarrassing gas problems, appliance loosening and leakage, and cosmetic difficulties.

Patients who develop social bowel continence can venture into public without fear of malodorous embarrassment and unpredictable social disaster that humiliates as well as requires substantial clean-up time. When such fears persist, full social and vocational reintegration is impeded. A major hurdle that many patients with neuromuscular compromise can overcome is control of the seemingly automatic neurogenic functions of defecation and bowel elimination. Such patients should not needlessly suffer because inadequate attention has been paid by care providers to this potentially functionally impairing and socially disabling deficit.

Many solutions are yet to come for the large number of persons who cope with neurogenic bowel dysfunction. The colon will continue to be a fertile area for research.[48]

REFERENCES

1. Aaronson MJ, Freed MM, Burakoff R: Colonic myolectric activity in persons with spinal cord injury. Dig Dis Sci 1985; 30:295–300.
2. Banwell JG, Creaswey GH, Aggarwal AM, et al: Management of the neurogenic bowel in patients with spinal cord injury. Urol Clin North Am 1993; 20:523.
3. Bartolo DC, Read NW, Jarratt JA, et al: Differences in anal sphincter function and clinical presentation in patients with pelvic floor descent. Gastroenterology 1983; 85:68–75.
4. Beuret-Blanquart F, Weber J, Gouverneur JP, et al: Colonic transit time and anorectal manometric anomalies in 19 patients with complete transection of the spinal cord. J Auton Nerv Syst 1990; 30:199–208.
5. Boss BJ, Pecanty L, McFarland SM, et al: Self-care competence among persons with spinal cord injury. SCI Nursing 1995; 12: 48–53.

6. Brindley GS, Rushton DN: Long-term follow-up of patients with sacral anterior root stimulator implants. Paraplegia 1990; 28: 469–475.
7. Cameron K, Nyulasi I, Collier G, et al: Assessment of the effect of increased dietary fibre intake on bowel function in patients with spinal cord injury. Spinal Cord 1996; 34:277–283.
8. Caroscio JT: Amyotrophic Lateral Sclerosis: A Guide to Patient Care. New York, Thieme, 1986, p 126.
9. Chia YW, Lee TK, Kour NW, et al: Microchip implants on the anterior sacral roots in patients with spinal trauma: Does it improve bowel function? Dis Colon Rectum 1996; 39:690–694.
10. Christensen J: The motor function of the colon. In Yamada T (ed): Textbook of Gastroenterology. Philadelphia, JB Lippincott, 1991, pp 180–196.
11. Cummings JH: Laxative abuse. Gut 1974; 15:758–766.
12. Deshmukh G, Barkel D, Sevo D, et al: Use or misuse of colostomy to heal pressure ulcers. Dis Colon Rectum 1996; 39:737–738.
13. Devroede G: Constipation. In Sleisenger MH, Fordtran JS (eds): Gastrointestinal Disease. Philadelphia, WB Saunders, 1993, pp 837–887.
14. Devroede G, Lamarche J: Functional importance of extrinsic parasympathetic innervation in the distal colon and rectum in man. Gastroenterology 1974; 66:273–280.
15. Dikenson VA: Maintenance of anal continence: A review of pelvic floor physiology. Gut 1978; 19:1163–1174.
16. Doughty DB, Jackson DB: Gastrointestinal Disorders. St Louis, Mosby–Year Book, 1993, p 268.
17. Frost F, Hartwig D, Jaeger R, et al: Electrical stimulation of the sacral dermatomes in spinal cord injury: Effect on rectal manometry and bowel emptying. Arch Phys Med Rehabil 1993; 74: 696–701.
18. Gore RM, Mintzer RA, Calenoff L: Gastrointestinal complications of spinal cord injury. Spine 1981; 6:538–544.
19. Goyal RK, Crist JR: Neurology of the gut. In Sleisenger MH, Fordtran JS (eds): Gastrointestinal Disease. Philadelphia, WB Saunders, 1989, pp 21–52.
20. Granger CV, Hamilton BB, Gresham GE, et al: The stroke rehabilitation outcome study: Part II. Relative merits of the total Barthel Index score and a four-item subscore in predicting patient outcomes. Arch Phys Med Rehabil 1989; 70:100–108.
21. Guyton AC: Textbook of Medical Physiology, ed 8. Philadelphia, WB Saunders, 1991, pp 731–735, 742.
22. Hammond MC, Umlauf RL, Matteson B, et al: Yes you can!: A guide to self-care for persons with spinal cord injury. Washington, DC, Paralyzed Veterans Organization of America, 1989, p 361.
23. Hanson R, Franklin M: Sexual loss in relation to other functional losses for spinal cord injured males. Arch Phys Med Rehabil 1976; 57:291–293.
24. King JC, Currie DM, Wright E: Bowel training in spina bifida: Importance of education, patient compliance, age, and anal reflexes. Arch Phys Med Rehabil 1994; 75:243–247.
25. King JC, Nelson R, Tuturro T, et al: Prescriptions, referrals, and the rehabilitation team. In Delisa JA: Rehabilitation Medicine Principles and Practice, ed 3. Philadelphia, JB Lippincott, 1998.
26. King R, Biddle A, Braunschweig C, et al: Neurogenic bowel management in adults with spinal cord injury. J Spinal Cord Med 1998; 21:248–293.
27. Kirshblum SC, Gulati M, O'Connor KC, et al: Bowel care practices in chronic spinal cord injury patients. Arch Phys Med Rehabil 1998; 79:20–23.
28. Koyle M, Kaji D, Duque M, et al: The Malone antegrade continence enema for neurogenic and structural fecal incontinence and constipation. J Urol 1995; 154:759–761.
29. Levi R, Hulting C, Nash M, et al: The Stockholm spinal cord injury study: 1. Medical problems in a regional SCI population. Paraplegia 1995; 33:308–315.
30. Liptak GS, Reveli GM: Management of bowel dysfunction in children with spinal cord disease or injury by means of the enema continence catheter. J Pediatr 1992; 120:190–194.
31. Longo WE, Ballantyne GH, Modlin IM: The colon, anorectum, and spinal cord patient. Dis Colon Rectum 1989; 32:261–267.
32. MacDonagh R, Sun W, Smallwood R: Anorectal function in patients with complete supraconal spinal cord lesions. Gut 1992; 33:1532–1538.
33. MacDonagh RP, Sun WM, Smallwood R, et al: Control of defecation in patients with spinal injuries by stimulation of sacral anterior nerve roots. Br Med J 1990; 300:1494–1497.
34. Madoff RD, Williams JG, Caushaj PF: Fecal incontinence. N Engl J Med 1992; 326:1002–1007.
35. Malone P, Ransley P, Kiely E: Preliminary report: The antegrade continence enema. Lancet 1990; 336:1217–1218.
36. Martelli H, Devroede G, Arhan P, et al: Mechanisms of idiopathic constipation: Outlet obstruction. Gastroenterology 1978; 75:623–631.
37. Martelli H, Devroede G, Arhan P, et al: Some parameters of large bowel motility in normal man. Gastroenterology 1978; 75:612.
38. Menardo G, Baujano G, Corazziari E: Large bowel transit in paraplegic patients. Dis Colon Rectum 1987; 30:924–928.
39. Meshkinpour H, Nowroozi F, Glick M: Colonic compliance in patients with spinal cord injury. Arch Phys Med Rehabil 1983; 64:111–112.
40. Nino-Murcia M, Stone J, Chang P, et al: Colonic transit in spinal cord-injured patients. Invest Radiol 1990; 25:109–112.
41. Pedersen E: Regulation of bladder and colon-rectum in patients with spinal lesions. J Auton Nerv Syst 1983; 7:329–338.
42. Rendtorff RC, Kashgarian M: Stool patterns of healthy adult males. Dis Colon Rectum 1967; 10:222.
43. Saltzstein R, Romano J: The efficacy of colostomy as a bowel management alternative in selected spinal cord injured patients. J Am Paraplegia Soc 1990; 13:9–13.
44. Schiller LR: Fecal incontinence. In Sleisenger MH, Fordtran JS (eds): Gastrointestinal Disease. Philadelphia, WB Saunders, 1993, pp 934–953.
45. Shandling B, Gilmour RF: The enema continence catheter in spina bifida: Successful bowel management. J Pediatr Surg 1987; 22:271–273.
46. Smith B: Effect of irritant purgatives on the myenteric plexus in man and mouse. Gut 1968; 9:139–143.
47. Stiens S, Goetz L: Neurogenic bowel dysfunction. In O'Young B, Young M, Stiens S (eds): Physical Medicine and Rehabilitation Secrets. Philadelphia: Hanley & Belfus, 1997, pp 460–464.
48. Stiens SA, Biener Bergman S, Goetz LL: Neurogenic bowel dysfunction after spinal cord injury: Clinical evaluation and rehabilitative management. Arch Phys Med Rehabil 1997; 78:S-86–S-102.
49. Stiens SA, Braunschweig C, Cowel F, et al: Neurogenic Bowel: What You Should Know. A Guide for People with Spinal Cord Injury. Washington, DC, Consortium for Spinal Cord Medicine, 1999, p 53.
50. Stiens SA, Piddie T, Veland B, et al: Accidents Stink. Video, Bowel Care 202 video. Washington, DC, Paralyzed Veterans of America Education and Training Foundation, in press.
51. Stone J, Nino-Murcia M, Wolf V, et al: Chronic gastrointestinal problems in spinal cord injury patients: A prospective analysis. Am J Gastroenterol 1990; 85:114–119.
52. Stone J, Wolfe V, Nino-Murcia M: Colostomy as treatment for complications of spinal cord injury. Arch Phys Med Rehabil 1990; 71:514–518.
53. Suckling P: The ball-valve rectum due to impacted feces. Lancet 1962; 2:1147.
54. Swash M: New concepts in the prevention of incontinence. Practitioner 1985; 229:895–899.
55. Teichman JMH, Barber DM, Rogenes VJ, et al: Malone antegrade continence enemas for autonomic dysreflexia secondary to neurogenic bowel. J Spinal Cord Med 1998; 160:1278–1281.
56. Tobin GW, Brocklehurst JC: Faecal incontinence in residential homes for the elderly: Prevalence, aetiology and management. Age Aging 1986; 15:41–46.
57. Varma J: Autonomic influences on colorectal motility and pelvic surgery. World J Surg 1992; 16:811–819.
58. White J, Verlot M, Ehrentheil O: Neurogenic disturbances of the colon and their investigation by the colonmetrogram. Ann Surg 1949; 112:1042–1057.
59. Wingate DL, Ewart WR: The brain-gut axis. In Yamada T (ed): Textbook of Gastroenterology. Philadelphia, JB Lippincott, 1991, pp 50–60.
60. Wrenn K: Fecal impaction. N Engl J Med 1989; 321:658–662.
61. Yang CC, Stiens SA: Antegrade continence enema for the treatment of neurogenic constipation and fecal incontinence after spinal cord injury. J Spinal Cord Med, in press.

29 CHAPTER

Richard T. Katz, M.D., Julius P.A. Dewald, P.T., Ph.D., and Brian D. Schmit, Ph.D.

Spasticity

Spasticity is more difficult to characterize than to recognize, and still more difficult to quantify. Occurring in a variety of central nervous system disorders, spastic hypertonia has both diagnostic and therapeutic significance. Diagnostically, it is a hallmark of an upper motor neuron disorder; therapeutically, it represents one of the most important impairments for individuals who care for patients with central nervous system disease. The following discussion of spastic hypertonia is divided into three parts: (1) pathophysiology, (2) methods of quantifying spasticity, and (3) therapeutic management.

PATHOPHYSIOLOGY

According to a widely accepted definition, spasticity is "a motor disorder characterized by a velocity-dependent increase in tonic stretch reflexes (muscle tone) with exaggerated tendon jerks, resulting from hyperexcitability of the stretch reflex, as one component of the upper motor neuron syndrome."[31] Muscle tone may be characterized as "the sensation of resistance felt as one manipulates a joint through a range of motion, with the subject attempting to relax."[32] Although this definition is adequate for the bedside clinical examination, a more rigorous analysis indicates that the sensation of resistance is likely to result from several distinct components: (1) physical inertia of the extremity, (2) altered viscoelastic characteristics of muscular and connective tissues, and (3) reflex muscle activation due to hyperactive stretch reflexes. Because inertia of the limb does not change after an upper motor neuron lesion, it is clear that the heightened resistance on bedside examination represents changes in the musculotendinous unit (e.g., contracture), and/or changes within the segmental reflex arc (hyperactive stretch reflexes).

Changes in Passive Muscle Properties

The passive stiffness of a muscle is one contributor to muscle tone. Passive stiffness is defined as the slope of a curve relating joint torque to the angle of joint displacement with the test subject relaxed and without reflex or voluntary activation of relevant muscles. This stiffness can be estimated by studying the tension elicited when a joint is extended through a given arc at low stretch velocities. Changes in passive stiffness could be mediated by permanent structural changes in the mechanical properties of muscle connective tissues, or could be variable in character. In either case, the changes in passive stiffness would appear as an increase in the resistance to limb extension, without a commensurate increase in muscle excitation as measured by the electromyogram.

It has been proposed that *changes in the muscle mechanical properties* (rather than stretch reflex enhancement) are largely responsible for spastic hypertonia.[16] These claims are based on electromyographic and tension analysis of leg muscles of hemiplegic adults and cerebral palsy children during ambulation. Abnormally high tension developed in the spastic triceps surae during passive stretch without a parallel increase in electromyographic activity. Arguably, these EMG findings, coupled with observations of temperature effects on muscle response, suggest a change in the mechanical response of muscle to stretch.

Although this idea is highly interesting and provocative, this observation may be explained equally well by some form of degenerative or atrophic change in muscle structure, such as precipitous muscle atrophy with collagenous and elastic tissue infiltration. There are no present grounds to propose an anomalous change in the physiological muscle response to stretch. Moreover, this

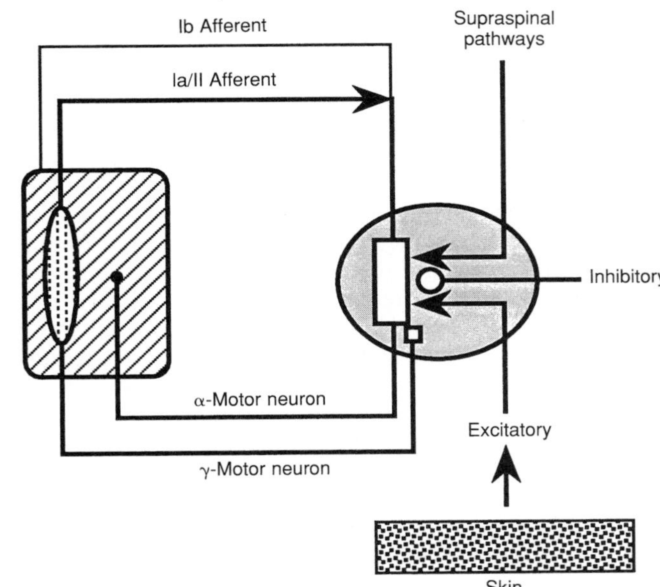

FIGURE 29–1. The basic neural circuitry is the segmental reflex arc, which consists of muscle receptors, their central connections with spinal cord neurons, and the motoneuronal output to muscle. This outflow is the summation of a host of different synaptic and modulatory influences, including (1) excitatory post-synaptic potentials from group Ia and II muscle spindle afferents; (2) inhibitory post-synaptic potentials from interneuronal connections from antagonistic muscles and Golgi tendon organs; and (3) presynaptic inhibition initiated by descending fiber input.

"intrinsic" muscle hypothesis does not easily account for many established findings—such as hyperexcitable stretch reflexes and increased tendon jerks—which indicate that motoneuron excitability is also markedly increased.

Neural Mechanisms for Stretch Reflex Hyperactivity

The basic neural circuit on which to build a framework for understanding spastic hypertonia is the segmental reflex arc. This arc consists of muscle receptors, their central connections with spinal cord neurons, and the motoneuronal output to muscle (Fig. 29–1). Within this arc, the alpha motor neuron may be likened to a final conduit for motoneuronal outflow. This outflow is the summation of many synaptic and modulatory influences, including (1) excitatory post-synaptic potentials from group Ia and II muscle spindle afferents, (2) inhibitory post-synaptic potentials from interneuronal connections from antagonistic muscles and Golgi tendon organs, and (3) presynaptic inhibition via interneurons modulated by descending fiber input. Presynaptic inhibition is exerted via interneurons which end on primary afferent nerve terminals and which reduce the ability of sensory afferents to depolarize the post-synaptic membrane (by changing calcium and/or potassium conductances). Exteroceptive (e.g., cutaneous) and interoceptive (e.g., visceral) afferent information can also provide important input into the spinal segmental reflex arc.

Within this framework, there are two distinct ways in which stretch reflex hyperexcitability could be explained. The first is by selectively increasing motoneuronal excitability, which is reflected as an increased motoneuronal response to a particular level of stretch-evoked synaptic input. The second is by *increasing the amount of excitatory synaptic input elicited by muscle extension.* Various mechanisms can be responsible for such changes, as summarized in Table 29–1. While both mechanisms may co-exist, it is useful to examine the possibilities independently.

Increased Motoneuronal Excitability. *Alpha motoneuron hyperexcitability* implies that increased motor neuron recruitment and/or increased discharge are elicited with lower than normal levels of excitatory input. That is, either a smaller stretch amplitude or a slower than usual stretch velocity would excite motoneurons. Similarly, synaptic input elicited by synchronous electrical excitation of Ia afferent fibers (e.g., the H reflex) or mechanical excitation (muscle stretch reflex) would result in an augmented evoked response in muscle. The

TABLE 29–1 Possible Neural Mechanisms for Spastic Hypertonia

- I. Increased motoneuronal excitability
  - A. Excitatory synaptic input is enhanced
    1. Segmental afferents
    2. Regional excitatory interneurons
    3. Descending pathways, i.e., lateral vestibulospinal tract
  - B. Inhibitory synaptic input is reduced
    1. Renshaw cell recurrent inhibition
    2. Ia Inhibitory interneurons
    3. Ib Afferent fibers
  - C. Change in the intrinsic electrical properties of the neuron
    1. Changes in passive membrane electrical properties
    2. Changes in voltage sensitive membrane conductance
- II. Enhanced stretch-evoked synaptic excitation of motoneurons
  - A. Gamma efferent hyperactivity
  - B. Excitatory interneurons more sensitive to muscle afferent
    1. Collateral sprouting
    2. Denervation hypersensitivity
    3. Decrease in presynaptic inhibition

evidence for enhanced motoneuronal excitability in spasticity is very strong.

Increased excitability could arise if motoneurons are more depolarized than usual, so that they are perched close to their threshold for recruitment. Increased depolarization could arise either (1) because *tonic excitatory input is enhanced* (e.g., from segmental afferents, regional excitatory interneurons, or monosynaptic descending pathways such as the lateral vestibulospinal tracts), or (2) because there is a *reduction of inhibitory synaptic input* from regional inhibitory interneurons (such as Renshaw cell recurrent inhibition, Ia inhibitory interneurons, or Ib afferent interneurons). There is substantial evidence for an increased tonic drive of α-motoneuron as an important contributor to spasticity.

Motor neurons could also exhibit increased excitability because of a *change in the intrinsic electrical properties of the neurons.* Possible mechanisms could include a change in passive membrane electrical properties (such as resistance and/or capacitance), or change in the normal ionic conductance mechanisms. Both types of disturbance could result in a larger than normal voltage change and a resulting increase in motoneuronal activity, without commensurate change in stretch reflex threshold. To date, no convincing evidence supports the notion of a change in the intrinsic membrane properties in chronic spastic animals.

Increased Stretch-Evoked Synaptic Excitation of Motoneurons. An increased motor neuron response to stretch might also arise by virtue of an augmented synaptic input resulting from muscle stretch. That is, spasticity could arise if muscle afferent discharges were to increase the excitatory synaptic current flowing to the motor neuron—either directly from muscle afferent terminals or via interposed interneurons. This increased synaptic current could arise (1) if muscle spindle afferents were to exhibit enhanced response to stretch due to changes in spindle properties, (2) if there were a reduction in presynaptic or Renshaw (autogenic) inhibition, or (3) if there were changes in force feedback via Ib afferents.

Previously, spastic hypertonia was attributed to hyperactivity of the gamma efferent fibers (*gamma spasticity* in older nomenclature), causing an increased sensitivity of the muscle spindle receptor to change in muscle length. This hypothesis was based on the observation that spasticity diminished when nerves were infiltrated with dilute local anesthetic at concentrations appropriate for blocking fusimotor input. Although stretch reflexes can be diminished by gamma efferent blockade, this does not prove that spasticity is due to hyperactivity within afferent limbs of the reflex arc. If this were true, blockade of gamma fibers would induce loss of tone in normal as well as abnormal muscle, since voluntary alpha motor neuron activation is normally accompanied by significant gamma activation. To determine whether the level of gamma activity is abnormal in spastic muscle would require that the effects of gamma blockade be compared in normal and spastic muscle at equivalent levels of motor output, a prohibitively difficult experimental protocol to implement.

Experimental evidence to date does not support the concept of enhanced gamma efferent hyperactivity. Microneurographic recordings of spindle afferent discharge have been used to evaluate the levels of gamma activation. Microneurography, in which a tungsten steel microelectrode is used to impale human peripheral nerves, has also failed to confirm fusimotor hyperactivity. Similarly, studies of spindle responses in monkeys after cortical ablation also fail to reveal an excess of fusimotor activity after the development of spastic hypertonia.

Three mechanisms have been proposed whereby interposed excitatory interneurons become more responsive to muscle afferent input: (1) collateral sprouting, (2) denervation hypersensitivity, and (3) changes in presynaptic inhibition. First, in the course of post-injury recovery, muscle afferents could undergo sprouting of their terminal branches, to accommodate synaptic sites vacated by destruction of supraspinal tracts. *Collateral sprouting* has been observed in spinal cord and autonomic nervous systems, as well as in several specific regions of the brain. In principle, sprouting could also help explain the significant delay before spastic hypertonia appears after a spinal cord injury (SCI). However, there is little support for the view that collateral sprouting is an important process in spinal cord reorganization following partial deafferentation. Models of sprouting in the mammalian central nervous system typically require much more radical removal of afferent input to a spinal neuron than is likely to arise in most supraspinal lesions.

Second, synapses that lose their presynaptic terminals may become more sensitive to ambient transmitter effects. Studies utilizing chemical destruction of descending spinal cord tracts mediated by monoamines (serotonin and norepinephrine) lend support to the idea of *denervation hypersensitivity* as a contributing factor to spastic hypertonia. Exaggerated extensor hind limb reflexes are observed after administration of serotonergic agonists in animals whose serotonergic systems were chemically destroyed, and similarly exaggerated flexor reflexes were noted in animals with noradrenergic destruction. Histochemical studies of serotonergic and noradrenergic receptor density have demonstrated a nearly complete degeneration of these receptors approximately two weeks after axonotomy, followed by a regeneration of terminal density to 50% to 66% of original levels after three to six months. The regeneration of these terminals suggests that surviving fibers may have produced new sprouts by the mechanisms of collateral sprouting, and reinnervated the empty synaptic sites.

Finally, enhanced synaptic excitation could also arise if the *level of baseline presynaptic inhibition were reduced,* since this would result in a greater than normal release of transmitter for each incoming afferent impulse. Evidence for this has been based largely on the failure of the tonic vibration reflex (TVR) to suppress the H reflex in the spastic patient. In this paradigm a tonic vibratory stimulus is applied to a limb, usually the lower extremity. Tonic vibration has been shown to preferentially and repetitively drive Ia afferent fibers. They exert their inhibitory characteristics by way of an interneuron which is both excited by Ia afferent input, then acts on terminal Ia fiber arborizations. This interneuron is strongly modulated by descending pyramidal (corticospinal) and extrapyramidal (vestibulospinal, reticulospinal) tracts; hence the TVR can help to elucidate the role of these descending fibers on the segmental reflex arc.

When an electrical stimulus is applied to the tibial nerve in normal subjects, the predominantly monosynaptic Hoffman (H) reflex is noted approximately 30 msec later in the triceps surae. This H reflex is partially suppressed in normal subjects when the TVR is applied to the limb. The *failure* of the TVR to effectively inhibit the H reflex in those with spasticity has been a strong argument implicating diminished presynaptic inhibition as a mechanism contributing to spastic hypertonia. Presynaptic inhibition may act (1) by limiting the magnitude of calcium current moving into primary afferent terminals, or (2) by increasing potassium conductances and thereby hyperpolarizing the resulting primary axon terminals. The net result is a reduction in transmitter release. Recent investigation of the H reflex in the spastic hind limbs of a chronic spinal hemisectioned rat demonstrated a reduced dependence on H reflex stimulus frequency, supporting the concept of alteration in presynaptic inhibition.[51]

Supraspinal Mechanisms

Descending tracts contribute to spastic muscle hypertonia either via monosynaptic excitatory projections to lower motoneurons (e.g., from the corticospinal tracts), or indirectly by inhibition or facilitation of interneurons within spinal reflex pathways.

Changes in Motoneuron Excitability. Changes in motoneuronal excitability might be contingent primarily on changes in the "baseline" levels of depolarization of the motoneuron, rather than on changes in intrinsic motor neuron properties. The increased baseline depolarization depends on the net *tonic* excitatory synaptic input that is converging on the neuron from descending pathways or segmental interneuronal input.

The lateral vestibulospinal pathway is important for the development of the increased excitability in axial and extensor muscle alpha motor neurons that characterizes supraspinal forms of spastic hypertonia. Most excitatory contributions from the vestibulospinal system are likely provided via local excitatory interneurons. It is also likely that the excitation or inhibition mediated by descending reticulospinal fibers originating in the medulla and pons is mediated largely by segmental interneurons.

Changes in Segmental Reflex Function. Loss of the supraspinal inhibition on regional interneurons, especially from reticulospinal tracts, is also likely to be very important in spinal forms of spasticity. The loss of inhibition may result from direct pathway interruption (as in spinal or brainstem injury), or secondary to the loss of supraspinal facilitation of brainstem reticulospinal neurons (whose discharge can be reduced or even silenced). These reductions in descending input release powerful segmental reflexes that are normally suppressed.

The Babinski reflex, which inevitably accompanies spastic hypertonia, represents a transition from the normal plantar reflex to a more diffusely organized flexion withdrawal response. The normal plantar reflex promotes postural stability by increasing the grip of the digits on the terrain, not unlike the feline plantar cushion reflex. The Babinski reflex is a more diffusely organized flexion withdrawal reflex in which toes, ankles, and even more proximal joints are progressively flexed.

The clasp-knife reflex is a second and less common manifestation. It is characterized by an abrupt reduction of EMG activity and force once a spastic muscle is stretched through a particular length. The term "clasp-knife" is used because the initial high resistance to stretch is interrupted by the onset of inhibition. The resistance declines abruptly, similar to an old-fashioned clasp-knife. Recent evidence suggests that the clasp-knife is a reflection of the activity of group III and IV mechanoreceptors, which become pronounced due to the reduced descending inhibition of segmental interneurons. Yet another example of the alteration in reflex responsiveness is the facilitation of flexor reflexes coupled with the inhibition of antagonist extensors, presumably via the Ia reciprocal inhibitory interneuron. The clasp-knife reflex is again illustrative, as inhibition of triceps and quadriceps is accompanied by an excitation of the opposing flexors.

In summary, spasticity can be characterized by a combination of two major disturbances, both mediated by alterations in the balance of descending pathway activity. The first induces an increase in excitability of motoneurons innervating antigravity muscles (which are physiological extensors in the legs, and flexors in the arms), and the second changes the patterns of reflex responsiveness of many segmental reflexes, often promoting flexor muscle activity and reduced extensor activity.

Pathways Responsible for Modifications in Descending Control in Spasticity. Cortex, basal ganglia, and cerebellum all provide important modulation of brainstem structures in normal motor control. Selective destruction of corticospinal tracts does not result in spastic hypertonia, but rather hypotonia and loss of fine hand movements. Interruption of extrapyramidal fibers is needed before spastic hypertonia develops. Lesions of particular premotor cortical sites (Brodman areas 4 and 6) result in hypotonia followed by hypertonic hemiparesis. Bilateral premotor damage causes spasticity that is more severe.

It is not yet clear which pathways are instrumental in mediating the increase in motor neuron excitability. However, it seems likely that the alterations in segmental interneuronal responsiveness follow loss of activity in the dorsal reticulospinal system. This pathway appears to require substantial facilitation from corticobulbar projections. After extensive white matter lesions, which diminish the excitatory inflow to the brainstem, there is a reduction of the descending inhibition of segmental interneurons.

It is also possible that descending monoaminergic systems from the locus ceruleus pathways are involved in regulating the excitability of segmental circuits. These pathways may be damaged directly in spinal cord injury, or lose cortical excitatory drive, causing them to reduce their inhibitory control of segmental interneurons. This reduced inhibition may (1) release segmental interneurons subserving cutaneous or muscle-based inhibitory pathways, and/or (2) release excitatory interneurons receiving input from secondary spindle afferents.

Upper Motor Neuron Syndrome

Patients with lesions of cortical, subcortical, and spinal cord structures exhibit a wide variety of abnormal behaviors beyond those attributable to hypertonia. We use the term *upper motor neuron (UMN) syndrome* to describe such changes. Careful study of patients with UMN syndrome reveals that motor difficulties can be divided into abnormal behaviors (positive symptoms) and performance deficits (negative symptoms) (Table 29–2).

Positive symptoms are easily recognized in disorders of the spinal cord. Symptoms include exaggerated flexion reflexes and a positive Babinski response. Release of reflexes from descending inhibitory control causes flexor or adductor spasms. Flexor spasms may become so severe that a paraplegic person requires the help of restraints in order to remain in a wheelchair. "Scissoring" due to spastic hip adductors can limit a spastic person's ability to ambulate effectively. Clonus, cyclical hyperactivity of antagonistic muscles in response to stretch, may become so severe as to prevent functional muscle groups from performing effectively.

Another frequently overlooked component of the UMN syndrome is the loss of precise autonomic control. Loss of UMN modulation of spinal autonomic mechanisms can produce a disorganization of autonomic function below the level of SCI. When spinal cord lesions are above the mid-thoracic level, seemingly innocuous sensory input can result in a potential hypertensive crisis. This response is one component of autonomic dysreflexia, a gross nonselective "mass response." Disorganization of sympathetic activity below the level of SCI may be responsible for autonomic dysreflexia, but mechanisms other than exaggerated sympathetic outflow may contribute as well.

Negative symptoms are performance deficits and are more frequently observed in hemiparetic patients than in spinal cord forms of spasticity. Movements are often weak, easily fatigued, and lacking in dexterity. Several physiological factors may contribute to these performance deficits. The loss of orderly recruitment and rate modulation of motoneurons results in inefficient muscle activation, early loss of force, augmented subject effort, and the clinical perception of weakness. High-threshold motor units with rapid rates of adaptation are recruited early, and these "fast twitch" units are poorly suited to maintain sustained muscle contractions. Changes in mean motor unit discharge rates in paretic muscles may produce abnormal EMG-force relationships, where surface EMG activity is augmented per unit force generated. Twitch-contraction time of fast motor units has also been shown to change in hand muscles of hemiplegic limbs.

TABLE 29–2 Upper Motor Neuron Syndrome

Abnormal Behaviors (positive symptoms)
Reflex release phenomena
Hyperactive proprioceptive reflexes
Increased resistance to stretch
Relaxed cutaneous reflexes
Loss of precise autonomic control
Performance Deficits (negative symptoms)
Decreased dexterity
Paresis/weakness
Fatiguability

EMG recordings from spastic persons demonstrate disturbances of spatial patterns of muscle selection in hemiparetic limbs. EMG recordings from normal limbs during isometric torque generation at the elbow reveal an orderly pattern of recruitment of different muscles that contribute to movement at that joint. Each muscle is activated over a broad angular range in a symmetrical pattern, and the EMG pattern increases with escalating force. The peak EMG value occurs at the angle of maximum mechanical advantage. In contrast, spastic paretic limbs exhibit severe disturbances in the pattern of muscle activation. The angular range and spatial orientation are radically disturbed. For example, normal elbow flexor muscles are activated maximally in flexion. In the hemiparetic flexors show a substantial shift in the angle of peak EMG away from the normal angle.[15] More importantly, abnormal muscle co-activation patterns (synergies) arise between elbow flexors and shoulder adductors, elbow extensors and shoulder adductors.[15] These abnormal co-activation patterns likely have a greater detrimental impact on functional arm use after stroke then spasticity.

Finally, there is an alteration in the time-course of EMG activation in agonist and antagonist muscles. In normal limbs, rapid flexion of a joint is associated with a so-called triphasic pattern of EMG activation, in which the agonist muscle is activated in two sequential bursts and the antagonist is activated in the intervening interval. In the UMN syndrome the orderly timing may be lost, so that only a portion of the triphasic pattern is expressed. In the extreme, there is a poorly timed and ineffective simultaneous co-contraction of agonist and antagonist.

The evidence implicating hyperexcitable stretch reflexes to disturbances in voluntary movement subsequent to stroke is limited and contradictory. Some studies attribute a portion of the motor disturbance to an inappropriate stretch reflex response in the antagonist muscle on the basis of the velocity-dependent nature of the activation. In contrast, it has been suggested that upper extremity movement dysfunction after stroke may be more attributable to prolongation of agonist activation[48] or abnormal signal command.[35] This might help explain why anti-spastic therapies and surgical procedures may fail to produce significant improvements in motor performance.

Kinesiological analysis of hemiplegic ambulation offers valuable insight into abnormal motor behaviors. Spastic reflexes tested in a passive limb are not identical with those in movements actively performed by the patient. In some patients a low threshold for stretch reflex activation can be found at bedside examination in muscles that are not activated by the stretch imposed by ambulation. Such studies have demonstrated that there is a wide inter-individual variation in gait patterns among affected patients. However, all patients demonstrated varying degrees of (1) lowered stretch reflex threshold, (2) inadequate muscular activation, and (3) stereotyped co-activation of muscles in primitive locomotor patterns.[30]

In summary, relief of the hypertonic "spastic" components of the UMN syndrome does not necessarily imply enhanced performance. Synergy patterns, flexors spasms, paresis, loss of dexterity, and agonist/antagonist co-contraction are probably more disabling than the hypertonic response to stretch.

QUANTIFICATION OF SPASTIC HYPERTONIA

The quantification of spasticity is a challenging problem, made even more difficult because measurements tend to be highly observer-dependent.[28] The lack of effective measurement techniques has been quite restrictive, since quantification is necessary to evaluate various modes of treatment.[24] Measurement of day-to-day torque variations for a particular joint in one subject is probably valuable in quantifying the effects of a therapeutic intervention such as a drug or surgical procedure.

Efforts have included tabulation of functional activities, electromyographic and biomechanical analysis of limb resistance to mechanical displacement, rectified surface electromyographic responses to perturbation or voluntary movement, gait analysis, and a host of electrophysiological reflex studies. For a variety of reasons, no uniformly useful clinical measurements have yet emerged. Quantification has been hampered by changes in performance due to training effects, emotional status, and various systemic factors.

TABLE 29–3 Clinical Scale for Spastic Hypertonia

0	No increase in tone
1	Slight increase in muscle tone, manifested by a catch and release or by minimal resistance at the end of the range of motion when the affected part(s) is moved in flexion or extension
1+	Slight increase in muscle tone, manifested by a catch, followed by minimal resistance throughout the remainder (less than half) of the range of motion
2	More marked increase in muscle tone through most of the range of motion, but affected part(s) easily moved
3	Considerable increase in muscle tone, passive movement difficult
4	Affected part(s) rigid in flexion or extension

From Bohannon RW, Smith MB: Interrater reliability on a modified Ashworth scale of muscle spasticity. Phys Therapy 1987; 67:206–207.

TABLE 29–4 Fugl-Meyer Scale of Functional Return After Hemiplegia

Movement of the shoulder, elbow, forearm, and lower extremity

I	Muscle stretch reflexes can be elicited
II	Volitional movements can be performed within the dynamic flexor/extensor synergies
III	Volitional motion is performed mixing dynamic flexor and extensor synergies
IV	Volitional movements are performed with little or no synergy dependence
V	Normal muscle stretch reflexes

Wrist function—stability, flexion, extension, circumduction
Hand function
Mass flexion, mass extension, 5 different grasps
Coordination and speed—assess tremor, dysmetria, speed
Finger-to-nose test; heel-to-shin test
Balance
Sit without support
Parachute reaction—nonaffected side, affected side
Stand—supported, unsupported
Stand on nonaffected side, affected side
Sensation—light touch, position sense
Passive joint motion, joint pain

Clinical Scales

A clinical scale from 0 (normal muscle tone) to 4 (severe spasticity) was first proposed by Ashworth.[4] It offers ease of measurement, but may lack temporal and inter-examiner reproducibility. The Ashworth scale suffers from "clustering" of most patients within the middle grades. The patient is usually examined supine, and muscle stretch reflexes and passive muscle tone are assessed for the upper and lower extremities. A modification of the Ashworth scale that added an additional intermediate grade has high interrater reliability when testing elbow flexors (Table 29–3).[5] Clinical scales offer only qualitative information, but they the most widely used yardstick of spasticity.

The *Fugl-Meyer scale* (Table 29–4) is an accurate and objective method of assessing function (but not necessarily spastic hypertonia) in hemiplegic patients, based on the natural progression of functional return.[18] Hemiplegic patients often have recurrence of muscle stretch reflexes before volitional motor action, followed by synergistic movement patterns, return of voluntary selective motor function, and finally a decrease in hyperreflexic stretch reflexes. Evaluation in the upper extremity assesses movement within and independent of synergistic patterns, including coordination and speed of movement. The intricate movements of the hand and wrist are assessed separately, as is the patient's ability to maintain body posture. Light touch, position sense, joint movement, and pain-free movement add critical sensory observations as they contribute to motor function. The Fugl-Meyer scale has been demonstrated to have high intra-tester and inter-tester reliability, and can be completed in 10 to 20 minutes. Decline of function of the Fugl-Meyer scale has been shown to correlate closely with the severity of spastic tone.[27] Scales with similar purpose have been reported, but do not appear to have any clear advantage.

Electromyographic Analysis of Spastic Hypertonia

Several studies have identified reduced EMG levels in the spastic muscle as an indicator of reduced spasticity. However, the inherent variability and high level of noise associated with muscle EMG recordings and poor correlation with intensity of spasticity make this approach a suboptimal choice for spasticity quantification. Furthermore, this is an indirect measure of joint stiffness (spasticity) and does not provide a quantitative and reliable measure of limb impedance.

Biomechanical Measures of Spastic Hypertonia

Biomechanical measures quantify changes in stretch reflex activity in limbs of spastic patients. They are an extension of the Ashworth scale, in which the clinician applies a stretch to the limb and feels the resistance to stretch. Biomechanical measures use a controlled perturbation while quantifying the mechanical response to the movement with torque and position transducers and EMG. The motor-induced perturbation is critical to ensure that the applied joint deflection is constant in amplitude and velocity. The joint perturbation may be implemented either by controlling the applied torque while measuring the resulting change in position, or by applying a controlled position perturbation and measuring the resulting torque. Many different types of perturbations have been used, and the application of different types of perturbation has led to some confusion in interpreting and comparing the resulting results from different studies.

When interpreting torque responses to controlled mechanical perturbations, it is critical to distinguish between what is due to the stretch reflex and what is due to the "passive" or nonreflexive aspects of the limb. Clinicians are similarly faced with the dilemma of distinguishing contracture from spastic hypertonia on clinical exam. This problem is generally addressed by applying a mechanical perturbation to the limb that does not evoke a stretch reflex, and is believed to represent the mechanical properties of the limb. This response is then compared to a stretch that does evoke a reflex response, as reflected by the EMG response.

Reflex Threshold and Reflex Gain. An important concept that has evolved from biomechanical measurements is the distinction between reflex threshold and reflex gain. *Reflex threshold* implies that there is a certain threshold input above which a reflex is evoked. *Reflex gain* is the relationship between the size of the input as compared to the size of the output. These parameters have important implications for the neurophysiological disturbances outlined earlier (Fig. 29–2).

A decreased reflex threshold would be the result of motor neurons that are perched close to depolarization. This depolarization can result from an increase in tonic excitatory synaptic drive via descending or interneuronal input. Alternatively, an increase in stretch reflex gain would occur if afferent input elicited a greater change in membrane potential. This could result from afferent terminal sprouting (increasing the number of active terminals), postsynaptic receptor hypersensitivity (increasing the impact of released transmitter), or reductions in presynaptic inhibition (increasing the amount of transmitter released for each incoming action potential).

When interpreting the results of studies of the stretch reflex response in spastic patients, it is helpful to understand that the stretch reflex is sensitive to two types of inputs—velocity of the stretch and the joint angle

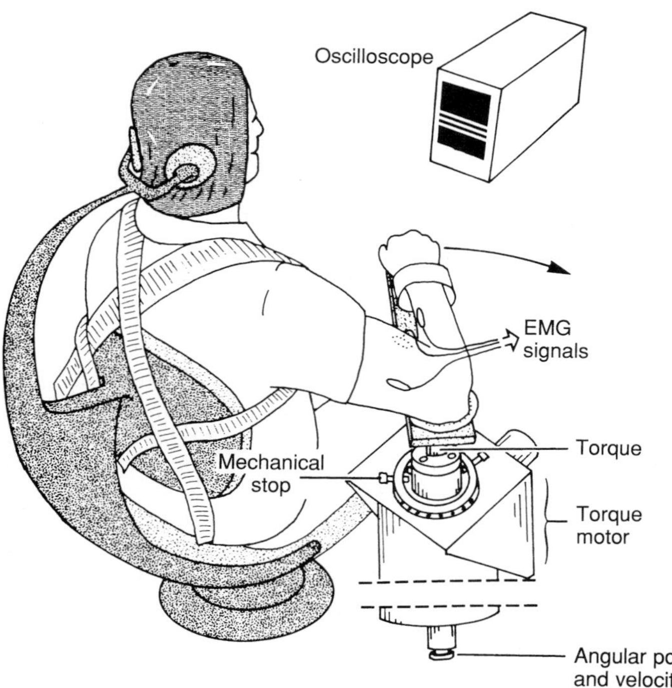

FIGURE 29–2. Possible stretch reflex abnormalities in spasticity. As a joint is extended, torque elicited by muscle stretch begins to increase after a certain threshold angle (θ) is reached. The amount of torque per unit angle, or muscle stiffness, is the slope of the curve. θ_2 denotes a "normal" threshold angle; θ_1 denotes a reduced threshold for motoneuron recruitment. Curve *a* represents a state in which both reduced threshold and increased stiffness exist. Curves *b* and *c* represent cases in which reduced threshold or increased stiffness exists alone, respectively. Curve *d* represents the normal state of reflex threshold and stiffness.

(which changes muscle length). The reflex threshold may be expressed either as (1) a velocity threshold or (2) an angular threshold. Angular threshold is manifested clinically as the catch point at which the resistance to manual stretch abruptly increases. The reflex gain may be defined either as the change in reflex torque as a function of velocity or joint angle.

Results of some studies using sinusoidal and step perturbations suggest that reflex gain is enhanced in spastic patients in comparison to control subjects. This conclusion is based on a possibly inflated increase in velocity sensitive gain, because measured reflex torques did not account for changes in angular threshold. Conversely, protocols utilizing constant velocity ramp stretches have not considered velocity threshold or velocity gain. In these studies, reflex gain is unchanged in the spastic limb, but reflex threshold is decreased. Perturbation studies have led to confusion about the pathophysiology of spastic hypertonia, and have raised the question of whether changes in threshold or gain are most representative of the severity of spasticity.

Fortunately, this distinction is not critical to the clinical applicability of biomechanical measures of spasticity. Changes in both reflex gain and threshold can contribute to increases in stretch reflex responses. Ultimately, any type of mechanical perturbation can be useful for quantification, provided the perturbation remains uniform across patients and across sessions. Similarly, changes in stretch reflex excitability are ultimately reflected in a change in the torque response, whether interpreted as a change in gain or as a change in threshold.

While biomechanical measures have been correlated with clinical measures,[27] they have not become standard in clinical practice, despite their resolution, objectivity, and repeatability. The advantages of mechanical measures of spasticity are increased resolution, objectivity, and repeatability. The use of these devices for spasticity quantification is clearly feasible and the measures may be useful for clinical studies investigating the effects of pharmacological and physical interventions.

Pendulum Test

The pendulum test uses gravity for the assessment of spasticity. The relaxed limb's impedance to imposed movement reflects the degree of spastic hypertonia in the quadriceps and hamstring muscles and has been evaluated in supine normal and spastic patients.[52] Stiffness of the lower limb is assessed by placing the patient in a supine position with both legs extending over the edge of a table which supports them only as far as the distal thigh. In this way the knee joint can be easily flexed and extended. When the lower limb segment falls from a fully extended position, it sways about the vertical like a pendulum, and its movement is damped or "braked" by the viscoelastic elements of the limb (Fig. 29–3). Knee movement is assessed by an electrogoniometer and rate of movement by a tachometer. These instruments usually show sinusoidal patterns of angular motion on which a mathematical model has been created to differentiate a spastic from a normal limb.

Although easy to use, the mathematical analysis of the pendulum biomechanical model suffers from the questionable assumption that mechanical properties of knee extensor and flexor musculature are equal, and that the model can be treated as a simple linear "second-order" system (in which elements can be simulated by various masses, springs, and variable resistors). In fact, muscle stiffness and viscosity vary with the level of muscle excitation, and with muscle length. In contrast to biomechani-

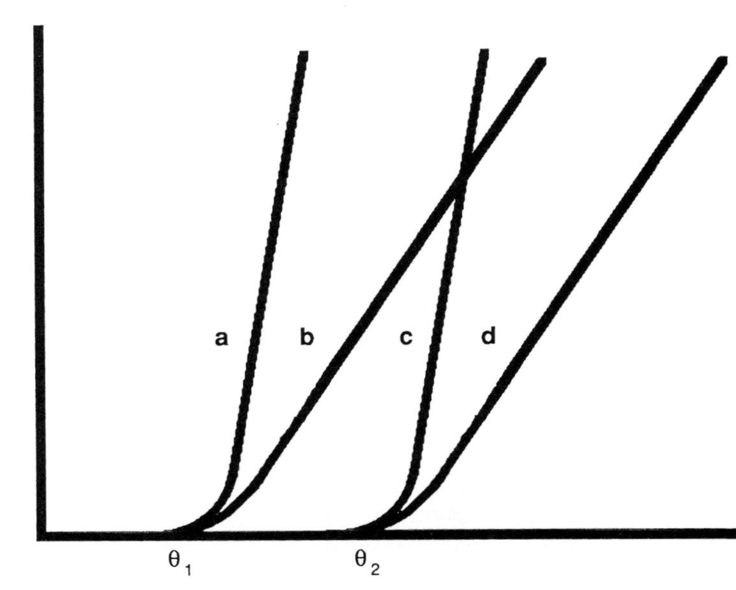

FIGURE 29–3. Pendulum test for spastic hypertonia used to assess spastic hypertonia of the quadriceps and hamstring muscle groups. Stiffness of the limb is assessed by placing the patient in a supine position with both legs extending over the edge of a table which supports them only as far as the distal thigh. A_0 represents the amplitude of the damped sinusoidal curve as it falls from the extended position to the final resting angle. A_1 represents the amplitude of the plotted waveform from full extension to its first absolute minimum. The upper tracing depicts a normal subject. The lower tracing depicts a moderately spastic subject. Notice that the initial swing from full extension (A_1) does not reach the vertical, while the normal subject obtains 27° of flexion beyond the vertical. The marked damping of the altered sinusoidal curve is evident in the spastic subject.

cal perturbation, the pendulum test includes no explanation for threshold and stiffness variation.

Electrophysiological Testing

A wide variety of electrophysiological reflex studies have been performed to assess spasticity and explore neuronal circuits within the spinal cord. While they are easily recorded, analyzed, and quantified, they have yet to be proven clinically useful. Readers are referred to other sources for a full description of these tests,[25] which are summarized in Table 29–5.

Electrophysiological testing has been a fascinating tool to examine changes in spinal cord function and

TABLE 29–5 Electrophysiological Tests for Quantifying Spasticity

Reflex Study	Description	Purported Use & Limitation
H Reflex	Submaximal stimulus delivered to tibial nerve in popliteal fossa while recording over soleus. Can also be recorded in other sites, especially in UMN patients. Analagous to the muscle stretch reflex arc bypassing the muscle spindle. Stimulus duration 0.5–1.0 ms.	Riddled with methodological difficulties: electrode placement, contributions of neighboring muscles to the evoked response, effects of patient relaxation or limb position, effects of head and neck position. Amplitude changes dramatically with stimulus duration.
H(max)/M(max)	Ratio of the maximal H reflex and M response (compound muscle action potential from supramaximal orthodromic response).	Assesses excitability of the motor nucleus by comparing % of motoneurons activated by H reflex in comparison to direct activation. Ratios increase after UMN injury. Ratio normalizes after treatment with intrathecal baclofen. Correlates poorly with clinical assessment.
T/M Ratio	Ratio of mechanically-induced muscle stretch reflex (via reflex hammer) with the direct M response.	Similar to H(max)/M(max).
Inhibition of H reflex by muscle contraction	Tibialis anterior contraction during H reflex.	Assesses reciprocal inhibition. In normal subjects contraction inhibits H reflex recorded from triceps surae. Less inhibition seen in spastic subjects.
Inhibition of H reflex by stimulation of peroneal nerve	Peroneal nerve stimulation during H reflex.	Electrical stimulation of peroneal nerve serves as substitute for voluntary contraction. Less inhibition of H reflex seen in spastic subjects.
H reflex recovery curves	Paired equal stimuli of the tibial nerve applied in varying intervals.	First H reflex inhibits or facilitates amplitude of the second depending on the interval. Poorly reproducible and unknown significance. Alterations in inhibitory and facilitatory periods noted in spastic individuals.
Paired H reflex studies utilizing collision technique	Normally, supramaximal stimulus of a mixed nerve eliminates the H reflex due to antidromic cancellation of the efferent volley. This cancellation can itself be nullified by giving a conditioning electrical stimulus sufficient to generate an H reflex *prior* to the supramaximal M response (collision technique). The volley of the *conditioning* H reflex volley collides with the *antidromic* volley of the M stimulus, which subsequently allows the *afferent* volley from the supramaximal stimulus to generate an H reflex.	Purports to assess Renshaw cell activation and recurrent inhibition. Spastic patients demonstrate an increase in the second H reflex amplitude.
IB inhibition using H reflexes and conditioning stimulus	Conditioning stimulus applied to the nerve to the medial head of the gastrocnemius which inhibits subsequent H reflex.	Assesses short-latency autogenic inhibition from IB fibers. Inhibition of subsequent H reflex in normals, facilitation in plegics.
F wave	Supramaximal stimulation of a mixed nerve while recording over a distal muscle.	Assesses alpha motor neuron excitability. F/M ratio is increased in spastic patients.
Tonic vibration reflex	Discussed above. Vibrator applied to Achilles tendon normally inhibits the soleus H reflex.	Assesses presynaptic inhibition. Failure of tonic vibration to suppress the H reflex noted in spastic individuals.
$H(max)_{(vib)}/H(max)$	Ratio of maximal H reflex during vibration and without vibration	Increases in spastic patients. Wide normal values, poor correlation with intensity of spasticity.
Flexor withdrawal a responses	Automatic withdrawal of the lower extremity upon electrically stimulating the sole of the foot.	Reflects global interneural activities. Early phase responses disappear after UMN lesion.
Lumbosacral spinal evoked response	Submaximal stimulation of tibial nerve yields triphasic evoked response recorded over T12.	Reflects presynaptic inhibition in dorsal horn. Change in positive and negative peaks in spastic patients.

segmental reflexes in spastic patients. The premises for use of these techniques are based on animal models, which may or may not be applicable to intact human subjects. Most of these studies also assess the neural circuitry of the spastic individual at rest, ignoring the biomechanical and neurophysiological features of movement. As any clinician would aptly point out, much of the disability present in a spastic patient is associated with human movement. Consequently, electrophysiological studies are hampered by taking neural mechanisms out of the milieu of the behavioral motoric complex, studying them as an isolated event. As these scales correlate poorly with clinical severity, it is unclear what significance these changes in electrophysiological parameters reflect.

THERAPEUTIC MANAGEMENT OF SPASTIC HYPERTONIA

Before treatment for spasticity is initiated, the clinician must address several important questions:

- Does hypertonia exacerbate a functional impairment, or does it threaten to cause disability if left unchecked? Is it causing discomfort? Is it making care of the person by others more difficult?
- Is the disability specifically a result of spastic hypertonia or another motor disorder, such as rigidity, muscle "spasms," or weakness? Are several disorders contributing to the disability?
- Is the spastic hypertonia useful to the patient? Is increased lower extremity tone utilized for standing or walking? Is spasticity or disordered motor control the primary detriment to the gait pattern? Is it inappropriate to routinely reduce or inhibit the reflex response to improve functional movement in stroke rehabilitation[1]?
- What are the static (i.e., contracture) and dynamic (reflex) contributions to the problem? How do they affect other areas of function?
- What are the overall functional abilities of the individual—motor, sensory, cognitive, and behavioral? How will these be affected as the goals for treatment of spasticity are achieved?
- Are there other medical issues that might be contributing to the problem? Might these conditions be exacerbated by spasticity treatment?
- How much time has elapsed since the onset of the condition that was the cause of spasticity? What is the prognosis?

Addressing these questions allows a rational approach to the treatment of spasticity, as outlined in Figure 29–4.

Good nursing care can reduce the nociceptive and exteroreceptive stimuli that can exacerbate the patient's hypertonia. The avoidance of noxious stimuli is an important initial management step. This includes such measures as prompt treatment of urinary tract complications (infections, stones), prevention of pressure sores and contractures, release of tightly wrapped leg bags and clothes, proper bowel and bladder management to prevent fecal impaction and bladder distension, and prophylaxis of deep venous thrombosis. Heterotopic bone has been suggested as an exacerbant of spasticity, but the prevention of this complication can be difficult.

Proper bed positioning early after spinal cord injury has been suggested as an important step in the long-term reduction of spastic hypertonia, but this assertion has never been systematically evaluated. A daily stretching program is an integral component of any spasticity management program. A common bedside observation is that limb resistance progressively diminishes as the limb is repeatedly ranged.

Physical Modalities

Stretching is probably an essential component for relieving muscle stiffness in spastic patients, although there are few quantitative reports demonstrating spasticity relief following muscle stretch. In fact, the long-term efficacy of stretch for reducing spasticity has been challenged.[8, 54] Conceivably, the lack of spasticity reduction in these early studies is related to the inadequate quantification techniques; or perhaps cost-prohibitive, repeated daily treatments are needed in order to see a meaningful treatment effect.

Ranging can reduce the severity of spastic tone for several hours. The reason for the "carry-over" is not completely clear, but it could be related to mechanical changes in the musculotendinous unit or to plastic changes within the central nervous system. These plastic events may correlate with short- and long-term modulation of synaptic efficacy associated with neurotransmitter changes on a cellular level. Habituation of reflex activity has been studied in the marine snail *Aplysia californica,* which has a simple nervous system. The snail has a reflex for withdrawing its respiratory organ and siphon, which is similar to the leg-flexion withdrawal reflex in humans. Repetitive activation results in a decrease in synaptic transmission, partly due to an inactivation of calcium channels in the presynaptic terminal. The decrease in calcium influx diminishes the release of neurotransmitter, probably owing to the calcium-dependent exocytosis of neurotransmitter vesicles.[11] Recently, quantification of the torque response to repeated movements has indicated that a significant adaptation of the stretch reflex occurs over 30 movements of the elbow in spastic, hemiparetic brain-injured patients.

The therapeutic benefit of repeated ranging and stretch is incorporated into the Neurodevelopment Technique of Bobath, and more recently into proprioceptive neuromuscular facilitation.[12] The original Bobath technique made use of "reflex inhibitory patterns"—joint positions that stretch the most spastic muscles—with the goal of reducing tone by inhibition of exaggerated reflexes. Proprioceptive neuromuscular facilitation also uses stretch in combination with contraction of either the stretched or antagonist muscle, and is often used to improve range of motion. Although stretch therapy reduces spasticity, the reduction is tem-

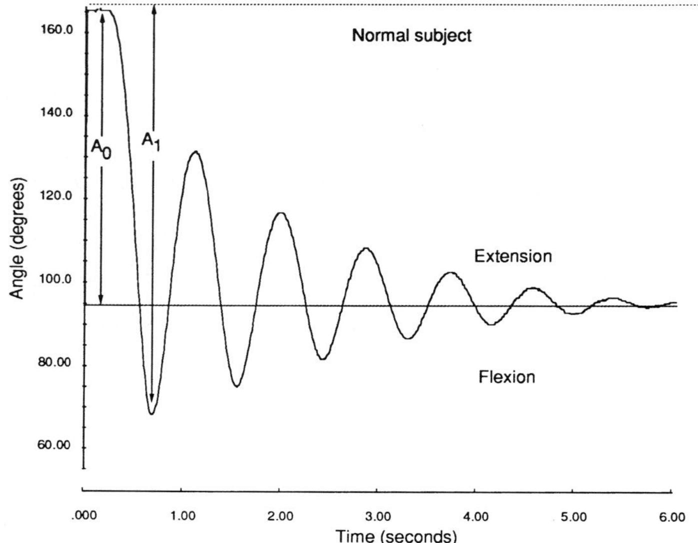

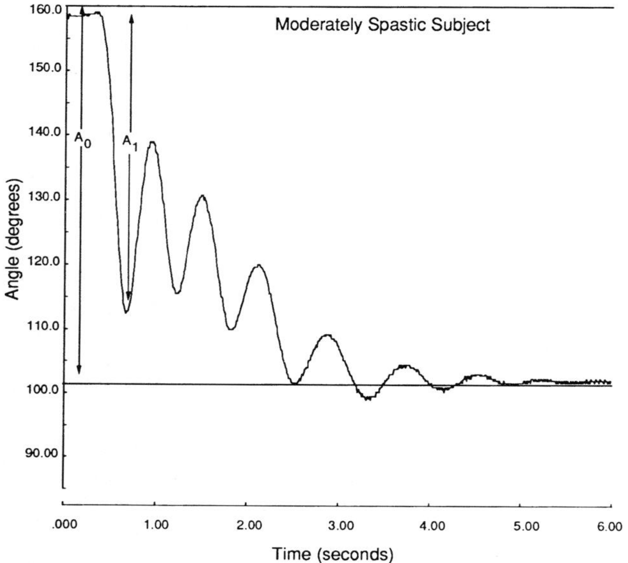

FIGURE 29–4. Flowchart for the treatment of spastic hypertonia.

porary and may not affect voluntary movements in a useful manner. The long-term effects of stretch and its effect on voluntary movement need to be more carefully examined.

Cryotherapy. Topical cold has been reported to decrease muscle stretch reflex excitability, reduce clonus, increase range of motion of the joint, and improve power in the antagonistic muscle group. These effects can be used to facilitate improved motor function for short periods of time. Tone may be decreased very shortly after the application of ice, probably due to decreased sensitivity in cutaneous receptors and slowing of nerve conduction. Changes in central nervous system excitability may take longer to occur. A therapist might apply a cold pack for twenty or more minutes to obtain maximum effect. Topical anesthesia may have similar effects.

Casting and Splinting. Casting or splinting techniques can improve the range of motion in a joint due to hypertonic contracture, and positioning the limb in a tonic stretch has been observed to decrease reflex tone. In one study, long-term but not short-term casting resulted in a significant decrease in both dynamic and static reflex sensitivity. Elongation of the series elastic component of the musculotendinous unit and an increase in the number of sarcomeres within muscle fibers each may have contributed to the decrease in tone.[43]

Biofeedback. EMG biofeedback may be useful for the treatment of spasticity and associated synergies. In general, biofeedback has been used initially to train the subject to relax the spastic extremity, and then to regain active control. Protocols utilizing biofeedback have involved retraining of the upper extremity of hemiplegics, some with aphasia. Biofeedback has been reported to be successful in improving dorsiflexion of the ankle in persons with stroke, multiple sclerosis, cerebral palsy, brain injury, and SCI. Despite great initial enthusiasm, however, biofeedback techniques have not found widespread acceptance.

Electrical Stimulation. The use of electrical stimulation to improve patient function—functional electrical stimulation (FES)—has received wide medical and lay press.[13] Electrical stimulation of peripheral nerves offers a potential adjunct to traditional rehabilitation therapeutics for paraplegic patients during standing, walking, and exercise training. Cyclical use of electrical stimulation has been shown to decrease upper extremity contractures, improve motor activity in agonistic muscles, and reduce tone in antagonistic muscle groups of the hemiplegic and quadriplegic patient.

Stimulation of the sural nerve, a flexor reflex afferent, has resulted in decreased extensor tonus and increased strength of ankle dorsiflexion. The therapeutic effect may last for an hour or more after stimulation has been discontinued, perhaps due to neurotransmitter modulation within the segmental reflex. Peroneal nerve stimulation can suppress ankle clonus in ambulatory hemiplegic patients via reciprocal inhibition. Electrical stimulation has limited but defined applications as an ankle dorsiflexor-assist during hemiplegic gait, and as a hand-opening device in the plegic upper extremity. Significant decrements in spastic hypertonia for up to thirty minutes have been demonstrated in rigorous studies utilizing cutaneous stimulation in a hemiplegic population.[13] Rectal probe stimulation, employed to induce ejaculation in spinal cord–injured men, has been associated with a significant reduction in spasticity lasting up to twenty-four hours.[23] Such reductions could arise because of changes in the effectiveness of synaptic transmission due to such mechanisms as short-term facilitation, short-term depression, long-term potentiation, and long-term depression.

Spinal cord stimulation (Fig. 29–5), also known as dorsal column stimulation, was initially embraced enthusiastically in the treatment of spinal hypertonia. A short chain of stimulating electrodes is threaded into the epidural space, resting in the vicinity of the spinal cord dorsal columns. Maximal improvement depends upon finding the ideal combination of electrode placement, stimulation intensity, and stimulation frequency. A critical analysis of the beneficial effects of dorsal column stimulation has questioned its efficacy in improving motor and bladder function. In a carefully performed study where examiners were blinded as to whether stimulation was on or off, measures of joint compliance and standardized neurological examination were no better than chance in determining whether spinal cord stimulation was being received.[20]

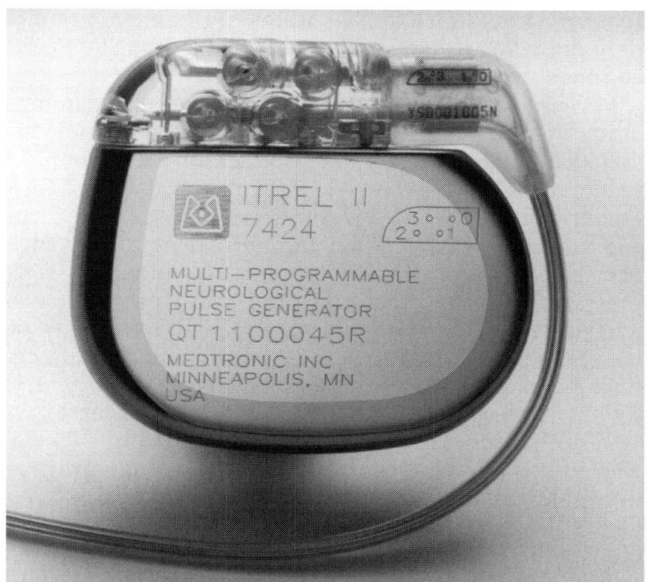

FIGURE 29–5. A subcutaneous stimulation unit can directly neuromodulate the spinal cord by threading a short chain of stimulating electrodes into the epidural space to rest beside the dorsal columns. (Medtronic Itrel II Spinal Cord Stimulator. Itrel II Spinal Cord Stimulator is a product of Medtronic Neurological, 800 53rd Ave. NE, POB 1250 Minneapolis, MN 55440-9087. Courtesy of Medtronic Neurological, with permission.)

Pharmacologic Intervention

Oral Medications. No medication (Table 29–6) has been uniformly useful in the treatment of spastic hypertonia.[26] Considering the variety of problems associated with spasticity—flexor spasms in the spinal patient, dystonic posturing in the hemiplegic, spastic diplegia in the cerebral palsy child—it is unlikely that one agent will be beneficial to all parties. More importantly, all drugs have potentially serious side effects, and these negative

TABLE 29–6 Drug Treatment of Spastic Hypertonia

Agent	Daily Dosage (mg)	Half-Life (hours)	Mechanism of Action
Baclofen	10–80+	3.5	Presynaptic inhibitor by activation of GABA "B" receptor
Diazepam	4–60+	27–37*	Facilitates post-synaptic effects of GABA, resulting in increased presynaptic inhibition
Dantrolene	25–400	8.7	Reduces calcium release, interfering with excitation-contraction coupling in skeletal muscle
Clonidine	0.1–0.4 (po) 0.1–0.3 (patch)** 12–16 (oral)		Alpha-2 adrenergic agonist
Tizanidine	4–36	8.4	Alpha-2 adrenergic agonist

* Half-life of active primary metabolite is significantly longer
** Patch is changed weekly

features should be carefully weighed when beginning a patient on any drug. Continued use of a drug should be contingent on a clearly beneficial effect.

Baclofen. Baclofen (Lioresal®) is an analog of gamma-aminobutyric acid (GABA), a neurotransmitter involved in presynaptic inhibition. Baclofen does not bind to the classical GABA "A" receptor, but rather to a recently discovered and less well-characterized "B" receptor. Agonism at this site inhibits calcium influx into presynaptic terminals and suppresses release of excitatory neurotransmitters. Baclofen inhibits both mono- and polysynaptic reflexes, and also reduces activity of the gamma efferent. Although therapeutic effects have been shown to occur when plasma levels exceed 400 ng/mL, optimal responses have been obtained at very different plasma and cerebrospinal fluid levels. Baclofen is completely absorbed after oral administration, and is eliminated predominantly by the renal route. Its half-life is approximately 3.5 hours. Baclofen readily crosses the blood-brain barrier, in contrast to GABA.

While baclofen is probably the drug of choice in spasticity following spinal cord injury, its role in the treatment of spasticity due to supraspinal injury remains unsettled. It may interfere with attention and memory in elderly and brain-injured patients. Baclofen is particularly effective for the flexor spasms with spinal cord lesions. Baclofen may improve bladder control by decreasing hyperreflexive contraction of the external urethral sphincter. It has been shown to be safe and effective in long-term use. Baclofen also has an anxiolytic effect, which probably contributes to its anti-spasticity actions.

Initial adult dosage is approximately 5 mg po, b.i.d. or t.i.d., and may be slowly titrated up toward a recommended maximum dose of 80 mg/day. This "recommended maximum dose" may not, however, be the most effective dose for the patient, and higher doses may be well tolerated by the patient and be additionally therapeutic. There is a low incidence of side effects, which include hallucinations, confusion, sedation, hypotonia, and ataxia. Sudden withdrawal of the drug can lead to seizures and hallucinations. Stereospecific L-baclofen has been shown to be more effective than the commonly used racemic form in treatment of headache pain. L-Baclofen deserves evaluation for treatment of spastic hypertonia.

Safe use of baclofen has not been adequately studied in children, and the Food and Drug Administration (FDA) has not approved its use in this age group. However, physicians have used baclofen in this age group with dosages initiated at 2.5 to 5 mg/day, with maximum dosages of 30 mg (children 2 to 7 years of age) to 60 mg (children 8 years or older).

Diazepam. Diazepam (Valium) facilitates postsynaptic effects of GABA, resulting in an increase in presynaptic inhibition. It has no direct GABA-mimetic effect, but exerts indirect mimetic effect only when GABA transmission is functional. In addition to its known effects in the brain, it has been shown to be effective in persons with demonstrated spinal cord division.

Diazepam has been a successful treatment for spastic hypertonia in spinal cord injury, and is generally well tolerated except for its sedative effect. Diazepam is generally unsuitable in patients with brain injury due to deleterious effects on attention and memory. Other side effects include intellectual impairment and reduced motor coordination. Evidence of abuse and addiction is rare, but true physiological addiction can occur. Withdrawal symptoms can appear if diazepam is tapered too rapidly. There is some synergistic depression of the central nervous system when it is administered with alcohol. Although the potential for overdose exists, the benzodiazepines have an extremely large index of safety. Dosage begins at approximately 2 mg po b.i.d., and may be slowly titrated up to 60 mg or more per day, in divided dosages. Pediatric dosages range from 0.12 to 0.8 mg/kg per day in divided doses.

Dantrolene Sodium. Dantrolene sodium (Dantrium) reduces muscle action potential–induced release of calcium from the sarcoplasmic reticulum, decreasing the force produced by excitation-contraction coupling. Dantrolene is the only drug that intervenes in spastic hypertonia at a "muscular" rather than a segmental reflex level. It reduces the activity of phasic stretch reflexes more than tonic ones. Dantrolene affects fast more than slow muscle fibers and, for unknown reasons, seems to have little effect on smooth and cardiac muscle tissues. It is metabolized largely in the liver, and eliminated in urine and bile. Its half-life is approximately 8 to 9 hours.

Dantrolene is preferred for spasticity subsequent to supraspinal injury such as hemiplegia or cerebral palsy, but may be a useful adjunct for the treatment of spasticity after spinal cord injury. It is less likely to cause lethargy or cognitive disturbances than are baclofen or diazepam. Although dantrolene can weaken muscles, the effects on spastic hypertonia are generally without impairment of motor performance. Its most pronounced effect is possibly the reduction in clonus and muscle spasms resulting from innocuous stimuli.

Dantrolene is mild to moderately sedative, and can cause malaise, nausea and vomiting, dizziness, and diarrhea. The most commonly considered side effect is that of hepatoxicity, which can occur in approximately 1% of patients. Liver function tests should be monitored periodically, and the drug can be tapered or discontinued if enzyme elevations are noted. Early on, fatal hepatitis was reported in 0.1 to 0.2% of patients treated for longer than sixty days, but this rate of fatalities occurred before enzyme monitoring was standard practice. Dosage begins at 25 mg/day, and may be slowly increased to 400 mg/day. Higher dosages are occasionally effective and can be tried provided monitoring for hepatotoxicity and other side effects is assured. Clinical results are not clearly related to dose, however, and may plateau at a dosage of 100 mg/day. Pediatric doses begin at 0.5 mg/kg twice daily, increasing the frequency and dosage until maximum effect is reached. The maximum dosage is generally 3 mg/kg q.i.d. or less than 100 mg q.i.d.

Tizanidine. Tizanidine (Zanaflex) is an imidazoline derivative that has an agonistic action at central alpha-2 adrenergic receptor sites.[55] Unlike clonidine, it is much less potent in lowering blood pressure. It may facilitate the action of glycine, an inhibitory neurotransmitter, and prevents the release of excitatory amino acids—i.e., L-glutamate and L-aspartate—from the presynaptic terminal of spinal interneurons. It reduces tonic stretch reflexes and enhances presynaptic inhibition in animals. It enhances vibratory inhibition of the H reflex and reduces abnormal co-contraction. It has been shown to be equivalent to baclofen as an antispastic agent (but may be better tolerated) in spastic patients after spinal and supraspinal injury in divided dosages up to 36 mg/day.[37] It has similarly been shown to be equally efficacious and better tolerated than diazepam in patients with chronic hemiplegia. Multiple sclerosis patients have shown significant benefit in several large double-blinded studies.

Common side effects include dry mouth, somnolence, asthenia, dizziness, headache, and insomnia. Liver function abnormalities have been noted only sporadically; nonetheless, the manufacturer recommends checking liver function tests periodically. Daytime somnolence may be secondary to nighttime insomnia, which was reported more frequently by patients receiving tizanidine than those receiving baclofen. Both tizanidine and baclofen are more effective in extensor than flexor musculature.

The usual initial starting dosage of tizanidine is 4 mg, usually started in the evening. This dosage can be titrated slowly upward in 2-mg increments. The medication is generally prescribed on a t.i.d. schedule. The average daily dosage is 24 mg/day, and the maximum dosage recommended is 36 mg/day. Dosage should be reduced in patients with renal impairment. In the United States, 4-mg tablets are available, while in Europe a 6- and 12-mg modified release formulation can be used. The half-life of tizanidine is just 2.5 hours, and the clinical effects of the drug peak 1 to 2 hours after each dose, disappearing by 6 hours. Thus, even with t.i.d. dosing, it does not remain effective around the clock. It may be used together with baclofen with additive effect.

Gabapentin. Although approved by the FDA only as an antileptic agent, gabapentin (Neurontin) has been shown to be an effective treatment in the treatment of spasticity as well. Gabapentin, which is a cyclohexane acetic acid derivative, was synthesized as an analog of GABA. It does not act at any known GABA receptor, and it does not affect the re-uptake or degradation of GABA. It is excreted by the kidneys, and has a relatively short half-life of 5 to 7 hours. Its common side effects include somnolence, dizziness, ataxia, fatigue, and nystagmus. It has recently been shown to be effective in the treatment of spastic hypertonia secondary to spinal cord injury[22] and multiple sclerosis.[41] It is generally necessary to treat with dosages greater than 1200 mg/day in three divided dosages. Maximum recommended dosage per day is 2400 mg, but one study noted increased effect with dosages up to 3600 mg/day.[45] Pediatric dosages have not been determined.

Benzodiazepines and Derivatives. *Ketazolam,* a benzodiazepine, has been shown to be equally effective and less sedating than diazepam in spinal forms of spasticity; it may have a similar pharmacologic action. An additional benefit is that ketazolam can be administered in a single dosage of 30 to 60 mg/day. It is not currently approved for use in the United States. *Tetrazepam* (Myolastan), a benzodiazepine derivative, is reported to reduce the tonic component of spastic hypertonia, with little effect on tendon hyperreflexia and no influence on muscle strength. *Clorazepate,* a benzodiazepine analog which is transformed into desmethyldiazepam (the major metabolite of diazepam), has been shown to be effective in normalizing phasic but not tonic stretch reflexes.

Chlorpromazine and Phenytoin. Chlorpromazine has been applied to the treatment of hypertonia because of its alpha-adrenergic blocking effect. Clinical and electrophysiological studies in humans before and after administration of alpha and beta blocking agents suggest descending adrenergic and noradrenergic pathways may have important modulatory effects on spastic hypertonia. However, the depression of motor function by phenothiazines is thought to be due largely to their effects upon the brainstem reticular formation. A small double-blinded study of *chlorpromazine with phenytoin* suggests that a combination of these drugs may be beneficial in the treatment of spastic hypertonia. Neither drug alone was as efficacious as the combination of the two, although chlorpromazine alone was nearly as effective. Phenytoin serum levels did not correlate with therapeutic effect as long as the concentration was above 7 μg/mL. The addition of phenytoin lowered the needed optimally therapeutic dose of chlorpromazine, decreasing its sedative effect. However, because of the danger of tardive dyskinesia, chlorpromazine should not generally be used to treat spasticity.

Clonidine. Clonidine, an alpha-2 adrenergic agonist, has been used with fair success in spinal cord injury patients. Clonidine, in combination with desipramine, improved the vibratory inhibition of the H reflex after spinal cord injury. Co-activation of antagonist muscle decreased, allowing improved locomotor function in a spastic paraparetic patient with clonidine therapy. Syncope, hypotension, and nausea and vomiting are the most common side effects. Most patients who benefit from the drug note acceptable relief with dosage of 0.1 mg twice a day or less.[17] Clonidine is now available in an adhesive patch (Catapres-TTS) for week-long transdermal delivery. Initial studies have demonstrated favorable results, starting with 0.1-mg patch and titrating up to 0.3-mg patch as needed. Adverse effect rates were similar to those reported with oral clonidine.[53]

Vigabatrin. Vigabatrin is an epileptic drug specifically designed to increase brain GABA levels by inhibiting catabolism of this neurotransmitter. It replaces GABA as a substrate for GABA transaminase, the enzyme responsible for the first step in GABA breakdown. Vigabatrin was developed as an antiepileptic agent and has shown promise in the treatment of refractory cases of epilepsy. In placebo-controlled trials vigabatrin in doses of 2 to 3 g/day improved spasticity in patients with spinal cord injury and multiple sclerosis. The most common adverse reactions were drowsiness, fatigue, and weight gain, but behavioral disturbances have been reported to be uncommon.[21]

Intrathecal Medications. Intrathecal administration of baclofen has been successfully attempted in the treatment of spastic hypertonia related to spinal cord dysfunction and cerebral palsy.[9] A pump can be planted subcutaneously in the abdominal wall, with a catheter surgically placed into the subarachnoid space. In this manner, higher dosages of these medications can be placed near the spinal cord—the desired site for action of the drug—while largely avoiding the central nervous system side effects associated with increased oral intake. The pump can be refilled on a monthly basis by transcutaneous injection. Complications include tube dysfunction (dislodgement, disconnection, kinkage, and blockage), pump failure, infection, and baclofen overdosage.

The first application for intrathecal baclofen infusion was spasticity after spinal cord insult from SCI or multiple sclerosis with some preserved function below the level of the lesion allowing the patient to be ambulatory.[9] Recently, success with intrathecal baclofen has been reported in patients with cerebral forms of spasticity. Benefits have included a decrease in upper and lower extremity spasticity, improvement in hamstring motion, upper extremity function, and activities of daily living.[2] Intrathecal baclofen infusion treatment decreases the need for lower extremity contracture surgery in spastic cerebral palsy. Indeed, it might be prudent to consider this treatment before orthopedic procedures are performed.[19] Intrathecal baclofen has been prospectively evaluated in patients with acquired brain injury. When administered as a bolus, there is significant improvement in spastic tone as compared with placebo.[38] The reduction in tone is maintained once continuous infusion of baclofen is initiated.[39]

Intrathecal baclofen dosage is adjusted to provide maximal spasm relief while minimizing weakness. The prospective patient should be free from active infection and pressure sores. Skin over the back should be intact, and the anterior abdominal wall should be a suitable site for pump placement. Multiple abdominal procedures such as colostomies, ileal conduits, or feeding tubes must be separated from the pump site. In patients who have a potential block of cerebrospinal fluid flow, myelography may be required to ensure that there is communication between the proposed site of infusion and the source of spasticity. As pumps are expensive (approximately $7000 for the pump alone, another $3000 per year for the drug, plus surgical costs of approximately $8500), a short trial run with intrathecal baclofen via percutaneous lumbar catheter (preferably in combination with an external continuous infusion pump) is suggested. Medicare covers the implantation of infusion pumps for spasticity.

Two types of pump are available. The Infusaid Corporation (Infusaid Inc., 1400 Providence Highway, Norwood, MA 02062) manufactures a gas-powered bellows device which is purely mechanical and has no battery. Unfortunately, it can infuse drug only at a constant rate, and thus offers changes of titration of dose primarily at time of refill. The electronic pump (Fig. 29–6) can be programmed to deliver drug several times daily via an on-board computer. It allows precise titration of drug. The computer can be adjusted by an external laptop computer equipped with a programming wand. Battery life is currently about 4 to 5 years.

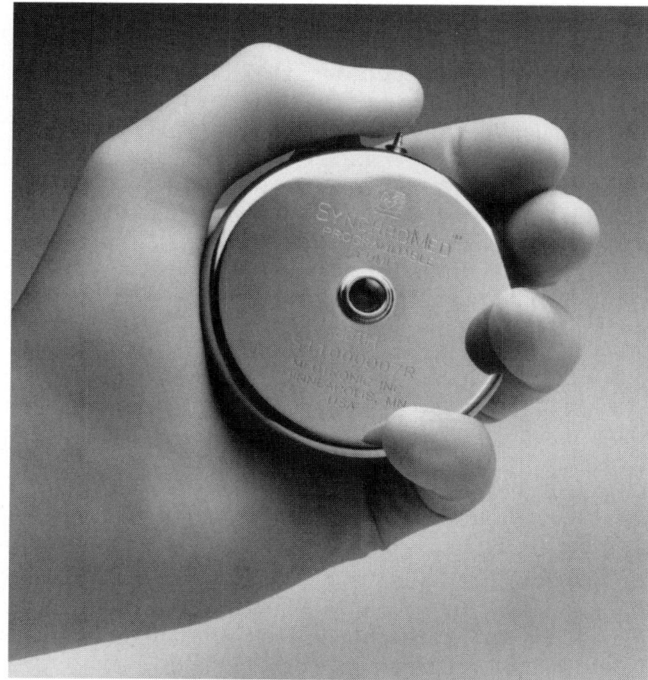

FIGURE 29–6. Intrathecal baclofen can be administered via a pump planted subcutaneously in the abdominal wall via a catheter placed into the subarachnoid space (Medtronic SynchroMed Drug Infusion Pump. SynchroMed Drug Infusion Pump is a product of Medtronic Neurological, 800 53rd Ave. NE, POB 1250 Minneapolis, MN 55440-9087. Courtesy of Medtronic Neurological, with permission.)

Baclofen is initially infused continuously at 25 μg/day. The most common side effects are drowsiness, dizziness, nausea, hypotension, headache, and weakness. The dosage is titrated up to an average of 400 to 500 μg/day or until satisfactory reduction in spasticity has been achieved. Some authors report experience with doses as high as 1500 μg/day.[36] While dosages can escalate early in the course of intrathecal baclofen use, it generally reaches a plateau six months following implantation. In addition to beneficial effects on limb spasticity, intrathecal baclofen may have a beneficial effect on bladder management. Caution concerning inadvertent overdose should be exercised, as reversible coma due to baclofen toxicity has been reported. Respiratory depression secondary to accidental intrathecal bolus injection has been reversed upon intravenous administration of 2 mg of physostigmine. The half-life of intrathecal baclofen is approximately 5 hours.

The administration of 1 to 2 mg of intrathecal morphine has similarly caused a dramatic reduction in spasticity and pain in spinal cord patients. Patients do not seem to develop drug tolerance nor lose the beneficial effect of the morphine in long-term follow-up. Despite its efficacy, intrathecal morphine is rarely used.

Nerve Blocks. Nerve blocks involve the application of a chemical agent to a nerve to impair the function of the nerve, either temporarily or permanently. This can result in improved range of motion, lessening of clonus, increase in speed and dexterity of movement (due to blockade of inappropriately firing antagonists), improved crawling/sitting/standing in children, and even diminished spasticity in contralateral extremities.

Commonly used agents include local anesthetics (e.g., lidocaine), phenol, alcohol, and botulinum toxin. Local anesthetics temporarily block conduction by interfering with the increase in permeability to sodium ions that normally occurs when the membrane is depolarized. The effects are short-lived (several hours) and are usually used in the assessment of the potential effect of a longer-acting nerve block or surgical procedure. Ethyl alcohol is also a potent neurolytic agent, but offers no particular advantage over phenol, and has not been as extensively evaluated.

Aqueous phenol solutions (2% to 7%) are the most commonly used agents to produce chemical neurolysis when applied to a mixed sensorimotor nerve, motor nerve, or its terminal nerve fibers (motor point block). ("Motor point" actually refers to electrosensitive sites along a motor branch, but it is not a useful term. In common parlance, it is used in several ways; so it is best avoided.) Concentrations of phenol greater than 5% cause protein coagulation and necrosis of axons of all sizes. Nerve blocks may be quite effective, and can last months to years when performed using electrophysiological guidance and a Teflon-coated needle (Fig. 29–7). Axons destroyed by phenol gradually regenerate, with some increase in fibrous tissue at the site of injection. Mixed sensorimotor blocks are more quickly and easily performed in some locations and may be more effective than motor branch blocks. Motor branch blocks can be as or nearly as effective as mixed blocks.

Blocks of the musculocutaneous nerve or its branches can be helpful in the hemiplegic patient with severe elbow flexion contracture, or in the C5 quadriplegic, with flexor contractures due to loss of triceps function. Elbow flexion is preserved through the action of the brachioradialis muscle, which, unlike other elbow flexors, is innervated by the radial nerve. Median nerve blocks help relax the tightly flexed hemiplegic wrist and fingers. An obturator block decreases lower extremity scissoring during gait, and facilitates hip abduction to ease personal hygiene. Hip flexor spasticity may be diminished by paravertebral block of the upper lumbar spinal nerves. Owing to the proximity of important visceral and vascular structures, lumbosacral paravertebral nerve blocks require special caution. Tibial nerve block can reduce severe equinovarus ankle posturing or painful clawing of the toes. Perineal nerve block can significantly reduce post-void residual volumes when the external urethral sphincter is very spastic.

As both sensory and motor nerve fibers are damaged, mixed sensorimotor nerve blocks with phenol can be associated with burning and discomfort. Dysesthesias, usually lasting one to three weeks, have been reported in approximately 10% of subjects. Although usually mild, the patient should be advised of this before the block is administered. Severe persistent dysesthesias can be treated with tricyclic antidepressants, carbamazepine, oral steroids, transcutaneous nerve stimulation, or repetition of the phenol block. Dysesthesias do not occur when motor nerves or branches are injected. Unwanted weakness may acutely complicate a phenol block, but often resolves in the first hours or days after nerve block. Care should be used in planning nerve blocks, as some patients harness their hypertonia for functional use. Overdosage with phenol can result in convulsions, central nervous system depression, and cardiovascular collapse. However, the usual dosages (e.g., 20 mL of 5% phenol) are well below the lethal range of the drug (>8.5 g). Venous thrombosis is a rare complication of phenol injection for chemical neurolysis.

Botulinum Toxin Injection. Botulinum toxin has been used to diminish spasticity and has been evaluated in prospective clinical trials involving patients with multiple sclerosis, cerebral palsy, head injury, spinal cord injury, and stroke.[49] Botulinum toxin was originally developed for clinical use by an ophthalmologist treating

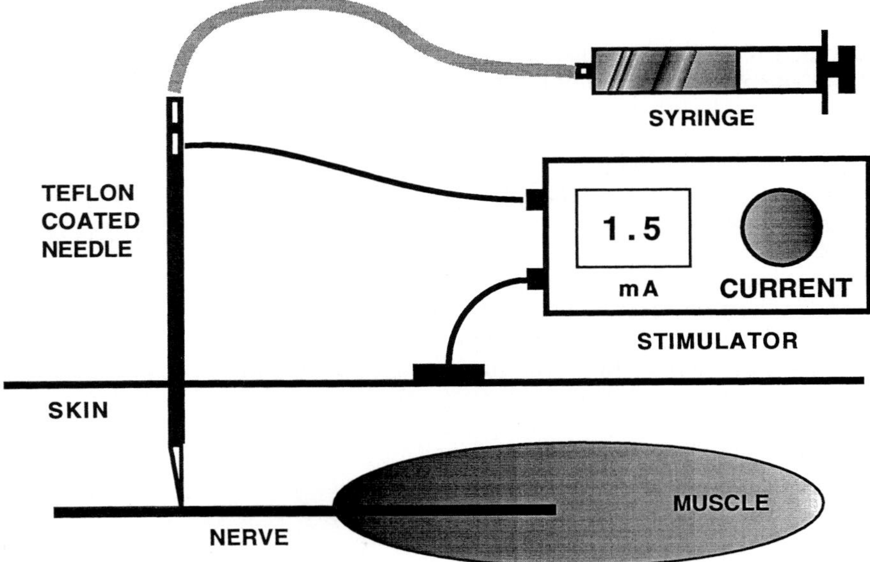

FIGURE 29–7. Nerve blocks can be performed using a 22-gauge Teflon-coated needle with a bared bevel. The hub of the needle is connected to a stimulator which delivers a square pulse of approximately 0.1 msec once or twice per second. Surface stimulation can be used to approximate the site of the nerve, watching for a visible twitch in the desired muscle. After the needle is inserted, the needle is gradually moved until only the minimal current (approximately 1 mA) is necessary to obtain a maximal twitch in the desired muscle(s). At this point the phenol is injected. Motor point blocks may require multiple injections into a single muscle. As commonly practiced, aspiration should be carried out before injection to avoid intravascular administration of the drug.

disorders such as blepharospasm and strabismus. Its use spread to the treatment of movement disorders such as torticollis and focal dystonias, and most recently to patients with spastic hypertonia.[6]

Clostridium botulinum produces seven serologically distinct toxins designated A, B, C, D, E, F, and G. Commercially available preparations of botulinum toxin A (BTX-A) include BOTOX (Allergan), which is marketed worldwide, and Dysport (Speywood), which is marketed in Europe but not yet available in the United States. Botulinum toxin works at the neuromuscular junction by inhibiting the release of acetylcholine.[6] BTX-A is internalized into the axon terminal by endocytosis and is then fully activated by disulfide reduction once inside the cell. The toxin targets key proteins on the inner membrane surface which inhibit neurotransmitter release, resulting in reversible denervation atrophy. Collateral sprouting from adjacent axons limits the clinical effects of BTX-A to 2 to 6 months. The extent of denervation is largely determined by the dosage and volume of BTX-A used, as well as the proximity to the motor end-plate band.

BTX-A is available in vials of 100 (BOTOX) or 500 (Dysport) "mouse" units (U), where the unit is that amount of drug that will kill 50% of animals in a specific mouse model.[6] Some evidence suggests that BOTOX is approximately 3 to 5 times more potent per unit than Dysport. While the lethal parenteral dose in humans is not known, it has been estimated to be 3000 U. The maximum recommended dose per treatment session is 400 U. Antitoxin is available to treat accidental overdose.

Increasing evidence suggests that certain patients, as many as 3%, may develop significant neutralizing antibodies with chronic treatment. This immunoresistance, as well as suboptimal technique, may be two important reasons why some patients are treatment-resistant. Available antibody assays may underestimate the true incidence of significant immunoresistance, but certain strategies can be used to minimize this problem: (1) The minimal effective dosage should be utilized; (2) treatment sessions should be separated by a period of three months; and (3) "booster" injections should be avoided. Patients who develop resistance may benefit from injection with other botulinum toxin serotypes. Reported side effects include unwanted weakness, as well as transient fatigue, nausea, and headache. Rare side effects have included gall bladder attacks, immunologically mediated brachial plexopathy, and urinary incontinence. Administration is contraindicated in pregnant or lactating women, and patients with neuromuscular disease.

As in the case of phenol injections, electrical stimulation and electromyographic evaluation can help localize optimal site of injection. Localization of motor end points, however is difficult, but theoretically attempts to place the needle near the motor end-plate band. The greatest likelihood of targeting a sufficient number of motor end points to significantly reduce muscle activity occurs in smaller muscles or in the pediatric population.

Effective dosage per muscle varies widely and has continued to escalate—a serious concern in light of the high cost of the drug. Trials in multiple sclerosis demonstrated significant improvement when 400 U of BTX-A was injected into spastic thigh adductors. Use of BTX-A in the hemiplegic upper extremity has shown significant improvement in Ashworth scores with injections of 75 to 300 U into elbow and wrist flexors.[49] Similar improvements have been noted in the lower extremities with dosages of 40 to 800 U, depending on the size of muscle injected. Injections of BTX-A reduce foot inversion in spastic equinovarus foot alone,[10] or in conjunction with ankle-foot taping.[46] Injection of 20 to 80 U of BTX decreased urethral pressure and post-void residuals in SCI patients.

Injections of 1 to 4 U/kg of BTX-A into medial and lateral gastrocnemius in cerebral palsy children resulted in significant improvement in gait patterns. Injection may also diminish spasticity in scissoring adductors and overactive knee flexors. The "ideal" cerebral palsy patient has hypertonia which (1) interferes with function, (2) is expected to develop fixed contracture, and (3) involves only a few muscles.[47] Dosage varies from 1 to 2 U/kg per visit to 3 to 6 U/kg per visit in small and large muscles, respectively. The respective roles of BTX-A versus intrathecal baclofen in the amelioration of spasticity in cerebral palsy children is not yet clear.

The "Spasticity Study Group" dosing recommendations are included in Table 29–7. For most muscles, a concentration of 5 to 10 U/0.1 mL is appropriate to avoid diffusion beyond the target area. Higher concentrations may be appropriate for tiny muscles. Treatment effects may be noted after one to three days, and peak at approximately two weeks.

Spinal Blocks. Intrathecal chemical neurolysis is another method of decreasing spastic hypertonia. Spinal root neurolysis may be carried out via spinal administration of 5% to 7% phenol in water or absolute alcohol, but control over affected fibers is rather imprecise. Patients must be carefully immobilized to allow precise layering of the neurolytic material, so that damage is limited to the desired spinal roots. Complications of this procedure include urinary and fecal incontinence, paresis, paresthesias, and even death. Complication rates have varied from 1% to 10% in various series of patients. Given the potential complications and the alternatives available, intrathecal neurolysis should rarely, if ever, be necessary.

Surgical Interventions

Orthopedic Procedures. Orthopedic surgery may be a useful adjunct in the management of selected patients.[29] Surgical procedures are generally reserved for adult patients who have been refractory to more conservative measures including ranging and/or casting, but have also found widespread use in the pediatric cerebral palsy population (Table 29–8). Several considerations should be addressed before surgery is considered:

(1) *When was the insult to the central nervous system?* It is important to schedule surgical intervention only when the plastic changes of recovery have more or less plateaued. This may be at least six

TABLE 29–7 Suggested Adult Botulinum Toxin A Dosing

Clinical Pattern	Potential Muscles Involved	Average Starting Dose/Units	BOTOX® Dose Units/Visit	Number of Injection Sites
Upper Limbs				
Adducted/internally rotated shoulder	Pectoralis complex	100	75–150	4
	Latissimus dorsi	100	50–150	4
	Teres major	50	25–75	1
	Subscapularis	50	25–75	1
Flexed elbow	Brachioradialis	50	25–75	2
	Biceps	100	50–200	4
	Brachialis	50	25–75	2
Pronated forearm	Pronator quadratus	25	10–50	1
	Pronator teres	40	25–75	1
Flexed wrist	Flexor carpi radialis	50	25–100	2
	Flexor carpi ulnaris	40	10–50	2
Thumb in palm	Flexor pollicis longus	15	5–25	1
	Adductor pollicis	10	5–25	1
	Opponens	10	5–25	1
Clenched fist	Flexor digitorum superficialis	50	25–75	4
	Flexor digitorum profundus	15	25–100	2
Intinsic plus hand	Lumbricals and Interossei	15	10–50/hand	3
Lower Limbs				
Flexed hip	Iliacus	100	50–150	2
	Psoas	100	50–200	2
	Rectus femoris	100	75–200	3
Flexed knee	Medial hamstrings	100	50–150	3
	Gastrocnemius (as knee flexor)	150	50–150	4
	Lateral hamstrings	100	100–200	3
Adducted thighs	Adductor brevis/longus/magnus	200/leg	75–300	6/leg
Stiff (extended) knee	Quadriceps mechanism	100	50–200	4
Equinovarus foot	Gastrocnemius medial/lateral	100	50–200	4
	Soleus	75	50–100	2
	Tibialis posterior	50	50–200	2
	Tibialis anterior	75	50–150	3
	Flexor digitorum longus/brevis	75	50–100	4
	Flexor hallucis longus	50	25–75	2
Striatal toe	Extensor hallucis longus	50	20–100	2
Neck				
	Sternocleidomastoid	40	15–75	2
	Scalenus complex	30	15–50	3
	Splenius capitis	60	50–150	3
	Semispinalis capitis	60	50–150	3
	Longissimus capitis	60	50–150	3
	Trapezius	60	50–150	3
	Levator scapulae	80	25–100	3

The dose should be reduced by 50% if both SCM muscles are injected.
Total maximum dose per visit = 400 U
Maximum dose per injection site = 50 U
Maximum volume per site = p.5 ml, except in select situations
Reinjection > 3 months
(From Brin MF, Spasticity Study Group: Dosing, administration, and a treatment algorithm for use of botulinum toxin A for adult-onset spasticity. Muscle Nerve 1997; 20(suppl 6):S208–S220. Reprinted by permission of John Wiley & Sons, Inc.)

months after a stroke, but 12 to 24 months after a traumatic brain injury.

(2) *Are the "spastic" changes dynamic or static in nature? Dynamic* refers to dysfunction that appears with movement, such as scissoring of the lower extremities during ambulation in an individual with cerebral palsy. *Static* deformities are fixed contractures, present both at rest and with movement, such as the clenched flexed hand of the hemiplegic upper extremity. This differentiation is based on examination of the patient, and can often be augmented with a diagnostic block with lidocaine or similar anesthetic. For example, a median nerve block at the elbow is useful in determining the dynamic versus static contribution of finger and wrist flexion in the hemiplegic.

(3) *What are the goals of surgery?* Is it to increase function (e.g., hand opening/closing or gait), or simply to increase range of motion to facilitate self-care or nursing care? For example, hip adduction can be lessened to diminish scissoring during gait in a cerebral palsy child, or to facilitate perineal hygiene in a patient with traumatic brain injury.

TABLE 29–8 Treatment Protocol for Spastic Cerebral Palsy

1. Surgery to improve gait in the CP child should await maturation of gait (approximately age 6–10 years). Temporize with appropriate orthotics (e.g., abduction splint, ankle foot orthosis), inhibitory casting, physical therapy, positioning (e.g., lying prone), and a home maintenance program.
2. Consider the roles of rhizotomy, botulinum toxin injection, and intrathecal baclofen before initiating surgery.
3. Perform gait analysis to help plan surgical procedures once gait is mature. Consider relative contributions of surgery and orthotics.
4. Try to avoid staging of surgical procedures. If necessary, stage two procedures close together to avoid multiple periods of extended recovery.
5. Minimize post-surgical casting and rapidly mobilize the patient.
6. Continue physical therapy as long as gait continues to improve (approximately 12 months).
7. Continue night splinting, tone management, and home maintenance program to avoid contractures.

Adapted from Russman BS, Tilton A, Gormley ME: Cerebral palsy: A rational approach to a treatment protocol, and the role of botulinum toxin in treatment. Muscle Nerve 1997; 20(suppl 6):S181–S193. Reprinted by permission of John Wiley & Sons, Inc.

(4) *What is the residual sensory and motor function of the limb in question?* Sensory input is vital to useful function in the upper extremity, and can be assessed with a variety of tools including two-point discrimination. Residual motor function in the upper extremity can be assessed with clinical scales, a vital component of which is the degree of remaining trunk and shoulder stability. A functioning hand and wrist is useless unless one can place them meaningfully, permitting interaction with oneself and the environment. Gait analysis with polyelectromyography is frequently used as an adjunct in planning procedures in the lower extremity. There are occasions when intervention can be rationally performed only after analysis of muscle firing during the gait cycle (see, for example, the discussion of stiff knee gait below).

(5) *What type of procedure will best restore the abnormal forces acting on muscles and joints?* Deforming forces can be eliminated with a tenotomy or neurectomy, redirected with a tendon transfer, diminished with tendon lengthening procedures, or stabilized by a fusion procedure when soft tissue procedures alone would be inadequate (e.g., triple arthrodesis of the foot).

(6) *What pre-existing complications may interfere with surgery?* Preoperative plain films and bone scans are useful to assess the patient for fractures, dislocations, arthritis, and heterotopic ossification. Care should be taken on the physical examination to assess that weakness is due to upper motor neuron insult, and not to undiscovered lower motor neuron injury (e.g., undiscovered brachial plexopathy or peripheral nerve injury).

Orthopedic surgery for the upper extremity (Table 29–9) may be useful in selected spastic patients.[44] The spastic posturing of the hemiplegic shoulder (adduction and internal rotation) can be treated with release of the pectoralis major and subscapularis tendons, followed by a sling and passive stretching program. Inferior subluxation is a frequent problem in the paretic shoulder. When a sling gives inadequate symptomatic/functional relief, the biceps tendon can be looped over the coracoid process of the shoulder to serve as a static sling.

Dynamic flexion deformities of the elbow can be treated by step-cut lengthening of the biceps and fractional musculotendinous lengthening of the brachialis. The rare patient with triceps spasticity may benefit from V-Y lengthening of the triceps (V-Y refers to the shapes of the proximal and distal end of the tendon after a V-shaped incision). Occasionally, when simple lengthening is not adequate, a more extensive release may be necessary.

When flexor spasticity is not too severe, the patient with inadequate hand opening may benefit from fractional lengthening (Fig. 29–8) of the flexor digitorum sublimis and profundus tendons combined with step-cut lengthening of the flexor pollicis longus, and over-lengthening of the flexor carpi radialis and flexor carpi ulnaris. Patients are splinted in neutral, with active range of motion beginning on the third postoperative day. Overlengthening of the finger flexors can result in a loss of grip strength. An alternative procedure for patients with voluntary control but overpowering flexors is to perform a flexor-pronator origin release. For the nonfunctional spastic hand, the superficialis to profundus tendon transfer of finger flexors provides sufficient flexor tendon lengthening with preservation of a passive tether to prevent hyperextension deformity.

Procedures for hand deformities include release of the thenar and thumb adductor muscles for thumb-in-palm deformity, release of hand intrinsics, and wrist arthrodesis. While these procedures may improve cosmesis, the functional improvement after these procedures in hemiplegics is unclear, as patients frequently

TABLE 29–9 Orthopedic Intervention for the Spastic Upper Extremity

Shoulder

Adducted/internally rotated shoulder: pectoralis major/subscapularis tendon release

Painful shoulder subluxation: biceps tendon sling

Elbow

Flexor spasticity: step-cut lengthening of brachioradialis, biceps, and brachialis

Extensor spasticity: V-Y lengthening of triceps

Wrist and Hand

Flexor spasticity:

- Fractional lengthening of FDS/FDP
- Step-cut lengthening of FPL
- Overlengthening of FCR/FCU
- Flexor-pronator origin release
- Sublimis to profundus transfer

Thumb-in-palm deformity: release of thenar and adductors

FDS, flexor digitorum superficialis; FDP, flexor digitorum profundus; FPL, flexor pollicis longus; FCR, flexor carpi radialis; FCU, flexor carpi ulnaris.

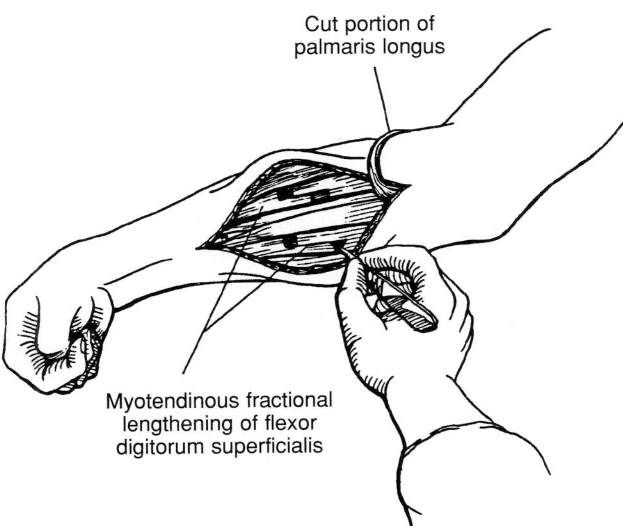

FIGURE 29–8. When upper extremity flexor spasticity of the wrist and fingers is not too severe, the patient who cannot adequately open the hand may benefit from fractional lengthening of the flexor musculature. (Modified, with permission, from Keenan MA, Kozin S, Berlet A: Manual of Orthopaedic Surgery for Spasticity. New York, Raven Press, 1993.)

continue to carry out most activities with the uninvolved upper extremity.

There are five common dynamic clinical scenarios in the lower extremities for which surgery may be considered (Table 29–10): (1) limb scissoring, (2) crouched gait, (3) stiff-knee gait, (4) equinovarus foot, and (5) spastic valgus foot.[3]

(1) *Limb scissoring* is often treated with obturator neurectomy, which improves the base of support during ambulation. If a static component complicates the picture, a hip adductor release may also be needed. No immobilization or abduction splinting is needed following surgery, and early gait training with weight bearing as tolerated should follow.

(2) *Crouched gait* results from spastic hip flexors with compensatory knee flexion and lumbar hyperlordosis. This results in a very energy-inefficient gait. The iliopsoas tendon is removed from the lesser trochanter while maintaining its capsular insertions. This allows the iliopsoas to recess proximally and diminish its pull. There is no need for postoperative immobilization, and range of motion and gait training (weight bearing as tolerated) are initiated early. Distal hamstring lengthening may also improve the crouched gait; however, care must be taken to extend the flexed knee deformity only very gradually, for fear of over-stretching the neurovascular bundle. Postoperatively, the patient is immobilized in a long leg cast, and the cast can be changed weekly to promote further extension. Transfers and gait training can be started once the cast is applied.

(3) *Stiff-knee gait* results from inappropriate firing of the quadriceps muscle, preventing adequate knee flexion during the gait cycle. Gait analysis with EMG of the various heads of the quadriceps is important so that the offending muscle groups can be selectively released (often the rectus femoris and/or vastus intermedius). Postoperative management includes a knee immobilization splint for five days followed by postoperative ambulation with weight training as tolerated. Range of motion and strengthening are begun approximately five days postoperatively.

(4) *Equinovarus foot* is the most common deformity seen in the lower extremity, with flexed ankle and turned-in foot often accompanied by excessive toe curling. The SPLATT [*spl*it *a*nterior *t*ibial *t*ransfer] Procedure is a procedure to help reduce excessive supination at the subtalar joint due to the spastic tibialis anterior muscle (Fig. 29–9). The tibialis anterior tendon is split along its length, and the distal end of the lateral half is tunneled into the third cuneiform and cuboid bones. This creates an eversion force which is slightly greater than the varus pull of the remaining medial portion. It is generally performed in combination with tendo-Achilles lengthening (Fig. 29–10), often using the Hoke triple hemisection technique. Occasionally, the tibialis posterior may be the offending muscle for the turned-in foot. Toe clawing or curling is often simultaneously treated with release of the intrinsic and extrinsic toe flexors. Postoperative management includes a short leg walking cast for six weeks followed by a molded ankle foot orthosis for an additional 4½ months. The SPLATT, tendo-Achilles lengthening, and toe flexor release are some of the most successful and rewarding procedures for the hemiplegic patient.

(5) *Valgus foot* results from overactivity of the peroneus longus muscle. This may occur in concert with an equinovarus deformity during swing

TABLE 29–10 Orthopedic Intervention for the Spastic Lower Extremity

Functional Deformities

Limb scissoring: obturator neurectomy
Crouched gait: iliopsoas recession, hamstring lengthening
Stiff knee gait: selective quadriceps release in select patients
Equinovarus foot: tendo-Achilles lengthening, split anterior tibial tendon transfer, release of extrinsic/intrinsic toe flexors
Spastic valgus foot: release and transfer of peroneus longus

Static Deformities

Hip adduction contracture: release adductor longus, gracilis
Hip flexion contracture: release of sartorius, rectus femoris, tensor fascia lata, iliopsoas, pectineus
Hip extension: release proximal hamstrings
Knee flexion contracture: release distal hamstrings
Knee extension: V-Y-plasty to lengthen quadriceps
Foot: as for functional deformities; other options include release of plantar fascia and triple arthrodesis

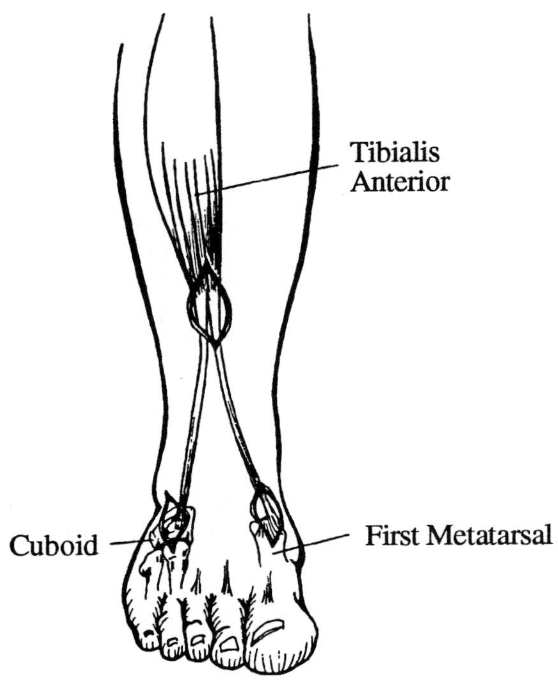

FIGURE 29–9. The SPLATT procedure helps reduce excessive supination at the subtalar joint due to the spastic tibialis anterior muscle. The tibialis anterior tendon is split along its length, and the distal end of the lateral half is tunneled into the cuboid and sometimes the third cuneiform bones. This creates an eversion force which is slightly greater than the varus pull of the remaining medial portion. (Modified, with permission, from Keenan MA, Kozin S, Berlet A: Manual of Orthopaedic Surgery for Spasticity. New York, Raven Press, 1993.)

phase. Spastic valgus is corrected by release and transfer of the peroneus longus across the dorsum of the foot into the navicular bone. Postoperative management involves a short leg walking cast in neutral position for six weeks, with immediate ambulation and weight bearing as tolerated. A molded AFO is worn for an additional 4½ months.

Static contractures in the lower extremity are treated with muscle release and lengthening. In patients with a static adductor contraction, hip adductor release (adductor longus, gracilis) is performed, followed by four weeks of forced abduction with casts or an abduction pillow splint. Hip flexion contracture is corrected with release of the sartorius, rectus femoris, tensor fascia lata, iliopsoas, and pectineus. Wound care is especially important in wounds near the perineum. The patient is placed prone three times a day with limited time in a seated position. Hip extension contractures (sometimes seen in patients with prolonged decerebrate posturing) may be treated by releasing proximal hamstrings, followed by gentle hip range of motion and sitting.

Knee flexion contractures are improved with release of the distal hamstrings. The knee is cast postoperatively and progressively extended with weekly cast changes. The extension contracture of the knee is treated with V-Y plasty of the quadriceps tendon, followed by casting in flexion for three weeks. Therapy is initiated once the cast is removed. Fixed equinovarus posturing of the foot with clawing of the toes is treated as above. In addition, it may be necessary to perform a release of the plantar flascia and/or triple arthrodesis of the ankle.

Neurosurgical Procedures. Rhizotomies, the interruption of spinal roots, can be performed for the remediation of spasticity in severe cases. Rhizotomies may be

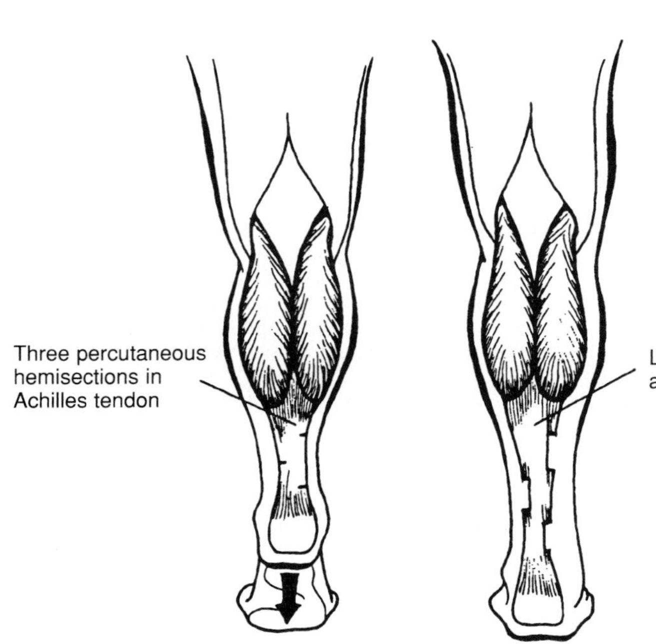

FIGURE 29–10. The tendo-Achilles lengthening is often performed in conjunction with the SPLATT procedure using the Hoke triple hemisection technique. (Modified, with permission, from Keenan MA, Kozin S, Berlet A: Manual of Orthopaedic Surgery for Spasticity. New York, Raven Press, 1993.)

categorized as open (requiring laminectomy) or closed, complete or selective, and anterior or posterior. Anterior rhizotomies are associated with severe denervation-type atrophy of all innervated muscles, and can place the patient at increased risk of skin breakdown. The recent work in surgical management of spasticity focuses largely around the issue of posterior rhizotomy.

Radiofrequency rhizotomy utilizes a radiofrequency wave to heat a needle which burns individual dorsal roots localized under fluoroscopy. It can cause significant sensory loss, so is best reserved for patients with complete sensory loss or those who are so impaired that they rely on others for turning and monitoring their skin. Because of the proximity of the cervical roots to the vertebral arteries, radiofrequency rhizotomy is not performed in the cervical area. The reduction of muscle tone usually recurs, but may last for years.

Selective dorsal rhizotomy (SDR), the neurosurgical ablation of a select proportion of dorsal rootlets, has been most often applied to children with cerebral palsy.[34] While selective rhizotomy is most often carried out in the lumbosacral roots, success has also been reported for treatment of spasticity and pain in the hemiplegic upper extremity. The term "selective" refers to the sectioning of particular segmental rootlets or fascicles, generally chosen because of their abnormal neurophysiological characteristics. The preferred subjects for this procedure are young children with spastic (not athetoid, ataxic, dystonic, rigid) cerebral palsy with good motor control and some degree of forward locomotion whose function is primarily limited due to the spastic hypertonia (Table 29–11). However, other forms of spasticity have also been treated with SDR.

The dorsal aspect of the thecal sac is exposed by laminectomy, although surgical approaches toward the spine may differ. Dorsal roots are stimulated with an insulated bipolar stimulator, and responses are recorded with polyelectromyogram (surface or intramuscular) from ipsilateral and contralateral muscles of various myotomes. Neurophysiological assessment is used to distinguish afferent rootlets that cause "spastic" responses in muscles from those that do not. The electrophysiological criteria for determining "abnormal" rootlets remains controversial, however. Investigators have stimulated rootlets at frequencies from 1 to 50 Hz, observing the "spread" of the evoked response to various muscle groups. Various parameters of the H reflex—H reflex recovery curves and ratios of initial and subsequent H reflexes—have also been employed. It remains unclear whether the neurophysiological direction for rootlet section makes a significant difference in outcome as compared with a more random rootlet selection. Part of the problem may be related to lack of standardization of stimulation and recording techniques.[42]

TABLE 29–11 Favorable Selection Criteria for Selective Dorsal Rhizotomy

Pure spasticity (limited dystonia/athetosis)
Function limited primarily by spasticity
Not significantly affected by primitive reflexes/movement patterns
Absence of profound underlying weakness
Selective motor control
Some degree of spontaneous forward locomotion
Adequate truncal balance/righting responses
Spastic diplegia
History of prematurity
Age 3–8 years
Minimal joint contractures or spine deformity
Adequate cognitive ability to participate in therapy
No significant motivational/behavioral problems
Supportive and interactive family

Adapted from MacDonald CM: Selective dorsal rhizotomy. *In* Katz RT (ed): Spasticity. State of the Art Reviews in Physical Medicine and Rehabilitation, vol 8, no 3. Philadelphia, Hanley & Belfus, 1994.

The proportion of dorsal rootlets sectioned varies from 25% to 80% in different reports. Complete section of all dorsal rootlets at a given level is generally avoided to preserve sensory function. L5 and S1 are the most frequently abnormal roots. Most reports of outcome have been based on the modified Ashworth Scale. While most surgical series offer favorable outcomes, there is still considerable controversy whether SDR makes a significant contribution to the range of functional motor performance deficits seen in cerebral palsy. Subjective improvements have been noted in range of motion and gait, while difficulties in motor control persist. Intensive therapy appears necessary to maximize long-term functional gains. The most common unwanted post-surgical effects have included hypotonia (usually transitory) and weakness. Sensory changes, bladder dysfunction, and hip subluxation/dislocation have also been reported. There is also concern that a laminectomy in a young child may predispose to later spinal deformity. Most agree that there is great need for a randomized long-term clinical trial in the evaluation of SDR.[33] Ten-year follow-up in one group suggested that lasting improvements in gait can be obtained.[50]

Microsurgical dorsal route entry zone selective destruction has been performed for the treatment of spasticity and pain in the lower limbs. However, it is not clear what advantage this procedure offers over selective posterior rhizotomy.

Myelotomy, severance of tracts in the spinal cord, has been advocated as a treatment modality in the most severe cases of spastic hypertonia. Bischoff introduced a myelotomy to interrupt the reflex arc in which the cord was approached through the lateral funiculus on one side, extending through the middle of the cord to traverse through the gray matter on the other side. Only segmental analgesia resulted from the procedure, and all long tracts except the pyramidal tract remained intact. A modification of this procedure was the posterior longitudinal myelotomy, which similarly cut through the gray matter on each side using a T-shaped myelotome via a median sulcus approach. This improvement preserved lateral funiculus white matter tracts bilaterally. Loss of bowel and bladder function must be considered as possible complications of myelotomy. Sectioning or excision of portions of the cord, cordotomy and cordectomy, causes severe muscle wasting, frequent voiding difficulties, loss of erectile function, and are rarely practiced.

SUMMARY AND CONCLUSIONS

Spastic hypertonia has been defined as "a motor disorder characterized by a velocity-dependent increase in tonic stretch reflexes (muscle tone) with exaggerated tendon jerks, resulting from hyperexcitability of the stretch reflex, as one component of the upper motor neuron syndrome." Heightened muscle tone may result from changes intrinsic to the muscle or from altered reflex properties. Increased motoneuronal excitability and/or enhanced stretch-evoked synaptic excitation of motoneurons are mechanisms whereby stretch reflexes could be enhanced.

Two distinct parameters may be altered in the pathological stretch reflex—the "set point," or angular threshold of the stretch reflex, and the reflex "gain," the amount of force required to extend the limb in proportion to the increasing joint angle. Previous studies of spastic hypertonia may be limited by the failure to dissociate the contributions of reflex threshold and reflex gain. Recent investigations suggest that spastic hypertonia may be the result of a decrease in stretch reflex threshold without significant increase in reflex gain, as was previously believed. Various clinical scales, biomechanical paradigms, pendulum models, and electrophysiological studies have been used to quantify spastic hypertonia. Biomechanical methods seem to correlate most closely with the clinical state.

Spastic hypertonia is but one component of the upper motor neuron syndrome, whose features also include loss of dexterity, weakness, and fatigability, as well as various reflex release phenomena. These other features of the upper motor neuron syndrome may well be more disabling to the patient than the changes in muscle tone. The functional impairment due to spasticity must be carefully assessed before any treatment is considered. Therapeutic intervention is best individualized to a particular patient.

Treatment to ameliorate spastic hypertonia has two basic principles: (1) avoid noxious stimuli, and (2) provide frequent range of motion. Therapeutic exercise, cold, or topical anesthesia may decrease reflex activity for short periods of time in order to facilitate minimal motor function. Casting and splinting techniques are extremely valuable to extend joint range diminished by hypertonicity.

Baclofen, diazepam, dantrolene, and, more recently, tizanidine are the most commonly used pharmacologic agents in the treatment of spastic hypertonia. Baclofen is generally the drug of choice for spinal cord types of spasticity, while sodium dantrolene is the only agent that acts directly on muscle tissue. Tizanidine has become a significant addition to the pharmacologic armamentarium for both spinal and supraspinal forms of spastic hypertonia. Intrathecal administration of anti-spastic medications delivers high concentrations of drug near the site of action, which limits systemic side effects. This form of treatment is the most exciting recent development in the treatment of spastic hypertonia.

Peripheral electrical stimulation may have limited use in diminishing tone and facilitating paretic muscles. Dorsal column stimulation via electrodes within the spinal column was initially hailed as a therapeutic advance, but has subsequently been shown to be minimally effective. Phenol and botulinum toxin injections provide a valuable transition between short-term and long-term treatments, and offer remediation of hypertonia in selected muscle groups.

Tenotomies and tendon transfers offer significant benefit to carefully chosen patients. The SPLATT procedure—transfer of the lateral portion of the tibialis anterior tendon to the lateral part of the foot—is one of the most successful rehabilitative surgeries. Hamstring tenotomies, Achilles tendon lengthening, and release of long toe flexors may all benefit selected patients with spastic hypertonia.

Surgical neurectomies can release spastic muscles in selected patient groups. Obturator neurectomies can substantially improve scissoring of gait in cerebral palsy patients. Lesions of spinal roots can decrease hypertonic reflexes; selective rhizotomies are most invasive, but offer the most precise control of neural destruction. While selective dorsal rhizotomies have enjoyed a swell of enthusiasm, especially in children with cerebral palsy, their efficacy remains to be clearly defined. Closed radiofrequency rhizotomies are performed under fluoroscopic guidance, but may only have temporary effect.

REFERENCES

1. Ada L, Vattanaslip W, O'Dwyer NJ, et al: Does spasticity contribute to walking dysfunction after stroke? J Neurol Neurosurg Psych 1998; 64:628–635.
2. Albright AL, Barron WB, Fasick MP, et al: Continuous intrathecal baclofen infusion for spasticity of cerebral origin. JAMA 1993; 270:2475–2477.
3. Anmuth CJ, Esquenazi A, Keenan MAE: Lower extremity surgery for the spastic patient. In Katz RT (ed): Spasticity. State of the Art Reviews in Physical Medicine and Rehabilitation, vol 8, no 3. Philadelphia, Hanley & Belfus, 1994.
4. Ashworth B: Preliminary trial of carisoprodol in multiple sclerosis. Practitioner 1964; 192:540–542.
5. Bohannon RW, Smith MB: Interrater reliability on a modified Ashworth scale of muscle spasticity. Phys Therapy 1987; 67:206–207.
6. Brin MF: Botulinum toxin: Chemistry, pharmacology, toxicity, and immunology. Muscle Nerve 1997; 20(suppl 6):S146–S168.
7. Brin MF, Spasticity Study Group: Dosing, administration, and a treatment algorithm for use of botulinum toxin A for adult-onset spasticity. Muscle Nerve 1997; 20(suppl 6):S208–S220.
8. Brown RA, Lawson DA, Leslie GC, et al: Observations on the applicability of the Wartenberg pendulum test to healthy elderly subjects. J Neurol Neurosurg Psych 1988; 51:1171–1177.
9. Bucholz RD: Management of intractable spasticity with intrathecal baclofen. In Katz RT (ed): Spasticity. State of the Art Reviews in Physical Medicine and Rehabilitation, vol 8, no 3. Philadelphia, Hanley & Belfus, 1994.
10. Burbaud P, Wiart L, Dubos JL, et al: Randomized, double blind, placebo controlled trial of botulinum toxin in the treatment of spastic foot in hemiparetic patients. J Neurol Neurosurg Psych 1996; 61:265–260.
11. Castellucci VF, Carew TJ, Kandel ER: Cellular analysis of long-term habituation of the gill withdrawal reflex of *Aplysia californica.* Science 1978; 202:1306–1308.
12. Dewald JPA: Sensorimotor neurophysiology and the basis for neurofacilitation therapeutic techniques. In Brandstater ME, Basmajian JV (eds): Stroke Rehabilitation. Baltimore, Williams & Wilkins, 1987, pp 109–182.

13. Dewald JPA, Given JD, Rymer WZ: Long-lasting reductions of spasticity induced by skin electrical stimulation. IEEE Trans Rehab Eng 1996; 4:231–242.
14. Dewald JPA, Given JD: Electrical stimulation and spasticity reduction: Fact or fiction. In Katz RT (ed): Spasticity. State of the Art Reviews in Physical Medicine and Rehabilitation, vol 8, no 3. Philadelphia, Hanley & Belfus, 1994.
15. Dewald JPA, Pope PS, Given JD, et al: Abnormal muscle coactivation patterns during isometric torque generation at the elbow and shoulder in hemiparetic subjects. Brain 1995; 118: 495–510.
16. Dietz V, Berger W: Normal and impaired regulation of muscle stiffness in gait: A new hypothesis about muscle hypertonia. Exp Neurol 1983; 79:680–687.
17. Donovan WH, Carter RE, Rossi D, et al: Clonidine effect on spasticity: A clinical trial. Arch Phys Medicine Rehab 1988; 69:193–194.
18. Fugl-Meyer AR, Jaasko L, Leyman I, et al: The post-stroke hemiplegic patient: A method for evaluation of physical performance. Scand J Rehab Med 1975; 7:13–31.
19. Geszten PC, Albright AL, Johnstone GF: Intrathecal baclofen infusion and subsequent orthopedic surgery in patients with spastic cerebral palsy. J Neurosurg 1998; 88:1009–1013.
20. Gottlieb GL, Myklebust BM, Stefoski D, et al: Evaluation of cervical stimulation for chronic treatment of spasticity. Neurology 1985; 35:699–704.
21. Grant SM, Heel RC: Vigabatrin: A review of its pharmacodynamic and pharmacokinetic properties and therapeutic potential in epilepsy and disorders of motor control. Drugs 1991; 41(6):889–926.
22. Gruenthal M, Mueller M, Olson WL, et al: Gabapentin for the treatment of spasticity in patients with spinal cord injury. Spinal Cord 1997; 35:686–689.
23. Halstead LS, Seager SWJ, Houston JM, et al: Relief of spasticity in SCI men and women using rectal probe electrostimulation. Paraplegia 1993; 31:715–721.
24. Hinderer SR, Gupta S: Functional outcome measures to assess interventions for spasticity. Arch Phys Med Rehabil 1996; 77:1083–1089.
25. Katz RT: Electrophysiological quantification of spastic hypertonia. In Katz RT (ed): Spasticity. State of the Art Reviews in Physical Medicine and Rehabilitation, vol 8, no 3. Philadelphia, Hanley & Belfus, 1994.
26. Katz RT, Campagnolo DI: Pharmacologic care of the spastic patient. In Katz RT (ed): Spasticity. State of the Art Reviews in Physical Medicine and Rehabilitation, vol 8, no 3. Philadelphia, Hanley & Belfus, 1994.
27. Katz RT, Rovai G, Brait C, et al: Objective quantification of spastic hypertonia: Correlation with clinical findings. Arch Phys Med Rehab1992; 73:339–347.
28. Katz RT, Rymer WZ: Spastic hypertonia: Mechanisms and measurement. Arch Phys Med Rehab 1989; 70:144–155.
29. Keenan MA, Kozin S, Berlet A: Manual of Orthopaedic Surgery for Spasticity. New York, Raven Press, 1993.
30. Knutsson E, Richards C: Different types of disturbed motor control in gait of hemiparetic patients. Brain 1979; 102: 405–430.
31. Lance JW: Symposium synopsis. In Feldman RG, Young RR, Koella WP (eds): Spasticity: Disordered Motor Control. Chicago, Year Book Medical Publishers, 1980.
32. Lance JW, McLeod JG: Disordered muscle tone. In Physiological Approach to Clinical Neurology, Boston, Butterworth Publishers, 1981.
33. Landau WM, Hunt CC: Dorsal rhizotomy, a treatment of unproven efficacy. J Child Neurology 1990; 5:174–178.
34. MacDonald CM: Selective dorsal rhizotomy. In Katz RT (ed): Spasticity. State of the Art Reviews in Physical Medicine and Rehabilitation, vol 8, no 3. Philadelphia, Hanley & Belfus, 1994.
35. McLellan DL, Hassan N, Hodgson JA: Tracking tasks in the assessment of spasticity. In Delwaide PJ, Young RR (eds): Clinical Neurophysiology in Spasticity. Amsterdam, Elsevier, 1985, pp 131–139.
36. Medical Letter: Intrathecal baclofen for spasticity. 1994; 36(917): 21–22.
37. Medical Letter: Tizanidine for spasticity. 1997; 39(1004):62–63.
38. Meythaler JM, DeVivo MJ, Hadley M: Prospective study on the use of bolus intrathecal baclofen for spastic hypertonia due to acquired brain injury. Arch Phys Med Rehabil 1996; 77:461–466.
39. Meythaler JM, Guin-Renfroe S, Grabb P, Hadley MN: Long-term continuous infused intrathecal baclofen for spastic-dystonic hypertonia in traumatic brain injury: 1-year experience. Arch Phys Med Rehabil 1999; 80:13–19.
40. Miller JF, Paul KD, Lee RH, et al: Restoration of extensor excitability in the acute spinal cat by the 5HT2 agonist DOI. J Neurophysiol 1996; 75:620–628.
41. Mueller ME, Gruenthal M, Olson WL, et al: Gabapentin for relief of upper motor neuron symptoms in multiple sclerosis. Arch Phys Med Rehabil 1997; 78:521–524.
42. Ojemann JG, Park TS, Komanetsky R, et al: Lack of specificity in electrophysiological identification of lower sacral roots during selective dorsal rhizotomy. J Neurosurg 1997; 86:28–33.
43. Otis JC, Root L, Kroll MA: Measurement of plantar flexor spasticity during treatment with tone-reducing casts. J Ped Ortho 1985; 5:682–686.
44. Pinzur MS: Upper extremity surgery for the spastic patient. In Katz RT (ed): Spasticity. State of the Art Reviews in Physical Medicine and Rehabilitation, vol 8, no 3. Philadelphia, Hanley & Belfus, 1994.
45. Priebe MM, Sherwood AM, Graves DE, et al: Effectiveness of gabapentin in controlling spasticity: A quantitative study. Spinal Cord 1997; 35:171–175.
46. Reiter F, Danni M, Lagalla G, et al: Low-dose botulinum toxin with ankle taping for the treatment of spastic equinovarus foot after stroke. Arch Phys Med Rehabil 1998; 79:532–535.
47. Russman BS, Tilton A, Gormley ME: Cerebral palsy: A rational approach to a treatment protocol, and the role of botulinum toxin in treatment. Muscle Nerve 1997; 20(suppl 6):S181–S193.
48. Sahrmann SA, Norton BJ: The relationship of voluntary movement to spasticity in the upper motor neuron syndrome. Ann Neurol 1977; 2:460–465.
49. Simpson DM: Clinical trials of botulinum toxin in the treatment of spasticity. Muscle Nerve 1997; 20(suppl 6):S169–S175.
50. Subramanian N, Vaughan CL, Peter JC, et al: Gait before and ten years after rhizotomy in children with cerebral palsy spasticity. J Neurosurg 1998; 88:1014–1019.
51. Thompson FJ, Reier PJ, Lucas CC, et al: Altered patterns of reflex excitability subsequent to contusion injury of the rat spinal cord. J Neurophys 1992; 68:1473–1486.
52. Wartenberg R: Pendulousness of the legs as a diagnostic test. Neurology 1951; 1:18–24.
53. Weingarden SI, Belen JG: Clonidine transdermal system for treatment of spasticity in spinal cord injury. Arch Phys Med Rehab 1992; 73:876–877.
54. Wright T, Nicholson J: Physiotherapy for the spastic child: An evaluation. Dev Med Child Neurol 1973; 15:146–163.
55. Young RR (ed): Role of tizanidine in the treatment of spasticity. Neurology 1994; 44(11, suppl 9):S1–S80.

30 CHAPTER

Diane M.-L. Gilbert, M.D.

Sexuality Issues in Persons with Disabilities

A virtually universal concern of rehabilitation patients, regardless of their impairment, is the impact their disability has on their sexual function and sexuality. It is not uncommon for patients, upon grasping the seriousness of their disability, to experience significant if often unexpressed anxiety over the prospects for their sexual life. Yet, despite the ubiquity of patient sexual concerns, medical schools pay little attention to training physicians in methods of patient sexual education. As early as 1900, Lewis chided his colleagues for this oversight and urged reform: "It is, therefore, proper for medical men, in their deliberations, to take cognizance of this great factor in human life. They should know its relationship to health and happiness. They should not be deterred from its scientific investigation by false modesty or by the fear of being accused of sensationalism."[73] Ende et al[45] noted that physicians generally report discomfort in discussing sexual issues with their patients. Teal and Athelstan[126] reported that 65% of patients with spinal cord injuries (SCIs) did not discuss sex with anyone during their acute hospitalization and that 85% did not discuss these matters with their physician. In the late 1980s Blake[12] found that only 22% of 169 patients with arthritic disorders had been asked by their physicians about their sexual adjustment, even though 80% believed such inquiry to be important.[12] Since physiatrists value holistic functional return to independence, they are remiss when omitting this area in the rehabilitation program.

This chapter serves as an introduction to sexual functioning and sexuality in persons with disabilities and discusses new research developments. It should be noted from the outset that the emphasis in this chapter is on "sexual intercourse," defined broadly as communication involving sexual self-expression and associated pleasuring, with or without genital involvement, to which everyone is entitled (Fig. 30–1). When sexuality is viewed from this encompassing perspective, it becomes apparent what a vital part knowledge in this area plays in developing the rehabilitation team's care plan and how important it is to incorporate discussions of sexual issues in that plan.

The first section of this chapter concentrates on *sexual function,* with a summary of normal function and detailed coverage of the many changes that accompany impairments. The second section deals with the impact of impairment on the *sexuality* of the patient. The discussion emphasizes that sexuality is not confined to the performance of sex acts but involves a much broader concept of identity and self-image. The third section addresses interactions between the rehabilitation team and the patient during the *process of assessment and recommendation for sexual satisfaction.* The goal of this chapter is to familiarize any member of a rehabilitation team with the common sexual concerns faced by patients and to provide a guide to better care in this often-neglected area.

SEXUAL FUNCTION

Anatomy and Physiology

Normal. Masters and Johnson have described four phases of sexual response: excitement, plateau, orgasm, and resolution[78] (Table 30–1; Figs. 30–2 and 30–3).[78] Arousal or excitement occurs at multiple levels and is associated with the various senses: vision, smell, hearing, memory, fantasy, and touch. Men's arousal pattern is more direct than women's, usually ending with climax. Women have varying patterns with prolonged plateau phases: no climax, single climax, or multiple climaxes (Fig. 30–3). Although our focus is on physiological sexual changes, sexual education must include other impor-

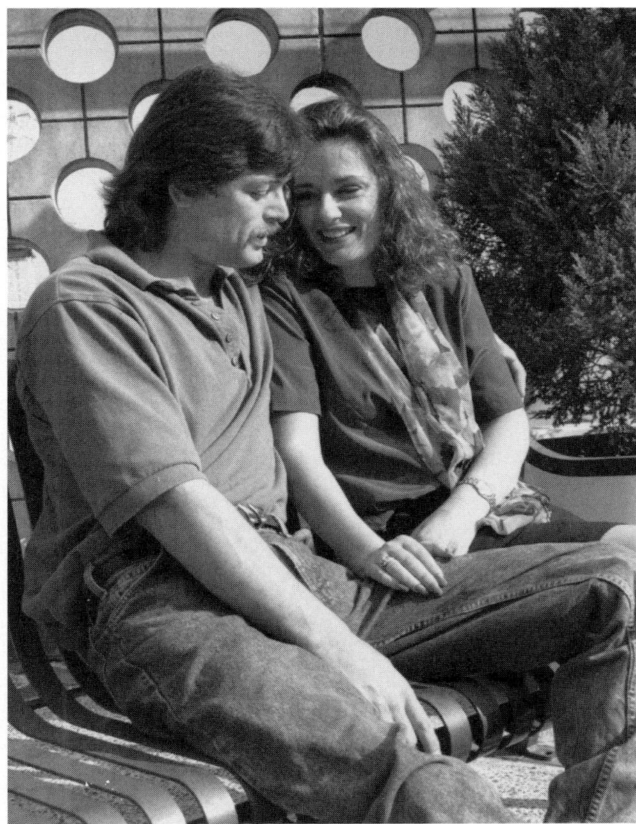

FIGURE 30–1. Sexuality is a form of communication to which all are entitled.

tant issues. Educating patients about sexually transmitted diseases and their prevention, and fertility issues such as birth control, should be an integral part of the curriculum.

Excitement or Arousal. The neurological components of the sexual response are summarized in Figure 30–4, while Figure 30–5 delineates the vascular anatomy. The sympathetic pathways involved in male erections have been intensively studied.[112] In the penile flaccid state, tonic sympathetic discharge (probably via postsynaptic alpha-receptors) causes contraction of the smooth muscles of the penile arterioles and sinusoids, which keeps blood from entering the corpora cavernosa.[1]

With sexual stimulation, nitric oxide (NO) is released by nerve cells and endothelial cells within the corpus cavernosum.[28] NO stimulates the formation of cyclic guanosine monophosphate (GMP), which causes relaxation of the corpus cavernosal smooth muscle cells and dilation of the arteries, arterioles, and sinusoids of the corpus cavernosum, causing it to fill with blood and stiffen. Cyclic GMP is then degraded by phosphodiesterase-5 (PDE-5), an enzyme that is highly concentrated in genital tissue.[43, 66] The predominant theory of venous outflow occlusion is passive veno-occlusion as the sinusoids dilate and the trabecular walls are forced against the tunica albuginea (see Fig. 30–5).[6, 84]

Excitement or arousal occurs in response to sexual stimulation either due to touch (reflexogenic) or imagination (psychogenic). In the male, the normal result is an erection and in the female, vaginal lubrication, swelling of the labia, and clitoral erection. This phase may last several minutes to hours.

The brain is the most important sexual organ in the body, with multiple loci responsible for sexual activity. Considering the importance of sexual function to species survival, it is not surprising that the cerebral tissue that results in erection and vaginal lubrication is related to the brain's phylogenetically oldest area, the limbic system.[58] Psychogenic stimuli can be both facilitory or inhibitory, and the degree of tactile stimulation necessary to produce reflex lubrication or erection can be diminished by psychic stimulation.[143] Libido is affected by concentrations of neurotransmitters, and is decreased by serotonin or stimulated by dopamine.[10] Libido is affected by depression and medications affecting the neurotransmitters (Table 30–2).[42] For patients who need antidepressant therapy, medications should be chosen carefully to prevent a lessening of sexual desire. Selective serotonin reuptake inhibitors have roughly a 50% to 70% chance of delaying orgasm even if neurological disease is absent.[4, 87]

Reflexogenic erections are those mediated via sensory input elicited by direct stimulation of the genital area through the sensory fibers of the dorsal nerve through the pudendal nerve to the sacral spinal cord. The sacral parasympathetic (S2–S4) response travels via the nervi erigentes to the cavernosal nerves and into the corporal trabeculae via autonomic fibers (see Fig. 30–4).[143] Psychogenic erections are believed to originate in the cerebral cortex from stimuli passing through the different senses such as visual stimuli like movies, pictures, or fantasizing. The impulses producing psychogenic erection travel through the hypothalamic and thalamic centers to the sympathetic thoracolumbar cord and the parasympathetic sacral cord. Studies have demonstrated cholinergic fibers within the hypogastric nerves coming from the thoracolumbar spinal cord that transmit psychic impulses responsible for erection.[125] Erections can occur even if the sacral segments are destroyed or separated from suprasacral structures, as seen in paraplegics with reported complete lower motor neuron lesions and abolished reflexogenic erections.[143] Supraspinal mechanisms are complex and can facilitate or inhibit erections.[68]

Many studies have been done documenting the type and frequency of erections in SCI males (Table 30–3).[16] Animal studies demonstrate the sympathetic outflow. Cats whose sacral cord was resected were still able to attain erection in the presence of female cats in estrus. There is sympathetic discharge to genitals as long as there is no disruption above L2 (T11–L2).[68] It was postulated that the erections in the 26% of patients with complete lower motor neuron lesions studied by Comarr (see Table 30–3) were possible because sympathetic nerves mediate erections, but they may have had incomplete lesions.[63] There is little evidence to support the role of only *thoracolumbar* sympathetic outflow in erec-

TABLE 30–1 Physiological Changes Seen in Men and Women During Sexual Activity

	Phases			
	I. Excitement	*II. Plateau*	*III. Orgasm*	*IV. Resolution*
Description	Occurs in response to sexual stimulation either due to touch (reflexogenic) or imagination (psychogenic) in both female and male	The high level of sexual arousal that precedes the threshold levels required to trigger orgasm	Believed to be a cortical experience; seems to depend mainly on intactness of sensation associated with muscles of ejaculation	Return to prearousal state over a period of 5–15 min
Duration	May be seconds, minutes, or hours	2 min to a much more prolonged duration	10–20 sec	Depends on length of excitement phase and sensory stimulation
Cardiovascular	HR and BP increase	HR continues to increase (110–175), as does BP (SBP up 20–80 mm Hg, and DBP up 10–40 mm Hg); RR begins to rise; hyperventilation begins	HR: 110–180; BP: SBP increases 40–100 mm Hg; RR: 40	RR, HR, and BP return to normal; one-third of men and women have perspiratory reaction of soles of feet, palms of hands, or entire body
Female				
Skin	No change	Sexual flush: inconstant; may appear on abdomen, breasts, neck, face, thighs	No change	Flush disappears in reverse order
Breasts	Nipple erection, venous congestion, areolar enlargement	Venous pattern prominent; size may increase one fourth over resting state; areolae enlarge, impinge on nipples so they seem to disappear	No change	Return to normal
Clitoris	Glans diameter increased; shaft: variable increase in diameter; elongation occurs in only 10% of subjects	Retraction: shaft withdraws deep into swollen prepuce	No change (shaft movements continue throughout if thrusting maintained)	Shaft returns to normal position in 5–10 sec; full detumescence in 5–10 min
Labia majora	Nullipara: thin down, flatten against perineum	Nullipara: may swell if phase II unduly prolonged	No change	Nullipara: increase to normal size in 1–2 min or less; multipara: decrease to normal in 10–15 min
Labia minora	Color change: bright pink in nullipara and red in multipara; size: increase 2–3 times normal	Color change: bright red in nullipara, burgundy red in multipara; size: enlarged labia form a funnel into vaginal orifice	Proximal areas contract with contractions of lower third	Return to resting state in 5 min
Vagina	Transudate appears 10–30 sec after onset of arousal; drops of clear fluid coalesce to form a well-lubricated vaginal barrel	Copious transudate can continue to form; quantity of transudate generally increased by prolonging preorgasm stimulation	No change	Some transudate collects on floor of upper two thirds formed by its posterior wall (in supine position)
Upper two-thirds	Balloons: dilates as uterus moves up, pulling anterior vaginal wall with it; fornices lengthen; rugae flatten	Further ballooning occurs, then wall relaxes in a slow tensionless manner	No change; fully ballooned-out and motionless	Cervix descends to seminal pool in 3–4 min
Lower one-third	Dilation of vaginal lumen occurs; congestion of walls proceeds gradually	Maximum distention reached rapidly; contracts lumen of lower third; contraction around penis aids thrusting traction on clitoral shaft via labia and prepuce	3–15 contractions of lower third and proximal labia minora at 0.75-sec intervals	Congestion disappears in seconds (if no orgasm, congestion persists for 20–30 min)

TABLE 30–1 Physiological Changes Seen in Men and Women During Sexual Activity *Continued*

	Phases			
	I. Excitement	*II. Plateau*	*III. Orgasm*	*IV. Resolution*
Uterus	Ascends into false pelvis in phase I	Contractions: strong sustained contractions begin late in phase II	Contractions strong throughout orgasm; strongest with pregnancy and masturbation	Slowly returns to normal position
Rectum			Inconstant rhythmic contractions	All reactions cease within a few seconds
Male				
Physiology	Coordinated interaction of nervous, arterial, venous, and sinusoidal systems[1] Need intact neuronal innervation, intact arterial supply, appropriately responsive corporal smooth muscle, and intact venous mechanics[141] Exact nature of venous control still not clear Phases of erection 1. Flaccid phase 2. Latent (filling) phase 3. Tumescent phase 4. Full erection phase 5. Skeletal or rigid erection phase (elicit BCB reflex) 6. Detumescent phase	*Ejaculation*—SNS, PS, and somatic systems involved synchronously *Emission* of semen Prostatic secretions, sperm from distal vas deferens and ampulla expressed through ejaculatory ducts Traverse the prostatic urethra posteriorly and join the fructose-rich contents of the seminal vesicles Development of a pressure chamber in the posterior urethra Expulsion of ejaculate through the urethra with contractions of periurethral and pelvic floor muscles[18] *Orgasm*—the sensory appreciation of this muscle response		Back to baseline *Refractory period* Time period immediately after ejaculation when further ejaculation cannot occur but erection may occur Length of period varies and tends to increase with age
Skin	No change	Sexual flush; inconsistently appears on abdomen and spreads to chest, face, and neck; can include shoulders and forearms	Widely spread flush if present, persists	Flush disappears in reverse order of appearance
Penis	Erection within 10–30 sec	Increase in size of glans and diameter of penile shaft; deepened coronal and glans coloration	Ejaculation: marked by 3–4 major contractions at 0.8-sec intervals followed by minor contractions	Partial involution of erection in 5–10 sec with variable refractory period; complete detumescence in 5–30 min
Scrotum and testes	Elevation of testes toward perineum and tightening and lifting of scrotal sac	Marked increase in size of testes over unstimulated state due to vascongestion	No change	Return to normal size due to loss of vasocongestion; testicular and scrotal descent within 5–30 min
Other	Inconsistent nipple erection	A preejaculate of a few drops of mucoid fluid which may contain viable sperm; this is not the ejaculate	Partial loss of voluntary muscular control along with ejaculation; rhythmic contractions of rectal sphincter may be noted	Return to quiescent state in 5–10 min

Abbreviations: HR, heart rate; BP, blood pressure; SBP, systolic blood pressure; DBP, diastolic blood pressure; RR, respiratory rate; BCB, bulbocavernosus reflex; SNS, sympathetic nervous system; PS, parasympathetic system.

Adapted from Masters WH, Johnson VE, Kolodny RC: Human Sexuality. Boston, Little, Brown, 1982.

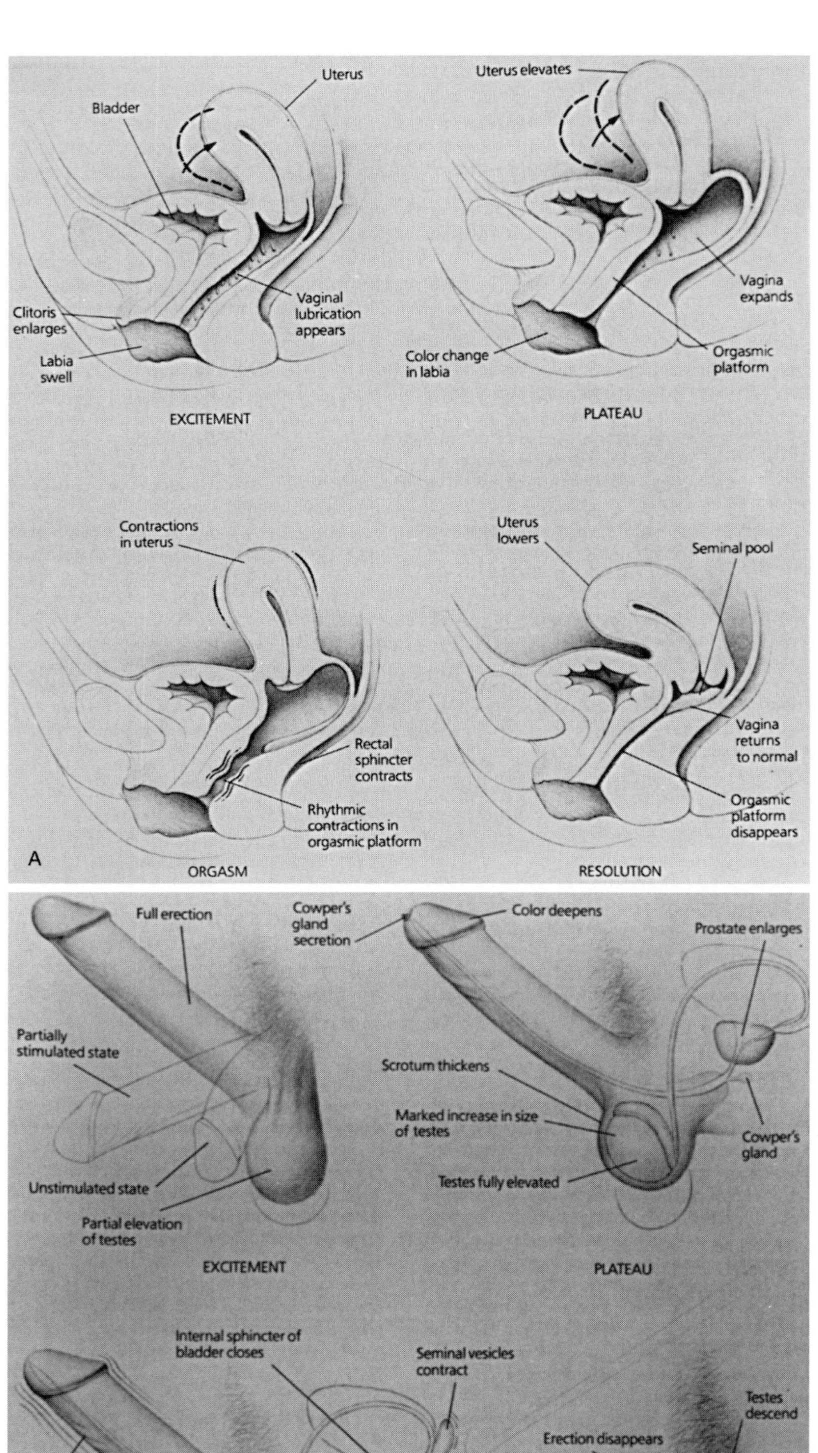

FIGURE 30–2. *A.* Internal changes in the female sexual response cycle (explained in detail in Table 30–1). *B.* External and internal changes in the male sexual response cycle (explained in detail in Table 30–1). (From Masters WH, Johnson VE, Kolodny RC: Human Sexuality. Boston, Little, Brown, 1982, pp 60–61.)

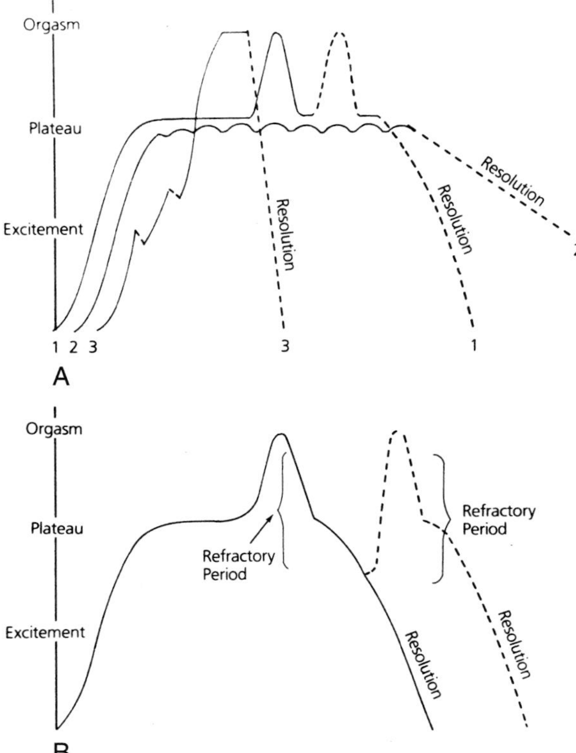

FIGURE 30–3. The sexual phases of women (*A*) and men (*B*) as described by Masters and Johnson: excitement, plateau, orgasm, and resolution, (From Masters WH, Johnson VE, Kolodny RC: Human Sexuality. Boston, Little, Brown, 1982, p 58.)

tion development. Erections are now believed to occur only rarely with complete lower motor neuron lesions.

Male erectile dysfunction (ED) has been defined as the inability of a man to achieve an erect penis as part of the overall multifaceted process of male sexual function. ED refers to attaining and maintaining penile erection sufficient for satisfactory sexual performance.[95]

Plateau. The plateau phase can be very brief (seconds) or prolonged (minutes) and is described as a pleasurable sense of well-being.[78] A number of sexual dysfunctions can occur in this stage. With *anorgasmy* the individual does not progress further than the plateau stage. *Premature ejaculation* refers to emission or ejaculation that is accompanied by loss of erection before or immediately upon penetration.

Ejaculation. Male ejaculation requires a coordinated series of muscular and neurophysiological events involving the sympathetic, parasympathetic, and somatic nervous supply that cause the constituents of the ejaculate to be deposited in the posterior urethra, then evacuated through the urethra and urethral meatus in an antegrade fashion. It is generally agreed that no anatomical sphincter exists within the posterior urethra in the area of the bladder neck, but rather the neck has inherent tension in postpubertal males that is augmented during ejaculation by sympathetic input to prevent retrograde flow.[93] The tension corresponds to the sense of inevitability of ejaculation where cerebral control is minimal, described by Masters et al[78] Emission and ejaculation are reflexive and can occur independently, and erection is not an absolute prerequisite. The emission center of the spinal cord is T10 to L2, and Sato et al have proposed three routes for the efferent signal transmission for seminal emission from the L1 paravertebral sympathetic ganglion.[114] The three routes are (1) through the hypogastric nerves, (2) sympathetic nerve fibers through the lumbosacral sympathetic trunk, and (3) through the spermatic nerves.[25]

Female ejaculation is not as easily a quantifiable response as is the male norm and remains a more controversial subject. When it occurs, the ejaculate has been

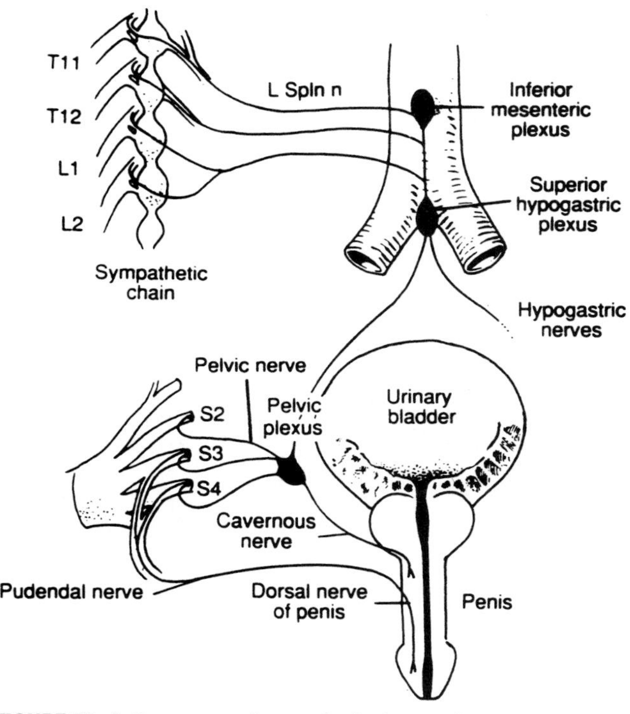

FIGURE 30–4. Summary of neurological sexual anatomy. Parasympathetic innervation: originates in the anterior divisions of spinal roots S2 to S4; preganglionic fibers enter the pelvis as the nervi erigentes or pelvic nerves course in close proximity to the hypogastric vessels, terminating in the pelvic plexus; the cavernous nerve then travels to the corpora, and other fibers to the scrotum and pubis. Sympathetic innervation: T10 to L2 supply the sympathetic fibers to the penis and female genitalia; preganglionic fibers course to the superior hypogastric plexus, join the pelvic plexus via the hypogastric nerves, and travel via the cavernous nerve to the genitalia; postganglionic nerves in the hypogastric nerves travel to the vas deferens, seminal vesicle, ampulla, bladder neck, musculature of the prostate, and blood vessels of the prostate and penis. Somatic innervation: pudendal nerve is formed from the anterior divisions of S2 to S4; it supplies both sensory innervation (to penis, scrotum, and pubis) and motor innervation (to bulbocavernosus, ischiocavernosus, striated urethral sphincter, and perineal muscles). (From Melman A, Christ GJ, Hirsch MS: Anatomy and physiology of the penis. In Bennett AH (ed): Impotence: Diagnosis and Management of Erectile Dysfunction. Philadelphia, WB Saunders, 1994, p 21.)

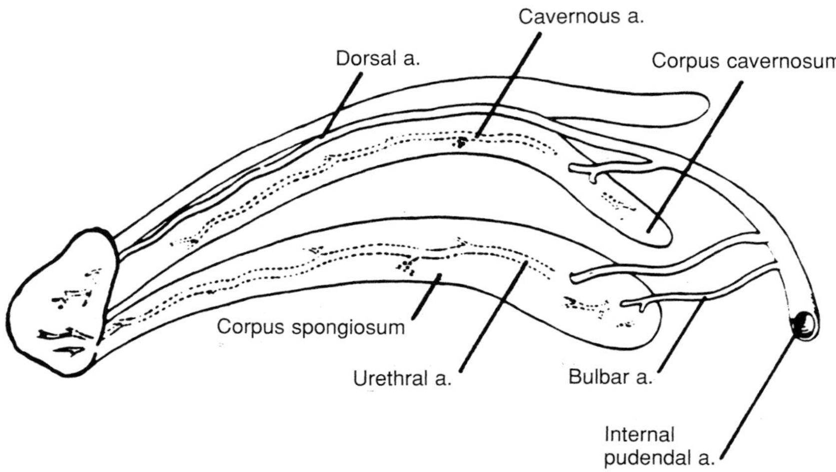

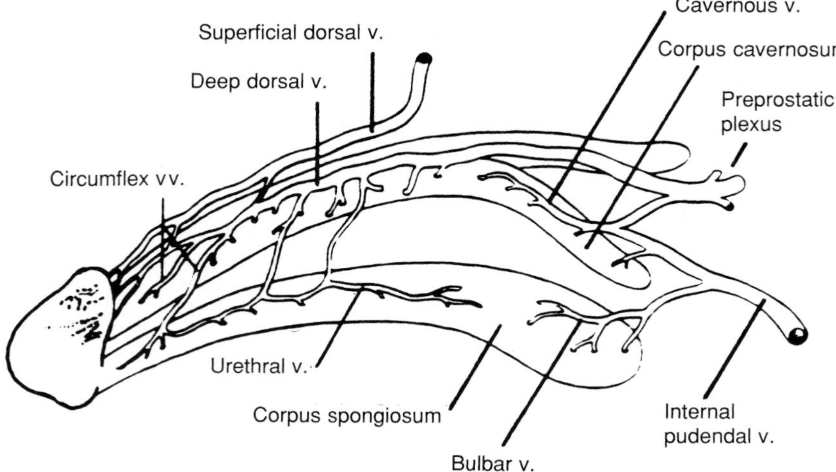

FIGURE 30–5. There are four paired arteries: (1) dorsal, which supply the glans; (2) cavernosal (corporal), which are responsible for tumescence; (3) spongiosal (ventral), which supply the spongiosa, urethral tissue, and glans; and (4) bulbar, which supply the Cowper's gland and proximal urethral bulb. The venous system is composed of the superficial, intermediate, and deep systems. (From Aboseif SR, Lue TF: Hemodynamics of penile erection. Urol Clin North Am 1988; 15:2.)

traced to the motor response of the above routes and the anterior portion of the vagina (G-spot). Vaginal transudates accumulate throughout the arousal process and can give the appearance of an ejaculate.

Orgasm. Orgasm is believed to be a cortical experience of "supreme pleasure followed by a feeling of well-being and satiation."[144] It occurs in the limbic system. In the majority of men, orgasm seems to depend on intactness of sensation associated with the muscles of ejaculation. That orgasm can be experienced separate from ejaculation is very important in those with ejaculatory disorders. The relatively long waiting period between ejaculations for men is related to the time required to build up seminal ejaculate. The intensity of orgasms varies from person to person and often from each encounter to the next.

Women have described orgasm on a continuum from a "mild stimulation [to] a sensation of ecstasy so overwhelming that a [woman] momentarily loses consciousness."[144] The muscles involved in orgasm produce a biphasic motor response involving sympathetic contraction of the smooth muscles of the fallopian tubes, uterus, and paraurethral glands of Skene: somatic contraction of striated pelvic floor muscles; perineum; and anal sphincter.

Resolution. Resolution is the return to the pre-arousal physiological state, usually occurring over a period of 5 to 15 minutes (see Table 30–1). Sympathetic tonic discharge resumes in the penis, resulting in contraction of the smooth muscles around the sinusoids and arterioles. Arterial blood flow is decreased and venous channels are reopened.[1] Presumably, the analogous situation occurs in the female.

Normal Age-Related Physiological Changes. These occur in women most dramatically at the onset of menopause, when the relative steroid deficit reduces the ra-

TABLE 30–2 Sexual Dysfunction Side Effects Associated with Medication

Medication	Sex	Type of Sexual Dysfunction
Cardiovascular agents		
Chlorothiazide	M	Impotence, failed ejaculation
Clonidine	M	Impotence in ~24%
Guanethidine	M/F	Diminished libido, dose-related
	M	Delayed ejaculation, libido impairment, potency impairment, retrograde ejaculation
Hydrochlorothiazide	M/F	Decreased erection in ~9%; in combination with β-blockers, 23%
Labetalol	M	Changes in erection, delayed tumescence, delayed ejaculation, priapism
Methyldopa	M/F	Sedation, depression, sexual dysfunction in ~32%
Prazosin	M	Priapism
Propranolol	M	Decreased potency, impotence, failed ejaculation
	M/F	Decreased libido
Reserpine	M	Impotence, failed ejaculation, dose-related in ~60%
Spironolactone	M	Gynecomastia, impotence
	F	Menstrual irregularity
Digoxin	M/F	Decreased libido and arousal
Psychotherapeutic agents		
Phenothiazine, MAO, TCA	M/F	Sedation, anticholinergic, sympatholytic
Serotonin uptake inhibitors	M/F	Decreased libido; impotence/anorgasmia
Lithium, diazepam	M/F	Sedation, decreased libido
Anxiolytics	M/F	Decreased libido/anorgasmia
Other		
Phenytoin	M/F	Decreased libido
Cimetidine	M	Impotence
Naproxen	M	Impaired ejaculation
Alcohol	M/F	Prominent libido suppression, impotence, dysfunction with orgasm, relationship problems
Tobacco	M	Impotence
Marijuana	M/F	Delayed orgasm
Cocaine, heroin	M/F	Autonomic dysfunction with excessive use

Abbreviations: MAO, monoamine oxidase inhibitor; TCA, tricyclic antidepressant.

Data from Deamer RL, Thompson JF: The role of medications in geriatric sexual function. Clin Geriatric Med 1991; 7:95–111; Murphy JB, Lipshultz LI: Abnormalities of ejaculation. Urol Clin North Am 1987; 14:583–595; Relf MV: Sexuality and the older bypass patient. Geriatr Nurs 1991; 34:294–296; Seidl A, Bullough B, Haughey B, et al: Understanding the effects of a myocardial infarction on sexual functioning: A basis for sexual counseling. Rehabil Nurs 1991; 16:255–264.

pidity and intensity of the physiological sexual response. There is a decrease in the frequency of vaginal and uterine contractions during orgasm.[52] The vaginal canal becomes thinner and shorter secondary to decreased estrogen. Lubrication diminishes or takes longer, and non-petroleum-based lubricating jelly can be helpful. There is an increased incidence of vulvovaginitis and urethritis, atrophy of the external genitals, changes in the size of the clitoris and labia, and pubic hair loss. These changes are greatly ameliorated with estrogen replacement.[76] Prolapse and stress incontinence are also seen in multiparous aging women but they can be managed well surgically. Changes seen in men are summarized in Table 30–4.[65, 115, 137]

TABLE 30–3 Erectile Functioning After Spinal Cord Injury: Observations in Several Large Series

Study*	Subjects	Overall (%)	Reflex (%)	Psychogenic (%)	C-T (%)	L-S (%)
Munro, 1948	84	74			83	50
Talbot, 1949	200	64	43	21	75	53
Kuhn, 1950†	25	88			88	
Talbot, 1955	208	69	49	20	75	60
Comarr, 1977‡	679	80	73	7	73§	31¶
Zeitlin, 1957	100	86			86	86

Abbreviations: C-T, cervicothoracic; L-S, lumbosacral.

*Munro D, Horne HW, Paull DP: N Engl J Med 1948; 239:903; Talbot HS: Sexual function in paraplegia. J Urol 1955; 73:91–100; Kuhn RA: Functional capacity of the isolated human spinal cord. Brain 1950; 73:1–51; Zeitlin AB, Cottrell TL, Lloyd FA: Fertil Steril 1957; 8:337

†All T2–T12.

‡Summary of reference 16 and Comarr AE: Sexual function in patients with spinal cord injury. In Pierce PS, Nickel VH (eds): The Total Care of Spinal Cord Injury. Boston, Little, Brown, 1977, p 171–185.

§Upper motor neuron lesions all reflexogenic.

¶Lower motor neuron lesions all psychogenic.

From Yarkony GM: Enhancement of sexual function and fertility in spinal cord-injured males. Am J Phys Med Rehabil 1990; 69:81–87.

TABLE 30–4 Normal Age-Related Physiological Changes in Men

Phase	Change
Excitement	Develop erections 2–3 times slower than younger men Tactile stimulation may be necessary Erection is not as firm, approaches full ridigity only seconds before ejaculation
Plateau	Able to maintain erection for longer period prior to ejaculation Less discernible nipple swelling and erection Testicular elevation is reduced
Ejaculation/ orgasm	Ejaculation lacks the well-defined sense of impending orgasm because accessory organs fail to secrete and create the welling of semen in the prostatic urethra One to two expulsive contractions of the urethra occur instead of the usual four major contractions Seepage can occur rather than expulsion, which dimishes the sensation through the urethra
Resolution	More rapid detumescence Refractory period increases in length (>55 yr ~ 12–24 hr)

Data from Kaiser FE: Sexuality and impotence in the aging man. Clin Geriatr Med 1991; 7:63–71; Schiavi RC, Schreiner-Engel P, Mandeli J, et al: Healthy aging and male sexual function. Am J Psychiatry 1990; 147:766–771; Weiss JN, Mellinger BC: Sexual dysfunction in elderly men. Clin Geriatr Med 1990; 6:185–196; LoPiccolo J: Counseling and therapy for sexual problems in the elderly. Clin Geriatr Med 1991; 7: 161–179.

Changes with Impairments

From a physiological point of view, normal sexual function depends on the interaction of libido and potency.[65] *Sexual dysfunction* can be defined as any sexual behavioral problem that makes sexual expression consistently unsatisfying for the individual or partner (Table 30–5).[116] Eighty percent of sexual complaints can be successfully managed in the office setting.[65] The sudden onset of disability or the more chronic issues of malaise, pain, fatigue, or stress can contribute to decreased libido.

The Massachusetts Male Aging Study showed that among 1290 men ages 40 to 70 years, 52% complained of some degree of ED.[46] Ten to 30 million men in the United States are affected, and this is age-associated, with estimated prevalence rates of 39% among men 40 years old and 67% among those 70 years old.[99] Sixty percent of all male sexual dysfunction at a performance level is physical in origin and this dysfunction increases with age. Dysfunction is most common in patients with diabetes, circulatory changes, autonomic nervous disorders, venous leakages or arteriovenous shunting, alcoholism, or from effects of medications.[39] There is evidence to indicate that it is frequently associated with depression, increased anxiety, and poor self-esteem in affected patients.[102]

Some 14% to 20% of women over 15 years of age have a long-term disability. The most common sexual concern for women with or without disabilities is low desire. This must be distinguished from biological sexual drive and lack of privacy, misinformation, concerns about birth control, lack of sexual skills in the partner, or interruption of the physiological sexual response.[4] Sadoughi et al[111] studied 34 males and 21 females with emphysema, arthritis, stroke, and amputation. Disability-related physical limitations were the most frequently cited reasons for fear and feelings of discomfort in carrying out sexual activity, with 78% reporting a decline in frequency of sexual activity, and greater than 50% reporting a change in pattern. Thirty-six percent desired more satisfaction, and 42% believed their spouses presently desired more sexual satisfaction. Just as in SCI patients, 50% would have liked to discuss sexual problems with a member of the hospital staff prior to discharge, preferably with a physician of the same sex.[81]

Sildenafil (Viagra). On March 27, 1998, the FDA approved sildenafil (Viagra) as the first oral agent specifically indicated for the treatment of male ED. This drug is now widely used for ED in the normal male and has begun to change the sexual landscape in the United States, much as the birth control pill did in the 1960s.[66] Sildenafil is an orally active, potent, selective inhibitor of cGMP-specific PDE-5, resulting in higher concentra-

TABLE 30–5 Types of Sexual Dysfunction

Dysfunction	Characteristics
Decreased libido	Decline in sexual drive or desire; may be conscious or subconscious
Decreased vaginal lubrication	Reduction in lubrication fluid in vagina
Delayed orgasm	Prolonged time for orgasm to occur
Anorgasmia	Inability to achieve orgasm
Breast hyperplasia	May adversely affect self-esteem and body image, especially as adolescent
Gynecomastia	Enlargement or excessive development of male breast; may be unilateral or bilateral
Impotence	Inability to achieve or maintain erection sufficient for penetration and intercourse
Priapism	Prolonged, painful erection caused by lack of drainage of corpus cavernosum
Retarded ejaculation	Delayed ejaculation or inability to ejaculate
Retrograde ejaculation	Ejaculation into urinary bladder caused by insufficient tightening of internal urethral neck
Premature ejaculation	When emission/ejaculation is accompanied by loss of erection, before or immediately upon vaginal penetration

Adapted from Seidl A, Bullough B, Haughey B, et al: Understanding the effects of a myocardial infarction on sexual functioning: A basis for sexual counseling. Rehabil Nurs 1991; 16:255–264.

tions of cGMP, better vasodilation, and hence an erection that it is easier to get and maintain.[66, 91] In men with ED, the problem is often that cGMP is not present in high enough concentrations either to develop or to maintain an erection. There has been an 80% rate of improved erections in the studies looking at a general population use.[50, 102]

The current recommended dose is one 50-mg tablet taken 1 hour before sexual activity. The drug is absorbed rapidly and reaches peak levels in 30 to 120 minutes. The effect usually lasts 4 hours. It is primarily cleared by hepatic enzymes. The drug should not be taken more than once a day. It is not an aphrodisiac and therefore will not work without sexual stimulation. The risk of priapism is therefore minimal. This is a valuable advantage over the injectable vasoactive medications. The side effects and warnings are related to other autonomically involved areas of anatomy and physiology. The primary side effects are headache, facial flush, upset stomach, and visual color distortion (a shift toward blue).

Sildenafil when taken alone can cause small (usually clinically imperceptible) drops in systolic blood pressure and does not have a synergistic effect when taken with common antihypertensive drugs. The drug is *absolutely contraindicated* in patients on organic nitrates, as this combination can lead to severe drops in blood pressure.[66] The FDA advises caution for men who have suffered a heart attack, stroke, or life-threatening arrhythmia within the previous 6 months, have resting hypotension (blood pressure 90/50 mm Hg) or hypertension (blood pressure more than 170/110 mm Hg), have a history of cardiac failure or coronary artery disease causing unstable angina, or have retinitis pigmentosa. Patients with heart disease, suspected heart disease, and risk factors for heart disease should discuss with their physician the safety of resuming sexual activity. A cardiac workup, including exercise treadmill testing, should be considered in appropriate patients.[60, 92]

Additional oral forms of therapy for ED (e.g., oral phentolamine, apomorphine) are being studied, but as yet none has been approved by the FDA.[66]

Spinal Cord Injury

Patients with SCI constitute less than 5% of a typical physiatrist's practice, but much of the sexuality literature on rehabilitation has focused on this subset of patients. This is probably because function is greatly changed in SCI patients and more than half are 15 to 25 years old (a time of usual sexual awareness). The 15% of SCI patients who are female have unfortunately been largely ignored in the literature. White found in a survey of female SCI patients that only 37% indicated they had received information on sexual issues since their injury.[139] Rates of attempted suicide for female patients were double those for comparable male subjects and were thought to be due to self-destructive lifestyles. It is now clear that sexual activity after injury is indeed related to the neurological level and the completeness of the lesion in females as well as males.[134] For a more detailed look at SCI, the reader is referred to the excellent reviews by Linsenmeyer and Perkash[74] Yarkony,[43] Sipski and Alexander (men),[117] Bérard,[7] Charlifue et al (women),[32] and Rabin.[106]

Neurological injury can affect either upper motor neurons (e.g., tetraplegia) or lower motor neurons (e.g., cauda equina). These lesions usually involve motor and sensory pathways, and the patient has to deal with motor weakness, loss of sensation, and changes in erection or lubrication, ejaculation, orgasm and fertility. Incomplete lesions might spare some sexual function, but genital sensation is lost with injury to the spinal cord above S2. Males with complete lower motor neuron disease involving the S2–S4 segments (i.e., cauda equina) will have poor erectile function as the S2–S4 reflex is interrupted. The motor deficits can interfere with mobility and impair social contact, both of which can affect sexual function.

After SCI, previous erogenous zones may be insensate, which can affect the excitement phase. The demarcation between insensate and sensate skin may become the new erogenous zone. Incomplete SCI patients often have erogenous sensation in the perianal area, but cultural attitudes toward anal stimulation can prevent patients from benefiting from this erogenous area.[14] Patients must be encouraged to experiment with their bodies to learn and understand the new changes and effectively communicate their needs to their partners.

Achieving Erections. Reflexogenic erection can occur with stroking, oral stimulation, vibration, pulling pubic hair, or a full bladder. The degree of stimulation required may decrease or increase with psychogenic stimulation. The genitals might need continuous physical stimulation to maintain their arousal. Experimentation is encouraged to discover individual stimulation techniques. Education by the staff can help prevent uncomfortable or embarrassing situations, such as when a male patient has an erection while a nurse performs a bladder catherization. Psychogenic erections can occur with incomplete lower motor neuron lesions, as previously described. The importance of a secure, private location for the patient's experimentation must be emphasized.

The results of several large studies on erectile functioning after SCI help predict what can be expected with various lesion levels. These studies should be viewed with caution since the studies generally relied on patient report (see Table 30–3).[143] Psychogenic erections are typically lost with lesions between T10 and T12, while both reflexogenic and psychogenic erections are possible with lesions between L2 and S1. Talbot[124] reported that erections (both types) are most common in males with injury levels higher than T11 and in those with incomplete lesions. Kuhn[69] found that erections could always be induced if there was reflex activity (bulbocavernosus reflex) below the lesion level. There is a sharply circumscribed reflexogenic area on the penis that includes the corona of the glans and the penile frenulum.[143]

Patients should be evaluated carefully and individually to assess their deficits. The evaluation should follow the PARSS model (discussed later) with a thorough history and general neurological examination. Patients with bilateral sphincterotomies have a 2% to 56% incidence of ED, while those with the more recent anteromedian sphincterotomy approach have a less than 5% incidence.[142] Neurogenic causes of ED can be confirmed by testing with vasoactive substances injected into the corpora. During the period of spinal shock, which can last from a few hours to several weeks, it is impossible to predict sexual impairment. In all deliberations regarding sexual function, it is important to note that function might not return for 6 to 24 months (in 80% of cases it does so within 1 year of injury, and in another 5% within 2 years).[142] Clinicians should not overlook the possibility of a nonorganic cause (i.e., psychogenic impotence) as the primary cause of erectile dysfunction.[125] Aggressive (especially invasive) intervention should be limited during this time period.

Techniques to Restore Erection. Restoring erection in the SCI male may be accomplished using one of the following four options.

Neuropharmacotherapy: Oral Agents. Oral sildenafil (Viagra), taken as required (not more than once daily), significantly improves the quality of erections and satisfaction with sex life in men with ED caused by SCI between T6 and L5. Patients selected had to be able to achieve at least a partial reflexogenic erectile response to penile vibratory stimulation. No patients discontinued treatment due to adverse events; however, the risk of priapism in SCI patients with vasodilator chemicals of all types may be greater, and this type of patient should be started on a lower dose.[43, 80]

Well-controlled double-blind studies of yohimbine hydrochloride, an oral alpha-2-adrenergic blocking agent, have shown it to have only limited efficacy in ED when used singly or in combination with methyltestosterone and a variety of vitamins and caffeine-based stimulants.[15] Oral levodopa has also been used, with 55% to 60% of patients reported to achieve rigid erection.[142]

Intracavernous Injection of Vasoactive Substances.[3, 113, 142] Injection into the corpora of papaverine (a nonspecific smooth muscle relaxant producing vasodilation and relaxation of the sinusoidal spaces), a combination of papaverine and phentolamine (an alpha-adrenergic blocker producing vasodilation), or prostaglandin E_1 produces an erection. The patients are typically managed by a urologist, who carefully titrates the doses of the vasoactive substances, as there is a risk for priapism, even with small doses. This risk is increased in the SCI patient because neurogenic-based ED requires lower doses. The vasoactive agents are injected sterilely into the lateral aspect of the base of the penile shaft, avoiding midline neurovascular structures. Hematomas are prevented by compressing the injection site for 2 to 5 minutes. Sympathomimetic agents such as phenylephrine and epinephrine can be used to treat drug-induced priapism.[3] Our institution has a policy of treating patients with injection therapy only if they comply with their bladder, bowel, and skin management. This form of therapy is effective but is associated with a high rate of withdrawal from treatment, which in one series was 41% at 12-month follow-up because of the invasiveness and lack of spontaneity.[66] Intraurethral application of alprostadil via urethral suppository seemed like an attractive option, but its inability to produce consistently rigid erections has been disappointing.[71, 99, 109] Topical papaverine gel may augment reflex erections by enhancing penile arterial flow.[64]

Vacuum Tumescence Constriction Therapy.[94, 141] VCTC refers to the use of external devices that create a vacuum and cause an erection-like state that is maintained by a constricting band (Fig. 30–6). The flaccid penis is placed in a rigid cylinder. A pump creates the vacuum needed to fill the corpora with blood. A constricting band is placed at the base of the penis, after the cylinder is removed, to prevent blood from leaving the penis (partners may complain of a cold penis) (Fig. 30–7). This can maintain an erection for up to 30 minutes. Detumescence follows rapidly after the band is removed. The ErecAid (ErecAid Osbon Medical Systems, Augusta,

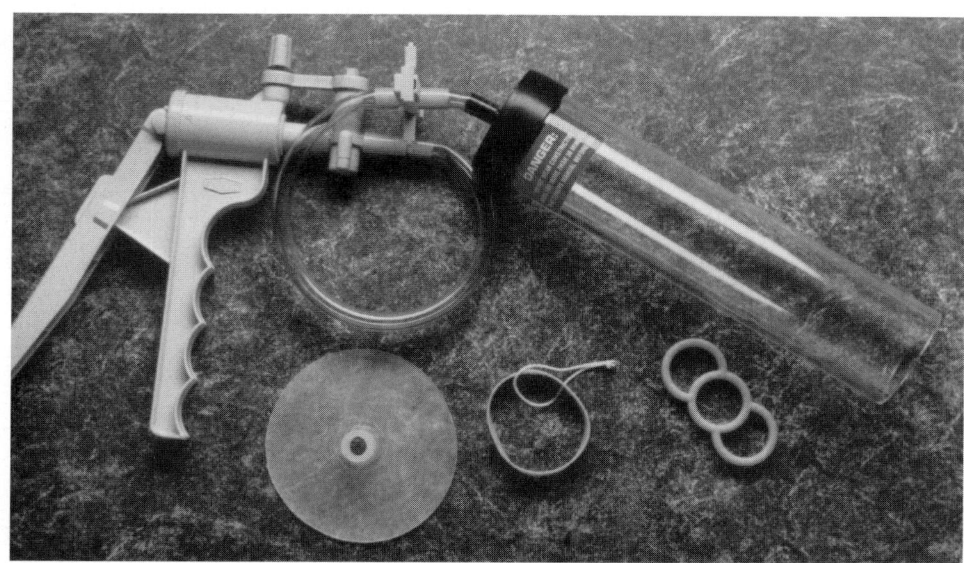

FIGURE 30–6. Assembled vacuum tumescence constriction device, with two types of constriction bands displayed.

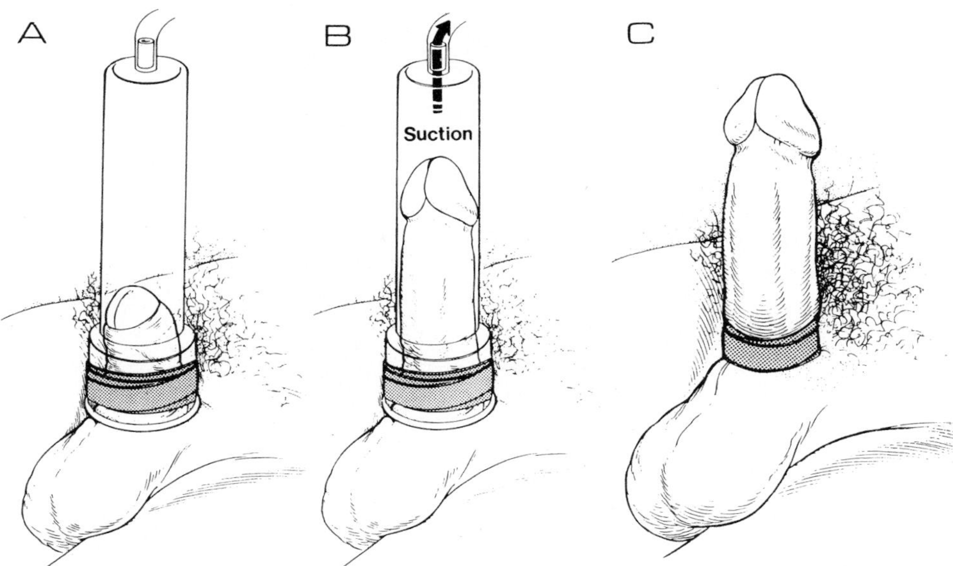

FIGURE 30–7. *A.* Cylinder with constriction bands around base placed over flaccid penis. *B.* Suction applied, creating negative pressure within cylinder and resulting in penile engorgement. *C.* Constriction bands guided from cylinder to base of penis. (From Witherington R: External aids for treatment of impotence. J Urol Nurs 1987; 6:10.)

Ga.), originally marketed as the Youth Equivalent Device, has been available since 1917.[143] These devices can be found in many shops that sell sex-related paraphernalia for far less cost than from a medical vendor. The constricting band prevents urinary leakage but also antegrade ejaculation. Reliability of the patients is important, since the constricting band should not be left in place longer than 30 minutes because of a risk of penile ischemia and necrosis. Patients taking anticoagulant medication or those with bleeding disorders should not use VTCT.[142]

Penile Prosthesis.[89] Implantable penile prostheses are available in numerous designs, including fixed, semirigid (flexible), or inflatable. Semirigid prostheses can be hinged, malleable, or articulated. Inflatable penile prostheses can be multicomponent or self-contained (Fig. 30–8).[143] With the inflatable prosthesis, the penis is inflated to full erection by means of a pump located in the scrotum. When a valve is opened, the penis deflates. The multicomponents of the inflatable prosthesis make it more difficult and costly to insert than the fixed or flexible rods.[131] Indications for these devices in SCI patients include both ED and maintenance of external catheters. Their use has recently declined in SCI males. The reason for this decrease is twofold: the frequency of complications and the simpler, safer, cost-effective injection and vacuum techniques. The problem with the fixed prosthesis is that the malleable rods that are placed in the corpus callosum can sometimes cause problems such as infection and erosions, especially in the insensate. The rate of postoperative infection in the general population is 2%, but it is 7% in the SCI population. The erosion rate is as high as 11% in the SCI population, but only 1% in the general population (Table 30–6).[37, 143] An artificial penis (dildo) can be strapped on the groin to simulate a natural erection.[131]

Transcutaneous Agents.[90] Transcutaneous nitroglycerin has been used as topical therapy for ED in SCI patients. It produced an erection sufficient for coitus in 25% of patients in whom papaverine injections had induced rigid erections.[121, 142] Nitroglycerin has frequent side effects, including hypotension and headaches.

Achieving Vaginal Lubrication. Much of what was said in the Achieving Erection section applies to females with respect to vaginal lubrication and engorgement. There is both reflexogenic and psychogenic lubrication. A sensation similar to that of a full bladder is described by some women with reflexogenic lubrication, while the sensation with psychogenic lubrication is often attenuated. Those with complete lesions involving T10 to T12 do not have lubrication and benefit from vaginal lubricants such as saliva, Replens, or K-Y jelly.

Coitus. *Coitus* is defined as intromission and intravaginally sustained erection. To accomplish this an erection must occur at the right time, be sufficiently hard for penetration, and last long enough to satisfy the partner.[143] Talbot[124] studied 208 SCI patients and found that only 23% of those who attained an erection were able to achieve successful coitus (see Table 30–3). It is important not to overemphasize the need for an erection in sexual relationships, and to ensure that the patients are aware that more than 50% of well-adjusted women do not reach orgasm with vaginal stimulation alone. The "stuffing technique" can be used if the patient or his partner desire vaginal intromission.[131] Loss of lubrication in the female patient can interfere with coitus. Pelvic floor and adductor muscle spasticity can restrict penile penetration.[6] Premedication with benzodiazepines can help reduce this spasticity. Both male and female SCI patients must learn to empty their bladder and bowel prior to sexual activity and remember to void or catheterize themselves after sexual activity to lessen the chances of urinary tract infection (UTI). The level of concern regarding incontinence during sex is very high in both males and females.[138, 139]

Ejaculation.[5] Failure of synchronous activity involving deposition of ejaculate constituents and antegrade

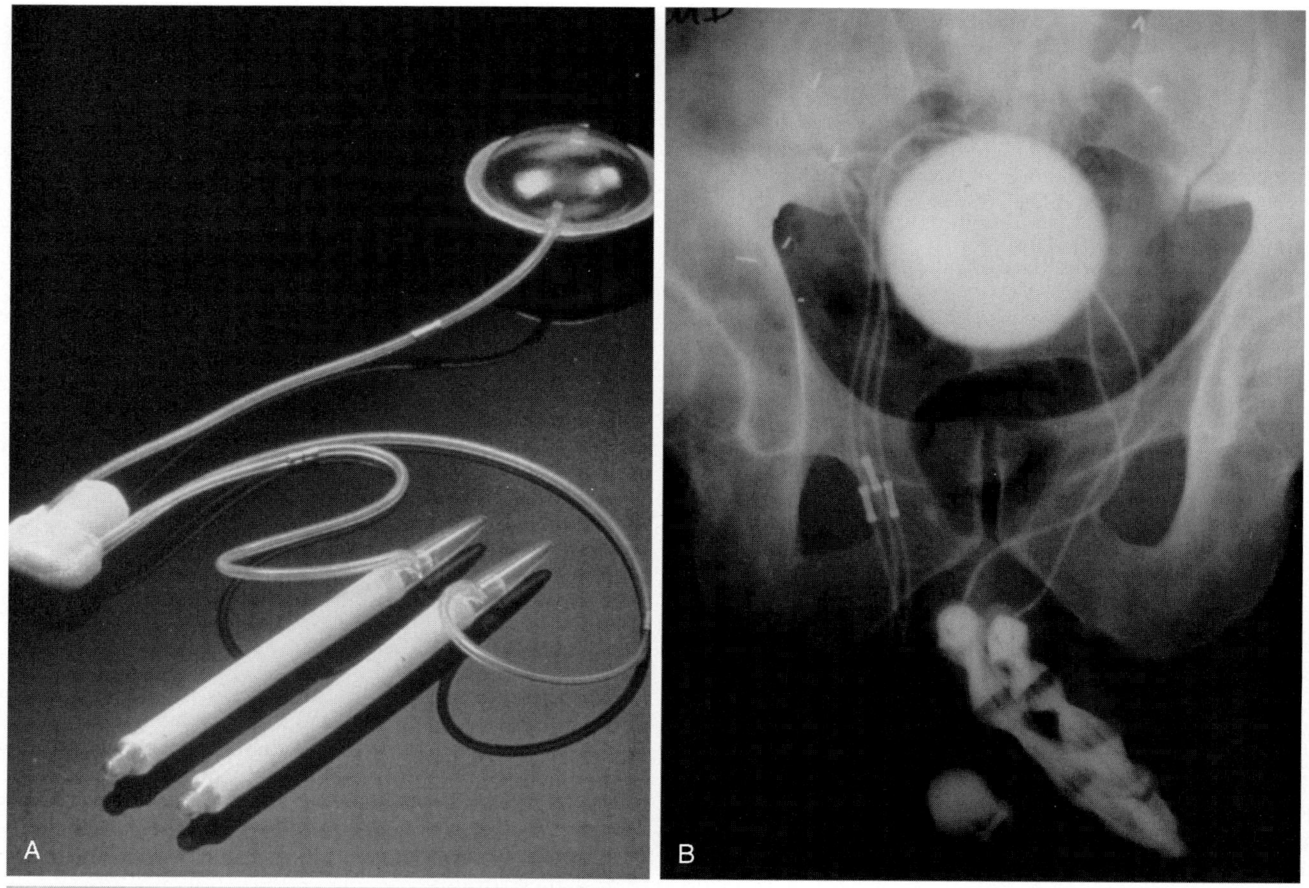

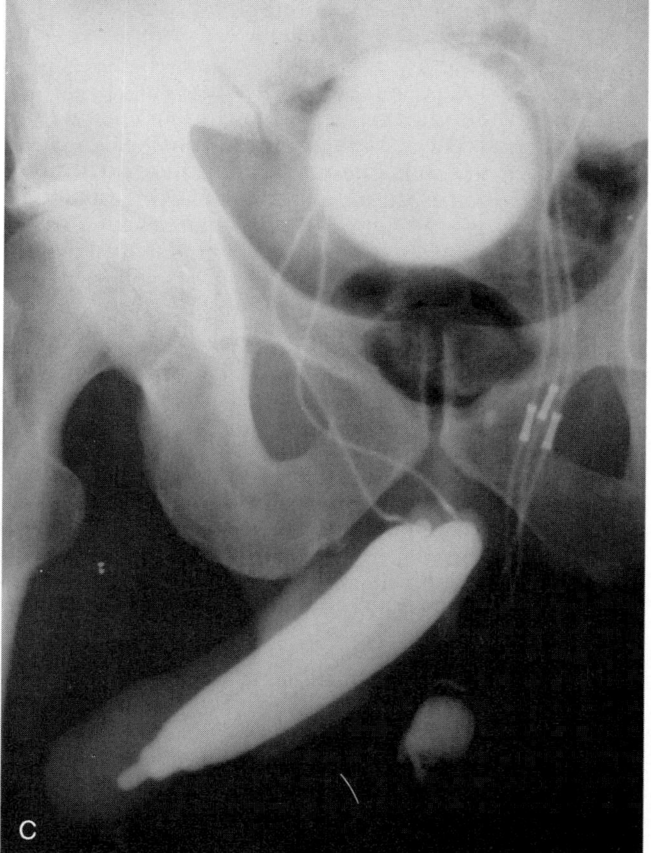

FIGURE 30–8. *A.* Inflatable prosthesis with the paired cylinders scrotal pump, and an abdominal fluid reservoir. *B.* Three-piece inflatable prosthesis viewed by x-ray prior to full inflation. *C.* Inflatable prosthesis at full inflation.

TABLE 30–6 Complications Reported with Penile Prostheses in Spinal Cord-Injured Men

Study	Type of Prostheses	Complication	Comments
Van Arsdalen et al	20 noninflatable	25% erosion rate	Decrease in skin problem in 70% due to maintenance of condom catheter
Rossier and Fam	36 semirigid	Removal in 19.5%, infection in 11%	
Yarkony	Semirigid	22% erosion	
	29 inflatable	8% erosion	Minor surgical repair in 31%
Collins and Hackler	53 semirigid	33% extrusion	After reimplantation, 83% function rate
	10 inflatable	40% lost	

Data From Van Arsdalen KN, Klein FA, Hackler RH, et al: Penile implants in spinal cord injury patients for maintaining external appliances. J Urol 1981; 126:331–332; Rossier AB, Fam BA: Indication and results of semirigid penile prosthesis in spinal cord jury patients: Long term followup. J Urol 1984; 131:59–62; Yarkony GM: Enhancement of sexual function and fertility in spinal cord-injured males. Am J Phys Med Rehabil 1990; 69:81–87; Collins KP, Hackler RH: Complications of penile prostheses in the spinal cord injury population. J Urol 1988; 140:984–985.

evacuation through the urethra constitutes *retrograde ejaculation* or *ejaculatory failure.* Retrograde ejaculation can be secondary to an abnormal state (sympathetic nervous system damage) preventing adequate closure of the bladder neck, leading to retrograde semen flow. After sexual activity, males may complain of dry ejaculate (sensation of orgasm with no explusion of semen) or cloudy urine at the time of their next void or catherization. Ejaculatory failure also occurs in up to 90% of patients after transurethral prostatectomy (TURP).[93] The higher the spinal cord lesion, the more likely the patient is to have an erection, but the less likely to have ejaculation. Twenty percent of all SCI males retain some ability to ejaculate in either antegrade or retrograde fashion. Ejaculatory failure is seen least often in those with lower lesions or incomplete lesions.[143]

Orgasm. We have previously emphasized the importance of the brain in the experience of orgasm. All the issues discussed in the sexuality section play a vital role in the patient's libido and responsiveness to the sexual experience. There is a correlation between the richness of the individual's sexual fantasy and fulfillment of sexual life, which may be even more important when genital impairments exist.[7, 105] Phantom orgasm was described by Money as an occasional culmination of vivid fantasies or dreams with no physical stimulation.[88] The brain can work independent of genitalia in the generation of erotic experience, just as the genitalia of SCI patients can work reflexively independent of the brain. Surveys of able-bodied females report that approximately 10% have never achieved orgasm and that up to 75% do not routinely achieve orgasm with penile thrusting alone.[144] It should not be surprising to find that, with SCIs, female orgasms are typically experienced differently than they were premorbidly. They are described as pleasurable feelings of intense excitement or as sudden enhancement of spasticity followed by prolonged relaxation.[51] The extragenital responses during orgasm include "headache, warm sensation, physical pleasure, and sexual excitement."[51] It is important to educate the patient that the orgasms are real, just different.[127]

Orgasm is conveyed in the anterior spinothalamic and pyramidal tracts and can easily be tested in an office setting. A normally appreciated cold stimulus to the clitoris or penis and the ability to voluntarily contract the external anal sphincter indicates intact orgasmic pathways. This allows the patient to know that given the right mental and physical stimuli, he or she could experience orgasm.[4]

If SCI males anticipate pleasurable feelings (orgasm) only if they ejaculate, they will be disappointed, as the percentage of successful ejaculation is low. Education about the importance of the mind and awareness of other body changes will enhance their sensation. Orgasms are practically nonexistent in patients with complete upper motor neuron lesions. Persons with complete lower motor neuron injuries occasionally perceive pleasurable sensation lower in the abdomen, pelvis, or thighs.

Autonomic Dysreflexia.[128] All patients with SCIs at or above T4 to T6 are at risk for autonomic dysreflexia. Patients are advised to evacuate their bowel and bladder prior to sexual activity, thus avoiding incontinence and reducing the risk of autonomic dysreflexia during sexual activity. In the event of dysreflexia, the patient should be educated to stop, and to sit up to elevate the head (to help lower blood pressure). Medical assistance should be sought if the headache does not subside. Prophylactic medication can be used if autonomic dysreflexia is not otherwise manageable.

Male Fertility.[74] The etiology of infertility in the SCI population is the subject of much research. Less than 10% of SCI patients retain the ability to impregnate their partner spontaneously.[5, 51] A successful pregnancy requires the male to achieve complete and adequate spermatogenesis, ductal transport of sperm, erection, emission, and ejaculation.[93] Problems arise from ejaculatory failure, obstruction of genital passages, impairment of spermatogenesis, or a combination of these.[130]

Techniques to restore ejaculation are usually aimed at restoring fertility.[107] A review of the patient's medication and prior sexual function is required. The techniques involve stimulation of the intact neurological center below the SCI through chemical, vibratory, or transrectal electrical ejaculation.[93] These techniques are most successful when the T10 to T11 spinal segments are intact. Alpha-adrenergic agonists (pseudoephrine and imipramine) are used to attempt to convert retrograde ejaculation to anterograde ejaculation. If this is not successful, harvesting and processing of the retrograde ejaculate should be attempted. One method is to have the patient void (almost completely) prior to masturbation and then collect the postejaculatory voided urine. To ensure optimal sperm survival, the second method involves washing the bladder with sperm-processing buffer, leaving 30 mL of the buffer in the bladder; masturbation; and collection of the post-ejaculate fluid. The ejaculate must be processed carefully to obtain a concentrated healthy sample.[25] Chen[34] found no statistically significant differences between antegrade and retrograde samples in sperm count, motility, and normal morphology, while Brackett[19] found a lower percentage of dead sperm in the antegrade samples. Level of injury did not correlate with any differences in the samples.[19, 34] Intrathecal physostigmine was used by Guttmann and Walsh[53] to elicit ejaculation chemically, but this lost favor because of complications, including autonomic dysreflexia. Subcutaneous physostigmine was also rejected because of its dangerous side effects.[31, 142]

Vibratory stimulation of the glans penis has been used successfully by various groups to collect semen via antegrade and retrograde ejaculation (successful in about 50% of SCI males) as it requires an intact reflex arc.[8, 23] Ejaculatory success is better with high-amplitude vibration.[18] The advantages are noninvasiveness, home use, possibility of "natural" fertilization, and that retrograde emission is less likely than with transrectal electrical stimulation. Improvement in quantity and quality of sperm with weekly use of the vibratory ejaculatory technique may occur.[8, 39] The disadvantages are an unpredictable response in many patients and the risk of autonomic dysreflexia.[25, 142]

Transrectal electrical stimulation or electroejaculation involves stimulation of the myelinated preganglionic efferent sympathetic fibers of the hypogastric plexus to obtain seminal emission into the posterior urethra (Fig. 30–9).[5] The semen is obtained from the posterior urethra by milking the urethral bulb and by catheterization. This technique was first introduced in humans in 1948, but until recently experience and further research were acquired mainly through veterinary use. It is currently the most common method used in the United States. Buch and Zorn[26] found that semen could be obtained from up to 90% of all patients evaluated. There appears to be a decrease in sperm motility in the semen collected by transrectal stimulation, with normal fertility seen in only 25%.[26] The decrease in motility is slightly more than is seen with vibratory ejaculation, but patient preference is much higher with vibration.[20, 96] Electroejaculation is an office- or hospital-based procedure because of the need to monitor for autonomic dysreflexia and the anoscopy performed to evaluate the rectal mucosa. Pretreatment with sublingual nifedipine has decreased the risk of autonomic dysreflexia in both techniques.[142] Anesthesia may be required in some patients with incomplete lesions due to pain. Perkash and co-workers[100] have been successful in simplifying the equipment, lowering the current required, and therefore increasing the patient's tolerance.

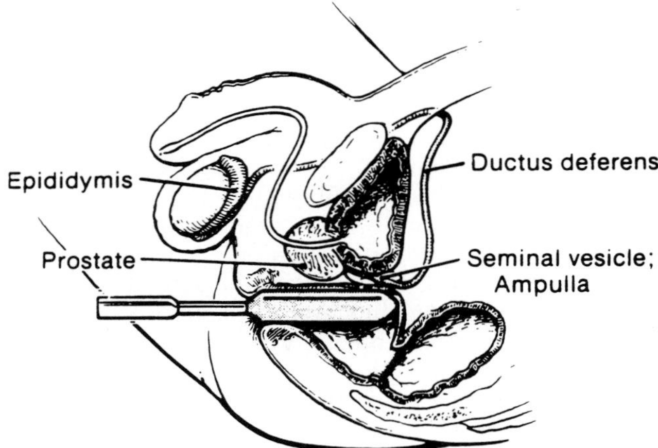

FIGURE 30–9. Sagittal view of rectal probe placement for electroejaculation. (From Buch JP: Disorders of ejaculation. In Bennett AH (ed): Impotence: Diagnosis and Management of Erectile Dysfunction. Philadelphia, WB Saunders, 1994, p 193.)

Assisted reproductive technologies such as IVF (in vitro fertilization) and GIFT (gamete intrafallopian transfer) have been used to achieve pregnancy. Another study looking at fertilization rates after electroejaculation found them to be significantly lower and recommended consideration of epididymal or testicular fine needle aspiration.[59] ICSI (intracytoplasmic sperm injection) has revolutionized the treatment of male fertility. High fertilization rates are usually achieved with ICSI independent of semen parameters.[36]

With the advent of ICSI, standard sperm retrieval now includes microepididymal sperm aspiration, percutaneous sperm aspiration, modified percutaneous sperm aspiration and testicular sperm extraction.[8, 24, 29]

Fertility problems can also stem from obstructed passages of the vas deferens, epididymis, and seminiferous tubules, most likely from repeated infection involving the bladder. Duct obstruction can be treated only by surgical resection. Spermatogenesis may be impaired, resulting in a decrease in number of sperm, decrease in normal motility, and increase in abnormal morphology. Sperm contact with urine, medication, antisperm antibodies, or raised scrotal temperature may be explanations for the poor semen quality typically seen in patients with SCI.[74] The local testicular temperature is normally 2.2°C lower than the intra-abdominal temperature, but the lifestyle of sitting with thighs together or crossed, not shifting position frequently, or wearing tight clothes can raise the temperature. Lowering the testicular temperature can reverse the maturation arrest caused by the increased temperature.[22] Temperature sensitivity is also seen in sperm from SCI men to be used for insemination.[17] This emphasizes the importance of patient education. SCI men are predisposed to the development of antisperm antibodies because of blockage of ductal tracts and UTIs. It is not known what contribution antisperm antibodies make to impaired spermatogenesis.[57, 130] Weakness with marked debility is commonly associated with testicular atrophy. There are numerous articles regarding testicular biopsies in the literature, but insufficient data exist to correlate testicular abnormalities with potentially contributing factors such as SCI level, urological management, history of urological complications, and medications.[74, 143] Studies seem to indicate close to normal levels of testosterone and an intact hypothalamus-pituitary-testicular axis.[143] Medications such as nitrofurantoin cause temporary spermatogenesis arrest in rats. This has been reviewed by Linsenmeyer and Perkash.[74]

As in vitro fertilization and present methods of semen collection are improved, and as even better methods are developed, the chances of an SCI male fathering a biological offspring are increased. Physiatrists must work with urologists and fertility specialists to provide the best possible opportunity to induce pregnancy. Counseling of the patient and partner is an integral part of any assisted reproductive program.

Female Fertility. Amenorrhea occurs in most women acutely after traumatic SCI, and lasts from 6 months to 1 year. The first ovulation cycle is unpredictable and therefore contraception must be considered from the beginning. There are a number of contraceptive methods that can be used (Table 30–7).[49, 135]

Although the ability to bear children is usually not affected, pregnancy presents many challenges to the SCI female.[7, 140] Self-care must be heightened to avoid the complications of UTIs, thrombophlebitis, edema of the legs, pressure ulcers, premature labor, and immobiliza-

TABLE 30–7 Female Fertility and Contraception

Type	Side Effects	Comments
Periodic abstinence or coitus interruptus	None	A woman must be well instructed in her biological rhythms to avoid unplanned pregnancy
Condoms	Decreased effectiveness if not properly used Must be reapplied for second sexual activity Taste may be offensive	Ready availability, increased acceptability, increased effectiveness Need dexterity Indwelling catheter may tear condom; therefore, lubricate Protects against sexually transmitted diseases
Foam and sponge	None	Ready availability, increased acceptability, increased effectiveness
Diaphragm/foam	Weakened pelvic muscles may not hold diaphragm in place	Requires dexterity Partner may be trained to insert the diaphragm
Intrauterine device (IUD)	May be unable to feel early signs of pelvic inflammatory disease Manual dexterity is needed to check for placement	Inserted by physician Insertion may be easier with paralysis Teach the patient to look for spotting, irregular periods, increased spasticity, fever, increased or different vaginal discharge
Oral contraceptive pill	Studies of the early use (estrogen, 50–150 μg; progestin) revealed an association with cardiovascular, thromboembolic, cerebrovascular, and thrombophlebitic disease Studies of low-dose estrogen (35 μg) and progestin suggest only individual situations of hypertension and thrombophlebitis Both are aggravated by smoking Spinal cord–injured women must be taught the warning signs of thrombophlebitis	Most common reason for unplanned pregnancy is improper dosing Need sufficient cognition and reliability as well as the manual dexterity to take pill as required
Subdermal hormonal implants (Norplant)	Has not been shown to produce thromboembolic, cerebrovascular, or cardiovascular disease Monitor for hypertension and thrombophlebitis Side effects include irregular vaginal bleeding, changes in weight, and psychic symptoms similar to menopause or premenstrual syndrome	Good option for women who do not desire children for a period of years Added benefit of reducing or totally eliminating menstrual bleeding, which can facilitate hygiene
Medroxyprogesterone acetate (Depo-Provera)	Same as above	Added benefit of reducing or totally eliminating menstrual bleeding, which can facilitate hygiene
Sterilization by tubal ligation or vasectomy	Permanent	Continue to menstruate
Therapeutic abortion		Prior to sexual activity, patient and partner should discuss family planning and options

Data from Bérard EJJ: The sexuality of spinal cord injured women: Physiology and pathophysiology: A review. Paraplegia 1989; 27:99–112; Goddard LR: Sexuality and spinal cord injury. J Neurosci Nurs 1988; 20:240–243.

tion-induced osteoporosis.[40, 142] Repeated UTIs increase the risk of developing toxemia of pregnancy.

The uterus is innervated by spinal cord levels T10 to T12; therefore patients with complete lesions above T10 will not appreciate uterine contractions or fetal movement. Although the discomfort of labor is not felt as in able-bodied women, the onset of labor is typically detected but as a different sensation. The contractions may be stronger, more prolonged, and more frequent, but the duration of labor is shorter than for the non-SCI women.[145] Although the abdominal muscles may be paralyzed, the uterus will contract due to hormonal influence. Delivery of the fetus may require the use of forceps or episiotomy. Cesarean section should be performed for the same indications as in the able-bodied. Patients with lesions above T6 are at risk for autonomic dysreflexia during childbirth.[132] The treatment of choice is epidural anesthesia, as it allows continuous medication administration. Oral premedication can be tried as an alternative.

Breast-feeding may require adaptation of wheelchairs or assistance from others. Women with lesions above T6 usually experience a decrease in milk production after 6 weeks. One of the major concerns of SCI women during their pregnancy is the loss of control and consequent sense of helplessness. This is exacerbated by a decrease in level of functioning, fear of the unknown, and lack of knowledge, all of which can be addressed by a well-organized rehabilitation team.[40]

Cortical Involvement

With cortical involvement, one may be required to cope with aphasia (communication), left- or right-sided neglect (disinhibition, impulsivity, poor social interaction), or apraxias (motor planning difficulty). Sexuality and sexual function are related to understanding and communication between the patient and partner, which are affected by these neurological sequelae.

Cerebrovascular accidents (CVAs) affect 600,000 persons in the United States every year. The mean age of the 400,000 who survive is 60 years. Most led an active life prior to the disability and want sexuality issues to be addressed during hospitalization. There is a general decline in sexual activity and libido in both sexes after stroke, but there is little evidence of organic causes for the sexual dysfunction.[13, 27] The comorbidity associated with CVA, such as diabetes, hypertension, and cardiac problems, contributes to sexual dysfunction.[48] Psychological factors seem to be important in determining changes in sexual life after stroke. These factors may be a result of change in the sex role, dependence on a partner for activities of daily living, or attitudes of partners. The patient might be forced into a more passive role but the partner might be unwilling to become more aggressive or to use new sexual positions.[81] The more dependent the patient is on the spouse, the more likely there will be a decrease in sexual activity.[118] The partner may fear a recurrence of the event, may resent loss of income, or may infantilize the patient. These phenomena produce dysfunction in other disabilities as well. Impairment of cutaneous sensibility, neurogenic bladder, fatigue, depression, and aphasic disorders have been found to play a role in sexual changes.[13] With the decrease in verbal communication and decrease in spontaneous touching, establishing successful "sexual intercourse" becomes more difficult. There are discrepancies in the literature regarding the incidence of arousal, ejaculation, and orgasmic dysfunction after strokes, which may be partly explained by the methodology used (most frequently questionnaires).[13, 21]

Traumatic brain injury (TBI) patients share many of the epidemiological characteristics of SCI patients.[146] The severity of disability varies from case to case, depending on the injury, premorbid status, family support, and extent of rehabilitation.[58] Therefore, the rehabilitative process must be adaptable.[11] When 19 male patients with postconcussive syndrome were studied for sexual dysfunction, 58% reported difficulty.[67] Cerebral involvement can lead to sexual disinhibition, hyposexuality, and hypersexuality (Klüver-Bucy syndrome), in that order of frequency.[147] Cortical motor deficits can lead to spasticity, paresis, paralysis, heterotopic ossification, contractures, and neurogenic bowel and bladder. Cortical involvement can result in dysphasia, dysarthria, dysprosody, and oromotor apraxias, which can interfere with communication and oral sexual contact. In addition to the objective impairments listed, TBI patients may have significant personality changes that adversely affect their relationships and appear to deteriorate over time rather than improve.[97] The sexuality of women with cognitive disabilities tends to be overlooked, and inappropriate or misguided sexual remarks made may provoke anxiety in her caregivers but are often ignored rather than being met with a helpful response.[4]

Multiple sclerosis is a chronic illness that affects many aspects of sexuality (often in young adults) (see Chapter 52).[129, 136]

Diabetic Neuropathy

Peripheral neuropathies, such as in diabetes mellitus, have many effects on the peripheral somatic and autonomic nervous systems affecting the expression of sexuality. Diabetes mellitus is a chronic illness and affects psychological aspects of sexuality through changes in body image and control issues.[61] Within 5 years of the onset of diabetes mellitus, one-third to one-half of males experience some sexual dysfunction. This is usually impotence secondary to a combination of physiological (neurological and vascular) and psychological factors. The physiological factors can involve erectile problems, including the vasodilation necessary for increased arterial inflow, relaxation of muscles necessary for the spaces in the corpora cavernosa to fill, and possibly the venous outflow or the sensory input that facilitates obtaining and maintaining an erection. Oral sildenafil (Viagra) is an effective and well-tolerated treatment for ED in men with diabetes. Patient age and duration of diabetes or ED did not affect the efficacy of sildenafil, with 56% in the sildenafil group reporting improved erections, compared with 10% in the placebo group. Sexual intercourse was possible in 61% of those in the sildenafil group, compared with 22% of the placebo group.[109, 133]

Female diabetic patients experience sexual dysfunction with impaired lubrication, impaired sensation, increased vaginal infections leading to dyspareunia, and changes in sexual desire.[70]

Vascular Disease

Cardiovascular disease has a high prevalence in American culture, especially in men more than 50 years old.[108] Research is now demonstrating a much higher incidence of the disease than previously estimated in females. Coronary disease resulting in myocardial infarction and peripheral vascular disease leading to amputation have a significant impact on patients and their sexual functioning.[55] Vascular disease can cause a loss of the ability to maintain an erection from a "venous leakage." Risk factors for atherosclerotic vascular disease are known contributors to ED. These include smoking, diabetes, low levels of high-density lipoprotein (HDL) cholesterol, high levels of total and low-density lipoprotein (LDL) cholesterol, and hypertension.[66] Viagra has proved to be effective in this population, but once again the precautions are emphasized.

Medications used for treatment often interfere with libido or sexual function. For example, long-term digoxin use in men causes estradiol levels three times higher than in controls, while testosterone decreases by two-thirds (correlating with an increased incidence of impotence). Hypertension interferes with sexual function most directly because of the medications used to treat it (see Table 30–2). It is important to evaluate sexual function prior to initiating therapy, if possible. Sexual dysfunction is one of the main reasons for noncompliance with antihypertensive medication regimens.

The frequency of sexual activity often decreases dramatically after myocardial infarction or coronary bypass. Survivors of myocardial infarction often experience anxiety and depression even 1 year after insult, and their sexual concerns frequently are not adequately addressed during the acute hospitalization.[55] Energy expenditure during sexual activity is similar to that of walking on a treadmill at 3 to 4 miles per hour (5 to 6 METS [metabolic equivalents of oxygen consumption]).[47] The amount of energy expenditure during sexual activity has been compared to climbing two flights of stairs at a brisk rate, or climbing 20 steps in 10 seconds. It is now recommended that counselors advise patients to use their usual sexual position(s), as these are generally less stressful than learning a new position (Table 30–8).[116]

TABLE 30–8 Patient Guidelines for Sexual Intercourse

1. Resume sexual intercourse in familiar surroundings. Strange environments add to psychological stress.
2. Provide a room with a comfortable temperature for intercourse. Extreme room temperatures and extremely hot or cold showers or baths add to heart stress.
3. Remember that foreplay is desirable and helps prepare your heart gradually for the increased activity of intercourse.
4. Use positions that are comfortable and relaxing and permit unrestricted breathing.
5. Usual positions are the most desirable because they are the least stressful.
6. If inclined, oral-genital sex causes no undue strain and may be a satisfactory means of sexual expression with appropriate attention to disease prevention.
7. Obtain rest before intercourse; morning is an ideal time for lovemaking.
8. Postpone intercourse for 3 hours after eating a heavy meal or drinking alcohol.
9. Remember that sex with someone other than your usual partner may increase stress to your heart.
10. See that clothing, if worn, is loose-fitting.
11. Take medications, such as nitroglycerin or isosorbide dinitrate, before intercourse to prevent chest pain.
12. Consider masturbation because it requires less energy than intercourse.

From Seidl A, Bullough B, Haughey B, et al: Understanding the effects of a myocardial infarction on sexual functioning: A basis for sexual counseling. Rehabil Nurs 1991; 16:255–264.

Physical Disfigurement

Physical disfigurement can arise from a wide variety of conditions, including amputations, burns, cancer, and arthritis. Often genital sexual function is not affected, but other factors affecting sexuality may be severely affected. Resuming sexual activity helps those with amputations incorporate their prostheses into their body image, increases self-esteem, and facilitates rehabilitation.[82]

Oncology patients have multiple issues, including body image (as in breast cancer post mastectomy) and mortality. Chemotherapy-induced nausea, malaise, or weakness may compromise sexual frequency.[119] Although 3% to 12% of men are impotent after TURP, appropriate counseling can result in continued satisfactory sexual relationships. Impotence occurs in 15% of prostatectomy patients, in 67% of cystoprostatectomy cases, in 15% of men less than 50 years old after abdominoperineal resection, and in 100% of men older than 70 years. There is strong evidence to encourage urologists to continue to perform and perfect the nerve-sparing approach with prostatectomy, as 80% of patients with resulting ED responded to sildenafil citrate (Viagra) while no patient who had undergone a non-nerve-sparing procedure responded.[148] Patients with an ileostomy or colostomy often have secondary erectile failure due to decreased self-esteem and depression.[132]

Arthritis is a chronic disease and, as with diabetes mellitus, chronic obstructive pulmonary disease,[54] and renal disease, increased age, severity of illness, and depression are associated with decreased sexual function.[75] Some 38% to 80% of patients with chronic renal failure requiring dialysis have reduced or partial erectile function, but 20% to 55% are completely impotent.[38] Chronic diseases seen in children, such as juvenile rheumatoid arthritis, cystic fibrosis, or myelomeningocele, affect many of the sexuality issues all adolescents face.[41]

With the dramatic improvement in burn survival, attention must be directed to the quality of life for the patient. Physiological function is usually intact and the concerns are body image, self-esteem, and interpersonal relationships. Following the models described in the following pages allows sexual issues to be integrated into the comprehensive, often lengthy rehabilitation of the burn patient.[140]

Terminal Illness

When dealing with the terminally ill, physicians do not typically consider the consequences to the patient's sexuality. Patients can get mired in the grieving process and not be able to move forward to the enjoyment of their modified sexuality. Physicians view the more obvious medical problems to be more worthy of attention than sexuality. This is not the case with the majority of such patients, however, and education of both clinicians and patients can help ameliorate this discrepancy. The rehabilitation of the human immunodeficiency virus (HIV)–positive patient or the patient with acquired immunodeficiency syndrome (AIDS) underscores the importance of treating the whole patient.[72, 120]

SEXUALITY

We have previously defined sexuality as a form of communication and self-expression to which everyone is entitled. Sexuality is a "combination of sex drive, sex acts and all those aspects of personality concerned with learned communications and relationship patterns . . . rooted in the human need to relate to others, to receive and share pleasure, to love and to be loved."[110] The patient, his or her relationships, and the environment reflect the wide spectrum of beliefs and attitudes encompassed by sexuality.[35]

Sexuality is an integral part of a person's psychological makeup and self-concept. We know that psychological health can positively or negatively affect the course of rehabilitation. It should come as no surprise that impairments affect sexuality and that sexuality issues affect a patient's ability to deal with the rigors of rehabilitation. We must incorporate sexuality in the rehabilitation process. In a recent Swedish study, sexual information was given to only 6 of 62 female SCI patients.[134] None received target-oriented counseling by a sexual counselor, and at no stage was the partner included.

Sexual Development

Clinicians attempting to assist patients to return to healthy sexual function must be careful not to convey their biases or prejudices to the patient. This requires being fully informed about the physiological and psychological aspects of sexuality. Of course, clinicians need to be comfortable with their own sexuality. It is incumbent upon the physiatrist to allow patients the opportunity to address sexual issues. However, it is also appropriate to refer those patients whose issues are outside one's expertise or values to a trained clinician.

Our culture abounds with myths and taboos about sexual function, performance, and expression. For example, pre- or extramarital sexual activity, masturbation, aging,[39] homosexuality, and birth control are differently defined and accepted intraculturally and cross-culturally. These form one's construction of norms that are communicated by family, educators, and peers across the life span. This is no less true for persons with disabilities and their families. The physician could explain that in some cultures the norm is to explore the sexual potential of the whole body, mind, and spirit as the couple touches, talks, caresses, kisses and only sometimes purposefully stimulates to actual orgasm. We can discuss how creative bodily positioning, minimizing the focus on penile-vaginal contact and fostering eroticism, can lead to greater pleasure and intimacy.[4]

Parental attitudes toward the developing sexuality of children can be facilitative or inhibitive, affecting adult options of sexual expression.[79] These attitudes may be extremely repressive, controlling, and overprotective. Assumptions may be made by the family that a child with a disability will never marry, reproduce, or have intimate relationships.[83] A more supportive stance parallels the stance that the parent of an able-bodied child would be advised to take. The child's sexual identity should be acknowledged. When intimate relationships are formed in late adolescence and early adulthood the parent's response should be neutral or positive.

Shielding and overprotecting children and adolescents with disabilities prevents them from experiencing the sexual banter that goes on, the verbal and nonverbal communication with another person in whom they are sexually interested. Placing these limitations on a disabled child can lead to a more socially disabled adult. Supporting the child's or adolescent's participation in peer groups is critical for the development of interpersonal skills, including the socially appropriate communication skills associated with sexual development. A healthy adjustment is becoming "sexually assertive," such as by using a wheelchair or brace as an introduction to a conversation rather than allowing it to be a barrier to interactions.[79]

Myths that the elderly are asexual, or should be, pervade the culture and enforce incongruity between what many elderly persons experience and what is considered normal.[77] Elderly patients undergoing rehabilitation deserve the same consideration of their sexuality issues as younger patients.[65] The sexual interest of the elderly is affected by many factors of which clinicians should be aware. These include the following:[65]

- General health (including mental health)
- Availability of a partner and opportunity to be alone with a partner
- Personality and attitude
- Educational level
- Social status
- Degree of satisfaction with life
- The attitude of others
- Sexual beliefs, activity, interests, and practices earlier in life (especially those of the patient when between the ages of 20 and 40)

The most common sexual problem in older couples is male erectile difficulties. Disease, drug reactions, and disability can contribute to emotional upset, decreased libido, decreased erectile function, and consequently decreased sexual activity. Roughly 50% to 75% of all marriages among older persons can be affected by some sexual disability.[77] Some patients (mostly women) continue sexual activity for their partners rather than for self-gratification. Knowing they can still please others sexually can improve their morale and self-concept. Those most likely to discontinue all sexual activity after a disabling accident or illness are widowed or single persons.[131]

Factors Affecting Sexuality

When patients are confronted with serious illness or disability, a central task of coping is a redefinition of self that incorporates the limitations of or adjustments to the illness or disabling condition.[38]

Unfortunately, because of the nature of hospitals, patients are denied privacy, and social permission for sexual questioning and exploration is withheld. Patients often share the negative societal stereotypes of disabled people as pathetic, unhappy, unproductive, and asexual.[135] Physiatrists can counteract these images by supporting patients in reconstructing their sexual identities. In order to assist them, it is imperative that we understand not only biological but also psychosocial factors affecting sexuality.[96] These include body image, self-esteem, gender identity, and role compliance.[135] Each of these factors involves a composite of the patient's personal cognitions based on the messages construed from family, peers, culture, and, of course, from the clinicians assigned to their care. Through education, support, and normalization, physicians (especially physiatrists) and the team of rehabilitation professionals are uniquely positioned to enhance their patients' lives in each of these domains. Since the focus of rehabilitation medicine is to maintain and increase a patient's function, our practice is solution-based: relationships with patients are long term and our therapeutic stance with patients is supportive. We serve as a partner to our patients and their families by fostering their reintegration into the lifestyles that they choose. Our goal is to add life to years, not just years to life (see Figs. 30–1 and 30–10).

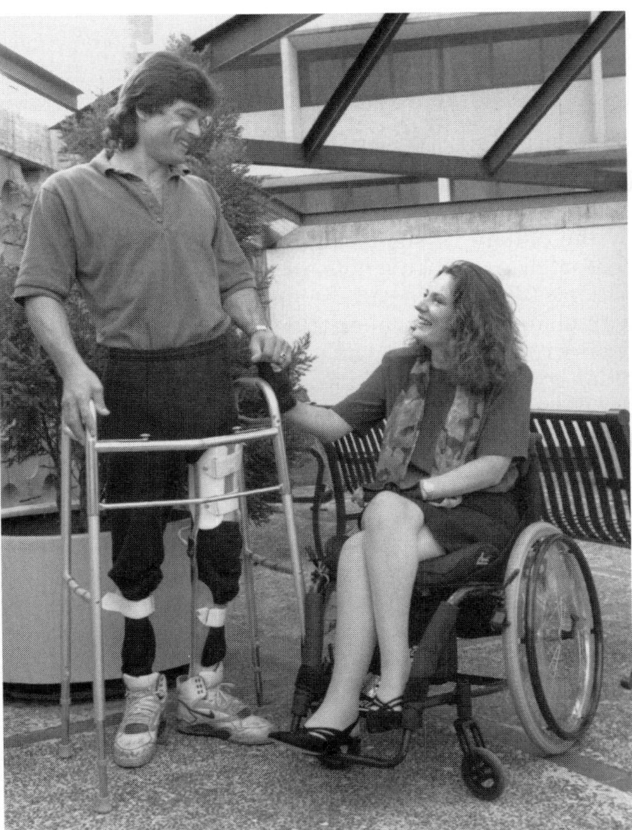

FIGURE 30–10. Factors affecting sexuality include impaired body image; decreased self-esteem; difficulty with gender identity and role; difficulty with decisions about sexuality and parenthood; personal and observed sexual experience; value system, morality, religion, prohibition, and taboos; personal, cultural, and societal attitudes; and health status and physical capabilities.[110] What was your reaction to the "romantic" portrait in Figure 30–1 vs. your reaction to this portrait? Did you make assumptions? It is easy to comprehend how the visible factors can affect sexuality, but we carry an entire host of hidden factors.

Body Image

Body image is one of the most essential components of self, incorporating "feelings and attitudes toward one's own body, body parts, and body functions."[110] Prostheses, wheelchairs, scars, or adaptive equipment all have to be incorporated into a new body image.[104] If this is viewed negatively by the patient or society, a spiral of loss of confidence and body shame can result. The term "body shame" was coined by Kaufman in discussing shame associated with aging. These experiences with bodily changes are often similar to those of persons with disability. The decline in appearance, bodily function, and vitality becomes a source of increasing shame and frustration. This change is experienced as a loss, and loss activates distress and grieving.

To illustrate the point, picture yourself with a third-degree burn covering your face, or with an eruption of Kaposi's sarcoma across your body as a result of being HIV-seropositive. Failure to accept one's body as is, in the presence of disability, can lead to feelings not only of shame but also of dissociation from one's body and a perceived loss of control. Such feelings can be exacerbated in women by perceptions that their self-worth is associated with physical appearance and sexual attractiveness (a perception that is consistent with societal expectations). Some disabilities are hidden (bladder/bowel and sexual difficulties), which poses the extremely difficult question of when to disclose the problem to a potential partner.[4] In addition, hygiene and use of associated devices (catheters, ostomy bags, menstrual products) may require the assistance of another person. If a partner assists with such intimate personal care, it may be difficult for the partner and the patient to readjust to sexual intimacy. The uncertainty and anxiety created by a progressive disability could compromise spontaneity and forward planning.[56] Clinicians should not assume that patients will inevitably have body image distortions or problems, but should be ready to treat them when they occur.[110]

Self-Esteem

Self-esteem, the personal sense of one's inherent worth, is essential to mental health and identity. As with other components of self, self-esteem develops interactively over the course of the life span. The presence of impairments and physical disabilities can be an assault on one's self-esteem, particularly if these are perceived by the patient or significant others as a diminution of competence, attractiveness, or intrinsic value. In some patients, diminished self-esteem can exist concurrently with inadequate sexual relationships and feelings of inferiority, weakness, and helplessness.[35] Disabled women more commonly experienced sexual abuse and sexual harassment than nondisabled women, and this can be particularly devastating in view of their already vulnerable self-esteem. Moreover, some men who do credit disabled women as sexual make inappropriate, unwanted, and exploitative advances.[4] Concerns about not satisfying a partner ranked number one in a study of 79 SCI males.[138] Loneliness and isolation can emerge in combination with a fear of humiliation that leads to avoidance of sexual situations.[9]

Other patients react to diminished self-esteem by displaying hypersexuality, apparently seeking assurance or validation from others that they are still attractive.[147] It is important to understand the insecurity that underlies these inappropriate displays so as not to further undermine the patient's self-esteem with negative reactions. Physicians are often viewed by the patient as being very powerful and should use this position to assist the team with dealing with such issues. The patient's feelings should be acknowledged, and then the patient should be redirected to a more appropriate expression (rephrasing an offensive statement, suggesting a more appropriate expression). Patients need to learn to express their needs and desires with family, partner, and clinicians. Assertiveness training has been used successfully to assist with this expression and subsequently has increased patients' self-esteem.[135] For example, in vivo and in vitro situational behavior rehearsals, essentially practice sessions, can make it easier the next time a potential real-life "sexual intercourse" occasion presents itself.

Gender Identity

One's gender identity exists along a continuum of femininity and masculinity that is consistent or inconsistent with societal assumptions based on the individual's sex. Both gender identity and gender role develop in socially interactive processes. For disabled patients, gender identity can be compromised by an impairment in their ability to express their assumed gender role. How this is negotiated is greatly influenced by the patient's interaction with clinicians, family, peers, and intimate partners. Patients might test their identity by acting out an exaggeration of their assumed gender role. For example, a male who has been raised to value assertiveness, dominance, and strength and then finds himself with quadriplegia is forced to accept a more passive physical role. He may attempt to compensate through verbal abuse of family, therapists, or nursing staff.

Literature as recent as the 1970s gave the opinion that SCI was not as devastating to women because they could continue their passive role.[122] Yet females, particularly those who value a more traditional feminine role, are much more sensitive to their perceived loss of sexual attractiveness and perceived loss of fertility in defining their female identity.[40] For women with cognitive disabilities, particularly if insight and self-awareness are impaired, relationships may be a challenge. Behaviors that promote acceptance by other people have to be learned, and awareness of social subtleties such as eye contact and a sense of personal space may be inadequate.[4]

Children with disabilities encounter many unique challenges in the struggle to develop their own gender identity and role. Often these develop because parents avoid sexual subjects and limit participation in the normal sexual developmental activities, such as dances, parties, dating, and sports. Rehabilitation specialists can assist with family training and with providing safe environments for social experimentation.

PARSS MODEL (*P*ROCESS OF *A*SSESSMENT AND *R*ECOMMENDATION FOR *S*EXUAL *S*ATISFACTION)

History and Physical Examination

Sexuality is central to the patient's health and quality of life. Physiatrists are comfortable asking patients very personal questions to assist with skin integrity, physical strength, bowel and bladder programs, and to reintegrate the patient's independence. However, they are frequently uncomfortable with sexual issues. This section details the processes of history taking and physical examination in the context of providing the patient maximum opportunity to voice sexual concerns. The goals of the *p*rocess of *a*ssessment and *r*ecommendation for *s*exual *s*atisfaction (PARSS) are to enable patients to express their concerns openly and to offer them counseling and education, whenever possible, in order to minimize sexual dysfunction and maximize sexual satisfaction (Table 30–9).[33] More than 80% of sexual complaints can be successfully managed in the office setting, but only if they are addressed (see Table 30–5).[65]

In a study of patient-physician interactions, physicians stated they did not include sexual issues in their evaluation because of lack of knowledge and training, discomfort and embarrassment, and lack of research in connection with sex and disability. Experimentally trained physicians obtained a sexual history 82% of the time, compared with 32% of the time by the untrained physicians. Many physicians assumed sexual function was not important to the patient, but without confirmation from the patient, that assumption is invalid.[45] Patients whose physician had asked sexual questions as a part of the initial history assessment thought the subject was more appropriate in an examination than those whose physician has not broached the subject.[85] All patients with impairments have some type of sexual concern, whether

TABLE 30–9 Goals of the Process of Assessment and Recommendation for Sexual Satisfaction (PARSS)

To minimize sexual dysfunction and maximize sexual satisfaction:
Give the patient permission to discuss sexual issues and establish these as legitimate concerns
Obtain important information needed for the medical care of the patient:
- Insight into family and social support
- Potential risks of infection or injury
- Side effects of medication
- Functional impact on the patient's life of chronic diseases and disabilities
- Symptoms such as impotence, dyspareunia, and angina, which may lead the clinician to investigate previously undiagnosed medical problems

Discovery of sexual misconceptions, anxieties, or dysfunctions
- Myths about masturbation, different sexual activities, genital size
- Anxiety about cardiovascular problems, performance

Adapted from Cheadle MJ: The screening sexual history: Getting to the problem. Clin Geriatric Med 1991 7:9–13.

physiological, physical, social, or psychological. A good example of this is in adolescents with cancer, who have many concerns their peers do not.[30] History taking that includes questions about sexuality is critical to learning about their concerns.

During the initial evaluation, the physician must establish rapport and present himself or herself as approachable. Spica[122] emphasizes that "a knowledgeable, nonjudgmental clinician [nurse] with good communication skills can play an important role in enhancing a patient's quality of life through effective sexual counseling." In re-educating patients with impairments, we need to discuss not only the physiological aspects of sex but also the more subtle expressions of sexuality such as caring, touching, holding, and being held.

The physiatrist should initiate these discussions with patients throughout their care. At a minimum, these topics should be broached during the screening sexual history, admission physical examination, and discharge planning sessions. Several factors facilitate the PARSS process: attention to the topic throughout therapy, privacy, confidentiality, awareness of sociosexual variation with generations, and appreciation of the difficult nature of the topic for patients and many physicians. In considering outlines to clarify various clinical situations and thus to enhance positive outcomes and limit negative outcomes, a simple model is used to guide history taking. It goes beyond the traditional set of standard questions—often cold and at "arm's length"—and emphasizes the clear need to update the history and information throughout the process (PARSS).

The ENIGMA model is orderly and open-ended. First, one should *engage* the patient in conversation, providing an opening and opportunity to talk. It need not be directly about sexual matters. The first contact may be solely with the patient, but the partner should be included as soon as the patient gives permission. *Normalize* sexual interest and activity in a matter-of-fact way that makes the subject standard and legitimate. *Inform* the patient and partner about sexual physiology and anatomy. This leads to answering questions in a more natural fashion. *Guide* the patient and his or her partner by responding in the same language and metaphors. (A common error made by clinicians is to use medical terminology instead of the vernacular.) *Maximize* problem-solving ability by encouraging experimentation, reading, and peer counseling. *Assess and reassess* the sexual issues at the next visit and make it an ongoing subject, not a one-time thing (Table 30–10). For example, with the SCI patient, I routinely review a problem list (skin, bowel, bladder, mobility, sexual function). By the third visit the patient is usually waiting with a sexual question, but the patient typically does not bring it up on his or her own. The pertinent physical examination, which should be performed when assessing sexual function, is described in Table 30–11. This should be a routine part of the physical examination, addressing concerns raised during the screening history.[65] After the sexual history, physical examination, and psychosocial evaluation, a diagnostic formulation should be made which delineates the sexual dysfunction, distress, and disability.[86]

Table 30–12 summarizes the findings of a Canadian SCI rehabilitation program developed in 1975, in which a nonphysician specialist was trained to diagnose and treat the sexual dysfunction of disabled persons in acute, rehabilitation, and extended care settings.[86] Such a specialist would be invaluable in a general rehabilitation practice as well. Results of patients' sexual satisfaction surveys showed a positive correlation with active, varied, and satisfying sexual relationships prior to injury, as well as with having an available interested and adventurous partner. A negative correlation was noted with anger. Appropriate clinical training is important as counseling without knowing the sexual diagnosis and without understanding the dynamics of the sexual rehabilitation process can harm the patient.[86]

PLISSIT Model (*P*ermission, *L*imited *I*nformation, *S*pecific *S*uggestions, *I*ntensive *T*herapy)[2]

The goals of the patient-clinician interaction should be to develop trusting relationships, support gender identity, maintain body image, and teach socialization (Table 30–13).[49] The entire rehabilitation team should be particularly adept at handling the first phase, permission, and understand how to lead patients through the appropriate phases. Personal attitudes and beliefs about one's own sexuality and the expression of such attitudes and beliefs by disabled patients must be examined.

The patient's interest in sexuality often comes out in a subtle way as an expression of poor self-image, hostile humor, profanity, or sexual aggressiveness.[101] Clinicians should recognize these subtleties and respond appropriately. This might include acknowledgment of the patient's sexual need with the suggestion that it be directed toward more appropriate partners, or by setting firm limits.[123] Not all patients want sexual information, and

TABLE 30–10 ENIGMA—Model of Assessment and Recommendation for Sexual Satisfaction

E—engage	*Engage* the patient in conversation by providing an opening and opportunity to talk	Need not directly address sexual issues History of surgery, presence of other significant medical conditions Assess interpersonal skills for expression of need Is sexual partner(s) present or absent and what is current relationship to patient? If no partner, is masturbation a release option?
N—normalize	*Normalize* sexual interest and activity in a matter-of-fact way that makes the subject standard and legitimate	Open discussion acknowledging individual variations Clarify sexual concerns, preferences, interest, experience, values Clarify satisfaction with sexual functioning as well as the existence and nature of any problem with sexual functioning Leads to acceptance of self and validation of interest
I—inform	*Inform* the patient and partner about sexual physiology and anatomy, thus naturally answering their questions	Establish current sexual knowledge regarding normal body anatomy and physiological function of both patient and partner Thorough, frank but sensitive education of function and response, both physical and emotional, of the disabling condition and its effects on motor and sensory function, communication, cognition, and fertility Discuss health issues relevant to patient's sexual behavior (e.g., risk factors for human immunodeficiency virus) Re-educate about masturbation Discuss health issues relevant to patient's medications
G—guide	*Guide* the patient and partner by responding in the same language and metaphors	The clinician is a powerful role model and can set the stage by understanding the patient's language, (e.g., "hard-on," for erection, "come" for experiencing orgasm) Problems such as pain, spasticity, decreased endurance and bowel and bladder function may require introduction by clinician
M—maximize	*Maximize* their problem-solving ability by encouraging experimentation, reading, and peer counseling	Discuss experimentation such as masturbation, sexual aids such as vibrators, couple-play Provide list of reading, medical and lay
A—assess/reassess	*Assess and reassess* the sexual issues at the next visit and make it an ongoing subject, not a one-time thing	At each visit a checklist through the ENIGMA model should be briefly reviewed to monitor progress, hang-ups or anxiety, acceptance of each area There are frequent anxieties and misconceptions after heart attack, hysterectomy, stroke, or life-altering medical condition Discuss the patient's sexual experience since the onset of the disability Assess interpersonal and psychosocial factors that may enhance or interfere with sexual relationships

it should not be pushed on them. Patients can use their impairment as an excuse for avoiding sexuality in their life, perhaps because of fear of rejection, failure, or unavailability of a partner. Table 30–14 lists precautions that should be followed when counseling patients. The single most important factor in improving sexual relationships between people is communication.

The PLISSIT model is simplistic and has been critiqued as providing a way for clinicians (especially physicians) to pass on their patient's sexual concerns to other clinicians. However, the rehabilitation model is interdisciplinary, and the PLISSIT model provides the basis for addressing sexual issues in a comprehensive manner.[2] Counselors should have factual information about sexuality, sexual physiology and function, and changes caused by disabling conditions. This knowledge can be gained through in-service programs, professional workshops,[44] seminars, and by availing oneself of topical literature and audiovisual materials.[122] Discussing feelings, concerns, and questions with colleagues and experienced patients is a method that can be used to increase counseling competence and comfort level.[110]

SUMMARY

Full and positive understanding and achievement of sexuality and sexual experience are accepted by most social components in both Eastern and Western civilization as a valuable, creative, recreative, and stress-releasing part of the quality of life. This can be no more true than in the health and medical processes of rehabilitation, in acquired physical or mental disabilities, and in rehabilitation of those with congenital or lifelong limitations.

The rules and religions of various social and cultural groups can add strength to or undermine the individual's sexual self-concept. When a patient is confronted by a physical or mental disability, an adequate or optimal sexual rebuilding must include not only an education of normal and modified sexual function and physiology, of acceptable options, and of ways to see his or her new physique and brain function as desirable, but also a process to expand positively sexuality and moral beliefs.

The plumbing of sexual function—the mechanics of how to make what is present work to the fullest extent—is the challenge to the physiatrist. Sexuality is a

TABLE 30–11 Suggested Physical Examination for Assessing Sexual Function

System		Examination
Mental health	Cognition	Competence to consent to sexual activity Judgment to make safe decisions regarding high-risk sexual activity and contraception
	Mood	Depressed Abusive
Neurological	Sensation	Evaluate sensate distribution Assess for decubitus ulcers *Educate regarding possible new erotic areas (insensate-sensate border) *Instruct patient and partner to concentrate on sensate skin
	Dysesthesia	*Positions to avoid stimulating sensitive areas *Techniques for desensitization
	Strength	Assess potential for touching, caressing, receiving touch Review positioning that allows for above
	Communication	Assess for aphasias, dysarthria
Musculoskeletal	Contractures	Assess for evidence of arthritis Does patient demonstrate knowledge of stretching? Is surgical intervention necessary?
	Spasticity	In females, evaluate adductor spasms as these may interfere with coitus
Genitalia	Hygiene	Examine for general hygiene, odors suggestive of yeast infection Is there need for attendant care?
	Sensation	Sensate distribution Evidence of reflexogenic erection or lubrication
	General	Evidence of sexually transmitted disease—condyloma, herpes In females, pelvic examination may need modified positioning[103]
Urological	Continence	Evidence of epididymitis If indwelling catheter, evidence of scrotal fistula; may wear condom over the folded catheter If external catheter, is there a good seal? If incontinent, skin breakdown
Gastrointestinal	General	Evaluate any ostomy sites
	Rectal	Assessment of anal wink, sphincter tone, voluntary control Assesment of bulbocavernosus reflex (manual compression of glans penis/clitoris or pulling on Foley catheter should elicit a reflex contraction of the anal sphincter) *Provides an opportunity to instruct patient regarding reflexogenic erection or lubrication
General	Vascular	Evidence of peripheral vascular disease or diabetes may alert clinician to presence of difficulty with erectile or lubrication function
	Cardiac	Assess for arrhythmias, pulse rate, blood pressure
	Pulmonary	Evidence of rales, shortness of breath

* Opportunities to instruct the patient.

TABLE 30–12 Role of a Sexual Health Care Program

Clinician role	1. Patient care services—contact with family and patient, assessment, diagnosis, prognosis, treatment. 2. In-service and professional education. 3. Liaison with hospital community agencies—involved with national and local associations. 4. Administration and research—statistical analysis, evaluation.
Stages of program	1. Begins on admission to acute unit as more than two-thirds of patients have sexual concerns and more than half experiment with some form of genital exploration or sexual activity before discharge from acute unit. Early acknowledgment to patient and family that sexually related problems occur with spinal cord injury (SCI) but that sex life is not over. 2. Introductory visits with the patient and family where potential problems and concerns are outlined and discussed. 3. Assessment and diagnostic formulation, history, physical, and psychosexual examination. 4. Series of follow-up visits to clarify areas of confusion, misinformation, and monitor changes. Encourage experimentation. May return months or years after finding a partner.
Patient concerns	1. Sexual disabilities exist after SCI patients want and need information about their future sexual potential. 2. Patient concerns are often present soon after injury.[74] It is not surprising to find patients more concerned about loss of sexual function than ambulation. 3. Concerns surface in many ways other than planned consultation. 4. When professionals do not inquire about patient's sexual concerns, they confirm to the patient suspicions that sexual life is over.
Benefits	1. Early legitimization of sexually related concerns. 2. Crystallization of physiological, emotional, and social capabilities and needs. 3. Specific instructions for experimentation with various sexual alternatives. 4. Patients not treated in the acute setting indicate long-standing sexual conerns, difficulty relating to partner, and negative attitude toward sexual abilities.

Adapted from Miller S, Szasz G, Anderson L: Sexual health care clinician in an acute spinal cord injury unit. Arch Phys Med Rehabil 1981; 62:315–320.

TABLE 30–13 PLISSIT Model for Sexual Counseling

	Goals	Responsibility	Example	References
P *p*ermission	Assure the patient that sexuality is a legitimate concern in the rehabilitation process.[49, 110] Provide a positive climate in which patients feel comfortable to ask questions, seek advice, and experiment. Do not expect the patient to initiate the discussion! Open the door with your questions.	Should be addressed by any team member in any discussion.	If sexual history is included as a routine part of *every* intake examination, it signals to the client that sexuality is considered an integral part of rehabilitation. The initial interaction can also serve to set the stage for further discussion and questions. "Being a good listener, attending to and acknowledging spoken or body language, asking leading questions, initiating discussion of sensitive subjects, and making observations about physical manifestations, such as reflex erections in the male client with spinal cord injury."[110] Telling people that their thoughts, feelings, and behaviors are "normal."[116]	The clinician is directed to read general textbooks and review articles.[38, 78]
LI *l*imited *i*nformation	Deals with the disability and its implications for sexual health in a general fashion.[110] Used to change relevant attitudes and behavior. Can serve as the means for dispelling general sexual myths relating to breast and genital size, masturbation, oral-genital contact, anal intercourse.	May be provided to the patient in a private impersonal manner by way of educational material or by any comfortable team member.	This level of information is easily provided during the initial examination. While eliciting the bladder-bowel history or examining the genitalia, one can provide vital information. For example, performing the bulbocavernosus reflex test can be very intimidating or embarrassing for the patient but can be an easy steppingstone to a more in-depth discussion regarding sexual function. Clients should be encouraged to seek out new areas of hypersensitivity. This information should also be provided to family and significant others.	Pamphlets or educational handouts on head injury, stroke,[110] or spinal cord injury. (Sexuality After Spinal Cord Injury: Fact Sheet no 3. National Spinal Cord Injury Association, 1987; Male Reproductive Function After Spinal Cord Injury: Fact Sheet no 10. National Spinal Cord Injury Association, 1988).

SS *s*pecific *s*uggestions	Patient and partner are actively assisted by staff to set and reach specific goals to address sexual concerns and dysfunctions.[110]	Rehabilitation team member knowledgeable about sexuality and the particular physical disability affecting the patient.	Therapists can assist patients with positioning for comfortable lovemaking like using the partner for a backboard, sensual ways to undress, technqiues of foreplay, the use of fantasy, types of mechanical devices available, how to deal with urinal and bowel mishaps. Pipe-cleaner figures can be useful in demonstrating alternative sexual positions. "You'll have to try it and see" is not good enough. Use peer counseling.	Excellent books and videos depicting different lovemaking options. (Mooney TO, Cole TM, Chilgren RA: Sexual Options for Paraplegics and Quadriplegics. Boston, Little, Brown, 1975; Bregman S: Sexuality and the Spinal Cord Injured Woman. Minneapolis, Sister Kenny Foundation, 1975; Rabin BJ: The Sensuous Wheeler. Long Beach, CA, 1980.)
IT *i*ntensive *t*herapy	When is it time to refer? Psychological problems General sexual dysfunction Overall low sexual interest Primary orgasmic dysfunction Vaginismus Primary impotence Ejaculatory incompetence Destructive paraphilias	Requires assistance of a specially trained professional or professional sexual therapist since harm may be done to the patient if a clinician is inexperienced.	"Injury is likely to magnify any sexual difficulties that the patient and the partner have (interpersonal and psychological issues) and these must be overcome before progress can be made."[131]	American Association of Sex Educators, Counselors and Therapists, 435 N. Michigan Ave., Suite 1717, Chicago, IL 60611 (312) 644–0828.

Adapted from Annon JS, Robinson CH: Treatment of common male and female sexual concerns. In Ferguson JM, Taylor CB (eds): The Comprehensive Handbook of Behavioral Medicine, Vol 1. New York, SP Medical & Scientific Books, 1980, pp 273–296.

TABLE 30–14 Sexual Counseling Precautions

1. Do not put persons in conflict with their God.
2. Avoid extreme pressure on the patient to discuss sexuality.
3. Avoid forcing your morality and convictions on the patient.
4. Do not threaten the patient with your own sexuality.
5. Do not make sex an all-or-none sort of experience.
6. Do not assume that once the topic is discussed that you can leave it alone.
7. Do not conclude that there is only one way to convey information.
8. Be sure that the conjoint nature of sexual relationships is held paramount.
9. Do convey the notion that all relationships, including the sexual one, are a matter of compromise.

From Rieve JE: Sexuality and the adult with acquired physical disability. Nurs Clin North Am 1989; 24:265–276. Information compiled by Rieve from Hohmann GW: Sexual dysfunction associated with physical disabilities. Arch Phys Med Rehabil 1975; 56:1, and other sources.

primary example of head, heart, and body interaction. Positive issues must be encouraged. Negative issues must be examined and addressed. All this must be done in the full knowledge and understanding of the patient, partner, family, and support by the rehabilitation team. Any individual therapist can rehabilitate, but in this complex area especially, it is typically best done by a well-coordinated team.

In looking at the complete individual patient, a thorough history, physical evaluation, assesssment of self-concept and formation of goals must all be inculcated into sexuality rehabilitation. It must be accepted by all involved—patient included—that the acquisition of a disability requires a reexamination of the patient's sexuality. Treatment of an acquired disability should include sexual therapy.

REFERENCES

1. Aboseif SR, Lue TF: Hemodynamics of penile erection. Urol Clin North Am 1988; 15:1–7.
2. Annon JS, Robinson CH: Treatment of common male and female sexual concerns. In Ferguson JM, Taylor CB (eds): The Comprehensive Handbook of Behavioral Medicine, vol 1. New York, SP Medical & Scientific Books, 1980, pp 273–296.
3. Barada JH, McKimmy RM: Vasoactive pharmacotherapy. In Bennett AH (ed): Impotence: Diagnosis and Management of Erectile Dysfunction. Philadelphia, WB Saunders, 1994, pp 229–250.
4. Basson R: Sexual health of women with disabilities. Can Med Assoc J 1998; 159(4):359–362.
5. Bennett CJ, Seager SW, Vasher EA, et al: Sexual dysfunction and electroejaculation in men with spinal cord injury: Review. J Urol 1988; 139:453–456.
6. Benson GS, McConnell J, Lipshultz LI: Neuromorphology and neuropharmacology of the human penis: An in vitro study. J Clin Invest 1980; 65:506–513.
7. Bérard EJJ: The sexuality of spinal cord injured women: Physiology and pathophysiology. A review. Paraplegia 1989; 27:99–112.
8. Beretta G, Chelo E, Zanollo A: Reproductive aspects in spinal cord injured males. Paraplegia 1989; 27:113–118.
9. Berkman AH, Weissman R, Frielich MH: Sexual adjustment of spinal cord injured veterans living in the community. Arch Phys Med Rehabil 1978; 59:29–33.
10. Bitran D, Hull EM: Pharmacological analysis of male rat sexual behavior. Neurosci Biobehav Rev 1987; 11:365–389.
11. Blackerby WF: A treatment model for sexuality disturbance following brain injury. J Head Trauma Rehabil 1990; 5:73–82.
12. Blake DJ, Masiak R, Brown S, et al: Acceptance by arthritis patients of clinical inquiry into their sexual adjustment. Psychosomatics 1986; 27:576–579.
13. Boldrini P, Basaglia N, Calanca MC: Sexual changes in hemiparetic patients. Arch Phys Med Rehabil 1991; 72:202–207.
14. Bolling RD: Prevalence, goals and complications of heterosexual anal intercourse in a gynecologic population. J Reprod Med 1977; 19:120–124.
15. Boolell M, Gepi-Attee S, Gingell JC, et al: Sildenafil, a novel effective oral therapy for male erectile dysfunction. Br J Urol 1996; 78:257–261.
16. Bors E, Comarr AE: Neurologic disturbances of sexual function with special reference to 529 patients with spinal cord injury. Urol Surv 1960; 10:191–222.
17. Brackett NL, Santa-Cruz C, Lynne C: Sperm from spinal cord injured men lose motility faster than sperm from normal men: The effect is exacerbated at body compared to room temperature. J Urol 1997; 157:2150–2153.
18. Brackett NL, Ferrell SM, Aballa TC, et al: An analysis of 653 trials of penile vibratory stimulation in men with spinal cord injury. J Urol 1998; 159:1931–1934.
19. Brackett NL, Bloch WE, Lynne CM: Predictors of necrospermia in men with spinal cord injury. J Urol 1998; 159:844–847.
20. Brackett NL, Padron OF, Lynne CM: Semen quality of spinal cord injured men is better when obtained by vibratory stimulation versus electroejaculation. J Urol 1997; 157:151–157.
21. Bray GP, DeFrank RS, Wolfe TL: Sexual functioning in stroke survivors. Arch Phys Med Rehabil 1981; 62:286–288.
22. Brindley GS: Deep scrotal temperature and the effect on it of clothing, air temperature, activity, posture and paraplegia. Br J Urol 1982; 54:49–55.
23. Brindley GS: The fertility of men with spinal injuries. Paraplegia 1984; 22:337–348.
24. Brindley GS: The actions of parasympathetic and sympathetic nerves in human micturation, erection and seminal emission, and their restoration in paraplegic patients by implanted electrical stimulators. Proc R Soc Lond 1988; 235:111.
25. Buch JP: Disorders of ejaculation. In Bennett AH (ed): Impotence: Diagnosis and Management of Erectile Dysfunction. Philadelphia, WB Saunders, 1994, pp 186–196.
26. Buch JP, Zorn BH: Evaluation and treatment of infertility in spinal cord injured men through rectal probe electroejaculation. J Urol 1993; 149:1350–1354.
27. Burgener S, Logan G: Sexuality concerns of the post-stroke patient. Rehabil Nurs 1989; 14:178–181.
28. Burnett AL: Nitric oxide in the penis: Physiology and pathology. J Urol 1997; 157:320–324.
29. Cha KY, Oum KB, Kim HJ: Approaches for obtaining sperm with male factor infertility. Fertil Steril 1997; 67:985–995.
30. Chambas K: Sexual concerns of adolescents with cancer. J Pediatr Oncol Nurs 1991; 8:165–172.
31. Chapelle PA, Blanquart F, Peuch AJ, et al: Treatment of anejaculation in the total paraplegic by subcutaneous injection of physostigmine. Paraplegia 1983; 21:30–36.
32. Charlifue SW, Gerhart KA, Menter RR, et al: Sexual issues of women with spinal cord injuries. Paraplegia 1992; 30:192–199.
33. Cheadle MJ: The screening sexual history: Getting to the problem. Clin Geriatr Med 1991; 7:9–13.
34. Chen D, Hartwig DM, Roth EJ: Comparison of sperm quantity and quality in antegrade v retrograde ejaculates obtained by vibratory penile stimulation in males with spinal cord injury. Am J Phys Med Rehabil 1999; 78:46–51.
35. Chicano LA: Humanistic aspects of sexuality as related to spinal cord injury. J Neurosci Nurs 1989; 21:366–369.
36. Chung PH, Palermo G, Schlegel PN, et al: The use of intracytoplasmic sperm injection with electroejaculates from anejaculatory men. Hum Reprod 1998; 13:1854–1858.
37. Collins KP, Hackler RH: Complications of penile prostheses in the spinal cord injury population. J Urol 1988; 140:984–985.
38. Comfort A: Sexual Consequences of Disability. Philadelpha, GF Stickley, 1978.
39. Comfort A, Dial LK: Sexuality and aging: An overview. Clin Geriatr Med 1991; 7:1–7.
40. Craig DI: The adaptation to pregnancy of spinal cord injured women. Rehabil Nurs 1990; 15:6–9.

41. Cromer BA, Enrile B, McCoy K, et al: Knowledge, attitudes and behavior related to sexuality in adolescents with chronic disability. Dev Med Child Neurol 1990; 32:602–610.
42. Deamer RL, Thompson JF: The role of medications in geriatric sexual function. Clin Geriatr Med 1991; 7:95–111.
43. Derry FA, Dinsmore WW, Fraser M, et al: Efficacy and safety of oral sildenafil (Viagra) in men with erectile dysfunction caused by spinal cord injury. Neurology 1998; 51:1629–1633.
44. Eisenberg MG, Rustad LC: Sex education and counseling program on a spinal cord injury service. Arch Phys Med Rehabil 1976; 57:135–140.
45. Ende J, Rockwell S, Glasgow M: The sexual history in general medicine practice. Arch Intern Med 1984; 144:558–561.
46. Feldman HA, Goldstein I, Hatzichristou DG, et al: Impotence and its medical and psycholosocial correlates: Results of the Massachusetts Male Aging Study. J Urol 1994; 151:54–61.
47. Fletcher GF, Johnston BL, Cantwell JD: Dynamic electrocardiographic monitoring during coitus in patients post myocardial infarction and revascularization. Circulation 1978; 57(suppl 2):204.
48. Freda M, Rubinsky H: Sexual function in the stroke survivor. Phys Med Rehabil Clin North Am 1991; 2:643–658.
49. Goddard LR; Sexuality and spinal cord injury. J Neurosci Nurs 1988; 20:240–243.
50. Goldstein I, Lue TF, Padma-Nathan H, et al: Oral sildenafil in the treatment of erectile dysfunction. N Engl J Med 1998; 338:1397–1404. [Published erratum appears in N Engl J Med 1998; 339:59].
51. Griffith ER, Tomko MA, Timms RJ: Sexual function in spinal cord-injured patients: A review, Arch Phys Med Rehabil 1973; 54:539–542.
52. Gupta K: Sexual dysfunction in elderly women. Clin Geriatr Med 1990; 6:197–203.
53. Guttmann L, Walsh JJ: Prostigmine assessment test of fertility in spinal man. Paraplegia 1971; 9:39–50.
54. Hahn K: Sexuality and COPD. Rehabil Nurs 1989; 14:191–195.
55. Hamilton GA, Seidman RN: A comparison of the recovery period for women and men after an acute myocardial infarction. Heart Lung 1993; 22:308–315.
56. Harrison J, Glass CA, Owens RG, et al: Factors associated with sexual functioning in women following spinal cord injury. Paraplegia 1995; 33:687–692.
57. Hirsch IH, Sedor J, Callahan HJ, et al: Antisperm antibodies in seminal plasma of spinal cord–injured men. Urology 1992; 39:243–247.
58. Horn LJ, Zasler ND: Neuroanatomy and neurophysiology of sexual function. J Head Trauma Rehabil 1990; 5:1–13.
59. Hovav Y, Kafka I, Dan-Goor M, et al: Electroejaculation in combination with intracytoplasmic sperm injection in patients with psychogenic anejaculation results in lower fertilization rates. Fertil Steril 1998; 69:561–563.
60. Hutter AM, Cheitlin MD, et al: Summary statement of the American College of Cardiology and the American Heart Association on the use of sildenafil (Viagra) in patients at clinical risk from cardiovascular effects. Cardiology 1999; 33(1):273–282.
61. Jensen SB: Sexual relationships in couples with a diabetic partner. J Sex Marital Ther 1985; 11:259–270.
62. Kaiser FE: Sexuality and impotence in the aging man. Clin Geriatr Med 1991; 7:63–71.
63. Kedia KR, Markland C, Fraly EE: Sexual function following high retroperitoneal lymphadenectomy. J Urol 1975; 114:237.
64. Kim ED, El-Rashidy R, McVary KT: Papaverine topical gel for treatment of erectile dysfunction. J Urol 1995; 153:361–365.
65. Kligman EW: Office evaluation of sexual function and complaints. Clin Geriatr Med 1991; 7:15–39.
66. Klomer RA: Viagra: What every physician should know. ENT J 1998; 77:783–786.
67. Kosteljanetz M, Jensen T, Norgard B, et al: Sexual and hypothalamic dysfunction in the post-concussional syndrome. Acta Neurol Scand 1981; 63:169–180.
68. Krane RJ, Siroky MB: Neurophysiology of erection. Urol Clin North Am 1981; 8:91–101.
69. Kuhn RA: Functional capacity of the isolated human spinal cord. Brain 1950; 73:1–51.
70. LeMone P: Human sexuality in adults with insulin-dependent diabetes mellitus. Image J Nurs Scholarship 1993; 25:101–105.
71. Levine SB, Althof SE, Turner LA, et al: Side effects of self-administration of intracavernous papverine and phentolamine for the treatment of impotence. J Urol 1989; 141:54–57.
72. Levinson SF, O'Connell PG: Rehabilitation dimensions of AIDS: A review. Arch Phys Med Rehabil 1991; 72:690–696.
73. Lewis D: The gynecologic consideration of the sexual act. JAMA 1983; 250:222–227.
74. Linsenmeyer TA, Perkash I: Infertility in men with spinal cord injury. Arch Phys Med Rehabil 1991; 72:747–754.
75. Lipe H, Longstreth WT Jr, Bird TD, et al: Sexual function in married men with Parkinson's disease compared to married men with arthritis. Neurology 1990; 40:1347–1349.
76. LoPiccolo J: Counseling and therapy for sexual problems in the elderly. Clin Geriatr Med 1991; 7:161–179.
77. Marsiglio W, Donnelly D: Sexual relations in later life: A national study of married persons. J Gerontol 1991; 46:S338–S344.
78. Masters WH, Johnson VE, Kolodny RC: Human Sexuality. Boston, Little, Brown. 1982.
79. Mayers KS: Sexual and social concerns of the disabled: A group counseling approach. Sex Disability 1978; 1:100–111.
80. Maytom MC, Derry FA, Dinsmore WW, et al: A two-part pilot study of sildenafil (Viagra) in men with erectile dysfunction caused by spinal cord injury. Spinal Cord 1999; 37:110–116.
81. McCormick GP, Riffer DJ, Thompson MM: Coital positioning for stroke afflicted couples. Rehabil Nurs 1986; 11:17–19.
82. Medhat A, Huber PM, Medhat MA: Factors that influence the level of activities in persons with lower extremity amputation. Rehabil Nurs 1990; 15:13–18.
83. Meeropol E: One of the gang: Sexual development of adolescents with physical disabilities. J Pediatr Nurs 1991; 6:243–249.
84. Melman A, Christ GJ, Hirsch MS: Antomy and physiology of the penis. In Bennett AH (ed): Impotence: Diagnosis and Management of Erectile Dysfunction. Philadelphia, WB Saunders, 1994, pp 18–30.
85. Merrill JM, Laux LF, Thornby JI: Why doctors have difficulty with sex histories. South Med J 1990; 83:613–617.
86. Miller S, Szasz G, Anderson L: Sexual health care clinician in an acute spinal cord injury unit. Arch Phys Med Rehabil 1981; 62:315–320.
87. Modell J, Katholi C: Comparative sexual side effects of buproprion, fluoxetine, paroxetine and sertraline. Clin Pharmacol Ther 1997; 61:476–487.
88. Money J: Phantom orgasm in the dreams of paraplegic men and women. Arch Gen Psychiatry 1960; 3:373–382.
89. Montague DK, Lakin MM: Penile prostheses. In Bennett AH (ed): Impotence: Diagnosis and Management of Erectile Dysfunction. Philadelphia, WB Saunders, 1994, pp 257–295.
90. Morales A: Nonsurgical management options in impotence. Hosp Pract. 1993, March, pp 16–23.
91. Moreland RB, Goldstein I, Traish A: Sildenafil, a novel inhibitor of phosphodiesterase type 5 in human corpus cavernosum smooth muscle cells. Life Sci 1998; 62:309–318.
92. Muller JE, Mittleman MA, Maclure M, et al: Triggering myocardial infarction by sexual activity: Low absolute risk and prevention by regular physical exertion, for the Determinants of Myocardial Infarction Onset Study Investigators. JAMA 1996; 275:1405–1409.
93. Murphy JB, Lipshultz LI: Abnormalities of ejaculation. Urol Clin North Am 1987; 14:583–595.
94. Nadig PW: Vacuum therapy and other devices. In Bennett AH (ed): Impotence: Diagnosis and Management of Erectile Dysfunction. Philadelphia, WB Saunders, 1994, pp 251–256.
95. National Institute of Health Consensus Development Panel on Impotence Conference. Impotence. JAMA 1993; 270:83–90.
96. Nosek M, Rintala D, Young ME, et al: Sexual functioning among women with physical disabilities. Arch Phys Med Rehabil 1996; 77:107–115.
97. O'Carroll RE, Woodrow J, Maroun F: Psychosexual and psychosocial sequelae of closed head injury. Brain Injury 1991; 5: 303–313.
98. Ohl DA, Sonksen J, Menge AC, et al: Electroejaculation versus vibratory stimulation in spinal cord injured men: Sperm quality and patient preference. J Urol 1997; 157:2147–2149.

99. Padma-Nathan H, Hellstrom WJG, Kaiser FE, et al: Treatment of men with erectile dysfunction with transurethral alprostadil. N Engl J Med 1997; 336:1–7.
100. Perkash I, Martin DE, Warner H, et al: Electroejaculation in spinal cord injury patients: Simplified new equipment and technique. J Urol 1990; 143:305–307.
101. Pervin-Dixon L: Sexuality and the spinal cord injured. J Psychosoc Nurs Ment Health Surv 1988; 26:31–34.
102. Pfizer: Viagra (Sildenafil Nitrate): Full Prescribing Information (monograph). Pfizer US Pharmaceuticals, April 1998.
103. Phelps G, Brown M, Chen J, et al: Sexual experience and plasma testosterone levels in male veterans after spinal cord injury. Arch Phys Med Rehabil 1983; 64:47–52.
104. Pilsecker C: Starting out: the first six months posthospital for spinal cord-injured veterans. Am J Phys Med Rehabil 1990; 69:91–95.
105. Purifoy FE, Grodsky A, Giambra LM: The relationship of sexual daydreaming to sexual activity, sexual drive, and sexual attitudes for women across the life-span. Arch Sex Behav 1992; 21: 369–385.
106. Rabin BJ: The Sensuous Wheeler: Sexual Adjustment for the Spinal Cord Injured. Long Beach, CA, Rabin, 1980.
107. Rawicki HB, Hill S: Semen retrieval in spinal cord injured men. Paraplegia 1991; 29:443–446.
108. Relf MV: Sexuality and the older bypass patient. Geriatr Nurs 1991; 34:294–296.
109. Rendell MS, Rajfer J, Wicker PA, et al: Sildenafil for treatment of erectile dysfunction in men with diabetes: A randomized controlled trial. JAMA 1999; 281:421–426.
110. Rieve JE: Sexuality and the adult with acquired physical disability. Nurs Clin North Am 1989; 24:265–276.
111. Sadoughi W, Leshner M, Fine HL: Sexual adjustment in a chronically ill and physically disabled population: A pilot study. Arch Phys Med Rehabil 1971; 52:311–317.
112. Saenz de Tejada I, Goldstein I, Krane RJ: Local control of penile erection. Urol Clin North Am 1988; 15:9–15.
113. Sarosdy MF, Hudnall CH, Erickson DR, et al: A prospective double-blind trial of intracorporeal papaverine versus prostaglandin El in the treatment of impotence. J Urol 1988; 141: 551–553.
114. Sato K, Kihara K, Ando M, et al: Seminal emission by electrical stimulation of the spermatic nerve and epididymis. Int J Androl 1991; 14:461.
115. Schiavi RC, Schreiner-Engel P, Mandeli J, et al: Healthy aging and male sexual function. Am J Psychiatry 1990; 147:766–771.
116. Seidl A, Bullough B, Haughey B, et al: Understanding the effects of a myocardial infarction on sexual functioning: A basis for sexual counseling. Rehabil Nurs 1991; 16:255–264.
117. Sipski ML, Alexander CJ: Sexual function and dysfunction after spinal cord injury. Phys Med Rehabil Clin North Am 1992; 3:811–828.
118. Sjogren K: Sexuality after stroke with hemiplegia: II. With special regard to partnership adjustment and to fulfillment. Scand J Rehabil Med 1983; 15:63–69.
119. Smith DB, Babaian RJ: The effects of treatment for cancer on male fertility and sexuality. Cancer Nurs 1992; 15:271–275.
120. Smith LL, Lathrop LM: AIDS and human sexuality. Can J Public Health 1993; 84:S14–18.
121. Sonksen J, Biering-Sorensen F: Transcutaneous nitroglycerin in the treatment of erectile dysfunction in spinal cord injured. Paraplegia 1992; 30:554–557.
122. Spica MM: Sexual counseling standards for the spinal cord-injured. J Neurosci Nurs 1989; 21:56–60.
123. Stockard S: Caring for the sexually aggressive patient. Nursing 1991; 11:72–73.
124. Talbot HS: Sexual function in paraplegia. J Urol 1955; 73:91–100.
125. Tay HP, Juma S, Joseph AC: Psychogenic impotence in spinal cord injury patients. Arch Phys Med Rehabil 1996; 77:391–393.
126. Teal JC, Athelstan GT: Sexuality and spinal cord injury: Some psychosocial considerations. Arch Phys Med Rehabil 1975; 56:264–268.
127. Thornton CE: Sexuality counseling of women with spinal cord injuries. Sex Disabil 1979; 9:267–277.
128. Trop CS, Bennett CJ: Autonomic dysreflexia and its urological implications: A review, J Urol 1991; 146:1461–1469.
129. Valleroy ML, Kraft GH: Sexual dysfunction in multiple selerosis. Arch Phys Med Rehabil 1984; 65:125–128.
130. VerVoort SM: Infertility in spinal-cord injured male. Urology 1987; 29:157–165.
131. Walbroehl GS: Sexuality in the handicapped. Am Fam Physician 1987; 36:129–133.
132. Wanner MB, Rageth CJ, Zäch GA: Pregnancy and autonomic hyperreflexia in patients with spinal cord lesions. Paraplegia 1987; 25:482–490.
133. Ware CJ: Impotence and aging. Clin Geriatr Med 1989; 5: 301–314.
134. Westgren N, Hultling C, Levi R, et al: Sexuality in women with traumatic spinal cord injury. Acta Obstet Gynecol Scand 1997; 76:977–983.
135. Weinberg JS: Human sexuality and spinal cord injury. Nurs Clin North Am 1982; 17:407–419.
136. Weiss J: Multiple sclerosis: Will it come between us? Sexual concerns of clients and their partners. J Neurosci Nurs 1992; 24:190–193.
137. Weiss JN, Mellinger BC: Sexual dysfunction in elderly men. Clin Geriatr Med 1990; 6:185–196.
138. White MJ, Rintala DH, Hart KA, et al: Sexual activities, concerns and interests of men with spinal cord injury. Am J Phys Med Rehabil 1992; 71:225–231.
139. White MJ, Rintala DH, Hart KA, et al: Sexual activities, concerns and interests of women with spinal cord injury living in the community. Am J Phys Med Rehabil 1993; 72:372–378.
140. Whitehead TL: Sexual health promotion of the patient with burns. J Burn Care Rehabil 1993; 14:221–226.
141. Witherington R: Vacuum constriction device for management of erectile impotence. J Urol 1989; 141:320–322.
142. Yalla SV, Vickers MA, Sullivan MP, et al: Sexual dysfunction and spinal cord injury. In Bennett AH (ed): Impotence: Diagnosis and Management of Erectile Dysfunction. Philadelphia, WB Saunders, 1994, pp 175–185.
143. Yarkony GM: Enhancement of sexual function and fertility in spinal cord-injured males. Am J Phys Med Rehabil 1990; 69: 81–87.
144. Yoffe E: Women and sex. Health 1994; 4:53–60.
145. Young BK, Katz M, Klein SA: Pregnancy after spinal cord injury: Altered maternal and fetal response to labor. Obstet Gynecol 1983; 62:59–62.
146. Zasler ND, Horn LJ: Rehabilitative management of sexual dysfunction. J Head Trauma Rehabil 1990; 5:14–24.
147. Zencius A, Wesolowski MD, Burke WH, et al: Managing hypersexual disorders in brain-injured clients. Brain Injury 1990; 4:175–181.
148. Zippe CD, Kedia AW, Kedia K, et al: Treatment of erectile dysfunction after radical prostatectomy with sildenafil citrate (Viagra). Urology 1998; 52:963–966.

31

CHAPTER

Richard Salcido, M.D., and Robert Goldman, M.D.

Prevention and Management of Pressure Ulcers and Other Chronic Wounds

Disease management is shifting from inpatient to outpatient care, from invasive to noninvasive therapies, from treatment to prevention. There is an economic imperative to create Disease Management Models of outpatient or skilled-care programs, utilizing prevention and early intervention to replace expensive acute-hospital–based treatment. According to the federal government, prevention and early intervention with chronic wounds could reduce amputations by 40% between 1990 and 2000.[40] Chronic wound care fits well into an outpatient and skilled-care model.

The financial burden of chronic wound care is immense: In the United States, the chronic wound care bill, including professional expenses, hospital costs, and complications (direct costs only), ranges from $7 billion to $15 billion. Moreover, the costs of all chronic wound types are increasing at 10% per year, driven by the aging of the "baby boomers." Four basic ulcer types present significant economic burden: pressure ulcers ($3 to 6 billion), ischemic/neuropathic ulcers ($3 to 5 billion), and venous ulcers (>$2 billion). Because prevention and aggressive treatment of early ulcers reduces costs, there is an economic impetus for growth of outpatient wound centers. In the past 15 years, the number of wound care treatment centers has risen from very few to more than 200.[36, 108]

Another trend in wound care derives from the current revolution in molecular biology, with direct application to conservative closure of chronic wounds. Chronic wound products are now FDA-approved in two novel areas: (1) topical growth substances[128] and (2) artificial skin grafts.[43] Both promise good outcomes for the most intractable wounds in the outpatient setting, and are only the beginning in terms of future therapies.

Physiatrists should be interested and involved in chronic wound care because they are invested in optimizing function, employ team management, have a wound-healing knowledge base, and are trained in the biomechanics of gait and the functional aspects of protected weight bearing. Physiatrists also prescribe durable medical equipment, orthoses, and special shoes, all of which are critical components of chronic wound care. Because physiatrists do not do surgery, they are well positioned to practice the noninvasive wound management outlined in this chapter. This chapter elaborates the emerging field of outpatient and skilled-care chronic wound practice for physiatrists, who are urged to adopt a proactive role in saving limbs.

SCOPE OF THE PROBLEM

Definitions

The National Pressure Ulcer Advisory Panel (NPUAP) defines a *pressure ulcer* as an area of unrelieved pressure over a defined area, usually over a bony prominence such as the greater trochanter of the femur, sacrum, or occiput, resulting in ischemia, cell death, and tissue necrosis.[102] Pressure ulcers are associated with impaired sensorium or sensation, poor hygiene or nutrition, and chronic illness. High standards of nursing and medical management are key to prevention of ulcers in immobilized patients.

Chronic venous or edematous ulcers of the leg typically arise above the medial malleolus (the origin of the saphenous vein), but could arise anywhere on the leg or foot dorsum. They are associated with impaired venous return, incompetence of venous perforators, or loss of fascial integrity of the leg (e.g., from trauma) in patients with normal arterial inflow. The cornerstone of treatment is compression.

Neuropathic ulcers are multifactoral, but typically follow repetitive trauma to hyposensate distal extremities (e.g., feet), usually on weight-bearing bony prominences, such as metatarsal heads. For uncomplicated neuropathic ulcers, the circulation is usually clinically intact.[63] A cornerstone of treatment is mitigating the axial repetitive pressure and shear.

Ischemic ulcers occur on limbs with impaired arterial inflow due to atherosclerotic disease. Often initiated by minor trauma or shoe pressure on the malleoli, heels, or lateral metatarsal heads, they are typically painful and blanched. Ischemic ulcers are frequently associated with neuropathy or edema. Healing primarily depends on re-establishing arterial circulation, either or medically or surgically.

Epidemiology of Chronic Wounds

Persons with spinal cord injury (SCI) and associated comorbidity are at increased risk for the formation of pressure ulcers.[10] The incidence of pressure ulcers in this population ranges from 25% to 66%.[51]

The incidence of pressure ulcers in acutely hospitalized patients ranges from 2.7%[54] to 29%[30] (prevalence, 3.5%[123] to 69%[4, 91]). Patients in critical care units run a higher risk of developing pressure ulcers, as evidenced by 33% incidence[15] and 41% prevalence[115] in this population. Elderly patients admitted to acute care hospitals for nonelective, orthopedic procedures such as hip replacement and long bone fractures are at even greater risk for developing pressure ulcers[114, 135] (66% incidence).

Long-term facilities are frequently the disposition for patients with pressure ulcers sustained during acute hospitalization. About 25% of residents admitted from an acute care hospital have pressure ulcers.[109] In addition, patients with pre-existing pressure ulcers are predisposed to form new ones. Unfortunately, 26% of residents with a pressure ulcer form a new one over a 6-month period. However, while 33% of those admitted to a chronic care hospital have pressure ulcers,[17] long-term follow-up demonstrates that the majority of ulcers healed within a year[17, 21]; thus the incidence in chronic care hospitals is reported to be 10.8%.[8] Unfortunately, approximately 60,000 people die each year from complications of pressure ulcers.[2] Pressure ulcer development has been associated with a 4.5 times greater risk of death than for persons with the same risk factors but without pressure ulcers.[126]

Pressure ulcers develop or do not develop depending on our ability to handle issues of incontinence, inspection, turning, positioning, range of motion, and nutrition. Variable implementation of these care practices might explain the wide variation in the prevalence of pressure ulcers in long-term care facilities of 2.6% to 24%.[21, 109] Because of this wide disparity, the prevalence of pressure ulcers is an important index of care quality and is monitored by federal and state governments in the Minimum Data Set (MDS).

Diabetes Mellitus

Neuropathy, arteriosclerosis, and microvascular disease combine in diabetes, creating a high risk for chronic wounds of the lower extremities. These foot complications often result in amputation. There were 54,000 amputations in diabetic patients in 1990, preceded in 85% of cases by foot ulcers. Amputations are ten times more prevalent among diabetic individuals than in the general population. The first major limb amputation for diabetics is often followed by a second major amputation, and 28% to 51% have a contralateral amputation within 5 years.[110]

The cost of a single major amputation is conservatively estimated at $100,000, including the acute hospital stay, surgeries, rehabilitation, and prostheses (unpublished data[140]). Multiplying the cost per amputation and number of amputations among those with diabetes, there is a likely cost burden of $5.4 billion. Because of this cost burden, The U.S. Public Health Service called for a 40% reduction in diabetic-related amputations by the year 2000, and urged prevention and earlier treatment to achieve this goal.[40] Unfortunately, recent estimates indicate that the number of amputations has actually increased from 1990 estimates.

Chronic Venous Disease

Venous stasis ulcers occur in up to 1% of the population, and it is estimated that 2.5 million Americans suffer from venous ulcers. Only 600,000 per year are treated, however, so it is likely that chronic venous disease is underdiagnosed. The cost estimate for healing an uncomplicated ulcer is $2,500.[105] Intractable ulcers are much more expensive, and 20% to 30% of ulcers present as intractable. Intractable ulcers are those that are present for more than one year or those whose area exceeds 10 square centimeters. The cost can approach $10,000 for each of these intractable cases.[100] At an average cost of $3,000 per ulcer, the total direct cost is estimated at $2 billion, which does not factor in the hidden costs of undiagnosed ulcers. In addition to the hidden cost of untreated ulcers, there are two million lost workdays from this condition.[106]

WOUND PHYSIOLOGY AND PATHOPHYSIOLOGY

Definitions

The Wound Healing Society defines *healing* as complete closing of the integument. Skin wounds that heal by *primary intention* are similar to incisions that are created by a scalpel blade and then heal rapidly and without complication. More complicated are the wounds that heal by *secondary intention.* Secondary intention wounds are large tissue defects that fill by granulation followed by epitheliazation. Wound closure occurs to some extent because of wound contraction.

Process of Normal Healing

There are four major phases of wound healing: inflammation, provisional matrix formation, repair, and remodeling. The sequence begins with wound formation. After wound formation, hemostasis is achieved as a plug of fibrin and cellular debris fills the defect. Platelets release growth substances and cytokines, which are chemotactic for neutrophils and monocytes, and yield a nonspecific inflammatory response. This response is enhanced by monocyte release of cytokines interleukin-1 (IL-1) and tumor necrosis factor (TNF), which in turn induce complement factors by fibroblasts.

As the general inflammatory response subsides, polypeptide growth factors platelet derived growth factor (PDGF), epidermal growth factor (EGF), and basic fibroblast growth factor (b-FGF) gradually replace cytokines in the wound fluid. These growth substances down-regulate inflammatory protein production and up-regulate fibroblast collagenase[29] to degrade the existing extracellular matrix. A provisional matrix of fibronectin and glycosaminoglycans is synthesized by fibroblasts,[107] partially in response to PDGF in wound fluid.[73]

After provisional matrix formation, transforming growth factor-beta (TGF-beta) peaks between day 7 and day 14 and partially directs the repair phase,[28] wherein wound fibroblasts synthesize and secrete type I collagen. The secreted collagen fibrils self-assemble into fibers that form (in a vitamin C-dependent process) cross-links between lysine residues and collagen fibrils. These are randomly laid down during the repair phase of wound healing within granulation tissue. Also within granulation tissue, b-FGF induces neo-angiogenesis.[107] Later, during the remodeling phase, the dermis becomes stronger, turning over collagen fibers so they are retained preferentially along lines of stress.

Simultaneously with early dermal healing, wounds re-epithelialize. Fibroblast-secreted keratinocyte growth factor (KGF) and IL-6 help cause keratinocytes to proliferate and then differentiate into the epidermis.[124] Epidermis at the wound edge, from which nascent keratinocytes arise, also directs keratinocytes to cover the opening. This is done by way of the skin battery. The skin battery, which is contained within the stratum spinosum, is an amiloride-blocked sodium pump that induces electrical currents at the wound edge sufficient to cause keratinocytes to migrate purposefully in the direction of wound closure.[9] Water-loss and bacterial contamination cease with the closure of the epidermal layer.

Normal healing of a wound by primary intention takes 3 to 14 days to complete. The 14-day interval is for deeper, sutured surgical incisions. The process takes longer for secondary intention wounds. These wounds form granulation tissue consisting of a loose connective tissue framework with fibroblasts actively synthesizing and secreting extracellular matrix, and there is a high density of immature neo-vessels engorging the repairing region with oxygen and nutrients.

Pathophysiology of Chronic Wounds

Chronic wounds appear to be in a chronic inflammatory state synonymous with healing-arrest. Five easily identified factors dynamically interact to arrest healing and perpetuate wound status: (1) pathomechanics; (2) reperfusion injury; (3) chronic hypoxia; (4) growth factor derangement, and (5) chronic inflammation.

Pathomechanics

Pathomechanics implies noxious application of shear (force tangential to the skin surface) and axial pressure (perpendicular to the skin). Unrelieved static axial pressure[78, 79] is a critical factor in development of pressure ulcers of the buttocks. Prolonged pressure leads to ulcers if tissue capillary pressure is exceeded.[79] The pressure that exceeds capillary pressure was first quantified by Landis (1930), then confirmed by others[85, 120, 121] to be 32 mm Hg in the arteriolar limb. This benchmark is further defined as interface pressure: Although critically influenced by body contour, tissue stiffness, and composition, pressures under 32 mm Hg are assumed by many clinicians to be safe.[119] Products aimed at reducing or relieving pressure have tended to use interface pressure as the standard for judging product efficacy.[82, 119, 120]

The critical interface pressure is the pressure above which a tissue cannot be loaded for an indefinite period without resulting ulceration. There is an inverse, hyperbolic relationship between pressure and the duration of pressure application necessary to cause ulcers. Unrelieved axial pressure 4 to 6 times systolic causes necrosis in less than an hour. However, pressure below systolic might require 12 hours to produce a similar lesion. Kosiac,[78] Husain, and Dinsdale qualitatively verified this hyperbolic relationship to be true for dogs, rats, and pigs, respectively. However, the critical interface pressure is animal-model–specific. This animal research prompted the practice of turning patients every two hours, which originated with the work of Reswick and Rogers[112] and is the mainstay of prevention strategies.

Shear exacerbates the tendency to ulcerate as a result of axial forces. Dinsdale determined that continuous shear directed to a site of constant axial pressure lowered the ulceration threshold sixfold.[41] Shear forces, for example, can be important for sacral pressure ulcer formation. It is logical to conclude that the angular and vertical force downward while patients are in the semi-upright position in bed tends to distort the tissues and blood vessels near the sacrum, placing this region at risk for tissue breakdown.[20, 111]

Neuropathic ulcers develop due to both shear and very high transient axial pressure. Repeated noxious pressure causes an inflammatory response, with pain, redness, and heat. Using thermography, Brand and colleagues[31] have observed temperature increase. Brand has suggested that areas at risk be monitored for temperature in patients at risk for neuropathic ulcers to compensate for the absence of pain.

Once ulcers form, they are empirically more sensitive to transient or static pressure and shear than is intact skin. Much more time and effort must be devoted to pressure and shear relief to obtain healing than is required just to prevent an ulcer from forming. In fact, wounds once formed might, in response to pathomechanics, paradoxically get larger.[142]

Reperfusion Injury

Ischemia from pressure-induced capillary collapse is associated with buildup within the microvasculature of supraoxide free radicals. Supraoxide rises during periods of ischemia, and an excess causes neutrophils to marginate and traverse the endothelial cell, inducing an inflammatory response.[120, 121] Salcido and colleagues noted histopathologic changes in experimentally derived pressure ulcers. Foci of this damage appeared to be associated with high concentrations of neutrophils in muscle. Recurrent ischemia-reperfusion events exhibit a cumulative effect on muscle.[120, 121] Muscle and subdermal injury for the fuzzy rat model follows the clinical pattern of pressure ulcers of the buttocks, which are typically cavernous, with disproportionate erosion of muscle and subcutaneous tissue but with skin relatively spared.

Reperfusion injury can be potentiated by (1) chronic hypoxia, which causes ulceration well below interface pressure and shorter-than-usual ischemic time, and (2) conditions that impair microvessel nitric oxide (NO) production. Such conditions include diabetes, as NO is a potent vasodilator which protects endothelium from reperfusion injury.[131] Both impaired NO production and excess supraoxide from chronic hypoxia might occur among the acutely ill with systemic hypoperfusion, increasing risk of heel ulcer formation. Heel or forefoot ischemic ulcers can also arise outside the hospital. Patients with arteriosclerosis are at risk, as are persons suffering foot hypoxia from wearing shoes that are too tight.

Chronic Hypoxia

Chronic hypoxia results from poor inflow of blood typically due to arteriosclerotic narrowing proximal to hypoxic skin. In addition, if steady-state oxygen is too low, wounds will not heal. Goldman[58] has observed an inverse relationship between oxygen in the dermis, measured by transcutaneous oxygen (TcPO2) and the healing rate. The literature consistently reports that healing is not expected when TcPO2 is less than 15 mm Hg, but proceeds normally when TcPO2 exceeds 40 mm Hg. There are mixed results between these values.[7, 101, 113]

For ischemic wounds, there is biochemical and histological derangement of the wound healing process. New granulation tissue deposition and mononuclear cell infiltration are dramatically lower in ischemic wounds compared with nonischemic controls.[141] For the moderately hypoxic wound condition, there is actually an increase in TGF-beta transcription, as well as collagen synthesis and deposition.[48] This underscores the complexity of the relationship between oxygen tension and healing.

Edema and Impaired Oxygen and Nutrient Exchange

Edema of the leg is a hallmark of venous stasis disease, and stasis ulceration is the end result of longstanding venous congestion. In venous congestion there is breakdown of the ankle pump mechanism. The ankle pump is powered by the contraction of calf muscles during gait within an unyielding leg fascial envelope, creating cyclic pressure peaks, which can reach 100 mm Hg.[86] Normally, this pressure drives venous blood cephalad, with back-flow prevented by valves within veins. However, veins can become incompetent due to presence of old clot or proximal vein occlusion (e.g., from organized deep venous thrombosis, pelvic mass, or fibrosis), which leads to gravity-induced high static pressure and loss of the ankle-pump pressure cycle. The pressure cycle can also be disrupted by traumatic or surgical loss of the fascial envelope, such as from fasciotomies associated with remote compartment syndrome.

Edema is one of the major factors associated with the pathogenesis and maintenance of chronic wounds. Venous ulcers, due to venous congestion and backpressure, extravasate fibrinogen and fluid across the microvasculature endothelium, leading to excess protein-rich interstitial fluid. This fluid is thought to sequester growth factors, which are then unavailable to heal the edematous skin.[47]

Venous congestion can also lead to endothelial damage, causing neutrophils to marginate. This ultimately causes the release of free radicals and collagenases, which promote cell death and make the endothelial layer more permeable to macromolecules. This alters osmotic pressure and shifts fluid to the extravascular space, resulting in worsening edema.[46] Less well recognized is the fact that edematous skin can reduce diffusion of oxygen from capillaries to the dermal and epidermal layer. Measured empirically at the skin surface, edematous skin has low transcutaneous oxygen (TcPO2), and often the TcPO2 is less than 15 mm Hg. The resulting surface hypoxia further supports tissue breakdown.

Growth Factor Abnormalities

Growth factor abnormalities might occur in one of four categories: (1) reduced synthesis; (2) increased protein or matrix sequestration; (3) increased breakdown, or (4) insensitivity of target cells. For example, consider alterations in TGF-beta. TGF-beta is critical in directing extracellular matrix formation during the repair phase of healing. TGF-beta concentration at the wound edge of venous ulcers is directly related to the probability of wound closure within a six-month period.[84] Some venous stasis ulcers that are especially chronic do not respond to TGF-beta.[64] Some chronic venous ulcers appear to have an excess of proteases, which might digest TGF-beta and other growth factors.[62] Growth factor alterations in chronic wounds are the subject of active and ongoing research.

Chronic Inflammation

Noxious mechanical stimulation contributes to the clinical persistence of pain, edema, warmth, and redness. Inflammation can also result from local infection, which is very common in untreated chronic wounds. Wounds that have greater than 10^5 organisms per gram of tissue do not heal. Pseudomonas toxin applied to animal wounds blunts or stops wound contraction.[65] Inflamma-

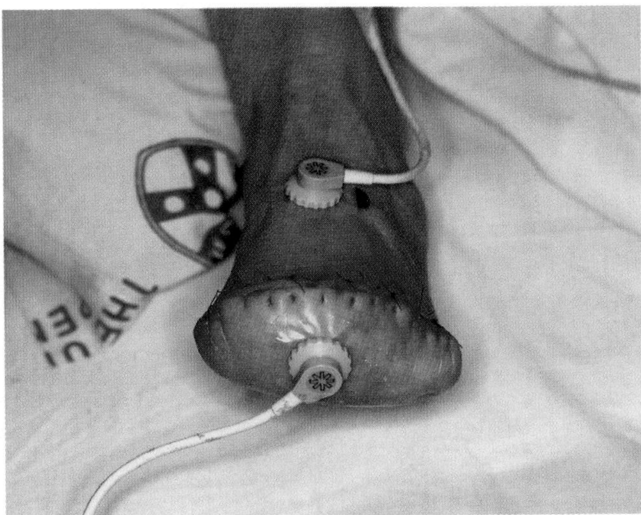

FIGURE 31–2. Placement of polarographic TcPO2 electrodes on two areas of interest on the foot dorsum (TcPO2 = 12) and transmetatarsal residuum (TcPO2 = 2). Note livido on the forefoot. This placement avoids TcPO2 measurement pitfalls: (1) TcPO2 is artefactually low for skin with subcutaneous edema or hyperkeratosis; (2) TcPO2 will be low or not stabilize over callus; (3) the TcPO2 electrode seal to the skin is easily compromised if the electrode is placed over a bony prominence, or if there is traction on the lead. Because of these variables, multiple measurements should be obtained in the same region if there is any question about edema, hyperkeratosis, or air leak.

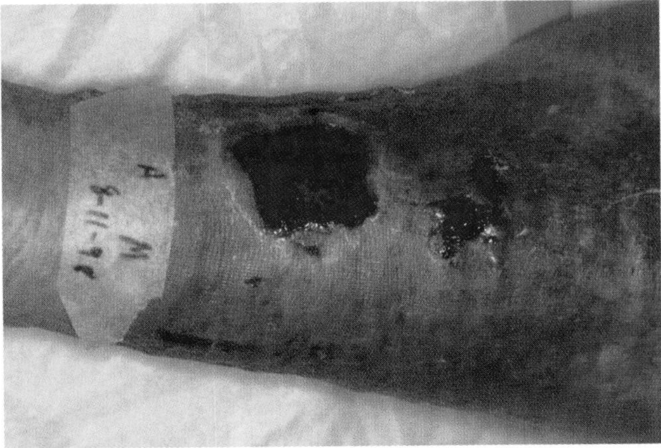

FIGURE 31–5. A venous stasis ulcer in an otherwise healthy 71-year-old male, demonstrating hyperpigmentation and "wine bottle" leg shape. Ulcers have irregular borders.

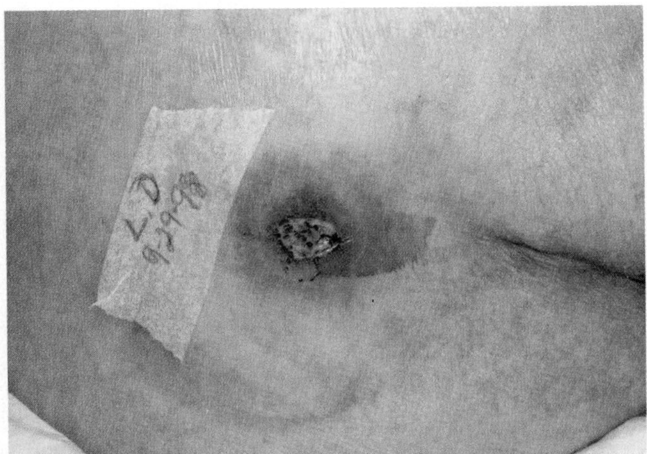

FIGURE 31–3. A stage III pressure ulcer in a homebound 89-year-old female with Parkinson's disease, osteoporosis, kyphosis, and pressure ulcer at the sacral bony prominence.

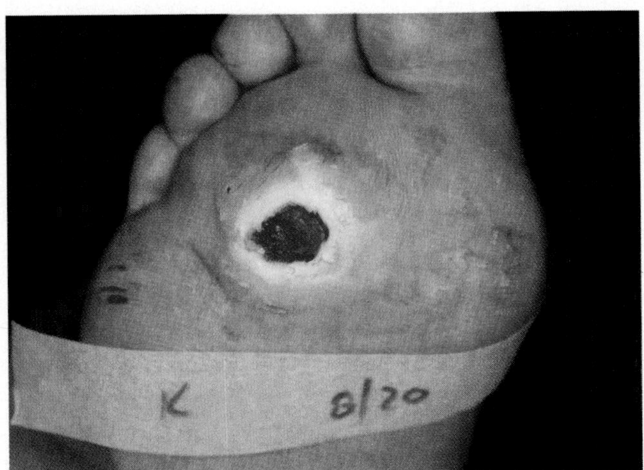

FIGURE 31–6. A neuropathic ulcer in a 56-year-old male with insulin-dependent diabetes and forefoot insensitivity. (His circulation is normal; the MRA shown in Figure 31–1 is his.)

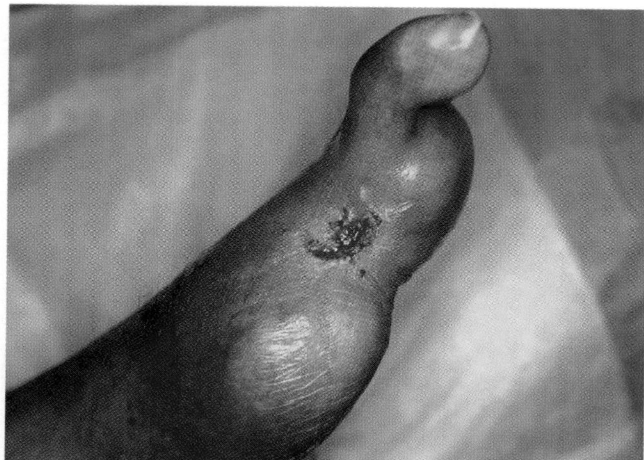

FIGURE 31–7. An ischemic ulcer in a 44-year-old female with severe coronary artery disease, pacemaker placement, renal insufficiency, right above-knee amputation, and left minor foot amputation; ischemic ulcer is long-standing (TcPO2 = 5 to 15 mm Hg of peri-wound margin).

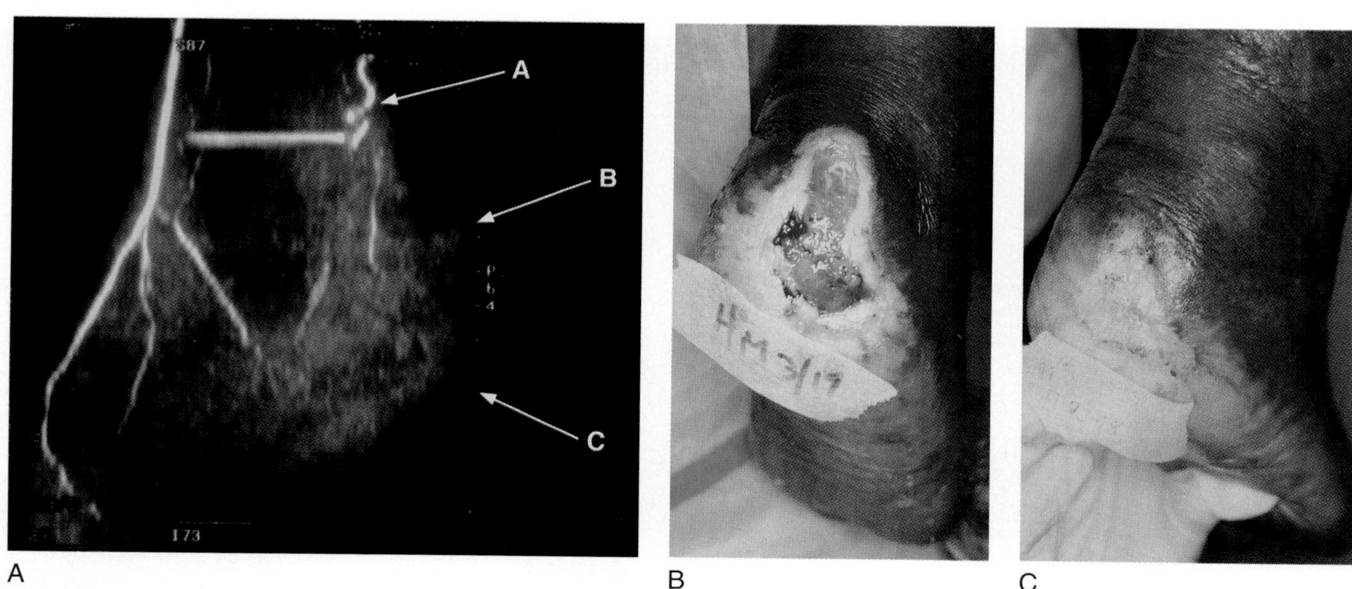

FIGURE 31–8. The patient is a 70-year-old male with insulin-dependent diabetes, insensate peripheral neuropathy, congestive heart failure (ejection fraction = 20%), venous stasis disease and multi-infarct dementia with bradykinesia. While hospitalized for urosepsis, he sustained a worsening of a right heel pressure ulcer. After OR debridement, the wound diameter was 7.5 cm in diameter, with granulating base. The patient was followed up at our wound clinic. We assessed peri-wound transcutaneous oxygen at <5 mm Hg, so his prognosis for healing was guarded. Consistently, magnetic resonance angiography revealed no flow through named arteries through the heel region. *A.* MRA: collateral remnant of the posterior tibial artery (A); upper (B) and lower (B) borders of the ulcer. As an outpatient, this ischemic wound began to heal only after weight bearing in a DH walker, which optimally distributes both the axial pressure and the shear forces that occur during ambulation. Gait force-vector reduction allowed the wound to improve and heal over 12 months. *B.* Healing wound, with hypopigmented new skin. *C.* Complete healing. This case study highlights healing of a complex ischemic pressure ulcer, for a patient not a candidate for surgical bypass and at high initial risk of limb loss, by skillful application of limiting weight bearing.

tion associated with autoimmunity perpetuates vasculitic ulcers. Long-standing skin ulcers are inflamed to a greater or lesser degree by vasculitis, mechanical irritation, or chromic local injection.

Pathophysiological Factors

The factors that contribute to chronic wound persistence are diverse, interactive, and cumulative, and they affect the whole organism. Predisposing conditions include aging, spinal cord injury, and diabetes, among many others (Table 31–1). These predisposing conditions interact at many levels to promote pathomechanics, reperfusion injury, static hypoxia, and local inflammation; and, speculatively, they may lead to growth factor abnormalities within wounds.

CLINICAL WOUND ASSESSMENT

Wound Area and Volume Assessment

Wound Appearance. For wound care, the adage is true: A picture is worth a thousand words. Color photography dramatically reveals infection, eschar, exudate, complete granulation, and epithelialization. To obtain sufficient detail, we suggest low-speed slide film (e.g., ASA 100), macro lens, and ring flash on a good-quality automatic 35-mm camera.

TABLE 31–1 Systemic Conditions Associated with Chronic Wounds

Condition	Pathophysiological Effect Related to Wound Healing
Spinal cord injury	Vasomotor instability (>T6 level), insensitivity, denervation atrophy, spasticity, contractures, bowel/bladder alterations
Elderly	Reduced skin elasticity and altered skin microcirculation,[130] co-morbidities, reduced healing rate noted clinically and in animal models[59]
Diabetes	Insensitivity, microangiopathy and altered inflammatory response,[93] foot deformities (intrinsic minus, Charcot), blunted reactive hyperemia, reduced incision breaking strength,[104] and contraction[60] in animal models
Malnutrition	Negative nitrogen balance, cachexia, immunosuppression
Anemia	Local hypoxia
Arteriosclerosis	Local hypoxia
End-stage renal disease	Transient dialysis-related hypoperfusion distal to atherosclerotic plaques, co-morbidities
Steroid medications	Reduced healing rate in animal models, immunosuppression
Transplant recipients	Immunosuppression, co-morbidities
Smoking	Vasoconstriction, increased blood viscosity
Parkinson's disease	Immobility
Osteoporosis	Bony prominences
Upper motor neuron disease	Immobility, contractures, bowel/bladder alterations
Dementia	Immobility, malnutrition, contractures, bowel/bladder alterations
Acutely ill (ICU related)	Hypotension, immobility, bowel/bladder alteration, malnutrition, fever, increased metabolic demands
Noncompliance, abuse and neglect	Multifactoral

Wound Outline. For lower-extremity ulcers (ischemic, neuropathic, or venous), a useful, inexpensive technique is drawing outlines on clear plastic with a "laundry marker"; these drawings then become part of the patient's permanent record. Inspection allows immediate appraisal of progress; and if the wound has increased in size, the clinician can modify treatment without delay. For consistency, one person should do the outlines. These outlines can also be analyzed in terms of overall area and graphed with respect to time for research purposes.

Wound Volume. Pressure ulcers of the buttocks tend to be undermined, so the wound outline can underestimate volume. For a first approximation of volume, depth and direction of tracks are measured in centimeters and included on the outline. However, for a quantitative measure suitable for careful clinical or research use, volume is assessed by adding a measured amount of saline or moist alginate gel, then removing and measuring the volume of this saline or gel.

Computerized Area and Volume Measurement. The VistaMed™ wound measurement system[134] quantifies shape, outline, area, color, and appearance of the clinician-defined image areas.

Perfusion Assessment

It is exceedingly rare that large vessel disease contributes to the formation of pressure ulcers of the trunk, occiput, hips, or buttocks. For more distal wounds of the leg and foot, however, perfusion must be assessed because: (1) in the setting of poor perfusion, therapeutic compression might cause pressure necrosis; and (2) perfusion prognosticates wound closure. (See also Chapter 56.)

Macrocirculation. Macrocirculation refers to blood flow through named anatomic arteries, such as the iliac, femoral, posterior tibial, and plantar.

Ankle Brachial Index and Pulse Volume Recording. Ankle brachial index (ABI) is the ratio of systolic blood pressure of the ankle to that of the arm (brachium). Normal ABI is greater than 0.8. The ABI is similar to pulse volume recording (PVR), which is continuous monitoring of small blood pressure changes within cuffs over the thigh, calf, and ankle. These segmental measurement traces are checked for bilateral symmetry and a dicrotic notch. Asymmetric pressure-amplitude abnormalities or absence of a notch suggest proximal flow compromise.

Conventional Angiography. Angiography typically involves injecting a radio-opaque dye into the proximal arterial tree. Conventional dye angiography precedes flow-promoting angioplasty or stenting of stenotic arteries. However, conventional angiography has two important disadvantages: (1) It is less useful for visualizing very distal arteries, because dye becomes dilute farther from the site of injection. It also might fail to show distal

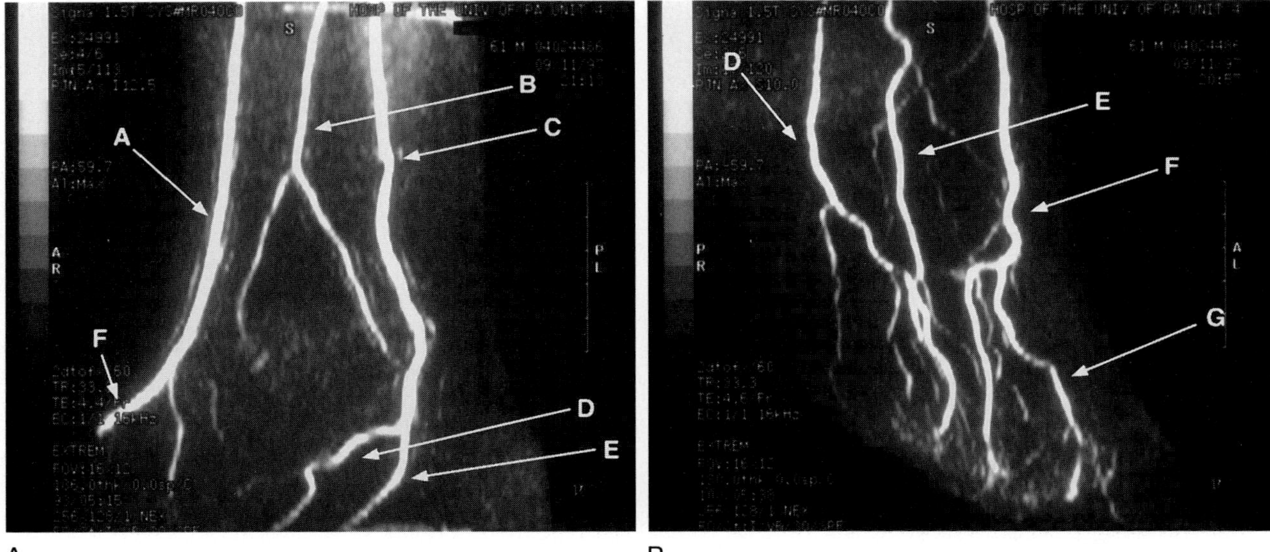

FIGURE 31–1. Magnetic resonance angiography (MRA) by time-of-flight technique, of the ankle (*a*) and foot (*b*) of a 56-year-old male with insulin-dependent diabetes but normal circulation to and below the ankle. *A.* The ankle projection (*a*) reveals the peroneal artery (B) ending at the ankle, the anterior tibial artery (A) extending into the foot as the dorsalis pedis (F), and the posterior tibial artery (C) dividing into the medial (D) and lateral (E) plantar arteries. *B.* On the foot projection, the lateral plantar (D) and dorsalis pedis (F) arteries are connected by the plantar arterial arch, with the plantar arch giving off digital arteries (G).

arteries beyond blockages or stenoses. (2) Nonionic dye-load remains problematic for patients with renal insufficiency, which is not uncommon in the population with significant arteriosclerosis.

Magnetic Resonance Angiography (MRA). Magnetic resonance angiography (MRA) requires no contrast dye and is superior to conventional angiography in visualizing arteries of the ankle and foot.[90] MRA directly visualizes flow as low as 2 cm/sec. For these reasons, MRA is better at discerning infra-popliteal and infra-malleolar flow than conventional angiography (Fig. 31–1). MRA independently guides surgical revascularization.[26] Where arteries are patent but there is no net flow, however, MRA might be falsely negative. This is noted to occur most often in the plantar arterial arch. Not only can MRA determine presence or absence of flow, it can image subtle flow defects such as focal or segmental arteriosclerotic disease. It can also image the reconstitution of an anatomic artery with aberrant up-stream feeders.

Microcirculation. Having traversed named arteries, blood reaches the skin. In the skin, blood flows through arterioles, capillaries, and venules in the papillary and reticular dermis. Skin microcirculation assessment is being increasingly performed in wound centers, and is recognized as a wound healing benchmark. There are three well-published methods to measure skin microcirculation: TcPO2, laser Doppler flow, and vital capillarioscopy.[45] Vital capillarioscopy visualizes capillaries, while the laser Doppler flow measures relative movement of red blood cells through the upper millimeter of living dermis. Both are relative flow measures. Transcutaneous oxygen is an absolute measure of oxygen tension, and is in essence a "blood gas" of the skin. The normal TcPO2 is greater than 50 mm Hg.

TcPO2 prognosticates the success of amputation residual limb healing and predicts the healing rate of neuropathic and ischemic ulcers (Fig. 31–2). Its predictive value is uniquely strong for diabetic individuals, who have distal arterial calcinosis. This makes segmental ar-

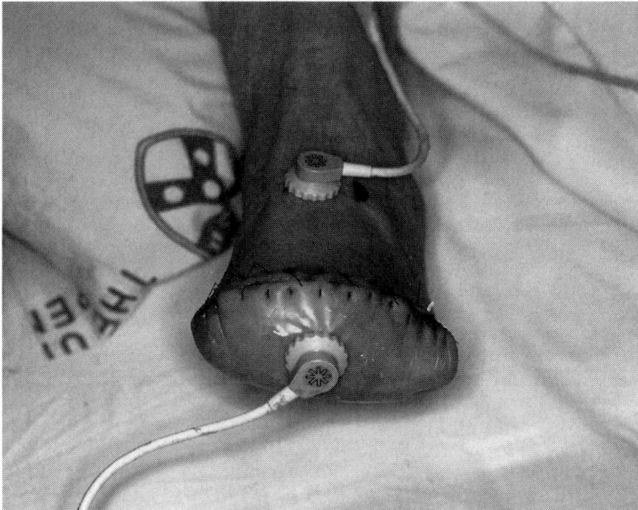

FIGURE 31–2. Placement of polarographic TcPO2 electrodes on two areas of interest on the foot dorsum (TcPO2 = 12) and transmetatarsal residuum (TcPO2 = 2). Note livido on the forefoot. This placement avoids TcPO2 measurement pitfalls: (1) TcPO2 is artefactually low for skin with subcutaneous edema or hyperkeratosis; (2) TcPO2 will be low or not stabilize over callus; (3) the TcPO2 electrode seal to the skin is easily compromised if the electrode is placed over a bony prominence, or if there is traction on the lead. Because of these variables, multiple measurements should be obtained in the same region if there is any question about edema, hyperkeratosis, or air leak.

terial measurements (i.e., pulse volume recording and ankle brachial index) artefactually high.[101] The surgical literature reports that TcPO2 also prognosticates success of healing incisions of amputation residual limbs.[113] Below the knee, where the disease state is defined as no flow of an artery as assessed by MRA, overlying TcPO2 is 80% sensitive and 83% specific (where TcPO2 measure of "no flow" is set at TcPO2 < 15 mm Hg).

TcPO2 is also a measure of integrity of local macrocirculation. As the distal-most capillary bed of the arterial tree, skin microcirculation indirectly assesses flow through upstream arterial feeders. In diabetic patients, upstream feeders are better assessed by TcPO2 than by PVR. PVR is insensitive to collaterals, which are multiple minute, unnamed arteries that bridge across large-vessel stenoses to re-establish flow. Owing to collateralization, TcPO2 can be normal very distal to regions that have been interpreted by PVR to be stenosed. Where TcPO2 is normal, healing prognosis is favorable.

Pressure and Shear Assessment

Although pressure and shear are critical in the pathogenesis of chronic wounds, pressure and shear are not routinely measured in chronic wound practice. There are several important reasons. Transducers are thick, bulky, rigid, or expensive.[56] In addition, shear transducers have yet to be perfected and are not available for clinical use. Although relatively expensive, axial pressure transducers provide accuracy and high resolution of axial forces on an area at risk of ulceration (e.g., Teckscan, Emed). Systems have been developed for pressure ulcers of the buttocks and neuropathic ulcers of the plantar surface of the foot. For measuring point pressures, such as that between a wheelchair cushion and a bony prominence, one can use balloons (e.g., Roho) that provide output of pressure, and measure pressure reduction with therapeutic cushioning.

GENERAL PRINCIPLES OF TREATMENT

Debridement

Sharp Debridement. Sharp debridement is surgical removal of the eschar and any devitalized tissue within it. The removal of devitalized tissue is prerequisite for new tissue growth. Surgical debridement is well established as an approach to pressure ulcer care.

Sharp debridement can be done in the operating room under an anesthetic. Although this level of sharp debridement is the most effective and quickest method of removing necrotic tissue, it is contraindicated in certain patients, particularly those who cannot withstand the loss of blood that can occur during the procedure. Surgical sharp debridement is relatively indiscriminate in the removal of vital and devitalized tissue: Tissue is debrided back to tissue bleeding. To minimize removal of viable tissue, a great deal of clinical skill and judgment is needed.[18, 34]

Less aggressive sharp debridement is commonly performed in the outpatient setting as part of routine wound care, usually with minimal blood loss or pain. Pain is usually not a problem for patients with neuropathic ulcers. These ulcers develop a copious callus that is "saucerized" in an inverted-cone pattern. Venous ulcers frequently develop peri-wound hyperkeratosis, which can be removed in a straightforward manner (e.g., with mineral oil and forceps). In addition, if necrosis is not excessive, the base of venous and pressure ulcers can be debrided carefully with curette, forceps, and scalpel (if necessary with application of 5% Lidocaine ointment per package insert) in the outpatient setting. Debridements should be performed at regular intervals to ward off infection. Devitalized tissue supports the proliferation and growth of pathogens. Outpatient debridements are clean, but not sterile. Elderly and diabetic patients often have leathery, blackened pressure ulcers of the heel that should not be mechanically debrided if there is any question of depth: If eschar is contiguous with bone, that bone will likely not heal if exposed. In this circumstance, eschar should be left to auto-debride unless infection supervenes.

Mechanical Nonselective Debridement. Mechanical nonselective debridement is accomplished by whirlpool treatments (although, owing to cost, this practice is less popular than in the past), forceful irrigation, or use of wet-to-dry dressings. Wet-to-dry dressings involve placing unraveled, moist gauze into the lesion so that all sections of it are touching the dressing, then allowing the dressing to dry. When the dressing is removed, necrotic tissue is removed with it. This is typically done on each shift in the hospital or long-term care setting, or once or twice a day at home. Normal saline solution is commonly used as the wetting agent. Other wetting agents for wet-to-dry dressings include 0.25% acetic acid solution (where pseudomonas is suspected) and dilute povidone-iodine solution or hydrogen peroxide. However, hydrogen peroxide and povidone-iodine are not recommended for long-term use because they are toxic to fibroblasts in vitro.[72, 116] Hydrotherapy is typically used for debridement of post-surgical wounds and abscesses in the acute hospital setting. Hydrotherapy performs both irrigation and debridement.

Enzymatic Debridement. Enzymatic debridement uses various chemical agents (e.g., Elase) that act by attacking collagen and liquefying necrotic wound debris without damaging granulation tissue. Proteolytic enzymes are used to chemically debride wounds. The action of these enzymes is aimed specifically at necrotic tissue.[13, 75] As a safeguard, enzymatic agents should be removed after 12 to 24 hours.

Autolytic Debridement. Proteases and collagenase expressed by wound cells digest eschar in contact with wound fluid. Dressings that maintain a moist wound environment and peri-wound seal (e.g., hydrocolloid) promote autolytic debridement.

Dressings

Winter and colleagues[139] demonstrated that the closure rate of wounds doubled in a moist environment as compared to controls. In a moist environment, epithelium advances and adjoins without having to digest eschar. Wound fluid beneath occlusive dressings also has several other important features: (1) It is well supplied with growth factors and self-expressed digestive enzymes; (2) it is conductive and enables wound closure to be at least partially directed by the skin battery.[9] Moist wounds do not become infected if the bacterial load is kept low.

Gauze Dressings. Gauze pads and nonadherent gauze (e.g., Telfa) and bulky pads (e.g., ABD pads) might well be considered the foundation of wound care. These wound dressings are combined with antibiotic ointments to create a moist environment. Antibiotic ointments (e.g., Mupirocin) especially are useful when dressings are changed infrequently, as is the case for venous ulcers under compressive dressings or neuropathic plantar ulcers within casts. Bulky pads or anti-shear pads are especially protective of somewhat transudative wounds in areas subject to excessive friction, such as those over the malleoli or Achilles tendon.

Transparent Adhesive Dressings. Transparent adhesive dressings (e.g., Tegaderm, OpSite) are semipermeable and occlusive, and are typically indicated for nontransudative stage I or II wounds without necrotic debris. Transparent dressings allow gaseous exchange and transfer of water vapor from the skin and prevent maceration of the healthy skin around the wound. They are not absorptive. They reduce the incidence of secondary infection, and they eliminate the risk of traumatic removal. They do not function well on diaphoretic patients or in wounds that have significant exudate.[42, 50]

Hydrocolloid Wafer Dressings. Hydrocolloid wafer dressings (e.g., Duoderm) contain hydro-active particles that interact with wound exudate to form a gel. These dressings provide absorption of minimal to moderate amounts of exudate and keep the wound surface moist. This gel can have fibrolytic properties that enhance wound healing, protect against secondary infection, and insulate the wound from contaminants.[42, 67] In fact, hydrocolloid dressings form a seal with peri-wound skin, causing the dressing and skin to move together to minimize shear. For this reason, hydrocolloid dressings are good for shallow, clean, stage III ulcers in an easily contaminated environment such as the sacrum. Hydrocolloid can be applied to clean venous stasis ulcers.

Gel Dressings. Gel dressings (e.g., NuGel, Vigilon) are available in sheet form, in granules (Intrasite), and as liquid gel (e.g., Curasol). All forms of gel dressings, as long as they are not allowed to dehydrate, keep the wound surface moist. Some gel dressings provide limited to moderate absorption, some provide insulation, some provide protection against bacterial invasion, and all provide nontraumatic removal.[13, 42, 80] Gel dressings provide a moist, nontraumatic environment for clean wounds. Some gel dressings are expensive, however; and gel sheets utilize no adhesive to provide a barrier or prevent shear.

Calcium Alginate Dressings. Calcium alginate dressings (e.g., Sorbsan)[55] are semi-occlusive, highly absorbent, and easy to use. They are natural, sterile, nonwoven dressings derived from brown seaweed. Calcium alginate dressings are extremely effective in treating wet (exudative) wounds and can be used on wounds that are contaminated or infected.[55] Dressings need to be frequently changed for very transudative wounds to prevent maceration of fragile epithelium.

DIAGNOSIS AND TREATMENT OF SPECIFIC ULCER TYPES

Pressure Ulcers

Presentation

Only a patient who can act to relieve a noxious stimulus can prevent pressure ulcers. Patients who are comatose or severely demented, or who are insensate (e.g., spinal cord–injured patients) are at increased risk. Spasticity, contractures, incontinence, cachexia, diabetes, and advanced age also increase risk. It has been suggested that patients with darkly pigmented skin are at higher risk, because nonblanching erythema of stage I pressure ulcers might not be visible on casual inspection.

Sites of occurrence vary in different studies and with different diagnoses.[1–3, 51–53, 102] The most common sites of pressure ulcer formation are the ischium (28%), the sacrum (17 to 27%), the trochanter (12 to 19%), and the heel (9 to 18%). The sacrum is the site of a Stage III pressure ulcer in a homebound bradykinetic elderly female (Fig. 31–3). The pressure ulcer staging system is illustrated in Figure 31–4. There is no consensus on generalizing the Shea index to leg ulcer types.

Treatment

The mainstay of pressure ulcer treatment is good medical and nursing care.[1, 68, 132] In the long-term care setting or at home, the debilitated or partially dependent patient with a pressure ulcer should be turned every two hours[112] and have frequent dressing changes to reduce bacterial count and to keep the wound moist. Wound size should be assessed at least weekly and treatment modified as necessary to maintain healing rate.

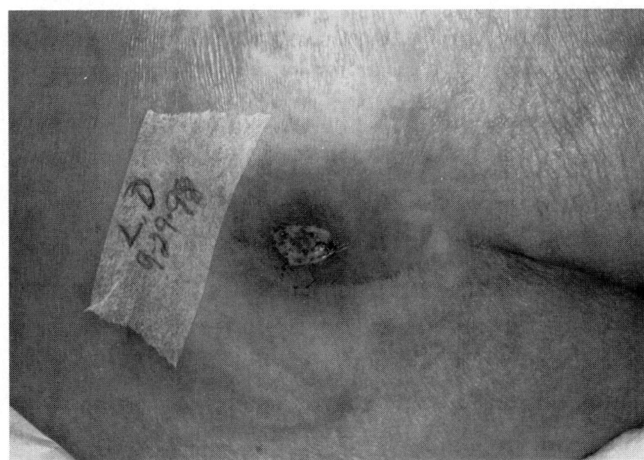

FIGURE 31–3. A stage III pressure ulcer in a homebound 89-year-old female with Parkinson's disease, osteoporosis, kyphosis, and pressure ulcer at the sacral bony prominence.

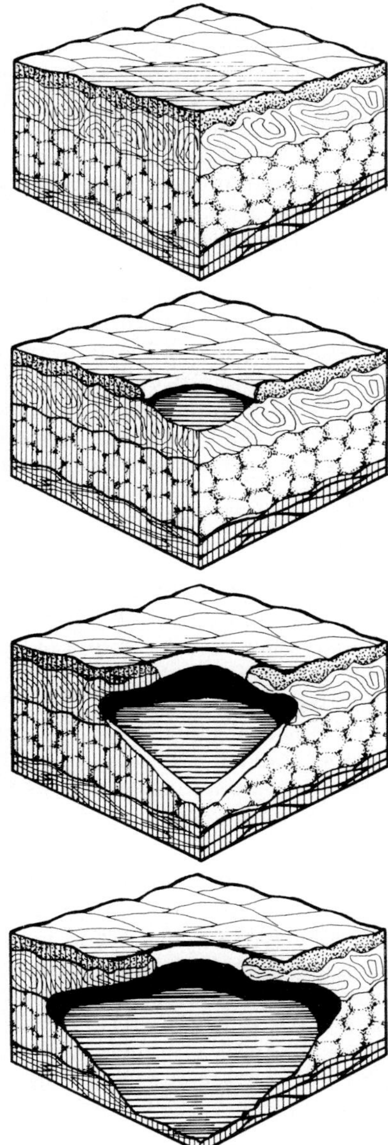

FIGURE 31–4. National Pressure Ulcer Advisory Panel (NPUAP) classification: Identification and staging of pressure ulcers. *Stage 1:* Nonblanchable erythema not resolved in 30 min; epidermis intact; reversible with intervention. *Stage 2:* Partial-thickness loss of skin involving epidermis, possibly into dermis; may appear as blisters with erythema. *Stage 3:* Full-thickness destruction through dermis into subcutaneous tissue. *Stage 4:* Deep tissue destruction through subcutaneous tissue to fascia, muscle, bone, or joint. (Used with permission from the NPUAP.)

Wounds with necrosis or fibrin must first be debrided (e.g., sharp, mechanical, enzymatic). Once the wound has been debrided and is granulating, moist dressings (e.g., hydrogel, alginate) are appropriate. It is important to seal the wound with surrounding skin. Variable moisture barrier and shear protection is available from hydrocolloid (e.g., Duoderm) or flexible, porous, adhesive gauze (e.g., Coverderm, Medapore). In addition to these conservative measures, pressure surface relief is critical.

Pressure Relief

Table 31–2 describes the selected characteristics as well as the advantages and disadvantages of separate classes of support surfaces.[24] The mattress overlay is designed to be effective when applied directly over a mattress. Mattress replacements are designed for use on an existing hospital bed frame. Specialty beds are entire units used in place of hospital beds.

TABLE 31–2 Advantages and Disadvantages of Support Surfaces

Surface	Advantages	Disadvantages
Static overlays		
Air	Low maintenance Inexpensive Multi-patient use Durable	Can be punctured Requires proper inflation
Gel	Low maintenance Easy to clean Multi-patient use Resists puncture	Heavy Expensive Little research
Foam	Lightweight Resists puncture No maintenance	Retains heat Retains moisture Limited life
Water	Readily available in community Easy to clean	Requires heater Transfers are difficult Can leak Heavy Difficult maintenance Procedures difficult
Dynamic overlays	Easy to clean Moisture control Deflates for transfers Reusable pump	Can be damaged by sharp objects Noisy Assembly required Requires power
Replacement mattresses	Reduced staff time Multi-patient use Easy to clean Low maintenance	High initial cost May not control moisture Loses effectiveness
Low air loss	Head and foot of bed can be raised Less frequent turning required Pressure relieving Reduces shear and friction Moisture control	Noisy Difficulty with transfers Expensive Requires energy source Restricts mobility Skilled setup required Rental charge
Air-fluidized	Reduces shear and friction Lowest interface pressure Low moisture Less frequent turning required	Expensive Noisy Heavy Dehydration can occur Electrolyte imbalances can occur May cause disorientation Difficulty with transfers Hot

Adapted from Bryant R: Acute and Chronic Wounds: Nursing Management. St Louis, Mosby–Year Book, 1992.

Each device can be further described as a pressure-reducing or pressure-relieving device. Pressure-relieving devices are those that consistently reduce pressure below capillary closing pressure (32 mm Hg). Pressure-reducing devices keep pressures lower than with the standard hospital bed but not consistently below capillary closing pressure. Mediums used in mattress overlays and replacements include water, gel, foam, air, and composite products. Each type of device can be subdivided into dynamic systems (which require an energy source to alternate pressure points and static systems) and static systems (which rely on passive pressure redistribution). Most overlays and replacement mattresses, whether static or dynamic, are considered pressure-reducing devices.

Specialty beds that are truly pressure-relieving include low–air-loss beds (e.g., Flexicare) and air-fluidized beds (e.g., Clinitron). Low–air-loss beds use separate air-filled cushions that are individually monitored to reduce pressures below capillary closing pressures. Air-fluidized therapy uses warm air forced through silicone beads to simulate a fluid environment in reducing pressures. Although there is evidence that these surfaces can provide an environment in which ulcers can be prevented or improved,[3, 44, 49, 69] there is no evidence that one support surface consistently performs better than all others in all circumstances.[3, 32, 49, 70, 96, 129, 137, 138] Therefore, patients should be actively managed on an individual basis to reduce specific risk factors.

The guidelines developed by the AHCPR Pressure Ulcer Panel for managing existing pressure ulcers include the following:

- Use positioning devices to raise a pressure ulcer off the support surface. If the patient is no longer at risk for developing pressure ulcers, these devices may reduce the need for pressure-reducing overlays, mattresses, and beds. Avoid using donut-type devices.[35]
- Assess all patients with existing pressure ulcers to determine their risk for developing additional pressure ulcers. If the patient remains at risk, use a pressure-reducing surface.[15, 98, 99] If patients can assume a variety of positions without bearing weight on the lesion and without "bottoming out," a static support surface should be used.[32, 49, 125, 137, 138] If, however, the patient cannot assume a variety of positions without bearing weight on the ulcer, if the patient fully compresses the static support surface, or if the pressure ulcer does not show evidence of healing, a dynamic surface should be used.[49]
- If the patient has large stage III or stage IV pressure ulcers on multiple turning surfaces, a pressure-relieving product is warranted.[3, 33, 49, 95, 97, 125, 137, 138]

Uncomplicated Chronic Venous Ulcers

Presentation

There is usually a history of previous venous ulcer, dependent edema, previous deep venous thrombosis, pelvic surgery or manipulation, vein stripping, vein harvest for coronary artery bypass graft, or leg graft. Peripheral pulses are typically intact (although it is sometimes difficult to palpate pulses through edematous skin). A well granulating ulcer with irregular borders positioned about the medial malleolus is typical of saphenous vein dysfunction. However, venous ulcers can be located anywhere on the lower leg, ankle, or edematous foot dorsum. Frequently associated with the venous ulcer are lower leg hyper-pigmentation and an induration of subcutaneous tissue called lipidermosclerosis. Extensive lipidermosclerosis gives the leg an "inverted wine bottle" appearance[46] (Fig. 31–5).

The differential diagnosis of venous leg ulcers is a long one. Congestive heart failure could lead to pedal edema with subsequent ulceration (i.e., not related to venous congestion). Besides pedal edema, an important cause of intractable ulceration is epitheliomas, including squamous and basal cell types. If a wound does not respond within three months, a biopsy is indicated to rule out malignancy.[105]

Diagnostic Tests

It is frequently useful to determine arterial perfusion in anticipation of compression therapy, especially if there is a history of claudication, absent pulses, or other cues of arterial insufficiency. Pulse volume recordings are adequate for nondiabetics. For diabetic individuals, TcPO2 is determined on nonedematous areas, such as the upper leg, foot dorsum, and plantar arch.[101] Venous Doppler is useful to rule out acute venous thrombosis.

Treatment

Compression therapy is the mainstay of treatment for venous or lower extremity edematous ulcers. Edema reduction clinically typically results in pain reduction and wound healing. Nonelastic compression, classically the Unna Paste Boot, has been used effectively for more than 100 years to treat venous ulcers.[86] Edema is reduced by the inelastic dressing, which serves as a substitute "fascial envelope" against which calf muscles can increase pressure during ambulation. Ambulators ob-

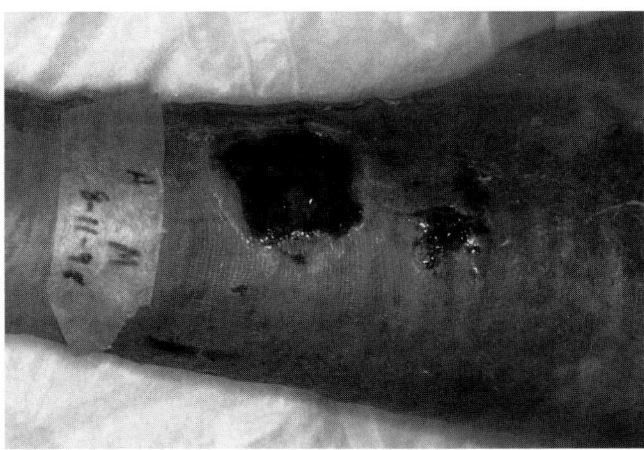

FIGURE 31–5. A venous stasis ulcer in an otherwise healthy 71-year-old male, demonstrating hyperpigmentation and "wine bottle" leg shape. Ulcers have irregular borders.

tain the best edema reduction.[86] Unna's boots are wrapped from toe to knee and are frequently left intact for a week or longer, once it is clear that there is no local infection.

Elastic compression supplies compression of 30 to 40 mm Hg continuously, depending on the elastic compression brand. Brands include Coban (3M) or Cetapress (Convatec). A middle gauze layer (e.g., Kling) can be wrapped from toe to knee for comfort and to reduce shear. Over-the-counter elastic wraps tend not to supply the adequate compression needed to heal venous ulcers.

If infection is suspected and is being treated, compression therapy can be used with frequent dressing changes and debridements. Frequent dressing changes are also required for draining wounds to prevent maceration and shear. Shear can dislodge delicate epithelium, causing venous ulcers to increase in size, even with adequate compression.

Most venous ulcers (70 to 80%) close with compression and good wound care. Wounds that do not close typically have these characteristics in common: ulcer size greater than 10 cm^2, wound present more than 12 months, and ABI less than 0.8. These hard-to-heal ulcers may need additional measures, depending on the decision of the patient and wound care team. Split-thickness skin grafts have been employed to close intractable venous ulcers.[105]

Apligraft is FDA-approved as a laboratory-prepared dermal-epidermal construct. This construct is prepared with neonatal human dermal fibroblasts that are cultured in media with bovine type I collagen. As a living tissue preparation, Apligraft serves as a split-thickness skin graft without the donor-site pain or post-surgical "downtime." Neonatal cells are nonimmunogenic, so tissue sloughing does not occur as would occur with an allograft. Apligraft can increase complete healing of intractable venous ulcers from 25% to 50%.[43] A disadvantage is cost; currently, a 9-cm^2 piece costs $1000. Apligraft should be reserved for venous ulcers that remain open after 24 weeks of conventional treatment.

Compression Stockings

Once venous ulcers heal, the patient remains at risk for recurrence since the underlying venous or fascial anatomic defect remains. Compression must be a lifelong habit. Compression garments come in many sizes, colors, and pressures. Most have the appearance of stiff stockings (e.g., Jobst). Some are segmental and are applied with Velcro straps (e.g., Circ-aide). Compression garments, when used as directed, prevent most ulceration recurrences. Getting patients to use compression garments faithfully is often difficult. Noncompliance stems mainly from difficulty in donning and doffing these very stiff stockings and (to many patients) their distasteful appearance. The appearance has improved in the past 5 to 10 years, with increasing availability of stockings that match most skin pigments. The new varieties have better stretch characteristics and are sheerer, while still retaining therapeutic compression. Most patients do well with 20 to 30 mm Hg, while some will need 30 to 40 mm Hg. Most garments are off-the-shelf and only a few, very obese patients or those with unusual-shaped legs (post-trauma) require custom stockings. Several pairs of stockings should be purchased to allow washing, and stockings should be replaced at six-month intervals. Patient education and "buy-in" are key to long-term ulcer prevention.

Uncomplicated Neuropathic Ulcers

Presentation

Neuropathic or "insensate" foot ulcers are most often (in the United States) related to diabetes; however, they also occur in the setting of infection (e.g., leprosy), as well as traumatic and congenital sensory neuropathy. The sensorimotor neuropathy of diabetes is a "dying-back" distal neuropathy leading to preferential denervation-atrophy of intrinsic foot muscles. This results in an unbalanced pull of long flexors and extensors leading to pes cavus, claw toes, and subluxation of the metatarsal heads. This "intrinsic minus" deformity increases the pressure on bony prominences on already insensate feet. Insensitivity most often affects the plantar forefoot first, so neuropathic ulcers commonly affect plantar toes, hallux, or metatarsal heads. Neurotrophic osteoarthropathy, or Charcot foot, frequently causes midfoot collapse and plantargrade subluxation of navicular or cuboid, leading to especially problematic neuropathic midfoot ulcers.[63]

The physical exam of an uncomplicated ulcer typically shows peripheral pulses to be intact, but sensation is diminished or absent in the vicinity of the ulcer as measured by the Simmes 5.07 or 6.10 monofilaments. Ulcers most frequently are located on bony prominences of the plantar metatarsals, midfoot, or heel. Ulcers might also be associated with digital abnormalities such as claw toes or hallux rigidus. Ulcers usually have regular borders and copious surrounding callus (Fig. 31–6).

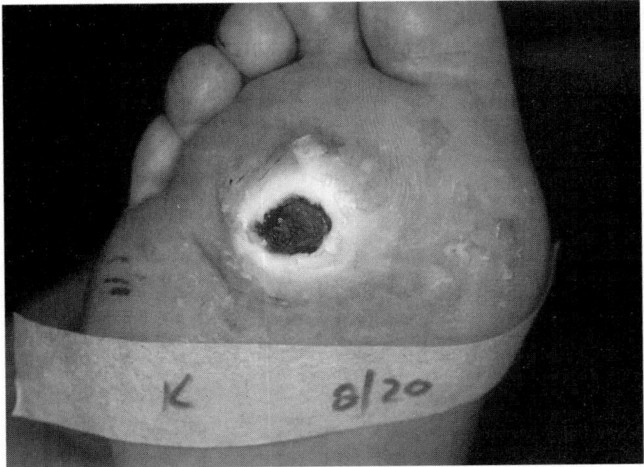

FIGURE 31–6. A neuropathic ulcer in a 56-year-old male with insulin-dependent diabetes and forefoot insensitivity. (His circulation is normal; the MRA shown in Figure 31–1 is his.)

Diagnostic Tests

TcPO2 should be used to assess perfusion. Because conservative wound management focuses on local wound conditions, transcutaneous oxygen has value to reveal local macrocirculation. There are several caveats in measuring TcPO2 in patients with neuropathic ulcers. Neuropathic ulcers usually occur in the setting of hyperkeratosis over bony prominences. Therefore, TcPO2 should not be assessed over bony prominences or metatarsal heads, but rather at the instep or plantar arch.

Treatment Strategies

Treatment strategies usually involve "off-weighting" the ulcer, which reduces mechanical irritation, inflammation, and edema and promotes healing. Neuropathic patients do not feel pain on ambulation, and hence may be challenged to adhere to weight-bearing restrictions. Limited weight bearing must be implemented after a complete physiatric assessment that incorporates inspection, range of motion, muscle testing, and sensory testing. This assessment should also encourage decision making concerning orthoses, assistive devices, weight relief shoes, physical therapy, and facilitate periodic patient education by nursing staff at the clinic and/or in the home.

Local care of neuropathic ulcers follows general "good wound care" principles. The moist wound environment can be maintained by antibiotic ointments such as Bactroban or Bacitracin. These antibiotic ointments also reduce the bacterial count around an area that is easily contaminated.

Debridement is also regularly employed, both to reduce the burden of dead tissue and to make the wound margin more flexible. Callus is removed by "saucerization." In this procedure, the rim of the callus is debrided in the manner of an inverted cone, using a scalpel and forceps. Debridements should be done weekly, as neuropathic ulcers readily form callus even with very little weight bearing, and a callus paradoxically increases mechanical tension in the wound.

Regranex, a formulation of rh-PDGF-BB (recombinant platelet derived growth factor, BB isoform), has been approved by the FDA for healing of foot ulcers of neuropathic and diabetic etiology. In a multicenter, randomized, prospective, double-blind, parallel-group, placebo-controlled trial, there was a significant overall 30% increase in wound closure after 20 weeks of treatment with rh-PDGF-BB,[128] as compared to placebo and "good wound care" alone. There is some evidence, not conclusive, that the best results with PDGF-BB are obtained if wounds are also aggressively debrided.[127] Based on these and other studies, rh-PDGF-BB was approved by the FDA for nonhypoxic (i.e., TcPO2 $>$ 30 mm Hg) neuropathic diabetic foot ulcer healing.

Non–weight bearing is the cornerstone of treating neuropathic ulcers. Patients on strict bedrest tend to rapidly close well-perfused neuropathic ulcers. However, patients tend to "cheat," and only a few steps can defeat healing. So a patient who becomes a low-level in-house ambulator, for bathroom trips only, still might not heal.[31]

Sometimes, bevels or reliefs are set in shoe insoles to "off-weight" an area of high pressure and neuropathic ulcer. Although axial pressure may be reduced in the immediate vicinity of the ulcer, shear might be increased. For this reason, "healing shoes" are not recommended.[25]

Canvas cast boots have specific off-weighted regions that are useful in some situations: Darco forefoot relief shoes are low, with the ulcer set against a raised insole. IPOS heel relief shoes are canvas boots with openings for the frequently ulcerated lateral heel. Heel pain on ambulation can be markedly reduced, and this shoe also helps resolve ulceration in many cases.

The IPOS forefoot relief shoe has a raised heel with the forefoot "hanging in space": Although it is not clear if shear is eliminated, axial pressure is clearly reduced. Pressure reduction with the forefoot relief shoe reduces ulceration-related hospitalization, and causes a trend toward healing rate increase.[27] After a while, however, the elevation may lead to tendinitis, muscle sprain, or a worsening of pre-existing arthritis.

Another boot available is the DH walker. The heart of the DH walker is the insole. The insole has several hundred hexagonal pieces that form the surface, each 1.5 to 2 cm thick, and connected to a base plate by Velcro. Because each hexagon has a small area of attachment to the base relatively far from the skin interface, it moves freely, both up and down and side to side, to reduce shear pressure. By reducing both shear and axial pressure, the DH walker has empirically yielded good results, especially for heel ulcers in some patients that were otherwise without options. However, the DH walker boot significantly reduces step length and gait velocity, and finds limited acceptance from some patients for these reasons.

A very effective treatment for recalcitrant neuropathic ulcers with good circulation is total contact casting.[31, 66, 94] The total contact cast has very little padding, usually only around the toes, the malleoli, and the tibial crest. The leg and foot are literally encased in plaster and there is no room for movement inside the cast. Pressure is distributed axially by virtue of the custom-contour of the set plaster. There is no shear because there is no space inside the cast in which to move. The disadvantage of the cast is that it is time- and labor-intensive. It is best reserved until other, simpler methods are used and the wound plateaus (i.e., healing rate drops to zero). The total contact cast is contraindicated where TcPO2 is less than 35 mm Hg or ABI is less than 0.45 in the affected leg.

Recurrence Prevention

Neuropathic ulcers often recur in the absence of careful and persistent follow-up.[27] Even if the shoe prescription is filled correctly so that axial pressure and shear are minimized, there is a recurrence rate of up to 30% per year. Every effort should be made to optimize the shoe prescription. After healing, it is frequently best to let the former wound "mature" (i.e., develop a stronger dermal layer and a thicker epidermal layer). During this maturation process, callus buildup should be kept to a minimum by careful debridements.

During the period of skin maturation, a shoe prescription can be filled by a certified pedorthist. (Contact Pedorthic Footwear Association, 9861 Broken Land Parkway, Suite 255, Columbia, MD, 21046). A pedorthist has been specifically trained and certified in specialty shoes, and is well versed in insole and outsole modifications. A typical accommodative shoe prescription is for "orthopedic oxford shoes with high toe box and removable PPT-plastizote insoles." Each element is important. The diabetic foot has claw toes that require space. A two-layer insole allows some "bottoming out," but PPT is a foam without memory, so some resiliency is always maintained. If the former wound is at a metatarsal head, the best deweighting strategy is to apply a lift just behind (proximal) to the bony prominence with a cork metatarsal bar. The outsole rocker bottom is modified or rigid, with apex set just behind the metatarsal heads. (Rocker bottoms reduce pressure at the metatarsal heads[11]). Insoles tend to "bottom out" and should be replaced at three-month intervals. Patient education involves daily inspection of the feet and legs to make sure there are no echymoses or excessive callus, which are harbingers of re-ulceration. Emollients such as lanolin or lac-hydrin help prevent the drying and cracking of skin, especially between toes, that can be portals for entry of infection.[92]

Ischemic Ulcers

Ischemic leg ulcers seen in outpatient practice most often occur as mixed disease: neuropathic/ischemic or venous/ischemic. However, simple ischemic ulcers related to proximal occlusion in patients without comorbidities should be evaluated for angioplasty or bypass surgery.

Presentation

Patients with ischemic ulcers usually have the same risk factors that would cause coronary artery disease and myocardial infarction: hypertension, diabetes, smoking, and hypercholesterolemia. In addition to these risk factors, patients with ischemic ulcers often have significant arteriosclerosis, history of myocardial infarction, ischemic cardiomyopathy, cerebrovascular accident, dysrhythmias, or pre-existing amputation. Patients may or may not have a history of claudication, as those with diabetes might have peripheral neuropathy and be relatively insensate. Because of their multiple comorbidities, patients with ischemic ulcers are most often low-level ambulators, who for this reason do not claudicate.

Ulcers typically occur at areas of trauma or static or transient repeated pressure. Static pressure necrosis is most common at the lateral outer heels, which commonly press against the hospital mattress. Not infrequently, such pressure ulcers occur during hospitalization and result in a contralateral amputation. A minor or major amputation incision site might not heal and undergo ischemic change. Ischemic pressure ulcers can also occur at the lateral malleolus. Excessively tight shoes can create pressure necrosis at the lateral fifth toe, medial hallux, or medial forefoot at the metatarsal prominence.

The distal plantar transmetatarsal residuum is a common site for ischemic ulceration, perhaps created and worsened by transient repeated pressure. Ischemic ulcers tend to be exceedingly painful for patients without neuropathy, and pain is worsened by leg elevation. Some patients with painful ischemic ulcers are able to sleep only in the sitting position.

Patients frequently share pre-existing toe or ray amputations or a contralateral major amputation. The skin over the affected area is hairless and appears friable. The ischemic ulcer frequently (but not always) has a blanched base, has a "punched out" appearance, is painful to probe, and the area surrounding the ulcer might have a bright or dusky red hue that has been termed ischemic livido (Fig. 31–7). The color can be purple or black, signaling the onset of gangrene. The onset of gangrene or cellulitis requires immediate surgical referral.

Assessment

Vascular studies are critical to establish a prognosis for conservative healing. Pulse volume recordings might show an asymmetrically low index at a proximal level, such as the calf, indicating superficial femoral artery disease. Healing is not likely in this case, or in the case of a diabetic patient with TcPO2 less than 15 mm Hg. Healing requires getting more oxygen to the wound. Because there are nonsurgical protocols for limb rescue that involve inframalleolar perfusion enhancement, MRA of the ankle and foot might be warranted to delineate arteriosclerosis at the ankle and below.

Treatment

If the wound is truly ischemic, a vascular surgical referral is standard to determine if proximal flow can

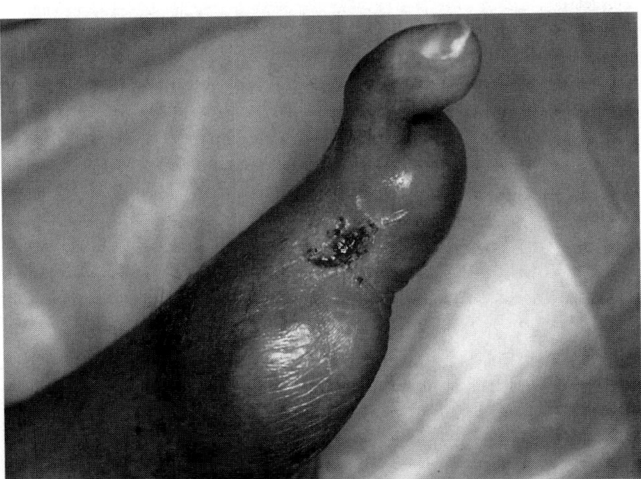

FIGURE 31–7. An ischemic ulcer in a 44-year-old female with severe coronary artery disease, pacemaker placement, renal insufficiency, right above-knee amputation, and left minor foot amputation; ischemic ulcer is long-standing (TcPO2 = 5 to 15 mm Hg of peri-wound margin).

be re-established by angioplasty or bypass. If the surgical consultant concludes that bypass or angioplasty is not indicated, noninvasive methods should be used to save the limb. Of course, conservative "good wound care" must be maximized, including liberal use of padding and weight relief strategies such as the DH walker. A case study is described in Figure 31–8.

Other than conventional "good wound care" for limb salvage, few nonsurgical methods have been independently validated. This gap in management is now being explored in a number of studies on adjunctive therapies. One such study combines the use of high-volt pulsed galvanic stimulation electrotherapy (known to promote microcirculation[89]) with growth factor for treatment of ischemic ulcers. Another novel treatment now being studied in clinical trials involves vascular endothelial growth factor (VEGF), with VEGF-induced lower extremity ischemia resolution.[87]

Paradoxically, hyperbaric oxygen is not often employed for ischemic ulcers. Hyperbaric oxygen is itself a vasoconstrictor, so it is frequently avoided when there is very distal arteriosclerosis, because it could reduce the perfusion of a compromised region.[74] A trial of 100% O_2 while the ischemic site is monitored with TcPO2 might help determine the efficacy for a particular patient.

INFECTION, SURGICAL REPAIR, AND THE TRANSITION FROM OUTPATIENT TO ACUTE INPATIENT MANAGEMENT

Presentation

All infected ulcer types have a similar presentation: A foul smell, greenish or copious drainage, scant granulation, and dull whitish base (rather than bright red granulation tissue). Infected ischemic wounds can present with acute onset of gangrene or eschar of a digit, or cellulitis. Cellulitis is an invasion of organisms beyond 1 to 2 cm of the ulcer margin, and is marked by erythema, warmth, swelling, or tenderness. Systemic bacteremia often produces symptoms of fever, chills, sweats, nausea, vomiting, or loss of appetite. Signs of bacteremia also include elevated or depressed temperature, elevated white count, change in mental status, or glucose intolerance in patients with diabetes. Locally infected lesions on patients without systemic signs can usually be managed on an outpatient basis. The presence of cellulitis, necrotizing cellulitis, painful fluctuance, or signs of bacteremia are considered limb- or life-threatening, necessitating an acute hospital admission for intravenous antibiotics and consideration of surgical debridement.[57]

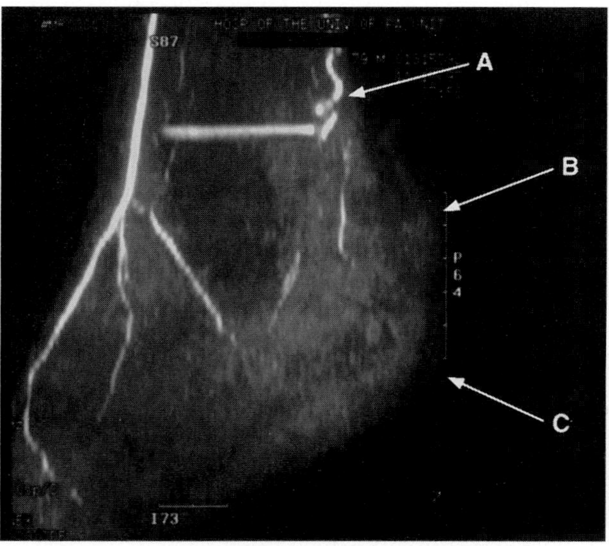

A

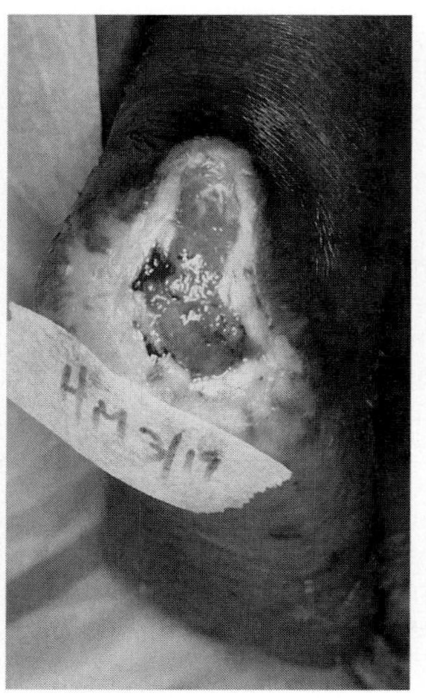

B

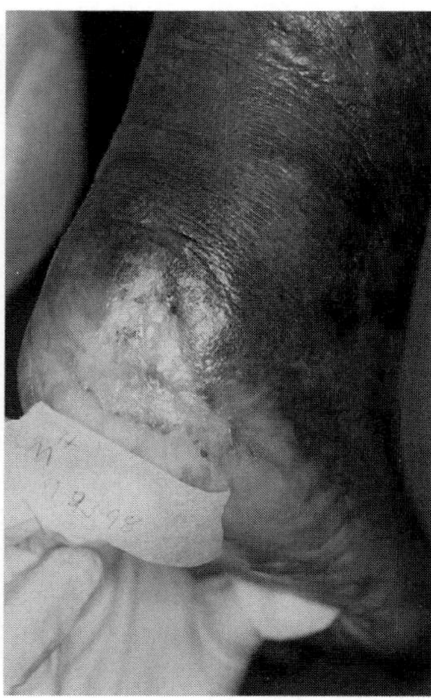

C

FIGURE 31–8. The patient is a 70-year-old male with insulin-dependent diabetes, insensate peripheral neuropathy, congestive heart failure (ejection fraction = 20%), venous stasis disease and multi-infarct dementia with bradykinesia. While hospitalized for urosepsis, he sustained a worsening of a right heel pressure ulcer. After OR debridement, the wound diameter was 7.5 cm in diameter, with granulating base. The patient was followed up at our wound clinic. We assessed peri-wound transcutaneous oxygen at <5 mm Hg, so his prognosis for healing was guarded. Consistently, magnetic resonance angiography revealed no flow through named arteries through the heel region. *A.* MRA: collateral remnant of the posterior tibial artery (A); upper (B) and lower (B) borders of the ulcer. As an outpatient, this ischemic wound began to heal only after weight bearing in a DH walker, which optimally distributes both the axial pressure and the shear forces that occur during ambulation. Gait force-vector reduction allowed the wound to improve and heal over 12 months. *B.* Healing wound, with hypopigmented new skin. *C.* Complete healing. This case study highlights healing of a complex ischemic pressure ulcer, for a patient not a candidate for surgical bypass and at high initial risk of limb loss, by skillful application of limiting weight bearing.

Soft Tissue Infections: Wound Culture, Microbiology, and Antibiotic Therapy

Since the surfaces of all ulcers are colonized by bacteria, ulcer cultures should not be routinely performed, even for locally infected wounds. Cultures can be performed, however, if antiseptic preparation (e.g., Betadine application) precedes local debridement, which exposes a sequestered abscess or fluid collection (which is immediately cultured).

Surgical debridement under "sterile" conditions provides the opportunity to aspirate or swab deep tissue from previously unexposed regions, and more reliably isolates causative organisms. Occasionally, quantitative culture is performed, especially for infected burn wounds. Quantitative culture results are described as colony-forming units (CFU) per gram of tissue. At levels above 10^5 CFU, wounds do not heal[65].

A patient need not be diabetic or immunosuppressed to have mixed bacterial infections. Clinical infection is almost always polymicrobial, including strict anaerobes and facultative aerobes. Aerobic organisms are usually found in surface swabs, whereas anaerobes are more often isolated from deep tissue or in larger pressure ulcers. Deep tissue isolates reveal *Proteus mirabilis,* group B or D *streptococci, Escherichia coli, Staphylococcus aureus, Pseudomonas aeruginosa, Peptostreptococcus species, Clostridia, and Bacteroides fragilis.*[22] *Bacteroides fragilis* is often found in blood cultures associated with clinical sepsis.

Locally infected wounds are frequently associated with eschar. Eschar should be debrided mechanically if possible, using acetic acid, Dakin's solution, or dilute Betadine wet-to-dry. If the patient cannot tolerate wet-to-dry dressings, or if wet-to-dry is not feasible from a nursing standpoint, an antibiotic ointment that permeates eschar, such as Silvidine, can be employed.

Outpatient infections can also be treated with broad-spectrum oral antibiotics that cover gram-positives, gram-negatives, and anaerobes.[25] Choices for aerobes include cephalexin (Keflex), sulfamethoxazole-trimethoprim (Bactrim), and quinilone (e.g., Ciprofloxicin or Levofloxicin). For anaerobes, choices include metronidazole (Flagyl) and clindamycin (Cleocin). Clindamycin also covers some gram-positives and can be used in simple infections as a single agent.[22] Another choice as a single agent is amoxicillin trihydrate-clavulanate potassium (Augmentin). Intravenous antibiotics for inpatient infections are typically best determined in conjunction with infectious disease or internal medicine consultants.

Osteomyelitis

Osteomyelitis requires a high index of suspicion on initial presentation of ulcers of any etiology. This is especially true if the ulcer occurs over a bony prominence, or is a pressure ulcer stage IV,[38, 39] whether or not tracts to bone are clinically apparent. Subclinical untreated osteomyelitis often leads to nonhealing ulcers. Approximately 25% of all nonhealing ulcers contain bone infection,[57] and osteomyelitis should be ruled out on the initial presentation. Although bone biopsy is 96% sensitive,[38, 39] it is usually performed only as part of aggressive operating room debridement for treatment of life or limb threatening infection. Osteomyelitis is most easily diagnosed in the outpatient setting by imaging studies.

Imaging Studies

Plain films are positive for osteomyelitis if they show reactive bone formation and periosteal elevation. Plain films are the least expensive imaging study, but have a sensitivity of 78% and specificity of just 50%. Because of the deficiencies of plain films, test combinations have been suggested. A combination of the leukocyte count, erythrocyte sedimentation rate, and plain films provided a sensitivity of 89% and specificity of 88%. If all three test results are positive, the positive predictive value of this combination is 69%. If all are negative, the negative predictive value is 96%.[38, 39] The combination is less helpful if only one or two tests are positive.

Conventional three-phase bone scan is more sensitive for osteomyelitis than plain films, but specificity is still just 50%. Specificity is low because bone scans are poor at differentiating osteomyelitis from soft tissue infection contiguous with bone.[11, 93] Indium leukocyte scanning has been reported to overcome this deficiency, with a sensitivity of 89%. When combined with a three-phase bone scan, the sensitivity of indium white blood cell scanning is 100% and the specificity is 81%.[22] Radionuclide tests either singly or in combination have the drawback of not revealing anatomic detail.

Magnetic resonance imaging (MRI) reveals anatomic detail and is now recognized as an effective tool for diagnosis of osteomyelitis. MRI is extremely sensitive to the presence of marrow edema on the T2 weighted image. An analysis of eleven studies investigating the diagnosis of osteomyelitis by MRI showed a sensitivity of 95% and a specificity of 88%. One study that used histopathologic findings as the "gold standard" found a sensitivity of 98% and specificity of 78%. Because the specificity rating of MRI is not 100%, other entities that cause marrow edema, such as resolving fracture, have to be considered. MRI also offers the advantage of spatial resolution. MRI can highlight sinus tracts to bone abscesses of the long flexor tendons, septic arthritis, periurethral or perirectal fistula, and other soft tissue abnormalities with a single test[117] (Fig. 31–9).

Outpatient Treatment of Osteomyelitis

The advent of home infusion therapy has enabled patients with osteomyelitis to acquire "good wound care" at home. This must be preceded by wound and bone culture, and appropriate antibiotic selection. The management of antibiotics and potential adverse reactions often becomes the responsibility of the wound specialist. The physiatric wound specialist seeks to maximize the antibiotic management, combining modalities to yield the highest possibility of cure in the outpatient setting.

For "aggressive," conservative treatment of osteomyelitis, antibiotics are typically administered to diabetic patients up to 16 weeks, twice as long as for conventional osteomyelitis treatment.[25] For recurrent osteomyelitis

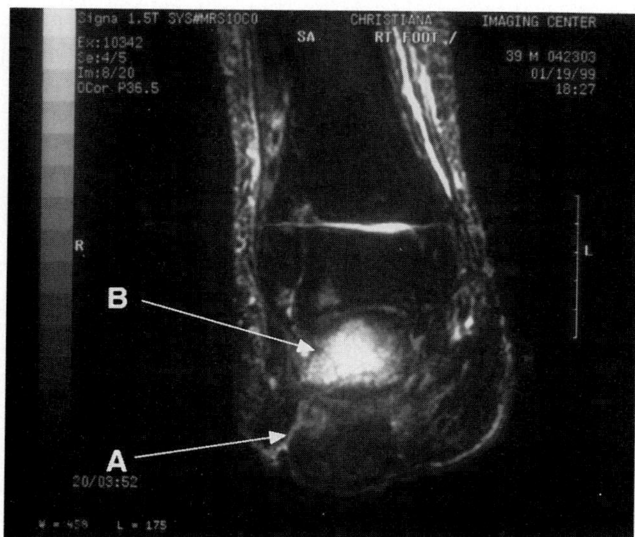

FIGURE 31–9. MRI (T2 weighted image) of the hindfoot of a 38-year-old male with right leg traumatic neuropathy and calcaniovarus heel, with neuropathic ulcer extending to bone (A), revealing osteomyelitis of the calcaneus (B).

or an initial presentation of osteomyelitis in an immunosuppressed patient (i.e., transplant recipient), hyperbaric oxygen therapy is considered in parallel with home antibiotic infusion. An oxygen-rich environment in bone is synergistic with antibiotics, and combining conservative therapies maximizes the opportunity for limb salvage.

Surgical Management

Surgical repair achieves rapid closure and improves vascularity to promote deep soft tissue healing.[5, 12, 23] When considering operative repair, however, the health of the entire patient must be considered by the team and the patient. If the surgery is likely to result in prolonged bedrest, this too must be considered. If the pressure defect that led to ulcer in the first place is not corrected, the ulcer is likely to recur post-operatively. Operative procedures often result in blood loss and prolonged exposure to general anesthesia, which is a relative contraindication for patients with coronary artery disease, ischemic cardiomyopathy, end-stage renal disease, or other high-risk co-morbidities.

Soft Tissue Reconstruction

Patients often ask, "Why not just close the wound?" Although direct closure is the simplest procedure, there is likely to be excessive tension on the incision and a paucity of soft tissue coverage. Direct closure has been advocated, however, for intractable venous ulcers unlikely to generate growth factors. Tissue expanders have recently been used to provide more skin surface in selected cases.[19] Split-thickness skin grafts can also be used to repair recalcitrant venous ulcers.[122]

Musculocutaneous flaps are usually the best choice for pressure ulcers of the buttocks in spinal cord–injured patients, or when the concomitant loss of muscle function does not contribute to co-morbidity. For ambulatory patients, the choice is less clear, since the improved blood supply and reliability of the muscle flap must be balanced against the need to sacrifice functional muscle units.[77, 81, 136] Musculocutaneous flaps are also occasionally employed for well-vascularized pressure ulcers of the heel. Musculocutaneous flaps can help heal osteomyelitis and limit the damage caused by shearing, friction, and pressure.[37, 88, 133] Musculocutaneous flaps have a significant recurrence rate in ulceration, with short-term failure rate (most commonly due to suture line dehiscence) from 5% to 36%. The long-term recurrence rate can be as high as 61%.[117]

Orthopedic Surgical Management

The diabetic foot has deformities that predispose to ulceration. If optimal conservative management has failed to close an otherwise well-vascularized neuropathic ulcer, or if the ulcer heals and then recurs, the orthopedic surgeon should be consulted to evaluate surgical approaches to pressure relief. These include consideration of osteotomies and tendon recessions.

Vascular Surgical Management

The ischemic ulcers that should be treated surgically are more associated with rest pain and have proximal arterial occlusion with limited collaterals. Recent strides have been made in bypass of infra-popliteal stenoses via femoral-distal bypass.[25] The potential for bypass surgery or angioplasty should be assessed.

WOUND CARE CENTERS

The wound care center concept is probably more than a century old, but it was not until recently that this clinic concept was implemented nationwide. This dissemination was fueled, not by physicians, but by the private sector. Curative Technologies is a "biotech" firm that patented a process for rendering growth substances from autologous blood platelets. The result was platelet-derived wound healing factor (PDWHF) marketed as Procurin. Curative Technologies developed a wound clinic model in the 1980s, partially to render and dispense Procurin under controlled conditions. Although two initial studies with PDWHF demonstrated efficacy,[6, 76] a prospective, randomized controlled trial could not replicate these results.[83] Even though the efficacy of Procurin is controversial, the wound center concept is robust: Applying "good wound care" on outpatients and apparently achieving good results (although not published), Curative Technologies has helped in the evolution of the concept of the chronic wound care center, and manages more than 100 wound care centers in the United States.

Outpatient Wound Clinic Principles and Logistics

Close periodic follow-up of individual patients is a necessity. Patients with open wounds typically have co-morbidities that tend to result in limb- or life-threatening infections without close (at least weekly) follow-up. Follow-up by "visiting nurses" is consistent with this principle: The international literature reports that wounds that get regular nursing follow-up have an amputation rate 40% lower that expected.[61, 103, 118]

The clinic often coordinates home care for complex patients needing durable medical equipment and/or having psychosocial issues. Consistent with physiatric principles, the team concept is utilized. Teams are made up of visiting nurses, home physical and occupational therapists, vendors, and case managers. Other professionals consulted by the wound clinic on- or off-site include nutrition specialists and weight loss and smoking cessation counselors. The certified pedorthist has been trained in methods to mitigate noxious foot pressure for patients with previous neuropathic ulcers. Clinical psychology and psychiatry have a role to play for patients with recalcitrant ulcers, which can be a manifestation of depression and displaced anger. In these cases behavioral techniques for wound management often give good results.

PREVENTION

Education, inspection, and continued pressure and shear optimization are the keys to preventing the first or recurrent ulcerations. In the long-term care setting, assessment by the Braden[14–16] or Norton[98, 99] index, pressure support selection, and continued good nursing care are critical. For chronic venous or edematous ulcers, compression stockings should be used indefinitely. All diabetic patients should be screened with the Simmes 5.07 monofilament.[63] Insensitivity to this puts the patient at increased risk for skin breakdown, and orthopedic oxford shoes with high toe box and removable two-layer insoles should be prescribed.[71] The removable insoles should be replaced every three months. Skin and nail care must be lifelong for patients at risk for buttock or leg ulcers. Emollients (e.g., lanolin, lac-hydrin) prevent "cracking" of the skin and consequent entry of bacteria.[92] Inspection and care of skin and nails is also performed by professionals on routine follow-up in more severe cases. For additional information, see Chapter 56.

CONCLUSION

Prevention and early, aggressive intervention are the cornerstones of outpatient and skilled-care chronic-wound management. Wound management that utilizes the principles outlined in this chapter balances cost with quality of care. Individual functional outcomes are inextricably linked with patient satisfaction, and are optimized if wounds are healed with a minimum of complications in the outpatient setting. Outpatient physiatric practice is compatible with outpatient chronic wound care, and chronic wound practice offers new opportunities for practicing physiatrists in the 21st century.

ACKNOWLEDGEMENTS

Our thanks to the following: NIH K08HD01065-01, NIH HD07425, University of Pennsylvania Research Foundation, and Hartford Foundation 91009-G.

REFERENCES

1. Abrussezze R: Early assessment and prevention of pressure ulcers. In Lee BY (ed): Chronic Ulcers of the Skin. New York, McGraw-Hill, 1985, pp 1–9.
2. Allman RM: Pressure sores among the elderly. New Engl J Med 1989; 320:850–853.
3. Allman RM, Walker JM, Hart MK, et al: Pressure ulcers among hospital patients. Ann Intern Med 1987; 107:337–342.
4. Ameis A, Chiarcossi A, Jimenez J: Management of pressure sores. Comparative study in medical and surgical patients. Postgrad Med 1980; 67:177–184.
5. Anthony J, Huntsman W, Mathes S: Changing trends in the management of pelvic pressure ulcers: A 12 year review. Decubitus 1992; 5.
6. Atri SC, Misra J, Bisht D, et al: Use of homologous platelet factors in achieving total healing of recalcitrant skin ulcers. Surgery 1990; 108:508–512.
7. Bacharach JM, Rooke T, Osmundson PJ, et al: Predictive value of transcutaneous oxygen pressure and amputation success by use of supine and elevation measurements. J Vasc Surg 1992; 16:558–562.
8. Barbenel J, Jordan M, Nicol S, et al: The incidence of pressure sores in the Greater Glasgow Health Board area. Lancet 1977; 2:548–550.
9. Barker A: Glaboris epidermis of the cavy contains a powerful battery. Am J Physiol 1982; 242:R358.
10. Basson M, Burney R: Defective wound healing in patients with paraplegia and quadriplegia. Surg Gynecol Obstet 1982; 155:9–12.
11. Bauman JH, Girling JP, et al: Plantar pressures and trophic ulceration: An evaluation of footware. J Bone Joint Surg [Br] 1963; 45:652–673.
12. Becker H: The distally-based gluteus maximus muscle flap. Plast Reconstr Surg 1979; 63:653–656.
13. Bergstrom N, Bennett M, Carlson C: Treatment of Pressure Ulcers. Rockville, MD, Agency for Health Care Policy and Research, Public Health Service, U.S. Department of Health and Human Services, 1994.
14. Bergstrom N, Braden B: A prospective study of pressure sore risk among institutionalized elderly. J Am Geriatr Soc 1992; 40:747–758.
15. Bergstrom N, Braden B, Laguzza A, et al: The Braden scale for predicting pressure sore risk. Nurs Res 1987; 36:205–210.
16. Bergstrom N, Demuth P, Braden B: A clinical trial of the Braden Scale for Predicting Pressure Sore Risk. Nurs Clin North Am 1987; 22:417–428.
17. Berlowitz D, Wilking S: Risk factors for pressure sores. A comparison of cross-sectional and cohort-derived data. J Am Geriatr Soc 1989; 37.
18. Black JM, Black SB: Surgical management of pressure ulcers. Nurs Clin North Am 1987; 22:429–438.
19. Braddom R, Leadbetter M: The use of a tissue expander to enlarge a graft for surgical treatment of a pressure ulcer in a quadraplegic. Am J Phys Med Rehabil 1989; 68:70–72.
20. Brand P: Pressure Sores the Problem. London, MacMillan Press, 1976.
21. Brandeis GH, Morris JN, Nash DJ, et al: Epidemiology and natural history of pressure ulcers in elderly nursing home residents. JAMA 1990; 264:2905–2909.
22. Bridges R, Deitch E: Diabetic foot infections: Pathophysiology and treatment. Surg Clin North Am 1994; 74:537–555.
23. Bruck J, Buttenmeyer R, Grabosch A, et al: More arguments in favor of myocutaneous flaps for the treatment of pelvic pressure sores. Ann Plast Surg 1991; 26:85–88.
24. Bryant R: Acute and Chronic Wounds: Nursing Management. St Louis, Mosby-Yearbook, 1992.

25. Caputo G, Cavanagh P, Ulbrecht J, et al: Assessment and management of foot disease in patients with diabetes. New Engl J Med 1994; 331:854–860.
26. Carpenter JP, Baum RA, Holland GA, et al: Peripheral vascular surgery with magnetic resonance angiography as the sole preoperative imaging modality. J Vasc Surg 1994; 20:861–871.
27. Chantaleau E, Breuer U, Leisch A, et al: Outpatient treatment of unilateral diabetic foot ulcers with "Half Shoes." Diabetic Med 1993; 10:267–270.
28. Chen T, Bates R, Xu Y, et al: Human recombinant transforming growth factor—Beta1 modulation of biochemical and cellular events in healing of ulcer wounds. J Invest Dermatol 1992; 98:428–435.
29. Circolo A, Welgus H, Pierce G, et al: Differential regulation of the expression of proteinases/antiproteinases in fibroblasts. J Biol Chem 1991; 266:12283–12288.
30. Clarke M, Kahdom H: The nursing prevention of pressure sores in hospital and community patients. J Adv Nurs 1988; 13:365–373.
31. Coleman WC, Brand PW, Birke JA: The total contact cast: A therapy for plantar ulceration on insensitive feet. J Am Podiatry Assoc 1984; 548–552.
32. Conine T, Daechsel D, Lau M: The role of alternating air and silicone overlay in preventing decubitus ulcers. Int J Rehabil Res 1990; 13:317–321.
33. Containment NCfC: National Specialized Bed Study and Other Support Surface Guidelines. Washington, DC, U.S. Department of Veterans Affairs, 1992.
34. Cooper D: Challenge of open wound assessment in the home setting. Prog Dev Ostomy Wound Care 1990; 2:11–18.
35. Crewe R: Problems of rubber ring nursing cushions and a clinical survey of alternative cushions for ill patients. Care Sci Pract 1987; 5:9–11.
36. Curative I: http//www.curative.com. In Curative, Inc., 1998.
37. Daniel R, Hall E, MacLeod M: Pressure sores: A reappraisal. Ann Plast Surg 1979; 3:53–63.
38. Deloach E, Christy R, Ruf L: Osteomyelitis underlying severe pressure sores. Contemp Surg 1992; 40:25–32.
39. Deloach E, DiBenedetto R, Womble L, et al: The treatment of osteomyelitis underlying pressure ulcers. Decubitus 1992; 5: 32–41.
40. Department of Health and Human Services: Healthy People 2000: National health promotion and disease prevention objectives, vol 91-50213. Washington, DC, Government Printing Office, 1991.
41. Dinsdale S: Decubitus ulcers: Role of pressure and friction in causation. Arch Phys Med Rehabil 1974; 55:147–152.
42. Doughty D: The process of wound healing: A nursing perspective. Prog Dev Ostomy Wound Care 1990; 2:3–12.
43. Eaglstein WH, Falanga V: Tissue engineering and the development of Apligraf, a human skin equivalent. Adv Wound Care 1998; 11:1–8.
44. Exton-Smith A, Overstall P, Wedgwood J, et al: Use of the air wave system to prevent pressure sores in hospital. Lancet 1982; 1:1288–1290.
45. Fagrell B: Advances in microcirculation network evaluation: An update. Int J Microcirc 1995; 15:34–40.
46. Falanga V: Venous ulceration. Dermatol Surg Oncol 1993; 19:764–771.
47. Falanga V, Eaglstein W: The "trap" hypothesis of venous ulceration. Lancet 1993; 341:1006–1008.
48. Falanga V, Qian S, Danielpour D, et al: Hypoxia upregulates the synthesis of TGF-beta1 by human dermal fibroblasts. J Invest Dermatol 1991; 97:634–637.
49. Ferrell B, Osterweil D, Christenson P: A randomized trial of low-air-loss beds for treatment of pressure ulcers. JAMA 1993; 269:494–497.
50. Fowler E, Papen J: Evaluation of alginate dressing for pressure ulcers. Decubitus 1991; 4:47–52.
51. Fuhrer M, Garber SDR: Pressure ulcers in community-resident persons with spinal cord injury: Prevalence and risk factors. Arch Phys Med Rehabil 1993; 74:1172–1177.
52. Garber S, Campion L, Krouskop T: Trochanteric pressure in spinal cord injury. Arch Phys Med Rehabil 1982; 63:549–552.
53. Garber S, Krouskop T, Carter R: A system for clinically evaluating wheelchair pressure-relief cushions. Am J Occup Ther 1978; 32:565–570.
54. Gerson L: The incidence of pressure sores in active treatment hospitals. Int J Nurs Stud 1975; 12:201–204.
55. Gilchrist T, Martin A: Wound treatment with Sorbsan™: An alginate fibre dressing. Biomaterials 1982; 4:317–320.
56. Goldman R: Capacitive biofeedback sensor with resilient polyurethane dielectric for rehabilitation, in. US Patent Number 5,449,002, September 12, 1995.
57. Goldman R (ed): Pressure Ulcers. Philadelphia, Hanley & Belfus, Inc, 1996.
58. Goldman RJ: Relationship between transcutaneous oxygen and healing rate of diabetic foot ulcers. Arch Phys Med Rehabil 1997; 78:1055.
59. Goodson WH: Wound healing and aging. J Invest Dermatol 1990; 73:88–91.
60. Greenhalgh DG, Sprugel KH, Murray MH, et al: PDGF and FGF stimulate wound healing in the genetically diabetic mouse. Am J Pathol 1990; 136:1235–1245.
61. Griffiths GD, Weiman TJ: Meticulous attention to foot care improves the prognosis in diabetic ulceration of the foot. Surg Gynecol Obstet 1992; 174:49–51.
62. Grinnel F, Ho CH, Wystocki A: Degradation of fibronectin and vitronectin in chronic wound fluid: Analysis by cell blotting, immunoblotting and cell adhesion assays. J Invest Dermatol 1992; 98:410–416.
63. Grunfeld C: Diabetic foot ulcers: Etiology, treatment, and prevention. Adv Int Med 1991; 37:103–132.
64. Hasan A, Murata H, et al: Dermal fibroblasts from venous ulcers are unresponsive to the action of transforming growth factor beta 1. J Dermatol Sci 1997; 16:59–66.
65. Heggers J, Haydon S, Ko F, et al: Pseudomonas aeruginosa exotoxin A: Its role in retardation of wound healing. J Burn Care Rehabil 1992; 13:512–518.
66. Helm PA, Walker SC, Pulliam G: Total contact casting in diabetic patients with neuropathic foot ulcerations. Arch Phys Med Rehabil 1984; 65:691–693.
67. Hutchinson J, McGuckin M: Occlusive dressings: A microbiologic and clinical review. J Infect Control 1990; 18:257–268.
68. International Association of Enterostomal Therapy: Dermal wounds: Pressure sores. Philosophy of the IAET. J Enterostomal Ther 1988; 15:4–17.
69. Inman K, Sibbald W, Rutledge F, et al: Clinical utility and cost-effectiveness of an air suspension bed in the prevention of pressure ulcers. JAMA 1993; 269:1139–1143.
70. Jackson B, Chagare R, Nee N, et al: The effect of a therapeutic bed on pressure ulcers: An experimental study. J Enterostomal Ther 1988; 15:220–226.
71. Janisse D: Pedorthic care of the diabetic foot. In Levin M, O'Neal L, Bowker J (eds): The Diabetic Foot, ed 5. St. Louis, Mosby–Year Book, 1993, pp 549–575.
72. Johnson A, White A, McNalley B: Comparison of common topical agents for wound treatment: Cytotoxicity for human fibroblast in culture. Wounds 1989; 1:186–192.
73. Katz M, Alvarez A, Kirsner R, et al: Human wound fluid from acute wounds stimulates fibroblast and endothelial cell growth. J Am Acad Dermatol 1991; 25:1054–1058.
74. Kindwall E: Uses of hyperbaric oxygen therapy in the 1990's. Cleve Clin J Med 1992; 59:517–528.
75. Knauer C: Management of malignant fungating breast lesions. Prog Dev Ostomy Wound Care 1990; 2:3–11.
76. Knighton DR, Ciresi K, Fiegel VD, et al: Stimulation of repair in chronic, nonhealing, cutaneous ulcers using platelet-derived wound healing formula. Surg Gynecol Obstet 1990; 170:56–60.
77. Koshima I, Moriguchi T, Soeda S: The gluteal perforator-based flap for repair of sacral pressure sores. Plast Reconstr Surg 1993; 91:678–683.
78. Kosiak M: Etiology and pathology of ischemic ulcers. Arch Phys Med Rehabil 1959; 40:62–69.
79. Kosiak M: Prevention and rehabilitation of pressure ulcers. Decubitus 1991; 4:60–68.
80. Krasner D: Shifting paradigms for wound care: Dressing decisions; multidisciplinary care; effectiveness. In Portnow J (ed): Wound Care. Durable Medical Equipment Review, vol 1, 1994.
81. Kroll S, Rosenfield L: Perforator-based flaps for low posterior midline defects. Plast Reconstr Surg 1988; 81:561–566.

82. Krouskop T, Noble P, Garber S, et al: The effectiveness of preventive management in reducing the occurrence of pressure sores. J Rehabil Res Dev 1983; 20:74–83.
83. Krupski WC, Reilly LM, Perez S, et al: A prospective randomized trial of autologous platelet-derived wound healing factors for treatment of chronic nonhealing wounds: A preliminary report [see comments]. J Vasc Surg 1991; 14:526–532.
84. Lagattolla NR, Stacey MC, Burnand KG, et al: Growth factors, tissue and urokinase-type plasminogen activators in venous ulcers. Ann Card Angeiol 1995; 44:299–303.
85. Landis E: Micro-injection studies of capillary blood pressure in human skin. Heart 1930; 15: 209–228.
86. Lippmann H, Fishman L, Farrar R, et al: Edema control in the management of disabling chronic venous insufficiency. Arch Phys Med Rehabil 1994; 75:436–441.
87. Majesky M: A little VEGF goes a long way: Therapeutic angiogenesis by direct injection of vascular endothelial growth factor-encoding plasmid DNA. Circulation 1996; 94:3062–3064.
88. Mathes S, Feng L, Hunt T: Coverage of the infected wound. Ann Surg 1983; 198:420–429.
89. Mawson AR, Siddiqui FH, Connolly BJ, et al: Effect of high voltage pulsed galvanic stimulation on sacral transcutaneous oxygen tension levels in the spinal cord injured. Paraplegia 1993; 31:311–319.
90. McDermott VG, Meakem JP, Carpenter JP, et al: Magnetic resonance angiography of the distal lower extremity. Clin Radiol 1995; 50:741–746.
91. Meehan M: Multisite pressure ulcer prevalence survey. Decubitus 1990; 3:14–17.
92. Miller OF: Essentials of pressure ulcer treatment: The diabetic experience. J Dermatol Surg Oncol 1993; 19:759–763.
93. Morain WD, Colen LB: Wound healing in diabetes mellitus. Clin Plast Surg 1990; 17:493–501.
94. Mueller JJ, Diamond JE, Sinacore DR, et al: Total contact casting in treatment of diabetic plantar ulcers. Diabetes Care 1989; 12:384–388.
95. Mulder G, Seeley J: The effectiveness of specialty beds in the treatment of severe pressure ulcers in nursing home patients: A preliminary report. Unpublished research report, 1991.
96. Munro B, Brown L, Heitman B: Pressure ulcers: One bed or another? Geriat Nurs 1989; 10:190–192.
97. Nimit K: Public health service assessment guidelines for home air-fluidized bed therapy. Health Technol Assess Rep 1989; 5:1–11.
98. Norton D: Calculating the risk: Reflections on the Norton scale. Decubitus 1989; 2:24–31.
99. Norton D, McLaren R, Exton-Smith A: An Investigation of Geriatric Nursing Problems in Hospital. London, Churchill Livingstone, 1975.
100. Olin J, Beusterien K, Childs MB, et al: Medical costs of treating venous statis ulcers: Evidence from a retrospective cohort study. Vasc Med 1999; 4:1–7.
101. Padberg F, Back T, Thompson P, et al: Transcutaneous oxygen (TcPO2) estimates probability of healing in the ischemic extremity. J Surg Res 1996; 60:365–369.
102. Panel NPUA: Pressure Ulcers: Incidence, Economics, Risk Assessment. Consensus Development Conference Statement. West Dundee, IL, S-N Publications, 1989.
103. Partl M: After-care of patients with diabetic feet by general practitioners or special ambulatory care—effect on rate of amputation. Gesundheitswesen 1994; 56:215–219.
104. Phillips L, Abdullah K, Geldner P, et al: Application of basic fibroblast growth factor may reverse diabetic wound healing impairment. Ann Plast Surg 1993; 31:331–334.
105. Phillips T, Dover J: Leg Ulcers. J Am Acad Dermatol 1991; 25:965–985.
106. Phillips T, Stanton B, Provan A, et al: A study of the impact of leg ulcers on quality of life: Financial, social, and psychologic implications. J Am Acad Dermatol 1994; 31:49–53.
107. Pierce GF, Tarpley JE, Yanagihara D, et al: Platelet-derived growth factor (BB homodimer), transforming growth factor-beta 1, and basic fibroblast growth factor in dermal wound healing. Neovessel and matrix formation and cessation of repair. Am J Pathol 1992; 140:1375–1388.
108. Provider MH: Modern Healthcare Provider's Survey, 1998.
109. Reed J: Pressure ulcers in the elderly: Prevention and treatment utilizing the team approach. Md State Med J 1981; 30:45–50.
110. Reiber G, Boyko E, Smith D (eds): Lower Extremity Foot Ulcers and Amputations in Diabetes. Washington, DC, U.S. Government Printing Office, 1997
111. Reichel S: Shearing force as a factor in decubitus ulcers in paraplegics. JAMA 1958; 166:762–763.
112. Reswick JB, Rogers JE: Experience at Rancho Los Amigos Hospital with devices and techniques to prevent pressure ulcers. In Kenedi R, Cowden J, Scales J (eds): Bedsore Biomechanics. London, University Park Press, 1976, p 300.
113. Rhodes GR: Uses of transcutaneous oxygen monitoring in the management of below-knee amputations and skin envelope injuries. Am Surg 1985; 51:701–707.
114. Roberts B, Goldstone L: A survey of pressure sores in the over sixties on two orthopaedic wards. Int J Nurs Stud 1979; 16:355–364.
115. Robnett M: The incidence of skin breakdown in a surgical intensive care unit. J Nurs Qual Assur 1986; 1:77–81.
116. Rodeheaver G, Kurtz L, Kircher B, et al: Pluronic F-68: A promising new skin wound cleanser. Ann Emerg Med 1980; 9:572–576.
117. Ruan C, Escobedo E, Harrison S, et al: Magnetic resonance imaging of nonhealing pressure ulcers and myocutaneous flaps. Arch Phys Med Rehabil 1998; 79:1080–1087.
118. Runyan JW: The Memphis chronic disease program. JAMA 1975; 231:264–267.
119. Russ G, Motta G: Eliminating pressure: Is less than 32 mm Hg enough for wound healing? Ostomy Wound Manage 1991; 34:60–63.
120. Salcido R, Carney J, Fisher S: A reliable animal model of pressure sore development: The role of free radicals. J Am Paraplegia Soc 1993; 16:61.
121. Salcido R, Donofrio JC, Fisher SB, et al: Histopathology of pressure ulcers as a result of sequential computer-controlled pressure sessions in a fuzzy rat model. Adv Wound Care 1994; 7:23–28.
122. Sanchez S, Eamegdool S, Conway H: Surgical treatment of decubitus ulcers in paraplegics. Plast Reconstr Surg 1969; 43: 25–28.
123. Shannon M, Skorga P: Pressure ulcer prevalence in two general hospitals. Decubitus 1989; 2:38–43.
124. Smola H, Theikotter G, Fusenig N: Mutual induction of growth factor gene expression by epidermal-dermal cell interaction. J Cell Biol 1993; 122:417–429.
125. Smoot E: Clinitron bed therapy hazards [letter]. Plast Reconstr Surg 1986; 77:165.
126. Staas WJ, LaMantia J: Decubitus ulcers and rehabilitation medicine. Int J Dermatol 1982; 21:437–444.
127. Steed DL, Donohoe D, Webster MW, et al: Effect of extensive debridement and treatment on the healing rate of diabetic foot ulcers. J Am Coll Surg 1996; 183:61–64.
128. Steed DL, Group DUS: Clinical evaluation of recombinant human platelet-derived growth factor for the treatment of lower extremity diabetic ulcers. J Vasc Surg 1995; 21:71–81.
129. Strauss M, Gong J, Gary B: The cost of home air-fluidized therapy for pressure sores: A randomized controlled trial. J Fam Pract 1991; 33:52–59.
130. Van den Brande P, von Kemp K, De Coninck A, et al: Laser Doppler flux characteristics at the skin of the dorsum of the foot in young and in elderly healthy human subjects. Microvasc Res 1997; 53:156–162.
131. van Marum RJ, Meijer JH, Bertelsmann FW, et al: Impaired blood flow response following pressure load in diabetic patients with cardiac autonomic neuropathy. Arch Phys Med Rehabil 1997; 78:1003–1006.
132. VanEtten N, Sexton P, Smith R: Development and implementation of a skin care program. Ostomy Wound Manage 1990; 27:40–54.
133. Vasconez L, Schneider W, Trukiewicz MJ: Pressure sores. Curr Probl Surg 1977; 24:23.
134. Verg, Inc: Wound Measurement System. Verg, Inc., 633 Wellington Crescent, Winnepeg, Manitoba, Canada, R3M 0A8.
135. Versluysen M: How elderly patients with femoral fractures de-

velop pressure sores in hospital. Br Med J Clin Res Ed 1986; 292:1311–1313.
136. Vyas S, Binns J, Wilson A: Thoracolumbar-sacral flaps in the treatment of sacral pressure sores. Plast Reconstr Surg 1980; 65:159–163.
137. Warner D: A clinical comparison of two pressure-reducing surfaces in the management of pressure ulcers. Decubitus 1992; 5: 52–64.
138. Wiersema L, Lueckenotte A: Determination of the effectiveness of four sleep surfaces in the treatment of stage 2 and 3 pressure sores (unpublished research report). Batesville, IN, Barnes Hospital, St. Louis, and Hill-Rom, 1992.
139. Winter G (ed): Epidermal Regeneration in the Domestic Pig. Chicago, Year Book Medical Publishers, 1970.
140. Wu F: Relative cost of amputation and total contact casting. In Rehabilitation Medicine. Philadelphia, University of Pennsylvania, 1996, p 20.
141. Wu L, Brucker M, Gruskin E, et al: Differential effects of platelet-derived growth factor BB in accelerating wound healing in aged versus young animals: The impact of tissue hypoxia. Plastic Reconstr Surg 1997; 99:815–822.
142. Yamaguchi M, et al: Effect of tension-force on plasminogen activator activity from human periodontal ligament cells. J Periodont Res 1997; 32:308–314.

32

CHAPTER

Jonathan R. Moldover, M.D., and Matthew N. Bartels, M.D., M.P.H.

Cardiac Rehabilitation

The two primary goals of any cardiac rehabilitation program are to increase the functional capacity of the patient and to change the natural history of the disease in order to reduce morbidity and mortality. Improvement in functional capacity has been repeatedly demonstrated and accepted for many years. More recently the second goal of reduced morbidity and mortality has been shown to be achievable. A number of studies have indicated that a comprehensive program of risk factor reduction, lifestyle alteration, and exercise training can lower morbidity and mortality and even produce regression of atherosclerotic stenoses.[42, 71, 72, 74]

EPIDEMIOLOGY OF HEART DISEASE

Despite a steady, two-decade decline, cardiac disease remains the leading cause of morbidity and mortality in the adult population of the United States. Approximately 1.5 million people each year suffer an acute myocardial infarction (MI).[2] With increased public awareness of cardiac risk factors, better management of cardiac disease, and risk intervention by the medical community, these rates have been steadily decreasing. Reductions in cigarette smoking, decreasing red meat consumption, and increasing exercise have all contributed to the decrease in coronary artery disease (CAD). The major risk factors are outlined in Table 32–1. The death rate of CAD was 228.1 per 100,000 population in 1970 but diminished to 102.6 per 100,000 by 1990.

CAD is the number-one cause of mortality in men aged 45 years and older, and in women aged 75 and older. CAD is the overall number-one cause of death in the United States, with more than 72,000 deaths in 1990. The estimated mortality cost of cardiac disease in 1990 was more than $70 billion, with an estimated 8.2 million life-years lost.[91]

Cardiac disease accounts for a large proportion of total health-care expenditures. In 1992, cardiovascular disease was the single greatest cause of hospital admissions (3.9 million). Myocardial ischemia accounted for more than 2.1 million of these hospital admissions, and congestive heart failure (CHF) accounted for approximately 800,000 admissions. Cardiac arrhythmias cause nearly 550,000 admissions each year.

Cardiac surgery accounts for the third largest number of surgical procedures for inpatients. More than a million cardiac catheterizations and more than 300,000 coronary artery bypass grafts (CABGs) were performed in 1992.[40]

With new technologies, congestive heart disease patients are living longer, and more patients are surviving myocardial infarction (MI). Improved survival rates after cardiac transplant have increased the number of cardiac transplant procedures performed. More than 2100 heart transplants were performed in 1990, and more than 2200 people were on the waiting list.[91]

TYPES OF HEART DISEASE

Physiatrists practicing cardiac rehabilitation have been encountering an increased variety of heart disease in recent years. "Standard" cardiac rehabilitation of the post-MI patient comprises the bulk of the practice, but post-CABG, post-transplant, and post-valve replacement surgery patients are now being referred for cardiac rehabilitation in increasing numbers. Patients with chronic CHF are now also being referred for cardiac rehabilitation, as are patients with life-threatening arrhythmias.

TABLE 32–1 Risk Factors for Coronary Artery Disease (CAD)

Irreversible Risks	Reversible Risks
Male gender	Cigarette smoking
Family history of premature CAD (before age 55 yr in a parent or sibling)	Hypertension
Past history of CAD	Low HDL cholesterol [<0.9 mmol/L (35 mg/dL)]
Past history of occlusive peripheral vascular disease	Hypercholesterolemia [>5.20 mmol/L (200 mg/dL)]
Past history of cerebrovascular disease	High lipoprotein A
	Abdominal obesity
	Hypertriglyceridemia [>2.8 mmol/L (250 mg/dL)]
	Hyperinsulinemia
	Diabetes mellitus
	Sedentary lifestyle

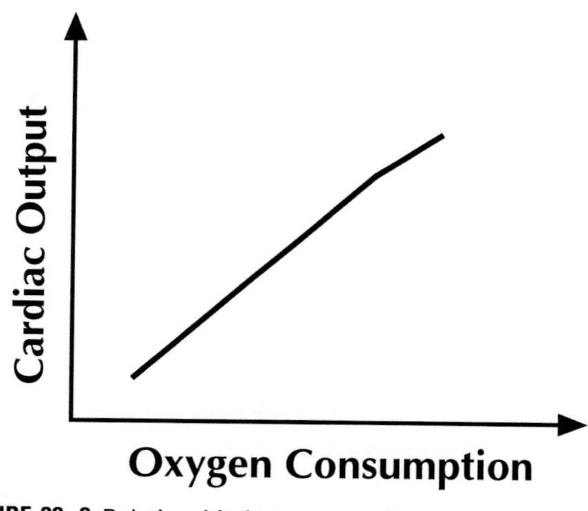

FIGURE 32–2. Relationship between cardiac output and oxygen consumption.

EXERCISE PHYSIOLOGY

The clinician needs to understand the cardiac response to exercise and the effects of aerobic training in order to design a safe and effective rehabilitation program for any given patient.[66]

Aerobic Capacity. *Aerobic capacity* is a physiological term used to measure the work capacity of an individual. It is represented by the maximum oxygen consumption ($\dot{V}O_{2max}$), which is usually expressed in milliliters of oxygen consumed per kilogram of body weight per minute. If the total oxygen consumption ($\dot{V}O_2$) of the exercising individual is measured and plotted against the workload (Fig. 32–1), the $\dot{V}O_2$ increases linearly until it levels off in a short plateau. This plateau represents the point at which the $\dot{V}O_2$ cannot increase further despite further increases in the workload. This is the $\dot{V}O_{2max}$ (or aerobic capacity) of the individual. The total $\dot{V}O_2$ provides a measure of the increasing metabolic work of the peripheral skeletal muscles, not of the heart itself. The $\dot{V}O_2$ is useful as a measure of the physical work being performed. In research studies the work being performed is often expressed as a percentage of the $\dot{V}O_{2max}$. Since physiological responses to exercise are typically proportional to the relative workload for any individual rather than the absolute workload, using the percentage of $\dot{V}O_{2max}$ allows us to normalize the data for a population of subjects.

Cardiac Output. Cardiac output (CO) increases with increasing work. In early exercise, CO increases due to augmented stroke volume via the Frank-Starling mechanism. In late exercise, CO is increased primarily through an increase in ventricular rate.[29] Plotting CO against $\dot{V}O_2$ (Fig. 32–2), we see that this increase is essentially linear. The break in the slope of the line represents a lessening of the rate of increase caused by shifts in the oxyhemoglobin dissociation curve due to increasing temperature, acidity, and carbon dioxide in the working muscles. The maximum CO is the primary determinant of the $\dot{V}O_{2max}$. The CO in turn has two determinants: the heart rate and the stroke volume (SV).

Heart Rate. Heart rate (HR) increases in linearly when plotted against the $\dot{V}O_2$ or other measures of physical work (Fig. 32–3). The HR is limited by the person's age. Even with regular exercise there is a linear

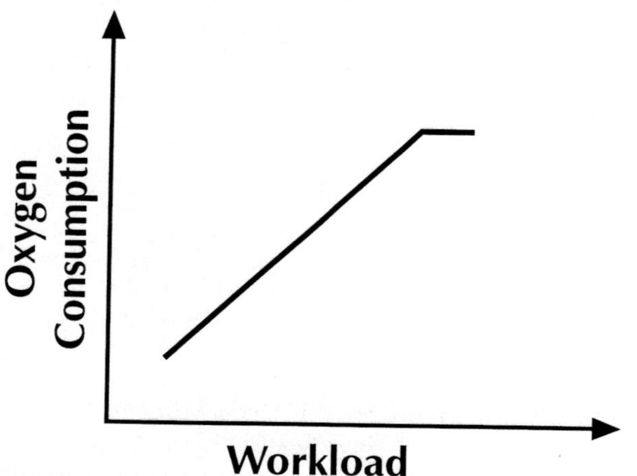

FIGURE 32–1. Relationship between oxygen consumption and intensity of work being performed.

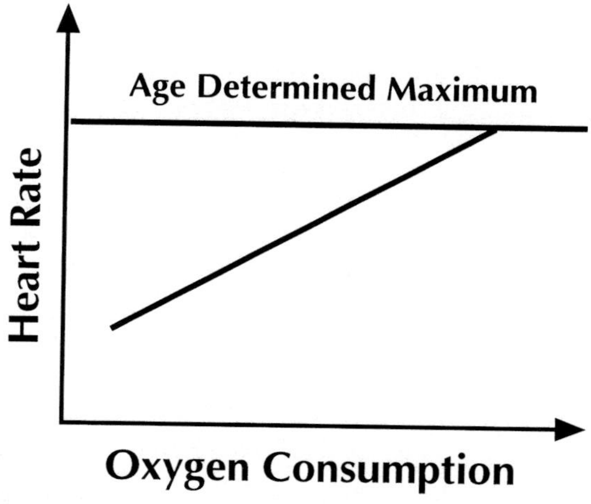

FIGURE 32–3. Relationship between heart rate and oxygen consumption.

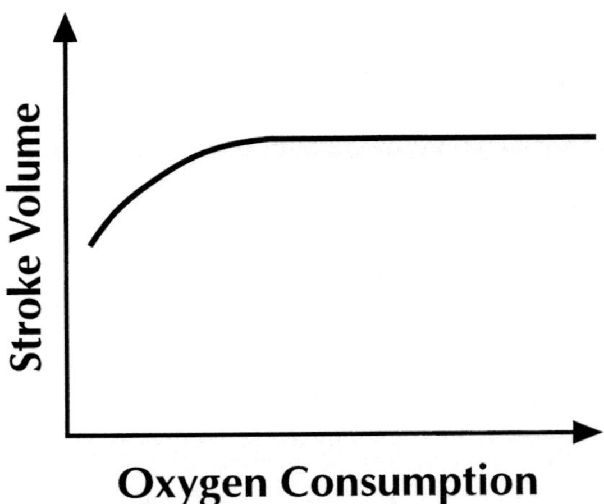

FIGURE 32–4. Relationship between stroke volume and oxygen consumption.

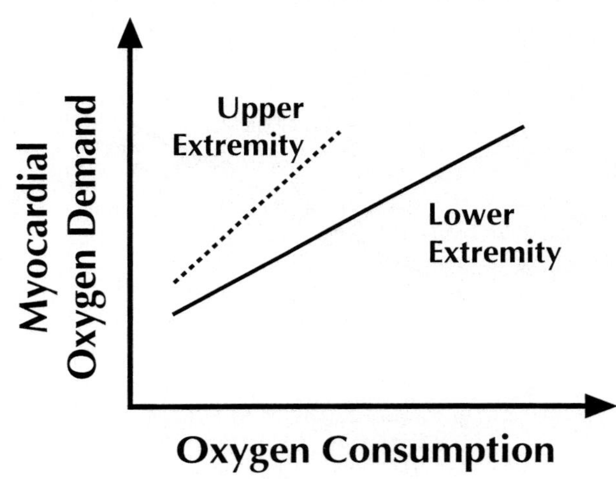

FIGURE 32–6. Comparison of the myocardial oxygen demand for upper extremity vs. lower extremity exercise.

decrease in the maximum HR with age.[4] For practical purposes a person's maximum HR can be estimated by subtracting the age in years from 220.

Stroke Volume. Stroke volume represents the quantity of blood pumped with each heartbeat. It increases in a curvilinear fashion (during exercise done in an upright position) until it reaches a plateau at about 40% of the $\dot{V}O_{2max}$ (Fig. 32–4). In the supine position the SV is close to maximal from the beginning of exercise, with increases in CO being due to increasing HR. A major determinant of SV is the diastolic filling volume, which is inversely related to the HR.

Myocardial Oxygen Consumption. The myocardial oxygen consumption ($M\dot{V}O_2$) is the actual oxygen consumption of the heart. The $\dot{V}O_2$ represents the oxygen consumption of the whole body (mainly due to the work of the skeletal muscles). The $M\dot{V}O_2$ rises in a linear fashion when plotted against the $\dot{V}O_2$ or other measure of workload (Fig. 32–5). It is limited by the anginal threshold, if one exists, or by the $\dot{V}O_{2max}$ if there is no CAD. The *anginal threshold* is defined as the point where the myocardial oxygen demand exceeds the ability of the coronary circulation to meet that demand. At the anginal threshold the patient can experience typical anginal chest pain, ischemic changes on the electrocardiogram (ECG), or arrhythmias. Although the $M\dot{V}O_2$ can be measured directly with cardiac catheterization, this is rarely practicable in a clinical setting. It has been shown that the HR and systolic blood pressure (BP) correlate well with the actual $M\dot{V}O_2$ and can be used as a clinical guide. The usual measure is the rate pressure product (RPP), which is calculated by multiplying the HR by the systolic BP and dividing the product by 100.

The linear relationship between the $M\dot{V}O_2$ and the $\dot{V}O_2$ suggests that the relative cardiac stress of various activities can be compared by measuring the $\dot{V}O_2$ produced by the activities. However, it should be noted that the linear relationship holds true only for a single activity performed under identical circumstances with varying intensity (e.g., pedaling a bicycle ergometer at different workloads or walking on a treadmill at different speeds). Activities performed with the upper extremities as opposed to the lower extremities generate a higher $M\dot{V}O_2$ at the same $\dot{V}O_2$ (Fig. 32–6). Activities performed supine as opposed to upright generate a higher $M\dot{V}O_2$ at low intensities and a lower $M\dot{V}O_2$ at

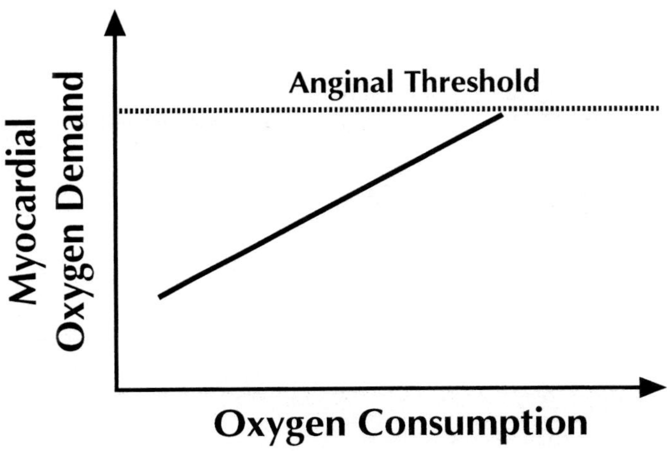

FIGURE 32–5. Relationship between myocardial oxygen demand and total body oxygen consumption.

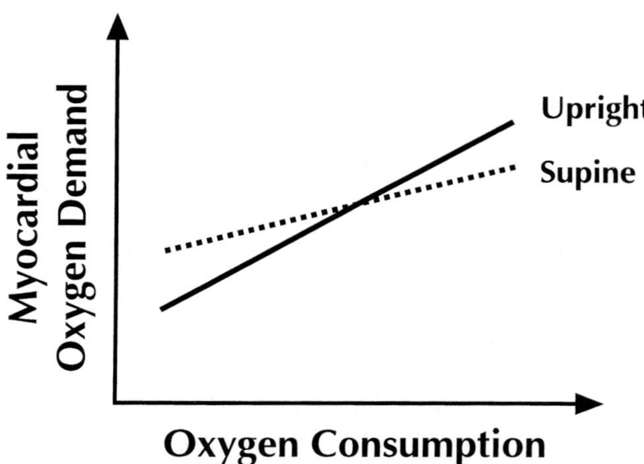

FIGURE 32–7. Comparison of the cardiac response to lower extremity exercise performed in upright and supine positions.

higher intensities (Fig. 32–7). Activities performed under emotional stress, after smoking a cigarette, after eating, or in cold weather all generate a higher $M\dot{V}O_2$ at the same $\dot{V}O_2$ than do activities performed at baseline. Activities that have an isometric component generate a higher $M\dot{V}O_2$ than a similar activity at the same $\dot{V}O_2$ without the isometric component (e.g., ambulating while gripping a cane or carrying a briefcase compared with ambulation without anything in the hands).

AEROBIC TRAINING

Aerobic training refers to an exercise program that involves dynamic exercise with large muscle groups of sufficient intensity, duration, and frequency to alter the cardiopulmonary response to exercise.

Principles

Intensity. The *intensity* of aerobic exercise can be defined either in terms of the individual's physiological response (HR or RPP) or in terms of exercise intensity (speed or resistance setting). A typical exercise prescription might be written with a target HR to be sustained after an appropriate warm-up period. The usual target HR is approximately 85% of the maximum HR achieved during a pretraining exercise tolerance test (ETT). If the individual is very frail or deconditioned, or if the limiting factor on the ETT was a dangerous arrhythmia, an intensity as low as 60% of maximum can be prescribed and a training effect can still be expected. Alternatively, if the training exercise is to be the same as the testing exercise, the prescription can be written in terms of the workload on a bicycle ergometer, or speed and grade on a treadmill.

Duration. The duration of each exercise session in the typical aerobic training program is 20 to 30 minutes. The actual training period is preceded by a warm-up phase at lower intensity and followed by a cool-down phase at a lower intensity. In general, training at a lower intensity of exercise requires a longer duration to achieve a training effect, and training at a relatively higher intensity requires a shorter duration.

Frequency. Aerobic training schedules usually involve exercise 3 days a week. Programs involving exercise at lower intensities should be performed at least 5 days a week.

Specificity. A key concept in all exercise training is that of specificity of training. The changes in the cardiac response to exercise apply only to exercise with muscles that have been involved in the training program. Training with a walking program or on a bicycle does not affect the cardiac response to upper extremity work. Training a carpenter with a vigorous treadmill program does nothing to change his cardiac response to strenuous woodworking activities performed with the arms. All muscle groups that the person needs for vocational or avocational pursuits should be included in the training program.

Effects

Aerobic Capacity. The defining characteristic of a successful aerobic training program is an increase in the aerobic capacity ($\dot{V}O_{2max}$), as shown in Figure 32–8. Note that while the $\dot{V}O_{2max}$ increases, there is no change in the resting $\dot{V}O_2$ or in the $\dot{V}O_2$ at any given submaximum workload. It should also be noted that the effect is seen only if both the pre-test and the post-test use the same muscle groups that are used in the training program.

Cardiac Output. The maximum CO increases with aerobic training, as seen in Figure 32–9. As with the $\dot{V}O_2$, note that while the CO at maximum exercise increases, the resting and the submaximum CO remain the same.

Stroke Volume. Although the CO at any given submaximum workload remains the same, there are significant changes in the way that the CO is generated. The SV is higher at rest, submaximum work, and maximum work after aerobic training (Fig. 32–10). This increase in SV is mostly due to a combination of increased blood volume and prolonged diastolic filling time.

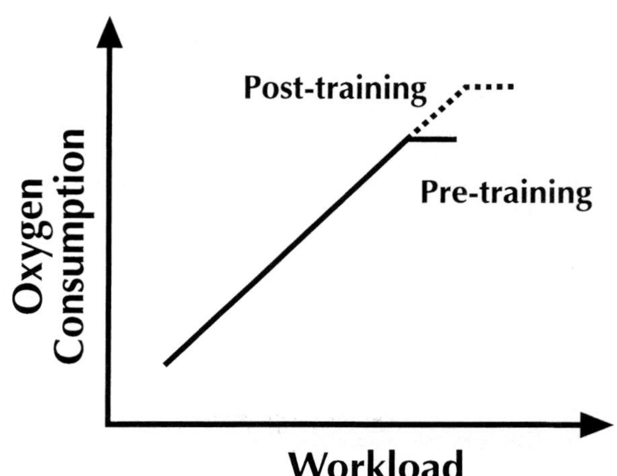

FIGURE 32–8. Effect of training on relationship between oxygen consumption and workload.

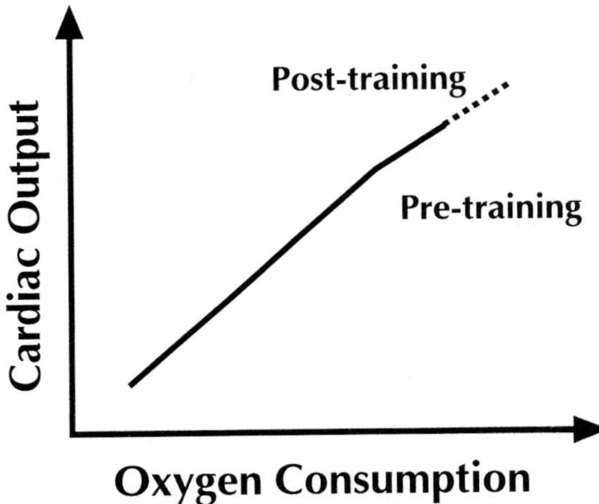

FIGURE 32–9. Effect of training on relationship between cardiac output and oxygen consumption.

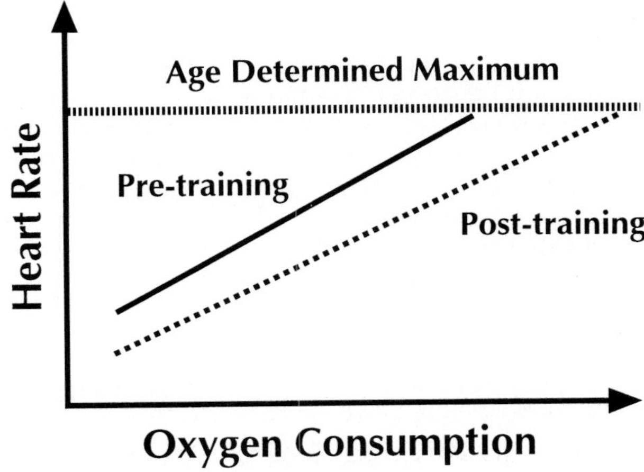

FIGURE 32–11. Effect of training on relationship between heart rate and oxygen consumption.

Heart Rate. The HR following aerobic training is lower at rest and at any given submaximum workload but remains unchanged at maximum work (Fig. 32–11). As noted earlier, the maximum HR is determined by the person's age, not level of fitness. Of course, if the ETT is prematurely limited by a noncardiac endpoint, one might see an increase in the maximum HR obtained during the post-test.

Myocardial Oxygen Consumption. From the point of view of cardiac rehabilitation, it is the effect of aerobic training on the $M\dot{V}O_2$ that makes exercise training such an important part of any rehabilitation program. Note that in Figure 32–12 there is a decrease in the $M\dot{V}O_2$ at rest and at any submaximum workload, but there is no change in the maximum $M\dot{V}O_2$. The maximum level is still determined by the anginal threshold, which is not affected by aerobic conditioning. Consequently, exercise training does not appear to have a significant effect on the coronary circulation. Pharmacological interventions also have an effect on resting and submaximum, but not maximum $M\dot{V}O_2$. Only angioplasty or bypass surgery can raise or eliminate the anginal threshold.

Benefits

Even though aerobic training does not change the anginal threshold, the change in the cardiac response to exercise is extremely beneficial. The workload that can be tolerated before the anginal threshold is reached increases significantly. Patients can now do more activities because they can perform them without overtaxing the coronary circulation. In addition, activities that could be performed previously now require a lower percentage of the maximum, making them less stressful and creating a wider margin of safety between the cardiac response to that activity and the anginal threshold.

In addition to the reduced relative stress of specific activities provided by the increased physical work capacity, there is a growing body of evidence that aerobic training has a beneficial effect on the natural history of CAD that can be isolated from other lifestyle alterations. Paffenbarger et al[74] demonstrated that beginning

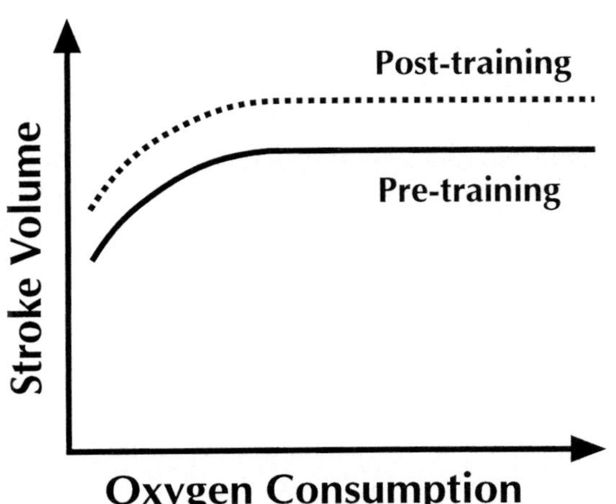

FIGURE 32–10. Effect of training on relationship between stroke volume and oxygen consumption.

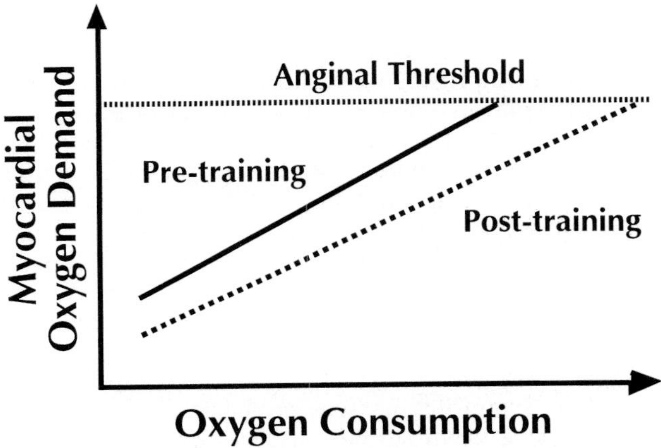

FIGURE 32–12. Effect of training on relationship between myocardial oxygen demand and oxygen consumption.

moderate physical activity in or after middle age resulted in a significant reduction in mortality from all causes and from CAD in particular, and that this effect was separable from the benefits of smoking cessation, BP normalization, and weight control. Hambrecht et al[42] used quantitative coronary angiography to show that regression in artery stenosis correlated with the level of physical activity. Aerobic training is an integral part of other, more comprehensive studies of lifestyle alteration that have shown regression of atherosclerotic plaques.[71, 72]

ASSESSMENT OF CARDIAC FUNCTION

History and Physical Examination

The cardiac history and physical examination are important in the evaluation of the patient with cardiac disease who is to undergo cardiac rehabilitation. The history often reveals important issues and gives the treating physiatrist the information needed to develop and direct a rehabilitation program. Some of the most pertinent details and important aspects of a patient's disability can be obtained from the physician-directed history as the patient establishes a relationship of trust, and the examiner can also get the nuances of the history from verbal and nonverbal cues. The patient can express concerns and goals to the physician. This helps the patient and physician to establish mutual goals and often encourages patient compliance with the treatment program.

History

Historical information can help direct further testing and help interpret the real meaning of the test results. The physician can observe the patient's emotional state, and make an assessment of concurrent illnesses and disabilities. The functional history, occupational history, social history, and personal habits should be verified. Family members can provide additional information. Family dynamics and functional disability from cardiac disease should be evaluated. Table 32–2 summarizes the key issues of the history. Special attention should be paid to the nature of the symptoms at rest and with activity. Several important symptoms specific to the cardiac history are discussed separately below.

Dyspnea. Shortness of breath (SOB) or dyspnea is often the central symptom in cardiac disease. A complete description of dyspnea should be obtained. This can help to differentiate cardiac and noncardiac causes of dyspnea. Among the common causes of exertional dyspnea are congestive heart failure, ischemic cardiac disease, chronic pulmonary disease, and deconditioning. Several of these can be present simultaneously, with or without cardiac disease. These issues require consideration in the design of the exercise program.

Chest Pain. Chest pain, tightness, and burning are the classic symptoms of ischemic heart disease. Other causes include valvular heart disease, arrhythmia, pleural irritation, chest wall pathology, and musculoskeletal pain. The cause of the pain can often be clarified by noting the duration, quality, provocation, location of the pain, and any ameliorating factors (Table 32–3). The precipitating factors and nature of chest pain create functional limitations for the patient and influence the design of the therapy program.

TABLE 32–2 Key Issues to Address in the History of a Patient with Cardiac Disease

Key Elements of the History
Family History
Premature CAD (before age 55 yr in first-degree relative)
Family history of familial hypercholesterolemia or hyperlipidemia
Family history of sudden death
Family history of arrhythmias
Family history of Marfan disease
Family history of hypertrophic cardiomyopathy
Social History
Cigarette use, cigar/pipe use
Sedentary lifestyle
Alcohol abuse history
Symptom History
Chest pain: duration, location, character, precipitating and relieving factors, pain radiation
Shortness of breath: duration, precipitating and relieving factors, day or night, position
Dizziness/lightheadedness
Syncope
Presence of nausea/vomiting, anorexia
Cyanosis/pallor
Palpitations
Edema
Cough
Hemoptysis
Fatigue
Functional History
Level of activity prior to cardiac event
Present level of activity
Exercise tolerance level
Level of activity required at home and at work
Level of function, stable or progressively worse
Extent and rate of activities performed
Patient Goals
Vocational plans
Leisure activities
Emotional adaptation to the cardiac condition
Medications
Complete Review of Systems and Past Medical History

Palpitation. Palpitation is the subjective sensation of an irregular or forceful heartbeat. It is often benign, but can be indicative of serious tachyarrhythmias. It should be noted that it is not always a reliable indicator of the presence of arrhythmias.

Syncope. In a patient with CAD, syncope can be associated with serious cardiac events. Cardiac syncope is usually abrupt in onset, occurring with little or no warning. Causes of cardiac syncope include aortic stenosis, idiopathic hypertrophic subaortic stenosis (IHSS), primary pulmonary hypertension, ventricular arrhythmias, reentrant arrhythmias, high-degree atrioventricular (AV) block, or sick sinus syndrome. Postural syncope can be due to autonomic dysfunction, neurological

TABLE 32–3 Cardiac vs. Noncardiac Chest Pain by Symptoms

Cardiac Pain Symptoms	Noncardiac Pain Symptoms
Pain Quality	
Constricting/squeezing	Dull aching
Visceral quality	Sharp, stabbing, piercing, knife-like
Burning	Muscular
Heaviness	
Pain Location	
Substernal	Left submammary area, apex of heart
Across precordium	Superficial tissues of the left chest
Neck	Right lower chest
One or both shoulders, arms	Very discrete localization possible
Intrascapular region	
One or both forearms, hands	
Epigastrium	
Pain Duration	
Angina, 2–10 min	Infarction, >20 min to 24 hr
<20 sec	Persistent without change for >24–48 hr
Precipitating and Aggravating Factors	
Exercise, particularly with hurrying	After completion of exercise
Excitement	With specific body positions, chest wall movement, and respiration
Cold temperature exposure	With direct palpation of chest wall
Stressful stimuli	Spontaneous
Postprandially, after heavy meal	Head and neck movement
	During fasting, with cold liquids
Relieving Factors	
Rest	Antacids
Nitroglycerin	Food
	Nonsteroidal analgesia

disease, vagal stimuli, or psychological stimuli. These differences can usually be determined by the history.

Edema. Peripheral edema can be an indication of CHF. Other causes of edema include postural edema, liver disease, renal disease, or lymphatic obstruction. Edema can have implications for individuals with multiple disabilities, as the satisfactory use of braces or prostheses might be impaired.

Fatigue. This is a nonspecific symptom with multiple causes. Depression, medications, physical exhaustion, and deconditioning are common noncardiac causes of fatigue. Cardiac fatigue is usually seen in severe heart failure. Cardiac fatigue is typically relieved with rest and occasionally presents as a form of atypical angina.

Cough. Cough is also a nonspecific symptom. Most causes are related to pulmonary or upper airway irritation. Cardiac cough is often initiated by assuming a recumbent position. Typically, a cardiac cough is nocturnal and episodic. There is little or no sputum production and the cough is relieved by resuming an upright position.

Limitations of the History. Despite the importance of the history, it has limitations. The design of a cardiac rehabilitation program cannot be assessed by history alone in patients with known CAD. Cardiac stress testing and other techniques to permit cardiac risk assessment should also be done. Table 32–4 lists historical features that can help indicate the overall prognosis. However, true risk assessment requires the detection of subclinical features that can be obtained only through testing.

Physical Examination

Every cardiac rehabilitation patient requires a complete examination by the prescribing physician. Specific findings can provide a clue to interventions. For example, exophthalmos might be a clue to hyperthyroidism, or xanthelasma can indicate hypercholesterolemia. There are associations between conditions such as ankylosis with aortic valve disease and conduction defects, and Down syndrome with cardiac abnormalities. Myasthenia or neuromuscular disease can indicate the cause of cardiomyopathy or conduction disease.

The details of the cardiac examination are described in basic physical examination textbooks. There are specific findings that physiatrists should be aware of in individuals with multiple disabilities. Cardiac auscultation revealing a fixed splitting of the second heart sound can indicate an atrial septal defect. Aortic valve stenosis can be detected via a systolic murmur. Pulmonary hypertension typically produces a heightened second heart sound in the pulmonic valve area. A mid-systolic click can be heard in mitral valve prolapse. The presence of a noncompliant ventricle with diastolic dysfunction is often indicated by an atrial gallop at the cardiac apex. A left ventricular gallop can be heard in patients with heart failure. Aortic and pulmonary valve disease can be detected. IHSS can be detected in younger patients. Diastolic murmurs can indicate the presence of mitral stenosis or pulmonary hypertension with pulmonary valve regurgitation. Continuous murmurs need further investigation to rule out a ventricular septal or atrial septal defect. A complete description of all of the important findings in a cardiac examination is beyond the scope of this chapter, but can lead to detection of cardiac disease and the prevention of complications during cardiac rehabilitation.

Summary

The basic history and physical examination is an important tool for the detection of patients at risk for complications in a cardiac rehabilitation program. They

TABLE 32–4 Historical Data That Indicate Increased Cardiac Risk

Postinfarction angina
Symptomatic congestive heart failure
Age >70 yr
Severe exercise limitation
Diabetes
History of hypertension, or loss of hypertension
Palpitation
Syncope
Fatigue

should be performed regularly on all individuals who are to begin an exercise program. While the history and physical examination are critical, you should not overlook the importance of new imaging and cardiac testing techniques. These now offer the most reliable assessment of the patient's true risk and functional status.

EXERCISE TOLERANCE TESTING

Exercise tolerance testing (ETT) is essential in the exercise design of any cardiac rehabilitation program. It is used to create an individualized exercise prescription, allowing an optimal level of training stimulus without exposing the patient to undue risk. Many new techniques are available in addition to the classic exercise treadmill test. These alternative tests can be used for patients with physical impairments as well as for other challenging patients. In exercise testing, the methods of application of the stress can vary, as can the evaluation of the response of the myocardium. With the new evaluations, the physiatrist can evaluate and rehabilitate both the able-bodied and the physically impaired patient with cardiac disease.

Electrocardiographic Exercise Tolerance Testing

Although more modern tests have taken over the diagnostic role for cardiac ischemia, the exercise stress test is still the most commonly used evaluation technique for determining cardiac risk stratification and functional capacity. The contraindications to exercise stress testing are summarized in Table 32–5. Some non-

TABLE 32–5 Contraindications to Exercise Tolerance Testing

Absolute Cardiac Contraindications to Exercise Testing

1. Unstable angina with recent chest pain
2. Untreated life-threatening cardiac arrhythmias
3. Uncompensated congestive heart failure
4. Advanced atrioventricular block
5. Acute myocarditis or pericarditis
6. Critical aortic stenosis
7. Severe hypertrophic obstructive cardiomyopathy
8. Uncontrolled hypertension
9. Acute myocardial infarction
10. Active endocarditis

Absolute Noncardiac Contraindications to Exercise Testing

1. Acute pulmonary embolus or pulmonary infarction
2. Acute systemic illness

Relative Contraindications

1. Significant pulmonary hypertension
2. Significant arterial hypertension
3. Tachyarrhythmias or bradyarrhythmias
4. Moderate valvular heart disease
5. Myocardial heart disease
6. Electrolyte abnormalities
7. Left main coronary obstruction
8. Hypertrophic cardiomyopathy
9. Psychiatric disease

TABLE 32–6 Bruce Protocol*

Stage	Grade (%)	Speed (mph)	Time (min)	Total Time (min)
1	10	1.7	3	3
2	12	2.5	3	6
3	14	3.4	3	9
4	16	4.2	3	12
5	18	5.0	3+	15+

* For each stage, both the grade and the speed are increased every 3 min.

cardiac contraindications can be overcome with some of the newer techniques of applying cardiac stress or recording methods. The basic principle of all exercise stress testing is to cause an increase in the $M\dot{V}O_2$ through the physiological response to exercise, which can induce myocardial ischemia, which can then be detected via the electrocardiogram (ECG).

Exercise Protocols. Exercise protocols are normally designed with 3 to 5-minute stages in order to achieve a steady-state response.[35] Protocols usually include a warm-up period of low-intensity exercise, and end with a cool-down period of suitable length. The exercise protocol needs to be tailored to the individual patient and should allow testing of patients with very limited cardiac reserve, as well as patients with excellent aerobic conditioning.

Treadmill Protocols. The most commonly used treadmill protocol is the Bruce protocol[26, 34] (Table 32–6). The main limitations of this protocol include the large increases in $\dot{V}O_2$ [5 METs; 1 MET is defined as the resting metabolic rate (approximately 3.5 mL O_2/kg body weight/min)] between stages, and the additional cost of energy in running that occurs in Bruce stage III and above.[13] Other protocols are available to overcome these limitations in patients with disability or limited cardiac reserve. The Naughton, Weber, and Balke-Ware protocols use 1 to 2-minute stages that have 1-MET increments. These protocols are sometimes better tolerated by patients with CHF, deconditioning, or other causes of limited exercise tolerance. The Cornell protocol is a modification of the Bruce protocol with increments in 2-minute stages, allowing a better estimate of ST segment-HR measurements.[70] A comparison of the various protocols is found in Table 32–7.

Bicycle Ergometry. The most common alternative to treadmill protocols is bicycle ergometry. The advantages include better ECG and blood pressure recording, chiefly because the patient's chest and arms remain relatively stable. The influence of the patient's weight is less, and a bicycle often takes up less room in the laboratory than a treadmill. Bicycle ergometry can also be performed with the patient lying supine. Disadvantages include difficulty with bicycle pedaling owing to incoordination or fatigue.[69] Another limitation is the artificial elevation of RPP and systolic BP at a given level of submaximum $\dot{V}O_2$, while maximum $M\dot{V}O_2$ is approximately 10% greater on the treadmill.[68] Table 32–8 is a comparison of the alternative tests discussed in this chapter.

TABLE 32–7 Comparison of Exercise Tolerance Testing Protocols

	Bruce	Cornell	Weber	Balke-Ware	Naughton
Time of stages	3 min	2 min	2 min	1 min	2 min
MET level	2 to >16	2–16	1–10	4–16	2–7 at 2 mph 3–16 at 3 mph 4–16 at 3.4 mph
Step changes	2 MET steps from 2 to 7 MET 3 MET steps from 7 to >16 MET	2 MET	1 MET	1/2 MET	1 MET
Changes grade	Yes	Yes	Yes	Yes	Yes
Range of grade	0–20%	0–18%	0–15%	1–26%	0–17.5% at 2 mph 0–32.5% at 3 mph 0–26% at 4 mph
Step changes	5% from 0% to 10% 2% from 10% to 20%	5% from 0% to 10% 1% from 10% to 18%	3.5% from 0% to 10.5% (2 mph) 2.5% from 7.5% to 15% (3 mph) 14% fixed at 3.4 mph	1% from 1% to 26%	3.5% from 0% to 17.5% (2 mph) 2.5% from 0% to 32.5% (3 mph) 2% from 2% to 26% (3.4 mph)
Changes speed	Yes	Yes	Yes	No	No
Range of speed	1.7–5.5 mph	1.7–5.0 mph	1.0–3.4 mph	Constant 3.3 mph	2, 3, or 4 mph
Step changes	0.8 mph	0.4 mph	0.5 mph		
NYHA functional classes tested	Normal, I, II, III	Normal, I, II, III	Normal, I, II, III, IV	Normal, I, II, mild III	Normal, I, II, III

In all forms of ETT, it is important that the patient not hold the handrail or handlebars, since an exaggerated cardiac response is caused by the isometric hand grip. This can cause the functional capacity to be overestimated by as much as 20%.[13]

Upper Extremity Ergometry. The main advantage of this type of ETT is that it can be used for patients who have orthopedic, vascular, or neurological disabilities and cannot perform the standard treadmill or bicycle test. Typical subjects for this type of testing include patients with amputation, spinal cord injury, arthritis, and recent orthopedic procedures. The physiological effects of upper extremity ergometry are different from those seen in treadmill exercise testing. The RPP is elevated in upper extremity ergometry due to a greater increase in the systolic BP than HR. This effect is thought to be due to the increase in vascular tone seen in the non-exercising vascular beds. There is also less increase in CO during upper extremity ergometry than in treadmill exercise testing.[3]

Preparation for Stress Testing. Although the techniques of stress testing vary slightly from laboratory to laboratory, there are some basic rules that generally apply. Patients should not eat or have caffeinated beverages for at least three hours before a stress test. Patients should wear comfortable, loose-fitting clothes and comfortable walking shoes. A 12-lead ECG is taken before the test and a limited physical examination is performed. Supine and erect ECGs with the torso electrodes are typically obtained to ensure that there are no changes in the ECG based solely on position changes. The patient is taught how to ambulate on the treadmill or use the ergometer. Vital signs and ECGs are taken before, at each stage of the test, at the conclusion of the exercise, and during the recovery period.

ECG Criteria. The normal lead placement in cardiac stress testing is the modified 12-lead system. The hallmark of ischemia on the exercise cardiogram is ST segment depression. ST depressions of 2 mm or more in one lead is a positive test[13] (Fig. 32–13). Not all ST

TABLE 32–8 Advantages and Disadvantages of Alternative Test Devices

Test	Bicycle Ergometry	Upper Extremity Ergometry	Treadmill	Pharmacological Agents
Advantages	Has good correlation with treadmill testing Thorax and arms remain stable Less effect of patient body weight	Useful for patients with orthopedic, vascular, or neurological conditions who cannot perform leg exercise	Readily available Well standardized Multiple protocols available Can be used for ramp protocols	Can be used in all patients, even the most deconditioned or impaired Good reliability Well standardized
Disadvantages	Patient may not be able to learn to bicycle MV_{O_2} 6–25% less than in treadmill exercise Greater cardiac stress (rate pressure product) for a given V_{O_2} Bicycle takes up space in laboratory	Less increase in cardiac output than in treadmill testing Greater rate pressure product increase than in treadmill testing	Overweight, orthopedic, neurological, vascular, or arthritic patients may not be able to reach acceptable exercise levels	Not physiological Some risks involved, depending on the agent Invasive Need to have special imaging equipment and properly equipped and staffed laboratory

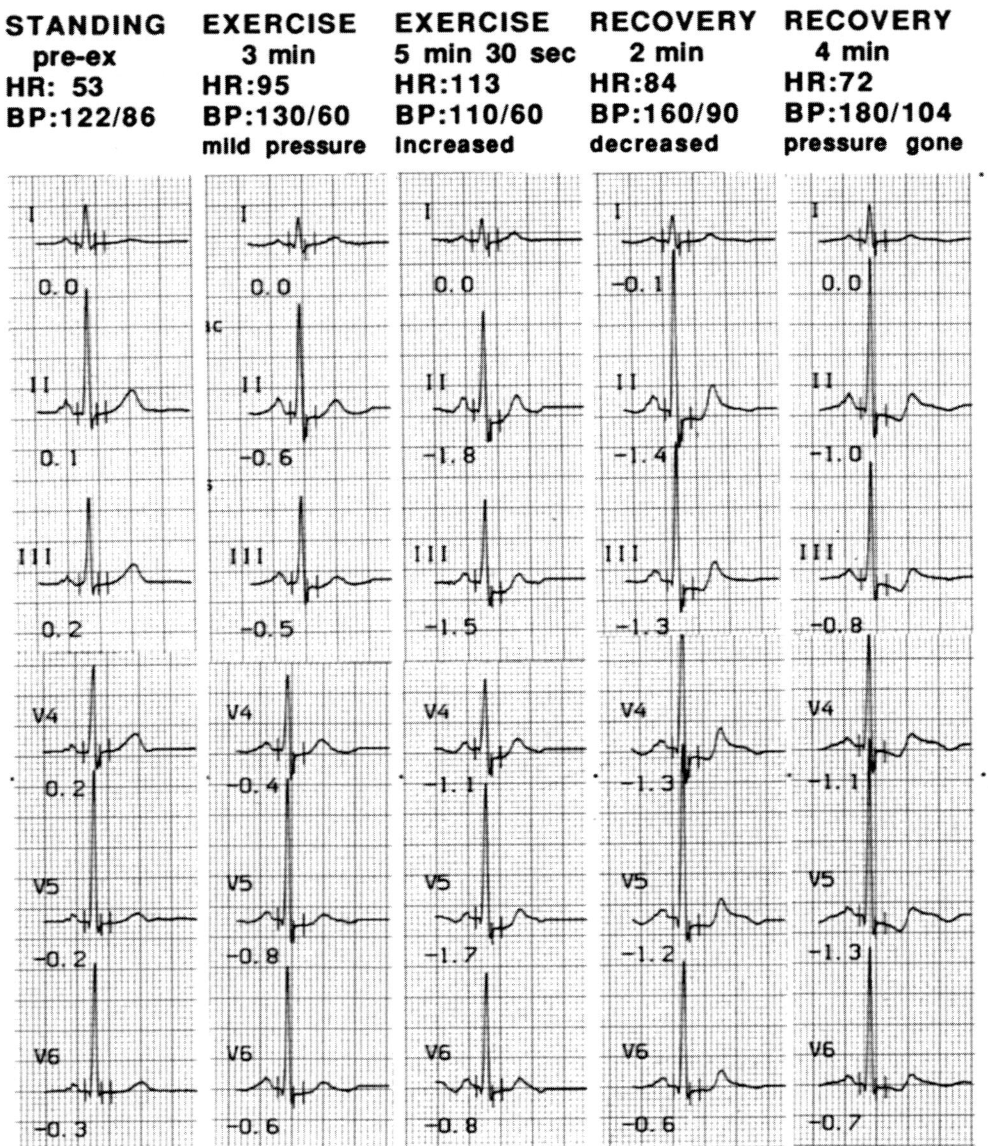

FIGURE 32–13. Electrocardiographic changes of ischemia during exercise testing in a 71-year-old man with exertional chest pain: progressive ST segment depression with upsloping contour is noted during exercise. The ST depression becomes horizontal during recovery with partial T wave inversion. (Courtesy of David Blood, M.D.)

depression is of cardiac origin.[13] Other abnormalities can also be seen in patients during exercise stress testing, such as ST elevation, upsloping ST segments, and variation of the R wave amplitude. In the absence of a previous MI or Q wave, ST elevation is a marker of high-grade stenosis or coronary vasospasm causing transmural ischemia. ST segment elevation in a lead with an abnormal Q wave can be seen in patients with poor left ventricular function.[16] It is also seen in up to 30% of patients with anterior wall MI and 15% of patients with inferior wall MI tested within 2 weeks of MI (it decreases after six weeks). ST segment elevation in these Q wave leads is not a marker of cardiac ischemia.[41] Upsloping of ST segments is a normal finding in the ECG during maximum exercise. The finding of a slowly upsloping ST segment after a 1.5-mm ST depression is an indicator of probable ischemia.[19] The changes in R wave amplitude during exercise are relatively nonspecific. When the R wave meets the criteria for left ventricular hypertrophy (LVH), ST segment response is not usable for the diagnosis of ischemia, and loss of R wave in a lead after MI reduces the prognostic use of that particular lead for ischemic changes after MI.

Non-ECG Criteria. In addition to the ECG, there are other clinical factors to observe during the performance of the ETT. Blood pressure and symptoms of chest discomfort are also important. The important data that need to be determined during the stress test include the maximum work capacity, the RPP, and the HR response. The BP in normal exercise increases progressively with increasing workload. The failure of systolic BP to increase appropriately can be a sign of ischemia or of left ventricular dysfunction.[26, 34] A fall in the systolic BP with increasing load is an indication for aborting the ETT. Nonischemic causes of fall in systolic BP in ETT include cardiomyopathy, cardiac arrhythmias, vasovagal reaction, left ventricular outflow tract obstruction, use of antihypertensive drugs, hypovolemia, and prolonged vigorous exercise. The diastolic BP does not change significantly in normal patients during exercise. A rise in diastolic BP in a stress test can be associated with ischemia.

There should be a gradual decline in the systolic BP after exercise. In up to 3% of healthy normal adults, profound post-exercise hypotension can occur that is not due to CAD.[30]

Although chest pain starts after the onset of ST depression in most cases, chest pain can be the only indicator of ischemia in some patients.[58] The presence of pain with no ECG changes is often an indication that nuclear or echocardiographic testing is needed.

The maximum work capacity can be determined during the ETT and serves as an important prognostic measurement, as well as a target for the maximum work during a rehabilitation program.[10, 62, 96] A limited exercise capacity in a patient with a known cardiac disease is associated with an increased risk of cardiac events and worse prognosis. The amount of work performed or the level reached is the best estimate of functional capacity. The time exercised is not as useful, as it is dependent on the test protocol used. Exercise impairment is determined by comparing the patient's performance to a table of normal levels adjusted for age, which is available in the literature for the specific exercise protocol employed[94] (Table 32–9). If serial determinations of exercise capacity are to be determined, the patient needs to have exactly the same protocol done each time, preferably administered by the same testing team in the same laboratory to minimize variation.

TABLE 32–9 Examples of Some Age-Adjusted Normal Fitness Levels

Study	Predicted MET	Age Range (yr) (Mean)	Protocol
Bruce	13.7–0.08 (age)	NA (44.4)	Bruce
Wolthius	13–0.05 (age)	25–54 (37)	Balke-Ware
Morris (<54 yr old)	18.8–0.17 (age)	21–53 (42)	USAFSAM
Morris	18.1–0.17 (age)	21–89 (57)	USAFSAM
Dehn	16.2–0.11 (age)	40–72 (52.2)	Mixed
Froelicher	13.1–0.08 (age)	20–53 (NA)	Balke-Ware

Abbreviations: USAFSAM, United States Air Force School of Aerospace Medicine; NA, not applicable.

Adapted from Froelicher VF: Exercise and the Heart. St Louis, Mosby–Year Book, 1987.

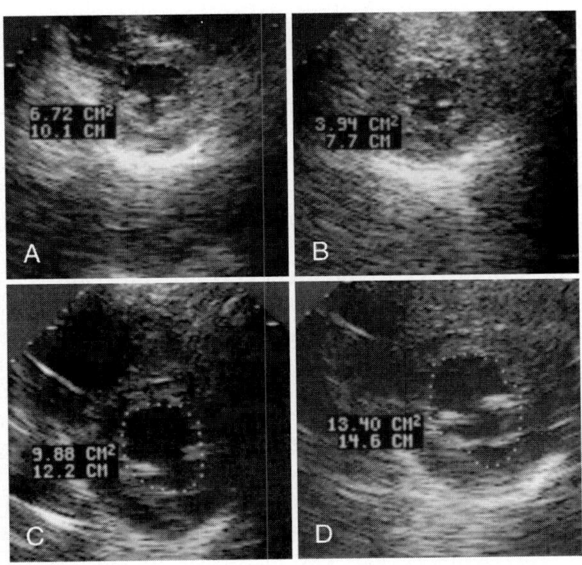

FIGURE 32–14. Echocardiographic changes of ischemia during exercise. *A.* End-systolic size of normal left ventricle at rest. *B.* Note smaller end-systolic size of the same heart during exercise. *C.* Resting end-systolic size of left ventricle of patient with coronary artery disease. *D.* Note increase in end-systolic size of ischemic ventricle during exercise. (Courtesy of ECHO Dx, Inc.)

Other Cardiac Stress Testing Techniques

Numerous alternatives procedures are now available for cardiac stress testing. These alternative techniques facilitate the cardiac stress testing of physically impaired or debilitated persons. They can also be used in situations in which the standard protocols are limited by patient anxiety or poor effort. New techniques for detecting cardiac ischemia allow testing in patients who previously had obstacles to assessment, such as left bundle branch block and abnormal baseline ECG.

Echocardiographic Stress Testing. Exercise echocardiography is one of the more commonly used techniques in exercise testing. There are three basic assumptions that underlie the use of echocardiography in stress testing: (1) Induction of ischemia will result in an area of ventricular dyssynergy; (2) these regional wall motion abnormalities are specific for ischemia; (3) changes in wall motion can be accurately seen on two-dimensional echocardiography[84] (Fig. 32–14). The evidence for the first two assumptions has been long-standing, and the improvement in technique and the addition of digital echocardiography have now verified the third assumption.[28] The exercise can be performed either on a treadmill or with a bicycle ergometer. Scanning can be done only before and after exercise with treadmill testing, while the bicycle allows for continuous monitoring and the detection of transient ischemic changes.[25, 44] Exercise echocardiography using newer techniques and digital imaging has a diagnostic sensitivity of 74% to 97% and specificity of 64% to 100%. This compares favorably with the results of stress ECG.[84] The test is particularly useful in situations in which the stress ECG is ambiguous or nondiagnostic, in women (who have a higher likelihood of a false-positive ECG test), and in those having an abnormal resting ECG.

Nuclear Stress Testing. Thallium-201 perfusion scintigraphy is widely accepted for the detection of ischemia in CAD. It is more accurate than the use of stress echocardiography alone.[45, 81] The imaging is typically performed in conjunction with a treadmill test.[60] It can also be done with dipyridamole and adenosine pharmacological stress testing (see below).[38, 56] Comparisons of findings on ECG, radionuclide ventriculography, and thallium-201 scanning during exercise on a treadmill or bicycle ergometer have demonstrated that the diagnosis with scintigraphy is more accurate than when done by ECG alone.[8, 11]

The physiological basis behind the use of thallium-201 scintigraphy is the uptake of thallium-201 in the cardiac myocyte via the Na^+,K^+-ATPase pump. The first-pass extraction of thallium-201 from the blood is 85%, and it is continuously exchanged.[95] This means that images taken early and late after injection provide different pathophysiological data. The immediate images give information about regional myocardial blood flow, while the delayed images (2 to 24 hours) show distribution of the potassium pool and reflect myocardial viability[13] (Fig. 32–15). Thallium-201 testing offers the advantage of being able to image all patients regardless of habitus, and can often be done in patients in whom echocardiography cannot be performed. It can also be used during both exercise and pharmacological types of stress testing. The disadvantages of thallium-201 scanning are that it is an invasive procedure, it is a radioactive agent with a long half-life, and it requires expensive and complex imaging equipment.[102] Because of the poor sensitivity of ECG recording alone with upper extremity ergometry, the test is usually performed with thallium-201 scintigraphy.[5, 6]

Pharmacological Stress Testing. Among the most common and perhaps the best types of diagnostic stress testing available for the physically impaired are the pharmacological stress tests. Although their usefulness for functional evaluation and for exercise prescription in rehabilitation programs is questionable, they can be used for diagnosis of CAD and for risk stratification. The earliest tests used dipyridamole, but in recent years other agents have been tested and have gained acceptance. The main advantage of the use of these agents for cardiac stress testing is that a patient can be tested regardless of ability to perform adequate levels of exercise. The usual methodologies call for simultaneous use of cardiac imaging and follow distinct protocols.

Dipyridamole has been well studied as a pharmacological agent to induce cardiac stress, most often when used in conjunction with thallium-201 scintigraphy.[1, 56] It has been used for detection of CAD, cardiac risk stratification, and peri-operative risk evaluation. There have been proposed protocols for the use of thallium-201 scintigraphy with dipyridamole and the simultaneous application of isometric hand grip or low-level exercise to increase the accuracy of those tests.[14, 18] The mechanism of action of dipyridamole is via its activity as a coronary artery vasodilator, especially of the smaller arterioles.[27] The development of ischemia in the cardiac vessels results from differential vasodilation of the cardiac arteries and arterioles. Dipyridamole causes normal vessels to dilate, but the diseased vascular beds do not have the capacity to further dilate. This phenomenon

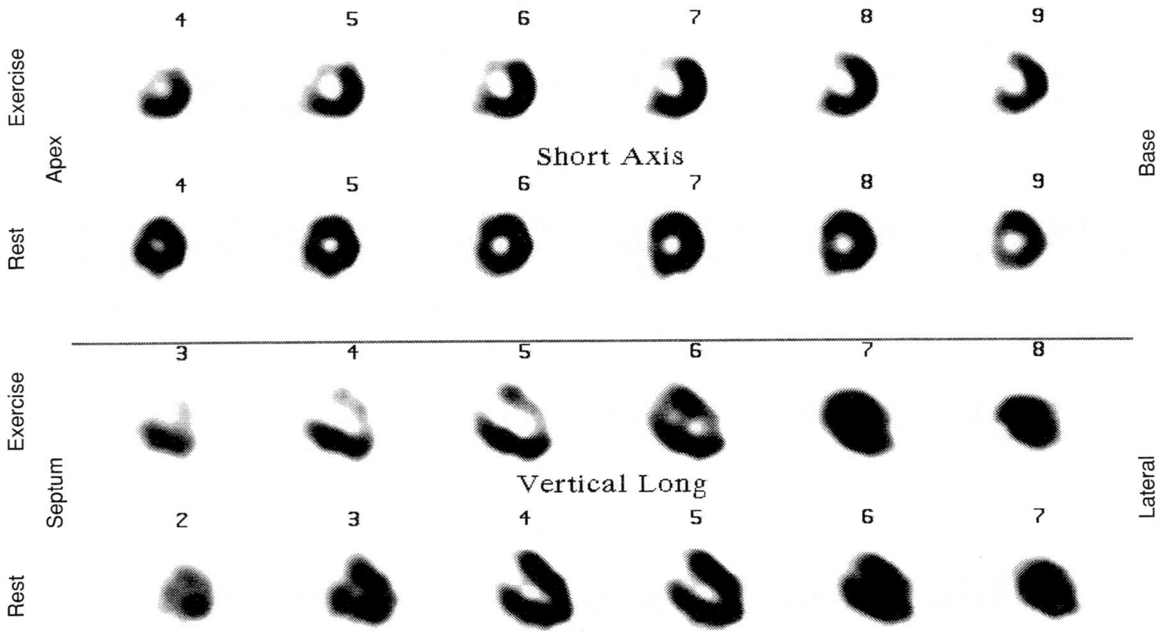

FIGURE 32–15. Exercise and redistribution myocardial perfusion SPECT scans using thallium-201: diminished thallium uptake in the septum, anterior wall, and apex of the left ventricle is seen after exercise injection of thallium-201. The thallium uptake normalizes at rest (redistribution), reflecting exercise-induced ischemia in the distribution of the left anterior descending artery. (Courtesy of David Blood, M.D.)

TABLE 32–10 Sample Dipyridamole Protocol

Thallium-201 Imaging

0.142 mg/kg/min infusion intravenously over 4 min (0.568 mg/kg total dose)
Thallium imaging performed at 10 min, 4 hr, and, depending on protocol, 12–24 hr
Isometric hand grip exercises may be performed simultaneously with the infusion
Continuous ECG and vital sign monitoring is done throughout the test

Echocardiography

High-dose protocol may be followed
0.142 mg/kg/min infusion intravenously over 4 min (0.568 mg/kg total dose), followed by 4 min of no infusion, followed by 0.142 mg/kg/min infusion intravenously over 2 min (0.282 mg/kg supplemental dose) for a total of 0.850 mg/kg over 10 min
2-Dimensional echocardiography is performed continuously throughout the infusion and for 10 min after the infusion is completed
Continuous ECG and vital sign monitoring is done throughout the test

is described as cardiac steal. A typical dipyridamole protocol is shown in Table 32–10. The dosage of dipyridamole in this protocol increases blood flow 3 to 5 times the resting level. Continuous ECG and BP monitoring is done during the procedure. Initial imaging is done at 12 to 35 minutes, followed by delayed imaging at 180 to 240 minutes[39] (Fig. 32–16).

The use of echocardiography with dipyridamole stress testing is gaining popularity. The same basic instructions pertain to the performance of the test, but a "high-dose" protocol for the administration of dipyridamole has been developed to increase the sensitivity.[61, 78] A positive test is one in which areas of transient asynergy arise or worsen from baseline on the echocardiogram.

Adenosine is a powerful vasodilator and causes its effects by its action on receptors in blood vessels, including both a vascular smooth muscle receptor and an endothelial cell receptor.[7] Dipyridamole and adenosine work similarly in the cardiac circulation. The major advantage of adenosine via intravenous (IV) administration is that it has a rapid onset of action and a brief half-life of only 10 to 30 seconds. This short duration of action allows for repeated measurements, which is an advantage over dipyridamole testing. Adenosine raises coronary blood flow by a factor of 4.4 times, which is close to the maximum coronary blood flow reserve.

The mechanism of action of *dobutamine,* a synthetic catecholamine, is via the β_1-, β_2-, and α_1-adrenergic receptors. Dobutamine has strong β_1, moderate β_2, and mild α_1 stimulation.[83, 90] In the heart, β_1 stimulation leads to increased inotropy and chronotropy while α_1 stimulation causes only a mild increase in inotropy, and β_2 stimulation yields moderate coronary vasodilation. As a result, IV dobutamine causes increased SV and CO, increasing the RPP. Dobutamine also increases SV and ejection fraction, resulting in decreased end-systolic volume, decreasing wall stress and $M\dot{V}O_2$. BP usually remains relatively constant with dobutamine infusion, as β_2 stimulation decreases systemic vascular resistance and sympathetic tone decreases owing to the increased CO. The rationale for the use of dobutamine as a pharmacological stressor lies in its ability to elevate the RPP by raising both inotropy and chronotropy. Dobutamine

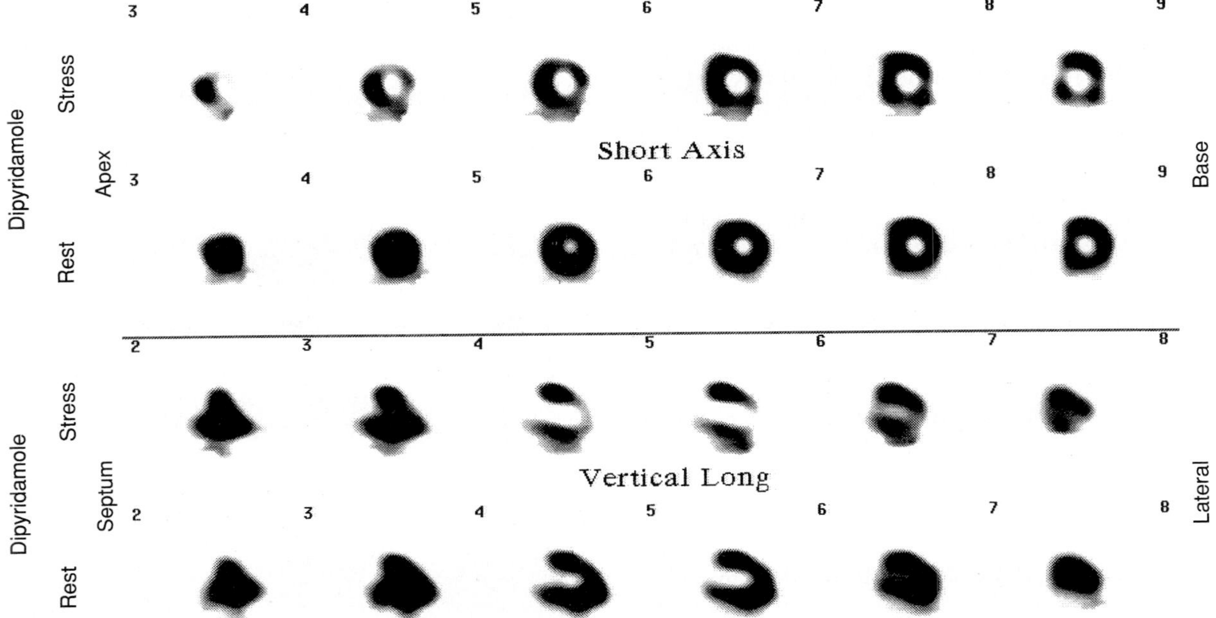

FIGURE 32–16. Pharmacological stress and redistribution myocardial perfusion SPECT scans using thallium-201: diminished thallium uptake in the anterolateral wall and apex of the left ventricle after injection of thallium-201 during dipyridamole coronary vasodilatation (stress). The thallium uptake normalizes at rest (redistribution). These findings reflect severe stenosis of a large diagonal branch of the left anterior descending artery. (Courtesy of David Blood, M.D.)

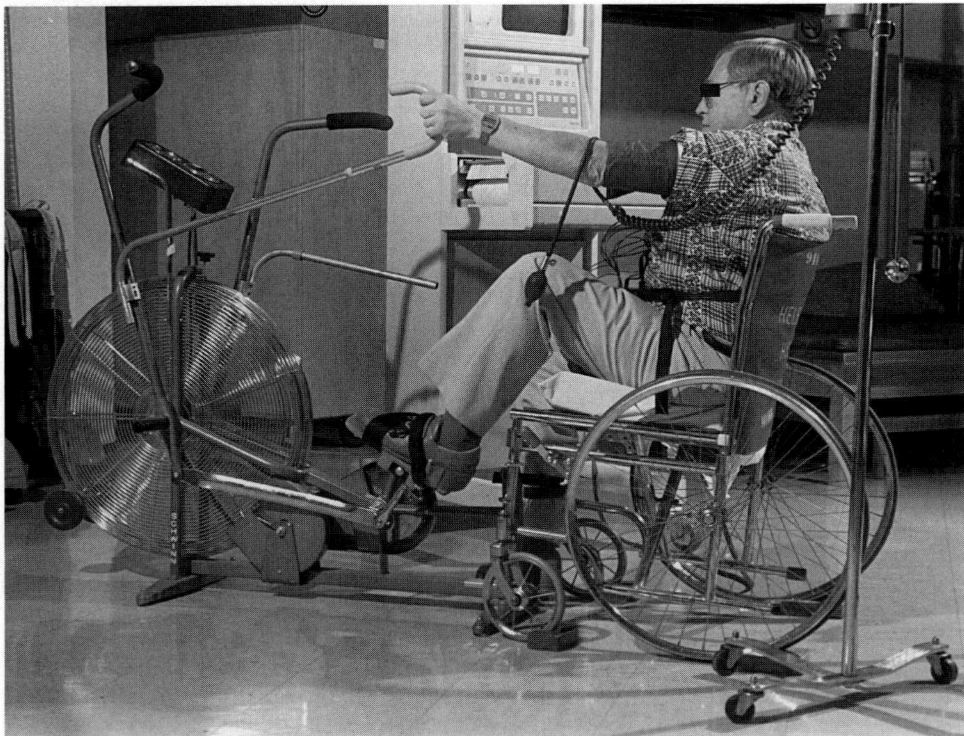

FIGURE 32–17. Exercise tolerance testing with an adapted Airdyne bicycle ergometer (Schwinn).

has been shown to be relatively safe in patients with CAD, even in the perimyocardial infarction period.[21, 99]

The final determination of the best agent to test any given patient still must be decided on a case-by-case basis. All of the various agents described previously have their advantages and offer the ability to test the severely impaired or deconditioned patient who might be encountered in a physiatric practice.

Isometric Hand Grip Test. This test uses the isometric contraction of the upper extremity with a dynamometer to provide an exercise stress. Typically, the test is performed with the patient squeezing the dynamometer at one-fourth to three-fourths of maximum hand strength for as long as tolerated.[26] The isometric exercise increases the RPP by increasing both HR and BP. The ejection fraction does not normally change, and some studies show that a decline of 5% in the ejection fraction can occur in some patients.[14, 77] This variation in the ejection fraction response means that some of the major imaging studies used to assess the heart for ischemia are of limited use after this type of cardiac stress. In addition, since this technique does not provoke ischemia as effectively as some of the other available tests, it should be used only in select cases.[52]

Modifications for the Physically Disabled

Exercise tolerance testing for the physically disabled is especially challenging because of the restrictions created by weakness, limb availability, balance problems, and spasticity. Echocardiographic and nuclear testing increase the sensitivity of testing performed on various exercise devices, partially compensating for the reduced workloads achieved. Devices which have been used successfully include the arm crank ergometer, an adapted Schwinn Airdyne (Fig. 32–17),[12, 53] a supine bicycle ergometer (Fig. 32–18),[65] and a wheelchair ergometer (Fig. 32–19).[36]

Assessment of Cardiac Demands of Activities

Direct assessment of the cardiac demands of various activities is technically difficult. The use of the RPP or HR gives a reasonable estimate of the relative stress on the coronary circulation by correlation with $M\dot{V}O_2$, and these numbers can be used in conjunction with the patient's ETT to judge the safety of the activity in relation

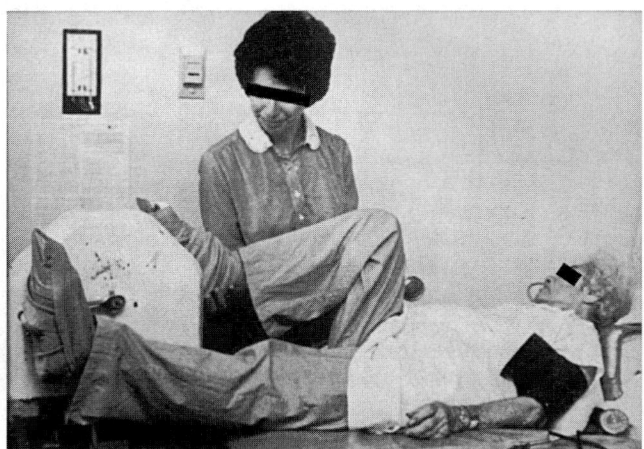

FIGURE 32–18. Exercise tolerance testing with a supine bicycle ergometer.

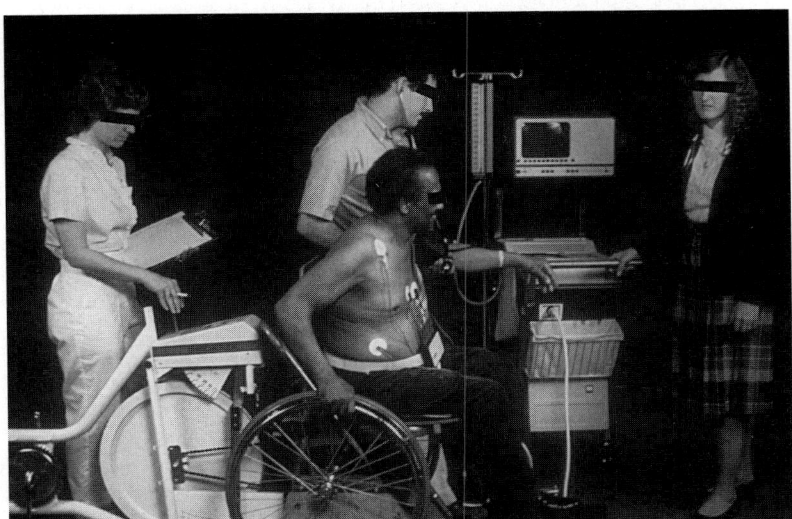

FIGURE 32–19. Exercise tolerance testing with a wheelchair ergometer. (Courtesy of Majorie King, M.D.)

to the anginal threshold. The information obtained in this manner is highly individualized and can be correlated to functional activities through the use of tables of metabolic demands of various self-care, mobility, vocational, and avocational activities[37] (Table 32–11). These tables usually express the metabolic demands of the activities in METs (1 MET = approximately 3.5 mL O_2/kg body weight/min).

The rationale for using these tables for cardiac patients is the linear relationship between the $M\dot{V}O_2$ and the $\dot{V}O_2$, as noted above. The fallacy in the use of these tables comes from ignoring the fact that the linear relationship holds true only for a single activity performed at varying intensities under the same conditions. A MET level achieved safely on a treadmill ETT doesn't always correlate with the MET level that might be achieved during upper extremity activities without crossing the anginal threshold. A treadmill test cannot be used to evaluate a subject who must perform at a high MET level with the upper extremities (e.g., a carpenter). The $M\dot{V}O_2$ is also higher for any given activity if performed under conditions of emotional or physiological stress. The use of MET tables can give useful information about the relative metabolic demands of various activities, but they must be used with caution and an awareness of the physiological limitations involved.

TABLE 32–11 A Typical MET Table

Activity	MET
Lying quietly	1.0
Sitting at ease	1.2–1.6
Sitting writing	1.9–2.2
Standing at ease	1.4–2.0
Walking 1 mph	2.3
Standing, washing, and shaving	2.5–2.6
Standing, dressing, and undressing	2.3–3.3
Light housework	1.7–3.0
Heavy housework	3.0–6.0
Office work	1.3–2.5
Walking 2 mph	3.1
Light industrial work	2.0–5.0
Walking 3 mph	4.3

CARDIAC REHABILITATION PROGRAMS

Risk Factor Modification

In addition to exercise training, all cardiac rehabilitation programs should emphasize patient and family education for risk factor reduction and lifestyle modification. The material must be presented in a format suitable for the patient's learning style, and material must be repeated as necessary until the patient gains mastery of the techniques. These patients are under a great deal of stress related to their medical illnesses, and should not be expected to assimilate major lifestyle recommendations with a single series of lectures or brochures. In the past, the goal of this part of the program was only to slow the progression of the disease; however, Ornish et al and Hambrecht et al, reporting on a very low-fat vegetarian diet[71, 72] and a more vigorous exercise program with less severe fat restriction, respectively,[42] have actually shown regression of stenotic lesions. In both of these studies, control groups showed progression of the stenoses.

Smoking cessation is an essential ingredient of cardiac rehabilitation. For those who discontinue smoking, the risk of recurrent cardiac events falls by about 50% in one year and approaches that of nonsmokers in two years.[64] Elevated BP should be normalized. Other pharmacological interventions including beta-blockers or angiotensin-converting enzyme inhibitors can be helpful, especially for patients with low ejection fractions.[63] Physical activity should be encouraged with a regular aerobic conditioning program. As noted above, a relatively short-term exercise program can increase work capacity and exercise safety. A more prolonged program can, in some instances, increase myocardial perfusion.[85]

Elevated blood lipids should be lowered by pharmacological or dietary intervention. A number of pharmacological trials have demonstrated clear benefit, as indicated by reduction in cardiac events and by angiographic measurement of stenoses.[64] Of particular note is the observation that the reduction in cardiac events exceeds the reduction in stenosis size, suggesting an effect on plaque stabilization which reduces the risk of plaque rupture.[64] Although reduction of dietary fat from the average of 37% of caloric intake to 30% is estimated to have only limited benefit in terms of life expectancy,[15] more significant fat reduction does have clear benefit.[71, 72] The Ornish diet consists of just 10% of caloric intake as fat. While many Americans might not find this palatable, further studies on diets consisting of 10% to 30% intake as fat could help to find a generally acceptable compromise.

Stress management has been recognized as an important component of these programs since Friedman first described the type A behavior pattern.[33] In later refinements of his diagnostic criteria, he has emphasized impatience and free-floating hostility as the key elements of this behavior pattern, rather than ambition and competitive drive. He reports that counseling directed toward these behavior patterns can produce a significant reduction in coronary morbidity and mortality.[33] The Ornish program includes the following stress management techniques: stretching exercises, breathing techniques, meditation, progressive relaxation, and imagery.[71] A similar approach is used in Kabat-Zinn's Stress Reduction Clinic at the University of Massachusetts Medical Center.[47] Recent studies of the effects of the addition of psychosocial interventions for individuals with CAD have demonstrated significant reductions in morbidity and mortality in the first two years post MI.[57] In these studies maintenance of stress management practice is as important as maintenance of exercise training. The protective effect is lost within six months if the practice is discontinued.[32] The mechanism of the protective effect is presumably through a reduction in the activation of the sympathetic nervous system.[64]

Primary Prevention Programs

Programs designed to intervene before the clinical onset of CAD have the greatest opportunity for producing major alterations in the natural history of the disease. The program should consist of identification and modification of risk factors, dietary counseling, stress management training, and instruction in a sustainable exercise regimen. Evaluation of the long-term benefits of such a program is difficult due to the self-selection process typically involved in entering and maintaining such a program. Based on the results reported by Paffenbarger,[74] Hambrecht,[42] and Ornish[71, 72] and their coworkers, it would seem reasonable to expect significant benefit from the application of the same principles in this setting with little risk of harm. The American Heart Association in their recent position papers advocate primary prevention through the institution of exercise programs. Moderate-intensity activities (40 to 60% of maximum $\dot{V}O_2$) performed for 20 to 30 minutes 3 to 4 times a week are sufficient.[31]

Rehabilitation Following Myocardial Infarction

The rehabilitation program following MI is the classic model for cardiac rehabilitation. It can be divided into four phases: (1) the acute in-hospital phase beginning in the cardiac care unit (CCU); (2) the convalescent phase continuing the program at home until a strong scar has formed on the damaged myocardium; (3) the training phase using aerobic conditioning to increase the patient's physical work capacity; and (4) the maintenance phase, where the gains achieved by training are sustained by regular exercise. Patient education aimed at risk factor reduction and lifestyle modification is included during each of these phases.

Acute Phase. Early mobilization of the patient with an acute MI was introduced by Wenger.[97] Instead of the traditional 4 to 6 weeks of bed rest after acute MI (longer in some countries), her program took patients from bed rest in the CCU to climbing two flights of stairs in 14 days. A Swiss study compared outcomes of two groups of patients: one mobilized early with a modified Wenger program, while the other managed with the then-accepted six months of rest.[9] At the end of one year, there was no difference in mortality and morbidity between the two groups, demonstrating the safety of early mobilization. Although there was no difference in physical work capacity between the two groups, there was a significantly higher return-to-work rate in the group of patients who were mobilized early. The authors' suggestion that the difference was mostly due to an improved psychological adjustment was confirmed by later studies.

Early mobilization programs have been modified dramatically during the past decade due to the effects of more aggressive interventional cardiology and the pressure of managed care for shorter lengths of stay. Many patients with uncomplicated infarctions have cardiac catheterization followed by angioplasty or bypass surgery. Those who do not have procedures are often discharged in 3 to 6 days, which greatly modifies the original Wenger program. Table 32–12 shows the original program and a shortened version. There is a gradual daily increase in exercise intensity, which progresses as long as there are no arrhythmias, congestive heart failure, or ischemia. Patients are monitored with ECG telemetry during each increase in exercise level. The schedule obviously has to be altered if complications occur. In this phase, the goal is to progress the patient gradually and safely from the initial bed rest of the CCU to a level consistent with most activities of daily living. By mobilizing the patient early, deconditioning from excessive bed rest and psychological invalidism are reduced or eliminated. Actual exercise training for a higher work capacity is not a goal of this phase. It is imperative that the educational programs for risk factor modification be introduced at this time.

Convalescent Phase. During the convalescent phase, the goal is to maintain early mobilization and gradually to increase the endurance for exercise at the same intensity used at the end of the acute phase program. This is usually walking or bicycling using a target HR taught

TABLE 32–12 Summary of Early Mobilization Program

Day	Wenger	Beth-Israel
1	Passive range of motion (ROM), active ankle exercise; self-feeding, orientation to program.	Sit at edge of bed, dangle, AAROM, wash to waist with assist, use commode, in chair for 30 min.
2	Same exercise; legs dangling at side of bed.	Wash to waist without assist, AROM, sit in chair for 60 min 2×, eat independently, ambulate with PT 30–50 feet.
3	Active assisted ROM; sitting in chair, bedside commode; more detailed explanation of program; light recreation.	All of above, plus increase ambulation to 100 feet 2× per day, bathroom privileges.
4	Minimal resistance; increase sitting time; patient education; light craft activities.	Continue all of above, increase ambulation to 150 feet 2× per day.
5	Moderate resistance; unlimited sitting, sitting for meals, seated ADL activities; continued patient education.	Add stairs, ½ to 1 flight if indicated as part of discharge plan.
6	Increase resistance, walking to bathroom; standing ADL; group meetings up to 1 hr.	
7	Standing warm-up exercises, walking 100 ft at comfortable pace; tub bath; walking to group meetings.	
8	Increase active standing exercise, increase ambulation, walk down stairs (take elevator up); continue education program.	
9	Increase exercise program; review energy-conservation and pacing techniques.	
10	Increase exercises with light weights and increase walking distance; increase craft activities; discuss home exercise program.	
11	Increase duration of each activity.	
12	Increase walking down stairs to 2 flights; increase resistance used in exercises.	
13	Continue same activities.	
14	Walk up 1 flight of stairs and down; complete instructions for home exercise program and pacing of activities.	

at the end of the acute phase and known to be within the patient's safe capacity. In an uncomplicated case, this phase lasts for about six weeks from the time of the infarction. This allows time for a firm scar to form on the infarcted area, thereby reducing the risk of ventricular aneurysm or wall rupture.

Training Phase. This is the actual exercise training program—the program most people associate with cardiac rehabilitation. It begins with a symptom-limited ETT to screen out patients with contraindications for exercise training. These include dangerous arrhythmias or a drop in BP with increasing exercise intensity. The results of the ETT are also used to determine a target HR for exercise training. If the maximum HR achieved on the ETT is limited only by a relatively benign endpoint such as fatigue, musculoskeletal pain, or angina preceding ECG changes, a target HR as high as 85% of the maximum HR can be used. If the endpoint is a serious arrhythmia or ECG changes without chest pain, a lower target HR should be chosen. Target heart rates as low as 60% of maximum can result in effective training. It is critical for patient safety that target heart rates in this population be based on actual ETTs, not tables or equations estimating maximum rates from the patient's age. Monitoring with ECG telemetry is usually used with each upgrading of the exercise prescription, but continuous monitoring is not necessary for each session. The patient can be taught to monitor HR (using the carotid pulse) or to use the Borg scale (Table 32–13).

As noted, the improvements in the cardiac response to exercise that result from aerobic training occur only when the muscles involved with the training are used. It is necessary to individualize each patient's program to include the muscle groups necessary for vocational and avocational goals. A generic treadmill or bicycle exercise program cannot meet everyone's needs.

The usual training program calls for three sessions a week for 6 to 8 weeks. Each session should start with a stretching program, followed by an aerobic program. The aerobic program can use equipment such as treadmills, upper or lower extremity ergometers, Airdynes, rowing machines, walking, running, and calisthenics. Each exercise should have a warm-up period, a training period at target HR, and a cool-down period.

TABLE 32–13 The Borg Scale of Perceived Exertion

Score	Perceived Exertion
6	Very very light
7	
8	Very light
9	
10	Fairly light
11	
12	Somewhat hard
13	
14	Hard
15	
16	Very hard
17	
18	Very very hard
19	
20	

Maintenance Phase. The maintenance phase is probably the most important phase of all—if it is neglected, the benefits of the training phase are lost within a few weeks. This part of the program needs to be addressed before the patient starts training, and a commitment to continue with the maintenance program must be obtained from the patient in order to justify the time and expense of the training program. The actual exercises included should reflect the selection of muscles trained in the preceding period and should fit within the interests and lifestyle of the individual patient. The minimum requirement is exercise at least twice a week and preferably three times a week for at least 30 minutes. ECG monitoring is not necessary during this phase.

Rehabilitation of the Patient with Angina Pectoris

Rehabilitation of the patient with stable angina can begin once the medical regimen has been optimized. As explained above (see Fig. 32–12), an aerobic training program results in an improved work capacity for these patients, even though there is no effect on the anginal threshold. An educational program for risk factor modification should be an integral part of the overall program. The exercise program begins with the ETT and then progresses with the training and maintenance programs as outlined above for the post-MI patient.

Rehabilitation Following Bypass Surgery

In the post-bypass surgery patient, cardiac rehabilitation can provide benefit by several mechanisms[46] (Table 32–14). Since patients who have just undergone CABG usually have not had a recent MI and have just been revascularized, they make excellent candidates for cardiac rehabilitation.[98] Complicating issues to remember in the post-CABG patient include the fact that the patient might have incomplete revascularization. With recent advances in surgical technique, there are now many patients with low ejection fractions who are undergoing the procedure. This means that the rehabilitation program must be individualized to meet each patient's needs. A symptom-limited ETT can be safely performed at 3 to 4 weeks after surgery to determine the level of exercise that a patient can tolerate.[24, 79, 93]

Cardiac rehabilitation after CABG can be thought of in two phases: the immediate postoperative period and the later maintenance phase. The in-hospital first phase is usually in the first week or so postoperatively, as patients are typically sent home after that period of time. The initial period can be thought of in three stages: (1) mobilization in the immediate postoperative period; (2) progressive ambulation and daily exercises; (3) discharge planning and exercise prescription for the maintenance stage.[46] Mobilization in the intensive care unit on postoperative day 1 (POD 1) includes sitting upright, active leg exercises, and mobilization out of bed. Only an unstable postoperative course or severe CHF should interfere with this early mobilization. This aggressive early intervention has several benefits, including decreasing the deleterious effects of bed rest such as deep venous thrombosis (DVT), pulmonary embolus (PE), pulmonary complications, and cardiac deconditioning.

The POD 2 to 5 program should include progressive ambulation and daily exercise. Ambulation begins with supervision for distances of 150 to 200 feet, followed by gradually progressive ambulation until most patients are starting independent ambulation by POD 3. Monitoring with ECG telemetry is usually used during the early mobilization. In the last few days prior to discharge, the patient and physician should develop a self-monitored home program that allows for gradual progression to previous levels of activity.

The second stage of a program for the post-CABG patient is conducted at home for the usual patient, or in an inpatient rehabilitation center for the high-risk patient or those who need more intensive interventions and monitoring.

Each patient can be in one of three types of programs: low, moderate, or high intensity. A low-intensity program is a progressive walking program with energy expenditures in the range of 2 to 4 METs, and a target HR of 65% to 75% of maximum HR. A moderate-intensity program is a progressive walk to walk-jog program from 3.0 to 6.5 METs, with target HR 70% to 80% of maximum HR. A high-intensity program is a progression from walk-jog to jogging from 5.0 to 8.5 METs, with a target HR of 75% to 85% of maximum HR. For a patient on a beta-blocker, the target HR is set at 20 beats per minute above the resting HR. Both objective criteria and patient observation in the postoperative period determine the assignment of patients to a level of exercise. A submaximum stress test before discharge is an important way to evaluate physiological response to submaximum effort.[46] The inpatient program has to be tailored to the specific needs of the patient and is best designed in cooperation with the patient's cardiologist.

TABLE 32–14 Benefits of Cardiac Rehabilitation After Bypass Surgery

Increased ischemic threshold
Improved left ventricular function
Increased coronary collaterals
Ameliorated serum lipids
Decreased serum catecholamines
Decreased platelet aggregation and increased fibrinolysis
Improved psychological status

Rehabilitation Following Cardiac Transplantation

As the techniques of cardiac transplantation have improved, the number of patients receiving transplants has increased. Five- and ten-year survival rates are now 82% and 74%, respectively.[43] Cardiac transplant patients are typically middle-aged, have suffered from months of preoperative invalidism, have generalized muscle weakness, and suffer from depression and anxiety. The transplant itself usually resolves the cardiac disability, but a comprehensive approach to the patient is necessary. The physiology of the post-transplant patient is unique. There is a loss of vagal inhibition to the sinoatrial node, with a resulting resting HR of about 100 beats per minute.[22] With increased exercise, the circulating catecholamine-induced chronotropic and inotropic responses increase CO.[17, 101] Post-transplant, there is a blunted HR response to an incremental exercise test, with peak HR 20% to 25% lower than in age-matched controls. Resting hypertension is common, due to the renal effects of cyclosporine, prednisone, and other medications.[88]

Transplant recipients usually have a 10% to 50% loss of lean body mass from inactivity and high-dose steroids in the perioperative period, with a resultant decrease of maximum work output and $\dot{V}O_{2max}$ by two-thirds.[51] At submaximum exercise levels, perceived exertion, minute ventilation, and the ventilatory equivalent for oxygen are all increased. $\dot{V}O_2$ is the same, however, implying earlier onset of anaerobic metabolism. At maximum effort there is lower work capacity, CO, HR, systolic BP, and $\dot{V}O_2$.

The cardiac training regimen in transplant patients should address overall conditioning as well as cardiac function. Walking, jogging, cycling, and swimming are commonly used exercises. The initial postoperative period encourages sitting upright, lower extremity exercises, and mobilization from the bed. The patient then starts ambulation, just as with the post-CABG patient. After discharge the patient uses self-monitoring to increase ambulation to one mile. The goal of the exercise program is to achieve a pace of 60% to 70% of peak effort for 30 to 60 minutes 3 to 5 times weekly.[49] The Borg level of perceived effort (see Table 32–13) should be maintained at 13 to 14, with activity increasing incrementally to stay at this level.

Other important aspects of the rehabilitation of cardiac transplant patients include the complicated medical regimen, psychological needs, vocational rehabilitation, and exercises for generalized weakness. There are significant musculoskeletal and neurological complaints (weakness, fatigue, low back pain).[82] The exercise conditioning program is aimed at helping to alleviate these complaints and to help prevent the accelerated atherosclerosis seen after transplantation.

The outcomes of rehabilitation in the cardiac transplant population have been generally favorable. The usual reports are of increased work output and improved exercise tolerance.[51, 54] Some transplant patients can even resume competitive-level athletics.[50] General well-being and quality of life have been demonstrated to be on the level of cardiac arrest survivors and post-MI patients: less than that of normals, but better than that of chronic low back pain patients[82] (see also Chapter 61).

Rehabilitation of the Patient with Cardiomyopathy

With increasingly aggressive cardiac care, the number of patients with a left ventricular ejection fraction of less than 30% has increased, and this group represents one of the fastest-growing subsets of the cardiac rehabilitation population.[75] Because these patients have poor left ventricular function, their complications and expectations are different from those of the post-CABG or post-MI population. They are at higher risk of sudden death and often are emotionally depressed because of their chronic cardiac disability.[20, 48, 73] Patients with heart failure demonstrate inconsistent responses to exercise.[89] Limited exercise capacity is one of the earliest findings in heart failure. The hemodynamic alterations seen with exercise do not always correlate with the overall exercise capacity.[59] The normal response to exercise is often absent. Exercise in heart failure can cause a drop in ejection fraction, a decrease in SV, and exertional hypotension. In the worst cases, CO might not be increased sufficiently to generate a dynamic exercise response.

Low endurance and fatigue are also a problem. After achieving a high aerobic workload, fatigue can persist for hours to days after the session.[23] Atrial fibrillation, fluid overload, or medication noncompliance can also decrease exercise tolerance. Despite these problems, there is documented benefit from exercise in this patient population.[23, 86] A gradual program of increasing the HR above resting level can be safely done, and increases oxygen extraction efficiency. Patients who have participated in cardiac rehabilitation programs have lower HRs during submaximum exercise, and increased maximum workloads.[55] The return to the ability to sustain activity at a low MET level can mean the difference between independent living and dependency.

The evaluation of the CHF patient consists of a graded ETT and can include measurements of left ventricular ejection fraction by multiple gated acquisition scanning (MUGA) or echocardiography during exercise. Unstable angina, decompensated CHF, and unstable arrhythmias are contraindications to cardiac rehabilitation. In the design of the rehabilitation program, certain aspects specific to the failure patient need to be kept in mind. Prolonged warm-ups and cool-downs are appropriate since these patients can increase the duration of exercise, but are unable to tolerate more than a limited workload. Dynamic exercise is preferable to isometrics, and the target HR should be 10 beats per minute below any significant endpoint, such as exertional hypotension, significant dyspnea, or sustained arrhythmia seen in the pretraining exercise test.[76] The exercise program is best done initially under supervision, at least until the patient is able to self-monitor and prevent complications during exercise. Patients with severe left ventricular dysfunction need telemetry during warm-up, exercise, and cool-down. The clinical status and progress can be monitored with body weight, BP, and HR response to exercise.

Rehabilitation of the Patient with Valvular Heart Disease

The major problems in patients with valvular heart disease include deconditioning and CHF. The management of the valvular heart disease patient in CHF is essentially as outlined in the section on CHF. After surgical correction, the patient improves in cardiac fitness as measured by improved $\dot{V}O_2$.[67] Training can increase physical work capacity by 60% and decrease perceived exertion and the RPP by 15%.[87] A complicating feature is the fact

TABLE 32–15 Patients at High Risk During Cardiac Rehabilitation

Risk of Ischemia
Postoperative angina
Left ventricular ejection fraction <35%
NYHA grade III or IV congestive heart failure
Ventricular tachycardia or fibrillation in the postoperative period
Systolic BP drop of 10 points or more with exercise
Excessive ventricular ectopy with exercise
Incapable of self-monitoring
Myocardial ischemia with exercise
Risk of Arrhythmia
Acute infarction within 6 wk
Active ischemia
Significant left ventricular dysfunction (LVEF <30%)
History of sustained ventricular tachycardia
History of sustained life-threatening supraventricular arrhythmia
History of sudden death, not yet stabilized on medical therapy
Initial therapy of patients with automatic implantable cardioverter defibrillator
Initial therapy of a patient with rate-adaptive cardiac pacemaker

Abbreviations: BP, blood pressure; LVEF, left ventricular ejection fraction.

that many of these patients are on anticoagulants postoperatively and need to be on low-impact exercises to avoid hemarthroses and bruising. They also need special education to avoid injury.[75] The training program is similar to that followed for the post-CABG patient.

Cardiac Arrhythmias. The risk of death from cardiac arrhythmia during rehabilitation exercises is very low. From 1980 to 1984, one cardiac arrest per 112,000 patient-hours of cardiac rehabilitation was reported.[92] Therefore, it might be prudent to continually monitor only those patients who are at high risk (Table 32–15). For patients with life-threatening arrhythmias, the automatic implantable cardiac defibrillator (AICD) has become a common treatment.[100] The modifications to the cardiac rehabilitation program in these patients are few. The AICD devices are rate-sensitive, so it is essential to ensure that this rate is not exceeded during the exercise stress test and that the HR achieved with exercise does not exceed this threshold. The support and reassurance that can be given to these patients during an exercise program is important, as anxiety about arrhythmia is a significant concern.[80]

Modifications for the Physically Disabled

Little attention has been paid to the problem of cardiac rehabilitation programs for the physically disabled. The risk factor modification programs are easily adapted for any patient population. The exercise training can be accomplished with the same adapted equipment described above for modified exercise testing. The same training principles can be applied. This is an area where physiatrists can take a leadership role, as most existing programs are limited in the ability to compensate for physical impairments.

REFERENCES

1. Albro PC, Gould KL, Westcott RJ, et al: Noninvasive assessment of coronary stenoses by myocardial imaging during pharmacologic vasodilation. III. Clinical trial. Am J Cardiol 1978; 42:751.
2. American Heart Association. Heart and Stroke Facts: 1995 Statistical Supplement. Dallas, TX, American Heart Association, 1995.
3. Ästrand P-O, Ekblom B, Messin R, et al: Intra-arterial blood pressure during exercise with different muscle groups. J Appl Physiol 1965; 20:253.
4. Ästrand P-O, Rodahl K: Textbook of Work Physiology, ed 3. New York, McGraw-Hill, 1986.
5. Balady GJ, Weiner DA, McCabe CH, et al: Value of arm exercise testing in detecting coronary artery disease. Am J Cardiol 1985; 55:37.
6. Balady GJ, Weiner DA, Rothendler JA, et al: Arm exercise thallium imaging testing for the detection of coronary artery disease. J Am Coll Cardiol 1987; 9:84.
7. Belardinelli L, Linden J, Berne RM: The cardiac effects of adenosine. Prog Cardiovasc Dis 1989; 32:73–97.
8. Beller GA, Gibson RS: Sensitivity, specificity, and prognostic significance of non-invasive testing for occult or known coronary disease. Prog Cardiovasc Dis 1987; 29:241.
9. Bloch A, Maeder JP, Haissly JC, et al: Early mobilization after myocardial infarction. A controlled study. Am J Cardiol 1974; 34:152–157.
10. Bogaty P, Dagenais GR, Cantin B, et al: Prognosis in patients with a strongly positive exercise electrocardiogram. Am J Cardiol 1989; 64:124.
11. Borer JS, Kent KM, Bacharach SL, et al: Sensitivity, specificity and predictive accuracy of radionuclide cineangiography during exercise in patients with coronary artery disease: Comparison with electrocardiography. Circulation 1979; 60:572.
12. Bostom AG, Bates E, Mazzarella N, et al: Ergometer modification for combined arm-leg use by lower extremity amputees in cardiovascular testing and training. Arch Phys Med Rehabil 1987; 68:244–247.
13. Braunwald E (ed): Heart Disease, a Textbook of Cardiovascular Medicine. Philadelphia, WB Saunders, 1993.
14. Brown BG, Josephson MA, Peterson RB, et al: Intravenous dipyridamole combined with isometric handgrip for near maximal acute increase in coronary flow in patients with coronary artery disease. Am J Cardiol 1981; 48:1077–1085.
15. Browner WS, Westenhouse J: What if Americans ate less fat? JAMA 1991; 265:3285–3291.
16. Bruce RA, Fischer LD, Pettinger M, et al: ST segment elevation with exercise: A marker for poor ventricular function and poor prognosis. Coronary Artery Surgery Study (CASS) confirmation of Seattle Heart Watch results. Circulation 1988; 77:97.
17. Cannom DS, Rider AK, Stinson EB, et al: Electrophysiologic studies in the denervated transplanted human heart. Am J Cardiol 1975; 36:859.
18. Casale PN, Guiney TE, Strauss HW, Boucher CA: Simultaneous low level treadmill exercise and intravenous dipyridamole stress thallium imaging. Am J Cardiol 1988; 62:799–802.
19. Chaitman BR: The changing role of the exercise electrocardiogram as a diagnostic and prognostic test in chronic ischemic heart disease. J Am Coll Cardiol 1986; 8:1195.
20. Christopherson LK: Cardiac transplantation: A psychological perspective. Circulation 1987; 75:57–62.
21. Cillespie TA, Ambos HD, Sobel BE, Roberts R: Effects of dobutamine in patients with acute myocardial infarction. Am J Cardiol 1977; 39:588–594.
22. de Marneffe M, Jacobs P, Haardt R, Englert M: Variations of normal sinus node function in relation to age: Role of autonomic influence. Eur Heart J 1986; 7:662.
23. Dubach P, Froelicher VF: Cardiac rehabilitation for heart failure patients. Cardiology 1989; 76:368–373.
24. Dubach P, Froelicher V, Klein J, et al: Use of the exercise test to predict prognosis after coronary artery bypass grafting. Am J Cardiol 1989; 63:530.
25. Duchak J, Ryan T, Sawada SG, et al: Bicycle stress echocardiography for the detection of coronary artery disease (abstract). J Am Soc Echocardiogr 1990; 3:225.

26. Ellestad MH: Stress Testing, Principles and Practice, ed 3. Philadelphia, FA Davis, 1986.
27. Elliot EC: The effect of Persantine on coronary flow and cardiac dynamics. Can Med Assoc J 1961; 85:469–476.
28. Feigenbaum H: Exercise echocardiography. J Am Soc Echocardiogr 1988; 1:161–166.
29. Flamm SD, Taki J, Moore R, et al: Redistribution of regional and organ blood volume and effect on cardiac function in relation to upright exercise intensity in healthy human subjects. Circulation 1990; 18:1550.
30. Fleg JL, Lakatta EG: Prevalence and significance of post-exercise hypotension in apparently healthy subjects. Am J Cardiol 1986; 63:81.
31. Fletcher GF, Balady G, Blair SN, et al: Statement on exercise: Benefits and recommendations for physical activity programs for all Americans. A statement for health professionals by the Committee on Exercise and Cardiac Rehabilitation of the Council on Clinical Cardiology, American Heart Association. Circulation 1996; 94(4):857–862.
32. Frasure-Smith N, Prince R: Long-term follow-up of the Ischemic Heart Disease Life Stress Monitoring Program. Psychosom Med 1984; 51:485–513.
33. Friedman M: Type A behavior: Its diagnosis, cardiovascular relation and the effect of its modification on recurrence of coronary artery disease. Am J Cardiol 1989; 64:12C–19C.
34. Froelicher VF: Exercise and the Heart. Clinical Concepts. St Louis, Mosby–Year Book, 1987.
35. Froelicher VF, Marcondes GD: Manual of Exercise Testing. St Louis, Mosby–Year Book, 1989.
36. Glaser RM, Sawka MN, Laubach LL, Suryaprasad AG: Metabolic and cardiopulmonary responses to wheelchair and bicycle ergometry. J Appl Physiol 1979; 46:1066–1070.
37. Gonzalez EG, Corcoran PJ: Energy expenditure during ambulation. In Downey JA, Myers SJ, Gonzalez EG, Lieberman JS (eds): The Physiological Basis of Rehabilitation Medicine, ed 2. Boston, Butterworth-Heinemann, 1994.
38. Gould KL: Noninvasive assessment of coronary stenoses by myocardial perfusion imaging during pharmacologic coronary vasodilation. I. Physiologic basis and experimental vasodilation. Am J Cardiol 1978; 41:267–278.
39. Gould KL, Westcott RJ, Albro PC, Hamilton GW: Noninvasive assessment of coronary stenoses by myocardial imaging during pharmacologic coronary vasodilation. II. Clinical methodology and feasibility. Am J Cardiol 1978; 41:279–287.
40. Graves EJ: 1992 Summary: National Hospital Discharge Survey. Advance data from vital and health statistics; no. 249. Hyattsville, MD, National Center for Health Statistics, 1994.
41. Haines DE, Beller GA, Watson DD, et al: Exercise induced ST segment elevation 2 weeks after uncomplicated myocardial infarction: Contributing factors and prognostic significance. J Am Coll Cardiol 1987; 9:996.
42. Hambrecht R, Niebauer J, Marburger C, et al: Various intensities of leisure time physical activity in patients with coronary artery disease: Effects on cardiorespiratory fitness and progression of coronary atherosclerotic lesions. J Am Coll Cardiol 1993; 22: 468–477.
43. Heck CF, Shumway SJ, Kaye MP: The registry of the International Society for Heart Transplantation: Sixth official report 1989. J Heart Transplant 1989; 8:271–276.
44. Heng MK, Simard M, Lake R, Udhoji VH: Exercise two dimensional echocardiography for the diagnosis of coronary artery disease. Am J Cardiol 1984; 54:502–507.
45. Iskandrian AS, Wasserman LA, Anderson GS, et al: Merits of stress thallium-201 myocardial perfusion imaging in patients with inconclusive exercise electrocardiograms: Correlation with coronary arteriograms. Am J Cardiol 1980; 46:553–558.
46. Juneau M, Geneau S, Marchand C, Brosseau R: Cardiac rehabilitation after coronary bypass surgery (review). Cardiovasc Clin 1991; 21:25–42.
47. Kabat–Zinn J: Full Catastrophe Living. New York, Delta, 1990.
48. Kannel WB, Plehn JF, Cupples LA: Cardiac failure and sudden death in the Framingham Study. Am Heart J 1988; 115:869–875.
49. Kavanagh T: Exercise training in patients after heart transplantation. Herz 1991; 16:243–250.
50. Kavanagh T, Yacoub MH, Campbell R, Mertens D: Marathon running after cardiac transplantation: A case history. J Cardiac Rehabil 1986; 6:16–20.
51. Kavanagh T, Yacoub M, Mertens DJ, et al: Cardiorespiratory responses to exercise training after orthotopic cardiac transplantation. Circulation 1988; 77:162–171.
52. Kerber RE, Miller RA, Najjar SM: Myocardial ischemic effects of isometric, dynamic, and combined exercise in coronary artery disease. Chest 1975; 67:388.
53. King ML, Guarracini M, Lennihan L, et al: Adaptive exercise testing for patients with hemiparesis. J Cardiopulmonary Rehabil 1989; 9:237–242.
54. Kobashigawa JA, Leaf DA, Lee N, et al: A controlled trial of exercise rehabilitation after heart transplantation. N Engl J Med 1999; 340:272–277.
55. Lee AP, Ice R, Blessey R, et al: Long-term effects of physical training in coronary patients with impaired ventricular function. Circulation 1979; 60:1519.
56. Leppo JA: Dipyridamole thallium-201 imaging: The lazy man's stress test. J Nucl Med 1989; 30:281–287.
57. Linden W, Stossel C, Maurice J: Psychosocial interventions for patients with coronary artery disease. Arch Int Med 1996; 156: 745–752.
58. McCance AJ, Forfar JC: Selective enhancement of the cardiac sympathetic response to exercise by anginal chest pain in humans. Circulation 1989; 80:1642.
59. McKirnan MD, Sullivan M, Jensen D, et al: Treadmill performance and cardiac function in selected patients with coronary heart disease. J Am Coll Cardiol 1984; 3:253–261.
60. Mahmarian JJ, Verani MS: Exercise thallium-201 perfusion scintigraphy in the assessment of coronary artery disease. Am J Cardiol 1991; 67:2D–11D.
61. Margonato A, Chierchia S, Cianflone D, et al: Limitations of dipyridamole echocardiography in effort angina pectoris. Am J Cardiol 1987; 59:225–230.
62. Mark DB, Hlatky MA, Harrel FE, et al: Exercise treadmill score for predicting prognosis in coronary artery disease. Ann Intern Med 1987; 106:793.
63. Mehta RH, Eagle KA: Fortnightly review: Secondary prevention in acute myocardial infarction. Br Med J 1998; 316:838–842.
64. Merz B, Noel C, Rozanski A, Forrester JS: The secondary prevention of coronary artery disease. Am J Med 1997; 102:572–581.
65. Moldover JR, Daum MC, Downey JA: Cardiac stress testing of hemiparetic patients with a supine bicycle ergometer: Preliminary study. Arch Phys Med Rehabil 1984; 65:470–473.
66. Moldover JR, Stein J: Cardiopulmonary physiology. In Downey JA, Myers SJ, Gonzalez EG, Lieberman JS (eds): The Physiological Basis of Rehabilitation Medicine, ed 2. Boston, Butterworth-Heinemann, 1994.
67. Newell JP, Kappagoda CT, Stoker JB, et al: Physical training after heart valve replacement. Br Heart J 1980; 44:638–649.
68. Niederberger M, Bruce RA, Kusumi F, Whitkanak S: Disparities in ventilatory and circulatory responses to bicycle and treadmill exercise. Br Heart J 1974; 36:377.
69. Niemeyer MG, van der Wall EE, D'Haene EG, et al: Alternative stress methods for the diagnosis of coronary artery disease. Netherlands J Med 1992; 41:284–294.
70. Okin PM, Klingfeld P: Effect of exercise protocol and lead selection on the accuracy of heart rate adjusted indices of ST-segment depression for the detection of three vessel coronary artery disease. J Electrocardiol 1989; 22:187.
71. Ornish D, Brown SE, Scherwitz LW, et al: Can lifestyle changes reverse coronary artery disease? The Lifestyle Heart Trial. Lancet 1990; 336:129–133.
72. Ornish D, Scherwitz LW, Billings J, et al: Intensive lifestyle changes for reversal of coronary heart disease. JAMA 1998; 280: 2001–2007.
73. Packer M: Sudden unexpected death in patients with congestive heart failure: A second frontier. Circulation 1985; 72:681–685.
74. Paffenbarger RS Jr, Hyde RT, Wing AL, et al: The association of changes in physical-activity level and other lifestyle characteristics with mortality among men. N Engl J Med 1993; 328: 538–545.
75. Pashkow F: Rehabilitation strategies for the complex cardiac patient. Cleve Clin J Med 1991; 58:70–75.

76. Pashkow FJ: Complicating conditions. In Pashkow FJ, Pashkow P, Schafer M (eds): Successful Cardiac Rehabilitation: The Complete Guide for Building Cardiac Rehabilitation Programs. Loveland, CO, Heart Watchers, 1988, pp 228–247.
77. Peter CA, Jones RH: Effect of isometric handgrip and dynamic exercise in left ventricular function. J Nucl Med 1980; 21:1131.
78. Picano E, Lattanzi F, Masini M, et al: High dose dipyridamole echocardiography test in effort angina pectoris. J Am Coll Cardiol 1986; 8:848–854.
79. Pollock ML, Foster C, Anholm JD, et al: Diagnostic capabilities of exercise testing soon after myocardial revascularization surgery. Cardiology 1982; 69:358.
80. Pycha C, Gulledge AD, Hutzler J, et al: Psychological response to the implantable defibrillator. Psychosomatics 1986; 27:841–845.
81. Ritchie L, Trobaugh GB, Hamilton GW, et al: Myocardial imaging with thallium-201 at rest and during exercise: Comparison with coronary arteriography and resting and stress electrocardiography. Circulation 1977; 56:66–71.
82. Rosenblum DS, Rosen ML, Pine ZM, et al: Health status and quality of life following cardiac transplantation. Arch Phys Med Rehabil 1993; 74:490–493.
83. Ruffolo RR Jr: The pharmacology of dobutamine. Am J Med Sci 1987; 294:244–248.
84. Ryan T, Feigenbaum H: Exercise echocardiography. Am J Cardiol 1992; 69:82H–89H.
85. Sebrechts CP, Klein JL, Ahnve S, et al: Myocardial perfusion changes following 1 year of exercise training assessed by thallium-201 circumferential count profiles. Am Heart J 1986; 112:1217–1226.
86. Shabetai R: Beneficial effects of exercise training in compensated heart failure. Circulation 1988; 78:775–776.
87. Sire S: Physical training and occupational rehabilitation after aortic valve replacement. Eur Heart J 1987; 8:1215–1220.
88. Starling RC, Cody RJ: Cardiac transplant hypertension. Am J Cardiol 1990; 65:106–111.
89. Sullivan MJ, Higginbotham MB, Cobb FR: Exercise training in patients with severe left ventricular dysfunction. Circulation 1990; 81(suppl 2):II5–II13.
90. Tuttle RR, Mills J: Dobutamine: Development of a new catecholamine to selectively increase cardiac contractility. Circ Res 1975; 36:185–196.
91. US Bureau of the Census: Statistical Abstract of the United States, ed 113. Washington, DC, 1993.
92. Van Camp S, Peterson R: Cardiovascular complications of outpatient cardiac rehabilitation programs. JAMA 1986; 256:1160–1163.
93. Wainright RJ, Brennand-Roper DA, Maisey MN, et al: Exercise thallium-201 myocardial scintigraphy in the follow-up of aorto-coronary bypass graft surgery. Br Heart J 1980; 43:56.
94. Wasserman K, Hansen JE, Sue DY, Whipp BJ: Principles of Exercise Testing and Interpretation. Philadelphia, Lea & Febiger, 1987.
95. Weich HF, Strauss HW, Pitt B: The extraction of thallium-201 by the myocardium. Circulation 1977; 56:188.
96. Weiner DA, Ryan TJ, McCabe CH, et al: Prognostic importance of a clinical profile and exercise test in medically treated patients with coronary artery disease. J Am Coll Cardiol 1984; 3:772.
97. Wenger NK: Physiological basis for early ambulation after myocardial infarction. Cardiovasc Clin 1978; 9:107–115.
98. Wenger NK: Rehabilitation of the coronary patient. Status 1986. Prog Cardiovasc Dis 1986; 29:181.
99. Willerson JT, Hutton I, Watson JT, et al: Influence of dobutamine on regional myocardial blood flow and ventricular performance during acute and chronic ischemia in dogs. Circulation 1976; 53:828–833.
100. Winkle RA, Mead RH, Ruder MA, et al: Long term outcome with the automatic implantable cardiac-defibrillator. J Am Coll Cardiol 1989; 13:1353–1361.
101. Yusuf S, Aikenhead J, Theodoropoulos S, et al: Mechanism of cardiac output during dynamic exercise in cardiac transplant patients (abstract). J Am Coll Cardiol 1986; 7:225A.
102. Zaret BL, Wackers FJ, Soufer R: Nuclear Cardiology. In Braunwald E (ed): Heart Disease, a Textbook of Cardiovascular Medicine. Philadelphia, WB Saunders, 1993.

33 CHAPTER

Augusta S. Alba, M.D.

Concepts in Pulmonary Rehabilitation

PRINCIPLES

Statistics regarding smoking and respiratory disease with chronic airway obstruction (CAO) are shown in Table 33–1.[2, 18, 44] Restrictive pulmonary disease is most commonly caused by neuromuscular orthopedic disorders, such as spinal cord injury (SCI). The annual incidence of SCI in developed countries is 11.6 per 1 million.[31] Diseases can also result in restrictive pulmonary dysfunction, such as Duchenne muscular dystrophy (DMD), which has an incidence of 21/100,000 in the United States.

Pulmonary rehabilitation (PR)[70] is defined as a comprehensive team approach that provides patients with the ability to adapt to their chronic lung disease. It includes medical management, training in coping skills, and exercise reconditioning. Fear of dyspnea can lead to panic, which increases the work of breathing, and to progressive inactivity, which further weakens the patient. PR addresses this fear and uses exercise reconditioning to increase strength and endurance, which leads to greater tolerance of dyspnea. When exercise reconditioning is no longer possible in a progressive disorder, mechanical ventilation, partial lung resection, and lung transplants become options. The guidelines for PR when exercise reconditioning is still possible are straightforward. A candidate should have a decrease in functional capacity due to pulmonary disease, relative stability of the underlying pulmonary disease, absence of other significant diseases including orthopedic limitations, adequate motivation to undergo a rigorous program, and a pattern of continued improvement in the course of the program.[54]

PRIMARY MODALITIES

General Medical Management

Pharmacological therapy includes vaccination against influenza and pneumococcal pneumonia, inhaled quaternary anticholinergic or beta$_2$-agonist bronchodilators, or both. Oral theophylline can improve respiratory muscle endurance and provide ventilatory stimulation. The new leukotriene receptor antagonist (LTRA) zafirlukast has proved valuable in asthma. Persistent airway obstruction may be an indication for a trial of oral or inhaled steroid therapy. If hypoxemia is present, long-term oxygen therapy (LTOT) will improve survival and quality of life.[18] Environmental and occupational pollution must be prevented and eliminated.

Chest Physical Therapy

A good understanding of pulmonary function tests (Figs. 33–1 and 33–2) and the mechanics and work of breathing in normal and diseased states[41] is essential in planning an effective physical therapy program for persons with pulmonary disease. Breathing exercises include relaxation techniques, which then become the foundation for breathing retraining. Some of these exercises are pursed-lips breathing, head-down and bending-forward postures, slow deep breathing, diaphragmatic breathing, and localized expansion exercises or segmental breathing.[29] The other component utilized to reduce fatigue is respiratory muscle endurance training, which usually concentrates on inspiratory resistance training.

Clearance of secretions is mandatory to reduce the work of breathing and to limit infection and atelectasis. In order for chest physical therapy to be effective, mucoactive medications must be given.[65] These include expectorants, mucolytics, bronchodilators, surfactants, and mucoregulatory agents which reduce the volume of mucus secretion. Techniques for clearing secretions are postural drainage, manual or device-induced chest percussion and vibration, device-induced airway oscillation, incentive spirometry, and various measures that improve the ability to cough. These measures include methods to control coughing, since an uncontrolled

TABLE 33–1 Statistics Regarding Smoking and Respiratory Disease

American youth, aged 12–17: 2.2 million smoke
Children under age 5: 9 million live with a smoker
Annual deaths from tobacco-related illness: 417,000
Mothers who smoke 10 or more cigarettes per day: 26,000 new cases of asthma among their children
Persons with asthma in the United States: 11.6 million
Persons with chronic bronchitis in the United States: 12 million
Persons with emphysema in the United States: 2 million
Fifth leading cause of death in North America: COPD
Only leading cause of death increasing in prevalence: COPD

cough can precipitate dynamic airway collapse, bronchospasm, or syncope. In a manually assisted cough, the patient's abdomen is compressed while the patient controls the depth of inspiration and the timing of opening and closing of the upper airway. Intermittent positive pressure ventilation (IPPV) or glossopharyngeal breathing (GPB) or both are used, if needed, to increase the depth of inspiration. Similarly, in persons with an upper motor neuron lesion affecting the abdominal muscles, as in SCI with a lesion above the midthoracic level, a cough can be produced by electrical stimulation of the abdominal muscles.[46]

Positive expiratory pressure (PEP) mask therapy followed by "huff coughing" is a useful technique when other methods of raising secretions are not tolerated.[52] Autogenic drainage (AD) is a secretion clearance technique that combines variable tidal breathing at three distinct lung volume levels, controlled expiratory airflow, and huff coughing. The In-exsufflator machine (Fig. 33–3), manufactured by the J.H. Emerson Company (Cambridge, MA) provides a deep inspiration either through a mask or a tracheostomy attachment followed rapidly by a controlled suction. It has been shown to provide highly effective secretion removal.[9] A recent study[30] on a normal subject has compared the mechanical effects of devices that create airway oscillation, chest wall oscillation, expiratory positive airway pressure (EPAP) with a threshold resistor, and positive expiratory pressure (PEP) with a fixed orifice resistor. Considerable variation in flow and pressure patterns was found between devices, even in the same general classification. Because of this variation, these devices may have markedly different effects on patients and further study is necessary.

Exercise Conditioning

If the cardiovascular, respiratory, and neuromuscular systems have adequate reserve to undergo a program of progressive exercise, skeletal muscles can develop an increased ability to perform aerobic exercise. After training, a given level of heavy exercise results in lower levels of blood lactate. This also means that the requirement for oxygen uptake, carbon dioxide production, and ventilation for a given level of work is less. Healthy subjects must train for at least 30 minutes a day, 3 to 5 days per week, for 4 to 8 weeks to achieve this effect. Whether a critical training intensity exists and how to measure it are more controversial. Moss and Make[59] have reviewed the pulmonary response to exercise in health and disease. Once the training effect has been achieved, regular exercise must be continued or the gains will be lost.[19]

Cardiopulmonary exercise testing is necessary for the selection and evaluation of patients with chronic obstructive pulmonary disease (COPD) for exercise training. Exercise testing is carried out as a baseline measurement and as a measurement of progress. It also helps to define the cause of dyspnea, the need for supplemental oxygen, and the status of the preoperative patient.[28] The parameters of inspiratory vital capacity (IVC), forced

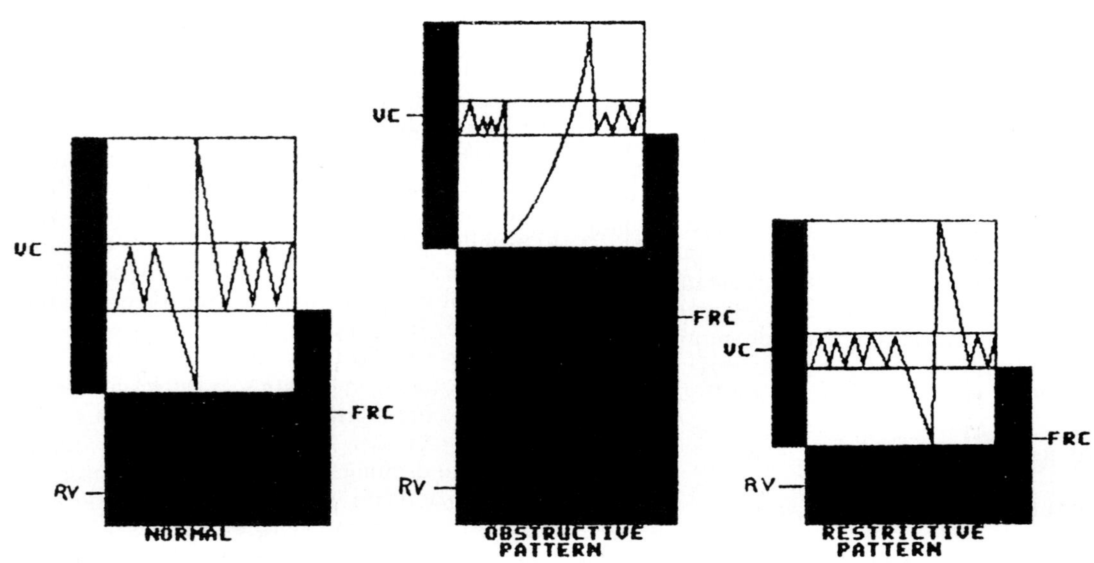

FIGURE 33–1. Lung volumes in disease. VC, vital capacity; FRC, functional residual capacity; RV, residual volume.

TEST	OBSTRUCTIVE DISEASE	RESTRICTIVE DISEASE
VC	↔ ↓	↓ ↓
FEV	↓ ↓	↔ ↓
MMF	↓ ↓	↔ ↓
MVV	↓ ↓	↔ ↓
RV	↑ ↑	↓ ↓
FRC	↑ ↑	↓ ↓
TLC	↑ ↑	↓ ↓

FIGURE 33–2. Typical results of disease on ventilatory function. VC, vital capacity; FEV, forced expiratory volume; MMF, midmaximal flow; MVV, maximal voluntary ventilation; RV, residual volume; FRC, functional residual capacity; TLC, total lung capacity.

expiratory volume in 1 second (FEV_1), maximum minute ventilation (VEmax), and maximum oxygen consumption ($\dot{V}O_{2max}$) have the greatest clinical potential for functional assessment of patients because they show the least variability over time in stable COPD patients.[60]

Types of exercise include lower extremity training on a bicycle ergometer or treadmill, respiratory muscle training using a threshold inspiratory pressure trainer, and unsupported versus supported arm exercise. Unsupported exercise is carried out with free weights; supported exercise is performed on the arm ergometer with the arms supported by the handgrip on the ergometer pedals. Ventilatory muscle endurance exercise, muscle rest therapy, and ventilatory support by nasal intermittent positive pressure ventilation (NIPPV) during exercise can also be used.

Exercise in COPD

A study of COPD patients with hypercapnia subjected to intensive inpatient exercise conditioning of all extremities has shown that even this group with severe ventilatory impairment can benefit from exercise.[34] Ambulation distances on a 6-minute walk (6-minute distance or 6 MD) doubled in a eucapnic group as well as in a group with moderate hypercapnia (partial pressure of carbon dioxide [pCO_2] = 45–54 mm Hg). They were almost doubled in a group with severe hypercapnia ($pCO_2 > 54$ mm Hg).

A study of 317 COPD patients with severe impairment and 32 non-COPD patients who were given a 4-week inpatient PR program showed that both groups doubled the 6 MD.[35] There was no difference among the diagnostic subgroups of the non-COPD patients. No patient had walked more than 500 feet in 6 minutes before the program or more than 900 feet in 6 minutes afterward.

In COPD, NIPPV during exercise can effectively support ventilation, decrease dyspnea, and prolong endurance time.[55] The results of exercise from several studies[20, 24, 62, 78] are summarized in Table 33–2. It has been

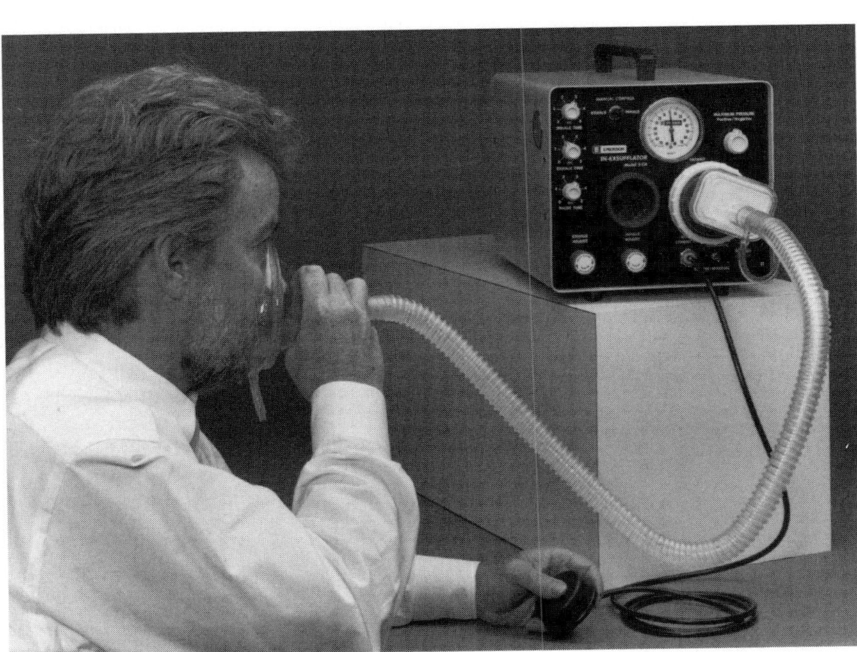

FIGURE 33–3. In-exsufflator cough machine in use with face mask.

TABLE 33–2 Improvements Seen in Exercise Reconditioning in Moderate COPD

IMT
Maximal inspiratory mouth pressure ↑
EMG fatigability of the diaphragm ↓
PR with or without IMT
Maximal workload ↑
ADL scores ↑
Anxiety and depression scores ↓
12 MD ↑
PR (cycle ergometry, 70 W)
V_E decrease of 2.5 L/min per blood lactate decrease of 1 mEq/L (normal, VE decrease of 7.2 L/min per blood lactate decrease of 1 mEq/L)

Abbreviations: IMT, inspiratory muscle training; EMG, electromyography; PR, pulmonary rehabilitation; ADL, activities of daily living; 12 MD, 12-minute walking distance; V_E, minute volume.

demonstrated that high work rates above pretraining anaerobic threshold (AT) reduce the production of lactate at any given work rate to a considerably greater degree than a low work rate above AT.[20, 62]

Hypertensive patients who participate in a PR program typically show no change in the hypertension.[57] Medical treatment of the hypertension is necessary. The main hemodynamic abnormality in COPD is raised pulmonary vascular resistance and pulmonary hypertension.[64] Pulmonary hypertension worsens with the increased demand of exercise because of the absence of reserve collateral vessels. This increases afterload and reduces right ventricular ejection fraction and stroke volume, forcing cardiac output to be maintained by a relative tachycardia. Few studies have been done on the effects of PR on pulmonary hemodynamics, but those done to date have not shown significant improvement. Using a single-exhalation maneuver that analyzes CO and C_2H_2 uptake, it has been possible to calculate pulmonary diffusion (DL) and pulmonary capillary blood flow (Qc) in normal volunteers. This can be done not only during rest, but also during maximal exercise.[12] Both increase substantially during mild to moderate exercise, but appear to plateau at higher levels. This method will be applied to patients in the future.

Exercise in Asthma

Moderate asthma is defined as asthma in which there is no pulmonary impairment during symptom-free intervals. *Severe asthma* is defined as asthma with persistent airway obstruction. Studies of young asthmatic patients in a stable state have shown that the $\dot{V}O_{2max}$ is limited in the severe asthmatic group by decreased cardiac output and stroke volume. It is hypothesized that the high tidal volume leads to decreased left ventricular performance. Aerobic training is recommended because it can decrease VE and hence the tidal volume for any given workload.[74] Aerobic dance is an example of this type of therapeutic exercise.[77]

Exercise in Cystic Fibrosis

An estimated 30,000 persons in the United States suffer from cystic fibrosis (CF), which is a hereditary autosomal recessive disorder. The basic defect is one of chloride transport, which produces a viscid mucus that inhibits the capability of the lungs to clear infection. The patient ultimately suffers from severe combined obstructive-restrictive pulmonary disease, which leads to hypoxia, pulmonary hypertension, and death. However, the number of CF sufferers reaching adulthood and living productive lives is increasing by 10% per year, the median age of survival having increased to 29.4 years.[36] These improved statistics reflect (1) a multidisciplinary team approach to management in accredited CF centers; (2) a better understanding of antimicrobial treatment, including the liberal use of aerosolized antibiotics; and (3) the recent addition of daily long-term nebulization of dornase alfa (Pulmozyme). Dornase alfa, or human recombinant deoxyribonuclease (DNase), is an enzyme capable of digesting extracellular DNA. The abnormal viscosity of the CF secretions is caused to a great extent by degenerating neutrophils which produce extracellular DNA. Dornase alfa is used for patients older than 5 years or for those with a forced vital capacity (FVC) greater than 40%.

Chest physical therapy of all pulmonary segments from one to four times daily is indicated, with increased frequency during exacerbations. Such therapy is rarely available with the necessary frequency in a long-term care setting because patient/staff ratios do not permit it. The person with CF is best cared for in a home setting with personal caregivers who have been trained to deliver the therapy.

Exercise in Disorders of Chest Wall Function

Ankylosing spondylitis, kyphoscoliosis or scoliosis, pectus excavatum, obesity, the sequelae of thoracoplasty or phrenic nerve crush for the treatment of pulmonary tuberculosis, neuromuscular diseases with weakness of the respiratory bellows mechanism, and superimposed spinal curvatures are all disorders in which respiratory muscle fatigue can be reduced by ventilatory muscle training. Hornstein and co-workers[45] outlined this approach for kyphoscoliosis. Persons with Parkinson's disease show improvement with PR.[19]

Spinal cord–injured (SCI) patients can benefit from PR techniques. The SCI child as young as three years can learn neck breathing as a form of voluntary respiration.[37] In children with levels as high as C2 with no diaphragmatic function, this technique produces enough tidal volume that the child can spend some time off the respirator. With some ability to breathe without aid, the child has less fear of accidental disconnection of the respirator and can have some degree of privacy and independence in the home.

Vital capacity (VC) and VE during exercise can be improved even in chronic tetraplegia. The low cervical or incomplete tetraplegic person can perform resistance exercise by pedaling an arm ergometer (AE) for 30 minutes three times a week. Incentive spirometry is a technique in which a patient trains to perform regular deep insufflations by inspiring through a handheld apparatus that gives visual feedback of inspiratory flow. It should be performed for 15 minutes 3 to 5 times a week.[76]

Glossopharyngeal breathing (GPB) (Fig. 33–4) is another technique a patient can use to perform or supplement regular deep insufflations. Like neck breathing, it can be used as an alternative form of respiration. Air is pumped into lungs by the patient using the tongue as a piston. The ball of the tongue strokes boluses of air at the rate of 100 per minute into the throat. The lips, soft palate, and vocal cords open and close in rhythm during each stroke. The patient usually obtains a full tidal breath by stacking gulps of 60 to 90 mL over a period of 10 to 15 seconds, then exhales. Full inflation of the lungs requires stacking for a period of 30 to 40 seconds. Tetraplegic patients, whose resting $\dot{V}O_2$ is approximately half-normal (150 mL/min, personal observation), are able to obtain adequate VE by this method if their lungs have no major abnormalities. This enables them to breathe without artificial ventilation for hours. If the lungs are abnormal, as in severe scoliosis, a person may only be able to frog-breathe for minutes because the VE is not adequate to prevent hypoxia. As soon as the oxygen saturation falls to 85% to 90%, the patient will typically ask for mechanical ventilatory assistance. GPB improves vocal volume and the flow of speech, allows the patient to call for help, and provides the deep breath needed for an assisted cough.

Patients with midthoracic and lower thoracic paraplegia have aerobic and anaerobic capacities that are primarily limited by available muscle mass rather than impaired cardiovascular (CV) or cardiopulmonary function.[27] A study of four subjects using AE and functional neuromuscular stimulation (FNS) of the hips and lower extremities showed mean METS (metabolic equivalents of oxygen consumption) during FNS of 4.8, during FNS + AE of 10.3, and during AE of 7.2.[27] VE and $\dot{V}O_2$ for the three midthoracic subjects were greater than 90% of those observed in sedentary normals. In only one subject, a T11 paraplegic patient, was CV limitation due to excessive lactic acid production noted.[27]

Nutrition

In acute respiratory failure, a fat emulsion (Pulmocare) can be given as 20% to 30% of total daily calories to reduce carbon dioxide production and to provide a volume-concentrated source of calories in the fluid-restricted patient. Dietary fat has a lower level of carbon dioxide production per kilocalorie of energy extracted. This is evident in the respiratory quotient, which is 0.7 for fat and 1.0 for carbohydrate.[67]

In 40% to 50% of persons with COPD with either chronic hypoxemia or severe airflow obstruction ($FEV_1 < 35\%$ of predicted) and in 25% of persons with moderate airflow obstruction ($FEV_1 < 50\%$ of predicted), there is depletion of body weight, of fat-free mass, and of muscle mass.[72] A threshold value of

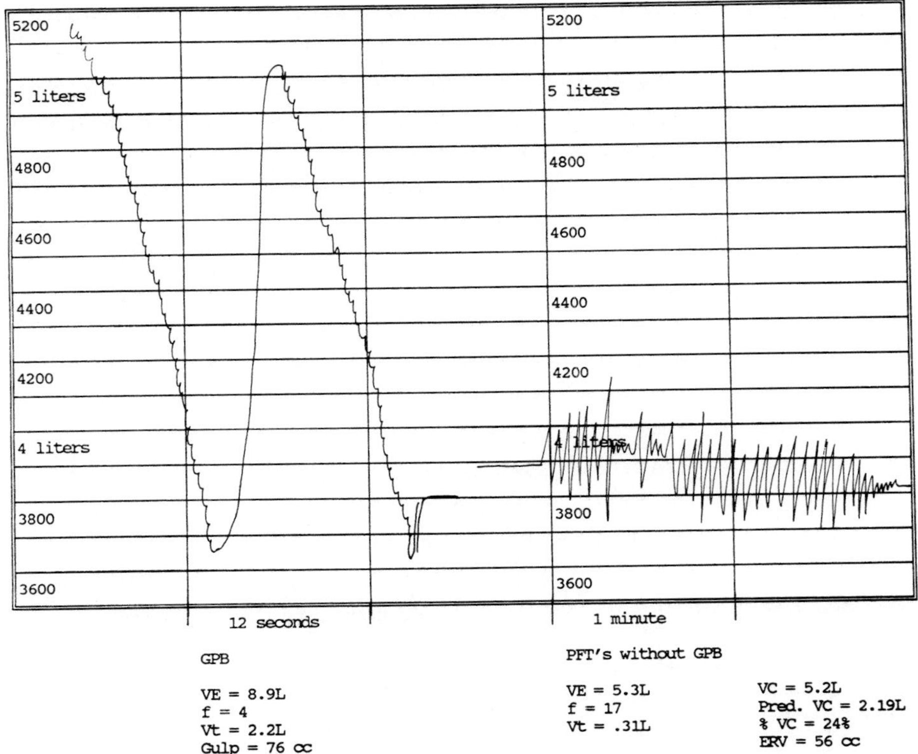

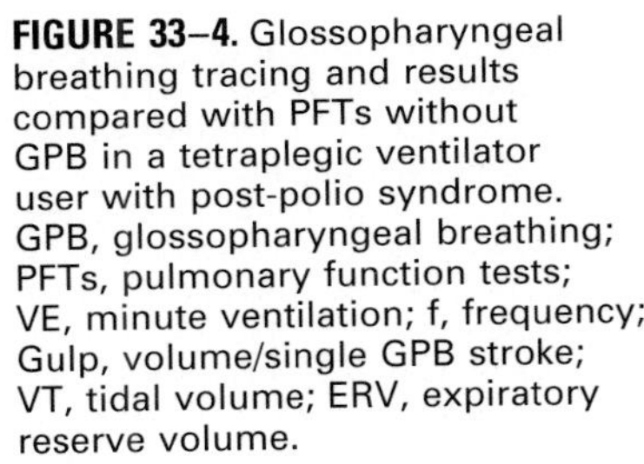
FIGURE 33–4. Glossopharyngeal breathing tracing and results compared with PFTs without GPB in a tetraplegic ventilator user with post-polio syndrome. GPB, glossopharyngeal breathing; PFTs, pulmonary function tests; VE, minute ventilation; f, frequency; Gulp, volume/single GPB stroke; VT, tidal volume; ERV, expiratory reserve volume.

25 kg/m^2 has been identified below which mortality risk increases. On nutritional therapy a weight gain of over 2 kg/8 wk in depleted and nondepleted patients with COPD is a significant predictor of survival.[66]

Mechanical Ventilation

In the patient whose respiratory status is compromised, there may be alterations in the central drive for breathing, obstructive changes in the upper airway, and restrictive and obstructive changes in the lungs. These conditions can exist alone or in various and changing combinations. Assessment of the central drive for breathing and the upper airway is best done at a sleep disorders center with specialized staff and equipment for diagnosis and therapy. Portable polysomnography has allowed this valuable information to be obtained in the intensive care unit (ICU) and in the home.

A reduction in the central drive for breathing results in central sleep apnea (CSA). Obstruction at any site in the upper airway produces obstructive sleep apnea (OSA). Both forms of apnea frequently coexist and are generally more severe during sleep, especially during rapid eye movement (REM) sleep, when there is the greatest degree of muscle relaxation. OSA is treated most commonly by continuous positive airway pressure (CPAP) or bilevel positive airway pressure (BIPAP). CSA is treated with mechanical ventilation.

The physician and the patient should decide jointly what type of mechanical ventilation to use as well as the frequency and duration of its use. Cost, availability, portability, and preference are factors to consider. The choice of ventilators can be confusing. However, if the basic features of ventilators are kept in mind, the prescription is readily generated (Fig. 33–5). Given the answers to four basic questions, one can readily master the intricacies of any ventilator: (1) Does the ventilator act on the body or the airway? (2) Does the ventilator produce positive or negative pressure or both? (3) Does the machines's pressure(s) produce active inspiration or

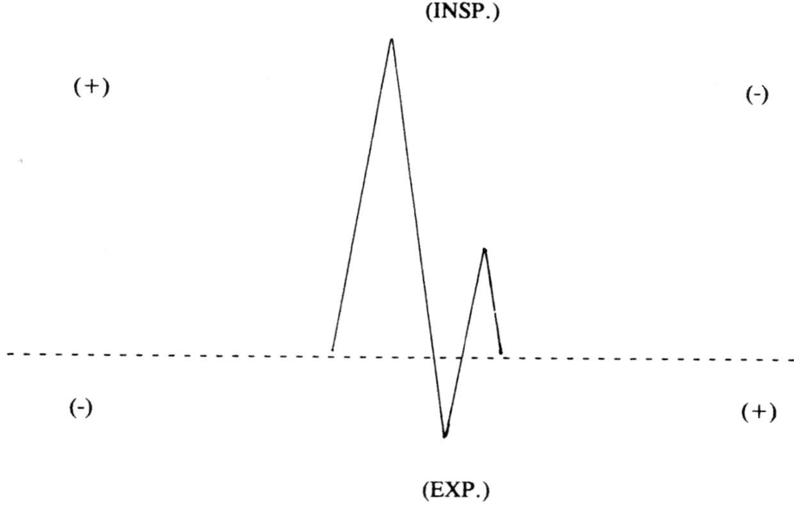

FIGURE 33–5. Respiratory assistive devices superimposed on a graphic representation of the vital capacity. IPPV, intermittent positive-pressure ventilation; INSP, full inspiration; GPB, glossopharyngeal breathing; EXP, forced expiration; airway(+), ventilation by positive pressure on airway, producing inspiration; airway(−), ventilation by negative pressure on airway, producing suctioning; body(−), ventilation by negative pressure on body, producing inspiration; body(+), ventilation by positive pressure on body, producing expiration.

active expiration or both? (4) Does the ventilator have a cycling device?

Noninvasive artificial ventilation is the use of a ventilator without an endotracheal or tracheostomy tube. There are numerous advantages to a noninvasive approach (Table 33–3). One of the most important is the avoidance of respiratory nosocomial infection. Noninvasive approaches such as nasal intermittent positive pressure ventilation (NIPPV) are now being used even in the emergency room and ICU for patients in acute respiratory failure (Fig. 33–6). The concomitant use of the In-exsufflator is necessary for removal of tracheobronchial secretions.[9]

Two of the most acceptable forms of noninvasive ventilation for daytime use are mouth intermittent positive-pressure ventilation (MIPPV) with a small mouthpiece held between the teeth (Fig. 33–7) and the pneumobelt (Fig. 33–8). The pneumobelt holds a bladder that produces a forced expiration when inflated. This expiration is followed by a passive inspiration. The inspiration may be supplemented by the use of the remaining inspiratory muscles or GPB, or a combination of these. MIPPV can be used at night by using a mouthpiece with a lip seal (Fig. 33–9). The patient can use a rocking bed (Fig. 33–10) or a chestpiece (Fig. 33–11) at rest or during sleep. Body ventilators comprise no more than 10% of ventilator usage.

When a decision has been made to retain a tracheostomy in a ventilator-user, a cuffless tracheostomy tube or a tube with a partially deflated cuff can generally be used.[7] Tubes without a fully inflated cuff require adequate pulmonary compliance and sufficient oropha-

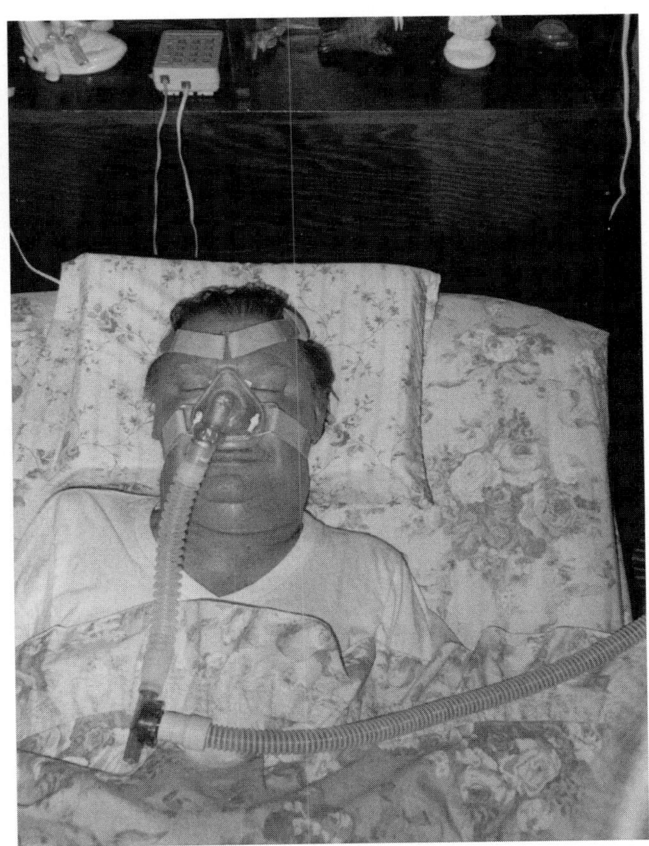

FIGURE 33–6. Nasal intermittent positive-pressure ventilation in a tetraplegic ventilator user with post-polio syndrome.

TABLE 33–3 Respiratory Assistive Devices: Pros and Cons

Type	Use	Pro	Con
Airway Positive Pressure			
Intermittent Positive-Pressure Ventilation			
Console	Bedside; generally hospital setting, acute care, via tracheostomy	Sophistication (alarms; %O_2)	Stationary; high cost
Compact	Long-term; generally noninvasive	Portability; generally AC/DC; lower cost	Some models bulky
Body Negative Pressure			
Iron lung	Replaces bed; long-term	Reliable; good ventilation	Weight; size; confining
Porta-Lung	Same as iron lung	Same as iron lung	Light weight; relative portability
Poncho (wrap)	In bed; long-term	Same as iron lung	May restrict upper chest expansion
Chest shell (cuirass)	In bed; rarely in wheelchair; long-term	Less confining than iron lung	Restricts upper and lateral chest expansion
Diaphragmatic pacemaker	Long-term; relatively intact phrenic nerve, diaphragm muscle, and lower lobes	Very light weight; easy operation	Surgery; initial cost very high; moves only diaphragm
Body Negative/Positive Pressure			
Rocking bed	Replaces bed; requires healthy lower lobes; "movable abdomen"; long-term	Less confining than iron lung; passive movement of body	Weight; size; moves only diaphragm
Body Positive Pressure			
Pneumobelt	Long-term; generally requires sitting position of at least 45 degrees; "movable abdomen"	Good cosmetic effect	Moves only diaphragm

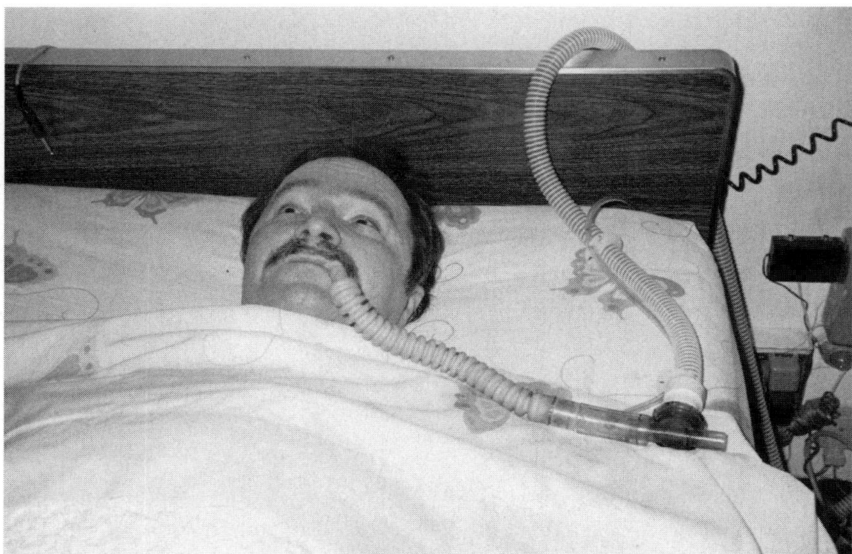

FIGURE 33–7. Mouth intermittent positive-pressure ventilation with mouthpiece in a tetraplegic ventilator user with post-polio syndrome.

ryngeal strength for functional swallowing and articulation. If the patient has a progressive disorder, periodic monitoring with continuous overnight oximetry and capnography is indicated to ensure that leakage through the nose or mouth during sleep is not excessive. When a fully inflated cuff must be used, the lowest possible cuff pressure needed to achieve a seal should be used (preferably <15 mm Hg). If the pressure exceeds the critical pressure for perfusion of the tracheal mucosa (25 mm Hg), destruction of the tracheal wall can occur. Ulceration, bleeding, perforation, loss of tracheal cartilage, localized trachiectasis or stenosis, and granulation tissue are potential complications.

Types of tracheostomy tubes include metal tubes and disposable tubes made of plastic or silicone. Specialized tubes include fenestrated tubes, talking tubes, and tubes for the laryngectomized person. Some speech pathologists have gained extensive experience in communication in tracheostomized and ventilator-dependent patients.[25] Both pneumatic and electrical devices are available to assist vocalization in the presence of a tracheostomy tube. Speaking valves can be attached to the tracheostomy tube adapter. Currently, the most frequently used valve is the Passy-Muir. When vocalization is not possible, nonvocal communication can be provided by a manual or electronic communication system. Numerous systems for nonvocal communication are available today, and a speech pathologist should be consulted before choosing the most appropriate system in each case.

In cases of advanced COPD, mechanical ventilation via a tracheostomy is often necessary for survival. More

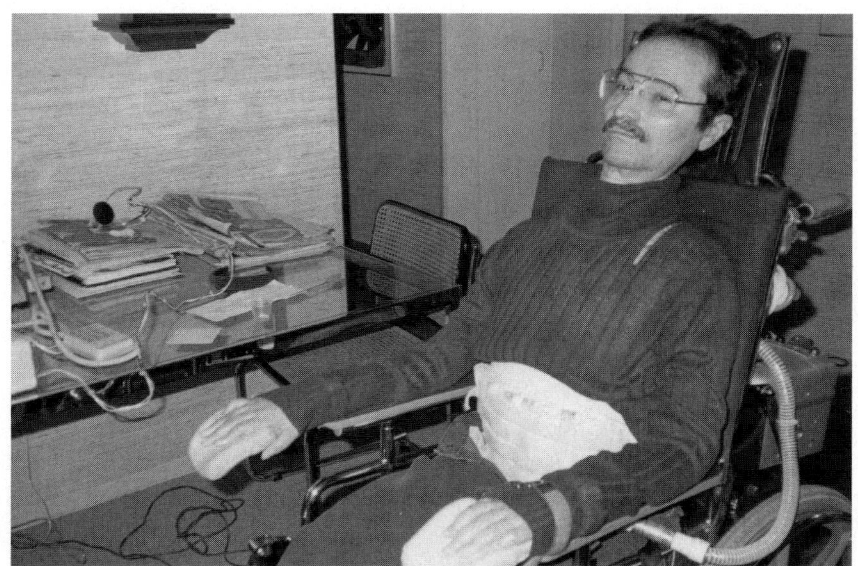

FIGURE 33–8. Pneumobelt ventilation in a tetraplegic ventilator user with post-polio syndrome.

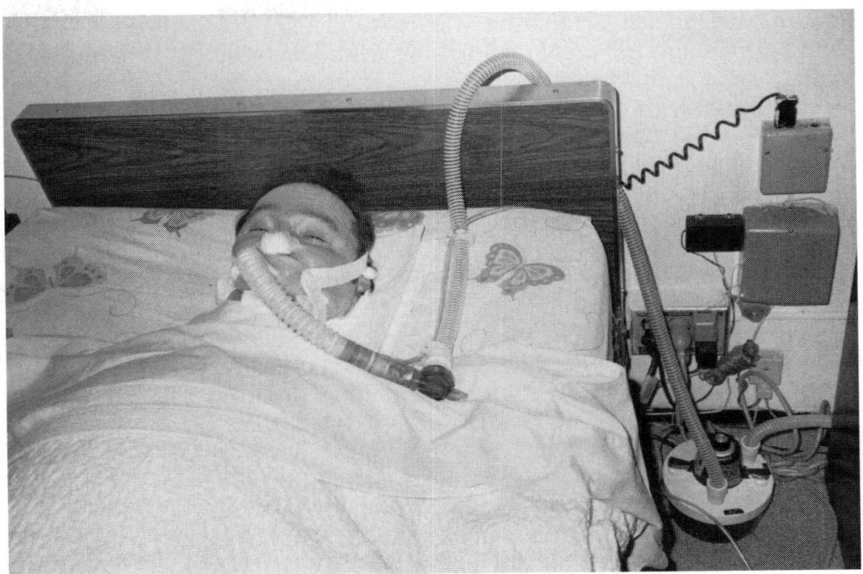

FIGURE 33–9. Mouth intermittent positive-pressure ventilation with lip seal, mouthpiece and nose taped, in a tetraplegic ventilator user with post-polio syndrome.

controversial, however, is the use of mechanical ventilation to reduce respiratory muscle fatigue. Patients with diffuse bronchiectasis and severe chronic respiratory failure have a reduction of hospitalizations and improvement of functional status on NIPPV added to LTOT.[10]

Mechanical ventilation in patients with neuromusculoskeletal disorders has been facilitated in the past 15 years by the development of portable volume ventilators and BIPAP used as a ventilator. In the ICU the increased sophistication of console volume ventilators has aided the survival of persons with these disorders. The critically ill patient in the ICU with sepsis and multiple organ failure can develop a primary axonal form of polyneuropathy, which delays weaning as well as overall recovery and mobilization.[65] Early diagnosis with the aid of electrodiagnostic studies facilitates the rehabilitation process. Tetanus has to be quickly recognized in its early stage with prompt ventilator support, vigorous treatment of infection, and management of the muscle rigidity with benzodiazepines, narcotics, and neuromuscular blockers. With this regimen patients can usually be ready for rehabilitation within 4 weeks.[61]

The halo brace is frequently used for patients with SCI if surgical stabilization has not been carried out after fracture of the cervical spine.[13] The halo brace permits early patient mobilization and early admission to a rehabilitation setting. Early mobilization helps prevent the pulmonary complications associated with prolonged bedrest and paralysis, the most serious of which are atelectasis and pneumonia.

Persons with high and midcervical tetraplegia will invariably require mechanical ventilation during the initial hospitalization. At least one in five tetraplegics who

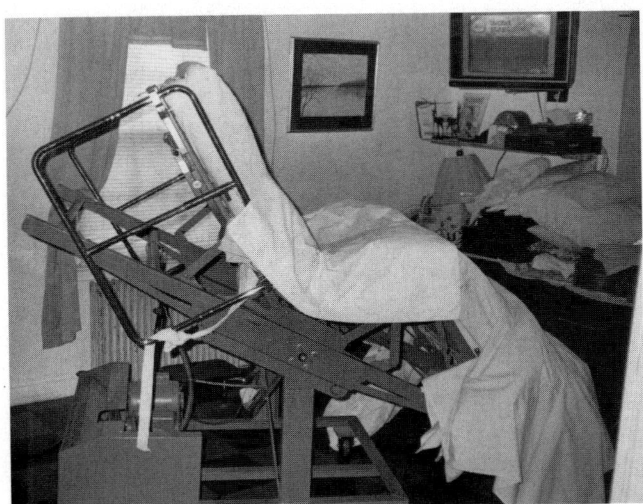

FIGURE 33–10. Rocking bed in head-up position with elevation of the head of bed.

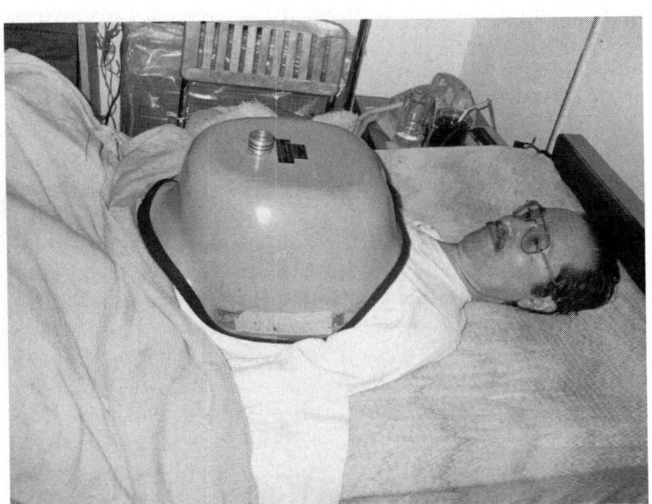

FIGURE 33–11. Chestpiece without hose applied to a tetraplegic ventilator user with post-polio syndrome.

require mechanical ventilation will be discharged on ventilator support. Persons with low tetraplegia frequently require mechanical ventilation during the acute hospitalization. Financial support for hospitalization, rehabilitation, and long-term care is a serious national health issue. Bach[6] describes conversion of high-level tetraplegic patients to noninvasive ventilatory support or providing such support from the onset as a means of simplifying care and reducing cost.

Other common neurological disorders in which long-term mechanical ventilation is used include amyotrophic lateral sclerosis (ALS), syringomyelia, multiple sclerosis, muscular dystrophies, and poliomyelitis. Bach[4] found that ALS patients can survive a mean of 4.4 (SD 3.9) years (range, 1 month to 26.5 years) using respiratory support. Survival was comparable for patients maintained at home or in long-term care facilities. The use of noninvasive respiratory aids not only simplified care, but also gave patients and families time for decision-making regarding tracheostomy. Duchenne muscular dystrophy (DMD) patients, once on ventilator assistance, tend to increase its use approximately 1 hour/day per year.[23] The average length of survival in DMD patients is increased by six years with respiratory assistance.

Postpoliomyelitis patients on long-term nocturnal ventilation have also been studied. Curran and Colbert[23] found that these patients showed no significant decrease in muscle strength or increase in the number of hours of nocturnal ventilation over a 12-year period. However, over a period of 30 to 40 years, postpoliomyelitis ventilator-users invariably show an increase in the number of hours of assisted ventilation (personal observation). Increased weakness of oropharyngeal muscles over time can also occur, with resulting new problems of swallowing and obstructive apnea.

The use of mechanical ventilation in patients post cardiac surgery is a "crutch" that can facilitate the rehabilitation process, as has been described by Sivak.[69]

Weaning from mechanical ventilation is an important aspect of PR, both in terms of reduced cost and patient satisfaction. Due to advances made in detecting the earliest point at which a person can breathe without a ventilator following respiratory failure, weaning has been described as the science of liberation from mechanical ventilation.[56] Weaning techniques include CPAP, blow-by systems or T piece, pressure support, and the use of the Passy-Muir ventilator speaking valve. The use of manual and mechanical exsufflation to clear airway secretions and the use of noninvasive positive airway pressure ventilatory assistance by nasal or oral interfaces speed weaning in the patient on tracheal intermittent positive-pressure ventilation. Weaning of the SCI patient is best carried out in a SCI center where staff can alleviate anxiety and depression, enlist family support, solve problems as a team, and prevent infections. Diaphragmatic strengthening and endurance training can be used to facilitate weaning in the high tetraplegic patient in whom there is only partial involvement of the anterior horn cells of the phrenic nerve at the C3–C5 levels.[51]

Patients on mechanical ventilation in the home or in an alternative setting benefit from those aspects of PR that promote a quality lifestyle of independence and autonomy. International conferences on PR and home mechanical ventilation have been held during the past two decades. An international resource directory 1998/1999 for ventilator-users is now available.[38] It has been demonstrated that a chronic ventilator unit in an acute hospital is cost-effective.[40] Because of the multidisciplinary approach, weaning can be performed with greater success in such a unit. COPD was the most frequent diagnosis. In the study of Gracey et al, almost 90% of the patients admitted to the unit over an 18-month period were weaned and more than 70% were discharged home.[40] A small number required nocturnal mechanical ventilation at home. Success in weaning in a ventilator unit in a long-term care facility is less probable because the resident has already failed to be weaned in a hospital setting. However, a success rate of almost 50% has been achieved.[32]

Diaphragmatic pacing (Fig. 33–12) is a highly sophisticated form of mechanical ventilation. It has been available in the clinical setting for more than 25 years, but has attained a higher level of reliability and broader application in the past decade.[26] Infection and failure of components are now rare complications. The need to retain a tracheostomy because of obstructive sleep apnea is more common. Worldwide, there have been more than 1400 phrenic nerve implants in patients whose ages ranged from a few months to 80+ years. Many of these patients have been successfully paced for more than 20 years. Diaphragmatic pacing is indicated in patients who have damage to the respiratory control centers or their pathways in the brainstem and spinal cord. The pacing system consists of an external transmitter and antenna and implanted electrodes and receiver. The working life expectancy of the receiver is for the lifetime of the patient and batteries last for two to three weeks. A bipolar electrode is available for use in persons who already have demand cardiac pacers. There is advanced warning of transmitter battery failure via a gradual decrease in tidal volume over several days. The pacer is thermal-stabilized to allow full outdoor activities while pacing. The cervical implant is now recommended in the older child and adult, with "customized" stimulation parameters that enable pacing with small numbers of residual fibers. The surgery is simple and the hospitalization brief. Thoracic implants requiring bilateral thoracotomies are still needed for infants. The physician can use transtelephonic monitoring (TTM) for remote assessment of stimulation effectiveness and diagnosis of problems. The most common impairments for which the pacer is used are idiopathic central hypoventilation syndrome (CHS) or Ondine's curse, acquired CHS, and high SCI.

Krieger and associates[50] have developed a technique to reinnervate the recently denervated diaphragm by intercostal nerve-to-phrenic nerve anastomosis with implantation of a pacing electrode. The phrenic nerve lies in close proximity to the intercostal nerves in the thoracic cavity. They are related in size and have similar functions.

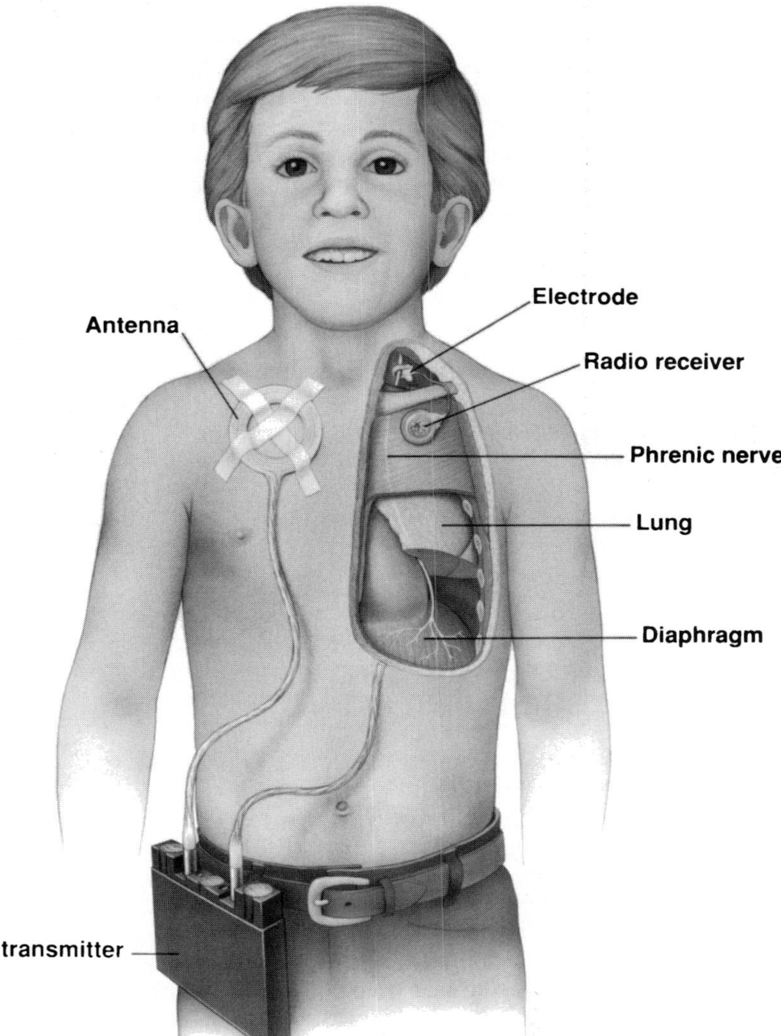

FIGURE 33–12. Diaphragmatic pacemaker use in child with central hypoventilation syndrome.

Oxygen Therapy

Oxygen therapy with or without mechanical ventilation can be administered on a long-term basis. The physician should provide a prescription to the vendor who furnishes oxygen in the home.[70] The physician must include on the prescription the diagnostic reasons for oxygen, results of blood gas studies, type of delivery system, and specific liter flow for the patient during rest, sleep, and/or exertion. For the hypoxemic patient, oxygen should be administered continuously to improve mortality and morbidity. Oxygen therapy is most easily monitored by pulse oximetry during the different activity conditions of the patient.

Estimates of the number of supplemental oxygen users in the United States range from 600,000 to 800,000. The Americans With Disabilities Act of 1991 contains no specific references to oxygen users, but its provisions still apply, even aboard major airlines or ocean liners. Home oxygen systems include high-pressure compressed gas cylinders in several sizes, transfilling liquid oxygen systems with both a stationary reservoir and a portable device weighing 11 lbs when full, and oxygen concentrators that require an electrical outlet. The liquid oxygen canister can provide up to 9 hours of oxygen at 2 L/min. Methods of conservation include devices that either cause the oxygen to flow only during inspiration (pulse oxygen systems) or that store oxygen during the expiratory phase. Both as a method of conservation and for the cosmetic effect, transtracheal oxygen can be used. Nasal cannulas can be concealed in the eyeglasses.

BIOPSYCHOSOCIAL CONSIDERATIONS

Biopsychosocial considerations for persons with pulmonary dysfunction include education of the patient and family, psychotherapy, disability evaluation, vocational counseling, and availability of resources. Education must be ongoing in all clinical settings and in the home. It is the responsibility of all team members. A format should be utilized that simplifies documentation of what has been taught, and makes it readily available to the other team members. Janelli and co-workers[47] studied the effect of group teaching programs in a PR setting on the COPD patient. They found that they increased knowledge, but did not change coping strategies unless the patients were specifically taught how to incorporate appropriate strategies into their lifestyles. Psychotherapy includes the assessment of neurocognition, which can be affected by hypoxemia and hypercapnia, and of the individual's self-concept. Stress management includes cognitive restructuring, progressive relaxation, breathing exercises, and visual imagery. Biofeedback and sexual counseling are additional psychotherapeutic approaches.

Resources in the community should include financial support, home health-care agencies with personnel trained to care for the person with respiratory disability, and support groups. Burns[14] found that support groups helped overcome the isolation, depression, and irritability associated with chronic respiratory disease. However, such groups require a large investment of time and energy on the part of volunteers and patients to be self-sustaining.

SURGICAL APPROACHES TO PULMONARY REHABILITATION

Lung volume reduction surgery (LVRS), in which 20% to 30% of one or both lungs is removed, is now an option prior to or in lieu of lung transplantation for COPD patients. Areas of the lungs with the most severe lesions (usually the apices) are removed. This technique is believed to restore pulmonary elastic recoil, and correct over-distention of the thorax and depression of the diaphragm. This results in better respiratory mechanics and relief from severe dyspnea. Improvements in lung function begin to decline in two years. Since the safety, benefits, and cost of this surgery are not clear, a National Emphysema Treatment Trial (NETT) was begun in 18 centers nationwide in 1997 to evaluate optimal medical therapy as compared to optimal medical therapy plus LVRS.[53]

In the past 20 years lung transplantation has become increasingly accepted as the treatment of choice in numerous end-stage pulmonary diseases. More than 6400 lung transplants have been performed worldwide.[58] Single or bilateral lung transplants and heart-lung transplants are available to patients less than 55 to 65 years old, including children. Living donor lobar transplantation is being used in CF. Overall survival rates are between 60% and 65% at two years and approximately 40% at five years. In selected patients long-term mechanical ventilatory support has not been shown to be a contraindication to lung transplantation. A program of physical training prior to and following surgery expedites postoperative recovery. Survivors are typically able to return to an active lifestyle within two months of discharge from the hospital. Cardiac transplant candidates waiting for a donor heart often benefit from a left ventricular assist device.[15] The device can be used up to several months prior to the transplantation. This device reverses multiorgan failure, including pulmonary dysfunction, and the candidate can participate in a cardiac rehabilitation program prior to transplantation.

LONG-TERM RESULTS OF PULMONARY REHABILITATION

Long-Term Results in Lung Disease

Programs of PR are usually either short-term hospital inpatient[39, 75] or short-term outpatient programs. The program needs a proper team structure, adequate space, knowledge of the services to be provided, a marketing plan, and reimbursement for services.[43] Services may include medical and nutritional management, addressing of psychosocial issues, education, physical rehabilitation, recreational therapy, and occupational therapy. The way the participants define their health is a major consideration in the program because their definition typically parallels their goals.[33] When the providers of a program fail to listen to the participants, communication is not optimal and participants tend to be dissatisfied. Following twenty-five years of PR, it has been possible for evidence-based guidelines to be developed for its use in COPD.[1] There is certainty that lower extremity training improves exercise tolerance, and a PR program improves the symptom of dyspnea. Results of PR are somewhat less consistent for the following propositions: that upper extremity training improves arm function; that ventilatory muscle training is of value when there is decreased respiratory muscle strength and dyspnea; that PR improves health-related quality of life and reduces both the number and duration of hospitalizations. Short-term psychosocial interventions have not been shown to be beneficial. Longer-term interventions may be helpful in a setting of a comprehensive PR program. PR might also improve survival.

A component of education that provides the resident with a feasible method of tracking respiratory status is scoring dyspnea once daily and measuring PEFR twice daily, before and after bronchodilators.[16] The gains from a comprehensive PR program tend to diminish after one year.[63]

Cox and colleagues[22] studied 44 persons with asthma or mild COPD who participated in a 3-month comprehensive rehabilitation program and were followed for a 2-year period along with a control group. The treatment group showed improvement in endurance, decreased body fat percentage, an increase in working days, more active life, and a decrease in consumption of medical care. However, bronchial hyperreactivity, need for pulmonary drugs, degree of coughing, and sputum production were not affected. Boyers[11] reported on the presence of all three entities of CAO-asthma, chronic bronchitis, and emphysema in the elderly. PR had gratifying results even in this group.

Van-der-Schoot and Kaptein described the stabilization of respiratory symptoms in asthmatics, whose symptoms could not be otherwise controlled.[73] They used interdisciplinary treatment in a high-altitude climate with low air humidity and low allergen concentration. However, six months later, approximately 35% of patients had been readmitted to a hospital for an exacerbation. Psychological factors played a key role in the readmissions.

As with COPD, guidelines for the management of asthma are now available.[72]

Long-Term Results in Pneumonia

Asauliuk[3] reviewed more than 1000 cases of acute pneumonia in young adult patients. At the time of discharge, approximately 50% were normal clinically, by laboratory studies including VC measurement, and radiologically. Moderate deficits in pulmonary function tests were found in 17% before discharge. An asthenic syndrome that was retained after discharge in 30% of patients required 3 to 10 months of PR to reverse.

Long-Term Results in Neuromuscular Disorders

Koch and colleagues[48] have shown that an outpatient neuromuscular disease clinic is cost-effective. In a total of 210 patients over a one-year period, ancillary services were utilized as follows: pulmonary (11% of patients), orthopedic (10%), social service (43%), formal occupational therapy (7%), and physical therapy (6%). Seventy percent of the annual costs of the clinic were for equipment, 11% for laboratory testing, and 8% for physician costs. The total mean per capita cost of outpatient rehabilitation in this population was $750 per year. In muscular dystrophy patients, prevention of morbidity over time has been demonstrated through the use of a respiratory management protocol including inspiratory and expiratory aids and oximetry monitoring during acute respiratory infections.[8]

Bach[5] has shown that persons with SCI who are weaned despite having a significant restrictive pulmonary problem can develop ventilatory decompensation weeks to decades after weaning. Their course can be complicated by multiple pulmonary complications, including bouts of acute respiratory failure. Noninvasive mechanical ventilation is an option when ventilatory aid is needed again. Chawla[21] reported that although there has been an increased survival rate among persons with high SCI, ideal rehabilitation for those who remain paralyzed and in need of partial or complete ventilator support is frequently not available because of cost factors. This includes the cost of delivery of home care, reliable portable ventilators, phrenic nerve stimulators, environmental controls, specialized wheelchairs, and alternative communication aids. Outcomes and problems in pediatric pulmonary rehabilitation have been reported with emphasis on the success rate of weaning in bronchopulmonary dysplasia (BPD) and in non-BPD children.[17]

Although disability in adductor spastic dysphonia (ASD) is limited to a severe communication disability, Harrison and co-workers[42] noted that the presence of phonatory spasm during speech can be so extreme that the use of inspiratory speech is preferable. Blood gas measurements showed no change during extended speaking periods. More recently Botulinum Type A Neurotoxin Complex is also being used for this problem.

SUMMARY

The physiatrist requires a basic knowledge of the anatomy and pathophysiology of the cardiovascular and respiratory systems, as well as exercise physiology to be able to practice PR. Patient assessment skills include proficiency in electrodiagnosis as it applies to the respiratory muscles, and in the interpretation of radiological studies of the lungs.

The practice of PR can be in a setting limited to this subspecialty, or in a broader setting where patients with neurological or musculoskeletal disabilities have pulmonary dysfunction as a complication of the disease or as a medical co-morbidity. In either setting general rehabilitative therapeutic approaches apply.

Health policy, legislation, and regulations, including new health-care delivery systems, must take into account the need for PR at all ages in society. A well-informed public can facilitate change. On-line interest groups, bulletin boards, and more then 3500 titles concerning pulmonary rehabilitation on the Web are helping to make this possible.

REFERENCES

1. ACCP/AACVPR Pulmonary Rehabilitation Guidelines Panel. Pulmonary Rehabilitation: Joint ACCP/AACVPR Evidence-Based Guidelines. Chest 1997; 112:1363–1396.
2. American Heart Association: Heart and Stroke Facts: 1994 Statistical Supplement. Dallas, American Heart Association.
3. Asauliuk IK: The rehabilitation of young patients with a history of acute pneumonia. Vrach Delo 1989; 7:53–55.
4. Bach, JR: Amyotrophic lateral sclerosis: Communication status and survival with ventilatory support. Am J Phys Med Rehabil 1993; 72:343–349.
5. Bach JR: Inappropriate weaning and late onset ventilatory failure of individuals with traumatic spinal cord injury. Paraplegia 1993; 31:430–438.
6. Bach JR: New approaches in the rehabilitation of the traumatic high level quadriplegic. Am J Phys Med Rehabil 1991; 70:13–19.
7. Bach JR, Alba A: Tracheostomy ventilation: A study of efficacy with deflated cuffs and cuffless tubes. Chest 1990; 97:679–683.
8. Bach JR., Ishikawa Y, Heakyyung K: Prevention of pulmonary morbidity for patients with Duchenne muscular dystrophy. Chest 1997; 112:1024–1028.
9. Bach J, Smith WH, Michael J, et al: Airway secretion clearance by mechanical exsufflation in post poliomyelitis ventilator assisted individuals. Arch Phys Med Rehabil 1993; 74:170–177.
10. Benhamou D, Muir JF, Raspaud C, et al: Long-term efficiency of home nasal mask ventilation in patients with diffuse bronchiectasis and severe chronic respiratory failure. Chest 1997; 112:1259–1266.
11. Boyars MS: COPD in the ambulatory elderly: Management update. Geriatrics 1988; 43:29–40.
12. Brown CD, MacIntyre NR, Huang YC: Diffusing capacity and pulmonary capillary blood flow during maximal exercise. Chest 1998; 114(suppl 4):335S.
13. Browner CM, Hadley MN, Sonntag VK, et al: Halo immobilization brace care: An innovative approach. J Neurosci Nurs 1987; 19:24–29.
14. Burns M: Outpatient pulmonary rehabilitation. A new lease on life. Postgrad Med 1989; 86:129–130.
15. Burnett CM, Duncan JM, Frazier OH, et al: Improved multiorgan function after prolonged univentricular support. Ann Thorac Surg 1993; 55:63–71.
16. Busby HK, Murata GH, Lium DJ, et al: Patient compliance with peak flow monitoring in chronic obstructive pulmonary disease. Chest 1997; 112(suppl 3):81S.
17. Buschbacher R: Outcomes and problems in pediatric pulmonary rehabilitation. Am J Phys Med Rehabil 1995; 74(4):287–293.

18. Canadian Thoracic Society Workshop Group: Guidelines for the assessment and management of chronic obstructive pulmonary disease. Can Med Assoc J 1992; 147:420–428.
19. Casaburi R: Principles of exercise training. Chest 1992; 101 (suppl 5):263S–267S.
20. Casaburi R, Pastesio A, Loli F, et al: Reductions in exercise lactic acidosis and ventilation as a result of exercise training in patients with obstructive lung disease. Am Rev Respir Dis 1991; 143:9–18.
21. Chawla JC: Rehabilitation of spinal cord injured patients on long term ventilation. Paraplegia 1993; 31:88–92.
22. Cox NH, Hendricks JC, Binkhorst RA, et al: A pulmonary rehabilitation program for patients with asthma and mild chronic obstructive pulmonary disease (COPD). Lung 1993; 171:235–244.
23. Curran FJ, Colbert AP: Ventilator management in Duchenne muscular dystrophy and post poliomyelitis syndrome: 12 years experience. Arch Phys Med Rehabil 1989; 70:180–185.
24. Dekhuijzen PN, Beek MM, Folgering HT, et al: Psychological changes during pulmonary rehabilitation and target-flow inspiratory muscle training in COPD patients with a ventilatory limitation during exercise. Int J Rehabil Res 1990; 13:109–117.
25. Dikeman KJ, Kazandjian MS: Communication and Swallowing Management of Tracheostomized and Ventilator-Dependent Adults. San Diego, Singular Publishing Group, 1995.
26. Dobelle WH, D'Angelo MS, Goetz BF, et al: 200 cases with a new breathing pacemaker dispel myths about diaphragm pacing. ASAIO J 1994; 40:M244–M252.
27. Edwards BG, Marsolais EB: Metabolic responses to arm ergometry and functional neuromuscular stimulation. J Rehabil Res Dev 1990; 27:107–114.
28. Epstein SK, Celli BR: Cardiopulmonary exercise testing in patients with chronic obstructive pulmonary disease. Cleve Clin J Med 1993; 60:119–128.
29. Faling LJ: Pulmonary rehabilitation–physical modalities. Clin Chest Med 1986; 7:599–618.
30. Fink JB, Fahey PJ: A comparison of common bronchial hygiene devices and their effects on esophageal pressure. Chest 1998; 114(suppl 4):293S.
31. Flavel H, Marshall R, Thorton A, et al: Hypoxia episodes during sleep in high tetraplegia. Arch Phys Med Rehabil 1992; 73: 623–627.
32. Fleming R, Sobol E: Weaning outcomes and survival on a ventilator unit in a long-term care facility. Chest 1997; 112(suppl 3):129S.
33. Folden SL: Definitions of health and health goals of participants in a community-based pulmonary rehabilitation program. Pub Health Nurs 1993; 10:31–35.
34. Foster S, Lopez D, Thomas HM: Pulmonary rehabilitation in COPD patients with elevated PCO_2. Am Rev Respir Dis 1988; 138:1519–1523.
35. Foster S, Thomas HM: Pulmonary rehabilitation in lung disease other than chronic obstructive pulmonary disease. Am Rev Respir Dis 1990; 141:601–604.
36. Franz MN, Cohn RC, Wachnowsky-Diakiw DM, et al: Management of children and adults with cystic fibrosis: One center's approach. Hosp Formul 1994; 29:364–378.
37. Gilgoff IS, Barras DM, Jones MS, et al: Neck breathing: A form of voluntary respiration for the spine-injured ventilator-dependent quadriplegic child. Pediatrics 1988; 82:741–745.
38. G.I.N.I. International Ventilator Users Network Resource Directory 1998/1999. St. Louis, Gazette International Networking Institute.
39. Glassman SJ: Pulmonary rehabilitation in the acute inpatient rehabilitation hospital. Respir Care Clin North Amer 1998; 4(1): 47–57.
40. Gracey DK, Viggiano RW, Naessens JM, et al: Outcomes of patients admitted to a chronic ventilator-dependent unit in an acute care hospital. Mayo Clin Proc 1992; 67:131–136.
41. Haas F, Axen K (eds): Pulmonary Therapy and Rehabilitation. Principles and Practice, ed 2. Baltimore, Williams & Wilkins, 1991, pp 29–42.
42. Harrison GA, Davis PJ, Troughear RH, et al: Inspiratory speech as a management option for spastic dysphonia. Case study. Ann Otol Rhinol Laryngol 1992; 101:375–382.
43. Hodgkin JE: Organization of a pulmonary rehabilitation program. Clin Chest Med 1986; 7:599–618.
44. Hodgkin JG, Connors GL, Bell CW: Pulmonary Rehabilitation. Guidelines to Success, ed 2. Philadelphia, JB Lippincott, 1992, p xiii.
45. Hornstein S, Inman S, Ledsome JH: Ventilatory muscle training in kyphoscoliosis. Spine 1987; 12:859–863.
46. Jaeger R, Turba RM, Yarkony GM, et al: Cough in spinal cord injured patients: Comparison of three methods to produce cough. Arch Phys Med Rehabil 1993; 74:1358–1361.
47. Janelli LM, Scherer YK, Schmieder LL: Can a pulmonary health teaching program alter patients' ability to cope with COPD? Rehabil Nurs 1991; 16:199–202.
48. Koch SJ, Arego DE, Bowser B: Outpatient rehabilitation for chronic neuromuscular diseases. Am J Phys Med 1986; 65: 245–257.
49. Koseoglu F, Inan L, Ozel S, et al: The effects of a pulmonary rehabilitation program on pulmonary function tests and exercise tolerance in patients with Parkinson's disease. Funct Neurol 1997; 12(6):319–325.
50. Krieger AJ, Gropper MR, Adler RJ: Electrophrenic respiration after intercostal to phrenic nerve anastomosis in a patient with anterior spinal artery syndrome: Technical case report. Neurosurgery 1994; 35(4):760–763.
51. Lerman RM, Weiss MS: Progressive resistive exercise in weaning high quadriplegics from the ventilator. Paraplegia 1987; 25: 130–135.
52. Mahlmeister MJ, Fink JB, Hoffman GL, et al: Positive-expiratory-pressure mask therapy: Theoretical and practical considerations and a review of the literature. Respir Care 1991; 36:1218–1229.
53. Make BJ: Lung volume reduction surgery and the National Emphysema Treatment Trial. Update of the National Jewish Medical and Research Center 1998; 15(3).
54. Mall RW, Medeiros M: Objective evaluation of results of a pulmonary rehabilitation program in a community hospital. Chest 1988; 94:1156–1160.
55. Maltais F, Reissmann H, Gottfried SB: Pressure support reduces inspiratory effort and dyspnea during exercise in chronic airflow obstruction. Am J Resp Crit Care Med 1995; 151:1027–1033.
56. Manthous CA, Schmidt GA, Hall JB: Liberation from mechanical ventilation. A decade of progress. Chest 1998; 114:886–901.
57. Marchman HB, Skolnick JL: Blood pressure changes in patients with chronic obstructive pulmonary disease and hypertension completing phase II pulmonary rehabilitation. J Ky Med Assoc 1992; 90:503–505.
58. Maurer JR, Frost AE, Estenne M, et al: Coordinating Committee. International guidelines for the selection of lung transplant candidates. Heart & Lung 1998; 27(4):223–228.
59. Moss M, Make BJ: Pulmonary response to exercise in health and disease. Semin Respir Med 1993; 14:106–120.
60. Noseda A, Carpiaux JP, Prigogine T, et al: Lung function, maximum and sub-maximum exercise testing in COPD patients: Reproducibility over a long interval. Lung 1989; 167:24.
61. Olesen KM, Hiller FC: Management of tetanus. Clin Pharm 1987; 6:570–574.
62. Patessio A, Carone M, Loli F, et al: Ventilatory and metabolic changes as a result of exercise training in COPD patients. Chest 1992; 101:274S–278S.
63. Ries AL, Kaplan RM, Limberg TM, et al: Effects of pulmonary rehabilitation on physiologic and psychosocial outcomes in patients with chronic obstructive pulmonary disease. Ann Int Med 1995; 122(11):823–832.
64. Rogers TK, Howard P: Pulmonary hemodynamics and physical training in patients with chronic obstructive pulmonary disease. Chest 1992; 101(suppl 5):289S–292S.
65. Rubin BK, van der Schans CP, Kishioka C, et al: Mucus and mucoactive therapy in chronic bronchitis. Clin Pulm Med 1998; 5(1):1–13.
66. Schols AM, Slangen J, Volovics L, et al: Weight loss is a reversible factor in the prognosis of chronic obstructive pulmonary disease. Am J Respir Crit Care Med 1998; 157(6 Pt 1):1791–1797.
67. Schols AM, Soeters PB, Dingemans AM, et al: Prevalence and characteristics of nutritional depletion in patients with stable COPD eligible for pulmonary rehabilitation. Am Rev Respir Dis 1993; 147:1151–1156.
68. Seiser A, Schwartz S, Brainin M: Critical illness polyneuropathy: Clinical aspects and long-term outcome. Wien Klin Wochenschr 1992; 104:294–300.

69. Sivak ED: Management of ventilator dependency following heart surgery. Semin Thorac Cardiovasc Surg 1991; 3:53–62.
70. Tiep BL: Long-term home oxygen therapy. Clin Chest Med 1990; 11:505–521.
71. Tiep BL: Reversing disability of irreversible lung disease. West J Med 1991; 154:591–597.
72. U.S. National Institutes of Health. National Asthma Education and Prevention Program Expert Panel Report 2: Guidelines for the Diagnosis and Management of Asthma. Bethesda, MD, NIH, 1997.
73. Van-der-Schoot TA, Kaptein AA: Pulmonary rehabilitation in an asthma clinic. Lung 1990; 168(suppl):495–501.
74. Varray A, Mercier J, Savy-Pacaux AM, et al: Cardiac role in exercise limitation in asthmatic subjects with special reference to disease severity. Eur Respir J 1993; 6:1011–1017.
75. Votto J, Bowen J, Scalise P, et al: Short-stay comprehensive inpatient pulmonary rehabilitation for advanced chronic obstructive pulmonary disease. Arch Phys Med Rehabil 1996; 77(11):1115–1118.
76. Walker J, Cooney M, Norton S: Improved pulmonary function in chronic quadriplegics after pulmonary therapy and arm ergometry. Paraplegia 1989; 27:278–283.
77. Wolf SI, Lampl KL: Pulmonary rehabilitation: The use of aerobic dance as a therapeutic exercise for asthmatic patients. Ann Allergy 1988; 61:357–360.
78. Zu-Wallack RL, Patel K, Reardon JZ, et al: Predictors of improvement in the 12-minute walking distance following a six-week out-patient pulmonary rehabilitation program. Chest 1991; 99: 805–808.

34 CHAPTER

Ralph M. Buschbacher, M.D., and C. Douglas Porter, M.D.

Deconditioning, Conditioning, and the Benefits of Exercise

Since civilization began, it has been recognized that exercise is good for the body, whereas inactivity promotes its decline. Perhaps Maimonides said it best in his *Treatise of Hygiene* (1199): "Anyone who lives a sedentary life and does not exercise, even if he eats good foods and takes care of himself according to proper medical principles—all his days will be painful ones and his strength shall wane." Physicians from ancient Greece and China to medieval Europe all espoused one form of exercise or another to treat and prevent illness and infirmity. Nor was this belief limited to physicians; it was also the province of poets and philosophers. As John Dryden wrote: "Better to hunt in fields, for health unbought, /Than fee the doctor for a nauseous draught. /The wise, for cure, on exercise depend; /God never made his work, for man to mend."

Yet somehow, in the mid-1800s, medicine turned its back on promoting activity and began recommending long periods of bed rest and immobilization for a variety of disorders. Hugh Owen Thomas and John Hunter were among the first to recommend (per Thomas) "enforced, uninterrupted, and prolonged" rest.[68] In 1863, John Hilton published his book, *On the Influence of Mechanical and Physiological Rest in the Treatment of Accidents and Surgical Diseases, and the Diagnostic Value of Pain,*[92] in which he described a series of cases successfully treated with enforced rest. Hilton's work was very influential, eventually going through six editions and numerous printings. He did not, in fact, see rest as a panacea; but his teachings were misunderstood and misapplied by several generations of physicians taught to view bed rest as a desirable treatment rather than an occasionally necessary evil.

In various medical specialties, particularly in obstetrics and gynecology, and in surgery, prolonged bed rest became a mainstay of treatment. It was once considered routine to prescribe a week or more of bed rest after simple back strain. When White and colleagues[193] and Mallory and others[128] noted that it took approximately 8 weeks for large myocardial infarctions to heal (5 weeks for small infarcts), they recommended at least 1 month of bed rest (2 weeks absolute) followed by 1 month of limited activity after infarction. At least 3 weeks of bed rest was advocated for even the smallest infarcts.

Clearly, much has changed since this method of treatment was considered routine. Through the pioneering efforts of Cuthbertson,[46] Dietrick and colleagues,[51] Saltin and colleagues,[160] Taylor and colleagues,[184] and many others, we have come to understand the deleterious effects of immobility. In addition, the space program has provided much information about the effects of bed rest, immobilization, and weightlessness. One by one, the outdated tenents of the past have been refuted, and today exercise is viewed as a positive mode of treatment while bed rest is a negative. But even in this modern era, misperceptions abound in the lay press. In 1994, for example, a *U.S. News & World Report* article contained the following statement: "While prolonged bed rest can cause emotional and financial hardships, it doesn't have the side effects that drugs do. So doctors have believed that at least bed rest does no harm. . . ."[157]

This chapter explores the fundamental physiological changes that occur with deconditioning and examines the benefits of exercise. *Deconditioning* as a rehabilitation diagnosis is also discussed.

Many of the data presented here are the result of research in the space program. As the effects of weightlessness might not be directly applicable to the person on bed rest, every effort has been made to cite the most clinically useful references. Similarly, much of the information on the consequences of immobility, especially at the cellular level, comes from animal studies. Again, where possible, the emphasis is on appropriate human models.

CONSEQUENCES OF DISUSE

The functional capacity of the body and of the body organs depends on the previous stresses placed on the body and its organs. Within certain physiological limits, the body can be trained to be stronger, quicker, better conditioned, and more fit. It can also be "trained" to deteriorate. The physiological maximum potential is the upper limit of function, which cannot be altered through activity or use. Age, illness, and injury can cause a decline in the maximal limit, but need not portend a corresponding decline in functional ability. As depicted in Figure 34–1, most persons operate at a level well below their maximum. With training, they can move closer to this limit. With disuse they move farther away. But as long as the limit is not lowered excessively, the person can maintain and even increase function. As a result, we see persons who, having started training after a myocardial infarction, are now "in the best shape of their lives."

Obviously, such a scenario is not realistic in all cases. But in rehabilitation, we strive to maximize function: Even when the physiological maximum is decreased, a person is better off if operating at or near this (lowered) limit (see Fig. 34–1).

Bed rest, immobilization, or relative rest is unfortunately necessary in some situations. These include some acute injuries, especially fractures and dislocations, acute myocardial infarction or pulmonary disease, and severe medical or surgical disorders. Yet even when rest is properly prescribed, we should be aware of its deleterious effects. The consequences of such disuse on the body organs and systems are described in the following section and summarized in Table 34–1.

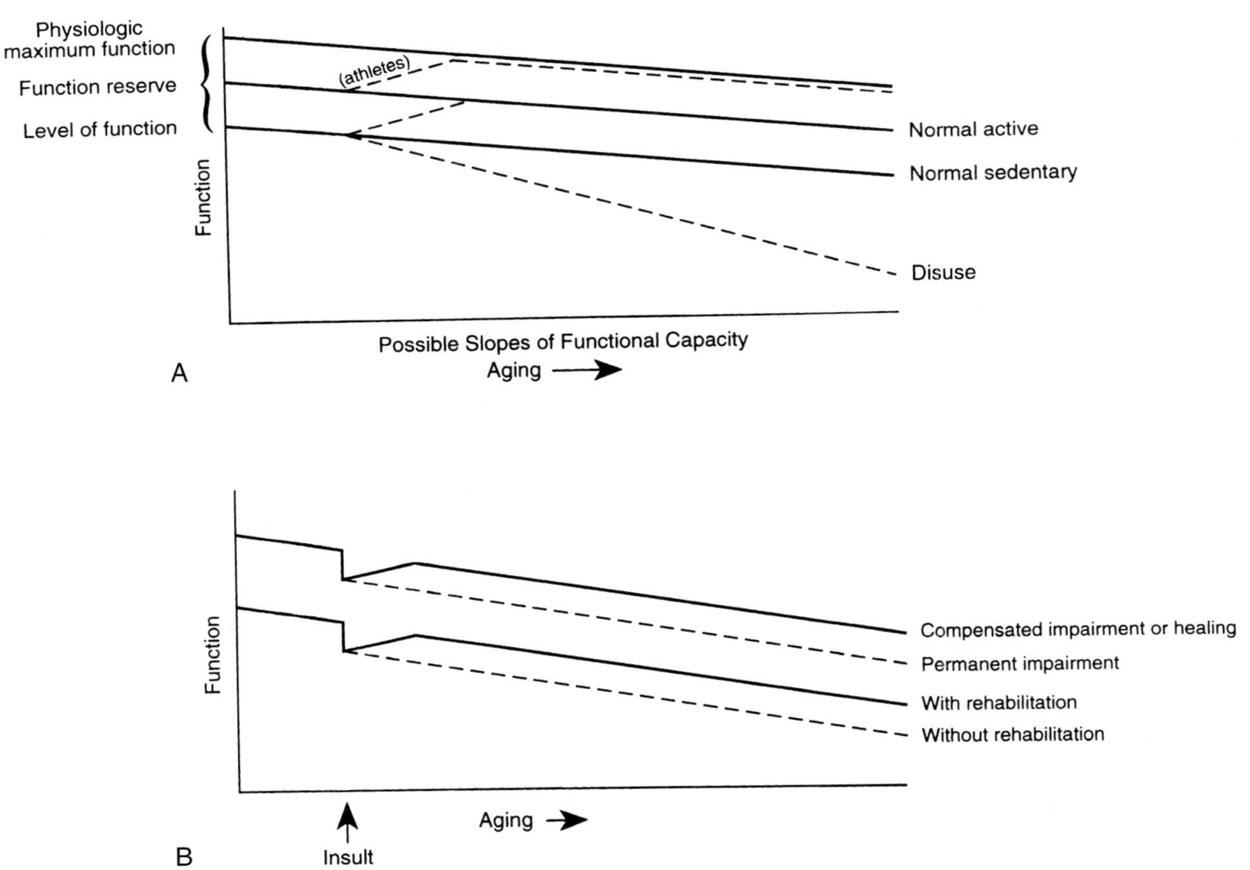

FIGURE 34–1. Physiological maximum is the maximal theoretic functional level attainable by a person. For most body systems, this value decreases somewhat with age. *A*. Athletes operate near their physiological maximum. Normal sedentary persons operate at a level below that of the normal active individual. Through exercise or disuse it is possible to change the slope of the line representing a given person's physiological maximum. This will affect function regardless of the maximal attainable level. *B*. When a body system (or the whole body) sustains an insult, its level of function is lowered. This might lead to a permanent impairment (*top dotted line*). If the insult is healed or compensated for, the previous functional level can be regained. The *lines below* indicate that rehabilitation may raise a person's capacity back to the higher level. However, prolonged inactivity can permanently alter the maximum physiological potential that can be obtained.

TABLE 34–1 Major Complications of Immobility by Body System

Musculoskeletal

- Muscles
  - Atrophy; decreased strength and endurance
  - Contracture
  - Altered electrical activity/excitation
  - Weakened myotendinous junction
  - Contractures
  - Decreased strength of tendons and ligaments and their insertions on bone
- Bone
  - Osteoporosis
- Joints
  - Cartilage degeneration
  - Fibrofatty tissue infiltration
  - Synovial atrophy
  - Ankylosis

Cardiovascular

- Cardiac (at rest)
  - ↑ Heart rate
  - ↓ Stroke volume
  - Cardiac output unchanged or slightly decreased
  - $\dot{V}O_2$ unchanged
  - ↓ Cardiac size/volume
  - ↓ Left ventricular end-diastolic volume
  - Systolic/diastolic blood pressure unchanged
  - Arteriovenous oxygen difference unchanged or slightly increased
- Cardiac (with exercise)
  - ↑ Heart rate response to submaximal exercise
  - Maximum heart rate unchanged
  - ↓ $\dot{V}O_{2max}$
  - ↓ Stroke volume (submaximal/maximal)
  - ↓ Cardiac output (submaximal/maximal)
  - ↑ Arteriovenous oxygen difference (submaximal) (maximal is unchanged)
- Neurovascular
  - Orthostatic intolerance
- Fluid balance
  - ↓ Plasma volume
  - ↓ Total blood volume
  - ↓ Red blood cell mass
  - Mineral and plasma protein loss (mainly isocontent)
- Blood coagulation
  - ↑ Venous thrombosis
  - ↓ Calf blood flow (possible)
  - ↑ Blood fibrinogen

Skin

- Pressure ulcer
- Edema
- Subcutaneous bursitis

Body Composition, Metabolism, Nutrition

- ↓ Lean body mass
- ↑ Body fat
- Minerals
  - Nitrogen loss
  - Calcium loss
  - Phosphorus loss
  - Sulfur loss
  - Potassium loss

Endocrine

- Impaired glucose tolerance
- Altered circadian rhythm
- Altered temperature and sweating response
- Altered regulation of parathyroid hormone, thyroid hormones, adrenal hormones, pituitary hormones, growth hormone, androgens, and plasma renin activity

Respiratory

- ↑ Forced vital capacity
- ↑ Total lung capacity (slight)
- Residual volume unchanged
- Functional residual capacity unchanged
- ↑ Respiratory rate
- Vital capacity unchanged (possibly decreases in time owing to contractures of chest wall)
- Maximal minute ventilation unchanged
- Possible ventilation/perfusion mismatch
- Pulmonary embolism (possible)

Genitourinary

- Diuresis
- ↑ Mineral excretion
- Difficulty voiding
- ↑ Postvoid residual volume (possible)
- ↑ Urinary tract infection (possible)
- ↑ Overflow incontinence (possible)
- ↑ Calculus formation (possible)
- ↓ Glomerular filtration rate
- ↓ Ability to concentrate urine

Gastrointestinal

- ↓ Fluid intake
- ↓ Appetite
- ↓ Bowel motility
- ↓ Gastric secretion
- Constipation (possible)

Neurological, Emotional

- Compression neuropathies
- Sensory deprivation (attention span, altered time awareness, hand-to-eye coordination, depression, anxiety)
- ↓ Balance
- ↓ Coordination
- Sleep disturbance
- ↑ Auditory threshold
- ↓ Visual acuity

Abbreviations: $\dot{V}O_2$, rate of oxygen consumption; $\dot{V}O_{2max}$, rate of maximum oxygen consumption.

The Musculoskeletal System

The primary functions of the musculoskeletal system are to support the body, to transport the body, and to use the body to accomplish physical tasks. It is affected by both activity and inactivity, and disorders of the system in turn affect the activity level that is possible.

Muscles

Disuse leads to muscle weakness. In the classic studies by Mueller,[140] the muscles of persons on strict bed rest lost 1.0% to 1.5% of their initial strength (torque about a joint) per day (over a 2-week period, with a sampling of 17 muscles tested). With cast immobilization of the upper extremity, 1.3% to 5.5% of strength was lost per day, over a 2-week period.[140] This corresponds to a 10% to 20% loss of strength per week for most persons. The loss was greatest during the first week of inactivity and gradually plateaued at a 25% loss.[140] In other studies of immobilization, up to a 40% loss of strength has been recorded.[127] In a compilation of data from other studies Greenleaf et al[79] concluded that there is a loss of about

0.7% of strength per day. Mueller's studies (and most others) were performed by testing isometric strength, and this might not be as functionally relevant as other methods of testing strength and endurance. In addition, the generalizability of his results is limited because loss of strength can be different in previously sedentary versus trained subjects.

Loss of strength varies among muscle groups. In a classic study by Dietrick et al,[51] healthy volunteers were placed on bed rest in bivalved casts from the umbilicus to the toes, with a 30- to 40-minute break per day. They were immobilized in this fashion for six to seven weeks. On average, the subjects lost 6.6% of their elbow flexor strength, 8.7% of their shoulder flexor strength, 13.3% of their dorsiflexor strength, and 20.8% of their plantar flexor strength. They experienced about a 2% loss of girth in the upper arms and forearms. Thigh circumference decreased between 2.1% and 5%, and calf circumference decreased between 5.5% and 6.3%. This corresponded to a loss of cross-sectional area of 4.2% to 10% in the thighs and 9.7% to 12.5% in the calves, a loss attributed primarily to atrophy of muscle tissue (Fig. 34–2). In more recent studies measuring muscle circumference, one month of bed rest caused an 8–13% loss of cross-sectional area of selected leg muscles measured by magnetic resonance imaging,[20] and quadriceps cross-sectional area declined by 27% with four weeks of cast immobilization as measured by computed tomography (CT).[189] One patient who was immobilized after an ankle fracture had a 25% reduction of gastrocnemius-soleus cross-sectional area over an eight-week period.[187] Others were demonstrated to have a 10–18% loss of muscle mass in various leg muscles, measured by MRI, after 30 days of bedrest.[57, 72] Such atrophy is not necessarily to be viewed as an abnormal response. In fact, it is most likely a normal reaction to an activity level that does not require the tissues to be present; the body does not needlessly support redundant tissues.

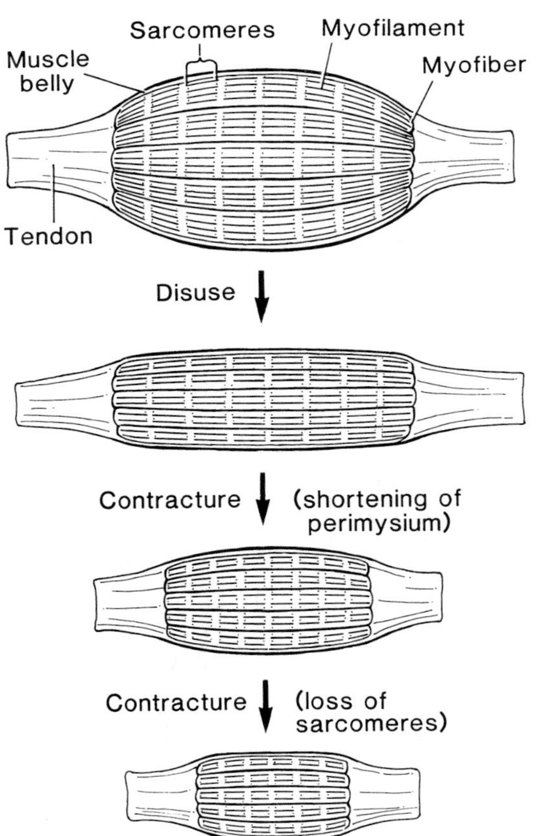

FIGURE 34–2. Progression of muscle atrophy and contracture. In early disuse, a loss of muscle mass occurs through a reduction in myofilaments (muscle cross-section). The total number of myofibers (muscle cells) is unchanged, and sarcomere number remains constant. With contracture, however, a shortening of the perimysial connective tissue, and later a loss of sarcomeres (in series), occurs.

Antigravity muscles, such as the gastrocnemius-soleus and the back muscles, appear to lose strength disproportionately, and large muscles seem to lose strength twice as quickly as smaller ones.[79] Handgrip strength is not affected by prolonged bed rest,[79, 184] although grip endurance does seem to be reduced.[79] The loss of strength can vary with different speeds of muscle contraction.[11]

It is commonly reported that type I, slow-twitch muscle fibers are more subject to immobilization atrophy than are type II, fast-twitch fibers.[11] Many of the data supporting this contention come from animal studies. Animals often have a more homogeneous fiber-type preponderance in various muscles than do humans, and these observations might not be directly applicable to humans. Nevertheless, it appears that in muscles that have been trained to have a relatively high cross-sectional area of type I fibers (such as the antigravity muscles predominantly affected by disuse) atrophy can selectively affect these fibers.[87, 105] This preferential atrophy is most likely influenced by the location and function of the involved muscles.[91] The affected fibers degenerate and develop an increased noncontractile connective tissue content.[91, 134] The total number of fibers is unchanged.[33, 142]

Immobilization appears to affect some parts of the muscle fiber substructure more than others. In one study of eight human subjects on 17 days of bedrest, the soleus type I fibers were found to have a disproportionate loss of thin filaments (16% to 23% decrease) with no change in thick filament density. Interestingly, when immobilization is combined with a shortened muscle position, the thick filaments are also lost.[155]

Muscle fiber atrophy has been shown to begin after as little as one day of immobilization,[134] and in rats there are signs of decreased protein synthesis within only six hours.[25] Positioning is important in the development of atrophy, at least in animal studies. Stretching of the muscles seems to delay the atrophy (and can even cause growth). Immobilization in a shortened position promotes a more rapid deterioration (primarily due to a loss of muscle length).[12, 90, 99, 173] Immobilization has been shown to cause changes in muscle electrical activity[14, 55] and in the myoneural junction.[70, 146, 152] There is also a decrease in strength of the myotendinous junction,[103] and an alteration in intramuscular vasculature.[145]

There might be some protective effect of training before immobilization,[11, 79, 104] especially in untrained persons. Trained subjects, however, lose the most absolute muscle strength when they are immobilized.[11]

After remobilization, it can take two or more times the period of immobilization to recover muscle strength.[94] In some cases, residual deficits from a period of disuse have lasted for months or years, especially after injury or surgery.[83, 158] Consequently, it is desirable, when possible, to prevent the disuse weakening from developing. Muscle strength can be maintained by performing daily muscle contractions, though the optimal type and amount of exercise are not known. Hettinger showed that isometric muscle strength can be maintained by performing daily isometric contractions of 10% to 20% of maximal tension for 10 sec.[140] His subjects were placed in bivalved arm casts and were otherwise free to go about their daily activities. Undoubtedly they experienced a training effect from incidental activity, and it is difficult to generalize his results to persons on bed rest. In another study, subjects on 14 days of bedrest were found to maintain knee extensor strength with five sets of leg presses performed at 80% to 85% of their one-repetition maximum strength every other day.[14] Cycle ergometry and isokinetic strength training have been shown to maintain muscle strength and mass of some, but not all, muscle groups during bedrest.[57, 74] A combination of exercise types is most likely best,[72] but it is still unclear exactly what exercise regimen is required to prevent a decline in function. It appears to be advisable to maintain as near normal activity as possible, even during periods of immobilization or hospitalization. In patients with casts, muscle contraction within the cast, either voluntary or through electrical stimulation, might also be beneficial.

Periarticular Soft Tissues

Contracture is an abnormal limitation of passive joint range of motion. It is usually due to a restriction of the periarticular connective tissue, but in more advanced cases also involves tendons, ligaments, muscles, and joints. If not treated, it can lead to bony ankylosis of the joint. While there are many possible causes of contractures (Table 34–2), the primary cause (and the one pertinent to this chapter) is lack of normal joint mobilization. Joints must periodically be put through their full range of motion to prevent a tightening of the surrounding soft tissues and muscles.

TABLE 34–2 Major Causes of Joint Contracture

Muscular	*Joints*
Muscle strength imbalance	Connective tissue disease
Neuromuscular disease	Pain
Burn tracts	Inflammation
Degenerative disease	Congenital disorders
Inflammation	Sepsis
Trauma	Ankylosis
Skin, Soft Tissues	
Scleroderma	
Scar	
Burns	

The mobile tissues of the body are typically separated by thin layers of loose areolar connective tissue. This allows tendons, ligaments, muscles, and joint capsules to glide on one another during normal motion. With immobilization, the loose connective tissue is reorganized and is replaced by more dense material containing a greater abundance of collagen cross-links (the type of collagen is probably unchanged).[3, 7, 59] This process can begin after as little as one week of immobilization[114] and is aggravated in conditions of increased collagen turnover. It is complemented by an active fibroblast-mediated contraction within these tissues.[197] It is also believed to be accelerated in the presence of superimposed local trauma, hemorrhage, impaired circulation, pre-existing degeneration, or edema.[113] Once the other soft tissues have become involved in contracture formation, the muscles may become shortened as well (see Fig. 34–2).

In the early phase of this muscular shortening, the primary contribution to the loss of length comes from the intrinsic muscle-supporting tissues, mainly the perimysium.[196] Only later does actual muscle fiber shortening occur. When it does occur, it is due to a loss of sarcomere number (in series),[12, 173, 195] mainly at the ends of the muscle fibers.[12]

As the affected body part loses normal range of motion, other parts of the body must compensate for the loss. This leads to increased stress on adjacent and distant joints. Increased energy expenditure due to abnormal biomechanics may lead to even more immobility. Ultimately, function is lost. The abnormal range of motion also makes the nursing care of bedridden patients more difficult.

A number of conditions predispose patients to contractures. Spasticity, paralysis, or muscle strength imbalance hastens their development. Patients with amputations tend to develop contractures, mainly because of position and strength imbalances. The below-knee amputee, for instance, often sits with the knee flexed. This leads to a hip and knee flexion contracture. The above-knee amputee loses strength of the hip adductors, some of which insert below the knee. This can lead to a fixed hip flexion and abduction deformity.

In conditions of joint pain and inflammation, the patient tends to position the joint in the least painful position (to minimize intra-articular pressure). The most common of these positions are flexion and external rotation of the hip, flexion of the fingers and knees, and plantar flexion of the ankles. Similar positions are taken by patients on bed rest (Fig. 34–3). They also tend to position the shoulders in internal rotation. Common joint contractures and their sequelae are described in Table 34–3.

Inactive persons eventually develop contractures, whether their inactivity is due to illness or they are sedentary by choice. These can be mild and seemingly insignificant, but often affect the ability to reach, to take long strides, to comb one's hair, etc.

Contractures are likely to affect muscles that cross multiple joints, because stretching of only one joint or the other may not adequately stretch the entire muscle. Where and how contractures develop depends on the

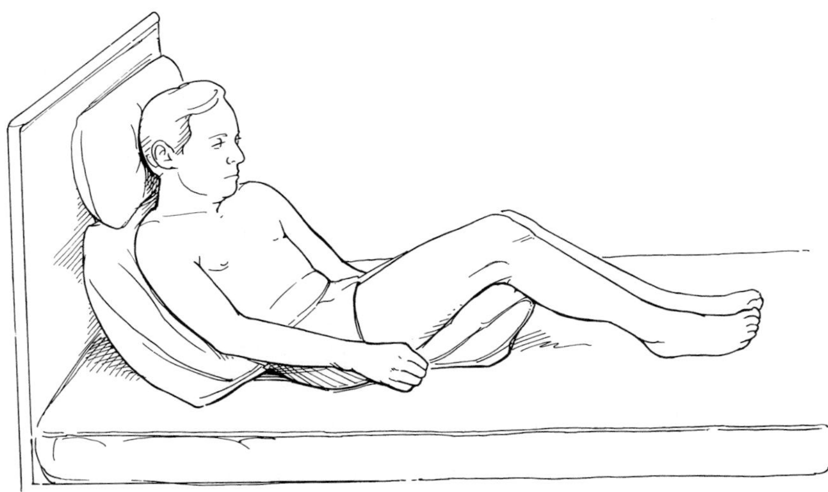

FIGURE 34–3. Common bed position and the areas susceptible to contracture: neck, flexed; shoulders, internally rotated; thorax, flexed; arms, flexed; forearms, pronated; fingers, flexed; hips, flexed; knees, flexed; and ankles, plantar flexed.

position of the joint and the length of time that position is maintained (as well as predisposing factors). They may be precipitated by painful conditions. For instance, a "frozen shoulder," in which the inferior axillary fold of the joint capsule is reduced, often follows tendonitis, surgery, or trauma to the shoulder. The shoulder is particularly susceptible to loss of range of motion because of its normally great mobility. The only major contracture with little functional disability is a mild-to-moderate elbow flexion contracture. Such a contracture maintains this joint in a position of function, such as for eating. Elbow extension contractures are actually more limiting than flexion contractures (Fig. 34–4).

It is not clear how often the soft tissues must be passed through a complete range of motion to prevent contracture. Normal living and motion cause compound motions that most likely stretch nearly all parts of the body multiple times a day. It is commonly believed that contractures can be prevented by daily or twice-daily range-of-motion exercise. This is especially important in the hospitalized patient, in the elderly, and in arthritic joints, which are believed to develop contractures relatively rapidly.

In the presence of risk factors predisposing to contractures (such as muscle strength imbalances or paralysis), proper positioning and possibly intermittent splinting (or dynamic splinting) might be necessary. Too soft a bed can aggravate abnormal positioning and should be avoided. It is important for patients to lie prone occasionally, especially to stretch the hip joint. Even lying prone, however, doesn't always stretch the hips adequately, so a pillow under the knees while in the prone position might be advisable, especially in persons who are sitting or lying for prolonged periods of time. Standing upright is also an effective stretch of the anterior hip, as well as of the posterior knee. In bed, pillows or trochanteric rolls applied to the lateral surfaces of the thighs may help prevent external rotation deformity of the legs. Proper active dorsiflexion exercise and possibly a footboard can help prevent plantar flexion contractures.

Once contractures have developed, they are treated with range-of-motion exercise (Table 34–4). Voluntary active range-of-motion exercise is preferred, but in some cases assisted range-of-motion exercise is needed. When stretching a contracted area, it is important to make sure that there is no bony block or other mechanical limitation to motion (Table 34–5). If such a condition is present, it can be a contraindication to range-of-motion exercise. It is also important not to be overly aggressive when stretching. If the tissues are torn and damaged during stretching, they are more likely to develop an even thicker connective tissue barrier to normal mobility. Overly aggressive stretching can also lead to joint dislocation or damage, especially in the knee or elbow.

When manual stretching is inadequate, or in cases of advanced contractures, deep heating to the involved connective tissue can help increase range of motion.[192] In some cases, motor point or nerve blocks can be used

TABLE 34–3 Common Joint Contractures and Their Sequelae

Contracture	Sequelae
Hip joint flexion	Compensatory lordosis (back pain), knee flexion, short steps
Hip joint external rotation	Stiff-legged gait, excessive stress on medial knee ligaments
Knee flexion	Plantar flexion (toe-walking), crouch gait
Ankle plantar flexion	Genu recurvatum, absence of heel-strike
Shoulder flexion, adduction, and internal rotation	Cannot reach back pocket, comb hair, or reach above shoulder level
Elbow flexion	If mild, little function loss; if severe, interferes with dressing, weakens triceps position
Wrist flexion	Weakened grip
Finger flexion	Cannot open hand to grasp

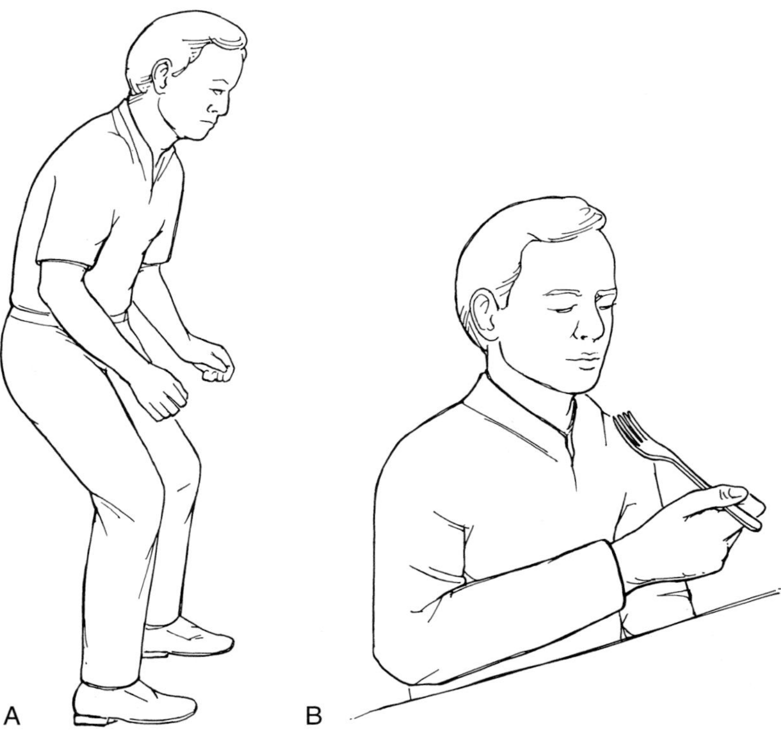

FIGURE 34–4. Similar contractures of knee (*A*) and elbow (*B*) cause vastly different functional outcomes. In fact, the elbow contracture might be virtually unnoticed.

to weaken an overpowering muscle imbalance. (This also helps to differentiate a true contracture from abnormal tone or spasticity.) In refractory cases, serial casting might be necessary. The joint is stretched maximally and a cast is applied. The process is repeated, with a cast change every 2 to 3 days to progressively stretch the connective tissues. Care must be taken not to cause pressure sores to the skin or circulatory compromise to the limb when performing the casting. If such casting still does not reduce the contracture, surgical treatment might be necessary. This can include capsular release, tenotomy, or tendon-lengthening procedures. In conditions of muscle strength imbalance, tendon transfer might be indicated as well. (In conditions of muscle imbalance, strengthening of the weak muscles might also be helpful.) Postsurgical contractures can often be prevented by using continuous passive range-of-motion machines.

Ligaments and Tendons

Ligaments and tendons are composed primarily of longitudinally arranged, parallel, type I collagen fibers. This gives them great strength in the direction of pull. This parallel alignment of collagen fibers is fostered by longitudinal stress applied to these connective tissues. When this stress is lacking, as during immobilization, the newly formed collagen is laid down in a haphazard array (Fig. 34–5) and the function of the structures deteriorates.[8] Immobilization causes an increase in collagen turnover,[8] a decrease in collagen mass,[3] a decrease in glycosaminoglycan and water content,[4] an increase in soft tissue stiffness,[143] and an alteration in fibroblast function.[141] In addition to a deterioration of the soft tissues themselves, there is a loss of strength at the collagen-bone interface, with bone resorption directly below the insertion site.[109, 118, 143]

TABLE 34–4 Progression of Treatment of Contractures from Least to Most Aggressive Methods

Proper positioning
Active range of motion exercise
Active assisted range of motion exercise
Passive range of motion exercise
Static splinting
Dynamic splinting
Nerve/motor point blocks
Serial casting
Surgery

TABLE 34–5 Mechanical Limitations to Joint Range of Motion That May Be Contraindications to Stretching

Bony block
Cartilage damage
Loose body in joint
Joint incongruity
Synovial thickening
Severe bony degenerative disease
Fracture
Dislocation

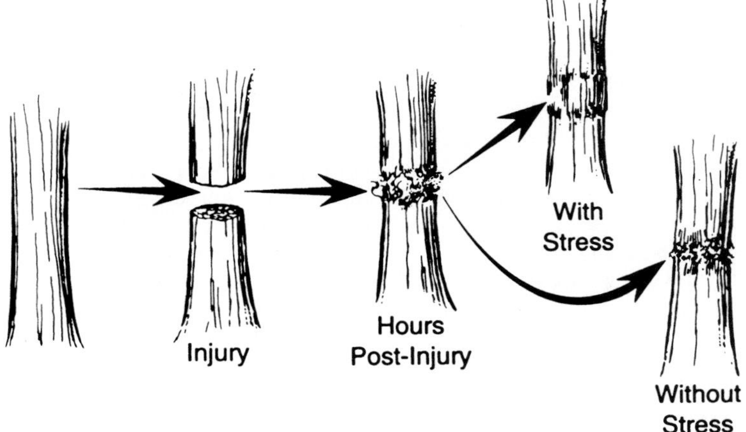

FIGURE 34–5. Normal recovery progression of a tendon after laceration. If the tendon is not stressed, the collagen scar remains unorganized instead of the fibers' being arranged in parallel. Similar haphazard collagen orientation is promoted through immobilization, though weakening is not as rapid or dramatic. (From Buschbacher RM: Tissue injury and healing. *In* Buschbacher RM (ed): Musculoskeletal Disorders: A Practical Guide for Diagnosis and Rehabilitation. Stoneham, MA, Butterworth-Heinemann, 1994, p 21.)

As mentioned above, longitudinal stress is required to achieve proper collagen orientation.[8] Even in the absence of weightbearing stress on the joint, movement can prevent soft tissue deterioration, although bone atrophy is not necessarily retarded.[109] It is important to continue to stress the tendons and ligaments in all persons, both healthy and ill, and as soon as is clinically feasible, in those recovering from injury or surgery. Ligaments have been shown, in a primate model, to lose up to one-third of their strength in just eight weeks of immobilization.[143] Once weakness of these tissues has developed, it takes months to years to recover.[2, 143]

Bones

Bone is normally in a state of dynamic equilibrium in which the rate of bone formation and resorption is held in balance. The ratio of formation to resorption is influenced by the stresses on bone, in accordance with what is commonly known as Wolff's law. Weightbearing is the primary stress on most of the bones of the body, and it causes a buildup of bone. Other activities in which the pull of muscles stresses the bone also increase bone mass.

Lack of stress on the bones leads to a predominance of bone resorption (osteoclastic activity), which decreases bone mass and causes osteoporosis (see Chapter 41 on osteoporosis). In rats this loss of bone mass can start to occur in as little as 30 hours after immobilization.[185] The rate of loss of bone varies with the type of disuse and by body part, with weightbearing bones being relatively more affected. During bed rest there can be an almost 1% loss of vertebral mineral content per week.[117, 121] With immobilization in animal studies, the bone mass generally drops until it plateaus at approximately 50% of the original mass.[124, 186] In human studies of the calcaneus, losses of 25% to 45% were documented after 30 to 36 weeks of bed rest.[54] There was a loss of 4.2% of total body calcium during this same time period.[54] The remaining bone was histologically normal, with a normal ratio of mineral to matrix, although the organization of the bone may be altered. The bone is less massive.

In addition to generalized osteoporosis, there can also be local bone loss in conditions of partial immobilization, as after casting of fractures. In persons with paralysis, osteoporosis is often severe, and fractures can occur with relatively nontraumatic events such as transfer activities.

Osteoporosis is a slowly advancing disease which can show little or no outward sign of its progression until pathological fractures occur. It is not easily diagnosed radiographically, since a large loss of bone is required before it can be detected on plain films. In the early stages, special bone density measurement techniques, such as photon absorptiometry or CT scanning,[124] are needed to make the diagnosis. It commonly affects trabecular bone more than cortical bone in the early stages. Cortical bone loss occurs later as well, especially in the midcortical layer.[198]

Osteoporosis is best treated with preventive measures such as active weightbearing exercise and active muscle contraction. Exercise in bed, even if intense, might not be effective in preventing or treating the disorder.[136] In women, postmenopausal estrogen supplementation is also an option, and proper calcium intake is important as well.

Proper exercise is also advocated once osteoporosis has developed (after any fractures have healed). If the osteoporosis is related to a short duration (less than 3 to 6 months) of immobilization, as for casting of a fracture, it is likely to be reversed nearly completely. Longer-standing disuse osteoporosis, or that due to years of sedentary living, is not as easily reversed.[136] In a study of primates immobilized for 7 months, there was evidence of renewed bone formation after 2 months of resumption of activity. Normal bone formation was seen after 6 months, but it was thought that the trabecular bone would never completely recover its normal architecture.[200] While exercise might not reverse the bone loss that has already occurred, it will slow the progression of the disorder.[117]

Immobilization hypercalcemia is a condition often associated with osteoporosis, especially in adolescent males who have had traumatic injuries. As their bones are resorbed, serum calcium levels rise. They may become symptomatic, usually 2 to 4 weeks after the immobilization began. Signs and symptoms include nausea, vomiting, abdominal pain, lethargy, muscle weakness, and anorexia. If not treated, death can occur. Treatment is with intravenous furosemide and hydration. Etidronate disodium, intravenous pamidronate,[108] and calcitonin can be used as well, especially in refractory cases.[133]

Heterotopic ossification is a condition of bone growth in abnormal locations, usually around joints. It is not caused by immobility, but is generally found in persons who have experienced trauma. The trauma can be neurological (such as spinal cord injury) or a direct muscle contusion. It can also be seen in persons immobilized because of other injuries.

Joints

During embryonic development joints are formed in response to movement. It should not be surprising, then, that movement is required to maintain their integrity.

The hyaline cartilage in synovial joints is not supplied by vascular blood flow. It receives its nutrition from the synovial fluid by a regular loading and unloading of pressure, which draws fluid into and out of the cartilage in a process known as imbibition. During immobilization imbibition ceases, and the cartilage is dependent on simple diffusion to obtain nutrients. This diffusion is not adequate to the needs of the cartilage, and the joints begin to deteriorate.

Immobilization-induced cartilage degeneration affects both the opposing joint surfaces that are in contact with each other and those that are not. The areas in contact develop pressure necrosis and erosions.[58] The noncontact surfaces develop fissures and lose their smoothness[2, 102] (Fig. 34–6). Proteoglycan balance is altered,[18] and the cartilage becomes stiffer. As the joints attempt to repair themselves, there is a compensatory cartilage proliferation and osteophyte formation.[58] In addition, there is a fibrofatty infiltration of the joint cavity, and the synovium becomes atrophic. There is deterioration of the subchondral bone as well.[171] This is accompanied by extra-articular connective tissue contracture, which exacerbates the condition,[58] and can eventually lead to ankylosis.

These changes can occur in some joints, not only with cast immobilization, but also when weightbearing is restricted.[148] As little as 2 weeks of immobilization begins the process, at least in rabbits.[62] The cause of the joint changes is believed to be an attempt to repair tissues damaged by inadequate nutrition.[58] In the early stages this degeneration can be reversible to some extent,[147] but later it most likely is not.

Nevertheless, in some arthritic conditions a short period of joint immobilization is indicated and can help reduce synovitis and pain caused by even passive range-of-motion exercise.[132] Such short-term immobilization can, however, worsen cartilage destruction.[188] As a rule, it should be kept to a minimum.

Patients with paralysis sometimes develop knee joint effusions of unknown cause. This has been termed "benign knee joint effusion of paralysis," and is seen predominantly in persons with spinal cord injury. It can also occur in Guillain-Barré syndrome and other neuromuscular diseases.[31] It has been hypothesized that these effusions are due to inadequate muscular control of the intra-articular knee joint structures, namely the meniscus and the plica. As passive range-of-motion exercise is performed, these structures are irritated and cause an effusion, making the cause not true immobilization, but rather muscle weakness.

The Cardiovascular System

Disuse (especially bed rest) causes a number of cardiovascular adaptations that are generally deleterious. These adaptations include (1) cardiac deconditioning, (2) an impaired response to the upright position (neurovascular deconditioning), (3) changes in fluid balance, and (4) decreased ability to prevent venous thrombosis. In general, long-term inactivity is comparable to hypertension, smoking, and an elevated serum cholesterol level as a risk factor for coronary heart disease.[151]

Cardiac Deconditioning

It is a common observance for athletes to develop a resting bradycardia. Elite athletes can have heart rates in the 50s. Their heart rates increase less with submaximal exercise than is the case in untrained persons, whereas their maximal heart rates are essentially unchanged. Deconditioned persons have a resting tachycardia and an abnormally high heart rate with submaximal exercise. A severely deconditioned person can reach maximal heart rate with a seemingly trivial workload.

When a normal person assumes the recumbent position, a number of changes occur. First, venous return increases because there is less pooling of blood in the venous system of the legs. This causes an increase in cardiac contractility and output, a decrease in heart rate, and an increase in cardiac work. There is a shift of fluid from the extravascular spaces to the intravascular circulation. This stimulates diuresis to reduce the blood volume. Ordinarily, these effects are mild and rapidly reversible, but during periods of prolonged bed rest they progress.

Deconditioning-Induced Changes Occurring at Rest. After a period of bed rest, the resting heart rate starts to rise.[51, 160, 184] It is generally believed to rise by about one-half beat per minute each day for the first 3 to 4 weeks of immobilization.[160, 184] The reason for this rise is unclear, but it appears to be due to an imbalance of autonomic nervous system function.[154] Resting stroke volume is decreased for most persons,[160] while cardiac output is not changed significantly.[77, 160, 184] Cardiac size falls by up to 11%,[160, 184] and cardiac muscle atrophy may occur.[106] Resting systolic and mean blood pressures are not changed, nor is total peripheral resistance.[40, 51, 72, 80, 160] There is no change in oxygen uptake ($\dot{V}O_2$) at rest and no significant change in the arteriovenous oxygen difference.[77, 160]

Deconditioning-Induced Changes Occurring During Exercise. After prolonged bed rest the normal heart rate response to exercise is altered. Deconditioning causes a

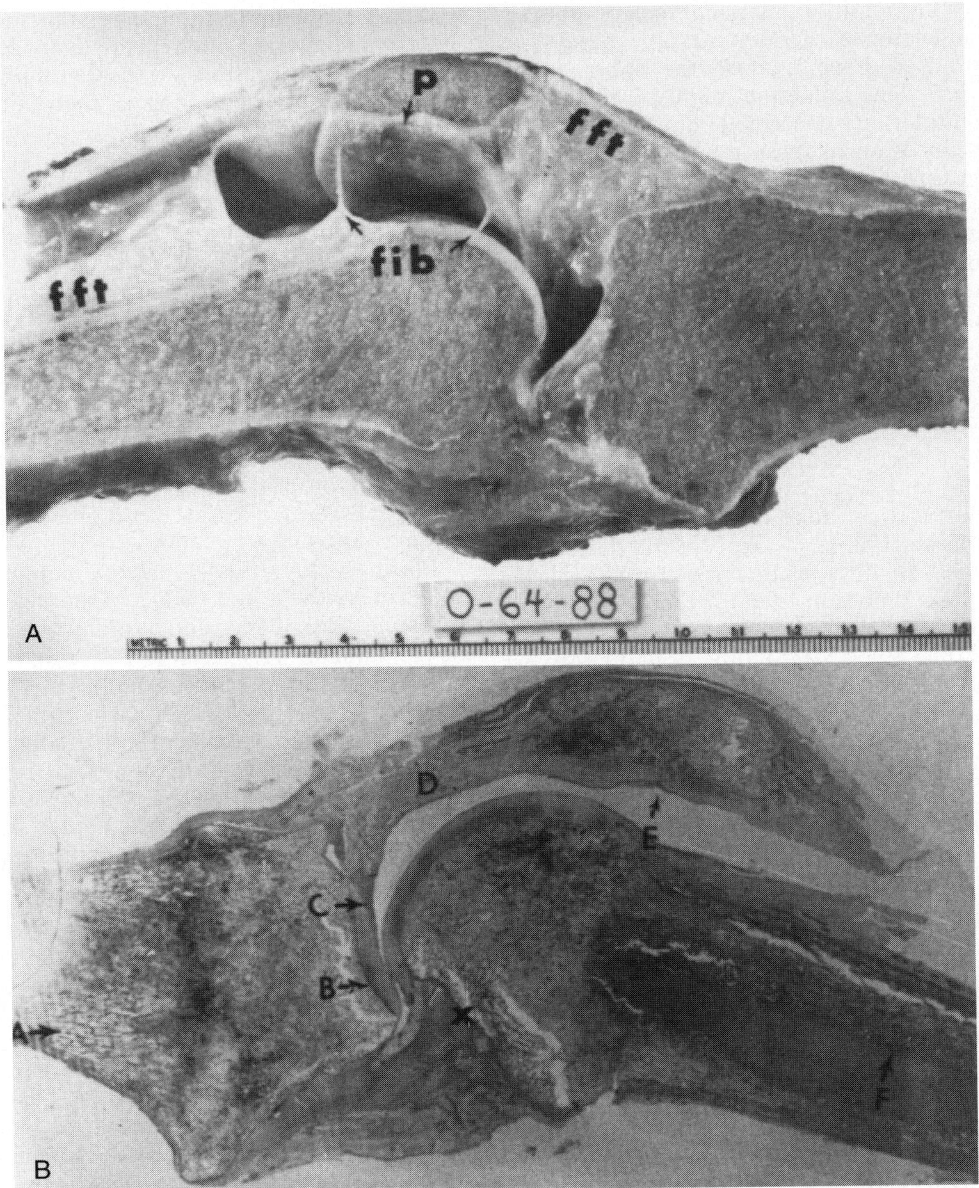

FIGURE 34–6. Cartilage degeneration with immobilization. The knees were obtained from human subjects whose knees had been immobilized and who later underwent proximal amputation. *A.* Sagittal section demonstrates fibrofatty tissue (*fft*) filling the inferior portion of the joint cavity. Fibrous septa (*fib*) extend from the femoral condyle to the patella. The articular cartilage of the patella (*p*) is irregular. *B.* There is a fibrofatty infiltration from the inferior fat pad (*D*) covering the distal pole of the patella. This has become adherent to the articular surface of the tibia (*C*). Fibrofatty tissue from the suprapatellar pouch covers the proximal patella. The posterior cruciate ligament (*x*) has been completely enveloped by fibrofatty tissue. The articular cartilage of the patella (*E*) has been compressed and replaced by fibrous connective tissue. (From Enneking WF, Horowitz M: The intra-articular effects of immobilization on the human knee. J Bone Joint Surg Am 1972; 54:973–985.)

higher heart rate at any given level of submaximal exercise, although maximal heart rate is unchanged or only slightly increased.[40, 81, 160] The heart rate response to submaximal exercise can be as much as 30 to 40 beats per minute greater than expected after only three weeks of bed rest.[77, 81, 160] With this faster heart rate, the diastolic filling period of the cardiac cycle is shortened and myocardial perfusion is decreased. When combined with an increase in the rate-pressure product,[40] this can precipitate angina in the person with pre-existing coronary artery disease. In a small study of senior athletes who refrained from training for 3 months, it was also found that these individuals developed asymptomatic ischemic-appearing exercise-induced ST-segment depression during exercise testing. This resolved in almost all subjects after training was resumed.[107]

After deconditioning there is a decrease in stroke volume at submaximal and maximal exercise (30%).[160] Cardiac output declines slightly at submaximal exercise and more significantly (26% mean drop) at maximal exercise.[77, 160] In addition, maximal oxygen uptake ($\dot{V}O_{2max}$), an indicator of general aerobic fitness, is reduced (mean, 28% lower), as is the submaximal $\dot{V}O_2$.[40, 75, 160, 177, 184] This reduction might be related to the orthostatic intolerance described below.[40] Deconditioning also produces an increase in the arteriovenous oxygen difference with submaximal, although not with maximal, exercise.[160] There is no significant difference in total peripheral resistance. In the deconditioned person it takes longer for the heart rate to return to the resting state after a period of exercise.[51]

Recovery from Deconditioning. It is difficult to state the exact rate of recovery from cardiovascular deconditioning because the studies to date have used different patient populations and different methods of enforcing disuse. A number have also assessed the effects of training in the recovery period. For most parameters it seems to take at least as long to recover from the disuse as it took to deteriorate. It can take up to twice as long or more (with intensive training) to reverse the decline in $\dot{V}O_{2max}$ caused by 20 days of bed rest in previously active subjects. Less time is needed for recovery in previously sedentary persons.[160, 181] Resting heart rate returns to near normal levels after a time period approximately equal to the duration of disuse, at least for 7 weeks of immobilization in the study of Dietrick and co-workers.[51] After 3 to 4 weeks of immobilization, heart rate recovery (after exercise) is only 50% of normal by 16 days and is again normal by 36 days.[184] Submaximal $\dot{V}O_2$ recovers to normal between 16 and 36 days.

Hemodynamic and Neurovascular Deconditioning

As described earlier, lying down causes a shift in blood volume to the thorax. Conversely, standing up causes blood to pool in the lower extremities. This causes an immediate drop in venous return which reduces stroke volume and cardiac output. In a normal person, immediate vasoconstriction and a rise in heart rate and systolic blood pressure compensate for these effects. The person who has been on prolonged bed rest, however, loses this adaptation and develops an orthostatic intolerance.[36, 40, 51, 149, 184] Blood pools in the legs, venous return drops, stroke volume is diminished, and the systolic blood pressure is not maintained. This may be due, at least in part, to an altered carotid baroreflex.[41, 42] or a change in autonomic balance.[149] When a deconditioned person stands up there is an abnormally large increase in heart rate, as much as 37 beats per minute in the study of Taylor and others.[184] This is accompanied by the common signs and symptoms of orthostatic hypotension, including a feeling of lightheadedness, nausea, dizziness, sweating, pallor, tachycardia, and a drop in systolic blood pressure. In severe cases, syncope or angina can occur.

Most of the effects of neurovascular deconditioning appear to occur in the first 4 to 7 days of bed rest.[73, 149] They can become evident in as little as 3 days of immobilization in a normal person.[36] They develop much more rapidly in the elderly and in persons with associated medical problems, although persons more conditioned before undertaking bed rest appear to have the greatest absolute deterioration. After remobilization these effects can take twice as long, or more, to reverse as they took to develop.[184]

Fluid Balance

As described earlier, when assuming recumbency there is an immediate shift in blood volume to the thorax and a delayed shift of extravascular fluid into the circulation. This causes a compensatory diuresis, which leads to a decreased plasma volume.[76] Because red blood cell mass remains unchanged, hematocrit rises[71] and blood viscosity can be increased. Over the course of 2 to 4 weeks, red blood cell mass decreases and hematocrit begins to fall. During this time period, the loss of plasma volume is proportionally greater than the loss of red blood cells.[64, 71, 72, 76] Later, red blood cell losses exceed plasma losses.

Plasma volume loss is approximately 10% after one week of bed rest and 15% by four weeks.[72, 80] The decrease in plasma and blood volume continues and most likely plateaus around 70% of normal plasma volume and 60% of normal blood volume.[73, 76] It is accompanied by a proportionate loss of plasma proteins. There also appears to be an isocontent loss of albumin, creatinine, chloride, phosphorus, calcium, potassium, and glucose. Urea nitrogen, globulin, sodium, and osmotic concentrations are increased, while uric acid is decreased.[76] It is unclear what, if any, clinical significance is attached to these changes.

Thrombotic Disease

In 1899 Welch, summarizing previous work, described what is now known as Virchow's triad.[5] He thought that three factors might contribute to clot formation: (1) factors intrinsic to the blood, (2) blood vessel injury, and (3) stasis of blood flow. It is easy to appreciate that immobility causes stasis due to reduced muscular pumping of the blood out of the venous plexus of the legs, and it can reduce blood flow through the calves.[21] By increasing blood viscosity, immobility also may increase the intrinsic predisposition of the blood to clot.[73] Platelet aggregation may be stimulated,[28] and blood fibrinogen may be increased as well.[73] Therefore, disuse is a significant risk factor for developing thrombotic complications. This is often seen in patients acutely hospitalized. It is also seen in patients with paralysis, particularly in the early stages of spinal cord injury and stroke.

Prevention and Treatment of the Cardiovascular Complications of Immobility

Prevention is obviously the best way to deal with cardiovascular deconditioning. Avoiding prolonged bed rest and immobility is important. Even just sitting in a chair prevents a large amount of the deterioration in $\dot{V}O_{2max}$ and orthostatic tolerance that occurs with bed rest.[23] Isometric exercises have also been shown to minimize the decline of $\dot{V}O_{2max}$ as well as the loss of plasma volume.[177] Leg ergometer exercise has been shown to maintain $\dot{V}O_{2max}$ and to reduce the decrease in plasma volume and red blood cell volume while on bedrest.[72, 75, 80, 81, 177] Supine exercise does not appear to prevent orthostatic intolerance,[22, 43, 81] even when plasma volume is maintained.[72]

Cardiovascular deconditioning can be reversed by progressively increasing activity and regaining the upright posture (as tolerated). This can be done initially with passive and active range-of-motion exercise in bed and with a tilt table. Later, more aggressive activity is promoted. Deep venous thrombosis (DVT) is obviously associated with bed rest as well as surgery, trauma, and paralysis. It may be prevented with active calf contractions to pump the blood out of the venous plexus of the legs, subcutaneous or low-molecular-weight heparin, intermittent pneumatic compression of the legs, gradient pressure stockings, and in high-risk patients, with anticoagulation. Proper position, active exercise, and proper leg elevations are also used. Treatment of DVT requires anticoagulation. The most serious complication of DVT is pulmonary embolism, which needs to be prevented to reduce morbidity and mortality.

Integumentary System

Pressure ulcer formation (see also Chapter 31) is a leading health problem in immobilized or bedridden patients. It is a particular problem in persons with insensate skin or mental status deterioration. It is also a major health problem among the elderly nursing home population. Factors that predispose to the development of pressure sores are listed in Table 34–6. Of these, the intrinsic risk factors cannot necessarily be modified. Other factors that cause pressure ulcers that can be modified by intervention are the position of the patient, the patient handling procedure, proper skin care, and the length of time the patient is kept in one position.

Capillary blood pressure is approximately 30 mm Hg. Sitting can cause a pressure in excess of this amount over the ischial tuberosities, whereas supine lying causes an excess of pressure over the sacrum. Such excess pressures are also found over the heels and occiput (especially in children because of their proportionally greater head size) while supine, and over the greater trochanter while side-lying. These pressures can completely occlude the capillaries; and if sustained long enough, they lead to skin necrosis. In the presence of a shear force, as when slumping in a chair or during improper patient transfers, necrosis is even more likely to occur.

TABLE 34–6 Risk Factors for Developing Pressure Sores

Intrinsic
Abnormal skin sensation
Abnormal mental status or altered consciousness
Advanced age
Increased local tissue metabolic rate
Previous pressure sore
Muscle and skin atrophy
Scars
Edema
Malnutrition
Anemia
Sedative medication
Obesity
Skin grafts
Infection
Extrinsic
Pressure
Duration of pressure
Shear force
Skin maceration

Prevention of pressure ulcers is much more desirable than having to treat them. Proper turning of hospitalized patients, especially those with abnormal sensorium or sensation, the judicious use of a pressure-relieving bed when indicated, proper skin care and toileting, proper seating, and proper nutrition are all important. If pressure sores still develop, they can be treated with enzymatic, mechanical, or surgical debridement; in severe cases, they might require surgical excision. It is imperative that all patients with abnormal skin sensation be taught adequate pressure relief and skin care procedures.

Dependent edema and subcutaneous bursitis can also occur with immobilization. The edema can generally be prevented with adequate mobilization and elevation. In some cases elastic stockings or gloves, pressure gradient compression, or massage may be indicated. Care should be taken to investigate cardiac or metabolic causes of edema. Such edema can predispose to cellulitis and should be minimized if possible.

Subcutaneous bursitis is the result of excessive pressure on the bursae. This commonly occurs as "housemaid's knee," a prepatellar bursitis obviously not caused by immobilization (except occasionally, when a person is restricted to lying prone to treat a pressure ulcer on the buttock). *Student's elbow,* an olecranon bursitis, is also due to prolonged pressure, as can be seen in students who study for prolonged periods of time with their elbows propped on armrests. Bursitis is best treated by removing the aggravating pressure, but it can also be treated with nonsteroidal anti-inflammatory agents, percutaneous drainage, and instillation of corticosteroid. In refractory cases, surgical drainage or excision might be necessary.

Body Composition, Metabolic, and Nutritional Changes

In addition to the fluid balance changes described earlier, there are a number of metabolic and body composition changes that occur with bed rest or immobilization. There is a decrease in lean body mass and an increase in body fat content.[115, 160] In one study of five weeks of bed rest, lean body mass decreased by 2.3% and body fat increased by 12%.[115] Total body weight was not changed.[115, 160]

The body appears to become less efficient at storing excess calories as fat while on bed rest, because the increase in fat percentage is actually less than would be predicted by caloric intake.[115] Energy absorption from food is unchanged,[115] but appetite and water intake are lowered. Bed rest does not cause increased protein breakdown, but if dietary protein is low, total body protein synthesis is decreased.[178] There may be a decrease in basal metabolic rate,[51, 184] probably related to loss of muscle mass, although this is not evident in all studies.[73] There are also a number of changes in body minerals and metabolites seen with immobilization.

Nitrogen. Nitrogen is lost during immobilization. This loss occurs through urinary excretion and basically parallels the loss of muscle. The loss begins 5 to 6 days after the start of immobilization and peaks in the second week. When activity is resumed (after 6 to 7 weeks of immobility), nitrogen loss continues for another week, but excretion is normalized by the second week. Later, nitrogen excretion falls to below-normal levels to recapture the amount that was lost. Maximum nitrogen retention occurs four weeks after resumption of activity and is back to a normal balance by around the sixth week.[51]

Calcium. Like all other body components, calcium is normally in a dynamic equilibrium, with absorption, distribution, and excretion being balanced by the needs of the body (Fig. 34–7). During periods of disuse there is loss of this mineral. This loss parallels the loss of bone mass described above. Calcium is excreted in both urine and feces. Fecal excretion is somewhat variable and increases progressively, at least through the 6 to 7 weeks of immobility that have been studied.

Urinary calcium excretion begins to rise after 2 to 3 days of immobility. It peaks in 3 to 7 weeks[51, 54, 163] at approximately twice the normal rate of excretion.[22] It then plateaus, at least through 6 to 7 weeks. By approximately 16 weeks, excretion drops to a new plateau, which is maintained at least through 36 weeks.[163] Throughout this time total body calcium is lost at a rate of about 0.5% per month.[163] This loss can be prevented to some extent by weightbearing activity, even standing.[97]

When activity is resumed, calcium excretion initially remains high, but gradually returns to normal by 3 weeks. Excretion continues to fall to reach a trough below the normal excretion level at 5 to 6 weeks, and then gradually normalizes.

Phosphorus. Phosphorus loss with immobilization is primarily through the urine, although a small amount is also lost fecally. The loss begins during the first week of immobility and peaks at 2 to 3 weeks (along with nitrogen). Excretion then falls, but peaks again at 6 to 7 weeks (along with calcium). On resumption of activity, phosphorus excretion returns to normal by the third week. This is followed by below-normal excretion for weeks 3 through 5 and normalization of excretion by week 6.[51]

Other Losses. Sulfur loss during immobilization basically parallels nitrogen loss, and is believed to result from loss of muscle mass.[51] Other minerals such as sodium, potassium, magnesium,[69] and zinc[69, 116] are also lost during immobilization. This is due in part to the loss of plasma volume, but there may also be an excess excretion. Sodium and chloride loss is greatest during early immobilization (as is plasma loss).[36] Potassium loss increases progressively through 2 to 3 weeks of bed rest,[36] and recovery of this mineral during remobilization is twice the amount that was lost.[51]

Endocrine and Receptor Function

Prolonged bed rest causes a decrease in glucose tolerance. This is primarily due to changes in peripheral muscle sensitivity to circulating insulin,[125, 179] though some adaptation is also believed to occur in the cells of the pancreas.[135] The glucose intolerance caused by bed rest can, to some extent, be ameliorated with both isotonic and isometric exercise.[52] Following 2 weeks of bed rest approximately 2 weeks of resumed activity is required for the glucose response to return to normal.[125]

Another immobility-induced change in endocrine function is in parathyroid hormone production. In the rat model, immobilization causes a suppression of parathyroid hormone and a decrease in intestinal calcium absorption.[199] This has been supported in human studies,[174] and is believed to be a response to the calcium released from bone resorption. In persons with immobilization hypercalcemia, however, the parathyroid hormone level can be elevated.[122]

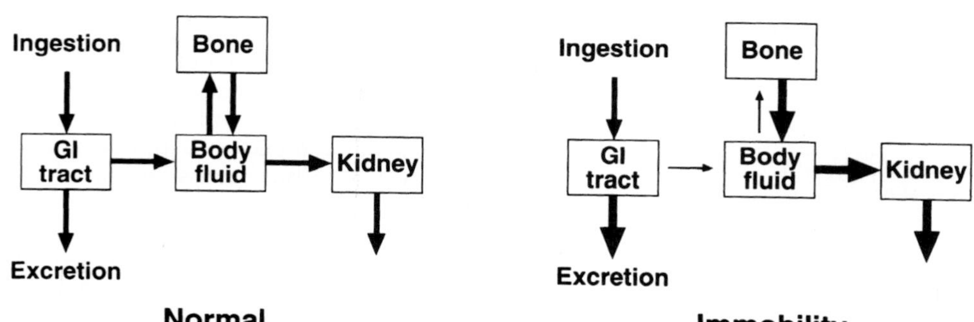

FIGURE 34–7. Calcium homeostasis and flux. Normally, the calcium balance of intake and excretion is fairly equal and changes only slowly over the course of years. With immobilization, less calcium absorption occurs from the gastrointestinal tract, accompanied by a net resorption from bone and an increased renal excretion of the mineral.

Other immobility-induced changes may include an increase in urinary hydrocortisone excretion (at least in a very long bed rest study),[120] increased plasma renin activity,[35, 131, 190] increased aldosterone secretion,[35, 131] altered growth hormone production,[191] and altered spermatogenesis[39] and androgen secretion.[27, 60, 190] Changes may also occur in adrenal[120] and pituitary function,[176, 190] although such changes may not be directly attributable to the immobility.[156] There is also an increased body temperature response to exercise.[73, 78] Central nervous system function and receptors may be altered, as is the circadian rhythm.[161] There appears to be no change in thyroid hormone degradation, although blood levels may be altered.[13, 60, 191, 202]

Respiratory System

There are both immediate and long-term consequences of bed rest on the respiratory system. Immediately after assuming a supine or forward-slumped position, the diaphragm and intercostal muscles are restricted in their normal motion and breathing is impaired (an exception could be in spinal cord injured patients in whom the supine position can place the diaphragm into a biomechanically advantageous position [see Chapter 55]). The work of breathing is increased in the slumped or supine position due to increased mechanical resistance. Because of blood pooling in the thorax, there is also an immediate decrease in lung volume and residual volume.

Although not proven, it is commonly held that if the recumbent position is maintained, gravity-induced changes will occur within the lungs. There is thought to be a pooling of mucus in the lower (dependent) parts of the airway, while the upper segments tend to dry out. This is believed to create an environment predisposing to respiratory infection, mucous plugging, and atelectasis. This situation is aggravated by a decrease in respiratory activity and an impaired cough mechanism. In addition, there can also be a mismatch between lung ventilation and perfusion.

Both Dietrick and co-workers[51] and Saltin and co-workers[160] found no major changes in pulmonary tests after immobilization. But Beckett and colleagues,[16] in a study of normal subjects placed on bed rest for 11 to 12 days, found an increase in forced vital capacity and a small increase in total lung capacity. Residual volume and functional residual capacity were unchanged.[16] Other studies have not shown demonstrable changes in maximal ventilatory volume or maximal minute volume, at least in normal subjects on a relatively short period of bed rest.[76, 177] Convertino et al[40] reported that the ventilatory volume was elevated during maximal and submaximal exercise in middle-aged men exposed to 10 days of bed rest. Finding that the respiratory exchange ratio was significantly increased during upright submaximal exercise, they concluded that orthostatic stress, not pulmonary function, was the main limiting factor in exercise tolerance after bed rest.[40]

With prolonged bed rest, the intercostal muscles and costal joints develop contractures, breathing becomes shallower, and respiratory rate increases. In addition, the immobilized patient is at risk of developing pulmonary embolism due to DVT in the lower extremities.

The pulmonary deterioration induced by bed rest can be prevented to a large extent by frequent changes in position, incentive spirometry, deep breathing, coughing, and pulmonary toilet. The only definitive solution to the problem is mobilization.

Genitourinary System

Genitourinary effects of bed rest and immobility include the increased diuresis and mineral excretion described above. There are also other changes, which are primarily mechanical in nature. While one study in rats demonstrated early bladder distention and relatively rapid increase in bladder tissue growth,[9] the main problems encountered in humans include urinary stasis and calculus formation.

Voiding is more difficult when supine, so patients tend to wait longer before emptying their bladders. There is also a lack of gravity assistance in voiding, and postvoid residual volume may be increased. This predisposes to urinary tract infection, and in severe cases, to overflow incontinence.

In addition, there may be gravity-induced urinary stasis in the renal pelves. Together with increased calcium excretion, this can increase the incidence of calculus formation—another factor predisposing to urinary tract infection. Calculus formation is especially common in patients with fractures and spinal cord injury.

Long-term consequences of immobilization can lead to a sustained (up to 9 months) decrease in glomerular filtration rate and (greater than 4 weeks) decreased ability to concentrate urine.[10]

Reproductive effects of immobility have not been studied adequately to date, but there appears to be a decrease in spermatogenesis, at least in primates.[39] Androgen secretion might be altered as well.[27, 60, 190]

The genitourinary consequences of immobility can most likely be prevented by assuming the upright posture as frequently as possible and by ambulation. Adequate fluid intake is important, and voiding while supine should be discouraged. In select cases postvoid residual volumes should be measured. In some cases, catheterization is needed.

Gastrointestinal Tract and Digestion

Bed rest causes mechanical effects on the gastrointestinal tract similar to those undergone by the genitourinary system. There is an increased risk of constipation due to decreased mobility, decreased peristalsis (possibly due to an increased adrenergic state), and decreased fluid intake. Gastrointestinal secretion decreases and "heartburn" symptoms increase.[73] There is also a decrease in or loss of appetite,[73] which can lead to impairment of nutrition. The supine position can also interfere with eructation and can increase gastroesophageal reflux. The potential embarrassment of using a bedpan often causes people to delay defecating. Persons on bed rest should ingest adequate protein, fiber, and fluid. Stool softeners can be helpful, but enemas and laxatives should be avoided, if possible.

Neurological System, Emotions, and Intellectual Function

There are few true neurological sequelae of bed rest that affect either the central or peripheral nervous systems. Instead, there are disorders of coordination, balance, and emotions that may have a component of physiological deterioration as well as a predominant integrative component. *Critical illness neuropathy* is a neurological process that mimics the weakness of immobility/deconditioning. Painless weakness can be associated with this symmetrical axonal sensorimotor neuropathy. This condition can exacerbate any concurrent deconditioning in the critically ill patient.[98]

One potential complication of bed rest is the occurrence of compression neuropathies. Peroneal nerve compression below the fibular head and ulnar nerve compression at the retrocondylar groove are probably the most common such compression neuropathies. They are specifically due to bed rest rather than immobilization. Ulnar nerve compression was found in 23% of patients in a small study of orthopedic, neurological, neurosurgical, and rehabilitation inpatients.[38] Other compression neuropathies can occur as well, especially in obtunded patients or in those with sensory or motor deficits. They can also occur in patients who are restrained. The integrative components of emotions and cognitive function are affected by bed rest and immobilization, most likely due to sensory deprivation and boredom, and not specifically due to the lack of mobility.[49] Anxiety also results from being restricted to bed.[159] Medications and "ICU [intensive care unit] psychosis" play a role as well in medically ill patients. Affected persons can experience a lowered pain threshold and a decrease in coordination[201] and balance.[56, 88, 184] They can have emotional disturbances such as depression, anxiety, withdrawal, apathy, incontinence, and sleep disturbance,[159, 201] and might even develop paranoia and dementia. Intellectual function is impaired, as is orientation and the perception of time.[170] Patients with these problems become emotionally labile, irritable, and uncooperative. They can suffer from headache, dizziness, general discomfort, nightmares, and even hallucinations, primarily because of sensory deprivation.[170, 201] They may also have a decreased visual acuity and a raised auditory threshold.[73] Proprioception does not appear to be impaired, at least not with 4 weeks of bedrest.[19, 72]

DECONDITIONING AS A REHABILITATION DIAGNOSIS

There are six basic conditions causing disuse: (1) a sedentary lifestyle that is a result of personal choice; (2) rest that is imposed because of a medical or surgical illness; (3) medical or caregiver "neglect," with a person needlessly restricted from mobility, usually in a hospital or nursing home; (4) immobilization of the body or part of the body by casts or braces, usually after trauma or fracture; (5) disuse due to paralysis or neuromuscular disorder; and (6) disuse due to weightlessness.

Weightlessness is germane to this chapter mainly because many of the studies of immobility were performed to assess the effects of weightlessness in astronauts.

Disuse due to paralysis or weakness, as well as casts and braces used to treat an injury, can cause local, regional, or systemic complications, depending on the extent of the problem. Physical medicine and rehabilitation consultation in such patients is typically aimed at aiding in recovery from injury, maximizing function, and preventing long-term health hazards (such as cardiovascular deconditioning).

The abundance of persons who suffer from disuse because of a sedentary lifestyle is, in large part, a consequence of modern life, with people relying on machines to perform their work. Deconditioning due to rest is largely associated with hospitalization or being in a nursing home. In the past, it was seen in women in the peripartum period and in patients with back injuries. In some cases, bed rest is indicated for such patients; often, it is not.

Inpatient Rehabilitation Interactions

A recent survey of a large inpatient rehabilitation unit revealed that over a 6-month period, nearly 20% of admissions were for the diagnosis of deconditioning. In a consult service at a large tertiary care hospital, 21% of adult consultations were for patients with deconditioning. These patients were typically older, and had longer hospital stays and more serious medical complications than other patients who received a physical medicine and rehabilitation consult.[30]

Most of the deconditioned patients were hospitalized with a variety of medical and surgical illnesses, were treated successfully, but were left with residual weakness and other complications of immobility. These residual impairments were often more disabling than the problem for which they were admitted. These patients had what is known as *deconditioning syndrome.* They were unable to function as before, could not be returned home safely, and required a short inpatient rehabilitation stay to regain their lost independence.

Treatment of inpatients with deconditioning syndrome includes adequate sensory and intellectual stimulation, regaining an upright posture as tolerated, regaining and maintaining proper joint range of motion with active (preferred) or passive (if needed) exercise, and increasing strength and coordination with a combination of isometric, isotonic, and functional activities. All the other interventions described above (incentive spirometry, proper fluid intake, etc.) are also incorporated.

Prevention of deconditioning involves these same principles. In addition, it is important to allow the patient to sit upright, if possible, to "see the world." Lying in bed, staring at the ceiling, distorts a normal perspective on life. It is also important that health-care workers avoid "talking down" to the patient. Often, adults are treated like children just because they are in bed and require help with their activities of daily living (ADL). Little wonder that these patients become anxious and uncooperative. Excessive use of medications is to be avoided, and proper sleep-wake cycles should be fostered. Patients who nap out of boredom during the day and then develop a reliance on nighttime sleep medications risk increased emotional and intellectual deterioration. Proper nutrition, proper positioning and turning, and exercise are important as well. It is somewhat unclear which type of exercise is best in the immobilized patient, as studies have mainly been done on young healthy volunteers. Pending further data, it is probably reasonable to encourage a variety of isotonic, isometric, and aerobic exercises, as tolerated.

Outpatient Rehabilitation Interactions

Deconditioning in the outpatient physical medicine and rehabilitation setting centers mainly on persons who have had an injury and who have been off work long enough to develop muscle weakness and inflexibility. This can put them at risk of further injury if they return to work without proper conditioning. Such patients often benefit from a work-conditioning or work-hardening program prior to return to activity. Viewing them as "occupational athletes" is helpful, as many principles of sports rehabilitation can be incorporated into their care.

Aging Versus Disuse Effects on the Body

It is common knowledge that as we age, we deteriorate to a certain extent. But aging is often compounded by disease, and it appears that disuse and aging synergistically accelerate the decline in maximal physiological capacity of virtually every body system. The increased incidence of medical illness in the elderly necessarily enforces a certain amount of disuse. Nevertheless, it is clear that active persons can prevent a large amount of the physical decline seen in aging.

TABLE 34–7 Major Benefits of Exercise

Musculoskeletal
↑ Muscle strength and endurance
↑ Bone mass
Obesity
Sustained weight loss
Cardiovascular
↓ Hypertension
Improved blood lipids
↑ $\dot{V}O_{2max}$
↑ Maximal cardiac output
↓ Resting and submaximal heart rate
↑ Peripheral oxygen extraction
Endocrine
Improved glucose tolerance
Emotional
Improved sense of well-being
Neurological
Improved balance and coordination
↑ Pain threshold
Elderly
May help to prevent falls (improved margin of safety)
↑ Functional capacity
Women
↓ Premenstrual syndrome
↓ Symptoms of endometriosis
Lessened stress of labor
Disabled
↑ Quality of life
↑ $\dot{V}O_{2max}$
↓ Medical complications (possible)

Abbreviations: $\dot{V}O_{2max}$, maximum rate of oxygen consumption.

THE BENEFICIAL EFFECTS OF EXERCISE

Muscle Strength and Endurance

Since strength is ultimately proportional to the cross-sectional area of muscle, muscle-building exercise increases the strength available to a person to meet the physical demands of living. Muscular endurance is similarly enhanced by endurance training. The major benefits of exercise are summarized in Table 34–7. Chapter 19 describes the benefits of exercise in more detail. For the purposes of this chapter, it is important to remember that excessive muscle weakness, even of local or regional muscle groups, can prevent a person from leading a normal lifestyle. This is, of course, exaggerated in the elderly or otherwise impaired. Strength and endurance training will not increase the maximal physiological potential, but can certainly increase a person's fitness and function.

Obesity

Obesity is usually defined as a state in which ideal body weight is exceeded by more than 20%. It is common in the United States, with up to 25% of the population being affected. Most obese persons have a long-term battle with their weight. They commonly choose to attack the problem by dieting, even though exercise can be more effective. Regular aerobic exercise helps reduce body weight even while maintaining fat-free weight.[162] It brings about a more sustained weight loss than does dieting alone. In general, any form of aerobic exercise is beneficial for weight loss, although swimming does not seem to help decrease weight as much as walking, running, and bicycling.[84]

Hypertension

Aerobic exercise training can be valuable in the treatment of mild-to-moderate essential hypertension.[123] It can cause a decrease of up to 10 mm Hg in blood pressure[86] and appears to lower both systolic and diastolic blood pressures.[123] The blood pressure response to such exercise can also be used to screen normotensive persons for the risk of later developing elevated blood pressure.[183]

The first line of treatment for mild hypertension is usually pharmacological, but aerobic exercise and lifestyle changes such as weight loss, diet changes, and cessation of smoking are probably a better choice. Exercise alone might normalize blood pressure, but if it doesn't, pharmacological treatment can still be instituted at a later date. In moderate-to-severe essential hypertension, exercise should probably be combined with lifestyle changes and antihypertensive medication for first-line treatment. When exercise starts to decrease the blood pressure, lower doses of medication are often possible.

According to the American College of Sports Medicine, in normal healthy adults, aerobic exercise is recommended at 60% to 85% of the maximum heart rate, three to four times per week, for 20 to 60 minutes per session.[6] Since exercise at the upper limit of this level of intensity might actually worsen hypertension,[182] aerobic exercise of more moderate intensity is recommended in the hypertensive patient.[86] Such low-to-moderate training intensity has been shown to be as effective as high-intensity training in lowering blood pressure.[123]

It has generally been recommended that isometric exercise (approximated by heavy weightlifting) be avoided in the hypertensive population, as it can increase blood pressure both during exercise and for a sustained period afterward. Isometrics, or heavy resistance exercise, can increase myocardial oxygen demand out of proportion to the physical work being performed.[53] Despite these caveats, it is not entirely clear that isometrics are harmful, and moderate weightlifting might be helpful even in patients with coronary artery disease and mild hypertension.[93, 175] Lighter weights used for more repetitions may help the hypertensive patient gain strength with less risk. Because heart rate and systolic blood pressure (and hence myocardial oxygen demand) are higher in upper-extremity than in lower-extremity exercise for a constant workload[137] (Fig. 34–8), caution should be exercised in prescribing upper extremity activities. It should also be kept in mind that a variety of antihypertensive agents can alter the heart rate response to exercise as well as cause dehydration or hypokalemia.

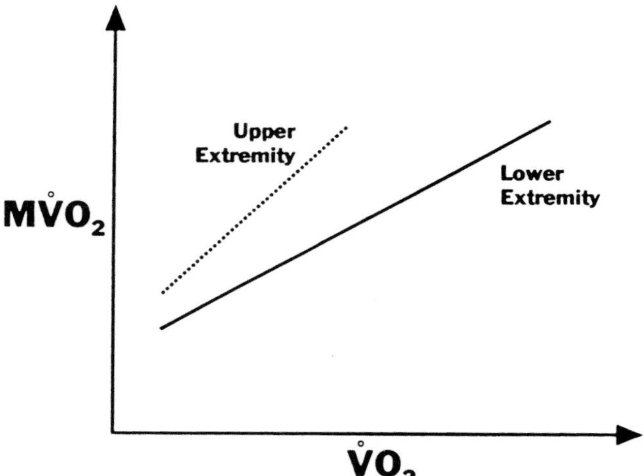

FIGURE 34–8. A comparison of the relationship between myocardial oxygen demand and total oxygen consumption for upper and lower extremity work. (From Downey JA, Myers SJ, Gonzales EG, Lieberman JS (eds): The Physiologic Basis of Rehabilitation Medicine, ed 2. Stoneham, MA, Butterworth-Heinemann, 1994.)

Cardiovascular Disease

Aerobic exercise has long been used as part of cardiac rehabilitation in patients who have suffered from myocardial infarction or who have had cardiac surgery. It is also useful in helping prevent the atherosclerosis that causes so much morbidity and mortality in the western world. The mechanism of action of exercise is not fully understood, but exercise can modify the risk factors for atherosclerosis.[129] It also appears to have both peripheral and cardiac benefits in patients with coronary artery disease.[85] As described earlier, it can reduce hypertension and obesity. It also lowers serum triglycerides and can alter serum cholesterol levels to increase the high-density/low-density lipoprotein (HDL/LDL) ratio.[85, 166, 180] In some persons, these benefits might be due to weight loss or other changes, and not directly due to the exercise. Aerobic exercise may be particularly effective at increasing the HDL_2 subfraction, which is thought to be an especially important anti-atherogenic factor. It is unclear whether these benefits to the lipid profile require a threshold amount of exercise. Superko[180] noted that jogging at least 15 miles per week is needed to produce a beneficial change in blood lipids. Kokkinos et al,[112] however, did not detect a threshold (though the lipid changes reached statistical significance at 7 miles per week). They noted that runners who ran 7 to 14 miles per week (mild to moderate intensity) had an increase in HDL levels, although a causal relationship was not established. Haskell[89] reported that at least 1000 kcal/week must be expended to obtain these benefits. Above this level he reported a "dose-related" increase in benefit up to 4500 kcal/week, and above this, a plateau. He believed that the beneficial effects on the lipid profile were evident only if accompanied by weight loss.[89] They do not appear to occur in resistance exercise.[95]

In addition to the benefits of reducing atherogenic risk factors, regular aerobic exercise helps to increase the body's aerobic endurance, as demonstrated by a higher $\dot{V}O_{2max}$ (Fig. 34–9*A*). There is an increase in maximal cardiac output (Fig. 34–9*B*), an increase in stroke volume for a given level of $\dot{V}O_2$ (Fig. 34–9*C*), and an increase in peripheral oxygen extraction (this peripheral skeletal muscle adaptation has been identified as the primary cause of increased peak aerobic capacity in older patients with coronary artery disease[1]). Resting heart rate drops. The intensity of the exercise should most likely be moderate; high intensity is not necessarily more beneficial.[65]

Persons who regularly participate in an aerobic exercise program have an increased life expectancy and a decreased risk of coronary artery disease.[151] They have a decreased heart rate (Fig. 34–9*D*) and blood pressure response to submaximal exercise, an increase in $\dot{V}O_{2max}$, a decreased myocardial oxygen demand for a given workload, and decreased angina for a given workload (though anginal threshold for a given myocardial oxygen demand is unchanged)[48] (Fig. 34–10). Ideally,

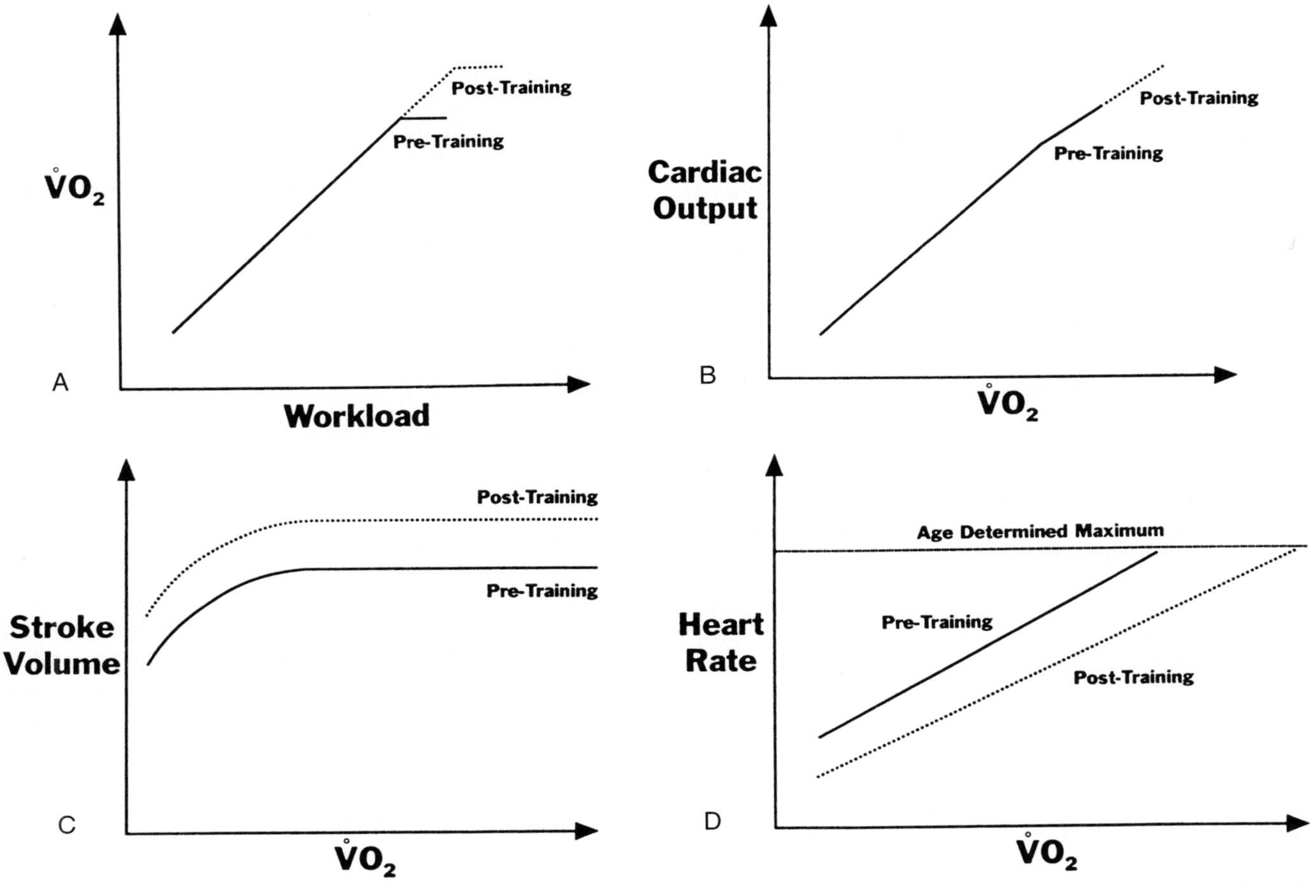

A
$\dot{V}O_2$
Workload
Post-Training
Pre-Training

B
Cardiac Output
$\dot{V}O_2$
Post-Training
Pre-Training

C
Stroke Volume
$\dot{V}O_2$
Post-Training
Pre-Training

D
Heart Rate
$\dot{V}O_2$
Age Determined Maximum
Pre-Training
Post-Training

FIGURE 34–9. *A.* Effect of training on relationship between oxygen consumption and workload. *B.* Effect of training on relationship between cardiac output and oxygen consumption. *C.* Effect of training on relationship between stroke volume and oxygen consumption. *D.* Effect of training on the relationship between heart rate and oxygen consumption. (From Downey JA, Myers SJ, Gonzales EG, Lieberman JS (eds): The Physiologic Basis of Rehabilitation Medicine, ed 2. Stoneham, MA, Butterworth-Heinemann, 1994, p 135.)

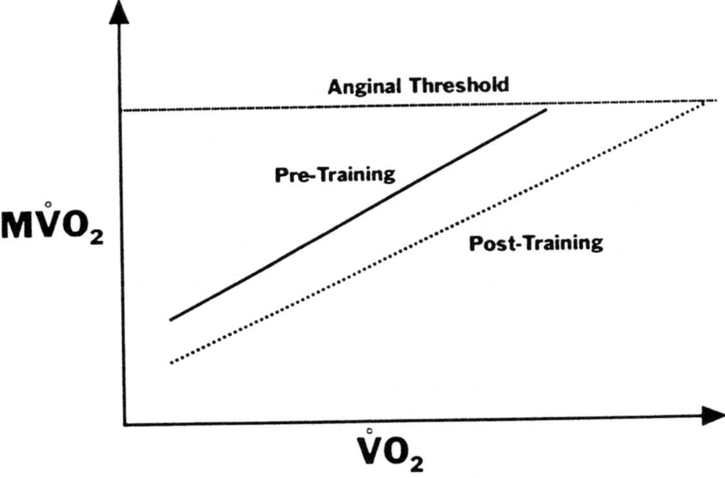

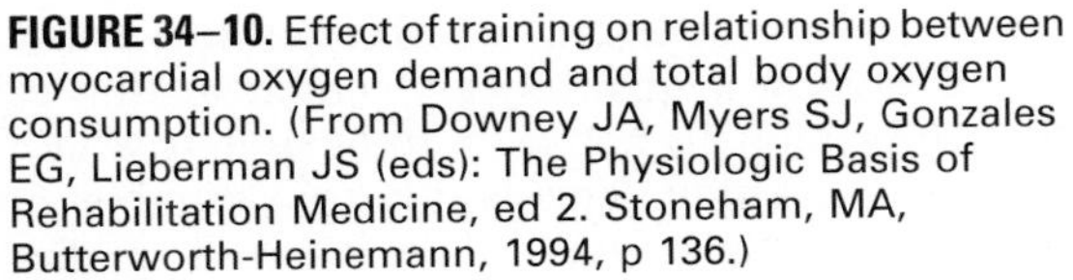
FIGURE 34–10. Effect of training on relationship between myocardial oxygen demand and total body oxygen consumption. (From Downey JA, Myers SJ, Gonzales EG, Lieberman JS (eds): The Physiologic Basis of Rehabilitation Medicine, ed 2. Stoneham, MA, Butterworth-Heinemann, 1994, p 136.)

exercise should be combined with healthy lifestyle changes and a proper diet. Such risk factor modification has been shown to reverse atherosclerosis to some extent.[194]

Diabetes

Inactivity causes a decreased peripheral sensitivity to insulin. Conversely, aerobic exercise increases the end organ cell receptor sensitivity to insulin,[24, 111] primarily in the regions being exercised.[50] This can be an important benefit in those with non–insulin-dependent diabetes mellitus (NIDDM). It may also reduce the other risk factors for diabetes. In insulin-dependent diabetes mellitus (IDDM), exercise has little effect, except that it lowers insulin requirements by utilizing circulating glucose.

When a person is first diagnosed as having glucose intolerance or mild diabetes, exercise may be combined with diet changes as the first mode of treatment. This may obviate the need for oral hypoglycemic medication in some, although many patients will probably eventually need such medication. Exercise can also be used as part of the treatment program in patients with more severe diabetes and in gestational diabetes.[29] Care should be taken when exercising, however, not to cause post-exercise hypoglycemia. This can be a problem in persons who exercise in the evening, as they can become hypoglycemic during sleep. Diabetics can also suffer from silent myocardial ischemia during exercise, so they should have an appropriate cardiac screening evaluation before initiating an exercise program.

Osteoporosis

As described above, immobility causes a loss of bone mass, primarily in the weightbearing bones. Conversely, exercise can help to maintain bone mass, and more active elderly women have been shown to have a lower rate of hip and vertebral fractures than their sedentary counterparts.[82] In early adulthood weightbearing exercise can help to increase bone mass, which generally peaks in the early 30s. After the fourth decade, exercise probably does not increase bone mass, but can help slow down the normal decline in bone mass with aging.

Exercise can have beneficial effects even on bones not involved in a loading stress,[47, 100] but it has its primary benefit on the bones being stressed. Intermittent bone compression appears to be more beneficial than static stress.[32] It is probably reasonable to perform some weightlifting exercise to benefit bones not directly involved in weightbearing.

The exercises that are most beneficial for maintaining bone mass are walking and running, rather than swimming.[26] The exercise should be combined with adequate calcium intake, proper diet, and treatment of hypoestrogenemia, if appropriate (in young and postmenopausal women).

Sense of Well-Being, Pain Threshold, Sleep, and Immune Function

Regular aerobic exercise is generally believed to raise the pain threshold, probably by stimulating the release of endogenous opiates.[67, 165] It is useful in conditions such as fibromyalgia, myofascial pain syndrome, chronic pain syndrome, and back pain. It also increases the general sense of well-being and helps to reduce anxiety, depression, and neuroticism.[26, 37, 110, 130, 138] Some evidence suggests that regular physical activity can be useful in reducing daytime sleepiness and in improving the quality of sleep; however, the data for this are not yet conclusive.[144] Moderate endurance exercise can have a beneficial effect on the immune system, but more intense exercise might have the opposite effect.[168]

Balance, Coordination, and Proprioception

As described earlier, immobility decreases balance,[88] and there is some evidence to support the clinical observation that exercise improves balance.[126] Exercise has also been shown to increase function and the velocity of gait.[34, 101] Exercise seems to improve proprioception,[19, 150] but there is little direct evidence that it specifically improves coordination. But by promoting general fitness, strength, and health habits, it increases the functional reserve of persons going about their daily activities. This allows the fit person to better compensate for the natural stresses and potentially risky incidents that arise in normal life. In essence, it creates a buffer of safety.

Exercise in the Older Population

As most of the medical conditions described earlier are more prevalent in the elderly, exercise can be especially important in this age group. Exercise earlier in life may help prevent some of the disorders, while later in life it may slow their progression. This can be true for osteoporosis, obesity, coronary artery disease, diabetes, and hypertension. In addition, exercise can increase strength in the elderly, even in frail persons.[61] This occurs primarily through a more advantageous neural recruitment of muscles rather than hypertrophy,[139] though hypertrophy also occurs.[66] The increase in strength can help prevent falls and other injuries, and exercise appears to improve the quality of life in the elderly.[167] Before prescribing exercise in the older population, a proper screening evaluation is indicated (Fig. 34–11). A proper exercise prescription, tailored to the appropriate activity level, is important as well.

Exercise in Women

The effect of aerobic exercise on the cardiovascular endurance of women is qualitatively similar to that of men, although women do not seem to be able to attain as high a $\dot{V}O_{2max}$ as men. This is due to a number of factors, including a higher body fat content, a smaller heart,[96] lower hematocrit,[45] and other, as yet unknown, factors.[172] The reaction of women to strength training is also qualitatively similar to that of men. Due to low levels of testosterone, women are unable to build as much muscle mass as men and thus do not generally attain as great a strength. Women are especially lacking in upper body strength compared with men.[119] They do

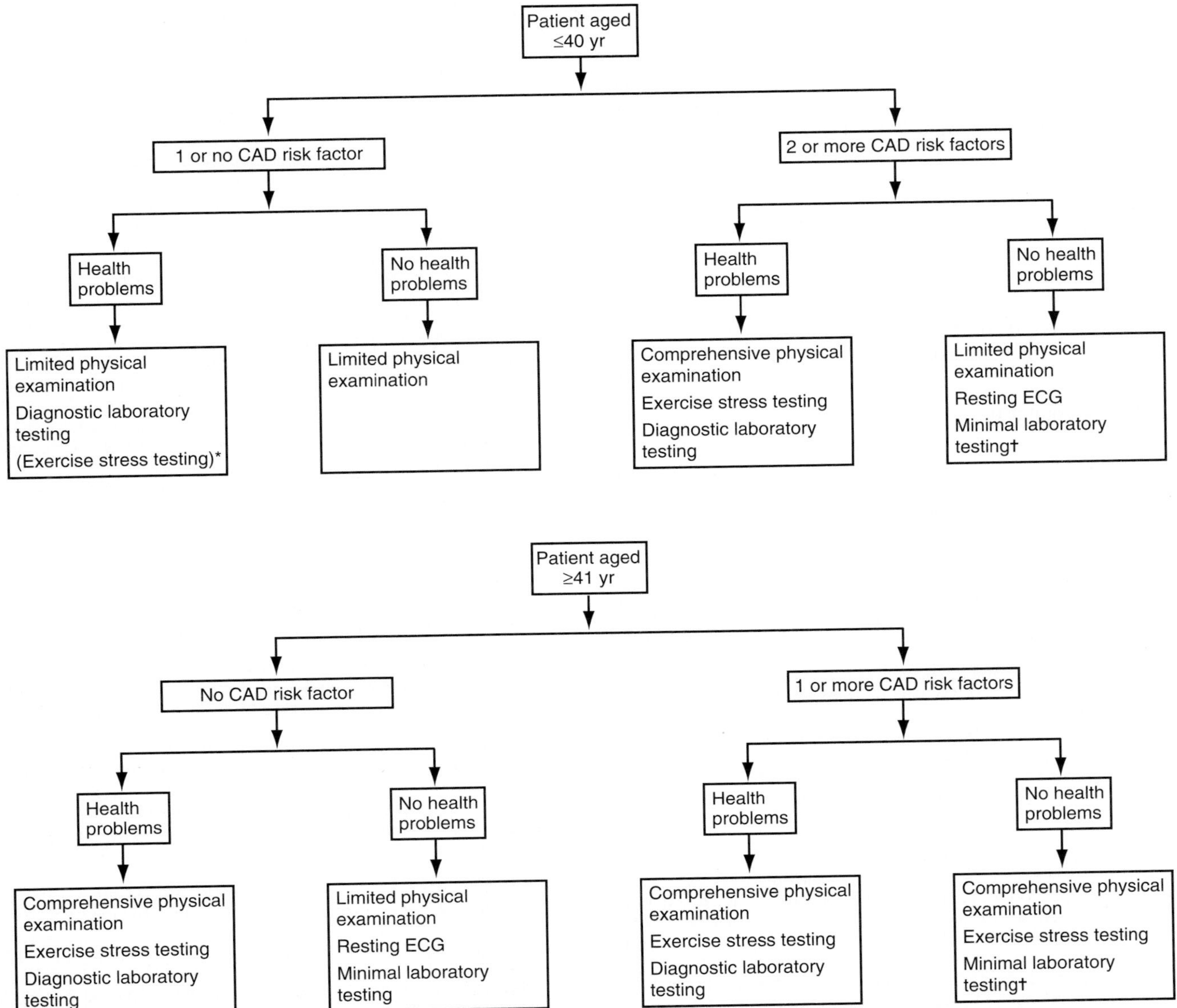

FIGURE 34–11. Preparticipation screening evaluation for persons wishing to begin an exercise program. *Risk factors* for coronary artery disease (CAD) include hypertension, smoking, diabetes, hypercholesterolemia, previous CAD, strong family history, and obesity or sedentary lifestyle. *Health problems* include cardiopulmonary disease, neurological disease, endocrinopathy, musculoskeletal disorder, psychiatric disorder, renal or hepatic disease, anemia, current drug use, and other chronic or acute diseases. Diagnostic laboratory testing can include fasting chemical survey, complete blood cell count, urinalysis, and lipid profile. Minimal laboratory testing can include a chemical survey.* Exercise stress testing is recommended if the patient has cardiopulmonary disease. †Diagnostic laboratory testing is indicated if coronary heart disease risk factors include hyperlipidemia, hyperglycemia, or hyperuricemia. (From Putukian M, McKeag D: The preparticipation physical examination. *In* Buschbacher R, Braddom RL: Sports Medicine and Rehabilitation: A Sports-Specific Approach. Philadelphia, Hanley & Belfus, 1994.)

gain strength with weight training—both through some hypertrophy and through neural factors such as improved recruitment.

In addition to the physiological effects just described, aerobic exercise can lessen the effects of premenstrual syndrome (PMS)[153] and endometriosis.[15, 44] It also tends to normalize the menstrual cycle, though very heavy endurance exercise can adversely affect the cycle. Exercise in moderation has been shown to be safe for women with routine pregnancies. While women should probably be counseled not to try to markedly increase their exercise load during pregnancy, moderate exercise is believed to be safe for both mother and fetus,[17, 63] and can even improve the process of labor and postlabor recovery. It is important when exercising during pregnancy to avoid dehydration and hyperthermia. Hyperthermia is a teratogen.[169]

Other beneficial effects of exercise that are particularly important in women include the slowing or prevention of osteoporosis described earlier.

Special Issues in the Disabled Population

Sports are becoming increasingly available to persons with physical impairments. This is especially true for wheelchair athletes, mainly those with paraplegia. Exercise in wheelchair athletes has been shown to increase $\dot{V}O_{2max}$, decrease cardiovascular disease and respiratory infection, improve self-image, improve psychological function, and decrease time hospitalized. These benefits come at a price: namely, an increase in traumatic and overuse injuries, shoulder pain and degeneration, compression neuropathies, and bladder and skin problems. When done carefully, however, the benefits outweigh the risks in most persons.[164]

REFERENCES

1. Ades PA, Waldmann ML, Meyer WL, et al: Skeletal muscle and cardiovascular adaptations to exercise conditioning in older coronary patients. Circulation 1996; 94:323–330.
2. Akeson WH, Amiel D, Abel MF, et al: Effects of immobilization on joints. Clin Orthop 1987; 219:28–37.
3. Akeson WH, Amiel D, Mechanic GL, et al: Collagen cross-linking alterations in joint contractures: Changes in the reducible cross-links in periarticular connective tissue collagen after nine weeks of immobilization. Connect Tissue Res 1977; 5:15–19.
4. Akeson WH, Woo SLY, Amiel D, et al: The connective tissue response to immobility: Biochemical changes in periarticular connective tissue of the immobilized rabit knee. Clin Orthop 1973; 93:356–362.
5. Allen EV, Barker NW, Hines EA Jr: Peripheral Vascular Diseases, ed 2. Philadelphia, WB Saunders, 1955, p 490.
6. American College of Sports Medicine: Guidelines for Graded Exercise Testing and Exercise Prescription. Philadelphia, Lea & Febiger, 1990.
7. Amiel D, Akeson WH, Harwood FL, Mechanic GL: The effect of immobilization on the types of collagen synthesized in periarticular connective tissue. Connect Tissue Res 1980; 8:27–32.
8. Amiel D, Woo SLY, Harwood FL, Akeson WH: The effect of immobilization on collagen turnover in connective tissue: A biochemical-biomechanical correlation. Acta Orthop Scand 1982; 53:325–332.
9. Anderson RL, Lefever FR, Francis WR, Maurer JK: Urinary and bladder responses to immobilization in male rats. Food Chem Toxicol 1990; 28:543–545.
10. Andrews PI, Rosenberg AR: Renal consequences of immobilization in children with fractured femurs. Acta Paediatr Scand 1990; 79:311–315.
11. Appell H: Muscular atrophy following immobilization. Sports Med 1990; 10:42–58.
12. Baker JH, Matsumoto DE: Adaptation of skeletal muscle to immobilization in a shortened position. Muscle Nerve. 1988; 2:231–244.
13. Balsam A, Leppo LE: Assessment of the degradation of thyroid hormones in man during bed rest. J Appl Physiol 1975; 38:216–219.
14. Bamman MM, Clarke MSF, Feeback DL, et al: Impact of resistance exercise during bed rest on skeletal muscle sarcopenia and myosin isoform distribution. J Appl Physiol 1998; 84:157–163.
15. Barbieri RL: Etiology and epidemiology of endometriosis. Am J Obstet Gynecol 1990; 162:565–567.
16. Beckett WS, Vroman NB, Nigro D, et al: Effect of prolonged bed rest on lung volume in normal individuals. J Appl Physiol 1986; 61:919–925.
17. Beckmann CRB, Beckmann CA: Effect of a structured antepartum exercise program on pregnancy and labor outcome in primiparas. J Reprod Med 1990; 35:704–709.
18. Behrens F, Kraft EL, Oegema TR Jr: Biochemical changes in articular cartilage after joint immobilization by casting or external fixation. J Orthop Res 1989; 7:335–343.
19. Bernauer EM, Walby WF, Ertl AC, et al: Knee-joint proprioception during 30-day 6 degree head-down bed rest with isotonic and isokinetic exercise training. Aviat Space Environ Med 1994; 65:1110–1115.
20. Berry P, Berry I, Manelfe C: Magnetic resonance imaging evaluation of lower limb muscles during bed rest—a microgravity simulation model. Aviat Space Environ Med 1993; 64:212–218.
21. Bird AD: The effect of surgery, injury, and prolonged bed rest on calf blood flow. Aust N Z J Surg 1972; 41:374–379.
22. Birkhead NC, Blizzard JJ, Daly JW, et al: Cardiodynamic and Metabolic Effects of Prolonged Bed Rest. Ohio Aerospace Medical Research Laboratories, Wright-Patterson Air Force Base. AMRL-TDR-63-37, May 1963.
23. Birkhead NC, Blizzard JJ, Daly JW, et al: Cardiodynamic and metabolic effects of prolonged bed rest with daily recumbent or sitting exercise and with sitting inactivity. Ohio Aerospace Medical Research Laboratories, Wright-Patterson Air Force Base, AMRL-TDR-64-61, August 1964.
24. Bjorntorp P, Krotkiewski M: Exercise treatment in diabetes mellitus. Acta Med Scand 1985; 217:3-7.
25. Booth FW, Seider MJ: Early change in skeletal muscle protein synthesis after limb immobilization of rats. J Appl Physiol 1979; 47:974–977.
26. Bravo G, Gauthier P, Roy PM, et al: A weight-bearing, water-based exercise program for osteopenic women: Its impact on bone, functional fitness, and well-being. Arch Phys Med Rehabil 1997; 78:1375–1380.
27. Briggs MH, Garcia-Webb P, Cheung T: Androgens and exercise. BMJ 1973; 3:49–50.
28. Buczynski A, Kedziora J, Wachowicz B, Zolynski K: Effect of bed rest on the adenine nucleotides concentration in human blood platelets. J Physiol Pharmacol 1991; 42:389–395.
29. Bung P, Bung C, Artal R et al: Therapeutic exercise for insulin-requiring gestational diabetics: Effects on the fetus—results of a randomized prospective longitudinal study. J Perinat Med 1993; 21:125–137.
30. Buschbacher R: Unpublished results, January 1994.
31. Buschbacher R, Coplin B, Buschbacher L, McKinley W: Noninflammatory knee joint effusions in spinal cord-injured and other paralyzed patients. Am J Phys Med Rehabil 1991; 70:309–312.
32. Camay A, Tschantz P: Mechanical influences in bone remodeling: Experimental research on Wolff's law. J Biomechanics 1972; 5:173–180.
33. Cardenas DD, Stolov WC, Hardy MR: Muscle fiber number in immobilization atrophy. Arch Phys Med Rehabil 1977; 58: 423–426.
34. Chandler JM, Duncan PW, Kochersberger G, Studenski S: Is lower extremity strength gain associated with improvement in physical performance and disability in frail, community-dwelling elders? Arch Phys Med Rehabil 1998; 79:24–30.
35. Chaviari M, Ganguly A, Luetscher JA, Zager PG: Effect of bedrest on circadian rhythms of plasma renin, aldosterone, and cortisol. Aviat Space Environ Med 1977; 48:633–636.
36. Chobanian AV, Lille RD, Tercyak A, Blevins P: The metabolic and hemodynamic effects of prolonged bed rest in normal subjects. Circulation 1974; 49:551–559.
37. Choi PYL, Van Horn JD, Picker DE, Roberts HI: Mood changes in women after an aerobics class: A preliminary study. Health Care Women Int 1993; 14:167–177.
38. Chuman MA: Risk factors associated with ulnar nerve compression in bedridden patients. J Neurosurg Nurs 1985; 17:338–342.
39. Cockett ATK, Elbadawi A, Zemjanis R, Adey WR: The effects of immobilization on spermatogenesis in subhuman primates. Fertil Steril 1970; 21:610–614.
40. Convertino V, Hung J, Goldwater D, DeBusk RF: Cardiovascular responses to exercise in middle-aged men after 10 days of bedrest. Circulation 1982; 65:134–140.
41. Convertino VA, Doerr DF, Eckberg DL, et al: Carotid baroreflex response following 30 days exposure to simulated microgravity. Physiologist 1989; 32:S67–S68.
42. Convertino VA, Doerr DF, Guell A, Marini JF: Effects of acute exercise on attenuated vagal baroreflex function during bed rest. Aviat Space Environ Med 1992; 63:999–1003.
43. Convertino VA, Goldwater DJ, Sandler H: $\dot{V}O_2$ kinetics of constant-load exercise following bed-rest–induced deconditioning. J Appl Physiol 1984; 57:1545–1550.

44. Cramer DW, Wilson E, Stilman RJ, et al: The relation of endometriosis to menstrual characteristics, smoking, and exercise. JAMA 1986; 225:1904–1908.
45. Cureton K, Bishop P, Hutchison P, et al: Sex difference in maximal oxygen uptake. Eur J Appl Physiol 1986; 54:656–660.
46. Cuthbertson DP: The influence of prolonged muscular rest on metabolism. Biochemistry 1929; 23:1328–1345.
47. Dalen N, Olsson E: Bone mineral content and physical activity. Acta Orthop Scand 1974; 45:170–174.
48. DeBusk RF, Hung J: Exercise conditioning soon after myocardial infarction: Effects on myocardial perfusion and ventricular function. Ann N Y Acad Sci 1982; 382:343–354.
49. DeRoshia CW, Greenleaf JE: Performance and mood-state parameters during 30-day 6 degree head-down bedrest with exercise training. Aviat Space Environ Med 1993; 64:522–527.
50. Devlin JT: Effects of exercise on insulin sensitivity in humans. Diabetes Care 1992; 15(suppl 4):1690–1693.
51. Dietrick JE, Whedon GD, Shorr E: Effects of immobilization upon various metabolic and physiologic functions of normal men. Am J Med 1948; 4:3–36.
52. Dolkas CB, Greenleaf JE: Insulin and glucose responses during bed rest with isotonic and isometric exercise. J Appl Physiol 1977; 43:1033–1038.
53. Donald KW, Lind AR, McNichol GW, et al: Cardiovascular responses to sustained (static) contractions. Circulation 1967; 20(suppl 1):115–130.
54. Donaldson CL, Hulley SB, Vogel JM, et al: Effect of prolonged bed rest on bone mineral. Metabolism 1970; 19:1071–1084.
55. Duchateau J, Hainaut K: Effects of immobilization on contractile properties, recruitment and firing rates of human motor units. J Physiol 1990; 422:55–65.
56. Dupui P, Montoya R, Costes-Salon M, et al: Balance and gait analysis after 30 days-6° bed rest: Influence of lower-body negative-pressure sessions. Aviat Space Environ Med 1992; 63:1004–1010.
57. Ellis S, Kirby LC, Greenleaf JE: Lower extremity muscle thickness during 30-day 6 degree head-down bed rest with isotonic and isokinetic training. Aviat Space Environ Med 1993; 64:1011–1015.
58. Enneking WF, Horowitz M: The intra-articular effects of immobilization on the human knee. J Bone Joint Surg Am 1972; 54:973–985.
59. Evans EB, Eggers GWN, Butler JK, Blumel J: Experimental immobilization and remobilization of rat knee joints. J Bone Joint Surg Am 1960; 42:737–758.
60. Farabollini F, Lupo Di Prisco C, Carli G: Changes in plasma testosterone and in its hypothalamic metabolism following immobility responses in rabbits. Physiol Behav 1978; 20:613–618.
61. Fiatarone MA, Marks EC, Ryan ND, et al: High intensity strength training in nonagenarians: Effects on skeletal muscle. JAMA 1990; 263:3029–3034.
62. Finsterbush A, Friedman B: Early changes in immobilized rabbits knee joints: A light and electron microscopic study. Clin Orthop 1973; 92:305–319.
63. Fishbein EG, Phillips M: How safe is exercise during pregnancy? J Obstet Gynecol Neonatal Nurs 1990; 19:45–49.
64. Fortney SM, Hyatt KH, Davis JE, Vogel JM: Changes in body fluid compartments during a 28-day bed rest. Aviat Space Environ Med 1991; 62:97–104.
65. Franklin BA, Gordon S, Timmis GC: Amount of exercise necessary for the patient with coronary artery disease. Am J Cardiol 1992; 69:1426–1432.
66. Frontera WR, Meredith CN, O'Reilly KP, et al: Strength conditioning in older men: Skeletal muscle hypertrophy and improved function. J Appl Physiol 1988; 64:1038–1044.
67. Fuller AK, Robinson ME: A test of exercise analgesia using signal detection theory and a within-subjects design. Percept Mot Skills 1993; 76:1299–1310.
68. Ghormley RK: The abuse of rest in bed in orthopedic surgery. JAMA 1944; 125:1085–1086.
69. Giannetta CL, Castleberry HB: Influence of bedrest and hypercapnia upon urinary mineral excretion in man. Aerospace Med 1974; 45:750–754.
70. Grana EA, Chiou-Tan F, Jaweed MM: Endplate dysfunction in healthy muscle following a period of disuse. Muscle Nerve 1996; 19:989–993.
71. Greenleaf JE: Energy and thermal regulation during bed rest and spaceflight. J Appl Physiol 1989; 67:507–516.
72. Greenleaf JE: Intensive exercise training during bed rest attenuates deconditioning. Med Sci Sports Exerc 1997; 29:207–215.
73. Greenleaf JE: Physiological responses to prolonged bed rest and fluid immersion in humans. J Appl Physiol 1984; 57:619–633.
74. Greenleaf JE, Bernauer EM, Ertl AC, et al: Isokinetic strength and endurance during 30-day 6 degrees head-down bed rest with isotonic and isokinetic exercise training. Aviat Space Environ Med 1994; 65:45–50.
75. Greenleaf JE, Bernauer EM, Ertl AC, et al: Work capacity during 30 days of bed rest with isotonic and isokinetic exercise training. J Appl Physiol 1989; 67:1820–1826.
76. Greenleaf JE, Bernauer EM, Young HL, et al: Fluid and electrolyte shifts during bed rest with isometric and isotonic exercise. J Appl Physiol 1977; 42:59–66.
77. Greenleaf JE, Ertl AC, Bernauer EM: Submaximal exercise $\dot{V}O_2$ and Q_c during 30-day 6 degree head down bed rest with isotonic and isokinetic exercise training. Aviat Space Environ Med 1996; 67:314–319.
78. Greenleaf JE, Reese RD: Exercise thermoregulation after 14 days of bed rest. J Appl Physiol 1980; 48:72–78.
79. Greenleaf JE, Van Beaumont W, Convertino VA, Starr JC: Handgrip and general muscular strength and endurance during prolonged bedrest with isometric and isotonic leg exercise training. Aviat Space Environ Med 1983; 54:696–700.
80. Greenleaf JE, Vernikos J, Wade CE, Barnes PR: Effect of leg exercise training on vascular volumes during 30 days of 6 degree head-down bed rest. J Appl Physiol 1992; 72:1887–1894.
81. Greenleaf JE, Wade CE, Leftheriotis G: Orthostatic responses following 30-day bed rest deconditioning with isotonic and isokinetic exercise training. Aviat Space Environ Med 1989; 60:537–542.
82. Gregg EW, Cauley JA, Seeley DG, et al: Physical activity and osteoporotic fracture risk in older women. Ann Intern Med 1998; 129:81–88.
83. Grimby G, Gustafsson E, Peterson L, Renstrom P: Quadriceps function and training after knee ligament surgery. Med Sci Sports Exerc 1980; 12:70–75.
84. Gwinup G: Weight loss without dietary restriction: Efficacy of different forms of aerobic exercise. Am J Sports Med 1987; 15:275–279.
85. Hagberg JM: Physiologic adaptations to prolonged high-intensity exercise training in patients with coronary artery disease. Med Sci Sports Exerc 1991; 23:661–667.
86. Hagberg JM, Seals DR: Exercise training and hypertension. Acta Med Scand Suppl 1986; 711:131–136.
87. Häggmark T, Eriksson E, Jansson E: Muscle fiber type changes in human skeletal muscle after injuries and immobilization. Orthopedics 1986; 9:181–185.
88. Haines RF: Effect of bed rest and exercise on body balance. J Appl Physiol 1974; 36:323–327.
89. Haskell WL: The influence of exercise training on plasma lipids and lipoproteins in health and disease. Acta Med Scand Suppl 1986; 711:25–37.
90. Herbert RD, Balnave RJ: The effect of position of immobilization on resting length, resting stiffness, and weight of the soleus muscle of the rabbit. J Orthop Res 1993; 11:358–366.
91. Herbison GJ, Jaweed MM, Ditunno JF: Muscle fiber atrophy after cast immobilization in the rat. Arch Phys Med Rehabil 1978; 59:301–305.
92. Hilton J: On the Influence of Mechanical and Physiological Rest in the Treatment of Accidents and Surgical Diseases, and the Diagnostic Value of Pain. London, Bell & Daldy, 1863.
93. Hirth VA, Schwartz RS: The effects of endurance exercise and resistance training on blood pressure. Phys Med Rehabil Clin North America 1994; 5:317–336.
94. Houston ME, Bentzen H, Larsen H: Interrelationships between skeletal muscle adaptations and performance as studied by detraining and retraining. Acta Physiol Scand 1979; 105:163–170.
95. Hurley BF: Effects of resistive training on lipoprotein-lipid profiles: A comparison to aerobic exercise training. Med Sci Sports Exerc 1989; 21:689–693.
96. Hutchinson PL, Cureton K, Outz H, et al: Relationship of cardiac size to maximal oxygen uptake and body size in men and women. Int J Sports Med 1991; 12:369–373.

97. Issekuts B Jr, Blizzard JJ, Birkhead NC, Rodahl K: Effect of prolonged bed rest on urinary calcium output. J Appl Physiol 1966; 21:1013–1020.
98. Jarrett SR, Mogelof JS: Critical illness neuropathy: diagnosis and management. Arch Phys Med Rehabil 1995; 76:688–691.
99. Jarvinen MJ, Einola SA, Virtanen EO: Effect of the position of immobilization upon the tensile properties of the rat gastrocnemius muscle. Arch Phys Med Rehabil 1992; 73:253–257.
100. Jones HH, Priest JD, Hayes WC, et al: Humeral hypertrophy in response to exercise. J Bone Joint Surg Am 1977; 59:204–208.
101. Judge JO, Underwood M, Gennosa T: Exercise to improve gait velocity in older persons. Arch Phys Med Rehabil 1993; 74:400–406.
102. Jurvelin J, Helminen HJ, Lauritsalo S, et al: Influences of joint immobilization and running exercise on articular cartilage surfaces of young rabbits. Acta Anat 1985; 122:62–68.
103. Kannus P, Josza L, Kvist M, et al: The effect of immobilization on myotendinous junction: An ultrastructural, histochemical and immunohistochemical study. Acta Physiol Scand 1992; 144: 387–394.
104. Karpakka J, Vaananen K, Orava S, Takala TES: The effects of preimmobilization training and immobilization on collagen synthesis in rat skeletal muscle. Int J Sports Med 1990; 11: 484–488.
105. Kasper CE, McNulty AL, Otto AJ, Thomas DP: Alterations in skeletal muscle related to impaired physical mobility: An empirical model. Res Nurs Health 1993; 16:265–273.
106. Katsume H, Furukawa K, Azuma A, et al: Disuse atrophy of the left ventricle in chronically bedridden elderly people. Jpn Circ J 1992; 56:201–206.
107. Katzel LI, Busby-Whitehead J, Hagberg JM, Fleg JL: Abnormal exercise electrocardiograms in master athletes after three months of deconditioning. J Am Geriatr Soc 1997; 45:744–746.
108. Kedlaya D, Brandstater ME, Lee JK: Immobilization hypercalcemia in incomplete paraplegia: Successful treatment with Pamidronate. Arch Phys Med Rehabil 1998; 79:222–225.
109. Klein L, Heiple KG, Torzilli PA, et al: Prevention of ligament and meniscus atrophy by active joint motion in a non–weight-bearing model. J Orthop Res 1989; 7:80–85.
110. Koeppl PM, Heller J, Bleecker ER, et al: The influence of weight reduction upon the personality profiles of overweight males. J Clin Psychol 1992; 48:463–471.
111. Koivisto VA, DeFronzo RA: Exercise in the treatment of type II diabetes. Acta Endocrinol Suppl 1984; 262:107–111.
112. Kokkinos PF, Holland JC, Narayan P, et al: Miles run per week and high-density lipoprotein cholesterol levels in healthy, middle-aged men. Arch Intern Med 1995;155:415–420.
113. Kottke FJ: Deterioration of the bedfast patient. Public Health Rep 1965; 80:437–447.
114. Kottke FJ, Pauley DL, Ptak RA: The rationale for prolonged stretching for correction of shortening of connective tissue. Arch Phys Med Rehabil 1966; 47:345–352.
115. Krebs JM, Schneider VS, Evans H, et al: Energy absorption, lean body mass, and total body fat changes during 5 weeks of continuous bed rest. Aviat Space Environ Med 1990; 61:314-318.
116. Krebs JM, Schneider VS, LeBlanc AD: Zinc, copper, and nitrogen balances during bed rest and fluoride supplementation in healthy adult males. Am J Clin Nutr 1988; 47:509–514.
117. Krolner B, Toft B: Vertebral bone loss: An unheeded side effect of therapeutic bed rest. Clin Sci 1983; 64:537–540.
118. Laros GS, Tipton CM, Cooper RR: Influence of physical activity in the knees of dogs. J Bone Joint Surg Am 1971; 53:275–286.
119. Laubach LL: Comparative muscular strength of men and women: A review of the literature. Aviat Space Environ Med 1976; 47:534–542.
120. Leach CS, Hulley SB, Rambaut PC, Dietlein LF: The effect of bedrest on adrenal function. Space Life Sci 1973; 4:415–423.
121. LeBlanc AD, Schneider VS, Evans HJ, et al: Bone mineral loss and recovery after 17 weeks of bed rest. J Bone Miner Res 1990; 5:843–850.
122. Lerman S, Canterbury JM, Reiss E: Parathyroid hormone and the hypercalcemia of immobilization. J Clin Endocrinol Metab 1977; 45:425–428.
123. Levine DM, Cohen JD, Dustan HP, et al: Behavior changes and the prevention of high blood pressure. Workshop II. AHA Prevention Conference III. Behavior change and compliance: Keys to improving cardiovascular health. Circulation 1993; 88:1387–1390.
124. Li XJ, Jee WSS, Chow S, Woodbury DM: Adaptation of cancellous bone to aging and immobilization in the rat: A single photon absorptiometry and histomorphometry study. Anat Rec 1990; 227:12–24.
125. Lipman RL, Schnure JJ, Bradley EM, Lecocq FR: Impairment of peripheral glucose utilization in normal subjects by prolonged rest. J Lab Clin Med 1970; 76:221–230.
126. Lord SR, Caplan GA, Ward JA: Balance, reaction time, and muscle strength in exercising and nonexercising older women: A pilot study. Arch Phys Med Rehabil 1993; 74:837–839.
127. MacDougall JD, Elder GCB, Sale DG, et al: Effects of strength training and immobilization on human muscle fibres. Eur J Appl Physiol 1980; 43:25–34.
128. Mallory GK, White PD, Salcedo-Salgar J: The speed of healing of myocardial infarction: A study of the pathologic anatomy in seventy-two cases. Am Heart J 1939; 18:647.
129. Marti B, Suter E, Riesen WF, et al: Effects of long-term, self-monitored exercise on the serum lipoprotein and apolipoprotein profile in middle-aged men. Atherosclerosis 1990; 81:19–31.
130. Martinsen EW: Benefits of exercise for the treatment of depression. Sports Med 1990; 9:380–389.
131. Melada GA, Goldman RH, Luetscher JA, Zager PG: Hemodynamics, renal function, plasma renin, and aldosterone in man after 5 to 14 days of bedrest. Aviat Space Environ Med 1975; 46:1049–1055.
132. Merritt JL, Hunder GG: Passive range of motion, not isometric exercise, amplifies acute urate synovitis. Arch Phys Med Rehabil 1983; 64:130–131.
133. Meythaler JM, Tuel SM, Cross LL: Successful treatment of immobilization hypercalcemia using calitonin and etidronate. Arch Phys Med Rehabil 1993; 74:316–319.
134. Michelsson J, Aho HJ, Kalimo H, Haltia M: Severe degeneration of rabbit vastus intermedius muscle immobilized in shortened position. APMIS 1990; 98:336–344.
135. Mikines KJ, Dela F, Tronier B, Galbo H: Effect of 7 days of bed rest on dose-response relation between plasma glucose and insulin secretion. Am J Physiol 1989; 257:E43–E48.
136. Minare P: Immobilization osteoporosis: A review. Clin Rheumatol 1989; 8:95–103.
137. Moldover JR, Downey JA: Cardiac response to exercise: Comparison of 3 ergometers. Arch Phys Med Rehabil 1983; 64: 155–159.
138. Morgan WP: Affective beneficence of vigorous physical activity. Med Sci Sports Exerc 1985; 17:94–100.
139. Moritani T, deVries HA: Neural factors versus hypertrophy in the time course of muscle strength gain in young and old men. J Gerontol 1981; 36:294–297.
140. Mueller EA: Influence of training and of inactivity on muscle strength. Arch Phys Med Rehabil 1970; 51:449–462.
141. Newton PO, Woo SLY, Kitabayashi LR, et al: Ultrastructural changes in knee ligaments following immobilization. Matrix 1990; 10:314–319.
142. Nicks DN, Beneke WM, Key RM, Timson BF: Muscle fiber size and number following immobilization atrophy. J Anat 1989; 163:1–5.
143. Noyes FR: Functional properties of knee ligaments and alterations induced by immobilization. Clin Orthop 1977; 123: 210–242.
144. O'Connor PJ, Youngstedt SD: Influence of exercise on human sleep. Exerc Sport Sci Rev 1995:23; 105–134.
145. Oki S, Itoh T, Desaki J, et al: Three-dimensional structure. Arch Phys Med Rehabil 1998; 79:31–32.
146. Pachter BR, Eberstein A: Neuromuscular plasticity following limb immobilization. J Neurocytol 1984; 13:1013–1025.
147. Palmoski M, Perricore E, Brandt KD: Development and reversal of a proteoglycan aggregation defect in normal canine cartilage after immobilization. Arthritis Rheum 1979; 22:508–515.

148. Palmoski MJ, Colyer RA, Brandt KD: Joint motion in the absence of normal loading does not maintain normal articular cartilage. Arthritis Rheum 1980; 23:325–334.
149. Pavy-Le Traon A, Sigaudo D, Vasseur P, et al: Orthostatic tests after a 4-day confinement or simulated weightlessness. Clin Physiol 1997; 17:41–55.
150. Petrella RJ, Lattanzio PJ, Nelson MG: Effect of age and activity on knee joint proprioception. Am J Phys Med Rehabil 1997; 76:235–241.
151. Powell KE, Thompson PD, Caspersen CJ, Kendrick JS: Physical activity and the incidence of coronary heart disease. Annu Rev Public Health 1987; 8:253–287.
152. Prakash YS, Miyata H, Zhan WZ, Sieck GC: Inactivity-induced remodeling of neuromuscular junctions in rat diaphragmatic muscle. Muscle Nerve 1999; 22:307–309.
153. Prior JC, Vigna Y, Alojado N: Conditioning exercise decreases premenstrual symptoms: A prospective controlled three month trial. Eur J Appl Physiol 1986; 55:349–355.
154. Raab W, De Paula E, Silva P, et al: Cardiac adrenergic preponderance due to lack of physical exercise and its pathogenic implications. Am J Cardiol 1960; 5:300–320.
155. Riley DA, Bain JLW, Thompson JL, et al: Disproportionate loss of thin filaments in human soleus muscle after 17-day bed rest. Muscle Nerve 1998; 21:1280–1289.
156. Roberts NA, Barton RN, Horan MA, White A: Adrenal function after upper femoral fracture in elderly people: Persistence of stimulation and the roles of adrenocorticotrophic hormone and immobility. Age Aging 1990; 19:304–310.
157. Rubin R: Pregnant? Go to bed. US News & World Report 61, Jan 10, 1994; p 61.
158. Rutherford OM, Jones DA, Round JM: Long-lasting unilateral muscle wasting and weakness following injury and immobilisation. Scand J Rehabil Med 1990; 22:33–37.
159. Ryback RS, Lewis OF, Lessard CS: Psychobiologic effects of prolonged bed rest (weightlessness) in young, healthy volunteers (study II). Aerospace Med 1971; 42:529–535.
160. Saltin B, Blomquist G, Mitchell JH, et al: Response to exercise after bed rest and after training. A longitudinal study of adaptive changes in oxygen transport and body composition. Circulation 1968; 38(suppl 7):VII1–VII78.
161. Samel A, Wegmann H, Vejvoda M: Response of the circadian system to 6° head-down tilt bed rest. Aviat Space Environ Med 1993; 64:50–54.
162. Saris WH: The role of exercise in the dietary treatment of obesity. Int J Obesity 1993; 17(suppl 1):S17–S21.
163. Schneider VS, McDonald J: Skeletal calcium homeostasis and countermeasures to prevent disuse osteoporosis. Calcif Tissue Int 1984; 36:S151–S154.
164. Schutz LK: The wheelchair athlete. In Buschbacher RM, Braddom RL (eds): Sports Medicine and Rehabilitation: A Sports Specific Approach. Philadelphia, Hanley & Belfus, 1994.
165. Schwarz L, Kindermann W: Changes in β endorphin levels in response to aerobic and anaerobic exercise. Sports Med 1992; 13:25–36.
166. Seip RL, Moulin P, Cocke T, et al: Exercise training decreases plasma cholesteryl ester transfer protein. Arteriosclerosis Thromb 1993; 13:1359–1367.
167. Shephard RJ: Exercise and aging: Extending independence in older adults. Geriatrics 1993; 48:61–64.
168. Shephard RJ, Rhind S, Shek PN: The impact of exercise on the immune system: NK cells, interleukins 1 and 2, and related responses. Exerc Sport Sci Rev 1995; 23:215–241.
169. Smith DW, Claren SK, Harvey MAS: Hyperthermia as a possible teratogenic agent. J Pediatr 1978; 92:878–883.
170. Smith MJ: Changes in judgement of duration with different patterns of auditory information for individuals confined to bed. Nurs Res 1975; 24:93–98.
171. Smith RL, Thomas KD, Schurman DJ, et al: Rabbit knee immobilization: Bone remodeling precedes cartilage degeneration. J Orthop Res 1992; 10:88–95.
172. Sparling PB: A meta-analysis of studies comparing maximal oxygen uptake in men and women. Res Q Exerc Sport 1980; 51:542–552.
173. Spector SA, Simard CP, Fournier M, et al: Architectural alterations of rat hind-limb skeletal muscles immobilized at different lengths. Exp Neurol 1982; 76:94–110.
174. Stewart AF, Adler M, Byers CM, et al: Calcium homeostasis in immobilization: An example of resorptive hypercalciuria. N Engl J Med 1982; 306:1136–114.
175. Stewart KJ: Weight training in coronary artery disease and hypertension. Prog Cardiovasc Dis 1992; 35:159–168.
176. Stolk JM, Harris PQ: Differentiation of adrenomedullary catecholamine synthesizing enzyme responses to repeated immobilization in hybrid rats. Life Sci 1980; 26:2099–2104.
177. Stremel RW, Convertino VA, Bernauer EM, Greenleaf JE: Cardiorespiratory deconditioning with static and dynamic leg exercise during bed rest. J Appl Physiol 1976; 41:905–909.
178. Stuart CA, Shangraw RE, Peters EJ, Wolfe RR: Effect of dietary protein on bed-rest-related changes in whole-body-protein synthesis. Am J Clin Nutr 1990; 52:509–514.
179. Stuart CA, Shangraw RE, Prince MJ, et al: Bed-rest–induced insulin resistance occurs primarily in muscle. Metabolism 1988; 37:802–806.
180. Superko HR: Exercise training, serum lipids, and lipoprotein particles: Is there a change threshold? Med Sci Sports Exerc 1991; 23:677–685.
181. Suzuki Y, Kashihara H, Katagiri A, et al: Effects of moderate physical training after 10 days horizontal bed-rest on peak $\dot{V}O_2$ and cardio-respiratory functions during submaximal supine and sitting exercise in young subjects. Physiologist 1992; 35(suppl 1):S198–S199.
182. Tanji JL: Hypertension part I: How exercise helps. Phys Sports Med 1990; 18:77–82.
183. Tanji JL, Champlin JJ, Wong GY, et al: Blood pressure recovery curves after submaximal exercise: A predictor of hypertension at ten-year follow-up. Am J Hypertens 1989; 2:135–138.
184. Taylor HL, Henschel A, Brozakek J, Keys A: Effects of bed rest on cardiovascular function and work performance. J Appl Physiol 1949; 2:223–239.
185. Thompson DD, Rodan GA: Indomethacin inhibition of tenotomy-induced bone resorption in rats. J Bone Miner Res 1988; 3:409–414.
186. Uhtoff HK, Jaworski ZFG: Bone loss in response to long-term immobilization. J Bone Joint Surg Br 1978; 60:420–429.
187. Vandenborne K, Elliott MA, Walter GA, et al: Longitudinal study of skeletal muscle adaptations during immobilization and rehabilitation. Muscle Nerve 1998; 21:1006–1012.
188. van Lent P, Wilms FHA, van den Berg WB: Interaction of polymorphonuclear leucocytes with patellar cartilage of immobilised arthritic joints: A scanning electron microscopic study. Ann Rheum Dis 1989; 48:832–837.
189. Veldhuizen JW, Verstappen FTJ, Vroemen JPAM, et al: Functional and morphological adaptations following four weeks of knee immobilization. Int J Sports Med 1993; 14:283–287.
190. Vernikos J, Dallman MF, Keil LC, et al: Gender differences in endocrine responses to posture and 7 days of 6° head-down bed rest. Am J Physiol 1993; 265:E153–161.
191. Vernikos-Danellis J, Leach CS, Winget CM, et al: Changes in glucose, insulin, and growth hormone levels associated with bedrest. Aviat Space Environ Med 1976; 47:583–587.
192. Warren CJ, Lehmann JF, Koblanski JN: Elongation of rat tail tendon: Effect of load and temperature. Arch Phys Med Rehabil 1971; 52:465–474.
193. White PD, Mallory GK, Salcedo-Salgar J: The speed of healing of myocardial infarcts. In Transactions of the American Clinical and Climatological Association. Framingham, MA, Lakeview Press, 1937; pp 97–104.
194. Whitney EJ, Ashcom TL, Hantman RK, et al: Reversibility of fixed atherosclerotic lesions with aggressive risk factor modification: Milit Med 1991; 156:422–429.
195. Williams PE: Use of intermittent stretch in the prevention of serial sarcomere loss in immobilized muscle. Ann Rheum Dis 1990; 49:316–317.

196. Williams PE, Goldspink G: Connective tissue changes in immobilized muscle. J Anat 1984; 138:343–350.
197. Wilson CJ, Dahners LE: An examination of the mechanism of ligament contracture. Clin Orthop 1988; 227:286–291.
198. Yagan R, Radivoyevitch M, Khan M: Double cortical line in the acetabular roof: A sign of disuse osteoporosis. Radiology 1987; 165:171–175.
199. Yeh JK, Aloia JF: Effect of physical activity on calcitropic hormones and calcium balance in rats. Am J Physiol 1990; 258:E263–E268.
200. Young DR, Niklowitz WJ, Brown RJ, Jee WSS: Immobilization-associated osteoporosis in primates. Bone 1986; 7:109–117.
201. Zorbas YG, Andreyev VG, Popescu LB: Fluid-electrolyte metabolism and renal function in men under hypokinesia and physical exercise. Int Urol Nephrol 1988; 20:215–223.
202. Zorbas YG, Naexu KA, Federenko YF: Blood serum biochemical changes in physically conditioned and unconditioned subjects during bed rest and chronic hyperhydration. Clin Exp Pharmacol Physiol 1992; 19:137–145.

35 CHAPTER

Donna Jo Blake, M.D., and Dan D. Scott, M.D.

Employment of Persons with Disabilities

In the United States, disability is a significant public health and social issue. The number of Americans who experience disability, activity limitations secondary to chronic illnesses, or impairments has risen while mortality has declined. Approximately 54 million noninstitutionalized Americans—almost one person in five—have a mental or physical disability, nearly half of whom can be considered to have a severe disability. And 37.7 million noninstitutionalized Americans—almost one person in seven—have limitations severe enough to prevent them from playing, attending school, working, maintaining a household, or caring for themselves. Given these two measures, disability ranks as the nation's largest public health problem.[5, 16, 18, 20, 24, 27, 43]

The growing numbers of Americans with disabilities present new medical, social, and political challenges. The major activity limitations found in those with disabilities include an inability to manage personal care, inability to work and be financially self-supporting, and the inability to integrate socially and enjoy leisure.[31] These limitations have medical, behavioral, social, and economic implications. In order to help those with disabilities restore functional capacity, prevent further deterioration in functioning, and maintain or improve their quality of life, programs of any type should emphasize rehabilitation and prevention of secondary conditions.[24] These programs must respect disability as multifaceted and foster an interdisciplinary approach to treatment.

Within the medical arena, the specialty of Physical Medicine & Rehabilitation has been concerned with the establishment of physiological, psychological, and social equilibrium for persons with disabilities.[15] According to Rusk,[27] "A rehabilitation program is designed to take a disabled person from his bed back to his job, fitting him for the best life possible commensurate with his disability and more importantly with his ability." In order to help all persons with disabilities achieve their maximum level of independence, avert further deterioration in functioning, and maintain or improve their quality of life, the physiatrist and the medical rehabilitation team must appreciate the multifaceted character of disability. We must accept the responsibility to initiate appropriate referrals to other collaborating programs that can support these goals beyond the medical arena. One such program is *vocational rehabilitation.*

In this chapter, we examine the subject of employment of people with disabilities. Specifically, we:

- Discuss the concept of disability
- Review national data on disability and employment
- Consider the economic impact of disability
- Review policies supporting employment of persons with disabilities
- Discuss economic assistance strategies
- Discuss vocational rehabilitation strategies
- Enumerate the incentives and disincentives for returning to work
- Postulate that vocational rehabilitation serves as an actual rehabilitation treatment as well as a disability prevention strategy for people with disabilities

CONCEPT OF DISABILITY

Disability itself is not always precise and quantifiable. The concept of disability is not agreed upon by persons who consider themselves to have a disability, professionals who study disability, or the general public.[18] This lack of agreement is an obstacle to all studies of disability and to the equitable and effective administration of programs and policies intended for people with disabilities.[8, 9, 18, 23, 24]

The World Health Organization (WHO) has a mandate to develop a global common health language—one that is understood to include physical, mental, and social well-being. The International Classification of Impairments, Disabilities, and Handicaps (ICIDH) was first published by WHO in 1980 as a tool for classification of the "consequences of disease." The new version, ICIDH-2 beta-1 draft is now being field-tested. The ICIDH-2 beta-1 draft is designed to provide a common framework for understanding the dimensions of disablement and functioning at three different levels: the body, the person, and society.

The ICIDH-2 reflects the biopsychosocial model of disablement. In this model, disablement and functioning are viewed as outcomes of an interaction between a person's physical or mental condition and the social and physical environment. Human functioning is characterized at three levels: the body or body part, the whole person, and the whole person in social context. Disablements are the dimensions of dysfunctioning that result for an individual at these three levels; these include *impairment,* losses or abnormalities of bodily function and structure; *limitations of activities;* and *restrictions of participation.*

This biopsychosocial model regards functioning and disablement as outcomes of interactions between health conditions (disorders/diseases) and conceptual factors such as social and physical environmental factors and personal factors. The interactions in this paradigm are dynamic, complex, and bidirectional (Fig. 35–1).

Dimensions of dysfunctioning are defined as follows:

Impairment is the loss or abnormality of body structure or of a physiological or psychological function.

Activity is the nature and extent of functioning at the level of the person.

Participation is the nature and extent of a person's involvement in life situations in relation to impairment, activities, health conditions, and contextual factors and may be restricted in nature, duration, and quality.[45]

The concept of disability or disablement continues to be one about which there are many interpretations and opinions. This lack of agreement about the concept of disablement affects epidemiological studies of disablement and the development of effective treatment and prevention strategies. The biopsychosocial model and the common language of the ICIDH-2 can help to define the need for health care and related services; define health outcomes in terms of body, person and social functioning; provide a common framework for research, clinical work, and social policy; ensure the cost-effective provision and management of health care and related services; and characterize physical, mental, social, economic, or environmental interventions that will improve lives and levels of functioning.[45]

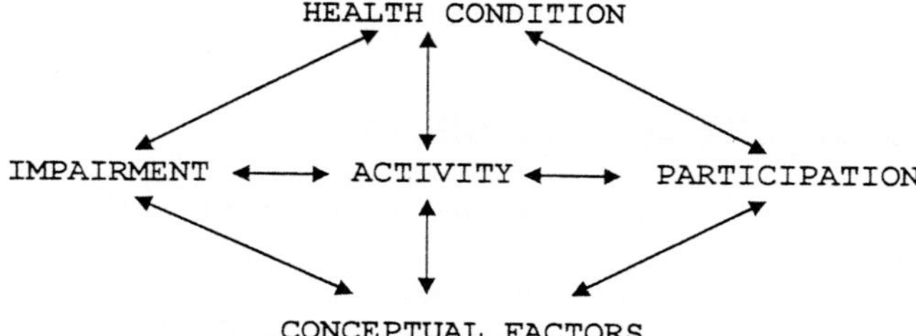

FIGURE 35–1. Biopsychosocial model of disablement.

DATA: IMPAIRMENT AND DISABILITY

Estimates of impairment and disability come from many sources. In 1990, the National Health Interview Survey (NHIS) found at least 120 million persons with impairments and 33.8 million people with disabilities living in households. Estimates from the 1990 Census indicate that 2.3 million residents of institutions can be considered to have a disability. An estimate of the number of people with limitations in life activities, according to the NHIS (1992) is 37.7 million, or 15% of the U.S. population.[16]

The Survey of Income and Program Participation (SIPP) from the U.S. Bureau of the Census provides extensive information on the number and characteristics of people with disabilities. SIPP information excludes people living in institutions. Data from SIPP (1994) indicate that 54 million people, or 20.6% of the U.S. population, have some level of disability.[20] Inability to walk without an assistive device was reported in 1.8 million using a wheelchair, and 5.2 million using another gait aid. Requiring help with one or more activities of daily living was reported in 4.1 million. The International Center for the Disabled (ICD) surveyed 12,500 households in 1986 and found the prevalence of disability to be 15% among Americans aged 16 years and older.[10] While the concept of disability was different for each survey, the results indicate that at least 54 million Americans have disabilities.

Impairments due to chronic disease have become increasingly significant as risk factors of disability.[5, 18] Table 35–1 lists the 15 conditions with the highest prevalence of functional compromise or disability.[18] The prevalence of disability with these conditions appears to be due to the prevalence of the condition itself and the chance that the condition will cause a disability. Table 35–2 shows the ranking of persons by percent of specific conditions who have functional limitations secondary to that condition.[18] In general, many of the conditions that are significant risk factors for disability are low in prevalence. For example, multiple sclerosis has a low overall prevalence, but is a significant risk factor for disability. Examination of this ranking shows seven out of the top ten disabling conditions to be conditions frequently managed by the physiatrist and the rehabilitation team. These conditions or diseases are typically chronic, requiring a lifetime of rehabilitative

TABLE 35–1 Conditions with Highest Prevalence of Activity Limitation

Main Cause	%	All Causes	%
Orthopedic impairments	16.0	Orthopedic impairments	21.5
Arthritis	12.3	Arthritis	18.8
Heart disease	22.5	Heart disease	17.1
Visual impairments	4.4	Hypertension	10.8
Intervertebral disc disorders	4.4	Visual impairments	8.9
Asthma	4.3	Diabetes	6.5
Nervous disorders	4.0	Mental disorders	5.6
Mental disorders	3.9	Asthma	5.5
Hypertension	3.8	Intervertebral disc disorders	5.2
Mental retardation	2.9	Nervous disorders	4.9
Diabetes	2.7	Hearing impairments	4.3
Hearing impairments	2.5	Mental retardation	3.2
Emphysema	2.0	Emphysema	3.1
Cerebrovascular disease	1.9	Cerebrovascular disease	2.9
Osteomyelitis/bone disorders	1.1	Abdominal hernia	1.8

From La Plante MP: The demographics of disability. Milbank Q 1991; 69:55–77.

management in order to have an effect on the disabling process, prevent secondary conditions, and maintain quality of life.

SOCIOECONOMIC EFFECT OF DISABILITY

Disablement has significant socioeconomic consequences for the individual with disabilities and for society. When a person is unable to participate in his or her social role as a worker or homemaker because of a physical or mental condition, that person is said to have a work disability or a work participation restriction.[4, 45] Work participation restriction results in dependency and loss of productivity for that person. Society, in turn, incurs direct and indirect costs.

Direct expenditures include those for medical and personal care, architectural modification, assistive technology, and institutional care as well as income support for the person with a disability. For the individual, these expenses contribute to impoverishment.[3, 38] Society's response to the expenditures related to disablement includes disability-related programs such as Social Security Disability Insurance (SSDI), Supplemental Security Income (SSI), Medicare, and Medicaid. Direct expenditures incurred by our economy in 1986 totaled $169.4 billion.[4]

TABLE 35–2 Conditions with Highest Risk of Disability[18]

Chronic Condition	No. of Conditions*	% Causing Activity Limitation	Rank	% Causing Major Activity Limitation	Rank	% Causing Need for Help in Basic Life Activities	Rank
Mental retardation	1202	84.1	1	80.0	1	19.9†	9
Absence of leg(s)†	289	83.3	2	73.1	2	39.0†	2
Lung or bronchial cancer	200	74.8	3	63.5	3	34.5†	4
Multiple sclerosis†	171	70.6	4	63.3	4	40.7†	1
Cerebral palsy†	274	69.7	5	62.2	5	22.8†	8
Blind in both eyes	396	64.5	6	58.8	6	38.1†	3
Partial paralysis in extremity†	578	59.6	7	47.2	7	27.5†	5
Other orthopedic impairments†	316	58.7	8	42.6	8	14.3‡	12
Complete paralysis in extremity†	617	52.7	9	45.5	9	26.1†	6
Rheumatoid arthritis†	1223	51.0	10	39.4	12	14.9†	11
Intervertebral disc disorders†	3987	48.7	11	38.2	14	5.3†	—
Paralysis in other sites (complete/partial)†	247	47.8	12	43.7	10	14.1‡	13
Other heart disease disorders§	4708	46.9	13	35.1	15	13.6†	14
Cancer of digestive tract	228	45.3	14	40.3	11	15.9‡	15
Emphysema	2074	43.6	15	29.8	—	9.6†	15
Absence of arm(s)/hand(s)†	84	43.1	—	39.0	13	4.1‡	—
Cerebrovascular disease†	2599	38.2	—	33.3	—	22.9†	7

* In thousands.
† Conditions frequently managed by physiatrists.
‡ Figure has low statistical reliability or precision (relative standard error >39%).
§ Heart failure (9.8%), valve disorders (15.3%), congenital disorders (15.0%), other ill-defined heart conditions (59.9%).

Disablement is also costly to the individual and society because of the loss of productivity. The indirect monetary costs for the individual are reckoned in terms of losses in job earnings and homemaker services. People with disabilities are less likely to be employed. The employment rate for people 21 to 64 years of age in 1994 without a disability was 82.1%; for those with a nonsevere disability, the employment rate was 76.9%; and for those with a severe disability, the employment rate was 26.1%[20] (Table 35–3).

Disablement is also associated with lower earnings. Thirty percent of persons with a restriction in work participation in 1994 were below the poverty line, while only 8% of nondisabled persons were at the same level.[19] In 1986, the ICD survey found that 50% of all people with disabilities reported household incomes of $15,000 or less as compared to 25% of nondisabled with incomes in that range.[10] In 1994, men 21 to 64 years of age without a disability had median monthly earnings of $2,190. Those with a nonsevere disability had $1,857 median monthly earnings, and those with a severe disability had $1,262 median monthly earnings[20] (Table 35–3). The indirect monetary cost to society is loss from the labor force.[3] For example, in 1988, spinal cord injury alone was estimated to have cost our economy $2.4 billion in lost productivity.[11]

Disablement imposes indirect nonmonetary costs to the individual and to society. Fifty-seven percent of persons with disabilities surveyed by Harris[10] in 1986 believed their disability prevented them from reaching their full potential. Restriction in work participation, in particular, places the individual in a position of dependency on insurance payments or government benefits for income support and medical care. Dependency affects people's feelings about themselves and their overall satisfaction with life.

Pressure from various customers and especially the third-party payers for accountability in medical care focuses attention on outcome and cost-effectiveness. Interventions directed at disablement should be assessed with measures of both outcome and cost-effectiveness. Disablement is more than a medical phenomenon—it is a complex socioeconomic process. Assessment of the outcome and cost-effectiveness of an intervention should take into consideration the quality of life and indirect monetary costs, as well as direct expenditures.

Vocational rehabilitation is an intervention that can limit restrictions in work participation. In 1993, the Social Security Administration estimated that for every dollar spent on vocational rehabilitation services, five dollars in future direct expenditures was saved.[19] While employment is the expected outcome of vocational rehabilitation, the impact of this intervention goes beyond simple employment and saving of direct expenditures. The positive effects of working are demonstrated when the characteristics of working and nonworking persons with disabilities are compared. Those who work are better educated, have more money, are less likely to consider themselves disabled, and, in general, are more satisfied with life.[10]

Comprehensive rehabilitation of persons with disabilities should include strategies such as vocational rehabilitation that reduce work restrictions. The outcomes will include increased independence and increased productivity. The cost-effectiveness of comprehensive rehabilitation should be measured in direct and indirect monetary and nonmonetary costs over the lifetime of the individual.[2]

DISABILITY-RELATED PROGRAMS AND POLICIES

Programs

There is a plethora of disability-related programs and policies. Each program and policy has its own definition of disablement and/or disability, and therefore differs in the eligibility and application criteria. The programs can be characterized as ameliorative or corrective.[12] *Ameliorative programs* provide payment for income support and medical care. *Corrective programs* facilitate the individual's ability to return to work and to reduce or remove the disablement. Whether ameliorative or corrective, all programs influence the biopsychosocial model of disablement.

Disability-related programs can be categorized into three basic types: (1) cash transfers, (2) medical care programs, and (3) direct service programs. Table 35–4 presents specific programs within these three basic types.[4] Estimates of the expenditures of these disability-related programs provide insight into expenditure trends. In 1970, 61.4% of the disability dollar went for cash transfers, 33% for medical care, and 5.4% for direct services. By 1986, the proportion of the disability dollar for direct services had decreased to 2.1% as the proportion for medical care had increased.[4]

The trend toward ameliorative programs' capturing more resources is a concern. Studies of the socioeconomic consequences of disability support the utility of rehabilitating people with disabilities, allowing them to enter the labor market and thereby decrease their dependency and loss of productivity. The physiatrist has an important supportive role in initiating referrals to

TABLE 35–3 Employment and Earnings[20] (1994)

	Employment Rate People 21–64 Years of Age	Median Monthly Earnings Men 21–64 Years of Age	Median Monthly Earnings Women 21–64 Years of Age
No disability	82.1%	$2,190	$1,470
Nonsevere disability	76.9%	$1,857	$1,200
Severe disability	26.1%	$1,262	$1,000

TABLE 35–4 Disability-Related Programs

Type of Program	Specific Programs
Cash transfer	Social insurance: Social Security Disability Insurance Private insurance Indemnity compensation Income support: Supplemental Security Income, veterans' pensions, Aid to Families with Dependent Children
Medical care	Medicare Private disability insurance Veterans' programs Workers' compensation Tort settlements Medicaid
Direct services	Rehabilitation and vocational education Veterans' programs Services for persons with specific impairments General funded programs, e.g., food stamps, developmental disabilities, blind, mentally ill Employment assistance programs, i.e., Comprehensive Employment Training Program

From Berkowitz M, Hill MA: Disability and the labor market: An overview. In Berkowitz M, Hill MA (eds): Disability and the Labor Market: Economic Problems, Policies, and Programs. New York, ILR Press, 1989, pp 1–28.

the corrective programs. These programs are in keeping with the philosophy of rehabilitation, which is to maximize individual functioning and lessen disability.

Public Disability Policies

Public policy in the United States has begun to recognize that many barriers to integration faced by persons with disabilities are the result of discriminatory policy and practices. There is also the view that disability is an interaction between an individual and the environment. This has played a fundamental role in shaping public policy toward disability over the last 20 years. Since the late 1960s, Congress has passed a series of laws aimed at enhancing the quality of life for persons with disabilities. These laws have mandated that housing and transportation be accessible, that education for children with disabilities be appropriate, and that employment practices be nondiscriminatory.[6, 7, 40]

Three legislative actions deserve to be highlighted. The Rehabilitation Act of 1973 extended civil rights protection to persons with disabilities. This legislation included antidiscrimination and affirmative action in employment. The Rehabilitation Act Amendments of 1978 broadened the responsibility of the Rehabilitation Services Administration (RSA) to include independent living programs, and created the National Council of the Handicapped (the National Council of the Handicapped became the National Council on Disability in January of 1989). The capstone of this legislative tradition is the Americans with Disabilities Act of 1989. This legislation established a clear and comprehensive prohibition of discrimination on the basis of disability.[6, 36, 40, 41] Table 35–5 reviews the federal disability laws since 1968.[6, 36]

VOCATIONAL REHABILITATION

The objective of vocational rehabilitation is to allow persons with physical disabilities to engage in gainful employment. Historically, formal vocational rehabilitation services were instituted to provide returning World War II veterans with disabilities assistance in obtaining suitable occupations.[40]

Before the 1970s, jobs earmarked for persons with disabilities were provided through government-subsidized sheltered workshops. The Comprehensive Employment Training Act of 1973 (CETA) provided public service jobs for persons with disabilities and for the disadvantaged, along with training programs for this population. At its peak in 1980, CETA and sheltered workshops provided more than a million jobs for a broadly defined "disabled" population. The CETA program lasted from 1973 to 1982, whereupon the federal government subsequently returned to state-run vocational rehabilitation agencies for provision of these services to persons with disabilities.

The Rehabilitation Act of 1973 authorized federal funding for state rehabilitation agencies to provide a variety of services to qualified persons with disabilities. Table 35–6 lists the services provided. The federal government supplies 80% of the funding for state vocational rehabilitation agencies, while the states must provide the remaining 20%. State agencies administer the programs under the Rehabilitation Services Administration (RSA) in the Department of Education. The intent of the Rehabilitation Act was to provide services to persons with disabilities with emphasis placed on serving those with more severe disabilities (General Accounting Office [GAO] testimony).[37] State agencies are usually located in the state division or bureau of vocational rehabilitation. The state division provides direct services, and also refers individuals to private rehabilitation agencies and training programs when indicated.

Traditional Approaches to Vocational Rehabilitation

A variety of approaches to vocational rehabilitation have been developed over the years. The traditional approach begins with referral of a person with a disability to a vocational rehabilitation counselor. This referral can be generated by the person with a disability, a physician, a social worker, or a case manager. The initial referral includes medical records, documentation of disabilities and capabilities, and neuropsychological testing (if available).

The initial interview between the counselor and the client (person with a disability) establishes rapport and provides background information about previous job skills and experiences. The interview also provides information about the individual's educational level, motivation, perceived abilities and disabilities, and areas of interest. If the client was employed prior to the onset

TABLE 35–5 Federal Disability Laws

Year	Public Law No.	Title of Law	Key Provisions
1968	90–480	Architectural Barriers Act	Requires that buildings built with federal funds or leased by the federal government be made accessible
1970	91–453	Urban Mass Transportation Act	Requires eligible local jurisdictions to plan and design accessible mass transportation facilities and services
1973	98–87	Federal Aid Highway Act	Requires that transportation facilities receiving federal assistance under the act be made accessible; allows highway funds to be used to make pedestrian crosswalks accessible
1973	93–112	Rehabilitation Act	Prohibits discrimination against qualified people with disabilities in programs, or receiving services and benefits, that are federally funded; created Architectural and Transportation Barriers Compliance Board
1975	93–391	Department of Transportation Appropriations Act	Prohibits purchase of mass transit equipment or construction of facilities unless they are accessible to elderly and people with disabilities
1975	94–103	Developmental	Establishes protection and advocacy systems for developmentally disabled people; establishes representative councils in each state for developmentally disabled people
1975	94–142	Education for All Handicapped Children Act	Provides for a free appropriate education for handicapped children in the least restrictive setting possible
1975	94–173	National Housing Act Amendments	Provide for the removal of barriers in federally supported housing; establish Office of Independent Living for disabled people in Department of Housing and Urban Development
1978	95–602	Rehabilitation, Comprehensive Services, and Developmental Disability Amendments	Establish independent living as a priority for state vocational rehabilitation programs; provide federal funding for independent living centers
1980	96–265	Social Security Disability Amendments	Remove certain disincentives to work by allowing people with disabilities to deduct independent living expenses in computing income benefits
1990	101–336	Americans with Disabilities Act	Establishes a clear and comprehensive prohibition of discrimination on the basis of disability

Data from DeJong G, Lifchez R: Physical disability and public policy. Sci Am 1983; 248:40–50; and U.S. Equal Employment Opportunity Commission and the U.S. Department of Justice: Americans with Disabilities Act Handbook (EEOC-BK-19). Washington, DC, US Government Printing Office, 1991.

of disability, there is often potential for placement with the former employer. This previous employer should be contacted to learn of employment opportunities for the person with a disability. The vocational rehabilitation counselor also assesses the skills the person had premorbidly and the skills needed prior to placement in a suitable position. If no positions are available, vocational testing is performed.

Aptitude Matching versus Work Sample

Vocational testing is performed to assess the client's level of general intelligence, achievement, aptitudes, interests, and work skills. Formal testing consists of administering a battery of paper-and-pencil standardized tests, examples of which are listed in Table 35–7. This type of approach is known as "aptitude matching." It determines the client's aptitudes or traits in the areas of general intelligence, visuospatial perception, eye-hand coordination, motor coordination, and dexterity. Performance on the tests is compared against a list of essential aptitudes, grouped by occupation, in the *Dictionary of Occupational Titles* (DOT) published by the Department of Labor.[21] When a client's aptitudes match a particular occupation, a job search is undertaken by the counselor.

TABLE 35–6 Services Provided by Vocational Rehabilitation Specialists

Diagnosis and Evaluation	Adjustment Training
Counseling and guidance	Business or vocational training
Restoration*	Miscellaneous training
Transportation	Placement
College or university training	Referrals
Income maintenance	On-the-job training

* Includes medical treatment, prosthetic devices, or medically necessary services to correct or modify a physical or mental disorder.

TABLE 35–7 Tests Administered by Vocational Rehabilitation Counselor or Neuropsychologist

Test	Type
Wechsler Adult Intelligence Scale-Revised (WAIS-R)	Intelligence
General Aptitude Test Battery (GATB)	Aptitude
Differential Aptitude Test (DAT)	Aptitude
Wide Range Achievement Test (WRAT)	Achievement
Strong-Campbell Interest Inventory (SCII)	Interest
Career Assessment Inventory (CAI)	Interest
Minnesota Multiphasic Personality Inventory (MMPI)	Personality
Halstead-Reitan	Cognitive evaluation
Luria-Nebraska	Cognitive evaluation

A work sample approach is often used in conjunction with aptitude batteries. The work sample approach measures general characteristics such as size discrimination, multilevel sorting, eye-hand-foot coordination, and dexterity. The Valpar Component Work Sample Series (VCWSS) is a good example of the work sample approach. The VCWSS uses complex work apparatus to measure almost exclusively motor responses. There is less focus on general intelligence, aptitude, or academic performance. Work samples can also evaluate the type of "work group" in which the client is most skilled. This simulated work requires performance of a series of tasks, such as drill press operation or circuit board or bench assembly.[21]

Once the client's skills have been evaluated and interests explored, a vocational goal is developed. The requirements of the potential position must first be determined. This is accomplished by performing a job analysis of the position, then identifying the physical and mental requirements and any necessary job site modifications (e.g., adaptive equipment). If training is proposed, it must be accessible and available to the client. Transportation should be arranged and can be paid for by the vocational rehabilitation agency. Tuition, books, and adaptive equipment to allow performance of the position can also be provided by the agency.

Training programs vary in length depending on the potential vocational goal. They can last from a few weeks to several years. Training can be conducted at a trade school, college, university, or on the job with state vocational rehabilitation agency funding.

On-the-job training requires job development. The counselor or the client explores community business resources to develop suitable positions. Tax incentives for potential employers can help convince industry to offer training. Sliding-scale wages can be arranged to assist in developing positions. For example, the state rehabilitation agency may fund 100% of salary for 3 to 6 months. The employer gradually assumes that responsibility over the next 3 to 6 months as the new employee becomes trained. Many employers want to keep the employees they have trained, but some prefer to act in the capacity of trainers for a series of persons with disabilities. In this case, the counselor still has the task of placing the newly trained people.

Once an individual has completed training and has been placed for 60 days, the state vocational rehabilitation agency considers the case a "success" and closes its file. No follow-up is typically provided.

Sheltered Workshops

One of the problems with the traditional approach of the vocational rehabilitation agency has been its poor record of success, especially for persons with severe disabilities. There were 45% fewer people successfully vocationally rehabilitated in 1988 than in 1974, despite increased financial support and larger numbers of persons with disabilities.[40] A 1987 GAO survey found that of SSDI recipients receiving vocational rehabilitation, less than 1% left the SSDI rolls.[30] The ICD survey reported that although 60% of persons with disabilities knew about vocational rehabilitation services, only 10% took advantage of those services. Of those using the services, more than 50% felt they were not useful in securing gainful employment.[10]

As a result of the poor placement record, alternative strategies have been developed for enabling persons with disabilities to obtain gainful employment. These include sheltered workshops, day programs, transitional and supported employment, projects with industry, independent living center–directed employment, and others. Funding for these programs has come from public nonprofit and private industry, state and federal social service programs, religious entities, corporate and foundation contributions, and individual donations.

A sheltered workshop is a "public non-profit organization certified by the U.S. Department of Labor to pay 'sub-minimum' wages to persons with diminished earning capacity."[13] There are more than 5000 of these workshops, including Goodwill, Inc., serving approximately 250,000 persons with disabilities. This form of employment serves persons with severe disabilities, including limited vision, mental illness, mental retardation, and alcoholism. While sheltered workshops provide job experience and income, critics report that sheltered workshops rarely lead to competitive, integrated employment. People with severe disabilities can be competitively employed in the community through the use of some modern strategies, as outlined below.

Day Programs

Day programs have existed since before the 1970s and are meant to provide supervised vocational activity for persons with severe disabilities, usually those with mental retardation or mental illness. These programs are funded by private and corporate sponsors, as well as by state and federal agencies. They are not designed as a transition into competitive employment, nor do they allow community integration. They are geared toward providing supervised day activities while the caretakers of these persons work or perform their own daily routines. Activities are performed in facilities that serve only persons with disabilities.

Home-Based Programs

Another more traditional method for assisting persons with severe disabilities to obtain employment is the home-based program. Home-based programs can be funded by state vocational rehabilitation, insurance carriers, foundations and societies, or by other agencies. The person with a disability can perform a variety of jobs, including telephone solicitation, typing, or computer-assisted occupations. Some examples include graphics, accounting, or drafting.

Of these programs—sheltered workshops, day programs, and homebound programs—none emphasizes gainful employment in a nonsheltered integrated setting. It was the failure of these programs to reintegrate their clients into competitive community employment that resulted in the emergence of transitional and supported employment models.

Other Programs for Employment

Projects with Industry

Projects with Industry (PWI) is a federally sponsored collaborative program established by the Vocational Rehabilitation Act. Employers design and provide training projects for specific job skills in cooperation with rehabilitation agencies. The goal of PWI is competitive employment for the participants.

Job fairs have been somewhat successful in matching vacant positions with capable individuals with disabilities. Businesses in a community spend one day interviewing applicants with disabilities who have been prescreened by a participating placement agency. The placement agency might provide further services such as transportation for the potential employee and make recommendations for work accommodations to the potential employer.

Transitional and Supported Employment

Transitional and supported employment are two newer strategies for returning disabled persons to competitive, integrated gainful employment. Transitional employment consists of providing the job placement, training, and support services necessary to help persons move into independent or supported employment.[32] Independent employment provides at least a minimum wage to the employee and requires no job subsidy or ongoing support. Transitional employment is a short-term provision of services for a period not to exceed 18 months, and culminates in an independent or supported employment position.

Supported employment has been utilized as a successful strategy for placing or returning the most severely disabled individuals to competitive, integrated community employment. It requires ongoing support after placement, including counseling for the employee and co-workers, and assistance with transportation, housing, and other non–work-related activities.

It began as an alternative to sheltered workshops or day programs and has grown to have modest federal funding and broad community support. This support comes from groups of persons with disabilities, state vocational rehabilitation agencies, and state departments for the developmentally disabled. This concept became a permanent part of the Rehabilitation Act of 1973 with the passage of the 1986 amendments, and final regulations published in June 1992.[42]

Supported employment is meant to provide ongoing support for persons with severe disabilities. According to Wehman and co-workers,[42] it must meet five critical criteria (Table 35–8). The first is that all interventions, including training, placement, and counseling, be provided at the job site rather than in a therapy room or vocational school. Second, the intervention and services are provided on a permanent or long-term basis as the individual requires them. Third, these programs are intended to serve only those individuals with the most severe disabilities who have been unable to enter the competitive labor market with their disability in the past. Fourth, the work provided is real and meaningful for the employee, and compensation is received equal to that of an able-bodied co-worker for the same duties. Fifth, work must occur in an integrated setting allowing interaction with co-workers without disabilities.[42]

TABLE 35–8 Critical Criteria for Supported Employment

Interventions provided at the job site
Assistance will be long-term or permanent
Programs will serve only severely disabled
Real pay for real work
Work is performed in an integrated setting

From Wehman P, Sherron P, Kregel J, et al: Return to work for persons following severe traumatic brain injury: Supported employment outcomes after five years. Am J Phys Med Rehabil 1993; 72:355–363.

The Department of Education's operational definition of supported employment requires that employees be paid for working an average of at least 20 hours per week in a position that provides interactions with persons who are not disabled and are not paid caregivers. There must be eight or fewer people with disabilities working together at the job site, and there must be ongoing public funding for providing intervention directly related to sustaining employment. Supportive employment defines the type and level of support needed by an individual to be employable now, not after a nonintegrated training program.

Four models of supported employment have been developed. The "enclave" model consists of a small group of persons with disabilities working together at an integrated job site. The "mobile work crew" model uses a small group of workers who travel from job to job and offer contractual services under the direction of a supervisor. The "small business or entrepreneurial" model creates a new small business which produces goods or services using both workers with disabilities and those without them. The most frequently used model is the "job coach with individual placement."[13]

The job coach, or employment specialist, is an employee of the agency providing supported employment services. The coach works with an individual at the job site to provide interpersonal and coping skills as well as job skills. The coach performs job development prior to placement. Once placement occurs, job training and ongoing job retention services are provided. Job coaches might initially be required to complete the duties not yet mastered by the worker with a disability.

Depending on the disability, behavior modification or cognitive training might be required to enable learning of vital skills. These become the responsibility of the job coach. The job coach should be able to evaluate the ecology of the job site, that is, attitudes of co-workers, accessibility of the job site, and the necessity for adaptive equipment. The job coach should then be able to educate co-workers and ensure implementation of appropriate accommodations for the person with a disability.

Job coach intervention time can be very significant (almost 8 hours/day) initially. Wehman and others conducted a 5-year study of supported employment for persons with traumatic brain injury (TBI).[42] They documented an average requirement of 249.1 hours per person of job coach time over 6 months. The job coach's intervention time decreased steadily with time on the job to an average of less than 3 hours per week per person after 30 weeks of employment.

Some persons require continued significant intervention to assist them in meeting difficulties that arise from changes at the job site, that is, new job duties or changes in personnel or goods produced. Some workers are able to depend on support from employers and co-workers, however, and require little or no further direct job coach support. Supportive employment has been highly successful in allowing persons with severe disabilities to participate competitively in the job market and improve their quality of life and economic situation.

Independent Living Centers

The independent living center (ILC) movement has traditionally provided a core of nonvocational services such as housing, independent living skills, advocacy, and peer counseling. Just as supported employment has broadened its scope, so has the ILC movement. Both provide a combination of nonvocational and vocational services to persons with severe disabilities. ILCs often employ workers with disabilities as peer counselors and program administrators. The small business approach of supported employment has been successfully implemented by ILCs to place their clients in competitive community employment. As these two philosophies continue to merge and provide similar services to persons with severe disabilities, cooperative ventures between them will allow persons with severe disabilities to fully achieve their maximum level of independence.

Provision of vocational rehabilitation services to persons with disabilities requires a diversity of strategies. The more severe the disability, the more intensive the support and services have to be. Full participation in society is a right of all people. This participation includes being employed in a meaningful job that both gives satisfaction to the worker and contributes to society as a whole. The methods for returning persons with disabilities to work vary, but creative strategies have proved significantly more successful than noncreative strategies.

DISINCENTIVES FOR VOCATIONAL REHABILITATION

Public and political opinion has changed in recent years regarding the ability of persons with disabilities to work. Both persons with disabilities and policymakers have demonstrated a desire to return persons with disabilities to gainful employment. Statements of past presidents of the United States reflect the change of opinion. In 1973 Richard M. Nixon spoke concerning the Rehabilitation Act of 1973, saying it "would cruelly raise the hopes of the handicapped [for gainful employment] in a way that we could never hope to fulfill."[13] Advocacy by groups for the rights of persons with disabilities has achieved significant policy changes, as reflected by Ronald Reagan's November 1983 proclamation of the "Decade of Disabled Persons" in which the economic independence of all people with disabilities was to become a "clear national goal."[32] With the passage of the Americans with Disabilities Act (ADA) in July 1990, George Bush proclaimed the "end to the unjustified segregation and exclusion of people with disabilities from the mainstream of American life."[13]

Despite the obvious changes in public and political policies and attitudes, disincentives to entering "the mainstream" abound for persons with disabilities. In order to become eligible for cash and medical benefits through SSI and SSDI, persons with disabilities must prove that they have total and permanent or long-term disability and must meet strict eligibility criteria. Prior to meeting those criteria, the individual and the family typically must have suffered a series of indignities including exhausting all personal resources and submitting to significant bureaucratic red tape. "Red tape" means completing substantial paperwork, obtaining medical reports verifying disability, and enduring long waiting periods for commencement of benefits. This is usually a long and arduous process. Once the person with a disability finally achieves a modest degree of security, an "opportunity" to give it all up and enter the work force is made available. Naturally, the person with a disability is suspicious about the assurance that benefits will be preserved and eligibility will not be taken away because of returning to or entering the job market.

Stereotypes about persons with disabilities being unproductive in society are pervasive. Individuals with disabilities often come to view themselves as totally dependent and unable to work. After all, they are placed in a position to prove their dependency and inability to be productive. The government disability entitlement policies state that if you are unable to work, the government will take care of you. In fact, many government policymakers believe that the person with a disability cannot and should not be expected to work. Some even believe that sending a person with a disability a check is much simpler than implementing the provisions of the ADA.

Employers' attitudes serve as another disincentive. Obstacles to qualified applicants with disabilities who want to participate in the work force include employers' ignorance about the capabilities of a potential employee with a disability, inaccessible work sites, transportation inaccessibility, and discrimination in hiring. The ADA will be instrumental in changing much of this behavior, and removing some of these disincentives. As disabled employees take their places, employers and co-workers will become educated, and attitudes will change.

The physiatrist and other physicians can also provide disincentives for persons with disabilities by labeling them as "totally and permanently disabled" or by restricting their activities. Emphasis should be on the capabilities of persons with disabilities and documentation of their functional abilities, both mental and physical.

INCENTIVES FOR VOCATIONAL REHABILITATION

In an effort to overcome disincentives, government policymakers have created incentives for persons with disabilities and for potential employers. These incentives often have a long list of requirements and are very specific in wording in order to prevent abuse.

Incentives for the Individual

Incentive programs are applicable depending on whether the person with a disability receives SSDI or SSI benefits, or both. SSDI work incentives will be discussed first. Table 35–9 presents a summary of the terminology and abbreviations for easy reference. Additional references are given here for those wanting more detailed information.[22, 25, 26, 29, 30, 33, 35]

The initial incentive toward a return to work involves a trial work period (TWP). The TWP lets people test their ability to work or run a business without affecting their benefits. This TWP maintains cash benefits for 9 months (not necessarily consecutive) of trial work in a 60-month period.

Upon completion of the TWP and continued employment at or above the substantial gainful activity (SGA) level, benefits continue to be paid for three more months and are then terminated.[22, 33, 35] Any earnings from work below the monetary limit of the SGA level described in Table 35–9 are excluded when figuring monthly benefit amounts.

The extended period of eligibility (EPE) is a period of 36 consecutive months during which cash benefits can be reinstated if, during that period, the individual's earnings fall below the SGA level. If the individual is unable to maintain earnings at the SGA level, benefits resume automatically, and no waiting periods are required.

Benefits cease at the end of the EPE, but Medicare continues for three additional months.[22, 33, 35] The elimination of a second waiting period for both cash benefits and Medicare benefits is also an incentive to perform a trial of work.

Under certain circumstances, the person might be able to participate in a Medicare "buy-in." The client must have completed both the TWP and the EPE. In addition, the extended three months of Medicare benefits must have passed. Once these conditions are met, Medicare A and B coverage can be purchased. This medical coverage is for those who cannot otherwise obtain health insurance because of pre-existing conditions.[22]

Another major incentive program for those receiving SSDI or SSI is for impairment-related work expenses (IRWE). This allows the cost of certain items and services to be deducted from earnings when determining the SGA level. Examples include attendant care, medical devices, equipment, and prostheses.[22]

For those persons with disabilities receiving SSI benefits, a different, but often similar, set of incentives applies. These incentives provide SSI recipients with assurances that working will not disadvantage them. Section 1619 of the Social Security Act was made permanent by the Employment Opportunities for Disabled Americans Act passed in November 1986. The incentive of Section 1619 allows receipt of SSI cash benefits, even though earned income exceeds the SGA level. Cash benefits are calculated using the earned income exclusion discussed below. Medicaid benefits continue as an additional incentive even after wages become high enough to cause cessation of SSI cash benefits, provided their continuation is needed to allow the recipient to maintain employment.[22, 33, 35]

The earned income exclusion (EIE) allows most of a recipient's earned income to be excluded, including pay received from a sheltered workshop or day activity center, when figuring the SSI monthly amount.[30] "Blind" work expenses (BWE) is an incentive that allows a person who has visual impairment to pay for work expenses, such as visual aids, guide dogs, or Braille translations. These allowable expenses are then excluded when calculating benefit amounts.

In an effort to prevent work disincentives, benefit caps have been implemented to decrease excessively generous benefits. These caps utilize various formulas to reduce or limit maximum benefits paid by Social Security. These formulas take into account other sources of income, such as workers' compensation benefits, but do not exclude veterans' benefits or disability pensions from government jobs.

Another incentive program, Plans for Achieving Self-Support (PASS), allows an SSI recipient to set aside income and resources necessary to achieve a work goal. The plan must be approved by the Social Security Administration.[25, 33, 35]

TABLE 35–9 Summary of Incentives for the Individual Receiving Benefits to Enter Work Activities

Social Security Disability Insurance (SSDI)	Disability benefits program based on medical disability and a worker's earnings covered by Social Security (Title II—Social Security Act)
Supplemental Security Income (SSI)	Disability benefits program based on medical disability and the amount of income a person receives (Title XVI—Social Security Act)
Trial work period (TWP)	Allows trial return to work to test work ability without affecting benefits (SSDI)
Substantial gainful activity (SGA)	Performance of significant and productive physical or mental work for pay or profit (over $500/mo for nonblind [SSDI and SSI] and $810/mo for blind recipients [SSDI only])
Extended period of eligibility (EPE)	Allows reinstatement of cash benefits without a waiting period if the worker's earnings fall below SGA level within 36 mos after TWP (SSDI)
Impairment-related work expenses (IRWE)	Allows costs for certain items to be deducted from earnings when figuring SGA level (SSI and SSDI)
Earned income exclusion (EIE)	Allows exclusion of a portion of earned income when figuring an individual's monthly benefit (SSI)
Blind work expenses (BWE)	Allows work-related expenses when figuring benefits (SSI)

Incentives for Industry

Government policymakers have made various attempts to offer tax incentives to business and industry. In the main, these incentives have been directed at making the workplace accessible. Section 190 of the Internal Revenue Code, enacted in 1976 and revised by the Revenue Reconciliation Act of 1990, allows a set amount per year to be deductible for any expenses incurred in barrier removal (making a business or public transportation accessible).[28]

The Revenue Reconciliation Act of 1990 (which was passed three months after the ADA) allows an "access" tax credit with Section 44 of the Internal Revenue Code for small businesses. It allows credit against income taxes for eligible expenditures (auxiliary services for the disabled employee and aids are covered). This access credit is only allowed for expenses incurred for the purpose of enabling a business to comply with the ADA.[28]

Tax credits have also been used as incentives to encourage hiring of target groups, including the "hard-core" unemployed—persons with disabilities and the homeless. The Targeted Jobs Tax Credit (TJTC), originally enacted in 1978, is meant to encourage employers to hire members of these groups. It provides a tax credit for targeted persons, including those persons receiving SSI benefits and vocational rehabilitation referrals (both groups containing large numbers of persons with disabilities). This credit only provides benefits to an employer for one year per employee. Many employers use the credit as a windfall, that is, hiring anyone they want and later checking to see if the new employee falls into a targeted group. This practice is called "retroactive certification."[28]

The TJTC has, unfortunately, not been particularly useful in increasing the number of disabled people hired. In fact, legislative incentives in general have not been very successful in achieving the goal of vocationally rehabilitating persons with disabilities. There are ongoing efforts in the U.S. Congress, however, to improve the incentives for persons with disabilities to return to work. For example, The Work Incentives Improvement Act of 1999 (S.331) provides adequate and affordable health insurance when a person on SSI or SSDI goes to work by expanding Medicaid options for states and by continuing access to Medicare after returning to work. It encourages SSDI beneficiaries to return to work by assuring that cash benefits remain available if employment proves unsuccessful. An expedited eligibility process is proposed for SSDI beneficiaries who lose benefits due to work and need reinstatement of benefits later. A "ticket" program would provide a new payment system for SSDI and SSI beneficiaries for employment services. It reimburses vocational rehabilitation, training, and employment service providers a portion of benefit payments saved when the beneficiary earns more than the SGA level, currently $500 per month ($1000 for blind beneficiaries).[15]

Approximately 80% of SSI recipients work prior to applying for SSI, and 20% work after they start receiving payments.[29] Scott Muller of the Social Security Administration performed a retrospective analysis of a cohort of over 4000 people who were initially entitled to benefits.[22] Approximately 10% worked during the initial period of entitlement. Of those, 84% were granted a TWP, and of that group, over 70% completed the TWP. More than 50% did not leave the rolls as a result of their efforts. Less than 3% had benefits terminated as a result of return to work.[22]

It is clear from the research conducted by the Social Security Administration that legislating incentives is not the complete answer to rehabilitating persons with work disability. Potential employers and persons with disabilities alike must take the initiative.

DISABILITY PREVENTION

With disability ranking as the nation's largest public health problem, it seems reasonable to interface the public health model of prevention with the ICIDH-2 model of disablement. The public health model defines three categories of prevention: primary, secondary, and tertiary.

Primary prevention is intended for healthy persons, helping them to avoid the onset of a pathological condition. In persons with disabilities, primary prevention comprises efforts toward preventing a worsening of impairments.

Secondary prevention is aimed at early identification and treatment of a pathological condition and reduction of risk factors for disablement. For persons with disabilities, there are many opportunities for preventing an impairment from limiting one or more activities. The ameliorative and corrective programs discussed above, including vocational rehabilitation strategies, are aimed at reducing activity limitation. Interventions in medical rehabilitation focused on the enhancement of activity, such as provision of assistive technology, can be considered secondary prevention.

Tertiary prevention focuses on arresting the progression of a pathological condition and on limiting further disablement. For people with disabilities, tertiary prevention is designed to limit the restriction of a person's participation in some area by the provision of a facilitator or the removal of a barrier.[45] Environmental modifications, provision of services, removal of physical barriers, changes in social attitudes, or reform in legislation and policy are tertiary prevention strategies. Medical rehabilitation is traditionally considered a tertiary prevention strategy. The public disability policies, such as the Americans with Disabilities Act, are also efforts to reduce environmental and social barriers to participation.[24, 39, 45]

Considering functioning and disablement as outcomes of interactions between health conditions (disorders/diseases) and conceptual factors (social/environmental/personal), there are many opportunities for the physiatrist and the medical rehabilitation team to intervene. Rehabilitation interventions aimed at prevention of activity limitation or prevention of participation restriction are secondary and tertiary prevention strategies that push the dynamic model of disablement in the direction of function. The physiatrist has a responsibility to be actively involved in therapeutic and public health management of disablement.[14]

CONCLUSION

Comprehensive rehabilitation is an intervention directed at human functioning. The desired outcome is to maximize the physical, mental, social, and economic function of the individual with disabilities. The physiatrist as team leader has the responsibility of encouraging the team to take a holistic approach to the person with disabilities. The holistic approach includes collaboration with professionals outside of the traditional medical rehabilitation team, such as those who can facilitate vocational rehabilitation for persons with disabilities.

Vocational rehabilitation is an intervention aimed at preventing an impairment from limiting activities and limiting participation in work. Limitation in work participation has significant socioeconomic consequences for the individual and for society. Employment of persons with disabilities supports a better quality of life and promotes function. Even for people with severe disabilities, vocational rehabilitation strategies have been successful in facilitation of work participation.

Disability is the largest public health problem in the United States. The demands of this public health issue have captured the attention of public policymakers. This has resulted in implementation of significant federal disability laws. The nation's public policies on disability reflect the policymakers' acceptance of disability as a complex process. Disablement is considered to be the result of a dynamic, complex, and bidirectional interaction between health conditions and conceptual factors for each individual.

The physiatrist is positioned to serve a primary role in the functioning and disablement paradigm. As persons with disabilities become a greater segment of our society, the opportunities for physiatrists' involvement are expanded. It is the physiatrists' responsibility to be active in disability prevention, in care and advocacy for persons with disabilities, and in the development of public policy on disablement.

REFERENCES

1. Adams PF, Benson V: Current estimates for the national health interview survey. Vital Health Stat [10] 1989.
2. Anderson TP: Quality of life of the individual with a disability. Arch Phys Med Rehabil 1982; 63:55.
3. Berkowitz M: The socioeconomic consequences of SCI. Paraplegic News 1994; January, pp 18–23.
4. Berkowitz M, Hill MA: Disability and the labor market: An overview. In Berkowitz M, Hill MA (eds): Disability and the Labor Market: Economic Problems, Policies, and Programs. New York, ILR Press, 1989, pp 1–28.
5. Colvez A, Blanchet M: Disability trends in the United States population 1966–76: Analysis of reported causes. Am J Public Health 1981; 71:464–471.
6. DeJong G, Lifchez R: Physical disability and public policy. Sci Am 1983; 248:40–50.
7. Funk R: Disability rights: From caste to class in the context of civil rights. In Gartner A, Joe T (eds): Images of the Disabled, Disabling Images. Westport, CT, Praeger, 1987, pp 7–30.
8. Haber LD: Identifying the disabled: Concepts and methods in the measurement of disability. Soc Secur Bull 1988; 51:11–28.
9. Haber LD: Issues in the definition of disability and the use of disability survey data. In Daniel LB, Aitter M, Ingram L (eds): Disability Statistics, An Assessment: Report of a Workshop. Washington, DC, National Academy Press, 1990, pp 1–71.
10. Harris L: The ICD Survey of Disabled Americans: Bringing Disabled Americans into the Mainstream. New York, Louis Harris and Associates, 1986.
11. Harvey C: The business of employment: employment after traumatic SCI. Paraplegic News 1993; October, pp 10–14.
12. Haveman RH, Halberstandt V, Burkhauser RV (eds): Public Policy Toward Disabled Workers: Cross-National Analyses of Economic Impacts. New York, Cornell University Press, 1984.
13. Hearne PG: Employment strategies for people with disabilities: A prescription for change. Milbank Q 1991; 69:111–128.
14. Joe TC: Professionalism: A new challenge for rehabilitation. Arch Phys Med Rehabil 1981; 62:245–250.
15. Kennedy EM, et al: The Work Incentives Improvement Act of 1999, Senate Bill 331, February, 1999.
16. Kraus LE, Stoddard S, and Gilmartin D: Chartbook on Disability in the United States, 1996; US Department of Education, National Institute on Disability and Rehabilitation Research, Washington, DC.
17. Kottke FJ: Philosophic considerations of quality of life for the disabled. Arch Phys Med Rehabil 1982; 63:60–63.
18. La Plante MP: The demographics of disability. Milbank Q 1991; 69:55–77.
19. La Plante MP, Kennedy J, Kaye S, et al: Disability and Employment, no 11. Disability Statistics Abstract Series 1997; Disability Statistics Rehabilitation Research and Training Center, Institute for Health & Aging, University of California, San Francisco.
20. McNeil JM: Current Population Reports, Household Economic Studies, Series P70-61, US Department of Commerce, Bureau of the Census, Washington, DC, 1994–95.
21. Menchetti BM, Flynn CC: Vocational evaluation. In Rusch FR (ed): Supported Employment. Sycamore, IL, Sycamore, 1990, pp 111–131.
22. Muller LS: Disability beneficiaries who work and their experience under program work incentives. Soc Secur Bull 1992; 55:2–19.
23. Nagi SZ: Disability concepts revisited: implication to prevention, appendix A. In Pope AM, Tarlov AR (eds): Disability in America: Toward a National Agenda for Prevention. Washington, DC, National Academy Press, 1991, pp 306–327.
24. Pope AM, Tarlov AR (eds): Disability in America: Toward a National Agenda for Prevention. Washington, DC, National Academy Press, 1991.
25. Rigby DE: SSI work incentive participants. Soc Secur Bull 1991; 54:22–29.
26. Rocklin SG, Mattson DR: The employment opportunities for disabled Americans act: legislative history and summary of provisions. Soc Secur Bull 1987; 50:25–35.
27. Rusk HA: The growth and development of rehabilitation medicine. Arch Phys Med Rehabil 1969; 50:463–466.
28. Schaffer DC: Tax incentives. Milbank Q 1991; 69:293–312.
29. Scott CG: Disabled SSI recipients who work. Soc Secur Bull 1992; 55:26–36.
30. Social Security Administration: Report of Disability Advisory Council: Executive Summary. Soc Secur Bull, 1988; 51:13–17.
31. Symington DC: The goals of rehabilitation. Arch Phys Med Rehabil 1984; 65:427–430.
32. Thornton C, Maynard R: The economics of transitional employment and supported employment. In Berkowitz M, Hill MA (eds): Disability and the Labor Market: Economic Problems, Policies, and Programs. New York, ILR Press, 1989, pp 142–170.
33. US Department of Health and Human Service. Social Security Administration: Social Security Handbook, ed 13. Washington, DC, Government Printing Office, 1997.
34. US Bureau of the Census: Disability, Functional Limitation, and Health Insurance Coverage: 1984–85. Current Population Reports, series P70, no. 8. Washington, DC, Government Printing Office, 1986.
35. US Department of Health and Human Service. Social Security Administration: Redbook on Work Incentives. Washington, DC, Government Printing Office, 1992.

36. US Equal Employment Opportunity Commission, US Department of Justice: Americans with Disabilities Act Handbook (EEOC-BK-19). Washington, DC, Government Printing Office, 1991.
37. US General Accounting Office: Testimony Before the Subcommittee on Select Education, Committee on Education and Labor, House of Representatives. Vocational Rehabilitation Program: Client Characteristics, Services Received, and Employment Outcomes. Washington, DC, Government Printing Office, November 1991.
38. Vachon RA: Inventing a future for individuals with work disabilities: The challenge of writing national disability policies. In Woods DE, Vandergoot D (eds): The Changing Nature of Work, Society and Disability: The Impact on Rehabilitation Policy. New York, World Rehabilitation Fund, 1987, pp 19–45.
39. Vachon RA: Employment assistance and vocational rehabilitation for people with HIV or AIDS: policy, practice, and prospects. In O'Dell MW (ed): HIV-Related Disability: Assessment and Management. Physical Medicine and Rehabilitation: State of the Art Reviews. Philadelphia, Hanley & Belfus, 1993, pp s203–s224.
40. Vachon RA: Employing the disabled. Issues Sci Technol 1989–90; winter: 44–50.
41. Verville R: The rehabilitation amendments of 1978: What do they mean for comprehensive rehabilitation? Arch Phys Med Rehabil 1979; 60:141–144.
42. Wehman P, Sherron P, Kregel J, et al: Return to work for persons following severe traumatic brain injury: Supported employment outcomes after five years. Am J Phys Med Rehabil 1993; 72:355–363.
43. Wilson RW: Do health indicators indicate health? Am J Public Health 1981; 71:461–463.
44. World Health Organization: International Classification of Impairments, Disabilities and Handicaps: A Manual of Classification Relating to the Consequences of Disease. Geneva, World Health Organization, 1980.
45. World Health Organization: Towards a Common Language for Functioning and Disablement: ICIDH-2, The International Classification of Impairments, Activities, and Participation. Geneva, World Health Organization, 1998.

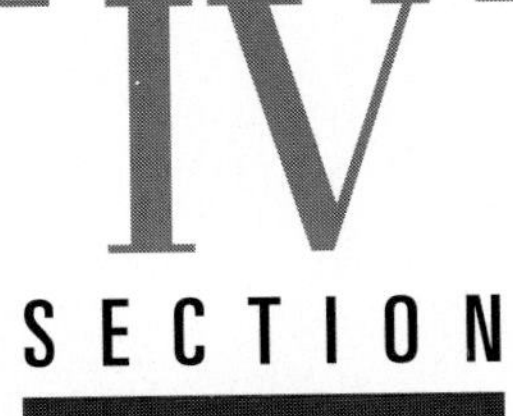

SECTION

ISSUES IN SPECIFIC DIAGNOSES IN PHYSICAL MEDICINE AND REHABILITATION

36 CHAPTER

John J. Nicholas, M.D.

Rehabilitation of Patients with Rheumatological Disorders

The rehabilitation of patients with rheumatic diseases has changed dramatically over the last few decades. These changes have been due to new medical and surgical treatments and to economic developments that affect the provision of rehabilitation care to rheumatic disease patients.

From about 1940 to the 1970s, a classic protocol of medical, surgical, and rehabilitation care was developed to treat arthritic patients.[11, 41, 56, 103, 105, 136, 137, 148, 179, 206, 240] This treatment program provided comprehensive care in medical centers and rehabilitation hospitals, and some outpatient facilities, utilizing an almost unlimited length of stay. The treatment included the careful prescription of rest, both at home and in hospitals, various forms of exercise, the applications of casts and splints, instruction in work simplification and energy conservation, prescription of heat and cold, and many medical treatments. Improvement was noted in most cases. It was demonstrated that bedrest and casts for as long as fourteen days did not permanently diminish the active range of motion of joints of patients with rheumatoid arthritis (RA).[192] It was further demonstrated that those patients with RA who had the most severely involved joints, benefited most from inpatient treatment and rest.[6] Generally, inpatient care was shown to be more effective than outpatient care in providing these treatments.[132]

Various physical modalities were widely used. Studies documented patients' appreciation and acceptance, but few studies demonstrated improvement in the patient's disease or function following the application of modalities.[169]

Beginning in the 1950s, the use of adrenocorticosteroids (ACS) provided great relief from joint pain for patients with RA, but ACS were subsequently shown to frequently lead to myopathy, cataracts, gastrointestinal bleeding, osteoporosis, compression fractures, and other complications. Patients suffering from these complications were often hospitalized in rehabilitation centers so that other treatment modalities could be substituted for the discontinuation of the steroids. Nowadays, ACS are rarely given in large enough doses, or long enough, to cause these complications. Thus, such patients are no longer admitted to rehabilitation centers. In addition, intramuscular gold, hydroxychloroquine, azathioprine, and, most recently, methotrexate have provided better suppression of joint inflammation than was previously possible. Currently, patients with RA and other inflammatory joint diseases seem, on balance, to be doing better, with less destructive inflammation, and hence less need to be hospitalized in an inpatient rehabilitation hospital or unit.[23]

Joint replacement (arthroplasty) has provided physiatrists a whole new range of therapeutic challenges, and patients with remarkable relief from pain and functional deficits. Many patients, however, require rehabilitation care to maximize the gains from their surgical procedure. Those without complications frequently leave the hospital within their diagnostic-related group (DRG)–designated length of stay, but those with severe RA or osteoarthritis in nonoperated joints, or with comorbidity (strokes, amputations, congestive heart failure, persistent pain, bilateral arthroplasties, lack of knee flexion, bone grafts, arthroplasty revision) require hospitalization on rehabilitation units (Table 36–1). Rehabilitation of these postoperative orthopedic patients has become quite frequent, and the postarthroplasty patient

TABLE 36–1 Causes for Comprehensive Rehabilitation Following Arthroplasty Procedures

Complex medical problems
Multiple joint involvement
Severe contralateral joint disease
Stroke
Amputation
Congestive heart failure
Persistent pain
Bilateral arthroplasties
Arthroplasty revision
Bone grafting
Cementless prostheses
Lack of knee flexion
Slow progress
Concurrent hemodialysis
Fractures
Infections

These are some of the conditions or medical problems that suggest a need to hospitalize post-arthroplasty patients in a comprehensive rehabilitation unit or center.

TABLE 36–2 Typical Reasons for Physiatric Consultation for Acutely Hospitalized Rheumatic Patients

1. Heel lift for leg-length discrepancy secondary to severe ankle degeneration
2. Flexion contracture treatment suggestions
3. Footwear and appropriate modifications for metatarsalgia
4. Management of neurogenic bladder secondary to lupus vasculitis, spinal cord involvement
5. Pressure gradient stockings for
   a. lower extremity edema and ulcers
   b. postphlebitic syndrome
6. Ankle-foot orthoses for neuropathy
7. Upper extremity splinting
8. Spinal jacket for vertebral compression fractures
9. Pressure sore treatment suggestions
11. Aerobic training recommendations for polymyositis patients
12. Cervical collar prescriptions for severe rheumatoid arthritis

now is more common in many rehabilitation care settings than the patient with a stroke.[186]

Since the advent of the DRG-based hospital reimbursement for Medicare patients, the acute hospital length of stay has become shorter, and admissions for treatment of rheumatic diseases less frequent. The Health Care Financing Administration (HCFA), however, will fund formal rehabilitation care for rheumatological patients provided they meet the criteria for admission to a DRG-exempt rehabilitation unit.

Surveys have demonstrated that rheumatologists receive relatively little education in rehabilitation techniques during their training,[101] and, conversely, physiatrists have little exposure to education in the treatment and diagnosis of rheumatic disease patients in their residency programs.[102] Further education will be necessary. Cooperative treatment seems optimal.

In the past, a classic analogy for the description of the application of treatments to rheumatic disease patients was the therapeutic pyramid.[116, 149] This analogy placed surgical treatments at the apex of the pyramid, and rehabilitation treatments at the base or at the initial onset of the disease. A more recent analogy suggests that various treatments should be added as the severity of the disease increases. The model places the patient in the center and various treatments around the periphery.[196] Again, it is recommended that rehabilitation treatments should be applied early, at the onset of the various rheumatic diseases.

Where should treatments be performed? Certainly at the present time, inpatient rehabilitation units and centers have been shown to provide exemplary care.[46] In addition, Finestone has demonstrated many opportunities for the physiatrist to provide consultation and patient services to patients hospitalized in an "acute" general hospital or on a rheumatology service (Table 36–2).[69] Alternative treatment sites include comprehensive outpatient rehabilitation facilities (CORFs), outpatient units, subacute rehabilitation units, skilled nursing facilities (SNFs), nursing homes, and home health services. Many of these provide care in a less costly setting. The physiatrist must become involved in the provision of rehabilitation services to rheumatic disease patients in these settings, and he should participate in the decision of the appropriate site of treatment. Some of the reasons to admit rheumatic disease patients to a rehabilitation unit include a marked decline in activities of daily living, inability to get around due to steroid myopathy, the development of quadriparesis (atlantoaxial subluxation), mononeuritis multiplex (vasculitis), severe anemia, out-of-control inflammation, and amputations (Table 36–3).

In addition, there are circumstances under which a rheumatologist should be involved in the daily care of these patients. The rheumatologist is needed to manage medications in difficult situations, initiate disease-modifying antirheumatic drugs, and help with the diagnostic dilemmas of anemia, mononeuritis multiplex, renal disease, unexplained weakness, and on occasion to solve a diagnostic dilemma (Table 36–4).

The physiatrist must determine when to hospitalize postoperative orthopedic patients in the rehabilitation unit or center. It is generally acknowledged that the patients with best results go home directly from the rehabilitation unit or center, but many others require an additional step of admission to nursing homes or "subacute units." These patients should be hospitalized for the comprehensive intensive rehabilitation services

TABLE 36–3 Typical Reasons for Hospitalization of Rheumatic Disease Patients on a Comprehensive Rehabilitation Unit

Decline in ADL
Steroid myopathy
Quadriparesis
Vasculitis
Severe anemia
Uncontrolled inflammation
Amputations

TABLE 36–4 Typical Reasons for Concurrent Care by a Rheumatologist

Medication management
Initiate DMARDs (disease modifying antirheumatic drugs)
Diagnostic Treatment Problems:
Anemia
Vasculitis
Peripheral neuropathy
Unexplained weakness
GI bleeding, renal disease
Determination of the specific type of arthritis

Almost any rheumatic disease patient who experiences a severe decrease in function will require consultation from a rheumatologist upon admission to a comprehensive rehabilitation unit or freestanding center.

provided in a rehabilitation unit or center under such circumstances as listed in Table 36–1. To date, no data demonstrate a better result following hospitalization on an inpatient unit rather than in a skilled nursing home or "subacute" rehabilitation unit; however, the physician must be an advocate, insisting on admission to a rehabilitation unit or center when it is clinically clear that such an admission is likely to provide a quicker and/or better outcome.

The effectiveness of the comprehensive rehabilitation team has been demonstrated, but it must be a genuine therapeutic team.[46] A team is not just a group of skilled persons playing the same game. There must be a coach, a captain, position players, and a clearly defined game plan. These interdisciplinary teams have traditionally been available only in inpatient settings; but they can be developed for day hospital, outpatient, or home care as well, provided there is proper leadership.

This chapter describes the modern rehabilitation techniques that are appropriate for patients with rheumatic diseases. The reader is referred to current rheumatology textbooks for detailed information about specific rheumatic diseases and the latest diagnostic techniques. The rheumatic diseases that are most appropriately treated by rehabilitation techniques include rheumatoid arthritis (RA), osteoarthritis (OA), ankylosing spondylitis (AS) and the other spondyloarthropathies, systemic lupus erythematosus (SLE), progressive systemic sclerosis (PSS), polymyositis/dermatomyositis (DM/PMD), and postoperative arthroplasty patients.

EVALUATION OF PATIENTS

Specific Historical Details

The rheumatic disease patient requires attention to details of the history and physical examination that are specific to the rheumatic diseases.[158, 197] Before prescribing a comprehensive rehabilitation program, the physiatrist must obtain specific information regarding rheumatological patients.

Functional screen: Can the patient perform such ADL tasks as dressing, bathing, feeding, toileting hygiene and transfers, and walking (see Chapter 1)?

Vocational screen: Can the patient get into and out of a car and get into and out of a parking place? Are ergonomic changes required at work, or is a different job necessary?

Physical Examination Techniques

Range-of-Motion Testing. In patients with rheumatic disease the range of motion (ROM) is frequently limited in one or more joints. At times, the joint surfaces and supporting structures are damaged so badly that the joint will not perform a normal arc of motion. The examiner should estimate and record the active and passive range of motion of involved joints and determine whether subluxation or dislocation is present. The examiner also records if pain limits motion or if there is a pain-free limit to the motion. Each joint having limited motion should be compared with its plain radiographs and to the joints on the opposite side. The degree of inflammation should be recorded for each joint that is abnormal. It should also be noted if a joint is swollen, deformed, hot, or unstable.

Manual Muscle Testing. The manual muscle test cannot be performed accurately at a joint in which muscle contraction causes pain. The examiner should record whether or not pain is present during muscle contraction and should estimate strength (see Chapter 1). The examiner should also take into account strength training, conditioning, sex, age, diagnosis, and degree of patient *effort* when assessing strength. Muscle weakness should be noted together with a characterization of its distribution as proximal, distal, lateral, or generalized pattern. The examiner should also take note of any muscle-affecting medications (ACS, lovastatin, hydroxychloroquine, etc.) that have been administered.

THERAPEUTIC MODALITIES

Heat and Cold

For thousands of years, various methods of applying superficial heat have been used to treat rheumatic disease (see Chapter 21). All over the Old and New Worlds, there are hot springs (e.g., the pool at Bath in England and the hot springs in Arkansas) that patients have visited in the hope of relieving various ailments, including arthritis. In modern times, Elkayam[61] described patients with both RA and OA who were treated in a controlled study with mineral baths and mud packs. No statistical evaluations were performed, but grip strength increased in treated subjects. Sukenik and co-workers[221] and Helliwell[98] also provided a review of spa therapy. When Verhagen et al[230] reviewed all available literature describing the effects of spa therapy in arthritis, they concluded that efficacy was not substantiated by careful scientific data.

Superficial heat is more commonly used than deep heat for treating rheumatic conditions. It has also been considered more beneficial and appropriate than deep heat.[67] This belief is due in part to reported patient discomfort from deep heat, and to Harris's study, which demonstrated that heating to therapeutic levels increased the activity of synovial collagenase obtained from a rheumatoid joint.[94]

When moist superficial hot packs are applied over arthritic joints, the joint temperature falls by as much as 2.2°F.[106] Furthermore, the use of microwave diathermy (12.2 Hz) increases the temperature at the skin surface and within the knee joint as much as 5°F.[104] Spiegal demonstrated that heating RA patients' knee joints with diathermy at 13.56 Hz for as long as 60 minutes did not increase pain.[216] Falconer showed that ultrasound treatment of OA knee joints did not appear to cause any improvement.[66] In a series of studies, Weinberger and associates[234, 235, 236] have shown, both in experimental animals and in humans, that diathermy at 9.15 Hz for 1 hour decreased chronic knee effusions of RA patients. They demonstrated in rabbits that zymosan synovitis was improved by this treatment. While these findings need to be confirmed, this "thermal synovectomy" seems to hold promise. Additional data on the use of superficial versus deep heat in rheumatic disease patients are both incomplete and inconclusive.[92] There was no improvement with ultrasound or shortwave diathermy in osteoarthritic patients' knees in a study using functional capacity score and Cybex testing as end points.[110] A classic 1949 study by Frankel showed that prolonged rest (4 weeks) and application of electric heating blankets below the waist was followed by a fall in sedimentation rate, diminution in soft tissue swelling, and improvement in ROM.[78] Mainardi demonstrated that heating the hands of patients with RA in an electric mitten raised the intra-articular temperature, and did not cause radiographic evidence of progression or destruction of the joints.[143]

Pegg et al[194] and Kirk et al[123] described the application of ice packs to patients with RA. Many patients preferred cold to heat. Some patients thought cold was followed by better ROM than hot packs. Trial and patient preference should direct the prescription of heat or cold for rheumatic disease.

It is apparent from clinical observation of patients with various types of inflammatory arthritis that the application of moist heat packs, moist heating pads, hot showers, paraffin baths, and the like produces at least temporary diminution in pain and increased ability to move and exercise inflamed joints. There is no scientific evidence to demonstrate that heat improves or increases joint erosions. Therefore, superficial heat should be applied before exercising. The dose is determined by cost, custom, and convenience rather than by scientific data. For example, moist heating packs should be applied as early in the day as possible, to help relieve morning stiffness, and then repeated once or twice during the day.

Other Modalities for Patients with Rheumatic Disorders

Various other modalities have been tried in the treatment of patients with rheumatic disease, and some scientific evidence supports their efficacy. Culic[50] treated RA patients with nylon spandex compression gloves. Patients reported feeling better after wearing these gloves, but there was little measurable change except for reduced finger circumference. These compression gloves are particularly helpful if finger stiffness is excessive.

Topical counterirritant ointments have been reported by White and Sage[237, 238] to provide relief, as judged by patients. In addition, McCarthy and McCarty[150] and Schnitzer[209] found that topical capsaicin reduced OA finger pain as determined by a dolorimeter and subjective scales. It was not possible to demonstrate improvement in RA patients with capsaicin. Rothacker et al[207] found that topical trolamine salicylate diminished OA hand pain and stiffness to a greater degree than placebo.

The use of transcutaneous electronic nerve stimulation (TENS) has been reported for many conditions (see Chapter 22). Improved wrist and hand function with TENS was reported for RA patients by Mannheimer[145, 146] and confirmed by Kumer and Redford.[129] Application of TENS to hands and wrists is awkward, however, limiting its use.

TENS has also been applied for OA of the knees.[135, 224] The results were not very dramatic, but selected patients reported considerable pain relief. A 1994 publication reviewed the use of TENS and acupuncture for rheumatic diseases, and in general found the results of treatment not very remarkable.[169]

The wide use of "complementary" or "alternative" forms of treatment by arthritic patients has been known for years. Boisset and Fitzcharles[26] have provided a review of a French clinic experience and the literature.

Relief of Joint Contractures

Patients with various forms of inflammatory rheumatic diseases or OA can lose full ROM. Historically, such joint contractures have been a great problem, but in contemporary medicine are now commonly relieved by surgical arthroplasty. The causes and treatments of these contractures were recently reviewed.[195, 172] Adhesions across the joint surfaces have not been shown to be the cause. Studies (beginning with that of Ely and Mensor in 1933) in both animals and patients have shown that surgical muscle release relieves contractures in the early stages.[62] After about two weeks, however, capsular and pericapsular structures must be released to regain motion. The changes in these capsular and pericapsular structures include a loss of water and glycosaminoglycans (4% to 6% loss of water and 30% to 40% glycosaminoglycans). There was no increase in total collagen, but there was an alteration in cross-linkages and the organization of the collagen fibers, which was thought to affect the ability to glide under tension. There was an ingrowth of fibrofatty connective tissue into the joint space and degenerative changes in the collagen.[3, 4, 5, 7, 8, 29, 63, 65, 68, 91]

Many authors have reported successful treatment of contractures, usually at the knee, with casts and splints. Modalities include wedge casting[19]; casts plus traction[57, 58]; serial casting, traction, weights and exercise, and manipulation under anesthesia[199]; splints for knees and wrists[222]; casts, exercise, and traction[115]; plaster casts and splints[44]; plaster splints with cuff[90]; and plaster casts, posterior splints, and a unique knee-straightening device.[96] In addition, casts have been used in an unsuccessful attempt to correct deformities of PSS.[213] Casts have been used to correct burn scar contractures[203] and elbow fractures or contractures.[214, 244] Relief of contractures through use of a constant passive motion machine (CPM) has been described anecdotally. Keenan has described the surgical release of contractures due to spasticity.[118, 119]

When joint contractures secondary to rheumatic disorders are treated with serial casting or splinting, the results are directly related to the severity of the joint destruction as demonstrated by radiographs (the better the x-ray appearance, the better the result) (Table 36–5). Treatment can be provided with various materials (e.g., plaster, fiberglass, plastic). Full cylinder casts, posterior splints, and splints with cuffs have all been used successfully when applied in a position of maximum extension without excessive force and removed for hygiene every day. At the end of 5 to 7 days, the casts or splints are replaced and more extension is noted. The last 10 degrees of extension is typically the most difficult to achieve. The total ROM usually does not change, but the ROM shifts toward the extension limits rather than the flexion limits of joint motion.[178]

APPROACHES TO SPECIFIC RHEUMATIC DISEASES

Rheumatoid Arthritis

Sir William Osler (1849–1919) considered syphilis the prototypical disease to study: "I often tell my students that [syphilis] is the only disease which they require to study thoroughly. Know syphilis in all its manifestations and relations, and all other things clinical will be added unto you."[187] Rheumatoid arthritis occupies a similar position in modern medicine. If physiatrists can apply rehabilitation techniques to patients with RA, they should be able to treat the manifestations of any of the other rheumatic diseases.

Pain Relief

The time-honored treatment of joint pain in RA has been application of moist heat. This has been accomplished through various devices, including moist heating packs, electric mittens, hot showers, hot water, and spas. It has been demonstrated in normal subjects that hot packs provide heat (lasting for about 15 minutes), to a depth of 1 to 1.5 cm.[134] The frequency of application is guided by cost, custom, and convenience, but should be at least twice daily. Because burns can occur with moist heat, the patient must be tested for sensory deficits before moist heat is used. Additional contraindications to heat are listed in Chapter 21.

TABLE 36–5 Technique for Cast Correction of Joint Flexion Contractures

Assess radiological status
Cast in maximum voluntary extension
Remove cast for daily hygiene
Recast weekly
Last 10 degrees will be the most difficult to get
ROM migrates but does not increase

The use of microwave has been thought to increase synovial collagenase activity,[94] possibly causing joint destruction, and to be ill-tolerated by patients.[67] However, Weinberger has advocated "thermal synovectomy" through diathermy treatment—a modality that needs further study.[234, 235, 236]

It is appropriate to treat joints with moist heat in preparation for ROM, stretching, and most muscle-strengthening exercises. Heat is usually a pain reliever; it also reduces stiffness and serves as a preparation to an exercise program. The most painful joints should be treated first. At least part of the treatment time in physical or occupational therapy should be used to make certain the patient knows how to use the modality at home. Moist heat treatments are no more temporary than nonsteroidal anti-inflammatory drugs (NSAIDs); they are, however, more inconvenient.

The application of splints, mostly for wrists and knees, has been shown to relieve pain in inflamed RA joints.[120, 121, 178] Gault demonstrated that splints universally diminished the signs of inflammation in RA-involved hands as compared to the opposite nonsplinted hand.[82] The chief drawbacks that decrease the use of splints for pain relief are poor cosmesis and inconvenience. Patients often choose to wear them despite these drawbacks. They are particularly helpful during heavy-use activities.[175, 176]

Prevention and Correction of Deformities

Most deformities in RA are predictable (Table 36–6).[218] For example, knee deformities occur in a position of flexion and shoulders in adduction. Hand deformities (e.g., swan's neck or boutonnière) are much less predictable.

Routine examination demonstrates whether or not there is loss of such joint motion as abduction at the shoulder, extension at the hip, knee, or wrist, or flexion of the fingers. Once a deformity has been detected, patient, physician, and therapist must enter into a cooperative venture in order to eliminate it, or at least prevent it from getting worse. This requires persistent, tedious compliance on the part of the patient. Initially, the application of moist heat to the joints followed by ROM active stretching exercises helps reduce the contracture if the inflammation is relieved or is not too severe. In more severe cases, protective splints should be applied. Joint mobilization, as described by Maigne—gentle manipulation of joints past the range normally reached by active ROM exercises—probably will not benefit patients with RA.[142] Spinal and other joint manipulation (see Chapter 20) has not been shown to prevent or correct these deformities.

Knees and wrist splints are most easily fitted. Gerber[84] described a hindfoot orthosis for preventing further progression of pronation and valgus deformity of the foot and ankle. Several varieties of resting wrist and hand splints are available (Fig. 36–1). Molded shoe insoles of materials such as plastizote can be used in combination with "extra-depth" shoes to provide support and spread of pressure. This can relieve pain, extend walking range, and slow progression of such deformities as pro-

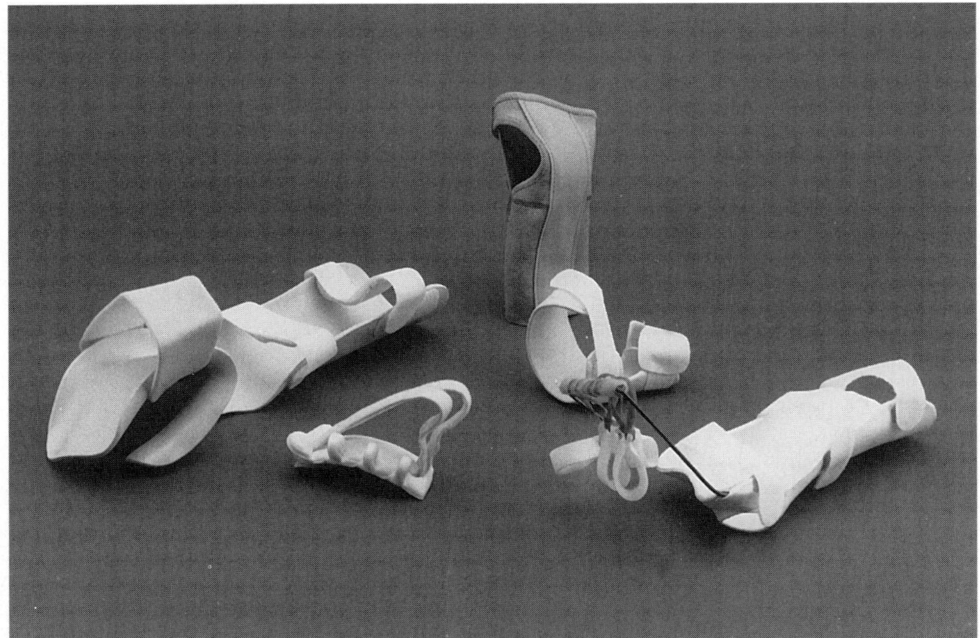

FIGURE 36–1. Molded wrist and hand splints can provide pain relief and support for painful, inflamed wrists.

TABLE 36–6 Predictions of Deformities* in Rheumatoid Arthritis

Joint	Deformity	Position of Splinting
Head and neck	Flexion, rotation	Full extension, cervical spine, chin forward
Dorsal spine	Flexion, chest flat	Full extension
Shoulder	Adduction, internal rotation	90 degrees abduction, neutral rotation
Elbow	Flexion, pronation	90 degrees flexion, 10 degrees supination
Wrist	Palmar flexion	30 degrees dorsiflexion
Thumb	Flexion	Extension, apposition
Finger	Flexion, ulnar deviation	Extension, no lateral deviation
Hips	Flexion, adduction, external rotation	Extension; in line with body; foot pointing upward
Knee	Flexion	Extension
Ankle	Plantar flexion	Right angle to leg
Foot	Valgus, spread of forefoot	No varus or valgus, upward pressure beneath second, third, and fourth metatarsal bones
Toe	Plantar flexion in phalangeal joints, flexion at metatarsophalangeal joints	In line with plantar surface of foot

* The deformities consequent to chronic rheumatoid arthritis have not changed since Dr. Steinbrocker first recorded them, and are thus quite predictable.

From Steinbrocker O: Arthritis in Modern Practice. Philadelphia, WB Saunders, 1947.

truding metatarsal heads. These shoes are somewhat unattractive and costly and often have to be refitted every few years, but they can be very effective (Fig. 36–2).

The "joint preservation" and "work simplification" techniques promulgated by Cordery and colleagues are thought also to help prevent deformities.[45] Many devices are available (Fig. 36–3). The concept is that if the patient does not overstress or overuse a joint and avoids biomechanical torques that excessively bend the wrist and fingers, these deformities can be prevented or limited.[154] Certainly, there are no serious side effects to these energy-saving techniques, which probably would benefit even able-bodied persons.

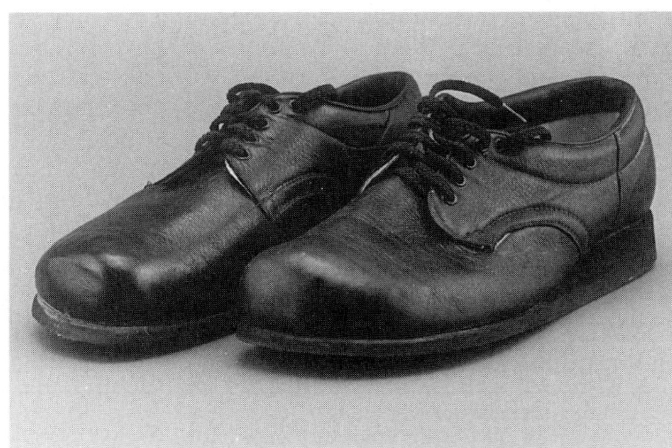

FIGURE 36–2. Extra depth shoes: These shoes provide space to accommodate cock-up toes or hallux valgus deformities and protruding metatarsal heads. They also allow room for custom-molded inserts.

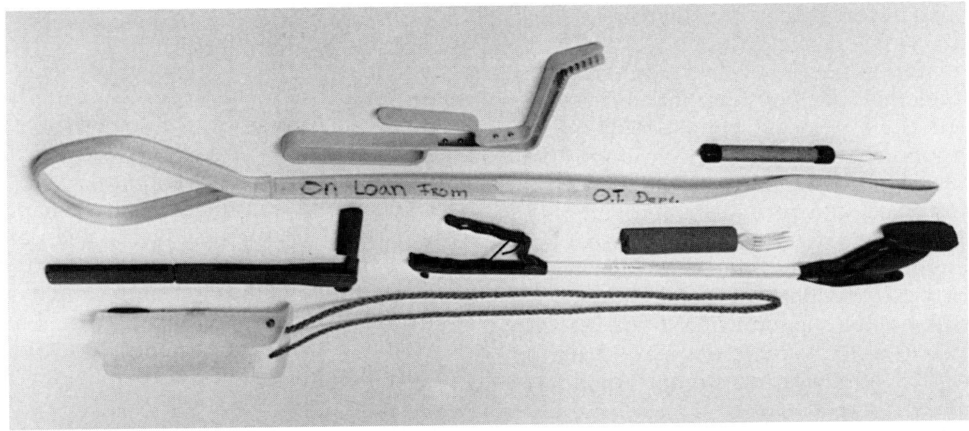

FIGURE 36–3. Devices that substitute for deformed joints and conserve energy. These devices enable patients with hand and arm arthritis to perform ADL more readily and completely. The *top* item is a clamp with enlarged handle for perineal care; *next right* is a large-handled buttonhook. *Beneath* it is a leg lifter for arthroplasty patients. *Middle left* is a comb extender; *center* is a large-handled reacher; and *just above,* a large-handled fork. The *bottom* item is a sock aid.

Increasing Strength and Endurance

Most patients with RA complain of weakness, feel chronically tired, and frequently do not want to exercise. Their lack of strength and endurance has been documented.[59, 156, 185] The clinician can usually demonstrate these deficiencies, which range from diminished ($\dot{V}O_{2max}$) to decreased strength on manual muscle testing. There are only minimal changes on microscopic examination of muscles of patients with RA, and even steroid-induced myopathy is amenable to improvement by strengthening exercises.[81]

Exercise can also be harmful to patients with RA. A patient who has been on a shopping spree or has cleaned the house for guests is a likely candidate for general and specific joint flareups. Many patients know this and often ask for joint injections before undertaking extra work or special activity. Multiple studies have demonstrated that patients with hemiplegia, peripheral nerve injury, and polio develop gout, RA, or OA more severely (unilaterally) on the sound side as opposed to the neurologically involved or rested side.[22, 86, 87, 88, 217, 225] Merritt and Hunder demonstrated in rats,[155] and Agudelo in dogs,[2] that in crystalline-induced arthritis the total synovial fluid and white cell count was increased after exercise but not after rest. Merritt and Hunder also demonstrated that isometric exercise did not increase the number of synovial fluid white cells or volume of fluid, whereas passive ROM exercises did. Other animal experiments have confirmed these studies.[89, 163]

Because patients complained of weakness and fatigue, several investigators exercised patients with RA and discovered that both strength and endurance can be increased. Machover and Sapecky demonstrated in 1966 that the isometric strength of the quadriceps muscle improved on both the exercised side and the opposite rested side of RA patients following isometric exercise.[139] Nordemar and others[60, 182, 183, 184] demonstrated that not only can patients with RA increase their strength, but their type II muscle fibers increase in size on serial biopsy, their ADL are performed with less effort, and the $\dot{V}O_{2max}$ increases. Banwell and colleagues have shown that aerobic exercise on a treadmill or bicycle is followed by an increase in aerobic and ADL capacity and gets an enthusiastic response from their patients.[17, 93] Danneskiold-Samsøe and colleagues have demonstrated that in-water exercises increase both strength and endurance in patients with RA.[51] In all these studies, there was no report of marked increase in joint pain or signs of inflammation following exercise. While little radiographic evidence was presented, it is presumed that the radiographic changes in the exercised joints were also relatively mild. There are no long-term follow-up studies other than those of Nordemar and his group, and these showed continuing improvement without subsequent joint damage with exercise.

It should be remembered, however, that the most inflamed joints are often those that have been exercised the most (especially in nature's experiments with hemiplegia). It would seem prudent for the physician to suppress the inflammation as thoroughly as possible before prescribing exercise. The exercise should be performed under careful, controlled conditions, and the patient and the physician should monitor the exercised joints for an increase in joint inflammation. Since long-term follow-up studies are not now available, the patient should be cautioned that moderation must be used. A review of the effects of exercise in arthritic patients has recently been published.[173]

Psychosocial Counseling

Patients with RA may well be depressed or suffer multiple social problems, mood swings, fatigue, and frustration.[14, 42, 153, 159, 215, 220, 227] These can affect the patient's entire family. Early detection of social and interpersonal problems allows early referral for treatment.[226] Often, social service or psychological evaluation on a rehabilitation unit can help such problems. Patients may or may not accept psychotherapy or drug treatment. A trial of antidepressants and referral to a psychiatrist is often necessary.

A discussion of the patient's job is pertinent. Many times, patients find that the physical demands of the workplace exceed their physical capability. Minimal changes in the ergonomics of their workstation, or perhaps something as simple as obtaining a permit to park closer to the workplace, can prolong employment. In general, the employment rate diminishes in direct proportion to the length of time a patient has RA. This is especially true of those who perform demanding physical tasks.[171] The physician encountering a patient with early RA is well advised to evaluate the work situation and suggest that the patient begin training for lighter work immediately.

Discussion of sexual function in patients with RA is helpful. One survey among upper socioeconomic, highly educated, university-associated persons described a high proportion of "dysfunction" among "normal" couples.[77] RA only makes the "normal dysfunction" situation worse. It is likely that sexual difficulties can arise due to mechanical problems and problems with medication.[223, 243] Mechanical problems related to disease of the hip joint can be treated, if necessary, with total hip arthroplasty.[12] Other difficulties often respond to a change in medication or counseling. A frank discussion of sexual function is more likely to be accepted by RA patients if a caring relationship between the patient and the practitioner has been established[174] (see Chapter 30).

Osteoarthritis

In patients with OA, typically only one or a few joints are involved. The pathological process begins with histological changes and ends in frank destruction of joint cartilage. There is an increase in the density of the bone adjacent to the joint, and bony excrescences (*osteophytes*) occur at the margins of the joints. Osteoarthritis occurs most commonly in older patients, but it can affect younger ones as well. It is frequently associated with conditions of previous joint damage, excessive wear, or obesity; and the relationship to exercise and work is probable but not clear.[33, 34, 35, 109, 131, 189, 190] Although OA is frequently termed *degenerative arthritis,* it can also be described as a misguided repair effort. Patients typically note pain on use or weight bearing, but sometimes after rest.

Shoulders

Osteoarthritis of the shoulders occurs usually in older patients and can be associated with excessive joint destruction or rotator cuff wear or rupture. Patients should be taught isometric exercises to strengthen the shoulder musculature, including the deltoid and rotator cuff muscles. Intra-articular steroid injections of the glenohumeral joint can also help. It is important to gain the patient's cooperation in trying to prevent adhesive capsulitis through active ROM exercises. The clinician must also be alert to the presence of other shoulder problems, such as biceps tendonitis, subdeltoid bursitis, and acromioclavicular arthritis, that can compound or mimic the symptoms of shoulder OA.

Elbows

Osteoarthritis of the elbow occurs after trauma, joint overuse, or inflammatory joint disease. Injections often provide symptomatic relief (see Chapter 24), and full ROM is not totally necessary. The patient needs only to be able to flex the elbow sufficiently to get the hand to the mouth and face for eating and hygiene. Neoprene elbow sleeves help diminish pain, but should be removed and cleaned frequently to avoid moisture buildup and fungal growth.

Hip

Osteoarthritis of the hip is common. While it can be due to congenital dislocation, previous infections, or aseptic necrosis, it is generally idiopathic. Initially, the pain may be relieved by having the patient ambulate with a cane in the contralateral hand.[24] Isometric gluteus medius and gluteus maximus exercises can increase hip pain, so they are not practical for some patients. Steroids are difficult to inject into the joint without fluoroscopic guidance. Most patients now receive total hip arthroplasty for intractable hip OA. Before or after surgery, a shoe lift may be required to correct leg-length discrepancies. Patients who have difficulties performing ADL or ambulation often need admission to a rehabilitation unit or center to maximize their recovery and function (see Table 36–1).

Knee

Osteoarthritis of the knee is associated with obesity in women, but has not been shown to result from osteochondritis dissecans or athletic activities. Quadriceps muscle strength in patients with OA of the knees has been shown to be consistently weak, and electrical stimulation testing has revealed additional inhibited strength or arthrogenous inhibition.[13, 107] Intra-articular steroid injections temporarily diminish pain and may increase the ability to perform exercises, as does the application of a moist heating pad. Many braces have been manufactured for arthritis of the knee, especially OA, but they are not generally useful. The use of elastic bandages, neoprene sleeves, or canvas braces has been shown to improve proprioception about the knee and to diminish arthrogenous muscle inhibition.[13] Many patients note an increased sense of stability and strength and diminished pain with these knee orthoses.

Use of a cane or crutches helps by relieving some of the weight-bearing stress in the knee. The cane should be held in the patient's hand of choice. There is no clear evidence to demonstrate that a cane in the contralateral hand gives consistent relief of pain for OA of the knee more frequently than one held in the ipsilateral hand.[228] Wearing shoes with soft soles such as those of Vibram diminishes knee pain in many patients with OA of the knees. Studies have demonstrated that TENS has relieved pain of OA of the knee, but the results across studies have not been consistent.[111, 135, 224]

Recent studies confirmed the notion that multiple-angle isometric exercises performed at the knee increase strength throughout the knee ROM and relieve the pain of OA. Fisher and co-workers demonstrated in a series of elegant papers that patients with OA of the knee have diminished muscular strength, especially with the hip in extension. They subsequently demonstrated that, in a specially designed machine, multiple-angle isometric exercises increased muscle strength, improved ability to perform ADL, and decreased the use of analgesics. The improvement was in excess of that following the usual active exercises.[71, 72, 73, 74, 75] Rejeski et al demonstrated that elderly patients with OA of the knees were more likely to comply with exercise if they had previously performed exercise and were prescribed exercise three times weekly in short sessions.[201]

Base of the Thumb

Osteoarthritis of the base of the thumb (carpometacarpal and metacarpophalangeal joints) is a common cause of pain. In this case, a thumb spica that immobilizes these two joints of the thumb can be helpful (Fig. 36–4). While it is somewhat awkward and interferes with some ADL activities, it does provide consistent relief of pain.[28]

Cervical Spine

Osteoarthritis of the cervical spine, which is common in the elderly, can cause symptoms of radiculopathy, due to osteophytes that impinge on nerve roots, and myelopathy, due to bony overgrowth that causes spinal cord compression. The x-ray evidence of OA of the cervical spine is frequent; nevertheless, symptoms of OA are rare. If bony osteophytes can be determined to be a cause of radiculopathy, treatment with a cervical collar or traction with the neck in flexion to hold open the interforaminal spaces can help. Cervical myelopathy from OA usually requires surgical treatment (see Chapter 37).

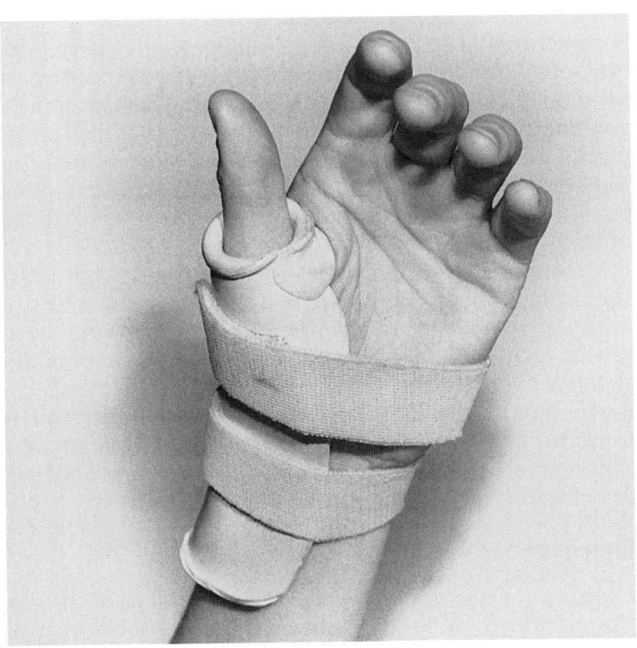

FIGURE 36–4. This thumb spica immobilizes the carpometacarpal and metacarpophalangeal joints of the thumb, but still allows fairly dexterous use of the hand.

Lumbosacral Spine and Spinal Stenosis

Spinal stenosis has been shown to be a common cause of lumbosacral myelopathy and polyradiculopathy, especially involving the L_3 and L_4 roots. The pain of lumbosacral spinal stenosis is brought on by walking or standing and relieved by sitting or lying. It can occur at night if congestive heart failure is present. Epidural injections and a brace to hold the spine in slight lumbosacral flexion can provide temporary relief. NSAIDs are also helpful in many patients. Frequently patients with a compromised spinal canal become more symptomatic because of an acute lumbar disc herniation. As time passes and the disc is absorbed or retracts, symptoms improve. Exercises have a small part to play in the treatment of this condition, but extension of the spine increases symptoms. If polyradiculopathy is significant and the patient does not wish surgery, a plastic ankle-foot orthosis for foot-drop may help. Spinal stenosis in mature adults is usually caused by OA rather than a congenitally small spinal canal.

Radiologic OA of the lumbosacral spine is almost universal in middle-aged to elderly persons. Myelopathy and radiculopathy, however, are rare in these patients. Symptoms of back pain in adults at an age when OA is prevalent should be carefully studied to find the exact cause, which may be cancer, infection, osteoporosis, or compression fracture. Osteoarthritis is diagnosed in this age group only by exclusion.

Foot

Hallux valgus of the great toe and cock-up deformity of digits II-V are the most common expressions of OA in the feet. A deep-toe box shoe (extra depth) with a molded insole to accommodate dropped metatarsal heads is helpful (see Fig. 36–2). However, rocker-bottom sole, to compensate for a stiffened great toe (hallux rigidis), often makes walking difficult and unstable. Surgical procedures are often helpful for this deformity.

Psoriatic Arthritis

Psoriatic arthritis occurs in a small subgroup of patients who have psoriasis. The arthritis is characterized by tendonitis, enthesitis, and synovitis of both peripheral and spinal joints in various clinical pictures. In a recent review, Veale described 100 consecutive patients with psoriatic arthritis admitted to both inpatient and outpatient clinics who met the criteria of having at least one psoriatic skin lesion, more than 20 fingernail pits and/or onycholysis, and a rheumatoid factor titer of less than 1 : 80.[229] Of these patients, 43% had the asymmetrical oligoarthritis type, 33% had symmetrical arthritis and more bony erosions, 16% had arthritis predominantly of the distal interphalangeal joints, 4% had spondylitis, 2%

had arthritis mutilans, and 2% had the synovitis-acne-pustulosis-hyperostosis-osteomyelitis syndrome.[229] The physician should look for psoriatic lesions in all of these patients, and examination of the scalp, anal area, and umbilicus may reveal hidden psoriatic plaques.

The rehabilitation of psoriasis patients requires detailed attention to the joints most severely involved. Patients with tendonitis and synovitis of the toes should be supplied with high-toe box shoes having soft leather uppers. A heel lift and a longitudinal arch support are helpful for associated plantar fascitis. Intra-articular injections may help individual finger joint and others. Paraffin baths provide moist heat to inflamed fingers for pain relief. Splinting individual proximal or distal interphalangeal joints can relieve pain, but will not prevent deformity in the long run.

Inflammation and pain in the costochondral joints may require individual injections and the use of superficial heat. If significant spondylitis is present with stiffness and progressive deformity, spinal extension exercises, such as walking into the corner with abducted arms and performing push-ups, should be emphasized. The spinal joint involvement in psoriatic arthritis, however, is often asymmetrical, and as a result, the spine becomes less stiff than in ankylosing spondylitis—in which case, exercises will be more successful and should be encouraged more strongly.

Ankylosing Spondylitis

Ankylosing spondylitis (AS) is inflammation of the enthesis (the tissue attaching tendons and joint capsules to bone) plus synovitis of the spinal joints. Inflammation of the synovial joints and tendons of the spine heals by ossification, causing the spine to become progressively more rigid and stiff. The spine usually becomes stiff in flexion rather than extension, probably because of the posture of the patient. This can leave the patient unable to see straight ahead, as the face is directed toward the floor during standing and walking. Inflammation of the uveal tract (iritis) and aortic valve disease also occur in AS. The condition is similar in some ways to Reiter's syndrome and psoriatic arthritis, but is distinguished because it is predominantly a disease of the spine.

No studies to date have demonstrated that exercises, braces, or medications preserve the flexibility of the spine or prevent stiffening. The physician's job is to keep the spine as functional as possible, despite gradual stiffening. An extension deformity of the spine is better for most purposes than extreme flexion. The physician must make certain that the spine is becoming stiff in extension rather than flexion by measuring the patient at each visit with Schober's test, measuring the distance from the patient's occiput to the wall when standing in maximum extension with heels against the wall, and measuring the expansion of the thoracic cage at the third to the fourth intercostal spaces.

Exercises thought to maintain the erect posture include push-ups and "walking into corners" with the hands on the occiput and the shoulders abducted. The patient must be constantly reminded to attempt to maintain an erect posture and to sleep on a firm mattress with the spine extended as much as possible. Kraag and co-workers[127] demonstrated that exercise therapy only twice monthly helps maintain posture, and Fisher and associates[70] found that those who exercised maintained greater aerobic capacity (although it was unrelated to chest expansion). Other individual synovial joints can be involved, and NSAIDs, other systemic medication, or intra-articular steroids may be required.

The physiatrist should assist the patient with AS in the battle to maintain upright posture and not allow the patient to slip into noncompliance with daily exercises. If an arthroplasty is performed, it should be remembered that postoperative heterotopic ossification is more common in patients with AS than in RA or OA.

Scleroderma and Progressive Systemic Sclerosis

Patients with progressive systemic sclerosis (PSS) form excessive amounts of abnormal collagen, which causes thickening of the skin and difficulty moving the joints, especially those of the fingers, shoulders, and knees. Systemic involvement can occur, with the fibrosis affecting motility of the gastrointestinal tract, air exchange in the lungs, and expansion or motion in the pericardium; and there can be infiltration of muscles (myopathy), which decreases strength. The kidneys are frequently affected by a particular kind of vasculitis, and kidney disease is a leading cause of death in patients with PSS. A large percentage of PSS patients have Raynaud's phenomenon, in which blood flow to the fingers is markedly constricted on an episodic basis, and ulcers, sores, and pain can ensue. A variant of PSS called the CREST syndrome consists of subcutaneous *c*alcinosis, *R*aynaud's phenomenon, *e*sophageal dysfunction, *s*clerodactyly, and *t*elangiectasia, often of the lips and fingers. These patients usually have less joint restriction.

The rehabilitation techniques for preventing joint contractures of PSS have been only partially successful, but must not be ignored. Patients with myopathy or localized myopathy frequently respond to exercise therapy and decrease of ACS doses, but the creatine phosphokinase levels must be monitored. Finger function is not typically helped by splinting; but plaster casts can be used to cover painful ulcers, and patients can be offered finger exercises to maintain strength.[213]

Speech pathologists and occupational therapists should become involved in treating dysphagia and can help the patient by determining the appropriate swallowing technique and food consistency (see Chapter 26). It has recently been shown that patients with scleroderma who have amputations of the lower extremities tolerate standard prostheses as well as other patients do. Appropriate prostheses, therefore, should be prescribed for all patients (see Chapter 14).[202]

Dermatomyositis/Polymyositis

Dermatomyositis/polymyositis (DM/PM) is a disease characterized by inflammation of the muscle, with or without a rash. It has been divided into five varieties by Bohan and co-workers[25]: PM in adults, DM in adults, PM/DM in adults with malignancy, childhood PM/DM, and DM/PM with collagen vascular disease. Regardless of the variety, the physiatrist is faced with a patient who has weakness, usually of the proximal muscles, although distal muscle involvement has been described. Joint disease is rare, but bony erosions have been reported. Subcutaneous calcinosis occurs frequently in children and can limit joint ROM. Weakness of the respiratory muscles and the muscles of swallowing can result in aspiration pneumonia and subsequent lung dysfunction, which has been negatively linked to survival in this disease (see Chapters 11, 12, and 48 for further information on myopathy diagnosis).

Preserving and increasing muscle strength are main rehabilitation goals. Hicks described a 4-week course of isometric muscle contractions, six per muscle on 6 days weekly for 6 seconds each.[99] Patients who had DM/PM for less than 2 years had better results, so it was recommended that exercises be performed early in the course of DM/PM.

Escalante and others described five patients with DM/PM, persistent muscle weakness, and elevated serum muscle enzymes of less than one year's duration who were treated with alternating periods of exercise.[64] These consisted of functional activities plus resistive exercises (two to three sets of five to ten repetitions each), alternating with periods of functional activities only. The patients had only mild increases in CPK levels following exercise. Responses were not uniform, and one patient with severe weakness did not improve. A second patient demonstrated functional improvement but little strength improvement. The third and fourth patients improved considerably, and the fifth patient improved remarkably. Hicks and colleagues described an additional patient with DM/PM of less than two years' duration who gained strength in the quadriceps and biceps without creatine phosphokinase elevations following an isometric exercise program.[100]

A dilemma frequently occurs when it must be decided whether the patient with increasing weakness has an exacerbation of DM/PM or has steroid myopathy from ACS treatment. The evaluation of serum muscle enzymes, electromyography, muscle biopsy, or a trial of steroids is often required to resolve this dilemma. Often a trial of increased oral ACS increases strength if active DM/PM is the problem.

If persistent or chronic weakness cannot be improved, the patient may require fitting with a plastic ankle-foot orthoses to stabilize the knees and ankles and prevent foot-drop (see Chapter 16). In addition, assistive living devices to help with toileting, hygiene, eating, and dressing are often required (see Chapter 25). Wheelchairs or electrically powered wheel carts are helpful in many patients (see Chapter 18). The patient with suspected dysphagia should be referred for a swallowing evaluation and proper dietary precautions taken (see Chapter 26).

It is still controversial whether or not the physician should extensively test all DM/PM patients for possible malignancy. If any suggestions of malignancy are present, consultation with the primary care physician should be enlisted and a search for occult malignancy carried out. Adults with a rash are thought most likely to have a malignancy.

Systemic Lupus Erythematosus

Systemic lupus erythematosus (SLE) is a systemic immune-mediated disorder, but one of its major manifestations is a mild but painful synovitis that resembles RA. The synovitis results in weakening of tendinous and capsular structures, so that the hands demonstrate the deformities characteristic of RA, such as ulnar deviation and subluxation of the metacarpophalangeal joints and boutonnière and swan's neck deformities of the proximal interphalangeal joints. These joint findings are termed *non-erosive deforming arthritis* or *Jaccoud's arthritis* and are not RA.[36, 55] Because bony erosions are not a feature, the joints are not destroyed as in RA, but they can have reduced function because of the deformities. Lively splints (powered by springs or rubber bands) to help hold the hands and fingers in place during activities, if tolerated, can be helpful.

A second form of joint disease, avascular necrosis, occurs with increased frequency in SLE patients, independent of treatment with steroids.[125] The knees, hips, shoulders, and other joints are frequently involved. At initial diagnosis, consideration must be given to orthopedic surgery, but the pain can often be relieved by causing less weight to be distributed to the involved joint through the use of a walker, canes, crutches, or other ambulation aids.

Patients with SLE also have ruptures of the patellar and Achilles tendons, with or without association with ACS. Following repair and diminution of steroid dose, muscle-strengthening exercises must be initiated. Both functional electrical stimulation and biofeedback can help to train patients to once again contract these weak muscles after tendon repair.

Patients with SLE can also have systemic involvement—wolf-like skin rash, renal failure, central and peripheral nervous system abnormalities, hematological problems (including hemolytic anemia and idiopathic thrombocytopenic purpura), and systemic cutaneous vasculitis. Pleurisy is a frequent accompaniment of lung disease, and it has been suggested that TENS can help manage the pain of this transient phenomenon.[83] Other neurological problems can occur, such as stroke or a foot-drop from peripheral neuropathy.

SLE patients often have a bland vasculitis of the central nervous system. Psychological testing and counseling are appropriate, and the psychological status must be considered when prescribing exercise or splints, because of potential compliance problems.

MAXIMIZING COMPLIANCE WITH TREATMENT

Treatment can be successful only if the patient complies with the treatment. Unfortunately, rehabilitation modalities, exercises, aids, and devices do little good if the patient neglects them. Patient noncompliance with treatment programs, which has been widely documented in the medical literature, has also been demonstrated in the rehabilitation literature with arthritic patients.[18, 21, 52, 97] Parker and Bender administered a questionnaire to 56 patients regarding a home treatment program and found only 54% persisted in following it at 12 months.[191] Carpenter and Davis questioned 54 patients about an exercise program and found only about half continued to follow instructions.[38] Belcon has reviewed a number of studies describing compliance with splint use (Table 35–7).[18] Compliance rates varied from 28% to 78%, and the reasons for noncompliance also varied widely. The noncompliance rate is so high that it is difficult to assess the actual efficacy of splint wear in these studies.

There are numerous studies describing medication compliance in arthritis patients. Joyce studied 60 women with rheumatoid arthritis[114]; Geertson, Gray, and Ward studied 123 patients with rheumatoid arthritis[85]; Wright and Hopkins studied 200 rheumatic patients[241]; and Lee and Tan studied 100 patients with RA.[133] The high level of noncompliance described in these studies was attributed to lack of physician-patient interaction time, protracted waiting room periods, impersonal doctors, poor communication, preference for capsules or tablets, dislike of side effects, dislike of taking pills, forgetfulness, and amelioration of symptoms. In a study of 66 RA patients, 41 OA patients, 27 gout patients, and 14 ankylosing spondylitis patients, it was found that the more drugs patients were prescribed, the better was their compliance.[53] The highest compliance rate was 80% for prednisone. Wasner, who studied 33 patients with RA and 32 with ankylosing spondylitis, found, conversely, that the more pills prescribed, the less the patients complied.[233] Bond and Monson studied 81 rheumatic disease patients and found that intervention by a clinical pharmacist and nurse clinician helped educate patients and increased their compliance by solving problems.[27] Another study of 178 RA patients showed that the ones who complied tended to have more severe rheumatoid disease.[188]

It is not yet possible to formulate a definitive list of reasons why patients do not comply with exercise, splint wearing, and other modalities. It has been suggested that the physician or other health professional discuss frankly with all patients whether or not they are compliant and attempt to discover the specific reasons in each case. The use of a Compliance Card or other device that lists reasons for noncompliance can help gather appropriate information.[170] Once the patient discloses the reason for noncompliance, there is an opportunity to rectify the situation. It is difficult for the patient to improve if a treatment program is not followed, and it is difficult for the physician to assess the efficacy or failure of a treatment program if the patient does not comply with it.

It may or may not be easier for patients to comply with physical medicine and rehabilitation treatments than with surgical or medical programs. The physiatrist, however, must be tenacious in monitoring patients' compliance, monitoring the efficacy of treatment, and making changes and adaptations when necessary. Most of the rheumatic conditions dealt with by physiatrists are chronic and persisting and require patience and persistence on the part of *both* the patient and the physician.

REHABILITATION FOLLOWING ARTHROPLASTY

Approximately 800,000 joint replacement arthroplasties are performed annually world-wide.[79] These procedures have become more and more successful, with improvement in activities of daily living (ADL), survival, freedom from pain, improved function, and increased duration of satisfactory function of the implants.[15, 40, 117, 124, 147, 204, 208, 210, 211] The length of stay following surgery has decreased from an original 10 to 15 days to less than 5, and even 3, days for primary procedures in some centers. Patients who fall outside these lengths of stay often require rehabilitation treat-

TABLE 36–7 Compliance Rates for Splinting

Subjects (*N*)	Study Design	Intervention or Disease Feature	Compliance Measure	Compliance Result (%)	Compliance Definition	Disease Definition	Regimen Definition	Duration of Observation
56	Cross-sectional analytic survey	Home physiotherapy	Interview	39	0	0	0	0
218	Cross-sectional analytic survey	Home physiotherapy	Interview	65	0	0	0	+
40	Cross-sectional analytic survey	ASA use	Interview + serum assay	78	+	0	0	0
		Exercise	Interview	40	+	0	0	0
		Splint wear	Interview	25	+	0	0	0
12	Time series	Exercise/visual feedback	Electronic counter	Enhancement	+	0	+	+
46	Cross-sectional analytic survey	Splinting	Weighted-index	28	+	0	0	0
36	Cross-sectional analytic survey	Splinting	Interview	50	0	0	0	0
50	Cross-sectional analytic survey	Splinting	Interview	62	+	+	0	+
66	Prospective analytic survey	Splinting	Interview	65	0	+	+	+

Key: +, presence; 0, absence of feature; ASA, acetylsalicylic acid.
Adapted from Belcon MC, et al: A critical review of compliance studies in rheumatoid arthritis. Arthritis Rheum 1984; 27:1230.

ment. Table 36–1 lists reasons for such continued hospitalization for rehabilitation. There is a wide variation in the length of time for patients to meet their expected length of stay milestones.[245] Living alone, older age, increased co-morbidity, greater pain levels, diminished range of motion, and low strength level will often predict which patients will require further rehabilitation.[162] Nonetheless, persons 80 years of age or older have been shown to do quite well following arthroplasty.[30] There is preliminary evidence to suggest that the centers and surgeons who perform the greatest volume of arthroplasty procedures typically have the best results.[128]

Hip Arthroplasty

Descriptions of rehabilitation techniques following hip arthroplasty are infrequent,[39, 76, 80, 177, 180] but a consensus has developed as experience has increased. The essentials are that the physiatrist must determine the weight-bearing status of each patient. With a cemented prosthesis, patients are immediately allowed to bear weight. With an uncemented prosthesis, weight bearing may be limited to touch-down for as long as eight weeks.[95] Touch-down weight bearing is preferred over non–weight bearing so that the patient may go through the motions of walking without actually bearing significant weight in order to maintain walking reflexes and muscular proprioception. Patients are immediately taught range-of-motion exercises and mild isometric exercises to re-educate muscles that have been inactive and to avoid contractures. Patients are taught to walk with crutches or a walker prior to going home to maintain weight-bearing status. They generally do not cease use of a walking device until they can walk without a limp or Trendelenburg gait.

Patients must also be taught precautions in order to avoid dislocating their hip prosthesis. With the standard posterolateral incision (capsular weakness posterior), they must avoid hyperflexion, hyperadduction, and excessive internal rotation or they may lever the head of the femoral component out through the posterior capsule. Patients with anterior incisions must avoid hyperextension. Hip dislocations usually occur shortly after surgery, and this incidence diminishes over the course of time. The occupational therapist must carefully instruct the patient in ADL techniques designed to diminish the likelihood of dislocation. Patients who have undergone revision frequently are fitted with an abductor brace with an adjustable hip hinge (Newport brace) to limit adduction, internal rotation, and flexion while healing takes place. Conditions associated with increased postoperative dislocation are small femoral head, previous surgery, posterior approach, component malposition, osteotomy of the greater trochanter, a short femoral component, alcoholism, older age, and organic brain disease.[16, 32, 48, 161, 193, 239]

Postoperative activities should be limited in the sense that high-impact activities and vigorous sports must be avoided.[122, 151] Scuba diving, sailing, bowling, cycling, swimming, and golfing are allowed by most surgeons. Jogging, racquetball, football, baseball, water skiing, hockey, basketball, etc., are not recommended after hip replacement. Reaction time has been found to be slowed as long as eight months postoperatively,[138] and patients with hip or knee arthroplasty should probably get permission from their insurance companies prior to driving a car. Previous health status, race, education, and number of co-morbid conditions have been found to be directly associated with a less favorable outcome in hip arthroplasty.[140]

Complications

Heterotopic ossification may be prevented by low-dose radiation and possibly nonsteroidal anti-inflammatory agents.[212] Nerve injuries following hip arthroplasty occur in the common peroneal in the leg and the ulnar nerve in the hand most commonly.[168] Femoral, obturator, lateral femoral cutaneous, brachial plexus, ulnar, axillary, and median nerve injuries have been described. If the leg is lengthened, the sciatic nerve may be damaged. Compartment syndrome and hematomas (potentially curable causes) can also be involved in postoperative neuropathies.

Deep venous thrombosis following arthroplasty is common and is usually prevented with prophylactic coumadin. Low-molecular-weight heparin and compression stockings have also been advocated.[108]

Postoperative pain gradually subsides over a few days. If pain persists or there is an acute exacerbation, radiographs should be taken to attempt to discover a dislocation. Signs of inflammation around the wound and drainage should be brought to the attention of the orthopedic surgeon. If superficial infection is suspected, a culture should be obtained and antibiotics started. Deep infections ordinarily are not clinically obvious until after rehabilitation has been completed.

Leg length discrepancies often appear due to contractures around the hip or to extremity shortening. The prescription of a shoe lift should be delayed until any contractures have been eliminated.

Failure of the total hip arthroplasty sufficient to require revision has become common even as the duration of successful outcomes has increased.[9] Mahomed and Katz have provided a description of indications for revision and the expected outcomes.[141]

Knee Arthroplasty

Total knee arthroplasty has become much more successful than in the past.[37] Hemi- and unicompartmental and constrained arthroplasties have been less successful.[37] Rehabilitation following *bilateral* cemented total knee arthroplasties is a frequent occurrence, and the outcome is typically quite successful. While morbidity and cost is increased in bilateral knee procedures, it is not doubled.[130, 157]

Rehabilitation

The most difficult rehabilitation problems are obtaining full flexion and extension of the knee. Vigorous passive exercises are prescribed almost immediately postoperatively, and some surgeons bandage the knee in flexion rather than extension in order to facilitate increased flexion. The physiatrist should know the weight-bearing condition immediately following surgery. Most knee prostheses are now cemented; therefore, partial weight bearing is necessary only when grafting or tendon or muscle tears have occurred and been repaired. Weight bearing is allowed very promptly, and most patients are able to bear weight. An exception is bilateral knee arthroplasties, performed when the patient does not have a good knee. Bilateral total knee arthroplasties have been shown to increase the likelihood of referral to a rehabilitation unit, increasing—but not doubling—the costs.[130] Costs have also not diminished, although LOS for unilateral knee arthroplasties has fallen significantly.[219] In spite of postoperative pain, patients must be encouraged to flex and extend their knees and utilize their muscles. Sometimes biofeedback or FES may help, but usually the services of a skilled and persistent therapist will suffice. Patients typically note pain after a total knee arthroplasty for a much longer period than after total hip arthroplasty.[1]

The use of passive motion machines postoperatively is quite controversial. Unless the patient utilizes the machine for an unusually long length of time, no improvement has been demonstrated.[112, 113, 144, 152, 160, 164, 198, 231, 232, 242] Preoperative exercise has not been shown to shorten the length of stay or decrease the complication rate.[54]

Activity limitations following total knee arthroplasty are similar to those following hip arthroplasty. McGroy's survey[151] revealed a consensus that golfing, swimming, cycling, sailing, bowling, and cross-country skiing are preferable to karate, soccer, water skiing, hockey, basketball, running, and baseball. Both singles and doubles tennis received an intermediate evaluation.

Driving following total knee arthroplasty depends upon each individual patient's recovery. The physiatrist should become informed about the rules for driving after surgery in his/her own state.

Complications

Complications following knee arthroplasty have been well described.[10] Peroneal palsy may occur and surgical exploration may be indicated if direct compression from a hematoma is suspected. Reflex sympathetic dystrophy is rare and requires aggressive treatment. Fractures can occur proximal to the total knee prosthesis, and x-rays are again required for patients who have persistent pain. Deep infections are associated with the use of constrained prostheses, previous surgery, open skin lesions, and rheumatoid arthritis. The orthopedic surgeon must be consulted for their treatment. Superficial infections are to be suspected when increased signs of inflammation and drainage occur. Again, cultures should be obtained, and antibiotics should be given intravenously if appropriate. Wound dehiscence from physical therapy or other reasons should be treated with closure and rest.

Deep venous thrombosis occurs with alarming frequency following total knee arthroplasty. Anticoagulation with coumadin or heparin is appropriate, and ultrasound Doppler studies should be ordered whenever they seem indicated.

There are also problems associated with the knee extensor mechanism following knee arthroplasty. Some of these include an unstable patella, a patellar "clunk" or patellar tendon rupture.

Shoulder Arthroplasty

The rehabilitation of the patient with a shoulder arthroplasty was initially quite individualized, tedious, and prolonged. It was carefully outlined by Dr. Neer,[165] who developed the technique.[49, 166, 167] A current review of complications of shoulder arthroplasty[181] includes technical error, instability, rotator cuff tears, heterotopic ossification, loosening, modular component dislocation, sepsis, humeral fracture, and nerve injuries.

Rehabilitation should begin on the first postoperative day,[31] and each surgeon probably will recommend his/her own individual protocol. Initial active assisted exercise should be prescribed, avoiding excessive shoulder internal rotation and adduction. Minimal abduction and external rotation is performed until a relatively pain-free arc of motion occurs, and then the activity is extended to approximately 140° of flexion and 40° of external rotation. When near full ROM has been achieved, isometric exercises, assistive exercises, and pulley exercises should be employed to strengthen muscles. Weight training is sometimes advised at 12 weeks postoperatively.

Complications can occur, including superficial infection, brachial plexus stretches, humeral fractures, hematomas, glenoid component loosening, and humeral component loosening.[43, 205] The complication of heterotopic ossification has not been reported.

A recent symposium describes the techniques, design, indications, complications, and results.[20] Shoulder arthroplasty has been shown to provide long-lasting pain relief in patients with RA.[126]

Elbow and Wrist Arthroplasty

The historical development, indications, techniques, complications, and results of the total elbow arthroplasty have been recently reviewed. The device is still evolving,[200] and is not currently routinely used in clinical practice.

Costi et al have provided a description of recent developments in wrist arthroplasty.[47]

REFERENCES

1. Aarons H, Hall G, Hughes S, et al: Short-term recovery from hip and knee arthroplasty. J Bone Joint Surg Br 1996; 78:555–558.
2. Agudelo CA, Schumacher HR, Phelps P: Effect of exercise on urate crystal-induced inflammation in canine joints. Arthritis Rheum 1972; 15:609–616.
3. Akeson WH, Amiel D, Woo SL: Immobility effect on synovial joints. The pathomechanics of joint contracture. Biorheology 1980; 17:95–110.
4. Akeson WH, Amiel D, Abel MF, et al: Effects of immobilization on joints. Clin Orthop 1987; 219:28–37.
5. Akeson WH, Woo SL, Amiel D, et al: Value of 17beta-oestradiol in prevention of contracture formation. Ann Rheum Dis 1975; 35:429–436.

6. Alexander GJ, Hortas C, Bacon PA: Bed rest, activity and the inflammation of rheumatoid arthritis. Br J Rheumatol 1983; 22:134–140.
7. Amiel D, Woo SL, Harwood FL, et al: The effect of immobilization on collagen turnover in connective tissue: A biochemical-biomechanical correlation. Acta Orthop Scand 1982; 53:325–332.
8. Amiel D, Akeson WH, Harwood FL, et al: Stress deprivation effect on metabolic turnover of the medial collateral ligament collagen. A comparison between nine- and 12-week immobilization. Clin Orthop 1983; 172:265–270.
9. Aufranc OE, Harris SM, McKay SJ, Dinardo DM: Revision Hip Arthroplasty. In Turner RH, Scheller AD (eds): Rehabilitation in Revision Arthroplasty. New York, Grune and Stratton, 1982, pp 379–396.
10. Ayers DC, Dennis DA, Johanson NA, et al: Common complications of total knee arthroplasty. J Bone Joint Surg Am 1997; 79:278–311.
11. Bach F: Physical medicine and the rheumatic diseases. Br J Phys Med 1947; 10:66–69.
12. Baldursson H, Brattstrom H: Sexual difficulties and total hip replacement in rheumatoid arthritis. Scand J Rheumatol 1979; 8:214–216.
13. Barrett DS, Cobb AG, Bentley G: Joint proprioception in normal osteoarthritic and replaced knees. J Bone Joint Surg Br 1991; 73:53–56.
14. Baum J: A review of the psychological aspects of rheumatic diseases. Seminars Arthritis Rheum 1982; 11:352–361.
15. Bayley KB, London MR, Grunkemeier GL, Lansky DJ: Measuring the success of treatment in patient terms. Med Care 1995; 33:AS226–235.
16. Beabout JW: Radiology of total hip arthroplasty. Radiol Clin North Am 1975; 13:3–19.
17. Beals CA, Lampman RM, Banwell BF, et al: Measurement of exercise tolerance in patients with rheumatoid arthritis and osteoarthritis. J Rheumatol 1985; 12:458–461.
18. Belcon MC, Haynes RB, Tugwell P: A critical review of compliance studies in rheumatoid arthritis. Arthritis Rheum 1984; 27:1227–1233.
19. Bell BT: The prevention and correction of deformities in arthritis. Med Clin N Amer 1940; 24:1735–1743.
20. Bigliani LU: Shoulder arthroplasty. Sem Arthroplasty 1997; vol 8.
21. Blackwell B: Drug therapy—patient compliance. N Engl J Med 1973; 289:249–252.
22. Bland JH, Eddy WM: Hemiplegia and rheumatoid hemiarthritis. Arthritis Rheum 1968; 11:72–80.
23. Blocka KL: Changing trends in the hospitalization of patients with rheumatoid arthritis and the future of the inpatient rheumatic disease unit. J Rheumatol 1994; 21:587–590.
24. Blount WP: Don't throw away the cane. J Bone Joint Surg 1956; 2:695–698.
25. Bohan A, Peter JB: Polymyositis and dermatomyositis. N Engl J Med 1974; 292:344–347.
26. Boisset M, Fitzcharles MA: Alternative medicine use by rheumatology patients in a universal health care setting. J Rheumatol 1994; 21:148–152.
27. Bond CA, Monson R: Sustained improvement in drug documentation, compliance, and disease control. A four-year analysis of an ambulatory care model. Arch Intern Med 1984; 144:1159–1162.
28. Bongi SM, Guidi G, Cencetti A, Zoppi M: Treatment of carpometacarpal joint osteoarthritis by means of a personalized splint. Pain Clinic 1991; 4:119–123.
29. Botte MJ, Nickel VL, Akeson WH: Spasticity and contracture. Physiologic aspects of formation. Clin Orthop 1988; 233:7–18.
30. Brander VA, Malhotra S, Jet J, et al: Outcome of hip and knee arthroplasty in persons aged 80 years and older. Clin Orthop 1997; 345:67–76.
31. Brems JJ: Rehabilitation following total shoulder arthroplasty. Clin Orthop 1994; 307:70–85.
32. Brien WW, Salvati EA, Wright TM, et al: Dissociation of acetabular components after total hip arthroplasty. Report of four cases. J Bone Joint Surg Am 1990; 72:1548–1550.
33. Bunning RD, Materson RS: A rational program of exercise for patients with osteoarthritis. Sem Arthritis Rheum 1991; 21:33–43.
34. Bunning RD, Materson RS: Exercise and osteoarthritis. (Letter). Ann Intern Med 1992; 117:697–698.
35. Burry HC: Sport, exercise and arthritis. Br J Rheumatol 1987; 26:386–388.
36. Bywaters E: Jaccoud's syndrome: Today's view. Clin Rheumatol Practice 1986; Winter:148–152.
37. Callahan CM, Drake BG, Heck DA, et al: Patient outcomes following tricompartmental total knee replacement. A meta-analysis. JAMA 1994; 271:1349–1357.
38. Carpenter JO, Davis LJ: Medical recommendations—followed or ignored? Factors influencing compliance in arthritis. Arch Phys Med Rehabil 1976; 57:241–246.
39. Chandler HP: Postoperative rehabilitation of the total hip patient. In Stillwell W (ed): The Art of Total Hip Arthroplasty. New York, Grune and Stratton, 1987, pp 371–401.
40. Charnley J: Total hip replacement. JAMA 1974; 230:1025–1028.
41. Clark WS, Case HB, Furey JG: Rehabilitation of patients with rheumatoid arthritis. J Chron Dis 1957; 5:712–722.
42. Cobb S: Contained hostility in rheumatoid arthritis. Arthritis Rheum 1959; 2:419–425.
43. Cofield RH, Frankle MA, Zuckerman JD: Humeral head replacement for glenohumeral arthritis. Sem Arthroplasty 1995; 6:214–221.
44. Convery FR, Conaty JP, Nickel, VL: Flexion deformities of the knee in rheumatoid arthritis. Clin Orthop 1971; 74:90–93.
45. Cordery JC: Joint protection: A responsibility of the occupational therapists. Am J Occ Ther 1965; 19:285.
46. Cosgrove JL, Nicholas JJ, Barmak J, et al: Team treatment. Does a specialized unit improve team performance? Am J Phys Med Rehabil 1988; 67:253–260.
47. Costi J, Krishnan J, Pearcy M: Total wrist arthroplasty: A quantitative review of the last 30 years. J Rheumatol 1998; 25:451–458.
48. Coventry MB: Late dislocations in patients with Charnley total hip arthroplasty. J Bone Joint Surg Am 1985; 67:832–841.
49. Craig EV: Total shoulder replacement. Orthopedics 1988; 11:125–136.
50. Culic DD, Battagalia MC, Wichman BS, et al: Efficacy of compression gloves in rheumatoid arthritis. Am J Phys Med 1979; 58:278–284.
51. Danneskiold-Samsøe B, Lyngberg K, Risum T, et al: The effect of water exercise therapy given to patients with rheumatoid arthritis. Scand J Rehabil Med 1987; 19:31–35.
52. Deyo RA: Compliance with therapeutic regimens in arthritis: Issues, current status, and a future agenda. Sem Arthritis Rheum 1982; 12:233–244.
53. Deyo RA, Inui TS, Sullivan B: Noncompliance with arthritis drugs: Magnitude, correlates, and clinical implications. J Rheumatol 1981; 8:931–936.
54. D'Lima DD, Colwell CW Jr, Morris BA, et al: The effect of preoperative exercise on total knee replacement outcomes. Clin Orthop 1996; 326:174–182.
55. Dorwart BB, Schumacher HR: Hand deformities resembling rheumatoid arthritis. Sem Arthritis Rheum 1974; 4:53–71.
56. Duthie JJ: The fundamental treatment of rheumatoid arthritis. Practitioner 1951; 166:22–32.
57. Edström G: Kinesotherapy and extension treatment in rheumatoid arthritis. Br J Phys Med 1947; 10:4–8.
58. Edström G: Rehabilitation and treatment by movement of contractures in rheumatoid arthritis. Ann Rheum Dis 1952; 2:196–203.
59. Ekblom B, Lovgren O, Alderin M, et al: Physical performance in patients with rheumatoid arthritis. Scand J Rheumatol 1974; 3:121–125.
60. Ekblom B, Lovgren O, Alderin M, et al: Effect of short-term physical training on patients with rheumatoid arthritis. I. Scand J Rheumatol 1975; 4:80–86.
61. Elkayam O, Wigler I, Tishler M, et al: Effect of spa therapy in Tiberias on patients with rheumatoid arthritis and osteoarthritis. J Rheumatol 1991; 18:1778–1779.
62. Ely LW, Mensor MC: Studies on the immobilization of the normal joint. Surg Gyn Obstet 1933; 57:212–215.
63. Enneking WF, Horowitz M: The intra-articular effects of immobilization on the human knee. J Bone Joint Surg Am 1972; 54:973–985.

64. Escalante A, Miller L, Beardmore TD: Resistive exercise in the rehabilitation of polymyositis/dermatomyositis. J Rheumatol 1993; 20:1340–1344.
65. Evans EB, Eggers GWN, Butler JK, et al: Experimental immobilization and remobilization of rat knee joints. J Bone Joint Surg Am 1960; 42:737–758.
66. Falconer J, Hayes KW, Chang R: Effect of ultrasound on mobility in osteoarthritis of the knee. A randomized clinical trial. Arthritis Care Res 1992; 5:29–35.
67. Feibel A, Fast A: Deep heating of joints: A reconsideration. Arch Phys Med Rehabil 1976; 57:513–514.
68. Finsterbush A, Friedman B: Early changes in immobilized rabbits knee joints: A light and electron microscopic study. Clin Orthop 1973; 92:305–319.
69. Finestone HM: Rheumatology rehabilitation: The role of a physical medicine and rehabilitation liaison consultation service. Am J Phys Med Rehabil 1992; 71:191–192.
70. Fisher LR, Cawley MI, Holgate ST: Relation between chest expansion, pulmonary function, and exercise tolerance in patients with ankylosing spondylitis. Ann Rheum Dis 1990; 49: 92–95.
71. Fisher NM, Gresham GE, Abrams M, et al: Quantitative effects of physical therapy on muscular and functional performance in subjects with osteoarthritis of the knees. Arch Phys Med Rehabil 1993; 74:840–847.
72. Fisher NM, Gresham G, Pendergast DR: Effects of a quantitative progressive rehabilitation program applied unilaterally to the osteoarthritic knee. Arch Phys Med Rehabil 1993; 74:1319–1326.
73. Fisher NM, Pendergast DR, Calkins EC: Maximal isometric torque of knee extension as a function of muscle length in subjects of advancing age. Arch Phys Med Rehabil 1990; 71:729–734.
75. Fisher NM, Pendergast DR, Calkins E: Muscle rehabilitation in impaired elderly nursing home residents. Arch Phys Med Rehabil 1991; 72:181–185.
75. Fisher NM, Pendergast DR, Gresham GE, Calkins E: Muscle rehabilitation: Its effect on muscular and functional performance of patients with knee osteoarthritis. Arch Phys Med Rehabil 1991; 72:367–374.
76. Foster RR, Khalifa S: Total knee replacement rehabilitation. Sports Med Arthroscopy Rev 1996; 4:83–91.
77. Frank E, Anderson C, Rubinstein D: Frequency of sexual dysfunction in "normal" couples. N Engl J Med 1978; 299:111–115.
78. Frankel E: Electric blanket treatment of rheumatoid arthritis. Lancet 1949; 2:1084–1085.
79. Galante JO, Rosenberg AG, Callaghan JJ: Total Hip Revision Surgery. New York, Raven Press, 1995, p 13.
80. Garden FH: Rehabilitation following total hip arthroplasty. J Back Musculoskel Rehabil 1994; 4:185–192.
81. Gardner DL: Pathological basis of the connective tissue diseases. London, Lea & Febiger, 1992, pp 509–510.
82. Gault SJ, Spyker JM: Beneficial effect of immobilization of joints in rheumatoid and related arthritides: A splint study using sequential analysis. Arthritis Rheum 1969; 12:34–44.
83. Gerber LH, Hicks JE: Rehabilitation management of rheumatic diseases. In Hicks JE, Nicholas JJ, Sweazey RL (eds): Handbook of Rehabilitative Rheumatology, Atlanta, American Rheumatism Association, 1988, p 95.
84. Gerber LH, Hunt G, Hurwitz S: Ankle orthosis for rheumatoid disease. Arthritis Rheum 1985; 28:S47.
85. Geertsen HR, Gray RM, Ward J Jr: Patient non-compliance within the context of seeking medical care for arthritis. J Chron Dis 1973; 26:689–698.
86. Glick L: Asymmetrical rheumatoid arthritis after poliomyelitis. Br Med J 1967; 3:26.
87. Glyn JH, Sutherland I, Walker GF, et al: Low incidence of osteoarthritis in hip and knee after anterior poliomyelitis: A late review. Br Med J 1966; 2:739–742.
88. Glynn JJ, Clayton ML: Sparing effect of hemiplegia on tophaceous gout. Ann Rheum Dis 1976; 35:534–535.
89. Glynn LE: The chronicity of inflammation and its significance in rheumatoid arthritis. Ann Rheum Dis 1968; 27:105–121.
90. Guess VA: Plaster cuff-in splints to reduce knee flexion contracture in patients with chronic rheumatoid arthritis. Phys Ther 1972; 52:634–638.
91. Hall, MC: Cartilage changes after experimental immobilization of the knee joint of the young rat. J Bone Joint Surg Am 1963; 45:36–44.
92. Hamilton DE, Bywaters EGL, Please NW: A controlled trial of various forms of physiotherapy in arthritis. Physiotherapy 1959; 45:139–142.
93. Harkcom TM, Lampman RM, Banwell BF, et al: Therapeutic value of graded aerobic exercise training in rheumatoid arthritis. Arthritis Rheum 1985; 28:32–39.
94. Harris ED Jr, McCroskery PA: The influence of temperature and fibril stability on degradation of cartilage collagen by rheumatoid synovial collagenase. N Engl J Med 1974; 290:1–6.
95. Harris WH: The case for cementing all femoral components in total hip replacement. Can J Surg 1995; 38(suppl 1):S55–S60.
96. Hawkes J, Fogden J, Wright V: Straightening the knees in rheumatoid arthritis. Physiotherapy 1972; 58:226–229.
97. Haynes RB, Taylor DW, Sackett D (eds): Compliance in Health Care. Baltimore, Johns Hopkins University Press, 1979.
98. Helliwell PS: An appraisal of medicinal spa therapy for rheumatological disorders. J R Soc Health 1989; 109:3–7.
99. Hicks JE, Miller F, Plotz P, Chen TH: Strength improvement without CPK elevation in a polymyositis patient on an isometric exercise program. Arthritis Rheum 1988; 31(suppl):S59.
100. Hicks JE, Miller F, Plotz P, et al: Osometric exercise increases strength and does not produce sustained creatine phosphokinase increase in a patient with polymyositis. J Rheumatol 1993; 20:1399–1401.
101. Hicks JE, Nicholas JJ: Rehabilitative rheumatology content in current rheumatology training programs. Arthritis Rheum 1984; 27:1076–1078.
102. Hicks JE, Nicholas JJ: Rehabilitative rheumatology content in current rehabilitation medicine training programs. Arch Phys Med Rehabil 1985; 66:631–633.
103. Hill D: Basic treatment in rheumatoid arthritis. Med Clin N Am 1955; 39:393–403.
104. Hollander JL, Horvath SM: The influence of physical therapy procedures on the intra-articular temperature of normal and arthritic subjects. Am J Med Sci 1949; 218:543–548.
105. Holt PJ: Management of rheumatoid arthritis. Br Med J 1969; 3:514–518.
106. Horvath SM, Hollander JL: Intra-articular temperature as a measure of joint reaction. J Clin Invest 1949; 28:469–473.
107. Hurley MV, Newham DJ: The influence of arthrogenous muscle inhibition on quadriceps rehabilitation of patients with early, unilateral osteoarthritic knees. Br J Rheum 1993; 32:127–131.
108. Imperiale TF, Speroff T: A meta-analysis of methods to prevent venous thromboembolism following total hip replacement. JAMA 1994; 271:1780–1785.
109. Isdale A, Helliwell PS: Athletes and osteoarthritis—Is there any relationship? (Letter). Br J Rheumatol 1991; 30:67–68.
110. Jan MH, Lai JS: The effects of physiotherapy on osteoarthritic knees of females. J Formosan Med Assoc 1991; 90:1008–1013.
111. Jensen H, Zesler R, Christensen T: Transcutaneous electrical nerve stimulation (TNS) for painful osteoarthrosis of the knee. Int J Rehabil Res 1991; 14:356–358.
112. Johnson DP: The effect of continuous passive motion on wound-healing and joint mobility after arthroplasty. J Bone Joint Surg Am 1990; 72:421–426.
113. Johnson DP, Eastwood DM: Beneficial effects of continuous passive motion after total condylar knee arthroplasty. Ann R Coll Surg Engl 1992; 74:412–416.
114. Joyce CR: Patient co-operation and the sensitivity of clinical trials. J Chronic Dis 1962; 15:1025–1036.
115. Karten I, Koatz AO, McEwen C: Treatment of contractures of the knee in rheumatoid arthritis. Bull N Y Acad Med 1968; 44:763–773.
116. Kantor TG: Order out of chaos—The primary mission of the pyramid (editorial). J Rheumatol 1990; 17:1580–1581.
117. Kavanaugh BF, Hassen AD, Coventry MB: Cemented hip replacement. In Morrey BF (ed): Joint Replacement Arthroplasty. New York, Churchill Livingstone, 1991, pp 639–646.
118. Keenan MA: Surgical decision making for residual limb deformities following traumatic brain injury. Orthop Rev 1988; 17:1185–1192.

119. Keenan MA, Ure K, Smith CW, et al: Hamstring release for knee flexion contracture in spastic adults. Clin Orthop 1988; 236:221–226.
120. Kelly M: The prevention of deformity in rheumatic disease. Med J Australia 1990; 2:1–8.
121. Kelly M: Rheumatoid arthritis. The active immobilization of acutely inflamed joints. NZ Med J 1961; 60:311–315.
122. Kilgus DJ, Dorey FJ, Finerman GA, et al: Patient activity, sports participation, and impact loading on the durability of cemented total hip replacements. Clin Orthop 1991; 269:25–31.
123. Kirk JA, Kersley GD: Heat and cold in the physical treatment of rheumatoid arthritis of the knee. A controlled clinical trial. Ann Phys Med 1968; 9:270–274.
124. Kirwan JR, Currey HL, Freeman MA, et al: Overall long-term impact of total hip and knee joint replacement surgery on patients with osteoarthritis and rheumatoid arthritis. Br J Rheumatol 1994; 33:357–360.
125. Klippel JH, Gerber LH, Pollack L, et al: Avascular necrosis of bone in systemic lupus erythematosus, silent symmetric osteonecroses. Am J Med 1979; 67:83–87.
126. Koorevaar RC, Merkies ND, de Waal Malefijt MC, et al: Shoulder hemiarthroplasty in rheumatoid arthritis. 19 cases reexamined after 1–17 years. Acta Orthop Scand 1997; 68:243–245.
127. Kraag G, Stokes B, Groh J, et al: The effects of comprehensive home physiotherapy and supervision on patients with ankylosing spondylitis—A randomized controlled trial. J Rheumatol 1990; 17:228–233.
128. Kreder HJ, Deyo RA, Koepsell T, et al: Relationship between the volume of total hip replacements performed by providers and the rates of postoperative complications in the state of Washington. J Bone Joint Surg Am 1997; 79:485–494.
129. Kumar VN, Redford JB: Transcutaneous nerve stimulation in rheumatoid arthritis. Arch Phys Med Rehabil 1982; 63:595–596.
130. Lane GJ, Hozack WJ, Shah S, et al: Simultaneous bilateral versus unilateral total knee arthroplasty. Outcomes analysis. Clin Orthop 1997; 345:106–112.
131. Lane NE, Buckwalter JA: Exercise: A cause of osteoarthritis? Rheum Dis Clin North Am 1993; 19:617–633.
132. Lee P, Kennedy AC, Anderson J, et al: Benefits of hospitalization in rheumatoid arthritis. Q J Med 1974; 43:205–214.
133. Lee P, Tan LJ: Drug compliance in outpatients with rheumatoid arthritis. Aust NZ J Med 1979; 9:274–277.
134. Lehmann JF, Silverman DR, Baum BA, et al: Temperature distributions in the human thigh, produced by infrared, hot pack and microwave application. Arch Phys Med Rehabil 1966; 47: 291–299.
135. Lewis D, Lewis B, Sturrock RD: Transcutaneous electrical nerve stimulation in osteoarthrosis: A therapeutic alternative? Ann Rheum Dis 1984; 43:47–49.
136. Lowman EW, Solomon WM, Hill F, Martin GM: Panel on rehabilitation in rheumatoid arthritis. GP 1955; November:69–86.
137. Lowman EW, Lee P, Rusk HA: Total rehabilitation of the rheumatoid arthritic cripple. JAMA 1955; 158:1335–1344.
138. Macdonald W, Owen JW: The effect of total hip replacement on driving reactions. J Bone Joint Surg Br 1988; 70:202–205.
139. Machover S, Sapecky AJ: Effect of isometric exercise on the quadriceps muscle in patients with rheumatoid arthritis. Arch Phys Med Rehabil 1966; 47:737–741.
140. MacWilliam CH, Yood MU, Verner JJ, et al: Patient-related risk factors that predict poor outcome after total hip replacement. Health Serv Res 1996; 31:623–638.
141. Mahomed N, Katz JN: Revision total hip arthroplasty. Indications and outcomes. Arthritis Rheum 1996; 39:1939–1950.
142. Maigne R: Manipulations and mobilizations of the limbs. In Rogoff JB (ed): Manipulation, Traction and Massage. Baltimore, Williams & Wilkins, 1980.
143. Mainardi CL, Walter JM, Spiegel PK, et al: Rheumatoid arthritis: Failure of daily heat therapy to affect its progression. Arch Phys Med Rehabil 1979; 60:390–393.
144. Maloney WJ, Schurman DJ, Hangen D, et al: The influence of continuous passive motion on outcome in total knee arthroplasty. Clin Orthop 1990; 56:162–168.
145. Mannheimer C, Lunds S, Carlsson CA: The effect of transcutaneous electrical nerve stimulation (TNS) on joint pain in patients with rheumatoid arthritis. Scand J Rheum 1978; 7:13–16.
146. Mannheimer C, Carlsson CA: The analgesic effect of transcutaneous electrical nerve stimulation (TNS) in patients with rheumatoid arthritis. A comparative study of different pulse patterns. Pain 1979; 6:329–334.
147. Martell JM, Pierson RH, Jacobs JJ, et al: Primary total hip reconstruction with a titanium fiber-coated prosthesis inserted without cement. J Bone Joint Surg Am 1993; 75:554–571.
148. Martin GM: Physical medicine in rheumatoid arthritis. Arthritis Rheum 1963; 6:177–185.
149. McCarty DJ: Treatment of rheumatoid arthritis in arthritic and allied conditions. In McCarty DJ, Koopman WJ (eds): Arthritis and Allied Conditions, ed 12, Philadelphia, Lea & Feibiger, 1993, pp 878–880.
150. McCarthy GM, McCarty DJ: Effect of topical capsaicin in the therapy of painful osteoarthritis of the hands. J Rheumatol 1992; 19:604–607.
151. McGrory BJ, Stuart MJ, Sim FH: Participation in sports after hip and knee arthroplasty: Review of literature and survey of surgeon preferences. Mayo Clin Proc 1995; 70:342–348.
152. McInnes J, Larson MG, Daltroy LH, et al: A controlled evaluation of continuous passive motion in patients undergoing total knee arthroplasty. JAMA 1992; 268:1423–1428.
153. Medsger AR, Robinson J: A comparative study of divorce in rheumatoid arthritis and other rheumatic disease. J Chronic Dis 1972; 25:269–275.
154. Melvin JL: Rheumatic disease. In Occupational Therapy and Rehabilitation. Philadelphia, FA Davis Co, 1982, pp 351–372.
155. Merritt JL, Hunder GG: Passive range of motion, not isometric exercise, amplifies acute urate synovitis. Arch Phys Med Rehabil 1983; 64:130–131.
156. Minor MA, Hewett JE, Webel RR, et al: Exercise tolerance and disease related measures in patients with rheumatoid arthritis and osteoarthritis. J Rheumatol 1988; 15:905–911.
157. Minter JE, Dorr LD: Indications for bilateral total knee replacement. Contemp Orthopaedics 1995; 31:108–111.
158. Moder KG, Hunder GG: Examination of the joints. In Kelley WN, Harris ED Jr, Ruddy S, et al (eds): Textbook of Rheumatology, ed 5. Philadelphia, WB Saunders, 1997, pp 353–370.
159. Moldofsky H, Chester WJ: Pain and mood patterns in patients with rheumatoid arthritis: A prospective study. Psychosom Med 1970; 32:309–318.
160. Montgomery F, Eliasson M: Continuous passive motion compared to active physical therapy after knee arthroplasty. Acta Orthop Scand 1996; 67:7–9.
161. Morrey BF: Joint replacement arthroplasty. New York, Churchill Livingstone, 1991, pp 667–672.
162. Munin MC, Kwoh CK, Glynn N, et al: Predicting discharge outcome after elective hip and knee arthroplasty. Am J Phys Med Rehabil 1995; 74:294–301.
163. Murray D: Modification of experimental arthritis in rabbits by tenotomy. J Surg Res Clin Lab Invest 1966; 6:488.
164. Nadler SF, Malanga GA, Zimmerman JR: Continuous passive motion in the rehabilitation setting. A retrospective study. Am J Phys Med Rehabil 1993; 72:162–165.
165. Neer CS II: Articular replacement for the humeral head. J Bone Joint Surg Am 1955; 37:215–228.
166. Neer CS II: Unconstrained shoulder arthroplasty. Instr Course Lect 1985; 34:278–286.
167. Neer CS: Shoulder Reconstruction. Philadelphia, WB Saunders, 1990, p 498.
168. Nercessian OA, Macaulay W, Stinchfield FE: Peripheral neuropathies following total hip arthroplasty. J Arthroplasty 1994; 9:645–651.
169. Nicholas JJ: Physical modalities in rheumatological rehabilitation. Arch Phys Med Rehabil 1994; 75:994–1001.
170. Nicholas JJ: Compliance Card, University of Pittsburgh, 1985.
171. Nicholas JJ: Vocational capacity with arthritis. In Scheer SJ (ed): Medical Perspectives in Vocational Assessment of Impaired Workers. Gaithersburg, MD, Aspen Publishers, 1991, pp 101–117.
172. Nicholas JJ: Joint contractures. Phys Med Rehabil Clin N Am 1994; 5:803–813.
173. Nicholas JJ: Exercise prescription for the arthritic patient. In Exercise Prescription. Philadelphia, Hanley & Blefus, 1998, pp 277–296.

174. Nicholas JJ (unpublished data).
175. Nicholas JJ, Gruen H, Weiner G, et al: Splinting in rheumatoid arthritis. I. Factors affecting patient compliance. Arch Phys Med Rehabil 1982; 63:92–94.
176. Nicholas JJ, Gruen H, Weiner G, et al: Splinting in rheumatoid arthritis. II. Evaluation of lightcast fiberglass polymer splints. Arch Phys Med Rehabil 1982; 63:95–96.
177. Nicholas JJ, Rosenberg AN: Arthritis and arthroplasty in the elderly. In Felsenthal GF, Garrison SJ, Steinberg FU (eds): Rehabilitation of the Aging and Elderly Patient. Baltimore, Williams & Wilkins, 1994, pp 101–106.
178. Nicholas JJ, Ziegler G: Cylinder splints: Their use in the treatment of arthritis of the knee. Arch Phys Med Rehabil 1977; 58:264–267.
179. Nickel VL, Kristy J, McDaniel L: Physical therapy for rheumatoid arthritis. J Am Phys Ther Assoc 1965; 45:198–204.
180. NIH Consensus Conference. Total hip replacement. JAMA 1995; 273:1950–1956.
181. Noble JS, Bell RH: Failure of total shoulder arthroplasty: Why does it occur? Sem Arthroplasty 1995; 6:280–288.
182. Nordemar R, Edstrom L, Ekblom B: Changes in muscle fibre size and physical performance in patients with rheumatoid arthritis after short-term physical training. Scand J Rheumatol 1976; 5:70–76.
183. Nordemar R, Berg U, Ekblom B, Edstrom L: Changes in muscle fibre size and physical performance in patients with rheumatoid arthritis after 7 months' physical training. Scand J Rheumatol 1976; 5:233–238.
184. Nordemar R: Physical training in rheumatoid arthritis: A controlled long term study. II. Functional capacity and general attitudes. Scand J Rheumatol 1981; 10:25–30.
185. Nordesjo LO, Nordgren B, Wigren A, Kolstad K: Isometric strength and endurance in patients with severe rheumatoid arthritis or osteoarthrosis in the knee joints. Scand J Rheumatol 1983; 12:152–156.
186. Opitz JL: Total joint arthroplasty: Principles and guidelines for postoperative physiatric management. Mayo Clin Proc 1979; 54:602–612.
187. Osler W: Aequanimitas with Other Addresses, ed 3, Philadelphia, Blakistor's Son, 1932, pp 133–135.
188. Owen SG, Friesen WT, Roberts MS, Flux W: Determinants of compliance in rheumatoid arthritic patients assessed in their home environment. Br J Rheumatol 1985; 24:313–320.
189. Panush RS, Brown DG: Exercise and arthritis. Sports Med 1987; 4:54–64.
190. Panush, RS: Does exercise cause arthritis? Long-term consequences of exercise on the musculoskeletal system. Rheum Dis Clin North Am 1990; 16:827–836.
191. Parker LB, Bender LF: Problem of home treatment in arthritis. Arch Phys Med Rehabil 1957; 38:392–394.
192. Partridge RH, Duthie JJ: Controlled trial of the effect of complete immobilization of the joints in rheumatoid arthritis. Ann Rheum Dis 1963; 22:91.
193. Paterno SA, Lachiewicz PF, Kelley SS: The influence of patient-related factors and the position of the acetabular component on the rate of dislocation after total hip replacement. J Bone Joint Surg 1997; 79:1202–1210.
194. Pegg SMH, Littler TR, Litten EN: A trial of ice therapy and experience in chronic arthritis. Physiotherapy 1969; 55:51–56.
195. Perry J: Contractures. A historical perspective. Clin Orthop 1987; 219:8–14.
196. Pincus T, Callahan LF: Remodelling the pyramid or remodelling paradigms concerning rheumatoid arthritis—Lessons from Hodgkin's disease and coronary artery disease (editorial). J Rheumatol 1990; 17:1582–1585.
197. Polly HF, Hunder GG: Rheumatologic Interviewing and Physical Examination of the Joints, ed 2. Philadelphia, WB Saunders, 1978, p 286.
198. Pope RO, Corcoran S, McCaul K, Howie DW: Continuous passive motion after primary total knee arthroplasty. Does it offer any benefits? J Bone Joint Surg Br 1997; 79:914–917.
199. Preston RL: The rehabilitation of the patient with rheumatoid arthritis. New York J Med 1955; 55:2887–2896.
200. Ramsey ML: Management of elbow arthritis. Sem Arthroplasty 1998; vol. 9.
201. Rejeski WJ, Brawley LR, Ettinger W, et al: Compliance to exercise therapy in older participants with knee osteoarthritis: Implications for treating disability. Med Sci Sports Exerc 1997; 29:977–985.
202. Riedy ME, Steen V, Nicholas JJ: Lower extremity amputation in scleroderma. Arch Phys Med Rehabil 1992; 23:811–813.
203. Ridgway CL, Daugherty MB, Warden GD: Serial casting as a technique to correct burn scar contractures: A case report. J Burn Care Rehabil 1991; 12:67–72.
204. Rissanen P, Aro S, Slätis P, et al: Health and quality of life before and after hip or knee arthroplasty. J Arthroplasty 1995; 10:169–175.
205. Romeo AA: Total shoulder arthroplasty: Pearls and pitfalls in surgical technique. Sem Arthroplasty 1995; 6:265–272.
206. Ropes MW: Conservative treatment in rheumatoid arthritis. Pub. no. 293, Robert W. Lovett Memorial Unit for the Study of Crippling Diseases, Harvard Medical School, Massachusetts General Hospital, 1960.
207. Rothacker DQ, Lee I, Littlejohn TW III: Effectiveness of a single topical application of 10% trolamine salicylate cream in the symptomatic treatment of osteoarthritis. J Clin Rheumatol 1998; 4:6–12.
208. Salvati EA, Wilson PD, Jolley MN, et al: A ten-year follow-up study of our first one hundred consecutive Charnley total hip replacements. J Bone Joint Surg Am 1981; 63:753–767.
209. Schnitzer TJ, Posner M, Lawrence ID: High strength capsaicin cream for osteoarthritis pain. J Clin Rheumatol 1995; 1:268–273.
210. Schulte KR, Callaghan JJ, Kelley SS, et al: The outcome of Charnley total hip arthroplasty with cement after a minimum twenty-year follow-up. The results of one surgeon. J Bone Joint Surg Am 1993; 75:961–975.
211. Scott WW Jr, Riley LH Jr, Dorfman HD: Focal lytic lesions associated with femoral stem loosening in total hip prosthesis. Am J Roentgenol 1985; 144:977–982.
212. Seegenschmiedt MH, Goldmann AR, Martus P, et al: Prophylactic radiation therapy for prevention of heterotopic ossification after hip arthroplasty: Results in 141 high-risk hips. Radiology 1993; 188:257–264.
213. Seeger MW, Furst DE: Effects of splinting in the treatment of hand contractures in progressive systemic sclerosis. Am J Occup Ther 1987; 41:118–121.
214. Shewring DJ, Beaudet M, Carvell JE: Reversed dynamic slings: Results of use in the treatment of post-traumatic flexion contractures of the elbow. Injury 1991; 22:400–402.
215. Spergel P, Ehrlich GE, Glass D: The rheumatoid arthritic personality. Psychosomatics 1978; 19:79–86.
216. Spiegel TM, Hirschberg J, Taylor J, et al: Heating rheumatoid knees to an intra-articular temperature of 42.1°C. Ann Rheum Dis 1987; 46:716–719.
217. Stecher RM, Karnash LJ: Herberden's nodes: VI. The effect of nerve injury upon formation of degenerative joint disease of the fingers. Am J Med Sci 1947; 213:181.
218. Steinbrocker O: Arthritis in Modern Practice. Philadelphia, WB Saunders, 1947, p 485.
219. Stern SH, Singer LB, Weissman SE: Analysis of hospital cost in total knee arthroplasty. Does length of stay matter? Clin Orthop 1995; 321:36–44.
220. Stitt FW, Frane M, Frane JW: Mood changes in rheumatoid arthritis: Factor analysis as a tool in clinical research. J Chronic Dis 1977; 30:135–145.
221. Sukenik S, Buskila D, Neumann L, et al: Sulphur bath and mud pack treatment for rheumatoid arthritis at the Dead Sea area. Ann Rheum Dis 1990; 49:99–102.
222. Swanson N: The prevention and correction of deformity in rheumatoid arthritis. Canad Med Assoc J 1956; 75:257–261.
223. Swinburn WR: Sexual counselling for the arthritic. Clin Rheum Dis 1976; 2:639–651.
224. Taylor P, Hallett M, Flaherty L: Treatment of osteoarthritis of the knee with transcutaneous electrical nerve stimulation. Pain 1981; 11:233–240.
225. Thompson J, Bywaters EGL: Unlimited rheumatoid arthritis following hemiplegia. Ann Rheum Dis 1962; 21:370.
226. Udelman HD, Udelman DL: Group therapy in rheumatoid arthritis patients. Am J Psychotherapy 1978; 32:288–299.

227. Udelman HD, Udelman D: Emotions in rheumatologic disorders. Am J Psychotherapy 1981; 35:576–587.
228. Vargo MM, Robinson LR, Nicholas JJ: Contralateral vs. ipsilateral cane use: Effects on muscles crossing the knee joint. Am J Phys Med Rehabil 1992; 71:170–176.
229. Veale D, Rogers W, Fitzgerald O: Classification of clinical subsets in psoriatic arthritis. Br J Rheumatol 1994; 33:133–138.
230. Verhagen AP, de Vet HC, de Bie RA, et al: Taking baths: The efficacy of balneotherapy in patients with arthritis. A systemic review. J Rheumatol 1997; 24:1964–1971.
231. Walker RH, Morris BA, Angulo DL, et al: Postoperative use of continuous passive motion, transcutaneous electrical nerve stimulation, and continuous cooling pad following total knee arthroplasty. J Arthroplasty 1991; 6:151–156.
232. Wasilewski SA, Woods LC, Torgerson WR Jr, et al: Value of continuous passive motion in total knee arthroplasty. Orthopedics 1990; 13:291–295.
233. Wasner C, Britton MC, Kraines RG, et al: Nonsteroidal anti-inflammatory agents in rheumatoid arthritis and ankylosing spondylitis. JAMA 1981; 246:2168–2172.
234. Weinberger A, Fadilah R, Lev A, et al: Treatment of articular effusions with local deep microwave hyperthermia. Clin Rheumatol 1989; 8:461–466.
235. Weinberger A, Fadilah R, Lev A, et al: Deep heat in the treatment of inflammatory joint disease. Med Hypotheses 1988; 25:231–233.
236. Weinberger A, Abramonvici A, Fadila R, et al: The effect of local deep microwave hyperthermia on experimental zymosan-induced arthritis in rabbits. Am J Phys Med Rehabil 1990; 69:239–244.
237. White JR, Sage J: Effects of a counterirritant on muscular distress in patients with arthritis. Phys Ther 1971; 51:36–42.
238. White JR: Effects of a counterirritant on perceived pain and hand movement in patients with arthritis. Phys Ther 1973; 53:956–960.
239. Wilson AJ, Monsees B, Blair VP III: Acetabular cup dislocation: A new complication of total joint arthroplasty. AJR 1988; 151:133–134.
240. Wright V: The treatment of rheumatoid arthritis. J Chron Dis 1963; 16:83–103.
241. Wright V, Hopkins R: Administration of antirheumatic drugs. Ann Rheum Dis 1978; 35:174.
242. Yashar AA, Venn-Watson E, Welsh T, et al: Continuous passive motion with accelerated flexion after total knee arthroplasty. Clin Orthop 1997; 345:38–43.
243. Yoshino S: Sexual problems of women with rheumatoid arthritis. Arch Phys Med Rehabil 1981; 62:122–123.
244. Zander CL, Healy NL: Elbow flexion contractures treated with serial casts and conservative therapy. J Hand Surg Am 1992; 17:694–697.
245. Zavadak KH, Gibson KR, Whitley DM, et al: Variability in the attainment of functional milestones during the acute care admission after total joint replacement. J Rheumatol 1995; 22:482–487.

37 CHAPTER

Francis P. Lagattuta, M.D., and Frank J. E. Falco, M.D.

Assessment and Treatment of Cervical Spine Disorders

Cervical spine disorders have been described since ancient times. The Papyrus written more than 5000 years ago by the Egyptian physician Imhoptep, of the Third Dynasty, describes cervical sprains and dislocations.[100] Hippocrates, who was born in 460 BCE, developed the cervical traction concept and recognized that vertebral injuries to the cervical spine could result in paralysis. The Greek physician Paul of Aeginia (625 to 690 CE) was the first to perform cervical laminectomies.[1] In the second century, Galen, the physician to the Roman emperor Marcus Aurelius, performed cervical surgery on gladiators.[113, 233] Galen separated the spinal cord at different cervical root levels and recorded the subsequent motor and sensory effects. In 1828 Alban Smith performed the first laminectomy in America.[211] The term "whiplash" was first introduced in 1928 by Crowe.[62]

Neck complaints are commonly encountered in clinical practice. The prevalence of neck pain with or without arm pain is approximately 13% of females and 9% of males in the general population.[139, 154] One out of every three individuals can recall an incident of neck pain at least once in their lifetime.[139] The occurrence is greater in the workplace, where 51% to 80% of laborers can recall an episode of neck and arm pain.[114, 116] The frequency of neck complaints increases with age in the workplace. In the 25 to 29 age group, 25% to 30% complain of neck stiffness and 5% to 10% complain of pain radiating into the upper limb. In those over 45 years of age, 50% complain of neck stiffness and 25% to 40% complain of pain radiating into the upper limb.[115] Overall, 45% of working men have experienced at least one episode of neck discomfort, 23% remember at least one episode of upper limb pain, and 51% complain of both symptoms.[115]

Chronic neck pain has a statistically significant correlation with previous neck, back, or shoulder injury; work-related mental distress; and physical stress.[154] Chronic neck pain is rare in those with a high education level, white-collar workers, and housewives.[154] There is no association between chronic neck pain and smoking.[154]

Conditions affecting the neck that can lead to pain and other associated symptoms are listed in Table 37–1. The history and physical examination are still the most important elements in making the diagnosis.[99] Recent advances in diagnostic testing have improved the clinician's ability to make the appropriate diagnosis, as well as determine the presence or absence of serious complications.

This chapter outlines the clinical evaluation and treatment of cervical spine disorders after a review of the cervical anatomy and biomechanics. A discussion of the most common cervical spine conditions encountered in clinical practice is also presented.

ANATOMY AND BIOMECHANICS

The cervical spine is a discrete part of the axial skeleton.[29, 30, 79, 110, 180] The neck is the most mobile portion of the spine and serves three major functions: (1) It supports and provides stability for the head; (2) it enables the head to move in all planes of motion; (3) it protects the structures that pass through it, specifically the spinal cord, nerve roots, and the vertebral artery. Restriction of these basic cervical spine functions by injury or disease can lead to impairment, disability, and handicap.

TABLE 37–1 Disorders Affecting the Neck

- Mechanical
  - Cervical sprain
  - Cervical strain
  - Herniated nucleus pulposus
  - Osteoarthritis
  - Cervical spondylosis
  - Cervical stenosis
- Rheumatologic
  - Ankylosing spondylitis
  - Reiter's syndrome
  - Psoriatic arthritis
  - Enteropathic arthritis
  - Rheumatoid arthritis
  - Diffuse idiopathic skeletal hyperostosis (DISH)
  - Polymyalgia rheumatica (PMR)
  - Fibrositis (fibromyalgia)
- Infectious
  - Vertebral osteomyelitis
  - Discitis
  - Herpes zoster
  - Infective endocarditis
  - Granulomatous process
  - Epidural, intradural, and subdural abscesses
  - Retropharyngeal abscess
  - Acquired immunodeficiency syndrome (AIDS)
- Endocrinological and metabolic
  - Osteoporosis
  - Osteomalacia
  - Parathyroid disease
  - Paget's disease
  - Pituitary disease
- Tumors
  - Benign tumors
    - Osteochondroma
    - Osteoid osteoma
    - Osteoblastoma
    - Giant cell tumor
    - Aneurysmal bone cyst
    - Hemangioma
    - Eosinophilic granuloma
    - Gaucher's disease
  - Malignant tumors
    - Multiple myeloma
    - Solitary plasmacytoma
    - Chondrosarcoma
    - Ewing's sarcoma
    - Chordoma
    - Lymphoma
    - Metastases
  - Extradural tumors
    - Epidural hemangioma
    - Epidural lipoma
    - Meningioma
    - Neurofibroma
    - Lymphoma
  - Intradural tumors
    - Extramedullary, intradural
      - Neurofibroma
      - Meningioma
      - Ependymoma
      - Sarcoma
    - Intramedullary
      - Ependymoma
      - Astrocytoma
  - Arteriovenous malformations
  - Syringomyelia

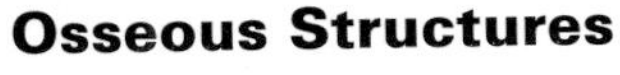

Osseous Structures

The cervical column is made up of seven vertebrae, which are divided into an upper (C1–C2) and lower (C3–C7) region (Fig. 37–1). There are distinct anatomical and functional differences between these two sections of vertebrae.[18]

The C1 (atlas) and C2 (axis) are considerably different from other vertebrae in the spinal column (Fig. 37–2). The atlas is a ring-like structure without a vertebral body. There are two lateral atlanto masses that articulate with the occipital condyles above and the axis below. The axis has a vertebral body, bifid spinous process, and an upward projecting odontoid process, which is the congenitally fused atlas body. The odontoid articulates with the anterior arch of the atlas. This normal relationship allows for less than 3 mm separation between the anterior arch and odontoid.[239] This joint can be weakened by trauma or by disease, such as rheumatoid arthritis.[20, 22, 24, 40, 41] A separation of 3 mm or more in flexion and extension is considered to be unstable and evidence of instability.[239]

The atlas and axis in combination with the cranial occiputs assist in flexion, extension, and rotation. The atlanto-occipital (CO–C1) articulation permits 10 degrees of flexion and 25 degrees of extension. The greatest amount of rotation in the cervical spine occurs at the C1–C2 joint with 45 degrees of rotation in either direction. A few degrees of flexion-extension are also seen at the C1–C2 joint.[72, 73, 74] A true synovial joint is located between the lateral masses of the atlas and axis between the interior arch of the atlas and odontoid process.

The lower cervical region vertebrae are similar to one another in shape and function (Fig. 37–3). The C3–C7 vertebrae have small bodies, with the longest dimension

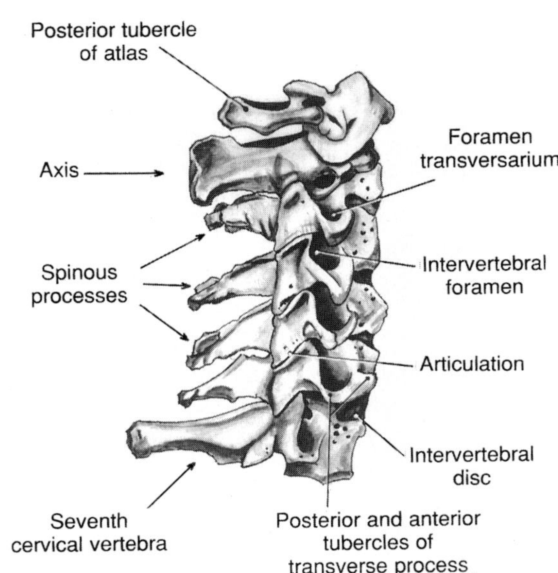

FIGURE 37–1. Lateral view of the cervical spine. (From Crafts RC: Textbook of Human Anatomy, ed 2. New York, John Wiley & Sons, 1979. Reprinted by permission of John Wiley & Sons, Inc.)

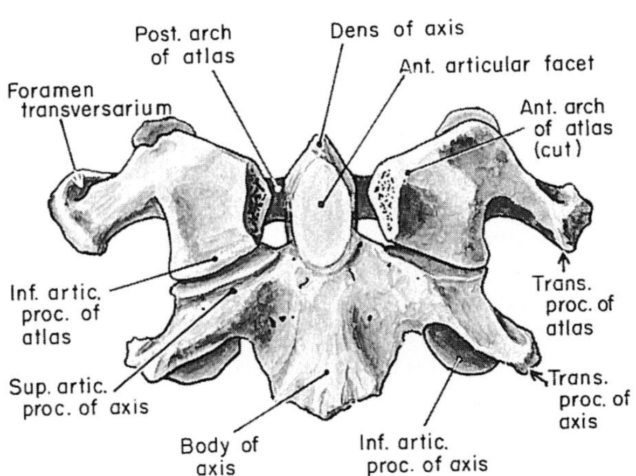

FIGURE 37–2. Anterior view of the atlas and axis. The anterior tubercle of the atlas has been removed to reveal the odontoid process of the axis. (From Crafts RC: Textbook of Human Anatomy, ed 2. New York, John Wiley & Sons, 1979. Reprinted by permission of John Wiley & Sons, Inc.)

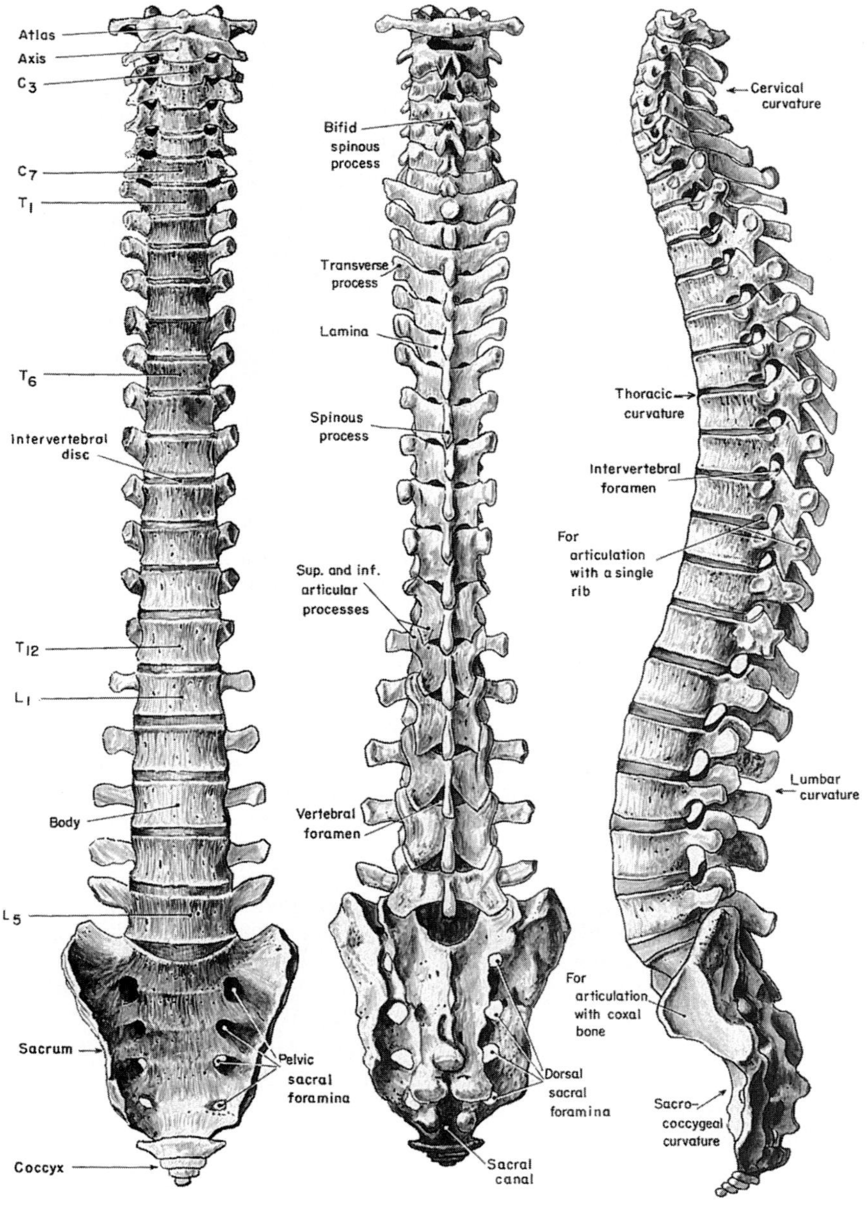

FIGURE 37–3. Anterior, posterior, and lateral views of the entire human spine. (From Crafts RC: Textbook of Human Anatomy, ed 2. New York, John Wiley & Sons, 1979. Reprinted by permission of John Wiley & Sons, Inc.)

in the coronal plane. The spinous processes are bifid from C3–C6, and C7 has the longest process, which is easily palpable on examination in most individuals. The cervical zygapophyseal joints are more concave than convex, as compared to the thoracic and lumbar spines.[71] Cervical facet orientation is at 45 degrees, rather than the 60 degrees in the thoracic spine or the 90 degrees in the lumbar spine. The spinous processes, transverse processes, and lamina serve as areas for muscle attachments.

At the C2–C3 junction there is a change in the shape of the articulating joints, permitting a distinct difference in function. This is a transitional area for the cervical spine, where the permitted motion changes from rotation to flexion, extension, and lateral bending. There is approximately 10 degrees of flexion per segment, with the greatest amount of flexion occurring at C4–C5 and C5–C6.[86, 143] Lateral bending occurs primarily at C3–C4 and C4–C5. Horizontal displacement of the vertebrae during flexion and extension greater than 3.5 mm or angular deformity greater than 11 degrees indicates spinal instability.[239]

All cervical spine motions are coupled such that rotation is associated with lateral bending and vice versa. Restriction of range of motion in a particular plane helps the clinician determine which segment is involved

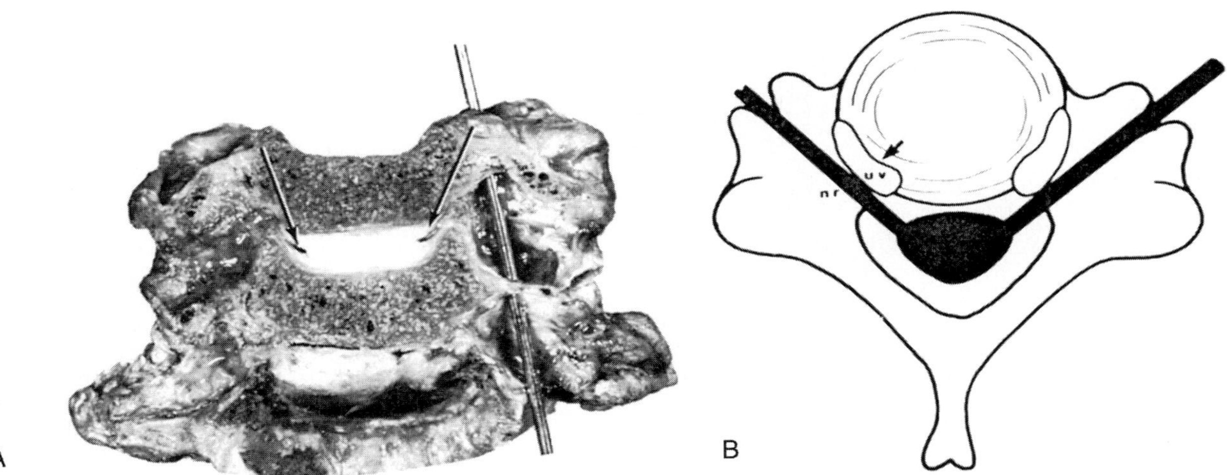

FIGURE 37–4. Luschka's (uncovertebral) joints. *A.* Coronal dissection of cervical spine displaying Luschka's joints (*arrows*). *B.* Proximity of uncovertebral joints to cervical nerve roots. (*A* from Parke WW: Applied anatomy of the spine. In Rothman RH, Simone FA (eds): The Spine, ed 3. Philadelphia, WB Saunders, 1992. *B* from Macnab I, McCulloch J: Neck Ache and Shoulder Pain. Baltimore, Williams & Wilkins, 1994.)

and especially whether it is in the upper or lower cervical spine.

The lower cervical vertebrae (C3–C7) have unique articulations called uncovertebral joints, which are also known as joints of Luschka or neurocentral joints[57–59] (Fig. 37–4). They arise from the posterolateral margins of the vertebral bodies and lie anterior to the exiting nerve roots. These joints are not present at birth, but develop by the end of the first decade. Although the distinction is controversial, these "joints" are not considered true joints since they do not possess synovium.[105, 177, 182] The uncovertebral articulations are thought to develop from degenerative clefts or from fibrous tissue resorption within the supraposterolateral margins.[105, 177, 182] These articulations can degenerate by undergoing hypertrophy and calcification with associated disc degeneration. This process can ultimately lead to encroachment on the intervertebral canal, causing nerve root or even spinal cord compression.

Soft Tissue Structures

Intervertebral discs are located in the cervical spine between the C2 through T1 vertebrae. There is no disc between C1 and C2, and only the ligaments and joint capsules resist excessive motion.[42] The intervertebral discs provide shock absorption, accommodate movement, and separate the vertebral bodies to give height to the intervertebral foramina. The disc is made up of the eccentrically located nucleus pulposus and the surrounding annulus fibrosus (Fig. 37–5). Intervertebral disc degenerative changes and/or herniation can lead to spinal cord or nerve root injury.

There are several ligaments found at each vertebral level that give strength and stability to the cervical spine (Fig. 37–6). The transverse, alar, and accessory atlantoaxial ligaments help maintain the integrity of the odontoid and C1 articulation. The anterior (ALL) and posterior longitudinal ligaments (PLL) run along the anterior and posterior surfaces of the vertebrae and discs, providing stability during flexion and extension. The PLL also reinforces the posterior annulus. The facet capsule ligaments, supraspinous, interspinous, and ligamentum flavum ligaments provide flexion stability. The ligamentum nuchae spans from the occiput to the C7 spinous process and adds support to the posterior neck.

The neck muscles give support and provide movement for the cervical spine and the head. The musculature can functionally be divided into the anterior flexors and the posterior extensors. The posterior muscles are

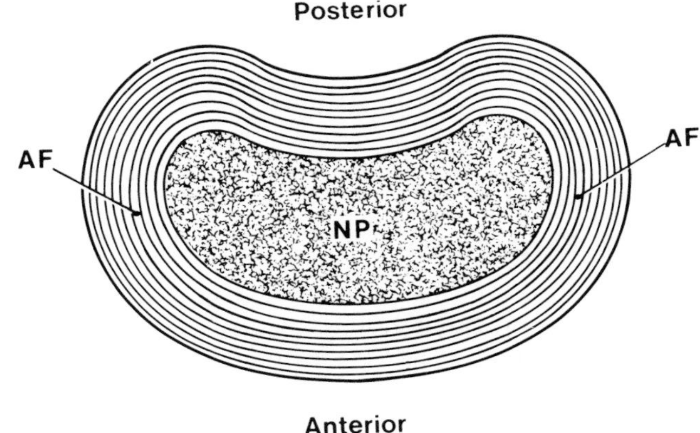

FIGURE 37–5. Structural components of the intervertebral disc. NP, nucleus pulposus; AF, annulus fibrosus. (From Bogduk N, Twomey LT: Clinical Anatomy of the Lumbar Spine. New York, Churchill Livingstone, 1988.)

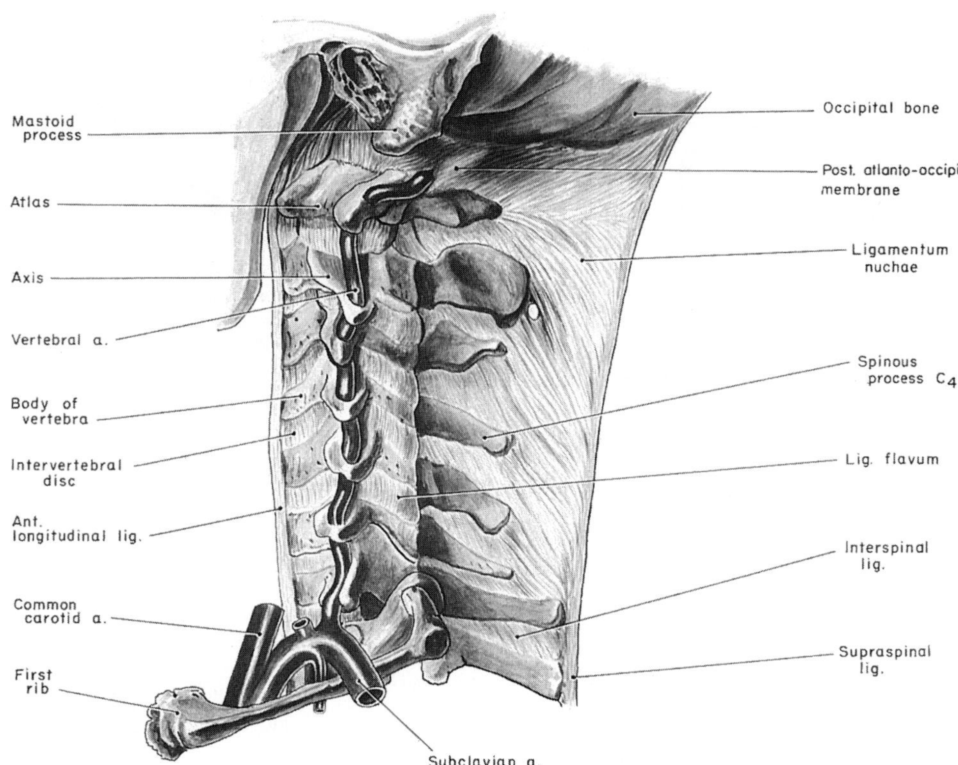

FIGURE 37–6. Anatomical relationship of cervical spine ligaments to other structures in the neck. (From Crafts RC: Textbook of Human Anatomy, ed 2. New York, John Wiley & Sons, 1979, p 55. Reprinted by permission of John Wiley & Sons, Inc.)

arranged with the longer groups superficial and the shorter groups closest to the vertebral column. For example, the iliocostalis and longissimus muscles span many vertebral levels and are superficial, whereas the deeply located short cervical rotators pass from only one vertebra to the next. These muscles produce extension of the spine and/or head when contracting bilaterally, or rotation when acting ipsilaterally. The anteriorly placed scalene and sternocleidomastoid muscles are important flexors and additional rotators of the neck and/or head.

Some of the extrinsic shoulder muscles such as the trapezius, rhomboid, levator scapulae, and latissimus dorsi muscles have attachments to the cervical spine. An injury to these structures can lead to neck pain because of this anatomical relationship.[135]

Neural Structures

The spinal cord begins at the foramen magnum and extends to approximately the L2 vertebral level. The spinal cord is about 10 mm in diameter and the vertebral canal averages 17 mm in sagittal diameter.[34, 179] The spinal canal is the widest at C3–C5, and rapidly decreases in size to a small circular lumen throughout the thoracic area. In the cervical region, the transverse diameter of the spinal canal is almost twice that of the anteroposterior diameter. As a result of this, the spinal cord has ample room to expand laterally, but has considerably less room in the anteroposterior direction.

The union of the ventral motor and dorsal sensory roots (Fig. 37–7) forms spinal nerves. All of the cervical nerves contain motor and sensory fibers except for the C1 nerve, which has only motor fibers. The first cervical nerve emerges from the vertebral canal at the atlanto-occipital junction, while the eighth nerve exits between the seventh cervical and the first thoracic vertebrae. In the cervical spine below C2, the segmental nerves progress from the entrance of the thecal sac to the tubercles of the transverse process. The cervical nerves run over the upper border of the pedicles and slope laterally and anteroinferiorly along the upper surface of the transverse process. Cervical spinal nerves exit through the root canals, dividing into anterior and posterior rami. The anterior rami supply the prevertebral and paravertebral muscles, and form the brachial plexus to provide innervation for the upper limbs. The posterior rami divide into muscular, cutaneous, and articular branches for the posterior neck structures, including the postvertebral muscles.

The cervical intervertebral discs receive innervation to the outer third of the annulus anteriorly, posteriorly, and laterally (Fig. 37–8).[33] The disc receives branches anteriorly from the vertebral nerve which accompanies the vertebral artery. The vertebral nerve is derived from the gray rami communicans of the sympathetic trunk at midcervical levels, and branches of the stellate ganglion at lower cervical levels. Posterolateral innervation is provided by the sinuvertebral nerve, also known as the recurrent nerve of Luschka, which is formed by a branch

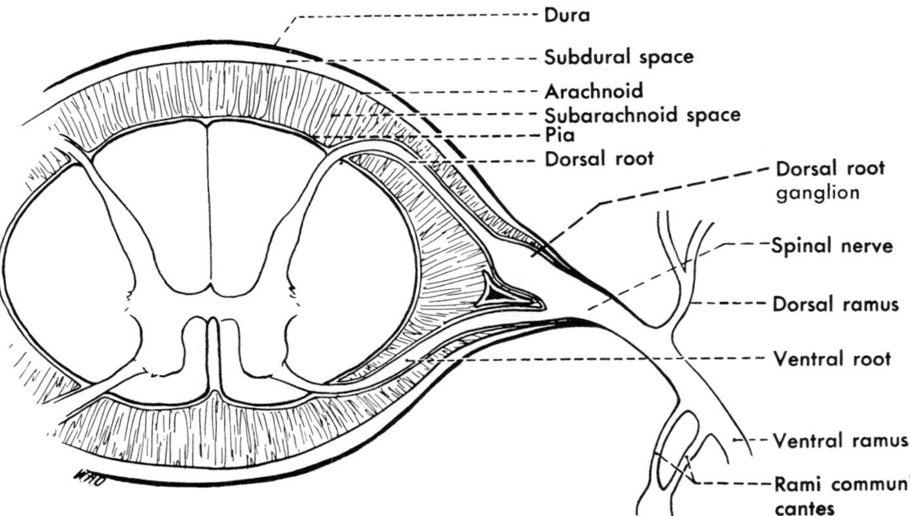

FIGURE 37–7. Formation of spinal nerves from the spinal cord. (From Hollinshead WH, Jenkins DB: Functional Anatomy of the Limbs and Back, ed 5. Philadelphia, WB Saunders, 1981, p 218.)

of the vertebral nerve and ventral ramus at each level. The sinuvertebral nerve supplies the posterior segmental disc and the disc above, as well as innervating the posterior longitudinal ligament, pedicle, posterior vertebral periosteum, epidural veins, and dorsal dura mater.

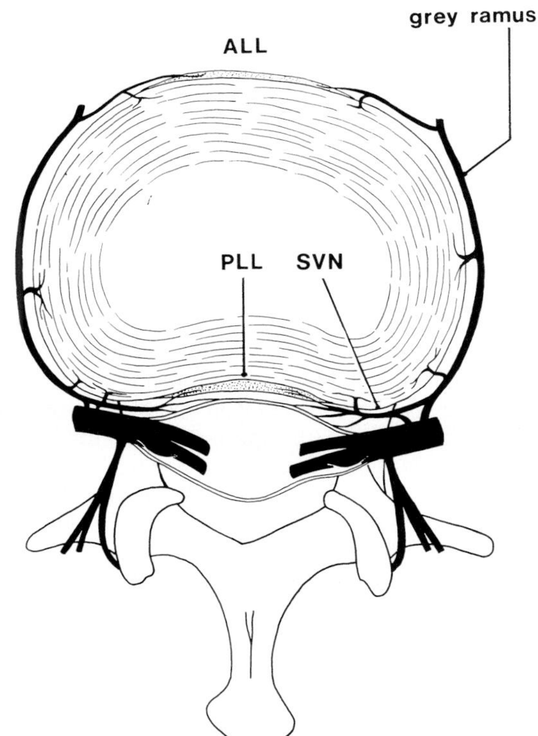

FIGURE 37–8. Nerve supply of the cervical intervertebral disc. PLL, posterior longitudinal ligament; ALL, anterior longitudinal ligament; SVN, sinovertebral nerve. (From Bogduk N, Twomey LT: Clinical Anatomy of the Lumbar Spine. New York, Churchill Livingstone, 1991, p 117.)

The cervical zygapophyseal joints are innervated by the medial branches from the posterior cervical rami. The joints from C3–C4 to C6–C7 are supplied by the medial branches that run above and below the joints.[22, 46, 141] The medial branch of the C3 dorsal ramus, which is the third occipital nerve, innervates the C2–C3 joints.[22, 46, 141] The atlanto-occipital and atlantoaxial joints are respectively supplied by the C1 and C2 ventral rami.[21, 22, 141]

Pain Generators

Many structures in the neck can be potential pain generators. Pain can also be referred to the neck from other structures such as the upper limbs. Identification of the nociceptive site is important in order to make the correct diagnosis and plan the appropriate treatment.

Any structure that receives innervation can be a potential pain generator. Injury or compromise of the cervical nerves can cause radicular pain as well as weakness and sensory loss. Nerve injuries can be due to a disc herniation, an uncovertebral joint impingement, brachial plexopathy, tumor, hematoma, infection, and metabolic or direct trauma.[134] Radicular symptoms include pain into the shoulder and beyond, sensory loss, paresthesias, and weakness.[31, 35, 83, 84, 222] There can also be injuries to the sympathetic nerves, which may precipitate disorders such as fibromyalgia.[92, 229] Specific peripheral nerves can be injured, an example being an injury to the occipital nerve producing occipital neuralgia with headaches.[21, 136, 178]

The cervical vertebrae can also be nociceptive sources. This can be seen with cervical zygapophyseal joint injury secondary to a fracture, from trauma, or from osteoporosis with microscopic fractures.[18, 22, 24, 28, 148, 202, 207] Pain can originate solely from the intervertebral disc if there is disruption of the outer annular fibers.[23, 33, 50, 240]

Cervical muscles and ligaments are also potential sources of pain. The musculature can generate pain when injured from direct trauma or from the relatively common traumatic flexion-extension injuries ("whiplash").[83, 84, 119] The highly innervated ligaments can be stretched or even torn during flexion-extension injuries, resulting in pain.[68, 216, 221, 238]

HISTORY

The history of a patient with neck pain should have the usual format: chief complaint; history of the present illness; review of past medical and pharmacological history; family, social, functional, and occupational histories; and review of organ systems (see Chapter 1). As with most illnesses, the history provides more information about the underlying condition than any other single part of the evaluation.

Chief Complaint

Cervical conditions can present with a chief complaint involving the neck or the upper limb. An individual might complain of upper limb pain, numbness, or weakness. There can be similar symptoms involving the lower limbs. The patient can have headaches, visual disturbances, dizziness, or jaw pain. Difficulty in performing activities of daily living, bladder dysfunction, or bowel incontinence can also be the presenting concern.

History of Present Illness

The history is used to generate a differential diagnosis from a chronological account of the current disorder. Potential conditions leading to neck pain are then included or excluded with subsequent history, and later confirmed with physical examination and/or diagnostic testing. The clinician attempts to identify the nociceptive site and determine whether there is a serious neurologic problem.[225–228] This information has a significant impact on the initial management and timing of diagnostic testing.

The onset, duration, origin, and distribution of symptoms, as well as the mechanism of injury, can provide significant clues to the pathophysiology of the disorder. For example, acute onset of localized posterior neck pain after a motor vehicle accident without neurologic symptoms is most indicative of musculoligamentous or posterior element injury. An insidious onset of slowly progressive symptoms might indicate the presence of an expanding mass or development of a systemic disease process. On the other hand, subacute onset of neck pain with discretely referred arm pain in a laborer after years of repetitive lifting is consistent with cervical radiculopathy.

Documentation of modifying activities can give additional diagnostic information. For example, the aggravation of neck and upper limb symptoms by lifting, sneezing, and/or coughing typically implies the presence of a disc abnormality. Radicular symptoms from foramenal stenosis usually intensify with positions that further reduce foramenal size, such as cervical extension.

The temporal relationship of symptoms also helps identify the cervical condition. For example, neck discomfort that is worse at the end of the day in an elderly individual, suggests a degenerative process. Pain that is worse at night is often suggestive of malignancy. The presence of constitutional symptoms is very important when considering malignancy or infection.

There are many neurologic symptoms associated with cervical pathology that seem unrelated to the neck, including headaches,[118] dizziness, nausea, vomiting, upper limb paresthesias, concentration difficulties, memory disturbances, and weakness. These are important details of the history, which should not be overlooked by the clinician. Limb weakness, bowel dysfunction, and bladder incontinence can indicate serious neurological compromise, which warrants aggressive evaluation and treatment.

Previous neck injuries or problems need to be documented and compared to the current disorder. This is especially important when dealing with a personal or work-related injury. The presence or absence of litigation should be noted, since this has been shown to have a bearing on treatment and outcome.[7, 37, 96]

Past Medical History

The main purpose of the past medical history is to determine the presence of an existing disease process or prior surgical procedure that might have contributed to the present neck complaints or that could affect treatment. Any history of a rheumatologic, metabolic, endocrine, or oncologic process needs to be investigated as a possible cause of neck pain. Prior cervical surgery, such as a fusion, raises important issues such as fusion integrity and stability, as well as work limitations and treatment precautions. The presence of general medical conditions such as diabetes, chronic obstructive pulmonary disease, coronary artery disease, depression, or other mental disorders needs to be documented because of their potential impact on therapy and recovery. Information that can affect the prescription of medication is listed, including drug allergies or sensitivities, present medications, and gastrointestinal intolerance.

Social History

The patient's personal life, childhood experiences, social status, and cultural background all influence treatment and outcome. Stress—disruption in the tranquility of home life, marital strife, disciplinary problems with children, occupational pressures—has been shown to affect recovery.[188, 229] Financial difficulties can limit treatment options or motivate conscious malingering. The custodial care of elderly parents, loss of parents, or molestation as a child can lay down psychological barriers to successful treatment of any type.[203] Cultural differences have been linked to pain tolerance.[15, 188, 214, 248, 249] Use of tobacco can lead to disc degeneration, presumably by affecting nutrient transport.[128, 160] Tobacco has also been associated with poor operative outcome and a decreased response to therapeutic epidural injections.[102, 111, 213] Alcohol and drug abuse have been linked to a poor treatment outcome, as well as to having a greater risk for medication dependency and addiction.[163, 186, 187] Elaboration on hobbies might identify recreational activities that should be avoided while treating the cervical disorder.

Family/Occupational/Functional History

The clinician needs to be aware of any family history of diabetes, disability, rheumatological disorders, cancer, neck pain, psychological illness, or fibromyalgia. This information is important in determining the differential diagnosis. A family tradition of pain and disability can adversely affect treatment and outcome.

The current employment status is important information especially in work-related injuries. Knowledge of the individual's job requirements and responsibilities and an understanding of the work environment enable the physician to appropriately determine work status and applicable restrictions. The ergonomics of the job, such as static positioning and overuse, are important factors regarding employment. Other nonphysical factors related to work also have an impact on the clinical condition. For example, an uncertain employment status and a poor perception of job security have been shown to be risk factors for pain—as much so as heavy lifting.[5, 16, 64] While the cited studies were for back pain, they appear no less relevant for neck pain.

The person's quality of life with the cervical disorder can be evaluated by determining if there are any restrictions on social activities or limitations on activities of daily living (ADL). Treatment and outcome goals are then modified for each person to progress toward a return to prior recreational activities and to achieve independence in ADL.

Review of Organ Systems

The review of systems should be similar to that for any patient, but certain aspects need to be emphasized in patients with cervical disorders. Bowel and bladder function, difficulty sleeping, psychological problems, extremity weakness, recent weight loss, and night sweats are all important indicators. A previous history of peptic ulcer disease, renal insufficiency, or liver dysfunction is critical information to have before prescribing certain medications. The clinician should inquire about any systemic or metabolic problem that could be causing the neck pain either primarily or secondarily.

Pain Diagrams

The history is often supplemented with pain diagrams that the patient completes after instruction. The visual analog scale (VAS) and pain drawing can provide useful information to the clinician (Fig. 37–9). The VAS quantifies pain intensity by placing a point on a line that represents a continuum of pain from none to incapacitating.[117] The completed pain drawing can reveal characteristic symptom patterns consistent for particular disorders and give information regarding the patient's psychological status.[169, 189]

PHYSICAL EXAMINATION

The patient is asked to identify any neurologic deficit and to locate the pain generator site. The examination typically includes observation and inspection, range of motion (ROM), neurologic evaluation, palpation, and provocative maneuvers.

Observation/Inspection

The examination begins as soon as there is patient contact. Gait, facial expressions, and body language are noted during the evaluation. These observations help identify pain behaviors and body mechanics. The neck is inspected for masses, such as from adenopathy or goiter, surgical scars, erythema, lesions, or any skin aberrations. The presence of abnormal cervical positioning is recorded, such as forward posturing, absent cervical lordosis, kyphosis, or listing.

Range of Motion

The evaluation of cervical range of motion includes flexion, extension, rotation, and lateral bending. An inclinometer method is currently the most reliable for documenting ROM.[131, 230] Normal range of motion of the neck is 60 degrees of flexion, 75 degrees of extension, 45 degrees of lateral flexion, and 80 degrees of rotation (Table 37–2).[143] Clinical evaluation of ROM can be done without an inclinometer. The patient with normal neck ROM is able to rest the chin on the chest, look straight up at the ceiling, touch each ear to the shoulder, and tap the chin against each shoulder. Patients accomplishing these movements have normal range of motion. These ROM tests are reliable only if the patient does not move the shoulders, the rest of the spine, or the hips.[131]

The cervical spine is assessed for both active and passive ROM. The patient is asked to actively move the neck and then the examiner gently tries to passively increase the range. The neck should not be forced into a nonphysiological or painful range that can cause an increase in symptomatology. Range-or-motion testing is contraindicated in the presence of spinal instability. The lack of active motion can be secondary to pain or muscle guarding. Decreased active and passive ROM can be secondary to spondylosis or ankylosis.

Shoulder ROM testing is included in cervical spine evaluations to detect any loss that may affect cervical spine function. Disorders such as adhesive capsulitis, rotator cuff tendonitis, or shoulder impingement often lead to decreased passive and active shoulder range of motion, which leads to altered biomechanics and increased mechanical stress to cervical spine structures.

Neurologic Evaluation

The neurologic examination involves testing of the peripheral and central nervous system to determine the presence or absence of neurologic deficits. Strength, muscle stretch reflexes, sensation, and reflex tests for upper motor neuron lesions are performed on every patient presenting with neck problems.

The motor examination can determine the presence of a root, trunk, or peripheral nerve injury when there is involvement of motor fibers. Knowledge of the peripheral nervous system and upper limb innervation patterns allows for localization by eliciting muscle weakness

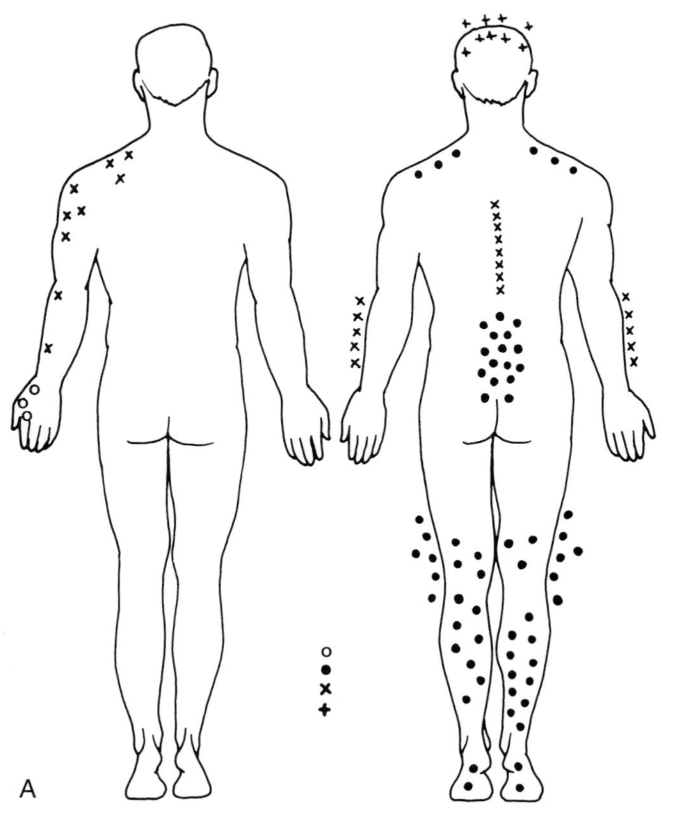

No pain — Severe pain

B

FIGURE 37–9. Pain diagrams. *A.* Pain drawing. Pain drawing on *left* represents an organic cervical radicular syndrome. Pain drawing on *right* is a diffuse nonorganic pain reaction. *Open circle:* tingling; *solid circle:* burning; *times sign:* pain; *plus sign:* numbness. *B.* Visual analog scale. The patient is instructed to place a mark on the line that represents the intensity of the pain. (*A* and *B* from Macnab I, McCulloch J: Neck Ache and Shoulder Pain. Baltimore, Williams & Wilkins, 1994, p 138.)

in a root or peripheral nerve distribution (Table 37–3). Neck strength is tested in flexion, extension, and rotation to detect neck weakness that is typically present in myasthenia gravis, myopathy, and some rheumatologic conditions.

Reflex testing is useful in evaluating nerve root function and in localizing the lesion. While any level of reflex amplitude can be normal, hyporeflexia is consistent with lesions at the root level, plexus, or peripheral nerve. Hyperreflexia is more associated with lesions from the

TABLE 37–2 Cervical Spine Range of Motion at Each Segmental Level

	Combined Flexion/Extension (± x-axis rotation)		*One-Side Lateral Bending (z-axis rotation)*		*One-Side Axial Rotation (y-axis rotation)*	
Interspace	**Limits of Ranges (degrees)**	**Representative Angle (degrees)**	**Limits of Ranges (degrees)**	**Representative Angle (degrees)**	**Limits of Ranges (degrees)**	**Representative Angle (degrees)**
Middle						
C2–C3	5–16	10	11–20	10	0–10	3
C3–C4	7–26	15	9–15	11	3–10	7
C4–C5	13–29	20	0–16	11	1–12	7
Lower						
C5–C6	13–29	20	0–16	8	2–12	7
C6–C7	6–26	17	0–17	7	2–10	6
C7–T1	4–7	9	0–17	4	0–7	2

From White AA, Panjabi MM: Biomechanics of the Spine, ed 2. Philadelphia, JB Lippincott, 1990, p 98.

TABLE 37–3 Nerve Root Levels, Peripheral Nerves, and Muscles of the Upper Limb Commonly Evaluated in the Patient with Neck Pain

Nerve Root Level	Nerve	Muscle
C5, C6	Axillary	Deltoid
C5, C6	Musculocutaneous	Biceps brachii
C5, C6	Suprascapular	Supraspinatus
	Suprascapular	Infraspinatus
C7	Radial	Triceps
	Median	Pronator teres
C8, T1	Median	Abductor pollicis brevis
	Ulnar	First dorsal interrossei

brain to the spinal cord. Hyporeflexia and hyperreflexia can be present together if the lesion involves both the central and peripheral nervous system. Asymmetric hyporeflexia at a specific root level is typical of unilateral radiculopathy, whereas generalized symmetric hyperreflexia with long tract signs is consistent with a myelopathic process.

When assessing an upper limb reflex, it is important that the correct reflex be elicited and not an inverted reflex. An inverted reflex can occur, for example, if there is a large disc herniation. This could result in elbow flexion rather than extension when checking for the triceps reflex. The unwary clinician might note this as a normal reflex. Actually, the stimulus from the reflex at the C7 level is blocked and travels cephalad one level to produce a biceps response.[156] This often indicates a more serious problem of myelopathy, in addition to a concurrent C7 radiculopathy.

Another significant point about muscle stretch reflex testing is that it must be established whether a decrease in the reflex really represents a diminution. For example, a tense patient might not be able to relax, resulting in a diminished or absent reflex. Reflexes should be obtained carefully and repeated with and without facilitation. Facilitation in the upper limbs, similar to Jendrassik's maneuver for the lower limbs, is best done by asking the patient to tense muscles outside the limb. The patient can bite down hard, squeeze the knees together, or make a fist with the opposite hand. The reflex examination should include attempts to elicit pathological reflexes which typically include the Babinski and Hoffmann tests. These testing methods are conducted to assess the integrity of the long tracts within the central nervous system. The presence of these superficial reflexes is suggestive of a central nervous system lesion such as a central cervical disc herniation, cervical spinal stenosis, or other pathology resulting in myelopathy.

The sensory exam is designed to test the competence of the dorsal roots. Figure 37–10 shows the classic dermatomal pattern of the upper limbs. Pain, tested by pinprick, is usually the last sensory modality to be decreased and is not the most sensitive indication of sensory loss.[93] Vibration fibers are affected more often than the smaller pain fibers in a radiculopathy. Position sense is also likely to be abnormal before pain sensation. Although pain testing is more convenient, vibratory and position sense testing are likely to be the first involved in a radiculopathy.[93] The only problem with vibration is that it cannot be well localized to one dermatome. Specific patterns of sensory change must be documented and assessed to see whether or not these changes actually follow a dermatomal pattern. Cervical spine soft tissues also refer pain and unusual sensations into the limbs.[24, 119] These "sclerotomal" symptoms should not be confused with actual dermatomal sensory loss. Sensa-

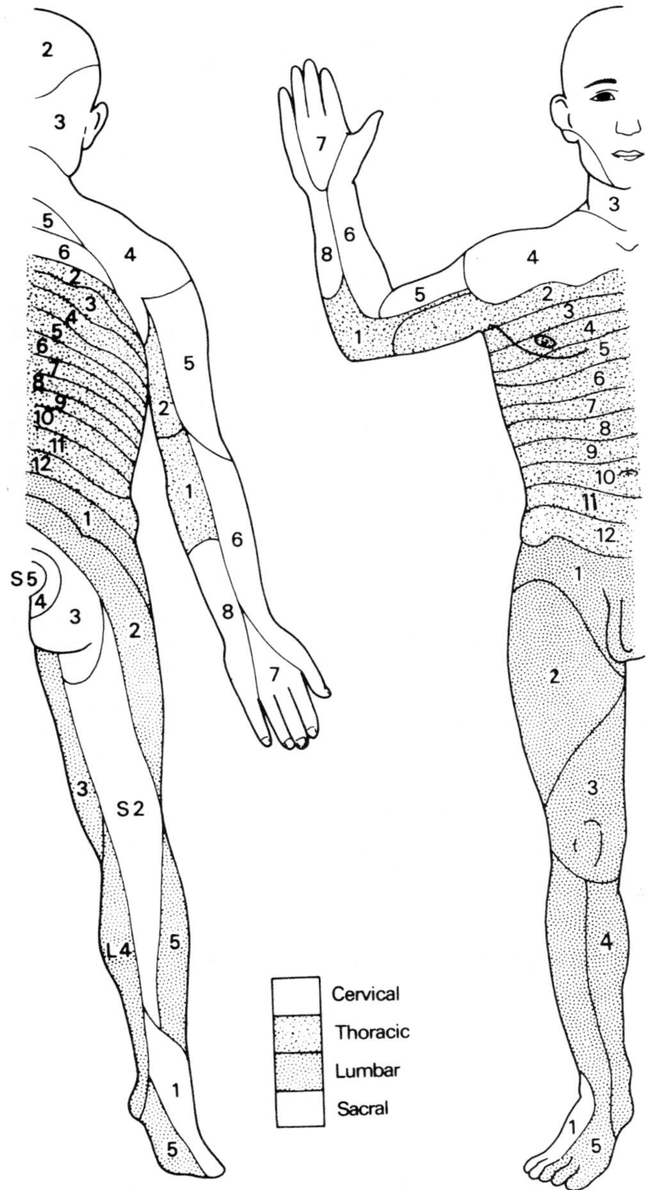

FIGURE 37–10. Dermatomal distribution of the cervical nerve roots. (From Ellis H: Clinical Anatomy: A Revision and Applied Anatomy for Clinical Students, ed 6. London, Blackwell, 1976, p 205.)

tions referred by sclerotomal sources do not actually produce real sensory deficit.

A cranial nerve evaluation is incorporated in the neurologic assessment of patients with cervical spine disorders. Cranial nerve injuries can be associated with traumatic or nontraumatic cervical spine conditions. Barrd-Lieou syndrome is a condition associated with cervical spine hyperextension injuries to the vertebral artery, cervical sympathetic chain, or brainstem nuclei, leading to symptoms such as tinnitus, facial numbness, aphonia, hoarseness, vertigo, ocular pain, and blurry vision.[220]

Palpatory Examination

Palpation of the osseous structures of the anterior aspect of the neck should include the hyoid bone and the thyroid cartilage. The hyoid bone should move from side to side as the patient swallows. The carotid tubercles of C6 can be palpated and they are important structures used to identify cervical ganglion sites for sympathetic blocks. The posterior osseous structures of the neck are examined by palpating the occiput, inion, superior nuchal line, mastoid processes, zygapophyseal joints, and the spinous processes. These structures are palpated to identify any painful sites. Cervical spine osseous structures such as the facet joints and the spinous processes can be palpated during motion to identify dysfunction in movement, especially in non-obese patients.

Soft tissue palpation is an important part of the cervical spine examination. The cervical and shoulder musculature are evaluated to identify trigger/tender points that can cause muscular-related referred headache and upper extremity pain patterns.[229] Tenderness of the ligamentum nuchae often indicates a stretched ligament resulting from a neck flexion or direct injury. Lymph nodes in the region of the sternocleidomastoid can indicate infection in the oropharynx or upper respiratory tract. The consistency and size of the thyroid and parotid glands are evaluated to assess for any abnormalities. The greater occipital nerves are commonly affected in flexion/extension injuries, resulting in occipital neuralgia with occipital headaches.[136] Palpation of the nerves commonly causes an increase in the patient's headache, if it is due to occipital neuralgia. The greater occipital nerves are located at one third of the distance from the occipital protuberance to the ipsilateral mastoid process.[38]

Provocative Maneuvers

The Spurling test looks for foramenal encroachment on an inflamed cervical nerve root. The patient's head is extended, laterally flexed, and held down for up to one minute.[40, 41, 151] The sign is present if there is increased symptomatology into the shoulder and hand in a radicular pattern.

Lhermitte's sign was first described in patients with multiple sclerosis. It is elicited by briskly flexing the patient's neck.[151] Electric-like pain or shock sensations shooting down through the spine as a result of this maneuver are often indicative of spinal cord pathology. This sign is also positive in some patients with herniated cervical discs.

Adson's maneuver is a test for neurovascular compromise due to a thoracic outlet problem from a cervical rib or a tight scalenus anterior medius muscle.[151] The symptomatic arm is placed in extension and lateral rotation. The radial pulse is monitored as the patient takes a deep breath and turns the head toward the ipsilateral side. The presence of subclavian artery compression is confirmed if there is a marked diminution or absence of the radial pulse. This test is sensitive but not very specific, resulting in many false positives.

Cervical spine pathology can cause difficulty with swallowing. The swallowing test assesses the patient's ability to swallow normally on command. Swallowing dysfunction can be secondary to protruding osteophytes, soft tissue swelling from hematomas, infection, or tumors located in the anterior portion of the cervical spine. (See Chapter 26 for more information on swallowing dysfunction.)

DIAGNOSTIC STUDIES

Imaging is an important asset in the evaluation and treatment of cervical spine problems. The clinician should remember that imaging techniques evaluate anatomy rather than physiology or function. Imaging has the inherent problem of false positive or negative results. In Boden's cervical magnetic resonance (MR) study, nearly 20% of asymptomatic individuals had demonstrable abnormalities.[17] The physician needs to interpret diagnostic studies only in the context of each clinical case (see Chapter 7).

Plain films provide useful information in evaluating the cervical spine for chronic degenerative changes, metastatic disease, infection, spinal deformity, and stability. Cervical spine films in trauma cases typically incorporate seven views, including anterior-posterior (AP), lateral, bilateral obliques, open-mouth, flexion, and extension views (Fig. 37–11). Flexion-extension views can help identify subluxation or cervical spine instability.[181] An open-mouth view is important in evaluating the status of the odontoid process and instability between the first two cervical vertebrae (Fig. 37–12). The AP view helps in the evaluation of the spine for tumors, osteophytes, and fractures. The lateral views check for stability as well as for signs of spondylosis including spurring and disc space narrowing (Fig. 37–13). The oblique views are necessary for evaluating degenerative disc disease and foramenal encroachment by osteophytes of uncovertebral joints or the facet joints (Fig. 37–14).[164, 195]

Computed Tomography (CT)–Myelography

The CT scan and myelogram individually or in combination continue to be important diagnostic studies in the evaluation of cervical spine problems. The CT scan is particularly helpful when a fracture of the cervical spine is suspected. One advantage of helical or spiral CT over conventional CT scanning is the infinite number of im-

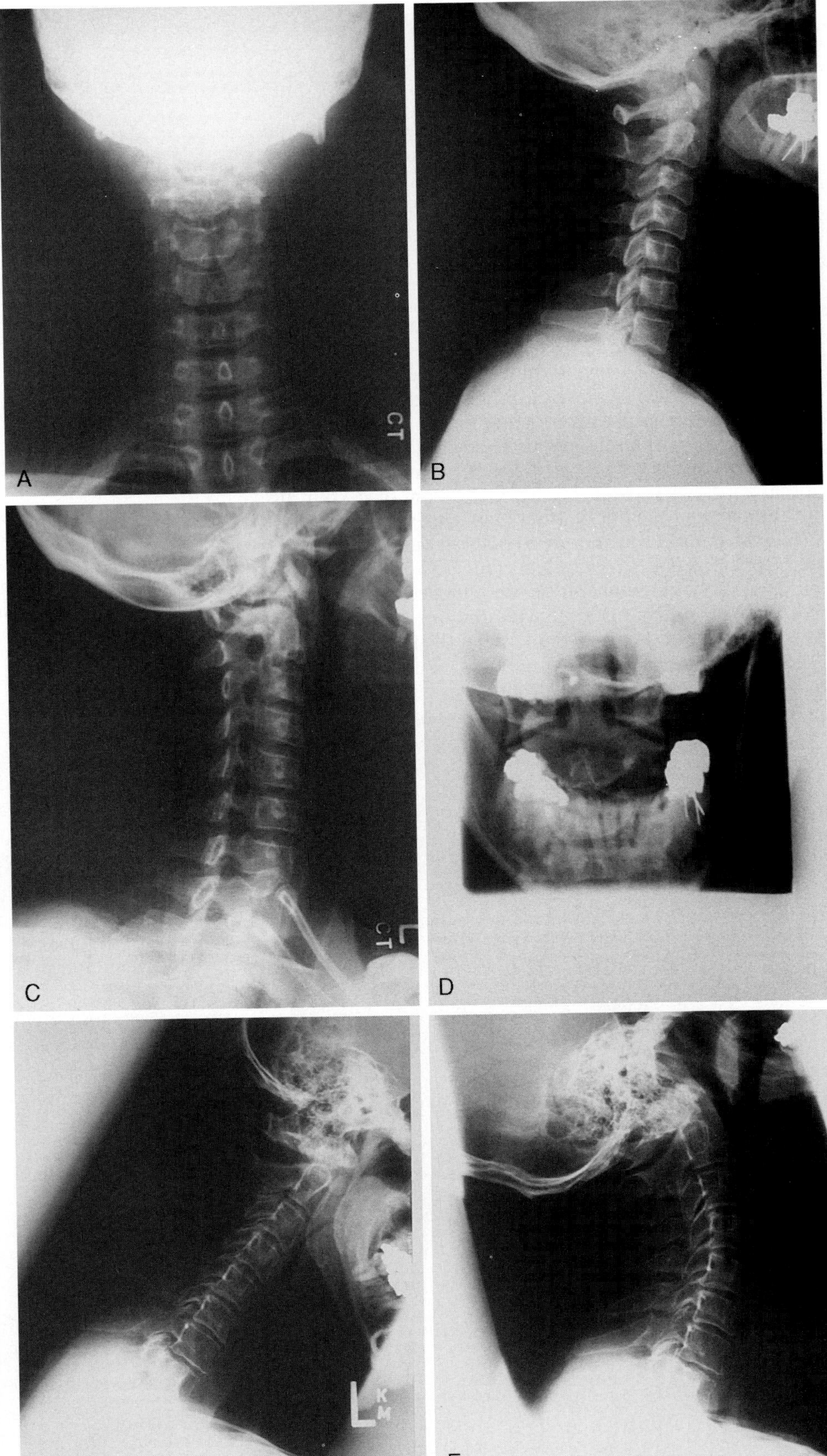

FIGURE 37–11. Complete cervical spine radiograph series. Anteroposterior (*A*), lateral (*B*), oblique (*C*), open-mouth (*D*), flexion (*E*), and extension (*F*) views.

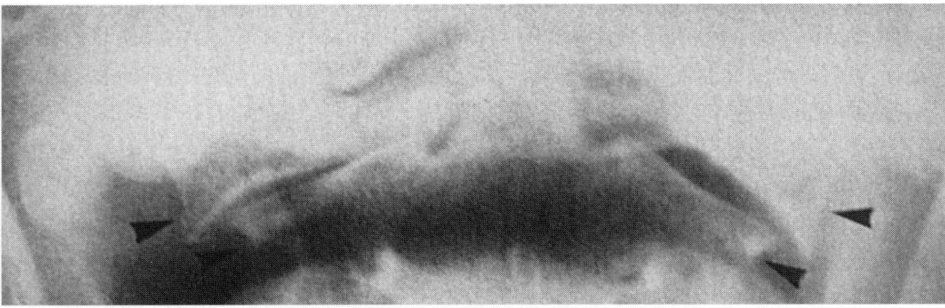

FIGURE 37–12. Open-mouth view of cervical spine demonstrating a burst fracture of the atlas (Jefferson fracture). Offsetting of the lateral masses of the atlas with those of the axis (*arrowheads*) confirms the burst fracture. (From Pavlov H, Torg JS: Roentgen examination of cervical spine injuries in the athlete. Clin Sports Med 1987; 6:761.)

ages that can be produced after data acquisition, allowing for a more detailed evaluation of a suspected fracture.[124, 172, 205] A myelogram followed by a CT scan is often the imaging study of choice prior to cervical surgery for decompression of the spinal cord or nerve root(s).[15, 34, 179] This study provides a comprehensive evaluation of the spinal canal and its relationship to the spinal cord. Nerve root impingement from disc, spur, or foramenal encroachment is best assessed in this manner. CT-myelography is superior to MRI in detecting lateral and foramenal encroachment (Fig. 37–15).[166, 195, 196] However, CT-myelography is often more expensive and has a higher morbidity than MR imaging.[144] Therefore, CT-myelography is usually not one of the initial diagnostic studies performed to evaluate the cervical spine; typically, it is reserved for surgical cases.

Magnetic Resonance Imaging (MRI)

MRI has become the imaging technique of choice in the cervical spine for ruling out a herniated disc (Fig. 37–16).[63, 65, 88, 176, 195, 245] The major strength of the MRI is the definition of soft tissue structures, including cervical discs, spinal cord, and cerebrospinal fluid. This soft tissue definition is not possible with other imaging methods. The MRI is noninvasive and does not expose the patient to radiation. Newer MRI pulse sequences and higher field magnets have recently been introduced, pro-

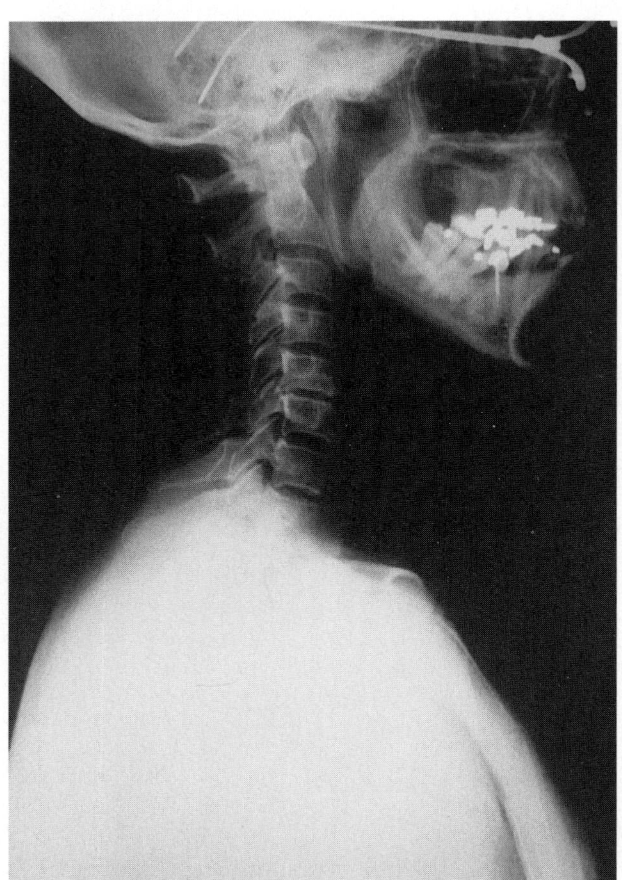

FIGURE 37–13. Lateral cervical spine radiograph revealing disc space narrowing at C5 to C6 with vertebral spurring.

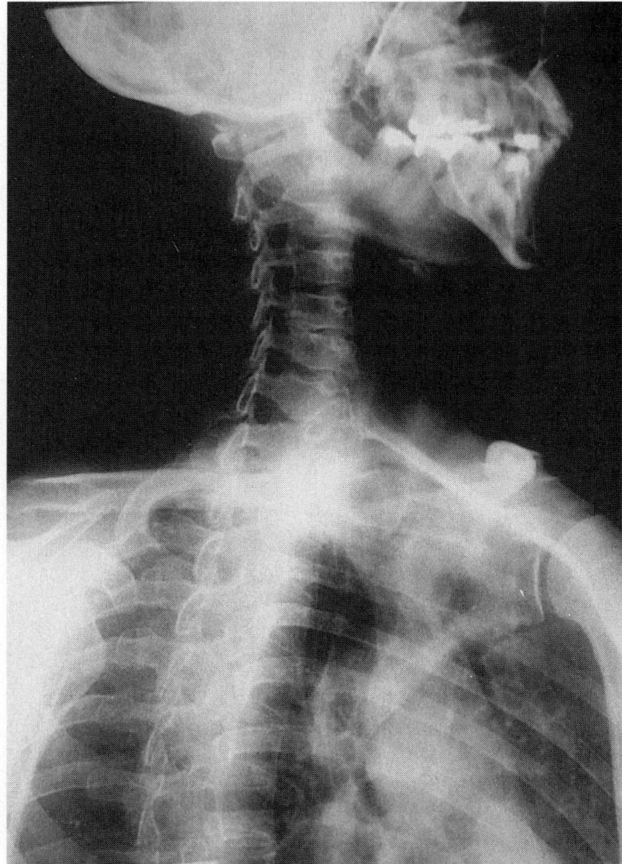

FIGURE 37–14. Oblique cervical spine radiograph showing uncovertebral spurring at the C5 to C6 intervertebral foramen, possibly encroaching on the cervical nerve root.

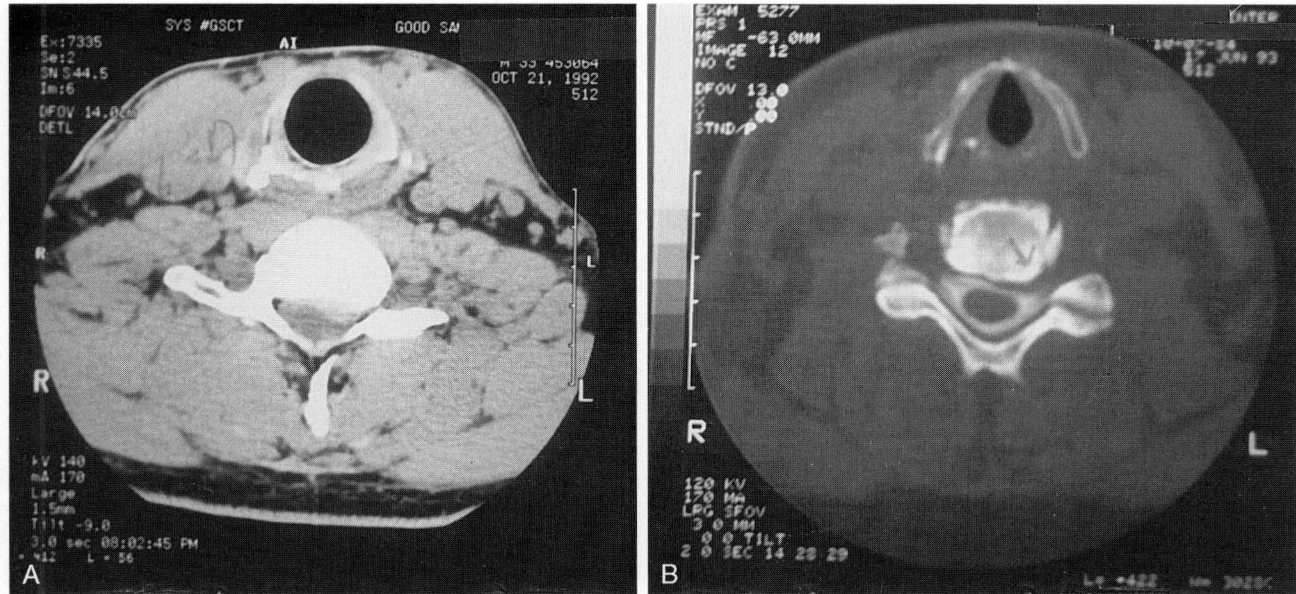

FIGURE 37–15. Cervical spine CT scan. *A.* Abnormal study demonstrating left posterolateral cervical disc herniation with nerve root impingement. *B.* Postmyelogram CT scan defailing thecal sac and nerve root compression from left posterolateral cervical disc herniation in a different patient.

viding for faster and more detailed imaging. Unfortunately, some of the sequencing, such as spin echo, can cause pathology to appear larger than actual size while obscuring other abnormalities.[205]

Although MRI is widely used and provides useful information, it has some shortcomings. The test is fairly expensive, not tolerated by claustrophobic patients, requires that a patient cooperate to minimize artifact, and can have false-positive results.[17, 223] The MRI is not as sensitive as the CT scan in evaluating bony structures such as spurs and bony impingements.[166, 195, 196, 242] Individuals with embedded metallic objects such as pacemakers, surgical clips, or prosthetic heart valves cannot be scanned by MR imaging since the powerful magnets can dislodge these items.

As with any imaging modality or diagnostic test, the MRI has to be interpreted in relation to the patient's symptoms. Many anatomical lesions seen on MRI scans are not functionally important. In a study of asymptomatic subjects by Boden, 25% of those under the age of 40 and 60% of those older than 40 had at least one degenerative cervical spine segment by MRI.[17]

Discography

Cervical discography has remained controversial since Smith introduced it in 1957.[212] The test involves the placement of spinal needles under sterile technique into the cervical intervertebral discs. Care is taken to avoid puncture of soft tissue structures such as the trachea, carotid artery, lung, and esophagus when employing an anterolateral technique. Once the spinal needles are properly placed within the center of the disc nucleus, contrast is injected to determine the internal disc architecture and, more importantly, any pain response that is provoked during the injection. Discography has demonstrated a 60% prevalence of concordant disc pain in a patient population with posttraumatic chronic neck pain.[23] The discomfort and invasiveness of this test makes it less desirable than a cervical MRI, which provides most of the anatomical information that a discogram provides.[55] Cervical discography (Fig. 37–17) has a role in identifying the symptomatic disc(s), which can be useful in the evaluation of patients with inconclusive diagnostic tests and in the planning of cervical fusions.[23, 240] Large disc herniations and midsagittal spinal canal diameters less than 11 mm are contraindications to discography at any level.[3]

Electrodiagnostic Evaluation

Electrodiagnostic evaluation continues to be a mainstay for evaluating the cervical spine. Electrodiagnostic studies have the advantage of being relatively inexpensive as well as low in morbidity. Nerve conduction studies and electromyography (EMG) provide physiologic information regarding cervical nerve root and peripheral nerve function.

Acute, subacute, and chronic radicular features can be detected by needle EMG when there is involvement of motor fibers.[136, 137, 231] Abnormal spontaneous potentials and changes in motor unit action potentials in two or more muscles innervated by the same nerve root are highly suggestive of a radiculopathy (see Table 37–3). The compound muscle action potential (CMAP) amplitude from nerve conduction studies can be helpful in determining the degree of axonotmesis. A 50% drop or more in CMAP amplitude is indicative of significant axonal loss.[121]

Ulnar nerve entrapment, carpal tunnel syndrome, and peripheral neuropathy can be confused with cervical radiculopathy.[120, 121] Electrodiagnostic testing is very

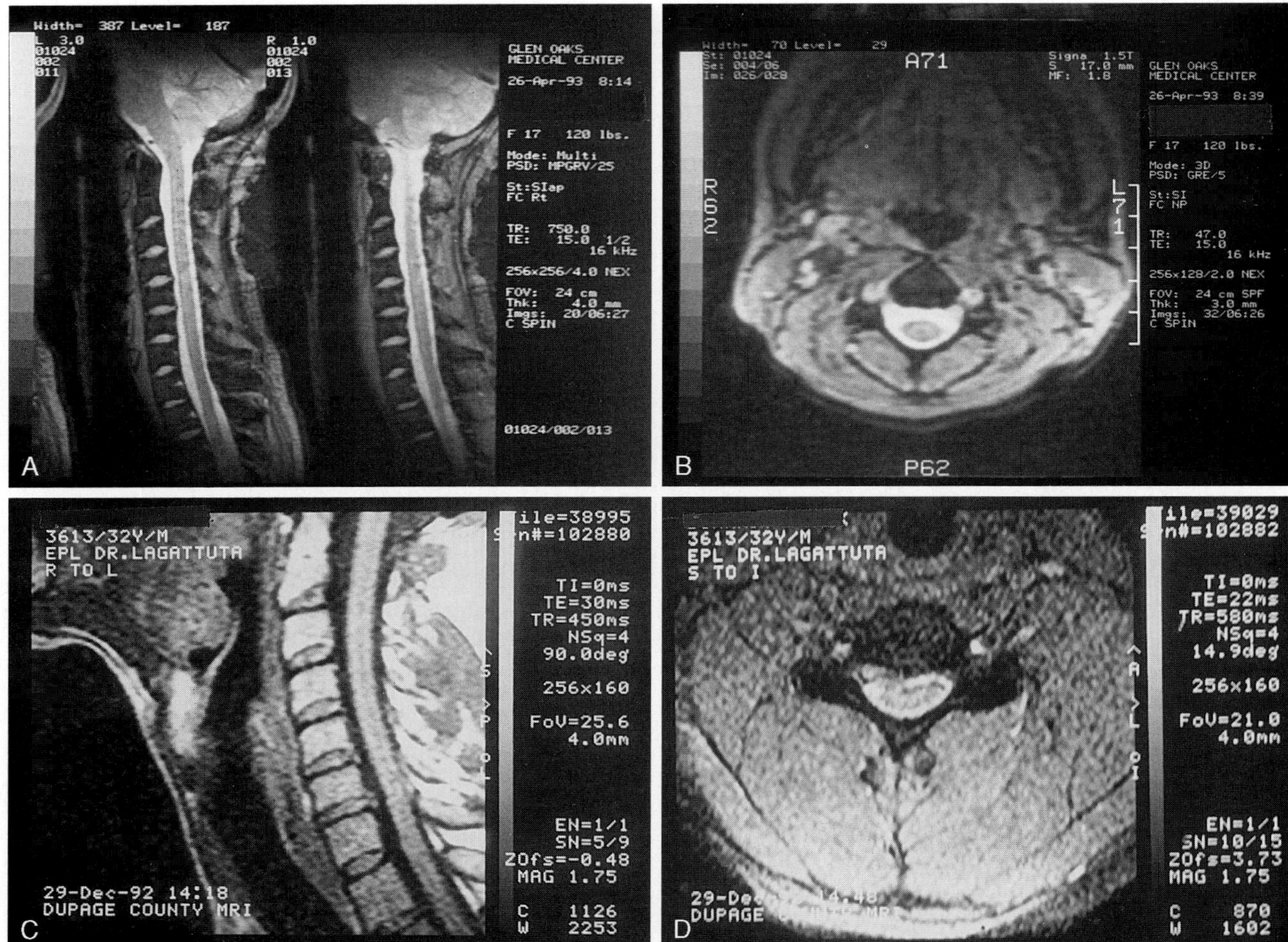

FIGURE 37–16. Cervical spine MRI. *A.* Normal sagittal image. *B.* Normal axial image. *C.* Abnormal sagittal image reveals C6 to C7 posterior disc herniation. *D.* Abnormal axial image in same patient shows right lateral projection of the posterior C6 to C7 disc herniation compromising the right C7 nerve root.

helpful in diagnosing these conditions, and separating them out from cervical radiculopathy.

Somatosensory evoked potentials (SEP) are important in evaluating sensory conduction both peripherally and centrally. Lower limb nerve testing, such as of the tibial and peroneal nerves, has been shown to be helpful in diagnosing a myelopathy by assessing spinal cord conduction. Lower limb SEPs are more sensitive than upper limb SEPs in detecting cervical myelopathy.[244, 246] Dermatomal evoked potentials have been performed for cervical radiculopathy, but are of questionable value.[201] (See Chapters 10, 11, and 12 for more detailed information on electrodiagnostic testing.)

TREATMENT

Modalities

Physical modalities should typically be used only in the acute phase of the condition to help with pain control. Once the patient is past the acute phase, modalities are used only on an as-needed basis. Superficial heat modalities can relax muscles and relieve pain in many cervical disorders. On the other hand, deep heating modalities like ultrasound should be avoided in acute cervical radiculopathy, since this could increase the inflammation of a swollen nerve, leading to more pain or nerve injury.[142] (See Chapter 21 for more information on modalities.)

Traction

Cervical traction can be helpful in relieving symptoms associated with nerve root compression and mild to moderate soft tissue neck injuries.[51, 219] Hot packs, massage, and/or electrical stimulation should be done prior to traction to help relieve pain and relax the muscles.[51, 52, 53] Cervical traction can be performed using either a heavy weight–intermittent or a light weight–continuous regime in a clinic or home environment.[52, 53, 54, 219] The neck should be positioned in 15 to 20 degrees of flexion rather than extension during traction.[51] The use of light weight–continuous home

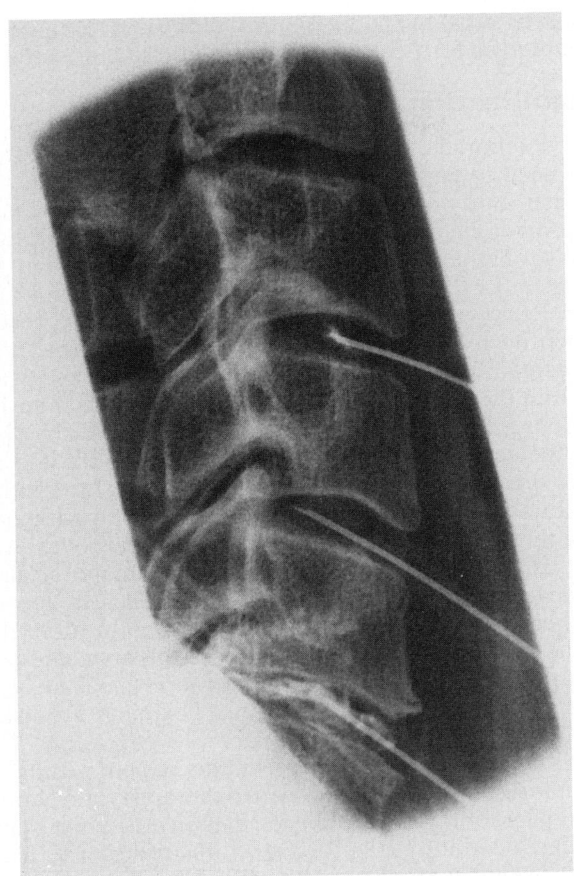

FIGURE 37–17. Cervical discogram. Lateral radiograph view showing needle placement in the C4 to C5, C5 to C6, and C6 to C7 discs. Contrast was injected into the normal C4 to C5 and abnormal C6 to C7 discs. Only a small amount of contrast could be injected into the painless C4 to C5 disc. The C6 to C7 disc revealed significant degenerative changes with spread of contrast throughout the disc. The patient's symptoms were reproduced when the C6 to C7 disc was injected during the study.

traction is a cost-effective alternative and gives the patient more autonomy. (See Chapter 20 for more information on traction.)

Cervical Orthoses

A soft collar is recommended only in acute soft tissue neck injuries and for a short period of time, not to exceed three or four days of continued use. There is a risk of limiting cervical ROM or losing neck strength if collars are worn continuously for longer periods, even though a patient can move the neck in a soft collar.[161, 162, 184] When used for radiculopathy management, the wide part of the collar is placed posteriorly and the thin part anteriorly (Fig. 37–18). This allows the patient to flex the spine and open the intervertebral foramena while discouraging neck extension. The collar can also be used intermittently for a longer period during certain activities, such as sleeping or driving. A Philadelphia collar can be used at night to give more rigid positioning. This helps prevent foramenal narrowing by keeping the neck out of extension. (See Chapter 17 for more information on spinal orthoses.)

Medications

Nonsteroidal anti-inflammatory drugs (NSAIDs) are the first line of pharmacologic intervention in treating most cervical conditions. They provide pain relief at low doses and reduce inflammation at high doses. The patient has to have a therapeutic NSAID level in order to get an anti-inflammatory effect. NSAIDs requiring only once-a-day dosing improve compliance and increase the likelihood of reaching therapeutic levels. Decreasing inflammation is very important when treating cervical radiculopathies.

Aspirin is not recommended because of the large doses needed for an anti-inflammatory effect, longer time to action onset, gastrointestinal toxicity, and irreversible binding to cyclo-oxygenase. The traditional NSAIDs have a long history of multi-organ toxicity such as peptic ulcers, renal insufficiency, and hepatic dysfunction. The discovery and recent release of cyclo-oxygenase isomer type 2 (COX 2) NSAID inhibitors provides for the same analgesic/anti-inflammatory properties without as much associated toxicity.[104] All NSAIDs have a dose-related ceiling point for analgesia above which higher dosing does not provide additional pain relief.

Oral steroids are used when a potent anti-inflammatory effect is needed in cervical radiculopathy. Treat-

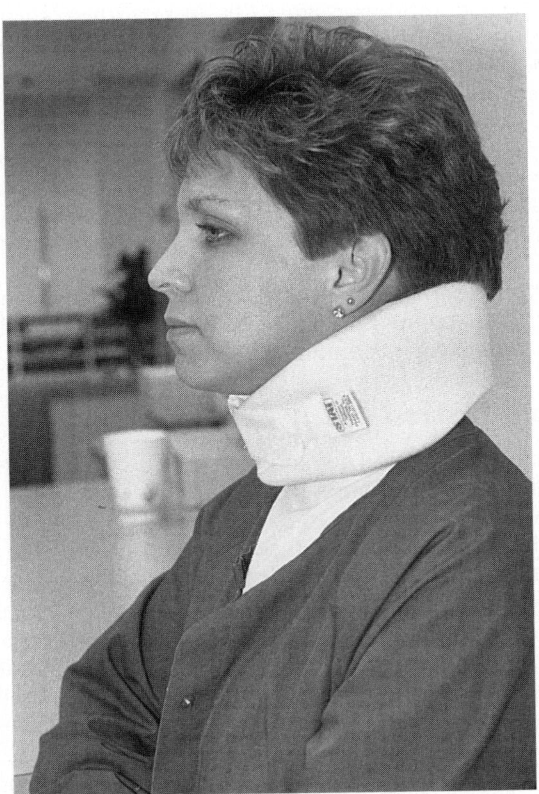

FIGURE 37–18. Cervical orthosis. Cervical soft collar with widest side posteriorly and narrowest side anteriorly.

ment with steroids is typically initiated when an inflammatory etiology for the radiculopathy is suspected and there are no contraindications, such as the presence of infection or history of peptic ulcer disease.[91, 200] The dosage for prednisone should begin at about 70 mg per day and decrease 10 mg each day for a total course of 280 mg. One of the most feared complications of steroid use is avascular necrosis, such as that of the head of the femur. However, there is no documented case to date in the literature of avascular necrosis occurring when the total dose of prednisone or its corticosteroid equivalent is under 550 mg.[106]

Muscle relaxants, opioids, and antidepressants are other medications that can be helpful for cervical disorders. Muscle relaxants should be used to potentiate the pain-relieving effects of NSAIDs, and not necessarily for the reduction of muscle guarding. The only major effect of muscle relaxants in the doses typically used in humans is sedation (they appear to relax muscles by relaxing the patient). Analgesics are a better choice in most cases and are typically of the opioid type.[69] They should be used orally on a scheduled dose basis for a short period of time. Dependency is a concern with long-term use of these medications, particularly in those with an addiction history such as alcoholism.[163, 186, 187] A narcotic contract between the patient and physician should be used when anticipating long-term consumption. The contract restricts the patient to one pharmacy, prescription by one physician, scheduled use of the medication, no unscheduled refills, and no sharing or selling of medications.

Tricyclic antidepressants (TCAs) can help decrease pain and improve sleep. Tricyclics appear to decrease pain by affecting Substance P and improve sleep by increasing stage IV (non-REM) sleep.[44, 168, 197, 232] TCA side effects—especially dry mouth, constipation, and weight gain—can unfortunately limit their use in some individuals. The serotonin reuptake inhibitor antidepressants (SRIs) do not have the side effects associated with TCAs, and can be used in patients intolerant to the TCAs. Although the SRIs are not as effective as TCAs in treating pain due to diabetic peripheral neuropathy, their comparative effectiveness has not yet been determined for neck and back pain.[157]

Manipulation

Spinal manipulation and mobilization are treatment modalities used to restore normal range of motion and decrease pain. There is no clear explanation of how manipulation works, but some believe that "adjustments" to zygapophyseal joints improve afferent signals from mechanoreceptors to the peripheral and central nervous system.[191] The normalization of afferent impulses results in better muscle tone, decreased muscle guarding, and more effective local tissue metabolism. These physiologic modifications lead to improved range of motion and pain reduction.

Spinal manipulation has been shown to have beneficial short-term results in the acutely injured patient.[39, 82, 98, 108] There is no evidence that manipulation provides long-term benefits, improves chronic conditions, or alters the natural course of the disorder.[171] (See Chapter 20 for further information on manipulation.)

Stabilization

Cervicothoracic stabilization is a rehabilitation program designed to limit pain, maximize function, and prevent further injury.[217, 218] The stabilization program includes improving cervical spine flexibility, posture reeducation, and strengthening. This program emphasizes patient responsibility through active participation. Restoring normal ROM and good posture is necessary to prevent repetitive microtrauma to cervical structures from poor movement patterns.[40] Full range of motion is necessary to train the cervicothoracic spine in stabilization during various activities. Pain-free ROM is determined by placing the cervical spine in positions that produce and relieve symptoms. The stabilization programs starts within the established pain-free ROM and is then applied outside this ROM as the patient's condition improves. Any soft tissue or joint restriction present is treated to help achieve normal cervical spine ROM. This is accomplished through passive ROM, spine mobilization, soft tissue mobilization techniques, self-stretching, and correct posturing. The anterior and posterior neck muscles that are stretched to maintain full flexibility are listed in Table 37–4.

Postural training begins with the patient sitting or standing in front of a mirror with a therapist. The patient then performs various transfer maneuvers while maintaining a "neutral spine" (correct posturing) with feedback from the mirror and the therapist. The goal is to teach the patient to maintain a neutral spine position while performing daily activities. These proprioceptive skills are implemented during strengthening exercises designed to help the patient keep the cervical spine in a stable, pain-free, and safe position during strenuous activities.

Cervicothoracic stabilization requires training and coordination of the muscles in the neck area. The neck and shoulder girdle muscles, especially the scapular muscles, need to be individually strengthened (see Table 37–4).[97, 199, 216] The regional muscles of the cervical

TABLE 37–4 Muscle Groups and Individual Muscles Utilized in Cervicothoracic Stabilization

Anterior Muscles	Posterior Muscles
Sternocleidomastoid	Rectus capitis posterior major
Scaleni	Rectus capitis posterior minor
Pectoralis major	Obliquus capitis inferior
Pectoralis minor	Obliquus capitis superior
Biceps (long head)	Levator scapulae
	Superior trapezius
	Latissimus dorsi
	Teres major
	Subscapularis
	Rhomboids
	Middle trapezius
	Lower trapezius
	Serratus anterior

From Sweeney T, Prentice C, Saal JA, et al: Cervicothoracic muscular stabilizing technique. Phys Med Rehabil 1990;4:339.

spine include cervical spine extensors as well as flexors, the rectus capitis anterior, rectus capitis lateralis, longissimus cervicis, and longissimus capitis. The primary thoracic stabilizers are the abdominal and lumbar paraspinal extensor muscles and latissimus dorsi muscles. The scapular muscles include the middle and lower trapezius, serratus anterior, and rhomboids. The chest wall muscles include the pectoralis major and minor muscles.

The exercises used for stabilization proceed from the simple to more advanced techniques (Table 37–5). A variety of isometric and isotonic resistance exercises are used to train the cervicothoracic muscles. Elastic bands, weight machines, and free weights are used in a progressive manner. The patient is instructed to maintain a neutral spine position at all times during stabilization exercises. Advanced exercises challenge the patient to maintain this position during dynamic activities. An engram is achieved through repetition, which eventually enables the patient to stabilize the cervical spine automatically.

Stabilizing the cervical spine using muscular control and enhanced proprioceptive feedback allows the patient to perform activities safely by balancing forces around the cervical spine. Conditioning and training the thorax and upper extremities help to distribute forces away from the cervical spine. The cervicothoracic spine and upper extremities cannot be trained in isolation. Successful treatment with stabilization requires that the lumbar spine and lower extremities be incorporated in the program.[216] The lumbar spine and lower extremities provide a base for the cervicothoracic area and cannot be neglected during training.

Functional Restoration

Functional restoration programs are designed for patients disabled by chronic cervical pain. These medically directed interdisciplinary programs have successfully returned workers' compensation patients with chronic cervical pain to work.[243] These programs typically use an occupational and/or physical therapist, athletic trainer, or nurse to instruct patients in cervical anatomy, biomechanics, pathology, and ergonomics. This accomplishes several goals, including teaching the patient preventive measures against further injury in all activities. Wright and colleagues have shown that those patients

TABLE 37–5 Cervicothoracic Stabilization Exercises

	Cervicothoracic Stabilization Levels		
	I Basic	II Intermediate	III Advanced
Direct cervical stabilization exercises	Cervical active range of motion Cervical isometrics	Cervical gravity Resisted isometrics	Cervical active Range gravity resisted
Indirect cervical stabilization exercises			
Supine, head supported	Theraband chest press Bilateral arm raise Supported dying bug	Unsupported dying bug	Chest flies Bench press Incline dumbbell press
Sit	Reciprocal arm raise Unilateral arm raise Bilateral arm raise Seated row Latissimus pulldown	Swiss ball reciprocal Arm raises Chest press	Swiss ball bilateral Shoulder shrugs Supraspinatus raises
Stand	Theraband reciprocal Chest press Theraband straight Arm latissimus Pulldown Theraband: Chest press Latissimus pulldown Standing rowing Crossovers Triceps press	Standing rowing Biceps pulldown	Upright row Shoulder shrugs Supraspinatus raises
Flexed hip–hinge position	0–30 degrees Reciprocal arm raise Unilateral arm raise Bilateral arm raise Interscapular flies	30–60 degrees Incline prone flies Reciprocal deltoid raise Cable crossovers	60–90 degrees Bilateral anterior Deltoid raises Interscapular flies
Prone	Reciprocal arm raise Unilateral arm raise Bilateral arm raise	Quadruped Head unsupported Swiss ball bilateral Anterior deltoid raises Swiss ball prone Rowing Swiss ball prone flies	Head supported Prone flies Latissimus flies
Supine, head unsupported	Not advised for level I	Partial sit-ups Arm raises	Swiss ball chest flies Swiss ball reciprocal

From Sweeney T, Prentice C, Saal JA, et al: Cervicothoracic muscular stabilizing technique. Phys Med Rehabil 1990; 4:345.

with cervical spinal disorders that successfully complete a functional restoration program have lower rates of recurrent injury, less new surgery in the injured area, and lower use of health care resources.[243]

Selective Spinal Injections

Cervical epidural,[45] selective nerve root (transforamenal), facet, and sympathetic blocks can be used both diagnostically and therapeutically. These procedures can be very helpful in finding the pain generator site and allow for "aggressive conservative" treatment. Cervical epidurals and selective nerve root blocks can be used when there are radicular features associated with a cervical disorder.[85, 234] Cervical sympathetic blocks can be performed when sympathetic mediated pain is suspected, such as in the case of chronic regional pain syndrome (CRPS) type I or II.

An anesthetic and steroid preparation can be injected into the epidural space (translaminar) or along the nerve root (transforamenal) after precise localization under fluoroscopy with radiopaque contrast (Figs. 37–19, 37–20). The anesthetic in the epidural injectant decreases or resolves symptoms in cases of irritation or injury to the nerve root. Long-term relief can be expected from the steroid if the pathophysiology is secondary to an intense inflammatory process.[18, 47, 85, 208, 234] Relief typically lasts no longer than the duration of the anesthetic if the problem is secondary to mechanical compression, such as foramenal stenosis. Selective nerve root blocks are more precise than the "shotgun" approach of the epidural and can identify the symptomatic root or roots. Selective cervical nerve root blocks have been shown by one study to have a low morbidity without permanent sequelae when performed under fluoroscopic guidance with contrast enhancement.[210]

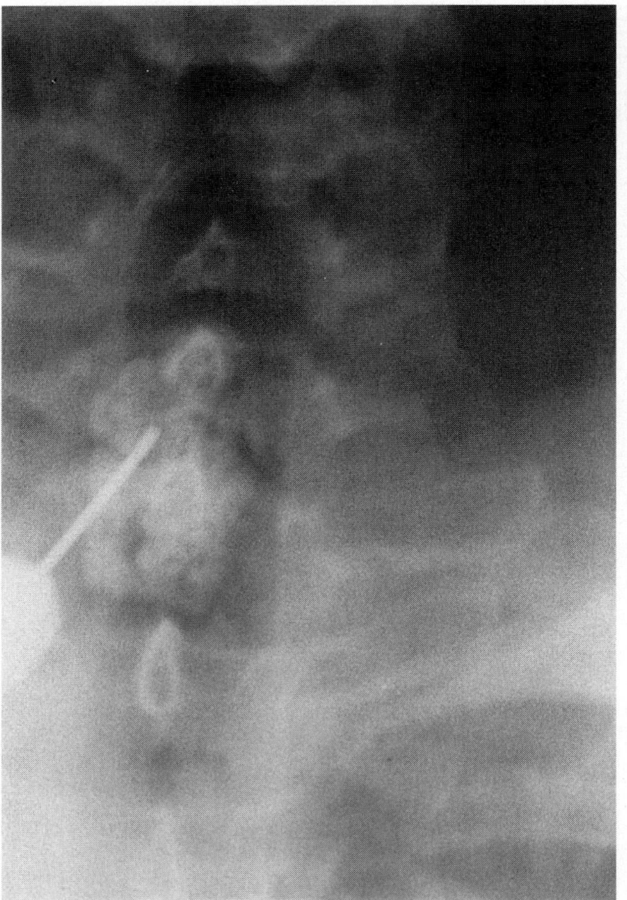

FIGURE 37–19. Cervical epidurogram. Anteroposterior cervical spine radiograph showing contrast within the epidural space and confirming correct needle placement prior to injecting medication.

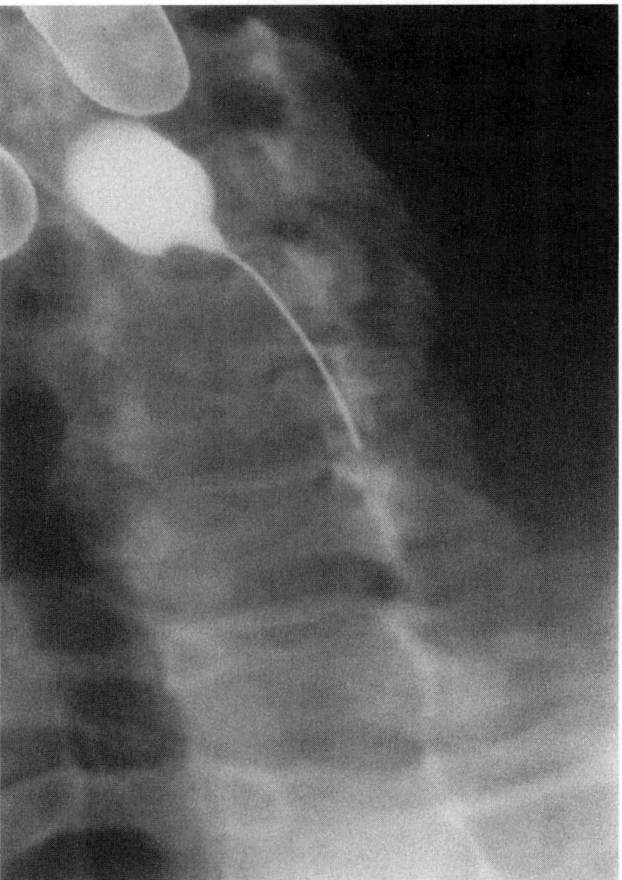

FIGURE 37–20. Cervical perisheathogram. Oblique cervical spine radiograph displaying a small amount of contrast in the C6 to C7 neuroforamen to establish proper needle position before injection of medication.

Facet blocks are performed in one of two different ways. Either the intra-articular joint or the medial branch nerves are injected with medication (Fig. 37–21). Usually intra-articular injections are done for diagnostic and therapeutic effects with an anesthetic and steroid when synovitis is suspected (as in osteoarthritis). Facet joint (medial branch) nerve blocks are diagnostic injections performed with an anesthetic, usually when there has been a mechanical injury to the posterior elements such as with "whiplash" type injuries.[20, 24, 28, 40] A higher diagnostic sensitivity and specificity is obtained if medial branch blocks are performed on different occasions with anesthetics possessing different durations of action.[11, 13]

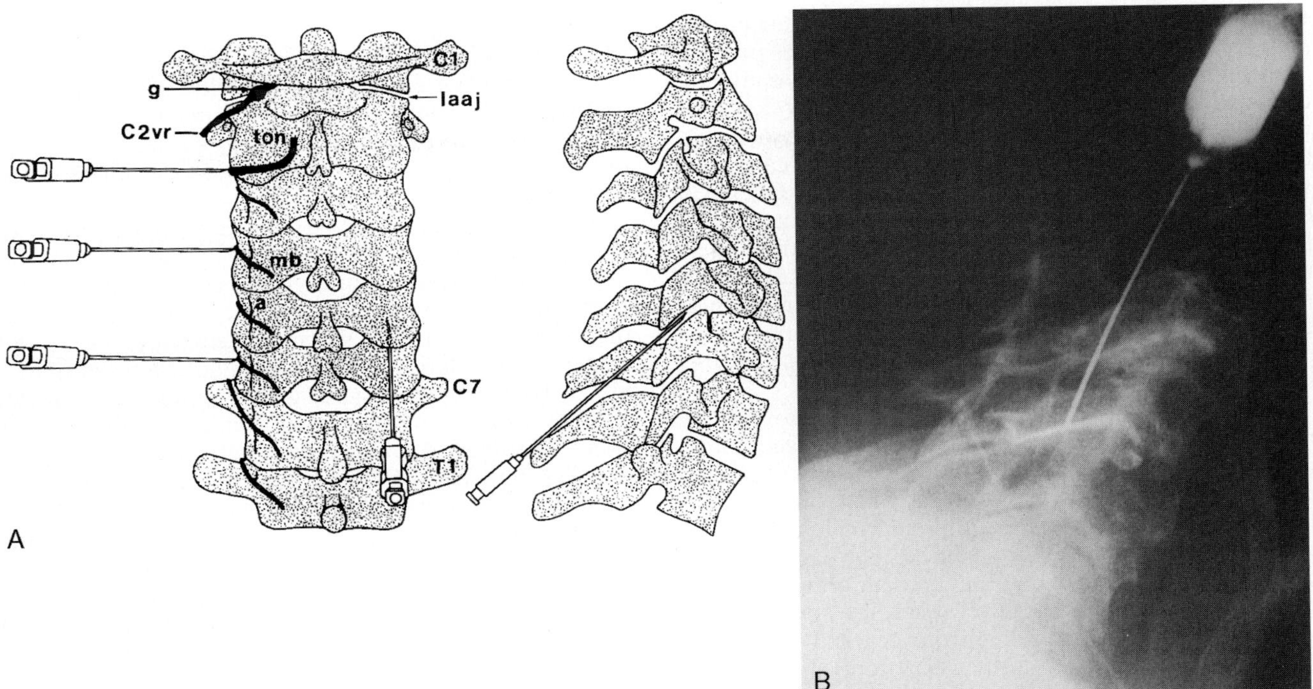

FIGURE 37–21. Cervical facet injections. *A.* Needle placement for medial branch nerve and intra-articular zygapophyseal injections. *Left:* Posterior view of cervical spine showing location of the C2 ganglion (g) behind the lateral atlantoaxial joint (laaj), the C2 ventral ramus (C2vr), location of the medial branches of the cervical dorsal rami (mb), their articular branches (a), and the third occipital nerve (ton). Needles are positioned for injection of the C4 and C6 medial branches and the third occipital nerve. The articular pillar of C7 may be obscured by the shadow of the large C7 transverse process, in which case the C7 medial branch can be located midway between the lateral convexities of the C6 to C7 and C7 to T1 zygapophyseal joints. *Right:* Lateral view of cervical spine shows course of needle in facet joint cavity of the C5 to C6 facet joint using a posterior approach. *B.* Lateral cervical radiograph demonstrates precise needle placement into the zygapophyseal joint, producing a characteristic arthrogram. The joint was entered using a lateral approach to the cervical spine. (*A* and *B* from Bogduk N: Back pain: Zygapophyseal joint blocks and epidural steroids. In Cousins MJ, Bridenbaugh PO (eds): Neural Blockade in Clinical Anesthesia and Pain Management, ed 2. Philadelphia, JB Lippincott, 1988, p 939.)

Those patients who experience pain relief from either intra-articular injections or medial branch blocks are considered to have a facet disorder. These patients often benefit from a medial branch nerve rhizotomy procedure.[129, 190, 209] Studies have clearly demonstrated the effectiveness and long-term benefit of radiofrequency denervation of the cervical medial branch nerve in treating cervical facet pain.[146, 147]

All of the spinal injection procedures described in this section are best done with fluoroscopic guidance and contrast dye. The major advantage of performing these procedures in this manner is proper localization for the injection. Close attention to needle placement allows for more accurate injections with smaller volumes of anesthetic, which leads to more exact identification of pain generators. The use of radiopaque dye also can help prevent complications by avoiding errant injections into structures such as the subarachnoid space or vascular system.

These injection procedures can enhance rehabilitative efforts in two ways. Identification of the pain generator allows for a more specifically designed treatment protocol, and pain relief from the procedure gives a pain-free window of opportunity for more aggressive rehabilitation.

There are risks involved with performing these procedures, including side effects from the anesthesia, the steroids themselves, and the noniodizing contrast media. Blood clotting parameters should be studied prior to epidural procedures in anyone suspected of having a bleeding diathesis. Significant complications can result if bleeding occurs in the presence of relative spinal stenosis (midsagittal diameter <12 mm). This is due to the fact that there is little room to accommodate a space-occupying lesion such as a blood clot without producing spinal cord compression. There is potential risk of seizures, vertebral artery spasm, and temporary quadriparesis from the anesthetic and respiratory arrest. Proper monitoring and emergency equipment should be present for any complications that might arise so that permanent sequelae do not follow from a temporary complication.[14, 18, 32, 33, 47, 48, 56, 61, 67, 85, 193, 234]

Rhizotomy

Percutaneous rhizotomy procedures can be done by radiofrequency electrocoagulation (hyperthermia), cryoanalgesia (hypothermia), or chemical neurolysis. As compared to the other techniques, radiofrequency rhizotomy completely destroys the nerve and provides a relatively large denervation area with longer-lasting pain relief.[2, 25, 145, 209] Cryoanalgesia procedures provide a shorter period of pain relief due to less complete destruction of the nerve and a smaller area of denervation.[36, 80, 173, 204] One advantage of cryoanalgesia is that there is no risk of neuroma formation, which can occur with the radiofrequency technique.[36, 80, 173, 204] Chemical denervation is typically performed by injecting a sterile phenol preparation on the facet joint nerve. This method of denervation is not as specific as the other two methods because there is little control over injection flow patterns. There is also a risk of potential complications due to the phenol spreading to nearby structures in the neck during the injection.

Percutaneous rhizotomies are usually performed in the cervical spine to denervate symptomatic facet joints identified at an earlier time by either intra-articular or medial branch nerve injections. The facet joint nerve is localized under fluoroscopy using anatomic landmarks when performing these procedures. The facet joint is denervated by destroying the medial branch nerves which supply the joint.[26] Several studies have demonstrated long-term pain relief from cervical facet pain using this modality.[146, 147] Other rhizotomy applications for cervical pain using the radiofrequency electrocoagulation technique include cervical dorsal ganglionotomy, disc annular denervation, and sympathectomy.[129]

Surgery

Surgical intervention for cervical conditions is typically thought to be indicated when there is neurogenic bowel or bladder dysfunction, deteriorating neurologic function, or intractable pain.[151] The majority of cervical surgeries are performed because of intractable radicular arm or discogenic neck pain. Cervical spine surgery results are best in the presence of radicular pain, spinal instability, progressive myelopathy, or upper extremity weakness.[95, 236, 241] In the case of chronic discogenic axial neck pain, recent literature demonstrates favorable cervical spine fusion results when utilizing cervical discography.[240, 241]

Implantable Devices

Implantable devices such as spinal cord stimulation (SCS) and intrathecal drug delivery systems (IDDS) are typically used in failed back and neck surgeries, complex regional pain syndromes (CRPS), and chronic painful conditions of benign or malignant origin. The implantable devices are used as a last resort for painful conditions after all other nonsurgical and surgical treatments have failed to provide substantial and long-lasting pain relief. Refractory CRPS or chronic radiculopathy involving the upper limb(s) is the condition most often treated with SCS in the cervical spine region.[138, 175] A stimulating electrode is placed percutaneously within the cervical epidural space for SCS trials and permanent implantation. The electrode position within the epidural space is adjusted together with stimulation parameters (amperage, pulse wide, and stimulation rate) until there is optimal coverage of limb pain during both trials and permanent procedures. During ambulatory trials the electrode is connected to an external battery-operated generator. After a successful trial, the tail end of a permanent epidural electrode is tunneled subcutaneously and surgically connected to a subcutaneous generator with an internal or external battery source. A 50% reduction in pain in half of those treated with SCS ten years after the procedure is the best long-term pain result that can be expected from this procedure with current technology.[138, 175]

Intrathecal drug delivery systems consist of a subcutaneous reservoir pump and catheter that travels from the pump to and into the intrathecal sac. There are essentially two types of pumps available: a programmable, battery-operated type, and a nonprogrammable, continuous-infusion pump that utilizes gas-liquid diffusion technology. Although SCS is effective primarily in treating limb pain, IDDS is effective in treating both axial and extremity pain using a number of different intrathecal medicines such as morphine, bupivicaine, sulfentanyl, dihydromorphone, and clonidine. At the present time the Food and Drug Administration (FDA) has approved only intrathecal morphine for treating pain in this manner. IDDS has been shown to be effective in relieving malignant as well as nonmalignant pain.[133] After the initial 22 months of intrathecal therapy, IDDS is more cost-effective than conventional medical management for treating chronic nonmalignant (benign) pain.[103] Potential complications associated with SCS and IDDS include infection, hematoma, seroma, respiratory depression, and paralysis.

COMMON CERVICAL SYNDROMES

Cervical Sprain and Strain

Epidemiology

Sprain and strain injuries to cervical spine structures are the most commonly encountered cervical disorders. A sprain is an overstretching or tearing of ligaments and/or tendons secondary to joint trauma. A strain is an injury to the muscles. "Whiplash" injuries are the most frequent cause of cervical sprain and strain, with more than one million cases in the United States every year.[81, 153] The typical mechanism is a hyperextension injury to the cervical spine from a rear-end motor vehicle collision.[20, 148] This condition is more common in western societies and metropolitan areas where there is a greater concentration of automobiles. The incidence is higher in women and in those 30 to 50 years old.[215] Approximately one third of subjects develop neck pain within 24 hours of the injury.[206] The natural history of whiplash injuries is that 60% get better within the first year, 32% get better in the next year, and 8% have permanent problems.[9, 174, 235] Litigation, psychological factors, and personality traits may or may not have an effect on treatment outcome.[6, 96, 158, 188]

Pathophysiology

Whiplash is caused by a hyperextension injury to the cervical spine, typically by a rear-end collision. The impact produces cervical extension followed by flexion because of elevated G-forces (Fig. 37–22). This acceleration and deceleration causes injuries to ligaments, facet joints, and muscle.[10, 49, 68, 89, 90, 126, 202, 207] Nerve root injuries can also occur with radicular features, presumably from a stretch injury or from focal hemorrhages.[49, 125] The C2 dorsal root ganglia are vulnerable to injury between the axis and atlas vertebral arches during hyperextension, which can lead to occipital neuralgia.[27] In rare instances, there can be an injury to the descending portion of the cranial V nerve sensory nucleus resulting in facial sensory disturbances. Temporomandibular joint injuries can also occur with whiplash injuries.[194]

Diagnosis

The history usually includes both neck pain and headaches. Symptoms can also be referred into the upper limbs (Fig. 37–23). The patient typically complains of neck fatigue, stiffness, and pain associated with movement. Pain patterns should be evaluated carefully to differentiate sclerotomal from radicular features.[28, 75, 119, 134] Other symptoms include dizziness, lightheadedness, difficulty with concentration and memory, unusual skin sensations over the face, blurred vision, difficulty hearing, tinnitus, and other cranial nerve problems.[8, 28, 35, 66, 87, 109, 149, 150, 178, 183, 221, 222]

The physical exam shows decreased neck ROM with poor quality of movement. Spurling's and Lhermitte's signs are typically negative. Patients frequently show tenderness to palpation in both the anterior and posterior structures of the neck. Facet joint tenderness on palpation is common with injuries to the facet joints, ligaments, and/or capsules.[123] Structural defects can occur with dysfunction of cervical facet movement. The neurologic exam is usually normal. Sensation abnormalities in most cases are sclerotomal rather than radicular. Radicular signs are sometimes present early after injury, but usually resolve within the first two weeks.

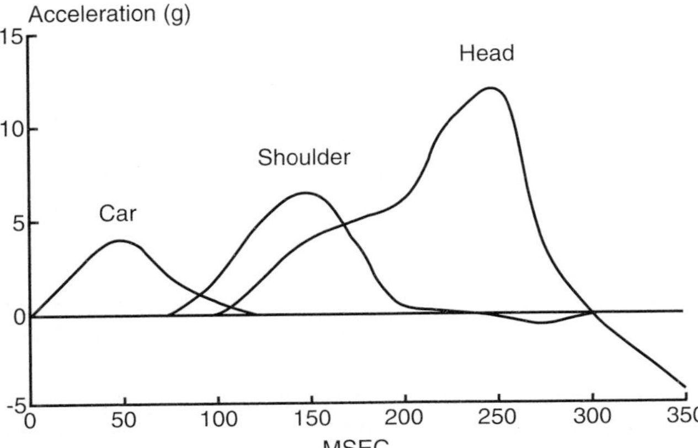

FIGURE 37–22. Idealized graph showing acceleration curves of the head, shoulders, and vehicle following a rear-end impact at 5 mph. Note that peak acceleration of the head is considerably greater than that of the car, followed by significant deceleration. (From Barnsley L, Lord S, Bogduk N: Pathophysiology of whiplash. Rev Spine 1993; 7:330.)

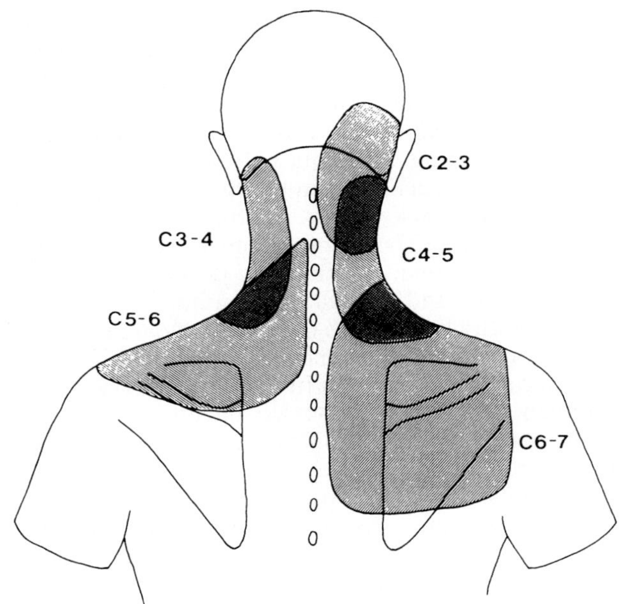

FIGURE 37–23. Pain referral from C2 to C3 through C6 to C7 facet joints. (From Dwyer A, Aprill C, Bogduk N: Cervical zygapophyseal joint pain patterns. I. A study in normal volunteers. Spine 1990; 15:456.)

Plain neck films can show loss of the normal cervical lordotic curvature. MRIs and CT scans are typically normal, but can show disc herniations, ligamentous injury, and hemorrhage.[65] Electrodiagnostic studies can help rule out radiculopathy in patients with continued pain and unusual referred limb sensations.

Treatment

Initial care involves the use of NSAIDs and analgesics to control pain. Tricyclics can also be used to help decrease pain and lessen sleep disturbances. There is usually no need for muscle relaxants when there is sufficient use of analgesics.

Physical therapy modalities can include mobilization, which can be effective acutely after the injury.[39, 82, 98, 108] Before performing mobilization, the clinician should rule out cervical instability in patients of all ages and vertebral insufficiency in the elderly. There is a rare risk of stroke with high-velocity movements.[43, 165] Massage is beneficial in increasing circulation, decreasing pain, and facilitating the exercises that will be the mainstay of treatment. Ultrasound and electrical stimulation are also beneficial, as is postural reeducation.[142] Orthotic devices should not be used continuously for more than 72 hours, since they can delay healing and lead to soft tissue tightening.[161, 162, 184]

Proper movement patterns need to be reestablished within the cervical segments. Poor posture can lead to rounding of the shoulders, dorsal thoracic kyphosis, and forward head thrusting from the lower cervical spine.[40] Poor neck posture can cause microtrauma to the cervical facets, disc, ligaments, and muscles.[40] This can result in bony hypertrophy, ligamentous laxity, and breakdown of the disc and facet articulations. Correct segmental movement depends on balancing the head, cervical spine, and thoracic spine. This provides optimal biomechanical balance within all three structures, and is achieved through increased cervical flexibility and proprioception. Flexibility is achieved with mobilization and self-stretching techniques. Proprioception is improved with instruction from the therapist or physician and visual feedback from a mirror. The stabilization exercises in Table 37–5 allow the muscles to self-correct the neck into proper position and posture, resulting in decreased pain and trauma to the joints.[130, 199, 216]

There is a high incidence of facet joint pain in patients with chronic neck pain and headaches.[4, 23, 112] These patients can be identified with facet joint nerve blocks. Although intra-articular steroid injections have been shown not to provide significant relief,[12] rhizotomy of the facet joint nerves in properly identified patients can provide longer relief of symptoms.[2, 25, 145, 209] This provides an opportunity to aggressively rehabilitate these individuals if they do not respond to more conservative measures.

Cervical Disc Disorders

Epidemiology

Internal disc disruption (IDD), herniated nucleus pulposus (HNP), and degenerative disc disease (DDD) are the three general types of cervical disc disorders encountered in clinical practice. The anatomical presence of these disorders in the asymptomatic population is common and degenerative disc changes are considered part of the natural spine aging process. Herniated discs are found in 10% of asymptomatic individuals under 40 years old and 5% in those older than 40 by MR imaging.[17] Degenerative discs are present in 25% of asymptomatic persons under 40 and nearly 60% in those older than 40 by MRI.[17] Younger individuals tend to have herniated discs, while older persons tend to have degenerative disc changes.

Cervical radiculopathy is a relatively common consequence of a herniated nucleus pulposus (see Fig. 37–16C,D) or due to spurring associated with degenerative disc disease (see Fig. 37–14). A radiculopathy is any sensory, motor, or reflex abnormality secondary to nerve root injury. Although there are no data on the true incidence or prevalence of cervical radiculopathy, 51% of the adult population at some time experience neck and arm pain.[115] Job activities and smoking are other factors in addition to abnormal anatomy that predispose to the development of radiculopathy.[5, 16, 64]

Pathophysiology

Internal disc disruption is a term used to describe pathological changes of the internal structure of the disc.[60] IDD is characterized as an abnormality of the nucleus pulposus or annulus fibrosus without any external disc deformation. This disorder is believed to result from either nuclear degradation related to trauma, or isolated annular injury from a combination of cervical flexion and rotation movements. Some have implicated cervical whiplash injuries as a cause of cervical IDD.[101] The outer annulus of the cervical disc is innervated and is a source of pain and pain referral.[23, 33, 240]

Intervertebral disc herniations are generally classified into three categories based upon the pathoanatomy.[17, 167] The protruding disc is described as nuclear material that penetrates asymmetrically through the annular fibers without escaping beyond the outside margin of the annulus. If nuclear material extends outside the periphery of the annulus, it is called an extruded disc. A sequestered disc is an extruded disc in which a fragment of nuclear material has separated from the rest of the disc and lies in the spinal canal. Disc herniation typically occurs through a weakening of the posterolateral annulus from repetitive stress. Only rarely does herniation occur as a result of a single traumatic incident.

Cervical radiculopathy can be secondary to mechanical compression or to an intense inflammatory process.[200] In acute disc herniation, the pain is induced by chemical inflammation from proteoglycans of the nucleus pulposus as well as any compression on the nerve root.[91, 94, 155, 159] Acute demyelination of the nerve can result from the herniation.[155]

Disc degeneration is a normal part of the aging process. Age-related cervical disc changes are indistinguishable from symptomatic degenerative discs. Degenerative disc changes on radiographic studies are simply a reflection of the natural aging process and are not necessarily indicative of a symptomatic process.[152]

The disc begins to degenerate in the second decade of life. Circumferential tears begin in the annulus after recurrent strains, particularly in the posterolateral portion. Several tears often consolidate to form radial tears, which eventually progress to form radial fissures that extend to the nucleus. The disc then becomes completely disrupted, with tears passing through the disc. There is also loss of disc height with subsequent annular bulging at the periphery. Proteoglycans and water from nuclear degradation are lost through the fissures. Finally, the disc space becomes thin and is associated with vertebral sclerotic changes and osteophyte formation (see Fig. 37–13).

Diagnosis

Discogenic pain is typically vague and diffuse in an axial distribution. Pain referred from the disc to the arm is usually in a nondermatomal pattern. Symptoms can vary according to changes in intradiscal pressure. Activities such as lifting and vasalva maneuvers that increase disc pressure can intensify symptoms, whereas lying supine can provide relief by decreasing intradiscal pressure. Vibration also has a tendency to exacerbate discogenic pain.

On physical examination the discogenic patient typically has decreased cervical range of motion. Neurologic examination is usually normal. The pain is made worse by axial compression and better with distraction. Myofascial tender or trigger points are commonly present and palpable.

Radicular pain is deep, dull and achy, or sharp, burning, and electric in quality depending on whether there is primarily motor or dorsal root involvement.[83, 84] The pain associated with radiculopathy generally follows a dermatomal or myotomal pattern in the shoulder, arm, and hand.[198, 200] The most common site of cervical radicular pain is the interscapular region, although pain can also radiate to the occiput, shoulder, or arm. Neck pain is not necessarily associated with radiculopathy and frequently can be absent. Patients with radiculopathy may have upper limb numbness or weakness in addition to pain.

The radicular patient typically displays decreased cervical range of motion. Pain is usually worse with extension and rotation or during Spurling's maneuver, and improved with neck flexion or abduction of the symptomatic upper limb. There can be decreased sensation to pain, light touch, or vibration. Upper limb weakness can be present when there is significant motor root compromise, but must be differentiated from pain-related weakness. The presence of increased lower extremity reflexes or other upper motor neuron signs suggests the possibility of a myelopathy and needs an aggressive work-up.

Plain films help evaluate the disc space and vertebral body height, and can reveal degenerative osseous and disc changes. Electrodiagnostic studies are helpful in determining the presence and extent of radiculopathy, as well as peripheral or focal neuropathy. MRI can provide an in-depth anatomical evaluation of the intervertebral discs. Clinical correlation must always be used to interpret the results of diagnostic testing and in particular when using anatomical studies such as imaging techniques.

Treatment

Conservative treatment is generally the same for discogenic pain with or without radiculopathy. Initially, the patient is placed on NSAIDs for pain control. An oral steroid used in a rapidly tapering dosage schedule provides a powerful anti-inflammatory effect and can be used in treating a radiculopathy that does not initially respond to NSAIDs. Steroids should not be given concomitantly with NSAIDs or aspirin products, in order to avoid gastric and other potential side effects. Most patients with DDD are elderly; and NSAIDs, like many other medications in this age group, have to be prescribed cautiously. Muscle relaxants can be used as adjuncts to analgesics. Narcotics are used sparingly and only for short periods of time.

Physical modalities are initially used for acute pain control and later used on an as-needed basis only. Cervical traction is beneficial in discogenic pain and also with radicular symptoms. Cervical spine range of motion is actively and passively performed to help restore normal function. As the acute episode subsides, the patient is advanced from a passive program to an active stretching and flexibility routine for the cervical spine. Strengthening and stabilization comprise the next part of the rehabilitation process. The patient should go through a neck school program and be independent in a home program at the time of discharge from rehabilitation. The use of neck education to prevent recurrent episodes is very important.

Those individuals who progress slowly sometimes require the use of selective spinal injection procedures. Cervical epidurals and selective nerve root blocks in radiculopathy patients provide diagnostic and therapeutic benefits. An epidural can provide enough relief to allow for an aggressive rehabilitation program. Patients with discogenic pain alone typically do not respond well to epidural procedures. In DDD patients without radicular symptoms, there can be a significant amount of segmental facet pain resulting from poor articulation mechanics due to the DDD. These patients can benefit from facet rhizotomy after an appropriate response to facet injections.

Those patients who fail with conservative treatment (including the use of spinal injection procedures) might benefit from surgery. Individuals with neck pain alone and no radicular features typically do not benefit from surgery unless there is instability or a myelopathic process. The best results of cervical disc surgery are in those patients with clear-cut radicular pain.[95, 237, 241]

Cervical Spondylosis and Stenosis

Epidemiology

Some use the terms *spondylosis* and *osteoarthritis* interchangeably. Others define them as separate conditions: While spondylosis is described as the degenerative changes in the intervertebral disks and vertebral bodies, osteoarthritis (OA) is considered to be exclusive to the zygapophyseal and uncovertebral joints (closely resembling OA in other joints). For the purposes of this chapter, both terms are considered to be synonymous with a degenerative cervical spine. Factors that contribute to degenerative changes of the spine include aging, trauma, work activities, and genetics.

Degenerative changes of the cervical spine are very common with advancing age. In asymptomatic individuals under the age of 40, 25% have DDD and 4% have foramenal stenosis by MRI.[17] In those over 40, almost 60% have DDD and 20% have foramenal stenosis by MRI.[17] Seventy percent of asymptomatic individuals over 70 have degenerative cervical spine changes in one form or another.[127, 140] Spondylytic changes can result in spinal canal, lateral recess, and foramenal stenosis. The former can result in myelopathy, whereas the latter two can present with radiculopathy.

Pathophysiology

Intervertebral discs lose hydration and elasticity with age, leading to cracks and fissures. The disc subsequently collapses due to biomechanical incompetence, causing the annulus to bulge outward. The surrounding ligaments also lose their elastic properties and develop traction spurs. Uncovertebral spurring occurs as a result of the degenerative process in which the facet joints lose cartilage, become sclerotic, and develop osteophytes (see Fig. 37–14).

Acquired cervical stenosis more commonly results from degenerative changes such as spur formation, disc protrusion, ligamentum hypertrophy, and/or facet joint hypertrophy (Fig. 37–24). Disorders such as Paget's disease and gout can also result in cervical stenosis. Neurologic sequelae from central canal stenosis typically develops when the diameter becomes less than 12 mm in the midsagittal plane.[34, 179] Spinal stenosis with myelopathic symptoms can include neurogenic bowel and bladder dysfunction, gait disturbances, impotence, and altered sexual function. Leg weakness or spasticity can also occur. Weakness and numbness may have a specific level that coincides with the location of the most severe stenosis.[156, 195] Radiculopathy can develop from degenerative changes to the joints of Luschka and facet joints, leading to lateral or foramenal stenosis.

Congenital and developmental stenosis are two other types of cervical spinal canal stenosis. Congenital stenosis is commonly due to short pedicles, which causes the cervical canal to be smaller than normal. The average midsagittal AP diameter is 10 mm for the spinal cord and 17 mm for the spinal canal.[34, 179] Relative stenosis is considered to be present when the diameter is less than 12 mm, and absolute stenosis when it is less than 10 mm.[34, 156, 179, 195] Although cervical spinal stenosis usually comes on insidiously, it can develop acutely in the presence of congenital or developmental stenosis, since there is little room for space-occupying lesions such as an acute large central disc herniation.

Diagnosis

Cervical spondylosis can cause radicular pain due to nerve root impingement, but it can also cause cervical zygapophyseal joint pain.[185] Patients having only facet joint pain typically have pain confined to the neck and shoulder.[76, 77] The pain is worse at different positions[122] and can interfere with sleep. They do not complain of numbness or weakness in the upper limbs. Those individuals with myelopathic symptoms such as neurogenic bowel and bladder dysfunction need aggressive investigation.[15]

Physical exam typically shows decreased ROM of the cervical spine, especially with neck extension. The neurologic exam concentrates on detecting long tract signs consistent with myelopathy, as well as signs of radiculopathy. Positive findings for myelopathy include hyperreflexia, Babinski's sign, and weakness at and below the involved levels. Positive signs for radiculopathy are decreased sensation, diminished reflexes, and weakness in a segmental distribution. Spurling's and Lhermitte's signs can both be present in either case.

Diagnostic testing includes cervical spine films to evaluate the uncovertebral joints, facet joints, foramen, and intervertebral disc spaces. MRI permits evaluation of the spinal canal and foramen in relation to the spinal cord, thecal sac, and nerve roots. SEP responses from lower limb peripheral nerve stimulation are delayed or of low amplitude in the presence of myelopathy. SEPs can be performed serially to evaluate the ongoing status of myelopathies. In cases of radicular symptoms, needle EMG can confirm motor nerve root involvement. CT scans and myelography are usually the imaging tests of choice to document spinal and foramenal stenosis. MRI alone is not as sensitive and can give false positive and negative results.[17, 166, 195, 196]

Treatment

The treatment for cervical spondylosis pain that occurs with or without radicular features begins with NSAIDs. Analgesics can also be used in a scheduled manner, but usually only for six weeks or less. Tricyclic antidepressants can be used for pain relief and sleep dysfunction.

Physical therapy modalities in this situation can include a trial of careful traction. Cervical orthoses are typically not helpful. Ultrasound, electrical stimulation, and massage can all be very helpful.[78] Mobilization such as muscle energy techniques can be of benefit.[43] Extreme mobilization can cause myelopathy and should be closely monitored. The exercise program is the same as for cervical radiculopathy, including flexibility, strengthening, stabilization, and aerobic conditioning.

A cervical zygapophyseal intra-articular steroid injection can be helpful in the presence of an active synovitis.

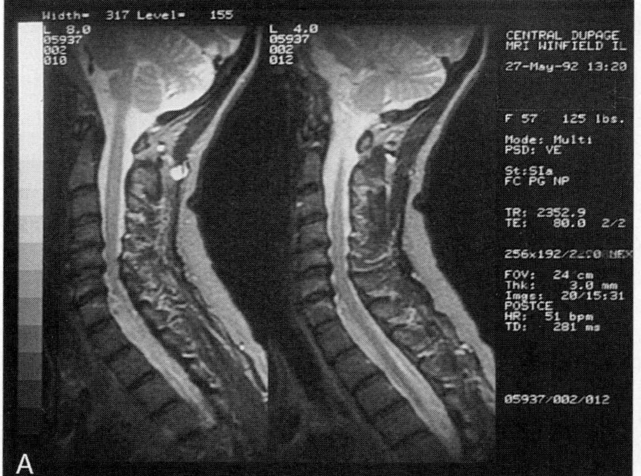

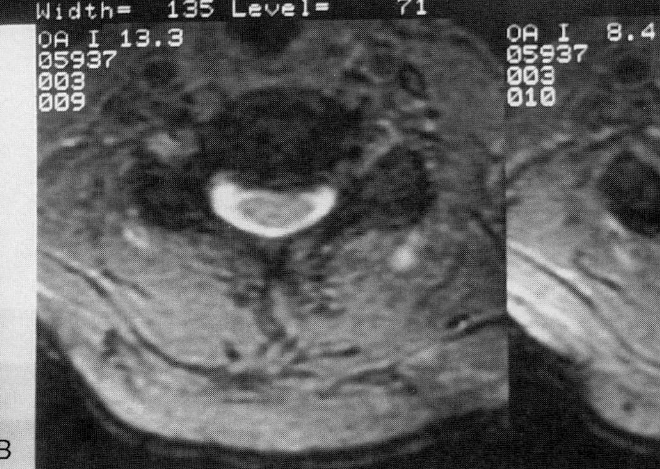

FIGURE 37–24. Cervical stenosis. Cervical MRI sagittal (*A*) and axial (*B*) views demonstrating degenerative spinal stenosis.

The facet injections can be both diagnostic and therapeutic.[18–20, 24, 28, 70, 75, 88, 107, 170] Mechanical facet pain is better evaluated with facet joint nerve blocks. Long-term relief can often be accomplished with a rhizotomy procedure. Cervical epidurals might be of benefit in cervical spondylosis, especially if there is an inflammatory component. Epidurals and selective nerve root blocks can be diagnostically and therapeutically helpful in cases of radiculopathy.

Surgical referral is needed immediately when the clinical evaluation and neurodiagnostic tests are positive for myelopathy.[176] Conservative treatment is generally used when there are no myelopathic findings on clinical evaluation, even if anatomical tests show cervical stenosis.

Myofascial Pain Syndrome

Myofascial pain syndrome is discussed in detail elsewhere in this text (see Chapter 43), but deserves mention here. Myofascial pain syndrome often mimics cervical radiculopathy and cervical facet syndrome. A thorough understanding of particular muscles and their referral zones is important, especially when the diagnostic tests do not demonstrate a clear-cut localization of the problem. Myofascial pain or fibromyalgia should be considered as a possible etiology when imaging studies are normal in an individual with neck pain and referred pain into the shoulders and upper limbs.[132, 192, 224, 247]

CONCLUSION

The cervical spine is a complicated structure that can develop pathology leading to pain and impairment. Success in treating cervical conditions depends upon making the correct diagnosis, providing appropriate treatment, and practicing prevention. More accurate diagnosis for cervical disorders through the use of advanced imaging modalities and fluoroscopically guided, contrast-enhanced spinal injection procedures have allowed for specific rehabilitation programs for specific diagnoses. Improved technologies such as the COX-2 NSAID inhibitors, radiofrequency denervation, and implantable devices are giving clinicians better and safer options for controlling pain. Once the pain has decreased or resolved, diagnosis-related treatment progresses to flexibility, strengthening, and endurance exercises. Prevention of future pain episodes is emphasized during the recovery process through education in proper body mechanics, posture, and exercise. Ergonomic modifications at work and at home are also important to prevent further injury.

REFERENCES

1. Adams F: Paulus Aeginata, vol 2. London, Sydenham Society, 1816, pp 155–156, 193, 197.
2. Anderson KH, Mosdal C, Vaernet K: Percutaneous radiofrequency facet denervation in low-back and extremity pain. Acta Neurochir 1987; 87:48–51.
3. Aprill CN: Diagnostic disc injection. In Frymoyer JW (ed): The Adult Spine: Principles and Practice. New York, Raven Press, 1991, pp 403–442.
4. Aprill C, Bogduk N: The prevalence of cervical zygapophyseal joint pain. A first approximation. Spine 1992; 17:744–747.
5. Astrand NE: Medical, psychological, and social factors associated with back abnormalities and self reported back pain. Br J Ind Med 1987; 44:327–336.
6. Awerbuch MS: Whiplash in Australia: Illness or injury? Med J Aust 1992; 157:193–196.
7. Balla A, Moraitis S: Knights in armour: A follow up study of injuries after legal settlement. Med J Aust 1970; 335–361.
8. Balla JI: The late whiplash syndrome. Aust Nz J Surg 1980; 50:610–614.
9. Bannister G, Gargan M: Prognosis of whiplash injuries. In A Review of the Spine: State of the Art Reviews. Philadelphia, Hanley & Belfus, 1993, pp 557–570.
10. Barnsley L, Lord S, Bogduk N: Pathophysiology of whiplash. In Spine. State of the Art Reviews, vol 7. Philadelphia, Hanley & Belfus, 1993, p 330.
11. Barnsley L, Lord S, Bogduk N: Comparative local anaesthetic blocks in the diagnosis of cervical zygapophyseal joint pain. Pain 1993; 55:99–106.
12. Barnsley L, Lord SM, Wallis BJ: Lack of effect of intraarticular corticosteroids for chronic pain in the cervical zygapophyseal joints. N Engl J Med 1994; 330:1047–1050.
13. Barnsley L, Lord SM, Wallis BJ, et al: The prevalence of chronic cervical zygapophyseal joint pain after whiplash. Spine 1995; 20:20–25.
14. Benzon HT: Epidural steroids for lumbosacral radiculopathy. Adv Pain Res Ther 1990; 13:231.
15. Bernhardt M, Hynes R, Blune H, et al: Cervical spondylitic myelopathy. J Bone Joint Surg [Am] 1993; 75:119–128.
16. Bigos SJ, Spengler DM, Martin NA, et al: Back injuries in industry: A retrospective study. III. Employee-related factors. Spine 1986; 11:252–256.
17. Boden SD, McCowin PR, Davis DO, et al: Abnormal magnetic–resonance scans of the cervical spine in asymptomatic subjects. J Bone Joint Surg [Am] 1990; 72:1178–1184.
18. Bogduk N: Back pain: Zygapophyseal joint blocks and epidural steroids. In Cousins MJ, Bridenbaugh PO (eds): Neural Blockade in Clinical Anesthesia and Pain Management, ed 2. Philadelphia, JB Lippincott, 1988, pp 935–954.
19. Bogduk N: Back pain: Zygapophyseal joint blocks and epidural steroids. In Cousins MJ, Bridenbaugh PO (eds): Neural Blockade in Clinical Anesthesia and Pain Management, ed 2. Philadelphia, JB Lippincott, 1988, p 939.
20. Bogduk N: The anatomy and pathophysiology of whiplash. Clin Biomech 1986; 1:92–101.
21. Bogduk N: The anatomy of the occipital neuralgia. Clin Exp Neurol 1980; 17:167–184.
22. Bogduk N: The clinical anatomy of the cervical dorsal rami. Spine 1982; 7:319–330.
23. Bogduk N, Aprill C: On the nature of neck pain, discography and cervical zygapophyseal joint blocks. Pain 1993; 54:213–217.
24. Bogduk N, Aprill C, Dwyer A: Cervical zygapophyseal joint pain patterns II: A clinical evaluation. Spine 1990; 15:458–461.
25. Bogduk N, Long DM: Percutaneous lumbar medial branch neurotomy. A modification of facet denervation. Spine 1980; 5:193–201.
26. Bogduk N, Macintosh J, Marsland A: Technical limitations to the efficacy of radiofrequency neurotomy for spinal pain. Neurosurgery 1976; 20:529–535.
27. Bogduk N, Marsland A: On the concept of third occipital headache. J Neurol Neurosurg Psychiat 1986; 49:775–780.
28. Bogduk N, Marsland A: The cervical zygapophyseal joints as a source of neck pain. Spine 1988; 13:610–617.
29. Bogduk N, Twomey LT: Clinical Anatomy of the Lumbar Spine, ed 2. New York, Churchill Livingstone, 1991, p 12.
30. Bogduk N, Twomey LT: Clinical Anatomy of the Lumbar Spine, ed 2. New York, Churchill Livingstone, 1991, p 117.
31. Bogduk N, Valencia F: Innervation and pain patterns of the thoracic spine. In Grant R (ed): Physical Therapy of the Neck and Thoracic Spine. New York, Churchill Livingstone, 1988, pp 27–37.

32. Bogduk N, Wilson AS, Tynan W: The human lumbar dorsal rami. J Anat 1982; 134:383–397.
33. Bogduk N, Windsor M, Inglis A: The innervation of the cervical intervertebral discs. Spine 1988; 13:2–8.
34. Bohlman HH, Emery SE: The pathophysiology of cervical spondylosis and myelopathy. Spine 1988; 13:844.
35. Braaf MM, Rosner S: Symptomatology and treatment of injuries of the neck. NY J Med 1955; 55:237.
36. Brechner T: Percutaneous cryogenic neurolysis of the articular nerve of Luschka. Reg Anesth 1981; 6:18–22.
37. Breck LW, Van Norman RW: Medicolegal aspects of cervical spine strains. Clin Orthop 1982; 74:124–128.
38. Brown DL: Atlas of Regional Anesthesia. Philadelphia, WB Saunders, 1992, pp 129–132.
39. Brunarski DJ: Clinical trials of spinal manipulation. J Manip Physiol Ther 1984; 7:4.
40. Cailliet R: Neck and Arm Pain, ed 3. Philadelphia, FA Davis, 1991.
41. Cailliet R: Soft Tissue Pain and Disability, ed 2. Philadelphia, FA Davis, 1988, pp 123–169.
42. Cailliet R: Soft Tissue Pain and Disability, ed 2. Philadelphia, FA Davis, 1988, pp 179–208.
43. Cantu R, Grodin A: Soft tissue mobilization. In Basmajian JV, Nyberg R (eds): Rational Manual Therapies. Baltimore, Williams & Wilkins, 1993, pp 199–221.
44. Carette S, McCain GA, Bell DA, et al: Evaluation of amitriptyline in primary fibrositis. A double blind, placebo control study. Arthritis Rheum 1986; 29:655–659.
45. Catchlove RF, Braha R: The use of cervical epidural nerve blocks in the management of chronic head and neck pain. Can Anaesth Soc J 31:188–191.
46. Cave AJE: The innervation and morphology of the cervical intertransverse muscles. J Anat 1927; 71:497–515.
47. Cicala RS, Thoni K, Angel JJ: Long-term results of cervical epidural steroid injections. Clin J Pain 1989; 5:10–15.
48. Cicala RS, Westbrook LL, Angel JJ: Side effects and complications of cervical epidural steroid injections. J Pain Symptom Manage 1989; 4:64–66.
49. Clemens HJ, Burow K: Experimental investigation on injury mechanisms of cervical spine and frontal and rear-frontal vehicle impacts. In Proceedings of the Sixteenth STAPP Car Crash Conference. Warrendale, Society of Automotive Engineers, 1972, pp 76–104.
50. Cloward RB: Cervical discography: A contribution to the etiology and mechanism of neck, shoulder, and arm pain. Ann Surg 1959; 150:1052.
51. Colachis S, Strohm B: A study of tractive forces and angle of pull on vertebral interspaces; in the cervical spine. Arch Phys Med Rehabil 1965; 46:820.
52. Colachis S, Strohm B: Cervical traction: Relationship of traction time to varied tractive force with constant angle of pull. Arch Phys Med Rehabil 1965; 46:815.
53. Colachis SC, Strohm BR: Effect of duration of intermittent cervical traction on vertebral separation. Arch Phys Med Rehabil 1966; 47:353–359.
54. Colachis SC, Strohm BR: Effect of intermittent traction on separation of lumbar vertebrae. Arch Phys Med Rehabil 1969; 50:251.
55. Connor PM, Darden BV: Cervical discography complications and clinical efficacy. Spine 1993; 18:2035–2038.
56. Cousins MJ: Epidural neuronal blockade. In Cousins MJ, Bridenbaugh PO (eds): Neuronal Blockade in Clinical Anesthesia and Pain Management. Philadelphia, JB Lippincott, 1980, pp 183–185.
57. Crafts RC: Textbook of Human Anatomy, ed 2. New York, John Wiley & Sons, 1979, p 55.
58. Crafts RC: Textbook of Human Anatomy, ed 2. New York, John Wiley & Sons, 1979, p 76.
59. Crafts RC: Textbook of Human Anatomy, ed 2. New York, John Wiley & Sons, 1979, p 77.
60. Crock HV: A reappraisal of intervertebral disc lesions. Med J Aust 1970; 1:983–989.
61. Cronen M, Waldman S: Cervical steroid epidural nerve blocks in the palliation of pain secondary to intractable tension-type headaches. J Pain Symptom Manage 1990; 5:379–381.
62. Crowe H: Injuries to the cervical spine. Presented at the Annual Meeting of the Western Orthopedic Association, San Francisco, 1928.
63. Czervionke L, Daniels D, Ho P, et al: Cervical neural foramina: Correlative anatomic and MR imaging study. Radiology 1988; 169:753–759.
64. Damkot DK, Pope MH, Lord J, et al: The relationship between work history, work environment and low-back pain in men. Spine 1984; 9:395–399.
65. Davis SJ, Teresi LM, Bradley WG, et al: Cervical spine hyperextension injuries: MR findings. Radiology 1991; 180:245–251.
66. Deans GT, Magalliard JN, Kerr M: Neck sprain—A major cause of disability following car accidents. Injury 1987; 18:10–12.
67. Delaney TJ, Rowlingson JC, Carron H, et al: Epidural steroid effects on nerves and meninges. Anesth Analg 1980; 58:610.
68. Deng YC: Anthropomorphic dummy neck modeling and injury considerations. Accid Anal Prev 1989; 21:85–100.
69. De Vries HA, Adams GM: Electromyographic comparisons of single doses of exercises and meprobamate as to effects on muscular relaxation. Am J Phys Med 1972; 51:130–141.
70. Dory M: Arthrography of the cervical facet joints. Radiology 1983; 148:379–382.
71. Dussault RG, Nicolet VM: Cervical facet joint arthrography. J Can Assoc Radiol 1985; 36:79–80.
72. Dvorak J, Panjabi M, Gerber D, et al: Functional diagnostics of the rotary instability of the upper cervical spine: An experimental study in cadavers. Spine 1987; 12:197.
73. Dvorak J, Panjabi MM, Grob D, et al: Validation of flexion extension radiographs of cervical spine. Spine 1987; 18:120–127.
74. Dvorak J, Panjabi M, Novotny J, et al: In vivo flexion/extension of the normal cervical spine. J Orthop Res 1991; 9:828–834.
75. Dwyer A, Aprill C, Bogduk N: Cervical zygapophyseal joint pain patterns I: A study in normal volunteers. Spine 1990; 15:453–457.
76. Dwyer A, Aprill C, Bogduk N: Cervical zygapophyseal joint pain patterns I: A study in normal volunteers. Spine 1990; 15:456.
77. Eisenstein SM, Parry CR: The lumbar facet arthrosis syndrome. J Bone Joint Surg [Br] 1987; 69:3–7.
78. Eldred E, Lindsky D, Buchwald J: The effect of cooling on mammalian muscle spindles. Exp Neurol 1960; 2:144–157.
79. Ellis H: Clinical Anatomy: A Revision and Applied Anatomy for Clinical Students, ed 6. London, Blackwell Scientific Publications, 1976, p 205.
80. Evans PJD: Cryoanalgesia. The application of low temperatures to nerves to produce anaesthesia or analgesia. Anaesthesia 1981; 36:1003–1013.
81. Evans RW: Some observations on whiplash injuries. Neurol Clin 1992; 10:975–997.
82. Farrell JB, Twomey LT: Acute low back pain. Comparison of two conservative treatment approaches. In Proceedings of Manipulative Therapists Association of Australia, Perth, Western Australia, 1983, p 162.
83. Feinstein B: Referred pain from paravertebral structures. In Buerger AA, Tobis JS (eds): Approaches to the Validation of Manipulative Therapy. Springfield, IL, Charles C Thomas, 1977, pp 139–174.
84. Feinstein B, Langton JNK, Jameson RM, et al: Experiments on pain referred from deep somatic tissues. J Bone Joint Surg [Am] 1954; 36:981–997.
85. Ferrante MF, Wilson SP, Lacobo C, et al: Outcome predictions after cervical epidural steroid injection. Spine 1993; 18:1736–1745.
86. Fielding JW: Cineroentgenography of the normal cervical spine. J Bone Joint Surg [Am] 1957; 39:1280–1288.
87. Fisher CM: Whiplash amnesia. Neurology 1982; 32:667–668.
88. Fletcher G, Haughton V, Ho K, et al: Age-related changes in the cervical facet joints: Studies with cryomicrotomy, MR and CT. Am J Neurol Res 1990; 11:27–30.
89. Fornage BID, Touche DH, Segal P, et al: Ultrasonography in the evaluation of muscular trauma. J Ultrasound Med 1983; 2:549–554.
90. Frankel VH: Temporomandibular joint pain syndrome following deceleration injury to the cervical spine. Bull Hosp Joint Dis 1969; 26:47.
91. Franson R, Saal J: Human disc phospholipase A2 in inflammatory disease. Spine 1992; 17(suppl 6):S129–S132.

92. Garvey TA, Marks MR, Wiesel SW: A prospective double-blind evaluation of trigger-point injection therapy for low-back pain. Spine 1989; 14:962–964.
93. Ganong WF: Review of Medical Physiology, ed 13. New York, Appleton & Lange, 1987.
94. Garfin SR, Rydevik BL, Brown RA: Compressive neuropathy of spinal nerve roots. A mechanical or biological problem? Spine 1991; 16:162–165.
95. Gore D, Sepic S: Anterior cervical fusion for degenerated or protruded discs. Spine 1984; 9:667.
96. Gotten N: Survey of one hundred cases of whiplash injury after settlement of litigation. JAMA 1956; 162:865–867.
97. Gracovetsky S, Farfan H: The optimum spine. Spine 1986; 10:543–573.
98. Hadler NM, Curtis P, Gillings DB, et al: A benefit of spinal manipulation as adjunctive therapy for acute low-back pain: A stratified controlled trial. Spine 1987; 12:7.
99. Haldeman CW: Guideline factors for evaluation of neck and back injuries. Spine 1993; 18:1736–1745.
100. Hamada G, Rida A: Orthopaedics and orthopaedic diseases in ancient and modern Egypt. (Letter). Clin Orthop 1972; 89:253.
101. Hamer J, Gargan MF, Bannister GC: Whiplash injury and surgically treated cervical disc disease. Injury 1993; 24:549–550.
102. Hanley EN, Shapiro DE: The development of low-back pain after excision of a lumbar disc. J Bone Joint Surg [Am] 1989; 71:719–721.
103. Hassenbusch SJ, Paice JA, Patt RB, et al: Clinical realities and economic considerations: Economics of intrathecal therapy. J Pain Symptom Manage 1997; 14(suppl):S36–S48.
104. Hawkey CJ: Cox-2 inhibitors. Lancet 1999; 353:307–314.
105. Hayashi K, Yabuki T: Origin of the uncus and of Luschka's joint in the cervical spine. J Bone Joint Surg [Am] 1985; 67:788–791.
106. Heller B: Correspondence to Francis Lagatutta, MD, regarding literature search on oral corticosteroids, 1986.
107. Hildebrandt J, Argyrakis A: Percutaneous nerve block of the cervical facets—A relatively new method in the treatment of chronic headache and neck pain. Pathological anatomical studies and clinical practice. Manual Med 1986; 2:45–52.
108. Hoehler FK, Tobis JS, Buerger AA: Spinal manipulation for low back pain. JAMA 1981; 245:1835.
109. Hohl M: Soft tissue injuries of the neck in automobile accidents: Factors influencing prognosis. J Bone Joint Surg [Am] 1974; 56:1675–1681.
110. Hollinshead WH, Jenkins DB: Functional Anatomy of the Limbs and Back, ed 5. Philadelphia, WB Saunders, 1981, p 218.
111. Hopwood MB, Abram S: Factors associated with failure of lumbar epidural steroids. Regional Anesth 1993; 18:238–243.
112. Hove B, Gyldensted C: Cervical analgesic facet joint arthrography. Neuroradiology 1990; 32:456–459.
113. Howorth B, Petrie G: Injuries to the Spine. Baltimore, Williams & Wilkins, 1964.
114. Hult L: Cervical, dorsal, and lumbar spinal syndromes. Acta Orthop Scand 1954; 17(suppl 1).
115. Hult L: Frequency of symptoms for different age groups and professions. In Hirsch C, Zotterman Y (eds): Cervical Pain. New York, Pergamon Press, 1971, pp 17–20.
116. Hult L: The munkford investigation. Acta Orthop Scand Suppl 1954; 17:1.
117. Huskisson EC: Visual Analogue Scales. In Melzack R (ed): Pain Measurement and Assessment. New York, Raven Press, 1983, pp 33–40.
118. Hunter CR, Mayfield FH: Role of the upper cervical root in the production of pain in the head. Am J Surg 1949; 78:743–749.
119. Inman VH, Saunders JB de CM: Referred pain from skeletal structures. J Nerv Ment Dis 1944; 99:660–667.
120. Johnson EW: Carpal tunnel syndrome. In Johnson EW (ed): Practical Electromyography, ed 2. Baltimore, Williams & Wilkins, 1988, pp 187–205.
121. Johnson EW: Practical Electromyography, ed 2. Baltimore, Williams & Wilkins, 1988.
122. Johnson EW, Wolfe CV: Bifocal spectacles in the etiology of cervical radiculopathy. Arch Phys Med Rehabil 1972; 53: 201–205.
123. Jull G, Bogduk N, Marsland A: The accuracy of manual diagnosis for cervical zygapophyseal joint pain syndromes. Med J Aust 1988; 148:233–236.
124. Kaiser A, Holland BA: Imaging of the cervical spine. Spine 1998; 23:2701–2712.
125. Kallieris D, Mattern R, Schmidt G, et al: Kinematic and spinal columnar injuries in active and passive passenger protection: Results of simulated frontal collisions. In Proceedings of the 1984 International Conference on Biomechanics of Impact. Bron, France, IRCOBI, 1984, pp 279–295.
126. Kaplan PA, Anderson JC, Norris MA, et al: Ultrasound of post traumatic soft tissue lesions. Radiol Clin North Am 1989; 27:973–982.
127. Kellegren JH, Lawrence JS: Osteoarthritis and disk degeneration in an urban population. Ann Rheum Dis 1958; 17:388–397.
128. Kelsey JL, Githens PB, O'Conner T, et al: Acute prolapsed lumbar intervertebral disc. An epidemiologic study with special reference to driving automobiles and cigarette smoking. Spine 1984; 9:608–613.
129. Kline MT: Stereotactic Radiofrequency Lesions as Part of the Management of Pain. Orlando, FL, Paul M Deutsch Press, 1992.
130. Knott M, Voss D: Proprioceptive Neuromuscular Facilitation: Patterns and Techniques. New York, McGraw-Hill, 1956.
131. Kottke FJ, Mundale MO: Range of mobility of the cervical spine. Arch Phys Med Rehabil 1959; 40:379.
132. Kraft GH, Johnson EW, LaBan MM: The fibrositis syndrome. Arch Phys Med Rehabil 1968; 49:155–162.
133. Krames ES: Intraspinal opioid therapy for chronic nonmalignant pain: Current practice and clinical guidelines. J Pain Symptom Manage 1996; 11:333–352.
134. Kurz LT: The differential diagnosis of cervical radiculopathy. In Herkowitz HN (ed): Seminars in Spinal Surgery. Philadelphia, WB Saunders, 1989, pp 194–199.
135. Kvist M, Jarvenen M: Clinical, histochemical and biochemical features in repair of muscle and tendon injuries. Int J Sports Med 1982; 3:12–14.
136. LaBan M: "Whiplash": Its evaluation and treatment. In Saal JA (ed): Neck and Back Pain. Physical Medicine and Rehabilitation. State of the Art Reviews, vol 4. Philadelphia, Hanley & Belfus, 1990, pp 293–308.
137. LaBan MM: Electrodiagnosis in cervical radicular and myelopathic syndromes. In Herkowitz HN (ed): Seminars in Spinal Surgery. Philadelphia, WB Saunders, 1989, pp 222–228.
138. Law JD, Kirkpatrick AF: Update: Spinal cord stimulation. Am J Pain Med 1992; 2:34–42.
139. Lawrence JS: Disc degeneration. Its frequency and relationship to symptoms. Ann Rheum Dis 1969; 28:121.
140. Lawrence JS, Brenner JM, Bier F: Osteoarthrosis: Prevalence in the population and relationship between symptoms and x-ray changes. Ann Rheum Dis 1966; 25:1–24.
141. Lazorthes G, Gaubert J: L'innervation des articulations interapophysiares vertebrales. C R Ass Anat 1956; 43:488–494.
142. Lehmann J, deLateur BJ: Diathermy and superficial heat and cold therapy. In Kottke EJ, Stillwell GK, Lehmann JF (eds): Krusen's Handbook of Physical Medicine and Rehabilitation, Philadelphia, WB Saunders, 1982, pp 275–350.
143. Und B, Schlbom H, Nordwall A, et al: Normal range of motion in cervical spine. Arch Phys Med Rehabil 1989; 70:692–695.
144. Lipman JC, Wang AM, Brooks ML, et al: Seizure after intrathecal administration of lopamidol. Am J Neurol Res 1988; 9:787–788.
145. Lora J, Long D: So-called facet denervation in the management of intractable back pain. Spine 1976; 1:121–126.
146. Lord SM, Barnsley L, Bogduk N: Percutaneous radiofrequency neurotomy in the treatment of cervical zygapophyseal joint pain: A caution. Neurosurgery 1995; 36:732–739.
147. Lord SM, Barnsley L, Wallis BJ, et al: Percutaneous radiofrequency neurotomy for chronic cervical zygapophyseal-joint pain. N Engl J Med 1996; 5:1721–1726.
148. Macnab I: Acceleration injuries of the cervical spine. J Bone Joint Surg [Am] 1964; 46:1797–1799.
149. Macnab I, McCulloch J: Neck Ache and Shoulder Pain. Baltimore, Williams & Wilkins, 1994, p 8.
150. Macnab I, McCulloch J: Neck Ache and Shoulder Pain. Baltimore, Williams & Wilkins, 1994, p 138.
151. Magee DJ: Orthopedic Physical Assessment, ed 2. Philadelphia, WB Saunders, 1992, pp 34–70.

152. Maigne J, Deligne L: Computed tomographic follow-up study of cases of non-operatively treated cervical intervertebral soft disc herniation. Spine 1994; 19.
153. Maimaris C, Barnes MR, Allen MJ: "Whiplash injuries" of the neck: A retrospective study. Injury 1988; 19:393–396.
154. Makela M, Heliovaara M, Sievers D, et al: Prevalence, determinants, and consequences of chronic neck pain in Finland. Am J of Epidemiol 1991; 134:1356–1367.
155. Marshall L, Trethewie E, Curtain C: Chemical irritation of nerve root in disc prolapse. Lancet 1973 (Aug. 11); 2(7824):320.
156. Matsunaga S, et al: Dissociated motor loss in the upper extremities. Spine 1993; 18:1964–1967.
157. Max MB, Lynch SA, Muir J, et al: Effects of desipramine, amitriptyline and fluoxetine on pain in diabetic neuropathy. N Engl J Med 1992; 326:1250–1256.
158. Mayou R, Bryant B, Duthie R: Psychiatric consequences of road traffic accidents. Br Med J 1993; 307:1047–1050.
159. McCarron RF, Wimpee MW, Hudkins PG: The inflammatory effect of nucleus pulposus. A possible element in the pathogenesis of low-back pain. Spine 1987; 12:760–764.
160. McFadden JF: Smoking cigarettes and lumbar disc pain. A preliminary report on 400 patients. J Neurol Orthop Med Surg 1985; 6:125–128.
161. McKinney LA: Early mobilization of acute sprain of the neck. Br Med J 1989; 299:1006–1008.
162. Mealy K, Brennan H, Fenelon GC: Early mobilization of acute whiplash injury. Br Med J 1986; 292:1656–1657.
163. Medina JL, Diamond S: Drug dependence in patients with chronic headaches. Headache 1977; 17:12–14.
164. Miles A, Maimaris C, Finlay D, et al: The incidence and prognostic significance of radiological abnormalities in soft tissue injuries to the cervical spine. Skeletal Radiol 1988; 17:493–496.
165. Miller R, Burton R: Stroke following chiropractic manipulation of the spine. JAMA 1974; 229:189.
166. Modic MT, Masaryk TJ, Mulopulos GP, et al: Cervical radiculopathy: Prospective evaluation with surface coil MR imaging: CT with metrizamide and metrizamide myelography. Radiology 1986; 161:753–759.
167. Modic MT, Masaryk TJ, Ross JS: Magnetic Resonance Imaging of the Spine. Chicago, Year Book Medical Publishers, 1990, pp 83–90.
168. Moldofsky H, Scarisbrick P, England R, et al: Musculoskeletal symptoms and non-REM sleep disturbance in patients with "fibrositis syndrome" and healthy subjects. Psychosom Med 1975; 37:341–351.
169. Mooney V, Cairns D, Robertson J: A system for evaluation and treatment of chronic back disability. West J Med 1976; 124:370–376.
170. Mooney V: Injection studies: Role in pain definition. Adult Spine 1991; 25:527–539.
171. Moritz U: Evaluation of manipulation and other manual therapy. Criteria for measuring the effect of treatment. Scand J Rehab Med 1979; 11:173.
172. Muroff LR: Optimizing the performance and interpretation of bone scans. Clin Nucl Med 1981; 6:68–76.
173. Myers BR, Powell HC, Heckman HM, et al: Biophysical and pathological effects of cryogenic nerve lesion. Ann Neurol 1981; 10:478–485.
174. Norris SH, Watt I: The prognosis of neck injuries resulting from rear-end vehicle collisions. J Bone Joint Surg [Br] 1983; 65: 608–611.
175. North RB, Kidd DH, Zahurak M, et al: Spinal cord stimulation for chronic, intractable pain: Experience over two decades. Neurosurg 1993; 32:384–395.
176. Okada S, et al: Magnetic resonance imaging study on the results of surgery for cervical compression myelopathy. Spine 1993; 18:2024–2029.
177. Orofino C, Sherman MS, Schechter D: Luschka's joint—A degenerative phenomenon. J Bone Joint Surg [Am] 1964; 42: 853–858.
178. Pand LQ: The otological aspects of whiplash injuries. Laryngoscope 1971; 81:1381–1387.
179. Park WW: Correlative anatomy of cervical spondylotic myelopathy. Spine 1988; 13:831.
180. Parke WW: Applied anatomy of the spine. In Rothman RH, Simone FA (eds): The Spine, ed 3. Philadelphia, WB Saunders, 1992, p 49.
181. Pavlov H, Torg JS: Roentgen examination of cervical spine injuries in the athlete. Clin Sports Med 1987; 6:761.
182. Payne EE, Spillane JD: The cervical spine. An anatomicopathological study of 70 specimens (using a special technique) with particular reference to the problem of cervical spondylosis. Brain 1957; 80:571–596.
183. Pennie B, Agambar L: Patterns of injury and recovery in whiplash. Injury 1991; 22:57–59.
184. Pennie BH, Agambar LJ: Whiplash injuries. Trial of early management. J Bone Joint Surg [Br] 1990; 72:277–279.
185. Penning L: Differences in anatomy, motion development and aging in the upper and lower cervical disk segments. Clin Biomech 1991; 3:37–47.
186. Perry S, Heidrich G: Management of pain during debridement: A survey of U.S. burn units. Pain 1982; 13:267–280.
187. Porter J, Jick H: Addiction rare in patients treated with narcotics. N Engl J Med 1980; 302:123.
188. Radanov BP, Stefano G, Schnidrig A, et al: Role of psychosocial stress in recovery from common whiplash. Lancet 1991; 338:712–715.
189. Ransford AO, Cairns D, Mooney V: The pain drawing as an aid to the psychologic evaluation of patients with low-back pain. Spine 1976; 1:127–134.
190. Rashbaum RF: Radiofrequency facet denervation. A treatment alternative in refractory low back pain with or without leg pain. Orthop Clin North Am 1983; 14:569–575.
191. Roeske R: The new vertebral subluxation. J Chirop 1993; 30:19–24.
192. Rogers EJ, Rogers R: Fibromyalgia and myofascial pain: Either, neither, or both? Orthop Rev 1989; 18:1217–1224.
193. Rowlingson JC, Kirschenbaum LP: Epidural analgesic techniques in the management of cervical pain. Anesth Analg 1986; 65:938–942.
194. Roydhouse RH: Torquing of the neck and jaw due to belt restraint in whiplash type accidents. Lancet 1985; 1:1341.
195. Russell E: Cervical disc disease. Radiology 1990; 177:313–325.
196. Russell E, D'Angelo C, Zimmerman R, et al: Cervical disc herniation: CT demonstration after contrast enhancement. Radiology 1984; 152:703–712.
197. Russell IJ, Bowden CL, Michlek JE, et al: Imipramine receptor density on platelets on patients with fibrositis syndrome: Correlation with disease severity and response to therapy (Abstract). Arthritis Rheum 1987; 30.
198. Rydevik B, Brown M, Lundborg G: Pathoanatomy and pathophysiology of nerve root compression. Spine 1984; 9:7–15.
199. Saal JS: Flexibility Training. Physical Medicine and Rehabilitation. State of the Art Reviews. Philadelphia, Hanley & Belfus, 1987, pp 537–554.
200. Saal JS, Saal JJ, Herzog R: The natural history of lumbar intervertebral disk extrusions treated nonoperatively. Spine 1990; 15: 683–686.
201. Schmid LID, Hess CW, Ludin HP: Somatosensory evoked potentials following nerve and segmental stimulation do not confirm cervical radiculopathy with sensory deficit. J Neurol Neurosurg Psychiatry 1988; 51:182–187.
202. Schneider LW, Foust DR, Bowman BM, et al: Biomechanical properties of the human neck in lateral flexion. In Proceedings of the 19th STAPP Car Crash Conference. Warrendale, Society of Automotive Engineers, 1975, pp 453–485.
203. Schofferman J, Anderson D, Smith G, et al: Childhood psychological trauma and chronic low back pain. In Proceedings of the 7th Annual NASS Meeting. Boston, North American Spine Society, 1992, p 148.
204. Schuster GD: The use of cryoanalgesia in the painful facet syndrome. J Neurol Orthop Surg 1982; 3:271–274.
205. Schwartz RB: Helical (spiral) CT in neuroradiologic diagnosis. Radiol Clin North Am 1995; 3:981–995.
206. Selecki BR: Whiplash. Aust Fam Phys 1984; 13:243–247.
207. Severy DM, Mathewson JH, Bechtol CO: Controlled automobile rear end collisions: An investigation of related engineering and medical phenomena. Can Serv Med J 1955; 11:727–759.

208. Shulman M: Treatment of neck pain with cervical epidural steroid injection. Regional Anesth 1986; 11:92–94.
209. Silvers HR: Lumbar percutaneous facet rhizotomy. Spine 1990; 15:36–40.
210. Slipman CW, Plastaras CT, Palmitier RA, et al: Symptom provocation of fluoroscopically guided cervical nerve root stimulation. Are dynatomal maps identical to dermatomal maps? Spine 1998; 15:2235–2242.
211. Smith AG: Account of a case in which portions of three dorsal vertebrae were removed for the relief of paralysis from fracture, with partial success. N Am Med Surg J 1829; 8:94.
212. Smith GW, Nichols P: The technique of cervical discography. Radiology 1963; 68:163–165.
213. Spengler DM: Lumbar discectomy: Results with limited disc excision and selective foraminotomy. Spine 1982; 7:604–706.
214. Sternbach RA, Tursky B: Ethnic differences among housewives in psychophysical and skin potential responses to electric shock. Psychophysiology 1965; 1:241.
215. Su HC, Su RK: Treatment of whiplash injuries with acupuncture. Clin J Pain 1988; 4:233.
216. Sweeney T, Prentice C, Saal JA, et al: Cervico thoracic muscular stabilizing technique. In Physical Medicine and Rehabilitation. State of the Art Reviews, vol 4. Philadelphia, Hanley & Belfus, 1990, pp 335–360.
217. Sweeney T, Prentice C, Saal JA, et al: Cervico thoracic muscular stabilizing technique. Physical Medicine and Rehabilitation. State of the Art Reviews, Philadelphia, Hanley & Belfus, 1990, p 339.
218. Sweeney T, Prentice C, Saal JA, et al: Cervico thoracic muscular stabilizing technique. Physical Medicine and Rehabilitation. State of the Art Reviews, vol 4. Philadelphia, Hanley & Belfus, 1990, p 345.
219. Swezey RL, Swezey AM, Warner K: Efficacy of home cervical traction therapy. Am J Phys Med Rehabil 1999; 78:30–32.
220. Tamura T: Cranial symptoms after cervical injury. Aetiology and treatment of the Barrd-Lieou syndrome. J Bone Joint Surg [Br] 1989; 71:283–287.
221. Taylor JR, Womey T: Acute injuries to cervical joints. Spine 1993; 18:1736–1745.
222. Teasell RW, McCain G: The clinical spectrum and management of whiplash injuries. In Tollison CID (ed): Painful Cervical Trauma: Diagnosis and Rehabilitation Treatment of Neuromuscular Injuries. Baltimore, Williams & Wilkins, 1992, pp 292–318.
223. Teresi LM, Lufkin RB, Reicher MA: Asymptomatic degenerative disk disease and spondylosis of the cervical spine: MR imaging. Radiology 1987; 164:83–88.
224. The American College of Rheumatology 1990 criteria for the classification of fibromyalgia: Report of the multicenter criteria committee. Arthritis Rheum 1990; 33:160–172.
225. Torg J: Injuries to the cervical spine and spinal cord resulting from water sports. In Torg JS (ed): Athletic Injuries to the Head, Neck, and Face, ed 2. St Louis, Mosby–Year Book, 1991, pp 157–173.
226. Torg J: The epidemiologic, biomechanical, and cinematographic analysis of football-induced cervical spine trauma and its prevention. In Torg JS (ed): Athletic Injuries to the Head, Neck, and Face, ed 2. St Louis, Mosby–Year Book, 1991, pp 97–111.
227. Torg J: Trampoline-induced cervical quadriplegia. In Torg JS (ed): Athletic Injuries to the Head, Neck, and Face, ed 2. St Louis, Mosby–Year Book, 1991, pp 85–96.
228. Torg JS, Fay CM: Cervical spinal stenosis with cord neurapraxia and transient quadriplegia. In Torg JS (ed): Athletic Injuries to the Head, Neck, and Face, ed 2. St Louis, Mosby–Year Book, 1991, pp 533–552.
229. Travell JG, Simons DG: Myofascial Pain and Dysfunction—The Trigger Point Manual. Baltimore, Williams & Wilkins, 1983.
230. Tucci SM, Hicks JE, Gross EG, et al: Cervical motion assessment: A new, simple and accurate method. Arch Phys Med Rehabil 1986; 67:225–230.
231. Uematsu S, Hendler N, Hungerford D, et al: Thermography and electromyography in the differential diagnosis of chronic pain syndromes and reflex sympathetic dystrophy. Electromyogr Clin Neurophysiol 1982; 21:165.
232. Vaeroy H, Helle R, Forre O, et al: Elevated CSF levels of substance P in high incidence of Raynaud's phenomenon in patients with fibromyalgia: New features for diagnosis. Pain 1988; 32:21–26.
233. Walker EA: A history of neurological surgery. New York, Hafner Publishing, 1967.
234. Warfield CA, Biber MP, Crews DA, et al: Epidural steroid injection as a treatment for cervical radiculitis. Clin J Pain 1988; 4:201–204.
235. Watkinson A, Gargan MF, Bannister GC: Prognostic factors in soft tissue injuries of the cervical spine. Injury 1991; 22:307–309.
236. White A, Southwick W, Deponte RJ: Relief of pain by anterior cervical spine fusion for spondylosis. J Bone Joint Surg [Am] 1973; 55:525.
237. White AA, Panjabi MM: Biomechanics of the Spine, ed 2. Philadelphia, JB Lippincott, 1990, p 98.
238. White AA, Panjabi MM: Biomechanics of the Spine, ed 2. Philadelphia, JB Lippincott, 1978, pp 199–235.
239. White AA, Panjabi MM: Update on the evaluation on instability of the lower cervical spine. In AAOS Instruction Course Lectures, XXXVI. St Louis, Mosby, 1987, pp 513–520.
240. Whitecloud TS, Seago RA: Cervical discogenic syndrome: Results of operative intervention in patients with positive discography. Spine 1987; 12(4):313–316.
241. Williams J, Allen M, Harkess J: Late results of cervical discectomy and interbody fusions: Some factors influencing the results. J Bone Joint Surg [Am] 1968; 50:227.
242. Woolfenden JM, Pitt MJ, Durie BGM, et al: Comparison of bone scintigraphy and radiography in multiple myeloma. Radiology 1980; 134:723–728.
243. Wright A, Mayer TG, Gatchel RJ: Outcomes of disabling cervical spine disorders in compensation injuries. A prospective comparison to tertiary rehabilitation response for chronic lumbar spinal disorders. Spine 1999; 24:178–183.
244. Yiannikas C, Shahani BT, Young RR: Short-latency somatosensory-evoked potentials from radial, median, ulnar and peroneal nerve stimulation in the assessment of cervical spondylosis. Arch Neurol 1986; 43:1264–1270.
245. Youssen D, Atlas S, Goldberg H, et al: Degenerative narrowing of the cervical spine neural foramina: Evaluation with high-resolution 3DFT gradient-echo MR imaging. Am J Neurol Res 1991; 12:229–236.
246. Yu YL, Jones SJ: Somatosensory evoked potentials in cervical spondylosis: Correlation of median, ulnar and posterior tibial nerve responses with clinical and radiological findings. Brain 1985; 108:273–300.
247. Yunus MB, Kalyan-Raman UP, Kalyan-Raman K: Primary fibromyalgia syndrome and myofascial pain syndrome: Clinical features and muscle pathology. Arch Phys Med Rehabil 1988; 69:451–454.
248. Zborowski M: Cultural components in response to pain. J Soc Issues 1952; 8:16.
249. Zola IK: Culture and symptoms—An analysis of patients presenting complaints. Am Sociol Rev 1966; 31:615.

38 CHAPTER

Jeffrey A. Strakowski, M.D., J. William Wiand, D.O., and Ernest W. Johnson, M.D.

Upper Limb Musculoskeletal Pain Syndromes

Musculoskeletal pain syndromes of the upper limb are among the most common and challenging diagnostic and treatment problems facing the practitioner. A variety of physical problems present with a common symptom of pain. These include limitations of joint motion, soft tissue changes, and weakness, all of which can significantly compromise normal physiological function. Effective physiatric care requires an accurate diagnosis, a complete assessment of functional impairments, and an appropriate rehabilitation program. Treatment includes pain control, activity modification, and minimizing functional loss.

SHOULDER PAIN

Rotator Cuff Disease

Impingement, also called "painful arc syndrome," is a poorly defined term that encompasses a variety of disorders that manifest with anterior shoulder pain. These disorders have in common a pathological course that includes tendinitis of the rotator cuff, which can progress to complete rupture. Impingement ordinarily involves pain that occurs through the arc of motion as the arm is raised overhead. Impingement syndrome includes the conditions subacromial and subdeltoid bursitis, as well as rotator cuff tendinitis.

Many entities other than rotator cuff disease present with pain or decreased range of motion of the shoulder. These entities include adhesive capsulitis, calcific tendinitis, dynamic functional instability, acromioclavicular (AC) degenerative joint disease, glenohumeral joint degenerative disease, tumors of the shoulder girdle and lung apex, crystalline and rheumatoid arthropathies, and cervical radiculopathy.[73]

A growing body of primary research and literature has led to better understanding of the biomechanics and etiology of rotator cuff disease. Consequently, management, both operative and nonoperative, has improved.[26, 55, 61] To have a complete understanding of these mechanisms, the physician should have an in-depth knowledge of the three-dimensional anatomical and spatial relationships of the rotator cuff (Fig. 38–1).

There is considerable evidence in the literature for a multifactorial etiology of rotator cuff disease and impingement syndrome.[18, 45] Impingement itself denotes the physical compression and shearing of the rotator cuff tendon between the closed space of the rigid coracoacromial (CA) arch and the humeral head. Not all rotator cuff disease is a direct result of this specific extrinsic process, particularly in the elderly. Many feel that the term impingement syndrome fails to reflect the multiple possible causes and the spectrum of treatment options.[4]

In addition to categorizing rotator cuff disease on the basis of extrinsic vs. intrinsic etiologies, some also divide impingement into primary and secondary.[18] Primary impingement is due to the rigid CA arch (stenotic), and secondary impingement is defined as a relative decrease in the supraspinatus outlet caused by instability of the glenohumeral joint (nonstenotic).[45]

Stenotic Impingement

The subacromial impingement syndrome reported by Meyer[39] and Neer[43] suggests that rotator cuff degeneration and subsequent tears are produced extrinsically by the rigid CA arch. Neer states that 95% of rotator cuff tears are associated with extrinsic impingement,[43] and he describes three stages of progression (Table 38–1). Partial tears can extend to complete tears with relatively minor trauma. The stages are not discrete but evolve

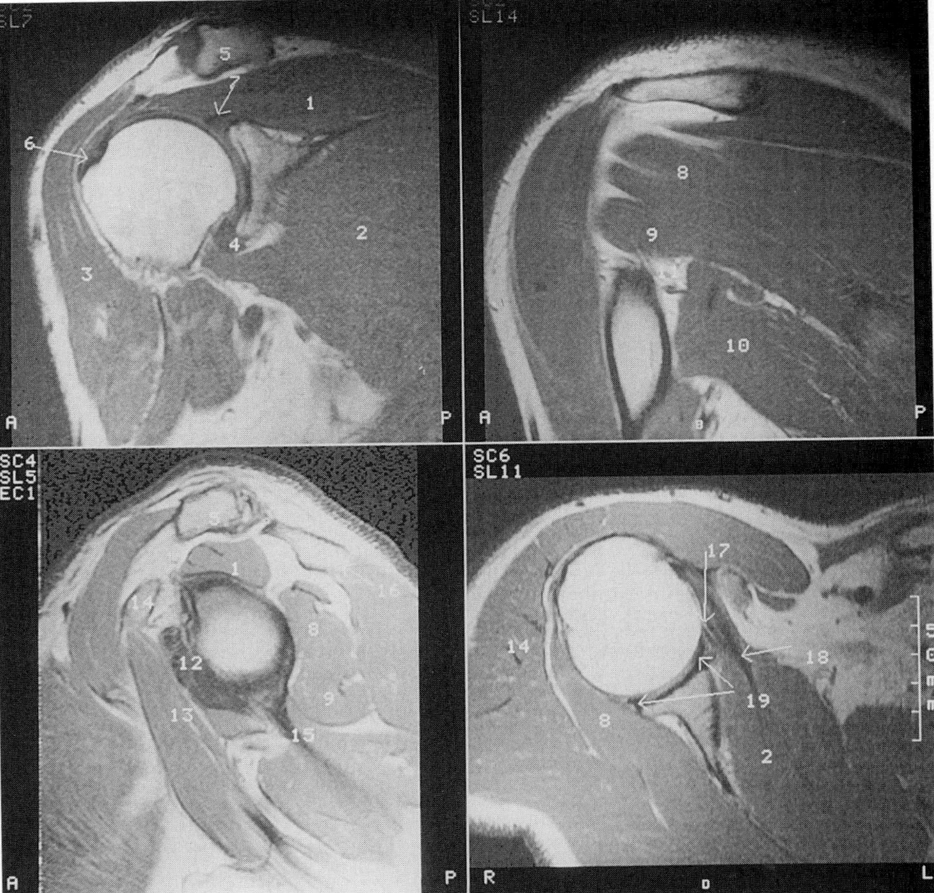

FIGURE 38–1. MRI of a normal shoulder showing anatomical relationships. Shown is the supraspinatus muscle (m.) (*1*), subscapularis m. (*2*), deltoid m. (*3*), axillary recess (*4*), and clavicle (*5*). Also seen are the normal cuff insertion (*6*), infraspinatus m. (*8*), teres minor m. (*9*), and latissmus dorsi m. (*10*), as well as the coracobrachialis and short head of the biceps m. (*13*) and subscapularis tendon (*19*).

as a continuum over time. Progression can also involve problems with the biceps tendon, subscapularis tendon, subacromial bursa, AC joint, and glenohumeral joint.

Virtually all complete rotator cuff tears manifest as distal midsubstance tears. Bone-tendon junction disruptions occur but are less common.[18] Acute cuff avulsion injuries are also rare in the shoulder.

There are a number of anatomical relationships and variations that contribute to reducing the available space for the rotator cuff tendon and result in stenosis. In addition to the rigid bony structures (humeral head, anterior third of the acromion, and the AC joint), there is the coracoacromial ligament (CAL), which constitutes the anterior third of the CA arch and contributes to confinement of the tendon in a fixed space.

Variations in shape and orientation of the acromion significantly affect stenosis and subsequently impingement (Fig. 38–2). The main variations are the flat type (type I), the smoothed curve (type II), and the angled curve (hook) (type III). Morrison and Bigliani, who described these variations, noted that the hook-type acromion was most common in patients with a complete rotator cuff tear.[42, 51]

Impingement can also lead to tendinitis and rupture of the long head of the biceps tendon. Neer showed that the functional arc of elevation of the shoulder is forward, not lateral, and that the impingement occurs predominantly against the anterior edge of the acromion and the CAL.[43] Poorly healed greater tuberosity fractures and a thickened CAL can also contribute to stenosis.

TABLE 38–1 The Stages of Rotator Cuff Disease

Stage I:	Rotator cuff inflammation—edema and hemorrhage
Stage II:	Progression to tendinitis—fibrosis and tendinitis
Stage III:	Partial or full-thickness tear—tendon degeneration and rupture
Stage IIIA:	Tears <1 cm in length
Stage IIIB:	Tears >1 cm in length
Stage IV:	Multiple tendon tears

Data from Neer CS: Anterior acromioplasty for chronic impingement syndrome in the shoulder. A preliminary report. J Bone Joint Surg Am 1972; 54:41–50.

Nonstenotic Impingement

Rotator cuff disease is not always due to stenosis. Subdeltoid bursitis is a common cause of anterior shoulder pain. It frequently develops in throwing athletes and is usually associated with the acceleration phase of throwing. Direct palpation over the subdeltoid bursa

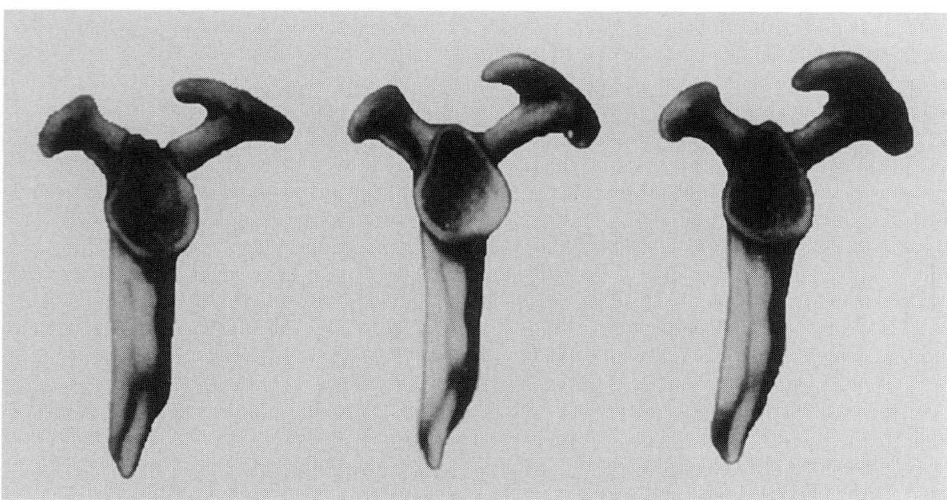

FIGURE 38–2. Acromial variation. *Left to right:* type I, Bigliani, flat acromion; type II, gentle anterior curve; type III, marked hooking. In addition, the acromion can be upsloping, horizontal, or downsloping.

to localize the area of tenderness is essential for the diagnosis (Fig. 38–3). It ordinarily responds well to rest, ice, and anti-inflammatory medications. In refractory cases, local injection of a steroid into the subdeltoid bursa might be necessary.

Subdeltoid adhesions occasionally develop. These typically present as limitation in range of motion and result from repetitive mechanical trauma, chronic bursal inflammation, crystalline disease, and rheumatologic causes. Adhesions are primarily manifested in external rotation and should be suspected when chronicity, loss of motion, and calcific deposits are present.

Primary glenohumeral instability should also be considered when evaluating rotator cuff disease. Abnormal excursion of the shoulder joint due to laxity results in fatigue and traction of the shoulder girdle musculature.[27] The resulting muscular dysfunction can allow even greater humeral head motion, including proximal migration of the head under the CA arch, which subsequently leads to the development of impingement and cuff disease. Affected individuals are typically younger adults (less than 35 years old) and involved in throwing or repetitive overhead activities such as tennis, swimming, and baseball. Recurrent anterior subluxation is occasionally seen with the overhead phase of throwing in these individuals.[28] The clinical signs and symptoms of instability are discussed elsewhere in this chapter. The difficulty with instability associated with rotator cuff disease is that the often dramatic signs of rotator cuff pathology can obscure the more subtle signs of instability. Every effort should be made to identify shoulder instability as a component of the shoulder pathology, particularly in younger patients and those with persistent symptoms. Imprecise diagnosis of this shoulder instability can lead to unnecessary and unsuccessful repeated injections and occasionally even to acromioplasties.

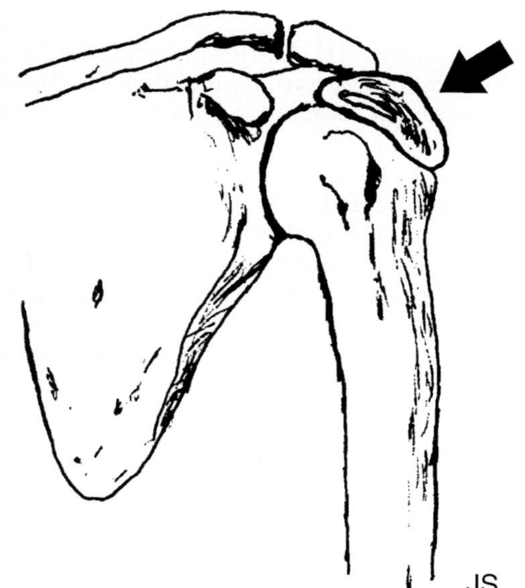

FIGURE 38–3. Anatomical position of the subdeltoid bursa.

The frequent performance of overhead activities can place enormous stresses on the dynamic and static stabilizers of the shoulders. Repetitive stresses of this nature can, over the course of time, lead to microtrauma of the glenohumeral ligaments, with eventual attenuation of these structures. Without normal functioning of these static stabilizers, a pattern of mild instability can develop, placing further demands on the dynamic stabilizers of the rotator cuff.[18, 55]

Anterior shoulder pain and impingement syndrome can also result from adhesive capsulitis at any time during its course. The many other causes of anterior shoulder pain should be excluded before it is attributed to capsulitis.

It has also been demonstrated that scapular stabilizers are important factors in humeral head control. The important relationship of the scapulohumeral complex to glenohumeral stabilization has been discussed by Kibler and Chandler.[18] In a test they referred to as the lateral scapular slide, they measured the distance between the medial border of the scapula and the spinous processes and found that this distance was increased in symptomatic throwing athletes, suggesting scapulothoracic instability. The muscle groups specifically involved include

TABLE 38–2 Conditions with Clinical Appearances Potentially Similar to Primary Rotator Cuff Disease

Acute traumatic bursitis
Instability
Primary acromioclavicular disease
Cervical radiculopathy
Arthritides of the glenohumeral joint
Calcific tendinitis
Adhesive capsulitis

the trapezius, rhomboids, and serratus anterior. Deficiencies in the strength or flexibility of these muscles can affect the synchrony of scapular motion. This disruption of the normal scapulohumeral rhythm due to abnormal motion on the chest wall leads to excessive stress on the glenohumeral joint. This then leads to impingement of the rotator cuff underneath the CA arch, and is an important consideration when designing an exercise program for throwing athletes.

In a somewhat different vein from the extrinsic stress theories proposed by Meyer and Neer, Codman[11] in 1934 suggested an intrinsic theory of rotator cuff disease. He postulated that intrinsic ischemic degenerative changes within the cuff itself lead to tears. He proposed the concept of the "critical zone" near the insertion of the supraspinatus tendon.[11] Nirschl[48] described "angiofibroblastic hyperplasia" as the initial change in the cuff that leads to more permanent change. Uhthoff et al[68] in 1987 found in a study of cadaveric specimens that the majority of cuff tears began on the articular side, and they proposed that the extrinsic findings were actually a secondary process. This relationship has since been confirmed by others.[4] The severity of the degenerative acromial changes seems to correlate with the severity of the rotator cuff disease in these specimens. Despite considerable controversy, there is often no evidence of extrinsic factors in persons with rotator cuff pathology.[51]

Several investigators have discussed the implications of the rotator cuff vascular supply in primary disease. The rotator cuff musculature is richly supplied by the suprascapular, the anterior and posterior circumflex humeral, and the axillary arteries. Nevertheless, there are hypovascular zones in the rotator cuff tendons that are thought to coincide with commonly observed areas of degeneration, such as the site of the humeral insertion.[58] These areas may play an important role in the development of tendon degeneration and inability to heal. If the injury outstrips the blood supply, progression will occur.

Rathbun and Macnab[58] also found that a distinct and characteristic vascular pattern can be related to the position of the arm. By injecting micro-opaque spheres into the subclavian artery supplying the rotator cuff, they found the vessels supplying the supraspinatus tendon completely filled while the shoulder was in the abducted position. However, they found a constant area of avascularity extending from 1 cm proximal directly to the point of insertion into the greater tuberosity with the shoulder in the adducted position. Similar studies have shown a similar avascular zone in the intracapsular portion of the biceps tendon as it passes over the head of the humerus.[20]

The list of clinical conditions that can resemble primary rotator cuff disease is extensive (Table 38–2). Acute traumatic bursitis usually results from a direct blow to the cuff severe enough to produce hemorrhage and edema. Acute traumatic bursitis is ordinarily a self-limiting condition that resolves with appropriate rest and time. It can occasionally initiate a continuing impingement syndrome. The temporal relationship to trauma and the physical findings suggest the diagnosis. Instability should be distinguished from primary rotator cuff disease.

With primary AC joint disease a history of previous trauma is usually present, in addition to the findings being restricted primarily to the AC joint itself. Physical findings include tenderness and pain reproduced on forcible adduction and internal rotation of the humerus. These findings can be mistaken for subacromial impingement.

Cervical radiculopathy is discussed elsewhere in this text (see Chapter 37). It can frequently be distinguished from rotator cuff dysfunction by posterior shoulder pain, by pain extending below the elbow, or by weakness, sensory loss, and reflex changes.

Calcific tendinitis is thought to represent a separate pathological process. Calcification is seldom seen with degenerative rotator cuff disease, and its radiological demonstration generally precludes the diagnosis of impingement syndrome, although occasionally capsular ruptures into the bursa result in calcification.

Diagnosis

A comprehensive history is essential to accurately identify the disease process. Age, occupation, avocations, and the presence of systemic disease all can provide clues to the appropriate diagnosis. Medical conditions such as diabetes mellitus, arthritides, crystalline disease, cervical spine disorders, and neuromuscular disease can all contribute to rotator cuff disease and should be appropriately treated. A history of previous treatment, including the specific type of treatment, its duration, and the response, offers important insights into the likely origin of the present disorder and suggests management steps.

Although the clinical picture of rotator cuff disease is more of a continuum, Hawkins and Kennedy[20] described characteristic signs and symptoms that correlate with the stage of disease (Table 38–3). Stage I disease is more common in patients under 25 years of age. These patients typically complain of a toothache-like discom-

TABLE 38–3 Clinical Stages of Rotator Cuff Disease

Stage I:	Minimal pain with activity; no weakness and no loss of motion
Stage II:	Marked tendinitis with pain and no loss of motion
Stage III:	Pain and weakness (cuff tear)

Data from Hawkins RJ, Kennedy JC: Impingement syndrome in athletes. Am J Sports Med 1980; 8:151–157.

fort radiating laterally to the middle of the arm. Point tenderness is noted over the greater tuberosity and occasionally over the anterior acromion and CAL. Pain is often induced with flexion and abduction to 90 degrees.

The classic impingement test has been described as a complaint of pain when the examiner flexes the shoulder anteriorly while stabilizing the scapula to prevent scapulothoracic compensation.[73] This maneuver, when positive, reproduces pain and apprehension as it jams the greater tuberosity against the anteroinferior surface of the acromion. This may be the most reliable physical sign in establishing the diagnosis. Internal rotation of the shoulder into this forward flexed position typically accentuates the discomfort (Fig. 38–4). An alternative test for impingement was described by Hawkins and Kennedy (Fig. 38–5).[20] For clarity, the specific maneuver used should be specified and the physical examination findings reported. An injection of 10 mL of 1% lidocaine directly into the subacromial bursa often eliminates or reduces pain and helps to confirm the diagnosis.

Stage II disease is most frequently seen in the 25- to 40-year-old age group but can occur at any age. The pain is described as toothache-like and increases with overhead activities. It is often worse at night and frequently limits sleep. It can progress to limit daytime activities that aggravate the discomfort. The tenderness is more severe than in stage I and can secondarily involve the AC joint. Range of motion often becomes painful and difficult at this stage. There can be a particularly painful catching sensation as the arm is brought down from the abducted position. This sensation is believed by some to represent catching of the scar under the impingement area.[20]

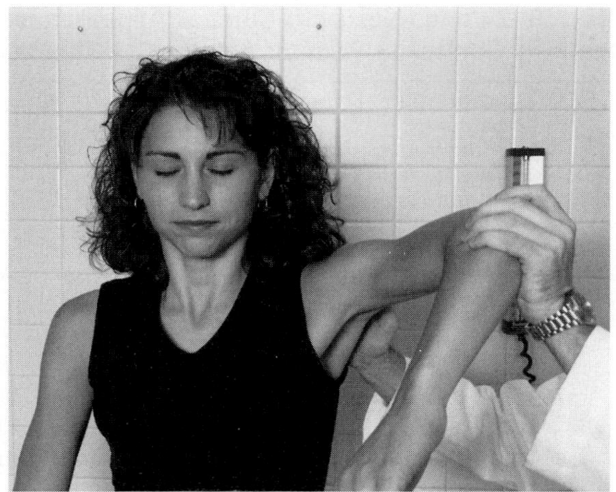

FIGURE 38–5. Impingement sign described by Hawkins and Kennedy.[20] Pain is elicted on forced internal rotation of the shoulder with the elbow flexed to 90 degrees.

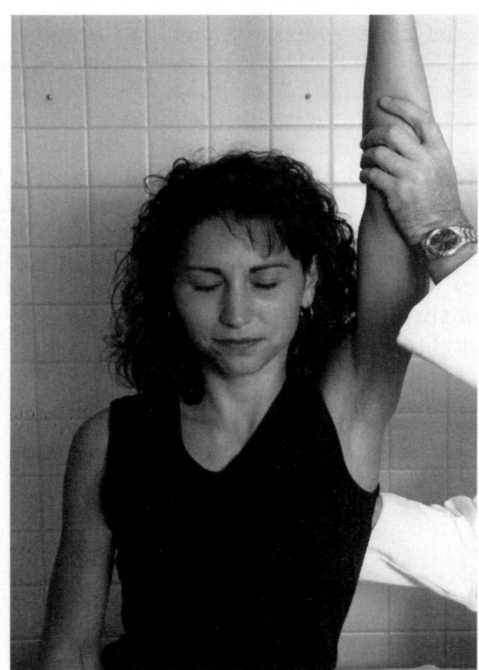

FIGURE 38–4. Positioning for the impingement test. The scapula is stabilized posteriorly while the arm is elevated, taking the shoulder through its range of foward flexion. Reproducible pain with apprehension, including grimacing, is characteristic of the positive impingement sign.

Stage III disease is ordinarily seen in patients more than 40 years old and is usually associated with a long history of intermittent or progressive shoulder problems, including the signs and symptoms seen in stages I and II. Symptoms are usually worse with overhead activity and at night. Affected individuals typically exhibit weakness secondary to pain (Fig. 38–6). Decreased range of motion and shoulder stiffness are also noted.

The clinical findings in complete rotator cuff tendon rupture may differ little from the clinical findings of earlier stages; or there may be a dramatic clinical change (such as sudden inability to elevate the arm) as a result of an acute event that finally causes rupture. However, there is virtually always a long history of shoulder problems. Complete or partial tears occur at an average age of 50 years. Several signs indicative of full-thickness

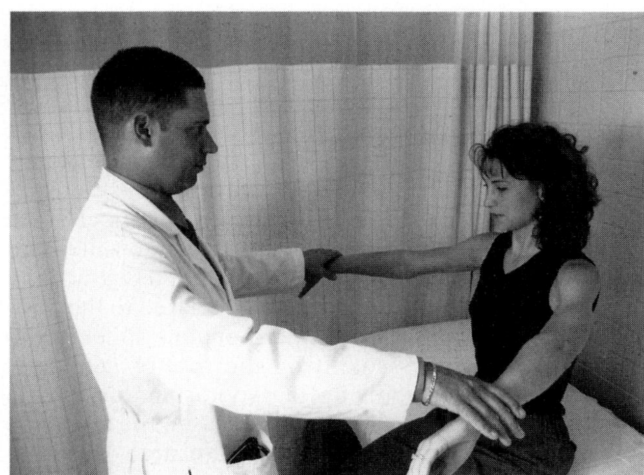

FIGURE 38–6. A positive supraspinatus test. Pain and/or weakness is elicted with downward pressure on the arm with the shoulder abducted to 90 degrees, 30 degrees anterior to the coronal plane.

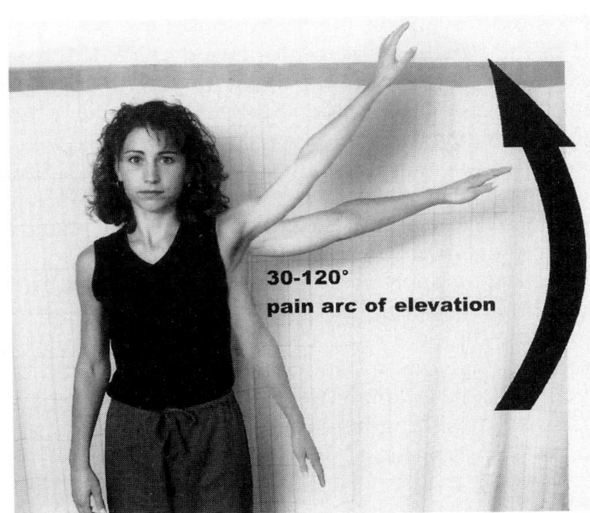

FIGURE 38–7. Painful arc of abduction in rotator cuff disease. Impingement occurs, somewhat variably, in the range of motion from approximately 45 degrees to 120 degrees. Relief of pain typically occurs with continued abduction beyond 120 degrees, in the absence of concomitant pathology such as acromioclavicular joint arthritis.

rotator cuff tears have been described.[20] These include infraspinatus and supraspinatus wasting, tenderness over the greater tuberosity and anterior acromion, AC joint tenderness, painful arc of motion at 90 degrees of abduction (Fig. 38–7) or forward flexion, passive range of motion greater than active range of motion (particularly in abduction and external rotation), and weakness of abduction and external rotation.

Plain film evaluation is the first step in radiological imaging of the shoulder. It is most sensitive for osseous lesions, including fractures, metastatic lesions, and developmental or degenerative variations. Plain radiography most often yields positive findings in stage III disease. These findings include sclerosis and osteophyte formation on the anteroinferior acromion and greater tuberosity (which also might exhibit cystic degeneration). Osteophyte formation may be present, and the distance between the acromion and humeral head may be reduced. Osteolysis manifests as demineralization of the distal clavicle and widening of the AC joint. Plain radiography, however, is of limited use in demonstrating abnormal calcifications and soft tissue disease. Whereas calcific bursitis and tendinitis often have recognizable radiographic appearances, most soft tissue lesions of the shoulder do not.

Although ultrasonography (US) is used in some centers for evaluating rotator cuff disease, most centers in the United States have limited experience with this modality, and there is difficulty with reproducibility of findings.[16, 50]

Arthrography is similarly of limited use in evaluating rotator cuff disease. It has good sensitivity only for complete tears or high-grade partial undersurface tears. In full-thickness tears, the contrast medium leaks through the defect and pools outside the cuff, ordinarily adjacent to the undersurface of the acromion (Fig. 38–8).

Arthrograms are ordinarily normal in partial-thickness tears or earlier stages of degeneration. Some obvious drawbacks to the use of this imaging modality are that approximately 70% of tears are partial and that the bursal surface is more commonly involved than the undersurface.[26] Further lowering its sensitivity are situations in which a complete tear is partially fibrosed or healed. Another limitation is the inability to distinguish muscle pathology by arthrography.

The primary role of radionuclide scintigraphy is in characterizing patterns of disease in patients with known or suspected malignancies or arthritides. Its high sensitivity but low specificity limits its role in the evaluation of monoarticular disease.

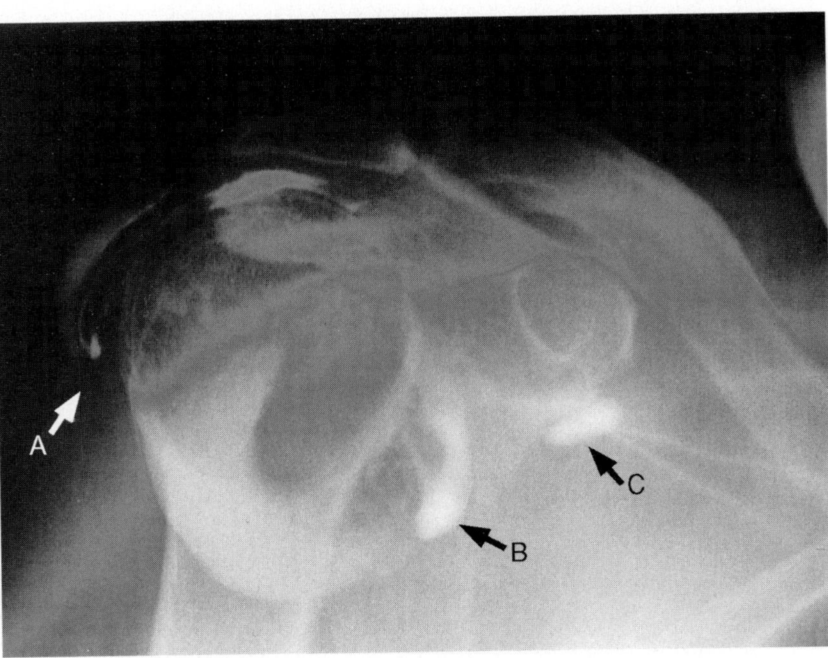

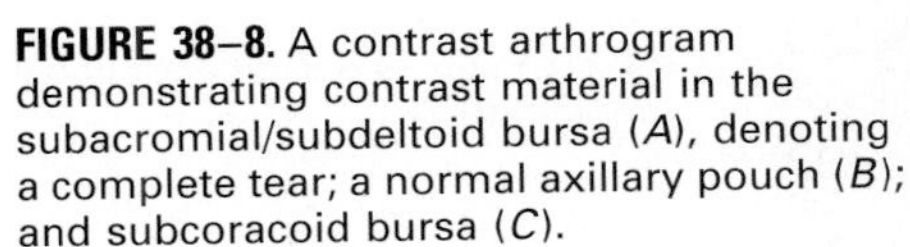
FIGURE 38–8. A contrast arthrogram demonstrating contrast material in the subacromial/subdeltoid bursa (*A*), denoting a complete tear; a normal axillary pouch (*B*); and subcoracoid bursa (*C*).

Magnetic resonance imaging (MRI) has become the primary imaging modality of choice. Its three-dimensional capabilities provide more specific characterization of incomplete tears and afford three-dimensional characterization of complete tears (Fig. 38–9); it also yields important information on the status of muscle groups. Examples of its use are in the identification of ganglia in the spinoglenoid fossa and in locating focal suprascapular nerve palsies.

Treatment

Precise etiological diagnosis is the foundation for appropriate and effective treatment of rotator cuff disease. Whereas surgically enlarging the CA space through partial acromioplasty and CAL lysis provides symptomatic relief in some patients, recently physiatric rehabilitation of the dynamic stabilizers has been emphasized as the most effective therapeutic modality. Physiatric treatment should be individualized for each patient. Many of the early rehabilitation techniques employed are similar for all patients and have the goal of promoting healing and returning the physiological motion and normal scapulothoracic rhythm of the shoulder girdle. The training techniques employed beyond this point, however, must be consistent with the goals and needs of the individual patient (e.g., throwing athlete, laborer, sedentary person).

Primary prevention should be considered an integral part of the treatment of rotator cuff disease. Educating persons at risk can do much to circumvent the development of rotator cuff disease. Athletes, particularly those involved in throwing and overhead sports, as well as laborers who incur repetitive shoulder stress should be instructed in proper warmup techniques, specific strengthening techniques, and the warning signs of early impingement.

Tailoring an appropriate therapeutic prescription requires understanding the stage of the rotator cuff disease. Most stage I disease is reversible.[45] Treatment for this stage includes modalities such as ice, alteration of activity, anti-inflammatory medications, therapeutic exercises for strengthening the dynamic stabilizers, and, rarely, the use of intra-articular steroids. Anti-inflammatory measures are taken to reduce cuff edema and hemorrhage. Local ice massage for 10 to 20 minutes is indicated following activity that exacerbates symptoms. US can be helpful. A typical US regimen for the supraspinatus tendon is 1.2 to 1.5 W/cm^2 for 8 minutes per day for 10 days. Total joint rest is to be avoided in favor of symptom-limited activity and specific therapeutic exercises.

A technique suggested to correct deficiencies in strength, flexibility, and coordination is proprioceptive neuromuscular facilitation (PNF).[18] This is performed

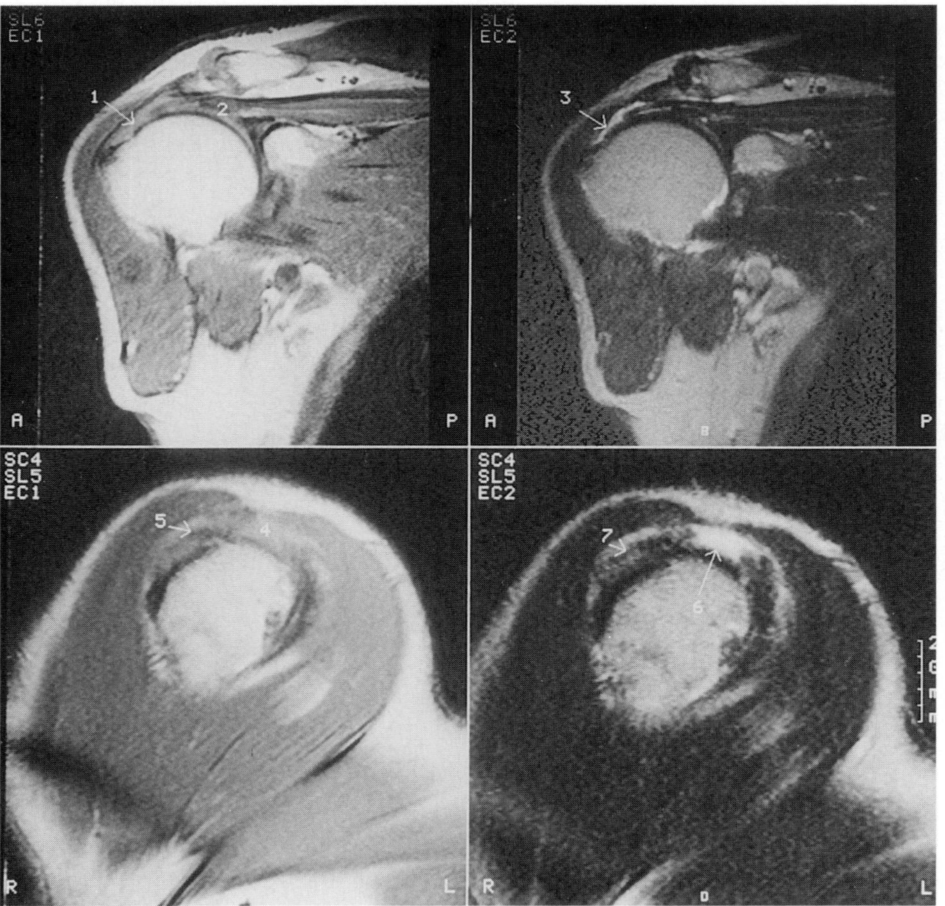

FIGURE 38–9. T1-weighted (*left panels*) and matching T2-weighted (*right panels*) MR images demonstrating a full-thickness rotator cuff tear. The coronal images demonstrate gray signal in the supraspinatus portion of the cuff (*1*), a retracted tendon (*2*), and fluid in the distal tear (*3*). The sagittal images show the torn cuff (*4* and *6*) and viable cuff (*5* and *7*).

by selective exercise patterns ordinarily led by a therapist. The neurophysiological basis for the facilitation is believed to involve the stretch reflex. This facilitates or inhibits agonist and antagonist muscle groups in a rate-dependent fashion and attempts to redevelop normal scapulohumeral rhythm with joint distraction and compression techniques. The effectiveness of this technique can depend on the experience of the therapist.

After symptomatic relief has been obtained, a program of active exercise is initiated with the goal of strengthening both the internal and external shoulder rotators in the nonabducted position.

The supraspinatus is strengthened by the patient moving the hand from the straight adducted position to abduction at approximately 90 degrees, with the hand in the thumb-down position after the arm is placed in a position of 30 degrees anterior to the straight abducted position (Fig. 38–10).

These exercises can be initially performed with just the weight of the hand, with eventual progression to external weights (ordinarily 2.5 to 10 lb). Isotonic strengthening of all of the rotator cuff musculature has also been found to be useful. The basic goal of rotator cuff strengthening is to restore its function as a humeral head stabilizer. This can reduce the degree of impingement and accelerate the return to pain-free activities. Strengthening of the scapulothoracic musculature can also provide clinical improvement. One-third of shoulder abduction is due to scapular rotation. With an increased scapulothoracic component of shoulder motion, there is a more favorable positioning of the scapula and acromion to alleviate tendon impingement. The strength and flexibility of all of the muscles involved in the dynamic stabilization of the humerus should be continually assessed as the rehabilitation process progresses. This includes the deltoid and biceps, as well as the rotator cuff and scapulothoracic muscles.

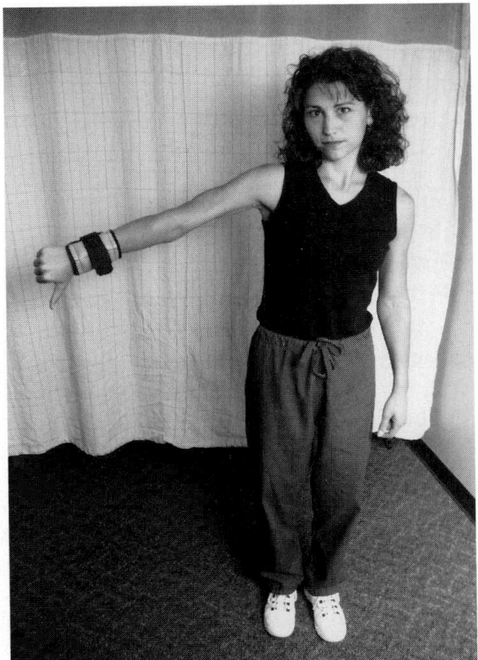
FIGURE 38–10. Demonstration of supraspinatus strengthening. The shoulder is abducted in the scapular plane with resistance while in internal rotation.

The use of intra-articular steroids is controversial because of the well-known risks to the tendon structure,[69] which include collagen necrosis, weakness, and possible rupture. Repetitive injections increase these risks. Selective use of a well-performed single injection in the subacromial space, however, has been shown to hasten the recovery process by reducing pain and inflammation, allowing more rapid advancement to an exercise program.

Current treatment trends limit the role of surgical decompression to symptomatic relief of pain, primarily in elderly patients with more advanced disease. Widespread, indiscriminate surgical decompression in early stages of disease does not reflect the current pathophysiological understanding of the disease process. Patients with early-stage disease that is refractory to appropriate physiatric treatment protocols need to be reconsidered to ensure accurate diagnosis. Further diagnostic modalities such as MRI, electromyography (EMG), and arthroscopy should be considered so that any unsuspected disorder can be diagnosed and addressed. Meyers[40] reports that spurs on the undersurface of the clavicle or acromion should be removed.

Conservative treatment protocols for stages II and III disease are the same as for stage I. Surgical decompression is entertained in patients with stage II or III disease that does not respond to appropriate physiatric treatment protocols. Some feel that a general principle in the absence of a cuff tear is to consider surgery if pain has persisted for more than 1 year. The purpose of decompression by anterior acromioplasty and CAL release, with preservation of the deltoid by reattachment and repair of the cuff, is to reduce or eliminate impingement pain, improve function, and prevent recurrence. In successful surgical decompression, the anterior inferior acromial edge, the undersurface of the AC joint, and the CAL are surgically modified.

Bicipital Tendinitis

Bicipital tendinitis is an inflammation of the long head of the biceps where the tendon passes through the bicipital groove (Fig. 38–11). Although often a manifestation of progressive cuff disease, particularly in the elderly, it is also frequently seen in younger persons as a result of chronic repetitive motion. Recurrent subluxation of the long head of the biceps tendon is also a consideration, particularly in throwing athletes. It has also been theorized that the long head of the biceps tendon plays a role in controlling superior subluxation of the humeral head,[1] which can contribute to secondary impingement.

Bicipital tendinitis as a manifestation of repetitive motion disorders occurs most often as an occupational disorder in laborers and others who use frequent overhead motions. There can be a spectrum from acute myositis and tenosynovitis to chronic tendinopathy, which may or may not include calcification.

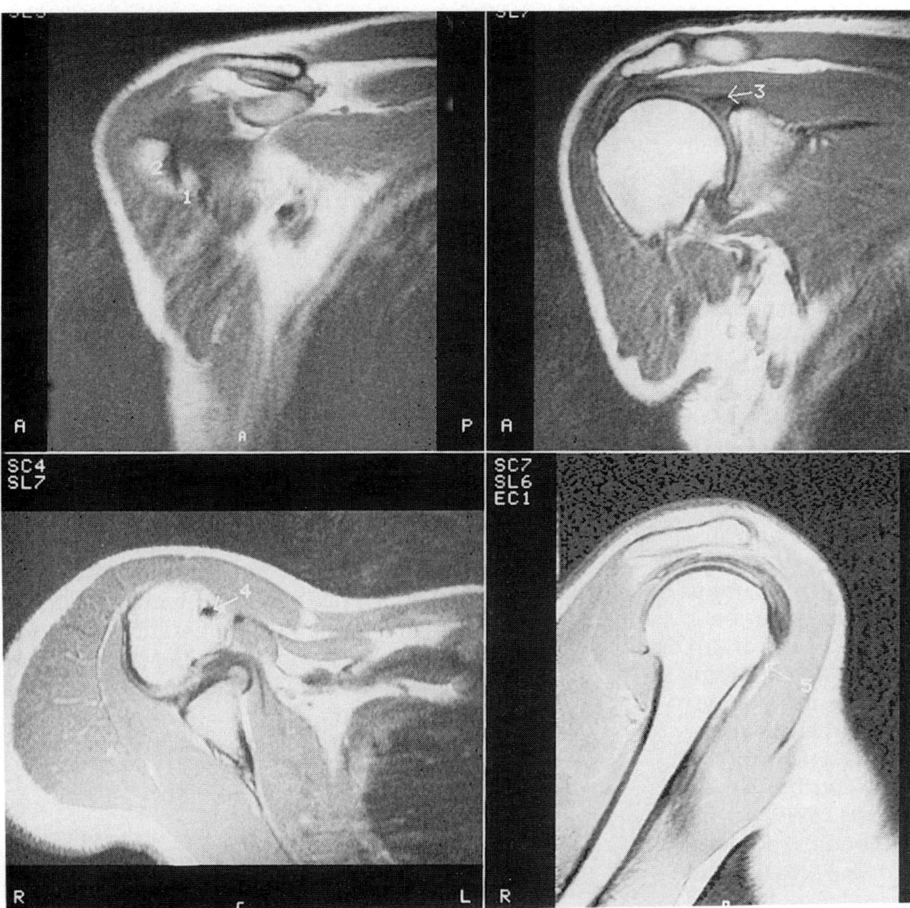

FIGURE 38–11. The spatial anatomical relationships of the long head of the biceps are demonstrated on MRI. The position in its groove (*1*) is shown on coronal section in close proximity to the greater tuberosity (*2*). Its insertion site is also shown on the coronal (*3*), axial (*4*), and sagittal views (*5*).

Although less common, recurrent subluxation can lead to bicipital tendinitis. It occurs most frequently during maximum muscular tension, as during the cocking phases of throwing when the shoulder goes from extremes of external rotation into internal rotation. Persons who are most predisposed to this include those with congenitally shallow or posttraumatic bicipital grooves. These medial subluxations can be palpated by the examiner with a finger placed over the bicipital groove.

Inflammation of the intracapsular portion of the biceps tendon is a frequent manifestation of stage II and III rotator cuff disease. It is often seen with associated cuff tendinitis. Its anatomical location close to the supraspinatus and subscapularis tendon predisposes it to the inflammatory and degenerative processes of severe rotator cuff disease. This is particularly true in the elderly, who, after a complete rotator cuff tear, may place undo strain on the bicipital tendon, owing to its increased role in controlling superior subluxation of the humeral head. This contributes to a form of "secondary impingement."[1] This is the most common cause of a complete bicipital tendon rupture in elderly individuals.

Diagnosis

Patients often present with anterior shoulder pain and palpable tenderness of the biceps tendon in the bicipital groove. The bicipital groove can be palpated by internally rotating the humerus 30 degrees with the patient supine. The groove will be located directly anterior.

Other diagnostic tests include pain on straight-arm raising (performed with resisted forward flexion of the shoulder at approximately 80 degrees with the elbow extended) or resisted supination of the forearm (Fig. 38–12).[20] On both of these maneuvers pain is felt in the area of the bicipital groove. Complete ruptures are often apparent on inspection and palpation of the biceps muscle (Fig. 38–13).

Treatment

The treatment of patients with an intact tendon is physiatric therapy similar to that described for rotator cuff disease. Emphasis is placed on the dynamic stabilizers of the shoulder, with treatment primarily entailing progressive resistance exercises of the internal and external shoulder rotators. Use of a Theraband is a convenient means of achieving this (Fig. 38–14). Nonsteroidal anti-inflammatory drugs (NSAIDs), heat and cold modalities, and activity modification are also essential components of the treatment plan. US applied over the relatively superficial biceps tendon can be useful in reducing pain, and should be administered at a dosage of 0.8 to 1.2 W/cm^2 for 8 minutes per day for 10 days. Steroids should not be injected into the bicipital groove because of the possibility of promoting eventual tendon

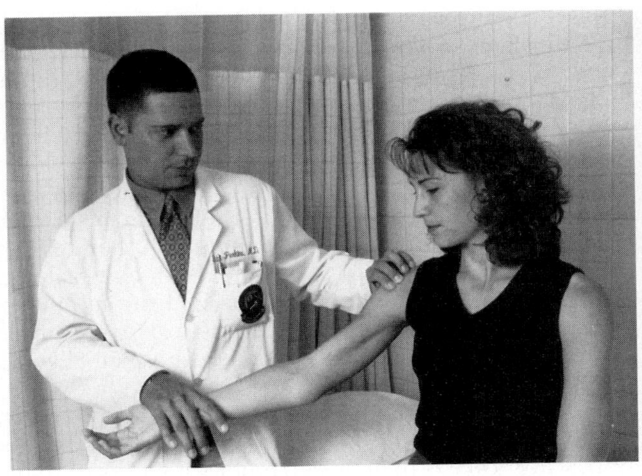
A

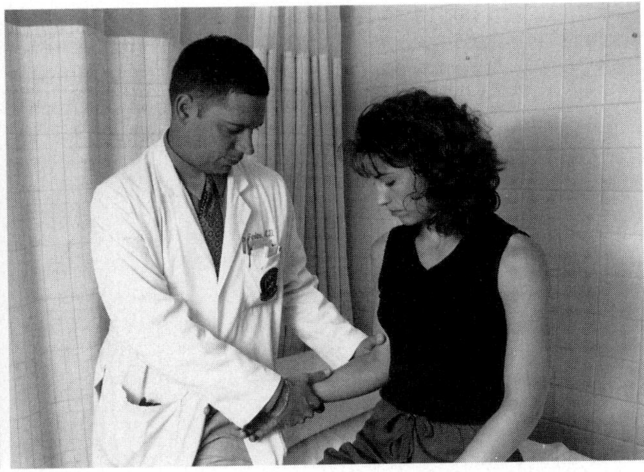
B

FIGURE 38–12. Tests for bicipital tendonitis. *A.* Straight arm raising performed with resisted forward flexion of the shoulder at approximately 80 degrees. *B.* Resisted supination of the forearm.

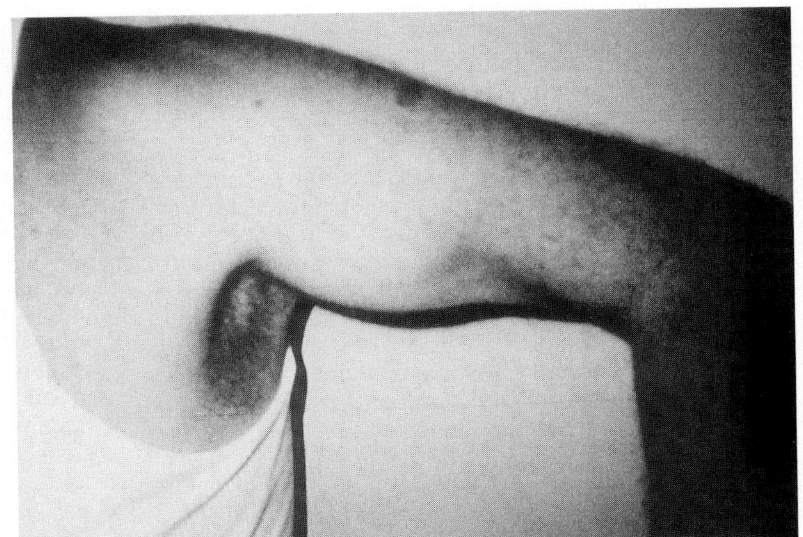

FIGURE 38–13. Distal biceps tendon rupture in a 38-year-old man. The biceps muscle has migrated proximally.

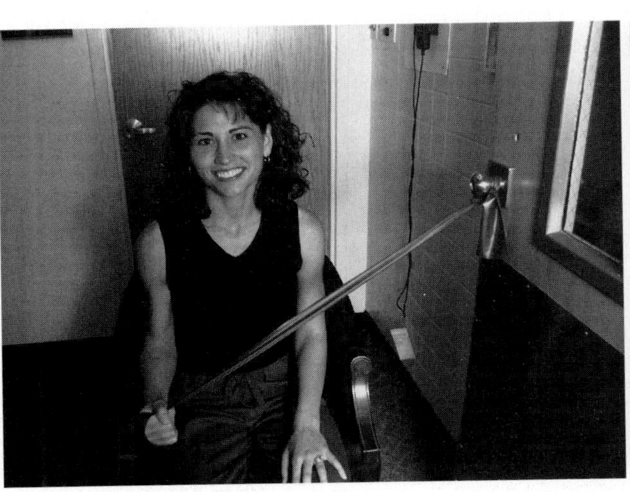
A

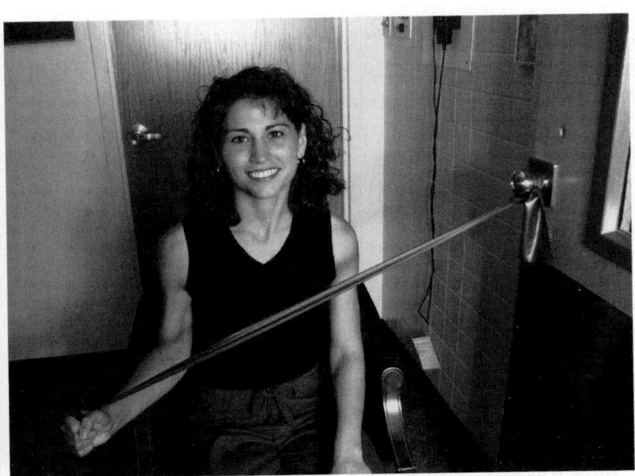
B

FIGURE 38–14. A Theraband is a convenient aid to performing internal and external rotation resistance exercises.

rupture.[69, 73] In light of the importance of the biceps tendon as a dynamic stabilizer of the glenohumeral joint, indiscriminate surgical transfer for chronic biceps tendinitis should be avoided.

Biceps Rupture

In a younger person, violent trauma is ordinarily needed to tear the biceps brachii at the musculotendinous junction, a circumstance often requiring surgical repair (see Fig. 38–13). In most cases, particularly in individuals more than 40 years old, biceps rupture occurs in the intra-articular area and is frequently associated with rotator cuff disease and often even a full-thickness tear of the rotator cuff. Neer reported that in 300 cuff tears in older people, one-third involved the biceps.[45] Biceps rupture most frequently manifests as a partial or complete avulsion of its insertion from the superior rim of the anterior labrum.

Instability

The shoulder joint has the greatest range of motion of any joint in the body. Stability has been sacrificed for range of motion. Instability of the shoulder is essentially defined as excessive translation of the humeral head on the glenoid, and subsequent labral disease.

Although instability can be congenital, as in Marfan syndrome or Ehlers-Danlos syndrome, it is seen most frequently after trauma or in chronic degenerative fatigue syndromes. As the dynamic stabilizers fatigue or fail, the glenohumeral labral complex (static stabilizers) is stretched or torn. The most common dislocation by far is traumatic anterior dislocation with labral injury, the "Bankhart complex" (Fig. 38–15B). Less common, and more frequently associated with overuse syndromes, are posterior subluxations (so-called Bennett lesions) and multidirectional instability.[17]

Diagnosis

Diagnosis requires detecting a range of problems from obvious dislocation to subtle multidirectional instability associated with fatigue. A thorough medical history is necessary to properly identify the disorder and its cause. A history of trauma, recurrent dislocation, chronic overuse, and multijoint instability can assist in properly identifying the disorder. Other problems such as nerve palsies, radiculopathies, or glenohumeral fractures should be considered and pursued if the history is suggestive.

Physical examination in these cases is often insensitive or inaccurate. The dynamic stabilization of this joint and the effects of fatigue are critical elements in the development of instability, which might not be adequately evaluated at rest or under anesthesia. Instability in throwers is often difficult for the examiner to accurately assess, including distinguishing between anterior and posterior instability. Both can be seen in the same phase of throwing, and both present with pain.

The shoulder examination includes visual inspection for gross bony deformity and muscle wasting. The shoulder should be palpated for glenohumeral relationships, and evaluation of the AC joint and coracoclavicular relationships should also be routinely performed to rule out AC separation or focal bone or muscle trauma. The shoulder should be taken through its full range of motion both actively and passively and limitation in any plane should be noted.

Specific tests for instability include Lachman's test and the relocation test.[4] To perform Lachman's test, the examiner positions the patient supine on the table and abducts the shoulder to 90 degrees with external rotation. An anterior force is then applied to the humeral head. A positive test is indicated by excessive anterior translation, which can be associated with pain (Fig. 38–16A).

In the relocation test the patient is positioned supine and the shoulder is abducted and externally rotated. Posterior force is then placed on the humerus to reduce the subluxation of anterior glenohumeral instability (Fig. 38–16B). The most important factor in both tests is patient apprehension when the arm is abducted and externally rotated.

Radiography plays an even greater role in the evaluation of instability than in rotator cuff disease. Plain film evaluation of the shoulder, in internal and external rotation, is complemented by an axillary projection. These views will often show the anterior labral injuries of the Bankhart complex and the notch-like defect on the superior greater tuberosity (Hill-Sachs lesion) characteristic of anterior dislocations. Also evaluated are joint surfaces that provide clues to chronic degenerative glenohumeral disease (see Fig. 38–15).

When the initial workup is inconclusive, the next level of testing typically involves arthrography with computed tomography (CT). Although invasive, this test provides valuable information on the labrum, glenoid, and humeral head. Increasingly, however, MRI is replacing this invasive procedure. In addition to the information gleaned with CT-arthrography, MRI allows a noninvasive evaluation of the rotator cuff, impingement, and occasionally nerve palsies.

Treatment

The initial management for an acute shoulder dislocation is reduction. The mechanism of injury should be identified and the patient evaluated for neurovascular compromise before reduction is initiated. Axillary nerve palsies are common with anterior dislocations. Closed reduction for acute dislocations is frequently performed in emergency room settings. There are multiple techniques for performing closed reduction. The most important factor is that it be performed with gentle steady pressure to avoid further injury. Contraindications to closed reduction include severe osteoporosis or suspected fracture.

A thorough neurovascular examination should be performed after reduction. The joint is then protected to prevent recurrent dislocation. This is accomplished primarily by activity modification. Younger persons, particularly those less than 20 years old, are less likely to get adhesive capsulitis and more predisposed to redislocation. Immobilization of the shoulder is better toler-

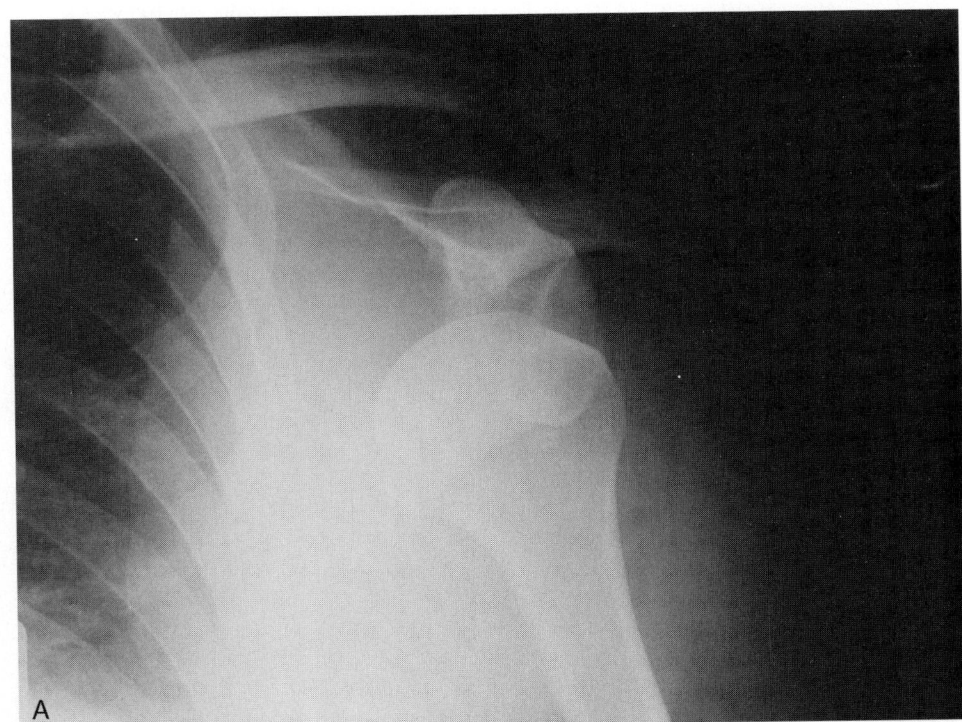

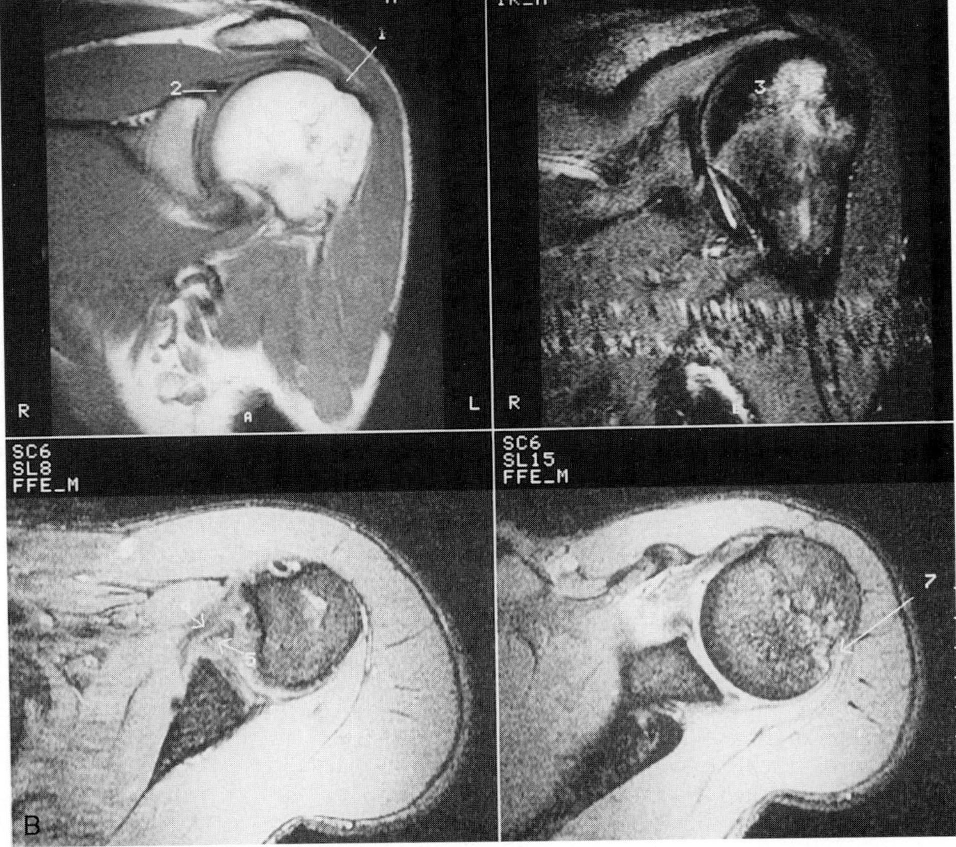

FIGURE 38–15. Radiological series of an acute shoulder dislocation in a 42-year-old man. *A.* The anterior dislocation is easily recognizable on plain film. *B.* MRI demonstrates a normal rotator cuff (*1*) and superior labrum (*2*). The bone compression characteristic of Hill-Sachs lesions are well demonstrated on the water-weighted images (*3* and *7*). Also seen is the avulsed labral-capsular complex of the Bankhart lesion (*4* and *5*).

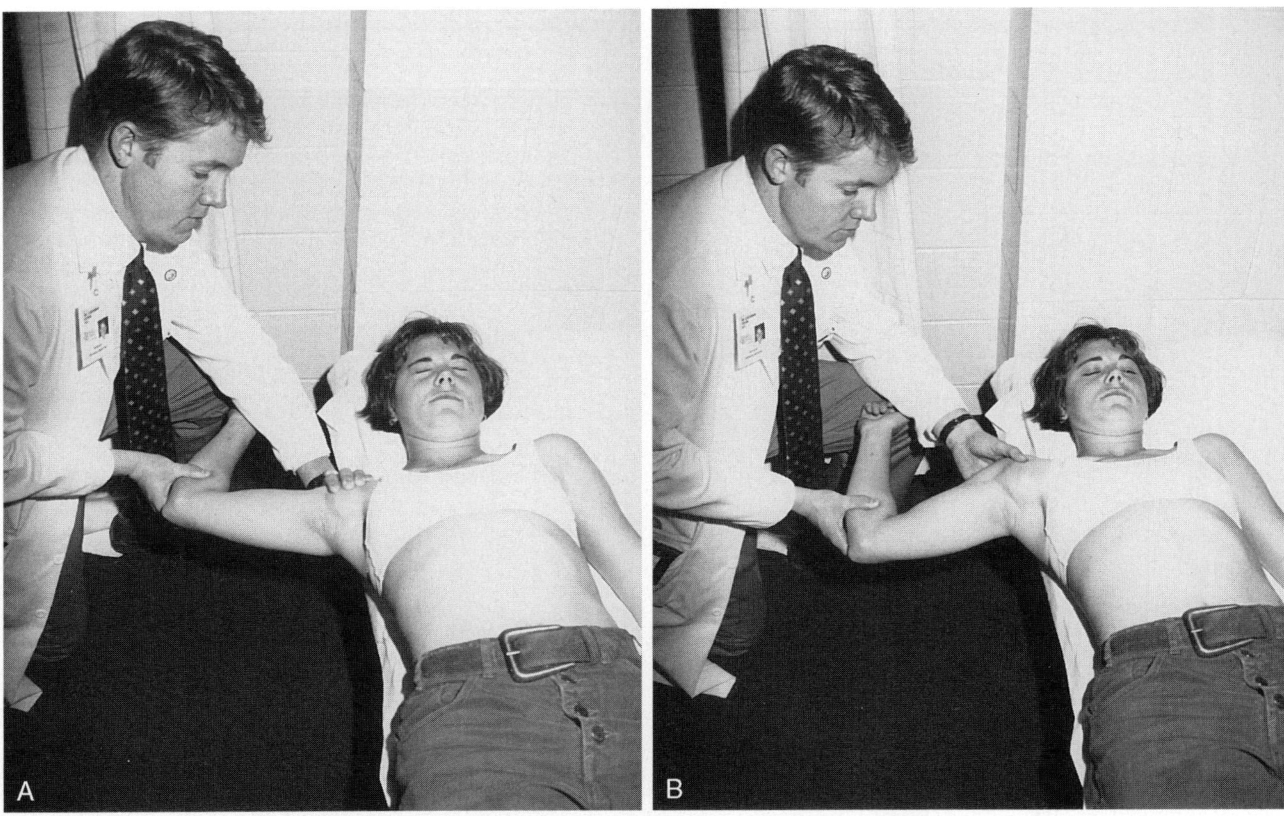

FIGURE 38–16. Tests for shoulder instability. *A.* Lachman test. *B.* Relocation test.

ated and indicated for a longer period of time in this group than in more elderly patients. Use of a sling for approximately 6 weeks[72] is more appropriate for a younger individual than the 2-week time period used for patients over the age of 40.

Isometric exercises are begun within days following an acute dislocation. The rehabilitation program begins with active assisted exercises to increase range of motion. Progressive resistance exercises are then incorporated to strengthen the dynamic stabilizers of the shoulder. Emphasis is also placed on the periscapular musculature, including the rhomboids, trapezius, and serratus anterior, to improve control of scapular motion. Acute surgical intervention for an initial dislocation is rare unless the dislocation is accompanied by a complete rotator cuff tear.

Hemiplegic Shoulder Pain

Shoulder pain is a frequent complication of individuals with hemiplegia. Its presence can compromise rehabilitation efforts. Unfortunately, it is a syndrome that is not completely understood and is somewhat controversial. Although the presentation is variable and symptoms can appear anytime in the first year, they ordinarily appear within the first few weeks after a stroke or other neurological insult. Hemiplegic shoulder pain is more frequently associated with spastic than with flaccid hemiplegia, but it can be seen in both.[56, 70]

The overall function, including stability and flexibility, of the shoulder depends less on the movement of the humeral head in the glenoid cavity than on the musculotendinous sleeve that surrounds it. Impairment of these neuromuscular components in a situation of hemiplegia or tetraplegia, therefore, greatly disrupts the usual functioning of this poorly balanced joint. There is considerable controversy regarding the precise cause of this common problem, but it most likely is multifactorial. Contributing factors are listed in Table 38–4.[19, 30, 35, 36, 54, 59]

Anteroinferior subluxation is the most frequently cited concomitant condition in patients with hemiplegia who have shoulder pain. Although it is seen more frequently in flaccid shoulders, it is more often associated with shoulder pain in conditions with spasticity.[70]

Diagnosis

The maximal site of tenderness can often be located near the subacromial space. The degree of subluxation

TABLE 38–4 Factors Cited for the Multifactorial Basis of Hemiplegic Shoulder Pain

Rotator cuff and biceps tendon disease
Anteroinferior subluxation
Spasticity
Capsular constriction
Suprascapular neuropathy
Reflex sympathetic dystrophy
Ganglia
Hemineglect

should be evaluated, but a valid, standardized method of measuring this has not been adequately developed.[57]

The radiographic evaluation is similar to the protocols previously described for rotator cuff disease and instability. Three-phase bone scanning is often utilized if shoulder-hand syndrome or complex regional pain syndrome is being considered. Electrodiagnosis can be helpful in ruling out peripheral nerve compromise, radiculopathy, or plexopathy.

Treatment

The management of patients with hemiplegic shoulder pain is frequently difficult and often unsatisfactory. A primary consideration for treatment should be combating spasticity if present, as this can play an important role. Strategies should begin with the onset of shoulder plegia with the goal of prevention. Commonly used medications for this include baclofen, dantrolene sodium, and diazepam, for which each patient should be evaluated individually. Heat and cold modalities can also be helpful. Lidocaine or phenol motor point blocks are sometimes indicated in patients with uncontrolled spasticity.

Proper positioning should begin early. The shoulder should be positioned in abduction and external rotation while the patient is in bed. Gentle, passive range-of-motion exercises should be instituted early. Subluxation frequently occurs in the shoulder that is flaccid. An axillary cushion, attached with a harness bandage, can be used to correct the subluxation while the patient is sitting or standing. A hemisling or wheelchair arm support can also serve this function. Use of the hemisling has been questioned by some authors.[24] Regardless, any material used should be one that is easily manipulated by the patient with the unaffected hand. An axillary cushion or hemisling can also be used to correct subluxation in patients with spasticity, but caution must be exercised, because these devices can increase spasticity or contribute to an elbow flexion contracture.

Adhesive Capsulitis

Adhesive capsulitis, also referred to as "frozen shoulder," is an abnormality that ordinarily develops gradually, with increasing pain and decreasing range of motion. Pain and limited motion occur particularly in glenohumeral internal and external rotation as well as in abduction. There are three clinical phases in the classic description of adhesive capsulitis—pain, progressive stiffness, and then a phase of gradual improvement with return of motion.

The most commonly identified factor predisposing to adhesive capsulitis is a period of immobility of the shoulder,[23] but other clinical conditions are associated (Table 38–5).

TABLE 38–5 Factors Predisposing to the Development of Adhesive Capsulitis

Immobility
Age between 40 and 60 yr
Female
Diabetes
Thyroid disease
Humeral lesions
Personality disorder

Neviaser[46] describes adhesive capsulitis as a distinct entity with four identifiable stages that are arthroscopically distinct. Stage 1 is clinically similar to early impingement syndrome and is often confused with rotator cuff disease. Shoulder motion is restricted little if at all during this stage. Arthroscopy shows an erythematous fibrinous pannus over the synovium, primarily around the dependent fold. The articular cartilage is normal in this condition. Treatment protocols for this entity, such as that utilized for rotator cuff disease, often fail. Inappropriate acromial arch decompression often accelerates the disease process owing to postoperative immobility.

Stage 2 is characterized by pain with associated loss of motion in all planes. Arthroscopically, the synovium appears red, thickened, and inflamed. Adhesions across the dependent fold can be seen. There is loss of the space between the humeral head and glenoid as well as between the humeral head and biceps tendon.

Stage 3 is characterized by the transition from inflammatory synovitis to chronic fibrosis and by a markedly decreased size of the dependent fold. There is complete obliteration of the space between the humeral head and glenoid and between the humeral head and biceps tendon.

There is no longer synovitis present in stage 4. The dependent fold has become severely contracted by this stage, and clinically, shoulder motion is severely limited.

Diagnosis

An adequate history is essential for evaluation of the painful and stiff shoulder. Bilaterality can suggest an underlying systemic disorder. The differential diagnosis includes hemarthrosis, aseptic necrosis of the humeral head, infection (to be strongly considered in elderly or immunocompromised persons), rotator cuff tears and anterior capsular tear. The usual history is the insidious onset of a stiff, painful shoulder. The pain is ordinarily poorly localized but frequently most intense at the posterior and superior aspects of the shoulder.

Initially the motion limitation might appear secondary to guarding from pain, but eventually, measurable limitation in both active and passive range of motion in different planes is demonstrated. The patient often attempts to overcome the restricted glenohumeral movement with the use of accessory muscles and excessive compensatory scapular rotation. In normal scapulohumeral rhythm there is a 2:1 ratio of movement of the humerus to the scapula during 180 degrees of abduction. Of this 180 degrees, 120 degrees occurs at the glenohumeral joint and 60 degrees at the scapulothoracic joint.[62] This normal ratio (codman's ratio) is frequently disrupted in adhesive capsulitis because of excessive compensatory scapular rotation. The addition of accessory muscle strain can lead to additional painful cervical and shoulder musculature. Tenderness over the

AC joint and biceps tendon is a frequently associated finding.

Radiography is of limited value in diagnosing adhesive capsulitis. The findings are inconsistent and nonspecific. Often mild degenerative changes of the glenohumeral joint and AC joint are seen as well as osteopenia. Bone scans have been studied and have also been found to have limited usefulness.[3]

Although the diagnosis is ordinarily made clinically, if in doubt, it can be confirmed with arthrography. This can demonstrate loss of the ordinarily loose dependent fold of the joint and a dramatic decrease in the volume of contrast material that can be injected. A reduction of the normal 25 to 35 mL of joint volume to less than 10 mL is seen.[46] An irregular joint outline with incomplete filling of the axillary fold, subacromial bursa, and biceps tendon sheath is frequently seen. The pain can often be reproduced by distending the joint and relieved by withdrawing some of the contrast fluid. The findings at athrography are not useful for prognosis or staging, however. Subacromial injection of 10 mL of lidocaine can be used to differentiate adhesive capsulitis from rotator cuff disease, as previously described.

The role of arthroscopic evaluation in this condition is unclear. Although Neviaser used arthroscopic findings to develop the staging system, arthroscopy is not considered a standard diagnostic procedure for this condition, and its role is limited to the detection of other possible shoulder disorders.

Treatment

There is some disagreement in the literature regarding the natural course of adhesive capsulitis. Some report it to be a self-limited condition that will improve spontaneously over a 1- to 2-year period.[5, 21, 36] Others think there is a significant subset of patients who, if not adequately treated, will develop persistent symptoms and disability. Irrespective of this opinion, few people can accept a full year of such a disability, and therefore aggressive treatment is warranted to accelerate recovery.

When the diagnosis has been established, the treatment goal is to control pain to facilitate progressive range of motion. NSAIDs, analgesics, heat modalities, and intensive physical therapy are utilized, with progression to a home exercise program. The emphasis in therapy is on passive stretching of the shoulder capsular contracture in all planes of motion. Many modalities have demonstrated limited efficacy, including transcutaneous electrical nerve stimulation (TENS), pulley traction, corticosteroid injections, ice, and heat. Most have shown limited value in altering the course of the disease[23, 60] when used by themselves. Their value lies in reducing pain in the primary stages to facilitate increased range of motion.

Corticosteroid injections, although popular, have little supportive literature to demonstrate their efficacy. Accurate location of the glenohumeral joint with the injecting needle is a problem when there is a severe contracture. Rizk and colleagues[60] showed no significant difference in outcome between the use of lidocaine and steroid injections, but pain was temporarily relieved with steroid injections. The same study also found no significant difference between intrabursal and intraarticular injection. Although one to two steroid injections might have a beneficial effect early in the course of rehabilitation, repeated injections can have an adverse effect on tissue healing and are to be discouraged.

Codman's exercises are the exercises most frequently used to improve range of motion. Efficacy can be increased with the use of wrist weights. These exercises can be easily performed by the patient at home after proper instruction (Fig. 38–17).

Some advocate the use of distention arthrography or infiltration brisement. With this technique, a combination of local anesthetic and saline is injected into the glenohumeral joint to produce hydraulic distention of the capsule and lysis of adhesions. This is ordinarily performed under general anesthesia. Many authors have reported good results.[23]

Manipulation under anesthesia is considered if the patient has made poor progress with the therapy program. Manipulation is performed with forced abduction of the humerus while fixing the scapula. This is performed with the shoulder in pure glenohumeral abduction because most of the contracture and capsular adhesions are in the dependent fold.[46] The goal is to obtain a range of motion as close to that of the normal opposite shoulder as possible.

Physiatric care should begin the day of the procedure, with attention to positioning in bed. The patient is placed in bed with the arm restrained to maintain abduction of 90 degrees and external rotation as far as that obtained during the manipulation. Emphasis is placed on achieving range of motion in internal and external rotation with abduction maintained at 90 degrees, as well as on increasing elevation and flexion. For the next

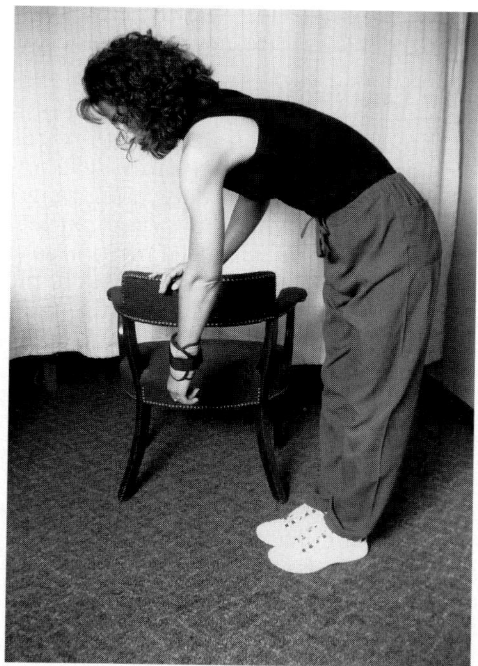

FIGURE 38–17. Codman's pedulum exercises. The patient uses the body to range the passive dependent upper limb.

few days the arm is maintained above 90 degrees to avoid approximation of the dependent fold edges. After this, the arm is allowed down only for short periods, primarily to perform pendulum exercises. During this period the patient should sleep in a sling that maintains the arm in the abducted position, and should participate in a formal daily physical therapy program and a home exercise program. Proper patient education and close follow-up in the home setting are essential to success.

Posterior capsulitis is a common cause of posterior shoulder pain. The posterior capsule can sustain repeated microtrauma and tearing during the follow-through phase of throwing. The capsule can remain inflamed, become calcific, and result in decreased internal rotation of the shoulder. Posterior capsulitis is frequently associated with inflammation of the long head of the triceps tendon at its attachment to the inferior glenoid rim. It might respond to a single steroid injection. Injection should be performed with the patient prone and the arm hanging off the table in 90 degrees of shoulder flexion.

ELBOW PAIN

Lateral

Lateral Epicondylitis

Lateral epicondylitis, also known as "tennis elbow," is a common clinical condition. A significant number of people who participate in tennis are afflicted with this ailment at one time or another.[49] The vast majority of individuals seen with this condition, however, are manual laborers, office workers, or homemakers who engage in repetitive manual activities.

There is considerable controversy in the literature regarding the precise cause as well as the pathological changes that occur in lateral epicondylitis. A widely accepted belief is that an inflammatory lesion with degeneration occurs at the insertion of the extensor tendons, primarily the extensor carpi radialis brevis (ECRB), with eventual fibrous adherence to the capsule (Fig. 38–18).[47] This is an area where Sharpey's fibers enter the periosteum on the lateral epicondyle of the humerus. Also closely involved is the origin of the superficial part of the supinator, which is in very close proximity to the origin of the ECRB at the lateral epicondyle, as well as the elbow joint capsule. Other muscles that are felt to possibly contribute are the extensor carpi radialis longus and the extensor digitorum communis, which originate in close proximity. Continued inflammation and fraying occur at this area with ongoing repetitive use of the wrist extensors. Hypervascularity, granulation tissue, and fibrosis in the extensor aponeurosis and in the subaponeurotic space of the elbow can develop, as can contracture of the anterolateral elbow capsule.[7]

Lateral epicondylitis usually occurs in persons over 35 years of age. Patients often present with a history of

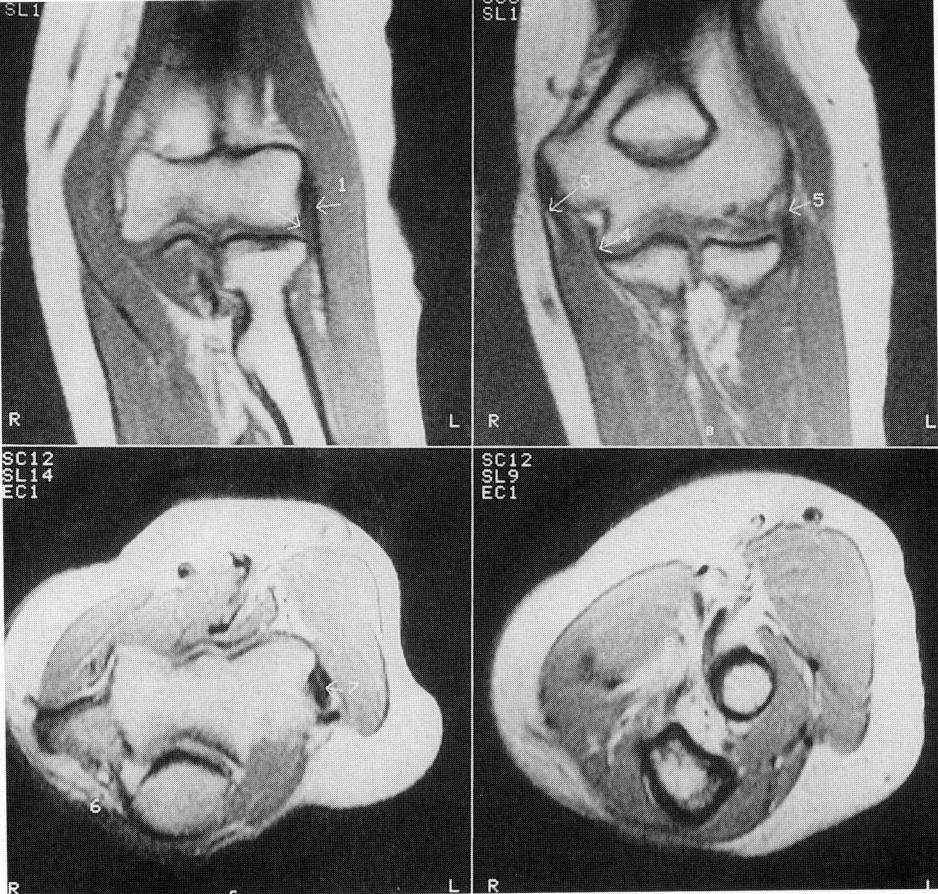

FIGURE 38–18. MRI series depicting the anatomical relationships about the elbow. The coronal views demonstrate the common extensor tendon (*1*), the lateral collateral ligament (*2*), the common flexor tendon (*3*), and the medial collateral ligament (*4*). The biceps insertion is shown on the axial view (*8*).

chronic activity involving repetitive flexion and extension of the wrist or pronation and supination of the forearm. However, in many instances no predisposing event is established. The onset can be gradual or sudden.

In tennis players, it is believed that an incorrect tennis stroke can lead to the development of lateral epicondylitis. Poor technique can place excessive stress on the forearm muscles and tendons and ligaments around the elbow joint.[25] The backhand is the most common stroke that elicits symptoms. When performed with the arm in full pronation and the trunk leaning backward at the point of impact, further stress is placed on the elbow extensors, as compared with a high-quality backhand with the forearm in mid-pronation with forward lean (Fig. 38–19).[48]

On examination there is tenderness over the lateral epicondyle, usually at the origin of the ECRB. There is increased pain with resisted wrist extension; the pain is greater with a straight elbow. Pain can be maximally reproduced by having the patient make a fist, pronate the forearm, and radially deviate the wrist while performing this maneuver.

The middle finger test can also be performed. This involves resisting the extension of the proximal interphalangeal joint of digit 3. This places stress on the extensor digitorum and ECRB. The test is considered positive if pain is elicited over the lateral epicondyle.

Routine anteroposterior (AP) and lateral radiographs are of little help in evaluating this condition. Oblique views of the lateral epicondyle can show irregularity or punctate calcification around the origin of the ECRB. EMG is not helpful in the evaluation of lateral epicondylites, except in identifying entrapment neuropathies.

Primary in treatment of this condition is decreasing repetitive stress. Avoidance of painful activities, particularly repetitive wrist flexion-extension and forearm pronation-supination, is important. For athletes or laborers in whom complete elimination is not a reasonable option, activity modification should be developed to minimize stress on the lateral epicondyle. An example of this is the previously discussed stroke modification in tennis players. Equipment modification can also provide some benefit. In tennis, the proper handle size should be ensured (usually enlarging it) and the string tension should be reduced.

Anti-inflammatory medication can be a useful adjunct to reducing inflammation when initiating therapy. Heat modalities such as hot packs, short-wave diathermy, or heat lamps might provide symptomatic relief. US can be applied directly to the inflamed area at the lateral epicondyle at 1.5 to 2.0 W/cm^2 in a continuous fashion once to twice per day for up to 10 days. Ice is useful to minimize the inflammatory response and should be applied after the inciting activity. An injection of cortisone and Xylocaine can be helpful for temporary relief and confirmation of the diagnosis. Injection is made directly over the point of maximal tenderness with care not to enter the tendon itself.

Forearm bands (lateral elbow counterforce braces) have become popular in recent years (Fig. 38–20). The

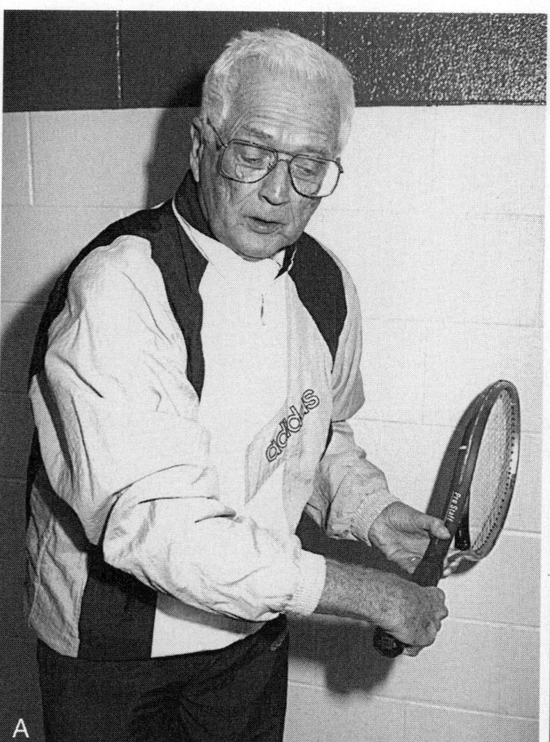

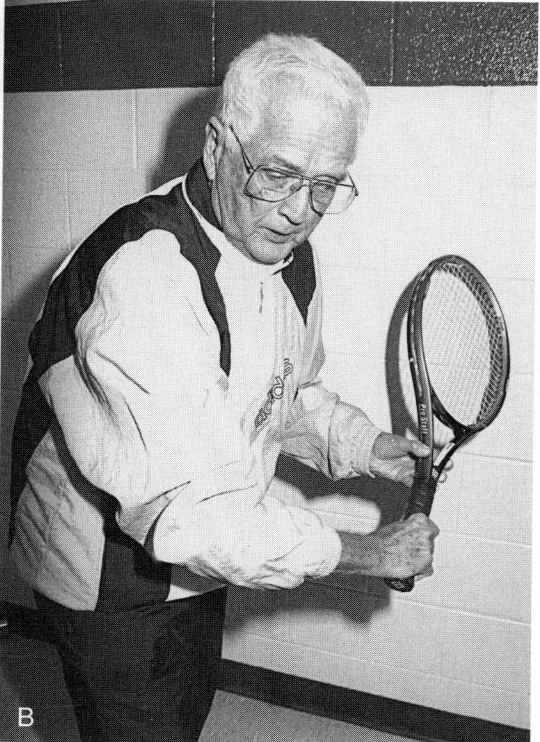

FIGURE 38–19. *A.* Demonstration of incorrect tennis form. Note the flexed and pronated wrist, improper foward lean, and lead with the elbow. This position places greater stress on the extensor mechanism with ball strike. *B.* Proper tennis form, with a straight wrist and appropriate body positioning.

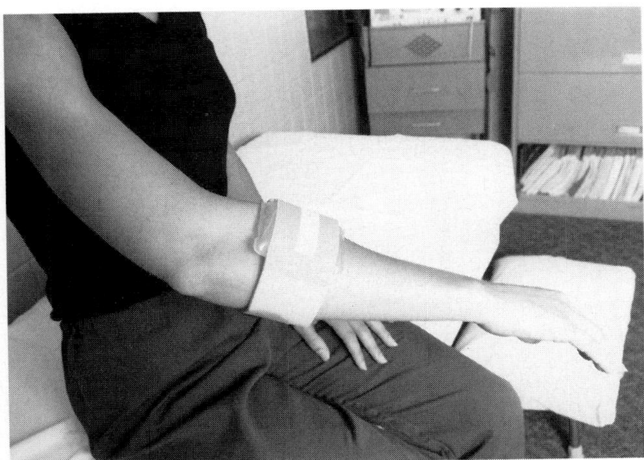

FIGURE 38–20. "Tennis elbow" band.

purpose is to prevent full muscular forearm expansion and alleviate tension on the attachment site at the lateral epicondyle.

Proper exercise is probably the most significant intervention to produce long-term benefit. We suggest a technique of using 10 repetitive maximum (10 RM) of the wrist extensors with the elbow flexed to 90 degrees, and then repeated with the elbow extended to 180 degrees. One set of 10 is done with the elbow extended to 180 degrees and the wrist over the end of a table and one set with the elbow flexed to 90 degrees. The specific technique is the slow wrist extension followed by slowly allowing the wrist into full flexion (Fig. 38–21). The eccentric, or lengthening, contraction as the weight is lowered is most important. The RM weight is determined after clinical evaluation. It ordinarily should start at 6 to 10 lb and increase gradually each week. The cycle should be repeated 10 times slowly, with the elbow first in the 90-degree flexed position and then with the elbow extended. This series of exercises should continue for 4 to 8 weeks. The exercises should be performed both in the morning and at night. The weights can be dumbbells or another form of improvised weights. Discomfort might increase during the first week or two, but continuation can be facilitated by appropriate use of heat modalities and a 10-day course of NSAIDs.

Many operative procedures have been described for this condition. Lateral extensor release is considered by some to be the surgical procedure of choice.[71]

Bone Trauma

Osteochodritis dissecans of the capitelum is commonly seen in patients younger than 25 years old who present with joint pain and occasional locking. Plain films often demonstrate fragmentation of the capitelum associated with an elbow effusion.

Similarly, a history of trauma, often a direct blow or fall on an extended arm with the elbow locked, can lead to suspicion of an occult radial head fracture. Directly palpable tenderness is noted when the examiner's thumb is placed over the radial head as the forearm is moved through pronation and supination.

Avulsion of the distal biceps tendon at the elbow is an uncommon injury. It is ordinarily without a prerupture syndrome and it is usually due to a single, acute event, often a traumatic or heavy lifting episode done with the elbow flexed to 90 degrees.

Medial

Medial Epicondylitis

Pain localized to the medial aspect of the elbow suggests other diagnostic entities, often related to valgus distraction forces on the medial joint structures. Medial epicondylitis, also known as "pitcher's elbow" or "golfer's elbow," develops as a result of a medial stress overload on the flexor musculature and medial collateral ligament (MCL) at the elbow. It is seen frequently in the skeletally immature, primarily in 9- to 15-year-old boys, as a physeal injury resulting from throwing stresses (Little Leaguer's elbow).[48]

Critical components of the history include an acute onset or exacerbation of symptoms, which can suggest

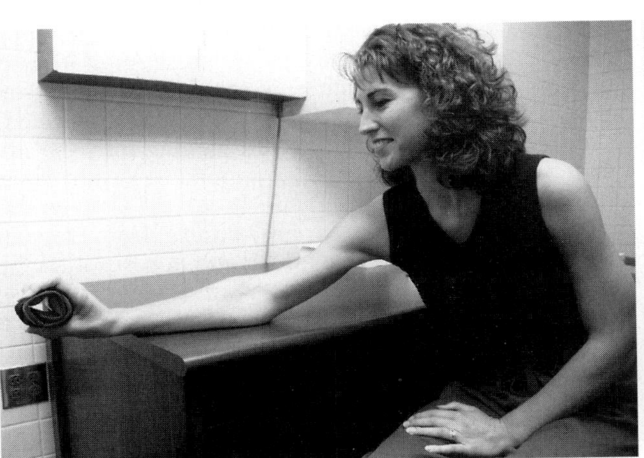

A

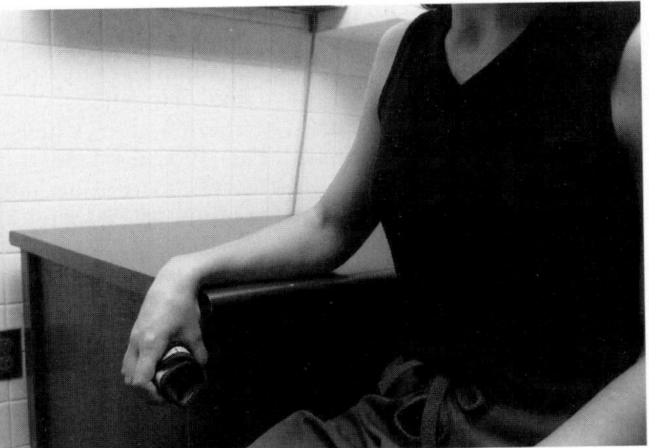

B

FIGURE 38–21. Resistance exercises for lateral epicondylitis.

an MCL tear, epiphyseal fracture, or flexor tendon tear. An insidious onset of medial elbow pain is more typical of medial epicondylitis. Bony spurring or ulnar neuropathy at the elbow should be considered in the cases that chronically progress. Identification of detailed activity patterns and their relationship to pain is necessary not only to assist with the diagnosis but also to determine appropriate long-term management.

The specific site of tenderness should be identified on physical examination to rule out injury of the triceps insertion or posterior elbow. The characteristic pain can be elicited by stressing the flexor tendons with resisted flexion at the wrist or forced wrist extension. The elbow should also be evaluated for limited or excessive range of motion in comparison with the uninjured side, and should be examined for laxity with varus and valgus stress.

Avulsion fractures and osteochondral defects are often identified on a standard series of AP, lateral, and oblique plain radiographs. Physeal separation in adolescents is difficult to identify and can require comparison views of the noninjured elbow or the use of higher-technology imaging.

Treatment for this entity is essentially the same as that previously described for lateral epicondylitis, only with the emphasis on the strengthening of the flexor muscles of the forearm as well as the use of modalities for pain relief.

Common flexor tendon avulsions are rare, whereas chronic tendinopathy is frequently seen with repetitive motion disorders. Chronic flexor tendinopathy typically presents in manner similar to medial epicondylitis. These entities are difficult to distinguish clinically. The point of maximal tenderness may be located more distally, although this is not a reliable sign. MRI can be used for more precise anatomical localization.

Medial Collateral Ligament Trauma

MCL rupture is seen in skeletally mature throwers and is believed to be due to excessive valgus force on the medial compartment. The late-cocking and acceleration phases of throwing produce the most significant stress on this area.[33] Flexor and pronator muscle tears, as well as ulnar neuropathy, can also be associated in this condition.

MCL damage ordinarily is accompanied by a history of chronic and repetitive trauma and pain, but it can be the result of acute trauma. On examination, valgus instability is invariably present. This should be determined by gently applying valgus stress to the medial aspect of the elbow while flexing the elbow to 25 degrees and externally rotating the humerus (Fig. 38–22).[41]

The ligament is most frequently torn off at the medial aspect of the coronoid process, and therefore the palpable tenderness is more severe on the ulnar aspect than the humeral side of the MCL. Ecchymosis can be present in an acute rupture.

Treatment consists of rest, ice, and a short course of NSAIDs until swelling and inflammation subside. Pain should be resolved and full range of motion should be attained before the individual gradually resumes throwing activities. This might require 6 weeks to 3 months.

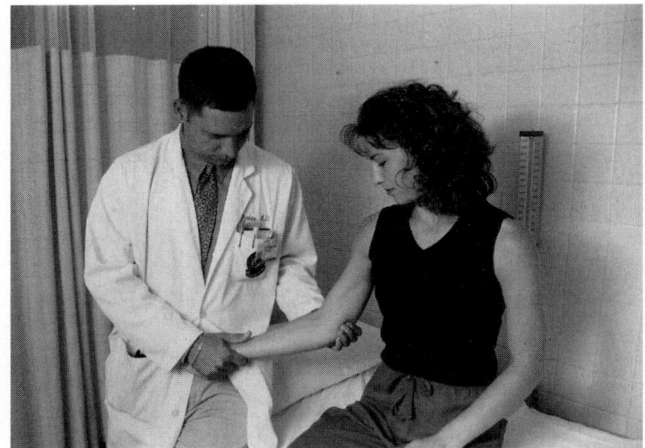

FIGURE 38–22. Evaluation for valgus instability.

In patients with MCL injury refractory to treatment beyond 6 months, surgical ligament repair might be considered.

Posterior

Olecranon Bursitis

The olecranon bursa is one of the most frequently inflamed bursae in the human body. Inflammation is seen very commonly in athletes engaged in contact sports and in laborers.[10] Of all of the bursae around the elbow, inflammation of the superficial olecranon bursa is that most frequently seen. It can present as acute, chronic, or infectious.

Acute bursitis usually results from a direct blow to or prolonged pressure on the area. Tenderness and distention of the bursa are noted on physical examination. Bursitis should be differentiated from cellulitis. Tendinitis, acute arthritis (including crystalline arthropathies), and ligamentous injury are also included in the differential diagnosis. Joint motion is ordinarily not limited with olecranon bursitis unless extreme flexion causes increased skin tension over the painful, swollen bursa. Treatment involves primarily prevention of recurrence and might consist of wearing elbow pads or other appropriate covering, especially in athletes. Aspiration can be considered if the bursa is severely distended and painful. Compression and cold packs can be applied in the first 72 hours to minimize bleeding into the area. After this period, heat can be applied to hasten resorption of the bursal fluid.

Chronic olecranon bursitis occurs from repeated trauma and results in thickening and fibrosis of the bursal lining. It commonly occurs as an occupational disorder. Medical attention may be sought after an acute traumatic episode has been superimposed on a more chronic inflammation. Examination findings are similar to those seen in acute trauma, but fibrous trabeculation of the bursal sac can often be palpated. Aspiration is frequently indicated and should be followed by a compressive dressing to minimize the tendency of the bursa to refill. Steroid injections are not indicated for acute bursitis as they tend to inhibit the normal protective

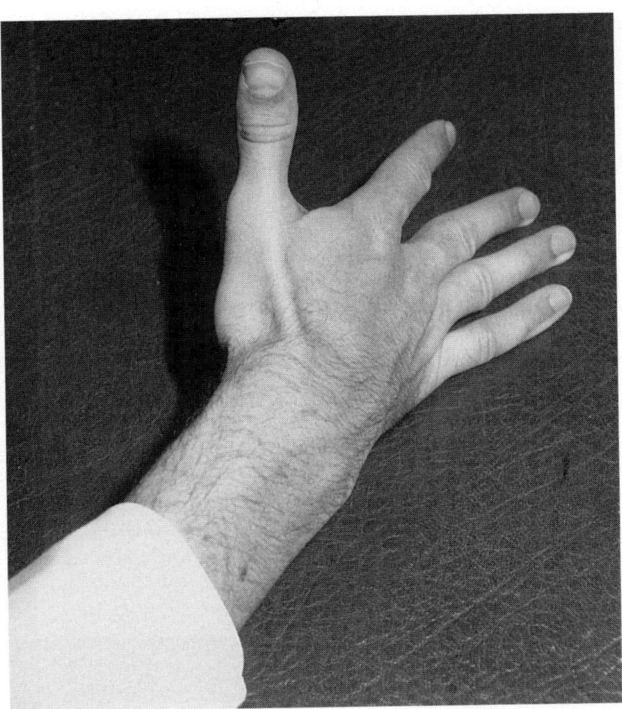

FIGURE 38–23. Demonstration of the surface anatomy of the anatomical snuffbox. The dorsal aspect is the extensor pollicis longus tendon, and the volar aspect is the extensor pollicis brevis tendon in close proximity to the abductor pollicis longus tendon.

mechanisms against infection. They have only limited success in chronic bursitis. Surgical removal of the bursa is an option in severe refractory or chronic bursitis.

Septic bursitis is diagnosed with aspiration and culture.[22] It should be suspected in the setting of warmth and erythema. Septic fluid can appear purulent or bloody. The fluid should be sent for Gram stain, crystal determination, cell count, and culture. Septic joint fluid shows a predominence of polymorphonuclear cells, whereas mononuclear cells tend to predominate in nonseptic fluid. The most common infectious organism is *Staphylococcus aureas.* Treatment involves appropriate antibiotics.

Triceps Tendinitis

Another common cause of posterior elbow pain is triceps tendinitis.[48] This is seen frequently in persons who engage in activities requiring rapid elbow extension, such as throwers and fly fisherman, and in those with repetitive motion occupations, such as carpentry. Triceps tendinitis is managed similarly to the lateral and medial epicondylitides, with the mainstay of treatment involving reduction of inflammation and activity modification.

WRIST

De Quervain's Tenosynovitis

In 1895 de Quervain[14] originally noted a condition of stenosing tenosynovitis. He described five women who had pain and swelling of the tendon sheath of the abductor pollicis longus (APL) and extensor pollicis brevis (EPB) muscles near the area of the radial styloid at the wrist. He noted localized thickening of the tendon sheath in that area, which he attributed to increased friction at that point.

This syndrome has become widely recognized and is called, appropriately enough, de Quervain's tenosynovitis. In this condition, swelling and palpable tenderness of the APL and EPB tendon sheaths at the lateral border of the anatomical snuffbox are characteristically described (Fig. 38–23).

This disorder of the first dorsal compartment is often associated with a history of rapid repetitive movements of occupational and avocational stresses and less commonly with rheumatoid arthritis. The diagnosis is confirmed by eliciting localized tenderness and by a positive Finkelstein's test (Fig. 38–24). In the absence of a history of predisposing activities, rheumatoid arthritis should be considered, with appropriate serologic and rheumatologic testing.

Treatment focuses on reducing inflammation by means of activity alteration (which can include the use of splinting in severe cases), NSAIDs, and local steroid injection into the tendon sheath. Surgical release of the tendons sheaths is considered in severe cases refractory to treatment.

Acute and Occult Wrist Injuries

Acute wrist injuries with their attendant osseous, ligamentous, and tendinous manifestations usually are treated by emergency medicine or orthopedic specialists. Physiatrists are often involved when undiagnosed pain persists more than 4 to 6 weeks, at which time subtle fractures and their complications have to be included in the differential diagnosis. Repeat plain radiography or bone radionuclide scintigraphy can often demonstrate occult bony pathology. Complications of radial fractures (Colles fracture) typically present at this time and are the most commonly seen wrist injuries of this nature.

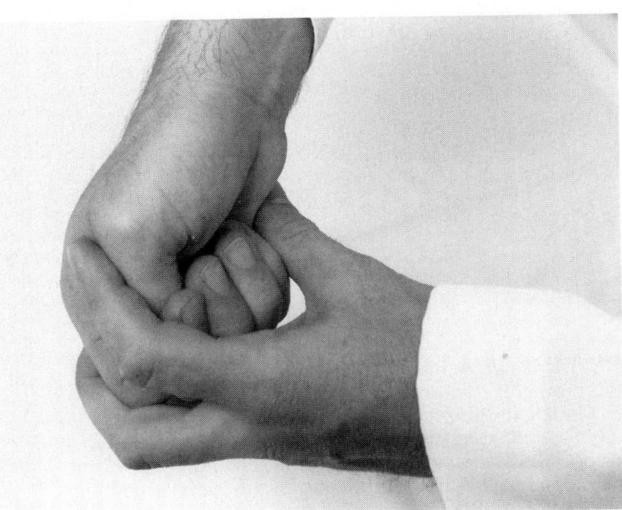

FIGURE 38–24. Finkelstein's test for de Quervain's tenosynovitis. The wrist is forced into ulnar deviation with the thumb flexed and abducted. Pain is exacerbated in a positive test.

Scaphoid Injuries

The scaphoid is the most commonly injured carpal bone.[9] It transfers axial load from the distal radius to the distal carpal row. A common mechanism of injury involves a direct fall on an outstretched arm with a dorsiflexed wrist. The degree of dorsiflexion and the amount of radial or ulnar deviation influence the specific site of fracture (distal, waist, proximal).

The diagnosis of a scaphoid fracture is made from the classic traumatic history described, in the presence of pain and tenderness over its location at the anatomical snuffbox. There is ordinarily little outward visible evidence of this fracture. A plain radiographic series with AP, lateral, and radial and ulnar oblique views should be obtained if this fracture is suspected (Fig. 38–25B). Views that image the carpal bones should be obtained to evaluate for scapholunate dissociation if the problem is of long standing. A bone scan should be considered in patients with normal radiographs but in whom there remains a strong clinical suspicion of bone trauma.

The patient with normal radiographs but a classic history and physical findings should be placed in a short arm-thumb spica cast and re-evaluated in 2 weeks. Meticulous follow-up for this condition is imperative because of the high incidence of scaphoid non-union after fracture.

Understanding anatomical considerations such as fracture pattern and blood supply is essential for appropriate management. The frequency of non-union increases as the location of the fracture moves from distal to proximal and correlates directly with the amount of blood supply, which is quite variable over the length of the scaphoid.

Nondisplaced fractures in the distal third, which has an excellent blood supply, frequently heal effectively within a 6-week period with proper immobilization. Fractures in the middle third or the waist or the scaphoid are reported to have up to a 30% incidence of non-

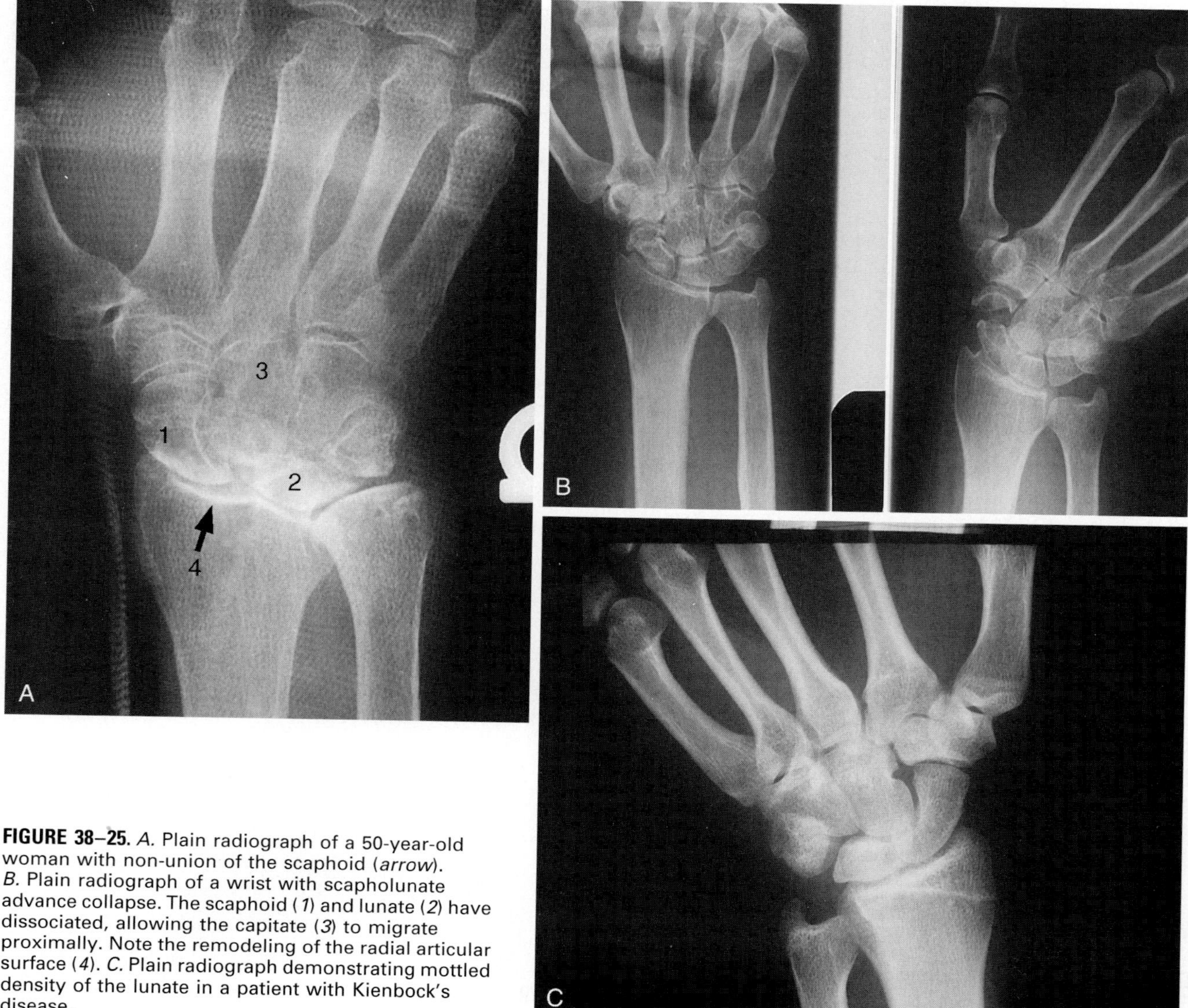

FIGURE 38–25. *A.* Plain radiograph of a 50-year-old woman with non-union of the scaphoid (*arrow*). *B.* Plain radiograph of a wrist with scapholunate advance collapse. The scaphoid (*1*) and lunate (*2*) have dissociated, allowing the capitate (*3*) to migrate proximally. Note the remodeling of the radial articular surface (*4*). *C.* Plain radiograph demonstrating mottled density of the lunate in a patient with Kienbock's disease.

union despite adequate immobilization. Non-union can occur in as many as 90% of patients with fracture in the proximal third of the scaphoid, which has the poorest blood supply.[9] Scaphoid non-union can be relatively asymptomatic, but it is associated with a high incidence of the late development of osteoarthritis or carpal collapse.[38] The fracture can be treated with pulsed electromagnetic stimulation to promote healing if it is less than 5 years old and relatively asymptomatic, and if no significant degenerative changes are present. Surgical intervention of open reduction and internal fixation, including possible bone grafting, is considered in patients with long-lasting symptoms or degenerative carpal changes.[12]

Kienbock's Disease

Another common source of occult bone pain was first described by Kienbock in 1910.[31] Kienbock's disease presents as wrist pain with sclerosis and collapse of the lunate secondary to avascular necrosis (Fig. 38–25C).

The precise cause of this condition is not well understood, but it is most common in the dominant wrist in 15- to 40-year-old men, most of whom have a history of preceding trauma. Surgical treatment is indicated when satisfactory relief of pain is not obtained with conservative management.[34]

Osteoarthritis of the Carpometacarpal Joint of the Thumb

Another common source of pain about the wrist and hand occurs at the carpal-metacarpal joint of the thumb. It is the most frequent site of osteoarthritis in the upper limb and commonly the most disabling, particularly in persons over 60 years old.

Scapholunate Advance Collapse

The most common form of chronic wrist arthritis is scapholunate advance collapse (SLAC). This is a posttraumatic rotary subluxation that causes the scaphoid and lunate to separate and the capitate to migrate proximally. The ensuing impingement and osteoarthritic change can result in neuropathies and extensive arthropathic changes. This entity is readily identified with plain radiography (Fig. 38–25B).

Other focal pain syndromes of the wrist are often associated with the presence of ganglia, intercarpal ligament tears, and failed carpal tunnel surgery.

HAND PAIN

Dupuytren's Contracture

Fibrous contracture of the palmar fascia leading to flexion contractures of the fingers was originally described by Clive in 1808. The condition has subsequently become known as Dupuytren's contracture, after the surgeon who first described an operation for its treatment.[8] The causative factors are unknown. The condition is more prevalent in men than in women and is seen most frequently in the fifth to seventh decades. It is often unilateral but can be bilateral. It most frequently involves the fourth or fifth digit.

Thickening of the palmar fascia is the hallmark of this condition (Fig. 38–26). As the fascia progressively thickens, the penetrating nutrient arteries are compromised, leading to further thickening, contracture, and atrophy of the overlying skin.

A classification system proposed by Shaw[8, 65] distinguishes the progression of a nodule of the palmar fascia (stage 1), to a nodule with involvement of the skin (stage 2), to subsequent flexion contractures of one or more fingers (stage 3), to the final stage (stage 4) with fixed tendon and joint contractures.

Failure to establish the proper diagnosis can lead to inappropriate attempts at progressive stretching, which are typically of no benefit. Continued extensor stress may cause progression of the syndrome. Surgical release is the treatment of choice. However, it might only be indicated with severe digital contracture.

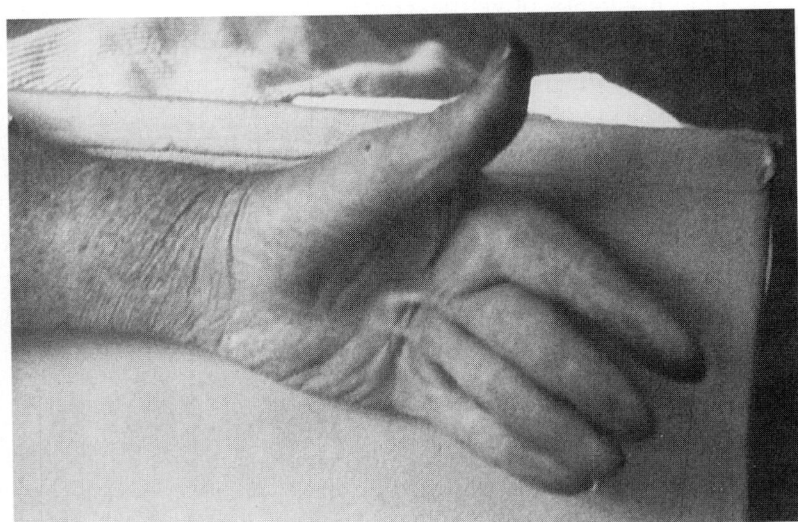

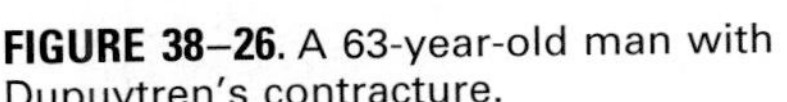

FIGURE 38–26. A 63-year-old man with Dupuytren's contracture.

Gamekeeper's (Skier's) Thumb

Gamekeeper's thumb is characterized by an injury to the ulnar collateral ligament and insertion of the adductor pollicis. It is seen frequently in skiers and is associated with resultant instability. It can occur with acute trauma or can develop gradually with acute stress. This condition is identified on physical examination by swelling and tenderness over the metacarpophalangeal joint of the thumb, pain elicited by passive motion, and weakness in pinch. It can occasionally be identified radiographically. Surgical repair is typically the treatment of choice.

Trigger Finger

Acute or chronic inflammation and flexor tendinitis can result in a disproportion between the flexor tendon and its sheath. Subsequent constriction at the pulley near the level of the metacarpal head is associated with painful snapping of the flexor tendons. This condition is called trigger finger or stenosing tenovaginitis.

Treatment consists of a local steroid injection, which can be repeated once if the condition is refractory. Splinting following the injections can also be beneficial. In highly resistant cases, surgery may be needed. Complications such as postoperative bowstringing, painful scarring, and digital nerve injuries can occur.

Mallet Finger

Mallet finger occurs as a result of a tear of the extensor tendon from its attachment on the distal phalanx. This is usually due to an acute flexion injury when the extensor tendon is taut. In the majority of cases, the tendon itself is torn from the insertion, but a significant percentage sustain a bone avulsion.

Conservative treatment includes immobilization of the distal phalanx in hyperextension with the middle phalanx in flexion for approximately 6 to 10 weeks. Surgical repair is considered if functional recovery is inadequate.

Raynaud's Phenomenon

Vasomotor instability, often triggered by cold or stress, results in a syndrome of pain, a burning sensation, cyanosis, numbness, and swelling of the upper extremities. This is referred to as Raynaud's phenomenon and is believed to be a result of increased sympathetic response to stress.

Raynaud's phenomenon is ordinarily bilateral and is most frequently seen in women in their 40s. The classic color changes from white to blue to red are often observed. The pattern is sudden pallor of the fingers, progressing to cyanosis, and eventually hyperemia with reflex dilation. Although the pattern is most frequently seen alone (primary vascular instability), it occasionally is the first clinical sign of scleroderma, other collagen-vascular disorders, or vasculitides (secondary).

Management of this condition consists of patient reassurance and avoidance of precipitating factors such as a cold environment and handling cold objects. Nicotine is a known precipitant, and smoking should be discontinued. Biofeedback has been reported to be effective in many patients.[64] Medical management with beta-blockers or sympathectomies can be considered, but produces inconsistent results.

Heterotopic Ossification

The abnormal formation of mature lamellar bone in soft tissue is called heterotopic ossification. It is characterized by a matrix and crystalline form of true bone that develops outside the confines of normal periosteum and with a distinct vascular supply (Fig. 38–27). There are multiple precipitating factors, which include neurological insult, burns, direct trauma, surgery, and hereditary disorders. In neurogenic diseases, such as spinal cord injury, it typically develops below the level of the lesion.

Its development is initiated by a nonspecific inflammatory phase with symptoms generally beginning 1 to 3 months after the inciting event. Osteoid deposition follows the inflammatory phase.

Diagnosis

In the upper limb, heterotopic ossification is most often seen in the shoulder and elbow. It is generally characterized by swelling, moderate pain, joint limitation, localized warmth and tenderness, and occasionally low-grade fever. Alkaline phosphatase levels can be ele-

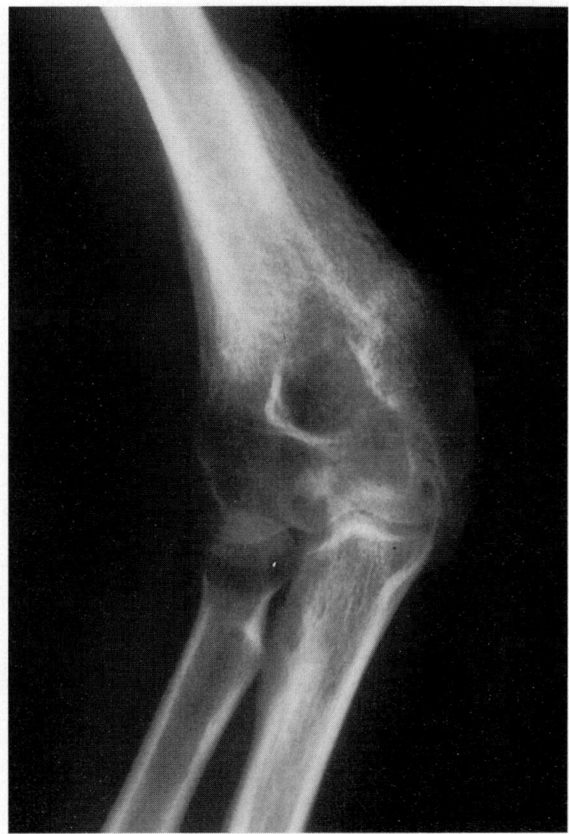

FIGURE 38–27. Heterotopic ossification about the elbow in a 26-year-old woman with a prior traumatic brain injury.

vated early in this condition.[32] The specificity is increased if the levels are fractionated. Radiological studies performed early in the course of the disease often are negative, with calcifications appearing later. Bone scanning is more sensitive early in the process and shows increased uptake before any diagnostic findings become discernible on plain radiography. The increased uptake of tracer reflects the increased vascularity and ongoing calcium deposition.

Treatment

Treatment consists of range-of-motion exercises to maintain joint function as the ectopic bone matures. Modalities for pain relief and the use of NSAIDs for their anti-inflammatory effect, with indomethacin being the most studied,[63] are helpful. Etidronate disodium has been extensively described for use early in the course of the disease to minimize eventual ossification. Its long-term benefit remains in doubt.[6] Criteria for its use include early recognition prior to ossification becoming evident on plain films. Its detractors believe its use at best merely delays the inevitable ossification.

Although the prophylactic perioperative use of local radiation treatment can be effective for prevention of the process,[2] its indications and uses are complex and controversial, and beyond the scope of this discussion.

Surgical removal in the acute phases prior to the completion of the ossification process is contraindicated. Aggressive recurrence is likely if surgical intervention is undertaken prematurely. Bone scanning should be performed to ensure that no active process is ongoing. Fractionated alkaline phosphatase levels can also help in this determination.

COMPLEX REGIONAL PAIN SYNDROME

Complex regional pain syndrome (CRPS) is a syndrome involving a chronic painful condition of the upper limb associated with neurovascular disturbance and dystrophic changes of the skin and bones. Typically there is painful impairment of the shoulder and swelling and tenderness of the hand, with sparing of the elbow. Other names that have been given to this constellation of signs and symptoms include reflex sympathetic dystrophy (RSD), Sudek's atrophy, causalgia, and shoulder-hand syndrome.

This syndrome is traditionally attributed to autonomic, particularly sympathetic, instability. Recently the term CRPS has been substituted for RSD, however, because it is not certain that sympathetic hyperactivity is the cause. The appearance of this condition in a typical physiatric practice is high. CRPS is thought to be present in up to 10% to 15% of all patients with hemiplegia and painful shoulders.[13] Stroke is a common predisposing event. Other predisposing conditions include trauma of any severity, thoracic surgery, cervical radiculopathy, and myocardial infarction. Some cases occur without any known precipitating event.[67] A psychological basis for predisposition to this condition is possible but not well substantiated in the literature.[37, 52, 53]

The disease process ordinarily progresses through different stages. Stage 1 typically lasts a few weeks to 6 months and is characterized by significant pain and increased blood flow, with resultant pitting edema, redness, and warmth. Reduced range of motion of the wrist, hand, and shoulder often begins to develop at this stage and is related in part to pain inhibition. Hyperhydrosis may begin. The skin can be hyperestetic and tender. The development of osteoporosis is thought to begin at this stage but is usually not detectable on plain films.

Stage 2 typically lasts 3 to 6 months following stage 1. The edema is often less predominant and is described as brawny or spreading. However, pain and further impairment in range of motion are prominent features. Blood flow is decreased, and the temperature of the extremity falls. Hair and nail growth is diminished at this stage and hyperhydrosis persists. Atrophy of muscle and the subcutaneous tissue develops. Plain films can reveal localized patchy osteoporosis as well as periarticular thickening. A "causalgia personality" has been described[15] and can be a feature during this stage.

Stage 3 can persist for additional months. This stage is characterized by less pain but progression to irreversible changes of atrophic soft tissue, muscle atrophy, severe loss of motion, and extensive osteoporosis. The skin appears smooth and glossy and is dry and cool. Other common features include coarse upper limb hair and ridged nails.

Diagnosis

The diagnosis is ordinarily made on a clinical basis, primarily from the history and observation and physical signs outlined above. The patient typically reports pain out of proportion to the injury and extending beyond the confines of dermatomal patterns. Descriptions such as burning, numbness, and tingling are often used. The patient is evaluated for swelling, dystrophic changes, muscle atrophy, and tenderness (Fig. 38–28).

Radiological evaluation can be helpful, but changes might not be seen on plain films until the later stages of the disease (ordinarily after 3 or more months). Triple-phase bone scan can show increased uptake in the involved limb early in the process, possibly reflecting increased blood flow from localized bone turnover due to sympathetic vasoconstriction.[56] This is most significantly seen in the carpal and metacarpal joints in the hand. The findings do not, however, correlate accurately with the degree of vasomotor disturbances.

Treatment

Graded activities are encouraged to facilitate a "desensitization" of the hypersensitive tissues. Aggressive activity to "overload" the painful input is the basic treatment for this condition.[29] Isotoner gloves are also beneficial for this purpose. Other techniques of desensitization include increasingly vigorous massage. Use of contrast baths has been also shown to be beneficial for this purpose. A reduction in distal edema can also occur with use of these modalities. Some have reported symptomatic improvement with the use of US[54]; however, the mechanism is not clear. Other modalities that have

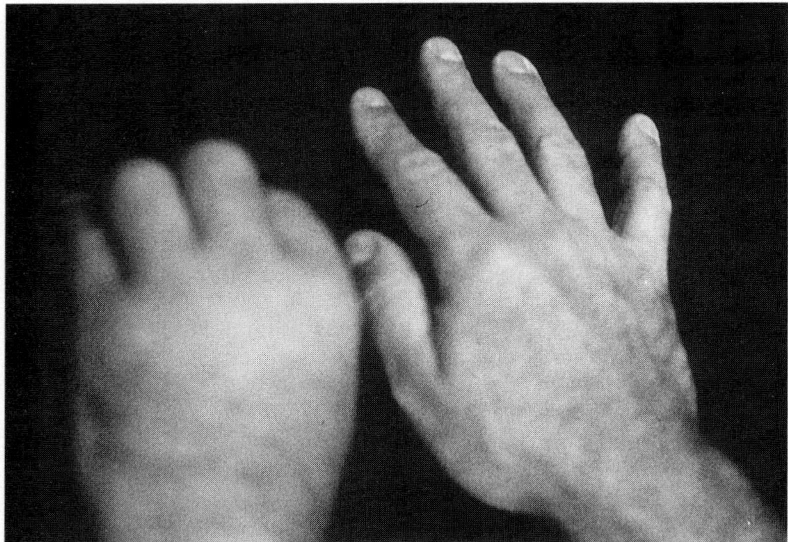

FIGURE 38–28. Reflex sympathetic dystrophy in the left hand of a 52-year-old man. Edema and dystrophic changes of the affected extremity are noted.

been reported to provide symptomatic relief include TENS, paraffin baths, and pneumatic pumps.

A large majority of patients respond to systemic corticosteroids instituted in the acute phase of the disease. This underscores the importance of early recognition. Prednisone is used most frequently, in doses up to 100 mg/day or 1 mg/kg and tapered over 2 weeks. In the face of relapse, this treatment can be repeated. A wide range of drug interventions have been suggested and include NSAIDs, anticonvulsants, tricyclic antidepressants, beta-blockers, calcium channel blockers, calcitonin, and even topical capsaicin. These treatments are occasionally beneficial, but most often are not helpful.

A local anesthetic block of the second or third sympathetic ganglia can often confirm the diagnosis as well as provide symptomatic relief. Other clinical signs reflecting response to injection include improvement in cyanosis and a rise in temperature of the affected limb of 1°C. Temporary procedures sometimes utilized other than stellate ganglia blockade include Bier block and peripheral nerve blocks. Sympathectomy is utilized when the chemical blocks have been transiently effective.

Following invasive procedures, emphasis must be placed on aggressive and progressive activity of the affected limb for optimal results. Early recognition is critical for intervention prior to the development of trophic changes seen in stages 2 and 3. After this time, the prognosis for satisfactory and complete recovery is poor.[66]

REFERENCES

1. Andrews JR, Broussard TS, Carson WG: Arthroscopy of the shoulder in the management of partial tears of the rotator cuff: A preliminary report. Arthroscopy 1985; 1:117.
2. Ayers DC, Evarts CM, Parkinson JR: The prevention of heterotopic ossification in high risk patients by low dose radiation after total hip arthroplasty. J Bone Joint Surg Am 1986; 68:1423.
3. Binder AT, Bulgen DY, Hazelman BL, et al: Frozen shoulder: An arthrographic and radionuclide scan assessment. Ann Rheum Dis 1984; 43:365–369.
4. Beach WR, Caspari RB: Arthroscopic management of rotator cuff disease. Orthopedics 1993; 16:1007–1015.
5. Bulgen DY, Binder AI, Hazelman BL, et al: Frozen shoulder: Prospective clinical study with an evaluation of three treatment regimens. Ann Rheum Dis 1984; 43:353–360.
6. Buschbacher R: Heterotopic ossification: A review. Crit Rev Phys Rehabil Med 1992; 4:199–213.
7. Cabot A: Tennis elbow, a curable affliction. Orthop Rev 1987; 16:69–73.
8. Cailliet R: Hand Pain and Impairment, ed 4. Cailliet Pain Series, Philadelphia, FA Davis, 1994, pp 179–182.
9. Calandra JJ, Goldner RD, Hardaker WT: Scaphoid fractures: Assessment and treatment. Orthopedics 1992; 15:931–938.
10. Canoso JJ: Idiopathic or traumatic olecranon bursitis. Arthritis Rheum 1977; 20:1213–1216.
11. Codman EA: The Shoulder: Rupture of the Supraspinatus Tendon and Lesions in or about the Subacromial Bursa. Boston, Thomas Todd, 1934, pp 65–177.
12. Cooney WP, Dobyns MD, Linscheid RL: Nonunion of the scaphoid: Analysis of the results from bone grafting. J Hand Surg 1980; 5:343–354.
13. Davis SW, Petrillo CR, Eichberg RD, et al: Shoulder-hand syndrome in a hemiplegic population: A 5-year retrospective study. Arch Phys Med Rehabil 1977; 58:353–356.
14. de Quervain F: Ueber eine form von chronischer tendovaginitis. Cor-VI: Schweiz Aerzte Basel 1895; 25:389–394.
15. DeGood DE, Cundiff GW, Adams LE, et al: A psychosocial and behavioral comparison of reflex sympathetic dystrophy, low back pain, and headache patients. Pain 1993; 54:317–322.
16. Drakeford MK, Quinn MJ, Simpson SL, et al: A comparative study of ultrasonography and arthrography in evaluation of the rotator cuff. Clin Ortho Rel Res 1990; 253:118–122.
17. Fischbach TJ, Seeger LL: Magnetic resonance imaging of glenohumeral instability. Topics Magn Reson Imaging 1994; 6:121–132.
18. Fu FH, Harner CD, Klein AH: Shoulder impingement syndrome: A critical review. Clin Orthop Rel Res 1991; 269:162–173.
19. Hakuno A, Sashika H, Ohkawa T, et al: Arthrographic findings in hemiplegic shoulders. Arch Phys Med Rehabil 1984; 65:706–711.
20. Hawkins RJ, Kennedy JC: Impingement syndrome in athletes. Am J Sports Med 1980; 8:151–157.
21. Hazelman BL: The painful stiff shoulder. Rheumatol Rehabil 1972; 11:413–421.
22. Ho G, Tice AD, Kaplan SR: Septic bursitis in the prepatellar and olecranon bursae. Ann Intern Med 1978; 89:21–27.
23. Hulstyn MJ, Weiss AC: Adhesive capsulitis of the shoulder. Orthop Rev 1993; 22:425–432.
24. Hurd MM, Farrell KH, Waylonis GW: Shoulder sling for hemiplegia: Friend or foe? Arch Phys Med Rehabil 1974; 55:519–522.

25. Ilfeld FW: Can stroke modification relieve tennis elbow? Clin Orthop Rel Res 1992; 276:182–186.
26. Itoi E, Tabata S: Conservative treatment of rotator cuff tears. Clin Orthop Rel Res 1992; 275:165–173.
27. Jobe FW: Impingement problems in the athlete. Instructional Course Lectures, no 38, 1989, pp 205–209.
28. Jobe FW, Jobe CM: Painful athletic injuries of the shoulder. Clin Orthop 1983; 173:117–124.
29. Johnson EW, Pannozzo AN: Management of shoulder hand syndrome. JAMA 1966; 195:108–110.
30. Joynt RL: The source of shoulder pain in hemiplegia. Arch Phys Med Rehabil 1992; 73:409–413.
31. Kienbock R: Uber treumatische Malazie des Mondbeins und ihre Folgezustande: Entartungsformen und kompressionsfrakturen. Fortschr Geb Rontgen 1910; 16:78–103.
32. Kim SW, Charter RA, Chai CJ, et al: Serum alkaline phosphatase and inorganic phosphorus value in spinal cord injury patients with heterotopic ossification. Paraplegia 1990; 28:441–447.
33. King JW, Brelsford JH, Tullos HS: Analysis of the pitching arm of the professional baseball pitcher. Clin Orthop 1969; 67:116.
34. Kuschner SH, Brien WW, Bindiger A, et al: Review of treatment results for Kienbock's disease. Orthop Rev 1992; 21:717–728.
35. Lee KH, Khunadorn F: Painful shoulder in hemiplegic patients: Study of the suprascapular nerve. Arch Phys Med Rehabil 1986; 67:818–820.
36. Lee M, Haq AM, Wright V, et al: Periarthritis of the shoulder: A controlled trial of physiotherapy. Physiotherapy 1973; 59:312–315.
37. Lynch ME: Psychological aspects of reflex sympathetic dystrophy: A review of the adult and paediatric literature. Pain 1992; 49:337–347.
38. Mack GR, Boss MJ, Gelberman RH, et al: The natural history of scaphoid nonunion. J Bone Joint Surg Am 1984; 66:504–509.
39. Meyer AW: The minute anatomy of attrition lesions. J Bone Joint Surg 1931; 13:341–360.
40. Meyers JF: Arthroscopic management of the impingement syndrome in rotator cuff tears. Sports Med Fitness 1989; 2:243–260.
41. Morrey BF, An KN: Stability of the elbow joint: A biomechanical assessment. Am J Sports Med 1984; 12:315–319.
42. Morrison DS, Bigliani LU: Variations in acromial shape and its effect on rotator cuff tears. In: The Shoulder. Tokyo, Professional Postgraduate Services, 1987, pp 213–214.
43. Neer CS: Anterior acromioplasty for chronic impingement syndrome in the shoulder: A preliminary report. J Bone Joint Surg Am 1972; 54:41–50.
44. Neer CS: Shoulder Reconstruction. Philadelphia, WB Saunders, 1990, pp 422–427.
45. Neer CS: Impingement lesions. Clin Orthop Rel Res 1983; 173:70–77.
46. Neviaser TJ: Adhesive capsulitis. Orthop Clin North Am 1987; 18:439–443.
47. Neviaser TJ, Neviaser RJ, Neviaser JS, et al: Lateral epicondylitis: Results of outpatient surgery and immediate motion. Contemp Orthop 1985; 11:43–46.
48. Nirschl RP: Prevention and treatment of elbow and shoulder injuries in the tennis player. Clin Sports Med 1988; 7:289–308.
49. Nirschl RP, Pettrone FA: Tennis elbow: The surgical treatment of lateral epicondylitis. J Bone Joint Surg Am 1979; 61:832–839.
50. Olive RJ, Marsh HO: Ultrasonography of rotator cuff tears. Clin Orthop Rel Res 1992; 282:110–113.
51. Ozaki J, Fujimoto S, Nakagawa Y, et al: Tears of the rotator cuff of the shoulder associated with pathological changes in the acromion: A study in cadavers. J Bone Joint Surg Am 1988; 70:1224.
52. Pak TJ, Martin GM, Nagness JL, et al: Reflex sympathetic dystrophy: Review of 140 cases. Minn Med 1970; 53:507–512.
53. Pollock FE Jr, Koman LA, Smith BP, et al: Patterns of microvascular response associated with reflex sympathetic dystrophy of the hand and wrist. J Hand Surg 1993; 18A:848–852.
54. Portwood MM, Lieberman JS, Taylor RG: Ultrasound treatment of reflex sympathetic dystrophy. Arch Phys Med Rehabil 1987; 68:116–118.
55. Post M, Silver R, Singh M: Rotator cuff tear: Diagnosis and treatment. Clin Orthop Rel Res 1983; 173:78–91.
56. Poulin de Courval L, et al: Painful shoulder in the hemiplegic and unilateral neglect. Arch Phys Med Rehabil 1990; 71:673–676.
57. Prevost R, Arsenault AB, Dutil E, et al: Shoulder subluxation in hemiplegia: A radiologic correlational study. Arch Phys Med Rehabil 1987; 68:782–785.
58. Rathbun JB, Macnab I: The microvascular pattern of the rotator cuff. J Bone Joint Surg Br 1970; 52:540–553.
59. Rizk TE, Christopher RP, Pinals RS, et al: Arthrographic studies in painful hemiplegic shoulders. Arch Phys Med Rehabil 1984; 65:254–256.
60. Rizk TE, Pinals RS, Talaiver AS: Corticosteroid injections in adhesive capsulitis: Investigation of their value and site. Arch Phys Med Rehabil 1991; 72:20–22.
61. Rockwood CA, Lyons FR: Shoulder impingement syndrome: Diagnosis, radiographic evaluation, and treatment with a modified Neer acromioplasty. J Bone Joint Surg Am 1993; 75:409–424.
62. Rowe C: The Shoulder. New York, Churchill Livingstone, 1988.
63. Schmidt SA, Kjaersgaard-Anderson P, Pedersen NW, et al: The use of indomethacin to prevent the formation of heterotopic bone after total hip replacement. J Bone Joint Surg Am 1988; 70: 834–838.
64. Sedlacek K: Biofeedback treatment of primary Raynaud's disease. In Basmajian JV (ed): Biofeedback: Principles and Practice for Clinicians, ed 3. Baltimore, Williams & Wilkins, 1989.
65. Shaw MH: Treatment of Dupuytren's contracture. Br J Plast Surg 1951; 4:218–223.
66. Steinbrocker O: The shoulder-hand syndrome: Present perspective. Arch Phys Med 1968; 49:388.
67. Subbarao J, Stillwell GK: Reflex sympathetic dystrophy syndrome of the upper extremity: Analysis of total outcome of management of 125 cases. Arch Phys Med Rehabil 1981; 62:549–554.
68. Uhthoff HK, Loehr J, Sarkar K: The Pathogenesis of Rotator Cuff Tears. The Shoulder. Tokyo, Tokyo Professional Postgraduate Services, 1987, p 211.
69. Unverferth LJ, Olix ML: The effect of local steroid injections on tendon. J Sports Med 1973; 1:31–37.
70. Van Ouwenaller C, Laplace PM, Chantraine A: Painful shoulder in hemiplegia. Arch Phys Med Rehabil 1986; 6:23–36.
71. Verhaar J, Walenkamp G, Kester A, et al: Lateral extensor release for tennis elbow. J Bone Joint Surg Am 1993; 75:1034–1043.
72. Warner J, Caborn DN: Overview of shoulder instability. Crit Rev Phys Rehabil Med 1992; 4:145–198.
73. Zuckerman JD, Mirabello SC, Newman D: The painful shoulder: Part II. Intrinsic disorders and impingement syndrome. Am Fam Physician 1991; 43:497–512.

39 CHAPTER

Brian A. Casazza, M.D., Jeffrey L. Young, M.D., M.A., and Kirsten K. Rossner, M.S., P.T., A.T.C.

Musculoskeletal Disorders of the Lower Limbs

The overwhelming majority of musculoskeletal problems can be solved nonsurgically. In order for aggressive conservative treatment to be successful, however, the physician must have the skills to make an accurate diagnosis, generate a logical differential diagnosis, and formulate a precise rehabilitation program. The physician should also be able to recognize when other interventions, including physical therapy and surgery, are the best solution to restore prior function. The ability to recognize ailments combined with the capacity to refer and communicate with other health care practitioners will ensure quality care for the patient, and reduce cost as well. The purpose of this chapter is not to be encyclopedic, but to provide the foundation for assessing a variety of musculoskeletal problems in the lower limbs, emphasizing injuries that arise from repetitive musculotendinous overload.

MUSCULOSKELETAL HISTORY

A careful history is required to identify the diagnosis and mechanism of injury (see Chapter 1). The following is an overview of basic questions that need to be asked of the patient presenting with a musculoskeletal injury of the lower limbs.

Chronology of the Injury. When did the pain first appear? Was the onset of pain sudden or gradual? Has this happened before? Has the patient just begun an exercise program?

Mechanism of Injury. Was trauma involved? Was the foot planted or in the air at the time of injury? Did the foot invert or evert? Was there a valgus or varus moment at the knee or was there a sense of rotational strain? Did the patient feel or hear a "pop" or a "snap"? Was there a sudden inability to bear full body weight? A noncontact knee injury occurring with the foot planted and accompanied by a valgus moment, rotation, and a pop is classic for an acute disruption of the anterior cruciate ligament (ACL). A noncontact, non-weight-bearing injury in the posterior thigh occurring with the hip flexed, the knee extended, and accompanied by a pop suggests a hamstring tear.

Nature of the Pain. Is the pain constant or intermittent? What makes it more tolerable and what exacerbates it? Is it associated with weight bearing? If so, how soon does the pain occur after beginning activity? Is the pain highly localized or does it radiate to or from another area? Is the pain associated with inflammation? Pain associated with compartmental syndromes is often less apparent at rest and at the onset of exercise, but becomes worse after a relatively consistent amount of activity. Pain from a fracture is present at rest or provoked by minimal activity. Achy anterior knee pain worsened by squatting or prolonged sitting (the "theater sign") alerts the clinician to patellofemoral joint dysfunction, while anterior knee pain aggravated by maintaining full knee extension suggests infrapatellar fat pad irritation.[25, 34] A "pulled" calf muscle during a tennis match usually reflects musculotendinous overload of the medial gastrocnemius, while calf pain unassociated with exertion but worsened with forward spine flexion suggests lumbosacral radiculopathy. Tendinitis exhibits the cardinal signs of inflammation (redness, swelling, and increased warmth) within a painful tendon. Tendinosis is painful, but lacks signs of inflammation.[86]

Injury Inventory. How many other injuries have been sustained? What were the locations? Were they managed nonsurgically or surgically? The current injury can often be preceded by a previous injury to that area, one that did not undergo proper rehabilitation.

Age Considerations. The differential diagnosis of distal Achilles tendon pain in the skeletally immature runner must include calcaneal apophysitis (Sever's disease). In the elderly runner it is much more likely to involve pathological changes within the tendon itself.[9, 10] Hip pain in the young athlete should raise suspicion of a femoral stress fracture or traction apophysitis, while the same symptoms in the elderly runner can indicate fracture or symptomatic spinal stenosis.[9, 10]

Exercise Habits. How much does the patient exercise? Has there been a sudden increase in frequency, intensity, or duration of workouts? Does the patient routinely stretch before and after exercising? The patient who trains intensively every day, does not vary the muscle groups exercised, and does not stretch is an obvious candidate for both musculotendinous overload and overtraining.

Equipment. What type of shoes does the patient use? How often are new pairs purchased and old pairs discarded? Does the patient wear shoe orthotic inserts? When were the inserts originally constructed and for what purpose? These questions offer insight into potential errors of training and biomechanical imbalances. Shoes or inserts that have broken down and no longer serve their original intent are commonly seen and easily corrected problems. (Refer to articles by Subotnick[151] and Newell and Bramwell[112, 113] for excellent reviews of evaluating the foot and the role of foot orthoses.) Orthotic devices are especially useful when placed to correct biomechanical imbalances that are not correctable by specific stretching and strengthening programs. In one survey study of 347 symptomatic runners whose average training was approximately 40 miles/week, 75% reported marked improvement or resolution of their symptoms with the use of orthotic inserts.[56]

Exercise Environment. Where does the patient typically train? Does the runner train on a level dirt path, on a banked concrete surface, on a treadmill, or on a flat circular track? Poor running course selection can create imbalances at the level of the foot and ankle—imbalances that are transmitted up the biomechanical chain to the more proximal structures. For example, running on a banked surface causes pronation of the "uphill" foot, stressing the medial ankle and creating a knee valgus force, hip abduction, and elevation of that hemipelvis. The "downhill" foot supinates more, which stresses the lateral ankle and creates a knee varus force, hip adduction, and lowering of that hemipelvis.[23, 132]

Review of Systems. Is there a nonmusculoskeletal process contributing to the current problem? Does the middle-aged club tennis pro who presents with calf pain have signs of vascular claudication? Is the young female runner who presents with pelvic stress fractures amenorrheic and exhibiting signs of disordered body image? What medications are being used? Are anabolic steroids being taken? Has the patient been using narcotics for pain relief? These and other factors can weigh heavily on the runner's overall health and hence should be identified.

Function. How has his injury affected this person's life? Is the patient still working? Is this person still capable of performing all activities of daily living independently?

Coping Skills. Can this person tolerate relative or complete rest? How will this person react if true rest is required for an undetermined amount of time? Are there secondary gain issues at hand, and is there reason to be concerned about this patient's developing a chronic pain problem? In a holistic approach, input from a psychologist or psychiatrist can be essential to the successful rehabilitation of a person with a musculoskeletal injury. By taking time to understand the patient as well as the ailment and by choosing the best line of treatment, the clinician has the best chance of alleviating symptoms in the most time-efficient and cost-effective way.

PHYSICAL EXAMINATION

Establishing a diagnosis-specific rehabilitation program requires a thorough physical examination. It is critical to adhere to the concept of the kinetic chain and to recognize that biomechanical dysfunction in one body region is capable of causing "injury at a distance." Consequently, it should be routine to examine the low back, hip, knee, and ankle regions in virtually all patients presenting with lower extremity complaints. The following section serves as an overview of the basic components of a physical examination. More specific tests are discussed within the region-specific problem sections.

It is important for the clinician evaluating the patient to take into consideration non-weight-bearing structural abnormalities and to correlate these findings with a dynamic assessment. Structures that must be evaluated statically include scoliosis, lumbar spine lordosis, pelvic bony landmarks, genu varum/valgum, femoral and tibial torsion, foot/ankle structure, relative muscle bulk bilaterally, calluses, and visible evidence of inflammation. A gait analysis should be performed to evaluate how these structural problems affect dynamic motion.

Often structural abnormalities are compensated for at other sites in the biomechanical chain. For example, the clinician might note a leg length discrepancy in non-weight bearing, a discrepancy that is compensated for in the longer limb by hyperextension at the knee and overpronation at the foot. Gluteus medius weakness might cause sidebending toward the affected side during gait (compensated Trendelenburg's sign).

Coupling the static and dynamic evaluation with the patient's history is imperative. Muscle fatigue might not be immediately evident in the clinic, but can play a significant role in dysfunction. For instance, a younger high-school aged girl in a growth spurt might not have the eccentric muscle control of the hip and pelvis to endure many miles of running without loss of hip/pelvic control. Statically, the clinician might note a slight internal femoral torsion, but she might appear normal during a relatively brief gait analysis. With longer running, however, she might develop excessive internal rotation of the lower extremity due to eccentric weakness of the hip external rotators and tightness of the adductors. This can manifest itself as medial knee, hip, or lower back pain.

For running athletes, video analysis of treadmill running at varying speeds with and without shoes, and with and without orthotic devices, is recommended. This enables the clinician to identify more subtle biomechanical imbalances, as well as flaws in running style. Video recordings are not only a useful diagnostic aid but can also be a vehicle for patient education. The recording and projecting system should be capable of high resolution when played at normal, fast-forward, or slow-motion speeds.

Just as the entire lower extremity is evaluated both statically and dynamically, each component part is also evaluated.[66] The effect of foot structure and function on lower extremity dysfunction is not entirely clear. Studies that attempt to correlate static measures of the lower extremity with pathology have not been conclusive. While some have found correlations between static measures and lower extremity dysfunction,[94, 125, 145] others have not.[102, 144, 160] The clinician must become adept at identifying major structural abnormalities and neutralizing these effects when possible. Foot assessment in non-weight bearing should begin with the identification of callus, and with viewing static forefoot position with the foot in subtalar joint neutral position. For this evaluation, the patient should be in the prone position, with the feet hanging over the edge of the plinth. The head of the talus is palpated between the thumb and index finger anteriorly with one hand while the other hand applies a dorsiflexion force through the fourth and fifth ray. The talar head should be palpated equally between the thumb and index finger. A posterior-to-anterior view down the foot will reveal either a varus, neutral, or valgus alignment of the forefoot and rearfoot relative to the horizontal plane. Evaluation of foot motion and relative laxity in the talocrual, subtalar, or midfoot joints, as well as of the first ray, are also important in assessing the non-weight-bearing position. With the patient standing, the clinician should note the amount of motion from the subtalar joint neutral position to a relaxed standing position (Fig. 39–1). With the patient standing, the clinician should note the amount

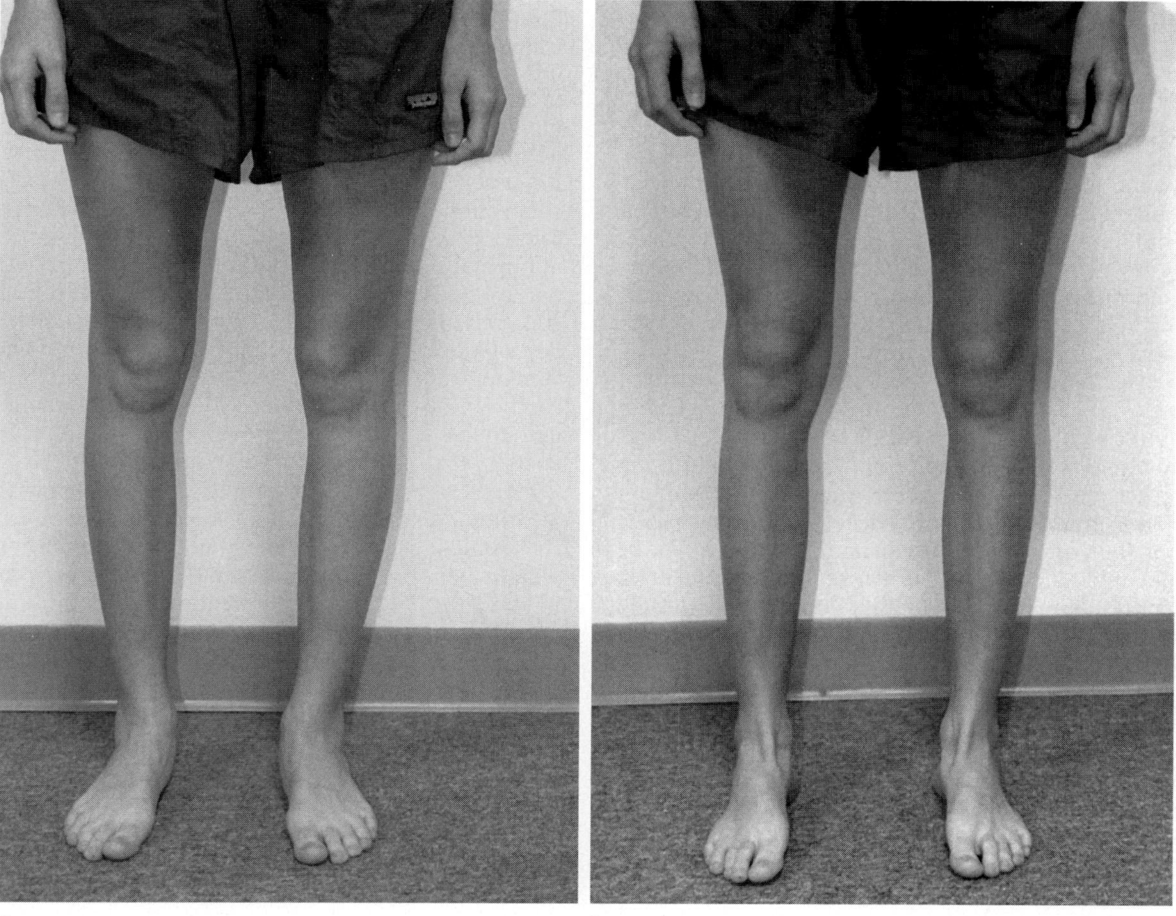

A B

FIGURE 39–1. *A.* Subtalar joint relaxed position: Note the valgus orientation of the great toes, overpronation through the rearfoot, and subsequent relative internal rotation of the lower extremities causing the patellae to face inward. *B.* Subtalar joint neutral position: After the subtalar joint has been positioned in neutral, note the relative neutral position of the great toes, rearfoot, and alignment of the lower extremities with the patellae facing forward.

of motion from a subtalar joint neutral position to a standing relaxed position. The standing subtalar joint neutral position is when the talar head is felt equally between the thumb and index finger as the patient inverts and everts their foot.[24] The navicular drop test is also used in this position. The prominence of the navicular is marked in standing subtalar joint neutral to a relaxed standing position. We have noted clinically that an overly pronated foot may have a combination of callus along the medial edge of the great toe, forefoot and/or a rearfoot varus, a navicular drop of over 10 to 12 millimeters and relative laxity through the joints. Our observations have also noted that an underpronated foot often has callus at the base of the fourth and fifth metatarsals, neutral to valgus rearfoot/forefoot alignment, less than 8 millimeters of navicular drop and minimal joint laxity.

The navicular drop test is also performed in the standby position. The vertical descent of the navicular bone is noted when going from a foot touch to a full weight-bearing posture. We have noted clinically that an overly pronated foot can have a combination of callus along the medial edge of the great toe, forefoot, and/or a rearfoot varus deformity, a navicular drop of over 10 to 12 millimeters, and relative laxity through the joints. Our observations have also noted that an underpronated foot often has callus at the base of the fourth and fifth metatarsals, neutral to valgus rearfoot/forefoot alignment, less than 8 millimeters of navicular drop, and minimal joint laxity.

The knee is first examined statically. Femoral anteversion, femoral and tibial torsion, patellar position in weight bearing and non-weight bearing, and Q-angle are important measures. The Q-angle (Fig. 39–2) is usually in the range of 10 to 15 degrees and is considered to be excessive if it exceeds 20 degrees.[21, 72, 95, 132] Next the range of motion in the knee joint, proximal tibiofibula joint, and patellofemoral joint should be assessed. Patellar mobility and tracking should be assessed passively and with an active quadriceps contraction in both non-weight-bearing and weight-bearing positions. The presence of lateral tracking of the patella, patella baja, and patella alta should be noted. Hypermobility of the patella, external tibial torsion, increased Q-angle, femoral neck anteversion, a broad pelvis, and overpronation can combine to form the "malalignment syndrome," which can be associated with medial knee pain.[21, 23, 84, 100, 132] Assessment of the ligaments including the anterior cruciate ligament (ACL), posterior cruciate ligament (PCL), medial collateral ligament (MCL), and lateral collateral ligament (LCL) as well as the menisci is also indicated. Since nonacute knee dysfunction is often the result of muscular inflexibility and connective tissue restriction in the lower extremity, it is important to do a flexibility assessment of the hamstrings, hip rotators, gastroc/soleus complex, and iliotibial band.

Static measures of the hip in non-weight bearing should include observing for femoral torsion and femoral anteversion/retroversion. Femoral torsion is evaluated by palpating the greater trochanter with one hand and passively rotating the femur internally and externally at the level of the femoral condyles. When the greater trochanter is most easily palpated, the relative position of the femur can be noted by the orientation of the femoral condyles. Weight-bearing assessment should include noting the degree of toe-out, which is directly affected by femoral anteversion/retroversion as well as tibial/malleolar torsion.

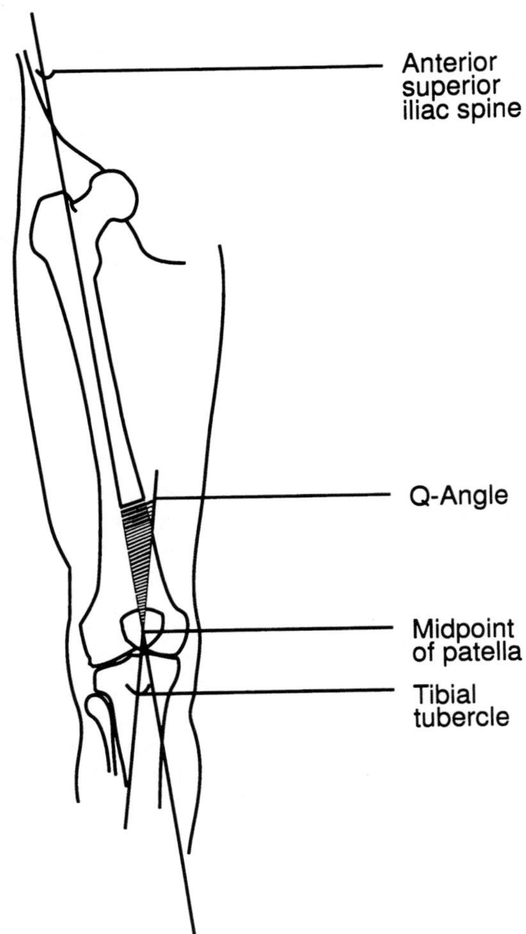

FIGURE 39–2. The Q-angle: the angle formed between the line of pull of the quadriceps and the center line of the patellar tendon (*hatched area*). A line is drawn from the anterior superior iliac spine through midpoint of the patella, and a second line is drawn through the midaxis of the patella to the tibial tubercle for determination.

The hip should also be evaluated for the presence of tight flexors, extensors, rotators, and adductors. Loss of mobility in this region can be a factor in the development of the patient's injury.[122, 158] The Thomas test assesses hip flexor flexibility. For this test the patient lies supine and brings both knees up to the chest. The patient then lowers one knee down to the level of the plinth while continuing to hold the other to the chest. If the leg cannot be brought in line with the plinth or if the lumbar spine must arch to do so, there is indication of hip flexor restriction.[64] Hamstring flexibility can be measured in the supine position with the hip flexed to 90 degrees while the lower leg is passively extended by the clinician. Tissue restriction is noted at the point where the clinician can no longer extend the lower leg. External/internal rotation of the hip can be evaluated by rotating the hip while the hip and knee are flexed and the patient lies supine. Adductor tightness can be assessed by abducting the patient's leg in the supine position. If the adductors are restricted, the entire body appears to pivot and rotate about the pelvis instead of just the leg abducting. The hip joint capsule can be assessed by placing the hip in flexion in addition to abduction and external rotation. This is called Patrick's test or the FABER test. FABER is an acronym for flexion, abduction, and external rotation of the hip. The grind test can also be done to assess for the possibility of an arthritic condition. The patient lies supine with the knee drawn to the chest and flexed while the clinician provides a compressive and rotational force to the femur. This test should not produce discomfort.

The sacroiliac joint can be a source of pain for a number of reasons. Leg length discrepancies uncompensated for in the lower extremity can place increased shear force through the joint, causing localized pain and surrounding soft tissue spasm. Muscular imbalances can also cause increase sacroiliac joint irritation. For example, iliopsoas tightness can cause increased lumbar lordosis and affect sacroiliac joint motion. Evaluation of the sacroiliac joint should begin with the palpation of the bony landmarks, including the posterior superior iliac spine (PSIS), the anterior superior iliac spine (ASIS), iliac crests, sacral base, inferior lateral angle (of the sacrum), and ischial tuberosities. For a comprehensive evaluation of the sacroiliac joint, bony landmarks should be assessed in non-weight bearing (supine and prone), standing, and sitting. Static asymmetries give only one dimension of possible dysfunction. Further motion testing in standing and sitting should also be incorporated in the evaluation.

The March test evaluates sacroiliac joint motion relative to the opposite side. The evaluator stands behind the patient and palpates the PSIS with one hand and the sacral base with the other. The patient then draws one knee up to the chest while balancing on the other limb. The relative posterior motion of the PSIS is compared bilaterally, with the restricted joint revealing relatively less range of motion. An additional standing test includes the forward flexion test where the evaluator palpates the PSIS bilaterally and has the patient slowly bend to touch the toes. The evaluator looks for increased motion of one PSIS relative to the other. Often the restricted sacroiliac joint is the one that shows greater range of motion in forward flexion. With the patient sitting with feet supported, the clinician can evaluate the sit-to-slump test. For this test the evaluator palpates the PSIS bilaterally and asks the patient to sit in a neutral pelvic position. The patient is then instructed to alternately "slump" and extend the lower back. Relative movement of each PSIS is compared in all three positions.

A quick but effective screen of the back incorporates all the observations from the lower body segments, since the concept of the kinetic chain must not be forgotten. Lumbosacral spine motion is intimately related to motion at the level of the hip and pelvis. Tightness of lower extremity muscles attaching to the pelvis can interfere with the normally smooth combination of spine flexion–pelvic rotation and spine extension–pelvic derotation (lumbopelvic rhythm) observed during trunk flexion and extension.[28] During spine flexion and extension, it is essential to identify the major motion segments. Approximately 80% to 90% of the motion in the lumbosacral spine should be at L4 to L5 and L5 to S1.[28] Migration of the motion up toward the thoracolumbar junction with altered tone of the paraspinal muscles suggests spinal segment dysfunction. A "springing sensation" in the lower spine during anterior glides (placement and release of pressure along the spine while the patient is in a relaxed prone-lying position) also suggests spinal segmental dysfunction. Abdominal muscle weakness and weakness of the muscles attaching to the thoracolumbar fascia further indicate that the spine is in need of conditioning.[136] Many persons who appear to be otherwise highly fit from constant aerobic exercise fail to perform regular exercise that promotes conditioning of the supportive spinal musculature. In the young runner with back pain, provocative tests such as extending the spine while standing on one leg help identify active posterior element irritation or symptomatic spondylolysis.

A brief neurological examination is recommended regardless of whether the patient appears to present with a neurogenic problem or not. The elderly patient with "hip pain" can have unrecognized spinal stenosis. The young runner with a chronic "hamstring strain" can have an unrecognized S1 radiculopathy.[12] Cutaneous nerve injuries need to be considered as well. Careful evaluation of a persistently painful ankle that appears to have healed from an inversion sprain might reveal ongoing irritation of the superficial peroneal nerve. Persistent medial leg pain in the presence of a negative bone scan can be related to saphenous nerve irritation rather than to shin splints.

The person's shoes should be inspected for signs of breakdown. Wearing away of the leather along the distal toecap region can imply subtle anterior tibial weakness. Excessive medial or lateral wear can indicate increased pronation or supination, respectively. Matching up regions of wear on the shoe with regions on the foot (a blister or callus) might convince the patient that new shoes are needed. As a general rule, pronation control is best achieved with a straight board-lasted shoe having good rearfoot control. Persons predisposed to supination do better with a flexible and curve-lasted shoe.[23, 56, 150] It is more important for the athlete to pay close attention to the appropriate components of the shoe than to buy the latest style. Since shoe companies change the components of shoes every few months, finding a store with a knowledgeable shoe specialist is very helpful.

INJURY ANALYSIS AND REHABILITATION

Proper rehabilitation requires a thorough understanding of applied anatomy, biomechanics, and the kinetic chain. The effects of a musculoskeletal injury are rarely confined to a single joint, and rehabilitation programs should take into account the alterations in anatomy and biomechanics that have occurred proximal, distal, and contralateral to the site of acute injury. The physician must also be able to recognize the adaptations that have occurred in response to errors of training, particularly those induced by chronic musculotendinous overload. This section details a "template" for rehabilitation of musculotendinous overload injuries. Application of the template to specific lower extremity musculoskeletal problems follows.

Step 1: Establish an Accurate Diagnosis. Inherent to this task is recognizing how muscle overload injuries and tendon injuries present. The vicious circle model for analysis of musculotendinous injury induced by repetitive overload is presented in Figure 39–3. To aid those unfamiliar with this model, some clarification of the terminology is provided:

Tissue injury complex—the area of actual tissue disruption[78–81, 126]

Clinical symptom complex—the symptoms associated with the dysfunction and injury[78–81, 126]

Tissue overload complex—the tissue group being subjected to tensile overload[78–81, 126]

Functional biomechanical deficit—inflexibilities or muscle strength imbalances that create altered mechanics[78–81, 126]

Functional adaptation complex—functional substitutions used by the patient in order to try to maintain activity[78–81, 126]

When the musculotendinous unit is subjected to tensile overload, damage occurs at a cellular level.This typically produces symptoms of pain, dysfunction, and instability. It also impairs athletic performance.[78–80] If the extent of that overload is small (microtear) and nutrition and healing time are adequate, activities can be safely resumed. However, if the injury is not adequately treated and is allowed to progress (macrotear), healing is accompanied by development of scar tissue, with the onset of subclinical adaptations such as loss of flexibility, loss of strength, or strength imbalances.[78–80] This leads to further decrements in performance and biomechanical substitutions that perpetuate this "negative-feedback vicious circle" (Fig. 39–3B), creating the chance for more overload and injury.[78–80]

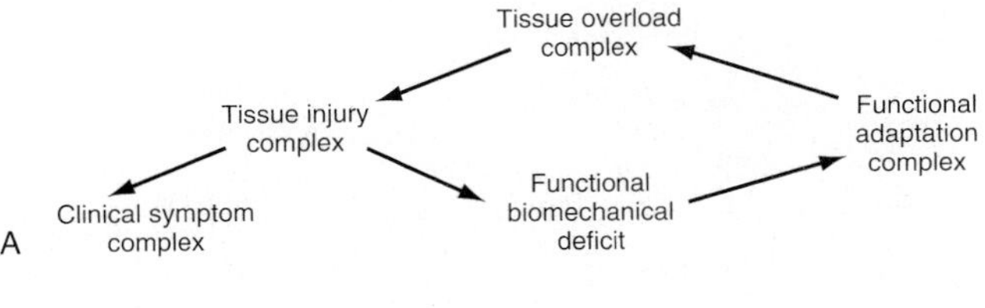

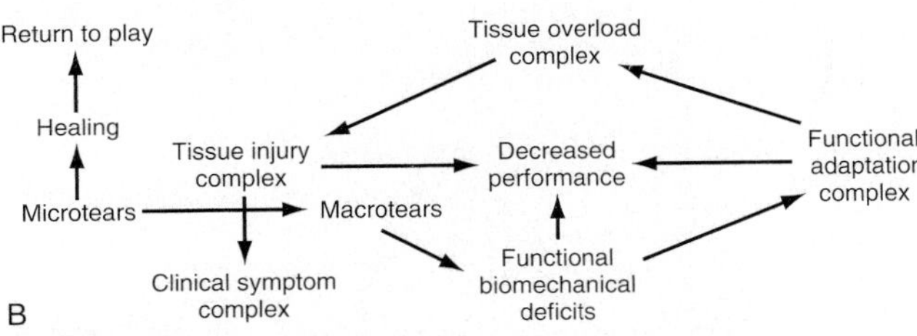

FIGURE 39–3. *A.* and *B.* Model for vicious cycle of musculotendinous overload.

Muscle injury can present as acute or chronic injury, as exacerbation of a chronic injury, or as a subclinical injury.[80] Muscle "strain"-type injuries typically manifest themselves microscopically as a zone of myonecrosis confined to within 500 μm of the myotendinous junction.[128] Tendon injuries present as either an acute inflammatory process superimposed upon acute or chronic injury (tendinitis) or as a product of maladaptation and intratendinous degeneration unaccompanied by mediators of inflammation (tendinosis).[80, 86] In tendinitis, the immediate treatment goal is relief of symptoms, while in tendinosis the immediate goal is restoration of function.[80] Identification of the components of musculotendinous injury within the vicious circle facilitates understanding the functional consequences of the injury that need to be addressed in the rehabilitation program.

Step 2: Acute Management. Efforts are directed toward minimizing the effects of inflammation and controlling pain. The PRICE principle (*p*rotection, *r*elative rest, *i*ce, *c*ompression, and *e*levation) is followed. This is usually a period for judicious use of anti-inflammatory medications and pain-relieving modalities.[62, 80, 126, 132, 162]

Step 3: Initial Rehabilitation. This phase continues to focus on promotion of proper healing. Restoration of motion helps to reduce the effects of immobilization, with controlled tensile loading promoting ordered collagen growth and alignment. Identification of correctable biomechanical imbalances is initiated. Many rehabilitation programs fail by not progressing beyond this step.

Step 4: Correction of Imbalances. Development of symmetric motion and symmetric strength is a twofold goal. When the patient is pain-free, and when nearly full concentric strength has been achieved, it is essential that an eccentric strengthening program be initiated. This is a critical step in developing a musculotendinous unit that is less likely to fail in the face of future tensile stresses. It is also important to understand the difference between *closed kinetic chain* (CKC) and *open kinetic chain* (OKC) exercises. If, for instance, during knee flexion or extension, the foot is allowed to move freely through space, the system is called "open." In an OKC system, the hamstrings dominate in flexion while the quadriceps dominate in extension. During CKC exercise for the lower limbs, the foot is kept immobile or maintains contact with a ground reactive force, thus creating a multi-articular closed chain. Rather than the near isolation of the large muscle groups seen during OKC exercises, performance of CKC knee flexion and extension results in "co-activation" of both hamstrings and quadriceps groups.[43, 140] Examples of CKC exercises are leg presses or partial squats (Fig. 39–4). These types of exercises strengthen agonist and antagonist simultaneously via co-contraction, and are more physiological for lower limb sporting activities such as running. An OKC knee extension is shown in Figure 39–5. One can begin to identify flaws in exercise technique and training prac-

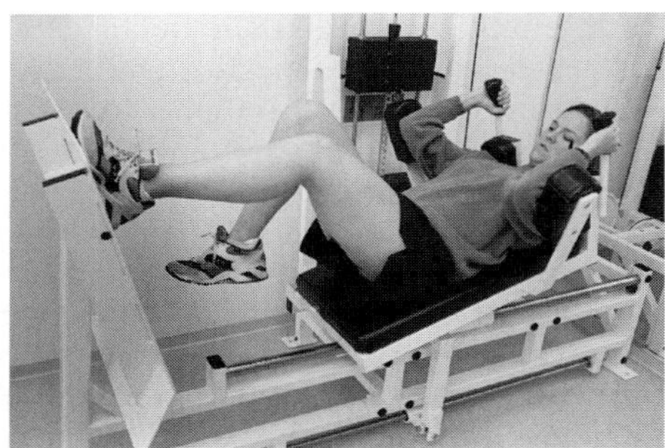

FIGURE 39–4. Example of a closed kinetic chain knee extension.

tices when the patient is capable of full weight bearing under controlled conditions. Structure of the lower extremity can influence function, so the movement patterns adopted by the athlete are important. If these movement patterns predispose an athlete to injury, they must be identified and remedied. This includes strengthening of weak musculature and stretching tight tissues. Additionally, proprioception and balance exercises must not be overlooked. Proprioceptive aids such as taping into external rotation for an individual with weak hip external rotators can give input for improved proprioceptive feedback. Alternative aerobic conditioning exercises are encouraged. Other than local icing, treatment modalities are rarely indicated during this phase.

Step 5: Return to Normal Function. Cross-training, aqua training, and the use of alternative conditioning schemes give way to a gradual increase in activity-specific training and eventual resumption of full activity. Endurance performance, power, and agility should be restored to baseline.

Injuries About the Hip

Applied Anatomy and Biomechanics

The hip is functionally constructed to provide stable weight bearing through a wide variety of lower limb movements. The hip joint encounters forces equivalent to more than three times body weight during walking, and nearly five times body weight during running.[135]

The femoral head approximates two-thirds of a sphere and is contained within the deep acetabular fossa (ball-and-socket joint). Containment of the femoral head is enhanced by a fibrocartilaginous labrum at the outer rim of the acetabulum. Most of the hip joint's stability comes from the articular capsule of the joint itself rather than the surrounding musculature. The primary stabilizers of the hip consist of a very strong synovial capsule reinforced by three ligaments arising from the bony components of the pelvis. The iliofemoral ligament, also called the *Y ligament of Bigelow,* arises from the anterior inferior iliac spine (AIIS) and divides, forming two femoral insertions at the greater trochanter and on the anterior femur inferior to the intertrochanteric line. This ligament resembles an inverted Y and restrains hyperextension at the hip.[64] Two additional ligamentous supports include the pubofemoral (which checks abduction and extension of the femur) and ischiofemoral (which checks extension) ligaments. The spiral direction of the ligaments also serves to limit internal rotation of the femur, as all three get wrapped tighter with medial femoral rotation. Functioning as a group, they contribute to hip stability by restraining extension, abduction, and internal rotation of the femur. The hip joint is consequently the least stable in flexion, adduction, and external rotation (the most frequent position of hip dislocation).[159]

The mature femoral neck is angled at 120 to 130 degrees to the central axis, and is positioned in approximately 15 degrees of anteversion (medial femoral torsion). An increase in the neck-shaft angle is termed *coxa valga,* and a decrease is called *coxa vara.*

The vascular supply to the femoral head and neck is somewhat tenuous. In the center of the head there is a slight flattening, called the *fovea,* where the ligamentum teres attaches. The femoral head receives vascularity from a small artery within the ligamentum teres, and through the medial and lateral circumflex arteries, which pierce the capsule. This architecture renders the vascular supply vulnerable to disruption during dislocation (loss of flow to the head through the ligamentum teres) and fracture (interference with flow through the circumflex vessels).

Some of the key muscles surrounding the hip joint include the piriformis, gluteus maximus, and gemelli. The piriformis runs from the anterior sacrum through the greater sciatic foramen, inserting on the greater tro-

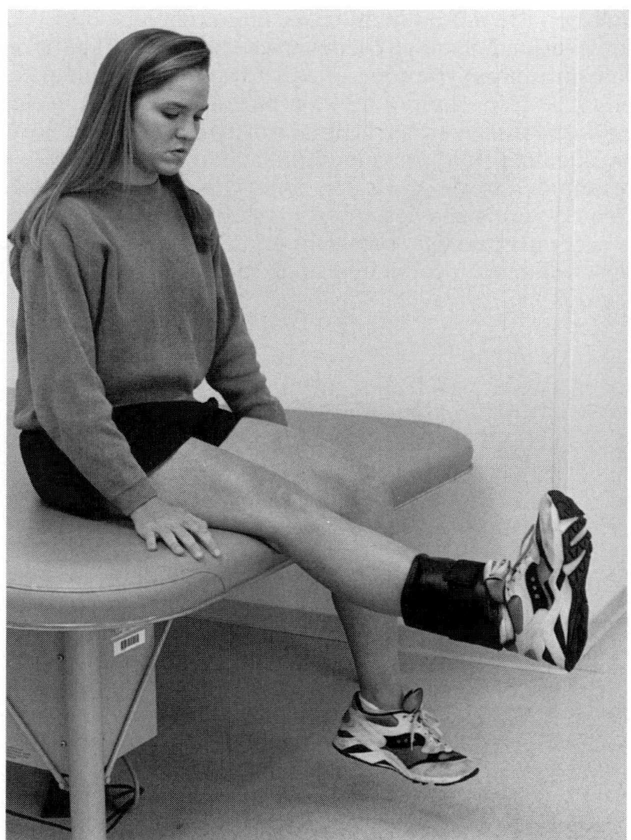

FIGURE 39–5. Example of an open kinetic chain knee extension.

chanter, and functions as an external rotator. The gluteus maximus has its origins at the posterolateral sacrum, sacrotuberous ligament, and posterior ilium, and inserts on the iliotibial tract and gluteal tuberosity. It functions as a hip and spine extensor and as a hip external rotator. The gemelli are short muscles that run from the ischial spine to the greater trochanter; they function as minor external rotators. The majority of neurovascular structures emerging from the sciatic foramen exit inferior to the piriformis muscle (the superior gluteal nerve and artery exit above), creating a potential point of entrapment or irritation.

Specific Problems in the Hip Region

Piriformis Syndrome. This syndrome is both underrecognized and overdiagnosed. As mentioned previously, there is the potential for sciatic nerve entrapment beneath the piriformis as the nerve exits the sciatic foramen. In Agur's review[3] of 640 limbs, the tibial and peroneal divisions passed beneath the muscle 87% of the time. In slightly more than 12% of the cases, the peroneal division passed through the muscle, and in less than 1% the peroneal division emerged above the piriformis.[3] Sciatic nerve compression by this muscle leads to complaints of dysesthesias down the posterior thigh and often into the calf or foot. Buttock pain and tenderness through the piriformis can be found. Side-to-side comparisons of piriformis tightness (i.e., allowable internal rotation of the hips) should be made either with the person in a prone-lying position with the hips adducted and knees flexed to 90 degrees, or in a supine lie with 60 degrees of hip flexion and slight hip adduction while introducing the internal rotation stress.[51] Electrodiagnostic testing can reveal involvement of tibial and peroneal innervated muscles, with sparing of superior and inferior gluteal nerve-innervated structures and absence of abnormal electromyographic activity in the paraspinal musculature. Magnetic resonance imaging (MRI) can demonstrate injury or edema within the piriformis muscle, but is rarely a necessary procedure.

The clinical symptom complex in piriformis syndrome consists of buttock (and possibly leg) pain, and dysesthesias aggravated by sitting or lower limb exertion.[16] The tissue injury complex comprises myotendinous breakdown within the piriformis and possible focal demyelination within the tibial and peroneal divisions of the sciatic nerve. The structures within the tissue overload complex are the piriformis, gluteal muscles, gemelli, quadratus lumborum, the sacroiliac ligaments, and the sciatic nerve. The functional biomechanical deficits include a tight piriformis and external rotators, hip abductor weakness, sacroiliac joint hypomobility or hypermobility, and lower lumbar spine dysfunction.[16, 51] Functional adaptations consist of ambulating with an externally rotated thigh, shortened stride length, and functional limb length shortening.

Rehabilitation efforts are geared toward stretching of the piriformis and associated external rotators and evaluation of the sacrum and pelvis for other imbalances. Once sacral and pelvic abnormalities have been defined and corrected, strengthening and stabilization exercises should be incorporated into the home exercise program. These include pelvic tilts, minibridges, and hip external rotation strengthening in a variety of positions. Although many patients have tenderness, tightness, or pain in the region of the piriformis, it is essential to be sure that a lumbar spine-based problem with secondary referral to the piriformis is not being missed.

Snapping Hip Syndrome. This is associated with a variety of extra-articular and intra-articular phenomena. The most common cause appears to be the snapping or popping of the iliotibial band (ITB) across the greater trochanter, although involvement of the iliopsoas tendon snapping over the iliopectineal eminence can also be seen.[51, 107, 129] Less commonly, loose bodies, labral tears, and osteochondritis dessicans can be intra-articular sources of the snap. Treatment typically consists of muscle rebalancing with stretching and myofascial release to promote return of muscles and tendons to their normal length.[51] Correction should take only a few weeks. Should symptoms persist despite an adequate stretching program, evaluation of intra-articular pathological changes by computed tomography (CT), MRI, or arthroscopy is recommended.[129]

Trochanteric Bursitis. This is commonly seen in the elderly and manifests as pain in the lateral thigh during ambulation and decreased tolerance for lying on the affected side. The trochanteric bursa lies beneath the tendon of the gluteus maximus and is located posterolateral to the trochanter. Patients can describe a pseudoradicular pattern with the pain extending down the lateral aspect of the lower extremity and into the buttock.[154] The clinical symptoms can be elicited by placing the lower extremity in external rotation and abduction. Direct palpation or deep pressure applied posterior and superior to the greater trochanter will reproduce the pain.[138] Functional biomechanical deficits consist of shortening of the tensor fascia lata (TFL), rectus femoris, hamstrings, and weakness of the adductors.[126] Functional adaptations include increased hip external rotation with an altered gait or running pattern.[126] Treatment should be geared toward restoration of flexibility and strength imbalances. Injecting the bursa with corticosteroid and anesthetic can be helpful if the flexibility and conditioning exercises are unsuccessful.[120] Hip pain that persists despite comprehensive rehabilitation and injection therapy should alert the physician to alternative sources of pain including the lumbar spine and adjacent joints throughout the kinetic chain.[31, 156]

Ischial Bursitis. The ischial bursa lies between the ischial tuberosity and the gluteus maximus. Irritation of this bursa is not common. Classically, *ischial bursitis* (tailor's or weaver's bottom) occurs with friction and trauma after prolonged sitting on a hard surface. It can also be seen in adolescent runners, often in conjunction with ischial apophysitis. Pain can be aggravated during uphill running. The pain is distributed down the posterior aspect of the thigh and occurs with activation of the hamstring muscles. Initial treatment approaches involve modification of the patient's activity, such as a decrease in the duration and frequency of running. If an alternative to running includes cycling, the patient should be advised to avoid the use of toe clips, which increase activation of the hamstrings. When the cause is prolonged sitting, the patient's workstation should be modified to allow for activities to be conducted in a standing position and a cushion should be used during sitting. Ice and nonsteroidal anti-inflammatory drugs (NSAIDs) are helpful in controlling symptoms. The adolescent athlete might require a radiological series to screen for callus formation secondary to ischial apophysitis if the pain does not resolve with conservative measures. Corticosteroid injections can be helpful in cases of persistent pain. The use of fluoroscopy to demonstrate a bursogram minimizes the possibility of improper needle location and avoids unnecessary repeat injections.

Avascular Necrosis of the Femoral Head. Most clinicians have little difficulty determining if an overt hip fracture has occurred, but often neglect to aggressively evaluate the patient with groin (hip joint) pain and negative plain films. As discussed previously, the blood supply to the femoral head is fragile and subject to compromise with hip dislocation or femoral neck fracture. Disruption of this supply can have catastrophic results. Even if initial plain radiographs are negative, there should be a high index of suspicion for *avascular necrosis* (AVN) of the femoral head if the hip is painful with joint loading and no source of pain coming from outside the hip can be identified. Although a bone scan can show a stress reaction within days, MRI scanning is preferable. MRI is sensitive to the early signs of AVN, and also provides information about the integrity of the bony cortex (necrosis and surrounding edema can be clearly seen in Figure 39–6). As bone death occurs, the plain films show destruction of the femoral head, but onset of treatment this late in the course is sure to have a poor outcome. If the MRI shows evidence of necrosis, immediate surgical consultation and non-weight-bearing status are recommended.

Specific Problems in the Thigh

The thigh consists of the heavily muscled region about the shaft of the femur. The structures in this region are extremely vulnerable both to tensile overload and to direct trauma. The majority of thigh injuries adhere to the overload vicious circle as previously described.

Anterior Thigh

Relevant Anatomy and Biomechanics. The majority of the mass of the anterior thigh is formed by the quadriceps muscle group (Fig. 39–7). All of these muscles are innervated by the femoral nerve (L2–L4). The vastus lateralis, vastus intermedius, and vastus medialis all have their origin along the shaft of the femur and insert on the proximal patellar pole (via the quadriceps tendon), and therefore act solely as knee extensors. The fourth muscle of this group, the rectus femoris, originates at the anterior inferior iliac spine, and acts as both a hip flexor and knee extensor. Although often thought of as part of the quadriceps group, the vastus medialis obliquus is functionally distinct—it does not act like the other four muscles. The sartorius, which is also less commonly involved in disorders of the thigh than the knee, has its origin at the ASIS and terminates at the pes anserinus along the inferomedial knee.

The quadriceps is capable of providing explosive force, such as that needed for jumping, vertical leaping, and kicking. It is also essential in its role as a shock attenuator during landing from jumps and in the control of knee flexion during the single-leg loading response and early stance phase of the gait cycle. The rectus femoris, along with the iliopsoas, also serves to initiate forward motion of the femur during early swing phase.

There are two common mechanisms of anterior thigh injuries: tensile overloading of the musculotendinous

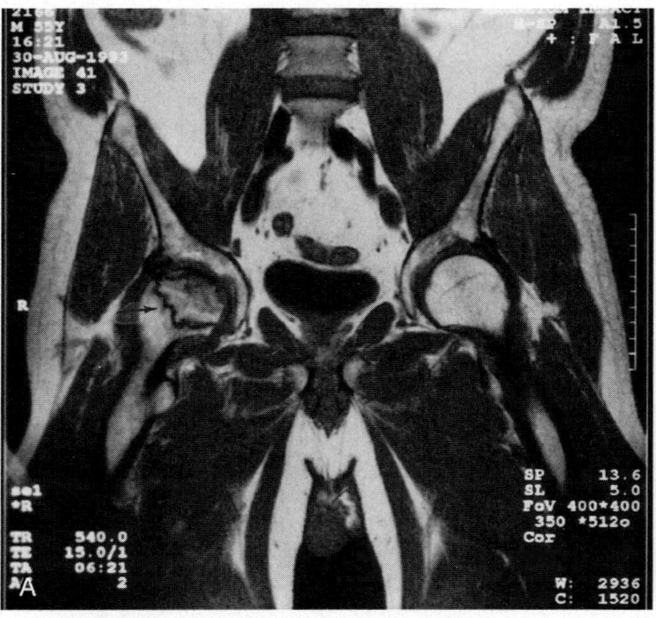

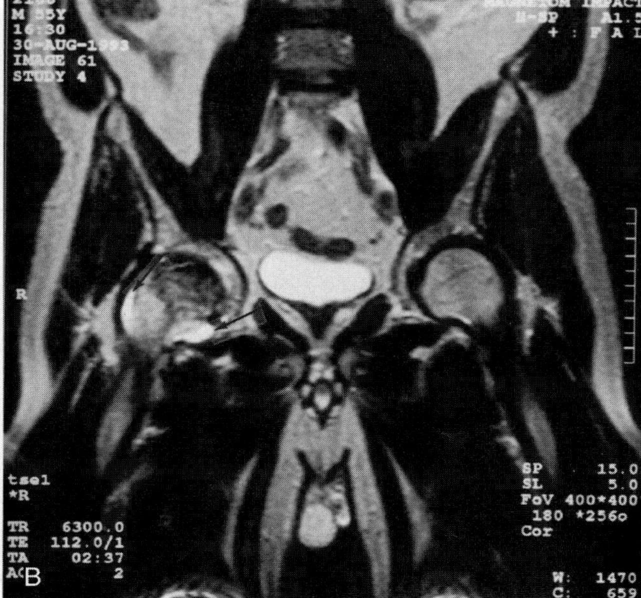

FIGURE 39–6. Avascular necrosis of the femoral head. *A.* T1-weighted image. *B.* Edema present on T2-weighted image.

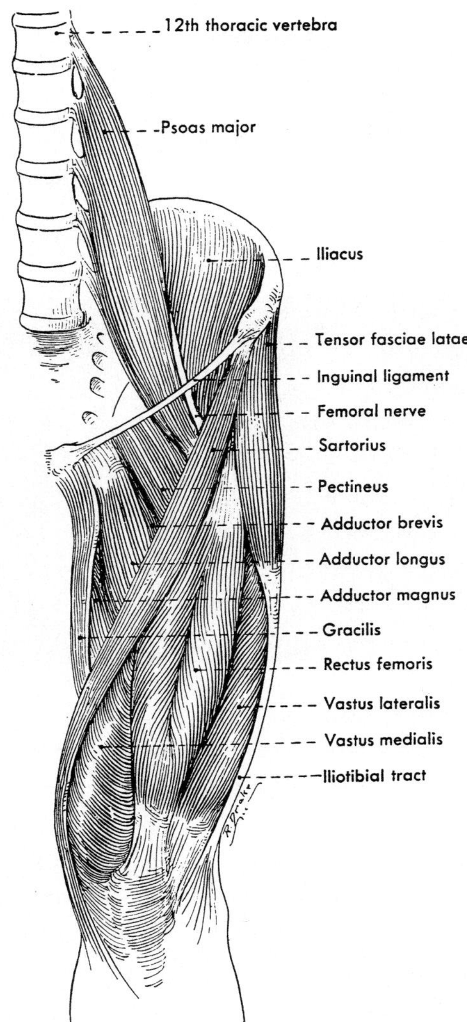

FIGURE 39–7. Muscles of the anterior and medial thigh. (From Hollinshead WH, Jenkins DB: Functional Anatomy of the Limbs and Back, ed 5. Philadelphia, WB Saunders, 1981.)

unit with induction of a "strain," or high-velocity compressive forces resulting in a "contusion." Persons particularly prone to anterior thigh injuries include football, soccer, and rugby players.

Quadriceps Strains. Strain injuries are graded as follows:

1. First degree (mild)—an overstretch with minimal disruption of musculotendinous unit integrity. There is probably less than 5% fiber disruption, and the patient experiences soreness with motion but has only minimal strength loss.[73, 162, 164]
2. Second degree (moderate)—an actual (although incomplete) muscle tear (Fig. 39–8). There is intramuscular bleeding with hematoma formation, and muscle strength is clearly compromised.[73, 162, 164]
3. Third degree (severe)—a complete rupture. Muscle function is essentially lost. Avulsion injuries are included in this category.

The rectus femoris is the most commonly strained of the quadriceps group.[93] *Ely's test* (passive flexion of the knee with the patient prone) is useful for isolation of the rectus. A tight rectus induces elevation of the ipsilateral hemipelvis as maximum allowable knee flexion is approached, as the hip-flexing component of the rectus femoris is blocked.

The signs and symptoms of quadriceps strain vary depending on the severity of the injury. Lower-grade injuries might have only pain on deep palpation or passive stretch. Higher-grade injuries are typically accompanied by swelling and discoloration. Total rupture of the muscle typically results in a palpable mass in the zone of muscle injury.

Functional biomechanical deficits and other factors that can increase the risk of quadriceps strain include tightness or weakness of the quadriceps musculature, hamstring tightness, lack of sufficient warm-up or stretching prior to exercise, previous injury without rehabilitation, and overtraining. The functional adaptations that persist when the return to activity is too early include greater reliance on the unaffected leg for upward propulsion in jumping activities, shortened running stride with reduced hip flexion, and reduced running velocity. Occasionally, the patient tries to maintain an externally rotated femur so the adductor group can be used to advance the thigh.

Acute rehabilitation follows the PRICE principle. Ice is generally preferable to heat, and interferential current can be useful as an adjunct in pain control.[162] However, the role of NSAIDs as modifiers of the inflammatory response to acute injury makes them extremely valuable in the acute management of all first- and most second-degree strains. The early use of NSAIDs in high-degree strains should be weighed carefully as antiplatelet activities can increase local bleeding.

Initial rehabilitation includes pain-limited stretching to achieve progressive increases in muscle length. The patient should be taught the proper technique and instructed to continue the stretching program on a long-term basis. The vastus muscles can be stretched by flexing the knee at any hip angle, but the rectus femoris is stretched only if the hip is in a neutral or extended position. An example of a combined hip flexor and knee extensor stretch is shown in Figure 39–9. In more chronic or recurrent cases, soft tissue mobilization can be instituted. Mobilization of scar can break up scar tissue and improve flexibility, especially when immediately followed by gentle passive stretching.

Strengthening should be initiated only after range of motion is pain-free and complete. The progression should be from either isometric or low-resistance dynamic contractions to full-range progressive resistance exercises (PREs). The PRE regimen should include both concentric and eventually eccentric exercise, and care should be taken to ensure that movements are smooth and without muscle substitutions. Eccentric work against maximal or supramaximal loads should be avoided early in the rehabilitation program to lessen the likelihood of further structural damage. Aerobic conditioning can be maintained initially by upper body ergometry, swimming with a pull buoy between the legs,

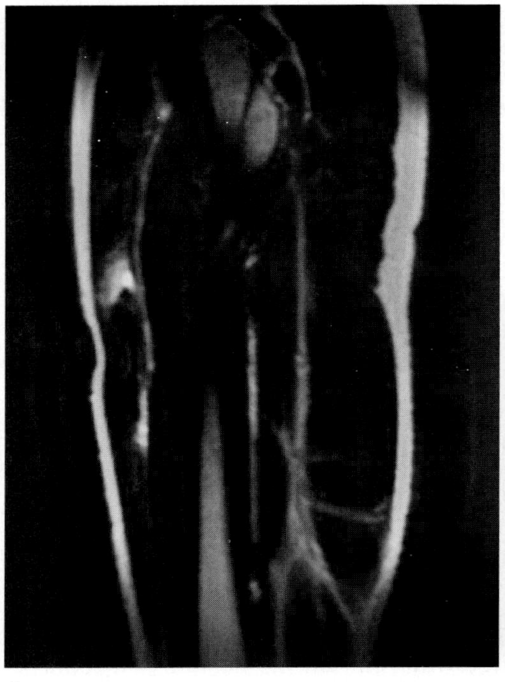

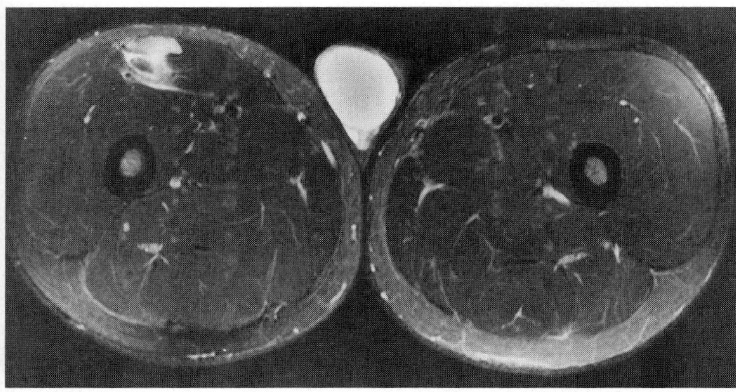

FIGURE 39–8. Second-degree tear of the rectus femoris (quadriceps group). *A.* Sagittal T2-weighted image with increased signal on left indicative of edema within the rectus femoris. *B.* Axial T2-weighted image with increased signal within the rectus femoris indicative of edema.

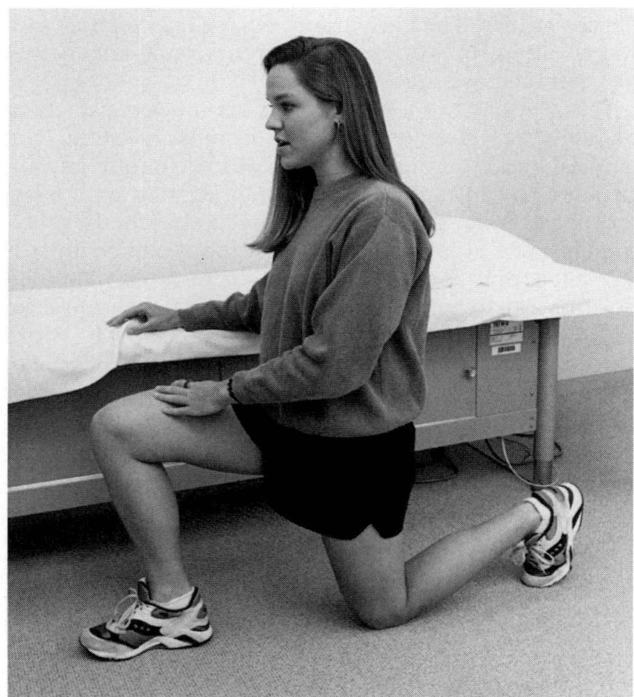

FIGURE 39–9. Stretching of the hip flexors. To obtain additional stretch for the knee extensors, the patient must grab the ankle and increase the knee flexion angle. Note that the spine must maintain a neutral position to avoid the development of lumbar injury.

or via tri-limb exercise with the affected limb kept at rest. When full range of motion is achieved, stationary two-legged bicycling, skiing, or rowing can be attempted. Full-weight-bearing exercises with axial loading of the affected limb (treadmill, stair climber, etc.) are gradually added, with eventual progression to faster-paced activities, agility drills, and finally, sport-specific training when applicable.

Quadriceps Tendon Rupture. This represents an extreme form of overload to the quadriceps and is often the end result of repeated strain injuries.[49, 84] In contrast to quadriceps strains, which are more common in younger athletes, tendon ruptures tend to occur in older athletes. As with strains, the rectus femoris is the most vulnerable of the quadriceps group.[118] A typical presentation is a 40-year-old basketball player landing off balance and on one leg, with sudden giving way and pain, and rapid development of a palpable defect at the site of injury. This is often at the site of tendon insertion at the proximal patellar pole.[84, 132] Incomplete tears can be treated conservatively with initial splinting and use of crutches for protected weight bearing. Full rehabilitation and reconditioning of the remaining muscles is required to prevent residual strength deficits. Complete tears require surgical repair.

Quadriceps Contusions. These are characterized by capillary rupture, edema, inflammation, and infiltrative bleeding. The severity of the contusion is proportional to the extent of blood vessel breakdown and muscle crush. The more relaxed the quadriceps is at the time of impact, the greater the ultimate injury.[84] Clinical grading of the contusion is related to the available passive, pain-free knee flexion 12 to 24 hours post injury. Flexion of less than 45 degrees usually indicates a severe injury; 45 to 90 degrees, a moderate injury; and greater than 90 degrees flexion, a mild injury.[69, 132, 134]

It is important to begin treatment with PRICE as close to the time of injury as possible. The thigh and lower leg should be wrapped or strapped into maximally tolerated knee flexion (Fig. 39–10). Crutch walking is advised. As with strains, NSAIDs are used judiciously. Attempted aspiration of the hematoma is not recommended, particularly since blood is usually clotting by the time the physician examines the injury. Corticosteroid and proteolytic enzyme injections probably do more harm than good. Steroid injections theoretically weaken already stressed connective tissue fibers and collagen, while use of enzymes has never been conclusively shown to be of benefit.[20, 117] Ice is perhaps the only modality that can be used safely. Local heating, soft tissue mobilization, shortwave, and ultrasound have all been implicated in the possible development of the most undesirable complication of a contusion, myositis ossificans traumatica.[8, 20, 58, 111, 151, 162, 164]

Early rehabilitation focuses on re-establishing normal pain-free range of motion through a progressive stretching program. Aerobic conditioning is started as soon as possible, with upper body or tri-limb exercises. As knee flexion returns to normal, isometrics and then CKC strengthening of the knee flexors and extensors are instituted. Criteria for resumption of full activity include minimal thigh tenderness, as well as symmetric range of motion and quadriceps strength. If the patient participates in a contact sport, the use of custom-molded protective padding is recommended.[162] When using off-the-shelf types of padding, it is important to be sure that the entire front of the thigh is covered. A hip spica wrap may also be utilized to limit full motion and provide soft tissue stability. The recovery time for contusive injuries varies greatly. Although recovery from most mild injuries takes less than two weeks, there is considerable overlap in healing times between mild, moderate, and severe injuries (a range of 2 to 60 days of disability[134]).

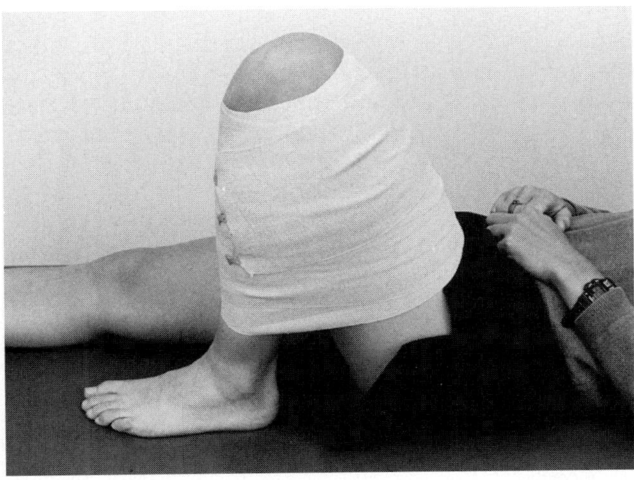

FIGURE 39–10. Compressive dressing applied to the thigh following an acute quadriceps contusion. Note the knee is kept in maximally tolerated flexion.

Myositis Ossificans Traumatica. One of the most vexing complications of contusive injuries is *myositis ossificans traumatica* (MOT) or the formation of nonneoplastic cartilage or bone in connective tissue.[20] MOT is the most common type of extraskeletal bone-forming lesion.[1, 20, 162] It is most common in football and rugby, but has been reported in hockey, soccer, baseball, wrestling, and martial arts.[8, 134, 157, 162] The quadriceps is the most common site of involvement. Initial symptoms are nonspecific, and include local pain, warmth, and tenderness. This usually progresses to a soft tissue swelling and ultimately to a discrete mass with an associated loss of range of motion at the surrounding joints.[20, 162] MOT develops rapidly and can be evident within 3 weeks on plain films.[1] Even earlier detection is possible with three-phase bone scan or ultrasonography.[82, 104]

MOT tends to stabilize in size in 3 to 6 months, and there is great likelihood of spontaneous resorption, particularly when the MOT is near the muscle belly and not lying near the tendon.[84, 91] In Jackson's series of 71 patients with MOT, 69 recovered without residual symptoms.[71]

Recommended treatment following detection of MOT is adherence to the PRICE principle, with immobilization of the affected area while it is overtly inflamed to facilitate the natural sequence of resorption. Prophylactic use of diphosphonates does not seem warranted due to the low likelihood of a persistent lesion. The use of NSAIDs such as indomethacin is common among clinicians, but this has not been conclusively shown to halt the progression of the lesion. Follow-up radiographs showing corticated MOT borders, and "cold" bone scans are useful in determining if the lesion has become "mature." Activity is gradually increased after maturity has been determined. On rare occasions, surgical excision of a mature MOT lesion is necessary. This should generally be reserved for those patients with pain and loss of range of motion persisting 6 to 12 months after the lesion has matured.

Acute Compartment Syndrome. Far less common than the above entities is an *acute compartment syndrome* of the anterior thigh. Patients present with a palpably tense thigh and exhibit decreased sensation in the front of the thigh or in the saphenous nerve distribution, or both. They typically also have pain, pallor, and a progressive loss of quadriceps strength.[7, 162] A key symptom is pain that is seemingly disproportionate to the injury. The patient might also report that the leg feels better in a dependent position. If a compartment syndrome is suspected, surgical consultation should be obtained. Intracompartmental pressure measurements should be made; when the pressure exceeds 40 mm Hg, a fasciotomy is typically necessary.

Medial Thigh

Relevant Anatomy and Biomechanics. The bulk of the medial thigh musculature is composed of the adductor group. The adductor longus, adductor brevis, and adductor magnus all originate along the ischiopubic ramus and insert along the linea aspera of the femur (see Fig. 39–7). The adductor brevis and longus, which are more anteriorly situated, can function as weak hip flexors. The posteriorly positioned adductor magnus is a large muscle that can "double" as an accessory hamstring. The gracilis shares the same origin as the other adductors but crosses the medial knee joint, where it meets the sartorius and the semitendinosis as part of the pes anserinus. The obturator externus is a minor muscle that runs from the obturator foramen to the greater trochanter. All the adductor muscles are innervated by the obturator nerve (L2–L4). The posterior portion of the adductor magnus, in keeping with its role as an accessory hamstring, has tibial innervation as well.

The adductor muscles function as pelvic stabilizers, femoral rotators, and femoral accelerators during the gait cycle. Their peak electromyographic activity occurs shortly after heel-strike and in the mid- to late-stance phase of gait.

Adductor Strain. Adductor injuries are relatively common in soccer and other kicking sports, horseback riding, gymnastics, and ice hockey. The most common of the medial thigh injuries is *adductor strain* due to tensile overload. The adductor longus and magnus are the most frequently affected.[164] High-grade strains can result from sudden femoral abduction in external rotation (e.g., a place-kicker's plant leg slipping on a muddy field so that the kicking leg is subjected to a sudden abduction force). Another common mechanism is repetitive forceful adduction, as when hockey players or roller bladers push off and shift their weight from one leg to the other to propel themselves forward.[105, 142]

The adductor strain clinical symptom complex typically consists of medial thigh and groin pain that is worsened by abduction. The tissue injury complex and overloaded structures include the musculotendinous units of the adductor muscles. Associated biomechanical deficits that can precede the acute event include loss of adductor and psoas flexibility, loss of external rotation of the femur, hamstring tightness and weakness, and gluteus medius weakness. Functional adaptations to injury include shortened stride with less crossover, and an attempt to maintain a relatively internally rotated position of the femur (which accentuates the gluteus medius weakness).

Acute management involves application of the PRICE principle with use of NSAIDs as needed. Interferential current can be a useful adjunct in pain management as well. The patient with a high-degree strain might need crutches, since any attempt to advance the femur forward can induce pain. Spica wraps with elastic bandage can be of benefit early on to remind the patient not to suddenly abduct or flex the thigh. Some athletes continue to use the spica wrap throughout the entire rehabilitation process. If a complete disruption of the adductor longus has occurred, surgical consultation to evaluate the possibility of repair is highly recommended.

Initial rehabilitation emphasizes establishment of a stretching program for the adductor group. Adductor stretching after injury can be quite painful and the stretching should be kept within a pain-free zone. The gluteal muscles and external rotators of the thigh need to be stretched as well, since loss of external rotation and anterior hip capsular tightness frequently coexist with adductor inflexibility.

Correction of imbalances begins with the stretching outlined above and progresses to more aggressive adductor stretching. Using a partner to help stretch in the manner shown in Figure 39–11 or via a "contract/relax" method (a proprioceptive neuromuscular facilitation technique) helps to achieve greater gains. Contract/relax stretching consists of having a partner passively move the limb into a position of stretch. The patient then gently performs an isometric contraction against the resistance of the partner for approximately 10 to 15 seconds. The patient then relaxes the isometric hold at the same time that the partner gently pushes/pulls the patient into more of a stretch. This is repeated 4 to 5 times. "Butterfly" stretches can be used for self-stretching of the adductors. (The person sits on the floor with the soles of the feet together, knees flexed, and with

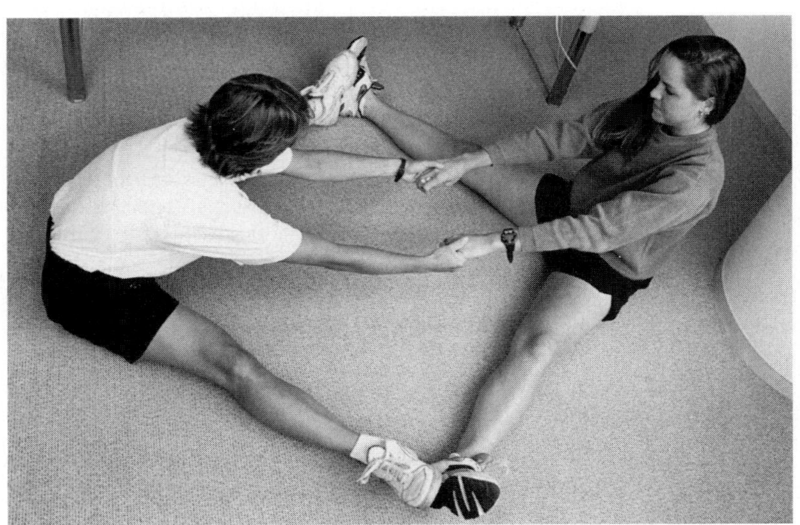

FIGURE 39–11. Assisted adductor stretch.

the hips externally rotated and abducted. Downward pressure is then applied along the inside of the thigh until a pulling sensation is felt within the adductor group.) This technique does not provide good adductor stretch unless the anterior hip capsule has previously been mobilized. Strengthening of all muscles about the hip is necessary. This is particularly true for the external rotators, which usually have been working through a limited range prior to the stretching program. Isometrics and then elastic or rubber tubing for dynamic strengthening can be used early on for adductor strengthening. It can be 1 to 3 weeks post-injury before the patient can safely tolerate higher-resistance weights or aggressive CKC strengthening exercises, particularly in the high-grade adductor strains.

Osteitis Pubis. The diagnosis of *osteitis pubis* should be considered when pain in the groin or symphysis pubis region persists beyond a month. Inflammation in the symphysis pubis generally results from repetitive microtrauma or persistently abnormal mechanics. During mid-stance, when the unsupported hemipelvis attempts to drop, the symphysis encounters increased shear forces from the pull of the adductors below and the rectus abdominis above. Runners and cross-country skiers who abruptly increase their mileage (and who have weak gluteal muscles) are particularly prone to this problem. Definitive diagnosis is made with radiographs or bone scan. A bone scan can show findings before radiographs. Typical radiographic findings include periosteal reaction, demineralization, and sclerosis along the pubis, although these might not be present for 2 to 3 weeks.[84, 143]

The treatment of choice for osteitis pubis is rest for 1 to 2 months with avoidance of lower extremity exercise. Upper extremity conditioning is emphasized, and resumption of a lower extremity rehabilitation and conditioning program is permitted only when there is no tenderness to palpation of the symphysis pubis and hip abduction is pain-free.

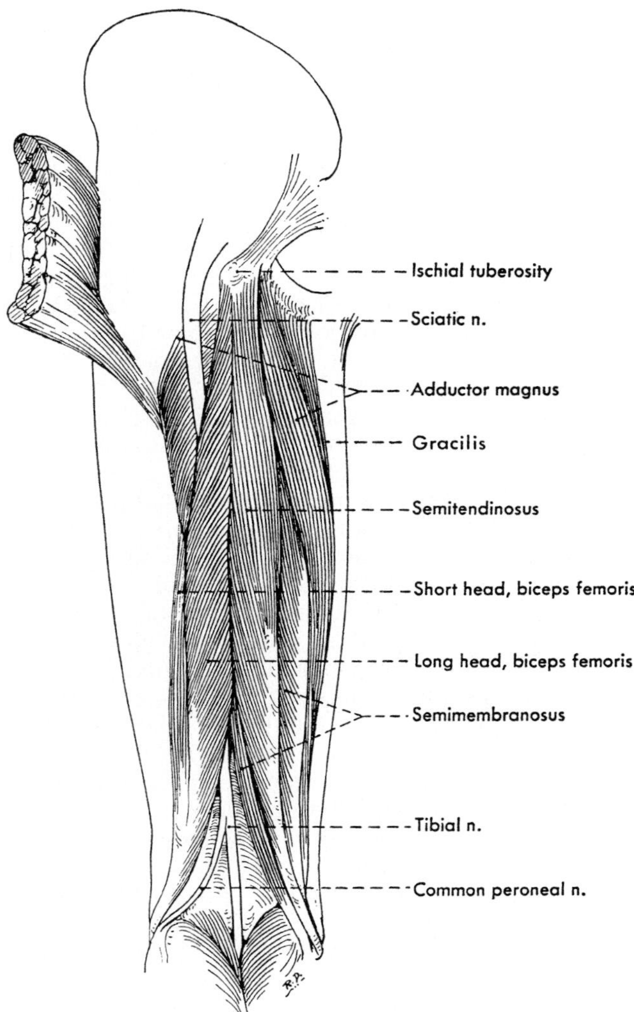

FIGURE 39–12. Muscles of the posterior thigh. (From Hollinshead WH, Jenkins DB: Functional Anatomy of the Limbs and Back, ed 5. Philadelphia, WB Saunders, 1981.)

Posterior Thigh

Relevant Anatomy and Biomechanics. The bulk of the posterior thigh is comprised of the hamstrings group (Fig. 39–12). The long head of the biceps femoris, semimembranosus, and semitendinosus all arise from the ischial tuberosity. The short head of the biceps arises from the linea aspera of the femur. The semimembranosus and semitendinosus descend medially with the semimembranosus, inserting on the posteromedial tibial condyle and the semitendinosus, meeting the gracilis and sartorius at the anteromedial tibia. The long and short heads of the biceps become confluent as they descend and both insert laterally along the proximal fibula. All hamstrings except the short head of the biceps function as hip extensors and knee flexors. The short head is a knee flexor only. The semimembranosus and semitendinosus are also internal rotators of the flexed knee, whereas the biceps can act as an external rotator. All of these muscles are innervated by the tibial division of the sciatic nerve (L5–S1) except for the short head of the biceps, which receives peroneal innervation. The hamstrings are critical for control of swing phase deceleration, control of knee rotation, and (via CKC mechanisms) prevention of knee buckling at heel-strike.

Hamstring Strains. These are among the most common of all thigh injuries. The short head of the biceps is the most frequently involved.[60, 132] This has been theorized to be due to its different innervation from the other hamstrings, which potentially results in asynchronous firing at high recruitment frequencies.[2, 26, 84, 132] Injuries are more likely to occur at higher running speeds. The higher the running speed, the less time spent in stance phase. This shorter interval subjects the hamstrings to greater angular velocities and increased eccentric (decelerating) forces at the time of heel-strike and initial loading of that limb. The remaining hamstrings, being two-joint muscles, are vulnerable to injury under conditions of extreme hip flexion combined with knee extension. Hurdlers and football punters are at risk for this type of injury mechanism.

The clinical symptom complex generally consists of pain in the proximal thigh with the onset associated with a popping sensation in the posterior thigh. By the time of examination, there might be a palpable mass, presence of ecchymosis, and extreme tenderness over the injured site. The musculotendinous junctions of the hamstrings are the primary sites of tissue injury. These junctions occur throughout the gross length of these muscles, and it should not surprise the examiner to find a focal site of injury anywhere along the length of the muscle. As with other strains, eccentric overload is the major mechanism of injury. (See Chapter 19 for an explanation of why eccentric forces are typically greater than concentric).

Functional biomechanical deficits include decreased knee extension, reduced hamstring-to-quadriceps strength ratio (normally about 0.6), and increased hip flexion.[60, 126, 163] Pre-existing conditions that predispose to this injury include insufficient warm-up, poor muscle coordination, fatigue, and other muscle strength and flexibility imbalances. These should be corrected owing to the high recurrence rate of this type of injury. The functional adaptations in response to the injury include shortened walking or running stride length.[126, 163]

Acute management consists of PRICE, cane or crutch walking (especially with the higher-grade injuries), NSAIDs, and gentle passive stretching as tolerated. Isometric and dynamic strengthening begins only when the patient is pain-free. For full stretching of the hamstrings, the hip must be flexed with maintenance of complete knee extension. Stretching should be performed in a supine position, and a towel can be used to facilitate this stretching maneuver (Fig. 39–13). Sustaining a low-grade stretch for 30 to 60 seconds in a pain-free range is recommended. This can help elongate scar tissue in its plastic stage[83] (see Chapters 31 and 58 for an explanation of wound healing and scar formation). Rehabilitation can proceed more rapidly once full muscle length is achieved. Aerobic conditioning exercises applicable during hamstring healing include bicycling without toe clips (which reduce the role of the hamstrings), upper body ergometry, kayaking, swimming breaststroke, or swimming with a pull buoy between the thighs. Resumption of activity is allowed when motion is restored and is pain-free, strength is at least 90% of the uninjured side, and the hamstrings/quadriceps strength ratio has normalized.[132, 162, 163] The use of a neoprene thigh sleeve to keep muscles warm when active might also be helpful upon return to sport or full activities.

Lateral Thigh

Relevant Anatomy and Biomechanics. The primary lateral thigh structure most subject to injury is the tensor fascia lata (TFL). The TFL has its origin at the ASIS and becomes part of the iliotibial band (ITB) inserting into Gerdy's tubercle on the anterolateral tibia. It functions as a hip flexor and internal rotator of the hip. It is innervated by the superior gluteal nerve (mainly L5 fibers). The gluteus medius and minimus are also innervated by the superior gluteal nerve. They originate from the lateral ilium and insert on the greater trochanter. Due to their wide origin and fan-shaped structure, they not only function as the major hip abductors but also play a role in hip rotation, flexion, and extension.

The most common problems related to the TFL are related to inflexibility. It is not a structure frequently contused or strained. Tightness of the TFL has been associated with a number of clinical entities including snapping hip (see above), ITB syndrome, patellofemoral pain, and lumbar spine dysfunction. TFL tightness is usually seen in conjunction with gluteal muscle inflexibility and weakness. TFL shortening can be demonstrated using *Ober's test* (see Fig. 39–14). A tight TFL causes failure of the thigh to easily resume or maintain an adducted or neutral position while the hip is in extension.

TFL tightness responds reasonably well to a stretching program, but the appropriate stretching program is difficult for the patient to learn without careful instruction. Stretches can be done initially by simulating the Ober's test position (Fig. 39–15) with the help of a

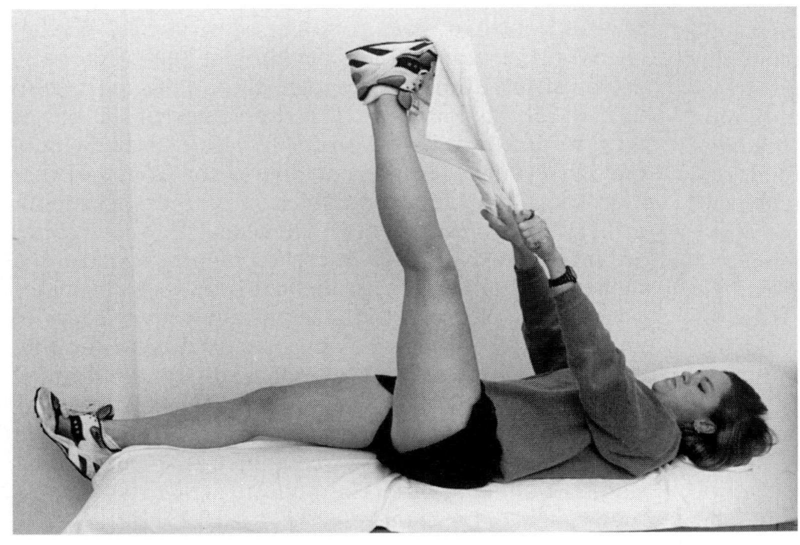

FIGURE 39–13. Hamstring stretch. Note that the spine is kept in a neutral position to avoid injury to the lumbar region.

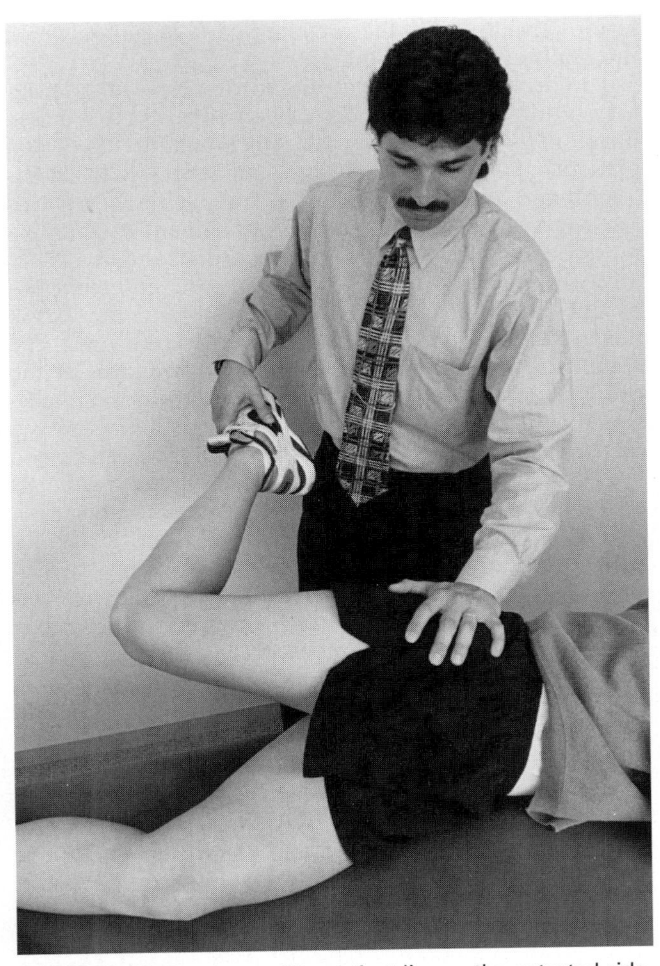

FIGURE 39–14. Ober's test. The patient lies on the untested side, with the lower (untested) leg maintained in mild to moderate hip and knee flexion for stability. The clinician extends and abducts the patient's upper thigh while maintaining the pelvis in a neutral position. The test leg is then slowly lowered.

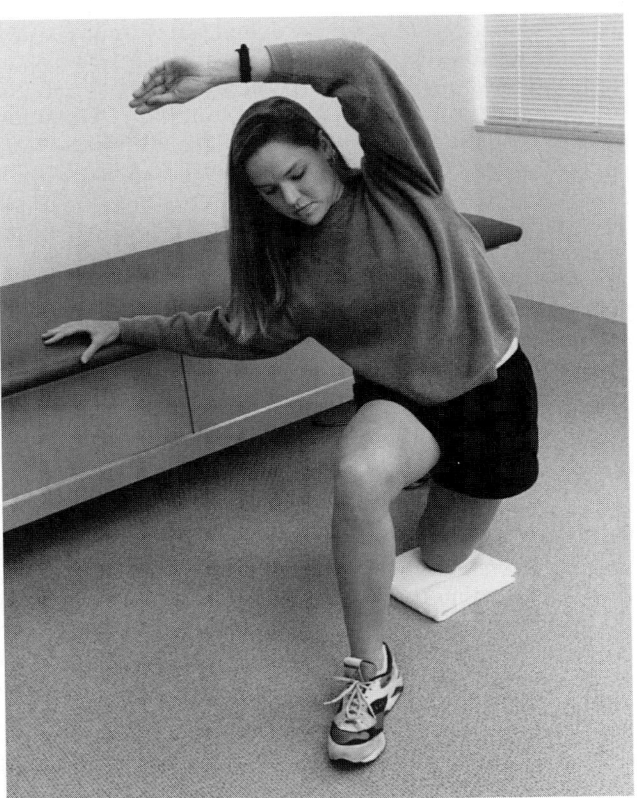

FIGURE 39–16. Self-stretching of the tensor fascia lata (TFL). The patient is stretching the left TFL.

therapist, or the patient can perform a self-stretch as demonstrated in Figure 39–16.

Meralgia Paresthetica. This consists of pain and dysesthesias in the lateral thigh typically caused by entrapment of the lateral femoral cutaneous nerve (L2–L3) underneath the inguinal ligament. Less likely sites of entrapment are within the TFL, or after it emerges from the psoas muscle. Since this nerve is purely sensory,

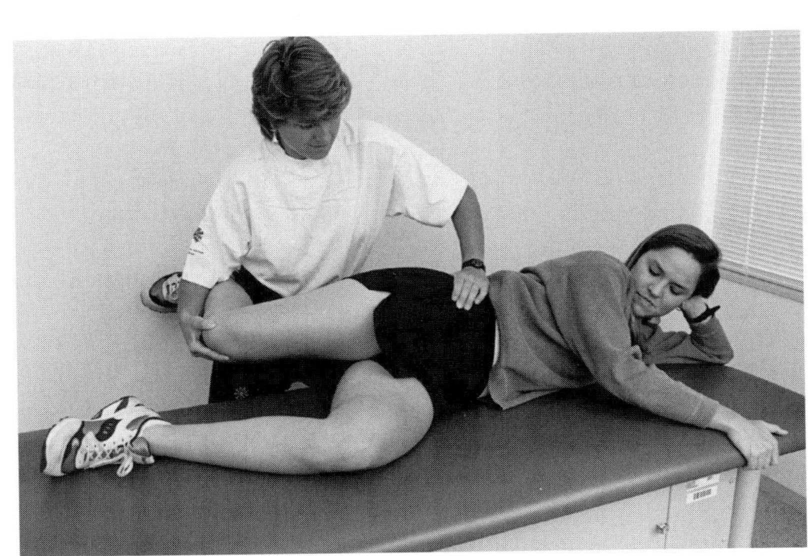

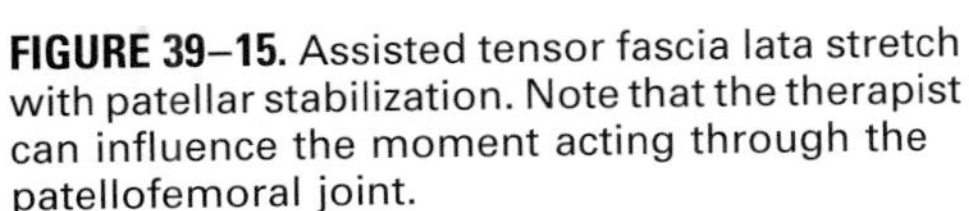

FIGURE 39–15. Assisted tensor fascia lata stretch with patellar stabilization. Note that the therapist can influence the moment acting through the patellofemoral joint.

there is no resulting motor deficit. Like many other nerve irritation or entrapment syndromes, the nerve is more vulnerable if "already sick" due to diabetes or other neuropathy-producing condition. Common sources of irritation of this nerve include abdominal distention from pregnancy or obesity, wearing a tight lumbar corset, and sudden hip hyperextension.[39, 44, 74] Treatments include weight reduction, avoidance of binding clothing, local injection of anesthetic agents at the level of the inguinal ligament, and oral medications such as amitriptyline and carbamazepine (Tegretol).

Disorders of the Knee

Applied Anatomy and Biomechanics

The knee should not be viewed as a simple "hinged joint." The knee actually consists of three joints—the tibiofemoral, the patellofemoral, and the tibiofibular.[161] Actions at these joints are determined by local forces and by events occurring above and below the knee. Actions affecting the knee can occur above the knee in the hip, pelvis, and thigh; and below the knee at the levels of the leg, ankle, and foot. Knee joint structures are frequently injured because of muscular imbalances and mechanical flaws existing elsewhere along the kinetic chain.

The structural integrity of the knee is maintained by way of a complex system of static and dynamic restraints. The knee joint is enveloped by an extensive synovial capsule. The capsule is an important secondary restraint to joint destruction and can be injured in combination with high-grade damage to the primary ligamentous structures. The capsule is confluent with expansions of the patellar tendon anteriorly, the ITB laterally, and the semimembranosus tendon and the deep fibers of the tibial collateral ligament medially. Laterally the fibular collateral ligament remains separate from the synovium. On the posteromedial corner, the capsule is reinforced by the blending of the semimembranosus and the oblique popliteal ligament. In the fibular region the posterior capsule forms the arcuate ligament below which the popliteus enters the knee.

The primary static restraints to tibiofemoral translatory motion are the cruciate ligaments. Each cruciate ligament is described by its attachment to the tibial plateau. The anterior cruciate ligament (ACL) arises lateral and anterior to the tibial spine, and its fascicles fan out to form a broad-based attachment to the posteromedial aspect of the lateral femoral condyle. There are two primary groups of fascicles—the anteromedial bundle, which is taut in knee flexion, and the larger posterolateral band, which tightens in extension.[97] The ACL functionally prevents forward translation of the tibial plateau relative to the femur and aids in rotational control.

The posterior cruciate ligament (PCL) arises between the posterior junction of the tibial condyles and attaches to the lateral aspect of the medial femoral condyle. The PCL is composed of an anterior band and a smaller posterior bundle.[97] The PCL prevents forward translation of the femur on the tibial condyles and provides secondary rotational stability. Both cruciate ligaments are intra-articular but extrasynovial.

The menisci are cartilaginous structures that assist the motion of the femoral condyles at the tibiofemoral joint. They deepen the articular surfaces, provide a thin layer of lubrication, and assist in shock absorption. The menisci guide the femur through a rolling and gliding type of motion combined with rotation. They also limit the extremes of knee flexion and extension. They have been shown to transmit approximately 50% of weight-bearing moments in extension and 85% in flexion.[4, 48] Viewed from above (Fig. 39–17), the menisci approximate incomplete circles, open at their central borders. The medial meniscus is firmly attached to the medial collateral ligament and the synovial capsule, while the lateral meniscus has a less significant bond to the capsule and is separate from the collateral ligament. This strong medial anchor restricts the mobility of the medial meniscus and might account for the high frequency of injuries

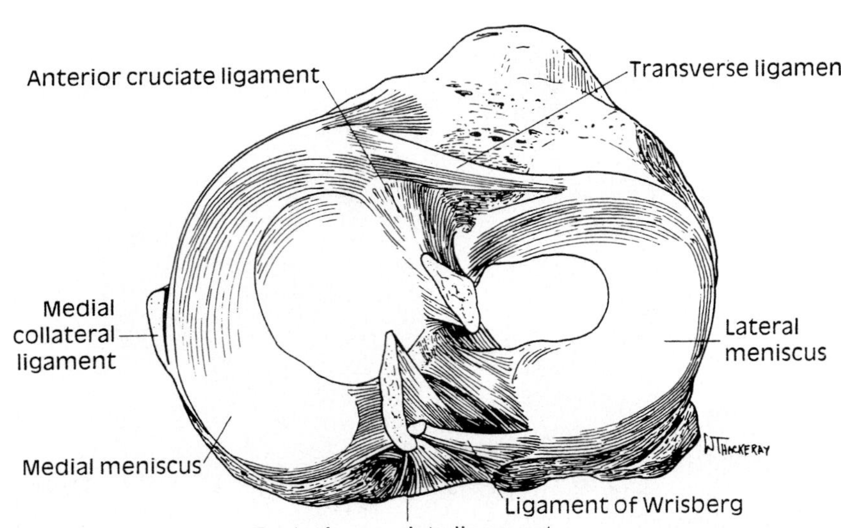

FIGURE 39–17. Attachments of menisci and ligaments at the level of the tibial plateau. (From Warren R, Arnoczky SP, Wickiewicz TL: Anatomy of the knee. *In* Nicholas JA, Hershman EB (eds): The Lower Extremity and Spine in Sports Medicine. St Louis, Mosby–Year Book, 1991.)

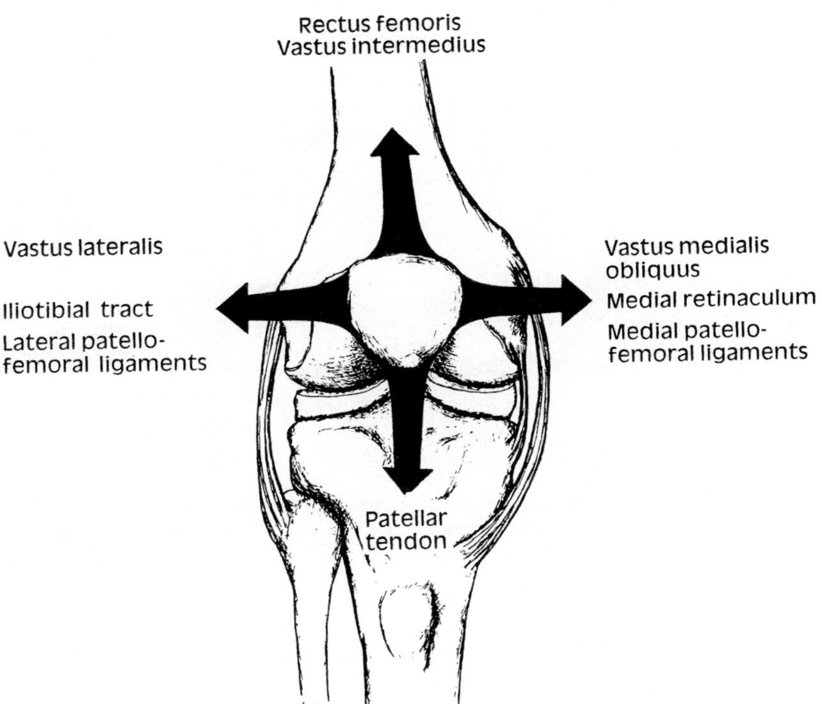

FIGURE 39–18. Forces about the patella. (From Striazk AM, Stroberg AJ: Knee injuries in the skeletally immature athlete. *In* Nicholas JA, Hershman EB (eds): The Lower Extremity and Spine in Sports Medicine. St Louis, Mosby–Year Book, 1991.)

in the posterior horn. Meniscal vascular support consists of a capillary plexus located in the thicker, peripheral third.[11] The central portion of the meniscus is thinner and relies on the synovial fluid for diffusion of nutrients.

The two collateral ligaments control valgus and varus moments acting at the knee and help limit rotation of the tibia.[42] The medial collateral ligament (MCL) consists of superficial and deep layers separated by a bursa. Superiorly the MCL arises from the medial epicondyle and is anchored in the medial proximal tibia with its deep layer attaching to the meniscal periphery. The lateral collateral ligament (LCL) courses from the lateral femoral condyle to the fibula, free of the meniscus and the synovial capsule.

The patellofemoral joint is essentially a soft tissue joint under the control of numerous muscular and fascial structures. The patella is the centerpiece of all the static and dynamic stabilizing forces about the patellofemoral joint (Fig. 39–18). The extensor mechanism consists of the quadriceps group, the patella, and the quadriceps and patellar tendons. The hamstrings act as antagonists to the anterior group. Laterally directed pull is provided by the iliotibial tract, lateral retinaculum, and patellofemoral ligaments. Medially directed pull is provided by the vastus medialis obliquus (VMO), medial retinaculum, and medial patellofemoral ligaments. These stabilizing forces, by compressing the patella against the femur, create a patellofemoral joint reaction force (PFJRF). The PFJRF becomes greater with increases in quadriceps tension and with increased knee flexion (Fig. 39–19). The PFJRFs for walking, ascending stairs, and squatting approximate 0.5, 3.3, and 6 to 7 times body weight, respectively.[46] The patellofemoral joint reaction stress (PFJRS) refers to the PFJRF per unit

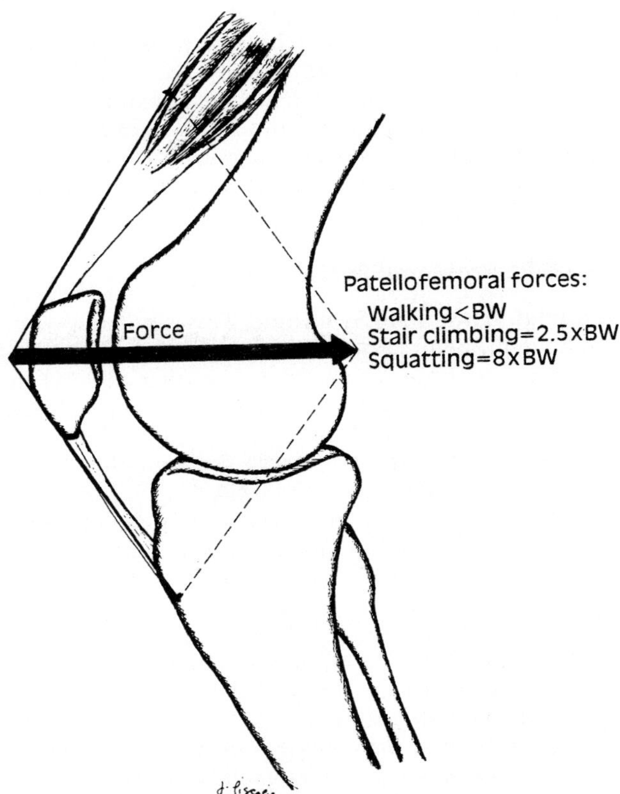

FIGURE 39–19. Patellofemoral joint reaction forces during different activities (BW is body weight). (From Striazk AM, Stroberg AJ: Knee injuries in the skeletally immature athlete. *In* Nicholas JA, Hershman EB (eds): The Lower Extremity and Spine in Sports Medicine. St Louis, Mosby–Year Book, 1991.)

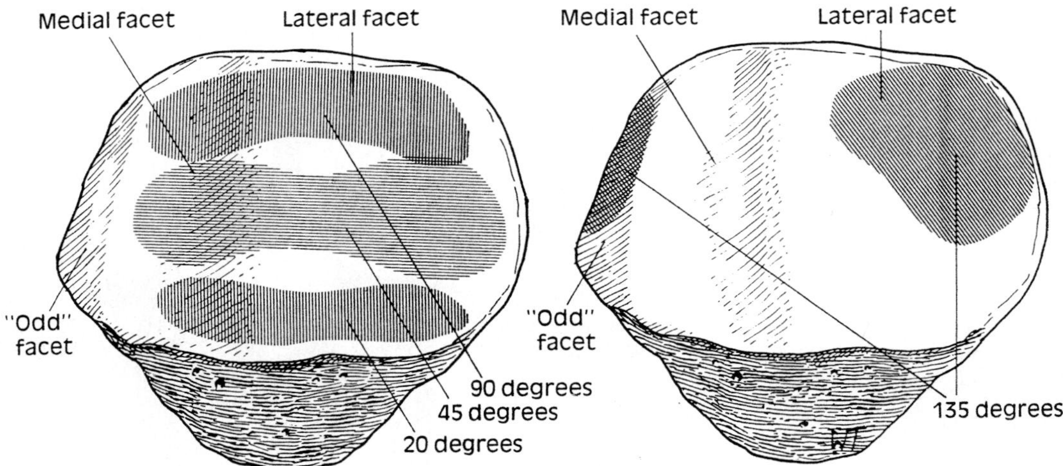

FIGURE 39–20. Areas of patellar contact at different knee flexion angles. Note that the odd facet does not effectively encounter forces until deep knee flexion. (From Warren R, Arnoczky SP, Wickiewicz TL: Anatomy of the knee. *In* Nicholas JA, Hershman EB (eds): The Lower Extremity and Spine in Sports Medicine. St Louis, Mosby–Year Book, 1991.)

contact area. A large PFJRF distributed over a large contact area produces a relatively lower degree of articular stress. A large PFJRF over a smaller area yields high articular stresses and heightens the chances of subchondral degenerative changes. The amount of patellofemoral contact area changes with knee flexion, as shown in Figure 39–20. From full extension through the first 10 to 20 degrees of flexion there is little contact. Trochlear engagement then begins, with the inferior margin of both medial and lateral facets sharing the load.[67] Between 20 and 90 degrees of flexion, there is increased proximal patellar and lateral edge contact. Beyond 90 degrees of flexion, the odd facet makes contact.[67] The patellofemoral contact areas are the greatest in the mid-range (30 to 90 degrees).

Specific Problems in the Knee

Patellofemoral Pain Syndrome. This is the most common knee problem in outpatient physical medicine and rehabilitation (PM&R) practice. It is also cited as the most common knee problem in runners.[127] The differential diagnosis of anterior knee pain includes, but is not restricted to, infrapatellar bursitis, synovial plica, patellar tendinitis, quadriceps tendinitis, Osgood-Schlatter syndrome, osteochondritis dissecans, patellofemoral tracking disorder, and meniscal disorders. Factors that predispose to patellofemoral pain include the presence of patella alta, increased Q-angle, femoral anteversion, and excessive pronation.[63, 101] The clinician should look for all of these as well as attempt to mobilize the patella superiorly, inferiorly, medially, and laterally to uncover any soft tissue restrictions.

The clinical symptom complex consists of pain, crepitation, and occasionally swelling, all typically worsened by prolonged knee flexion. The previously mentioned "theater sign" might also be present. Pain with knee extension should alert the clinician to the possibility of infrapatellar fat pad impingement between the inferior pole of the patella and the femoral condyle.

The tissue injury complex consists of the patellar cartilage and synovium, and the insertion site of the patellar tendon.[126] Functional biomechanical deficits include all the factors above and below the knee joint that contribute to abnormal tracking. These factors include (1) medial quadriceps insufficiency; (2) inflexibility of the lateral retinacula, ITB, hamstrings, and gastrocnemius muscles (all of which either increase effective knee flexion or cause lateral tracking of the patella); (3) gluteus medius and hip external rotator weakness (leading to increased medial rotation of the femur and furthering stress on the patellofemoral joint); (4) imbalance of hip internal and external rotators (leading to increased torque at the knee); and (5) excessive pronation.[126] Tightness of the lateral retinacula and ITB creates excessive lateral tilt of the patella, as demonstrated in Figure 39–21.

The functional adaptation complex consists of knee flexion contracture (loss of terminal extension), lateral patellar tracking, and altered stride to avoid full loading of the knee. The overloaded structures include the patellar tendon and lateral retinaculum, the hip external rota-

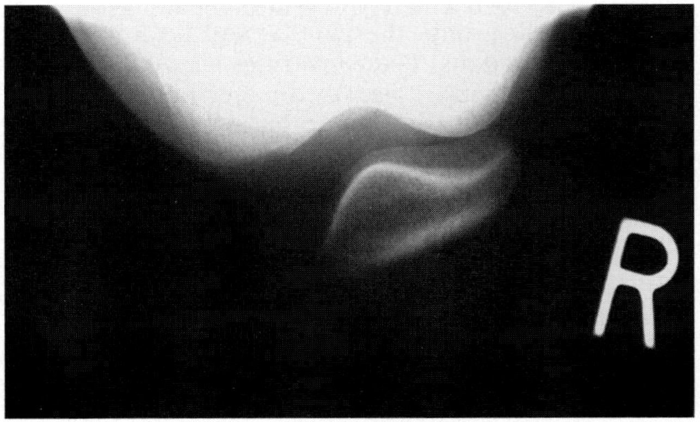

FIGURE 39–21. Sunrise view of the patella demonstrating lateral patellar tilt with elevation of the medial patellar border.

tors, the medial longitudinal arch of the foot, and the synovium of the first metatarsophalangeal joint (from excessive pronation and uneven load bearing at the foot).

Following acute management, problems with the malalignment syndrome should be corrected. Biomechanical deficits should be minimized by restoring full flexibility of the gastrocnemius-soleus complex, hamstrings, ITB, and VMO. Strength training of these muscles is needed as well. If biomechanical deficits persist after this program, the patient (particularly if a runner) might require the fitting of foot orthotic devices to correct pronation. Taping of the patella to simulate proper patellar alignment accompanied by neuromuscular reeducation of the knee musculature (McConnell technique) can also be beneficial.[63, 101] Her techniques involve looking at the static position of the patella tilt and glide (both anterior/posterior and medial/lateral of each), and rotation (internal/external). This information is then combined with assessment of the dynamic motion of the patella in open and closed chain. Tape is then utilized to correct for any excessive deviations from the norm. McConnell has reported improvement rates of better than 90% with her technique.[63, 101] Critics of her program have pointed out the lack of data showing actual change in patellar position as measured radiographically. However, the clinically observed improvement rates and reduction in pain scale ratings, even among those without radiological improvement, show the clinical utility of McConnell's technique.

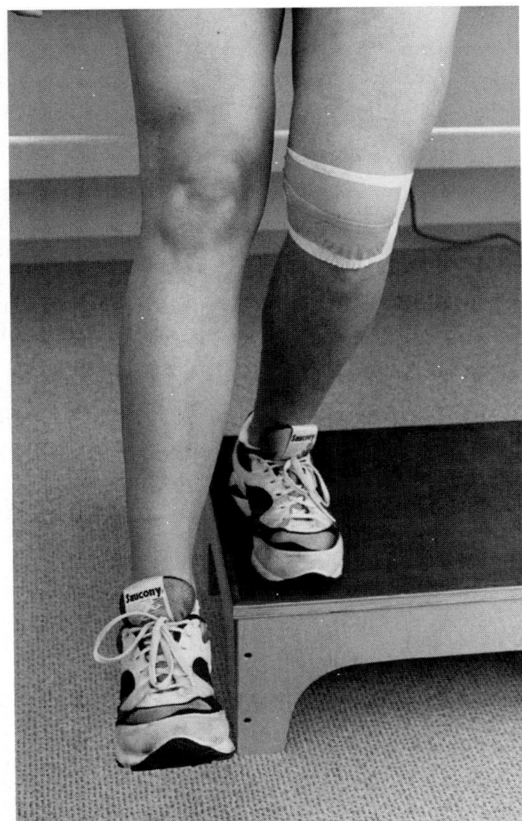

FIGURE 39–22. Patellofemoral rehabilitation. McConnell taping of the patient's knee is combined with dynamic gluteal and adductor strengthening as the patient slowly steps down.

A dynamic strengthening exercise for the hip stabilizers and the adductor magnus-VMO complex is demonstrated in Figure 39–22. A strong adductor magnus-VMO complex is needed to prevent lateral tracking of the patella. Note that the patient is instructed to keep the affected knee over the middle toe to avoid excessive internal rotation of the lower extremity, and to keep the hips level as the knee is flexed. Strengthening of the quadriceps mechanism is typically performed in the last 30 degrees of knee extension, but the selectivity of this method for strengthening only the VMO is debatable.[52] Recent work by Steinkamp et al[147] indicates that the best method to strengthen the quadriceps group while incurring the least PFJRFs and PFJRS is via short-arc (<45 degrees flexion to extension) CKC exercises. Hip adductor squeezes and CKC short-arc knee extension exercises also help with VMO training. Patellar stabilizing braces can also be considered, but should not be the first methodology utilized.

The ITB Syndrome. The iliotibial band is the extension of the TFL that extends down the lateral leg to insert into Gerdy's tubercle along the lateral tibia. The *ITB syndrome* (also known as the ITB friction syndrome) is associated with painful sensation when the ITB slides back and forth over the lateral femoral condyle as the knee flexes and extends.[106, 114, 152] Risk factors include running on beveled surfaces, limb length discrepancies, tibia vara, foot hyperpronation, and ITB contracture.[106, 152] The Noble compression test is a useful maneuver when an ITB syndrome is suspected. With the patient supine, and after positioning the knee in 90 degrees of flexion, the examiner presses on or just proximal to the lateral epicondyle. The knee is then gradually extended. Pain occurring at about 30 degrees (as the ITB crosses the bony prominence) is a positive finding.[114]

The tissue injury complex is typically the ITB over the femoral condyle or at Gerdy's tubercle. The clinical symptom complex consists of localized pain over the lateral femoral condyle, worsened with running. The functional biomechanical deficit is the inflexible ITB, while the functional adaptation complex consists of functional pronation of the foot, external rotation at the hip, internal rotation of the lower leg, and lateral patellar tracking.[126]

Rehabilitation of ITB syndrome consists of attempts to stretch the ITB, hip flexors, and gluteus maximus. Correction of foot pronation is needed and the runner should discontinue running or run only on level surfaces. Swimming and stationary ski machines can help maintain fitness. Strengthening of the hip adductors, gluteus maximus, and TFL is emphasized. The adductors counter the pull of the tight ITB. The other muscles that give rise to the ITB (gluteus maximus and TFL) should be strengthened to avoid overuse.[126] Symptoms can take 2 to 6 months to resolve.[152] Local injection of a combination of anesthetic agent and corticosteroid placed in the region of the lateral femoral condyle is sometimes helpful.[126]

Pes Anserinus Bursitis. The anserine bursa separates the three conjoined tendons of the pes anserinus (semitendinosus, sartorius, and gracilis muscles) from the MCL and the tibia. *Pes anserinus bursitis* is commonly seen in women with heavy thighs and osteoarthritis of the knees. The bursa can also become inflamed after direct trauma in athletes, especially soccer players. Patients complain of pain inferior to the anteromedial surface of the knee with ascension of stairs. The examiner can reproduce the symptoms by moving the knee in flexion and extension while holding the leg in an internally rotated position. Resistance testing of the hamstring in hip internal rotation with the patient seated can also elicit pain at the pes anserine. Palpation localizes the pain to the anserine bursa. Steroid injection is typically effective in reducing the inflammatory symptoms. The athlete at risk for direct trauma can benefit from padded protection around the knee. The rehabilitation program should emphasize stretching of the medial hamstring and adductor muscles.

Prepatellar Bursitis. Prepatellar bursitis, colloquially referred to as housemaid's knee, is often the result of frequent kneeling, producing an effusion of the subcutaneous bursa at the anterior surface of the patella. The patient rarely complains of pain, unless direct pressure is applied to the bursa. Occupational modifications should include patient education, avoidance of kneeling, and the use of kneepads when pressure must be applied to the patella. Rehabilitation should correct any flexibility deficits in the quadriceps, hamstrings, and triceps surae. The bursal enlargement is reduced with the application of ice.[120]

Acute Ligamentous Injuries of the Knee

Primary and secondary restraints of the knee are frequently injured in occupational and recreational activities. It is beyond the scope of this chapter to provide a detailed description of all the surgical and nonsurgical management schemes for collateral and cruciate ligament injuries. However, regardless of surgical or nonsurgical routes of treatment, the patient will benefit from a rehabilitation program that emphasizes maximizing function at the lowest cost. Once an acceptable level of function has been achieved, the patient should be directed to continue a maintenance program to prevent reinjury. There is no single best "cookbook" for success; what is presented here is but one rehabilitation scheme.

Anterior Cruciate Ligament Injuries. Partial or complete disruption of the ACL can be a disabling event for the athlete or worker. Frequently the patient describes an audible snap or pop while the lower limb undergoes hyperextension or rotational strain. The injury is painful and an acute hemarthrosis usually develops in the first few hours following the insult. It is common to damage additional restraints of the knee at the same time. If the patient complains of "locking" or "clicking" and there is an associated restriction of range of motion, the clinician should be suspicious of an associated meniscal tear. An accurate diagnosis should be established to include each structure damaged, so an appropriate treatment plan can be initiated.

Examination should begin with the uninvolved lower limb and progress to include all the joints in the kinetic chain on the involved extremity. Functional limitations should be observed in standing, during ambulation, and in the squatting position. Palpation should localize tenderness and grade any effusion present. Careful examination for range-of-motion deficits is needed, using the uninvolved limb for comparison. Limitation of full extension can be seen with capsular distention, but this also raises the possibility of a meniscal tear. Loss of ACL integrity can be demonstrated with *Lachman's maneuver.*[57] The examiner attempts to introduce anterior tibial translation while the limb is kept in 15 to 20 degrees of knee flexion. Complete tears of the ACL reveal significant anterior tibial translation and a loss of a distinctive end feel. A partial tear will maintain a "soft" end feel, but tibial translation will be greater than on the uninvolved side. Quantification of the tibial translation can be done with the use of an arthrometer. The *anterior drawer test,* although technically easier for many clinicians to perform than Lachman's test, has significant limitations. For one, in this position, the hamstrings are at a mechanical advantage, and tibial translation will not be appreciated if there is any degree of hamstring activity. For another, an associated meniscal tear can act like a "door jam" and provide a block to tibial motion in this position. Finally, if there is a PCL tear, a false-positive drawer might ensue as the tibia is actually being brought back to its proper position from a position of tibial "sag" rather than truly being translated forward. The *pivot-shift test* further indicates anterolateral rotatory instability, and represents increased risk for cartilaginous injury acutely or at a later date.[42, 50, 92] (Please see the work of Losee et al[92] for a detailed explanation of this test.) MRI is excellent for visualizing the disrupted ACL, as well as for assessing the presence of other injuries (Fig. 39–23).

Acute treatment includes aggressive reduction of joint swelling, either via Cryocuff compression or aspiration of the hemarthrosis. Even if surgical reconstruction is planned, there is evidence to suggest that early repair within the first three weeks is not advisable. This is due to an increased chance of developing graft arthrofibrosis.[139] An appropriate "prehabilitation" should be initiated after the injury and continued until the time of surgery or entry into an aggressive nonsurgical rehabilitation program. Gentle passive stretching of the lower extremity musculature, isometric co-contraction of the quadriceps and hamstrings, straight leg raises, and protected weight bearing are encouraged early on. Hyperextension of the knee should be avoided. Regular icing should continue as long as any effusion persists during the acute stage.

A number of materials and techniques can be used for surgical reconstruction. The most common is the patellar tendon autograft using the middle third of the patellar tendon. The bone-patellar-bone graft offers excellent fixation and has been shown to be stronger than the original ACL.[42, 115] While the graft might be "stronger," it never ultimately performs at the same functional level as the original ACL. Following reconstruction, safe restoration of motion and weight bearing

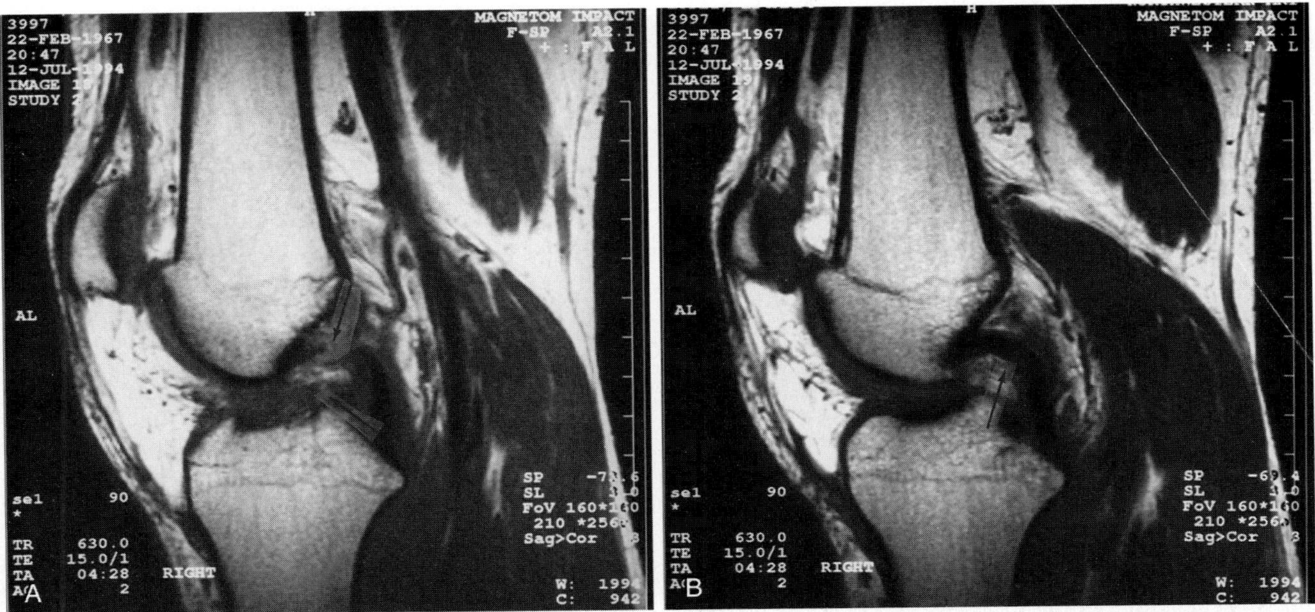

FIGURE 39–23. *A.* Disruption of the anterior cruciate ligament (ACL) viewed on sagittal MRI. *B.* The posterior cruciate ligament (PCL) is seen to be intact in the next view.

is emphasized. During the immediate postoperative period, passive range of motion is begun. In order to maximize the patient's compliance, it is necessary to provide adequate pain relief. The first step is to control the effusion with compression, ice, and elevation. Electrical stimulation of the quadriceps to help prevent atrophy can be considered. Soft tissue mobilization about the patella should be employed to restore patellar mobility and lessen the chance of adhesion formation.

It is important to gain full extension at the tibiofemoral joint during the first postoperative week to avoid a persistent "extension block." Weight bearing is done in extension while wearing an immobilizer. If swelling and other soft tissue restrictions preclude immediate extension, it can be helpful to have the patient lie prone with a towel beneath the knee while wearing an ankle weight to provide a passive stretch. Soft tissue mobilization at the origin of the medial and lateral head of the gastrocnemius can also assist in gaining extension. The patient can cycle on a stationary bike without resistance to facilitate motion as well.

Once the swelling is controlled and extension is achieved, the next goal is re-establishment of a normal gait pattern. Crutch walking progresses from two crutches with partial weight bearing to one crutch and then none by the end of the first month. By this time most patients no longer need the knee immobilizer. CKC exercises to promote strengthening of the lower extremity are then begun. CKC exercises are theoretically preferable to the OKC type because of their reported lessening of tibiofemoral shear forces.[140] However, even with CKC exercises, hyperextension and dynamic pivot shifting must be avoided. Leg presses at submaximal load, bicycles, and stair climbers can be used safely. Arm ergometry and tri-limb exercises are useful in maintaining cardiovascular fitness during this period. By the end of the first month, the bony plugs from the graft should be healed and fixed into the surrounding tibial and femoral tunnels constructed at the time of surgery.[42] The goals of the first month are summarized in Table 39–1.

During the weeks that follow, the program emphasizes further increases in range of motion, restoration of baseline strength in both hamstring and quadriceps groups, and progression to functional activities.[42, 140] Exercises to develop appropriate strength and flexibility in hip abduction, adduction, extension, and flexion are essential for maintaining control of the affected limb. Cardiovascular efforts are continued on a stationary bike, and the position of the seat should be adjusted to avoid knee hyperextension. As the patient gains proprioceptive and muscular control of the lower extremity, progression to a cross-country ski machine, stair climber, or slide board is encouraged. Hyperextension at the knee should be avoided, and the entire kinetic chain should show the proper synergistic pattern for each exercise to avoid unnecessary stresses at the reconstructed knee. Reviewing proprioceptive neurofacilitation patterning can be helpful in restoring proper me-

TABLE 39–1 Rehabilitation Goals After Anterior Cruciate Ligament Reconstruction—Weeks 0–4

1. Control pain to maximize effort in rehabilitation
2. Rapidly reduce effusion
3. Avoid development of extension block
4. Improve flexion to 90 degrees by weeks 3–4
5. Promote wound healing and mobilize adhesions
6. Activate quadriceps mechanism
7. Begin closed kinetic chain exercises
8. Maintain general cardiovascular conditioning and body strength

chanics in these functional skills. During the second to third month, the rehabilitation program should include unidirectional jogging. Once thigh circumference approximates the size of the uninvolved limb (typically by the fourth to sixth month), functional bracing with a derotation brace might be a consideration. The brace provides some mechanical restraint and probably enhances proprioceptive feedback as well.[15]

Agility drills include jumping rope, lateral shuffling around cones, figure-of-8 drills, and carioca. When the quadriceps, hamstrings, and primary movers of the hip show strength that is 90% or better in comparison with the uninvolved limb, and there is no evidence of clinical pivot shifting, the patient can return to full sporting and occupational activities. Although isokinetic testing provides some level of objectivity, functional ability is our preferred method to measure the effectiveness of a successful rehabilitation program and return to full activity. Once patients begin running in the third month, they often feel ready to return to sport. Returning at that time to sport should be discouraged, however, since this is possibly one of the weakest points for the healing graft.[33, 121] Functional tests such as bilateral jumping, single-limb hopping for distance, and single-limb hopping for time can be used. A comparison between the affected and unaffected limbs can often vividly demonstrate to the patient any remaining deficits.

Some patients elect to pursue a nonoperative course. The exercise program is virtually identical to that following surgery, but the use of a functional brace is instituted earlier to protect the tibiofemoral joint and the menisci from potential damage. Patients who are candidates for nonoperative management include those who are not motivated for postsurgical rehabilitation, those who want to modify their lifestyle to accommodate the ligamentous injury, those who do not have any other associated ligamentous or meniscal injuries, and those whose lifestyle is already sedentary.[116] There are individuals who, through aggressive exercise, can often return to high levels of athletic competition without surgery. Unfortunately, at the time of injury, it is difficult to predict which patients will gain this successful outcome. Under any circumstance, the success of a nonoperative treatment requires both hard work and extensive patient education.[115]

Posterior Cruciate Ligament Injuries. Acute *tears of the PCL* are not as common as ACL injuries. Isolated PCL injury occurs with direct trauma forcing the tibia posteriorly (as when the knee hits a car dashboard during an automobile accident), a fall on a flexed knee, or from knee hyperflexion.[40] Unlike ACL injuries, the patient's symptoms can be vague. There is less pain, less restriction of motion, and generally less hemarthrosis.[40] Visual inspection typically shows posterior tibial translation with a positive "sag sign." The *reverse Lachman's test* (directing the tibia posteriorly while the knee is in approximately 15 to 20 degrees of flexion) is positive. Roentgenographic examination should be done to exclude a bony avulsion from the tibial insertion of the PCL. Presence of an avulsed bony fragment requires immediate surgical fixation. MRI can clearly demonstrate the presence of the PCL injury.

Treatment of isolated injury to the PCL remains controversial. Most studies have shown good functional outcomes with nonoperative treatment and aggressive rehabilitation.[37, 47, 123, 155] Since there are relatively few reports with long-term follow-up, patients treated conservatively should be monitored for premature tibiofemoral joint degeneration due to instability. PCL insufficiency is frequently accompanied by other ligamentous, meniscal, or capsular damage, necessitating surgical reconstruction[133] to manage joint instability. The MCL and the oblique popliteal ligament are commonly injured in conjunction with the PCL.

The treatment plan should be congruent with the patient's preinjury lifestyle, functional goals, and motivation for postoperative rehabilitation. Whether or not the patient undergoes surgery, it is essential to reduce the effusion and regain full range of motion as the patient re-establishes neuromuscular control to normalize gait. Exercises should initially focus on CKC strengthening of the quadriceps and then progress to include the musculature of the hip and the hamstrings. As strength returns and atrophy is reduced, the patient should begin sport-specific agility drills and be able to return to full activity approximately two months post injury.

Medial Collateral Ligament Injuries. MCL injuries are quite common and are seen in direct trauma or as overuse syndromes. Swimmers who use the breaststroke undergo repeated valgus strain and can develop irritation of the MCL. There are three grades of damage. Grade I (mild) and grade II (moderate) injuries have good functional results with a nonsurgical approach and appropriate rehabilitation.

Grade I (mild) MCL strains demonstrate pain with palpation, but there is no evidence of valgus instability. Treatment is based on the type of injury and the demands of the patient's activity. In the case of a traumatic injury, pain and inflammation should be controlled with cryotherapy and possibly a limited course of NSAIDs. The patient should be placed in a locked brace for the first few days and then progressed to a hinge brace. A strengthening and flexibility program should be used to stabilize the knee and limit further injury. Athletes attempting a return to sports can wear the hinged brace for 1 to 2 months following injury.

Grade II (moderate) injuries to the MCL are characterized by inability to fully extend the knee because of pain and inflammation. The extracapsular fibers of the MCL are ruptured. There is mild-to-moderate instability when a valgus stress is applied in knee flexion, and there is swelling and hemorrhage. When implementing a treatment plan, it is important to recall that the ligament tightens in extension and is most relaxed in flexion. Consequently, a knee orthosis should restrict the last 20 to 30 degrees of extension for the first week while the effusion is reduced with the application of ice and compression. After the first week, a limited arc of motion (20 to 75 degrees) is permitted. Early mobilization is encouraged within pain-free limits, and range of motion should be regained over a 3 to 4-week period. Near the end of the first month, the patient can be full weight bearing in a brace that allows full flexion and extension. Strengthening of the hip girdle muscles and knee stabilizers is integrated into the rehabilitation program as the effusion is reduced and there is no exacerbation of pain. After 4 to 5 weeks the patient should advance to agility drills and sport-specific activities that include lateral movements. Return-to-play criteria include 90% strength or better, minimal or no thigh atrophy, and no inhibition during agility drills.[42]

Severe grade III MCL tears demonstrate instability to valgus stress in both flexion and extension. Hemarthrosis usually develops within a few hours due to rupture of both the deep and superficial fibers. Treatment for grade III insufficiency remains controversial. It is essential that the knee be examined to rule out associated meniscal or cruciate ligament damage, which increases the chance that surgical repair is needed. It has been reported that isolated rupture of the MCL can undergo nonoperative treatment similar to that for a grade II tear.[59, 68, 137] Conversely, Kannus[75] reported deterioration of the knee after long-term follow-up of nonoperative treatment. Closer review of this work, however, reveals that one-third of his population with insufficiency of the MCL also had a Lachman's maneuver of at least grade II. This could account for some of the unsatisfactory results with nonoperative care. However controversial the decision for surgical care, the development of an appropriate treatment plan should focus on the patient's preinjury demands and motivation to return to biomechanically stressful activities. In the case of a young, aggressive person wanting to return to previous activities, surgical reconstruction with appropriate postoperative rehabilitation might be warranted. For patients who are able to modify their lifestyles, a nonoperative approach can achieve satisfactory functional results.

Lateral Collateral Ligament Injuries. The treatment program for *isolated LCL injuries* is similar to the nonoperative approach described for the MCL. However, the vulnerability of the peroneal nerve at the level of the fibular head must be kept in mind. The peroneal nerve can be injured during the initial trauma or can be subjected to pressure with improper taping or bracing or frozen during cryotherapy. Grade III injuries are often associated with capsular or cruciate ligament insufficiency, giving rise to a rotational instability as well. These combination injuries require surgical reconstruction to avoid later degeneration of the joint and allow return to more demanding activities.[41]

Meniscal Lesions. These are common in both sport and industry. Tears in the semilunar cartilages are most common in the posterior horn of the medial meniscus. Injury usually follows forceful rotation of the lower extremity while the foot is firmly placed on the ground. An effusion usually develops within 24 to 48 hours, in contrast to the rapid development of hemarthrosis seen in an acute ligament rupture. Damage can range from a small peripheral tear to a larger bucket-handle tear presenting with intense pain. The patient might describe a sensation of giving way or mechanical locking. Clinical examination often reveals tenderness on palpation of the joint line. *McMurray's test* is performed with varying degrees of tibial internal and external rotation combined with valgus or varus moment while the limb is moved from full flexion to extension. The test is positive if a "click" is produced or if pain is reproduced. Care must be taken to avoid being fooled by clicking from within the patellofemoral joint or the pseudomeniscal clicking produced by a plica. The posterior meniscus can be further loaded by having the patient attempt to squat or by the examiner taking the knee into deep flexion and introducing rotation. Intermittent locking can be subtle or obvious, as in the case of a large bucket-handle tear.

MRI can be used to demonstrate a meniscal tear, but if mechanical symptoms exist, arthroscopy is probably the diagnostic test of choice. Arthroscopic evaluation is required when range of motion is severely limited or if the knee joint is locked. Locking can be observed with osteochondral lesions, cruciate ligament rupture, bony avulsions, or meniscal impingement.

Treatment of meniscal lesions is dependent on the severity of the injury to the meniscus and the possibility of combined damage. In the absence of a locked knee, a period of observation to allow for pain control and reduction of the effusion can help delineate the most appropriate treatment. The presence of associated ligamentous tears or inability to bear weight after 2 to 3 days suggests the need for arthroscopic evaluation. If the swelling goes down and the patient is able to regain full joint motion and full strength (and high-intensity athletic competition is not planned), a nonoperative approach can be successful.

The surgical approach to meniscal tear management has changed significantly in the last 15 to 20 years. Total meniscectomy is no longer an acceptable treatment, and efforts are geared toward preserving as much of the cartilage as possible. The degenerative effects of meniscectomy described by Fairbanks[45] include joint space narrowing, ridging, and squaring of the condyles. Preservation of the meniscus reduces the likelihood of such degenerative changes.[36, 90, 96] Currently, surgeons make an attempt to repair the meniscus when possible, and remove as little of the meniscus as possible.[109]

For the nonsurgically treated patient, early rehabilitation consists of pain and swelling reduction with institution of hamstring and ITB stretching and short-arc CKC activities. Swimming pool exercise can facilitate recovery and allow the patient to maintain endurance. Use of a cane or crutches to unload the affected side is strongly recommended. Once symptoms are reduced, the intensity of the program is increased, but activities involving loading with rotation are avoided.

For the surgically treated patient, postoperative rehabilitation depends on the complexity of the repair. Once pain-free range of motion has been established, and there is no joint line tenderness, the patient should return to full weight bearing. Too early a return to weight-bearing activities or overaggressive strengthening can induce effusion and an exacerbation of pain. If this occurs, the program should be modified and the patient returned to a partial weight-bearing status. Deep squatting should be avoided during the first six months.[48] Progressive strengthening should focus on the quadriceps and hamstrings, and include the entire lower extremity.

Osteochondritis Dissecans. This is a lesion of subchondral bone with or without articular cartilage involvement.[55] In the knee, the most common site for a subchondral lesion occurs at the interior portion of the medial femoral condyle. Lesions in the lateral condyle and under the patellar articular cartilage occur with less frequency. Chondral flaps and chondral loose bodies might also be present.[22, 30] Patients experience intermittent mechanical symptoms with or without pain. An effusion can be present. Radiographs should include a tunnel view to evaluate the intracondylar notch. CT is helpful in evaluating the bony lesions, while MRI can provide a more accurate view of the articular cartilage. Treatment is based on the staging of the lesion, and the patient's symptoms.[55] Arthroscopic evaluation is indicated when there is separation of the lesion from the femur, mechanical locking, or chronic pain and effusion.

The Leg

Relevant Anatomy and Biomechanics

The tibia and fibula and associated structures make up the leg. All muscles are innervated by the tibial or peroneal nerves. The crural structures are encased in a tight connective tissue fascia, with separation of the muscles of this region into four compartments. The anterior compartment consists of the anterior tibial, extensor hallucis longus, extensor digitorum, peroneus tertius, and deep peroneal nerve. The lateral compartment consists of the peroneus longus and brevis muscles, and the superficial peroneal nerve. The superficial posterior compartment consists of the gastrocnemius-soleus complex, plantaris, and sural nerve. The deep posterior compartment includes the posterior tibialis, flexor digitorum longus, flexor hallucis longus, and posterior tibial vessels and nerve. The gastrocnemius-soleus complex blends distally into the Achilles tendon. The anterior tibial muscle functions as a dorsiflexor and invertor, the posterior tibial muscle as a forefoot flexor and invertor, while the peroneus longus and brevis muscles serve as the only major evertors and provide some plantar flexion as well.

Achilles Tendinitis (Tendinosis). This is perhaps the most common injury of the lower leg. Repeated episodes of microtrauma result in the development of microtearing of the tendon in the region of least vascularity, approximately 2 to 6 cm above the tendon insertion.[86, 126] Contributing factors include excessive pronation, supination, tight heel cords, and rearfoot or forefoot varus.[126] Overtraining, a single excessively strenuous workout, and hill running can create this problem as well. It is important to recognize that while the majority of patients feel they have an acute inflammatory problem (tendinitis), they actually have a chronic problem (tendinosis), in which asymptomatic intratendinous degeneration has been occurring over time.[79] This can eventually lead to frank rupture of the tendon.

The tissue injury complex is generally confined to the myotendinous junction of the Achilles tendon. In more chronic cases, this can extend throughout the midsubstance of the tendon. The clinical symptom complex is pain located typically 6–8 cm proximal to the insertion on the calcaneus that is worsened by dorsiflexion.[126] The functional biomechanical deficits consist of weak dorsiflexors and tight plantar flexors, while the functional adaptation complex includes increased knee flexion and increased pronation (both particularly influenced by the tight gastrocnemius which crosses both knee and ankle joints).

The rehabilitation program is initiated with the PRICE principle and anti-inflammatory medications. The tendon is never injected. Heel lifts often provide some relief in early rehabilitation, but should not be used indefinitely (this promotes shortening of the heel cord). Ultrasound can be useful in chronic cases if loosening of old, scarred connective tissue is needed and stretching is difficult.[126] Reduction in weight-bearing activity is mandatory. These patients are good candidates for aquatic-based conditioning. In chronic cases, additional aggressive soft tissue mobilization to promote an initial inflammatory response, coupled with a controlled passive stretching regime, can help break up scar tissue. As pain is reduced, the patient should go through a gradual program of first concentric and ultimately eccentric strengthening of the plantar flexors. Chronic cases of Achilles tendonitis can be debilitating and every effort should be made to educate the patient on the hazards of returning to running too early. If the pain continues despite all the above measures, an MRI study of the Achilles tendon can help identify previously undetected partial tendon tears, musculotendinous tears, retrocalcaneal bursitis, or stress fractures.[79, 80, 126]

Stress Fractures. A *stress fracture* is defined as a partial or complete fracture of a bone that results from that bony region's inability to withstand a repetitively applied subthreshold and nonviolent mechanical stress.[100] Persons most at risk are those who have asymmetrical limb lengths, who pronate or supinate excessively, or who run on rigid surfaces.[38, 100] Common sites of stress fractures in runners include the tibia, fibula, navicular bone, metatarsals, and femur.[100] The tibia is the most common site (34%), followed by the fibula (24%), metatarsals (20%), and femur (14%).[100] Well localized pain is a major clinical feature.[100] Stress fracture can also be suggested by pain produced over the suspected fracture site by application of a vibrating tuning fork or with percussion of the bone away from the affected site.[136, 163] Because they frequently do not produce a full cortical defect, stress fractures are difficult to detect by routine radiographs[18] early in their course. Clinicians sometimes use ultrasound for diagnosis of stress fractures, but this has not been proven to be effective.[19, 131] Bone scans are recommended in cases of increased clinical suspicion when the plain film study is negative.[18] An example of a fibular stress fracture in a runner that did not show up on plain films is shown in Figure 39–24.

Local bone represents the tissue injury complex. The clinical symptom complex consists of localized pain that tends to worsen with a reproducible amount of activity and is relieved by rest.[126] The functional biomechanical deficits and adaptations are dictated by the site of fracture.

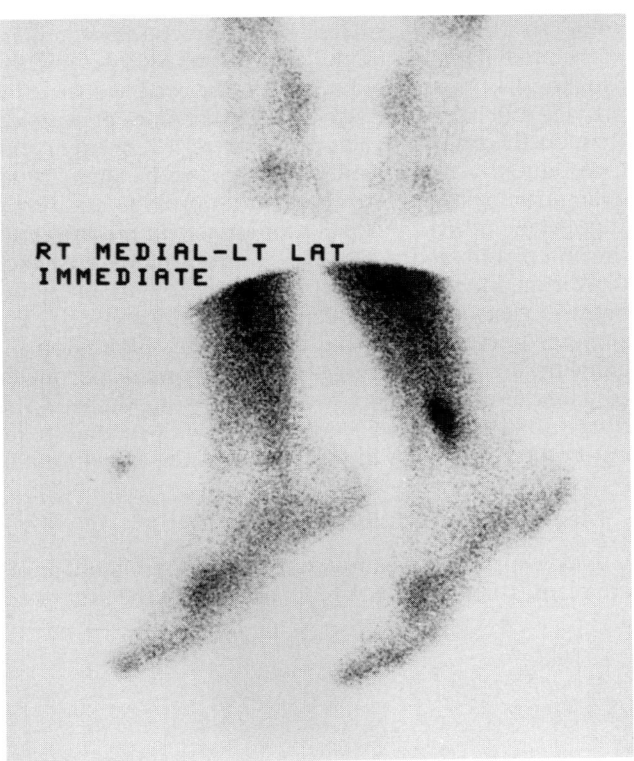

FIGURE 39–24. Bone scan, revealing a stress fracture.

During rehabilitation of a stress fracture, the first principle is to have the patient reduce activity to stay below the level of activity that induces symptoms. Running on dry land is prohibited until an adequate amount of time for healing has passed. Healing time is approximately 3 weeks for the fibula, 4 to 8 weeks for the tibia (although considerably longer if the tibial plateau has been affected), and several months (with limited weight bearing) for the neck of the femur.[100, 126] In the past, runners with stress fractures were primarily restricted to alternative forms of aerobic exercises such as swimming and bicycling, which were of general conditioning value but not particularly specific to running. In recent years, aqua running has become available. During aqua running, the runner, wearing an inflatable vest, is placed into the deep end of the pool so that the feet are not in contact with the bottom. The athlete is then tethered to a side of the pool and begins to "run." The viscosity and drag of the water provide resistance proportional to the effort, while the buoyancy effect maintains non-weight-bearing conditions.[153] This is an excellent way to maintain condition while protecting the injured area.

Compartment Syndromes. In *dynamic compartment syndromes* of the leg, elevated tissue pressure in any of the four compartments transiently reduces the capillary perfusion below the level needed for tissue viability. The anterior compartment is most frequently affected. Dysesthesias in the distribution of the deep peroneal nerve, foreleg pain, dorsiflexor weakness, and hypoperfusion are common. The syndrome can be confirmed with intracompartmental pressure measurements.[99, 150] Postexertional MRIs can also be of value.[6] Although fasciotomy is often seen as the definitive treatment for this problem, recent evidence suggests that cycling produces lower anterior compartment pressures than does running, implying that for athletes willing to modify their training regimens, an alternative to surgery, with maintenance of fitness, is possible.[17]

Bursal Syndromes of the Foot. The retrocalcaneal, subtendinous bursa lies between the posterior surface of the calcaneus and the tendon of the triceps surae. Inflammation of the bursa can result from training errors, as in a runner who increases mileage too rapidly, and from ill-fitting shoes, which can create excessive pressure in the heel counter region. Discomfort occurs when the examiner places the thumb and index finger on the anterior edges of the Achilles tendon and applies pressure. Footwear modification is an important first step. Symptoms are controlled with ice and antiinflammatory medications. When the pain begins to resolve, the patient should stretch the triceps surae complex daily to avoid recurrence. Injections into the bursa are done only with caution, as corticosteroids can weaken the Achilles tendon, increasing the risk for tendon rupture.

Subcutaneous bursitis, or Achilles bursitis, involves the bursa lying subcutaneous to the posterior surface of the Achilles tendon. The patient develops midline swelling where the upper edge of the heel counter comes in contact with the heel cord. Subcutaneous bursitis is commonly seen in women who wear high heels that apply direct pressure on the bursa. The mainstay of treatment is to change the patient's shoes. Ice and antiinflammatory medications can provide symptomatic relief.

Ankle Injuries

Ankle injuries are probably the most common sports-related injury and one of the most frequently seen musculoskeletal problems presenting to the outpatient physiatrist's office. Inversion sprains alone account for at least 85% of isolated ankle injuries.[27, 35, 61, 148] As with many of the entities previously discussed, without appropriate rehabilitation the likelihood of recurrent injury is high.

Relevant Anatomy and Biomechanics

The ankle can be described as a hinge joint with a mortise (the tibia and fibula) and tenon (talus). The distal tibia forms the medial malleolus, while the fibula, which extends further distally, forms the lateral malleolus. There is approximately 20 degrees of ankle dorsiflexion and 50 degrees of available plantar flexion under normal conditions. The talocrural joint is widest anteriorly, so the joint has its maximum osteological stability in dorsiflexion (when the wide portion of the talus becomes wedged into the narrower portion of the mortise) and minimal osteological stability in plantar flexion. The joint is obliquely placed relative to the knee joint axis and the line of progression, creating an external tibial torsion of approximately 20 degrees. The subtalar (talocalcaneal) and midtarsal (talonavicular and calcaneocuboid) joints both permit the additional motions of inversion and eversion, and influence hindfoot-to-midfoot load transfer.

The critical ligamentous structures on the lateral side include the posterior talofibular ligament (PTFL), anterior talofibular ligament (ATFL), and the calcaneofibular ligament (CFL) (Fig. 39–25B). Of the three lateral ligaments, the PTFL is the strongest and the ATFL is the weakest. On the medial side the deltoid ligament is composed of the anterior tibiotalar, posterior tibiotalar, tibionavicular, and tibiocalcaneal ligaments (Fig. 39–25A). Anterolaterally, between the fibula and the tibia, is the tibiofibular syndesmosis. The lateral ligaments tend to check inversion and stabilize against posterior talar displacement, while the medial complex guards against eversion injuries. The hinge motion of the talar joint has a direct effect on the tautness of the LCLs. Dorsiflexion promotes ATFL laxity and CFL tautness, whereas plantar flexion results in ATFL tautness and CFL laxity. The PTFL is the restraint against posterior displacement. Inversion sprains typically occur when the ankle is plantar-flexed, so the ATFL is the most vulnerable of the lateral ligaments. Given the broadness of the medial malleolus, the angle of the mortise, and the toughness of the deltoid complex, the medial structures provide much greater restriction to extremes of eversion than do the lateral structures to extremes of inversion. Consequently, medial injuries are far less frequent. Muscular structures about the ankle that provide additional support include the peroneus longus and brevis laterally, the anterior tibial dorsally, the posterior tibial, the flexor digitorum longus and flexor hallucis longus medially, and the gastrocnemius-soleus complex posteriorly. Peripheral nerves vulnerable to injury in this region include the sural (laterally), deep and superficial peroneals (dorsolaterally), and saphenous (dorsomedially). The distal tibial nerve may be damaged with medial ankle injury or compressed in the region of the tarsal tunnel.

Mechanisms of Injury

Ankle sprains typically occur when the foot and ankle are plantar-flexed. The ATFL is generally the first struc-

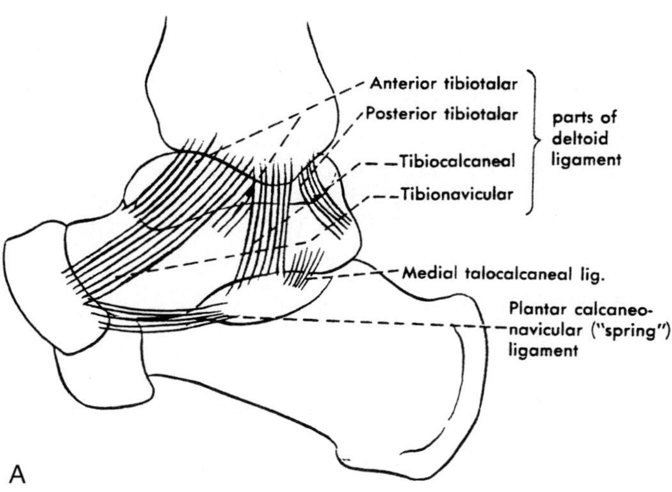

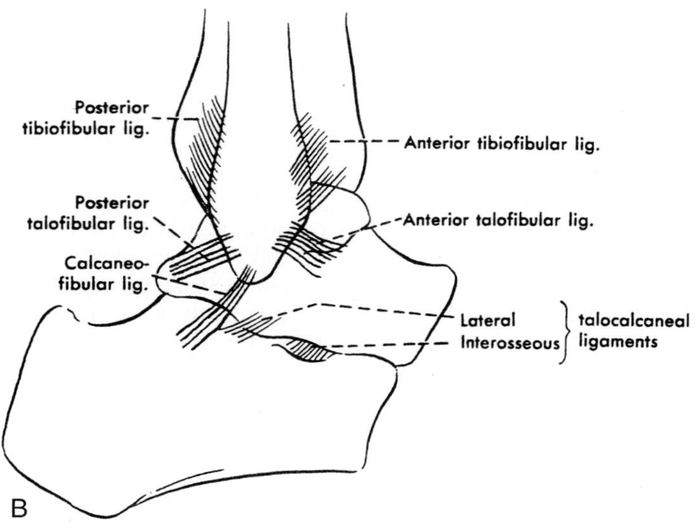

FIGURE 39–25. *A.* Medial ligaments of the ankle. *B.* Lateral ligaments of the ankle. (From Hollinshead WH, Jenkins DB: Functional Anatomy of the Limbs and Back, ed 5. Philadelphia, WB Saunders, 1981.)

ture injured with a combined inversion–plantar flexion stress. The CFL is the second structure injured as the inversion stress increases. For the PTFL to become injured, either inversion must continue further or some posterior displacement of the talus must occur.[130] Inversion in neutral dorsiflexion primarily stresses the CFL. The deltoid ligament is injured with eversion stress. Addition of any rotatory stress to the above, or inversion in dorsiflexion leads to syndesmosis injury.[130, 132]

Classes of Injury

The most common site of injury in a ligament tends to be within the midsubstance of the ligament.[130] Tears occurring closer to the insertion are often accompanied by avulsion fractures. More violent forces are often associated with multiligamentous injury or fractures of bones about the ankle mortise. Each ligament is graded separately. The following system combines the categorizations of a number of authors[14, 29, 76, 130]:

Grade I (mild)—minor ligamentous disruption (essentially a stretch) with maintenance of integrity and no signs of instability.

Grade II (moderate)—near complete disruption with macroscopic tearing and swelling. There is a moderate amount of functional loss such as difficulty with toe-walking and there is mild or moderate instability.

Grade III (severe)—complete ligamentous rupture with obvious swelling, discoloration, and tenderness. There is significant functional loss with limited range of motion due to swelling, limited weight-bearing tolerance due to pain, and reduced stability due to the ligamentous disruption.

The mechanism and consequences of the acute ankle injury can be obtained from the history and physical examination. Sensation of a tear or pop with a "rolling over" of the ankle are highly suggestive of an ATFL or CFL tear. Anteriorly based pain with inability to bear weight following the foot's "getting stuck" while the leg continues to rotate suggests syndesmosis injury.

The examination should be done in a methodical manner. The fibular head region is palpated to detect defects and tenderness suggestive of fracture and to check for irritability over the peroneal nerve. The fibular shaft is percussed throughout its length to identify possible fracture sites. The distal tibia and fibula and the talar dome region are similarly inspected for overt fracture. The foot must not be ignored since metatarsal fractures (e.g., the Jones fracture of the fifth metatarsal) often accompany higher-grade sprains. Points of maximal tenderness are commonly elicited over the ATFL and CFL. Careful deep palpation underneath the distal lateral malleolus can reveal a defect consistent with complete CFL tear. A complete sensory examination and light percussion over the superficial nerves are important to identify stretch injuries which can cause superimposed dyesthetic pain. Examination of the injured ankle should be preceded by examination of the uninjured side. This gives the examiner a sense of the "baseline" and helps put the patient a bit more at ease.

The *anterior drawer* test is the hallmark test for integrity of the ATFL. The patient's calf muscles should be relaxed and the foot should be in approximately 10 degrees of plantar flexion. The calcaneus is grasped firmly and drawn forward while the tibia is pushed posteriorly with the other hand. Under normal conditions, the translation of the talus is no more than 4 mm.[130, 132] A drawer of more than 8 mm is indicative of at least an ATFL tear.[54, 130, 132]

The *talar tilt* (inversion) test is more sensitive for CFL tears. The lower leg is held firmly by one hand while applying an inversion stress to the talus and calcaneus with the other hand. Separation of the surface of the talus from the tibia (i.e., a tilting) is considered a positive test. The ankle should be kept in neutral during this maneuver, since plantar flexion stresses the ATFL.

The *clunk test* (side-to-side) is a gross assessment of mortise widening, as when there is a tibiofibular ligament complex injury. Grasping the calcaneus with one hand and surrounding the distal third of the tibia and fibula with the other, the examiner attempts to move the talus from side to side. A "clunk" or "thud" is felt as the talus hits the tibia or fibula. Care must be taken not to allow inversion or eversion to occur during this maneuver, or a false-positive result will be obtained.

When there is true tibiofibular diastasis due to complete syndesmosis injury, the *squeeze test* can be helpful. Proximal compression of the tibia and fibula together produces pain at the level of the interosseous membrane.[65] Diastasis compromises load bearing at the ankle joint severely and requires surgical consultation.

The *eversion test* assesses the integrity of the deltoid ligament complex. The lower tibia is grasped in one hand and the heel in the other. If the tibiotalar joint widens medially with eversion stress, the test is positive.

If a sprain is thought to be grade II or more, radiographs should be obtained to rule out a coexisting fracture. Standard views include an anteroposterior, a lateral, and a "mortise" view, taken with the lower leg in 20 degrees of internal rotation. The mortise view is necessary to fully evaluate the talar dome surface as well as to adequately examine the distal tibial and fibular surfaces. If the mortise is not disrupted, the distances between the lateral talus and fibula and between the medial talus and the tibia are equal.[130] A medial clear space (the distance between the medial tibia border and the talus border) of greater than 5 mm suggests deltoid ligament injury, while a distance of 5 mm or more between the medial fibular cortex and the incisura fibularis of the talus indicates a syndesmosis tear.[87]

When examining radiographs of the ankle, it is important to remember the "ring concept."[54] When the mortise is viewed directly, the lateral malleolus, the tibial plafond superiorly, the medial malleolus, and the talus inferiorly form a ring which is held together by the lateral and medial ligaments and the syndesmosis (Fig. 39–26). Disruption of any of these support structures tends to alter the shape of the ring. If the ring is deformed on one side (e.g., a distal fibular fracture), one should look for a coexisting injury somewhere else along the ring (e.g., a deltoid ligament injury with widening of the medial mortise).

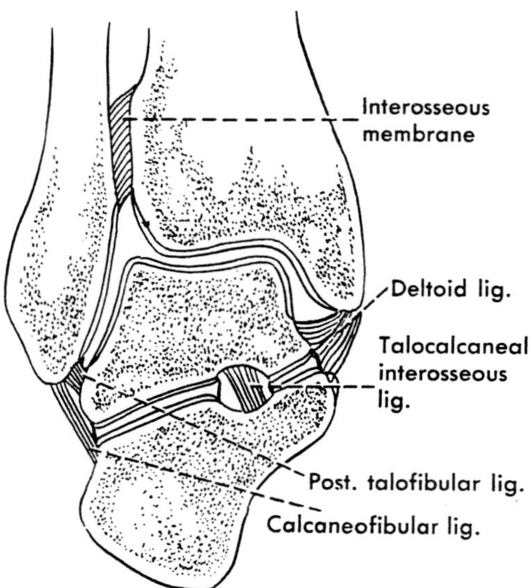

FIGURE 39–26. The "ring" of the ankle.

Occasionally "stress views" of the ankle are performed.[53] These can be helpful in determining completeness of a ligamentous tear, or more importantly, can help determine the presence of avulsed fragments of bone. Traction forces are applied to the ankle to promote a tilt or drawer effect, and comparisons are made between injured and uninjured sides for asymmetry. For the "tilt stress," the angle between the talar dome and tibial plafond is measured. Although controversy exists as to the exact angle constituting a significant widening, lateral opening of more than 10 degrees suggests either a CFL or ATFL injury, while greater than 20 degrees is highly suggestive of a combined CFL and ATFL injury.[35, 130, 132]

There are many types of fractures associated with ankle sprains, and it is beyond the scope of this chapter to discuss them all. The *spiral fracture of the distal fibula* is one of the most common fractures of the ankle region. When seen, the proximal fibula must also be examined as forces might have been transmitted up the interosseous membrane. The *Jones fracture* is a fracture at the base of the fifth metatarsal associated with inversion sprain and pulling of the peroneus brevis. *Osteochondral talar dome fractures* may follow almost any type of ankle injury and should be considered in "slow-healing" cases and where the region over the talus is tender. *Mortise disruption* follows syndesmosis or deltoid ligament injury; the ring of the mortise should immediately be inspected for evidence of bimalleolar (or trimalleolar) fractures.[35, 84, 130, 132] With the exception of the nondisplaced Jones fracture, all of these problems can require surgical consultation.

Ankle Rehabilitation

Acute treatment of all sprains includes icing and compressive wrapping of the injured site (tissue injury complex). Cryocuffs or aggressive icing and elevation can be particularly helpful in minimizing the amount of post-injury swelling, which facilitates the rehabilitation process. Early mobilization of the sprained but nonfractured ankle is the preferred treatment. The ankle should be protected with elastic support, air stirrup splints, lace-up braces, or plastic-molded supports. Casting of the uncomplicated sprain actually slows recovery, even in grade III sprains.[27, 70, 76] Crutches are used only when gait is affected enough to increase the chance of further injury or when pain precludes full weight bearing. Ankle pumping, "writing the alphabet" with the feet, and stretching of the gastrocnemius-soleus complex (tightness is a typical accompanying biomechanical deficit) can all be started during this period. Once the patient is able to bear full weight on the affected ankle, a single-limb balance program should be instituted. The patient begins by balancing on the affected side for 30 to 60 seconds on a hard floor. Difficulty of the activity is increased by having patients close their eyes, and by changing the surface to carpeting, grass, or a foam cushion. During the next phase, strengthening of the evertors, invertors, plantar flexors, and dorsiflexors can be performed dynamically with elastic tubing, and then via heel raises and partial squats. Hip abductor muscle strengthening should be done as well. Balance boards are an essential part of the rehabilitation, as these help with proprioceptive retraining and with strengthening (Fig. 39–27). Bicycle exercise is a safe way to maintain or increase endurance without subjecting the ankle to excessive stress. As the patient progresses, more dynamic training is introduced, including slide board, figure-of-8 running drills, hexagon drills, and carioca drills. Functional tests to determine readiness to return

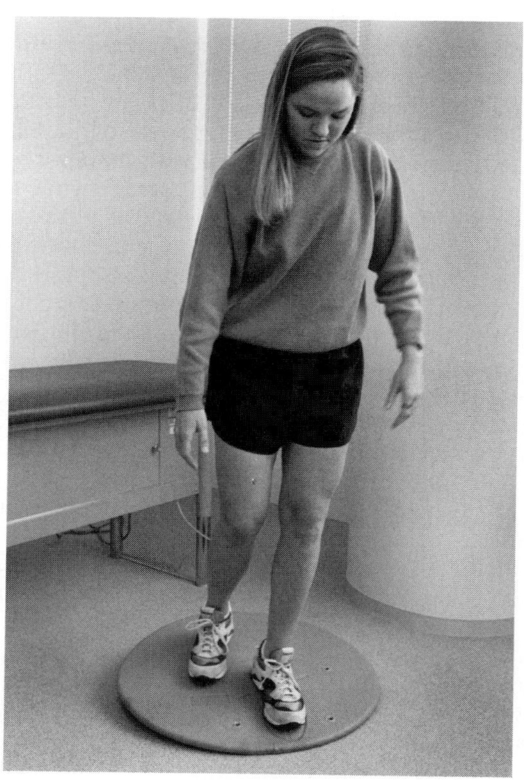

FIGURE 39–27. Dynamic ankle rehabilitation with a balance board.

to activity include "shuttle runs" and single-leg hopping. Side-to-side comparisons for hop height or time to cover a given distance can be made. In our experience, the majority of sprains treated in this manner are ready to return to activity within 1 to 3 weeks. The use of postrehabilitation bracing is not mandatory, but athletes in higher-risk sports such as basketball, soccer, and football might elect to use hightop shoes, lace-up braces, or taping for injury prophylaxis.

Foot Injuries

Plantar Fasciitis. This consists of traction-induced microtears of the plantar fascia and its associated structures at the insertion on the calcaneus.[85] The fascia tightens passively with toe extension, creating a stiffer midfoot with arch elevation. This "windlass effect" and the transition from pronation to supination are critical for transforming the foot from a deformable structure suited for surface accommodation and shock absorption to one that is rigid and suited for use as a lever during push-off. Limited ankle dorsiflexion, excessive pronation, and a tight gastrocnemius-soleus complex all increase the chance of developing plantar fasciitis, because prolonged pronation during the stance phase decreases the chances of achieving the rigid, closed, packed midtarsal joint needed to push off. This subjects other medial support structures, such as the plantar fascia, to increased tensile forces and excessive overload. The patient with plantar fasciitis typically presents with progressively worsening pain during exertion and dreads taking the first step out of bed in the morning. It is worth noting that although plantar fasciitis is usually seen in persons with high or normal arches, it can also be seen in the person with flat feet.

Symptoms of plantar fasciitis consist of point tenderness along the medial fascia, inability to run, and a painful first step of the morning.[81] The functional biomechanical deficits include decreased plantar flexor flexibility and strength, and functional pronation.[81] Functional adaptations include attempted inversion to reduce medial structure overload and, in the case of runners, forefoot running with a choppy stride.[81, 126]

Acute management consists of the PRICE principle and use of anti-inflammatory medications as needed. Ice massage is a particularly useful modality. If the diagnosis is clear, radiographs are not needed. If they are obtained, it is important to realize that heel spurs on the calcaneus are a common radiographic finding (up to 30% of the asymptomatic population) and are likely to represent repetitive plantar ligament traction rather than a site of true pathological changes.[126] Similarly, spurs might not be found in patients with profound symptoms. Consideration is given to steroid injection into the calcaneal attachment, although this is rarely our approach.[126, 163] Arch supports, counterforce taping, and heel pads might be helpful.[81, 126] A full evaluation of the foot in non-weight-bearing and in a weight-bearing position is critical when making shoe and insert recommendations. A structurally rigid insert might alleviate symptoms for an athlete who overpronates, but might exacerbate symptoms for an individual with a rigid high arched foot. The critical measures are stretching of the gastrocnemius-soleus complex, hamstrings, and plantar fascia, together with strengthening of foot intrinsic muscles.[81, 126] Chronic cases can take up to 3 to 4 months to resolve. Formulation of a temporary alternative training program such as rowing, swimming, or aqua running can maintain fitness without delaying resolution of the plantar fasciitis.

Calcaneal Bursitis. This often develops in elderly patients with a calcified spur, subjecting the bursa to trauma after prolonged walking or running. Evaluation of the footwear often reveals poor shock-absorbing capacity. Selecting the appropriate walking or running shoes supplemented with a heel cup is often enough to relieve the symptoms. Restoration of normal flexibility and strengthening of the foot intrinsics can help prevent recurring symptoms. Athletes should be encouraged to change running shoes every 200 to 300 miles due to the midsole breakdown.[163]

Morton's Neuroma. This represents the entrapment of interdigital nerves in the foot. The structure most often implicated is the transverse metatarsal ligament, but surrounding bursal structures can also cause local irritation.[5] The neuromas are most frequently found between the third and second interspaces. Patients complain of an aching forefoot, with at times lancinating foot pain. It is exacerbated by wearing tight shoes, high heels, and athletic activities requiring repetitive forefoot weight bearing (e.g., bicycling, step aerobics). Patients obtain almost immediate relief when they take their shoes off and often prefer to walk barefoot. During physical examination, grasping the foot in one hand and squeezing the metatarsals together reproduces the symptoms. Along with this maneuver, the examiner must examine each metatarsal ray individually to be sure that the pain is not coming directly from the shaft of the metatarsals. If there is even the slightest question of an overt fracture or a stress fracture, radiographs or a bone scan should be obtained. Intermediate-to-long-term relief can be obtained with footwear modification (increased width), orthotic inserts, and corticosteroid injection. For those who do not respond to conservative measures, neuroma excision can provide relief.[98]

Common Pediatric Injuries—Traction Apophysitises

In the skeletally immature, the physis is the weakest part of the skeleton. The apophyseal growth plate, where the musculotendinous unit inserts into bone, is at particular risk for injury. This site is often subject to repetitive traction forces and microtrauma. Microtrauma, possibly caused by a relatively inflexible musculotendinous unit, leads to inflammation and an apophysitis. With continued microtrauma, the macrotrauma resulting from a single rapid and forceful contraction of the musculotendinous unit can produce an avulsion fracture.[13, 88] These injuries occur in adolescents, but can start in children as young as eight. Growth spurts can play a large role in the development of these injuries. Due to the more rapid bony growth and development compared to muscle-tendon growth, there is a measurable increase in tightness of the musculotendinous unit around the joint. This appears to cause increased tension at the apophysis. With continued microtrauma and inflammation, injury can lead to marked enlargement of the apophysis and spur formation.

Several sites in the lower extremities are at particular risk and account for the majority of these injuries. These include the hip (iliac crest, ischial tuberosity, lesser trochanter), the tibial tubercle (Osgood-Schlatter disease), the inferior patella (Sindig-Larsen-Johansson syndrome), and the posterior calcaneous (Sever's disease).

Apophyseal Injuries at the Hip. Five sites in the adolescent hip and pelvis are at particular risk for injury. These sites include the ischium, the anterior superior iliac spine (ASIS), the anterior inferior iliac spine (AIIS), and the lesser trochanter of each femur. Injuries at these sites typically occur in runners and dancers.[108, 124] The adolescent presents with a dull, aching pain with activity, often with a history of worsening over weeks to months. Pain is accompanied by tenderness at the site of injury. Apophysitis typically does not produce abnormalities on plain films unless an avulsion has occurred.

Iliac crest apophyseal injuries commonly occur with either sudden or repetitive abdominal contraction opposed by forceful contraction of the tensor fasciae latae and the gluteus medius with a planted leg. A direct blow can also cause injury. This injury, a "hip pointer," can occur in football from a hit from another player or in basketball due to a fall to the hardwood floor. Pain and tenderness are seen at the iliac crest as well as painful active hip abduction. The adolescent might walk with a gluteus medius lurch, leaning toward the affected site when stepping with that foot.[32]

ASIS and AIIS apophyseal injuries are usually acute, with a sudden sharp pain in the hip and groin region occurring during sprinting. This is often referred to as "the sprinter's fracture."[32] Distance running can also lead to injuries at these sites. However, these injuries are less acute and often give dull aching pain.[77] The mechanism of injury is forceful contraction of the sartorius and/or hyperextension of the spine in ASIS injury, and forceful contraction of the rectus femoris in AIIS injury. Pain and swelling are seen at the site of injury, often with painful active hip flexion and an antalgic gait.

Sports involving sprinting, jumping, and kicking can lead to apophyseal injury at the lesser trochanter due to the powerful contraction of the iliopsoas against resistance. The patient typically complains of anterior hip pain. Pain can radiate to the groin or flank. Deep palpation of the anterior hip is painful, as is active hip flexion. Passive extension and internal rotation are also painful. An antalgic gait is observed with a shortened stance phase on the affected side. Differentiation from iliac spine injuries can be usually made by site of tenderness and by radiographic findings (if present).

Ischial apophyseal injury is the most frequently reported apophyseal injury at the hip and pelvis.[32] Forceful and powerful contraction of the hamstrings with the pelvis in a flexed position and an extended knee can be the mechanism for injury. Injury can be acute with sprinting or hurdling, or chronic with distance runners. Pain is seen in the buttock region, often radiating into the posterior thigh. Tenderness occurs at the ischial tuberosity. Stretching or contraction of the hamstrings elicits discomfort. Most patients with ischial apophyseal injury walk with an antalgic gait, and some cannot walk without crutches.

Treatment for each of the hip apophysitises and minimally separated avulsion fractures includes relative rest followed by a progressive restoration of strength and flexibility of the entire hip and pelvic region. Initial treatment should include protected ambulation with crutch walking until the gait pattern is normal. If crutch walking is painful, 2 to 4 days of bedrest might be required in a position of hip flexion and knee flexion. Once gait has normalized (usually 7 to 10 days), gentle stretching and strengthening of the involved musculotendinous unit can begin. By 3 weeks, pain is usually minimal, and more aggressive strengthening can be started for the entire lower extremities (focused on the injured musculotendinous unit). Limited athletic activity can be started by week 4, with a progression to full activity by week 6. Running form should also be evaluated to correct any significant errors that might place the involved structures at risk. Some cases, particularly injury to the lesser trochanter, might take up to 12 weeks for full recovery. Very few patients with these injuries have any residual symptoms beyond 12 weeks.

Osgood-Schlatter Disease. The most common traction apophysitis and one of the most common problems in the adolescent athlete is Osgood-Schlatter disease. The etiology is believed to be microtraumatic with multiple avulsions and healing at the tibial tubercle.[119] The injury, frequently bilateral, commonly occurs between the ages of 10 to 15 years, with males more often affected.[146] However, as more young females are participating in athletics, the ratio appears to be balancing. Symptomatic onset often coincides with the beginning of a growth spurt.

The young athlete complains of pain at the tibial tubercle with running or jumping. Often by the time the patient seeks medical attention, there is swelling at the tibial tubercle and pain with daily activities such as climbing stairs or even walking. Examination typically shows a prominence of the tibial tubercle without a knee effusion. Active knee extension is painful, but an isometric quadriceps contraction with a straight leg raise is not painful. Inflexibility of the quadriceps muscle is also common. Plain radiographs can range from a normal appearance to multiple areas of irregular calcification.

Treatment varies depending on the severity of symptoms. Milder cases often respond to ice, a compressive wrap,[89] or a knee brace.[108] More severe cases might require crutch walking. Immobilization should be avoided, as this can prolong the symptomatology.[108, 149] If a compressive wrap or a brace does not alleviate symptoms, a period of rest from sports is recommended. Pain-free straight leg raises should be started almost immediately. Stretching of the quadriceps group is imperative and should be started as soon as tolerated. Often all the musculotendinous groups in the lower extremities are tight, particularly the hamstrings and the gastrocnemius-soleus complex. These require an appropriate stretching program as well. Pain can persist for months, particularly pain on pressure palpation of the tibial tubercle. Residual deformity at the tibial tubercle persists after symptomatic improvement. Even in problematic cases, skeletal maturity leads to cessation of symptoms. Only a very small number of adolescents have symptoms beyond skeletal maturity, and these cases frequently require surgery for improvement.[110]

Sindig-Larsen-Johansson Syndrome. Sindig-Larsen-Johansson syndrome, though less common than Osgood-Schlatter disease, presents with similar symptomatology. Rather than pain and tenderness at the tibial tubercle, however, signs and symptoms are seen at the inferior pole of the patella. This condition is most commonly caused by repetitive microtrauma in sports that require frequent kicking, running, and/or jumping. It has also been reported to result from a single episode of macrotrauma, such as a kick of a ball or a jump.[108] Radiographic findings are similar to those of Osgood-Schlatter, ranging from normal to bony irregularity or avulsion at the distal patella.

Treatment and outcome are very similar to those of Osgood-Schlatter disease. For cases involving a single episode of macrotrauma, some advocate a cylinder cast in full extension for 3 to 4 weeks to aid healing.[103, 108] This is followed by a progressively increased stretching and strengthening program.

Sever's Disease. This condition usually presents with heel pain in the adolescent athlete.[141] Similar to the other traction apophysitises, the injury is due to repetitive microtrauma with resulting inflammatory changes. In this case the injury is at the calcaneal insertion of the Achilles tendon. Like other apophysitises, pain occurs during a growth spurt, can be bilateral in up to 60% of the cases, and is almost always associated with sports involving a lot of running.[108] Examination shows tenderness at the Achilles tendon insertion, tightness of the gastrocnemius-soleus complex, and relative weakness of the ankle dorsiflexors. There is often genu varum, and subtalar and forefoot varus. Radiographs can be helpful in ruling out other causes of heel pain such as stress fracture, infection, or neoplasm. A bone scan is necessary in some cases to make certain of the diagnosis.

Treatment is similar to other apophysitises. In severe cases, 1 to 2 days of crutch walking might be necessary, with initial activity modification needed in most other cases. Ice and massage are useful initially with shoe modification. Heel cups or lifts can be helpful. In cases with significant biomechanical foot abnormalities, orthoses might be necessary. Stretching of the entire gastrocnemius-soleus complex is essential and should be started as early as possible. Strengthening of the ankle dorsiflexors is also important. When the adolescent is asymptomatic, begin dynamic strengthening of the foot-ankle complex with a wobbleboard for dynamic stability. Heel cups or lifts should be discontinued when the patient becomes asymptomatic. Good athletic shoe fit is then imperative, with the addition of an over-the-counter shoe insert if necessary. Most cases resolve within 3 to 6 weeks.

REFERENCES

1. Ackerman L, Ramamurthy S, Jablokow V, et al: Case report 488. Skeletal Radiol 1988; 17:310–314.
2. Agre JC: Hamstring injuries: Proposed aetiologic factors, prevention and treatment. Sports Med 1985; 2:21–33.
3. Agur AMR: Grant's Atlas of Anatomy, ed 9. Baltimore, Williams & Wilkins, 1991.
4. Ahmed AM, Burke DL: In vitro measurement of static pressure distribution in synovial joints in the tibial surface of the knee. J Biomech Eng 1983; 105:216–225.
5. Alexander IJ, Johnson KA, Parr JW: Morton's neuroma: A review of current concepts. Orthopedics 1987; 10:103–106.
6. Amendola A, Rorabeck CH, Vellet D: The use of magnetic resonance imaging in exertional compartment syndromes. Am J Sports Med 1990; 18:29–34.
7. An HS, Simpson JM, Gale S, et al: Acute anterior compartment syndrome in the thigh: A case report and review of the literature. J Orthop Trauma 1987; 1:180–182.
8. Antao NA: Myositis of the hip in a professional soccer player: A case report. Am J Sports Med 1988; 16:82–83.
9. Apple DF Jr: Adolescent runners. Clin Sports Med 1985; 4:641–655.
10. Apple DF Jr: End stage running problems. Clin Sports Med 1985; 4:657–670.
11. Arnoczky SP, Warren RF: Microvasculature of the human meniscus. Am J Sports Med 1982; 10:90–95.
12. Bach DK, Green DS, Jensen GM, et al: A comparison of muscular tightness in runners and nonrunners and the relation of muscular tightness to low back pain in runners. J Orthop Sports Phys Ther 1985; 6:315–323.
13. Bak K: Separation of the proximal tibial epiphysis in a gymnast. Acta Orthop Scand 1991; 62:293–294.
14. Balduni FC, Vegso JJ, Torg JS, et al: Management and rehabilitation of ligamentous injuries to the ankle. Sports Med 1987; 4:364–380.
15. Barrack RL, Skinner HB, Buckley SL: Proprioception in the anterior cruciate deficient knee. Am J Sports Med 1989; 17:1–6.
16. Barton PM: Piriformis syndrome: A rational approach to management. Pain 1991; 47:345–352.
17. Bechham SG, Grana WA, Buckley P, et al: A comparison of anterior compartment pressures in competitive runners and cyclists. Am J Sports Med 1993; 21:36–40.
18. Belkin SC: Stress fractures in athletes. Orthop Clin North Am 1980; 11:735–742.
19. Boam WD, Miser WF, Yuill SC, et al: Comparison of ultrasound examination with bone scintiscan in the diagnosis of stress fractures. J Amer Board Fam Pract 1996; 9:414–417.
20. Booth DW, Westers BM: The management of athletes with myositis ossificans traumatica. Can J Sports Sci 1989; 14:10–16.
21. Bourne MH, Hazel WA, Scott SG, et al: Anterior knee pain. Mayo Clin Proc 1988; 63:482–491.
22. Bradley J, Dandy DJ: Osteochondritis dissecans and other lesions of the femoral condyles. J Bone Joint Surg Am 1983; 65:193.
23. Brody DM: Running injuries. Clinical Symp 1987; 39:2–36.
24. Brody DM: Techniques in the evaluation and treatment of the injured runner. Orthop Clin North Am 1982; 13(3):541–558.
25. Brukner P, Khan K: Clinical Sports Medicine. Sydney, Australia, McGraw-Hill, 1993, p 522.
26. Burkett LN: Causative factors in hamstring strains. Med Sci Sports Exerc 1970; 2:39–42.
27. Buschbacher R: The use and abuse of ankle supports in sports injuries. J Back Musculoskeletal Rehabil 1993; 3:57–68.
28. Cailliet R: Low Back Pain Syndrome. Philadelphia, FA Davis, 1989.
29. Chapman MW: Part II. Sprains of the ankle. Instruct Course Lect 1975; 24:294–308.
30. Clanton TO, Delee JC: Osteochondritis dissecans: History, pathophysiology and current treatment concepts. Clin Orthop 1982; 167:50.
31. Collee G, Dijkmans BAC, Vandenbroucke JD, et al: Greater trochanteric pain syndrome (trochanteric bursitis) in low back pain. Scand J Rheumatol 1991; 20:262–266.
32. Combs J: Hip and pelvis avulsion fractures in adolescents. Phys Sports Med 1994; 22(7):41–49.

33. Corsetti JR, Jackson DW: Failure of anterior cruciate ligament reconstruction: The biologic basis. Clin Orthop 1996; 325:42–49.
34. Cox JS: Patellofemoral problems in runners. Clin Sports Med 1985; 4:699–715.
35. Cox JS: Surgical and nonsurgical treatment of acute ankle sprains. Clin Orthop 1985; 198:118–126.
36. Cox JS, Nye CE, Schaeffer WW, et al: The degenerative effects of partial and total resection of the medial meniscus in dogs' knees. Clin Orthop 1975; 109:178–183.
37. Cross MJ, Powell JF: Long-term follow up of posterior cruciate ligament rupture: A study of 116 cases. Am J Sports Med 1984; 12:292–297.
38. Daffner RH: Stress fractures: Current concepts. Skeletal Radiol 1978; 2:221–229.
39. Deal CL, Canoso JJ: Meralgia paresthetica and large abdomens. Ann Intern Med 1982; 96:787–788.
40. Delee JC, Bergfeld JA, Drez D Jr, et al: The posterior cruciate ligament. In Delee JC, Drez D Jr (eds): Orthopaedic Sports Medicine. Philadelphia, WB Saunders, 1994, pp 1374–1400.
41. Delee JC, Riley MB, Rockwood CA: Acute straight lateral instability of the knee. Am J Sports Med 1983; 11:404.
42. Dillingham MF, King WD, Gamburd RS: Rehabilitation of the knee following anterior cruciate ligament and medial collateral ligament injuries. Phys Med Rehabil Clin North Am 1994; 5:175–194.
43. Draganich LF, Jaeger RJ, Kralj AR: Coactivation of the hamstrings and quadriceps during extension of the knee. J Bone Joint Surg Am 1989; 71:1075–1081.
44. Ecker AD, Woltman HW: Meralgia paresthetica: A report of 150 cases. JAMA 1938; 110:1650–1652.
45. Fairbanks TJ: Knee joint changes after meniscectomy. J Bone Joint Surg Br 1948; 30:664–670.
46. Ficat RP, Hungerford DS: Disorders of the Patellofemoral Joint. Baltimore, Williams & Wilkins, 1977.
47. Fowler PJ, Messieh SS: Isolated posterior cruciate ligament injuries in athletes. Am J Sports Med 1987; 15:553–557.
48. Fu FH, Baratz M: Meniscal injuries. In Delee JC, Drez D Jr (eds): Orthopaedic Sports Medicine. Philadelphia, WB Saunders, 1994, pp 1146–1248.
49. Funk FJ Jr: Injuries of the extensor mechanism of the knee. Athletic Training 1975; 10:141–145.
50. Galway RD, Beaupre A, MacIntosh DL: Pivot shift: A clinical sign of symptomatic anterior cruciate ligament insufficiency. J Bone Joint Surg Br 1972; 54:763.
51. Geraci MC: Rehabilitation of pelvis hip and thigh injuries in sports. Phys Med Rehabil Clin North Am 1994; 5:157–174.
52. Grabiner MD, Koh TJ, Draganich LF: Neuromechanics of the patellofemoral joint. Med Sci Sports Exerc 1994; 26:10–21.
53. Grace DL: Lateral ankle ligament injuries. Inversion and anterior stress radiography. Clin Orthop 1984; 183:153–156.
54. Grana WA: Acute ankle injuries. In Renstrom PAFH (ed): Clinical Practice of Sports Injury Prevention and Care. London, Blackwell, 1994, pp 217–227.
55. Green W, Banks H: Osteochondritis in children. J Bone Joint Surg Am 1958; 14:26.
56. Gross ML, Dalvin LB, Evanski PM: Effectiveness of orthotic shoe inserts in the long distance runner. Am J Sports Med 1991; 19:409–412.
57. Gurtler RA, Stine R, Torg JS: Lachman test revisited. Contemp Orthop 1990; 20:145–154.
58. Hait G, Boswick JA Jr, Stone NH: Heterotopic bone formation secondary to trauma (myositis ossificans traumatica): An unusual case and a review of current concepts. J Trauma 1970; 10:405–411.
59. Hastings DE: The non-operative management of collateral ligament injuries of the knee joint. Clin Orthop 1980; 147:22–28.
60. Heiser TM, Weber J, Sullivan G, et al: Prophylaxis and management of hamstring injuries in intercollegiate football players. Am J Sports Med 1984; 12:368–370.
61. Henry J: Lateral ligament tears of the ankle, 1–6 years after follow up: Study of 202 ankles. Orthop Rev 1983; 10:31–39.
62. Herring SA, Kibler WB: Rehabilitation. In Cantu RC, Micheli LJ (eds): ACSM's Guidelines for the Team Physician. Philadelphia, Lea & Febiger, 1991, pp 191–195.
63. Hilyard A: Recent developments in the management of patellofemoral pain: The McConnell programme. Physiotherapy 1990; 76:559–565.
64. Hollinshead WH, Jenkins DB: Functional Anatomy of the Limbs and Back, ed 5. Philadelphia, WB Saunders, 1981.
65. Hopkinson WJ, St. Pierre P, Ryan JB, et al: Syndesmosis sprains of the ankle. Foot Ankle 1990; 10:325–330.
66. Hoppenfeld S: Physical Examination of the Spine and Extremities. Norwalk, CT, Appleton-Century-Crofts, 1976.
67. Hungerford DS, Barry M: Biomechanics of the patellofemoral joint. Clin Orthop 1979; 144:9–15.
68. Indelicato PA: Non-operative treatment of complete tears of the medial collateral ligament of the knee. J Bone Joint Surg Am 1983; 65:323–329.
69. Jackson DW: Managing myositis ossificans in the young athlete. Phys Sports Med 1975; 3:56–61.
70. Jackson DW, Ashley RL, Powell JW: Ankle sprains in young athletes. Relation of severity and disability. Clin Orthop 1974; 101:201–215.
71. Jackson DW, Feagin JA: Quadriceps contusions in young athletes: Relation of severity of injury to treatment and prognosis. J Bone Joint Surg Am 1973; 53:95–105.
72. James SL, Bates BT, Osterning LR: Injuries to runners. Am J Sports Med 1978; 6:40–50.
73. Jarvinen M: Muscle injuries. In Renstrom PAFH (ed): Clinical Practice of Sports Injury Prevention and Care. London, Blackwell, 1994, pp 115–124.
74. Jones RK: Meralgia paresthetica as a cause of leg discomfort. Can Med Assoc J 1974; 111:541–542.
75. Kannus P: Long-term results of conservatively treated medial collateral ligament injuries of the knee joint. Clin Orthop 1988; 226:103–112.
76. Kannus P, Renstrom P: Treatment for acute tears of the lateral ligaments of the ankle. J Bone Joint Surg Am 1991; 73:305–312.
77. Karlin LI: The skeletally immature athlete: Injuries to the hip and pelvis. In Nicholas JA, Hershman EB (eds): The Lower Extremity & Spine in Sports Medicine. St. Louis, Mosby–Year Book, 1995.
78. Kibler WB: Clinical aspects of muscle injury. Med Sci Sports Exerc 1990; 22:450–452.
79. Kibler WB, Chandler TJ, Pace BK: Principles of rehabilitation after chronic tendon injuries. Clin Sports Med 1992; 11:661–671.
80. Kibler WB, Chandler TJ, Stracener ES: Musculoskeletal adaptations and injuries due to overtraining. Exerc Sports Sci Rev 1992; 20:99–126.
81. Kibler WB, Goldberg C, Chandler TJ: Functional biomechanical deficits in running athletes with plantar fasciitis. Am J Sports Med 1991; 19:66–71.
82. Kirkpatrick JS, Koman LA, Rovere GD: The role of ultrasound in the early diagnosis of myositis ossificans: A case report. Am J Sports Med 1987; 15:179–181.
83. Kujala UM: Hamstring injuries. Current trends in treatment and prevention. Sports Med 1997; 23(6):397–404.
84. Kuland DN: The Injured Athlete, ed 2. Philadelphia, JB Lippincott, 1988, pp 428–453.
85. Kwong PK, Kay D, Voner RT, White MW: Plantar fasciitis: Mechanics and pathomechanics of treatment. Clin Sports Med 1988; 7:119–127.
86. Leadbetter WB: Cell-matrix response in tendon injury. Clin Sports Med 1992; 11:533–578.
87. Leeds HC, Ehrlich MG: Instability of the distal tibiofibular syndesmosis after bimalleolar and trimalleolar ankle fractures. J Bone Joint Surg Am 1984; 66:490–503.
88. Lepse PS, McCarthy RE, McCullough FL: Simultaneous bilateral avulsion fracture of the tibial tuberosity. Clin Orthop 1988; 229:232–235.
89. Levine J, Kashyap S: A new conservative treatment of Osgood-Schlatter disease. Clin Orthop Rel Res 1981; 158:126–128.
90. Levy M, Torzilli PA, Warren RF: The effect of medial meniscectomy on anterior-posterior motion of the knee. J Bone Joint Surg Am 1982; 64:883–888.
91. Lipscomb AB, Thomas ED, Johnston RK: Treatment of myositis ossificans traumatica in athletes. Am J Sports Med 1976; 4:111–120.

92. Losee RE, Johnson TR, Southwick WO: Anterior subluxation of the lateral tibial plateau: A diagnostic test and operative repair. J Bone Joint Surg Am 1978; 60:1015.
93. Lotke PA: Soft tissue lesions affecting the hip joints. In Tronzo R (ed): Surgery of the Hip Joint. New York, Springer-Verlag, 1973, pp 368–377.
94. Loudon JK, Jenkins W, Loudon KL: The relationship between static posture and ACL injury in female athletes. J Orthop Sports Phys Ther 1996; 24(2):91–97.
95. Lutter LD: The knee and running. Clin Sports Med 1985; 4:685–698.
96. Lynch MA, Henning CE, Glick KR: Knee joint surface changes: Long term follow-up of meniscus tear treatment in stable anterior cruciate ligament reconstructions. Clin Orthop 1983; 172: 148–153.
97. Main WK, Scott NW: Knee anatomy. In Scott NW (ed): Ligament and Extensor Mechanism Injuries of the Knee: Diagnosis and Treatment. St Louis, Mosby–Year Book, 1991, pp 17–18.
98. Mann RA, Reynolds JC: Interdigital neuroma: A critical clinical analysis. Foot Ankle 1984; 3:238–243.
99. Matsen FA, Winquist RA, Krugmire RB: Diagnosis and management of compartmental syndromes. J Bone Joint Surg Am 1980; 62:286–291.
100. McBryde AM: Stress fractures in runners. Clin Sports Med 1985; 4:737–752.
101. McConnell J: The management of chondromalacia patellae: A long term solution. Aust J Physiother 1986; 32:215–219.
102. McPoil TG, Cornwall MW: The relationship between static lower extremity measurements and rearfoot motion during walking. J Orthop Sports Phys Ther 1996; 24(5):309–314.
103. Medler RC, Lyne ED: Sinding-Larsen-Johansson disease. J Bone Joint Surg 1978; 60A:1113–1116.
104. Mellerowicz H, Stelling E, Kefenbaum A: Diagnostic ultrasound in the athlete's locomotor system. Br J Sport Med 1990; 24:31–39.
105. Merrifield HH, Cowan RF: Ice hockey groin pulls. Am J Sports Med 1973; 1:41–42.
106. Messier SP, Pittala KA: Etiologic factors associated with selected running injuries. Med Sci Sports Exerc 1988; 20:501–505.
107. Micheli LJ: Overuse injuries in children's sports: The growth factor. Orthop Clin North Am 1983; 14:337–361.
108. Micheli LJ: The traction apophysitises. Clin Sports Med 1987; 6(2):387–404.
109. Miller MD, Ritchie JR, Harner CD: Meniscus surgery: Indications for repair. Operative Tech Sports Med 1994; 2:164–171.
110. Mital MA, Matza RA, Cohen J: The so-called unresolved Osgood-Schlatter's lesion. J Bone Joint Surg 1981; 62(A): 732–739.
111. Nalley J, Jay MS, Durant RH: Myositis ossificans in an adolescent following sports injury. Adolesc Health Care 1985; 6:460–462.
112. Newell SG: Functional neutral orthoses and shoe modifications. Phys Med Rehabil Clin North Am 1992; 3:193–222.
113. Newell SG, Bramwell ST: Overuse injuries to the knee in runners. Phys Sports Med 1984; 12:81–92.
114. Noble CA: Iliotibial band friction syndrome in runners. Am J Sports Med 1980; 8:232–234.
115. Noyes FR, Butler DL, Paulos LE, et al: Inter-articular cruciate reconstruction. Perspectives on graft strength, vascularization, and immediate motion after replacement. Clin Orthop 1983; 172:710–717.
116. Noyes FR, Matthews DS, Moor PK, et al: The symptomatic anterior cruciate deficient knee. II: The results of rehabilitation activity modification and counseling on functional disability. J Bone Joint Surg Am 1983; 65:163–174.
117. O'Brien M: Functional anatomy and physiology of tendons. Clin Sports Med 1992; 11:505–520.
118. O'Donoghue DH: Treatment of Injuries to Athletes, ed 4. Philadelphia, WB Saunders, 1984, pp 433–444.
119. Ogden JA, Southwick WO: Osgood-Schlatter's disease and tibial tubercle development. Clin Orthop Rel Res 1976; 116:180–189.
120. Olsen NK, Press JP, Young JL: Bursal injections. In Lennard TA (ed): Physiatric Procedures in Clinical Practice. Philadelphia, Hanley & Belfus, 1995, pp 36–43.
121. O'Meara PM: Rehabilitation following reconstruction of the anterior cruciate ligament. Orthopedics 1993; 16(3):301–306.
122. O'Toole ML: Prevention and treatment of injuries to runners. Med Sci Sports Exerc 1992; 24:S360–S363.
123. Parolie JM, Bergfeld JA: Long term results of nonoperative treatment of isolated posterior cruciate ligament injuries in the athlete. Am J Sports Med 1986; 14:35–38.
124. Peck, DM. Apophyseal injuries in the young athlete. Amer Fam Phys 1995; 51(8):1891–1898.
125. Powers CM, Maffucci R, Hampton S: Rearfoot posture in subjects with patellofemoral pain. J Orthop Sports Phys Ther 1995; 22(4):155–160.
126. Press JM, Herring SA, Kibler WB: Rehabilitation of Muculoskeletal Disorders. United States Army Publication, in press.
127. Putnam CA, Kozey JW: Substantive issues in running. In Vaughn CL (ed): Biomechanics of Sport. Boca Raton, FL, CRC Press, 1989, pp 2–33.
128. Reddy AS, Reedy MK, Seaber AV, et al: Restriction of the injury response following an acute muscle strain. Med Sci Sports Exerc 1993; 25:321–327.
129. Renstrom PAFH: Groin and hip injuries. In Renstrom PAFH (ed): Clinical Practice of Sports Injury Prevention and Care. London, Blackwell, 1994, pp 97–114.
130. Renstrom PAFH, Kannus P: Injuries of the foot and ankle. In Delee JC, Drez D Jr (eds): Orthopedic Sports Medicine. Philadelphia, WB Saunders, 1994, pp 1705–1767.
131. Romani WA, Perrin DH, Dussault RG, et al: The efficacy of therapeutic continuous ultrasound in the diagnosis of tibial stress fractures. Doctoral dissertation, University of Virginia, April, 1998.
132. Roy S, Irvin R: Sports Medicine: Prevention, Evaluation, Management and Rehabilitation. Englewood Cliffs, NJ, Prentice-Hall, 1983, pp 299–305.
133. Rubinstein RA Jr, Shelbourne DK: Diagnosis of posterior cruciate ligament injuries and indications for nonoperative and operative treatment. Operative Tech Sports Med 1993; 1:99–103.
134. Ryan JB, Wheeler JH, Hopkinson WJ, et al: Quadriceps contusions (West Point update). Am J Sports Med 1991; 19:299–304.
135. Rydell N: Biomechanics of the hip joint. Clin Orthop 1973; 92:6–19.
136. Saal JA: Rehabilitation of sports related lumbar spine injuries. Phys Med Rehabil 1987; 1:613–638.
137. Sandberg R, Balkfors B, Nilsson B, et al: Operative versus non-operative treatment of recent injuries to the ligaments of the knee. J Bone Joint Surg Am 1987; 69:1120–1126.
138. Schumacher RH: Primer on the Rheumatic Diseases. Atlanta, Arthritis Foundation, 1988, pp 263–274.
139. Shelbourne KD, Nitz P: Arthrofibrosis in acute anterior cruciate ligament reconstruction: The effect of timing of reconstruction and rehabilitation. Am J Sports Med 1991; 19:332–335.
140. Shelbourne KD, Wilckens JH, Mollabashy A, et al: Accelerated rehabilitation after acute anterior cruciate ligament reconstruction. Am J Sports Med 1990; 18:292–299.
141. Shuster R: Children's foot survey. J Podiatr Soc N Y 1956; 17:13.
142. Sim FH, Scott SG: Injuries of the hip and pelvis in athletes: Anatomy and function. In Nicholas JA, Hershman EB (eds): The Lower Extremity and Spine in Sports Medicine. St Louis, Mosby–Year Book, 1986, pp 1119–1169.
143. Sim FH, Simonet WT, Scott SG: Ice hockey injuries: Causes, treatments, and prevention. J Musculoskeletal Med 1989; 6:15–44.
144. Smith J, Szczerba JE, Arnold BL, et al: Role of hyperpronation as a possible risk factor for anterior cruciate ligament injuries. J Athl Training 1997; 32(1):25–28.
145. Sommer HM, Vallentyne SW: Effect of foot posture on the incidence of medial tibial stress syndrome. Med Sci Sports Exerc 1995; 27(6):800–804.
146. Soren A, Fetto JF: Pathology, clinical findings, and treatment of Osgood-Schlatter's disease. Orthopedics 1984; 7:230.
147. Steinkamp LA, Dillingham MF, Markel MD, et al: Biomechanical considerations in patellofemoral joint rehabilitation. Am J Sports Med 1993; 21:438–444.
148. Stormont DM, Morrey B, An K, et al: Stability of the loaded ankle. Am J Sports Med 1985; 13:295–303.
149. Striazk AM, Stroberg AJ: Knee injuries in the skeletally immature athlete. In Nicholas JA, Hershman EB (eds): The Lower

Extremity and Spine in Sports Medicine. St Louis, Mosby–Year Book, 1991.
150. Styf J: Diagnosis of exercise-induced pain in the anterior aspect of the leg. Am J Sports Med 1988; 16:165–169.
151. Subotnick SI: The biomechanics of running. Sports Med 1985; 2:144–153.
152. Sutker AN, Barber FA, Jackson DW, Pagliano JW: Iliotibial band syndrome in distance runners. Sports Med 1985; 5:447–451.
153. Svedenhag J, Seger J: Running on land and in water: Comparative exercise physiology. Med Sci Sports Exerc 1992; 24:1155–1160.
154. Swezey RL: Pseudo-radiculopathy in subacute trochanteric bursitis of the subgluteus maximus bursa. Arch Phys Med Rehabil 1976; 57:387–390.
155. Tietjens BB: Posterior cruciate ligament injuries. J Bone Joint Surg Br 1985; 59:15–19.
156. Traycoff RB: "Pseudotrochanteric bursitis": The differential diagnosis of lateral hip pain. J Rheumatol 1991; 12:1810–1812.
157. Tredget T, Godberson CV, Bose B: Myositis ossificans due to hockey injury. Can Med Assoc J 1977; 116:65–66.
158. Van Mechelen W, Hlobil H, Zijlstra WP, et al: Is range of motion at the hip and ankle joint related to running injuries? Int J Sports Med 1992; 13:605–610.
159. Walsh ZT, Micheli L: Hip dislocation in a high school football player. Phys Sports Med 1989; 17:112–115.
160. Warren BL: Anatomical factors associated with predicting plantar fasciitis in long-distance runners. Med Sci Sports Exerc 1984; 16(1):60–63.
161. Warren R, Arnoczky SP, Wickiewicz TL: Anatomy of the knee. In Nicholas JA, Hershman EB (eds): The Lower Extremity and Spine in Sports Medicine. St Louis, Mosby–Year Book, 1991.
162. Young JL, Laskowski ER, Rock M: Thigh injuries in athletes. Mayo Clin Proc 1993; 68:1099–1106.
163. Young JL, Press JM: Rehabilitation of Running Injuries. In Buschbacher R, Braddom R (eds): Sports Medicine and Rehabilitation: A Sports Specific Approach. Philadelphia, Hanley & Belfus, 1994.
164. Zarins B, Ciullo JV: Acute muscle and tendon injuries in athletes. Clin Sports Med 1983; 3:167–182.

40
CHAPTER

Mehrsheed Sinaki, M.D., M.S., and Bahram Mokri, M.D.

Low Back Pain and Disorders of the Lumbar Spine

EPIDEMIOLOGY OF BACK PAIN

In the industrialized world, low back pain is second only to headache as a cause of pain. It is the leading cause of expenditure for Workers' Compensation. Although it is often a self-limiting symptom, it costs at least $16 billion a year.[59, 146] and disables 5.4 million Americans.[48, 52]

According to estimates of the U.S. Census Bureau, 1.8 million Americans were unable to work at some time during 1984 to 1985 because of low back pain. One study reported that 2% of all U.S. workers have a compensable back injury each year. Another study[154] suggested that 25 million Americans lost 1 or more days of work annually because of low back pain. About 2% of workers each year submit claims for disability due to low back pain.

Low back pain is a symptom that can be caused by various disease entities and can be affected by various psychosocial factors. Furthermore, in the absence of specific anatomical and pathological findings, the pain is not objectively verifiable. Thus, applying the science of epidemiology to the subject of low back pain is difficult. The available survey studies have to be analyzed with attention to several factors, including the presence or absence of specific anatomical change or pathological process, whether the pain is severe or trivial, whether the report of pain is through questionnaires or through direct evaluation of the patient, whether the patient is referring to low back pain or to spine pain in general, and the accuracy of the patient's report (a pre-employment health survey typically does not reveal the same prevalence of low back pain as does an anonymous survey).

Some 50% to 80% of adults will have low back pain at some time in their lives.[18, 19, 65, 66, 72, 73, 78] In 1985, the Nuprin Pain Report,[154] conducted through telephone interviews of 1254 Americans, revealed that 56% of the adult population had some low back pain in the year preceding the survey, and 3% of them had had low back pain for more than 1 month. The U.S. population in 1985 was approximately 180 million, and one can conclude from this study that approximately 100 million persons had some low back pain and 6 million had low back pain for more than 1 month during that year.[85] In a study conducted in Finland,[65, 66] about 75% of both men and women reported having had at least one episode of low back pain, 45% recalled at least six episodes of low back pain, and 18% reported having low back pain in the previous month. Prevalence was greatest in the 55- to 64-year age group.

Current studies[20, 53, 124, 147, 151] suggest a lifetime rate of low back pain of about 60% to 90% and an annual rate of about 5%. The overall incidence is equal in men and women, but women report more low back pain after age 60 years.[20] This difference is likely due to the development of osteoporosis in women. Only 1% of patients with acute low back pain have lumbar radiculopathy. This rate is probably even lower for those with chronic low back pain. Lumbar radiculopathies often occur in patients during the fourth and fifth decades of life. The average age of patients who undergo lumbar laminectomy and discectomy is 42 years.[52, 147]

Risk Factors

Epidemiological studies also point to certain risk factors that influence the incidence or prevalence of low back pain. These can be divided into two major groups: occupational and patient-related.[124]

Occupational Factors

Hard labor and heavy exertions have been claimed as the cause of pain by more than 60% of patients with low back pain.[21, 124, 127] Lifting, pulling and pushing, twisting, slipping, sitting for an extended period, and exposure to prolonged vibration, in isolation or in various combinations, have been attributed to development of low back pain. Persons who view their occupations as boring, repetitious, or dissatisfying might also report a higher rate of low back pain.[5, 157]

Patient-Related Factors

Age

The likelihood of developing low back pain gradually increases up until approximately 55 years of age.[12, 18, 19]

Gender

Men and women have similar risks of low back pain up until age 60 years. Thereafter, women are at greater risk, probably because of the development of osteoporosis.

Anthropometric Factors

There are no strong correlations between height, weight, or body build and low back pain. However, there is a higher risk of low back pain in very obese persons[76] and possibly in tall persons.[18, 79, 82, 153]

Postural Factors

The effect of scoliosis on spine pain is discussed in Chapter 17. The role of other postural changes such as kyphosis, increased or decreased lumbar lordosis, and discrepancy in the length of the lower limbs in the production of back pain is controversial. Although these factors might contribute to back pain in some patients, no generally accepted hard evidence exists of a true association.

Spine Mobility

Most subjects with low back pain have at least some limitation of range of motion of the lumbar spine. One study[18] found more pronounced reduction of flexibility of the lumbar spine in subjects who went on to experience recurrence of low back pain during the year after the examination.

Muscle Strength

Several studies[1, 2, 16, 17, 64, 93, 104, 112, 113, 120, 128] have shown decreased strength of abdominal and spinal muscles in patients with low back pain. Some studies[135] have shown comparatively weaker extensors, whereas others[18, 125] have shown comparatively weaker flexors.

Physical Fitness

A study conducted in Los Angeles firefighters found that physical fitness and conditioning had a preventive effect on low back injuries. Another study[16] found no difference in the rate of recovery from acute low back pain with improved physical fitness. One study[121] found no correlation between cardiovascular physical fitness and back strength in a group of healthy, normal women aged 29 to 40 years.

Smoking

Persons who smoke seem to have an increased likelihood of developing low back pain.[35, 65, 66] Smoking is also known to increase the incidence of osteoporosis.

Psychosocial Factors

Depression, anxiety, hypochondriasis, hysteria, alcoholism, divorce, chronic headaches, and other factors have been reported with higher frequency in patients with chronic low back pain.[54] Whether these are the cause or the result of the low back pain is unclear.

Most adults in the United States will have low back pain at some time in their lives. As it stands, low back pain is the most frequent cause of lost work days in the United States, surpassing the combination of acquired immunodeficiency syndrome (AIDS), cancer, and stroke as a cause of disability among persons of working age.

Etiology

Various disease entities can cause low back pain. The causes of low back pain are many, most of which can be categorized according to the classification provided in Table 40–1. Some of the common entities are listed with each classification. Several of these disease entities are discussed later in the chapter.

ANATOMY AND KINESIOLOGY OF THE LUMBAR SPINE

The vertebrae increase in size distally in the spine. Vertebrae are most massive in the lumbar region, which constitutes 25% of the height of the entire vertebral column. The "shock absorbers" of the spine are the intervertebral disks. In young persons, they constitute 25% of the height of the spine, but this percentage decreases significantly with age, as the disks lose water and collapse. The orientation of the facet joints varies at different levels of the spine. The superior and inferior articular facets are in frontal planes in the midthoracic regions. The lumbar facets are almost in sagittal planes, allowing the facet joints to glide anteroposteriorly and facilitating most of the flexion and extension movements of the lower spine. The contribution from thoracic vertebral segments to these movements is negligible. Seventy-five percent of lumbar flexion and extension occurs in the lumbosacral joint, 20% at L4–5, and the remaining 5% at the other levels.

The lumbar vertebrae are composed mainly of cancellous bone that is susceptible to collapse under trauma or from osteoporosis. The thin but dense cortical layer can proliferate with aging at the sites of ligamentous

TABLE 40–1 Causes of Low Back Pain

Cause	Common Diseases
1. Degenerative	Degenerative joint disease (DJD), osteoarthritis, lumbar spondylolysis Facet joint disease, facet DJD Degenerative spondylolisthesis Degenerative disk disease Diffuse idiopathic skeletal hyperostosis
2. Inflammatory (noninfectious)	Spondyloarthropathies (ankylosing spondylitis) Rheumatoid arthritis
3. Infectious	Pyogenic vertebral spondylitis Intervertebral disk infection Epidural abscess
4. Metabolic	Osteoporosis or osteopenia Paget's disease of bone
5. Neoplastic	Benign Spinal (benign bony tumors of spine) Intraspinal (meningiomas, neurofibromas, neurilemmomas, low-grade ependymomas) Malignant Spinal (malignant bony or soft tissue tumors, metastasis) Intraspinal (metastasis, high-grade ependymomas, astrocytomas, meningeal carcinomatosis)
6. Traumatic	Fractures or dislocations Sprains (lumbar, lumbosacral, sacroiliac)
7. Congenital or developmental	Dysplastic spondylolisthesis Scoliosis
8. Musculoskeletal	Acute or chronic lumbar strain Mechanical low back pain Myofascial pain syndromes Fibromyalgia, tension myalgia Tension myalgia of the pelvic floor, coccygodynia Postural abnormalities, pregnancy
9. Viscerogenic	Upper genitourinary disorders Retroperitoneal disorders (often neoplastic)
10. Vascular	Abdominal aortic aneurysm or dissection Renal artery thrombosis or dissection Stagnation of venous blood (nocturnal back pain of pregnancy)
11. Psychogenic	Compensation neurosis Conversion disorder
12. Postoperative and multiply operated-on back	

attachments and lead to osteophyte formation. The vertebral body is attached to the neural arch, which is composed of pedicles, superior and inferior facet joints, and the lamina (Fig. 40–1). The superior facet joint is smaller than the inferior one. It has a concave cartilaginous articular surface and forms the roof of the lateral recess. This is where the nerve root leaves the central canal to enter the neural foramen. Pedicles form the floor and the roof of the neural foramina. The laminae unite posteriorly to complete the neural arch. They protect the neural elements and are the sites of paraspinal muscle attachments. However, the laminae contribute little to the stability of the spinal column, and unilateral fracture or surgical removal of the laminae (laminectomy) does not cause spinal instability. The pedicle facet complex normally bears only 20% of the intervertebral vertical load; the remaining 80% is absorbed by the intervertebral disk.[102] The posterior longitudinal ligament extends along the posterior aspects of vertebral bodies and is attached to the lumbar disks and vertebral body margins. This ligament is not attached to the periosteum; a potential space is thus left between the ligament and periosteum that can expand with purulent material, tumor, or hematoma. The posterior longitudinal ligament, along with the anterior longitudinal ligament, helps maintain the axial stability of the vertebral column.[77, 162]

Intervertebral disks are remnants of the notocord that act as cushions between vertebral bodies and are composed of fibrocartilaginous elements. The nucleus pulposus is an ovoid, yellowish, gelatinous, and paracentrally located middle portion of the disk made of mucoprotein. This is surrounded by a firm, concentric meshwork of collagenous fibers called the *annulus fibrosus.* The lumbar disk is normally thicker anteriorly, a shape that partly explains the normal lumbar lordosis. Tiny blood vessels enter and exit the disk in the early decades of life, but these are obliterated during the first

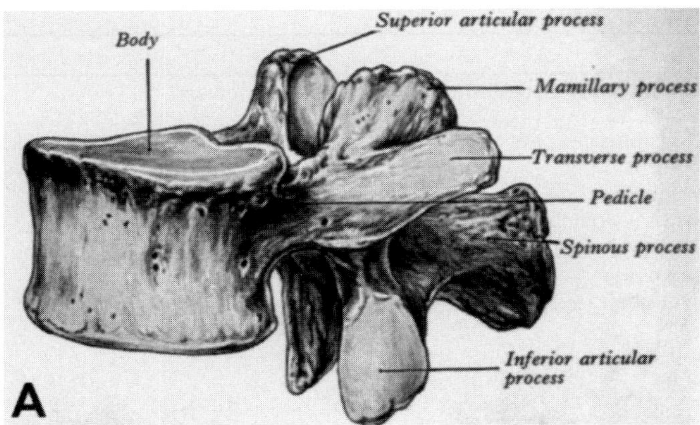

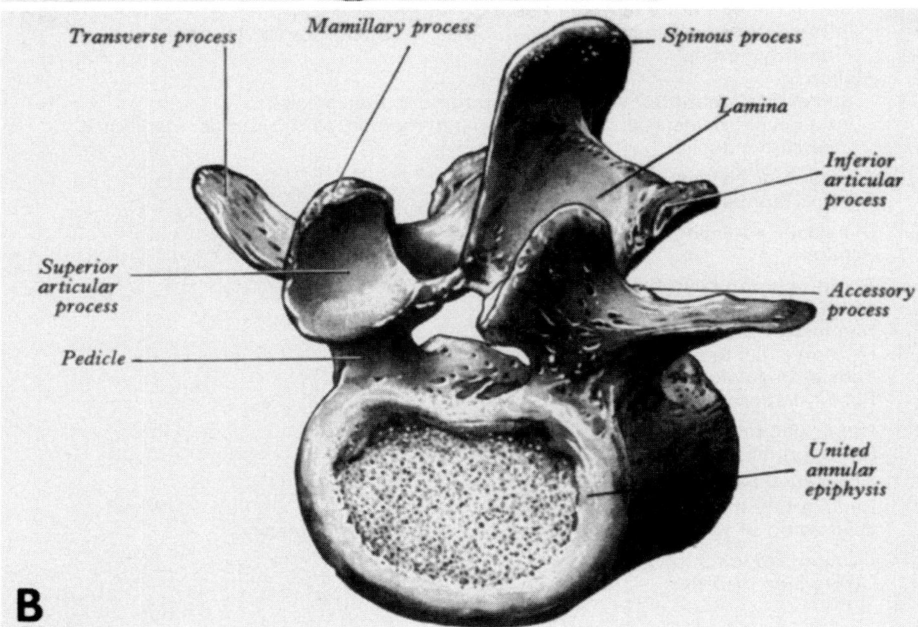

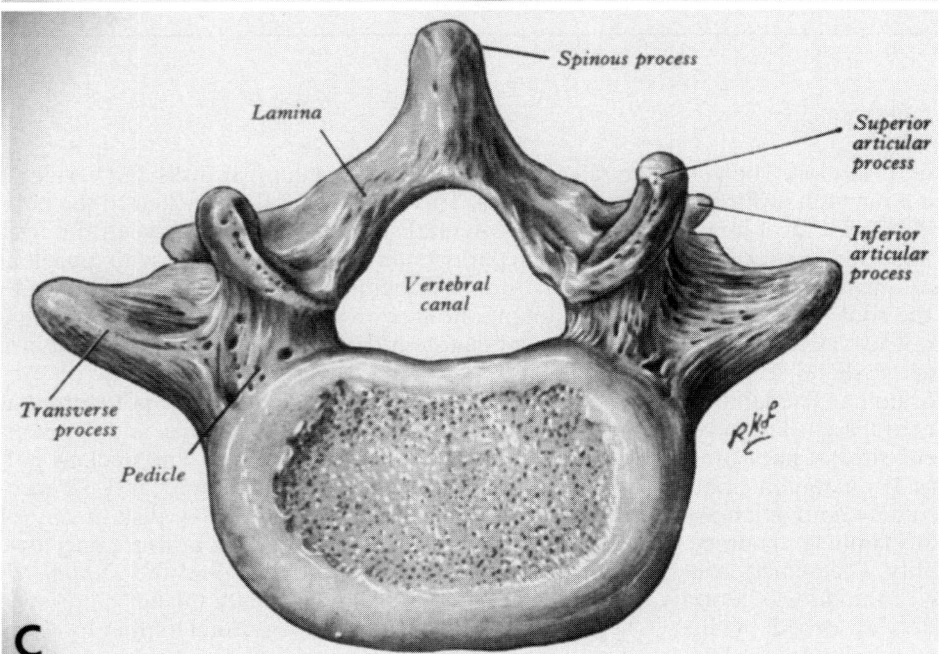

FIGURE 40–1. Lumbar vertebra. *A.* Left lateral aspect. *B.* Posterosuperior aspect, viewed obliquely from the left side. *C.* Superior aspect of the fifth lumbar vertebra. (From Williams PL, Warwick R: Gray's Anatomy, ed 36. Edinburgh, Churchill Livingstone, 1980, p 277. By permission of Longman Group.)

three decades. Thereafter, the disk nutrition is supported only through the lymphatics and by extracellular fluid osmosis. This lack of support may be responsible, at least in part, for loss of water from disks with advancing age. The water content of a disk in young persons is 88%, but it is reduced to less than 70% in the elderly.[68]

Functionally, the spine is composed of a series of mechanical units. Each unit consists of an anterior segment (two adjacent vertebral bodies and the intervertebral disks between them) and a posterior segment (neural arches). The anterior segment is primarily the weight-bearing and shock-absorbing component, whereas the posterior segment protects the neural structures and directs movements of the units in flexion and extension. The amount of force exerted on the spine can vary depending on the type of activity and posture. Figure 40–2 demonstrates relative changes in L3 disk pressures in various positions and during various muscle-strengthening exercises.[105, 106]

MUSCLES SUPPORTING THE SPINE AND THEIR FUNCTION

Muscle Groups

Four groups of muscles provide support to the spine: the extensors, the flexors, the lateral flexors, and the rotators of the spine. Normally, the extensors and rotators are the main supportive muscles of the spine.[13, 129] The massive musculotendinous bulk over the upper sacral and lower lumbar vertebrae is the origin of the erector spinae muscles, which extend the vertebral column. Deep to the erector spinae lie the semispinalis muscles (Fig. 40–3). The interspinal muscles are between spinous processes. The main role of the back muscles in erect posture is to resist gravity. When a movement of the spine is initiated, and once the vertebral column is bent far enough in any direction, the muscles of the back that resist this movement must actively contract to provide smooth and controlled movements and also to prevent falling. Some muscles that have no vertebral attachments also participate in movements of the spine. The abdominal muscles are the significant flexors and lateral flexors of the trunk and also participate in rotation.

Normal Posture

In normal posture, the line of gravity passes from C1 to C7 vertebral bodies to T10 and the lumbosacral junction and passes through the common axis of the hip joint or slightly behind it. It passes in front of the sacroiliac articulation and knee joint and then in front of the ankle joint. An increase in lumbar lordosis causes an increase in pelvic inclination, which can produce a protrusion of the abdominal wall. If pelvic inclination is reduced through flattening of the lumbar curve, the line of gravity is shifted forward. Any shift from standard alignment of the spine requires increased muscular activity to maintain posture as close to the line of gravity as possible. Posture is maintained through backward and forward swaying of the line of gravity. Normally, this sway has only a limited range.[148] Therefore, in comparison with other postural changes, normal posture requires the least amount of paraspinal muscular recruitment.

EVALUATION OF THE PATIENT WITH LOW BACK PAIN

Clinical Evaluation

History

At the very least, the following information should be gathered:

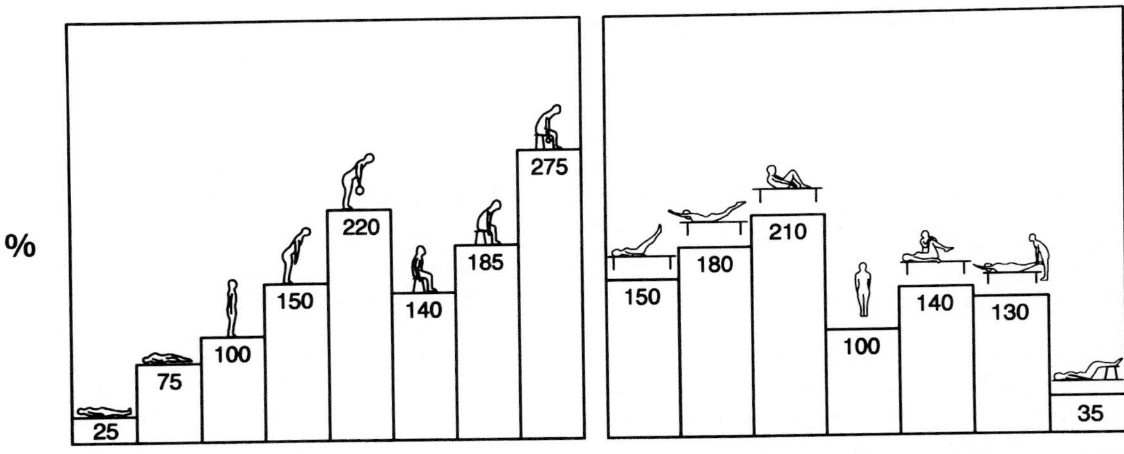

FIGURE 40–2. *Left.* Relative change in pressure (or load) in the third lumbar disk in various positions in living subjects. *Right.* Relative change in pressure (or load) in the third lumbar disk during various muscle strengthening exercises in living subjects. Neutral erect posture is considered 100% in the figures; other positions and activities are calculated in relationship to this. (From Nachemson AL: The lumbar spine: An orthopaedic challenge. Spine 1976; 1:59. By permission of Harper & Row.)

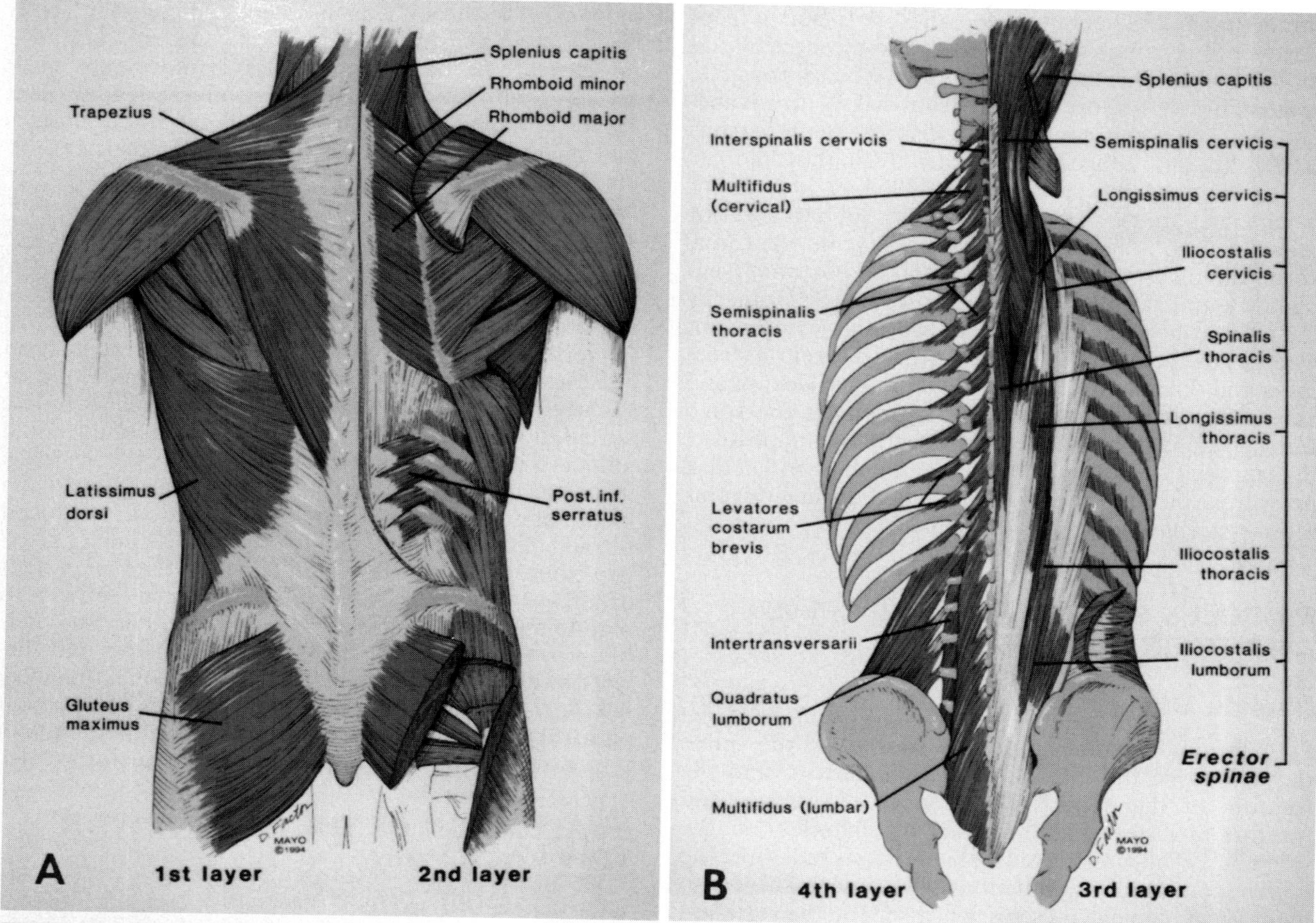

FIGURE 40–3. Muscle anatomy of spine. *A.* First and second layers. Post. inf., posterior inferior. *B.* Third and fourth layers. (By permission of Mayo Foundation.)

Mode of onset of low back pain (abrupt or insidious).
Provoking, aggravating, and relieving factors.
Effect of posture, inactivity, exertion, and rest.
Effect of cough, sneeze, or strain on the low back pain, especially if these cause pain down the lower limbs.
Presence or absence of pain at night and interference with sleep.
Course—whether the pain has been progressive, decreasing, fluctuating, or episodic.
History of similar or different back or lower limb pains.
Associated limb symptoms (pain, paresthesias, numbness, weakness, atrophy, cramps, fasciculations).
Presence or absence of urinary frequency, urgency, or retention; bowel or bladder incontinence; or constipation.
History of lumbar surgery (such as laminectomy or fusion).
Types of treatments implemented, medications used, and the effects of these medications on the symptoms.
Presence or absence of litigation or compensation issues.

Examination

Inspection

Look for deformities, paraspinal spasm, birthmarks, unusual hair growth, listing to one side, corkscrew deformity, decrease or increase in lordosis, presence of scoliosis, muscular atrophy, or asymmetries.

Palpation and Percussion

Determine whether there are tender or trigger points, local tenderness or pain on percussion, spasm, or tightness of the paraspinal muscles. Observe the patient's reaction to pain, whether there is a "touch-me-not" withdrawal to palpation or touch.

Range of Motion

Range of motion should be determined for flexion, extension, lateral bending, and rotation. Values for normal range of motion of the lumbar spine are as follows: flexion, 40 degrees; extension, 15 degrees; lateral bending, 30 degrees; lateral rotation, 40 degrees to each side. Several techniques and instruments can be used for measurement of range of motion of the spine. These range from simple and inexpensive methods to the use of expensive and complicated machines:

Tape Measure Method. Originally described by Schober,[134] this method is a simple and practical way to determine the amount of flexion of the lumbar spine. A line is drawn that connects the "dimples of Venus."

Then, two marks are made along a line that perpendicularly bisects the first line. One mark is 5 cm below and the other 10 cm above the point of bisection, with the distance between these two marks being 15 cm. The patient is then asked to bend forward maximally. The measured distance beyond the original 15 cm gives an estimate of the degree of spinal flexion (Fig. 40–4).[67]

Inclinometers. These were initially introduced by Asmussen and Heebøll-Nielsen[7] for measuring spinal motions and later were further developed by Loebl[84] (Fig. 40–5). This method fails to separate hip motion from spine motion. It is also subject to variability with the subject's effort.[91]

Various electronic and computerized gadgets are available for measurement of spinal range of motion, and many of them also measure muscle strength.

The representative rotations for flexion and extension, lateral bending, and axial rotation are shown in Figure 40–6. This is a composite of what Panjabi et al,[118] on the basis of their studies and extensive review of the literature, consider to be the most representative values for rotation at different levels of the spine in the traditional planes of motion.

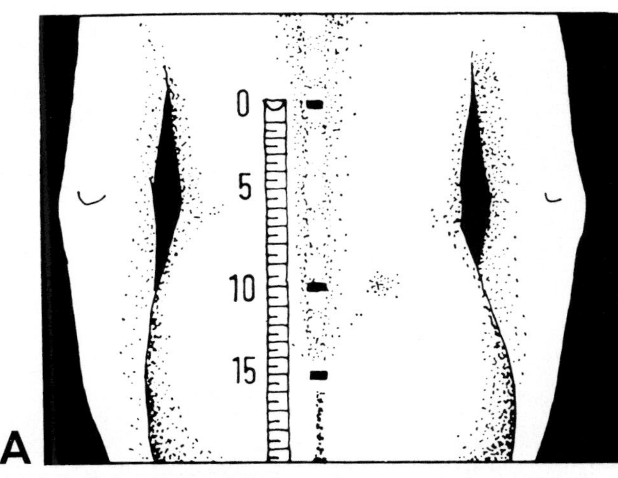

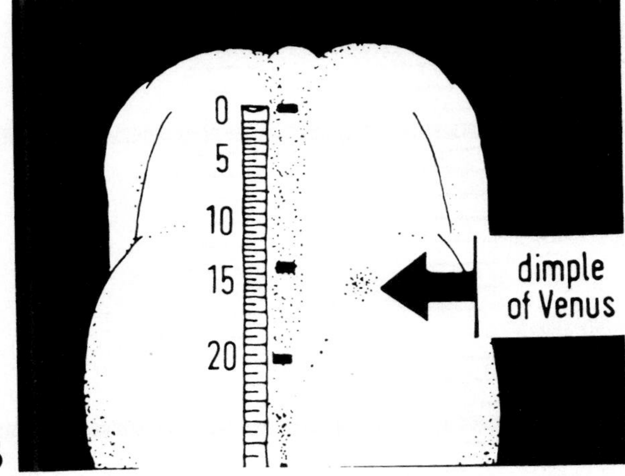

FIGURE 40–4. Modified Schober method to measure anterior flexion. *Top.* Position 1: placing of skin marks. *Bottom.* Position 2: distraction of upper and lower marks on anterior flexion. (From Helliwell P, Moll J, Wright V: Measurement of spinal movement and function. In Jayson M (ed): The Lumbar Spine and Back Pain, ed 4. New York, Churchill Livingstone, 1992, pp 173–205. By permission of the publisher.)

Neurological Examination

This is a very important part of the evaluation of patients with low back pain.[34]

Gait, Station, and Coordination

Gait is a complex activity that depends on the integration of several neural mechanisms, but it can also be affected by disturbed posture, disorders of joints, pain, or functional overtone. One should look for antalgic gait, footdrop, and functional or hysterical features. The patient should do toe-walking, heel-walking, and tandem gait. It should be determined whether the patient can stand on either foot or can squat and rise. Alternate-motion rates are to be done rapidly and regularly. They depend on an intact sensory motor system. These can also be affected by pain, diseases of joints, insufficient effort, poor cooperation, and functional factors.

Muscle Stretch Reflexes

An increase, decrease, or absence of muscle stretch reflexes should be recorded. Neither a decrease nor an increase of these reflexes in itself can be interpreted as definitely abnormal. Neurologically normal persons can have exaggerated, diminished, or even absent reflexes. A patient's reflexes must be compared with other muscle stretch reflexes, particularly of the corresponding opposite side. Reflex asymmetry, however, is most often significant.

Muscle Bulk

Inspect for muscle atrophy. Comparison of the circumference of the lower limbs, determined with a tape measure, at different levels (such as mid-calf level) is sometimes useful. One should also look for muscle fasciculations.

Muscle Strength

It is important to determine whether the muscle weakness is genuine or whether it is a giving-way as the result of pain, functional factors, or poor effort. It should be noted whether the distribution of the weakness corresponds to a single root or multiple roots or to a peripheral nerve or plexus, or whether the weakness is of upper motor neuron type.

Sensory Examination

This is the least reliable part of the neurological examination. It should be done at the end of the examination, when the examiner typically already has some impression about the disorder affecting the patient. Asking the patient to outline areas of sensory loss may help orient the examiner and save time. The nature of the

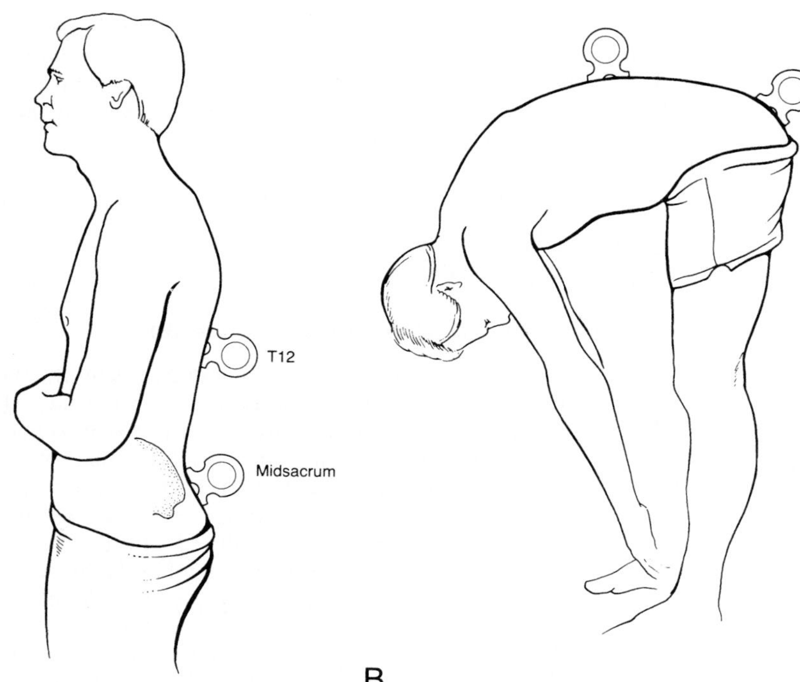

FIGURE 40–5. Loebl measurements. *A.* Double-inclinometer method: zero starting position. The inclinometers are aligned over T12 and the sacrum and their gauges are set at 0 degrees. *B.* The subject positions the spine in maximal flexion. The degrees recorded on the sacral inclinometer are subtracted from the degrees recorded on the inclinometer positioned over the T12 spinous process. (From Greene WB, Hackman JD: The Clinical Measurement of Joint Motion. Rosemont, IL, American Academy of Orthopaedic Surgeons, 1994, p 86. By permission of the Academy.)

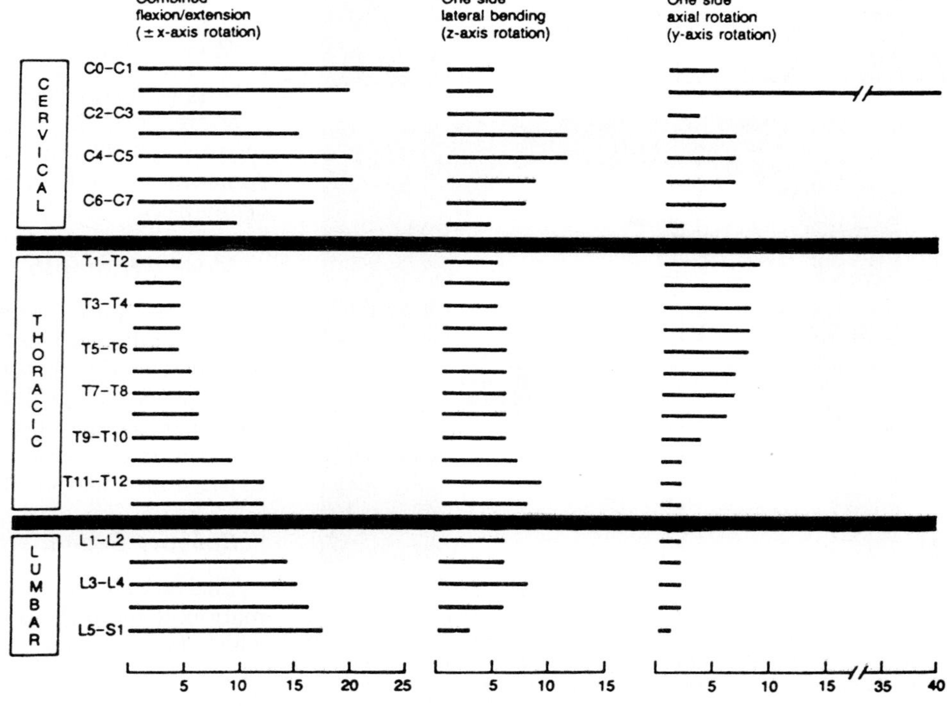

FIGURE 40–6. Representative values for rotation at different levels of the spine in traditional planes of motion. (From Panjabi MM, Hult JE, Crisco JJ III, et al: Biomechanical studies in cadaveric spines. In Jayson MIV (ed): The Lumbar Spine and Back Pain, ed 4. New York, Churchill Livingstone, 1992, pp 133–155. By permission of the publisher.)

sensory tests should be carefully explained to the patient. Determine whether the reported sensory changes are consistent and reproducible, and whether they follow anatomical dermatomal patterns (although they may be noted in only part of a dermatome).

Straight-Leg-Raising Test

At least one of the variations of this test should be done in all cases. The test (also called the Lasègue test) is done with the patient supine in bed or on an examining table. The relaxed lower limb in extension is gently and gradually elevated, and the patient is instructed to inform the examiner when the pain occurs and also to report the location of the pain. Sometimes, if the patient is sitting on an examining table or a chair (and therefore the hips and knees are flexed, each at about 90 degrees), gently bringing the knee into extension often produces the same type of pain as does the straight-leg-raising test in a patient with L5 or S1 radiculopathy. Sometimes elevation of the asymptomatic lower extremity causes pain in the symptomatic side ("well-leg" or crossed straight-leg-raising sign). This is often a reliable sign of root irritation.

The fabere test, an acronym for *f*lexion, *ab*duction, *e*xternal *r*otation, and *e*xtension, is done to look for any associated hip disease. It is also known as Patrick's test.

Diagnostic Studies

Plain Radiography

Despite the increasing availability and use of computed tomography (CT) and magnetic resonance imaging (MRI), plain radiography is still useful as a quick and less costly screening study. It is helpful for detecting fractures, dislocations, degenerative joint disease, spondylolisthesis, narrowing of intervertebral disk space, and many bony diseases and tumors of the spine. Oblique views are helpful for visualizing the neural foramina. Flexion and extension views are useful for studying subluxations and stability. Changes of degenerative joint disease are fairly common, especially in persons past middle age. Therefore, this finding might not necessarily explain the patient's symptoms. Clinical judgment is required to determine any causal relationship (Fig. 40–7).[92]

Radioisotope Bone Scanning

Radioisotope scanning is a valuable test for screening the entire or a large part of the skeleton. It is useful for the detection of tumors, particularly bony metastases. Gallium scanning is used if infection is suspected.

CT and MRI

Both CT and MRI are useful for detecting disk disease, herniated or extruded disk, or tumors (vertebral, epidural, meningeal, intradural, or cord). Overall, MRI (especially with gadolinium enhancement) is superior to CT. MRI can image the entire lumbar spine in a single scanning session and shows the soft tissues better than CT. It is an excellent method for detecting epidural, intradural, and some of the intra-axial spinal cord lesions, such as tumor, cyst, or even demyelinating plaques. CT can define or demonstrate bony lesions better.

Myelography

The use of CT and, especially, MRI has decreased the use of myelography. This test is, however, still used by many surgeons before a final decision is made regarding lumbar surgery. CT-myelography has added to the accuracy of the test by detecting more subtle intraspinal

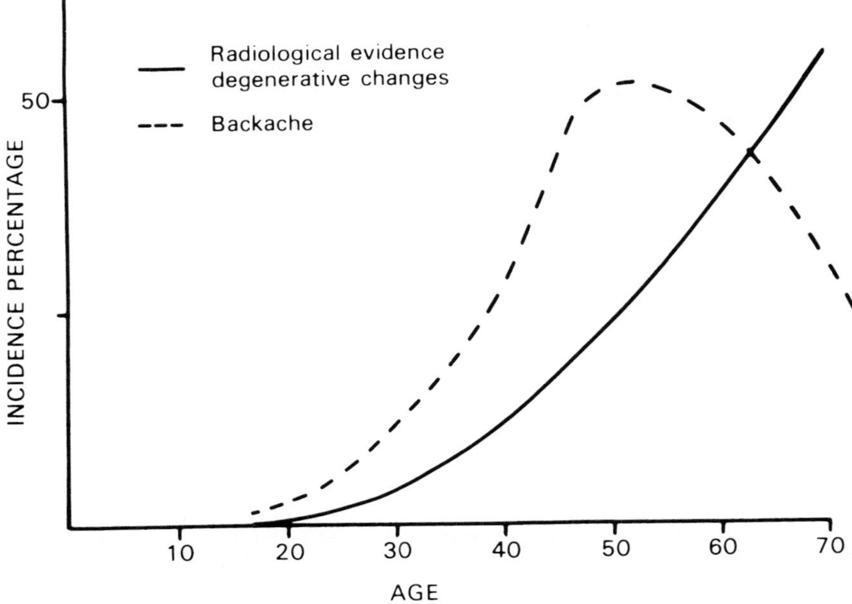

FIGURE 40–7. Incidence of radiologically demonstrable degenerative changes in lumbar spine and back pain with age. Although changes in lumbar spine increase with age, maximal incidence of back pain has a peak at age 45 years, and thereafter tends to decline. (From Macnab I: Backache, Baltimore, Williams & Wilkins, 1977, p 90. By permission of Lippincott Williams & Wilkins.)

lesions. CT-myelography remains the most accurate imaging method for the diagnosis of disk herniations and extrusions.

Electromyography

Electrodiagnostic studies are useful for detecting neurogenic changes and denervation, as well as for evaluating the extent of these changes and the level of involvement. Unlike imaging studies, electrodiagnostic studies provide physiological information (see Chapters 10, 11, and 12).

SOME COMMONLY ENCOUNTERED PAINFUL DISORDERS OF THE SPINE

Mechanical Low Back Pain

Mechanical low back pain is a descriptive term commonly used for nondiscogenic back pain that is provoked by physical activity and relieved by rest. It does not point to a single or particular cause. Although sometimes over-used, the term is practically useful. This type of pain is often due to stress or strain to the back muscles, tendons, and ligaments and is usually attributed to strenous daily activities, heavy lifting, or prolonged standing or sitting. Mechanical low back pain is often a chronic, dull, aching pain of varying intensity that affects the lower spine and might spread to the buttocks. The pain often progressively worsens during the day because daily physical activities such as bending, twisting, lifting, prolonged sitting, and standing often aggravate the pain. There are no associated neurological symptoms or signs, nor is there a cough or sneeze effect on the lower limbs.[97]

Deconditioning and decompensation can also cause a mechanical type of low back pain. Indeed, this decompensation syndrome is one of the most common causes of low back pain. The onset is often insidious, the patients are usually obese and display manifestations of chronic inactivity, and the back and abdominal muscles are weak. These patients demonstrate much difficulty or even inability in performing a situp, a hook-lying situp, a leg lift for 10 seconds at 30 degrees, a prone torso lift for 10 seconds, a prone leg lift for 10 seconds, or one slow toe touch in the standing position. Patients with deconditioning or decompensation syndrome fail at least one of these maneuvers and often fail several of them. Overall, for the management of mechanical low back pain, correction of static or dynamic postural abnormalities is helpful. An exercise program consisting of abdominal and back strengthening exercise is necessary, and patients often improve quickly (Fig. 40–8).

Osteoarthritis

Osteoarthritis, also known as degenerative joint disease, occurs with aging and can begin during the third decade of life.[42] Lumbar osteoarthritis can remain asymptomatic. If the disease is symptomatic, the associated pain is centered in the lower back and is often increased with movement of the spine. Stiffness, morning stiffness, and stiffness after having been in one position for an extended period are common. Range of motion of the spine may be limited. Pain is often relieved by rest. Hypertrophic changes and spurs can compress nerve roots and cause additional radicular pain. Radiographs, particularly after the early stages, are diagnostic. Improvement in spinal muscle support through proper strengthening exercises can alleviate pain. Improvement and provision of proper static and dynamic posture principles, such as bending one knee during prolonged standing (such as by placing one foot on a low stool), provide pain relief and decrease the risk of further strain (Fig. 40–9). When muscle support is poor, the application of an elastic support to control pain is advisable. The back support can be used for 6 weeks while attempts are made to improve the strength of the supporting muscles. The back support enables the patient to be more mobile and prevents prolonged immobility due to pain. Exercises include abdominal and back muscle strengthening exercises (preferably isometric exercises).

Osteoarthritis of the Facet Joints

Osteoarthritis of the facet joints results in localized spine pain, often episodic, that sometimes extends to the limb and can mimic radicular pain. The onset of each attack is usually abrupt. Range of motion, especially with extension, is often limited. In some cases, facet joint osteoarthritis, more diffuse osteoarthritis, and even degenerative disk disease can coexist. Pain is increased with activity and relieved by rest. Surgery is rarely indicated. Nonsteroidal anti-inflammatory drugs (NSAIDs) often help, and manipulation can at times give dramatic relief. Some patients may benefit from facet joint injection. Spontaneous improvement is not unusual. Most patients can achieve relief of pain to a tolerable level with a carefully adjusted program of weight control, rest, analgesics, or NSAIDs. Back pain in patients with degenerative disease of the facet joints can be induced with lumbar extension maneuvers. Conservative treatment is directed toward reducing the hyperextension. Therefore, hyperextension exercises are not recommended for these patients (see Fig. 40–8E). Improvement in abdominal muscle strength and isometric contraction of the quadratus lumborum with pelvic tilt exercises place the sacrum in a more vertical position. If flexion contractures of the hips are present, they need to be reduced through Thomas stretch maneuvers.

Patients with facet joint pain are instructed to avoid sleeping in the prone position. When bending over a wash basin, slightly elevating one foot by placing it on a low stool with the knee bent can decrease lumbar strain (see Fig. 40–9A). In general, the objective of exercise is to develop the supportive muscles of the lumbosacral spine. The properly prescribed exercises are performed once or twice a day (see Figs. 40–8A through C). The maximal effect of strengthening exercises appears in 6 weeks.[100] After 6 weeks, exercises may be performed three times per week to maintain the achieved level of strength. In cases of severe low back pain, application of a lumbosacral support can

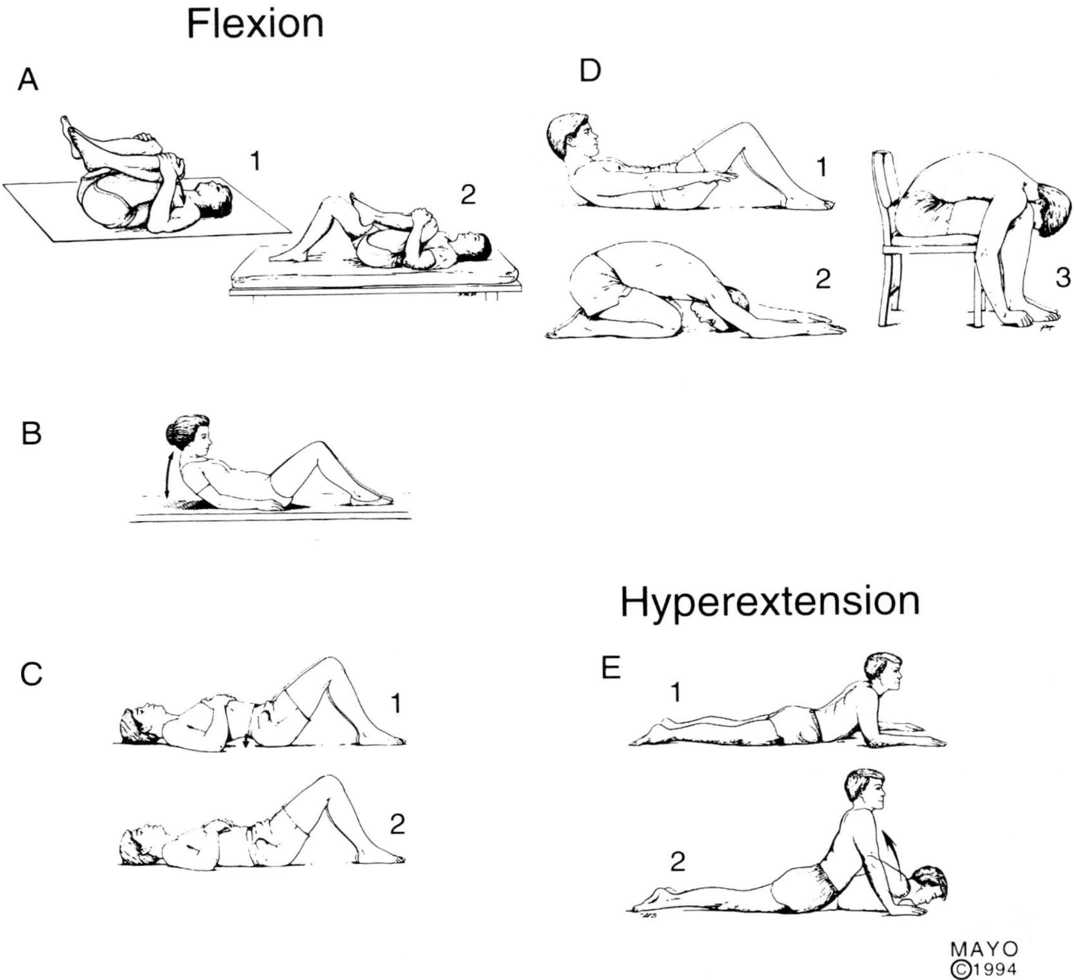

FIGURE 40–8. Back-strengthening exercises. *A–D.* Flexion exercises. *A.* Knee to chest—both knees (*1*) or one knee at a time to avoid strain (*2*). *B.* Isotonic abdominal strengthening. *C.* Pelvic tilt to reduce lumbar lordosis. *D.* Flexion exercises for spondylolisthesis. *E.* Extension exercise. Prone passive extension—on elbows (*1*) or hyperextension (*2*). (*A* from Low Back Stretches, handout no. MC 1899/R38, Mayo Foundation for Medical Education and Research, 1990. By permission of Mayo Foundation for Medical Education and Research. *B* from Sinaki M: Exercise and physical therapy. In Riggs BL, Melton LJ III (eds): Etiology, Diagnosis, and Management. New York, Raven Press, 1988, pp 457–479. By permission of Mayo Foundation. *D1* and *D3* from Sinaki M, Lutness MP, Ilstrup DM, et al: Lumbar spondylolisthesis: Retrospective comparison and 3-year follow-up of two conservative treatment programs. Arch Phys Med Rehabil 1989; 70:594. By permission of Mayo Foundation. *D2* from Sinaki M: Metabolic bone disease. In Sinaki M (ed): Basic Clinical Rehabilitation Medicine, ed 2. St Louis, Mosby–Year Book, 1993, pp 209–236. By permission of Mayo Foundation. *E* from Low Back Extension Exercises, handout no. MC 2032/R789. Mayo Foundation for Medical Education and Research, 1989. By permission of Mayo Foundation for Medical Education and Research.)

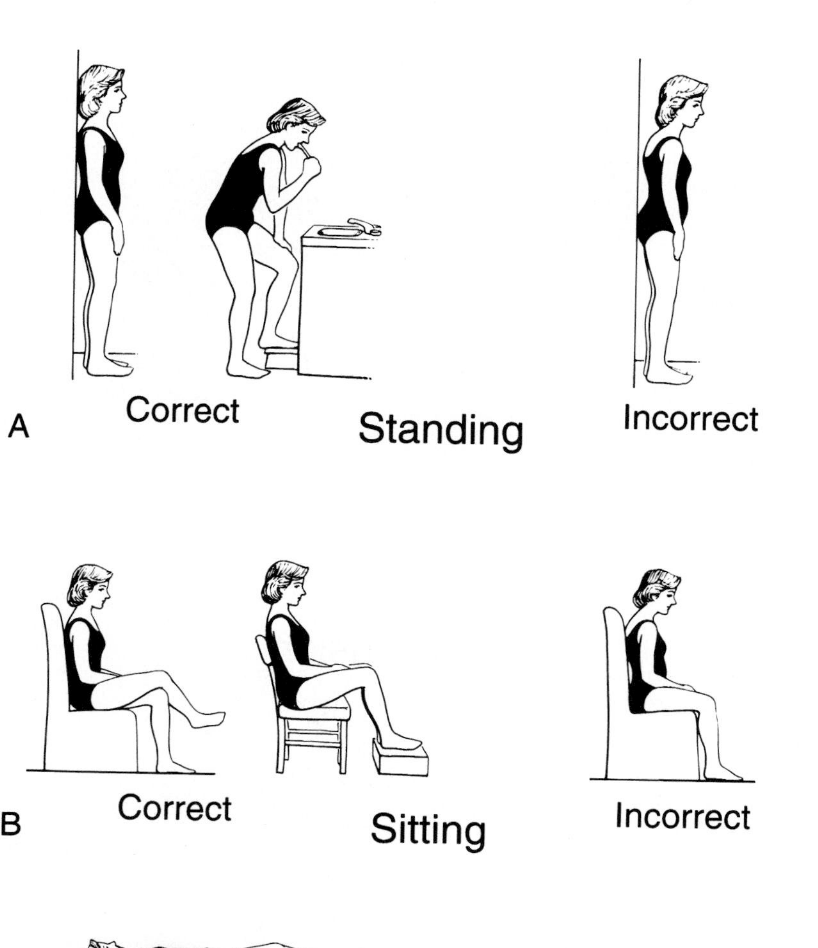

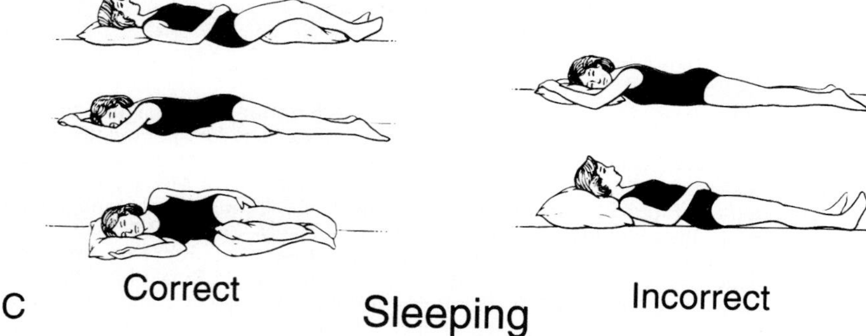

FIGURE 40–9. *A*–I. Static and dynamic correct and incorrect postures (developed by M. Sinaki). (By permission of Mayo Foundation.)

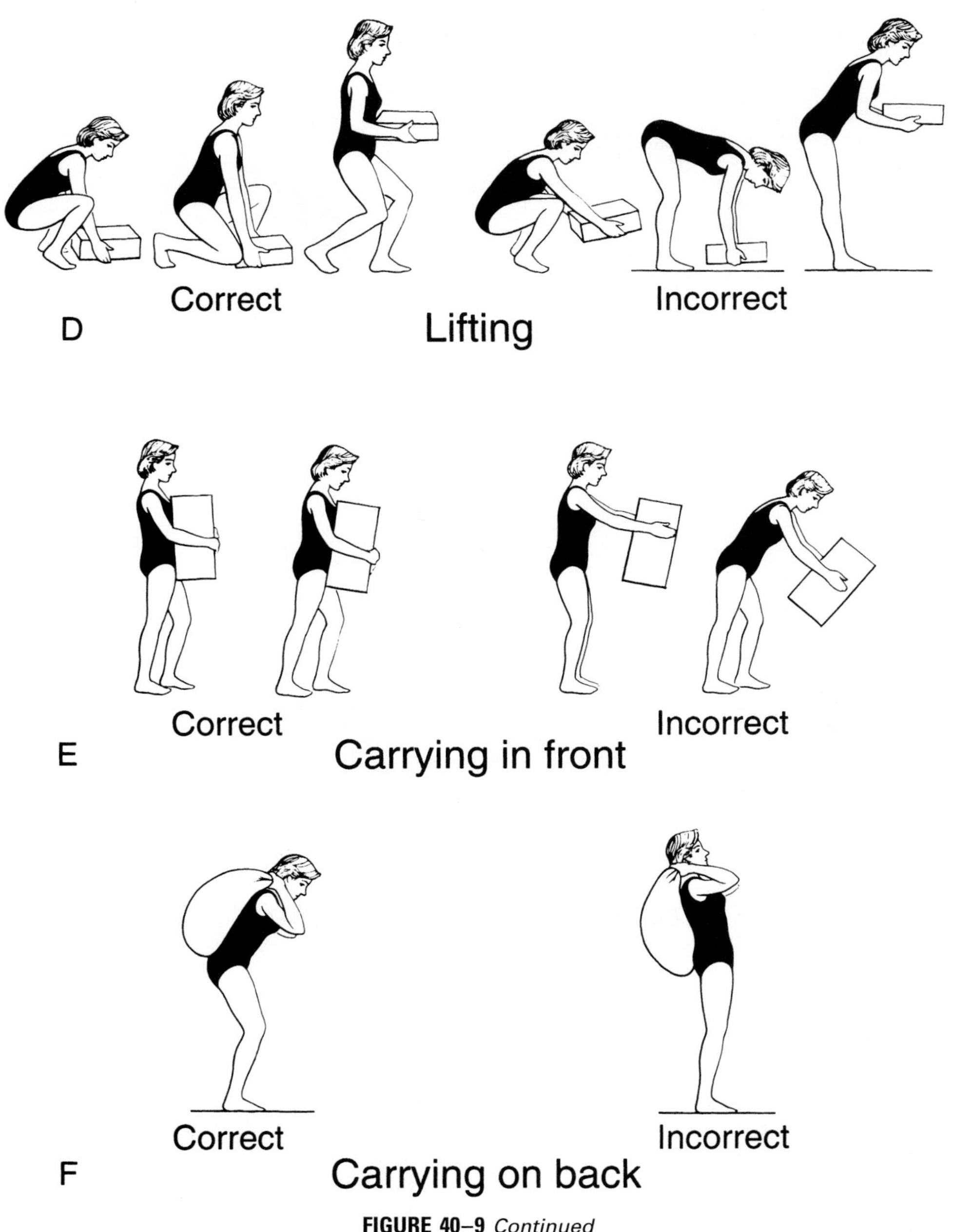

FIGURE 40–9 *Continued*

Illustration continued on following page

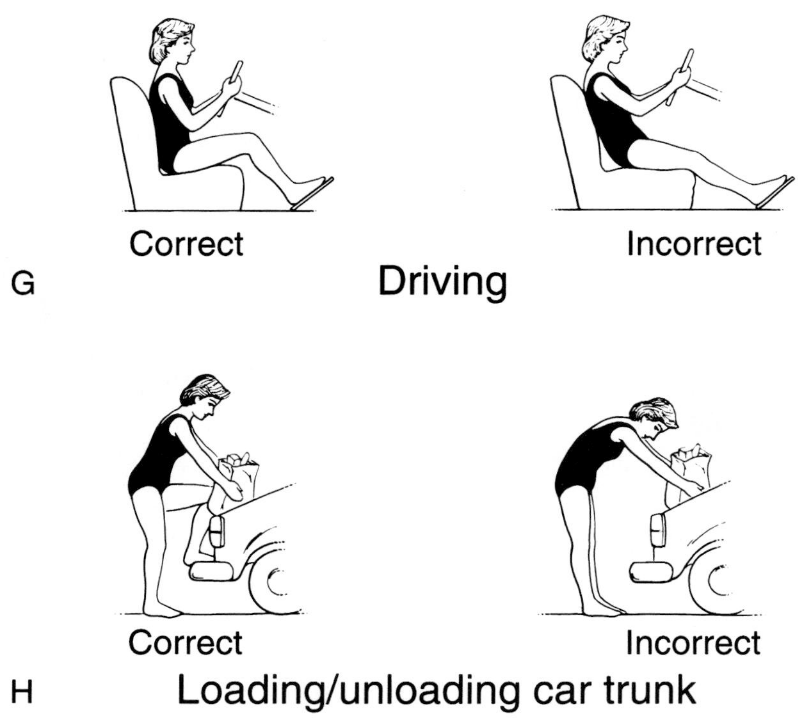

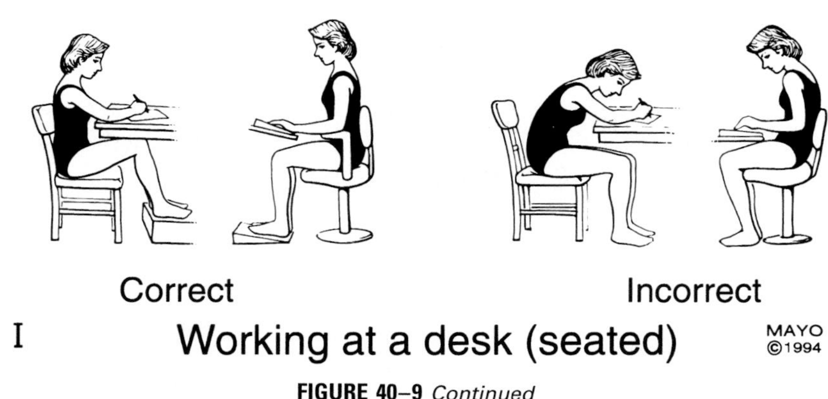

FIGURE 40–9 *Continued*

decrease pain and improve compliance with the exercise program. However, prolonged use of a back support (more than 3 weeks) is discouraged because muscle disuse can result.

Lumbar Disk Syndrome and Lumbosacral Radiculopathies

Lumbar disk syndrome is a common cause of acute, chronic, or recurrent low back pain,[52, 136] particularly in young to middle-aged men, but it also occurs in women, older persons, and even adolescents, especially if they are involved in strenuous physical activity. Overall, the mean age of the patient with lumbar disk herniation is the early 40s. Disk herniation can occur in the midline, but it often occurs to one side. Pain may be unilateral, bilateral, or bilateral but more prominent on one side. The cause is usually a flexion injury. Repetitive injury results in degeneration of the posterior longitudinal ligaments and annulus fibrosus.

Irritation or compression of an adjacent nerve root can occur, as is often the case with laterally extruded ("squeezed toothpaste") disk herniations (Figs. 40–10 and 40–11). Different degrees and types of disk herniation can occur. Macnab's classification is useful, and it indeed correlates well with MRI findings.[90, 159]

Bulging Disk. A bulge and convexity of the disk beyond the adjacent vertebral disk margins, but with an intact annulus fibrosus and Sharpey's fibers (Fig. 40–12A).

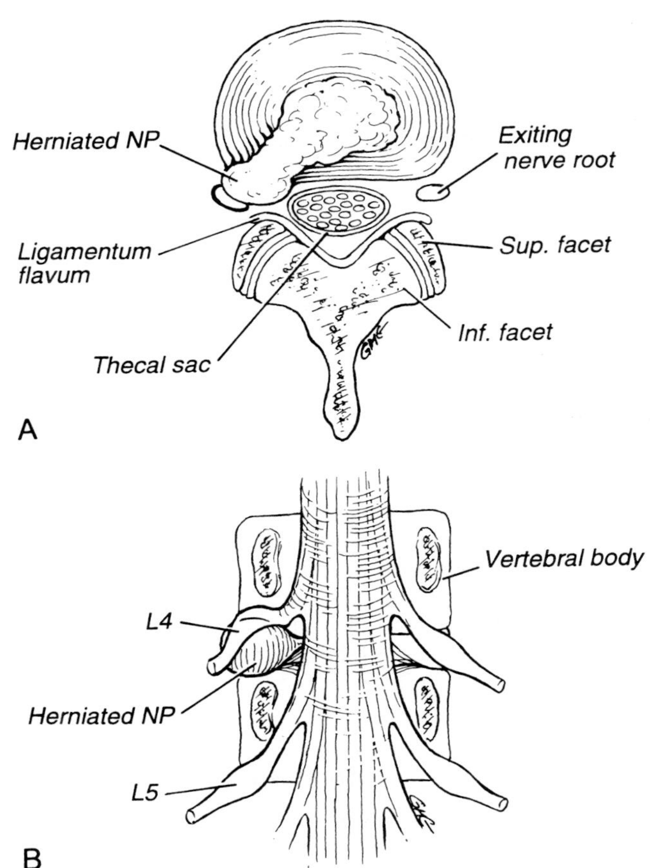

FIGURE 40–10. Lateral disk herniation. *A* and *B*. Lateral disk herniation, impinges on exiting nerve root, causing radicular symptoms. Inf., inferior; NP, nucleus pulposus; Sup., superior. (From Vanderburgh DF, Kelly WM: Radiographic assessment of discogenic disease of the spine. Neurosurg Clin North Am 1993; 4:13.)

Prolapsed Disk. The disk herniates posteriorly through an incomplete defect in the annulus fibrosus (see Fig. 40–12B).

Extruded Disk. The disk herniates posteriorly through a complete defect in the annulus fibrosus (see Fig. 40–12C).

Sequestered Disk. Part of the nucleus pulposus is extruded through a complete defect in the annulus fibrosus and has lost continuity with the present nucleus pulposus (see Fig. 40–12D).

The pain often radiates into the buttock, the posterior thigh, and lateral calf or to lateral or medial malleoli (in cases of L5 or S1 radiculopathies). This pain follows the path of the sciatic nerve and is often referred to as *sciatica.* The pain radiates to the anterior thigh in L3 or L4 radiculopathies. When the disk is extruded, the low back pain is sometimes decreased or even relieved, but the radicular limb symptoms become more prominent. About 5% to 10% of patients with root lesions do not have associated back pain. In these cases, a mononeuropathy (such as sciatica, femoral neuropathy, or obturator neuropathy) or a lumbosacral plexus lesion has to be ruled out. Diabetic lumbar polyradiculopathy sometimes is also part of the differential diagnosis.

The most common levels of lumbar disk protrusion, herniation, or extrusion, in decreasing order of frequency, are L5–S1, L4–L5, L3–L4, and L2–L3. Therefore, the most common lumbosacral radiculopathies related to lumbar disk herniation are L3, L4, L5, and S1 radiculopathies. Lower lumbar and S1 radiculopathies are usually a result of degeneration or herniation of intervertebral disks[43, 86, 147] and are usually unilateral. Midline disk protrusion may cause low back pain but no significant radiculopathy. Large midline disk herniations can cause bilateral radiculopathies or cauda equina syndrome severe enough to produce sphincter problems. Upper lumbar radiculopathies are less commonly caused by disk disease. When upper lumbar radiculopathy is evaluated, other etiologic factors, particularly neoplastic disease, should be ruled out.

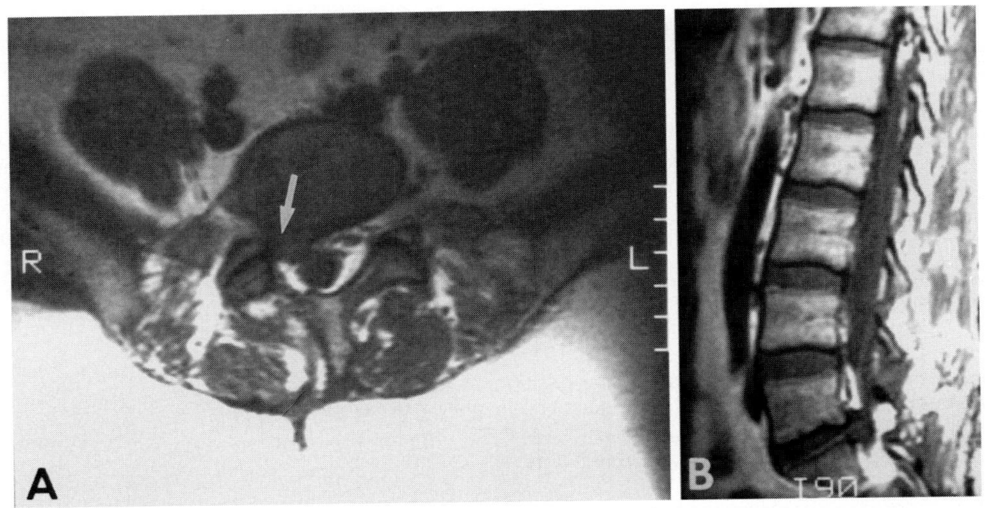

FIGURE 40–11. Recurrent extruded L5 disk, as seen on axial (*A*) and sagittal (*B*) images. Extrusion of disk to the right is well seen on axial image (*arrow* in *A*).

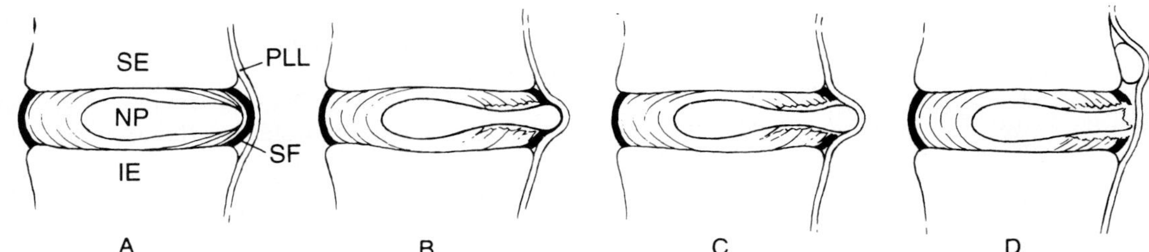

FIGURE 40–12. Classifications of disk herniation. *A.* Bulging annulus fibrosus. *B.* Prolapse. *C.* Extrusion. *D.* Sequestration. IE, inferior end-plate; NP, nucleus pulposus; PLL, posterior longitudinal ligament; SE, superior end-plate; SF, Sharpey's fibers. (From Vanderburgh DF, Kelly WM: Radiographic assessment of discogenic disease of the spine. Neurosurg Clin North Am 1993; 4:13.)

Examination of the back often shows paraspinal muscle spasm, loss of lumbar lordosis, listing of the spine away from the side of root pain, limitation of motions of the lumbar spine with the "corkscrew phenomenon" on flexion and straightening, positive straight-leg-raising test, and, sometimes, crossed straight-leg-raising sign in cases of L5 or S1 radiculopathies. The chin-chest maneuver might cause low back pain because of upward traction on the cord and lower nerve roots. Dorsiflexion of the foot can also cause stretching of the sciatic nerve and therefore stretching of the attached tendon nerve root, leading to pain. The same findings may be noted when the patient tries to perform heel-walking or tries to bend forward. Coughing, sneezing, or straining causes an increase in abdominal pressure leading to distention of epidural and intervertebral veins. These distentions directly compress and put traction on the nerve roots and cause pain, particularly radiation down the involved lower extremity.

When radiculopathy occurs, several features, including distribution of pain, reflex changes, distribution of weakness, and sensory alterations, provide reliable information that enables the clinician to localize the level of disc protrusion or root irritation. Changes in these features as they pertain to each lumbar and sacral nerve root are outlined in Table 40–2.[98]

Laboratory Tests for Lumbosacral Radiculopathies

MRI has become a major diagnostic tool in the diagnosis of herniated lumbar disks (Fig. 40–13). It is also

TABLE 40–2 Clinical Features of Lumbosacral Radiculopathies

Root	Distribution of Pain	Paresthesias or Sensory Loss	Weakness	Decreased or Absent Reflexes
L1	Lower abdomen, groin, or upper anterior medial thigh	Lower abdomen, inguinal region	Iliopsoas (±)	Hypogastric and cremasteric
L2	Groin, anterior or medial thigh	Anterior and medial thigh	Iliopsoas or adductors of thigh or both	
L3	Anterior thigh or knee	Anterior thigh and knee	Quadriceps and thigh adductors	Quadriceps
L4	Can extend below knee, often to inner leg or medial malleolus	Inner leg	Quadriceps and thigh adductors and tibialis anterior (±)	Quadriceps and medial hamstring
L5	Posterolateral thigh, lateral calf to dorsum of foot	Outer leg and dorsum of foot to great toe	Tibialis anterior, toe extensors, and extensor hallucis longus (therefore impaired heel-walking), hamstrings, perinei, and tibialis posterior, gluteus medius	Medial hamstring; ankle jerk often normal, sometimes decreased but not absent because only L5 root lesion
S1	Posterior thigh, calf, and lateral malleolus	Posterior leg, lateral foot, last two toes	Gastrocnemius-soleus and toe flexors (therefore impaired toe-walking), hamstring, gluteus maximus	Ankle jerk and lateral hamstring
S2	Posterior thigh and occasionally calf	Variable posterior thigh and saddle area	Intrinsic foot muscles (±), rectal sphincter (±)	Anal
S3 to S4	Buttock and upper posterior thigh or perianal region	Saddle and perineal area, perianal area	Rectal sphincter	Anal

Abbreviation: ±, weakness may or may not be present due to variability of innervation.

From Mokri B, Sinaki M: Lumbar disk syndrome, lumbosacral radiculopathies, lumbar spondylosis and stenosis, spondylolisthesis. In Sinaki M (ed): Basic Clinical Rehabilitation Medicine, ed 2. St Louis, Mosby–Year Book, 1993, pp 503–513. By permission of Mayo Foundation.

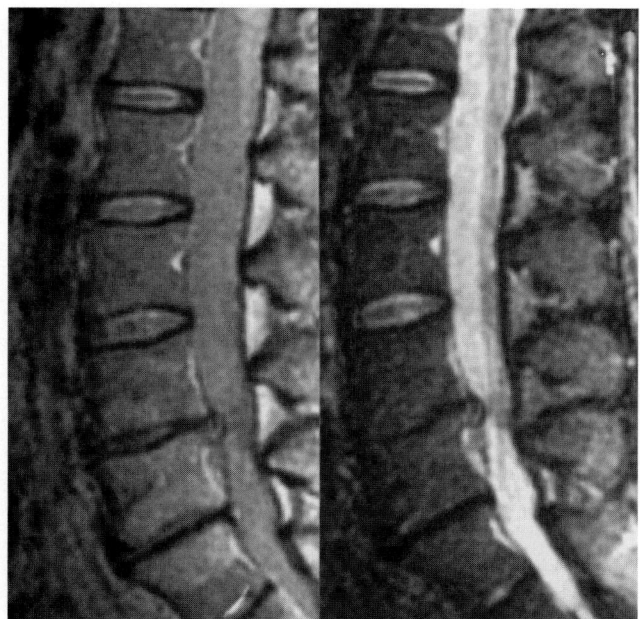

FIGURE 40–13. Magnetic resonance imaging of lumbar spine. T1-weighted (*left*) and T2-weighted (*right*) sagittal images demonstrate extruded L1 disk. (From Mokri B, Sinaki M: Lumbar disc syndrome, lumbosacral radiculopathies, lumbar spondylosis and stenosis, spondylolisthesis. In Sinaki M (ed): Basic Clinical Rehabilitation Medicine, ed 2. St Louis, Mosby–Year Book, 1993, pp 503–513. By permission of Mayo Foundation.)

very useful for demonstrating several nondiscogenic entities that may cause root lesions or enter in the differential diagnosis, including bone disease, vertebral or epidural intraspinal tumors, scar tissue formations, infections, and even some forms of meningeal disease. However, some herniated disks may be missed by MRI.

Myelography still maintains much of its significance. When coupled with CT (CT-myelography), it is still the most accurate imaging test for documentation of herniated disks (Fig. 40–14). Electromyography is very helpful for localizing the level of involvement, determining whether root involvement is single or multiple, and differentiating a multiple root from a plexus lesion.[166]

Treatment

Most patients with discogenic low back pain respond to conservative management. Studies by Saal and Saal[131] and others[39] have shown that most patients with herniated lumbar disk can be treated nonsurgically. The principles of conservative management of back pain are addressed at the end of the chapter.

Operation is considered when definite radiculopathy and neurological deficits are present, especially when they are persistent or progressive. However, in the spectrum of discogenic low back pain, patients in this group are a definite minority. Progressive and significant neurological deficits justify early surgical intervention. Large midline disk protrusions with cauda equina syndrome require urgent treatment and decompression. The success of surgical treatment is greatest when there are bona fide objective neurological deficits. With proper patient selection, about two-thirds have excellent results, and half of the remaining one-third have improvement to some extent. However, in many patients with lumbar disk syndrome, the major difficulty is low back pain with only mild, slight, or no evidence of radiculopathy. Most of these patients respond to conservative management. Lumbar laminectomy and discectomy for the sole complaint of low back pain are often unjustified.[136]

The standard surgical procedure is open laminectomy and discectomy. When there is spondylitic encroach-

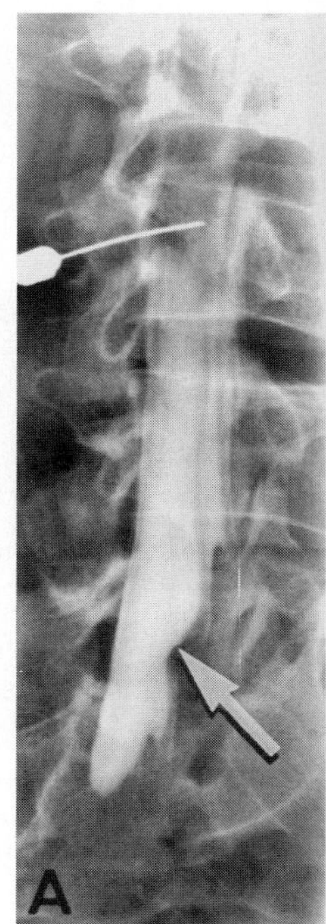

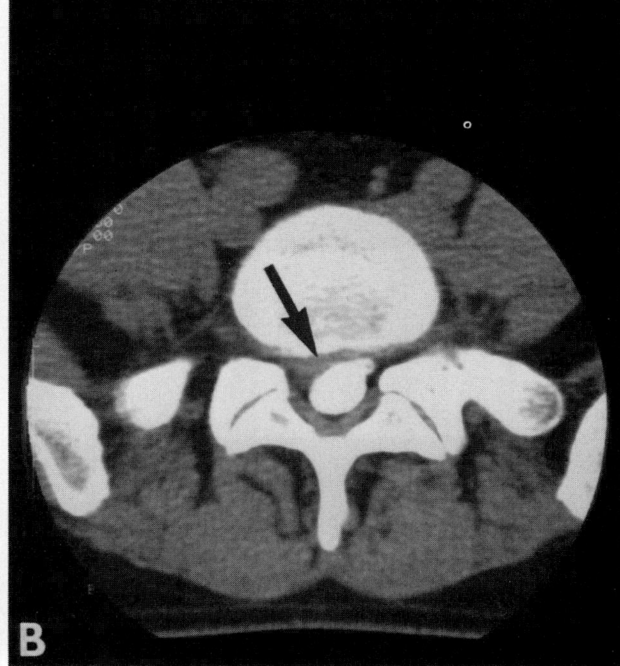

FIGURE 40–14. Extruded L5 disk on right (*arrows*). *A.* Myelogram. *B.* CT-myelogram.

ment, facetectomy and foraminectomy may be necessary, and when there is instability, spinal fusion might be needed.

Microdiscectomy

Microdiscectomy is a generic term without a specific definition and essentially means the use of an operative microscope to accomplish posterior approaches for removal of a herniated lumbar disk through the smallest possible skin incision.[74] The skin incision is usually about 2 cm long. Long-term results from microdiscectomy are not necessarily better than those from standard operation. The initial concerns regarding increased risk of infection with the use of a microscope do not seem to be substantiated by the subsequent experience. The recurrence rate after microdiscectomy is higher than that after standard operation. Proponents of this technique argue that this increase possibly is related to earlier return of the patients to higher levels of activity. As minimally invasive surgical procedures are gaining momentum, an increase in microdiscectomy can be expected.

Percutaneous Lumbar Discectomy

This is another procedure used to treat lumbar disk herniations less invasively and to reduce morbidity.[89] The technique has been claimed to be effective for treating patients with small to moderate-sized, well-contained disk herniation who show clinical and imaging evidence of nerve root compression. A nucleotome is guided into the disk space with precise radiographic control. The disk material is then aspirated, and because the disk is avascular, the aspirated contents should be essentially free of blood. The claimed advantages are use of local anesthesia, minimal tissue disruption, performance on an outpatient basis, earlier return to usual activities, and minimizing the possibility of development of epidural fibrosis and scarring. Misplacement of the probe and serious neurological and vascular complications are feared sequelae. The rate of recurrent symp-

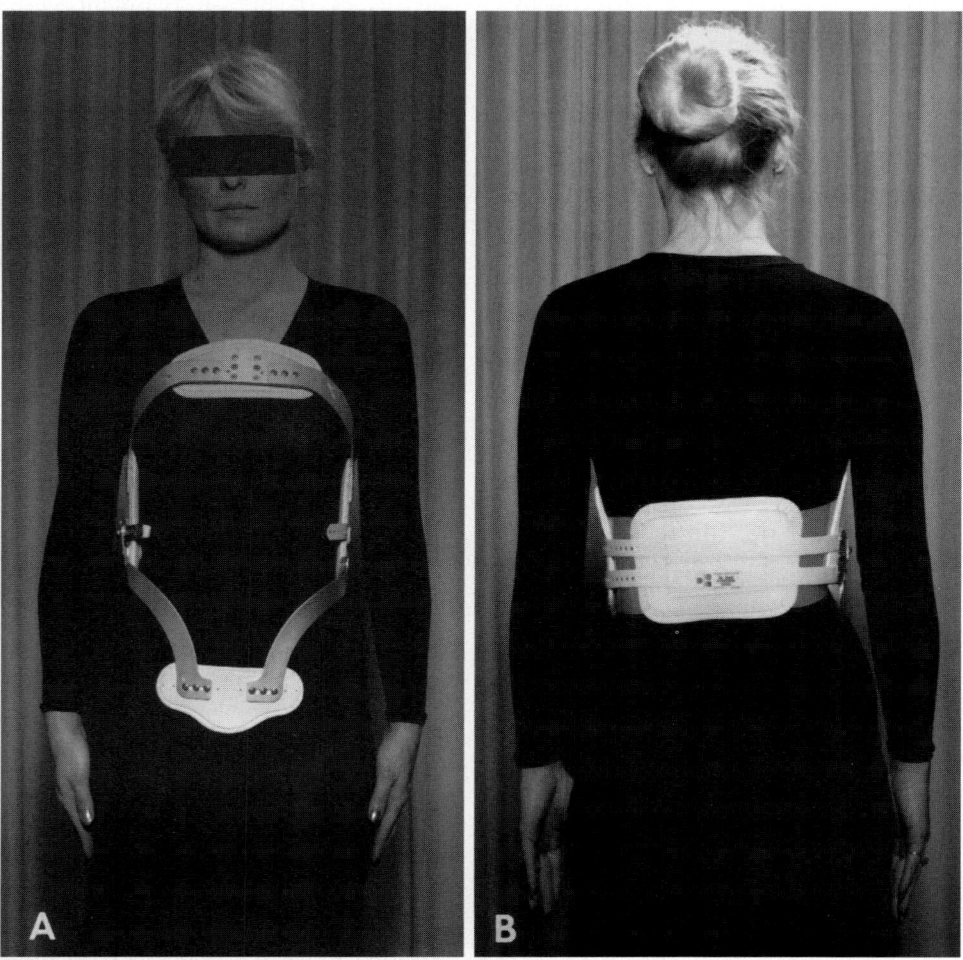

FIGURE 40–15. Jewett brace, used to prevent lumbar and thoracic flexion when patient has acute pain due to recent compression fracture of spine. Proper fitting requires proper contact at base of sternum and over pubic bone. *A.* Anterior view. *B.* Posterior view. (From Sinaki M: Exercise and physical therapy. In Riggs BL, Melton LJ III (eds): Osteoporosis: Etiology, Diagnosis, and Management. New York, Raven Press, 1988, pp 457–479. By permission of Mayo Foundation.)

toms may be high because of missed disk fragments and because of collapse of disk space and exacerbation of spondylitic nerve root compression.[49] The potential for effective treatment with this technique may prove to be limited.

Chemonucleolysis

Chemonucleolysis is less efficacious than open discectomy. Furthermore, it is associated with a significant incidence of anaphylaxis. In a study of 151 patients with L4–5 or L5–S1 disk herniations who were evenly divided between treatment with open discectomy or chemonucleolysis,[158] 22% of the chemonucleolysis group and 0% of the discectomy group had increased radicular pain. Twenty-five percent of the chemonucleolysis group required open discectomy as the result of treatment failure. The resolution of pain in patients who have chemonucleolysis may be related to prolonged inactivity after the procedure and during convalescence.

In a search for less invasive techniques, investigators have utilized laser fiberoptics passed through small-gauge needles to vaporize the herniated disks. More experience is required to determine the practical validity and efficacy of these approaches compared with more established approaches. They may present some of the same problems and limitations associated with percutaneous discectomy.

Posttraumatic Compression Fracture

Posttraumatic compression fracture usually results from compressive flexion trauma. It can also occur spontaneously in patients with osteoporosis, osteomalacia, multiple myeloma, hyperparathyroidism, and metastatic cancer. The upper lumbar spine or the middle to lower thoracic spine is most commonly affected. The pain usually is present immediately after the fracture and is often localized. There may be accompanying paraspinal muscle spasm, and the range of motion of the related level of the spine is limited. Plain radiography, CT, MRI, or bone scanning may be needed to establish the diagnosis.

Sedative rehabilitative measures, especially in the acute phase, including application of cold for the first 24 to 48 hours, analgesics, and muscle relaxants, are often necessary. The pain can be managed with use of a back support, such as a thoracolumbar support that functions on the basis of three-point contact. For provision of extension in cases of thoracic compression fractures, the three points of contact are the base of the sternum, the symphysis pubis, and the lumbar spine, as in the Jewett brace (Fig. 40–15) (see Chapter 17). When therapeutic exercises are to be prescribed, extension rather than flexion exercises should be utilized.[143] Flexion exercises can increase the incidence of vertebral body wedging and compression fractures (see Fig. 40–8C). Extension exercises are effective for strengthening back muscles at any age.[137, 138, 140]

Spondylolysis and Spondylolisthesis

General Considerations

Spondylolysis refers to a bony defect in the pars interarticularis. Bilateral spondylolysis of the lumbar spine can lead to anterior slipping of the vertebral body on its adjacent vertebra and cause spondylolisthesis (in Greek, *spondylo* means "vertebra" and *listhesis* means "sliding on a slippery surface").[14] Even in the absence of all soft tissue attachments, spondylolisthesis does not occur unless there is a defect of the pars interarticularis or unless the pars is elongated.[4, 23, 69, 108, 111, 167] Newman,[111] Wiltse,[167] and Wiltse and associates[168] described five types of spondylolisthesis: (1) dysplastic, (2) isthmic, (3) degenerative, (4) traumatic, and (5) pathological (Table 40–3). To these categories, a sixth category is sometimes added: postsurgical or iatrogenic spondylolisthesis.

Symptoms and Signs

Spondylolysis or spondylolisthesis may cause back pain. However, the presence of a pars defect (spondylolysis) or even spondylolisthesis in a patient with back pain does not necessarily indicate a cause-and-effect relationship (Fig. 40–16). Spondylolisthesis is two to four times more common in males. The pars defect is at L5 in 67% of persons, at L4 in 15% to 30%, and at L3 in 2%. It is rare in the cervical region. In patients with back pain and spondylolisthesis, the back pain is more likely to be due to the pars defect if the patient is younger than 25 years. A pars defect is an uncommon cause of back pain in patients older than 40 years. Pain is common in children and adolescents who have spondylolysis and spondylolisthesis. Spondylolisthesis can also cause compression of nerve roots and lead to radicular pain or neurological deficits in the lower extremities. By narrowing the spinal canal, it can cause pseudoclaudication or compression of the cauda equina and

TABLE 40–3 Classification of Spondylolisthesis

Type	Criteria
I	*Dysplastic:* The only truly congenital form of spondylolisthesis. The defect is a congenital dysplasia in the superior sacral facet or inferior L5 facet that allows L5 on S1 subluxation.
II	*Isthmic:* Defect (spondylosis) in pars interarticularis; the most common form of spondylolisthesis; typically involves L5–S1. a. Lytic type, probably a fatigue fracture with hereditary predisposition. b. Elongated (attenuated) but intact pars, similar to type IIa, but the fatigue fractures have healed, resulting in elongated but intact pars. c. Acute fracture or pars due to trauma.
III	*Degenerative:* Secondary to degenerative changes at the disk and facet joints, most frequent at L4–5, followed by L3–4.
IV	*Traumatic:* Due to fracture of posterior elements other than pars (fractures of facet joints, lamina, pedicles).
V	*Pathological:* Due to pathological changes in posterior elements as a result of malignancy, primary bone disease, or infection.

From Mokri B, Sinaki M: Painful disorders of the spine and back pain syndromes. In Sinaki M (ed): Basic Clinical Rehabilitation Medicine, ed 2. St Louis, Mosby–Year Book, 1993, pp 489–502. By permission of Mayo Foundation.

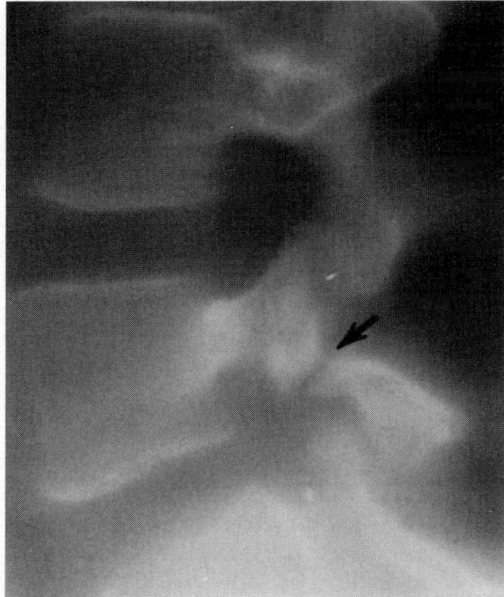

FIGURE 40–16. Incidental finding of unilateral spondylolysis in a 24-year-old woman with Ewing's sarcoma (*arrow*).

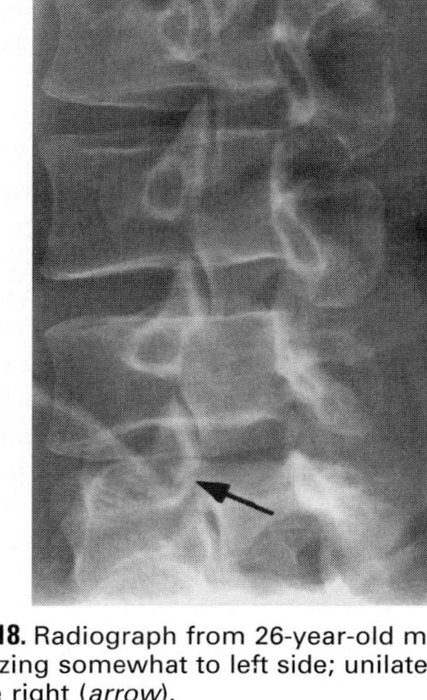

FIGURE 40–18. Radiograph from 26-year-old man with low back pain lateralizing somewhat to left side; unilateral spondylolysis at L5 on the right (*arrow*).

can even lead to sphincter or sexual dysfunction. The lumbar lordosis is often exaggerated in patients with spondylolisthesis, and range of motion of the lumbar spine may be limited. Scoliosis and rotation of the pelvis may be noted. The hamstrings may be tight and, when standing, patients may hold their knees slightly flexed. The frequency of pars defects (spondylolysis) in children is about 4.5% (in adolescents it is about 6%), but it increases to 12% in gymnasts. In children, the most common types are dysplastic and isthmic (Fig. 40–17).[14] Strenous athletic activity in children may lead to fracture of a congenitally weak pars intra-articularis.

Radiographic and Imaging Studies

The defect in the pars intra-articularis, known as *spondylolysis,* is often visible on lateral lumbosacral radiographs and can be noted as a break in the neck of the "Scottie dog" on oblique views of the lumbar spine (Fig. 40–18). Radioisotope bone scan may show increased activity on one or both sides.[87] Sometimes, single-photon emission computed tomography (SPECT) shows a pars defect that is not apparent on radiographs or bone scans.[14]

Spondylolisthesis is graded according to Meyerding's classification[96] as grades 1 to 4, depending on the degree of displacement (Fig. 40–19). In advanced cases of dis-

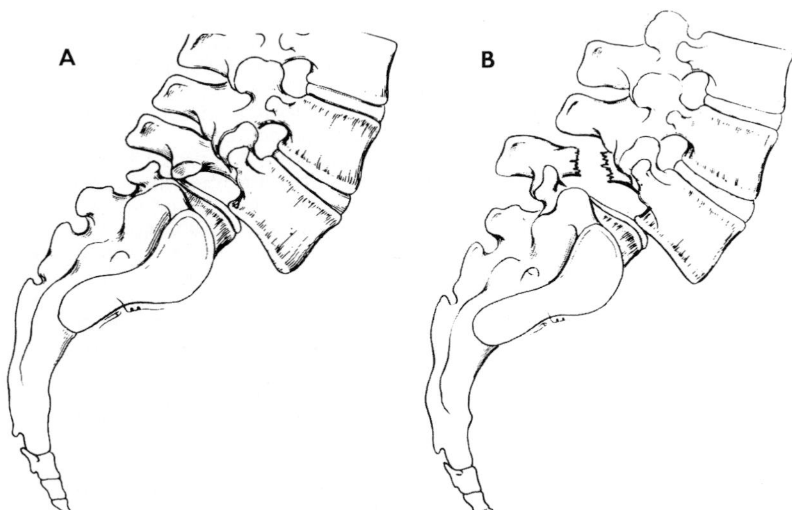

FIGURE 40–17. Dysplastic and isthmic spondylolisthesis. *A.* Dysplastic congenital spondylolisthesis. Note that neural arch of L5 is intact, although somewhat elongated. The primary defect is a deficiency in the development of the superior sacral facet, allowing anterior slippage of L5 on S1. *B.* Isthmic spondylolisthesis. Note that anterior slippage of L5 on S1 occurs because of a defect in the pars interarticularis. (From Hensinger RN: Spondylolysis and spondylolisthesis: Part I. Spondylolysis and spondylolisthesis in children. Instr Course Lect 1983; 32:132.)

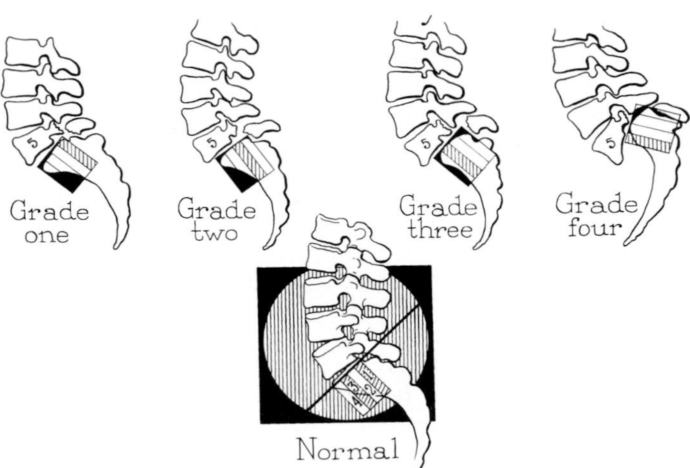

FIGURE 40–19. Meyerding's classification. The degree of subluxation is divided into four groups: grade 1, slipping on the vertebra less than one-fourth the distance of the lumbosacral angle: grade 2, less than half; grade 3, less than three-fourths; and grade 4, more than three-fourths. (From Mokri B, Sinaki M: Painful disorders of the spine and back pain syndromes. In Sinaki M (ed): Basic Clinical Rehabilitation Medicine, ed 2. St Louis, Mosby–Year Book, 1993, pp 489–502. By permission of Mayo Foundation.)

placement, L5 slips completely off S1. Flexion and extension views of the lumbosacral spine are obtained to determine any segmental instability. Evaluation of patients with root symptoms, neurological deficits, or pseudoclaudication calls for further studies, such as CT, MRI, myelography, and electrodiagnostic testing.

Treatment

In posttraumatic cases of spondylolisthesis, after healing of the fracture and resolution of the pain, provision of immobilization for 10 to 12 weeks with application of a custom-made body jacket is the recommended treatment. In cases of chronic back pain, the patient should be instructed in abdominal muscle strengthening, lumbar flexion exercises, and static and dynamic body mechanics. In cases of persistent pain, the application of a lumbosacral brace or corset is recommended. In children, once the symptoms resolve, normal activities can be resumed, although a return to vigorous spine flexion or hyperextension athletic activities (such as football or gymnastics) is controversial.

For grades 1 and 2 spondylolisthesis (Fig. 40–20) and in older patients, nonsurgical treatment is recommended.[58] The physical therapeutic procedures consist of application of heat and massage for reduction of pain

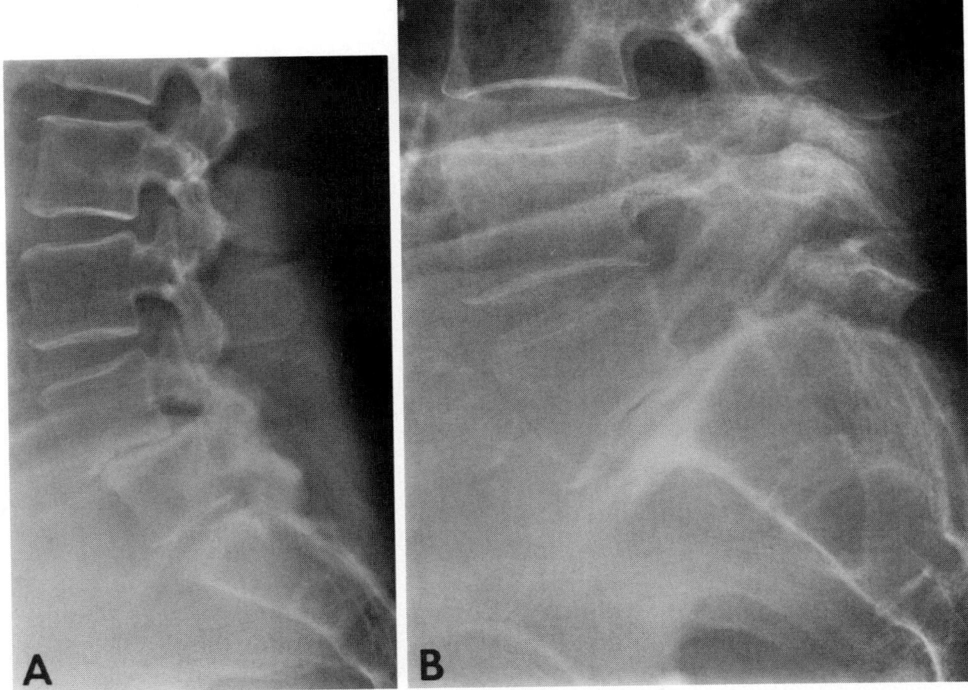

FIGURE 40–20. Grades 1 and 2 spondylolisthesis. *A.* Grade 1. Degenerative disk disease at L4 interspace with anterior subluxation of L4 on L5 due to facet joint degenerative joint disease. *B.* Grade 2, L5 on S1.

and stiffness. Special attention can be given to reducing the tightness of the hip flexors, hamstrings, and Achilles tendons. A program of stretching exercises is recommended. During stretching of the back and lower extremities, flexion of one hip (related knee) at a time helps reduce the strain on the lumbar spine (Fig. 40–21).

In a study to determine the efficacy of conservative management of lumbar spondylolisthesis, two groups of subjects were compared.[142] One group followed a back flexion exercise program (see Figs. 40–8A through C, D1, and D3), and the other group performed extension exercises. At the end of 3 years, 62% of the flexion group considered themselves recovered, whereas none in the extension group did so. The goals of an exercise program should be reduction of lumbar lordosis through stretching of the lumbar paraspinal muscles and other tight structures and strengthening of the lumbar flexors (see Figs. 40–8C1, C2, and D2). Strengthening of abdominal muscles is also of significant benefit. In cases of severe weakness of the abdominal muscles and poor response to strengthening (often seen with significant obesity or previous abdominal operations), application of an elastic lumbosacral support can decrease pain until other measures (such as weight loss or improvement of posture) contribute to reduction of pain.[142]

Spondylolisthesis can become more symptomatic during the advanced months of pregnancy. In such cases, application of an abdominal pregnancy support may help significantly. Flexion exercises are also effective for conservative management of spondylolisthesis in children.[122] In some cases, severe osteoporosis of the spine occurs with degenerative changes of ligamentous structures and spondylolisthesis. In these instances, a therapeutic exercise program that combines dynamic and static posturing along with isometric strengthening of spinal flexors and extensors without inducing strain on the osteoporotic spine has been shown to be helpful.[139]

In younger patients or persons who are involved in heavy physical jobs or strenuous sports activities, and when severe symptomatic slips with neurological symptoms or deficits are present, surgical treatment should be considered. Surgical management includes fusion of the unstable segment. Patients with advanced spondylolisthesis beyond grade 2 may need surgical intervention to decrease the symptoms.[31] Adolescents who have spondylolisthesis of grade 2 or more have a greater risk for progression of the defect.[23] In these patients, serial evaluations must be done to monitor the progress of the listhesis. Once patients experience symptoms of spondylolisthesis, they should not perform heavy work or participate in high-performance, competitive sports. The patients should restrict activities such as heavy lifting, repetitive flexion of the spine, or strenuous pulling activities. Segmental fusion results in relief of pain but does not warrant resumption of strenuous activity, and surgical intervention should not be undertaken for this expectation.

Lumbar Spinal Stenosis

Stenosis of the lumbar spine may involve the central canal at a single level or multiple levels and may jeopardize the cauda equina. Sometimes the stenosis involves

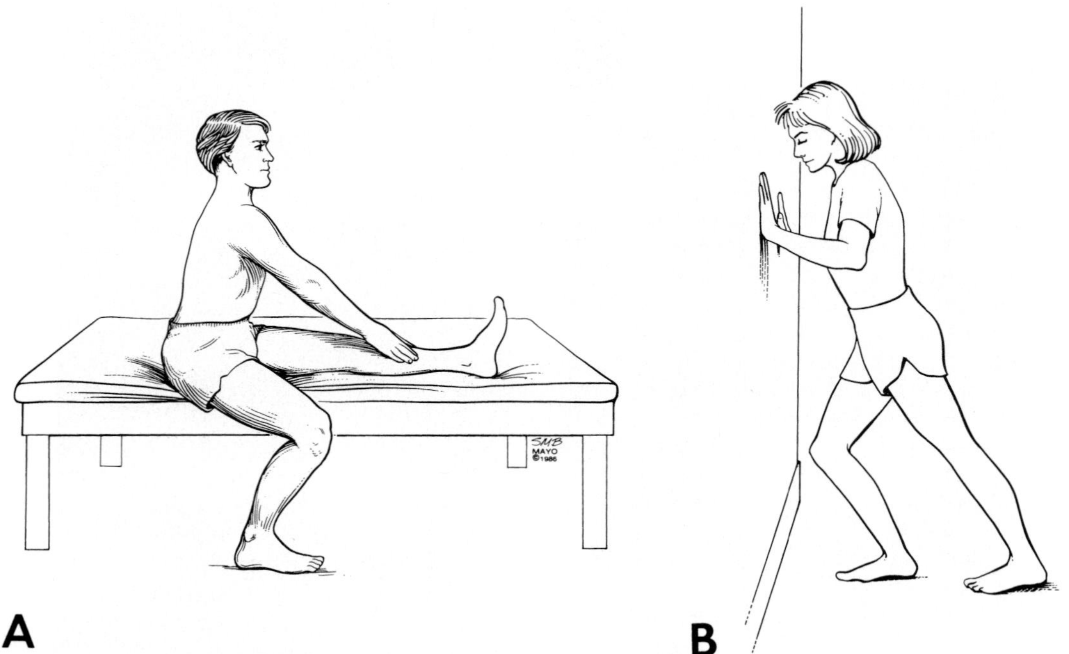

FIGURE 40–21. *A.* Hamstring stretches. For a single-leg stretch, the back is kept straight and the patient leans forward until a gentle stretch is felt behind the knee. Hold for 5 to 20 minutes as needed or as tolerated. *B.* Stretches for Achilles tendons. Patient stands at arm's length from wall with palms flat against the wall. Involved leg is kept back with knee straight and heel flat on floor as tolerated. (From Mokri B, Sinaki M: Painful disorders of the spine and back pain syndromes. In Sinaki M (ed): Basic Clinical Rehabilitation Medicine, ed 2. St Louis, Mosby–Year Book, 1993, pp 489–502. By permission of Mayo Foundation.)

TABLE 40–4 Different Forms of Spinal Stenosis

- I. Primary
  - A. Congenital
  - B. Developmental (various forms of dwarfism)
- II. Secondary
  - A. Degenerative spondylolysis (with or without spondylolisthesis)
  - B. Late sequelae of fracture
  - C. Late sequelae of infection
  - D. Systemic bone disease (Paget's disease of bone)
- III. Mixed
  - A. Spinal stenosis due to degenerative joint disease in an individual with a congenitally narrow spinal canal

From Postacchini F: Lumbar Spinal Stenosis. New York, Springer-Verlag, 1989, p 54. By permission of the publisher.

only the lateral recess or root canal at single or multiple levels and jeopardizes one or more nerve roots. At times, a combination of both may be present. Lumbar spinal stenosis clinically leads to the syndrome of neurogenic claudication (pseudoclaudication). When the stenosis is limited to the lateral recess or root canal, the lateral recess syndrome of root claudication (a variant of spinal stenosis) is produced. Sometimes the two syndromes coexist, but one usually dominates the clinical picture.

Pathophysiology

Spinal stenosis may be congenital, developmental, or acquired[38, 126] (Table 40–4). Because degenerative joint disease is the most common cause of spinal stenosis, the resulting clinical syndromes occur most commonly after middle age.

Degenerative disk disease and narrowing of the intervertebral spaces, spur formation, ligamentous hypertrophy, facet hypertrophy, and subluxation all contribute to the decreased caliber of the central spinal canal, lateral recess, and root canal. Development of degenerative spondylolisthesis and subluxations may further compromise the central spinal canal.[170] With a gradual increase in stenosis, gait endurance is gradually decreased. The caliber of the central spinal canal varies; some persons have congenitally narrow canals and are predisposed to symptoms.

Clinical Manifestations

Lumbar spinal stenosis clinically manifests as pseudoclaudication (neurogenic claudication), with unilateral or bilateral discomfort in the buttocks, thighs, or legs. Symptoms are produced by standing or walking and are relieved within a few minutes by sitting, lying down, or adopting a posture of flexion at the waist. The symptoms can include pain, numbness or paresthesias, or weakness. Combinations of these frequently exist, and low back pain may also be present. The waist-flexion posture is achieved by such maneuvers as backing up to a wall and leaning forward, or leaning forward on a shopping cart or a church pew.[63]

The anteroposterior diameter of the lumbar spinal canal is increased during flexion because of separation of the laminae and a consequent decrease in the thickness of the ligamenta flava. At the same time, as the result of stretching of the posterior aspect of the annulus, particularly in young patients, the bulge of the disk toward the spinal canal is decreased. Lumbar flexion also leads to an increase in the caliber of the intervertebral foramina. The opposite occurs with extension of the lumbar spine (Fig. 40–22).

It is assumed that compression of the roots or cauda leads to ischemic changes in these neural structures and to the development of neurological symptoms. These are reversed when the compression is alleviated and adequate circulation is restored.

Patients frequently prefer to walk in a stooped manner rather than with a straight, erect posture, in distinction to patients with vascular claudication. For the former patients, walking uphill (waist-flexion posture) may be easier than walking downhill (straight, erect posture). In some patients, pain and discomfort are worsened by lying supine with the lower limbs extended, and relieved

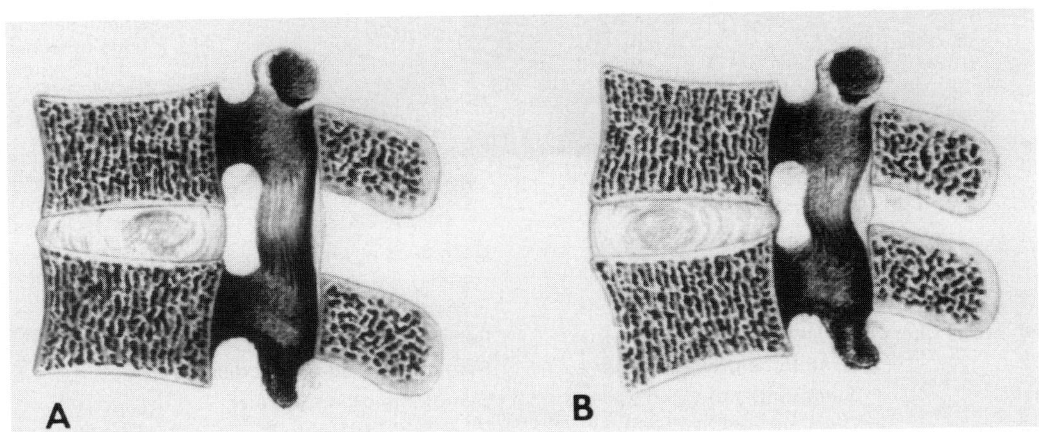

FIGURE 40–22. Functional changes of vertebral canal in spinal flexion and extension. *A.* In flexion, spinal canal lengthens and increases in width in sagittal plane, due both to separation of the laminae and the consequent decrease in thickness of the ligamenta flava and to distention of the posterior annulus fibrosus. *B.* Opposite changes occur in extension. (From Postacchini F: Lumbar Spinal Stenosis. New York, Springer-Verlag, 1989, p 41. By permission of the publisher.)

by elevating the knees or by lying on one side in a fetal position.

Symptoms are bilateral in more than two-thirds of patients, but a significant asymmetry often exists. The low back pain that is present in two-thirds of patients is typically mild and nondiscogenic and has essentially the same features as low back pain associated with lumbar spinal degenerative joint disease.

An absence or decrease in muscle stretch reflexes is noted in about 50% of patients. Weakness can be detected in about 40% of patients. This is usually mild, unilateral, and often in the distribution of L5 or S1 roots.

The clinical features of lateral recess syndrome and root claudication are different from those of central canal stenosis.[28] Patients usually report a unilateral intense sciatic pain (L5 or S1 root irritation) that is provoked by standing or walking and is relieved by sitting, lying down, or flexing the lumbar spine. Neurological deficits, if present, are mild. The straight-leg-raising test is usually negative.[44] There is little or no low back pain.

Differentiation of Vascular Claudication from Neurogenic Claudication

Vascular claudication occurs when exertion of the lower limb muscles results in energy consumption that exceeds the amount that can be provided by the circulation. Walking (especially fast or uphill), climbing stairs, or riding a bicycle (regular or stationary) induces the pain. This pain is relieved when exercise is discontinued, and low back pain and frank neurological symptoms are not present. Overall, in vascular claudication, the lower limb pain is relieved by rest. The limb pain resulting from spinal stenosis (pseudoclaudication) is relieved only when the spine is flexed or when the patient sits down. Some of the factors that are useful for differentiating vascular from neurogenic claudication are listed in Table 40–5.

Laboratory Tests

Electromyography

Electromyographic abnormalities are noted in more than 90% of patients and are more frequent than the abnormalities detected on neurological examination. Findings include evidence of denervation in the distribution of a single root or multiple roots, often bilaterally.[63]

Plain Radiography

Most patients have degenerative joint or disk disease with or without spondylolisthesis. In some patients, the lumbar spinal canal appears congenitally narrow. In certain congenital syndromes, such asachondroplastic dwarfism, spinal stenosis can be significant.

Myelography and Imaging Studies

Myelography shows complete or partial obstruction to the flow of contrast at one or more levels (Figs. 40–23

TABLE 40–5 Differentiation of Vascular and Neurogenic Claudication

Factor	Neurogenic Claudication (Pseudoclaudication)	Vascular Claudication	Pitfalls and Remarks
Low back pain	Frequently present	Absent	Sometimes, coincidental degenerative joint disease can be present in patients with vascular claudication
Effect of standing	Provokes symptoms	Does not provoke symptoms	
Direction of radiation of pain in lower limbs	Usually downward	Usually upward	
Sensory symptoms	Present in 66% of patients	Absent	Some patients with vascular claudication can have distal sensory symptoms due to ischemic or diabetic neuropathy
Muscle weakness	Present in more than 40% of patients	Absent	
Reflex changes	Present in about 50% of patients	Absent	In older patients, especially if there is associated neuropathy, reflexes may be decreased or absent
Arterial pulses	Normal	Decreased or absent	In older patients, pulses may be reduced
Arterial bruits	Absent	Frequently present	
Effect of rest while standing	Does not relieve symptoms	Relieves symptoms	
Walking uphill	Symptoms produced later	Symptoms produced earlier	
Walking downhill	Symptoms produced earlier	Symptoms produced later	
Bicycling (stationary or regular)	Does not provoke symptoms	Provokes symptoms	

From Mokri B, Sinaki M: Lumbar disk syndrome, lumbosacral radiculopathies, lumbar spondylosis and stenosis, spondylolisthesis. In Sinaki M (ed): Basic Clinical Rehabilitation Medicine, ed 2. St Louis, Mosby–Year Book, 1993, pp 503–513. By permission of Mayo Foundation.

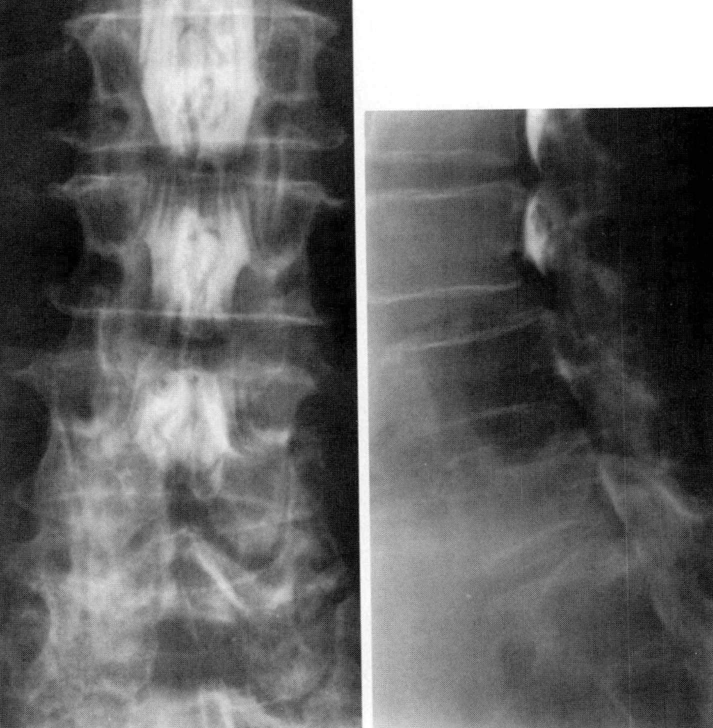

FIGURE 40–23. Lumbar myelograms. Anteroposterior (*left*) and lateral (*right*) views demonstrate multiple lumbar stenosis. (From Mokri B, Sinaki M: Lumbar disc syndrome, lumbosacral radiculopathies, lumbar spondylosis and stenosis, spondylolisthesis. In Sinaki M (ed): Basic Clinical Rehabilitation Medicine, ed 2. St Louis, Mosby–Year Book, 1993, pp 503–513. By permission of Mayo Foundation.)

and 40–24). CT and MRI show stenosis of the central canal, lateral recess, root canal, or a combination of these. CT-myelography is a very accurate test for evaluation of stenosis of these regions.[26, 27, 169]

Levels of stenosis (in decreasing order of frequency) are L4–5 (55%), L3–4 (44%), L2–3 (26%), L5–S1 (14%), and T12–L1 (3%).[126]

Treatment

The natural history of pseudoclaudication is not entirely clear. The symptoms of canal stenosis either remain unchanged or gradually worsen. The symptoms of root claudication are thought to either remain unchanged or perhaps gradually improve in some patients, but in an unpredictable time frame. Many patients, however, experience marked reduction in their activities and seek a solution. For cases in which progressive neurological deficits occur, surgical decompression should be seriously considered.[41]

Conservative Management

Reduction of lumbar lordosis is effective for reducing lumbar stenosis. Exercises that are aimed at strengthening the abdominal muscles and lumbar flexors are helpful. For patients in whom it is not possible to strengthen the abdominal muscles or in those with a protuberant abdomen and extensive body weight, an elastic abdominal binder is recommended. A program consisting of knee-to-chest exercises, pelvic tilt, and standing against a wall while attempting to contract the lumbar flexors to decrease lumbar lordosis may be beneficial. Patients should be instructed to avoid exercises that result in hyperextension of the spine. NSAIDs can help in managing the pain, particularly pain related to the associated degenerative joint disease.

Surgical Management

When patients are properly selected, decompressive single-level or multilevel laminectomy, with or without foraminotomies, alleviates manifestations of pseudoclaudication in most patients. However, the effect of this surgery on any associated low back pain is often less satisfactory. When low back pain rather than pseudoclaudication is the dominant feature, the expectations for an overall good recovery should be less. Although the patients with low back pain may obtain relief from the symptoms of pseudoclaudication, they may still continue to suffer from the pain.

Overall, the more pronounced the degree of spinal canal compromise and neural compression, the better the chance of obtaining a good surgical result. When long-standing and pronounced neurogenic atrophy and weakness have developed, patients may get relief from the leg pain resulting from the pseudoclaudication, but they typically have only a partial or negligible recovery of the muscle weakness and atrophy.[38]

Low Back Pain in Pregnancy

In 50% to 90% of pregnant women, low back pain develops at some point during pregnancy.[15, 45, 46, 117, 130] The back pain in 10% to 33% of these women is severe enough to reduce their activities of daily living significantly and, frequently, to require bedrest. The prevalence of low back pain during pregnancy increases 5%

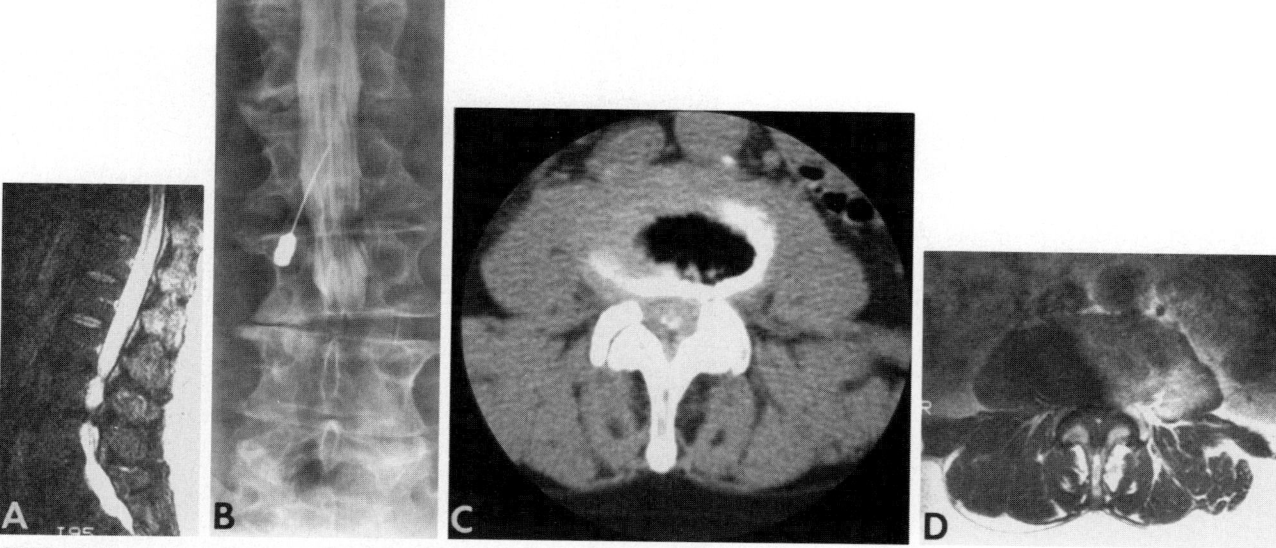

FIGURE 40–24. Lumbar spinal stenosis in a 73-year-old man. A very tight central canal stenosis is seen at L3–4 interspace and a moderate stenosis at L2–3 interspace, as noted in the sagittal T2-weighted MRI (*A*) and in the myelogram (*B*), which shows block to the flow of contrast dye at L3–4. CT-myelogram at this level shows a very tight canal (*C*), and axial T2-weighted MRI shows only a tiny cerebrospinal fluid signal (*D*).

for every 5 years of the pregnant woman's age. Other than age, such factors as heavy labor, smoking, parity, and a previous history of low back pain have been cited as risk factors for back pain during pregnancy.[15, 116, 152] Alternatively, several studies[45–47, 130] have not found any correlation between the development of back pain during pregnancy and age, race, parity, occupation, baby's weight, mother's prepregnancy weight, weight gain during pregnancy, exercise habits, or sleeping posture.

Low back pain is frequent in pregnancy, and women with a history of back pain often fear that pregnancy will activate or aggravate their back pain. Physicians are apprehensive about treating pregnant patients who have back pain because of the fear of interfering with the pregnancy or adversely affecting the fetus.

Clinical Manifestations

Pregnant women obviously are not immune to the back pains of various causes that can develop in others. Additionally, they frequently also have back pains directly related to pregnancy. Essentially four types of pain can be recognized: (1) nocturnal back pain, which occurs in more than one-third of patients; (2) low dorsal pain (Fig. 40–25A); (3) lumbar pain, which may or may not extend to one or both lower limbs (Fig. 40–25B); and (4) sacroiliac region pain (Fig. 40–25C).

Nocturnal back pain of pregnancy occurs 1 to 2 hours after lying down and is thought to be related to stagnation of venous blood in the vertebral venous plexus due to return of fluid of dependent edema of pregnancy to the circulation during recumbency, on one hand, and the venous blockage caused by pressure of the fetus on the vena cava on the other.

Sacroiliac pain is probably the most common type of back pain in pregnancy.[15, 30, 133] It may be unilateral or bilateral, may extend to the upper thigh, and might not be substantially relieved by lying down. Normally, the sacroiliac joint moves only minimally. During pregnancy, the production of relaxin (a hormone secreted by the corpus luteum) leads to articular laxity that can result in sacroiliac inflammation, pain, and discomfort.

The other low dorsal and lumbar pains of pregnancy have mechanical features, are increased by physical activity, and are decreased by rest. The leg pain and radicular symptoms that can accompany the low back pain of

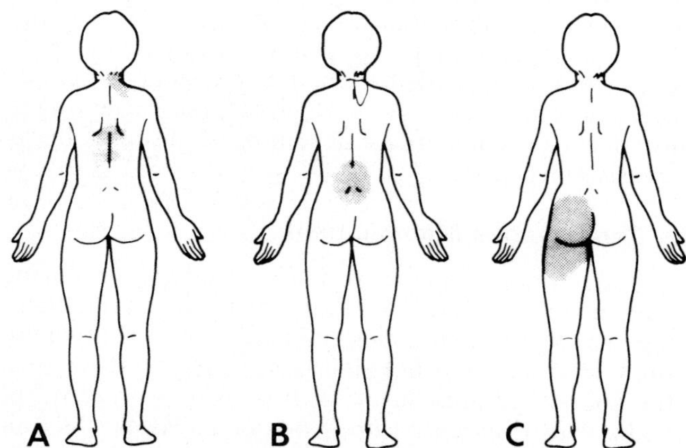

FIGURE 40–25. Areas of back pain during pregnancy. *A.* Low dorsal pain. *B.* Lumbar pain, which may or may not extend to both lower extremities. *C.* Sacroiliac region pain. (From Ostgaard HC, Andersson GBJ, Karlsson K: Prevalence of back pain in pregnancy. Spine 1991; 16:549.)

pregnancy are frequently caused by the direct pressure of the gravid uterus on components of the lumbosacral plexus. These cases actually are lumbosacral plexopathies or proximal sciatic neuropathies rather than true radiculopathies.

The back pain of pregnancy may not disappear with delivery, and in 20% to 25% of cases the pain may linger for some time.

Other causes of low back pain, such as herniated lumbar disk, tumors, and infections, can occur in pregnant women just as in the nonpregnant population. Pregnancy can induce a remission of rheumatoid arthritis, with frequent flareups after delivery.

Prophylaxis

Measures that prevent low back pain are less effective during pregnancy. The options are few but can be helpful. These include (1) reducing the load on the spine by appropriate changes in lifestyle and work environment, especially in women with a past history of back pain or back pain with previous pregnancies; (2) avoidance of excessive weight gain during pregnancy; and (3) educating the patient regarding proper posture to decrease lumbar lordosis; proper techniques for lifting, working positions, and resting positions (Fig. 40–26); and techniques for avoidance of aggravating factors. Pregnancy back supports and exercise instructions for abdominal muscle and pelvic floor contraction (see Fig. 40–8C), lateral bending, and rotational trunk exercises performed in a standing position may be helpful. Situps requiring a supine position and Valsalva's maneuver should be avoided, particularly after the fourth month of pregnancy.[3]

Treatment

In most cases, when pregnant women are reassured of the benign nature of the back pain, they find the discomfort tolerable and typically manage the problem symptomatically by rest and modification of their activities. For more bothersome low back pain, application of an abdominal pregnancy support with shoulder suspenders, physical therapy, and massage may help. For pain in the sacroiliac region, a trochanteric belt or a sacroiliac corset may offer reasonably good relief.[15, 40] Severe sacroiliac pain may require a period of bedrest (see Fig. 40–26) and physical therapy consisting of application of cold or superficial heat and sedative massage. Nocturnal pain of pregnancy might be difficult to manage. The use of venous support stockings to reduce the dependent edema during the waking hours and proper posturing at night can help. Acetaminophen is the analgesic of choice for management of low back pain during pregnancy.[24] Nonsteroidal agents are relatively contraindicated, and aspirin can increase the incidence of fetal intracranial hemorrhage in premature infants.[9] Medication for back pain in pregnancy should be used only as a last resort, with the approval of the obstetrician and with the informed consent of the patient.

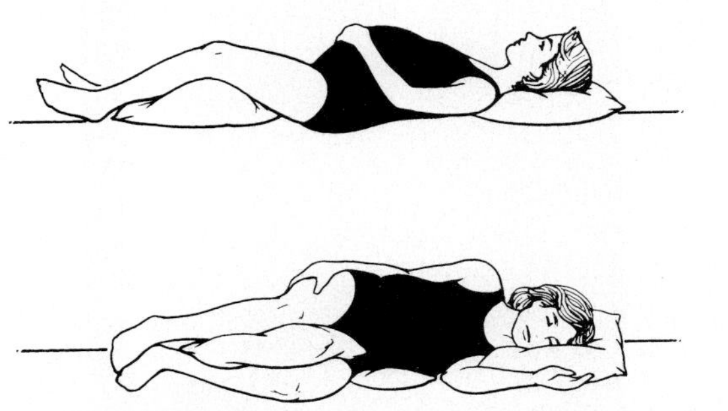

FIGURE 40–26. Proper positioning through use of cushions in bed helps decrease patient's nocturnal discomforts during pregnancy.

Paget's Disease

Paget's disease of bone is a rather common disease, particularly in elderly patients. It is marked by focal disturbance of bone architecture due to abnormally increased osteoblastic activity. It may involve a single bone (monostotic) or several bones (polyostotic), including the pelvis or vertebral bones. The alkaline phosphatase level is typically elevated, except in some early, limited, or monostotic forms. The disease may be asymptomatic or may cause focal pain. Involvement of the posterior pelvis or lumbar spine causes low back pain in some patients. Malignant transformation of Paget's lesion can occur, but this is uncommon. The lesions should be differentiated from those of hyperparathyroidism, fibrous dysplasia, myeloma, and metastatic tumors, particularly metastases from prostate cancer. The involved vertebral bone typically shows generalized enlargement and increased width. There is increased trabeculation (corduroy pattern), and a thickened rim of cortex may cause a picture-frame appearance. Dense sclerosis of vertebral bodies can give a pattern of "ivory vertebrae" and may simulate osteoblastic metastases. The involved area shows significant uptake on radioisotope bone scan, but MRI findings can be surprisingly unremarkable.

Treatment is needed only in symptomatic cases. Aspirin or nonsteroidal agents can reduce the pain. In active disease and when the pain is clearly related to the Paget's disease and not to other conditions (degenerative joint or degenerative disk disease), treatment with etidronate sodium (5 to 10 mg/kg/day orally for 6 months) can be considered. In a recent clinical trial, risedronate (one 30-mg tablet daily for a period of 2 months) was highly effective and well tolerated.[96a] Alendronate, an amino-bisphosphonate, is taken as a single dose on arising in the morning and at least 30 to 45 minutes before breakfast (40 mg/day orally for 6 months). Pamidronate is infused over 4 hours for 3 consecutive days (30 to 90 mg/day intravenously). Systemic calcitonin (50 to 100 IU [0.25 to 0.5 mL] per day) is given subcutaneously or intramuscularly. The dose may be tapered to 50 IU twice a week. Calcitonin also may be given as a nasal spray. Among these pharmacological trials, alendronate has been demonstrated to be more potent than etidronate for inhibiting osteoclastic-mediated bone resorption without being associated with abnormal mineralization.[145] Continuous treatment with etidronate can result in side effects of osteomalacia with increased bone fractures and pain. Consequently, drug holiday periods of 3 to 6 months should be interspersed between the treatment courses. Calcitonin is also effective but has to be given subcutaneously or intramuscularly. Ambulatory assistive devices (cane, walker) reduce the accompanying weight-bearing pain. For associated focal muscle pain with tenderness, application of superficial heat and massage can be helpful.[144]

Low Back Pain due to Neoplastic Disease

Primary spinal cord tumors such as astrocytomas, and particularly spinal ependymomas, can cause low back pain. Extramedullary intraspinal tumors such as meningiomas or neurilemmomas, as well as primary tumors of the vertebral bones (whether benign or malignant), can also cause low back pain. The most common neoplastic diseases causing low back pain are the metastatic spinal or epidural cancers (multiple myeloma and malignant lymphomas included) (Figs. 40–27 through 40–32). The low back pain related to neoplastic disease can be steady or may be provoked by physical activity or change in posture. However, one of the hallmarks of cancer pain is pain at rest, particularly nocturnal pain.

With advances in radiation therapy and chemotherapy, patients with primary malignant tumors are living longer; as a result, metastases, such as spinal epidural metastases, have more time to develop. Spinal cord compression due to metastatic cancer is found in about 5% to 10% of patients with bony metastases. At the lumbar and low dorsal level, most of these are also associated with low back pain. The tumors that most frequently metastasize to the spine include cancers of the lung, prostate, breast, kidney, and colon, and malignant melanoma, myeloma, and lymphoma. Sometimes spinal metastasis is the first clinical manifestation of the cancer.

Radiation is the palliative treatment of choice (often 3000 cGy in 10 fractions). In cases of cord compromise, in addition to the radiation therapy, high-dose dexamethasone is also often administered (with a subsequent quick tapering of dose). Such treatments do not necessarily prolong survival, but they are effective for relieving pain and lessening neurological deficits and disability. In selected cases, surgical decompression or even

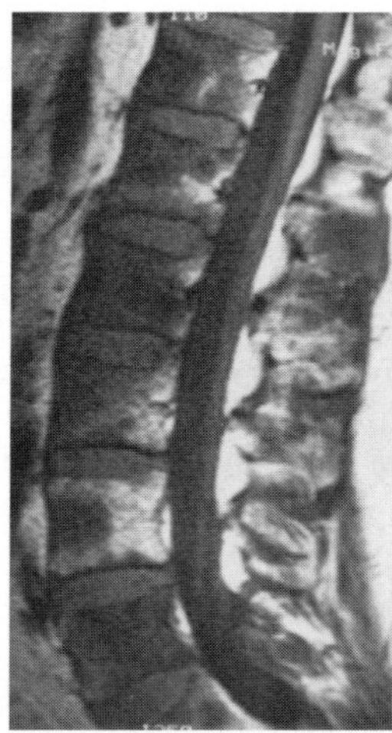

FIGURE 40–28. Multiple metastases to lumbar spine in a 66-year-old man with prostate cancer.

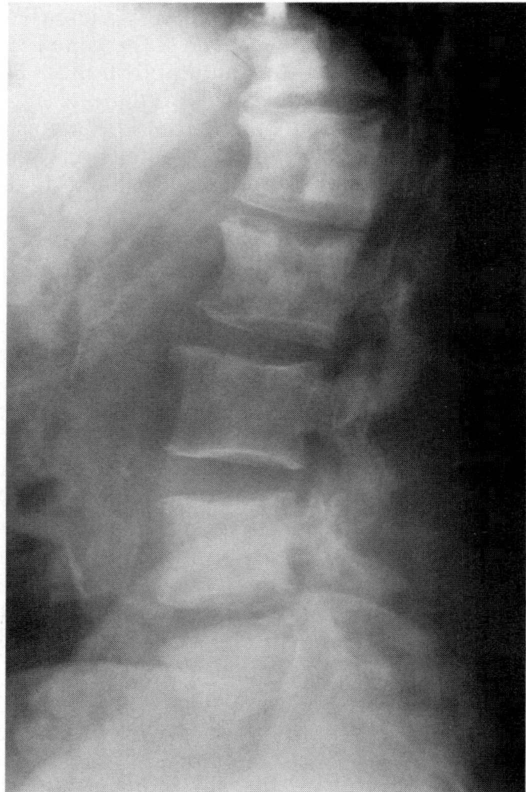

FIGURE 40–27. Spinal metastases with osteoblastic features in a 63-year-old man with prostate cancer.

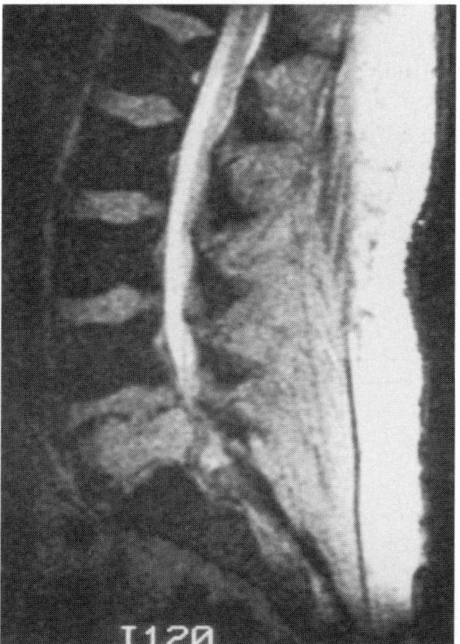

FIGURE 40–29. Metastatic carcinoma involving L5, with epidural extension, compressing the thecal sac and cauda equina.

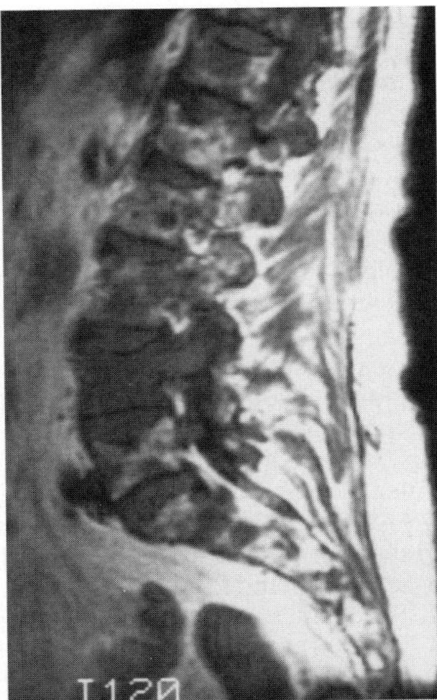

FIGURE 40–30. Extensive involvement of vertebrae in multiple myeloma; marrow replacement by infiltrating cells, deossification, and destructive and punched-out lesions. Pedicles, which are frequently involved in metastatic disease, are often spared in multiple myeloma (pedicles lack red marrow).

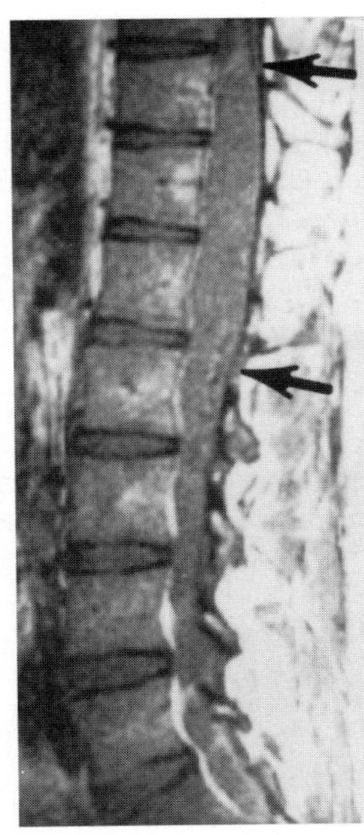

FIGURE 40–32. Magnetic resonance image of spine demonstrating large fusiform tumor extending from T10 to L3 (*arrows*) in a 30-year-old man. Tumor was found to be a low-grade ependymoma. This patient had had unexplained low back pain for several years before neurological deficits began to appear.

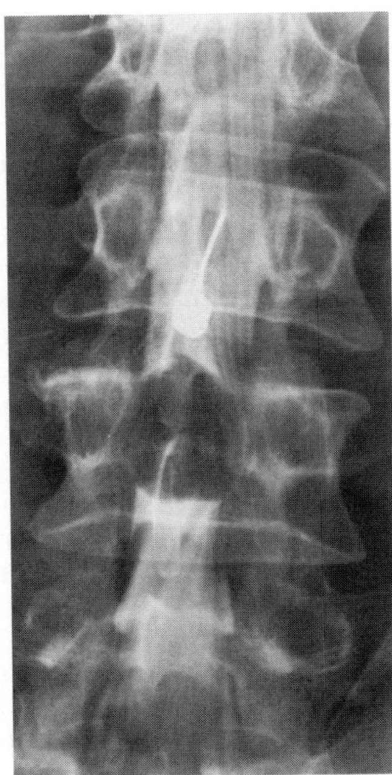

FIGURE 40–31. Lumbar myelogram showing intraspinal neurilemoma. A sharply circumscribed, round myelographic defect is displacing elements of the cauda equina. Note the cuplike upper and lower margins of the defect with the concavity facing the tumor.

corpectomy has been considered. Imaging studies, particularly MRI, are helpful for detection of spinal and epidural metastases, for determining the field of radiation therapy, and for post-treatment follow-up.

Analgesic medications are often required, particularly for the acute pain. Proper bracing and spinal immobilization and support should be provided if they help to decrease the pain or if there is a suggestion of spinal instability. Application of a spinal orthosis to decrease the pain due to weight bearing increases the patient's ability for ambulatory activities and reduces the risks of bone loss and muscle atrophy caused by immobility. Participation in physical activities often improves the patient's feeling of well-being. Ambulatory assistive devices such as a wheeled walker can also reduce weight-bearing pain.

Ankylosing Spondylitis

Ankylosing spondylitis is a chronic inflammatory seronegative rheumatic spondyloarthropathy that affects skeletal and extraskeletal tissues. It mainly affects the spine and invariably involves the sacroiliac joints. Eighty percent to 90% of patients are HLA-B27–positive. The prevalence is about 1 per 1000 in the white population. Males predominate, but the frequently stated ratio of 10:1 is definitely too high.[164] Although the true ratio is unknown, a ratio of 3:1 is more realistic. The disease often is milder in females and frequently presents with involvement of one of the appendicular joints before the appearance of sacroiliitis. The disease usually begins at age 20 to 35 years. Sacroiliitis is usually the first manifestation, presenting as unilateral or bilateral low back pain of insidious onset. Classically, significant morning stiffness and pain in the lower back are noted. These symptoms typically improve with activity during the day and return after rest or immobility. Many patients are awakened from sleep because of pain and stiffness of the lower back. To get relief, they often have to get up and move around. Pain may extend to the buttocks and posterior thighs. Lumbar lordosis may be lost (Fig. 40–33). Recurrent iritis, aortitis, and carditis are some of the peripheral manifestations of the disease.[6, 80] Cauda equina syndrome may occur in long-standing cases.[11]

The diagnosis must be confirmed by radiography. The earliest radiographic findings are almost invariably in the sacroiliac joints and include blurring of the margins of the lower two-thirds of these joints, especially on the iliac side, and widening of the joint space. With advance of sacroiliitis, increase in erosions and joint space destruction, and progression of sclerosis, total ankylosis and obliteration of the joint may finally occur. Early changes in the lumbar spine include squaring of the lumbar vertebral body and demineralization and spotty ligamentous calcification. In advanced cases with diffuse paraspinal ligamentous calcification, the classic picture of "bamboo spine" is produced. This change occurs only in a minority of patients and takes many years to develop; therefore, in reality, it has no value in the early diagnosis of the disease. Myelography and CT, especially in long-standing ankylosing spondylitis with cauda equina syndrome, show characteristic enlargement of the cul de sac, enlarged and often multiloculated dorsal arachnoid diverticula, and erosion of laminae and spinous processes. These changes can be clearly seen with MRI (Fig. 40–34).

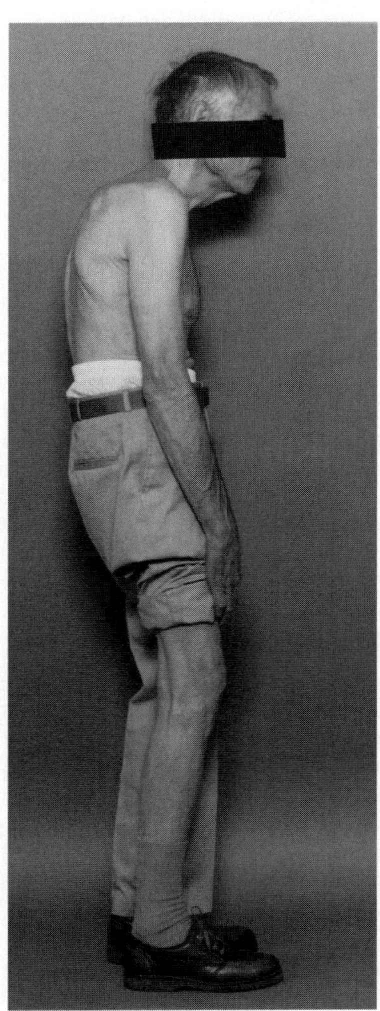

FIGURE 40–33. Ankylosing spondylitis; kyphotic posturing with contractures of hamstrings and hip flexors from compensating to maintain erect posture.

The prognosis is variable. *Osteitis condensans ilii,* a benign condition in women, should be differentiated from ankylosing spondylitis. It is particularly common in postpartum women, and the lesions likely develop as a result of mechanical strain placed on the sacroiliac joint during pregnancy. The radiographic features that differentiate the typical osteitis condensans ilii from ankylosing spondylitis include preservation of the sacroiliac joint and confinement of the sclerotic changes to the iliac side of the joint. Overall, women have less severe spinal disease but may have more peripheral joint involvement. The prognosis is less favorable in patients with refractory iliitis. Overall, most patients have mild disease and can lead full and productive lives.

Conservative treatment is the basis of management of patients with ankylosing spondylitis. NSAIDs can help diminish the pain and stiffness. Surgical intervention (such as extension osteotomies for excessive thoracic and cervical kyphosis) only very rarely becomes necessary.

Evaluation should include periodic measurements (in centimeters) of height, chest expansion, and C7 to S1 spinal flexion. A back extension exercise program (see Fig. 40–21), deep-breathing exercises, posture training, range of motion of the proximal joints (shoulders and hips), range-of-motion exercises to the cervical spine (if possible), and stretching exercises for the pectorals, hamstrings, Achilles tendons, hip flexors, and low back are important and should be included in the overall management program. The patient needs to have periodic measurement of height. Flexed posture needs to be avoided on the job, while driving, and during rest. Application of heat and massage before exercise can facilitate pain relief. Evaluation of chest expansion through periodic measurement of chest circumference at the level of T5 with a tape measure is recommended (this value is usually more than 5 to 7 cm). If chest expansion is reduced to less than 5 cm, respiratory function tests and encouragement for the patient to improve diaphragmatic breathing are recommended. Again, every effort should be made to avoid a flexed posture because there is no cure for subsequent fusion in a flexed position. Certain assistive devices facilitate daily activities despite limited spine motion. These include prism glasses, reachers, and wide-angle rear view mirrors for the car. Activities that may unduly strain the spine (such as contact sports, motorcycle riding, jumping) should be avoided because they could result in vertebral fractures. Most NSAIDs are of value in the management of ankylosing spondylitis. They need to be prescribed according to the patient's tolerance with the least drug toxicity. The lowest effective daily dose needs

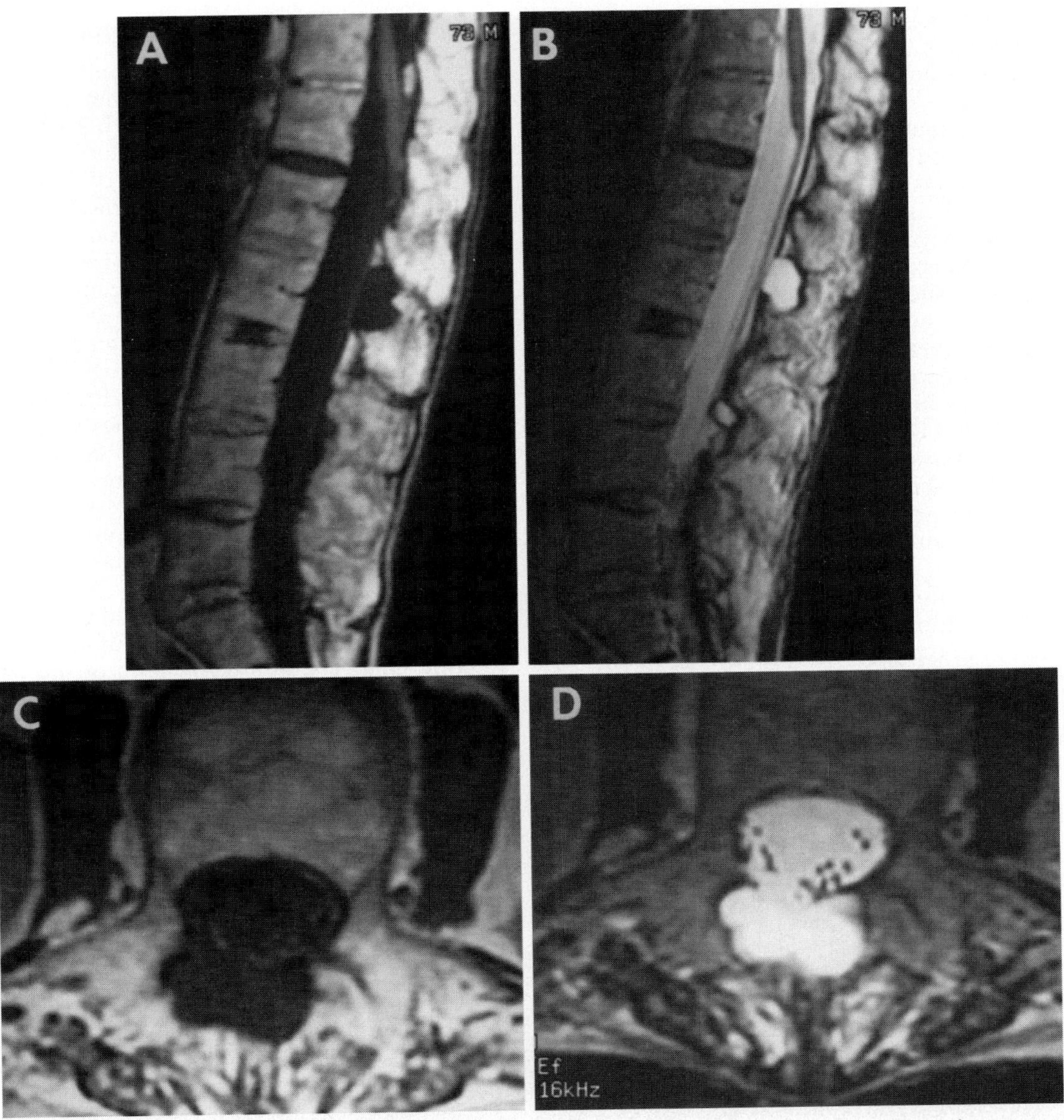

FIGURE 40–34. Ankylosing spondylitis associated with cauda equina syndrome in a 73-year-old man. Magnetic resonance images of lumbar and lower thoracic spine: sagittal T1 (*A*) and T2 (*B*) images and axial T1- (*C*) and T2-weighted (*D*) images. Note multiple arachnoid diverticula in lower thoracic and upper lumbar canal, deviation of conus medullaris, and straightening of spine.

to be recommended. Several NSAIDs, referred to as COX-2 drugs because they inhibit cyclo-oxygenase 2, are promising and may provide efficacy equal to that of drugs that inhibit cyclo-oxygenase-1 (COX-1) because the former have fewer adverse effects on the gastric mucosa and kidneys.

Diffuse Idiopathic Skeletal Hyperostosis (DISH)

Described by Forestier and Rotes-Querol in 1950,[50] Forestier's disease, also known as ankylosing hyperostosis, is a fairly common nondeforming, ossifying disease that occurs in elderly and middle-aged patients, particularly men. Ossification occurs along the anterior and lateral spinal ligaments without disk narrowing, apophyseal joint ankylosis, sacroiliac joint erosions, sclerosis, fusion, or vertebral body marginal sclerosis.[156] The ossification may also involve peripheral muscular tenderness at insertions. Any level of the spine may be involved, but thoracic involvement is more common, followed by involvement of the lumbar region. The involvement may be unilateral. The condition may be asymptomatic or cause stiffness, pain, and some limitation of motion, but significant functional inability is rare. Management is conservative; nonsteroidal agents may also be helpful. Application of infrared heat and massage decrease the accompanying myalgias and stiffness.

Pyogenic Vertebral Spondylitis

This condition includes infectious discitis (intervertebral disk infection) and infectious vertebral osteomyelitis. Although these can occur postoperatively, the focus here is on childhood and adult pyogenic infectious spondylitis that occurs without a history of spinal surgery.

These cause low back pain and enter into the differential diagnosis of back pain. The mechanism is from a contiguous infection or by hematogenous or lymphatic seeding from a remote site.[8, 32, 57, 62, 70, 75, 95, 99] Common sources of infection are pneumonia; urinary tract, cutaneous, and dental infections; and abdominal surgery. The source of infections is not apparent in more than one-third of cases.[8, 95] It is more common in patients with diabetes, malignancy, renal failure, alcoholism, and AIDS; in intravenous drug abusers; and in immunocompromised patients. Thoracic and lumbar spines are more frequently involved, but back pain is more common with lumbar spine involvement because the thoracic cage splints the spine and can mute the localized back pain.[115] The most common infectious agent is *Staphylococcus aureus,* but other bacteria, especially gram-negative agents and anaerobes, have been implicated.[29, 60, 161] Pyogenic vertebral spondylitis may become associated with spinal epidural abscess, which may cause compression of the spinal cord or cauda equina and create a surgical emergency.

The clinical features are often different in children and adults. In children, the onset is often abrupt, with fever, malaise, back pain, and spine tenderness. The diagnosis is typically not difficult.[115] In adults, the onset is more gradual; there is little or no fever and malaise is generally absent. Point tenderness is evident at the involved site, but in a small percentage of patients, back pain may not be evident, and it can take up to 3 months to reach a diagnosis.[149, 150] The erythrocyte sedimentation rate is usually elevated, but leukocytosis is more evident in acute cases (therefore, it is generally noted in children and might not be evident in adults).

Radiographic and Imaging Findings

Radiographic abnormalities significantly lag behind the actual pathological changes that are taking place. The radiographic findings include narrowing of the intervertebral disk space in discitis, loss of definition and destruction of the cortical margins of the vertebral bodies facing the disk, bone loss and rarefaction, vertebral body collapse, and gibbus formation (Fig. 40–35).

Myelography does not directly visualize epidural abscesses but demonstrates the associated mass effect on the thecal sac and neural structures. Myelography also carries the risk of introducing the infection to the spinal subarachnoid space and creating meningitis.

CT may show the pathological alterations, including the epidural abscesses, although they might appear isodense or hypodense compared with the adjacent musculature. CT can also demonstrate paravertebral soft tissue components of the infectious process. The presence of an epidural mass centered on an intervertebral disk is a helpful CT feature that differentiates the process from a neoplastic cause. MRI is clearly superior to CT for evaluation of epidural abscesses and paraspinal masses. Its ability to image long segments of the spinal canal in multiple planes allows delineation of the pathological process.[160, 165] MRI is more sensitive than plain radiography or CT for the diagnosis of discitis and osteomyelitis.[56]

Treatment

The infection should be treated with antibiotics. Ideally, the diagnosis is established before neurological deficits develop. In general, nonsurgical therapy is con-

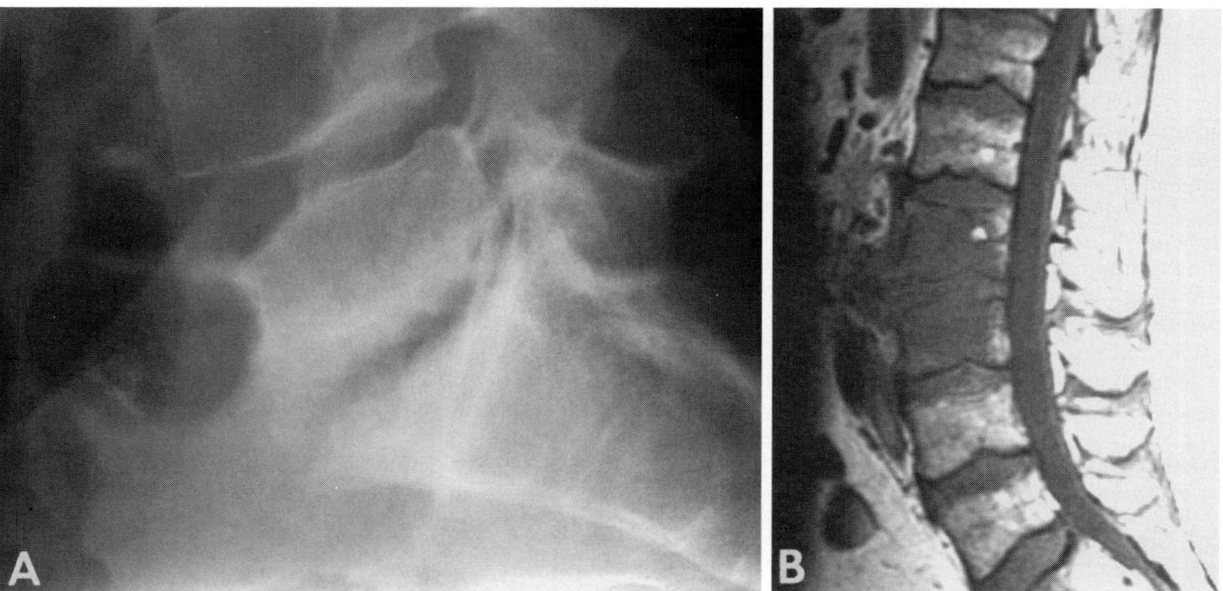

FIGURE 40–35. Pyogenic vertebral osteomyelitis and intravertebral disk infection. *A.* Radiograph of lumbar spine in a patient with L5–S1 intervertebral disk infection. Note narrowing of the disk space and irregularities of the adjacent end-plates associated with reactive sclerosls. *B.* Magnetic resonance image of lumbar and lower thoracic spine of another patient, demonstrating involvement of L2–3 intervertebral disk, especially anteriorly, and involvement of adjacent vertebral bodies and soft tissues anterior to these vertebrae.

sidered for patients without neurological deficits. Surgery for decompression and drainage of pus should be considered when pressure effects and neurological deficits develop. Undue delays should be avoided, because the chances of full recovery diminish with progression of neurological impairment. Childhood disk space infection often responds well to antibiotics and immobilization with application of a rigid orthosis for 6 to 12 weeks.

BACK PAIN IN CHILDREN

Children are not small adults. Low back pain in childhood is quite different from the low back pain in adults. Although low back pain in adults is very common, in children it is uncommon to rare. Children are less likely to report their back pain early and may provide a vague or incomplete history. Very young children, obviously, can provide no history. Therefore, the diagnosis and evaluation of back pain in children may be delayed for several months.[88]

There is also a significant difference in the frequency of causative factors between children and adults. Degenerative diseases, which are the most common cause of low back pain in adults (see Table 40–1), are rare in children, whereas strains, developmental disorders, infection or inflammation, or neoplasms are relatively more common. Overall, back pain in childhood frequently, but not always, can result from a serious underlying cause (Table 40–6).

Helpful Hints in the History

Children may be poor historians or give no history. Parents might not remember the details, including the onset of the pain. The physician should use certain

TABLE 40–6 Causes of Low Back Pain in Children

Etiological Factor	Comments
Trauma	
Strain	Ligamentous or muscle strain. Probably the most common cause of low back pain (LBP) in this group. Look for a history of fall, strenuous exercise, or other trauma. Localized tenderness and paraspinal spasm may be present.
Disk herniation	Uncommon in children and often posttraumatic. LBP alone or with radicular symptoms in lower limbs.
Infections	
Urinary tract infection	Back pain may be the primary complaint.
Discitis	Most common at age 2–6 years (when disk space is still vascularized). Young children may refuse to walk. Back motion is limited. Low-grade fever and irritability may be present. May be associated with epidural abscess or vertebral osteomyelitis.
Inflammatory	
Ankylosing spondylitis	Usually affects boys. Loss of back mobility; arthritis in hips or knees.
Juvenile rheumatoid arthritis	Outlook typically better than in adults.
Neoplastic	
Vertebral bones	
Benign	Osteoid osteoma, benign chondroblastoma, eosinophilic granuloma, aneurysmal bone cyst.
Malignant	Ewing's sarcoma, osteogenic sarcoma, metastases.
Spinal cord and roots	Astrocytoma, ependymoma, hemangioblastoma, teratomas, lipomas, neurilemomas, neurofibromas.
Bony abnormalities	
Scheuermann's disease	Osteochondritis of upper and lower cartilaginous end-plate of several vertebrae, causing anterior wedging and kyphosis, "round back deformity," and back pain; often presents in adolescence.
Spondylolisthesis	
Spondylolysis	Defect of pars interarticularis, probably due to stress fracture.
Scoliosis	
Psychogenic	Reaction to stressful situations; affect may be inconsistent with symptoms; findings may be unexplainable. Can be risky diagnosis. Thorough workup may be needed to rule out organic disease.
Extraspinal	
Retrocecal appendicitis	
Pyelonephritis	
Hydronephrosis	
Psoas abscess	
Retroperitoneal mass	
Miscellaneous	
Tethered cord	
Cord AVM/dural AVF	
Diastematomyelia	

Abbreviations: AVF, arteriovenous fistula; AVM, arteriovenous malformation; LBP, low back pain.
Modified from Tunnessen WW Jr: Signs and Symptoms in Pediatrics, ed 2. Philadelphia, JB Lippincott, 1988, pp 467–470. By permission of the publisher.

events, such as holidays, birthdays, or school events, to obtain an estimate of the date of onset of pain, any particular aggravation of pain, or any additional developments. Determine whether there is additional limb pain, neurological defects or symptoms (such as weakness, paresthesias, numbness, footdrop, or unsteadiness), or sphincter trouble. Determine whether a relationship with trauma can be established and whether aggravating or relieving factors have been noted.

Nocturnal pain responding to aspirin or NSAIDs may suggest osteoid osteoma, and a higher than expected family history of spondylolysis or scoliosis may have diagnostic significance. A history of uveitis or iritis can suggest juvenile ankylosing spondylitis or juvenile rheumatoid arthritis. Improvement in morning stiffness (and uveitis) as the day progresses suggests ankylosing spondylitis, whereas stiffness that worsens as the day progresses suggests juvenile rheumatoid arthritis.[119] In a young child with back pain and a history of fractures, the possibility of child abuse should be kept in mind. Persistent pain unresponsive to analgesics and rest, increasing pain, weight loss, fever, the appearance of neurological symptoms and signs, or sphincter trouble calls for an urgent workup.

Helpful Hints on Physical Examination

Many of the principles described for adults are applicable to children, but signs of spinal anomalies (skin lesions, café-au-lait spots, tufts of hair, dimples, dermal cyst) should be particularly sought. Curvatures of the spine, a paraspinal mass, asymmetry, or spasm (including on flexion and extension) should be sought. Hamstring tightness is common in children with low back pain,[119] including in spondylolysis, spondylolisthesis, discitis, and epidural abscess. Percussion may help differentiate spine pain from flank pain (often of renal origin).

Back pain in children also can be related to lack of physical activity and deconditioning of truncal supportive muscles. Studies have shown that the level of physical activity correlates with the rate of increase in back strength.[110, 132]

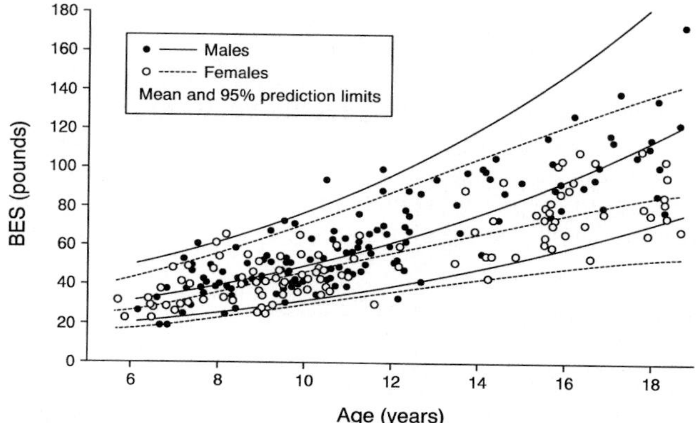

FIGURE 40–37. Correlation of back extensor strength (BES) and age in 246 healthy children (137 boys and 109 girls). (From Sinaki M, Limburg PJ, Wollan PC, et al (eds): Correlation of trunk muscle strength with age in children 5 to 18 years old. Mayo Clin Proc 1996; 71:1047. By permission of Mayo Foundation for Medical Education and Research.)

Evaluation of muscle strength in healthy children aged 5 to 18 years has demonstrated that back strength in boys and girls is approximately the same until age 9 to 10; after age 10, the disparity develops. After age 11 boys' muscle strength varies from that of girls, and by age 18 girls' muscle strength is about 70% that of boys.[141]

The ratio of back extensor strength to back flexor strength is known to decrease with advancing age.[141] One study showed this ratio to change from 2.0 in young children to about 1.5 in 18 year olds (Fig. 40–36). In the clinical evaluation of children with back pain, muscle strength testing is important. The lack of ability in children age 5 or younger to perform a sit-up is not considered abnormal. In one study, the ages at which children experienced the greatest increase in their back extensor strength was 13.2 years for girls and 15.8 years for boys (Fig. 40–37). For back flexor strength, this increment was at age 11.3 in girls and 15.7 in boys (Fig. 40–38).

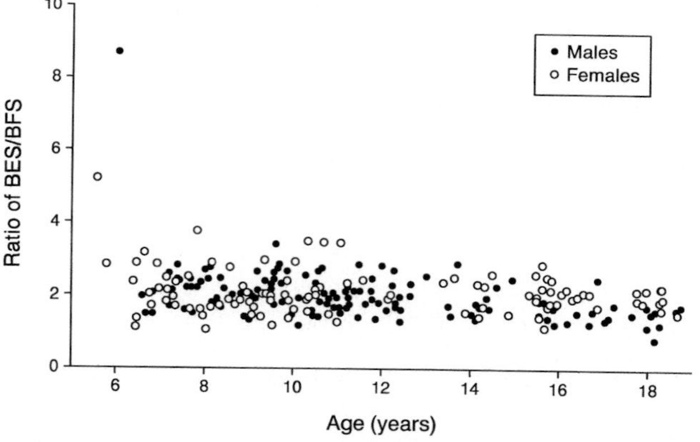

FIGURE 40–36. Ratio of back extensor strength to back flexor strength, by age, in 246 healthy children (137 boys and 109 girls). (From Sinaki M, Limburg PJ, Wollan PC, et al (eds): Correlation of trunk muscle strength with age in children 5 to 18 years old. Mayo Clin Proc 1996; 71:1047. By permission of Mayo Foundation for Medical Education and Research.)

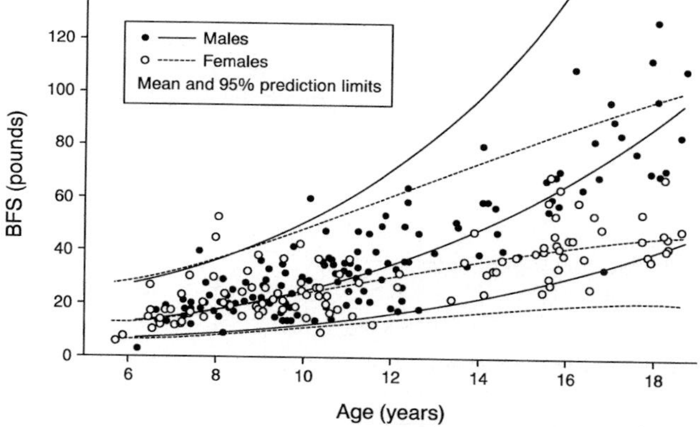

FIGURE 40–38. Correlation of back flexor strength (BFS) and age in 246 healthy children (137 boys and 109 girls). (From Sinaki M, Limburg PJ, Wollan PC, et al (eds): Correlation of trunk muscle strength with age in children 5 to 18 years old. Mayo Clin Proc 1996; 71:1047. By permission of Mayo Foundation for Medical Education and Research.)

Increased physical activity without proper development of strength in the back extensors as compared with flexors can be associated with back pain.[109]

Lumbar Disk Disease

About 1% of children presenting with low back pain have lumbar disk disease. Two percent of all operations on lumbar discs are in children.[55, 88] Overall, lumbar disk disease is an uncommon condition in children, and the vast majority of the patients are 10 years or older. Practically all patients have back pain, and 90% have radicular symptoms; in about 50% of the patients, the radicular symptoms develop sometime after establishment of the low back pain. The straight-leg-raising test is frequently positive, and neurological deficits are noted in more than half of the patients.[22, 33, 61, 155, 171] Despite a trial of conservative measures, more than 60% of patients need surgery. In 95% of the cases, the involved disk is at L4–5 and L5–S1. A history of trauma is more commonly elicited in adolescents with lumbar disk disease than in adults. A family history of lumbar disk disease is five to seven times more common in children and adolescents than in adults. Results of surgical therapy are encouraging. The cure rate is about 90% to 95%. It is not uncommon for children who have undergone treatment for lumbar disk disease to have disk disease at a different level in the future.

Scheuermann's Disease

Scheuermann's disease is another cause of low back pain in adolescents. It is more frequent in boys and is characterized by herniation of a disk through the end-plate into the vertebral body. Osteochondritis of the upper and lower vertebral end-plates and trauma might play a role. Some patients have marfanoid features, and a familial tendency is present in some. The back pain typically responds to rest and immobilization through application of a proper spinal orthosis.

Spondylolysis and Spondylolisthesis

In the pediatric age group, spondylolysis and spondylolisthesis are the most common causes of back pain associated with structural change. Spondylolysis is likely related to injury to the pars interarticularis.[163] Older children and adolescents are more frequently affected than younger ones. In acute cases, a pars fracture may actually heal with immobilization for 10 to 12 weeks in a plaster body jacket. Restriction of activity and occasional bracing aid in resolution of the pain. In chronic cases, instructions in back care, abdominal muscle strengthening, and stretching of paraspinal muscles, hip flexors, hamstrings, and Achilles tendons are helpful. After resolution of symptoms, normal activities can be resumed, but a return to vigorous athletic events involving the spine (such as gymnastics and football) is controversial.[123]

Congenital Diseases

With modern neuroimaging techniques, congenital spine and spinal cord problems and dysraphic anomalies are relatively easily detected in children with back pain. About 10% of patients have more than one spinal lesion, and imaging of the entire spine is therefore prudent.

Infections

Infectious vertebral osteomyelitis and discitis have been addressed, and the differences in various features of these entities in adults and children have been outlined.

Tumor

Nocturnal pain, pain at rest, and pain on awakening are symptoms that may draw attention to tumors of the spinal column. Metastatic tumors of the spine may occur, but in contrast to the case in adults, they are uncommon in children. The most frequent tumors of the spinal column in children include osteoid osteoma, osteoblastoma, histiocytosis X, and aneurysmal bone cyst. The pain of osteoid osteoma is typically nocturnal and responds to aspirin. Osteoblastoma has features similar to those of osteoid osteoma, but it is usually of larger size. Histiocytosis X may cause vertebral body collapse.[88]

CONSERVATIVE MANAGEMENT OF BACK PAIN: GENERAL CONSIDERATIONS

Conservative treatment of back pain traditionally has included rest, avoidance of stressful activities, use of back supports in some cases, and exercise. We prefer to divide the conservative management of back pain into two categories: (1) management of acute low back pain syndromes and (2) management of chronic low back pain syndromes.

Acute Low Back Pain Syndromes

Acute back pain is usually accompanied by anxiety and fear of possible debilitating causes. Conservative treatment is indicated for each case of acute back pain (Table 40–7). However, this option should at times be modified by other factors, such as the accompanying neurological loss, repeated hospitalization, and economic hardship imposed on the patient by the situation.

Acute back pain is most commonly related to a traumatic injury or a mechanical strain that is beyond the biomechanical competence of low back structures. As in any acute injury, the contributing factors to pain are not only the injury to the structures involved but also the soft tissue edema at the location.

As in any acute injury, cold packs decrease edema and should be applied immediately after injury. The patient is encouraged to comply with physical therapy measures, such as application of cold packs during the first 48 hours after strain or sprain and, thereafter, application of heat or cold to the area for pain relief. Heat is applied to the lower back through an infrared heat lamp or an electric heating pad for 20 to 35 minutes (continuous heat application is not recommended).[83] Application of light stroking massage can decrease the

TABLE 40–7 Some Causes of Acute Low Back Pain and Their Treatment

Cause	Treatment
Musculoskeletal	
Muscle strain or ligamentous sprain	Symptomatic treatment (bedrest, corset, cold [first 48 hr]/heat, massage)
Herniated disk	
Nonprogressive	Conservative treatment, injection
Progressive neurological signs	Laminectomy and disk excision
Traumatic fracture	
Stable	Spinal orthoses, analgesics
Unstable	Fusion, bone graft, or instrumentation
Inflammatory disease (acute spondyloarthropathies)	Conservative management, treatment of underlying disease
Infections (pyogenic, vertebral spondylitis, intervertebral disk infection)	Immobilization, antibiotics, surgery and drainage of pus if pressure effect and neurological deficits are present
Compression fracture (osteopenia, osteoporosis)	Bedrest (1–2 days), back support, simple analgesics, treatment of underlying disease
Degenerative joint disease with or without facet abnormality	Conservative treatment Posture instructions Back support
Malignancy, pathological compression fractures	Radiation therapy, usually high-dose dexamethasone at onset if cord compromise is present; orthosis for stabilization; surgical decompression and stabilization in selected cases

superficial soft tissue edema induced by the use of heat and also provide more relaxation to the paraspinal muscles. The practice of manipulation in an attempt to reposition the displaced spine is controversial.

For acute discogenic disorders, the use of simple analgesics every 4 to 6 hours is also helpful. Adequate analgesia with acetaminophen, NSAIDs, or a short course of sedative muscle relaxants or even synthetic opiates may be recommended. Simple sedatives are given to reduce muscle spasm even further. In severe cases, the use of narcotics may be necessary for a short time (1 week to 10 days). Only minor concern of addiction is present with short-term use of narcotics, and the benefits surpass the risks. It is better to avoid codeine and its derivatives because constipation induced by these agents aggravates back pain as a result of straining and elevation of intraspinal pressure.

In the acute stage of back pain it is helpful to provide support for the spine during weight bearing and ambulatory activities to decrease pain related to paraspinal muscle co-contraction. As has been demonstrated through measurement of pressure of the intervertebral disks during different positions of the spine,[105] flexing the hips and the knees with the patient in a supine or a lateral position can decrease the intervertebral pressure (see Fig. 40–2). This position reduces the lumbar lordotic curve and opens the posterior intervertebral disk interspaces. A firm mattress with a soft top-layer covering is required for any prolonged immobilization in bed.

The optimal duration of bedrest is uncertain, and for many patients without neuromotor deficits, 2 days of bedrest may suffice without any significant difference for clinical outcome.[36] Therefore, a period of bedrest for 2 to 3 days is helpful and does not result in excessive bone loss or debilitation. The duration of bedrest varies from a few days to 2 weeks before the acute symptoms subside. Prolonged bedrest is not recommended. In a reported study[81] of 34 adults who were hospitalized for low back pain and required therapeutic bedrest, the lumbar spine bone mineral content decreased about 0.9% per week, as assessed with dual-photon absorptiometry.

Patients benefit from the application of a well-fitted spinal orthosis during the acute stage. Depending on the extent or severity of injury, the back support may consist of an elastic lumbosacral corset or a rigid support in the form of a brace or a plaster cast that is applied before the patient is allowed to start ambulatory activities. During recumbency the support is removed. The reduction of motion in the lumbar spine can be achieved only if the support is extended from the lower thoracic spine to the greater trochanteric areas.[10] This reduction of mobility in the involved area significantly decreases the pain and reduces the duration of bedrest required. Restriction of back motion results in weakness of the low back supportive muscles; therefore, prolonged use of a back support is discouraged. It should be discarded as soon as low back pain symptoms have subsided. Scientific studies of spinal orthoses and functional units of the spine have suggested that muscle atrophy, accelerated osteopenia, and osteoarthritic changes result from use of rigid orthoses.[51, 107, 114] These studies were based on long-term use of orthoses in patients with spinal cord injury who used body jackets or halopelvic fixation devices. Performing isometric strengthening exercises in conjunction with application of a back support reduces the effect of immobility on muscles. A progressive, nonstrenuous back strengthening exercise program should be started as soon as tolerated by the patient. This is initiated with isometric exercises and can be advanced to flexion or extension or combined exercise programs. By the end of 6 weeks, the effects of a muscle strengthening course should be evident.[100] When the patient is pain-free, normal daily activities can be gradually resumed. Recreational and athletic activities may have to be curtailed. If slight recurrence of low back pain or sciatica is noticed, the back support can be reapplied and periodic bedrest is ordered.

Treatment of acute back sprain (defined as soft tissue injury of an otherwise normal back) should permit the patient to return to normal activities with 2 to 4 weeks. Often, busy professional patients return to work in 1 to 2 weeks. Patients involved in occupations that require heavy manual labor are usually able to return to work by 6 weeks after injury and should be encouraged to do so. Mild symptoms may persist while the patient is applying physical therapy measures. Hyperextension exercises, such as the McKenzie program, have also been advocated[37] for the management of herniated disk and, in some cases, seem to be helpful. Although hyperextension exercises might be beneficial in some instances for treatment of low back pain, we have not had favorable results. The McKenzie exercises are *hyperextension* exercises, which should not be confused with the *spinal extension* exercises that are prescribed for osteoporotic back pain.

Repetition of acute episodes of back pain associated with progressive disk degeneration, localized instability, and degenerative arthritis can result in prolonged immobility. In selected cases, spinal manipulation can result in immediate relief of pain after the first treatment. In a randomized trial,[71] patients were selected for randomization after eligibility was established through inclusion criteria. One group received manipulation therapy and the other group received soft tissue massage. The outcome was not significantly different between the two groups, and both groups showed substantial improvement.

Chronic Low Back Pain Syndromes

Back pain that has been present for more than 6 months is chronic and usually is accompanied by changes in the patient's lifestyle and behavior. The longer the pain has been present, the more resistive it becomes to therapeutic intervention. Table 40–8 lists some common causes of chronic low back pain and their management. For patients who are unable to perform any back strengthening exercises because of chronic pain, transcutaneous electrical nerve stimulation (TENS) can be tried in an attempt to control the pain and enable the patient to proceed with exercises.

In a controlled trial[94] of the effect of low-frequency electrical stimulation of back extensor muscles, a significant improvement in back strength was demonstrated. One study[101] has shown that, overall, patients with acute back pain who complained of pain over a wider area of the body were highly anxious, had a lower activity level, and had more tendency for chronic pain syndrome. After careful evaluation of the patient's physical status, assessment of the patient's environment, work incentive and disability status, and financial loss or gain is mandatory. The multidisciplinary evaluation and approach is very helpful.

Patients can also develop a behaviorally based type of chronic low back pain known as chronic pain syndrome. For treatment of this condition, see Chapter 42.

TABLE 40–8 Some Causes of Chronic Low Back Pain and Treatment

Cause	Treatment
Osteoarthritis; degenerative joint disease (DJD) Lumbar spondylosis Diffuse idiopathic skeletal hyperostosis, Forestier's disease	Improve muscular back support Corset Weight loss Improve posture
Facet pain syndrome Facet DJD	Avoid lumbar hyperextension Improve muscular support Consider injection Dynamic, static posture principles
Spondylolisthesis Stable	Flexion exercise program Spinal orthosis Activity precautions
Progressive neurological deficit	Decompression and fusion
Spinal stenosis Pseudoclaudication Lateral recess syndrome	Spinal flexion exercises Weight reduction Correction of posture Decompression
Metabolic bone disease Osteopenia Osteoporosis Paget's disease	Isometric back extension program Treat underlying disease Avoid heavy lifting (5 to 10 lb) Weight-bearing exercise program
Malignancy (multiple myeloma, metastatic) Stable spine	Conservative treatment Orthosis Gait-assistive devices Wheelchair Avoid strenuous activities Radiation therapy with or without steroids
Unstable spine	Surgical stabilization and orthotics
Chronic inflammatory disease (ankylosing spondylitis, chronic spondyloarthropathies)	Conservative treatment Nonsteroidal agents Back extension and stretching exercises Deep breathing exercises
Fibromyalgia	Conservative treatment Biofeedback Relaxation Correction of posture
Chronic pain syndrome	Multidisciplinary behavioral approach Psychological testing (MMPI*) Stretching Stress management to consider antidepressants Electromyographic biofeedback

* Minnesota Multiphasic Personality Inventory.

PREVENTIVE MEASURES AND BACK SCHOOLS

Episodes of acute low back pain usually subside within a few days to 3 months.[25] Low back pain becomes problematic in many patients in whom it is recurrent. Prevention of recurrence is of major importance in the management of low back pain syndromes.

During the acute phase, the patient should be instructed in proper positioning techniques to decrease low back pain during dynamic or static posturing and to avoid reinjury. At this stage, pain is managed with the use of sedative physical therapeutic measures and analgesics. Meanwhile, the patient should be introduced to progressive isometric exercise programs to improve muscular support of the spine. Provision of a back education program (back school) very early in the patient's treatment program is helpful. Back school programs vary from small classes (six to eight patients) with a physical therapist instructor to one-on-one instruction with either a physician or physical therapist. Back schools are often supported by companies that provide back education programs for their employees. Typically, employees' performances are videotaped before participation in the back school. A back program, including audiovisual presentation, is then set up to meet the specific needs of the employees' jobs. The objective of any preventive or therapeutic rehabilitation program is to teach patients how to help themselves. They are taught how to be "kind to one's back." Figure 40–9 demonstrates correct and incorrect postures that should be provided as preliminary training for an individual.

Patients with low back pain should be instructed in basic body mechanics and the following measures:

1. If prolonged sitting is required for an occupation, one should get up every 20 minutes. In addition, to decrease strain on the low back during sitting, the patient can be instructed to perform pelvic tilt exercises, to sit with knees bent and one or both feet slightly elevated on a footrest, and to support the low back with a small cushion (see Figs. 40–9B and I).
2. For driving a car, the seat should be brought close to the steering wheel so that the knees are slightly higher than the hips (see Fig. 40–9G). In the presence of lumbar degenerative disk disease, getting out of the car frequently (every 20 to 30 minutes) to stretch is helpful.
3. Before coughing or sneezing, the stomach muscles should be tightened.
4. Begin a progressive low back isometric strengthening exercise program and perform stretching exercises to increase flexibility for performing daily activities.
5. Forward bending increases intradiskal pressure.[103] Therefore, certain precautions such as kneeling when trying to pick an object up from the floor (see Fig. 40–9D) or when making a bed are advisable to decrease intradiskal pressure.
6. To decrease low back strain when getting into bed, one should sit on the edge of the bed, turn and roll slightly to one hip, bring the knees up with the feet hanging over the edge of the bed, and slowly recline, pushing up with the arms on the bed to support the body during this procedure. For getting out of bed, one needs to reverse this sequence.

In more advanced programs, the patient's physical status is evaluated, including range of motion of the spine and measurement of body weight and back and upper and lower extremity strengths. For postmenopausal women who are involved in heavy physical labor, it is wise to keep in mind the biomechanical competence of the spine to avoid spinal compression fractures due to involutional osteopenia or osteoporosis. When avoidance of heavy lifting is not possible, provision of a rigid dorsolumbar support is recommended.

In summary, every effort should be made to prevent low back pain or to avoid its recurrence through education and instruction in proper body mechanics.

ACKNOWLEDGMENTS

Supported in part by a research grant from the Donaldson Trust. The authors would like to thank LeAnn Stee and the Section of Scientific Publications for service, John Hagen for the illustrations, and Sandy Fitzgerald for secretarial assistance.

REFERENCES

1. Addison R, Schultz A: Trunk strengths in patients seeking hospitalization for chronic low-back disorders. Spine 1980; 5:539.
2. Alston W, Carlson KE, Feldman DJ, et al: A quantitative study of muscle factors in the chronic low back syndrome. J Am Geriatr Soc 1966; 14:1041.
3. American College of Obstetricians and Gynecologists: Pregnancy and the postnatal period. In ACOG Home Exercise Program. Chicago, American College of Obstetricians and Gynecologists, 1985, pp 1–5.
4. Amundson G, Edwards CC, Garfin SR: Spondylolisthesis. In Rothman RH, Simeone FA (eds): The Spine, ed 3, vol. 1. Philadelphia, WB Saunders, 1992, pp 913–969.
5. Anderson GBJ, Svensson H-O, Odén A: The intensity of work recovery in low back pain. Spine 1983; 8:880.
6. Arnett FC: Seronegative spondyloarthropathies. Bull Rheum Dis 1987; 37(1):1.
7. Asmussen E, Heebøll-Nielsen K: Posture, mobility and strength of the back in boys 7 to 16 years old. Acta Orthop Scand 1959; 28:174.
8. Baker AS, Ojemann RG, Swartz MN, et al: Spinal epidural abscess. N Engl J Med 1975; 293:463.
9. Barron WM: Medical evaluation of the pregnant patient requiring nonobstetric surgery. Clin Perinatol 1985; 12:481.
10. Bartelink DL: The role of abdominal pressure in relieving the pressure on the lumbar intervertebral discs. J Bone Joint Surg Br 1957; 39:718.
11. Bartleson JD, Cohen MD, Harrington TM, et al: Cauda equina syndrome secondary to long-standing ankylosing spondylitis. Ann Neurol 1983; 14:662.
12. Battie MC, Bigos SJ, Fisher LD, et al: Anthropometric and clinical measures as predictors of back pain complaints in industry: A prospective study. J Spinal Disord 1990; 3:195.
13. Beimborn DS, Morrissey MC: A review of the literature related to trunk muscle performance. Spine 1988; 13:655.
14. Bell GR: Spondylolisthesis. In Hardy RW (ed): Lumbar Disc Disease, ed 2. New York, Raven Press, 1993, pp 209–223.
15. Berg G, Hammar M, Möller-Nielson J, et al: Low back pain during pregnancy. Obstet Gynecol 1988; 71:71.
16. Bergquist-Ullman M, Larsson U: Acute low back pain in industry: A controlled prospective study with special reference to therapy and confounding factors. Acta Orthop Scand Suppl 1977; 170:1.
17. Berkson M, Schultz A, Nachemson A, et al: Voluntary strengths of male adults with acute low back syndromes. Clin Orthop 1977; 129:84.
18. Biering-Sørensen F: Low back trouble in a general population of 30-, 40-, 50-, and 60-year-old men and women: Study design, representativeness and basic results. Dan Med Bull 1982; 29:289.
19. Biering-Sørensen F: A prospective study of low back pain in a general population: I. Occurrence, recurrence and aetiology. Scand J Rehabil Med 1983; 15:71.
20. Biering-Sørensen F: Physical measurements as risk indicators for low-back trouble over a 1-year period. Spine 1984; 9:106.
21. Boden SD, Davis DO, Dina TS, et al: Abnormal magnetic-resonance scans of the lumbar spine in asymptomatic subjects. J Bone Joint Surg Am 1990; 72:403.
22. Børgesen SE, Vang PS: Herniation of the lumbar intervertebral disk in children and adolescents. Acta Orthop Scand 1974; 45:540.

23. Boxall D, Bradford DS, Winter RB, et al: Management of severe spondylolisthesis in children and adolescents. J Bone Joint Surg Am 1979; 61:479.
24. Briggs GG, Freeman RK, Yaffe SJ: Drugs in Pregnancy and Lactation: A Reference Guide to Fetal and Neonatal Risk. Baltimore, Williams & Wilkins, 1990.
25. Cailliet R: Low Back Pain Syndrome, ed 4. Philadelphia, FA Davis, 1988.
26. Carrera GF, Haughton VM, Syvertsen A, et al: Computed tomography of the lumbar facet joints. Radiology 1980; 134:145.
27. Carrera GF, Williams AL, Haughton VM: Computed tomography in sciatica. Radiology 1980; 137:433.
28. Ciric I, Mikhael MA, Tarkington JA, et al: The lateral recess syndrome: A variant of spinal stenosis. J Neurosurg 1980; 53:433.
29. Collert S: Osteomyelitis of the spine. Acta Orthop Scand 1977; 48:283.
30. Daly JM, Frame PS, Rapoza PA: Sacroiliac subluxation: A common, treatable cause of low-back pain in pregnancy. Fam Pract Res J 1991; 11:149.
31. Dandy DJ, Shannon MJ: Lumbo-sacral subluxation (group I spondylolisthesis). J Bone Joint Surg Br 1971; 53:578.
32. Danner RL, Hartman BJ: Update of spinal epidural abscess: Thirty-five cases and review of the literature. Rev Infect Dis 1987; 9:265.
33. DeOrio JK, Bianco AJ Jr. Lumbar disc excision in children and adolescents. J Bone Joint Surg Am 1982; 64:991.
34. Department of Neurology, Mayo Clinic and Mayo Foundation: Clinical Examinations in Neurology, ed 6. St Louis, Mosby–Year Book, 1991.
35. Deyo RA, Bass JE: Lifestyle and low-back pain: The influence of smoking and obesity. Spine 1989; 14:501.
36. Deyo RA, Diehl AK, Rosenthal M: How many days of bed rest for acute low back pain? A randomized clinical trial. N Engl J Med 1986; 315:1064.
37. Dimaggio A, Mooney V: The McKenzie program: Exercise effective against back pain. J Musculoskel Med 1987; 4:63.
38. Duvoisin RC, Yahr MD: Compressive spinal cord and root syndromes in achondroplastic dwarfs. Neurology 1962; 12:202.
39. Ellenberg MR, Ross ML, Honet JC, et al: Prospective evaluation of the course of disc herniations in patients with proven radiculopathy. Arch Phys Med Rehabil 1993; 74:3.
40. Epstein JA (moderator): Treatment of low back pain and sciatic syndromes during pregnancy. NY State J Med 1959; 59:1757.
41. Epstein JA, Epstein NE: Lumbar spondylosis and spinal stenosis. In Wilkins RH, Rengachary SS (eds): Neurosurgery, vol 3. New York, McGraw-Hill, 1985, pp 2272–2278.
42. Fahrni WH: Conservative treatment of lumbar disc degeneration: Our primary responsibility. Orthop Clin North Am 1975; 6:93.
43. Falconer MA, McGeorge M, Begg AC: Observations on cause and mechanism of symptom-production in sciatica and low-back pain. J Neurol Neurosurg Psychiatry 1948; 11:13.
44. Fast A: Low back disorders: Conservative management. Arch Phys Med Rehabil 1988; 69:880.
45. Fast A, Shapiro D, Ducommun EJ, et al: Low-back pain in pregnancy. Spine 1987; 12:368.
46. Fast A, Weiss L, Ducommun EJ, et al: Low-back pain in pregnancy: Abdominal muscles, sit-up performance, and back pain. Spine 1990; 15:28.
47. Fast A, Weiss L, Parikh S, et al: Night backache in pregnancy: Hypothetical pathophysiological mechanisms. Am J Phys Med Rehabil 1989; 68:227.
48. Feller BA: Prevalence of Selected Impairment, United States, 1977, Hyattsville, MD, DHHS publication (PHS) 81-1562. Washington, DC, US Department of Health and Human Services, Public Health Service, Office of Health Research and Technology, National Center for Health Statistics, 1981.
49. Fischer DK, Simpson RK Jr, Baskin DS: Spinal spondylosis and disc disease. In Evans RW, Baskin DS, Yatsu FM (eds): Prognosis of Neurological Disorders. New York, Oxford University Press, 1992, pp 335–351.
50. Forestier J, Rotes-Querol J: Senile ankylosing hyperostosis of the spine. Ann Rheum Dis 1950; 9:321.
51. Freehafer AA: Orthotics in spinal cord injuries. In Bunch W (ed): Atlas of Orthotics: Biomechanical Principles and Application, ed 2. St Louis, Mosby–Year Book, 1985, pp 287–296.
52. Frymoyer JW: Back pain and sciatica. N Engl J Med 1988; 318:291.
53. Frymoyer JW, Pope MH, Clements JH, et al: Risk factors in low-back pain: An epidemiological survey. J Bone Joint Surg Am 1983; 65:213.
54. Frymoyer JW, Rosen JC, Clements J, et al: Psychologic factors in low-back-pain disability. Clin Orthop 1985; 195:178.
55. Garrido E: Lumbar disc herniation in the pediatric patient. Neurosurg Clin North Am 1993; 4:149.
56. Gellin BG, Weingarten K, Gamache FW Jr, et al: Epidural abscess. In Scheld WM, Whitley RJ, Durack DT (eds): Infections of the Central Nervous System. New York, Raven Press, 1991, pp 499–514.
57. Gilmour WN: Acute haematogenous osteomyelitis. J Bone Joint Surg Br 1962; 44:841.
58. Gramse RR, Sinaki M, Ilstrup DM: Lumbar spondylolisthesis: A rational approach to conservative treatment. Mayo Clin Proc 1980; 55:681.
59. Grazier KL, Holbrook TL, Kelsey JL, et al (eds): The Frequency of Occurrence, Impact and Cost of Selected Musculoskeletal Conditions in the United States. Chicago, American Academy of Orthopaedic Surgeons, 1984.
60. Griffiths HED, Jones DM: Pyogenic infection of the spine: A review of 28 cases. J Bone Joint Surg Br 1971; 53:383.
61. Grobler LJ, Simmons EH, Barrington TW: Intervertebral disc herniation in the adolescent. Spine 1979; 4:267.
62. Hakin RN, Burt AA, Cook JB: Acute spinal epidural abscess. Paraplegia 1979; 17:330.
63. Hall S, Bartleson JD, Onofrio BM, et al: Lumbar spinal stenosis: Clinical features, diagnostic procedures, and results of surgical treatment in 68 patients. Ann Intern Med 1985; 103:271.
64. Hasue M, Fujiwara M, Kikuchi S: A new method of quantitative measurement of abdominal and back muscle strength. Spine 1980; 5:143.
65. Heliövaara M: Risk factors for low back pain and sciatica. Ann Med 1989; 21:257.
66. Heliövaara M, Sievers K, Maatela J, et al: Descriptive epidemiology and public health aspects of low back pain. Ann Med 1989; 21:327.
67. Helliwell P, Moll J, Wright V: Measurement of spinal movement and function. In Jayson MIV (ed): The Lumbar Spine and Back Pain, ed 4. New York, Churchill Livingstone, 1992, pp 173–205.
68. Hendry NGC: The hydration of the nucleus pulposus and its relation to intervertebral disc derangement. J Bone Joint Surg Br 1958; 40:132.
69. Hensinger RN: Spondylolysis and spondylolisthesis in children. Instructional Course Lecture, no 32. 1983, p 132.
70. Heusner AP: Nontuberculous spinal epidural infections. N Engl J Med 1948; 239:845.
71. Hoehler FK, Tobis JS, Buerger AA: Spinal manipulation for low back pain. JAMA 1981; 245:1835.
72. Holt EP Jr: The question of lumbar discography. J Bone Joint Surg Am 1968; 50:720.
73. Horal J: The clinical appearance of low back disorders in the city of Gothenberg, Sweden: Comparisons of incapacitated probands with matched controls. Acta Orthop Scand Suppl 1969; 118:1.
74. Hudgins WR: Microdiscectomy. In Hardy RW Jr (ed): Lumbar Disc Disease, ed 2. New York, Raven Press, 1993, pp 139–145.
75. Hulme A, Dott NM: Spinal epidural abscess. Br Med J 1954; 1:64.
76. Ikata T: Statistical and dynamic studies of lesions due to overloading on the spine. Shikoku Acta Med 1965; 40:262.
77. Jenkins DB: Hollinshead's Functional Anatomy of the Limbs and Back, ed 6. Philadelphia, WB Saunders, 1991.
78. Kellgren JH, Lawrence JS: Osteo-arthrosis and disk degeneration in an urban population. Ann Rheum Dis 1958; 17:388.
79. Kelsey JL: An epidemiological study of the relationship between occupations and acute herniated lumbar intervertebral discs. Int J Epidemiol 1975; 4:197.
80. Khan MA: An overview of clinical spectrum and heterogeneity of spondyloarthropathies. Rheum Dis Clin North Am 1992; 18:1.
81. Krølner B, Toft B: Vertebral bone loss: An unheeded side effect of therapeutic bed rest. Clin Sci 1983; 64:537.
82. Lawrence JS, Molyneux MK, Dingwall-Fordyce I: Rheumatism in foundary workers. Br J Indust Med 1966; 23:42.

83. Lehmann JF, De Lateur BJ: Diathermy and superficial heat, laser, and cold therapy. In Kottke FJ, Lehmann JF: Krusen's Handbook of Physical Medicine and Rehabilitation, ed 4. Philadelphia, WB Saunders, 1990, pp 283–367.
84. Loebl WY: Measurement of spinal posture and range of spinal movement. Ann Phys Med 1967; 9:103.
85. Loeser JD, Volinn E: Epidemiology of low back pain. Neurosurg Clin North Am 1991; 2:713.
86. Love JG, Walsh MN: Protruded intervertebral disks: Report of 100 cases in which operation was performed. JAMA 1938; 111:396.
87. Lowe J, Schachner E, Hirschberg E, et al: Significance of bone scintigraphy in symptomatic spondylolysis. Spine 1984; 9:653.
88. Mapstone TB: Back pain in children. In Hardy RW Jr (ed): Lumbar Disc Disease, ed 2. New York, Raven Press, 1993, pp 255–259.
89. Maroon JC, Onik G, Quigley M, et al: Automated percutaneous lumbar discectomy: Indications, technique, and results. In Hardy RW Jr (ed): Lumbar Disc Disease, ed 2. New York, Raven Press, 1993, pp 147–153.
90. Masaryk TJ, Ross JS, Modic MT, et al: High-resolution MR imaging of sequestered lumbar intervertebral disks. AJR 1988; 150:1155.
91. Mayer TG, Tencer AF, Kristoferson S, et al: Use of noninvasive techniques for quantification of spinal range-of-motion in normal subjects and chronic low-back dysfunction patients. Spine 1984; 9:588.
92. McCulloch JA, Transfeldt E (eds): Macnab's Backache, ed 3. Baltimore, Williams & Wilkins, 1997.
93. McNeill T, Warwick D, Andersson G, et al: Trunk strengths in attempted flexion, extension, and lateral bending in healthy subjects and patients with low-back disorders. Spine 1980; 5:529.
94. McQuain MT, Sinaki M, Shibley LD, et al: Effect of electrical stimulation on lumbar paraspinal muscles. Spine 1993; 18:1787.
95. Menelaus MG: Discitis: An inflammation affecting the intervertebral discs in children. J Bone Joint Surg Br 1964; 46:16.
96. Meyerding HW: Spondylolisthesis. Proc Staff Meet Mayo Clin 1934; 9:666.
96a. Miller PD, Brown JP, Siris ES, et al: A randomized, double-blind comparison of risedronate and etidronate in the treatment of Paget's disease of bone. Am J Med 1999; 106:513.
97. Mokri B, Sinaki M: Painful disorders of the spine and back pain syndromes. In Sinaki M (ed): Basic Clinical Rehabilitation Medicine, ed 2. St Louis, Mosby–Year Book, 1993, pp 489–502.
98. Mokri B, Sinaki M: Lumbar disk syndromes, lumbosacral radiculopathies, lumbar spondylosis and stenosis, spondylolisthesis. In Sinaki M (ed): Basic Clinical Rehabilitation Medicine, ed 2. St Louis, Mosby–Year Book, 1993, pp 503–513.
99. Mooney RP, Hockberger RS: Spinal epidural abscess: A rapidly progressive disease. Ann Emerg Med 1987; 16:1168.
100. Müller EA: Influence of training and of inactivity on muscle strength. Arch Phys Med Rehabil 1970; 51:449.
101. Murphy KA, Cornish RD: Prediction of chronicity in acute low back pain. Arch Phys Med Rehabil 1984; 65:334.
102. Nachemson A: Lumbar intradiscal pressure: Experimental studies on post-mortem material. Acta Orthop Scand Suppl 1960; 43:1.
103. Nachemson A, Elfström G: Intravital dynamic pressure measurements in lumbar discs: A study of common movements, maneuvers and exercises. Scand J Rehabil Med Suppl 1970; 1:1.
104. Nachemson A, Lindh M: Measurement of abdominal and back muscle strength with and without low back pain. Scand J Rehabil Med 1969; 1:60.
105. Nachemson AL: The lumbar spine: An orthopaedic challenge. Spine 1976; 1:59.
106. Nachemson AL: Disc pressure measurements. Spine 1981; 6:93.
107. Nachemson AL: Orthotic treatment for injuries and diseases of the spinal column. Phys Med Rehabil 1987; 1:11.
108. Neugebauer FL: A new contribution to the history and etiology of spondylolisthesis. Select Monographs, no 8. London, 1888, pp 1–64.
109. Newcomer K, Sinaki M: Low back pain and its relationship to back strength and physical activity in children. Acta Paediatr 1996; 85:1433.
110. Newcomer K, Sinaki M, Wollan PC: Physical activity and four-year development of back strength in children. Am J Phys Med Rehabil 1997; 76:52.
111. Newman PH: The etiology of spondylolisthesis. J Bone Joint Surg Br 1963; 45:39.
112. Nordgren B, Schéle R, Linroth K: Evaluation and prediction of back pain during military field service. Scand J Rehabil Med 1980; 12:1.
113. Nummi J, Järvinen T, Stambej U, et al: Diminished dynamic performance capacity of back and abdominal muscles in concrete reinforcement workers. Scand J Work Environ Health 1978; 4 (suppl 1):39.
114. O'Brien JP: The halo-pelvic apparatus: A clinical, bio-engineering and anatomical study. Acta Orthop Scand Suppl 1975; 163:1.
115. Onofrio BM: Spine and intraspinal infections. In Horwitz NH, Rizzoli HV (eds): Postoperative Complications of Extracranial Neurological Surgery. Baltimore, Williams & Wilkins, 1987, pp 169–206.
116. Ostgaard HC, Andersson GBJ: Previous back pain and risk of developing back pain in a future pregnancy. Spine 1991; 16:432.
117. Ostgaard HC, Andersson GBJ, Karlsson K: Prevalence of back pain in pregnancy. Spine 1991; 16:549.
118. Panjabi MM, Hult JE, Crisco JJ III, et al: Biomechanical studies in cadaveric spines. In Jayson MIV (ed): The Lumbar Spine and Back Pain, ed 4. New York, Churchill Livingstone, 1992, pp 133–155.
119. Payne WK III, Ogilvie JW: Back pain in children and adolescents. Pediatr Clin North Am 1996; 43:899.
120. Pedersen OF, Petersen R, Staffeldt ES: Back pain and isometric back muscle strength of workers in a Danish factory. Scand J Rehabil Med 1975; 7:125.
121. Petrie RS, Sinaki M, Squires RW, et al: Physical activity, but not aerobic capacity, correlates with back strength in healthy premenopausal women from 29 to 40 years of age. Mayo Clin Proc 1993; 68:738.
122. Plucinski T, Sinaki M, Currier B, et al: Sports and spondylolisthesis in children. In Proceedings of Advances in Idiopathic Low Back Pain Congress. Vienna, Blackwell Scientific Publications, June 1993.
123. Plucinski T, Sinaki M, Rizzo T, et al: Spondylolisthesis in children: Surgery, symptoms and physical findings. In Official Program of the Spring Meeting of the Association of Academic Physiatrists, Naples, FL, January 1994.
124. Pope MH: Risk indicators in low back pain. Ann Med 1989; 21:387.
125. Pope MH, Wilder DG, Stokes IAF, et al: Biomechanical testing as an aid to decision making in low-back pain patients. Spine 1979; 4:135.
126. Postacchini F: Lumbar Spinal Stenosis. New York, Springer-Verlag, 1989.
127. Riihimäki H, Tola S, Videman T, et al: Low-back pain and occupation: A cross-sectional questionnaire study of men in machine operating, dynamic physical work, and sedentary work. Spine 1989; 14:204.
128. Rowe ML: Preliminary statistical study of low back pain. J Occup Med 1963; 5:336.
129. Rudins A, Sinaki M, Miller JL, et al: Significance of back extensors versus back flexors in trunkal support (abstract). Arch Phys Med Rehabil 1991; 72:824.
130. Rumgee JL: Low back pain during pregnancy. Orthopedics 1993; 16:1339.
131. Saal JA, Saal JS: Nonoperative treatment of herniated lumbar intervertebral disc with radiculopathy: An outcome study. Spine 1989; 14:431.
132. Salminen JJ, Oksanen A, Maki P, et al: Leisure time physical activity in the young. Correlation with low-back pain, spinal mobility and trunk muscle strength in 15-year-old school children. Int J Sports Med 1993; 14:406.
133. Sands RX: Backache of pregnancy: A method of treatment. Obstet Gynecol 1958; 12:670.
134. Schober P: Ledenwirbelsäule and Kreuzschmerzen. Munchen Med Wochnschr 1937; 84:336.
135. Schultz A, Andersson G, Örtengren R, et al: Loads on the lumbar spine: Validation of a biomechanical analysis by measurements

of intradiscal pressures and myoelectric signals. J Bone Joint Surg Am 1982; 64:713.
136. Simeone FA: Lumbar disk disease. In Wilkins RH, Rengachary SS (eds): Neurosurgery, vol 3. New York, McGraw-Hill, 1985, pp 2250–2259.
137. Sinaki M: Exercise and physical therapy. In Riggs BL, Melton LJ III (eds): Osteoporosis: Etiology, Diagnosis, and Management. New York, Raven Press, 1988, pp 457–479.
138. Sinaki M (ed): Basic Clinical Rehabilitation Medicine, ed 2. St Louis, Mosby–Year Book, 1993, pp 209–236.
139. Sinaki M, Chan C, Plucinski T, et al: Spondylolisthesis of the osteoporotic spine. In Proceedings of the Fourth International Symposium on Osteoporosis and Consensus Development Conference. Hong Kong, March 27–April 2, 1993, p 106.
140. Sinaki M, Grubbs NC: Back strengthening exercises: Quantitative evaluation of their efficacy for women aged 40 to 65 years. Arch Phys Med Rehabil 1989; 70:16.
141. Sinaki M, Limburg PJ, Wollan PC, et al: Correlation of trunk muscle strength with age in children 5 to 18 years old. Mayo Clin Proc 1996; 71:1047.
142. Sinaki M, Lutness MP, Ilstrup DM, et al: Lumbar spondylolisthesis: Retrospective comparison and 3-year follow-up of two conservative treatment programs. Arch Phys Med Rehabil 1989; 70:584.
143. Sinaki M, Mikkelsen BA: Postmenopausal spinal osteoporosis: Flexion versus extension exercises. Arch Phys Med Rehabil 1984; 65:593.
144. Sinaki M, Nicholas JJ: Metabolic bone diseases and aging. In Felsenthal G, Garrison SJ, Steinberg FU (eds): Rehabilitation of the Aging and Elderly Patient. Philadelphia, Williams & Wilkins, 1994, pp 107–122.
145. Siris E, Weinstein RS, Altman R, et al: Comparative study of alendronate versus etidronate for the treatment of Paget's disease of bone. J Clin Endocrinol Metab 1996; 81:961.
146. Snook SH: Low back pain in industry. In White AA III, Gordon SL (eds): American Academy of Orthopaedic Surgeons: Symposium on Idiopathic Low Back Pain. St Louis, Mosby–Year Book, 1982, pp 23–38.
147. Spangfort EV: The lumbar disc herniation: A computer-aided analysis of 2,504 operations. Acta Orthop Scand Suppl 1972; 142:1.
148. Steindler A: Kinesiology of the Human Body Under Normal and Pathological Conditions. Springfield, IL, Charles C Thomas, 1965.
149. Stern WE, Balch RE: Surgical aspects of nonspecific inflammatory and suppurative disease of the vertebral column. Am J Surg 1966; 112:314.
150. Stone DB, Bonfiglio M: Pyogenic vertebral osteomyelitis: A diagnostic pitfall for the internist. Arch Intern Med 1963; 112:491.
151. Svensson H-O, Andersson GBJ: Low-back pain in 40- to 47-year-old men: Work history and work environment factors. Spine 1983; 8:272.
152. Svensson H-O, Andersson GBJ, Hagstad A, et al: The relationship of low-back pain to pregnancy and gynecologic factors. Spine 1990; 15:371.
153. Tauber J: An unorthodox look at backaches. J Occup Med 1970; 12:128.
154. Taylor H, Curran NM: The Nuprin Pain Report. New York, Louis Harris & Associates, 1985.
155. Turner PG, Green JH, Galasko CSB: Back pain in childhood. Spine 1989; 14:812.
156. Utsinger PD, Resnick D, Shapiro R: Diffuse skeletal abnormalities in Forestier disease. Arch Intern Med 1976; 136:763.
157. Vällfors B: Acute, subacute and chronic low back pain: Clinical symptoms, absenteeism and working environment. Scand J Rehabil Med Suppl 1985; 11:1.
158. Van Alphen HAM, Braakman R, Bezemer PD, et al: Chemonucleolysis versus discectomy: A randomized multicenter trial. J Neurosurg 1989; 70:869.
159. Vanderburgh DF, Kelly WM: Radiographic assessment of discogenic disease of the spine. Neurosurg Clin North Am 1993; 4:13.
160. Wagner DK, Varkey B, Sheth NK, et al: Epidural abscess, vertebral destruction, and paraplegia caused by extending infection from an aspergilloma. Am J Med 1985; 78:518.
161. Waldvogel FA, Medoff G, Swartz MN: Osteomyelitis: A review of clinical features, therapeutic considerations and unusual aspects. N Engl J Med 1970; 282:316.
162. Weinstein PR: Anatomy of the lumbar spine. In Hardy RW Jr (ed): Lumbar Disk Disease, ed 2. New York, Raven Press, 1993, pp 5–11.
163. Weir MR, Smith DS: Stress reaction of the pars interarticularis leading to spondylolysis: A cause of adolescent low back pain. J Adolesc Health Care 1989; 10:573.
164. Weisman MH: Spondyloarthropathies. In Stein JH (ed): Internal Medicine, ed 4. St Louis, Mosby–Year Book, 1994, pp 2454–2462.
165. Whelan MA, Naidich DP, Post JD, et al: Computed tomography of spinal tuberculosis. J Comput Assist Tomogr 1983; 7:25.
166. Wilbourn AJ: The value and limitations of electromyographic examination in the diagnosis of lumbosacral radiculopathy. In Hardy RW Jr (ed). Lumbar Disc Disease, New York, Raven Press, 1982, pp 65–109.
167. Wiltse LL: Common problems of the lumbar spine: Spondylolisthesis and its treatment. J Cont Educ Orthop 1979; 7:13.
168. Wiltse LL, Newman PH, Macnab I: Classification of spondylolysis and spondylolisthesis. Clin Orthop 1976; 117:23.
169. Witt I, Vestergaard A, Rosenklint A: A comparative analysis of x-ray findings of the lumbar spine in patients with and without lumbar pain. Spine 1984; 9:298.
170. Yong-Hing K, Kirkaldy-Willis WH: The pathophysiology of degenerative disease of the lumbar spine. Orthop Clin North Am 1983; 14:491.
171. Zamani M, MacEwen GD: Herniation of the lumbar disc in children and adolescents. J Pediatr Orthop 1982; 2:528.

41

CHAPTER

Mehrsheed Sinaki, M.D., M.S.

Prevention and Treatment of Osteoporosis

Bone, to be maintained, needs to be mechanically strained—within its biomechanical limits.

Mehrsheed Sinaki, M.D.

Through a multidisciplinary approach, we can add quality to the years of life with osteoporosis. Osteoporosis, the most prevalent metabolic bone disease in the United States, is a major public health problem. The direct and indirect cost of osteoporosis in the United States is estimated to be more than $14 billion annually.[35] Much of this expense relates to hip fractures. In 12% to 20% of hip fracture cases, the outcome is fatal.[37, 42]

Osteoporosis consists of a heterogeneous group of syndromes in which there is reduced bone mass per unit volume in otherwise normal bone, resulting in fragile bone. The increment in bone porosity results in architectural instability of bone and increases the likelihood of fracture. The ratio of mineral to matrix is normal in osteoporosis, but in osteomalacia the mineral content is significantly reduced. The World Health Organization has defined osteoporosis as bone mineral density 2.5 standard deviations below the peak mean bone mass of young normal adults.[71]

In the asymptomatic stage of the disease, it is characterized simply by a low bone mass without fractures. Osteoporosis becomes clinically problematic only when the bone fractures.

BONE FUNCTION AND STRUCTURE

Bone serves as a mechanical support for musculoskeletal structures, as protection for vital organs, and as a metabolic source of ions, especially calcium and phosphate. Despite its appearance, bone is very active tissue. To maintain its biomechanical competence, bone tissue undergoes continuous change and renewal so that older bone tissue is replaced by newly formed bone tissue. Approximately 20% of bone tissue is replaced annually by this cyclic process. There are two types of bone cells: osteoclasts, which resorb the calcified matrix, and osteoblasts, which synthesize new bone matrix.[45]

Osteoclasts are localized on the endosteal bone surfaces; their origin is hematopoietic, and they share a common precursor with the monocyte macrophage. Osteoclasts are large multinucleated cells with an average of 10 to 20 nuclei. Osteoclasts have a special cell membrane with folds and invagination at the interface with bone surface, called the "ruffled border." To induce resorption of bone and the mineralized bone matrix, osteoclasts produce proteolytic enzymes in this ruffled border.

Osteoblasts are derived from mesenchymal cells. The role of osteoblasts is mineralization of the matrix through budding of vesicles from their cytoplasmic membrane. These vesicles are rich in alkaline phosphatase. Osteoblasts secrete all the growth factors that are trapped in the matrix.

BONE REMODELING

Bone is continuously being turned over by the two processes of modeling and remodeling. This process allows maintenance of the biomechanical integrity of the skeleton, and it supports the role of bone in provision of an ionic bank for the body and mechanical support. Bone remodeling is a process that allows removal of old bone and replacement with new bone tissue.

Bone remodeling has five phases: (1) activation—osteoclastic activity is recruited; (2) resorption—osteoclasts erode bone and form a cavity; (3) reversal—osteoblasts are recruited; (4) formation—osteoblasts replace the cavity with new bone; and (5) quiescence—bone tissue remains dormant until the next cycle starts. This process is cyclical, starting with bone resorption and finishing with bone formation. In adult human bone, each cycle of remodeling lasts 3 to 12 months. The signal that stops osteoclastic activity is not yet completely defined. After bone resorption, the reversal phase starts, which involves osteoblastic activity. Then the osteoblasts start to fill the resorption cavity. During the process of osteoclastic activity, the growth factors, stored in the bone matrix, are released and subsequently can stimulate osteoblastic proliferation. This process of bone resorption and formation is called "coupling." The ideal situation in the coupling process is equilibrated bone formation and resorption. In osteoporosis, however, there is a disequilibrium between resorption and formation, favoring resorption that results in bone loss.

The number of active remodeling units in trabecular bone is about three times higher than that in cortical bone. The physical endurance of any bone is affected by the percentage of cortical bone involved in its structure. Trabecular bone is more active metabolically than cortical bone because of the significant surface exposure areas. Consequently, more bone loss occurs at the trabecular areas when resorption is greater than formation. The vertebrae consist of 50% trabecular bone and 50% cortical bone, whereas the femoral neck consists of 30% trabecular bone and 70% cortical bone. When bone turnover increases, bone loss and osteoporosis occur in the vertebrae before the femoral neck.

PATHOGENESIS

Peak adult bone mass is achieved between ages 30 and 35 years. Thereafter, bone mass at any point in life is the difference between the peak adult bone mass and the amount that has been lost since the peak was reached. Age-related bone loss is a universal phenomenon in humans. Any circumstances that limit bone formation or increase bone loss increase the likelihood that osteoporosis will develop later in life. Measures that can maximize peak adult bone mass are clearly desirable.

Trabecular (or cancellous) bone represents about 20% of skeletal bone mass and makes up 80% of the turnover media. The cortex, which is made of compact bone and represents 80% of skeletal bone mass, makes up only 20% of the turnover media. In both cortical and trabecular bone, bone remodeling is initiated with activation of osteoclasts, which erode the bone, resulting in bone resorption. The resorption sites are then refilled by osteoblastic activities, which is called bone formation. If the amount of bone resorbed equals the amount formed, the bone loss is zero. The remodeling process does not result in zero balance after age 30 to 35 years. After this age, the normal process of remodeling results in bone loss.[44]

In the normal aging process, there is deficit between resorption and formation because osteoblastic activity is not equal to osteoclastic activity. The net result of the remodeling process is bone loss during each cycle of remodeling. Bone loss occurs even when the remodeling process is not increased. In fact, activation of skeletal remodeling is decreased as a result of the process of aging. This gives rise to the concept of low-turnover osteoporosis, which occurs concomitantly with the aging process.

Certain conditions, such as hyperparathyroidism or thyrotoxicosis, can increase the rate of bone remodeling. These conditions increase the rate of bone loss, which results in high-turnover osteoporosis. The secondary causes of osteoporosis are associated with an increased rate of activation of the remodeling cycle. Although environmental factors such as calcium intake, smoking, alcohol, physical exercise, and menopause are important factors in determining bone mineral density, genetic factors are the major determinant and contribute to 80% of the variance in peak bone mineral density.[9] Fracture incidence related to osteoporosis is lower in men than in women because the diameter of vertebral bodies and long bones is greater in men at maturity and bone loss is less (about half that of women) throughout life in men.[48]

HORMONES AND PHYSIOLOGY OF BONE

The rate of bone remodeling can be increased by parathyroid hormone, thyroxine, growth hormone, and vitamin D [$1,25(OH)_2D_3$]; it can be decreased by calcitonin, estrogen, and glucocorticoids.[27]

The major hormone for calcium homeostasis is *parathyroid hormone* (PTH). PTH is secreted by the parathyroid glands, located behind the thyroid glands. The level of plasma calcium is the major moderator of the secretion of PTH. PTH regulates the plasma calcium ion (Ca^{2+}) concentration in three ways: (1) In the presence of active vitamin D, it stimulates bone resorption and the release of calcium and phosphate; (2) through production of calcitriol in the kidneys, it indirectly increases intestinal absorption of calcium and phosphate; and (3) it increases active reabsorption of calcium ions in the renal distal tubal area. PTH also reduces proximal tubular reabsorption of phosphate. In general, PTH increases serum calcium and mostly tends to lower serum phosphate.

Calcitonin is a hormone secreted by the parafollicular cells of the thyroid gland. The major stimulus of calcitonin is the serum level of calcium. Through inhibition of osteoclastic activity, calcitonin directly prohibits calcium and phosphate resorption, lowering the serum calcium level.

The main regulators of vitamin D synthesis are the serum concentrations of $1,25(OH)_2D_3$ itself, calcium, phosphate, and PTH. PTH is the major inducer of the active form of vitamin D formation in the kidney. This function is accomplished through the effect of the enzyme 1α-hydroxylase, which transforms the inactive form of vitamin D to the potent form. The active form of vitamin D increases intestinal absorption of calcium and phosphate. Vitamin D also is required for appropriate bone mineralization. The effect of the active form of vitamin D is both a direct stimulation of osteoblastic activity and indirect through increasing the intestinal absorption of calcium and phosphorus.

SEX STEROIDS

The main endocrine function that occurs at menopause is loss of secretion of estrogen and progesterone from the ovaries.[22, 28, 48] The premenopausal ovary produces primarily estradiol. Progesterone secretion, which occurs cyclically after ovulation in the premenopausal state, also declines to very low levels at the postmenopausal stage. These changes in circulating sex steroids are gradual in a woman's sexual reproductive life. The premenopausal ovary also produces androgens, especially testosterone. The circulating testosterone levels decrease after menopause. The major source of estrogen in postmenopausal women is conversion from dihydroepiandrostenedione. This is converted into androstenedione, which changes into estrone in fat cells. Estrone is the major source of estrogen in postmenopausal women. Men do not have the equivalent of menopause, but in some elderly men, bone mass decreases along with decline in gonadal function. The testosterone level in men decreases with age as a result of a decreased number of Leydig cells in the testes. Male hypogonadism is typically associated with bone loss.

OTHER FACTORS AFFECTING BONE MASS

Several other factors can contribute to the reduction of gender-related steroids. In hyperprolactinemia, which is due to a prolactin-secreting pituitary tumor, failure of the gonadal axis results in a significant loss of bone. Amenorrheic athletes who exercise excessively (such as high-mileage runners) and have lower than normal body weight have lower circulating estradiol, progesterone, and prolactin levels. Their amenorrhea is associated with hypothalamic hypogonadism, which leads to excessive bone loss. This bone loss can be partly reversible when training distances are decreased.[8, 26]

Reduction of sex steroids is not the only cause of bone loss. Other factors such as race, genetics, nutrition, physical exercise, and lifestyle can also contribute to the rate of bone loss after ovariectomy or natural menopause.[55] It is well known that bone must be physically stressed to be maintained. A significant body of data shows that the rate of strain change also influences bone growth and remodeling.[34]

EFFECT OF AGING

Age plays a significant role in the rate of bone turnover. It has been clearly determined that bone turnover increases in women at menopause, but bone turnover does not increase significantly in men with aging. Most studies have shown that plasma levels of $1,25(OH)_2D_3$ decrease with age by about 50% in both men and women.

Growth hormone stimulates renal production of the active form of vitamin D [$1,25(OH)_2D_3$] and growth hormone decreases with age. It appears that vitamin K therapy in the elderly is associated with a decrease in the rate of bone resorption, as demonstrated by decreased excretion of urinary hydroxyproline. Further studies are needed to support this. Studies have shown that calcium absorption is less efficient in the elderly.[20] Bone loss also has been related to deficiencies in trace metal elements such as copper, zinc, and magnesium, but this issue is not fully resolved.

Plasma calcitonin levels are higher in men than in women. Calcitonin levels do not change with age. Studies have shown that estrogens stimulate calcitonin secretion.[67, 68] Thyroid hormone levels typically show no change or are slightly decreased with age. Growth hormone secretion is reduced in osteoporotic patients. Growth hormone and insulin-like growth factor I have several positive effects on calcium homeostasis, including synthesis of $1,25(OH)_2D_3$, osteoblast proliferation, osteoclast differentiation, and bone resorption.

PTH level increases with age, perhaps due to mild hypocalcemia and decreased $1,25(OH)_2D_3$. This reduction in the active form of vitamin D can be due to lower consumption of dietary vitamin D, lower exposure to sunlight, lower skin capacity for vitamin D conversion, reduced intestinal absorption, and reduced 1α-hydroxylase activity.

Several studies have demonstrated that the level of physical activity decreases with aging.[55] Physical strain and mechanical load also affect bone mass.[14] Exercise is known to stimulate the release of growth hormone or other trophic factors that can stimulate osteoblastic activity.[12] Optimal nutrition and physical activity are necessary to achieve the genetic potential for bone mass. The peak bone mass attained by young adulthood is a major determinant of bone mass in later life. Female gymnasts, both children and college-aged athletes, reportedly have higher bone mineral density than swimmers.[2, 11] Nutrition also can affect both bone matrix formation and bone mineralization. The recommended adequate calcium intake for ages 9 to 18 years is 1300 mg/day (see Table 41–7).[31]

CLASSIFICATION OF OSTEOPOROSIS

Osteoporosis can be primary or secondary. Primary osteoporosis is also known as idiopathic osteoporosis because no specific etiologic mechanism is recognized. This type of osteoporosis is either postmenopausal (type I) or senile, or age-related (type II).[41] Another type of primary osteoporosis is the rare disorder of idiopathic juvenile osteoporosis, the cause of which is unknown. This typically occurs before puberty (between ages 8 and 14 years), and patients present with osteoporosis that is progressive over a period of 2 to 4 years with the occurrence of multiple fractures, axial or axioappendicular. Remission usually occurs by the end of the 2 to 4 year course.[23] In this type of osteoporosis, the process of bone formation is normal, but there is an increase

TABLE 41–1 Common Causes of Osteoporosis

Hereditary, congenital: osteogenesis imperfecta, neurologic disturbances (myotonia congenita, Werdnig-Hoffmann disease), gonadal dysgenesis
Acquired (primary and secondary)
1. Generalized
    - Idiopathic (premenopausal women and middle-aged or young men; juvenile osteoporosis)
    - Postmenopausal (type I)
    - Senile (type II)
    - Secondary (type III):
        - Nutrition: malnutrition, anorexia/bulimia, vitamin deficiency (C or D), vitamin overuse (D or A), calcium deficiency, high sodium intake, high caffeine intake, high protein intake, high phosphate intake, alcohol abuse
    - Sedentary lifestyle, immobility, smoking
    - Gastrointestinal diseases (liver disease, malabsorption syndromes, alactasia, subtotal gastrectomy) or small bowel resection
    - Nephropathies
    - Chronic obstructive pulmonary disease
    - Malignancy (multiple myeloma, disseminated carcinoma)
    - Drugs: phenytoin, barbiturates, cholestyramine, heparin
    - Endocrine disorders: acromegaly, hyperthyroidism, Cushing's syndrome (iatrogenic or endogenous), hyperparathyroidism, diabetes mellitus (?), hypogonadism
2. Localized: inflammatory arthritis, fractures and immobilization in cast, limb dystrophies, muscular paralysis

From Sinaki M: Rehabilitation in metabolic bone disease. In Sinaki M (ed): Basic Clinical Rehabilitation Medicine, ed 2. St Louis, Mosby, 1993, pp 209–236. By permission of Mayo Foundation.

in osteoclastic activity resulting in increased bone resorption. This type of osteoporosis is most evident in the thoracic and lumbar spine and needs to be distinguished from juvenile epiphysitis or Scheuermann's disease. This disorder is usually self-limiting, but the radiographic appearance might not return to normal. The laboratory values are typically normal, and the diagnosis is made by exclusion. The most common causes of osteoporosis are listed in Table 41–1.

CLINICAL MANIFESTATIONS OF OSTEOPOROSIS

Osteoporosis is typically a "silent disease" until fractures occur. Osteoporotic vertebral fractures can go unnoticed until incidentally seen on a chest radiograph. Appendicular fractures, however, require immediate attention. The fact that the fracture results from osteoporosis should not affect the orthopedic method of management. The most common areas for osteoporotic fractures are the mid-thoracic and upper lumbar spine (Fig. 41–1),[63] hip (proximal femur), and distal forearm (Colles' fracture). The highest incidence of fractures is in white females. The female : male ratio is about 7 : 1 for vertebral fractures, 2 : 1 for hip fractures, and 5 : 1 for Colles' fractures. It has been estimated that after menopause, a woman's lifetime risk of sustaining an osteoporotic fracture is 1 in 2 or 3.[33]

The most concern is for hip fracture because the risk of death with osteoporotic hip fracture is 15% to 20%, despite all the developments in surgical and nonsurgical intervention. The management of an osteoporotic spine fracture requires immobilization of the involved vertebral bodies and analgesia. Fortunately, these fractures heal through becoming more condensed and do not require any specific treatment process, as is usually needed for the appendicular fractures. If there is nonunion of the appendicular fracture, one needs to look for conditions other than osteoporosis, such as osteomalacia or hyperparathyroidism. The duration of immobilization should be for only a limited time, sufficient to ensure the primary fracture healing process. Prolonged immobilization is discouraged because it can contribute to osteoporosis.

The orthopedic management for most osteoporotic fractures is generally noncontroversial, except for the management of hip fracture. The management of femoral neck fracture creates a great deal of controversy because of the high complication rate. There is an ongoing effort to try to solve these controversies through prospective studies. Despite these efforts, the treatment of hip fracture remains a challenge, and each case creates an emergency situation. Shoulder fracture, espe-

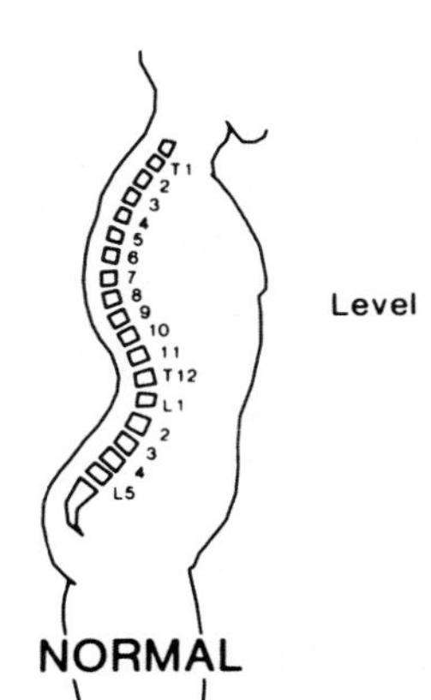

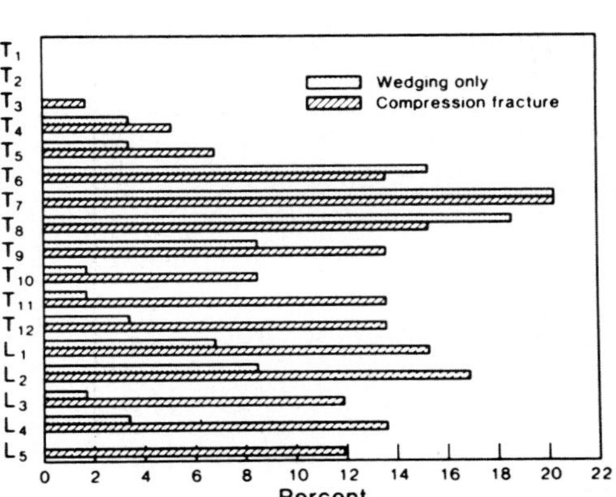

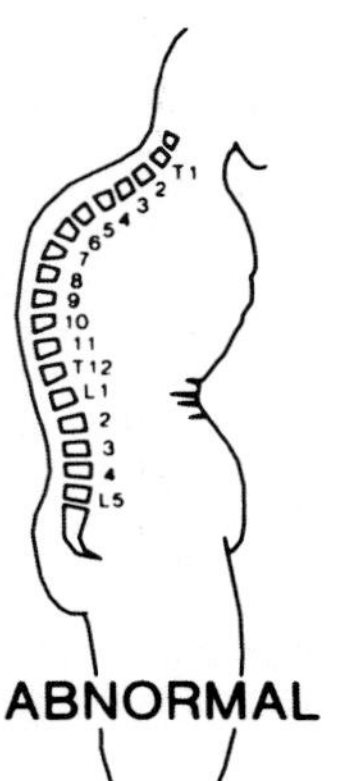

FIGURE 41–1. Incidence of wedging and compression fractures at various levels of spine. (From Sinaki M, Mikkelsen BA: Postmenopausal spinal osteoporosis: Flexion versus extension exercises. Arch Phys Med Rehabil 1984; 65:593. By permission of the American Congress of Rehabilitation Medicine and the American Academy of Physical Medicine and Rehabilitation.)

cially the surgical neck of the proximal humerus, is not uncommon in elderly women. This type of fracture usually occurs from an impact force directly onto the shoulder during a fall. In most cases, this fracture is not dislocated and a conservative treatment regimen suffices.

FRACTURES AND MANAGEMENT

The relationship between bone mass and spinal fractures has been studied extensively. As bone mass decreases, fracture risk increases. For every standard deviation of decrease in bone mineral density, the risk of osteoporotic fracture of the spine increases 1.5- to 2-fold, and the risk of hip fracture increases 2.6-fold.[19] Another predictor of fracture risk is age itself. The risk of fracture due to osteoporosis doubles every 5 to 7 years.[19] It is not clear whether age-related changes in bone density and bone quality are factors that increase the risk of fractures due to falls.

Vertebral Fracture

The incidence of vertebral fractures is poorly understood because 50% of these fractures can be subclinical and the patient might not seek medical attention. Vertebral fractures can create two types of pain: acute and, later, chronic pain.

Acute pain that occurs in the absence of a previous fracture is usually due to compression fractures in the vertebrae. Sometimes a minor fall or even an affectionate hug can lead to a compression fracture. The compressed vertebrae might not be apparent on radiographs for up to four weeks after the injury.[36] Compression fracture usually results in acute pain that later resolves (Table 41–2).[52] The spinal deformity as a result of these fractures can produce chronic pain.[53]

Kyphotic postural change is the most physically disfiguring and psychologically damaging effect of osteoporosis.[60] The incidence of osteoporosis can be substantially decreased only by early detection and subsequent intervention in the high-risk patient population. Disproportionate weakness in back extensor musculature relative to body weight or flexor strength considerably increases the possibility of compressing vertebrae in the fragile osteoporotic spine. Recognition and improvement of decreased back extensor strength enhance the ability to maintain proper vertical alignment.[50] The geriatric population has an increased risk for debilitating postural changes because of several factors, the two most apparent being a greater prevalence of osteoporosis and involutional loss of functional muscle motor units.[17, 32] Development of kyphotic posture not only can predispose to postural back pain, but also can increase the risk of falls.[30, 66] Several other factors can also contribute to the risk of falls (Table 41–3).[56]

TABLE 41–2 Management of Acute Pain in Patients with Osteoporosis

Bedrest (2 days). Significant bone loss is not likely to occur with 2 days of bedrest
Analgesics (avoid codeine derivatives)
Avoidance of constipation
Physical therapy: initially cold packs, then mild heat and stroking massage
Avoidance of exertional exercises
Teach lifting and standing principles to avoid excessive spinal strain
Back supports, if needed, to decrease pain and expedite ambulation
Gait aids if needed

Modified from Sinaki M: Rehabilitation in metabolic bone disease. In Sinaki M (ed): Basic Clinical Rehabilitation Medicine, ed 2. St Louis, Mosby, 1993, pp 209–236. By permission of Mayo Foundation.

TABLE 41–3 Contributing Factors to Risk of Falling

Visual impairment
Vestibular changes
Impaired proprioceptive feedback
Cognitive changes
Poor coordination
Postural changes, balance disorder, unsteady gait
Reduced muscle strength
Reduced flexibility
Respiratory, orthopnea
Postural hypotension
Cardiovascular deconditioning
Iatrogenically reduced alertness
Inappropriate footwear
Insufficient ambulatory aids
Environmental (such as poor illumination, uneven surface, loose carpeting, slippery floor, pets)

From Sinaki M: Prevention of hip fracture: Physical activity. In Ringe JD, Meunier JP (eds): Osteoporotic Fractures in the Elderly: Clinical Management and Prevention. Stuttgart, Georg Thieme Verlag, 1996, pp 99–115. By permission of Georg Thieme Verlag.

Chronic pain can be due to the development of deformity caused by vertebral wedging, compression, and ligamentous strain. The intervertebral disks undergo the most dramatic age-related changes of all connective tissues.[1] With aging, the number and diameter of the collagen fibril portion of the disk increase. This change is accompanied by a progressive decrease in disk compliance. Loss of distinction between the nucleus pulposus and the annulus fibrosus occurs eventually.

Chronic back pain is related to postural changes due to vertebral fractures.[60] Strong back muscles contribute to good posture and skeletal support (Fig. 41–2).[21, 65, 66] The pain and skeletal deformity associated with osteoporosis might secondarily reduce muscle strength. The reduction in muscle strength can further exacerbate the postural abnormalities associated with this condition (Fig. 41–3). Chronic pain can also be due to microfractures that are visible only on bone scanning and that occur continuously. Management of chronic osteoporosis-related pain is outlined in Table 41–4. One should be hesitant about using strong analgesics such as codeine sulfate or its derivatives because they can cause constipation.[49]

Hip Fracture

Hip fracture is an emergency situation. In typical cases, the extremity is rotated outward (externally rotated)

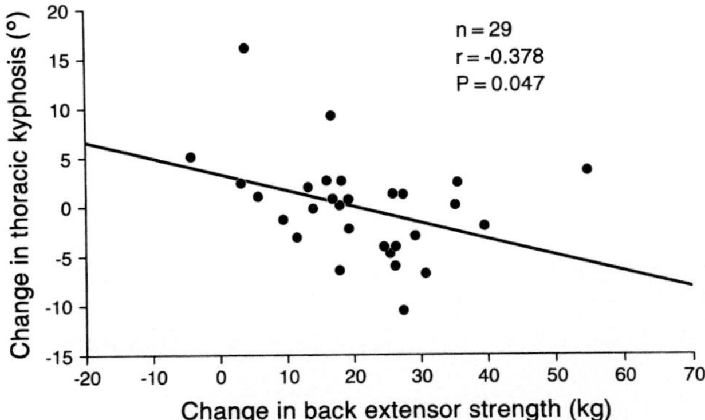

FIGURE 41–2. Correlation between change in back extensor strength and change in thoracic kyphosis in patients with hyperkyphosis (34.1° or more) of 29 healthy estrogen-deficient women. A significant negative correlation was found. (From Itoi E, Sinaki M: Effect of back-strengthening exercise on posture in healthy women 49 to 65 years of age. Mayo Clin Proc 1994; 69:1054. By permission of Mayo Foundation.)

and shortened. It is difficult to tell from the clinical evaluation whether the fracture is intracapsular (femoral neck fracture) or extracapsular (trochanteric fracture). Radiographs are necessary to make this distinction because the operative treatment and the outcome of intracapsular versus extracapsular hip fractures differ considerably. The consensus is that surgery is the treatment of choice for femoral neck fracture and trochanteric hip fracture. However, in some unusual cases of impacted fracture, particularly in a patient who is severely debilitated and has impaired general health, conservative treatment might be advisable. Femoral neck fracture requires fixation, and the type of fixation varies among surgeons. Because of the high incidence of operative failures after internal fixation of these fractures, most orthopedists prefer performing arthroplasties. Some orthopedists prefer total joint replacement, whereas some prefer hemiarthroplasty only for the femoral neck and head. The rationale is that total hip arthroplasties are considered to stay intact longer than

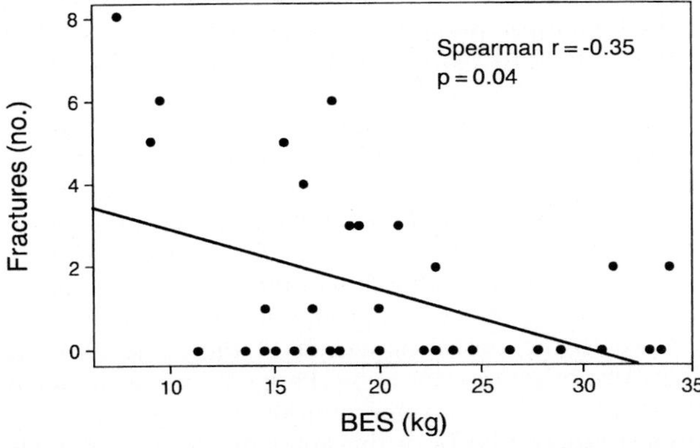

FIGURE 41–3. Correlation of number of vertebral fractures with back extensor strength (BES) in women with osteoporosis. (From Sinaki M, Wollan PC, Scott RW, et al: Can strong back extensors prevent vertebral fractures in women with osteoporosis? Mayo Clin Proc 1996; 71:951. By permission of Mayo Foundation.)

TABLE 41–4 Management of Chronic Pain in Patients with Osteoporosis

Improve faulty posture, may need Posture Training Support (PTS)
Manage pain (ultrasound, massage, or transcutaneous electrical nerve stimulation [TENS])
If beyond correction, apply back support to decrease painful stretch of ligaments
Avoid physical activities that exert extreme vertical compression forces on vertebrae
Prescribe a patient-specific therapeutic exercise program
Start appropriate pharmacologic intervention

From Sinaki M: Rehabilitation in metabolic bone disease. In Sinaki M (ed): Basic Clinical Rehabilitation Medicine, ed 2. St Louis, Mosby, 1993, pp 209–236. By permission of Mayo Foundation.

hemiarthroplasties. The only concern is that the hemiarthroplasty is a considerably smaller surgical trauma for the patient, and hence is advocated in the very old or frail patient with a prognosis of limited mobility.

The trochanteric hip fracture creates lesser problems despite the fact that the fracture engages more bone than does the femoral neck fracture. The operative treatment of choice is internal fixation (Fig. 41–4). The postoperative course for all hip fractures, regardless of whether internal fixation or joint arthroplasty is done, is less eventful if physical therapeutic measures are used postoperatively, such as use of gait aids with partial weight bearing on the operative side. Only in severely comminuted fractures or fractures in which the operative result has been unsatisfactory is the restriction of weight bearing to no weight bearing needed.

Sacral Insufficiency Fracture

Other axial skeletal fractures such as fractures of the sacral alae and pubic rami also can occur (Fig. 41–5). Pelvic fractures are particularly common in patients with osteoporosis. Fractures of the pubic rami can occur with minimal strain, and most patients can hardly recall having a severe strain. Healing typically occurs without invasive procedures. Ambulatory activities are reduced temporarily, and a wheeled walker is initially recommended for decreasing pain. Later in the treatment, crutches and a cane can be used. Weight bearing is limited, as dictated by the level of pain in the pelvic area. Fracture of the sacrum with minimal trauma also can occur, and the goal of management is to decrease weight-bearing pain with the use of proper assistive devices for ambulation.[54] For management of pelvic pain, sedative physical therapeutic measures are recommended.

DIAGNOSTIC STUDIES IN OSTEOPOROSIS

The diagnosis of osteoporosis requires a thorough history and physical examination, including family history of osteoporosis, type and location of musculoskeletal pain, general dietary calcium intake, level of physical

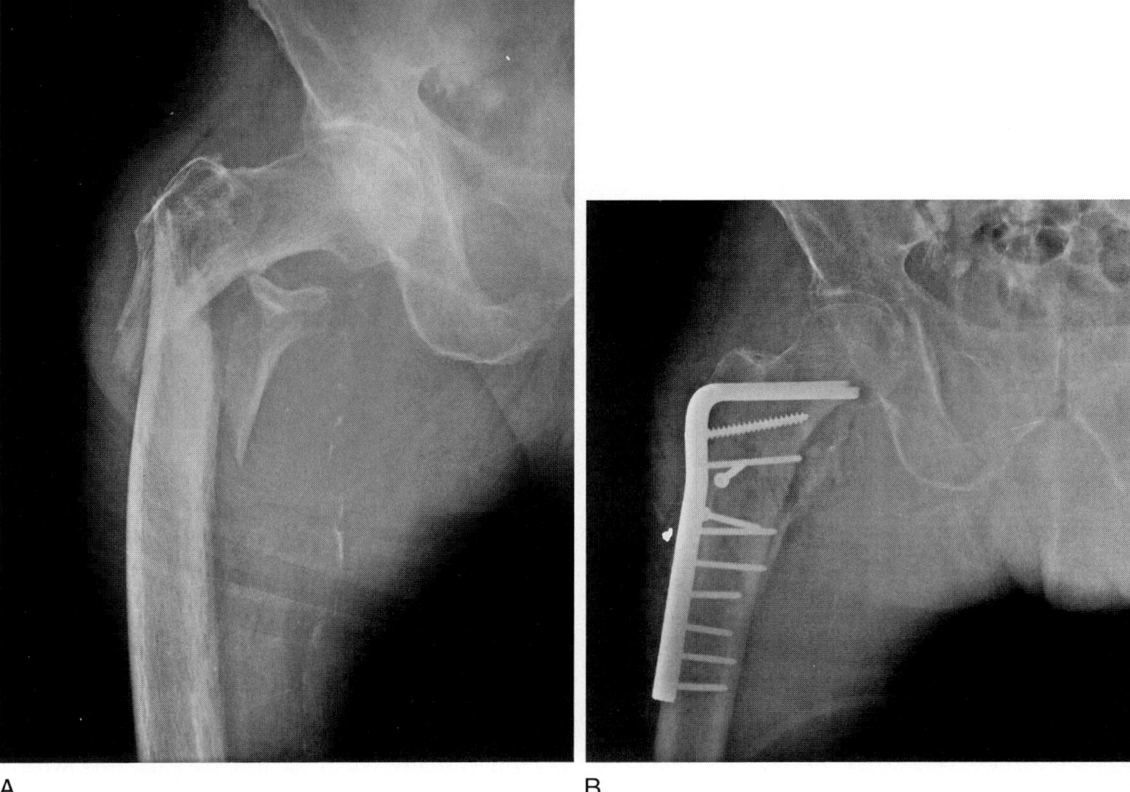

FIGURE 41–4. *A.* A 92-year-old man with intertrochanteric fracture of the right femur with medial displacement of a large fragment containing lesser trochanter and lateral angulation across the fracture. *B.* Internal nail, plate, and screw fixation in same patient.

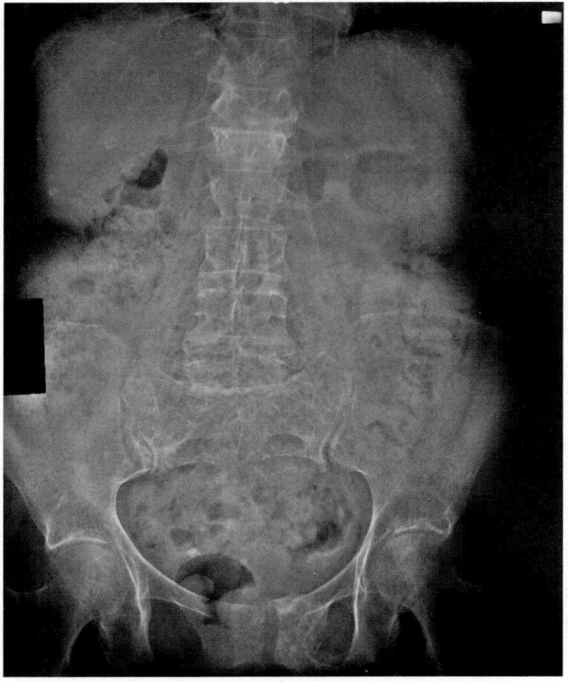

FIGURE 41–5. A 75-year-old woman with osteoporosis who had insufficiency fractures of left pubic bone and in both sacral alae. (From Sinaki M: Musculoskeletal challenges of osteoporosis. Aging Clin Exp Res (Milano) 1998; 10:249.)

activity, and height and weight measurements (Table 41–5).

Several biochemical indices also are used in the differential diagnosis of metabolic bone disease or, in some instances, for therapeutic follow-up. For example, biochemical markers for bone formation are bone-specific alkaline phosphatase and serum osteocalcin. Resorption markers include urinary calcium corrected by creatinine excretion, hydroxyproline, and pyridinium cross-links (in urine).[15] Unfortunately, the interpretation of these tests is clouded in patients with osteoporosis because of the high intra- and inter-individual variations of these parameters. Indices of bone turnover show seasonal and circadian variations (Table 41–5).

Radiographic findings consist of increased lucency of the vertebral bodies with loss of horizontal trabeculae and increased prominence of the cortical end plates and vertically oriented trabeculae, reduction in cortex thickness, and anterior wedging of vertebral bodies.[7, 16] The degree of wedging that indicates a true fracture varies from a 15% to 25% reduction in anterior height relative to the posterior height of the same vertebra. There are other morphologic changes, such as biconcavity of vertebral bodies and complete compression fractures (reduction in both the anterior and the posterior height by at least 25% compared with the adjacent normal vertebrae).[16, 47] Bone scan and magnetic resonance imaging can further define the cause of bone loss (Fig. 41–6), if needed.

TABLE 41–5 Some of the Diagnostic Evaluations for Osteoporosis

History and physical examination	Family history of osteoporosis, type and location of pain, general dietary calcium intake, level of physical activity, height and weight
Radiography of chest and spine	To rule out lymphomas, rib fractures, compression fractures, etc.
Bone mineral density (spine and hip)	At menopause and every 2 years for high-risk patients and every 5 years for low-risk patients
Complete blood cell count	To rule out anemias associated with malignancy, etc.
Chemistry group	To assess the level of alkaline phosphatase, which can be increased in osteomalacia, Paget's disease, bony metastasis and fracture, intestinal malabsorption, vitamin D deficiency, chronic liver disease, alcohol abuse, phenytoin (Dilantin) therapy, hypercalcemia of hyperparathyroidism, hypophosphatemia of hyperparathyroidism and osteomalacia, malabsorption, malnutrition. (These tests will also demonstrate an increase in calcium in hyperparathyroidism.)
Erythrocyte sedimentation rate and serum protein electrophoresis	To determine changes indicative of multiple myeloma or other gammopathies
Total thyroxine	Increased total thyroxine may be a cause of osteoporosis because of increased bone turnover
Immunoreactive parathyroid hormone	Hyperparathyroidism (accompanied by hypercalcemia)
25-Hydroxyvitamin D and 1,25-dihydroxyvitamin D	Gastrointestinal diseases, osteomalacia
Urinalysis and 24-hour urine	To check for proteinuria due to nephrotic syndrome and for low pH due to renal tubular acidosis. A 24-hour urine test can exclude hypercalciuria (normal calcium value in men is 25 to 300 mg/specimen; in women, 20 to 275 mg/specimen)[51]
Optional: Bone scan, iliac crest biopsy	After tetracycline double-labeling for bone histomorphometry, bone marrow biopsy may be indicated to exclude multiple myeloma and metastatic malignancy
Biochemical markers of bone turnover	*Formation:* Serum osteocalcin, alkaline phosphatase (bone), procollagen peptides *Resorption:* Serum acid phosphatase, pyridinoline, deoxypyridinoline, urinary calcium/creatinine

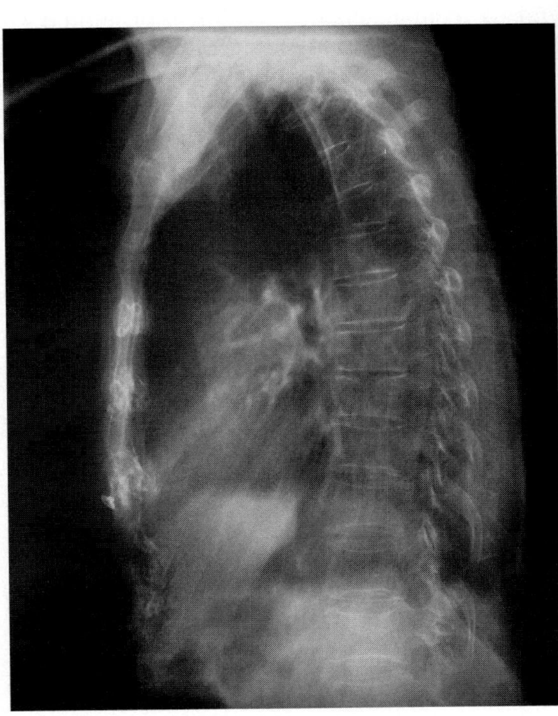

A

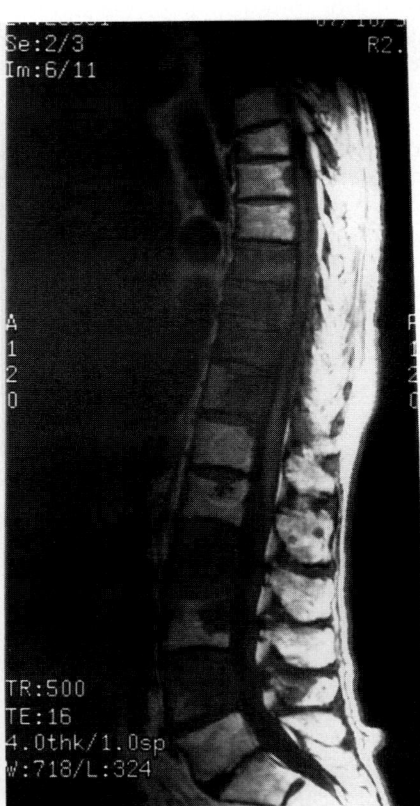

B

FIGURE 41–6. *A.* Lateral radiograph of spine in a 77-year-old man with persistent back pain. No evidence of metastatic lesion identified. *B.* Magnetic resonance imaging demonstrates extensive skeletal metastases from T3 through lower lumbar spine with involvement of nearly every vertebral body. The most extensive involvement is at T3, T8 through T11, T12, and L4.

Osteoporosis is typically not visible on conventional radiographs until at least 25–30% of bone mineral has been lost. Consequently, evaluation of bone mineral density through absorptiometry techniques is recommended.[69] These are also helpful in treatment because calculated bone loss or gain is required in therapeutic trials of agents affecting bone mass. The different methods for evaluation of bone mass have different levels of precision.[70] Available methods include photon absorptiometry (single or dual), finger x-ray spectrometry, ultrasound densitometry, qualitative computed tomography, and dual x-ray absorptiometry. The most commonly used technique is dual-energy absorptiometry. Dual-energy x-ray absorptiometry (DEXA) has high precision and is commonly used for research and clinical evaluations to measure the bone mineral density of the spine and hips (Fig. 41–7). More commonly measured is the bone mineral density of the femoral neck because that of the spine can be erroneously high as a result of osteoarthritis of the spine. It also can be used to measure total-body bone mass. It is x-ray–based and has a precision of about 1%. The amount of radiation is less than 3 mrad.[69]

TREATMENT

Osteoporosis is a multifactorial condition and its treatment has several facets, so it requires a team approach. Endocrine consultation, physical medicine and rehabilitation, pharmacological and psychological interventions, and nutrition are concomitant methods of management. The World Health Organization has devised definitions for osteoporosis as follows: bone mineral density T-score > 1 to −1 SD, normal; T-score −1 to −2.5 SD, osteopenia; and T-score of −2.5 SD or more, osteoporosis. (SD = standard deviation below the peak, normal young adult mean.) These definitions facilitate decision-making for therapeutic trials. They are also helpful for prescription of a proper exercise program.

Exercise

The efficacy of exercise for improving bone mass is supported by hormonal and nutritional factors (Table 41–6). To meet the challenge of mechanical load, skeletal tissue must have enough bone mass and proper architecture to withstand the physical strain that is imposed on it. Fortunately, normal musculoskeletal structure is highly adaptable and can meet the challenge of usual mechanical loads. In osteopenia and osteoporosis, the challenge from mechanical load and strain might not be tolerated without damage to the architecture of bone. A supervised nonstrenuous, progressive, resistive exercise program can improve bone mass in inactive individuals.[64] By understanding both the benefits and the shortcomings of nutritional and exercise approaches for musculoskeletal management of osteoporosis, we can create a better prophylactic program for osteoporosis.

High rates and magnitude of bone strain are produced during high-impact sports activities such as gymnastics, badminton, tennis, volleyball, and basketball. The high-impact bone loading results in site-specific increases in bone mineral density. One study showed a significant difference in bone mineral density between gymnasts and volleyball players. The upper extremities are loaded differently in these two athletic activities.[11] Gymnasts had higher bone mineral density than volleyball players, except for the pelvic bone.

According to Frost's theory, a minimum threshold of mechanical loading is needed to evoke an increased level of bone mineral density.[13] This theory is referred to as the minimum effective strain stimulus (MESS). Lanyon[24] suggested that the greatest osteogenic effect from mechanical loading is promoted when the strain is vigorous enough to produce high strain, repeated daily, short in duration, and applied to a specific bone site. Mechanical loading, when applied properly, can stimulate osteogenic activity. Axial loading of the skeleton during lifting activities at one's job or in the care of children can be as osteogenic as working out in a gym

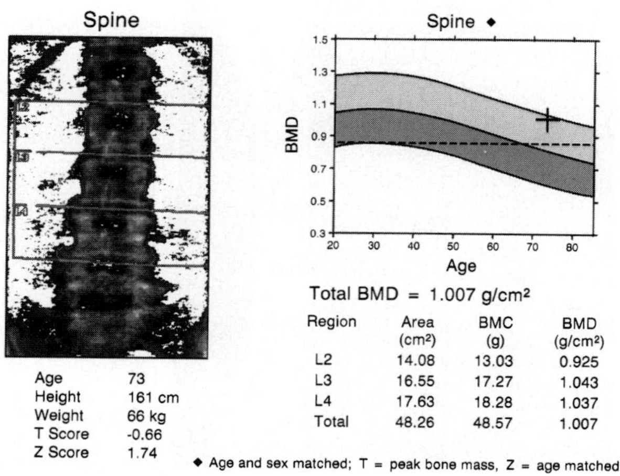

Region	Area (cm2)	BMC (g)	BMD (g/cm2)
L2	14.08	13.03	0.925
L3	16.55	17.27	1.043
L4	17.63	18.28	1.037
Total	48.26	48.57	1.007

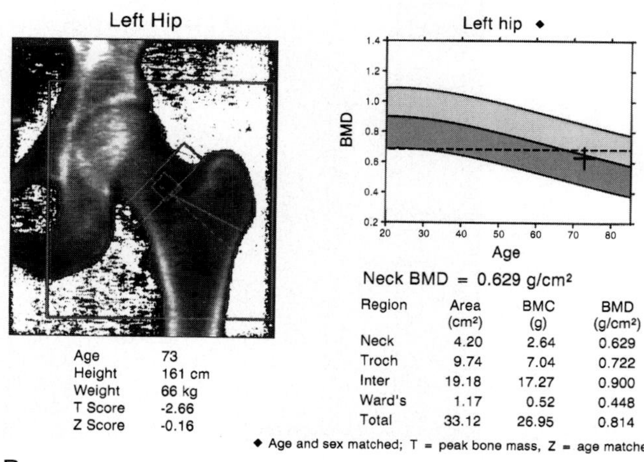

Region	Area (cm2)	BMC (g)	BMD (g/cm2)
Neck	4.20	2.64	0.629
Troch	9.74	7.04	0.722
Inter	19.18	17.27	0.900
Ward's	1.17	0.52	0.448
Total	33.12	26.95	0.814

FIGURE 41–7. Reports of bone mineral density (BMD) studies with dual-energy x-ray absorptiometry of spine and hip in a patient with osteoporosis. *A.* Lumbar spine BMD. *B.* Femoral neck BMD. BMC, bone mineral content; Inter, intertrochanteric; Troch, trochanter. BMD of the spine can be erroneously high due to osteoarthritis of the spine.

TABLE 41–6 Suggested Rehabilitation Guidelines on the Basis of Bone Mineral Density T-Scores*

Reduction to −1 SD (normal)	−1 to −2.5 SD (osteopenia)†	−2.5 SD or more (osteoporosis)†
No treatment	Consultation for treatment	Pharmacologic intervention
Patient education, preventive measures	Patient education, preventive interventions	Pain management
Lifting techniques	Pain management	Range of motion, strengthening, coordination
Proper diet (calcium and vitamin D)	Back strengthening exercises	Mid-day rest, heat/cold, stroking massage if needed
Jogging (short distances)	Limit load lifting (≤10–20 pounds)	Back extensor strengthening
Weight training	Aerobic exercises, walking 30 min/day	Walking 30 min/day, Frenkel exercises
	Exercises: weight training 3 times a week	Aquatic exercises 1–2 times a week
	Postural exercises: Posture Training Support combined with pelvic tilt and back extension	Fall prevention program (Table 41–3)
		Postural exercises: Posture Training Support combined with pelvic tilt and back extension
Aerobics	Frenkel exercises, prevention of falls	Prevention of vertebral compression fractures (orthoses, as needed)
	T'ai chi, if desired	
Abdominal and back strengthening exercises‡	?Hormone replacement	Prevention of spinal strain (lifting ≤ 5–10 pounds)
Postural exercises	?Other antiresorptive agents	Evaluation of balance, gait aid
		Safety and facilitation of self-care through modification of bathroom (grab bars), kitchen (counter adjustment), occupational therapy consultation
		Start strengthening program with 1–2 pounds and increase as tolerated to 5 pounds in each hand
		Hip protective measures

* T-score: Standard deviation below peak normal young adult bone mass.
† Osteopenia/osteoporosis as defined by the World Health Organization.[71]
‡ See Figures 41–9 and 41–10 for proper exercise program and posture.

(Fig. 41–8).[59] Individuals with normal bone mineral density can perform high-impact exercises such as aerobics, jogging, and skiing. For persons with osteoporosis, nonstraining exercises such as walking for 45 minutes three times a week or daily walking for 30 minutes are recommended. In-water exercises are recommended for patients who are unable to perform antigravity exercises

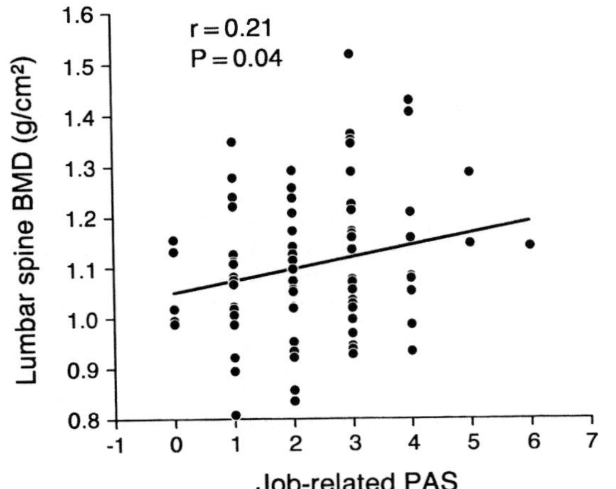

FIGURE 41–8. Physical activity score (PAS; job) significantly correlated with spinal bone mineral density (BMD). (From Sinaki M, Fitzpatrick LA, Ritchie CK, et al: Site-specificity of bone mineral density and muscle strength in women: Job-related physical activity. Am J Phys Med Rehabil 1998; 77:470. By permission of Williams & Wilkins.)

because of pain or weakness. The nonstrenuous, low-resistance exercises can be advanced to antigravity and strengthening exercises as permitted by a patient's musculoskeletal status.

Spinal extension exercises should be used along with exercises to reduce lumbar lordosis.[61] Weakness in abdominal muscles adds to the problems of poor posture and protruded abdomen. To complement a posture training exercise program, isometric abdominal muscle strengthening exercises should be included (Figs. 41–9 and 41–10).

Certain exercises should be avoided in patients with osteoporosis, especially spinal flexion exercises (Fig. 41–11).[63] Osteoporotic women, in general, have weaker back extensors than normal women of comparable age (Fig. 41–12). The choice of physical activity is important and has to be individualized. Fitness programs, such as swimming, fast walking, or short periods of stationary biking, are not significantly osteogenic[10, 38] but can fulfill the need for cardiovascular fitness without straining the osteoporotic frame. Knowledge of the bone mineral density is helpful before recommending a weight-training program.

Posture Training Program and the Osteoporotic Skeletal Frame

Any support that can improve posture and decrease pain-related paraspinal muscle co-contraction is desirable. With aging, the number and diameter of collagen

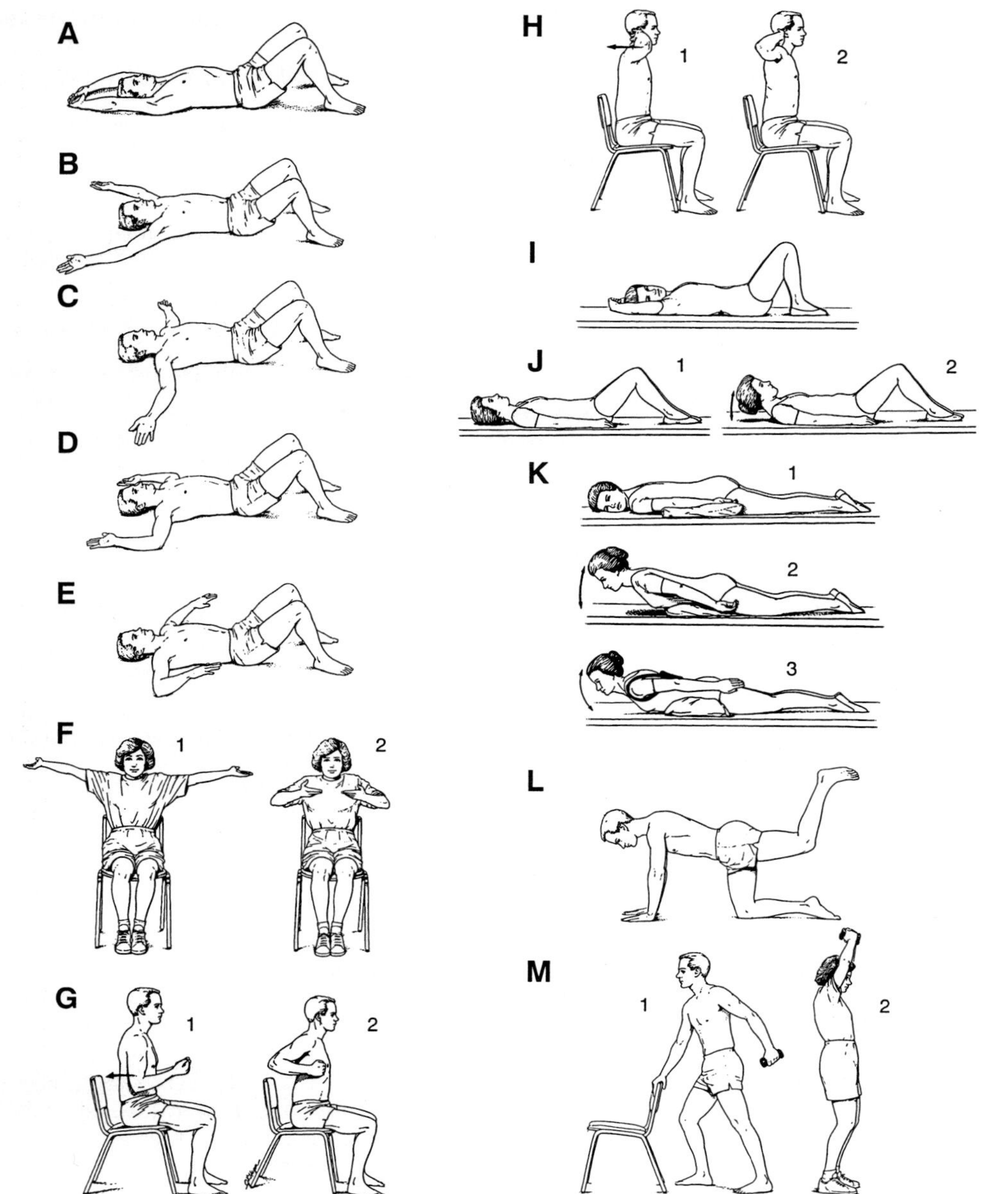

FIGURE 41–9. Nonstrenuous exercises for patients with severe osteoporosis. *A* through *C.* Upper back and shoulder extension exercise performed with spine supported. *D* and *E.* Flexibility of shoulder joint may contribute to improvement of upper back posture. To avoid upper back and neck strain in a fragile skeleton, shoulder rotation exercises can be performed in supine position. *F1,2.* Pectoral stretching exercise performed in sitting position. This is used to reduce kyphotic posturing. *G1,2.* Back extension exercise in sitting position. This position avoids or minimizes pain in patients with severe osteoporosis. *H1,2.* Deep-breathing exercise combined with pectoral stretching and back extension exercise. Patient sits on a chair, places hands at the level of head, and inhales deeply while gently extending the elbows backward. While exhaling, patient returns arms to the starting position. This is repeated 10 to 15 times. (*A* through *H2:* From Sinaki M: Rehabilitation in metabolic bone disease. In Sinaki M (ed): Basic Clinical Rehabilitation Medicine, ed 2. St Louis, Mosby, 1993, pp 209–236. By permission of Mayo Foundation.) *I.* Exercise to decrease lumbar lordosis with isometric contraction of lumbar flexors. *J1,2.* Isometric exercise to strengthen abdominal muscles. *K1,2,3.* Extension exercises in prone position with pillow under abdomen (to avoid hyperextension). *K3.* To increase the effect of back extension strengthening, weight is added. (*K3:* From PTS [developed by M. Sinaki]: Posture Training Support brochure Y32255, 1993, Jackson, Michigan, Camp International. By permission of Mayo Foundation.) *L.* Exercise for improving strength in lumbar extensors and gluteus maximus muscles. *M1,2.* Specificity of exercises: Muscle-strengthening and weight-loading exercises that may decrease bone loss. (These exercises were developed for the osteopenic spine by M. Sinaki through a grant from the Retirement Research Foundation. These techniques are designed to decrease strain on the spine despite weight lifting.) *M1.* Shoulder extensors contribute to reduction of kyphotic posturing. Shoulder extensors can be strengthened with a proper combination of weight-lifting and weight-bearing exercises while balance is maintained. One knee is bent to avoid lumbar strain. To avoid straining the spine and to maintain balance, leaning or holding onto a steady object for support is recommended. *Note:* The amount of weight lifted is about 1 to 2 pounds in each hand, not to exceed 5 pounds in each hand. The amount of weight needs to be prescribed according to the patient's bone mineral density (status of osteoporosis) and the condition of the upper extremities. *M2.* Bilateral or unilateral spine and hip weight-loading exercise. When weight is lifted above the head, knees should be bent slightly to avoid straining the lumbar spine. *Note:* The amount of weight lifted is about 1 to 2 pounds in each hand, not to exceed 5 pounds in each hand. The amount of weight needs to be prescribed according to the patient's bone mineral density (status of osteoporosis) and the condition of the upper extremities. (*I, J1,2, K1,2:* From Sinaki M: Exercise and physical therapy. In Riggs BL Jr, Melton LJ III (eds): Osteoporosis: Etiology, Diagnosis, and Management. New York, Raven Press, 1988, pp 457–479. By permission of Mayo Foundation.) (*L, M1,2:* From Sinaki M: Rehabilitation in metabolic bone disease. In Sinaki M (ed): Basic Clinical Rehabilitation Medicine, ed 2. St Louis, Mosby, 1993, pp 209–236. By permission of Mayo Foundation.)

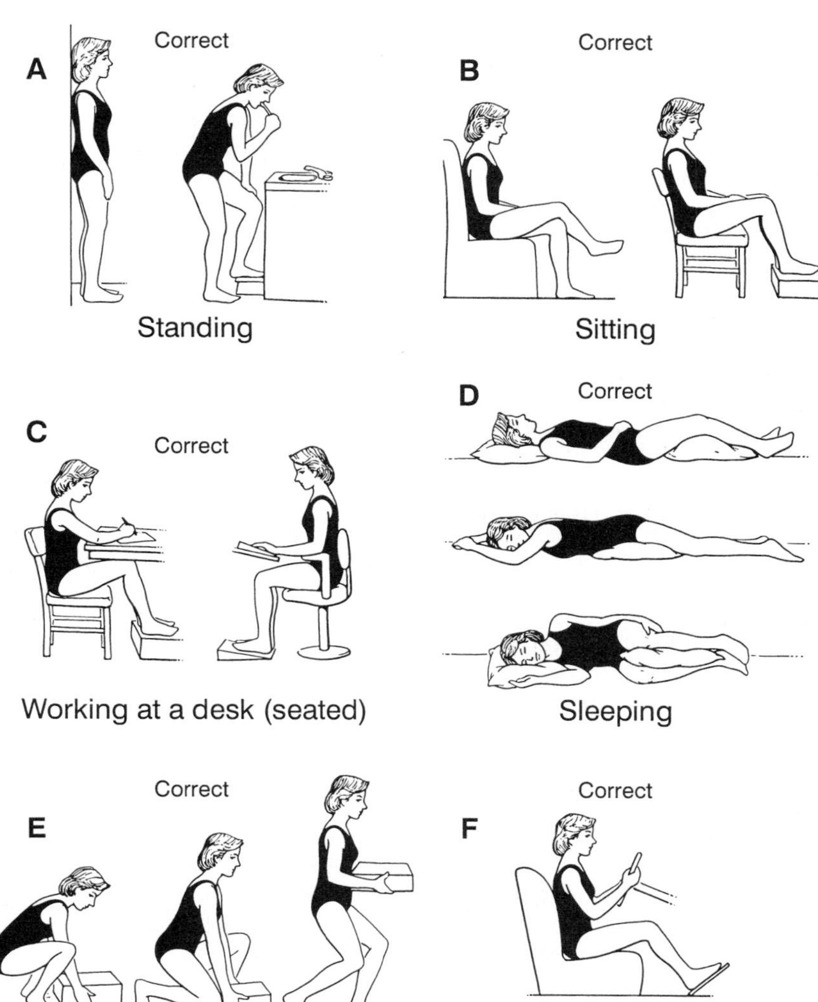

FIGURE 41–10. Static and dynamic correct postures. (From Sinaki M, Mokri B: Low back pain and disorders of the lumbar spine. In Braddom RL (ed): Physical Medicine & Rehabilitation. Philadelphia, WB Saunders, 1996. By permission of WB Saunders.)

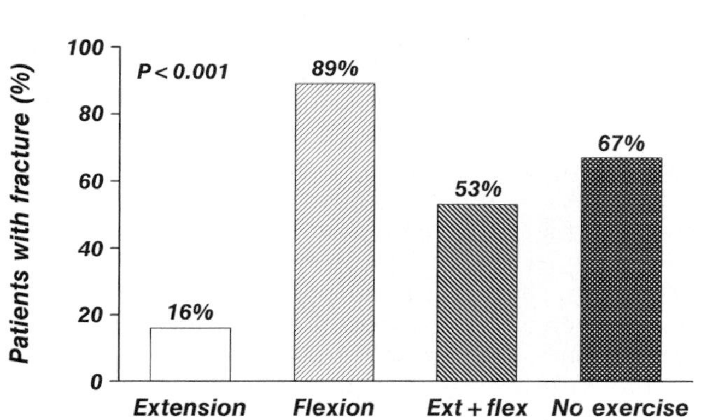

FIGURE 41–11. Percentage of patients with fracture with extension exercise, flexion exercise, extension and flexion exercise, and no exercise. (Data from Sinaki M, Mikkelsen BA: Postmenopausal spinal osteoporosis: Flexion versus extension exercises. Arch Phys Med Rehabil 1984; 65:593.)

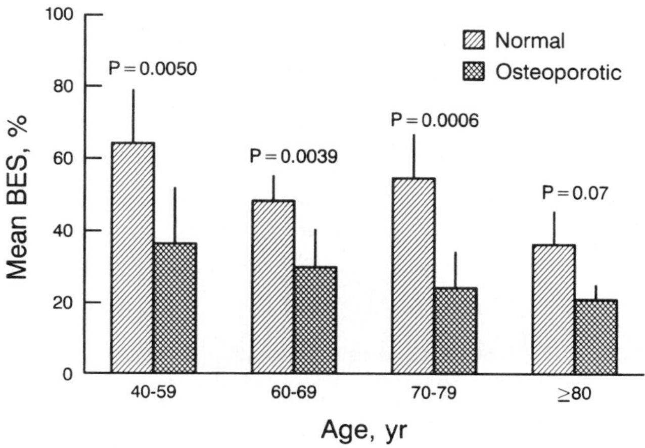

FIGURE 41–12. Back strength in normal women and women with osteoporosis. BES, back extensor strength. (Data from Sinaki M, Khosla S, Limburg PJ, et al: Muscle strength in osteoporotic versus normal women. Osteoporosis Int 1993; 3:8.)

fibrils of the intervertebral disks decrease. This results in loss of resiliency of the disks. In addition, reduced paraspinal muscle strength[63a] and forward tendency of head and trunk related to the effect of gravity can cause iliocostal friction syndrome and flank pain. This pain does not respond to the use of conventional orthoses. Indeed, orthoses such as corsets can make the pain worse through pressure over the lower rib cage (Fig. 41–13). Posture training programs that can decrease kyphosis can also subsequently reduce iliocostal friction syndrome.[23a, 58] Posture training programs such as the application of a weighted kypho-orthosis for half an hour twice a day or for one hour twice a day while trying to contract back extensors can provide re-education for improvement of kyphotic posturing and reduction of the risk of falls[62] (Fig. 41–14).

Orthotics and the Osteoporotic Spine

Acute compression fracture usually results in severe pain and, if not managed well, can lead to prolonged immobility. The final outcome is creation of chronic pain behavior and subsequent psychological consequences. Acute pain needs to be actively managed with proper physical measures. Sedative physical therapy including application of cold and later heat and isometric muscle contractions of the paraspinal muscles can be helpful. Rigid thoracolumbar orthoses to promote extension of the spine are helpful (Fig. 41–15) (also see Chapter 17). If thoracolumbar orthoses are not tolerated because of postural changes, a thoracic weighted kypho-orthosis (Fig. 41–16) or a combination of a kypho-orthosis and lower back support (elastic abdominal support) might suffice. In some cases, long-distance ambulatory activities can require use of a cane or a wheeled walker. Temporary use of a wheelchair with a supportive back cushion is indicated in some cases. Every effort needs to be taken to prevent the patient's confinement to one room or prolonged bedrest. Every effort should be made to limit immobility and its resulting reactive depression. Safety during ambulation is paramount, and prevention of falls and fracture should be taught in the rehabilitative program for patients with osteoporosis.

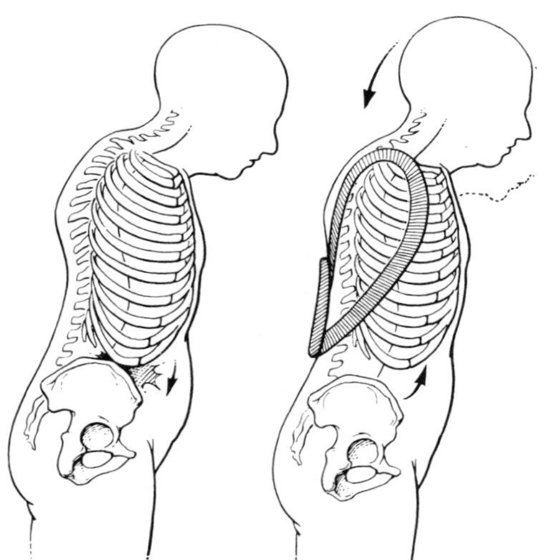

FIGURE 41–13. Severe kyphosis can result in iliocostal contact or iliocostal friction syndrome (*left*). Application of a weighted kypho-orthosis provides counteracting forces, which enable users to contract their erector spinae muscles better and decrease kyphotic posturing (*right*). (From Sinaki M: The influence of exercise on bone and the rehabilitation of osteoporotic patients. In Passeri M (ed): The Opinion of the Orthopedist and Physiatrist. Pavia, Italy, EDIMES Publishing, 1995.)

Pharmacological Interventions

Several agents can be used for treatment of osteoporosis. Estrogen, calcium, and vitamin D are the most commonly advocated pharmacological treatments for involutional osteoporosis. Antiresorptive agents include estrogens, androgens, calcitonin, and bisphosphonates. Osteoblast stimulator agents include fluoride and PTH. PTH is still an investigational supplement, and fluoride is not approved by the Food and Drug Administration at this time for the treatment of osteoporosis. Studies are currently in progress evaluating new agents that can improve bone mass.

Needless to say, cessation of tobacco and alcohol abuse is necessary. An adequate calcium intake is required (Table 41–7) to permit normal bone development and potentially to decrease bone loss. Adequate calcium intake appears to have only a modest effect on bone loss after menopause. Inadequate intakes of calcium and vitamin D are common, especially in elderly nursing home residents. The efficacy of supplementation of calcium and vitamin D for reduction of the risk of hip fracture has been substantiated.[3] Typical recommendations are 1500 mg of elemental calcium daily in divided doses (Table 41–7). The recommended vitamin D dosage is between 400 and 800 IU/day. The dose of vitamin D varies and depends on the patient's exposure to the sun and dietary intake of vitamin D. In some cases, it is necessary to determine the serum level of $1,25(OH)_2D_3$ (the normal levels are at least 20 ng/mL and preferably 30 ng/mL). These values can differ in different laboratories. In the upper midwestern region of the United States, they are 15 to 80 ng/mL in the summer and 14 to 42 ng/mL in the winter.

Estrogen acts directly on bone cells and is an antiresorptive agent that has been shown to decrease the rate of bone loss and fractures in postmenopausal women whether the menopause is natural or surgical. Estrogen is the most widely prescribed agent in the United States (except for calcium) for the treatment of established osteoporosis.[25] When a patient with an intact uterus is treated with estrogen, progestogen also should be used under proper regimen to prevent the development of endometrial hyperplasia and possibly endometrial carcinoma. There are several regimens for estrogen and progestogen use. They can be used concurrently (combination pills) or cycled. The proper regimen needs to be individualized.

Minimal effective doses of some forms of oral estrogen are usually used (conjugated equine estrogens, 0.625 mg; estradiol 50 μg/day). Parenteral estrogens can be administered in the form of patches, implants, or

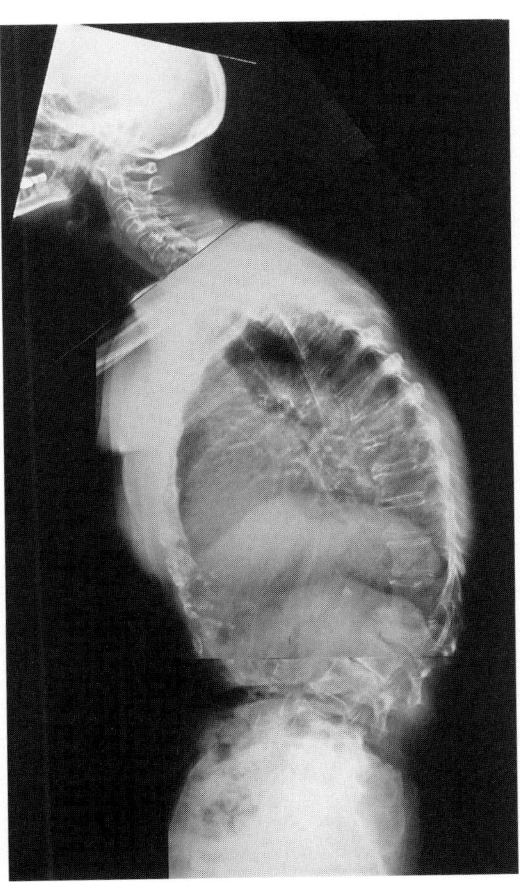

A

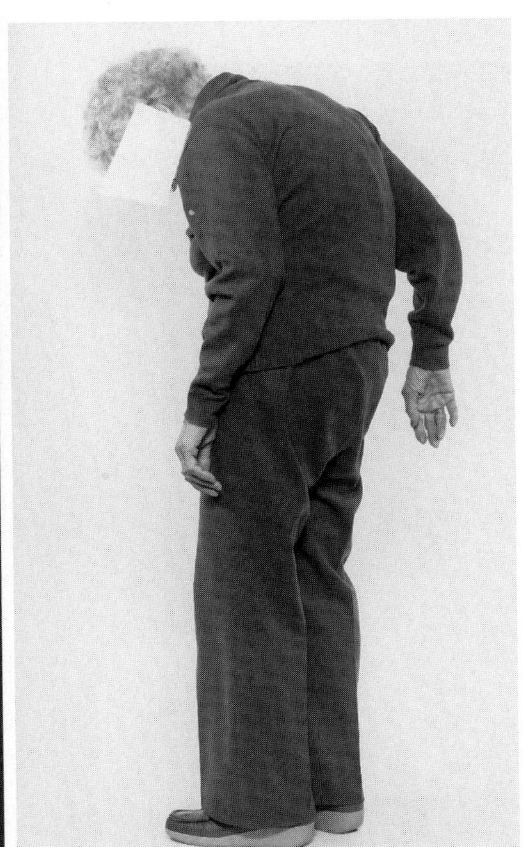

B

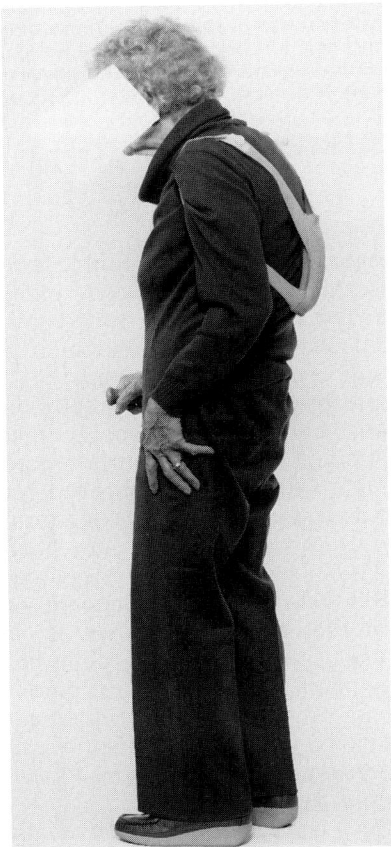

C

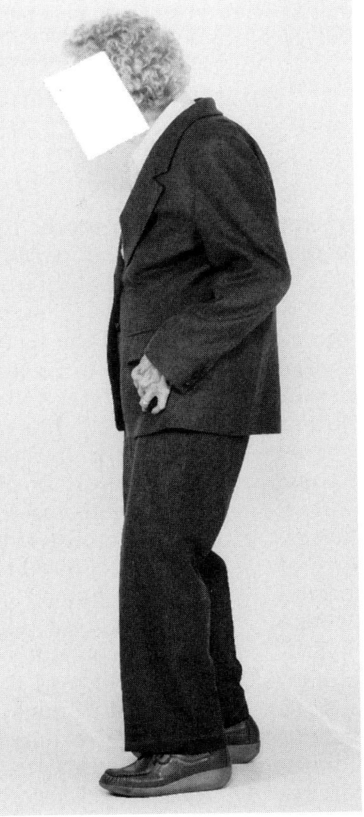

D

FIGURE 41–14. An 86-year-old woman with osteoporosis. *A.* Radiograph of spine depicts osteoporotic and postural changes. *B.* Severe kyphotic posturing, which made ambulation difficult. *C.* Same patient wearing weighted kypho-orthosis. (*B* and *C:* From Sinaki M: Rehabilitation of osteoporotic fractures of the spine. In Physical Medicine and Rehabilitation: State of the Art Reviews, vol 9. Philadelphia, Hanley & Belfus, 1995, pp 105–123.) *D.* Same woman's postural correction at age 92 after 6-year trial with weighted kypho-orthosis and posture training program: patient is not wearing kypho-orthosis. (*A, D:* From Sinaki M: Musculoskeletal challenges of osteoporosis. Aging Clin Exp Res (Milano) 1998; 10:249.)

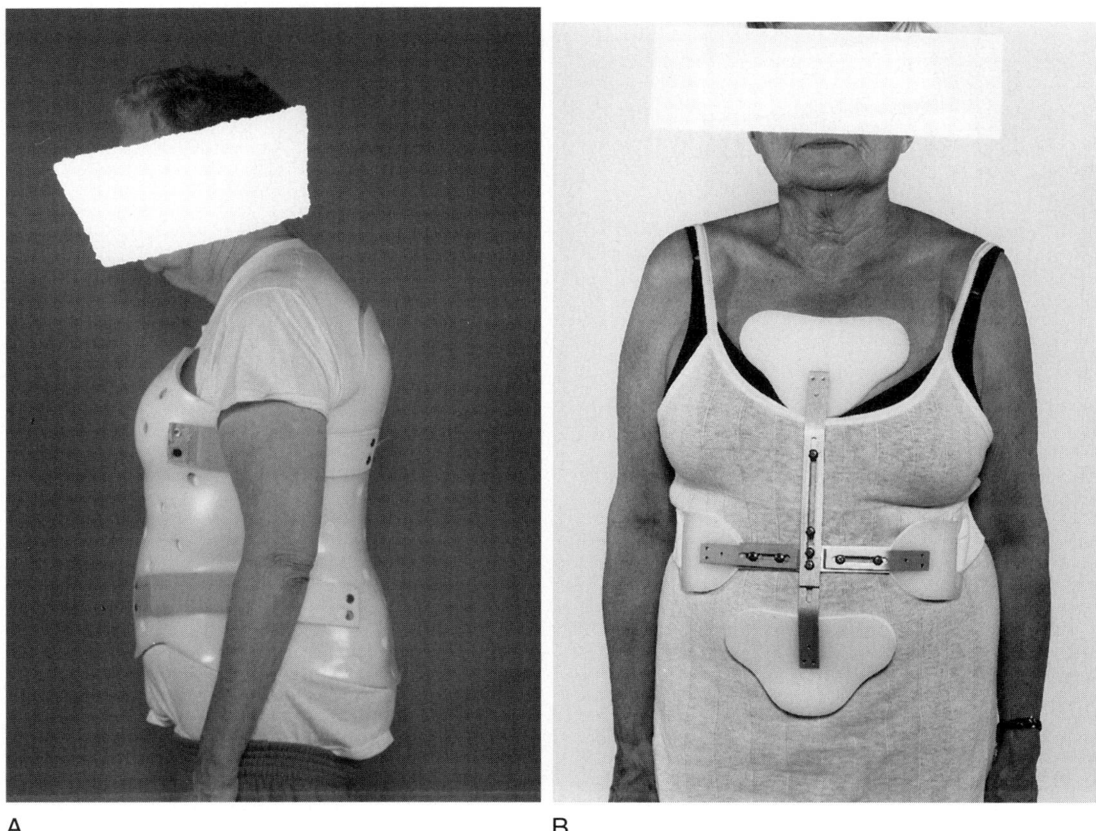

FIGURE 41–15. *A.* Rigid back support; bivalved body jacket. Brace is made of polypropylene and is custom-fitted. (From Sinaki M: Prevention of hip fracture: Physical activity. In Ringe JD, Meunier JP (eds): Osteoporotic Fractures in the Elderly: Clinical Management and Prevention. Stuttgart, Georg Thieme Verlag, 1996, pp 99–115.) *B.* CASH brace. Patient with osteoporosis of spine and compression fractures was unable to tolerate increased intra-abdominal pressure with use of abdominal back support because of hiatal hernia. Patient was fitted with cruciform anterior spinal hyperextension (CASH) brace satisfactorily. (From Sinaki M: Exercise and physical therapy. In Riggs BL Jr, Melton LJ III (eds): Osteoporosis: Etiology, Diagnosis, and Management. New York, Raven Press, 1988, pp 457–479. By permission of Mayo Foundation.)

gels. Estrogen patches deliver estradiol through the skin. The implants are inserted subcutaneously, where they slowly release estradiol. Patches are changed once or twice weekly, and implants are usually inserted every six months. Implants are not popular in the United States. The advantage of parenteral estrogen is that metabolism in the liver is bypassed and, consequently, smaller doses are sufficient. The commonly used transdermal estradiol 17 (patch) strength can vary from 0.05 mg (usual dose) to 0.1 mg (high dose). In some instances a low dose of 0.025 mg is used.

Contraindications to estrogen replacement therapy include liver or gallbladder disease, recent history of thromboembolism or thrombophlebitis, and suspected breast or endometrial carcinoma. Estrogens also can have an adverse effect on existing hypertension, hyperlipidemia, migraine headaches, chronic thrombophlebitis, and endometriosis. Administration of progestins can result in uncomfortable side effects such as fatigue, depression, breast tenderness, bloating, menstrual cramps, and headaches.[39] Progesterone in the form of medroxyprogesterone acetate (Provera) at a dosage of 2.5 to 5 mg/day is often used for the first 10 days at the beginning of the cycle. Estrogen protects against both osteoporosis and cardiovascular disease. However, many postmenopausal women remain skeptical or noncompliant because of increased risk of breast and endometrial cancer and the inconvenience of menstruation.[5, 46]

Calcitonin, an antiresorptive agent, acts directly on the osteoclasts. Calcitonin has a few disadvantages that limit its use.[40] It is most effective in patients whose rate of bone turnover is high. Calcitonin is approved for therapy of established osteoporosis, but the long-term fracture-reducing efficacy of calcitonin has not been clearly demonstrated. The subcutaneous or intramuscular injection of 50 to 100 units of salmon calcitonin, or 0.5 mg of human calcitonin, given every other day is commonly used. The use of nasal calcitonin might improve the patient's compliance. Side effects of parenteral use such as flushing or nausea and development of antibodies might limit its use. The nasal spray can cause nasal irritation, crusting, and ulcerations, which require discontinuation of its use.

Bisphosphonates affect trabecular bone, especially the lumbar spine, where bone mineral density increases of 5% to 10% occur during the first two years of treat-

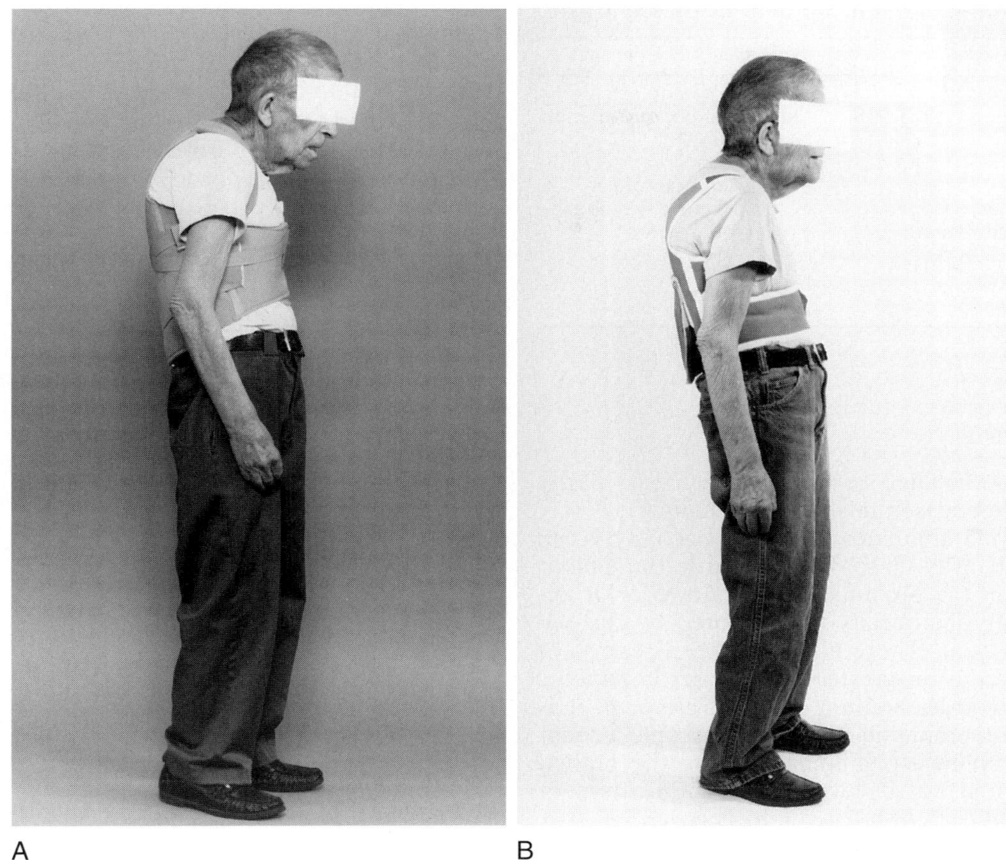

A B

FIGURE 41–16. *A.* Thoracolumbar support (rigid stays). Problem with fitting due to spinal deformities. *B.* Posture Training Support Thoracic (vest) sometimes is tolerated better than conventional thoracolumbar support. Weight in the pouch may range from 1 to 2½ pounds, as required.

TABLE 41–7 Optimal Calcium Intake*

	Calcium (mg/day)
Infants, children, and young adults	
Birth to 6 months	400
6 months to 1 year	600
1–10 years	800–1200
11–24 years	1200–1500
Adult women	
>24 years, pregnant and lactating	1200–1500
<24 years, pregnant and lactating	1200
25–49 years (premenopausal)	1000
50–64 years (postmenopausal), taking estrogen	1000
50–64 years (postmenopausal), no estrogen	1500
>65 years	1500
Adult men	
25–64 years	1000
>65 years	1500

* National Institutes of Health recommendations for calcium intake. Modified from Optimal Calcium Intake. NIH Consensus Statement June 6–8 12:1, 1994.

ment. Alendronate sodium, an amino-bisphosphonate, has been shown to normalize the rate of bone turnover and increase bone mass.[4] Alendronate must be taken with a full glass of water upon awakening. The patient should not eat or recline for 30 to 45 minutes after taking the medication. Patient education and compliance are very important for treatment with alendronate. One potential adverse effect of alendronate is esophageal irritation, particularly in patients with reflux or other esophageal dysfunction. Risedronate is another bisphosphonate that has been more recently introduced for the treatment of osteoporosis. Treatment with risedronate, 5 mg per day, was shown to significantly decrease the incidence of vertebral and nonvertebral fractures in postmenopausal osteoporosis.[18]

Anabolic steroids have an osteoblastic effect. However, because they have significant androgenic effects and induce liver function abnormalities, they are used only under the most extreme circumstances. Thiazide diuretics inhibit urinary excretion of calcium and can retard bone loss and reduce the rate of fractures in patients with osteoporosis. PTH can have an anabolic effect on bone when administered parenterally. Treatment with small doses of synthetic PTH and $1,25(OH)_2D_3$ has been shown to increase spinal bone

TABLE 41–8 Pharmacologic Options in Osteoporosis

Antiresorption	Formation
Acts on osteoclasts	Acts on osteoblasts
Stabilizes bone	Increases bone formation
Calcium	Vitamin D
Estrogen	Fluoride*
Calcitonin	Anabolic steroids
Bisphosphonates	Parathyroid hormone*
Selective estrogen receptor modulators (SERMs)	Growth factors*
Thiazide diuretics	
Ipriflavone*	

* Investigational.

mineral density. Further studies are needed to clarify the proper dose and administration technique.

Sodium fluoride stimulates osteoblastic activity. It can increase bone density up to 8% per year in the lumbar spine and 4% in the proximal femur. However, it decreases cortical bone density in the radius by approximately 2% per year. There also have been reports of an increased rate of nonvertebral fractures in patients treated with fluoride. Sodium fluoride, although it is being used as a therapeutic measure in European countries, remains an investigational agent in the United States and should not be used as a routine form of treatment in patients with osteoporosis.[43]

The estrogen-receptor mixed agonists/antagonists tamoxifen and raloxifene protect against bone loss in ovariectomized rats. They have an anti-estrogenic effect on breast tissue. These agents also are known as selective estrogen-receptor modulators (SERMs).[6] However, the mechanism by which these compounds affect bone is not completely defined. Recent studies in humans have been promising,[29] but the percentage increment in bone mineral density has not been as much as that with alendronate sodium. One of the side effects related to tamoxifen is uterine hyperplasia, but this is not a concern in treatment with raloxifene. Raloxifene decreases total cholesterol and serum low-density lipoprotein levels. Raloxifene is currently used only in the postmenopausal stage of osteoporosis (Tables 41–8 and 41–9).

Treatment of osteoporosis in men includes the usual supplementation with calcium and vitamin D, limitation of alcohol use, and cessation of smoking. In cases of hypogonadism in men, endocrine consultation is necessary, and testosterone replacement therapy is a possibility.

Management of steroid-induced osteoporosis requires calcium and vitamin D supplementation, use of antiresorptive agents such as alendronate sodium (10 mg/day orally), and implementation of a proper exercise program. In advanced stages of bone loss and muscle weakness, the use of assistive devices or a wheelchair might be necessary.[49] If hyperparathyoidism or thyrotoxicosis is present, proper management should be implemented.

A balanced diet is needed for maintenance of musculoskeletal health. Excessive dietary intake of sodium and phosphorus should be avoided. Studies of young women with malnutrition due to anorexia nervosa have demonstrated poor muscle strength, significant loss of bone mass, irregularity of menstrual periods, and estrogen deficiency.

In regard to osteoporosis, one cannot separate the effects of nutrition, exercise, hormones, and lifestyle; they indeed intertwine.[57] The patient's quality of life can certainly be affected by musculoskeletal changes related to osteoporosis. Practical management of patients with osteoporosis requires not only pharmacological interventions, physical and rehabilitative measures, and good nutrition but also consideration of the psychological consequences and reactions experienced by the patients.[59] Public education can contribute to preven-

TABLE 41–9 Commonly Used Agents in Osteoporosis

Agent	Common Dosage	Potential Side Effects
Calcium (type depends on patient's needs)	1000–1500 mg/day (Table 41–7)	
Vitamin D (multivitamin)	400–800 IU/day	
Estrogen		Headache, weight gain, change of mood or depression, increased blood pressure, gallbladder or liver disease, thrombophlebitis and increased blood clotting, increased serum triglycerides and blood glucose levels, abnormal vaginal bleeding, endometrial hyperplasia/cancer, breast cancer
Conjugated equine (Premarin)	0.625 mg (oral)/day	
Transdermal estradiol 17 (patch)	0.05–0.1 mg	
Progesterone (Provera), oral	2.5–5 mg (days 1–10 of cycle)	
Alendronate sodium (Fosamax)	5–10 mg/day	Esophageal irritation
Calcitonin	200 units nasal spray (Miacalcin) or 50 to 100 mg every-other-day injections	Nasal irritation/ulceration
Raloxifene (Evista)	60 mg/day (oral)	Leg cramps, hot flashes, deep vein thrombosis

tion, better understanding, and management of the consequences of osteoporosis.

REFERENCES

1. Adams P, Eyre DR, Muir H: Biochemical aspects of development and ageing of human lumbar intervertebral discs. Rheumatol Rehabil 1977; 16:22.
2. Cassell C, Benedict M, Specker B: Bone mineral density in elite 7- to 9-yr-old female gymnasts and swimmers. Med Sci Sports Exerc 1996; 28:1243.
3. Chapuy MC, Arlot ME, Duboeuf F, et al: Vitamin D_3 and calcium to prevent hip fractures in the elderly woman. N Engl J Med 1992; 327:1637.
4. Chesnut CH III, McClung MR, Ensrud KE, et al: Alendronate treatment of the postmenopausal osteoporotic woman: Effect of multiple dosages on bone mass and bone remodeling. Am J Med 1995; 99:144.
5. de Lignieres B: Hormone replacement therapy: Clinical benefits and side-effects. Maturitas 1996; 23(suppl):S31.
6. Delmas PD: Clinical use of selective estrogen receptor modulators. Bone 1999; 25:115.
7. Doyle FH, Gutteridge DH, Joplin GF, et al: An assessment of radiological criteria used in the study of spinal osteoporosis. Br J Radiol 1967; 40:241.
8. Drinkwater BL, Nilson K, Ott S, et al: Bone mineral density after resumption of menses in amenorrheic athletes. JAMA 1986; 256:380.
9. Econs MJ, Speer MC: Genetic studies of complex diseases: Let the reader beware (editorial). J Bone Miner Res 1996; 11:1835.
10. Emslander HC, Sinaki M, Muhs JM, et al: Bone mass and muscle strength in female college athletes (runners and swimmers). Mayo Clin Proc 1998; 73:1151.
11. Fehling PC, Alekel L, Clasey J, et al: A comparison of bone mineral densities among female athletes in impact loading and active loading sports. Bone 1995; 17:205.
12. Felsing NE, Brasel JA, Cooper DM: Effect of low and high intensity exercise on circulating growth hormone in men. J Clin Endocrinol Metab 1992; 75:157.
13. Frost HM: A determinant of bone architecture. The minimum effective strain. Clin Orthop 1983; 175:286.
14. Frost HM: Why do marathon runners have less bone than weight lifters? A vital-biomechanical view and explanation. Bone 1997; 20:183.
15. Garnero P, Darte C, Delmas PD: A model to monitor the efficacy of alendronate treatment in women with osteoporosis using a biochemical marker of bone turnover. Bone 1999; 24:603.
16. Genant HK, Vogler JB, Block JE: Radiology of osteoporosis. In Riggs BL Jr, Melton LJ III (eds): Osteoporosis: Etiology, Diagnosis, and Management. New York, Raven Press, 1988, pp 181–220.
17. Gutmann E: Age changes in the neuromuscular system and aspects of rehabilitation medicine. In Buerger AA, Tobis JS (eds): Neurophysiologic Aspects of Rehabilitation Medicine. Springfield, Charles C Thomas, 1976, pp 42–61.
18. Harris ST, Watts NB, Gerant HK, et al: Effects of risedronate treatment on vertebral and nonvertebral fractures in women with postmenopausal osteoporosis: A randomized controlled trial. JAMA 1999; 282:1344.
19. Hiu SL, Slemenda CW, Johnston CC Jr: Age and bone mass as predictors of fracture in a prospective study. J Clin Invest 1988; 81:1804.
20. Ireland P, Fordtran JS: Effect of dietary calcium and age on jejunal calcium absorption in humans studied by intestinal perfusion. J Clin Invest 1973; 52:2672.
21. Itoi E, Sinaki M: Effect of back-strengthening exercise on posture in healthy women 49 to 65 years of age. Mayo Clin Proc 1994; 69:1054.
22. Jackson JA, Kleerekoper M: Osteoporosis in men: Diagnosis, pathophysiology, and prevention. Medicine (Baltimore) 1990; 69:137.
23. Jones ET, Hensinger RN: Spinal deformity in idiopathic juvenile osteoporosis. Spine 1981; 6:1.

23a. Kaplan RS, Sinaki M, Hameister MD: Effect of back supports on back strength in patients with osteoporosis: A pilot study. Mayo Clin Proc 1996; 71:235.

24. Lanyon LE: Using functional loading to influence bone mass and architecture: Objectives, mechanisms, and relationship with estrogen of the mechanically adaptive process in bone. Bone 1996; 18(suppl 1):37S.
25. Lindsay R: Osteoporosis and its relationship to estrogen. Contemp Obstet Gynecol 1984; 63:201.
26. Lindsay R: Estrogen deficiency. In Riggs BL Jr, Melton LJ III (eds): Osteoporosis: Etiology, Diagnosis, and Management, ed 2. Philadelphia, Lippincott-Raven, 1995, pp 133–160.
27. Lindsay R, Cosman F, Herrington BS, et al: Bone mass and body composition in normal women. J Bone Miner Res 1992; 7:55.
28. Lindsay R, Hart DM, Sweeney A, et al: Endogenous oestrogen and bone loss following oophorectomy. Calcif Tissue Res 1977; 22(suppl):213.
29. Lufkin EG, Whitaker MD, Nickelsen T, et al: Treatment of established postmenopausal osteoporosis with raloxifene: A randomized trial. J Bone Miner Res 1998; 13:1747.
30. Lynn SG, Sinaki M, Westerlind KC: Balance characteristics of persons with osteoporosis. Arch Phys Med Rehabil 1997; 78:273.
31. Matkovic V, Heaney RP: Calcium balance during human growth: Evidence for threshold behavior. Am J Clin Nutr 1992; 55:992.
32. McComas AJ, Fawcett PR, Campbell MJ, et al: Electrophysiological estimation of the number of motor units within a human muscle. J Neurol Neurosurg Psychiatry 1971; 34:121.
33. Melton LJ III, Kan SH, Frye MA, et al: Epidemiology of vertebral fractures in women. Am J Epidemiol 1989; 129:1000.
34. Mosley JR, Lanyon LE: Strain rate as a controlling influence on adaptive modeling in response to dynamic loading of the ulna in growing male rats. Bone 1998; 23:313.
35. National Osteoporosis Foundation: Capitol Hill rallies Americans to take a walk! America Walks for Strong Women. National Osteoporosis Foundation, Washington, DC, August 5, 1998.
36. Nordin BE, Horsman A, Crilly RG, et al: Treatment of spinal osteoporosis in postmenopausal women. Br Med J 1980; 280:451.
37. Peck WA, Riggs BL, Bell NH, et al: Research directions in osteoporosis. Am J Med 1988; 84:275.
38. Petrie RS, Sinaki M, Squires RW, et al: Physical activity, but not aerobic capacity, correlates with back strength in healthy premenopausal women from 29 to 40 years of age. Mayo Clin Proc 1993; 68:738.
39. Prelevic GM, Bartram C, Wood J, et al: Comparative effects on bone mineral density of tibolone, transdermal estrogen and oral estrogen/progestogen therapy in postmenopausal women. Gynecol Endocrinol 1996; 10:413.
40. Riggs BL: Overview of osteoporosis. West J Med 1991; 154:63.
41. Riggs BL, Melton LJ III: Evidence for two distinct syndromes of involutional osteoporosis. Am J Med 1983; 75:899.
42. Riggs BL, Melton LJ III: Involutional osteoporosis. N Engl J Med 1986; 314:1676.
43. Riggs BL, Melton LJ III (eds): Osteoporosis: Etiology, Diagnosis, and Management. New York, Raven Press, 1988.
44. Riggs BL, Wahner HW, Melton LJ III, et al: Rates of bone loss in the appendicular and axial skeletons of women. Evidence of substantial vertebral bone loss before menopause. J Clin Invest 1986; 77:1487.
45. Rodan GA, Rodan SB: The cells of bone. In Riggs BL Jr, Melton LJ III (eds): Osteoporosis: Etiology, Diagnosis, and Management, ed 2. Philadelphia, Lippincott-Raven, 1995, pp 1–39.
46. Salamone LM, Pressman AR, Seeley DG, et al: Estrogen replacement therapy. A survey of older women's attitudes. Arch Intern Med 1996; 156:1293.
47. Sartoris DJ, Clopton P, Nemcek A, et al: Vertebral-body collapse in focal and diffuse disease: Patterns of pathologic processes. Radiology 1986; 160:479.
48. Seeman E: The dilemma of osteoporosis in men. Am J Med 1995; 98:76S.
49. Sinaki M: Exercise and physical therapy. In Riggs BL Jr, Melton LJ III (eds): Osteoporosis: Etiology, Diagnosis, and Management. New York, Raven Press, 1988, pp 457–479.
50. Sinaki M: Beneficial musculoskeletal effects of physical activity in the older woman. Geriatr Med Today 1989; 8:53.

51. Sinaki M: Exercise and osteoporosis. Arch Phys Med Rehabil 1989; 70:220.
52. Sinaki M: Rehabilitation in metabolic bone disease. In Sinaki M (ed): Basic Clinical Rehabilitation Medicine, ed 2. St Louis, Mosby, 1993, pp 209–236.
53. Sinaki M: Musculoskeletal rehabilitation. In Riggs BL Jr, Melton LJ III (eds): Osteoporosis: Etiology, Diagnosis, and Management, ed 2. Philadelphia, Lippincott-Raven, 1995, pp 435–473.
54. Sinaki M: Rehabilitation of osteoporotic fractures of the spine. In Physical Medicine and Rehabilitation: State of the Art Reviews, vol 9. Philadelphia, Hanley & Belfus, 1995, pp 105–123.
55. Sinaki M: Effect of physical activity on bone mass. Curr Opin Rheumatol 1996; 8:376.
56. Sinaki M: Prevention of hip fracture: Physical activity. In Ringe JD, Meunier JP (eds): Osteoporotic Fractures in the Elderly: Clinical Management and Prevention. Stuttgart, Georg Thieme Verlag, 1996, pp 99–115.
57. Sinaki M: Spectrum and management of musculoskeletal changes in osteoporosis. In The Official Program, IX Congresso Nazionale Societa Italiana dell' Osteoporosi e delle Malattie Metaboliche dell' Osso. Parma, Italy, October 1-4, 1997.
58. Sinaki M: Musculoskeletal challenges of osteoporosis. Aging Clin Exp Res (Milano) 1998; 10:249.
59. Sinaki M, Fitzpatrick LA, Ritchie CK, et al: Site-specificity of bone mineral density and muscle strength in women: Job-related physical activity. Am J Phys Med Rehabil 1998; 77:470.
60. Sinaki M, Grubbs NC: Back strengthening exercises: Quantitative evaluation of their efficacy for women aged 40 to 65 years. Arch Phys Med Rehabil 1989; 70:16.
61. Sinaki M, Itoi E, Rogers JW, et al: Correlation of back extensor strength with thoracic kyphosis and lumbar lordosis in estrogen-deficient women. Am J Phys Med Rehabil 1996; 75:370.
62. Sinaki M, Lynn S: Effect of posture training and exercise on balance versus exercise alone in osteoporotic women: A pilot study. 21st Annual Meeting of the American Society for Bone and Mineral Research. J Bone Miner Res 1999; 14:S419.
63. Sinaki M, Mikkelsen BA: Postmenopausal spinal osteoporosis: Flexion versus extension exercises. Arch Phys Med Rehabil 1984; 65:593.
63a. Sinaki M, Nwaogwugwu NC, Phillips B, et al: Effect of gender, age, and anthropometry on axial and appendicular muscle strength. (Submitted for publication.)
64. Sinaki M, Wahner HW, Bergstralh EJ, et al: Three-year controlled, randomized trial of the effect of dose-specified loading and strengthening exercises on bone mineral density of spine and femur in nonathletic, physically active women. Bone 1996; 19: 233.
65. Sinaki M, Wahner HW, Offord KP, et al: Efficacy of nonloading exercises in prevention of vertebral bone loss in postmenopausal women: A controlled trial. Mayo Clin Proc 1989; 64:762.
66. Sinaki M, Wollan PC, Scott RW, et al: Can strong back extensors prevent vertebral fractures in women with osteoporosis? Mayo Clin Proc 1996; 71:951.
67. Stevenson JC: Regulation of calcitonin and parathyroid hormone secretion by oestrogens. Maturitas 1982; 4:1.
68. Stevenson JC, Abeyasekera G, Hillyard CJ, et al: Calcitonin and the calcium-regulating hormones in postmenopausal women: Effect of oestrogens. Lancet 1981; 1:693.
69. Wahner HW: The Evaluation of Osteoporosis: Dual Energy X-Ray Absorptiometry in Clinical Practice. London, M Dunitz, 1994.
70. Wahner HW, Dunn WL, Brown ML, et al: Comparison of dual-energy x-ray absorptiometry and dual photon absorptiometry for bone mineral measurements of the lumbar spine. Mayo Clin Proc 1988; 63:1075.
71. WHO Study Group: Assessment of fracture risk and its application to screening for postmenopausal osteoporosis. Technical Report Series/World Health Organization 843. Geneva, Switzerland, 1994.

42

CHAPTER

Donna Bloodworth, M.D., Octavio Calvillo, M.D., Ph.D., Kevin Smith, M.D., and Martin Grabois, M.D.

Chronic Pain Syndromes: Evaluation and Treatment

Chronic pain is difficult and frustrating to manage, and patients who experience it are often viewed as being undesirable.[35] We in the field of Physical Medicine and Rehabilitation, however, frequently have the opportunity to work with these patients. The approach we advocate for these patients is one that is both comprehensive and interdisciplinary.

This chapter covers chronic pain, the evaluation and treatment of chronic pain, the role of pain clinics, and the outcomes obtainable with appropriate treatment.

DEFINITION

Perhaps the best way to define chronic pain is to compare and contrast it with acute pain (Table 42–1). Chronic pain syndrome is an abnormal condition in which pain is no longer a symptom of ongoing tissue injury, but one in which pain and pain behavior become the primary disease processes.[95] You can have chronic pain without having chronic pain "syndrome." Chronic pain syndrome is distinct from chronically or intermittently painful disease in which the patient experiences pain, but manifests function and behavior appropriate to the degree of tissue injury. In chronic pain syndrome, subjective and behavioral manifestations of pain persist beyond objective evidence of tissue injury. Not all persons with chronically painful conditions manifest chronic pain behavior and disability. Patients with chronic pain syndrome have been characterized by Brena and Chapman as demonstrating the following characteristics: dramatic pain complaints which are diffuse; dysfunction manifested by misuse of braces, collars, or ambulatory devices, together with poor posture and inactivity; drug misuse/overuse (usually of drugs prescribed for acute pain and anxiety); dependency on the health care system and family; disability that far exceeds underlying identifiable pathology or impairment; and dependency for source of income contingent upon continuing pain complaints.[105] Some of the conditions that can cause chronic pain are listed in Table 42–2.[3, 98]

In chronic pain syndrome the original causes are often blurred by subsequent complications of multiple procedures, compensation factors, medication dependency, inactivity, and psychosocial behavior changes[9] (Fig. 42–1). The Brena and Chapman model (Fig. 42–2) takes into account the chronicity and behavioral components in a nociceptive spectrum[11] and relates it to a rehabilitation medicine algology.

EPIDEMIOLOGY

Bonica[8] distinguishes chronic pain from chronic pain syndrome. From knowledge about the incidence of chronically painful disease, he extrapolates the number of persons who develop chronic pain syndrome and estimates that one third of all Americans have a chronically painful condition (including headache, back pain, and degenerative joint disease). He notes that 50% to 60% of these individuals are partially or totally disabled by pain, either transiently or permanently.[8] It is estimated that in the United States approximately $79 billion is spent annually on health care, workers' compensation, and litigation, while 40 million visits to the doctor are due to chronically painful conditions.[8]

TABLE 42–1 Acute vs. Chronic Pain

Acute	Chronic
Physicians trained in evaluation and diagnosis	Physician typically less interested and less trained
Short evaluation and treatment course	Long evaluation and treatment course
Pain is a biological symptom	Pain is a disease
Pain plus anxiety	Pain plus depression
Medications as needed	Nonnarcotic analgesics, antidepressants preferred
Little addiction concern	Polyaddiction concern
Diagnosis straightforward	Diagnosis complex
Cure likely	Cure usually not achieved

Adapted from Grabois M: Chronic pain. Evaluation and treatment. *In* Goodgold J (ed): Rehabilitation Medicine. St Louis, Mosby–Year Book, 1988.

Data on the disability, handicap, and social impact associated with low back pain and headache are available, but the chronicity of these conditions is not clear. Aronff[3] studied the personal and social impact of back pain, and found that 80% of all persons at some time experience low back pain severe enough to interfere with activity. Back pain accounts for expenditures of $14 billion per year, 19 million physician visits, and half of all workers' compensation cases. Approximately 10 million Americans are disabled by chronic low back pain and 250 million workdays are lost per year.[52] Ten million people seek treatment each year for back pain, and it is the most common cause of disability in those under the age 45 years.[98] Bonica notes that headache has a higher incidence, disables more persons, and causes more lost workdays than low back pain, but low back pain produces higher medical costs.[8]

ETIOLOGY

Chronic pain can be caused by ongoing pathological processes (e.g., arthritis), chronic nervous system dysfunction (e.g., phantom limb pain), or a combination of both processes. The patient's perception of the pain is modified by psychological, social, and environmental factors to yield the presenting complaint. The evaluation of a chronic pain patient should focus on defining the pain sources as nociceptive, neuropathic, or neuropsychological,[26] while recognizing potential modifiers of the complaints.

In an effort to optimize the care of patients with chronic pain, the International Association for the Study of Pain (IASP) Subcommittee on Taxonomy has developed a scheme for the coding of chronic pain syndromes.[70] Codification of chronic pain presentations should enhance communication between treating physicians and provide direction to research efforts in this field. The pain diagnoses are separated into somatic, neuropathic, and psychological etiologies. The IASP classification system further defines five axes based on (1) the anatomical region affected, (2) systemic etiology, (3) temporal characteristics (4) intensity, and (5) initiating etiology. Each of these factors plays an important role in defining the treatment of pain.

Somatic Etiology

For a somatic structure to be a source of pain, it must be innervated. Degenerative disc changes that do not affect the annulus fibrosus are usually painless because the outer annulus is the only portion of the disc that is innervated in adults.[42, 58]

Since nerve endings are stimulated by either mechanical or chemical irritation, any pathological process producing chronic stretching of connective tissues or inflammation of these innervated structures can lead to chronic somatic pain. This is usually manifested as aching, dull, or throbbing pain. Examples of this include rheumatoid arthritis, vertebral facet disease, and fibromyalgia.[64, 65]

Neuropathic Etiology

Neuropathic pain results from alterations in nerve structure or function with or without associated deafferentiation.[55] It is characteristically described as burning, shooting, or electrical in nature and is not associated with any ongoing nociceptive process. Trauma to or disease of the peripheral nerves can lead to chronic neuropathic pain.[55] This can be the result of neuromas, phantom pain, causalgia,[18] or other sympathetically maintained pain syndromes.[18, 44, 46] Spinal cord injury or dorsal root ganglion injury can lead to various deafferentiation pain syndromes, with pain being experienced in an area of sensory loss.[58] Chronic postlaminectomy back pain can, in some cases, be due to immobilization of dorsal root ganglia by scar tissue. Because of their mechanical sensitivity, the dorsal root ganglia can initiate high-frequency pain signals when stretched. This can perpetuate radicular-type pain.[55]

Thalamic infarcts can cause "central pain,"[60] and postherpetic neuralgia can result from inflammatory injury with resultant deafferentiation of the dorsal root ganglia and dorsal horn.[54] Metabolic derangement, as seen in diabetes, alcoholism, amyloidosis, and hypothyroidism, can lead to painful peripheral neuropathies.

Psychological Etiologies

Psychogenic pain is often referred as a somatization disorder. The cause lies in an underlying emotional disturbance or stressor that often goes unrecognized by the patient. While the pain can present in any area of the body, the most common forms are tension headaches, angina-like symptoms, colitis, nonspecific vaginal pain, and myofascial pain involving the shoulder and upper and lower extremities.[95]

CHRONIC PAIN MANAGEMENT

Swanson and colleagues[96] remarked that when pain becomes chronic, it increases in complexity and the patient becomes more resistant to treatment. It is widely accepted that continuation of the sequential outpatient-inpatient approach of the medical model is not successful for the typical chronic pain patient.[38]

Since chronic pain syndrome is a complex problem with medical and psychosocial aspects, it requires a com-

TABLE 42–2 Diagnoses Characterized by Intermittent, Recurrent, or Chronic Pain

Afferent Loss Syndromes

Diabetic mononeuropathy
Diabetic polyneuropathy
Nerve root avulsion
Central poststroke pain
Phantom pain
Postherpetic neuralgia
Ramsey-Hunt syndrome of the seventh cranial nerve

Headache

Classic migraine
Common migraine
Complicated migraine
Cluster headache
Ophthalmoplegic migraine
Hemiplegic migraine
Lower-half headache (atypical facial neuralgia)
Tension
Combined
Psychogenic
Nonmigrainous vascular
Dialysis headache
Hypertension headache
Rheumatoid atlantoaxial arthritis headache
Traction headache
Temporomandibular joint headache
Vasculitic
Cranial neuralgic
Post-traumatic
Ocular headache
Tolosa-Hunt syndrome

Causalgia

Causalgia
Sympathetic dystrophy

Low Back Pain

Psychosomatic
Psychogenic
Modified behavior with or without organic disease
Low back pain with radiation to leg

Low Back Pain (*continued*)

Mechanical low back pain
Bilateral radicular pain
Facet arthropathy
Metabolic disorders (rare)
Osteoarthritis
Fibrositis
Myofascial pain
Extra-articular pain sources

Failed Back Syndrome

Persistent disc herniation
Lateral stenosis
Central stenosis
Arachnoiditis
Epidural fibrosis
Instability

Erectile Dysfunction and Male Genital Pain

Referred pain from kidney or ureter
Referred pain from kidney, ureter, psoas, retroperitoneal mass, cauda mass
Bladder obstruction
Prostatic causes
Prostatic inflammation
Prostatodynia
Urethral pain
Urethral stricture, infection
Testicular causes
Testicular trauma or infection
Testicular cancer
Testicular torsion
Intermittent testicular torsion
Torsion of testicular appendage
Testicular pain of polyarthritis nodosa
Epididymo-orchitis
Orchialgia with negative examination
Cellulitis of the scrotum
Varicocele
Phimosis and paraphimosis
Peyronie's disease
Penile prosthesis pain
Priapism, balanitis, penile cancer

Erectile Dysfunction and Male Genital Pain (*continued*)

Penile pain after vasectomy
Anal fistula
Pelvic floor tension myalgia
Scar entrapment of ilioinguinal nerve
Illioinguinal, genitofemoral, iliohypogastric neuralgia

Painful Neuropathles

Guillian-Barré syndrome
Chronic inflammatory demyelinating neuropathy
Porphyric polyneuropathy
Alcoholic polyneuropathy
Toxic, drug-related neuropathy
AIDS sensory neuropathy
Diabetic polyneuropathy
Mononeuritis multiplex
Cryoglobulin neuropathy
Brachial neuritis
Lateral femoral cutaneous entrapment
Other entrapment neuropathies
Amyloidosis
Tic douloureux (trigeminal neuralgia)
Glossopharyngeal neuralgia
Dorsal root ganglionopathy

Facial Pain

Trigeminal neuraglia
Glossopharyngeal neuralgia
Nervus intermedius neuralgia (Ramsey-Hunt syndrome)
Sphenopalatine neuralgia
Paratrigeminal neuralgia
Vidian
Atypical face pain
Sinus disease
Carotiditis
Hyoid bone syndrome
Temporal tendonitis
Temporomandibular dysfunction pain syndrome

Joint Pain

Rheumatoid arthritis
Other systemic inflammatory disease
Autoimmune disorders
Rheumatic fever
Infectious arthritis
Granulomatous
Crystal arthritides

Painful Metabolic Bone Disease

Osteomalacia
Osteoporosis
Hyperparathyroidism
Renal osteodystrophy
Paget's disease

Cancer Pain

Cervical Spine Pain

Spinal cord compression
Extrinsic spinal cord compression
Osteoarthritis
Cervical spondylosis
Cervical radiculitis
Syringomyelia
Cervical trauma
Rheumatic atlantoaxial
Ankytosis spondylitis infection

Gynecological Pain

Ectopic pregnancy
Uterine causes: dysmenorrhea
Adenomyosis
Benign tumors: leiomyoma
Malignant tumors
Ovarian causes: inflammatory, infectious
Follicular cyst
Corpus luteum cyst
Theca luteum cyst
Ovarian malignancy
Endometriosis
Chronic pelvic congestion

Adapted from Aronoff GM: Evaluation and Treatment of Chronic Pain, Baltimore, Williams & Wilkins, 1992; Tollison CD, Satterthwaite JR, Tollison JW: Handbook of Pain Management. Baltimore, Williams & Wilkins, 1994.

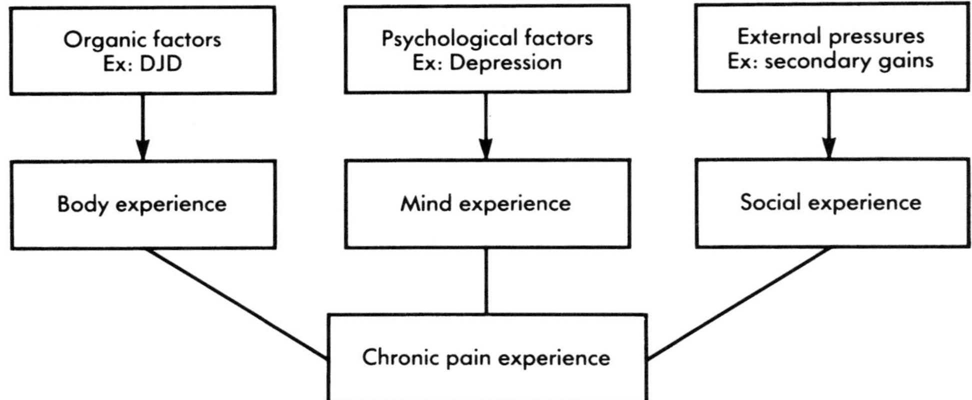

FIGURE 42–1. Chronic pain: interaction of organic, psychological, and social factors. *Abbreviation:* Ex, example. (From Grabois M: Chronic pain. Evaluation and treatment. *In* Goodgold J (ed): Rehabilitation Medicine. St Louis, Mosby–Year Book, 1988.)

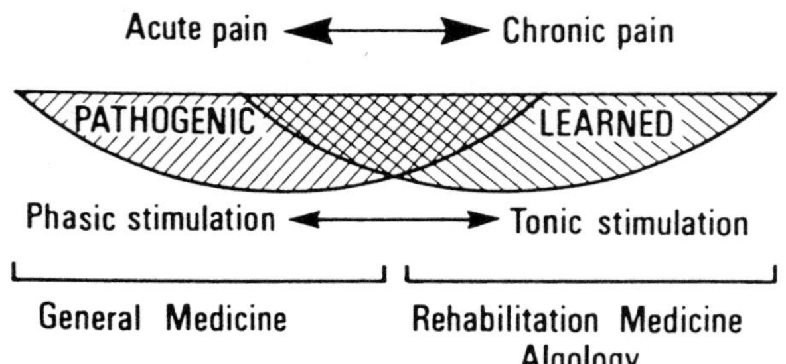

FIGURE 42–2. Nociceptive spectrum. (From Brena SF, Chapman SL: Management of Patients with Chronic Pain. New York, SP Medical & Scientific Books, 1983.)

prehensive and multidisciplinary approach to evaluation and treatment.[38] If the patient is to have the best chance of reaching the highest functional goals possible within medical and psychological limitations, practitioners need to consider chronic pain syndrome as seriously as alcoholism, stroke, or spinal cord injury.[36] In an attempt to maximize the treatment outcomes, pain programs have developed comprehensive and interdisciplinary approaches to evaluating and treating patients with chronic pain.[35]

Programs for chronic pain management like those for Physical Medicine and Rehabilitation are relatively new developments, having their beginnings during World War II.[37] Originated by Alexander and popularized by Bonica,[9] these programs have multiplied in recent years and now number in the thousands.

More recently, with the advent of managed care, approval for evaluation and treatment of patients with chronic pain in an interdisciplinary or multidisciplinary chronic pain program has become more difficult. It is important that we develop pain strategies to overcome this increasing problem. Managed care leaders at a roundtable sponsored by the American Pain Society recently outlined some concepts that appear to help the third party payer better understand and be in a better position to approve patients with chronic pain for evaluation and treatment by pain clinics. Winning strategies seem to center around low price, customer satisfaction, demonstrated exceptional outcome, prestige, ease of access, and the development of practice parameter and/or clinical pathways. Having an appropriate utilization review program can control costs and still provide patients with good outcomes. Involvement in a vertically integrated health care network with access and referral mechanism for patients is very helpful in sustaining a multidisciplinary pain clinic.

Pain management is becoming an important issue in health care delivery in the United States. Both regulators (e.g., the Joint Commission on Accreditation of Health Care Organizations) and practitioners perceive the need for guidelines to strike a balance between the judicious use of opioids and the constraints imposed by side effects, potential diversion, and possible misuse. Pain is often managed inadequately, despite readily available treatments. Much of the conventional wisdom surrounding the medical use of opioids is unfounded folklore, and little progress has been made in dispelling the myths. Regulatory changes are occurring in response to public awareness of the need for better pain management.

Ideally, a pain clinic should be comprehensive and interdisciplinary, capable of offering a wide range of treatment techniques.[35] However, there are several types of pain clinics. The International Association for the Study of Pain has identified three such types, classifying pain clinics as modality-oriented, disease-oriented, or multidisciplinary.

In the organization of a typical pain clinic (Fig. 42–3), the director provides overall leadership while the coordinator is responsible for day-to-day management. The patient's case manager is often the attending physician. The clinical team regularly evaluates patients, sets goals, treats patients, and evaluates treatment outcomes. The

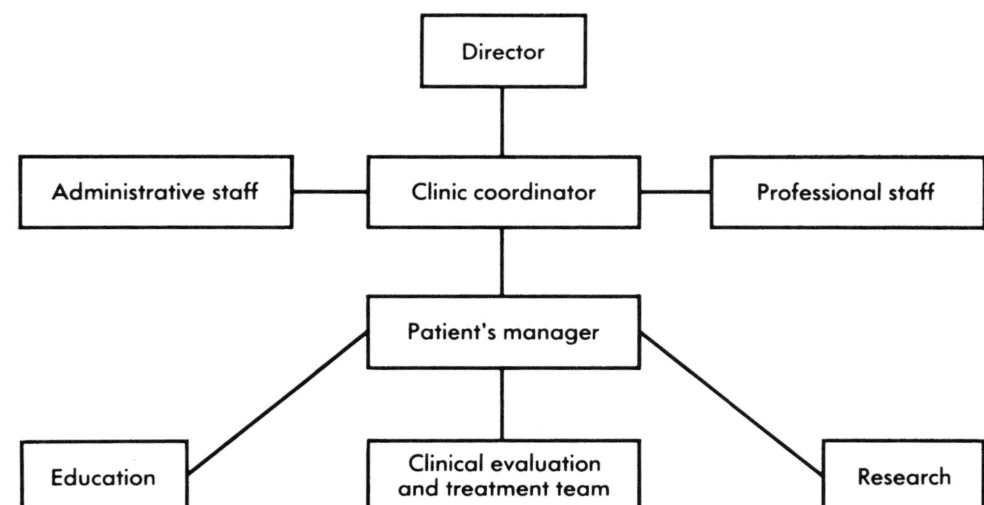

FIGURE 42–3. Organization of multidisciplinary pain clinic. (From Grabois M: Pain clinics: Role in rehabilitation of patients with chronic pain. Ann Acad Med 1983; 12:428.)

TABLE 42–3 Chronic Pain Management Team

Core Personnel	Consultant Personnel
Physician	Medical subspecialists
Psychologist	Anesthesiologist
Physical therapist	Neurosurgeon
Occupational therapist	Physical medicine and rehabilitation professional
Social services counselor	Psychiatrist
Rehabilitation nurse	Recreational therapist
Vocational counselor	Biomedical engineer
Pharmacist	
Dietitian	

team members typically include a physician, a psychologist, a physical therapist, a vocational counselor, an occupational therapist, a social services counselor, a pharmacist, a dietitian, and a nurse (Table 42–3). Other medical subspecialists are usually available on a consultative basis. They attend regular team conferences that select patients to be accepted for further evaluation treatment and monitor patients' progress.[35]

The physician leads the team, coordinates the program, and provides overall medical management. The psychosocial-vocational team, consisting of the psychologist, social worker, and vocational counselor, provides leadership in the evaluation and treatment of the behavioral changes that are a result of chronic pain, as well as appropriate vocational intervention.[35] The therapy team typically consists of nurses, pharmacists, dieticians, physical therapists and occupational therapists. They provide daily therapy to control medication levels, modulate the pain level, and increase patient activity.[1] The flowchart of patient care in a typical pain management program is depicted in Figure 42–4.

Referrals are typically accepted from both medical and nonmedical sources. An appropriate history must be supplied, and the patient should complete a pain questionnaire. The most appropriate patients are chronic pain patients who are motivated to participate in the program, who have no overwhelming secondary gain issues that might inhibit improvement, and who accept the concepts of goals of the program.

Opioids should be considered only after all other reasonable analgesic therapy has failed. Opioid therapy should be considered complementary to other analgesic and rehabilitative approaches. Contraindications to chronic opioids use can include a history of substance abuse, severe character disorder, or chaotic home environment. A single practitioner should take primary responsibility for treatment. Fully informed consent should be obtained and a written contract can be considered. Medication should be given orally except in rare circumstances. Long-acting opioids are preferred for ease of administration. Fixed-schedule dosing is preferable for continuous or frequently recurring pain. "Rescue" doses can be used under clearly defined circumstances, but total (weekly/monthly) dose must be constant. Patients should initially be seen monthly for monitoring their improvement in function. Periodic assessment should specifically address degree of analgesia, adverse effects, functional status (physical, social, psychological), and indications of aberrant drug-related behaviors. Evidence of aberrant behavior—hoarding, multiple sources of supply, repeated "lost" prescriptions or medications, unauthorized dosage escalation, use of unauthorized medicine or alcohol—should be carefully assessed. Consideration should be given to referral to an addiction specialist or discontinuing (tapering) the opioid. Failure to obtain partial analgesia at low doses should trigger a reassessment.

CLINICAL EVALUATION

Patients referred for chronic pain treatment have usually been seen by a number of specialists, undergone numerous diagnostic tests, and tried various therapeutic procedures, largely without obtaining the results they anticipated or expected. They might be labeled as "professional patients" or medical system failures. It is important to obtain a complete history and physical examination (see Chapter 1) to assess the factors contributing to the patient's complaints, and to assess the impact of the pain on the patient's functional capacity. Searching for a single cause to explain all of the patient's symptoms is typically futile. It can also be counterproductive, because it reinforces the patient's perception that "there's something seriously wrong with me and they just can't figure out what it is."

History

The history should focus on the time course, intensity, and location of the pain. The functional state of the patient prior to the onset of the problem should be established, as it is usually unrealistic to obtain improvement beyond this level. Reactions to diagnostic and therapeutic interventions should be noted, as they can be predictors of responses to future treatment. Have

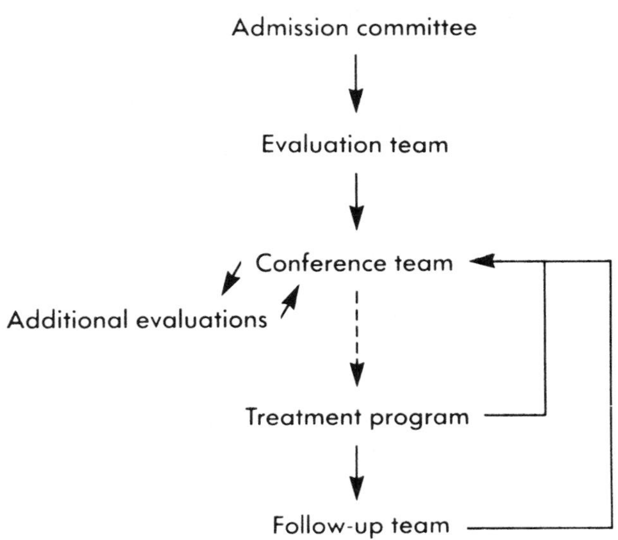

FIGURE 42–4. Pain clinic: flowchart. (From Grabois M: Chronic pain: Evaluation and treatment. *In* Goodgold J (ed): Rehabilitation Medicine. St Louis, Mosby–Year Book, 1988.)

iatrogenic problems resulted from inappropriate or unnecessary procedures? Is there a past history of substance abuse or addictive behavior (a negative prognostic indicator)? What exacerbates and what relieves the pain? Is litigation a factor to be considered? All responses to prior and current medications should be noted.

Physical Examination

A complete physical examination should be done, focusing on the neurological and musculoskeletal systems. The cranial nerves should be assessed, and exteroceptive sensations of pain, temperature, and touch documented. Anatomical patterns of pain and sensory loss often provide clues to the level of a lesion or to the lack of an organic basis for the complaint. For example, loss of light touch in a hand and arm, but with retained ability to identify objects and perform fine motor movement (which require intact sensory input), suggests a functional, overly malingering or somatization.

While motor system examination might be limited by pain, the assessment of strength, muscle bulk, and muscle tone should provide valuable diagnostic clues. Autonomic dysfunction, such as vasomotor instability, can be assessed by comparison of skin temperature, perspiration, and hair and nail changes in the extremities. These abnormalities can be signs of ongoing sympathetic overactivity, especially if localized to painful areas. Changes in reflex responses can be one of the earliest signs of central nervous system (CNS) dysfunction, and reflex testing is often one of the most objective parts of the examination of pain patients. In addition to these standard evaluation techniques, it is important to use other assessment and diagnostic tests as indicated, bearing in mind that endless repetition of tests is generally not very likely to turn up a previously undiagnosed problem.

FUNCTIONAL EVALUATION

As with any patient requiring rehabilitation, an appropriate functional evaluation should be performed before, during, and after the completion of the program, and at follow-up evaluations. Walsh et al[108] report that functional evaluation measures the appropriateness of the patient's functional capabilities for the level of impairment. Objective, quantitative measurements give a baseline with which to evaluate the patient's progress and long-term outcome.

Functional capacity evaluations (FCE) have existed in one form or another since the 1940s, although their use and application have changed over the decades. Employers used pre-vocational FCEs in the 1940s to determine if a worker had the physical capacity to perform a job.[89] Ranchos Los Amigos Hospital in California evaluated workers with coronary heart disease for return to employment using an FCE tool as early as 1972.[40] The Carl Perkins Vocational Education Act (1984) legislatively required the assessment of all students with disabilities in public schools.[106] It was vocational counselors who developed and began using vocational assessment evaluations.[106] The components of a vocational assessment include a survey of the client's vocational interests, an evaluation of aptitudes and achievements, and evaluation of motor skills and a work sample.[106] Therapists and other health care workers administer functional capacity evaluation to injured workers to quantify the injured worker's remaining physical capacity for work.

Tests of pain assessment, psychological distress, and self-perception of abilities and limitations describe the person's symptomatology but do not specifically assess the person's physical capacity for work.[106] Researchers commonly use four test batteries for assessing personal functional status: the Roland disability questionnaire, the Oswestry disability questionnaire, the Million visual analog scale, and the Waddell disability index.[6] Beurskens reviewed these four tools for their clinical and research applications to measure improvement or decline in low back patients over time and during treatment.[6] The four tests correlate highly with each other, suggesting that they are valid measures of personal disability. The Oswestry questions the patient in the context of function lost due to pain. The Million asks about the influence of activity pain.[6] The Roland, Million, and Waddell batteries ask about performance activity, while the Oswestry allows more room for recalled ability and limitation.[6] The Roland Disability Index is a derivative of the Sickness Impact Profile, and asks specifically about current functional ability.[6]

When evaluating an injured worker, the physician should establish the medical impairment and translate that impairment into functional limitation, including an estimate of work capacity (limited by appropriate restrictions).[24] Physicians and patients have great difficulty estimating functional limitation and physical ability.[24, 99] Complaints of chronic low back pain correlate poorly with objective pathology and measurable impairment.[41] The patient's subjective reporting of his or her disability correlates poorly with actual physical ability.[99] Despite the scientific limitations of functional capacity evaluation testing, the literature supports obtaining an objective measure of the injured worker's physical abilities when indicated.[24, 40, 50, 99] The limitations of FCE include the finding that an injured person's physical capacity or ability does not predict return to work,[41] and that FCEs lack the ability to predict a worker's success in actual job-related tasks.[99] The validity and reliability of FCEs have not been established, and a two- to six-hour choreographed evaluation might not have much correlation with an actual eight- to twelve-hour work day with distractions.[50] (see also Chapter 45.)

According to Harten, an FCE is indicated when: (1) the patient's rehab progress plateaus, (2) a difference exists between the patient's reported and observed function, (3) vocational planning calls for an accounting of the patient's physical abilities, or (4) case closure is indicated by judgment or statute.[40] Third parties and allied health care personnel use FCEs as: (1) an objective independent medical evaluation, (2) a baseline of function for a work hardening or functional restoration program, and (3) a screening device for return to work.[40]

The primary use of FCEs is the industrial medicine field, particularly by those professionals returning injured workers to the job site. Other users of FCEs include personal injury attorneys and other injury and disability compensation parties.[99]

An FCE can be used in the industrial medicine setting to help determine: (1) rate and release of the injured worker; (2) a foundation of ability for vocational rehabilitation; and (3) a job-specific evaluation before, during, or after rehabilitation.[99] In the field of litigation and disability assessment, FCEs provide a relatively objective assessment of the extent of damages.[99] Contraindications to FCE mainly relate to medical instability.[40] Tramposh notes that lack of a payment source artificially limits the application of FCEs in cases where they might otherwise be useful.[85, 99]

Harten estimates that more than 100 protocols for FCE are used, but only three protocols are standardized.[40] Publication of these protocols in peer-reviewed journals is rare or nonexistent.[85] FCEs typically last 1–3 days, and usually require 2–6 hours per day to carry out.[40, 50, 85, 99] Tramposh divides FCEs into four types: (1) simulation of the job requirements using trained observers, (2) simulation of the job requirements with no qualifications required for the observer, (3) generic evaluations of lifting and carrying abilities with a requirement for trained observers, or (4) generic evaluations of lifting and carrying abilities with no qualifications required for the observer.[99]

FCEs typically contain an interview, akin to a medical history, a psychological test battery, a musculoskeletal evaluation, functional testing, validation of sincerity of effort by various methods, and report and summary with specific comparisons to a specific job requirement.[40, 50, 85, 114] The musculoskeletal evaluation of the patient includes assessment of posture, flexibility, range of motion, endurance, dexterity, attitude, and consistency of effort during activity performance.[114] Functional testing includes material handling, tasks, holding of static postures, and repetitive task performance.[85] Many FCE protocols assess only lifting and carrying, but patient abilities can be identified and employment possibilities broadened by testing all Dictionary of Occupational Titles (DOT) job factors (Table 42–4), using a tool called the DOT-REC.[24]

Several indicators and tools are available to help assess the patient's effort and sincerity of performance during FCE. These include a patient's refusal to cooperate, performance limited solely by physical complaints, presence of three or more Waddell signs, inconsistency of performance, and degree of increase in heart rate.[85] The therapist or FCE observer also monitors the patient's performance during FCE for signs of fatigue. The indications for a pause or discontinuation of the FCE include modification of body mechanics, especially to an unsafe posture, excessive increase in heart and respiratory rate, perspiration, and decline in performance speed.[85]

TABLE 42–4 Dictionary of Occupational Titles Job Factors

Standing	Kneeling
Walking	Crouching
Sitting	Crawling
Carrying	Reaching
Pushing	Handling
Pulling	Fingering
Lifting	Feeling
Climbing	Talking
Balancing	Hearing
Stooping	Seeing

TABLE 42–5 Dictionary of Occupational Titles Job Intensity

Sedentary
Light
Medium
Heavy
Very Heavy

Other tests related to the FCE include the physical capacity evaluation used in the context of sports medicine, and the work capacity evaluation.[106] The physical capacity evaluation examines an isolated body part (e.g., lumbar strength), while the work capacity evaluation assesses several functional units to complete a whole body task (e.g., lifting).[106]

Velozo and Wyman both note that work capacity evaluations and FCEs should take into account the work environment.[106, 114] The specific job criteria as defined by the DOT job factors should be known.[85, 114] The degree of intensity of the job as defined by the DOT must also be quantified (Table 42–5), based on the maximum amount of weight lifted and carried. The employer should be able to provide this information, or it can be determined by observation on the job site. The factors that help determine whether a patient can return to a specific job include the patient's abilities and limitations, as well as specific job requirements including movements and intensity.

Velozo points out that issues other than just the physical ones should be considered in returning an injured worker to work.[106] The evaluation of work readiness should consider the "meaning" of work to the injured worker, as well as the psychological and social issues that might prevent successful return to employment. For example, in the study of Hazard and colleagues, psychosis significantly predicted inability to maintain employment at one year after a functional restoration program.[41] High pain reporting and pain intensity and elevated values on some MMPI psychological scales correlated significantly with noncompletion of a three week program.[41] Fear of work activities, fear of recurrent injury, and motivation and secondary gain can affect performance during the FCE; moreover, such factors can affect the likelihood of a successful return to work regardless of the patient's performance on the FCE.[40, 99]

FCEs have scientific limitations in regard to standardization, validity, and reliability; but they do provide useful information about the injured worker's ability, as well as insight into effort and evoked symptomatology.

Functional capacity testing does not predict return to work; but for the motivated patient who is returning to work or beginning a rehabilitation program, it can be a useful tool for scripting work restrictions or initial rehabilitation orders.

PSYCHOLOGICAL EVALUATION

The perception of chronic pain is influenced by psychological factors, and a patient's overall psychological status is in turn influenced by chronic pain. A psychological evaluation is useful in all cases in which pain causes significant impairment in psychological, vocational, or social functioning.[72] The goal of the psychological evaluation is to determine the emotional, cognitive, behavioral, social, or vocational factors that are potentially affecting the patient's perception of the pain being experienced. While it is true that patients with primary psychiatric disease can present with complaints of chronic pain that are largely psychogenic in nature, the use of the psychological evaluation solely for the purpose of determining whether pain is due to an organic or psychogenic cause is problematic.

Turk and Rudy[103] present the following questions to illustrate the problems with this unidimensional approach:

What medical evidence has to be present for us to say there is in fact an organic basis for a pain complaint?
Are medical and diagnostic procedures 100% effective at identifying all sources of physical pathology likely to cause the pain reported by the patient?
Are there other factors beyond psychopathology which could influence the perception of pain?
Is it possible that the psychological difficulties expressed by the patient are a result of their pain?
Could there be individual rather than psychological characteristics that could account for the differences expressed in pain reports?
Is it possible for a psychiatric problem and a pain condition to coexist in the same patient?

TABLE 42–6 Appropriate and Inappropriate Uses of Psychological Assessment

Appropriate Uses	Inappropriate Uses
To determine specific psychological and behavioral contributions to a patient's pain and concomitant behaviors, disability, and suffering	To determine if pain is organic or functional (i.e., real or psychogenic)
To determine appropriate treatment strategies	To detect malingerers
To provide essential information on particular aspects of a patient's psychosocial background and current situation that may be affecting the pain problem	To justify dumping of more difficult patients

Adapted from Turk DC: Psychological assessment of patients with persistent pain: I. Traditional views. Pain Manage 1990; 3:167–172.

TABLE 42–7 Guidelines for Psychological Services Referral

Clearly identify nonmedical consultants
Acknowledge that problem is legitimate
Provide a positive rationale for referral
Inform other staff of rationale
Avoid making cynical comments about referral
Let patient know if referral is routine
Personalize the referral
Inform patient that referral does not imply transfer

Adapted from Cameron R, Shepel LF: The process of psychological consultation in pain management. *In* Holzman AD, Turk DC (eds): Pain Management: A Handbook of Psychological Treatment Approaches. New York, Pergamon Press, 1986.

These questions illustrate the need to conceptualize chronic pain beyond the unidimensional construct of organic versus psychogenic, and to embrace a broader and more comprehensive scheme. Practitioners should be sensitive to the multifaceted aspects of chronic pain, and not confuse the emotional consequences of pain with causation when no readily apparent medical explanation is available. A person without a readily diagnosable organic cause of pain is often treated as if it is "all in his/her head." The patient might react to this by dramatization and symptom magnification in an attempt to convince the clinician that the pain is real. The cycle typically worsens with each specialist the patient sees.

Once the patient has been referred to a chronic pain program, it is important to prepare him or her for psychological evaluation. Many patients with chronic pain are defensive and concerned about the hidden meaning of a referral for a psychologist's evaluation. It is important to provide the patient with the rationale for psychological evaluation in a manner that minimizes misunderstanding and defensiveness. The patient should know that the psychological evaluation and the use of psychological interventions in no way implies that the pain is not "real." Getting the patient's "buy-in" greatly facilitates an accurate and effective evaluation. Providing the patient with appropriate information about the outcome of the evaluation and testing can also prove helpful (Tables 42–6, 42–7).

A wide variety of instruments can be used in clinical settings to assess pain patients in different dimensions, including pain intensity, pain sensation, psychopathology, coping strategies, beliefs, behaviors, and social functioning. The primary components of the initial psychological evaluation include the clinical interview(s) with the patient and family members, health questionnaires, pain inventories (e.g., McGill Pain Questionnaire, Multidimensional Pain Inventory), and measures of psychological and behavioral dysfunction (e.g., Minnesota Multiphasic Personality Inventory [MMPI],[83] Symptoms Checklist-90, Beck Depression Inventory, State-Trait Anxiety Inventory). Turk and Melzack[102] have published an excellent review of pain assessment instruments.

For the initial clinical interview, many clinicians utilize a structured interview format. At a minimum, a pain-specific inventory (e.g., McGill Pain Questionnaire, Multidimensional Pain Inventory) and a general measure of psychopathology (i.e., MMPI-II, Personality Assessment Inventory) are needed to assess patients with chronic pain. The conceptualizing of pain is multidimensional and necessarily requires more than one type of assessment instrument and approach.[86] The psychological evaluation of patients with chronic pain should be conducted by clinicians who are sensitive to and knowledgeable about the psychological aspects of chronic pain.

PAIN MEASUREMENT

Pain measurement is a vital part of chronic pain evaluation and treatment.[79] Without adequate methods of measurement, pain treatments will continue to be adopted for use without proper scientific evaluation.[79] Cost-effectiveness is becoming more important in pain rehabilitation, and scientifically established and reliable assessment techniques are necessary to determine the treatment techniques that are the least invasive, least extensive, and least expensive.

Measurement of induced acute pain is easier than measurement of chronic pain.[35] In laboratory-induced acute pain emotional or cognitive factors are minimal, and the quantity of the pain stimulus is easily controlled. In the measurement and assessment of chronic pain, there is, unfortunately, no generally accepted laboratory model. A clear linear relationship between the quantity of noxious input and the intensity of pain experience is not readily apparent in chronic pain. It is difficult to capture what is ultimately a personal and private sensory experience. In many cases all we have are the patients' words, their recollections of the experience, and the behavior exhibited when they have the pain experience.[35] In a very real sense all pain is "in the head" and measuring it objectively is difficult. For all these reasons, a pain scale should, at a minimum, include ease of administration and scoring, the potential for consistently accurate use by a variety of health-care professionals, high inter-rater reliability, and validity.[35]

Sternbach and co-workers[95] noted that pain is a complex experience, and evidence of its presence involves several dimensions that depend on changing states which are continuously influenced by a multitude of extrinsic and intrinsic stimuli. Fordyce[30] described four main components of pain: (1) nociception, (2) sensation, (3) suffering, and (4) behavioral reactions.

Using the concepts of Sternbach[95] and Fordyce,[31] three components of chronic pain measurement are noted: (1) the subjective, (2) the physiological, and (3) the behavioral. The interaction between these components is dynamic and involves a balanced appraisal of sensory input and the degree to which this is modulated by psychological factors (including other determinants of verbal and overt behavior). The subjective component of chronic pain management is reflected in rating scales, questionnaires, and diary cards. The visual analog scale (1–10) is the most commonly used rating scale.

Questionnaires have gained wide acceptance, with the McGill Pain Questionnaire being the most popular.[66] It evaluates three major classes of word descriptions (sensory, affective, and evaluative) that patients use to specify their subjective pain experience. It has a built-in intensity scale. Multiple literature studies have evaluated this method of pain measurement, and it has been used extensively in clinical evaluation and treatment trials. Melzack[67] and others believe it provides a quantity of information that can be treated statistically, and that it is sufficiently sensitive to detect outcome differences that allow judgments about the effectiveness of various pain relief treatments. Although physiological techniques such as measurement of cortical evoked potentials, muscle tension, vasodilation, heart rate, and blood pressure have a firm scientific basis in the measurement of acute pain in the laboratory, they have not yet been adequately evaluated in the clinical (or chronic) pain setting.

Behavioral measurements of pain, as advocated by Fordyce,[31] are logical techniques for measuring pain, since people in pain must engage in behavior indicative of their state. Most behavior measurement techniques use three categories of behavior: (1) somatic intervention, (2) impaired functional capacity, and (3) pain complaints. The University of Alabama Behavioral Measurement of Pain Scale is based on 10 behaviors, including vocalization and the frequency and intensity of these expressions.[82] Although inter-observer reliability of behavioral aspects of pain is good, it is very important to use trained observers to obtain accurate and valid information.

Clearly there is no current ideal method for evaluating and measuring chronic pain and the effectiveness of treatment techniques. Those measurements that reflect subjective, physiological, and behavioral components with independent and direct monitoring are the most appropriate.[35] Reading[79] reports that behavioral indices can assume greater importance as chronicity increases, since the question of how much the patient is able to do rather than how much it hurts can be the more important question in a chronic pain management setting. This is especially true when considering the cost-effectiveness of pain management programs, since functional outcome is often more important to third-party payers than the patient's perceived level of pain.[79]

DIAGNOSTIC TESTING

Diagnostic testing should be undertaken with care in patients with chronic pain syndromes. Careful review of old records can save time and expense by preventing repetition of prior studies, especially invasive studies. The use of diagnostic testing should always be based on clinical findings or changes noted in the examination. If symptoms and findings have remained static since the last evaluation, the likelihood of finding a significant change in a repeated diagnostic test is low.

Laboratory Tests

Chronic pain states usually do not produce distinct laboratory findings, other than those that result from any

TABLE 42–8 Diagnostic Studies Commonly Utilized in Chronic Pain Syndrome Patients

Imaging Study	Comment
Spinal plain films	Low specificity and predictive value
Computed tomogram (with myelography)	Demonstrates over 90% of herniated disks, but can have false-positives
Magnetic resonance imaging	Excellent soft tissue and disc images
Thermography	Can be used for confirmation of autonomic dysfunction in conditions such as reflex sympathetic dystrophy
Electromyography and nerve conduction studies	Objectively assess severity, location, and extent of nerve and muscular lesions
Bone scan	One of the few imaging techniques that detects physiological changes
Three-phase bone scan	Sensitive and specific for reflex sympathetic dystrophy

underlying disease. Routine monitoring for drug effects is performed for patients taking anticonvulsants or other medications known to have adverse effects on specific organ systems. Urine or blood screening should be considered in any drug detoxification program. The evaluation and treatment of specific connective tissue syndromes requires routine monitoring of appropriate laboratory indicators, such as the use of the erythrocyte sedimentation rate to assess the response to some types of therapeutic interventions.

Imaging Studies

Radiographic studies are used extensively in the evaluation of patients with chronic pain because of their relative simplicity and lack of invasiveness. Magnetic resonance imaging, computed tomography, and plain radiographs are generally a part of every chronic pain patient's workup. They rarely need be repeated, and for the most part these patients have already been adequately diagnosed and treated in the medical model before referral to the chronic pain program. In the event that the patient's workup has not been complete, other evaluations such as electrodiagnostic studies, bone scanning, or even thermography, are indicated (Table 42–8).

TREATMENT GOALS

The cause of the chronic pain syndrome should be determined from a medical and psychosocial point of view and the location of "pain generator" should be noted. Attempts to decrease or eliminate the "pain generator(s)" are important and should be carried out first, followed by consideration of other treatment options (see Table 42–9).

The goals of treatment in an interdisciplinary program center on moderating pain, increasing function, and decreasing health care utilization.[84] These goals can be achieved by modifying pain medication and pain behavior, decreasing reliance on medical care utilization, and increasing activity through exercise.

The Fordyce model of behavioral modification is a useful one in treatment patients with chronic pain syndrome.[55] The goal in these patients is not to "cure the pain" but to interrupt the pain behavioral reinforcement cycle by rewarding healthy behavior and setting appropriate goals that the patient must achieve. These goals include reduction in the use of medicines, modulation of pain response, increased activity, and reduction in pain behaviors.[36]

Behavioral Treatment

More recent developments in the theory and practice of pain management have led to the development of the cognitive-behavioral approach. In contrast to the behavioral approach, which emphasizes only the environmental factors, the cognitive-behavioral model of pain management emphasizes the reciprocal interaction between the individual and the environmental factors. The primary assumption from the cognitive-behavioral perspective is that the individual has learned maladaptive ways of thinking, feeling, and behaving. Cognitive-behavioral treatment (CBT) interventions are designed to change both the thoughts and behaviors of the individual to improve adjustment with chronic pain. Cognitive-behavioral interventions teach patients effective coping strategies, provide patients an opportunity

TABLE 42–9 Classification of the Chronic Nonmalignant Pain Patient with Examples and Treatment Strategies

Class	Symptoms	Objective Findings	Social and Vocational Components	Example	Treatment Strategies
IA	High	High correlation	High	Rheumatoid arthritis	Behavior modification approach with emphasis on medication and modalities
IB	High	High correlation	Low	Rheumatoid arthritis	Medication and modalities approach
IIA	High	Low correlation	High	Musculoskeletal/low back pain	Behavioral modification approach
IIB	High	Low correlation	Low	Musculoskeletal/low back pain	Modalities

to rehearse these new strategies, and work to prevent relapse following treatment.[33, 39]

What are some of these coping skills?

1. Patients learn to be more active and informed participants in their health care.
2. Patients are given information about medications to promote treatment compliance.
3. Patients learn how to pace their activities.
4. Patients learn to think differently about their pain, life goals, and available treatment options.
5. Patients learn to recognize what kinds of thoughts are maladaptive and how to change them.
6. Patients gain an awareness of how they can tense and brace in response to pain, leading to an increase in muscle tension and even more pain.
7. Patients learn effective ways to reduce muscle tension and to relax.
8. Patients learn how to cope with and manage feelings like anger.
9. Patients learn how to resolve conflict and improve communication with family members.
10. Patients are encouraged to set realistic functional and vocational goals to promote meaningful activity in their lives.

In the last several years, an effort has been made to identify specific cognitive-behavioral factors that can promote more successful patient outcome. Having better information about critical factors would allow the development of more effective cognitive-behavioral treatment strategies and more successful treatment outcomes. One of the factors identified by researchers is a patient's "readiness to change."[48, 49] This concept was borrowed from the substance abuse literature, but it appears to have important utility for clinicians interested in identifying those patients who are most likely to benefit from cognitive-behavioral treatments for pain.[48] Anger management style[12, 13, 14] and pessimism[57] are two other cognitive-behavioral factors thought to influence outcomes for pain patients. Promising research in this area is ongoing.

CBT can be applied on an individual basis or in a group format,[80] but CBT is believed to be most effectively implemented in the context of a fully integrated multidisciplinary pain management program (MPC).[5] In spite of some skepticism, the effectiveness of MPCs has been widely demonstrated. Several recent research studies[5, 43, 57, 80] and one meta-analysis study[27] have demonstrated that MPCs that emphasize cognitive-behavioral methods do show significant positive outcomes on a variety of measures (i.e., cost-effectiveness, reduced medication use, improved return to work rates, lower disability rates, and reduced health care utilization). The cognitive-behavioral approach to pain management is an effective approach and an important component to any multidisciplinary pain practice.

Medication Management Philosophy

Physicians have a long history of prescribing, and chronic pain patients have a long history of using, inappropriate medications (Fig. 42–5), particularly narcotic medications. Studies show that patients are usually inadequately treated for acute pain syndromes, and overtreated for chronic ones.[81] In addition, some physicians mistakenly believe that giving medication on an as-needed basis rather than on a scheduled dosage results in less addiction. Physicians also tend to incorrectly label patients who respond to placebo as having a nonorganic type of pain.

The philosophy of health care professionals regarding the use of opioid medication for treating chronic pain has gradually evolved over the years. At one time it was felt that patients with chronic noncancer pain should not be on opioid medication. However, with enlightened thinking and research, it is now felt that appropriate utilization of opioid medication can be a helpful strategy in some patients with chronic pain.[78] The American Pain Society and the American Academy of Pain Medicine have developed a position paper for appropriate utilization of opioids medication in patients with chronic pain.[2]

In spite of this changing philosophy, physicians have been reluctant to prescribe opioid medications for chronic pain because of fear of retribution from state medical boards. The Federation of State Medical Boards of the United States has now adopted model guidelines for the use of controlled substances for the treatment of pain.[20] Wilson noted that this consensus statement defines the broad principles of the use of opioids in the treatment of chronic pain.[113] Many physicians utilize a medication management agreement that delineates the responsibilities of the health care team and patient in the use of opioids for chronic pain.[16]

When the goal of pharmacological management of a patient with chronic pain is to moderate or eliminate possible use of narcotics, tranquilizers, and hypnotic

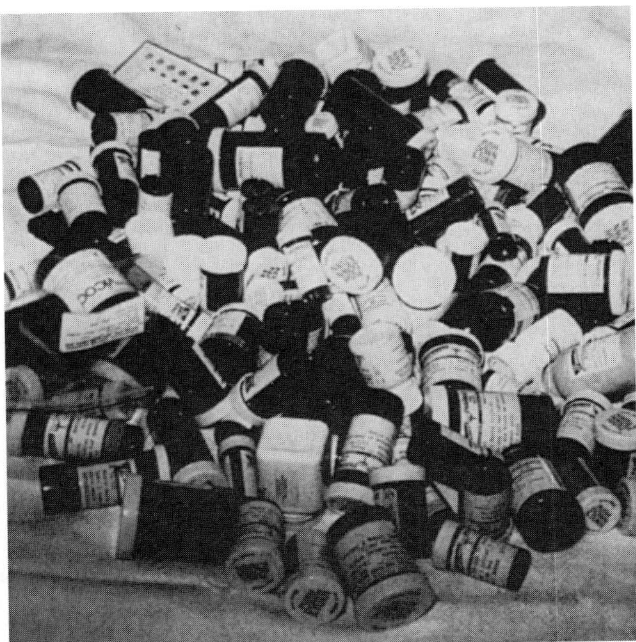

FIGURE 42–5. Medication usage of chronic pain patient over 1-year period.

medications,[35] it usually requires detoxification in an organized treatment program. No new narcotics, tranquilizers, or hypnotic drugs should be prescribed. Once the daily requirement for the patient is obtained over a few days, a "pain cocktail" approach is used on a time-contingent basis (Table 42–10).

The pain cocktail typically consists of methadone or a similar preparation in a dose equivalent to the currently used narcotic medication.[6] It is mixed with a masking vehicle such as cherry syrup. The patient is fully informed in advance that the drug will gradually be withdrawn, but is not told the daily dose of the active ingredient. The cocktail is given at the dosage and on the time schedule the patient demonstrated in the daily requirement. Gradual reduction of the active ingredient with an equal increase in the masking vehicle is carried out over 3 to 6 weeks. Decrements are made slowly so as not to elicit withdrawal signs and symptoms. Eventually, the patient is receiving only the masking vehicle, and the cocktail is discontinued. Figure 42–6 compares the pain cocktail approach with the medication-as-needed method. The cocktail approach of gradual withdrawal can be used for tranquilizers and hypnotics as well as for narcotic medications. Kanner[46] believes that judiciously used antidepressants, particularly the tricyclic antidepressants, often offer a smoother treatment course for the patient with chronic pain.

Pharmacological Management

Nonopioid analgesics can be subdivided into aspirin-like drugs (nonsteroidal anti-inflammatory drugs, [NSAIDs]) and acetaminophen. NSAIDs have analgesic, antipyretic, anti-inflammatory, and antithrombotic actions. Inhibition of prostaglandin synthesis appears to explain their analgesic, antithrombotic, and antipyretic actions, while interference with neutrophil function might account for their anti-inflammatory properties. These medications are well-absorbed, but demonstrate an analgesic ceiling. Gastropathy is the most common side effect and can be neutrophil- or prostaglandin-mediated.[107] Renal complications include the nephrotic syndrome and interstitial nephritis, which are reversible. Irreversible papillary necrosis can occur, but is exceed-

TABLE 42–10 Sample Pain Cocktail Regimen

Inpatient Days		Pain Cocktail Format
1–6	*Baseline:*	Patient reports preadmission pattern of "one or two of the 50-mg tablets of Demerol [meperidine] two or three times a day, as needed, at home."
		Physician orders to nurse: "May have Demerol, *prn* pain, not to exceed three 50-mg tablets q3h. Carefully record amount taken."
		Analysis of baseline data: Patient averaged 600 mg of Demerol/24 hr, averaging of 3- to 4-hr intervals between requests.
7–9 First cocktail		
	℞ *to pharmacist:*	Demerol, 1920 mg Bevisol, Plebex, or other liquid B complex, 12 mL; cherry syrup qs 240 mL
	Sig:	Pain cocktail, 10 mL po q3h, day and night, not *prn*
	Nursing order:	Pain cocktail, 10 mL po q3h, day and night, not *prn*
	Since the contents of the pain cocktail are not on the label, a copy of the prescription must be kept in a separate pain cocktail book.	
10–12	Decrease each daily total by 64 mg, to 1/10 of original amount. A 3-day ℞ is decreased by 64 × 3 or 192 mg.	
	℞ *to pharmacist:*	Demerol, 1728 mg Bevisol, Plebex, or other liquid B complex, 12 mL; cherry syrup qs 240 mL
	Sig:	Pain cocktail, 10 mL po q3h, day and night, not *prn*
	Nursing order:	Pain cocktail, 10 mL po q3h, day and night, not *prn*
13–15	℞ *to pharmacist:*	Demerol, 1536 mg Bevisol, Plebex, or other liquid B complex, 12 mL; cherry syrup qs 240 mL
	Sig:	Pain cocktail, 10 mL po q3h, day and night, not *prn*
	Nursing order:	Pain cocktail, 10 mL po q3h, day and night, not *prn*
16–18	℞ *to pharmacist:*	Demerol, 1344 mg Bevisol, Plebex, or other liquid B complex, 12 mL; cherry syrup qs 240 mL
	Sig:	Pain cocktail, 10 mL po q3h, day and night, not *prn*
	Nursing order:	Pain cocktail, 10 mL po q3h, day and night, not *prn*
19–21	℞ *to pharmacist:*	Demerol, 1152 mg Bevisol, Plebex, or other liquid B complex, 12 mL; cherry syrup qs 240 mL
	Sig:	Pain cocktail, 10 mL po q3h, day and night, not *prn*
	Nursing order:	Pain cocktail, 10 mL po q3h, day and night, not *prn*
22–24	℞ to pharmacist:	Demerol 960 mg Bevisol, Plebex, or other liquid B complex, 12 mL; cherry syrup qs 240 mL
	Sig:	Pain cocktail, 10 mL po q3h, day and night, not *prn*
	Nursing order:	Pain cocktail, 10 mL po q3h, day and night, not *prn*
37–39	℞ *to pharmacist:*	Demerol, 0 mg Bevisol, Plebex, or other liquid B complex, 12 mL; cherry syrup qs 240 mL
	Sig:	Pain cocktail, 10 mL po q3h, day and night, not *prn*
	Nursing order:	Pain cocktail, 10 mL po q3h, day and night, not *prn*
(Maintain patient on vehicle for 2–10 days; if all is going well, inform patient and ask if continuation of vehicle is desired.)		

Modified from Fordyce WE: Behavioral Methods for Chronic Pain and Illness. St Louis, Mosby–Year Book, 1979.

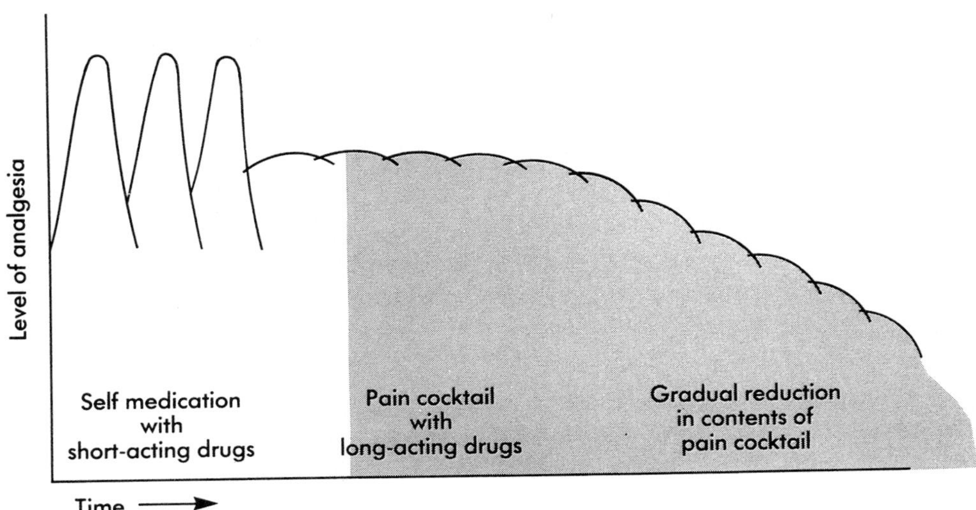

FIGURE 42–6. Pain cocktail approach: comparison of as-needed and around-the-clock approaches.

ingly rare.[110] NSAIDs should be used cautiously or avoided in patients with a past history of peptic ulcer disease or with decreased renal function.

Acetaminophen's analgesic properties are equipotent with aspirin. While it is antipyretic, it is not anti-inflammatory and does not affect platelet function. Doses exceeding 4 to 6 g/day can be hepatotoxic, and caution should be taken when using combination medications that contain this amount of acetaminophen.

Opioid analgesics are generally not indicated for the treatment of nonmalignant chronic pain.[112] While efficacy without dependence has been reported for opioid treatment of somatic pain,[29] opioid use for sympathetic pain and other chronic neuropathic pain disorders has been shown to have poor efficacy. For chronic somatic pain, opioids have improved efficacy, but dependence and tolerance remain a problem in some patients. Chronic malignant pain of somatic origin can be treated effectively with long-term opioid management. It should be noted that caffeine can increase the analgesic effects of aspirin-like drugs in the treatment of headaches and other pain syndromes.[29]

Several adjuvant medications have independent analgesic effects or enhance the effects of opioids. Tricyclic antidepressants have been shown in controlled trials to have analgesic effects independent of their antidepressant properties.[61, 109] They have also been shown in laboratory animals to enhance the effects of opioid analgesics with an efficacy 70 times that of aspirin.[90] These effects were not reversed with naloxone. They were reversed by central serotonin depletion, implicating serotonin reuptake blockade as an analgesic mechanism.[38] Amitriptyline is the best studied of the tricyclics, but its anticholinergic side effects (dry mouth, sedation, blurred vision, urinary retention, constipation, or delirium) can make this drug undesirable in some patients. Doses required to achieve analgesic effects are below those needed to relieve depression (usually in a range of 10 to 100 mg per day).[10, 21] It can be given at night to take advantage of its sedative properties to normalize sleep patterns and thus improve compliance. Caution should be taken in patients with hypertension or coronary artery disease, since amitriptyline can cause a precipitous rise in blood pressure.

Benzodiazepines are useful in relieving anxiety, but they have no intrinsic analgesic properties. Long-term use can lead to dependence and withdrawal effects, including seizures, muscle cramps, and dysphoria. If given in combination with opioids, they can potentiate respiratory depression, even in small doses.

Steroids, in bolus doses, have been shown to be effective in the treatment of reflex sympathetic dystrophy[51] (now often referred to as complex regional pain syndrome) and can be helpful in cancer pain.[29] Side effects with long-term use include Cushing's syndrome, weight gain, myopathy, psychosis, and gastrointestinal bleeding. Steroids should not be used in conjunction with NSAIDs. Abrupt withdrawal of steroids after long-term use can precipitate an Addisonian crisis with nausea, vomiting, hypotension, and hypoglycemia.

The anticonvulsants carbamazepine, phenytoin, and valproic acid can also be effective in the treatment of neuropathic pain. Carbamazepine has been found to be useful in the treatment of trigeminal neuralgia,[8, 35] posttraumatic neuropathies,[36] and phantom limb pain.[34] Side effects that require routine monitoring with these medications include bone marrow suppression and hepatotoxicity.

Clonidine, an α_2-adrenergic agonist, has been shown to enhance the effects of opioids and has independent analgesic properties when administered intrathecally.[19] Potential side effects of clonidine include orthostatic hypotension and rebound hypertension upon withdrawal.

Pain Modulation

The complete eradication of chronic pain is rarely achieved and is not the goal of most interventions. The goal is the modification of pain to a more tolerable level.

TABLE 42–11 Pharmacological and Nonpharmacological Pain Interventions

Pharmacological Interventions	Nonpharmacological Interventions
NSAIDs	Behavior modifiers
Antidepressants (TCAs)	Relaxation
Anticonvulsants	Biofeedback
Carbamazepine	Guided visual imagery
Phenytoin (Dilantin)	Music therapy
Invasive pain modulators	Distraction
Spinal opioids	Hypnosis
Peripheral nerve stimulators	Pain modulators
Dorsal column stimulators	TENS
Epidural and deep brain stimulators	Acupuncture
Invasive pain relievers	Conditioning exercises
Sympathetic nerve blocks	Stretching/flexibility
Epidural anesthetics/steroids	Myofascial release
Root sleeve injections	Spray and stretch
Trigger point injections	

Abbreviations: NSAIDs, nonsteroidal anti-inflammatory drugs; TCAs, tricyclic antidepressants; TENS, transcutaneous electrical nerve stimulation.

One way of explaining this to patients is to tell them that the pain program is designed to make them more "comfortable." A comprehensive pain management program utilizes an array of modalities to accomplish this goal. Nonpharmacological methods are usually adjunctive therapies and do not necessarily substitute for pharmacological interventions.[75] For the chronic pain population, the optimal techniques are those that can be used by the patient in the home setting, are active rather than passive, and can be used for the shortest time possible or gradually weaned.[68] Transcutaneous electrical nerve stimulation (TENS), biofeedback, and thermal modalities fulfill these criteria. Table 42–11 lists commonly used pharmacological and nonpharmacological pain-modulating interventions.

Pain modulation techniques take advantage of the body's endogenous pain-modulating abilities first postulated and implied by the gate theory of pain of Melzack and Wall.[68] This theory supports the observation that a direct correlation does not always exist between the extent of organic injury and the expression of pain.[104] Melzack and Wall proposed that pain information was modulated at the level of the "target cell" in the substantia gelatinosa, or laminae II and III of the dorsal horn, by afferent information from A delta and C sensory fibers.[68] This "gating" effect on the target cell modulates input before it evokes pain perception.[29] Since the description of the gate theory, modulation events higher in the neuraxis and modulation by descending or efferent mechanisms have been proposed. Basbaum and Fields[4] proposed that pain modulation occurs at the periaqueductal gray area of the midbrain by descending efferent tracts. The modulation of pain information and pain perception occurs at multiple sites along the neuraxis and by afferent and efferent pathways.

The pain modulation network can be activated by the administration of spinal opiates. It can also be activated by electrical stimulation (transcutaneously or percutaneously) to peripheral nerves, or epidurally at the level of the spinal cord or brain.[74]

Transcutaneous Electrical Nerve Stimulation

TENS at rates of 50 to 100 Hz produces analgesia that is not reversible by naloxone.[74] Stimulation of large myelinated fibers presumably blocks nociceptive transmission at the level of the spinothalamic tract cell bodies.[68] TENS can produce neuromodulation by three routes: (1) presynaptic inhibition of the spinal cord, (2) direct inhibition of an excited, abnormally firing nerve, or (3) restoration of afferent input.[32]

TENS is helpful in the treatment of many painful conditions.[52, 71, 75] A recent blinded and controlled trial of TENS and exercise showed a significant benefit only in the exercise group.[9] However, double-blinded, controlled trials of TENS have shown it to be of significant benefit in the treatment of rheumatoid arthritis and osteoarthritis.[1, 88, 97] Proponents of TENS recommend its use early in a pain treatment program.[59] The patients who respond best to TENS typically have neurogenic or musculoskeletal pain (Table 42–12).

The patient should learn to apply the TENS electrodes over or near the area of pain with the dipole parallel to major nerve trunks.[53] Patients have to determine by trial and error the optimal electrode placement and stimulus intensity, and the therapist or physician should encourage the patient to adjust the unit as needed for optimal relief. TENS variables that can be adjusted include the stimulus amplitude, rate, pulse width, and location of the electrodes.[73] There is no current research to support the use of one type of TENS over another (e.g., conventional, burst, modulated, brief-intense, acupuncture-like, strength-duration).[59] Adverse reactions to TENS are infrequent; the most common is skin hypersensitivity.[53] TENS should be avoided over the carotid sinus, in patients with demand-type pacemakers and during pregnancy.

Heat and Cold

The use of hot and cold modalities, particularly those which the patient can safely use at home, should be encouraged (see Chapter 21). The use of devices or treatments that require the help of other persons or professional settings, such as ultrasound or massage, are best reserved for acute pain syndromes or intermittently painful chronic conditions.

TABLE 42–12 Indications for Transcutaneous Electrical Nerve Stimulation

Musculoskeletal Pain	Neurogenic Pain
Rheumatoid arthritis pain	Deafferentiated pain syndromes (phantom limb)
Osteoarthritis pain	Sympathetically mediated pain
Myofascial pain	Tension headache
Dysmenorrhea	Acute postoperative pain
Visceral pain	

Biofeedback

Relaxation training and biofeedback are behavioral treatment methods that have been successfully used to treat a wide variety of pain syndromes, including myofascial and sympathetically maintained pain syndromes.[28, 34, 56, 101] There are several relaxation techniques that are used for chronic pain. The two most commonly utilized are autogenic training and progressive muscle relaxation.[103] Biofeedback utilizes instrumentation to provide feedback on a variety of physiological responses (e.g., hand temperature, muscle tension, and sweat gland activity). It is typically used to facilitate relaxation and enhance self-regulation. Relaxation training and biofeedback are thought to be equally effective in pain modulation.[86]

Interventional Procedures

Interventional procedures are an important component of the therapeutic armamentarium for chronic pain management. Some of these techniques play an especially important role when used as diagnostic procedures. Interventional procedures can be powerful tools when used and interpreted intelligently in the context of a multidisciplinary approach to chronic pain. They can also help prevent the development of chronic pain syndromes. The most commonly employed interventional techniques are listed in Table 42–13.

A common interventional procedure is neural blockade, which can be performed using anatomical landmarks. Other technologies offer more precise nerve blocks: A nerve stimulator can be used to evoke either a motor or sensory response, a doppler can identify blood vessels in proximity to a nerve, and fluoroscopy can be used when bony landmarks are available. Diagnostic blocks are used to determine the afferent pathway and the source of pain and as a tool in differential diagnosis. Prognostic blocks let the patient become aware of the consequences of prolonged blockade of afferent input, and are often used before neuroablative procedures.

TABLE 42–13 Commonly Utilized Interventional Treatments in Chronic Pain Syndrome

Treatment	Use/Comment
Nerve blocks	As diagnostic, prognostic, or therapeutic procedures
Diagnostic blocks	To ascertain source of pain, nerve pathway, or as tools for differential diagnosis
Prognostic blocks	Before neuroablative or neurolytic procedures to assess their possible effects
Therapeutic blocks	Can be performed with local anesthetics or with neurolytic agents
Trigger point injections	Treatment of myofascial pain
Facet or zygapophyseal blocks	Diagnostic or therapeutic
Epidural blocks	Useful especially when prolonged analgesia might be required for physical therapy, not for days but for weeks
Spinal blocks	Differential pain diagnosis
Neurolytic, epidural, and spinal techniques	Specific indications for the treatment of some intractable chronic pain syndromes
Sympathetic nerve blocks	Effective therapeutic tools in dealing with sympathetically maintained pain
Chemoneurolysis	Very effective in treatment of sympathetically maintained pain and cancer or noncancer chronic pain
Cryoneurolysis/ cryoanalgasia	

Sympathetic blocks are particularly effective as diagnostic and therapeutic tools in chronic pain management. Sympathetic blockade is useful in various pain syndromes, and is of particular importance in determining the degree of sympathetic mediation in complex regional pain syndrome type I [reflex sympathetic dystrophy] and type II [causalgia]. When dealing with sympathetic mediated pain, a series of sympathetic blocks can be an effective therapeutic approach.

The sympathetic chain can be blocked in many locations, including the cervical [stellate ganglion], thoracic, and lumbar sympathetic ganglia. Splanchnic and celiac plexus blockade plays a special role in pain due to malignancies of upper abdominal organs, particularly the pancreas. Pelvic pain of various origins can often be managed by blocking the superior hypogastric plexus.

Chemoneurolysis

The injection of agents capable of interfering with neural conduction for prolonged periods of time is another common technique for pain control. Neurolytic agents include alcohol, phenol, ammonium sulfate, and chlorocresol. There is active research for the development of local anesthetic agents with long duration of action measured sometimes in months or even years. The most commonly used neurolytic agent is probably phenol, followed by alcohol. Chemoneurolysis can be done intrathecally and epidurally, as well at various plexuses or in some peripheral nerves.

Sympathetic chemoneurolysis has a special indication in complex regional pain syndrome, either type I or II, with evidence of sympathetically maintained pain. Somatic neurolytic techniques are used in the control of cancer and noncancer pain. Gasserian alcohol gangliolysis has been used extensively in trigeminal neuralgia, although this technique has been largely replaced by radiofrequency thermocoagulation of the Gasserian ganglion.

Chemoneurolysis, even when meticulously performed, can be associated with serious complications such as neuritis. This can lead to increased pain, sexual dysfunction, or other serious side effects. Patients should be informed about such possibilities and informed consent must be obtained prior to any neurolytic procedure.

Cryolysis

Another technique commonly used in pain management is cryoanalgesia. This technique is based on the fact that freezing can induce a nerve lesion. This modality was introduced in 1961 when the first cryoprobe was developed. This probe employed the principle of phase change using liquid nitrogen to produce temperatures in the vicinity of −196°C. A probe was subsequently developed that used nitrous oxide, applying the principle of gas expansion, reaching temperatures of −70°C. There are other probes of various sizes that have also incorporated thermocouples and nerve stimulators.

Freezing causes removal of pure water from a solution, isolating it as ice crystals. All subsequent anatomical, biochemical, and physiological consequences of freezing are directly or indirectly related to this single event. Inducing cryogenic neural lesions, when done carefully, can be a powerful technique. Frustratingly, its effectiveness cannot be predicted; moreover, pain relief can last from 3 to 1000 days, with a mean of 60 to 90 days. Indications for cryolysis include facial pain, and cryolysis of the trigeminal nerve or its branches has been described in the literature. Thoracic pain such as acute post-thoracotomy pain or post-thoracotomy intercostal neuralgia can be treated by cryolysis. Spinal pain originating in the facets is often treated by cryolytic lesioning of the medial branch of the posterior primary ramus of symptomatic facets. Pelvic pain can be a particularly good indication for cryolysis, and it is often indicated in coccygodynia, or perineal pain from cancer of the rectum.

Radiofrequency Thermocoagulation

Electrical current has been used to produce neural lesions for many years. Radiofrequency thermocoagulation [RFTC] has been used to ablate pain pathways in the trigeminal ganglion, sympathetic chain, spinal cord, dorsal root entry zone, dorsal root ganglion, and peripheral nerves.

A lesion is produced when neural temperatures exceed 45°C. This temperature is the result of frictional heat that is generated by molecular motion in a field of alternating current at 250 kHz. Currents in the radiofrequency range produce an electromagnetic field around an active electrode. There is some evidence that a neural lesion can be produced by inducing an electromagnetic field around the nerve without having to raise the temperature at the tissue level above 40°C, but this is experimental and remains to be proven.

Since the neural lesion produced by RFTC is irreversible, it has to be considered an end-of-the-line procedure to be used only when other, more conservative modalities have failed. One complication that has been reported is the development of painful neuroma formation.

Steroid Injections

Injection of steroids has been used widely for the treatment of chronic pain[3, 52] (see Chapter 24). Injections of steroids into the epidural space, onto peripheral nerves, and into joints have been done for many years with variable degrees of success. This variability of the success rate appears to depend on the condition being treated. The injection of steroids to treat pain due to irritation of spinal segmental nerves secondary to intervertebral disk herniations has been used to avoid spinal surgery. A large number of patients experience significant relief of pain after epidural injection of steroids. This technique has survived the test of time despite criticism.[47] It is unfortunate that despite its extensive clinical use, there are few controlled studies to validate the use of steroids in nerve pain such as sciatica.

Lidocaine Challenge

Neuropathic pain responds well at times to carbamazepine and sometimes to antiarrhythmic agents that are structurally similar to lidocaine, such as mexiletine[17] and tocainide. The usefulness of a treatment with mexiletine can be tested by a lidocaine challenge. For this challenge, lidocaine is injected intravenously with a constant infusion pump over 1 to 2 hours. The maximum dose should not exceed 7 mg/kg. Cardiorespiratory function is monitored during the infusion, and if pain relief is obtained the patient might be a candidate for mexiletine.

Spinal Opiates

Spinal opiates are used extensively for the management of chronic benign pain as well as cancer pain.[115] Opiates can be delivered epidurally or intrathecally. The delivery system can be fully implantable or use external pumps. The fully implantable system is preferable for chronic use except when life expectancy is less than 6 months. Cancer pain can be treated efficaciously, thus providing adequate quality of life.

Noncancer pain has been treated extensively with spinal opiates, and it has a special application in failed back syndrome and any type of orthopedic intractable pain. Even though neuropathic pain and complex regional pain syndrome are relatively insensitive to opiates, they can be managed successfully with spinal opiates. The myth and fear of addiction has limited the use of spinal opiates, but efforts to educate the public and the medical profession have proved beneficial and this technique is becoming more popular.

Neuroaugmentation (Spinal Cord and Nerve Stimulation)

Central and peripheral neuroaugmentation can be used in selected patients. Its mechanism of action is based on the notion that afferent input along low-threshold, large-diameter nerve fibers can exert a powerful inhibitory effect on nociceptive input conveyed along C fibers. This therapeutic modality is indicated when other, more conservative measures have failed.

Failed back syndrome with radicular pain in either one or both extremities can be reasonably treated with spinal cord stimulation. It is important to mention that axial pain is not an indication for neuroaugmentation. Patients with complex regional pain syndrome of the upper or lower extremity are typically good candidates for spinal cord stimulation. Patients with neuropathic pain or causalgia limited to a well defined peripheral major nerve can benefit greatly from peripheral nerve stimulation.

Increasing Activity Level

Therapeutic exercises are intended to improve physical condition and functional capacities. They also indirectly provide pain relief and a better quality of life.

Patients with chronic pain conditions tend to reduce or discontinue their activities because of fear of increased pain or harm. This can result in joint stiffness, decreased endurance, decreased muscle strength, muscle wasting, and even a general state of decompensation. The aim of therapeutic exercises for these patients should be reconditioning, improved muscle strength and length, and attainment of optimal joint range of motion.

Appropriate exercises that are specific for the pain area (e.g., Williams's flexion exercises for low back pain), and general conditioning exercises such as bicycling, walking, and swimming are usually indicated. Fordyce[31] noted that appropriate exercise in a behavior modification program must be relevant to the patient's pain and limitations, and quantifiable, visible, and accessible. The patient's baseline exercise level is determined by asking the patient to exercise to tolerance (until pain, weakness, or fatigue necessitates stopping) over a few days. Once the baseline has been established, the initial exercise goal is set within the patient's tolerance and then gradually increased, with new goals being set every few days (Fig. 42–7). Rewards and reinforcement are given for accomplishing the established goals without demonstrating pain behavior. In some patients, however, it is necessary to reduce excessive activity levels by teaching them to pace themselves more appropriately.

Psychosocial Interventions

Recent evidence suggests that the use of psychological modalities in conjunction with medical interventions and physical therapy increases the effectiveness of the chronic pain treatment program. Psychological treatments of chronic pain include psychoeducation, psychotherapy, biofeedback and relaxation training, and vocational counseling. Cognitive behavioral approaches to chronic pain rely heavily on skills training and psychoeducational interventions. Group psychotherapy has been used successfully to enhance the functioning of patients in a pain rehabilitation program.[45] Individual[102] and family therapy[7] are other interventions frequently used with chronic pain patients to treat underlying psychosocial stresses. Recently a compelling case has been made for including family members and significant others in the evaluation and treatment process.[69]

Relaxation training and biofeedback are behavioral treatment methods that have been successfully used to treat a wide variety of pain syndromes, including myofascial and sympathetically maintained pain syndromes.[93, 101] Several relaxation techniques can be used for chronic pain, the two most common being autogenic training[23] and progressive muscle relaxation.

Vocational Rehabilitation

Vocational counseling is an important component of the psychological approach to chronic pain. Each patient is evaluated to determine work history, educational background, vocational skills and abilities, and motivation to return to work. The vocational counselor can determine whether past work skills and current aptitudes can be transferred to alternative occupations if necessary. The vocational counselor works with the patient regarding legal rights and obligations for each state (e.g., worker's compensation), and helps the patient set realistic vocational goals. They also help the patient improve overall vocational functioning. Vocational counseling is also used to reduce functional impairment and disability, improve coping strategies, enhance effective use of pain medications, and decrease use of health care resources.

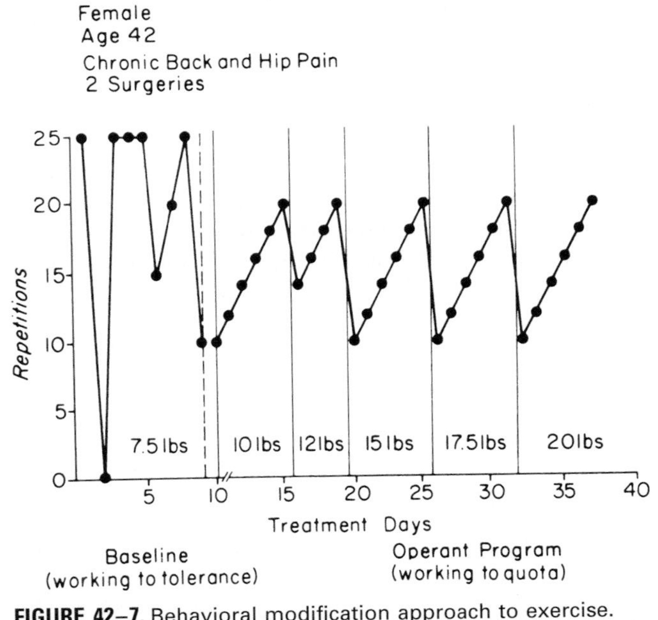

FIGURE 42–7. Behavioral modification approach to exercise. (From Fordyce WE: Behavioral Methods for Chronic Pain and Illness. St Louis, Mosby-Year Book, 1976.)

RESULTS

While clinical judgment represents a significant contribution to the rationale for current clinical practices, it does not replace scientific evidence of efficacy. However, much of the existing literature pertaining to rehabilitation of chronic pain syndromes consists of retrospective record reviews, surveys, or review articles. Although numerous experimental or quasi-experimental studies have been published, in many cases the inferences that can be drawn from this literature are compromised by the lack of control groups, nonequivalent control groups, weak statistical analysis, and other limitations to internal and external validity.

Several general and meta-analytic review articles have been published on the evaluation and treatment of chronic pain syndromes, as well as the efficacy of multidisciplinary pain treatment centers. Flor et al[27] conducted a meta-analysis of reports of the efficacy of multidisciplinary pain treatment centers and found 65 to 300 published studies to be suitable for including in their analysis. The preponderance of these papers supported the value of multidisciplinary pain centers. The investigators further noted that the beneficial effects of treatment by pain clinics are maintained over an extended period of time. The improvements have been documented both by subjective ratings of pain, and by more objective measures such as return to work and reduced use of the health care system.[27] The investigators noted that their results have to be interpreted cautiously because the quality of the study designs and descriptions of how the studies were performed was sometimes marginal. Improvements in future research design and reporting were recommended.

Cutler et al,[15] in a review and meta-analysis study, examined the return to work of patients treated by nonsurgical pain centers. Of the 171 studies reviewed, seven fulfilled the selection criteria for inclusion in their analysis. In spite of methodological problems, the statistical evidence was overwhelmingly in favor of major and significant benefits to the patients participating in the programs. These results indicated that (1) nonsurgical treatment of chronic pain returns patients to work; (2) increased rates of return to work are due to treatment; and (3) the benefits of treatment are not temporary.

Turk[100] commented that, in spite of these favorable findings, pain clinics continue to be viewed with skepticism—especially by third-party payers. Admittedly, there is no perfect study of multidisciplinary pain center treatment outcomes, but the data taken as an aggregate should not be summarily dismissed.

Turk[100] summarized the results of selected studies,[15, 25, 27] and reported the following facts about the efficacy of multidisciplinary pain centers: (1) Following treatment at a typical multidisciplinary pain center, the patients reported a reduction in pain ranging from 16% to 60%—comparable to the pain reduction reported following surgery. The pain reductions were reasonably maintained up to five years following treatment. (2) More than 65% of patients treated at multidisciplinary pain centers discontinued use of opioid medications and were still medication-free one year following discharge from the program. In contrast, patients not treated at such facilities reported an average reduction in medication of only 6% one year following treatment. (3) On average, 65% of patients treated in multidisciplinary pain centers report increased activity at termination of treatment compared to 35% of patients not treated at these facilities. (4) The average return-to-work rate following treatment at multidisciplinary pain centers is 67% compared to 24% for patients not treated at those facilities. Approximately 43% more patients were working following treatment at multidisciplinary pain centers than prior to treatment. (5) Patients treated at multidisciplinary pain centers are three to six times less likely to be hospitalized later and have significantly fewer surgeries for pain than those patients not treated at those facilities. (6) Studies that have investigated the closure rate of disability cases indicate that 64%[77] to 89%[22] of claims were settled by 3 months following discharge from multidisciplinary pain centers. This can be compared with 39% closure of claims following surgery.[111] (7) Up to 86% of pending litigation cases have been reported as being resolved following treatment at a multidisciplinary pain center.[62, 63]

A study by Stieg et al[94] in association with the Colorado Department of Labor demonstrated potential savings in medical and disability costs for a group of patients who were treated in an interdisciplinary pain treatment program. Most of these patients were judged to be permanently and totally disabled at the start of treatment. A formula for estimated future cost-benefit savings was derived.[91, 92]

Simmons et al[87] discussed practical measures that demonstrate cost-effectiveness, such as: (a) return to gainful employment measured at 3-month intervals for 2 years; (b) decreased narcotic usage measured at discharge, compared to initial baseline; (c) decreased use of medical care, as measured by the cost of care for 1 year prior to treatment compared to the cost for 1 year following treatment in a pain treatment center; (d) increased function measured isokinetically on equipment such as the rehabilitation trainer, determined at discharge and compared to admission baseline recordings; (e) return to school, if school is preparation for work.

Outcome measurements for treatment of chronic pain can include use of medication, walking distance, strength, flexibility, sitting tolerance, pain behaviors, vocational placement, and use of health care resources.[35] The American Academy of Pain Medicine has developed an online computerized outcome program called digimed.com to help demonstrate results of treatment by pain programs.[76] When comparing one program with another, it is important to evaluate each program in terms of types of patients accepted, types of treatments offered, criteria for improvement, and follow-up time. "Ideal" pain rehabilitation candidates can achieve an 80 to 90% success rate. As the incidence of psychosocial problems and secondary gain issues increases, however, this rate drops to 40 to 50%. With major psychiatric or secondary gains, the success rate drops to 20% or less.[37]

CONCLUSION

Patients with chronic pain syndrome are often difficult and frustrating to manage, especially for the solo practitioner trying to use the medical model of care. These patients combine traditional clinical problems with psychosocial, vocational, and behavioral issues. The "pain clinic" concept, which utilizes a comprehensive, multidisciplinary approach with knowledgeable personnel devoted to treating chronic pain syndrome, is most appropriate for evaluation and rational treatment of these patients. The evaluation should consist of an independent history and physical examination with emphasis on the pain experience, past evaluations, and past treatment(s). The psychosocial, vocational, and behavior aspects of the pain experience should be independently evaluated through interviews and psychological testing. Previously completed medical diagnostic tests should be reviewed, and ordered or reordered only if considered absolutely necessary to complete the evaluation.

The treatment of the patient with chronic pain syndrome should emphasize four components: (1) modification of medication, (2) modification of pain, (3) increase in activity, and (4) treatment of psychosocial and vocational issues. "Pain generators" should be identified and treated, when possible. The Fordyce model of behavioral modification[30] is an appropriate one to consider in organizing and carrying out a treatment program for patients with chronic pain syndrome. With appropriate evaluation and treatment, patients with chronic pain syndrome can achieve reasonable success in improving their quality of life.

REFERENCES

1. Ableson K, Langley GB, Sheppeard H, et al: Transcutaneous electrical nerve stimulation in rheumatoid arthritis. NZ Med J 1983; 96:156–161.
2. American Academy of Pain Medicine: The use of opioids for treatment of chronic pain, 1999. (Available online at www.painmed.org)
3. Arnoff GM: Evaluation and Treatment of Chronic Pain. Baltimore, Williams & Wilkins, 1992.
4. Basbaum AI, Fields HL: Endogenous pain control mechanism. Review and hypothesis. Ann Neurol 1978; 4:452–455.
5. Bendix AF, Bendix T, Lund C, et al: Comparison of three intensive programs for chronic low back pain patients: prospective, randomized, observer-blinded study with one-year follow up. Scand J Rehab Med 1997; 29(2):81–89.
6. Beursken AJ, deVet HC, Koke AJ, et al: Measuring the functional status of patients with low back pain. Spine 1995; 20(9):1017–1028.
7. Blumenthal SM: Vocational rehabilitation with the industrially injured worker. J Hand Surg Am 1987; 12:926–930.
8. Bonica JJ: General considerations of chronic pain. In Bonica JJ (ed): The Management of Pain, vol 1. Philadelphia, Lea & Febiger, 1990.
9. Bonica JJ: Preface. In Ng LKY (ed): New Approaches to Treatment of Chronic Pain: A Review of Multidisciplinary Pain Clinics and Pain Centers. National Institute on Drug Abuse Research monograph 36, Rockville, MD, 1981.
10. Botney M, Field H: Amitriptyline potentiates morphine analgesia by a direct action on the central nervous system. Ann Neurol 1983; 13:160–164.
11. Brena SF: Pain control facilities: Root, organization and function. In Chapman SL (ed): Management of Patients with Chronic Pain. New York, Spectrum, 1983.
12. Burns JS: Anger management style and the prediction of treatment outcome among male and female chronic pain patients. Behav Res Therapy 1998; 36(11):1051–1062.
13. Burns JW: Anger management style and hostility: Predicting symptom-specific physiological reactivity among chronic low back pain patients. J Behav Med 1997; 20(6):505–522.
14. Burns JW, Johnson BJ, Mahoney N, et al: Anger management style, hostility and spouse responses: Gender differences in predictors of adjustment among chronic pain patients. Pain 1996; 64(3):445–453.
15. Cutler RB, Fishbain DA, Rosomoff HL, et al: Does nonsurgical pain center treatment of chronic pain return patients to work? Spine 1994; 19(6):643–652.
16. Dalessio DJ: Management of the cranial neuralgias and atypical facial pain. Clin J Pain 1989; 5:55–59.
17. Dejgard A, Peterson P, Kastrup J: Mexiletine for treatment of chronic painful diabetic neuropathy. Lancet 1988; 1:9–11.
18. Devor M: Nerve pathophysiology and mechanisms of pain in causalgia. J Auto Nerv Syst 1983; 7:371–384.
19. Eisenach JC, Lysak SZ, Niscomi CM: Epidural clonidine analgesia following surgery: Phase 1. Anesthesiology 1989; 71:40–646.
20. Federation of State Medical Boards of the United States: Model guidelines for the use of controlled substances for the treatment of pain, 1998. (Available online at www.fsmb.org/pain.htm)
21. Feinmann C: Pain relief by antidepressants: Possible modes of action. Pain 1985; 23:1–8.
22. Fey SG, Williamson-Kirkland TE, Fraugione R: Vocational restoration in injured workers with chronic pain. Pain 1987; 4(suppl):S379.
23. Fine PG: The nociceptive system and persistent pain syndromes. Prob Anesth 1990; 4:452–456.
24. Fisbain DA, Abdel-Moty E, Cutler R, et al: Measuring residual functional capacity in chronic low back pain patients based on the dictionary of occupational titles. Spine 1994; 19(8):872–880.
25. Fishbain DA, Rosomoff HL, Goldberg M, et al: The prediction of return to work to the workplace after multidisciplinary pain center treatment. Clin J Pain 1993; 9:3–15.
26. Fishman PS: Retrograde changes in the corticospinal tract of posttraumatic paraplegics. Arch Neurol 1987; 44:1082–1084.
27. Flor H, Fydrich T, Turk D: Efficacy of multidisciplinary pain treatment centers: A meta-analytic review. Pain 1992; 49(2): 221–230.
28. Flor H, Turk DC, Rudy TE: Pain and families II: Assessment and treatment. Pain 1987; 30:29–45.
29. Foley KM: Adjuvant analgesic drugs in cancer pain management. In Aronoff GM (ed): Evaluation and Treatment of Chronic Pain. Baltimore, Urban & Schwartzenberg, 1985.
30. Fordyce WE: The validity of pain behavior measurement. In Melzack R (ed): Pain Measurement and Assessment. New York, Raven Press, 1983.
31. Fordyce WE, Lansky D, Calsyn DA, et al: Pain measurement and pain behavior. Pain 1984; 18:53–69.
32. Frampton V: Transcutaneous electrical nerve stimulation and chronic pain. In Wells PE, Frampton V, Borosher D (eds): Pain Management in Physical Therapy. Norwalk, CT, Appleton & Lange, 1988.
33. Gatchel RJ, Turk DC: Psychological Approaches to Pain Management: A Practitioner's Handbook. New York, Guilford Press, 1996.
34. Getto CJ, Heaton RK, Lehmann RA: PSPI: A standardized approach to the evaluation of psychosocial factors in chronic pain. Adv Pain Res Ther 1985; 5:885–889.
35. Grabois M: Chronic pain. Evaluation and treatment. In Goodgold J (ed): Rehabilitation Medicine. St Louis, Mosby–Year Book, 1988.
36. Grabois M: Comprehensive evaluation and management of patients with chronic pain. Cardiovasc Res Center Bull 1981; 133–117.
37. Grabois M: Pain clinics: Role in rehabilitation of patients with chronic pain. Ann Acad Med Singapore 1983; 12:428–433.
38. Greehott JD, Sternbach RA: Conjoint treatment of chronic pain. Adv Neurol 1974; 4:595–603.
39. Hanson RW, Gerber KE: Coping with Chronic Pain: A Guide to Patient Self-Management. New York, Guilford Press, 1990.
40. Harten JA: Functional capacity evaluation. Occup Med: State Art Rev 1998; 13(1):209–212.
41. Hazard RG, Bendix A, Fenwick JW: Disability exaggeration as a predictor of functional restoration outcomes for patients with chronic low back pain. Spine 1991; 16(9):1062–1067.
42. Jackson HC, Winkelman RK, Bickel WH: Nerve endings in the human lumbar spinal column and related structures. J Bone Joint Surg Am 1966; 48:1272–1281.
43. Jankus WR, Park TJ, VanKeulen M, Weisensel M: Interdisciplinary treatment of the injured worker with chronic pain: Long-term efficacy. Wis Med J 1995; 94(5):244–249.
44. Jensen TS: Phantom pain and related phenomena after amputation. In Wall P, Melzack R (eds): Textbook on Pain. London, Churchill Livingstone, 1989.
45. Kanfer FH, Karoly P: The psychological self-management: Abiding issues and tentative directions. In Karoly P, Kanfer FH (eds): Self-Management and Behavior Change. Elmsford, NY, Pergamon Press, 1982.
46. Kanner R: Psychotropic drugs in the management of pain. Curr Concepts Pain 1983; 1:11.
47. Keepes ER, Duncalf D: Treatment of backache with spinal injections of local anesthetics, spinal systemic steroids. A review. Pain 1985; 22:33–47.
48. Kerns RD, Rosenber R, Jamison RN: Readiness to adopt a self-management approach to chronic pain: The Pain Stages of Change Questionnaire (PSOCQ). Pain 1997; 72(1–2):227–234.

49. Keefe FJ, Caldwell DS: Cognitive behavioral control of arthritis pain. Med Clin North Am 1997; 81(1):277–290.
50. King PM, Tuckwell N, Barrett TE: A critical review of functional capacity evaluations. Phys Therapy 1998; 78(8):852–866.
51. Kozin F, McCarthy DJ, Sims J, Genant H: The reflex sympathetic dystrophy syndrome, I. Clinical and histologic studies: Evidence for bilaterality, response to corticosteroids and articular involvement. Am J Med 1976; 60:321–331.
52. Kreigler JS, Ashenberg ZS: Management of chronic low back pain. A comprehensive approach. Sem Neurol 1987; 7:303–312.
53. Landau B, Levy RM: Neuromodulation techniques for medically refractory pain. Annu Rev Med 1993; 44:279–287.
54. Loeser JD: Herpes zoster and post-herpetic neuralgia. Pain 1986; 25:149–164.
55. Loeser JD: Pain due to nerve injury. Spine 1985; 10:232–235.
56. Love AW, Peck CL: The MMPI and psychological factors in low back pain. A review. Pain 1987; 28:1–12.
57. Lynch RT, Agre J, Powers JM, Sherman J: Long-term follow-up of outpatient interdisciplinary pain management with a no-treatment comparison group. Am J Phys Med Rehabil 1996; 75(3):213–222.
58. Malinsky J: The onogenetic development of nerve terminations in the intervertebral discs of man. Acta Anat 1959; 38:96–113.
59. Mannheimer JS, et al: Pain and TENS in pain management. In Mannheimer JS, Lampe GN (eds): Clinical Transcutaneous Electrical Nerve Stimulation. Philadelphia, FA Davis, 1984.
60. Mauguiere F, Desmedt JE: Thalamic pain syndrome of Dejerine-Roussy: Differentiation of four subtypes assisted by somatosensory evoked potential data. Arch Neurol 1988; 34:1312–1320.
61. Max MB, Culnane M, Schafer SC, et al: Amitriptyline relieves diabetic neuropathy pain in patients with normal or depressed mood. Neurology 1987; 37:589–596.
62. Mayer TG, Gatchel RJ, et al: Objective assessment of pain function following industrial low back injury. JAMA 1985; 258:1763–1767.
63. Mayer TG, Gatchel RJ, Kishino N, et al: Objective assessment of spine function following industrial injury. A prospective study with comparison group and one-year follow-up. Spine 1985; 10:484–493.
64. McCain GA, Scudds RA: The concept of primary fibromyalgia (fibrositis): Clinical value, relation and significance to other chronic musculoskeletal pain syndromes. Pain 1988; 33:272–287.
65. McCall IW, Park WM, O'Brien J: Induced pain referral from posterior lumbar spinal elements in normal subjects. Spine 1979; 4:441–446.
66. Melzack R: The McGill Pain Questionnaire. In Melzack R (ed): Pain Measurement and Assessment. New York, Raven Press, 1983.
67. Melzack R: Measurement of the dimensions of pain experience. In Bram EV (ed): Pain Measurement in Man: Neurophysiological Correlates of Pain. New York, Elsevier, 1984.
68. Melzack R, Wall PD: Pain mechanism: A new theory. Science 1965; 150:971–979.
69. Merskey H: Traditional individual psychotherapy and psychopharmacotherapy. In Holman AD, Turk DC (eds): Pain Management: A Handbook. New York, Pergamon Press, 1986.
70. Merskey H, Bogduk N: Classification of Chronic Pain, ed 2. Seattle, ISAP Press, 1994.
71. Meyer GA, et al: Causalgia treated be selective large fiber stimulation of peripheral nerve. Brain 1972; 95:163–168.
72. Morey LC: Personality Assessment Inventory Professional Manual. Psychological Assessment Resources, Odessa, FL, 1991.
73. Nolan MF: Selected problems in the use of transcutaneous electrical nerve stimulation for pain control. An appraisal with proposed solutions. Phys Ther 1988; 1694.
74. North RB: Electrical stimulation for pain relief. Transcutaneous peripheral nerve, spinal cord and deep brain stimulation. In Swerlow M, Charlton JE (eds): Relief of Intractable Pain. Amsterdam, Elsevier, 1989.
75. Owens MK: Literature review of non-pharmacologic methods for the treatment of chronic pain. Holistic Nurs Pract 1991; 6:24–31.
76. Pain Medicine Network: American Academy of Pain Medicine 1998; vol 13, no. 5.
77. Painter JR, Seres JL and Newman RI: Assessing benefits of the pain center: Why some patients regress. Pain 1980; 8:101–113.
78. Portenoy RK, Dole V, Joseph H, et al: Pain management and chemical dependency—Evolving perspectives. JAMA 1997; 278(7):591–593.
79. Reading AE: Testing pain mechanisms in persons with pain. In Wall PD, Melzack R (eds): Textbook of Pain. New York, Churchill Livingstone, 1984.
80. Rose MJ, Reilly JP, Pennie B, et al: Chronic low back pain rehabilitation programs: A study of the optimum duration of treatment and comparison of group and individual therapy. Spine 1997; 2246–2251.
81. Reuler J, Girard D, Nardone D: The chronic pain syndrome: Misconceptions and management. Ann Intern Med 1980; 93:588–596.
82. Richards JS, Nepormuceno C, Riles M, Suer Z: Assessing pain behavior: The UAB pain behavior scale. Pain 1982; 14:393–398.
83. Rook JC, Pesch RN, Keeler EC: Chronic pain and the questionable use of the Minnesota Multiphasic Personality Inventory. Arch Phys Med Rehabil 1981; 62:373–376.
84. Sanders SH, Rucker KS, Anderson KO, et al: Clinical practice guidelines for chronic non-malignant pain syndrome patients. J Back Musculoskel Rehab 1995; 5:15–120.
85. Saunders RL, Beissner KL, McManis BG: Estimates of weight that subjects can lift frequently in functional capacity evaluations. Phys Ther 1997; 77(12):1717–1728.
86. Silver BV, Blanchard EB: Biofeedback and relaxation training in the treatment of psychophysiological disorders: Or, are the machines really necessary? J Behav Med 1978; 1:217–239.
87. Simmons JW, Avant WS, Dermski J, Parisher D: Determining successful pain clinic treatment through validation of cost-effectiveness. Spine 1988; 13:342–344.
88. Smith CR, Lewith GT, Machin D: TNS and osteoarthritic pain. Preliminary study to establish a controlled method assessing transcutaneous nerve stimulation as treatment of the pain caused by osteoarthritis of the knee. Physiotherapy 1983; 69:266–268.
89. Smith SL, Cunningham S, Weinberg R: The predictive validity of the functional capacities evaluation. Am J Occup Ther 1986; 40:564–567.
90. Spiegel K, Kalb R, Pasternak GW: Analgesic activity of tricyclic antidepressants. Ann Neurol 1983; 13:462–465.
91. Steig RL: The cost-effectiveness of pain treatment: Who cares? Clin J Pain 1990; 6:301–304.
92. Steig RL, Turk DC: Chronic pain syndrome: The necessity of demonstration the cost-benefit treatment. Pain Management 1988; 1:58–63.
93. Steig RL, Williams RC, Gallagher LA: Multidisciplinary pain treatment centers. J Occup Med 1981; 23:94–102.
94. Steig RL, Williams RC, Timmerman-Williams G, et al: Cost-benefits of interdisciplinary, chronic pain treatment. Clin J Pain 1986; 1:189–193.
95. Sternbach RA: Psychophysiology pain syndromes. In Bonica JJ (ed): The Management of Pain. Philadelphia, Lea & Febiger, 1990.
96. Swanson DW, Floreen AC, Swenson WM: Programs for managing chronic pain II. Short term results. Mayo Clin Proc 1979; 51:409–411.
97. Taylor P, Hallet M, Flaherty L: Treatment of osteoarthritis of the knee with transcutaneous electrical nerve stimulation. Pain 1981; 11:233–240.
98. Tollison CD, Satterthwaite JR, Tollison JW: Handbook of Pain Management. Baltimore, Williams & Wilkins, 1994.
99. Tramposh AK: The functional capacity evaluation: Measuring maximal work abilities. Occup Med: State Art Rev 1992; 7(1):113–124.
100. Turk DC: Multidisciplinary Pain Centers: Foibles, Fallacies and Facts. SPS News 1995, pp 6–8.
101. Turk DC, Flor H, Rudy TE: Pain and families I. Etiology, maintenance, and psychosocial impact. Pain 1987; 30:3–27.
102. Turk DC, Melzack R: Handbook of Pain Assessment. New York, Guilford, 1992.
103. Turk DC, Rudy TE: A cognitive-behavioral perspective on chronic pain. Beyond the scalpel and syringe. In Tollison CD(ed): Handbook of Chronic Pain Management. Baltimore, Williams & Wilkins, 1989.
104. VanDalfsen RJ, Syrjala KL: Psychologic strategies in acute pain management. Crit Care Clin1990; 6:421–431.

105. Vasudevan SV, Lynch NT: Pain centers—Organization and outcome. W J Med 1991; 154:532–535.
106. Velozo CA: Work evaluations: Critique of the state of the art of functional assessment of work. Am J Occup Ther 1993; 47(3):203–209.
107. Wallace JL, Granger DN: Pathogenesis of NSAID gastropathy: Are neutrophils the culprits? TIPS 1992; 32:671–673.
108. Walsh NE, Dumitru D, Ramamurthy S, Schoenfeld LS: Treatment of patients with chronic pain. In DeLisa JA (ed): Rehabilitation Medicine: Principles and Practice, ed 2. Philadelphia, J.B. Lippincott, 1993.
109. Watson CP, Evans RJ, Reed K, et al: Amitriptyline versus placebo in post-herpetic neuralgia. Neurology 1982; 32:671–673.
110. Whelton A, Hamilton CW: Nonsteroidal anti-inflammatory drugs effect on kidney function. J Clin Pharmacol 1991; 31: 588–598.
111. White AWM: The compensation back. Appl Therapeutic 1966; 8:871–874.
112. Wilson P: Pain mechanism: Anatomy and physiology. In Raj P (ed): Practical Management of Pain. St Louis, Mosby-Year Book, 1992.
113. Wilson PR: Opioids and chronic pain (editorial). Clinical J Pain 1997; 13:1–2.
114. Wyman DO: Evaluating patients for return to work. AFP 1999; 59(4):844–848.
115. Yaksh TL: The principles behind the use of spinal narcotics. Clin Anesth 1983; 1:219–232.

43 CHAPTER

Jeffrey M. Thompson, M.D.

The Diagnosis and Treatment of Muscle Pain Syndromes

Muscle pain is a universal human experience. The muscle pain syndromes, however, have yet to achieve universal acceptance in the medical community. Muscles make up 40% of the mass of the human body. The forces muscles generate and the mechanical stresses they are subjected to are tremendous. It is not surprising, therefore, that many causes of muscle pain exist (Table 43–1). Those disorders with obvious pathological or laboratory findings are fairly easily defined and are well established as diagnostic entities. The muscle pain syndromes described in this chapter remain controversial largely because of the lack of such objective findings.

More than in most areas of medicine, a complete understanding of the muscle pain syndromes requires review of their derivations (Fig. 43–1) (the serious student of history is referred to two excellent and comprehensive reviews of the origins of muscle pain syndromes—one focusing on the concept of "fibrositis"[80] and the other addressing muscle pain syndromes in general[87]). After a quick look at the history of muscle pain, this chapter discusses the basic science of muscle nociception, outlines the proposed mechanisms for pain generation in general, examines the concept of muscle dysfunction, and addresses the diagnosis and treatment of the most common muscle pain syndromes.

HISTORICAL REVIEW

Early German Literature: Myelogelosis

The medical world did not distinguish between joint pain (rheumatism) and muscle pain (muscular rheumatism) until the early 1700s.[87] In Germany physicians focused on the presence of hardenings or nodules within painful muscles. The popularity of massage as a diagnostic and therapeutic tool likely heightened awareness of these nodules, although a special technique of palpation was often necessary to identify the characteristic hardenings. Physicians blamed a change in the "colloidal state" of muscle cytoplasm for these nodules, thus giving rise to the term "myelogelosis." This term is still in use today and refers to localized muscle pain associated with a poorly characterized pathological area within the muscle (the tender point or nodule).

In Germany and Scandinavia the mainstay of treatment for muscle pain associated with nodules was massage, with the goal of breaking up the muscle hardenings. Massage types ranged from "decongestive" to a technique called *Gelotripsie,* a traumatic massage involving beating the nodules with a stick.[87] The less frightening forms of massage remained the major form of physical therapy treatment for muscle pain syndromes well into this century.[60]

Early British Literature: The Concept of Fibrositis

In Great Britain, physicians identified nonarticular rheumatism as a disorder of connective tissue rather than muscle. In 1815, William Balfour of Edinburgh described nodules in rheumatic muscles. He ascribed the nodules to the products of inflammation in the connective tissue—edema and exudate—rather than to the German theory of a change in the muscle cytoplasm. In the 1850s, Thomas Inman proposed that nodules resulted from neuromuscular dysfunction manifest by local hypertonus or spasm. However, researchers found

TABLE 43–1 Causes of Muscle Pain

Causes of Focal Muscle Pain	Causes of Generalized Muscle Pain
With Swelling or Induration	*With Muscle Weakness*
Neoplasm	Inflammation (polymyositis, dermatomyositis)
Trauma (hematoma)	Infection
Ruptured tendon	Toxoplasmosis
Ruptured Baker's cyst	Trichinosis
Thrombophlebitis	Toxic myopathy (influenza or other viral infections, leptospirosis, gram-negative infections, toxic shock syndrome, Kawasaki's syndrome)
Infection	Poliomyelitis
Streptococcal myositis	Toxic and metabolic disorders
Gas gangrene	Acute alcoholic myopathy
Pyomyositis	Hypophosphatemia
Trichinosis, hydatid cysts, sparganosis	Potassium deficiency
Painful leg weakness in children with influenza	Total parenteral nutrition (essential fatty acid deficiency)
Inflammation	Necrotic myopathy stemming from carcinoma
Localized nodular myositis	Hypothyroid myopathy
Proliferative myositis	Drugs (ε-aminocaproic acid, clofibrate, emetine)
Pseudomalignant myositis ossificans	Carnitine palmityltransferase deficiency
Eosinophilic faciitis	Amyloidosis
Sarcoidosis (nodular form)	Bone pain and myopathy (osteomalacia, hyperparathyroidism)
Ischemia	Acute polyneuropathy (Guillain-Barré syndrome, porphyria)
Muscle necrosis following relief of large artery occlusion	*Without Muscle Weakness*
Diabetes (infarction of thigh muscle)	Polymyalgia rheumatica
Embolism (marantic endocarditis)	Muscle pain-fasciculation syndrome
Azotemic hyperparathyroidism (muscle and skin necrosis)	Myalgia in infection or fever
Toxic and metabolic disorders	Myalgia in collagen-vascular disease
Acute alcoholic myopathy	Steroid withdrawal
Myoglobinuria in drug-induced coma	Hypothyroidism
Exertional muscle damage	Primary fibromyalgia (fibrositis)
Normal persons (e.g., military recruits)	Fabry disease
Metabolic myopathies	Parkinsonism
Motor unit hyperactivity states (stiff-man syndrome, tetanus, strychnine poisoning)	
No Swelling or Induration	
Exertional myalgia	
Normal persons	
Vascular insufficiency (intermittent claudication)	
Metabolic myopathies	
Acute brachial neuritis	
Ischemic mononeuropathy	
Parkinsonism	
Resting leg pain of obscure cause	
Growing pains	
Restless legs	
Painful legs and moving toes	
Idiopathic leg pain	

Adapted from Layzer RB: Muscle pain, cramps, and fatigue. In Engel AG, Banker BQ (eds): Myology. New York, McGraw-Hill, 1986, pp 1907–1922.

that these nodules persisted under anesthesia and after death, which cast some doubt on any theories involving nervous action.

Many physicians had trouble finding nodules in patients with muscular rheumatism while others reported finding them in asymptomatic persons. Such discrepancies lowered the status of the nodule as a diagnostic sign. In 1824, Balfour described tender points in muscular rheumatism as distinct from nodules,[80] but the tender points were often found in locations typical for nodules. In 1841, Valleix hypothesized that these pain points arose from the pressure of diseased tissue on nerves. This began the shift from the nodule to the tender point as the primary diagnostic feature in muscle pain syndromes.

In 1904, Sir William Gowers wrote a paper in which he speculated on the etiology of "lumbago" (lumbar area muscular rheumatism).[38] He noted the frequent association of "sciatica" (posterior thigh pain) with lumbago and reasoned that, since sciatica was inflammatory in origin (according to the prevailing theory at that time), then lumbago too must be an inflammatory disorder. He generalized this logic to all soft tissue rheumatism and called it "fibrositis."

Also in 1904, Ralph Stockman[97] at the University of Glasgow published pathological studies of nodules he had excised from painful muscle. He described "edematous fibrous tissue" and, although no leukocytes were seen, he labeled these nodules inflammatory. This seemed to confirm Gowers' "fibrositis" hypothesis and served to combine the German-Scandinavian concept of the painful nodule with the British concept of inflamed connective tissue. Unfortunately, the concept of inflamed connective tissue dominated thinking about mus-

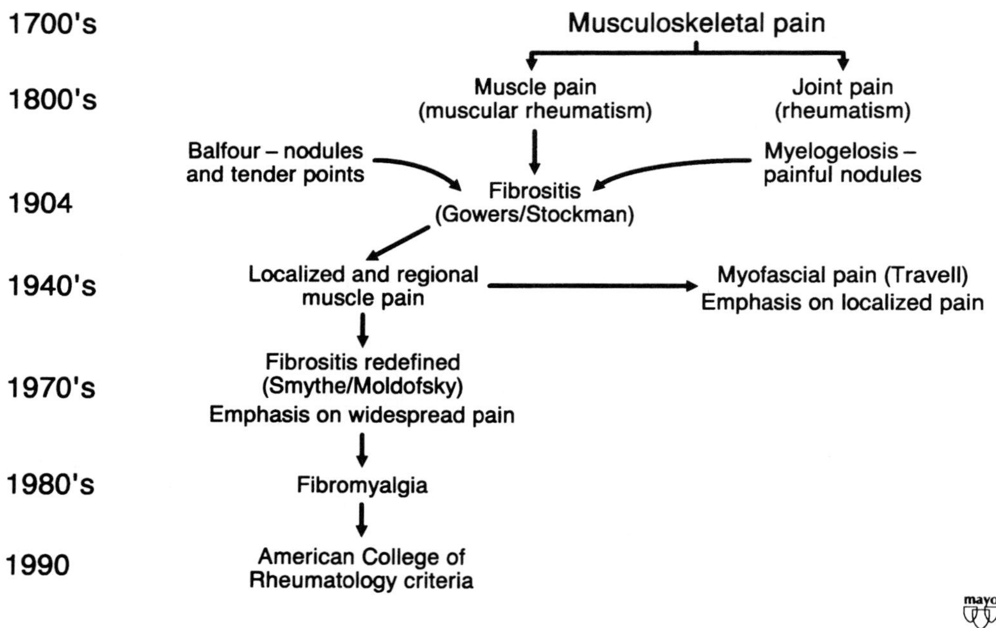

FIGURE 43–1. Muscle pain syndrome family tree—a simplified time line depicting the derivation of two of the muscle pain syndromes (fibromyalgia and myofascial pain syndrome).

cle pain syndromes for decades to come despite a dearth of corroborating studies.

Over the course of time, the lack of clear diagnostic criteria allowed fibrositis to be used as the label for a wide variety of pain disorders. The vast majority of the early literature dealt with localized or regional muscle pain, usually secondary to trauma. In a 1943 review, Slocumb[90] at the Mayo Clinic stated that "fibrositis can affect any part of the body" and listed the various anatomical types as follows: intramuscular, periarticular, tendinous, bursal, perineural, and panniculitis. Slocumb and many others found only normal tissue on biopsy of palapable nodules, discrediting the notion of inflammation as the cause of pain in fibrositis. Many clinicians began to realize that the term "fibrositis" was a misnomer, but its widespread use and the lack of an alternative mechanism to explain muscle pain syndromes has allowed the term to survive to this day.

Early Theories of Etiology

As noted above, when nodules were believed to be the characteristic feature of "muscular rheumatism," theories of etiology focused on explaining their presence (products of inflammation, changes in muscle cytoplasm, local muscle spasm). As tender points became a more important diagnostic feature, theories of etiology were required to explain these points and their tendency to refer pain to distant sites. Examiners found tender points over muscles or their insertions, with a consistent predilection for certain sites. Most authors invoked various reflex mechanisms to explain these findings.

J. H. Kellgren,[52, 53] expanding on work done by Sir Thomas Lewis, investigated experimentally produced muscle pain by injecting 1 to 3 mL of 6% saline into various muscles. He concluded that (1) pain from muscle is very diffuse (whereas fascia gives rise to sharply localized pain); (2) the pain has a predictable distribution for a given muscle that varies only slightly from person to person; (3) the distribution of pain generally follows a segmental pattern but differs from the segmental innervation of the skin; (4) a stimulus can cause pain that spreads over several segments; and (5) the referred pain is perceived as coming from deep structures, not the skin (Fig. 43–2).

Kellgren postulated that pain impulses from the muscle and these "deep structures" traveled a common pathway in the central nervous system (CNS) and that pain from one might be confused with pain from the other. This explained many of the findings in muscular rheumatism but not what initiated the muscle pain (presumably not surreptitious saline injections).

In 1945 and 1946, Kelly[54, 55] published two reports that attempted to explain many of the features common to fibrositis. He described his reflex theory for fibrositis as follows. Impulses from tissue injury (either somatic or visceral) travel to the CNS, where they have direct connections with other cells in the CNS. Impulses from the other cells travel antidromically and cause pain in the "myalgic spot" (tender point). These myalgic spots then produce their own impulses, which, again via CNS connections and antidromic spread, travel to the areas of referred pain. Kelly believed that an underlying increased excitability of the nervous system (brought about by stress or illness) facilitated the development of myalgic spots. (Sorenson et al recently revisited the concept of increased central excitability.[96]) The "antidromic spread" described by Kelly has never been shown to exist, however.

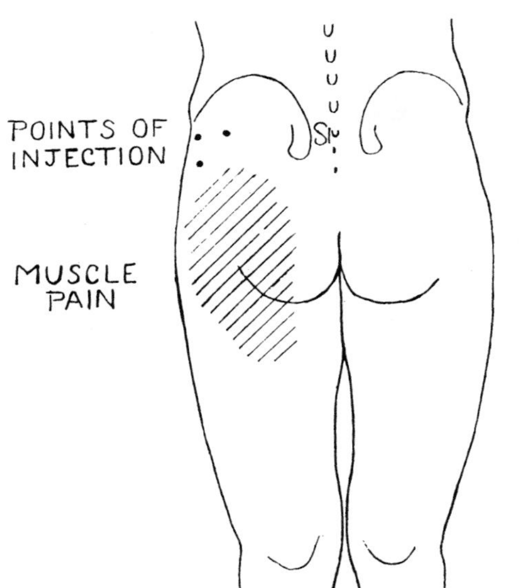

FIGURE 43–2. Kellgren's depiction of referred muscle pain after injection of 6% saline. (From Kellgren JH: On the distribution of pain arising from deep somatic structures with charts of segmental pain areas. Clin Sci 1939; 4:35–46.)

As the 20th century wore on, fibrositis came to be increasingly identified with chronic widespread pain and less so with localized muscle pain (at least among rheumatologists).

The Redefinition of Fibrositis

In the early 1970s, the concept of fibrositis was redefined, largely through the efforts of Hugh Smythe and Harvey Moldofsky. In 1972, Smythe's chapter on fibrositis in a major rheumatology text[92] emphasized chronic, widespread pain and the presence of multiple tender points. The concepts of local muscle trauma and referral of pain to distant sites, central to Kelly's description of fibrositis, were hardly mentioned. In 1977, Smythe together with Moldofsky[94] wrote an influential paper further refining the "fibrositis syndrome" to include nonrestorative sleep and tenderness at 12 of 14 specific sites. Thus fibrositis came to be defined by rheumatologists as a chronic systemic disorder. Palpatory findings such as nodules or taut muscle bands, prominent features in the early history of soft tissue rheumatism, were left out entirely.

The Concept of Myofascial Pain

About the same time that Kelly[54, 55] wrote about fibrositis, Janet Travell formulated a theory for the cause of localized muscle pain.[15] She described the sometimes insidious onset of localized muscle spasm which led to muscle pain and, through a reflex vicious circle, to more spasm and pain. Travell uses "spasm" to describe muscle hyperactivity or guarding. Trauma was believed to be the most common cause—often such subtle trauma that the "spasm" might develop over several days before becoming evident as pain. Chronic muscular strain was deemed an equally important causative factor, often brought on by fast movements or "hurry at work." Other causes described by Travell included chilling of the body, visceral disease, and psychogenic factors. She found that the pain often radiated to distant sites from "trigger points" within the muscle (so named because they cause effects at a distance, as does the trigger of a gun). Travell advocated "local block therapy," including trigger point injections and cooling with ethyl chloride spray, to interrupt the pain-spasm cycle. The various manifestations of localized muscle pain described by Travell became known as the "myofascial pain syndromes" and attracted a fervent following.

PHYSIOLOGY OF MUSCLE PAIN

Muscle pain is so common one would think its physiological basis would be well delineated. Such is not the case. Although much has been learned through extensive experimentation in both animals and humans, the exact mechanism of muscle pain and the nature of stimuli adequate to cause it remain a mystery. Nevertheless, an understanding of what is known about muscle nociception is essential to an understanding of the muscle pain syndromes.

Interestingly, the massive muscle tissue damage found in Duchenne muscular dystrophy is pain-free, yet a single sprint to first base by an unconditioned weekend athlete can result in several days of muscle pain. Obviously, simple muscle cell damage is not the stimulus for muscle pain. Mechanical damage to the connective tissue surrounding muscle cells or changes in the chemical milieu, or both, are the prime candidates for the role of muscle pain stimulators. The interaction of these stimuli with the nerve fibers purported to subserve nociception has been the topic of extensive research, well described in several reviews.[22, 64, 67, 68] The essentials are highlighted in this section.

Classification of Nociceptors

The small-diameter, slowly conducting (less than 30 m/sec) afferent fibers transmit the pain signals from muscle. These include the thin myelinated group III fibers (A delta fibers) and the unmyelinated group IV fibers (C fibers).[67] In a typical nerve to a locomotor muscle, two-thirds of the fibers are unmyelinated, with 50% of these being sensory nerves. In turn, 43% of these sensory nerves are nociceptive.[67] Thus muscles are richly supplied with pain-sensing fibers. All of these group IV fibers begin as free nerve endings, mostly near the wall of muscle arterioles and in the surrounding connective tissue.[67] This location may explain why vascular changes (ischemia) greatly affect muscle pain (see the following section). Muscle sensory fibers terminate in laminae I and V of the dorsal horn, whereas skin sensory fibers terminate mostly in laminae II to IV.[67]

The group III and IV afferent fibers can be classified functionally as well. Those responding only to mechanical stimuli in the range that would cause tissue damage are termed high-threshold mechanosensitive (HTM). Those that respond to weak mechanical stimuli are called low-threshold mechanosensitive (LTM).[68] The HTM receptors are most likely the true muscle nociceptors. Mense and co-workers delineated the properties of these muscle nociceptors in an elegant series of experiments on the cat gastrocnemius muscle.[67] They functionally defined the receptive fields of nociceptor units and then subjected them to various other stimuli while recording the activity of the nociceptive unit. It became clear that these pain receptors could be activated in multiple ways. One receptor type was activated only during ischemic muscle contractions. It was postulated that these fibers transmit the pain of claudication.[68]

Mechanisms of Nociceptor Activation and Sensitization

The most potent stimulator of muscle nociceptors identified to date is bradykinin.[67] Damaged tissue releases this nonapeptide in response to lowered pH, ischemia, or blood clotting. It is likely that it is directly responsible for the muscle pain that accompanies inflammation and muscle strain (as in the weekend athlete).

The indirect effects of bradykinin can play an equally important role, however (Fig. 43–3). At lower concentrations bradykinin "sensitizes" nociceptors without activating them and lowers the threshold to mechanical stimuli of some HTM receptors. The bradykinin-sensitized HTM receptors can be activated by even gentle pressure, which may explain the tenderness of damaged (or maybe even undamaged) muscle.[67] Bradykinin also causes the release of prostaglandins from tissue cells, which in turn sensitizes nociceptors to the effects of bradykinin, leading to a positive feedback loop. Aspirin, by blocking prostaglandin production, interrupts this self-perpetuating loop and thereby blocks much of the nociceptor-activating effects of bradykinin. Increased temperature and lowered pH lead to sensitization of nociceptors as well, and may partially explain the beneficial effects of therapeutic cold on inflammatory pain.

Hypoxia and epinephrine also activate muscle nociceptors.[67] Nociceptors in damaged tissue are the most sensitive to activation by epinephrine, which may indicate one mechanism by which the sympathetic nervous system affects the pain experience. Other activators of nociceptors include serotonin and potassium ions.

Spinal Mechanisms of Muscle Pain

Stimulation of muscle nociceptors is only one step in the very complex physiological system that subserves the experience of muscle pain. There are several mechanisms at the spinal level that further influence muscle nociception. These include convergence of peripheral input on dorsal horn neurons, descending inhibition of the dorsal horn, distribution of muscle afferents over several spinal segments, and neuroplasticity.

Neurons that receive input from nociceptors in muscle and other deep structures are located in laminae I and IV to VI in the dorsal horn. Dorsal horn cells that receive input only from muscle nociceptors are extremely rare. The vast majority of cells that respond to stimulation of muscle nociceptors respond to skin stimulation as well.[67] In fact, these cells often respond to stimulation of several "receptive fields" located both deep and on the skin (Fig. 43–4). This convergence of several receptive fields from the periphery on a single dorsal horn cell explains the poorly localized nature of muscle pain and other deep sensations, affirming the theories of Kellgren (see earlier section, Early Theories of Etiology). These convergent dorsal horn cells are also under strong tonic descending inhibition which preferentially inhibits the input from deep structures, further decreasing the accuracy of localization.

Another cause of the poor localization of muscle pain could be the distribution of afferents from a specific muscle over several spinal segments.[68] This, combined with the multiple deep receptive fields found for many dorsal horn neurons, could explain the spread or referral of muscle pain to other areas. Strong stimulation of

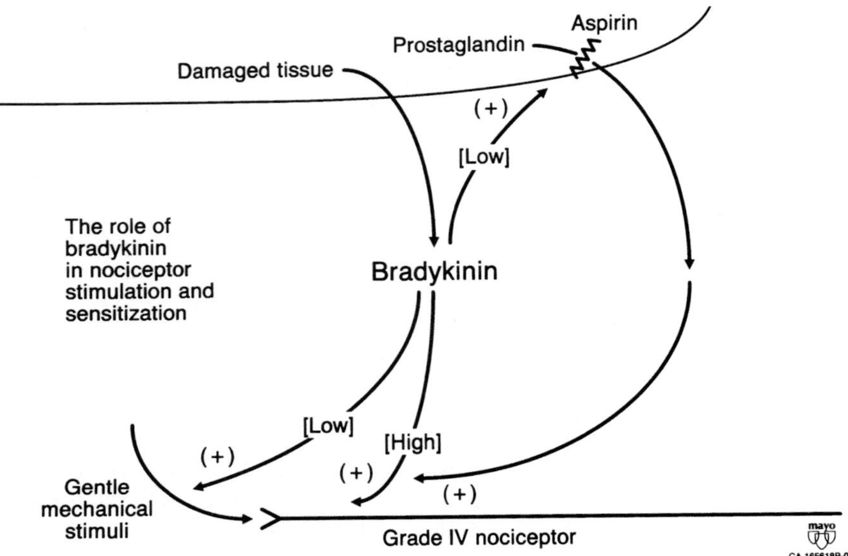

FIGURE 43–3. The role of bradykinin in nociceptor stimulation and sensitization. Bradykinin is released by damaged tissue. The arrow labeled [*high*] depicts its influence at high concentrations. The arrows labeled [*low*] depicts its influence at low concentrations. The (+) signifies activation or facilitation.

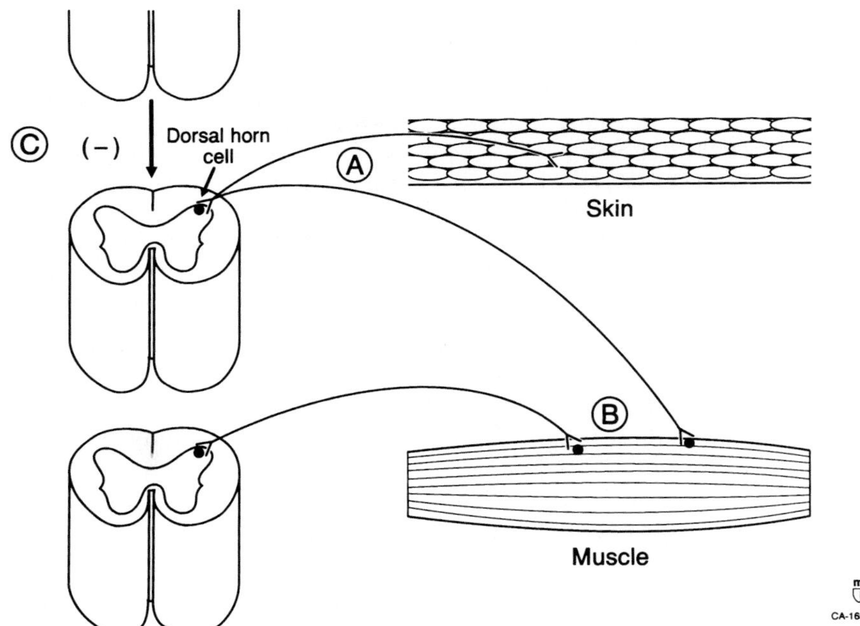

FIGURE 43–4. Spinal mechanisms of nociception. *A.* Convergence of deep and skin nociceptors on a single dorsal horn neuron. *B.* Afferents from one muscle can spread over several spinal segments. *C.* Descending inhibitory pathways also terminate on nociceptive dorsal horn cells.

distal motor nerve fascicles leads to deep cramping pain not only in the muscles innervated by that nerve, but also in other muscles innervated at the same root level.[64] This "radicular pattern" of pain referral does not follow the cutaneous distribution of the nerve roots, confirming Kellgren's observation that referred muscle pain follows a myotome rather than a dermatome.

Neuroplasticity at the spinal level refers to the finding that dorsal horn cells can have long-lasting changes in their response characteristics and morphology after a triggering stimulus.[67] Bradykinin stimulation of skeletal muscle in animals lowers the threshold to mechanical stimuli of the injected receptive field and increases the size of this field. It also causes a prolonged lowering of the threshold in other receptive fields. Researchers believe this results from a sensitization of the dorsal horn neuron by a neuropeptide (such as substance P) released from the spinal terminals of muscle afferents.[46] In a rat model, substance P unmasked previously ineffective dorsal horn synaptic connections. Some of these unmasked connections might include afferents from low-threshold mechanosensitive receptors, allowing these low-threshold receptors to activate nociceptive cells in the dorsal horn.[67] In this way, strong activation of muscle nociceptors could release substance P at their dorsal horn terminals, thereby inducing such changes in the dorsal horn neurons. The unmasking of previously ineffective connections to allow non-nociceptive nerve fibers to activate nociceptive dorsal horn cells may explain allodynia—the perception of pain caused by nonpainful stimuli.[65]

Supraspinal Mechanisms of Muscle Pain

Little knowledge exists about the processing of muscle nociception at the subcortical and cortical levels of the brain, although the thalamic nuclei and somatosensory cortex are apparently involved to some degree. Recent studies using single-photon emission computed tomography (SPECT) to measure cerebral blood flow have indicated increased activity in the thalamus, primary (SI) and secondary (SII) somatosensory cortex, and the cingulate cortex in experimental acute pain. The SI and SII appear to be involved in encoding the sensory-discriminative dimensions of pain, while the anterior cingulate cortex assists in encoding the aversive-emotional dimension of pain. Chronic pain patients, however, have decreased cerebral blood flow in the thalamus, possibly indicating a functional change brought on by the barrage of input from peripheral nociceptors.[73] Cutaneous pain and muscle pain may well be processed in different areas, since some patients with thalamic lesions have insensate skin but perceive the deep pain of saline injections.[67]

Evidence also exists for both inhibiting and facilitating pathways from supraspinal structures affecting the dorsal horn.[68] Serotonin appears to be one of the major neurotransmitters of the inhibitory system. Dysfunction of these central pain mechanisms forms the basis of at least one theory of widespread muscle pain.

The Concept of Motor Dysfunction

"Motor dysfunction" is a vague term used by practitioners of manual medicine. Examples of motor dysfunction include contractures, "tight" muscles, muscle "spasm," and incoordination of muscle firing patterns (including co-contraction). Most clinicians dealing with muscle pain patients describe various degrees of muscle "spasm," including the common finding of the patient who moves en bloc because of axial muscle pain. According to the manual medicine literature, this motor dysfunction leads to muscle overuse and microtrauma, which in turn lead to muscle pain. At least one study found that manual medicine to correct the motor dysfunction relieved the pain with a success rate similar to that found with traditional physical therapy.[57]

Demonstration of muscle dysfunction is largely subjective, relying on palpation and often subtle deficiencies of range of motion. Recently, dynamic surface electromyographic (EMG) monitoring has been used to more objectively measure motor dysfunction. One application of this technique monitors the activity of an individual muscle and its contralateral counterpart (e.g., right and left sternocleidomastoid) while the subject performs symmetrical movements (flex and extend, turn right and left). The "dysfunctioning" muscle often has a higher level of activity or does not return to baseline at the end of a movement[29] (Fig. 43–5). Studies of EMG activity in static postures or with prolonged ambulatory recordings do not differentiate patients with pain from those without pain, however.[11] Actually, when muscle pain is experimentally produced, the EMG activity at rest is decreased, as is the maximal voluntary muscle strength.[40] Another important finding in these studies is increased co-contraction and loss of coordination between agonists and antagonists. This loss of normal dynamic muscle coordination might be much more important than static muscle activity levels for the production of muscle pain. Both clinical and experimentally produced muscle pain cause these changes in muscle firing patterns. If not a primary cause of chronic muscle pain, these disordered motor patterns are at least major contenders as perpetuating factors.[2, 26, 81]

Surface EMG monitoring has also demonstrated a decrease in the number and length of pauses in EMG activity between contractions[24, 25] and higher activity

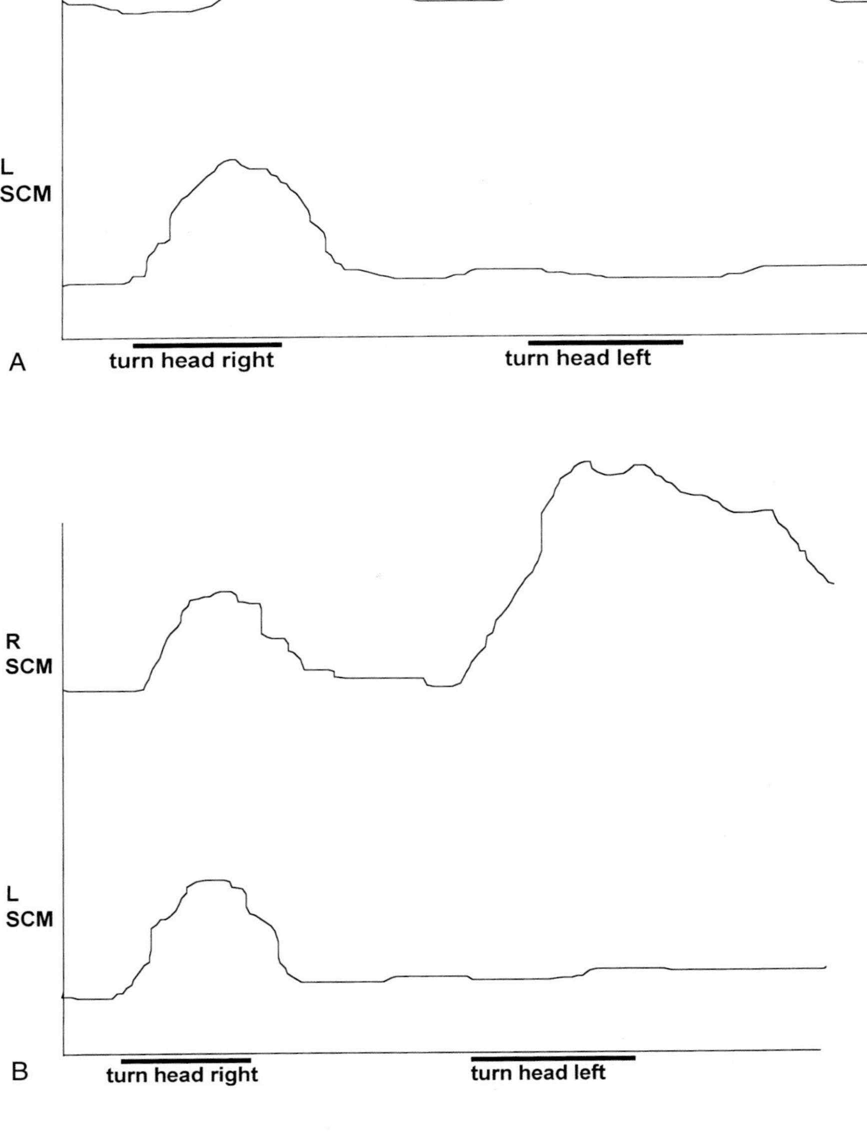

FIGURE 43–5. Surface EMG recording from the right and left sternocleidomastoid (SCM) in a subject without neck pain, showing normal reciprocal activation (*A*), and in a subject with neck pain, showing "dysfunction" of the right SCM (*B*). Note the excessive activation and the failure of the right SCM to return to baseline after the movement. (The lines under the graphs labeled "turn head right" and "turn head left" depict the duration of the respective movements.)

during a functional task or during contraction of distant muscles.[29] In a prospective study, workers who had fewer "gaps" in their EMG activity developed localized muscle pain in the monitored muscle.[105] This implies that lack of rest between contractions leads to muscle pain. Sleep disturbance further disrupts the muscles' ability to "rest."[23]

Treatment of motor dysfunction involves restoration of normal length and tension relationships in muscle and normal range of motion around joints. Surface EMG biofeedback is a common and often effective way to accomplish the neuromuscular re-education required to treat disordered muscle firing patterns. This typically involves teaching the patient to achieve muscular relaxation at rest and to eventually maintain this relaxation without feedback. Another common strategy teaches the patient to work for symmetry of EMG activity in paired muscles by increasing activation in the "hypoactive" muscle. Pain relief often coincides with resumption of EMG symmetry.[51]

MUSCLE PAIN SYNDROMES

Table 43–1 lists the many causes of muscle pain. The muscle pain syndromes are those entities that have muscle pain as a major component but do not have an established cause and therefore do not qualify as diseases. The following are descriptions of the most common muscle pain syndromes, roughly ordered from localized to more generalized, systemic disorders.

Postexercise Muscle Soreness

Most people experience postexercise muscle soreness at one time or another. However, its cause is still not fully understood. Clinically, the pain is most common following unaccustomed exercise using untrained muscles and peaks 24 to 48 hours after the exercise. Serum muscle enzymes reach their peak at about the same time.[62] Eccentric (lengthening) contractions provoke this pain much more efficiently than concentric (shortening) contractions. A few weeks of training can reduce or prevent this type of muscle soreness.

The cause of postexercise muscle pain may be a clue to muscle pain in general. Unfortunately, it remains an enigma. With eccentric exercise (e.g., going downstairs), the external forces acting on the muscle are greater than the forces generated by the muscle itself. These external forces are spread over a smaller percentage of motor units, leading to damage in the muscle fibers and connective tissue.[67] The release of nociceptor-sensitizing substances during repair of this damage may lead to the delayed muscle soreness. The pain probably is not caused by the mechanical muscle fiber damage directly, since serum enzyme levels do not rise immediately. Since type I (oxidative) fibers are preferentially damaged, and since training can have a protective effect, disordered metabolism is probably a contributing component.[62] Excessive eccentric exercise also leads to neuromuscular dysfunction, with an increase in tremor amplitude and decreased proprioception.[81] The strengthening that occurs during the first few weeks of training is attributed to neural factors such as coordination of motor unit firing. This could explain how training of similar duration protects against postexercise muscle soreness.

Treatment of postexercise muscle soreness is simple and effective. Rest and a more gradual approach to exercise cures most patients. Nonsteroidal anti-inflammatory drugs do not help, which eliminates prostaglandin from contention as a sensitizing agent.

Overuse Syndromes

The terms "overuse injury" and "repetitive strain injury" encompass a wide variety of musculoskeletal pain problems. Nerve entrapments, stress fractures, tendinitis and bursitis, and muscle pain have all been labeled overuse injuries. These are covered in more detail in Chapter 45 (occupational rehabilitation) and in Chapters 38 and 39 (upper and lower limb musculoskeletal disorders). This section focuses briefly on the place of overuse injuries in the spectrum of muscle pain.

In contrast to postexercise muscle pain, overuse muscle pain often occurs in well-trained muscles. Overuse pain arises from the repetitive use of a muscle, not from a single bout of exercise. These injuries are most common in athletes, musicians, and factory-line workers, where precise repetition of motor tasks is frequently a requirement for success.

The cause of overuse muscle pain is thought to be microtrauma that outpaces the capacity of the muscle for repair. Edwards[23] describes the final common pathway of muscle pain beginning with an excessive force per muscle fiber leading to hypoxia, acidosis, and metabolic depletion, followed by calcium-mediated cellular damage. In laborers, continued use of fatigued muscles causes mechanical damage that is directly related to the heaviness of the work. Again, eccentric work seems to subject small numbers of muscle fibers to excessive loads.

Many occupations, however, require precise manipulations, leading to excessive contraction of the proximal stabilizers that is unrelated to the heaviness of the task. The forces required to perform the task are not large enough to overload the muscles and cause damage. Rather, the conflict of motor control between the postural stabilizers and the muscles needed for precise manipulation or movement leads to the fiber damage.[23]

The combination of mental stress and precise manipulations experienced by musicians can lead to occupational cramps believed to be of central origin (focal dystonia). These cramps may be just an extreme example of the muscle pain that can occur with disordered motor planning. They occur more commonly early in the career of the artist, before the smooth, seemingly effortless motor patterns are established.[23]

Incoordination of movements and co-contraction of agonist-antagonists are often seen in the context of muscle pain. An example is the trapezius myalgia found in factory workers (see the discussion of motor dysfunction, above).

Myofascial Pain Syndromes

The myofascial pain syndromes owe their ever-widening acceptance (if not their existence) to the pioneering work of Travell[15] and her later collaboration with Simons.[101] In 1983, they combined their clinical experience in a detailed description of the multiple pain syndromes attributed to this disorder.[101] In doing so, they further defined the major clinical components characteristic of myofascial pain, the most important being the trigger point, the "taut band," and the local "twitch" response.

The Trigger Point

As noted earlier, the trigger point got its name from its propensity to cause pain at a distant site. These points play a central role in the definition of myofascial pain syndromes and appear in predictable locations, usually in the midportion or belly of the affected muscle. Flat palpation of a relaxed muscle under passive stretch best locates these small (less than 1 cm^2), discrete tender spots (Fig. 43–6). Sustained pressure (10 seconds) or penetration by a needle usually causes referral of pain into the "zone of reference" typical of that muscle. There may or may not be a palpable nodule at the site. Often the trigger point is located within a taut band in a muscle with decreased range of motion.

The significance of these trigger points is not clear. Some researchers believe they arise from localized areas of muscle trauma, but biopsy studies show mostly normal muscle. Uncontrolled studies have found non-specific changes suggestive of localized ischemia (ragged red fibers, decreased adenosine triphosphate [ATP]).[117, 118] Others believe these findings are secondary to a local "energy crisis" in the muscle. Such an energy crisis is postulated to cause release of substances that sensitize nociceptors to respond to innocuous pressure.[45] When controlled for level of deconditioning, however, patients and controls have the same subtle muscle changes.[85]

A recent study using monopolar needle EMG found spontaneous electrical activity on penetration of trapezius trigger points.[48] The electrical activity was usually of low amplitude and was accompanied by aching pain in the same referral pattern as that found with sustained pressure on the trigger point. The electrical activity described is identical to that attributed to "end-plate noise" during routine EMG. The authors theorized that spontaneous activity from the muscle spindle is being recorded.[48] Sustained activity in the intrafusal fibers of the muscle spindle (due to sympathetic activity) is thought to bring about an increase in the resting tone of the muscle. Pain is attributed to damage to the spindle capsule. On the other hand, the researchers may have recorded only end-plate noise. Others, using similar techniques,[22] have found no such activity attributable to trigger points.

The inter- and intratester reliability of the trigger point examination has not been adequately investigated. In fact, in one pilot study, even expert examiners varied widely in trigger point count.[113] Less well trained examiners performed even more poorly.[75] Pressure algometers improve the objectivity of the examination and may be useful in clinical studies or in documenting response to treatment[14, 21, 64] (although the relationship between the number and sensitivity of trigger points and disease severity has not been established).[21, 28, 78]

Thermography is another tool used for documentation of trigger points. However, in a blinded study, patients without trigger points had as many hot spots as those with trigger points.[98] Whether trigger points differ from the tender points of fibromyalgia remains unclear. Rheumatologists generally do not apply sustained pressure to tender points or needle them, and therefore are not likely to elicit the major differentiating feature—referred pain. There is likely a large amount of overlap between the two types of points.[103]

The Taut Band

Trigger points are characteristically found within taut bands of muscle. The taut band is a shortened group of muscle fibers and can be best palpated by sliding the skin and subcutaneous tissues perpendicularly across the fibers of the muscle. These bands are electrically silent and therefore not due to "spasm." Localized contracture of a few muscle fibers is one proposed mechanism. Today's taut bands may be identical to the fibrositic nodules of the early muscle pain literature. Once the taut band is found, palpation along it will lead to the most tender point—the trigger point. "Snapping palpa-

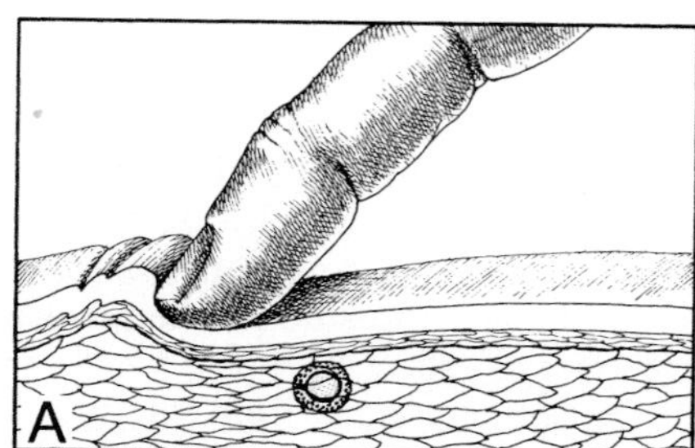

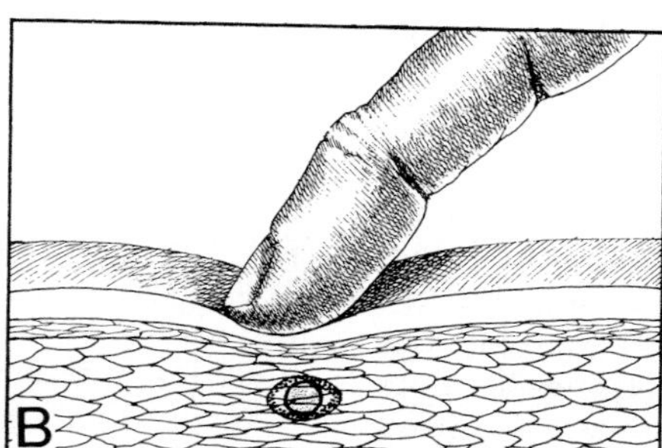

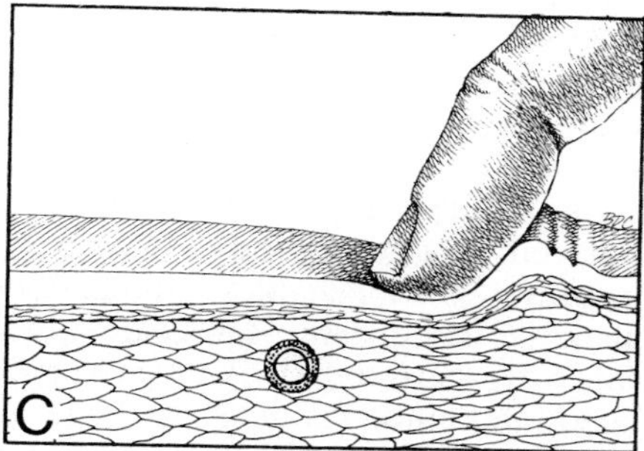

FIGURE 43–6. Cross-sectional schematic drawing of the technique of flat palpation of a trigger point. The dark ring represents a taut band and the circle within it is the trigger point. *A.* Skin is pushed to one side to begin palpation. *B.* Fingertip sliding across the muscle fibers to feel the taut band rolling beneath it. *C.* Skin pushed to other side at completion of "snapping" palpation (see also Fig. 43–7). (From Travell JG, Simons DG: Myofascial Pain and Dysfunction: The Trigger Point Manual. Baltimore, Williams & Wilkins, 1983.)

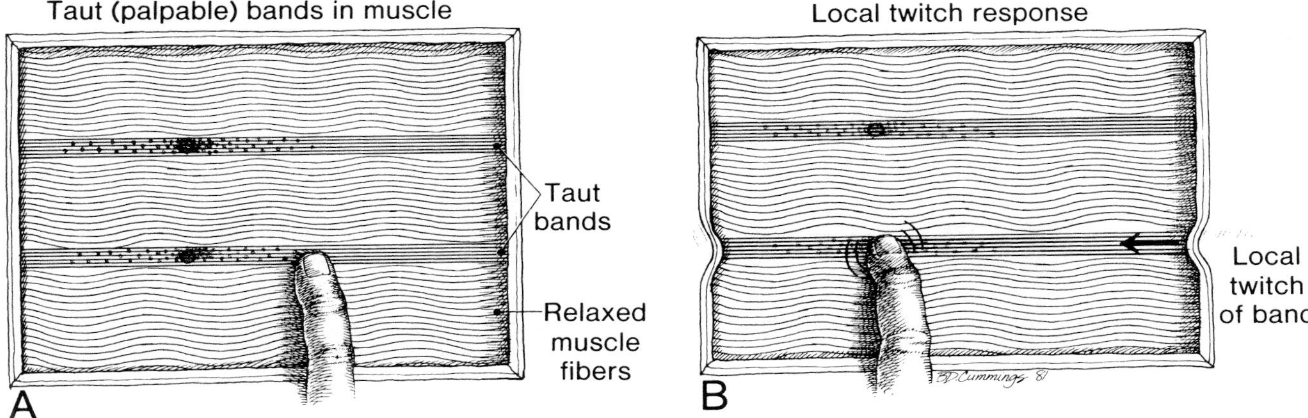

FIGURE 43–7. Schematic drawing of taut bands and myofascial trigger points. *A.* Straight lines represent the cord-like taut band of muscle within normal, relaxed muscle (*wavy lines*). The density of the stippling within the taut band corresponds to the degree of tenderness to palpation. The most tender spot (*dark ring*) is the trigger point. *B.* Rolling the taut band under the fingertip at the trigger point (snapping palpation) often produces a "local twitch response" with shortening of the band of muscle. (From Travell JG, Simons DG: Myofascial Pain and Dysfunction: The Trigger Point Manual. Baltimore, Williams & Wilkins, 1983.)

tion" of the band gives rise to another cardinal sign of myofascial pain, the local twitch response (Fig. 43–7).

The Local Twitch Response

When one "snaps" the taut band containing a trigger point, a transient contraction of the band's muscle fibers occurs. This sign is diagnostically important, as noted below, but its pathophysiological significance is unclear. EMG studies document electrical activity during the twitch[30] that is not blocked by total motor and sensory anesthesia. Needling of a trigger point also produces a twitch response. The technique of snapping palpation requires significant skill, and its validity as a diagnostic sign has not been established.

Clinical and Research Criteria

The first international symposium on myofascial pain and fibromyalgia was held in 1989. It marked one of the first meetings of the principal proponents of the two major muscle pain syndromes. In the proceedings of that symposium, Simons[88] listed the clinical criteria for diagnosis of myofascial pain syndrome (Table 43–2). The required features include regional pain, referred pain or disturbed sensation in a predicted location, a taut band, a tender point along the taut band, and restricted range of motion. One of three "minor criteria" must also be present: (1) pain complaint reproduced by pressure on the tender spot, (2) a local twitch response, or (3) relief of the pain by stretching or injecting. At the same time Simons listed research criteria for the identification of trigger points. To qualify, the point must be exquisitely tender, located in a taut band of a muscle with restricted range of motion, refer pain when pressed or needled, and exhibit a twitch response when needled.

These criteria are obviously derived from many years of clinical experience, but their validity has not been tested. Simons suggests that, in the absence of a gold standard, these criteria should be tested against clinical expert opinion. Four such experts found taut bands and twitch responses with equal frequency in fibromyalgia patients, myofascial pain patients, and controls. The experts also differed significantly among themselves in their determinations of trigger point count, taut bands, and twitch responses.[113] Although these criteria can be clinically useful as guidelines, they likely will not show enough validity for strict diagnostic criteria.

Pathophysiology

The myofascial pain syndromes remain largely a clinical construct based more on case studies, anecdote, and clinical experience than on basic science. The applica-

TABLE 43–2 Clinical Criteria for the Diagnosis of Myofascial Pain Syndrome Caused by Active Trigger Points

To make the clinical diagnosis of myofascial pain syndrome, the findings should include five major criteria and at least one of three minor criteria. The five *major criteria* are the following:

1. Regional pain complaint.
2. Pain complaint or altered sensation in the expected distribution of referred pain from a myofascial trigger point.
3. Taut band palpable in an accessible muscle.
4. Exquisite spot tenderness at one point along the length of the taut band.
5. Some degree of restricted range of motion, when measurable.

The three *minor criteria* are the following:

1. Reproduction of clinical pain complaint, or altered sensation, by pressure on the tender spot.
2. Elicitation of a local twitch response by transverse snapping palpation at the tender spot or by needle insertion into the tender spot in the taut band.
3. Pain alleviated by elongating (stretching) the muscle or by injecting the tender spot (trigger point).

Note: Additional symptoms such as weather sensitivity, sleep disturbance, and depression are often present but are not diagnostic because they may be attributable to chronic severe pain perpetuated by multiple mechanical and/or systemic perpetuating factors.

From Simons AG: Muscular pain syndromes. Adv Pain Res Ther 1990; 17:18.

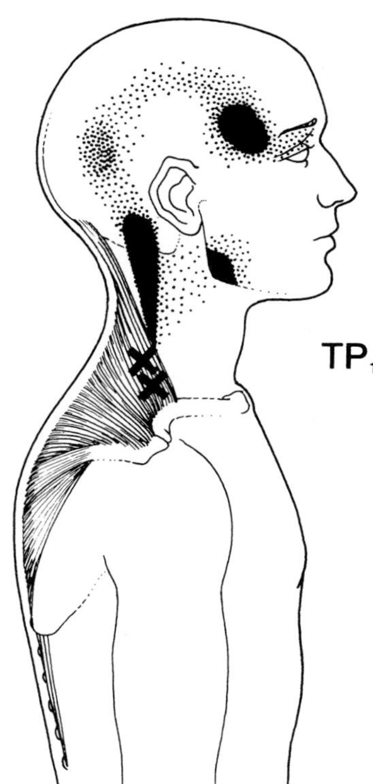

FIGURE 43–8. Location (*X*) and referred pain pattern for the most common trapezius trigger point, referred to as trigger point 1 (TP1). *Dark areas* show the main pattern of pain referral; *stippling* maps the spillover areas. (From Travell JG, Simons DG: Myofascial Pain and Dysfunction: The Trigger Point Manual. Baltimore, Williams & Wilkins, 1983.)

tion of EMG to the study of myofascial pain forced a redefinition of the syndrome. Since EMG studies failed to find "spasm" in the involved muscles,[58] the spasm-pain-spasm theory was abandoned. In its place Travell and Simons[101] combined facts of muscle physiology with some conjecture and arrived at the following sequence: acute muscle strain → tissue damage in a very localized area of muscle → tears in the sarcoplasmic reticulum → free calcium ions → sustained contraction → increased strain on vulnerable areas of muscle → free calcium ions, etc.

Travell and Simons further proposed that the free calcium ions plus ATP leads to sustained contraction of fibers, causing a hypermetabolic state locally and local vasoconstriction (possibly via the sympathetic nervous system). Local vasoconstriction causes local ischemia, which, combined with increased energy demands, leads to the histological changes mentioned previously (see the discussion under The Trigger Point [ragged red fibers]).

Travell and Simons postulated that depletion of ATP leads to a contracture state with electrical silence (as in McArdle's disease or rigor mortis). In addition, the tissue damage releases serotonin, histamine, and kinins, which also lead to local ischemia as well as nerve sensitization.[101]

Even with the difficulties outlined above, the myofascial pain syndromes remain a useful clinical paradigm, often leading to successful treatment of muscle pain problems. They are also very common. Thirty percent of patients attending a general medical clinic with the chief complaint of pain were found to have myofascial pain.[89] Several of the most common single muscle syndromes are presented in Figures 43–8 through 43–11. Shown are the locations of trigger points and the pattern of referred pain.

Chronic Regional Myofascial Syndromes

The single-muscle myofascial pain syndromes are usually acute and follow an episode of muscle overload. In some cases the pain persists and spreads to other, usually synergistic, muscles. This is referred to as a chronic regional myofascial syndrome.[88] Many perpetuating factors encourage transformation to a more widespread muscle pain problem. Mechanical factors include postural stress, muscle imbalances, and skeletal asymmetries. These can put additional stress on surrounding muscles, leading to spread of dysfunction and pain. Systemic perpetuating factors purportedly include anything jeopardizing the energy supply to muscle (i.e., anemia, endocrine imbalances, low thyroid function, vitamin deficiencies).[101] Chronic regional myofascial syndromes are conceptually close to the "malignant, metastasizing fibromyalgia" referred to by Bennett.[5]

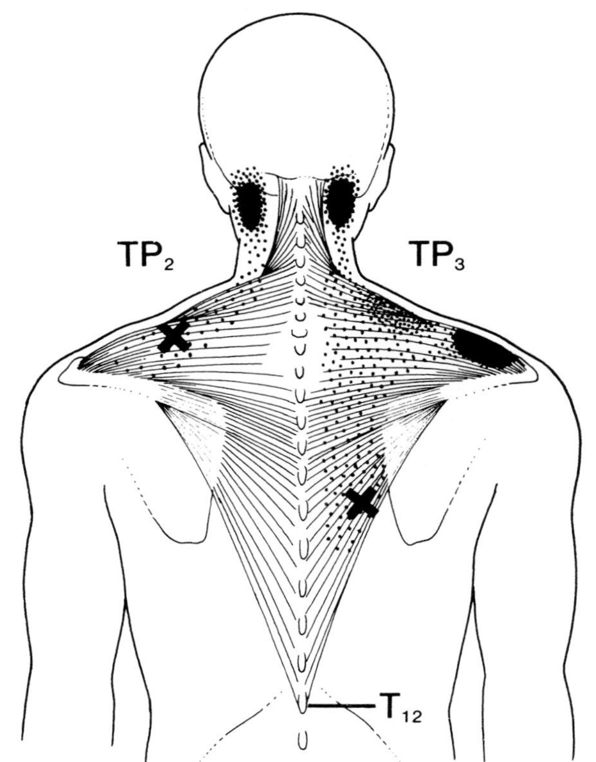

FIGURE 43–9. Locations (*X*) and referred pain patterns of trigger point 2 (TP2), in the left upper trapezius, and trigger point 3 (TP3), in the right lower trapezius, (Conventions are as in Fig. 43–8.) (From Travell JG, Simons DG: Myofascial Pain and Dysfunction: The Trigger Point Manual. Baltimore, Williams & Wilkins, 1983.)

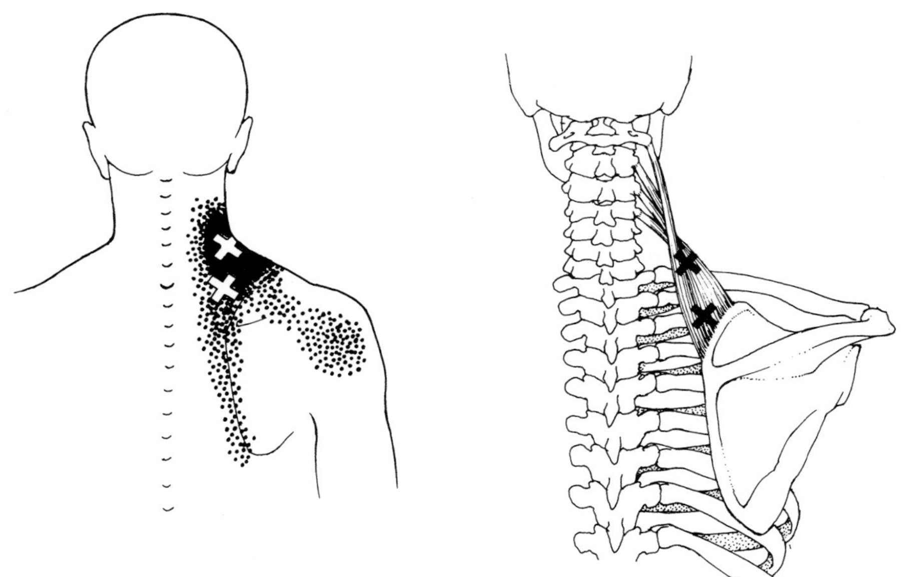

FIGURE 43–10. Trigger points (*X*) of the right levator scapulae muscle. The *dark area* shows the pattern of referred pain and the *stippling* locates the spillover zone. (From Travell JG, Simons DG: Myofascial Pain and Dysfunction: The Trigger Point Manual. Baltimore, Williams & Wilkins, 1983.)

Fibromyalgia

The Search for a Definition

As mentioned earlier, Smythe and Moldofsky redefined fibrositis to include only the widespread form of muscle pain. Table 43–3 lists their criteria, which include widespread aching for 3 months, 12 of 14 tender points, and disturbed sleep, along with several other attempts at a definition for widespread muscle pain.

Yunus et al[119] further refined Smythe's original criteria with the addition of commonly found associated symptoms. They reduced the required number of tender points to five and allowed as few as three tender points if five of the minor criteria were present. A later update allowed as few as two of 14 tender points.[115] Yunus et al[119] also changed the name from fibrositis to fibromyalgia (borrowing from Hench) because of the lack of inflammation. Most subsequent studies have used the Yunus criteria to define fibromyalgia, allowing for the inclusion of regional and even localized muscle pain. Recognizing the problem the Yunus criteria posed when trying to differentiate fibromyalgia from myofascial pain and other localized muscle pain syndromes, Wolfe[110] raised the tender point count to seven of 14. He also eliminated associated symptoms and modulating factors from the definition because they did not improve the sensitivity of the criteria.[110]

In 1990, the Multicenter Criteria Committee of the American College of Rheumatology (ACR 90) pub-

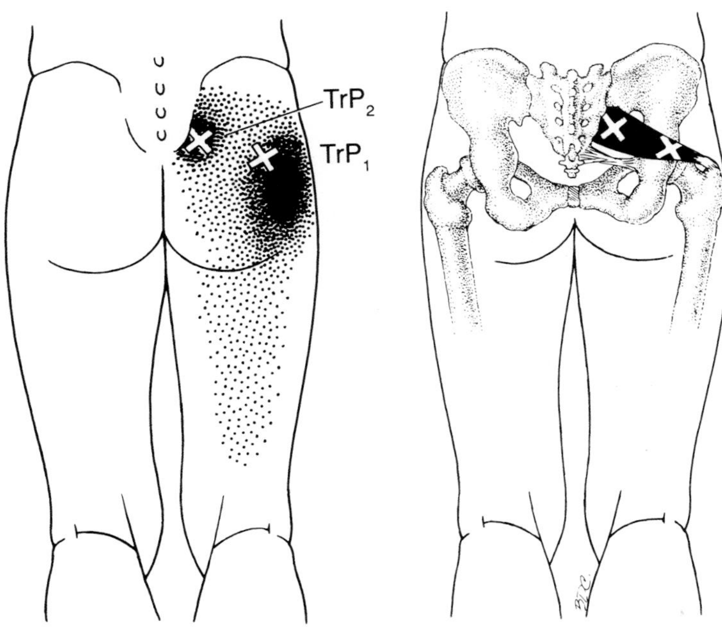

FIGURE 43–11. Locations of trigger points (*X*) in the piriformis muscle. The lateral *X* marks the most common location within the piriformis. The *dark area* shows the pattern of referred pain and the *stippling* locates the spillover zone. (From Travell JG, Simons DG: Myofascial Pain and Dysfunction: The Trigger Point Manual. Baltimore, Williams & Wilkins, 1983.)

TABLE 43–3 Reported Diagnostic Features of Muscle Pain Syndromes

Feature	Fibrositis (Smythe[92])	Nonrestorative Sleep (Moldofsky[72])	Fibromyalgia		
			Wolfe[110]	*Yunus et al.[119]*	*1990 ACR[114]*
Widespread aching (3 mo)	X	X	X	X	X
Tender points (no.)	X (12/14)	X	X (7+)	X (5 +)	X (11/18)
Skin roll tenderness	X	—	—	—	—
Disturbed sleep	X	X	—	X	—
Normal x-ray and laboratory findings	X	X	X	X	—
"Type A" personality	X	—	—	—	—
Relief with heat	—	X	—	—	—
Dermatographia	—	X	—	—	—
Emotional distress	—	X	—	X	—
Effects of weather	—	X	—	X	—
No trauma or rheumatic disease	—	—	—	X	—
Relief with physical activity	—	—	—	X	—
Irritable bowel syndrome	—	—	—	X	—

lished its criteria for classification of fibromyalgia[114] (Table 43–4). Once again, emphasis was placed on the widespread nature of fibromyalgia, with the requirement of 11 of 18 tender points.

Prevalence and Epidemiology

Few epidemiological studies have used the ACR 90 criteria. Nevertheless fibromyalgia is common in the community, found in 2% to 4% of the general population.[109] Widespread pain as defined by the ACR 90 criteria is found in 11.2% of the adult population of northern England.[20] Eight percent of general medical patients meet previous definitions of fibromyalgia,[10] as do about 15% to 20% of rheumatology clinic patients, making fibromyalgia the third most common diagnosis made by rheumatologists.[112, 119] Women make up 73% to 90% of those diagnosed with fibromyalgia,[7, 109] although this may represent a selection bias. Regardless of the definition, fibromyalgia appears to be a very common entity.

Throughout all of the definitions, the major clinical features of fibromyalgia have remained relatively constant but with varying degrees of emphasis. The best way to differentiate patients with fibromyalgia appears to be by widespread pain and high tender point count. Other important features include sleep disturbance, fatigue, headaches, irritable bowel syndrome, and paresthesias.

Clinical Features

Widespread Pain and Tenderness

Widespread pain of 3 months' duration is required for the diagnosis of fibromyalgia and is defined as pain both above and below the waist, on both the right and left sides of the body, along with axial pain (low back pain is considered below the waist).[114] As noted earlier, this may include more than 10% of the population, making the tender point count very important in the diagnosis of fibromyalgia. The point count required was set at 11 to maximize the specificity of the classification for study purposes. There appears to be a continuous spectrum of increasing numbers of tender points coinciding

TABLE 43–4 The American College of Rheumatology 1990 Criteria for Classification of Fibromyalgia*

1. History of widespread pain
   Definition: Pain is considered widespread when all the following are present—pain in the left side of the body, pain in the right side of the body, pain above the waist, and pain below the waist. In addition, axial skeletal pain (cervical spine, anterior chest, thoracic spine, or low back) must be present. In this definition, shoulder and buttock pain is considered as pain for each involved side. "Low back" pain is considered lower segment pain.
2. Pain in 11 of 18 tender point sites on digital palpation
   Definition: On digital palpation, pain must be present in at least 11 of the following 18 tender point sites:
   - *Occiput*—Bilateral, at the suboccipital muscle insertions
   - *Low cervical*—Bilateral, at the anterior aspects of the intertransverse spaces at C5 to C7
   - *Trapezius*—Bilateral, at the midpoint of the upper border
   - *Supraspinatus*—Bilateral, at origins, above the scapular spine near the medial border
   - *Second rib*—Bilateral, at the second costochondral junctions, just lateral to the junctions on upper surfaces
   - *Lateral epicondyle*—Bilateral, 2 cm distal to the epicondyles
   - *Gluteal*—Bilateral, in upper outer quadrants of buttocks in anterior fold of muscle
   - *Greater trochanter*—Bilateral, posterior to the trochanteric prominence
   - *Knee*—Bilateral, at the medial fat pad proximal to the joint line

   Digital palpation should be performed with an approximate force of 4 kg

   For a tender point to be considered "positive," the subject must state that the palpation was painful. "Tender" is not to be considered "painful."

* For classification purposes, patients will be said to have fibromyalgia if both criteria are satisfied. Widespread pain must have been present for at least 3 months. The presence of a second clinical disorder does not exclude the diagnosis of fibromyalgia.

From Wolfe F, Smythe HA, Yunus MB, et al: The American College of Rheumatology 1990 criteria for the classification of fibromyalgia. Arthritis Rheum 1990; 33:160–172.

with increasing numbers of painful body segments in the general population.[19] Many of those with fewer points are also likely to have fibromyalgia. How low the count should be allowed to go is a matter of debate.

The reliability of the tender point count is somewhat better established than is the trigger point examination. In the study mentioned earlier the fibromyalgia experts were fairly consistent in the point count, largely owing to the predetermined examination sites and the sole requirement of tenderness.[113] The test-retest and inter-rater reliability of the tender point examination using a pressure algometer was quite good (.85 generalizability coefficient), but the points were marked ahead of time.[102] Even so, the two examiners differed significantly at the most common tender point site—the upper trapezius.

The sites in the ACR 90 criteria were chosen based on their utility in separating fibromyalgia patients from those with other painful conditions. It is implied that they are discrete points of tenderness. A study of 75 unilateral points found 19 that best discriminated between patients and controls.[86] Only three of the ACR 90 points were included in the 19 best points. The significant tender points clustered in regions—the anterior shoulder, anterior chest, scapula, and medial knee—suggesting that tenderness in a region may be more useful clinically than tenderness at specific points.

Three interpretations, singly or in combination, are possible regarding tender points: (1) they represent specific areas of pathological change; (2) they identify multiple regions of pain; or (3) they signify a generalized increase in tenderness. This has implications for the etiology of fibromyalgia. Those who have found increased tenderness at tender points but no difference between patients and controls at usually nontender control sites favor a peripheral mechanism for the production of pain.[10] Those who have found a generalized increase in sensitivity to pressure proclaim the importance of central modulating factors as a cause of increased pain in fibromyalgia.[39, 86, 96, 111]

Sleep Disturbance

Almost all descriptions of fibromyalgia include poor sleep as a feature. In 1975, Moldofsky and associates[71] proposed the term "non-restorative sleep syndrome" to replace fibrositis. They studied 10 patients with the diagnosis of fibrositis and found that seven had intrusion of alpha rhythms into stage 4 delta sleep. At one time, and even recently,[7] the alpha-delta sleep pattern was thought to be diagnostic, and possibly the cause of fibromyalgia.[72] This alpha-delta sleep pattern was originally described by Hauri and Hawkins[43] and correlates with subjective fatigue. The presence of poor sleep in the diagnostic criteria used for patient selection in the study of Moldofsky et al likely influenced the results, since fibromyalgia patients who claim to be good sleepers do not differ from controls in alpha-delta sleep.[47] Other investigators have been unable to confirm the correlation of alpha-delta sleep with fibrositis (fibromyalgia).[33] The finding is very nonspecific and can be found in any chronically painful condition.[42]

Nonetheless, disturbed sleep is common in fibromyalgia, with reports of incidence ranging from 60% to 90%.[35] Patients with myofascial pain have similar degrees of sleep disturbance,[84] with the incidence of sleep disturbance correlating better with duration of pain than with diagnosis.[50]

Associated Symptoms

Multiple associated features commonly appear in reports of fibromyalgia. The most common are fatigue (75% to 100%), stiffness (75% to 90%), subjective swelling (30% to 100%), tension-type headache (45% to 75%), anxiety (40% to 70%), and irritable bowel syndrome (35% to 50%).[50] Other common features include aggravation of symptoms by cold, humidity, change of weather, and physical activity. The frequency of these features in regional and localized muscle pain syndromes and other chronic pain syndromes remains unclear. The prevalence of many of these features likely increases as the number of regions involved with pain increases and as the pain becomes more chronic.

Psychological Aspects

Partly because of the high number of somatic complaints voiced by patients with fibromyalgia, many clinicians view the patients as psychologically disturbed. In fact, one clinician refers to the disorder as a "psychophysiologic" state.[107] Many early studies reporting psychopathological findings used the Minnesota Multiphasic Personality Inventory (MMPI), which is poorly suited to the study of patients with pain.[93] Although some studies find no difference between fibromyalgia patients and controls using other standardized tests (Beck Depression Inventory, Spielberger State and Trait Anxiety Inventory, SCL-90-R),[12] or DSM-III (*Diagnostic and Statistical Manual of Mental Disorders*) diagnoses,[1] a review concluded that psychological disturbance is associated with fibromyalgia syndrome.[8] The majority of fibromyalgia patients do not have an active psychiatric disorder, but there is a greater prevalence of major depression and panic disorder.[49, 74] A multinational primary care survey found an association between persistent pain and psychological disorders (anxiety or depression) across all 15 sites on five continents.[41] It may well be that the psychological aspects of fibromyalgia simply result from chronic pain and its effect on central pain modulation systems.[6, 61, 79]

Another view is that patients with a primary psychiatric disorder and symptoms of fibromyalgia represent one end of the spectrum of fibromyalgia disorders.[74] In these patients the symptoms of fibromyalgia wax and wane with the psychiatric disorder and with psychosocial stressors. A particularly difficult differentiation is that between fibromyalgia and somatization disorder or somatoform pain disorder. Both of these require the presence of multiple symptoms or pain without causative organic pathological findings, or that the complaint or impairment be out of proportion to the physical findings. As muscle pain persists and becomes more widespread, the incidence of these psychiatric disorders increases.

Pathophysiology: Proposed Mechanisms

The pathophysiology of fibromyalgia remains a mystery. The few abnormalities found in various studies tend to be nonspecific and lend themselves to various interpretations. These have been combined liberally with conjecture to arrive at the leading theories of pathophysiology. The theories can be divided into three groups based on the location of the proposed mechanism: (1) primarily central, (2) a combination of central and peripheral, or (3) primarily peripheral.

One "central mechanism" theory hypothesizes that fibromyalgia is a variation of an affective disorder.[49] This is based primarily on the frequent co-morbidity of fibromyalgia with major depression, migraine, irritable bowel syndrome, chronic fatigue syndrome, and panic disorder—all of which are thought to share a common pathophysiology. No causal link exists between the disorders, but rather an underlying abnormality exists that is necessary but not sufficient for these disorders to occur. This predisposition (genetic?) combines with environmental factors to produce the particular disorder.

Another "central" theory identifies the alpha electroencephalographic (EEG) sleep anomaly as the root cause of fibromyalgia.[70, 71] Anything that disrupts sleep—an emotionally stressful event, sleep apnea, or flulike illness—can cause the alpha sleep anomaly. The sleep disorder in turn alters the brain chemistry of substances associated with both sleep arousal and pain modulation, such as serotonin and substance P.

Yunus[116] adds peripheral modulation to aberrant central pain mechanisms, combining central with peripheral components (Fig. 43–12). He blames "central neurohormonal dysfunction" for a functional deficiency of inhibitory neural transmitters or overactivity of excitatory neurotransmitters. Decreased serotonin is one possible mechanism. Peripheral factors such as microtrauma and referred pain are thought to play a minor role. The presence of a generalized decrease in pain tolerance points to the importance of central factors. The "central neurohormonal dysfunction" may be triggered by nonspecific stress from trauma, viral infection, or mental stress.[17]

Smythe,[91, 95] on the other hand, favors the preeminence of peripheral factors such as mechanical problems in neck and low back areas as the primary cause of fibromyalgia. Local injury leads to sleep disturbance, fatigue, more pain, stiffness, and deconditioning. In regional pain the local mechanical factors predominate. Centrally acting modulating factors (along with poor sleep and deconditioning) become more important as the pain becomes more widespread.

Others point to the presence of the tender point as evidence for a predominant peripheral mechanism. Bennett,[4, 5] borrowing from the myofascial pain syndrome model, proposes that muscle microtrauma leads to activation of muscle nociceptors and is the initial event in the pathogenesis of fibromyalgia. A genetic and acquired (through alpha sleep anomaly and its effect on the hypothalamic-pituitary axis) predisposition to muscle microtrauma at low levels of exertion leads to muscle pain with eccentric contractions. The pain leads to inactivity and deconditioning, which perpetuates the microtrauma. Elements of central pain enhancement also play a role (Fig. 43–13).

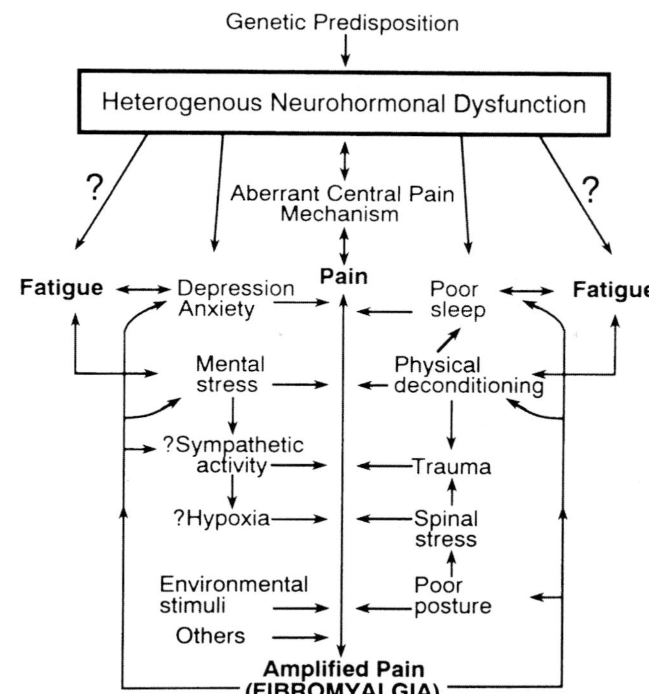

FIGURE 43–12. The pathophysiology of fibromyalgia according to Yunus. The primary defect is thought to be a poorly characterized central "neurohormonal dysfunction," which leads to an "aberrant central pain mechanism." Pain is amplified by numerous factors, including many in the periphery (trauma, hypoxia), leading to fibromyalgia. (From Yunus MB: Towards a model of pathophysiology of fibromyalgia: Aberrant central pain mechanisms with peripheral modulation. J Rheumatol 1992; 19:846–850.)

Another prominent theory focuses on localized ischemia due to disturbed microcirculation.[44, 45] This theory relies on the interpretation of the equivocal findings on muscle biopsy mentioned earlier (see the discussion under The Trigger Point [ragged red fibers]). Studies using phosphorus-31 MR spectroscopy have found decreased levels of ATP and phosphocreatine in muscles both at rest and with exercise in fibromyalgia patients compared to controls. This supports the notion of focal ischemia.[77] Critics claim that these findings are due to the use of healthy controls with higher levels of cardiovascular fitness and point to similar studies that find no differences between patients and controls.[85] The proponents of the disturbed microcirculation theory suggest that discrete muscle tension caused by gamma reflexes, emotional stress, or insufficient relaxation combines with the disturbed microcirculation to cause muscle pain (Fig. 43–14). To explain widespread pain at rest, characteristic of fibromyalgia, this theory invokes disturbed pain modulation in the CNS.

Some investigators champion abnormalities of the neuroendocrine system as an etiological factor in fibromyalgia. Disruptions of the hypothalamic-pituitary-adrenal (HPA) axis are found in many stress-related

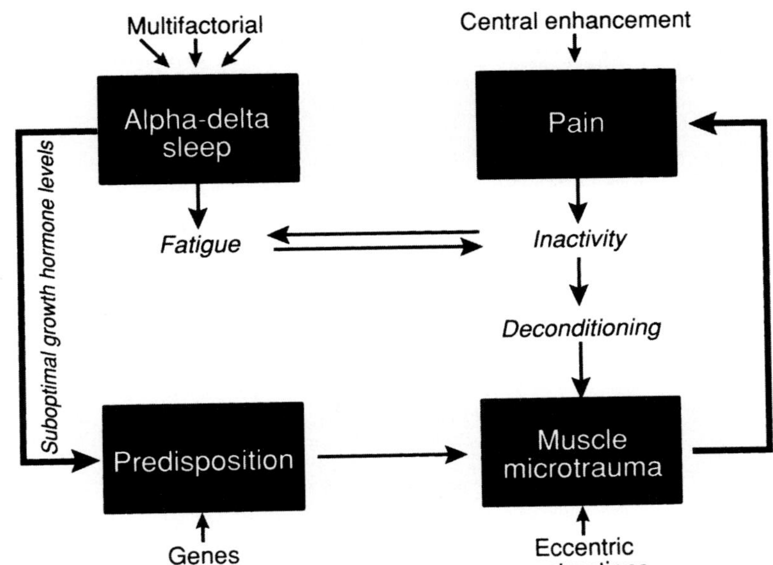

FIGURE 43–13. The pathophysiology of fibromyalgia according to Bennett. Muscle microtrauma is thought to be the primary event leading to muscle pain. Central factors play a role in enhancing the pain and in predisposing the individual to muscle microtrauma, creating several feedback loops, as shown. (From Bennett RM: Fibromyalgia and the facts: Sense or nonsense. Rheum Dis Clin North Am 1993; 19:45–59.)

somatic and psychiatric syndromes, however, and are not specific for fibromyalgia. Recent proposals suggest that perhaps alterations in the HPA axis predispose to the development of stress-related syndromes. Which specific syndrome develops (fibromyalgia, chronic fatigue, or irritable bowel) depends on yet unidentified triggers.[18]

Weigent et al[106] have integrated many aspects of previous theories along with recent research findings, resulting in a theory of the pathophysiology of fibromyalgia that combines interactions among the musculoskeletal, neuroendocrine, and central nervous systems. Several precipitating factors (e.g., trauma, stress, infections) eventually lead to increased dorsal horn spinal neuron excitability and a barrage of nociceptive input to the brain. This in time causes functional changes centrally that lead to abnormal pain thresholds and chronic pain (Fig. 43–15).

Myofascial Pain Syndrome versus Fibromyalgia

Although fibromyalgia and myofascial pain syndrome have many similarities, most investigators maintain that they are two distinct entities. In general, myofascial pain is thought to be a local or regional problem due to acute muscle trauma, whereas fibromyalgia is a widespread pain problem affecting more than just muscle and has systemic features. The presence of taut bands, referred pain, and twitch responses is often cited to differentiate myofascial pain. As noted earlier (see discussion under Myofascial Pain Syndrome), these have not been shown to be reliable findings, even in the hands of experts.[75, 113] The distinction becomes more artificial when one considers that fibromyalgia can begin as a localized pain disorder and later become widespread, and that persistent myofascial pain syndromes can involve multiple sites and cause systemic symptoms.[5, 110]

Myofascial pain and fibromyalgia might be labels for the two extremes of a single disorder.[50, 19] Bennett[5] proposed that they could well have the same pathogenic mechanism. In its simplest form, a myofascial pain syndrome consists of the acute onset of pain in one muscle after trauma to that muscle. It is more than the generalized ache of a muscle after exertion but less than the

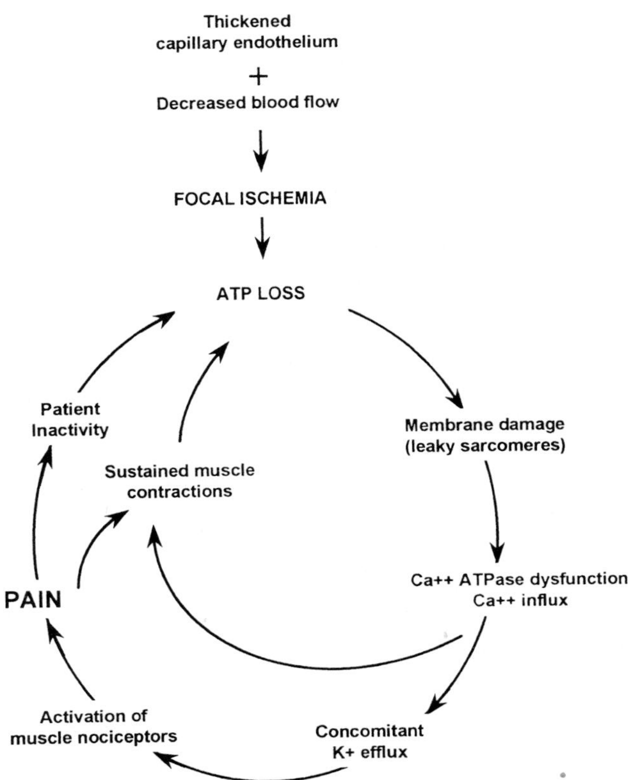

FIGURE 43–14. Diagram of proposed interactions of various muscle abnormalities leading to pain and muscle dysfunction. (From Olsen NJ, Park JH: Skeletal muscle abnormalities in patients with fibromyalgia. Am J Med Sci 1998; 315:351–358.)

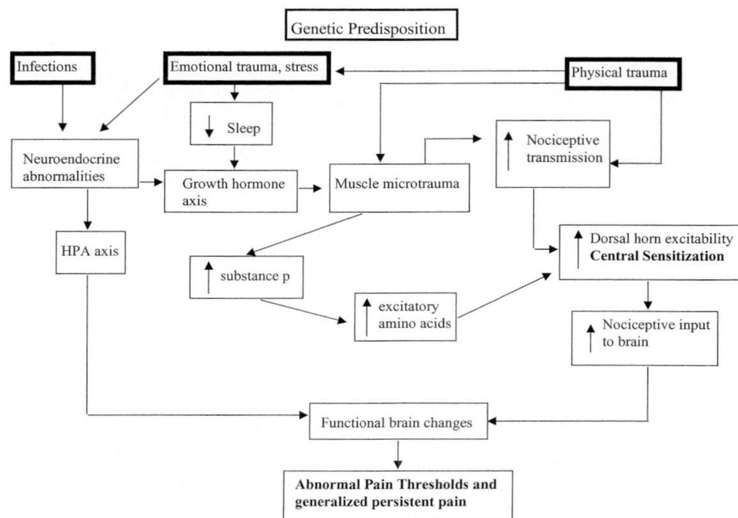

FIGURE 43–15. Simplified model of the pathophysiology of abnormal pain perception in fibromyalgia as proposed by Weigent et al. Several precipitating factors (in *bold boxes*) may lead to abnormalities in neuroendocrine axes, muscle tissue, sleep, and peripheral nociceptors. These abnormalities lead to hyperexcitability of dorsal horn spinal neurons, which in turn produce excessive nociceptive input to the brain, leading to functional alterations in the areas that process the sensory-discriminative and affective-emotional dimensions of pain. The result is abnormal pain thresholds and widespread persistent pain. HPA, hypothalamic-pituitary-adrenal. (Modified from Weigent DA, Bradley LA, Blalock JE, et al: Current conceptions in the pathophysiology of abnormal pain perception in fibromyalgia. Am J Med Sci 1998; 315:405–412.)

obvious trauma of a muscle strain. Under the right conditions, trigger points can develop in nearby muscles until widespread chronic pain involves multiple muscle sites associated with systemic features such as disturbed sleep, generalized fatigue, and anxiety, the characteristic features of fibromyalgia. At what point did the disorder change from myofascial pain to fibromyalgia? Is fibromyalgia myofascial pain plus chronic pain syndrome? Is myofascial pain simply localized fibromyalgia? These are questions yet to be answered.

Chronic Fatigue Syndrome

Chronic fatigue syndrome (CFS) has recently emerged as a popular diagnostic label for "a centuries-old disorder of fatigue and multiple somatic complaints."[56] It has also been termed "yuppie flu" by the lay press. Because it shares many features with fibromyalgia—including the lack of objective physical or laboratory abnormalities—Goldenberg[34] classified CFS as a subset of fibromyalgia. Others believe the two conditions may well be the same disorder.[49]

The 1987 Centers for Disease Control and Prevention (CDC) definition of CFS included fatigue of at least 6 months' duration in the absence of a known cause, and the presence of eight of 11 symptoms that included sleep disturbance, muscle pain, postexertional fatigue, and migratory myalgias[56] (Table 43–5). The large number of symptoms required tended to select patients with psychiatric disorders. Because of this, the CDC criteria were modified to specifically exclude patients with psychoses and substance abuse.[82] The criteria also excluded many patients with what were thought to be overlap syndromes. These confounding syndromes were made exclusion criteria and included fibromyalgia, nonpsychotic depression, somatoform disorders, and generalized anxiety disorder. In a general medical practice, 21% met the criteria for CFS.[56] Twenty-six percent of CFS patients met the criteria for fibromyalgia, and 70% to 80% were women. As in fibromyalgia, there is a high lifetime incidence of major depression (46% to 75%) and somatization disorder,[63] with current depression found in up to 42%.[32]

The cause of CFS is unknown. It most commonly begins suddenly after an infectious-like illness, but no link to any specific pathogen has been established. Initial

TABLE 43–5 Centers for Disease Control's Case Definition of the Chronic Fatigue Syndrome (CFS)

A case of CFS must fulfill both major criteria as well as either eight symptom criteria or six symptom criteria plus two physical criteria.

Major Criteria

1. New onset of fatigue lasting 6 mo reducing activity to <50%
2. Other conditions producing fatigue must be ruled out

Minor Criteria

Symptom Criteria—beginning at or after onset of fatigue and persisting or recurring for at least 6 mo

1. Low-grade fever, temperature of 37.5°C–38.6°C (99.5°F–101.5°F) orally or chills
2. Sore throat
3. Painful cervical or axillary lymph nodes
4. Generalized muscle weakness
5. Muscle pain
6. Postexertional fatigue lasting 24 hr
7. Headache
8. Migratory arthralgias
9. Neuropsychological complaints (photophobia, transient visual scotomata, forgetfulness, excessive irritability, confusion, difficulty thinking, inability to concentrate, or depression)
10. Sleep disturbance
11. Acute onset of symptoms over a few hours to a few days

Physical Criteria—documented by a physician twice, at least 1 mo apart

1. Low-grade fever, temperature of 37.6°C–38.6°C (99.7°F–101.5°F) orally or 37.8°C–38.8°C (100.0°F–101.8°F) rectally
2. Nonexudative pharyngitis
3. Palpable cervical or axillary lymph nodes up to 2 cm in diameter

Adapted from Klonoff DC: Chronic fatigue syndrome. Clin Infect Dis 1992; 15:812–823.

findings in support of such a role for Epstein-Barr virus, cocksackie B virus, and the human herpesvirus 6 have all been contradicted in more recent studies.[32, 63]

There continues to be some discussion as to whether CFS is an organic or psychiatric illness. It is likely a combination of the two, with a link between organic and psychiatric factors similar to that found in chronic pain. In both, the symptoms and functional deficits are out of proportion to the identifiable pathological findings. In CFS, an underlying hyperresponsive immune system might provide the organic half of the link. Inappropriate release of cytokines in response to certain infections can cause CFS symptoms. Psychiatric disturbance (depression) could magnify this deranged immune response.[56]

The recommended treatment for CFS is very similar to that for fibromyalgia (see below). Gantz and Holmes[31] recommend (1) exclusion of other conditions, (2) reassurance about the benign nature of the disorder, (3) use of antidepressants to treat both the depression and the sleep disorder, if present, (4) a graduated exercise program, (5) stress reduction, and (6) use of counseling and support groups.

Tension Myalgia

Starting in about 1950, patients at the Mayo Clinic presenting with multiple areas of muscle pain and high levels of psychological tension or stress received the diagnosis "tension myalgia."[99] The use of the term grew as the term "fibrositis" and its incorrect implication of inflammation fell out of favor. Over the years the application of the diagnosis evolved to the point where it is now used to describe the spectrum of muscle pain syndromes from localized to regional to generalized. In this way the term *tension myalgia* covers the patients who do not meet the strict criteria for fibromyalgia or myofascial pain, that is, the majority. With the recent resurgence of interest in muscle pain disorders nationally and the more widespread use of the terms *fibromyalgia* and *myofascial pain* (and the expansion of these terms to cover "localized fibromyalgia" and "generalized myofascial pain"), use of the diagnosis tension myalgia has declined. The concept of a continuum of muscle pain disorders remains, however, and tension myalgia remains a useful paradigm.

The major utility of the term tension myalgia lies in patient education. Most patients have seen multiple health care providers without a specific diagnosis, resulting in the often less than subtle implication that it is "all in their head." They are concerned that something has been overlooked and that they may have cancer or some other debilitating disease. This situation often adds to the already stressful fact of chronic pain. Receiving a definite diagnosis and an understandable explanation for their symptoms allays these fears and is the first step in successful treatment.

"Myalgia" refers to the most characteristic symptom—local, regional, or widespread muscle pain, including pain at musculotendinous junctions and muscle attachments. "Tension" has two connotations. First, it suggests that a common finding (and possibly a causative factor) is muscle under tension, whether it be from "spasm," postural stress, overuse, or disordered motor sequencing. As mentioned above, there have been mixed findings in EMG studies of muscle pain syndromes. Some find no activity in muscles at rest,[58] whereas others find increased activity.[14, 27] Needle EMG of painful muscles can be silent when surface EMG reveals increased activity over the same muscles with the patient in the relaxed seated position. The presence or absence of "spasm" is not significant. Rather, these patients misuse their muscles by habitually cocontracting them, by failing to fully relax them, by overusing them, by subjecting them to unrelenting postural stress, or by a combination of these. This misuse ties in with the concept of motor dysfunction mentioned earlier.

Second, the word *tension* suggests that psychological tension or stress may play a major role, especially in patients with more widespread pain. When the diagnosis is presented in this way, patients more willingly accept the possibility of psychological influences on their muscle pain disorder and are more likely to take the necessary steps to address them. This also allows the physician to acknowledge that a psychological disturbance is not the primary cause.

Diagnostic Approach to Muscle Pain Syndromes

The approach to the diagnosis of muscle pain is fairly straightforward (Table 43–6). Despite a lengthy differential diagnosis (see Table 43–1), distinguishing these entities is seldom difficult in clinical practice. One difficulty can arise, however, if tension myalgia and another chronic disorder, such as rheumatoid arthritis, are present. In these cases, tension myalgia may be confused with a flare of the underlying disorder, resulting in unnecessary treatments and medications.

A study of 109 consecutive patients referred with a chief complaint of muscle pain found a specific diagnosis in only one-third of the patients.[69] The majority of the rest likely had tension myalgia (fibromyalgia, myofascial pain syndrome). The most useful laboratory screening tests were the erythrocyte sedimentation rate and serum creatine kinase activity. An abnormal result on either test prompted further evaluation with EMG and muscle biopsy. The initial evaluation should also include a complete blood cell count, thyroid function tests, and per-

TABLE 43–6 Suggested Laboratory Evaluation for Muscle Pain

Erythrocyte sedimentation rate
Serum creatine kinase
Complete blood count
Thyroid function tests
Also consider:
Electromyography
Rheumatoid factor
Antinuclear antibody
Muscle biopsy

haps tests for rheumatoid factor and antinuclear antibody.[35, 99]

As with most diagnoses in medicine, the most important aspect is a complete history and careful physical examination, in this case emphasizing the musculoskeletal and neurological components. Points to remember include the following: the pain of tension myalgia is within or over muscles or their attachments, not in the joints; the results of the neurological examination, including strength, sensation, and reflexes, are normal, as are results of the joint examination; and laboratory findings, including those noted above, are within normal limits.

Treatment of Muscle Pain Syndromes

Specific treatment usually follows specific delineation of pathophysiology. Along with the multiple theories of etiology for muscle pain syndromes come multiple, mostly unproven, methods of treatment. This section describes one approach to treatment, combining what little has been shown to be useful with what appears empirically to be useful (Fig. 43–16).

The first step in treatment is establishing the diagnosis with the patient and spending the time to help the patient understand what the diagnosis is and is not (see Tension Myalgia, above). Such education and reassurance takes time but may put an end to the constant "doctor shopping" and help the patient focus on self-management of his or her disorder.

Elimination of Contributing Factors

The next step in treatment is the elimination of contributing factors. Travell and Simons[101] reported a host of perpetuating factors for myofascial pain syndrome, including various vitamin deficiencies. A good diet is certainly important, including plenty of B vitamin sources. However, more common contributing factors include poor posture and poor body mechanics, which should be corrected to eliminate unnecessary muscle use. Anatomical variations such as a leg-length discrepancy should also be sought and corrected.

Vocational and avocational muscle overuse is a common contributing factor and must be specifically pursued. This more commonly appears with the more localized forms of muscle pain. Even so, patients with widespread pain benefit from principles such as frequent breaks for stretching and changes of position or task. It is important to specifically ask about hobbies, sports, daily tasks, and sleeping position. An ergonomic evaluation of the workplace is often valuable.

The more chronic and widespread the muscle pain syndrome, the more likely that psychological stress plays a role. Instruction in stress management techniques can be useful but if a major psychopathological disorder is suspected, formal psychiatric evaluation may be warranted. Often the more involved patients benefit from the cognitive-behavioral treatment approach[3, 76, 108] used in comprehensive pain management centers (see Chapter 42).

Poor sleep is another feature found more often in the more chronic cases. If present, it often responds to low-dose tricyclic antidepressant medications (e.g., amitriptyline, 10 to 25 mg nightly). This is one of the few treatments shown to be useful for the reduction of pain and improvement of sleep in double-blind controlled studies of patients with widespread muscle pain.[13, 36, 83]

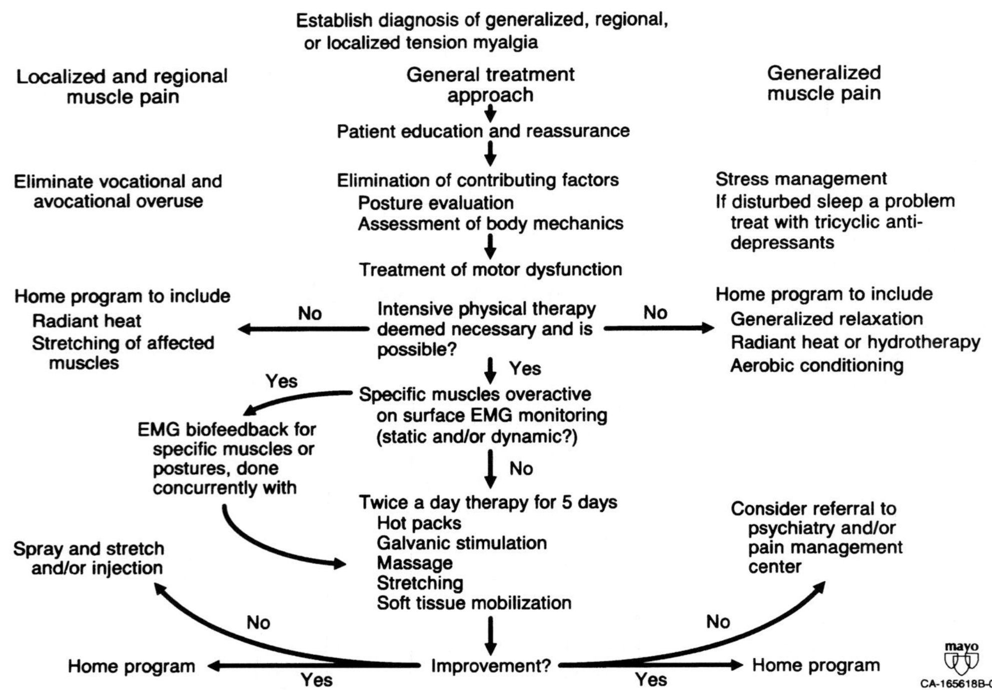

FIGURE 43–16. Treatment algorithm for tension myalgia (myofascial pain/fibromyalgia). *Central column* lists approaches useful in both localized and generalized muscle pain problems. The approaches more specific to generalized muscle pain (fibromyalgia) are in the *right column,* and the approaches more specific for localized muscle pain (myofascial pain syndromes) are in the *left column.*

Trazodone, 25 to 75 mg nightly, appears to work equally well and is better tolerated. I recommend taking it 1 hour prior to retiring to help avoid morning drowsiness. Even greater improvement may result from combination treatment with a selective serotonin re-uptake inhibitor (SSRI) in the morning and a tricyclic at night to improve sleep (e.g., 20 mg of fluoxetine in the morning and 10 to 25 mg of amitriptyline in the evening).[37] Whether these medications help in the absence of sleep disturbance remains unclear. Be sure to explain the rationale of treatment so the patient is not put off by being placed on an antidepressant.

Treatment of Motor Dysfunction

The next major category of treatment addresses the problem of motor dysfunction. This often requires specific physical therapy. The goals of treatment are to decrease pain, restore normal range of motion, restore normal neuromuscular functioning, and improve fitness.

Reducing pain will increase the patient's confidence in the treatment plan. It is also a necessary prerequisite to establishing normal motor function. One method combines hot packs and high-voltage "galvanic" stimulation to the most symptomatic area. This can be followed by deep sedative massage or gentle soft tissue mobilization. The use of these passive modalities should be limited to the early treatment phase to avoid patient dependence and the persistent notion that something must be done *to* them in order to get "fixed."

A general stretching program with special emphasis on muscle groups found to be "tight" on examination is a basic part of treatment. The patient should learn to do this several times a day. Using heat before gentle prolonged stretching may improve its effectiveness and lessen its discomfort.

The goal of neuromuscular re-education lies in restoring normal resting tone and fluid movement without co-contraction of agonists and antagonists. Surface EMG biofeedback over specific areas can be helpful, especially with the postural muscles, which often function subconsciously. Multiple muscle sites can be quickly sampled by "scanning" with hand-held post-style electrodes.[16, 100] Areas of increased activity are targeted for specific relaxation exercises. Attached surface electrodes give information about the activity of muscles in dynamic situations. This type of biofeedback helps train patients to eliminate co-contraction, and teaches them to return their muscles to electrical silence after contraction. This resting state is often missing in patients with muscle pain.[25, 105]

A short, intense course of biofeedback training (e.g., twice a day for 1 week) is often necessary in chronic, more widespread muscle pain. An excellent textbook describing specific EMG biofeedback approaches is now available.[51] Since it is difficult to relearn correct motor function after prolonged dysfunction, low-intensity biofeedback (three times a week) is likely of little utility, but this has not been studied. More acute, localized muscle pain likely will not require this labor-intensive, and therefore costly, intervention.

Once pain has been reduced and motor dysfunction minimized, a very graduated aerobic fitness program can be instituted. Again, the extent and chronicity of the muscle pain problem parallel the need for this treatment step. A controlled study of widespread muscle pain patients found an aerobic program more beneficial than stretching alone.[66] The combination of biofeedback for relaxation and a moderate exercise program (stretching and aerobic walking) maintained significant improvement for 2 years.[9] It is important to stress a very gradual return to activity to avoid fatigue and increased muscle pain. I instruct patients to start at a level that seems ridiculously easy and slowly advance from there.

Local Treatments

Localized and regional muscle pain syndromes often respond to specific localized therapies. None of these have been proved effective in adequately controlled studies. Many practitioners have great success employing them, however.

Spray and stretch is the mainstay of myofascial pain syndrome treatment (see Fig. 43–17).[101] The vapocoolant spray is used to reflexively relax the muscle to allow an adequate stretch. One maintains a sweeping pattern of spray in the direction of the muscle fibers as the muscle is passively stretched by the patient or the clinician's free hand. The coolant spray serves to distract the patient and possibly relax the treated muscle to allow for a more effective stretch. The prolonged stretch is the key element and is what provides pain relief through an as yet unknown mechanism.

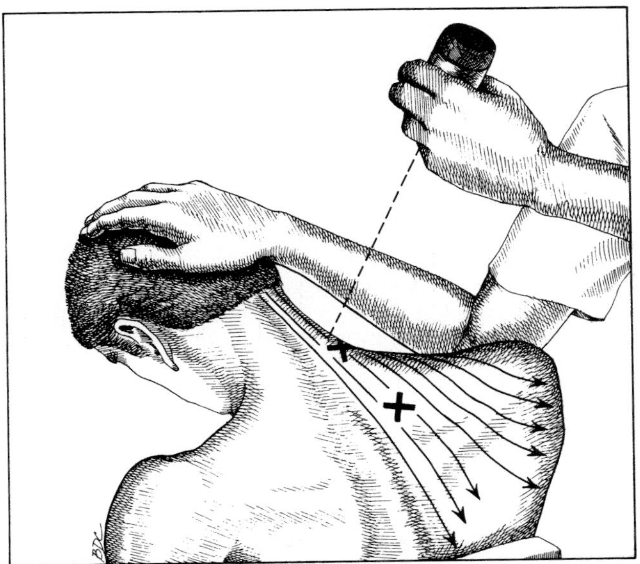

FIGURE 43–17. Technique of "spray and stretch" treatment for right levator scapulae trigger points (*X*). The *arrows* indicate the direction and pattern of the vapocoolant spray. During the "distraction" of the spray, the operator presses the patient's head forward and to the opposite side while using the elbow to press the patient's shoulder down and back. Similar techniques are applied to most other trigger points. The key ingredient is the prolonged stretch of the affected muscle. (From Travell JG, Simons DG: Myofascial Pain and Dysfunction: The Trigger Point Manual. Baltimore, Williams & Wilkins, 1983.)

The second most commonly used treatment for localized muscle pain is injection. Some practitioners simply inject the general area of the most intense pain. Others take great care in locating the "trigger point," watching for the "twitch response" on entering it with the needle. Dry needling appears to work as well as any other type, but most physicians use a local anesthetic for the sake of patient comfort. The addition of corticosteroids to the injection has many advocates but likely adds little but cost to the procedure. This has not been well studied, however. Proponents of injection focus on finding the primary trigger point, which, when treated successfully, leads to resolution of many of the secondary trigger points. Treating only the secondary points without finding the primary point is one reason for treatment failure.

Even less well studied is the use of ischemic compression to treat trigger points.[101] The theory is that sustained pressure over the pathological area induces increased blood flow on release of pressure with hyperemia of the skin. This in turn reverses the assumed localized ischemia in the underlying muscle. The digitally applied pressure lasts for about 1 minute at gradually increasing pressure as tolerated up to 30 lb.

Medications

Both amitriptyline and cyclobenzaprine have provided short-term relief in controlled studies of fibromyalgia patients[36] as noted above in the discussion of contributing factors. Anti-inflammatory agents (including corticosteroids) and analgesics are generally not useful[13, 36] and should be avoided.

The most important component of any treatment approach is the patient. The ultimate goal is to educate patients and provide them with the means to manage their own muscle pain disorder, eliminating dependence on (and overutilization of) health care providers.

REFERENCES

1. Ahles TA, Kahn SA, Yunus MB, et al: Psychiatric status of patients with primary fibromyalgia, patients with rheumatoid arthritis, and subjects without pain. Am J Psychiatry 1991; 148:1721–1726.
2. Arendt-Nielsen L, Graven-Nielsen T, Svarrer H, et al: The influence of low back pain on muscle activity and coordination during gait: A clinical and experimental study. Pain 1995; 64:231–240.
3. Bennett R, Burckhandt C, Clark S, et al: Group treatment of fibromyalgia: A 6 month outpatient program. J Rheumatol 1996; 23:521–528.
4. Bennett RM: Fibromyalgia and the facts: Sense or nonsense. Rheum Dis Clin North Am 1993; 19:45–59.
5. Bennett RM: Myofascial pain syndromes and the fibromyalgia syndrome: A comparative analysis. Adv Pain Res Ther 1990; 17:43–65.
6. Birnie DJ, Knipping AA, vanRijswijk MH, et al: Psychological aspects of fibromyalgia compared with chronic and nonchronic pain. J Rheumatol 1991; 18:1845–1848.
7. Boissevain MD, McCain GA: Toward an integrated understanding of fibromyalgia syndrome: I. Medical and pathophysiological aspects. Pain 1991; 45:227–238.
8. Boissevain MD, McCain GA: Toward an integrated understanding of fibromyalgia syndrome: II. Psychological and phenomenological aspects. Pain 1991; 45:239–248.
9. Buckelew S, Conway R, Parker J, et al: Biofeedback/relaxation training and exercise interventions for fibromyalgia: A prospective trial. Arthritis Care Res 1998; 11:196–209.
10. Campbell SM, Clark S, Tindall EA, et al: Clinical characteristics of fibrositis: I. A "blinded" controlled study of symptoms and tender points. Arthritis Rheum 1983; 26:817–824.
11. Carlson C, Wynn K, Edwards J, et al: Ambulatory electromyogram activity in the upper trapezius region: Patients with muscle pain vs pain free control subjects. Spine 1996; 21:595–599.
12. Clark S, Campbell SM, Forehand ME, et al: Clinical characteristics of fibrositis: A "blinded" controlled study using standard psychological tests. Arthritis Rheum 1985; 28:132–137.
13. Clark S, Tindall E, Bennett RM: A double blind crossover trial of prednisone versus placebo in the treatment of fibrositis. J Rheumatol 1985; 12:980–983.
14. Cobb CR, deVries HA, Urban RT, et al: Electrical activity in muscle pain. Am J Phys Med 1975; 54:80–87.
15. Conferences on Therapy: Treatment of painful disorders of skeletal muscles. NY State J Med 1948; 48:2050–2059.
16. Cram JR, Steger JC: Muscle scanning and the diagnosis of chronic pain. Biofeedback Self Regul 1983; 8:229–241.
17. Crofford L: Neuroendocrine abnormalities in fibromyalgia and related disorders. Am J Med Sci 1998; 315:359–366.
18. Crofford L, Demitrack M: Evidence that abnormalities of central neurohormonal systems are key to understanding fibromyalgia and chronic fatigue syndrome. Rheum Dis Clin North Am 1996; 22:267–284.
19. Croft P, Burt J, Schollum J, Thomas E, et al: More pain, more tender points: Is fibromyalgia just one end of a continuous spectrum? Ann Rheum Dis 1996; 55:482–485.
20. Croft P, Rigby AS, Boswell R, et al: The prevalence of chronic widespread pain in the general population. J Rheumatol 1993; 20:710–713.
21. Delaney GA, McKee AC: Inter- and intra-rater reliability of the pressure threshold meter in measurement of myofascial trigger point sensitivity. Am J Phys Med Rehabil 1993; 72:136–139.
22. Dunnette MR, Rodriquez AA, Agre JC, et al: Needle electromyographic evaluation of patients with myofascial or fibromyalgic pain. Am J Phys Med Rehabil 1991; 70:154–156.
23. Edwards RHT: Hypotheses of peripheral and central mechanisms underlying occupational muscle pain and injury. Eur J Appl Physiol 1988; 57:275–281.
24. Elert JE, Rantapaa-Dahlqvist SB, Almay B, et al: Muscle endurance, muscle tension and personality traits in patients with muscle or joint pain: A pilot study. J Rheumatol 1993; 20:1550–1556.
25. Elert JE, Rantapaa-Dahlqvist SB, Henriksson-Larsen K, et al: Increased EMG activity during short pauses in patients with primary fibromyalgia. Scand J Rheumatol 1989; 18:321–323.
26. Elert JE, Rantapaa-Dahlqvist SB, Henriksson-Larsen K, et al: Muscle performance, electromyography and fibre type composition in fibromyalgia and work-related myalgia. Scand J Rheumatol 1992; 21:28–34.
27. Elliott FA: Tender muscles in sciatica: Electromyographic studies. Lancet 1944; 1:47–49.
28. Fischer AA: Documentation of myofascial trigger points. Arch Phys Med Rehabil 1988; 69:286–291.
29. Fowler RS, Kraft GH: Tension perception in patients having pain associated with chronic muscle tension. Arch Phys Med Rehabil 1974; 55:28–30.
30. Fricton JR, Auvinen MD, Dykstra D, et al: Myofascial pain syndrome: Electromyographic changes associated with local twitch response. Arch Phys Med Rehabil 1985; 66:314–317.
31. Gantz NM, Holmes GP: Treatment of patients with chronic fatigue syndrome. Drugs 1989; 38:855–862.
32. Gold D, Bowden R, Sixby J, et al: Chronic fatigue: A prospective clinical and virologic study. JAMA 1990; 264:48–53.
33. Golden H, Weber SM, Bergen D: Sleep studies in patients with fibrositis syndrome (abstract). Arthritis Rheum 1983; 26(suppl):S32.
34. Goldenberg DL: Fibromyalgia, chronic fatigue syndrome, and myofascial pain syndrome. Curr Opin Rheumatol 1991; 3: 247–258.
35. Goldenberg DL: Fibromyalgia syndrome: An emerging but controversial condition. JAMA 1987; 257:2782–2787.
36. Goldenberg DL, Felson DT, Dinerman H: A randomized, controlled trial of amitriptyline and naproxen in the treatment of patients with fibromyalgia. Arthritis Rheum 1986; 29:1371–1377.

37. Goldenberg D, Mayskiy M, Mossey C. et al: A randomized double blind crossover trial of fluoxetine and amitriptyline in the treatment of fibromyalgia. Arthritis Rheum 1996; 39:1852–1859.
38. Gowers WR: Lumbago: Its lessons and analogues. Br Med J 1904; 1:117–121.
39. Granges G, Littlejohn G: Pressure pain threshold in pain-free subjects, in patients with chronic regional pain syndromes, and in patients with fibromyalgia syndrome. Arthritis Rheum 1993; 36:642–646.
40. Graven-Nielsen T, Svensson P, Arendt-Nielsen L: Effects of experimental muscle pain on activity and coordination during static and dynamic motor function. Electroencephalogr Clin Neurophysiol 1997; 105:156–164.
41. Gureje O, Von Korff M, Simon G, et al: Persistent pain and well being. JAMA 1998; 280:147–151.
42. Hauri P: Personal communication, February 1994.
43. Hauri P, Hawkins DR: Alpha-delta sleep. Electroencephalogr Clin Neurophysiol 1973; 34:233.
44. Henriksson KG: Pathogenesis of fibromyalgia. J Musculoskel Pain 1993; 1:3–16.
45. Henriksson KG, Bengtsson A: Fibromyalgia: A clinical entity? Can J Physiol Pharmacol 1991; 69:672–677.
46. Hoheisel U, Mense S, Ratkai M: Effects of spinal cord superfusion with substance P on the excitability of rat dorsal horn neurons processing input from deep tissues. J Musculoskel Pain 1996; 3:23–43.
47. Horne JA, Shackell BS: Alpha-like EEG activity in non-REM sleep and the fibromyalgia (fibrositis) syndrome. Electroencephalogr Clin Neurophysiol 1991; 79:271–276.
48. Hubbard DR, Berkoff GM: Myofascial trigger points show spontaneous needle activity. Spine 1993; 18:1803–1807.
49. Hudson JI, Goldenberg DL, Pope HG, et al: Comorbidity of fibromyalgia with medical and psychiatric disorders. Am J Med 1992; 92:363–367.
50. Jacobsen S, Petersen IS, Danneskiold-Samsoe B: Clinical features of patients with chronic muscle pain: With special reference to fibromyalgia. Scand J Rheumatol 1993; 22:69–76.
51. Kasman G, Cram J, Wolf S: Clinical Applications in Surface Electromyography: Chronic Musculoskeletal Pain. Gaithersburg, MD, Aspen, 1998.
52. Kellgren JH: Observations on referred pain arising from muscle. Clin Sci 1938; 3:174–190.
53. Kellgren JH: On the distribution of pain arising from deep somatic structures with charts of segmental pain areas. Clin Sci 1939; 4:35–46.
54. Kelly M: The nature of fibrositis: Part I. The myalgic lesion and its secondary effects: A reflex theory. Ann Rheum Dis 1945; 5:1–7.
55. Kelly M: The nature of fibrositis: Part II. A study of the causation of the myalgic lesion (rheumatic, traumatic, infective). Ann Rheum Dis 1946; 5:69–77.
56. Klonoff DC: Chronic fatigue syndrome. Clin Infect Dis 1992; 15:812–823.
57. Koes BW, Bouter LM, van Mameren H, et al: The effectiveness of manual therapy, physiotherapy, and treatment by the general practitioner for nonspecific back and neck complaints. Spine 1992; 17:28–35.
58. Kraft GH, Johnson EW, LaBan MM: The fibrositis syndrome. Arch Phys Med Rehabil 1968; 49:155–162.
59. Kravitz E, Moore ME, Glaros A: Paralumbar muscle activity in chronic low back pain. Arch Phys Med Rehabil 1981; 62:172–176.
60. Krusen FH: Physical therapy of fibrositis. Arch Phys Ther 1937; 18:687–697.
61. Kuch K, Cox B, Evans R, et al: To what extent do anxiety and depression interact with chronic pain? Can J Psychiatry 1993; 38:36–38.
62. Layzer RB: Muscle pain, cramps, and fatigue. In Engel AG, Banker BQ (eds): Myology. New York, McGraw-Hill, 1986, pp 1907–1922.
63. Manu P, Lane TJ, Matthews DA: The pathophysiology of chronic fatigue syndrome: Confirmations, contradictions and conjectures. Int J Psychiatry Med 1992; 22:397–408.
64. Marchettini P: Muscle pain: Animal and human experimental and clinical studies. Muscle Nerve 1993; 16:1033–1039.
65. Marchettini P, Simone D, Caputi G, et al: Pain from excitation of identified muscle nociceptors in humans. Brain Res 1996; 740:109–116.
66. McCain GA: Role of physical fitness training in fibrositis/fibromyalgia syndrome. Am J Med 1986; 81(suppl 3A):73–77.
67. Mense S: Nociception from skeletal muscle in relation to clinical muscle pain. Pain 1993; 54:241–289.
68. Mense S: Physiology of nociception in muscle. Adv Pain Res Ther 1990; 17:67–85.
69. Mills KR, Edwards RHT: Investigative stategies for muscle pain. J Neurol Sci 1983; 58:73.
70. Moldofsky H: Sleep-wake physiology and fibromyalgia. Adv Pain Res Ther 1990; 17:227–238.
71. Moldofsky H, Scarisbrick P, England R, et al: Musculoskeletal symptoms and non-REM sleep disturbance in patients with "fibrositis syndrome" and healthy subjects. Psychosom Med 1975; 37:341–351.
72. Moldofsky H, Warsh JJ: Plasma tryptophan and musculoskeletal pain in non-articular rheumatism ("fibrositis syndrome"). Pain 1978; 5:65–71.
73. Mountz J, Bradley L, Alarcon G: Abnormal functional activity of the CNS in fibromyalgia syndrome. Am J Med Sci 1998; 315:385–396.
74. Mufson M, Regestein QR: The spectrum of fibromyalgia disorders (editorial). Arthritis Rheum 1993; 36:647–650.
75. Nice DA, Riddle DL, Lamb RL, et al: Intertester reliability of judgments of the presence of trigger points in patients with low back pain. Arch Phys Med Rehabil 1992; 73:893–898.
76. Nielson WR, Walker C, McCain GA: Cognitive behavioral treatment of fibromyalgia syndrome: Preliminary findings. J Rheumatol 1992; 19:98–103.
77. Park J, Phothimat P, Oates C, et al: Use of P-31 magnetic resonance spectroscopy to detect metabolic abnormalities in muscles of patients with fibromyalgia. Arthritis Rheum 1998; 41:406–413.
78. Reeves JL, Jaeger B, Graff-Redford SB: The reliability of the pressure algometer as a measure of myofascial trigger point sensitivity. Pain 1986; 24:313–321.
79. Reilly PA, Littlejohn GO: Fibrositis/fibromyalgia syndrome: The key to the puzzle of chronic pain. Med J Aust 1990; 152:226–228.
80. Reynolds MD: The development of the concept of fibrositis. J Hist Med Allied Sci 1983; 38:5–35.
81. Saxton J, Clarkson P, James R, et al: Neuromuscular dysfunction following eccentric exercise. Med Sci Sports Exerc 1995; 27:1185–1193.
82. Schluederberg A, Straus SE, Peterson P, et al: Chronic fatigue syndrome research: Definition and medical outcome assessment. Ann Intern Med 1992; 117:325–331.
83. Scudds RA, McCain GA, Rollman GB, et al: Improvements in pain responsiveness in patients with fibrositis after successful treatment with amitriptyline. J Rheumatol 1989; 16(suppl 19):98–103.
84. Scudds RA, Trachsel LC, Luckhurst BJ, et al: A comparative study of pain, sleep quality and pain responsiveness in fibrositis and myofascial pain syndrome. J Rheumatol 1989; 16(suppl 19):120–126.
85. Simms R: Fibromyalgia is not a muscle disorder. Am J Med Sci 1998; 315:346–350.
86. Simms RW, Goldenberg DL, Felson DT, et al: Tenderness in 75 anatomic sites: Distinguishing fibromyalgia patients from controls. Arthritis Rheum 1988; 31:182–187.
87. Simons DG: Muscle pain syndromes (in two parts). Am J Phys Med 1975; 54:289–311; 1976; 55:15–42.
88. Simons DG: Muscular pain syndromes. Adv Pain Res Ther 1990; 17:1–41.
89. Skootsky SA, Jaeger B, Oye RK: Prevalence of myofascial pain in general internal medicine practice. West J Med 1989; 151:157–160.
90. Slocumb CH: Fibrositis. Clinics 1943; 2:169–178.
91. Smythe HA: Links between fibromyalgia and myofascial pain syndromes (editorial). J Rheumatol 1992; 19:842–843.
92. Smythe HA: Non-articular rheumatism and the fibrositis syndrome. In Hollander JL, McCarty DJ Jr (eds): Arthritis and Allied Conditions, ed 8. Philadelphia, Lea & Febiger, 1972, pp 874–884.
93. Smythe HA: Problems with the MMPI (editorial). J Rheumatol 1984; 11:417–418.
94. Smythe HA, Moldofsky H: Two contributions to understanding of the "fibrositis" syndrome. Bull Rheum Dis 1977; 28:928.

95. Smythe HA, Sheon RP: Fibrositis/fibromyalgia: A difference of opinion. Bull Rheum Dis 1990; 39:1–3.
96. Sorenson J, Graven-Nielsen T, Henrickson K, et al: Hyperexcitability in fibromyalgia. J Rheumatol 1998; 25:152–155.
97. Stockman R: The causes, pathology, and treatment of chronic rheumatism. Edinburgh Med J 1904; 15:107–116.
98. Swerdlow B, Dieter JNI: An evaluation of the sensitivity and specificity of medical thermography for the documentation of myofascial trigger points. Pain 1992; 48:205–213.
99. Thompson JM: Tension myalgia as a diagnosis at the Mayo Clinic and its relationship to fibrositis, fibromyalgia, and myofascial pain syndrome. Mayo Clin Proc 1991; 65:1237–1248.
100. Thompson JM, Madson TJ, Erickson RP: EMG muscle scanning: Comparison to attached surface electrodes. Biofeedback Self Regul 1991; 16:167–179.
101. Travell JG, Simons DG: Myofascial Pain and Dysfunction: The Trigger Point Manual. Baltimore, Williams & Wilkins, 1983.
102. Tunks E, Crook J, Norman G, et al: Tender points in fibromyalgia. Pain 1988; 34:11–19.
103. Tunks E, McCain G, Hart L, et al: The reliability of examination for tenderness in patients with myofascial pain chronic fibromyalgia and controls. J Rheumatol 1995; 22:944–952.
104. Turk D, Okifuji J, Sinclair D, et al: Interdisciplinary treatment for fibromyalgia syndrome: Clinical and statistical significance. Arthritis Care Res 1998; 11:186–195.
105. Veierstad KB, Westgaard RH, Andersen P: Electromyographic evaluation of muscular work pattern as a predictor of trapezius myalgia. Scand J Work Environ Health 1993; 19:284–290.
106. Weigent D, Bradley L, Blalock J, et al: Current concepts in the pathophysiology of abnormal pain perception in fibromyalgia. Am J Med Sci 1998; 315:405–412.
107. Weinberger LM: Fibrositis (letter). West J Med 1981; 135:425.
108. White K, Nielson W: Cognitive-behavioral treatment of fibromyalgia syndrome: A follow-up assessment. J Rheumatol 1995; 22:717–721.
109. Wolfe F: The epidemiology of fibromyalgia. J Musculoskel Pain 1993; 1:137–148.
110. Wolfe F: Fibrositis, fibromyalgia, and musculoskeletal disease: The current status of the fibrositis syndrome. Arch Phys Med Rehabil 1988; 69:527–531.
111. Wolfe F: What use are fibromyalgia control points? J Rheumatol 1998; 25:546–550.
112. Wolfe F, Cathey MA: Prevalence of primary and secondary fibrositis. J Rheumatol 1983; 10:965–968.
113. Wolfe F, Simons DG, Fricton J, et al: The fibromyalgia and myofascial pain syndromes: A preliminary study of tender points and trigger points in persons with fibromyalgia, myofascial pain syndrome and no disease. J Rheumatol 1992; 19:944–951.
114. Wolfe F, Smythe HA, Yunus MB, et al: The American College of Rheumatology 1990 criteria for the classification of fibromyalgia. Arthritis Rheum 1990; 33:160–172.
115. Yunus MB: Diagnosis, etiology and management of fibromyalgia syndrome: An update. Compr Ther 1988; 14:8–20.
116. Yunus MB: Towards a model of pathophysiology of fibromyalgia: Aberrant central pain mechanisms with peripheral modulation. J Rheumatol 1992; 19:846–850.
117. Yunus MB, Kalyan-Raman UP: Muscle biopsy findings in primary fibromyalgia and other forms of nonarticular rheumatism. Rheum Dis North Am 1989; 15:115–134.
118. Yunus MB, Kalyan-Raman UP, Kalyan-Raman K: Primary fibromyalgia syndrome and myofascial pain syndrome: Clinical features and muscle patholgy. Arch Phys Med Rehabil 1988; 69;451–454.
119. Yunus MB, Masi AT, Calabro JJ, et al: Primary fibromyalgia (fibrositis): Clinical study of 50 patients with matched normal controls. Semin Arthritis Rheum 1981; 11:151–171.

44 CHAPTER

Edward R. Laskowski, M.D.

Concepts in Sports Medicine

Kraus and Conroy[80] estimated that 3 to 5 million sports-related injuries were treated in the United States in 1984. Women's sports participation is now at an all-time high. Many medical specialties now include sports medicine as a practice domain, for example, internal medicine, family practice, pediatrics, emergency medicine, orthopedics, and physical medicine and rehabilitation. Physiatrists are in a unique position to be important providers of care for musculoskeletal sports injuries. Because most sports injuries are musculoskeletal and do not require surgical treatment, appropriate care is best provided by someone who understands the anatomy, biomechanics, kinesiology, and rehabilitation principles related to a particular sport and injury. Physiatrists have the most comprehensive training and background in each of these realms. Furthermore, the physiatric focus on a team concept of medical care is perfectly suited to the interdisciplinary care often required in sports medicine. For example, for any given sport, the team might include athletic trainers, physical therapists, coaches, team owners, a sports psychologist, physicians, and, of course, athletes. Physiatric training provides much experience in the leadership and effective coordination necessary for these multidisciplinary team members to function for the maximum benefit of the patient. In addition, the prescription of therapeutic and prophylactic exercise should be considered similar to the prescription of a medication. Exercise has indications, contraindications, side effects, optimal uses, and suboptimal uses. The physiatrist has a unique knowledge base to prescribe exercise appropriately. In essence, physiatrists are ideally suited for the practice of sports medicine, and sports medicine is becoming an increasingly popular part of residency and post-residency training.[49]

Physiatrists are also well equipped to address the sport-specific and disability-specific requirements of physically challenged athletes. The Americans with Disabilities Act (ADA) mandates equal opportunity for sports and recreation for persons with physical disabilities. The use of sports and conditioning-training exercises to prepare for sports is an excellent way of continuing therapeutic exercise. Unique considerations with respect to physically challenged athletes and young athletes are considered later in this chapter.

GENERAL CONCEPTS OF THE MUSCULOSKELETAL SYSTEM

Muscle

A detailed description of the anatomy and structure of muscle fibers is beyond the scope of this chapter. However, it is important to understand the mechanism and ramifications of muscle injury. Muscle injury can occur from direct macrotrauma, tissue invasion (via laceration), and repetitive microtrauma (overuse).[95] Failure often occurs when a muscle reaches overload at the myotendinous junction.[10, 57] During the healing process of a muscle injury—and after the inflammatory phase subsides and tissue healing, repair, and remodeling occur—concomitant changes take place in muscle function unless appropriate treatment is undertaken. Deficits in absolute strength, strength balance (i.e., agonist vs. antagonist muscle groups), flexibility, and proprioception (via cutaneous, muscle, and joint receptors) can occur.[73, 139] If treatment is not initiated, these deficits are likely to predispose the patient to further injury at the same site or at a distal site in the kinetic chain. The *kinetic chain,* which is referred to frequently in this chapter, can be thought of as the linked system of muscles, joints, and body segments involved in a particular biomechanical movement or task. Often, the site of pain may not be the actual origin of the problem; thus, the patient should be carefully evaluated for biomechanical, strength, and/or flexibility problems, both proximal and distal to the site of injury.

Tendons

Tendons connect muscle to bone. Their primary function is to transmit muscle force to the osseous skeleton, with minimal change in their inherent length. Tendons consist of densely packed collagen fibers that have a high tensile strength. The fibers are arranged in parallel with one another and are oriented toward the tensile pull of the muscle.[7] Herring and Nilson[64] and Barfred[22] indicate that tendons can be damaged if (1) a force is applied rapidly and obliquely through the tendon, (2) the tendon is under tension before the load is applied, (3) the musculotendinous group is stretched, (4) the attached muscle is maximally contracted, or (5) the tendinous structure itself is weak in comparison with the muscle.

Tendon healing basically occurs in three phases. The first 48 to 72 hours of healing is known as the *inflammatory phase* and is characterized by an influx of vasoactive substances, chemotactic factors, and degradative enzymes.[127] The second phase is reparative and entails collagen production. The collagen fibers laid down during this phase have little strength because they occur in a random, haphazard pattern. During the final phase of healing, the mechanical strength of the healing tendon increases with the maturation and remodeling of fiber architecture. This increase in strength occurs along the direction of muscle force. The latter principle is crucial in injury rehabilitation; it is the basis for early mobilization and is the reason why soft tissue is not immobilized for a prolonged period unless absolutely dictated by the injury. The tensile strength of the scar tissue is not optimum unless specific and gradually applied stressors are placed on the healing tissue.[4, 5, 123, 146, 147]

It is important to note that beyond the acute inflammation and repair response, chronic repetitive microtrauma to the tendon can lead to a condition of degenerative change and damage. This pathological condition has been called *tendinosis*.[84] Conditions in which tendinosis is common include plantar fasciitis, lateral epicondylitis, patellar tendinitis, and Achilles tendinitis.[36, 83, 119] In tendinosis, cell degeneration and tissue changes, rather than an active inflammatory response, are the principal causes of pain and dysfunction. Tendinosis requires a complete analysis of kinetic chain function, including flexibility, muscle balance, and proximal and distal mechanics and kinesiology, rather than mere control of inflammation. "Weak links" in kinetic chain biomechanics and function must be corrected to avoid repetitive tissue stress and damage. In addition, prolonged use of nonsteroidal anti-inflammatory drugs (NSAIDs) in a tendinosis condition must seriously be questioned.

Ligaments

Ligaments consist of dense connective tissue and connect bone to bone. They have a mechanical stabilizing effect on joints. Ligaments contain proprioceptive afferents that provide feedback to the musculoskeletal system. Injuries to ligaments usually result from a large overload force. As with tendons, early motion is important to maximize tensile strength of a healing ligament.[6, 106] Continued research is needed on the time course of revascularization and recovery of strength in various ligaments after injury. With respect to patellar tendon grafts used for anterior cruciate ligament reconstruction, it is theorized that the graft tissue revascularizes more quickly with controlled stress, becoming stronger through hypertrophy during revascularization and, consequently, reducing the likelihood of complications.[130]

The neuromuscular role of ligaments should not be ignored. It has been emphasized that in addition to the role of ligaments in mechanical restraint, their role in neurosensory function could be just as important.[26, 158] Palmer[109] was perhaps the first to propose that ligaments supply the central nervous system with input that enables neuromuscular control of the knee joint. Cohen and Cohen[39] coined the term *arthrokinetic reflex* and suggested that the knee joint capsule is the origin of protective afferent input and that co-contraction of the quadriceps and hamstring muscles is necessary for knee joint stability. Abbott and colleagues[1] stated that ligaments are the first link in the kinetic chain and provide rich sensory input to the central nervous system. Recent studies seem to indicate that when an injury occurs to the passive mechanical constraint system, new demands are placed on the dynamic restraints because of a loss of afferent feedback. Retraining of dynamic stability becomes a key to adaptation and complete rehabilitation.

Bursae

Bursae are sacs formed by two layers of synovial tissue. The sacs usually contain a thin layer of synovial fluid. Bursae are located at sites of friction between tendon and bone. Often, they can communicate with an adjacent synovial sac. With overuse or repetitive trauma, bursae can be injured by friction or external pressure. They also can become inflamed through the degeneration and calcification of an overlying tendon (e.g., subacromial bursitis due to calcific supraspinatus tendinitis). The response of bursae to injury usually consists of inflammation, with resultant effusion and thickening of the bursal wall.

GENERAL CONCEPTS OF THE CARDIOVASCULAR SYSTEM

The importance of maintaining appropriate cardiovascular conditioning during sports participation and injury rehabilitation is well known. The deleterious effects of bed rest and activity limitation have been well documented. Complications of inactivity include cardiovascular and musculoskeletal deconditioning, bone loss, orthostatic hypotension, deep venous thrombosis, contracture, and pressure ulceration (see Chapter 32).[27, 98, 117, 131] A 50% reduction in gains of aerobic capacity due to exercise has been shown in only 4 to 12 weeks of "detraining."[56, 72, 122] Convertino,[40] Saltin,[126] and Taylor[143] and their colleagues have shown decrements in aerobic capacity and related cardiovascular variables when subjects remain on bed rest for an extended period. Oxygen uptake decreases, as do cardiac output, stroke volume, and heart volume. In any musculoskeletal sports injury the principle of "relative rest" applies. This principle dictates that the injured body part should be "rested" and protected from further trauma or injury while the remaining muscle mass is used to provide appropriate stress to the cardiovascular system for maintaining optimal aerobic conditioning (see Chapter 32). In addition, strength training should continue in uninvolved body parts. "Crossover" training effects have been documented in the rested limb when the contralateral limb is exercised.[102]

INJURY PREVENTION AND PRE-REHABILITATION

The origin of the term pre-rehabilitation, or *prehabilitation (prehab)*, which has become popular in recent years, is unclear. The term refers to rehabilitative exercises that are performed preoperatively to enhance the postoperative outcome. Theoretically, pre-rehabilitation can enhance the neuromuscular engram and hasten motor learning of the rehabilitative program after the surgical procedure. In addition, pre-rehabilitation can refer to exercises that are used to prevent injury or to prevent previously delineated biomechanical or kinetic chain deficits from contributing to musculoskeletal injury. The current scientific support for the role of a specific exercise in prevention of a specific injury is minimal. Instead of being able to truly "prevent" (keep from happening) injury, we might be able to "protect" (shield) against injury with prophylactic programs.

The seven main components of a hypothetical protective exercise program are listed in Table 44–1. They include flexibility, strength training, aerobic training, analysis of kinetic chain function, proprioception, sport-specific and higher level skills training, and the incorporation of these elements into a practical training program.

TABLE 44–1 Main Components of a Protective Exercise Program

Flexibility
Strength training
Aerobic training
Analysis of kinetic chain functions
Proprioception
Sport-specific and higher level skills
Practical training program

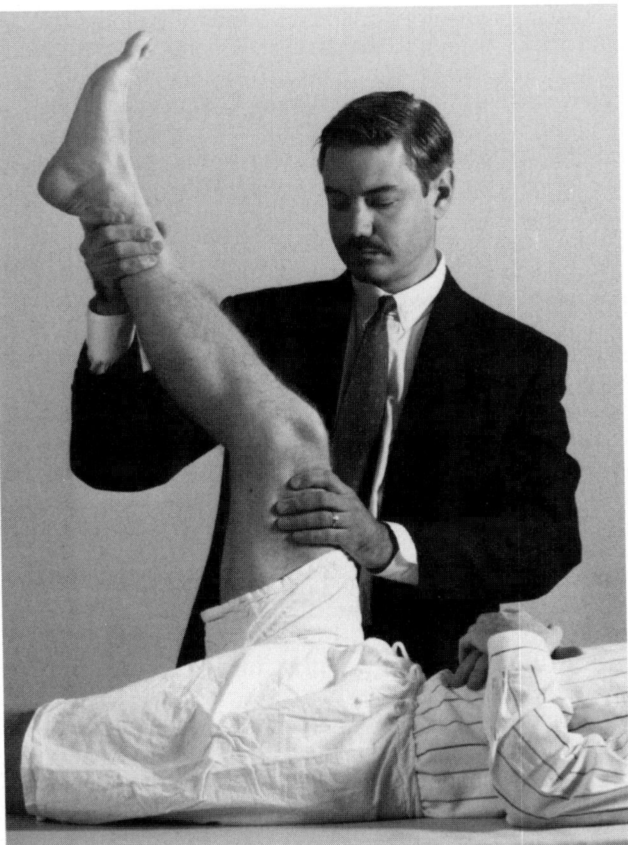

FIGURE 44–1. The popliteal angle is an objective measure of hamstring tightness. The angle is measured while the hip is flexed at 90 degrees.

Flexibility

Historically, emphasis has been placed on an appropriate and comprehensive stretching program to reduce injuries. Data that indicate a direct association between objective measures of flexibility and either increased or decreased risk of musculoskeletal injury are few. Poor flexibility could contribute to injury,[81] but optimal flexibility has not been defined. Protection from injury probably does not require the flexibility of a ballet dancer, but a certain base level (not yet determined) might be necessary to prevent tensile overload of the muscles in all range-of-motion planes, especially at the extremes.

There are also differing opinions about the relative contribution of the muscular and neurologic systems to muscle flexibility. Relaxation strategies to affect the neurophysiologic tone of the muscle may play a role comparable to stretching of the viscoelastic elements.

Muscles that cross two joints can have an especially powerful impact on kinetic chain function. Tightness of these muscles can have more wide-ranging sequelae than for muscles crossing only one joint. In the lower extremities, hamstring flexibility can be measured objectively by measuring the popliteal angle (Fig. 44–1). In performing this test, the hip must first be flexed to 90 degrees; the knee is then gradually extended toward full extension. Performing only a straight-leg raise can give a false impression of adequate hamstring flexibility, because the proximal hamstrings will not be "hooked" around the ischial tuberosity if the leg is directly elevated without the hip first being flexed.

Quadriceps flexibility (specifically, the rectus femoris) can be measured with the Ely test (Fig. 44–2), and the distance from the buttock to the heel (or the knee flexion angle) can be recorded to gauge improvement as the flexibility program progresses. Flexibility of the Achilles tendon can be gauged by measuring the degree of dorsiflexion that can be attained with the foot in a partially supinated position (Fig. 44–3). Iliotibial band tightness can be measured with the Ober test (Fig. 44–4), although there is no reliable objective measurement for this maneuver.

In the upper extremities, range of motion at the wrists and elbows can be measured goniometrically. With respect to the shoulder, external and internal rotation have special significance (discussed later) and should be measured bilaterally.

Asymmetry, rather than "perfect" geometry, might be the most important clinical aspect of flexibility, especially after an injury. One of the most important predictors of future injury is a history of past injury, and any flexibility deficit and asymmetry can increase the risk of musculoskeletal injury or reinjury.[77] Even without previous injury, stretching can help physiologically to prevent injury in many ways. Janda and associates[69] have shown that tight and inflexible muscles can act like an effusion and have an inhibitory effect on antagonist muscle groups. This inhibitory effect probably occurs through the afferent proprioceptive arc, and preparticipation stretching might decrease facilitation of muscle spindle afferents and assist the facilitation of Golgi tendon organs.[47] In addition, Noonan and colleagues[105] have shown that stretching can increase the temperature of the tendon, which can have a protective effect via increased skeletal muscle tensile strength.

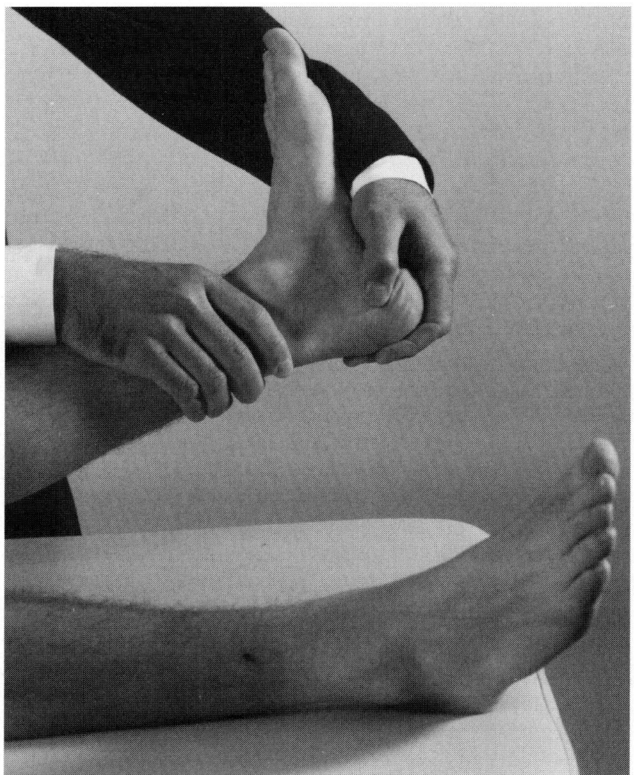
FIGURE 44–3. Testing foot dorsiflexion as a measure of tightness of the Achilles tendon. Note that the examiner's forearm keeps the subject's heel in partial supination.

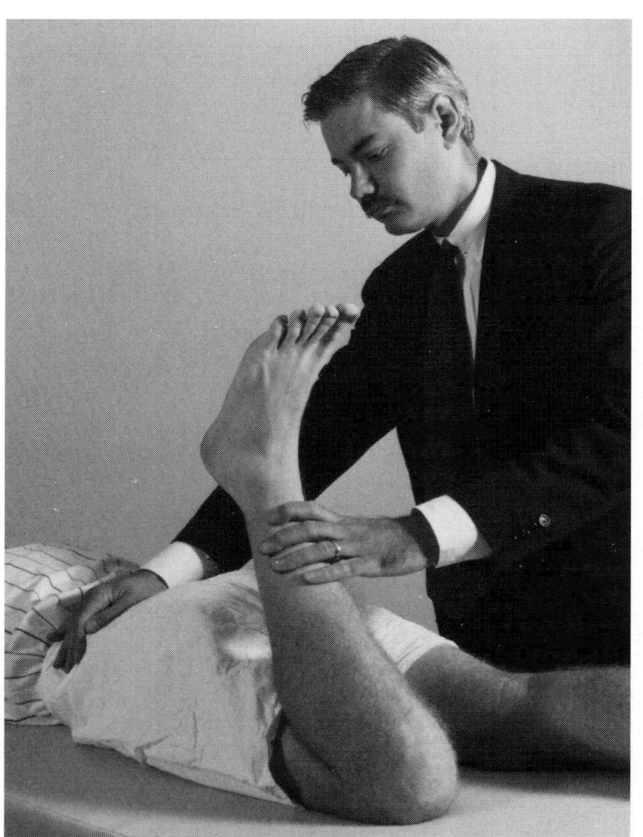
FIGURE 44–2. Ely test for evaluating tightness of the rectus femoris.

Proper stretching technique is crucial, because both the positioning of the body during the stretch and the duration of hold are important in maximizing the result of the stretch. For example, a common mistake in the gastrocnemius-soleus stretch occurs when the patient externally rotates the rear foot (Fig. 44–5). This takes the vector of stretch off the main bulk of the Achilles tendon. Ballistic, aggressive stretching without previously warming up is likely to contribute to muscle microtrauma and, subsequently, to contracted scar tissue—results that are opposite to the goal of stretching. Conversely, sport-specific, gradually progressive dynamic stretching (i.e., progressive high kicks in martial arts) can be beneficial to reset proprioceptors and to prepare the muscle for the demands of the sport or exercise. Proper positioning of the body while stretching is essential to ensure that the muscle group being stretched is isolated while the rest of the musculoskeletal system is protected. For example, there are many ways

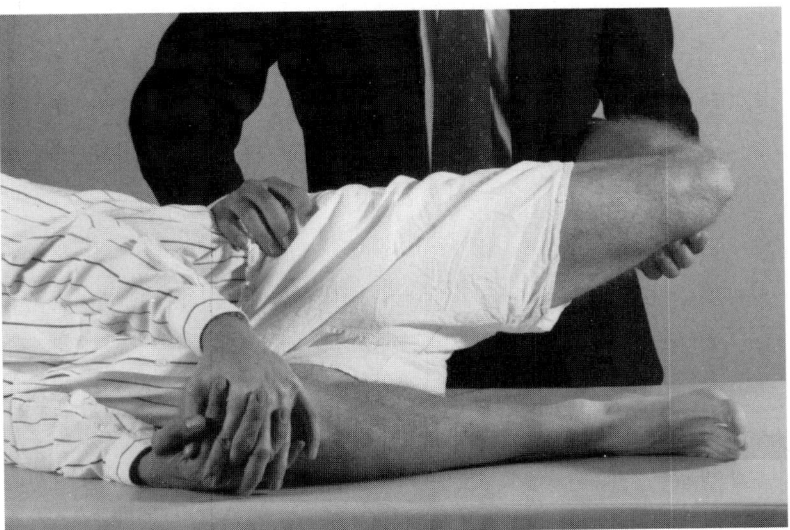

FIGURE 44–4. In the Ober test of the iliotibial band, the hip is passively extended with the pelvis in a neutral position to ensure that the tensor fascia lata passes over the greater trochanter. Tightness of the iliotibial band is present if the leg remains elevated above the horizontal.

to stretch the hamstrings, but some of these could be injurious to the low back.

The duration of the stretch is also important, because stretches of short duration (5 to 10 seconds) probably do not provide enough stimulus to cause the temporary elongation, or creep, of tissue that promotes permanent changes in muscle length. If the central nervous system influences muscular flexibility, improved relaxation may also contribute to increasing muscle length. The optimal duration for a stretch is still a matter of controversy, but the evidence favors holding the stretch for 15 to 30 seconds and repeating it three to five times.[142] This probably is much longer than most people are accustomed to holding a stretch. It is advisable for the novice to look at the second hand of a watch or to use a stop watch to make sure that the stretch is held for an adequate time. Ideally, the stretch should be performed before and after the competition or exercise period. If stretching is going to be done only once, it should be *after* the exercise session. Lehmann and associates[87] have shown in an animal model that the percentage increase in tendon length is greater when the tendon is stretched at a temperature of 45°C than at 25°C (Fig. 44–6). After a session of exercise, increased deep muscle

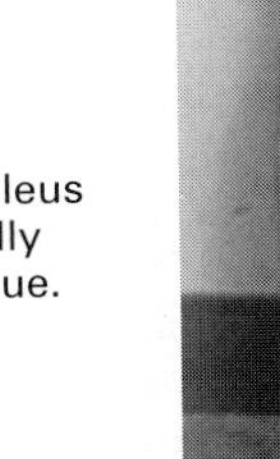

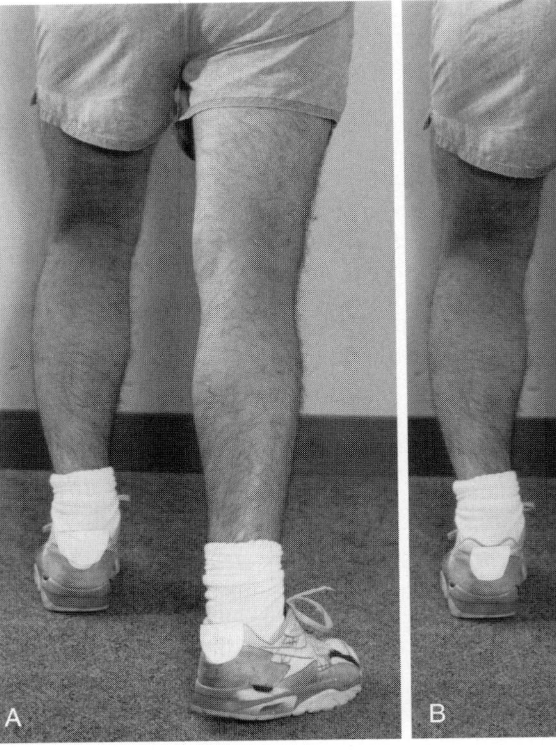

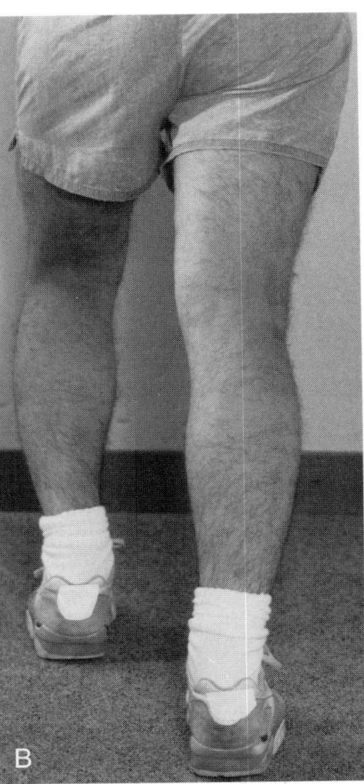

FIGURE 44–5. Technique for gastrocnemius-soleus stretch. *A.* Incorrect technique. Note externally rotated and elevated foot. *B.* Correct technique.

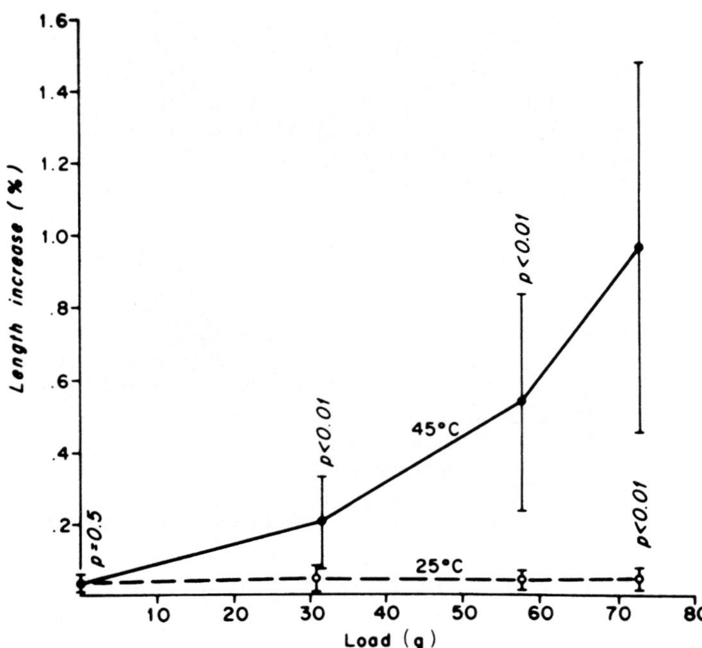

FIGURE 44–6. Percentage increase in tendon length as function of load (in grams) at 45°C and at 25°C. (From Lehmann JF, Massock AJ, Warren CG, et al: Effect of therapeutic temperatures on tendon extensibility. Arch Phys Med Rehabil 1970; 51:481. By permission of WB Saunders.)

blood flow can increase tissue temperature far greater than superficial heat can. Jogging for even a short time can increase tissue temperature and aid in facilitating stretches.[92]

There are also age-specific and sport-specific stretching concerns. For example, specific muscle tightness (i.e., quadriceps) during adolescence can have an impact on growth-related musculoskeletal problems, such as Osgood-Schlatter disease. More concentrated stretching on two-joint muscles (such as the hamstrings, hip flexors, and rectus femoris) is important during this stage. Older adults have specific flexibility concerns with respect to posture and biomechanics. Hamstring and hip flexor flexibility are particularly important as a person ages. Stretching the muscles that are used in specific sports (and in playing specific positions in a sport) should also be considered. The hip adductors and shoulder rotators, for example, are especially important in tennis, the hamstrings in running (especially sprints), and the hip flexors and hip adductors in soccer. When an active person changes sports during the year, requirements for stretching can also change. For example, someone who bicycles during the summer can develop tightness in the rectus femoris from the relatively constrained hip extension during cycling. When the same person begins cross-country skiing (a sport that requires hip extension) in the winter, the risk of straining a hip flexor may increase.

Finally, one of the most effective means of stretching a chronically tight muscle is to strengthen the antagonist muscle. As an example, tight gastrocsoleus muscles can often be passively stretched by strengthening the anterior tibialis, and tight hamstrings can be passively stretched by strengthening the quadriceps group. Correcting these strength imbalances may contribute to increased static and dynamic flexibility.

Protective Strength Training

The role of strength training in preventing injury depends primarily on two mechanisms. First, a stronger muscle is able to absorb more tensile loading and force before breakdown occurs either in the muscle itself or at the musculotendinous junction.[21] Second, it is important clinically to address any relative muscle weakness, asymmetry, or imbalance (discussion follows).[32] Some examples of muscle deficiency that lead to musculoskeletal problems include weakness of the oblique fibers of the vastus medialis and patellofemoral pain, weakness of the scapular stabilizers and shoulder pain or dysfunction, and weakness of abdominal muscles and back or lower extremity (or both) problems.

Aerobic Training

Aerobic exercise can be a key component of a preventive musculoskeletal exercise program. The cardiovascular protective effects of aerobic exercise are well known, and for endurance athletes, aerobic exercise is essential in improving maximum oxygen uptake ($\dot{V}_{O_2}$ max).[13, 19, 28, 63, 93, 129] Less well delineated are the benefits of aerobic exercise that can accrue to the musculoskeletal system. Strength and some components of flexibility depend on a solid aerobic base, because the ability of the muscles to generate and to absorb force depends on the availability of adequate adenosine triphosphate (ATP). Aerobic conditioning can ensure good aerobic metabolism and maximize production of ATP. The documented muscle effects of aerobic exercise include increased capillary density, increased number of mitochondria and mitochrondrial oxidative enzymes, improved usage of free fatty acids, and increased percentage of type IIA muscle fibers (i.e., the fibers capable of adapting to endurance or short-burst activities).[2, 15, 41, 42, 66, 67, 104, 112] These alterations in skeletal muscle with aerobic training favor improvement in the "lactate threshold," or onset of blood lactate accumulation. This is favorable for endurance sports because muscle fatigue is lessened, but these alterations can also favor and enhance musculoskeletal performance.

Decreased muscular fatigue could lead to a decrease in the number of musculoskeletal injuries. Nygaard and colleagues[107] have shown that in the vastus lateralis muscle there is an average 50% decrement of glycogen on day 5 compared with day 1 of consecutive daily alpine skiing. These authors also noted that most skiing injuries occur toward the end of the ski week and at the end of a ski day, and are likely related to muscle fatigue caused by glycogen depletion. Endurance athletes generally use fats more efficiently and effectively during exercise and, in essence, are able to "spare glycogen."[93] This occurs in part because endurance athletes accumulate less lactic acid via the above mechanisms than untrained persons at the same work output.

Aerobic exercise should be an essential component of training to prevent early musculoskeletal fatigue, since this might help prevent injury. Increased capillary density also helps combat the relative ischemia of a tight muscle group, perhaps contributing to earlier washout of lactic acid. Strength training can negate some of the beneficial effects of increased capillary density,[19, 42, 93, 140, 144] and a regular aerobic component can help balance this seemingly counterproductive effect.

With respect to sport-specific upper extremity training for exercises or sports that primarily use the arms (e.g., swimming and kayaking), the onset of lactate accumulation occurs earlier during arm exercise than during leg exercise.[114, 115] When subjects pursue endurance training with the arms, they have less accumulation of lactate and higher values of $\dot{V}_{O_2}$ max.[30]

For sports specificity, for decreasing fatigue, and for avoiding musculoskeletal injury, aerobic training should be considered an essential component of the exercise prescription. Of course, sport-specific training orients most of the work toward the predominant energy system that the sport requires. The energy systems include ATP-phosphocreatinine, anaerobic, and aerobic systems.

ATP-Phosphocreatinine Energy System. The ATP-phosphocreatinine system provides for explosive power and is extremely short-lived (5 to 10 seconds).[63] Training in this system helps to improve speed and quickness. Traditionally, this system has been thought to be enhanced through plyometric-type activities that stress muscle power (discussion follows). Lower-weight, higher-repetition weight training that emphasizes speed and explosiveness of movement is thought to enhance this energy system. To exploit maximal power, however, one desires maximal recruitment of motor units "on demand." Rather than plyometric activities, one-repetition maximal resistance training sessions might also help to neuromuscularly train the development and availability of maximal motor unit activity.

Anaerobic Energy System. Intermediate-duration (60 to 90 seconds) power comes from the anaerobic energy system (glycolysis).[63] Training of this type enables high-speed, high-intensity activity to be sustained over short periods of time. Exercises that enhance this energy system include 220- and 440-yard sprints, stair runs, and interval training on a bicycle, running, or with in-line skates.

Aerobic Energy System. Aerobic training enables sustained intervals of higher intensity exercise and quicker recovery between exercise sessions. It also allows more frequent periods of high-intensity exercise.[63] In aerobically fit persons, the transport of oxygen to the tissues and muscles is more efficient and recovery from a strenuous day of sport or exercise is quicker.

Kinetic Chain Function

The importance of analyzing kinetic chain mechanics cannot be overstated. Attending only to the local area of pain and treating this area exclusively can contribute to perpetuation of symptoms. For example, lateral epicondylitis (tennis elbow) is manifested as tenderness to palpation at the lateral epicondyle and forearm extensor muscle mass. This area can be iced and anti-inflammatory medication can be given, but if the biomechanical deficits of suboptimal wrist or shoulder strength, flexibility, or mechanics are not addressed, and if potential problems with sports equipment (such as high tension of the strings in a graphite racquet) are not considered, the problem will continue. Another frequent example is shoulder pain in a baseball pitcher. Local modalities and shoulder exercises can be attempted for pain relief, but unless the biomechanics of the throwing motion are analyzed to ensure that kinetic chain function is normal, the problem might not be entirely addressed. For example, a pitcher might "open up" (hips facing toward home plate) early during delivery, increasing the force load and stress on the shoulder and elbow. Furthermore, the spine and proper spine mechanics and function are essential for effectively transmitting ground reaction force into the upper extremities, and the scapular stabilizer muscles are important in ensuring that the humeral head maintains its center of rotation in the glenoid fossa during the throw.

With respect to overuse and macrotraumatic musculoskeletal injuries, a therapeutic intervention must occur to make the person "different" before he or she returns to the sport or activity that originally caused the problem. This "different" transformation occurs during rehabilitation, as suggested by Gray.[61] The injured tissue must be modified to deal more effectively with the loads and mechanics of the sport or activity and be reintegrated into the functional kinetic chain through a logical progression of sport-specific exercises. Gray[61] coined the term "integrated isolation" to describe the importance of understanding the site of injury, tightness, malalignment, or strength deficit, and how integration of this region into the kinetic chain can contribute to excessive loading, overuse, or injury.

There are many ways of incorporating kinetic chain exercises that occur in a proprioceptively enriched environment and that can be specific for integration of various upper extremity and lower extremity biomechanical movements. Various functional upper extremity and lower extremity exercises include the use of multiple joints and muscle co-contraction (Fig. 44–7). These exercises are sport- and life-specific and use muscle groups in a coordinated fashion rather than in an isolated one.

Building on the concept of "integrated isolation," Gray[61] pointed out that we probably should stretch in a kinetic chain fashion because this is the way that the tissue is normally used. Isolated stretches can help to heal and to modify tissue at the site of injury, but true functional stretch can occur only when the tissue is incorporated into the loads it will be experiencing in the kinetic chain (Fig. 44–8).

Proprioception

A new frontier in musculoskeletal medicine is the development and expansion of knowledge about the afferent

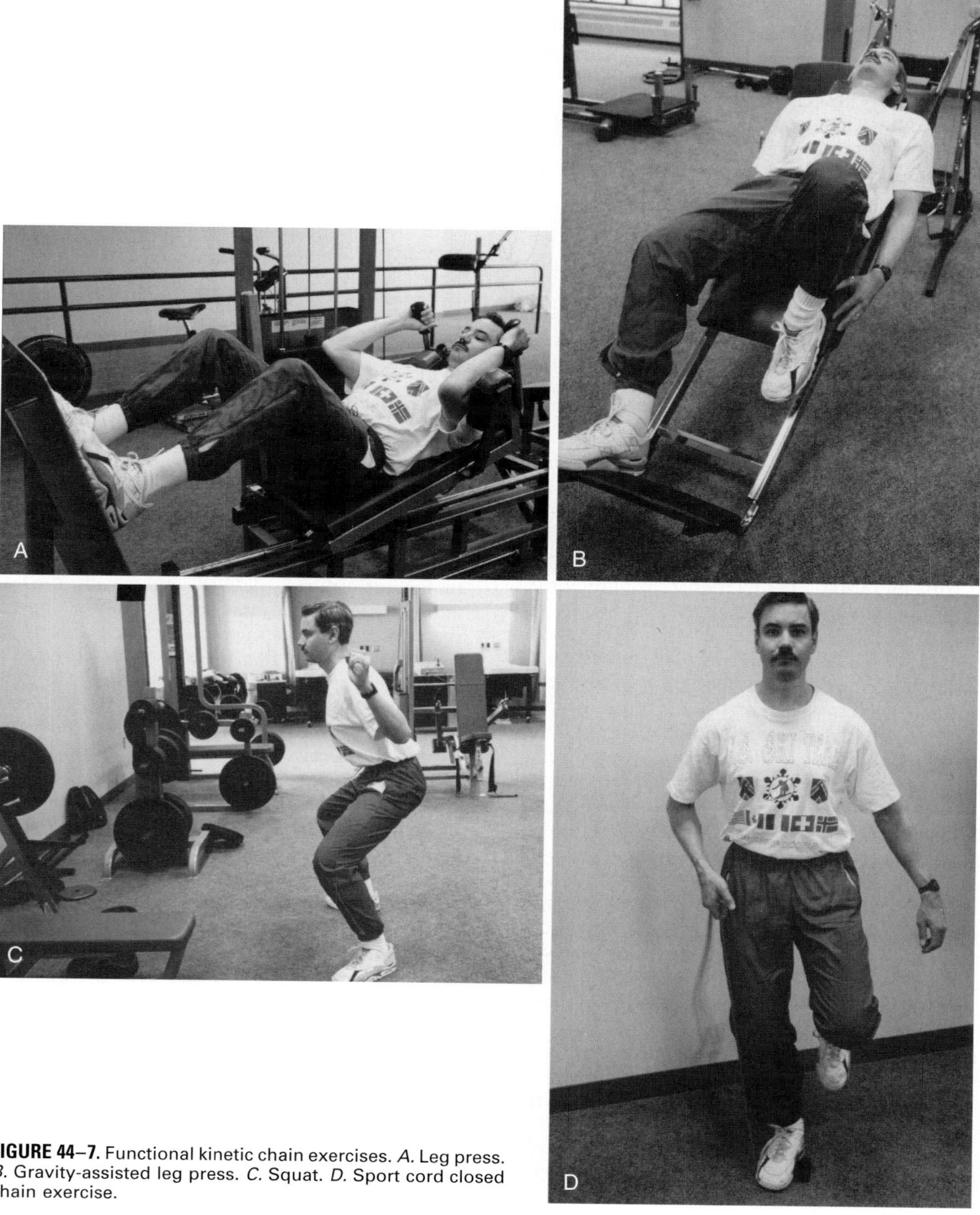

FIGURE 44–7. Functional kinetic chain exercises. *A.* Leg press. *B.* Gravity-assisted leg press. *C.* Squat. *D.* Sport cord closed chain exercise.

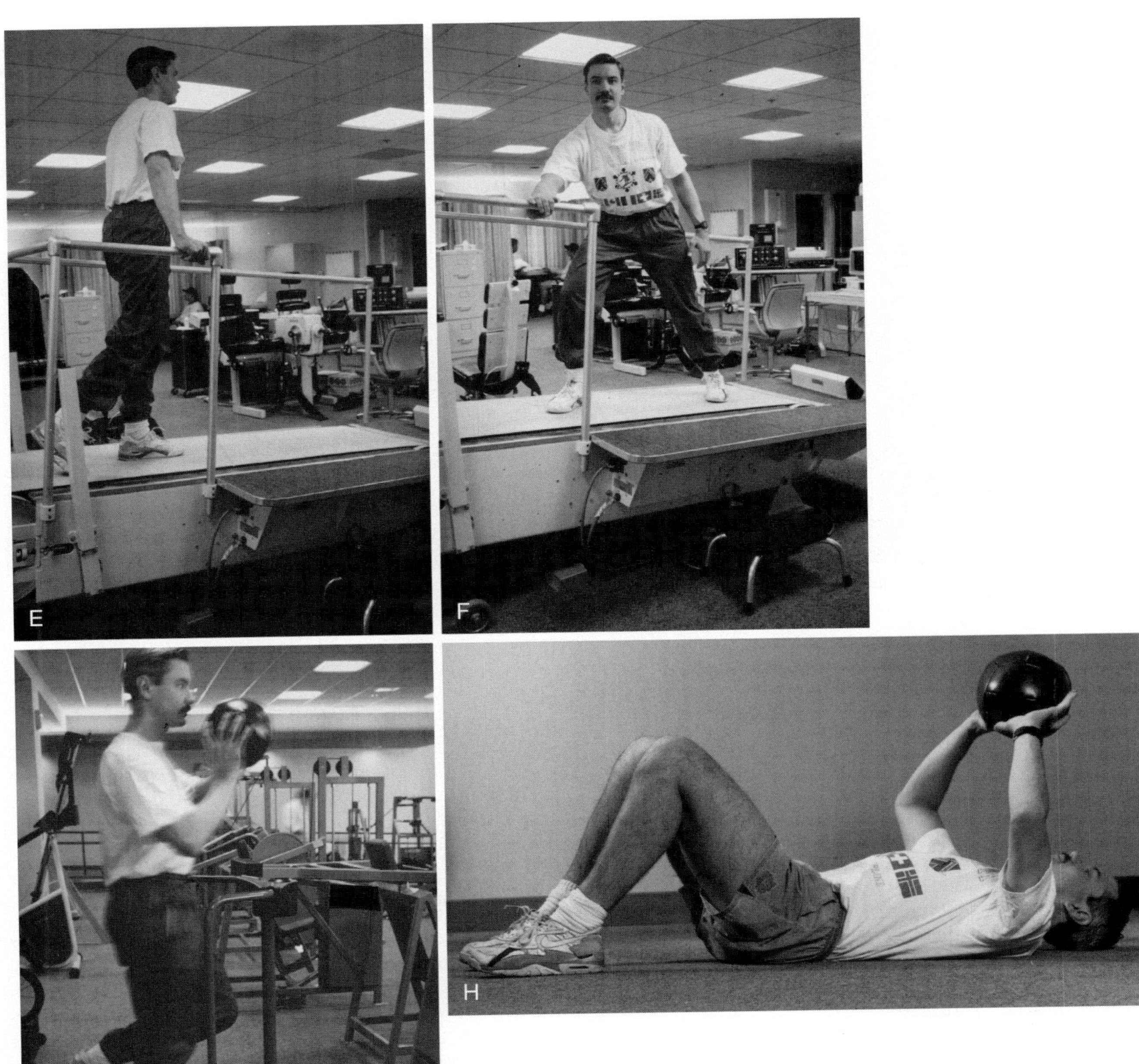

FIGURE 44–7 *Continued. E.* Retrowalking. *F.* Lateral walking. *G.* Combined upper and lower extremity exercises (proprioceptively enriched). *H.* Upper extremity medicine ball.

sensory pathway for movement: proprioception. The term *proprioception* is controversial because there is no agreement about its definition.[16, 17, 51, 118, 136] Proprioception can be thought of as a complex neuromuscular process that allows the body to maintain proper stability and orientation whether moving or standing still. Injury to a joint can cause direct or indirect alterations in the innervation of mechanoreceptors. As a consequence, messages to and from these joint receptors are disrupted, and deafferentation (disruption of input information) leads to insufficient or uncoordinated activation of muscle groups. For example, an ankle sprain might heal, but because of deafferentation, a patient might still complain of looseness without gross mechanical instability. This looseness, which can be termed "functional instability," can impair performance and increase the risk of reinjury. One of the most important predictors of future injury is a history of previous injury.[151]

With stabilometry (the quantitative measurement of postural equilibrium based on changes in the center of

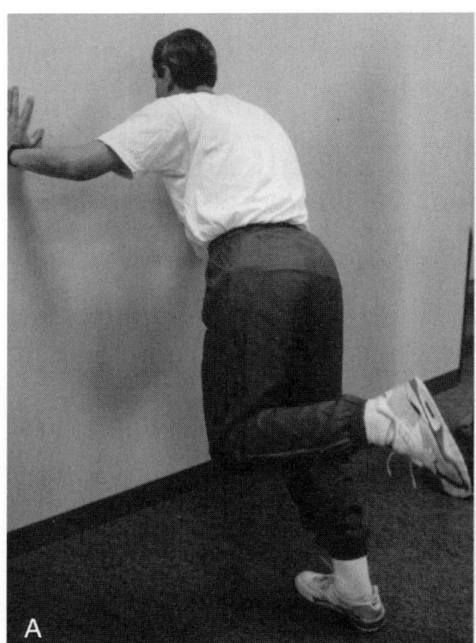
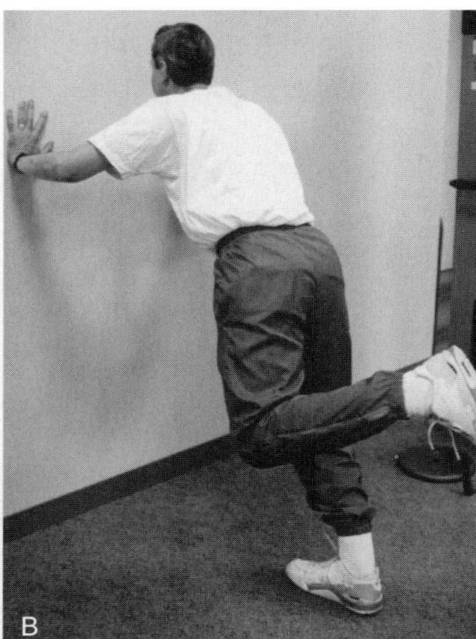
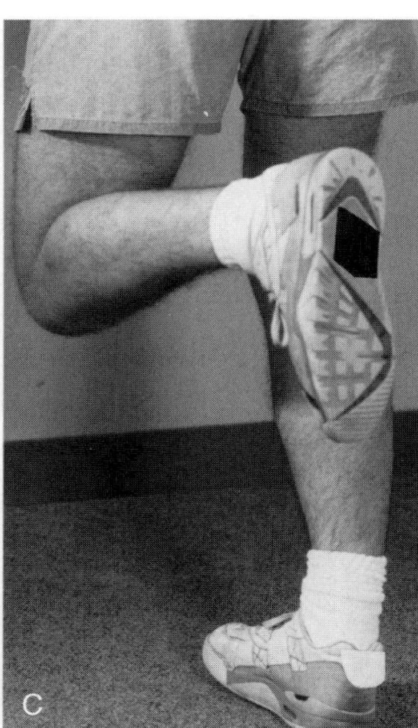

FIGURE 44–8. Stretching of Achilles tendon in kinetic chain. *A.* Pronated position. *B.* Supinated position. *C.* Close-up of supinated kinetic chain stretch.

pressure), Tropp et al[150] found that previously injured soccer players whose postural sway values were greater than two standard deviations above normal had a higher risk of injury during the following season. In a prospective study[149] of the value of wobble board training and injury reduction, Tropp et al demonstrated improved stabilometry values and lower injury rates in soccer players who underwent 10 weeks of ankle disk training. Such training can also affect more proximal joints. In soccer players, prospective training on balance boards has also been shown to significantly reduce the incidence of injury to the anterior cruciate ligament.[29] In situations that challenge joint stability, balance retraining theoretically reduces the risk of future injury.

After an injury, "pain free" does not mean "cured" and, unless the proprioceptive deficit has been addressed, complete rehabilitation has not been accomplished. To improve dynamic joint stability, the proprioceptive system must in some way be challenged. Balance training (e.g., single-leg stance exercises) and closed kinetic chain exercises are effective ways to challenge the dynamic and reflexive aspects of proprioception in the lower extremities. Functional testing (e.g., figure-eight cuts, vertical jumps, single leg hops) and sport-specific testing (e.g., timed, backward running for a defensive back in football) are ways to ensure that the proprioceptive neuromuscular system has been sufficiently retrained for safe participation in sports.

Often with proprioceptively challenging exercises, we can measure only the results of proprioception (i.e., dynamic stability). From these measures, however, we can infer how interventions affect the proprioceptive system. For example, a study[132] simulated ankle sprains in normal persons with a platform that has a hinged trap door that produces sudden lateral ankle inversion of 20 degrees. The study revealed that after 8 weeks of using a wobble board, a remodulation of the ankle group muscles occurred to provide maximal dynamic ankle stability. Muscles that would create a greater inversion moment were slowed, which indirectly improved the efficiency of the peroneus longus to decelerate the foot during unexpected ankle inversion.

Sport-Specific Higher Level Skills

Before a person returns to a sport after an injury or before initial participation in a sport, sport- and position-specific skills are necessary to ensure that the skills related to a sport are performed with the greatest facility and dexterity. In essence, one should not "play a sport to get in shape," but rather should "get in shape to play a sport." These exercises include higher-order gait and coordination exercises, plyometrics, and sport-specific drills. In addition to sports specificity, position specificity is important. The job description for a lineman on a football team is different from that for a wide receiver, and each of these jobs requires a specific exercise program.

The key purpose of sport-specific practice is to solidify and to hardwire the neuromuscular engrams required for the execution of sport movements. Integral to this principle is the concept that "only perfect practice makes perfect." In essence, the foundational movement patterns and skills for a particular sport and sport position must be learned and practiced to avoid potential musculoskeletal injuries. The great athletes of a sport are often those who have what is considered classic technique (e.g., Nolan Ryan, Bob Gibson, and Steve Carlton in baseball). Variations around the ideal (e.g., change in pitching mechanics) might seem harmless in the short term, but long-term complications can result from musculoskeletal overload and kinetic chain dysfunction. Alternatively, the institution of a prophylactic training program emphasizing technique issues specific to the sport may help to decrease the risk of musculoskeletal injury. A recent prospective study has demonstrated a decreased incidence of knee injury in female athletes after a specific jump training program.[65a]

The sports medicine physiatrist and physical therapist should understand the essential technique element of the major sports, such as the baseball pitch, the tennis ground stroke and serve, and the golf swing. A valuable liaison to the sports medicine team can be the local golf or tennis pro or pitching coach. They can help refine and develop correct foundational skills, which then can be enhanced by practice. It is especially important to establish appropriate technique and mechanics when first beginning a sport. Suboptimal neuromuscular engrams are difficult to modify after many years of incorporation into a sport movement pattern. This is crucial for younger athletes, because the pressure is great to continue with a special pitch or swing that might be successful and contribute to winning but, in the long term, be detrimental to the musculoskeletal system. In addition, in times of neuromuscular fatigue and stress (times of intense competition), athletes tend to revert to their original neuromuscular patterns, which might not be optimal.

Incorporation of Components into a Practical Training Program

None of the components of injury protection and prehabilitation mentioned previously are effective unless they can be incorporated into an individual or group training program. Education is essential and can be incorporated on three levels. The person should receive information from the sports medicine team (e.g., physician, physical therapist, athletic trainer, coach, and others, as applicable). At local and regional levels, high school and college sports programs can have considerable impact by implementing the above prehabilitation or injury protection elements into their programs. On a national level, organizations such as the American College of Sports Medicine, the American Medical Society for Sports Medicine, the American Orthopedic Society for Sports Medicine, and the Physiatric Association of Spine, Sports, and Occupational Rehabilitation can contribute by formulating consensus and position statements.

EXTRINSIC CONTRIBUTORS TO INJURY AND SUBOPTIMAL SPORTS PERFORMANCE

The major factors that contribute to injury can be grouped into extrinsic and intrinsic factors. Extrinsic factors consist primarily of elements external to a person, whereas intrinsic factors are related to a person's anatomical and biomechanical characteristics.

Extrinsic factors that can contribute to injury or suboptimal sports performance are listed in Table 44–2.

Conditioning and Preparation

It is important to analyze an athlete's training history (e.g., the types of terrain on a runner's running route, the volume of training, and the intensity of training). The *terrible too's*—"too much, too soon, too fast, and too hard"—contribute to many overuse injuries. The classic example is medial tibial stress syndrome seen in springtime high school track participants.[103] These athletes usually progress from winter sports and activities that do not require sustained long-duration running or impact loading to training and competition that suddenly demand sustained high-impact exercise. It is also important to ensure that sport-specific conditioning and sport preparation have taken place, as outlined above in the section on sport-specific practice.

Climate, Fluids, and Hydration

Climatic extremes can be a factor in thermal injuries. The importance of adequate hydration and fluid replacement should be stressed for persons competing in endurance events. In hot conditions, water loss from the skin and lungs can be greater than 2 L per hour. Because water constitutes most of the fluid that is lost in events lasting less than 90 minutes, water replacement is the best mode of restoring fluid status. You should drink at least 16 ounces of fluid approximately 2 hours before starting physical activity and 20 to 40 ounces per hour of a cool, noncarbonated beverage during exercise. Drink 16 ounces of fluid for each pound of weight lost during physical activity. Carbohydrate supplementation can be helpful during exercise that lasts longer than 90 minutes.[43] Athletes who use creatine supplementation should pay special attention to adequate hydration, because creatine draws water inside muscle cells and can lead to a relative extracellular volume depletion.

Kinesiology of the Sport

Understanding the kinesiology of the sport and sports task is important for optimal performance and efficiency, as discussed above. This is true for every sport-specific movement. Each sport places unique kinesiological and biomechanical stresses on the components of the kinetic chain that are involved in performing the sport. If training focuses on optimizing the mechanics of the sport, injuries might be prevented. A video camera recording can often help delineate the suboptimal components of the kinetic chain and provide feedback for technique correction.

TABLE 44–2 Contributors to Injury: Extrinsic Factors

Training errors—conditioning and preparation
Climate, fluids, and hydration
Kinesiology of the sport
Epidemiology
Equipment
Playing field

Epidemiology

Certain sports have an inherent risk and predispose to injury of specific parts of the body, and each sport has certain risk factors that pretraining can help minimize. The seemingly innocuous and frequently prescribed step aerobic exercise was found by one study to cause injury in a large percentage of persons.[120] This is likely because the exercise made apparent previously unmanifested anatomical, biomechanical, strength, or flexibility problems as the kinetic chain was stressed. It is important to identify injuries that are specific for a sport or activity and to maximize the kinetic chain function related to the particular part of the body at risk.

Equipment

Equipment can play a significant role in injury. For example, appropriate release settings for ski binding and binding maintenance are essential to protect a skier in the event of a fall. Inadequate release settings increase the risk of injury many times.[78] Similarly, tennis racquets strung at an excessively high tension can contribute to the development of lateral epicondylitis.

Playing Field

The playing field should be considered an extrinsic contributor to injury. Various artificial turf surfaces can alter foot and lower limb torque, and certain injuries (e.g., "turf toe" in football) seem to be more prevalent on artificial surfaces. However, every surface has a unique effect on transmitting reaction force up through the lower extremities. The composition of the playing surface should be considered in relation to the particular sport training and game requirements. For example, cross-country runners should not be trained exclusively on concrete surfaces.

INTRINSIC CONTRIBUTORS TO INJURY AND SUBOPTIMAL SPORTS PERFORMANCE

The intrinsic contributors to injury are listed in Table 44–3. Malalignments and anatomical variations such as excessive forefoot pronation, cavus foot, varus/valgus malalignment, excessive tibial torsion, excessive leg-length discrepancy (more than 2 cm), and excessive femoral anteversion can contribute to numerous biomechanical problems that can cause injury. Orthotic interventions, such as supports to preserve the longitudinal arch of the foot, can help to optimize foot biomechanics and to improve the distribution of force throughout the lower extremity. In addition, adequate shock absorption can help reduce the incidence of overuse injury in such sports as running.[100, 128]

TABLE 44–3 Contributors to Injury: Intrinsic Factors

Malalignment/Anatomical variation
Leg-length discrepancy
Poor flexibility
Muscle weakness
Muscle imbalance
Decreased neuromuscular skills
Kinetic chain dysfunction

Ensuring symmetrical and sport-specific flexibility is important, as is maintaining balanced muscle group strength. Signs of incomplete or improper rehabilitation from a previous injury, such as strength asymmetries or deficits, flexibility asymmetries, or a poor aerobic base, should be addressed. For example, it previously was believed that the relative lack of internal rotation of the shoulder in many tennis players was acceptable, and that it resulted from "resetting the thermostat." Essentially, this lack of internal rotation was assumed to be adequately compensated for by excessive external rotation. This assumption is incorrect. Internal rotation deficits have been found over time to predispose to shoulder and rotator cuff injury.[33, 34] Muscle imbalances can also prove problematic, as evidenced in the shoulder muscles. Many persons concentrate heavily on anterior shoulder exercises (such as the bench press and pectoral strengthening) during strength training. If the scapular stabilizers (primarily serratus anterior, latissimus dorsi, trapezius, and rhomboids) are neglected, an imbalance results that can place the rotator cuff at risk.

Lack of appropriate neuromuscular skills for a particular sport or position within a sport can contribute to an increased risk of injury. There have been many instances of players injured after a change in position (e.g., baseball player José Canseco attempting to pitch after playing in the outfield) or during competition at a high level in a sport outside their field. If an athlete returns to competition after an injury before sport-specific skills are gained, the risk of reinjury is also increased.

Generalized ligamentous laxity is often discussed as an independent risk factor for musculoskeletal injury. No study clearly validates this assumption, however, and laxity might, in some instances, protect from injury. Asymmetry is again a more likely contributor to injury, and if preinjury range is not reestablished, the immediate area and related kinetic chain components are at risk.

Gait, stance, and the biomechanics of a particular sport movement should be examined for possible dysfunction of the kinetic chain. It is important to look at static and dynamic alignment as well as at function. In a case of suspected patellofemoral pain, not only should the knee be thoroughly examined with the patient supine, but patellofemoral tracking and activation of the oblique portion of the vastus medialis should be assessed with the patient in weight-bearing and squatting positions.

Principles of sports psychology are important in injury prevention because they can help a person to focus his or her concentration. They also provide techniques for relaxation and stress management. Neuromuscular engrams and motor learning can be facilitated through the use of such techniques as imagery.

GENERAL PRINCIPLES OF MUSCULOSKELETAL REHABILITATION

Assessment of Injury

Most musculoskeletal injuries can be divided into two broad categories: (1) acute and (2) subacute, or chronic. Acute injuries are often related to macrotrauma and a breach of integrity of the musculoskeletal system, such as bone fracture or ligamentous disruption. The range of severity is broad and includes everything from a mild inversion ankle sprain to a devastating spinal cord injury. For this reason, the diagnostic acumen of an evaluator should be wide-ranging. The evaluator must be capable of recognizing the signs and symptoms of a neurological problem. It is equally important to know the indications for and use of spinal stabilization and transport techniques to prevent spinal cord injury.[148, 153] Some sports injuries and conditions benefit from early surgical intervention to maximize function, to enable early return to activity, and to prevent reinjury. Early identification of these conditions is crucial. Delays in diagnosis can lead to slow recovery and possibly further injury.

The age of the patient should be considered when an injury is evaluated. For example, a high school football player who has vague left-sided abdominal pain after being tackled and has a history of viral illness should be thoroughly evaluated for splenic involvement due to possible mononucleosis. Similarly, older athletes should be evaluated in the context of concurrent medical problems such as cardiac disease, respiratory compromise, or severe degenerative changes.

Subacute or chronic injury can usually be thought of as repetitive damage to or overuse of the musculoskeletal system. Examples are the repetitive microtrauma sustained by the forearm extensor muscle mass and tendon group in lateral epicondylitis (tennis elbow) and by the tibia in medial tibial stress syndrome. Treatment of these injuries typically involves the principle of relative rest, in which the injured body part is protected from further trauma and then gradually rehabilitated to normal function. During the treatment, aerobic fitness is maintained by using other, noninjured parts of the body. Essential to the successful treatment of chronic injury is an understanding of the factors that put the injured tissue at risk and contributed to musculoskeletal stress. These factors could include inadequate strength training or flexibility, suboptimal ergonomics or sport technique, or inappropriate training.

Treatment

The basic principles of rehabilitation after musculoskeletal injury include pain reduction by means of various modalities (i.e., ice, superficial and deep heat, interferential current) and appropriately prescribed medications, restoration of range of motion and flexibility, therapeutic strengthening, and maximization of sport-specific agility, coordination, and proprioception before return to sports. Another basic principle is the use of relative rest to maintain aerobic conditioning and cardiovascular fitness.

Relative Rest

A significant decrease in aerobic capacity can occur in as short a time as 4 weeks of detraining.[56, 72, 122] The principle of relative rest means that the injured part of the body is rested and protected from further trauma or injury while the remaining muscle mass is used to provide appropriate stress to the cardiovascular system for maintaining optimal aerobic conditioning. The injured part can be protected by a brace, cast, or limited weight-bearing status. The patient might need to be instructed about the appropriate use of crutches or a cane. Initially, the injured part should be rested, with little movement beyond a pain-free range. Strength training should continue in the uninjured parts of the body because crossover training effects occur in the rested limb when the contralateral limb is exercised.[102]

Relative rest of an injured part of the body is achieved with splinting, bracing, taping, or specialized adaptive equipment that permits performance of aerobic exercise. (Aerobic exercise is defined by the American College of Sports Medicine as any exercise that uses large muscle groups, can be maintained continuously, is rhythmic and aerobic in nature, and lasts from 20 to 60 minutes.[14]) A resting hand splint (prescribed for a person with wrist pain from carpal tunnel syndrome or elbow pain due to lateral epicondylitis) and an elbow hyperextension block brace (which can be used for a person who is recovering from an elbow dislocation) permit the aerobic component of training to be continued while the injured part is rehabilitated. Lower extremity injuries can be protected while the upper extremities and possibly even the noninvolved lower limb are used in the aerobic program. Exercise of the contralateral limb can be continued by use of devices such as resistance bicycles that provide for both upper extremity and lower extremity movement for bi- and tri-limb work (Fig. 44–9A).Wet-vest running (running in deep water with a buoyancy vest to keep the head above water) is also an effective method of non-weight-bearing training (Fig. 44–9B). The resistance of the water contributes to strengthening of the lower limb and to aerobic fitness. The water also provides a "proprioceptive corset" and can enhance truncal stability. Similar benefits with minimal weight-bearing stress can be achieved by walking in water that is only waist deep.

Pain Relief and Inflammation Control

The initial goals of the treatment of a sports injury should be to limit as much as possible the extent of the initial injury, to aid healing, and to provide for early institution of rehabilitation measures. The mainstay of early treatment (i.e., 24 to 48 hours after the injury) follows the principles of PRICE, as listed in Table 44–4.

Ice is efficacious for decreasing pain and swelling by producing local vasoconstriction. Ice packs can safely be applied for 20 minutes of every hour. For focal injuries, ice massage is easy to apply and it can be particularly

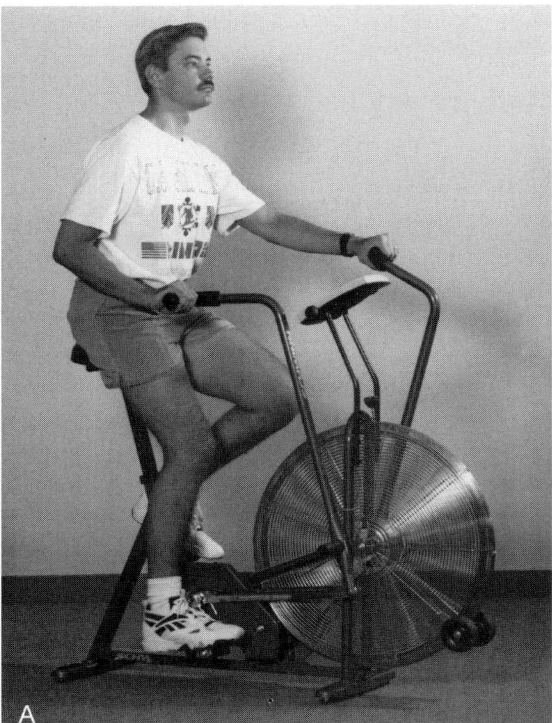

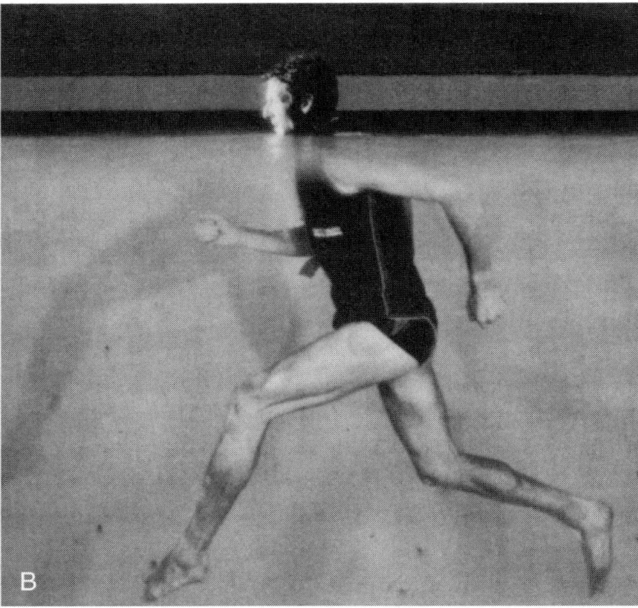

FIGURE 44–9. *A.* Resistance bicycle (Airdyne) enables exercise of upper and lower extremity muscles. *B.* Wet-vest running. (*B* from McWaters G: Aquatic rehabilitation. In Andrews JR, Harrelson GL (eds): Physical Rehabilitation of the Injured Athlete. Philadelphia, WB Saunders, 1991, pp 473–503. By permission of Bioenergetics Inc., Pelham, Al [1–800–938–8378].)

time-effective. Compression around the injured area also helps to limit swelling and enhances comfort and earlier range of motion. Physiologically, this can improve outcome, because early tensile stress to tissue causes more linear collagen formation and enables stronger tensile strength. If compression initially is instituted with elastic wraps (e.g., Ace bandages), rewrapping should be performed every 4 hours to ensure appropriate compression. The elastic wrap should first be stretched to its fullest extent and then be reduced to two-thirds of this length, to provide appropriate tension during wrapping and to prevent circulatory compromise. Alternative means of compression include elastic fabric, which can be customized to fit the injured body part, and neoprene sleeves. Compression and cold can be applied simultaneously with an intermittent pneumatic compression pump (Fig. 44–10). The injured extremity should be raised to a level higher than the heart to facilitate venous return. Controversy exists about the role of electrical stimulation as an independent factor in the resolution of swelling.

TABLE 44–4 PRICE Principles

P:	protection
R:	relative rest
I:	ice
C:	compression
E:	elevation

Superficial ice (acute and chronic) and heat (subacute and chronic) modalities are likely to continue to be the mainstays of pain relief because of the low risk of complications, the ease of application, and the therapeutic efficacy. Ultrasound treatment, short-wave diathermy, interferential current, and transcutaneous electric nerve stimulation can also be used safely with the usual precautions and with appropriate prescription (see Chapters 21 and 22). Physiatrists need to ensure appropriate selection of therapeutic modalities to avoid misuse and abuse. For example, ultrasound treatment is most effective at sites with the greatest change in absorption characteristics of the tissue, such as at the interface of bone and soft tissue. In these regions, the temperature can increase more than 5°C.[85, 86] Ultrasound treatment is inappropriate and ineffective for use with diffuse and uniformly absorptive tissue, for example, the lumbar paraspinal muscle mass.

Other modalities such as electrical stimulation are often applied inappropriately to a wide range of musculoskeletal injuries. The clinical efficacy of electrical stimulation, apart from its neuromuscular reeducation value, has not been validated, and in this era of cost-containment and outcome efficacy, its random, widespread use has been questioned (see Chapter 22).

Overuse Injury

Early treatment of an overuse injury is different from that of an acute injury. Because significant swelling usually is not a permanent component, a compression gar-

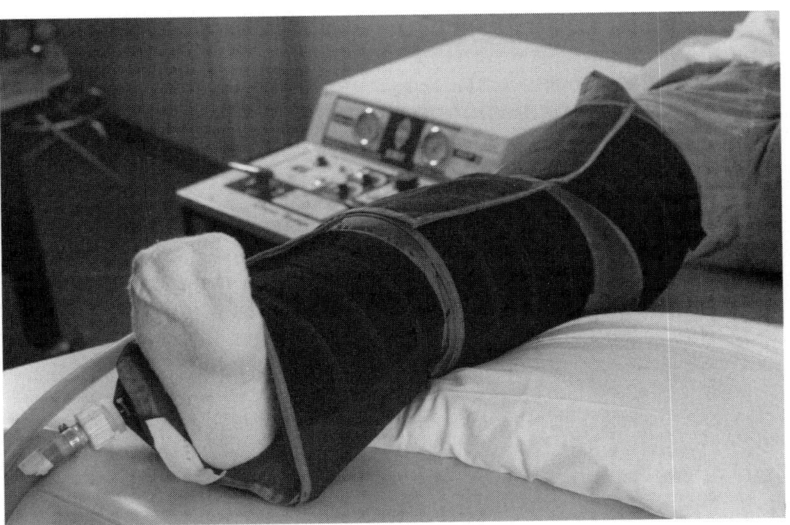

FIGURE 44–10. Intermittent pneumatic compression pump applies cold and compression simultaneously.

ment or elevation might not be needed. However, protection and ice are essential. The activity that contributed to the microtrauma must be avoided or at least greatly modified, especially with respect to frequency. Patients must be educated about appropriate biomechanical and kinesiological principles of the sport-related movement. Ice can be an effective method of pain control, but heat might be especially beneficial. Heat can be delivered as superficial heat or deeper heat at the bone-tendon interface (ultrasound treatment). Heat causes blood vessel dilation, provides pain relief, and can help decrease muscle tightness. Heat can be used in combination with gentle prolonged stretching to increase range of motion by promoting collagen extensibility.[87] General and muscle-specific relaxation and stretching techniques can help diminish muscle tightness and enhance whole body relaxation. Massage techniques, appropriately used, can be a beneficial adjunct, and cross-fiber or friction massage can be used to help mobilize contracted scar tissue. Aggressive cross-fiber massage and techniques such as dry needling might in fact help bring the inflammatory response to completion, in concert with the concept that overuse is actually underhealing. Myofascial interventions such as strain/counterstrain can also be useful tools in an attempt to reset chronically altered muscle proprioceptors.

Biofeedback is effective for reeducating the patient regarding the kinesthetic sensation of achieving and maintaining relaxation in a particular muscle. This can be helpful in cases of painful muscle splinting that are refractory to other treatment. Biofeedback can also enhance activation of a specifically inhibited muscle group. In tandem with functional electrical stimulation, it can be effective in neuromuscular reeducation. For example, the effort of the quadriceps (particularly the oblique portion of the vastus medialis) can be inhibited up to 60% by a small (20 mL) knee effusion.[159] This inhibition can cause deactivation of the neuromuscular pathway and a relative shutdown of the muscle group because of nociceptive stimuli. Pain affects the afferent neuromuscular arc by causing neural inhibition that hinders muscle activation ("deafferentation" or "alienation"). Athletes might find it difficult, if not impossible, to produce a voluntary contraction of the oblique portion of the vastus medialis in such circumstances. Electrical stimulation can help athletes regain kinesthetic awareness of a particular muscle group, and biofeedback can verify voluntary activation and be effective in learning to enhance selective muscle use. The latter program is particularly efficacious in entities such as patellofemoral pain, in which an afferent nociceptive stimulus causes neuromuscular inhibition or asynchronous firing of the oblique portion of the vastus medialis.

Whether NSAIDs have any direct effect on the rehabilitative course is unclear. If used initially and for a short time, these drugs can assist in starting the rehabilitation process by decreasing the level of pain. However, in the early stages of macrotrauma with significant bleeding, NSAIDs may increase bleeding by decreasing platelet aggregation. Pain can be a great inhibitor, and muscle co-contraction and substitution are just two of the suboptimal biomechanical effects that can result from "going through the pain." Long-term use of NSAIDs is not advisable for either able-bodied or physically challenged athletes, and special care must be taken for those with spinal cord injury because they are particularly vulnerable to renal injury. For those who have been taking NSAIDs for a long time, it is often the case that a specific etiological problem (e.g., biomechanical deficit, flexibility or strength deficit, or asymmetry) has not been correctly identified.

Range of Motion, Flexibility, and Muscle Balance

Restoring joint range of motion, establishing symmetric flexibility, and regaining strength often can be facilitated concurrently in the rehabilitation program. Muscles are mechanically most efficient when they can shorten and lengthen maximally, especially during isotonic exercise.[117] Depending on the injury, range of motion might need to be protected, passive, or limited in the initial stages, but should progress to full range as tolerated. Joint motion provides nutrition to articular cartilage through hydrostatic pressure. It also prevents the formation of soft tissue contractures and provides proprioceptive joint and muscle feedback.[4] To achieve full range of motion, gentle terminal stretching might be necessary, especially after treatment with superficial heat or ultrasound. During the healing process, specific stresses must be applied to the tissue by range of motion and stretching to promote linear alignment of collagen.[58] Collagen produced in this manner is more effective with respect to load-bearing and has greater tensile strength.[36, 83, 119] Without stress, collagen fibers tend to be arranged in a chaotic fashion.

Stretching in combination with a strengthening program that emphasizes muscle balance is essential in athletic rehabilitation. Because of different levels of weakness and dysfunction, many persons have a relative dominance of one muscle group over another. Dominance of an agonist over a weakened or nonfunctioning antagonist group can produce contracture and joint dysfunction. Dominance of one muscle group can result from strength imbalances, for example, greater development of anterior shoulder muscle groups than of posterior shoulder muscle groups.[74] This pattern is often seen in baseball pitchers and in persons who stress the anterior muscle groups in weight training (pectorals, anterior deltoid, and biceps). The important posterior shoulder group and scapular stabilization musculature (rhomboids, serratus anterior, latissimus dorsi, and trapezius) are unfortunately neglected. Consequently, relative tightness of the anterior capsule occurs. In conjunction with the relative weakness of the posterior group, this can predispose a person to shoulder problems.[73] This unbalanced system creates a potential for overuse and stress at the weak link (i.e., the point of imbalance). The entire kinetic chain mechanics must be assessed in relation to the particular task or movement of a sport.

Strength Training

Strength training can begin in some fashion early in rehabilitation, with progression as tissue healing and joint range of motion permit. The strength that is gained in the first few weeks is due to the neural effect of enhanced synchronization and recruitment of motor units.[101] Muscle fiber hypertrophy does not occur until after 2 to 4 weeks or more of strengthening exercise.[102] The more efficient use of muscle provided by strengthening exercises has a positive effect on early return of function and performance. The various types of strength training include isometric, isotonic, isokinetic, resistance band, variable resistance, plyometric, and kinetic chain exercise (see Chapter 19). Of paramount importance in strength training is proper technique. There are few inherently poor exercises, but many exercises are poorly performed with bad technique and form, which predisposes to musculoskeletal injury. Technique, form, safety, the risk-benefit ratio of the exercise, and the ability of the person to stabilize himself or herself and control the resistance should be carefully considered in the strength training prescription.

Isometric

Isometric, or equal length, exercise is essentially a static muscular contraction. In essence, both ends of the muscle are fixed, with no motion in the muscle as a result of the contraction. It entails exerting a maximal force against a relatively immovable object, with no appreciable change in muscle length. No mechanical work is performed during the contraction, and consequently the energy is dissipated as heat.

The most effective way to perform isometric exercise to gain strength has not been clearly defined.[20] Hettinger[65] showed strength gains of 5% per week with one 6-second contraction per day at 67% maximal effort. He later concluded that maximal contractions produced better results. Clarke[37] stated that the best results were obtained with maximal contractions held for 6 seconds, five to ten times per day. According to Atha,[20] isometric contraction should be "near maximal, long enough for total fiber recruitment, and repeated several times per day." The problem with incorporating this advice into practical strength training is obvious.

Among the problems with isometric training is that the strength gains are specific to the angle of the joint.[60] Furthermore, isometric training does not change the ability of a muscle to exert force rapidly, and it provides little stimulus for hypertrophy or endurance in dynamic activity. Thus, isometric training is not a functional type of exercise. It does, however, protect the joint from undue stress, and it creates less inflammatory response in the joint than does isotonic exercise.[96] Isometric exercise can prepare the muscle for functional kinetic chain strengthening at a later stage.

The most important role of isometric contractions might be in body stabilization. Without a stable platform, muscle strength cannot be used effectively. We are constantly performing isometric stabilizing contractions to maintain body position when standing, and we must have a stable platform from which to throw or to use the lower extremities. Isometric contractions are consequently ubiquitous in both everyday life and in sport. Proper training of stabilization, as when training with free weights, is essential to ensure that we can use muscles effectively in an isolated fashion and that we do not put other elements of the kinetic chain at risk because of an excessive or unbalanced load.

Isotonic

Isotonic, or equal tension, exercise ideally consists of constant muscle contraction with constantly applied tension. Isotonic exercise is dynamic and occurs when the muscle contraction itself is used to move a joint that ultimately moves a load through a range of motion. Initially the load might be no more than the weight of the limb, with later progression to resistance exercises. Isotonic strength depends on the contractile force and mechanics of movement about a joint (Fig. 44–11).[156] The muscle is not contracting at constant capacity or a specific percentage thereof throughout the entire range of motion. For this reason, the term *isotonic* technically is not accurate, because equal tension is not exerted throughout the joint range of motion. Isotonic exercise

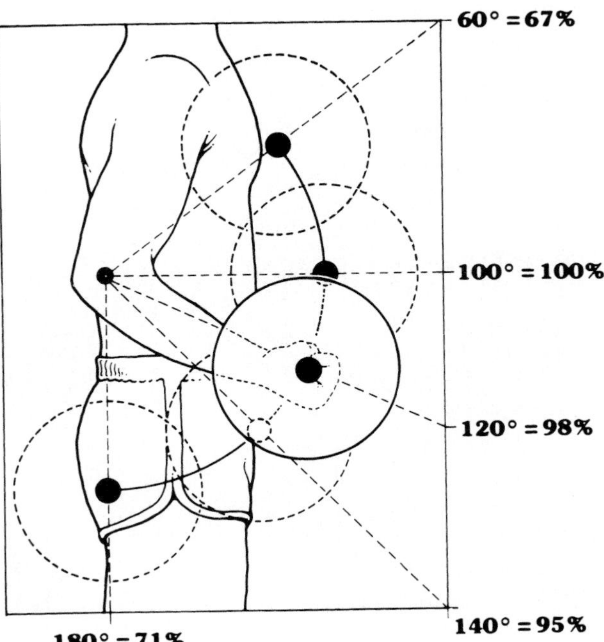

FIGURE 44–11. Percentage of force production as a muscle moves through its range of motion (From Wilmore JH, Costill DL: Training for Sport and Activity. The Physiological Basis of the Conditioning Process, ed 3. New York, McGraw-Hill, 1988. By permission of publisher.)

can further be divided into concentric and eccentric components. Concentric contractions require the loading of the muscle while it is shortening, whereas eccentric contractions load the muscle while it is lengthening. An example of each type occurs in a biceps curl: lifting the weight is a concentric contraction and lowering it slowly is an eccentric contraction.

The traditional belief is that eccentric exercise is more likely to cause muscle damage. Asmussen[18] demonstrated that eccentric exercise resulted in muscle soreness 24 to 48 hours after exercise. Others have shown that eccentric exercise produces muscle soreness, but the soreness dissipates after 1 week.[79] Clarkson and Ebbeling[38] pointed out that an increase in plasma levels of creatine kinase seems unrelated to the development of muscle soreness, loss of strength after exercise, fitness level of the subject, or lean body weight. According to Evans and Cannon,[53] this exercise-induced skeletal muscle "damage" causes a release of intracellular proteins, delayed-onset muscle soreness, and an increase in turnover of skeletal muscle protein. These adaptations appear to be integral to the repair of the damaged muscle. They can also be essential for hypertrophy, because chronic exercise causes adaptations in skeletal muscle that result in an increased capacity of oxidative metabolism. The repair of damaged muscle resulting in the hypertrophy seen in eccentric exercise might be a mechanism for protection against further exercise-induced damage.[53] Eccentric exercise might offer an opportunity to delineate signals and modulators during repair of damaged muscle. Much might be learned about the response to and adaptation of muscle to chronic exercise by further investigation of this topic.

Isokinetic

Isokinetic, or equal speed, exercise was introduced by Perrine.[116] It allows maximal force production through full range of motion (e.g., Cybex machines; Ronkonkoma, NY) (Fig. 44–12). Isokinetic exercise consists of exercising at a predetermined constant velocity of joint motion. Isokinetic strength is the maximal torque that can be developed at any given velocity of contraction.[48] This type of exercise provides objective information about peak muscle torque, power, and endurance at reproducible velocities. Side-to-side data for comparison with an uninjured limb are easily obtained.

The velocities that can be achieved with isokinetic equipment are greater than those attained with traditional weight-training equipment. These velocities, however, are much slower than those of certain sports movements (e.g., a maximum of 300 degrees/sec on a machine compared with 7000 degrees/sec in the overhand throwing motion).[111] This type of exercise for strength training purposes is also nonfunctional because only one joint and one muscle system are used at maximal contraction. Isokinetic exercise does not simulate the way we use our muscles either during a sport or in activities of daily living.

Although objective data are obtained, athletes still must regain agility, coordination, and sport-specific skills before returning to competition. There is also no direct correlation between machine scores and athlete performance. One can have a good score on machine testing but significantly limited sport performance, and vice versa. It is preferable to rely on isokinetic measurements as a rough estimate of progression and rehabilitation, but use more functional testing for return-to-play criteria. Isokinetic exercise can cause increased patellofemoral shear and compression forces and is contraindicated early on in knees with a reconstructed anterior

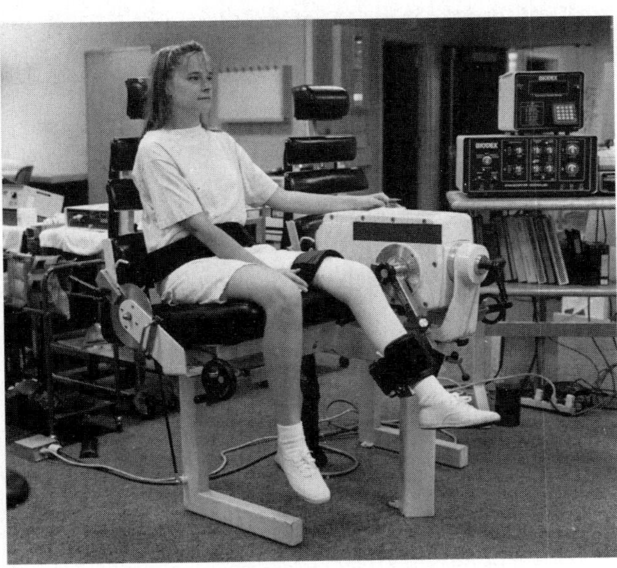

FIGURE 44–12. Isokinetic exercise machine.

cruciate ligament.[113, 136] This type of exercise can excessively load the secondary restraints in knees with a deficient anterior cruciate ligament.[62]

Resistance Band

Resistance-band exercise usually involves the use of a progressive resistance band (e.g., Theraband) that provides gradually increasing resistance when stretched. The band can be used in multiple planes of motion. It can also be used to simulate functional and sport-specific activities, such as the throwing motion of a baseball pitcher (Fig. 44–13) or the kicking motion of a soccer player. This type of exercise uses muscles in more of the complex and diagonal/spiral movement planes that sport movements require. With this type of resistance, it must be remembered that the most resistance occurs at the extreme of joint range of motion. At low levels of resistance, this might not be a problem, but with higher loads and healing tissue, care must be taken to ensure optimal technique to prevent excessive shear or compressive force across a joint. The apparatus is inexpensive and easily portable. Latex-free bands are available for those with a latex allergy.

Particularly for the upper extremities, manual resistance strengthening is a variation on resistance-band strengthening and is a way of providing carefully graded resistance in multiple dynamic movement planes (Fig. 44–14). Therapists can adjust the applied resistance according to the patient's pain and limitations of range of motion and strength.

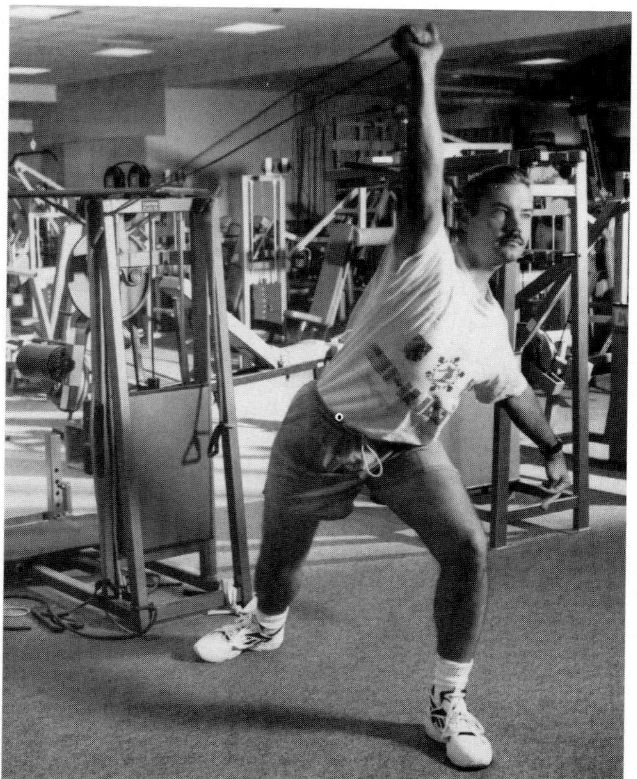

FIGURE 44–13. Resistance band exercise for "pitching-specific" strengthening.

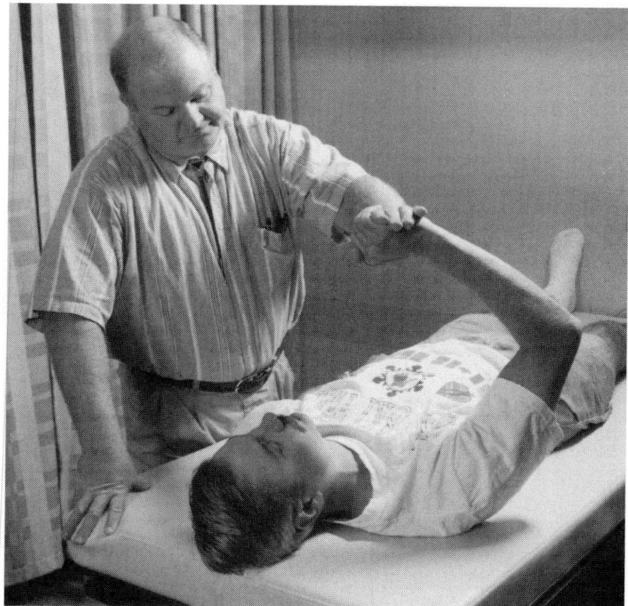

FIGURE 44–14. Manual resistance strengthening. The therapist provides resistance in functional planes of movement.

Variable Resistance

Variable resistance training means that the resistance is altered through the use of cams or pulleys in an attempt to match the force-producing capability of the muscle throughout the full range of motion (e.g., Cybex or Nautilus machines) (Fig. 44–15). This training attempts to compensate for the previously mentioned practical inability of a muscle to contract at a constant capacity throughout the entire range of motion. It is an isolated and nonfunctional exercise and does not stimulate associated proximal and distal components of the kinetic chain. Velocity and acceleration are variables in this type of exercise training, which is more useful for isolated strengthening than for sport-specific training.

Plyometric Exercise and Power Training

Plyometric exercises emphasize speed and power. They consist of concentric muscle contractions after a previous stretch of the same muscle groups. Theoretically, this helps provide neuromuscular facilitation, releases neural inhibition, and enables stronger and more forceful muscle contractions.[35, 152, 157] Plyometric exercises contain both eccentric and concentric components and load both the elastic and the contractile elements of a muscle. Examples of higher-level plyometrics include jumping rapidly onto and off different-sized boxes, jumping back and forth over a low object (Fig. 44–16), and performing specified weight-training maneuvers such as the "power clean." The power clean maneuver involves lifting a barbell from the ground in a rapid fashion, using coordinated kinetic chain movements of the lower extremities, trunk, and upper extremities. In general, sports-specific plyometric exercises should be performed on an appropriate surface (e.g., grass rather than concrete), under careful supervision, and with an

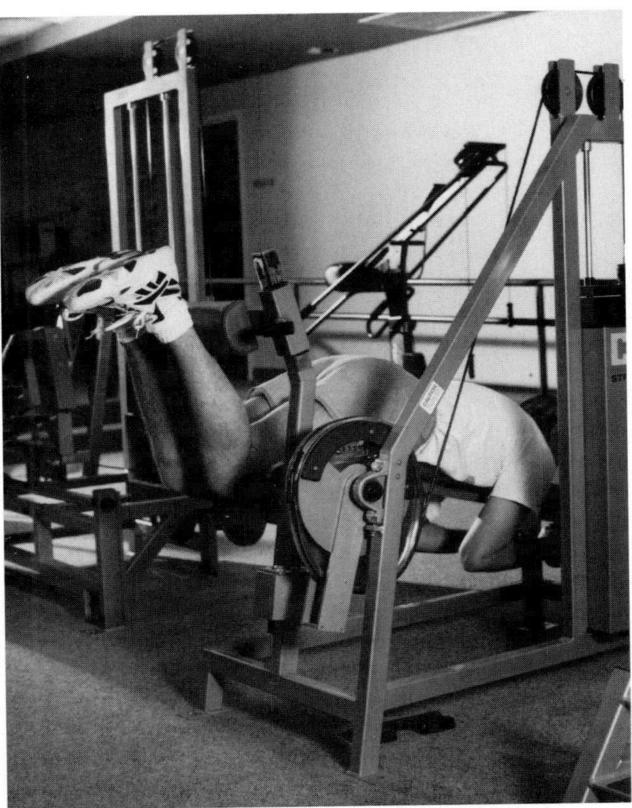

FIGURE 44–15. Variable resistance strength training equipment: prone hamstring curl.

adequate foundation of strength in the muscle groups used. The high-speed, high-impact nature of advanced-level plyometrics theoretically creates a greater potential for injury. Low-level plyometrics (e.g., skipping, hopscotch variations, high stepping) can be performed safely by most persons.

Power is work performed over time:

$$\text{Power} = (\text{Force} \times \text{Distance})/\text{Time}$$

and enhancement of power has implications for many areas in rehabilitation. For example, an elderly person not only needs to use lower extremity hip and knee muscle group strength to get up from a chair but also needs to use that strength over a specific period of time to be successful in the transfer. Muscle "power" also is needed when a person tries to cross the street before the light turns red. It is uncertain, however, whether plyometric exercises are the best method for developing power in the athlete. Theoretically, true power maximization would entail maximal recruitment of all available muscle motor units on demand for a particular sport movement. Consequently power development has a large neuronal component. Weight training with "power cleans" can enhance this specific skill task, but it might not contribute to increased recruitment. In addition, the effects of momentum and deceleration can be destructive. Perhaps a one-repetition maximum leg press, in which all available motor units are recruited to perform the exercise, is a more effective means of enhancing power output of the lower extremities. The sports-specificity aspect of functional plyometrics, which rely on movement patterns similar to the sport in the absence of applied load (i.e., jumping back and forth across a tape line for snow ski preparation [Fig. 44–16A]), likely is of significant benefit in enhancing and refining the neuromuscular engram.

Kinetic Chain Exercise

The concept and terminology of kinetic chain exercise were originally introduced by Steindler.[138] The term *closed kinetic chain* has become popular in recent years. Steindler pointed out that link system segment connections are considered closed if both ends are connected to an immovable framework, preventing translation of either proximal or distal joint centers. A true closed kinetic chain exists only during isometric exercise, because by definition neither the proximal nor the distal segments can move in a closed system.

Closed and Open Kinetic Chain Exercises

Closed kinetic chain exercises involve predictable coordinated muscle contractions with motion at multiple joints and a limb whose segment meets fixed or constrained resistance (i.e., leg press or squat [see Fig. 44–7]). In the upper extremities, a push-up can be considered a closed chain exercise. Squats and leg presses can each be closed chain exercises, and shear forces are generally less with these exercises at the tibiofemoral joint, although a recent study has suggested that maximal strain on the anterior cruciate ligament is similar in both open and closed chain exercises.[24] One of the key words in the closed kinetic chain definition is "predictable," because all joints must move in a predictable fashion for a true closed or constrained system to be present. A narrow grip barbell bench press, in which the person has to orchestrate stability of the upper arm and forearm during the maneuver, is technically not consistent with a closed chain exercise. If this same exercise were performed on a machine that controlled the upward and downward movement plane of the weights, a more specific closed chain exercise would be obtained. In general, closed chain exercises are more function-based and sport-specific for the lower extremities. For example, squats involve co-contraction of the quadriceps, hamstrings, and gastrocnemius-soleus muscle groups in a functional manner similar to that used in many sports and general daily living activities (e.g., getting up from a chair). If performed properly, squats can also provide joint and ligament safety. They are one of the primary exercises in rehabilitation of the anterior cruciate ligament.[90] Because co-contraction can be a stabilizing factor, shear force and compression force at the knees are diminished with closed chain as compared with open chain exercise.[23, 89, 110] In addition, closed chain exercises, as opposed to isolated quadriceps or hamstring exercises, more closely approximate the neuromuscular engrams used in lower-extremity-dominant sports. Closed kinetic chain exercise should be the predominant type of exercise for the lower extremities in

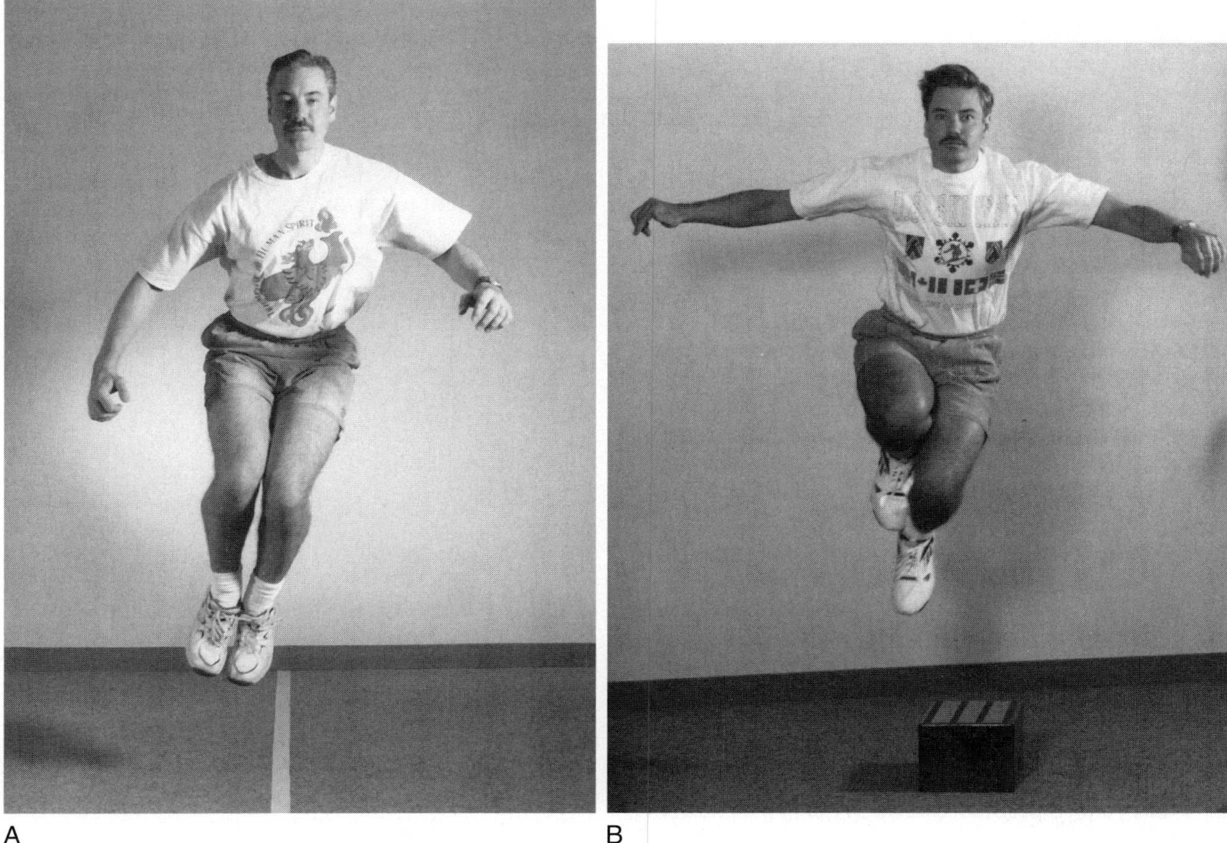

FIGURE 44–16. *A.* Side-to-side jumping across a tape line, a ski-specific preparation drill. *B.* Side-to-side low-level box jumping, an example of plyometric exercise.

sports medicine and in rehabilitation of the lower extremities in general. However, there are still many appropriate indications for use of open kinetic chain exercise.

Open kinetic chain exercises such as knee extensions tend to isolate a particular muscle group (in the case of knee extensions, the quadriceps) and involve motion distal to the axis of the joint. For the upper extremities, open kinetic chain exercises are essential before return to sports because these exercises are similar to the limb movements used in most sports (e.g., the throwing motion). These exercises for the lower extremities have been strongly criticized recently in favor of closed kinetic chain exercise because they are thought to involve significantly more harmful shear forces. As in any exercise, the way the exercise is performed is important in maximizing its safety and efficacy. During knee extensions, potentially damaging tibiofemoral shear force at the completion of the knee extension is greater during the last 5 to 10 degrees of extension and if the knee is hyperextended. In addition, at the extremes of knee flexion (greater than 60 degrees), there are increased patellofemoral compression forces that are potentially harmful.[23, 110] If one avoids excessive extension of the knee at the completion of knee extension and trains in a range that avoids extreme knee flexion and extension, especially if the load is decreased, knee extension is a safe and effective exercise for isolated quadriceps strengthening (Fig. 44–17). It appears that isolated strength training is essential to ensure side-to-side symmetry and to provide a base level of strength in the isolated muscle group before integrated strength training can occur. In addition, the quadriceps is still the major stabilizer of the knee, and adequate isolated strength is essential to maximize knee stability.

Shelbourne and Nitz[130] reported that reconstruction grafts of the anterior cruciate ligament did not stretch out with early, full-range, open chain quadriceps resistive exercise. The graft might revascularize more quickly with open chain exercise, and because ligaments respond to tensile stress through hypertrophy, the graft could become stronger during the revascularization period.[50] Shelbourne and Nitz[130] claimed that the number of complications decreased with open chain exercise. Others have noted a decreased incidence of joint stiffness, patellofemoral pain, and muscle atrophy and an early return of quadriceps strength.[50] Furthermore, compliance might be improved and return to sports or work might be more rapid.

Joint Isolation/Integration

Instead of using the terms *open* and *closed* chain exercise exclusively, it can be helpful to think of the former

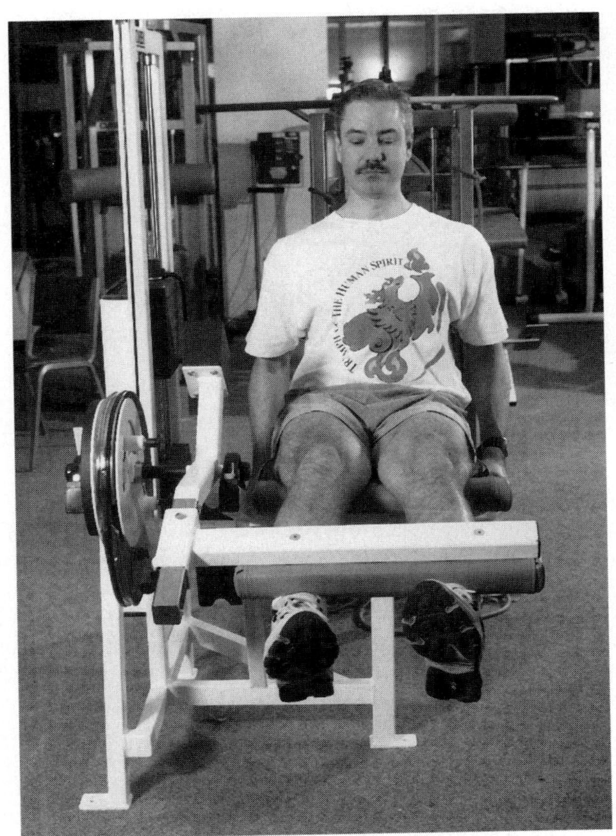

FIGURE 44–17. Knee extension, an open kinetic chain exercise.

exercises as *joint isolation* and the latter as *joint integration* exercises. Both are important. If an athlete has inadequate isolated strength of, for example, the quadriceps muscle, no matter how much he or she tries to perform a closed chain exercise (e.g., squat), they might be unsuccessful because of the isolated deficiency. Strength asymmetries and absolute deficits should be addressed before or concurrently with integrated exercises. It appears that the template for strength training should consist of isolated strength training, integrated strength training (closed chain exercise for lower extremities), and, finally, skill-specific "perfect" practice (Table 44–5).

As with any exercise and rehabilitative measure, no single protocol or exercise can be applied to all persons and to all situations. All of the previously mentioned exercises should be in the armamentarium of physiatrists who prescribe therapeutic exercise, and further research is needed to validate specific exercise applications (see Chapter 19).

TABLE 44–5 Template for Strength Training

1. Isolated strength training
2. Integrated strength training
3. Skill-specific "perfect" practice

AGILITY, PROPRIOCEPTION, AND SPORT-SPECIFIC SKILLS

Athletes should work to regain optimal agility and coordination either after strength has been maximized or in tandem with strength training. In many injuries, a muscle, tendon, or ligament and a joint are "detuned," and the proprioceptive feedback that the muscle or joint capsule normally provides is disrupted. Mechanoreceptors, muscle spindles, and Golgi tendon organs can be affected to various degrees. Examples of exercises that help regain this function include wobble board exercises, which help maximize balance and refine coordinating movements of lower extremity muscles, especially at the ankle (Fig. 44–18). Ankle group muscles are retrained to make the minute postural adjustments that are required for a person to maintain balance and remain upright. Knee proprioception can be better maximized with both standing and supine exercises involving a pediatric ball (Swiss ball) and knee-specific movements (Fig. 44–19). If lower extremity ambulation has been hindered by the injury, therapy should focus on higher-order gait activities, including carioca or crossover walking, and balance activities specific to the athlete's sport. For example, a football halfback could practice timed runs in tires or in a rope-maze course.

Evidence strongly supports specificity in training. Sale and MacDougall[124] stated that training should simulate

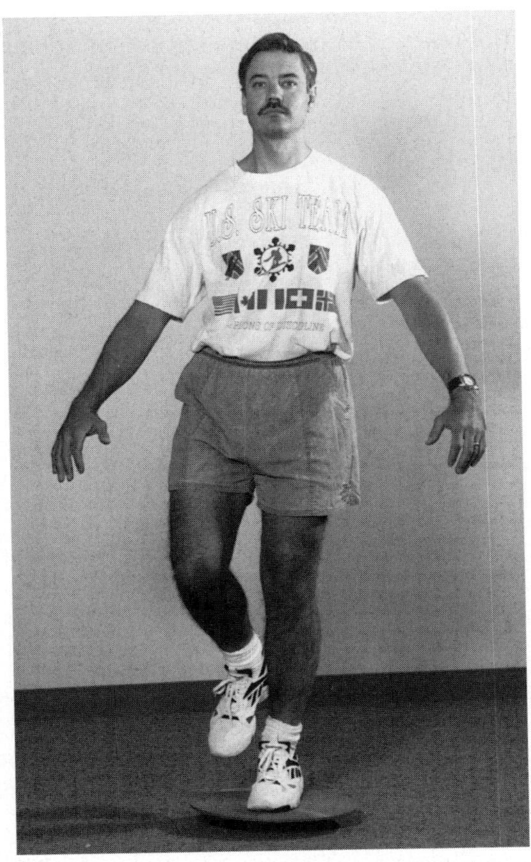

FIGURE 44–18. Wobble board exercise to enhance dynamic ankle stability.

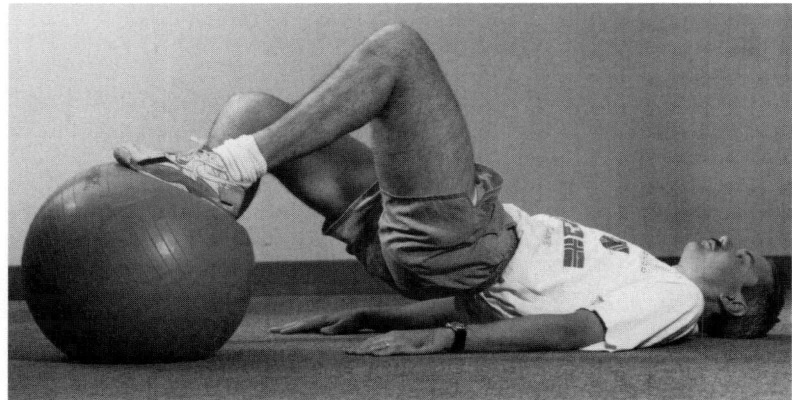

FIGURE 44–19. Supine knee-specific proprioceptive exercises with a pediatric ball (Swiss ball).

the movement desired as closely as possible with respect to anatomical movement pattern, velocity, and type and force of contraction. Exercise gains are specific to the type and pattern of movement addressed by training,[145] the velocity of training,[44] and the range of motion and angle at which training occurs.[60] Thorough knowledge of an athlete's sport and kinesiological demand is essential in designing an appropriate rehabilitation program for return to sports. Also essential is functional testing of these skills before competition. An athlete might have followed a comprehensive and thorough program of exercise, but rehabilitation is incomplete unless exercises specific to the sport and the athlete's position in the sport can be performed maximally and without pain or loss of function. These exercises also must be reprogrammed, and general exercises alone do not suffice. The ultimate goal is for an athlete to be at maximal strength and agility to maximize performance and to prevent recurrence of injury.

YOUTH SPORTS MEDICINE CONSIDERATIONS

Resistance training in young athletes must be used judiciously before closure of the growth plates occurs. These areas of growth are relatively weak in comparison with the surrounding ligamentous and fibrous supports, and if this "weak link" is injured, bony deformity and unequal growth can result.[121] Proper technique prevents these problems by not overloading any bone or muscle and joint complex. In this regard, prepubescent weight lifters should be encouraged to emphasize lower weight and higher repetitions, with impeccable technique, instead of trying to see how much weight they can lift. During periods of rapid growth, strength training should be decreased and flexibility exercises should be emphasized.[97] Nevertheless, strength training can be beneficial, and increased strength can be achieved in prepubescent children without an appreciable increase in muscle mass,[154] likely through improved synchronization in the recruitment of motor units.[125]

Children and adolescents are entering organized sports at earlier ages, resulting in increased musculoskeletal injuries and a change in distribution of injuries among young athletes.[97, 108] Traveling sports teams, training camps, pressure from coaches, peers, and parents, and year-round sports participation with inadequate recovery time have resulted in the dramatic increase in the frequency of pediatric overuse injuries.[137] As in adult athletes, overload injuries occur when an inadequately conditioned athlete experiences high load demands or when a highly conditioned athlete overtrains. As a result, there can be involvement of the bone (stress fractures), tendon (tendinitis), and bursa (bursitis). Skeletally immature athletes have growth centers that are susceptible to repetitive microtrauma or more acute injuries. Gross injuries include compression epiphysis and traction epiphysis (apophysis) injuries.[99] The apophysis is an area of major muscle-tendon insertion and undergoes maturational changes similar to that of the epiphysis, although at a slower rate. The treating physician should have a high level of awareness of these injuries and should be familiar with the characteristic patterns of appearance of fusion of each apophysis to differentiate normal variance from bony involvement. Most commonly, comparison radiographs of the uninjured side are obtained to judge asymmetries. Avulsion injuries can occur when tensile forces through the muscle-tendon units or ligaments cause separation of the vulnerable cartilaginous zone between the apophysis and bone. The ischial apophysis and the anterior superior iliac spine (ASIS) apophysis are common areas where avulsions can occur; if there is significant displacement of the ischial avulsion, surgical fixation may be indicated. Pediatric articular surface injuries can also occur as an osteochrondritis of the knee or osteochrondritis of the talar dome.

As in adult athletes, determining the etiological factors in overload injuries is necessary for successful treatment and prevention. Usually a combination of intrinsic and extrinsic factors contributes to a specific injury. Intrinsic factors can include the athlete's conditioning and be related to the athlete's growth rate, flexibility, and strength status (including asymmetries and imbalances), alignment issues, overall conditioning, and suboptimal kinetic chain issues. Extrinsic factors include equipment, training schedule and environment, and inappropriate training strategies. In general, training errors are thought to be the most common factor predisposing to overload injury.[97, 108] In the majority of overload injuries, the causative factors are similar to those in adult athletes and include increased intensity, increased volume or frequency of training, and inadequate rest that fails to allow adequate musculoskeletal anabolic activity. The pediatric examination should focus on identifying the developmental stage, strength and flexibility asymmetries or imbalances, malalignment issues, and equipment deficiencies.

The preparticipation examination for school sports is an excellent opportunity for physicians to help affect injury prevention and to assess at-risk areas in young athletes. Musculoskeletal and cardiovascular concerns are two areas in which intervention and identification of problems can contribute to reducing morbidity and, possibly, mortality. Several excellent publications can be consulted concerning the preparticipation evaluation.[11, 52, 75, 94]

UNIQUE CONSIDERATIONS FOR PHYSICALLY CHALLENGED ATHLETES

It is estimated that 2 to 3 million athletes with physical and mental disabilities participate in organized athletic activities in the United States.[25, 45] The importance of understanding the requirements and nature of the sports of physically challenged athletes cannot be overemphasized. Most sports for physically challenged persons have assimilated the rules and regulations of sports for able-bodied persons, with minimal exceptions. Some sports, however, are unique to the physically challenged and warrant further investigation by the medical professional to optimize training and injury rehabilitation programs. The groups that make up the Committee on Sports for the Disabled, a standing committee of the United States Olympic Committee, are excellent resources with respect to sports for physically challenged persons and participation requirements. These groups include the American Athletic Association for the Deaf, the Dwarf Athletic Association of America, Disabled Sports USA (DS/USA), the National Wheelchair Athletic Association, the Special Olympics, the United States Association of Blind Athletes, and the United States Cerebral Palsy Athletic Association.

Individuals who treat and advise physically challenged athletes should understand how the adaptive equipment required for the sport can affect injury risk. New aerodynamic body positions in wheelchair racing can increase the risk of pressure ulcers, and if the splash guards on high-performance wheelchairs are not adjusted properly, they can cause skin breakdown (Fig. 44–20). With respect to downhill snow skiing, monoskiers can risk skin breakdown if seating positions create too much ischial shear. Amputees can require special residual limb protectors or warmers (or both) if tissue blood flow is compromised. They might also need padding when downhill skiing. Athletes with cerebral palsy, multiple sclerosis, or spasticity require special containment provided by straps to enable more isolated limb movement, especially during resistance training. Wheelchair road racers benefit greatly from the use of gloves

Cisco Jeter,
Paralympics gold and
bronze medalist,
World record holder.

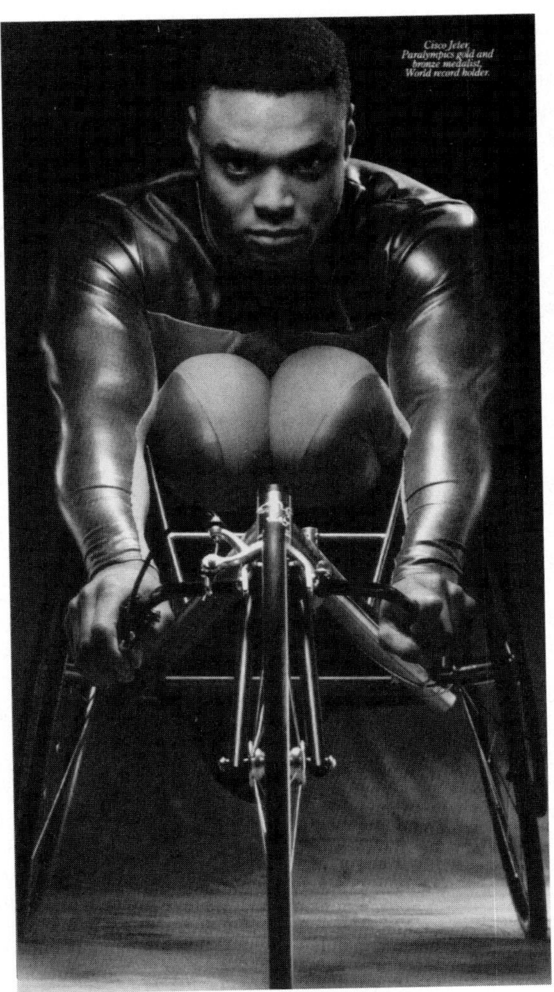

FIGURE 44–20. Aerodynamic wheelchair positioning. (From Sports 'N Spokes. 18:3, March/Apr 1993. By permission of Hall's Wheels.)

and from wearing friction-reducing material on the biceps and triceps regions of the arms and on the chest wall region of the axilla. The latter is necessary because of incidental contact with or intentional pressure on the wheels (e.g., for braking) with the axillary region.[91]

Equipment can also have an impact on the physiological benefits gained from exercise. Kinzer and Convertino[76] showed that a greater accumulation of fluid in the legs of paraplegic persons decreased cardiac preload and diminished the central cardiovascular training response. Wearing appropriately fitting compressive garments on the lower extremities during exercise can enhance the cardiovascular training effect.

Another external factor is the environment, which can pose risk of thermal injury to physically challenged athletes. Guidelines have been established for safe participation in sports in hot and humid environments.[12] In addition, wind-chill charts provide information about limits on outdoor exposure time during cold weather. The main group of athletes who need to use extra caution during temperature extremes are those with spinal cord injuries, especially with lesions above the T8 level.

In these persons autoregulation is impaired, and the body temperature tends to equalize with that of the ambient environmental temperature. Athletes with ischemia or vascular dysfunction and those who are insensate are also at risk in a cold environment, and frequent skin checks are necessary to ensure that skin damage is not occurring.

One of the key concepts in rehabilitation of physically challenged athletes, as in rehabilitation of able-bodied athletes, is appropriate training and injury prevention measures. Because shoulder injuries and carpal tunnel syndrome[9] seem to be prevalent among persons using wheelchairs, prophylactic programs of rotator cuff strengthening, scapular stabilization, and shoulder muscle endurance should be implemented early in conjunction with wrist stretches, wrist strengthening, and appropriate use of ice for inflammation control. It is essential to understand the biomechanics of a sport and the kinetic chain as they apply to a person's physical disability. Whiting and associates[155] showed that members of the U.S. men's water polo team throw the ball in the water with half of the velocity with which they can throw on land. This principle should be remembered for an athlete who is unable to make full use of ground reaction force because of a disability. Trunk restriction also causes a significant reduction in the velocity of throwing a ball.[8] In compensating for these deficiencies, other components of the kinetic chain should not be overused or misused biomechanically. Joints and muscle groups that are proximal and distal to the injury should be examined and treated to ensure that they are as biomechanically correct as possible with respect to flexibility, strength, balance, and kinesiological movement patterns. The kinetic chain for each athlete varies depending on functional ability, and it must be uniquely applied to the specific sport.

An aerobic exercise program for physically challenged athletes is essential. Numerous studies have shown that physical training can markedly enhance cardiovascular and aerobic fitness in those with spinal cord injury,[46, 59, 68] postpolio sequelae,[71, 82] traumatic brain injury,[70] or amputation.[3] The effects of exercises that use the arms only can translate into improved endurance for wheelchair propulsion, making it easier to complete activities of daily living, including school and work.[159] It appears that many of the same metabolic benefits can be derived from arm exercises as from lower extremity exercises. Taylor and colleagues[141] showed that slow-twitch fiber area increased with arm ergometer training, and Skrinar and associates[133] showed that glycogen utilization has the same pattern in the upper arm muscles of wheelchair athletes as in the legs of able-bodied athletes.

SPORTS PSYCHOLOGY

Physicians, athletic trainers, physical therapists, and coaches are the most visible members of the sports medicine team. The sports counselor or sports psychologist has recently had a larger presence as a member of the treatment team. Sports medicine professionals should be aware that the response of an athlete to injury can differ from that of other patients, and early identification and treatment of concurrent psychological issues by appropriate professionals often facilitate rehabilitation and maintenance of health. Many studies suggest that severe depression, tension, and anger are common among seriously injured athletes.[31, 134] As early as 1969, Little[88] found that about 75% of athletes who had symptoms of depression and anxiety had a preceding injury or illness. These symptoms were present in only 11% of nonathletes with injuries. This raises interesting questions about appropriate intervention to minimize psychological trauma and participation time lost due to injury. Many techniques have been advocated to provide psychological assistance and to facilitate rehabilitation, including visualization, relaxation, goal-setting, prioritization, and elimination of negative thoughts. However, there are not sufficient data to judge the effectiveness of any of these methods. Flint[55] suggested that modeling, or observational learning, could be a prime method for dealing with emotions that are detrimental to the recovery process. Athletes learn motor skills and social behaviors from coaches and teachers who use modeling as an instructional tool. Pride, determination, and hard work are intangible qualities possessed by many athletes, and during rehabilitation, these attributes can be used to help overcome injury.

Reinstilling self-confidence is another key aspect of the rehabilitation process. It has been shown by Smith and colleagues[135] that perceived severity of injury is often a major determinant of postinjury depression. Even though the physiological damage might not be severe, athletes who perceive an injury as serious are likely to experience more intense depression and to have a slower recovery than those who do not perceive an injury as serious. Three aspects of self-confidence that influence the recovery process have been suggested by Fisher[54]: competence, control, and commitment. Treatment programs that encompass these three elements are likely to increase compliance and outcome success. Athletes should believe that they will be able to resume competitive sports, take command of their rehabilitation, and commit time and effort to the sometimes long and arduous rehabilitation process.

Strategies for performance enhancement and stress management are ways in which sports psychology professionals can help to improve focus in competition and to maximize physical execution. Visualization and imagery also can be used in training to enhance neuromuscular engrams and to assist in rehabilitation. For example, an ice skater with a tibial stress fracture can substitute for the lack of ice time and training and augment alternative conditioning by observing videotapes that depict specific jumps and routines. This approach can expedite a return to competition because routines can be memorized and incorporated into a neuromuscular engram that might ultimately facilitate training on the ice. Control of pain can also be enhanced by imagery and relaxation techniques.

For optimal rehabilitation, athletes need the services of a multidisciplinary team that functions in an interdisciplinary manner. Each contributor plays an important role in helping an injured athlete to resume sports activities and to return to other activities of daily living.

REFERENCES

1. Abbott LC, Saunders JB, Bost FC, et al: Injuries to the ligaments of the knee joint. J Bone Joint Surg 1944; 26:503.
2. Acevedo EO, Goldfarb AH: Increased training intensity effects on plasma lactate, ventilatory threshold, and endurance. Med Sci Sports Exerc 1989; 21:563.
3. Adler JC, Mazzarella N, Puzsier L, et al: Treadmill training program for a bilateral below-knee amputee patient with cardiopulmonary disease. Arch Phys Med Rehabil 1987; 68:858.
4. Akeson WH: An experimental study of joint stiffness. J Bone Joint Surg Am 1961; 43:1022.
5. Akeson WH, Amiel D, LaViolette D: The connective-tissue response to immobility: A study of the chondroitin-4 and 6-sulfate and dermatan sulfate changes in periarticular connective tissue of control and immobilized knees of dogs. Clin Orthop 1967; 51:183.
6. Akeson WH, Woo SL, Amiel D, et al: The connective tissue response to immobility: Biochemical changes in periarticular connective tissue of the immobilized rabbit knee. Clin Orthop 1973; 93:356.
7. Akeson WH, Woo SL-Y, Amiel D, et al: The biology of ligaments. In Hunter LY, Funk FJ Jr (eds): Rehabilitation of the Injured Knee. St Louis, Mosby–Year Book, 1984, pp 93–148.
8. Alexander RM: Optimum timing of muscle activation for simple models of throwing. J Theor Biol 1991; 150:349.
9. Aljure J, Eltorai I, Bradley WE, et al: Carpal tunnel syndrome in paraplegic patients. Paraplegia 1985; 23:182.
10. Almekinders LC, Garrett WE Jr, Seaber AV: Pathophysiologic response to muscle tears and stretching injuries. Trans Orthop Res Soc 1984; 9:307.
11. American Academy of Pediatrics Committee on Sports Medicine: Recommendations for participation in competitive sports. Pediatrics 1988; 81:737.
12. American College of Sports Medicine: American College of Sports Medicine position stand on the prevention of thermal injuries during distance running. Med Sci Sports Exerc 1987; 19:529.
13. American College of Sports Medicine: Guidelines for Exercise Testing and Prescription, ed 4. Philadelphia, Lea & Febiger, 1991.
14. American College of Sports Medicine: The recommended quantity and quality of exercise for developing and maintaining cardiorespiratory and muscular fitness in healthy adults. The Official Position Papers of the American College of Sports Medicine. American College of Sports Medicine, Indianapolis, 1990.
15. Andersen P, Henriksson J: Training induced changes in the subgroups of human type II skeletal muscle fibres. Acta Physiol Scand 1977; 99:123.
16. Andersson S, Stener B: Experimental evaluation of the hypothesis of ligamento-muscular protective reflexes: II. A study in the cat using the medial collateral ligament of the knee joint. Acta Physiol Scand 1959; 48(suppl 166):27.
17. Andrew BL: The sensory innervation of the medial ligament of the knee joint. J Physiol 1954; 123:241.
18. Asmussen E: Positive and negative muscular work. Acta Physiol Scand 1953; 28:364.
19. Åstrand P-O, Rodahl K: Textbook of Work Physiology. New York, McGraw-Hill, 1986.
20. Atha J: Strengthening muscle. Exerc Sport Sci Rev 1981; 9:1.
21. Baker BE: Prevention of ligament injuries to the knee. Exerc Sport Sci Rev 1990; 18:291.
22. Barfred T: Experimental rupture of the Achilles tendon: Comparison of various types of experimental rupture in rats. Acta Orthop Scand 1971; 42:528.
23. Beynnon BD, Fleming BC, Johnson RJ, et al: Anterior cruciate ligament strain behavior during rehabilitation exercises in vivo. Am J Sports Med 1995; 23:24.
24. Beynnon BD, Johnson RJ, Fleming BC, et al: The strain behavior of the anterior cruciate ligament during squatting and active flexion-extension: A comparison of an open and a closed kinetic chain exercise. Am J Sports Med 1997; 25:823.
25. Birrer RB: The Special Olympics: An injury overview. Phys Sports Med 1984; 12:95.
26. Brand RA: Knee ligaments: A new view. J Biomech Eng 1986; 108:106.
27. Brooks GA, Fahey TD: Exercise Physiology: Human Bioenergetics and Its Application. New York, Wiley, 1984.
28. Brooks GA, Fahey TD: Fundamentals of Human Performance. New York, Macmillan, 1987.
29. Caraffa A, Cerulli G, Projetti M, et al: Prevention of anterior cruciate ligament injuries in soccer: A prospective controlled study of proprioceptive training. Knee Surg Sports Traumatol Arthrosc 1996; 4:19.
30. Cerretelli P, Pendergast D, Paganelli WC, et al: Effects of specific muscle training on $\dot{V}_{O_2}$ on-response and early blood lactate. J Appl Physiol 1979; 47:761.
31. Chan CS, Grossman HY: Psychological effects of running loss on consistent runners. Percept Mot Skills 1988; 66:875.
32. Chandler TJ, Kibler WB: A biomechanical approach to the prevention, treatment and rehabilitation of plantar fasciitis. Sports Med 1993; 15:344.
33. Chandler TJ, Kibler WB, Kiser AM, et al: Shoulder strength, power, and endurance in college tennis players. Am J Sports Med 1992; 20:455.
34. Chandler TJ, Kibler WB, Uhl TL, et al: Flexibility comparisons of junior elite tennis players to other athletes. Am J Sports Med 1990; 18:134.
35. Chu DA: Jumping Into Plyometrics. Champaign, IL, Leisure Press, 1992, pp 1–11.
36. Clancy WJ Jr: Tendinitis and plantar fasciitis in runners. In D'Ambrosia RD, Drez D Jr (eds): Prevention and Treatment of Running Injuries. Thorofare, NJ, Slack, 1989, pp 121–131.
37. Clarke DH: Adaptations in strength and muscular endurance resulting from exercise. Exerc Sport Sci Rev 1973; 1:73.
38. Clarkson PM, Ebbeling C: Investigation of serum creatine kinase variability after muscle-damaging exercise. Clin Sci 1988; 75:257.
39. Cohen LA, Cohen ML: Arthrokinetic reflex of the knee. Am J Physiol 1956; 184:433.
40. Convertino V, Hung J, Goldwater D, et al: Cardiovascular responses to exercise in middle-aged men after 10 days of bedrest. Circulation 1982; 65:134.
41. Costill DL, Daniels J, Evans W, et al: Skeletal muscle enzymes and fiber composition in male and female track athletes. J Appl Physiol 1976; 40:149.
42. Costill DL, Fink WJ, Pollock ML: Muscle fiber composition and enzyme activities of elite distance runners. Med Sci Sports 1976; 8:96.
43. Coyle EF, Coggan AR, Hemmert MK, et al: Muscle glycogen utilization during prolonged strenuous exercise when fed carbohydrate. J Appl Physiol 1986; 61:165.
44. Coyle EF, Feiring DC, Rotkis TC, et al: Specificity of power improvements through slow and fast isokinetic training. J Appl Physiol 1981; 51:1437.
45. Curtis KA, Dillon DA: Survey of wheelchair athletic injuries: Common patterns and prevention. Paraplegia 1985; 23:170.
46. Davis G, Plyley MJ, Shephard RJ: Gains of cardiorespiratory fitness with arm-crank training in spinally disabled men. Can J Sport Sci 1991; 16:64.
47. Day RW, Wildermuth BP: Proprioceptive training in the rehabilitation of lower extremity injuries. Adv Sports Med Fitness 1988; 1:241.
48. deLateur BJ, Lehmann JF: Strengthening exercise. In Leek JC, Gershwin ME, Fowler WM Jr (eds): Principles of Physical Medicine and Rehabilitation in the Musculoskeletal Diseases. Orlando, FL, Grune & Stratton, 1986, pp 25–60.
49. DeLisa JA: Academic physiatry: Trends, opportunities and challenges. Am J Phys Med Rehabil 1993; 72:113.
50. Dillingham MF, King WD, Gamburd RS: Rehabilitation of the knee following anterior cruciate ligament and medial collateral ligament injuries. Phys Med Rehabil Clin North Am 1994; 5:175.
51. Ekholm J, Eklund G, Skoglund S: On the reflex effects from the knee joint of the cat. Acta Physiol Scand 1960; 50:167.
52. Epstein SE, Maron BJ: Sudden death and the competitive athlete: Perspectives on preparticipation screening studies. J Am Coll Cardiol 1986; 7:220.

53. Evans WJ, Cannon JG: The metabolic effects of exercise-induced muscle damage. Exerc Sport Sci Rev 1991; 19:99.
54. Fisher AC: Adherence to sports injury rehabilitation programmes. Sports Med 1990; 9:151.
55. Flint FA: Seeing helps believing: Modeling in injury rehabilitation. In Pargman D (ed): Psychological Basis of Sport Injuries. Morgantown, WV, Fitness Information Technology, 1992, pp 183–198.
56. Fringer MN, Stull GA: Changes in cardiorespiratory parameters during periods of training and detraining in young adult females. Med Sci Sports 1974; 6:20.
57. Garrett WE Jr: Muscle strain injuries: Clinical and basic aspects. Med Sci Sports Exerc 1990; 22:436.
58. Gelberman RH, Woo SL, Lothringer K, et al: Effects of early intermittent passive mobilization on healing canine flexor tendons. J Hand Surg Am 1982; 7:170.
59. Glaser RM: Arm exercise training for wheelchair users. Med Sci Sports Exerc 1989; 21(suppl 5):S149.
60. Graves JE, Pollock ML, Jones AE, et al: Specificity of limited range of motion variable resistance training. Med Sci Sports Exerc 1989; 21:84.
61. Gray GW: Chain Reaction. Adrian, MI, Wynn Marketing, 1991, pp 80–98.
62. Grood ES, Suntay WJ, Noyes FR, et al: Biomechanics of the knee-extension exercise: Effect of cutting the anterior cruciate ligament. J Bone Joint Surg Am 1984; 66:725.
63. Guyton AC: Textbook of Medical Physiology, ed 8. Philadelphia, WB Saunders, 1991.
64. Herring SA, Nilson KL: Introduction to overuse injuries. Clin Sports Med 1987; 6:225.
65. Hettinger T: Physiology of Strength. Springfield, IL, Charles C Thomas, 1961.
65a. Hewett TE, Lindenfeld TN, Riccobene JV, et al: The effect of neuromuscular training on the incidence of knee injury in female athletes. Am J Sports Med 1999; 27:699.
66. Hickson RC, Heusner WW, Van Huss WD: Skeletal muscle enzyme alterations after sprint and endurance training. J Appl Physiol 1976; 40:868.
67. Hickson RC, Rennie MJ, Conlee RK, et al: Effects of increased plasma fatty acids on glycogen utilization and endurance. J Appl Physiol 1977; 43:829.
68. Hooker SP, Wells CL: Aerobic power of competitive paraplegic road racers. Paraplegia 1992; 30:428.
69. Janda DH, Wojtys EM, Hankin FM, et al: A three-phase analysis of the prevention of recreational softball injuries. Am J Sports Med 1990; 18:632.
70. Jankowski LW, Sullivan SJ: Aerobic and neuromuscular training: Effect on the capacity, efficiency, and fatigability of patients with traumatic brain injuries. Arch Phys Med Rehabil 1990; 71:500.
71. Jones DR, Speier J, Canine K, et al: Cardiorespiratory responses to aerobic training by patients with postpoliomyelitis sequelae. JAMA 1989; 261:3255.
72. Kendrick ZV, Pollock ML, Hickman TN, et al: Effects of training and detraining on cardiovascular efficiency. Am Correct Ther J 1971; 25:79.
73. Kibler WB: Concepts and exercise rehabilitation. In Leadbetter WB, Buckwalter JA, Gordon SL (eds): Sports-Induced Inflammation: Clinical and Basic Science Concepts. Park Ridge, IL, American Academy of Orthopaedic Surgeons, 1990, pp 759–771.
74. Kibler WB: The role of the scapula in the throwing motion. Contemp Orthop 1991; 22:525.
75. Kibler WB: The Sport Preparticipation Fitness Examination. Champaign, IL, Human Kinetics Books, 1990.
76. Kinzer SM, Convertino VA: Role of leg vasculature in the cardiovascular response to arm work in wheelchair-dependent populations. Clin Physiol 1989; 9:525.
77. Knapik JJ, Jones BH, Bauman CL, et al: Strength, flexibility and athletic injuries. Sports Med 1992; 14:277.
78. Kok G, Bouter LM: On the importance of planned health education: Prevention of ski injury as an example. Am J Sports Med 1990; 18:600.
79. Komi PV, Buskirk ER: Effect of eccentric and concentric muscle conditioning on tension and electrical activity of human muscle. Ergonomics 1972; 15:417.
80. Kraus JF, Conroy C: Mortality and morbidity from injuries in sports and recreation. Annu Rev Pub Health 1984; 5:163.
81. Krivickas LS, Feinberg JH: Lower extremity injuries in college athletes: Relation between ligamentous laxity and lower extremity muscle tightness. Arch Phys Med Rehabil 1996; 77:1139.
82. Kriz JL, Jones DR, Speier JL, et al: Cardiorespiratory responses to upper extremity aerobic training by postpolio subjects. Arch Phys Med Rehabil 1992; 73:49.
83. Leach RE, Paul GR: Running injuries of the knee. In D'Ambrosia RD, Drez D Jr (eds): Prevention and Treatment of Running Injuries. Thorofare, NJ, Slack, 1989, pp 98–119.
84. Leadbetter WB: Physiology of tissue repair. In Athletic Training and Sports Medicine. Park Ridge, IL, American Academy of Orthopedic Surgeons, 1991, pp 43–55.
85. Lehmann JF, deLateur BJ, Stonebridge JB, et al: Therapeutic temperature distribution produced by ultrasound as modified by dosage and volume of tissue exposed. Arch Phys Med Rehabil 1967; 48:662.
86. Lehmann JF, deLateur BJ, Warren CG, et al: Heating of joint structures by ultrasound. Arch Phys Med Rehabil 1968; 49:28.
87. Lehmann JF, Masock AJ, Warren CG, et al: Effect of therapeutic temperatures on tendon extensibility. Arch Phys Med Rehabil 1970; 51:481.
88. Little JC: The athlete's neurosis: A deprivation crisis. Acta Psychiatr Scand 1969; 45:187.
89. Lutz GE, Palmitier RA, An KN, et al: Comparison of tibiofemoral joint forces during open-kinetic-chain and closed-kinetic-chain exercises. J Bone Joint Surg Am 1993; 75:732.
90. Lutz GE, Stuart MJ, Sim FH, et al: Rehabilitative techniques for athletes after reconstruction of the anterior cruciate ligament. Mayo Clin Proc 1990; 65:1322.
91. Mangus BC: Sports injuries, the disabled athlete, and the athletic trainer. Athlet Training 1987; 22:305.
92. Martin BJ, Robinson S, Wiegman DL, et al: Effect of warm-up on metabolic responses to strenuous exercise. Med Sci Sports 1975; 7:146.
93. McArdle WD, Katch FI, Katch VL: Exercise Physiology: Energy, Nutrition, and Human Performance, ed 3. Philadelphia, Lea & Febiger, 1991.
94. McKeag DB: Preseason physical examination for the prevention of sports injuries. Sports Med 1985; 2:413.
95. McMaster PE: Tendon and muscle ruptures: Clinical and experimental studies on the causes and location of subcutaneous ruptures. J Bone Joint Surg 1933; 15:705.
96. Merritt JL, Hunder GG: Passive range of motion, not isometric exercise, amplifies acute urate synovitis. Arch Phys Med Rehabil 1983; 64:130.
97. Micheli LJ: Overuse injuries in children's sports: The growth factor. Orthop Clin North Am 1983; 14:337.
98. Micheli LJ: Thromboembolic complications of cast immobilization for injuries of the lower extremities. Clin Orthop 1975; 108:191.
99. Micheli LJ, Fehlandt AF Jr: Overuse injuries to tendons and apophyses in children and adolescents. Clin Sports Med 1992; 11:713.
100. Milgrom C, Finestone A, Shlamkovitch N, et al: Prevention of overuse injuries of the foot by improved shoe shock attenuation: A randomized prospective study. Clin Orthop 1992; 281:189.
101. Milner-Brown HS, Stein RB, Yemm R: The orderly recruitment of human motor units during voluntary isometric contractions. J Physiol 1973; 230:359.
102. Moritani T, deVries HA: Neural factors versus hypertrophy in the time course of muscle strength gain. Am J Phys Med 1979; 58:115.
103. Mubarak SJ, Gould RN, Lee YF, et al: The medial tibial stress syndrome: A cause of shin splints. Am J Sports Med 1982; 10:201.
104. Noakes TD: Implications of exercise testing for prediction of athletic performance: A contemporary perspective. Med Sci Sports Exerc 1988; 20:319.
105. Noonan TJ, Best TM, Seaber AV, et al: Thermal effects on skeletal muscle tensile behavior. Am J Sports Med 1993; 21:517.
106. Noyes FR: Functional properties of knee ligaments and alterations induced by immobilization: A correlative biomechanical and histological study in primates. Clin Orthop 1977; 123:210.

107. Nygaard E, Andersen P, Nilsson P, et al: Glycogen depletion pattern and lactate accumulation in leg muscles during recreational downhill skiing. Eur J Appl Physiol 1978; 38:261.
108. Outerbridge AR, Micheli LJ: Overuse injuries in the young athlete. Clin Sports Med 1995; 14:503.
109. Palmer I: Plastic surgery of ligaments of the knee. Acta Chir Scand 1944; 91:37.
110. Palmitier RA, An KN, Scott SG, et al: Kinetic chain exercise in knee rehabilitation. Sports Med 1991; 11:402.
111. Pappas AM, Zawacki RM, Sullivan TJ: Biomechanics of baseball pitching: A preliminary report. Am J Sports Med 1985; 13:216.
112. Pate RR, Branch JD: Training for endurance sport. Med Sci Sports Exerc 1992; 24(suppl 9):S340.
113. Paulos L, Noyes FR, Grood E, et al: Knee rehabilitation after anterior cruciate ligament reconstruction and repair. Am J Sports Med 1981; 9:140.
114. Pendergast D, Cerretelli P, Rennie DW: Aerobic and glycolytic metabolism in arm exercise. J Appl Physiol 1979; 47:754.
115. Pendergast DR: Cardiovascular, respiratory, and metabolic responses to upper body exercise. Med Sci Sports Exerc 1989; 21(suppl 5):S121.
116. Perrine JJ: Isokinetic exercise and the mechanical energy potentials of muscle. J Health Phys Educ Rec 1968; 39:40.
117. Pollock ML, Wilmore JH: Exercise in Health and Disease, ed 2. Philadelphia, WB Saunders, 1990.
118. Pope DF, Cole KJ, Brand RA: Physiologic loading of the anterior cruciate ligament does not activate quadriceps or hamstrings in the anesthetized cat. Am J Sports Med 1990; 18:595.
119. Puddu G, Ippolito E, Postacchini F: A classification of Achilles tendon disease. Am J Sports Med 1976; 4:145.
120. Requa RK, DeAvilla LN, Garrick JG: Injuries in recreational adult fitness activities. Am J Sports Med 1993; 21:461.
121. Rians CB, Weltman A, Cahill BR, et al: Strength training for prepubescent males: Is it safe? Am J Sports Med 1987; 15:483.
122. Roskamm H: Optimum patterns of exercise for healthy adults. Can Med Assoc J 1967; 96:895.
123. Saal JA: General principles and guidelines for rehabilitation of the injured athlete. Phys Med Rehabil Clin North Am November 1987; 1:523.
124. Sale D, MacDougall D: Specificity in strength training: A review for the coach and athlete. In Science Periodical on Research and Technology in Sport. Ottawa, Canada, The Coaching Association of Canada, 1981.
125. Sale DG: Neural adaptation to resistance training. Med Sci Sports Exerc 1988; 20(suppl 5):S135.
126. Saltin B, Blomqvist G, Mitchell JH, et al: Response to exercise after bed rest and after training. Circulation 1968; 38(suppl 5):VII1.
127. Schumacher HR Jr: Primer on the Rheumatic Diseases, ed 9. Atlanta, Arthritis Foundation, 1988, pp 24–30.
128. Schwellnus MP, Jordaan G, Noakes TD: Prevention of common overuse injuries by the use of shock absorbing insoles: A prospective study. Am J Sports Med 1990; 18:636.
129. Sharkey BJ: Training for sport. In Cantu RC, Micheli LJ (eds): ACSM's Guidelines for the Team Physician. Philadelphia, Lea & Febiger, 1991, pp 34–47.
130. Shelbourne KD, Nitz P: Accelerated rehabilitation after anterior cruciate ligament reconstruction. Am J Sports Med 1990; 18:292.
131. Shephard RJ: Physiology and Biochemistry of Exercise. New York, Praeger, 1982.
132. Sheth P, Yu B, Laskowski ER, et al: Ankle disk training influences reaction times of selected muscles in a simulated ankle sprain. Am J Sports Med 1997; 25:538.
133. Skrinar GS, Evans WJ, Ornstein LJ, et al: Glycogen utilization in wheelchair-dependent athletes. Int J Sports Med 1982; 3:215.
134. Smith AM, Scott SG, O'Fallon WM, et al: Emotional responses of athletes to injury. Mayo Clin Proc 1990; 65:38.
135. Smith AM, Stuart MJ, Wiese-Bjornstal DM, et al: Competitive athletes: Preinjury and postinjury mood state and self-esteem. Mayo Clin Proc 1993; 68:939.
136. Solomonow M, Baratta R, Zhou BH, et al: The synergistic action of the anterior cruciate ligament and thigh muscles in maintaining joint stability. Am J Sports Med 1987; 15:207.
137. Stanitski CL: Combating overuse injuries: A focus on children and adolescents. Phys Sportsmed 1993; 21:87.
138. Steindler A: Kinesiology of the Human Body Under Normal and Pathological Conditions. Springfield, IL, Charles C Thomas, 1973, p 63.
139. Stone MH: Muscle conditioning and muscle injuries. Med Sci Sports Exerc 1990; 22:457.
140. Stone MH, Wilson GD: Resistive training and selected effects. Med Clin North Am 1985; 69:109.
141. Taylor AW, McDonell E, Brassard L: The effects of an arm ergometer training programme on wheelchair subjects. Paraplegia 1986; 24:105.
142. Taylor DC, Dalton JD Jr, Seaber AV, et al: Viscoelastic properties of muscle-tendon units: The biomechanical effects of stretching. Am J Sports Med 1990; 18:300.
143. Taylor HL, Henschel A, Brožakek J, et al: Effects of bed rest on cardiovascular function and work performance. J Appl Physiol 1949; 2:223.
144. Tesch PA: Skeletal muscle adaptations consequent to long-term heavy resistance exercise. Med Sci Sports Exerc 1988; 20(suppl 5):S132.
145. Thorstensson A, Sjodin B, Karlsson J: Enzyme activities and muscle strength after "sprint training" in man. Acta Physiol Scand 1975; 94:313.
146. Tipton CM, James SL, Mergner W, et al: Influence of exercise on strength of medial collateral knee ligaments of dogs. Am J Physiol 1970; 218:894.
147. Tipton CM, Schild RJ, Tomanek RJ: Influence of physical activity on the strength of knee ligaments in rats. Am J Physiol 1967; 212:783.
148. Torg JS: Problems and prevention. In Torg JS (ed): Athletic Injuries to the Head, Neck, and Face. St Louis, Mosby–Year Book, 1982, pp 3–13.
149. Tropp H, Askling C, Gillquist J: Prevention of ankle sprains. Am J Sports Med 1985; 13:259.
150. Tropp H, Ekstrand J, Gillquist J: Stabilometry in functional instability of the ankle and its value in predicting injury. Med Sci Sports Exerc 1984; 16:64.
151. Van Mechelen W, Twisk J, Molendijk A, et al: Subject-related risk factors for sports injuries: A 1-yr prospective study in young adults. Med Sci Sports Exerc 1996; 28:1171.
152. Verkoshanski Y: Perspectives in the improvement of speed-strength preparation of jumpers. Track Field 1966; 9:11.
153. Watkins RG, Dillin WM: Cervical spine and spinal cord injuries. In Fu FH, Stone DA (eds): Sports Injuries: Mechanisms, Prevention, Treatment. Baltimore, Williams & Wilkins, 1994, pp 853–876.
154. Webb DR: Strength training in children and adolescents. Pediatr Clin North Am 1990; 37:1187.
155. Whiting WC, Puffer JC, Finerman GA, et al: Three-dimensional cinematographic analysis of water polo throwing in elite performers. Am J Sports Med 1985; 13:95.
156. Wilmore JH, Costill DL: Training for Sport and Activity: The Physiological Basis of the Conditioning Process, ed 3. Dubuque, William C Brown, 1988.
157. Wilt F: Plyometrics: What it is—how it works. Athlet J 1975; 55:89.
158. Wroble RR, Brand RA: Function of knee ligaments: A historical review of two perspectives. Iowa Orthop 1988; J8:67.
159. Young A, Stokes M, Iles JF: Effects of joint pathology on muscle. Clin Orthop 1987; 219:21.

45 CHAPTER

John A. Schuchmann, M.D.

Occupational Rehabilitation

Prior to the 1700s, most workers toiled at home in small shops or worked in the fields. Work was performed with crude hand tools rather than machines. Rural life was the norm, with fewer than 10% of Europeans living in cities. The development of automated machinery and factories, however, dramatically changed the way in which people lived and worked. The industrial revolution began in Great Britain in the 1700s and spread to North America in the early 1800s. Industrialization dramatically increased the production of many types of goods, but it also brought about many changes for workers.

Industrialization required the relocation of many workers into towns and cities. Skilled workers and craftsmen were often relegated to tedious, degrading jobs. Workers were required to produce at the "machine rate" rather than at their own pace. They were often required to work long hours for meager wages. The profit motive encouraged industrialists to search for even more rapid methods of production. Industrialists were often hard-working and ambitious, demanding the same from their employees.

By 1900, nearly 10 million Americans lived in poverty, despite the common 10-hour, 6-day work week. Little attention was paid to worker safety, and industrial accidents and deaths were common.

Unionization of labor, which began between 1860 and 1900, helped balance the demands on the worker while ensuring adequate compensation, reasonable working hours, and safe, adequate working conditions.[34, 35]

The labor movement was often stormy and violent, but ultimately conditions for the worker began to improve. Despite these improvements, the injured worker in the early 1900s had little recourse or compensation. Injured workers had to use the courts to recover any damages from employers. They had to prove both that the employer was negligent and that the employer's negligence resulted in their injury. With employer defenses such as "assumption of risk" and "contributory negligence," workers usually recovered little; 80% of cases were lost or the injured worker was left uncompensated.[2]

By 1910 it was recognized that industrialization benefited the whole country. Injury and even death, however, were still inevitable components of even the most progressive and sophisticated industrial activities. Workers' compensation programs were begun as a means of providing wage replacement and medical care for injured workers. New York was the first state to adopt compulsory workers' compensation in 1910. That law was later found unconstitutional. In 1911, Wisconsin passed the first workers' compensation act that remained in force. Other states gradually enacted workers' compensation plans. Mississippi was the final state to pass such a plan, in 1948.[2]

The risk of death from work accidents has decreased dramatically over the years. Between 1912 and 1996, the rate of unintentional work deaths decreased by 90%, from 21 to 2 deaths per 100,000 population. Despite major advances in industrial technology and safety, work today still poses considerable risk of injury.[20, 29, 40, 53, 60] There were 5.7 million occupational injuries in private industry in the United States in 1997. Workplace injuries resulted in an estimated 80 million lost work days in 1996, with the rate of occupational injuries and illnesses about 7.1 per 100 full-time workers.

Ten industries reported at least 100,000 injury cases each: (1) eating and drinking establishments, (2) hospitals, (3) nursing and personal care facilities, (4) grocery stores, (5) motor vehicles and equipment, (6) department stores, (7) air transportation, scheduled, (8) trucking and carrier services (except air), (9) meat products, and (10) hotels and motels. These industries accounted for 30% of all injury cases reported nationwide during 1997.[8a, 67]

The cost of workplace injuries in 1996 was estimated to be $121 billion. This figure includes $60.2 billion for wage and productivity losses, $19 billion for medical costs, and $25.6 billion for administrative costs. The yearly mean cost for each employed worker was $960, with a mean cost of $26,000 for each disabling injury.[44] A sampling of studies indicates that work-related injuries are certainly not unique to the United States but are ubiquitous throughout the world.[16, 21, 25, 26, 30, 35, 37, 46]

Industrial injuries are costly because the industry loses productivity and sales and the worker loses wages. Health care costs, as well as costs for retraining and replacing workers, add to the loss. These costs are ultimately reflected in higher prices of products for the consumer. With current profit margins slim and health care costs rising rapidly, industries and businesses are becoming proactive rather than reactive in trying to prevent and minimize the impact of injuries on their overall operations and profitability. This increased attention to safety is reflected in decreasing rates of injuries and illnesses in the workplace (Fig. 45–1).

Throughout the United States, there is a shortage of physicians trained in the comprehensive evaluation and treatment of the complex musculoskeletal problems often seen in injured workers. Many physicians in the field of physical medicine and rehabilitation are becoming involved in the early evaluation, treatment, and rehabilitation of workers to help them recover and return to the work site. Physiatrists possess the skills needed to help restore and enhance the injured worker's job performance. A team effort is often required to ensure the successful outcome of returning the injured worker to work. The physiatrist's team orientation and training in musculoskeletal disorders provides an excellent background to spearhead industrial rehabilitation efforts. The physiatrist is also able to evaluate and quantify any residual impairment once the worker has reached maximum medical improvement.

COMMON MEDICAL PROBLEMS SEEN IN A REHABILITATIVE INDUSTRIAL PRACTICE

Low Back Pain

Low back pain is a major expense to industry because of lost productivity, high medical costs, and compensation payments. Low back pain is so frequent in our society that 70% to 80% of persons will experience low back pain at some time in their lives.[43] Low back pain is second only to upper respiratory illnesses as the most common cause of time missed from work. Chronic low back pain has a major economic and personal impact, as it is the leading cause of disability for individuals between the ages of 19 and 45 years.[31] On any given day nearly 6.5 million people in the United States are receiving treatment for low back pain. The National Safety Council estimated that 370,000 disabling work-related back injuries occurred in the United States in 1991, at a cost of approximately $50 billion. In 1990, Liberty Mutual Insurance Co. Workers' Compensation claims showed a mean cost of $6807, with a median cost of $391. The large spread in costs was due to the fact that 25% of the cases consumed 95% of the costs.[63] By 1995, compensation claim costs had risen to $11,321 per case.[44] Lost work days attributable to low back pain have been reported to be 1400 lost days per 1000 workers.[42]

Low back pain is most prevalent in heavy industry. Some 50% to 80% of workers in heavy industry report having suffered from back pain in the past 12 years.[68]

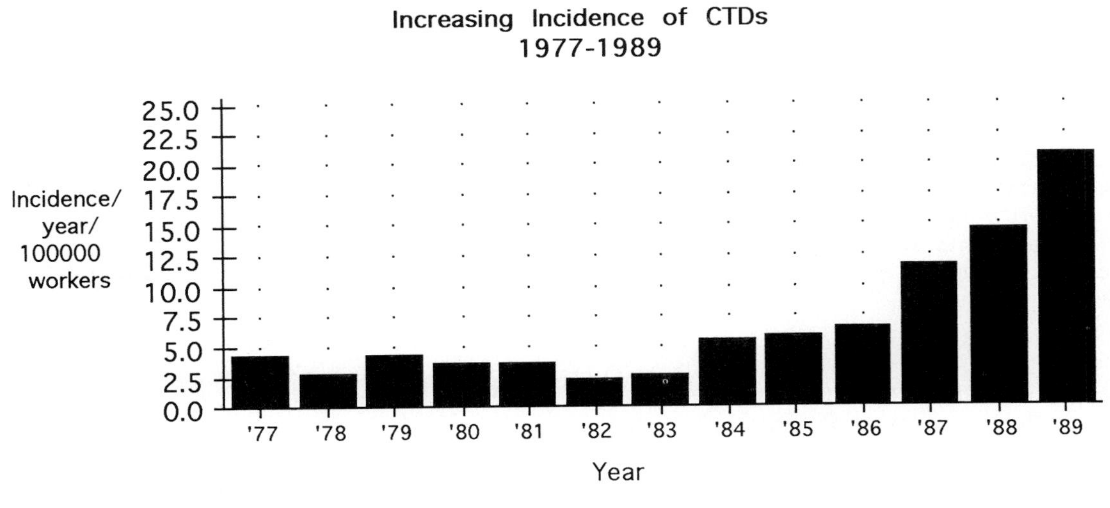

FIGURE 45–1. Injuries and illnesses have decreased in recent years as industries and businesses have become more proactive in early identification and treatment of work-related health problems. In the chart, incidence rate = injury and illness rate per 100 full-time workers. (Adapted from Bureau of Labor Statistics, Occupational Safety and Health Administration: Workplace Injuries and Illnesses in 1997. Washington, DC, US Department of Labor, Dec 17, 1998. http://stats.bls.gov/oshhome.htm)

The low back injury rate has been found to be about three to five per 1000 employees per year in light industries, as compared to 200 per 1000 employees per year in heavy industries.

Despite advances in automation, humans are still required by many industries to perform considerable manual material handling. Stresses on the spine vary depending on the lifting techniques utilized as well as on the load handled. Improper handling of work materials can precipitate back injuries. Overuse can also result in muscular fatigue and lead to a possible back injury. Repetitive vibratory stresses on the back, from such activities as driving vehicles or using vibrating tools such as jackhammers, can produce microtrauma.

Only 1% to 2% of patients with low back pain usually require surgical treatment.[38, 39] Approximately 90% of patients with extruded lumbar disks have good to excellent outcomes with nonoperative management, with return-to-work rates of more than 90%.[54] Overall, about 90% of patients with low back pain improve with minimal or no medical intervention. A small percentage of cases, however, become chronic, leading to long-term disability associated with increased medical expenses and compensation costs. Recurrence of low back pain is also quite common, with a recurrence rate of approximately 70%. (See Chapter 40 for additional information about low back pain.)

Cumulative Trauma Disorders

Cumulative trauma disorders, also referred to as repetitive motion disorders, repetition strain injuries, or occupational overuse injuries, have recently gained more attention throughout industry and in the health care sector.[19, 50] Cumulative trauma disorders are not a new entity or type of disorder, but the name indicates an awareness that overuse might be a causative factor. Cumulative trauma disorders increased at a rapid rate during the mid- to late 1980s and in the early 1990s. In the United States, such disorders accounted for 40% to 50% of all workers' compensation claims.[50] The increase in these problems was thought to have a number of causes (Table 45–1). More recent statistics point to a slow and progressive decrease in the number of cases of cumulative trauma disorders reported as industries aggressively institute preventive ergonomic and early intervention programs. Between 1992 and 1995, injuries and illnesses requiring days off work decreased by 19% for overexertion injuries and by 14% for repetitive motion injuries.[4]

A variety of tissues can be affected by cumulative trauma disorders:

- Muscles
- Tendons
- Bursae
- Ligaments
- Peripheral nerves
- Bones
- Cartilage
- Intervertebral disks

Many clinical problems fall under the category of cumulative trauma disorder, including:

- Muscle strains
- Tendinitis
- Bursitis
- Ligamentous injuries
- Compression neuropathies
- Fractures
- Cartilage damage
- Disk disease

The musculotendinous unit is most often affected by cumulative trauma disorders because of the relatively poor blood supply at the bone-tendon interface, which produces delayed, incomplete, or partial healing.

Repetitive motion and stress in cumulative trauma disorders lead to microtrauma of the tissue. An acute inflammatory response ensues that can become chronic. Chronic inflammation can lead to more tissue damage. The common etiological feature of these disorders is that repetitive trauma occurs faster than the tissue's ability to heal itself. Cumulative trauma disorders usually develop slowly and gradually over many weeks, months, or years. A number of activities and related equipment have been implicated as etiological and aggravating factors for the development of cumulative trauma disorders;[50] some of these are listed in Table 45–2.

In the workplace, upper extremity cumulative trauma disorders far outnumber lower extremity disorders. Some of the more common disorders seen in clinical practice are listed in Table 45–3.

Chronic muscle soreness in a worker might be an early warning sign of the development of a cumulative trauma disorder. Workers are often sore and stiff the first week or two after beginning a job, as a result of new physical demands. In most cases physical conditioning gradually occurs and the soreness subsides. The prolonged persistence of symptoms can indicate that tissues are not able to adapt to the stress. Continuing the activity could lead to tissue damage and the development of a cumulative trauma disorder.

TABLE 45–1 Causative Factors for Increase in Number of Cumulative Trauma Disorders Reported

More repetitive and faster-paced jobs
Job dissatisfaction
Increased awareness of signs and symptoms by employees, employers, and medical and legal professionals
Improved accuracy in identifying and reporting cumulative trauma disorders
Compensation coverage by workers' compensation carriers

PREVENTION

Back Injury

On-the-job back injuries are extremely expensive.[61] In a classic study reported in 1958, Krusen and Ford[33] noted that individuals receiving workers' compensation for back injuries demonstrated 33% less objective evidence of impairment, received nearly twice as many physical therapy treatments, and experienced long-term

TABLE 45–2 Sampling of Etiological or Aggravating Factors and Activities in Cumulative Trauma Disorders

Activities
Forceful grasping
Highly repetitive work
Activities causing rapid or extreme joint movements
Overhead work
Maintaining static work positions for prolonged times
Occupations
Assembly line worker
Carpenter
Butcher
Typist/data entry worker
Cashier
Driver
Factory worker performing repetitive activity
Food preparer
Postal worker
Musician
Electrician
Professional athlete
Tools and Equipment
Repetitive assembly lines, on which worker performs at "machine pace"
Undampened pneumatic tools
Hammers
Screwdrivers
Pliers
Scissors
Knives
Keyboards
Musical instruments
Use of gloves

improvement in 44% fewer cases compared with similar back pain patients not receiving compensation.

Sander and Meyers[55] also showed that railroad workers injured on the job were off work much longer than those who were hurt during off-duty hours. Workers with lumbosacral strains averaged 14.9 months off work when hurt on the job, but only 3.6 months off work when hurt during off-duty hours. Those who needed surgery returned to work more quickly if the injury was incurred during off-duty time (4.4 vs. 9.3 months from the time of surgery). As industries became aware of the cost of acute and chronic back injuries, attempts were made to lessen the incidence of back injuries in industry.[11, 24, 62]

X-Ray Screening

Initial attempts at low back injury prevention by industry focused on lumbar spine screening with x-rays. Individuals were required to obtain pre-employment lumbar spine radiographs, and employment was denied if abnormalities were detected. This practice was widespread until additional evidence brought it into question. It was subsequently discovered that there was generally no definite correlation between an abnormality seen on a lumbar x-ray and the chance of an individual's sustaining an on-the-job back injury.[22] The only radiographic abnormalities that seemed to have any predictive value were spondylolysis and spondylolisthesis, when found in individuals who performed very strenuous jobs. This abnormality is not seen often enough in the general population (about 5% to 6%) to justify routine back x-rays.[36] Osteophytes were not found to correlate with back pain. With the advent of computed tomography (CT) and magnetic resonance imaging (MRI), it has been found that disk abnormalities, including disk bulges and herniations, occur in 30% to 50% or more of asymptomatic individuals.[6, 48, 64] The use of pre-employment or preplacement spine radiographic studies is now in disrepute, and some consider the practice a violation of the Americans With Disabilities Act.

Education: The Back School Approach

Most individuals learn how to lift by trial and error. Proper lifting, however, is something that must be taught. In the past, industries trained workers to specific job requirements but did not always teach the worker how to lift properly and how to use the back. Today, many industries realize that an investment in a "back school" for employees can help decrease on-the-job back injuries.

An effective back school program incorporates individual or small group instruction along with actual practice and skill development. Items actually lifted and manipulated at work are used for training, and the worker is coached and reinforced in proper lifting and handling techniques. Supervisory personnel are also taught proper lifting and handling along with their workers. Without the full support of management, training is not likely to decrease the number of injuries. Managers must also be willing to structure and pace jobs in a way that will allow the use of proper material handling techniques.

The recommended lifting technique generally requires the worker to be positioned directly in front of and as close to the load as is feasible. The worker is taught to squat while keeping the shoulders back and the low back in a neutral position, with the lumbar lordosis maintained. Loads should be held close to the body to decrease stress on the low back. Footing should be secure, and the lift should be performed in a slow and controlled fashion.[18]

Jobs that require repetitive lifting by flexing at the waist place much more stress on the back than do similar manual materials-handling jobs that allow proper squat-

TABLE 45–3 Common Cumulative Trauma Disorders Related to Work Activities

Tendinitis and tenosynovitis at wrist and in forearm
Epicondylitis
Rotator cuff tendinitis and shoulder bursitis
Myofascial syndromes
Hand-arm vibration syndrome
Median nerve-carpal tunnel syndrome, nerve trauma in palm
Ulnar nerve compression in elbow, hand, or wrist
Thoracic outlet syndrome

ting and lifting postures. Proper and improper lifting techniques are illustrated in Figures 45–2 and 45–3.

Workers often revert to poor lifting techniques because their quadriceps are weak and fatigue with repetitive squatting. The back school education can also emphasize the value of quadriceps exercises, such as the wall slide exercise (Fig. 45–4).

Healthy lifestyle choices, such as proper diet and the avoidance of drugs, alcohol, and tobacco, and the value of regular exercise can be reinforced during back school educational programs.

Back school programs can result in cost savings and fewer injuries. In one study, back school education was provided to a plastics-related manufacturer with 800 employees and to a woodworking firm with 400 employees. The workers were observed for 2 years. Direct compensation and medical cost savings were 74% and 80%, respectively, and the incidence of back injuries decreased by 49% and 68%, respectively.[57] Much of the success was due to extensive education of managers and their subsequent positive reinforcement of the program.

Evaluation and Enhancement of Strength, Flexibility, and Fitness

It has been hypothesized that a more fit worker is less likely to be injured on the job. Cady and colleagues[10] assessed fitness in 1652 firefighters by measuring flexibility, isometric lifting strength, and aerobic capacity on a bicycle. Individuals were grouped according to fitness into thirds: least fit, middle fit, and most fit. Back injury rates varied depending on fitness: for the least fit group it was 7.1%; for the middle fit group, 3.2%; and for the most fit group, 0.8%.

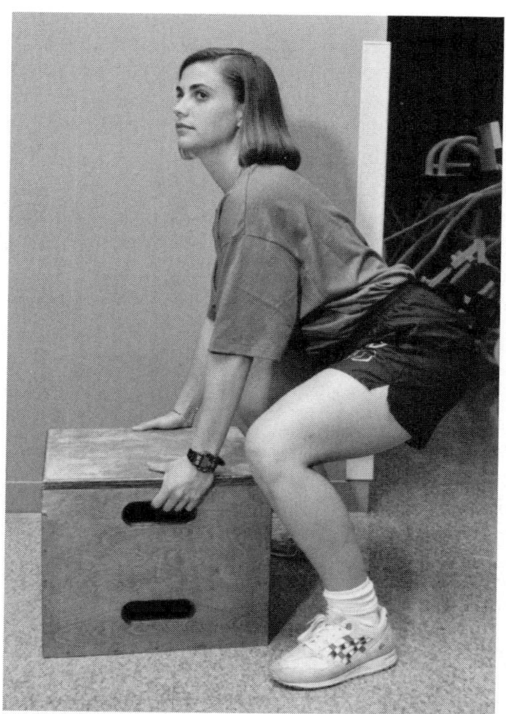

FIGURE 45–2. Proper lifting technique with the back in a neutral position.

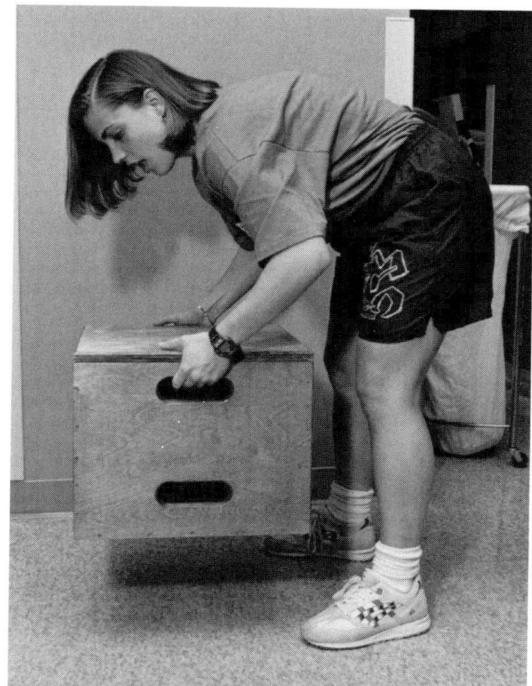

FIGURE 45–3. Faulty lifting technique with the back in a forward flexed posture.

Keyserling et al[32] conducted isometric strength tests on workers at a tire and rubber plant. The study showed an injury rate in the group hired after a screening strength test to be one-third that in the group hired without undergoing strength testing. Isometric strength testing was shown to be safe, but it has now been replaced in many facilities with job-specific testing that measures the ability to safely perform specific job tasks. A criticism of isometric strength testing as an employment screening tool is that it is considered by some to be discriminatory against women, older individuals, and persons with disabilities.

Some industries, especially those that require much physical work, are now realizing the importance of emphasizing physical fitness in their work force. The military has for many years realized the necessity of soldiers' maintaining physical fitness and combat readiness. Regular physical training and periodic fitness evaluations are a regular part of military life. Other professions, such as police and firefighters, have also emphasized fitness in their workers. Cady et al[9] showed that a program to improve firefighter fitness (physical work capacity, strength, and flexibility) resulted in lower injury rates and workers' compensation costs.

Other interventions, such as flexibility programs, have been used to try to improve performance on the job and to decrease injuries. The flexibility program of Hilyer and colleagues[28] was shown to help reduce the severity and cost of musculoskeletal injuries in firefighters. Some industries have established their own fully staffed fitness centers. Smaller industries typically find it more feasible and cost-effective to encourage the

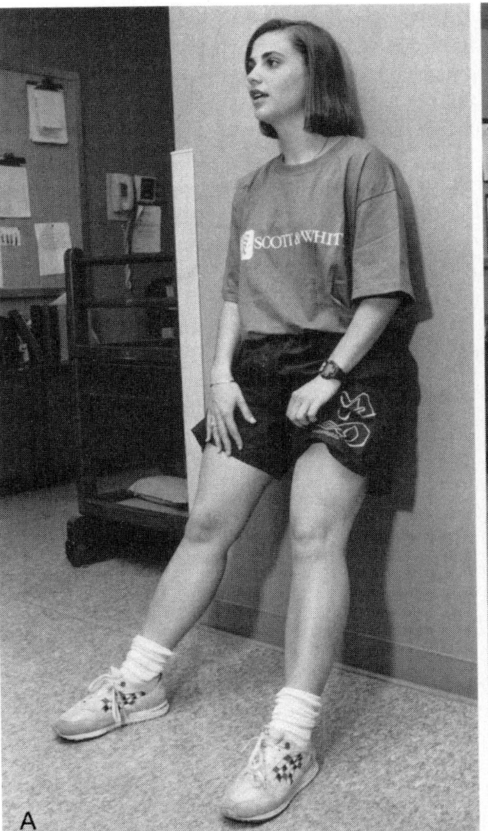

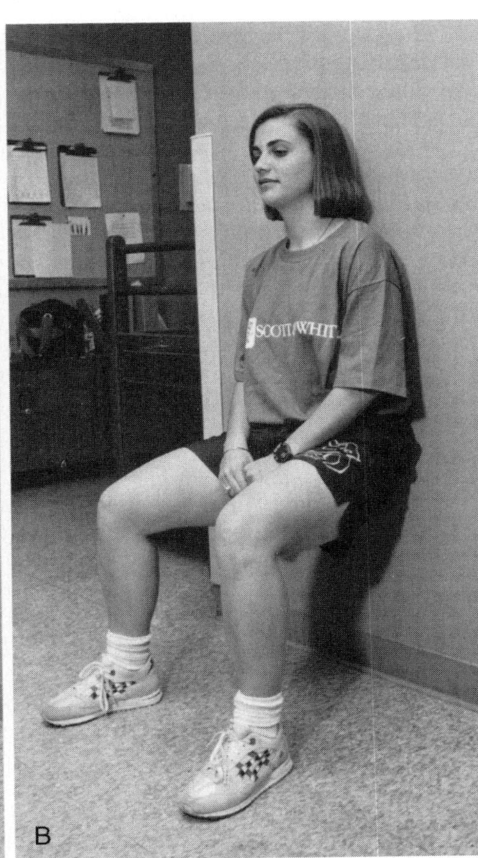

FIGURE 45–4. The wall slide exercise is excellent for strengthening the quadriceps and hip extensors. These important muscles facilitate lifting with proper technique when they have adequate strength and endurance. The worker is instructed to gradually increase the time interval maintained in the squatted-down position.

use of existing community fitness facilities and programs.

Ergonomic Assessment and Intervention

Injuries often occur because a worker is mismatched with a job, such as when a physically deconditioned worker is placed in a job that is very strenuous and demanding. Without adequate conditioning and training, that individual might be at a higher risk of injury. Physiatrists are often called on to help industries better understand specific physical requirements and demands of jobs to help ensure a better employee-job fit.

Ergonomics, or human factors engineering,[51, 52, 56] refers to the study of the "fit" between the worker, the job tasks, the tools and equipment used, and the work environment. The goal is to enhance the match between the worker's physical, emotional, and mental capabilities and the job. An ideal match should lessen the incidence of work injuries and errors, reduce the worker's fatigue and physical stress, and enhance overall productivity.

Lifting is often implicated as a factor that contributes to the development of low back pain. Jobs should be analyzed ergonomically to determine the amount and frequency of lifting required. Postures utilized by workers on the job should be noted. Other factors to be considered include the following: (1) What are the sizes and the shapes of the objects lifted? (2) Can the worker get a firm grasp on the object? (3) Is twisting required along with the lifting? (4) What speed of lifting is required to keep up with the expected productivity? (5) Does awkward placement of bins (or other equipment) require the worker to flex the spine into a position that creates a higher back injury risk?

Other work factors should be assessed, such as the amount of pushing or pulling. Are handles present that allow pushing and pulling in a biomechanically favorable position? If a wheeled cart is pulled or pushed, are wheels sufficiently maintained and large enough to allow smooth movement and to easily clear obstacles and irregularities in the workplace floor?

Proper lifting and materials-handling techniques are impossible to utilize in some circumstances. In these cases, an assessment should be performed to ascertain whether the load can be subdivided into lighter loads, whether a mechanical lifting device can be utilized, whether loads can be positioned to allow lifting without concomitant spine rotation, or whether help from another individual can produce a safer lift. The pace of lifting should also be sufficiently slow and deliberate to allow the use of good biomechanics.[18]

Low back pain is also common in sedentary workers such as secretaries and drivers. Properly fitting and supportive seating is essential to minimize stress on the back. Industries have traditionally purchased furniture in bulk on the one-size-fits-all principle. Today, many industries are realizing that workers come in all sizes and shapes. The purchase of higher-quality seating is often a prudent investment. Chairs can be properly fitted and adjusted to meet the specific needs of the workers who will occupy them for 8 or more hours per day.

Analysis of specific jobs is essential to ascertain the physical requirements and demands necessary for successful performance of the job. Job descriptions that actually quantify the amount and frequency of lifting, pushing, pulling, climbing, stooping, and squatting are helpful when trying to make a successful fit between a prospective worker and a specific job. Dynamometers and push-pull gauges can be helpful in assessing jobs, and occupational or physical therapists can often be helpful resources in establishing job descriptions and in evaluating specific job tasks.

Lumbar Support Orthoses

Lumbar support orthoses are widely marketed to industry as aids to help decrease the incidence of low back injuries. Studies validating the efficacy of back supports are limited at this time.[49] There might be some value in using back supports to prevent initial back injuries, but their across-the-board use for all workers in manual industries has not yet been shown to decrease overall injuries, injury severity, or overall cost per injury.[41]

Back supports can serve several useful functions. They are visible reminders of the need to lift properly. They also provide an increase in intra-abdominal pressure when properly fitted and worn, and they can help lessen intradiskal pressure during lifting. However, lumbar supports are secondary in importance to comprehensive training of the worker in appropriate body mechanics, and the provision of an ergonomically appropriate, safe job in a favorable working environment.

Preplacement Screening: ADA Approach

The Americans With Disabilities Act (ADA) (Public Law 101-336)[1, 58] became effective on July 26, 1992. This act changed the way in which job placement can be legally performed. Under this act, an employer can require an employee to undergo *job-specific* preplacement testing only after a job offer has been made to the prospective employee. This preplacement examination can test the ability to safely perform the *usual tasks* of the specific job. The goal of testing is to ensure that the employee is physically and emotionally capable of performing the job safely so that the worker or coworkers will not be endangered. If the employee is unable to successfully perform the testing due to some functional limitation, the employer is obliged to determine whether job accommodations could reasonably be implemented that would allow the successful performance of the required job tasks.

The goal of the preplacement testing should be to assess for the presence and severity of:

1. Stable impairments that could affect job performance and safety. (For example, a person with a traumatic amputation typically has a stable impairment. The examination should determine whether this employee could safely perform the job duties with the impairment.)
2. Impairments that could be worsened or aggravated by the job requirements. (For example, an individual with stage II spondylolisthesis would be at higher risk for back re-injury in a job that required frequent, repetitive bending and heavy lifting.)
3. Progressive conditions that would ultimately require job reassignment to a more sedentary occupation. (For example, an individual with ankylosing spondylitis would have limited ability to perform heavy labor and bending and would ultimately require placement in a more sedentary and less vigorous position.)
4. Intermittent problems that would impair performance safety. (For example, a history of a seizure disorder in an individual with a previous head injury. If seizure control is less than complete, placement considerations need to be taken to ensure the safety of the employee and co-workers.)

Preplacement examinations cannot be performed randomly. If they are used, the following requirements must be fulfilled:

1. All new employees for the same job must be examined using the same tests.
2. Results from the medical preplacement examination must be treated as a medical record and must be maintained confidentially.
3. Supervisors and managers can be informed about any specific accommodations or work restrictions that will be necessary for the worker's safety and success on the job.
4. Any investigation about a disability or impairment must be "job-related and consistent with business necessity."
5. Future risk cannot be considered when determining whether the individual can perform the specific offered job.

Preplacement testing should ideally help place an employee in a specific job in which the employee has the physical and emotional ability to successfully and safely complete the assigned work tasks. Proper placement should help ensure a healthy and contented worker and a safer work site.

Cumulative Trauma Disorders

Cumulative trauma disorders, such as tendinitis, bursitis, muscle strains, and peripheral nerve compression, are usually the result of repetitive stresses applied to the body at sufficient force or frequency to slowly and progressively lead to tissue damage. Injuries can be treated and improvements will occur; however, if the worker is reassigned to the same job, recurrence is likely.

Cumulative trauma disorders should be actively sought out in industry. Specific jobs that are found to pose a high risk of producing injury should be thoroughly analyzed to determine whether ergonomic changes could be made to enhance job tolerance and safety. Site visits and job analyses can be very helpful in pinpointing specific job modifications or job rotations that could be implemented to lessen risk to the workers. At-risk jobs might require such factors as excessive

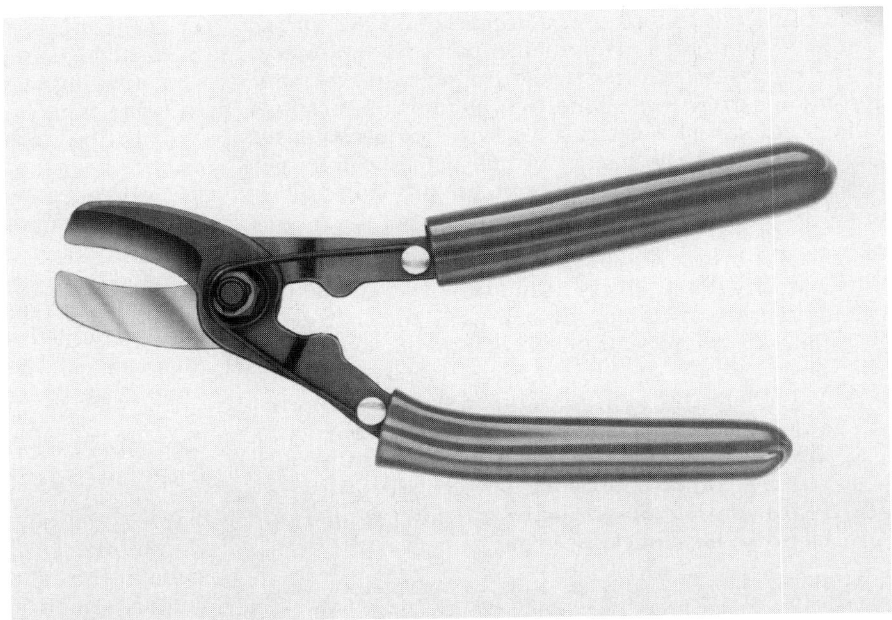

FIGURE 45–5. Ergonomic cutter features a cushioned and contoured grip with spring opening. It is designed to reduce local pressure on the hand and fatigue. (Courtesy of Torvaal Ergonomic Power Curve Tools, Chagrin Falls, OH.)

force, rapid speed (often machine paced), uncomfortable and poorly fitting tools, awkward working postures, or excessive joint motion. At times, ergonomic tools designed for the worker and the specific job can help decrease risk of injury (Fig. 45–5). Handle sizes about 1.5 inches (3.75 cm) in diameter often aid comfort. Comfortable, cushioned, and adequate-length grips can be useful. Vibratory and oscillating tools might need vibration dampening. Altering the work posture and job rotation can also facilitate safer job performance. Job rotation allows the worker to perform different work tasks and use different muscle groups. This can help minimize tissue overuse and prevent the development of cumulative trauma disorders.[52]

EVALUATION OF THE INJURED WORKER

Despite the best safety awareness and preventive programs, accidents occur. Appropriate early evaluation and treatment should be seamlessly integrated with efficient management and rehabilitation of more chronic and persistent injuries. A well-integrated program can help minimize lost time and productivity as well as help prevent the development of chronic disability.

The Detailed History

It is very important for the examining physiatrist to obtain a complete history from the worker. A description of the overall job tasks and requirements is helpful, as is a detailed history of what happened at the time of the accident. Incurring an injury on the job is often an emotionally charged event for both the employee and employer. The attitude and response that the injured worker perceives at the time of injury are vitally important. Occasionally, in the "heat of the battle," one or both parties say things that affect the long-term outcome. The injured worker should be treated with kindness and compassion. If he or she is treated abruptly or if there are accusations or insinuations that the worker was to blame for the accident, the worker can become angry and less motivated to return to work. When handled properly, the initial response can help develop a cooperative relationship between the worker and the employer. When handled poorly, the initial response can distance the employee from the employer and result in a chronic adversarial relationship. Part of history taking is to learn the worker's perception of how he or she has been treated.

The outline presented in Table 45–4 can be helpful when taking the history of the injury. By obtaining a thorough initial history, the physiatrist can obtain a

TABLE 45–4 Important Historical Facts to Assess in the Initial Interview

1. Ask the worker to describe the accident in detail.
2. What was the worker's position/posture at the time of the accident?
3. If the injury occurred during lifting, was there twisting or turning associated with the lifting motion?
4. What was being handled at the time? Ask the worker to describe the weight, size, and shape of the material and the frequency of handling.
5. Did a slip, fall, or other unusual event occur?
6. What was the worker's footing like?
7. Is this the worker's usual job, or were these new tasks?
8. How long has the worker been on this specific job?
9. Have other workers had injuries on this job?
10. Is there any problem with the equipment being utilized on the job?
11. At what time of day and what day of week did the accident occur?
12. Was anyone else injured?
13. What was the initial response by management to the injury?

more complete picture of the accident and the job, as well as of management's initial response to the injury.

The physiatrist is often asked by the workers' compensation carrier to respond to a number of questions to help determine whether a work-related problem really did occur.[50] The history should be sufficiently detailed to be able to answer these frequently asked questions:

1. Do the history and physical findings clearly support a work-related illness or injury?
2. Is there consistency between the history of the illness or injury and the clinical findings and diagnosis?
3. Was there sufficient job-related exposure to provide a clear cause-and-effect relationship between the work activities and the clinical presentation?
4. Are any other preexisting problems or causative factors present that could have led to the development of this clinical problem?

Some workers are seen by the physiatrist soon after the accident, but others are not seen for evaluation for weeks, months, or even years after the accident. In these more chronic cases, it is important to extend the history to include additional information (Table 45–5).

The worker's perception of and satisfaction with his or her job can strongly influence the course of the initial injury as well as the ultimate recovery and return to work. In one study, workers who "hardly ever" enjoyed their job tasks were 2.5 times more likely to report a back injury than workers who "almost always" enjoyed their jobs.[5]

It is also important to assess the individual's current lifestyle and plans for the future. What is his or her typical day? Is the worker being passive and inactive, or is there evidence that the worker is making efforts to stay active and productive? If he is not working now, is he making plans for the future that include a return to some type of reasonable, productive employment? What is the worker's outlook for the future? Does she see hope for the future or only despair? Some workers focus on keeping productive, taking the necessary steps to return to work, and maintaining favorable relationships with their employers. Others, however, blame the employer for all their problems and take a passive or even a passive-aggressive role in returning to any meaningful productivity. Litigation that is pending is also important, because it often slows down recovery and limits response to treatment.

TABLE 45–5 Important Areas to Assess with Chronic Injuries

1. Ask the worker to describe the initial medical examination and treatment. What did the worker understand the diagnosis to be? What was the response to initial treatment? Did the worker attempt to return to work? If so, what happened?
2. If improvement did not occur, what other testing, treatments, and physicians have been involved? Has surgery been performed? If so, how many operations, and how effective were they in providing relief?
3. Has the worker been involved in rehabilitative efforts such as active physical therapy, work conditioning, or work hardening?
4. Does the worker have a job to return to? What is the worker's current relationship with the employer? Does the employer seem willing to accept the worker back on the job?
5. How is the worker currently spending a typical day? How much time does the worker spend in bed every day? In front of the television? Does the worker get out of the house regularly? Does the worker participate in hobbies and recreation?
6. Does the worker participate in any regular exercise? This includes specific exercises to correct the condition as well as general exercises to improve overall aerobic fitness. What is the worker's estimate of his or her own level of physical fitness?

Concurrent Medical or Psychological Illnesses

The evaluation should include an assessment of the worker's overall health. Preexisting problems are occasionally present that could have contributed to the accident or injury or that can affect the recovery process. Such medical conditions as diabetes, arthritis, heart disease, and pulmonary disease should be considered. Occasionally, an occupational injury occurs because of such factors as leg weakness due to diabetic neuropathy or loss of balance due to pain in an arthritic joint. Obesity can also be a significant factor if its presence makes it difficult to use proper body mechanics during physical tasks or if its presence prolongs the recovery period.

The patient should be evaluated for the abuse of drugs, alcohol, and tobacco. Accidents and injuries can occur from working under the influence of these substances. Prescription medication overuse should also be considered. Workers often slip into such overuse gradually. The worker has pain and therefore takes medications. With time, tolerance often develops and medication use increases, with more potent medications and more frequent doses being taken. Tobacco use should also be addressed, as a number of studies[3, 24, 47] have shown a correlation between tobacco use and back pain, disk degeneration, and slower healing.

Physical Examination

A meticulous physical examination is essential for optimal management of injured workers. They should be undressed sufficient that the injured areas can be fully evaluated. Palpation can be difficult when working around clothing. Important findings such as winging of a scapula, muscle atrophy, or pertinent scars and rashes can be easily overlooked if the patient is not undressed.

A general assessment of the worker's health, as well as a thorough assessment of the musculoskeletal system, should be performed. It is useful to assess the freedom and smoothness of movement with the patient standing. How much pain behavior is present during this portion of the examination? Is the individual able to walk on toes and heels, to squat, and to forward flex and touch the toes? If appropriate, it is helpful to assess the individual's ability to hop on one foot or to run in place.

The amount of spine mobility and flexibility should be assessed, including forward flexion, extension, lateral bending, and rotation. Do any specific movements aggravate the symptoms? Leg-length inequalities or spinal deformities should be noted.

Palpation is helpful to evaluate for areas of local tenderness (trigger points or local areas of injury) or widespread tenderness. If tenderness is discovered, it should be mapped out as carefully as possible to identify the triggering tissue or source of pain (e.g., muscle, tendon, ligament, joint).

For shoulder girdle problems, the shoulder region should be observed from all sides. Is there any scapular winging with either forward flexion or abduction of the upper extremities, with or without resistance? Is pain produced at any point in the arc of motion? Are the shoulders symmetrical? Is any atrophy present? These findings are often overlooked if patients are evaluated only from the front while they are seated in a chair. (For additional information, see Chapter 38.)

Range of motion of the spine and joints in the affected area should be measured (see Chapter 1). Limitation of motion should be noted, as well as pain produced with movement.

A systematic evaluation of spinal and extremity strength is useful to identify areas of weakness. Muscle atrophy, either focal or generalized, should be noted. True organic weakness results in a smooth "giving way" during muscle testing. Muscle giving way in a ratchety pattern often suggests a possible "functional" nonorganic component to the symptoms. This ratchety response occasionally occurs despite the presence of actual organic disease. The examiner should also avoid mistakenly ascribing true weakness to a patient who actually has only pain inhibition of function.

Measurement of hand grip strength can be helpful during the evaluation. A hand-held dynamometer can be utilized to assess grip strength in various positions. Grip strength is normally strongest in the dominant upper extremity by about 5 to 10 lb and is greater in the mid-position of grip. These measurements can be useful in assessing the amount of weakness present, as well as in following progress during treatment. Multiple trials allow assessment of inconsistencies that can be useful in determining the degree of effort the patient is exhibiting.

Sensation should also be addressed to assess whether deficits follow specific peripheral nerve, nerve root, or neuropathic patterns. Sensory deficits that incorporate the whole leg or the whole arm often suggest the presence of a nonphysiological, functional sensory deficit. Vibratory sensation measured with a tuning fork can be used to help determine the validity of otherwise questionable sensory findings. When a vibrating tuning fork is placed over various sites in a single bone, the perception of vibration should be similar over all areas of the bone. For example, vibratory sensation should be similar on both sides of the forehead or both sides of the sternum. A right-to-left difference in vibratory sensation in a midline bone strongly suggests a functional, nonorganic deficit.

Muscle stretch reflexes need to be evaluated to assess integrity of the reflex arc. Straight-leg raising can be measured in both the sitting and supine positions to assess for consistency. Special tests such as Tinel's sign, Phalen's wrist flexion test, Spurling's test, Finkelstein's test, Patrick's test, and tests for thoracic outlet syndrome can provide helpful information at times. Unfortunately, these tests and others that are commonly used do not have perfect sensitivity and specificity. It should be remembered that the findings should be cautiously evaluated in light of the remainder of the history and physical findings.

The examiner needs to continually analyze the findings as the examination progresses. Findings should be reassessed several times during the examination using a variety of techniques to ensure consistency. Injured workers can occasionally demonstrate "symptom magnification," with inconsistencies in findings being common in these examinations. Tests such as those described by Waddell and co-workers[59] (Table 45–6) can help to differentiate nonorganic from organically mediated physical findings. Other findings, such as the presence of dirt under the nails and calluses on the hands, should be noted. Exaggerated pain behavior can indicate some degree of symptom magnification by the patient. Pain behavior and inconsistencies are important to recognize to ensure that the patient is not medically overevaluated or subjected to potentially risky tests or treatments. Identifying functional issues also allows for the institution of appropriate psychologically and behaviorally based intervention.

Appropriate testing (including radiography, CT, MRI, radionuclide scintigraphy, laboratory testing, or electrodiagnostic testing) can also be useful in confirming the diagnosis. These tests should not be used in an automatic "shotgun" fashion but only when each is specifically indicated.

Diagnosis

After the evaluation is completed, a working diagnosis should be formulated and explained to the worker in clear and understandable terms. It is important to try to avoid emotionally charged words such as "ruptured" disk or "degenerative" arthritis, which might frighten

TABLE 45–6 Nonorganic Findings in the Low Back Evaluation: Waddell's Signs

1. Tenderness of the skin to light pinch over a widespread area
2. Deep tenderness in a nonanatomical distribution
3. Reproduction of back pain with axial loading by pressing down on the worker's head while he or she is standing
4. Reproduction of back pain when the shoulders and pelvis are rotated together as a unit
5. Inconsistencies between straight-leg testing done when the worker is otherwise distracted vs. that done when worker is aware of the test being performed
6. "Giving way" weakness in a widespread and nonanatomical pattern
7. Inconsistent and nonanatomical sensory deficits
8. Overreaction (disproportionate verbalization, facial expression, muscle tension and tremor, collapsing, or sweating) during the examination

Adapted from Waddell G, McCulloch JA, Kummel E, et al: Nonorganic physical signs in low-back pain. Spine 1980; 5:117–125.

the worker. The overall prognosis and treatment plan should be clearly provided to the worker. In low back pain due to radiculopathy, for example, it should be explained that the vast majority of cases improve with conservative measures, and that only a small percentage require surgical intervention.[14, 17] Approximate time frames for treatment and return to work should be provided to the patient. These time frames are also helpful for the employer and insurer.

TREATMENT

In working with injured workers, it is necessary to have access to a spectrum of treatment approaches to meet the needs of each individual worker. Most workers respond to acute treatment quite readily and return to work quickly. Others have more protracted courses of recovery and need organized reconditioning efforts to achieve return-to-work fitness. Still others might not have jobs to return to and need more comprehensive programs with specific vocational planning and rehabilitation emphases. Some work-related injuries are resistant to virtually all standard methods of treatment and are best addressed with a chronic pain approach (see Chapter 42).

Early Intervention

Early treatment of the injured worker can occur in a number of settings, including (1) an on-site clinic at work, (2) the company physician's office, (3) an occupational medicine clinic, (4) a minor emergency clinic, or (5) the emergency department of a hospital. The goals of early intervention are accurate diagnosis and appropriate treatment to facilitate the worker's return to work as soon as possible, in a manner consistent with safety and quality medical care. The worker needs to be seen promptly after the injury and followed up closely with scheduled, short-interval follow-up appointments. In some instances, even daily appointments are appropriate. It is important that the worker does not feel abandoned or get lost in the system.

Pain is the major symptom of most acute injuries and is usually reflective of some degree of tissue damage. The early treatment of an acute injury focuses on control of pain and tissue damage. Often a sports medicine orientation using the RICE (*r*est, *i*ce, *c*ompression, *e*levation) approach can be initially helpful. Rest should be limited in duration for most musculoskeletal injuries, with 2 days of bedrest often being preferable to 7 days of bedrest for back injuries.[13] Specific rest of an injured part for other injuries can be provided with appropriate casts, splints, or braces. Prolonged bedrest or immobilization can perpetuate disability by causing deconditioning.[23] Appropriate analgesics can help control pain, as can physical modalities such as heat, cold, transcutaneous electrical nerve stimulation (TENS), massage, and gentle stretching. Physical modalities are often underutilized for acute treatment. They have advantages over medications in that they are often more effective, safer, and have fewer side effects (see Chapters 21, 44).

During the early intervention phase, it is often possible and desirable to provide treatment while the worker is still performing light duty or a modified job. As long as the medical outcome will not be compromised and no further tissue damage will occur, it is usually best to facilitate early return to work. This helps to avoid both physical and mental deconditioning.

As acute symptoms subside, use of medications and physical modalities should decrease. The worker should be instructed in specific flexibility and strengthening exercises that will improve conditioning and lessen the chance of recurrence. A common reason for recurrence is that the acute symptoms were treated and improved, but the causative factors underlying the injury were not addressed. The worker might have been in a deconditioned state prior to the injury and had inadequate strength and endurance to do the specific job tasks in a safe manner. Identification of this preexisting deconditioning gives the physician an opportunity to recondition the worker more extensively and to return a worker to the workplace in better condition than before the injury. In other instances, the job is poorly designed from an ergonomic perspective or the worker is using poor biomechanics in the performance of the job tasks. Prior to returning the worker to work, it is helpful to fully understand the worker's job. Ergonomic modifications or worker training in proper biomechanics could be helpful in avoiding recurrence of the injury.

Any identified problems with drug or alcohol overuse should be addressed, with referral to appropriate treatment programs. Cessation of smoking should also be encouraged, as recent studies show a correlation between back pain, disk degeneration, slower healing, and tobacco use.[3, 27, 47]

About 80% to 85% of workers with acute work injuries experience improvement and return to productive work. In others, symptoms persist longer than expected and progress to a subacute phase. It is important to intensify treatment efforts with these patients. Persistent stiffness or weakness often occurs and can be treated with a structured and regularly scheduled therapy program focused on reconditioning.

Chronic Treatment

About 10% of workers still have pain complaints and physical disability that prevent return to work after the completion of acute and subacute care programs.[8] These workers might be candidates for more highly structured treatment programs, such as work conditioning, work hardening, vocational rehabilitation, or chronic pain therapy.

It is well recognized that the longer workers are off the job, the more difficult it becomes to return them to work. This appears to be an independent factor, and occurs regardless of the type of impairment. There is about a 50% chance of return to work when a worker is off for 6 months, with the rate dropping to 25% when the worker is off for 1 year. After being off work for 2 years, the return-to-work rate is minimal unless a worker is highly motivated and participates in a comprehensive rehabilitation program.

When cases enter the chronic stage, the initial injury is often resolved, but the worker is left with chronic weakness, deconditioning, loss of flexibility, and poor endurance. This is typically the result of weeks or even months of inactivity. In addition to being physically deconditioned, the worker is often psychologically deconditioned. The worker has been removed from the role of being a productive worker and does not have to get up and be ready for work by a certain hour each day. The worker does not have to perform work tasks regularly and may even be relieved of normal responsibilities at home. The worker usually is much more sedentary at home, and physical deconditioning and weight gain often occur. It is common for such workers to let other positive health habits deteriorate, and they often increase the use of tobacco, alcohol, and medications. Prolonged absence from work can also be reinforced by a number of factors (see Table 45–7).[12, 61] Such an individual can be a candidate for a more intense program of work conditioning, work hardening, chronic pain treatment, or structured vocational rehabilitation.

Work Conditioning: A Sports Medicine Approach

Work conditioning (Fig. 45–6) is a program of progressive structured reconditioning to prepare the worker for return to the job. These programs are often provided by physical and occupational therapists in coordination with the primary physician, the employer, and the injured worker. The essential criteria for inclusion in a work conditioning program are that the worker has a job to return to and the employer is willing to accept the worker back on the job.

The treatment focus for work conditioning shifts away from passive modalities and medications and toward more active rehabilitation and physical restoration. This stage of care is often best presented to the worker as a "sports medicine" model of treatment. For example, an injured athlete might require a period of rest after an acute injury. After the period of rest is completed, it is often necessary to return the athlete to the training room to restore fitness prior to return to competition. The worker might be considered an "occupational athlete," as many workers perform vigorous repetitive physical activities on a daily basis. The goal is to return them to their game, which is their job. Restoring and enhancing fitness is often necessary prior to safe return to the job.

Understanding the physical requirements of a specific job should start with an analysis of the job description. Even more useful are job site visits (Table 45–8), if they can be arranged. These visits allow direct inspection of the specific job(s) performed by the worker. A clear understanding of the job allows a specific physical reconditioning program to be designed that most efficiently prepares the worker for return to work. A job that primarily involves upper body strength or flexibility would have different conditioning goals than a job that requires squatting or bending. Evaluation of the job and the job site can also help enhance the injured worker's confidence in the rehabilitative team and in his or her ability to return to work. The worker and rehabilitative staff should have a common understanding of the job and its requirements. They should speak a common language about the job, the equipment used, and the work environment.

Communicating with the worker's employer during job site visits can help overcome obstacles to returning the employee to the job. Management can outline whether light duty is available and what specific light duty tasks are available. Employers can also be educated about the value of light duty programs and about how they can help return workers to productivity earlier, while helping to minimize injury-related compensation costs.[15]

Work conditioning often begins on a three- to five-times-a-week schedule. The fitness level and work capacity of the worker are periodically assessed. When the worker is sufficiently conditioned to meet the requirements of light duty, the worker is usually returned to a light duty job. Arrangements are made to continue the conditioning until the worker has maximally improved or has met the requirements for returning to the original job.

Work conditioning treatment usually lasts 3 to 6 weeks. The outcome is that the vast majority of workers return to their jobs at the completion of the program.[8] In addition to improving physical fitness, the worker's confidence about being able to successfully perform the job requirements is enhanced.

TABLE 45–7 Factors Inhibiting Return to Work

Relief from responsibility
Relief from responsibility of getting up and going to work for a job that is not enjoyed
Relief from other jobs and chores at home and in the community because of illness or injury
Attention and support from family and friends
Financial rewards, such as disability income
Use of the illness as a tool of control in the family and against the employer
Progressive deconditioning, both physical and psychological, from being off work
Adversarial relationship between employer and employee
Unwillingness of employer to make reasonable accommodations or to consider temporary light-duty work for the employee

Work Hardening

Workers who have been off work for long periods of time, such as 3 months or more, might need a more comprehensive program than can be provided by work conditioning. These individuals are often even more deconditioned than those treated in work conditioning programs. If these individuals have a job to return to, they might well benefit from a work hardening program. Work hardening programs focus on physical conditioning, but also address psychological issues and vocational issues that often interfere with return to the job.

Success is facilitated if the work hardening team has a complete understanding of the worker's job and work conditions. This allows the provision of an appropriate

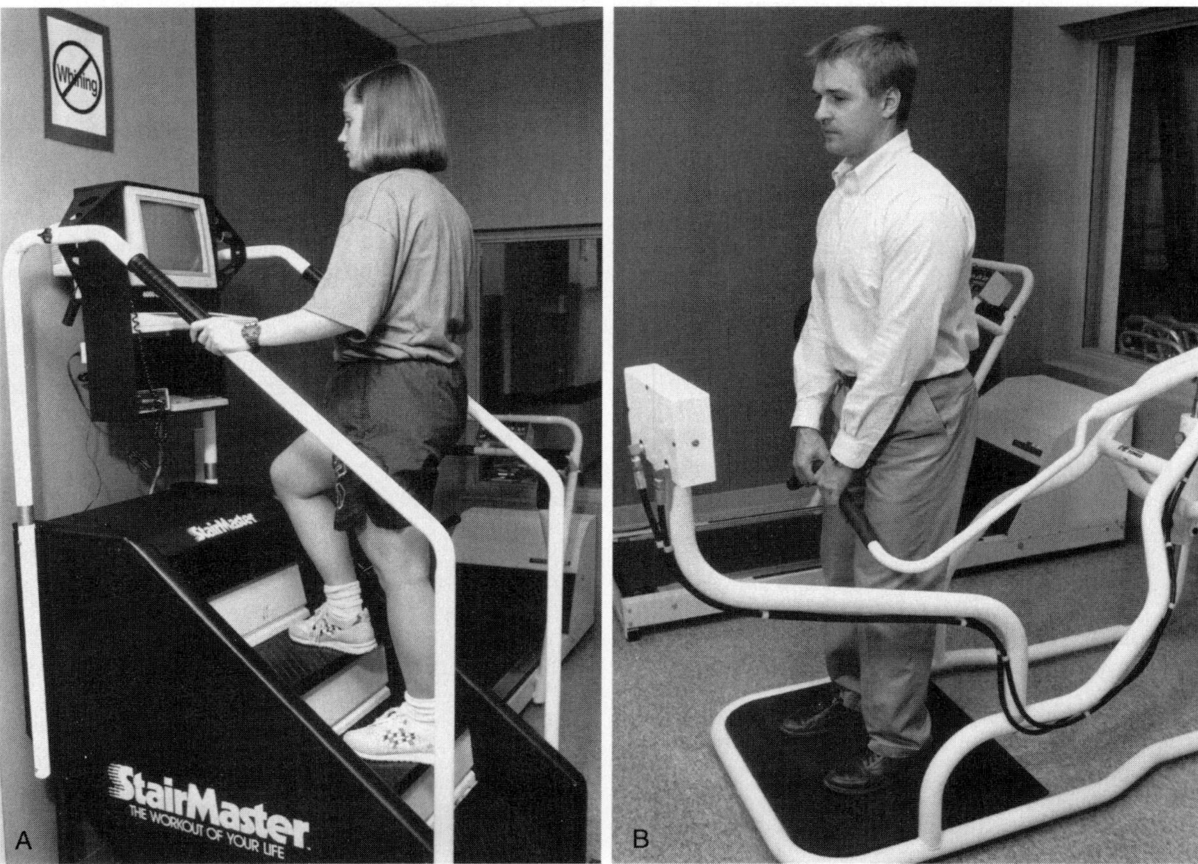

FIGURE 45–6. Work conditioning focuses on enhancing general aerobic fitness as well as on strengthening specific muscle groups that are used regularly in work activities.

program of reconditioning and work simulation for the worker. Work hardening (Figs. 45–7 through 45–10) usually incorporates general as well as job-related physical conditioning. The general conditioning is quite similar to that provided by the work conditioning program. To be most successful, the conditioning should focus on areas of weakness as well as on areas that require additional conditioning for the worker to successfully meet the job requirements.

Work hardening programs also incorporate job-specific work simulation activities. If the worker is required to lift boxes, for example, the program includes lifting boxes. If the worker uses a specific tool in a certain position, the program tries to simulate this activity.

The program also tries to simulate actual work conditions. The worker is often required to clock in and out daily. To minimize the worker's perception of illness and sickness, the program is often housed in a warehouse or other work-like setting, rather than in a medical clinic or hospital. The treatment duration is usually 5 half-days or whole days per week for up to 6 weeks.[8]

The goal is to progressively increase exercise tolerance and work activities until they simulate a typical day on the job. The program strives to enhance both physical capabilities and work skills, as well as to help

TABLE 45–8 The Job Site Analysis: Things to Observe

The Job

1. Objects handled (weight, size, shape, surface texture, presence or absence of handles)
2. Frequency of physical tasks (lifts per hour, objects handled per time period)
3. Positions and postures used to successfully perform the job
4. Tools used (handle size, weight, vibration, position of use)
5. Layout of work site (height of workbench, arrangement of tools used)

The Work Environment

1. Amount of lighting present (type and intensity of lighting, windows, color of walls, ceiling)
2. Temperature of the facility
3. Amount of noise present. Are hearing protectors available and used if excess noise is present?
4. Cleanliness of floor surface. Note any spills, greasy spots, clutter, or obstacles present on floor that could lead to stumbles and falls.
5. General ambience of the facility—pleasant, relaxed, clean, organized, and orderly? Or hurried, hostile, hectic, and cluttered?

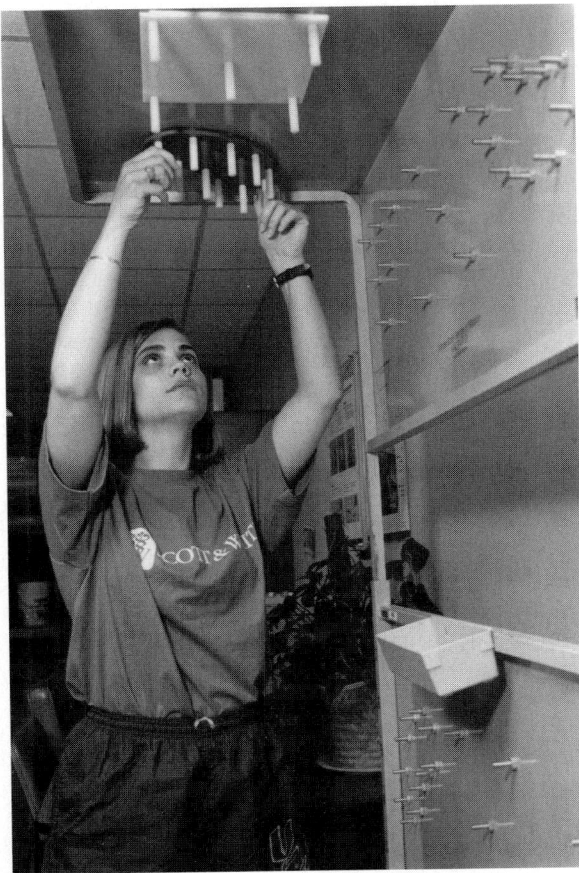

FIGURE 45–7. Work hardening continues to emphasize generalized conditioning, but it also simulates usual work activities. A job involving overhead tasks could require the redevelopment of strength, endurance, and flexibility. Work simulation helps to redevelop these abilities.

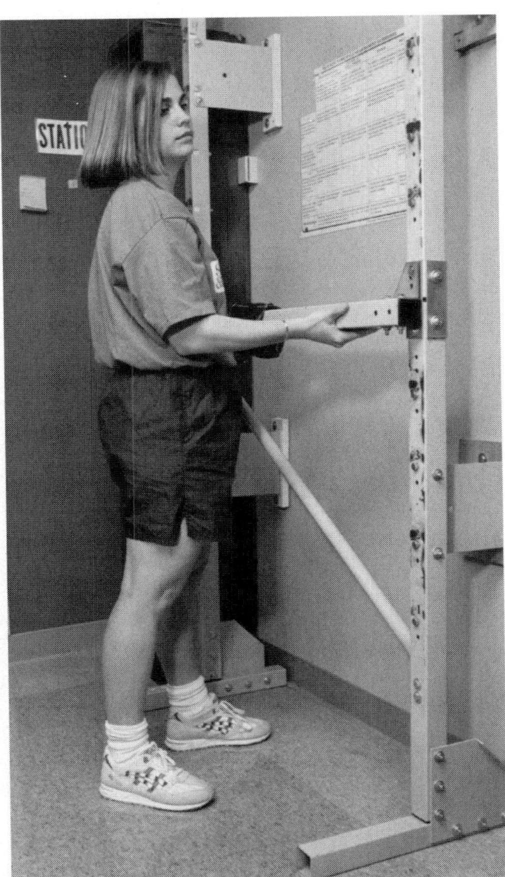

FIGURE 45–8. Lifting graded weights to various heights can simulate manual materials handling, as in stocking shelves or working in a warehouse.

the worker psychologically adjust to being a productive employee again. Education is an important part of the program, and should include such areas as

1. Proper use of the body to avoid re-injury.
2. Proper pacing on the job.
3. Relaxation and stress management skills.
4. Assertiveness training.
5. Interpersonal skills to facilitate conflict avoidance and resolution.
6. Healthy lifestyle.

Psychological counseling can help the worker overcome fears and anxieties about returning to work. Addressing possible unresolved anger about the injury is also important, as is evaluating for the presence of depression or other psychopathological conditions.

The work hardening team usually consists of the physician, physical therapist, occupational therapist, psychologist, vocational counselor, exercise physiologist, and other specialists as needed, including ergonomists and industrial engineers.

The cost of these programs is relatively high, but well-organized programs often have favorable success rates. Return-to-work rates of about 80% to 85% occur with

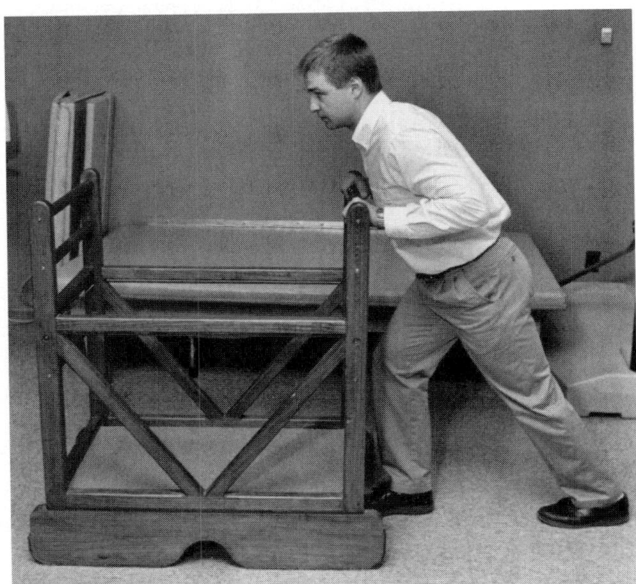

FIGURE 45–9. Simulated pushing can prepare workers for jobs requiring pushing of carts, skids, boxes, or other materials.

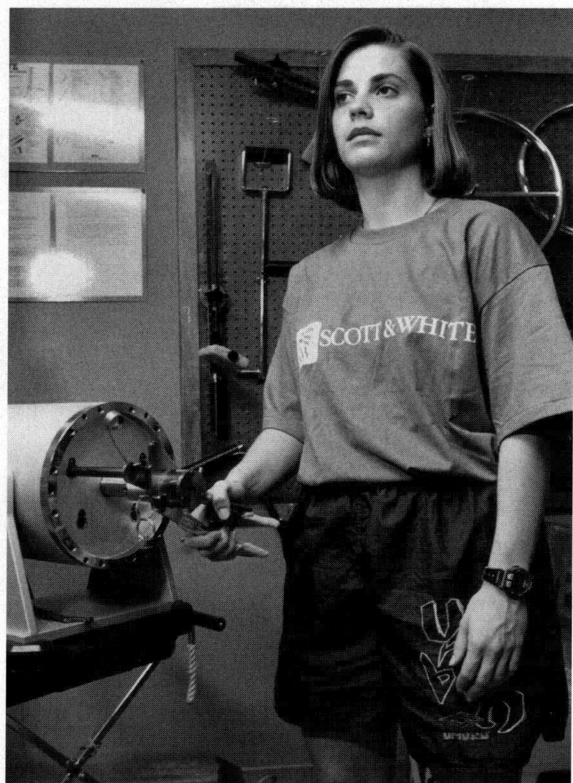

FIGURE 45–10. Use of a work simulator helps to develop strength and tolerance during the repetitive use of hand tools.

programs that carefully select their clients.[8] Individuals selected for these programs should be motivated to return to work, should have jobs available, and should be free of overwhelming psychological or secondary gain issues that can undermine successful return to work.

Vocational Rehabilitation

If at all possible, it is preferable to assist the injured worker to return to work with the previous employer in some capacity. If the employee had a favorable work history with the employer, it is usually much easier to work with that employer rather than to go out and try to find the patient a totally new job. Close communication between the worker, the employer, and the rehabilitation team can help achieve this goal and help to avoid misunderstandings that can inhibit the employer's willingness to accept the worker back on the job. The case manager can play a vital role in promoting this communication and facilitating return to the job.

Many injured workers return to former jobs after appropriate medical treatment and rehabilitation, but some workers do not have the option of returning to their former jobs. This might be the case for a number of reasons, such as the worker's inability to physically meet the job demands despite rehabilitative measures, poor worker-job match that would increase the risk of re-injury, lack of desire on the worker's part to return to the former job, or lack of willingness on the former employer's part to accept the worker back on the job. With no available job to return to, a more comprehensive vocational rehabilitation approach can be needed. Return to work is more difficult for patients with limited education and work skills. They might have little knowledge of the marketplace, of what jobs are available, or even of how to apply for a job.

The process starts with a thorough assessment of the individual. It is helpful to survey areas of interest and aptitude to help ascertain the appropriate vocational possibilities. Psychological testing can be helpful to determine aptitude for specific vocations, as well as for various levels of vocational or educational training (e.g., vocational school, junior college, college). Physical evaluation is helpful to determine the individual's work capacity and whether this level can be enhanced with physical reconditioning programs such as work conditioning.

The vocational counselor should be familiar with job options in the geographic area and able to assist the individual with formulating a reasonable plan for vocational rehabilitation. Vocational counseling can be provided by individual rehabilitation facilities. In many instances the resources of the state vocational rehabilitation services can be called on to assist with the vocational rehabilitation effort.

A successful vocational rehabilitation plan usually requires consideration of specific job adaptations or modifications to enable success in the work force. The prospective worker with a physical impairment, such as a previous brain or spinal cord injury, might need ergonomic adaptations. These might include modification of the worktable, tools, or the use of special seating. Assistive equipment such as lifts, hoists, and adapted control panels can occasionally help the worker maintain acceptable productivity and safety (see Chapter 35).

Job coaching and education are important for the individual who has been out of the work force for some time. The prospective worker might need coaching on

1. How to fill out a job application.
2. How to prepare a résumé.
3. How to dress for and act at a job interview as well as on the job.
4. How to deal effectively with authority figures and co-workers.
5. How to deal with stress or conflict in the work situation.
6. How to manage finances.

Vocational rehabilitation is a team effort. The vocational counselor usually coordinates the effort, with assistance provided as needed by physicians, psychologists, neuropsychologists, physical and occupational therapists, ergonomists, industrial engineers, employers, and educational facilities.

The vocational rehabilitation process is often a difficult one, but with a motivated patient, a return to gainful employment is frequently possible.

Chronic Pain Treatment

Some individuals with work-related injuries develop chronic pain. The chronic pain might be related to the original injury, or it can be an aftermath of the treatment efforts. For example, chronic pain due to arachnoiditis can develop after back surgery. In otherwise psychologically well-adjusted individuals, chronic pain can sometimes be treated effectively using the traditional medical model of care. Treatment modalities such as physical therapy, epidural blocks, TENS, or even implanted stimulators or pumps can be helpful and allow increased activity and productivity.

Many other individuals have chronic pain but no specific medical condition that can be readily treated or cured. This is often referred to as chronic pain syndrome. Psychological factors such as depression, somatization, hypochondriasis, or passive dependency can be present. There is frequently overuse of medications, alcohol and tobacco, and medical and surgical services. Secondary gain issues are often prominent. In such cases, individuals seem to have disability far in excess of any actual organic pathological findings that are present.[65] Such patients also are usually physically deconditioned and live sedentary and even dependent lifestyles. Return to work is not the initial priority with these individuals. Initial pain management efforts typically revolve around medication detoxification, psychological counseling, and progressive reconditioning. Such patients might be best treated in an interdisciplinary program that focuses on the behavioral treatment of chronic pain syndrome. If the chronic pain program proves successful, patients might later qualify for one of the programs more strictly focused on preparation for returning to the work force, such as work conditioning or vocational rehabilitation. (For more information on chronic pain and chronic pain syndrome, see Chapter 42.)

WRAPPING IT UP: RETURN-TO-WORK ISSUES

Case Management

Case management can play a useful role in assisting the worker and the treatment team during the treatment process. Case managers can be employed by the rehabilitation facility, the employer, the insurance carrier, or even the physician. They can communicate with the health care team, the insurer, the employer, and the worker to ensure that smooth, unhindered communications take place. This communication facilitates the worker's rehabilitative program.

The case manager assesses job availability with the current employer and investigates the existence of light-duty alternatives. The case manager communicates with the insurer to be sure that prompt coverage is provided for the necessary diagnostic, therapeutic, and rehabilitative efforts and to be certain that the insurer fully understands the proposed program, expected outcome, and time frames.

The case manager can also be valuable in maintaining lines of communication with the worker to help prevent any misunderstandings about diagnosis, treatment plans, and return-to-work options. The case manager can help ensure that the worker does not get lost in the system. The case manager can monitor attendance by the injured worker at appropriate therapy sessions and help ensure compliance with the program. Through these case coordination efforts, many patients have successful return to productive work in a reasonable time frame.

Functional Capacity Evaluation

After completion of medical treatment, the physician is often required to make a determination about whether the worker is capable of returning to the full-duty job or if specific limitations in performance remain. This is often a difficult determination, as most medical offices are not set up in a way that enables testing of the worker's abilities. The physician often simply eyeballs the worker and makes an estimate, or asks the worker if he or she thinks the job can be performed safely. A more rigorous approach is to assess the worker with a functional capacity evaluation.

Functional capacity evaluations are typically performed by physical or occupational therapists. The therapist needs the worker's specific job description to individualize the testing. The therapist then methodically tests the worker with actual or simulated job tasks to determine the worker's capabilities for performing the required job tasks. Such physical skills as lifting, bending, pushing, pulling, stooping, and carrying are measured. Assessments should include measures of strength, flexibility, and endurance factors (muscular as well as aerobic) that are also involved in the routine performance of the worker's specific job.

During performance of the work capacity evaluation it is helpful to learn from the worker the amount of energy and effort being expended. The Rating of Perceived Exertion Scale (Table 45–9) outlined by Borg[7] can be useful in making this determination. If return to light duty is a possibility, the functional capacity evaluation can be useful in outlining the worker's capabilities as well as restrictions. A comprehensive report is prepared for the referring physician and is extremely useful when communicating with the employer about job abilities and limitations. The work capacity evaluation helps

TABLE 45–9 Rating of Perceived Exertion

Rating	Description
0	Nothing at all
0.5	Very weak, just noticeable
1	Very weak
2	Weak (light effort)
3	Moderate
4	Somewhat strong
5	Strong (heavy effort)
>6	
7	Very strong
8	
9	
10	Very, very strong
>10	Maximal effort

From Borg GAV: Psychophysical bases of perceived exertion: Med Sci Sports Exerc 1982; 14:377–381.

ensure that the worker-job fit is appropriate and reduces the risk of re-injury.

Impairment Evaluation

After treatment is completed, and the patient's progress has plateaued and is not expected to change further, it is concluded that the maximum medical improvement has been achieved. In accordance with workers' compensation program rules in many states, an impairment evaluation must be performed when the worker reaches this plateau. (See Chapter 6 for more information on impairment rating.)

Litigation Resolution

After completion of treatment, it is important to document any residual impairment. Specific limitation of motion, sensory deficit, or muscle weakness is important to note in case the worker becomes involved in litigation about the injuries. Thorough documentation of the initial encounter and any preexisting injuries and disorders is important, as is documentation of diagnostic procedures and their results, working diagnoses, treatments rendered, response to treatment, and patient compliance and participation in the treatment program.

If litigation occurs, the physician might be called as a factual or expert witness. Documenting the case carefully as it progresses is extremely helpful in later establishing credibility and in accurately representing the facts. This contributes to a fair and equitable outcome for the injured worker as well as for the employer and compensation carrier.

OPPORTUNITIES FOR THE FUTURE

As we enter the new millennium, the cost of health care remains a major national concern (or crisis, as some have called it). Various measures have been developed to "fix" the system. Capitated, managed care plans are more pervasive around the country. With capitated care, the health provider receives a fixed amount of funding for each individual cared for under the plan. Under capitated systems, the more services provided to each individual, the less capital is available to the health care provider to meet expenses and to invest in new technology.

With a capitated system, there is a natural tendency to emphasize prevention—keeping people well, avoiding injuries, and keeping them out of hospitals. The emphasis shifts from treating episodes of illness to meeting individuals' health care needs over their lifetimes. There should develop a continuum of prevention and care, rather than illness-based episodic care. Communities need to realize that they have a responsibility to be active participants, rather than passive observers, in promoting health in their communities. Currently, some communities, as well as some industries, are addressing these issues by limiting smoking and sponsoring health promotion programs such as blood pressure screenings, cholesterol screening, drug and alcohol testing and treatment, and fitness promotion.

Physical medicine and rehabilitation has for many years been active in physical restoration and physical fitness enhancement as well as in the development of various programs for injury prevention, from back schools to the ergonomic analysis of specific jobs or industries. In the future, physical medicine and rehabilitation should expect to play a major role in enhancing worker fitness, preventing injuries, enhancing job safety, and restoring workers to full function in an expedient and cost-effective manner. Providers of care need to develop seamless programs that provide the appropriate level and intensity of care for the injured worker at the most reasonable cost. Outcome analysis will be essential for quantifying the success of various programs and for helping insurers, employers, and others decide where to use their scarce financial resources to provide acceptable, high-quality programs to the widest range of injured workers.

REFERENCES

1. Americans With Disabilities Act. Federal Register P. L. 101–336, (July 26) 1990, pp 327–378.
2. Babitsky S, Sewall HD: Understanding the AMA Guides in Workers' Compensation. New York, John Wiley & Sons, 1992.
3. Battie MC, Videman T, Gill K, et al: Smoking and lumbar intervertebral disc degeneration: An MRI study of identical twins. Spine 1991; 16:1015–1021.
4. Bernard BP (ed): Musculoskeletal Disorders (MSDs) and Workplace Factors. Cincinnati, OH, US Department of Health and Human Services, July 1997.
5. Bigos SJ, Battie M, Spengler DM, et al: A prospective study of work perceptions and psychosocial factors affecting the report of back injury. Spine 1991; 16:1–6.
6. Boden SD, Davis DO, Dina TS, et al: Abnormal magnetic-resonance scans of the lumbar spine in asymptomatic subjects. J Bone Joint Surg Am 1990; 72:403–408.
7. Borg GAV: Psychophysical bases of perceived exertion. Med Sci Sports Exerc 1982; 14:377–381.
8. Braddom RL: Industrial rehabilitation: An overview. Phys Med Rehabil Clin North Am 1992; 3:499–511.
8a. Bureau of Labor Statistics, U.S. Department of Labor, December 1999.
9. Cady L, Thomas P, Karawasky R: Increasing health and physical fitness of firefighters. J Occup Med 1985; 27:110–114.
10. Cady LD, Bischoff DP, O'Connell ER, et al: Strength and fitness and subsequent back injuries in firefighters. J Occup Med 1979; 21:269–272.
11. Daltroy LH, Larson MG, Wright EA, et al: A case-control study of risk factors for industrial low back injury: Implications for primary and secondary prevention programs. Am J Indust Med 1991; 20:505–515.
12. Derebery VJ, Tullis WH: Delayed recovery in the patient with a work compensable injury. J Occup Med 1983; 25:829–835.
13. Deyo RA, Diehl AK, Rosenthal M: How many days of bed rest for acute low back pain? N Engl J Med 1986; 315:1064–1070.
14. Deyo RA, Loeser JD, Bigos SJ: Herniated lumbar intervertebral disc. Ann Intern Med 1990; 112:598–603.
15. Dolney WP: Restricted work-activity programs minimize injury compensation cost. Occup Health Safety 1992; 61:75.
16. Doyle Y, Conroy R: The spectrum of farming accidents seen in Irish general practice: A 1-year survey. Fam Pract 1989; 6:38–41.
17. Ellenberg MR, Ross ML, Honet JC, et al: Prospective evaluation of the course of disc herniations in patients with proven radiculopathy. Arch Phys Med Rehabil 1993; 74:3–8.
18. Erdil M, Dickerson OB, Chaffin DB: Biomechanics of manual materials handling and low-back pain. In Zenz C, Dickerson OB, Horvath EP (eds): Occupational Medicine, ed 3, St Louis, Mosby–Year Book, 1994, pp 239–257.

19. Erdil M, Dickerson OB, Glackin E: Cumulative trauma disorders of the upper extremity. In Zenz C, Dickerson OB, Horvath EP (eds): Occupational Medicine, ed 3. St Louis, Mosby–Year Book, 1994, pp 48–64.
20. Feldstein A, Vollmer W, Valanis B: Evaluating the patient-handling tasks of nurses. J Occup Med 1990; 32:1009–1013.
21. Frumkin H, Camara VM: Occupational health and safety in Brazil. Am J Public Health 1991; 81:1619–1624.
22. Gibson ES, Martin JE, Terry CW: Incidence of low back pain and pre-placement X-ray screening. J Occup Med 1980; 22:515–519.
23. Gogia PP, Schneider VS, LeBlanc AD, et al: Bed rest effect on extremity muscle torque in healthy men. Arch Phys Med Rehabil 1988; 69:1030–1032.
24. Graveling RA: The prevention of back pain from manual handling. Ann Occup Hygiene 1991; 35:427–432.
25. Gutierrez-Fisac JL, Regidor E, Ronda E: Occupational accidents and alcohol consumption in Spain. Int J Epidemiol 1992; 21:1114–1120.
26. Harker C, Matheson AB, Ross JAS, et al: Occupational accidents presenting to the accident and emergency department. Arch Emerg Med 1992; 9:185–189.
27. Heliovaara M, Makela M, Knekt P, et al: Determinants of sciatica and low-back pain. Spine 1991; 16:608–614.
28. Hilyer JC, Brown KC, Sirles AT, et al: A flexibility intervention to reduce the incidence and severity of joint injuries among municipal firefighters. J Occup Med 1990; 32:631–637.
29. Howell E, Brown K, Atkins J: Trauma in the workplace. AAOHN J 1990; 38:467–474.
30. Jansson B, Eriksson C-G: Accident involvement and attitudes towards hazards and countermeasures in a Swedish rural population. Scand J Soc Med 1990; 18:139–142.
31. Kelsey JL, White AA: Epidemiology and impact of low-back pain. Spine 1980; 5:133–142.
32. Keyserling WM, Herrin GD, Chaffin DB: Isometric strength testing as a means of controlling medical incidents on strenuous jobs. J Occup Med 1980; 22:332–336.
33. Krusen EM, Ford DE: Compensation factor in low back injuries. JAMA 1958; 166:1128–1133.
34. Lampard EE: Industrial revolution. In The World Book Encyclopedia, vol 10, Chicago, World Book, 1985, p 186–195.
35. Low I, Holz A: Approach to risk reduction in manufacturing firms in Australia. Occup Med 1993; 43:43–46.
36. Magora A, Schwartz A: Relation between low back pain and X-ray changes. Scand J Rehabil Med 1980; 12:47–52.
37. Mathur N, Sharma KKR, Tiwari VK: Orthopaedic industrial injuries. J Indian Med Assoc 1990; 88:153–154.
38. Mayer TC, Gatchel RJ, Mager H, et al: A prospective 2-year study of functional restoration in industrial low back injury: An objective assessment procedure. JAMA 1987; 258:1763–1767.
39. McKenzie RA: Prophylaxis in recurrent low back pain. NZ Med J 1979; 89:22–23.
40. Merchant JA: Agricultural injuries. Occup Med 1991; 6:529–539.
41. Mitchell LV, Lawler FH, Bowen D, et al: Effectiveness and cost-effectiveness of employer-issued back belts in areas of high risk for back injury. J Occup Med 1994; 36:90–94.
42. Nachemson A: Work for all. Clin Orthop 1983; 179:77–82.
43. Nachemson AL: Advances in low-back pain. Clin Orthop 1985; 200:266–278.
44. National Safety Council: Accident Facts, 1997 Edition. Itasca, IL, National Safety Council, 1997.
45. Novak RD, Smolensky MH, Fairchild EJ, et al: Shiftwork and industrial injuries at a chemical plant in southeast Texas. Chronobiol Int 1990; 7:155–164.
46. Novek J, Yassi A, Spiegel J: Mechanization, the labor process, and injury risks in the Canadian meat packing industry. Int J Health Serv 1990; 20:281–296.
47. O'Conner FG, Marlowe SS: Low back pain in military basic trainees. Spine 1993; 18:1351–1354.
48. Paajanen H, Erkintalo M, Kuusela T, et al: Magnetic resonance study of disc degeneration in young low-back pain patients. Spine 1989; 14:982–985.
49. Perry GF: Lumbar support belts in occupational medicine forum. J Occup Med 1992; 34:679–680.
50. Rempel DM, Harrison RJ, Barnhart S: Work-related cumulative trauma disorders of the upper extremity. JAMA 1992; 267: 838–842.
51. Rodgers SH, Eggleton EM: Ergonomic Design for People at Work, vol 1, New York, Van Nostrand Reinhold, 1983.
52. Rodgers SH, Kenworthy DA, Eggleton EM: Ergonomic Design for People at Work, vol 2, New York, Van Nostrand Reinhold, 1986.
53. Ruckert A, Rohmert W, Pressel G: Ergonomic research study on aircraft luggage handling. Ergonomics 1992; 35:997–1012.
54. Saal JA, Saal JS: Nonoperative treatment of herniated lumbar intervertebral disc with radiculopathy: An outcome study. Spine 1989; 14:431–437.
55. Sander RA, Meyers JE: The relationship of disability to compensation status in railroad workers. Spine 1986; 11:141–143.
56. Scheer SJ: Ergonomics. Phys Med Rehabil Clin North Am 1992; 3:599–614.
57. Schuchmann JA: Low back pain: A comprehensive approach. Compr Ther 1988; 14:14–18.
58. Verville RE: The Americans with Disabilities Act: An analysis. Arch Phys Med Rehabil 1990; 71:1010–1013.
59. Waddell G, McCulloch JA, Kummel E, et al: Nonorganic physical signs in low-back pain. Spine 1980; 5:117–125.
60. Waller JA, Payne SR, Skelly JM: Disability, direct cost, and payment issues in injuries involving woodworking and wood-related construction. Accident Anal Prev 1990; 22:351–360.
61. Walsh NE, Dumitru D: Compensation and low back pain. Phys Med Rehabil 1991; 5:223–236.
62. Walsh NE, Schwartz R: Prevention of back injury in the work place. Phys Med Rehabil Clin North Am 1992; 3:553–561.
63. Webster B, Snook SH: The cost of compensable low back pain. J Occup Med 1990; 32:13–15.
64. Weinreb JC, Wolbarsht LB, Cohen JM, et al: Prevalence of lumbosacral intervertebral disk abnormalities on MR images in pregnant and asymptomatic nonpregnant women. Radiology 1989; 170:125–128.
65. Werneke MW, Harris DE, Lichter RL: Clinical effectiveness of behavioral signs for screening chronic low-back pain patients in a work-oriented physical rehabilitation program. Spine 1993; 18:2412–2418.
66. Williams TH, Current RN, Freidel F: A History of the United States, ed 2, New York, Knopf, 1965, pp 86–94.
67. Workplace Injuries and Illnesses in 1997. Washington, DC, Bureau of Labor Statistics, Department of Labor, December 1998.
68. Yu T, Roht LH, Wise RA, et al: Low-back pain in industry. J Occup Med 1984; 26:517–524.

A

Appendix

Internet Resource Guide

When dealing with injured workers, it is essential to practice in accordance with the appropriate workers' compensation rules and regulations for the jurisdiction. The following Internet sites are provided to help the practitioner obtain basic information and updates for various workers' compensation programs. Also, other pertinent sites of interest are provided. It should be noted that Internet site addresses do change periodically.

FEDERAL GOVERNMENT SITES

U.S. Department of Justice http://www.usdoj.gov
- Americans With Disabilities Act home page http://www.usdoj.gov/crt/ada/adahoml.htm
- Americans With Disabilities Act information on the web http://www.usdoj.gov/crt/ada/

U.S. Department of Labor http://www.dol.gov/
- Bureau of Labor Statistics http://stats.bls.gov/blshome.htm
- Occupational Safety and Health Administration http://www.osha.gov/index.html

National Institute for Occupational Safety and Health http://www.cdc.gov/niosh/homepage.html

STATE GOVERNMENT SITES

Alabama
- Department of Industrial Relations; Workers' Compensation Division http://www.dir.state.al.us/wc.htm

Alaska
- Department of Labor http://www.labor.state.ak.us/
- Workers' Compensation Division http://www.labor.state.ak.us/wc/wc.htm

Arizona
- State of Arizona http://www.state.az.us/
- Workers' Compensation Insurance—State Fund http://www.statefund.com/

Arkansas
- Arkansas Workers' Compensation Commission http://www.awcc.state.ar.us/

California
- Division of Workers' Compensation http://www.dir.ca.gov/
- Commission on Health and Safety and Workers' Compensation http://www.dir.ca.gov/DIR/OS&H/CHSWC/chswc.html

Colorado
- Division of Workers' Compensation http://workerscomp.cdle.state.co.us/default.htm

Connecticut
- State of Connecticut http://www.state.ct.us/
- Workers' Compensation Commission http://wcc.state.ct.us/

Delaware
- State of Delaware http://www.state.de.us/

District of Columbia http://www.ci.washington.dc.us/

Florida
- Department of Labor and Employment Security http://www.state.fl.us/dles/
- Division of Workers' Compensation http://www.wc.les.state.fl.us/DWC/

Georgia
- State of Georgia http://www.state.ga.us/

Hawaii
- State of Hawaii http://www.hawaii.gov/

Idaho
- Idaho Industrial Commission http://www.state.id.us/iic/index.htm

Illinois
Industrial Commission http://www.state.il.us/agency/iic/
Indiana
Workers' Compensation Board of Indiana
http://www.state.in.us/wkcomp/index.html
Iowa
State of Iowa http://www.state.ia.us/
Iowa Workforce Development
http://www.state.ia.us/government/wd/index.htm
Kansas
Kansas Workers' Compensation http://www.hr.state.ks.us/
Kentucky
Department of Workers' Claims
http://www.state.ky.us/agencies/labor/wrkclaim.htm
Louisiana
Louisiana Office of Workers' Compensation
http://www.ldol.state.la.us/homepage.htm
Maine
Workers' Compensation Board http://janus.state.me.us/wcb/
Maryland
Workers' Compensation Commission
http://www.charm.net/~wcc/
Massachusetts
Department of Industrial Accidents
http://www.state.ma.us/dia/index.htm
Michigan
Bureau of Workers' Disability Compensation
http://www.cis.state.mi.us/wkrcomp/bwdc/
Minnesota
Minnesota Department of Labor and Industry
http://www.doli.state.mn.us/
Mississippi
Workers' Compensation Commission
http://www.mslawyer.com/mwcc.html
Missouri
Department of Labor and Industrial Relations
http://www.dolir.state.mo.us/dolirla.htm
Montana
State of Montana http://www.mt.gov/
Workers' Compensation Court
http://jsd.dli.mt.gov/work_comp/tablel.htm
Nebraska
Nebraska Workers' Compensation Court
http://www.nol.org/home/WC/
Nevada
Department of Business and Industry
http://www.state.nv.us/b&i/
Division of Industrial Relations
http://www.state.nv.us/b&i/ir/
New Hampshire
Department of Labor http://www.state.nh.us/dol/index.html
Worker's Compensation Division
http://www.state.nh.us/dol/wc/index.html
New Jersey
Division of Workers' Compensation
http://www.state.nj.us/labor/wc/Default.htm
New Mexico
Workers' Compensation Administration
http://www.state.nm.us/wca/
New York
New York State Workers' Compensation Board
http://www.wcb.state.ny.us/
North Carolina
N.C. Industrial Commission http://www.comp.state.nc.us/
North Dakota
State of North Dakota http://www.state.nd.us/
Ohio
Bureau of Workers' Compensation
http://www.bwc.state.oh.us/
Oklahoma
Department of Labor http://www.oklaosf.state.ok.us/~okdol/
Workers' Compensation Division
http://www.oklaosf.state.ok.us/~okdol/workcomp/index.htm
Oregon
Workers' Compensation Division
http://www.cbs.state.or.us/external/wcd/index.html
Workers' Compensation Board
http://www.cbs.state.or.us/external/wcb/index.html
Workers' Compensation Ombudsman
http://www.cbs.state.or.us/external/wco/index.html
Pennsylvania
Department of Labor and Industry
http://www.li.state.pa.us/
Rhode Island
State of Rhode Island http://www.state.ri.us/
South Carolina
Workers' Compensation Commission
http://www.state.sc.us/wcc/
South Dakota
Division of Labor and Management
http://www.state.sd.us/state/executive/dol/dlm/dlm-home.htm
Tennessee
Department of Labor; Workers' Compensation Division
http://www.state.tn.us/labor/wcomp.html
Texas
Research and Oversight Council on Workers' Compensation
http://www.roc.capnet.state.tx.us/
Texas Workers' Compensation Commission
http://www.twcc.state.tx.us/
Utah
Industrial Accidents Division http://www.indcom.state.ut.us/indacc.htm
Vermont
Vermont Department of Labor and Industry
http://www.cit.state.vt.us/labind/
Workers' Compensation Division
http://www.state.vt.us/labind/wcindex.htm
Virginia
State of Virginia http://www.state.va.us/
Washington
Department of Labor and Industries http://www.wa.gov/lni/
Workers' Compensation Information
http://www.wa.gov/lni/workcomp/worker.htm

Handy Guide to Workers' Compensation http://www.wa.gov/lni/workcomp/wcquid.htm

West Virginia

Bureau of Employment Programs http://www.state.wv.us/bep/

Workers' Compensation Division http://www.state.wv.us/bep/WC/default.HTM

Wisconsin

Division of Workers' Compensation http://www.dwd.state.wi.us/WC/

Wyoming

Department of Employment http://wydoe.state.wy.us/

Workers' Safety and Compensation Division http://wydoe.state.wy.us/wscd/

OTHER SITES OF INTEREST

The Rehabilitation Accreditation Commission (CARF) http://www.carf.org/index.html

National Safety Council http://www.nsc.org

Nationwide Workers' Compensation Administrators Directory http://www.comp.state.nc.us/ncic/pages/wcadmdir.htm

Related web and gopher links http://www.comp.state.nc.us/ncic/pages/related.htm

State and local governments on the Net http://www.piperinfo.com/state/states.html

B
Appendix

Accreditation Issues

The Rehabilitation Accreditation Commission (CARF) helps ensure the quality of various occupational rehabilitation programs by surveying and accrediting programs that meet appropriate standards. CARF recognizes and accredits several different types of work-specific occupational rehabilitation programs. Appropriate standards exist for each type of program accredited, with these standards developed by experts in the respective fields with feedback provided from facilities that use that standards.

CARF categorizes "Work-Specific Occupational Rehabilitation Programs" as follows[1]:

Category one—This type of program is a "work-related, outcomes-oriented, interdisciplinary, and individualized treatment program that incorporates real or simulated work. Such a program is usually offered after an acute rehabilitation program, but may be offered without previous involvement in acute rehabilitation programs." Goals of the program include restoring physical, behavioral, functional, and vocational skills.

Category Two—This type of interdisciplinary program is similar but focuses primarily on functional restoration and return to work.

CARF also accredits programs in the area of Employment Services. These programs have varied goals, including (1) indentification of employment opportunities and resources in the local job market, (2) development of realistic employment goals, (3) establishment of service plans to achieve employment outcomes, and (4) identification of resources to achieve and maintain employment.

[1] 1998 Medical Rehabilitation Standards Manual. CARF—The Rehabilitation Accreditation Commission, 4891 East Grant Road, Tucson, AZ 85712, (520) 325-1044; web site http://www.carf.org.

46 CHAPTER

James C. Agre, M.D., Ph.D., and Dennis J. Matthews, M.D.

Rehabilitation Concepts in Motor Neuron Diseases

This chapter focuses on the rehabilitation of patients with motor neuron diseases, defined as diseases or conditions that produce dysfunction of the motor neurons, resulting in weakness and muscle wasting. These include diseases or conditions that affect the upper (corticobulbar and corticospinal) motor neurons, the bulbar and spinal lower motor neurons, or both.

Patients who have diseases or conditions affecting the motor neurons often benefit from rehabilitative care. As with all diseases and disorders, management of the patient with a motor neuron disease begins with a complete evaluation in order to establish as precise a diagnosis as possible. This allows the rehabilitation professional to determine the prognosis for progression or improvement of the disorder and assists the treatment team in determining the best course of therapeutic intervention.

A number of textbooks and chapters have considered these neuromuscular disorders in detail.* It is not the purpose of this chapter to provide all of the features of each disorder. Rather, the chapter briefly highlights these disorders, including their epidemiology, genetics, clinical features, and pathology, which should be of assistance to the treating clinician. The main focus is on the rehabilitation issues that arise in treating patients with these disorders and diseases.

CLASSIFICATION OF MOTOR NEURON DISEASES

Motor neuron diseases can be classified in a number of ways. The classification followed here is based on the location of pathophysiological involvement of these diseases and disorders as described in much greater detail by Hudson[59] (Table 46–1).

Upper Motor Neuron Disorders

Primary Lateral Sclerosis

Primary lateral sclerosis (PLS) is a rare, nonfamilial, slowly progressive corticobulbar and corticospinal tract disease of unknown cause.[59] In a review of 19 cases, Hudson reported an age at onset from 20 to 60 years, with men and women affected equally.[59]

Clinical Features. The onset of spasticity is usually noted in the lower limbs, although occasionally spasticity is first noted in the upper limbs or the bulbar musculature. As the disorder progresses, spasticity affects all limbs and the bulbar musculature. Urinary incontinence can occur, but usually not until late in the course. Survival is usually two to three decades or longer. Spastic dysphagia can be life-threatening in these patients. On physical examination, no signs of lower motor neuron dysfunction, such as muscle atrophy or fasciculations, are found. Electromyographic (EMG) examination of these patients does not reveal signs of denervation. These findings differentiate this disorder from classic amyotrophic lateral sclerosis (ALS).[59]

Pathology. The pathogenesis of PLS is unknown. Pathological findings include a reduced number or absence of Betz's cells in the primary motor cortex or precentral gyri accompanied by degeneration of the corticospinal pathways while other structures are spared.[59]

Tropical Spastic Paraparesis

Tropical spastic paraparesis is found in clusters in the tropics (in particular the Seychelles; Tumaco, Colombia;

* References 18, 19, 33, 41, 59, 68, 80, 87, 121, 127, 129.

TABLE 46–1 The Motor Neuron Diseases

Upper motor neuron disorders
Primary lateral sclerosis
Tropical spastic paraparesis
Lathyrism
Epidemic spastic paraparesis
Familial (hereditary) spastic paraplegia
Combined upper and lower motor neuron disorders
Amyotrophic lateral sclerosis (ALS)
Familial ALS
Western Pacific ALS–parkinsonism dementia complex
Groote Eylandt motor neuron disease
Postencephalitic (encephalitis lethargica) ALS
Juvenile inclusion body ALS
Lower motor neuron disorders
Spinal (bulbospinal muscular) atrophies
Monoclonal gammopathy and motor neuron disease
Cancer and motor neuron disease
Poliomyelitis and post-polio syndrome

Modified from Hudson AJ: The motor neuron diseases and related disorders. In Joynt RJ (ed): Clinical Neurology, vol 4. Philadelphia, JB Lippincott, 1991, pp 1–35.

and the West Indies) as well as in Central and South America, India, Africa, and Japan.[59, 106] All races are vulnerable to the disease, although it is primarily found in black populations. The disease is primarily found in adults and the incidence is approximately equal in males and females.[59] Details of the disease are described elsewhere.[59]

Lathyrism

Lathyrism is an upper motor neuron disorder produced by excessive consumption of the chickling pea (*Lathyrus sativus*) or its close relatives. The toxic agent thought to cause this disorder is β-*N*-oxalylamino-L-alanine (BOAA). This is an agonist of the excitatory neurotransmitter glutamate.[59, 117] Lathyrism is endemic to the Indian subcontinent, where the chickling pea is sometimes used as an emergency food. The disease is more common in men, who are also more severely affected by the disorder.[79] The age at onset ranges from 2 to 70 years in both sexes. The disorder usually manifests in males between the ages of 5 and 40 and in females between the ages of 6 and 20.[59] Details of the disease are described elsewhere.[59]

Epidemic Spastic Paraparesis

Epidemic spastic paraparesis is clinically similar to tropical spastic paraparesis but is considered to be etiologically different because the disorder affects children as well as adults and because patients are seronegative for human T-cell lymphotropic virus type 1 (HTLV-1).[107] The etiologic factor involved is unknown, but it may be infective or nutritional. Details of the disease are described elsewhere.[59]

Familial (Hereditary) Spastic Paraplegia

Familial spastic paraplegia can be transmitted as an autosomal dominant trait, occasionally as an autosomal recessive trait, and very rarely as an X-linked recessive disease.[59] The disorder can appear at any age, but usually occurs in childhood or early adult life.

Clinical Features. The onset of familial spastic paraplegia is accompanied by complaints of stiffness and unsteadiness of the legs and gradually results in a spastic paraplegia. Muscular atrophy has been reported, but often in only one or two members of a large pedigree.[59]

Pathology. The pathogenesis of familial spastic paraplegia is unknown. The pathological findings in this disease, reflecting its genetic transmission, are diverse. Symmetrical bilateral degeneration of the pyramidal pathway, spinocerebellar tract, and fasciculus gracilis has been reported.[59, 112] In the amyotrophic form of this disorder, a severe loss of anterior horn cells, particularly in the cervical and lumbar areas, has been reported.[43, 59]

Combined Upper and Lower Motor Neuron Disorders

Classic Amyotrophic Lateral Sclerosis

Amyotrophic lateral sclerosis is the benchmark of the motor neuron disorders. ALS encompasses two conditions, progressive bulbar palsy and progressive muscular atrophy, which differ only in their site of onset.[59] Progressive bulbar palsy initially affects the bulbar motor neurons, whereas progressive muscular atrophy initially affects the spinal motor neurons. These two diseases tend to overlap the longer the patient survives.

Epidemiology. The classic form of ALS is so named because it is the most prevalent motor neuron disease and because it was one of the first to be recognized.[59] The incidence of this disease is approximately 1.6 to 2.4 cases per 100,000 population, but incidence varies with age.[59] As reported by Hudson and colleagues, the average incidence of ALS in southwestern Ontario was 1.6 per 100,000 population, but it increased from the third decade of life (0.2 per 100,000 population) to the eighth decade (7.4 per 100,000 population).[59, 60] The average age at the time of diagnosis in this study was 62 years.[59] The average survival from time of diagnosis is approximately 2.5 years, but varies with age. Survival is reported to be somewhat shorter for patients over the age of 50.[59] The male-female ratio varies from 1.2:1 to 1.6:1.[59]

Clinical Features. Most patients with classic ALS complain of weakness. During the initial examination lower motor neuron signs of atrophy, weakness, and fasciculations are frequently noted. In addition to these signs, muscle stretch reflexes can be depressed in regions where there is primarily lower motor neuron involvement or where atrophy is so advanced that upper motor neuron signs cannot be demonstrated. Otherwise, it is common to find brisk muscle stretch reflexes in areas of muscle atrophy.[59] Occasional patients present with only mild spasticity, suggesting a purely upper motor neuron disorder. The most notable of these cases are patients who present initially with spastic dysarthria or facies (or both) with no detectable lower motor neuron signs.[59] Muscle cramping is a frequent complaint.

The most striking feature of ALS is the focal, often asymmetrical onset of weakness, which then spreads from the initial site to adjacent areas of the body.[59] Spasticity can be very disabling and can produce significant deformities of the hand.[59] Spasticity and clonus can make ambulation difficult. Except for constipation due to poor nutritional intake or inactivity, the bowel and bladder are spared in this disease. Sensation is generally spared, although subtle symptoms and signs of sensory involvement, complaints of paresthesias, and decreased vibratory sense occur in up to 25% of patients.[59, 89] A small percentage of individuals with classic ALS also show signs of dementia (about 3.5%) or parkinsonism (about 1.5%).[58–60, 76]

Pathology. The pathogenesis of classic ALS is unknown. Characteristic pathological findings in classic ALS include degeneration or complete loss of motor neurons in the brainstem and spinal cord areas corresponding to the muscle atrophy and degeneration of the large pyramidal neurons in the primary motor cortex and of the pyramidal tracts.[59] Onuf's nucleus (controlling the striated muscles of the pelvic floor and the bowel and bladder sphincters) is preserved.[59]

Familial Amyotrophic Lateral Sclerosis

Familial ALS is clinically identical to classic ALS except for a somewhat younger average age at onset. From a review of the world literature and their own cases, Strong and colleagues[120] reported a mean age at diagnosis of 46 years in familial ALS. They also found a bimodal distribution of survival in these patients, with peaks of survival at 2 years and 12 years from the time of initial diagnosis. The pattern of inheritance is reported to be autosomal dominant,[113] but a recessively inherited form of chronic juvenile ALS has been reported.[13]

Clinical Features. The clinical features of familial ALS are similar to those of classic ALS.[59]

Pathology. The pathogenesis of familial ALS is unknown. In addition to the degenerative changes in the pyramidal pathways and the lower motor neurons, as found in classic ALS, familial cases of ALS also show degenerative changes in the middle zones of the posterior columns, dorsal spinocerebellar tract, and the dorsal nucleus of Clarke.[59]

Western Pacific Amyotrophic Lateral Sclerosis–Parkinsonism Dementia Complex

The combination of ALS, parkinsonism, and dementia (ALS-PD complex) is found in a high incidence in some small populations in the western Pacific (as on the islands of Guam, Rota, and Tinian of the Mariana Islands).[59] These islands have a distinct population that differs from the population of other islands in their vicinity.

Epidemiology. The pathogenesis of western Pacific ALS is unknown, but several hypotheses have been made, including the lack of calcium in soil and water leading to secondary hyperparathyroidism and subsequently to neuronal damage,[39] a toxic substance in the cycad seed (used as food and medicine),[118] or that it is a sequel to encephalitis lethargica, which was pandemic in the 1920s.[61] Although neither of the last two hypotheses has been proved, both are supported by the significant decline in incidence of ALS on Guam from 50 to less than 5 cases per 100,000 population from the mid-1950s to the mid-1980s.[105]

Clinical Features. The clinical features of western Pacific ALS are the same as those of classic ALS; however, the ALS-PD complex adds the symptoms and signs of parkinsonism and dementia.[59]

Pathology. The pathological findings in western Pacific ALS are the same as for classic ALS, with the addition of neurofibrillary changes in certain neurons.[59]

Groote Eylandt Motor Neuron Disease

This is a very rare disorder that affects Australian aborigines and is found on Groote Eylandt in the Gulf of Carpentaria.[59]

Postencephalitic (Encephalitis Lethargica) Amyotrophic Lateral Sclerosis

The epidemic of encephalitis lethargica peaked in 1920 and 1924, and some of those who survived developed ALS.[59] The average interval between the acute encephalitis and the onset of ALS was 10 years, but in some cases ALS occurred up to 30 years later.[59]

Juvenile Inclusion Body Amyotrophic Lateral Sclerosis

Juvenile inclusion body ALS is a rare condition that is clinically identical to classic ALS but affects persons between the ages of 12 and 16 years.[59] The duration of the illness is also somewhat shorter than that of classic ALS, with survival between 1 and 1½ years from time of diagnosis.

Lower Motor Neuron Disorders

Infantile Forms of Spinal or Bulbospinal Muscular Atrophies

Acute Infantile Spinal Muscular Atrophy (Werdnig-Hoffmann Disease, Type I Spinal Muscular Atrophy, Acute Proximal Hereditary Motor Neuropathy)

The chronic form of acute infantile spinal muscular atrophy was first described by Werdnig[128] and by Hoffmann.[56] It is an autosomal recessive disorder[68] with an estimated incidence ranging from 1 in 15,000 to 1 in 25,000 live births.[94] The disease is already manifest in one-third of affected children by the time of birth through decreased fetal movements or congenital arthrogryposis.[96] The diagnosis is usually made by the age of 3 months and certainly by the age of 6 months. The average survival from time of diagnosis is 6 to 9 months; survival does not exceed 3 years.[22, 93]

Clinical Features. The clinical picture is dominated by severe hypotonia and weakness. There are resultant delays in motor milestones. At birth the baby is usually floppy (hypotonic), with generalized weakness and absence of reflexes. Feeding difficulty and poor breathing are soon apparent. Progressive muscle weakness, atrophy of the trunk and limbs, hypotonia, and feeding difficulties are the primary clinical features.[68] The infants characteristically lie motionless with the lower limbs abducted in the frog-leg position.[68] The face often lacks expression with an open mouth due to facial muscle weakness.[18] Intercostal muscle paralysis is evident and fasciculations are present. Fasciculations of the tongue are almost pathognomonic for the disease.[18] The cause of death is typically respiratory failure.[59]

Pathology. The pathogenesis of acute infantile spinal muscular atrophy is unknown. Severe loss of motor neurons throughout the brainstem and spinal cord is the primary pathological finding.[59]

Chronic Infantile Spinal Muscular Atrophy (Chronic Werdnig-Hoffmann Disease, Type II Spinal Muscular Atrophy, Chronic Proximal Hereditary Motor Neuropathy)

The chronic form of Werdnig-Hoffmann disease is much more slowly progressive than the acute form of this disease. This actually was the form of the disease initially described by Werdnig and Hoffmann.[56, 59, 128] Clinical signs indicative of this disease are usually present by age 3 years but occasionally are seen by 3 months of age.[95] This disease has variable progression, and the median age at death is about 12 years,[59] with some individuals surviving into the third decade.[18] This disease is autosomal recessive,[68] and the gene for chronic spinal muscular atrophy has been found on chromosome 5q.[85]

Clinical Features. Weakness and atrophy are predominantly proximal, with the lower limbs being more involved initially than the upper limbs. Muscle stretch reflexes are reduced or absent. Sensation is normal. Owing to the gradually progressive weakness, scoliosis, thoracic deformities, and equinus deformities of the feet usually develop as the disease progresses.[59]

Pathology. The pathogenesis of chronic infantile spinal muscular atrophy is unknown. The pathological findings are the same as for the acute infantile form.[59]

Juvenile and Adult Forms of Spinal or Bulbospinal Muscular Atrophies

Juvenile and Adult Proximal Spinal Muscular Atrophy (Kugelberg-Welander Disease, Type III Spinal Muscular Atrophy, Recessive Proximal Hereditary Motor Neuropathy; Type IV Spinal Muscular Atrophy, [Juvenile] Dominant Proximal Hereditary Motor Neuropathy; Type V Spinal Muscular Atrophy, [Adult] Dominant Proximal Hereditary Motor Neuropathy)

The juvenile and adult forms of spinal muscular atrophy (Kugelberg-Welander disease) are characterized by slowly progressive weakness and atrophy of the proximal limb and girdle musculature.[74] The disorder is genetically transmitted, usually as an autosomal recessive trait (type III proximal hereditary motor neuropathy), but an autosomal dominant inheritance (type IV juvenile and type V adult proximal hereditary motor neuropathy) is also possible.[9, 59, 124] The clinical onset of the disease can occur anytime between childhood and the seventh decade of life,[59] but is usually between the ages of 2 and 17 years.[123] The duration is also quite variable, ranging from 2 to more than 40 years.[42] It occurs predominantly in males.[59]

Clinical Features. Both the juvenile and the adult forms of proximal spinal muscular atrophy begin with symmetrical atrophy and weakness of the pelvic girdle and proximal lower limbs. This is followed by involvement of the shoulder girdles and upper arms. The leg and forearm musculature are affected later. Fasciculations are noted in about half of the cases. Dysphagia and dysarthria can occur late in the disease and are usually mild.[59]

Pathology. The pathogenesis of juvenile and adult proximal spinal muscular atrophy is presently unknown. Due to the chronicity of this disorder, the muscle biopsy shows a pattern similar to that found in primary myopathy with the presence of both atrophic and hypertrophic fibers. Postmortem studies have shown a loss of spinal motor neurons, but no degeneration of the corticospinal tract.[59]

Bulbar Disease of Childhood (Fazio-Londe Disease and Brown-Vialetto-van Laere Syndrome)

There are two forms of progressive bulbar paralysis of childhood: Fazio-Londe disease and Brown-Vialetto-van Laere syndrome. Both cause a slowly progressive weakness of the muscles of the face, tongue, and pharynx.[59] Most cases of Fazio-Londe disease were described between 1876 and 1925. The age at onset ranged from 2 to 12 years and the reported duration was as short as 9 months up to 8 years.[59] Inheritance appears to be autosomal recessive.[44] In the Brown-Vialetto-van Laere syndrome the first symptom is bilateral deafness, which occurs between the age of 18 months and 31 years (average onset at 12 years of age).[44] Cranial nerve palsies usually appear 4 to 5 years later. Survival may exceed two decades after onset. Inheritance is reported to be autosomal recessive.[44, 59]

Clinical Features. Most case reports describe only bulbar weakness, although the limbs have also been involved in a few instances.[40] In Fazio-Londe disease all of the bulbar motor neurons are affected.[44, 59] In Brown-Vialetto-van Laere syndrome cranial nerves VII through XII are affected in almost all cases, while cranial nerves III, V, and VI can be affected.[59]

Pathology. The pathogenesis of bulbar disease of childhood is unknown. Postmortem findings show a loss of motor neurons of the oculomotor, trochlear, abducens, facial, vagus, and hypoglossal nerves.[44]

Distal Spinal Muscular Atrophy (Distal Hereditary Motor Neuropathy)

Distal spinal muscular atrophy is also known as the spinal form of Charcot-Marie-Tooth disease and distal hereditary motor neuropathy.[59] There are a number of different forms of distal spinal muscular atrophy with different inheritance patterns: (1) autosomal recessive juvenile mild (onset between 2 and 10 years of age) and juvenile severe (onset between 4 months and 20 years), and (2) autosomal dominant in the juvenile (onset between 2 and 20 years) and in the adult (onset between

20 and 40 years).[52, 59, 83, 95] The majority of the cases reported, however, are sporadic, and a recessive inheritance is suspected.[59] Life expectancy is normal except in some severe juvenile cases.[59]

Clinical Features. Weakness and atrophy are most often initially noted distally in the legs, especially in the anterior tibial and peroneal muscles.[59] Usually the upper limbs are spared, but they are rarely predominantly affected.[53] Leg weakness in severe cases can also involve the thigh musculature.[59] Sensory examination and motor and sensory nerve conduction velocities are normal.[59]

Pathology. The pathogenesis of distal spinal muscular atrophy is unknown. Other than the findings of neurogenic muscular atrophy, the pathology of this entity is unknown.[59]

Adult Forms of Bulbar and Bulbospinal Muscular Atrophies

Scapuloperoneal (Facioscapuloperoneal) Muscular Atrophy

Scapuloperoneal muscular atrophy has an autosomal dominant inheritance. The atrophy begins between 30 and 50 years of age. The disease progresses slowly. Patients do not become incapacitated until at least 10 to 20 years after its onset and have a normal life expectancy.[59]

Clinical Features. Weakness and atrophy begin in the muscles of the legs, but the intrinsic muscles of the feet are spared.[59] Several years later the shoulder girdle musculature, and later the musculature of the thigh, pelvic girdle, upper arm, neck, and face, are affected.[59] At this stage the disorder appears similar to facioscapuloperoneal muscular dystrophy, but in the latter disorder the shoulder girdle musculature is affected first. In some cases dysphonia or dysphagia occurs.[59] There are no upper motor neuron or sensory findings on physical examination, but the EMG reveals fibrillation potentials and fasciculations.

Pathology. The pathogenesis of scapuloperoneal muscular atrophy is unknown. Other than findings consistent with chronic denervation, the pathology of this entity has not been explored.[59]

Chronic Bulbospinal Muscular Atrophy of Late Onset

Two families have been described in which a slowly progressive proximal spinal and bulbar muscular atrophy began between the third and sixth decades of life. Only males were affected, consistent with an X-linked recessive inheritance.[59, 67, 110] This disorder, also known as Kennedy's disease, has assumed importance because of the recognition of a specific chromosomal defect.[38] Studies using DNA probes have shown that this disorder is indeed an X-linked recessive rather than an autosomal defect with sex-limited expression, and the gene defect is localized to the proximal long arm of the X chromosome.[38] Life expectancy is normal.[59]

Clinical Features. Muscular weakness and atrophy are first noticed about the shoulder and pelvic girdle musculature. Distal muscular weakness becomes detectable later, but it is never as severe as in the proximal musculature. Bulbar changes, including dysarthria, dysphagia, and atrophy of the tongue, appear later. Bowel and bladder function are preserved, sensory examination is normal, and no evidence of upper motor neuron involvement is present.[59] EMG shows potentials consistent with denervation.

Pathology. The pathogenesis of chronic bulbospinal muscular atrophy of late onset is unknown. A postmortem examination in one case revealed loss of motor neurons and neurogenic atrophy of skeletal muscle. No other spinal cord degenerative changes were found.[59]

Monomelic (Segmental) Spinal Muscular Atrophy

Monomelic spinal muscular atrophy is not an inherited disorder. It has been reported to occur primarily in the Far East, most notably in India, Japan, and Malaysia.[55, 126] It occurs primarily in male juveniles or young adults and is segmental in its distribution. Often it affects only a portion of one limb, such as the forearm and hand, shoulder and upper arm, or thigh.[59] The corresponding contralateral limb may also be affected. It is insidiously progressive over a period of 1 to 3 years and almost always remains focal. Cranial nerves, upper motor neurons, bowel, bladder, and sensory systems are spared.[66] The pathogenesis is unknown. The spinal (bulbospinal) muscular atrophies are summarized in Tables 46–2, 46–3, and 46–4.

Monoclonal Gammopathy and Motor Neuron Disease

Motor neuron disease can occur in association with paraproteinemia.[59] A number of patients have been de-

TABLE 46–2 Spinal (Bulbospinal) Muscular Atrophies

Infantile
- Acute infantile spinal muscular atrophy (Werdnig-Hoffmann disease, type I spinal muscular atrophy, acute proximal hereditary motor neuropathy)
- Chronic infantile spinal muscular atrophy (Werdnig-Hoffmann disease, type II spinal muscular atrophy, chronic proximal hereditary motor neuropathy)

Juvenile and adult
- Juvenile and adult proximal spinal muscular atrophy (Kugelberg-Welander disease, type III spinal muscular atrophy, recessive proximal hereditary motor neuropathy; type IV spinal muscular atrophy, [juvenile] dominant proximal hereditary motor neuropathy; type V spinal muscular atrophy, [adult] dominant proximal hereditary motor neuropathy)
- Bulbar disease of childhood (Fazio-Londe disease, Brown-Vialetto-van Laere syndrome)
- Distal spinal muscular atrophy (distal hereditary motor neuropathy)

Adult
- Scapuloperoneal (facioscapuloperoneal) muscular atrophy
- Chronic bulbospinal muscular atrophy of late onset
- Monomelic (segmental) spinal muscular atrophy

Modified from Hudson AJ: The motor neuron diseases and related disorders: In Joynt RJ (ed): Clinical Neurology, vol 4. Philadelphia, JB Lippincott, 1991, pp 1–35.

TABLE 46–3 Spinal (Bulbospinal) Muscular Atrophies of Infancy and Childhood

Disease	Age at Onset	Weakness Distribution	Sit	Stand	Walk	Course
Werdnig-Hoffmann disease						
Type I	<2 mo	Proximal legs abducted; face, fingers, toes normal	–	–	–	Usually die by age 2–3 yr
Type II	2–12 mo	Proximal thigh and hip muscles	+	+	–	Most die during first decade; some live through second decade
Kugelberg-Welander disease	2–17 yr (mean: 9 yr)	Normal early development; shoulder and hip girdle atrophy (Gower's sign frequently present)	+	+	May walk for 20–40 yr after onset	

Symbols: +, ability present; –, ability not present.
Modified from Swaiman KF: Anterior horn cell and cranial motor neuron disease. In Swaiman KF (ed): Pediatric Neurology: Principles and Practice, vol 2. St Louis, Mosby–Year Book, 1989, pp 1083–1103.

scribed with IgG or IgM monoclonal gammopathy who had only lower motor neuron findings[91, 98, 108]; others have had combined lower and upper motor neuron signs identical to those of ALS.[12, 20, 23, 73, 109] In patients with exclusively lower motor neuron findings, diffuse muscle weakness and atrophy were seen. The time from onset of disease to death ranged from months to years.[59] The patients with both upper and lower motor neuron signs showed all of the signs of classic ALS, including nonsymmetrical muscle atrophy, fasciculation, and upper motor neuron findings.[59] The time from onset of disease to death in these patients ranged from 9 months to 4 years.[59]

Cancer and Motor Neuron Disease

The possibility of motor neuron disease occurring as an effect of cancer is difficult to evaluate at the present time because of the many other explanations for neurological signs, such as metastases to the nervous system and meninges, cachexia, and other factors.[59] However, there are reports of individuals who had apparent motor neuron disease related to cancer or lymphoma.[17, 21, 46, 59, 111, 131]

Acute Poliomyelitis

Acute poliomyelitis occurs as a result of a generalized viral infection that has an affinity for motor neurons. The virus is a single-stranded RNA enterovirus (picornavirus) and is comprised of three antigenically distinguishable viruses.[86] Acute poliomyelitis is presently very rare in the United States. It can occur in severely immunocompromised persons or in persons who did not receive the vaccination and were exposed to someone who recently received the oral vaccine, which has the live, attenuated virus. Although there is a worldwide attempt to eradicate poliomyelitis, acute poliomyelitis still occurs in developing nations with poor health care delivery systems.

The virus usually enters the body via the oral route. It replicates in the lymphoid tissues of the pharynx and the intestine. It then spreads to the regional lymphoid tissues and a viremia can follow, leading to a nonspecific illness.[69] Viremia is the most accepted mechanism for direct nervous system exposure to the virus. The reason for the selective vulnerability of certain cells, such as the motor neurons, to the poliomyelitis virus is unknown but may be related to specific receptors on their cell membranes.[100]

The poliovirus is an extremely infectious agent, but only a fraction of those infected have symptoms.[69] The disease progresses to central nervous system involvement and paresis or paralysis in 1% to 2% of cases, while in 90% to 95% of cases the infection is inapparent, and in 4% to 8% of cases only a nonspecific illness is noted.[57] With death of the motor neurons, Wallerian degeneration occurs, and the muscle fibers associated with those neurons become "orphaned," resulting in motor weakness.

In histological studies of motor neurons of monkeys with acute paralytic poliomyelitis, nearly all (96% to 97%) of the motor neurons of severely paralyzed limbs were affected by the virus during the acute infection.[16] About one-half of these motor neurons died during the early convalescent period and the other half survived. A good correlation was found between the proportion of destroyed motor neurons and the severity of paralysis.[15]

Clinical Features. The incubation period is from 1 to 2 weeks.[57, 103] The onset is usually accompanied by malaise, muscle aches, and low-grade fever lasting from 1 to 3 days. These findings may cease and no further symptoms might occur. Alternatively, a symptom-free period can be followed by recurrence of systemic symptoms.[69]

The potentially paralytic illness is characterized by fever, generalized headache, and neck and back stiffness. The illness may regress or may proceed, with paralysis appearing by the second to fifth day after onset. Muscle soreness and a sensation of tightness are present, as well as shooting pains and hyperesthesia.[69] Sensory loss is rare.[99] The weakness appears and evolves over hours to a few days. The lumbar area is more frequently involved than the cervical area or the cranial nerves.[69] Severe bulbar involvement is seen in 10% to 15% of

TABLE 46–4 Spinal (Bulbospinal) Muscular Atrophies (SMA), Hereditary Motor Neuropathies (HMN)

Distribution and Type	Synonyms	Inheritance	Age of Onset	Age Unable to Walk	Life Expectancy
Proximal					
Type I Acute infantile	Werdnig-Hoffmann disease, SMA type I, acute proximal HMN	AR	In utero to 6 mo	Never able to walk	7–18 mo
Type II Chronic childhood	Chronic Werdnig-Hoffmann disease, SMA type II, chronic proximal HMN	AR (some new dominant mutants)	3 mo–15 yr	Median ~12 yr (never to 5th decade)	18 mo–40 yr
Type III Juvenile, adult	Kugelberg-Welander disease, SMA type III, recessive proximal HMN	AR	15–60 yr	Rarely > 50 yr	Normal
Type IV Juvenile onset	SMA type IV, juvenile dominant proximal HMN	AD	6 mo–5 yr (rarely up to 15 yr)	Rare	Probably normal
Type V Adult onset	SMA type V, adult dominant proximal HMN	AD	25–65 yr	? 10 yr after diagnosis	20 yr after diagnosis
Bulbospinal					
	X-linked spinal and bulbar muscular atrophy	XLR	15–60 yr (usually 20–40 yr)	? 50 + yr	Minimally limited
Distal					
Type I Juvenile onset	Spinal form of Charcot-Marie-Tooth disease (CMTD)	AD	2–20 yr	Rare	Normal
Type II Adult onset	Spinal form of CMTD	AD	20–40 yr	Rare	Normal
Type III Mild juvenile	Spinal form of CMTD	AR	2–10 yr	Rare	Normal
Type IV Severe juvenile	Spinal form of CMTD	AR	4 mo–20 yr	~30 yr	?
Type V Upper limb predominance	—	AD	5–20 yr (Some sporadic)	Never	Normal
Scapuloperoneal					
Type I	—	AD	4–70 yr	? 50 + yr	? Reduced
Type II	—	AR	2–5 yr	?	?
Facioscapulohumeral		AD	Before 20 yr	?	?
Oculopharyngeal		AD	30–40 yr	?	?
Bulbar					
Type I With deafness	Brown-Vialetto-van Laere syndrome	AR	Before 20 yr (? males earlier)	—	20–40 yr (? males earlier)
Type II Without deafness	Fazio-Londe disease, progressive bulbar palsy of childhood	AR	1–12 yr		50% within 18 mo of onset

Abbreviations: AR, autosomal recessive; AD, autosomal dominant; XLR, X-linked recessive.

Modified from Harding AE: Inherited neuronal atrophy and degeneration predominantly of lower motor neurons. In Dyck PJ, Thomas PK, Lambert EH, Bunge R (eds): Peripheral Neuropathy, Pt 2. Philadelphia, WB Saunders, 1984, pp 1537–1556.

cases.[69] Atrophy of the involved muscle groups appears within the first week. Autonomic dysfunction with cardiac arrhythmia, hypertension, hyperhidrosis, urinary retention, and constipation can occur.[82] Changes in mental status ranging from anxiety to stupor can occur and are attributed to reticular formation or hypothalamic involvement.[11]

Death is usually the result of bulbar or respiratory involvement. Survivors commonly gradually recover muscle function in muscles not completely paralyzed, and some ultimately have minimal or no residua. Improvements begin in the first weeks, but can continue for several years after the acute illness.[2, 49] The mechanisms of recovery include both resolution of dysfunction of partially damaged motor neurons and reinnervation of denervated muscle fibers by surviving motor units.

Post-Polio Syndrome

A number of reports document the complaints registered by poliomyelitis survivors several decades after the acute poliomyelitis illness. In particular, new musculoskeletal and neuromuscular symptoms are reported by these patients.[5, 24, 26, 27, 48–51] Table 46–5 lists the most frequent new health and activities of daily living (ADL) problems of post-polio patients, whether they were seen in a post-polio clinic[5, 49] or had responded to a national survey.[48] The most prevalent new health-related complaints were fatigue, muscle or joint pain, and weakness. The most prevalent new ADL complaints were difficulties with walking and stair climbing. Fatigue was described by many (43% in one survey) as though they were "hitting the wall."[48] Of this group, 68% reported that this phenomenon occurred on a daily basis. Most commonly, this "wall" was experienced in the mid- to late afternoon. Fortunately, for almost all patients it could be ameliorated or aborted by increasing rest time,

TABLE 46–5 New Health Problems and New Problems in Activities of Daily Living in Post-Polio Patients in Three Studies

	Percent of Patients Affected, by Study		
Symptom	*Halstead and Rossi*[48] *(n = 539)*	*Halstead and Rossi*[49] *(n = 132)*	*Agre et al*[5] *(n = 79)*
New health problems			
Fatigue	87%	89%	86%
Muscle pain	80	71	86
Joint pain	79	71	77
Weakness			
Previously affected muscles	87	69	80
Previously unaffected muscles	77	50	53
Cold intolerance	—	29	56
Atrophy	—	28	39
New ADL problems			
Walking	85	64	—
Stair climbing	83	61	67
Dressing	62	17	16

napping, or reducing the overall level of activity during the day.[48]

The typical post-polio patient seen in a post-polio clinic had the acute poliomyelitis illness in childhood (average age at onset between 5 and 10 years), had gradually improving function over a period of 5 to 8 years after the acute illness, remained clinically stable for 25 to 30 years, and then noted the onset of new health or ADL problems that began 5 to 8 years before the individuals sought evaluation in a post-polio clinic.[5, 26, 49]

The percentage of post-polio survivors experiencing new symptoms that can be related to their previous poliomyelitis illness is not precisely known. The Sister Kenny Institute study reported that 41% of post-polio respondents to a questionnaire complained of progressive problems.[115] A Mayo Clinic study reported that approximately 25% of a cohort of 125 survivors were experiencing the late effects of poliomyelitis.[24] In an epidemiological study of 551 poliomyelitis survivors in Allegheny County, Pennsylvania, 28.5% of the patients acknowledged post-polio syndrome.[102] It can be estimated from these reports that approximately one-fourth to one-third of persons who had acute poliomyelitis in the past may be experiencing post-polio syndrome at the present time. This proportion may well increase as these persons age.

A number of terms have been used to describe the problems about which some poliomyelitis survivors complain many years after the acute illness. Such terms as "late-onset postpoliomyelitis progressive muscular atrophy," "late progressive postpoliomyelitis muscular atrophy," "late postpoliomyelitis muscular atrophy," "progressive postpolio atrophy," and "progressive postpoliomyelitis muscular atrophy" have been used.[14, 27–29, 75] Since there are no empirical research data to indicate progressive atrophy or rapid decline in strength, the term "post-polio syndrome" better describes the complaints and findings of polio survivors and does not make unfounded presumptions.

Post-polio syndrome is essentially a diagnosis by exclusion.[49] A good definition of post-polio syndrome has been given by Halstead and Rossi and is based on five criteria:

> (1) A confirmed history of paralytic polio; (2) partial to fairly complete neurologic and functional recovery; (3) a period of neurologic and functional stability of at least 15 years duration; (4) the onset of two or more of the following health problems since achieving a period of stability: unaccustomed fatigue, muscle and/or joint pain, new weakness in muscles previously affected and/or unaffected, functional loss, cold intolerance, new atrophy; and (5) no other medical diagnosis to explain these health problems.[49]

Many post-polio patients are apprehensive about the potential future loss of strength and function. A number of possible pathophysiological and functional causes have been suggested to explain the progressive loss of muscle strength in poliomyelitis survivors. Among the suggested causes are premature aging of motor neurons damaged by the poliovirus, premature aging of the motor neurons due to the increased metabolic demand, loss of muscle fibers within the surviving motor units, death of motor neurons due to the normal aging process, disuse weakness, overuse weakness, or weight gain.[6, 65]

Although the development of late-onset weakness in poliomyelitis survivors was first reported over a century ago,[25, 103] at the present time there is little objective evidence in the literature to indicate that the rate of loss in strength is greater than that expected as a result of the normal aging process. In several reports the determination of progressive loss in strength was made by patient report and not by longitudinal studies using valid and reliable measures. A recent 7-year follow-up study of 23 post-polio and 14 control subjects reported a loss of strength in the quadriceps muscles. There was no difference in the rate of strength loss in the post-polio and the control groups.[3] Further research is needed in this area.

Although a number of plausible hypothetical reasons have been suggested to explain a more rapid decline in strength in poliomyelitis survivors, there is no empirical evidence to date to indicate that the loss of strength is directly related to poliomyelitis. It may instead reflect the aging process in persons with impaired function.

EVALUATION OF THE PATIENT WITH MOTOR NEURON DISEASE

History

The initial phase in the management of a patient with a motor neuron disorder is, of course, to establish the diagnosis, which allows the clinician to better determine the progression of the disorder. Obtaining a detailed history is the first step in this process. The major complaints of the patients and their parents (in the case of children) should be noted. The pattern of weakness can be helpful in determining the specific motor neuron disease. It can be difficult at times to distinguish between some of the motor neuron disorders, muscular dystrophies, and neuropathies. A careful history is essential in this regard. In general, patients with neuropathic disorders usually give a history of distal rather than proximal weakness, often accompanied by sensory abnormalities (which are rare in the motor neuron disorders). It can be difficult, however, to separate the muscular dystrophies from the motor neuron disorders by history alone.

Significant elements to be obtained during the history include the age at onset of difficulties and the rate of progression of the disorder. The distribution of the weakness is also an important clue. The patient with distal weakness will, for instance, have difficulty holding objects. The patient with proximal lower limb weakness may have difficulty arising from a chair, whereas a patient with proximal upper limb weakness may have difficulty placing an object on a shelf. Muscle pain is very common in inflammatory neuropathies and myopathies but is uncommon in motor neuron disorders (except for acute poliomyelitis, where it is usually seen). A careful family history is also important, because a number of the motor neuron disorders are genetically transmitted. The history is very important in learning about the patient's social environment, such as support from family and friends. This is perhaps the most important factor in determining whether the patient will be able to live at home or need institutional care. Assessing the patient's living environment is also important in determining the assistive devices that might be needed to preserve function and independence.

Physical Examination

Visual inspection usually reveals areas of significant muscular atrophy, muscular hypertrophy (which can be found in some of the muscular dystrophies), and fasciculations. Visual inspection for atrophy assists in determining whether the disease involvement is greater in the proximal or the distal limb musculature. Palpation of the limbs can reveal the muscle tenderness that is found in inflammatory myopathies, but which is rare in motor neuron diseases other than acute poliomyelitis.

The sensory examination detects any sensory loss, which is very rare in motor neuron diseases but common in the neuropathic disorders. Muscle stretch reflexes can be increased in the upper motor neuron disorders or in the combined upper and lower motor neuron disorders, but such reflexes are reduced or absent in the lower motor neuron disorders. In the combined upper and lower motor neuron disorders, the muscle stretch reflexes can be increased or decreased, depending on the associated muscular weakness and atrophy. In the presence of significant weakness, the upper motor neuron component can be difficult to detect. Manual muscle testing demonstrates the level of residual muscle function and shows the distribution of the weakness (proximal, distal, or asymmetrical). Residual strength assessment allows for an estimation of residual functional capabilities and what assistive devices might be most helpful in improving or maintaining function.

Assessment of range of motion allows for the detection of contractures. It is important to determine passive range of motion in these patients, as muscle weakness can significantly limit active range of motion. Contractures can significantly limit the patient's functional abilities. For instance, mild flexion contractures of the elbows do not result in significant disability, but slight flexion contractures of the hips or knees can preclude ambulation in a patient with weak hip or knee extensor musculature.[63, 125]

A thorough functional assessment of the patient allows the rehabilitation team to determine the patient's present level of functional abilities including the patient's abilities to be mobile in bed, to transfer, to ambulate with or without assistive devices or be mobile in a wheelchair, and to perform all of the usual ADL. A functional assessment also allows the rehabilitation team to determine what assistive devices would help the patient be most functional and independent, now and in the future as the disorder progresses.

Laboratory Evaluation

In the evaluation of a patient suspected of having a motor neuron disease, it is important to carefully investigate laboratory studies to rule out other potentially remediable causes of motor neuron disorder.

Electrodiagnosis. Electrodiagnostic testing is an important part of the evaluation of the patient suspected of having a motor neuron disease. Nerve conduction studies can confirm the presence or absence of peripheral neuropathy (see Chapters 10 and 11).[123] The EMG can be of assistance in differentiating neuropathy and myopathy[123] and in determining loss of motor neurons, the amount of denervation, and the presence of collateral reinnervation.[8, 30, 129] An additional important role for EMG is to determine the muscle most appropriate for muscle biopsy. Because trauma to the muscle from the EMG needle can produce histological changes in the muscle that make interpretation difficult, it has been recommended that the EMG be limited to one side of the body. Because these disorders are usually symmetrical, an appropriate muscle from the other side of the body can then be recommended for the biopsy.[123]

Muscle Biopsy. The best muscle for biopsy depends on the experience of the clinician. The EMG can help to select a muscle that is definitely involved, but not so severely involved that it represents only end-stage disease, which would limit its diagnostic utility. The muscle biopsy can confirm whether the muscle is normal or abnormal and can help classify the abnormal muscle as myopathic or neuropathic in origin.[123] The muscle biopsy can also be of significance in determining whether the disorder is an inflammatory myopathy, since most inflammatory myopathies are amenable to treatment.[123]

Other Laboratory Evaluations. Depending on the clinical presentation of the patient, the clinical laboratory investigation can consist of a number of other evaluations, including serum protein electrophoresis (looking for evidence of monoclonal gammopathy or paraproteinemia), anti-acetylcholine receptor antibodies (looking for evidence of myasthenia gravis), various antiviral antibody titers (such as HLTV-1 and human immunodeficiency virus [HIV]), serum hexosaminidase A determination (looking for GM_2 gangliosidosis), of anti-GM_1 and GD_{1a} ganglioside IgM antibodies (which may be elevated in ALS and motor neuropathy), endocrine tests (looking for such disorders as diabetes mellitus or thyrotoxicosis), metabolic and blood cell studies (looking for amyotrophic choreic acanthocytosis), serum creatine kinase (usually normal in the motor neuron diseases but often elevated in myopathies), and heavy metal analysis of the urine (looking for such problems as lead and mercury intoxication).[59, 87] The spinal fluid evaluation of patients with motor neuron diseases is usually normal; any elevation of the spinal fluid protein above 80 mg/dL should lead the clinician to suspect another disorder.[130]

GENERAL PRINCIPLES OF REHABILITATION MANAGEMENT

Specific treatment for the pathophysiological processes in motor neuron disease is lacking at the present time. The best approach currently is prevention, with vaccination for the viral diseases, education to prevent toxic exposures, and genetic counseling for the hereditary diseases. Overall management should be divided into prospective care and expectant care.[97] The rehabilitation team should assist the patient in maximizing function and independence for as long as is possible.

Prospective care includes all the usual measures provided to all people regardless of their health status and includes such things as vaccinations and health screening tests.[97] *Expectant care* includes anticipation of complications that might be expected during the course of the patient's motor neuron disease. Aggressive measures can be taken to prevent or minimize these complications and maximize the patient's function and independence for as long as possible.[97] The expected complications include pain, muscle tightness, deformities of bones and joints, weakness, impaired ventilation, and impaired functional abilities.[97]

Pain

Pain is not usually a major problem in motor neuron diseases except for acute poliomyelitis. Patients with acute poliomyelitis complain of severe muscle pain.[70] Pain can usually be controlled by both physical treatments and pharmacological treatment. Hot packs, especially the Kenny hot packs (made from woolen blankets), applied at 5-minute intervals for 20 minutes, have been found to be useful in the acute stages.[70] Heat treatments in conjunction with stretching are useful in the acute stages to control pain and maintain range of motion.[70] Salicylates or other nonsteroidal anti-inflammatory medications (NSAIDs) can also be helpful. Narcotic analgesics should be used sparingly because of potential respiratory depression. For neuritic pain, the tricyclic antidepressant medications such as amitriptyline or carbamazepine can be used.[97] The combination of physical treatment and NSAIDs usually adequately controls the pain.

Muscle Tightness

Soft tissue contractures can occur at all stages in motor neuron disease. Muscles that span two joints are often the first to become tight, usually with the joint in the flexed position (contracture; Table 46–6).[97] Physical treatment includes passive, active-assistive, and active stretching, depending on the condition of the patient, usually after the application of superficial heat. A heated pool allows heat treatment and exercise to be com-

TABLE 46–6 Movements Frequently Affected by Tightness in Soft Tissue

Neck flexion	Hip flexion
Shoulder adduction	Hip internal rotation
Elbow flexion	Knee flexion
Forearm pronation	Ankle plantar flexion
Finger adduction	Foot inversion
Finger extension	

From Pease WS, Johnson EW: Rehabilitation management of diseases of the motor unit. In Kottke FJ, Lehmann JF (eds): Krusen's Handbook of Physical Medicine and Rehabilitation, ed 4. Philadelphia, WB Saunders, 1990, pp 754–764.

bined.[97] Appropriate positioning also facilitates prolonged stretching and prevents deformity.[72, 78] Bracing to aid in the prevention of contractures requires careful assessment of kinesiological factors. When preventing or correcting shortening of a muscle that spans two joints, the physiatrist must be certain that the muscles are stretched at both joints that they cross.[97]

Spasticity

In some motor neuron diseases, considerable spasticity can occur. This is treated in the same way as spasticity in other conditions (see Chapter 29).

Deformity

Malalignment of body segments leads to contracture and deformity.[72] Care must be taken in the prospective treatment of patients with motor neuron disease to prevent or minimize the development of contracture or deformity.[97] As briefly described above, appropriate stretching, bracing, and positioning help prevent contractures.

Care must also be taken in the prescription of equipment provided to patients to prevent contracture and progressive deformity wherever possible. Children are often placed in large wheelchairs to allow for growth, but such positioning does not properly support the child and can lead to contracture and subsequent deformity. For instance, a child sitting in a large wheelchair with a sling-type seat frequently ends up sitting with one hip higher than the other, with the hips internally rotated and adducted, and leaning on one elbow for support (Fig. 46–1A).[97] This postural asymmetry leads to contracture and subsequent deformity. The minimal wheelchair prescription should include a firm seat, with adequate lumbar, truncal, and arm support (Fig. 46–1B). Deformities can be prevented or minimized by the avoidance of malalignment by appropriate stretching, positioning, and bracing. If malalignments are fixed or rapidly advancing, they can be treated by aggressive stretching with serial casts or dynamic bracing, or both, and in some instances by surgical intervention.[97]

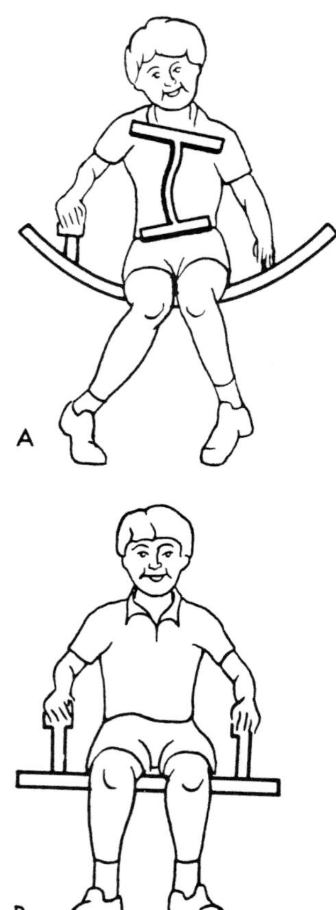

FIGURE 46–1. *A.* Wide hammock seat promotes deformity. *B.* Proper positioning includes a firm seat and correct arm height.

Management of Scoliosis

Preventing or managing scoliosis is one of the major rehabilitation goals in the management of neuromuscular disease. Abnormal spinal curvature occurs with increasing age and with advancing disability. The incidence and rate of progression of scoliosis vary with the type of disorder. Most children with motor neuron disease develop a collapsing, paralytic type of scoliosis. Initially, paraspinal muscular weakness is usually symmetrical, and if the child is still ambulatory, the development of scoliosis is uncommon. Once the weakness progresses sufficiently to prevent ambulation, scoliosis develops rapidly. Preventing scoliosis or limiting its effect is important because scoliosis alters sitting tolerance, leading to skin and pressure relief problems and a decrease in pulmonary function.

The initial approach to scoliosis management is to prescribe the most appropriate wheelchair for the individual child (see Chapter 18). The wheelchair must be measured for each child, after assessing the child's physical, social, and vocational-educational needs. The child must maintain a symmetrical sitting posture with adequate upper and lower extremity support. The sling seat should be avoided because it permits asymmetrical pelvic rotation. The pelvis provides the base of support for the spine, and any pelvic asymmetry permits the development of scoliosis. A solid foam-padded seat cushion can be used to level the pelvis during sitting in the early stages.

An erect spine is necessary for proper sitting balance. A variety of orthoses have been developed to manage the scoliosis curve from 20 to 40 degrees. Children tolerate the sitting support orthosis or the thoracolumbar orthosis well, until the curve reaches more than 40 degrees.[81] Once the curve is more than 40 degrees, a relatively rapid progression continues that generally cannot be managed orthotically.

Surgical stabilization of the spine has been advocated in a number of neuromuscular disorders.[119, 122] Various segmental instrumental and fusion techniques have been described. Postoperative complications are primarily pulmonary. It is believed that the earlier the spine is stabilized, the less likely are the secondary pulmonary and cardiac complications (see Chapters 32 and 33).[104]

Weakness

Motor weakness is a presenting problem in all motor neuron diseases, but it varies considerably in its presentation and location. Proximal weakness interferes with such activities as gait, transfers, and gross motor movements, while distal weakness interferes with more fine motor skills. Treatment of weakness, however, might include strengthening exercises, if prescribed judiciously and followed carefully. Although not well studied, it appears that vigorous, fatiguing progressive resistive exercise is contraindicated in most motor neuron diseases, as such exercise can lead to overuse weakness.[54, 123] Low-intensity, nonfatiguing exercise, however, may be quite beneficial for maintenance or improvement in muscle strength, as has recently been demonstrated in several studies on post-polio patients,[4, 34–37] and for enhancing cardiorespiratory fitness.[45, 64]

Respiratory Assistance

When motor weakness or deformity sufficiently limits the patient's ability to ventilate, mechanical ventilatory assistive devices are needed to allow for adequate ventilation. Early signs and symptoms of hypoxia include difficulty with sleeping, nighttime dyspnea, nightmares, and somnolence during the day.[10, 118] As these signs appear, appropriately prescribed ventilatory aids (such as a cuirass or plastic wrap) enhance gas exchange in the recumbent position.[118] In the later stages of motor neuron disease, oral positive pressure ventilation, a pneumobelt, or cuirass ventilators can be used throughout the day, energized by the wheelchair battery. Tracheostomy is rarely needed and its use is somewhat controversial. Although noninvasive management is preferable, tracheosomy may be useful if the patient has severe scoliosis or if control of aspiration is a major problem (see Chapter 33).[7, 97, 118]

Functional Ability

The primary goals of the rehabilitation team in treating a patient with motor neuron disease are to assist the patient in the maintenance of function, independence, and quality of life for as long as possible. This entails a coordinated effort by the entire rehabilitation team in prospective and expectant care of the patient (and family). Appropriate preventive and therapeutic interventions for the treatment of pain, soft tissue tightness, deformity, scoliosis management, motor weakness, and respiratory dysfunction can minimize complications and maximize the patient's ability to function. Functional training for locomotion, dressing, eating, and other ADL are practiced as developmentally appropriate (see Chapter 25).[97]

Assistive devices, substitution training, and selective surgical procedures (such as tendon transfers, releases, and arthrodeses) all represent management techniques that can be judiciously applied to improve the patient's ability to function.[97] Figure 46–2 demonstrates the util-

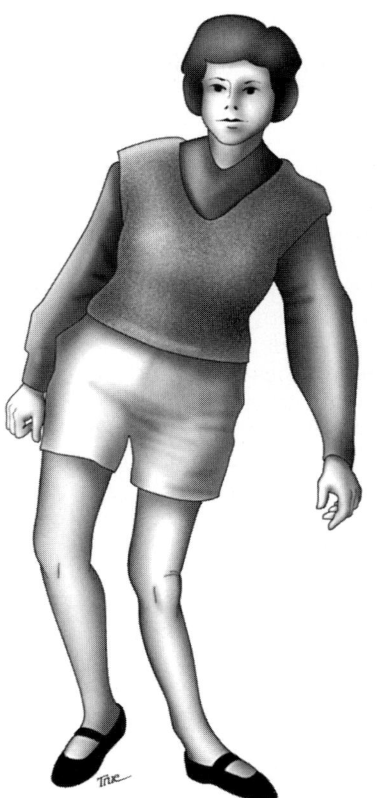

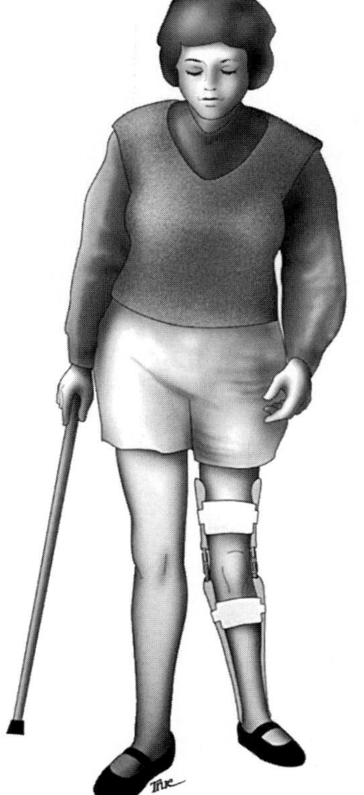

FIGURE 46–2. Post-polio patient ambulating without (*left*) and with (*right*) a knee-ankle-foot orthosis and cane.

ity of a knee-ankle-foot orthosis (KAFO) and cane in a post-polio patient who was seen in the clinic with complaints of left knee pain and fatigability while ambulating. The use of the KAFO and cane not only stabilized the patient's painful, unstable left knee (the patient had a 25-degree valgus deformity and a 30-degree hyperextension deformity) but also reduced the patient's energy expenditure during ambulation by more than 25%. In addition, this patient accepted the use of a motorized scooter for longer distances, which helped save energy in the performance of daily activities.

TREATMENT OF THE PATIENT WITH MOTOR NEURON DISEASE

As described earlier, motor neuron diseases include a number of disorders of the upper motor neuron, lower motor neuron, or both the upper and lower motor neurons. The success of the rehabilitation process depends on the active involvement of the patient. The treatment of two different syndromes or disease entities, post-polio syndrome and ALS, will be briefly discussed as examples of treatment for the patient with a motor neuron disease.

Treatment of Post-Polio Syndrome

The post-polio syndrome appears to be primarily related to overactivity and overuse in individuals with significant neuromuscular impairment attributable to their original poliomyelitis illness. Frequent clinical diagnoses made in these patients include muscle pain related to such factors as overactivity, muscle pain related to overuse or myofascial pain, joint pain related to arthritis, or mechanical problems in joints not well protected due to weakened musculature. The treatment for any particular patient, of course, depends on the evaluation of that individual's situation. Fatigue is a very common complaint of post-polio patients. As mentioned above, many patients describe this phenomenon as "hitting the wall."[48] The origin of this complaint is unknown but may be central in nature in at least some patients. Regardless of the cause, however, it has been reported that most post-polio patients have found that fatigue could be significantly reduced by increasing rest time, napping, or reducing the overall level of activity during the day.[48] Table 46–7 lists some of the more common interventions and recommendations made for post-polio patients as a result of their clinical evaluation. Most patients currently are getting many of the recommended treatments shown in the table. For instance, a large majority of patients in the two studies cited in the table were given advice or prescriptions regarding the type and amount of exercise, weight loss, and level of activity. Almost all were counseled on the need to reduce physical and emotional stress in their lives.[49] The use of new or modified aids (such as corsets, lumbar rolls, neck pillows, wheelchair positioners, canes, and crutches), energy conservation techniques, or the use of new orthotic devices enhances the patient's ability to function and minimizes overuse problems.[5, 49] Psychological counseling or participation in a post-polio support group to learn new coping skills was also recommended for many patients.[5]

TABLE 46–7 Common Clinical Interventions and Recommendations Made to Post-Polio Patients

	Percentage of Patients Given the Recommendation, by Study	
Intervention	*Halstead and Rossi[49] (n = 132)*	*Agre et al[5] (n = 79)*
New or modified aids*	87%	—
Energy conservation techniques	64	73%
Change in exercise program	64	—
Change in orthoses	52	34
Weight loss	52	27
New/modified wheelchair	26	—
Gentle exercise program		
Aerobic exercise	—	23
Stretching exercises	—	46
Strengthening exercises	—	43

*Durable products used to improve posture, diminish pain, and enhance comfort. These include corsets, lumbar rolls, neck pillows, wheelchair positioners, canes, and crutches.

Compliance with clinical recommendations made after physiatric evaluation for post-polio patients appears to be very helpful. For instance, Agre and colleagues[5] found that 78% of patients seen in follow-up reported an improvement in their symptoms. Improvements were noted in terms of decreased muscle and joint pain, decreased level of fatigue, improved gait pattern (with the use of an orthosis or cane), and improved coping abilities. The patients who did not report improvement also were not compliant with the recommendations made. Peach and Olejnik[92] also reported on the effects of treatment compliance in 77 patients seen in a post-polio clinic. These patients were divided into three groups, based on degree of compliance with clinical recommendations: compliers (n = 30), partial compliers (n = 32), and noncompliers (n = 15). Symptoms status at the time of follow-up (which averaged more than 2 years from the time of the initial evaluation) is shown in Table 46–8. In general, a significant proportion of patients in the compliant group noted resolution or improvement in their symptoms. Most of the partially compliant group noted improvement or no change in their symptoms, and only in the noncompliant group did the majority note no change or worsening of their symptoms. The compliant group had an increase in muscle strength, as measured by manual muscle testing, at an annualized rate of +0.6%. On the other hand, the partially compliant group lost muscle strength at an annualized rate of −1.3%, and the noncompliant group lost muscle strength at an annualized rate of −2.0%. It appears that patients who completely comply with clinical recommendations and successfully control the factors responsible for the neuromuscular overuse do not lose muscle strength and note an improvement in their symptoms.

The role of exercise in patients with post-polio syndrome has been somewhat controversial. Early reports

TABLE 46–8 Symptom Status of Post-Polio Patients at Time of Follow-up

Group/No. of Pts.		Resolved (%)	Improved (%)	Unchanged (%)	Increased (%)
Compliant group	(n = 30)				
Weakness	(n = 23)	17	83	0	0
Fatigue	(n = 28)	4	96	0	0
Muscle pain	(n = 25)	28	72	0	0
Joint pain	(n = 17)	41	53	6	0
Partially compliant group	(n = 32)				
Weakness	(n = 29)	0	79	21	0
Fatigue	(n = 31)	0	68	29	3
Muscle pain	(n = 32)	3	88	9	0
Joint pain	(n = 24)	4	83	13	0
Noncompliant group	(n = 15)				
Weakness	(n = 14)	0	0	64	36
Fatigue	(n = 14)	0	0	64	36
Muscle pain	(n = 14)	0	14	57	29
Joint pain	(n = 11)	0	0	82	18

From Peach PE, Olejnik S: Effect of treatment and non-compliance on post-polio sequelae. Orthopedics 1991; 14:1199–1203.

of exercise in post-polio patients yielded conflicting results. Some studies showed that muscle-strengthening exercises were beneficial,[32, 47, 90] whereas other reports indicated that vigorous exercise or activity was detrimental.[62, 71, 77, 88] It appears that a key difference between these studies was the intensity of the exercise program. It appears most probable that the exercise regimens in the studies reporting deleterious effects were too vigorous for the patients and subsequently led to overuse problems. Four studies have been conducted on muscle-strengthening exercise,[4, 34–36] two studies on general exercise or aerobic fitness training,[45, 64] one on efficiency of movement,[31] and one on aquatic exercise[101] in post-polio patients. These studies have shown that judicious exercise can improve muscle strength, cardiorespiratory fitness, and the efficiency of ambulation. These benefits occur when the patient's exercise program avoids excessive fatigue, muscle pain, and joint pain.

The difficulty in prescribing an exercise program for the post-polio patient has to do with the uniqueness of each patient. The physician needs to recognize each patient's particular circumstances, including the location and degree of muscle weakness and the location and degree of subsequent arthropathy or arthralgia. Muscle weakness from poliomyelitis is often asymmetrical and scattered, and the weakness in different muscles can vary considerably. It is important to protect the weakened muscles and affected joints of post-polio patients from overuse during exercise. At the same time, the patient needs to exercise those body areas that can tolerate exercise so that function is not reduced as a result of disuse. At present, it appears that muscles with antigravity or greater strength on manual muscle testing[84] can tolerate strengthening exercises.[4, 34–37] Swimming and aquatic exercise may be one of the best types of exercise in these persons as the buoyancy of the water reduces the effect of gravity on the patient's joints and limbs, protecting them from overuse. At present, it appears that judicious exercise in the appropriate post-polio patient (the patient who can exercise and avoid undue fatigue, muscle pain, and joint pain) is an important adjuvant in the patient's overall therapeutic program.[1]

Treatment of Amyotrophic Lateral Sclerosis

The progression of ALS is quite variable. It may be rapidly progressive or slowly progressive, with the patient surviving 15 to 20 years after the initial diagnosis is made. The rehabilitation treatment program of the patient with ALS is described elsewhere in more detail.[114] Briefly, most patients with ALS go through three phases.

In the first phase, the patient is independent. This phase can be separated into three distinct stages. In the first stage, the patient is ambulatory, independent in ADL, and has mild weakness or clumsiness. Treatment at this time includes encouraging the patient to perform range-of-motion exercises and strengthening exercises of the unaffected musculature to compensate for the weakened muscles. Strenuous exercise, however, is discouraged as it might lead to increased fatigue and disability. Psychological support is also very important at this stage. In the second stage the patient is still ambulatory but has moderate selective weakness and slightly decreased independence in the performance of ADL (e.g., difficulty with climbing stairs, raising arms overhead, or buttoning clothing). Treatment at this stage includes substituting Velcro closures for buttons, encouraging the use of ankle-foot orthoses, prescribing wrist-and-thumb splints, and encouraging selective strengthening for unaffected muscles and stretching exercises to avoid contractures. Patients are advised to avoid overuse and fatigue. In the third stage, the patient is still ambulatory but becomes easily fatigued with long-distance ambulation. There is severe selective weakness in the ankles, wrists, and hands with a moderate decrease in independence in ADL. Treatment in this stage is designed to keep the patient independent for as long as possible. Deep breathing exercises should be added in this stage and the patient should receive an appropriate wheelchair or motorized scooter for longer-distance mobility.

In the second phase, the patient is partially independent. This phase can be divided into stages 4 and 5 of the overall course of ALS. In the fourth stage, the patient is no longer ambulatory and is confined to a wheelchair. The patient has severe weakness in the lower limbs, with or without spasticity. The patient has moderate upper limb weakness but is able to perform many ADL independently or with partial assistance. The patient may have shoulder pain due to weakness about the shoulder girdle musculature and may have edema of the hand. Treatment at this time includes supporting the shoulder and using heat and massage for shoulder pain. Anti-edema preventive measures should be utilized. Passive range-of-motion exercises and stretching should be performed to prevent contracture. The patient should be encouraged to perform isometric exercises of the few remaining uninvolved muscles. In the fifth stage, the patient's strength continues to decline. The patient has severe lower limb weakness and moderate to severe upper limb weakness. The patient progressively needs more and more assistance with all ADL. The patient needs assistance in transferring into and out of the wheelchair. Pressure ulceration may also occur as a result of immobility and pressure. Treatment at this stage includes continuing with range-of-motion and stretching exercises to avoid contracture formation. The patient's family should be encouraged to learn proper transfer and positioning principles. Modifications of the home environment are needed to aid the patient's mobility and independence. Use of a water mattress may be helpful in preventing pressure ulcer formation.

In the third phase, the patient is totally dependent. The patient is essentially bedridden and is completely dependent in all ADL. Treatment includes continuance of range-of-motion and stretching exercises to prevent the formation of contractures. For dysphagia, a soft diet might be helpful; otherwise the patient may need tube feeding. For accumulation of saliva, the use of suction, medications, or surgery to decrease salivary flow may be helpful. For dysarthria, the use of palatal lifts or electronic speech amplification may be helpful. For breathing difficulty, the airway needs to be carefully monitored and cleared as needed. Tracheostomy or respirator use may be required. During this phase, the physical ability of the family to care for the patient at home needs to be considered.

SUMMARY

The overall aim in the treatment of a patient with a motor neuron disease is to prolong functional abilities, independence, and quality of life for as long as possible. A coordinated effort by the rehabilitation team to maintain mobility, prevent deformity, maintain or improve strength, and manage respiratory dysfunction can minimize complications and maximize function. Functional training, the use of assistive devices, and judicious surgical procedures may also be used.

ACKNOWLEDGMENT

We thank Donald W. Mulder, M.D., Emeritus Professor of Neurology, the Mayo Medical School, for reviewing this chapter and providing useful suggestions for revision.

REFERENCES

1. Agre JC: The role of exercise in the patient with post-polio syndrome. Ann NY Acad Sci, 1995; 753:321–334.
2. Agre JC, Rodriquez AA: Neuromuscular function: Comparison of symptomatic and asymptomatic polio subjects to control subjects. Arch Phys Med Rehabil 1990; 71:545–551.
3. Rodriquez AA, Agre JC, Franke TM: Electromyographic and neuromuscular variables in unstable post-polio subjects, stable post-polio subjects, and control subjects. Arch Phys Med Rehabil 1997; 78:986–991.
4. Agre JC, Rodriquez AA, Franke TM: Muscle strengthening exercise can increase strength, endurance, and work capacity in post-polio subjects. Arch Phys Med Rehabil 1997; 78:681–686.
5. Agre JC, Rodriquez AA, Sperling KB: Symptoms and clinical impressions of patients seen in a postpolio clinic. Arch Phys Med Rehabil 1989; 70:367–370.
6. Agre JC, Rodriquez AA, Tafel JA: Late effects of polio: Critical review of the literature on neuromuscular function. Arch Phys Med Rehabil 1991; 72:923–931.
7. Alexander MA, Johnson EW, Petty J, et al: Mechanical ventilation of patients with late stage Duchenne muscular dystrophy: Management at home. Arch Phys Med Rehabil 1979; 60:289.
8. American Association of Electrodiagnostic Medicine: Motor Neuron Diseases. 1990 AAEM Course C. Rochester, MN, American Association of Electrodiagnostic Medicine, 1990, pp 1–42.
9. Armstrong RM, Fogelson MH, Silberberg DH: Familial proximal spinal muscular atrophy. Arch Neurol 1966; 14:208–212.
10. Bach JR, O'Brien J, Krotenberg R, et al: Management of end stage respiratory failure in Duchenne muscular dystrophy. Muscle Nerve 1987; 10:177–182.
11. Baker AB, Cornwell S, Brown IA: Poliomyelitis: VI. The hypothalamus. Arch Neurol Psychiatry 1952; 68:16.
12. Bauer M, Bergström R, Ritter B, et al: Macroglobulinemia, Waldenström and motor neuron syndrome. Acta Neurol Scand 1977; 55:245–250.
13. Ben Hamida M, Hentati F, Ben Hamida C: Hereditary motor system diseases: Chronic juvenile amyotrophic lateral sclerosis. Brain 1990; 113:347–363.
14. Block HS, Wilbourn AJ: Progressive post-polio atrophy: The EMG findings (abstract). Neurology 1986; 36(suppl 1):137.
15. Bodian D: Pathologic anatomy. In Poliomyelitis: Transactions of the First International Poliomyelitis Conference. Philadelphia, JB Lippincott, 1949.
16. Bodian D: The virus, the nerve cell, and paralysis: Study of experimental poliomyelitis in the spinal cord. Bull Johns Hopkins Hosp 1948; 83:1–73.
17. Brain WR, Croft PB, Wilkinson M: Motor neurone disease as a manifestation of neoplasm (with a note on the course of classical motor neurone disease). Brain 1965; 88:479–500.
18. Brett EM, Lake BD: Neuromuscular disorders: I. Primary muscle disease and anterior horn cell disorders. In Brett EM (ed): Paediatric Neurology, ed 2. New York, Churchill Livingstone, 1991, pp 53–115.
19. Brooke MH: A Clinician's View of Neuromuscular Diseases, ed 2. Baltimore, Williams & Wilkins, 1986.
20. Brownell B, Oppenheimer DR, Hughes JT: The central nervous system in motor neurone disease. J Neurol Neurosurg Psychiatry 1970; 33:338–357.
21. Buchanan DS, Malamud N: Motor neuron disease with renal cell carcinoma and postoperative neurologic remission: A clinicopathologic report. Neurology 1973; 23:891–894.
22. Byers RK, Banker BQ: Infantile muscular atrophy. Arch Neurol 1961; 5:140–164.
23. Chazot G, Berger B, Carrier H, et al: Manifestations neurologiques des gammapathies monoclonales: Formes neurologiques

pures—Études en immunofluorescence. Rev Neurol 1976; 132:195–212.
24. Codd MB, Mulder DW, Kurland LT, et al: Poliomyelitis in Rochester, Minnesota, 1935–1955: Epidemiology and long-term sequelae. A preliminary report. In Halstead LS, Wiechers DO (eds): Late Effects of Poliomyelitis. Miami, Symposia Foundation, 1985, pp 121–134.
25. Cornil Lepine: Sur un cas de paralysie générale spinale antérieure subaiguë, suivi d'autopsie. Gaz Med Fr (Paris) 1875; 4:127–129.
26. Cosgrove JL, Alexander MA, Kitts EL, et al: Late effects of poliomyelitis. Arch Phys Med Rehabil 1987; 68:4–7.
27. Dalakas MB, Elder G, Hallat M, et al: A long-term follow-up study of patients with post-poliomyelitis neuromuscular symptoms. N Engl J Med 1986; 314:959–963.
28. Dalakas MC, Sever JL, Fletcher M, et al: Neuromuscular symptoms in patients with old poliomyelitis: Clinical, virological and immunological studies. In Halstead LS, Wiechers DO (eds): Late Effects of Poliomyelitis. Miami, Symposia Foundation, 1985, pp 73–90.
29. Dalakas MC, Sever JL, Madden DL, et al: Late post-poliomyelitis muscular atrophy: Clinical, virological and immunological studies. Rev Infect Dis 1984; 6(suppl 2):S562–567.
30. Daube JR: Electrophysiologic studies in the diagnosis and prognosis of motor neuron diseases. Neurol Clin 1985; 3:473–493.
31. Dean E, Ross J: Effect of modified aerobic training on movement energetics in polio survivors. Orthopedics 1991; 14:1243–1246.
32. DeLorme TL, Schwab RS, Watkins AL: The response of the quadriceps femoris to progressive resistance exercises in poliomyelitis patients. J Bone Joint Surg Am 1948; 30:834–847.
33. De Vivo DC, Hays AP: Disorders of the neuromuscular system. In Fishman MA (ed): Pediatric Neurology. Orlando, FL, Grune & Stratton, 1986, pp 111–135.
34. Einarsson G: Muscle conditioning in late poliomyelitis. Arch Phys Med Rehabil 1991; 72:11–14.
35. Einarsson G, Grimby G: Strengthening exercise program in post-polio subjects. In Halstead LS, Wiechers DO (eds): Research and Clinical Aspects of the Late Effects of Poliomyelitis. White Plains, NY, March of Dimes Birth Defects Foundation, 1987, pp 275–283.
36. Feldman RM, Soskolne CL: The use of nonfatiguing strengthening exercises in post-polio syndrome. In Halstead LS, Wiechers DO (eds): Research and Clinical Aspects of the Late Effects of Poliomyelitis. White Plains, NY, March of Dimes Birth Defects Foundation, 1987, pp 335–341.
37. Fillyaw MJ, Badger GJ, Goodwin GD, et al: The effects of long-term non-fatiguing resistance exercise in subjects with post-polio syndrome. Orthopedics 1991; 14:1253–1256.
38. Fischbeck KH, Ionasescu V, Ritter AW, et al: Localization of the gene for X-linked spinal muscular atrophy. Neurology 1986; 36:1595–1598.
39. Gajdusek DC: Foci of motor neuron disease in high incidence in isolated populations of East Asia and the western Pacific. In Rowland LP (ed): Human Motor Neuron Diseases. New York, Raven Press, 1982, pp 363–393.
40. Gallai V, Hockaday JM, Hughes JT, et al: Ponto-bulbar palsy with deafness (Brown-Vialetto-van Laere syndrome). A report on 3 cases. J Neurol Sci 1981; 45:259–275.
41. Gamstrop I, Sarnat HB (eds): Progressive Spinal Muscular Atrophies. New York, Raven Press, 1984.
42. Gardner-Medwin D, Hudgson P, Walton JN: Benign spinal muscular atrophy arising in childhood and adolescence. J Neurol Sci 1967; 5:121–158.
43. Gilman S, Romanul FCA: Hereditary dystonic paraplegia with amyotrophy and mental deficiency: Clinical and neuropathological characteristics. In Vinken PJ, Bruyn GW (eds): Handbook of Clinical Neurology, Fazio-Londe Disease, pt 2. Amsterdam, North-Holland, 1975, pp 445–465.
44. Gomez MR: Progressive bulbar paralysis of childhood. In Vinken PJ, Bruyn GW (eds): Handbook of Clinical Neurology. Fazio-Londe Disease, pt 2. Amsterdam, North-Holland, 1975, pp 103–109.
45. Grimby G, Einarsson G: Post-polio management. CRC Crit Rev Phys Med Rehabil 1991; 2:189–200.
46. Gritzman MCD, Fritz VU, Perkins S, et al: Motor neuron disease associated with carcinoma: A report of 2 cases. S Afr Med J 1983; 63:288–291.
47. Gurwitsch AD: Intensive graduated exercises in early infantile paralysis. Arch Phys Med 1950; 31:213–218.
48. Halstead LS, Rossi CD: New problems in old polio patients: Results of a survey of 539 polio survivors. Orthopedics 1985; 8:845–850.
49. Halstead LS, Rossi CD: Post-polio syndrome: Clinical experience with 132 consecutive outpatients. In Halstead LS, Wiechers DO (eds): Research and Clinical Aspects of the Late Effects of Poliomyelitis. White Plains, NY, March of Dimes Birth Defects Foundation, 1987, pp 13–26.
50. Halstead LS, Wiechers DO (eds): Late Effects of Poliomyelitis. Miami, Symposia Foundation, 1985.
51. Halstead LS, Wiechers DO (eds): Research and Clinical Aspects of the Late Effects of Poliomyelitis. White Plains, NY, March of Dimes Birth Defects Foundation, 1987.
52. Harding AE: Inherited neuronal atrophy and degeneration predominantly of lower motor neurons. In Dyck PJ, Thomas PK, Lambert EH, Bunge R (eds): Peripheral Neuropathy, pt 2. Philadelphia, WB Saunders, 1984, pp 1537–1556.
53. Harding AE, Thomas PK: Hereditary distal spinal muscular atrophy. A report of 34 cases and a review of the literature. J Neurol Sci 1980; 45:337–348.
54. Herbison GJ, Jaweed MM, Ditunno JF, Jr: Exercise therapies in peripheral neuropathies. Arch Phys Med Rehabil 1983; 64:201–205.
55. Hirayama K, Tomonaga M, Kitano K, et al: Focal cervical poliopathy causing juvenile muscular atrophy of distal upper extremity: A pathological study. J Neurol Neurosurg Psychiatry 1987; 50:285–290.
56. Hoffmann J: Über chronische spinale Muskelatrophie im Kindesalter, auf familiärer Basis. Dtsch Z Nervenheilk 1893; 3:427–470.
57. Horstmann DM: Epidemiology of poliomyelitis and allied diseases—1963. Yale J Biol Med 1963; 36:5–26.
58. Hudson AJ: Amyotrophic lateral sclerosis and its association with dementia, parkinsonism and other neurological disorders: A review. Brain 1981; 104:217–247.
59. Hudson AJ: The motor neuron diseases and related disorders. In Joynt RJ (ed): Clinical Neurology, vol 4. Philadelphia, JB Lippincott, 1991, pp 1–35.
60. Hudson AJ, Davenport A, Hader WJ: The incidence of amyotrophic lateral sclerosis in southwestern Ontario, Canada. Neurology 1986; 36:1524–1528.
61. Hudson AJ, Rice GPA: Similarities of Guamanian ALS/PD to post-encephalitic parkinsonism/ALS: Possible viral cause. Can J Neurol Sci 1990; 17:427–433.
62. Hyman G: Poliomyelitis. Lancet 1953; 1:852.
63. Johnson EW: Pathokinesiology of Duchenne muscular dystrophy: Implications for management. Arch Phys Med Rehabil 1977; 58:4–7.
64. Jones DR, Speier J, Canine K, et al: Cardiorespiratory responses to aerobic training by patients with postpoliomyelitis sequelae. JAMA 1989; 261:3255–3258.
65. Jubelt B, Cashman NR: Neurological manifestations of the post-polio syndrome. CRC Crit Rev Clin Neurobiol 1987; 3:199–220.
66. Kaeser HE: Scapuloperoneal muscular atrophy. Brain 1965; 88:407–418.
67. Kennedy WR, Alter M, Sung JH: Progressive proximal spinal and bulbar muscular atrophy of late onset: A sex-linked recessive trait. Neurology 1968; 18:671–680.
68. Kimura J: Electrodiagnosis in Diseases of Nerve and Muscle: Principles and Practice, ed 2. Philadelphia, FA Davis, 1989, pp 429–446.
69. Kincaid JC: Myelitis and myelopathy. In Joynt RJ (ed): Clinical Neurology, vol 4. Philadelphia, JB Lippincott, 1991, pp 1–36.
70. Knapp ME: The contribution of Sister Elizabeth Kenny to treatment of poliomyelitis. Arch Phys Med Rehabil 1955; 36:510–517.
71. Knowlton GC, Bennett RL: Overwork. Arch Phys Med Rehabil 1957; 38:18–20.
72. Kottke FJ: Therapeutic exercise to maintain mobility. In Kottke FJ, Lehmann JF (eds): Krusen's Handbook of Physical Medicine and Rehabilitation, ed 4. Philadelphia, WB Saunders, pp 436–451.
73. Krieger C, Melmed C: Amyotrophic lateral sclerosis and paraproteinemia. Neurology 1982; 32:896–898.

74. Kugelberg E, Welander L: Heredofamilial juvenile muscular atrophy simulating muscular dystrophy. Arch Neurol Psychiatry 1956; 75:500–509.
75. Kurent JE, Brooks BR, Madden DL, et al: CSF viral antibodies: Evaluation in amyotrophic lateral sclerosis and late-onset postpoliomyelitis progressive muscular atrophy. Arch Neurol 1979; 36:269–273.
76. Kurtzke JF, Beebe GW: Epidemiology of amyotrophic lateral sclerosis: 1. A case-control comparison based on ALS deaths. Neurology 1980; 30:453–462.
77. Lovett RW: The treatment of infantile paralysis: Preliminary report, based on a study of the Vermont epidemic of 1914. JAMA 1915; 64:2118–2123.
78. Lowenthal M, Tobis JS: Contractures in chronic neurologic disease. Arch Phys Med Rehabil 1957; 38:640–645.
79. Ludolph AC, Hugon J, Dwivedi MP, et al: Studies on the aetiology and pathogenesis of motor neuron diseases: 1. Lathyrism: Clinical findings in established cases. Brain 1987; 110:149–165.
80. Maloney FP, Burks JS, Ringel SP (eds): Interdisciplinary Rehabilitation of Multiple Sclerosis and Neuromuscular Disorders. Philadelphia, JB Lippincott, 1985.
81. Matthews DJ, Stempien LM: Orthopedic management of the disabled child. In Sinaki M (ed): Basic Clinical Rehabilitation Medicine. St Louis, Mosby–Year Book, 1993, pp 399–411.
82. McDowell FH, Plum F: Arterial hypertension associated with acute anterior poliomyelitis. N Engl J Med 1951; 245:241.
83. McLeod JG, Prineas JW: Distal type of chronic spinal muscular atrophy: Clinical, electrophysiological and pathological studies. Brain 1971; 94:703–714.
84. Medical Research Council: Aids to the Examination of the Peripheral Nervous System, ed 2, rev. War Memorandum no 7. London, HMSO, 1943.
85. Melki J, Abdelhak S, Sheth P, et al: Gene for chronic proximal spinal muscular atrophies maps to chromosome 5q. Science 1990; 344:767–768.
86. Melnick JL, Agol VI, Bachrach HL, et al: Picornaviridae. Intervirology 1974; 4:303–316.
87. Menkes JH: Textbook of Child Neurology, ed 4. Philadelphia, Lea & Febiger, 1990, pp 675–721.
88. Mitchell GP: Poliomyelitis and exercise. Lancet 1953; 2:90–91.
89. Mulder DW, Bushek W, Spring E, et al: Motor neuron disease (ALS): Evaluation of detection thresholds of cutaneous sensation. Neurology 1983; 33:1625–1627.
90. Müller EA, Bechmann H: Die Trainierbarkeit von Kindern mit gelähmten Muskeln durch isometrische Kontraktionen. Z Orthop 1966; 102:139–145.
91. Parry GJ, Holtz SJ, Ben-Zeev D, et al: Gammopathy with proximal motor axonopathy simulating motor neuron disease. Neurology 1986; 36:273–276.
92. Peach PE, Olejnik S: Effect of treatment and noncompliance on post-polio sequelae. Orthopedics 1991; 14:1199–1203.
93. Pearn JH: Genetics of the spinal muscular atrophies. In Gamstrop I, Sarnat HB (eds): Progressive Spinal Muscular Atrophies. New York, Raven Press, 1984, pp 19–30.
94. Pearn JH, Carter CO, Wilson J: The genetic identity of acute infantile spinal muscular atrophy. Brain 1973; 96:463–470.
95. Pearn JH, Hudgson P: Distal spinal muscular atrophy: A clinical and genetic study of 8 kindreds. J Neurol Sci 1979; 43:183–191.
96. Pearn JH, Wilson J: Acute Werdnig-Hoffmann disease: Acute infantile spinal muscular atrophy. Arch Dis Child 1973; 48: 425–430.
97. Pease WS, Johnson EW: Rehabilitation management of diseases of the motor unit. In Kottke FJ, Lehmann JF (eds): Krusen's Handbook of Physical Medicine and Rehabilitation, ed 4. Philadelphia, WB Saunders, 1990, pp 754–764.
98. Peters HA, Clatanoff DV: Spinal muscular atrophies secondary to macroglobulinemia: Reversal of symptoms with chlorambucil therapy. Neurology 1968; 18:101–108.
99. Plum F: Sensory loss with poliomyelitis. Neurology 1956; 6:166.
100. Price RW, Plum F: Poliomyelitis. In Vinken PJ, Bruyn GW (eds): Handbook of Clinical Neurology, vol 34. Amsterdam, North-Holland, 1978, p 93.
101. Prins JH, Hartung GH, Merritt DJ, et al: Effect of aquatic exercise training in persons with poliomyelitis disability. Sports Med Train Rehabil 1994; 5:29–39.
102. Ramlov J, Alexander M, LaPorte R, et al: Epidemiology of post-polio syndrome. Am J Epidemiol 1992; 136:769–786.
103. Raymond M (with contribution by Charcot JM): Paralysie essentiele de l'enfance: Atrophie musculaire consecutive. Gaz Med Fr (Paris) 1875; 4:225.
104. Rideau Y, Glovon B, Delaubier A: The treatment of scoliosis in Duchenne muscular dystrophy. Muscle Nerve 1984; 7:281–286.
105. Rodgers-Johnson P, Garruto RM, Yanagihara R, et al: Amyotrophic lateral sclerosis and parkinsonism–dementia on Guam: A 30-year evaluation of clinical and neuropathic trends. Neurology 1986; 36:7–13.
106. Román GC: The neuroepidemiology of tropical spastic paraparesis. Ann Neurol 1988; 23(suppl):S113–S120.
107. Rosling H, Gessain A, de The G, et al: Tropical and epidemic spastic parapareses are different. Lancet 1988; 1:1222–1223.
108. Rowland LP, Defendini R, Sherman W, et al: Macroglobulinemia with peripheral neuropathy simulating motor neuron disease. Ann Neurol 1982; 11:532–536.
109. Rudnicki S, Chad DA, Drachman DA, et al: Motor neuron disease and paraproteinemia. Neurology 1987; 37:335–337.
110. Schoenen J, Delwaide PJ, Legros JJ, et al: Motoneuropathie héréditaire: La forme proximale de l'adulte liéé au sexe (ou maladie de Kennedy). J Neurol Sci 1979; 41:343–357.
111. Schold SC, Cho E-S, Somasundaram M, et al: Subacute motor neuronopathy: A remote effect of lymphoma. Ann Neurol 1979; 5:271–287.
112. Schwarz GA, Liu C-N: Hereditary (familial) spastic paraplegia. Arch Neurol 1956; 75:144–156.
113. Siddique T, Figlewicz DA, Pericak-Vance MA, et al: Linkage of a gene causing familial amyotrophic lateral sclerosis to chromosome 21 and evidence of genetic-locus heterogeneity. N Engl J Med 1991; 324:1381–1384.
114. Sinaki M: Exercise and rehabilitation measures in amyotrophic lateral sclerosis. In Tsubaki T, Yase Y (eds): Excerpta Medica International Congress Series 769. Amsterdam, Elsevier, 1988, pp 343–368.
115. Speier JL, Owen RR, Knapp M, Canine JK: Occurrence of post-polio sequelae in an epidemic population. In Halstead LS, Wiechers DO (eds): Research and Clinical Aspects of the Late Effects of Poliomyelitis. White Plains, NY, March of Dimes Birth Defects Foundation, 1987, pp 39–48.
116. Spencer PS, Nunn PB, Hugon J, et al: Guam amyotrophic lateral sclerosis-parkinsonism-dementia linked to a plant excitant neurotoxin. Science 1987; 237:517–522.
117. Spencer PS, Nunn PB, Hugon J, et al: Motorneurone disease on Guam: Possible role of a food neurotoxin. Lancet 1986; 1:965.
118. Splaingard ML, Frates RC, Jefferson LS, et al: Home negative pressure ventilation: Report of 20 years of experience in patients with neuromuscular disease. Arch Phys Med Rehabil 1985; 66:239–242.
119. Staheli CT: Common orthopedic problems. Pediatr Clin North Am 1986; 33:269–280.
120. Strong MJ, Hudson AJ, Alvord WG: Familial amyotrophic lateral sclerosis, 1850–1989: A statistical analysis of the world literature. Can J Neurol Sci 1991; 18:45–58.
121. Swaiman KF: Anterior horn cell and cranial motor neuron disease. In Swaiman KF (ed): Pediatric Neurology: Principles and Practice, vol 2. St Louis, Mosby–Year Book, 1989, pp 1083–1103.
122. Tachdjiam MO: Scoliosis. In Tachdjiam MO (ed): Pediatric Orthopedics. Philadelphia, WB Saunders, 1990, pp 2265–2378.
123. Taylor RG, Lieberman JS: Rehabilitation of the patient with diseases affecting the motor unit. In DeLisa JA (ed): Rehabilitation Medicine: Principles and Practice. Philadelphia, JB Lippincott, 1988, pp 811–820.
124. Tsukagoshi H, Sugita H, Furukawa T, et al: Kugelberg-Welander syndrome with dominant inheritance. Arch Neurol 1966; 14: 378–381.
125. Vignos PJ: Physical models of rehabilitation in neuromuscular disease. Muscle Nerve 1983; 6:323–338.
126. Virmani V, Mohan PK: Non-familial, spinal segmental muscular atrophy in juvenile and young subjects. Acta Neurol Scand 1985; 72:336–340.
127. Walton J: Disorders of Voluntary Muscle. London, Churchill Livingstone, 1981.

128. Werdnig G: Zwei frühinfantile hereditäre Fälle von progressiver Muskelatrophie unter dem Bilde der Dystrophie, aber auf neurotischer Grundlage. Arch Psychiatr Nervenkrankheiten 1891; 22:437–480.
129. Wiechers DO, Warmolts JR: Anterior horn cell diseases. In Johnson EW (ed): Practical Electromyography. Baltimore, Williams & Wilkins, 1981, pp 135–154.
130. Windebank AJ, Mulder DW: Motor neuron disease in adults. In Engel AG, Franzini-Armstrong C (eds): Myology. New York, McGraw-Hill, 1994, pp 1854–1869.
131. Younger DS, Rowland LP, Latov N, et al: Lymphoma, motor neuron diseases, and amyotrophic lateral sclerosis. Ann Neurol 1991; 29:78–86.

A continually updated list of motor neuron diseases with the latest genetic information can be found on the Internet at http://www.neuro.wustl.edu/neuromuscular/index.html

47

CHAPTER

Lois Buschbacher, M.D.

Rehabilitation of Patients with Peripheral Neuropathies

Peripheral neuropathy includes any disorder of the peripheral nervous system involving either the axon or the myelin sheath. In some cases, both are affected, especially in the later stages of disease progression.

Peripheral neuropathies can be localized or generalized, proximal or distal. They can be due to compression, toxic exposure, metabolic derangements, neoplasm, infection, inflammation, amyloidosis, autoimmune phenomena, or hereditary causes. Usually they are generalized and produce diffuse peripheral weakness, impaired sensation, and hyporeflexia. Since many diseases cause similar neuropathies, the exact cause requires a thorough history and physical examination, electrodiagnostic studies, laboratory studies, and in some cases, a biopsy or genetic study.

NERVE ANATOMY AND PHYSIOLOGY

The peripheral nervous system begins as the neurons leave the brain and spinal cord. Peripheral nerves can have both afferent and efferent neurons. Figure 47–1 depicts the afferent and efferent tracts as they exit the spinal cord and join to form a spinal nerve. There are 12 cranial nerves and 31 spinal nerves, which together form the peripheral nervous system (Fig. 47–2). In the cervical and lumbosacral spine, these nerves intermingle with one another to form plexi (Fig. 47–3).

Each spinal nerve innervates a characteristic sensory area (dermatome) (Fig. 47–4) and muscle group (myotome) (Table 47–1). Peripheral nerves also innervate a characteristic set of muscles (see Table 47–1) as well as skin (Fig. 47–5). Knowledge of the usual paths of innervation is useful in determining the specific nerve or nerve root level of involvement in disease states. Individual patients do not always follow the usual innervation patterns, but variations are usually minor.

Each peripheral nerve is surrounded by an outer connective tissue sheath called the epineurium, which protects the nerve from compression. Inside the epineurium the nerve fibers are arranged in bundles, or fascicles, which are surrounded by a perineurium. The perineurium is the primary strengthening connective tissue of the nerve and also acts as a diffusion barrier. Nerve fibers can intermingle and cross from one fascicle to another along the course of the nerve. Each individual nerve fiber is surrounded by a membrane called the endoneurium[86] (Fig. 47–6).

The nerve roots are more vulnerable to injury than the rest of the peripheral nerve. This is because the roots lack perineurial and epineurial protection; moreover, the fibers are less "slack," and they are supported by less collagen.[86]

Axons are the long cellular processes of both motor and sensory nerves. They have an excitable membrane which causes an electrical current to propagate along the nerve to communicate with distal parts of the body, either to transmit sensory information or to activate the muscles or glands. Each segment of the axon must reach a threshold of electrical excitation, called depolarization, to propagate the impulse. The axonal membrane in isolation would lose current to the surrounding extracellular fluid. To counteract this and to increase the speed of nerve conduction, all axons are surrounded by an insulating layer of myelin (see Chapter 10). Some axons share myelin with other axons and are poorly insulated. These axons are commonly called "unmyelin-

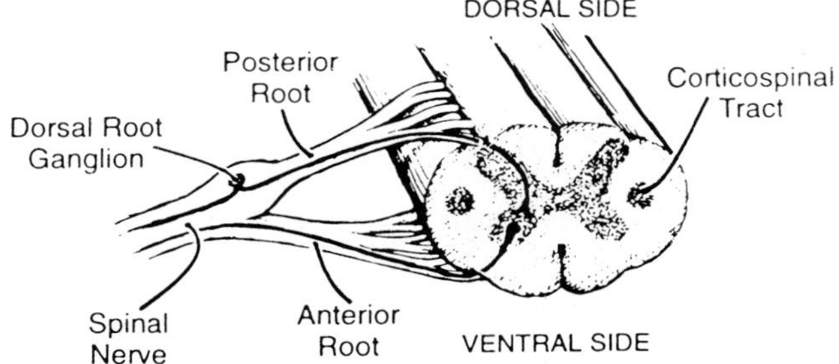

FIGURE 47–1. Cross-sectional segment of the spinal cord depicting afferent and efferent nerve roots, which combine to form a peripheral nerve. (From Buschbacher RM: Basic tissue organization and function. In Buschbacher RM (ed): Musculoskeletal Disorders: A Practical Guide for Diagnosis and Rehabilitation. Stoneham, MA, Butterworth-Heinemann, 1994, p 17.)

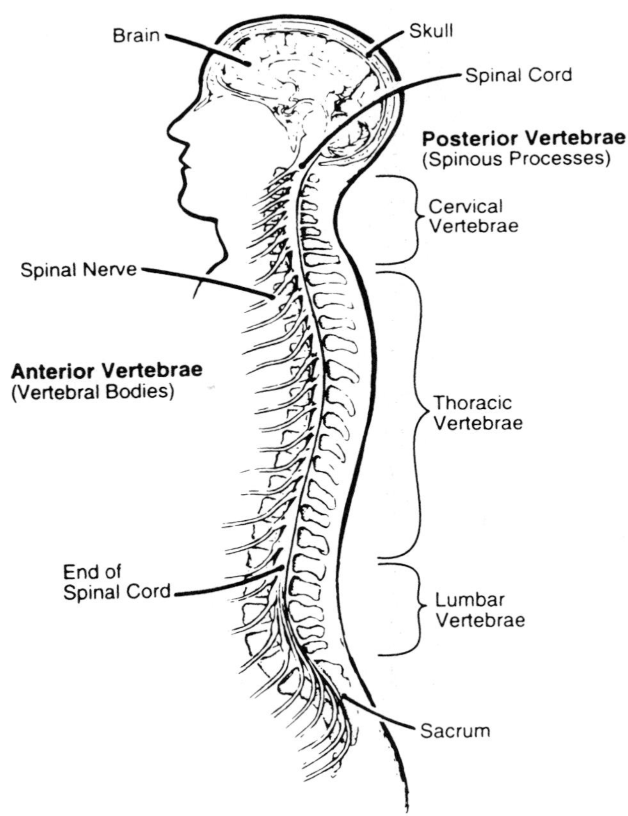

FIGURE 47–2. The central and peripheral nervous systems. Twelve cranial and 31 spinal nerves exit the brain and spinal cord to form the peripheral nervous system. (From Buschbacher RM: Basic tissue organization and function. In Buschbacher RM (ed): Musculoskeletal Disorders: A Practical Guide for Diagnosis and Rehabilitation. Stoneham, MA, Butterworth-Heinemann, 1994, p 17.)

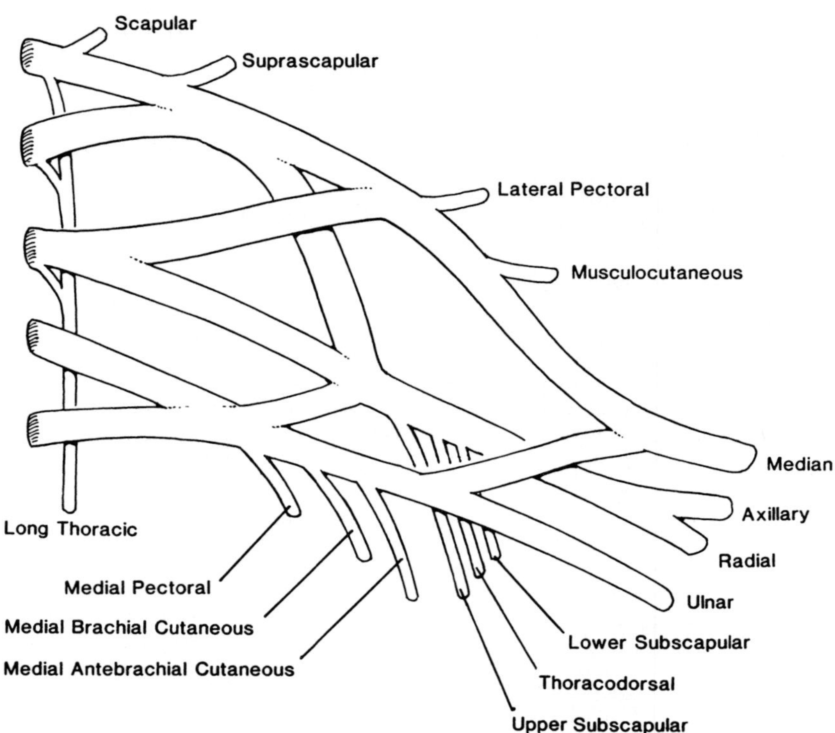

FIGURE 47–3. The brachial plexus. Ventral branches of the spinal nerves from C5 through T1 intermingle to form the peripheral nerves of the upper limb. (From Buschbacher RM: Basic tissue organization and function. In Buschbacher RM (ed): Musculoskeletal Disorders: A Practical Guide for Diagnosis and Rehabilitation. Stoneham, MA, Butterworth-Heinemann, 1994, p 18.)

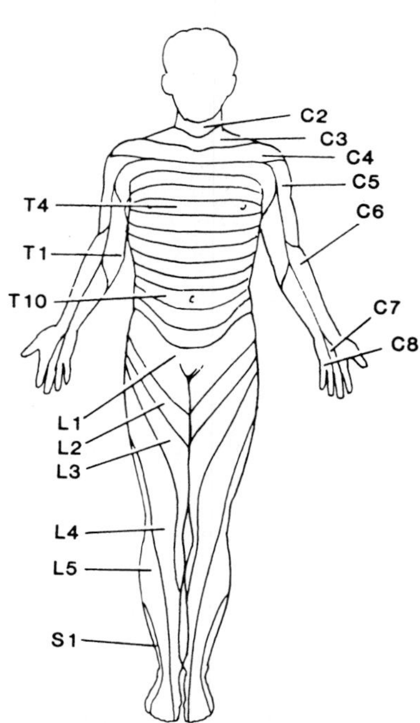

FIGURE 47–4. Dermatomal innervation pattern of the spinal nerves. Each spinal nerve goes on to provide sensation to a band of skin. This is done through a variety of peripheral nerves and is remarkably constant. (From Buschbacher RM: The musculoskeletal examination. In Buschbacher RM (ed): Musculoskeletal Disorders: A Practical Guide for Diagnosis and Rehabilitation. Stoneham, MA, Butterworth-Heinemann, 1994, p 88.)

TABLE 47–1 Common Spinal Nerve Level and Peripheral Nerve Innervation Patterns of Common Muscle Groups

	Major Cranial Nerve (CN) or Spinal Nerve Level	Peripheral Nerve
Upper Extremity		
Shoulder muscles		
Elevators	CN XI, C4, C5	Spinal accessory nerve; posterior branches of spinal nerves
Protractors	C5–C7	Long thoracic nerve; pectoral nerves
Retractors	C5–C8	Dorsal scapular nerve; spinal accessory nerve; thoracodorsal nerve
Upward rotators	CN XI, C5, C6	Long thoracic nerve; spinal accessory nerve
Downward rotators	C6–C8	Thoracodorsal nerve; pectoral nerves
Abductors	C5, C6	Axillary and suprascapular nerves
Extensors	C6–C8	Thoracodorsal, axillary, and pectoral nerves
Flexors	C5, C6	Axillary, musculocutaneous, and pectoral nerves
Internal rotators	C5, C6	Pectoral nerves; thoracodorsal and subscapular nerves
External rotators	C5, C6	Axillary and suprascapular nerves
Elbow flexors	C5, C6	Musculocutaneous nerve
Elbow extensors	C7	Radial nerve
Wrist extensors	C6, C7	Radial nerve
Wrist flexors	C7, C8	Median and ulnar nerves
Finger extensors	C7	Radial nerve
Finger flexors	C7, C8	Median and ulnar nerves
Intrinsic hand muscles	T1	Ulnar and median (thumb) nerves
Trunk and Back		
Abdominal muscles	T7-T12	Segmental innervation
Back muscles	C2–C5	Segmental innervation
Lower Extremity		
Hip flexors	T12, L1, L2	Lumbosacral plexus
Hip extensors	L5, S1, S2	Inferior gluteal nerve
Hip abductors	L4, L5, S1	Superior gluteal nerve
Hip adductors	L2–L4	Obturator nerve
Knee flexors	L5, S1	Sciatic nerve
Knee extensors	L2–L4	Femoral nerve
Foot dorsiflexors	L4, L5	Deep peroneal nerves
Foot plantarflexors	S1	Tibial nerve
Foot inverters	L4	Deep peroneal and tibial nerves
Foot everters	L5, S1	Superficial peroneal nerve

Modified from Buschbacher RM: Musculoskeletal Disorders: A Practical Guide for Diagnosis and Rehabilitation. Stoneham, MA, Butterworth-Heinemann, 1994, p 87.

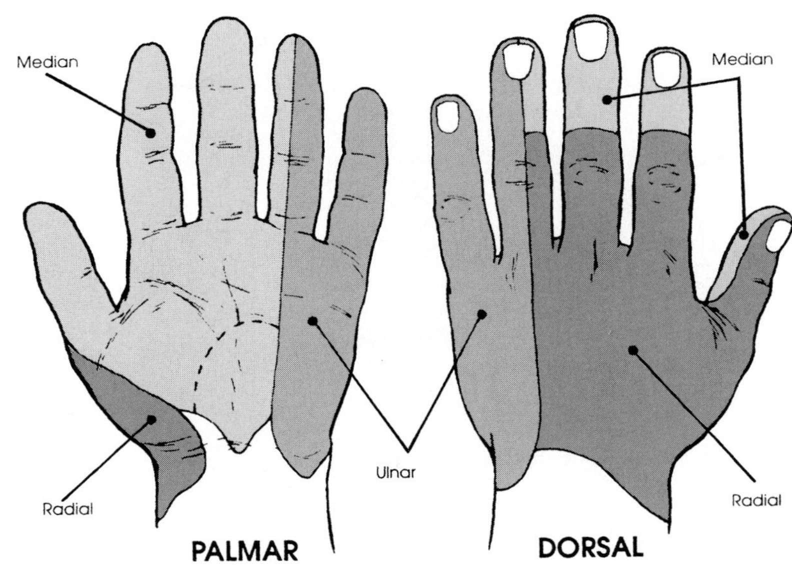

FIGURE 47–5. A sample of peripheral nerve patterns of innervation from the hand. Although overlap can occur with the dermatomal pattern, knowledge of both systems helps the examiner to distinguish spinal from peripheral nerve pathological features. (From McNeil BE, Buschbacher RM: Wrist and hand. In Buschbacher RM (ed): Musculoskeletal Disorders: A Practical Guide for Diagnosis and Rehabilitation. Stoneham, MA, Butterworth-Heinemann, 1994, p 175.)

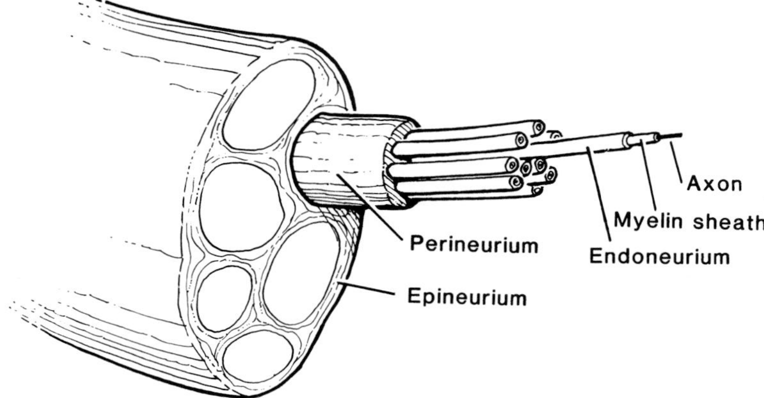

FIGURE 47–6. The internal anatomy of a nerve. The surrounding structure is called the epineurium. Internally, the nerve fibers are arranged in bundles, or fasciculi, surrounded by a perineurium. Each individual nerve fiber is enveloped by a sheath of myelin and an endoneurium. (From Buschbacher RM: Basic tissue organization and function. In Buschbacher RM (ed): Musculoskeletal Disorders: A Practical Guide for Diagnosis and Rehabilitation. Stoneham, MA, Butterworth-Heinemann, 1994, p 17.)

ated fibers" and are reserved for functions that do not require rapid transmission through the body. Other axons are surrounded by individual sheaths of the Schwann cells (Fig. 47–7). These axons are more effectively insulated, and transmit impulses much more rapidly. Between individual Schwann cells are gaps known as the nodes of Ranvier. These nodes depolarize while the intervening myelinated segments tend not to, and allow the nerve impulse to "jump" from one node to another in what is called saltatory propagation. Such propagation allows fast impulse transmission with minimal energy expenditure. These axons, which carry information that must be rapidly disseminated, are commonly called "myelinated fibers."

The fibers that must transmit impulses rapidly are, in general, larger in diameter, since larger fibers have less electrical resistance. There is a wide array of fibers of varying diameters and degrees of myelination. Larger fibers tend to be myelinated. Table 47–2 is a common classification scheme for all nerve fibers. Table 47–3 is an alternative classification system for sensory fibers only. Both classification schemes are in widespread use.

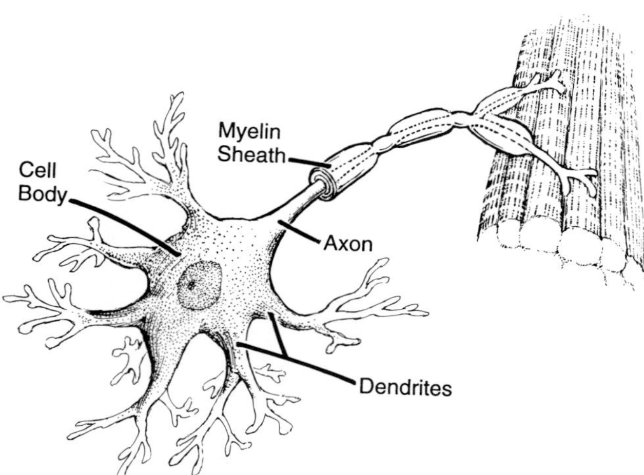

FIGURE 47–7. Schematic representation of a motor nerve from a cell body to the muscle it innervates. The nerve fiber is surrounded by myelin from the Schwann cells. (From Buschbacher RM: Basic tissue organization and function. In Buschbacher RM (ed): Musculoskeletal Disorders: A Practical Guide for Diagnosis and Rehabilitation. Stoneham, MA, Butterworth-Heinemann, 1994, p 16.)

TYPES OF NEUROPATHY

Peripheral neuropathies are divided into two major categories, demyelination and axonopathy, depending on whether they primarily affect the axon or the myelin sheath.[55] *Demyelination* occurs when the myelin sheath is disturbed. Guillain-Barré syndrome (GBS) and Dejerine-Sottas syndrome are examples of diseases that predominantly cause demyelination. The interruption of the myelin sheath causes a slowing in nerve conduction. This slowing can be localized (as in a focal neuropathy like carpal tunnel syndrome) or generalized (as in GBS).

Axonopathy can be caused by toxic or metabolic derangements, by trauma, compression, traction, or by transection. If the damage is severe enough to block nerve conduction, nerve conduction studies show a decrease in amplitude of the resulting motor unit action potential (MUAP) (see Chapter 10).

CLASSIFICATION SYSTEMS

Localized nerve injuries can be classified by degree of severity. There are two main classification schemes: the Seddon system[81] and the Sunderland system[86] (Table 47–4). The Sunderland system is an expansion on Seddon's divisions. Both are in common usage.

Seddon's Classification

Seddon proposed categorizing localized nerve injury into three divisions: (1) neurapraxia, (2) axonotmesis, and (3) neurotmesis.[81]

Neurapraxia. Neurapraxia is due to localized damage to the nerve that does not cause axonal death. It is often caused by nerve compression. It is characterized

TABLE 47–2 Nerve Fiber Types in Mammalian Nerve

Fiber Type	Function	Fiber Diameter (μm)	Conduction Velocity (m/sec)	Spike Duration (ms)	Absolute Refractory Period (ms)
A					
α	Proprioception; somatic motor	12–20	70–120		
β	Touch, pressure	5–12	30–70	0.4–0.5	0.4–1.4
γ	Motor to muscle spindles	3–6	15–30		
δ	Pain, temperature, touch	2–5	12–30		
B	Preganglionic autonomic	<3	3–15	1.2	1.2
C					
Dorsal root	Pain, reflex responses	0.4–1.2	0.5–2.5	2	2
Sympathetic	Postganglionic sympathetics	0.3–1.3	0.7–2.3	2	2

From Ganong WF: Review of Medical Physiology, ed 13. East Norwalk, CT, Appleton & Lange, 1987.

clinically by decreased vibratory and proprioceptive sensation and occasionally by decreased touch. Pain perception is seldom affected. Motor loss and paresthesias commonly result from neurapraxia. In neurapraxia impulse conduction is interrupted across the site of injury, but the damage is not severe enough to cause axonal death and Wallerian degeneration. In mild cases, as when a leg "falls asleep," the neurapraxia is most likely due to transient ischemia.[59, 71] In more severe cases such as "Saturday night palsy," there can be a compression injury to the myelin.[66] This causes a localized conduction block, but as the myelin recovers, the conduction across the affected segment is restored. Such recovery of motor and sensory function can take from a few seconds to six months.[81]

Axonotmesis. Axonotmesis is an injury of the axon that causes axonal death and subsequent Wallerian degeneration distal to the site of injury. The epineurium, perineurium, endoneurium, and Schwann cells remain intact. In Seddon's study,[81] these injuries most often occurred secondary to closed fractures or dislocations. Compressive injuries caused 18% of the axonotmetic injuries. Sensory, motor, and sudomotor function are all affected. The time course and completeness of recovery depend on the location of the injury and the age and condition of the patient. In general, axons regenerate at a rate of approximately 1.5 to 2.00 mm/day.[16] The more proximal the insult, the longer it takes to recover distal function. If the recovery is delayed excessively, the tract (endoneurial sheath) into which the axon regrows can deteriorate permanently and recovery may never be complete.[86] Nerve recovery is faster in younger patients and is slower in patients with metabolic conditions such as diabetes mellitus.

Neurotmesis. This most severe injury in Seddon's classification is a complete nerve transection involving the axon as well as the supportive structures, although on gross inspection the nerve can appear intact. These injuries have a poor prognosis, as axonal regrowth is problematic due to discontinuity of the neural tube. Neuroma formation is common and surgical excision of the damaged segment with reanastomosis can be indicated.

Sunderland's Classification

Sunderland expanded on Seddon's initial work and described five degrees of injury.[86] The third- through fifth-degree injuries are basically subcategories of Seddon's neurotmesis.

First-Degree Injury. First-degree injury is a focal conduction block in which the axon remains intact. This is essentially the same as neurapraxia.

TABLE 47–3 Numerical Classification Sometimes Used for Sensory Neurons

No.	Origin	Fiber Type
I		
a	Muscle spindle, annulospiral ending	Aα
b	Golgi tendon organ	Aα
II	Muscle spindle, flower-spray ending; touch, pressure	Aβ
III	Pain and temperature receptors; some touch receptors	Aδ
IV	Pain and other receptors	Dorsal root C

From Ganong WF: Review of Medical Physiology, ed 13. East Norwalk, CT, Appleton & Lange, 1987.

TABLE 47–4 The Seddon and Sunderland Classification Systems

Seddon[81]	Sunderland[86]	Description
Neurapraxia	First-degree injury	Focal conduction block; axons remain intact
Axonotmesis	Second-degree injury	Axonal damage and Wallerian degeneration; intact supporting structures
Neurotmesis	Third-degree injury	Interruption of axon and endoneurium
	Fourth-degree injury	Interruption of perineurium and endoneurium
	Fifth-degree injury	All supporting structures and axon damaged

TABLE 47–5 Hereditary Peripheral Neuropathies

Charcot-Marie-Tooth disease (hereditary motorsensory neuropathy [HMSN] types I and II)
Dejerine-Sottas disease (HMSN type III)
Refsum's disease (HMSN type IV)
Neuropathies associated with
Spinocerebellar degeneration (HMSN type V)
Optic atrophy (HMSN type VI)
Retinitis pigmentosa (HMSN type VII)
Friedreich's ataxia
Pressure-sensitive hereditary neuropathy
Acute intermittent porphyria
Familial amyloid neuropathy
Fabry's disease
Hereditary sensory neuropathy
Giant axonal neuropathies
Lipoprotein neuropathies
Roussy-Lévy syndrome
Riley-Day syndrome
Pelizaeus-Merzbacher disease
Metachromatic leukodystrophy
Krabbe's leukodystrophy
Tangier disease

TABLE 47–6 Toxic Peripheral Neuropathies

Drugs	*Heavy Metals*
Amiodarone	Antimony
Chloramphenicol	Arsenic
Corticosteroids	Gold
Dapsone	Lead
Diphenylhydantoin	Mercury
Disulfiram	Thallium
Halogenated hydroxyquinolones	***Organic Compounds***
Heroin	Acrylamide
Hydralazine	Carbon disulfide
Isoniazid	Dichlorophenoxyacetic acid
Lysergide (LSD)	Ethyl alcohol
Misonidazole	Ethylene oxide
Nitrofurantoin	Methyl butyl ketone
Pyridoxine	Triorthocresyl phosphate
Sodium cyanate	
Tetanus toxoid	
Thalidomide	

Second-Degree Injury. As in Seddon's axonotmesis, the axon in a second-degree injury is damaged with subsequent distal Wallerian degeneration. The supportive structures of the nerve, including the endoneurium, remain intact. The prognosis for nerve recovery is good since the nerve can grow down its original endoneurial tube.

Third-Degree Injury. In third-degree injury the axon and the endoneurium are both disrupted. The perineurium remains intact, but within the fascicle there is hemorrhage, edema, and subsequent fibrosis. The axon tips do not always follow their original pathway, but can grow into the distal endoneurial tubes randomly. Fibrosis can block their regrowth entirely. In general, the more proximal the level of injury, the less the likelihood of normal reinnervation's reaching the end-organ. The functional outcome of regrowth (rerouting) depends to some extent on whether the fibers within the fascicles share a similar common function. For example, a motor nerve is nonfunctional if it grows down to a sensory end-organ. As a rule, recovery is less complete than in second-degree injuries.

When axons regrow into different endoneurial tubes, they reach different end-organs. This process results in aberrant innervation[87] and can cause synkinesis. An example of this can occur in Bell's palsy wherein cranial nerve VII fibers, which previously innervated the salivary glands, can be rerouted to the tear glands, causing the salivating patient to experience "crocodile tears."[88] Similarly, proximal brachial plexus injury can cause fibers from the phrenic nerve to be rerouted so that during respiration the arm muscles contract.[87]

Fourth-Degree Injury. Both the perineurium and endoneurium as well as the axon are damaged in a fourth-degree injury. This allows recovering axons to sprout outside of their fascicles, which can lead to neuroma formation. Surgery is usually required to remove the damaged segment and reattach the healthy ends.

Fifth-Degree Injury. All supporting structures as well as the axon are damaged in a fifth-degree injury. Recovery depends on the mechanism of injury. Nerve lacerations can be treated with surgery and the outcome can be good, whereas injuries from stretch or compression have a poorer prognosis.

ETIOLOGY OF NEUROPATHY

There is a wide array of neuropathic disorders, which are usually categorized by etiology. These etiologies include hereditary (Table 47–5), toxic (Table 47–6; Fig. 47–8), those associated with diseases and inflammatory processes (Table 47–7), idiopathic (Table 47–8), entrapment (Table 47–9), nutritional (Table 47–10), and those secondary to infectious processes (Table 47–11; Figs. 47–9 and 47–10).

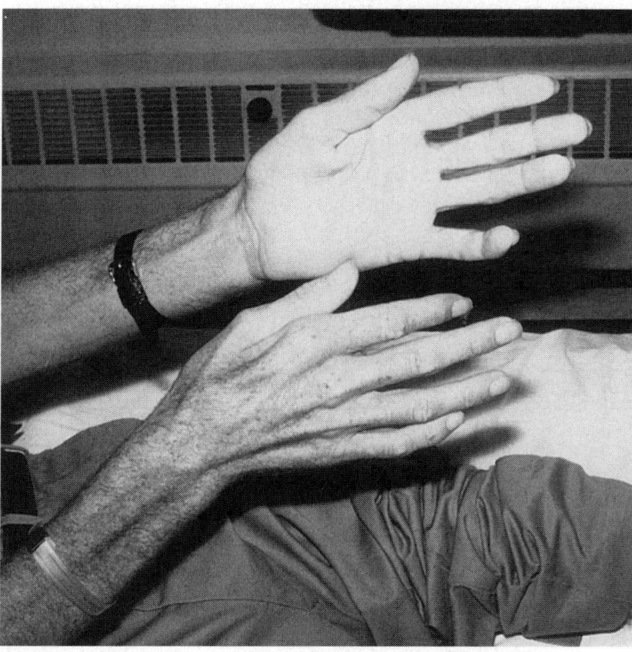

FIGURE 47–8. Hands of patient with arsenic peripheral neuropathy.

TABLE 47–7 Diseases Associated with Peripheral Neuropathy

Alcoholism
Amyloidosis
Benign monoclonal gammopathy (IgG, IgA, IgM)
Chronic liver disease
Chronic obstructive pulmonary disease
Cryoglobulinemia
Diabetes mellitus
  Distal symmetrical neuropathy
  Autonomic neuropathy
  Proximal asymmetrical painful motor neuropathy
  Cranial mononeuropathies
Giant cell arteritis
Gout
Hypothyroidism
Necrotizing angiopathy
Neuropathies in malignant diseases
  Lymphomas—focal and systemic
  Multiple myeloma
  Bronchogenic carcinoma
  Tumors of the ovary, testes, penis, stomach, or oral cavity
  Meningeal carcinomatosis
  Oat cell carcinoma
  Osteosclerotic myeloma
  Vasculitis/connective tissue disease

TABLE 47–9 Common Peripheral Nerve Injury and Entrapment Syndromes

Nerve	Entrapment
Radial nerve	At the radial groove of the humerus (Saturday night palsy) Posterior interosseous nerve syndrome
Ulnar nerve	At the olecranon groove Tardy ulnar palsy Cubital tunnel syndrome Injury at the wrist (can be at the canal of Guyon)
Median nerve	At the supracondylar ligament of Struthers (at elbow) Pronator teres syndrome Carpal tunnel syndrome Anterior interosseous syndrome
Sciatic nerve	Injection palsy—injury to lateral division Injury to medial division
Femoral nerve	Above or below the inguinal ligament
Peroneal nerve	At head of fibula
Tibial nerve	Tarsal tunnel syndrome

The inherited neuropathies have increasingly been linked to specific chromosomal abnormalities,[56, 60, 64, 69, 70, 74, 96, 101, 106] which are summarized in Table 47–12. The most common causes of diffuse peripheral neuropathy seen in the developed world are diabetes and alcoholism. Worldwide, however, the primary cause is leprosy. In up to one-third of cases a specific cause for peripheral neuropathy cannot be identified.[104]

While classification systems allow for a labeling framework, they do little to help diagnose and treat individual patients. A diagnostic algorithm is presented in Figure 47–11. What follows is a more practical clinical approach.

Evaluation of the Patient with Peripheral Neuropathy

History

As with any disease process, the physician must take a careful history to assess the patient with peripheral neuropathy. Was the onset sudden or gradual? Is the progression rapid or slow? Is there sensory or motor involvement, or both? Is the primary involvement distal or proximal, symmetrical or asymmetrical, focal or generalized? Is there pain or autonomic involvement? Does the patient have any associated diseases? An in-depth family and social history is useful, particularly if there have been familial occurrences or toxic exposures.[7]

Physical Examination

Sensory Examination

All sensory modalities should be tested, including pinprick, light touch, proprioception, vibration, graphesthesia, and temperature. If these are preserved, it is unlikely that a significant sensory deficit is present.

If sensory deficits are detected, the extent and pattern of the loss should be determined. This can help to chart the progression of the disease, and can assist in identifying patients who need to be counseled about protecting insensate or dysesthetic skin.

Motor Examination

Normal patients vary widely in their strength, owing both to variations in their absolute muscle mass and to varying motivation, understanding, and cooperation. Pain can also prevent a patient from exerting full muscle force (pain inhibition of function). Muscle strength should be graded by the make-and-break system and

TABLE 47–8 Idiopathic Neuropathies

Brachial neuritis (Parsonage-Turner syndrome)
Chronic inflammatory polyradiculopathy
Chronic relapsing polyneuropathy
Fisher syndrome
Acute inflammatory demyelinating polyradiculoneuropathy (Guillain-Barré syndrome)
Steroid-responsive polyneuropathy
Multifocal motor neuropathy

TABLE 47–10 Nutritional Neuropathies

Beriberi or pellagra—thiamine (vitamin B_1) deficiency
Riboflavin (vitamin B_2) deficiency
Pyridoxine (vitamin B_6) deficiency
Pernicious anemia (vitamin B_{12} deficiency)
Protein or calorie deficiency in children

TABLE 47–11 Infectious Causes of Peripheral Neuropathy

Cytomegalovirus in human immunodeficiency virus (HIV) infection
Diphtheria
Herpes zoster
Leprosy
Rabies

with functional tests of multiple muscles and muscle groups (see Chapter 1).

Reflex Testing

Muscle stretch reflex (MSR) testing, also known as deep tendon reflex (DTR) testing, causes a rapid stretch of the muscle that activates the muscle spindle fibers and generates a reflex contraction. This gives an indication of the state of the afferent and efferent fibers to the muscle as well as the local spinal cord level and descending central nervous system (CNS) control (see Chapter 1). In peripheral neuropathy the MSRs are usually depressed, especially distally. The patient must be relaxed, as an overly tense muscle will not respond to a tendon tap. Patients with bulky muscles can appear not to have reflexes because the heavy tendons and muscles are not stretched adequately by the usual hammer-strike technique. For these patients a heavier hammer should be used.

When the reflex is difficult to elicit, a facilitation technique should be used. Jendrassik's maneuver has the patient interlock the fingers and pull against them. This distracts the patient and removes suprasegmental inhibitory influences on the reflex. Other distracting techniques such as clenching the teeth or squeezing the eyelids can also be effective. The Queen's square hammer is heavier and can elicit reflexes that are, at times, not obtainable with the usual "hatchet"-style hammers. Reflexes are graded on a scale from 0 to 4+.

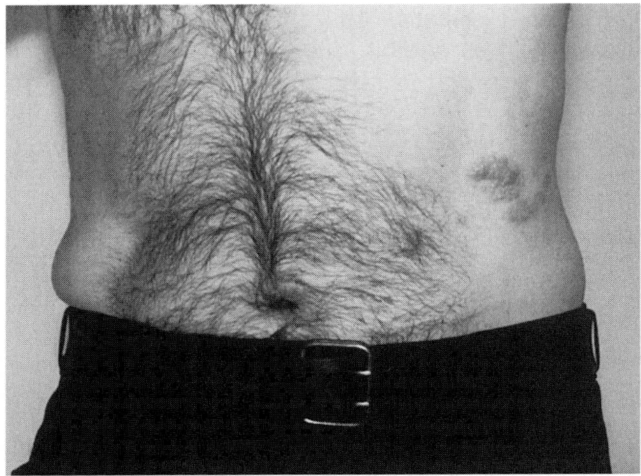

FIGURE 47–9. Patient with acute shingles (herpes zoster).

Superficial skin reflexes can also be evaluated. They are elicited by stroking the skin rather than striking a tendon. They include such normal reflexes as the abdominal and cremasteric reflexes. The presence of Babinski's, Hoffmann's, palmomental, grasp, suck, or glabellar reflex is usually considered abnormal in an adult. Abnormal superficial reflexes are usually signs of upper motor neuron disorders and are typically not present in peripheral neuropathy. Their presence can help differentiate a central from a peripheral condition.

Electrodiagnostic Examination in Peripheral Neuropathy

Nerve Conduction Studies

Nerve conduction studies (NCS) are the most helpful part of the electrodiagnostic examination for peripheral

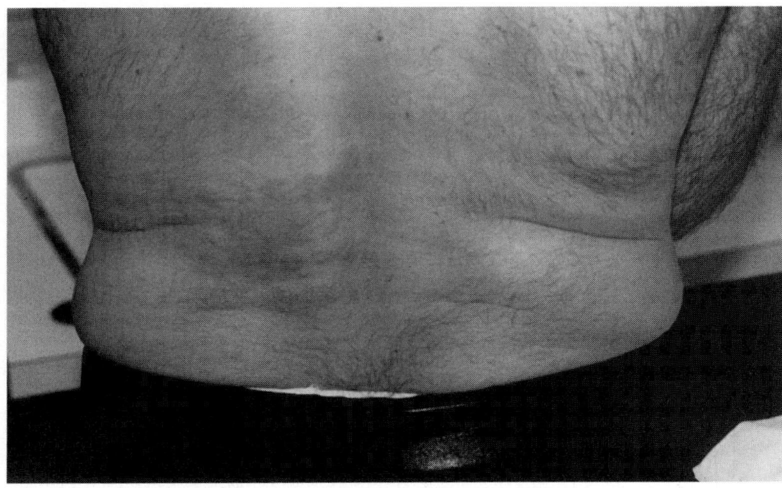

FIGURE 47–10. Patient with acute shingles (herpes zoster).

TABLE 47–12 Classification of Inherited Neuropathies

(1) Neuropathies in which the neuropathy is the sole or primary part of the disease	
Hereditary motor and sensory neuropathy (HMSN) [Charcot-Marie-Tooth disease (CMT)]	
HMSN I (CMT 1)	
HMSN IA (CMT 1A)	Duplication PMP-22; mutations PMP-22
HMSN IB (CMT 1B)	Mutations PO
HMSN IC	Location not known
X-linked (CMT X1)	Mutations connexin-32
X-linked (CMT X2)	Location unknown
Autosomal recessive	(see under CMT 4)
HMSN II (CMT 2)	
HMSN IIA (CMT 2A)	Locus on 1p35–p36
HMSN IIB (CMT 2B)	Locus on 3q13–q22
HMSN IIC (CMT 2C)	Location unknown
HMSN IID (CMT 2D)	Locus on 7p14
Autosomal dominant	Location unknown
Autosomal recessive	(see under CMT 4)
HMSN III (Dejerine-Sottas disease [DSD])	
DSD A	Mutations PMP-22
DSD B	Mutations PO
Autosomal dominant DSD	Locus on 8q23–q24
Autosomal recessive	Location unknown
CMT 4 (Autosomal recessive CMT)	
CMT 4A (demyelinating, basal lamina onion bulbs)	Locus on 8q13–21.1
CMT 4B (demyelinating, focally folded myelin sheaths)	Locus on 11q23.1
CMT 4C (normal motor conduction, no myelin changes)	Location unknown
CMT (demyelinating)	Locus on 5q23–q33
HMSNL (demyelinating, deafness, Balkan Gypsies)	Locus on 8q24
Complex forms of HMSN	Location unknown
Hereditary neuropathy with liability to pressure palsies (HNPP)	
HNPP	Deletion PMP-22; point mutations PMP-22; location unknown
Familial amyloid polyneuropathies (FAP)	
TTR-related FAP	Mutations transthyretin
Apolipoprotein A1-related FAP	Mutations apolipo protein A1
Gelsolin-related FAP	Mutations gelsolin
Hereditary sensory and autonomic neuropathies (HSAN)	
HSAN I (dominant sensory neuropathy)	Locus on 9q22.1–q22.3
HSAN II (recessive sensory neuropathy)	Location unknown
HSAN III (Riley-Day syndrome, familial dysautonomia)	Locus on 9q31–33
HSAN IV (congenital sensory neuropathy with anhidrosis)	Mutations TRKA gene
HSAN V (sensory neuropathy with loss of small myelinated fibers)	Location unknown
Hereditary motor neuronopathies (spinal muscle atrophy)	
X-linked bulbospinal neuronopathy	
(2) Neuropathies in which the neuropathy is part of a more widespread neurological or multisystem disorder	
Disturbance of lipid metabolism	
Leukodystrophies	
Metachromatic	
Globoid cell (Krabbe)	
Adrenoleukomyeloneuropathy	
Lipoprotein deficiences	
Alphalipoprotein deficiency (Tangier disease)	
Abetalipoproteinaemia (Bassen-Kornzweig disease)	
Phytanic acid storage diseases	
Classic Refsum disease	
Infantile Refsum disease	
Alpha-Galactosidase deficiency (Fabry disease)	
Cholestanolosis	
Spingomyelin lipidoses	
Porphyrias	
Acute intermittent	
Variegate	
Hereditary coproporphyria	
Ala dehydratase deficiency	
Disorders with defective DNA repair	
Xeroderma pigmentosum	
Ataxia telangiectasia	
Cockayne syndrome	
Neuropathies associated with defects of the mitochondrial respiratory chain and/or mitochondrial DNA	
Neuropathy in hereditary ataxias	
Spinocerebellar ataxias	
Friedreich's ataxia	
Miscellaneous, including	
Brachial plexus neuropathy	
Giant axonal neuropathy	
Neuroacanthocytosis	
Chediak-Higashi disease	

From Reilly MM: Genetically determined neuropathies. J Neurol 1998; 245:6–13.

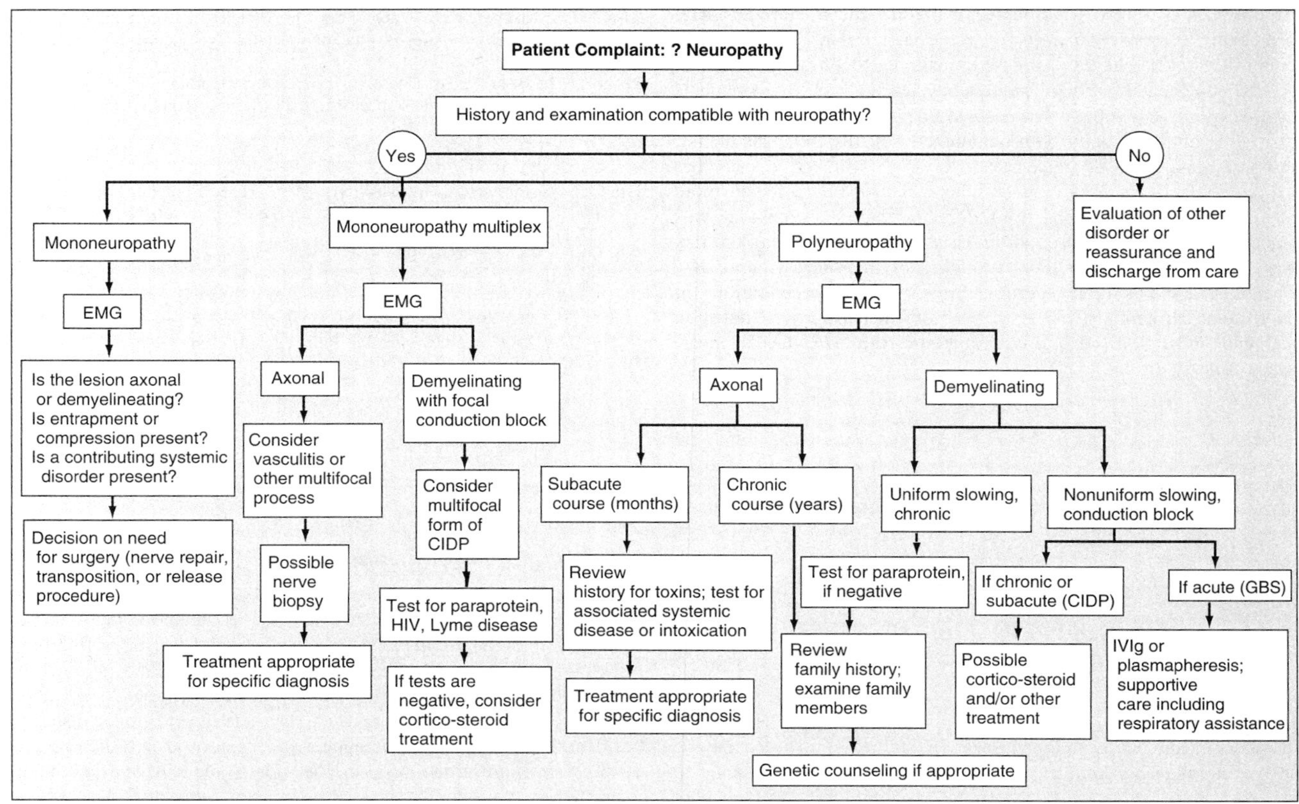

FIGURE 47–11. Diagnostic algorithm for neuropathies.

nerve disorders (Table 47–13). These studies determine the conduction velocity of the nerve as well as the amplitude of the propagated electrical waveform. In motor nerves, the NCS also provide distal latency information.[56] Both motor and sensory nerves can be evaluated by NCS.

The insulating layer of myelin can be impaired through thinning of the myelin sheath or through deterioration of the internodal segments.[55] When the internode is damaged, the electrical current "leaks," delaying depolarization. The time required for the next node to reach threshold is increased. This causes an overall slowing in the nerve conduction velocity as well as changes in other NCS parameters.

In severe demyelination the impulse can fail to excite the subsequent node, resulting in a conduction block. The conduction velocity is typically moderately to severely slowed, and the distal latency is prolonged, while the amplitude of the evoked responses is relatively preserved. These waveforms usually display a temporal dispersion. If conduction block is present in some fibers of a nerve, the amplitude of the evoked response is reduced (see Chapters 10, 11, and 12).

In diseases where axonal degeneration predominates, the conduction velocity generally remains normal or only slightly decreased. If the larger (faster) nerve fibers are predominantly involved, there can be more significant slowing. More typical of axonopathy, however, is

TABLE 47–13 Typical Electrodiagnostic Findings in the General Categories of Neuropathy*

Type	Motor Nerve Conduction Velocities	Amplitude of CMAP	Amplitude of Sensory Action Potential	EMG Findings
Hereditary	↓	NL/↓	↓	Usually denervation potentials
Toxic	NL/↓	NL/↓	NL/↓	Usually denervation potentials
Associated with disease	↓	↓	↓	Usually denervation potentials
Idiopathic	↓	↓	↓	Variable
Entrapment	↓	NL/↓	NL/↓	Variable; usually NL
Infectious	NL/slight ↓	Slight ↓	↓	Denervation potentials
Nutritional	↓	Slight ↓	↓	Denervation potentials

* Exceptions are common.
Abbreviations: CMAP, compound motor action potential; EMG, electromyography; NL, within normal limits.

a reduction in amplitude of the evoked responses. This is due to the fact that as some of the fibers die, they no longer contribute to the amplitude of these responses.[52] This is especially true when recording directly from nerves. When recording from the muscles, the remaining (fewer) axons can continue to innervate a constant number of muscle fibers (through reinnervation) and the evoked muscle response can be maintained well into the disease process. Temporal dispersion is usually minimal until well into the disease process.

Many peripheral neuropathies involve a component of both axonal degeneration and demyelination, and the resultant findings on nerve conduction studies suggest a mixed picture. There is slowed conduction and temporal dispersion, as well as decreased amplitude of the recorded responses (see Chapters 10, 11, and 12).

Electromyography

The electromyograph (EMG) needle records the electrical activity of muscle fibers. Since denervated muscle fibers display characteristic abnormalities in the needle examination (see Table 47–14), this part of the examination is useful in determining the extent of such loss and in localizing the nerve lesions. It can also aid in determining the time course of the disease to some extent, as it helps in analyzing the process of reinnervation. It is less useful in evaluating purely demyelinating lesions, as the muscle fibers retain their innervation in these disorders (see Chapter 11).

In mild peripheral neuropathy the EMG findings are generally minimal. The most affected muscles (usually distal ones) show the most obvious EMG findings. In mildly affected muscles the changes include increased polyphasicity of the MUAPs. In more severe neuropathies there is muscle membrane instability. As reinnervation progresses, polyphasic motor units of prolonged duration and high amplitude are seen. Demyelination typically causes little abnormal muscle membrane irritability, and fibrillation potentials and positive sharp waves are only occasionally seen[55] (see Chapters 10, 11, and 12).

COMMON COMPLICATIONS OF PERIPHERAL NEUROPATHY

Muscle weakness, sensory loss, and autonomic problems occur commonly in patients with peripheral neuropathies. Muscle weakness can lead to joint contractures and muscle shortening. Sensory loss can result in more frequent and severe injuries to insensate areas. Autonomic problems can affect many functions, including heart rate, blood pressure, and sweating, and can cause gastroparesis, neurogenic bladder, and impotence. Patients with peripheral neuropathy often complain of pain.

Muscle Weakness

Joint contractures and muscle shortening are associated with muscle weakness. They can be prevented with daily range-of-motion (ROM) and muscle-stretching exercises. Depending on the degree of weakness, this exercise can be passive, active-assistive, or active. When in bed or at rest, proper positioning is essential, as is splinting (if needed).

A program of gentle strengthening, which can include isometric, isotonic, isokinetic, manual-resistive, and progressive-resistive exercise, should be carefully tailored to the patient (see Chapter 19). While improvement of strength is desirable, the muscles should not be overworked, as this can result in paradoxical weakening (overwork weakness).[9, 44] Orthoses should be appropriately prescribed for the patient to increase function and aid in positioning. In the patient who is at bed rest or cognitively compromised, careful positioning is indicated to prevent injury to the peripheral nerves. Peripheral nerves can be compressed between bony prominences and the bed. Injury to the ulnar nerve at the elbow and compression of the common peroneal nerve at the head of the fibula are the injuries most commonly seen.

Sensory Loss

When protective sensation is compromised, patients should carefully examine the anesthetic or dysesthetic areas daily. Because they are the most distal body part, the feet are most commonly affected by loss of sensation in neuropathy. The patient can traumatize the skin and cause skin breakdown and ulceration. Repetitive joint trauma can lead to the development of neuroarthropathic (Charcot's) joints. In either case the prescription of extra-depth or custom-molded shoes might be indicated. A shoe insert helps to prevent foot trauma and ulcers.

In addition to careful daily skin examination, the patient should be instructed in thorough, gentle cleaning and soaking techniques. This should be followed by the application of a lubricant to help the foot resist fissuring and scaling. Such preventive care is much easier than treating a skin breakdown. Patients should be sure to rest and protect their skin at the earliest sign of trauma. Waiting too long to treat can lead to irreversible sequelae, which can ultimately result in amputation.

Autonomic Dysfunction

Autonomic problems are seen in a variety of peripheral neuropathies, but are perhaps most commonly associated with diabetes mellitus and Guillain-Barré syndrome. Cardiovascular symptoms can include orthostatic intolerance or cardiac arrhythmias. Genitourinary symptoms include a flaccid bladder and male impotence. Gastrointestinal symptoms can include vomiting, dysphagia, diarrhea, constipation, and many other problems.[105] Sweating abnormalities are seen with autonomic involvement as well.

The autonomic dysfunction in GBS can be life-threatening. These patients should have cardiac monitoring with close observation for dysrhythmias and postural hypotension in the early phases of their disease.

Pain

Pain is a common problem in peripheral neuropathy, and it can be difficult to treat. In addition to analgesics,

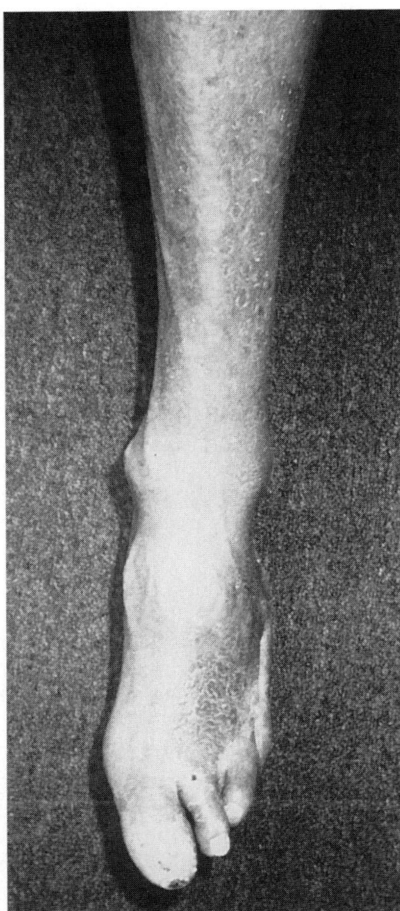

FIGURE 47–12. Typical appearance of a foot with changes of diabetic peripheral neuropathy and peripheral vascular disease.

which are often ineffective, the first line of treatment for neuropathic pain includes tricyclic antidepressants, starting at a low dose. The side effects of these drugs include orthostatic hypotension and worsening of urinary retention. Trazodone can be tried in patients who do not tolerate the tricyclics. The second line of treatment can include carbamazepine or gabapentin. If this does not control the pain, a third line of treatment including phenytoin and mexiletine can be instituted. Topical capsaicin can also be beneficial in some patients and transcutaneous electrical nerve stimulation (TENS) can be added as well.[7, 61, 62, 76, 77, 102] Often a multiple drug regimen is needed to control pain; care should be taken to avoid drug interactions.[99]

REHABILITATION MANAGEMENT OF THE MORE COMMON PERIPHERAL NEUROPATHIES

The following is a discussion of the rehabilitation management of several representative disorders. This list is not all-inclusive, but the principles described can readily be adapted to other, similar disorders.

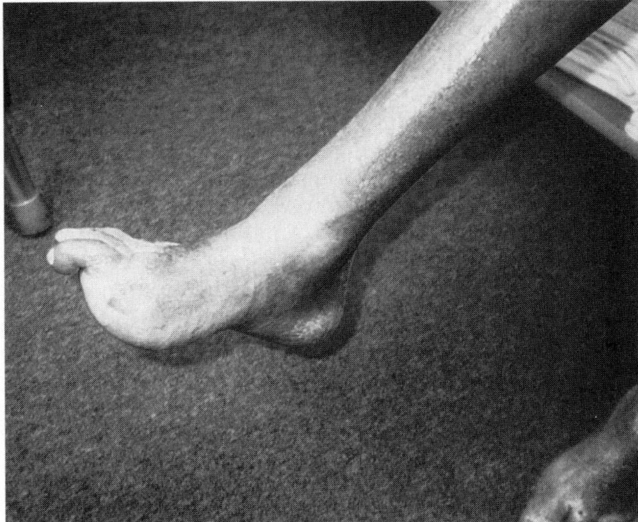

FIGURE 47–13. Foot with changes of diabetic peripheral neuropathy and peripheral vascular disease.

Diabetic Neuropathies

Both insulin-dependent (IDDM) and non–insulin-dependent diabetes mellitus (NIDDM) can cause neuropathies. These are subdivided into whether they are symmetrical or asymmetrical (Figs. 47–12 to 47–14). In the symmetrical group are polyneuropathies, including (1) a primarily sensory peripheral neuropathy, the most common of the diabetic neuropathies (acroneuropathy); (2) autonomic peripheral neuropathy, which is often seen in conjunction with the sensory form; (3) acute painful neuropathy; (4) subclinical neuropathy; and (5) proximal lower extremity motor neuropathy, also known by the less descriptive term *diabetic amyotrophy*.

The asymmetrical neuropathies include (1) neuropathy of individual nerves (mononeuropathy), (2) some painful neuropathies, (3) truncal neuropathy or radicu-

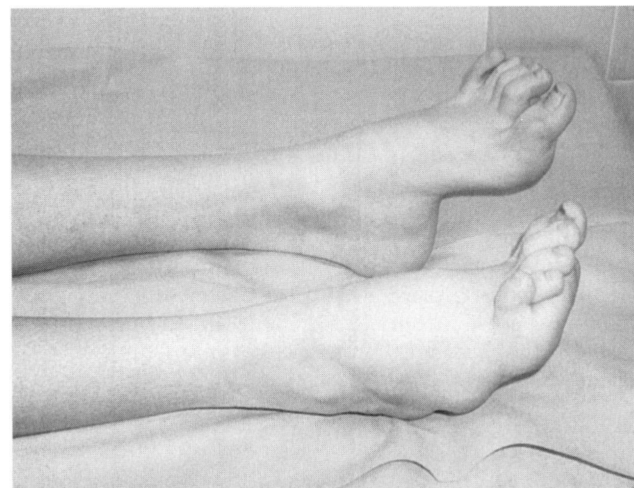

FIGURE 47–14. "Intrinsic minus" foot deformity in patient with diabetic peripheral neuropathy.

lopathy, and (4) entrapment neuropathies. Some cases of proximal lower extremity motor neuropathy are also asymmetrical.

It can easily be appreciated that these neuropathies might also be caused by other diseases, and every neuropathy in a diabetic patient should be separately evaluated and not automatically diagnosed as a diabetic neuropathy. Hyperglycemia in a newly diagnosed or poorly controlled diabetic can also cause a reduction in nerve conduction velocity. This is usually reversible.[91] Diabetes predisposes the patient to other neuropathies, especially focal neuropathies such as carpal tunnel syndrome.

Symmetrical Peripheral Neuropathy in Diabetes. The initial symptoms of diabetic symmetrical polyneuropathy are usually sensory. They include burning, itching, and a "pins-and-needles sensation." On physical examination the greatest abnormalities are in light touch and vibration, with preservation of conscious proprioception until late in the course. Patients complain of muscle cramping or tightness, especially at night. They also present with hypoesthesia or analgesia. Many patients have not noticed their "painless neuropathy" because of its gradual onset. The symptoms begin in the toes and progress proximally over the course of months to years. The longest nerves are affected first. Eventually the fingers and hands become involved, giving the typical stocking-and-glove distribution.[77]

Weakness is generally seen later in the course of diabetic complications. It starts distally and progresses proximally. A foot slap is a common result of this. Patients with diabetic polyneuropathy can also have an ataxic gait. This is due to abnormal proprioceptive sensation, which is involved typically only in the late stages of neuropathy.

If the diabetic patient with peripheral sensory impairment does not care for his or her affected areas meticulously, repeated trauma can result in skin ulceration, Charcot's joint, or even amputation.

Autonomic Peripheral Neuropathy. Autonomic symptoms are often seen together with sensory loss. They can involve various body functions including the cardiovascular, genitourinary, gastrointestinal, cutaneous,[2] and thermoregulatory systems. The primary cardiovascular abnormalities are orthostatic hypotension, cardiac arrhythmias, and impaired heart rate control.[45] The cause of the orthostatic hypotension is most likely an impaired vasoconstriction reflex.[45] Heart abnormalities include a resting tachycardia, fixed heart rate, and loss of sleep bradycardia.[27]

Gastrointestinal dysautonomia can manifest as esophageal dysmotility,[83] gastroparesis,[63] bowel incontinence,[80] and constipation or diarrhea.[79, 80]

Common genitourinary abnormalities are neurogenic bladder[51] and erectile dysfunction.[79] Diabetic impotence is common in the male and is usually irreversible.[29] The early signs of neurogenic bladder include decreased urinary frequency, followed by difficulties with initiating micturition. The bladder eventually becomes flaccid and urinary retention with overflow voiding occurs as the neuropathy worsens.[17, 28]

When the cutaneous system is also affected there can be impaired distal sweating. This often results in compensatory sweating of the trunk and face.[79]

Acute Painful Neuropathy. Acute painful diabetic neuropathy occurs rarely, and is characterized by severe pain in the distal lower extremities, described as a burning dysesthesia. It is often associated with depression, insomnia, and weight loss.[91] Examination reveals only a mild sensory loss, if any.[3] It is often referred to inappropriately as diabetic "neuritis."

Lower Extremity Proximal Motor Neuropathy. Lower extremity proximal motor neuropathy was earlier called "diabetic amyotrophy." It was initially described as being a unilateral proximal leg weakness.[93] Later, the term was used to describe bilateral leg weakness as well.[93] It was once thought that the cause of this disorder was a spinal cord lesion, but electrodiagnostic studies have shown that the dysfunction is in the proximal peripheral nerve (lumbosacral polyradiculopathy, plexus lesion, femoral neuropathy, or obturator nerve lesion).[93]

The onset of this neuropathy can be acute or subacute. The disorder is characterized by weakness of the quadriceps, iliopsoas, or thigh adductors, individually or in combination.[93] The gluteal muscles, hamstrings, and gastrocnemius can also be weak. Pain is often a prominent component of this problem and is worse at night.[93] The pain is described as severe, deep, and aching. Sensation is usually intact, but this disorder can coexist with a sensory neuropathy. Recovery occurs over a 12 to 24-month period and the prognosis for significant improvement is generally good.[93]

Mononeuropathy. Mononeuropathy, an asymmetrical form of diabetic peripheral neuropathy, can affect the cranial or peripheral nerves. The third cranial nerve is most commonly affected, although the abducens, trochlear, and facial nerves can be involved as well.[93] The pupil is usually spared in oculomotor palsy.[36] Multiple asymmetrical nerve involvements, referred to as mononeuropathy multiplex, can occur. In these cases, other causes of mononeuropathy multiplex (such as polyarteritis nodosa) have to be ruled out before attributing it to diabetes.

Truncal Neuropathy or Radiculopathy. Thoracoabdominal or truncal neuropathy or radiculopathy occurs most often in diabetic patients older than 50.[77] Onset can be acute or gradual. The distribution is usually unilateral, involving primarily T3 through T12.[84] The condition can be painful and includes a differential diagnosis of myocardial infarction, an intraspinal pathological process, abdominal disease, or malignancy.[77]

Entrapment Neuropathy. Persons with diabetes have long been thought to be at increased risk for entrapment neuropathies. Fraser et al[32] found no clear-cut relationship between the mononeuropathies and duration of diabetes, diabetic control, or the presence of other diabetic complications. Nevertheless, evidence seems to support the common belief that diabetes does indeed predispose to focal pressure neuropathies.[49, 91]

Electrodiagnostic Findings in Diabetic Neuropathy

In symmetrical peripheral sensory neuropathy nerve conduction, studies often show a mixed picture of an axonal and segmental demyelinating process.[93] Increased temporal dispersion of the sensory potential is one of the earliest signs of diabetic peripheral neuropathy.[93] The longest nerves are usually the first affected. They are slower distally than proximally. Sensory nerve amplitude is decreased and motor conduction velocity is slowed. Both axonal degeneration and segmental demyelination can occur. Single-fiber EMG studies indicate that the primary dysfunction is due to demyelination.[90] Moderate slowing occurs proximally and distally as determined by F-wave and other studies.[55]

Early needle examination reveals reduction in the number of MUAPs and only subtle changes of increased polyphasicity of the MUAP. There are few if any fibrillation potentials and the MUAP is close to normal in configuration, amplitude, and duration.[55] Later the needle EMG changes can be pronounced.

Lower extremity proximal motor neuropathy, thoracolumbar neuropathy, and acute painful diabetic neuropathy all have similar electrodiagnostic findings. Signs of muscle membrane instability (fibrillation potentials and positive sharp waves) are noted in the affected muscles or myotomes as well as in the paraspinal muscles. Nerve conduction studies are usually within normal limits unless there is concomitant peripheral sensory neuropathy.[3] Mononeuropathies are found most commonly in the peroneal nerve, with findings of slowed conduction in the segment of the nerve traversing the fibular head.[68] Other commonly affected nerves include the median and ulnar.[68] Kraft et al[56] found that approximately one half of diabetic patients have findings consistent with subclinical carpal tunnel syndrome.

Management of Diabetic Peripheral Neuropathy

Medical Management. The exact pathophysiology of diabetic neuropathy remains undetermined; therefore, no definitive treatment is available. Two current hypotheses are that the nerve injury is due to (1) metabolic or (2) ischemic processes.[14, 92] These processes are not mutually exclusive. Pathological studies provide evidence for ischemic microvascular disease,[92] while metabolic abnormalities include an accumulation of sorbitol and a reduction of myoinositol in the body.[34, 38] Because glucose is converted to sorbitol by aldose reductase, it was once thought that aldose reductase inhibitors might improve the course of the disease. They have not, however, been shown to be significantly helpful in the treatment of peripheral neuropathy.[50] Since there is a reduced myoinositol content, it was hypothesized that supplementation with this substance could be a useful treatment. In animal studies myoinositol has caused improvement of nerve conduction velocities,[38] but clinical trials in humans have not shown any significant benefit.[39]

The most important preventive measure for diabetic neuropathy is generally believed to be good glucose control. Although this has not been proven to prevent diabetic complications, there is evidence that better diabetic control lowers the incidence and severity of neuropathy.[19]

Sensory Changes. Sensory loss is the most common symptom of diabetic peripheral neuropathy. Since decreased protective sensation is frequently compounded by vascular insufficiency and dry skin (due to autonomic impairment), skin breakdown can occur. Careful daily inspection of the affected areas is necessary, with daily soaks followed by use of a good moisturizer. Toenails must be cut carefully straight across to prevent ingrown nails. Proper footwear, with appropriate in-shoe orthoses, is imperative. The patient should avoid use of heat on the affected limbs, and avoid foot trauma. When indicated, a podiatrist should be involved in the patient's care. If such preventive measures are not undertaken, ulceration and neuroarthropathy are common. Poor healing of ulcers can lead to gangrene and ultimately to amputation.

Pain. Neuropathic pain in diabetic patients is often a difficult and frustrating problem to control. In general, a treatment approach such as that described earlier is appropriate. Usually, the pain of diabetic neuropathy decreases spontaneously over time, and patients should be encouraged to remain active to avoid the complications of inactivity.

Autonomic Dysfunction. Autonomic neuropathy is a common complication of diabetes, and treatment should be directed to the specific system affected. Gastroparesis is typically treated with metoclopramide,[63] 10 mg four times daily. Diarrhea or constipation can be treated with a proper diet. A course of tetracycline or other broad-spectrum antibiotic can be used to alleviate diarrhea.[37] Postural hypotension should be managed with the least invasive measures. The initial treatment is to teach the patient to change position slowly and consider sleeping with the head of the bed elevated.[93] Compression stockings and an abdominal binder can improve venous return and decrease symptoms. When these fail, use of a mineralocorticoid such as fludrocortisone might benefit the patient.[93]

The management of neurogenic bladder depends on the severity of the condition. Postvoiding residual measurement often helps in determining the severity. In cases of mild to moderate impairment of bladder emptying, the patient should be encouraged to empty the bladder every 2 to 3 hours while awake. As severity increases, an intermittent catheterization program can be necessary to assure adequate drainage. Use of a parasympathomimetic agent can also be helpful (see Chapter 27).

Impotence is a common problem in diabetes. Treatment choices include counseling, medication, suction erection devices, and penile implants (see Chapter 30).

Sudomotor dysfunction is more pronounced over the distal extremities. It can leave the skin dry and subject to cracking and fissuring. Regular skin care and lubrication are necessary (see Chapter 56).

Alcoholic Neuropathy

The neuropathy of alcohol abuse appears to be, at least in part, related to malnutrition (especially the B vitamins).[20, 98] As with other toxic and metabolic disorders, the axons tend to "die back" from the periphery. The ensuing neuropathy is a mixed motor and sensory disorder,[55] with the symptoms first occurring in the lower extremities. Paresthesias are often present.

The affected patients have decreased sensation (especially of proprioception), distal muscle weakness and wasting, and depressed distal reflexes. As the disorder worsens, these changes appear more proximally in the lower extremities and begin to occur in the upper extremities.

Electrophysiological studies show decreased sensory action potential amplitudes. There is minimal slowing of motor conduction velocity, and distal latencies are minimally prolonged.[55] Needle examination typically shows positive sharp waves and fibrillation potentials in the distal muscles, with polyphasic units of increased amplitude[5] (see Chapter 12).

Management of Alcoholic Neuropathy

The primary treatment of alcoholic neuropathy is to stop the use of alcohol. Vitamins (especially B vitamins) and magnesium should be supplemented and a good diet instituted. Unlike diabetic polyneuropathy, alcoholic neuropathy has a good prognosis if treated promptly, or at least while it is not too advanced.[20]

The complications of alcoholic neuropathy are treated similarly to those of diabetes described above. Orthoses can be needed if significant weakness is a problem.

Acute Inflammatory Demyelinating Polyradiculoneuropathy

Acute inflammatory demyelinating polyradiculoneuropathy (AIDP), also known as Guillain-Barré syndrome (GBS), was first described by Landry in the 1860s, but derived its eponym from a description in 1916 by Georges Guillain and Jean Alexander Barré. Guillain and Barré noted that this was a paralyzing condition associated with an increased concentration of protein, but not cells, in the cerebrospinal fluid (CSF). This cytoalbuminological disassociation distinguished the condition from other common neuropathies, as well as from poliomyelitis. Since their description, other related disorders have been identified. They include a chronic or relapsing form, a steroid-responsive form, as well as the Miller-Fisher variant in which there is ataxia, ophthalmoplegia, and depressed muscle stretch reflexes.[31]

GBS is an acquired symmetrical polyneuropathy that usually affects the lower extremities initially.[30] It often begins with fine paresthesias in the toes or fingertips followed by an ascending weakness. The weakness progresses over days to weeks and can result in severe total body paresis, including the muscles of respiration. The facial muscles and oropharyngeal muscles are often involved, although the extraocular muscles and sphincters are generally spared. Pain is a common symptom. GBS can involve somatic, autonomic, and cranial nerves. Muscle stretch reflexes are typically absent or severely decreased.[75] The etiology is usually unknown, but the condition often follows a viral or bacterial infection, immunization, or surgery.[8]

Diagnostic criteria[75] for typical GBS include the required features of areflexia and progressive weakness in all extremities. Strong supporting features include a progression of the symptoms over a 4-week period, relative symmetry, mild sensory symptoms, cranial nerve involvement, recovery beginning 2 to 4 weeks after progression ceases, autonomic dysfunction, elevated concentration of protein in the CSF with less than 10 cells per cubic millimeter, and typical electrodiagnostic features. On physical examination there is symmetrical limb weakness, and bilateral facial weakness in one third of the patients. The muscle stretch reflexes are absent and there is minimal change in sensation. If the respiratory muscles are involved, the vital capacity is usually one half of the predicted value. The vital capacity should be carefully monitored as the patient might require ventilatory support. Autonomic function is often affected (71%)[35] and can precipitate abnormalities in heart rate, heart rhythm, and blood pressure. A period of observation in an intensive care unit (ICU) might be necessary. Patients who require ventilatory support generally have a longer period of recovery.[65]

Early histologic examination of the nerves reveals lymphocytes and macrophages surrounding the endoneurial vessels.[4] It was once thought that this was primarily an inflammatory neuropathy. More recent studies[43] propose that an early antibody attack on myelin occurs in some cases, with a mainly inflammatory process predominating in others. The nerves are affected earliest at the root level.[8] Later the most peripheral part of the nerve is damaged, with the intervening segments being affected last. The insult to the nerve appears to be primarily of a demyelinating type, but in more severe cases there can also be prominent axonal loss.[55]

Electrodiagnostic Findings in Guillain-Barré Syndrome

Since the earliest involvement of GBS is at the nerve root level, the earliest electrodiagnostic abnormalities are prolongation or absence of the late responses (F wave and H reflex). Later there can be a slowing of motor nerve conduction, but this is a less consistent finding. Temporal dispersion of the evoked responses, as well as significantly prolonged distal latencies, can also be noted. If serial studies are performed, the electrodiagnostic findings frequently lag behind the clinical course, both during worsening and during recovery of function.[6] Patients with weakness typically show a reduction in the number of motor units firing on maximal effort.

The best prognostic indicator is the needle EMG.[73] EMG signs of denervation indicate that the patient has axonopathy rather than just demyelination, and will have a slower recovery with poorer outcome.

Management of Guillain-Barré Syndrome

Patients with acute GBS should be hospitalized for observation and monitoring of the progression of the disease. It is particularly important to serially monitor the pulmonary and cardiovascular systems. If the vital capacity is rapidly declining, especially if it is less than 18 mL/kg of body weight,[75] or if there is cardiovascular dysautonomia, the patient should be monitored in an ICU. Mechanical ventilation might be necessary.

As these patients are immobile, they are at risk for developing deep venous thrombosis, pressure ulcers, and the other complications of immobility (see Chapter 34). Appropriate preventive and treatment measures should be undertaken.

Large randomized trials[33, 40] have shown the usefulness of plasmapheresis in treating GBS. The duration of mechanical ventilation can be halved with such treatment, and overall recovery time is significantly decreased. Contraindications to plasma exchange include recent myocardial infarction, angina, sepsis, or cardiovascular dysautonomia.[75] Patients should be warned about having surgery after recovery from GBS, as surgery can cause a recurrence, even years later. The recurrence is often worse than the original GBS episode. The exact part of the surgical experience that causes the recurrence is unknown. Even minor surgery such as oral surgery can trigger it.

Rehabilitation Methods. In the early stages of GBS the patient can be quadriplegic and bedridden. During this time prevention of contractures by ROM exercise, positioning, and the use of static splints is important. Careful positioning should also be done to prevent peripheral nerve compression and pressure ulcer formation. Meticulous pulmonary care is indicated to prevent atelectasis and pneumonia.

The rehabilitation program is gradually advanced in intensity as the patient improves. Since the patient with GBS is susceptible to overwork weakness, the strengthening program should initially be nonfatiguing. When muscles regain greater than antigravity strength, they can generally be stressed with more aggressive strengthening exercises. If the exercises are advanced too quickly, however, there can be a regression of strength (the so-called overwork weakness).[9] This should alert the clinician to reduce the activity level.

During recovery, GBS patients often benefit from the use of orthoses and assistive devices. Rocker feeders are helpful, as are clothing adaptations and other assistive devices. Ankle-foot and wrist orthoses can be useful in preventing contractures and enhancing function. It is more common for GBS patients to develop tightness of two-joint muscles than joint capsule contractures. Stretching of these muscles will alleviate this problem, and should include the hamstrings, tensor fascia lata, and gastrocnemius.

Gait retraining typically begins with the use of the tilt table. The tilt table is actually valuable well before gait training is possible, for it helps prevent deterioration in orthostatic tolerance. As soon as the patient is medically stable, tilt table training can be instituted. This can also be started in bed by having the patient sit upright for extended periods, as tolerated. There is a cardiovascular and autonomic adaptation as the patient is gradually elevated to the upright position. Patients are next allowed to stand in a standing table, which improves their muscular endurance and permits them to work on other tasks. Eventually the patient is advanced to the parallel bars, with the close assistance of the therapist to assist in movement and to prevent falls. As skills improve, the patient can be advanced to an assistive device for ambulation such as a walker, and then to crutches or canes. Eventually the patient is advanced to ambulation without assistance or with assistive devices. Lower extremity orthoses are used as indicated throughout the course of treatment (see Chapter 16).

In addition to progressive ambulation training, patients develop upper extremity strength and endurance through a combination of functional and weightlifting exercises. The goal is to achieve independent self-care, using assistive devices as needed (hopefully only temporarily). Most patients tolerate such a rehabilitation program and go on to an essentially complete recovery. The 5% to 10% or so who do not recover completely from GBS[75] benefit from the long-term use of assistive devices and rehabilitation strategies.

Uremic Neuropathy

Chronic renal insufficiency is associated with a sensorimotor peripheral neuropathy which causes a diffuse slowing of both motor and sensory conduction.[48] Symptoms of peripheral weakness and decreased sensation are often most severe in the lower extremities, despite an approximately equal slowing of conduction in both the upper and lower extremities.[46] The amplitude of the sensory nerve action potential and the H reflex latency are the most sensitive indicators of uremic neuropathy.[1, 42] Improvements in the electrodiagnostic findings are noted with dialysis and more significantly with kidney transplantation.[24, 89] Needle examination typically shows signs indicative of denervation in the weak muscles, with MUAPs decreased in number and increased in amplitude[25, 89] (see Chapters 11 and 12).

Medical treatment is aimed at compensating for the underlying disease. The special rehabilitation issues are similar to those encountered in diabetes (see above).

Charcot-Marie-Tooth Disease (Hereditary Motor Sensory Neuropathy, Types I and II)

Charcot-Marie-Tooth (CMT) disease includes a group of hereditary symmetrical distal polyneuropathies.[11] It is one of the most frequently inherited neurological diseases, with an estimated prevalence of 125,000 persons in the United States.[18] The inherited CMT defects have been mapped to chromosome 17 (CMT1A), chromosome 1 (CMT1B), the X chromosome (CMTX), and others.[10, 13, 18, 41, 47, 67, 97] The most common type is hereditary motor sensory neuropathy (HMSN), type HMSN-I (CMT1A). It is usually inherited in an autosomal dominant fashion.[74] CMT, type II (CMT-II) or HMSN-II is one third as common.[18]

CMT is usually detected in the first or second decade of life, although foot deformities can be noted even during infancy.[18] The initial symptoms include progressive distal lower extremity weakness and then atrophy. Pes cavus deformity is common, and is exaggerated (if not caused) by the distal motor dysfunction. The most severely affected muscles are the intrinsic foot muscles and peroneal muscles.[18] Distal sensory deficits are often present. Physical examination typically reveals notable peripheral weakness. The ankle muscle stretch reflexes are often absent and other reflexes can be hypoactive.[64] Gait abnormalities are common and include drop foot, foot slap, and steppage gait. As the disease progresses, the distal upper extremities can become involved, with atrophy and decreased strength and dexterity (Fig. 47–15). Nerves can be palpably enlarged.[18]

In HMSN-I there is a segmental demyelination with secondary Schwann cell proliferation. The Schwann cells form "onion bulbs"—concentric arrays around the demyelinated nerve—which account for the peripheral nerve enlargement.[21] HMSN-II is sometimes known as the "axonal" form of CMT. It is marked by axonal loss with subsequent Wallerian degeneration.[23]

CMT disease has variable penetrance.[12] A carrier might have only mild foot deformities, while members of the same family exhibit significant difficulties with ambulation, hand dexterity, and even diaphragmatic involvement.

The symptoms of CMT-I and CMT-II are remarkably similar, although they tend to be milder in type II.[23] In both conditions the symptoms generally progress slowly, with only gradual deterioration in function and a normal life span.[26] Despite distal weakness, these patients typically remain ambulatory throughout their lives.[23]

Electrophysiological studies are helpful in diagnosing CMT and in distinguishing type I from type II. In HMSN-I the motor nerve conduction velocities are significantly reduced (to about one-half of normal).[23] As the disease progresses, the muscle action potential amplitude decreases.[18] Sensory nerve action potential amplitudes are also significantly decreased.[18] Needle EMG examination can also show signs indicative of denervation in the affected muscles.[55] In HMSN-II the conduction velocity is normal or near normal, while both the motor and sensory action potential amplitudes are diminished and signs indicative of denervation are present.[55]

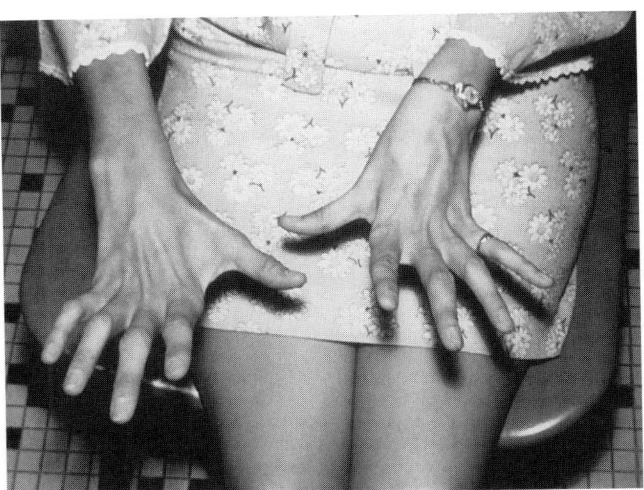

FIGURE 47–15. Hands in patient with advanced Charcot-Marie-Tooth disease.

Management of Charcot-Marie-Tooth Disease

Treatment of CMT is aimed primarily at maintenance of function, since currently there is no known way to alter the progression of the disease. Ankle-foot orthoses may be indicated if there is significant leg weakness or ankle instability or for protection if sensory symptoms are a significant issue. Careful selection of shoes is important. Custom-molded shoes might be necessary in some cases.

The patient with CMT is at risk for decreased ROM and contractures, especially loss of ankle dorsiflexion. The patient should be taught appropriate ROM and stretching exercises. Careful daily inspection of hypoesthetic areas should be encouraged.

Mononeuritis Multiplex

Mononeuritis multiplex is characterized by sensory and motor neuropathies[22, 90] that occur asymmetrically and asynchronously. It is most commonly due to multiple nerve infarction sites and is commonly seen in vasculitic conditions such as systemic vasculitides. These include polyarteritis nodosa and rheumatoid vasculitis, systemic lupus erythematosus, Lyme disease, Sjogren's syndrome, cryoglobulinemia, temporal arteritis, scleroderma, sarcoidosis, leprosy, acute viral hepatitis A, and acquired immunodeficiency syndrome (AIDS).[22, 72] It is also associated with diabetes mellitus and multiple nerve compressions, which are the most common causes.[72] Diagnosis is critical if mononeuropathy multiplex is due to a vasculitis, since treatment with steroids can arrest or limit the condition. Failure to recognize and treat vasculitis can have fatal consequences.

Electrodiagnostic studies show multiple nerve lesions. The rehabilitation management depends on the sites involved and generally includes positioning, bracing (static and functional), and a strengthening program, as tolerated. The precautions for insensate areas as described above should be instituted if appropriate.

Idiopathic Brachial Neuritis (Parsonage-Turner Syndrome)

Idiopathic brachial neuropathy, or brachial neuritis, is a peripheral neuropathy that most commonly affects the radial, long thoracic, phrenic, suprascapular, or spinal accessory nerves.[53, 100] Men are affected twice as frequently as women.[52] In approximately one third of the cases the shoulders are affected bilaterally.[55] This condition classically begins with a sharp pain in one shoulder followed by an aching sensation. Approximately one week later the patient notes weakness in the affected muscles. Atrophy typically develops later.[53, 55] The motor nerves are usually more affected than the sensory nerves; but if sensory nerves are affected, the most likely to have sensory deficits are the axillary, radial, or cutaneous nerves of the upper extremity.[55]

Electrodiagnostic studies show that motor conduction velocities are normal in the nerve fibers to the unaffected muscles. Latencies from Erb's point to the affected muscles can be slightly prolonged with decreased amplitude and temporal dispersion.[53] Needle EMG examination reveals signs of denervation in the affected muscles as well as polyphasic motor unit potentials and a reduced interference pattern.[15, 53]

Prognosis is generally good,[55] but recovery can take a few years in more severe cases.[53, 95] Rehabilitation management includes maintaining shoulder ROM and preventing contractures, so that the limb is functional when recovery eventually occurs. Orthotic prescription is also often appropriate.

Ischemic Monomelic Neuropathy

Ischemic monomelic neuropathy results from infarction of all the nerves of a distal extremity. It can be caused by spontaneous or iatrogenic arterial occlusion or embolization, such as during surgical procedures. The patient complains of a deep burning pain which persists even after arterial flow has been restored. Symptoms are predominantly due to a distal sensory loss in all nerve distributions. In more severe cases there is weakness as well, although the motor involvement is not usually as severe.[58] Symptoms can persist for months and are treated with antidepressants or anticonvulsants. Electrodiagnostic evaluation reveals sensory and motor axonal loss distally. Treatment is supportive with gait aids and orthoses as indicated. Sensory loss guidelines are to be followed as well.

CONCLUSION

Peripheral neuropathy is a common diagnosis with many causes and varied prognoses. It is of utmost importance to accurately diagnose the disease in order to be able to treat the patient with peripheral neuropathy appropriately and to give a reasonable prognosis. Much of the symptomatic treatment discussed in this chapter is similar for the different diseases and can be used for other forms of peripheral neuropathy which have not been discussed in detail. Rehabilitation treatment can significantly improve the patient's quality of life.

REFERENCES

1. Abers JW, Robers WC, Daube J: Electromyographic findings in porphyric neuropathy. Arch Phys Med Rehabil 1976; 57:595.
2. Archer AG, Roberts VC, Watkins PJ: Blood flow patterns in painful diabetic neuropathy. Diabetologia 1984; 27:563–567.
3. Archer AG, Watkins PJ, Thomas PK, et al: The natural history of acute painful neuropathy in diabetes mellitus. J Neurol Neurosurg Psychiatry 1983; 47:491–499.
4. Asbury AK, Arnason BG, Adams RD: The inflammatory lesion in idiopathic polyneuritis: Its role in pathogenesis. Medicine (Baltimore) 1969; 48:173–215.
5. Ballantyne JP, Hansen S, Weir A, et al: Quantitative electrophysiological study of alcoholic neuropathy. J Neurol Neurosurg Psychiatry 1980; 43:427–432.
6. Bannister RG, Sears TA: The changes in nerve conduction in acute idiopathic polyneuritis. J Neurol Neurosurg Psychiatry 1962; 25:321–328.
7. Barohn RJ: Approach to peripheral neuropathy and neuronopathy. Seminars Neurol 1998; 18:7–18.
8. Barohn RJ, Saperstein DS: Guillain-Barré syndrome and chronic inflammatory demyelinating polyneuropathy Seminars Neurol 1998; 18:49–62.
9. Bensman A: Strenuous exercise can impair muscle function in Guillain-Barré patients. JAMA 1970; 214:468–469.
10. Bergoffen J, Trofatter J, Pericak-Vance MA, et al: Linkage localization of X-linked Charcot-Marie-Tooth disease. Am J Hum Genet 1993; 52:312–318.
11. Bird TD: Hereditary motor-sensory neuropathies: Charcot-Marie-Tooth syndrome. Neurol Clin 1989; 7:9–23.
12. Bird TD, Kraft GH: Charcot-Marie-Tooth disease: Data for genetic counseling relating age to risk. Clin Genet 1978; 14:43–49.
13. Bird TD, Ott J, Giblett ER: Evidence for linkage of Charcot-Marie-Tooth neuropathy to the Duffy locus on chromosome 1. Am J Hum Genet 1982; 34:388–394.
14. Brown MJ, Asbury AK: Diabetic neuropathy. Ann Neurol 1984; 15:2–12.
15. Bradley WG, Madrid R, Thrush DC, Campbell MJ: Recurrent brachial plexus neuropathy. Brain 1975; 98:381–398.
16. Buchtal F, Kuehl V: Nerve conduction, tactile sensibility, and the electromyogram after suture or compression of peripheral nerve: A longitudinal study in man. J Neurol Neurosurg Psychiatry 1979; 42:436–451.
17. Buck AC, Reed PI, Siddiq YK, et al: Bladder dysfunction and neuropathy in diabetes. Diabetologia 1976; 12:251–258.
18. Chance PF, Pleasure D: Charcot-Marie-Tooth syndrome. Arch Neurol 1993; 50:1180–1184.
19. Committee on Health Care Issues, American Neurological Association: Does improved control of glycemia prevent or ameliorate diabetic polyneuropathy? Ann Neurol 1986; 19:288–290.
20. Dell PC, Guzewicz RM: Atypical peripheral neuropathies. Hand Clin 1992; 8:275–283
21. Dyck PJ: Histologic measurements and fine structure of biopsied sural nerve: Normal, and in peroneal muscular atrophy, hypertrophic neuropathy, and congenital sensory neuropathy. Mayo Clin Proc 1966; 41:742–774.
22. Dyck PJ, Benstead TJ, Conn DL, et al: Nonsystemic vasculitic neuropathy. Brain 1987; 110:843.
23. Dyck PJ, Chance PJ, Lebo RV, Carney JA: Hereditary motor and sensory neuropathies. In Dyck PJ, Thomas PJ, Griffin JW, et al (eds): Peripheral Neuropathy, vol 2. Philadelphia, WB Saunders, 1993, pp 1094–1136.
24. Dyck PJ, Johnson WJ, Lambert EH, et al: Comparison of symptoms, chemistry, and nerve function to assess adequacy of hemodialysis. Neurology 1979; 29:1361–1368.
25. Dyck PJ, Johnson WJ, Lambert EH, O'Brien PC: Segmental demyelination secondary to axonal degeneration in uremic neuropathy. Mayo Clin Proc 1971; 46:400–431.
26. Dyck PJ, Lambert EH: Lower motor and primary sensory neuron diseases with peroneal muscular atrophy: Neurologic, genetic and electrophysiologic findings in hereditary polyneuropathies. Arch Neurol 1968; 18:603.
27. Ewing DJ, Borsey DQ, Travis P, et al: Abnormalities of ambulatory 24-hour heart rate in diabetes mellitus. Diabetes 1983; 32:101–105.
28. Fagerberg S-E, Kock NG, Petersen I, Stener I: Urinary bladder disturbances in diabetics. A comparative study of male diabetics and controls aged between twenty and fifty years. Scand J Urol Nephrol 1967; 1:19–27.
29. Fairburn CG, Wu FCW, McCullock DK, et al: The clinical features of diabetic impotence: A preliminary study. Br J Psychiatry 1982; 140:447–452.
30. Feasby TE: Inflammatory-demyelinating polyneuropathies. Neurol Clin 1992; 10:651–670.
31. Fisher M: An unusual variant of acute idiopathic polyneuritis (syndrome of ophthalmoplegia, ataxia and areflexia). N Engl J Med 1956; 255:57–65.
32. Fraser DM, Campbell IW, Ewing DJ, Clarke BF: Mononeuropathy in diabetes mellitus. Diabetes 1979; 28:96–101.
33. French Cooperative Group on Plasma Exchange in Guillain-Barré Syndrome: Efficiency of plasma exchange in Guillain-Barré syndrome. Ann Neurol 1987; 22:753–761.
34. Gabbay KH, Merola LO, Field RA: Sorbitol pathway: Presence in nerve and cord with substrate accumulation in diabetes. Science 1966; 151:209–210.
35. Gibbels E, Giebisch U: Natural course of acute and chronic monophasic inflammatory demyelinating polyneuropathies

(IDP). A retrospective analysis of 266 cases. Acta Neurol Scand 1992; 85:282–291.
36. Goldstein JE, Cogan DG: Diabetic ophthalmoplegia with special reference to the pupil. Arch Ophthalmol 1960; 64:592–600.
37. Green PA, Berge KG, Sprague RG: Control of diabetic diarrhea with antibiotic therapy. Diabetes 1968; 17:385–387.
38. Greene DA, Lattimer SA, Sima AFA: Sorbitol, phosphoinositides and sodium-potassium-ATPase in the pathogenesis of diabetic complications. N Engl J Med 1987; 316:599–606.
39. Gregersen G, Borsting H, Theil P, Servo C: Myoinositol and function of peripheral nerves in human diabetics: A controlled clinical trial. Acta Neurol Scand 1978; 58:241–248.
40. Guillain-Barré Syndrome Study Group: Plasmapheresis and acute Guillain-Barré syndrome. Neurology 1984; 35:1096–1104.
41. Guiloff RJ, Thomas PK, Contreras M, et al: Linkage of autosomal dominant type 1 hereditary motor and sensory neuropathy to the Duffy locus on chromosome 1. J Neurol Neurosurg Psychiatry 1982; 45:669–674.
42. Halar EM, Brozovich FV, Milutinovic J, et al: H-reflex latency in uremic neuropathy: Correlation with NCV and clinical findings. Arch Phys Med Rehabil 1979; 60:174–177.
43. Hartung H-P, Hughes RAC, Taylor WA, et al: T cell activation in Guillain-Barré syndrome and in MS: Elevated serum levels of soluble IL-2 receptors. Neurology 1990; 40:215–218.
44. Herbison GJ, Jaweed M, Ditunno JF: Exercise therapies in peripheral neuropathies. Arch Phys Med Rehabil 1983; 64:201–205.
45. Hilsted J, Parving HH, Christensen NJ, et al: Hemodynamics in diabetic orthostatic hypotension. J Clin Invest 1981; 68:1427–1434.
46. Honet JC, Jebsen RH, Tenckhoff H: Comparison of motor and sensory nerve conduction velocity in early uremic polyneuropathy. Arch Phys Med Rehabil 1967; 48:209–212.
47. Ionasescu VV, Trofatter J, Haines JL, et al: Mapping of the gene for X-linked dominant Charcot-Marie-Tooth neuropathy. Neurology 1992; 42:903–908.
48. Jebsen RH, Tenckhoff H: Comparison of motor and sensory nerve conduction velocity in early uremic polyneuropathy. Arch Phys Med Rehabil 1969; 50:124–126.
49. Johnson EW: Sixteenth Annual AAEM Edward H. Lambert Lecture. Electrodiagnostic aspects of diabetic neuropathies: Entrapments. Muscle Nerve 1993; 16:127–134.
50. Judzewitsch RG, Jaspan JB, Polonsky KS, et al: Aldose reductase inhibition improves nerve conduction velocity in diabetic patients. N Engl J Med 1983; 308:119–125.
51. Kahan M, Goldberg PD, Mandel EE: Neurogenic vesical dysfunction and diabetes mellitus. NY State J Med 1970; 70:2448–2455.
52. Kimura J: Polyneuropathies. In Kimura J (ed): Electrodiagnosis in Diseases of Nerve and Muscle: Principles and Practice, ed 2. Philadelphia, FA Davis, 1989.
53. Kraft GH: Axillary, musculocutaneous and suprascapular nerve latency studies. Arch Phys Med Rehabil 1972; 53:383–387.
54. Kraft GH: Serial nerve conduction and electromyographic studies in experimental allergic neuritis. Arch Phys Med Rehabil 1975; 56:333–339.
55. Kraft GH: Peripheral neuropathies. In Johnson EW (ed): Practical Electromyography, ed 2. Baltimore, Williams & Wilkins, 1988, pp 246–318.
56. Kraft GH, Halvorson GA: Median nerve residual latency: Normal value and use in diagnosis of carpal tunnel syndrome. Arch Phys Med Rehabil 1983; 64:221–226.
57. Latour P, Fabreguette A, Ressot C, et al: New mutations in the X-linked form of Charcot-Marie-Tooth disease. Eur Neurol 1997; 37:38–42.
58. Levin KH: Ischemic monomelic neuropathy. Muscle Nerve 1985; 12:791–795.
59. Lewis T, Pickering GW, Rothschild P: Centripetal paralysis arising out of arrested blood flow to the limb including notes on a form of tingling. Heart 1931; 16:1–32.
60. Martini R, Zielasek J, Toyka KV: Inherited demyelinating neuropathies: From gene to disease. Curr Opin Neurol 1998; 11: 545–556.
61. Max MB, Culnane M, Schafer SC, et al: Amitriptyline relieves diabetic neuropathy pain in patients with normal or depressed mood. Neurology 1987; 37:589–596.
62. Max MB, Kishore-Kumar R, Schafer SC, et al: Efficacy of desipramine in painful diabetic neuropathy: A placebo-controlled trial. Pain 1991; 45:3–9.
63. McCallum RW, Ricci DA, Rakatansky H, et al: A multicenter placebo-controlled clinical trial of oral metoclopramide in diabetic gastroparesis. Diabetes Care 1983; 6:463–467.
64. Mendell JR: Charcot-Marie-Tooth neuropathies and related disorders. Seminars Neurol 1998; 18:41–48.
65. Meythaler JM, DeVivo MJ, Braswell WC: Rehabilitation outcomes of patients who have developed Guillain-Barré syndrome. Am J Phys Med Rehabil 1997; 76:411–419.
66. Miller RG: Acute vs. chronic compressive neuropathy. Muscle Nerve 1984; 7:427–430.
67. Mostacciuolo ML, Mueller E, Fardin P, et al: X-linked Charcot-Marie-Tooth disease: A linkage study in a large family by using 12 probes of the pericentromeric region. Hum Genet 1991; 87:23–27.
68. Mulder DW, Lambert EH, Bastron JA, Sprague RG: The neuropathies associated with diabetes mellitus. A clinical and electromyographic study of 103 unselected diabetic patients. Neurology 1961; 11:275–284.
69. Nelis E, Haites N, Van Broeckhoven C: Mutations in the peripheral myelin genes and associated genes in inherited peripheral neuropathies. Human Mutation 1999; 13:11–28.
70. Ouvrier R: Correlation between the histopathologic, genotypic, and phenotypic features of hereditary peripheral neuropathies in childhood. J Child Neurol 1996; 11:133–146.
71. Parry GJ, Cornblath DR, Brown MJ: Transient conduction block following acute peripheral nerve ischemia. Muscle Nerve 1982; 8:490–513.
72. Parry GJG: Mononeuropathy multiplex (AAEE case report #11). Muscle Nerve 1985; 8:493–498.
73. Raman PT, Taori GM: Prognostic significance of electrodiagnostic studies in the Guillain-Barré syndrome. J Neurol Neurosurg Psychiatry 1976; 39:163–170.
74. Reilly MM: Genetically determined neuropathies. J Neurol 1998; 245:6–13.
75. Ropper AH: The Guillain-Barré syndrome. N Engl J Med 1992; 326:1130–1136.
76. Ross DR, Varipapa RJ: Treatment of painful diabetic neuropathy with topical capsaicin. N Engl J Med 1989; 321:474–475.
77. Ross MA: Neuropathies associated with diabetes. Med Clin North Am 1993; 77:111–124.
78. Rull JA, Quibrera R, Gonzalez-Millan H, Castaneda OL: Symptomatic treatment of peripheral diabetic neuropathy with carbamazepine (Tegretol): Double blind crossover trial. Diabetologia 1969; 5:215–218.
79. Rundles RW: Diabetic neuropathy: General review with report of 125 cases. Medicine (Baltimore) 1945; 24:111–160.
80. Schiller LR, Santa Ana CA, Schmulen AC, et al: Pathogenesis of fecal incontinence in diabetes mellitus: Evidence for internal-anal-sphincter dysfunction. N Engl J Med 1982; 307:1666–1671.
81. Seddon HJ: Three types of nerve injury. Brain 1943; 66:17–288.
82. Skilman TG, Johnson EW, Hamwi GJ, Driskill HJ: Motor nerve conduction velocity in diabetes mellitus. Diabetes 1961; 10: 46–57.
83. Smith B: Neuropathology of the oesophagus in diabetes mellitus. J Neurol Neurosurg Psychiatry 1974; 37:1151–1154.
84. Stewart JD: Diabetic truncal neuropathy: Topography of the sensory deficit. Ann Neurol 1989; 25:233–238.
85. Sunderland S: The anatomy and physiology of nerve injury. Muscle Nerve 1990; 13:771–784.
86. Sunderland S: A classification of peripheral nerve injuries producing loss of function. Brain 1951; 74:491–516.
87. Swift TR, Leshner RT, Gross JA: Arm-diaphragm synkinesis: Electrodiagnostic studies of aberrant regeneration of phrenic motor neurons. Neurology 1980; 30:339–344.
88. Taverner D: Bell's palsy: A clinical and electromyographic study. Brain 1955; 78:209–235.
89. Taylor N, Halar EM, Tenckhoff H, et al: Effects of renal transplantation on motor nerve conduction velocity. Arch Phys Med Rehabil 1972; 53:227–231.

90. Taylor RA: Heredofamilial mononeuritis multiplex with brachial predilection. Brain 1960; 83:113–137.
91. Thomas PK: Classification, differential diagnosis, and staging of diabetic peripheral neuropathy. Diabetes 1997; 46(suppl 2): S54–S57.
92. Thomas PK: Diabetic neuropathy: Models, mechanisms and mayhem. Can J Neurol Sci 1992; 19:1–7.
93. Thomas PK, Thomlinson DR: Diabetic and hypoglycemic neuropathy. In Dyck PF, Thomas PK, Griffin JW (eds): Peripheral Neuropathy, vol 2. Philadelphia, WB Saunders, 1993.
94. Thorsteinsson G: Management of painful diabetic neuropathy. JAMA 1977; 238:2297.
95. Tsairis P, Dyck PJ, Mulder DW: Natural history of brachial plexus neuropathy: Report of 99 patients. Arch Neurol 1972; 27:109–117.
96. Valentijn LJ, Baas F: Genetic basis of peripheral neuropathies. Prog Brain Res 1998; 117:249–264.
97. Vance JM, Barker K, Yamaoka LH, et al: Localization of Charcot-Marie-Tooth disease type 1a (CMT1A) to chromosome 17p11.2. Genomics 1991; 9:623–628.
98. Victor M, Adams RD: Symposium on neurological and hepatic complications of alcoholism. On the etiology of the alcoholic neurologic diseases with special reference to the role of nutrition. Am J Clin Nutr 1961; 9:379–397.
99. Virani A, Mailis A, Shapiro LE, Shear NH: Drug interactions in human neuropathic pain pharmacotherapy. Pain 1997; 73:3–13.
100. Walsh NE, Dumitru D, Kalantri A, Roman AM: Brachial neuritis involving the bilateral phrenic nerves. Arch Phys Med Rehabil 1987; 68:46–48.
101. Warner LE, Garcia CA, Lupski JR: Hereditary peripheral neuropathies: Clinical forms, genetics, and molecular mechanisms. Annu Rev Med 1999; 50:263–275.
102. Wilton TD: Tegretol in the treatment of diabetic neuropathy. S Afr Med J 1974; 48:869–872.
103. Windebank AJ: Polyneuropathy due to nutritional deficiency and alcoholism. In Dyck PJ, Thomas PK, Griffin JW, (eds): Peripheral Neuropathy, vol 2. Philadelphia, WB Saunders, 1993, p 1313.
104. Wolfe GI, Barohn RJ: Cryptogenic sensory and sensorimotor polyneuropathies. Seminars Neurol 1998; 18:105–112.
105. Younger DS, Rosoklija G, Hays AP: Diabetic peripheral neuropathy. Seminars Neurol 1998; 18:95–104.
106. Zlotogora J: Dominance and homozygosity. Am J Med Genet 1997; 68:412–416.

48 CHAPTER

Maureen R. Nelson, M.D.

Rehabilitation Concerns in Myopathies

Myopathies are a group of muscle diseases whose most common primary symptom is proximal limb muscle weakness. There are a variety of myopathies which differ in etiology, course, specific muscle involvement, and associated problems. These include the muscular dystrophies and the myopathies that are congenital, metabolic, endocrine, infectious, collagen-vascular, toxic, or secondary to other etiologies. Most myopathy research has been done on Duchenne muscular dystrophy (DMD), which is in many ways a myopathy prototype. DMD is described in detail in this chapter, and the other myopathies are compared and contrasted with DMD. The majority of these disorders have no cure, although an extensive amount of research is underway. Treatment in these cases is focused on the prevention of secondary complications and maximizing function within each stage of the disease (Table 48–1).

DYSTROPHIES

Muscular dystrophies can be either hereditary or congenital disorders of muscle. The most common muscular dystrophy is DMD. This disease is more severe and progresses more quickly than other dystrophies. Other muscular dystrophies include Becker's, facioscapulohumeral, myotonic, the limb-girdle group, and the less common Emery-Dreifuss type (Table 48–2).

Duchenne Muscular Dystrophy

Duchenne muscular dystrophy is an X-linked recessive myopathy. DMD has an incidence of 1 in 3500 live male births[37] with a prevalence approximating 3 per 100,000 live males.[107] Approximately one-third of DMD cases are thought to occur secondary to a spontaneous mutation.[16] The absence or severe abnormality of the protein dystrophin is the cause of DMD. This is due to an abnormality on the short arm of the X chromosome at the Xp21 locus.[24, 69, 107] Dystrophin is a critical part of the cytoskeleton and its abnormality leads to membrane instability and injury.[90]

DMD typically becomes clinically evident at approximately 3 to 5 years of age.[68] Early difficulties noted are clumsiness, poor walking, and frequent falls. The weakness is generally symmetrical. It begins in the pelvic and then the shoulder girdle muscles, and finally progresses to the respiratory and distal limb muscles.[35, 39, 55] DMD progresses with a predictable pattern but with a variable rate of functional loss in different children.[55] Death is usually due to respiratory insufficiency and generally occurs at approximately 20 years of age unless ventilatory assistance is given.

There are several associated findings common in DMD. There can be muscle pain, particularly in the calves.[90] Restrictive pulmonary disease is frequently noted and progresses with the weakening of muscles. Scoliosis is also associated with progressive axial muscle weakness. Cardiac abnormalities are found as well, and cardiac failure is a common cause of death in patients whose life is prolonged by the use of respiratory devices.

DMD is seen rarely in females. Since this is an X-linked recessive disorder, it can occur in a girl with Turner's syndrome and an XO karyotype or with an X autosomal translocation and a break at the Xp21 locus.[107] Female carriers can also have varying degrees of mild muscle weakness and elevation of muscle enzymes, a phenomenon explained by the Lyon hypothesis.

Physical findings at the time of DMD diagnosis frequently include calf pseudohypertrophy, which is present in about 80% of patients.[107] This finding is believed to represent fatty and fibrotic replacement of muscle, which is rubbery to palpation. Another frequent sign is

TABLE 48–1 Types of Myopathies

Dystrophies	Endocrine myopathies
Duchenne muscular dystrophy	Hyperthyroidism
Becker's muscular dystrophy	Hypothyroid myopathy
Facioscapulohumeral dystrophy	Hyperparathyroidism
Limb-girdle dystrophy	Corticosteroid myopathy
Myotonic dystrophy	Inflammatory myopathies
Emery-Dreifuss muscular dystrophy	Polymyositis
Congenital myopathies	Dermatomyositis
Central core myopathy	Sarcoidosis
Nemaline myopathy	Infectious myopathies
Myotubular (centronuclear) myopathy	Trichinosis
Congenital fiber disproportion	Cysticercosis
Metabolic myopathies	HIV/AIDS
Muscle phosphorylase deficiency (McArdle's disease, type V glycogenosis)	Toxic myopathies
Phosphofructokinase (type VII) deficiency	Alcoholic myopathy
Acid maltase deficiency (type II glycogenosis; infantile [Pompe's disease])	Medications
Debranching enzyme deficiency	

Abbreviations: HIV, human immunodeficiency virus; AIDS, acquired immunodeficiency syndrome.

difficulty rising from the floor and demonstration of Gower's sign. As shown in Figure 48–1, the boy stabilizes his legs with his arms and pushes his arms up the front of his thighs to stand up. Proximal muscle atrophy might be detected. The child can also have difficulty raising his arms above his head. Predictable patterns of atrophy and hypertrophy show a linear depression of the posterior axillary fold with preserved muscles surrounding it when viewed from the back with the arms abducted to 90 degrees and the elbows flexed to 90 degrees.[114] The tongue can be enlarged, which is believed to lead to widening of the mandible and maxilla and separation of the teeth.[90] Pelvic girdle weakness is generally present earlier than shoulder girdle weakness. Gait is frequently wide-based and the child will progress to walking on tiptoe with tight Achilles tendons. The child might be unable to climb up the stairs or step up onto a low bench. Muscle stretch reflexes can be decreased or absent.[16]

Intelligence is affected by DMD, although the exact cause of this is unknown. Twenty-five percent of boys with DMD have intelligence quotients (IQs) lower than 75, which is not a progressive loss.[107] A recent small study revealed that with transcranial stimulation, central motor conduction time is normal, but the threshold for stimulation is higher in boys with DMD than in controls. This finding is possibly due to the deficiency of brain synaptic dystrophin.[34] Cardiac involvement initially involves the posterobasal area and contiguous left ventricular wall.[146] Arrhythmias and tachycardia can be present.[16] Upper gastrointestinal tract dysfunction can be present with dysphagia, heartburn, and nasal voice. Gastric hypomotility has also been noted.[63]

Patients with DMD and other myopathies have been reported as having malignant hyperthermia (MH) as an adverse response to general anesthesia. This is manifest by tachycardia, cardiac arrhythmia, tachypnea, unstable blood pressure, cyanosis, fever, and possibly convulsions. Seventy-five percent of the patients develop rigidity secondary to severe muscle contractures, frequently in the masseter muscles, with metabolic acidosis as a consequence. Myoglobinuria and renal failure can result with a mortality of 60%. MH can be induced by halothane and succinylcholine.[107] When the diagnosis is suspected, anesthetic agents should be immediately discontinued and 100% oxygen given. The patient is cooled, and bicarbonate is given for metabolic acidosis. Dantrolene is given to relax the muscles. Immediate treatment improves the outcome.[16] The classic MH defect is not present in muscular dystrophy, so the MH that clinically occurs in DMD is likely due to the defect of muscle cell membranes.[48]

The most useful laboratory finding in DMD is an elevated creatine kinase (CK), which can be 300 to 400 times normal.[107] This decreases with age as muscle mass declines with disease progression. CK is mildly elevated in 70% of female carriers.[107] Other muscle enzymes can also be elevated in DMD patients. The electrocardiogram (ECG) is abnormal in two-thirds of patients, usually demonstrating a tall right precordial R wave with deep Q waves in the limb and left precordial leads.

Needle electromyography (EMG) and nerve conduction studies (NCSs) are a useful part of the evaluation (also see Chapters 10–12). Sensory NCSs are normal. Motor NCSs have normal latencies, conduction velocities, and F-wave latencies, but the amplitude of the compound muscle action potential (CMAP) typically decreases as the disease progresses. The EMG shows an increase in insertional activity early in the disease, which can decrease later as fibrotic tissue replaces muscle. Fibrillations and positive sharp waves can be seen at rest. Complex repetitive discharges (CRDs) can also be observed.[81] Motor units in DMD show the classic short-duration, low-amplitude polyphasicity (often called "myopathic") accompanied by satellite potentials. Typically there is early motor unit recruitment.[81] Muscle fiber conduction velocity is slowed and variable.[87]

Muscle biopsy shows increased fibrosis with circular fibers. Muscle fiber necrosis and phagocytosis occur in association with small groups of basophilic fibers. There are also opaque fibers and an increase in undifferentiated fibers.[16] Dystrophin is noted to be virtually absent

TABLE 48–2 Muscular Dystrophies

Type	Genetic	Signs at Presentation	Age at Presentation	Associated Findings	Chromosome	Disease Course	Laboratory Studies	Electrodiagnosis	Biopsy
Duchenne muscular dystrophy	XLR	Poor walking Frequent falls Gower's maneuver Pseudohypertrophy of calves	3–5 yr	Cardiac disease Restrictive lung disease Scoliosis Decreased IQ	Xp21	Severe, progressive	Early: very high CK ECG abnormal	Positive sharp waves, fibrillations, CRDs, small-amplitude polyphasics	Fibrosis, circular fibers, basophilic fibers, abnormal or no dystrophin
Becker's muscular dystrophy	XLR	Decrease in walking Pseudohypertrophy of calves	10–15 yr—varies	Cardiac disease	Xp21	Slowly progressive—varies	Increased CK ECG abnormal	Positive sharp waves, fibrillations, CRDs small-amplitude polyphasics, paraspinal	Abnormal quality or quantity of dystrophin
Facioscapulohumeral dystrophy	AD	Facial weakness Shoulder weakness	Teenage—varies	Dry sclera Facial droop		Varies	Normal or mildly increased CK	CRDs early, may be normal Positive sharp waves, fibrillations, small-amplitude polyphasics	Tiny fibers "moth-eaten" fibers
Limb-girdle dystrophy	AR	Hip weakness	Teenage–20s	Cardiac disease Pulmonary disease		Varies	Increased LDH Increased CK	CRDs Small-amplitude polyphasics,	Varied fiber size, increased internal nuclei Fiber splitting, "moth-eaten" whorled fibers
Myotonic dystrophy	AD	Myotonia (cramping or stiffness) Long face Distal extremity weakness	Late teenage–20s	Cataracts Cardic conduction defects Endocrine abnormalities	Chromosome 19	Varies	Increased CK	Myotonic discharges (wax and wane) Small-amplitude polyphasics	Internal nuclei, type I fiber atrophy
Emery-Dreifuss muscular dystrophy	XLR	Early contractures Cardiac conduction defect	Childhood	Denial Cardiac disease	Xq28	Slowly progressive	CK normal to increased	Small- and large-amplitude polyphasics	Type I predominance and atrophy

* *Abbreviations:* IQ, Intelligence quotient; CK, creatine kinase; ECG, electrocardiogram; CRDs, complete repetitive discharges; LDH, lactic dehydrogenase; XLR, X-linked recessive; AD, autosomal dominant; AR, autosomal recessive.

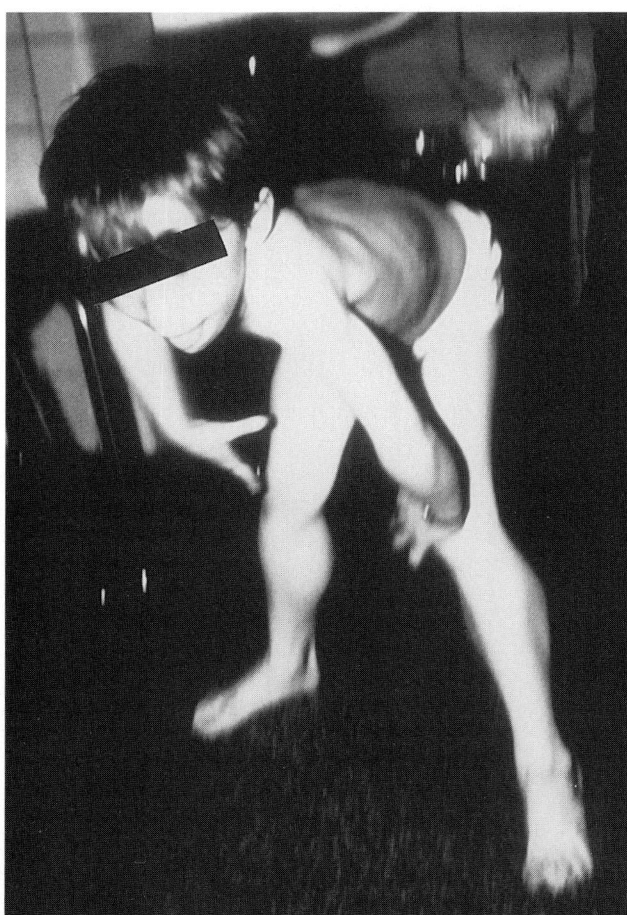

FIGURE 48–1. Boy with Duchenne muscular dystrophy demonstrating calf pseudohypertrophy and Gowers's maneuver in standing up. (Photograph courtesy of R. Braddom, M.D.)

in the sarcolemma of skeletal muscle fibers in DMD by microscopic immunochemistry.[24, 69]

The DMD gene is a large genetic locus including over 2.5 million base pairs of a human X chromosome.[76] This gene is approximately 10 times larger than the next largest identified gene. It encodes 79 exons of coding sequence.[119] The large size of the gene is believed to be the cause of the high mutation rate. Identifiable exon deletions are present in 55% of DMD and 65% of BMD patients. The size of the deletion does not correlate with disease severity.[99] If the patient does not have a deletion, he generally has a point mutation. The severity of weakness depends on whether the deletion or point mutation allows translation of a partially functional dystrophin.[1] Because the gene is so large and there are so many areas where a genetic mutation can occur, once the mutation is identified in a family member, the specific genetic lesion present in that family can be searched for in DNA prenatal diagnosis.[76] For deletion-positive patients, DNA screening of carriers and intrauterine diagnosis are recommended. For those families without a known deletion, genetic linkage analysis studies and muscle biopsy of a potential carrier or male fetus are available, as well as chorionic villus DNA analysis.[79]

The clinical course in DMD includes progressive respiratory and limb muscle weakness, contractures, and reduction of physical function. Ambulation ceases at approximately 10 years of age, ranging from 7 to 13 years. Ambulation past 14 years should lead to consideration of other diagnoses.[90] One study reported that boys who took 9 seconds to walk 30 feet lost ambulation in 2 years, and those who took 12 seconds lost walking in 1 year.[91] When the child can no longer climb four stairs in less than 5 seconds, it will be approximately 2.4 years until he will be unable to stand or walk without assistive devices. If it takes him longer than 12 seconds for that same stair climbing, he is on average 1.2 years from inability to walk independently.

Scoliosis is present in approximately 75% of patients. Contrary to common belief, scoliosis is not secondary to inability to walk, but in fact is present in many boys prior to this change in mobility.[20] This finding is supported by a study which shows that scoliosis and the cessation of ambulation are temporally, but not causally related.[83] Surgery for scoliosis is generally considered when the curve is greater than 35 degrees. Forced vital capacity (FVC) is generally improved or stable after surgery for scoliosis, particularly when the FVC is greater than 1.5 L at the time of surgery. Bracing of the spine is typically not indicated in DMD, as surgical treatment is much preferable. The boy will be more comfortable, be able to handle respiratory devices better, and be in a more cosmetic position in the wheelchair following scoliosis surgery.

There is a correlation between development of pneumonia and an FVC of approximately 1 L or less. Patients who are weaker tend to die from respiratory failure and pneumonia, while patients who are stronger have preserved respiratory function and might eventually die from cardiac failure.[20]

Treatment

There is currently no cure for DMD, although intensive research is underway. Medications are used in some patients to attempt to slow the progression of the disease (see below). There is treatment for minimizing the problem of contractures with bracing and stretching exercises. Surgical interventions are frequently undertaken to relieve contractures. Respiratory management is an area with a wide array of treatment options. Spinal fusion for scoliosis is a useful intervention for many of these children. Exercise to improve muscle strength is an area of controversy. Various braces are used to increase mobility. AFOs can be used as night or day splints to preserve normal ankle position after the patient becomes a wheelchair user. One of the main goals of treatment is to minimize medical complications.

Pharmacology

Pharmacological intervention has consisted primarily of steroids. Limited investigations have shown that strength, functional status, and pulmonary function improve with steroids.[19] A long-term study also demonstrated that the duration of independent ambulation was prolonged in boys treated with prednisone as compared to a control group.[31] Side effects include cushingoid facial appearance, increased appetite and excessive weight gain, hyperactivity, cataracts, gastritis, behavioral changes, bone loss leading to fracture, and acne.[19, 31] Studies have also investigated the possible beneficial effects on progression of DMD of amino acids,[93] allopurinol,[13, 61] calcium channel blockers,[106] methysergide,[113] and isaxonine,[52] but none of these was found to have any benefit.[53]

Deflazacort (a derivative of prednisone) was used in children with DMD in an attempt to have the benefits of steroids with fewer side effects than found with prednisone. It was used for a 2 year trial with positive outcomes.[3] Both an improvement in functional ability and a delay in the loss of ambulation were noted, along with fewer side effects than prednisone.[3] An experimental protocol of 10 days steroid treatment alternating with 10 days drug holiday is currently ongoing. The side effects and the long-term need for the steroids, once begun, make many experts hesitant to use steroids.[101] Deflazacort is not yet approved for use in the United States. Steroids cannot prevent the ultimate outcome in DMD.

Cyclosporines improve strength to a degree similar to prednisone, and also with the pattern of a decline in strength over time. Doses of 5 mg/kg/day taken orally are typically effective within two weeks, with transient, minor side effects.[101]

Ventilation

Maximizing ventilatory assistance in patients with DMD is critical. The median age of death in DMD is between 18 and 25 years of age.[10, 45, 118] Approximately 90% of these patients die secondary to chronic respiratory insufficiency.[10, 118] Contributory factors include restrictive pulmonary disease, chest wall muscle weakness, and scoliotic deformity.[10] Ventilatory assistance can extend the length of life and ventilation options are increasing as research in this area continues.[86]

Respiratory assistance is typically initiated when vital capacity (VC) decreases to approximately 20% of predicted normal and symptoms of hypercapnia begin.[10, 44] VC generally maximizes at approximately age 10 years in children with DMD. The maximal level that is attained can help predict the progression of the restrictive disease in each child. In the ensuing years, the VC decreases, generally to 30–50% of predicted by the mid-teenage years.[10] Some caregivers then recommend the use of mouth intermittent positive pressure breathing (MIPPB) with the use of an intermittent positive pressure breathing (IPPB) device. This intervention is designed to obtain maximal lung expansion, with a goal of minimizing the microatelectasis and maintaining the chest wall compliance. It is also used for management of acute respiratory infections.[10]

Glossopharyngeal breathing (GPB), or frog breathing, can be a useful tool for DMD patients. For persons who can learn to essentially breathe their swallowed air, the time of ventilatory assistance can be decreased. Additionally, GPB is a useful backup for any mechanical failure of ventilatory assistance. GPB can be used to take deep breaths, shout, and increase the effect of coughing, even in individuals who have no measurable VC. Intact oropharyngeal muscles are necessary for GPB. It is not possible to perform GPB with an open tracheostomy and rarely can it be done with a plugged tracheostomy.[7]

Respiratory assistance is usually considered when the VC falls to approximately 10% of the predicted normal, or when a patient begins to have symptoms of nocturnal hypoventilation. Symptoms of hypercarbia include irritability, daytime somnolence, morning headaches, nausea, restless sleep, palpitations, dysphoria, and decrease in daytime vigor.[26, 135, 137, 139] Respiratory drive decreases at night, so there is an increased risk at that time.[26] The workup of a patient with falling VC typically consists of admission to the hospital for continuous overnight capnography (measurement of partial pressure of carbon dioxide [PCO_2]). This measures the end-expiratory PCO_2. For those without significant intrinsic lung disease, this will be approximately equal to the arterial PCO_2. Arterial blood gases can also be done and oxygen saturation using pulse oximetry can be monitored. With a night PCO_2 of 55 mm Hg, the patient can have daytime symptoms, even if blood gases during the day are normal. If the PCO_2 levels are increased during the day, there is frequently severe nocturnal hypoventilation, with the PCO_2 as high as 80 to 95 mm Hg.[10] Treatment is initiated with the use of noninvasive negative or positive pressure ventilators.

The rationale for the use of negative pressure ventilation is that the ventilator actually performs part of the patient's work of breathing, resulting in rest for the respiratory muscles. The goal is to allow the respiratory muscles to work efficiently during the day after a night of relative rest.[137] Tank ventilators have been shown to reduce diaphragmatic and accessory muscle electrical activity in patients with restrictive lung disease, while maintaining adequate ventilation.[7, 120, 137]

Negative pressure ventilators work by an intermittent flow of negative pressure in a tank, resulting in a negative intrapleural pressure, generating airway flow to ventilate the lungs.[7] Commonly used types of negative pressure ventilation include the iron lung, Porta-Lung (Lifecare, Lafayette, Colorado), chest cuirass, negative pressure wrap, and rocking beds. All except the cuirass ventilator require the patient to be supine. These systems are driven by negative pressure pumps. The cuirass is convenient, and can be used while sitting. It is ineffective if there is poor pulmonary compliance or if there is any significant scoliosis.[7] Some patients use a cuirass during the day and an iron lung or other tank ventilator at night. Complications from using the iron lung or tank respirators are minimal. Pressure ulcers are rarely seen with the use of four-inch egg crate mattresses. Chafing of the neck from the rubber of the tank collar is generally no longer seen because of improved collar design. Other difficulties in using negative pressure ventilation occur in patients younger than 3 years of age, who tend to have recurrent atelectasis and pneumonia. Fortunately, DMD patients rarely need ventilatory assistance in this age group. Severe thoracic or cervical thoracic scoliosis can also prevent adequate fit of negative pressure ventilation devices.[137]

There are several forms of positive pressure ventilation (PPV) available. Noninvasive intermittent PPV (NIPPV, bipap) can be done with mouth or nasal access. Alternatively, the more commonly used PPV is the invasive method using a tracheostomy. NIPPV methods include the exsufflation belt or pneumobelt, which has an elastic inflatable bladder within an abdominal corset. Cyclic positive pressure inflation causes the bladder to compress the abdomen, pushing the diaphragm upward, which induces a forced expiration. When the bladder deflates, the diaphragm passively lowers and inspiration occurs. The patient can support this passive inspiration with any available active inspiratory efforts. This mechanism is effective only in the seated position, and ineffective in patients with severe scoliosis. When effective, however, it can increase the inspired volume by approximately 300 mL.[7]

Bipap is PPV noninvasively delivered with an oral or nasal interface. For oral PPV a mouth seal (Puritan-Bennett, Boulder, Colorado) is often used to keep the mouthpiece in place and prevent excessive leakage.[7] Both the PPV system devices and the negative pressure devices are generally initiated with nighttime use.[10]

Invasive PPV is done with a tracheostomy and positive pressure ventilator. Tracheostomy is deemed mandatory when oral pharyngeal muscle strength is inadequate to control secretions or speech, when patients are unreliable or uncooperative, when severe intrinsic lung disease is present, when there are seizures, or when there are severe orthopedic facial problems.[7] Tracheostomy intermittent positive pressure ventilation (IPPV) is the most common method of respiratory support offered to DMD patients requiring ventilatory assistance.[10] There are a number of potential problems associated with tracheostomy ventilation: airway colonization, increased risk of respiratory tract infection, tracheal necrosis, tracheoesophageal fistula, tracheostenosis, laryngeal complications, swallowing problems, food aspiration, cardiac arrhythmias, chronic granulation tissue formation, painful tracheostomy tube change, mucous plug, and death either from sudden respiratory arrest secondary to mucous plug or from accidental disconnection of the ventilator.[7] Additionally, the mere presence of a tracheostomy stimulates airway secretions, making more frequent suctioning and pulmonary toilet necessary. Most routine suctioning fails to clear the left mainstem bronchus and leads to an increased risk of pneumonia on the left. Speech is dependent on ventilator cycling and timing with inspiration. A tracheostomy is also an open wound, which makes the patient ineligible for certain activities and living situations.[7]

Patients without ventilatory assistance and a maximum plateau VC below 1200 mL die on average at age 15.3 years, while those with a plateau over 1700 mL live to approximately age 21.[10, 118] Patients with a peak FVC over 2500 mL have a slower progression: 4% of predicted FVC per year versus 9.6% FVC loss per year for those with peak FVC less than 1700 mL.[91] With maximal respiratory assistance and early optimal treatment of scoliosis to maintain lung position, these numbers may be greatly improved in the future. Patients with DMD have a progressive decrease in VC, even with ventilatory assistance. They can anticipate an increased use of assisted ventilation each year. The treatment is not giving oxygen; it is the mechanical work of ventilation. With assisted ventilation, survival is increased by approximately six years.[26]

Ventilatory assistance in DMD is controversial. In a 1985 survey of Muscular Dystrophy Association (MDA) clinics, Colbert and Schock[25] found that ventilatory aids were prescribed on a regular basis in just 33% of the 132 responding clinics. A similar survey in 1990 by Bach and colleagues[8] reported that ventilatory assistance was being offered on an elective basis in just 43 of 167 (26%) MDA clinics. Sixty-two clinics (37%) were not managing anyone on a ventilator. Sixty-one percent of the clinics reported that they followed regular pulmonary function tests, but the majority of them began initial ventilator use only during acute respiratory episodes. The 143 clinics that did not offer ventilatory aid or discuss ventilatory assistance stated that the main reason was poor quality of life on a ventilator. Other responses reported were financial problems, home environment, cognitive deficits, and family burden.[6] Of the 91 clinic directors who discouraged ventilatory assistance, only four had any experience with noninvasive ventilation.[6]

Patients note that physicians severely underestimate their quality of life. Both patients and families report deficits; and many patients indicate dissatisfaction with the information given about ventilatory assistance, maintaining that they should have received the information earlier and more completely.[97] When a group of DMD patients and a control group of medical professionals were surveyed with respect to satisfaction with their own lives, 12.5% of the patients reported dissatisfaction in general compared with 9.0% of the health-care professionals.[8] So the great majority of patients are indeed satisfied with their lives. The medical professionals' perception of the patients' self-satisfaction significantly underestimates the patients' responses.[8] Because of the inherently personal nature of the decision, information about ventilation and its consequences should be made available to patients and families early in the disease course. This will enable them to make an informed decision based on their own assessment, as opposed to their physician's assessment, of the quality of life.

Other aspects of pulmonary care include vaccination against influenza beginning at age 6 months and against *Haemophilus influenzae* and pneumococcus beginning at age 2 years.[35] During upper respiratory infections, antibiotics, chest physical therapy, postural drainage, and assisted cough with suction should be used. Supplemental oxygen might be necessary during these times. Careful monitoring of any spinal orthoses must be made to ensure that they do not impair respiratory muscle function. The orthoses can decrease VC, and consideration should be given to cutting out an anterior window to ease breathing.[40]

Contractures

Contractures are a severe problem in DMD. In a recent study of 230 patients with 11 different neuromuscular diseases, the highest percentage of contractures occurred in patients with DMD. Of these patients, 78% had ankle contractures; 67%, hip and knee; 65%, elbow; and 44%, iliotibial band (ITB) and wrist contractures.[66] Mild heel cord, ITB, and hip flexion contractures are typically present by age 6.[18] Significant contractures are rare before age 9.[90] Muscle imbalance around a specific joint is not associated with the severity of contractures present. There is an association of lower extremity and elbow flexion contractures with wheelchair reliance.[91] In 1960 Vignos and Archibald[145] described how contractures often progressed more rapidly than muscle weakness in DMD. They reported an association between lower limb contractures and loss of independent ambulation.[145] Another study, however, reports that weakness rather than contracture is the likely major cause of loss of ambulation.[90] In support of this position, McDonald and colleagues cite the finding of some rare boys with ankle plantarflexion contractures over 15 degrees prior to wheelchair reliance.[91] Nighttime use of bilateral ankle-foot orthoses (AFOs) along with a regular stretching routine has been shown to delay development of contractures of the Achilles tendon.[124] Boys who regularly wear AFOs and stretch their legs walk independently for a longer period of time, and children who do not stretch or use splints lose the ability to ambulate much earlier. Standing is described as an excellent stretching activity.[51, 124, 144] Stretching of the tensor fascia lata (TFL) is crucial. Good positioning includes lying prone to promote extension of the hip and knees.[43]

Mobility

Maintained mobility, particularly ambulation, is a focus of a good deal of attention and research in DMD. One recommendation for quantifying the difficulties of gait and predicting the decline of gait is using the double-support time.[71] The double-stance phase is a logical portion of gait to analyze because the center of gravity is in its lowest position and the body is most stable in this phase. Also, the gluteal muscles help to raise the center of mass during stance and these muscles are affected early in DMD. In this small study, the boys for whom the portion of double support was increased soon afterward lost the ability to ambulate independently, while the boys who did not have an increase in double-support time maintained their ambulation.[71]

Many attempts have been made to maximize ambulation time for boys with DMD. AFOs or ischial weight-bearing plastic knee-ankle-foot orthoses (KAFOs) are often used to maximize gait. The KAFOs are frequently used with locked knees.[40, 43, 138] Surgical intervention for contracture release has also been used to maximize and prolong ambulation. The timing for surgical intervention has been a frequent point of dispute, the concern being that surgery can prematurely halt ambulation.[9, 16, 46, 136] The commonly involved areas for surgical tendon release are the hip flexors, TFL and ITB, hamstrings, and Achilles tendons.[9, 20, 40, 43] The progression of weakness in DMD typically involves the hip girdle muscles first, with contracture of these muscles and of the Achilles tendon. This leads to difficulty in appropriately maintaining the weight line in relation to the center of gravity. This is particularly true as the extensor muscles continue to weaken and as the hamstrings contract. The TFL contracts when the patient attempts to walk with a wide-based gait to maintain balance. Usually by this time patients are in a position of hip flexion and abduction, with heel varus angulation and equinus of the foot. A compensatory increase in lumbar lordosis must occur to balance the weight line with respect to the center of gravity. The patients have to keep the weight line posterior to the hips and anterior to the knees to prevent falling. Shoulders also are weakened and the trunk becomes less stable.[43] Tendon releases are sometimes performed in an attempt to stop this cycle of contractures, worsening posture, and decreasing stability.

Contractures of the lower extremities decrease balance in standing and walking and contribute to the loss of walking ability, in conjunction with quadriceps weakness.[9, 127, 140] Bach and McKeon[9] showed that a single early procedure of tendon surgical releases with short-term intensive rehabilitation could prolong ambulation, reduce falls, and improve contractures. They found that children who were operated on while they were still ambulating well did better and were happier with their surgical results than children who were treated just prior to using, or after beginning to use, a wheelchair. Surgical release of the ITB, TFL, gluteus maximus, and hamstrings was performed, as well as Achilles tendon lengthening. Some of the children also underwent a transfer of the posterior tibial muscle to the dorsal surface of the foot. The children who had this procedure maintained active dorsiflexion of the ankle for several years. The children were up in the parallel bars and ambulating in short leg casts by the second day, and the children who had posterior tibial transfers had short leg casts for 3 to 6 weeks. Even these children had the cast bivalved after one week and began performing exercises for reeducation of the posterior tibial muscle at that time. The posterior tibial muscle is "out of phase" in this position, being asked to be a dorsiflexor. They also used stretching, general conditioning, mobility, hydrotherapy, and pool ambulation. All the children had a significant decrease in the number of falls, less lumbar lordosis and hip flexion, fewer abduction contractures, and a decrease in the width of their gait. The children who were treated at an early stage had a prolongation of their walking without bracing for approximately 1 year longer than predicted. Those who were operated on later had approximately 8 months longer walking time than expected. Bach and McKeon[9] recommend that this surgery be done while ambulation and stair climbing difficulties are minimal, and while quadriceps strength is at least antigravity, to minimize the need for bracing postoperatively. Immobilization can lead to a dramatic loss of strength and mobility. A fracture or other injury leading to immobilization can lead to loss of ambulation.[90]

Scoliosis

Scoliosis is an almost inevitable progressive problem in DMD. Between 12 and 15 years of age, there is onset of scoliosis in 50% of DMD patients. Ten percent of older DMD patients have no scoliosis.[90] The progression of scoliosis causes problems in several areas, including skin ulceration, back pain, decreased sitting balance, possible limitations on cardiopulmonary reserve, cosmetic difficulties, wheelchair seating problems, and limitations of the variety of assisted ventilation techniques that can be used.

Scoliosis progresses in patients without any spinal intervention until the time of death. The mean final scoliotic deformity has been shown to be approximately 90 degrees, with some curves greater than 100 degrees.[128, 134]

Bracing is not effective in the prevention of scoliosis or its progression.[20, 95, 128] Some bracing can be used to facilitate wheelchair seating. Scoliosis progression can require wheelchair seating alterations repeatedly as the curve progresses. For correcting the scoliosis, spinal fusion has been found to be effective. The most common procedure currently is the use of Luque rods with double sublaminar wires, unit rod fixation, and placement of bone grafts.[95, 128] The timing for surgery is based on the balance between scoliosis progression, remaining FVC, and spine growth.

The trend recently has been to operate on scoliosis earlier in an attempt to minimize the residual scoliosis left after surgical intervention, maximize seating and standing position postoperatively, and minimize respiratory complications.[40, 95, 128, 134] In one study[95] of 183 DMD patients, 91% of the children had scoliosis that reached 30 degrees before the FVC decreased to 35% of normal, and the scoliosis always progressed. In the group in whom the percentage of FVC was less than 35% before their curve reached 30 degrees, 50% developed severe deformities.[95] There was a correlation in the development of scoliosis and degree of decrease in FVC. The authors also noted that the risk of pulmonary complications during and after surgery significantly increased as the percentage of normal FVC decreased. Their recommendation was for spinal stabilization before the percentage of normal FVC is 45%, and a cutoff of 35% as the absolute minimum.[95] Other groups report FVC over 40% as ideal, with 30% as the minimum.[128] There is controversy over the impact of scoliosis surgery on future VC progression, with no hard evidence of stabilization or deterioration of VC. There is a known minimal decrease in FVC when the thoracic region is fused following fixation of the ribs.

Problems with spinal fusion include anesthesia risks, blood loss, respiratory problems, and potential neurological injury. It is important to have anesthesiologists who are familiar with the complications that can arise in a child with DMD, particularly the restrictive ventilatory limitations, MH, and potential cardiac problems. If somatosensory and motor evoked potentials are being done as intra-operative monitoring to assess spinal cord function, the anesthesiologist needs to be aware of this and adjust the medications used accordingly. There is significant blood loss during these procedures, averaging between 3400 and 3700 mL.[95, 128] Many centers are using a "cell saver" to treat and reinfuse the patient's own red blood cells during the procedure.

Mobilization should begin as quickly as possible postoperatively. Children are generally able to move about initially on the second day postoperatively. They begin in physical therapy for mobility and strengthening exercises immediately. A plastic body jacket is frequently used for sitting in a wheelchair approximately one week postoperatively and for several months afterward.[128] In the studies by Shapiro et al, none of the 27 spinal fusion patients required intubation beyond the second postoperative day,[128] whereas 11 of the 183 spinal fusion patients reported by Miller et al required more than five days of mechanical ventilation and were treated in the intensive care unit for approximately 12 days.[95] Those 11 patients had a lower FVC (32% vs. 50% of normal) than those who had no complications. Fifty percent of those with an FVC of less than 35% had pulmonary complications, with only 11% of those with an FVC greater than 35% having any pulmonary difficulties.[95]

In considering surgical intervention for scoliosis in an adult with a muscular dystrophy (not Duchenne), one must take into account the adaptations that the person makes in ambulation. Spinal fixation can later prevent some of the postural adaptations that allow patients to ambulate. This frequently occurs with destabilization of the knee joint, with subsequent inability to walk. A preoperative evaluation of this can be performed by using a firm brace around the spine to see if balance and posture are maintained.[36]

Other Complications

Other complications in DMD include osteoporosis secondary to disuse, and with it, the risk of pathological fractures. Fractures should be treated with minimal immobilization to encourage continued ambulation and mobility. Immobilization must also be avoided to prevent additional weakness due to disuse.[40]

Obesity also becomes a frequent problem once patients become nonambulatory. The change in calorie expenditure from walking to wheelchair mobility is the major contributing factor. Food sometimes becomes a substitute for decreased opportunities for activities and pleasures. The weight of DMD patients is variable, with half within normal limits, approximately a third overweight, and about 15% underweight.[40] Weight management for obesity consists of a low-calorie, well balanced diet, taking care to monitor calorie intake and output. Weight loss can become a problem in later stages, likely due to hypercatabolic protein metabolism,[90] and is most commonly reported in those 17 to 21 years old.[91, 152]

Loss of Strength

The natural history of the progression of weakness in DMD has been analyzed in an attempt to establish a baseline from which to interpret the effectiveness of early intervention. Muscle strength declines with age with a predictable pattern.[72, 125] There is a fairly steady decrease of strength with symmetrical weakness, most severe proximally and in the extensor muscles. Muscle strength, motor ability, and performance are closely correlated.[125] Neck flexor weakness is the earliest reported, often in the preschool years.[152] Ankle dorsiflexors are weaker than plantarflexors, ankle everters are weaker than inverters, hip abductors are weaker than adductors, and hip and knee extensors are weaker than flexors.[152] Some studies report that ambulation ceases when muscle strength is decreased by 50%.[125, 145] Others report that quantitative testing shows a 40 to 50% loss of strength by 6 years of age.[152] The strength levels of knee extensors and hip abductors are key in maintaining ambulation, along with the degree of contractures and the problem of maintaining balance. Treatment is directed at maintaining range of motion, strength, and the use of earlier involved muscles.[125] Knee flexor strength has been described as less than 60% of normal during the transition from ambulation to wheelchair use, which is believed to indicate that the hip and knee are passively stabilized by the patient's shifting his center of gravity.[72]

Quantitative computed tomography (CT) offers a method of quantifying muscle damage. It measures the degree of muscle fiber loss and fatty replacement using percent cross-sectional area (%CSA) of muscle and fat. The %CSA of muscle is decreased as muscle strength decreases and as disability progresses. The rate of progression varies with different muscles.[82]

A study of fatigability in boys with DMD showed that their muscle force generation was less than that in controls, but the decline in force during a sustained contraction was similar.[129]

Exercise

The effect of exercise on muscle in DMD—both its beneficial effects and possible detrimental side effects—has long been the subject of research and a source of controversy. Maintaining muscle strength requires repetitive contractions that produce tension (see Chapter 19). If the tension produced in a day is less than 20% of the maximum possible, a decrease in strength occurs.[75, 144] A major concern in trying to prevent a decrease in muscle function in DMD is that of overwork weakness.[144] Bennett and Knowlton[12] defined *overwork weakness* as a prolonged decrease in both absolute strength and endurance of a muscle. This must be differentiated from a transient decrease postexercise, as well as from progression of the muscle disease. Overwork weakness is reversible if noted early and corrected by rest.[12] Overwork weakness was first reported in myopathy in members of a family with facioscapulohumeral dystrophy. This led to an understanding that excessive overwork can have a long-term detrimental impact on muscle function.[67] Several prospective studies of prescribed daily strengthening programs for DMD patients showed no adverse effects on muscles. These studies have also shown either short-term improved strength or no significant increase in strength, but less of a decrease in strength than in controls.[30, 56, 123]

In supervised resistive exercise programs there is no negative effect on muscle in DMD. Objective increases in muscle strength are found, but these diminish as the disease advances. The pre-exercise strength level determines the amount of increase possible, with stronger muscles able to increase more. The overall gain in strength noted in DMD is the strength increase from the exercise program offset by the progression of disease and loss of strength. Patients maintaining ambulation have larger increases in strength with exercise. Exercise programs should be carried out early in the course of DMD when more relatively healthy muscle fibers are present.[144] Braddom[15] describes overwork weakness quickly occurring in muscles with 60% or less strength, with muscles of 80% or greater strength resistant to these adverse changes.

Electrical Stimulation

Low-frequency electrical stimulation (LFES) of fast-twitch muscle fibers can transform them into slow-twitch muscle fibers.[60, 121] Degenerative processes in dystrophic muscle affect fast-twitch fibers preferentially.[21] Zupan[156] stimulated muscles in DMD patients with LFES twice daily in an attempt to confer a protective effect on the muscle fibers of DMD and prevent degeneration. Half of the children in this small study had no significant changes in 3 months, and the remaining children demonstrated short-term increased strength that was greatest after 5 months of stimulation. There was no change in the level of fatigue with stimulation and no adverse effects.[156] Scott et al also found increases in maximal contractions in stimulated versus nonstimulated muscles in boys with DMD.[126] Milner-Brown and Miller[103] studied 10 children having various types of muscular dystrophies with unilateral electrical stimulation, with active weight training added in some muscles. There was a greater rate of increase with the combination of electrical stimulation and weight training, but the absolute gain of muscle strength was greater in the group with weight training alone.[103]

Muscle and Gene Research

Current areas of DMD research include myoblast implantation and gene transfer. Myoblast transfers have been attempted in patients with DMD, but without success to date.[49, 57, 58, 59] Part of the failure in these attempts can be secondary to immune rejection problems.[58, 59] Human myoblast clones are capable of fusing to form new muscle fibers and hybrid muscle fibers even after replications of more than 10 million myoblasts per clone.[59] Because only the relatively few muscle fibers injected pick up the dystrophin, attempts are underway to obtain more widespread results.[154] Pilot studies with donor myoblasts from male relatives showed slightly increased dystrophin in a minority of boys. Increased strength has been documented, although both the myoblast-implanted leg and placebo leg showed improvement; hence the increase was believed to be secondary to the use of cyclosporine.[102] The limitations of myoblast implantation include barriers to myoblast migration, cell rejection, and the inability to treat cardiac or brain deficits.[100]

Researchers are attempting gene transfers by transplanting portions of a dystrophin copy DNA (cDNA) into skeletal muscle fibers. If the dystrophin is produced, then the muscle fibers are protected from necrosis. This has been experimentally performed in animals, but it is not ready for trial in humans. If gene transfers and long-term expression of the gene product dystrophin do occur in the future, the skeletal fibers would acquire a normal phenotype. Areas under study include direct injection of dystrophin cDNA; viral vectors for transfer of a minigene of the large dystrophin gene or utrophin, a smaller, related gene; and genetic engineering of myoblasts. These myoblasts receive recombinant dystrophin cDNA and are grown in culture and then reimplanted into the patient.[100] Even if some of these do become effective for skeletal muscle, however, cardiac muscle treatment might remain problematic.[70]

Dystrophin constitutes 2% of the total sarcolemmal protein and 5% of sarcolemmal cytoskeleton protein, making it a major structural component of the cytoskeleton.[23, 88, 109] Dystrophin is associated with a large complex of glycoproteins, known as the dystrophin associated proteins (DAPs).[88] DAPs are critical in dystrophin's interaction with the cytoskeleton. DAPs are reduced in all DMD patients of any age. DAPs are missing in all muscle fibers in DMD patients but are present in other neuromuscular diseases.[88, 110] This implies that any myoblast or dystrophin gene therapy for DMD can require replacement of DAP as well as dystrophin.[88]

Hand Function

Hand function is critical in DMD because the hands are useful not only for activities of daily living (ADL), but also for assistance in mobility as the disease progresses. The Vignos scale examines overall function in patients with DMD. There is some inclusion of upper limb function, but the major emphasis is on the lower limb. The Brook Upper Limb Functional Rating Scale consists of six functional levels, where 1 represents most useful and 6 designates no useful hand function.[42] The advantage of the Brook scale is that it looks at varying muscle groups covering the spectrum of upper limb function. The Jebson Hand Function Test assesses general upper limb function and consists of six timed subtests.[65] Lower Jebson scores reflect better hand function.[62] This has been demonstrated to be useful in children with DMD.[54, 147] The Jebson scale is advantageous because it does not require expensive equipment and can provide a more constant view of the patient over the course of time. This permits one to monitor the progression of disease and the need for intervention.[65]

ADL problems in older patients with DMD typically manifest as a limited ability to pick up heavy objects, whereas fine motor ability is relatively preserved.[148] Difficulty with fine motor tasks is often secondary to proximal muscle weakness.[64] It has also been reported that the difference between the functional ability of the dominant and nondominant hand becomes more significant with age and with wheelchair use. The nondominant hand typically becomes less involved in functional activity. This might be due to needing this hand more for balance, or it could be due to a combination of causes.[54] Functional deterioration of the arms begins around age 10, with the deterioration plateauing approximately 2.2 years later.[84]

Older children with DMD exhibit some common physical abnormalities in the wrist and hand that can contribute to decreased upper limb function. These abnormalities include extrinsic and intrinsic digital muscle shortness, swan neck and boutonniere deformities, and hyperextension of the interphalangeal joints, as well as wrist flexion and ulnar deviation contractures. Decreased wrist extensor strength occurs by age 8.[147, 148] Ability to perform ADL is influenced primarily by decreased strength of wrist extensors and decreased active radial deviation.[147] The goals of therapy are to maintain optimal range of motion of the wrist, prevent wrist ulnar deviation contractures, and maintain wrist extensors strength. Therapy includes stretching exercises and positioning of the wrist and fingers. Splint use is necessary in some cases. Boys with DMD are usually able both to write and turn the pages of a book throughout their disease. Picking up or holding heavy or large objects, including filled glasses and pieces of fruit, is difficult after age 15 years. Lighter and smaller objects should gradually replace heavier objects in the older child's environment.[147] Consideration of assistive device use and teaching of work simplification for all ADL tasks can be helpful. Balanced forearm orthoses (BFOs) can be used to compensate for proximal strength deficits when distal function remains intact. Minimal elbow flexion contractures of up to 15 degrees can actually be of benefit in initiating flexion and certainly are not a detriment to ADL function.[43]

Robotic arms have also been used to assist in daily activities. The weakness in DMD is progressive, but finger movement continues throughout the course of DMD. And with a small amount of finger manipulation, it is possible to run a wheelchair-mounted robotic arm. Thus a patient can operate a power wheelchair, a computer, or an environmental control system, or do simple daily activities.[11] A wheelchair-mounted mechanical arm can be used with a control transducer that is adapted to the patient's abilities. Industrial trainer robot manipulators, which have been modified for use with batteries, can be mounted on a wheelchair lapboard. The arm can be used for eating and recreation. Some patients use a robotic arm for manipulating books and turning pages, using the telephone, opening doors, using light switches, pushing elevator buttons, and even operating electric razors. It is reported to save over 2 hours a day in attendant care time. While the cost of a robotic arm is approximately $4000,[11] a robotic arm can be invaluable in increased independence. And as these devices become more sophisticated, they will likely offer even greater benefits.

Psychosocial Management

Psychosocial management is crucial in the care of a DMD patient and his family. When a child has an incurable progressive disease, his family requires varying amounts of support from and interaction with professionals (and others) from the time of diagnosis onward. Grief in the family tends to wax and wane with disease exacerbations, dramatic changes in the child's functional ability, and at other stressful times. It is important for physicians to anticipate medical changes and deterioration and to prepare the family for them. For example, the family should be prepared for such changes as using a wheelchair and ventilatory assistance—both of which are highly predictable occurrences.[40] Boys in the early stages of DMD often have a great deal of anxiety, along with fear of falling. Later there is a tendency toward social withdrawal, frustration, and anxiety secondary to a fear of dying.[43] Counseling services should be available for the children and families throughout the lifetime of the boys, and beyond that for the parents. Proper school placement can be extremely helpful in this regard. Communication should be facilitated with the school and the teachers, and therapy needs clearly delineated. Consideration should also be given to the fact that, as a group, DMD boys have lower intelligence quotients and approximately one-third are mentally retarded.[43, 54] Thus, many require special classes or tutoring.

Becker's Muscular Dystrophy

Becker's muscular dystrophy (BMD) is a milder variant of DMD and is caused by a mutation of the same gene as that in DMD.[155] It is a slowly progressive X-linked recessive disorder and has an incidence of approximately 1 in 50,000 live male births. The onset of weakness generally manifests between 10 and 15 years of age. Motor milestones are met, but the pattern of weakness follows that in DMD, although to a much milder degree, with a better prognosis. Pseudohypertrophy of the calves is commonly seen.[107] The presentation of BMD is much more variable than DMD, with variable age of onset, progression, distribution, and severity of muscle involvement[155] (Fig. 48–2). Some boys have a restricted area of weakness, mimicking metabolic or other myopathies.[103]

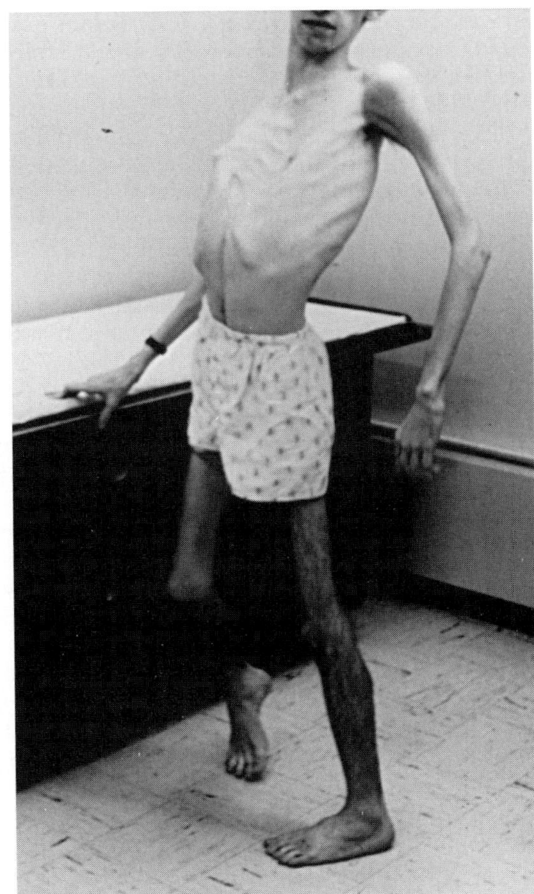

FIGURE 48–2. A 25-year-old man with Becker's muscular dystrophy demonstrating generalized atrophy, with calf pseudohypertrophy and difficulty in mobility. (Photograph courtesy of R. Braddom, M.D.)

Associated findings in BMD include cardiac disease, which can be noted at an early age or during adulthood. It is unrelated to the degree of musculoskeletal weakness. ECG changes identical to these in DMD are found in 45% of BMD patients, while 17% have echocardiagram changes consistent with a dilated cardiomyopathy.[155] In some patients cardiac failure is the presenting symptom.[34]

An elevated CK is noted in BMD, but it is usually lower than in boys with DMD.[34] Needle EMG can show primarily symmetrical changes in the proximal limb muscles, including positive waves, fibrillations, and CRDs. Paraspinal muscles can demonstrate CRDs earlier than limb muscles. Motor unit potentials (MUPs) generally are small, polyphasic, and have early recruitment.[73] Muscle biopsy shows an abnormal quantity and quality of dystrophin, but not as severe as in DMD.[107] Dystrophin levels are at least 5% or more of normal.[34]

The clinical course of BMD is similar to that of DMD, though it is milder, with later onset, and is more variable. Proximal weakness leads to difficulties in walking, climbing stairs, and rising from the floor. Contractures can develop late in the disease. Myocardial disease usually (but not always) presents in later years. Survival is generally into middle adulthood.[73] In mild cases a patient can live to 60 years of age, while in more severe cases death can occur in the 20s.[15]

Since the course of BMD is milder than that of DMD, the treatment is less aggressive. Medications are not used except in those persons with the most severe form of the disease. Steroids pose more of a problem than in DMD because of the side effect of stunted growth. (BMD patients and their families are usually not concerned about stunted growth). AFOs for ambulation and a wheelchair for mobility can become necessary as the disease progresses. Stretching to prevent contractures is important as independent mobility declines. Surgical treatment of severe contractures can be helpful when they interfere with gait or posture. Patients with BMD can gain significant increases in muscle strength, endurance, and work capacity with a weight training program.[104]

Facioscapulohumeral Dystrophy

Facioscapulohumeral dystrophy (FSH) is an autosomal dominant myopathy with complete penetrance but variable expressivity. There can be a spectrum of mild to severe cases within the same family.[16, 107] There is typically a normal life span. The incidence is approximately

3 to 10 cases per million.[16] When FSH is first noted in infancy, its course is more severe.[107] The age of onset is generally in the second decade, but can be later. A common presentation is facial weakness at approximately 15 years of age, with facial and proximal weakness progressing very slowly. The molecular defect is linked to chromosome 4q35 markers.[143]

The weakness is generally present in the face, shoulder girdle, and anterior portion of the leg[107] (Fig. 48–3). Facial weakness causes an inability to whistle, drink through a straw, and blow up a balloon. During sleep the eyes can remain open. Proximal upper limb muscles are weak; often patients are unable to hold heavy objects or lift above the shoulders, climb a rope, or perform a pushup. The hip musculature gradually weakens and drop foot can eventually occur. This progression usually occurs over decades. The face is characteristically smooth and unlined. There is loss of contour of the mouth with a horizontal appearance of the lower lip and a pouting expression of the lips. Neck muscles are often weak. The triceps and biceps brachii can be weak early, but the deltoid is relatively preserved, as are the forearm and the wrist flexor muscles. Wrist drop can be present. Hip weakness can lead to compensatory lumbar lordosis. The calf muscles are generally preserved to a greater degree than the dorsiflexors of the ankle, with a resultant drop foot. Limb weakness can be asymmetrical and reflexes can be decreased.[16]

There are no ECG or echocardiographic abnormalities, or any rhythm disturbances in FSH.[146] In some patients there is congenital absence of the pectoralis, biceps, and brachioradialis muscles.[73] Nerve deafness is associated with the infantile onset of FSH.[16]

In FSH the CK is elevated two to four times normal in 50% of the patients. The needle EMG is myopathic with fibrillations and repetitive discharges occasionally seen.[107] Early needle EMG in FSH can be normal even in clinically involved muscles. Later on, the motor units become small, polyphasic, and show increased recruitment relative to effort.[73] The biopsy in FSH usually shows an increased variability in the size of fibers, with small fibers called tiny fibers. Additionally there can be a moth-eaten appearance to the fibers.[16]

Treatment is focused on assistance in ADL with hand or foot orthoses (see Chapters 15 and 16). There has been concern about overwork weakness, as this was described in three generations of a family with FSH who had physical examination abnormalities and needle EMG changes in their most frequently used arms.[67] Subsequently, several studies have examined the effect of an exercise program on patients with FSH, looking at the possibility of muscle strength improvement and conversely, muscle damage. There is a lack of consensus regarding statistically significant improvement in muscle strength following exercise.[2, 89, 104] The studies show, however, that carefully supervised strength-training programs with a gradual increase in activity does not cause damage to the muscle or increase weakness.[2, 89, 104]

Some patients with FSH gradually develop scapular instability secondary to weakness of the scapular stabilizing muscles. Because of this, they cannot flex or abduct the arm. If they have deltoid and supraspinatus muscle sparing, they might be able to abduct the arm if the scapula is stabilized. In assessing the potential effectiveness of scapular surgical fixation to the thorax, a preoperative assessment can include manually holding

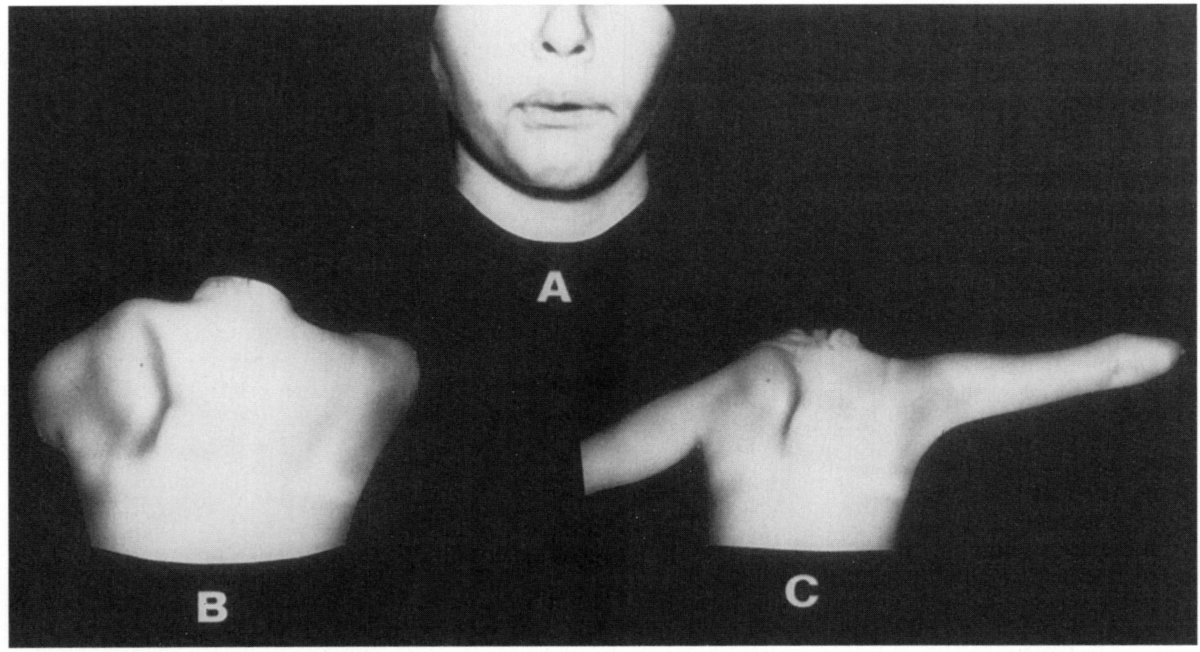

FIGURE 48–3. An 18-year-old woman with facioscapulohumeral muscular dystrophy demonstrating an inability to purse the lips (*A*) and winging of the left scapula (*B* and *C*). The patient is left-hand dominant. (From Johnson EW, Braddom R: Over-work weakness in facioscapulohumeral muscular dystrophy. Arch Phys Med Rehabil 1971; 52:333–336.)

the scapula stable bilaterally while the patient attempts to raise the arm above the head. If the patient can do so, it predicts that the stabilizing operation would be helpful. If weakness continues to preclude this maneuver, the surgery is unlikely to improve the patient's function.[36] Following surgery, isometric deltoid exercises are performed, with pendulum exercises and strengthening of the shoulder muscles. Preoperative strength has been noted to return within six months of surgery. Active shoulder abduction can be improved by approximately 60 degrees.[22] This often leads to an improvement in the strength needed to lift and carry objects.[22] There might, however, be a decrease in VC secondary to immobilization of the ribs.

FSH patients can have weak eye closure and drying of the sclera. This can be uncomfortable and also lead to conjunctivitis or even ulceration. Artificial tears can control this problem; but if artificial tears prove ineffective, plastic surgery should be considered. If FSH facial weakness leads to severe weakness of the mouth, there might be difficulties with eating, drinking, and cosmetic appearance. Plastic surgery can often alleviate these difficulties.[36]

Limb-Girdle Dystrophy

Limb-girdle dystrophy (LGD) is a group of disorders producing weakness about the hips and shoulders. It can be either autosomal recessive or dominant. LGD is a less well-defined myopathy which actually represents a heterogeneous spectrum of diseases. Genetic linkage studies have shown at least 12 different loci and gene products have been identified for five genes.[151] Sarcoglycan gene mutations have been identified in four forms of LGD.[80] The weakness most commonly begins in the second or third decade and affects the hips first, and then the shoulders. In later years there can be progression to involve other muscle groups. It has been reported as rarely involving only one limb. Facial muscles are generally spared.[73]

Associated findings can include cardiopulmonary difficulties, although cardiac conduction defects are rare. Intellect is normal.[16] Death can occur from cardiopulmonary complications, including pneumonia.[16]

Laboratory findings show an increase in CK and lactic dehydrogenase. The increase is generally mild, but can be up to 10 times normal. Needle EMG shows small-amplitude polyphasic MUPs of short duration and, rarely, CRDs. Muscle biopsy shows variation in fiber size with increased internal nuclei, fiber splitting, and "moth-eaten," whorled fibers.[16]

The clinical course is varied but classically is described as beginning with hip weakness (flexors and extensors), quickly followed by shoulder weakness. There also can be weakness of both neck flexors and extensors. Shoulder weakness includes the deltoid muscle. There is dramatic weakness and frequently atrophy of the biceps brachii[16] (Fig. 48–4).

Ventilatory assistance, including intermittent positive or negative pressure ventilation, can be helpful in the treatment of LGD.[36] A monitored strength training program has been shown to have no adverse effects and, in some cases, shows an increase in strength, at least for the short term.[2, 89, 104]

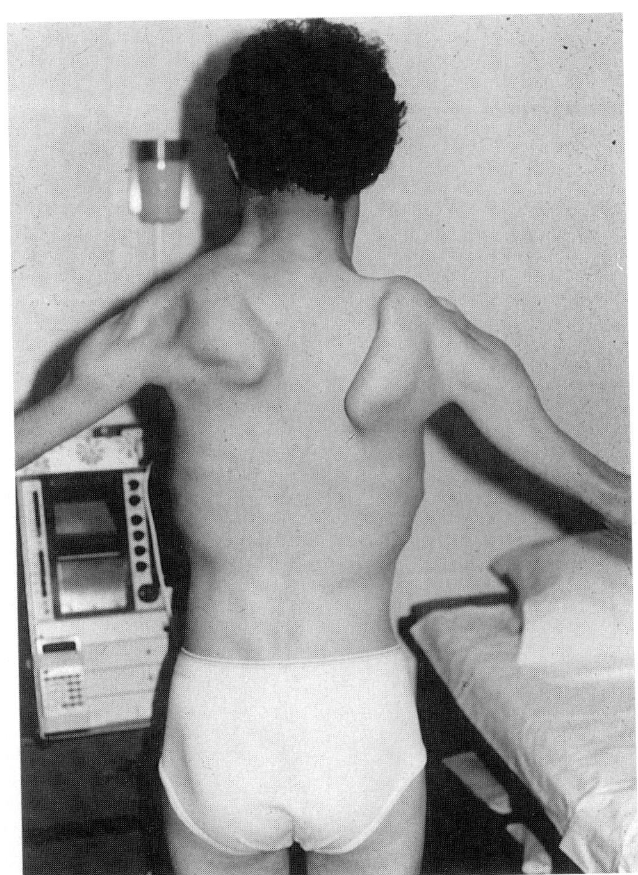

FIGURE 48–4. A 35-year-old man with limb girdle muscular dystrophy demonstrating shoulder weakness, including deltoid and biceps brachii atrophy. (Photograph courtesy of R. Braddom, M.D.)

Myotonic Dystrophy

Myotonic muscular dystrophy (MMD) is an autosomal dominant disease with a prevalence of 3 to 5 per 100,000, with complete penetrance but variable expression.[16, 107] The incidence is 13 per 100,000 live births.[16] In MMD there is progressive muscle weakness (generally worse distally) and atrophy with characteristic involvement of facial, jaw, anterior neck, and distal limb muscles, as well as myotonia. *Myotonia* is defined as a delayed relaxation of muscle contraction. Patients generally interpret myotonia as muscle stiffness. This can be worsened by cold. Patients with MMD frequently minimize or deny their weakness and myotonia. The onset of weakness is generally gradual in late teenage years or early adulthood. Distal muscle weakness is generally symmetrical and slowly progressive. A long face and slightly nasal voice[16] are often noted early in the course (Fig. 48–5). Patients with MMD can complain of muscle stiffness or cramps, but weakness of the feet and hands is usually their first complaint.[16] Myotonia of the muscle can be present with percussion, although this tends to decrease as the weakness progresses. The myotonic phenomenon

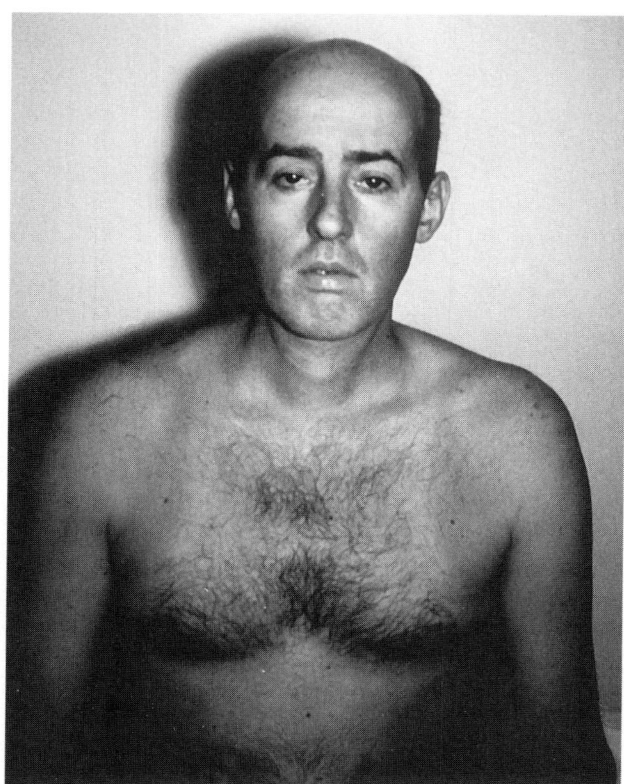

FIGURE 48–5. An adult man with myotonic dystrophy demonstrating an elongated face and balding. (Photograph courtesy of R. Braddom, M.D.)

can be elicited by striking the abductor pollicis brevis with a reflex hammer, which causes the thumb to move across the palm.[15]

MMD is described as a multisystem disease because of the many associated findings. Cataracts are noted in over 90% of patients, with characteristic multicolored lens opacities which are specific in the early stages. This can be noted by the early teenage years. Weak uterine contractions have been noted.[107] Smooth muscle abnormalities are also present which can cause dilation of the esophagus.[107] There is an increase in gallbladder problems.[16] Weakness in the bowel musculature can cause significant problems with constipation.[36]

Cardiac abnormalities in MMD include cardiomyopathy and conduction defects.[36, 107] Cardiac conduction disturbances are present in one-half to two-thirds of patients.[107] A pacemaker can be useful when the bundle of His is involved. Death can be due to sudden cardiac arrhythmia.[107] Arrhythmias and mitral valve prolapse are increased in MMD. Since an abnormal exercise response of the left ventricle has been reported in MMD patients, any exercise program should be closely prescribed and monitored.[16]

Males with MMD have degeneration of testicular tubular cells with low sperm formation and low testosterone levels. In females variable abnormalities are present including amenorrhea and menstrual irregularities. Infertility is common in MMD patients of both sexes.[107, 130] Glucose intolerance with hyperinsulinemia and a defect in insulin receptors are common, but there is no increased incidence of diabetes.[16, 107] Increased denial of abnormalities has been noted in patients with MMD, along with frequent mild mental retardation.[16]

Infants born to mothers having MMD can have a much more severe form of MMD; this form, which is present at birth, is called congenital myotonic dystrophy. Presumably, it is due to an intrauterine influence that is not strictly genetic (possibly a cell membrane change). In this group there is mental retardation as well as respiratory difficulties and motor delay.[130] In congenital MMD there is hypotonia and facial paralysis with the upper lip having an inverted V appearance (Fig. 48–6). Clubfeet and frequent respiratory infections are also common.[16]

Some MMD patients have a sleep disturbance, which is believed to be secondary to pulmonary hypoventilation. There is also an increased pulmonary risk associated with general anesthesia, and with use of barbiturates and other medications that depress respiratory drive.[16]

Evaluation of MMD patients typically shows facial weakness as described above, as well as weakness of the hands and feet. Percussion myotonia is present, and a slow handshake release can be the first indication of MMD. Needle EMG shows myotonic discharges that wax and wane in amplitude and frequency. The sound

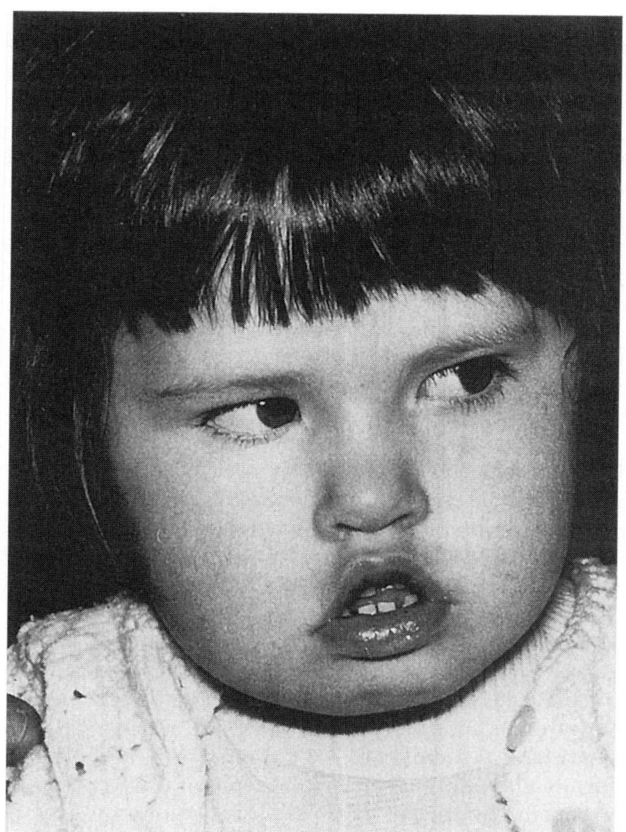

FIGURE 48–6. A toddler with facial paralysis and inverted-V appearance of the lip in congenital myotonic dystrophy. (From Eagel AG, Franzihi-Armstrong C (eds): Myology: Basic and Clinical, ed 2. New York, McGraw-Hill, 1994.)

is often described as similar to a dive bomber or motorcycle. There can also be brief, small polyphasic potentials[16] (see Chapters 10–12). CK is generally increased. Muscle biopsy shows internal nuclei and atrophy of type I fibers. The biceps brachii muscle tends to show more abnormalities on biopsy than the quadriceps or gastrocnemius muscles.[16] The myotonic dystrophy gene is on chromosome 19.[130] There is an unstable CTG trinucleotide repeat at 19q13.3.[150] The severity of the disease is typically related to the number of these repeats, which can be measured by a genetics laboratory. Some MMD families also show the genetic phenomenon of "anticipation," in which each succeeding generation tends to be clinically worse than the previous generation.

Treatment for patients with MMD includes orthoses for distal weakness, including AFOs or wrist-hand orthoses. When myotonia is a severe functional problem, medications can be tried to stabilize the muscle membranes. Quinine and procainamide have been used, although they can depress cardiac conduction. Phenytoin (Dilantin) can also be used, with less risk of cardiac conduction problems. Calcium channel blockers and carbamazepine (Tegretol) can also be used.[16, 107] As weakness is generally a more severe problem than myotonia, the success of these medications is variable and many patients choose not to use them.[16]

In attempting to demonstrate the cause of myotonia, Taylor et al[141] studied contractility measurements. They demonstrated that MMD patients had a failure of sarcolemmal activation, failure of contractile machinery, and altered excitation-contraction coupling mechanisms.[141] Some believe this is secondary to problems in membrane chloride conductance.

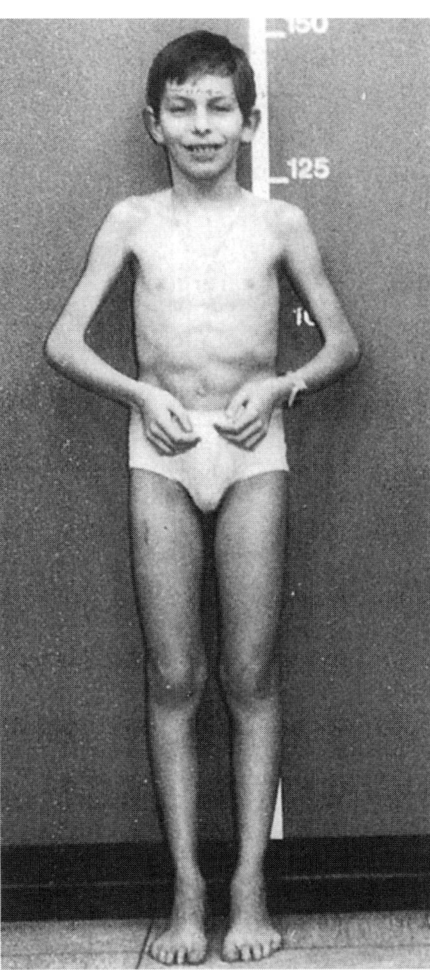

FIGURE 48–7. A 13-year-old boy with Emery-Dreifuss muscular dystrophy showing bilateral elbow flexion contractures and shoulder girdle atrophy. (From Eagel AG, Franzihi-Armstrong C (eds): Myology: Basic and Clinical, ed 2. New York, McGraw-Hill, 1994.)

Emery-Dreifuss Muscular Dystrophy

Emery-Dreifuss muscular dystrophy (EDMD) is an X-linked recessive dystrophy with a classic triad of findings. These include (1) early contractures, particularly of the elbows, Achilles tendon, and posterior cervical muscles; (2) cardiac conduction defects; and (3) a slowly progressive weakness and atrophy in a humeroperoneal distribution.[33, 38, 94] The incidence is estimated to be 1 in 100,000, but is not well defined.[47] This disorder is believed to be a slowly progressive myopathy, but the disease spectrum includes patients whose disease is much more severe. Some are unable to walk by the time they reach adulthood,[103, 121] but survival is generally into middle age.[60] Cardiomyopathy can present with heart block, frequently in late teenage or the early twenties, and all adult patients with EDMD have this disorder. Early signs are bradycardia and a prolonged PR interval on the ECG. Cardiac pacemakers are typically inserted as soon as the diagnosis is made.[133] The severity of the cardiac disease is much greater than the myopathy.[94] The early onset of contractures before the onset of any significant weakness is unique to this disease (Fig. 48–7). The elbows are generally held in a semiflexed position, and the child typically begins walking on tiptoe. The limitation of neck flexion is infrequently noticed except on specific physical examination.[38] There are also contractures of other ligaments, including the metacarpals and other smaller joints.[16]

In EDMD the CK is normal or moderately increased. Needle EMG is usually myopathic, although a more neurogenic pattern with high-amplitude, long-duration MUPs is combined in some patients.[30] Muscle biopsy is myopathic with type I predominance and atrophy.[16] The gene responsible for EDMD is on Xq28.33. The gene product is a nuclear protein, emerin.[108] Dystrophin is normal in EDMD.[33]

Treatment is primarily focused on the cardiac disease, with a pacemaker being the typical form of treatment. Bracing can also be helpful as the disease progresses. Early frequent range-of-motion exercise and positioning are also advisable.

CONGENITAL MYOPATHIES

The congenital myopathies are a group of nonprogressive or slowly progressive myopathies presenting with hypotonia or weakness in the neonatal period. These babies frequently have decreased spontaneous movement and delayed motor milestone achievement. Their muscles can feel flabby to palpation. Physical anomalies such as high palate, pectus excavatum, elongated face, and scoliosis can be present as an indication of long-standing weakness[14] (Table 48–3).

Central Core Myopathy

Central core myopathy (CCM) is an autosomal dominant myopathy with the gene involved located on the long arm of chromosome 19 at 19Q13.1. This is in the same area of the chromosome as the gene for MH, which can also be seen in CCM.[17]

The child with CCM is floppy at or shortly after birth, with frequent congenital hip dislocation. The milestones are delayed, although weakness never becomes a severe problem. The child is frequently clumsy, slender, and short. The diffuse weakness typically includes the face and neck, as well as the extremities. Reflexes are normal or decreased.[17] Skeletal deformities can be present, including lordosis, kyphoscoliosis, and clubfeet. The children generally are unable to jump.[16] There is relative sparing of the bulbar muscles. Significant muscle atrophy is not seen.[14]

The CK level is usually normal. Needle EMG shows small-amplitude, short-duration, polyphasic MUPs.[14, 17] Single-fiber EMG shows abnormalities due to an increased number of fibers innervated per anterior horn cell.[14] Biopsy shows a type I fiber predominance with central cores (unstained central area running through the center of the fibers) present in type I and some type II fibers.[14, 16, 17] Electron microscopy shows an absence of mitochondria in the central core.[16, 73] The disease course is very mild and the life span is normal. The weakness is generally so mild that no specific treatment is usually needed. If there is significant weakness, bracing can be helpful in some patients.

Patients with CCM have an increased risk of MH, as do their family members. This must be considered in any patient who is to undergo surgery.[14, 16, 17] MH is present in 1 per 15,000 anesthetic cases and is believed to be inherited in an autosomal dominant manner. Patients with MH (but with no other identifiable diseases) can demonstrate a subclinical weakness, CK elevation, and nonspecific muscle biopsy changes.

Nemaline Myopathy

Nemaline myopathy (NM) is a congenital myopathy that is distinguished by small, rodlike particles on muscle biopsy. These are noted on trichrome stain, with major components of the rod including actinin and desmin. The gene is located on the long arm of chromosome 1.[17, 18] There is an autosomal dominant pattern of inheritance with reduced penetrance and variable expressivity.[14]

In NM, hypotonia with diffuse mild weakness of the extremities and facial muscles with frequent dysmorphic appearance is noted. The face can be long and narrow with an abnormal mandible.[17] Facial muscle weakness often results in poor suck and swallow.[14] Clubfeet and kyphoscoliosis are present.[14] A more severe form of NM can arise which involves the respiratory muscles to a greater degree. This can actually cause death in young adulthood from respiratory failure. Cardiomyopathy is also present in severely affected patients.[17] The disease, however, is believed to be slowly progressive in the large majority of patients. The disease severity on presentation indicates the severity of the clinical course.[14]

In most chidren with NM, the disease is diagnosed before the age of 1 year. Walking occurs late, averaging 19 months, with a waddling gait evident in most children from their first step. There are frequent falls and Gower's maneuver is present. A nasal voice is observed in all children with NM. During preschool, two-thirds of the children are susceptible to respiratory infections; some require hospitalizations.

CK is normal to mildly elevated and needle EMG shows a nonspecific myopathic pattern.[16, 17, 73] The muscle biopsy reveals type I fiber predominance (up to 90%) as well as selective type I fiber atrophy and nemaline rods.[14, 16, 17, 73] The rods contain Z-band muscle fiber material and are noted in all involved muscles, including cardiac muscle. They are more prevalent at the periphery of muscle fibers.[14] The rods are not specific to NM and can be seen in unrelated diseases.[14, 16, 73]

Treatment includes appropriate bracing for weakness and limb function, surgery for severe skeletal anomalies, and close follow-up and treatment of cardiomyopathy. Respiratory care must be diligent, particularly during times of pulmonary infection. Therapy for improving strength, ADL, range of motion, and endurance is useful, and work simplification is important. Assistive devices such as AFOs and some hand orthoses can be useful. Wheelchairs are required for some patients. Early therapy for feeding assistance is helpful.[149]

Myotubular (Centronuclear) Myopathy

Myotubular (centronuclear) myopathy (MTM) is a congenital myopathy with two distinct forms. The first form is autosomal recessive and has delayed motor milestones and hypotonia, with weakness beginning early in life. There is also ptosis, ophthalmoplegia, slowly progressive weakness, generalized facial weakness, and equinovarus. Seizures can be present.[14, 17] This form is variable in severity.[26] Patients survive into adulthood with minimal motor deficits.[73]

The second form of MTM is an X-linked recessive disorder that leads to early respiratory failure. There is severe weakness of the face, poor suck and swallow, and weak neck muscles, but ptosis is not severe.[13, 16] The X-linked form has an 80% fatality rate in the first year,[14, 17] and there is also an increased incidence of spontaneous abortions and stillbirths.[29] Ventilatory support can decrease the early deaths. The gene is located on the long arm of the X chromosome.[14, 17]

In both forms of MTM, CK is normal or slightly elevated.[14, 16, 17, 73] Needle EMG can show low-amplitude polyphasic MUPs as well as fibrillations, positive sharp waves, and CRDs. Myotonic discharges can also be present.[4, 73] The muscle biopsy shows increased central nuclei with increased staining of the fiber with oxidative

TABLE 48–3 Congenital Myopathies

Types	Genetics	Course	Associated Findings	Biopsy	Electrodiagnostics	Laboratory Studies
Central core myopathy	AD Chromosome 19	Mild Normal life span	Frequent CDH MH	Type I predominance Unstained central areas	Small-amplitude polyphasics	CK normal
Nemaline myopathy	AD Chromosome 1	Slowly progressive	Respiratory muscles abnormal Cardiomyopathy	Small rodlike particles, more peripheral Type I fiber predominance and atrophy	Small-amplitude polyphasics	CK normal to mild increase
Myotubular (centronuclear) myopathy	AR XLR	AR—varies XLR—early death; 80% in first year	AR—seizures, ptosis XLR—severe respiratory disease	Internal nuclei Type I fiber predominance	Small-amplitude polyphasics, CRDs, fibrillations, positive sharp waves, myotonic discharges	CK normal to mild increase
Congenital fiber disproportion	Varied reports of AD, AR, or sporadic	Improves after weakness first 2 yr	Frequent CDH Short height and low weight	Small type I fibers Increased percentage of type I fibers	Small-amplitude polyphasics	CK normal to mild increase

Abbreviations: CDH, congenital dysplasia of hip; MH, malignant hyperthermia; CK, creatine kinase; CRDs, complex repetitive discharges; AD, autosomal dominant; AR, autosomal recessive; XLR, X-linked recessive.

enzymes, and a pale area centrally with adenosine triphosphatase (ATPase) reactions. There is type I fiber predominance.[16, 17, 73] The large plump nucleus in the center of many fibers resembles the fetal myotube stage.[17] An electroencephalogram (EEG) typically shows paroxysmal abnormalities in the patient with the autosomal form.[17]

Treatment is variable, depending on the type of MTM. Antiseizure medication is important for patients with the autosomal recessive form. Ventilatory assistance is important for survival in patients with the X-linked type of MTM. Therapy and bracing can be helpful, depending on the extent of weakness and deficits.

Congenital Fiber Disproportion

In congenital fiber type disproportion (CFTD), no classic structural abnormalities are noted, but there is abnormalities in the size of muscle fibers and fiber type predominance. In normal muscles, type I fibers make up 30% to 40% of the fibes, with type II constituting 60%. The sizes of the type I and II fibers are normally comparable. In CFTD, the type I fibers are at least 15% smaller than the type II fibers, with type II fibers having a more uniform size than type I.[14, 16, 73] It has recently been proposed that the difference should actually be greater than 45% in size between type I and II fibers, along with greater than 75% of the fibers being type I.[17]

Children with CFTD present with floppiness at birth, with weakness most severe in the first two years. The weakness subsequently improves or stabilizes. There are delayed motor milestones. Congenital hip dislocation is frequent and other skeletal abnormalities are frequently seen. The patients are short and frequently have low weight as well. Congnitive function is intact.[14, 16, 17, 73] The proximal muscles are more involved than the distal, but weakness is generally mild to moderate. Reflexes can be decreased or absent.[16] Respiratory infections and complications are common in the first two years of life.[14, 17] CK is normal or mildly elevated and needle EMG is myopathic.[14, 16, 17]

Treatment emphasizes respiratory care, particularly in the first two years of life. Subsequently therapy and bracing are used depending on individual patient status. Range of motion and stretching exercises are advisable early in the disease course because of the potential for contractures.

Over time the children demonstrate a decrease in muscle bulk, an onset of foot deformities and scoliosis. Patients often require some assistance with ADL, ranging from requiring help with heavy lifting to complete dependence.[149]

METABOLIC MYOPATHIES

There are a variety of myopathies that are secondary to metabolic abnormalities. Ten glycogen storage diseases have been well described, with four demonstrating significant muscle involvement: types II, III, V, and VII[73] (Table 48–4).

The glycogen storage diseases present in one of two ways. One is with progressive muscle weakness, as in acid maltase deficiency and debranching enzyme deficiency. The other presentation is with exertional cramps and myalgias, as in muscle phosphorylase deficiency (McArdle's disease).[99, 107]

Muscle Phosphorylase Deficiency (Type V Glycogenosis, McArdle's Disease)

Muscle phosphorylase deficiency (McArdle's disease) presents in a heterogeneous manner. Muscle phosphorylase normally makes the hexose sugar available from the glycogen chain so it can be used for metabolism and glycolysis. Glycogen is normally used during intensive short-term exercise.[16] Without this enzyme a person cannot use glycogen as an energy source. In McArdle's disease there is exercise intolerance, easy fatigability, and stiffness of the exercised muscles.[16, 73, 99, 115] Patients have symptoms brought on by bursts of exercise, the amount of which varies between patients and in the same patient over time. There also can be episodes of myoglobinuria and cramping after exercise. This cramping can proceed to the hallmark of full contracture with electrical silence.[16, 99]

McArdle's disease is generally inherited in an autosomal recessive manner, although some persons have an autosomal dominant form. This disease is more frequent in males than females, with a ratio of 3 : 1.[107] The disease is genetically heterogeneous, the most common mutation being a substitution of thymine for cytosine at codon 49. Thus, 90% of patients can be diagnosed from their leukocytes, avoiding the need for muscle biopsy.[142] There no other organs primarily involved in McArdle's disease, but renal involvement can occur secondary to myoglobinuria.[16]

Physical findings vary with age, but are typically normal between episodes. Proximal muscle weakness might develop late in the disease. Reflexes are normal.[16] CK is elevated at rest in more than 90% of patients,[99] and needle EMG frequently shows fibrillations and positive waves, as well as polyphasic MUPs. During a contracture episode the needle EMG shows no electrical activity, in contrast to the appearance of ordinary cramped muscle, which is very active. Repetitive nerve stimulation at 20 Hz can show a marked decremental response.[73, 99] The ischemic forearm exercise test (forearm muscles are exercised using an inflated cuff around the arm) is also abnormal in these patients. In normal muscles, venous lactate levels increase secondary to glycogen breakdown under ischemic conditions. In McArdle's disease there is no rise because patients cannot catabolize glycogen.[73, 99, 107]

Muscle biopsy typically shows excessive glycogen in vacuoles in the subsarcolemmal region. There is a variability of fiber size with degenerating and regenerating fibers noted.[99, 107] The histochemical reaction for phosphorylase is absent except in blood vessel walls and regenerating fibers.[99, 107] A biochemical test for phosphorylase shows no activity or up to 10% of normal activity.[99]

TABLE 48–4 Metabolic Myopathies

Types	Enzyme Abnormality	Muscle Presentation	Laboratory Studies	Lactate Response to Ischemic Exercise Test	Associated Findings	Genetics	Treatment
Type V (McArdle's disease)	Phosphorylase	Exertional cramps and myalgias	CK increased	No rise	Myoglobinuria	Generally AR; more males	Use of "second wind" with timing of exercise with rest High fructose diet
Type VII	Phosphofructokinase	Exertional cramps and myalgias	CK increased	No rise	Hemolysis Gout Jaundice Reticulocytosis Nausea and vomiting	AR	Gradual exercise and rest
Type II	Acid maltase	Muscle weakness; three forms—vary	CK increased	Able to utilize glycogen; increase	Three varieties: infantile (Pompe's disease)—fatal in first 2 years due to cardiac respiratory disease	AR	None
Type III	Debranching enzyme deficiency	Muscle weakness	CK increased	No rise	Hepatomagaly Cardiac disease	AR	Small, frequent meals

Abbreviations: CK, creatine kinase; AR, autosomal recessive.

McArdle's disease is usually first noticed late in the first decade when the child complains of fatigue and is unable to keep up with peers. In early adolescence there is typically mild aching of the legs, which increases in severity and gradually is produced by less vigorous activity. During the teenage years, painful cramps after exercise are noted which can last for hours. There is myoglobinuria after these episodes and the muscle pain can gradually become more severe. In later years there can be permanent proximal muscle weakness.[16] Approximately 25% of the patients have an episode of renal failure secondary to myoglobinuria.[99] "Second wind" is used by patients to increase their tolerance of activity. The patients rest immediately when they note muscle fatigue at the beginning of exercise. Taking a brief rest after first noting myalgia or muscle stiffness allows them to resume exercise at a somewhat lower level. This enables them to exercise for a longer period of time at an increased comfort level.[6, 99, 115]

Treatment for patients with McArdle's disease is through use of the second wind phenomenon and careful timing of exercise and rest. A graduated exercise program with aerobic activity is helpful. Some patients benefit from a high-fructose diet.[99]

Phosphofructokinase Deficiency

Phosphofructokinase deficiency glycogenosis (type VII, PFKD) is an autosomal recessive disease with symptoms closely resembling McArdle's disease. The episodic exercise-induced symptoms are similar to those of McArdle's disease except that they are frequently associated with nausea and vomiting. Permanent weakness generally does not occur.[99, 107] Gout may be a complication of PFKD.[99] There can be episodes of hemolysis and jaundice, with decreased erythrocyte survival time and a peripheral blood reticulocytosis.[99] CK, needle EMG, muscle biopsy, and glycogen accumulation are much like those in McArdle's disease. The diagnosis of PFKD can be made by direct measurement of muscle phosphofructokinase activity.[107] Three gene mutations have been identified in Ashkenazi Jews, with no correlation between specific mutations and symptoms. Male patients were found to be more symptomatic than female patients.[132] A molecular diagnosis is now possible to screen for the known allele mutations, which account for 95% of patients.[116] No treatment has been described, but the gradual exercise with intermittent rest, as in McArdle's disease, can be utilized.

Acid Maltase Deficiency

Acid maltase deficiency (type II glycogenosis, AMD) is an autosomal recessive disease that can occur in three different forms. In the first or infantile form (Pompe's disease), children have severe hypotonia which develops shortly after birth. These children die in the first 2 years from cardiac or respiratory failure. Abnormal glycogen deposition results in an enlarged tongue, heart, and liver.[73, 99, 107] The second or childhood-onset type produces proximal limb and trunk weakness with motor milestone delay. The liver and tongue can be enlarged. There is respiratory muscle involvement and death occurs approximately by age 20.[73, 99, 107] In the third or adult variety of AMD, there is a slow progression of proximal weakness beginning in the third or fourth decade. Bulbar musculature is spared, as are the heart and liver.[73, 99, 107] Respiratory failure is seen in one-third of the adults, with the diaphragm selectively involved. Pulmonary hypertension can also be present.[95]

The CK is elevated in AMD and needle EMG shows increased insertional activity with fibrillations and positive sharp waves, as well as complex repetitive discharges.[73, 107] There are small brief polyphasic MUPs with early recruitment, and myotonic discharges. Electrodiagnostic abnormalities can be more frequent in proximal muscles and lower paraspinal muscles.[73, 99] The ECG is abnormal in the infantile form of AMD with depressed ST segments and inverted T waves, along with a shortened PR interval. Acid maltase activity is deficient in all muscles, even those that are relatively clinically spared.[16] Prenatal diagnosis is available by fetal cell culturing, which shows absence of enzyme activity.[16, 99] There is an absence of lysosomal alpha-glucosidase in patients. Two mutations are frequently found in this group, a deletion of exon 18 and a single base pair deletion of delta T525.[74] Muscle biopsy shows abundant vacuoles with high glycogen content, affecting type I more than type II fibers.[73, 99, 107] Glycogen and glucose in AMD are utilized normally by muscles, unlike the other glycogen storage diseases.[99] Treatment with specific diet or medications has not been found to be effective.[99, 107]

Debranching Enzyme Deficiency

Debranching enzyme deficiency (type III glycogenosis, DED) is an autosomal recessive glycogen storage disease. The breakdown of glycogen in these patients can occur only in the outer straight glycosyl chains, so that glycogen with short branched outer chains accumulates in muscle and liver tissues.[73] Infants are hypotonic with proximal weakness noted.[73, 99] Hepatomegaly is present secondary to glycogen accumulation and there can be episodes of hypoglycemia.[73, 107] Symptoms tend to improve around puberty with myopathy appearing in adulthood and progressing as proximal muscle weakness. Some adult patients can have heart disease along with hepatomegaly.[107]

CK is elevated in DED. The forearm ischemic exercise test shows no increase in venous lactate.[99, 107] Despite this finding, there is no severe exercise intolerance or cramping.[99] EMG can show fibrillations, CRDs, and brief small polyphasic MUPs.[73] Biopsy shows subsarcolemmal periodic acid–Schiff positive vacuoles, particularly in type II fibers.[73, 99, 107] Biochemical muscle assay reveals an absence of the debranching enzyme.[99] Several mutations have been identified in the gene, but more than half of them remain unknown. Prenatal diagnosis with enzymatic marker methods is difficult and cannot distinguish carriers from affected patients.[131] Treatment is with small, frequent meals to avoid hypoglycemia. Cardiac status is also carefully monitored, since heart disease can be present.[99]

ENDOCRINE MYOPATHIES

Proximal muscle weakness can be seen with abnormalities of thyroid and parathyroid function as well as secondary to endogenous or exogenous steroids (Table 48–5).

Hyperthyroidism

Hyperthyroid or thyrotoxic myopathy is present in a large percentage of patients with thyrotoxicosis. Approximately half of these patients have some muscle atrophy and 80% have muscle weakness.[122] The myopathy is more common in men with thyrotoxicosis than in women.[73] Proximal weakness develops, most frequently about the shoulders.[16, 73, 122] Extraocular muscles can be tethered, causing exophthalmic ophthalmoplegia. Reflexes are normal or hyperactive.[16, 73] CK can be normal, with muscle biopsy demonstrating nonspecific abnormalities.[16] The EMG shows brief, small-amplitude MUPs with early recruitment.[73, 122] Successful treatment of the thyroid disease cures the muscle disease.[122]

Thyrotoxic patients have been reported to have episodes of periodic paralysis. In exercise tests of 2 to 5 minutes with serial measurements of compound MUP amplitude, an initial amplitude increase is noted immediately post-exercise with a subsequent decrease. When a patient is treated and becomes euthyroid, the above pattern remains but is less dramatic.[62] This test can be helpful for a diagnosis of periodic paralysis between episodes, in the absence of intercurrent muscle weakness.[62]

Hypothyroid Myopathy

Hypothyroid myopathy produces proximal muscle weakness, occasionally associated with muscle cramps. Muscle hypertrophy is also seen in some children. There is a slowed relaxation of muscle stretch reflexes.[16, 73] CK can be elevated and needle EMG shows increased insertional activity and repetitive discharges.[16, 73] Successful treatment of the thyroid disease causes subsequent improvement of muscle symptoms.

Parathyroid Disease

In *hypoparathyroidism,* tetany is a neuromuscular complication secondary to chronic hypocalcemia.[6, 73] *Hyperparathyroidism* can lead to proximal muscle weakness which is more severe in the pelvic girdle than in the shoulder region. Reflexes are normal to increased.[16, 73] Some patients show extensor plantar responses.[73] There may be fatigue and muscle aching, along with weakness and atrophy. Bulbar findings are also noted.[16] The severity of the disease is not correlated with calcium or phosphate levels.[16] On needle EMG there are brief small-amplitude MUPs and early recruitment, with no spontaneous activity. NCSs can show reduced amplitude of the compound MUP with normal conduction velocities.[73] Muscle biopsy shows changes indicative of denervation with type II atrophy.[16] Treatment is of the underlying hyperparathyroidism.

Corticosteroid Myopathy

Myopathy can be due to excessive corticosteroids, whether exogenous or endogenous. Weakness can occur in Cushing's syndrome as well as with corticosteroid treatment.[107, 122] The weakness generally begins in the hip and proximal lower limb muscles, later affecting the proximal upper limb muscles and, in severe cases, the distal limb muscles. Weakness gradually begins from a few weeks to several years after the onset of corticosteroid administration. Weakness is frequently, but not always, related to corticosteroid dose and time. Fluorinated steroids are most commonly linked with myopathy.[107]

Severe myopathies have recently been reported related to the use of high-dose intravenous corticosteroids in patients with asthma who required mechanical ventilation and neuromuscular blocking agents (pancuronium bromide and vecuronium). The neuromuscular blocking agents appeared to facilitate a steroid myopathy with an increase in severity.[5, 77] The myopathy is reversible, but the morbidity is significant.[77]

The CK is normal in steroid myopathy.[16] Needle EMG shows no spontaneous activity, but can reveal

TABLE 48–5 Endocrine Myopathies

Types	Presentation	Electrodiagnostics	Biopsy	Treatment
Hyperthyroidism	Proximal weakness EOM abnormal Atrophy	Brief, small polyphasics with early recruitment	Abnormal, nonspecific	Treat underlying disease
Hypothyroid myopathy	Proximal weakness Painful muscle spasms	Increased insertional activity Repetitive discharges		Treat underlying disease
Hyperparathyroidism	Proximal muscle weakness Fatigue and aching	Brief, small polyphasics with early recruitment NCSs—decreased CMAP	Signs of denervation and type II atrophy	Treat underlying disease
Hypoparathyroidism	Tetany			Treat underlying disease
Corticosteroid myopathy	Hip weakness; later, shoulder weakness	No spontaneous activity Brief, small polyphasics		Remove steroids

Abbreviations: EOM, extraocular muscle; NCSs, nerve conduction studies; CMAP, compound muscle action potential.

small polyphasic potentials which are recruited early.[122] The myopathy improves with a decrease or discontinuation of the steroid, after some days or weeks.[107]

INFLAMMATORY MYOPATHIES

Polymyositis and Dermatomyositis

Polymyositis (PM) and dermatomyositis (DM) are generally described together as variants of the same disease, but there is evidence that their etiologies are different. Clinically, however, they are expressed and evaluated in the same manner,[16, 73, 107] so we discuss them together. The HLA-DQA1*0501 allele is strongly associated with juvenile DM.[117] Autoinvasive CD8+T cells are present in PM, but not in DM.[27] PM and DM are acquired myopathies, each with an acute or subacute course (Table 48–6). Pain and muscle aches are sometimes present but certainly are not diagnostic.[16, 73] DM has a bimodal distribution, being more common in childhood and in middle age (the 40s and 50s). It can occur at any age, with an incidence of 5 to 10 cases per million.[76] PM or DM can be associated with neoplasms, vasculitis, or collagen-vascular diseases. Neoplasms are more commonly associated with dermatomyositis, except in children. Childhood dermatomyositis is more frequently associated with collagen-vascular disease.[16, 73, 107] DM is distinguished from PM by the rash that is present prior to, during, or subsequent to the muscle weakness. There is a violet rash over the upper and lower eyelids and cheeks with periorbital edema. An erythematous rash can also be present in any exposed part of the body[73, 107] (Fig. 48–8). Calcinosis can occur, particularly in children. It has been described in 50 to 75% of children with DM. Calcinosis tends to resolve spontaneously in some patients but can be a chronic problem in others[4, 111] (Fig. 48–9).

Associated findings can include vasculitis, especially in children, which can affect the gastrointestinal tract and myocardium. Myocarditis can present a serious risk during the acute phase.[4] Initial symptoms generally are nonspecific systemic complaints of malaise, fever, anorexia, and weight loss.[73] Raynaud's phenomenon is present in approximately 20% of patients. Dysphagia is common and can necessitate tube feeding. Neoplasms involving the breast, lung, ovary, or stomach are the classic diseases associated with the adult form of PM or DM. A neoplasm is found in 10 to 20% of PM and DM patients. Other collagen-vascular diseases are frequently present.[16]

Physical examination shows proximal weakness involving first the hips, then the shoulders, and also the anterior neck muscles.[73] As the disease progresses, it involves the distal limb muscles. In children the rash is almost invariably seen.

Reflexes are normal until depressed late in the course of the disease. Mild muscle atrophy can be noted. There is generally minimal tenderness to muscle palpation; if present, it is most frequently about the shoulder region.[73]

CK is elevated in 90% of patients. The myoglobin and erythrocyte sedimentation rate can also be increased. The needle EMG shows fibrillations, positive sharp waves, CRDs, and small, brief-duration polyphasic MUPs with early recruitment. Ten percent of patients have a normal EMG study.[73] Muscles with moderate weakness, especially the paraspinal muscles, show needle EMG abnormalities. There is no correlation between the severity of the PM or DM and the needle EMG findings. A correlation is noted of changes over a clinical course with the amount of spontaneous activity found in DM or PM, so that serial EMGs can be useful in following the course of disease and the treatment response.[73] Muscle biopsy shows necrosis, phagocytosis, inflammatory cells, and degeneration, along with regeneration.[73, 107] Abnormalities of swallowing in the distal esophagus can also be detected on cineradiography.[16]

The clinical course is variable and more severe in DM than in PM.[107] Unfavorable prognostic factors include an underlying malignancy, previous diagnosis of collagen-vascular disease, advanced age, and a delay in corticosteroid treatment. Conversely, the severity of weakness at the beginning of the disease, level of CK, and muscle biopsy findings do not correlate with outcome.[107] Some patients have a complete recovery after one episode, whereas others can have a remitting and relapsing course, with some weakness between severe episodes. A third type is a chronic form of DM or PM. In this last form pulmonary function can ultimately be compromised and the patient can die from respiratory failure. Mortality is believed to be approximately 15 to 30% in patients with chronic DM and PM.[16]

Improved treatment of DM and PM is currently an area of active research. The one point of agreement is that steroids must be instituted as early as possible for maximal effectiveness. Corticosteroids are the first line of treatment, most commonly oral prednisone. Prednisone is generally begun at 60 to 80 mg/day or 1 to 2 mg/kg/day in children.[16, 107] If steroids are ineffective, other immunosuppressants are generally used, such as methotrexate, cyclophosphamide, azathioprine, and chlorambucil. Cyclosporine has been shown to be effective in some patients resistant to steroid treatment.[50, 85, 92] Cyclosporine use decreases the amount of steroid needed in children who chronically use steroids.[50] Methotrexate is useful in combination with prednisone in some patients who are resistant to treatment with prednisone alone, but complications can be severe; recurrence has been noted after discontinuation of an apparently successful treatment with the medication.[98] Chlorambucil is effective in some patients who are resistant to prednisone, with leukopenia occasionally noted.[133] High-dose immunoglobulin monthly for three months can increase muscle strength and decrease neuromuscular symptoms.[28] Plasma exchange and leukopheresis are not effective.[96] Low-dose total body irradiation (150 rads) has been used in cases not responding to medications.[16, 107] Cataracts have been shown to occur as a side effect in approximately 30% of patients who use steroids for longer than 12 months.[16]

A critical element of treatment in DM or PM is range-of-motion and stretching exercises early in the course of disease. This regimen helps prevent contractures when muscles are at their weakest. When patients are better

TABLE 48–6 Inflammatory Myopathies

Type	Presentation	Age at Presentation	Laboratory Studies	Electrodiagnostics	Treatment	Associated Findings
Dermatomyositis	Rash Proximal weakness of gradual onset ± Muscle ache	Biomodal	Increased CK, ESR, myoglobin	Fibrillations, positive sharp waves Small-amplitude polyphasics CRDs (especially in paraspinal muscles) 10% normal	Prednisone Ongoing research on other medications ROM exercise	Neoplasms (in adults) Collagen-vascular disease Calcinosis (children) Raynaud's phenomenon
Polymyositis	Proximal weakness of gradual onset ± Muscle ache	Adults	Increased CK, ESR, myoglobin	Fibrillations, positive sharp waves Small-amplitude polyphasics CRDs (especially in paraspinal muscles) 10% normal	Prednisone Ongoing research on other medications ROM exercise	Neoplasms (in adults) Collagen-vascular disease Raynaud's phenomenon
Sarcoidosis	Generally asymptomatic Chronic proximal weakness Palpable nodules	Postmenopausal women most commonly affected		Small-amplitude polyphasics	Steroids ACTH	

Abbreviations: CK, creatine kinase; ESR, erythrocyte sedimentation role; CRDs, complex repetitive discharges; ROM, range of motion; ACTH, adrenocorticotropic hormone.

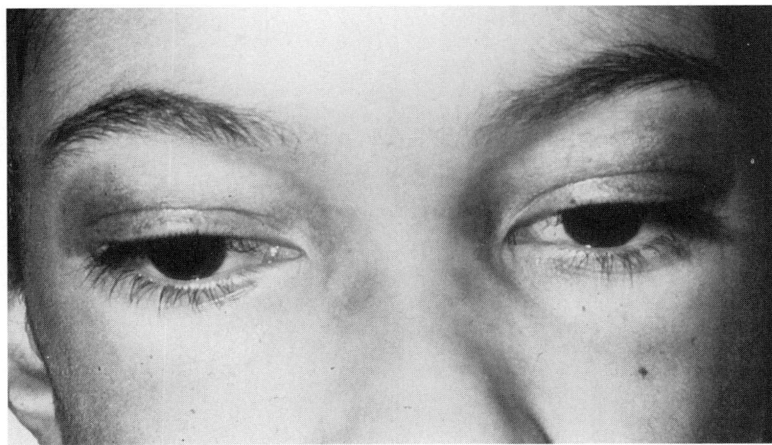

FIGURE 48–8. A teenage girl with chronic dermatomyositis demonstrating the classic rash over the eyelids. (Photograph courtesy of R. Braddom, M.D.)

clinically, monitored resistive exercises improve muscle strength without elevations in CK.[41]

Sarcoidosis

Sarcoidosis is a multisystem granulomatous disorder that commonly involves pulmonary, skin, and eye tissues. Hilar lymphadenopathy is present in many cases.[153] Muscle involvement in sarcoidosis is present in at least 50% to 80% of patients, but is most frequently asymptomatic.[16, 32, 153] Symptomatic muscle presentation is often one of chronic, slowly progressive proximal weakness, along with atrophy. There can also be acute myositis with myalgias and weakness. Palpable nodules in muscle are less common.[16, 32] Diaphragm muscle weakness has been reported in a few patients.[32] Postmenopausal women are more commonly affected.[16, 153] CK is generally normal to mildly elevated and needle EMG shows myopathic changes.[153] Muscle biopsy shows noncaseating granulomas. There is generally bilateral hilar

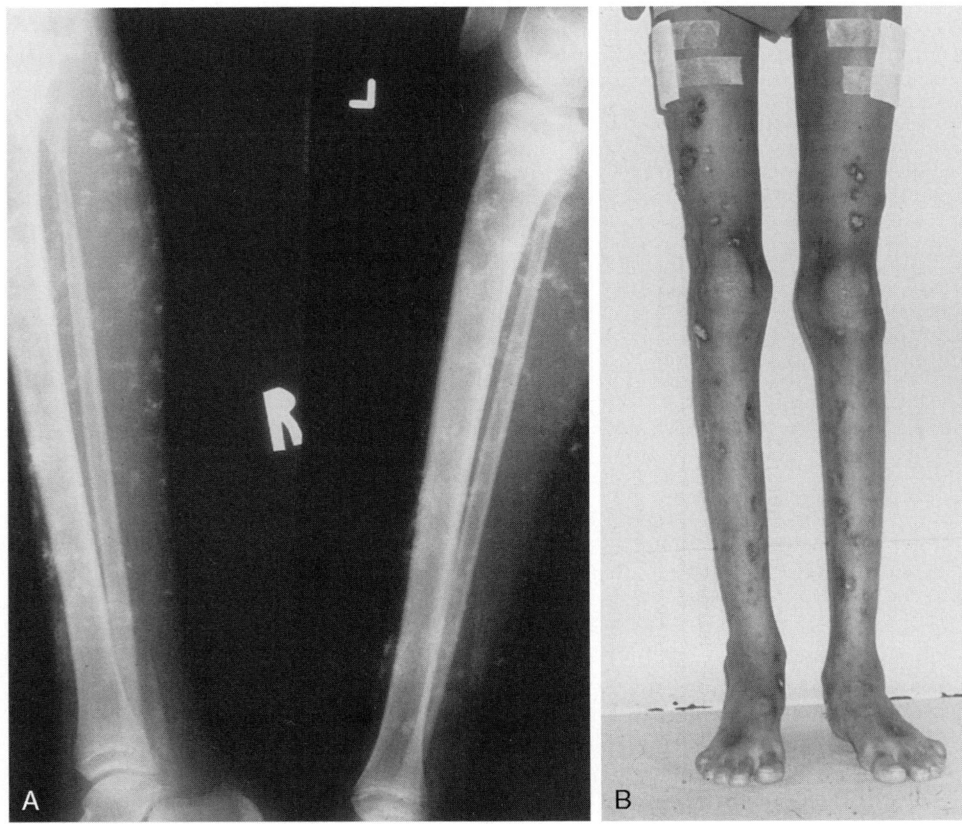

FIGURE 48–9. The same subject shown in Figure 48–8. *A.* X-ray of calcifications in the lower limbs. B. Severe calcifications extrude through skin. (Photograph courtesy of R. Braddom, M.D.)

lymphadenopathy on chest radiography, and a skin reaction to the Kveim-Siltzbach antigen can also be helpful in diagnosing sarcoidosis.[16] MRI shows abnormalities suggestive of a nodular type of muscular sarcoidosis, and Ga scintigraphy shows abnormalities in nodular muscular and myopathic types of sarcoidosis.[112] Treatment with steroids or adrenocorticotropic hormone (ACTH) is generally effective.[16, 33, 153]

INFECTIOUS MYOPATHIES

Documented parasitic infections of the muscle are uncommon outside of tropical areas.[73] Subclinical infection can be more common, however. *Trichinella* larvae can get into human muscle after infected pork is eaten. Fever can be present with muscle pain and stiffness, along with periorbital edema. The masseter muscle is commonly involved, causing painful chewing. Skin rash and retinal hemorrhages can be present.[16] *Trichinella* preferentially invade the extraocular muscles.[73] Muscle biopsy shows a parasite and frequently a hypersensitivity reaction. Treatment is with prednisone and thiabendazole.[16] *Cysticercosis* can also cause muscle aches and pains with palpable nodules. Rarely, it can cause a pseudohypertrophic change in muscle.[16]

Viral infections of muscles may be very common. It is probable that the muscular discomfort that often accompanies influenza might actually be a viral inflammation of the muscle. In influenza B virus infections, acute calf muscle pain is often present. Echovirus, influenza A virus, herpesvirus, coxsackievirus, and adenovirus 21 have all been associated with muscle pain. Muscle biopsies show necrosis, or if less severe, vacuolar degeneration.[16]

The *human immunodeficiency virus* (*HIV*), along with its treatment, can cause muscle disease[78, 122] (see Chapter 60). There are two separate myopathies noted in the HIV positive population. One type is in patients who are HIV-positive and the other is in patients taking zidovudine (AZT). The patients with AZT myopathy have early prominent proximal weakness and myalgia. They fulfill the criteria for *acquired immunodeficiency syndrome* (*AIDS*) and have generally taken AZT for more than nine months. Muscle biopsy shows ragged red fibers. Mitochondrial dysfunction is suggested as a cause of this weakness. Withdrawal of AZT results in reversal of the myopathy, but reducing the AZT does not. Improvement in muscle status and CK is generally noted several months after AZT is stopped. Full muscle recovery might not occur. Restarting AZT at a lower dose after recovery can prevent recurrence.[78] CK is generally markedly elevated.[78, 122]

The other form of myopathy is noted in HIV patients who are not taking AZT. This group does not generally meet the criteria of AIDS, and this type of inflammatory myopathy occurs early in the infection. There is a relatively painless, severe proximal weakness with elevated CK. Biopsy shows inflammation and nemaline rod bodies.[78, 122] The weakness is generally improved with use of steroids or plasmapheresis.[78] In both of these disorders, needle EMG shows spontaneous activity and short-duration MUPs.[78, 122]

TOXIC MYOPATHY

The most common toxic myopathy is *alcoholic myopathy*. There is an acute type and a chronic type. Acute alcoholic myopathy occurs after a bout of excessive drinking with an acute attack of muscle pain, weakness, and muscle swelling. This is generally most common in the thigh muscles, but can be present in any large muscle group. Muscles are tender to palpation. There can be myoglobinuria and subsequent renal failure. It can resolve completely or residual weakness might be present. In chronic alcoholic myopathy there is generally leg weakness, with the shoulders involved somewhat less frequently.[16] Vincristine and chloroquine have also been implicated in toxic myopathies.[16] Treatment for toxic myopathies is removal of the toxin, which allows for partial or complete improvement.

CONCLUSION

The myopathies are a broad group of muscle disorders, most of which share proximal muscle weakness as the primary problem. The myopathies include the dystrophies, congenital myopathies, and myopathies due to metabolic, endocrine, inflammation, and toxic causes. The causes are diverse and the extent of muscle disease varies, as do the muscle groups involved. These differences, along with associated findings in other body systems, help to make each diagnosis, in combination with laboratory studies, electrodiagnosis, and biopsy. Treatment for most is supportive, not curative, and therefore rehabilitation intervention plays a critical role in determining the patients' ability to function and their level of comfort. Orthoses, physical and occupational therapy interventions, and ventilatory assistance are vital in many of these areas. Surgical intervention can also be helpful in many diseases. The majority of research in myopathies has been on DMD. The evaluation and treatment approach to DMD is a basis for that of all other myopathies. The maximal rehabilitative intervention is made in patients with the severe effects of DMD. Patients with less severe myopathies require a variety of these interventions.

REFERENCES

1. Ahn AH, Kunkel LM: The structural and functional diversity of dystrophin. Nature Genet 1993; 3:283–291.
2. Aitkens SG, McCrory MA, Kilmer DD, et al: Moderate resistance exercise program: Its effect in slowly progressive neuromuscular disease. Arch Phys Med Rehabil 1993; 74:711–714.
3. Angelini C, Pegoraro E, Turella E, et al: Deflazacort in Duchenne dystrophy: Study of long-term effect. Muscle Nerve 1994; 17:386–391.
4. Ansell BM: Juvenile dermatomyositis. J Rheumatol 1992; 33 (suppl): 60–62.
5. Apte-Kakade S: Rehabilitation of patients with quadriparesis after treatment of status asthmaticus with neuromuscular block-

ing agents and high-dose corticosteroids. Arch Phys Med Rehabil 1991; 72:1024–1028.
6. Bach JR: Ventilator use by Muscular Dystrophy Association patients. Arch Phys Med Rehabil 1992; 73:179–183.
7. Bach JR: Ventilatory support alternatives to tracheostomy and intubation: Current status of the application of this technology. Conn Med 1991; 55:323–329.
8. Bach JR, Campagnolo DI, Hoeman S: Life satisfaction of individuals with Duchenne muscular dystrophy using long-term mechanical ventilatory support. Am J Phys Med Rehabil 1991; 70:129–135.
9. Bach JR, McKeon J: Orthopedic surgery and rehabilitation for the prolongation of brace-free ambulation of patients with Duchenne muscular dystrophy. Am J Phys Med Rehabil 1991; 70:323–331.
10. Bach JR, O'Brien J, Krotenberg R, et al: Management of end stage respiratory failure in Duchenne muscular dystrophy. Muscle Nerve 1987; 10:177–182.
11. Bach JR, Zeelenberg A, Winter C: Wheelchair-mounted robot manipulators: Long term use by patients with Duchenne muscular dystrophy. Am J Phys Med Rehabil 1990; 69:59–69.
12. Bennett RL, Knowlton GC: Overwork weakness in partially denervated skeletal muscle. Clin Orthop 1958; 12:22–29.
13. Bertorini TE, Palmieri GM, Griffin J, et al: Chronic allopurinol and adenine therapy in Duchenne muscular dystrophy: Effects on muscle function, nucleotide degradation, and muscle ATP and ADP content. Neurology 1985; 35:61–65.
14. Bodensteiner JB: Congenital myopathies. Muscle Nerve 1994; 17:131–144.
15. Braddom R: Written communication, 1994.
16. Brooke MH: A Clinician's View of Neuromuscular Diseases, ed 2. Baltimore, Williams & Wilkins, 1986, pp 117–154.
17. Brooke MH: Congenital muscular disorders. In 1992 AAEM Course C: Update of Myopathies. American Association of Electrodiagnostic Medicine, 15th Annual Continuing Education Course, Charleston, SC, Oct 15, 1992.
18. Brooke MH, Fenichel GM, Griggs RC, et al: Clinical investigation in Duchenne dystrophy. 2. Determination of the "power" of therapeutic trials based on the natural history. Muscle Nerve 1993; 16:91–103.
19. Brooke MH, Fenichel GM, Griggs RC, et al: Clinical investigation of Duchenne muscular dystrophy. Interesting results in a trial of prednisolone. Arch Neurol 1987; 44:812–817.
20. Brooke MH, Fenichel GM, Griggs RC, et al: Duchenne muscular dystrophy: Patterns of clinical progression and effects of supportive therapy. Neurology 1989; 39:475–481.
21. Brust M: Relative resistance to dystrophy of slow skeletal muscle of the mouse. Am J Physiol 1966; 210:445.
22. Bunch WH, Siegel IM: Scapulothoracic arthrodesis in facioscapulohumeral muscular dystrophy. J Bone Joint Surg Am 1993; 75A:372–376.
23. Carpenter S, Karpati G: Duchenne muscular dystrophy: Plasma membrane loss initiates muscle cell necrosis unless it is repaired. Brain 1979; 102: 147–161.
24. Carpenter S, Karpati G, Zubryzycka-Gaarn EE, et al: Dystrophin is localized at the plasma membrane of human skeletal muscle fibers by electron microscopic cytochemical study. Muscle Nerve 1990; 13:376–380.
25. Colbert AP, Schock NC: Respirator use in progressive neuromuscular disease. Arch Phys Med Rehabil 1985; 66:760–762.
26. Curran JF, Colbert AP: Ventilator management in Duchenne muscular dystrophy and postpoliomyelitis syndrome: Twelve years' experience. Arch Phys Med Rehabil 1989; 70:180–185.
27. Dalakas MC: Molecular immunology and genetics in inflammatory muscle diseases. Arch Neurol 1998; 55:1509–1512.
28. Dalakas MC, Illa I, Dambrosia JM, et al: A controlled trial of high-dose intravenous immune globulin infusions as treatment for dermatomyositis. N Engl J Med 1993; 329:1993–2000.
29. De Angelis MS, Palmucci L, Leone M, et al: Centronuclear myopathy: Clinical, morphological and genetic characters. J Neurol Sci 1991; 103:2–9.
30. DeLateur BJ, Giaconi RM: Effect on maximal strength of submaximal exercise in Duchenne muscular dystrophy. Am J Phys Med Rehabil 1979; 58:26–36.
31. De Silva S, Drachman DB, Mellits D, et al: Prednisolone treatment in Duchenne muscular dystrophy. Arch Neurol 1987; 44:818–822.
32. Dewberry RG, Schneider BF, Cale WF, et al: Sarcoid myopathy presenting with diaphragm weakness. Muscle Nerve 1993; 16:832–835.
33. Deymeer F, Oge AE, Bayindir C, et al: Emery-Dreifuss muscular dystrophy with unusual features. Muscle Nerve 1993; 16:1359–1365.
34. DiLazzaro V, Restuccia D, Servedei S, et al: Functional involvement of cerebral cortex in Duchenne muscular dystrophy. Muscle Nerve 1998; 21:662–664.
35. Dubowitz V: Some clinical observations on childhood muscular dystrophy. Br J Clin Pract 1963; 17:283.
36. Edwards RHT: Management of muscular dystrophy in adults. Br Med Bull 1989; 45:802–818.
37. Emery AE: Population frequencies of inherited neuromuscular diseases—A world survey. Neuromuscul Disord 1991; 1:19–29.
38. Emery AEH: Emery-Dreifuss muscular dystrophy and other related disorders. Br Med Bull 1989; 45:772–787.
39. Emery AEH, Skinner R: Clinical studies in benign (Becker type) X-linked muscular dystrophy. Clin Genet 1976; 10:189.
40. Eng GD, Binder H: Rehabilitation of infants and children with neuromuscular disorders. Pediatr Ann 1988; 17:745–755.
41. Escalante A, Miller L, Beardmore TD: Resistive exercise in the rehabilitation of polymyositis/dermatomyositis. J Rheumatol 1993; 20:1340–1344.
42. Florence JM, Pandya S, King WM, et al: Clinical trials in Duchenne dystrophy: Standardization and reliability of evaluation procedures. Phys Ther 1984; 64:41–45.
43. Fowler WM Jr: Rehabilitation management of muscular dystrophy and related disorders: II. Comprehensive care. Arch Phys Med Rehabil 1982; 63:322–328.
44. Fukunaga H, Okubo R, Moritoyo T, et al: Long-term follow-up of patients with Duchenne muscular dystrophy receiving ventilatory support. Muscle Nerve 1993; 16:554–558.
45. Gardner-Medwin D: Clinical features and classification of the muscular dystrophies. Br Med Bull 1980; 36:109–115.
46. Gibson DA, Roy L: Pseudohypertrophic muscular dystrophy and its surgical management: Review of 30 patients. Can J Surg 1970; 13:13–20.
47. Grimm T, Janka M: Emery-Dreifuss muscular dystrophy. In Engel AG, Franzini-Armstrong C (eds): Myology: Basic and Clinical, ed 2. New York, McGraw-Hill, 1994.
48. Gronert GA, Fowler W, Cardinet GH, et al: Absence of malignant hyperthermia contractures in Becker-Duchenne dystrophy at age 2. Muscle Nerve 1992; 15:52–56.
49. Gussoni E, Pavlath GK, Lanctot AM, et al: Normal dystrophin transcripts detected in Duchenne muscular dystrophy patients after myoblast transplantation. Nature 1992; 356:435–438.
50. Hamill G, Saunders C, Heckmatt J, et al: "Catch-up" growth in steroid dependent dermatomyositis treated with cyclosporin-A. Eur J Med 1992; 1:16–18.
51. Harris SE, Cherry DB: Childhood progressive muscular dystrophy and the role of physical therapy. Phys Ther 1974; 54:4–12.
52. Heckmatt JZ, Hyde SA, Gabain A, et al: Therapeutic trial of isaxonine in Duchenne muscular dystrophy. Muscle Nerve 1988; 11:836–847.
53. Heckmatt J, Rodillo E, Dubowitz V: Management of children: Pharmacological and physical. Br Med Bull 1989; 45:788–801.
54. Hiller LB, Wade CK: Upper extremity functional assessment scales in children with Duchenne muscular dystrophy: A comparison. Arch Phys Med Rehabil 1992; 73:527–534.
55. Hinge HF, Hein-Sorensen O, Reske-Nielsen E: X-linked Duchenne muscular dystrophy: Motor functions and prognosis. Scand J Rehabil Med 1989; 21:27–31.
56. Hoberman M: Physical medicine and rehabilitation: Its value and limitations in progressive muscular dystrophy. Am J Phys Med Rehabil 1955; 34:109–115.
57. Huard J, Bouchard JP, Roy R, et al: Human myoblast transplantation: Preliminary results of 4 cases. Muscle Nerve 1992; 15:550–560.
58. Huard J, Roy R, Bouchard JP, et al: Human myoblast transplantations between immunohistocompatible donors and recipi-

ents produce immune reactions. Transplant Proc 1992; 24:3049–3051.

59. Huard J, Roy R, Guerette B, et al: Human myoblast transplantation in immunodeficient and immunosuppressed mice: Evidence of rejection. Muscle Nerve 1994; 17:224–234.
60. Hudlicka O, Tyler KR: The effect of long-term high frequency stimulation on capillary density and fibre types in rabbit fast muscles. J Physiol 1984; 353:435–445.
61. Hunter JR, Galloway JR, Brooke MH, et al: Effects of allopurinol in Duchenne muscular dystrophy. Arch Neurol 1983; 40:1294–1299.
62. Jackson CE, Barohn RJ: Improvement of the exercise test after therapy in thyrotoxic periodic paralysis. Muscle Nerve 1992; 15:1069–1971.
63. Jaffe KM, McDonald CM, Ingman E, et al: Symptoms of upper gastrointestinal dysfunction in Duchenne muscular dystrophy: Case-control study. Arch Phys Med Rehabil 1990; 71:742–744.
64. James WV, Orr JF: Upper limb weakness in children with Duchenne muscular dystrophy—A neglected problem. Prosthet Orthot Int 1984; 8:11–13.
65. Jebsen RH, Taylor N, Trieschmann RB, et al: An objective and standardized test of hand function. Arch Phys Med Rehabil 1969; 50:311–319.
66. Johnson ER, Fowler WM, Lieberman JS: Contractures in neuromuscular disease. Arch Phys Med Rehabil 1992; 73:807–810.
67. Johnson EW, Braddom R: Over-work weakness in facioscapulohumeral muscular dystrophy. Arch Phys Med Rehabil 1971; 52:333–336.
68. Johnson EW, Kennedy JH: Comprehensive management of Duchenne muscular dystrophy. Arch Phys Med Rehabil 1971; 52:110–114.
69. Karpati G: Update in Duchenne/Becker dystrophy. In 1992 AAEM Course C: Update on Myopathies. American Association of Electrodiagnostic Medicine, 15th Annual Continuing Education Courses, Charleston, SC, Oct 15, 1992.
70. Karpati G, Acsadi G: The potential for gene therapy in Duchenne muscular dystrophy and other genetic muscle diseases. Muscle Nerve 1993; 16:1141–1153.
71. Khodadadeh S, McClelland MR, Nene AV, et al: The use of double support time for monitoring the gait of muscular dystrophy patients. Clin Biomech 1987; 2:68–70.
72. Kilmer DD, Abresch RT, Fowler WM: Serial manual muscle testing in Duchenne muscular dystrophy. Arch Phys Med Rehabil 1993; 74:1168–1171.
73. Kimura J: Myopathies. In Kimura J (ed): Electrodiagnosis in Diseases of Nerve and Muscle: Principles and Practice, ed 2. Philadelphia, FA Davis, 1988.
74. Kleiger WJ, van der Kraan M, Kroos MA, et al: Prenatal diagnosis of glycogen storage disease type II: Enzyme assay or mutation analysis? Pediatr Res 1995; 38:103–106.
75. Kottke FJ: The effects of limitation of activity upon the human body. JAMA 1966; 196:117–122.
76. Kunkel LM, Hoffman EP: Duchenne/Becker muscular dystrophy: A short overview of the gene, the protein, and current diagnostics. Br Med Bull 1989; 45:630–643.
77. Lacomis D, Smith TW, Chad DA: Acute myopathy and neuropathy in status asthmaticus: Case report and literature review. Muscle Nerve 1993; 16:84–90.
78. Lange DJ: Neuromuscular diseases associated with HIV-1 infection. Muscle Nerve 1994; 17:16–30.
79. Leshner RT: Diagnostic evaluation of Duchenne's muscular dystrophy and spinal muscular atrophy. In 1998 AAEM Course D: Updates in Neuromuscular Diseases in Children. American Association of Electrodiagnostic Medicine, 21st Annual Continuing Education Courses, Orlando, FL, Oct 15, 1998.
80. Lim LE, Campbell KP: The sarcoglycan complex in limb-girdle dystrophy. Curr Opin Neurol 1998; 11:443–452.
81. Litchy WJ: Electromyography and clinical neurophysiology: A high intensity review. In 16th Annual Course, Chicago, Rehabilitation Institute, March 1–4, 1993.
82. Liu M, Chino N, Ishihara T: Muscle damage progression in Duchenne muscular dystrophy evaluated by a new quantitative computed tomography method. Arch Phys Med Rehabil 1993; 74:507–514.
83. Lord J, Behrman B, Varzos N, et al: Scoliosis associated with Duchenne muscular dystrophy. Arch Phys Med Rehabil 1990; 71:13–17.
84. Lord JP, Portwood MM, Lieberman JS, et al: Upper extremity functional rating for patients with Duchenne muscular dystrophy. Arch Phys Med Rehabil 1987; 68:151–154.
85. Lueck CJ, Trend P, Swash M: Cyclosporin in the management of polymyositis and dermatomyositis. J Neurol Neurosurg Psychiatry 1991; 54:1007–1008.
86. Martin AM, Stern L, Yeates J, et al: Respiratory muscle training in Duchenne muscular dystrophy. Dev Med Child Neurol 1986; 28:314–318.
87. Martinez AC, Terradas JML: Conduction velocity along muscle fibers in situ in Duchenne muscular dystrophy. Arch Phys Med Rehabil 1990; 71:558–561.
88. Matsumura K, Campbell KP: Dystrophin-glycoprotein complex: Its role in the molecular pathogenesis of muscular dystrophies. Muscle Nerve 1994; 17:2–15.
89. McCartney N, Moroz D, Garner SH, et al: The effects of strength training in patients with selected neuromuscular disorders. Med Sci Sport Exerc 1988; 20:362–368.
90. McDonald CM: Clinical findings, measurement of impairment, and natural history of Duchenne's muscular dystrophy and spinal muscular atrophy. In 1998 AAEM Course D: Updates in Neuromuscular Diseases in Children. American Association of Electrodiagnostic Medicine, 21st Annual Continuing Education Courses, Orlando, FL, Oct 15, 1998.
91. McDonald CM, Abresch RT, Carter GT, et al: Profiles of neuromuscular diseases: Duchenne muscular dystrophy. Am J Phys Med Rehabil 1995; 74:S70–S92.
92. Mehregan DR, Su WP: Cyclosporin treatment for dermatomyositis/polymyositis. Cutis 1993; 51:59–61.
93. Mendell JR, Griggs RC, Moxley RT, et al: Clinical investigation of Duchenne muscular dystrophy: 4. Double blind controlled trial of leucine. Muscle Nerve 1984; 7:535–541.
94. Merlini L, Granata C, Dominici P, et al: Emery-Dreifuss muscular dystrophy: Report of five cases in a family and review of the literature. Muscle Nerve 1986; 9:481–485.
95. Miller F, Moseley CF, Koreska J: Spinal fusion in Duchenne muscular dystrophy. Dev Med Child Neurol 1992; 34:775–786.
96. Miller FW, Leitman SF, Cronin ME, et al: Controlled trial of plasma exchange and leukopheresis in polymyositis and dermatomyositis. N Engl J Med 1992; 326:1380–1384.
97. Miller JR, Colbert AP, Osberg JS: Ventilator dependency: Decision-making, daily functioning and quality of life for patients with Duchenne muscular dystrophy. Dev Med Child Neurol 1990; 32:1078–1086.
98. Miller LC, Sisson BA, Tucker LB, et al: Methotrexate treatment of recalcitrant childhood dermatomyositis. Arthritis Rheum 1992; 35:1143–1149.
99. Miller RG: Metabolic myopathies. In 1992 AAEM Course C: Update on Myopathies. American Association of Electrodiagnostic Medicine, 15th Annual Continuing Education Courses, Charleston, SC, Oct 15, 1992.
100. Miller RG: Pathogenesis and pharmacologic management of Duchenne's muscular dystrophy and spinal muscular atrophy. In 1998 AAEM Course D: Updates in Neuromuscular Diseases in Children. American Association of Electrodiagnostic Medicine, 21st Annual Continuing Education Courses, Orlando, FL, Oct 15, 1998.
101. Miller RG, Hoffman EP: Molecular diagnosis and modern management of Duchenne muscular dystrophy. Neurol Clin 1994; 12:699–725.
102. Miller RG, Pavlath G, Sharma K, et al: Myoblast implantation in Duchenne muscular dystrophy: The San Francisco study. Neurology 1992; 42:189.
103. Milner-Brown HS, Miller RG: Muscle strengthening through electrical stimulation combined with low-resistance weights in patients with neuromuscular disorders. Arch Phys Med Rehabil 1988; 69:20–24.
104. Milner-Brown HS, Miller RG: Muscle strengthening through high-resistance weight training in patients with neuromuscular disorders. Arch Phys Med Rehabil 1988; 69:14–19.
105. Mizuno Y, Yoshida M, Nonaka I, et al: Expression of utrophin (dystrophin-related protein) and dystrophin-associated glyco-

proteins in muscles from patients with Duchenne muscular dystrophy. Muscle Nerve 1994; 17:206–216.
106. Moxley RT, Brooke MH, Fenichel GM, et al: Clinical investigation in Duchenne dystrophy. VI. Double-blind controlled trial of nifedipine. Muscle Nerve 1987; 10:22–33.
107. Munsat TL: Review of neuromuscular diseases. Phys Med Rehabil 1988; 2:467–480.
108. Muntoni F, Lichtarowicz-Krynska EJ, Sewry CA: Early presentation of X-linked Emery-Dreifuss muscular dystrophy resembling limb-girdle dystrophy. Neuromuscul Disord 1998; 8:72–76.
109. Ohlendieck K, Ervasti JM, Snook JB, et al: Dystrophin-glycoprotein complex is highly enriched in isolated skeletal muscle sarcolemma. J Cell Biol 1991; 112:135–148.
110. Ohlendieck K, Matsummara K, Ionasescu VV, et al: Duchenne muscular dystrophy: Deficiency of dystrophin-associated proteins in the sarcolemma. Neurology 1993; 43:795–800.
111. Ostrov VE, Goldsmith DP, Eichenfield AH, et al: Hypercalcemia during the resolution of calcinosis universalis in juvenile dermatomyositis. J Rheumatol 1991; 18:1730–1734.
112. Otake S: Sarcoidosis involving skeletal muscle: Imaging findings and relative value of imaging procedures. Am J Roentgenol 1994; 162:369–375.
113. Patten BM, Zeller RS: Clinical trials of vasoactive and anti serotonin drugs in Duchenne muscular dystrophy. Ann Clin Res 1983; 15:164–165.
114. Pradhen S: New clinical sign in Duchenne muscular dystrophy. Pediatr Neurol 1994; 11:298–300.
115. Puig JG, DeMiguel E, Mateos FA, et al: McArdle's disease and gout. Muscle Nerve 1992; 15:822–828.
116. Raben N, Sherman JB, Adams E, et al: Various classes of mutations in patients with phosphofructokinase deficiency (Tarui's disease). Muscle Nerve 1995; 3(suppl):S35–S38.
117. Reed AM, Stirling JD: Association of the HLA-DQA1*0501 allele in multiple racial groups with juvenile dermatomyositis. Hum Immunol 1995; 44:131–135.
118. Rideau Y, Gatin G, Bach J, et al: Prolongation of life in Duchenne muscular dystrophy. Acta Neurol 1983; 5:118–124.
119. Roberts RG, Coffey AJ, Bobrow M, et al: Exon structure of the human dystrophin gene. Genomics 1993; 16:536–538.
120. Rochester DF, Braun NMT, Laine S: Diaphragmatic energy expenditure in chronic respiratory failure: Effect of assisted ventilation with body respirators. Am J Med 1977; 63:223–232.
121. Salmons S, Vrbova G: The influence of activity on some contractile characteristics of mammalian fast and slow muscle. J Physiol 1969; 201:535–549.
122. Sanders DB: Electromyographic evaluation of myopathies. In 1992 AAEM Course C: Update of Myopathies. American Association of Electrodiagnostic Medicine, 15th Annual Continuing Education Course, Charleston, SC, Oct 15, 1992.
123. Scott OM, Hyde SA, Goddard C, et al: Effect of exercise in Duchenne muscular dystrophy. Physiotherapy 1981; 67:174–176.
124. Scott OM, Hyde SA, Goddard C, et al: Prevention of deformity in Duchenne muscular dystrophy: A prospective study of passive stretching and splintage. Physiotherapy 1981; 6:177–180.
125. Scott OM, Hyde SA, Goddard C, et al: Quantitation of muscle function in children: A prospective study in Duchenne muscular dystrophy. Muscle Nerve 1982; 5:291–301.
126. Scott OM, Vrbova G, Hyde SA, et al: Responses of muscles of patients with Duchenne muscular dystrophy to chronic electrical stimulation. J Neurol Neurosurg Psychiatry 1986; 49:1427–1434.
127. Seigel IM, Miller JE, Ray RD: Subcutaneous lower limb tenotomy in the treatment of pseudohypertrophic muscular dystrophy. J Bone Joint Surg Am 1968; 50:1437–1443.
128. Shapiro F, Sethna N, Colan S, et al: Spinal fusion in Duchenne muscular dystrophy: A multidisciplinary approach. Muscle Nerve 1992; 15:604–614.
129. Sharma KR, Mynhier MA, Miller RG: Muscular fatigue in Duchenne muscular dystrophy. Neurology 1995; 45:306–310.
130. Shaw DJ, Harper PS: Myotonic dystrophy: Developments in molecular genetics. Br Med Bull 1989; 45:745–759.
131. Shen J, Liu HM, McConkie-Rosell A, Chen YT: Prenatal diagnosis and carrier detection for glycogen storage disease type III using polymorphic DNA markers. Prenat Diagn 1998; 18:61–64.
132. Sherman JB, Raben N, Nicastri C: Common mutations in the phosphofructokinase-M gene in Ashkenazi Jewish patients with glycogenesis VII—and their population frequency. Am J Hum Genet 1994; 55:305–313.
133. Sinoway PA, Callen JP: Chlorambucil. An effective corticosteroid-sparing agent for patients with recalcitrant dermatomyositis. Arthritis Rheum 1993; 36:319–324.
134. Smith AD, Koreska J, Moseley CF: Progression of scoliosis in Duchenne muscular dystrophy. J Bone Joint Surg Am 1989; 71:1066–1074.
135. Smith PEM, Coakley JH, Edwards RHT: Respiratory muscle training in Duchenne muscular dystrophy. Muscle Nerve 1988; 70:784–785.
136. Spencer GE Jr, Vignos PJ Jr: Bracing for ambulation in childhood progressive muscular dystrophy. J Bone Joint Surg Am 1962; 44:234–242.
137. Splaingard ML, Frates RC, Jefferson LS, et al: Home negative pressure ventilation report of 20 years of experience in patients with neuromuscular disease. Arch Phys Med Rehabil 1985; 66:239–242.
138. Stallard J, Henshaw JH, Lomas B, et al: The ORLAU VCG (variable centre of gravity) swivel walker for muscular dystrophy patients. Prosthet Orthot Int 1992; 16:46–48.
139. Stern LM, Martin AJ, Jones N, et al: Respiratory training in Duchenne dystrophy. Dev Med Child Neurol 1991; 33:648–649.
140. Sutherland DH, Olshen R, Cooper L, et al: The pathomechanics of gait in Duchenne muscular dystrophy. Dev Med Child Neurol 1981; 23:3–22.
141. Taylor RG, Abresch RT, Lieberman JS, et al: In vivo quantification of muscle contractility in humans: Healthy subjects and patients with myotonic muscular dystrophy. Arch Phys Med Rehabil 1992; 73:233–236.
142. Tsujino S, Shanske S, DiMauro S: Molecular genetic heterogeneity of myophosphorylase deficiency (McArdle's disease). N Engl J Med 1993; 329:241–245.
143. Tupler R, Barbierato L, Memmi M, et al: Identical de novo mutation at the D4F104S1 locus in monozygotic male twins affected by facioscapulohumeral dystrophy (FSHD) with different clinical expression. J Med Genet 1998; 35:778–783.
144. Vignos PJ: Physical models of rehabilitation in neuromuscular disease. Muscle Nerve 1983; 6:323–338.
145. Vignos PJ, Archibald KC: Maintenance of ambulation in childhood muscular dystrophy. J Chron Dis 1960; 112:273–290.
146. Visser M, Voogt WG, Riviere GV: The heart in Becker muscular dystrophy, facioscapulohumeral dystrophy, and bethlem myopathy. Muscle Nerve 1992; 15:591–596.
147. Wagner MB, Vignos PJ Jr, Carlozzi C, et al: Assessment of hand function in Duchenne muscular dystrophy. Arch Phys Med Rehabil 1993; 74:801–804.
148. Wagner MB, Vignos PJ Jr, Carlozzi C: Duchenne muscular dystrophy: A study of wrist and hand function. Muscle Nerve 1989; 12:236–244.
149. Wallgren-Pattersson C: Congenital nemaline myopathy: A clinical follow-up of twelve patients. J Neurol Sci 1989; 89:1–14.
150. Weglewski A, Jurynczyk J: Current problems in myotonic dystrophy. Neurol Neurochir Pol 1998; 32:903–911.
151. Weiler T, Greenberg CR, Zelinski T, et al: A gene for autosomal recessive limb-girdle dystrophy in Manitoba Hutterites maps to chromosome region 9q31–q33: Evidence for another limb-girdle muscular dystrophy locus. Am J Hum Genet 1998; 63:140–147.
152. Willig TN, Carlier L, Legrand M, et al: Nutritional assessment in Duchenne muscular dystrophy. Dev Med Child Neurol 1993; 35:1074–1082.
153. Wolfe SM, Pinals RS, Aelion JA, et al: Myopathy in sarcoidosis: Clinical and pathologic study of four cases and review of the literature. Semin Arthritis Rheum 1987; 16:300–306.
154. Yang J, Seelig M, Rayner S, et al: Increasing the proliferative capacity of muscular dystrophy myoblasts. Muscle Nerve 1992; 15:941–948.
155. Yoshida K, Ikeda S, Nakamura A, et al: Molecular analysis of the Duchenne muscular dystrophy gene in patients with Becker muscular dystrophy presenting with dilated cardiomyopathy. Muscle Nerve 1993; 16:1161–1166.
156. Zupan A: Long-term electrical stimulation of muscles in children with Duchenne and Becker muscular dystrophy. Muscle Nerve 1992; 15:362–367.

CHAPTER 49

Corwin Boake, Ph.D., Gerard E. Francisco, M.D., Cindy B. Ivanhoe, M.D., and Sunil Kothari, M.D.

Brain Injury Rehabilitation

This chapter covers the rehabilitation of persons with brain injury, which is defined as an acquired, nonprogressive injury to the brain. Traumatic brain injury (TBI) is the most frequent form of brain injury. Less frequently, brain injury may be caused by anoxia and certain types of strokes, infections, and brain tumors. Despite different etiologies, many patients with brain injury have a similar clinical course—that starts with a global impairment of brain function, progresses through a period of functional recovery, and terminates in a stable level of functioning without further deterioration. This similarity in clinical course is the rationale for treating these different etiologies of brain injury in the same rehabilitation programs, just as spinal cord injury rehabilitation programs treat different etiologies of paraplegia and tetraplegia.

This chapter summarizes the field of brain injury rehabilitation from the viewpoint of the physician who is responsible for the management of individuals with brain injury after discharge from acute care. The chapter emphasizes medical complications of brain injury rehabilitation inpatients. Topics related to brain injury rehabilitation that are covered in other chapters of this book are spasticity (Chapter 29), communication disorders (Chapter 3), outcome measurement (Chapter 8), ambulation (Chapter 5), and daily living skills (Chapter 25).

TBI was recognized early in recorded history,[96, 294] but it was in the twentieth century that rehabilitation programs for brain-injured patients were developed. During World War I,[44] such programs were initiated to help brain-injured war veterans. In the late twentieth century, growth in the field accelerated sharply, spurred on by at least four interrelated factors: (1) improvements in trauma systems and neurosurgical care, which increased the rate of survival from TBI[203, 317]; (2) a subsequent increase in the prevalence of brain injury survivors with long-term disabilities, which placed emotional and financial burdens on their families[351]; (3) public education by national advocacy organizations, notably the Brain Injury Association (formerly the National Head Injury Foundation) in the United States and Headway in the United Kingdom, which increased public recognition of the needs of brain injury survivors and their families; (4) growing recognition of the costs—estimated at $25.9 to $34.4 billion in the United States during 1986[184]—that TBI imposes upon society. The problem of brain injury is now a common focus of attention in many different fields, ranging from neuroscience to injury prevention. More detailed information about brain injury rehabilitation, and about TBI in general, can be found in a variety of books and monographs.[25, 52, 88, 114, 149, 154, 171, 207, 215, 232, 260, 261, 295, 345]

TERMINOLOGY OF BRAIN INJURY

Traumatic Brain Injury. The term *traumatic brain injury* (TBI) is endorsed as the general term for all injuries to the brain caused by external force.[207] Like *spinal cord injury,* TBI is a general term that does not imply a specific pathology. Alternative terms can be used when there is a need to describe the pathology of TBI. Table 49–1 presents commonly used terminology for TBI. While several older terms, chiefly *head injury* (or *head trauma*), are still used to refer to TBI, such terms can be misleading. "Head injury," for example, only implies the presence of injury to the brain. Moreover, this term is sometimes used to refer to injuries confined to the face or head, but without injury to the brain. Thus the term *traumatic brain injury* is preferred because it clearly denotes that injury to the brain is the

TABLE 49–1 Terminology of Traumatic Brain Injury

Term(s)	Definition
Blunt head injury	Traumatic brain injury caused by contact between the head and a blunt object; synonymous with *nonpenetrating traumatic brain injury*
Brain trauma	Synonymous with *traumatic brain injury*
Concussion* (*commotio cerebri*)	Synonymous with *closed head injury,* in particular, mild closed head injury
Craniocerebral injury	Synonymous with *traumatic brain injury*
Closed head injury Head injury (*trauma capitis*) Head trauma Traumatic head injury	Traumatic brain injury in which the dura remains intact
Open head injury	Traumatic brain injury in which dura is opened (e.g., assault with a weapon, struck by a moving object, crushing)
Missile wound	Type of penetrating traumatic brain injury (e.g., gunshot, bomb fragments from an explosion, nail gun)
Penetrating head injury Penetrating brain injury	Traumatic brain injury caused by a foreign object penetrating the dura and entering the brain (e.g., gunshot wound, knife wound, laceration by a moving object)
Stab wound	Type of penetrating traumatic brain injury (e.g., assault with a knife)

* The International Classification of Diseases −9 (ICD)[3] used this term for all levels of severity of traumatic brain injury, regardless of severity.

major cause of morbidity and mortality, and that the injury is caused by external force.[330]

Nontraumatic Brain Injuries. The terminology of nontraumatic brain injuries indicates a specific etiology and pathology, and is therefore readily understood. The term *anoxic brain injury* refers to injuries caused by decreased oxygen supply to the brain.[145] This term is equivalent to the terms *hypoxic brain injury* and *hypoxic encephalopathy.* Major causes of anoxic brain injury are cardiac arrest, respiratory arrest, and carbon monoxide poisoning. Terms for other nontraumatic brain injuries, such as stroke (Chapter 50), infection, tumor, and toxic-metabolic brain injury,[9] are already familiar.

PATHOPHYSIOLOGY OF BRAIN INJURY

This section discusses the pathophysiology of brain damage in TBI and anoxic brain injury. The pathophysiology of stroke is described in Chapter 50. Details of terminology and pathophysiology of other causes of brain injury are discussed elsewhere.[9, 224]

Traumatic Brain Injury

The pathophysiology of TBI differs between closed or open head injury, on the one hand, and penetrating head injury on the other. The large number of mechanisms that cause traumatic brain damage can be categorized into primary and secondary mechanisms. *Primary* mechanisms occur at the moment of impact; *secondary* mechanisms are triggered by primary mechanisms and, in turn, cause additional brain damage.[8]

Closed or Open Head Injury

In closed or open head injury, the brain can be damaged by contact between the head and another object, and/or by acceleration or deceleration of the brain within the skull.[146] In a fall, for example, the brain rapidly decelerates when the head hits the ground, and in an assault the brain rapidly accelerates when the weapon hits the head. Motor vehicle crashes typically involve both acceleration and deceleration.

Most of the primary mechanisms of brain damage in closed or open head injury are caused by acceleration-deceleration. The major mechanisms of primary brain damage produced by acceleration-deceleration are diffuse axonal injury, multiple petechial hemorrhages, contusions, and cranial nerve injury. *Diffuse axonal injury*[133] refers to the widespread stretching of axons caused by rotation of the brain around its axis. The distribution of axonal damage is consistent with the centripetal model of closed head injury,[268] which postulates that the force exerted by rotation of the brain is greatest at the brain's surface and weaker in deeper brain structures. The model correctly predicts that neuroimaging abnormalities in milder TBI tend to be located near the cortex, but in more severe TBI are located in deep as well as surface brain regions.[222] In severe TBI, axonal damage tends to be greater in longer fiber tracts (e.g., corpus callosum).[146] Regardless of the point of contact of the head against an external object, contusions are most frequently situated in the inferior frontal and anterior temporal lobes, where the adjacent skull surfaces are irregular.[146]

Secondary mechanisms of traumatic brain damage include intracranial hemorrhage (epidural, subdural, and intracerebral hematomas), brain swelling (vasogenic or cytogenic edema), excitotoxicity, oxidant injury, and hypoxia due to decreased cerebral perfusion pressure. Both primary and secondary brain damage can lead to increased intracranial pressure (ICP), which in turn can potentiate the mechanisms of secondary brain damage in a positive feedback loop.[146] Brain shift and herniation can be produced by mass effect from brain swelling or intracranial hemorrhage. Hydrocephalus is a treatable cause of secondary brain damage which can occur remotely post-injury. (See Fig. 49–1 for a case example of some of these injury mechanisms.)

Excitotoxicity refers to neuronal damage caused by above-normal release of excitatory neurotransmitters by injured neurons.[146] Excitotoxic brain damage can be reduced by moderate hypothermia.[80, 81, 234, 235] In a study of 82 patients with severe closed head injuries, Marion et al[235] demonstrated that early (average 10 hours post-injury) treatment with hypothermia hastened neurologic recovery and improved outcome in those with admission GCS scores of 5 to 7. The patients were maintained at 32 to 33°C for 24 hours, and then re-warmed.

Brain damage in TBI is therefore a summation of the effects of multiple primary and secondary mechanisms that generally result in diffuse rather than focal patterns of damage, especially in patients with closed head injury. The diffuse pattern of brain damage is consistent with the chronic picture of cerebral atrophy and ventricular enlargement that is commonly observed in neuroimaging of severe closed head injury survivors.[18] Despite these commonalities, individual differences in patterns of brain damage produce mixed patterns of neurologic and neuropsychologic impairments[14] in individual TBI survivors.

Recognizing the importance of delayed, or secondary, insults to the injured brain, the American Academy of Neurological Surgery (AANS) published the *Guidelines for the Management of Severe Head Injury*[16] to promote better treatment using evidence-based guidelines developed after a careful review of the literature. The document consists of recommendations for resuscitation of blood pressure and oxygenation, cerebral perfusion pressure, indications for ICP monitoring and treatment threshold, and ICP monitoring technology. Also discussed are the use of hyperventilation in acute management, the use of mannitol and barbiturates, the role of glucocorticoids, the treatment of elevated intracranial hypertension, nutritional support, and the role of anti-seizure prophylaxis.

Gunshot Wounds of the Brain

In gunshot wounds, most brain damage is located along the track of the bullet and indriven bone fragments.[333] A major rehabilitation implication is that gunshot wounds of the brain generally cause syndromes of focal brain damage (e.g., hemiplegia, hemianopsia), with relatively spared functioning of brain regions located away from the missile track. (See Fig. 49–2 for a case example of gunshot wound to the brain.)

Anoxic Brain Injury

The mechanism of brain damage in anoxic brain injury is ischemia due to hypoxemia or decreased cerebral perfusion.[145] Although anoxic brain injury typically causes diffuse neuronal death and injury, there is selective vulnerability of neurons in parts of the hippocampus, cerebellum, and basal ganglia, and in arterial boundary zones (i.e., watershed areas) of the cerebrum.[145] Neurons in parts of the hippocampus appear to be the most vulnerable, which correlates with the high frequency of amnesia following anoxic brain injury.[170] In addition, the frequency of movement disorders in this population correlates with the selective vulnerability to hypoxia of neurons in the basal ganglia and cerebellum. (See Fig. 49–3 for a case example of anoxic brain injury.)

EPIDEMIOLOGY OF TRAUMATIC BRAIN INJURY

This section discusses the epidemiology of TBI. The epidemiology of stroke is discussed in Chapter 50. The epidemiology of brain tumors and other nontraumatic brain injuries is discussed elsewhere.[9, 224] Relatively less is known about the epidemiology of anoxic brain injury.

TBI is one of the most common neurologic disorders resulting in death and disability. Recent reviews[30, 196, 197–199, 315] summarizing major epidemiological studies in the United States estimate that the annual incidence of hospitalized TBI is approximately 200 per 100,000 persons. Approximately 80% of new hospitalized TBI cases are graded as mild and have a survival rate of nearly 100%. The true incidence of mild TBI could be double the estimate based on hospital admissions because many mild TBI patients fail to seek medical attention or are discharged home from the emergency department.[87, 316] The remaining 20% of new hospitalized TBI cases can be divided evenly between moderate and severe TBI. However, severe TBI has a survival rate of approximately 40%, as compared to 90% to 95% for moderate TBI. See Table 49–2 for projected numbers of new TBI patients in the United States for the year 2000.[335]

The risk of TBI is highly predictable from demographic factors. Males are at higher risk in all age groups. The peak risk is during young adulthood and particularly between 18 and 25 years of age.[315] The annual incidence of males in this age group has been estimated at 350 to 700 per 100,000.[198] This explains the predominance of young adult males in TBI rehabilitation.[144] There are also smaller peaks in the incidence of TBI in the pediatric and geriatric age groups.

The single largest indirect cause of TBI is probably alcohol abuse.[92, 94] The single largest external cause of TBI is motor vehicle crashes, followed in frequency by auto-pedestrian accidents, falls, and assaults (including gunshot).[197, 199] The importance of these external causes differs widely among demographic groups. Motor vehicle crashes account for the largest proportion of young adult TBI cases. Auto-pedestrian and bicycle crashes are relatively more frequent among children than in other age groups. Falls are relatively more frequent among children and elderly persons than in young or middle-aged adults.[197, 199] The epidemiological features of TBI support the view that TBI represents a final common pathway of societal problems such as substance abuse, crime, environmental and workplace hazards, un-

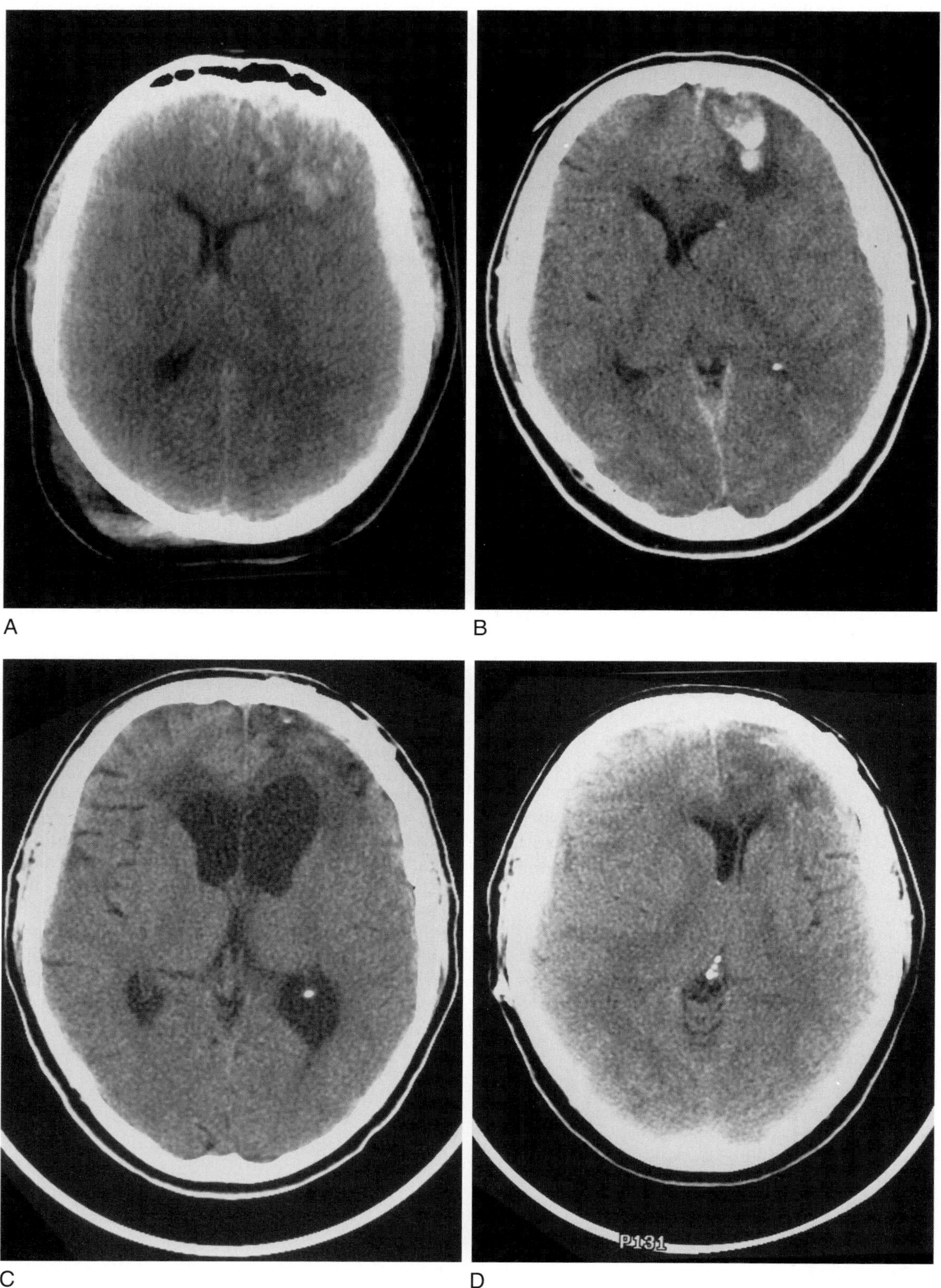

FIGURE 49–1. *See legend on opposite page*

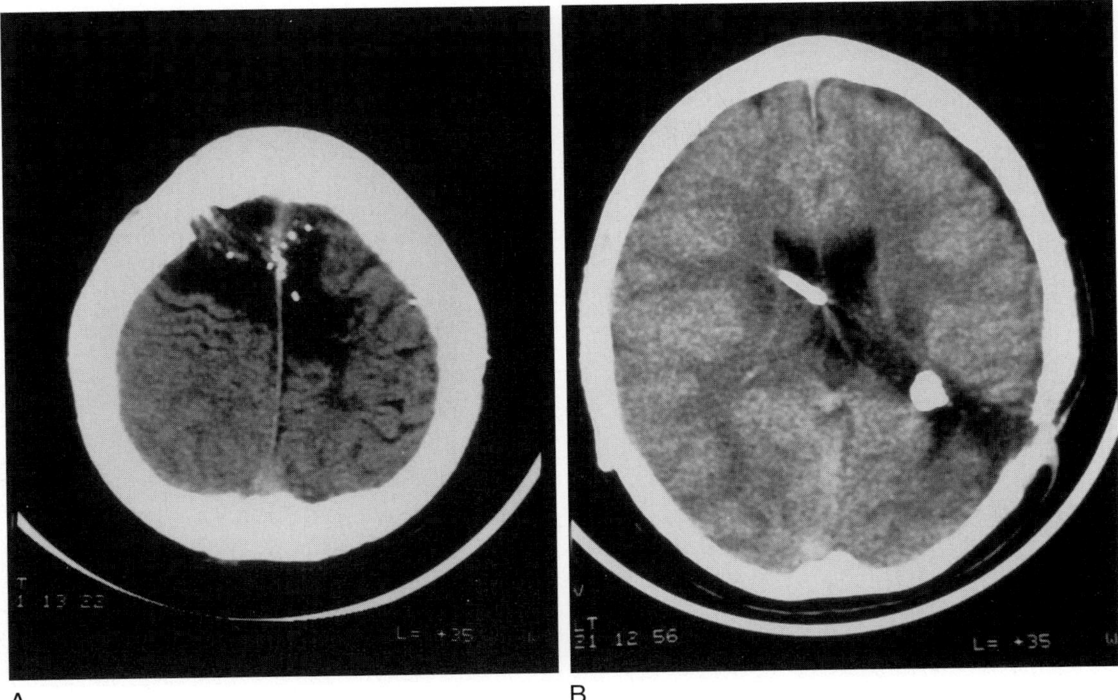

FIGURE 49–2. Penetrating Traumatic Brain Injury Caused by Gunshot. Initial CT scan images of the brain of a 14-year-old boy shot at close range during an assault involving a playground altercation with another teenager. *A.* Entry wound in the superior right frontal area with bullet track crossing the midline. Indriven bone fragments underlie the entry wound. *B.* Exit wound in the left temporal-parietal area. Destruction of brain tissue is seen along the bullet path. Focal injuries to the bilateral superior frontal area and to the left parietal-temporal area correlate with chronic bilateral lower-extremity paresis and written-language deficits. After extended physical and occupational therapy, the patient gained independence in feeding with setup and mobility using a motorized wheelchair.

safe driving, child abuse, and inadequate supervision of children and elderly persons.

ASSESSMENT TECHNIQUES AND PROGNOSIS

This section discusses assessment and outcome prediction of TBI and anoxic brain injury. Details of assessment and prognostication of stroke are discussed in Chapter 50. Other references discuss these topics in relation to nontraumatic brain injuries.[9, 224]

Measuring Severity of Brain Injury: Glasgow Coma Scale

Glasgow Coma Scale. Lacking a direct way to measure severity of brain injury, most centers use the Glasgow Coma Scale (GCS)[324] to measure brain injury severity, particularly during the early stages of recovery. Although the GCS was initially designed for TBI, it is also used with anoxic brain injury and other nontraumatic brain injuries that cause impairment of consciousness. The rationale of using the GCS as a severity measure is the relationship between brain injury severity,

←

FIGURE 49–1. Severe Traumatic Brain Injury Complicated by Hydrocephalus. CT scan images of the brain of a 47-year-old woman who suffered a severe traumatic brain injury in a fall from a horse. Glasgow Coma Scale score was 14 at the scene but later decreased to 8. *A.* Initial day-of-injury scan reveals hemorrhagic contusions in the left frontal lobe and swelling of the left cerebral hemisphere, with less extensive contusions in the right frontal and anterior left temporal lobes. *B.* Follow-up scan at 4 days post-injury reveals increased swelling of the left cerebral hemisphere causing early herniation and mass effect. Partial lobectomy of the left frontal lobe was then performed. She regained independence in ambulation and self-care but remained in posttraumatic amnesia (PTA). *C.* Follow-up scan at 2 months post-injury, obtained because of an early plateau in functional recovery, reveals generalized enlargement in the ventricular system consistent with communicating hydrocephalus. After placement of a ventriculoperitoneal (VP) shunt, she promply cleared from PTA. *D.* Follow-up scan at 7 months post-injury, obtained because of worsening cognitive and behavioral problems, reveals a chronic right frontal-parietal subdural hematoma. After drainage of the hematoma, functional recovery progressed for several more months. By 15 months post-injury, she had passed a driving evaluation and was independent in shopping and cooking, but had not returned to work. Neuropsychological evaluation revealed moderate, selective deficits in recent memory and right-hand coordination.

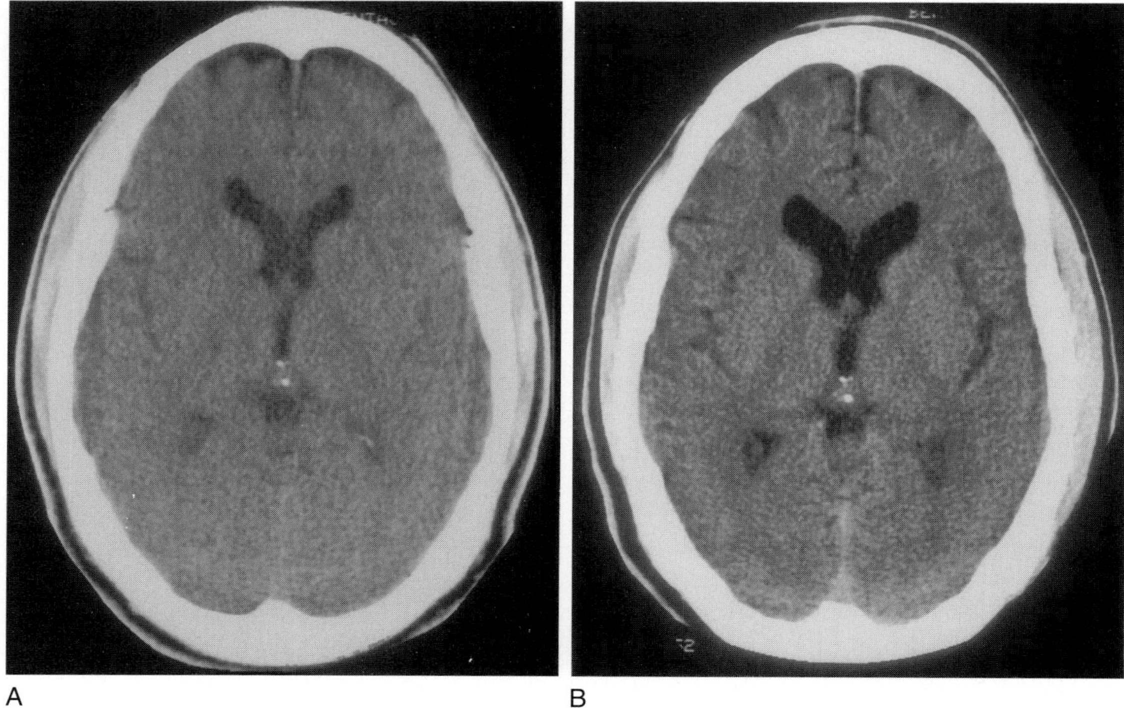

FIGURE 49–3. Anoxic Brain Injury. CT images showing anoxic brain injury in a 32-year-old man who sustained a mild traumatic brain injury and facial injury (zygomatic arch fracture) in a fall from a ladder, and then suffered a 10-minute cardiac arrest during facial surgery. Images are in the horizontal plane through the level of the lateral ventricles, performed before and after the brain injury. *A.* Day of injury scan, performed to clear him for surgery, revealed no intracranial abnormality. *B.* Follow-up scan, performed 20 days later, revealed atrophic changes predominantly in the frontal and temporal lobes. During the first month post-injury, he was agitated and confused, but he gradually recovered independence in ambulation and self-care. Follow-up at 4 months post-injury indicated severe amnesia for which he received full-time supervision. By 1 year post-injury, his level of functioning had improved to part-time supervision. The patient has never resumed working, driving, or going unsupervised for a 24-hour period.

which cannot be directly measured, and the level of consciousness, which can be observed and rated. The GCS, shown in Table 49–3, consists of rating the patient's best motor and speech responses and the weakest stimulus needed to elicit eye opening. Ratings of these

TABLE 49–2 Estimated Annual Incidence of Traumatic Brain Injury (TBI) in the United States in 2000

	U.S. Population (est. 274,634,000)	Per 1 Million
Total incidence	549,268	2000
Total pre-hospital deaths	54,927	200
Admitted alive		
Mild TBI	395,473	1440
Moderate TBI	49,434	180
Severe TBI	49,434	180
Discharged alive		
Mild TBI	395,473	1440
Moderate TBI	45,864	167
Severe TBI	20,872	76

Adapted from Kraus JF: Epidemiology of head injury. In Cooper PR (ed): Head Injury, ed 3. Baltimore, Williams & Wilkins, 1993. pp 1–25.

TABLE 49–3 Glasgow Coma Scale

Patients Response	Score
Eye opening	
Eyes open spontaneously	4
Eyes open when spoken to	3
Eyes open to painful stimulation	2
Eyes do not open	1
Motor	
Follows commands	6
Makes localizing movement to pain	5
Makes withdrawal movements to pain	4
Flexor (decorticate) posturing to pain	3
Extensor (decerebrate) posturing to pain	2
No motor response to pain	1
Verbal	
Oriented to place and date	5
Converses but is disoriented	4
Utters inappropriate words, not conversing	3
Makes incomprehensible nonverbal sounds	2
Not vocalizing	1

Instructions: Rate best response in the verbal and motor categories and the stimulus needed to elicit eye opening. Sum the three ratings to obtain the score.

three responses are summed to yield a GCS score that ranges from a minimum of 3 to a maximum of 15. Lower GCS scores indicate lower levels of consciousness and therefore imply greater severity of brain injury. Conversely, higher GCS scores indicate levels of consciousness that are closer to normal, implying less severe brain injury. It has been repeatedly demonstrated that the depth and duration of unconsciousness, as measured by the GCS score, is the single best predictor of outcome from TBI.[78, 337] A modification of the GCS is available for children.[339]

The lowest post-resuscitation GCS score, obtained at any time following resuscitation, is the preferred index of severity. The major advantage of using the lowest post-resuscitation GCS score is that it can reflect later deterioration that would not be reflected by a GCS score obtained at the scene or immediately upon hospital arrival.[110] The major disadvantage of using the pre-resuscitation GCS score is that the score might be depressed as a result of extracranial injuries (e.g., shock).

Apolipoprotein E4 and Prognosis of TBI. Interest in apolipoprotein E4 (APOE-4), previously linked to Alzheimer's disease, surged with reports suggesting that it may be a susceptibility marker for unfavorable outcome after TBI.[187, 325] APOE, which is the only significant lipid transporter in the brain and cerebrospinal fluid,[85] is believed to play a role in neural regeneration.[72] Studies suggest that the presence of the apolipoprotein ε4 allele (which produces APOE-4) increases the risk of Alzheimer's disease[116, 307] and severity of chronic neurologic deficits in certain TBI populations.[187, 325]

Classifying Severity of TBI

It is now accepted that the severity of TBI should be graded into the three categories—mild, moderate, and severe—based on the patient's GCS score (Table 49–4).

Severe TBI, defined by a lowest GCS score ≤ 8, implies that the patient was in coma. *Coma* is defined as the state in which the patient does not open the eyes and does not demonstrate evidence of cognition, such as following commands or communicating.[180, 279] In some studies, the criterion of coma duration > 6 hours has been added[110] in order to rule out the possibility of a depressed GCS score due to extracranial injury or sedation. Severe TBI accounts for the large majority of inpatients in acute brain injury rehabilitation units.[144] In terms of prognosis, the large majority of severe TBI survivors have permanent neurologic and neuropsychological impairments that result in functional disabilities.[218, 229, 299] The time needed to reach maximum neurologic recovery from severe TBI is approximately one year in the majority of cases,[79] but is probably longer in the most severe injuries.

Moderate TBI, which corresponds to a lowest GCS score in the range of 9 to 12, implies that the patient's level of consciousness is combative or lethargic. At a GCS score of 9 to 12, it is possible for the patient to follow commands, but not to answer questions appropriately. Moderate TBI accounts for a minority of inpatients in acute TBI rehabilitation.[144] With respect to prognosis, the majority of patients with moderate TBI and without complicating extracranial injuries are able to resume their preinjury activities, despite mild, permanent cognitive deficits in an undetermined proportion of this population.[106, 229, 290, 320] The time needed to reach maximal neurologic recovery from moderate TBI is shorter than for severe TBI.

Mild TBI, defined by a lowest GCS score ≥ 13, indicates that the patient might be confused or disoriented, but is awake (or wakes when spoken to), follows commands, and speaks coherently. The commonly used term *concussion* is equivalent to mild TBI. The diagnosis of mild TBI can be made despite a GCS score of 15 if there is neuroimaging evidence of brain trauma or if the injury caused altered mental status such as loss of consciousness, a period of confusion or disorientation, or amnesia for the injury itself. On the basis of studies showing that neuroimaging findings are the single best prognostic indicator for mild TBI, it is recommended that patients in the GCS 13 to 15 range be categorized according to whether computed tomography (CT) scanning of the head reveals any brain trauma. Specifically, it is recommended that mild TBI patients with evidence of brain trauma on CT scanning should be classified as *complicated mild TBI* or *high-risk mild TBI.*[173, 350] Conversely, TBI patients without evidence of brain trauma on CT scanning should be classified as *uncomplicated mild TBI* or *low-risk mild TBI.* Although mild TBI is not by itself an indication for inpatient rehabilitation, mild TBI often co-occurs with spinal cord injury and musculoskeletal injuries that do receive inpatient rehabilitation.[103] The long-term prognosis of mild TBI is controversial, as discussed later in this chapter. However, it has been demonstrated that the outcome of a single uncomplicated mild TBI to a child or young adult generally is return to preinjury activities, without detectable cognitive impairments.[210, 229, 306] Moreover, the time needed for neurologic recovery from mild TBI in such cases is at most 3 months,[212] and probably less than one month in most cases.

As an index of severity, the GCS has significant disadvantages that are important to consider. First, all or part of the GCS can be unscorable during the early acute care phase because of chemical paralysis or sedation, spinal cord injury, facial injury, or intubation.[110, 233] The sensitivity of the GCS to sedation can become a major

TABLE 49–4 Classifying Severity of Traumatic Brain Injury (TBI) Based on the Glasgow Coma Scale (GCS)

Mild TBI—GCS score of 13–15 at lowest point after resuscitation and no TBI-related abnormalities on neurologic examination.

- *Uncomplicated mild TBI*—normal CT scan of the brain.
- *Complicated mild TBI*—CT scan of the brain reveals brain trauma.

Moderate TBI—GCS score of 9–12 at lowest point after resuscitation

Severe TBI—GCS score of 3–8 at lowest point after resuscitation.

problem in grading brain-injury severity. Although the GCS score of a comatose patient is probably not affected by endotracheal intubation (which prevents the patient from making verbal responses), intubation can obscure the difference between moderate and mild TBI. The GCS score can be affected by intoxication. It is also unscorable in patients who do not understand the examiner's language.[180] Although GCS score are sometimes not recorded during acute care, it is generally possible to score the GCS retrospectively based on records of the patient's neurologic and mental status.

Neuroimaging of Brain Injury

CT scanning and magnetic resonance imaging (MRI) are the major neuroimaging modalities applied to brain injury and to TBI in particular.[131, 134, 174] In TBI, CT is the technique of choice during the acute-care stage because of its sensitivity to the presence of blood, facial or skull fractures, and most other intracranial injuries requiring emergency treatment. CT scans of the head can be obtained quickly and are not contraindicated by the presence of metallic material in the body or in life support equipment. Relationships between early results of CT brain scanning and later gross outcome (i.e., conscious survival vs. deceased or vegetative) are well understood. Normal CT findings point to the best prognosis, and CT findings of acute subdural hematoma, intracerebral hemorrhage, and massive bilateral hemispheric swelling point to a worse prognosis.[110, 337] The value of CT scan findings in predicting outcome of TBI survivors in rehabilitation remains to be defined.[90]

MRI of the brain is generally more sensitive than CT to traumatic brain lesions because of its greater resolution. MRI is selectively more sensitive than CT to nonhemorrhagic shear injuries and to contusions in certain areas, such as the inferior frontal region and brainstem, which are located near bony surfaces that produce artefacts in CT scanning.[131] Disadvantages of MRI are the relatively long time needed for scanning, inaccessibility of the patient during this time, and its contraindication by metallic materials in the patient's body or medical equipment. (See Fig. 49–4 for a case example of MRI scan of the brain in a patient with TBI.)

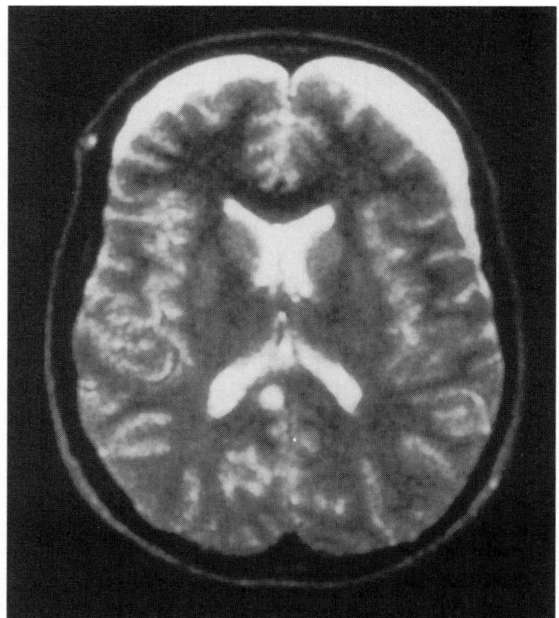

FIGURE 49–4. T2-Weighted MRI Scan of Severe Traumatic Brain Injury. T2-weighted MRI scan of a 32-year-old woman who was injured in an automobile-pedestrian accident 1 month earlier. Initial CT scan revealed a right frontal subdural hematoma. This image shows bifrontal subdural fluid collections and a shear injury in the splenium of the corpus callosum. The corpus callosum lesion, which is a classic sign of diffuse axonal injury, was not visualized on CT scans. In general, MRI can visualize a larger number of traumatic lesions than can CT, especially lesions that are nonhemorrhagic or are located near bony areas. The patient, who had an initial Glasgow coma scale score of 7, underwent inpatient and post-acute rehabilitation. She returned to work as a secretary and lives independently.

Attempts to expand the role of CT and MRI as prognostic indicators have been made, but their ability to predict outcome is variable. Early studies suggested poor outcome in those with CT abnormalities such as cisternal compression and herniation.[257, 332] Other studies[327, 365] did not find CT scans to have predictive value in determining functional outcome. The value of MRI in predicting the outcome of TBI rehabilitation appears promising in view of the relationship between MRI abnormalities and neuropsychological deficits in mild and moderate TBI patients.[223] MRI should be more useful than CT scanning in rehabilitation planning since MRI is more helpful in explaining patients' neurologic and neuropsychological deficits.

Finally, promising research results obtained with single proton emission CT (SPECT) scanning of the brain in TBI patients[143, 266] suggest the possibility that SPECT scanning could have an important role in evaluating unconscious or mild brain injury patients in the future. Another study demonstrated the utility of SPECT in identifying patients with poor outcomes.[6] The potential use of SPECT scanning in brain injury has been recently reviewed.[70, 166, 328, 367]

Neurophysiologic Studies

While CT and MRI provide structural information, electroencephalography (EEG) and other electrophysiologic assessment tools, such as evoked potentials, give information about neurophysiologic functions. EEG is more commonly used in seizure assessment. However, its usefulness as a predictor of posttraumatic seizures is limited since interictal EEG abnormalities can merely reflect the severity of the brain injury.[101, 176, 311] Focal slowing, a frequent EEG abnormality, can persist for a long time without clinical seizures.[95]

In the acute setting, EEG is a powerful predictor of survival from traumatic brain injury.[322] As a predictor of functional outcome, however, the role of conventional EEG and quantitative EEG is still being delineated.[331] Certain EEG patterns, such as abnormal sleep spindles and predominance of alpha waves, suggest poor prognosis.[60, 341] A review of this topic[242] suggested that in comatose patients, quantitative EEG might have a role in predicting survival and functional outcome and in continuous monitoring of neurologic status. A review of studies using evoked potentials to predict outcome from TBI[275] concluded that the bilateral absence of waves N20 to P22 in somatosensory evoked potentials of comatose TBI patients was a strong predictor of failure to recover consciousness. The same review[275] concluded that the absence of wave V or other components of the brainstem auditory evoked potential was also predictive of a poor outcome; however, the presence of normal brainstem auditory evoked potentials was not a valid predictor of good outcome.

Somatosensory evoked potentials (SEP) have also been shown to predict long-term outcome of severe brain injury.[99] Electrophysiologic assessment in brain injury is discussed extensively elsewhere.[284, 331]

Neuropsychological Testing

Neuropsychological tests are the major tools used to evaluate cognitive functions in brain-injured patients.[34, 209, 329] Table 49–5 presents cognitive deficits that are frequently caused by brain injury, together with commonly used neuropsychological tests (described by Lezak[227]), several of which are used in the TBI Model Systems project. Some advantages of neuropsychological testing in brain injury rehabilitation are:

1. Providing an understanding of patients' cognitive strengths and weaknesses that can be used to set rehabilitation goals; assessing competency to consent to medical procedures and make other decisions, assessing readiness to resume activities (e.g., work, school, driving); recommending modifications in order to improve safety and efficiency; and predicting outcome.
2. Providing standardized measures that can be repeated in order to monitor change due to recovery, interventions, or medical complications.
3. Providing a basis for differential diagnosis of cognitive and behavioral disorders where there are pre- or coexisting disorders (e.g., learning disability, dementia).
4. Detecting task performances that are invalid (e.g., malingering).

The disadvantages of neuropsychological testing include the time needed for testing, the difficulty of testing uncooperative patients, and the limited availability of tests for low-level and non–English-speaking patients.[218]

Summary of Acute Prognostic Indicators

Table 49–6 presents the major prognostic indicators for TBI available upon admission to acute rehabilitation.[78, 189, 274] The best predictors of outcome from TBI are the GCS score and other indicators of overall severity of brain injury.[78, 225] The GCS score is also a strong predictor of outcome from penetrating TBI.[13] It should be noted that the validity of many of these indicators as predictors of gross outcome from the acute stage has been demonstrated in multi-center neurosurgical studies.[110, 337] As there are relatively fewer predictive studies in rehabilitation patients, some of these indicators might be less valid in predicting functional outcome of TBI survivors than they are in predicting survival itself.[366]

Since duration of unconsciousness reflects the severity of brain injury, it is a prognostic indicator that can be used in combination with GCS scores, or in the absence of GCS scores, to predict outcome. For example, a patient with a lowest GCS score of 7 who was unconscious for just one day probably has a much lower degree of brain-injury severity than if the patient was unconscious for one week. The duration of posttraumatic amnesia is a strong prognostic indicator, but is not available in most TBI patients at the time of rehabilitation admission. There is a need for a procedure to combine available indicators to yield a predicted outcome category or score. Although Choi[78] has developed such procedures, they need to be evaluated in the rehabilitation setting.

Prognosis in anoxic brain injury is discussed below, in the section on coma management. Prediction of outcome from stroke is discussed in Chapter 50 and prognosis in brain tumors is discussed elsewhere.[225] Unfortunately, much less information is available on the rehabilitation prognosis of nontraumatic brain injuries and this remains an area for future research.[153, 264]

Measures of Outcome from Brain Injury

Since brain injury can affect different aspects of a person's life, measurement of the outcome of brain injury needs to be multidimensional. However, to avoid the need for multiple outcome measures, brain-injury researchers have favored rating scales that reduce different outcomes to a single rating of global outcome.[185] The Glasgow Outcome Scale (GOS),[178] shown in Table 49–7, is the most commonly used measure of outcome in brain injury research. Although the GOS has been criticized in the rehabilitation literature for insensitivity to change and other shortcomings,[185] it remains the primary outcome measure in acute-care clinical trials. Familiarity with this scale is necessary in order to read the brain injury outcome literature. The Disability Rating Scale (DRS)[286, 287] was designed to provide a more sensitive and comprehensive measure than the GOS. Table 49–8 compares major outcome measures used in brain injury rehabilitation.[156]

CONTINUUM OF BRAIN INJURY REHABILITATION SERVICES

Rehabilitation of the brain-injured patient is typically divided into acute rehabilitation and post-acute rehabilitation. The pathway of rehabilitation services of brain-injured patients is shown in Figure 49–5. *Acute rehabilitation* refers to the patient's inpatient treatment in a hospital-based unit, during early stages of recovery. *Post-acute rehabilitation* refers to treatment after hospital discharge during later stages of recovery.[230]

Acute Brain Injury Rehabilitation

Rehabilitation of the brain-injured patient should begin during critical care. At this stage the rehabilitation phy-

TABLE 49–5 Cognitive Deficits and Neuropsychological Tests

Cognitive Domain	Description	Examples of Related Neuropsychological Tests	Example of Test Procedure
Recent memory (also termed long-term memory, new learning)	Learning and retaining information from ongoing experiences *Example:* Remembering to take medications and where they are kept	Rey Auditory Verbal Learning Test Rey Complex Figure (recall) Selective Reminding Test Wechsler Memory Scale—Revised and III	For the Logical Memory subtest of the Wechsler Memory Scales, a new story is read aloud. The task is to recall the story immediately and after a 30-minute delay. Recognition is tested by discrimination of true from false details.
Working memory (also termed divided attention, information processing speed)	Holding information on-line in order to guide ongoing responses *Example:* Performing mental arithmetic	Paced Auditory Serial Addition Test (PASAT) Trailmaking Test	For the Trailmaking Test, a random array of digits and numbers is presented on a sheet of paper. The task is to connect them in sequence, alternating between letters and numbers.
Language	Although all aphasic syndromes may occur, difficulty in retrieving words (dysnomia) and in discourse coherence are most frequent in brain injury. *Example:* Narrating a recent experience	Boston Naming Test Multilingual Aphasia Examination Verbal Fluency Token Test	For verbal fluency, the task is to rapidly recall words that begin with a given letter or that are members of a category (e.g., animals).
Visual-spatial perception	Judging relationships between objects in space (e.g., distance) or guiding movements in space. *Example:* Following a route that involves changes of direction.	Block Design subtest of IQ test Rey Complex Figure (copy) Judgment of Line Orientation Visual Form Discrimination	For the Rey figure, the task is to a copy a geometric diagram with pencil and paper.
Executive functions	Planning responses or inhibiting habitual responses *Example:* Preparing to complete task by a deadline.	Wisconsin Card Sorting Test Tower of London Test	For the Wisconsin Card Sorting Test, the task is to learn the rule for sorting cards. The rule changes without warning during the test.

TABLE 49–6 Prognosis of Traumatic Brain Injury at Rehabilitation Admission

Predictor	Description
Glasgow Coma Scale (GCS)	Strongest predictor of survival and functional outcome from traumatic brain injury; basis for grading severity as mild, moderate, or severe[78]
Duration of unconsciousness	Interval from injury to following commands. Alternative to GCS as an injury severity indicator[107, 296]
Age	School-age children and young adults (<45 years) achieve better outcomes than infants or older adults (>45 years).[78, 113, 213, 297]
Posttraumatic amnesia (PTA) duration	PTA duration may be a stronger predictor than GCS score in survivors of moderate-severe TBI.[123] Predictive value of PTA in mild TBI is not established.[112, 368]
Pupillary light reflex	One or both nonreactive pupils predict a worse outcome because of association with brain swelling and/or herniation.[78, 213, 218]
Neuroimaging findings	CT scanning is a strong predictor of outcome from mild TBI. In severe TBI, worse prognosis is predicted by midline shift, herniation, or cisterns compressed by swelling.[111, 236, 350]
Multiple trauma	Musculoskeletal or internal injuries predict worse outcomes.[102, 107]

sician can intervene to prevent complications that could magnify later disability. For example, the unconscious patient without contraindications should undergo passive range of motion twice daily in order to prevent contractures and other joint abnormalities, and should be positioned to prevent pressure ulcers, edema, and contractures. Additional interventions can be recommended for spasticity, nutrition, and incontinence. Although definitive orthopedic management of fractures in TBI patients can often be delayed, early surgical treatment of orthopedic injuries can minimize later disability.[161]

The initial rehabilitation evaluation can determine whether the patient is appropriate for acute rehabilitation (in either a general rehabilitation unit or a specialized brain injury unit), for a subacute program, or for treatment in a post-acute program. Transfer to an acute rehabilitation program should be done at the point when the patient is medically stable and when the ongoing medical care will not substantially interfere with progress in rehabilitation.[250] The criterion of following commands before admission to rehabilitation is unjustifiable because, as shown in Table 49–9, the majority of surviving unconscious TBI patients eventually regain consciousness. Instead, the rehabilitation physician can use prognostic indicators to select unconscious patients with the highest probability of recovery. Direct transfer of the unconscious patient from acute care to a nursing home, without prior evaluation by the rehabilitation physician, should be avoided. This is because of the risk of overlooking developing complications or signs of improvement, and because of the risk of delaying or even preventing access to rehabilitation.

TABLE 49–7 Glasgow Outcome Scale

Category	Definition
Good recovery	Able to resume all preinjury activities despite mild deficits. Psychosocial factors may prevent return to work.
Moderate disability	Able to care for self for at least 24 hours and to travel by public transportation. May work at a noncompetitive level.
Severe disability	Needs on-site assistance during each 24-hour period. May require full-time supervision even if independent in self-care.
Persistent vegetative state	Spontaneous eye-opening without evidence of consciousness (e.g., following commands, speaking words, communicating by gesture).
Death	

Indications for admission to a specialized brain injury rehabilitation unit, instead of to a general rehabilitation unit, include (1) unconsciousness or inconsistent evidence of consciousness, (2) agitation requiring environmental modifications, (3) risk of complications (e.g., spasticity) requiring specialized management, and (4) severe cognitive impairment requiring modifications of therapy and nursing procedures. Dedicated brain injury rehabilitation units have the advantages of more experienced staff, a network of consultants with special expertise in brain injury, programs for family and public education, and protocols for typical brain injury rehabilitation problems. The therapy team of the acute brain injury rehabilitation unit typically includes the traditional rehabilitation disciplines, a rehabilitation physician with expertise in brain injury, and a neuropsychologist. The team also needs access to specialists in optometry and orthotics. Detailed descriptions of rehabilitation therapies for brain-injured patients are available.[43, 152, 206, 245, 355, 363]

Further research is needed to evaluate the efficacy of acute rehabilitation units dedicated to brain injury, as compared to treatment of brain-injured patients in general rehabilitation units.[289] Reviews of efficacy studies of acute TBI rehabilitation[74, 167] have found that, while TBI patients in these studies typically made great improvements during inpatient rehabilitation, these gains could not be uniquely attributed to rehabilitation because the studies failed to control for spontaneous recovery or for preexisting differences between the treatment and comparison groups. In addition, the outcome

TABLE 49–8 Measures of Functional Outcome from Brain Injury

Outcome Measure	Description	Advantages	Disadvantages
Glasgow Outcome Scale (GOS)[178, 179]	Rates global outcome on 5-point ordinal scale. Range = Good Recovery to Death.	All patients can be rated at any stage of recovery. Most widely used outcome measure in research.	May be sensitive only to major differences in outcome. Measures potential rather than actual independence.
Rancho Los Amigos Levels of Cognitive Functioning[231]	Rates level of recovery on 8-point ordinal scale representing levels of neurobehavioral functioning. Range = Level I (no response) to VIII (spontaneous-appropriate).	All survivors can be rated at any stage of recovery. Widely used in brain injury rehabilitation.	May be less useful with outpatients. Some patients do not progress through all levels.
Disability Rating Scale (DRS)[286, 287]	Rates 8 subscales measuring level of consciousness, cognitive independence in self-care, employability, and need for supervision. Subscale ratings are summed to yield a Total Score. Range = 0 (no disability) to 29 (vegetative state); death = 30.	All patients can be rated at any stage of recovery. Provides more scale points than GOS and is therefore potentially more sensitive.	Rates potential rather than actual independence (e.g., employability instead of employment status). Clinical trials have shown sensitivity no greater than GOS.
Community Integration Questionnaire (CIQ)[349]	Structured interview with patient or caregiver about independence in specific activities. Ratings of interview responses are summed to yield 3 subscale scores measuring independence in home, community, and work.	Measures multiple dimensions of outcome. Measures actual rather than potential independence.	More time-consuming than one-dimensional outcome measures.
Supervision Rating Scale (SRS)[46]	Rates amount of supervision that patient receives over 24 hours. Supervision is categorized into 5 levels (independent, overnight, part-time, full-time indirect, and full-time direct) or rated on a 13-point scale.	Measures actual independence. Supervision level should cumulatively reflect all sources of impairment and disability. Scale levels are clinically relevant.	Actual supervision level may be inappropriate (e.g., oversupervised, undersupervised).
Functional Assessment Measure (FAM)[155]	Rates independence in 13 activities (e.g., swallowing, community mobility) on a 7-point ordinal scale. Designed to extend the FIM to outcomes relevant to brain injury. "FIM + FAM" refers to combination of both scales.	7-point FIM ratings are already familiar. FIM + FAM covers most features relevant to brain injury.	FAM may not add to FIM's validity as an outcome measure.

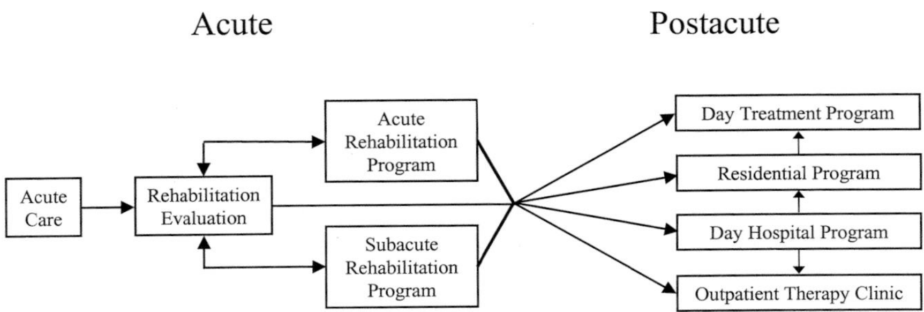

FIGURE 49–5. Rehabilitation Pathway Following Brain Injury. Flowchart showing typical pathways followed by patients from injury through the acute and post-acute phases of rehabilitation. Evaluation by a rehabilitation physician is the initial, necessary step before patients are transferred from acute care to rehabilitation programs. Patients may be transferred between acute and subacute rehabilitation programs depending on individual needs. Choice of post-acute program may depend on local availability.

measures used in these studies might have been inappropriate or not sufficiently sensitive or comprehensive to detect differences in improvement.[160] The majority of functional improvement in brain injury patients during acute rehabilitation is probably due to spontaneous neurologic recovery, with therapy playing the roles of preventing complications (e.g., contractures), reconditioning after inactivity during acute care, providing an enriched environment, teaching compensatory strategies (including environmental modifications), and possibly facilitating neurologic reorganization.[56, 263, 342]

Stages of Neurobehavioral Recovery from Brain Injury

Compared to other neurologic disorders treated in rehabilitation, brain injury has an unusually long course of recovery. For example, TBI patients generally make more functional progress during inpatient rehabilitation than do patients in other diagnostic groups.[69] The course of recovery from severe brain injury consists of distinct stages, as shown in Figure 49–6. The stages of neurobehavioral recovery from anoxic brain injury, anterior communicating artery aneurysm rupture, and many other nontraumatic brain injuries are similar to those of TBI. The Levels of Cognitive Functioning scale, shown in Table 49–10, was developed at Rancho Los Amigos Medical Center[231] to describe the sequence of neurobehavioral recovery from TBI and to provide a rationale for cognitive rehabilitation at each recovery stage. Although the Levels of Cognitive Functioning scale has been criticized because recovery from TBI is more variable than the scale implies, the scale has the advantage of distinguishing major stages of recovery and providing a basis for communication within the team. Rehabilitation strategies during acute rehabilitation are largely determined by the patient's stage of recovery, as described in the following sections.

Coma and Unconsciousness

The natural history of recovery from severe brain injuries begins with coma, a state in which the patient shows no evidence of cognition and does not open his or her eyes, even to painful stimulation.[180] In brain injury due to trauma, coma and unconsciousness are caused by the disruption of input to surface brain structures from deeper structures that subserve arousal and wakefulness.[279] This disruption can, in turn, be produced by disconnection of ascending fiber pathways due to diffuse axonal injury, or by compression of brainstem or diencephalic structures due to mass effect from supratentorial lesions. In surviving patients, there is a fairly consistent sequence of recovery of function from coma that begins with eye opening and sleep-wake cycles, and then progresses to following commands and, finally, to speaking.[59] This recovery sequence is consistent with the centripetal model of TBI, which predicts that functions subserved by deeper brain structures, such as sleep-wake cycles, should recover earlier than functions sub-

TABLE 49–9 One-Year Outcome of Traumatic Coma

Investigators	No. of Patients	Minimum Duration of Unconsciousness	*Outcome at 1 Year (% of Patients)*		
			Conscious	Unconscious	Dead
Bricolo et al[59]	135	2 wk	62	8	30
Pitts[278]	56	1 mo	61	7	32
Braakman et al[57]	140	1 mo	37	11	52
Sazbon and Groswasser[309]	134	1 mo	54	14	32
Levin et al[221]*	93	Discharge from acute care	58	18	24

* Data from 3-year follow-up.

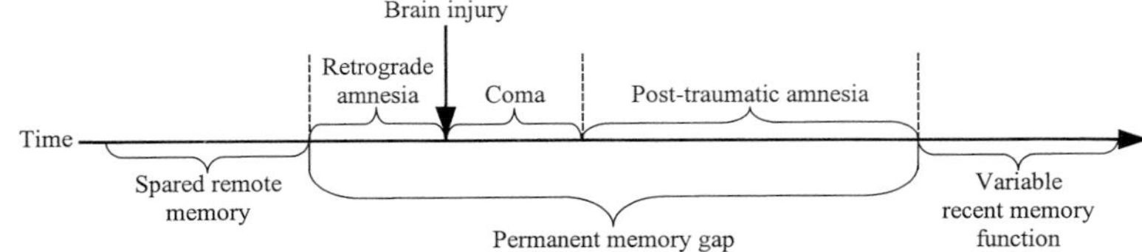

FIGURE 49–6. Recovery of Memory after Brain Injury. Timeline showing the stages of cognitive recovery that apply to most survivors of severe brain injury. Mild and moderate TBI will demonstrate the same stages as depicted, except for coma. Some survivors do not recover from unconsciousness or from posttraumatic amnesia (PTA). The majority of patients emerge from PTA and have a permanent memory gap for experiences that occurred during unconsciousness, PTA, and a shorter pre-injury period (retrograde amnesia).

served by surface brain structures, such as memory.[268] Cognition is usually first demonstrated by the patient's ability to communicate, such as following commands or gesturing. In patients who are recovering quickly, assessment of these early signs of cognition is usually straightforward and does not require special techniques. In slowly recovering patients, however, specialized techniques might be needed to detect progress, or even evidence of consciousness.[343]

In previous studies of severe TBI, 10% to 15% of survivors were still unconscious at the time of discharge from acute care.[221] Most patients who remain unconscious after one month have regained sleep-wake cycles, and therefore spontaneously open their eyes part of the time. They typically also exhibit pupillary reactivity and oculocephalic reflexes, primitive behaviors such as chewing and roving eye movements, and vegetative functions such as spontaneous respiration, all of which reflect preserved brainstem and hypothalamic functions. While there is general agreement on diagnostic criteria for coma, diagnostic inaccuracies and confusion attend attempts to distinguish vegetative from minimally conscious or minimally responsive states. The term *persistent vegetative state* (PVS) has been used to describe a state in which a previously comatose patient has recovered sleep-wake cycle and progressed to a state of wakefulness without awareness.[180, 279] Patients in PVS have no reproducible, purposeful, or voluntary behavioral response to stimuli, and no evidence of language comprehension or expression. Over the years, PVS has been incorrectly used as a prognostic term, leading to inaccurate diagnosis, inappropriate treatment recommendations, limitation of medical and rehabilitation services, and poor utilization and budgeting of resources. The Multi-society Task Force on PVS argued that, since PVS merely refers to "a condition of past and continuing disability with an uncertain future," PVS is a diagnosis rather than a prognosis.[255, 256] A related condition, *permanent vegetative state,* signifies irreversibility and is therefore a prognosis. The Task Force operationally defined PVS as a vegetative state present for one month after an acute nontraumatic or traumatic brain injury. The vegetative state should not be labeled permanent until a prognosis of irreversibility can be established with a high degree of clinical certainty, after 12 months of remaining vegetative post-TBI and 3 months following nontraumatic injuries. Table 49–11 presents terminology used for unconscious or low-level patients.[139]

Rehabilitation of Patients with Impaired Consciousness

Patients who remain unconscious upon discharge from acute care present difficult assessment and treatment problems, and should be admitted to a brain injury rehabilitation program. In the absence of treatments with proven efficacy to facilitate recovery of consciousness, the goals of rehabilitation of unconscious TBI patients are (1) to remove obstacles to recovery, thereby allowing patients who have the potential to regain consciousness to do so; (2) to treat medical complications that can increase disability in those patients who do recover; and (3) to provide education, counseling, and support to family members. Detailed reviews on the management of such patients are available.[38, 51, 138, 265, 304, 346]

The first step in assessing patients with severely impaired consciousness is to rule out the possibility that

TABLE 49–10 Rancho Los Amigos Medical Center Levels of Cognitive Functioning

Level	Name	Description
I	No response	Appears to be in deep sleep; no response to any stimulation
II	Generalized response	Appears to be resting quietly; makes gross movements in response to noxious stimulation
III	Localized response	Makes spontaneous, purposeful movements; may follow commands inconsistently
IV	Confused-agitated	Confused, amnestic, and inattentive; may be aggressive
V	Confused-inappropriate	Not agitated; confused and amnestic
VI	Confused-appropriate	Lacks initiative and problem solving; functional with structure and supervision
VII	Automatic-appropriate	Follows daily routines; needs supervision for home and community skills; independent in self-care within physical ability
VIII	Purposeful-appropriate	Independent in home and community skills; may have cognitive deficits

Instructions: Assign the patient to the level that most closely describes his or her level of cognitive functioning.

TABLE 49–11 Recommended Terminology for Describing Severe Alterations of Consciousness

Clinical Feature	Coma	Vegetative	Minimally Conscious
Spontaneous eye opening	None	Yes	Yes
Sleep-wake cycle	None	Resumes	Abnormal to normal
Arousal	None	Sluggish; poorly sustained	Obtunded to normal
Evidence of perception, communication ability, or purposeful motor activity	None	None	Reproducible but inconsistent
Visual tracking	None	None, but may have roving eye movements	Often intact
Yes/No responses, verbalizations and gestures	None	None	None to unreliable and inconsistent

failure to exhibit consciousness is an artifact of the examination techniques or due to reversible medical factors. Patients who fail to follow commands because of incomprehension of the examiner's language or because of aphasia or apraxia[217] might succeed if the examination techniques are properly modified. Most important, a patient's arousal and responsiveness can be impaired by sedating drugs, systemic illness, malnutrition, and other medical problems that may be correctable.

In particular, the problem of drug-induced sedation in unconscious patients is more serious than generally appreciated and needs to be emphasized. It should be recognized that sedative side effects can be magnified in the injured brain, and that even small changes in arousal can affect the patient's responsiveness. Medications given to the unconscious patient should be carefully reviewed in order to discontinue those that are unnecessary and, if possible, to replace necessary drugs with ones that are less sedating. Potentially sedating medications that are often given to unconscious patients are listed in Table 49–12. Anticonvulsant prophylaxis can be discontinued in many patients, as discussed below, or switched to less sedating anticonvulsants such as carbamazepine (Tegretol) or valproic acid. Treatment of hypertension with clonidine, angiotensin-converting enzyme inhibitors, calcium channel blockers, or diuretics might be possible instead of using antihypertensives with sedating side effects, such as propranolol, metoprolol, and methyldopa. The use of metoclopramide (Reglan) should be avoided in the treatment of delayed gastric emptying because of its sedating side effects. Benzodiazepines such as diazepam (Valium), which are often used for spasticity control, should also be avoided. Antidepressants such as amitriptyline (Elavil), which are sometimes given to increase the level of consciousness, can paradoxically decrease arousal because of their anticholinergic effects. There is no role for neuroleptics such as haloperidol (Haldol), chloropromazine (Thorazine), and thioridazine (Mellaril) in the medical management of unconscious patients.

The best predictors of whether unconscious patients will regain consciousness are etiology, age, and the duration of unconsciousness itself.[255, 256] Studies of outcome in TBI patients who were unconscious at approximately one month post-injury (summarized in Table 49–9) show that 40% to 50% regained consciousness by one year post-injury. These findings also support the recommendation that TBI patients who are unconscious upon discharge from acute care should be admitted to brain injury rehabilitation programs instead of transferred to nursing facilities, where there is a risk of never receiving specialized care even after recovering consciousness. A review of all verified cases of prolonged vegetative state following TBI concluded that, in patients who were unconscious at 3 months post-injury, the probability of regaining consciousness by one year post-injury was 36%; however, in patients who remained unconscious at 6 months post-injury, this probability decreased to 21%.[255, 256] In patients with nontraumatic brain injuries who remained unconscious at 3 months post-injury, the probability of regaining consciousness by one year post-injury was only 7% and, in nontraumatic patients who were still unconscious at 6 months post-injury, the probability was even lower.[255, 256] The same review reported

TABLE 49–12 Alternatives to Commonly Used Sedating Medications

	Sedating Medications	Less Sedating Alternatives
Antiepileptics	Phenytoin Phenobarbital	Carbamazepine Valproic acid Gabapentin
Drugs for excesses of behavior (e.g., agitation, episodic dyscontrol)	Haloperidol and other neuroleptics Lorazepam Diazepam	Risperidone Carbamazepine Valproic Acid Buspirone
Antidepressants	Tricyclic antidepressants	Selective serotonin reuptake inhibitors Venlafaxine
Antispasticity medications	Baclofen (oral) Diazepam	Botulinum toxin Baclofen (intrathecal)
Gastrointestinal drugs	Cimetidine iMetoclopramide	Antacids Erythromycin

fewer than twenty verified cases of TBI patients who recovered consciousness after remaining in a vegetative state longer than one year, and concluded that recovery of consciousness after one year was "extremely rare."[255, 256]

Age is a predictor of recovery from traumatic unconsciousness, with the best recovery seen in children, followed by adults under 40 years of age.[255, 256] However, age does not appear as strongly predictive of recovery from nontraumatic unconsciousness.[226] There is also evidence that recovery from traumatic unconsciousness is less likely in patients with neuroimaging evidence of severe cerebral atrophy or the bilateral absence of somatosensory evoked potentials.[255, 256, 275] Numerous other potential predictors of recovery from traumatic unconsciousness have been studied,[221] but none has been validated for use in clinical prediction.

In patients who are unconscious or who are not consistently responding selectively, there is a strong need for an assessment technique that can track recovery. The GCS and Rancho Los Amigos Levels of Coginitive Functioning Scale lack sensitivity in unconscious patients who have already regained spontaneous eye-opening.[51] Several rating scales have been developed to assess the responsiveness of unconscious or low-level patients.[172] Examples of such scales are the Coma/Near-Coma Scale,[285] Coma Recovery Scale,[140] Western Neuro Sensory Stimulation Profile,[24] and Sensory Stimulation Assessment Measure.[282] Although none of these scales can predict recovery in patients who are still unconscious, they can be useful in monitoring whether a conscious patient is losing responsiveness over time, which can be a sign of a sedation or a treatable complication. As a preferred alternative to these scales, techniques have recently been developed for detecting evidence of consciousness in patients with infrequent or ambiguous responses.[343]

Rehabilitation of unconscious patients remains controversial.[54, 244, 354, 372] In particular, the efficacy of *sensory stimulation* (also termed *coma stimulation*), in which patients are presented with directed stimulation in multiple modalities,[51] has not been supported by clinical trials. A review of published studies[354] found no evidence that sensory stimulation improved the recovery from chronic traumatic unconsciousness, although there was some evidence of a treatment effect in acute TBI patients who were still comatose.

Pharmacological treatment remains the most promising intervention to directly increase arousal and facilitate recovery of consciousness of these patients. Table 49–13 summarizes some medications used for neurostimulation. There have been numerous anecdotal reports of unconscious TBI patients who regained consciousness when treated with stimulants (e.g., methylphenidate, dextroamphetamine) or anti-parkinsonian agents (e.g., bromocriptine, amantadine).[50, 51, 118, 119, 201, 358, 369] Although controlled trials of these medications have not appeared, in our experience they are now widely used in neurotrauma care and acute brain injury rehabilitation.

Posttraumatic Amnesia and Agitation

Following recovery of consciousness, patients with brain injury typically pass through a period of confusion and disorientation termed *posttraumatic amnesia* (PTA).[214, 300] PTA is defined as the period during which the patient's ability to learn new information is minimal or nonexistent. For example, early in PTA, patients might not be aware of being in a hospital and may instead state that they are at home or at work. This false recall of fictitious events, termed *confabulation,* is an organic rather than a functional symptom. Toward the end of PTA, patients become less confabulatory but still fail to recall specific episodes (e.g., visitors received the previous day). After emerging from PTA, patients have a permanent memory gap for events that occurred during the period of PTA. They usually also have a memory gap for events that occurred a short period before the moment of injury (termed *retrograde amnesia*). Although the term PTA implies that the brain injury was due to trauma, patients with anoxic brain injuries and certain other nontraumatic brain injuries (e.g., rupture of anterior communicating artery aneurysm) pass through the same stage of recovery. Therefore, an alternative term is needed to refer to amnesia without specifying a traumatic etiology.

Different measures are available to assess whether a patient is in PTA or is recovering out of PTA. The most widely used measure is orientation to place and time, but this can be less suitable in rehabilitation units where patients are given frequent "reality orientation" drills.[93] A standard technique for assessing PTA is the Galveston Orientation and Amnesia Test (GOAT),[214] a brief structured interview that quantifies orientation and recall of recent events. The GOAT score can range from 0 to 100, with a score >75 defined as normal. The end of PTA can be defined as the date after which the GOAT score is consistently >75. The advantage of using the GOAT is that results can be directly compared to outcome studies that also used this scale.[112]

Duration of PTA is an indicator of the severity of brain injury and should be used to supplement the GCS score, duration of unconsciousness, and neuroimaging findings. In fact, the duration of PTA was the first such severity indicator to be widely accepted.[123] It should be noted that PTA duration, like duration of unconsciousness, can reflect factors other than severity of brain injury itself. Failure to clear from PTA can indicate a permanent amnesic disorder, such as produced by anoxic brain injury, or can signal preventable complications such as hydrocephalus.

During PTA many patients exhibit a neurobehavioral syndrome, termed *agitation,* which includes cognitive confusion, extreme emotional lability, motor overactivity, and physical or verbal aggression. The agitated patient is typically unable to sustain attention and effort long enough to perform simple tasks, such as dressing, and can overreact to frustration by crying or shouting. The patient can be easily frustrated and irritated, and show grossly inappropriate behavior toward staff or family members. To date, there is no consensus on the definition of agitation. Sandel and Mysiw,[303] based on their review of the literature, defined posttraumatic agitation as "a subtype of delirium, occurring during the period of posttraumatic amnesia, characterized by excessive behaviors, including some combination of ag-

TABLE 49–13 Neurostimulant Medications

Drug	Mechanism of Action	Dose	Side Effects	Comment
Methylphenidate	Promotes release of dopamine and norepinephrine; blocks reuptake of catecholamines	10–30 mg/day in 2–3 divided doses	Tachycardia Hyper- or hypotension Nausea, vomiting Insomnia Anorexia Nervousness and anxiety Headache Dizziness Exacerbation of tic and Tourette's Dysphoria	Peak effect in about 1–2 hours after administration Avoid late-afternoon or evening doses to avoid insomnia Sustained release form (20 mg-SR) to be given in the morning
Amantadine	Stimulates presynaptic dopamine release; possible direct agonist effect	100–400 mg/day, in 2–4 divided doses	Dizziness Insomnia Nervousness Anxiety Impaired concentration Nausea Anorexia Livedo reticularis Seizures Peripheral edema Orthostatic hypotension	Mean peak blood concentrations at 1–4 hr after an oral dose of 2.5 mg/kg Concerns about lowering seizure threshold at higher doses Adjust dose in hepatic or renal dysfunction
Bromocriptine	Direct D_2 receptor agonist	5–30 mg/day, in divided doses	Nausea, vomiting Reduced GI motility Hypotension Headache Dizziness Drowsiness Agitation, confusion Depression Hallucinations Nightmares	

Table continued on following page

TABLE 49–13 Neurostimulant Medications *Continued*

Drug	Mechanism of Action	Dose	Side Effects	Comment
Levodopa/carbidopa	Directly converted to dopamine	Start at 25/100 tid	Choreiform, dystonic, dyskinetic, and other movement disorders Orthostatic hypotension Psychosis Hallucination Depression Decreased attention span Memory loss Confusion Anxiety, nervousness Restlessness Insomnia Anorexia Episodic hyperventilation	Levodopa reduces side effects of carbidopa Therapeutic response usually consists of short-duration (up to 5 hours after a dose) and long-duration improvement associated with chronic therapy. Caution in patients with history of myocardial infarction and arrhythmias; history of psychosis; active peptic ulcer disease
Dextroamphetamine	Facilitates release of dopamine and norephinephrine; reduces catecholamine turnover; blocks reuptake of catecholamines		Tachycardia Hyper- or hypotension Insomnia Nervousness Hyperexcitability Anorexia Irritability Dysphoria Dizziness Headache Nausea, vomiting	Peak effect about 2–4 hr after administration Avoid late-afternoon or evening dosing to avoid insomnia Available in extended-release form
Atypical Neurostimulants				
Tricyclic antidepressants (TCAs)				
Protriptyline				
Selective serotonin reuptake inhibitors (SSRI)				
Fluoxetine				
Paroxetine				
Sertraline				
Others				
Bupropion				
Venlafaxine				

gression, akathisia, disinhibition, and emotional lability." Furthermore, they cautioned that mood and thought disorders must be diagnosed separately. In a survey of members of the Brain Injury Special Interest Group of the American Academy of Physical Medicine and Rehabilitation, Fugate et al[126] found that the majority did not use standardized techniques to measure agitation. Only 6% used the Agitated Behavior Scale (ABS), the most commonly used measure. The ABS is a 14-item scale that rates behavior in three interrelated realms: disinhibition, aggression, and lability.[91] It is simple to administer and has been shown to have good interrater reliability.

Agitation becomes critical if the patient becomes harmful to self or others (e.g., pulling out tubes, falling, or attempting to escape from the unit). Previously it was believed that most severe TBI patients exhibited agitation during PTA, as implied by the Rancho Los Amigos scale.[231] However, research showed that agitation with aggression occurs in a minority of these patients, that many more exhibit only agitation with motor restlessness,[63, 288] and that many others exhibit no agitation. Risk factors for agitation remain to be identified but experience suggests that severe cognitive deficits and frontal lobe damage might be predictive.

Rehabilitation of the Agitated Patient

Although agitation is commonly observed in brain injury, it should be a diagnosis of exclusion. Concurrent medical or neurologic problems can cause or aggravate delirium and agitated behavior. Obviously, these conditions are managed differently from agitation. Metabolic derangement, hyperthyroidism, infection and sepsis, hypoglycemia, hypoxemia, medications (e.g., anticholinergics), and drug withdrawal (e.g., baclofen, sedatives, hypnotics) are some medical causes of delirium and agitation. Among the neurologic complications that might present as delirium or agitation are seizures, hydrocephalus, intracranial mass lesions (e.g., hematoma, hygroma), and migraine. Pain, especially in a patient who is confused and unable to communicate, is a frequently overlooked cause of agitation. It is reasonable to perform various tests in the evaluation of the confused and agitated patient (Table 49–14). Only after medical and neurologic conditions have been ruled out should a diagnosis of agitation be made.

TABLE 49–14 Suggested Tests for the Evaluation of the Confused and Agitated Patient

Serum electrolytes
Blood urea nitrogen (BUN), serum creatinine
Glucose, calcium, magnesium, and liver enzymes
Thyroid function
CBC with differential
Urinalysis
Serum B-12 and folate levels
Drug and alcohol screen
Brain CT or MRI
EEG
Plain radiograph (to evaluate for occult fractures or heterotopic ossification causing pain)

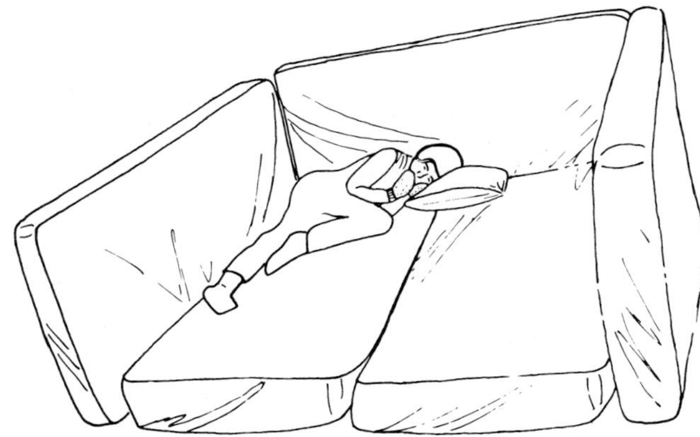

FIGURE 49–7. The Craig Bed. Agitated nonambulatory patients often benefit from the use of a floor (Craig) bed. Mattresses can be laid on the floor and 3- to 4-ft padded walls on four sides allow the patient to roll around. The use of a floor bed with close supervision together with the use of mittens and a helmet (if necessary) often eliminates the need for restraints.

Treatment of agitation involves medications, behavioral strategies, and environmental management. Severe physical restraints have fallen out of favor. Because of public concern, the Joint Commission on the Accreditation of Health Care Institutions (JCAHO) and the Health Care Financing Agency (HCFA) have recently toughened their guidelines for the use of restraints. Injuries related to use of vest restraints have been reported.[62] If needed, restraints should be applied to the minimal degree necessary, such as padded hand mittens and soft lap belts for wheelchair safety. The use of a floor bed (Fig. 49–7) provides a safe, controlling environment and can eliminate the need for restraints. Traditional behavioral modification techniques, such as using rewards for desired behaviors, are not considered effective for agitation since the patient is generally confused and amnestic. Nonpharmacological efforts are directed toward environmental management and restructuring of therapies (Table 49–15). The goal of environmental management is to lower the level of stimulation and cognitive complexity in the patient's immediate surroundings. In addition to staff education and strategy planing, families need to understand the management techniques being used and be involved in their implementation as appropriate. Agitated behavior by a loved one is often understandably distressing to families. It is important to reassure them that agitation is a predictable stage of recovery and that efforts are being exerted in identifying treatable causes of the behavior. Detailed discussions of environmental management of agitation are available in other publications.[61, 165, 272, 351]

No guideline exists in the use of medications for agitation. Sedation should be used only when environmental strategies have failed and in emergency situations. In the same survey by Fugate et al.[125, 126] it was found that the most frequently prescribed drugs by "TBI experts" were carbamazepine, tricyclic antidepressants (TCAs), trazodone, amantadine, and beta-blockers. These "ex-

TABLE 49–15 Environmental Management of Agitation

1. **Reduce the level of stimulation in the environment**
   - Avoid overstimulation by decreasing background noise (e.g., radio, television) and visual distraction in the patient's room and in therapy areas. Monitor room temperature for comfort.
   - Room should be in an area with low traffic but where the patient can be easily monitored.
   - Limit visitors. Orient visitors regarding strategies.
   - During therapies, eliminate or reduce activities that appear to cause annoyance, frustration, and overstimulation.
   - Avoid excessive touching and handling.
   - Provide frequent breaks during therapy sessions.
   - Staff needs to maintain calm demeanor. Keep voice volume and pitch low.
2. **Reduce the patient's confusion**
   - Provide consistent staffing.
   - Avoid moving rooms.
   - Allow one person to speak at a time.
   - Communicate clearly and concisely (i.e., one idea at a time).
   - Keep a consistent schedule for therapies and activities.
   - Reorient to place, time, and purpose through the day.
3. **Protect the patient from harming self or others**
   - Keep the patient in a locked unit or use an alarm system to prevent elopement.
   - Consider using a floor bed with padded walls (e.g., Craig bed).
   - Use stable wheelchair with appropriate safety straps.
   - Avoid use of physical restraints (e.g., Posey) that may heighten agitation.
   - Consider the option of a 1 : 2 or 1 : 1 sitter for close supervision.
   - Staff responsible for close supervision can wear a bracelet.
4. **Tolerate restlessness as much as possible**
   - Review with staff specific therapy and environmental strategies to be used for each patient and "crisis intervention" techniques.
   - Allow patient to thrash about in floor bed.
   - Allow ambulatory patient to pace around the unit, with supervision.
   - Allow confused patient to be verbally inappropriate.

perts" were also less likely than "nonexperts" to use sedating drugs, such as haloperidol and benzodiazpines. Table 49–16 lists some of these commonly used medications. Only a few of these medications have been evaluated for efficacy through clinical trials.[64] In situations where agitation is uncontrollable and has progressed to violent behavior, intramuscular lorazepam (Ativan), 1 to 2 mg, might be required. This is recommended only for emergency situations when there is immediate danger to the patient or others, and not as a substitute for environmental interventions and safer drugs. The physician should also be aware of a paradoxical increase in agitation, which can occur with the use of lorazepam.

Rehabilitation During and After Posttraumatic Amnesia

The rehabilitation program during PTA should be modified for the patient's severe memory impairments.

TABLE 49–16 Some Drugs Used to Treat Posttraumatic Agitation

Class	Drug
Beta-blockers	Propranolol
Antiepileptics	Carbamazepine
	Valproic acid
Dopamine agonist	Methylphenidate
	Amantadine
	Bromocriptine
Tricyclic antidepressants	Amitriptyline
	Nortriptyline
Benzodiazepine	Lorazepam
Others	Buspirone
	Risperidone

The rehabilitation unit should have a system (e.g., colored wristbands) for identifying how closely each patient needs to be supervised. Patients who are at high risk of eloping or of harming themselves or others might need a locked area or direct supervision by nursing staff. To reorient patients to their environment, the place and date and a daily schedule should be posted in patient rooms, and orientation information can be repeated through the day.[93] It might be helpful for patients to receive their meals and therapies on the rehabilitation unit, in order to avoid overstimulation. The team should avoid overstimulating the patient with a demanding therapy schedule, unrealistic therapeutic expectations, and unpleasant emotional interactions with family or staff. Patients who are capable of walking can require close supervision because of safety concerns and might be safer using a wheelchair when not in therapies. As the patient's safety awareness and endurance increase toward the end of PTA, the team can clear the patient for walking, toileting, and other activities at a reduced level of supervision.

After the patient emerges from PTA, a neuropsychological evaluation should be performed to plan rehabilitation and recommend activity restrictions. More realistic and demanding tasks can be presented in therapy, such as community outings. Behavior problems should be treated if they interfere with rehabilitation progress.[175] Noncompliance in therapies can be treated with behavioral management techniques.[228, 313] Mood disorders, which sometimes present as lack of willingness or motivation to participate in therapy, can be treated with antidepressants.[359] The family needs education about brain-injury symptoms and training in the physical and behavioral management techniques that need to be carried over at home. To facilitate family training, there should be an overnight pass (or at least day pass) before discharge to home in order to verify that the family has received proper training, to check whether the level of supervision at home will be adequate, and to evaluate equipment and home modifications.

Considerations for discharge from inpatient rehabilitation include the availability of necessary therapy and nursing services in a less restrictive environment and low probability that continued inpatient rehabilitation will result in or be necessary for functional progress. For patients who can be managed at home overnight but who still benefit from intensive therapy, the acute rehabilitation program can provide a day hospital program in which patients continue at the same level of therapeutic intensity and receive nursing care as needed.

Post-Acute Brain Injury Rehabilitation

Post-acute rehabilitation includes interventions designed to help patients reenter the community.[230] Most post-acute interventions are based on training patients to use compensatory strategies to overcome their permanent deficits (e.g., memory notebooks), or altering the environment so that the patient is more functional despite these deficits (e.g., following a routine schedule). There is a controversy in post-acute rehabilitation regarding the efficacy of *cognitive retraining,* the group of therapies directed at remediating deficits in memory, attention, and other cognitive functions.[7, 37, 163, 211, 238, 281, 314, 338, 352] The rehabilitation physician should be familiar with local post-acute programs in order to make appropriate referrals and monitor progress (see Table 49–17). It needs to be recognized that family members of brain-injured patients are placed under long-term emotional and financial stresses.[243, 351] The rehabilitation physician should be sensitive to the possibility of emotional distress and relationship problems,[66, 280] and be prepared to provide emotional support and help in advocating for needed services.

MEDICAL COMPLICATIONS OF BRAIN INJURY

In recent years there has been a trend toward shorter stays in acute care and, therefore, toward earlier admission to rehabilitation. In addition, studies of TBI patients during the 1980s showed that a significant number of medical complications were undiagnosed before the rehabilitation admission.[128, 188] Medical examination of brain-injured patients is typically made difficult because of inability to communicate or cooperate with procedures. For these reasons, a thorough evaluation by the rehabilitation physician is needed once the patient has been admitted to the rehabilitation unit. The following sections discuss the major medical complications encountered in brain injury rehabilitation and review the related interventions available to the rehabilitation physician. Some medical complications of brain injury are not common, such as endocrine and dermatologic abnormalities, and will not be discussed. More detailed information is available in specialized references.[158, 293]

Spasticity

Spasticity resulting from brain injury shares many similarities with spasticity associated with stroke. Moreover, the response of cerebral origin spasticity (COS) to interventions is often different from that of SCI spasticity, as is its presentation. For instance, COS characteristically presents with greater extensor tone in the lower extremities and a lesser tendency to "spasms."

Although spasticity can be beneficial, decreasing the risk of thrombophlebitis and in some cases aiding in function, it can also create impressive deformity, pain,

TABLE 49–17 Types of Post-Acute Rehabilitation Programs

Type of Program	Description of Program
Comprehensive (holistic) day treatment	Outpatient program accepting patients living in the community and not requiring full-time supervision. Team includes neuropsychologist and patient:staff ratio is approximately 2:1. Treatment emphasizes group interventions and job trials. Goals are awareness of deficits, acceptance of realistic goals, independence in home and community activities (e.g., transportation), family adjustment, and community re-entry into workforce or avocational activity.[36, 230]
Day treatment	Outpatient program that accepts patients living in the community, often after discharge from acute rehabilitation. Goal is to require less assistance or supervision. Team usually includes occupational therapist and speech-language pathologist. Usually clinic-based.
Vocational	Outpatient program that accepts patients living in the community. Goal is employment at supported or competitive level. Team may consist mostly of paraprofessionals supervised by vocational counselor. Licensed therapy services may be provided by consultants. Each patient proceeds through evaluation, training, and placement phases. In supported employment programs, job coaching is provided to facilitate placement.[340]
Residential	Program that accepts patients from acute rehabilitation or from the community. Goals are to require less assistance or supervision. Team may consist of therapists and paraprofessionals (e.g., life skills trainers).[45]
Neurobehavioral	Residential program that accepts patients with injury-related behavioral problems (e.g., physical aggression) which require intensive, full-time supervision. Goal is to reduce risk of harm and level of supervision. Treatment emphasizes behavior modification and psychopharmacology. Facility may restrict access to community by controlled exits or rural location. Team may consist mostly of paraprofessionals supervised by psychiatrist or neuropsychologist.[71, 356]

TABLE 49–18 Functional Goals of Spasticity Treatment

Improve hygiene
Decrease pain
Decrease deformity
Improve orthotic fit
Improve gait
Decrease energy expenditure of gait
Facilitate motor control

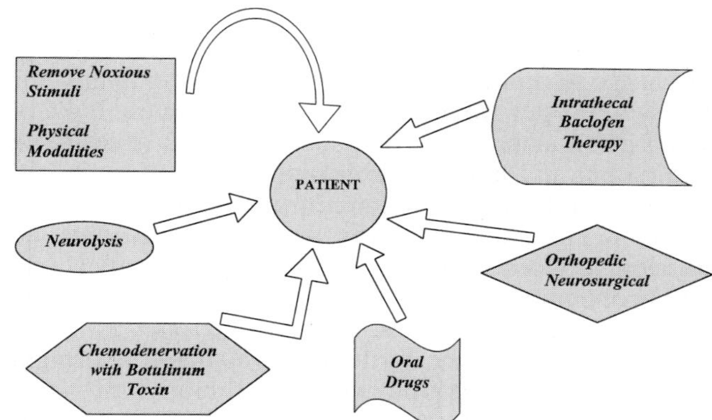

FIGURE 49–8. The complementary approach to the management of spasticity of cerebral origin.

and other medical complications. Spasticity that interferes with functional goals warrants treatment. Examples of functional goals are found in Table 49–18. The functional goals of spasticity treatment should be clearly defined, taking into account both the patient's and family's goals. In addition, potential complications of spasticity (heterotopic ossification, pressure ulcers, respiratory infections, etc.) should be considered. Basing treatments on specific goals assures that appropriate interventions are planned and instituted.

The evaluation of the patient with spasticity should include not only the usual neurologic examination, but also consideration of such factors as gait, balance, synergy patterns, speed of movement, distribution of tone, modified Ashworth scores (Table 49–19),[48] goniometric evaluation, and functional assessment.

In the past, a pyramid approach to spasticity treatment was advocated. This began with prevention of nociceptive stimuli and education and progressed to therapy (ROM, stretching, casting, orthoses, modalities), and then to more invasive options such as motor point blocks. Orthopedic and neurosurgical interventions were last to be considered. With changes in health care and advances in therapeutic options, this approach has lost popularity and become less practical. A "complementary approach," wherein various treatment strategies are employed concurrently based on therapeutic goals, is currently favored (see Fig. 49–8).

Oral medications used to treat spasticity due to other etiologies are generally not recommended for survivors of brain injury, since they might interfere with the goal of maximizing cognitive function. Diazepam and oral baclofen can be particularly cognitively impairing. Dantrolene sodium has been considered the oral medication of choice in the TBI population because it acts peripherally, at the muscle. Dantrolene reduces depolarization-induced calcium efflux into the sacroplasmic reticulum. It can also be sedating, however, and can lead to generalized weakness. Liver enzymes also need to be monitored when using dantrolene sodium. Tizanidine, which is an alpha 2 agonist like clonidine, has demonstrated effects in the multiple sclerosis and spinal cord injury populations.[32, 33, 39, 204, 318] It presumably increases presynaptic inhibition of motor neurons and probably reduces release of excitatory amino acids. Its effects are similar to those of oral baclofen.[39]

Serial casting refers to the practice of applying and removing casts to a limb as joint range of motion increases. Modalities such as heating and cooling can also be helpful for improving range in the short term, and can be used in conjunction with casting to allow for greater stretch. Patients might benefit from analgesia to improve their comfort level while the casts are in place. More than one limb can be casted at a time, but clinicians should consider the degree of agitation this may cause in each individual case. The skin should be monitored because patients might not be able to communicate their needs. Adequate padding within the casts is essential. In rare instances, tone is too great to allow for casting because of potential skin breakdown and behavioral issues. In these cases, injections of botulinum toxin and/or phenol should be considered to decrease the spasticity and thereby decrease this risk.

The role of positioning techniques in spasticity management is often underappreciated. Appropriate positioning should maximize muscle relaxation as well as improve alignment, symmetry, and function. Positioning can also be used to decrease the primitive reflexes that can recur in patients after brain injury. For example, lying supine can increase the tonic labyrinthine supine reflex (TLSR), thereby increasing extensor tone. One of the acceptable goals of rehabilitation can be providing equipment prescriptions to allow for optimal positioning. The antispasticity ball splint for the spastic hand is commonly used. Abduction of the thumb from the palm and spread of the digits can decrease flexor tone in the hand. Like casting, splinting techniques can also be used both to decrease tone and to stretch soft tissues. These techniques can also be combined. For instance, the inhibitory footplate fabricated into lower extremity casts

TABLE 49–19 Modified Ashworth Scale

Score	Description
0	= No increase in muscle tone
1	= Slight increase in tone, minimal resistance end of range
1+	= Slight increase in tone with minimal resistance throughout less than half the remainder range
2	= More marked increase in muscle tone through most of the range; affected part easily moved
3	= Considerable increase in tone, passive movement difficult
4	= Part fixed

Source: Bohannon RW, Smith MB: Interrater reliability of a modified Ashworth scale of muscle spasticity. Phys Ther 1987; 76:206–207.

improves support and alignment of the forefoot. These concepts can be incorporated into orthoses as well. Improving alignment of the foot and ankle frequently leads to a decrease in the presenting pattern of spasticity.

Other treatment options include injections such as neurolytic procedures and chemodenervation with botulinum toxin. Neurolytic procedures take a degree of technical skill to perform. Phenol, alcohol, or anesthetic agents are injected to impair conduction of impulses.[130] Chemical neurolysis refers to destruction of a portion of nerve with alcohol or phenol.[130] When injections are performed at nerves that are predominantly motor, they are referred to as motor point blocks or motor branch blocks. Overall tolerance of the procedure is good, although it can be challenging to perform in children and more agitated and active patients, as they need to remain at rest during injections. Sedation might be necessary in these cases. Reported side effects of neurolysis include swelling, pain, bleeding, dysesthesia, and deep venous thrombosis. After the procedure, patients should rest and elevate the injected extremity. Mild analgesics are beneficial and can be given prophylactically, especially for patients unable to communicate their needs.

Botulinum toxin A is also effective in the treatment of spasticity, although it is not FDA-approved for this indication.[273] It binds irreversibly at the neuromuscular junction, blocking contraction of muscle. Side effects are rare but include atrophy, pain, and infection. Unlike motor point blocks, there are no immediate restrictions on activity following injection. To minimize the potential for antibody production to the medication, it is recommended that injections not be repeated more often than every 3 months and that the total toxin dose be limited to 400 units per session.[318] However, these stipulations are evolving as more experience is gained with the medication and different strains become available for future use. The injection procedure is readily learned. Many clinicians prefer to inject with EMG guidance or electrical stimulation.[318] Results vary with the degree of spasticity, accuracy of injections, units of medication injected, and clinical assessment of the biomechanics contributing to the undesirable position.[76]

The FDA approved intrathecal baclofen therapy (ITB) for the treatment of cerebral origin spasticity in 1996.[12] It effectively reduces spasticity across the greatest number of joints and often produces a dramatic change in tone.[360] Administration of baclofen directly into the intrathecal space allows effective cerebrospinal fluid concentrations with plasma concentrations 100 times less than with oral administration.[12] The systemic side effects are decreased or absent and the clinical response is greater when used intrathecally. Effects of this treatment are greatest on the lower limbs, as the concentration of baclofen is four times greater in the lumbar region than in the cervical region. Changes in upper extremity spasticity are also seen, but this is not considered a primary indication for this treatment at this time.[135, 247] Response to previously attempted interventions should also be considered.

Patients should be carefully assessed and educated prior to undergoing a trial of ITB therapy. The more informed patients and families are about the potential benefits of the treatment, the better the outcome and patient satisfaction that will be obtained. Prior to undergoing a trial of intrathecal baclofen, the patient is assessed as described below. Psychosocial issues must be considered: Can the patient access appropriate therapies if indicated? Will he/she be able to undergo pump refills on time? Are patients and their families located within a reasonable proximity to health care services knowledgeable about ITB therapy?

Once someone is deemed an appropriate candidate, a trial is performed. Baclofen is injected intrathecally and the response is monitored for approximately 8 hours or until the effects wear off.[33] The trial is performed on consecutive days with 50, 75, and 100 micrograms (or 25, 50, and 75 micrograms in the pediatric population).[12, 246] If the patient responds on the first day, there is no reason to perform further trials. In our institution, therapists reassess patients at 4 and 6 hours after injection. Assessments can be videotaped and compared with the pretrial assessment. It is important to remember that the purpose of the trial is to assess whether or not the patient responds to the therapy; it is not to determine the patient's eventual dose and outcome. These will be determined over the first year or so following implant. If there is a favorable response, the pump is implanted. In our center, a neurosurgeon implants the pump and the patient is then managed by the physiatrist. This allows for continuity of care and a functional approach to dose titration and therapy prescriptions. There will often be a need for rehabilitation services as latent movement, motor control, and functional potential are unmasked.

Other surgical procedures available for spasticity management include tendon lengthenings and transfers. While surgeries can weaken spastic muscles, residual spasticity can lead to recurrent deformity.[136] More clinicians now recognize the inherent value in combining spasticity-reducing techniques. Adequate spasticity management with ITB therapy can decrease the need for surgical intervention.[135, 136] In our clinical experience, Achilles tendon lengthening (TAL) is accomplished relatively easily to correct plantarflexion contractures. The split lateral anterior tibialis tendon transfer (SPLATT) can correct forefoot inversion during ambulation. Rhizotomies are generally not performed on adult patients and their performance on children varies regionally. This is a permanently destructive procedure. Anterior rhizotomies provide denervation of the muscle whereas posterior rhizotomies interrupt IA and IB afferents from muscle spindles.

Posttraumatic Epilepsy

It is estimated that approximately 5% of all persons who are hospitalized for TBI will develop *late seizures,* defined as those that occur a week or more after the injury. However, the presence of certain risk factors can increase the probability of developing late seizures or posttraumatic epilepsy (PTE). In particular, penetrating injuries seem to significantly increase one's risk. Other factors that have been identified include seizures during the first week (*early seizures*), depressed skull fractures, acute intracranial hematomas, dural tearing, presence of foreign bodies, focal signs such as aphasia and hemiplegia, age of 65 years or older, loss of consciousness for more than one day, and posttraumatic amnesia present for longer than 24 hours.[22, 177]

In spite of our knowledge of these risk factors, determining the seizure risk of an individual patient is difficult. In 1979, Feeney and Walker[118] devised a mathematical model to estimate seizure risk based on a combination of risk factors. However, this has not proved to be helpful in most clinical situations. This has made decisions regarding prophylaxis against the development of late seizures more difficult.

In the past patients were placed on long-term seizure prophylaxis acutely. However, recent studies have shown that using phenytoin beyond the first week following a brain injury does not prevent the development of late PTE.[326] In addition, the neurobehavioral side effects of phenytoin and other sedating anticonvulsants, such as phenobarbital, can be detrimental to the patient with already slowed thinking and memory loss. These drugs appear to hamper the patient's overall rehabilitation program.[20, 108, 117, 237]

Therefore, seizure prophylaxis in patients with nonpenetrating injuries who have not demonstrated any seizure activity is no longer indicated. If a patient has a penetrating injury or if he/she had seizures during the first week (early seizures), then the decision on prophylactic medication needs to be based on the individual clinical situation. Figure 49–9 summarizes these suggestions, which are based partly on recently released clinical practice parameters.[58]

If late seizures develop, then the patient has PTE and the issue becomes treatment rather than prophylaxis. In these cases, carbamazepine appears to be the drug of choice.[142, 283] Most late seizures are of the partial variety, either simple partial or complex partial, which can secondarily generalize. Carbamazepine has been shown to be as effective as phenytoin and phenobarbital for generalized tonic-clonic seizures, and more effective in the control of partial seizures.[177, 239]

Carbamazepine is well tolerated and has few side effects (e.g., gastrointestinal distress, headaches, dizziness, diplopia), which are usually ameliorated by starting with a low dose and gradually building up to therapeutic range. The most limiting side effect of carbamazepine is bone marrow suppression. However, transient leukopenia, primarily a relative neutropenia, can usually be monitored as long as the white blood cell count is above 3000 cells/mm^8 (with 50% of the white blood cells being neutrophils).[277] The disadvantage of carbamazepine has been its relatively short half-life, which made three-times-daily dosing mandatory.[1] However, longer acting preparations are now available, making twice-a-day dosing and more consistent levels possible.

Valproic acid (Depakote, Depakene), although initially sedating, can be useful as well, since it can have fewer cognitive and behavioral side effects than carbamazepine. Gabapentin (Neurontin), another new antiepileptic medication, may prove to be helpful for patients with PTE. It is approved as adjunctive therapy, does not have significant cognitive side effects, and does not require monitoring of blood levels. Newer antiepileptics, whose benefits for PTE are unknown, include lamotrigine (Lamictal) and topiramate (Topamax).

Posttraumatic Hydrocephalus

Hydrocephalus is a well-recognized complication of traumatic brain injury. Differences in diagnostic criteria and patient populations studied may account for the wide range of estimated incidence (anywhere from 9 to 72%).[164, 220] The fundamental abnormality in hydrocephalus is an imbalance in the production and absorption of cerebrospinal fluid (CSF). Overall, impaired absorption accounts for most cases of hydrocephalus.

Traditionally, hydrocephalus is categorized as either communicating or noncommunicating. In the former, there is a free flow of CSF in the various portions of the ventricular system, the cisterns, and subarachnoid spaces. However, CSF flow from the cisterns to the arachnoid villi is blocked or CSF absorption by the villi is impaired. The latter occurs with inflammation or subarachnoid hemorrhage. Other commonly used terms to categorize hydrocephalus include obstructive hydrocephalus, which describes the pathomechanism, normal

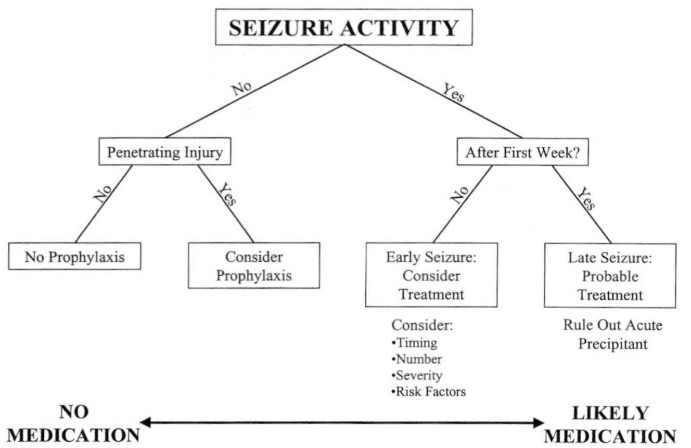

FIGURE 49–9. Guidelines for the initiation of antiepileptic medications.

pressure hydrocephalus (NPH), and hydrocephalus ex-vacuo. NPH is defined as a clinical triad of gait disturbance, mental deterioration, and urinary incontinence associated with ventricular enlargement and normal CSF pressure.[348] Despite radiographic evidence of ventricular enlargement, hydrocephalus ex-vacuo is not "true" hydrocephalus. Instead, it represents changes resulting from brain atrophy. Certain computerized tomography (CT) features that differentiate ex-vacuo from true hydrocephalus are listed in Table 49–20.[192]

Timely diagnosis and treatment are important during rehabilitation, since failure to do so may hamper recovery and minimize the chances of benefiting from therapies. Diagnosis in individuals with severe brain injuries is difficult, since the classic triad of NPH is already present as a direct result of brain trauma. The clinician often has to rely on atypical or more subtle symptoms (e.g., functional decline, failure to progress, seizures, emotional problems, abnormal posturing, or increased spasticity) and confirm the suspicion through CT.

If suspicion for the development of PTH is high, serial monthly CT scans for comparison can help make the diagnosis.[90, 192] In situations where the radiographic findings are equivocal, determining which patients might benefit from shunting is usually based on a constellation of findings. A lumbar puncture for craniospinal-axis pressure can be considered. Shunting is usually successful if the pressure is elevated above 180 mm of water or if the ventricles have progressively increased in size. The patient will also likely benefit from shunt placement if there is a clinical picture of normal pressure hydrocephalus.[259] CT cisternography and radionuclide cisternography can be helpful, but the reliability of these tests is not universally accepted.

The use of an adapted version of the cerebrospinal fluid tap test[348] has been helpful in some cases. This test involves utilization of psychometric measures and gait pattern observation before and after a lumbar puncture in which 50 cc of CSF is removed. Improvement in test results after the removal of fluid implies that successful results will occur if the patient is shunted.

CSF diversion, such as ventriculoperitoneal shunting, is the definitive treatment of hydrocephalus. Alternative methods of shunting include ventriculo-atrial, ventriculo-jugular, and lumboperitoneal. Complications may arise from mechanical failure of the shunt, functional failure resulting from an inadequate flow rate of a working shunt, and infection. Details about shunting are found in various neurosurgical textbooks.

TABLE 49–20 Computed Tomography (CT) Criteria to Define Hydrocephalus

1. "Distended" appearance of the anterior horns of the lateral ventricles
2. Enlargement of the temporal horns and third ventricle
3. Normal or absent sulci
4. If present, enlargement of the basal cisterns and fourth ventricle

Periventricular lucency was used as an indicator of communicating hydrocephalus.

Adapted from Kishore PRS, Lipper MH, Miller JD, et al.: Posttraumatic hydrocephalus in patients with severe head injury. Neuroradiology 1978; 16:261–265.

Cranial Nerve Damage

Cranial nerve damage is a common consequence of brain injury. The resulting impairments, such as compromise of sensation (sight, hearing, smell, taste) and swallowing, can lead to further impairment of function in an already confused patient.[190]

Patients injured in pedestrian-auto and motor vehicle crashes have a higher incidence of cranial nerve injuries than those injured by other causes. Nineteen percent of the patients examined recently in a multicenter study had impairment of one or more cranial nerves. Cranial nerve VII (9% of patients) was injured most frequently, followed by cranial nerve III (6% of patients); least frequently injured were IX and XI.[49, 50, 55] The true incidence of cranial nerve damage related to traumatic brain injury cannot be determined, however, since many studies and common clinical practice tend to ignore testing certain cranial nerves such as I (olfactory).

Cranial nerve I can be damaged directly as it goes through the cribiform plate by a frontal blow or via contra-coupe injury. Impaired olfaction, or dysosmia, can be complete (anosmia) or partial (hyposmia). Dysosmia frequently results in taste alterations and can cause patients to have strange or new food preferences. Patients with an impaired sense of smell might require cueing for hygiene, cooking, storage of food, and use of perfumes. They might need to install smoke detectors and natural gas detectors to compensate for their loss. Patients who work in the petrochemical industry can have significant problems returning to work safely, as they are unable to detect chemical leaks.[105]

Damage to cranial nerve II results in optic neuropathy that presents as visual loss of varying degrees. Injury to the motor system of the eye (i.e., cranial nerves III, IV, and VI) can occur at several levels, both centrally and peripherally. Secondary insults can occur after impact, as with temporal herniation due to edema (uncal herniation with cranial nerve III injury). The resulting strabismus can be due to cranial nerve injury, but some gaze deviations in the early stages after brain injury might not be due to cranial nerve injury. Objective testing to determine ocular alignment can be simply performed by noting symmetrical placement of the corneal reflection of a pen light in each of the cardinal eye positions (Hirschberg reflex). If the images on both corneas are centered, then the visual axes are usually well aligned. A cover/uncover test can generally determine the presence of misalignment of the visual axes when both eyes are viewing, but the need to ensure fixation might limit its utility and agitate uncooperative patients. Convergence and accommodation testing should be performed carefully. Side effects of drugs, most commonly phenytoin and phenobarbitol, can also impair these reflexes. Diplopia occurring at near-vision only can be the result of an impaired vergence system.[28]

Early neuro-ophthalmologic or neuro-optometric evaluation can be valuable in diagnosing subtle abnormalities, recommending corrective measures for visual abnormalities, and preventing secondary complications, such as exposure keratitis of the cornea. In our center, a weekly "Low Vision Rounds" run by a neuro-optometrist serves this purpose. It is unclear whether oculomotor exercises utilized by neuro-optometry specialists are of any value in this population, since there are no comprehensive studies. However, our experience indicates that such procedures might be helpful in enhancing vision during the rehabilitation phase. Certainly the use of corrective prisms, when a patient's alignment is several diopters off, is helpful for the patient who can utilize them.

Injury to the facial nerve most commonly occurs within its passage through the temporal bone. The most deleterious effect is inadequate lid closure and the patient may be susceptible to exposure keratitis of the cornea. If cranial nerve V has also been injured, resulting in the loss of corneal sensation, the problem is compounded. It is imperative that the eye be protected by the use of lubricants and taping the lid closed with eye pads. Unfortunately, this technique is not foolproof and, if not done properly, can cause further damage. Alternatively, occlusive transparent film (which covers the ocular area and creates a "wet chamber") has been utilized to keep the cornea lubricated with some success. Lid tarsorraphy might be necessary to prevent further damage, especially in a low-level patient.

Evaluation of cranial nerve VIII (vestibulo-cochlear nerve) usually occurs during the acute neurosurgical phase. Direct examination can reveal Battle's sign, mastoid fracture, otorrhea, bleeding from the ear, hemotympanum, and lacerations of the tympanic membrane. Hemorrhage from the ear and lacerations of the tympanic membrane might indicate a longitudinal fracture of the temporal bone. As the patient stabilizes, audiometry and the tuning fork test can be utilized. Brainstem auditory evoked potentials can provide further information about the integrity of the auditory system. If hearing loss is significant, hearing aids of the CROS [Contralateral Routing of Signal] type, which transfers sound to the intact ear, can help the patient compensate.

Vestibular disturbances can result in dizziness, impaired balance, ataxia, and nystagmus. The Barany test, a provocative test using head rotation, is useful in evaluating nystagmus. Patients will frequently compensate by tilting their heads to decrease the nystagmus. In patients complaining of dizziness, it is reasonable to implicate vestibular etiology. However, other possible etiologies need to be ruled out.[120] (See Table 49–21.)

TABLE 49–21 Some Common Causes of Dizziness in TBI

Brainstem involvement
Posterior circulation insufficiency
Vestibular impairment (cranial nerve VIII involvement)
Ocular abnormalities
Orthostatic hypotension
Benign paroxysmal positional vertigo
Perilymphatic fistula
Labyrinthine concussion
Meniere's syndrome
Cervical vertigo
Migraine
Medications

Common medications used for vestibular problems, such as meclizine or dimenhydrinate, are antihistamines and can cause sedation in patients with brain injuries. Vestibular therapy, employing habituation, is preferred.[312] The patient uses provocative exercises, which increase the symptoms, to decrease the sensitivity of the vestibular response.

The lower cranial nerves are only occasionally affected by brain injuries. They are more often damaged by direct trauma.[190]

Posttraumatic Hyperthermia

Hyperthermia is a common occurrence during recovery from trauma. It is tempting to attribute fever in an individual with brain injury to central dysfunction, especially if the results of the initial work-up do not suggest an infectious or inflammatory process. However, posttraumatic hyperthermia of central origin is relatively uncommon, occurring in just 4% in one series.[75] A thorough evaluation is usually needed to investigate other, more common etiologies. Although there are a number of potential inciting events, it is reasonable to consider infection as the most likely cause, since an individual with brain injury is susceptible to various complications such as urinary tract infection, aspiration pneumonia, and atelectasis. Associated injuries make the individual subject to multiple procedures and instrumentation, such as intracranial, abdominal, and orthopedic surgeries, ventriculostomy, intubation, central venous catheterization, and bladder catheterization. Immobility adds to the risk of infection. Other, less common causes of fever[75, 148] include medications (so-called "drug fever"), intracranial infection, deep venous thrombosis, paranasal sinusitis, heterotopic ossification, endocarditis, occult abscess, spasticity, hydrocephalus, and increased intracranial pressure. Figure 49–10[75] presents a suggested algorithm for the work-up of hyperthermia in an individual with brain injury.

When an extensive fever work-up fails to identify an etiology, the clinician is led to label the condition "fever of unknown etiology" or attribute the fever to central origin. Central fever usually results in a modest temperature elevation. In some cases, however, it can present as temperature lability. The goal of treatment is to prevent further complications, since elevation of body temperature is associated with increased metabolic demands, exacerbation of neuronal excitotoxicity, and disruption of the blood-brain barrier.[200] Management includes the use of cooling blankets and antipyretics, such as aspirin, acetaminophen, and nonsteroidal anti-inflammatory drugs.[35] Other medications that have been used include dopaminergics (bromocriptine, amantadine), dantrolene sodium, chlorpromazine, clonidine, and propranolol.[248]

Sleep Disorders

Although disturbance of sleep is a common observation in brain injury survivors, its exact incidence is not well known. One study reports an incidence of 73% and 52% in inpatient and outpatient settings, respectively.[84] Sleep

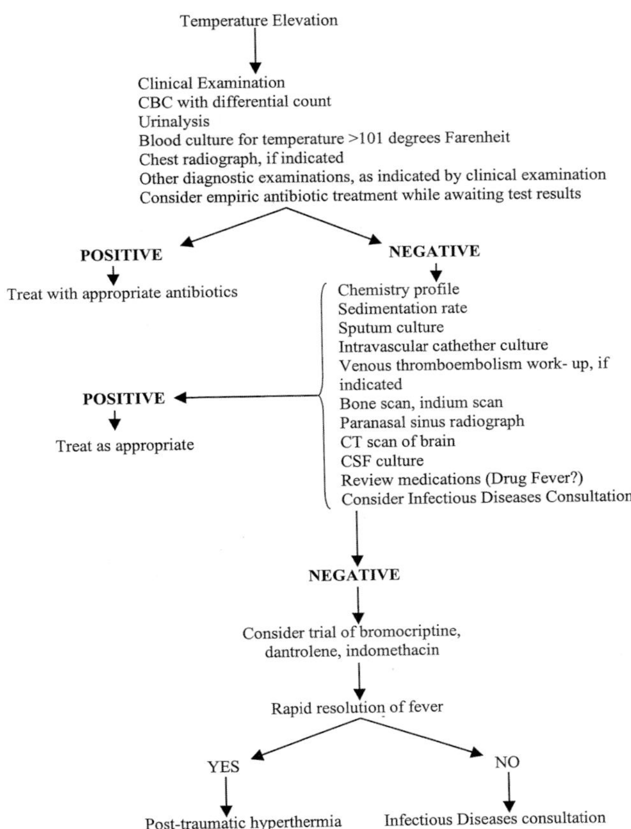

FIGURE 49–10. Suggested fever work-up algorithm for the patient with brain injury.

disorders following brain injury can be classified as either insufficient or excessive sleep. Insufficient sleep can be further categorized as a problem with either initiation or maintenance, or both. Excessive daytime sleepiness might be due to poor nighttime sleep, narcolepsy, or sleep apnea, among others. Too much or too little sleep can impair an individual's arousal, cognition, behavior, and ability to participate in therapies.

Various neurochemicals have been implicated in the sleep-wake cycle. Disruption of these chemicals following a brain injury might theoretically form the basis for posttraumatic sleep disturbance. However, other causes need to be identified in order to render the appropriate treatment. Causative or aggravating conditions include medications, pain, hypoxia, sleep apnea, stress, prior sleep history, poor environmental conditions, excessive caffeine intake, and nicotine use.

Various assessment scales, such as the Epworth Sleepiness Scale and the Pittsburgh Sleep Quality Index, can be used.[159] In the outpatient setting, a sleep log might suffice. However, self-report can be unreliable because of cognitive dysfunction. In the inpatient setting an observational sleep-wake cycle sheet can be used by the nursing staff.

Once other correctable etiologies have been identified, appropriate measures need to be instituted. Nonpharmacological strategies include environmental management (low noise and light, comfortable room temperature), discontinuation or change in administration time of alerting medications, and the avoidance of caffeine and nicotine. Table 49–22[159] lists some commonly used hypnotics.

Pulmonary Complications

Pulmonary complications associated with brain injuries can directly result from the trauma itself (e.g., pneumothorax), subsequent instrumentation (e.g., intubation), or associated neurologic deficits. Even when promptly managed, these problems prolong the need for acute intensive management, prevent early mobilization, and hinder full participation in rehabilitation.

Acute pulmonary complications resulting from trauma include pneumothorax, hemothorax, atelectasis, bacterial and chemical pneumonia, prolonged mechanical ventilation, and neurogenic pulmonary edema (NPE). In addition to complicating medical recovery, these conditions also increase the risk of secondary hypoxic injury. Neurogenic pulmonary edema, associated with isolated brain injury or hemorrhage, is probably related to adult respiratory distress syndrome (ARDS). Increased intracranial pressure, heightened sympathetic activity, and alteration in pulmonary capillary permeability are implicated in its causation. Clinical findings suggestive of NPE include dyspnea, hypoxia, decreased pulmonary vascular compliance, and appearance of

TABLE 49–22 Drugs for Sleep Disorders

Drug	Dose	Effect on Sleep	Side Effects	Comment
Trazodone	25–150 mg hs	Improved REM sleep latency Increased slow-wave sleep	Drowsiness Anticholinergic symptoms Nausea, vomiting Hypotension Musculoskeletal pain	Less anticholinergic and cardiotoxic than tricyclic antidepressants
Tricyclic Antidepressants				
Amitriptyline	25–100 mg hs	Increased stage 4 sleep Decreased percentage of REM sleep Prolonged REM latency Increased total sleep time Improved sleep quality Decreased number of awakenings	Same as nortriptyline	
Nortriptyline	25–150 mg hs		Anticholinergic symptoms Drowsiness Postural hypotension Various cardiac abnormalities Anorexia Nausea Weakness Lethargy Extrapyramidal symptoms Seizures	Monitor serum nortriptyline levels if dosage exceeds 100 mg/day
Zolpidem	5–10 mg hs	At low dose, preserves sleep stages; at high dose, increases slow wave sleep and decreases REM onset	Headache Drowsiness Dizziness Diarrhea Residual sedation or hangover	Higher doses (15–20 mg) may be associated with more adverse events Dose adjustment in those with hepatic impairment
Chloral hydrate	500–1000 mg hs (should not exceed 2000 mg/day)	Increased total sleep time Decreased sleep latency	Gastric irritation Nausea, vomiting, diarrhea Residual sedation or hangover	CNS effects may be due to metabolite, trichloroethanol Effective for short-term use as tolerance may develop after 2 weeks Used also as a sedative Caution when using in those with severe cardiac disease, mentally depressed, and marked hepatic or renal failure
Benzodiazepines				
Temazepam	15–30 mg hs	Decreased phasic interruptions Increased total sleep time Increased REM sleep latency Decreased early night REM sleep	CNS depression, amnesia, drowsiness, confusion, agitation, dizziness, vertigo, ataxia, fatigue, weakness, headache Paradoxical CNS stimulation Nausea, other GI symptoms	Use with caution in those with chronic pulmonary insufficiency, sleep apnea, depressive neurosis or psychotic reactions
Antihistamines				
Diphenhydramine	25–50 mg hs	Suppresses REM sleep Shortened latency to drowsy sleep and sleep onet Decreased number of awakenings	Hangover effect; daytime drowsiness and sleepiness Negative effects on cognition, memory and new learning Impaired motor performance	Not recommended for use in patients with brain injury

"fluffy" infiltrates on chest radiographs. It is usually a self-limiting complication treated with supportive measures. Sympatholytic and inotropic agents might also play a role in treatment.[347]

Pneumonia is a common complication of TBI. Up to 80% of patients with TBI develop early onset pneumonia during the first 7 days post-injury.[253] Early pneumonia is usually nosocomial. Intubated TBI patients are at particular risk because of instrumentation, mechanical ventilation, and compromise of the immune system. Common organisms include *Staphylococcus aureus, Haemophilus influenzae,* and *Pseudomonas aeruginosa.* Important risk factors include intubation at the scene of the injury, GCS score less than 5, evidence of aspiration, and swallowing dysfunction.[357]

In the rehabilitation setting, aspiration is a significant concern because it is a potential cause of pneumonia. Individuals with TBI are at risk of aspiration of stomach contents because of disruption of the normal cough reflex, decreased level of consciousness, decreased oropharyngeal sensation, and reduction in lower esophageal sphincter tone. In order to decrease complications, Nowak et al[262] recommended maintaining tracheostomy tubes in individuals at level III of the Rancho Los Amigos Cognitive Scale. Early tracheostomy plus percutaneous endoscopic gastrostomy has been shown to decrease the risk of clinically significant aspiration.[100] It is important for the clinician to recognize that the presence of an inflated tracheostomy tube is not an absolute protection against aspiration. Bypassing the oral route through a gastrostomy or jejunostomy tube also does not guarantee protection from aspiration. In fact, the presence of a feeding tube can decrease the lower esophageal sphincter tone. Moreover, there appears to be no significant difference in the occurrence of aspiration pneumonia in individuals with intragastric or transpyloric feeding tubes.

In most brain injury rehabilitation units, newly admitted patients are assessed for swallowing function by a speech pathologist. The appropriate fluid and diet consistency is then prescribed. This procedure is performed regardless of diet recommendations from the transferring hospital, since patients' swallowing abilities can change rapidly in the course of recovery. Bedside evaluation of oral motor strength and coordination, management of secretions, ability to swallow different fluid and diet consistencies, and estimation of laryngeal elevation can be helpful in identifying those at risk for aspiration. We have not found the "gag reflex" helpful for this purpose. The presence of a right middle or lower lobe infiltrate on the chest radiographs should raise the suspicion of aspiration pneumonia. Since some individuals are "silent aspirators" (i.e., have actual tracheal penetration or aspiration of food in the absence of clinical symptoms such as coughing or choking), modified barium swallow or videofluoroscopic study are important diagnostic adjuncts.

Early in recovery, an artificial airway is often necessary to prevent hypoxia and improve pulmonary toilet. As recovery progresses, the need for the artificial airway lessens; once this stage is reached, the clinician should consider decannulation (removal of the tracheostomy tube). In addition to pneumonia and other respiratory infections, prolonged use of tracheostomy tubes increases the risk for other complications. A prospective study of direct endoscopy prior to decannulation[262] showed that 32% of the patients had significant laryngeal and tracheal findings, including vocal cord paralysis, tracheal stenosis, subglottic stenosis, glottic stenosis, and tracheal malacia. It is unclear whether these complications resulted from intubation or polytrauma, or both. Granuloma formation has been observed in up to 56% of individuals with TBI who required a tracheostomy for more than one month. Up to 23% can develop tracheal malacia, or thinning and incompetence of the trachea, and up to 12% can suffer from tracheal stenosis. Other, less common complications include vocal cord paralysis and glottic and subglottic stenosis. Timely decannulation may prevent these complications, and is typically considered when the patient does not require oxygen support, is able to effectively manage secretions, and is at a low risk for aspiration.

Decannulation is commonly accomplished by first weaning down the tube size, then plugging the tracheostomy tube over a continuous 24-hour period, and finally by removal. In our center, we downsize the tube to a cuffless variety prior to plugging in order to prevent accidental suffocation. We begin tracheostomy tube plugging for about 2 hours. If the patient is able to tolerate this, that is, able to maintain good oxygenation (as gauged by symptoms and pulse oximetry) and able to handle their secretions, plugging is advanced by 2- to 6-hour intervals daily (depending on patient tolerance). This continues until the tube is plugged continuously for 24 hours. The tube is then removed.

Some authors advocate endoscopic examination of the larynx and trachea in all patients, to detect granulation tissue that can impair breathing once the tracheostomy tube is removed.[193, 262] Others recommend laryngoscopy only in patients who exhibit symptoms of airway obstruction or who are unresponsive.[347] Laryngoscopy can also be considered in those who have had the tracheostomy for more than a month. Decannulation is an important milestone in an individual's recovery from TBI. The tube can aggravate agitation in a recovering patient, cause apprehension in family members, and increase respiratory and nursing care requirements. In certain situations, the presence of a tracheostomy can influence discharge disposition, as some post-acute and long-term care facilities do not accept patients with tracheostomies.

Gastrointestinal and Nutritional Complications

Early Nutrition

The metabolic response to head injury is characterized by increased metabolism and catabolism. It is estimated that resting energy expenditure in patients with severe TBI increases by an average of 40%.[73, 82, 292, 353] In patients with isolated TBI, nitrogen loss is primarily due to an increase in the rate of whole body proteolysis for energy production.[121] Likewise, hyperglycemia with increased rates of glucose turnover and resistance to insulin are found in those with TBI, even in the absence of physical trauma.[121] Most trauma centers now take into account the nutritional needs of acutely injured patients by quickly initiating enteral tube feedings. Patients who have suffered severe visceral trauma can require supplementation by hyperalimentation.[147] Although total enteral nutrition (TEN) is preferred over total parenteral nutrition (TPN), TPN should be promptly given while increasing TEN to a goal of 2 to 2.5 g protein/kg/day and 25 to 35 nonprotein kcal/kg/day.[353] Early parenteral nutrition has been shown to affect immune function by improving T-lymphocyte responsiveness, increasing CD4 cells and preserving CD4:CD8 ratio.[302] Despite aggressive efforts at early nutritional support, it can take up to 3 weeks to achieve a positive nitrogen balance, even if positive caloric balance has been reached.[292, 364] Many TBI patients still need aggressive nutritional management upon admission to rehabilitation. The physiatrist and dietitian should also pay attention to fiber, vitamins, minerals, and isotonicity of enteral feedings, in addition to calories and protein. Weekly weights, as well as monthly measurements of serum prealbumin, are appropriate ways to monitor nutritional status during the rehabilitation phase.

Dysphagia

The incidence of dysphagia in patients with TBI at the time of transfer to rehabilitation is about 27%. In a study in which patients were evaluated via videofluoroscopy, 81% had a delay or absence of swallowing responses, roughly 50% showed reduced tongue control, about 33% had reduced pharyngeal transit, and 14% showed reduced laryngeal closure, elevation, or spasms. Most patients showed two dysfunctional aspects of swallowing, such as impaired tongue control and delayed triggering mechanisms.[205] Acutely, thin liquids are to be avoided, since they are typically the most difficult to handle from a swallowing perspective and, as a result, can lead to aspiration pneumonia.

Videofluoroscopy has become the gold standard for the evaluation of dysphagia. This technique allows the clinician to observe the anatomy and physiology of the swallowing mechanism as a bolus (a barium-impregnated liquid or cookie) travels from the mouth through the pharynx and into the esophagus. Various dysfunctions including aspiration can be documented on the video examination. Compensatory strategies can also be tried and tested during the evaluation.[152]

Patients with swallowing difficulties often have concomitant cognitive impairments. They typically need to be reminded and monitored to employ compensatory strategies. Their diets need to be changed in a sequential fashion (i.e., from pureed, to ground, to chopped, to soft, to regular) as their use of compensatory mechanisms increases and/or their swallowing improves. Treatment efforts primarily focus on compensatory mechanisms. The vast majority of patients improve spontaneously, although this can take several weeks. During this time, the patient is at high risk for developing aspiration pneumonia.

Patients who fail to progress cognitively, are unable to follow commands, have significant swallowing difficulties, and are documented to aspirate or are at high risk for aspiration, need to be fed via an enteral tube. If enteral feeding will be necessary for longer than three to four weeks, a gastrostomy or jejunostomy tube is preferable to a nasogastric tube. The tube can be placed through an open surgical procedure or using an endoscopic technique. Prolonged use of a nasogastric tube may lead to nasal ulceration, nasopharyngeal irritation, sinus infection, and discomfort. Nasogastric tubes can also aggravate agitation and cause the patient to pull out the tube. When this happens, frequent tube reinsertions might have to be done, increasing the risk for nasopharyngeal trauma.

Other Gastrointestinal Complications

Following TBI, stress gastritis can occur acutely in patients with TBI. Superficial mucosal erosions can extend beyond the muscularis mucosa and develop into ulcers. In contradistinction, the ulcers described by Cushing (Cushing's ulcers) are deeper and are associated with high gastrin levels and increased acid secretion. Prophylaxis with H_2 blockers and similar agents may help decrease the magnitude of this complication. One study[157] showed that even though cimetidine did not decrease the incidence of superficial gastric erosions, it reduced the severity of the lesions. Almost all patients are still on ulcer prophylaxis at the time of admission to rehabilitation. The clinician should discontinue the medication when feasible, to minimize adverse drug effects and drug-drug interactions, simplify the drug regimen, and save unnecessary expense.

Nausea and vomiting are frequently encountered gastrointestinal complications of TBI. Although these appear to be relatively minor symptoms, they can increase the risk of aspiration pneumonia, interrupt therapies, and cause distress to the patient and family. The etiologies of nausea and vomiting in TBI are multifactorial (see Table 49–23). Among the specific gastrointestinal abnormalities responsible for these symptoms are an incompetent lower esophageal sphincter (which can be aggravated by the presence of a feeding tube across the gastroesophageal junction) and delayed gastric emptying. In one study, about 50% of patients had delayed gastric emptying and intolerance of gastric feedings during the first week of injury. An improvement in gastric emptying was seen by week 3. The exact etiology of delayed gastric emptying in TBI remains obscure, but increased intracranial pressure, elevated levels of corticotropin-releasing factor, and medications have all been implicated.

Small bowel feeding through a jejunostomy is a treatment option. Jejunostomy was thought to decrease the risk of aspiration, since it bypasses the pylorus. A recent study, however, failed to demonstrate this purported advantage of a jejunostomy over a gastrostomy tube. Jejunostomy can give rise to problems with nutrition and medication administration, since the absorptive capacity of the small bowel is less than that of the stomach. Since jejunostomy also requires continuous feedings, it

TABLE 49–23 Some Causes of Nausea and Vomiting in TBI

Intracranial
- Increased intracranial pressure
- Space occupying lesion
- Hydrocephalus

Ophthalmologic
- Ocular muscle imbalance

Vestibular

Respiratory
- Associated with excessive gagging and coughing

Gastrointestinal
- Gastritis and ulcer
- Impaired LES (Lower Esophageal Sphincter) tone
- Impaired gastric emptying
- Constipation
- Pancreatitis
- Hepatitis

Infection

Iatrogenic
- Medications that cause gastric irritation
- Medications that directly induce nausea and vomiting
- Medication overdose

Migraine

Psychogenic

is not ideal during rehabilitation because it limits mobility and therapies. Unless the patient is suffering from severe reflux and aspiration, gastrostomy is the preferred route.[51]

There can be advantages to having both a jejunostomy and gastrostomy concurrently in those with impaired gastric emptying. The jejunostomy can be used for feeding and the gastrostomy for medication administration and decompression to prevent aspiration. Once gastric emptying improves, feeding can be switched to the gastrostomy route and be given in boluses. In the following weeks, aspirating the stomach for residuals is important in monitoring satisfactory gastric emptying. If reflux remains a concern, the head of the bed needs to be elevated and the patient should be tried on various formulas or smaller feedings.

In our practice, we use the "blue dye test" to help identify individuals with tracheostomies who aspirate oral secretions. This is performed on patients who have a good reflexive swallow and are able to tolerate tracheostomy cuff deflation. On the morning of the test, four drops of blue dye are placed orally and the tracheostomy cuff is deflated. More dye may be added at least every four hours. The night before the test, blue dye in the tube feedings is discontinued. The presence of blue dye in tracheal secretions is indicative of aspiration or tracheo-esophageal fistula.

Prokinetic agents can be used to facilitate gastric emptying. The use of metoclopramide (Reglan) should be avoided.[243] This drug is like the phenothiazines; while it can help initially with reflux by increasing gastric emptying in a small percentage of patients, it is not particularly useful in the long term. Moreover, it is known to cause significant cognitive difficulties for patients, especially for those regaining consciousness. It also has potential side effects of extrapyramidal movements and even permanent tardive dyskinesia. In addition to impeding cognitive recovery, metoclopramide can also cause swallowing difficulties. If the patient has to be on metoclopramide for any reason, it should be limited to two weeks or less.[51, 141] Cisapride (Propulsid) is a more attractive alternative because, unlike metoclopramide, it does not cause central dopaminergic blockade and extrapyramidal effects are rare. The Food and Drug Administration (FDA) has issued a warning on the concurrent use of cisapride and certain antibiotics, antidepressants, antifungals, and protease inhibitors, indicating that this combination could lead to serious cardiac arrhythmias and QT prolongation. In the event that cisapride cannot be used, erythromycin might be a useful alternative to improve gastric emptying.

Incontinence

Fecal incontinence following brain injury is fairly common, especially in patients with significant cognitive impairments. Following brain injury, patients can have an uninhibited neurogenic bowel and be unaware of the need to defecate in a timely and appropriate manner. Constipation or diarrhea can also be significant problems. The development of a daily bowel training program is appropriate regardless of the patient's cognitive status. This can be accomplished through the use of high-fiber enteral feedings or oral supplementation of fiber and the use of a glycerin rectal suppository daily or every other day.[344] Use of digital stimulation should be avoided as it can be misinterpreted by patients who have cognitive difficulties.

Diarrhea can be the result of impaction, osmolar overload from tube feeding, or *Clostridium difficile* colitis. Both osmolar overload and impaction can be prevented by the use of high-protein isotonic feedings that provide essential vitamins and minerals (e.g., Jevity or Enrich). Patients with brain injury are at an increased risk for the development of *C. difficile* colitis because of the frequent need for antibiotic treatment during the acute care phase. Screening for *C. difficile* toxin is indicated in the patient with a prior history of antibiotic administration and hospital-acquired diarrhea.[208] Treatment is usually successful with flagyl or oral vancomycin.

Gastrointestinal Bleeding

As with most polytrauma patients, the patient with a brain injury has an increased risk of gastrointestinal bleeding secondary to stress ulceration during the acute care phase.[73] It is not unusual for patients to be placed on prophylaxis with H_2 antagonists such as cimetidine or ranitidine.[157] Since cognitive and behavioral disturbances have been noted in patients on H_2 antagonists, these medications should be withdrawn once the risk of gastrointestinal bleeding has passed.

Thrombophlebitis

Deep venous thrombosis (DVT) is estimated to occur in up 40% to 54%[2, 132] of cases following major head trauma. Important risk factors for DVT following brain injury include immobility, muscle weakness, associated bone fracture, direct vascular trauma, and venous catheterization. Typical clinical signs, such as calf pain and leg swelling, are not present in all cases.[132] This is a concern because of the potential for pulmonary embolism (PE), which is the initial clinical presentation in up to 80%.[298] Early detection is important to avoid morbidities and potential fatal consequences (the incidence of fatal PE is estimated at 1%). Impedance plethysmography (IPG), doppler ultrasound, D-dimer assay,[188] I-fibrinogen scanning, and radionuclide and contrast venography are commonly used methods of DVT detection. Their sensitivities and specificities vary greatly, especially in the absence of clinical findings.

Commonly used prophylactic measures include intermittent pneumatic compression, graded compression elastic stockings, and anticoagulants (low-dose unfractionated and low–molecular-weight heparin, warfarin, and aspirin). The treatment of PE or DVT proximal to the calf includes anticoagulation. Following initiation of treatment with unfractionated heparin, warfarin is initiated once an activated partial thromboplastin time 1.5 times the control is reached. An initial dose of 5 mg of warfarin is recommended in order to avoid adverse effects, such as excessive anticoagulation and the development of a potential hypercoagulable state.[162, 168] The treatment goal with warfarin is an International Normalized Ratio (INR) between 2 and 3. In those at high risk for bleeding complications, inferior vena cava (IVC) filter placement (Greenfield Filter or Modified Bird's Nest Filter) should be considered.[49, 50, 73, 188] The use of anticoagulants following TBI with associated intracranial hemorrhage is controversial. It should also be used with caution in agitated or confused patients at significant risk for falls. Currently, there are no guidelines as to the optimal time of initiation of anticoagulation following trauma with associated intracranial bleeding.

Genitourinary Complications

Neurogenic bladder following TBI is quite rare; if it does exist, it is usually due to uninhibited detrusor hyperreflexia causing the patient to void small amounts frequently with complete bladder emptying. Patients can usually be adequately managed with an external collection device, such as a condom catheter in males or a diaper in females. These measures should be continued until patients are aware of their surroundings and have sufficient memory to benefit from being offered a commode or bed pan on a regular basis.[150, 183] Patients can also have detrusor hyporeflexia as a result of bladder overdistension that occurs with iatrogenic or traumatic outlet obstruction. These patients usually require prolonged intermittent catheterization (ICP) or an indwelling Foley catheter until this problem has resolved, which may take weeks to months. It is the rare, primarily brainstem-injured patient with detrusor sphincter dyssynergia who needs intermittent catheterization or prolonged Foley drainage and complete urologic studies.[19]

Musculoskeletal Complications

Heterotopic Ossification

Heterotopic ossification (HO) is the formation of mature lamellar bone in soft tissue and periarticular areas. The reported incidence of HO ranges from 11% to 76%, reflecting differences in study populations and detection methods. However, only 10% to 20% of cases have clinically significant HO.[129, 258, 310] Its exact pathophysiology is poorly understood; however, the presence of bone morphogenic protein and genetic susceptibility are implicated, but not proven, in its causation.[181] A related condition, myositis ossificans, is often confused with HO. In traumatic myositis ossificans the bone forms within soft tissues, while it occurs between fascial planes in HO.

Significant risk factors in TBI include prolonged coma (>1 month), immobilization, and limb spasticity.[319] Ectopic bone following TBI usually forms around major joints including elbows, shoulders, hips, and knees. HO frequently causes limitation of joint range of motion, joint deformity, and pain. It can also cause peripheral nerve compression,[65] vascular compression, and lymphedema. Diagnostic findings include transient depression in serum calcium in the early stages and elevated serum alkaline phosphatase, which reflects osteoblastic activity. Increased alkaline phosphatase is not specific for HO, since concurrent fractures or hepatic abnormalities can have a similar effect. Triple-phase bone scan demonstrates abnormalities sooner than plain radiographs.

Prophylaxis with etidronate disodium is controversial. This practice is not well supported in TBI by human and animal studies. It is likely that advocates of HO prophylaxis with etidronate disodium base the rationale of their practice on investigations conducted in the spinal cord and hip arthroplasty populations. By the time physiatrists receive these patients, typically a few weeks post-injury, HO might have started to develop, and prophylactic therapy becomes moot. In the presence of clinical findings suggestive of HO (such as loss of range of motion and joint or limb pain), efforts should be concentrated on early detection and treatment of HO. Although risk factors for HO have been identified, there are still no established criteria to determine which type of patients might benefit from prophylaxis.

Surgical excision is the definitive treatment of HO. In general, surgery should be considered after several months from the time of diagnosis to allow the HO to "mature," and therefore lessen the chances of excessive blood loss during the procedure. Decrease in serum alkaline phosphatase level and bone scan uptake can help indicate HO maturation. In certain cases, CT scanning might be necessary to delineate the extent of HO. Other reported treatments of HO include range of motion to counteract the effects of immobilization, nonsteroidal anti-inflammatory drugs (such as indomethacin), and etidronate disodium. Etidronate inhibits calcium precipitation and osteoid mineralization, but not the formation of the osteoid matrix. Warfarin and radiation[97] have also been reported to be helpful.

Sexual and Reproductive Functioning

Though well-recognized, the impact of TBI on sexual functioning is often neglected in the course of recovery.[137] In addition to physical impairments that might hinder sexual functioning and satisfaction, personality changes, impulsiveness and inappropriateness, and changes in libido can all contribute to the problem. Patients with frontal lobe lesions reported a higher level of sexual functioning and satisfaction than those without a similar lesion.[305] But patients with frontal lobe lesions are also more likely to display disinhibition and inappropriate sexual behavior,[373] which can pose difficulties not only for patients, but also for their interactions with families, the hospital staff, and the public at large. At the other extreme, some TBI patients appear to lose interest in sex. This can also be true of their partners, who may be affected by a change in their roles from partner to caregiver. Obviously, this has the potential to disrupt relationships, since many couples draw upon sex as an expression of love and intimacy.

It is important to address concerns about sexuality during or after acute rehabilitation if these issues appear to have a negative impact on the patient's reintegration into family life and the community. The PLISSIT Model[23] offers a comprehensive approach to identifying issues of particular concern to patients and their partners. Treatment interventions can include behavior modification and counseling. Medical treatment (e.g., drugs for erectile dysfunction, penile prostheses, etc.) are available, but contributing factors to loss of sexual drive, such as depression and medications, should be addressed first.

It is not uncommon for menstruation to cease after a TBI. In many cases, it can take up to one year for normal menses to return. In the event that resumption of menses is delayed, or if there are significant changes in menstrual characteristics (e.g., metromenorrhagia), it is reasonable to refer the patient to an obstetrician for further gynecologic, and possibly endocrinologic evaluation. For sexually active patients and their partners, counseling regarding birth control may also be carried out. It should be noted, however, that the use of oral contraceptives is a concern for those at risk for venous thrombosis.

In some cases,[271] pregnancy during TBI has affected therapeutic decisions during and after rehabilitation. Certain medications used to treat TBI complications have teratogenic potential, some documented (e.g., phenytoin) and others unknown (e.g., botulinum toxin for spasticity). For patients desiring to resume parenting after recovery, parenting activities (e.g., diaper change, breast feeding) can be incorporated into the various physical and occupational therapies. See Chapter 30 for further information on sexuality.

REHABILITATION OF PATIENTS WITH PEDIATRIC BRAIN INJURY

Pediatric brain injury differs in several important ways from brain injury in the adult. Pathologically, TBI in infants and children produces a higher frequency of diffuse cerebral swelling and a lower frequency of intracranial hemorrhage than seen in adults.[11, 194] A complicating epidemiological factor is that a proportion of pediatric TBI is caused by child abuse.[194] Special assessment techniques, such as pediatric coma scales and the Children's Orientation and Amnesia Test (COAT),[115] are needed to evaluate the level of consciousness and duration of PTA in infants and children. Severe childhood TBI appears to have a better prognosis for recovery of consciousness and mobility.[10, 255, 256] One unique feature of pediatric brain injury is that certain injuries suffered at younger ages can lead to functional outcomes worse than those arising from the same injuries suffered in adulthood (e.g., severe TBI during infancy producing mental retardation). This vulnerability has been attributed to disruption of the normal development process,[122] leading to a slower rate of skill acquisition.

A second unique component of pediatric brain injury rehabilitation is the need for long-term follow-up of the child's progress in school, since the child with brain injury is presented with increasing challenges at higher grades. The rehabilitation physician should be prepared to help advocate for the child's educational needs and to provide specific recommendations for modifications in the educational program.[186] The team should also be prepared to work closely with the parents on a long-term basis. Detailed information about pediatric rehabilitation is provided in specialized references.[83, 249, 336, 362]

MANAGEMENT OF MILD TRAUMATIC BRAIN INJURY

Management of mild TBI has undergone rapid change as a result of research on functional outcome, neuropsychological recovery, and the course of postconcussional symptoms. These findings are detailed in specialized references.[15, 31, 41, 42, 47, 212, 216, 240, 291, 370]

Diagnostic criteria for mild TBI are presented above in Table 49–4. Alternative criteria for mild TBI were proposed by a subcommittee of the American Congress of Rehabilitation Medicine (ACRM).[31] The ACRM definition defines mild TBI as a traumatic disruption of brain functioning manifested by at least one of the following: (1) loss of consciousness; (2) loss of memory for events occurring pre- or post-injury; (3) alteration in mental status at the time of injury; (4) physical symptoms attributable to brain injury such as tinnitus, visual changes, memory disturbances, fatigue, and anosmia; and (5) posttraumatic cognitive impairment. Since the ACRM criteria remain to be validated in outcome studies, research findings based on the mild TBI criteria in Table 49–4 should not be generalized to patients who meet the ACRM definition.

A rational strategy for managing mild TBI is based on chronicity, objective evidence of brain injury, and presence of extracranial injuries. During the acute stage following mild TBI, patients should receive a CT scan of the head, since the presence or absence of a traumatic brain lesion on CT scanning is the most reliable indicator of prognosis.[98, 173, 182, 223] In a healthy pediatric patient or young adult with mild TBI and without disability from associated injuries, the absence of brain trauma on CT scanning (i.e., uncomplicated mild TBI) should cause activity restrictions for a few days or weeks. However, when brain trauma is present on CT scanning (i.e., complicated mild TBI), the resumption of pre-injury activities might be delayed beyond this time and, in a minority of patients, some preinjury activities cannot be resumed. It is possible that the risk of failure to resume pre-injury activities is higher in elderly patients and those with preexisting neurologic or psychiatric disorders (e.g., previous TBI). In almost all mild TBI patients the prognostic question is not whether, but *when* activity restrictions can be lifted.

Techniques in the management of acute mild TBI are education and activity restrictions. Complaints of headache and dizziness are common for several months postinjury[301] and should be investigated.[334] The patient and family should be forewarned about cognitive and behavioral changes and about circumstances that might worsen them (e.g., inadequate sleep, substance abuse, stress). The likelihood of a rapid return to pre-injury activities should be emphasized to the patient and family.[15] Brief neuropsychological testing might be useful in identifying cognitive deficits during this stage. If injury-related cognitive deficits are present, the patient should be encouraged to temporarily limit activities and to resume them gradually. For example, a patient with memory deficits might be encouraged to delay returning to work until cleared to do so. Return to work can begin on a part-time or light-duty basis, possibly for only a few days before resuming full duty. In some cases it might be necessary to resume work duties through one or more intermediate steps.

Although isolated mild TBI is not usually seen in rehabilitation settings, it frequently co-occurs with orthopedic or spinal cord injuries that do require rehabilitation. In the case of mild TBI patients who are undergoing rehabilitation for other injuries, the strategy of recommending activity restrictions might be impossible to implement. Instead, it might be necessary to modify the rehabilitation program in order to avoid or circumvent problems related to TBI (e.g., minimize sedating antispasticity or analgesic medications, direct teaching toward family members, or extend the length of stay).

Management of mild TBI in the chronic stage remains controversial. The label of post-concussional syndrome[3] has traditionally been applied to multiple post-injury complaints of dizziness, headache, emotional instability, and cognitive difficulty. In recent years, it has been established that the frequency of secondary gain and somatoform disorders in causing chronic post-concussional complaints is greater than previously recognized.[40–42] The possibility of malingering needs to be considered in neuropsychological testing of chronic mild TBI patients with potential for secondary gain.[42, 251] Useful techniques in determining the validity of symptom complaints include specialized neuropsychological tests (e.g., forced choice recognition testing[169]). MRI of the brain detects traumatic lesions in a minority of mild TBI patients whose brain CT findings are normal,[219, 252] but the prognostic value of MRI findings in uncomplicated mild TBI patients is undetermined. SPECT imaging of mild TBI holds potential as a more sensitive diagnostic procedure, but the role of SPECT imaging in TBI remains to be defined.[166, 328]

POSTTRAUMATIC HEADACHE

Headache is a common complaint of patients after trauma to the head or neck. Packard[269] cited an incidence range of 30% to 80%. It can be as high as 44% six months post-injury[104] and is more prevalent in those with less severe injuries.[361] It must be emphasized that posttraumatic headache (PTH) is not a diagnosis. It is merely a symptom that can have various etiologies (Table 49–24). The International Headache Society[267] (IHS) criteria for posttraumatic headache requires that several conditions be met, such as loss of consciousness, posttraumatic amnesia lasting more than 10 minutes, and the headache beginning less than 14 days after the trauma or regaining consciousness. There must also be relevant abnormalities in at least two of the following: clinical neurologic examination, skull radiography, neuroimaging, evoked potentials, spinal fluid examination, vestibular function test, or neuropsychological testing. The latter is important, since cognitive difficulties are frequently associated with posttraumatic headache.[270] An acute posttraumatic headache becomes chronic if it persists longer than 8 weeks. Persistent posttraumatic headache, especially when associated with mental status or neurologic abnormalities,[202] may require further investigation, such as neuroimaging and CSF studies to rule out intracranial etiologies.

Treatment of posttraumatic headache is directed to correcting the underlying etiology. Some commonly used medications are listed in Table 49–25. Other treatment strategies, including biofeedback and relaxation training, were recently reviewed.[371]

SPORTS-RELATED TRAUMATIC BRAIN INJURY

Increased awareness of TBI resulting from sports and recreation parallels the continued popularity of sports

TABLE 49–24 Some Causes of Posttraumatic Headache

Intracranial

Injury to pain-sensitive structures (venous sinuses, dura in the base of the brain, blood vessels, cranial nerves)

Extracranial

Neuroma
Injury to skin, muscle, arteries
Injury to periosteum
Sinusitis
Temporomandibular joint dysfunction
Cranial nerve abnormalities (e.g., ophthalmoplegia)
Myofascial pain

Others

Adverse effect of medications and other substances (e.g., caffeine)
Co-morbid medical conditions (e.g., uncontrolled hypertension)
Seizures
Poor sleep
Psychological factors

TABLE 49–25 Some Medications Used to Prevent and Treat Headache

Nonsteroidal anti-inflammatory drugs
Antiepileptics
Serotonin-selective agonist (e.g., sumatriptan)
Selective serotonin reuptake inhibitors
Tricyclic antidepressants
Beta-blockers
Calcium channel blockers
Antihistamines
Steroids
Antiemetics

and growing attention from the media. It is estimated that up to 87% of boxers have either clinical or radiologic evidence of TBI. Indeed, the cognitive impairment in boxers has a special designation: *dementia pugilistica.* Nevertheless, boxing's popularity is unabated. Approximately 250,000 concussions have been attributed to football injuries per year. Practically every contact sport—basketball, soccer, and wrestling included—has the potential for TBI. The same is true for some recreational activities such as snow- and jet-skiing. Increased concerns about the "second impact syndrome" in young athletes were raised by studies suggesting that a second head injury sustained before symptoms associated with a previous head injury have fully cleared might result in cerebral swelling and death.[68, 308] However, a more recent investigation argued that when strict diagnostic criteria are applied, this syndrome might be less common than previously thought.[241]

The American Academy of Neurology recently published a report of its Quality Standards Subcommittee on practice parameters for the management of concussion in sports.[17] The common symptoms of concussion were categorized as either early, occurring minutes to hours after the event, or late (days to weeks). Among the early symptoms are headache, dizziness or vertigo, lack of awareness of surroundings, and nausea or vomiting. Late symptoms include persistent low-grade headache, lightheadedness, poor attention and concentration, memory dysfunction, easy fatigability, irritability and low frustration tolerance, intolerance of bright lights or difficulty focusing vision, intolerance of loud noises, anxiety, depressed mood, and sleep disturbance. Based on a review of the literature, a grading scale and treatment recommendations were established. These management recommendations were only considered *options,* as opposed to *standards,* since no class I evidence in the literature exists. The same report addressed recommendations for return to play after a concussion (see Table 49–26).[17, 191]

ETHICAL ISSUES

Brain injury raises many profound and difficult ethical issues. While some of these ethical issues can be addressed only at a collective level (e.g., how society allocates resources for people with brain injuries), others arise in the daily practice of rehabilitation professionals.[323] Clinicians are often confronted with ethical decisions that have significant consequences for those they care for. In what follows, we concentrate on several difficult ethical problems that have special relevance for physicians: assessing patient competency, making decisions to withhold or withdraw life-sustaining measures, and utilizing restraints.

One of the most commonly encountered problems in brain injury rehabilitation is the assessment of competency.[195] Determining a patient's competence to make decisions is crucial because, as clinicians, we have an obligation to honor the wishes of competent adult patients. At the same time, we are committed to preventing the harm that can result from decisions made by an incompetent patient. The practical question of whether or not to accede to a patient's wishes depends on our assessment of their competence to make decisions. Unfortunately, evidence suggests that clinicians working with people with brain injuries tend to neglect issues of competence and consent. These findings, documented by a congressional investigation earlier this decade,[86] were confirmed by a more recent study.[124]

Despite lingering areas of controversy, there is growing agreement in the bioethical and legal communities about the basic principles underlying the assessment of competence.[151] To begin with, the clinician should recognize that competence is domain-specific. That is, patients can be determined to be competent to make certain decisions (e.g., regarding medical treatment) but not others (e.g., regarding financial management). In

TABLE 49–26 Recommendations Regarding Return to Play After Sports-Related Concussion

Concussion Grade	Criteria	Guidelines for Return to Play*
Grade I	• Transient confusion • No Loss of consciousness (LOC) • Concussion symptoms or mental status abnormalities resolve in *less* than 15 minutes	15 minutes (single) 1 week (multiple)
Grade II	• Transient confusion • No loss of consciousness • Concussion symptoms or mental status abnormalities last *more* than 15 minutes	1 week (single) 2 weeks (multiple)
Grade III	Any loss of consciousness, either brief (seconds) or prolonged (minutes)	1 week (brief LOC) 2 weeks (prolonged LOC) 1 month or longer (multiple)

* Only after being asymptomatic with normal neurologic examination at rest and with exercise.

addition, recent commentators have emphasized evaluating the process by which a decision is made. That is, the focus is on how a decision is made, not what is decided.

The assessment of this process involves the direct examination of the abilities central to decision-making capacity. These include the abilities to *choose,* to *understand* relevant information, to *appreciate* its significance for one's own situation, and to *reason* logically with that information.[151] Consider, for example, patients who refuse a recommended treatment. In order to be determined competent to make the decision, they must appreciate their condition; understand the nature and rationale for the treatment as well as its risks, benefits, and alternatives; and be able to reason with this information in a logical manner. Whether or not the patient possesses the requisite capacities can usually be assessed on clinical interview; however, formal assessment tools incorporating these principles are also available.[151]

Despite the usefulness of this model of competency, there are limitations in its application to people with brain injuries.[195] In particular, the cognitive bias of the model can make it less sensitive to the affective and volitional sequelae of brain injury that can also compromise competence. In other words, a patient can appear to be clinically competent on interview and yet actually have significant impairments in making decisions in his/her everyday life.

If a person is found to be incompetent to make treatment decisions, substitute or *surrogate* decision-makers must be identified.[67, 276] Clinicians should be guided by the relevant laws in their states to determine who the surrogate may be and what sort of limits (if any) apply to their decision-making authority. Even after identifying the appropriate decision-maker (e.g., a family member), the clinician has an ongoing ethical responsibility to ensure that the decisions made by the surrogate are appropriate (i.e., represent the patient's prior preferences or best interests).[67]

One of the most difficult questions a family member or clinician is called upon to make is that of withholding or withdrawing life-sustaining treatments. This issue has dominated bioethics for the last two decades, and many of the most prominent cases have involved people with severe brain injuries.[127] Most often, the family of a severely injured patient makes the request to withhold or withdraw treatment. The patient is usually in a vegetative state. However, the number of similar requests for minimally conscious patients appears to be rising.[77]

Although controversy continues, a bioethical and legal consensus is beginning to coalesce around certain fundamental principles.[127] The primary obligation of the clinician in these situations is to ascertain what the patient's prior beliefs and preferences were. This information is most often obtained from the patient's family. A recent U.S. Supreme Court decision has confirmed that decisions regarding withholding or withdrawing life-sustaining treatments from incompetent patients can be guided by their previously expressed wishes.[4]

Despite this, questions remain. For example, several important court cases[4, 5] have focused on what constitutes sufficient evidence of an incompetent person's previous wishes; for instance, is anything short of a written directive acceptable? Even when a patient's previous wishes are well documented, the applicability of these prior wishes may still be problematic. For example, some minimally conscious people, although severely impaired, seem to be in no distress; they may even demonstrate the ability to derive pleasure from certain simple activities. Should we honor their prior wishes to discontinue life-sustaining interventions under such circumstances?[5, 29, 109]

The situation is even more complicated when a person's previous preferences are *not* known. In these circumstances, most jurisdictions recognize the authority of family members to make decisions for the patient.[127] However, the considerations that should guide these decisions remain controversial. Some have argued that, when a patient's prior wishes are unknown, the presumption should be to preserve life.[53] Others have argued that it is legitimate to base decisions in these situations on considerations of quality of life,[77] cost, or even the results of surveys indicating that most people would not want their lives preserved if they were in a persistent vegetative state.[21] A recent development has been the claim that considerations of quality of life are illegitimate and might even violate the Americans with Disabilities Act.[27] Confounding all of these issues is the considerable uncertainty about prognosis for recovery, especially soon after an injury.

Clearly, there is no societal consensus on how to proceed when a patient's previous wishes are not known. In these situations, clinicians should seek the guidance of hospital ethics committees as well as legal counsel. In addition, physicians who are uncomfortable with the decisions reached can consider transferring the care of the patient to another physician. Finally, it should be emphasized that hasty decisions are rarely necessary. Especially if a patient is in a vegetative state, little harm is done in taking time to address all considerations.

A less dramatic but far more common ethical issue confronting physicians involves the decision to initiate psychoactive medications[26, 89] or physical restraints.[254, 321] Some of the considerations that should guide the use of psychoactive agents were discussed in the section on the management of agitation. These same principles (i.e., obtaining consent, ensuring that the intervention is in the patient's best interest, exhausting less restrictive alternatives) apply when choosing to physically restrain a patient.

It is also important to recognize the disadvantages of physical restraints. Evidence is accumulating that restraints are not particularly effective (e.g., in preventing falls).[254, 321] Moreover, the restraints themselves pose a physical risk to the patient (including reported cases of death).[254] Finally, studies demonstrate that reducing restraint use does not necessarily increase the need for additional staff or cost to the institution.[321] For these reasons, and because of the ethical issues involved, many institutions are adopting a minimal-restraint or restraint-free policy.

ACKNOWLEDGMENTS

Preparation of this chapter was supported in part by grants H133A70015 (Traumatic Brain Injury Model System of TIRR) and

H133B40002 (Rehabilitation Research and Training Center on Rehabilitation Interventions Following Traumatic Brain Injury, PI: Walter M. High, Jr.) from the National Institute for Disability and Rehabilitation Research, U.S. Department of Education, Washington, D.C. The authors are grateful to Mary Nowak for preparing the manuscript, to Sean Little for entering references, and to Pam Cornell for library assistance. This chapter is dedicated to the memory of Catherine F. Bontke, M.D., who taught that our patients' outcomes should not be limited by our own lack of imagination.

REFERENCES

1. Drugs for epilepsy. Med Lett Drugs Ther 1986; 28:91–94.
2. Prevention of venous thrombosis and pulmonary embolism. NIH consensus development. JAMA 1986; 256:744–749.
3. The DRG ICD-9-CM codebook: A users guide. Washington, DC, St. Anthony Hospital, 1986.
4. Cruzan v. Director, Missouri Department of Health. 497 U.S. 261, 110 S. Ct. 2841, 111 L. Ed. 2d 224 (Supreme Court 1990).
5. In re Martin, 538 NW 2d 399 (Mich 1995).
6. Abdel DH, Sade K, Kouris K: Changes in cerebral perfusion after acute head injury: Comparison of TC with tc-99HMPAO SPECT. Radiology 1987; 165:221–226.
7. Adamovich BB, Henderson JA, Auerbach S: Cognitive Rehabilitation of Closed Head Injured Patients: A Dynamic Approach. San Diego, College-Hill, 1985.
8. Adams JH: Head injury. In Adams JH, Duchen LW (eds): Greenfield's Neuropathology, ed 4. London, E. Arnold, 1992.
9. Adams RD, Victor M, Ropper AH: Principles of Neurology, ed 6. New York, McGraw-Hill, 1997.
10. Adelson PD: Prognosis and recovery. In Marion DW (ed): Traumatic Brain Injury. New York, Thieme, 1999, pp 283–290.
11. Adelson PD, Kochanek PM: Head injury in children. J Child Neurol 1998; 13:2–15.
12. Albright AL, Barron WB, Fasick MP, et al: Continuous intrathecal baclofen infusion for spasticity of cerebral origin. JAMA 1993; 270:2474–2477.
13. Aldrich EF, Eisenberg HM: Prognostic factors. In Marion DW (ed): Traumatic Brain Injury. New York, Thieme, 1999, pp 223–229.
14. Alexander MP: Traumatic brain injury. In Benson DF, Blumer D (eds): Psychiatric Aspects of Neurologic Disease. New York, Grune & Stratton, 1982, pp 219–249.
15. Alexander MP: Mild traumatic brain injury: Pathophysiology, natural history, and clinical management. Neurology 1995; 45: 1253–1260.
16. American Academy of Neurological Surgery: Guidelines for the Management of Severe Head Injury. New York, Brain Trauma Foundation, 1995.
17. American Academy of Neurology Quality Standards Subcommittee: Practice parameter: The management of concussion in sports. Neurology 1997; 48:581–585.
18. Anderson CV, Bigler ED: Ventricular dilation, cortical atrophy, and neuropsychological outcome following traumatic brain injury. J Neuropsychiat Clin Neurosci 1995; 7:42–48.
19. Anderson JT: Neuro-urological investigation in urinary bladder dysfunction. Int Urol Nephrol 1977; 9:133–143.
20. Andrews DG, et al: The influence or carbamazepine and phenytoin on memory and other aspects of cognitive function in new referrals with epilepsy. Acta Neurol Scand 1984; 69(suppl 99):23–30.
21. Angell M: The dilemma of the persistent vegetative state. N Engl J Med 1994; 330:1524–1525.
22. Annegers JF, Hauser WA, Coan SP, Rocca WA: A population-based study of seizures after traumatic brain injuries. N Engl J Med 1998; 338:20–24.
23. Annon JS: The PLISSIT model: A proposed conceptual scheme for the behavioral treatment of sexual problems. J Sex Ed Ther 1976; 2:1–15.
24. Ansell B, Keenan J: The Western Neurosensory Stimulation Profile: A tool for assessing slow-to-recover head injured patients. Arch Phys Med Rehabil 1989; 70:104–108.
25. Ashley MJ, Krych DK (eds): Traumatic Brain Injury Rehabilitation. Boca Raton, FL, CRC Press, 1995.
26. Auerbach V, Jann B: Ethicolegal issues in pharmacotherapy for neurorehabilitation. Neurorehabil 1991; 1(1):58–63.
27. Avila D: The Americans with Disabilities Act and unconsciousness: A rejoinder. J Head Trauma Rehabil 1994; 9(1):103–105.
28. Baker RS, Epstein AD: Ocular motor abnormalities from head trauma: Major review. Surv Ophthalmol 1991; 35:245–267.
29. Banja JD: "You wouldn't want to live like that. . . ." J Head Trauma Rehabil 1997; 12(6):92–97.
30. Barth JT, Macciocchi SN, Diamond PT: Mild head injury: Current research and clinical issues. In Rosenthal M, Griffith ER, Kreutzer JS, Pentland B (eds): Rehabilitation of the Adult and Child with Traumatic Brain Injury, ed 3. Philadelphia, FA Davis, 1999, pp 471–478.
31. Barth JT, Macciocchi SN (eds): Mild traumatic brain injury. J Head Trauma Rehabil 1993; 8(3) [whole issue].
32. Bass B, Weinshenker B, Rice DP, et al: Tizanidine versus baclofen in the treatment of spasticity in patients with multiple sclerosis. Can J Neurol Sci 1988; 15:15–19.
33. Becker R, Bauer BL, Alberti O, et al: Continuous intrathecal baclofen infusion in severe spasticity after traumatic or hypoxic brain injury. J Neurol 1997; 244:160–166.
34. Bendixon BH, Benton AL: Cognitive and linguistic outcome. In Levin HS, Benton AL, Muizelaar JP, Eisenberg HM (eds): Catastrophic Brain Injury. New York, Oxford University Press, 1996, pp 121–151.
35. Benedek G, Toth-Daru P, Janaky J, et al: Indomethacin is effective against neurogenic hyperthermia following cranial trauma or brain surgery. Can J Neurol Sci 1987; 14:145–148.
36. Bergquist TF, Boll TJ, Corrigan JD, et al: Neuropsychological rehabilitation: Proceedings of a consensus conference. J Head Trauma Rehabil 1994; 9(4):50–61.
37. Berrol S: Issues in cognitive rehabilitation. Arch Neurol 1990; 47:219–220.
38. Berrol S: Persistent vegetative state. Phys Med Rehabil State Art Rev 1990; 4(3):559–567.
39. Bes A, Eyssette M, Pierrot-Deseilligny E, et al: A multi-centre, double blind trial of tizanidine—a new antispastic agent in spasticity associated with hemiplegia. Curr Med Res Opin 1988; 10:709–718.
40. Binder LM: Persisting symptoms after mild head injury: A review of the postconcussive syndrome. J Clin Exp Neuropsychol 1986; 8:323–346.
41. Binder LM: A review of mild head trauma part 2: Clinical implications. J Clin Exp Neuropsychol 1997; 19:432–457.
42. Binder LM, Rohling ML, Larrabee G: A review of mild head trauma part 1: Meta-analytic review of neuropsychological studies. J Clin Exp Neuropsychol 1997; 19:421–431.
43. Blanton S, Porter L, Smith D, et al: Strategies to enhance mobility in traumatic brain injured patients. Rosenthal M, Griffith ER, Kreutzer JS, Pentland B (eds): Rehabilitation of the Adult and Child with Traumatic Brain Injury, ed 3. Philadelphia, FA Davis, 1999, pp 219–241.
44. Boake C: A history of cognitive rehabilitation of head-injured patients, 1915 to 1980. J Head Trauma Rehabil 1989; 4(3):1–8.
45. Boake C: Transitional living centers in head injury rehabilitation. In Kreutzer JS, Wehman PH (eds): Community Integration Following Traumatic Brain Injury. Baltimore, Paul H Brookes, 1990, pp 115–124.
46. Boake C: Supervision Rating Scale: A measure of functional outcome from brain injury. Arch Phys Med Rehabil 1996; 77:765–772.
47. Boake C, Bobitec K, Bontke CF: Rehabilitation of the patient with mild traumatic brain injury. Neurorehabil 1991; 1(3):70–78.
48. Bohannon RW, Smith MB: Interrater reliability of a modified Ashworth scale of muscle spasticity. Phys Ther 1987; 67:206–207.
49. Bontke CF: Medical complications related to traumatic brain injury. Phys Med Rehabil State Art Rev 1989; 3(1):43–52.
50. Bontke CF: Medical advances in the treatment of brain injury. In Kreutzer JS, Wehman PH (eds): Community Reintegration Following Traumatic Brain Injury. Baltimore, Paul H Brookes, 1990, p 51.
51. Bontke CF, Baize C, Boake C: Coma management and sensory stimulation. Phys Med Rehabil Clin N Amer 1992; 3(2):259–272.
52. Bontke CF, Boake C, Zasler ND, et al: Rehabilitation of the head injured patient. In Narayan RK, Wilberger JE Jr, Povlishock JT (eds): Neurotrauma. New York, McGraw-Hill, 1996, pp 841–858.

53. Bontke CF, Dolan J, Ivanhoe CB: Should we withhold food from patients in persistent vegetative state? J Head Trauma Rehabil 1994; 9(4):62–69.
54. Bontke CF, Horn LJ, Sandel B: Sensory stimulation: Accepted practice or expected practice? J Head Trauma Rehabil 1992; 7(4):115–120.
55. Bontke CF, Lehmkuhl LD, Englander JS, et al: Medical complications and associated injuries of persons treated in Traumatic Brain Injury Model Systems programs. J Head Trauma Rehabil 1993; 8(2):34–46.
56. Boyeson MG, Jones JL: Theoretical mechanisms of brain plasticity and therapeutic implications. In Horn LJ, Zasler ND (eds): Medical Rehabilitation of Traumatic Brain Injury. Philadelphia, Hanley & Belfus, 1996, pp 77–102.
57. Braakman R, Jennett B, Minderhoud JM: Prognosis of the posttraumatic vegetative state. Acta Neurochir 1988; 95:49–52.
58. Brain Injury Special Interest Group of the American Academy of Physical Medicine and Rehabilitation. Practice parameter: Antiepileptic drug treatment of posttraumatic seizures. Arch Phys Med Rehabil 1998; 79:594–597.
59. Bricolo A, Turazzi S, Feriotti G: Prolonged posttraumatic unconsciousness: Therapeutic assets and liabilities. J Neurosurg 1980; 52:625–634.
60. Bricolo A, Turella G: Electroencephalographic pattern of acute traumatic coma: Diagnostic and prognostic value. J Neurosurg Sci 1973; 17:278–285.
61. Brigman C, Dickey C, Zegeer LJ: Agitated aggressive patient. Am J Nurs 1983; 83:1409–1412.
62. Bromberg MB, Vogel CM: Vest restraint palsy. Arch Phys Med Rehabil 1996; 77:1316–1319.
63. Brooke MM, et al: Agitation and restlessness after closed head injury: A prospective study of 100 consecutive admissions. Arch Phys Med Rehabil 1992; 73:320–323.
64. Brooke MM, et al: The treatment of agitation during initial hospitalization after traumatic brain injury. Arch Phys Med Rehabil 1992; 73:917–921.
65. Brooke MM, Heard DL, deLateur BJ, et al: Heterotopic ossification and peripheral nerve entrapment: Diagnosis and excision. Arch Phys Med Rehabil 1991; 72:425–429.
66. Brooks N: Head injury and the family. In Brooks N (ed): Closed Head Injury: Psychological, Social and Family Consequences. Oxford, Oxford University Press, 1984, pp 123–147.
67. Buchanan AE, Brock DW: Deciding for others: The ethics of surrogate decision making. New York, Cambridge University Press, 1989.
68. Cantu RC, Voy R: Second impact syndrome: A risk in any contact sport. Phys Sports Med 1995; 23:27–34.
69. Carey RG, Seiberg JH, Posavac EJ: Who makes the most progress in inpatient rehabilitation? An analysis of functional gain. Arch Phys Med Rehabil 1988; 69:337–343.
70. Caron M: PET/SPECT imaging in head injury. In Narayan RK, Wilberger JE Jr, Povlishock JT (eds): Neurotrauma. New York, McGraw-Hill, 1996, pp 163–168.
71. Cassidy JW: Pharmacological treatment of posttraumatic behavioral disorders: Aggression and disorders of mood. In Wood RL (ed): Neurobehavioral Sequelae of Traumatic Brain Injury. New York, Taylor & Francis, 1990, pp 250–273.
72. Chen YW, Lomnitski L, Michaelson DM, Shohami E: Motor and cognitive deficits in apolipoprotein E-deficient mice after closed head injury. Neurosurg 1997; 80:1255–1262.
73. Chestnut RM: Medical complications of the head injured patient. In Cooper PR (ed): Head Injury, ed 3. Baltimore, Williams & Wilkins, 1993, pp 459–501.
74. Chestnut RM, Carney N, Maynard H, et al: Summary report: Evidence for the effectiveness of rehabilitation for persons with traumatic brain injury. J Head Trauma Rehabil 1999; 14:176–188.
75. Childers MK, Rupright J, Smith DW: Post-traumatic hypothermia in acute brain injury rehabilitation. Brain Inj 1994; 8:335–343.
76. Childers MK, Stacy M, Cooke DL, et al: Comparison of two injection techniques using botulinum toxin in spastic hemiplegia. Am J Phys Med Rehabil 1999; 75:462–469.
77. Childs NL, Cranford RE: Termination of nutrition and hydration in the minimally conscious state: Contrasting clinical views. J Head Trauma Rehabil 1997; 12(4):70–78.
78. Choi SC: Predicting outcome in the head-injured patient. In Narayan RK, Wilberger JE Jr, Povlishock JT (eds): Neurotrauma. New York, McGraw-Hill, 1996, pp 593–611.
79. Choi SC, Barnes TY, Bullock R, et al: Temporal profile of outcomes in severe head injury. J Neurosurg 1994; 81:169–173.
80. Clifton GL, Hayes RL: Hypothermia for the treatment of head injury. In Narayan RK, Wilberger JE Jr, Povlishock JT (eds): Neurotrauma. New York, McGraw-Hill, 1996, pp 401–412.
81. Clifton GL, Jiang JY, Lyeth BG, et al: Marked protection by moderate hypothermia after experimental traumatic brain injury. J Cereb Blood Flow Metab 1991; 11:114–121.
82. Clifton GL, Ziegler MG, Grossman RG: Circulating catecholamines and sympathetic activity after head injury. Neurosurg 1981; 8:10–14.
83. Cockrell J: Pediatric brain injury rehabilitation. In Horn LJ, Zasler ND (eds): Medical Rehabilitation of Traumatic Brain Injury. Philadelphia, Hanley & Belfus, 1996, pp 171–196.
84. Cohen M, Oksenberg A, Snir D, et al: Temporally related changes of sleep complaints in traumatic brain injuries. J Neurol Neurosurg Psychiat 1992; 55:313–315.
85. Coleman M, Handler M, Martin C: Update on apolipoprotein E state of the art. Hosp Phys 1995:22–24.
86. Committee on Government Operations, House of Representatives, U.S. Congress: Fraud and abuse in the head injury rehabilitation industry: Twenty-fifth report. Washington, DC, Government Printing Office, 1992. U.S. Congress House, Report 102–1059.
87. Coonley-Hoganson R, Sachs N, Desai BT, Whitman S: Sequelae associated with head injuries in patients who were not hospitalized: A follow-up survey. Neurosurg 1984; 14:315–317.
88. Cooper PR (ed): Head Injury, ed 3. Baltimore, Williams & Wilkins, 1993.
89. Cope DN: Legal and ethical issues in the psychopharmacologic treatment of traumatic brain injury. J Head Trauma Rehabil 1989; 4(1):13–21.
90. Cope DN, Date ES, Mar EY: Serial computerized tomographic evaluations in traumatic head injury. Arch Phys Med Rehabil 1988; 69:483–486.
91. Corrigan JD: Development of a scale for assessment of agitation following traumatic brain injury. J Clin Exp Neuropsychol 1989; 11:261–277.
92. Corrigan JD: Substance abuse as a mediating factor in outcome from traumatic brain injury. Arch Phys Med Rehabil 1995; 76:302–309.
93. Corrigan JD, Arnett JA, Houck LJ, Jackson RD: Reality orientation for brain injured patients: Group treatment and monitoring of recovery. Arch Phys Med Rehabil 1985; 66:626–30.
94. Corrigan JD, Bogner JA, Lamb-Hart GL: Substance abuse and brain injury. In Rosenthal M, Griffith ER, Kreutzer JS, Pentland B (eds): Rehabilitation of the Adult and Child with Traumatic Brain Injury, ed 3. Philadelphia, FA Davis, 1999, pp 556–571.
95. Courjon J: A longitudinal electro-clinical study of 80 cases of posttraumatic epilepsy observed from the time of original trauma. Epilepsia 1970; 11:29–36.
96. Courville CB: Commotio Cerebri: Cerebral Concussion and the Post-concussion Syndrome in Their Medical and Legal Aspects. Los Angeles, San Lucas Press, 1953.
97. Coventry MB, Scanlon PW: The use of radiation to discourage ectopic bone. J Bone Joint Surg Am 1981; 63:201–208.
98. Culotta VP, Sementilli ME, Gerold K, Watts CC: Clinicopathological heterogeneity in the classification of mild head injury: Clinical studies. Neurosurg 1996; 38:245–250.
99. Cusumano S, Paolin A, Di Paola F, et al: Assessing brain function in post-traumatic coma by means of bit-mapped SEPs, BAEPs, CT, SPET and clinical scores. Prognostic implications. Electroencephalogr Clin Neurophysiol 1992; 84:499–514.
100. D'Amelio LF, Hammond JS, Spain DA, Sutyak JP: Tracheostomy and percutaneous endoscopic gastrostomy in the management of the head-injured trauma patient. Am Surg 1994; 60:180–185.
101. da Silva AM, Nunes B, Vaz AR, Mendonca D: Posttraumatic epilepsy in civilians: Clinical and electroencephalographic studies. Acta Neurochir Suppl 1992; 55:56–63.
102. Dacey R, Dikmen S, Temkin N, et al: Relative effects of brain and non-brain injuries on neuropsychological and psychosocial outcome. J Trauma 1991; 31:217–222.

103. Davidoff GN, Roth EJ, Richards JS: Cognitive deficits in spinal cord injury: Epidemiology and outcome. Arch Phys Med Rehabil 1992; 73:275–283.
104. De Benedittis G, De Santis A: Chronic post-traumatic headache: Clinical, psychopathological features outcome determinants. J Neurosurg Sci 1983; 27:177–186.
105. Deems DA, Doty RL, Settle G, et al: Smell and taste disorders: A study of 750 patients from the University of Pennsylvania Smell and Taste Center. Arch Otolaryngol Head Neck Surg 1991; 117:519–528.
106. Dikmen S, Machamer J, Savoie T, et al: Life quality outcome in head injury. In Grant I, Adams KM (eds): Neuropsychological Assessment of Neuropsychiatric Disorders, ed 2. New York, Oxford University Press, 1996, pp 552–576.
107. Dikmen SS, Temkin NR, Machamer JE, et al: Employment following traumatic head injuries. Arch Neurol 1994; 51:177–186.
108. Dikmen SS, Temkin NR, Miller B, et al: Neurobehavioral effects of phenytoin prophylaxis of posttraumatic seizures. JAMA 1991; 265:1271–1277.
109. Dresser R: Still troubled: In re Martin. Hastings Cent Rep 1996; 26:21–22.
110. Eisenberg HM: Outcome after head injury: General considerations and neurobehavioral recovery—part I, general considerations. In Becker DP, Povlishock JT (eds): Central Nervous System Trauma Status Report. Bethesda, MD, National Institute of Neurological and Communicative Diseases and Stroke, 1985, pp 271–280.
111. Eisenberg HM, Gary HE Jr, Aldrich EF, et al: Initial CT findings in 753 patients with severe head injury: A report from the NIH Traumatic Coma Data Bank. J Neurosurg 1990; 73:688–698.
112. Ellenberg JH, Levin HS, Saydjari C: Posttraumatic amnesia as a predictor of outcome after severe closed head injury: Prospective assessment. Arch Neurol 1996; 53:782–791.
113. Englander J, Cifu DX: The older adult with traumatic brain injury. In Rosenthal M, Griffith ER, Kreutzer JS, et al (eds): Rehabilitation of the Adult and Child with Traumatic Brain Injury, ed 3. Philadelphia, FA Davis, 1999, pp 453–470.
114. Evans RW (ed): Neurology and Trauma. Philadelphia, WB Saunders, 1996.
115. Ewing-Cobbs L, Levin HS, Fletcher JM, et al: The Children's Orientation and Amnesia Test: Relationship to severity of acute head injury and to recovery of memory. Neurosurg 1990; 27:683.
116. Farrer LA, Cupples LA, Haines JL, et al: Effects of age, sex and ethnicity on the association between apolipoprotein E genotype and Alzheimer diseases: A meta-analysis. JAMA 1997; 278:1349–1356.
117. Farwell JR, Lee YJ, Hirtz DG, et al: Phenobarbitol for febrile seizures—effects on intelligence and on seizure recurrence. N Engl J Med 1990; 322:364–369.
118. Feeney DM: Pharmacologic modulation of recovery after brain injury: A reconsideration of diaschisis. J Neurol Rehab 1991; 5:113–128.
119. Feeney DM, Sutton RL: Pharmacotherapy for recovery of function after brain injury. CRC Crit Rev Neurobiol 1987; 3:135–197.
120. Fitzgerald DC: Head trauma: Hearing loss and dizziness. J Trauma 1996; 40:488–496.
121. Flakoli PJ, Wentzel LS, Hyman SA: Protein and glucose metabolism during isolated closed-head injury. Am J Physiol 1995; 269(4 Pt 1):E636–E641.
122. Fletcher JM, Ewing-Cobbs L, Francis DJ, et al: Variability outcomes after traumatic brain injury in children: A developmental perspective. In Broman SH, Michel ME (eds): Traumatic Brain Injury in Children. New York, Oxford University Press, 1990, pp 3–21.
123. Forrester G, Encel J, Geffen G: Measuring post-traumatic amnesia (PTA): An historical review. Brain Inj 1994; 8:175–184.
124. Fowles GP, Fox BA: Competency to consent to treatment and informed consent in neurobehavioral rehabilitation. Clin Neuropsychol 1995; 9:251–257.
125. Fugate LP, Spacek LA, Kresty LA, et al: Definition of agitation following traumatic brain injury: I. A survey of the Brain Injury Special Interest Group of the American Academy of Physical Medicine and Rehabilitation. Arch Phys Med Rehabil 1997; 78:917–923.
126. Fugate LP, Spacek LA, Kresty LA, et al: Measurement and treatment of agitation following brain injury: II. A survey of the Brain Injury Interest Group of the American Academy of Physical Medicine and Rehabilitation. Arch Phys Med Rehabil 1997; 78:924–928.
127. Furrow BR, et al: Bioethics: Health Care Law and Ethics. St Paul, MN, West, 1997.
128. Garland DE, Bailey S: Undetected injuries in head-injured adults. Clin Orthop Rel Res 1981; 155:162–165.
129. Garland DE, Blum CE, Waters RL: Periarticular heterotopic ossification in head-injured adults. Incidence and location. J Bone Joint Surg 1980; 62:1143–1146.
130. Garland DE, Lilling M, Keenan MS: Percutaneous phenol blocks to motor points of spastic forearm muscles in head-injured adults. Arch Phys Med Rehabil 1984; 65:243–245.
131. Gean AD: Imaging of Head Trauma. New York, Raven, 1994.
132. Geerts WH, Code KI, Jay RM, et al: A prospective study of venous thromboembolism after major trauma. N Engl J Med 1994; 331:1601–1606.
133. Gennarelli TA: Cerebral concussion and diffuse brain injuries. Cooper PA (ed): Head Injury, ed 3. Baltimore, Williams & Wilkins, 1993, pp 137–158.
134. Gentry LR, Godersky JC, Thompson B: MR imaging of head trauma: Review of the distribution and radiopathologic features of traumatic lesions. AJR Am J Roentgenol 1988; 9:150–663.
135. Gerszten PC, Albright AL, Barry MJ: Effect on ambulation of continuous intrathecal baclofen infusion. Pediatr Neurosurg 1997; 27:40–44.
136. Gerszten PC, Albright AL, Johnstone GF: Intrathecal baclofen infusion and subsequent orthopedic surgery in patients with spastic cerebral palsy. J Neurosurg 1998; 88:1009–1013.
137. Gervasio AH, Griffith ER: Sexuality and sexual dysfunction. In Rosenthal M, Griffith ER, Kreutzer JS, Pentland B (eds): Rehabilitation of the Adult and Child with Traumatic Brain Injury, ed 3. Philadelphia, FA Davis, 1999, pp 479–502.
138. Giacino J (ed): Evaluation and management of low level neurologic states. Neurorehabil 1996; 6(1) [whole issue].
139. Giacino JT, et al: Development of practice guidelines for assessment and management of the vegetative and minimally conscious states. J Head Trauma Rehabil 1997; 12(4):79–89.
140. Giacino JT, Kezmarsky MA, DeLuca J, Cicerone KD: Monitoring rate of recovery to predict outcome in minimally responsive patients. Arch Phys Med Rehabil 1991; 72:897.
141. Glenn MB, Rosenthal M: Rehabilitation following severe traumatic brain injury. Semin Neurol 1985; 5:233–246.
142. Glenn MB, Wroblewski B: Anticonvulsants for prophylaxis of posttraumatic seizures. J Head Trauma Rehabil 1986; 1(1):73–74.
143. Goldenberg G, Oder W, Spatt J, Podreka I: Cerebral correlates of disturbed executive function and memory in survivors of severe closed head injury: A SPECT study. J Neurol Neurosurg Psychiat 1992; 55:362–368.
144. Gordon WA, Mann N, Willer B: Demographic and social characteristics of the Traumatic Brain Injury Model System Database. J Head Trauma Rehabil 1993; 8(2):26–33.
145. Graham DI: Hypoxia and vascular disorders. In Adams JD, Duchen LW (eds): Greenfield's Neuropathology, ed 5. New York, Oxford University Press, 1992, pp 153–268.
146. Graham DI: Neuropathology of head injury. In Narayan RK, Wilberger JE Jr, Povlishock JT (eds): Neurotrauma. New York, McGraw-Hill, 1996, pp 43–59.
147. Graham TW, Zadrozny DB, Harrington T: The benefits of early jejunal hyperalimentation in the head-injured patient. Neurosurg 1989; 25:729–735.
148. Green RJ, Clarke DE, Fishman RS, Raffin TA: Investigating the causes of fever in critically ill patients: Are you overlooking noninfectious causes? J Crit Illness 1995; 10(1):51–64.
149. Greenwood R, Barnes MP, McMillan TM, Ward CD (eds): Neurological Rehabilitation. London, Churchill Livingstone, 1993.
150. Grinspun D: Bladder management for adults following head injury. Rehabil Nurs 1993; 18:300–305.
151. Grisso T, Applebaum PS: Assessing Competence to Consent to Treatment: A Guide for Physicians and Other Health Professionals. New York, Oxford University Press, 1998.
152. Groher ME, Picon-Nieto L: Evaluation of communication and swallowing disorders. In Rosenthal M, Griffith ER, Kreutzer JS,

Pentland B (eds): Rehabilitation of the Adult and Child with Traumatic Brain Injury, ed 3. Philadelphia, FA Davis, 1999, pp 183–198.

153. Groswasser Z, Cohen M, Costeff H: Rehabilitation outcome after anoxic brain damage. Arch Phys Med Rehabil 1989; 70:186.
154. Guilmette TJ: Pocket Guide to Brain Injury, Cognitive, and Neurobehavioral Rehabilitation. San Diego, Singular, 1997.
155. Hall K: The Functional Assessment Measure (FAM). J Rehabil Outcomes Meas 1997; 1:63–65.
156. Hall KM: Functional assessment in traumatic brain injury. In Rosenthal M, Griffith ER, Kreutzer JS, Pentland B (eds): Rehabilitation of the Adult and Child with Traumatic Brain Injury, ed 3. Philadelphia, FA Davis, 1999, pp 131–146.
157. Halloran LG, Zfass AM, Gayle WE, et al: Prevention of acute gastrointestinal complications after severe head injury: A controlled trial of cimetidine prophylaxis. Am J Surg 1980; 139: 44–48.
158. Hammond FM, McDeavitt JT: Medical and orthopedic complications. In Rosenthal M, Griffith ER, Kreutzer JS, Pentland B (eds): Rehabilitation of the Adult and Child with Traumatic Brain Injury, ed 3. Philadelphia, FA Davis, 1999, pp 53–73.
159. Hammond FM, Zafonte RD: Drugs for management of sleep disorders. Phys Med Rehabil Clin N Amer 1997; 8:801–825.
160. Hannay HJ, Sherer M: Assessment of outcome from head injury. In Narayan RK, Wilberger JE Jr, Povlishock JT (eds): Neurotrauma. New York, McGraw-Hill, 1996, pp 723–747.
161. Hanscom DA: Acute management of the multiply injured head trauma patient. J Head Trauma Rehabil 1987; 2(2):1–12.
162. Harrison L, Johnston M, Massicotte MP, et al: Comparison of 5-mg and 10-mg loading doses in initiating warfarin therapy. Ann Int Med 1997; 126:133–136.
163. Hartley LL: Cognitive-Communicative Abilities Following Brain Injury: A Functional Approach. San Diego, Singular, 1994.
164. Hawkins TD, Lloyd AD, Fletcher GI, Hanka R. Ventricular size following head injury: A clinico-radiological study. Clin Radiol 1976; 27:279–289.
165. Herbel K, Schermerhorn L, Howard J: Management of agitated head-injured patients: A survey of current techniques. Rehabil Nurs 1990; 15:66–69.
166. Herscovitch P: Functional brain imaging—Basic principles and application to head trauma. In Rizzo M, Tranel D (eds): Head Injury and Postconcussive Syndrome. New York, Churchill Livingstone, 1996, pp 89–118.
167. High WM Jr, Boake C, Lehmkuhl LD: Critical analysis of studies measuring the effectiveness of rehabilitation following traumatic brain injury. J Head Trauma Rehabil 1995; 10(1):14–26.
168. Hirsh J, Dalen JE, Anderson DR, et al: Oral anticoagulants: Mechanism of action, clinical effectiveness, and optimal therapeutic range. Chest 1998; 114:S445–S469.
169. Hiscock M, Hiscock D: Refining the forced-choice method for the detection of malingering. J Clin Exp Neuropsychol 1989; 11:967–974.
170. Hopkins RO: Severe anoxia with and without concomitant brain atrophy and neuropsychological impairments. J Int Neuropsychol Soc 1995; 1:501–509.
171. Horn LJ, Zasler ND (eds): Medical Rehabilitation of Traumatic Brain Injury. Philadelphia, Hanley & Belfus, 1996.
172. Horn S, Shiel A, McLellan L, et al: A review of behavioral assessment scales for monitoring recovery in and after coma with pilot data on a new scale of visual awareness. Neuropsych Rehabil 1993; 3:121–137.
173. Hsiang JN, Yeung T, Yu AL, et al: High risk mild head injury. J Neurosurg 1997; 87:234–238.
174. Hughes M, Cohen WA. Radiographic evaluation. In Cooper PA (ed): Head Injury, ed 3. Baltimore, Williams & Wilkins, 1993, pp 65–89.
175. Jacobs HE: Behavior analysis and brain injury rehabilitation. In Rosenthal M, Griffith ER, Kreutzer JS, Pentland B (eds): Rehabilitation of the Adult and Child with Traumatic Brain Injury, ed 3. Philadelphia, FA Davis, 1999, pp 297–311.
176. Jennett B: EEG prediction of post-traumatic epilepsy. Epilepsia 1975; 16:251–256.
177. Jennett B: Posttraumatic epilepsy. In Rosenthal M, Griffith ER, Bond MR, Miller JD (eds): Rehabilitation of the Head-Injured Adult. Philadelphia, FA Davis, 1983, pp 119–124.
178. Jennett B, Bond M: Assessment of outcome after severe brain damage. Lancet 1975; i:480–487.
179. Jennett B, Snoek J, Bond MR, Brooks N: Disability after severe head injury: Observations on the use of the Glasgow Outcome Scale. J Neurol Neurosurg Psychiat 1981; 44:285–293.
180. Jennett B, Teasdale G: Management of Head Injuries. Philadelphia, FA Davis, 1981.
181. Jensen LL, Halar E, Little JW, Brooke MM: Neurogenic heterotopic ossification special review. Am J Phys Med 1988; 66: 351–363.
182. Jeret JS, Mandell M, Anziska B, et al: Clinical predictors of abnormality disclosed by computed tomography after mild head injury. Neurosurg 1993; 32:9–15.
183. Johnson JH: Rehabilitative aspects of neurologic bladder dysfunction. Nurs Clin N Amer 1980; 15:293–307.
184. Johnston MV: The economics of brain injury: A preface. In Miner ME, Wagner KA (eds): Neurotrauma: Treatment and Rehabilitation and Related Issues. Boston, Butterworths, 1989, pp 163–185.
185. Johnston MV, Hall K, Carnevale G, et al: Functional assessment and outcome evaluation in traumatic brain injury rehabilitation. In Horn LJ, Zasler ND (eds): Medical Rehabilitation of Traumatic Brain Injury. Philadelphia, Hanley & Belfus, 1996, pp 197–226.
186. Jones DM, Tilbury H: Parent Training Manual on Education Rights. Houston, HDI Publishers, 1994.
187. Jordan BD, Relkin NR, Ravdin LD, et al: Apolipoprotein E $\varepsilon 4$ associated with chronic traumatic brain injury in boxing. JAMA 1997; 278:136–140.
188. Kalisky Z, Morrison DP, Meyers CA, et al: Medical problems encountered during rehabilitation of patients with head injury. Arch Phys Med Rehabil 1985; 66:25–29.
189. Katz DI: Traumatic brain injury. In Gilchrist JM (ed): Prognosis in Neurology. Boston, Butterworth-Heinemann, 1998, pp 31–36.
190. Keane JR, Baloh RW: Posttraumatic cranial neuropathies. Neurol Clin 1992; 10(4):849–867.
191. Kelly JP: Diagnosis and management of concussion in sports. Neurology 1997; 48:575–580.
192. Kishore PRS, Lipper MH, Miller JD, et al: Post-traumatic hydrocephalus in patients with severe head injury. Neuroradiol 1978; 16:261–265.
193. Klingbeil GEG: Airway problems in patients with head injury. Arch Phys Med Rehabil 1988; 69:493–495.
194. Kochanek PM, et al: Pathophysiology. In Marion DW (ed): Traumatic Brain Injury. New York, Thieme, 1999, pp 233–256.
195. Kothari S, Kirschner K: Consent, assent, and empowerment: Assessing competence in people with brain injuries. In Adkins VK (ed): Treatment Perspectives on Head Injury Rehabilitation: A Focus on Practical Interventions. Westport, Greenwood, in press.
196. Kraus JF, McArthur DI: Incidence and prevalence of, and costs associated with traumatic brain injury. In Rosenthal M, Griffith ER, Kreutzer JS, Pentland B (eds): Rehabilitation of the Adult and Child with Traumatic Brain Injury, ed 3. Philadelphia, FA Davis, 1999, pp 3–18.
197. Kraus JF, McArthur DL: Epidemiologic aspects of brain injury. Neurol Clin 1996; 14:435–450.
198. Kraus JF, McArthur DL, Silverman TA, et al: Epidemiology of brain injury. In Narayan RK, Wilberger JE Jr, Povlishock JT (eds): Neurotrauma. New York, McGraw-Hill, 1996, pp 13–30.
199. Kraus JF, Sorenson SB: Epidemiology. In Silver JM, Yudofsky SC, Hales RE (eds): Neuropsychiatry of Traumatic Brain Injury. Washington, DC, American Psychiatric Press, 1994, pp 3–41.
200. Labi MLC: Neuroendocrine disorders after traumatic brain injury. In Horn LJ, Zasler ND (eds): Medical rehabilitation of traumatic brain injury. Philadelphia, Hanley & Belfus, 1995, pp 539–555.
201. Lal S, Merbitz CP, Grip JC: Modification of function in head-injured patients with Sinemet. Brain Inj 1988; 2:225.
202. Landy SH, Donovan TB, Laster RE: Repeat CT or MRI in posttraumatic headache. Headache 1996; 36:44–47.
203. Langfitt TW: Measuring the outcome from head injuries. J Neurosurg 1978; 48:673–678.
204. Lataste X, Emre M, Davis C, et al: Comparative profile of tizanidine in the management of spasticity. Neurol 1994; 44:S53–S59.

205. Lazarus C, Logemann JA: Swallowing disorders in closed head trauma patients. Arch Phys Med Rehabil 1987; 68:79–84.
206. Leahy P: Traumatic brain injury. In O'Sullivan SB, Schmitz TJ (eds): Physical Rehabilitation: Assessment and Treatment, ed 3. Philadelphia, FA Davis, 1994, pp 491–508.
207. Lehmkuhl LD: Brain Injury Glossary. Houston, HDI Press, 1993.
208. Lerman RM, Bontke CF: Clostridium difficile colitis: Nosocomial acquisition and cross infection among head injured patients. Curr Concepts Rehabil Med 1988; 4(2):1–5.
209. Levin H: A guide to clinical neuropsychological testing. Arch Neurol 1994; 51:854–859.
210. Levin HS: Neurobehavioral outcome of mild to moderate head injury. In Hoff J, Anderson T, Cole T (eds): Mild to Moderate Head Injury. Boston, Blackwell Scientific Publications, 1989, pp 152–185.
211. Levin HS: Cognitive rehabilitation: Unproved but promising. Arch Neurol 1990; 47:223–224.
212. Levin HS: Outcome from mild head injury. In Narayan RK, Wilberger JE Jr, Povlishock JT (eds): Neurotrauma. New York, McGraw-Hill, 1996, pp 749–754.
213. Levin HS, Aldrich EF, Saydjari C, et al: Severe head injury in children: Experience of the Traumatic Coma Data Bank. Neurosurg 1992; 31:435–443.
214. Levin HS, Benton AL, Grossman RG: Neurobehavioral Consequences of Closed Head Injury. New York, Oxford University Press, 1982.
215. Levin HS, Benton AL, Muizelaar JP, et al (eds): Catastrophic Brain Injury. New York, Oxford University Press, 1996.
216. Levin HS, Eisenberg HM, Benton AL (eds): Mild Head Injury. New York, Oxford University Press, 1989.
217. Levin HS, Gary HE, Eisenberg HM: Duration of impaired consciousness in relation to side of lesion after severe head injury. Lancet 1989; 2:1001–1003.
218. Levin HS, Gary HE, Eisenberg HM, et al: Neurobehavioral outcome one year after head injury: Experience of the Traumatic Coma Data Bank. J Neurosurg 1990; 73:699–709.
219. Levin HS, High WM, Goethe KE, et al: The Neurobehavioral Rating Scale: Assessment of the behavioural sequelae of head injury by the clinician. J Neurol Neurosurg Psychiat 1987; 50:183–193.
220. Levin HS, Meyers CA, Grossman RG, Sarwar M: Ventricular enlargement after closed head injury. Arch Neurol 1981; 38:623–629.
221. Levin HS, Saydjari C, Eisenberg HM, et al: Vegetative state after closed-head injury: A Traumatic Coma Data Bank report. Arch Neurol 1991; 48:580–585.
222. Levin HS, Williams D, Crofford MJ, et al: Relationship of depth of brain lesions to consciousness and outcome after closed head injury. J Neurosurg 1988; 69:861–866.
223. Levin HS, Williams DH, Eisenberg HM, et al: Serial MRI and neurobehavioral findings after mild to moderate closed head injury. J Neurol Neurosurg Psychiat 1992; 55:255–262.
224. Levin VA (ed): Cancer in the Nervous System. New York, Churchill-Livingstone, 1996.
225. Levin VA, Moser RP: Neoplasms. In Evans RW, Baskin DS, Yatsu FM (eds): Prognosis of Neurological Disorders. New York, Oxford University Press, 1992, pp 633–649.
226. Levy DE: Disorders of consciousness. In Evans RW, Baskin DS, Yatsu FM (eds): Prognosis of Neurological Disorders. New York, Oxford University Press, 1992, pp 353–358.
227. Lezak MD: Neuropsychological Assessment, ed 3. New York, Oxford University Press, 1995.
228. Light R: Behavioral management of the difficult neurologically impaired patient. J Neurol Rehabil 1989; 3:145–147.
229. Macciocchi SN, Reid DB, Barth JT: Disability following head injury. Curr Opin Neurol 1993; 6:773.
230. Malec JF, Basford JS: Postacute brain injury rehabilitation. Arch Phys Med Rehabil 1996; 77:198–207.
231. Malkmus D, Booth BJ, Kodimer C: Rehabilitation of Head Injured Adults: Comprehensive Cognitive Management. Downey, CA, Professional Staff Association of Rancho Los Amigos Hospital, 1980.
232. Marion DW (ed): Traumatic Brain Injury. Thieme, 1999.
233. Marion DW, Carlier PM: Problems with initial Glasgow Scale assessment caused by prehospital treatment of patients with head injuries: Results of a national survey. J Trauma 1994; 36:89–95.
234. Marion DW, et al: The use of moderate therapeutic hypothermia for patients with severe head injuries: A preliminary report. J Neurosurg 1993; 79:354–362.
235. Marion DW, Penrod LE, Kelsey SF, et al: Treatment of traumatic brain injury with moderate hypothermia. N Engl J Med 1997; 336:540–546.
236. Marshall LF, et al: A new classification of head injury based on computed tomography. J Neurosurg 1991; 75:S14–S20.
237. Massagli TL: Neurobehavioral effects of phenytoin, carbamazepine and valproic acid: Implications for use in traumatic brain injury. Arch Phys Med Rehabil 1991; 72:219–226.
238. Mateer CA, Raskin S: Cognitive rehabilitation. In Rosenthal M, Griffith ER, Kreutzer JS, Pentland B (eds): Rehabilitation of the Adult and Child with Traumatic Brain Injury, ed 3. Philadelphia, FA Davis, 1999, pp 254–270.
239. Mattson RH, Cramer JA, Collins JF, et al: Comparison of carbamazepine, phenobarbital, phenytoin, and primidone in partial and secondarily generalized tonic-clonic seizures. N Engl J Med 1985; 313:145–151.
240. McAllister TW: Mild traumatic brain injury and the postconcussive syndrome. In Silver JS, Yudofsky SC, Hales RE (eds): The Neuropsychiatry of Traumatic Brain Injury. Washington, DC, American Psychiatric Press, 1994, pp 357–392.
241. McCrory PR, Berkovic SF: Second impact syndrome. Neurology 1998; 50:677–683.
242. McDeavitt JT: Electroencephalographic technologies in traumatic brain injury. In Horn LJ, Zasler ND (ed): Medical Rehabilitation of Traumatic Brain Injury. Philadelphia, Hanley & Belfus, 1996, pp 317–332.
243. McKinlay WW, Brooks DN, Bond MR, et al: The short-term outcome of severe blunt head injury as reported by relatives of the injured persons. J Neurol Neurosurg Psychiat 1981; 44:527–533.
244. McMillan TM, Wilson S (eds): Coma and the persistent vegetative state. Neuropsych Rehabil 1995; 3(2) [whole issue].
245. McNeny R: Activities of daily living. In Rosenthal M, Griffith ER, Kreutzer JS, Pentland B (eds): Rehabilitation of the Adult and Child with Traumatic Brain Injury, ed 3. Philadelphia, FA Davis, 1999, pp 242–253.
246. Meythaler JM, Devivo MJ, Hadley M: Prospective study on the use of bolus intrathecal baclofen for spastic hypertonia due to acquired brain injury. Arch Phys Med Rehabil 1996; 77:461–466.
247. Meythaler JM, McCary A, Hadley MN, et al: Prospective assessment of continuous intrathecal infusion of baclofen for spasticity caused by acquired brain injury: A preliminary report. J Neurosurg 1997; 87:415–419.
248. Meythaler JM, Stinson AM: Fever of central origin in traumatic brain injury controlled with propranolol. Arch Phys Med Rehabil 1994; 75:816–818.
249. Michaud LJ, Duhaime A-C, Jaffe KM: Specific problems associated with pediatric brain injury. In Rosenthal M, Griffith ER, Kreutzer JS, Pentland B (eds): Rehabilitation of the Adult and Child with Traumatic Brain Injury, ed 3. Philadelphia, FA Davis, 1999, pp 345–355.
250. Miller JD, Pentland B: The neurologic evaluation. In Griffith ER, Bond MR, Miller JD (eds): Rehabilitation of the Adult and Child with Traumatic Brain Injury, ed 2. Philadelphia, FA Davis, 1990, pp 52–58.
251. Millis SR, Putnam SH: Detection of malingering in postconcussive syndromes. In Rizzo M, Tranel D (eds): Head Injury and Postconcussive Syndrome. New York, Churchill Livingstone, 1996, pp 481–498.
252. Mittl RL, Grossman RI, Hiehle JF, et al: Prevalence of MR evidence of diffuse axonal injury in patients with mild head injury and normal head CT findings. AJNR Am J Neuroradiol 1994; 15:1583–1589.
253. Morgan AS, Thomas LM, Barba C, et al: Respiratory management of the brain injured patient. In Chapman PE, Morgan AS, Mackay LE (eds): Maximizing Brain Injury Recovery: Integrating Critical Care and Acute Rehabilitation. Gaithersburg, MD, Aspen, 1997, pp 331–395.
254. Moss RJ, La Puma J: The ethics of mechanical restraints. Hastings Cent Rep 1991; 21:22–25.
255. Multi-society Task Force on PVS: Medical aspects of the persistent vegetative state (1). N Engl J Med 1994; 330:1499–1508.

256. Multi-society Task Force on PVS: Medical aspects of the persistent vegetative state (2). N Engl J Med 1994; 330:1572–1579.
257. Murphy A, Teasdale G, Matheson M, et al: Relationship between CT indices of brain swelling and intracranial pressure after head injury. In Intracranial Pressure, V. Berlin, Springer-Verlag, 1983; pp 562–566.
258. Najenson T, Groswasser Z, Stern JM, et al: Prognostic factors in rehabilitation after severe head injury. Scand J Rehabil Med 1975; 7:101–105.
259. Narayan R, Goskaslan Z, Bontke CF, et al: Neurologic sequelae of head injury. In Rosenthal M, Griffith ER, Bond MR, Miller JD (eds): Rehabilitation of the Adult and Child with Traumatic Brain Injury, ed 2. Philadelphia, FA Davis, 1990, pp 94–106.
260. Narayan RK, Wilberger JE Jr, Povlishock JT (eds): Neurotrauma. New York, McGraw-Hill, 1997.
261. NIH Consensus Conference on Rehabilitation of Persons with Traumatic Brain Injury: Rehabilitation of persons with traumatic brain injury. NIH Consensus Conference, 1999; 16:1–41.
262. Nowak P, Cohn AM, Guidice MA: Airway complications in patients with closed-head injuries. Am J Otolaryngol 1987; 8:91–96.
263. Nudo RJ, Wise BM, SiFuentes F, Milliken GW: Neural substrates for the effects of rehabilitative training on motor recovery after ischemic infarct. Science 1996; 272:1791–1794.
264. O'Dell MW, et al: Functional outcome of inpatient rehabilitation in persons with brain tumors. Arch Phys Med Rehabil 1998; 79:1530–1534.
265. O'Dell MW, Rigges RV: Management of the minimally responsive patient. In Horn LJ, Zasler ND (eds): Medical rehabilitation of traumatic brain injury. Philadelphia, Hanley & Belfus, 1996, pp 103–132.
266. Oder W, Podreka I, Spatt J, et al: Cerebral function following catastrophic brain injury: Relevance of single photon emission computed tomography and positron emission tomography. In Levin HS, Benton AL, Muizelaar JP, Eisenberg HM (eds): Catastrophic Brain Injury. New York, Oxford University Press, 1996, pp 51–76.
267. Olesen J, Headache Classification Committee of the International Headache Society: Classification of diagnostic criteria for headache disorders, cranial neuralgias, and facial pain. Cephalalgia 1988; 8:1–96.
268. Ommaya AK, Gennarelli TA: Cerebral concussion and traumatic unconsciousness: Correlation of experimental and clinic observation on blunt head injuries. Brain 1974; 97:633–654.
269. Packard RC, Ham LP: Posttraumatic headache. J Neuropsychiat Clin Neurosci 1994; 6:229–236.
270. Packard RC, Weaver R, Ham LP: Cognitive symptoms in patients with posttraumatic headache. Headache 1993; 33:365–368.
271. Patel M, Bontke CF: Impact of traumatic brain injury on pregnancy. J Head Trauma Rehabil 1990; 5(2):60–66.
272. Patterson TS, Sargent M: Behavioral management of the agitated head trauma client. Rehabil Nurs 1990; 15:248–253.
273. Penn RD, Kroin JS: Long-term intrathecal baclofen infusion for treatment of spasticity. J Neurosurg 1987; 66:181–185.
274. Penrod LE: Prognosis. In Marion DW (eds): Traumatic Brain Injury. New York, Thieme, 1999, pp 135–140.
275. Philip A, Philip M: Evoked potential in the prognosis of traumatic lesions of the central nervous system. Phys Med Rehabil Clin N Amer 1994; 5:643–656.
276. Phipps E, Whyte J: Medical decision-making with persons who are minimally conscious: A commentary. Am J Phys Med Rehabil 1999; 78:77–82.
277. Pisciotta AV: Carbamazepine: Hematological toxicity. In Woodbury DM, Penry JK, Pippenger CE (eds): Antiepileptic Drugs, ed 2. New York, Raven Press, 1982, pp 533–541.
278. Pitts LH, San Francisco General Hospital Medical Center Head Injury Data Bank. Cited in Bartowski M, Lovely MP: Prognosis in coma and the persistent vegetative state. J Head Trauma Rehabil 1986; 1(1):1–5.
279. Plum F, Posner JB: The Diagnosis of Stupor and Coma, ed 3. Philadelphia, FA Davis, 1982.
280. Prigatano GP, et al: Neuropsychological Rehabilitation after Brain Injury. Baltimore, Johns Hopkins University Press, 1986.
281. Prigatano GP, Ben-Yishay Y: Psychotherapy and psychotherapeutic interventions in brain injury rehabilitation. In Rosenthal M, Griffith ER, Kreutzer JS, Pentland B (eds): Rehabilitation of the Adult and Child with Traumatic Brain Injury, ed 3. Philadelphia, FA Davis, 1999, pp 271–283.
282. Rader RA, Ellis DW: Sensory Stimulation Assessment Measure. Camden, NJ, Mediplex Rehab-Camden, 1989.
283. Ramsey RE: Advances in the pharmacotherapy of epilepsy. Epilepsia 1993; 34(suppl 5):S9–S16.
284. Rappaport M: Electrophysiologic assessment. In Horn LJ, Zasler ND (eds): Medical Rehabilitation of Traumatic Brain Injury. Philadelphia, Hanley & Belfus, 1996, pp 271–316.
285. Rappaport M, Dougherty AM, Kelting DL: Evaluation of coma and vegetative states. Arch Phys Med Rehabil 1992; 73:628–634.
286. Rappaport M, Hall KM, Hopkins K, et al: Disability Rating Scale for severe head trauma: Coma to community. Arch Phys Med Rehabil 1982; 63:118–123.
287. Rappaport M, Herrero-Backe C, Rappaport ML, Winterfield KM: Head injury outcome up to ten years later. Arch Phys Med Rehabil 1989; 70:885–892.
288. Reyes RL, Bhattacharyya AK, Heller D: Traumatic head injury: Restlessness and agitation as prognosticators of physical and psychologic improvement in patients. Arch Phys Med Rehabil 1981; 62:20–23.
289. Ricker JH: Traumatic brain injury rehabilitation: Is it worth the cost? Appl Neuropsychol 1998; 5:184–193.
290. Rimel RW, Giordani B, Barth JT, et al: Moderate head injury: Completing the clinical spectrum of brain trauma. Neurosurg 1982; 11:344–351.
291. Rizzo M, Tranel D (eds): Head Injury and Post-Concussive Syndrome. New York, Churchill Livingstone, 1996.
292. Roberts PR: Nutrition in the head-injured patient. New Horiz 1995; 3(3):506–517.
293. Rogers RC: Heterotopic calcification in severe head injury: A prevention program. Brain Inj 1988; 2:169–172.
294. Rose FC: The history of cerebral trauma. In Evans RW (eds): Neurology and Trauma. Philadelphia, WB Saunders, 1996, pp 18–27.
295. Rosenthal M, Griffith ER, Kreutzer JS, Pentland B (eds): Rehabilitation of the Adult and Child with Traumatic Brain Injury, ed 3. Philadelphia, FA Davis, 1999.
296. Ross BL, Temkin NR, Newell D, Dikmen SS: Neuropsychological outcome in relation to head injury severity: Contributions of coma length and focal abnormalities. Am J Phys Med Rehabil 1994; 73:341–347.
297. Rothweiler B, Temkin NR, Dikmen SS: Aging effect on psychosocial outcome in traumatic brain injury. Arch Phys Med Rehabil 1998; 79:881–887.
298. Rubinstein I, Murray D, Hoffstein V: Fatal pulmonary embolism in hospitalized patients. Arch Int Med 1988; 148:1425–1426.
299. Ruff RM, Marshall LF, Crouch J, et al: Predictors of outcome following severe head trauma: Follow-up data from the Traumatic Coma Data Bank. Brain Inj 1993; 7:101–111.
300. Russell WR: The Traumatic Amnesias. London, Oxford University Press, 1971.
301. Rutherford WH: Postconcussion symptoms: Relationship to acute neurological indices, individual differences, and circumstances of injury. In Levin HS, Eisenberg HM, Benton AL (eds): Mild Head Injury. New York, Oxford University Press, 1989, pp 217–228.
302. Sacks GS, Brown RO, Teague D, et al: Early nutrition support modifies immune function in patients sustaining severe head injury. J Parenter Enteral Nutr 1995; 19:387–392.
303. Sandel EM, Mysiw WJ: The agitated brain injured patient. Part 1: Definitions, differential diagnosis and assessment. Arch Phys Med Rehabil 1996; 77:617–623.
304. Sandel ME, Ellis DW (eds): The coma emerging patient. Phys Med Rehabil State Art Rev 1990; 4(3) [whole issue].
305. Sandel ME, Williams KS, Dellapietra L, et al: Sexual functioning following traumatic brain injury. Brain Inj 1996; 10:719–728.
306. Satz P, Zaucha K, McCleary C, et al: Mild head injury in children and adolescents: A review of studies (1970–1995). Psych Bull 1997; 122:107–131.
307. Saunders AM, Strittmatter WJ, Schmechel D, et al: Association of apoplipoprotein E allele E4 with late onset familial and sporadic Alzheimer's disease. Neurology 1993; 43:1467–1472.

308. Saunders RL, Harbaugh RE: The second impact in catastrophic contact—Sports head trauma. JAMA 1984; 252:538–539.
309. Sazbon L, Groswasser Z: Outcome in 134 patients with prolonged posttraumatic unawareness: Part I: Parameters determining late recovery of consciousness. J Neurosurg 1990; 72:75–80.
310. Sazbon L, Najenson T, Tartakovsky M, et al: Widespread periarticular new-bone formation in long-term comatose patients. J Bone Joint Surg (Br) 1981; 63:120–125.
311. Scherzer E, Wessely P: EEG in posttraumatic epilepsy. Eur Neurol 1978; 17:38–42.
312. Shepard NT, Telian SA, Smith-Wheelock M: Vestibular and balance rehabilitation therapy. Ann Otol Rhinol Laryngol 1993; 102:198–205.
313. Silver BV, Boake C, Cavazos DI: Improving functional skills using behavioral procedures in a child with anoxic brain injury. Arch Phys Med Rehabil 1994; 75:742–745.
314. Sohlberg MM, Mateer CA: Introduction to Cognitive Rehabilitation: Theory and Practice. New York, Guilford, 1989.
315. Sorenson SB, Kraus JF: Occurrence, severity, and outcomes of brain injury. J Head Trauma Rehabil 1991; 6(2):1–10.
316. Sosin DM, Sniezek JE, Thurman DJ: Incidence of mild and moderate brain injury in the United States: 1991. Brain Inj 1996; 10:47–54.
317. Sosin DM, Sniezek JE, Waxweiler RJ: Trends in death associated with traumatic brain injury, 1979 through 1992: Success and failure. JAMA 1995; 273:1778–1780.
318. Spasticity Study Group: Spasticity: Etiology, evaluation, management, and the role of botulinum toxin type A. Muscle Nerve 1997; 6(suppl):S1–S231.
319. Spielman G, Gennarelli TA, Rogers CR. Disodium etidronate: Its role in preventing heterotopic ossification in severe head injury. Arch Phys Med Rehabil 1983; 64:539–542.
320. Stein SC: Outcome from moderate head injury. In Narayan RK, Wilberger JE Jr, Povlishock JT (eds): Neurotrauma. New York, McGraw-Hill, 1996, pp 755–766.
321. Strumpf NE, Evans LK: The ethical problems of prolonged physical restraint. J Gerontol Nurs 1991; 17:27–30.
322. Synek VM: EEG abnormality grades and subdivisions of prognostic importance in traumatic and anoxic coma in adults. Clin Electroencephalogr 1988; 19:160–166.
323. Tarvydas VM, Shaw L: Interdisciplinary team member perceptions of ethical issues in traumatic brain injury rehabilitation. Neurorehabil 1996; 6(2):97–111.
324. Teasdale G, Jennett B: Assessment of coma and impaired consciousness: A practical scale. Lancet 1974; 2:81–84.
325. Teasdale GM, Nicoli JA, Murray G, et al: Association of apolipoprotein E polymorphism with outcome after head injury. Lancet 1997; 350:1069–1071.
326. Temkin NR, Dikmen SS, Wilensky AJ, et al: A randomized, double-blind study of phenytoin for the prevention of posttraumatic seizures. N Engl J Med 1990; 323:497–502.
327. Thatcher RW, Cantor DS, McAlaster R, et al: Comprehensive predictions of outcome in closed head-injury patients. Ann N Y Acad Sci 1991; 620:82–101.
328. Therapeutics and Technology Assessment Subcommittee of the American Academy of Neurology: Assessment of brain SPECT. Neurology 1996; 46:278–285.
329. Therapeutics and Technology Assessment Subcommittee of the American Academy of Neurology. Neuropsychological testing of adults: Considerations for neurologists. Neurology 1996; 47:592–599.
330. Thurman DJ, et al: Guidelines for surveillance of central nervous system injury. Atlanta, Centers for Disease Control and Prevention, 1995.
331. Tippin J, Yamada T: The electrophysiologic evaluation of head injured patients: Value and limitations. In Rizzo M, Tranel D (eds): Head Injury and Postconcussive Syndrome. New York, Churchill Livingstone, 1996, pp 119–138.
332. Toutant S, Klauber M, Marshall L, et al: Absent or compressed basal cisterns in first CT scan: Ominous predictors of outcome in severe head injury. J Neurosurg 1984; 61:691–694.
333. Trask TW: Civilian penetrating head injury. In Narayan RK, Wilberger JE Jr, Povlishock JT (eds): Neurotrauma. New York, McGraw-Hill, 1996, pp 869–890.
334. Tursa RJ, Brown SB: Neuro-otologic trauma and dizziness. In Rizzo M, Tranel D (eds): Head Injury and Postconcussive Syndrome. New York, Churchill Livingstone, 1996, pp 177–200.
335. U.S. Bureau of the Census, Data User Services Division: Statistical abstract of the United States (CD-ROM). Washington, DC. U.S. Dept. of Commerce, Economics and Statistics Administration, Bureau of the Census, Data User Services Division, 1998 (http://www.census.gov/statab/www/).
336. Valko AS: Rehabilitation and disabilities. In Marion DW (ed): Traumatic Brain Injury. New York, Thieme, 1999, pp 269–282.
337. Vollmer DG: Prognosis and outcome of severe head injury. In Cooper PR (ed): Head Injury, ed 3. Baltimore, Williams & Wilkins, 1993, pp 553–581.
338. Volpe BT, McDowell FH: The efficacy of cognitive rehabilitation in patients with traumatic brain injury. Arch Neurol 1990; 47:220–222.
339. Ward JD: Pediatric head injury. In Narayan RK, Wilberger JE Jr, Povlishock JT (eds): Neurotrauma. New York, McGraw-Hill, 1996, pp 859–868.
340. Wehman P, West M, Johnson A, et al: Vocational rehabilitation for individuals with traumatic brain injury. In Rosenthal M, Griffith ER, Kreutzer JS, Pentland B (eds): Rehabilitation of the Adult and Child with Traumatic Brain Injury, ed 3. Philadelphia, FA Davis, 1999, pp 326–341.
341. Westmoreland BF, et al: Alpha coma. Arch Neurol 1975; 17: 278–285.
342. Whyte J: Mechanisms of recovery of function following CNS damage. In Rosenthal M, Griffith ER, Bond MR, Miller JD (eds): Rehabilitation of the Adult and Child with Traumatic Brain Injury, ed 2. Philadelphia, FA Davis, 1990, pp 79–88.
343. Whyte J, DiPasquale MC: Assessment of vision and visual attention in minimally responsive brain injured patients. Arch Phys Med Rehabil 1995; 76:804–810.
344. Whyte J, Glenn MB: The care and rehabilitation of the patient in a persistent vegetative state. J Head Trauma Rehabil 1986; 1(1):39–54.
345. Whyte J, Hart T, Laborde A, Rosenthal M: Rehabilitation of the patient with traumatic brain injury. In DeLisa J, et al (eds): Rehabilitation Medicine: Principles and Practice, ed 3. Philadelphia, Lippincott-Raven, 1998, pp 1191–1239.
346. Whyte J, Laborde A, DiPasquale MC: Assessment and treatment of the vegetative and minimally conscious patient. In Rosenthal M, Griffith ER, Kreutzer JS, Pentland B (eds): Rehabilitation of the Adult and Child with Traumatic Brain Injury, ed 3. Philadelphia, FA Davis, 1999, pp 435–452.
347. Wiercisiewski DR, McDeavitt JT: Pulmonary complications in traumatic brain injury. J Head Trauma Rehabil 1998; 13(1):28–35.
348. Wikkelso C, Andersson H, Bloomstrand C, et al: Normal pressure hydrocephalus: Predictive value of the cerebrospinal fluid tap test. Acta Neurol Scand 1986; 73:566–573.
349. Willer B, Ottenbacher KJ, Coad ML: The Community Integration Questionnaire: A comparative examination. Am J Phys Med Rehabil 1994; 73:103–111.
350. Williams DH, Levin HS, Eisenberg HM: Mild head injury classification. Neurosurg 1990; 27:422–428.
351. Williams JM, Kay T (eds): Head Injury: A Family Matter. Baltimore, Paul H Brookes, 1991.
352. Wilson BA: Cognitive rehabilitation: How it is and how it might be. J Int Neuropsychol Soc 1997; 3:487–496.
353. Wilson RF, Tyburski JG: Metabolic responses and nutritional therapy in patients with severe head injuries. J Head Trauma Rehabil 1998; 13(1):11–12.
354. Wilson SL, McMillan TM: A review of the evidence for the effectiveness of sensory stimulation treatment for coma and vegetative states. Neuropsych Rehabil 1993; 3:149–160.
355. Winkler PA: Head injury. In Umphred DA (ed): Neurological Rehabilitation, ed 3. St Louis, Mosby–Year Book, 1995, pp 421–453.
356. Wood RL: Brain Injury Rehabilitation: A Neurobehavioral Approach. Rockville, Aspen, 1987.
357. Woratyla SP, Morgan AS, Mackay LE, et al: Factors associated

with early onset pneumonia in the severely brain-injured patient. Conn Med 1995; 59(11):643–647.
358. Wroblewski BA, Glenn MB: Pharmacological treatment of arousal and cognitive deficits: J Head Trauma Rehabil 1994; 9(3):19–42.
359. Wroblewski BA, Joseph AB, Cornblatt RR: Antidepressant pharmacotherapy and the treatment of depression in patients with severe traumatic brain injury: A controlled, prospective study. J Clin Psychiat 1996; 57:582–587.
360. Yablon SA, Agana BT, Ivanhoe CB, Boake C: Botulinum toxin in severe upper extremity spasticity among patients with traumatic brain injury: An open-labeled trial. Neurology 1996; 47:939–944.
361. Yamaguchi M: Incidence of headache and severity of head injury. Headache 1992; 32:427–431.
362. Ylvisaker M (ed): Head Injury Rehabilitation: Children and Adolescents, ed 2. San Diego, Singular, 1998.
363. Yorkston KM, Kennedy MRT: Treatment approaches for communication disorders. In Rosenthal M, Griffith ER, Kreutzer JS, Pentland B (eds): Rehabilitation of the Adult and Child with Traumatic Brain Injury, ed 3. Philadelphia, FA Davis, 1999, pp 284–296.
364. Young B, Ott L: Nutrition and parenteral therapy. In Youmans JR (ed): Neurological Surgery, ed 4. Philadelphia, WB Saunders, 1996.
365. Zafonte R, Atty E, Dade R, et al: Neuroimaging classification of TBI: Predictors of functional status. Arch Phys Med Rehabil 1993; 74:1279.
366. Zafonte R, Hammond F, Mann N, et al: Relationship between Glasgow Coma Scale and functional outcome. Am J Phys Med Rehabil 1996; 75:364–369.
367. Zafonte RD: Neuroimaging in traumatic brain injury. In Horn LJ, Zasler ND (eds): Medical Rehabilitation of Traumatic Brain Injury. Philadelphia, Hanley & Belfus, 1996, pp 251–270.
368. Zafonte RD, Mann NR, Millis SR, et al: Posttraumatic amnesia: Its relation to functional outcome. Arch Phys Med Rehabil 1997; 78:1103–1106.
369. Zasler ND: Acute neurochemical alterations following traumatic brain injury: Research implications for clinical treatment. J Head Trauma Rehabil 1992; 7(2):102–105.
370. Zasler ND: Neuromedical diagnosis and management of postconcussive disorders. In Horn LJ, Zasler ND (eds): Rehabilitation of Post-Concussive Disorders. Philadelphia, Hanley & Belfus, 1992, pp 33–67.
371. Zasler ND (ed): Posttraumatic headaches. J Head Trauma Rehabil 1999; 14(1) [whole issue].
372. Zasler ND, Kreutzer JS, Taylor D. Coma stimulation and coma recovery: A critical review. Neurorehabil 1991; 1(3):33–40.
373. Zencius A, Wesolowski MD, Burke WH, et al: Managing hypersexual disorders in brain-injured clients. Brain Inj 1990; 4:175–181.

50

CHAPTER

Elliot J. Roth, M.D., and Richard L. Harvey, M.D.

Rehabilitation of Stroke Syndromes

Stroke has been described by Gresham[1] as a condition with a unique epidemiological profile, consisting of high incidence and mortality rates, and a large proportion of survivors who have significant but varying amount of residual disability. The clinical phenomena that result vary from stroke to stroke and from patient to patient. Most (but not all) patients who experience stroke can and do have improvement in functional status, but the amount, speed, pattern, and ultimate outcome of the improvements differ across patients and across situations. Therefore, the approach that is required for appropriate assessment and management of stroke patients demands specialized knowledge, skills, and attitudes.

Similar to the rehabilitation of patients with many other conditions, stroke rehabilitation is as much a philosophy of care as it is a set of tasks to carry out. Kottke[2] stated that the goal of rehabilitation in general is to "restore optimal physical function and psycho-social-vocational restoration to enable the patient to become a productive participant in the community." Referring specifically to care of the stroke patient, Bobath[3] defined stroke rehabilitation as "teaching the patient to manage his own life given the limitations of the damage to the central nervous system." Charness[4] pointed out several implications of this philosophy, emphasizing that rehabilitation does not consist of exercise alone; therapy involves returning control to the patient as soon as possible. It is critical that the managing clinical team involve the patient and family in the processes of setting goals, planning treatment, and implementing clinical activities. Stroke rehabilitation is done *with* the patient rather than *to* the patient.

While formal therapeutic exercise regimens usually comprise the most prominent components of the rehabilitation process, other aspects of the program are important as well; at times, the importance of these other activities exceeds that of the specific therapeutic exercise interventions. Many rehabilitation activities extend beyond the specific therapy treatment sessions. For example, repeating on an inpatient nursing care unit or in the home environment those skills that were learned in a formal therapy training session provides reinforcement of the learned activities. Dealing with psychological and social issues can be a major intervention. Interactions, both among patients and between patients and professionals, are important. The rehabilitation milieu typically provides the opportunity for these therapeutic interactions. Often, recreational programs serve as major therapeutic interventions.

The ultimate goal of the rehabilitation is long-term, safe, independent, energy-efficient, pleasurable, and high-quality functioning in the community. Achieving this goal requires addressing a wide variety of medical, functional, and psychosocial issues. Roth[5] enumerated five major functions of stroke rehabilitation:

1. Prevention, recognition, management, and minimizing the impact of preexisting medical conditions, ongoing general health functions, and secondary medical complications.
2. Training for maximal functional independence.
3. Facilitating optimal psychosocial adaptation and coping by both the patient and family.
4. Promoting community reintegration, resumption of prior life roles, and the return to home, family, recreational, and vocational activities.
5. Enhancing quality of life.

The major underlying theme of all rehabilitation interventions is the enhancement of quality of life of stroke patients. It is quality of life, and not simply functional independence or noninstitutional placement, that is the real goal. Indeed, it is important that for some stroke survivors, complete independence in ability to perform daily functional skills might be either undesirable or impractical for physical, psychological, or other reasons. The goal of enhancing quality of life is pervasive and affects both the choices of specific interventions and the manner in which clinical activities are performed. The comprehensive rehabilitation management program is characterized by a holistic approach in which the patient as a whole and his or her overall situation are considered, rather than focusing on isolated aspects of existence. This goal usually, but not always, includes helping the patient to achieve as much functional independence as possible.

Understanding stroke and the rehabilitation of patients who sustain stroke is important, not only because stroke is the most common diagnosis among patients in most rehabilitation programs, but also because it involves virtually all elements of rehabilitation activity and most or all of the members of the rehabilitation team. This chapter reviews the mechanisms and clinical features of stroke, the preventive, diagnostic, and acute management techniques, and the principles and practices of stroke rehabilitation assessment and intervention that enable rehabilitation providers to assist the patient in achieving the ultimate goal of enhancing quality of life. An important recurring theme during both acute management and rehabilitation care is the centrality of an attitude that replaces therapeutic nihilism with optimism and aggressiveness.[6]

DEFINITIONS

Stroke or Cerebrovascular Accident?

Ancient writers of history, science, and poetry used the word *apoplexy,* meaning a sudden strike of paralysis, dumbness, or fainting from which the victim frequently failed to recover. Such a stroke of illness, whether delivered by the gods or disease, was a spontaneous event of the same character as a "stroke of genius," a "stroke of luck," or a "stroke of misfortune." Today the term *stroke* connotes the sudden and surprising nature of symptomatic cerebrovascular disease and is preferred over the more scientific sounding phrase *cerebrovascular accident,* or CVA. The later term implies a nihilistic view, suggesting that the acute outcome cannot be modified by treatment. Many physicians who specialize in the care of patients with stroke prefer the historical term rather than the acronym *CVA*.

We define stroke as a nontraumatic brain injury caused by occlusion or rupture of cerebral blood vessels that results in sudden neurological deficit characterized by loss of motor control, altered sensation, cognitive or language impairment, disequilibrium, or coma. This definition includes an array of etiological sources but excludes nonvascular conditions that can present with stroke-like symptoms, such as seizure, syncope, traumatic brain injury, or brain tumor.

Pathophysiological Classification of Stroke

Stroke is a neurological syndrome caused by a heterogeneous group of vascular etiologies requiring different management.[7] The causes can be grossly categorized as hemorrhagic or ischemic. Intracranial hemorrhage accounts for 15% of all strokes and can be further divided into intracerebral (10%) and subarachnoid (5%) hemorrhage. Subarachnoid hemorrhages typically result from aneurysmal rupture of a cerebral artery with blood loss into the space surrounding the brain. Rupture of weakened vessels within brain parenchyma as a result of hypertension, arteriovenous malformation, or tumor causes intracerebral hemorrhage.

The remaining 85% of strokes are caused by ischemic brain injury resulting from large-vessel (40%) or small-vessel (20%) thrombosis, cerebral embolism (20%), and other less common causes (5%), such as cerebral vasculitis or cerebral hypoperfusion. Vessel occlusion from thrombosis in both large and small arteries occurs most commonly in the presence of atherosclerotic cerebrovascular disease. Vascular changes or lipohyalinosis found in small, deep, penetrating arteries as associated with chronic hypertension can lead to small-vessel thrombosis. Cerebral emboli are usually of cardiac origin and are frequently a result of chronic ischemic cardiovascular disease with secondary ventricular wall hypokinesis or atrial arrhythmia, both conditions that increase the risk for intracardiac thrombus formation.[8]

Temporal Classification of Stroke

The etiology of an acute stroke can often be inferred by classifying the temporal profile of the event using information gathered from the patient's initial history and physical examination. A transient ischemic attack (TIA) is an event in which neurological symptoms develop and disappear over several minutes and, by definition, completely resolve within 24 hours. TIAs are most frequently associated with atherosclerotic carotid artery disease and they should provoke an urgent diagnostic evaluation so that appropriate preventive care can be instituted.

A transient neurological event that lasts longer than 24 hours is called a reversible ischemic neurological deficit (RIND). Such events are clinically infrequent and their etiology is unknown. It is likely that RINDs result from small infarctions (lacunes) of the deep subcortical gray and white matter, resulting in only temporary impairment.

Embolic strokes generally have a quick onset and fully develop in a matter of minutes, whereas hemorrhagic strokes often evolve over 1 to 2 hours. Thrombotic strokes can have a rapid or a prolonged interval of onset, lasting many hours. *Stroke in evolution* denotes an unstable ischemic event characterized by the progressive development of more severe neurological impairment, and it is often associated with active occlusive thrombosis of a major cerebral artery. Once a stable neurological status is reached, clinicians refer to the event as a *completed stroke.* The therapeutic goal of many current acute stroke treatment protocols is to abort neurological deterioration and to limit the neurological impairment, in the hope of minimalizing the functional disability once the stroke is completed.

When a patient's neurological and medical status is stable, rehabilitation care should begin. Stroke rehabilitation is an interdisciplinary process whereby physical modalities and skill enhancement are used to maximize functional and psychosocial outcome in the presence of physical or cognitive impairment and simultaneously to prevent secondary medical complications that might impede recovery. Rehabilitation can begin during the acute medical hospitalization and continue until maximal functional recovery is achieved. Once a patient with stroke is discharged from acute hospital care, other rehabilitation settings may be chosen based on an individual's therapeutic need and tolerance for activity. These options include comprehensive inpatient rehabilitation, subacute rehabilitation care, rehabilitation day treatment programs, home therapy, or outpatient rehabilitation clinics.

EPIDEMIOLOGY

Stroke Mortality in the United States

Stroke was the primary cause of death in 159,942 persons in 1996 and it remains the third leading cause of death in the United States; it is exceeded only by cardiovascular disease and cancer.[9] However, a well-documented reduction in annual stroke mortality has taken place within the United States in the last century.[10, 11] In particular, there was a sharp decline in the annual stroke deaths for both men and women that began in the 1970s and continued well into the 1980s before the slope flattened (Fig. 50–1).[10, 12] Approximately 200,000 fewer fatal strokes occurred in this period than would have been predicted from data of the previous decade.[12] It can be argued that the improved detection and treatment of hypertension that began in the 1960s and escalated in 1973 with introduction of the National High Blood Pressure Education and Control Program is directly responsible for the steep decline in stroke mortality.[10, 12]

Although a cause-and-effect relationship between blood pressure control and stroke mortality cannot be verified in population studies, data from Rochester, Minnesota, have demonstrated a decline in annual incidence of new strokes during every 5-year period from 1950 to 1980, with a particularly sharp decline after 1970[11] that matches a similarly reduced incidence of hypertension in the same population.[13] It appears that the decline in stroke mortality is a result of reduced stroke incidence, possibly as a result of improved blood pressure control. In addition, direct evidence indicates that antihypertensive therapy reduces stroke risk, as shown in observational and randomized drug studies.[14–16]

Another explanation for reduced stroke mortality is improved survival. Hospital records from Allegheny County, Pennsylvania, demonstrated a decline in stroke-related coma from 1971 to 1980 that was responsible for 80% of the reduced stroke case fatality during that decade.[17] In contrast, data from the Minnesota Heart Survey showed no change in the severity of stroke or case fatality between 1970 and 1980, but hospitalization rates for stroke were significantly reduced in 1980.[18] Thus, the sharp decline in stroke mortality noted nationally was likely related to reduced stroke incidence and less likely to a result of improved acute survival during the 1970s, and can be attributed to an epidemiological improvement in hypertension detection and treatment.

Beginning in the 1980s the steep decline in mortality began to flatten, coincident with improved diagnostic sensitivity of cranial computed tomography (CT) and magnetic resonance imaging (MRI).[19–23] Improved stroke detection may explain the decline and more recent increase in stroke incidence, but there remains con-

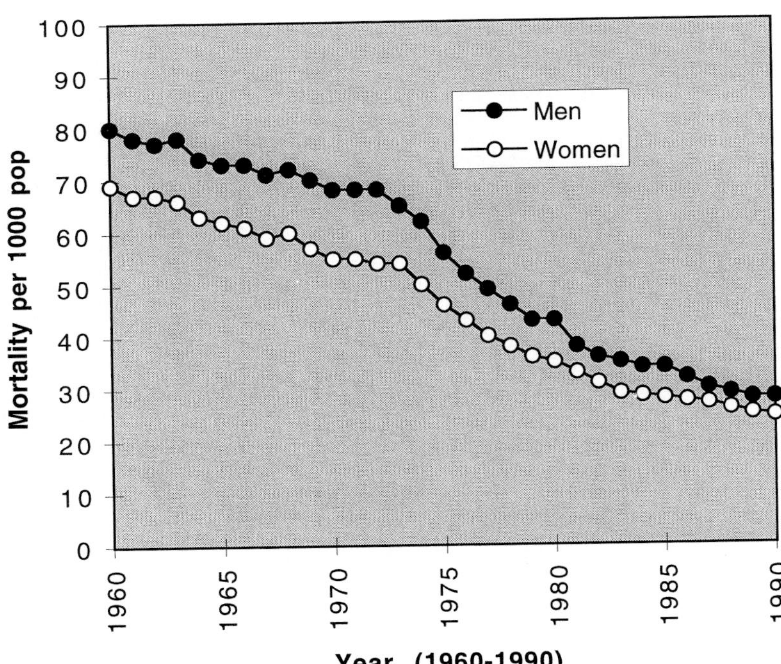

FIGURE 50–1. Annual U.S. stroke mortality for men and women.

cern that public health efforts to prevent stroke have not been fully effective.

Stroke Incidence in the United States: Age, Sex, and Race

Data from several population-based study cohorts estimate that the incidence of stroke in the United States is between 500,000 and 730,000 annually, resulting in significant morbidity, mortality, and disability, particularly among people older than 65 years.

Stroke is primarily a disease of older individuals, but 28% of strokes occur in persons younger than 65 years (Fig. 50–2). The incidence of stroke is 19% higher among men than women of all races. Among black men less than 65 years old, stroke incidence is two- to threefold higher than among whites. The relative incidence of stroke among black women compared to white women is even higher. Many important risk factors for stroke are found in higher frequency among blacks, including hypertension, diabetes mellitus, heart disease, smoking, excessive alcohol use, and sickle cell disease.

The rate of stroke in Asian countries is higher than in the United States, with a greater proportion of strokes caused by intracranial hemorrhage.

Stroke Survival

Stroke survivors, many of whom require rehabilitation services, presently number just over 4 million in the U.S. population. Still, the prevalence of stroke survivors has doubled over the past 25 years. Garraway and colleagues[24] compared survival patterns after first-time stroke for 5-year periods between 1945–1949 and 1975–1979. Twenty-one-day survival after intracerebral hemorrhage improved from 0% to 42%. Acute 30-day survival improved only modestly between 1945–1949 and 1975–1979 after ischemic stroke. Long-term survival up to 7 years improved significantly during the study period.

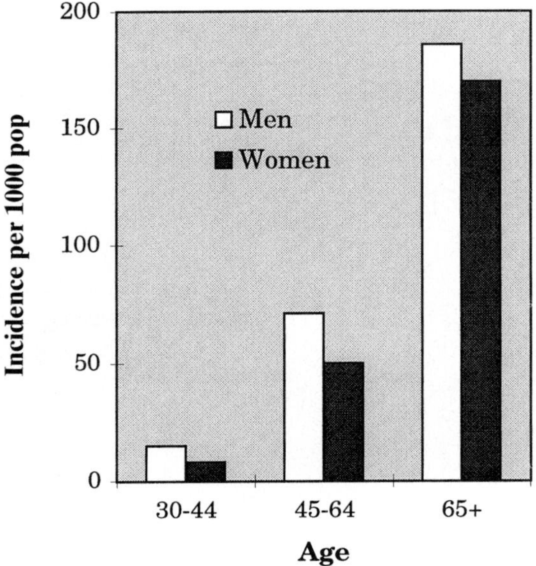

FIGURE 50–2. Annual U.S. incidence of stroke by age and sex.

Evidence from European studies on dedicated stroke units indicates that the major contributor to the increased proportion of stroke survivors is reduced short- and long-term mortality as a result of better management of medical co-morbidity and complications during acute care.[25] Better detection and management of coronary artery disease, prevention of aspiration pneumonia by identification and treatment of dysphagia, prevention of pulmonary embolism using prophylactic measures, and reduction of general disability and immobility by active rehabilitation care have improved long-term survival after stroke.

As our population ages, the incidence and prevalence of stroke will continue to rise. Stroke rehabilitation will have an important role in reducing the burden of long-term stroke care on society.

STROKE RISK FACTORS

Hypertension remains the most important public health concern today because it is the leading risk factor for two of the top three causes of death in the United States: coronary heart disease and stroke. Hypertension is treatable, and its control has the potential for widespread reduction in death and disability in this country. The combination of stroke and heart disease is not unusual and can have a significant impact on medical care and rehabilitation.[26] When faced with a patient with a recent stroke, TIA, or asymptomatic carotid bruit, the clinician must be concerned about the presence of coronary heart disease. Similarly, any patient who presents with known heart disease and chronic atrial fibrillation should be considered a candidate for stroke prophylaxis. A major but often neglected part of physiatric care for stroke survivors and their families is stroke and coronary heart disease prevention and risk factor reduction.

Hypertension

There is a 35% prevalence of hypertension within the U.S. adult population. Defined as a systolic pressure greater than 165 mm Hg or a diastolic pressure greater than 95 mm Hg, hypertension increases the relative risk of stroke by a factor of six. Among stroke survivors, 67% have chronic hypertension.[27] In a recent meta-analysis involving nine population-based observational studies, MacMahon and co-workers[15] noted that a 7.5 mm Hg reduction from the usual diastolic blood pressure (DBP) was associated with a 46% reduction in stroke risk in both hypertensive and normotensive subjects. Interestingly, no threshold diastolic value was found below which further pressure reduction lacked an additional effect on stroke risk. Thus, reductions in DBP below traditionally normotensive values contributed to further risk reduction in these studies.

The Hypertension Detection and Follow-up Program was the first major study to demonstrate a reduction in stroke incidence with antihypertensive treatment. This was a population-based randomized clinical trial with 5-year follow-up involving 11,000 hypertensive persons who were either provided with a stepped-care antihypertensive program or referred for traditional care. There was 1.9% incidence of stroke among patients on stepped-care treatment, compared with 2.9% on a referred-care program, equaling a 35% reduction in stroke incidence and a 44% reduction in fatal strokes.[14] In another study combining the results of 14 randomized antihypertensive drug treatment trials that included 35,000 persons over a 5-year period, subjects receiving blood pressure treatment had a 42% reduced risk of stroke compared with untreated controls.[16]

Isolated systolic hypertension is more common among individuals older than 60 years and is an independent risk factor for stroke and cardiovascular disease.[28] The Systolic Hypertension in the Elderly Program (SHEP)[29] randomized more than 4700 subjects age 60 years and older with systolic pressures greater than 160 mm Hg and diastolic pressure less than 90 mm Hg to antihypertensive treatment or placebo. Over the 5-year study period, subjects treated with antihypertensive medication had an average reduction in systolic blood pressure of 17 mm Hg and a 36% reduction in the incidence of stroke when compared with control subjects.

Ample evidence supports public health efforts aimed at reducing the prevalence of poorly controlled blood pressure, thereby reducing the risk of stroke and heart disease. Improved public education, detection, and treatment of hypertension will have a positive impact on the further decline of stroke incidence and mortality.

Risk Factors Modifiable by Lifestyle Changes

It has been known for many years that cigarette smoking is an important risk factor for cardiovascular disease, but its negative influence on stroke was questioned. More recently, community-based data from the Framingham Study has confirmed that smoking is independently associated with an increased risk of atherothrombotic stroke in both men and women. The relative risk of stroke for heavy smokers (>40 cigarettes per day) is twice that of light smokers (<10 cigarettes per day). Cessation of smoking reverses risk to that of nonsmokers within 5 years after quitting.[30] Twelve-year follow-up from the Honolulu Heart Program studying cardiovascular risk in men of Japanese descent has linked smoking to an increased risk of hemorrhagic stroke in addition to ischemic cerebral infarction.[31]

The role of elevated serum cholesterol has not been clearly linked to increased stroke incidence per se, but its strong influence on the development of coronary artery disease and atherosclerosis[32] indicates that hypercholesterolemia is at least an indirect risk factor for stroke. Indeed, an association between carotid artery atherosclerosis and increased serum cholesterol levels has been noted.[33–35] Reduced dietary intake of cholesterol and saturated fatty acids has been recommended for adults with total cholesterol levels greater than 200 mg/dL or low-density lipoprotein (LDL)-cholesterol levels greater than 160 mg/dL. If dietary measures are ineffective, cholesterol-reducing medications are recommended. There is interesting epidemiological evidence that a total serum cholesterol level less than 160 mg/dL is associated with higher risk of hemorrhagic stroke.[36, 37]

Whether obesity is a risk factor for stroke has been challenged. Hypertension and diabetes mellitus are more common in the obese and are strong influences for stroke risk. Weight loss has a positive influence on blood pressure and diabetic control and likely has a risk-reducing effect on stroke and cardiovascular disease. Although obesity may indirectly increase stroke risk, its independence as a risk factor remains questionable.

Heart disease, including electrocardiographic (ECG) evidence of left ventricular hypertrophy, cardiac failure, and nonvalvular atrial fibrillation, increases stroke risk by two to six times normal. Control of hypertension, cessation of smoking, and reduction of serum cholesterol can reduce the development of heart disease as well as prevent stroke. However, in the presence of established conditions such as atrial fibrillation or left ventricular failure, the use of medical means to reduce stroke risk can become important. Prevention of heart disease through lifestyle changes has a positive influence on stroke prevention.

Risk Factors Modifiable by Medical Means

Transient ischemic attacks are associated with intracranial and extracranial carotid artery disease and are an important sign of stroke risk. Approximately 35% of persons who experience a TIA will have a stroke within 5 years.[38] TIAs are considered physical warning signs of impending stroke and require urgent clinical attention. There is now substantial evidence that medical or surgical treatment for carotid artery disease in patients experiencing TIA can considerably reduce stroke incidence and mortality. But appropriate therapeutic measures can only be implemented after thorough diagnostic testing.

The presence of an asymptomatic carotid bruit due to carotid stenosis is a well-established risk factor for stroke, but it has only recently been considered efficacious to selectively modify this risk by surgical means.[39] More important, the presence of an asymptomatic carotid bruit is an indication of atherosclerotic disease in general, and is a strong predictor of myocardial infarction and cardiovascular death. Once carotid bruits are noted, diagnostic evaluation for coronary artery disease should be strongly considered.

Diabetes mellitus increases the relative risk of ischemic stroke to three to six times that of the general population. This risk can be partly attributed to the higher prevalence of hypertension and heart disease among diabetics, but even after controlling for these factors, diabetes independently doubles stroke risk.[40–42] The prevalence of diabetes among stroke survivors is 20%.[27, 42, 43] Although the data are not yet available, the Diabetes Control and Complications Trial, a prospective longitudinal study, will determine whether tight medical and dietary control of glucose level can reduce the incidence of stroke in diabetics.[44]

Two factors that increase blood viscosity, hematocrit and serum fibrinogen, have been implicated as risk factors for stroke.[45, 46] The mechanism by which stroke occurs in the presence of hyperviscous blood is unclear, but hypercoagulability or enhanced atherogenesis by microvascular damage from traumatic shearing forces against vessel walls are distinct possibilities.

Nonmodifiable Risk Factors

Certain important risk factors for stroke that are not modifiable include age, sex, race, and previous stroke. The epidemiology of age, sex, and race as they relate to stroke were reviewed earlier in the chapter. Once an individual has a stroke, the risk of recurrent stroke is significant. Although the presence of a stroke is not in itself modifiable as a risk factor, a careful workup to determine the cause of the stroke can provide valuable information for clinical decisions regarding secondary stroke prevention.

STROKE PREVENTION

The most effective means to diminish stroke-related morbidity, mortality, and disability is by further reducing the incidence of first-time and recurrent stroke. As emphasized thus far, public awareness of modifiable risk factors for stroke, medical management of risk factors, and the active promotion of lifestyle changes by physicians have the best potential to decrease the annual rate of new stroke occurrence. Physiatrists in particular can counsel patients with stroke and their families about risk factor reduction throughout the course of rehabilitation care. For selected patients who have significant risk for stroke, who have experienced a TIA, or who have had a stroke in the past, physicians can recommend additional medical interventions to minimize the risk of primary (first-time) and secondary (recurrent) stroke. These interventions include antiplatelet therapy, anticoagulation, and carotid endarterectomy.

Antiplatelet Therapy

Primary Prevention

Of the antiplatelet agents available, only aspirin has been studied for primary stroke and cardiovascular disease prevention. The Physicians Health Study[47] was a prospective, double-blind, placebo-controlled study to evaluate the effectiveness of low-dose aspirin for the prevention of cardiovascular mortality. Secondary end points included nonfatal stroke and myocardial infarction (MI). More than 22,000 healthy male physicians participated over the 5-year study period. A 325 mg every-other-day dose of aspirin showed no advantage over placebo for prevention of stroke. Hemorrhagic strokes were more prevalent in the aspirin group to nearly a statistically significant level ($P = 0.06$). This study did show that aspirin significantly reduced the incidence of fatal and nonfatal MI, with its greatest protection realized in men older than 50 years. The incidence of gastric ulcer was not significantly different in the aspirin group, but significantly more reports of bleeding and transfusion were noted in the treatment group.

The British Doctors Trial[48] is the only other study that has examined the use of antiplatelet therapy for primary stroke prevention. This study tested a 500 mg/day dose of aspirin in just over 5000 male subjects using a single-blind randomized design conducted over 6 years, but failed to show any effect of aspirin for the prevention of stroke or cardiovascular disease and mortality. These negative results have been attributed to the smaller sample size and reduced compliance with medication in the British project as compared to the U.S. study.

Currently, the *routine* use of aspirin for stroke and cardiovascular disease prophylaxis is not recommended. Decisions to use aspirin for primary prevention should be based on the patient's age, risk for stroke or MI, and risk for bleeding.[47, 49]

Secondary Prevention

An Oxford-based group called the Antiplatelet Trialists' Collaboration[49] has published a meta-analysis of pooled results from 145 trials of various antiplatelet agents for the prevention of vascular events, including nonfatal MI, nonfatal stroke, and vascular death. As a group, these studies include more than 70,000 subjects with risk factors for vascular disease who were randomized to receive various forms of antiplatelet therapy or placebo over 2 to 6 years. Antiplatelet agents were found to reduce the risk of nonfatal stroke by 31% in men and women. Subgroups of hypertensive and diabetic subjects also benefited from treatment. Although this study supports the benefit of antiplatelet agents have on the reduction of vascular disease in general, the use of and indications for these agents in stroke prophylaxis should be based on specific trials having clearly stated end points.

Aspirin is the most frequently prescribed antiplatelet agent for secondary stroke and cardiovascular disease prevention. By irreversibly inhibiting cyclooxygenase-dependent platelet aggregation, aspirin achieves a significant antiplatelet effect at fairly low serum concentrations.[50] Two large randomized controlled trials have compared aspirin with placebo in the prevention of death or recurrent infarct in nearly 40,000 patients hospitalized with acute ischemic stroke. In combined analysis the International Stroke Trial[51] and the Chinese Acute Stroke Trial[52] showed that aspirin (160 to 300 mg/day) administered early after acute stroke resulted in 9 fewer deaths and recurrent strokes per 1000 patients during the first few weeks, without significant complications. These studies justify the routine use of aspirin in patients with acute ischemic stroke.

Evidence for the long-term benefit of aspirin for secondary stroke prevention has been limited by insufficient sample size and a low overall incidence of recurrent stroke in various clinical trials. In general, these studies have supported the use of aspirin for stroke prophylaxis after TIA or mild stroke in men, but most lack the power to prove efficacy in women.[53–60] However, when studies that include women are pooled for meta-analysis, aspirin proves efficacious.[49] Controversy remains about the ideal aspirin dose. Trials have supported the use of doses between 30 and 1500 mg/day, but studies testing the most effective dose are lacking.[60] The principal advantage that aspirin has over other antiplatelet agents is its low cost and over-the-counter availability.

Clopidogrel and ticlopidine are newer agents that prevent platelet aggregation for the life of the cell by directly inhibiting adenosine diphosphate (ADP)-induced platelet aggregation, without affecting prostaglandin metabolism.[46] They both lack antipyretic, anti-inflammatory, and analgesic effects, and they do not affect the integrity of the gastric mucosa. Although both medications are effective antiplatelet agents and prevent secondary stroke, the use of ticlopidine is limited by the important side effects of rash and diarrhea (12% each), and reversible neutropenia (2.3%).[61, 62] Clopidogrel lacks these side effects and does not require monitoring of blood cell counts, making it a good choice for secondary stroke prevention in patients who cannot tolerate the gastric effects of aspirin.[63]

Anticoagulation and Antiplatelet Therapy in Atrial Fibrillation

Atrial fibrillation is commonly found among the elderly and is present in 15% of persons older than 75 years. Individuals with nonvalvular atrial fibrillation have five times the relative risk for cardioembolic stroke, and those with rheumatic heart disease have a 17-fold increase.[64] Other clinical factors, such as a history of TIA, stroke, hypertension, recent congestive heart failure, and ECG evidence of left ventricular dysfunction, are additional predictors of stroke when associated with atrial fibrillation. Clinical trials have supported the use of aspirin to prevent primary cardioembolic stroke in nonvalvular atrial fibrillation. In the Copenhagen AFASAK trial,[65] a 75 mg/day dose of aspirin reduced embolic stroke risk by 15% when compared with placebo. The U.S.-sponsored Stroke Prevention in Atrial Fibrillation (SPAF) trial[66] measured a 42% reduction in stroke risk using 325 mg of aspirin daily. However, in the SPAF study, aspirin was not clearly effective in men, and it was ineffective in women older than 75 years. The AFASAK and SPAF studies and two additional placebo-controlled trials[67, 68] have tested the use of warfarin anticoagulation for primary stroke prevention in nonvalvular atrial fibrillation. Warfarin reduces relative stroke risk by 58% to 86% over that in control subjects.

Although warfarin proved more effective than aspirin for stroke prevention in atrial fibrillation, a second phase of the SPAF trial (SPAF II)[69] compared warfarin to aspirin with the special intention of determining which medication provided superior stroke prevention for individuals older than 75 years with nonvalvular atrial fibrillation. The results of SPAF II are summarized in Figure 50–3. Care must be taken when considering

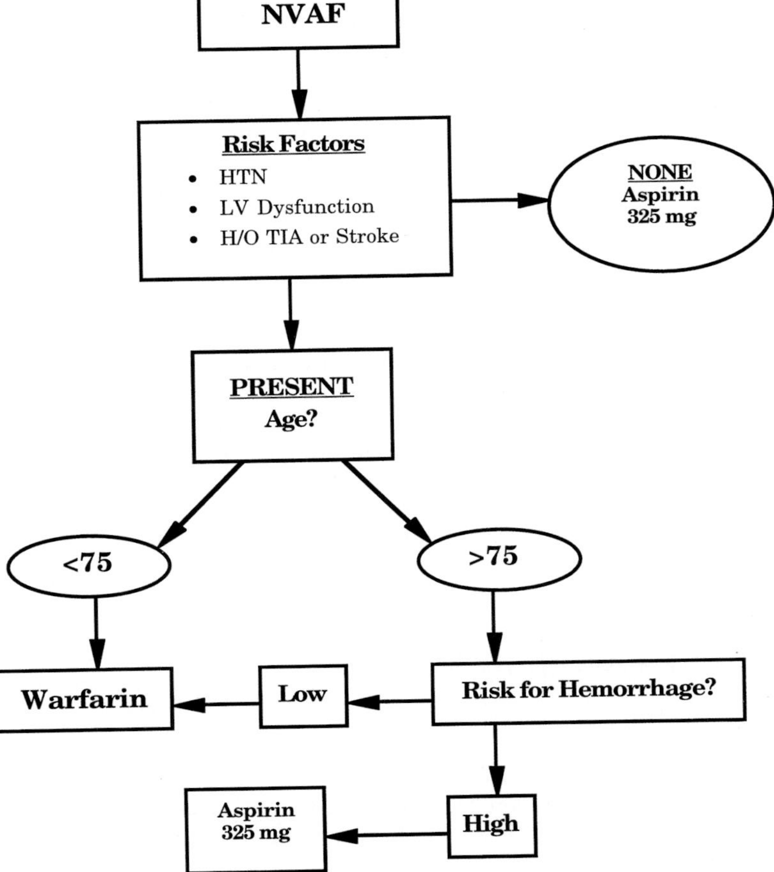

FIGURE 50–3. Stroke prevention in nonvalvular atrial fibrillation (NVAF). HTN, hypertension; LV, left ventricular; H/O TIA, history of transient ischemic attack.

anticoagulation in patients older than 75 years, as the risk of intracranial hemorrhage is higher in elderly persons. Recent results of the SPAF III trial have demonstrated that low-intensity, fixed-dose warfarin plus aspirin is inferior to adjusted-dose warfarin for stroke prevention in high-risk patients with nonvalvular atrial fibrillation.[70]

Individuals with rheumatic valvular disease and atrial fibrillation have a 17-fold increase in risk for embolic stroke. These patients benefit from anticoagulation with warfarin for stroke prevention.

Surgical Management of Carotid Artery Disease

For many years the benefits of surgical versus medical treatment in the management of TIA associated with carotid artery atherosclerosis was hotly debated. More recent evidence supports the use of carotid endarterectomy in combination with aspirin therapy as the treatment of choice for both symptomatic and asymptomatic high-grade carotid artery disease in centers with low surgical mortality and morbidity.

Data from the North American Symptomatic Carotid Endarterectomy Trial (NASCET)[71] revealed a 17% absolute reduction in stroke incidence with carotid endarterectomy over a 2-year follow-up in patients with critical stenosis of 70% to 99%. This represents a relative risk reduction of 65% for surgically treated patients. Perioperative mortality was less than 6% in the surgical group. Outcomes for patients with 30% to 69% carotid stenosis remain equivocal, and trials for moderate carotid artery disease are ongoing.

Carotid endarterectomy for asymptomatic carotid artery stenosis also results in reduced stroke occurrence and death compared with aspirin alone in centers with less than 3% perioperative mortality. Preliminary results from the Asymptomatic Carotid Atherosclerosis Study (ACAS)[39] have demonstrated a significant 5.8% absolute reduction in stroke for surgically treated patients with greater than 60% stenosis after a 5-year follow-up, representing a 55% reduction in relative risk of stroke.

Antiplatelet therapy after carotid surgery remains critical for successful overall outcome. Mild to moderate carotid stenosis (<60%) should be managed with antiplatelet medications, and patients should be monitored for signs of TIA or stroke. An asymptomatic carotid bruit discovered incidentally on physical examination is a sign of atherosclerotic disease and is more predictive of coronary artery disease than of stroke. A careful cardiovascular evaluation is indicated.[72]

STROKE PATHOPHYSIOLOGY

Ischemic Stroke

The unifying pathophysiology of thrombotic, embolic, and lacunar stroke is cerebral ischemia from compromise of cerebral blood flow. The location and temporal development of cerebral injury vary with the etiology.

Thrombosis

The entire pathophysiology of infarction from cerebral thrombosis remains controversial, but it is strongly associated with atherosclerotic cerebrovascular disease. Atherosclerotic plaque formation occurs frequently at major vascular branching sites, including the common carotid and vertebrobasilar arteries. The disease occurs often in the presence of chronic hypertension, with injury to the intimal surface followed by macrophage infiltration and cholesterol accumulation within the vascular media. Foam cells develop within the vessel wall and cholesterol streaks appear on the endothelial surface. Eventually, calcification and vessel wall thickening compromise blood flow, leading to turbulence. Cracking of the plaque and further intimal damage can promote initial thrombus formation by stimulating platelet aggregation and activation of the extrinsic pathway of the coagulation system. The loosely attached thrombus, or "white clot," that rapidly forms is composed of platelet cells and fresh fibrin.[73]

It is unclear whether symptoms of TIA are caused by transient thrombotic occlusion of major cerebral arteries or by microemboli that break away from a thrombus, but both phenomena might be important. Symptoms of transient monocular blindness, or amaurosis fugax, are likely due to microemboli from the internal carotid artery that cause a branch occlusion of the ispsilateral ophthalmic artery.[74] Similarly, other intracranial branch occlusions can result from microemboli arising in the extracranial vessels, leading to injury or infarction in focal regions.

In contrast, a large arterial thrombus can occlude a major extracranial artery, producing a low-flow state that causes ischemic injury to neural tissue supplied by the most distal arterial branches.[75] The volume of damage that results from such hemodynamic compromise can be quite large, but it is dependent on the length of time the vessel is occluded, the rate of flow through the occluded site, and the effectiveness of the collateral circulation. Fibrinolytic enzymes are released that control acute thrombus formation, potentially dissolving the clot within minutes to hours. However, recanalization might fail or be delayed, permitting the arterial thrombus to completely or partially occlude blood flow. Collateral circulation can support the compromised cortical zone, but it may be less effective in elderly persons or in those with diffuse atherosclerotic disease or diabetes.

Ischemic injury from a cerebrovascular thrombus likely results in simultaneous distal branch occlusions from microemboli and compromise of blood flow proximally. The neurological outcome of cerebral thrombi varies widely and can include brief TIAs, minor strokes without functional compromise, or major strokes resulting in significant impairment and functional disability.

Embolism

Beyond the microemboli produced by cerebrovascular thrombi, the majority of embolic strokes have a cardiac origin. Thrombus formation within the cardiac chambers is generally caused by structural or mechanical changes within the heart. Atrial fibrillation is a significant risk factor for embolic stroke as a result of poor atrial motility and outflow, with stasis of blood and atrial thrombus formation. Atrial fibrillation is often caused by rheumatic valvular disease or coronary artery disease, but it can be idiopathic. Mural thrombus within the left ventricle after MI, in the presence of cardiomyopathy or after cardiac surgery, is the other major cause of embolic stroke.[76, 77] Mechanical heart valves universally cause cerebral emboli if anticoagulation is insufficient. Infectious endocarditis can lead to septic emboli.

Paradoxical embolism is a rare cause of embolic stroke that occurs in the presence of a deep vein thrombosis (DVT) and an atrial or ventricular septal defect.[78] Typically, the DVT embolizes to the lung, causing a pulmonary embolus and an acute increase in pulmonary arterial resistance and right ventricular pressures. In the presence of a septal defect, the raised pulmonary pressure leads to a right-to-left shunt. Subsequent emboli cross through the septal defect into the left chambers and systemic circulation, resulting in peripheral emboli and stroke. On modern echocardiography, a patent foramen ovale is a frequent finding, indicating that paradoxical embolism might be more common than previously thought.[77]

Cerebral emboli lodge within arterial branches of the major arteries, causing single or multiple branch occlusions resulting in sudden focal neurological impairment. These branch occlusions significantly compromise flow distally, inducing ischemic injury to neural tissue, glia, and vascular endothelium. Reperfusion of the occluded vessel can occur in response to endogenous fibrinolysis, but because ischemic damage to the vascular bed is often significant, the capillaries become incompetent and secondary cerebral hemorrhage ensues.

In contrast to thrombotic stroke, microemboli probably do not precede cardioembolic strokes, as TIAs are uncommon. Frequently no cardiac thrombus can be found after the event, and the only clue to an embolic cause is the sudden neurological deficit without previous or progressive symptoms.

Lacunes

Lacunar infarcts are small, circumscribed lesions that measure less than 1.5 cm in diameter and are located in subcortical regions of the basal ganglia, internal capsule, pons, and cerebellum.[79] The area of a lacune (meaning "little lake") roughly corresponds to the vascular territory supplied by one of the deep perforating branches from the circle of Willis or major cerebral arteries. Lacunar strokes are strongly associated with hypertension, and pathologically associated with microvascular changes that often develop in the presence of chronic hypertension. Histological changes such as arteriolar thickening and evenly distributed deposition of eosinophilic material, called *lypohyalinosis* and *fibrinoid necrosis,* are commonly seen in the subcortical perforating arteries of hypertensive persons who have had lacunar strokes. Microatheromas within deep perforating arteries are also important causes of lacunar infarction. In addition to hypertension, diabetes mellitus is associated with lacunar stroke as a result of chronic microvascular changes.

Hemorrhagic Stroke

Intracerebral Hemorrhage

The deep perforating cerebral arteries are also the site of rupture preceding intracerebral hemorrhage (ICH). However, unlike lacunar strokes, ICH does not obey the anatomical distribution of a vessel but dissects through tissue planes. Such damage can be significant, resulting in increased intracranial pressure, disruption of multiple neural tracts, ventricular compression, and cerebral herniation. Acute mortality is high, but those who survive ICH often experience rapid neurological recovery during the first 2 or 3 months after the hemorrhage.

Nearly one-half of all ICHs occur within the putamen and the cerebral white matter.[80] Sudden hemorrhage into brain parenchyma is related to both acute elevations in blood pressure and chronic hypertension. Microvascular changes associated with hypertensive hemorrhages include lipohyalinosis and Charcot-Bouchard aneurysms.[81] The latter are not true aneurysms of the vessel wall but are pockets of extravasated blood or "pseudoaneurysms," a sign of previous microscopic ruptures within the vascular wall. Typically, the bleeding lasts no more than 1 or 2 hours, corresponding to the usual time course of acute symptom development. Late neurological decline is related to posthemorrhagic edema or rebleeding.

Cerebral amyloid angiopathy is unusual but is gaining recognition as an important cause of ICH in the elderly.[82] Superficially located hemorrhages that occur in patients older than 55 years who have some premorbid history of mild dementia are characteristic of this disease, but in the absence of tissue staining for Congo red amyloid deposits within the adventitia of cerebral vessels, diagnostic uncertainty remains.

Other notable causes of ICH include the use of anticoagulants, intracranial tumor, and vasculitis.

Subarachnoid Hemorrhage

Subarachnoid hemorrhage (SAH), or bleeding that occurs within the dural space around the brain and fills the basal cisterns, is most commonly caused by rupture of a saccular aneurysm or an arteriovenous malformation (AVM). Saccular aneurysms develop from a congenital defect in an arterial wall followed by progressive degeneration of the adventitia, which causes ballooning or outpouching of the vessel. The risk of bleeding from unruptured aneurysms is speculative but appears greatest for aneurysms greater than 10 mm in diameter.[83]

Saccular aneurysms often rupture during the fifth or sixth decade of life. When a rupture occurs, the extravasation of blood into the subarachnoid space is irritating to the dura and results in a severe headache often described as the "worst in my life." Because of a sudden drop in cerebral perfusion pressure, acute loss of consciousness is frequent. Focal neurological changes or coma can ensue. As many as one-third of patients with aneurysmal hemorrhage die immediately. Patients who present with coma, stupor, or severe hemiplegia have the worst prognosis for proximate survival. The risk of rebleeding from an unoperated aneurysm is as high as 30% within the first month after hemorrhage and declines thereafter. The risk for long-term rebleeding remains 3% per year.[84]

Saccular aneurysms are most often found in the anterior region of the circle of Willis, particularly near branches of the anterior communicating, internal carotid, and middle cerebral arteries, but they can also be found at the junction of almost any branch site within the cerebral circulation. Early surgical management using modern neurosurgical clipping techniques is as safe as late surgery, and it significantly reduces risk of rebleeding.

Arteriovenous malformations present with hemorrhage earlier in life than do aneurysms, often in the second or third decade. Although they cause nearly 9% of all SAHs, vascular malformations are also important causes of ICH and intraventricular hemorrhage.[85] An AVM is a congenital structure consisting of a tangled web of vascular tissue that contains multiple arteriovenous fistulas, which permit arterial-to-venous shunting of blood. They can be located anywhere in the CNS and may grow quite large, displacing normal neural structures, usually without disruption of function. Seizure, migraine, or hemorrhage are typical presenting symptoms.

The incidence of lifetime hemorrhage with AVM is 40% to 50%[86] with a rebleeding rate of 4% per year and a mortality rate of 1% per year.[87] Treatment options include neuroradiological embolization, surgical resection, and radiotherapy (gamma knife).

Hydrocephalus

Acute and chronic hydrocephalus can complicate both SAH and intraventricular hemorrhage by obstructing cerebrospinal fluid (CSF) outflow. Blood coagulum within the ventricular system can block the foramen of Sylvius or the fourth ventricle, causing acute obstructive hydrocephalus over minutes to hours after hemorrhage, leading to lethargy, coma, or death if not treated. Placement of an external ventricular drain can be life-saving, but if the obstruction does not resolve, a ventriculoperitoneal shunt is placed for long-term decompression.

Normal pressure hydrocephalus is very common after SAH and often develops during rehabilitation care. The pathophysiological cause is a functional disruption of CSF resorption due to fibrosis of the arachnoid granulations from subarachnoid blood.[88] The classical symptoms of subcortical dementia, incontinence, and gait disorder are clues to the presence of hydrocephalus, but the physiatrist should also have a high level of suspicion when a patient with recent hemorrhage is not making expected functional gains in a rehabilitation program. That suspicion is often confirmed when the patient makes a remarkable recovery after shunting.

STROKE-RELATED IMPAIRMENTS

Disability in stroke is a result of CNS injury by which physical, cognitive, and psychological functioning become impaired. Specific impairments appear when focal regions and neural systems within the brain are damaged by vascular compromise. Neurological brain mapping has been an active area of research dating back to 1800, when Franz Joseph Gall developed phrenology. He interpreted personality and mental capacity by studying the bumps on the human skull. Although phrenology has been discredited, the study of brain topography has proved quite useful for predicting neurological impairment after focal brain injury.

Motor Control and Strength

Anatomy

The primary motor area is located along the cortex of the precentral gyrus anterior to the central sulcus of both hemispheres, and extends from the paracentral lobule within the longitudinal fissure to the frontal operculum within the Sylvian fissure. The classic "motor homunculus" is useful for visualizing the topography of motor control along the precentral gyrus. Axons from these cortical cells descend via the internal capsule to the pyramidal tract in the brainstem and the corticospinal tract in the spinal cord.

Recovery

With hemiplegia, weakness and poor control of voluntary movement are present initially, associated with reduced resting muscle tone. As voluntary movement returns, nonfunctional mass flexion and extension of the limbs are first noted (Table 50–1). Synergy patterns, or mass contraction of multiple muscle groups, are seen.[89] Later, movement patterns can be independent of synergy.[90]

Motor Coordination and Balance

Trunk control and stability, coordination of movement patterns, and balance all involve complex extrapyramidal systems that are frequently disrupted by stroke. Extrapyramidal disorders can be a major impediment to

TABLE 50–1 Synergy Patterns in Motor Recovery After Stroke

Upper Limb	Lower Limb
Flexor Synergy	
Shoulder retraction	Hip flexion
Shoulder abduction	Hip abduction
Shoulder external rotation	Hip external rotation
Elbow flexion	Knee flexion
Forearm supination	Ankle eversion
Wrist flexion	Dorsiflexion
Finger flexion	Toe extension
Extensor Synergy	
Shoulder protraction	Hip extension
Shoulder adduction	Hip adduction
Elbow extension	Knee extension
Forearm pronation	Ankle inversion
Wrist extension	Plantar flexion
Finger flexion	Toe flexion

functional recovery but are often amenable to therapeutic exercise.

Anatomy

Anterior to the precentral gyrus within the frontal lobe is the premotor area, which is important in motor planning. Multiple fiber tracts from this region descend via the anterior limb of the internal capsule to the basal ganglia and the cerebellum, with input from the vestibular, visual, and somatosensory systems. Injury to either the efferent or afferent systems (or both) can cause poor static and dynamic balance as well as movement disorders such as ataxia, chorea, hemiballismus, and tremors.

Spasticity

Spasticity is a velocity-dependent increase in resistance to muscle stretch that develops after an upper motor neuron injury within the CNS. When severe, spasticity can cause reduced flexibility, posture, and functional mobility, as well as joint pain, contracture, and difficulty with positioning for comfort and hygiene. In stroke, an increase occurs in both tonic and phasic reflexes. Loss of upper motor neuron control causes disinhibited alpha and gamma motor neuron activity and heightened sensitivity to class 1a and II muscle spindle afferents.[91] Consequently, monosynaptic and multisynaptic spinal reflexes become hyperactive.

Spasticity develops shortly after completed stroke, and is initially manifested as an increased phasic response to tendon tap and a slight catch with passive ranging. Later, ranging can become difficult and the patient might show tonic positioning in flexion or extension. Often, as voluntary motor activity returns, a reduction in tone and reflex response is noted, but if recovery is incomplete, spasticity usually remains.

Sensation

Loss of sensation after stroke can have a significant effect on joint and skin protection, balance, coordination, and motor control.

Anatomy

Pain and temperature sensation are relayed centrally by fibers that enter the spinothalamic tract from the contralateral dorsal root ganglion and ascend to the ventral posterior lateral (VPL) nucleus of the thalamus. Some spinothalamic fibers enter the superior colliculus and ascending reticular formation.

Sensory fibers for joint proprioception and stereognosis ascend ipsilaterally from the dorsal root ganglion within the dorsal column and cross to the contralateral side within the lower medulla after synapsing with the nucleus gracilis and cuneatus. The fibers then ascend in the medial lemniscus to the VPL of the thalamus. The VPL relays sensory information to the primary sensory cortex, located posterior to the central sulcus in the postcentral gyrus.

Although injury to the sensory pathways typically causes hypoesthesia or reduced sensation, patients with lesions in the thalamus or spinothalamic tract occasionally experience severe pain that can interfere with functional recovery and rehabilitative care. Treatment options include tricyclic antidepressants, anticonvulsants, and physical modalities such as desensitization techniques or electrical stimulation.

Language and Communication

Aphasia is an impairment of language, but typical lesions that cause aphasia affect comprehension and the use of symbolic material for the purpose of communication and meaning (see also Chapter 3). Testing of language should include an examination of oral expression, verbal comprehension, naming, reading, writing, and repeating.[92] A simple and commonly used classification system for aphasia is listed in Table 50–2.

Although language is considered a function of the left or dominant hemisphere, some elements of communication such as *prosody* have nondominant hemisphere control. Prosody is the rhythmic pattern and vocal intonation of speech that adds emphasis and emotional content to language. There is some clinical and pathological evidence that prosody might have similar anatomical topography as verbal language in the nondominant hemisphere.[93]

Anatomy

Patients with Broca-type aphasia have lesions near the frontal operculum, anterior to the precentral gyrus. This location has been aptly named *Broca's area* and is considered a motor association area, as it is adjacent to the oral motor area of the primary motor cortex. However, the Broca-type aphasia is a primary language deficit with mildly compromised comprehension as well as impaired oral expression. It cannot be considered a

TABLE 50–2 Clinical Characteristics of the Common Aphasic Syndromes

Aphasia	Fluency	Expression	Comprehension	Repetition	Naming
Broca's	Impaired	Impaired	Mildly impaired	Impaired	Impaired
Wernicke's	Normal	Impaired	Impaired	Impaired	Impaired
Global	Impaired	Impaired	Impaired	Impaired	Impaired
Transcortical motor	Impaired	Moderately impaired	Minimally impaired	Normal	Impaired
Transcortical sensory	Normal	Minimally impaired	Moderately impaired	Normal	Impaired
Transcortical mixed	Impaired	Impaired	Impaired	Normal	Impaired
Conduction	Normal	Impaired in repetition	Normal	Impaired	Mildly impaired
Anomia	Normal	Normal	Normal	Normal	Impaired

purely motor impairment. The topographical location for the Wernicke type of aphasia is Wernicke's area, which is found in the posterior superior portion of the first temporal gyrus near the primary auditory cortex and is considered an auditory association area. Lesions near but not involving Broca's or Wernicke's area are associated with transcortical motor and sensory aphasias, respectively.[94]

Ross[93] has described aprosodia that is associated with lesions of the frontal operculum of the right or nondominant hemisphere. Patients who have aprosody speak at an even tempo with flat intonation when asked to express a sentence with an emotional tone. However, they are able to hear and comprehend the emotional content of language. In contrast, patients with a lesion in the temporoparietal region have an affective agnosia in that they are unable to recognize the emotional prosody of spoken language. Despite the agnosia, these patients express prosody without difficulty.

A conduction aphasia, with severely impaired repetition of language, is associated with a lesion of the arcuate fasciculus, which is a bundle of fibers that passes from the temporal to the frontal lobe.[95] Disorders of reading (alexia) and writing (agraphia) are associated with disconnection of the primary language area from the primary visual cortices, which correlates to lesions in the angular gyrus at the junction of the occipital and temporoparietal lobes.[96]

Apraxia

Disorders of skilled movement in the absence of motor, sensory, or cognitive impairment are called *apraxia.* Patients with apraxia often have difficulty performing simple functional activities, such as using a spoon or a comb, or they will perform them in a clumsy manner. It is often difficult to test for apraxia in the presence of a language deficit because the examiner must be assured that the patient understands the command. However, patients with apraxia can have difficulty waving goodbye or using a gesture for hitchhiking when asked to demonstrate these maneuvers. Apraxia is most commonly seen in left hemisphere strokes and affects the left nonhemiplegic limb. Geshwind[97] attributes apraxia in this situation to a disconnection of the right cortical motor association area from the left hemisphere due to an injury of the anterior callosal fibers. Under these circumstances, the right brain cannot know what the left brain wants to do!

Patients with right parietal strokes often have significant difficulty in dressing, despite adequate strength and flexibility. This has been called "dressing apraxia," but it is not a true apraxia, because it is not a disorder of skilled motor function. It is actually a disorder of spatial perception that impairs the patient's ability to find the sleeves and neck of a shirt. Similarly, patients with "constructional apraxia" have difficulty copying a figure due to visuospatial deficits consistent with right parietal stroke.

Neglect Syndrome

Heilman et al define hemispatial neglect as a failure to report, respond, or orient to novel or meaningful stimuli presented to the side opposite a brain lesion.[98] It is important to exclude visual, somatosensory, or motor impairments that would explain the lack of response before attributing it to neglect. Hemispatial neglect significantly contributes to disability after stroke because it has a negative impact on sitting balance, visual perception, wheelchair mobility, safety awareness, skin and joint protection, and fall risk. Patients with neglect have difficulty completing hygiene and self-care on the affected side, fail to eat food items in the neglected visual space, and frequently run into objects and walls. Neglect is a disorder of visual and spatial attention and is associated with temporoparietal strokes and lesions of the frontal eye fields, cingulate gyrus, thalamus, and reticular formation.

Dysphagia

Dysphagia is common after stroke, occurring in 30% to 65% of patients with unilateral or bilateral hemispheric and brainstem infarctions.[99–105] Risk for aspiration pneumonia is strongly associated with a delayed initiation of pharyngeal swallow and reduced pharyngeal transit times frequently seen on videofluoroscopic swallow evaluation.[106, 107] Other neurological factors that influence risk for aspiration after stroke include reduced labial and lingual mobility and sensation, unilateral neglect, pooling of pharyngeal residue within the vallecula and pyriform sinuses, and cricopharyngeal dysmotility. Laryngeal elevation during swallow normally declines with age and can have a negative influence on aspiration risk after stroke (see also Chapter 27).

Uninhibited Bladder and Bowel

Bladder and bowel incontinence are frequent consequences of stroke. Because the pontine micturition center is typically preserved, reflex voiding usually shows normal synchronous internal sphincter relaxation with detrusor contraction. Postvoid residual volumes are generally low in the absence of prostatic hypertrophy or other forms of bladder outlet obstruction. Incontinence is caused by a lack of voluntary inhibition to void from upper motor neuron injury and results in urgency of urination. In alert individuals, awareness of the need to void is unaffected, but immobility, unilateral neglect, and communication deficits often impair a patient's ability to use equipment or call for assistance when the need arises. Although most diabetic stroke survivors have uninhibited voiding, some might have a hypotonic bladder from a parasympathetic autonomic neuropathy to the detrusor muscle. Special care should be taken to check postvoid residual volumes in these patients. Bowel incontinence results from uninhibited reflex rectal emptying by the same mechanism as the uninhibited bladder.

NEUROANATOMICAL BASIS FOR CLINICAL STROKE SYNDROMES

Anatomical localization of lesions within the CNS predicts physical or cognitive impairment and disability.

Understanding the clinical syndromes associated with defined cerebrovascular lesions in ischemic stroke can be a valuable tool to the physiatrist leading the rehabilitation team.

Middle Cerebral Artery Syndromes

Strokes within the middle cerebral artery (MCA) distribution are very commonly seen within the inpatient rehabilitation setting. The anatomical distribution of the MCA includes a large proportion of cerebral cortex, and ischemia within the MCA imparts significant impairment and disability, often requiring intensive rehabilitation care. The MCA is particularly vulnerable to both cardioembolic and thrombotic disease, which can result in a variety of stroke syndromes.

Anatomy

The anterior circulation of the brain consists of both internal carotid arteries derived from the right and left common carotid arteries. The right carotid is usually a branch of the right subclavian; the left is a direct branch of the aorta. After the internal carotid artery passes intracranially through the carotid siphon, it provides the ophthalmic branch to the orbit and then bifurcates at the circle of Willis into the anterior cerebral artery and MCA. The MCA stem or M1 segment turns laterally, passing along the base of the brain to the sylvian fissure overlying the insular cortex, where it typically bifurcates into an upper and lower division. Along the path of the M1 segment, small, deep, perforating branches called *lenticulostriate arteries* are supplied to the putamen, globus pallidus, caudate, and internal capsule. The M2 segment comprises the upper and lower divisions of the MCA as they travel posteriorly and superiorly along the insular cortex. Branches of the divisions pass laterally along the frontal, parietal, and temporal opercula constituting the M3 segment. The M4 segment includes the branches supplying the frontal, parietal, and temporal convexities.

MCA Stroke

Main Stem. The impairments following occlusion of the MCA main stem (M1 segment) are listed in Table 50–3. The hemiplegia in a main-stem stroke is complete, affecting the upper and lower limbs and lower portions of the face equally. This results primarily from ischemia from within the deep lenticulostriate circulation to the posterior limb of the internal capsule through which the descending fibers of the primary motor cortex pass. In contrast, the hemisensory deficit is not as severe because the ascending sensory fibers are not affected, and only the inferior portion of the primary sensory cortex is supplied by the MCA. Although the MCA perforators supply only the upper half of the visual radiations, complete hemianopias are frequently described. Dysphagia and uninhibited voiding are commonly found, even in unilateral strokes.

TABLE 50–3 Middle Cerebral Artery Stroke: Main Stem

Contralateral hemiplegia
Contralateral hemianesthesia
Contralateral hemianopia
Head/eye turning toward lesion
Dysphagia
Uninhibited neurogenic bladder
Dominant hemisphere:
Global aphasia
Apraxia
Nondominant hemisphere:
Aprosody and affective agnosia
Visuospatial deficit
Neglect syndrome

TABLE 50–4 Middle Cerebral Artery Stroke: Upper Division

Contralateral hemiplegia*	Dominant hemisphere:
Contralateral hemianesthesia	Broca's (motor) aphasia
Contralateral hemianopia	Apraxia
Head/eye turning toward lesion	Nondominant hemisphere:
Dysphagia	Aprosody
Uninhibited neurogenic bladder	Visual-spatial deficit
	Neglect syndrome

* Leg relatively more spared than hand and face.

Upper Division. MCA upper division strokes are listed in Table 50–4. The clinical presentation is very similar to that of a main-stem infarction, but hemiplegia and language comprehension deficits are usually not as severe. Because the M1 segment of the MCA is spared, the vascular supply to the internal capsule is preserved and ischemia is limited to the inferolateral portion of the primary motor cortex. Thus, motor strength and control are better in the lower limb than in the hand and face. A classic Broca-type aphasia is typical in a dominant hemisphere stroke, and aprosodia without affective agnosia is found in nondominant hemisphere stroke.

Lower Division. Branch obstruction of the MCA lower division is much less common than upper division stroke, and is usually caused by an embolic event. Motor and sensory function are generally intact. Despite this, patients with stroke of the MCA lower division can have significant functional disability from impaired language and vision and poor awareness of deficits. Table 50–5 lists the impairments associated with lower division strokes.

TABLE 50–5 Middle Cerebral Artery Stroke: Lower Division

Contralateral hemianopia
Dominant hemisphere:
Wernicke's aphasia
Nondominant hemisphere:
Affective agnosia

Anterior Cerebral Artery Syndromes

Anatomy

The anterior cerebral artery (ACA) supplies the interhemispheric cortical surface of the frontal and parietal lobes. The A1 segment branches medially from the internal carotid bifurcation to the anterior communicating artery. Turning superiorly, the artery passes over the optic nerve, along the rostrum of the corpus callosum (A2), and around the genu (A3); it passes posteriorly to the coronal suture (A4) and terminates at the parietal lobe (A5). The ACA divides during its course into two major branches, the pericallosal and callomarginal branches, which provide smaller branches to the cortical surface. The recurrent artery of Heubner is a branch from the A1 or proximal A2 segment that deeply perforates to supply important structures such as the head of the caudate, the anterior limb of the internal capsule, the anterior putamen and globus pallidus, and the hypothalamus.

ACA Stroke

The disorders resulting from an ACA infarction are listed in Table 50–6. The hemiplegia in ACA strokes shows weakness of the shoulder and foot with relative sparing of the forearm, hand, and face, because the focus of ischemia is over the paracentral lobule of the interhemispheric cortex. Unilateral footdrop can be a long-term impairment requiring orthotic management. A left upper limb apraxia to verbal commands can also result from an infarction of the anterior corpus callosum, which disconnects the right hemisphere prefrontal area from the left hemisphere language area.

Occlusion involving the anterior communicating artery and the recurrent artery of Heubner can extend the infarction through the anterior limb of the internal capsule, causing complete hemiplegia. The proximity of such a stroke to Broca's area can also result in a transcortical motor aphasia.

Posterior Cerebral Artery Syndromes

Anatomy

The vertebral arteries typically branch from the right and left subclavian arteries, passing rostrally through the transverse foramina of the cervical vertebra and intracranially via the foramen magnum. At the junction of the medulla and pons, the vertebral arteries unite to form the basilar artery, which again divides into the two posterior cerebral arteries (PCAs) near the top of the midbrain. The P1 segment extends from the basilar to the posterior communicating artery, and the P2 segment extends beyond. Supplying the thalamus are the deep perforating arteries from the P1 and the stem of the P2 segments, called the *thalamoperforans* and *thalamogeniculates.* The branches of the P2 segment include the anterior and posterior inferior temporal, occipital temporal, calcarine, and occipitoparietal arteries.

TABLE 50–6 Anterior Cerebral Artery Stroke

Contralateral hemiplegia*	Grasp reflex—groping
Contralateral hemianesthesia	Disconnection apraxia
Head/eye turning toward lesion	Akinetic mutism (abulia)

* Hand relatively more spared than arm and leg.

TABLE 50–7 Posterior Cerebral Artery Stroke

Hemisensory deficit	Dyschromatopsia
Visual impairment	Alexia without agraphia
Visual agnosia	Memory deficits
Prosopagnosia	

PCA Stroke

The syndrome of PCA infarction is listed in Table 50–7. The blood supply of the thalamus is provided by the perforating arteries of the PCA. Infarcts in the region can cause hemisensory deficits, including hypoesthesia, dysesthesia, and, occasionally, hyperesthesia or pain. Thalamic pain syndrome was first described by Dejerine and Roussy in 1906,[108] but nearly any disruption of sensory afferent fibers within the CNS can cause a central poststroke pain syndrome. Visual disturbances result from injury to the lateral geniculate, temporal, and occipital visual radiations and the calcarine cortex of the occipital lobe. In addition, damage to visual association areas can cause dyschromatopsia, or altered color discrimination. A disorder of reading without impaired writing (alexia without agraphia) associated with a right visual field deficit results from an infarction of the left occipital cortex and posterior corpus callosum, disconnecting the intact right visual cortex from the primary language area of the left hemisphere. Impaired memory can result from infarction of the temporal lobe and the hippocampal gyri.

Vertebrobasilar Syndromes

Anatomy

The major arterial branches supplying the brainstem and cerebellum are the posterior inferior cerebellar artery (PICA), the anterior inferior cerebellar artery (AICA), and the superior cerebellar artery (SCA). The PICA originates from the distal vertebral artery and wraps dorsally around the medulla, whereas the AICA is a branch of the basilar artery circling around the pons. Both supply the inferior lobe of the cerebellum. The superior lobe of the cerebellum receives its blood supply from the SCA branching from the basilar artery at the level of the midbrain. Throughout the course of the basilar artery and its major tributaries, small, deep, perforating arteries branch to supply the brainstem. These branches include paramedian penetrators supplying the medial and basal portions of the brainstem, and the short and long circumferential arteries supporting the lateral brainstem.

Brainstem Stroke Syndromes

The brainstem is a complex structure containing cranial nerves, bulbar nuclei, and tracts. The bulbar nuclei

TABLE 50–8 Brainstem Syndromes and Their Anatomical Correlates

Syndrome	Location	Structural Injury	Characteristics
Weber's	Medial basal midbrain	Third cranial nerve	Ipsilateral third nerve palsy
		Corticospinal tract	Contralateral hemiplegia
Benedikt's	Tegmentum of midbrain	Third cranial nerve	Ipsilateral third nerve palsy
		Spinothalamic tract	Contralateral loss of pain and temperature sensation
		Medial lemniscus	Contralateral loss of joint position
		Superior cerebellar peduncle	Contralateral ataxia
		Red nucleus	Contralateral chorea
Locked-in	Bilateral basal pons	Corticospinal tract	Bilateral hemiplegia
		Corticobulbar tract	Bilateral cranial nerve palsy (upward gaze spared)
Millard-Gubler	Lateral pons	Sixth cranial nerve	Ipsilateral sixth nerve palsy
		Seventh cranial nerve	Ipsilateral facial weakness
		Corticospinal tract	Contralateral hemiplegia
Wallenberg's	Lateral medulla	Spinocerebellar tract	Ipsilateral hemiataxia
		Fifth cranial nerve	Ipsilateral loss of facial pain and temperature sensation
		Spinothalamic tract	Contralateral loss of body pain and temperature sensation
		Vestibular nuclei	Nystagmus
		Sympathetic tract	Ipsilateral Horner's syndrome
		Nucleus ambiguus	Dysphagia and dysphonia

form afferent and efferent cranial nerves that innervate the ipsilateral side of the body, whereas the ascending and descending bulbar and spinal tracts innervate contralaterally. Thus, unilateral brainstem strokes often cause loss of cranial nerve function ipsilaterally and sensorimotor dysfunction contralaterally.[109] Cerebellar strokes result in ipsilateral ataxia, whereas brainstem strokes can cause ipsilateral, contralateral, or bilateral limb ataxia. The common brainstem syndromes are listed in Table 50–8, along with their anatomical correlates.

The *Wallenberg* or lateral medullary syndrome is a commonly occurring stroke that frequently requires inpatient rehabilitation. It is characterized by ipsilateral limb ataxia, loss of pain and temperature sensation on the ipsilateral face and contrateral body, ipsilateral Horner's syndrome (myosis, ptosis, and anhydrosis), dysphagia, dysphonia, and nystagmus. Vertebral artery thrombosis near the PICA branch is the usual cause. The prognosis for functional improvement is excellent.

Most of the remaining brainstem syndromes occur with basilar artery thrombosis. The *locked-in* syndrome is a severe pontine stroke causing quadriplegia, oral motor and laryngeal weakness, and disruption of conjugate eye movements. Oral communication is impaired, but because upward gaze is controlled at the midbrain level within the tectum, patients usually have voluntary vertical eye movements that they can use for communication.

Cerebellar strokes are common and can cause life-threatening obstruction of the fourth ventricle and hydrocephalus if cerebellar edema develops. Such strokes occur with PICA, AICA, or SCA occlusion. PICA and AICA strokes are generally caused by arterial thrombosis of the vertebrobasilar system, but SCA strokes are more commonly cardioembolic.[110]

Lacunar Strokes

Lacunar strokes are located within the deep cerebral white matter, basal ganglia, thalamus, and pons, and result from occlusion of single, small, perforating arteries. These strokes are common and present with a wide variety of neurological and functional deficits. The most common syndromes are listed in Table 50–9.

ACUTE STROKE MANAGEMENT

Saving the Ischemic Penumbra

A basic pathophysiological understanding of cerebral ischemia clarifies the actions necessary to protect the brain during acute stroke. Cerebral tissue necrosis oc-

TABLE 50–9 Lacunar Syndromes and Their Anatomical Correlates

Syndrome	Anatomical Sites
Pure motor stroke	Posterior limb internal capsule
	Basis pontis
	Pyramids
Pure sensory stroke	Thalamus
	Thalamocortical projections
Sensory-motor stroke	Junction of internal capsule and thalamus
Dysarthria–clumsy hand	Anterior limb internal capsule
	Pons
Ataxic hemiparesis	Corona radiata
	Internal capsule
	Pons
	Cerebellum
Hemiballismus	Head of caudate
	Thalamus
	Subthalamic nucleus

curs when cerebral blood flow (CBF), normally under tight autoregulation, is compromised from either arterial thrombosis or embolism. Normal cerebral autoregulation maintains a cerebral perfusion rate of 50 mL/100 g of cerebral tissue per minute, which remains constant regardless of acute changes in systemic mean arterial pressure. During cerebrovascular compromise, normal neural activity can be sustained with a CBF as low as 20 mL/100 g/min, but a rate below 10 mL/100 g/min results in cellular death. Within the CBF range between 10 and 20 mL/100 g/min, basic cellular functions are supported, but the sodium-potassium pump fails, rendering the neural cells "electrically silent."[111] In an acute stroke, these surviving but inactive neural cells are located at the rim of the ischemic injury, where collateral circulation provides the minimal tissue perfusion needed. This rim has been called the *ischemic penumbra,* after the partial shadow surrounding a solar eclipse. Improved blood flow to the ischemic penumbra can theoretically restore normal neurological function. However, the longer the ischemic period before reperfusion, the less likely is the ischemic penumbra to survive. Recent acute stroke management protocols have focused on vascular reperfusion and neuropreservation of the ischemic zone in order to maximally save the ischemic penumbra. From the standpoint of public education regarding stroke, the National Stroke Association has emphasized that to reduce neural impairment, acute stroke management should be implemented within the first 6 hours of the event.[112]

The First 6 Hours

There are a number of ongoing and completed clinical trials investigating the efficacy of agents that can arrest, delay, or reverse cerebral ischemia and neural injury. Current research has focused mainly on four pharmacological treatments: thrombolytic agents, heparin, calcium channel blockers, and neuroprotective medications.

The National Institute of Neurological Disorders and Stroke (NINDS) sponsored the first trial of recombinant tissue plasminogen activator (rt-PA) for the treatment of acute ischemic stroke. Intravenous (IV) administration of rt-PA increases plasmin generation, resulting in significant thrombolytic activity. The NINDS rt-PA study randomized patients presenting to emergency departments within 3 hours of stroke symptom onset to receive either 0.9 mg/kg of IV rt-PA or placebo. Patients with recent surgery or bleeding, uncontrolled hypertension, hematological abnormalities, or any history of intracranial hemorrhage were excluded. Despite a significantly higher rate of symptomatic ICH at 36 hours post infusion, the study demonstrated a 12% absolute increase in patients with minimal or no disability at 3 months following rt-PA treatment compared to placebo.[113] Based on this study, the Food and Drug Administration (FDA) approved rt-PA for the treatment of acute ischemic stroke. Data from the European Cooperative Acute Stroke Study (ECASS) confirmed the safety of rt-PA in the first 3 hours but did not clearly show reduced disability with treatment.[114, 115] However, when combined with the NINDS results, it is clear that rt-PA can reduce unfavorable outcome in selected patients who present to the emergency department (ED) within the first 3 hours after acute stroke onset.

Despite its efficacy, rt-PA may not be effective in most community settings. In a recent study, only 6% of patients presenting with acute stroke to a major university medical center and only 1.1% presenting to community hospitals received rt-PA.[116] These low treatment rates can be partly attributed to a lack of public education about stroke symptoms and partly to insufficient responsiveness of emergency medical services (EMS). Better public education and a modified EMS infrastructure will improve the rapid identification and treatment of stroke in local communities.

Other thrombolytic agents have been studied as well. The use of IV streptokinase is associated with unacceptable rates of ICH and mortality in acute stroke.[117] On the other hand, there is preliminary evidence that intraarterial infusion of pro-urokinase can increase cerebral artery recanalization with an acceptable safety profile up to 6 hours following the onset of stroke symptoms.[118]

Heparin is frequently administered IV in the acute setting to arrest stroke progression or to prevent its recurrence, but there is little support for its efficacy, and clear guidelines for its use are lacking.[119] Subcutaneously injected heparin in dosages of 5000 and 12,500 units b.i.d. was studied in the large International Stroke Trial (N = 19,435). Neither dosage was effective in preventing death or disability at 14 days or 6 months following ischemic stroke. Significant bleeding was associated with the higher heparin dose, but not with 5000 units b.i.d. dosing.[51] In the only randomized placebo-controlled trial to date, IV infusion of danaparoid over 7 days failed to improve the 3-month Barthel Index score when compared to placebo.[120] The prevailing evidence supports the use of antiplatelet agents for the management of acute thrombotic stroke, whether or not thrombolytic agents are administered. Because the risk of recurrent cardioembolic stroke is 12% within the first 3 weeks without anticoagulation, the use of heparin followed by warfarin is warranted if the risk of bleeding is otherwise low.[75] Many clinicians advocate delaying initiation of anticoagulation by a minimum of 48 hours to avoid hemorrhagic transformation of the ischemic infarct. Low-dose subcutaneous heparin is safe to administer early following ischemic stroke and can be considered for prevention of venous thromboembolism.

Calcium channel–blocking agents, such as nimodipine, are effective in preventing death from vasospastic complications of SAH and are recommended for routine use during the first 21 days after hemorrhage.[121, 122] Several trials testing nimodipine for acute ischemic stroke treatment have had disappointing results. The vasodilating effect of these medications can hamper stroke recovery by increasing intracranial pressure.[123]

Another class of medications for the treatment of acute stroke are the neuroprotective agents. In particular, the *N*-methyl-D-aspartate (NMDA) receptor antagonists have shown the potential to delay neuronal injury. During ischemic injury, excitatory neurotransmitters such as glutamate and aspartate are released extracellularly. In high concentrations, these amino acids act on NMDA membrane receptors, causing an influx of cations, which results in rapid neuronal death. Several controlled studies testing the ability of NMDA antagonists to prevent cytotoxic injury during acute stroke have been discontinued because of safety concerns or lack of benefit. One solution may be to combine neuroprotective agents with thrombolytic therapy and improve delivery of medication to the ischemic penumbra.

Emergency Department Evaluation and Treatment

The modern era of acute stroke care requires that a rapid diagnosis be made so that early treatment options can be considered. Based on the need for rapid diagnosis, the NINDS has recommended that a physician assessment, laboratory testing, and cranial CT and its interpretation be completed within 45 minutes of arrival in the ED for all patients with acute stroke symptoms.[124] The goal of the initial physician evaluation is to establish medical stability, develop a differential diagnosis, and initiate the acute stroke management protocol if indicated by neurological assessment.

Laboratory tests performed in the ED include determining electrolyte, blood urea nitrogen, creatinine, glucose, and total cholesterol levels, obtaining a complete blood cell count with platelets, determining the prothrombin time, partial thromboplastin time, and erythrocyte sedimentation rate (ESR), and urinalysis. The purpose of these tests is to identify correctable abnormalities, screen for treatable risk factors, and determine whether thrombolytic agents are contraindicated.

Rapid performance and interpretation of cranial CT identifies whether the stroke is ischemic or hemorrhagic. In cases of ischemic infarct the CT findings are often negative for the first 24 to 48 hours after symptom onset. Early signs of a cortical infarct include loss of definition at the gray-white junction and effacement of the sulci overlying the infarcted region. Occasionally a bright area (or signal) is seen in the main stem of the MCA that is diagnostic of an acute thromboembolism.[125] During the first 48 hours following cerebral infarct the cranial CT image begins to show a hypodense area within the distribution of the vascular occlusion. Lacunar strokes appear as small punctate hypodensities within the basal ganglia, thalamus, and subcortical white matter. Strokes in the brainstem and cerebellum are more difficult to visualize using cranial CT because the thick bone of the skull base creates image artifacts that obscure soft tissue detail in the posterior fossa.

ICH has a hyperdense appearance on cranial CT and can be distinguished from infarction in the acute period. The location of the hemorrhage can provide cues to the etiology of the bleeding. Hemorrhage confined to the basal ganglia or thalamus is likely a result of hypertensive ICH. Saccular aneurysm and AVM should be considered if intraventricular or subarachnoid blood is seen. Within 1 or 2 weeks after hemorrhagic infarct, the appearance of blood on head CT becomes hypodense with soft tissue, and may be more difficult to differentiate. The late appearance of an ICH typically shows resolution of extravasated blood and edema, with only a small, residual, hypodense defect remaining.

The decision to use IV thrombolytic agents is not based only on the absence of hemorrhage on cranial CT. Patients with recent bleeding or surgery, a history of ICH, hemotological abnormalities, or uncontrolled hypertension should not be given rt-PA. Some debate remains about whether thrombolytic agents should be avoided in patients with severe stroke and early cranial CT changes such as edema or hypodensity. Subgroup analysis in both the NINDS and ECASS studies confirmed a higher rate of ICH in these patients[126, 127]; however, the NINDS study still showed a more favorable outcome among patients with baseline edema on cranial CT who were given IV rt-PA. What constitutes the best candidate for thrombolytic therapy is not settled, but experience to date shows that those with severe neurological deficit benefit the most and yet have the highest risk for hemorrhagic transformation.

Acute Medical Management

Initial medical care for a patient with acute stroke requires careful and frequent neurological monitoring to prevent and manage medical complications that compromise cerebral tissue perfusion. If the patient is obtunded, concern for airway protection is critical to maintain oxygenation, and an endotracheal tube should be placed, with ventilatory support if necessary. Cerebral edema and acute hydrocephalus may develop rapidly (particularly after ICH), requiring hyperventilation or placement of an external ventriculostomy device to relieve intracranial pressure. In cases of brainstem compression and hydrocephalus from cerebellar infarction or hemorrhage, surgical decompression of the posterior fossa can be life-saving.[128]

Blood pressure is often acutely elevated during stroke, usually as a response to cerebral injury, and often falls spontaneously over the following week.[129] Clinicians should resist the temptation to rapidly correct elevated blood pressure, because often it is a necessary compensatory response to impaired autoregulation after acute ischemic brain injury. Thus, a higher mean arterial pressure (MAP) is needed to maintain cerebral perfusion pressure to the ischemic area. A rapid drop in blood pressure can potentially enlarge an ischemic infarct. This is especially true in individuals with chronic hypertension, whose brains are accustomed to a higher perfusion pressure.[130, 131] Acute hypertension after stroke should be treated only if it is symptomatic, if there is evidence of end-organ injury, or if the diastolic pressure rises above 120 mm Hg.[132] When treated, elevated blood pressure should be lowered gently, and it is usually best to allow the systolic pressure to remain above 150 mm Hg and the diastolic pressure above 90 mm Hg. Calcium channel blockers are not ideal agents for acute hypertension management after stroke. These medications can cause cerebral vasodilation and increase intracranial pressure, resulting in reduced perfusion to the ischemic penumbra.[131] A better choice for acute blood pressure control are the mixed beta- and alpha-antagonists, such as labetolol, or alpha-2-receptor antagonists, like clonidine, which have no measurable effect on cerebral perfusion.[131, 133]

Hyperglycemia in response to acute physiological stress occurs in both diabetic and nondiabetic patients during stroke and is associated with increased levels of serum cortisol. Frequent monitoring and control of serum glucose levels during acute stroke have been recommended. Animal studies reveal that a high glucose concentration within partially perfused ischemic tissue provides the substrate for anaerobic cellular metabolism and lactic acid production.[134, 135] The accumulation of lactic acid is cytotoxic and can lead to further tissue injury.[135, 136] Thus, careful use of insulin and strict glucose control are potentially neuroprotective.

Further Diagnostic Evaluation

Following ED care and early acute stroke management, patients are admitted to the hospital for a complete diagnostic workup to determine the cause of the stroke and secondary preventive measures. Additional laboratory tests can be ordered as indicated, such as full lipid profile if the cholesterol level is elevated. In young patients with stroke it is important to consider hereditary diseases that increase the risk for hypercoagulability and stroke.[137] Serum hemoglobin electrophoresis can detect sickle cell disease or trait. Hypercoagulable states, such as deficiencies in protein C,[138] protein S, or antithrombin III, can be tested by measuring the plasma levels of each. An elevated ESR should stimulate an evaluation for vasculitis, anticardiolipin antibody, or lupus anticoagulant.

Cranial MRI is useful to determine the extent of brain injury and identify potential structural abnormalities. Standard two-dimensional spin-echo MRI is now available in most medical centers throughout the United States and has several advantages for the evaluation of stroke. Tissue density on MRI is dependent on the energy released in the presence of a strong magnetic field. On T1-weighted images, CSF appears dark, whereas gray and white matter are nicely differentiated. In contrast, T2-weighted images show a bright CSF signal, while the fat density is low. A third technique, in which CSF and soft tissue are isodense, is called "spin-density" weighting. With all techniques, bone is poorly imaged due to its low hydrogen content. The flow of blood within the cerebral circulation produces a signal void unless a static intravascular occlusion is present.

MRI is more sensitive than CT in demonstrating the changes of acute stroke in the first 48 hours.[139] Edema within an infarcted zone can appear as early as 2 to 4 hours after stroke onset and is best seen on T2-weighted images. Infarcts near the cortex or periventricular region are better seen on spin-density images, because the bright CSF signal of T2-weighting can otherwise obscure subtle changes. T1-weighted imaging is less sensitive for acute cerebral infarct but can show early effacement of gyri and occasionally a vascular thrombus. MRI is more sensitive than CT for lacunar strokes after the first 24 hours, and MRI is the test of choice for imaging the posterior fossa, where bone artifact is not a problem.[140] Newer diffusion-weighted MRI techniques are superior to conventional MRI for detecting early ischemic changes, and whole brain scans can now be performed quite rapidly.[141] Diffusion-weighted MRI may have a significant role in acute stroke management when it becomes more widely available.

MRI is nearly equivalent to CT for the detection of ICH in the acute setting. Cranial CT remains the test of choice for examination of hemorrhage because it is less costly than MRI. With subacute or chronic hemorrhagic stroke, MRI can differentiate methemoglobin from soft tissue and is better than CT for the detection of late hemorrhages.[139]

Magnetic resonance angiography is a noninvasive option for examining extra- and intracranial cerebral vessels. Using the two-dimensional "time-of-flight" technique, extracranial vessels can be visualized, often revealing the presence of carotid or vertibrobasilar atherosclerotic disease. The three-dimensional time-of-flight technique produces excellent images of the circle of Willis and the cerebral artery stems.[142] MR angiography is indicated as a screening test for extracranial and intracranial atherosclerotic disease, but has not yet exceeded the detail of conventional contrast-enhanced angiography. However, as the technology improves, it may soon be considered equivalent in accuracy.

Nuclear medicine scanning techniques, such as positron emission tomography (PET) and single-photon emission computed tomography (SPECT), detect the uptake of radiolabeled materials with a signal intensity dependent on blood flow to the soft tissue region. Changes can be detected within the ischemic zone immediately during acute cerebral infarct and hemorrhage. Currently, PET is not readily available and its use is limited to research settings, whereas SPECT continues to be evaluated for its clinical usefulness.[143]

Due to its noninvasive nature, ultrasonography (US) is gaining in popularity in many diagnostic areas, including stroke. Transthoracic echocardiography (TTE) imaging after suspected cerebral embolism is now standard practice and is simple to perform. Intraventricular thrombi and valvular vegetations are particularly easy to image using this technique. The detection of thrombi within the left atrium and the atrial appendage is unreliable with TTE because visualization of the left atrium is obscured by the left ventricle.[144] Transesophageal echocardiography (TEE) overcomes this limitation because the transducer is passed down the esophagus, posterior to the heart, where the left atrium and appendage can be directly visualized. This procedure is well tolerated and provides a tenfold improvement in left atrial thrombus detection.[145] Atrial septal defects are also well visualized with TEE, which can be important if paradoxical embolism is suspected.

Arterial duplex scanning combines either standard or color Doppler imaging with two-dimensional US and is a useful screening tool for carotid atherosclerosis. In practical use a negative carotid duplex scan excludes the need for carotid endarterectomy, but it does not rule out the presence of significant intracranial atherosclerosis. Similarly, a duplex scan that is positive for critical stenosis extracranially cannot exclude the presence of an arterial occlusion in the distal internal carotid artery, which is a contraindication to surgical treatment. Transcranial Doppler imaging can measure flow characteristics of the intracranial vessels, but it lacks imaging capability; it is most useful when serial measurements of CBF are needed, such as in the monitoring of cerebral vasospasm after SAH.[146] Although it is invasive and not without complications, conventional contrast-enhanced cerebral angiography is the most accurate method of detecting and anatomically defining extracranial or intracranial cerebrovascular disease when surgical treatment is considered. Contrast-enhanced angiography is the method of choice for detecting and defining the anatomy of cerebral aneurysms and AVMs.

NATURAL SPONTANEOUS NEUROLOGICAL RECOVERY

Patients improve after stroke in two different but related ways.[147] The first type of recovery, a reduction in the extent of neurological impairment, can result from natural spontaneous neurological recovery, from the effects of treatments that limit the severity or extent of the acute stroke, or from other interventions that enhance neurological functioning. This form of recovery presents clinically as improvements in motor control, language ability, or other primary neurological functions.[148]

The second type of recovery demonstrated by stroke patients is the improved ability to perform daily functions in their environment, within the limitations of their physical impairments.[149–152] A patient who has sensorimotor, cognitive, or behavioral deficits resulting from stroke may regain the capacity to feed himself or herself, dress, bathe, control elimination, walk, and carry out other activities of daily living (ADL), despite some degree of residual impairment. The ability to perform these tasks can improve through adaptation and training, in the presence or absence of natural neurological recovery. Although there is some controversy over the extent to which rehabilitation interventions might promote *remediation* of primary deficits, it is generally accepted that most rehabilitation activities are thought to exert their greatest effectiveness in providing compensatory training to reduce disability.

The recovery of independent functioning that occurs during rehabilitation has been found to differ in type and degree from that which might have been expected by a reduction in neural impairments alone.[153–162] This observation suggests that rehabilitation interventions by themselves probably play an important role in improvement. However, the two types of improvements are related to each other in subtle and complex ways.[147] Alternative compensatory functional strategies, such as one-handed dressing techniques for the hemiplegic patient, play a major role in the performance of functional tasks when neurological recovery is minimal or absent.

A recent study by Roth and associates[163] attempted to quantify the magnitude of improvement in functional skill performance (i.e., reduction of *disability*) in the small subgroup of patients who experienced no or minimal improvement in their neurological deficits (i.e., no or minimal reduction of *impairment*). This study was conducted to determine the "pure" or "isolated" effects of rehabilitation interventions, separated from functional improvements that might occur as a result of natural recovery. Of the 402 stroke patients who underwent comprehensive inpatient rehabilitation, the 342 (85%) who had substantial neurological recovery gained approximately 29% to 45% in their Functional Independence Measure (FIM) scores during rehabilitation, and the 60 (15%) patients who had no or minimal neurological recovery demonstrated reduced disability scores by as much as 22% to 38%. While those with neurological recovery experienced greater functional improvement, it is important to note that even patients with no or minimal neurological recovery significantly improved in their ability to carry out day-to-day skills.

The degree of natural recovery of neurological functioning is variable, but comparisons of figures on the relative frequencies of neurological deficits during the early and later stages following stroke offer some insight into the magnitude of recovery that might be seen. Generally, these deficits decline in frequency by about one-third to one-half.[27, 148, 164] For example, the prevalence of hemiparesis has been found to decline from 73% during initial presentation to 37% at 1-year follow-up, aphasia from 36% to 20%, dysarthria from 48% to 16%, dysphagia from 13% to 4%, and incontinence from 29% to 9%. The time course for recovery also is variable: although most improvements in physical functioning occur within the first 3 to 6 months, later recovery also is commonly seen.[154, 165–168] Although it is tempting to specify a definitive prognosis in a stroke patient who presents with a particular level of initial motor function, it is important to recognize that many variables determine ultimate outcome, and therefore expectations for recovery frequently are inaccurate.

Recovery of Motor Function

For most (but not all) stroke patients, the pattern of natural spontaneous recovery of motor function follows a relatively stereotypic sequence of events in which lower extremity function recovers earliest and most completely, followed by upper extremity and hand function. Return of tone usually precedes return of voluntary movement, proximal control precedes distal control, and mass movement patterns (or synergy patterns) precede specific isolated coordinated volitional motor functions (see Table 50–1).[89, 90, 169] There are many exceptions to these observations, however, primarily in patients who sustain strokes in distributions other than the common MCA area.

Although the prognosis for ultimate return of voluntary motor control cannot be provided with a strong degree of certainty to an individual patient, some degree of improvement in motor function usually can be expected following a stroke.[170–180] For example, one study[171] reported that lower extremity motor control improved by one Brunnstrom recovery stage in 39% and by two or more stages in 12% of patients, whereas upper extremity motor control improved by one stage in 24% and by two stages in 8%.

This sequence of recovery can stop at any stage. Some hemiparetic patients ultimately gain full or nearly complete use of all muscles in an isolated coordinated fashion, independent of synergy patterns. Others experience incomplete improvement with partial voluntary use of the recovering extremity, and a few patients demonstrate minimal or no recovery in motor control. One investigation[170] reported that moderate or severe motor weakness of the arm was present in about two-thirds of patients initially and in about one-fourth at 3-month follow-up.

Recovery of Language and Perceptual Functions

Language and perceptual functions tend to improve after stroke, but their recovery patterns can be more variable than those seen in motor function. The prevalence of aphasia declines from about one-fourth during the acute phase to about one-fifth or less during the later stages after stroke.[181] Recovery from aphasia usually occurs at a slower rate and over a more prolonged time course than does motor recovery.[167] Whereas most aphasia recovery occurs in the first 3 to 6 months,[181–183] at least one group has observed that patients with global aphasia show the greatest improvement during the latter half of the first year after stroke.[167, 181, 184] The amount and pattern of recovery are usually related to the initial severity of the aphasia and the specific aphasia type.[185, 186] Patients with nonfluent aphasia generally (but not always) have a less favorable prognosis than those with fluent aphasia, although both groups can and do improve. Comprehension usually returns earlier and to a greater extent than expression.[187]

Although most of the improvement in perceptual functioning occurs in the first 3 to 6 months after stroke,[188–194] some recovery occurs later. According to a study by Hier and associates,[194] most of the recovery of perceptual deficits, such as unilateral spatial neglect, denial of illness, loss of facial recognition, and motor impersistence, occurred within the first 20 weeks after stroke, but some improvement could be seen up to 1 year later.

Proposed Mechanisms of Recovery of Neurological Function

Several mechanisms have been proposed to explain the clinically observed phenomenon of spontaneous recovery of neurological functioning.[195–205] These mechanisms generally can be divided into two broad categories. The first mechanism is the resolution of local harmful factors, which usually accounts for early spontaneous improvement (usually within the first 3 to 6 months). These processes include resolution of local edema, resorption of local toxins, improved local circulation, and recovery of partially damaged ischemic neurons. The second mechanism to explain recovery is neuroplasticity, which can take place early or late after brain damage. The concept of brain plasticity refers to the ability of the nervous system to modify its structural and functional organization. The two most plausible forms of plasticity are collateral sprouting of new synaptic connections and unmasking of previously latent functional pathways. Other mechanisms of plasticity include assumption of function by undamaged redundant neural pathways, reversibility from diaschisis, denervation supersensitivity, and regenerative proximal sprouting of transected neuronal axons. Experimental evidence indicates that plasticity can be altered by several external conditions, including pharmacological agents, electrical stimulation, and environmental manipulation.[206] It is likely that this phenomenon has implications for the effectiveness of rehabilitation interventions. The reader is referred to several excellent references for additional information on the subject of natural neurological recovery.[196–198, 201, 205]

MEDICAL CO-MORBIDITIES AND COMPLICATIONS

Most patients with stroke who undergo rehabilitation have many other associated medical conditions that require professional attention. The Framingham Heart Study[27] reported that compared to age- and sex-matched controls, stroke survivors had significantly greater frequencies of hypertension, hypertensive heart disease, coronary heart disease, obesity, diabetes mellitus, arthritis, left ventricular hypertrophy, and congestive heart failure. Medical problems that are relevant in stroke patients undergoing rehabilitation can be categorized as (1) preexisting medical illnesses that necessitate ongoing care (such as hypertension and diabetes), (2) general health functions affected by the stroke (such as nutrition and hydration), (3) secondary poststroke complications (such as deep venous thrombosis and pneumonia), or (4) acute poststroke exacerbations of preexisting chronic diseases (such as an angina attack during physical exercise in a patient with a history of ischemic heart disease). Management of these conditions can take up major portions of the rehabilitation effort. It has been stated that some stroke patients can be more disabled by certain associated co-morbid diseases than by the stroke itself.[27, 207]

The occurrence of these associated conditions has several implications for stroke patient management during and after rehabilitation. First, these problems can detract from the benefits of rehabilitation. Some medical problems, such as heart disease, adversely affect the course of and outcome after a stroke.[27, 207–211] Intercurrent medical complications can limit the patient's ability to participate in a therapeutic exercise program, inhibit functional skill performance, and reduce the likelihood of achieving favorable outcomes from rehabilitation. The rehabilitation interventions also might adversely affect the medical condition, causing an exacerbation of the disease or a need to adjust medical management. Medical complications can occur during the rehabilitation program that demand diagnostic evaluation, prompt recognition, and appropriate medical management, which can be difficult to complete in the rehabilitation setting. A recent study by Harvey and associates[212] conducted on a large sample of stroke rehabilitation patients found that the presence of certain medical conditions, especially a tracheostomy, a feeding tube, a history of pneumonia, a history of coronary artery disease, and a history of renal failure, significantly increased the utilization of resources (as measured by average charge per day) during inpatient stroke rehabilitation.

Preventing and treating co-morbid medical conditions and medical complications are major components of the rehabilitation management of stroke patients, as they enable rehabilitation to take place and to be most effective. The clinical tasks in managing these problems are to prevent medical complications, to promptly and appropriately diagnose and treat complications when they occur, and to manage both preexisting medical illness and ongoing general health functions during rehabilitation. A few of the important complications are discussed briefly here. The reader is referred to several reviews of stroke co-morbidities[213–218] and to individual articles on several specific complications.[26, 219–226] for more complete discussions of associated medical problems as they relate to stroke patients and the rehabilitation process. Table 50–10 lists some of the common diagnoses that might accompany the stroke and that might require management.

Select Complications

Physiological deconditioning accompanies both acute medical illness and the prolonged bedrest that might be enforced immediately after its onset.[227–229] Deconditioning can contribute to fatigue, endurance limitations, poor exercise tolerance, orthostatic hypotension, lack of motivation, and depression. All of these problems can adversely affect the course of recovery and rehabilitation. Preventive techniques include early mobilization, early and gradually increasing participation in rehabilitation, and the development and implementation of a schedule that balances rest and activity. Interestingly, long-term stroke survivors, even those with nearly full neurological recovery, frequently report easy fatigability and endurance limitations.

TABLE 50–10 Common Medical Co-morbidities and Complications in Stroke Patients

Thromboembolic disease	Malnutrition
Pneumonia	Dysphagia
Ventilatory insufficiency	Shoulder dysfunction
Hypertension	Reflex sympathetic dystrophy syndrome
Orthostatic hypotension	Depression
Angina	Sexual dysfunction
Congestive heart failure	Seizure
Cardiac arrhythmias	Spasticity
Diabetes mellitus	Contracture
Prior stroke	Central poststroke pain syndrome
Recurrent stroke	Falls and injuries
Urinary tract infection	Medication overuse
Bladder dysfunction—incontinence or retention	Deconditioning and endurance limitations
Bowel dysfunction—incontinence or retention	Fatigue
Pressure sore	Insomnia
Dehydration	

The incidence of *venous thromboembolism* varies widely, depending on the specific investigator, but the average is between 40% and 50% for deep vein thrombosis and 10% for pulmonary embolism.[220] The National Institutes of Health Consensus Conference,[230] other investigators,[231] and extensive clinical experience[220] indicate that some form of prophylaxis for venous thromboembolism be instituted for all stroke patients. In patients in whom hemorrhagic stroke has been ruled out, repeated doses of low-dose heparin or low-molecular weight heparin compounds have been documented to be effective.

Pneumonia occurs in about one-third of patients with stroke, although the incidence is higher in the subset of patients who have subarachnoid hemorrhage. Dysphagia, present in about one-third to one-half of all stroke patients, can cause aspiration and pneumonia. This underscores the importance of evaluating swallowing function, instituting compensatory treatments such as positional changes during swallowing, and using alternative feeding methods if needed. Other factors that might predispose to pneumonia include abnormal central breathing patterns, general debility causing impaired immune response, and, especially, hemiparetic weakness of ventilatory muscles causing weakened cough.[213–215, 221]

Cardiac abnormalities can be causal, consequential, or coincidental in stroke,[26, 218] with rates of association of 75% for hypertension, 32% to 62% for coronary artery disease, 40% to 70% for various arrhythmias, and 12% to 18% for congestive heart failure. Since the presence of heart disease, and especially congestive heart failure, can adversely affect functional outcome, it may be necessary to more rigorously screen stroke patients prior to initiating exercise, to more closely monitor stroke patients during their participation in rehabilitation, or to modify their therapy somewhat.[219]

Central poststroke pain is relatively rare (estimated to occur in about 2% of patients), but often is highly problematic.[232, 233] It can be a limiting factor in functional recovery and often is refractory to treatment. Commonly used interventions include treatment of general medical conditions, proper positioning, the application of psychological techniques such as relaxation and imaging, the use of antiepileptic (with some recent favorable experience with gabapentin) and/or antidepressant medications, and, rarely, surgical intervention.

Preventing recurrent stroke is a key component of stroke rehabilitation care,[233] because patients who have had a stroke are at substantial risk for another stroke (about 7% to 10% per year). Although the choice of preventive therapy depends on the type of stroke, measures to prevent secondary stroke generally are directed toward controlling risk factors, which can be thought of in three broad categories: risk factors that are modifiable with lifestyle changes, such as smoking cessation, dietary alterations, and exercise; risk factors that are modifiable with medical-surgical interventions, such as carotid endarterectomy or the administration of anticoagulant or antiplatelet agents; and risk factors that cannot be modified. Surgical treatment of cerebral aneurysms after subarachnoid hemorrhage can be effective in reducing recurrences in most patients. Clearly, one of the major preventive interventions that a rehabilitation program can provide is education.

Bowel and bladder incontinence is seen in one-third to two-thirds of stroke survivors during the early post-stroke period and in about one-fifth to one-fourth after 6 months.[235–243] Continued incontinence in the stroke patient is often predictive of limited functional outcome. Urinary incontinence can result from urinary tract infection, neurogenic bladder dysfunction, causing detrusor hyperreactivity, cognitive or sensory dysfunction, causing inability to recognize bladder fullness or to know what to do when the bladder is full, or motor deficits, causing difficulty transferring to the toilet. Management of these problems focuses on addressing each of these problems as appropriate, with special emphasis on developing a timed planned toileting program. Bowel problems following stroke might be due to immobility and inactivity, inadequate fluid or nutritional intake, psychological depression, neurogenic bowel, lack of transfer ability, cognitive deficit, or reduced consciousness.

Shoulder pain, contracture, and other musculoskeletal disorders, resulting from glenohumeral subluxation, impingement syndromes, rotator cuff tears, frozen shoulder, brachial plexus injuries, complex regional pain syndromes, bursitis, or tendinitis, occur in about 70% to 80% of hemiplegic stroke patients.[244–254] Shoulder problems occur with greater frequency during the spasticity phase of recovery than during flaccidity. Treatment attempts to both support and mobilize the shoulder and includes the use of wheelchair arm troughs and lap trays, shoulder slings, physical modalities, medications, and, most important, aggressive and consistent ROM exercises.

Falls occur with striking frequency in stroke survivors, with most reports indicating that patients who sustain right hemisphere strokes are at substantially greater risk for falling than those with left hemisphere strokes (likely because of the associated cognitive-perceptual deficits, impulsivity, and lack of judgment).[255–258] Prevention approaches emphasize balance training, cognitive training, safety training (especially with caregivers), ensuring supervision during mobility activities, eliminating environmental hazards, and use of assistive devices.

Effective prevention and management of these and other medical complications of stroke are critical to enable effective rehabilitation to take place and to facilitate the achievement of optimal outcomes.

PRINCIPLES OF STROKE REHABILITATION

Because presentations, problems, recovery patterns, coping styles, social situations, and responses to treatment differ among individuals who sustain a stroke, it is necessary to individualize rehabilitation management programs. However, several common management principles are recognized by clinicians and observers in the field of stroke rehabilitation. Three views of the common features of stroke rehabilitation programs are enumerated in Table 50–11, and the most important ones are discussed here.

Holistic Care

Because the effects of stroke are broad, and because the course of stroke and the outcomes of care following stroke depend on a number of factors, it is extremely important that stroke rehabilitation professionals apply

TABLE 50–11 Three Views of the Features and Goals of Stroke Rehabilitation

Joint Committee for Stroke Facilities (1972)[258a]

1. Preventing deformities
2. Treating deformities, if they occur
3. Retraining the patient in ambulation activities
4. Teaching the patient to perform activities of daily living and working with the unaffected arm and hand
5. Retraining the affected arm and hand to its maximum capacity
6. Treating facial and speech disability if they are present
7. Compensation for sensory loss
8. Full social participation
9. Achievement of maximum patient motivation
10. Establishment of independent living post-discharge
11. Vocational placement, if appropriate

Goldberg (1986)[258b]

1. Preventing complications of inactivity
2. Preventing recurrent stroke
3. Identifying functional deficits and abilities
4. Improving overall physical functioning through conditioning exercises
5. Improving functional ability through training in specific daily living tasks, such as mobility, hand use, self-care, cognition, and communication
6. Assessing need for specialized equipment for mobility and daily living, and providing prescriptions for specific aids and orthoses and home modifications
7. Assessing and providing support to the patient and family in the process of social adjustment to a long-term change in the patient's overall state of health
8. Identifying and treating affective disorders and providing counseling and support to the patient
9. Preventing complications through evaluation and treatment of all associated medical conditions
10. Identifying and facilitating recreational activities, including leisure activities and hobbies
11. Ideally, returning the patient to complete self-support, including gainful employment

Brandstater (1987)[259]

1. Committed medical direction to provide continuity of care from acute phase through rehabilitation and long-term follow-up, to address medical problems during rehabilitation, and to provide leadership, supervision, and coordination of the rehabilitation team and its efforts
2. Use of a team approach, with staff that is knowledgeable of, experienced in, and dedicated to stroke patient care
3. Goal-directed treatment
4. Early initiation of treatment
5. Emphasis on patient education
6. Intensive focus on training of skills
7. Focus on facilitating adaptation
8. Early discharge planning
9. Heavy involvement of family members in the treatment program
10. Attention to psychosocial issues
11. A major goal of preparing the patient to resume optimal life roles at home, in the family, and in the community
12. Introduction of the patient to community resources

a holistic approach to the care of these patients. Social, vocational, and economic factors often play as important a role in determining rehabilitation participation and outcome as do physical and emotional issues. Neglecting to address those relevant issues can lead to failure of the rehabilitation effort.

Team Management

The multidimensional and interactive nature of the clinical consequences of stroke make interdisciplinary team care the most appropriate strategy for developing and implementing a complete and comprehensive approach to stroke patient management.[4, 251, 260] Coordination of care and good communication among team members help to avoid fragmentation and duplication of services. Among its many potential benefits, a comprehensive team approach allows treatment schedules to be tailored to patient needs. The team approach allows specialists from different backgrounds to treat the patient simultaneously and collaboratively with the goal of enhancing function, a concept that is particularly relevant for certain functional tasks that consist of several subroutines.

The composition of the team varies with the patient's needs and the available resources. In most comprehensive inpatient rehabilitation programs, team members usually include the rehabilitation physician, rehabilitation nurse, physical therapist, occupational therapist, psychologist, social worker, and often a therapeutic recreational specialist. A speech-language pathologist is included in the team if the patient has speech, language, or swallowing problems. Other potential team members include the vocational counselor, orthotist, rehabilitation engineer, chaplain, dietitian, and respiratory therapist. Success in a rehabilitation program is more likely to occur when the patient and family serve as members of the team, so that they gain an understanding of stroke and its potential outcomes, become involved in the setting of goals, and participate in care.

Effective teamwork can have problems because of the many and disparate clinical activities. Effective leadership, commitment to common goals, communication (often through team conferences), and collaboration are necessary to ensure coordination of activities and appropriate assumption of responsibilities and to avoid role confusion, conflict, and duplication of effort. Although the team approach has many clear-cut advantages, there is no concrete scientific evidence supporting its effectiveness.

Goal-Directed Treatment

An essential element of the rehabilitation treatment is that it is goal-directed. Physical interventions that do not aim to achieve specific objectives do not constitute therapy, although they may be valuable for other reasons, such as maintenance of current level of function. An early *and recurring* step in the treatment process is establishing realistic, practical, and feasible goals that are mutually agreed upon by the patient, family, and professionals.[259] Goals that are overambitious may lead to failure, depression, and misuse of rehabilitation resources. On the other hand, goals that are too modest may lead to inadequate fulfillment of rehabilitation potential. The fact that goal setting is done on an ongoing basis is important; since recovery and functional improvement are variable, goals should be re-evaluated and revised as needed.

Focus on Learning and Adaptation

Bleiberg and Merbitz[261] have pointed out that the rehabilitation process consists of learning and adaptation. Indeed, the design of many rehabilitation programs is based on principles of learning theory that suggest that patients re-acquire old skills or develop means to compensate for new impairments in a logical, coherent manner.[198] Supervised practice is a necessary component of this learning process. Ideally, rehabilitation training programs train patients in skills and knowledge that are meaningful to them. Concrete phrasing is used, and attempts are made to ensure that instructions are understood, sometimes through the use of return demonstrations. It is important that the tasks be tailored to meet the patient's level of skill, and that the level of difficulty of the tasks is progressively increased in a graded fashion. Another major component of the rehabilitation program is the frequent and timely provision of support, education, reassurance, direct physical assistance, and especially immediate feedback on progress as a means of enhancing performance. Rehabilitation has been described by one author as "the planned withdrawal of support."[262]

Therapy Environments

The environment in which the therapeutic program takes place should be conducive to learning, practice, and progress. Patients can benefit greatly from practice in therapy environments that closely reflect natural home or community settings. Some programs use mock kitchens, apartments, community shops, and other similar facilities to allow patient practice.

Learning can occur best in an environment in which the training effort can be focused. This is particularly important in the care of stroke patients, who are easily distracted by external stimuli or who may have other cognitive, perceptual, or behavioral abnormalities. In those situations, it is necessary to avoid overstimulation and frequent interruptions in the training regimen. These principles apply to rehabilitation programs provided in all environments, including hospital care units, long-term care settings, and the home.

A spectrum of types and intensities of rehabilitation programs and services is available, and the number and diversity of new entries into the field are changing rapidly. Comprehensive rehabilitation can be provided at a number of sites, including the hospital, long-term nursing care facility, outpatient clinic, and home. Program intensities also vary, depending on the situation, the patient, and the availability of appropriate services. A key element of the comprehensive rehabilitation program that distinguishes it from a group of individual therapy services is the coordinated nature of the interventions.

Timing of Therapy

Specific therapy schedules should be individualized for each patient. The stroke rehabilitation literature does not provide specific guidelines on the amount of therapy needed for specific problems, but it is reasonable to expect that patients should participate in functional activities at least once a day. Endurance, medical stability, mood, motivation, and other considerations affect the degree and duration of physical and cognitive activity that an individual patient can tolerate. The rate, pattern, and degree of remobilization efforts will be largely determined by these factors and others, including the duration of time since the stroke. The literature also is not clear regarding the optimal duration of formal rehabilitation or the specific methods or criteria for determining the optimal length of treatment for an individual patient, but generally, lack of significant functional progress on two successive measurements usually indicates that a change in treatment type or location is appropriate.

Attention to Psychosocial Issues

The new onset and persistence of disability can give rise to a variety of psychological reactions in patients who have sustained a stroke, including sadness, grief, anxiety, depression, despair, anger, frustration, and confusion. Addressing these issues is a critical component of the rehabilitation program. Although not unique to the specialty of medical rehabilitation, stroke care professionals have extensive experience in addressing the patient's level and method of coping and adaptation because of their involvement with engaging patients in active participation in care. For some patients, dealing with the emotional issues that accompany the stroke forms the major focus of the care activities. For others, addressing them facilitates improved participation in the rehabilitation program. In a substantial proportion of patients, the type and intensity of their reactions to the problems caused by the stroke are more dependent on their *prestroke* coping styles, levels of frustration tolerance, and ability and mechanisms used to deal with adversity. For most patients, dealing with psychological issues is an ongoing activity.

Dealing with family issues also is essential. Families might experience a variety of emotions, including grief, sadness, depression, anxiety, and guilt. In addition, families often serve as caregivers and therefore might experience the care as burdensome, and might feel guilt over their feelings. The complexity of these emotional reactions underscores the importance of ongoing counseling, support, and care for the family caregivers.

Focus on Families

To function optimally, rehabilitation programs require the involvement of families; family members serve as members of the rehabilitation team and participate actively in the rehabilitation process. In addition to providing psychological support, they also provide practical assistance to the patient in the treatment program. Engaging families to participate in the education program is essential to enable both a smooth transition to the community and safe functioning for the patient in the home environment. Family involvement includes encouraging them to ask questions, express concerns, make suggestions, develop rehabilitation goals and plans, observe and participate in the therapy sessions, and train in the performance of specific skills.

Emphasis on Community Issues

The focus of a rehabilitation hospitalization or outpatient episode of care cannot be only on the elements of the care during those professional interactions. The basis for the care provided is to enable smooth safe transition to community living. Therefore, medical rehabilitation includes planning for ways to meet the patient's needs in the home environment (including the development of contingency plans), educating family members on care techniques in the home, encouraging the practice of skills by patients and family members (including the use of therapeutic community passes or community recreation trips), providing instruction in medication administration and exercise technique, explaining potential medical complications and their warning signs, recruiting community resources and introducing these resources to the patient, training community members in functional care skills and equipment use, and other techniques.

REHABILITATION ASSESSMENT AND INTERVENTIONS DURING THE ACUTE PHASE

To consider rehabilitation as a philosophical approach that underlies all aspects of assessment and management throughout the continuum of care implies that rehabilitation is a component of the care that a stroke patient receives from the time of the acute admission. Many of the clinical problems that beset stroke patients are related to the immobility and deconditioning imposed by the prolonged bedrest that often accompanies acute stroke care. The maximum benefit of rehabilitation can be achieved when rehabilitation interventions are begun as early as possible after stroke. Early poststroke rehabilitation is both preventive and therapeutic. Table 50–12 lists some of the key clinical rehabilitation activities that should be performed during the acute poststroke phase. This list of evaluation and intervention measures closely resembles the list of specific interventions performed in formal comprehensive rehabilitation programs.[259, 260, 263–265]

Three controlled studies in humans[266–268] have examined the impact of developing and implementing a rehabilitation program in the early poststroke period during the acute hospitalization. The programs emphasized the value of early activation, education, remobilization, and training in independent performance of ADL.

During the acute poststroke phase, the patient should undergo an evaluation to determine the optimal type, level, setting, and timing of a continued rehabilitation and care program. In addition to the nature, pattern, and severity of physical impairments, some of the key

TABLE 50–12 Rehabilitation Activities During the Acute Poststroke Phase

Evaluate and manage medical problems
Monitor and adjust medications
Maintain hydration and nutrition
Facilitate rest and sleep
Venous thromboembolism prophylaxis (physical or pharmacological measures)
Proper bed and chair positioning
Frequent turns and position changes
Range-of-motion exercises
Deep breathing and cough exercises
Frequent skin inspections
Swallowing evaluation
Safety measures
Removal of indwelling catheter, if possible, with planned, timed toileting program
Bowel evacuation regimen
Sitting in chair
Supervised bedside exercises
Self-performance of activities of daily living
Mobilization exercises
Standing and gait training as able
Educational programs on stroke, recovery, and personal care
Communication evaluation and training
Psychological support to the patient
Family education and support
Evaluation of social supports and available resources
Evaluation for formal continued rehabilitation
Transition to rehabilitation

components of the assessment include health status, endurance level, and medical stability; functional capabilities and disabilities in the areas of mobility, self-care, and instrumental ADL; mood and coping ability; community resources and family supports; social situation and vocational/educational status; and cognitive, communicative, perceptual, and behavioral functioning.

Rehabilitation requires active participation by the patient and family members, who should be involved in identifying goals and developing rehabilitation strategies. Goal setting and treatment planning often take place during the assessment phase and serve as a means of focusing or directing the assessment procedures themselves. The evaluation and treatment-planning activities are ongoing processes.

Controversy exists in the literature concerning whether a delay in initiating transfer of the acute stroke patient from acute care to a formal rehabilitation program results in reduced outcomes. Although most studies[269–271] indicate that shorter stroke-to-rehabilitation latency periods are associated with better outcomes, other authors[207, 272] suggest that the interval between stroke onset and rehabilitation admission actually reflects severity of illness and co-morbidity, and that it may be more appropriate to aim for an "optimal time" to initiate therapy rather than a "shorter time," although a trend has occurred toward markedly shortened acute stays.

LEVELS OF POST-ACUTE STROKE CARE

Although the traditional view of rehabilitation relied on one or two types of settings (usually either inpatient or outpatient) for care to occur, more recent models emphasize a variety of types and levels of post-acute stroke services to better meet each stroke patient's specific needs.[273] Ideally, a complete and coordinated *system* of care provides services at each of several levels along a *continuum of care,* and also has a coordinated method to assess, direct (triage), and transfer patients to the setting that best meets their needs at the time the services are needed. Since care needs vary across patients and over time for individual patients, the quality of the system is extremely important. An integrated system requires a set of criteria to determine which patients qualify for which levels of care, a consistently applied patient assessment procedure, and exquisite communication and collaboration across the levels of the system of care to allow both smooth transfer of patients and information and a sharing of expertise.

Factors that are useful in determining the ideal setting of care for a patient at a particular point in time include the patient's cognitive ability, motivation level, prior and present level of functioning, medical stability, level of available social resources, medical and nursing needs, and likelihood of achieving significant functional gains during rehabilitation, as well as the availability of appropriate services and programs in the specific community. Unfortunately, the decisions as to which level or location of care a patient might be directed to are at times based on the preferences of third-party payers and on the availability of specific resources within the community, rather than solely on patient need.

There is considerable overlap among the post-acute stroke rehabilitation levels of care and among the patients who are cared for in each, but generally the levels of care delineated as acute inpatient rehabilitation, subacute inpatient rehabilitation, day rehabilitation, outpatient therapy, and home therapy. Each is discussed below.

Acute Inpatient Rehabilitation

Comprehensive acute inpatient stroke rehabilitation refers to the traditional interdisciplinary hospital-based coordinated program of medical, nursing, and therapy services. Care in this setting is directed by a physician and carried out by a team. This level of care is most appropriate for patients who need and can tolerate 3 or more hours of therapy a day, and who need both around-the-clock nursing care and at least daily physician supervision. Patients in intensive rehabilitation must have a reasonable likelihood of achieving significant functional gains from a comprehensive inpatient rehabilitation program.

Subacute Inpatient Rehabilitation

Subacute inpatient rehabilitation is appropriate for stroke survivors who need comprehensive and coordinated therapy services for functional training in an institutional setting, but in a less intensive program than is used at the acute level of rehabilitation. Patients in this level of care usually receive between 1 and 3 hours of therapy per day. Assessment of the intensity of therapy services that an individual patient needs is based primarily on his or her tolerance level and on the specific needs for functional training. Some patients are unable to tolerate the full course of intensive rehabilitation because of medical frailty or limited endurance. Some patients who receive subacute rehabilitation had strokes that were extremely severe, limiting their potential to participate in intensive rehabilitation. Others receive subacute rehabilitation because their strokes were so mild that the amount of therapy they need is small.

Subacute inpatient rehabilitation is usually conducted in a skilled nursing facility and occasionally in the hospital setting. In this level of care, patients receive 24-hour-a-day nursing care, but physician visits typically average only one to three times per week. Therefore, patients with more intensive medical needs may be more appropriately treated in an acute rehabilitation program.

Day Rehabilitation

In day rehabilitation, virtually all of the same therapy services that are provided in comprehensive inpatient rehabilitation are offered, but without the overnight stay. Day rehabilitation is a comprehensive and coordinated program of therapy that takes place in an outpatient setting. The rehabilitation is directed by a physician and facilitated by a team with regularly scheduled team conferences. Therapy services typically are provided between 3 and 8 hours a day. Relative medical stability is necessary, since patients live in their homes.

Outpatient Therapy

Many stroke patients need traditional outpatient therapy services. These services are also provided in an outpatient clinic setting, but they do not entail the coordination, comprehensiveness, and team conferences that characterize day rehabilitation. These services include single-modality training, such as physical therapy, occupational therapy, speech-language pathology services, or psychological support, for patients with focal deficits and for whom specific functional training might be useful.

Home Therapy

The home is the most familiar environment for the patient and family, and therapy in the home allows the patient and family to learn specific functional tasks in the setting in which those skills will be used most often. However, a potential disadvantage of home therapy is the limitation in available resources such as specialized equipment or experienced staff. Home therapy requires relative medical stability and the availability of social supports to enable the patient to live at home.

THERAPEUTIC INTERVENTIONS DURING REHABILITATION

The therapeutic interventions used to enhance functional and social recovery of the stroke patient include skills training, demonstration, providing opportunity for practice, offering feedback on quality of skills performance, therapeutic exercises, physical modalities, prescription of adaptive devices and training in their proper use, education, and supportive counseling. Medications and surgical techniques also can be used. These activities require conjoint evaluation and treatment planning, collaborative treatment, and communication among the team members, the patient, and the family.

Sensorimotor and Functional Training

Among the frequent and important interventions used to care for the stroke patient are therapeutic exercise programs. Several different types and components of exercise regimens are available for patients who are disabled by stroke.

Early programs of traditional therapeutic exercise regimens were developed and described by Clayton, Coulter, Deaver, and others, and later reviewed by Westcott[274] and others. Traditional therapeutic exercise programs consist of positioning, passive and active ROM exercises, and progressive resistive exercises. Endurance training, which at times can include aerobic fitness training, also can be implemented.

Functional training in the performance of self-care tasks, mobility skills, and advanced or instrumental ADL form the central focus of most standard rehabilitation programs. Compensatory functional training occurs when patients learn one-handed techniques to carry out personal care skills independently or learn to walk with a spastic hemiplegic lower extremity. The patient is encouraged to make use of residual abilities to develop new ways of achieving old goals and to perform routine tasks such as transferring and walking.

Several neuromuscular facilitation exercise approaches have been developed and used in the care of stroke patients. These were reviewed by Flanagan[275] and later by Lorish and colleagues[276] and Good.[277] Proprioceptive neuromuscular facilitation, developed by Kabat, Knott, and Voss, relies on several mechanisms such as quick stretch and spiral diagonal movement patterns of the extremities. Brunnstrom movement therapy encourages and facilitates the use of synergy patterns as a means of developing voluntary control. Cutaneous sensory stimulation in the form of superficial stroking, tapping, brushing, vibrating, or icing provides facilitatory or inhibitory inputs into the system, as proposed by Rood. In the commonly used Bobath neurodevelopmental treatment approach, inhibition of abnormal tone, synergies, and postures are combined with facilitation of normal automatic motor responses to develop skilled voluntary movements. One of the most recently developed methods, the motor relearning program of Carr and Shepard, emphasizes functional training for specific tasks, such as standing and walking, and carryover of those tasks. Many therapists use an eclectic approach, combining elements of various procedures from among these programs. Many resources exist that describe the specific goals and techniques of these functional training and neurofacilitation therapy programs.[3, 4, 90, 259, 277–283] Several studies have attempted to discern a relative advantage of one of these therapeutic approach over the others, but the results have been inconclusive and generally have failed to demonstrate greater neurological or functional improvements using one or another of these techniques.[234]

New Approaches for Sensorimotor and Functional Training

An exciting, new, and emerging method of training and improving quality of gait in hemiparetic stroke patients consists of a combination of providing partial body weight support to stabilize the trunk, by using a body harness suspended from the ceiling, together with enforced stepping movements, by using a motor-driven treadmill on the floor. Individual case reports[284, 285] have been followed by more formal studies of the effectiveness of this "partial weight-bearing treadmill training" (PWBTT) technique in restoring gait pattern in nonambulatory hemiparetic patients.[286, 287]

There is a recently renewed interest in behavioral approaches to motor control enhancement, including kinesthetic and positional biofeedback. Electromyographic biofeedback technology makes the patient consciously aware of his or her own muscle activity or lack of it[288–294] by using external auditory or visual cues as representations of internal neural control activity. This assists the individual to receive immediate feedback on performance, to experience and assume some level of voluntary control over muscle activity, and to monitor volitional activity as a means of modifying or enhancing muscle movement. Biofeedback therapy is usually considered adjunctive to standard voluntary exercise techniques, rather than an isolated treatment modality. Results of trials of biofeedback treatment studies are inconclusive.[234, 295, 296] Although some favorable results were noted by early investigators, these findings have not been substantiated on a consistent basis.

A potentially favorable effect of therapeutic exercise maneuvers that involve the hemiparetic extremity is to prevent or overcome "learned nonuse."[297] Taub[298] proposed that some of the disability seen in stroke survivors resulted in part from the patient's failure to use the affected limbs, as opposed to weakness of the limb itself. An important implication of this concept is its suggestion that all therapeutic attempts to use the affected limb should be reinforced, possibly by facilitation techniques. Another potential implication is that it could even be beneficial to inhibit or immobilize the function of the unaffected limb to encourage or "force" the use of the hemiplegic extremity. Some might even argue that the intensive focus on compensatory strategies that make heavy use of the nonhemiplegic limb to improve functional abilities is counterproductive, since it reinforces the failure to use the hemiplegic limb. Taub and colleagues,[298, 299] Wolf and associates,[300] and Barton and Wolf[301] have reported successful work with animals, and more recently in humans, that supports the usefulness of this "forced-use" approach, now known as "constraint-induced movement therapy."

Functional electrical stimulation of muscles that lack voluntary control could help facilitate their movement or compensate for their lack of voluntary movement.[234, 302]

An emerging body of literature demonstrates that sensory stimulation and acupuncture may have a beneficial effect on motor control following stroke.[303–305]

Spasticity Management

Muscle weakness is only one of the three types of motor dysfunction that typically occur in most hemispheric strokes; for some patients, the disordered motor control resulting in the predominance of synergy patterns and in muscle spasticity is as important as, or even more important than, the weakness or paresis. Spasticity following stroke, causing stiffness, tightness, and resistance to passive movement, can interfere with functional task performance such as dressing and walking, interfere with hygiene and positioning, cause muscle and joint contracture and pain, and result in skin breakdown.

Treatment of spasticity begins with good general medical care designed to prevent and treat infections or other secondary problems and is supplemented by aggressive and consistent manual stretch ROM exercises, positioning, and splinting. The use of oral medications is usually attempted but is generally unsuccessful, although dantrolene sodium may have a beneficial effect. Injections of neurolytic agents such as phenol have been used, with variable success. Most recently, the selective local intramuscular injection of extremely low doses of botulinum toxin A has been found to be effective in reducing local muscle tone for about 3 to 6 months, resulting in muscle relaxation, decreased pain, and improved function in selected patients.[234, 306]

Speech, Language, and Visuospatial Perceptual Disorders

Approximately one-third to one-half of stroke survivors experience speech and language disorders.[181] Many procedures have been developed to manage various aspects of these problems. Both remediation and compensation are used. One goal of therapy is to improve the patient's ability to speak, understand, read, and write. Another goal of speech therapy interventions is to assist patients to develop strategies that compensate for or circumvent speech and language problems that are not directly remediable. A final goal is to improve the quality of life for individuals with neuromotor speech impairments and their families.

For aphasia, a number of strategies and techniques have been developed.[307–323] One of these, melodic intonation therapy,[316] is an approach designed to use the noninjured functioning neural pathways in the nondominant hemisphere that carry musical information. Other techniques rely on encouraging verbalizations, conversational coaching, and oral reading. Probably the most important strategy is to encourage any vocalizations possible as a means of developing verbal communication of a more differentiated nature. Treatment of aphasia focuses on the most effective means by which the patient can communicate, including individual or group speech therapy with practice. Table 50–13 lists various treatment approaches for aphasia.[234]

For dysarthria, exercise modalities include sensory stimulation procedures, exercises designed to strengthen

TABLE 50–13 Selected Treatment Methods for Aphasia

Language-oriented treatment (LOT)
Direct stimulus-response treatment
Treatment of aphasic perseveration (TAP)
Visual action therapy (VAT)
Oral reading for aphasia (ORLA)
Conversational coaching
Promoting aphasic communicative effectiveness (PACE)
C-VIC (using alternative communication systems)
Programmatic combinations of approaches
Augmentative communication devices

oromotor speech muscles, respiratory training procedures, and retraining of articulatory patterns and sequences of gestures.[324–327]

Alternative forms of communication and augmentative devices can be used to enhance quality of life. These range from written or pictorial communication boards and books to electronic communication aids.

For some patients, visual-spatial perceptual deficits are the most troublesome problems that they experience. Potentially useful treatment methods include the use of prism glasses, providing visuospatial cueing to compensate for visuospatial perceptual losses, increasing awareness of deficits with cues, using computer-assisted training, using prism glasses, and providing compensatory strategies.[234, 308, 328–333]

There is increasing evidence of language problems resulting from right hemisphere strokes, including lack of organization and impaired use of language in social contexts. Treatment of these problems is aimed at improving organization of language, learning to use language within social contexts (language pragmatics), and learning to interpret figurative language.[234]

Swallowing Training

Dysphagia, or impaired swallowing, occurs in approximately one-third to one-half of all stroke survivors and places the stroke patient at risk for aspiration and pneumonia, malnutrition, and dehydration. Compensatory treatments for disordered swallowing function include changing posture and positioning for swallowing, learning new swallowing maneuvers, and changing food amounts and textures (generally smaller boluses of puréed foods and thick liquids are handled more easily). An observational study by Horner and colleagues[234, 334] found that treatment of swallowing dysfunction was effective.

Psychosocial Considerations

One of the major factors influencing both the degree of participation in a therapy program and the outcome achieved is patient motivation. Patients who cooperate with therapeutic efforts and who have the determination to improve are more likely to participate in a therapy program. However, the level of motivation and the amount of its specific direct effect on outcome are difficult to measure. A number of techniques can be used by the rehabilitation professional to enhance or direct motivation; examples include explanation, positive reinforcement, behavioral modification, and coaxing. Interestingly, it also has been found that the degree of family support favorably affects outcome.[335] Counseling interventions have proved to be consistently more effective in improving family functioning and patient adjustment than educational interventions alone.[336]

Depression can be a significant complication of stroke. It can be devastating and distressing on its own, and can limit patient participation and outcome by inhibiting patient motivation.[170, 337–345] Depression occurs in one-third to two-thirds of stroke survivors. Presenting features include loss of energy in 83%, sleep disorder in 67%, brooding in 60%, and hopelessness in 39%.[337] Although the organic component of poststroke depression may be significant,[340, 341] it is likely that most patients experience a combination of organic and reactive causes of mood disorders. Treatment consists of psychotherapy, psychosocial support, milieu therapy, and medications. To the extent that mood improves as the patient's physical independence improves and patient-family participation increases, the depression is likely to have been reactive. For some patients, especially those with significant disturbances in participation in daily activities or therapeutic exercise programs, antidepressant medications can be beneficial.[346, 347] Several studies have demonstrated the efficacy of various types of antidepressants in treating poststroke depression. These medications improve not only mood, but also functional performance. Their usefulness is limited only by their side effects.

Anxiety and fear are commonly reported and observed problems among stroke patients. A team of rehabilitation professionals who are sensitive to these issues, empathic toward the patient, and experienced in dealing with such problems can help to ease the distress associated with the disability and the rehabilitation experience, thereby possibly resulting in improved outcomes.

Sexual dysfunction has been reported in 40% to 70% of stroke survivors.[348–351] Its cause is largely psychological (e.g., fear, anxiety, depression, discomfort) rather than organic, although spasticity, pain, and sensory deficits may pose problems for some patients. Issues related to self-esteem, affection, and relationships should be emphasized, as should specific practical suggestions on positioning, timing, and techniques.[352]

Family reactions to the changes that result from the stroke are addressed by the team. This is particularly important in view of the need for the family's active participation in providing support to the patient during and after formal intensive rehabilitation. Lack of social supports or lack of available resources often are major problems for the patient and the rehabilitation team. In that situation, recruiting available resources and supports, securing appropriate entitlements, and advocating on behalf of the patient become major clinical tasks for the professional rehabilitation team. In general, family interventions include individual counseling, education, and support groups.[353] Evidence exists that both education and counseling interventions significantly improve caregiver knowledge and stabilize some aspects of family functioning, but that counseling is more effective than education alone.[336]

At times, problematic psychosocial functioning predominates among issues related to the recovery of physical function or motor skill performance. This underscores the importance of psychosocial, recreational, and vocational interventions.

Recreational activities often have the effect of improving affect, focusing therapy of meaningful activities and desirable goals, and facilitating a smooth transition to the community after discharge. Leisure evaluation, counseling on activities of interest, and educating the patient on community resources constitute some of the therapeutic recreation interventions for patients with stroke.

Peer support is one component of patient care activities that probably exerts a favorable effect on the successful rehabilitation of the stroke patient but is often overlooked in the description of interventions that affect patient progress and outcome. The presence of other patients with similar disabilities on the stroke rehabilitation unit can assist the patient in several ways. First, it can help to reduce the fear and anxiety often associated with the new onset of physically disabling or disfiguring conditions. Second, patients often can counsel and support each other in ways that even well-meaning and experienced professionals cannot. Finally, patients often not only gain insight into their disability, but also garner specific suggestions for functional skill performance or about adaptive equipment from other patients who have already been through the experience. Similar peer support may be available for families of patients as well, and could contribute favorably to the adjustment process after the stroke.

Specialized Equipment

Adaptive equipment and durable medical equipment can be used to assist the stroke patients to become more independent and to facilitate functional skill performance. It is important to consider the patient's functional level, level of adaptation to the disability, architecture of the living environment, and instruction in the use of all devices and equipment. Many types of devices are available to assist the stroke patient in achieving an improved level of independence. These include adaptive devices to assist in the performance of ADL, such as eating utensils, bathing and grooming aids, dressing devices, tub and shower equipment, assistive devices for walking, transfer aids, and wheelchairs. Fitting and providing a properly fitting wheelchair sometimes makes a huge difference for a patient with stroke; a wheelchair can greatly enhance quality of life by improving positioning and mobility. Generally, a wheelchair for a hemiplegic patient has a lowered base to allow the nonhemiparetic lower extremity to touch the floor and to allow the patient to use that limb in wheelchair propulsion. Likewise, there is usually also a one-arm drive mechanism to enable the patient to use the nonhemiplegic upper limb for wheelchair propulsion. Cushions, back rests, trunk supports, and head supports also can be beneficial.

Upper extremity resting hand splints are usually used to prevent deformity and to maintain the hemiplegic wrist in a functional, slightly extended position. Orthoses, especially ankle-foot orthoses, are used to improve the positioning of the foot to facilitate an optimal gait pattern.[354]

The various types of specialized equipment that are used for stroke survivors are summarized in the Table 50–14.

Caregiver Training

One of the most important interventions is the training of families and other caregivers in specific care techniques to prevent complications, perform physical functions, and encourage the patient to perform any activities he or she is capable of doing. Training in problem-solving techniques will help family members to provide effective support in the home environment. Additional teaching focuses on the dissemination of knowledge about strokes, their consequences, medications, and other care aspects. There is now evidence that both education and counseling significantly improve caregiver knowledge and stabilize some aspects of family functioning.[234, 355, 356] Family education has been found to contribute to the long-term maintenance of rehabilitation gains. It is possible to argue that education of the patient and family is the single most important interven-

TABLE 50–14 Specialized Equipment Used by Stroke Survivors

Eating Devices

- Utensils with built-up handles
- Universal cuff
- Rocking knife
- Nonskid mats
- Plate guards or scoop dishes
- Cup holder
- Adapted cups

Bathing and Grooming Devices

- Long-handled sponge
- Washcloth mitt
- Toothbrush, hairbrush, and comb with built-up handles or universal cuff
- Adapted shaving equipment
- Handheld shower nozzle
- Long-handled mirror

Tub and Shower Transfer Equipment

- Nonskid mat
- Grab bars
- Transfer seats
- Shower chair
- Hydraulic and motorized tub lifts

Dressing Devices

- Velcro closures
- Button hooks
- Long-handled reachers
- Long-handled shoehorn

Walking Devices

- Single-point cane
- Tripod cane
- Quad cane
- Walkers

tion that the stroke rehabilitation team performs. Important teaching points that should be included in the training program are listed in Table 50–15.

TRANSITION TO THE COMMUNITY, FOLLOW-UP, AND AFTERCARE

The effects of stroke can be enduring, and therefore rehabilitation is a lifelong activity involving the restoration of patients to their fullest physical, mental, and social capabilities on an ongoing basis. For this reason, medical rehabilitation for stroke survivors includes the many physical, social, and organizational aspects of the aftercare of stroke patients. Realizing the goal of optimal long-term quality of life is accomplished through an interdisciplinary approach that includes helping the patient to achieve maximal independent functioning in daily activities and training family members and other personal caregivers in the performance of specific physical skills. In this regard, it is important that family members be aware of the distinction between those skills patients can perform themselves and those tasks for which the patient needs assistance or supervision to carry out.

Major efforts toward preparation for discharge are directed toward securing community resources; these include competent and reliable professional or other attendant care, home nursing visits, outpatient or home therapy, and community transportation and recreational programs. Teaching patients about stroke, medications, fluid intake, diet, exercises, catheter care, feeding tube use, tracheostomy management, signs and symptoms of common complications such as infections, and specific functional task performance greatly facilitates a smooth transition to home and minimizes the likelihood of medical problems after discharge. Follow-up medical monitoring and care also is important.

TABLE 50–15 Patient and Family Education Issues

Etiology of stroke	Monitoring blood pressure
Effects of stroke on the patient	What to do for emergency or medical illness
Effects of stroke on the family	Safety; preventing falls
Medication administration	Behavioral issues
Medication side effects	Positioning and moving in bed
Swallowing technique training	Training in performance of specific skills for which the patient needs assistance (e.g., bed mobility, transfers, hygiene, dressing)
Maintenance of nutrition and hydration	Home exercise program
Bowel and bladder care	Optimizing social functioning
Sleep and rest	Depression
Prevention of blood clots	Lifestyle modification
Prevention of skin breakdown	Caregiver concerns
Respiratory complications	Family functioning
Tracheostomy, feeding tube, or catheter management	Sexual functioning
Signs and symptoms of common medical complications	Recreational activities
Signs of stroke	Driving
	Vocational counseling

Specific functional issues that are relevant around the time of transition to the community are the "higher level" community skills that are related to the postdischarge lifestyle. Important examples include sexual functioning, driving ability, grocery shopping, housekeeping, laundry management, safety considerations, socialization outside of the home, vocational pursuits, recreational activities, and others. Continuing mobilization exercises and maintaining an adequate activity level are important lifestyle adjustments that can enhance the likelihood of avoiding functional deterioration. The emphasis on education, mobilization, activity, independence, coping, family involvement, and especially quality of life should be incorporated into the patient's lifestyle, even long after completion of the formal rehabilitation program.[357, 358]

REHABILITATION OUTCOMES

More has been written in the medical rehabilitation literature about the functional outcomes after stroke than about outcomes following the occurrence of virtually any other disabling condition. The results described in some of these reports often are contradictory, misleading, and even confusing, because of differences in study design, methodology, sample criteria, rehabilitation practice, and outcome definitions.[1, 359] It is important to note that outcomes after stroke can be assessed in a number of ways, including medical morbidity, mortality, level of impairment, length of hospital stay, cost of care, functional ability (degree of disability), placement at the time of discharge and follow-up, amount of handicap or social functioning, quality of life, and life satisfaction. Functional outcomes can be measured either as absolute functional level at the time of discharge or community assessment or else as the amount of change or improvement in functional abilities between admission or onset and discharge or follow-up. Different conclusions can be reached, depending on the specific definitions used. Nonetheless, a few general principles emerge with some consistency.

Functional and Social Outcomes

One of the most striking aspects of caring for stroke patients is the common observation that their physical performance, functional abilities, and quality of life are considerably better after rehabilitation and during long-term care than immediately after the stroke. Most studies,[153–162] and extensive clinical experience, suggest that a substantial proportion of stroke survivors achieve independence in their ability to complete mobility and self-care skills, but that social and vocational outcomes are not as favorable as the functional independence figures. For example, data obtained from the Framingham Heart Study[27] indicated that 78% of 148 stroke survivors were independent in mobility skills, 68% were independent in the performance of self-care activities, and 84% were living in home environments. Unfortunately, however, 63% had reduced vocational function, 59% had decreased socialization outside the home, and 47% had decreased pursuit interests and hobbies.

Most other studies have yielded similar results. For example, Chin and colleagues[360] reported in a review that between 54% and 80% of stroke survivors were able to walk, but that only 15% were walking outside the home. Andrews and associates[154] found that only 13% of 1-year survivors were severely dependent and 27% were moderately dependent in performance of ADL. In general, about 75% to 85% of stroke patients are discharged home after formal acute rehabilitation care. Using data derived from a large number of stroke patients involved in inpatient rehabilitation, the Uniform Data System for Medical Rehabilitation reported that stroke patients improved in their average FIM scores from 63 on admission to 87 at discharge, with the greatest improvements occurring in locomotion, mobility, self-care, and sphincter control. Less improvement was noted to occur in communication and social cognition measures. Average length of stay in the rehabilitation facility was about 4 weeks and declining, and more than three-fourths of patients were reported to be discharged to the community. These figures match common clinical experience, although specific results vary, depending on the program.

Predictors of Outcome

Several factors might influence the specific outcome of an individual patient who is involved in a stroke rehabilitation program. Potentially important factors include the following:

- Type, distribution, pattern, and severity of physical impairment
- Cognitive, language, communication, and learning ability
- Number, types, and severity of co-morbid medical conditions and ongoing health functions
- Coping ability and coping style
- Nature and degree of family and other social supports
- Type and quality of specific rehabilitation training program

Numerous studies have examined and reported many diverse potential and actual predictors of favorable or unfavorable recovery of physical or psychosocial functioning. A large number of factors have been found to be statistically associated with outcome of stroke rehabilitation. The nature, type, and strength of the specific predictors depend to a great extent on the specific outcome measure being studied. Specific reported predictors are listed in Table 50–16. There now exist many reviews of those prognostic factors; some key references include those by Jongbloed,[361] Davidoff and associates,[362] and Johnston and co-workers.[363]

The strongest and most consistent predictor of discharge functional ability is admission functional ability.[361] Dombovy and colleagues[359] reviewed multiple studies and suggested that the strongest predictors of adverse outcomes are coma at onset, persistent incontinence, poor cognitive function, severe hemiplegia, lack of return of motor function after 1 month, prior stroke, visual-spatial perceptual deficit, unilateral hemineglect, significant cardiovascular disease, large cerebral lesion, and the presence of multiple neurological deficits. Wade and associates[364] studied 83 stroke patients and found that the best predictors of function after 6 months were sitting balance, age, hemianopsia, urinary incontinence, and motor deficit in the arm.

TABLE 50–16 Possible Predictors of Functional Outcome After Stroke

Age	Language function
Educational level	Hemianopia
Severity of stroke	Posture and balance
Type of stroke	Sensory function
Location of stroke	Bowel incontinence
Size of stroke	Bladder incontinence
Prior stroke	Interval elapsed from onset to rehabilitation admission
Multiple deficits	Congestive heart failure
Severity of plegia	Other medical co-morbidities
Initial functional status	Depression, emotional state
Coma at onset	Motivation
Cognitive function	Family involvement and support
Perceptual function	

It is important to note that although hundreds of articles describe numerous predictors of outcome after stroke rehabilitation, it is difficult to apply these predictors to individual patients in the clinical setting.[363] The multiplicity of variables that influence actual outcome, the degree to which the studies are flawed methodologically, and the unpredictable nature of certain aspects of poststroke functioning render the prediction of outcome for a specific patient by specific predictors incomplete or inadequate. Therefore, caution is needed in using the predictors for clinical purposes, such as assessing candidacy for rehabilitation. Identification of some of these factors, however, can help to better direct patient management activities.

EVIDENCE FOR EFFECTIVENESS OF STROKE REHABILITATION

The growing use of medical rehabilitation services by stroke patients, and the increasing awareness of rehabilitation within the medical community, have stimulated both a desire among clinicians and researchers and pressure from insurers and policy makers to demonstrate its effectiveness and to establish standards of stroke rehabilitation care to promote consistency of care to the extent possible. As a consequence, the medical literature has witnessed a recent heightened interest in the scientific investigation of the effectiveness of stroke rehabilitation.

Much of the early stroke rehabilitation effectiveness research consisted of observational descriptions of patient outcomes achieved after participation in rehabilitation programs, but more recent investigations have reported empirical results derived from prospectively conducted controlled clinical trials, the application of epidemiological principles to clinical research, the development and use of meta-analysis techniques, and, most recently, the publication of the U.S. Agency for Health Care Policy and Research (AHCPR) *Post-Stroke Rehabilitation Clinical Practice Guidelines.*[234]

The literature probably is better developed in the study of stroke rehabilitation than in the study of rehabilitation programs designed for the treatment of any other disabling condition, but the investigation of rehabilitation effectiveness is still fraught with numerous potential and real practical methodological problems that can diffuse the results of high-quality research trials on the effectiveness of rehabilitation. For example, it is necessary to control for natural recovery or else to demonstrate that the reduction in disability that occurs because of the rehabilitation program occurs to a greater extent than would be expected to occur by natural spontaneous recovery alone. The fact that multiple factors affect actual and measured patient outcomes following stroke also limits the ability to study the effectiveness of rehabilitation efforts.[359] There is considerable heterogeneity in patient presentations, since stroke can affect a variety of domains of physical, cognitive, communicative, emotional, social, vocational, and economic functioning, and in a variety of ways. There are considerable variations in the design and methodologies used in stroke rehabilitation research studies. Technical deficiencies in much of the research studies have included suboptimal study designs, small sample sizes, highly selected study populations, failure to control for time since onset, incompletely described interventions, use of unstandardized measures of outcomes, and inadequate statistical methodologies.[234] Ethical considerations are important in the conduct of randomized controlled trials, because these studies require an untreated control group, and it is not clear that it is appropriate to "deny" rehabilitation care to any stroke patient. Another difficulty is that many of the factors that affect outcome after stroke, such as motivation level, adaptability and coping style, learning ability, number and severity of comorbidities, family and social supports, and community resources, are specific to the individual and are unrelated to the rehabilitation intervention. It is difficult to control for these factors and to compare them across patient groups. Even diversity in the type, distribution, pattern, and severity of the neurological impairments may confound the results of the research.

Failure to provide detail on the type of rehabilitation intervention has limited the applicability of the results of some studies. A particularly difficult problem has been that of distinguishing the results of rehabilitation efforts from the effects of spontaneous neurological recovery. In addition, there is considerable subjectivity in the assessment of outcomes, and therefore comparing effectiveness may not be as unbiased or objective as desirable. Despite all of these methodological issues, results obtained from several randomized controlled clinical trials that compared the outcomes of stroke patients treated on stroke units by dedicated stroke teams with the outcomes of patients treated on general medical wards provide some indication of effectiveness.

Specific Effectiveness Trials

Garraway and colleagues[159] in 1980 reported one of the first randomized controlled trials of stroke rehabilitation. The 155 patients randomly admitted to a stroke unit began rehabilitation treatment significantly earlier, were significantly more likely to have received occupational and physical therapy, and were significantly more likely to achieve functional independence (50% versus 32%) at the time of discharge than the 156 patients admitted to general medical units. However, these improvements in functional outcomes for patients treated by the stroke unit group were found to have been lost at 1 year following stroke, possibly because of lack of appropriate family training.

Smith and colleagues[156] followed that report with a report of the results of a trial of three different types and intensities of rehabilitation. The 46 patients who received "intensive" therapy achieved better outcomes than the 43 patients who underwent "conventional" therapy, who in turn achieved better outcomes than the 44 patients who received encouragement to continue exercises but no formal rehabilitation. These reports were limited in the detail with which the program's interventions were described.

In another prospectively conducted, randomized controlled trial, Strand and colleagues[365] compared the clinical outcomes of 110 patients admitted to a nonintensive stroke unit and 183 patients admitted to general medical wards. Acute diagnostic workups and treatment programs were standardized. The stroke unit had a team approach to care, an education program directed toward the staff, early and focused rehabilitation efforts, active participation by family members, and education of patients and family members, while none of these characteristics were uniformly or consistently used on the general medical ward. Investigators found that patients who were admitted to the stroke unit were significantly more likely to be independent in personal hygiene and dressing and tended to be more likely to walk independently than patients admitted to the general medical wards. Notably, the 3-month hospitalization rate was only 15% for stroke unit patients but 39% for general medical ward patients, a statistically significant difference that persisted after 1 year.

In another well-done randomized controlled clinical trial conducted in Europe, Indredavik and associates[157] compared the clinical outcomes in 110 acute stroke patients who were assigned to treatment on a stroke unit with the outcomes in 110 stroke patients with similar characteristics who were assigned to treatment on general medical wards. Care on the stroke unit included both acute care and rehabilitation management. The early diagnostic and treatment interventions were standardized and focused. The rehabilitation program was organized with a team approach to care and was initiated shortly after arrival. Emphasis was placed on providing information to the patient and family. Treatment of patients admitted to general medical wards was not standardized. The maximum period of treatment for both patient groups was 6 weeks, at which time 56% of the stroke unit patients and 33% of the general medical ward patients were living at home. At 1 year, 63% of the stroke unit patients and 45% of the medical ward patients were living at home. Both of these differences were highly statistically significant. Functional status levels were significantly greater for stroke unit patients than for medical ward patients at both 6 weeks and 1 year. Interestingly, the 6-week mortality was 7% for stroke unit patients and 17% for medical ward patients, and the 1-year mortality was 25% for stroke unit patients and 33% for medical ward patients, differences that were statistically significant at 6 weeks but not at 1 year.

In another well-conducted prospective randomized controlled trial, Kalra and colleagues[366] studied three groups of stroke patients stratified according to prognosis, and compared 124 patients randomized to treatment on a stroke rehabilitation unit with 121 treated on general medical wards. Patients treated on the medical units were found to have received more physical therapy, but those on the stroke unit were found to have received more individualized therapy sessions. The findings were of particular interest. For patients with good prognoses, functional outcomes at discharge were found to be comparable in both settings. For patients with poor prognoses, functional abilities were comparable between the two units, but management on the general medical unit was associated with greater mortality and longer hospital stays than was treatment on the stroke unit. Patients with intermediate prognoses who were treated on the stroke unit had significantly better functional outcomes, a greater likelihood of returning home after hospitalization, a shorter length of hospital stay, and better functional abilities.

Another more recent trial by the same group[367] studied specifically 71 patients with severe disability after stroke and poor prognoses, randomizing 34 of those patients to a stroke rehabilitation unit and 37 to general medical wards. Compared to the patients treated on the general medical wards, the severe stroke patients who were treated on the stroke rehabilitation unit had significantly better mortality rates, home discharge placement rates, and lengths of hospital stay, and a trend toward significantly better improvement in functional scores.

In another recently published controlled clinical trial, Kaste and associates[368] studied the outcomes of 113 acute older stroke patients randomized to admission to a neurology department with an organized stroke care team that provided coordinated acute and rehabilitation care and 119 older stroke patients admitted to a medical department with no structured programs for diagnostic evaluation, acute treatment, or rehabilitation. Patients admitted to the focused stroke care unit were discharged an average of 16 days earlier and were more likely to have returned home (75% versus 62%) than those who were treated on the medical ward. Functional status at 1 year was significantly better for the neurological unit patients than for the medical ward patients.

Other controlled studies exist as well, including those by Sivenius et al,[369] Stevens et al,[370] and Wood-Dauphinee et al.[371] Methodological problems limit the applicability of the findings of these studies, and the results of these studies are variable and inconclusive. Studies on the effectiveness of rehabilitation programs are summarized and reviewed in the AHCPR document.[234]

In a meta-analysis of available literature on clinical trials in stroke rehabilitation research, Ottenbacher and Jannell[372] reported the results of 36 clinical trials in which 3717 patients participated. Their analysis indicated that the average stroke patient who underwent a focused stroke rehabilitation program performed better than approximately 65% of the patients in comparison groups. Rehabilitation had the largest effects on personal care skills, mobility activities, ambulation, and visuospatial-perceptual functions, while language and cognitive functions showed the smallest effects of rehabilitation. The authors found that the improvement in performance was related more to early initiation of treatment than to the duration of the intervention. Another meta-analysis, conducted by Langhorne and colleagues,[373] found reduced mortality in addition to improved functional outcomes among stroke patients who underwent a coordinated interdisciplinary rehabilitation program, although they noted considerable diversity among the studies in the type of functional outcome measures used to assess effectiveness, limiting to some extent the interpretation of these findings.

There is a growing number of trials of therapy interventions for patients who are in the post-acute stroke stage,[374, 375] and there are also several studies comparing the effectiveness of rehabilitation interventions performed in a variety of settings, such as home, outpatient departments, or day hospital programs.[376–381] In general, these studies indicate that long-term disabled stroke patients may attain significant functional improvement from rehabilitation, and that home physical therapy may be effective in improving outcome.

Common Themes of the Effectiveness Studies

In addition to early initiation of rehabilitation treatment, several other common characteristics of the intervention programs appear to have been important in the achievement of favorable outcomes by the experimental groups. These include focused personal care and mobility training; a comprehensive approach to care by a team of professionals, with coordination of treatment interventions, usually through team meetings and communication; education of patients and their families; active participation by family members; staff education on stroke and rehabilitation techniques; and care that is systematic, standardized, uniform, and consistent. While this does not diminish the importance of individualized treatment, ensuring that certain standards of care are met consistently is likely to improve the quality and outcome of that care. This consistency certainly supports the conduct of effective research and therefore enhances the usefulness of the results derived from that research.

Reding and McDowell[382] and Dobkin[383] argued in the scientific literature in 1989 as to whether there was convincing evidence concerning the usefulness and benefits of stroke rehabilitation. The scientific investigation of rehabilitation effectiveness has developed since that time, so that the current level of discussion about effectiveness has a somewhat more data-driven scientific basis. Despite limitations in the amount and quality of the research on the effectiveness of stroke rehabilitation, and despite several persisting questions on the effectiveness of the interventions that make up the programs, there is growing evidence that stroke rehabilitation programs improve the outcome of individuals who are disabled by stroke.

U.S. AGENCY FOR HEALTH CARE POLICY AND RESEARCH POSTSTROKE REHABILITATION CLINICAL PRACTICE GUIDELINES

The primary purpose of clinical practice guidelines is to assist clinicians in making decisions about care provided to patients. Guidelines also help to reduce practice variation, standardize management, improve quality, reduce costs, provide an educational tool, and serve as a platform for future research. In order to be successful the guideline should be useful, practical, and based on both the results of scientific trials and consensus reached by experts. The U.S. AHCPR Post-Stroke Rehabilitation Guidelines were designed to promote effective utilization of rehabilitation resources and to enhance outcomes. These guidelines focused on five major points:

1. The importance of thorough and consistent assessment of status at each stage of the recovery process to help guide treatment decisions and to monitor patient progress.
2. Early implementation of rehabilitation interventions during acute care to promote recovery and prevent complications.
3. Selection of the type of rehabilitation program and services best suited to meet the patient's needs.
4. Establishment of realistic rehabilitation goals and provision of treatment in accordance with a carefully developed rehabilitation management plan.
5. Combined follow-up and treatment during transition to a community residence.

Emphasis was also placed on the importance of active patient and family involvement.

In view of the support for these recommendations provided by the findings of research studies and the experience of clinician experts, adoption of these guidelines seems likely to lead to effective utilization of rehabilitation resources and to enhanced patient outcomes.

In making its recommendations, the AHCPR relied on evidence derived not only from an exhaustive literature review, but also from the development of consensus opinions by an expert panel. In view of the similarity of conclusions reached by that process and by the present review of controlled clinical trials, it seems sensible to adopt the AHCPR recommendations for implementation into practice.

According to the AHCPR Clinical Practice Guidelines, while several principles are important, several factors are critical to the appropriate implementation of a rehabilitation program, most of which have been reviewed in this chapter. First, there is a fundamental recommendation to use an interdisciplinary team approach to care. In addition, thorough, consistent, and fully documented patient assessment is key at several points in the poststroke course of care, including at the time of screening for rehabilitation, at rehabilitation admission, throughout the course of rehabilitation, at discharge, and during long-term follow-up. Continuity of care is also important; rehabilitation does not stop at the time of discharge from the formal program but continues throughout long-term follow-up.

Patient and family involvement in the rehabilitation process enhance the likelihood of achieving favorable outcomes. Principles derived from learning theory should be applied to ensure that appropriate training is occurring.

One of the most important recommendations is that stroke rehabilitation should begin as soon as the diagnosis of stroke is established, life-threatening problems are brought under control, and activity is deemed medically feasible. Specific measures should be taken to prevent recurrent stroke, to prevent secondary medical complications (such as venous thromboembolism, pneumonia, contracture, and pressure sores), and to address ongoing functional health issues (such as bowel and bladder function, nutrition, and hydration). The patient should be mobilized and encouraged to resume self-care activities as soon as it is medically feasible to do so.

During the acute phase after stroke, the patient should be screened for whether or not there is a need for rehabilitation, and if so, screened for the level, type, and setting. Rehabilitation is provided in a number of settings, including inpatient specialty rehabilitation hospitals, rehabilitation units in general hospitals, skilled nursing (or subacute) units, day hospitals, outpatient facilities, and home settings. Criteria for admission to specific levels or types of settings are not uniformly applied. However, the AHCPR guidelines attempt to provide threshold criteria for determining the need for rehabilitation, including medical stability, the presence of functional deficits, the ability to learn, enough physical endurance to allow the patient to sit up for at least 1 hour, and the ability to participate actively in the rehabilitation program. Within the group of patients who meet those criteria and who are candidates for rehabilitation, one criterion for admission to a comprehensive interdisciplinary program is the presence of at least two types of disability that would require at least two disciplines of professionals to assist in management.

Management during the rehabilitation program has several important components. One of the most important aspects of management is the performance of a thorough and accurate assessment. This assessment is then used to establish the goals of the rehabilitation program. The goals should be realistic, attainable, behavioral in nature, and mutually agreed upon by the patient, family, and professional team. The assessment is also used to drive the development of the management plan that is implemented to promote the attainment of those goals. Another reason for the assessment is to provide a baseline for comparing functional progress during the course of the rehabilitation program. Ongoing monitoring of progress allows the team to adjust the plan and the specific interventions to better meet the patient's needs. One of the most critical aspects of the recommendations is that the interventions in the treatment program be designed and implemented to *match* and meet the patient's specific needs.

Because the studies comparing the efficacy of various therapeutic modalities do not provide consistent and reliable results, specific recommendations cannot be made concerning the potential superiority of individual treatment methods or specific interventions to manage specific problems. However, a list of potentially useful modalities is available in the AHCPR guidelines and in other references. Specific recommendations should be made, however, concerning the need to manage sensorimotor deficits, provide compensatory training, evaluate and manage cognitive and perceptual deficits, diagnose and treat depression and other emotional issues, and manage speech and language disorders. Discharge planning should be performed during the rehabilitation program and should include family teaching and securing community resources.

Assistance should be provided to the patient and family to promote a smooth transition to the community at the time of discharge from the rehabilitation program. It is important to identify an individual to coordinate the post-discharge care. It is also important to monitor progress and status after discharge, as these often change over time. Specific attention should be paid to such important long-term "quality of life" issues as the availability of community supports, to safety and fall prevention, to health promotion, to sexuality issues, to leisure and recreational activities, to driving, and to return to work.

SPECIAL PATIENT CONSIDERATIONS

Pediatric Stroke

Stroke is unusual in children, with an estimated incidence of 2.5 per 100,000 children per year.[384] Although hemiparesis, aphasia, or isolated cognitive deficits can occur, the presentation of stroke in neonates and children often is different from that in older individuals; seizures, fever, and delayed achievement of developmental milestones are not uncommon. Causes of stroke also differ; these include hereditary conditions, congenital heart disease, metabolic disorders, coagulopathy, drugs, intracerebral vascular anomalies, and others. The prognosis after stroke in children is generally thought to be better than in adults. However, some residual deficit is present in the majority of children surviving a stroke. Rehabilitation emphasizes functional restoration and compensation, psychosocial support, and the attainment of normal developmental abilities.

Stroke in Young Adults

Although stroke is commonly considered a condition of aging, it is estimated that nearly one-third of all strokes occur in individuals less than 65 years old, and that 26% of strokes occur in persons between ages 45 and 65 years. Although early atherosclerosis, cardioembolism, and hemorrhages are common causes, the distribution of types of stroke in younger adults is somewhat different from that in older adults. Hemorrhagic strokes account for about one-third of all strokes in young adults (compared with one-fifth among all stroke survivors). Common causes of cerebral infarctions include atherosclerosis (usually in the setting of known atherogenic risk factors) in about 20%, cardiogenic embolism (usually from congenital heart defects or atrial fibrillation) in about 20%, cerebral vasculitis with or without known systemic collagen vascular disease in 10%, coagulopathy in about 10%, and others. The approach to the diagnostic workup of the younger stroke patient is aggressive, and often calls for procedures such as cerebral angiography, coagulation tests, collagen vascular disease evaluation, and cardiac workup, including transesophageal echocardiography.[384–389]

Young adults tend to present with unique rehabilitation needs and long-term issues. Table 50–17 lists many of the specialized problems and needs that are more prevalent and prominent among younger adults compared to older individuals. To address these specific patient needs, rehabilitation interventions should be directed toward the achievement of specific goals. Depending on the specific situation, functional therapy interventions should include training in complex instrumental ADL, such as shopping, homemaking, community level mobility, and child care. Communication and cognitive training should focus on money management skills and vocational activities. Psychological counseling of the patient and family should be instituted to address some of the issues that are specific to the age of the patient, such as self-image, interpersonal relationships, dating, sexuality, and stress management. Education of the patient and family should provide information on stroke, medications, nutrition, healthy lifestyle, and prevention measures. Driving evaluation and rehabilitation are important, as are vocational assessment, counseling, training, and referrals. Recreational and social programs, aerobic training or fitness exercise groups, and community reentry training all enhance the quality of life of young persons with stroke.[390–397]

Aggressive rehabilitation and continued care by specialized professionals who can recognize, understand, and address the specific physical and psychosocial considerations in young stroke patients can both facilitate the achievement of optimal outcomes in these patients and enhance their quality of life.

TABLE 50–17 Rehabilitation and Long-Term Issues in Young Stroke Survivors

1. Employment
2. Sexuality
3. Child care, parenting
4. Instrumental activities of daily living—homemaking, meal preparation, shopping
5. Psychological aspects of life-role changes
6. Spouse vs. personal caregiver role
7. Financial management
8. Driving
9. Relationship changes
10. Leisure planning, hobbies, socializing

Geriatric Stroke

The effect of age on recovery after stroke is variable and controversial. It has been found that young age at stroke onset has a favorable effect on long-term and short-term stroke survival,[385, 398] but the effect on functional recovery is less certain. In a review of 33 studies on functional outcome after stroke, Jongbloed[361] found that 18 studies evaluated the impact of age on stroke outcome. In 14 of the studies, younger patients tended to have better outcomes than older adults, but the overwhelming majority of these studies used functional status at discharge as the outcome measure. In four of the studies, no relationship was found between age and outcome, and in most of those studies, amount of functional improvement (rather than functional status at discharge) was used as the outcome measure under study. These findings suggest that younger adults tend to have less severe disability levels at presentation than older adults. It has been suggested that the adverse effect of increasing age on functional outcome is explained only by co-morbid conditions and frequency of prior stroke.

Age alone probably does not play a major role in determining the course and care of the patient with stroke. It is more likely that advancing age serves as a marker for the presence of medical co-morbidities, prior strokes, and limited social supports. Clinical experience indicates that many older adults successfully complete rehabilitation, return to their home and community, and contribute to their families and society. However, the frequency of multiple physical impairments and psychosocial problems is greater among older stroke patients than among younger individuals, and this most likely affects outcome.

As a consequence, older adults often require more medical monitoring, longer recovery times, reduced exercise intensities, or more psychosocial support during their rehabilitation program than do younger adults.

Ethical Considerations

Because of the complexity and severity of the problems with which stroke patients present, it is not surprising that ethical issues often arise during the evaluation and management of these patients. An issue that occurs somewhat frequently is whether and to what degree autonomy in decision making can be undertaken safely and reliably by patients, many of whom have cognitive, perceptual, emotional, or behavioral disturbances resulting from the stroke itself or from other conditions. Other problems arise when an individual insists on living independently when it is unsafe to do so, or when patients or their families insist on continued hospitalization or rehabilitation program participation when there is little or no clinical indication to do so. Many of these decisions involve the determination of the patient's competency and, possibly, establishment of guardianship. The latter two activities become critical components of the rehabilitation program for some patients. It is essential that patients and families be involved with the decision-making process. Involving members of the rehabilitation team in this process can be of value as well.

Decisions might have to be made about instituting resuscitative measures in the event of a cardiopulmonary arrest or whether to initiate or continue alternative measures for nutritional support, ventilatory support, or respiratory airway maintenance. These should be considered and acted on on an individual basis with the patient and family.

"Do not resuscitate" does *not* mean "do not treat." It often is appropriate for patients to receive therapy services and to participate in an intensive rehabilitation program even if the decision has been made to avoid resuscitative measures in the event of a cardiopulmonary arrest. Rehabilitation goals usually remain the same in these situations and include improving functional status, promoting psychosocial adaptation, providing caregiver education and support, and, especially, enhancing quality of life.

COMMENTS

Because many of the concepts and skills that are used to treat stroke patients are applicable to the management of the problems that result from many other medical conditions, stroke rehabilitation can be thought of as a prototypical rehabilitation activity. One of the most important aspects of treatment is avoiding a nihilistic attitude in caring for stroke patients. It is important to emphasize and to take advantage of the stroke patient's strengths and abilities, and to avoid focusing only on the disabilities. Initial and ongoing assessment is critical to the success of the interventions because of the changing nature of the patient's needs and the importance of matching professional services with specific patient needs. The interventions focus on functional enhancement through training, demonstration, supervision, suggestions, practice, and immediate feedback. Patient and family education play an extremely important role, and for some patients, caregiver training is the major focus of the program. It is generally found that psychological counseling and support facilitates better physical recovery and enhances quality of life, and that involving and supporting family members is critical to the process. Interdisciplinary collaboration and communication are the hallmarks of the rehabilitation program.

Stroke rehabilitation remains somewhat controversial and not universally or uniformly applied. Although the institution of a rehabilitation program after a stroke often is accepted as a common clinical practice and as a component of routine medical care, the specific methods and their investigations are still under scientific, clinical, and, more recently, fiscal scrutiny.

After reviewing available information about stroke rehabilitation, the British Department of Health[398] summarized several key points. They noted that stroke is a common clinical problem with a significant impact on its survivors and on society. It often presents as a disabling illness, involving many aspects of the patient's life and placing a substantial burden on family members and on others. The aims of rehabilitation are to minimize the impact of the disability resulting from the stroke and to optimize quality of life for both the patient and the personal caregiver. It was noted in the British report that although "there are very few well designed studies that assess the effectiveness of rehabilitation after stroke . . . , there is some evidence that formal rehabilitation after stroke is effective, and that it is best provided by well-organized interdisciplinary teams. . . ." Interpretation and extrapolation of the findings of most available investigations, and more important, of extensive clinical experience confirm those conclusions.

REFERENCES

1. Gresham GE: Stroke outcome research. Stroke 1986; 17:358.
2. Kottke FJ: Historica obscura hemiplegia. Arch Phys Med Rehabil 1974; 55:4–13.
3. Bobath B: Adult Hemiplegia: Evaluation and Treatment, ed 2. London, Heinemann, 1978.
4. Charness A: Stroke/Head Injury: A Guide to Functional Outcomes in Physical Therapy Management. Rockville, MD, Aspen Publishers, 1986.
5. Roth EJ: Medical rehabilitation of the stroke patient. Be Stroke Smart 1992; 8:8.
6. Biller J, Love BB: Nihilism and stroke therapy. Stroke 1991; 22:1105–1106.
7. Caplan LR: Diagnosis and treatment of ischemic stroke. JAMA 1991; 266:2413–2418.
8. WHO Task Force on Stroke and Other Cerebrovascular Disorders: Stroke—1989. Recommendations on stroke prevention, diagnosis, and therapy. Stroke 1989; 20:1407–1431.
9. American Heart Association: Heart and Stroke Facts: 1999. Statistical Supplement. Dallas, American Heart Association, 1999.
10. McGovern PG, Burke GL, Sprafka JM, et al: Trends in mortality, morbidity and risk factor levels for stroke from 1960 through 1990: The Minnesota Heart Survey. JAMA 1992; 26:753–759.
11. Whisnant JP: The decline of stroke. Stroke 1984; 15:160–168.
12. Klag MJ, Whelton PK, Seidler AJ: Decline in US stroke mortality: Demographic trends and antihypertensive treatment. Stroke 1989; 20:14–21.
13. Garraway WM, Whisnant JP: The changing pattern of hypertension and the declining incidence of stroke. JAMA 1987; 258:214–217.
14. Hypertension Detection and Follow-up Program Cooperative Group: Five-year findings of the hypertension and follow-up program: III. Reduction in stroke incidence among persons with high blood pressure. JAMA 1982; 247:633–638.
15. MacMahon S, Peto R, Cutler J, et al: Blood pressure, stroke, and coronary heart disease: 1. Prolonged differences in blood pressure: Prospective observational studies corrected for the regression dilution bias. Lancet 1990; 335:765–774.
16. Collins R, Peto R, MacMahon S, et al: Blood pressure, stroke, and coronary heart disease: 2. Short-term reductions in blood pressure: Overview of randomized drug trials in their epidemiological context. Lancet 1990; 335:827–838.
17. Ahmed OI, Orchard TJ, Sharma R, et al: Declining mortality from stroke in Allegheny County, Pennsylvania: Trends in case fatality and severity of disease, 1971–1980. Stroke 1988; 19:181–184.
18. Gillum RF, Gomez-Marin O, Kottke TE, et al: Acute stroke in a metropolitan area: 1970 and 1980: The Minnesota Heart Survey. J Chronic Dis 1985; 38:891–898.
19. Drury I, Whisnant JP, Garraway M: Primary intracerebral hemorrhage: Impact of CT on incidence. Neurology 1984; 34:653–657.
20. Gillum RF: Cerebrovascular disease morbidity in the United States, 1970–1983: Age, sex, region, and vascular surgery. Stroke 1986; 17:656–661.
21. Ingall TJ, Whisnant JP, Wiebers DO, et al: Has there been a decline in subarachnoid hemorrhage mortality? Stroke 1989; 20:718–724.
22. Broderick JP, Phillips SJ, Whisnant JP, et al: Incidence rates of stroke in the '80s: The end of the decline in stroke? Stroke 1989; 20:577–582.
23. Cooper R, Sempos C, Hsieh SC, et al: Slowdown in the decline of stroke mortality in the United States, 1978–1986. Stroke 1990; 21:1274–1279.
24. Garraway WM, Whisnant JP, Drury I: The changing pattern of survival following stroke. Stroke 1983; 14:699–703.
25. Indrevik B, Slordahl SA, Bakke F, et al: Stroke unit treatment. Long-term effects. Stroke 1997; 28:1861–1866.
26. Roth EJ: Heart disease in patients with stroke: Incidence, impact and implications for rehabilitation. 1. Classification and prevalence. Arch Phys Med Rehabil 1993; 74:752–760.
27. Gresham GE, Philips TF, Wolf PA, et al: Epidemiologic profile of long-term stroke disability: The Framingham Study. Arch Phys Med Rehabil 1979; 60:487–491.
28. Kannel WB, Wolf PA, McGee DL, et al: Systolic blood pressure, arterial rigidity and risk of stroke: The Framingham Study. JAMA 1981; 245:1225–1229.
29. SHEP Cooperative Research Group: Prevention of stroke by antihypertensive drug treatment in older persons with isolated systolic hypertension: Final results of the Systolic Hypertension in the Elderly Program (SHEP). JAMA 1991; 265:3255–3264.
30. Wolf PA, D'Agostino RB, Kannel WB, et al: Cigarette smoking as a risk factor for stroke: The Framingham Study. JAMA 1988; 259:1025–1029.
31. Abbot RD, Reed DM, Yin Y, et al: Risk of stroke in male cigarette smokers. N Engl J Med 1986; 315:717–720.
32. Ross R: The pathogenesis of atherosclerosis: An update. N Engl J Med 1988; 20:488–500.
33. Salonan R, Seppanen K, Rauramaa R, et al: Prevalence of carotid atherosclerosis and serum cholesterol levels in eastern Finland. Atherosclerosis 1988; 8:788–792.
34. O'Leary DH, Anderson KM, Wolf PA, et al: Cholesterol and carotid atherosclerosis in older persons: The Framingham Study. Ann Epidemiol 1992; 2:147–153.
35. The Expert Panel: Report of the National Cholesterol Education Program Expert Panel on Detection, Evaluation, and Treatment of High Blood Cholesterol in Adults. Arch Intern Med 1988; 148:36–69.
36. Yano K, Reed DM, MacLean CJ: Serum cholesterol and hemorrhagic stroke in the Honolulu Heart Program. Stroke 1989; 20:1460–1465.
37. Iso H, Jacobs DR, Wentworth D, et al: Serum cholesterol levels and 6-year mortality from stroke in 350,977 men screened for the Multiple Risk Factor Intervention Trial. N Engl J Med 1989; 320:904–910.
38. Whisnant JP, Matsumotoa N, Elveback LR: The effect of anticoagulant therapy on the prognosis of patients with transient cerebral ischemic attacks in a community: Rochester, Minnesota 1955 through 1969. Mayo Clin Proc 1973; 48:844–848.
39. Investigators of the Asymptomatic Carotid Atherosclerosis Study (ACAS): Clinical advisory: Carotid endarterectomy for patients with asymptomatic internal carotid artery stenosis. Stroke 1994; 25:2523–2524.
40. Kannel WB, McGee DL: Diabetes and cardiovascular disease: The Framingham Study. JAMA 1979; 241:2035–2038.
41. Barrett-Connor E, Khaw K: Diabetes mellitus: An independent risk factor for stroke? JAMA 1988; 258:116–123.
42. Abbott RD, Donohue RP, MacMahon SW, et al: Diabetes and the risk of stroke: The Honolulu Heart Program. JAMA 1987; 257:949–952.
43. Mohr JP, Caplan LR, Melski W, et al: The Harvard Cooperative Stroke Registry: A prospective registry. Neurology 1978; 28:754–762.
44. Nathan DM: Long-term complications of diabetes mellitus. N Engl J Med 1993; 329:2035–2038.
45. Kannel WB, Gordon T, Wolf PA, et al: Hemoglobin and the risk of cerebral infarction: The Framingham Study. Stroke 1972; 3:409–419.
46. Wilhelmsen L, Scardsudd K, Korban-Bengsten K, et al: Fibrinogen as a risk factor for stroke and myocardial infarction. N Engl J Med 1984; 311:501–505.
47. Steering Committee of the Physicians' Health Study Research Group: Final report on the aspirin component of the ongoing physicians health study. N Engl J Med 1989; 321:129–135.

48. Peto R, Gray R, Collins R, et al: Randomized trial of prophylactic daily aspirin in British male doctors. Br Med J 1988; 296:313–316.
49. Antiplatelet Trialists' Collaboration: Collaborative overview of randomised trials of antiplatelet therapy: I. Prevention of death, myocardial infarction, and stroke by prolonged antiplatelet therapy in various categories of patients. Br Med J 1994; 308:81–106.
50. Gilman AG, Rall TW, Nies AS, et al (eds): Goodman and Gilman's The Pharmacological Basis of Therapeutics, ed 8. New York, Pergamon Press, 1990, pp 1325–1326.
51. International Stroke Trial Collaborative Group: The International Stroke Trial (IST): A randomized trial of aspirin, subcutaneous heparin, both, or neither among 19435 patients with acute ischemic stroke. Lancet 1997; 349:1569–1581.
52. CAST Collaborative Group: CAST: Randomised placebo-controlled trial of early aspirin use in 20000 patients with acute ischemic stroke. Lancet 1997; 349:1641–1649.
53. Fields WS, Lemak NA, Frankowski RF, et al: Controlled trials of aspirin in cerebral ischaemia. Stroke 1977; 8:301–314.
54. The Canadian Cooperative Study Group: A randomized trial of aspirin and sulfinpyrazone in threatened stroke. N Engl J Med 1978; 299:53–59.
55. The Dutch TIA Trial Study Group: A comparison of two doses of aspirin (30 mg vs 283 mg a day) in patients after a transient ischemic attack or minor ischemic stroke. N Engl J Med 1991; 325:1261–1266.
56. The SALT Collaborative Group: Swedish Aspirin Low-dose Trial (SALT) of 75 mg aspirin as secondary prophylaxis after cerebrovascular ischaemic events. Lancet 1991; 338:1345–1349.
57. UK-TIA Study Group: United Kingdom Transient Ischaemic Attack (UK-TIA) aspirin trial: Final results. Br Med J 1991; 54:1044–1054.
58. ESPS Group: European Stroke Prevention Study. Stroke 1990; 21:1122–1130.
59. Bousser MG, Eschwege E, Hagrenau M, et al: "AICLA" controlled trial of aspirin and dipyridamole in the secondary prevention of athero-thrombotic cerebral ischemia. Stroke 1983; 14:5–14.
60. Dyken ML, Barnett HJM, Easton JD, et al: Low-dose aspirin and stroke: "It ain't necessarily so." Stroke 1992; 23:1395–1399.
61. Hass WK, Easton JD, Adams HP, et al: The TASS Group: A randomised trial comparing ticlopidine hydrochloride with aspirin for the prevention of stroke in high-risk patients. N Engl J Med 1989; 321:501–507.
62. Gent M, Easton JD, Hachinski V, et al: The CATS Group: The Canadian American Ticlopidine Study (CATS) in thromboembolic stroke. Lancet 1989; 1:1215–1220.
63. CAPRIE Steering Committee: A randomised, blinded, trial of clopidogrel versus aspirin in patients at risk of ischaemic events (CAPRIE). Lancet 1996; 348:1329–1339.
64. Wolf PA, Dawber TR, Thomas E, et al: Epidemiologic assessment of chronic atrial fibrillation and risk of stroke: The Framingham Study. Neurology 1978; 28:973–979.
65. Peterson P, Boysen G, Godtfredsen J, et al: Placebo-controlled, randomised trial of warfarin and aspirin for prevention of thrombotic complications in chronic atrial fibrillation: The Copenhagen AFA-SAK Study. Lancet 1989; 1:175–179.
66. Stroke Prevention in Atrial Fibrillation Investigators: Stroke Prevention in Atrial Fibrillation Study: Final results. Circulation 1991; 84:527–539.
67. Ezekowitz MD, Bridgers SL, James KE, et al: Warfarin in the prevention of stroke associated with nonrheumatic atrial fibrillation. N Engl J Med 1992; 327:1406–1412.
68. The Boston Area Anticoagulation Trial of Atrial Fibrillation Investigators: The effect of low-dose warfarin on the risk of stroke in patients with nonrheumatic atrial fibrillation. N Engl J Med 1990; 323:1505–1511.
69. Stroke Prevention in Atrial Fibrillation Investigators: Warfarin compared to aspirin for prevention of thromboembolism in atrial fibrillation: Stroke Prevention in Atrial Fibrillation II Study. Lancet 1994; 343:687–691.
70. Stroke Prevention in Atrial Fibrillation Investigators: Adjusted-dose warfarin versus low-intensity, fixed-dose warfarin plus aspirin for high-risk patients with atrial fibrillation: Stroke Prevention in Atrial Fibrillation III randomized clinical trial. Lancet 1996; 348:633–638.
71. North American Symptomatic Carotid Endarterectomy Trial Collaborators: Beneficial effect of carotid endarterectomy in symptomatic patients with high-grade carotid stenosis. N Engl J Med 1991; 325:445–453.
72. Hess DC, D'Cruz IA, Adams RJ, et al: Coronary artery disease, myocardial infarction, and brain embolism. Neurol Clin 1993; 11:399–417.
73. McGill HC: The pathogenesis of atherosclerosis. Clin Chem 1988; 34:B33–B39.
74. Pessin MS, Duncan GW, Mohr JP, et al: Clinical and angiographic features of carotid transient ischemic attacks. N Engl J Med 1977; 296:358–362.
75. Bogousslavsky J, Regli F: Borderzone infarctions distal to internal carotid artery. Ann Neurol 1986; 20:346–350.
76. Cerebral Embolism Task Force: Cardiogenic brain embolism: The second report of the Cerebral Embolism Task Force. Arch Neurol 1989; 46:727–743.
77. Caplan LR: Brain embolism, revisited. Neurology 1993; 43:1281–1287.
78. Jones HR, Caplan LR, Come PC, et al: Cerebral emboli of paradoxical origin. Ann Neurol 1983; 13:314–319.
79. Mohr JP: Lacunes. Stroke 1982; 13:3–11.
80. Furlan AJ, Whisnant JP, Elveback LR: The decreasing incidence of primary intracerebral hemorrhage: A population study. Ann Neurol 1979; 5:367–373.
81. Fisher CM: Pathological observations in hypertensive cerebral hemorrhage. J Neuropathol Exp Neurol 1971; 30:536–550.
82. Feldmann E, Tornabene J: Diagnosis and treatment of cerebral amyloid angiopathy. Clin Geriatr Med 1991; 7:617–630.
83. Sundt TM, Whisnant P: Subarachnoid hemorrhage from intracranial aneurysms. N Engl J Med 1978; 299:116–122.
84. Winn HR, Richardson AE, Jane JA: The long-term prognosis in untreated cerebral aneurysms: I. The incidence of late hemorrhage in cerebral aneurysm: A 10-year evolution of 364 patients. Ann Neurol 1977; 1:358–370.
85. Perret G, Nishioka H: Report on the Cooperative Study of Intracranial Aneurysms and Subarachnoid Hemorrhage: VI. Arteriovenous malformations: An analysis of 545 cases of cranio-cerebral arteriovenous malformations and fistulae reported to the cooperative study. J Neurosurg 1966; 25:467–490.
86. Mohr JP, Hilal SK, Stein BM: Arteriovenous malformations and other vascular anomalies. In Barnett HJM, Mohr JP, Stein BM, et al (eds): Stroke: Pathophysiology, Diagnosis, and Management, ed 2. New York, Churchill Livingstone, 1992.
87. Ondra SL, Troupp H, George ED, et al: The natural history of symptomatic arteriovenous malformations of the brain: A 24-year followup assessment. J Neurosurg 1990; 73:387–391.
88. Huckman MS: Normal pressure hydrocephalus: Evaluation of diagnostic and prognostic tests. Am J Neurol Res 1981; 2:385–395.
89. Twitchell TE: The restoration of motor function following hemiplegia in man. Brain 1951; 64:443–480.
90. Sawner K, LaVigne J: Brunnstrom's Movement Therapy in Hemiplegia: A Neurophysiological Approach, ed 2. Philadelphia, JB Lippincott, 1992.
91. Gordon J, Ghez C: Muscle receptors and spinal reflexes: The stretch reflex. In Kandel ER, Schwartz JH, Jessell TM (eds): Principles of Neural Science. New York, Elsevier Science Publishing, 1991, pp 564–580.
92. Benson DF: Aphasia. In Heilman KM, Valenstein E (eds): Clinical Neuropsychology. New York, Oxford University Press, 1985, pp 17–47.
93. Ross ED: Nonverbal aspects of language. Neurol Clin 1993; 11:9–23.
94. Albert ML, Helm-Estabrooks N: Diagnosis and treatment of aphasia: Part 1. JAMA 1988; 259:1043–1047.
95. Geshwind N: Disconnexion syndromes in animals and man. Part 2. Brain 1965; 88:237–294.
96. Friedman RB, Albert ML: Alexia. In Heilman KM, Valenstein E (eds): Clinical Neuropsychology. New York, Oxford University Press, 1985, pp 49–73.
97. Geshwind N: The apraxias: Neural mechanisms of disorders of learned movement. Am Sci 1975; 63:188–195.
98. Heilman KM, Watson RT, Valenstein E: Neglect and related disorders. In Heilman KM, Valenstein E: (eds): Clinical Neuro-

psychology. New York, Oxford University Press, 1985, pp 243–293.
99. Linden P, Siebens AA: Dysphagia: Predicting laryngeal penetration. Arch Phys Med Rehabil 1983; 64:281–284.
100. Gordon C, Hewer RL, Wade DT: Dysphagia in acute stroke. Br Med J 1987; 295:411–414.
101. Horner J, Massey EW, Riski JE, et al: Aspiration following stroke: Clinical correlates and outcome. Neurology 1988; 38: 159–162.
102. Horner J, Massey EW, Brazer SR: Aspiration in bilateral stroke patients. Neurology 1990; 40:1686–1688.
103. Barer DH: The natural history and functional consequences of dysphagia after hemispheric stroke. Neurol Neurosurg Psychiatry 1989; 52:236–241.
104. Horner J, Buoyer FG, Alers MJ, et al: Dysphagia following brainstem stroke: Clinical correlates and outcome. Arch Neurol 1991; 48:1170–1173.
105. Alberts MJ, Horner J, Gray L, et al: Aspiration after stroke: Lesion analysis by brain MRI. Dysphagia 1992; 7:170–173.
106. Johnson ER, McKenzie SW, Rosenquist J, et al: Dysphagia following stroke: Quantitative evaluation of pharyngeal transit times. Arch Phys Med Rehabil 1992; 73:419–423.
107. Johnson ER, McKenzie SW, Sievers A: Aspiration pneumonia in stroke. Arch Phys Med Rehabil 1993; 73:973–976.
108. Dejerine J, Roussy G: La syndrome thalamique. Rev Neurol (Paris) 1906; 14:521–535.
109. Gilman S, Newman SW: Manter and Gatz's Essentials of Clinical Neuroanatomy and Neurophysiology, ed 7. Philadelphia, FA Davis, 1987.
110. Amarence P: The spectrum of cerebellar infarctions. Neurology 1991; 41:973–979.
111. Siesjo BK: Pathophysiology and treatment of focal cerebral ischemia: 1. Pathophysiology. J Neurosurg 1992; 77:169–184.
112. Consensus Panel: Stroke: The first six hours. Stroke Clin Updates 1993; 4:1–12.
113. The National Institute of Neurological Disorders and Stroke rt-PA Stroke Study Group: Tissue plasminogen activator for acute ischemic stroke. N Engl J Med 1995; 333:1581–1587.
114. Hacke W, Kaste M, Fieschi C, et al: Intravenous thrombolysis with recombinant tissue plasminogen activator for acute hemispheric stroke (ECASS). JAMA 1995; 274:1017–1025.
115. Hacke W, Kaste M, Fieschi C, et al: Randomized double-blind placebo-controlled trial of thrombolytic therapy with intravenous alteplase in acute ischaemic stroke (ECASS II). Lancet 1998; 352:1245–1251.
116. Chiu D, Krieger D, Villar-Cordova C, et al: Intravenous tissue plasminogen activator for acute ischemic stroke: Feasibility, safety, and efficiency in the first year of clinical practice. Stroke 1998; 29:18–22.
117. The Multicenter Acute Stroke Trial—European Study Group: Thrombolytic therapy with streptokinase in acute ischemic stroke. N Engl J Med 1996; 335:145–150.
118. del Zoppo GJ, Higashida RT, Furlan AJ, et al: PROACT: A phase II randomized trial of recombinant pro-urokinase by direct arterial delivery in acute middle cerebral artery stroke. Stroke 1998; 29:4–11.
119. Korczya AD: Heparin in the treatment of acute stroke. Neurol Clin 1992; 10:209–217.
120. TOAST Investigators: Low molecular weight heparinoid, ORG 10172 (Danapariod), and outcome after acute ischemic stroke: A randomized controlled trial. JAMA 1998; 279:1265–1272.
121. Allen GS, Ahn HS, Preziosi TJ, et al: Cerebral arterial spasm: A controlled trial of nimodipine in patients with subarachnoid hemorrhage. N Engl J Med 1983; 308:619–624.
122. Pickard JD, Murray GD, Illingworth R, et al: Effect of oral nimodipine on cerebral infarction and outcome after subarachnoid hemorrhage: British Aneurysm Nimodipine Trial. Br Med J 1989; 298:626–642.
123. Frontoni DTM, Argentino C, Sacchetti ML, et al: Update on calcium antagonists in cerebrovascular diseases. J Cardiovasc Pharmacol 1991; 18:S10–S14.
124. Marler JR, Winters-Jones P, Emr M: Proceedings of a National Symposium on Rapid Identification and Treatment of Acute Stroke. Bethesda, MD, National Institute of Neurological Diseases and Stroke, 1997.
125. Gacs G, Fox AJ, Barnett HJM, et al: Visualization of intracranial arterial thromboembolism. Stroke 1983; 14:756–762.
126. The NINDS t-PA Stroke Study Group: Intracerebral hemorrhage after intravenous t-PA therapy for ischemic stroke. Stroke 1997; 28:2109–2118.
127. Larrue V, von Kummer R, del Zoppo G, et al: Hemorrhagic transformation in acute ischemic stroke: Potential contributing factors in the European Cooperative Acute Stroke Study. Stroke 1997; 28:957–960.
128. Waidhauser E, Hamburger C, Marguth F: Neurosurgical management of cerebellar hemorrhage. Neurosurg Rev 1990; 13:211–217.
129. Wallace JD, Levy LL: Blood pressure after stroke. JAMA 1981; 246:2177–2180.
130. Strandgaard S, Paulson OB: Regulation of cerebral blood flow in health and disease. J Cardiovasc Pharmacol 1992; 19:S89–S93.
131. Herpin D: The effects of antihypertensive drugs on the cerebral blood flow and its regulation. Prog Neurobiol 1990; 35:75–83.
132. Biller J: Medical management of acute cerebral ischemia. Neurol Clin 1992; 10:63–85.
133. Schroeder T, Schierbeck J, Howardy P, et al: Effect of labetolol on cerebral blood flow and middle cerebral arterial flow velocity in healthy volunteers. Neurol Res 1991; 13:10–12.
134. Nedergaard M, Diemer NH: Focal ischemia of the rat brain, with special reference to the influence of plasma glucose concentration. Acta Neuropathol 1987; 73:131–137.
135. DeCouten-Myers GM, Myers RE, Schoolfield L: Hyperglycemia enlarges infarct size in cerebrovascular occlusion in cats. Stroke 1988; 19:623–630.
136. Siesjo BK: Pathophysiology and treatment of focal cerebral ischemia: 2. Mechanisms of damage and treatment. J Neurosurg 1992; 77:337–354.
137. Schafer AI: The hypercoaguable states. Ann Intern Med 1985; 102:814–828.
138. Kohler J, Kasper J, Witt I, et al: Ischemic stroke due to protein C deficiency. Stroke 1990; 21:1077–1080.
139. Bryan RN, Levy LM, Whitlow WD, et al: Diagnosis of acute cerebral infarction: Comparison of CT and MR imaging. AJNR 1991; 12:611–620.
140. Matthews VP, Barker PB, Bryan RN: Magnetic resonance evaluation of stroke. Mag Res Q 1992; 8:245–263.
141. Warach S, Gaa J, Siewert B, et al: Acute human stroke studied by whole brain planar diffusion-weighted magnetic resonance imaging. Ann Neurol 1995; 37:231–241.
142. Fisher M, Sotak CH, Minematsu K, et al: New magnetic resonance techniques for evaluating cerebrovascular disease. Ann Neurol 1992; 32:115–122.
143. Hellman RS, Tikofsky RS: An overview of the contribution of regional cerebral blood flow studies in cerebrovascular disease: Is there a role for single photon emission computed tomography? Semin Nucl Med 1990; 20:303–324.
144. Tegeler CH, Downes TR: Cardiac imaging in stroke. Stroke 1991; 26:13–18.
145. Pop G, Sutherland GR, Koudstaal PJ, et al: Transesophageal echocardiography in the detection of intracardiac embolic sources in patients with transient ischemic attacks. Stroke 1990; 21:560–565.
146. Seiler RW, Grolimund P, Aaslid R, et al: Cerebral vasospasm evaluated by transcranial ultrasound correlated with clinical grade and CT-visualized subarachnoid hemorrhage. J Neurosurg 1986; 64:594–600.
147. Brandstater ME: An overview of stroke rehabilitation. Stroke 1990; 21(suppl II):II40–II42.
148. Kotila M, Waltimo O, Niemi M-L, et al: The profile of recovery from stroke and factors influencing outcome. Stroke 1984; 15:1039–1044.
149. Wade DT, Langton-Hewer R: Functional abilities after stroke: Measurement, natural history and prognosis. J Neurol Neurosurg Psychiatry 1987; 50:177–182.
150. Lehmann JF, DeLateur BJ, Fowler RS, et al: Stroke rehabilitation: Outcome and prediction. Arch Phys Med Rehabil 1975; 56:383–389.
151. Granger CV, Hamilton BB, Fiedler RC: Discharge outcome after stroke rehabilitation. Stroke 1992; 23:978–982.

152. Heinemann AW, Roth EJ, Cichowski K, et al: Multivariate analysis of improvement and outcome following stroke rehabilitation. Arch Neurol 1987; 44:1167–1172.
153. Ferrucci L, Bandinelli S, Guralnik JM, et al: Recovery of functional status after stroke: A postrehabilitation follow-up study. Stroke 1993; 24:200–205.
154. Andrews K, Brocklehurst JC, Richards B, et al: The rate of recovery from stroke—and its measurement. Int Rehabil Med 1981; 3:155–161.
155. Lehmann JF, DeLateur BJ, Fowler RS, et al: Stroke: Does rehabilitation affect outcome? Arch Phys Med Rehabil 1975; 56:375–382.
156. Smith DS, Goldenberg E, Ashburn A, et al: Remedial therapy after stroke: A randomized controlled trial. Br Med J 1981; 282:517–520.
157. Indredavik B, Bakke F, Solberg R, et al: Benefit of a stroke unit: A randomized controlled trial. Stroke 1991; 22:1026–1031.
158. Edmans JA, Towle D: Comparison of stroke unit and non-stroke unit in patients on independence in ADL. Br J Occup Ther 1990; 53:415–418.
159. Garraway WM, Akhtar AJ, Prescott RJ, Hockey L: Management of acute stroke in the elderly: Preliminary results of a controlled trial. Br Med J 1980; 280:1040–1043.
160. Wood-Dauphinee S, Shapiro S, Bass E, et al: A randomized trial of team care following stroke. Stroke 1984; 15:864–872.
161. Kalra L: The influence of stroke unit rehabilitation on functional recovery from stroke. Stroke 1994; 25:821–825.
162. Reding MJ, McDowell FH: Focused stroke rehabilitation programs improve outcome. Arch Neurol 1989; 46:700–711.
163. Roth EJ, Heinemann AW, Lovell LL, et al: Impairment and disability: Their relation during stroke rehabilitation. Arch Phys Med Rehabil 1998; 79:329–335.
164. Foulkes MA, Wolf PA, Price TR, et al: The Stroke Data Bank: Design, methods, and baseline characteristics. Stroke 1988; 19:547–554.
165. Skilbeck CE, Wade DT, Langton-Hewer R, et al: Recovery after stroke. J Neurol Neurosurg Psychiatry 1983; 46:5–8.
166. Bjorneby ER, Reinvang IR: Acquiring and maintaining self-care skills after stroke. Scand J Rehabil Med 1985; 17:75–80.
167. Sarno MT, Levita E: Some observations on the nature of recovery in global aphasia after stroke. Brain Lang 1981; 13:1–12.
168. Fugl-Meyer AR: Assessment of motor function in hemiplegic patients. In Buerger AA, Tobis JS (eds): Neurophysiological Aspects of Rehabilitation Medicine. Springfield, II, Charles C Thomas, 1976.
169. Gowland C, Stratford P, Ward M, et al: Measuring physical impairment and disability with the Chedoke-McMaster stroke assessment. Stroke 1993; 24:58–63.
170. Parker VM, Wade DT, Langton-Hewer R: Loss of arm function after stroke: Measurement, frequency, and recovery. Int Rehabil Med 1986; 8:69–73.
171. Gowland C: Recovery of motor function following stroke: Profile and predictors. Physiother Can 1982; 34:77–84.
172. Wade DT, Langton-Hewer R, Wood VA, et al: The hemiplegic arm after stroke: Measurement and recovery. J Neurol Neurosurg Psychiatry 1983; 46:521–524.
173. Bonita R, Beaglehole R: Recovery of motor function after stroke. Stroke 1988; 19:1497–1500.
174. Warabi T, Inoue K, Noda H, Murakami S: Recovery of voluntary movement in hemiplegic patients: Correlation with degenerative shrinkage of the cerebral peduncles in CT images. Brain 1990; 113:177–189.
175. Wing AM, Lough S, Turton A, et al: Recovery of elbow function in voluntary positioning of the hand following hemiplegia due to stroke. J Neurol Neurosurg Psychiatry 1990; 53:126–134.
176. Bohanon RW, Smith MB: Assessment of strength deficits in eight paretic upper extremity muscle groups of stroke patients with hemiplegia. Physical Therapy 1987; 67:522–525.
177. Shah S: Reliability of the original Brunnstrom recovery scale following hemipegia. Am Occup Ther J 1984; 31:144–151.
178. Bohanon RW: Muscle strength changes in hemiparetic stroke patients during inpatient rehabilitation. J Neurol Rehabil 1988; 2:163–166.
179. Shah SK, Harsymiw SJ, Stahl PL: Stroke rehabilitation: Outcome based on Brunnstrom recovery stages. Occup Ther J Res 1986; 6:365–376.
180. Shah SK, Corones J: Volition following hemiplegia. Arch Phys Med Rehabil 1980; 61:523–528.
181. Wade DT, Langton-Hewer R, David RM, et al: Aphasis after stroke: Natural history and associated deficits. J Neurol Neurosurg Psychiatry 1986; 49:11–16.
182. Kertesz A, McCabe P: Recovery patterns and prognosis in aphasia. Brain 1977; 100:1–18.
183. Pickersgill MJ, Lincoln NB: Prognostic indicators and the pattern of recovery in aphasic stroke patients. J Neurol Neurosurg Psychiatry 1983; 46:130–139.
184. Sarno MT, Levita E: Recovery in treated aphasia in the first year post-stroke. Stroke 1979; 10:662–670.
185. Kertesz A: What do we learn from recovery from aphasia? Adv Neurol 1988; 47:277–292.
186. Brust JCM, Shafer SQ, Richter RW, et al: Aphasia in acute stroke. Stroke 1976; 7:167–174.
187. Prins RS, Snow CE, Wagenaar E: Recovery from aphasia: Spontaneous speech versus language comprehension. Brain Lang 1978; 6:192–211.
188. Meerwaldt JD: Spatial disorientation in right hemisphere infarction: A study of the speed of recovery. J Neurol Neurosurg Psychiatry 1983; 46:426–429.
189. Stone SP, Patel P, Greenwood RJ, et al: Measuring visual neglect in acute stroke and predicting its recovery: The Visual Neglect Recovery Index. J Neurol Neurosurg Psychiatry 1992; 55:431–436.
190. Kotila M, Niemi M-L, Laaksonen R: Four-year prognosis of stroke patients with visuospatial inattention. Scand J Rehabil Med 1986; 18:177–179.
191. Egelko S, Simon D, Riley E, et al: First year after stroke: Tracking cognitive and affective deficits. Arch Phys Med Rehabil 1989; 70:297–302.
192. Sunderland A, Langton-Hewer R: The natural history of visual neglect after stroke: Indications from two methods of assessment. Int Rehabil Med 1987; 9:55–59.
193. Friedman PJ, Leong L: Perceptual impairment after stroke: Improvements during the first 3 months. Disabil Rehabil 1992; 14:136–139.
194. Hier DB, Mondlock J, Caplan LR: Recovery of behavioral abnormalities after right hemisphere stroke. Neurology 1983; 33:345–350.
195. Dombovy ML, Bach-y-Rita P: Clinical observations on recovery from stroke. Adv Neurol 1988; 47:265–276.
196. Bach-y-Rita P: Process of recovery from stroke. In Brandstater ME, Basmajian JV (eds): Stroke Rehabilitation. Baltimore, Williams & Wilkins, 1987, pp 80–108.
197. Bach-y-Rita P, Baillet R: Recovery from stroke. In Duncan PW, Badke MB (eds): Motor Deficits Following Stroke. Chicago, Year Book Medical Publishers, 1987, pp 79–107.
198. Bach-y-Rita P (ed): Recovery of Function: Theoretical Considerations for Brain Injury Rehabilitation. Baltimore, University Park Press, 1980.
199. Kaplan MS: Plasticity after brain lesions: Contemporary concepts. Arch Phys Med Rehabil 1988; 69:984–991.
200. Wainberg MC: Plasticity of the central nervous system: Functional implications for rehabilitation. Physiother Can 1988; 40:224–232.
201. Bach-y-Rita P: Brain plasticity as a basis of the development of rehabilitation procedures for hemiplegia. Scand J Rehabil Med 1981; 13:73–83.
202. Feeney DM, Baron JC: Diaschisis. Stroke 1986; 17:817–830.
203. Marshall JF: Neural plasticity and recovery of function after brain injury. Int Rev Neurobiol 1985; 26:201–247.
204. Boyeson MG, Bach-y-Rita P: Determinants of brain plasticity. J Neurol Rehabil 1989; 3:35–57.
205. Bach-y-Rita P: Central nervous system lesions: Sprouting and unmasking in rehabilitation. Arch Phys Med Rehabil 1981; 62:41–47.
206. Illis LS: The effects of repetitive stimulation in recovery from damage to the central nervous system. Int Rehabil Med 1982; 4:178–184.
207. Roth EJ, Mueller K, Green D: Stroke rehabilitation outcome: Impact of coronary artery disease. Stroke 1988; 19:42–47.
208. Sacco RL, Wolf PA, Kannel WB, et al: Survival and recurrence following stroke: The Framingham Study. Stroke 1982; 13:290–295.

209. Solzi P, Ring H, Najenson T, Luz Y: Hemiplegics after a first stroke: Late survival and risk factors. Stroke 1985; 4:703–709.
210. Dombovy ML, Basford JR, Whisnant JP, et al: Disability and use of rehabilitation services following stroke in Rochester, Minnesota, 1975–1979. Stroke 1987; 18:830–836.
211. Sheikh K, Brennan PJ, Meade TW, et al: Predictors of mortality and disability in stroke. J Epidemiol Commun Health 1983; 37:70–74.
212. Harvey RL, Roth EJ, Heinemann AW, et al: Stroke rehabilitation: Clinical predictors of resource utilization. Arch Phys Med Rehabil 1998; 79:1349–1355.
213. Roth EJ: Medical complications encountered in stroke rehabilitation. Phys Med Rehabil Clin North Am 1991; 2:563–578.
214. Roth EJ, Noll SF: Stroke rehabilitation: 2. Comorbidities and complications. Arch Phys Med Rehabil 1994; 75:S42–S46.
215. Roth EJ: Natural history of recovery and influence of comorbid conditions on stroke outcome. In Gorelick P (ed): Atlas of Cerebrovascular Disease. Philadelphia, Current Science Publishers, 1995.
216. Schmidt J, Reding M: Recognition and management of medical and specific associated neurological complications in stroke rehabilitation. Top Geriatr Rehabil 1991; 7:1–14.
217. Siegler EL, Whitney FW: Prevention and other special management issues in the postacute care of the geriatric stroke patient. Neurorehabil 1993; 3:1–11.
218. Brott T: Prevention and management of medical complications of the hospitalized elderly stroke patient. Clin Geriatr Med 1991; 7:475–482.
219. Roth EJ: Heart disease in patients with stroke: II. Impact and implications for rehabilitation. Arch Phys Med Rehabil 1994; 75:94–101.
220. Brandstater ME, Roth EJ, Siebens HC: Venous thromboembolism in stroke: Literature review and implications for clinical practice. Arch Phys Med Rehabil 1992; 73(suppl):S379–S391.
221. Couser JI: Diagnosis and management of pneumonia and ventilatory disorders in patients with stroke. Top Stroke Rehabil 1994; 1:106–118.
222. Harvey RL: Diabetes mellitus: Incidence and influence on stroke rehabilitation and outcome. Top Stroke Rehabil 1994; 1:91–108.
223. Saver JL: Poststroke seizures. Top Stroke Rehabil 1994; 1:109–130.
224. Teasell RW: Pain following stroke. Crit Rev Phys Med Rehabil 1992; 3:205–217.
225. Garrison SJ: Post-stroke pain. Phys Med Rehabil State Art Rev 1991; 5:83–88.
226. Boivie J, Leijon G: Clinical findings in patients with central poststroke pain. In Casey KL (ed): Pain and Central Nervous System Disease: The Central Pain Syndromes. New York, Raven Press, 1991, pp 65–75.
227. Steinberg FU: The Immobilized Patient: Functional Pathology and Management. New York, Plenum Press, 1980.
228. St Pierre D, Gardiner PF: The effect of immobilization and exercise on muscle function: A review. Physiother Can 1987; 39:24–36.
229. Reddy MP: A guide to early mobilization of bedridden elderly. Geriatrics 1986; 41:59–70.
230. Office of Medical Applications of Research, National Institutes of Health: Consensus Conference: Prevention of Venous Thrombosis and Pulmonary Embolism. JAMA 1986; 256:744–749.
231. Clagett GP, Anderson FA, Levine MN, et al: Prevention of venous thromboembolism. Chest 1992; 102(suppl):391S–407S.
232. Leijon G, Boivie J, Johansson I: Central post-stroke pain: Neurological symptoms and pain characteristics. Pain 1989; 36:13–25.
233. Holmgren H, Leijon G, Boivie J: Central post-stroke pain: Somatosensory evoked potentials in relation to location of the lesion and sensory signs. Pain 1989; 40:43–52.
234. Gresham GE, Duncan PW, Stason WB, et al: Post-Stroke Rehabilitation. Clinical Practice Guideline no 16. AHCPR Publication no 95-0662. Rockville, MD, US Department of Health and Human Services, Public Health Service, Agency for Health Care Policy and Research, 1995.
235. Brocklehurst JC, Andrews K, Richards B, et al: Incidence and correlates of incontinence in stroke patients. J Am Geriatr Soc 1985; 33:540–542.
236. Reding MJ, Winter SW, Hochrein SA, et al: Urinary incontinence after unilateral hemispheric stroke: A neurologic epidemiologic perspective. J Neurorehabil 1987; 1:25–30.
237. Gelber DA, Good DC, Laven LJ, et al: Causes of urinary incontinence after acute hemispheric stroke. Stroke 1993; 24:378–382.
238. Sedarat SM, Hecht JS: Urologic problems after stroke (parts I and II). Stroke Clin Updates 1993; 4:17–20, 21–24.
239. Linsenmeyer TA, Zorowitz RD: Urodynamic findings in patients with urinary incontinence after cerebrovascular accident. Neurorehabil 1992; 2:23–26.
240. Garrett VE, Scott JA, Costich J, et al: Bladder emptying assessment in stroke patients. Arch Phys Med Rehabil 1989; 70:41–43.
241. Barer DH: Continence after stroke: Useful predictor or goal of therapy? Age Ageing 1989; 18:183–191.
242. Hoogasian S, Walzak MP, Wurzel R: Urinary incontinence in the stroke patient: Etiology and rehabilitation. In Erickson RV (ed): Medical Management of the Elderly Stroke Patient. Phys Med Rehabil State Art Rev 1989; 3:581–594.
243. Borrie MJ: Urinary incontinence after stroke. In Teasell RW (ed): Long-Term Consequences of Stroke. Phys Med Rehabil State Art Rev 1993; 7:101–112.
244. Caillet R: The Shoulder in Hemiplegia. Philadelphia, FA Davis, 1980.
245. Najenson T, Yacubovich E, Pikielini S: Rotator cuff injury in shoulder joints of hemiplegic patients. Scand J Rehabil Med 1971; 3:131–137.
246. Griffin J, Reddin G: Shoulder pain in persons with hemiplegia: A literature review. Phys Ther 1981; 61:1041–1045.
247. Kozin F, et al: The reflex sympathetic dystrophy syndrome: Parts 1, 2, and 3. Am J Med 1976; 60:321–331, 332–338; 1981; 70:23–30.
248. Smith RG, Cruikshank JG, Dunbar S: Malalignment of the shoulder after stroke. Br Med J 1982; 284:1224–1226.
249. Tepperman PS, Greyson ND, Hilbert L, et al: Reflex sympathetic dystrophy in hemiplegia. Arch Phys Med Rehabil 1984; 65: 442–447.
250. Van Ouenaller C, Laplace PM, Chantraine A: Painful shoulder in hemiplegia. Arch Phys Med Rehabil 1986; 67:23–36.
251. Moodie NB, Brisbin J, Morgan AMG: Subluxation of the glenohumeral joint in hemiplegia: Evaluation of supportive devices. Physiother Can 1986; 38:151–157.
252. Totta M, Beneck S: Shoulder dysfunction in stroke hemiplegia. Phys Med Rehabil Clin North Am 1991; 2:627–641.
253. Werner RA, Priebe MM, Davidoff GN: Reflex sympathetic dystrophy syndrome associated with hemiplegia. Neurorehabil 1992; 2:16–22.
254. Teasell RW, Gillen M: Upper extremity disorders and pain following stroke. In Teasell RW (ed): Long-Term Consequences of Stroke. Phys Med Rehabil State Art Rev 1993; 7:133–146.
255. Poplingher AR, Pillar T: Hip fracture in stroke patients: Epidemiology and rehabilitation. Acta Orthop Scand 1985; 56:226–227.
256. De Vincenzo DK, Watkins S: Accidental falls in a rehabilitation setting. Rehabil Nursing 1987; 12:248–252.
257. Mion LC, Gregor S, Buettner M, et al: Falls in the rehabilitation setting: Incidence and characteristics. Rehabil Nursing 1989; 14:17–21.
258. Mayo NE, Korner-Bitensky N, Kaizer F: Relationship between response time and falls among stroke patients undergoing physical rehabilitation. Int J Rehabil Res 1990; 13:47–55.
258a. Peszczynski M, Benson F, Collins J, and the Joint Committee for Stroke Facilities: II. Stroke rehabilitation. Stroke 1972; 3:375–407.
258b. Goldberg G: Principles of rehabilitation of the elderly stroke patient. In Dunkle RE, Schmidley JW (eds): Stroke in the Elderly. New York, Springer-Verlag, 1987.
259. Brandstater ME, Basmajian JV (eds): Stroke Rehabilitation. Baltimore, Williams & Wilkins, 1987.
260. Roth EJ: The elderly stroke patient: Principles and practices of rehabilitation management. Top Geriatr Rehabil 1988; 3:27–61.
261. Bleiberg J, Merbitz C: Learning goals during initial rehabilitation hospitalization. Arch Phys Med Rehabil 1983; 64:448–450.
262. Hyams DE: Psychological factors in rehabilitation of the elderly. Gerontol Clin 1969; 11:129–136.
263. Whitney FW: Using physical and neuropsychological assessment in the nursing care of the acute stroke patient. In Dunkle RE,

Schmidley JW (eds): Stroke in the Elderly. New York, Springer-Verlag, 1987.
264. Frieden RA: Early rehabilitation after stroke. In Gordon WA (ed): Advances in Stroke Rehabilitation. Boston, Andover, 1993, pp 18–33.
265. McDowell FH: Rehabilitating patients with stroke. Postgrad Med 1976; 59:145–149.
266. Asberg KH: Orthostatic tolerance training of stroke patients in general medical wards. Scand J Rehabil Med 1989; 21:179–185.
267. Hamrin E: Early activation in stroke: Does it make a difference? Scand J Rehabil Med 1982; 14:101–109.
268. Hayes SH, Carroll SR: Early intervention care in the acute stroke patient. Arch Phys Med Rehabil 1986; 67:319–321.
269. Anderson TP, Bourestom N, Greenberg FR, et al: Predictive factors in stroke rehabilitation. Arch Phys Med Rehabil 1974; 55:545–553.
270. Feigenson JS, McDowell FH, Meese P, et al: Factors influencing outcome and length of stay in a stroke rehabilitation unit: 1. Analysis of 248 unscreened patients—medical and functional prognostic indicators. Stroke 1977; 8:651–656.
271. Novack TA, Satterfield WT, Lyons K, et al: Stroke onset and rehabilitation: Time lag as a factor in treatment outcome. Arch Phys Med Rehabil 1984; 65:316–319.
272. Johnston MV, Keister M: Early rehabilitation for stroke patients: A new look. Arch Phys Med Rehabil 1984; 65:437–441.
273. Roth EJ: Rehabilitation entails many levels of postacute stroke care. American Heart Association Stroke Council Newsletter, Summer 1996, pp 6–7.
274. Westcott EJ: Traditional exercise regimens for the hemiplegic patient. Am J Phys Med 1967; 46:1012–1023.
275. Flanagan EM: Methods for facilitation and inhibition of motor activity. Am J Phys Med 1967; 46:1006–1011.
276. Lorish TR, Sandin KJ, Roth EJ, et al: Stroke rehabilitation: 3. Rehabilitation evaluation and management. Arch Phys Med Rehabil 1994; 75:S47–S51.
277. Good DC: Treatment strategies for enhancing motor recovery in stroke rehabilitation. J Neurorehabil 1994; 8:177–186.
278. Duncan PW, Badke MB: Stroke Rehabilitation: The Recovery of Motor Control. Chicago, Year Book Medical Publishers, 1987.
279. Knott M, Voss DE: Proprioceptive Neuromuscular Facilitation, ed 2. New York, Harper & Row, 1968.
280. Davies PM: Steps to Follow: A Guide to the Treatment of Adult Hemiplegia. Berlin, Springer-Verlag, 1985.
281. Ernst E: A review of stroke rehabilitation and physiotherapy. Stroke 1990; 21:1081–1085.
282. Carr JH, Sheperd RB: A Motor Relearning Programme for Stroke. Rockville, MD, Aspen, 1987.
283. Swenson JR: Therapeutic exercise in hemiplegia. In Basmajian JV (ed): Therapeutic Exercise, ed 4. Baltimore, Williams & Wilkins, 1984, pp 357–380.
284. Waagfjord J, Levangle PK, Certo CME: Effects of treadmill training on gait in a hemiparetic patient. Phys Ther 1990; 70:549–560.
285. Malouin F, Potvin M, Prevost J, et al: Use of an intensive task-oriented gait training program in a series of patients with acute cerebrovascular accidents. Phys Ther 1992; 72:781–793.
286. Hesse S, Bertelt C, Schafftin A, et al: Restoration of gait in nonambulatory hemiparetic patient by treadmill training with partial body weight. Arch Phys Med Rehabil 1994; 75:1087–1093.
287. Hesse S, Bertelt C, Jahnke MT, et al: Treadmill training with partial body weight support compared with physiotherapy in nonambulatory hemiparetic patients. Stroke 1995; 26:976–981.
288. Barton LA, Wolf SL: Use of EMG feedback in stroke rehabilitation. In Gordon WA (ed): Advances in Stroke Rehabilitation. Boston, Andover, 1993, pp 88–99.
289. Wolf SL: Essential considerations in the use of EMG biofeedback. Phys Ther 1978; 58:25–31.
290. Wolf S, Baker M, Kelly J: EMG biofeedback in stroke: A 1-year follow-up of the effect on patient characteristics. Arch Phys Med Rehabil 1980; 61:351–355.
291. DeWeerdt W, Harrison M: Electromyographic biofeedback for stroke patients: Some practical considerations. Physiother Can 1986; 72:106–108.
292. Ince LP, Zaretsky HH, Lee MHM: Integrating EMG biofeedback treatment of the impaired upper extremity into the rehabilitation programs of stroke patients. Arch Phys Med Rehabil 1987; 68:645.
293. Kraft GH: New methods for the assessment and treatment of the hemiplegic arm and hand. Phys Med Rehabil Clin North Am 1991; 2:579–597.
294. Moreland J, Thomson MA: Efficacy of electromyographic biofeedback compared with conventional physical therapy for upper-extremity function in patients following stroke: A research overview and meta-analysis. Phys Ther 1994; 74:534–547.
295. Moreland JD, Thomson MA, Fuoco AR: Electromyographic biofeedback to improve lower extremity function after stroke: A meta-analysis. Arch Phys Med Rehabil 1998; 79:134–140.
296. Glanz M, Klawansky S, Stason W, et al: Biofeedback therapy in poststroke rehabilitation: A meta-analysis of the randomized controlled trials. Arch Phys Med Rehabil 1995; 76:508–515.
297. Wade DT, Langton-Hewer R, Skilbeck CE, et al: Stroke: A Critical Approach to Diagnosis, Treatment, and Management. Chicago, Year Book Medical Publishers, 1985.
298. Taub E: Somatosensory deafferentation research with monkeys: Implications for rehabilitation medicine. In Ince LP (ed): Behavioral Psychology in Rehabilitation Medicine: Clinical Applications. Baltimore, Williams & Wilkins, 1980.
299. Taub E, Miller NE, Novack TA, et al: A technique for improving chronic motor deficit after stroke. Arch Phys Med Rehabil 1993; 74:347–354.
300. Wolf SL, LeCraw DE, Barton LA, et al: Forced use of hemiplegic upper extremities to reverse the effect of learned nonuse among chronic stroke and head-injured patients. Exp Neurol 1989; 104:125–132.
301. Barton LA, Wolf SL: Learned nonuse in the hemiplegic upper extremity. In Gordon WA (ed): Advances in Stroke Rehabilitation. Boston, Andover, 1993, pp 79–87.
302. Glanz M, Klawansky S, Stason W, et al: Functional electrostimulation in poststroke rehabilitation: A meta-analysis of the randomized controlled trials. Arch Phys Med Rehabil 1996; 77:549–553.
303. Naeser MA, Alexander MP, Stiassny-Eder D, et al: Acupuncture in the treatment of hand paresis in chronic and acute stroke patients: Improvement observed in all cases. Clin Rehabil 1994; 8:127–141.
304. Johansson K, Lindgren I, Widner H, et al: Can sensory stimulation improve the functional outcome in stroke patients? Neurology 1993; 43:2189–2192.
305. Magnusson M, Johansson K, Johansson BB: Sensory stimulation promotes normalization of postural control after stroke. Stroke 1994; 25:1176–1180.
306. Lorish TR, Sandin KJ, Roth EJ, et al: Stroke rehabilitation: 3. Rehabilitation evaluation and management. Arch Phys Med Rehabil 1994; 75:S47–S51.
307. Morganstein S, Smith MC: Aphasia and right-hemisphere disorders. In Gordon WA (ed): Advances in Stroke Rehabilitation. Boston, Andover, 1993, pp 103–133.
308. Chapey R (ed): Language Intervention Strategies in Adult Aphasia, ed 2. Baltimore, Williams & Wilkins, 1986.
309. Sarno MT (ed): Acquired Aphasia. New York, Academic Press, 1981.
310. LaPointe L: Aphasia therapy: Some principles and strategies for treatment. In Johns DF (ed): Clinical Management of Neurogenic Communicative Disorders. Boston, Little, Brown, 1978.
311. Darley FL: The efficacy of language rehabilitation in aphasia. J Speech Hearing Dis 1972; 37:3–21.
312. Loverso FL, Prexcott TE, Selinger M: Cueing verbs: A treatment strategy for aphasic adults. J Rehabil Res Dev 1988; 25:47–60.
313. Howard D, Patterson K, Franklin S, et al: Treatment of word retrieval deficits in aphasia: A comparison of two therapy methods. Brain 1985; 108:817–829.
314. Shewan CM, Kertesz A: Effects of speech and language treatment on recovery from aphasia. Brain Lang 1984; 23:272–299.
315. Wertz RT, Collins MJ, Weiss D, et al: Veterans Administration Cooperative Study on Aphasia: A comparison of individual and group treatment. J Speech Hearing Res 1981; 24:580–594.
316. Sparks RW, Helm NA, Albert ML: Aphasia rehabilitation resulting from melodic intonation therapy. Cortex 1974; 10:203–216.
317. Therapeutics and Technology Assessment Subcommittee of the American Academy of Neurology: Assessment: Melodic intonation therapy. Neurology 1994; 44:566–568.

318. Helm-Estabrooks N, Emery P, Albert M: Treatment of aphasic perseveration (TAP): A new approach to aphasia therapy. Arch Neurol 1987; 44:1253–1255.
319. Wertz RT, Weiss DG, Aten JL, et al: Comparison of clinic, home, and deferred language treatment for aphasia: A Veterans Administration Cooperative Study. Arch Neurol 1986; 43: 653–658.
320. Shewan C, Bandur D: Treatment of Aphasia: A Language-Oriented Approach. San Diego, College Hill, 1982.
321. Holland A: Pragmatic aspects of intervention in aphasia. J Neurolinguistics 1991; 6:197–211.
322. Weinrich M, Steele R, Carlson G, et al: Processing of visual syntax by a globally aphasic patient. Brain Lang 1989; 36: 391–405.
323. Springer L, Glindemann R, Huber W, et al: How efficacious is PACE therapy when language systematic training is incorporated? Aphasiology 1991; 5:391–399.
324. Till JA, Yorkston KM, Beukelman DR (eds): Motor Speech Disorders: Advances in Assessment and Treatment. Baltimore, Paul H Brookes, 1994.
325. Yorkston KM, Beukelman DR, Bell KR: Clinical Management of Dysarthric Speakers. Austin, Pro-Ed, 1988.
326. Dworkin JP: Motor Speech Disorders: A Treatment Guide. St Louis, Mosby–Year Book, 1991.
327. Berry WR, Sanders SB: Environmental education: The universal management approach for adults with dysarthria. In Berry WR (ed): Clinical Dysarthria. Austin, Pro-Ed, 1983.
328. Gordon WA, Hibbard MR, Egelko S, et al: Perceptual remediation in patients with right brain damage: A comprehensive program. Arch Phys Med Rehabil 1985; 66:353–359.
329. Weinberg J, Diller L, Gordon WA, et al: Training sensory awareness and spatial organization in people with right brain damage. Arch Phys Med Rehabil 1979; 60:491–496.
330. Soderback I, Bengtsson I, Ginsburg E, et al: Video feedback in occupational therapy: Its effect in patients with neglect syndrome. Arch Phys Med Rehabil 1992; 73:1140–1146.
331. Butter CM, Kirsch N: Combined and separate effects of eye patching and visual stimulation on unilateral neglect following stroke. Arch Phys Med Rehabil 1992; 73:1133–1139.
332. Calviano R, Levine D, Petrone P: Elements of cognitive rehabilitation after right hemisphere stroke. Neurol Clin 1993; 11:25–57.
333. Weinberg J, Piasetsky E, Diller L, et al: Treating perceptual organization deficits in nonneglecting RBD stroke patients. J Clin Neuropsychol 1982; 4:59–75.
334. Horner J, Massey EW, Riski JE, et al: Aspiration following stroke: Clinical correlates and outcome. Neurology 1988; 38: 1359–1362.
335. Evans RL, Northwood L: Social support needs in adjustment to stroke. Arch Phys Med Rehabil 1983; 64:61–64.
336. Evans RL, Matlock A-L, Bishop DS, et al: Family intervention after stroke: Does counseling or education help? Stroke 1988; 19:1243–1249.
337. Robinson RG, Lipsey JR, Price TR: Depression: An often overlooked sequela of stroke. Geriatric Med Today 1984; 3:35–45.
338. Coll P, Erickson RV: Mood disorders associated with stroke. Phys Med Rehabil State Art Rev 1989; 3:619–628.
339. Binder LM: Emotional problems after stroke. Stroke 1984; 15:174–177.
340. Robinson RG, Szetela B: Mood change following left hemisphere brain injury. Ann Neurol 1981; 9:447–452.
341. Finkelstein S, Berkowitz LI, Baldessarini RJ: Mood vegetative disturbance, and dexamethasone suppression test after stroke. Ann Neurol 1982; 12:463–468.
342. Robinson RG, Starr LB, Kubos KL: A two-year longitudinal study of post-stroke mood disorders: Findings during the initial evaluation. Stroke 1983; 14:736–741.
343. Robinson RG, Kubos KL, Starr LB: Mood disorders in stroke patients: Importance of lesion location. Brain 1984; 107:81–93.
344. Robinson RG, Starr LB, Price TR: A two-year longitudinal study of mood disorders following stroke: Prevalence and duration at six months follow-up. Br J Psychiatry 1984; 144:256–262.
345. Parikh RM, Lipsey JR, Robinson RG: Two-year longitudinal study of post-stroke mood disorders: Dynamic changes in correlates of depression at one and two years. Stroke 1987; 18:579–584.
346. Reding MJ, Orto LA, Winter SW: Antidepressant therapy after stroke. Arch Neurol 1986; 43:763–766.
347. Lipsey JR, Robinson RG, Pearlson GD: Nortriptyline treatment of post-stroke depression: A double-blind study. Lancet 1984; 1:297–300.
348. Fugl-Meyer AR, Jaasko L: Post-stroke hemiplegia and sexual intercourse. Scand J Rehabil Med 1980; 7:158–166.
349. Monga TN, Lawson JS, Inglis J: Sexual dysfunction in stroke patients. Arch Phys Med Rehabil 1986; 67:19–22.
350. Bray GP, DeFrank PRS, Wolfe TL: Sexual functioning in stroke survivors. Arch Phys Med Rehabil 1981; 62:286–288.
351. Sjogren K, Fugl-Meyer AR: Adjustment to life after stroke with special reference to sexual intercourse and leisure. J Psychosom Res 1982; 26:409–417.
352. Freda M, Rubinsky H: Sexual function in the stroke survivor. Phys Med Rehabil Clin North Am 1991; 2:643–658.
353. Stein PN, Berger AL, Hibbard MR, et al: Intervention with the spouses of stroke survivors. In Advances in Stroke Rehabilitation. Boston, Andover, 1993, pp. 242–257.
354. Ragnarsson KT: Orthotics and shoes. In DeLisa JA (ed): Rehabilitation Medicine. Philadelphia, JB Lippincott, 1988, pp 307–329.
355. Friedland JF, McColl M: Social support intervention after stroke: Results of a randomized trial. Arch Phys Med Rehabil 1992; 73:573–581.
356. Evans RL, Matlock AL, Bishop DS, et al: Family intervention after stroke: Does counseling or education help? Stroke 1988; 19:1243–1249.
357. Poduri KR, Steimer SL: Comprehensive outpatient approach to stroke rehabilitation. J Stroke Cerebrovasc Dis 1993; 3:29–48.
358. Kamen LB: Issues in outpatient rehabilitation management of the stroke survivor. Phys Med Rehabil Clin North Am 1991; 2:615–626.
359. Dombovy ML, Sandok BA, Basford JA: Rehabilitation after stroke: A review. Stroke 1986; 17:363–369.
360. Chin PL, Rosie A, Irving M: Studies in hemiplegic gait. In Rose FC (ed): Advances in Stroke Therapy. New York, Raven Press, 1982.
361. Jongbloed L: Prediction of function after stroke: A critical review. Stroke 1986; 17:765–775.
362. Davidoff G, Keren O, Ring H, et al: Assessing candidates for inpatient stroke rehabilitation: Predictors of outcome. Phys Med Rehabil Clin North Am 1991; 2:501–516.
363. Johnston MV, Kirshblum S, Zorowitz RD, et al: Prediction of outcomes following rehabilitation of stroke patient. Neurorehabil 1992; 2:72–97.
364. Wade DT, Skilbeck CG, Hewer RL: Predicting Barthel ADL score at 6 months after an acute stroke. Arch Phys Med Rehabil 1983; 64:24–28.
365. Strand T, Asplund K, Eriksson S, et al: A non-intensive stroke unit reduces functional disability and the need for long-term hospitalization. Stroke 1985; 16:29–34.
366. Kalra L, Dale P, Crome P: Improving stroke rehabilitation. Stroke 1993; 24:1462–1467.
367. Kalra L, Eade J: Role of stroke rehabilitation units in managing severe disability after stroke. Stroke 1995; 26:2031–2034.
368. Kaste M, Palomaki H, Sarna S: Where and how should elderly stroke patients be treated? A randomized trial. Stroke 1995; 26:249–253.
369. Sivenius J, Pyorala K, Heinonen OP, et al: The significance of intensity of stroke: A controlled trial. Stroke 1985; 16:928–931.
370. Stevens RS, Ambler NR, Warren MD: A randomized controlled trial of a stroke rehabilitation ward. Age Ageing 1984; 13:65–75.
371. Wood-Dauphinee S, Shapiro S, Bass E, et al: A randomized trial of team care following stroke. Stroke 1984; 15:864–872.
372. Ottenbacher KJ, Jannell S: The results of clinical trials in stroke rehabilitation research. Arch Neurol 1993; 50:37–44.
373. Langhorne P, Williams BO, Gilchrist W, et al: Do stroke units save lives? Lancet 1993; 342:395–398.
374. Tangeman PT, Banaitis DA, Williams AK: Rehabilitation of chronic stroke patients: Changes in functional performance. Arch Phys Med Rehabil 1990; 71:876–880.
375. Dam M, Tonin P, Casson S, et al: The effects of long-term rehabilitation therapy on poststroke hemiplegic patients. Stroke 1993; 24:1186–1191.

376. Wade DT, Collin FM, Robb GF, et al: Physiotherapy intervention late after stroke and mobility. Br Med J 1992; 304:609–613.
377. Young J, Forster A: Day hospital and home physiotherapy for stroke patients: A comparative cost-effectiveness study. J R Coll Phys London 1993; 27:253–258.
378. Young J, Forster A: The Bradford community stroke trial: Eight week results. Clin Rehabil 1991; 5:283–292.
379. Gladman JRF, Lincoln NB, Barer DH: A randomised controlled trial of domiciliary and hospital-based rehabilitation for stroke patients after discharge from hospital. J Neurol Neurosurg Psychiatry 1993; 56:960–966.
380. Gladman JRF, Lincoln NB: Follow-up of a controlled trial of domiciary stroke rehabilitation (DOMINO Study). Age Ageing 1994; 23:9–13.
381. Gladman JRF, Whynes D, Lincoln N: Cost comparison of domiciary and hospital-based stroke rehabilitation. Age Ageing 1994; 23:241–245.
382. Reding MJ, McDowell FH: Focused stroke rehabilitation programs improve outcome. Arch Neurol 1989; 46:700–701.
383. Dobkin BH: Focused stroke rehabilitation programs do not improve outcome. Arch Neurol 1989; 46:701–703.
384. Biller J, Matthews KD, Love BB: Stroke in Children and Young Adults. Boston, Butterworth-Heinemann, 1994.
385. Weinfeld FD: The national survey of stroke. Stroke 1981; 12(suppl I):I1–I68.
386. Hart RG, Miller VT: Cerebral infarction in young adults: A practical approach. Curr Concepts Cerebrovasc Dis 1982; 17:15–20.
387. Hachinski V, Norris JW: The Acute Stroke. Philadelphia, FA Davis, 1985.
388. Coull BM: Stroke in the young patient: Coagulation disturbances. Stroke Clin Update 1990; 1:9–12.
389. Love BB, Biller J: Stroke in the young: Cardiac causes. Stroke Clin Update 1990; 1:13–16.
390. Black-Schaffer RM, Osberg JS: Return to work after stroke: Development of a predictive model. Arch Phys Med Rehabil 1990; 71:285–290.
391. Kertesz A, McCabe P: Recovery patterns and prognosis in aphasia. Brain 1977; 100:1–18.
392. van Zomeren AH, Brouwer WH; Minderhoud JM: Acquired brain damage and driving: A review. Arch Phys Med Rehabil 1987; 68:697–705.
393. Niemi M-L, Laaksonen R, Kotila M, et al: Quality of life 4 years after stroke. Stroke 1988; 19:1101–1107.
394. Oehring AK, Oakley JL: The young stroke patient: A need for specialized group support systems. Top Stroke Rehabil 1994; 1:25–40.
395. Black-Schaffer RM, Lemieux L: Vocational outcome after stroke. Top Stroke Rehabil 1994; 1:74–86.
396. Kempers E: Preparing the young stroke survivor for return to work. Top Stroke Rehabil 1994; 1:65–73.
397. Culler KH, Jasch C, Scanlan S: Child care and parenting issues for the young stroke survivor. Top Stroke Rehabil 1994; 1:48–64.
398. Andrews K, Brocklehurst JC, Richards B, et al: The influence of age on the clinical presentation and outcome of stroke. Int Rehabil Med 1984; 6:49–51.
399. Great Britain Department of Health: Stroke rehabilitation. Effective Health Care 1992; 2:1–11.

A

Appendix

Selected Interventions to Meet Specific Patient Needs

MEDICAL-PHYSIOLOGICAL FUNCTION

1. Prevent intercurrent complication
   - Position properly and turn frequently
   - Frequent passive range-of-motion exercises
   - Deep breathing and coughing exercises
   - Pharmacological and physical methods of preventing thromboembolic disease
   - Stroke prevention measures (e.g., anticoagulants or antithrombotic agents)
2. Treat medical complications (e.g., infections)
3. Treat spasticity and contracture
   - Prevent and treat medical complications
   - Stretching program
   - Positioning program
   - Splinting
   - Joint mobilization and manipulation
   - Forced weight bearing
   - Serial casting
   - Physical modalities, e.g., cold application
   - Injections: peripheral nerve and motor point blocks
   - Pharmacological measures
   - Biofeedback
   - Electrical stimulation
   - Tendon lengthening and contracture release surgery
   - Neurosurgical techniques
4. Treat pain (hemiplegic shoulder pain, reflex sympathetic dystrophy syndrome, other musculoskeletal pain, central poststroke pain)
   - Proper positioning, elevation, using slings, tray, armrests, supports
   - Edema reduction methods: elevation, massage, stockings, gloves, range-of-motion exercises
   - Tone reduction methods: stretching exercises, nerve or motor point blocks, medications
   - Physical modalities: ice, heat, ultrasound, others
   - Medications: analgesics, anti-inflammatory agents
   - Injections: peripheral nerve, motor point, sympathetic ganglion, etc.
   - Neurosurgical procedures
5. Manage co-morbid conditions, review and adjust medications (e.g., diabetes, hypertension, heart disease, arthritis)
6. Manage ongoing physiological functions
   - Nutrition assessment and management
   - Hydration assessment and management
   - Feeding tube management
   - Tracheostomy management
   - Timed, scheduled toileting program
   - Dietary fiber
   - Mobilization
   - Train toilet transfers
   - Catheterization program
   - Medication
   - Treat bladder and bowel infections
7. Prevent and treat fatigue, deconditioning, orthostatic intolerance, and endurance limitations
   - Treat medical conditions
   - Ensure adequate sleep, rest, nutrition, hydration, and appropriate medication use
   - Reassurance
   - Adjust therapy schedule to balance need for rest with need for mobilization and exercise

- Progressively increase mobilization times and amounts
- Endurance training

SENSORY-MOTOR DEFICITS

1. Prevent effects of prolonged immobility (e.g., contracture, orthostatic hypotension)
   - Early, cautious, and supervised exercise and remobilization
   - Early and frequent activation
   - Early and consistent performance of activities of daily living (ADL)
   - Conventional stretching exercises
   - Conventional strengthening exercises: active assistive, active, progressive resistive
2. Facilitate natural motor recovery of strength and control, including balance and fine motor control
   - Conventional strengthening exercises: active assistive, active, progressive resistive
   - Balance training
   - Trunk control exercises
   - Mat mobility exercises
   - Standing exercises
   - Weight-shifting exercises
   - Fine motor control finger exercises
   - Practice functional tasks requiring fine motor control
   - Exercise in specific positions: e.g., sitting, standing, kneeling
   - Neurophysiological facilitation and inhibition techniques
     - Neurodevelopmental treatment (Bobath)
     - Proprioceptive neuromuscular facilitation
     - Movement therapy (Brunnstrom)
     - Motor program for stroke (Carr and Shepherd)
     - Sensory facilitation (Rood)
     - Others
   - Use of facilitatory or inhibitory modalities simultaneously with volitional muscle contraction (e.g., quick stretch, stroking, tapping, vibration, brushing)
3. Teach compensatory functional strategies
   - Self-care; feeding, dressing, hygiene, grooming, toileting, bathing, telephone use
   - Mobility: sitting, bed mobility, rolling, transfers (bed, bath, toilet, car), wheelchair propulsion, walking, stairs
   - Community motor skills, instrumental ADL, laundry, meal preparation, shopping, housecleaning, child care, other community skills
4. Newer approaches to motor control enhancement
   - Behavioral techniques
     - Electromyographic-biofeedback
     - Positional biofeedback
     - Force biofeedback
     - Forced-use
   - Electrical stimulation
5. Orthotics, assistive devices, durable medical equipment, other aids
   - Dynamic orthoses
   - Tone-reducing orthoses
   - Static orthoses (e.g., resting hand splint)
   - Wheelchair
   - Bath bench
   - Reacher, other ADL aids
   - Walker, hemiwalker, quad cane, straight cane
   - Training in use of devices
6. Rehabilitation engineering and technology
7. Surgical intervention
   - Tendon releases
8. Family education

COGNITIVE-COMMUNICATION-OROMOTOR DEFICITS

1. Evaluate and treat dysarthria
   - Oromotor strengthening exercises
   - Enunciation practice
   - Alternative communication training
2. Evaluate and treat aphasia
   - Traditional modality-specific stimulus–response therapy
   - Language-oriented treatment
   - Treatment of aphasic perseveration
   - Visual action therapy
   - Conversational coaching
   - Functional communication therapy
   - Melodic intonation therapy
   - Programmed approaches
   - Response elaboration training
   - Auditory comprehension training
   - Computerized approaches
   - C-VIC
   - Promoting aphasic communicative effectiveness
   - Cognitive intervention
   - Augmentation approaches
   - Groups
   - Oral reading (reading aloud)
   - General stimulation
   - Compensatory/alternative communication training
   - Gestures
   - Writing
   - Electronic technology
3. Swallowing assessment and management
   - Thermal stimulation
   - Change head and neck position
   - Diet adjustment
   - Alter food quantity
   - Alternative nutrition routes if needed
   - Patient and family training
4. Cognitive evaluation and training (inattention, poor concentration, memory deficits, disorientation, concrete thinking, apraxia)
   - Cognitive skills training
   - Computer technology training
   - Memory strategy training
   - Memory book
   - Mnemonics
5. Perceptual evaluation and training (agnosias, unilateral neglect, right-left disorientation, impaired

sense of verticality, impaired time perception, impaired depth perception)
- Environmental adaptation
- Teaching of strategies
- Anchoring
- Pacing
- Density
- Feedback
- Scanning training
- Compensatory techniques
- Supplying cues and reminders
- Forced-use
- Eye patch use

PSYCHOLOGICAL AND SOCIAL ISSUES

1. Promote psychological adaptation and coping; treat poststroke mood disorders (depression, fear, anger, anxiety, lability)
   - Supportive counseling
   - Family involvement
   - Team approach
   - Positive reinforcement
   - Milieu therapy
   - Peer support
   - Social recreational activities
   - Antianxiety medications
   - Antidepressant medications
   - Relaxation training
   - Stroke support group
2. Evaluation and management of behavioral changes (impulsivity, aggressiveness, quick temper, rage, apathy)
   - Counseling
   - Redirection, refocusing
   - Low-stimulation environment
   - Safety education
   - Family education
   - Medication
3. Promote family and caregiver coping and stress management
   - Family education: team-family meetings, classes, brochures, books, videotapes
   - Functional skills training and practice
   - Family individual counseling
   - Family support groups

51 CHAPTER

Mary L. Dombovy, M.D., and Barbara A. Pippin, M.D.

Rehabilitation Concerns in Degenerative Movement Disorders of the Central Nervous System

The general category of movement disorders includes a number of central nervous system (CNS) neurodegenerative diseases such as Parkinson's disease and other brainstem-basal ganglia degenerations, the hereditary ataxias, and the dystonias (Table 51–1). Parkinson's disease is by far the most common, affecting 1% of the population 65 years old and over.[8] Many of the symptoms and signs of Parkinson's disease can be seen in other neurodegenerative disorders, as well as in anoxic encephalopathy, multiple lacunar infarcts, drug effects, and the normal aging process[34] (Table 51–2). "Parkinsonism" is commonly seen in patients on rehabilitation units. Unfortunately, the benefits of rehabilitation and specific therapy approaches for Parkinson's and other movement disorders remain unclear.

This chapter discusses the differential diagnosis of parkinsonism, the medical treatment of Parkinson's disease (Fig. 51–1), and rehabilitation of Parkinson's disease as a prototype for rehabilitation of parkinsonism in other disorders. Rehabilitation in the hereditary ataxias and the treatment of dystonia receive brief additional comment at the end of the chapter.

PARKINSON'S DISEASE

Pathophysiology, Clinical Presentation, and Differential Diagnosis

Parkinson's disease is characterized pathologically by degeneration of pigmented and other brainstem nuclei, particularly the substantia nigra, in association with the formation of eosinophilic neuronal inclusions called Lewy bodies.[5, 18] The primary biochemical defect in Parkinson's disease is the loss of striatal dopamine resulting from the degeneration of dopamine-producing cells in the substantia nigra. There is an associated hyperactivity of cholinergic neurons in the caudate nuclei contributing to the symptoms.[3] The four most prominent hypotheses regarding the etiology of Parkinson's disease are the theories of (1) accelerated aging, (2) toxin exposure, (3) genetic predisposition, and (4) oxidative stress. Although it is likely that all four processes contribute to the development of Parkinson's, the oxidative mechanism theory has received the most support to date.[27] Parkinson's disease is associated with increased activity of superoxide dismutase, which generates hydrogen peroxide, an oxygen radical. A decrease in radical scavengers, such as catalase and gluthathione, which break down hydrogen peroxide into water and hydrogen, is also seen in Parkinson's. All of these abnormalities are apparent only in the substantia nigra. Impaired mitochondrial respiratory mechanisms, manifested as reduced mitochondrial complex 1, results in increased oxygen-free radicals in patients with Parkinson's disease.[65]

Although Parkinson's disease can present with an array of clinical symptoms and signs (Table 51–3), the cardinal features of the disease are (1) resting or postural tremor, (2) bradykinesia, (3) rigidity, and (4) postural instability. In the early stages of Parkinson's disease, rigidity (often described as "stiffness" or "achiness" by patients) can be mistaken as a symptom

TABLE 51–1 Selected Central Nervous System Movement Disorders

Idiopathic	*Secondary*
Parkinson's disease	Birth injury
Progressive supranuclear palsy (Steele-Richardson-Olszewski syndrome)	Chorea gravidarum
Multiple system atrophy (Shy-Drager syndrome)	Neuroleptic medications
Corticobasal degeneration	Head injury
Most dystonias	Cerebral infarct/hemorrhage
Blepharospasm	Anoxia
Meige's disease	Carbon monoxide poisoning
Gilles de la Tourette's syndrome	Manganese poisoning
Genetic	Mercury poisoning
Huntington's disease	Basal ganglia tumor
Wilson's disease	Liver disease
Some dystonias	Oral contraceptives
Inherited ataxias	Hyperthyroidism and hypothyroidism
Numerous metabolic defects	Hypoparathyroidism
Ataxia telangiectasia	Alcohol
Olivopontocerebellar degeneration	Sydenham's chorea
Friedreich's ataxia (and others)	von Economo's encephalitis
Familial nonprogressive chorea	
Essential tremor	
Hallervorden-Spatz disease	

of arthritis. Masked facies and bradykinesia can lead to the most common early misdiagnosis, that of depression. The onset and progression of the disease are slow and insidious. The disease can begin either with tremor or with bradykinesia and rigidity as the initial presentation. Symptoms and signs typically begin in one extremity or one side but eventually spread to involve the other limbs and trunk. Lack of arm swing when walking and changes in handwriting (micrographia) are early signs.

Although tremor can become disabling, it usually does not impair function as much as bradykinesia and rigidity, which eventually lead to problems in all areas of mobility and activities of daily living (ADL). When ambulating, patients have difficulty in changing direction or moving around objects and can "freeze," unable to start again. Patients with Parkinson's disease have great difficulty in carrying out two simultaneous but unrelated motor acts, such as talking or taking notes while walking, throwing or reaching while walking, etc.

TABLE 51–2 Differential Diagnosis of Parkinsonism

Idiopathic Parkinson's disease*,†
Progressive supranuclear palsy*
Multiple system atrophy*
Oliropontocerebellar atrophy*
Striatonigral degeneration
Wilson's disease†
Westphal variant of Huntington's disease†
Corticobasal degeneration
Hallervorden-Spatz disease
Alzheimer's disease (late stages)
Parkinson-ALS-dementia complex
Post encephalitis
Drug-induced*,† (neuroleptics,*,† metaclopramide,*,† reserpine†)
Toxin-induced*,† (MPTP,† manganese,† carbon monoxide,*,† carbon disulfide,† cyanide†)
Metabolic*,† (anoxia,* hypothyroidism,*,† hypoparathyroidism*,†)
Multi-infarcts*,†
Subdural hemotoma*,†
Multiple head injuries (boxer's dementia†)
Basal ganglia tumor*,†
Normal-pressure hydrocephalus*,†

* Most common considerations.
† Important to consider and rule out.
Abbreviations: ALS, amyotrophic lateral sclerosis; MPTP, 1-methyl-4-phenyl-1,2,3,6-tetrahydropyridine.

Impairment of speech is one of the most frustrating disabilities for patients with Parkinson's disease. Speech becomes rapid, monotonous, and of low volume (hypokinetic dysarthria). Speech and handwriting can be affected by the same phenomenon that causes festinating gait.

Since the basal ganglia play an important role in motor planning and programming, Parkinson's disease patients display various degrees of difficulty with initiating an activity such as walking, reaching for objects, or changing course when walking. There is a loss of normal associated or preparatory movements such as arm swing in gait and positioning the feet back and inclining forward prior to rising from a chair.

As Parkinson's disease progresses, autonomic symptoms (slowed enteric mobility and constipation, urinary retention and incontinence, orthostatic hypotension), dysphagia, and postural instability become bothersome. Dementia is often a late feature and ultimately appears in about one-third of the patients. Depression can affect as many as 50% of the patients. Dementia and depression can be difficult to diagnose in the presence of psychomotor retardation (a slowness in producing the motor response). Hallucinations, insomnia, nausea, lack of appetite, weight loss, and dystonia are often encountered side effects of dopaminergic medications. Insomnia is also seen as the result of nocturnal bradykinesia.

Typically there is a gradual increase over time in all of the manifestations of Parkinson's disease. Before the advent of levodopa therapy, 25% of patients with symptom duration of less than 5 years were severely disabled, and 75% of survivors with symptom duration of 10 to

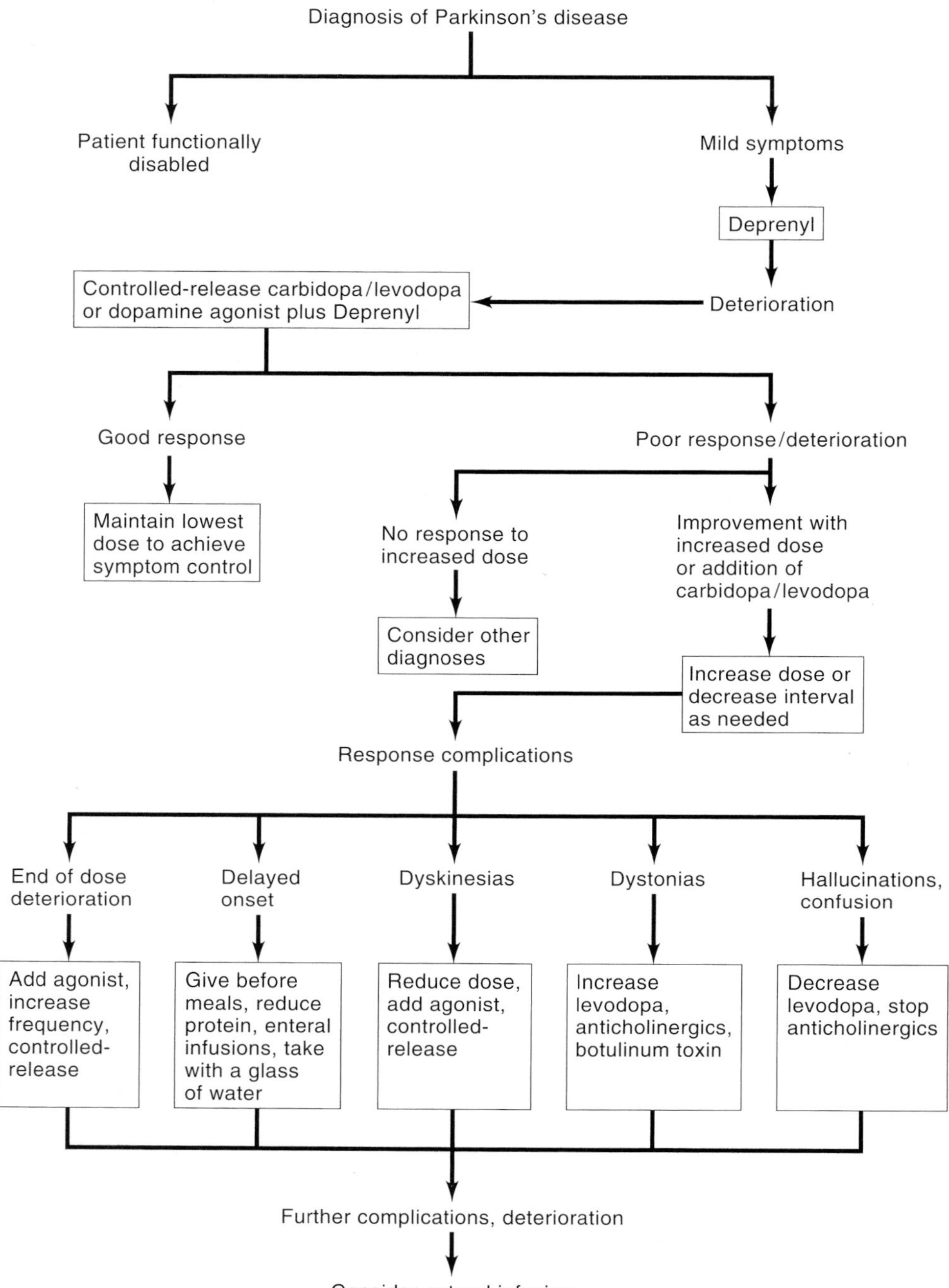

FIGURE 51–1. Sample of an algorithm for medical therapeutics in Parkinson's disease.

15 years were totally disabled. Patients having rigidity as the predominant initial symptom tend to experience disability earlier than those with tremor as the presenting feature. The introduction of levodopa, deprenyl (selegiline), and novel medication management strategies has prolonged independence and has allowed for continued employment in many cases.

Early Parkinson's disease can be difficult to distinguish from other subcortical degenerations. The hallmarks of Parkinson's disease are a definite response to levodopa treatment and the absence of symptoms and signs such as early vertical eye movement abnormalities (progressive supranuclear palsy [PSP]), early autonomic failure (Shy-Drager syndrome), hyperreflexia, Babinski's signs, ataxia, and peripheral neuropathy (multisystem degeneration). While other parkinsonian states sometimes show a mild to moderate response to levodopa, the beneficial effects are usually transient. One should always seek to exclude other nondegenerative causes such as drug and toxin exposure (see Table 51–2).

A number of medications are utilized in the management of Parkinson's disease (see Table 51–4). Levodopa

TABLE 51–3 Clinical Features of Parkinson's Disease

Symptoms and Signs	*Common Presenting Complaints*
Rigidity	Stiffness, aching muscular pain, slowed movements
Bradykinesia (slowness of movement)	Trouble getting out of a chair
Resting/postural tremor	Trouble rolling over in bed
Hypokinesia (small-amplitude movement)	Falling, tripping over objects on floor
Loss of postural reflexes	Tremor, "shaking"
Loss of preparatory and associated movements ("en bloc" movements, decreased arm swing, decreased blinking)	Depression
Akathisia (inability to sit still, relieved by walking about)	Memory loss
Dementia	Stooped posture
Autonomic dysfunction (orthostatic hypotension, slowed gastrointestinal motility, urinary retention, impotence)	Rapid or whispering speech
Hypokinetic dysarthria	Change in handwriting
Festinating gait	Slowness in activities, dressing, grooming
Masked facies (stare with decreased blinking)	Trouble walking
Dystonia	Slow to respond to questions and requests
Flexed posture	Drooling; trouble controlling saliva
Dysphagia	
Sudden "freezing" of motor activity	

combined with carbidopa (a peripheral dopa decarboxylase inhibitor, e.g., Sinemet) remains the cornerstone of pharmacological therapy for Parkinson's disease,[60] although controversy exists as to when treatment with levodopa should begin.[28] More than half of the patients with Parkinson's disease who receive treatment with conventional levodopa preparations later develop response complications, including a shortened response duration. The mechanisms of these complications are not completely understood, although emerging data seem to suggest the development of toxic oxygen free radicals with the use of levodopa. Dopamine, which is markedly elevated after the administration of levodopa, produces hydrogen peroxide by auto-oxidation and due to the effect of monoamine oxidase B (MAO-B).[42] Levodopa can also be converted to levodopa free radical. In addition, wide fluctuations in dopamine levels, disease-related changes in presynaptic handling of levodopa, and receptor alterations all might contribute.[49] Some treating physicians delay levodopa therapy until symptoms significantly interfere with function, or they begin treatment with a direct dopamine receptor agonist such as pergolide or bromocriptine.[60]

Since the late 1980s, results from the Parkinson Study Group suggest that monoamine oxidase B inhibitors such as deprenyl also exert a mild dopaminergic effect, which could also have produced the noted delay in disability in treated patients. Some treating physicians begin treatment of early Parkinson's disease with deprenyl due to its therapeutic effects and the potential that it might slow disease progression.[42, 43, 47, 63] Some of the effects of MAO-B antagonists such as deprenyl might be due to their inhibition of oxygen radical generation of dopamine by monoamine oxidase B. Deprenyl also can be used to smooth out levodopa-related fluctuations later in the disease.

Since the late 1980s, sustained-release levodopa combination preparations have become available (Sinemet CR, Madopar HBS). Peak dopamine levels are low and therapeutic levels are sustained, hence the potential for reducing symptom fluctuation. Bioavailability is less than with immediate-release preparations, and when switching from immediate release, the total levodopa dose usually needs to be increased. An additional advantage of sustained-release preparations is the reduction of the profound alterations in levodopa plasma concentrations that are thought to contribute to some of the later problems with dyskinesia and other dose-response fluctuations. Although the manufacturer indicates that twice-daily dosing is adequate with Sinemet CR, most patients achieve a smoother response dosing three times a day and eventually four times a day. The use of catechol *O*-methyltransferase (COMT) inhibitors has been shown to prolong the biologic half-life of levodopa. COMT metabolizes levodopa in the periphery to 3-*O*-methyldopa, effectively lowering functional brain levels of levodopa. COMT inhibitors increase the bioavailability of levodopa and smooth the fluctuations of plasma levels of levodopa.[31]

Variable gastric emptying is often a feature of advanced Parkinson's disease, and can lead to an apparent lack of response to oral medication. Jejunal infusion via a pump delivery system has been employed in some cases. Jejunal infusion has also been used in instances in which motor fluctuations and wearing-off effects are prominent even if gastric retention is not a problem.[11, 51] Enteral tubes are a consideration when dysphagia has progressed to the point of inadequate nutrition or there is a high risk of aspiration. Improvement in gastric emptying can also be achieved by administering a large glass of water with oral levodopa or carbidopa.

Direct dopamine agonists (DAs) such as bromocriptine and pergolide have emerged as a significant therapeutic addition to levodopa.[41] These compounds directly stimulate dopamine receptors independent of levodopa. The neurotoxic effects of levodopa are potentially avoided. DAs also scavenge oxygen radicals, suppress lipid peroxidation, and decrease dopamine release and turnover, all of which are neuroprotective. DA monotherapy has been shown to be effective for a majority of patients at 1 year, but was effective only for a small percentage (2% to 17%) at 5 years. A number of studies have shown that the combination of DA and levodopa is more effective than levodopa alone in preserving motor activity and minimizing dyskinesia at five-year follow-up. Some investigators suggest the use of DA monotherapy early, with addition of levodopa only when DA can no longer satisfactorily control the symptoms. The use of DA monotherapy and its timing is clearly still controversial.

Amantadine, which has both pre- and postsynaptic dopaminergic effects, is also used both as early treatment and later as an adjunct. Anticholinergics (e.g., trihexyphenidyl [Artane], benztropine [Cogentin]) are helpful when tremor is the predominant problem, but become less well tolerated as Parkinson's disease progresses. This is due to such side effects as sedation, impaired memory, and urinary retention. The use of anticholinergics to treat Parkinson's disease has decreased over the past 5 years.

Considering recent research and theory, a reasonable approach to initial treatment of Parkinson's disease[43] would be to: (1) introduce deprenyl at the time of early diagnosis; (2) begin a low dose of a dopamine agonist, either with or without a long-acting levodopa preparation, when symptomatic treatment becomes functionally indicated; and (3) titrate levodopa dosages as symptom control warrants, using the lowest dose required for adequate function. This approach is particularly reasonable for younger and middle-aged patients with Parkinson's disease. It should be noted that there appears to be declining enthusiasm for the use of deprenyl. Multiple drug approaches can produce significant side effects in the elderly, and can lead to decreased compliance with the medication program. Many treating physicians prefer to initiate the treatment of older patients with immediate release Sinemet and to titrate the dose depending on the patient's tolerance and the therapeutic response. The management of dose-response fluctuations, dyskinesia, and the "on/off" phenomenon is complex and can be frustrating. Consultation with a neurologist having expertise in the management of patients with advanced Parkinson's disease is usually required to provide optimal medication adjustment.

Most patients with Parkinson's disease experience varying degrees of side effects from the medications, particularly in later stages. Some patients are intolerant of levodopa on an empty stomach, in which case beginning with a smaller dose is helpful. If food must be taken, a high protein intake should be avoided. The potential side effects of these medications are numerous, and it is important to be aware of them in the rehabilitation setting. Table 51–4 lists the potential side effects by drug class.

TABLE 51–4 Common Side Effects of Medications Used in Parkinson's Disease

Carbidopa-levodopa compounds	Nausea, hypotension, arrhythmias, hallucinations, nightmares, hypomania, paranoid psychosis, delirium, insomnia, dystonia, dyskinesias
Deprenyl (selegiline)	Cardiac toxicity, hallucinations; potentiates side effects of levodopa
Amantadine	Hallucinations, insomnia, nervousness, edema, livedo reticularis, headache
Dopaminergic agonists	Hallucinations, vivid dreams, psychosis, paranoia
Anticholinergics	Impaired memory, confusion, urinary retention, blurred vision, dry mouth, constipation, orthostatic hypotension

The Rationale for Rehabilitation

Many experts in the treatment of Parkinson's disease recommend rehabilitative services as an adjunct to medical therapy[24, 37, 60] because it "intuitively" makes sense that these services can prevent complications and either maintain or assist with function. In addition, patients with Parkinson's disease often state that they "feel" or function better with a program of regular exercise. It is not clear whether this results from a general sense of well-being or the general conditioning effect that often occurs with exercise, from true improvement in function, or from actual improvement in some of the deficits of Parkinson's disease (e.g., bradykinesia, rigidity).

The literature on the benefits of rehabilitation services for patients is sparse. Most of the studies suffer from methodological problems such as lack of controls or blinding, inappropriate or nonvalidated assessment measures, and small numbers of subjects. The studies are not comparable because they use different therapy approaches with different levels of intensity over varying time frames. What outcome measures to choose is also a major question. Should the focus be on whether specific exercise programs, speech therapy techniques, etc., improve the neurological deficit? Or should the focus be on improved function, regardless of whether there has been any improvement in bradykinesia, hypokinesia, or rigidity? A few recent reviews have attempted to assess the efficacy of nonpharmacological therapy for patients with Parkinson's disease.[9, 12, 64] The reader is referred to them for a more detailed review.

The Parkinson's disease rehabilitation programs evaluated in studies range from home-based,[4, 26, 38] to outpatient physical (PT) or occupational therapy (OT),[13, 19, 22, 45, 62] or both, or from speech therapy (ST),[1, 23, 50, 53, 58, 59] to comprehensive inpatient programs.[12, 61] In general, the results suggest a benefit in patients with Parkinson's disease of an exercise program that focuses on improving range-of-motion (ROM), endurance, balance, and gait.[13, 19, 26, 38, 45] The efficacy of more functionally oriented programs has not been assessed, although Parkinson's disease patients report that the provision of equipment and instruction in adaptive techniques provided by OT in the home was helpful to them.[4] Small numbers of subjects and the lack of controls, as well as changes in medication, make the composite results less than conclusive. An enhanced sense of well-being can also contribute to the improvements noted in function.

Comella et al[13] recently conducted a prospective, randomized, single-blind crossover study of the effects of a 4-week outpatient physical rehabilitation program on mentation, ADL, and motor function, as measured by the Unified Parkinson's Disease Rating Scale (UPDRS).[17] Sixteen moderate to moderately severe Parkinson's disease patients were seen for 1 hour three times per week for 4 weeks by physical and occupational therapists. The program consisted of repetitive exercises directed at improving ROM, balance, fine motor dexterity, gait, and endurance. The intensity of the program was increased as endurance improved. The control group received no intervention. Two 4-week study periods were separated by 6 months. Medication changes were not allowed during the control or therapy phases, but adjustments were permitted during the 6-month interval between study periods as well as during the follow-up period.

Following the physical rehabilitation program there was a significant improvement in ADL and motor function (bradykinesia and rigidity), but no improvement in tremor, timed finger tapping, mentation, or mood. Despite instructions to the subjects to continue the exercise program at home at the completion of the rehabilitation phase, all resumed a more sedentary lifestyle; and at 6-month follow-up, the UPDRS scores returned to baseline. Continued exercise might be needed to maintain function, but permanently incorporating such a program into a patient's lifestyle without continuation of an organized program appears unlikely.

Interestingly, Palmer et al[45] found improvements in gait, tremor, motor coordination, and grip strength in Parkinson's disease patients in an exercise program, regardless of whether the program was that developed by the United Parkinson Foundation or a group in karate training! Such a program could be more easily continued in a group format at a community gymnasium or other facility in a more cost-effective fashion, with the additional benefit of increasing socialization.

Although speech and swallowing disorders are commonly a source of disability in Parkinson's disease,[14] speech therapy is likely underutilized.[40] Families often complain that speech is improved as long as the patient is receiving therapy, but as soon as the therapy ends, speech reverts to the previous pattern. This clinical experience is supported by the work of Sarno,[53] who noted in a study of 300 patients with Parkinson's disease that speech improved only during treatment. Allan[1] also reported rapid deterioration in formal speech therapy. The specific type of speech therapy might be important in terms of benefit and carryover. Another study[50] reported that intensive speech therapy (group and individual therapy lasting 3½ to 4 hours per day of 2 weeks duration) produced a positive effect on speech in Parkinson's disease patients, with some benefits lasting up to 3 months. Therapy focused on voice and respiratory control, loudness, pitch variation, and control of rate of speech.

In a series of studies, Scott and Caird[58, 59] demonstrated that speech therapy consisting of intonational and prosodic exercises produced improvements in speech, some of which lasted up to 3 months. The treatment program consisted of daily 1-hour sessions carried out in the patients home over 2 to 3 weeks. It appears that the types of motor deficits in Parkinson's disease resulting in both the physical symptoms and speech impairment improve with a program that provides regular and continuing intervention.

Another speech disorder common in Parkinson's disease and other neurological disorders (e.g., Alzheimer's disease, multi-infarct dementia) is palilalia. Palilalia is characterized by the repetition of a word or phrase with increasing rapidity and decreasing distinctiveness, and eventually becoming inaudible. The use of a pacing board has been noted to be helpful in decreasing palilalia.[38]

Studies addressing the benefits of inpatient rehabilitation in Parkinson's disease are few, as patients with Parkinson's disease are not commonly admitted to inpatient rehabilitation units. This likely reflects the societal view that patients with degenerative disorders are not candidates for inpatient rehabilitation because of resource utilization and cost concerns. Stern et al[61] studied 47 Parkinson's disease patients admitted to a rehabilitation center who received a course of intensive multidisciplinary rehabilitation in conjunction with the start of levodopa therapy. They noted good to excellent improvements in mobility in 66% and no improvement in 17%. A few patients not showing improvement in mobility did show improvement in ADL. Another study[32] initiated levodopa therapy in 100 outpatients with Parkinson's disease without any concomitant rehabilitation. Of these patients, 60% improved and 18% worsened or showed no change. The inference here is that the addition of an intensive inpatient rehabilitation program to the initiation of levodopa therapy does not appear to result in a superior outcome.

As part of a pilot study to develop appropriate measures to assess the impact of rehabilitation on patients with Parkinson's disease, Cedarbaum et al[12] looked at the changes in numerous tasks and activities following inpatient rehabilitation. Forty-five patients were studied in an unblinded, open fashion with medication adjustments allowed. Many patients came from acute care facilities following hospitalization for intercurrent illness or injury. Patients received an average of 4 hours of therapy per day, 5 days a week. Despite allowing for medication adjustment as dictated by the patient's condition, no significant overall average change in levodopa dosage occurred. No changes were noted in any of the timed tasks. Statistically significant improvements were noted in ambulation transfers, dressing, and personal hygiene. The large number of variables in this study raises the likelihood of some positive changes occurring by chance. Additionally, the lack of overall change in average levodopa dosage cannot be used to negate medication effects, as some patients might actually benefit from a decrease in levodopa and the addition of another agent. Many of these patients also might have been regaining function lost during a period of immobility that occurred during their acute hospital stay.

With future changes in healthcare delivery, it is unlikely that most Parkinson's disease patients will receive inpatient rehabilitation. It is also noted that continuation of an exercise program on a basis of two to three times a week can be necessary to optimize and maintain gains realized in formal therapy sessions. Future studies should focus on the effects of outpatient therapy programs that make use of a continued community-based group exercise and therapy program directed at maintaining mobility, function, and community involvement. Such studies should also take into account the natural history of Parkinson's disease, which typically results in a decline in function over 12 to 18 months.

Exercise and Muscle Physiology

In prescribing exercise programs for patients with Parkinson's disease, the ability of the patient to tolerate the exercise must be taken into account when there is evidence indicating differences in muscle physiology and response to exercise. It is not clear whether these effects are related to disuse, to altered central innervation, or to direct pathological involvement. Landin et al[32] looked at muscle metabolism and physiological response to exercise in six patients with Parkinson's disease and five healthy controls. On the basis of their results, the authors concluded that subjects with Parkinson's disease exercised with decreased efficiency. Their finding of reduced adenosine triphosphate (ATP) in muscles could mean a reduced efficiency in coupling between respiration and ATP generation by muscles. This could be the result of an altered metabolic state of muscle secondary to an abnormal pattern of innervation. This finding is also consistent with recent reports of alterations of mitochondrial respiration in brain tissue,[55] platelets,[46] and muscle tissue[6] in patients with Parkinson's disease. This suggests that there might be a systemic abnormality in mitochondrial function in Parkinson's disease.

Lowered mechanical efficiency in leg muscles has been demonstrated in Parkinson's disease patients, resulting in these patients' performing twice the work of normal controls.[52] The authors postulated that physical inactivity and deconditioning in subjects with Parkinson's disease might have been as important a factor as an altered metabolic state of muscle. However, Gersten et al[21] demonstrated that levodopa therapy reduced the externally measured work of walking in 46 subjects with varying stages of Parkinson's disease. When clinically appropriate, optimization of levodopa therapy is important to consider prior to embarking on an exercise program, since levodopa produces physiological changes that have an impact on the patient's ability to exercise and to benefit from the program.

Psychological and Social Aspects

Secondary to the predominance of motor symptoms in Parkinson's disease, psychological and cognitive impairments and their resultant impact on disability are often overlooked. Although severe dementia can occur late in the disease,[10] most patients with Parkinson's disease perform less well on a wide range of cognitive tests than age and education matched controls, even early in the course.[33, 39, 44] It appears that dementia in Parkinson's disease has both a cortical and a subcortical origin. Pathological changes similar to those found in Alzheimer's disease are commonly found in patients with Parkinson's disease. The changes do not always correlate with the presence of dementia and often overlap with the typical neural degeneration and Lewy body formation seen in Parkinson's disease.[2] In patients with Parkinson's disease with impaired intellect, choline acetyltransferase levels have been found to be reduced in the cortex.[48]

Adaptation to change in daily routine or environment can be difficult and result in undue anxiety. It is as if the same rigidity, bradykinesia, and difficulties with planning and adapting to change that affect the motor system in Parkinson's disease also affect the mind and thought processes. Patients with Parkinson's disease develop a sensitivity to drugs that affect the CNS, and often develop delirium when they are used.

Sleep disturbances are common, and difficulty falling asleep can occur early in the disease. In some patients, levodopa has a stimulant effect that prevents sleep. Early in the disease, one can avoid the use of levodopa late in the day. If there are no obvious cognitive impairments, diphenhydramine often works well and also tends to decrease tremor. Sleep problems can be accentuated by the vivid dreams and hallucinations that can occur as a side effect of dopaminergic medications. Fatigue and an increased tendency to daytime napping also contribute to what eventually can become a totally reversed sleep-wake cycle.

As noted earlier, depression is common in Parkinson's disease. It might be related to a deficit in serotonergic neurotransmission[36] or to the diminution of cortical levels of norepinephrine and dopamine.[54] Depression is difficult to treat in patients with declining mental function, because of the anticholinergic side effects of the tricyclic (noradrenergic-dopaminergic) antidepressants. A serotonergic agent might be the logical first choice in these patients. If that is ineffective, a tricyclic with low anticholinergic side effects, such as desipramine or nortriptyline, can be tried.

Social dysfunction is also quite common, with the most common problem being lack of socialization due to anxiety related to bodily symptoms. Patients with akinesia-rigidity tend to experience more emotional stress than those with tremor-predominant Parkinson's disease. Group-counseling activities involving both patients and caregivers were found in one study to be helpful in reducing stress in 74% of patients.[16]

Driving a motor vehicle is a complex cognitive-perceptual-motor task. Maintaining the ability to drive is also important to independence. When motor or cognitive function becomes impaired such that driving could be affected, the physician should suggest a detailed assessment, which can include retaking the driver's test. In many communities, driver screening is offered as part of a driver's training program for persons with disabilities.

A Practical Approach to Optimal Management

Optimal treatment of the patient with Parkinson's disease requires an interdisciplinary approach, using all needed therapies and community resources. The expertise of the rehabilitation physician is essential to the overall design of the program. An appropriately trained nurse-practitioner working under the supervision of a physician is very helpful in providing follow-up as well as coordination of care. Nurse-practitioners are often able to spend more time with the patient and family, as well as devote the time necessary to ensure true coordination of care. Consultation with a neurologist who has experience in the medical management of Parkinson's disease and who is versed in new treatment options is also essential.

Development of an interdisciplinary treatment team in the setting of a Parkinson's disease clinic works well in a large hospital or institutionally based multispecialty practice, or in tertiary care centers where most services are available. Many patients with Parkinson's disease, however, reside in small communities where the full spectrum of services is not available. Many patients are also not referred for neurological or rehabilitation consultation until late in the disease, when there is less opportunity to prevent some of the disease complications.

Emphasis should be placed on (1) educating consumers about optimal medical and rehabilitative management and the availability of resources, (2) educating primary care providers about the role of rehabilitation in treatment of Parkinson's disease (both early and late) and how to access services, and (3) further research on the benefits and costs of specific rehabilitation therapies.

Rehabilitation for Parkinson's disease is functionally based. The initial evaluation identifies the areas of disability experienced by the patient and prioritizes them. The ensuing assessment seeks to determine the underlying impairments and environmental barriers that result in the various disabilities. The treatment plan addresses the disabilities through (1) treatment of the impairments when feasible; (2) provision of aids and devices; (3) instruction in alternative approaches and a home maintenance program; (4) education of the patient and family, both about the disease process and the purpose of specific therapies and exercises; (5) provision of counseling and access to support groups as well as to other community services; and (6) appropriate periodic medical and rehabilitation follow-up to facilitate coordinated modification of both medical and rehabilitative treatment as the disease progresses. The treatment plan is developed with the participation of the patient and family. Table 51–5 is an example of a functionally based assessment and treatment program. Such an approach has the best chance of ensuring compliance and success.

Schenkman and Butler[56] provide an interesting and useful model for evaluation of Parkinson's disease based on separation of the impairments into three categories based on their origin: (1) those that are a direct result of nervous system pathological processes (e.g., rigidity, hypokinesia); (2) those that are an indirect result and not due to nervous system disorders (e.g., contracture, cardiopulmonary deconditioning); and (3) those that are a composite effect of nervous system and non-nervous system impairments (e.g., rigidity and loss of postural mechanisms facilitating and combining with the development of kyphosis and other fixed contractures leading to the composite of impaired balance). The composite impairments lead to disabilities affecting gait and other aspects of mobility and self-care. Such a model is useful in designing a PT approach, as it can be difficult or impossible for a physical therapist to correct impairments that are the direct result of neuronal and neurotransmitter changes. It is more realistic to prevent or lessen the impact that the CNS lesion has on impairments in other body systems and to teach the patient compensatory strategies, thus reducing potential sequelae. For additional details on this approach, the reader is referred to the work of Schenkman and Butler[56] and to an additional article by Schenkman et al[57] that focuses on management with case study examples.

Specific Therapy Approaches

Gait, Station, and Posture

The typical patient with moderate Parkinson's disease assumes a flexed posture, has difficulty initiating gait, and ambulates with short shuffling steps at an increasing rate. The base of support is usually narrow. Once walking begins, the patient has great difficulty changing di-

TABLE 51–5 Example of Rehabilitation Approach in Parkinson's Disease

Functional Problem	Underlying Impairments	Goals	Interventions
Slow and hesitant gait, problem reversing or changing direction, short steps	Bradykinesia, hypokinesia, loss of associated movements, loss of range of motion (ROM) in lower extremities	Decrease hesitancy; increase stride length; improve arm swing; allow for movement around obstacles	Mental rehearsal; marching to metronome and other external cues; exaggerate steps and arm swing; lower extremity ROM exercise and stretching
Kyphosis, reduced respiratory capacity	Rigidity, hip and knee flexion contractures, thoracic rigidity	Improve posture; improve respiration	Trunk extension exercises; breathing exercises; hip flexor and hamstring stretch
Rapid monotone speech with poor intelligibility	Hypokinesia, motor control disintegration	Improve intelligibility	Control breathing; pace rate; exaggerate enunciation
Falling	Rigidity, truncal and extremity contractures, loss of postural reflexes	Improve balance; decrease falls; improve safety	Stretching and ROM exercise of trunk, upper and lower extremities; balance training; instruction in falling and getting up from floor

rection, stepping over or moving around objects, or stopping (the festinating gait). Prior to beginning ambulation, the patient with Parkinson's disease does not make the normal preparatory movements of the trunk and extremities. During gait, associated movements such as arm swing, trunk rotation, and pelvic motion are reduced or absent. Postural reactions are impaired, so that the patient with Parkinson's disease is unable to correct for mild perturbations in the center of gravity (e.g., being brushed by another person or taking a slight misstep). The patient can topple over at times as if he or she were a statue. Sudden "freezing" can also occur and can precipitate a fall.

Although helpful in alleviating rigidity and bradykinesia, pharmacological therapy for Parkinson's disease usually does not help with postural instability, and will not be effective to the degree that fixed contracture contributes to the composite impairment. Later in the disease, as fluctuations in response to levodopa occur (the so-called on/off effect), performance can be extremely variable and unpredictable.

Useful approaches to these problems include exercises emphasizing trunk extension and lateral and rotational trunk mobility, weight shifting and balance training, and instruction in falling safely and getting up off the floor. Widening the stance provides a better base of support. Conscious strategies to initiate gait and maintain a cadence are often quite helpful and include mental rehearsal and counting or singing, either aloud or to oneself, and marching to the rhythm. The process can be begun with external cues, such as a metronome or music, that are gradually withdrawn. Exaggeration of arm swing and leg excursion is also helpful.

Balance activities can be made a part of other functional activities such as washing, grooming, and household activities. A cane can be of help, but it also can get in the way if not properly used. A rolling walker typically works better than a standard walker, since patients who are at a stage where a walker is needed usually cannot incorporate lifting a walker into their gait pattern. Care should be taken to set the walker at a higher height than usual so as not to further promote flexion. Inability to stop once started can be a problem with rolling walkers, and supervision is often required.

A visit to the patient's home by a physical or occupational therapist can result in environmental safety measures such as the removal of throw rugs, rearrangement of furniture, and installation of railings, grab bars, and other adaptive equipment. They can also help develop patient-specific home management strategies.

In the newly diagnosed patient, there is an opportunity to prevent loss of motion and the development of flexed posture. Vigorous exercise that improves coordination and balance and promotes general fitness is helpful. Walking, bicycling, dancing, low-impact aerobics, and other group exercise programs not only improve function but also provide the opportunity for socialization.

Tremor, Bradykinesia, Hypokinesia, and Rigidity

Although tremor does not usually cause the same degree of functional impairment as other aspects of Parkinson's disease, it can become a factor if it is severe. The tremor is typically a resting-postural tremor that often ceases (or at least does not become worse) during movement. Anticholinergic medications can be helpful if tolerated. Because the tremor becomes worse with anxiety or stress, relaxation techniques are often helpful. Distal weights have not been proven to be of benefit in improving function.

Bradykinesia (slowness of movement), hypokinesia (decreased movement), and rigidity affecting the flexor muscles more than the extensors are the key direct neurological impairments underlying the disability caused by Parkinson's disease. ROM exercises and stretching on a daily basis are important in preserving flexibility. Initiation of movement, larger excursions during movement, and coordination should be addressed as a part of functional activities. There is increasing evidence that exercise is most effective when it is task-specific.[20] Task-specific exercise might be especially important for the patient with Parkinson's disease, in light of the impairments in motor planning and programming that are characteristic of the disease. Helpful strategies and techniques include measures such as rocking to and fro in the chair before arising, and other preparatory motions to provide momentum. A raised chair and toilet seat and armrests also make arising easier.

One of the most difficult problems is the Parkinson's disease patient's inability to use automatic responses during willed functional movement. Clinical experience and the literature[20] suggest that repetition improves these responses and the resulting functional movements.

Rigidity can also result in musculoskeletal pain, which often responds to heat, massage, stretching, and ROM exercise.

Speech and Swallowing

Speech disturbances in patients with Parkinson's disease include initial hesitancy, low volume, rapid rate, monotone voice, poor articulation, hesitations or inappropriate periods of silence, stuttering, palilalia, and trailing off of the voice with an increasing rate. All of these combined are referred to as "hypokinetic dysarthria." The initial deficit is a failure to control respiration for the purpose of speech. Following this is gradual breakdown in the complex sensorimotor integration of speech production complicated by stiffness of facial and pharyngeal muscles.

Speech typically improves somewhat with levodopa treatment. Speech therapy interventions for speech disorders consist of exercises emphasizing breath and rate control, improved (often exaggerated) articulation, and increased volume.

Dysphagia tends to occur later in the disease and results in drooling, poor nutrition, and inability to take oral medications, and can lead to aspiration pneumonia. Common abnormalities include food-pocketing in the mouth and a delayed swallowing reflex. Aspiration pneumonia is a major cause of morbidity and mortality in Parkinson's disease. Therapeutic interventions include positioning of the neck in flexion, smaller amounts of food, thickened liquids, avoidance of foods with mixed consistencies (e.g., vegetable soup), and a double swallow (see Chapter 26). The caregiver should be instructed in the Heimlich maneuver. In later stages, placement of a gastrostomy tube and tracheostomy might be considered. Consultation with a dietitian is helpful to ensure adequate nutrition. A decrease in protein intake can be necessary to promote adequate levodopa absorption. Patients with frequent and severe dyskinetic reactions can require large amounts of calories.

A videofluoroscopic swallowing study is helpful in determining the cause of the swallowing difficulties and helps direct the treatment approach. The swallowing study is also able to assess the severity of the problem and the potential for and actual occurrence of aspiration (see Chapter 26). It is important to address the placement of a gastrostomy feeding tube before dysphagia progresses to the point of nutritional compromise or high risk of aspiration. Because Parkinson's disease is a progressive disorder, some patients choose to forego the placement of a feeding tube and continue with oral feedings despite the risk of aspiration. Beginning the discussion early gives the patient and family adequate time to think through their decision. It should be noted that there are patients with a variety of neurological disorders who chronically aspirate but do not routinely develop pneumonia.

Autonomic Dysfunction

Orthostatic hypotension becomes a problem in later stages of the disease. Arising slowly and pausing in the sitting position before standing, elevating the head of the bed, and using pressure garments are helpful conservative approaches. Mineralocorticoids can also be helpful.

Slowed gastric and intestinal motility lead to early satiety, vomiting, poor absorption of medications, and constipation. Useful strategies include frequent small meals, increased fiber intake, bulking agents, stool softeners, suppositories, and timed voiding. Metoclopramide facilitates gastric emptying but should generally be avoided because of its tendency to cause parkinsonian side effects. Cisapride, another such agent, might be a better choice.

Urinary incontinence, difficulty voiding, retention, and infections can also occur. Recurrent urinary infections frequently indicate neurogenic bladder dysfunction, although other causes such as prostatic hypertrophy are common in this age group. An appropriate investigation typically includes postvoid residual, cystoscopy, assessment of renal function, and in some cases cystometrogram-sphincter electromyography (CMG-EMG). The results of this workup can guide the practical and pharmacological interventions. An indwelling catheter should be used only as a last resort and if it will facilitate the care of a severely disabled patient (see Chapter 27).

Impotence can also occur as a result of autonomic dysfunction or psychological factors. This area deserves appropriate assessment and treatment as much as any other aspect of disability related to Parkinson's disease (see Chapter 30).

Sympathetic pain and reflex sympathetic dystrophy can be seen in Parkinson's disease. The pain is often alleviated by levodopa. If it is not, the use of a tricyclic antidepressant is often helpful and can also decrease tremor. In later stages, the anticholinergic effects on cognition are less well tolerated. The effectiveness of the serotonergic antidepressants in alleviating neurogenic pain is unclear.

Cardiopulmonary Function

Flexed posture leads to kyphosis, which reduces lung capacity. Rigidity can result in a "restrictive" pulmonary disease pattern, further complicating respiratory function. Endurance often decreases secondary to a sedentary lifestyle. A focus on breathing exercises, proper posture, and trunk extension early in Parkinson's disease is helpful in preventing these musculoskeletal complications which contribute to the high incidence of pulmonary dysfunction. Cardiopulmonary conditioning should also be a component of the early treatment program (see Chapters 32 and 33). Later in the course, breathing and extension exercise should be continued, with the addition of coughing, incentive spirometry, and respiratory therapy techniques as needed. Instruction in energy conservation techniques and pacing can preserve the ability to continue in a productive role.

Cognition and Depression

Management of declining cognitive function becomes a major issue in many cases. Although Parkinson's disease has its peak incidence in the sixth decade, the disease begins in some patients in their 40s or 50s. Most patients in this age group are either employed or responsible for management of the home. As noted above, patients with Parkinson's disease can have deficiencies in cognitive function very early in the disease that might not be apparent on a social level, but which can cause problems at work (particularly in highly technical, skilled, or professional occupations). Full neuropsychological assessment is prudent in such cases. In other cases more limited testing to assess for safety to continue independent living or driving is adequate. Making the family aware of safety issues and providing both the family and the patient with compensatory cognitive techniques are essential. The neuropsychologist or rehabilitation psychologist can provide the testing, interpretation, and recommendations (see Chapter 4).

A psychologist, psychiatrist, or experienced social worker can provide helpful input regarding the patient's emotional state. Counseling for both patient and family can be helpful in developing coping skills. It is essential that the patient and family be aware of and encouraged to use available community resources and support groups.

ADL and Adaptive Equipment

Since the primary purpose of rehabilitation is to improve or maintain function, a thorough functional assessment is key to the development of an integrated program for the patient with Parkinson's disease. The physical and occupational therapist should work together in their assessment of the patient and development of the program. While ideally the approach is to maintain or improve impairments, to the degree that this becomes impossible instruction in compensatory techniques and the use of various devices can allow the patient to remain functional for a prolonged period. A home visit not only helps in assessing the need for home modification, but also allows the therapist to see how the patient functions in the home. Numerous assistive devices are available (see Chapter 25).

The Home Program and Follow-up

As discussed earlier, patients with Parkinson's disease require a regular and ongoing exercise program to maintain or, in some cases, improve function. A specific exercise format does not appear to be as critical as covering the following areas: (1) relaxation and breathing; (2) posture principles; (3) active, active-assistive, and passive ROM exercises and stretching; (4) balance and gait activities; (5) coordination; (6) general conditioning; and (7) specific functional activities, including speech, ADL, and other tasks.

Since it is unlikely that reimbursement is available for continuous therapy, after individual assessment the patient and caregiver should be instructed in a program over three to five sessions that can be carried out at home on a regular basis. Early in the disease, and later whenever possible, participation in group exercise programs for the elderly that combine conditioning programs with socialization is an excellent option. Such programs are available in many communities. Some communities with an active Parkinson's disease support group have an ongoing exercise program specifically designed for patients with Parkinson's disease. The minimum exercise frequency is three times per week for the group programs and daily for a home program. In more severely involved patients, even twice-daily ROM exercise and stretching might not be sufficient to maintain mobility. There is almost always a tradeoff between the maximum benefit and the practicality of the exercise program.

As in patients with other chronic disabling conditions, patients with Parkinson's disease quickly lose ground when periods of illness restrict their activity or put them on bed rest. Care should be taken to provide ROM exercise, stretching, proper positioning, breathing exercises, and whatever mobility the patient can tolerate in these situations.

PARKINSON-LIKE SYNDROMES

The approach to the other degenerative disorders with features similar to or in common with Parkinson's disease, such as progressive supranuclear palsy and multiple system atrophy, is similar to that used with Parkinson's disease. Even though levodopa is not as effective in these disorders, it often has some benefit and should be given an initial trial. Many of these diseases have a more rapidly debilitating course, which needs to be considered when developing the rehabilitation plan.

Huntington's Disease

Huntington's disease is an autosomal dominant disorder caused by a genetic mutation which leads to an expanded CAG repeat in the coding sequence on chromosome 4. The mutation is ubiquitous although the striatum manifests the most severe neuropathological damage. New evidence suggests that this gene defect can result in an impairment of energy metabolism at the level of the mitochondria. The respiratory impairment, in turn, can lead to oxygen radical generation, further damaging neural tissue.

There is currently no effective treatment for Huntington's disease. Experiments in humans and animals with Coenzyme Q10,[30] which supplements the electron transport chain, or creatine kinase and cyclocreatinine,[35] which stabilize ATP, have shown limited effect.

Transplantation of allograft neural tissue remains an experimental but promising treatment of Huntington's disease. Successful integration of neural tissue has been established in rats[15] and more recently in primates.[29] Neural transplantation was able to almost completely reverse striatal lesion deficits in all monkeys transplanted. These findings promise clinical success for transplants in Huntington's disease.

Huntington's disease usually presents with chorea, dementia, and behavioral and mood disorders. In a small percentage of patients, hypokinesia and rigidity are the presenting features. This is referred to as the Westphal variant and tends to have its onset at an earlier age. It is now possible to identify patients while they are still asymptomatic with the use of genetic testing.

In addition to chorea and neuropsychological changes, dysarthria, dysphagia, and gait abnormalities can also occur. Rehabilitation efforts are functional and patient care and caregiver oriented. Chorea does not respond to PT, although dopaminergic blocking agents can be helpful. Chorea can consume a large amount of energy and calories, making nutrition a prime concern. Many communities have active support groups for patients and families affected by Huntington's disease.

Hereditary Ataxias

The hereditary ataxias include a wide variety of disorders. Some of these present with intermittent ataxia, and some have ataxia that is progressive and combined with other neurological features such as upper motor neuron signs (e.g., olivopontocerebellar atrophy) and peripheral nerve signs (e.g., absent ankle reflexes in Friedreich's ataxia). Ataxia can result from disorders of the cerebellum or its connections, the brainstem, the vestibular system, the dorsal columns and spinocerebellar tracts of the spinal cord, the dorsal root ganglia, or the peripheral nerves. Disorders resembling ataxia can also be seen following parietal or frontal lobe lesions. These disorders are rare, and when such a patient is referred for rehabilitation, it is important for the rehabilitation team to obtain full information of the projected course of the disease to ensure the development of an appropriate rehabilitation plan. Some of these disorders also have associated systemic involvement (e.g., cardiomyopathy and diabetes mellitus in Friedreich's ataxia), which also have an impact on the rehabilitation program.

A review of all of the hereditary ataxias is beyond the scope of this chapter, and the reader is referred to the review by Hurko.[25] The medical management of these disorders is based on accurate diagnosis that rules out treatable problems such as tumors, malformations, or metabolic defects (e.g., acoustic neuromas, Arnold-Chiari syndrome, Wilson's disease). Ataxia and ataxic (intention) tremor cannot be treated with medication in the same way that the symptoms of Parkinson's disease are diminished by levodopa. The mainstay of treatment is the provision of physical and occupational therapy directed at maintaining function for as long as possible. Gait training and instruction in the use of assistive devices to prevent falls and enhance mobility are useful. Distal weights can dampen the intention tremor. Speech therapy can be helpful in improving articulation dysphagia. Specific coordination exercises are rarely useful or practical in progressive disorders, at least as compared to their utility in static causes of ataxia (i.e., head injury or stroke). Social services and psychological support are especially important, as they are for all progressive disorders.

Dystonia

Dystonia is a syndrome characterized by sustained muscle contractions resulting in abnormal movements or sustained postures. These movements and postures are the result of sustained co-contraction of both the agonist and the antagonist. Dystonia can be focal, multifocal, segmental, or generalized. Dystonic syndromes can be primary (idiopathic) or associated with or caused by another disorder (e.g., in Parkinson's disease, anoxia, head injury, Wilson's disease, and inherited metabolic defects).

Most focal dystonias respond to injections of botulinum toxin.[7] Anticholinergics, levodopa, baclofen (Lioresal), carbamazepine, and clonazepam have all been used with some success in selected patients with more generalized forms. Thalamotomy is reserved for severe cases of generalized dystonia that have not responded to intensive pharmacological trials.

PT techniques, such as massage and slow stretching, and modalities such as ultrasound and biofeedback are sometimes helpful in the focal or regional dystonias. Patients with generalized dystonia often benefit from gait and mobility training and instruction in the use of assistive devices.

SUMMARY

Patients with Parkinson's disease and other neurodegenerative movement disorders often benefit from rehabilitation interventions. Careful evaluation, treatment planning, adequate follow-up, and patient and family education are required. As primary care physicians, neurologists, and others involved in the care of these patients might not be aware of the benefits of rehabilitation in Parkinson's disease, future educational efforts should also be directed at these professionals. Additional research is needed to develop more effective programs and to scientifically verify the impact of rehabilitation programs on disability.

REFERENCES

1. Allan CM: Treatment of nonfluent speech resulting from neurological disease: Treatment of dysarthria. Br J Disord Commun 1970; 5:3–5.
2. Alvord EC, Forno LS, Kusske JA, et al: The pathology of parkinsonism: A comparison of the degenerations in cerebral cortex and brain stem. Adv Neurol 1974; 5:175.
3. Atadzhanov M, Rakhimdhanov A: Dopamine deficiency and cholinergic models of the parkinsonian syndrome. Neurology 1993; 43(suppl 1):S126–S129.
4. Beattie A, Caird FI: The occupational therapist and the patient with Parkinson's disease. Br Med J 1980; 1:1354–1356.
5. Bethlem J, Den Hartog Jager WA: The incidence and characteristics of Lewy bodies in idiopathic paralysis agitans (Parkinson's disease). J Neurol Neurosurg Psychiatry 1960; 23:74–80.
6. Bindhoff LA, Birch-Machlin M, Cartlidge NEF, et al: Mitochondrial dysfunction in Parkinson's disease. Lancet 1989; 2:49.
7. Brin MF, Blitzer A, Stewart C, et al: Disorders with excessive muscle contraction: Candidates for treatment with intramuscular botulinum toxin (Botox). In DasGupta BR (ed): Botulinum and Tetanus Neurotoxins. New York, Plenum Press, 1993, pp 559–576.
8. Broe CA, Akhter AJ, Andrews CR, et al: Neurological disorders in the elderly at home. J Neurol Neurosurg Psychiatry 1976; 39:362–366.
9. Caird FI: Non-drug therapy of Parkinson's disease. Scott Med J 1986; 31:129–132.
10. Cedarbaum JM, McDowell FH: Sixteen-year follow up of 100 patients begun on levodopa in 1968: Emerging problems. Adv Neurol 1986; 45:469.
11. Cedarbaum JM, Silvestri M, Kutt H: Sustained enteral administration of levodopa increases and interrupted infusion decreases levodopa dose requirements. Neurology 1990; 40:995–997.
12. Cedarbaum JM, Troy L, Silvestri M, et al: Rehabilitation programs in the management of patients with Parkinson's disease. J Neurol Rehabil 1992; 6:7–19.
13. Comella CL, Stebbins GT, Brown-Toms N, et al: Physical therapy and Parkinson's disease: A controlled clinical trial. Neurology 1994; 44:376–378.
14. Critchley EMR: Speech disorders of parkinsonism: A review. J Neurol Neurosurg Psychiatry 1984; 47:751–758.
15. Dunnett SB, Kendall AL, Watts C, et al: Neuronal cell transplantation for Parkinson's and Huntington's disease. Br Med Bull 1997; 53(4):757–776.
16. Ellgring H, Seiler S, Perleth B, et al: Psychosocial aspects of Parkinson's disease. Neurology 1993; 43(suppl 6):S41–S44.
17. Fahn S, Elton RI: Unified Parkinson's disease rating scale. In Fahn S, Marsden CD, Calne D, Goldstein M (eds): Recent Developments in Parkinson's Disease, vol 2. Florham Park, NJ, Macmillan, 1987, pp 153–163.
18. Fearnley JM, Lees AJ: Ageing and Parkinson's disease: Substantia nigra regional selectivity. Brain 1991; 114:2283–2301.
19. Franklin S, Cohout LJ, Stern GM, et al: Physical therapy. In Rose F, Capildeo R (eds): Research Progress in Parkinson's Disease. London, Pitman, 1981, pp 397–400.
20. Gentile AM: Skill acquisition: Action, movement, and neuromotor processes. In Carr JH, Shepart RB (eds): Movement Science for Physical Therapy in Rehabilitation. Rockville, MD, Aspen, 1987, pp 1–30.
21. Gersten JW, Marshall C, Dillon T, et al: External work of walking and functional capacity in parkinsonian patients treated with L-dopa. Arch Phys Med Rehabil 1972; 53:547–553.
22. Gibbard FB, Page NGR, Spencer KM, et al: Controlled trial of physiotherapy and occupational therapy for Parkinson's disease. Br Med J 1981; 282:1196.
23. Helm N: Management of palilalia with a pacing board. J Speech Hear Disord 1979; 44:350–353.

24. Homberg V: Motor training in the therapy of Parkinson's disease. Neurology 1993; 43(suppl 6):S45–S46.
25. Hurko O: Hereditary cerebellar ataxia. In Johnson RT, Griffin SW (eds): Current Therapy in Neurologic Disease. St Louis, Mosby–Year Book, 1993, pp 254–261.
26. Hurwitz A: The benefits of a home exercise regimen for ambulatory patients with Parkinson's disease. J Neurosci Nurs 1989; 21:180–184.
27. Jankovic J: Theories on the etiology and pathogenesis of Parkinson's disease. Neurology 1993; 43(suppl 1):S121–S123.
28. Jankovic J, Shoulson I, Werner WJ: Early stage Parkinson's disease: To treat or not to treat. Neurology 1994; 44(suppl 1):S4–S5.
29. Kendall AL, Rayment FD, Torres EM, et al: Functional integration of striatal allografts in a primate model of Huntington's disease. Nature Med 1998; 4:727–729.
30. Koroshetz WJ, Jenkins BG, Rosen BR, et al: Energy metabolism defects in Huntington's disease and effects of enzyme Q10. Ann Neurol 1997; 41:160–165.
31. Kurth MC, Adler CH: COMT inhibition: A new treatment strategy for Parkinson's disease. Neurology 1998; 50:S3–S14.
32. Landin S, Hagenfeldt L, Saltin B, et al: Muscle metabolism during exercise in patients with Parkinson's disease. Clin Sci Mol Med 1974; 47:493–506.
33. Levin BE, Llabre MM, Weiner WJ: Cognitive impairments associated with early Parkinson's disease. Neurology 1989; 39:557.
34. ManKovskij N, Karaban I, Mialovickaig AD: Aging and its relation to parkinsonism. Neurology 1993; 43(suppl 1):29.
35. Matthews RT, Yang L, Jenkins BG, et al: Neuroprotective effects of creatine and cyclocreatine in animal models of Huntington's disease. J Neurosci 1998; 18(1):156–163.
36. Mayeux R, Stern Y, Cote L, et al: Altered serotonin metabolism in depressed patients with Parkinson's disease. Neurology 1984; 34:642.
37. McDowell FH, Cedarbaum JM: The extrapyramidal system and disorders of movement. In Joynt R (ed): Clinical Neurology. Philadelphia, JB Lippincott, 1991.
38. Mitchel PH, Mertz MA, Catanzaro M-L: Group exercise: A nursing therapy in Parkinson's disease. Rehabil Nurs 1987; 12:242–245.
39. Mortimer JA, Pirozzolo FJ, Hansch EC, et al: Relationship of motor symptoms to intellectual deficits in Parkinson's disease. Neurology 1982; 32:133.
40. Mutch WJ, Strudwick A, Roy SK, et al: Parkinson's disease: Disability, review, and management (medical practice). Br Med J 1986; 293:675–677.
41. Ogawa N: Early introduction of dopamine agonists in the long-term treatment of Parkinson's disease. Neurology 1998; 51: S13–S20.
42. Ogawa N: Neurodegeneration and free radical scavengers in Parkinson's disease. Prof Parkinson's Dis 1998; 2:10–12.
43. Olanow CW: The early treatment of Parkinson's disease. Neurology 1993; 43(suppl 1):S30–S31.
44. Oyebode LR, Barker WA, Blessed G, et al: Cognitive functioning in Parkinson's disease in relation to prevalence of dementia and psychiatric diagnosis. Br J Psychiatry 1986; 149:720.
45. Palmer SS, Mortimer JA, Webster DD, et al: Exercise therapy for Parkinson's disease. Arch Phys Med Rehabil 1986; 67:741–745.
46. Parker WD, Boyson SJ, Parks JK: Abnormalities of the electron transport chain in idiopathic Parkinson's disease. Ann Neurol 1989; 26:719–723.
47. The Parkinson Study Group: Effect of deprenyl on the progression of disability in early Parkinson's disease. N Engl J Med 1989; 321:1364–1371.
48. Perry EK, Curtis M, Dick DJ, et al: Cholinergic correlates of cognitive impairment in Parkinson's disease: Comparisons with Alzheimer's disease. J Neurol Neurosurg Psychiatry 1985; 48:413.
49. Poewe E: Clinical and pathophysiologic aspects of late levodopa failure. Neurology 1993; 43(suppl 6):S28–S30.
50. Robertson S, Thomson F: A study of the efficacy and long term effects of intensive treatment. Br J Disord Commun 1984; 19:213–224.
51. Sage JI, Trooskin S, Sonsalla PK, et al: Long-term duodenal infusion of levodopa for motor fluctuations in parkinsonism. Ann Neurol 1988; 24:87–89.
52. Saltin B, Landin S: Work capacity, muscle strength and SDH activity in both legs of hemiparetic patients and patients with Parkinson's disease. Scand J Clin Lab Invest 1975; 35:531–538.
53. Sarno MT: Speech impairment in Parkinson's disease. Arch Phys Med Rehabil 1968; 49:269.
54. Scatton B, Javoy-Agid F, Fouquier L, et al: Reduction of cortical dopamine, noradrenaline, serotonin and their metabolites in Parkinson's disease. Brain Res 1983; 275:321.
55. Schapira AHV, Cooper JM, Dexter D, et al: Mitochondrial complex I deficiency in Parkinson's disease. Lancet 1989; 1:1269.
56. Schenkman M, Butler RB: A model for multisystem evaluation treatment of individuals with Parkinson's disease. Phys Ther 1989; 69:932–943.
57. Schenkman M, Donovan J, Tsubota J, et al: Management of individuals with Parkinson's disease: Rationale and case studies. Phys Ther 1989; 69:944–955.
58. Scott S, Caird FI: The response of the apparent receptive speech disorder of Parkinson's disease to speech therapy. J Neurol Neurosurg Psychiatry 1984; 47:302–304.
59. Scott S, Caird FI: Speech therapy for Parkinson's disease. J Neurol Neurosurg Psychiatry 1983; 46:140–144.
60. Stern MB: Parkinson's disease. In Johnson RT, Griffin (eds): Current Therapy in Neurologic Disease, ed 4. St Louis, Mosby-Year Book, 1993, pp 242–246.
61. Stern PH, McDowell FH, Miller JM, et al: Levodopa and physical therapy in treatment of patients with Parkinson's disease. Arch Phys Med Rehabil 1970; 51:273–277.
62. Szekely BC, Kosanovich NN, Sheppard W: Adjunctive treatment in Parkinson's disease: Physical therapy and comprehensive group therapy. Rehabil Lit 1982; 43:72–76.
63. Tetrud JW, Langston JW: The effect of deprenyl (selegiline) on the natural history of Parkinson's disease. Science 1989; 245: 519–522.
64. Weiner WJ, Singer C: Parkinson's disease and nonpharmacologic treatment programs. J Am Geriatr Soc 1989; 37:359–363.
65. Wolters EC: The Pathogenesis of Parkinson's Disease. Prof Parkinson's Dis 1998; 2:18–20.

52

CHAPTER

Ronald S. Taylor, M.D.

Rehabilitation of Persons with Multiple Sclerosis

Multiple sclerosis (MS) is an inflammatory disease of the central nervous system (CNS) characterized by areas of demyelination. It is the third most common cause of disabling illness in individuals between the ages of 15 and 50.[48] Over 10,000 scientific articles have been published on this entity, but its exact cause remains uncertain and the pathogenesis profoundly debatable. Evidence supports, but does not substantiate, that MS is an illness of viral exposure during puberty that affects individuals with a genetically determined defect in their immune system. Functional and cognitive impairments develop in the majority of patients, with frequent involvement of gait, coordination, bladder, and sexual function. The full utilization of the rehabilitation team is critical to minimize the patient's level of disability.

EPIDEMIOLOGY

The geographic distribution of multiple sclerosis was first noted by Charcot.[14] The incidence of the disease, as well as its death rate, increases from the southern portions of the Western Hemisphere to the northern portions. Incidence rates are determined by where an individual lives before age 15 and are not affected by geographic changes beyond this age.[93] Studies from Olmstead County, Minnesota, indicate an incidence of 171 per hundred thousand population, with females accounting for approximately 70% of cases.[93] The average age at onset is 32.4 years for females, 34.3 for males.[71] The incidence of MS appears stable, with the apparent increase in number of cases explained by improved diagnostic techniques.

Human lymphocyte antigen (HLA) linkages to MS have been noted, but vary with different populations. In northern Europeans, MS is associated with HLA-A3, B7, DW2, and DR2, which are found in 70% of patients with MS but in only 25% of controls. There appears to be increased incidence of MS in families, but no true mendelian pattern of inheritance has been detected. No increase has been noted in the presence of consanguinity, as would be expected in a recessive pattern of inheritance. Rarely is MS diagnosed in three consecutive generations, as would be expected if the disease were transmitted as an autosomal dominant trait. In twin studies, concordance rates are 26% for monozygotic twins and 2.3% for dizygotic twins.[49] Because of its pleomorphic nature, MS can be confused with many other illnesses. A partial list of these illnesses is given in Table 52–1.

DIAGNOSTIC STUDIES

Cerebrospinal Fluid Examination

No cerebrospinal fluid (CSF) abnormalities are specific for MS. CSF protein is elevated in approximately one-fourth of patients during exacerbations.[42] Sixty percent to 75% of patients with MS have increased levels of CSF protein. Gamma-globulin is synthesized in the CNS,[22] and the ratio of IgG to albumin in the CSF divided by the ratio of these two factors in the serum often provides a more sensitive index. A value greater than 0.77 is found in 80% to 90% of patients with MS.[87] The oligoclonal nature of IgG in the CSF of patients with MS was recognized more than two decades ago

TABLE 52–1 Differential Diagnosis in MS

Disease	Clinical Features
Systemic lupus erythematosus	37% to 42% of patients with SLE present with neurological deficits; antinuclear antibody test is positive in 25% of MS patients
Sjögren's syndrome	Patients may have CNS symptoms, including a relapsing-remitting course, cerebellar findings, or internuclear ophthalmoplegia
AIDS	Often associated with progressive spastic paraparesis and sensory ataxia
Tropical spastic paraparesis	Sensory changes with pain in legs and neurogenic bladder, caused by HTLV-I
Sarcoidosis	CNS involvement in 5%
Lyme disease	Neurological changes may follow a relapsing-remitting course, with extremity and cranial involvement; oligoclonal bands in CSF. Serological testing helpful in sorting out the diagnosis
Cerebrovascular occlusive disease	Scattered lesions secondary to cardiac source of emboli may be confused with findings in MS
Remote effects of carcinoma	May have associated peripheral neuropathy; usually occurs in older people and has rapid downhill course
Diseases with single lesions and a relapsing course	Glioma, meningioma, arteriovenous malformation
Cervical spondylotic myelopathy	Usually affects an older population and characteristically produces more pain and less bladder involvement than MS; fasciculations may be present
Vestibular neuronitis	May be indistinguishable from an attack of MS; vestibular tests may be abnormal
Nonorganic symptoms	Often last less than 24 hours; dizziness without true vertigo; lack of correlating neurological abnormality

when these bands were demonstrated on agar gel electrophoresis. The CSF of patients with definite MS shows abnormalities by this technique in 90% of cases.[47, 88]

Magnetic Resonance Imaging

Magnetic resonance imaging (MRI) has been used as an adjunct in the diagnosis of MS since 1991, with positive findings seen in up to 95% of definite cases. Typical findings are multiple white matter lesions appearing as bright areas on T2-weighted (proton-density) sequences (Fig. 52–1). Lesions are often seen in the brainstem, periventricular region, and cerebellum, with lesions in the corpus callosum being relatively specific for MS.[28] Many other conditions are associated with similar changes on MRI. These conditions include aging, vasculitis, trauma, HIV infection, and irradiation. Paty et al[62] attempted to clarify this diagnostic dilemma by proposing the criterion of four lesions greater than 3 mm in size (three lesions, if one is periventricular in location) as necessary to make the diagnosis of MS. Fazenkas et al[24] reported a 100% specificity for MS when periventricular or infratentorial lesions greater than 6 mm are detected. Specificity might also be increased through the use of contrast agents or with the addition of spiral MRI.

The use of gadolinium adds to the utility of MRI. This tracer crosses the disturbed blood-brain barrier seen in MS exacerbations and allows the identification of acute inflammatory lesions and re-activated chronic plaques. In patients with undiagnosed neurological episodes, a negative contrast-enhanced MRI study virtually rules out the diagnosis of MS.

Sixty-five percent of patients with positive MRI findings go on to develop clinically definite MS within 5 years, whereas only 3% of those with negative studies are subsequently diagnosed as having the disease. It is also to be noted that in patients with MS, the lesions detected on 75% of MRI studies do not correlate with the patient's neurological status.

Evoked Potential Recordings

Evoked potentials are useful in the diagnosis of MS because of their ability to measure altered conduction time in the CNS myelinated pathways. Their primary diagnostic application lies in providing evidence of demyelination in clinically normal pathways. Visual-evoked potentials (VEP) are abnormal in 75% of patients with definite MS and in 15% to 60% of patients with possible MS. Subclinical abnormalities are detected in 20% to 30% of cases.[3]

Brainstem auditory-evoked potentials (BAEP) are also useful, with abnormalities seen in 67% of persons with definite MS, 41% of those with probable MS, and 30% of subjects with possible MS. Subclinical abnormalities are detected in 21% to 55% of studies.[15] Similar values are noted for somatosensory-evoked potentials (SSEPs), with higher rates of abnormality found in the lower extremities than in the upper extremities.[15] Combining all three potentials can be helpful when the diagnosis is questionable.

PATHOPHYSIOLOGY

Postmortem studies reveal areas of demyelination, with relative preservation of axons. Also noted are gliosis, a disappearance of oligodendrocytes, and inflammation.[85] These abnormal areas are called plaques and are found only in the CNS. They are irregular and can often be seen by the naked eye. They can occur anywhere in the CNS but have a predilection for the optic nerve, the perivenous areas, and the periventricular white matter of the cerebrum, brainstem, and spinal cord.[70]

These changes were first noted more than 100 years ago by Charcot.[14] More recently, MRI studies have shed light on the dynamic aspects of the MS process. The earliest abnormality typically detected is a localized breakdown in the blood-brain barrier. Such breakdown

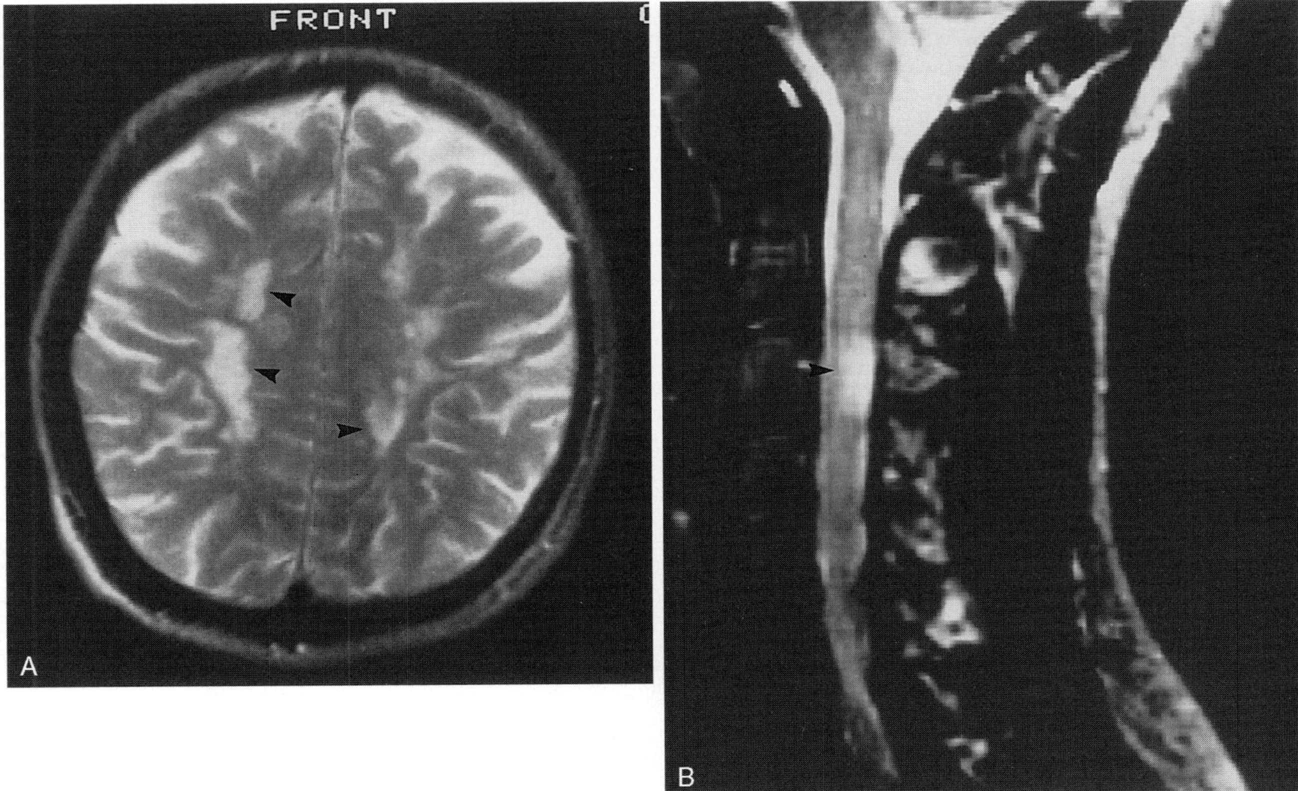

FIGURE 52–1. Brain (*A*) and spinal cord (*B*) MRIs indicating presence of MS plaques (*arrowheads*). (Courtesy of Ay Ming Wang, M.D.)

is seen as an area of enhancement on gadolinium-enhanced MRI and can precede the onset of neurological deficits.[79] In pathological studies, the endothelial cells of the blood-brain barrier can contain abnormal vesicles. Immune cells can often be detected in the surrounding brain parenchyma. The area of abnormality increases in size over an average of 6 weeks and eventually decreases down to the size of the original enhancing lesion.[51] The lesions disappear completely in approximately 6% to 20% of cases.[51] The decrease in size of the lesions is thought to be due to resolution of brain edema.[51] Serial MRI studies over a 6-month period in 12 patients with chronic progressive MS disclosed 109 new lesions. Enhancement on MRI was found in 87% of these, but only 17% actually progressed to clinically detectable neurological changes.[40]

Only about 20% of chronic lesions enhance with gadolinium. The extracellular spaces within the lesions are markedly narrowed.[19] Demyelination is the hallmark of MS, but it remains unknown whether it precedes or follows the changes in the blood-brain barrier discussed above. Signs of remyelination have been noted, but remyelination appears to take place predominantly in the early part of the illness.

Recent studies imply that axonal transection exists in patients with MS. Trapp and colleagues noted this finding in all 47 plaques they studied, with the densest concentration of transections in the center of the lesions.[89]

IMMUNOREGULATION

Recent clinical data indicate that MS could be an autoimmune disease triggered by an infectious agent. These findings are supported by an increase in CNS gammaglobulin with oligoclonal IgG production, perivenular lymphocytes in the CNS, abnormal cellular immune responses, and CNS autoantibodies against certain neuroviruses found in patients with MS.[45, 87] Abnormalities of T lymphocytes have been documented in MS patients since the early 1970s.[70] A 1980 study by Reinherz et al[70] showed a selective decrease in T8-positive suppressor cells in 11 of 15 patients with active MS but in only one of 18 patients with inactive MS. IgG has been shown to be increased in the CSF of patients with MS. This resolves into a series of oligocolonal bands when analyzed electrophoretically.[88] These bands represent antibody from B lymphocytes, but as yet the specific antigen to which they are directed is unknown. Various studies have implicated measles, rubella, or even "nonsense antibody" as their trigger.[71] Further theories postulate that these cells may have "escaped" more normal regulation and are synthesizing antibodies on their own.

Although the specific antibodies involved are unknown, recent studies of acute MS lesions have detected antibody against myelin-oligodendrocyte glycoprotein, a minor protein component of myelin. This is the first solid evidence of the presence of autoantibodies against myelin in patients with MS.[57] The basis for a proposed abnormal immune reaction in MS is provided in Table 52–2. T cells are thought to attach to endothelial cells in brain capillaries that have been exposed to cytokines, such as interferon-gamma and tumor necrosis factor.[10] The T cells cross the blood-brain barrier and enter the CNS, where they attach to specific antigens in the cleft of the HLA molecule. They then release tumor necrosis factor, lymphotoxin, and interferon-gamma, all of which destroy myelin. Cytokines are also released. They activate B cells to make antibodies directed not only at myelin, but also toward oligodendrocytes. Interferon also activates macrophages, with a resultant direct toxic effect on the myelin. Research is currently aimed at interrupting this process in hopes of finding a cure for MS.[10, 84]

Microglia are antigen-presenting cells found in the CNS and are capable of secreting various neurotoxic cytokines. Their exact role in MS is unclear but might be more important than was previously thought. Various viral studies have noted their presence in demyelinating lesions before T cells are detected.[84] It is interesting to speculate on the exact role of interferon-gamma, as clinical trials have shown this to exacerbate the symptoms of MS. Interferon-gamma is known to be increased in the presence of estrogen, which could explain the female preponderance of MS cases.[60] The recent success with interferon-beta in MS patients is based on its known anti-interferon-gamma capabilities.[67] Trials are also under way to specifically decrease the cells implicated in the autoimmune reaction, as well as to use various monoclonal antibodies to interrupt the inflammatory process.

SIGNS AND SYMPTOMS

The initial signs and symptoms of MS are quite variable. A general summary of these findings is provided in Tables 52–3 and 52–4. Fifty percent of patients have symptoms related to one site or system, and 40% present with weakness.[34] Optic neuritis is present at the onset in 20% to 48% of patients.[32] Reported signs and symptoms during the course of this illness vary significantly, depending on which patients are included in the study. If studies are limited to those symptoms present at the time of their death, all patients have had ocular symptoms and 93% have complained of weakness at one time in their illness. Table 52–4 provides a general summary of signs and symptoms seen in definite MS. Weakness is often accompanied by an increase in muscle stretch reflexes and is one of the more frequent symptoms found in patients with MS. The distribution of the weakness is most commonly in both lower extremities, with the next most common pattern being one leg, or one leg and the ipsilateral arm. Weakness confined to one or both upper extremities is unusual.[50]

Paresthesias can be present at any stage of the disease and often are described as painful. True radicular pain is unusual, and other causes should be sought when this occurs. Cerebellar signs increase during the course of the disease and often lead to marked disability.[50]

The general course of the illness in MS is variable but generally falls into a benign category (with one or two episodes followed by long periods of remission), a relapsing and remitting course, a relapsing-progressive course, or a chronic progressive course.

TABLE 52–2 Immune Basis for MS: Theory

Action	Effect
T cells release cytokines, damaging endothelial cells	Cytokines cause defects in blood-brain barrier
T cells attach to HLA receptor on myelin, releasing tumor necrosis factor (TNF) and interferon-gamma (INF-γ)	TNF and INF-γ destroy myelin sheaths
T cells attach to HLA receptor on macrophages	Macrophages release TNF, which directly attacks myelin
T cells activate B cells to secrete antibody	Antibody combines with complement to directly attack the oligodendrocyte

TABLE 52–3 Symptoms Present at Onset of Illness in Definite MS

Symptom	% of Patients
Weakness	40
Paresthesia	30
Gait difficulty	25
Optic neuritis	20
Diplopia	15
Ataxia	10
Disturbed nutrition	10
Vertigo	5

TABLE 52–4 Signs and Symptoms Present During the Course of MS

Sign/Symptom	% of Patients
Paresthesia	100
Weakness	100
Abnormal reflexes	80
Cerebellar signs	80
Spasticity	75
Fatigue	75
Decreased alternating movements	70
Heat intolerance	60
Nystagmus	50
Cognitive impairment	40
Erectile impotence	40
Lhermitte's sign	40
Pain	30
Depression	30
Muscle wasting	20
Dementia	10
Facial weakness	3
Unilateral hearing loss	3
Epilepsy	2
Visual failure	1
Trigeminal neuralgia	1

DIAGNOSIS AND COURSE

Because of the pleomorphic aspects of MS, the diagnosis depends on a skilled clinician's recognition of signs of demyelination. Visual, gait, and sensory disturbances are the most common presentations at the onset of the disease. Diagnostic criteria for MS established by Poser and colleagues are listed in Table 52–5.[66] In this schema an attack is defined as a neurological deficit lasting more than 24 hours. In 63% to 91% of patients MS begins with a relapsing and remitting course, with a majority of the exacerbations occurring in the first 5 to 10 years of the illness.[34] In many patients the disorder becomes stable or progresses only slowly after this point.[45] Chronic progressive MS is more likely to occur in patients with disease onset after age 40.[32] In many cases the disease is characterized by a long latent period, with minimal symptoms of progression. It is not clear whether the disease is active during these periods. Factors associated with an increase in MS exacerbations are listed in Table 52–6.

The course of MS is extremely variable, ranging from death within 5 years in 5% of affected people, to many cases that are manifested by only one episode. In some cases MS can be diagnosed only post mortem.[29] A decrease in life expectancy by 9½ years in men and 14 years in women has been reported,[45] but this is skewed by the rapid downhill course of a small percentage of patients. In the remainder of the MS population, life expectancy is not significantly affected. Severe disability is noted in 10% of patients within 5 years, in 25% of patients within 10 years, and in 50% of patients within 18 years. Approximately 20% of patients have no disability after 15 years of having MS.[49] Annual relapse rates in MS vary in different studies, ranging from 0.1 exacerbations per year to 1.5.[81] None of these indicators are absolute, and at best they can be used only as general predictors. Factors associated with poor prognosis in MS include[49]:

- Progressive course at onset
- Male sex
- Age at onset > 40 years
- Cerebellar involvement at onset
- Multiple system involvement at onset

TABLE 52–5 Diagnostic Criteria

Possible MS

History of relapsing and possibly remitting signs without prior neurogenic symptomatology.
Only one site of involvement in CNS determined by clinical, laboratory, or imaging studies.
No other diagnostic explanation.

Probable MS

Two documented attacks with clinical, laboratory, or imaging evidence of at least one lesion.
One documented attack with clinical, laboratory, or imaging evidence of two separate lesions.

Definite MS

Two attacks, separated by at least 1 month, with clinical, laboratory, or imaging evidence of at least two lesions.

TABLE 52–6 Factors Associated with an Increase in MS Exacerbations

Factors	Evidence
Infectious agents	Faroe islands epidemic Increase in measles antibodies in CSF of MS patients Seasonal fluctuations Increased number of exacerbations after infections
Pregnancy	Decreased risk during pregnancy, increased risk for 3–6 months post partum
Fatigue and heat	Can cause transient weakness; unlikely to cause actual exacerbation
Stress	Unproven; medico-legal implications
Trauma	Very controversial; described in 5% to 15% of cases; generally felt to be unrelated
Heavy metals	Reported after exposure to zinc (association not proved)
Diet	Association not proved; attempted diets include low-fat, gluten-free; megavitamins
Other autoimmune diseases	No clear linkage seen

SOME FEATURES

Cranial Nerve Involvement

Optic neuritis is more common early in the illness. It is usually associated with pain in the eye or forehead that can occasionally be severe. The visual field defect is typically a central scotoma. Bilateral simultaneous optic neuritis is not unusual and is especially common in patients of Japanese descent.[50] The visual-evoked potential after optic neuritis never returns to normal even if normal vision returns.

Trigeminal neuralgia is present in 1% of patients.[34] It can be bilateral and often is the presenting symptom. Facial palsy can be seen. Facial myokymia, manifested by rapidly firing muscular contractions of the facial muscles, is not unusual.[34] Vertigo is common and can be severe and associated with vomiting. This might be the only initial symptom in patients with MS, but it is almost always transient.

Epilepsy

Epilepsy occurs in 1% to 2% of patients with MS (making it perhaps no more common than in the general population). Tonic seizures are the most common seizures seen in MS. They are often triggered by movement. They generally involve one arm or leg. They typically last for a few seconds, although they can occur many times during the day. Other paroxysmal symptoms lasting for less than 1 to 2 minutes include dysarthria, ataxia, itching, and focal pain.[34]

Pain

Pain occurs in up to 50% of patients with MS. It is chronic in 90% of cases and manifests as dysesthetic extremity pain, chronic back pain, or painful leg cramps.[50] The dysesthetic pain is the most common and also the most difficult to treat.

Acute pain most frequently takes the form of trigeminal neuralgia or transient dysesthetic extremity pain.[49] All of these symptoms might respond to gabapentin (Neurontin), up to 2400 mg per day, or carbamazepine (Tegretol), up to 1200 mg per day.

DIFFERENTIAL DIAGNOSIS

The differential diagnosis in MS encompasses many entities, some of which are listed in Table 52–1. Care should be taken in diagnosing MS in the absence of eye findings, during a clinical remission, or in the presence of localized or atypical clinical features.

TREATMENT

Because of its variable presentations, the treatment of MS should be individualized for each patient. Treatments can be divided into symptomatic therapies and those that are designed to affect the natural course of the disease or to alter the length and severity of individual exacerbations. A sample of drug treatments is listed in Table 52–7. It is important to recognize and convey to the individual with MS that relapse rates decrease as the disease progresses, with the vast majority of relapses occurring in the first 5 to 10 years after the onset of initial symptoms.[43]

Treatment results in MS should be based on both objective findings and the subjective complaints of each patient. Objective findings with imaging techniques, evoked potentials, and morbid anatomy do not always correlate with the clinical presentation.

Many measurement devices have been proposed to monitor treatment efficacy. The most commonly used is the Kurtzke Disability Status Scale in either its original or expanded[45] forms (Tables 52–8 and 52–9).[44]

Treatment Designed to Alter the Course of the Disease

Steroids

Since 1970 the role of steroids in decreasing the length and severity of MS exacerbations has been documented in many articles.[13] The mechanism of action is unknown

TABLE 52–7 Sample Drug Treatments for MS

Medication	Dosage	Effects
Medications for Use in Exacerbations		
Prednisone	80–100 mg daily with taper over 7–21 days	Decreases length and severity of exacerbation
ACTH	40 units b.i.d. × 7 days	
Solumedrol	1000 mg IV over 2–4 hr, daily × 7 days, followed by 7–21 days of taper oral steroids	
Disease-Altering Medications		
Interferons	8 million units SQ, QD	
INF-β-1B	30 micrograms 1M qw	
INF-β-1A		
Copolymer-1	25 mg SQ qd	Decreases number of exacerbations
Medications for Chronic MS		
Cyclophosphamide with or without ACTH	By protocol	Slows progression in chronic MS
Azathioprine	By protocol	Slows progression in chronic MS
Cyclosporin A	By protocol	Slows progression in chronic MS
Medications for Fatigue		
Amantadine	200–300 mL/day	Decreases fatigue
Pemoline		Liver toxicity
Medications for Spasticity		
Baclofen	20–120 mg/day	Decreases spasticity
Dantrolene	75–250 mg/day	Decreases spasticity
Tizanidine	4–16 mg/day	Decreases spasticity
Valium	5–40 mg/day	Decreases spasticity
Medications for Paroxysmal Symptoms		
Carbamazepine	200 mg b.i.d. or TIW	Decreases pain and parynchemal spasms
Gabapentin	300–2400 mg/day	Decreases pain and spasticity
Phenytoin	200–400 mg 1 day	Decreases pain and parynchemal spasms
Medications for Ataxia		
Clonazepan	1–6 mg/day	Decreases ataxia
Isoniazid	900 mg/day	Decreases ataxia

TABLE 52–8 Neurological Assessment: Kurtzke Disability Status Scale (DSS)

0	Normal neurological examination (all grade 0 in functional systems*)
1	No disability and minimal signs such as Babinski sign or vibratory decrease
2	Minimal disability, for example, slight weakness or mild gait, sensory, visuomotor disturbance
3	Moderate disability though fully ambulatory (for example, monoparesis, moderate ataxia, or combinations of lesser dysfunctions)
4	Relatively severe disability though fully ambulatory and able to be self-sufficient and up and about for some 12 hours a day
5	Disability severe enough to preclude ability to work a full day without special provisions. Maximal motor function: walking unaided no more than several blocks
6	Assistance (canes, crutches, or braces) required for walking
7	Restricted to wheelchair but able to wheel self and enter and leave chair alone
8	Restricted to bed but with effective use of arms
9	Totally helpless bed-ridden patients
10	Death due to multiple sclerosis

* Excludes cerebral function grade 1.
From Hart RG, Sherman DO: The diagnosis of MS. JAMA 1982; 247:498–503.

but might relate to a decrease in CNS edema or to an effect on the immune system. Oral or intravenous steroids have been used more recently, with similar results. Oral prednisone, in a dose of 60 to 100 mg tapered over 1 to 3 weeks, is frequently used for the treatment of a documented exacerbation of MS.[72] Any existing infections should be treated before steroid treatments are started. If the exacerbation does not respond or is severe, intravenous doses of 500 to 1000 mg of methylprednisolone given daily for 3 to 7 days are recommended. The dose should be given over 2 to 3 hours to minimize the possibility of cardiac arrhythmias.[1] Large doses of methylprednisolone change the C9 and C8 T-cell indices as well as contribute to the abnormal IgG levels found in the CSF of MS patients during an exacerbation. These CSF effects have not been noted with lower oral doses.[17]

There is no definite measure of what constitutes an exacerbation of MS and when steroid treatment should be utilized. Each clinician has to make this decision based on the patient's specific pattern of MS, previous response to steroids, and overall condition. I consider an exacerbation to occur when the patient experiences a neurological change resulting in a decrease in functional capacity that lasts longer than 24 hours. Steroids can usually be safely administered two to three times per year. The patient must understand that although the length and severity of exacerbations can be affected by these treatments, the number of exacerbations and the ultimate course of the illness are in no way modified.[19, 71]

The use of steroids in the treatment of chronic progressive MS has not been shown to be effective. Drug management for this entity remains controversial and unsatisfactory, although recent studies with interferon-beta-1B might change this situation. Cyclophosphamide, with or without ACTH, has been shown to be beneficial by some investigators.[23] Castor and Huflei reported slowing of the illness in approximately 30% to 60% of their patients.[12] Others have been unable to duplicate these findings, however, and similar results have been found with low-dose methotrexate.[57]

Immunosuppressive Agents

Other attempts at immunosuppression in chronic MS have included the use of azathioprine[63, 76, 82] and, more recently, cyclosporin A.[55] Cyclosporin A has been shown to delay the time to becoming wheelchair dependent in patients with chronic progressive MS, but nephrotoxicity has limited its usefulness.[55] Plasmapheresis has also been used in addition to these medications, with mixed results.[33, 39] Studies of the use of these treatments are ongoing.

Disease-Modifying Treatment, Interferon and Copaxone

Three disease-modifing immunosuppressive therapy treatments are currently in widespread clinical use: two interferons, interferon-beta-1A (Avonex) and interferon-beta-1B (Betaseron), and glatirimer acetate (Copaxone). Each of these has been shown to be safe, to decrease the number of exacerbations by one-third, and possibly to slow the progression in chronic MS.[23]

Two other types of interferon, alpha and gamma, exist and also act as immunosuppressants. The use of interferon-alpha in the treatment of MS has been shown to be ineffectual.[11, 35, 41] Interferon-gamma has been shown to lead to an increase in the severity of the disease.[60] Interferons as a class impede viral replication, slow cell proliferation, and alter immune responses. Studies with interferon-beta have demonstrated a one-third decrease in incidence of exacerbations in patients with relapsing-remitting MS and a 50% decrease in severe exacerbations. A decreased accumulation of plaque has been measured on MRI in 60% of patients taking this medicine.

The two FDA-approved types of interferon for MS are interferon-beta-1A (Avonex) and interferon-beta-1B (Betaseron). They have been tested in double-blind, multicenter trials involving over 500 patients.[4, 49, 84] The major side effects include flu-like symptoms in approximately 60% of patients, which can usually be successfully treated with either anti-inflammatory medication or low-dose prednisone. Injection site reactions are also very common with interferon-beta, but rarely proceed to develop skin necrosis. Such reactions can usually be controlled by emphasizing proper injection technique, including rotating sites, injection to the proper depth using smaller-gauge needles, and emphasizing proper sterile technique.

Glatirimer acetate (Copaxone) is a synthetic polypeptide consisting of four amino acids. In a 2-year study of relapsing-remitting MS, glatirimer was found to decrease exacerbations by 29%. It also showed a significant slowing of cumulative disability.[38] Other studies, however, have demostrated a lack of response in patients with chronic progressive MS.[9] Major side effects include

TABLE 52–9 Neurological Assessment: Kurtzke Expanded Disability Status Scale (EDSS)

0	Normal neurological examination (all grade 0 in FS*)
1.0	No disability, minimal signs in one FS (i.e., grade 1)
1.5	No disability, minimal signs in more than one FS* (more than one FS grade 1)
2.0	Minimal disability in one FS (one FS grade 2; others 0 or 1)
2.5	Minimal disability in two FS (two FS grade 2; others 0 or 1)
3.0	Fully ambulatory but with moderate disability in one FS (one grade 3) and one or two FS grade 2; or two FS grade 3; or five FS grade 2 (others 0 or 1)
3.5	Fully ambulatory but with moderate disability in one FS (one grade 3) and one or two FS grade 2, or two FS grade 3; or five FS grade 2 (others 0 or 1)
4.0	Fully ambulatory without aid, self-sufficient, up and about some 12 hours a day despite relatively severe disability consisting of one FS grade 4 (others 0 or 1), or combinations of lesser grades exceeding limits of previous steps; able to walk without aid or rest some 500 meters
4.5	Fully ambulatory without aid, up and about much of the day, able to work a full day, may otherwise have some limitation of full activity or require minimal assistance; characterized by relatively severe disability usually consisting of one FS grade 4 (others 0 or 1) or combinations of lesser grades exceeding limits of previous steps; able to walk without aid or rest some 300 meters
5.0	Ambulatory without aid or rest for about 200 meters; disability severe enough to impair full daily activities (e.g., to work a full day without special provisions) (usual FS equivalents are one grade 5 alone, others 0 or 1; or combinations of lesser grades usually exceeding specifications for step 4.0)
5.5	Ambulatory without aid or rest for about 100 meters; disability severe enough to preclude full daily activities (usual FS equivalents are one grade 5 alone, others 0 or 1; or combination of lesser grades usually exceeding those for step 4.0)
6.0	Intermittent or unilateral constant assistance (cane, crutch, brace) required to walk about 100 meters with or without resting (usual FS equivalents are combinations with more than two FS grade 3+)
6.5	Constant bilateral assistance (canes, crutches, braces) required to walk about 20 meters without resting (usual FS equivalents are combinations with more than two FS grade 3+)
7.0	Unable to walk beyond approximately 5 meters even with aid, essentially restricted to wheelchair; wheels self in standard wheelchair and transfers alone; up and about in wheelchair some 12 hours a day (usual FS equivalents are combinations with more than one FS grade 4+; very rarely pyramidal grade 5 alone)
7.5	Unable to take more than a few steps; restricted to wheelchair; may need aid in transfer; wheels self but cannot carry on in standard wheelchair a full day; may require motorized wheelchair (usual FS equivalents are combinations with more than one FS grade 4+)
8.0	Essentially restricted to bed or chair or perambulated in wheelchair, but may be out of bed itself much of the day; retains many self-care functions; generally has effective use of arms (usual FS equivalents are combinations, generally grade 4+ in several systems)
8.5	Essentially restricted to bed much of day; has some effective use of arm(s); retains some self-care functions (usual FS equivalents are combinations generally 4+ in several systems)
9.0	Helpless bed-ridden patient; can communicate and eat (usual FS equivalents are combinations, mostly grade 4+)
9.5	Totally helpless bed-ridden patient; unable to communicate effectively or eat/swallow (usual FS equivalents are combinations, almost all grade 4+)
10.0	Death due to MS

Abbreviation: FS, functional system.
* Excludes cerebral function grade 1.
From Hart RG, Sherman DO: The diagnosis of MS. JAMA 1982; 247:498–503.

flu-like symptoms and occasional injection site reactions. These problems are generally well tolerated. A transient flushing associated with chest tightness and dyspnea lasting for 30 seconds to 30 minutes is experienced by 15% of patients. This typically resolves spontaneously.

Controversy exists as to the best time to begin immunosuppressive therapy in patients with MS. The physician must decide when the benefits of treatment outweigh the cost and side effects. In the case of stable MS or in patients who have had only one attack of the disease with good resolution, immunosuppressive therapy might not be beneficial. Original studies of interferon included only patients who were ambulating and were between the ages of 15 and 50, with Kurtkze disability scores of 5 or less. The Quality Standards Committee of the American Academy of Neurology has expanded this use to include patients older than 50, or nonambulating patients who are still losing function.[68]

A recent study in Europe of 700 patients with secondary progressive MS utilized 8 million units of interferon-beta subcutaneously every other day. The study was discontinued early because of the excellent response of treated patients when compared with those given placebo. Disease progressed in 38% of those treated with the medicine but in 50% of untreated patients. Relapse rate, hospitalization, and lesion volumes on T2-weighted MRI were similarly affected.[23] Further evidence pointing to the early use of interferon includes the significant decrease in plaque load on MRI,[65, 69, 83] especially in the corpus callosum and periventricular areas. Recent studies indicate that up to 70% of MS patients have cognitive deficits, and half of these have them early in the course of the disease.[65, 69, 83, 90] Early use of these medications will hopefully diminish further cognitive deterioration.

4-Aminopyridine

4-Aminopyridine (4-AP) has been shown to block potassium channel activation in animals, thus prolonging the duration of nerve action potentials and restoring conduction in previously blocked demyelinated fibers.[73, 74] VonDiemen and colleagues[91] treated 70 patients with relapsing-remitting MS with intravenous and oral 4-AP and placebo. Subjective improvement (defined as improvement in activities of daily living capabilities) was noted in 29% of the patients taking the medication but in only 1.6% of those taking placebo. At least a 1-point change in the Kurtkze disability score was seen in 16% of the patients. Patients with the most severe illness noted the most benefit from this medication.[91] Unfortunately, the clinical use of 4-AP has been delayed because of significant side effects, primarily seizures.[74]

Treatment Designed to Ameliorate the Course of the Disease

The overall goal of rehabilitation in MS is to maximize function, regardless of whether the impairment is stable or worsening. Since MS affects all phases of a patient's life, the skills of the entire rehabilitation team are needed to minimize this disability. Individuals with MS frequently present with problems in gait, sexuality, driving, shopping, cleaning house, urinary function, and socioeconomic stability. All of these factors lend themselves to intervention by the rehabilitation team. Providing assistance in these areas is extremely beneficial to the individual and the family and is critical to the maintenance of maximal function.

Ameliorating Weakness

Since weakness is often a significant problem in MS, it is important that general conditioning be maintained as long as possible. This has to be done in a way that does not increase fatigue or body temperature. Because elevated body temperature can worsen MS symptoms, it is important that these patients have air conditioning in their homes and cars, especially if they live in southern climates. They might even consider moving to a more temperate zone to alleviate these problems. An individualized exercise program should be developed by a physician or physical therapist and should be adapted to any ongoing changes in the patient's disease process.[21] The use of air resistance stationary bikes (air movement minimizes temperature fluctuation), cool therapeutic pools (84°F [29°C] or less), or upper extremity ergometers has proved beneficial in maintaining general aerobic conditioning. Such aerobic exercise has been shown by Petajan et al to have a significant impact not only on the patient's aerobic capacity, but also in decreasing depression, anger, and fatigue.[64]

If patients wish to do additional exercises, a light weight progressive resistance exercise program can be performed as tolerated. The use of weights, although often beneficial, is often not feasible, especially if the patient's primary disability relates to ataxia rather than weakness. Prior to embarking on any exercise program, a submaximal cardiovascular stress test should be performed to determine cardiac safety and an appropriate level of exercise intensity. Maintaining the optimal function of the musculoskeletal system is certainly helpful in minimizing the disability associated with MS. Not to be overlooked, however, is the significant psychological benefit and increase in overall self-esteem garnered from participating in a "can do" program.

Ameliorating Fatigue

The physician dealing with the patient with MS should be aware of the role that fatigue plays in resultant disability. The actual source of the fatigue is not well understood but might represent a combination of weakness, spasticity, ataxia, depression, and heat.[27] The Social Security Administration has recognized the disabling aspects of fatigue and has allowed it to be considered a major factor in the granting of disability benefits to people with MS. Patients with characteristic afternoon fatigue might benefit from Pemoline, 18.75 mg/day (up to 75 mg), as needed. Patients on this medicine must be watched closely for liver toxicity. Owing to the medication's stimulant and abuse potential, care should be taken to monitor the patient's response. The reason why a low dose of this stimulant often provides dramatic relief of fatigue is not clearly understood but might relate to a change in neurotransmitters in the area of brain from which the fatigue emanates. In my experience, this drug has one of the highest patient acceptance rates of all the medications used in the symptomatic treatment of MS. Amantadine (Symmetrel) in doses of 200 to 300 mg/day has also been documented to be useful.[16] The clinician might need to try each of these drugs in combination to determine the most beneficial regimen for any one patient.

Improving Mobility

Mobility problems are among the most common complaints voiced by individuals with MS. In a National Multiple Sclerosis Society survey, 60% of 122,000 patients reported the need for some assistance with mobility.[6] Maintaining mobility and functional independence is a constant challenge to the rehabilitation team, mainly due to the ever-changing clinical picture. Appropriate assistive devices should be prescribed to increase safety and decrease energy expenditure. Careful attention should be paid to psychological changes triggered by the need for these devices and the resultant implication that the disease is progressing. The experienced MS practitioner is constantly aware of these "crisis points" in the course of the patient's illness and deals with them on an individual basis, initiating medical and psychosocial interventions that are indicated. Patients should be informed that, on average, individuals with MS are still ambulating 27 years after diagnosis.[56] Proper prescription and instruction in the use of wheelchairs often prolongs and increases the patient's functional independence. Motorized three-wheeled scooters are frequently preferred by the patient with MS due to the perception of greater societal acceptance. Care should be taken to ensure that the patient does not lose remaining functional ambulation by becoming overly dependent on these aids (see Chapter 18). Such aids should initially be used for long distances and difficult tasks, with patients continuing to ambulate on their own when doing less stressful activity.

Habilitation in Activities of Daily Living

Activities of daily living are often affected in patients with MS. Brainstem lesions can result in dysphagia for liquids and solids. This can be evaluated by videofluoroscopy and treated by dietary management (see Chapter 26). Problems with balance, mobility, ataxia, spasticity, and weakness frequently lead to difficulty with hygiene, dressing, toileting, and communication. These problems are frequently amenable to the efforts of a rehabilitation team trained specifically to deal with the unique and variable patterns of MS.[26] Although rehabilitative management is often minimized by the medical community, it is critical to the successful adjustment of patients with MS and their families. Visits by a trained occupational therapist to a patient's home or office to recommend ergonomic considerations often lead to a marked increase in the patient's quality of life (see Chapter 25).

Assistance with Vocational and Avocational Activities

MS affects people in the prime of their lives, often after they have made and developed career choices. One-third of patients with MS are able to continue on their regular career path without modification, while another third can continue working with the help of the rehabilitation team and vocational counseling.[21] Economic problems are experienced by 83% of MS patients at some time in their illness. The average patient suffers a 40% decrease in total lifetime earning capacity.[56] Employers should be given information on the specific needs of the MS workers, including the elimination of architectural barriers and the role of fatigue in the patient's illness. The individual with MS should be counseled about the Americans With Disability Act and efforts required to accommodate the MS patient with disability. For most individuals with MS, having to discontinue working can engender great stress and torment. The physician should anticipate this and assist patients in this difficult transition (see Chapter 35).

Various home work situations, volunteer activities, and return to educational pursuits can ease these difficulties. The National Multiple Sclerosis Society is a reliable resource to assist the patient and physician in this regard. It can be reached at 1-800-295-1765.

OTHER PROBLEMS TO BE ADDRESSED IN TREATING MS

Cognitive and Psychiatric Aspects

Cognitive and psychiatric changes were once thought to be unusual in people with MS.[7] More recent data indicate that the problems are far more common than was previously suspected[83] and frequently contribute substantially to the patient's level of disability. Memory appears to be the most affected function, with conceptual and abstract reasoning diminished to a lesser extent.[65] One study of 108 patients reported mild intellectual deficits in 41% of people with MS, moderate deficits in 14%, and severe deficits in 6.5%. Although the severity tends to increase with duration, significant mental impairment can exist even in the presence of otherwise mild MS.[37] MRI studies have demonstrated that patients with more severe cognitive impairments typically have more extensive brain lesions, although disagreements exist as to which MRI abnormality best distinguishes cognitively impaired and unimpaired patients.[40]

Several authors characterize the dementia of MS as being of a subcortical type, marked by impaired manipulation of acquired knowledge, slowness of cognitive process, apathy, and lack of initiative. Vandenberg et al report that this leads to "slowness in acquiring new information from the outside world and in responding to its demands."[90] These cognitive problems are very important to identify, as patients with such deficits are also less likely to be employed and more likely to engage in fewer social and avocational activities, to have increased sexual difficulties, and to exhibit more psychopathology.[80, 83]

Psychiatric changes in MS have been described since the time of Charcot, with euphoria noted in 63% of patients in an early study by Cottrell and Wilson.[20] An increase in the incidence of depression has recently been noted that correlates with the degree of neurological impairment but not with functional disability, and is greater than that seen in other neuromuscular illnesses. One study of 108 patients with MS found depression that was mild in 17%, moderate in 7%, and severe in 4%.[37] Other authors indicate a depression rate of 27% to 54%, especially in patients who are older or who have more cognitive deficits.[7] It remains to be clarified whether these psychiatric changes are an organic result of the MS or are a reaction to the illness. This could be of clinical significance, as some patients with MS respond to very low doses of antidepressants and are thought to exhibit depression as a result of plaques in areas of the brain controlling emotions. Schizophrenia does not appear to be increased in MS compared to the general population, but both frequently have their onset in the same age groups. The treating physician should be aware of potential emotional problems and deal with them aggressively as soon as they are identified.

Neurogenic Bladder

Bladder dysfunction is a frequent complaint in MS patients. Early changes include either an increase or decrease in detrusor, bladder neck, or external sphincter control. Later stages of the disease are marked by bladder hyperreflexia and dyssynergia. The evaluation for these problems should include laboratory assessment of general renal function, with several determinations of postvoiding residuals. Cystometric evaluation with associated electromyographic monitoring of the pelvic floor musculature (see also Chapter 27) is helpful in categorizing bladder dysfunction. The constantly changing nature of the neurological and urological deficit in the patient with MS should be recognized before treatment is begun. Available treatments are summarized in Table 52–10.

Management of mild neurogenic bladder symptoms should begin with regulation of fluid intake to 1800 mL per 24-hour period and limiting intake after dinner. If postvoid residuals exceed 100 mL, consideration should be given to a program of intermittent catheterization.

TABLE 52–10 Treatment of Neurogenic Bladder in MS

Treatment	Background
Fluid restrictions	2000 mL/day with fluid restrictions after dinner
Intermittent catheterization	If postvoid residuals consistently greater than 100 mL
Sulfa or methenamine	Often used with intermittent catheterization
Medications	Probanthine Oxybutynin Bethanechol Ephedrine Prazosin Baclofen Indwelling catheter

Oxybutynin, 5 to 20 mg/day, can be used for its anticholinergic and direct smooth muscle relaxant effect on the bladder detrusor. Detrusor tone can be increased with the use of bethanechol. Alpha-adrenergic drugs such as ephedrine can be used to increase bladder tone. Alpha-adrenergic-blocking agents (prazosin or phenoxybenzamine) can decrease bladder neck tone. Baclofen can decrease external sphincter dyssynergia. Antibiotics such as sulfa or methenamine are often used prophylactically in conjunction with intermittent catheterization, but should be avoided when an indwelling catheter is utilized.

Neurogenic Bowel

Stool incontinence or constipation is often a disconcerting problem for the individual with MS. A bowel program that includes a high-fiber diet, a bulk former, a stool softener, and adequate fluid intake should be developed early in the course of the disease, before significant difficulties develop. The use of laxatives and enemas should be discouraged. It constipation becomes a problem, glycerin or dulcolax suppositories, taken 45 minutes after the day's major meal, can be useful in maintaining bowel function (see also Chapter 28).

Spasticity

Spasticity is a common problem in the management of the patient with MS. It can interfere with rehabilitation even when it is not associated with concurrent weakness. Severe spasticity can be totally disabling. Management options are outlined in Table 52–11 but should always begin with instructing the patient and family in a program of stretching the affected muscles and putting the involved joints through a full range of motion.[53] Attempts should be made to identify and correct sources of nociceptive input to the CNS, since they can worsen spasticity. Such irritating stimuli can include urinary tract infections, skin ulcers, constipation, deep venous thrombosis, or other irritative conditions. If spasticity remains a problem, the carefully monitored use of medications should be instituted. Baclofen is the initial drug of choice when spasticity is of spinal origin, but it is less useful in spasticity of supraspinal origin. The mechanism of action is both pre- and postsynaptic, and it is less likely to cause weakness and fatigue than either diazepam or dantrolene.[5] Baclofen treatment should begin at 10 to 20 mg/day in divided doses, with titration up to a dose of 80 to 100 mg/day if necessary. Care should be taken that the patient does not abruptly discontinue the medicine, as seizures can result. Tizanidine (Zanaflex), 8 to 16 mg/day, is another helpful drug, but its usefulness is often limited by sedation.

Benzodiazepines such as diazepam can be added if spasticity persists. They work at the spinal level but must be used cautiously as they can enhance previously existing fatigue, weakness, depression, and sedation.

In refractory cases, dantrolene can also be utilized. Its mechanism of action is peripheral (it prevents myofibrillar contraction).[54] Aggravation of previously existing weakness is often a problem. The dose should be gradually increased from 25 mg/day to 300 mg/day. Patients taking this medication should have close monitoring of their liver enzyme levels. Hepatotoxicity can occur, with the greatest incidence in women over 35 years of age.

Other drugs used with varying degrees of success for spasticity include phenytoin, carbamazepine, and phenothiazines. Recent trials have utilized localized botulinum toxin injection for a more specific and reversible treatment of intractable spasticity.[8] In refractory cases phenol nerve blocks can be attempted. The long-term nature of such blocks, as well as the possible side effect of painful paresthesias, limits their usefulness. If spasticity remains a problem, the use of intrathecal baclofen, neurectomy, rhizotomy, tenotomy, or myelotomy might be required. For further information about spasticity treatment, see Chapter 29.

Ataxia and Tremor

Ataxia and tremor are especially vexing symptoms in the person with MS, as they are often nonresponsive to rehabilitative or drug treatment. Light weights attached to the distal aspect of the extremities can decrease the appendicular component of ataxia. If exacerbated by weakness, appropriate strengthening can be beneficial. Repetitive coordinative exercises, such as those recommended by Frankel, are rarely useful, owing to the progressive nature of the illness. In patients with extremity ataxia that interferes with dressing or feeding, appropriate proximal splinting can be beneficial. Drug therapy is of limited usefulness. Clonazepam (1 to 6 mg/day)

TABLE 52–11 Treatment of Spasticity in MS

Decreased nociceptive input (bowel/bladder-skin, etc.)
Stretching the involved muscles
Baclofen
Dantrium
Valium
Intrathecal baclofen
Botulinum toxin nerve blocks
Phenol nerve blocks
Tenotomy, rhizotomy
Myelotomy

has been used with and without primidone (250 mg/day), with only slight success, and can cause drowsiness. Isoniazid (up to 900 mg/day) can be used in conjunction with pyridoxine (to reduce the resultant peripheral neuropathy). The mechanism of action for all of these drugs is unknown, and response rates of greater than 10% to 20% are unlikely.[26]

Sexual Function

In the early stages of MS there can be varied types of sexual dysfunction, most of which are usually transient. As the illness progresses, these symptoms typically become more frequent. In a study of 302 people with MS, 91% of men and 72% of women reported changes in their sexual life. Disturbances in erection were noted in 62% of males. Failure to achieve orgasm (33%), loss of libido (27%), and spasticity (12%) were the most common complaints in women.[46] Treatment involves identifying the problem as early as possible and providing appropriate counseling. Localized injections of papaverine or the use of penile implants can be beneficial for erection problems (see also Chapter 30). Sildenafil (Viagra) is often helpful in this population for erectile dysfunction.

Pregnancy

The effects of MS on pregnancy are very important, but remain controversial. In a recent study by Confavreux et al,[18] who followed 254 women with MS through 269 pregnancies, there were no excess pregnancy-related complications, with a mean pregnancy duration of 39 weeks and 27 pregnancies ending before the 36th week. In the year prior to becoming pregnant, the patients averaged 0.7 MS relapses. This number dropped to 0.5 relapses during the first trimester of pregnancy, 0.6 during the second trimester, and 0.2 during the third trimester. The relapse rate increased to 1.2 per year during the first 3 months post partum, however, leading to an overall relapse rate unchanged for the year dated from the onset of pregnancy to the first 3 months post partum. Epidural anesthesia and breast-feeding had no effect on the results. The authors postulate that the fetal placental units secrete downregulating cytokines, such as interleukin-10, resulting in the decreased exacerbation rate during pregnancy, with a reversal of this effect occurring immediately post partum.

The Effect of Trauma and Stress

Physicians involved in the treatment of patients with MS are often asked by patients or attorneys to comment on the possible association of trauma or stress on the onset or worsening of MS. This notion dates to 1897, when Mendel[52] reported four cases of MS after spinal cord injury or head trauma. Studies reported since that time have had mixed findings, with results showing a possible but not definite relationship. The proposed relationship assumes that trauma leads to a breakdown of the blood-brain barrier, thus triggering an exacerbation of MS. This presumed mechanism does not explain, however, why the abnormalities in MS are confined to the white matter and why MS is more common in women. Some studies reporting a link between trauma and the onset of MS contained small numbers of subjects and considered an exacerbation to be related to the trauma even if it occurred 1 year after the original episode. Other studies do not clearly define what constitutes significant trauma. The bulk of the studies[2, 42, 49, 75, 77] lead to the conclusion that there is no association between trauma and the course of MS.

The relationship of psychological trauma to the onset of MS is even more difficult to clarify. Several authors have reported an increase in life stress prior to the onset or exacerbation of MS. The significance of these concerns is still being debated.[30, 58]

Charlatanism

The chronic and variable nature of MS, coupled with the lack of a cure, makes the individual with this illness especially susceptible to medical quackery. Numerous miracle treatments have been proposed for MS, including calcium products, snake venom, bee pollen, removal of dental amalgams, megavitamins, and hyperbaric oxygen. None of these have been shown to be effective, and they are often nothing more than a hoax. The physician must be sensitive to the desire of the MS patient to "try anything" and counter these claims with education and the utilization of the full line of available rehabilitation resources.

RESEARCH DIRECTIVES

Physiatrists are well aware of the efficacy and benefit of rehabilitation techniques for the person with MS. Documented outcome studies, however, are critical to ensure future funding for these treatments. The impact on every aspect of life, including family, work, leisure, and physical function, mandates that psychosocial and rehabilitation studies become a major goal of MS research grants. Funding for such grants is strongly supported by the National Multiple Sclerosis Society, which in the past 15 years has provided $35 million for research. Research into the development of objective measures to track the course of MS and its response to various therapies are also critically needed. MRI and MR spectroscopy might prove useful in better enabling the research team to evaluate the effects of various interventions. Other areas of potential interest to the MS researcher include the following:

- Immunology
- Biology of glial cells
- Virology
- Therapy
- Genetics
- Utilization and availability of health services

INPATIENT REHABILITATION

With the current cost-containment pressures on rehabilitative facilities, patients with MS are often underserved in inpatient rehabilitation. This is despite the fact that rehabilitation, especially on an inpatient basis, can enhance the quality of a patient's life, improve functional status, and reduce overall health care costs.[25] In a study by Greenspan and co-workers,[31] two-thirds of patients admitted to the rehabilitation unit were transferred from an acute hospital, with the most common problems being mobility deficits and difficulty in performing activities of daily living. The average length of stay was 27 days, and follow-up visits at 90 days revealed excellent maintenance of gains made during hospitalization.[31] It appears that in patients whose functional capacities are significantly diminished, especially if they are going to have difficulty in maintaining independent living, an admission to an inpatient rehabilitation unit can often provide the skills necessary to avoid placement in a long-term care facility.

REFERENCES

1. Albruzzesi G, Gendolfo C, Loeb C: Bolus methylprednisone versus ACTH in the treatment for multiple sclerosis. J Neurosci 1983; 4:169–172.
2. Alter M, Speer J: Clinical evaluation of possible etiologic factors in MS. Neurology 1968; 18:109–115.
3. Aminoff MJ: Electrophysiologic evaluation of patients with multiple sclerosis. Neurol Clin 1985; 3:663–678.
4. Arnason GW: Interferon beta in MS. Neurology 1993; 43:641–643.
5. Basmajin J: Lioresal treatment of spasticity in multiple sclerosis: Further experience with double blind crossover studies. Am J Phys Med 1975; 54:175–177.
6. Baum HM, Rathschild BB: MS and mobility restrictions. Arch Phys Med Rehabil 1983; 64:591–596.
7. Beatty WA: Cognitive and emotional disturbances in MS. Neurol Clin 1993; 11:189–203.
8. Beorg-Stein J, Pine Z, Miller J, et al: Botulinum toxin in the treatment of spasticity in multiple sclerosis: New observations. Am J Phys Med Rehabil 1993; 32:364.
9. Borstein MB, Miller MA, Slagle S, et al: A placebo controlled, double-blind, randomized, two-center, pilot-controlled trial of Cop I in chronic, progressive MS. Neurology 1991; 41:189–204.
10. Brosnan CF, Selmay K, Raines L: A role for tumor necrosis factor in immune mediated demyelination and its relevance to multiple sclerosis. J Neuroimmunol 1988; 18:87–94.
11. Camenga DL, Johnson KP, Alter M, et al: Systemic recombinant alpha II interferon therapy in relapsing multiple sclerosis. Arch Neurol 1986; 43:1239–1246.
12. Castor JL, Huflei DA: Immunosuppression with high dose intravenous cyclophosphamide and ACTH in progressive multiple sclerosis: Cumulative six year experience in 164 patients. Neurology (Suppl) 1988; 2:914.
13. Cates JL, Rodriguez M: Immunosuppressive treatment of MS. Mayo Clin Proc 1989; 64:664–669.
14. Charcot JM: Lectures on Diseases of the Nervous System. Lecture 6. London, The New Sydenham Society, 1877.
15. Chiappa KH: Pattern shift, brainstem auditory and somatosensory evoked potentials in multiple sclerosis. Ann NY Acad Sci 1984; 436:315–326.
16. Cohn RA, Fisher M: Amantadine treatment of fatigue associated with multiple sclerosis. Arch Neurol 1989; 46:667–680.
17. Compston DA: Six double blind controlled trials of high dose methylprednisolone in patients with multiple sclerosis. J Neurol Neurosurg Psychiatry 1987; May, 50(5):517–522.
18. Confavreaux C, Hutchinson M, Auers MM, et al: Role of pregnancy-related relapse in MS. N Engl J Med 1998; 335(5): 285–291.
19. Confavreaux L, Armand G, Devic M: Course and prognosis of multiple sclerosis assessed by computerized data processing of 349 patients. Brain 1980; 103:281–300.
20. Cottrell SS, Wilson SA: The affective symptomatology of disseminated sclerosis: Study of 100 cases. J Neurol Psychother 1926; 7:1–30.
21. Erickson RP, Lie YR, Chiniger MA: Rehabilitation in multiple sclerosis. Mayo Clin Proc 1989; 64:818–828.
22. Esiri MM: Pathology in MS. In Swak M, Oxbury U (eds): Clinical Neurology. London, Churchill Livingstone, 1991, vol 2, pp 1117–1123.
23. European Study Group on Interferon Beta-1B in Secondary Progressive MS: Placebo-controlled, multi-center randomized trial of interferon beta 1B in treatment of secondary progressive MS. Lancet 1998; 352:1491–1497.
24. Fazenkas F, Offenbacher H, Fuoris S, et al: Criteria for an increased specificity of MRI interpretations for the elderly patient with suspected MS. Neurology 1988; 38:1822–1825.
25. Fergenson JS, Scheinberg L, Catalano A, et al: Cost effectiveness of MS rehabilitation: Model. Neurology 1981; 31:1316–1322.
26. Frankel D: Multiple sclerosis. In Umphrey DA (ed): Neurologic Rehabilitation, ed 2. St Louis, CV Mosby, 1990, pp 531–550.
27. Freal JE, Kraft GH, Coryell JK: Symptomatic fatigue in multiple sclerosis. Arch Phys Med Rehabil 1984; 65:135–138.
28. Gean-Norton AD, Vezina CG, Martonki G, et al: Abnormal corpus callosum MRI, a sensitive and specific indicator of MS. Neurology 1991; 180:213–221.
29. Gilfort JJ, Sade RM: Unexpected multiple sclerosis. Arch Neurol 1983; 40:533–536.
30. Grant I, Brown GW, Harris T, et al: Severely threatened events and markers presenting the onset or exacerbation of multiple sclerosis. J Neurol Neurosurg Psychiatry 1989; 52:8–13.
31. Greenspan B, Steineman M, Agri R: MS and rehabilitation outcome. Arch Phys Med Rehabil 1987; 68:434–440.
32. Hart RG, Sherman DO: The diagnosis of MS. JAMA 1982; 247:498–503.
33. House SC, Dawson DM, Lehiech JR, et al: Intensive immunosuppression and progressive multiple sclerosis with randomized 3 arm study of high dose intravenous cyclophosphamide and plasmapheresis, and ACTH. N Engl J Med 1983; 308:173–180.
34. Ivers RR, Goldstein ND: Multiple sclerosis: A current appraisal of symptoms and signs. Proc Staff Meet Mayo Clin 1963; 38:457–466.
35. Jacobs L, Salazar AM, Nerndon R, et al: Multicenter double-blind study of effect of intrathecally administered natural human fibroblast interferon in exacerbations of MS. Lancet 1986; 2:1411–1415.
36. Jacobs LD, Cookfair DL, Rudick RA, et al: Intramuscular interferon beta IA for disease progression in relapsing and remitting multiple sclerosis. Ann Neurol 1996; 39:285–294.
37. Joffe RT, Lippert GB, Gross TA, et al: Mood disorder and multiple sclerosis. Arch Neurol 1987; 44:376–378.
38. Johnson KP, Brooks BR, Cohen JA, et al: Cop I reduces relapse rate and improves disability in relapsing and remitting multiple sclerosis: Results of a Phase III multi-center, double-blind, placebo-conrolled trial. Neurology 1995; 45:1268–1276.
39. Khatri BO, McQuillen MP, Harrington GS, et al: Chronic progressive multiple sclerosis: Double blind controlled study of plasmapheresis in patients taking immunosuppressive drugs. Neurology 1986; 37:1754–1761.
40. Khoury SJ, Guttman CR, Orav EJ, et al: Longitudinal MRI and MS correlation of disability and lesion numbers. Neurology 1994; 44:2120–2124.
41. Knobles RC, Panitch HS, Braheny SL: Controlled clinical trial of systemic alpha interferon in MS. Neurology 1984; 34:1273–1279.
42. Kurland CT, Westland KB: Epidemiologic factors in the etiology and prognosis of MS. Ann NY Acad Sci 1954; 1958:682–701.
43. Kurtzke JF: A new scale for evaluating disabilities in MS. Neurology 1955; 5:580–583.
44. Kurtzke JF: Rating neurologic impairment in MS: An expanded disabilities status scan (EDSS). Neurology 1983; 33:1444–1453.
45. Kurtzke JF, Beebe GW, Nagel B, et al: Studies on the natural history of multiple sclerosis: Clinical and laboratory findings at first diagnosis. Acta Neurol Scand 1972; 48:19–46.
46. Lilius H, Valtonen E, Wikstrom J: Sexual problems in patients suffering from multiple sclerosis: J Chronic Dis 1976; 29:643–647.
47. Lowenthal A, Van Sande M, Koucher D: The differential diagnosis of neurological diseases by fractionating electrophoretically the CSF gamma-globulins. J Neurochem 1980; 6:51–56.

48. Lowry S: In Scheinberg L (ed): Multiple Sclerosis, ed 2. 1977, p 7.
49. Matthews WB: Clinical aspects of multiple sclerosis. In Matthews WB (ed): McAlpine's Multiple Sclerosis, ed 2. London, Churchill-Livingstone, 1991, pp 64–67.
50. Matthews WB: Clinical features of multiple sclerosis. In Swak M, O'Brien J (eds): Clinical Neurology. New York, Churchill Livingstone, 1993, vol 2, p 1098.
51. McDonald WI, Nielle DH, Barnes P: Pathologic evolution of MS. Neuropathol Appl Neurobiol 1988; 18:319–334.
52. Mendel K: Über Multiple Sclerosis in Thieren zur Trauma. Neurology 1897; 16:140–141.
53. Merritt JC: Management of spasticity in spinal cord injury. Mayo Clin Proc 1981; 56:616–622.
54. Mitchell G: Update in multiple sclerosis therapy. Med Clin North Am 1990; 77:233.
55. Multiple Sclerosis Study Group: The efficacy of cyclosporine immunosuppression in MS: A preliminary report of a randomized blinded placebo controlled clinical trial. Ann Neurol 1988; 24:119.
56. Multiple Sclerosis: A National Survey: NIH publication no 84-2479. Bethesda, MD, US Department of Health and Human Services, Public Health Service, National Institute of Medicine, 1984.
57. New research report of the role of antibodies in myelin destruction in MS. National Multiple Sclerosis Society Bulletin, January 1999.
58. Nisipeanu P, Korczyn A: Psychological stress as a risk factor for the exacerbation of MS. Neurology 1993; 43:1311–1312.
59. Padzlol DJ, Poclington PR: Course of MS: Results of a prospective study carried out on 102 patients from 1976 to 1980. Acta Neurol Scand 1982; 65:245–266.
60. Panitch HS, Hirsch RL, Schindler J, et al: Treatment of multiple sclerosis with gamma interferon: Exacerbations associated with the activation of the immune system. Neurology 1987; 37:1097–1102.
61. Paty DW, Ebers GC: Clinical features of multiple sclerosis. In Paty DW, Ebers GC (eds): Multiple Sclerosis. Philadelphia, FA Davis, 1998, pp 154–161.
62. Paty DW, Oger GF, Kastrukoff LF, et al: MRI in the diagnosis of MS: A prospective study with comparison of clinical evaluations, E.P. oligoclonal banding and CT. Neurology 1988; 38: 180–188.
63. Patzol DU, Hecker H, Peckington NP: Azathioprine in treatment of multiple sclerosis: Final results of a 4½ year controlled study of its effectiveness covering 114 patients. J Neurol Sci 1982; 54:377–394.
64. Petajan JH, Gappmaiere, White AT, et al: The impact of aerobic training on fitness and quality of life in multiple sclerosis. Ann Neurol 1996; 39:432–441.
65. Peterson RC, Koke NE: Cognitive and psychologic abnormalities in multiple sclerosis. Mayo Clin Proc 1989; 64:657–663.
66. Poser CW, Patty DW, Scheinber GL, et al: New diagnostic criteria for MS guidelines for research protocols. Ann Neurol 1983; 13:227–231.
67. Prime IFNB Multiple Sclerosis Study Group: Interferon beta 1B is effective in relapsing remitting multiple sclerosis. Neurology 1993; 43:655–661.
68. Quality Standards Committee of the American Academy of Neurology: Practice revision on treatment of patients with multiple sclerosis: Treatment with beta interferon. Neurology 1994; 44:1537–1540.
69. Rao SM, Leo GJ, Ellinston MS, et al: Cognitive dysfunction in MS: Impact on employment and social function. Neurology 1991; 41:691–697.
70. Reinherz EL, Weiner HL, Hauser SL: Loss of suppressor T cells in active multiple sclerosis. N Engl J Med 1980; 303:125–129.
71. Rodriguez M: Basic concepts and hypothesis in multiple sclerosis. Mayo Clin Proc 1989; 64:570–576.
72. Rudge P: Treatment of multiple sclerosis. In Swak M, Oxbury J (eds): Clinical Neurology. New York, Churchill Livingstone, 1993, vol 2, pp 1137–1151.
73. Sears TA, Postock H: Conduction failure in demyelination: Is it inevitable? Adv Neurol 1981; 51:357–375.
74. Sherratt RM, Bostock H, Leavis TA: Effects of 4-aminopyridine on normal and demyelinated mammalian nerve fibers. Nature 1980; 274:385–387.
75. Sibley WI, Banford CR, Clark K: Prospective study of physical trauma with multiple sclerosis. J Neurol Neurosurg Psychiatry 1991; 54:584–589.
76. Silberberg D, Lisak R, Sweiman B: Multiple sclerosis unaffected by azathioprine in a pilot study. Arch Neurol 1973; 28:210–212.
77. Siva A, Radhakrishnan K, Kurland LT, et al: Trauma in multiple sclerosis: A population-based cohort study from Olmstead, Minnesota. Neurology 1993; 43:1878–1882.
78. Steinman L: Autoimmune disease. Sci Am 1993; 269(3):107–114.
79. Stewart JM, Houser OW, Baker ML, et al: Magnetic resonance imaging and clinical relationships in MS. Mayo Clin Rev 1987; 62:174–184.
80. Surridge D: An investigation into some psychiatric aspects of multiple sclerosis. Br J Psych 1969; 115:749–762.
81. Swansen JW: Multiple sclerosis: Update in diagnosis and review of prognostic factors. Mayo Clin Proc 1989; 64:577–586.
82. Swinburn WR, Libersedge LA: Long term treatment of multiple sclerosis with azathioprine. J Neurol Neurosurg Psychiatry 1973; 36:124–126.
83. Taylor A, Taylor RS: Neuropsychologic aspects of multiple sclerosis. In Kraft G, Taylor RS (eds): Multiple Sclerosis: A Rehabilitative Approach. Philadelphia, WB Saunders, 1998, vol 9, pp 643–656.
84. Taylor RS: Immunologic aspects of multiple sclerosis. In Kraft G, Taylor RS (eds): Multiple Sclerosis: A Rehabilitative Approach. Philadelphia, WB Saunders, 1998, vol 9, pp 525–536.
85. Thompson AV, Kermode AG, Wieder D, et al: Major differences in the dynamics of primary and secondary progressive multiple sclerosis. Ann Neurol 1991; 29:53–62.
86. Thompson AV, McRonald WL: Pathophysiology of MS. In Osbury AK (ed): Diseases of the Nervous System, ed 2. Philadelphia, WB Saunders, 1992, p 1218.
87. Tourtellatte WW, Baumhefner RW, Potvin AR, et al: MS de novo: CNS IgG synthesis effect of ACTH and corticosteroids. Neurology 1980; 30:1155–1162.
88. Tourtellatte WW, Potvin AR, Fleming JO: MS: Measurement and quantitation of central nervous system IgG synthesis rate. Neurology 1980; 30:240–244.
89. Trapp BD, Peterson J, Ransohoff R, et al: Axonal transection in lesions of multiple sclerosis. N Engl J Med 1998; 338:278–285.
90. Vandenberg W, VanZomeren E, Minderhaud JM, et al: Cognitive impairment in patients with MS and mild physical disabilities. Arch Neurol 1987; 44:494–501.
91. VonDiemen HA, Polman CH, Pheom M, et al: The effect of four AP in clinical signs in multiple sclerosis: A randomized placebo controlled double blind crossover study. Ann Neurol 1992; 32:123–130.
92. Warren W, Warren KG, Cocherill K: Emotional stress in coping in MS exacerbations. J Psychosom Res 1991; 35:37–47.
93. Wynn NR, Rodriguez M, O'Fallan W: Update on the epidemiology of MS. Mayo Clin Proc 1989; 64:808–817.

53
CHAPTER

Lynne M. Stempien, M.D., and Deborah Gaebler-Spira, M.D.

Rehabilitation of Children and Adults with Cerebral Palsy

Cerebral palsy (CP) is a collection of diverse syndromes characterized by disorders of movement and posture caused by a nonprogressive injury to the immature brain.[170] The distinctive characteristic of these syndromes is the change in muscle tone and posture, both at rest and with voluntary activity.[177] The definition of cerebral palsy implies that the underlying pathologic process in the brain does not progress, and occurred in the early formation of the brain. The first year or two of life is included in most definitions, although some references include cases up to age 7 years. The wide range of normal neurological functioning, particularly in the first year of life, can make assessment of abnormalities difficult. Neurological maturation can also provide some improvement in the early years of life, thus causing overestimation of the number of children with permanent neuromotor dysfunction.[138]

EPIDEMIOLOGY

Cerebral palsy is one of the most common disabilities affecting children. The reported incidence varies but is approximately 2 to 3 per 1000 live births.[137] The incidence of CP in the United States in the 1940s and 1950s was estimated to be 1.6 to 5.8 per 1000 live births.[188] The larger, more recent Collaborative Perinatal Project measured a prevalence rate of 5.2 per 1000 live births at 1 year of age, but reported resolution in up to half of these children by 7 years of age.[180] The most recent studies in the United States match the average prevalence rate of CP in industrialized countries: 2 per 1000 live births.[23, 58]

There were hopes that recent improvements in neonatal care would decrease the incidence of CP. Several studies[134, 230] suggested a decrease in the 1970s, but this has been transient.[230, 232] CP prevalence in full-term infants has remained relatively constant. The improved neonatal survival has decreased the risk of CP for neonates weighing more than 2500 g.[146] In recent decades there has been a trend to higher survival rates for more immature, smaller, and premature infants with medical complications. Despite improved neonatal outcomes in general, the survival of these low–birth-weight (<2500 g) and very low–birth-weight (<1500 g) infants with higher CP risk has kept the prevalence of CP in childhood relatively constant.[22, 58, 98] In addition to birth weight less than 2500 g, a number of other factors predict increased risk for CP[58, 95, 247] (Table 53–1). Gestational age less than 32 weeks is one of the most powerful predictors of CP. Multivariate analysis reveals that maternal mental retardation, maternal seizure disorder, or hyperthyroidism; two or more prior fetal deaths; a sibling with motor deficit; third-trimester bleeding or increased urine protein excretion; and fetal bradycardia, chorionitis, low placental weight, fetal malformations, and neonatal seizures, all increase CP risk.[102, 179]

Other factors associated with CP are identified in epidemiological studies related to stages of pregnancy. Before pregnancy, long menstrual cycles or repeated fetal wastage during pregnancy; fetal growth retardation; twin gestation; congenital malformations; abnormal fetal presentation; or low socioeconomic class are associated with increased CP risk. During labor and delivery, only premature separation of the placenta poses an associated CP risk. In the early postnatal pe-

TABLE 53–1 Risk Factors Associated with Cerebral Palsy

General
Gestational age <32 wk
Birth weight <2500 g
Maternal history
Mental retardation
Seizure disorder
Hyperthyroidism
Two or more prior fetal deaths
Sibling with motor deficits
During gestation
Twin gestation
Fetal growth retardation
Third-trimester bleeding
Increased urine protein excretion
Chorionitis
Premature placenta separation
Low placenta weight
Fetal factors
Abnormal fetal presentation
Fetal malformations
Fetal bradycardia
Neonatal seizures

riod, newborn encephalopathy is the only epidemiological association.[145]

Despite these many associations, most children with these risk factors do not develop CP. Many of these abnormal characteristics can be consequences of the disease process and not the cause. Evidence is mounting for the postulate that CP is the result of processes causing problems with brain formation in utero. Many of the clinical associations such as preterm delivery and peripartum difficulties could be a consequence of this process.

ETIOLOGY

The brain injury that leads to CP can occur in the prenatal, perinatal, or postnatal period.[147] The causes of these lesions have been attributed to a wide variety of brain injury mechanisms. Currently, the most common causes are related to brain injury occurring in children born prematurely.[17, 58, 76, 144] The combination of immaturity, fragile brain vasculature, and the physical stresses of prematurity combine to predispose these children to compromise of cerebral blood flow.[35] The blood vessels are particularly vulnerable in the watershed zone next to the lateral ventricles in the capillaries of the germinal matrix. Bleeding in this area is often arterial in origin and can occur in differing degrees: cerebral intraventricular hemorrhage isolated to germinal matrix (grade 1), intraventricular hemorrhage[188] with normal ventricular size (grade 2), intraventricular hemorrhage with ventricular dilatation (grade 3), or intraventricular hemorrhage with parenchymal hemorrhage (grade 4) (Table 53–2).

Very low–birth-weight infants also have an increased incidence of periventricular hemorrhagic infarction, which is hemorrhagic necrosis lateral to the external angle of the lateral ventricle. This is thought to be bleeding of venous origin and is usually asymmetrical.[100, 167] With healing of this bleeding, symmetrical necrosis of white matter adjacent to the external angle of the lateral ventricles (periventricular leukomalacia) can develop[205] (Fig. 53–1). Periventricular leukomalacia is one of the strongest predictors of CP in the premature neonate.[145]

Fortunately, the large majority of children who are born prematurely do not develop CP, although they can have neuromotor and developmental abnormalities throughout the first year of life. Even the most sophisticated pediatric developmental assessment tools are not sufficiently sensitive to detect deficits that will persist until after 1 year of age.[109] Consequently, it is common for families to suspect motor problems long before diagnosis of CP is given at age 2 or more.

Almost half of all children with CP were not born prematurely. In term births that result in CP, the cause of brain injury is often elusive. Most known perinatal injuries that cause CP are due to severe anoxic or ischemic brain injury. This can occur with mechanical difficulties of the placenta, umbilical cord, or the actual delivery itself. Intrapartum asphyxia must be severe to be the cause of CP.[85, 178] Unfortunately, injuries of this type tend to be more global and are more likely to cause a more severe disability.[143]

Postnatal causes of CP can include any type of brain injury. Anoxia, ischemia, infection, or trauma can all cause injury that later results in a CP-type picture. Although these brain injuries might cause clinical consequences similar to CP, the clinical convention is to identify these children diagnostically by the specific insult (e.g., encephalitis, traumatic brain injury).

CLASSIFICATION

Cerebral palsy is often characterized by the type of muscle tone abnormality and the body parts involved (Table 53–3). The most common abnormality is that of increased muscle tone, or spasticity. Spastic disorders affect approximately three-fourths of all patients with CP.[143, 146] This spasticity can occur in either a consistent or velocity-dependent manner or both. When the resistance to passive movement is continuous and constant despite changes in limb velocity, the increased tone is called rigidity. This has often been compared to the feel of bending a lead pipe.

There are frequently signs of the upper motor neuron syndrome in CP (exaggerated muscle stretch reflexes and abnormal Babinski reflexes). There can be "overflow" of muscle stretch reflexes to adjacent joints such as the crossed adductor reflex (contraction of bilateral adductor muscles to unilateral adductor stretch).

TABLE 53–2 Grades of Intraventricular Hemorrhage in the Premature Brain

Grade 1	Isolated to germinal matrix
Grade 2	With normal ventricular size
Grade 3	With ventricular dilatation
Grade 4	With parenchymal hemorrhage

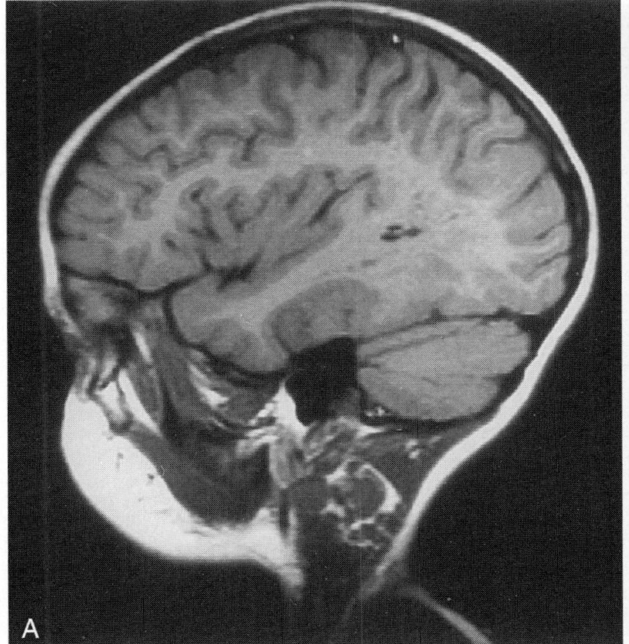

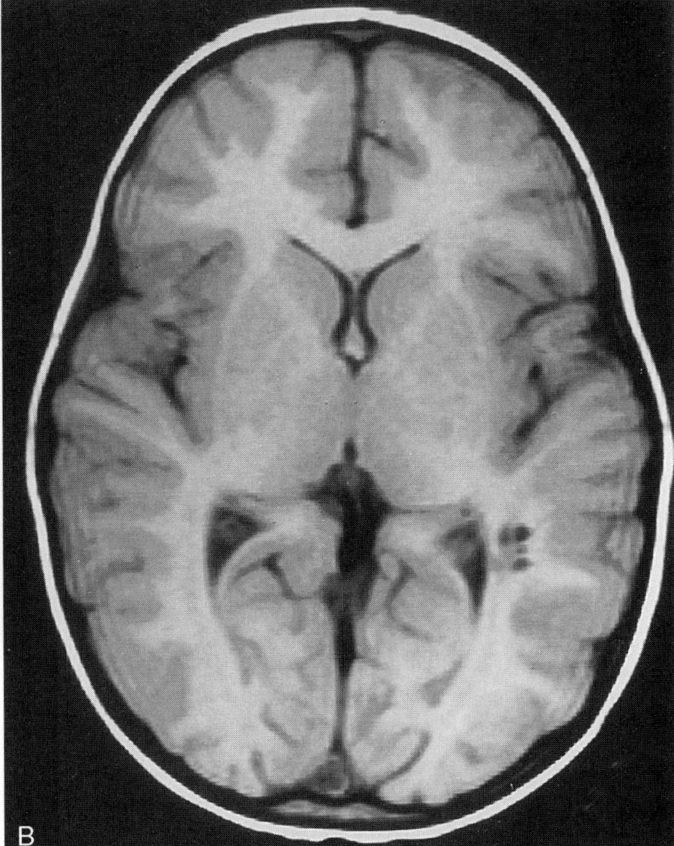

FIGURE 53–1. *A* and *B.* Periventricular leukomalacia.

Less common are dyskinetic disorders with involuntary movements. Classic athetoid movements which encompass large muscle groups are common. The involuntary, slow writhing posturing of athetosis is most easily detected in the movements of the head and face.[250] Dyskinetic disorders cause impairments in postural instability, and are sometimes reflected in "fluctuating tone" abnormalities. These patients often begin with hypotonia, and develop the discrete involuntary movements over the first few years of life. Athetoid disorders are most commonly caused by damage to the basal ganglia with hyperbilirubinemia or severe anoxia. Small muscle involuntary movements such as chorea can also be seen. Rarely, ballistic, rotary, and flailing movements have been described. Ataxic disorders that mimic cerebellar dysfunction with titubation, wide-based gait, and dysmetria are very rare in CP.

TABLE 53–3 Classification of Cerebral Palsy Types

By Tone Abnormalities	By Body Parts Involved
Spastic	Diplegia
Dyskinetic	Quadriplegia
Athetoid	Triplegia
Choreiform	Hemiplegia
Ballistic	
Ataxic	
Hypotonic	
"Mixed"	

A small percentage of patients have the hypotonic type of CP. These children need to be differentiated from those with more frequently identifiable causes of neonatal hypotonia such as muscle disease, metabolic disorders, and genetic syndromes. Many of these children develop spastic or extrapyramidal-type disorders after the first few months of life. All of these tone abnormalities can occur in mixtures. The most common combination is that of spasticity with athetosis. These patients are sometimes classified as "mixed-type" CP.

The distribution of body parts with disability is used to name the type of CP (Figs. 53–2 through 53–4). *Diplegia* refers to spastic paresis in the lower extremities more than in the upper extremities, and is the most common. *Quadriplegia,* involving abnormalities of both upper and lower extremities, is also frequent. In quadriplegia the disorder of motor control is typically worse in the legs.[231] Rarely, a child has obvious abnormalities of both legs and one arm, and is referred to as having *triplegia.* Patterns of abnormalities that involve an arm more than the ipsilateral leg (similar to a stroke) are labeled as *hemiplegia.* For unclear reasons, isolated right hemiplegia is twice as common as left hemiplegia.[100]

Diplegia, or leg-dominated symptoms, is most frequent in the low–birth-weight, premature groups. Quadriplegia is more frequent in those with normal

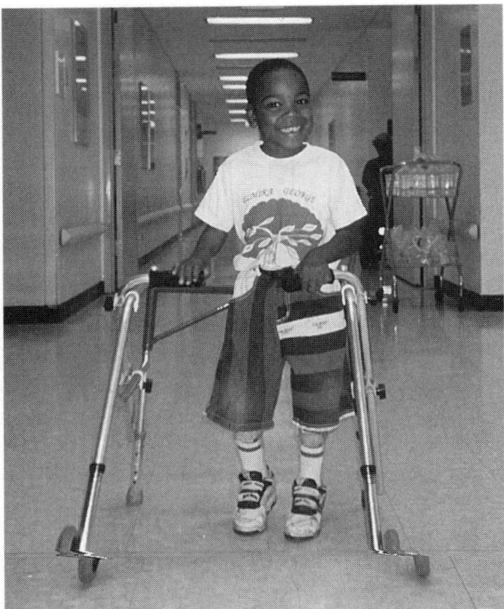

FIGURE 53–2. Patient with spastic diplegia.

birth weight.[143] It should be noted, however, that most children with CP are "total body–involved." Close examination of motor control in the more normal-appearing limbs, trunk, and oral-motor musculature often yields small abnormalities.

CLINICAL EFFECTS

The most striking difficulties in CP are disorders of neuromuscular control. Problems in infancy that suggest CP include irritability, lethargy, weak suck with tongue thrust, poor head control, high-pitched cry, oral hypersensitivity, tonic bite, and asymmetrical movements or unusual posturing. Motor delay can also be suggested by persistent abnormal motor activities, such as rolling for mobility, combat crawling, "W-sitting," "bunny hopping," or adopting a hand preference before the first birthday[74] (Figs. 53–5 and 53–6).

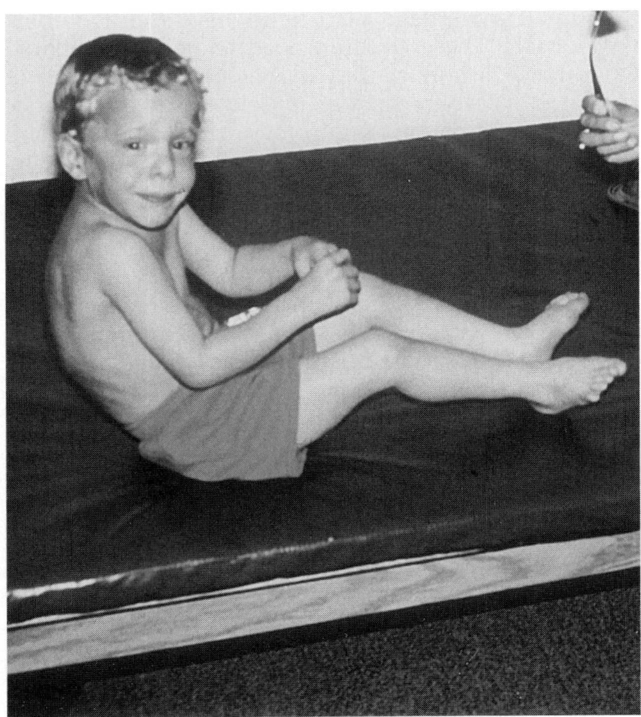

FIGURE 53–3. Patient with spastic quadriplegia.

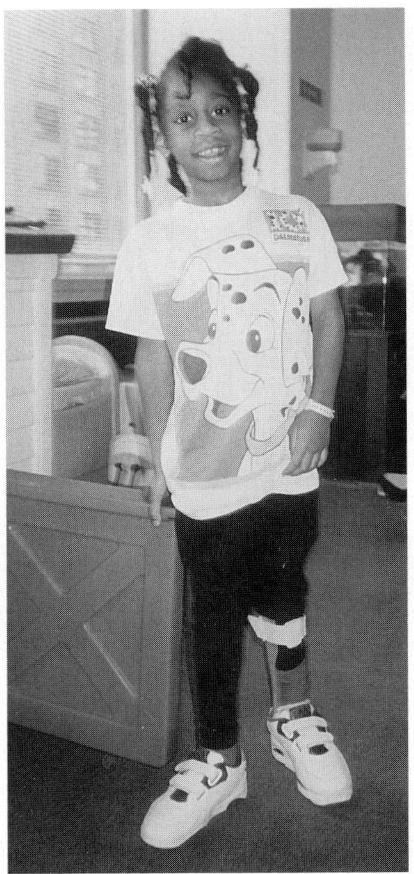

FIGURE 53–4. Patient with spastic hemiplegia.

Abnormalities of muscle tone are frequently accompanied by muscle weakness, which can cause certain strength imbalances at individual joints. This gives rise to a number of patterns of movement. Certain patterns occur frequently in children with CP, such as "scissoring," "guarding" of the upper extremities, extensor posturing, or proximal "fixing" (Figs. 53–7 through 53–9).

Scissoring is the simultaneous adduction, knee hyperextension, and plantar flexion of the lower extremities. Flexion synergy patterns of the upper extremities include flexion at the fingers, wrists, and elbows with shoulder abduction. As this upper extremity pattern becomes stronger, the child's hands rise from the waist, producing a low, mid, or high guard position (Fig. 53–10). Some patterns of movement can be recognized as components of persistent primitive reflexes, such as the asymmetric tonic neck reflex (ATNR), symmetric tonic neck reflex (STNR), or tonic labyrinthine reflex (TLR) (Figs. 53–11 through 53–13). These movement patterns can be seen in limbs as the child attempts voluntary

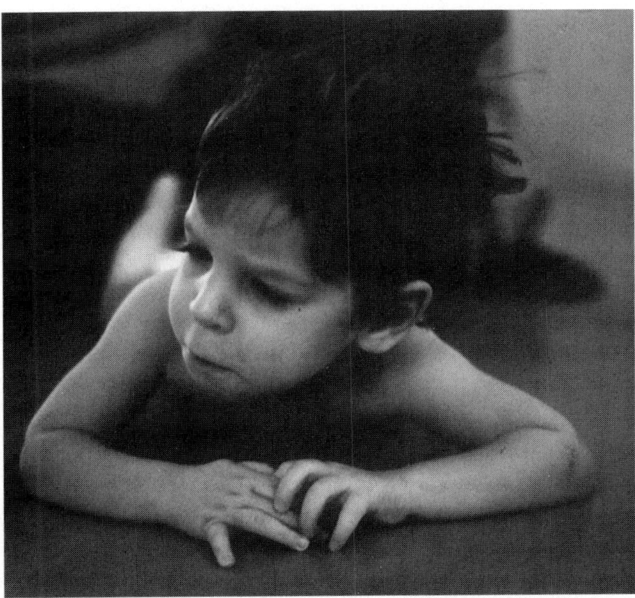

FIGURE 53–5. Combat, or belly crawl, with lower extremity extention and use of upper extremities for forward progression.

movement, triggered by passive positioning, in response to sensory stimuli, or as an "overflow" of uninvolved limbs.

These movement patterns are examples of a primary difficulty in CP—the inability to separate out individual movements. Children with CP often elicit motor activity in joints and limbs beyond the wanted action. These associated reactions or activation of muscles remote from where the child is trying to move is one of the major impediments to voluntary movement.

The abnormalities of muscle tone are often accompanied by weakness in individual muscles. Applying the traditional methods of measuring muscle strength is problematic in CP because the tone abnormalities mask the patient's ability to generate force.[84]

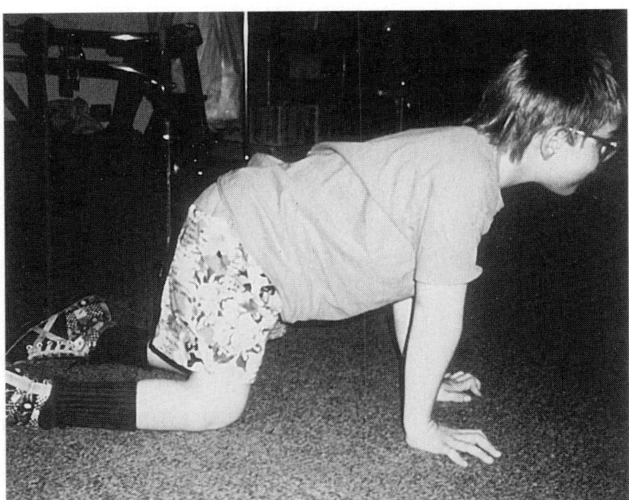

FIGURE 53–6. "Bunny hop."

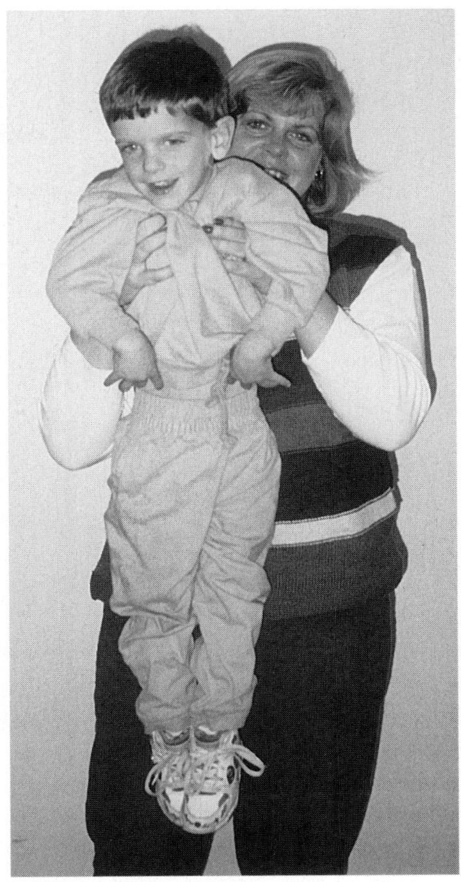

FIGURE 53–7. Scissoring on vertical suspension.

Difficulty with control of the midline structures such as the trunk and head interferes dramatically with a child's ability to develop good balance. This unbridled motor activity complicates the patient's ability to balance and coordinate movement. The development of appropriate, adequately implemented equilibrium and righting reactions is delayed or sometimes absent. Abnormal or inappropriate coordination patterns lead to limitations in acquiring, planning, executing, and correcting skillful actions. Even children with minimal involvement can exhibit apraxia when attempting high-level motor activities.

The combination of abnormal motor control and experience also contributes to a disordered kinesthetic sense. Children with CP are often sensitive to normally innocuous stimuli. The abnormal sensory experience of disordered motor control can contribute to disordered sensory perception, which further interferes with the child's ability to perform high-level motor activities.[39] Decreased ability to distinguish two-point discrimination has been found in the upper extremities of children with all types of CP.[150] Children with hemiparetic CP have also been found almost universally to have a decrease in stereognosis, with decreased proprioception in about half of patients tested.[241]

The major secondary effects of disordered muscle tone, control, and balance are changes in joint alignment

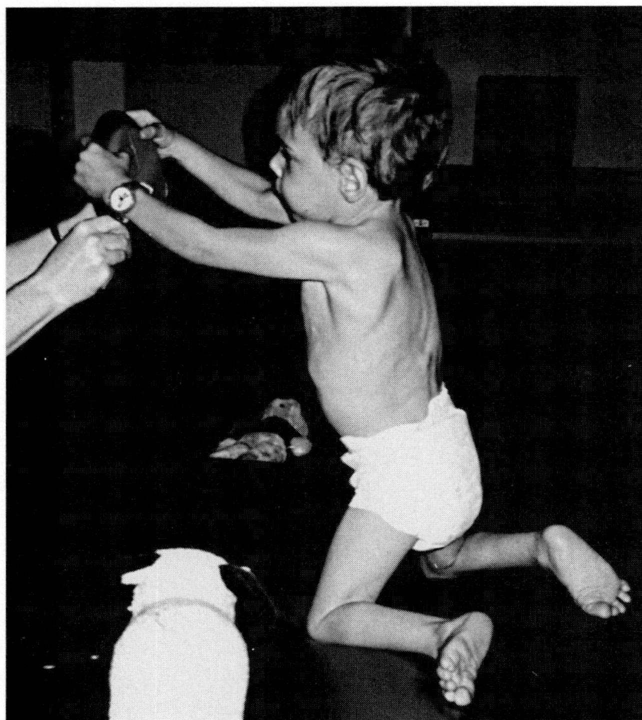

FIGURE 53–8. "Proximal fixing" with increased activity in shoulder girdle and neck muscles.

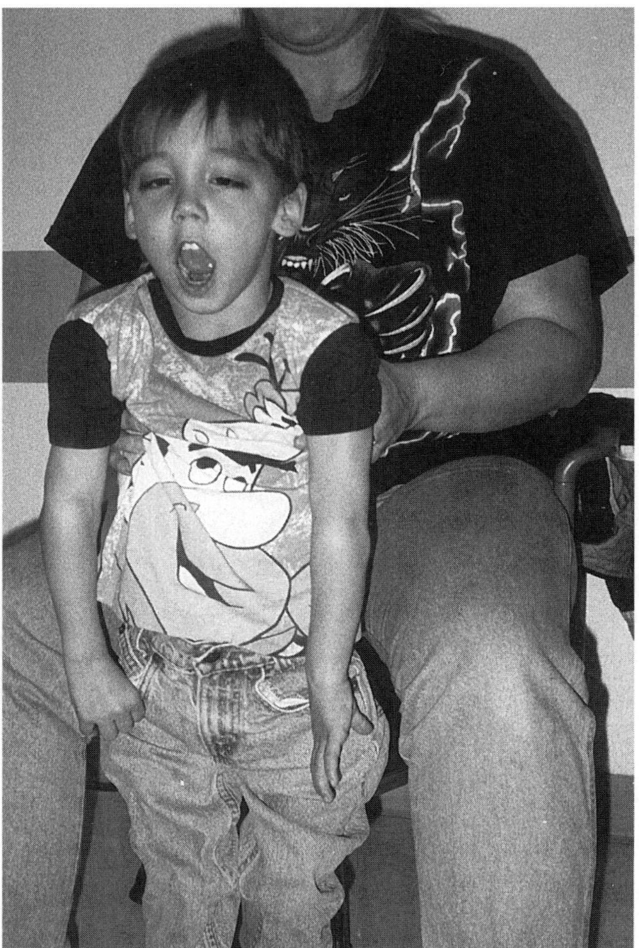

FIGURE 53–9. Patient with extensor posturing.

leading to contracture and deformity. Contracture, or passive shortening that can limit joint and soft tissue movement, frequently affects the adductor, hamstring, and plantar flexor muscles of the lower extremities and the flexors of the upper extremities. This reflects the presence of spasticity, scissoring, or upper extremity flexion patterns, individually or severally, which are present in the majority of children with CP.

Bony deformity can occur because the abnormal muscle forces of CP are acting on a growing skeleton. Of principal concern are the integrity of the hips and spine because of their primary role in weightbearing. The typical increase in hip flexion, adduction, and internal rotation of the femur acts to influence the femoral head in an upward posterolateral direction out of the acetabulum. The result is coxa valgus, malformed femoral head, and a shallow acetabulum, which causes the hip to be more prone to subluxation[26, 149] (Fig. 53–14).

Spinal deformities are not quite as common, but have more severe consequences. Asymmetrical muscle pull and immobility can contribute to significant deformity of the spine, including kyphosis, scoliosis, or rotational deformities. These spinal deformities can significantly affect comfort, tone, sitting and standing alignment, and balance. When these are severe, respiratory function can be compromised by the mechanical restriction of the chest combined with decreased efficiency of available respiratory muscle strength. This can have a significant impact on endurance, health, and longevity. Spondylolisthesis and spondylolysis are not increased in CP.[112]

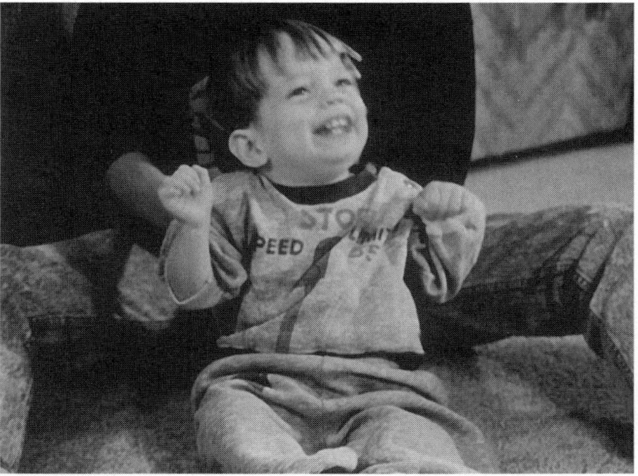

FIGURE 53–10. "High guard" position of upper extremities.

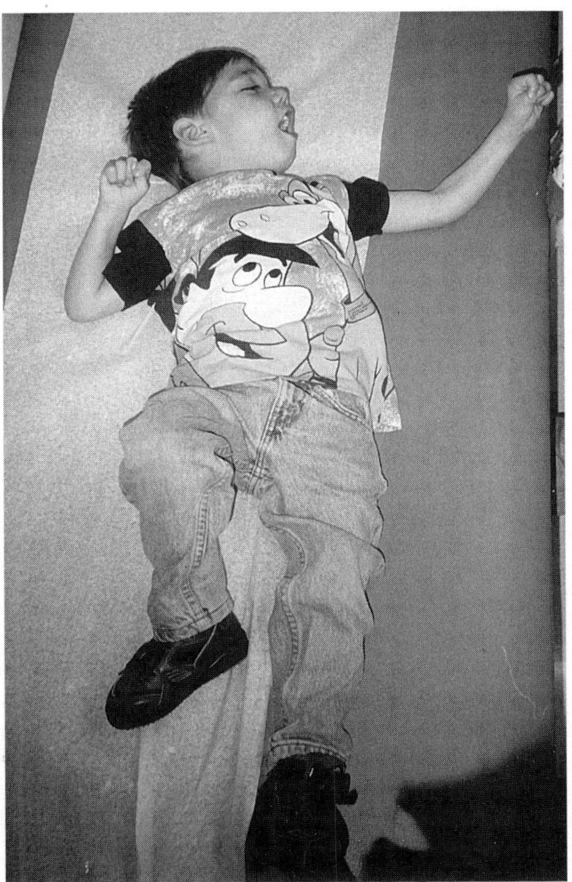

FIGURE 53–11. Patient with asymmetric tonic neck reflex.

Bony abnormalities of the feet can occur in a variety of patterns. The most common is deformity of the hindfoot with exaggerated heel valgus or varus. Hyperpronation occurs frequently with calcaneovalgus or cavus. Occasionally a rocker-bottom type of foot can be seen.

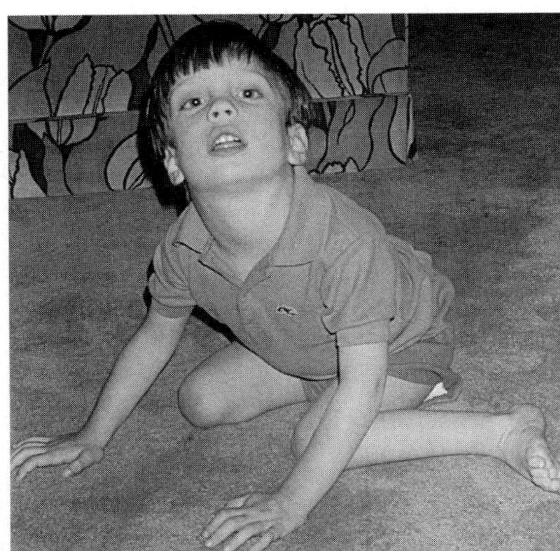

FIGURE 53–12. Symmetric tonic neck reflex (if neck is extended, upper extremities are extended and lower extremities are flexed).

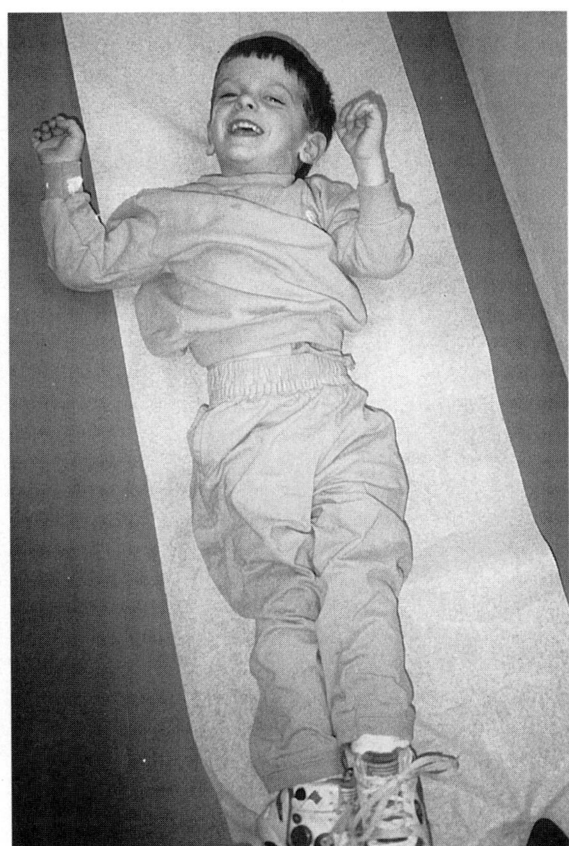

FIGURE 53–13. Patient with tonic labyrinthine reflex.

ASSOCIATED MEDICAL AND FUNCTIONAL PROBLEMS

The most common types of associated disabilities in CP are abnormalities in the oculomotor system. Esotropia, or exotropia, often requires strabismus surgery. Visual field deficits are less common but occur most frequently in the hemiplegic types. Visual impairments of acuity affect children with quadriplegia more than those with diplegia.

A large number of children with CP have abnormalities of oromotor function. This frequently leads to changes in their ability to feed well. Incomplete lip closure, low suction pressure, and delay between suction and propulsion cause inadequate bolus preparation.[152] In the more involved children, this can also interfere with their pharyngeal swallowing mechanism. Abnormalities in strength, tone, and coordination can be severe enough to cause difficulty protecting the airway. In one large study of patients with suspected oropharyngeal dysfunction, over half of those tested aspirated. Often the majority of patients have no effective cough during aspiration.[96, 209] Swallowing dysfunction is often present only with certain textures of food ingested, as detected by videoflouroscopy.[209] In severe cases, aspiration can cause hypoxemia.[210] Motor impairment can interfere with accessing food or communicating hunger.

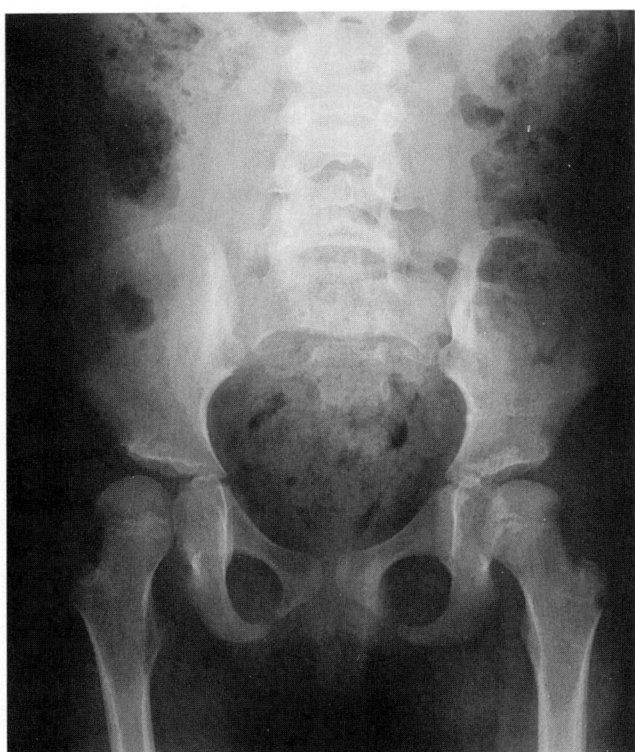

FIGURE 53–14. Dysplastic hip joints.

These feeding difficulties can contribute to substantial undernutrition or malnutrition.[81] Up to one-third of hemiplegic and diplegic CP patients and more than two-thirds of quadriplegic CP patients have been found to be undernourished.[129, 228, 229] This correlates with significantly reduced linear growth that is exclusive of the patient's motor disability.

Another unique growth disturbance can be asymmetry of linear growth, particularly in the limbs. The most severely motor-impaired limbs can have a decreased length and girth at maturity. Of interest is the effect of sensory disturbance, as there is a tendency for hemiplegic children with impaired sensation to have inadequate limb growth. This length deficiency seems to be worse the more severe the sensory deficit.[241]

Gastrointestinal symptoms are frequent in children with CP.[71] Gastroesophageal reflux can cause episodic emesis. It can also interfere with adequate ingestion and absorption of nutrients and compromise adequate nutrition and growth.[166, 191] Constipation, exaggerated by immobility and abnormal diet and fluid intake, can usually be managed with standard medical treatment.[3]

Physiological abnormalities of bowel and bladder control in CP have not been well studied. Incontinence is the most frequently reported urinary tract symptom. This increased incontinence as compared with that of peers has been attributed to decreased mobility, communication, and cognitive skills. Patients with dysfunctional voiding symptoms such as incontinence or dribbling studied by urodynamics revealed a continuum of disorders. The majority show upper motor neuron injury, but lower motor neuron disorders and vesicoureteral reflux have been described. Patients with complaints of fecal incontinence or defecation distress have been found to have anal sphincter or pelvic muscle incoordination, or both, without rectal dysfunction by anorectal manometry.[3] This dysfunction in the pelvic area appears to be related to abnormalities in neuromotor control (see Chapter 28).

Cognitive impairments are not obligatory with CP. The prevalence of mental retardation in all persons with CP is estimated to be 30%.[146] The risk increases with the severity of the motor disability.[163] Premature children with very low birth weight can have learning disabilities or mental retardation. Normal–birth-weight children with CP have had cognitive abnormalities reported in up to 40% to 50%.[144]

Seizure disorders can occur in up to a third of children with CP. Epilepsy is frequently active in the preschool and early school years. The highest incidence is in the most severely motor-affected children and those with mental retardation, reflecting the greater extent of brain injury in these cases.[144]

Hearing disabilities are rare in CP.[208] They are most commonly found in cases caused by congenital nervous system infections such as TORCH (toxoplasmosis, rubella, cytomegalovirus, and herpes). When hyperbilirubinemia was common and difficult to control secondary to maternal-fetal blood incompatibilities, bilirubin-induced sensorineural hearing loss often accompanied athetoid-type CP. Improvements in detecting and treating these conditions prenatally have now reduced this to a rare situation.

FUNCTIONAL PROGNOSIS

In the first few years of life, the child's neuromotor function can exhibit some evolution toward normal. The amount of tone abnormality and the importance of the reflexive movements can change over these years. Certain skills, such as sitting independently, are helpful in establishing an ultimate motor prognosis. Those children who will attain independent ambulation will achieve these skills during ages 2 to 7, rarely later. Seventy-five percent of children with spastic CP eventually ambulate, about 85% with diplegia, and 70% with quadriplegia. Most children with hemiplegic or ataxic CP ambulate independently, the majority by age 3 years. Unfortunately, those with hypotonic CP rarely walk.

Children who are able to sit independently before their second birthday eventually become independent walkers, with or without equipment. Those who cannot sit independently by age 4 years rarely walk. However, if the primitive reflexes (ATNR, STNR, tonic labyrinthine, Moro's, positive supporting reflex, or extensor posturing) still occur in an obligatory manner, the prognosis for independent ambulation is bleak.[25, 172] Obligatory reflexes occur consistently when the child's body is placed in certain positions passively or with voluntary movement. Most children who become ambulators have fewer than three of these reflexes present at age 18 months.[172]

Spasticity is a primary problem in at least 70% of children with CP. Other aspects of the upper motor neuron syndrome can be more disabling. Selective motor control, paresis, and retention of primitive reflexes can ultimately limit the motor potential. As the child grows, the spasticity interferes with the muscle length; hence alignment becomes altered. The biomechanical disadvantage of the child's altered skeletal system further impairs strength and function as "lever arm disease."

The most striking functional impact of this abnormal neuromotor control is a decrease in independence and mobility. One of the hallmarks of CP is motor delay, despite normal development in other areas. The increased muscle tone that is present with even small amounts of movement and during posture maintenance greatly increases the energy expended for motor activity. The ability to progress through motor milestones is greatly impeded. Children who do achieve ambulation typically have an inefficient gait, which includes much shorter step length, decreased range of motion at the hip and knee, more energy expenditure, and decreased velocity as compared with their peers. They also have impairment in coordination, and this becomes more apparent with more challenging motor activities.

Abnormalities affecting adequate motor control for speech, such as oromotor dysfunction and inadequate breath support, lead to dysarthria and can interfere with communication skills. Language-processing problems with reception or expression can occur, and correlate with cognitive impairments.[74] Difficulty controlling oral secretions can cause significant drooling.

All of these inefficiencies of muscle control contribute to decreased endurance.[212] Although endurance is difficult to measure with conventional methods because of the challenges of various impairments with CP, it seems to correlate with the overall gross motor capabilities of the individual.[190] Contractures and bone or joint deformities can greatly limit a child's function. Secondary pain can greatly worsen muscle tone and contribute to the inefficiency of movement.

EFFECTS OF AGING

The child with CP ages with a chronic, but not unchanging neuromuscular condition. Life expectancy for all but the most severely involved children is close to that for the unaffected population.[79, 146] Recently, there has been interest in defining the interaction of aging with the primary and secondary effects of CP.[13, 20, 59, 169, 201, 248] A person with CP can have ongoing medical issues that are exacerbated by aging such as dysphagia, gastroesophageal reflux, urinary incontinence, constipation, and painful musculoskeletal contractures that progress and cause a decline in function.[14, 28, 125] Problems of osteoporosis, fractures due to falls, deconditioning, and pressure sores are the expected potential consequences of the combined processes.

Spasticity can increase or decrease as the skeletal system matures. Painful sequelae of childhood deformity occur and become problematic for the adult. Dislocated hips and the chronic pull of asymmetric posture create uncomfortable sitting. The neck, particularly for the adult with athetoid CP, is vulnerable to excessive forces, which can narrow the disc spaces or compress the spinal cord.

Adults with CP often require new surgeries or a repeat of one they had during childhood.[198] Careful planning is needed, and rehabilitation is usually undertaken to address the deconditioning that ensues after postoperative immobilization. The orthopedic literature emphasizes that the adult with CP is frequently more motivated and able to participate in therapy than the child.[198]

Many of the adult pain problems can be sorted through and successfully treated. Positioning equipment, anti-inflammatory medication, bursal injections, mobilization by physical therapy, and spasticity treatment can improve activity tolerance and decrease pain.

Adults with CP rank communication, activities of daily living (ADL), and mobility as higher-priority goals than ambulation.[26] In the past, vocational rates among adults with CP were only 30% to 50%. The Americans with Disabilities Act, however, holds promise with respect to employment, housing, and accessibility to the community.[182]

THERAPEUTIC MANAGEMENT

The therapeutic management of the child with CP, whether by the physiatrist, orthopedist, or developmental pediatrician, emphasizes a functional aim- or goal-oriented approach.[42, 74, 107, 213, 249] The two major goals of rehabilitation, according to Molnar,[171] are to decrease complications of the CP and to enhance or improve the acquisition of new skills. Rothery and colleagues[214] include parent and caregiver education, decreasing skeletal deformity, and improving mobility. Promoting the child's assets offers a positive approach. Children should not be considered only in terms of potential deficits. Recommendations for management begin with an assessment of the child's and family's strengths and deficits. All associated problems should be correctly identified.[19, 85, 87]

From the first evaluation, the family and child should be encouraged to become active participants in the process of setting priorities and goals within the context of the impairment. The physician's role is to provide an accurate description of the therapies and interventions available to the child and family and the impact that these will have on the child's condition and function. The institution of therapy and other medical modalities should be approached and prescribed after a thorough discussion of efficacy. The following discussion represents the major therapeutic interventions for children with CP.

Early Intervention

Köng has suggested that early institution of physical therapy (PT) can decrease the impact of brain injury on the development of CP.[124, 143] There is a discrete group of children who initially appear to have manifestations of brain injury but appear to outgrow their CP at later age.[180] Whether or not early PT has an impact on brain injury, current thinking emphasizes early identification of the infant with developmental delay so that intervention can be instituted as soon as possible.[161] The Education of the Handicapped Act Amendments of 1986, Public Law (PL) 99-457, or IDEA (Individuals with Disabilities Education Act), mandated early intervention for infants and toddlers (0 to 3 years old) who demonstrate developmental delay. This federal law was established to provide educational and educationally related rehabilitative services to children who enter school with already identifiable problems. The law provides a downward extension of PL 94-142, which mandated that all states must provide a free and appropriate public education to eligible schoolchildren. One of the hallmarks of IDEA is the clearly identified role of the family as central to the goals of early intervention. The team acts not only to treat the child but also to empower the family. A mutual contract, the Individual Family Service Plan (IFSP), is developed actively by the team and parents. Unlike the IEP (Individual Education Plan) from PL 94-142, the IFSP must take the family's strengths and needs into account, as well as the child's goals.[107, 111, 114]

The rationale for early intervention is closely connected to concepts that stressed the importance of the early years for normally developing children and the role that environmental factors play in development. Parental characteristics, such as responsivity contingent on child initiations, the quality and quantity of verbal interactions, and the existence of a social support network and maternal sensitivity, have all been found to be associated with a child's concurrent or later developmental functioning.[21, 36, 149, 244]

There are two main models for the delivery of developmental early intervention: the direct therapy service model and the consultation model. In the direct model, service delivery can occur as a part of interdisciplinary, multidisciplinary, or transdisciplinary treatment in a center- or home-based program.[107] Traditionally, physical therapists and occupational therapists have been providers of therapeutic intervention for the child with CP. Many children are also seen by a speech-language pathologist for feeding difficulties and oromotor problems. A social worker, nurse, and developmental specialist constitute the members of a typical early intervention team. To reduce the number of therapists handling the child, Haynes[110] has advocated that one professional from the early intervention team integrate assessment data from all the members of the team, developing integrated strategies to meet the goals agreed upon in the IFSP. Given the shortage of pediatric physical therapists, occupational therapists, and speech-language pathologists, this transdisciplinary approach could assist in providing the number of therapists needed to deliver therapeutic input to the children eligible for treatment under Public Law 99-457.

Therapy Approaches

Children with CP who have motor problems that interfere with educational activities have the opportunity to participate in integrated therapy programs in school. The services should be delivered in the least restrictive environment, and are mandated to allow the child to participate in and benefit from the educational experience. The current philosophical trend in schools is to include disabled children as much as possible into the regular classroom, and few "pull-out" services are stressed. Mainstreaming has positive effects on the psychosocial aspects of schooling and increases the academic expectations of the disabled student.[49] Consultative models of PT, occupational therapy (OT), and speech therapy have provided a method of treating and involving more of the children with disabilities into regular education classes. Even though there is a move toward consultative services by PT, OT, and speech therapy in the school systems, direct service can be recommended to augment an overall therapy program.

There are a number of therapy systems that have influenced the management of children with CP (Table 53–4). Few therapists adhere strictly to a single therapy system. The following descriptions provide the basic principles of the most commonly used and influential therapies. Historically, the approach of Crothers remains a basic guide to involving patients in a meaningful program. He stressed the need for active movement and stimulation activities to prevent contractures and to encourage participation of severely involved children. Parents were counseled to avoid overprotection.[93] Phelps used an orthopedic approach with conventional techniques from poliomyelitis treatment regimens. He emphasized inhibiting abnormal movement.[197] Deaver[64, 65] emphasized functional ability rather than patterns of movement; this method is also known for its extensive use of bracing. Functional abilities were facilitated by intensive training efforts in residential units at frequent intervals of the child's life. Fay,[80] a neurophysiologist, postulated that motor developmental levels of the brain were comparable to the evolutionary process. This highly controversial concept is expressed by the well known aphorism "ontogeny recapitulates phylogeny." Doman, a physical therapist, integrated the concepts into the therapy known as patterning.[51, 69] Patterning has been subjected to critical review by the pediatric community and is not recommended.[7]

Rood,[211] an occupational and physical therapist, developed a sensorimotor approach to treatment. Rood's overall goal was to activate movement and postural responses at an automatic level while following a developmental sequence similar to the Bobath method of treatment. Rood used specific sensory stimulation to elicit movement.[211] The neurodevelopmental treatment (NDT) approach has been recommended for infants who display early signs of CP. This approach was developed by the Bobaths in England in the 1940s.[29–33] The main goals of NDT are to normalize tone, inhibit abnormal primitive reflex patterns, and to facilitate automatic reactions and subsequent normal movement. Therapists accomplish these goals by providing "key points of control" throughout the body.[32] Theoretically, this provides the child with kinesthetic normal feedback. The Bobaths emphasized family involvement and carryover of handling techniques in the home environment. For the older

TABLE 53–4 Similarities and Differences Between Neuromotor Therapy Approaches to Cerebral Palsy (CP)

	Neurodevelopmental Treatment (Bobaths)	Sensorimotor Approach to Treatment (Rood)	Sensory Integration Approach (Ayres)	Vojta Approach	Patterning Therapy (Doman-Delacato)
Central nervous system model	Hierarchical	Hierarchical	Hierarchical	Hierarchical	Hierarchical
Goals of treatment	1. To normalize tone 2. To inhibit primitive reflexes 3. To facilitate automatic reactions and normal movement patterns	1. To activate postural responses (stability) 2. To activate movement (mobility) once stability is achieved	1. To improve efficiency of neural processing 2. To better organize adaptive responses	1. To prevent CP in infants at risk 2. To improve motoric behavior in infants with fixed CP	1. To achieve independent mobility 2. To improve motor coordination 3. To prevent or improve communication disorders 4. To enhance intelligence
Primary sensory systems utilized to effect a motor response	1. Kinesthetic 2. Proprioceptive 3. Tactile	1. Tactile 2. Proprioceptive 3. Kinesthetic	1. Vestibular 2. Tactile 3. Kinesthetic	1. Proprioceptive 2. Kinesthetic 3. Tactile	All sensory systems are utilized
Emphasis of treatment activities	1. Positioning and handling to normalize sensory input 2. Facilitation of active movement	1. Sensory stimulation to activate motor response (tapping, brushing, icing)	1. Therapist guides, but child controls sensory input to get adaptive purposeful response	1. Trigger reflex locomotive zones to encourage movement patterns (e.g., reflex crawl)	Sensory and reflex stimulation, passive movement patterns, encouragement of independent movements
Intended clinical population	Children with CP Adults post cerebrovascular accident (CVA)	Children with neuromotor disorders such as CP Adults post CVA	Children with learning disabilities Children with autism	Young infants at risk for CP Young infants with fixed CP	Children with neonatal or acquired brain damage
Emphasis on treating infants	Yes	No	No	Yes	No
Emphasis on family involvement during treatment	Yes Handling and positioning for activities of daily living	No	No Supportive role encouraged	Yes Family administers treatment at home daily	Yes Family and friends administer treatment several times daily
Empirical support	Few studies Conflicting results	Very few studies Conflicting results	Many studies Conflicting results with school-age children Positive results for tactile and vestibular input with infants	Few studies Conflicting results	Few studies Conflicting results

From Harris SR, Atwater SW, Crowe TK: Accepted and controversial neuromotor therapies for infants at high risk for cerebral palsy. J Perinatol 1988; 8:3–13.

child, the Bobaths shift emphasis to ADL skills.[109] Two additional systems of therapy for CP practiced in Europe and not readily available in the United States are the Vojta and Peto methods.[57, 61]

Occupational therapy can also utilize defined systems or specialized treatment methods. Sensory integration (introduced by A. Jean Ayres[10, 11, 12] in the 1970s) is used to enhance the development of preschool and school age children who have learning disabilities. Ayres's premise is that "disordered sensory integration accounts for some aspects of learning disorders and . . . improving sensory integration will make academic learning easier."[12] This therapy is intended to enhance the child's ability to organize and integrate controlled sensory information, such as vestibular, proprioceptive, and tactile stimulation.[11, 134, 225]

Rarely does the clinical delivery of therapy services rely on any one system.[108] An eclectic approach is common—one that offers modalities from several schools of therapy. Such an approach provides the flexibility and individualization necessary to meet the child's and the family's goals.[18, 81, 154]

Sports as organized physical activities were once recommended only rarely for the child with CP. That has changed. There is no evidence that strengthening adversely affects muscle tone.[120, 126, 164] Neither is there evidence to preclude even vigorous activities, such as downhill skiing, that once were thought to increase orthopedic deformity.[83, 123] The therapeutic benefits of swimming and horseback riding for children with motor disabilities have been established.[43] While sports programs can improve endurance and strength, they also promote interpersonal growth and improve self-esteem—something that all children experience when appropriately supervised in a team sport with peers.[60, 222, 223] The established organizations for athletes with CP are the United States Cerebral Palsy Athletic Association and the Cerebral Palsy International Sports and Recreation Association.[130] Fitness programs that emphasize flexibility and endurance have been developed for both recreational and therapeutic use.[159, 161]

Equipment Concerns

For many families with a CP child, the physical therapist is the medical professional with whom they have the most frequent contact. The physical therapist recommends equipment to improve function, such as prone or supine standers, walkers, bathing equipment, wheelchairs, and, often, orthotic devices. All durable medical equipment should be considered in the context of the functional prognosis. The early introduction of independent mobility for children who are not yet able to negotiate at a household level increases exploration of the environment and has been proposed to improve self-esteem.[40] Use of a wheelchair for community mobility becomes a practical measure once a child has outgrown commercially available strollers. When standardized equipment does not meet the postural support needs of the severely involved child, adaptive seating is essential for the attainment of a sitting position.[37, 88, 235] Not only does a specialized seating system preserve a child's capacity to interact in a conventional posture but it can also improve pulmonary function tests[178] (see Chapter 33). The child who is comfortable and adequately seated typically has better feeding, digestion, and vocal production. Rehabilitation engineers working with therapists can address complex orthopedic and functional problems.[27, 201]

The early introduction of technology to improve communication, either written or oral, is warranted. The use of an augmentative communication device does not inhibit development of communication skills. In augmentative communication, speech is enhanced by the use of technology.[220] Occupational therapists and other adaptive specialists provide access to computers, environmental control units, and other ADL equipment[68, 136, 164] (see Chapter 25). In addition to specialized equipment, the child with CP is frequently assisted in mobility and ADL tasks by the use of splints or orthoses.[246] Splinting is a common conservative method of managing a spastic but flexible deformity. The physical therapist can provide low-temperature tone-reducing ankle-foot orthoses (TRAFOs) whose tone-reducing aspects are incorporated into their construction. TRAFOs have been useful in some children but are not universally recommended.[8, 245] The decision to brace and the type of orthosis to be used are dictated by the age of the child, functional level, motor control, type of deformity, and commitment to use. The availability of high-temperature material which can provide total contact allows an array of orthoses that can decrease energy expenditure when used in conjunction with therapy, surgery, and other treatment.[104] Other joint immobilizers can contribute to function and maintenance of range of motion for hygiene and dressing.[9, 246] Compression garments theoretically increase proprioceptive input to the neuromuscular system and improve motor function. Intermittent use is appropriate for tasks that are challenging and self-limited.

MEDICAL AND SURGICAL MANAGEMENT

Management of Spasticity

Medication to decrease spasticity is used in children, with the most commonly used drugs being baclofen (Lioresal) and dantrolene (Dantrium).[63, 66, 159, 170] The response to these drugs is unpredictable, and side effects often preclude long-term use. Studies have demonstrated clinically useful reduction in spasticity following the initiation of medication[48] (Table 53–5).

Reappraisal of spasticity in a growing child with CP every 6 months allows timely intervention.[171] Contractures develop over time and are a complex interaction of spasticity, growth, motor control deficits, weakness, and chronic positioning.[26]

Orthopedic Intervention

Nearly all children with CP develop an abnormality of physical form or function. The degree of the orthopedist's involvement with the child and family depends

TABLE 53–5 Comparison of Baclofen, Dantrolene, Diazepam

Feature	Baclofen	Dantrolene	Diazepam
Site of action	GABA "B" receptors in spinal cord	Intrafusal and extrafusal muscle fibers	Benzodiazepine sites in brainstem reticular formation and spinal cord
Mode of action	↓ Release of excitatory neurotransmitters from afferent terminals	↓ Release of calcium from sarcoplasmic reticulum	↑ GABA binding, potentiating presynaptic inhibition by GABA
Dose	Maximum: 20 mg qid (higher doses may be tolerated and therapeutic); start with 5 mg bid; increase by 5 mg/dose q3d	Maximum: 12 mg/kg/day (to 400 mg/day); start with 0.5 mg/kg bid; increase by 0.5 mg/kg q5–7d	Maximum: 40 mg qd; start with 2 mg bid; increase by 2 mg q2–3d
Half-life	3 to 4 hr	7 to 8 hr	8+ hr
Common side effects	Weakness, fatigue, confusion, depression, GI upset	Weakness, esp. if marginal strength; fatigue, drowsiness, diarrhea	Drowsiness, fatigue, urinary retention, constipation, impaired memory and recall
Precautions	May lower seizure threshold; abrupt withdrawal may precipitate seizures or hallucinations; additive side effects with other CNS depressants	May depress pulmonary function; reversible and irreversible hepatotoxicity (1.8%) in long-term (>2 mo) use, high dose (>300 mg/day), age >30 yr, but not reported in ≤16 yr	May develop tolerance and dependence; abrupt withdrawal may precipitate seizures; CNS effects more severe in MS and TBI and synergistic with other CNS depressants; can ↑ ataxia
Comments	Commonly recommended as drug of choice for MS and SCI; equal efficacy in complete and incomplete SCI; useful for flexor spasms	Commonly recommended as drug of choice for cerebral causes of spasticity but may be useful in SCI; little effect on cardiac or smooth muscle; monitor liver function tests before and during use	Possibly more useful in incomplete than complete SCI; effects more marked with IV that PO administration; other benzodiazepines also found useful including clorazepate and ketazolam; large index of safety; fatal overdose with diazepam alone almost unheard of

Abbreviations: CNS, central nervous system; GABA, γ-aminobutyric acid; GI, gastrointestinal; IV, intravenous; MS, multiple sclerosis; SCI, spinal cord injury; TBI, total body involvement.
Modified from Massagli TL: Spasticity and its management in children. Phys Rehabil Clin 1991; 2:867–890.

on the complexity and severity of the musculoskeletal system impairments.[69, 142] Children with CP should have regular orthopedic consultations. Follow-through with splinting, orthoses, PT, and recommendations made by the orthopedist are improved if the family and child have already built a relationship with the surgeon before the need for surgery arises. The physiatrist can facilitate this process by working in conjunction with the orthopedist and therapists involved with the child. Although the orthopedic management of the child with CP can show variations among different physicians, the fundamental goals of surgery should reflect a functional approach to problems of alignment.[116] If pain or discomfort is present, especially around the hip, surgical relief could be necessary. The following discussion addresses the surgical options for improvement in sitting, transfers, and ambulation (Table 53–6).

Surgery for Sitting

For every child, sitting is a realistic functional goal.[202] The necessary postural alignment for sitting includes a level pelvis and a reasonably straight spine.[117, 202] The loss of motion associated with hip dislocation can alter seating[53, 116] (see Chapter 18). Excessive pelvic obliquity reduces the sitting surface area and causes excessive pressure on the bony prominences of the pelvis.[142, 173, 203] The management of the hip is complex.[47, 227] Early detection of subluxation is possible with sequential radiographs of the pelvis. Physical examination of the hip is not sufficient to detect subluxation.[1]

If the hip is subluxed, the surgeon might be able to reduce the overpowering muscle forces by lengthening the iliopsoas and adductor muscles around the hip.[78, 122] This is a brief procedure that offers several benefits. It not only improves femoral head coverage under the acetabulum, but also allows easier dressing, diapering, cleaning, and positioning.[38] If the hip progresses to dislocation, then a more extensive procedure is necessary.[118] The femur and acetabulum need reconstruction, depending on the age and extent of the pathologic changes.[14, 199, 218] Commonly, excessive anteversion with a valgus orientation affects the femur. Acetabular dysplasia contributes to the inability of the femoral head to remain covered. A combination of muscle lengthenings, varus derotational osteotomy of the femur, and augmentation procedures of the acetabulum is complex and arduous; moreover, postoperative immobilization may be necessary for as long as 6 to 8 weeks.[142] Complications can arise following these procedures, including femoral fractures, heterotopic ossification, and peripheral neuropathy, depending on the concomitant surgeries.[144, 192] Rehabilitation plays an important role following cast removal.[90, 160] If the femoral articular cartilage is eroded and the hip becomes painful, the options for salvage are limited and fraught with problems. Hip fusion, artificial joint replacement, and finally resection of the femoral head can afford relief of the pain.[117] Painful hips are a chronic problem and need to be managed with multiple modalities.

The pelvis is also influenced by the hamstrings. The hamstrings act as hip extensors, but the major pull of this muscle is to tilt the pelvis in a posterior direction. Sacral sitting with constant sliding out of a wheelchair can be partially corrected by a hamstring release.[89, 116] Distal hamstring lengthening is the more common surgery, but a proximal lengthening can also be considered.[77] Other problems with sitting, which are addressed surgically less frequently, are extensor contractures of the hips and knee.

Scoliosis or kyphosis can be progressive.[206] Early treatment usually involves using a molded thoracic lumbar orthosis.[251] It is not thought that this prevents progression, but rather improves trunk support and slows the rate of progress. Total contact support can be incorporated into a contoured seating system. If a curve progresses beyond 40 degrees, fusion is considered to avoid compromise of the respiratory system.[5, 142, 215] If the deformity is rigid and extends over a long segment, staged procedures are performed. The risk of anesthesia, infection, blood loss, neurological compromise, and pseudarthrosis should be considered and planned for before surgery.[155]

Surgery for Standing

Supported standing and transfers are possible when the ankle can be held in the neutral position and the knee has less than 20 degrees of flexion contracture.[236] The surgical procedures used to improve alignment for these skills are hamstring lengthenings and Achilles tendon lengthenings.[87, 132, 204] Hip flexion contractures can also hinder standing and need attention if greater than 20 degrees.[205] Table 53–6 provides a description of procedures as well as the postoperative immobilization precautions.

Surgery for Ambulation

Surgery to improve ambulation remains problematic.[175] Difficulty in predicting outcome for the ambulator has led to caution in recommending orthopedic surgery.[70, 73, 75, 91] Close observation, aggressive bracing, and vigorous PT can temper the effect of dynamic tone and static contractures.[21] The tendency to scissor can hinder forward progression. Adductor myotomies in combination with hamstring lengthenings can create a better base of support and a more upright posture.[101, 119, 184] Recently, rectus femoris transfers and lengthenings have decreased the problem of stiff-knee gait following hamstring release.[62, 92] A braceable foot or a foot that allows for foot-flat or heel-strike is desirable for stance.[6, 15] Orthopedic surgery can affect balance, but the central processing of balance reactions remains the same after surgery. Assistive devices can play an important transitional role in household or community ambulation. A reverse walker can assist with upright posture better than the traditional forward walker.[153]

The use of gait analysis has refined the observation of components of the gait cycle and the combined effect of contractures on gait dynamics. Gait analysis defines cadence, velocity, stride length, and ranges of motion of the hip, knee, and ankle during various phases of the gait cycle and the timing of muscular activity. Some gait

TABLE 53–6 Common Orthopedic Surgeries in Cerebral Palsy

Surgical Procedure	Purpose	Positioning Considerations	Treatment
Hip flexor lengthening Usually iliopsoas Sometimes proximal rectus femoris Rarely sartorius	Increase extension ROM Decrease muscle imbalance—risk of hip subluxation Improve alignment stance, gait	Avoid prolonged sitting Prone wedge preferred Standing frame with foot control (casts/AFOs) Prone at night (with or without body splint)	Maintain length of hip flexor muscles Strengthen hip flexors (need for stairs, gait) Strengthen hip extensors
Hip adductor lengthening Usually proximal—origin Adductor longus, gracilis Sometimes adductor brevis	Increase hip abduction Decrease scissoring Decrease abnormal muscle imbalance—risk of hip subluxation Increase base of support Improve hygiene, positioning	Abduction at night, usually prone With/without night splint Abduction wedge on prone wedge/wheelchair	Maintain length of hip adductors (knees flexed and extended) Strengthen hip adductors and abductors
Hamstring lengthening Medial/lateral hamstrings Almost always distal	Increase knee extension Improve standing alignment Decrease crouch posture Increase stance-phase stability in gait, improved alignment Increase step length → increased terminal swing phase and heel-strike ability Increase positioning options	Avoid prolonged sitting Prone wedge preferred (consider soft knee splints) Standing frame with foot control Prone at night with soft knee splints or night splints	Maintain length of hamstrings (avoid knee hyperextension) Strengthen hamstrings and quadriceps (proximal and distal), especially terminal knee extension Monitor for overactive quadriceps, increase in extensor tone → knee hyperextension
Achilles tendon lengthening Five different types: Baker, percutaneous, sliding, fractional lengthening, vulpius	Increase dorsiflexion ROM Increase full-foot contact for standing and gait Increase ability for heel-strike in gait Allow for bracing	Initially no dorsiflexion beyond neutral Standing with neutral dorsiflexion only Temporary splint/cast initially to maintain ROM—begin early supportive weightbearing Sitting OK, if TALs only and other muscles not tight If prone wedge—feet off edge with AFO/cast/splint AFO approximately 6 mo (surgeon discretion) AFO/cast/splint at night	Maintain length of plantar flexors Strengthen plantar flexors and dorsiflexors Avoid overstretching—could lead to crouch posture (Special attention when considering hinged AFOs) (Repeat procedures common—especially if done at early age)

Abbreviations: ROM, range of motion; AFO, ankle-foot orthosis; TAL, tendoachilles lengthening.
From Feathergill B: Personal communications, 1993.

TABLE 53–7 Comparison of Botulinum Type A Toxin and Phenol

Blocking Agent	Administered	Effectiveness	Advantages	Drawbacks	Complications
Botulinum type A toxin	Injected into muscle	Lasts 12 to 30 wk	Easy to administer Diffuses readily into muscle Painless Can be administered without anesthesia	Effects are always transient Lasts only 12 to 30 wk Limited approval	No significant complications reported
Phenol block	Injected into motor points of involved muscle	Lasts 4 to 12 mo	Use is widely approved Lasts longer than botulinum toxin Cumulative effects often occur	Can be painful May require general anesthesia during administration Takes more skill to administer	Transient dysesthesias and numbness Hematomas may occur, which negate the effects of treatment If a large intravascular injection occurs, phenol can cause systemic effects such as muscle tremors and convulsions, as well as depressed cardiac activity, blood pressure, and respiration

From Gormley M: Personal communications, 1994.

laboratories also measure the forces generated at each joint. Gait analysis provides consistent objective information which enhances orthopedic decision-making and improves outcome studies[91] (see Chapter 5). Energy expenditure for some children with spastic CP can be as high as 350% of normal.[41] Energy expenditure is an important consideration for continued community ambulation.[91, 174]

Other Surgeries

Upper extremity surgery is uncommonly done to improve the function of the hand.[216] Flexor carpi ulnaris transfer has a place in reducing wrist flexion deformity. The active use of the hand, however, is dependent on stereognosis and two-point discrimination.[50, 237]

Neurosurgical procedures such as stereotactic ablation of selected thalamic nuclei and chronic electrical stimulation of the cerebellum or posterior columns have been unsuccessful in reducing spasticity in the child with CP.[52, 239] Selective posterior rhizotomy (SPR) and intrathecal baclofen pumps are two current neurosurgical procedures that hold promise in reducing spasticity.[2, 4, 193–195] Reduction in tone, as recorded by the modified Ashworth scale in both procedures, is improved[165, 196] (see Chapter 29). Gait analysis studies of children undergoing SPR have consistently shown an improved availability of range of motion at the knee and hip, resulting in an increased stride length.[34, 242, 243] Careful selection is critical because the subsequent weakness, which is an anticipated part of the postoperative recovery period, can reduce the level of independence of children who depend on their spasticity to transfer or stand.[159]

Other Interventions

In addition to surgical management of contractures, motor point blocks and, recently, botulism injections can be used as adjunct management of the spastic muscle.[46, 54, 72, 139, 219] These procedures are used to improve range of motion during the child's younger years when orthopedic surgery should be delayed. Indications for the use of each and the advantages are listed in Table 53–7.

Functional electrical stimulation and biofeedback can be helpful for training specific muscles.[16, 44, 45, 157] Another modality that is gaining attention for improving strength in the child with CP is therapeutic electrical stimulation. The use of low-voltage, high-frequency electrical stimulation increases blood flow and improves muscle growth and strength.[187]

The utilization of medication to reduce drooling and improve bladder control facilitates socialization. The most commonly used drugs are oxybutynin (Ditropan), scopolamine, and glycopyrrolate.[152, 224]

The effectiveness of any specific intervention for the child with CP is difficult to study owing to the multihandicapping nature of CP, lack of outcome measures, difficulty in obtaining control groups, and historically poor study designs. The American Academy of Cerebral Palsy and Developmental Medicine has approached CP outcome literature and evaluation with the National Center for Rehabilitation Research model of outcome. This model expands the World Health Organization model of impairment, disability, and handicap to include pathophysiology and functional limitations as multidimensional measures (Fig. 53–15). The encouraging development of appropriate evaluative measures, adherence to randomized control studies, and the use of meta-analysis portend improved understanding of the use of therapies on the outcome of the child with CP.[106, 128, 133, 183, 186, 214, 238] The use of gait analysis not only improves decision-making prior to surgeries, but allows objective analysis of outcome following surgery.[90, 221] Harris has provided a review of efficacy studies[109] (see Table 53–4).

Most studies of the effectiveness of PT and other treatment are inconclusive.[113, 161, 217, 233] Goldkamp[94] reviewed ADL outcome in children with CP and reported that few children after the age of 4 years achieved independence in their ADL. Investigators have found that the children most likely to improve in motor abilities were those children with higher intelligence quotients (IQs) and lesser involvement of the neuromuscular system.[94] Similar conclusions were obtained from a study by Perry and colleagues[197] in evaluating the use of Rolfing in CP. The use of a single-study design has demonstrated the positive effect of tone-reducing AFOs.[245] Cost containment provides the impetus for further study of the effects of therapy, including difficult issues such as frequency and duration.

SUMMARY

Successful rehabilitation of the child with CP includes the prevention of additional impairments, reduction of disability, and improved integration of the individual into the community. Total independence cannot be achievable or desirable for all patients. The pediatrician's primary interest for the child with CP is to provide preventive and diagnostic health care. The developmental pediatrician views the impact the cerebral palsy has on the child's development, while the pediatric or-

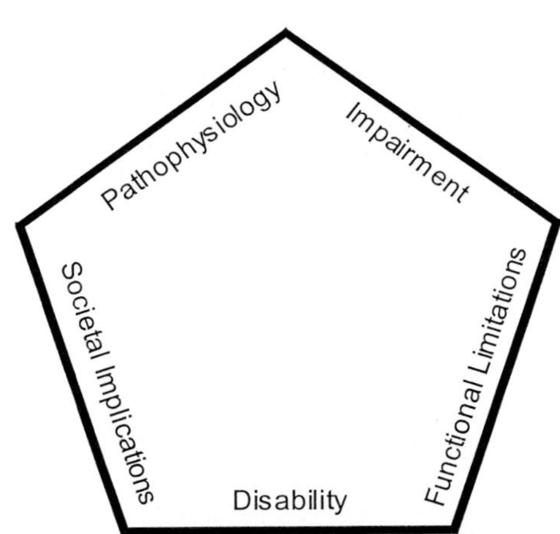

FIGURE 53–15. Model for measurements of outcomes based on NCMRR guidelines.

thopedist is interested in the impact of static and dynamic contractures on mobility. The pediatric physiatrist views the impact of CP on the child's overall medical, surgical, and therapeutic options. Facilitating the ability of the child and family to set functional goals is our primary responsibility. This process takes cooperation, prioritization of competing interests, and an advocacy position for the child. Physiatrists have an important place in assisting the person with CP to achieve the independence he or she desires within the constraints of the community environment.

REFERENCES

1. Abel MF, Wenger DR, Mubarak P, et al: Quantitative analysis in hip dysplasia in cerebral palsy: A study of radiographs and 3-D reformatted images. J Pediatr Orthop 1994; 14:283–289.
2. Abbott R, Johann SL: Selective posterior rhizotomy for the treatment of spasticity: A review. Childs Nerv Syst 1989; 5: 337–346.
3. Agnarsson U, Warde C, McCarthy G, et al: Anorectal function of children with neurological problems. II: Cerebral palsy. Dev Med Child Neurol 1993; 35:903–908.
4. Albright AL, Cervi A, Singletary J: Intrathecal baclofen for spasticity in cerebral palsy. JAMA 1991; 265:1418–1422.
5. Allen BL, Ferguson RL: L-rod instrumentation for scoliosis in cerebral palsy. J Pediatr Orthop 1982; 2:87.
6. Alman BA, Craig CL, Zimbler S: Subtalar arthrodesis for stabilization of valgus hindfoot in patients with cerebral palsy. J Pediatr Orthop 1993; 13:634–641.
7. American Academy of Pediatrics: The Doman-Delacato treatment of neurologically handicapped children. Pediatrics 1982; 70:810–812.
8. Anderson JP, Snow B, Dorey FJ, et al: Efficacy of soft splints in reducing knee flexion contractures. Dev Med Child Neurol 1988; 30:502–508.
9. Anderson L: Swimming to win. In Jones JA (ed): Training Guide to Cerebral Palsy Sports, ed 3. Champaign, IL, Human Kinetics, 1988.
10. Ayres AJ: The Development of Sensory Integration Theory and Practice. Dubuque, IA, Kendall/Hunt, 1974.
11. Ayres, AJ: Effect of sensory integrative therapy on the coordination of children with choreoathetoid movements. Am J Occup Ther 1977; 31:291–293.
12. Ayres AJ: Sensory Integration and Learning Disorders. Los Angeles, Western Psychological Services, 1972.
13. Bachrack S, Greenspun B: Care of the adult with cerebral palsy. Del Med J 1990; 62:1287–1295.
14. Bagg M, Farber J, Miller F: Long-term follow-up of hip subluxation in cerebral palsy patients. J Pediatr Orthop 1993; 13:32–36.
15. Banks HJ, Green WT: The correction of equinus deformity in cerebral palsy. J Bone Joint Surg Am 1958; 40:1359–1379.
16. Basmajian J: Biofeedback in therapeutic exercise. In Basmajian J (ed): Therapeutic Exercise. Baltimore, Williams & Wilkins, 1984.
17. Batshaw ML, Eicher PS: Cerebral palsy. Pediatr Clin North Am 1993; 40:537–551.
18. Bax M: Aims and outcomes of therapy for the cerebral palsied child. Dev Med Child Neurol 1986; 28:695–698.
19. Bax T, Coombes M, Bax M, et al: The health and social needs of physically handicapped young adults. Dev Med Child Neurol 1985; 15:27–37.
20. Bee HL, Barnard KE, Eyres SJ, et al: Prediction of IQ and language skill from perinatal status, child performance, family characteristics, and mother-infant interaction. Child Dev 1982; 53:1134–1156.
21. Bertoti DB: Effect of short leg casting on ambulation in children with cerebral palsy. Phys Ther 1986; 66:1522–1529.
22. Bhushan VB, Paneth N, Kiely JL: Impact of improved survival of very low birth weight infants on recent secular trends in the prevalence of cerebral palsy. Pediatrics 1993; 91:1094–1100.
23. Biether JK, Cummins SK, Nelson KB: The California Cerebral Palsy Project. Pediatr Perinatol Epidemiol 1993; 6:339–351.
24. Blair E, Ballantyne J, Horsman S, et al: A study of a dynamic proximal stability splint in the management of children with cerebral palsy. Dev Med Child Neurol 1995; 37:544–554.
25. Bleck EE: Locomotion prognosis in cerebral palsy. Dev Med Child Neurol 1975; 17:18–25.
26. Bleck EE: Orthopaedic Management of Cerebral Palsy. Philadelphia, WB Saunders, 1982.
27. Bleck EE: Severe orthopedic disability in childhood: Solutions provided by rehabilitation engineering. Orthop Clin North Am 1978; 9:509–526.
28. Bleck EE: Where have all the cerebral palsy children gone? The needs of adults. Dev Med Child Neurol 1984; 26:674–676.
29. Bobath B: Abnormal Posture Reflex Activity Caused by Brain Lesions, ed 2. London, Heinemann, 1971.
30. Bobath B: Motor development: Its effect on general development and application to the treatment of cerebral palsy. Physiotherapy 1971; 57:526.
31. Bobath K: Neurophysiological Basis for Treatment of Cerebral Palsy. Lavenham, England, Spastics International, 1980.
32. Bobath B: A neuro-developmental treatment of cerebral palsy. Physiotherapy 1963; 49:242–244.
33. Bobath B, Bobath K: Motor Development in the Different Types of Cerebral Palsy. London, Heinemann, 1975.
34. Boscarino LF, Ounpuu S, Davis RV, et al: Effects of selective dorsal rhizotomy on gait in children with cerebral palsy. J Pediatr Orthop 1993; 13:174–179.
35. Bozynski M, Nelson M, Genaze D, et al: Cranial ultrasonography and the production of cerebral palsy in infants weighing ≤1200 grams at birth. Dev Med Child Neurol 1988; 30:342–348.
36. Bradley R, Caldwell B: Early home environment and changes in mental test performance in children from 6–36 months. Dev Psychol 1976; 12:93–97.
37. Brown JK, Fulford GE: Position as a cause of deformity in children with cerebral palsy. Dev Med Child Neurol 1976; 18:305–314.
38. Brunner R, Baumann JU: Clinical benefit of reconstruction of dislocated or subluxated hip joints in patients with spastic cerebral palsy. J Pediatr Orthop 1994; 14:290–294.
39. Burton AW: Assessing the perceptual-motor interaction in the developmentally disabled and non-handicapped children. Adapted Phys Activity Q 1990; 7:325–337.
40. Butler C: Effects of powered mobility on self-initiated behaviors of very young children with locomotor disability. Dev Med Child Neurol 1986; 28:325–332.
41. Campbell J, Ball J: Energetics of walking in cerebral palsy. Orthop Clin North Am 1978; 9:374–377.
42. Capute AJ, Biehl R: Functional development evaluation. Pediatr Clin North Am 1993; 20:3–26.
43. Carlson L: Therapeutic riding and the rehabilitative process. Phys Ther Forum 1987; 6:4.
44. Carmick J: Clinical use of neuromuscular electrical stimulation for children with cerebral palsy: Part 1. Lower extremity. Phys Ther 1993; 73:505–513.
45. Carmick J: Clinical use of neuromuscular electrical stimulation for children with cerebral palsy: Part 2. Upper extremity. Phys Ther 1993; 7:514–522.
46. Carpenter EB: Role of the nerve block in the foot and ankle in the therapeutic management of cerebral palsy. Foot Ankle 1979; 4:164–166.
47. Carr C, Gage JR: The fate of the nonoperated hip in cerebral palsy. J Pediatr Orthop 1987; 7:262–267.
48. Carvalho O: A new objective method for evaluation of muscle relaxants in congenital spastic diplegia. Dev Med Child Neurol 1966; 8:34–36.
49. Center for Law and Education: Educational rights of children with disabilities under IDEA and Section 504 educational rights of children with disabilities: A primer for advocates. Cambridge, MA, Center for Law and Education.
50. Chakerian DL, Larson MA: Effects of upper extremity weight-bearing on hand-opening and prehension patterns of children with cerebral palsy. Dev Med Child Neurol 1993; 35:216–229.
51. Cohen HJ, Birch HG: Some considerations for evaluating the Doman-Delacato "patterning" method. Pediatrics 1970; 45:302.

52. Cooper I, Riklan M, Amin I, et al: Chronic cerebellar stimulation in cerebral palsy. Neurology 1976; 26:744–749.
53. Cooperman DR, Bartucci E, Dietrick E, et al: Hip dislocation in spastic cerebral palsy: Long-term consequences. J Pediatr Orthop 1987; 7:268–276.
54. Cosgrove AP, Corry IS, Graham HK: Botulinum toxin in the management of the lower limb in cerebral palsy. Dev Med Child Neurol 1994; 36:386–396.
55. Cosgrove AP, Graham HK: Botulinum toxin A prevents the development of contractures in the hereditary spastic mouse. Dev Med Child Neurol 1994; 36:379–385.
56. Costello AM de L, Hamilton P, Baudin J, et al: Prediction of neurodevelopmental impairment at four years from brain ultrasound appearance of very preterm infants. Dev Med Child Neurol 1988; 30:711–722.
57. Cottam P, McCartney E, Cullen C: The effectiveness of conductive education principles with profoundly retarded multiple handicapped children. Br Disord Commun 1985; 20:45–49.
58. Cummins SK, Nelson KB, Giether JK, et al: Cerebral palsy in four northern California counties, births 1983 through 1985. J Pediatr 1993; 123:230–237.
59. Currie DM, Gershkoff AM, Cifu DX: Geriatric rehabilitation. 3. Mid- and late-life effects of early-life disabilities. Arch Phys Med Rehabil 1993; 74(suppl 5):5413–5416.
60. Curtis K: Wheelchair sports medicine. In Klafs CE, Armheim DD (eds): Modern Principles of Athletic Training, ed 4. St Louis, Mosby-Year Book, 1977, pp 16–18.
61. d'Avignon M, Noren L, Arman R: Early physiotherapy and Vojta or Bobath in infants with suspected neuromotor disturbance. Neuropediatrics 1981; 12:232–237.
62. Damron TA, Breed AL, Cook T: Diminished knee flexion after hamstring surgery in cerebral palsy patients: Prevalence and severity. J Pediatr Orthop 1993; 13:188–191.
63. Davidoff R: Antispasticity drugs: Mechanisms of action. Ann Neurol 1985; 17:107–116.
64. Deaver G: Cerebral Palsy: Methods of Evaluation and Treatment. Rehabilitation Monograph 9, New York, Institute for Rehabilitative Medicine, 1952.
65. Deaver G: Methods of treating the neuromuscular disabilities. Arch Phys Med Rehabil 1956; 37:363–367.
66. Decter RM, Bauer SB, Khoshbin S, et al: Urodynamic assessment of children with cerebral palsy. J Urol 1987; 138:1110–1112.
67. Denhoff E, Feldman S, Smith GM, et al: Treatment of spastic cerebral palsied children with sodium dantrolene. Dev Med Child Neurol 1975; 17:736–774.
68. Dickey R, Shealey SH: Using technology to control the environment. Am J Occup Ther 1987; 41:717–721.
69. Doman R, Spitz E, Zucman E, et al: Children with severe brain injuries. Neurological organization in terms of mobility. JAMA 1960; 174:257–264.
70. Dormans JP: Orthopedic management of children with cerebral palsy. Pediatr Clin North Am 1993; 40:645–657.
71. Drvaric DM, Roberts JM, Burke SW, et al: Gastroesophageal evaluation in totally involved cerebral palsy patients. J Pediatr Orthop 1987; 7:187–190.
72. Easton JKM, Ozel T, Halpern D: Intramuscular neurolysis for spasticity in children. Arch Phys Med Rehabil 1979; 60:155–158.
73. Eggers GWN, Evans EB: Surgery in cerebral palsy. J Bone Joint Surg Am 1963; 45:1275.
74. Eicher PS, Batshaw ML: Cerebral palsy, the child with developmental disabilities. Pediatr Clin North Am 1993; 40:537–551.
75. Eilert RE, MacEwen GD: Varus derotational osteotomy of the femur in cerebral palsy. Clin Orthop 1977; 125:168.
76. Ellenberg JH, Nelson KB: Cluster of perinatal events identifying infants at high risk for death or disability. J Pediatr 1988; 113:546–552.
77. Elmer E, Wenger D, Mubarak S, et al: Proximal hamstring lengthening in the sitting cerebral palsy patient. J Pediatr Orthop 1992; 12:329–336.
78. Erken L, Einhard HW, Bischof FM: Iliopsoas transfer in cerebral palsy: The long-term outcome. J Pediatr Orthop 1994; 14:295–298.
79. Eyman RK, Grossman HJ, Chaney RH, et al: The life expectancy of profoundly handicapped people with mental retardation. N Engl J Med 1990; 323:584–589.
80. Fay T: The use of pathological and unlocking reflexes in the rehabilitation of spastics. Am J Phys Med 1954; 33:33–47.
81. Fee M, Charney E, Robertson W: Nutritional assessment of the young child with cerebral palsy. Infants Young Child 1988; 1:33–40.
82. Fernandez JE, Pitetti KH: Training of ambulatory individuals with cerebral palsy. Arch Phys Med Rehabil 1993; 74:468–472.
83. Ferrara MS, Buckley WE, et al: The injury experience of the competitive athlete with a disability: Prevention implications. Med Sci Sports Exerc 1992; 24:184–188.
84. Foley J: Dyskinetic and dystonic cerebral palsy. Acta Paediatr 1992; 81:57–60.
85. Freeman JM, Nelson KB: Special articles: Intrapartum asphyxia and cerebral palsy. Pediatrics 1988; 82:240–241.
86. Fremart A: Provision of related services for children with chronic disabilities. Pediatrics 1993; 92:879–881.
87. Fulford GE: Surgical management of ankle and foot deformities in cerebral palsy. Clin Orthop 1990; 253:55–61.
88. Fulford GE, Brown JK: Position as a cause of deformity in children with cerebral palsy. Dev Med Child Neurol 1976; 18:305–314.
89. Fulford GE, Cairns TP, Sloan Y: Sitting problems of children with cerebral palsy. Dev Med Child Neurol 1982; 24:48–53.
90. Gage JR: Gait analysis in cerebral palsy. Clin Dev Med 1991; 121:177–183.
91. Gage JR, Fabian D, Hicks R, et al: Pre- and post-operative gait analysis in patients with spastic diplegia: A preliminary report. J Pediatr Orthop 1984; 4:715–718.
92. Gage JR, Perry J, Hicks RR, et al: Rectus femoris transfer to improve knee function of children with cerebral palsy. Dev Med Child Neurol 1987; 29:159–166.
93. Gillette H: Systems of Therapy in Cerebral Palsy. Springfield, IL, Charles C Thomas, 1969.
94. Goldkamp O: Treatment effectiveness in cerebral palsy. Arch Phys Med Rehabil 1984; 65:232–234.
95. Graham M, Levene MI, Trounce JQ, et al: Prediction of cerebral palsy in very low birth weight infants: Prospective ultrasound study. Lancet 1987; 2:593–596.
96. Gramer R, Keller K, Baughman, J, et al: Data analysis on 600 pediatric videofluoroscopic swallow studies. Personal communication, 1994.
97. Greiner BM, Czerniecki JM, Deitz JC: Gait parameters of children with spastic diplegia: A comparison of effects of posterior and anterior walkers. Arch Phys Med Rehabil 1993; 74:381–385.
98. Griether JK, Cummins SK, Nelson KB: The California Cerebral Palsy Project. Pediatr Perinatol Epidemiol 1992; 6:339–351.
99. Griether JK, Nelson KB, Cummins SK: Twinning and cerebral palsy: Experience in four northern California counties' births 1983–1985. Pediatrics 1993; 92:854–888.
100. Guzzetta F, Shackelford GD, Volpe S, et al: Periventricular intraparenchymal echodensities in the premature newborn: Critical determinant of neurological outcome. Pediatrics 1986; 78: 995–1006.
101. Hadley N, Chambers C, Scarborough N, et al: Knee motion following multiple soft-tissue releases in ambulatory patients with cerebral palsy. J Pediatr Orthop 1992; 12:324–328.
102. Hagberg B, Hagberg G, Olow I, et al: The changing panorama of cerebral palsy in Sweden. V: The birth year period 1979–1982. Acta Paediatr Scand 1989; 78:283–290.
103. Halpren D: Therapeutic exercises for cerebral palsy. In Basmajian JV (ed): Therapeutic Exercise. Baltimore, Williams & Wilkins, 1984.
104. Harrington ED, Lin RS, Gage JR: Use of the anterior floor reaction orthosis in patients with cerebral palsy. Bull Orthot Prosthet 1984; 37:34–42.
105. Harris S: Early diagnosis of spastic diplegia, spastic hemiplegia, and quadriplegia. Am J Dis Child 1989; 143:1356–1360.
106. Harris SR: The effectiveness of early intervention for at-risk and handicapped children. In Guralnick MJ, Bennett FC (eds): The Effectiveness of Early Intervention for At Risk and Handicapped Children. San Diego, Academic Press, 1987, pp 175–212.
107. Harris SR: Efficacy of early intervention in pediatric rehabilitation. Phys Med Rehabil Clin North Am 1991; 2:725–742.
108. Harris SR, Atwater S, Crowe T: Accepted and controversial neuromotor therapies for infants at high risk for cerebral palsy. J Perinatol 1985; 8:3–12.

109. Harris SR, Tada WL: Providing developmental therapy services. In Garwood SG, Fewell RF (eds): Educating Handicapped Infants, Rockville, MD, Aspen 1983, pp 343–368.
110. Haynes UE: The National Collaborative Infant Project. In Tjossen TD (ed): Intervention Strategies for High Risk Infants and Children, Baltimore, University Park Press, 1976, pp 509–534.
111. Healy A: Pediatricians' role in the development and implementation of an Individual Education Plan (IEP) and/or an Individual Family Service Plan (IFSP). Pediatrics 1992; 89:340–342.
112. Hennrikus WL, Rosenthal RK, Kasser JR: Incidence of spondylolisthesis in ambulatory cerebral palsy patients. J Pediatr Orthop 1993; 13:37–40.
113. Herndon WA, Troup P, Yngve DA, et al: Effects of neurodevelopmental treatment on movement patterns of children with cerebral palsy. J Pediatr Orthop 1987; 7:395–400.
114. Hill AE: Problems in relation to independent living: A retrospective study of physically disabled school-leavers. Dev Med Child Neurol 1993; 35:1111–1115.
115. Hinderer KA, Harris SR, Purdy AH, et al: Effects of tone-reducing vs standard plaster casts on gait improvement of children with cerebral palsy. Dev Med Child Neurol 1988; 30: 370–377.
116. Hoffer M: Management of the hip in cerebral palsy. J Bone Joint Surg Am 1986; 68:629–631.
117. Hoffer M, Abraham E, Nickel VL, et al: Salvage surgery of the hip to improve sitting posture of mentally retarded, severely disabled children with cerebral palsy. Dev Med Child Neurol 1992; 14:51–59.
118. Hoffer M, Stein G, Koffman M, et al: Femoral varus-derotation osteotomy in spastic cerebral palsy. J Bone Surg Am 1985; 67:1229–1335.
119. Hoffinger SA, Rab GT, Abou-Ghaida H: Hamstrings in cerebral palsy crouch gait. J Pediatr Orthop 1993; 13:722–726.
120. Holland LJ, Steadward RD: Effects of resistance in flexibility training and strength, spasticity/muscle tone and range of motion of elite athletes with cerebral palsy. Palestra summer; 1990, pp 27–31.
121. Houle AM, Vernet O, Jednak R, et al: Bladder function before and after selective dorsal rhizotomy in children with cerebral palsy. J Urol 1998; 160:1088–1091.
122. Howard CB, Williams LA, Mackie I: Factors affecting the incidence of hip dislocation in cerebral palsy. J Bone Joint Surg Br 1985; 67:530–532.
123. Hueberman G: Organized sports activity with cerebral palsy adolescents. Rehabil Lit 1976; 37:103–106.
124. Irwin-Carruthers SH: Results of early intervention in the baby with cerebral motor disturbance. S Afr J Physiother 1981; pp 34–37.
125. Janicki M: Aging, cerebral palsy, and older persons with mental retardation. Aust N Z J Dev Disabilities 1989; 15:311–320.
126. Jankowski LW, Sullivan J: Aerobic and neuromuscular training: An effect of capacity, efficacy and fatigability of patients with traumatic brain injuries. Arch Phys Med Rehabil 1990; 71: 500–504.
127. Jarvis SN, Holloway JS, Hey EN, et al: Increase in cerebral palsy in normal birth weight babies. Arch Dis Child 1985; 60:1113–1121.
128. Jeffe AM: Using health-related quality of life measures. Physical therapy outcomes research. Phys Ther 1993; 73:523–527.
129. Jevsevar DS, Karlin LI: The relationship between preoperative nutritional status and complications after an operation for scoliosis in patients who have cerebral palsy. J Bone Joint Surg Am 1993; 75:880–884.
130. Johnstone K, Perrin J: Sports for the handicapped child. Phys Med Rehabil 1991; 5:331–350.
131. Jones ET, Knapp RB: Assessment and management of the lower extremity in cerebral palsy. Orthop Clin North Am 1987; 18:725–738.
132. Kalen V, Conklin M, Sherman F: Untreated scoliosis in severe cerebral palsy. J Pediatr Orthop 1992; 12:337–340.
133. Keller RB: Outcomes research in orthopaedics. J Am Acad Orthop Surg 1993; 1:523–527.
134. Kelly G: Vestibular stimulation as a form of therapy. Physiotherapy 1989; 75:136–140.
135. Khalili A, Betts HB: Peripheral nerve block with phenol in the management of spasticity. JAMA 1967; 200:1155.
136. Kibele A: Occupational therapy's role in improving the quality of life for persons with cerebral palsy. Am J Occup Ther 1991; 45:371–377.
137. Kiely M, Lubin RA, Kiely JZ: Descriptive epidemiology of cerebral palsy. Publ Health Rev 1984; 12:79–101.
138. Klapper ZS, Birch HG: The relation of childhood characteristics to outcome in young adults with cerebral palsy. Dev Med Child Neurol 1966; 8:645–656.
139. Koman LA, Mooney JF, Goodman A: Management of valgus hindfoot deformity in pediatric cerebral palsy. J Pediatr Orthop 1993; 13:180–183.
140. Koman LA, Mooney JF, Smith BP, et al: Management of spasticity in cerebral palsy with botulinum-A toxin: Report of a preliminary, randomized, double-blind trial. J Pediatr Orthop 1994; 14:299–303.
141. Köng E: Very early treatment of cerebral palsy. Dev Med Child Neurol 1966; 8:198–202.
142. Koop SE: Orthopedic aspects of static encephalopathies. In Miller G, Ramer J (eds): Static Encephalopathies of Infancy and Childhood. New York, Academic Press, 1992, pp 95–109.
143. Krageloh-Mann I, Hagberg G, Meisner C, et al: Bilateral spastic cerebral palsy—A comparative study between southwest Germany and western Sweden. I: Clinical patterns and disabilities. Dev Med Child Neurol 1993; 35:1031–1047.
144. Krum SD, Miller F: Heterotopic ossification after hip and spine surgery in children with cerebral palsy. J Pediatr Orthop 1993; 13:739–743.
145. Kuban KC, Leviton A: Cerebral palsy. N Engl J Med 1994; 330:188–195.
146. Kudrjavcev T, Schoenberg BB, Kurland LT, et al: Cerebral palsy: Survival rates, associated handicaps, and distribution by clinical subtype—Rochester, MN, 1950–1976. Neurology 1985; 35: 900–903.
147. Kudrjavcev T, Schoenberg BB, Kurland LT, et al: Cerebral palsy: Trends in incidence and changes in concurrent neonatal mortality—Rochester, MN, 1950–1976. Neurology 1983; 33:1433–1438.
148. Laplaza FJ, Root L, Tassanawipas A, et al: Femoral torsion and neck-shaft angles in cerebral palsy. J Pediatr Orthop 1993; 13:192–199.
149. Law M, King G: Parent compliance with therapeutic interventions for children with cerebral palsy. Dev Med Child Neurol 1993; 35:983–990.
150. Lesny I, Stehlik A, Tomasek J, et al: Sensory disorders in cerebral palsy: Two-point discrimination. Dev Med Child Neurol 1993; 35:402–405.
151. Lespargot A, Langevin MF, Muller S, et al: Swallowing disturbances associated with drooling in cerebral palsied children. Dev Med Child Neurol 1993; 35:298–304.
152. Lewis D, Fontana C, Mehallick L, et al: Transdermal scopolamine for reduction of drooling in developmentally delayed children. Dev Med Child Neurol 1994; 36:484–486.
153. Levangie PK, Guihan MF, Meyer P, et al: Effect of altering handle position of a rolling walker on gait in children with cerebral palsy. Phys Ther 1989; 69:130–134.
154. Levine MS, Kliebhan L: Communication between physician and physical and occupational therapists: A neurodevelopmentally based prescription. Pediatrics 1981; 68:208–214.
155. Lonstein JE, Akbarnia A: Operative treatment of spinal deformities in patients with cerebral palsy or mental retardation: An analysis of one hundred and seven cases. J Bone Joint Surg Am 1983; 65:33–55.
156. Lundberg A: Longitudinal study of physical working capacity of young people with cerebral palsy. Dev Med Child Neurol 1984; 26:328–334.
157. Mackey S: The use of computer-assisted feedback in a motor control task for cerebral palsied children. Physiotherapy 1989; 75:143–148.
158. Maltais D: Fit 'n Flex: A family-centered Saturday morning group exercise class for children with spastic diplegic cerebral palsy. Dev Med Child Neurol 1993; 35:41.
159. Massagli TL: Spasticity and its management in children. Phys Rehabil Clin 1991; 2:867–890.

160. Mathias A: Management of cerebral palsy: Physical therapy in relation to orthopedic surgery. Phys Ther 1967; 47:473–482.
161. Mayo N: The effect of physical therapy for children with motor delay and cerebral palsy: A randomized clinical trial. Am J Phys Med Rehabil 1991; 70:258–267.
162. McCarty SM, James PS, et al: Assessment of intelligence functioning across the life span in severe cerebral palsy. Dev Med Child Neurol 1986; 28:369–371.
163. McCuaig M, Frank G: The able self: Adaptive patterns and choices in independent living for a person with cerebral palsy. Am J Occup Ther 1991; 45:224–234.
164. McCubbin J, Shasby G: Effects of isokinetic exercise and adolescents with cerebral palsy. Adapted Phys Activity 1985; 2:56–64.
165. McDonald C: Selective dorsal rhizotomy: A critical review. Phys Med Rehabil 1991; 2:891–915.
166. McGrath S, Splaingard M, Alba H, et al: Survival and functional outcome of children with severe cerebral palsy following gastrostomy, abstract. Arch Phys Med Rehabil 1983; 73:133–137.
167. McMenamin JB, Shackelford GD, Volpe JJ: Outcome of neonatal intraventricular hemorrhage with echodense lesions. Ann Neurol 1984; 15:285–290.
168. McNeal DM, Hawtrey CE, Wolraich ML, et al: Symptomatic neurogenic bladder in a cerebral-palsied population. Dev Med Child Neurol 1983; 25:612–616.
169. Meadow R: Where have all the CP children gone? The needs of adults. Dev Med Child Neurol 1984; 26:669–676.
170. Molnar GE: Cerebral palsy. In Molnar GE (ed): Pediatric Rehabilitation. Baltimore, Williams & Wilkins, 1985, pp 481–533.
171. Molnar G: Long-term treatment of spasticity in children with cerebral palsy. In International Rehabilitation Medicine Association V Conference, 1987, pp 170–172.
172. Molnar GE, Gordon SU: Cerebral palsy: Predictive value of selected clinical signs of early prognostication of motor function. Arch Phys Med Rehabil 1976; 57:153–158.
173. Moreau M, Drummond D, Rogala E, et al: Natural history of the dislocated hip in spastic cerebral palsy. Dev Med Child Neurol 1979; 21:749–753.
174. Mossberg K, Linton K, Friske K: Ankle-foot orthoses: Effect on energy expenditure of gait in spastic diplegia children. Arch Phys Med Rehabil 1990; 70:490–494.
175. Mullaferoze P, Voro P: Surgery in lower limbs in cerebral palsy. Dev Med Child Neurol 1972; 14:45–50.
176. Murphy KP, Molnar GE, Lankasky K: Medical and functional status of adults with cerebral palsy. Dev Med Child Neurol 1995; 37:1075–1084.
177. Naeye R, Peters E, Bartholomew M, et al: Origins of cerebral palsy. Am J Dis Child 1989; 143:1154–1162.
178. Nelson KB: What proportion of cerebral palsy is related to birth asphyxia? J Pediatr 1988; 112:572–574.
179. Nelson KB, Ellenberg JH: Antecedents of cerebral palsy. Multivariate analysis of risk. Am J Dis Child 1986; 315:81–86.
180. Nelson KB, Ellenberg JH: Children who outgrew cerebral palsy. Pediatrics 1982; 69:529–535.
181. Nwaobi O, Smith PD: Effect of adaptive seating on pulmonary function of children with cerebral palsy. Dev Med Child Neurol 1986; 28:351–354.
182. O'Grady R, Nishimura D, Kohn J, et al: Vocational predictions compared with present vocational status of 60 young adults with cerebral palsy. Dev Med Child Neurol 1985; 27:775–784.
183. Ottenbacher KJ, Biocca Z, DeCrenter G, et al: Quantitative analysis of the effectiveness of physical therapy: Emphasis on the neurodevelopmental treatment approach. Phys Ther 1986; 66:1095–1105.
184. Ounpuu S, Muik E, Davis RB, et al: Rectus femoris surgery in children with cerebral palsy. Part II: A comparison between the effect of transfer and release of the distal rectus femoris on knee motion. J Pediatr Orthop 1993; 13:331–335.
185. Palmer FB, Shapiro BK, Wachtel RC, et al: The effects of physical therapy on cerebral palsy. A controlled trial in infants with spastic diplegia. N Engl J Med 1988; 13:803–808.
186. Paneth N, Kiely J: The frequency of cerebral palsy. A review of population studies in industrialized nations since 1956. In Stanley F, Alberman E (eds): The Epidemiology of Cerebral Palsies. Clinics in Developmental Medicine Series, No. 87. Philadelphia, JB Lippincott, 1984.
187. Pape KE, Kirsch SE, Galil A, et al: Neuromuscular approach to the motor deficits of cerebral palsy: A pilot study. J Pediatr Orthop 1993; 13:628–633.
188. Papile L, Munsick-Bruno G, Schaefer A: Relationship of cerebral intraventricular hemorrhage and early childhood neurologic handicaps. J Pediatr 1983; 103:273–277.
189. Park TS, Vogler GP, Phillips LH II, et al: Effects of selective dorsal rhizotomy for spastic diplegia on hip migration in cerebral palsy. Pediatr Neurosurg 1994; 20:43–49.
190. Parker DF, Carriere L, Hebestreit H, et al: Muscle performance and gross motor function of children with spastic cerebral palsy. Dev Med Child Neurol 1993; 35:17–23.
191. Patrick J, Boland M, Stoski S, et al: Rapid correction of wasting in children with cerebral palsy. Dev Med Child Neurol 1986; 28:734–739.
192. Payne LZ, DeLuca PA: Heterotopic ossification after rhizotomy and femoral osteotomy. J Pediatr Orthop 1993; 13:733–738.
193. Peacock WJ, Arens LJ, Berman B: Cerebral palsy spasticity: Selective posterior rhizotomy. Pediatr Neurosci 1987; 13:61–66.
194. Peacock WJ, Arens LJ, Peter J: Selective posterior rhizotomy: A long term follow up study. Childs Nerv Syst 1989; 5:148–152.
195. Peacock WJ, Staudt LA: Spasticity in cerebral palsy and selective posterior rhizotomy procedure. J Child Neurol 1990; 5:179–185.
196. Penn RD, Savoy SM, Corcos D, et al: Intrathecal baclofen for severe spinal spasticity. N Engl J Med 1989; 320:1517–1521.
197. Perry J, Jones M, Thomas L: Functional evaluation of Rolfing in cerebral palsy. Dev Med Child Neurol 1981; 23:717–729.
198. Peterson H, Coventry M: Long term results of surgical treatment of adults with cerebral palsy. Dev Med Child Neurol 1969; 11:35–43.
199. Petitt B: Surgery of the lower extremity in cerebral palsy: Considerations and approaches. Arch Phys Med Rehabil 1976; 57:443–447.
200. Phelps W: The rehabilitation of cerebral palsy. South Med J 1994; 34:770–775.
201. Rang M, Douglas G, Bennet G, et al: Seating for children with cerebral palsy. J Pediatr Orthop 1981; 1:279–286.
202. Rang M, Wright J: What have 30 years of medical progress done for cerebral palsy? Adv Cereb Palsy 1989; 247:55–60.
203. Rattey TE, Leahey L, Hyndman J, et al: Recurrence after Achilles tendon lengthening in cerebral palsy. J Pediatr Orthop 1993; 13:184–187.
204. Reid CJ, Borzyskowski M: Lower urinary tract dysfunction in cerebral palsy. Arch Dis Child 1993; 68:739–742.
205. Reimers J: Acetabular development after femoral osteotomy in cerebral palsy after age four years. J Pediatr Orthop 1992; 1:35–37.
206. Rinsky LA: Surgery of spinal deformity in cerebral palsy: Twelve years in the evolution of scoliosis management. Clin Orthop 1990; 253:100–109.
207. Robinson R: The frequency of other handicaps in children with cerebral palsy. Dev Med Child Neurol 1973; 15:305–312.
208. Rodriquez J, Claus D, Verellen G, et al: Periventricular leukomalacia and neuropathological correlations. Dev Med Child Neurol 1990; 32:347–352.
209. Rogers B, Arvedson J, Buck G, et al: Characteristics of dysphagia in children with cerebral palsy. Dysphagia 1994; 9:60–73.
210. Rogers BT, Srvedson J, Msall M, et al: Hypoxemia during oral feeding of children with severe cerebral palsy. Dev Med Child Neurol 1993; 35:3–10.
211. Rood M: Neurophysiological mechanisms utilized in the treatment of neuromuscular dysfunction. Am J Occup Ther 1956; 10:220–224.
212. Rose J, Haskell WL, Gamble JG: A comparison of oxygen pulse and respiratory exchange ratio in cerebral palsied and nondisabled children. Arch Phys Med Rehabil 1993; 74:702–705.
213. Rothery S, Benz H, Hoffer M, et al: Goal oriented approach to the physical therapy management of cerebral palsy. Contemp Orthop 1982; 5:59–64.
214. Russell DJ, Rosenbaum PL, Cadman DT, et al: The gross motor function measure: A means to evaluate the effects of physical therapy. Dev Med Child Neurol 1989; 31:341–352.
215. Samilson RL, Becharard R: Scoliosis in cerebral palsy: Incidence, distribution of curve patterns, natural history and thoughts on etiology. Curr Pract Orthop Surg 1973; 5:43–50.

216. Samilson RL, Green WL: Long-term results of upper limb surgery in cerebral palsy. Reconstr Surg Traumatol 1972; 13:43–50.
217. Scherzer AL, Mike V, Iison J: Physical therapy as a determinant of change in the cerebral palsied infant. Pediatrics 1979; 58:47–52.
218. Scrutton D, Baird G: Hip dysplasia in cerebral palsy. Dev Med Child Neurol 1993; 35:1028–1030.
219. Shaari CM, Sanders I: Quantifying how location and dose of botulinum toxin injections affect muscle paralysis. Muscle Nerve 1993; 16:964–969.
220. Shane H: Impact of AAC on natural speech production. NIDDR 1992, pp 92–105.
221. Shapiro A, Susak Z, Malkin C, et al: Preoperative and postoperative gait evaluation in cerebral palsy. Arch Phys Med Rehabil 1990; 71:236–240.
222. Sherrill C, Hinson M, Gench B, et al: Self-concepts of disabled young athletes. Percept Mot Skills 1990; 70:1093–1098.
223. Sherrill C, Rainbolt W: Self-actualization profiles of male able-bodied and cerebral palsied athletes. Adapted Phys Activity Q 1988; 5:108–119.
224. Siegel L, Klingbeil M: Control of drooling with transdermal scopolamine in a child with cerebral palsy. Dev Med Child Neurol 1991; 33:1013–1014.
225. Silver L: Acceptable and controversial approaches to treating the child with learning disabilities. Pediatrics 1975; 55:406.
226. Sola A, Piecuch RE: Prevalence of cerebral palsy: Estimations, calculations and neonatal care. Pediatrics 1994; 93:152–153.
227. Staheli L, Chew D: Slotted acetabular augmentation in childhood and adolescence. J Pediatr Orthop 1992; 12:569–580.
228. Stallings VA, Charney EB, Davies JC, et al: Nutritional status and growth of children with diplegic or hemiplegic cerebral palsy. Dev Med Child Neurol 1993; 35:997–1006.
229. Stallings VA, Charney EB, Davies JC, et al: Nutrition-related growth failure of children with quadriplegic cerebral palsy. Dev Med Child Neurol 1993; 35:126–138.
230. Stanley FJ, Alberman E (eds): The Epidemiology of the Cerebral Palsies. Clinics in Developmental Medicine Series, No. 87, Philadelphia, JB Lippincott, 1984.
231. Stanley FJ, Blair E, Hockey A, et al: Spastic quadriplegia in western Australia: A genetic epidemiological study. Dev Med Child Neurol 1993; 35:191–201.
232. Stanley FJ, Watson L: The cerebral palsies in western Australia: Trends 1968–1981. Am J Obstet Gynecol 1988; 158:89–92.
233. Stern FM, Gorga D: Neurodevelopmental treatment (NDT): Therapeutic intervention and its efficacy. Infants Young Children 1988; 23–32.
234. Sweetsor PM, Badell A, Schneider S, et al: Effects of sacral dorsal rhizotomy on bladder function in patients with spastic cerebral palsy. Neurolurol Urodynamics 1995; 14:57–64.
235. Taylor SJ: Evaluating the client with physical disabilities for wheelchair seating. Am J Occup Ther 1987; 711–716.
236. Tenuta J, Shelton VA, Miller F: Long-term follow-up of triple arthrodesis in patients with cerebral palsy. J Pediatr Orthop 1993; 13:713–716.
237. Thometz JG, Tachdjian M: Long-term follow-up of the flexor carpi ulnaris transfer in spastic hemiplegic children. J Pediatr Orthop 1988; 8:407–412.
238. Tirosh E, Rabino S: Physiotherapy for children with cerebral palsy. Am J Dis Child 1989; 143:552–555.
239. Trejos H, Araya R: Sterotactic surgery for cerebral palsy. Stereotact Funct Neurosurg 1990; 54–55:130–135.
240. UCP Research and Educational Foundation: Exercise principles and guidelines for persons with cerebral palsy and neuromuscular disorders. Distributed by United Cerebral Palsy Associations, Washington, D.C. Copyright 1999.
241. Van-Heest AE, House J, Putman M: Sensibility deficiencies in the hands of children with spastic hemiplegia. J Hand Surg Am 1993; 18:278–281.
242. Vaughn CL, Berman B, Peacock WJ: Gait analysis and rhizotomy: Past experience and future considerations. Neurosurgery 1989; 4:445–458.
243. Vaughn CL, Berman B, Staudt LA, et al: Gait analysis of cerebral palsy before and after rhizotomy. Pediatr Neurosci 1988; 14:297–300.
244. Wadsworth JS, Harper DC: The social needs of adolescents with cerebral palsy. Dev Med Child Neurol 1993; 35:1019–1022.
245. Watt J, Sims D, Harckham F, et al: A prospective study of inhibitive casting as an adjunct to physiotherapy for cerebral palsied children. Dev Med Child Neurol 1986; 28:480–488.
246. Waylett J, Barber L: Upper extremity bracing of the severely athetoid mental retardate. Am J Occup Ther 1971; 25:402–407.
247. Whyte HE, Fitzhardinge PM, Shennan AT, et al: Extreme immaturity: Outcome of 568 pregnancies of 23–26 weeks gestation. Obstet Gynec 1993; 82:1–7.
248. Winch R, Bengtson L, McLaughlin J, et al: Women with cerebral palsy: Obstetric experience and neonatal outcome. Dev Med Child Neurol 1993; 35:974–982.
249. Wright T, Nicholson J: Physiotherapy for the spastic child—An evaluation. Dev Med Child Neurol 1973; 15:146–163.
250. Yokochii K, Shimabukuro S, Kodama M, et al: Motor function of infants with athetoid cerebral palsy. Dev Med Child Neurol 1993; 35:54–60.
251. Zimbler S, Craig C, Harris J, et al: Orthotic management of severe scoliosis in spastic neuromuscular disease—Results of treatment. Orthop Trans 1985; 9:78–92.

54

CHAPTER

Ross M. Hays, M.D., and Teresa L. Massagli, M.D.

Rehabilitation Concepts in Myelomeningocele

More children in the United States are affected by myelomeningocele than by poliomyelitis, traumatic spinal cord injury, or muscular dystrophy. Physicians who care for these patients must appreciate the subtleties of a congenital defect that presents at birth, yet has signs and symptoms that change with time and with the development of the growing child. The clinical manifestations of the disorder include multiple organ systems in complicated and interdependent relationships. Many of the physical aspects of the disease produce both medical and psychological problems. Effective management requires a team of specialists cooperating with the child, family, and one another to deliver competent effective care. As the first large group of aggressively treated neonates is now entering middle age, an entirely new population—aging persons with myelomeningocele—is presenting clinical challenges that were previously unanticipated.

HISTORICAL BACKGROUND

Excavations in Morocco have disclosed spinal defects in bone remnants that are 10,000 to 12,000 years old.[21] Skeletons with lumbosacral defects have been found among Modoc Indian burial grounds in Arizona, and similar findings in skeletons from Roman Britain, where 7.3% were found to have openings in the spinal canal, provide a crude suggestion of the incidence of the disorder in ancient times.[70] Hippocrates described patients with myelomeningocele. Aristotle proposed to resolve with infanticide the burden that these children placed on society. Nicholas Tulpius wrote the first scientific description of the defect in Holland in 1652 and used the term *spina bifida.* In the 1860s both Lamarck and Darwin commented on the possibility of environmental influences in the etiology of the disease.[6] The advances in surgical technology leading to effective neonatal back closure in the 1940s and the invention of the one-way shunt valve by Holter, Nulsen, and Spitz in 1952 effectively reversed the survival curves from 10% survival in 1956 to 10% mortality in 1985. Lorber's proposed scheme for nontreatment of affected infants in Great Britain in 1971 and the subsequent "Baby Doe" legislation in the United States were watershed events in the application of modern bioethics to pediatric patients. The treatment of children with myelomeningocele continues to evolve and to reflect the changing face of medicine.

DEFINITIONS

Myelomeningocele (MMC) is the term used to describe the failure of fusion of the neural folds during the neurulation phase of embryologic development. It is also used interchangeably with *meningomyelocele* to describe both the embryologic defect of bone, meninges, and spinal cord, as well as the collection of clinical derangements—lower extremity paralysis, sensory loss, and neurogenic bowel and bladder—that results from damage to neuronal tissue in the open neural tube.

Meningocele describes a hernia of the meningeal membranes with little or no dysgenesis of the underlying nervous system. Most meningoceles contain all the neural elements within the neural canal, are skin-covered, and produce little paralysis.

Lipomeningomyeloceles, lipomeningoceles, and *lipomyeloceles* are lipomas that occur within the neural canal as a result of abnormal epidermal and mesodermal development. They most commonly accompany some degree of meningocele formation and interfere with neural function by increasing pressure on the lower spinal cord, either by adhesion or by growth.

Diastematomyelia is a splitting of the lower spinal cord in association with mesodermal elements, bone or cartilage spurs, and fibrous bands. It may occur alone or in association with meningomyelocele.

Myelocystocele describes a cystic defect that communicates with the central canal of the spinal cord. Myelocystoceles vary in size and may be either dorsal or ventral. They produce neurological symptoms by exerting pressure on the spinal cord during growth.

Spina bifida denotes the bony defect resulting from failure of mesodermal closure around the neural canal. Meningomyelocele and meningocele are examples of *spina bifida aperta. Spina bifida occulta* is a defect of the posterior bony element only with no involvement of the underlying meningeal or neural elements. Spina bifida occulta is not uncommon in the general public and is usually asymptomatic.

EPIDEMIOLOGY

Incidence

Both geographical and racial variations in the incidence of MMC have historically been reported. Rates in Ireland and Wales have been three to four times greater than the worldwide incidence of 1 case per 1000 live births. In Japan and several eastern European countries, rates have been much lower. In the United States, a gradient of decreasing rates from East Coast to West Coast was noted.[24]

Over the last 30 years, a decline in incidence has been reported in Great Britain and the United States.[64] This decrease cannot be entirely accounted for by prenatal diagnosis and termination of affected pregnancies and is suggestive of an important role for environmental factors.[61] From 1970 to 1989, the incidence of neural tube defects dropped from 1.3 to 0.6 per 1000 live births. About two-thirds of the neural tube defects are MMC cases, translating into about 2000 affected infants born each year in the United States.[86]

Etiology

Myelomeningocele occurs as a result of incomplete closure of the neural tube during fetal development. Morphological studies of embryonic development have shown that closure of the caudal neuropore normally occurs between 26 and 30 days after fertilization.[55] Any suspected cause of spina bifida must act prior to this time. One of the challenges to both determining cause and implementing prevention strategies is the fact that malformation occurs soon after conception, often before women are aware they are pregnant.

Genetics. Neural tube defects are believed to be multifactorial in origin. The multifactorial model implies (1) that the risk of a trait or disease is greater in relatives of affected persons than in members of the general population; (2) that the incidence of disease is higher in close relatives (who have more genes in common) than in distant relatives; and (3) that the risk to relatives increases with the number of affected relatives in the pedigree.[4]

Multifactorial diseases are influenced by genetic and environmental factors. However, the relative roles of each in MMC have not been settled. Open neural tube defects have occurred in multiple births and in infants with chromosomal disorders such as trisomy 13, but most occur as isolated defects, not associated with other malformations. There is a slight sex preference with a female to male ratio of 1.3 : 1.[10] Low sacral lesions are more common among males while thoracic lesions are more common among females.[64] MMC occurs in higher frequencies among relatives of children with MMC than in the general population. The recurrence rate appears to be related to the incidence of neural tube defects in the regional population. The recurrence risk in British Columbia and the United States for a second affected child is 2.4% to 3.0%, but in Ireland and Wales it is 5.0%.[15] Risks for a third affected child are approximately twice these. In children of maternal sisters, a frequency of 1% has been reported, and there is a similar risk for an affected child when one of the parents has a neural tube defect. Consanguinity between parents also increases the risk, and the high cousin marriage rate in Britain has been proposed as one of the contributors to the higher incidence there.[33]

The increased incidence of MMC in families, certain ethnic groups, and in cases of parental consanguinity suggests a strong role for inheritance, but the recurrence rates in siblings are not consistent with recessive, dominant, or cytoplasmic inheritance. It has been suggested that MMC and other neural tube defects arise from the interaction of many genes (polygenic inheritance), which may create a threshold whereby a fetus exposed at a certain time to certain environmental triggers becomes at risk for malformation.[10]

Environmental Factors. The observations of an increased incidence of MMC among people of low socioeconomic status and among children conceived in spring months has lent weight to theories of environmental contributors to etiology. Nutrition, drugs, and heat have been proposed as causes. The use of valproic acid during pregnancy is associated with the prevalence of MMC of 2.5% to 6.3%.[54]

Heat exposure has long been suspected of being a teratogen in humans, and strong associations between maternal heat exposure during early pregnancy and neural tube defects have been reported. Taking hot baths, having a febrile illness, or the use of hot tubs or saunas during the first trimester have been associated with twice the risk of fetal neural tube defects compared to women without such exposures.[48, 63] The amount of heat exposure necessary for teratogenicity in humans is unknown, as is the mechanism of action in preventing closure of the neural tube.

Folic acid supplementation is an important primary preventive measure against MMC. The evidence for folic acid supplementation to prevent tube defects has been steadily accumulating since the early 1980s. Folic acid supplementation was first shown to reduce the risk of recurrence in high-risk families.[33] These results were replicated using large doses of folate (4 mg/day), but were not found with general multivitamin supplementation without folate.[49] Only 5% of cases of neural tube defects represent recurrences, so further research examined whether or not vitamin supplementation could prevent first occurrences. Using smaller doses of folic acid (0.8 mg/day) in combination with multivitamins, researchers noted a very convincing reduction in the incidence of first occurrence of neural tube defects.[17] Based on these findings, the U.S. Public Health Service recommended that all women of childbearing age who are capable of becoming pregnant should consume 0.4 mg of folic acid per day to reduce their risk of having a pregnancy affected with MMC or other neural tube defects. Women who have had an affected child should consider periconceptional consumption of 4 mg of folate per day.[59] The mechanism of action of folate in preventing MMC is unknown.

MANAGEMENT

Early Management

Prenatal Management

Prenatal screening techniques have made it possible to identify the majority of cases of MMC. This information can be used to plan for termination of pregnancy, if parents so choose, or to enhance perinatal management if carried to term. Prenatal diagnosis begins with measurement of maternal serum alpha-fetoprotein (AFP) at 16 to 18 weeks after conception.

The presence of an open neural tube defect allows AFP and acetylcholinesterase to escape from the fetus into amniotic fluid. Peak levels of amniotic fluid AFP occur between the 13th and 15th postconception weeks and can be detected in maternal serum. Maternal serum levels rise at 15 weeks after conception and peak between 25 and 29 weeks. Elevated serum levels are confirmed by repeat studies. If still elevated, ultrasound (US) screening is performed.

High-resolution US can reveal the presence of MMC by 14 to 16 weeks of gestation. Because of advances in US technology and the skills of ultrasonographers, scanning alone may be sufficient to diagnose a neural tube defect.[64] The diagnosis should be confirmed by amniocentesis to measure the amount of AFP and acetylcholinesterase in amniotic fluid. Although elevated levels of AFP are seen in a number of conditions (e.g., anterior abdominal wall defects, fetal demise), isoenzymes of acetylcholinesterase are seen only in open neural tube defects and are independent of the length of gestation. Amniocentesis is best performed between 15 and 18 weeks after conception; earlier can be hazardous to the fetus, while later the AFP levels become more difficult to interpret and the opportunity for termination diminishes.[33]

There is marked regional variation in the acceptance of prenatal diagnosis and of pregnancy termination. In Australia, there has been no change in the total prevalence of neural tube defects from the mid-1960s to the early 1990s, but the number of terminations of pregnancy increased as a result of implementation of prenatal diagnosis programs, and the prevalence of live births of infants with neural tube defects dropped by 83%, from 2.01 to 0.35 per 1000 live births.[12] In contrast, only 50% of parents in Ireland elect termination of pregnancy after the diagnosis of a neural tube defect.[25]

Prenatal detection of MMC is important even for families who would not choose to terminate the pregnancy because it enhances perinatal management. Families have time to learn about the diagnosis and prepare for a safe delivery. High-resolution US can accurately predict functional motor outcome.[14] Infants with neural tube defects should be delivered in the medical center where surgical closure will occur, to minimize trauma to or infection of the sac during transportation. It has also been suggested that infants with MMC be delivered by cesarean section to avoid injury to the sac and contents. One group of researchers reported less severe lower extremity paralysis in infants born by cesarean section before the onset of labor than in infants delivered vaginally or by cesarean section after the onset of labor.[41] Levels of paralysis were no different in the infants exposed to labor, regardless of the method of delivery. Prenatal diagnosis allows physicians to plan for elective caesarean section prior to labor, when the fetus has achieved pulmonary maturation.

Neonatal Management

Back Defect. The first priority of medical treatment for the newborn with MMC is management of the open neural tube defect (Fig. 54–1). The treatment is a continuous sequence that includes delivery of the infant, protection of the back, closure of the defect, and stabilization of cerebrospinal fluid (CSF) flow. There are three goals in the management of the back defect: (1) to reduce the risk of infection, (2) to preserve existing neurological function, and (3) to decrease the deformity if severe kyphoscoliosis is present. Most centers advocate closure within the first hours after delivery. The risk of central nervous system (CNS) infection in lesions closed before 48 hours averages 7%; the infection risk for later closure rises to an average of 37%. The back defect must be carefully protected to prevent contamination or further damage due to trauma or desiccation. The surface of the lesion and CSF are cultured and the infant is treated with antibiotics at dosages sufficient to treat meningitis. Back closure is performed in three stages: (1) the neural plaque is returned to the canal and a watertight closure of dura and arachnoid is constructed; (2) the reformulated neural tube is then protected by myofascial closure; and (3) the skin is then closed with a tension closure.

Back repair may produce alterations in the CSF fluid dynamics by closing the open conduit at the caudal end of the central canal. In some cases, fluid pressures spontaneously readjust after closure. In others, hydrocephalus becomes more rapidly apparent. Kyphectomy to treat severe kyphoscoliosis in the newborn is difficult and often complicated by poor bone growth, high blood loss, and intraoperative mortality. Minimal osteotomy repair is a compromise that provides less immediate correction but is better tolerated by the infant.[71]

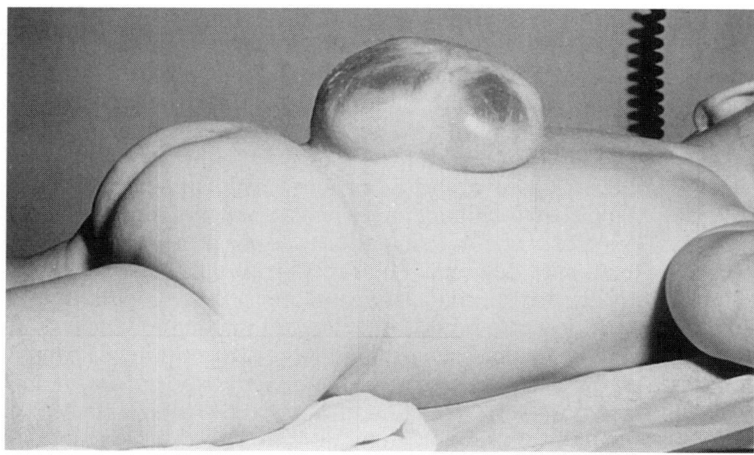

FIGURE 54–1. Typical appearance of a child with myelomeningocele lesion prior to surgical closure.

Hydrocephalus. Ninety percent of children with myelomeningocele will develop clinically significant hydrocephalus.[77] Some children have true aqueductal stenosis and others have communicating hydrocephalus that worsens after back closure. Nearly all children with MMC have displacement of the cerebellum caudally with elongation and kinking of the fourth ventricle and medulla. These combined defects are known as the Arnold-Chiari II malformation.[9] Recently, the term *constrictive hydrocephalus*[58] has been used to describe the relationship between Arnold-Chiari II malformation and the restricted flow of CSF that causes hydrocephalus in the majority of children with MMC.

Hydrocephalus is often present at birth or discovered prenatally on US. It usually does not progress immediately and may show no evidence of additional ventricular enlargement until 3 to 7 days of age. The onset of hydrocephalus in some patients does not require treatment for months or even years. Progressive hydrocephalus in the newborn manifests as increasing head size; older children with delayed-onset hydrocephalus develop signs and symptoms of increased intracranial pressure—vomiting, headache, somnolence, or irritability. Insidious onset of hydrocephalus may appear as lethargy, personality alterations, or subtle changes in intellectual performance.

Ventriculoperitoneal (VP) shunting is the treatment of choice for hydrocephalus. Technical advances have improved the results of hydrocephalus management from good results (better survival and intellectual performance) for 40% of patients in the 1950s to excellent results in over 90% of patients in the 1980s.[72] Half of all infants with shunts require replacement within the first year of life.[77] The likelihood of shunt failure and the need for shunt replacement decreases with each subsequent year.

Early Bladder Management. The status of the neurogenic bladder in the newborn period can be evaluated by physical examination. Babies with large distended bladders on abdominal examination are likely to have dyssynergia of the sphincter. A nonpalpable bladder and constant dribbling suggest weak or nonexistent sphincter tone. Abdominal US can detect the presence of a distended, poorly emptying bladder, hydronephrosis, or, more rarely, renal agenesis. US should be repeated after back closure to rule out any possibility of urinary tract obstruction resulting from damage to the spinal cord.

Postvoid residual urine volumes should be checked by US. A postvoid residual of 20 mL or greater in the newborn period indicates clinically significant urinary retention and requires intermittent catheterization, treatment with phenoxybenzamine, or both. Blood urea nitrogen (BUN) and creatinine levels must be monitored and routine urine cultures obtained during the first month of life. The first voiding cystourethrogram may be safely deferred until 6 months of age if all other tests suggest that bladder emptying is reasonable and the urine is infection-free.[30]

Assessment of Neurological Level. The actual pattern of voluntary motor innervation, that is, the motor level, is of some importance in predicting ambulation and intellectual potential, but it does not correlate well with the level of vertebral abnormality on radiographs, the anatomical site of the skin lesion, or the level of abnormality on sensory examination.[70] The best method of motor examination is careful inspection for muscle bulk and stimulation with postural challenges and gentle opposition of major muscle groups to elicit voluntary activity. The presence of considerable muscle bulk detected on palpation without any observed voluntary movement may indicate temporary spinal cord shock after delivery or back closure. In 37% of MMC newborns, motor strength improves within a week after delivery. Joint movement, especially hip and knee flexion in response to painful stimuli, may result from reflex-mediated activity below the level of the lesion rather than true voluntary control.

Therapy. Experienced therapists working with neonates can provide detailed motor examinations before and after back closure. They can also assist with positioning and handling of the newborn and provide anticipatory guidance for the parents in the transition of care from hospital to home. Children born with contractures of hips and knees benefit from a range-of-motion exercise program developed by the therapists and then implemented by the family. Babies with higher-level lesions may require custom-fabricated seating and support devices that protect the surgical site and assist with trunk and head control.

Family Counseling. The need for parents to be completely and accurately informed about all aspects of their infant's care, medical needs, and future potential cannot be overemphasized, nor can it be accurately delineated in this brief overview. Families are entitled to clinical opinions based on the most recent medical literature, regardless of their perceived ability to comprehend such a large body of technical material. Families who are overinformed and therefore given the opportunity to choose when and how much information to absorb maintain more control over their child's medical management. This attempt to respect a parent's autonomy in the midst of a catastrophic situation is aided by careful, competent repetition of information and the provision of detailed, accurate written material. The most successful centers have one physician and one nurse who act as the primary support for each family and child. Good communication among primary care physician, nurses, specialists, and the parents is the best assurance of achieving the desired medical outcome.

Long-Term Management

The Central Nervous System

Shunts. Approximately 90% of children with MMC need a VP shunt placed to manage hydrocephalus.[77] The two most common late complications associated with shunts are obstructions and infections. Of these, infections have the greater morbidity. The overall risk of shunt infection is 12% per child. The most common infections are caused by *Staphylococcus epidermidis* and are associated with the surgical insertion of the shunt. Each shunt placement or revision carries a 5% risk for infection. Delayed symptoms presenting 6 weeks after surgery with culture-proven *S. epidermidis* likely represent indolent, late postoperative infections.[71]

Children with hydrocephalus and shunts are at greater risk for epidemic meningitis caused by β-hemolytic streptococcus, meningococcus, pneumococcus, and, less often, *Hemophilus influenzae.* The other common source of infection is erosion of the VP shunt into intra-abdominal organs and resulting contamination with gram-negative organisms.[71]

Infections in the shunt downstream from the CNS are the least serious and the most easily treated. Low-grade ventriculitis is often associated with shunt obstruction; shunt infection with ventriculomeningitis carries the most severe morbidity. The relationship between shunt infection, CNS infection, and intellectual functioning in children with MMC is controversial,[77] several studies suggest, however, that a reduction in cognitive function is associated with the frequency and severity of infections.[47, 66]

Fifty percent of children with VP shunts experience obstruction and need shunt revision in the first year of life. Of those children whose shunts obstruct during the first 12 months, 31% need shunt replacement in the second year, and risk recurrence at a rate of 12% per year thereafter. In children who do not need shunt revision during the first year of life, the risk of obstruction is only 8% per year.

Complications of Arnold-Chiari II Malformation. Nearly all children with MMC have Arnold-Chiari II malformation of the hindbrain. The majority are asymptomatic. For those who do develop problems, the more severe symptoms—stridor, aspiration, periodic breathing with sleep, and central apnea—are grouped under the collective term *central ventilatory dysfunction* (CVD). This severe complication of Arnold-Chiari II malformation has been reported in 7% to 30% of children.[26] The most severe manifestations of CVD are upper airway obstruction due to vocal cord abductor paralysis (30%), vocal cord abductor paralysis with other cranial nerve involvement (17%), and central apnea (22%). The exact mechanism of action is probably a result of several factors, including traction on upper cervical nerves due to downward displacement of the medulla, brainstem compression with the abnormally located hindbrain, and increased intracranial pressure resulting from hydrocephalus.

The mainstays of treatment are management of increased intracranial pressure, treatment of CNS infection, and vigorous airway management. Decompression laminectomies to reduce local pressure on the brainstem have been helpful in some but not all cases. Placement or revision of CSF shunts to reduce intracranial pressure may provide improvement in some. The most effective treatment, regardless of underlying etiology, is aggressive attention to the airway obstruction and apnea.

CVD is not associated with the level of lesion, severity of hydrocephalus, or the presence of CNS bleeding and infection. Children with CVD who survive because of aggressive ventilatory support often experience remission of symptoms by 30 months of age. At the present time, the life-threatening consequences of CVD are the single most common cause of death in children with MMC.[26]

Hydromyelia. Hydromyelia or dilation of the central canal is analogous to the dilation of the ventricles in hydrocephalus and occurs in 50% to 80% of children with MMC. The most common symptoms are rapidly progressive scoliosis, weakness of the upper extremities, spasticity, and ascending motor strength changes in the lower extremities. Hydromyelia is best demonstrated by magnetic resonance imaging (MRI) of the brain and spinal cord. When symptoms warrant treatment, decompressing subclinical hydrocephalus may be effective. In more aggressive cases, decompressive laminectomy, plugging of the obex, and direct shunting of the hydromyelia may be required.

Tethered Cord Syndrome. *Tethered cord syndrome* refers to progressive neurological deficits resulting from traction of the conus medullaris and the cauda equina. It has been reported in 11% to 15% of children after myelomeningocele repair. The pathophysiology is related to decreased metabolism of nerve tissue in response to traction and deformation. The diagnosis is based on progressive symptoms, not the radiographic finding of a low-lying conus. Routine MRI studies have demonstrated that 80% to 90% of MMC patients have an abnormally low conus medullaris, most of whom never develop clinical symptoms.[29, 79]

Surgical release often halts the progression of symptoms but may not restore lost function. It is important to recognize the clinical presentation of tethered cord and consider surgery as early as possible to preserve function. The average age at diagnosis is 6 years.[27] Children with higher lesion levels, a shorter cord, and less tolerance for stretching may present as young as 4 years of age. Children with lower level lesions may not develop symptoms until after age 9.[56]

The most common symptom of tethered cord is change in motor strength (62%), followed by recent onset of spasticity (56%) and changes in mobility (43%). Back pain is reported in 37%, and 25% of patients report a recent change in bowel and bladder function or recent onset of scoliosis.[27] Because the diagnosis of tethered cord syndrome is clinical rather than radiographic and the symptoms described are either superimposed on or amplifications of existing pathological conditions, prospective screening with a high level of suspicion is required to diagnose the syndrome in children with MMC.

Neurologically stable children with MMC have been found to have a wide range of abnormalities on MRI, including low-lying cord, cavities within the cord, lipomeningoceles, diastematomyelia, and atrophy of the cord.[44]

Urological System

Patterns of Involvement. Unlike after traumatic spinal cord injury, the types of neurogenic bladder seen in children with MMC are not correlated with the lesion level. More than 80% have partial or complete denervation of the bladder with poor compliance and poor contractility, producing residual urine volumes. In 86%, the internal sphincter is incompetent, so that incontinence occurs when intravesical pressure exceeds urethral resistance. The external sphincter is usually at least partially functional, and in about one-third of patients detrusor-sphincter dyssynergia causes abnormally high intraluminal pressures.[45] Bladder function may change after birth or in a growing child experiencing tethered cord syndrome. Most changes occur in the first year after birth, and either deterioration or improvement in external sphincter function may be seen.[76] For these reasons, early assessment of bladder and kidney function followed by reassessment at least annually is necessary.

Preventing Renal Involvement. The goals of management of neurogenic bladder are prevention of urinary tract damage and achievement of continence. Urodynamic examination of intravesical and bladder neck pressures is a routine evaluation in newborn infants with MMC. About 75% of infants have normal upper tracts, while the rest have hydronephrosis due to such problems as vesicoureteral reflux (VUR), detrusor-sphincter dyssynergia, an enlarged bladder, or a structural abnormality. Infants with normal upper tracts and satisfactory bladder emptying are monitored twice a year by renal US during early childhood. If the bladder does not empty efficiently and there is no outlet resistance or reflux, parents can be taught the Credé maneuver to improve emptying. If detrusor-sphincter dyssynergia is present, there is a significant risk for development of hydronephrosis, and such infants are managed with anticholinergic medications and clean intermittent catheterization. The same management is used for infants who already have hydronephrosis. If clean intermittent catheterization fails to relieve hydronephrosis, a cutaneous vesicostomy can be done. It can be reversed after ureteral reimplantation or bladder augmentation when the child is old enough to perform clean intermittent catheterization.[46, 65]

If the child has VUR, prophylactic antibiotics are prescribed because VUR of infected urine can cause upper tract damage or even renal failure. Risk factors for upper tract damage and VUR include detrusor-sphincter dyssynergia, decreased bladder compliance, and elevated leak pressures. VUR is seen when detrusor pressure exceeds 40 cm H_2O before leakage of urine occurs.[46] If the child develops persistent febrile urinary tract infections or if hydronephrosis does not improve, antireflux surgery is indicated and includes options such as vesicostomy, reimplantation of ureters, or bladder augmentation.

One of the first surgical approaches to prevent upper tract injury was urinary diversion into an ileal conduit. This was often done prophylactically to prevent hydronephrosis. Follow-up studies have shown a disappointing frequency of complications, including renal deterioration, pyelonephritis, and stone disease. Many such patients have subsequently had reversal of the diversion.

Periodic monitoring of the upper urinary tract is essential. Renal US every 6 months for the first few years of childhood is common practice. If reflux is present, the child may periodically need an excretory urogram and voiding cystourethrogram. Urodynamic surveillance is also indicated because changes in the bladder do occur, most often in the first year of life or in later childhood, associated with tethered cord syndrome.[76] Asymptomatic bacteriuria is prevalent in children with MMC. Urine culture screening is indicated for those with VUR or when signs or symptoms of urinary tract infection occur. Prophylactic antibiotics have not been found to reduce the occurrence of clinical urinary tract infection.[82]

Continence. Less than 10% of children with MMC have normal urinary control.[34] Knowledge of bladder capacity and sphincter function is vital when considering options for management. For boys with reflex emptying, external collection devices may be feasible if they do not have VUR or large residual urine volumes. Applying condom catheters can be problematic in boys with a small penis, and requires careful attention to skin integrity when sensation is impaired.

There are no effective external collection devices for girls (excluding diapers). Girls and boys with incomplete emptying rely on clean intermittent catheterization and sometimes medications. Due to the high prevalence of small bladder capacity and low outlet resistance, only about one-fourth of children can become continent with clean intermittent catheterization alone.[81] Even adding anticholinergic medications (oxybutinin, propantheline) to inhibit contractions, alpha-adrenergic medications (ephedrine, phenylpropanolamine) to increase outlet resistance, and antibiotic instillations to reduce infection-induced bladder spasms achieved complete continence only in 49% of children in one study.[85] Long-term compliance may be a problem for such complicated regimens in this population. To maintain daily continence, such children need to empty their bladders very frequently, often at intervals of less than every 4 hours, and the entire daily bladder management can require more than 1.5 hours per day.[34]

Surgery may be considered for children who fail to become continent using medications and clean intermittent catheterization. The options depend on bladder size, sphincter competence, and the ability of the patient to perform clean intermittent catheterization. Augmentation of the size of the bladder may be necessary for the child with a small or noncompliant bladder and can be done in conjunction with an artificial sphincter if the outlet resistance is low. Ileum, sigmoid colon, and stomach have all been used for augmentation. Mucous production, urolithiasis, metabolic acidosis, and hypocalcemia can ensue after ileum or sigmoid patches, and gastrocystoplasty may be complicated by hematuria, dysuria, metabolic alkalosis, and hypokalemia. The most serious complication is spontaneous rupture, which may occur if the bladder becomes overdistended. Another long-term complication is development of a tumor in the bowel side of the cystoplasty. This risk may be associated with the chronic exposure of the bowel segment to urinary stasis, infection, or urinary *n*-nitrosamines.[65]

For those with low outlet resistance, implantation of an artificial urethral sphincter may be considered. The sphincter is placed around the bladder neck, and the procedure is commonly done in conjunction with bladder augmentation. About half of patients need to use clean intermittent catheterization after sphincter implantation, and overall success for long-term continence is over 60%.[5]

If the patient has difficulty performing urethral clean intermittent catheterization because of kyphoscoliosis, impaired fine motor skills, difficulty with hip abduction, or poor transfer skills, continent diversion is another option. The appendix can be used as a conduit to the bladder to create an abdominal stoma, which is easier for the patient to access.[65]

Development and Bladder Management. The accomplishment of independent toileting by children with MMC is delayed more than any other self-care task, even in those with normal intelligence. While most children with normal bladder and bowel function achieve independent control by 4 years of age, children with MMC may not accomplish this until 10 to 15 years of age.[53] The cause of this delay in developmental achievement is multifactorial, with likely contributors being level of paralysis, intelligence quotient (IQ), visual-spatial imperceptions, kyphoscoliosis, obesity, degree of parental support, degree of sensation, sphincter control, and bladder capacity.

Parents need to be trained not only in carrying out the child's bladder or bowel program but also in preparing the child to accept responsibility for these tasks once the child is physically and mentally capable.[75] Children can learn to catheterize themselves using clean technique as early as age 5 years, but will need help for many years to remind them to perform the task and to assist with cleaning the equipment. Unfortunately, as many as 30% of teenagers with MMC still need assistance from a caregiver for bladder management.[34]

Allergy to Latex. Children with MMC have recently been found to have high frequencies of allergy to latex products. This IgE-mediated allergic response can manifest as contact dermatitis, allergic rhinitis, asthma, angioedema, or intraoperative anaphylaxis.[73,78] Patients may encounter latex in such products as rubber balloons, rubber gloves, condoms, or ostomy bags. The allergens are thought to be small water-soluble antigens that can be eluted from the surface of latex products, transferred by direct contact with skin or mucous membranes or carried airborne by powder emitted from the latex product, and incompletely eliminated by washing the product.[83]

The most serious allergic manifestation, intraoperative anaphylaxis, has often occurred in patients who have safely undergone previous surgical procedures. It is thought that chronic exposure to rubber via catheters or gloves is the cause of the allergy. Patients with MMC who require surgery should be protected by a latex-free environment, regardless of latex reactivity.[80] Patients who exhibit allergic symptoms may need to avoid the use of latex products such as rubber gloves, rubber catheters, or latex condoms. Many clinics advocate nonlatex catheters for all MMC children.

Neurogenic Bowel

Description of Patterns. The key anatomical areas affecting fecal continence in children with MMC are the large intestine, rectum, and internal and external sphincters. The peristaltic movements of the large intestine differ from those of the small intestine in that they are not continuous but rather occur in mass movements several times a day. Fairly predictable mass movements occur in association with filling of the stomach and duodenum. This gastrocolic reflex is often strongest after the first meal each day. The rectum functions as a reservoir and is prevented from continuous emptying by the tone of the internal sphincter. When the rectum is full, reflex relaxation of the internal sphincter occurs. The external anal sphincter has both voluntary and reflex control and activates only when a bolus is present. It must relax to permit defecation.[84] Sacral parasympathetic and thoracolumbar sympathetic fibers innervate the lower colon, rectum, and sphincters, and the external anal sphincter has somatic innervation as well.

About 20% of children with MMC have normal bowel control.[34] Bowel continence may be compromised by impaired rectal sensation, impaired sphincter function, or altered colonic motility. Children with MMC may experience relative intestinal stasis due to loss of sacral parasympathetic input. It is not known whether the gastrocolic reflex is intact in patients with neurogenic bowel. If the external sphincter is partially or wholly denervated, incontinence results when the pressure in the rectum is high enough to produce reflex relaxation of the internal sphincter. In patients with MMC above L3, the tonic pressure of the internal sphincter is low, possibly due to loss of sympathetic input. Rectal sensation is also related to lesion level and is usually absent in those with lesions above L3 and more likely present, though often abnormal, with lower lesions.[1] It is important to know whether the child has any spasticity or voluntary control over the external anal sphincter, but the presence or absence of the anocutaneous reflex has not been shown to correlate with internal sphincter tone.[1] Although sphincter status can be determined with anorectal manometry, it is not clear that such knowledge alters the management plan. However, the presence of either a bulbocavernosus or anocutaneous reflex is associated with a greater likelihood of achieving continence.[31]

Management Strategies. To achieve bowel continence, the child with MMC needs efficient, regular, and predictable emptying of soft stool. The goal is to empty the rectum before it becomes full enough to stimulate reflex relaxation of the internal sphincter. If the child lacks rectal sensation, the emptying should be done according to a regular schedule. While clinicians often recommend that patients perform bowel programs after meals, to take advantage of the gastrocolic reflex, it is not known if this reflex is present in children with MMC, and owing to the length of time needed to complete the bowel program, this may not be convenient in the patient's or family's schedule.[18] Classic bowel programs often utilize stool softeners or bulking agents, but families often prefer dietary manipulations instead of medications and find that such programs are too time-consuming, often taking more than 30 minutes to complete.[18] Suppositories, digital anorectal stimulation, manual removal of stool, dolusate or glycerine mini-enemas, saline enemas, and use of biofeedback if the child has adequate rectal sensation are potentially useful; none is universally successful.

Surgical diversion may be helpful to children who suffer from intractable incontinence. One option is an antegrade continence enema procedure. In this procedure, the appendix is brought out to the skin to serve as a channel to the bowel. A catheter can be inserted into the cecum to deliver enema solution. Saline or tap water in the amount of 500 mL to 4 liters is used. Most children empty their colon in 15 to 45 minutes. Those who take longer may need pressure relief. Colostomy is another option when standard treatment or the antegrade continence enema procedure has failed.

Social Implications. It is important for parents to establish an effective program of bowel continence at an early developmental stage, usually around 3 years of age. Many children enter preschool or kindergarten shortly thereafter and can be subject to severe peer criticism if "accidents" occur. The child also needs to be encouraged to assume increasing responsibility for performing the bowel program. Clinicians can facilitate this learning experience for the child by keeping the program simple and as short as possible, so the child grasps cause and effect.

Unfortunately, substantial numbers of children with MMC do not attain the goal of independently managing bowel continence. In one study, up to 86% of teenagers 13 to 18 years old needed assistance from a caregiver for their bowel program.[34] As with bladder management, the reasons for this are not entirely clear, but probable contributors are physical limitations due to obesity or scoliosis, inconsistent parental expectations, and the fact that denervation of the external rectal sphincter makes continence more challenging than in upper motor neuron neurogenic bowel disorders. Children who are fearful of bowel accidents will try to avoid incontinence by staying constipated, but this strategy inevitably results in impaired bowel emptying.

Parents perceive urinary and fecal incontinence as more stressful than impaired motor function in their children with MMC,[34] and health care professionals must be persistent in their efforts to help these children achieve continence.

Musculoskeletal Complications

Motor Innervation. It is important to appreciate that the level of neurological lesion does not match the radiographic vertebral level in most cases. One percent of infants will have defects at the cervical levels and another 1% at the upper thoracic vertebral levels. Six percent of patients present with defects at the lower thoracic and upper lumbar vertebral levels. More than a fourth (27%) have mid-lumbar-level and 42% have lumbosacral-level vertebral lesions. One-fifth (21%) present with sacral-level involvement, and 2% will have large lesions encompassing the entire lumbosacral spine.

When patients are categorized by neurological impairment, 1% have severe lesions with cervical and upper thoracic impairment. Twenty-seven percent have lower thoracic level lesions with paralysis of the psoas and more distally innervated muscles. Almost one-fourth (23%) present with intact hip flexion but impaired quadriceps. Nearly half (45%) of all MMC children fall into the lower lumbar group where quadriceps are spared but lower segments are not. Only 4% present with lower sacral level paralysis with intact lower extremity strength and some degree of bowel and bladder dysfunction.

It is tempting to regard these lesion levels as a simple dichotomy, with normal voluntary motor control above the level of the lesion and flaccid paralysis below. Only one-third of children actually demonstrate flaccid paralysis. The majority of patients exhibit a variety of abnormal motor abnormalities, including incomplete flaccid paraplegia, spasticity, mixed paraplegia and spasticity, asymmetry of involvement on either side, intact regions of voluntary control below the other segments of paralysis, and combinations of these impairments within the individual.

The level of neurological impairment influences the types of musculoskeletal deformities and complications. Regardless of the characteristics of the motor disability, essentially half of all children have defects that include the L5 or S1 and lower levels and 92% have lesions at or below L2. This general pattern suggests that hip flexors and adductors are less often affected than hip extensors and abductors. The common finding of hip flexion contractures supports this theory. The same argument suggests that knee extensors would be more frequently spared than knee flexors. The relative rarity of knee extension contractures in this patient group illustrates the complex interplay of factors that leads to musculoskeletal deformity in MMC.

Hips. The majority of patients have some hip deformity that interferes with ambulation, seating, or bracing, but only those with functional deficits or pain need treatment. Muscle imbalance at the hip accounts for most of the hip flexion deformity. A small number of patients develop hip flexion contractures from spasticity in the iliopsoas, rectus femoris, or sartorius (Fig. 54–2). Any hip flexion contracture of 20 degrees or more will increase the anterior pelvic tilt, create excessive lumbar lordosis, and interfere with ambulation. Patients with lesions at a high level may require soft tissue releases and anterior capsulotomy to improve seating and comfort. Patients with lesions at lower levels who are over 10 or 11 years of age may require a subtrochanteric extension osteotomy to preserve ambulation. This approach is less successful in younger ambulatory patients, for whom continued growth is likely to result in bone remodeling. Younger patients may respond to hip flexor releases with free tendon grafting using the tensor fasciae latae.[36]

Hip flexion-abduction-external rotation deformity is seen in patients with higher lesion levels and may necessitate radical hip releases for seating. Iliotibial band and tensor fasciae latae strength may be asymmetrical and lead to hip abduction contracture and pelvic obliquity. Hip adduction contracture is the deformity that is most often associated with secondary hip dislocation. The goal in treating this deformity is to release the adductors to regain 45 to 60 degrees of passive abduction.[36]

Fifty percent of children with myelomeningocele have subluxated or dislocated hips at some time. Hip dislocation at birth occurs with lesions that are very high (thoracic level) or very low (sacral level). Some 50% to 70% of hip dislocations are associated with the muscle imbalance of mid-lumbar-level lesions, where flexors and adductors are innervated by L1 to L5, and L5 to S2 innervation to extensors and abductors is absent. When hip dislocation occurs in later childhood or adolescence it may signal new-onset, late neurological changes such as hydromyelia or tethered cord.

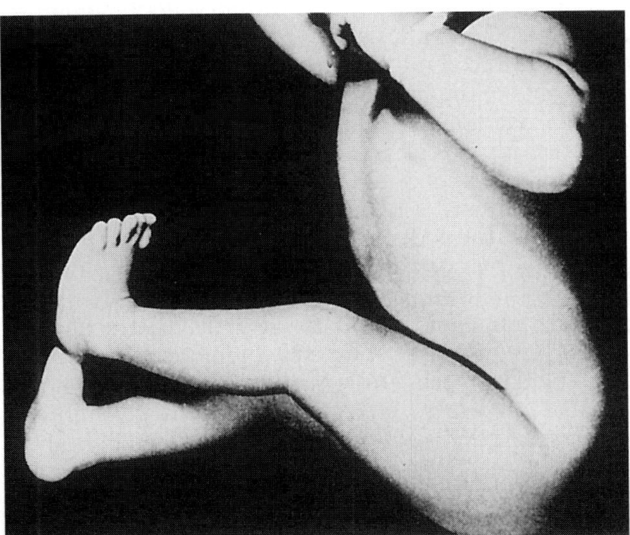

FIGURE 54–2. Hip flexion contracture is very common in infancy and early childhood.

There is some evidence that reducing dislocated hips in the active, ambulatory child may decrease dependence on assistive devices and reduce energy expenditure.[36] When the dislocations are bilateral and very high, reduction requires soft tissue releases and pelvic and femoral procedures and has such a high complication rate that the reduction is often contraindicated. Nonambulatory children with high lesion levels frequently need only soft tissue releases. Hip surgery must be carefully planned; the most common postoperative complication is hip flexion contracture that interferes with mobility in later life. Repeated procedures are associated with greater hip stiffness and greater disability.[36]

Knees. The most common deformity of the knee is flexion contracture. The development of knee flexion contracture is complex and incompletely understood. It may be caused by congenital joint stiffness due to decreased intrauterine movement, from spasticity in the knee flexors, or from progressive crouched posture with weak quadriceps and a need to keep the center of gravity over the midfoot during weight bearing. The incidence of knee flexion contractures is related to the neurological level of the lesion and the child's age. About 70% of patients with lesions at the level of L3 or higher develop knee flexion contractures by 8 years of age. Patients with lesions at the L4 to L5 level do better; only 25% have contractures by age 12 years. Most patients with sacral-level lesions do not suffer knee flexion contractures. Knee extension contractures and valgus and varus deformities occur rarely and are seen most often in the groups with higher level lesions.[68]

Feet. Foot deformities occur in 85% of children and are the most common orthopedic abnormality in children with MMC.[36] Both muscular imbalance and spasticity contribute to deformities. The muscular imbalance associated with the level of the neurological lesion interferes with the bony and cartilaginous growth of the hindfoot. Lack of sensation and autonomic dysfunction with vasomotor instability are responsible for secondary skin injury and poor wound healing. The goals of treatment are braceable plantigrade feet and balanced muscle control around the ankle joint.

Equinovarus, the rigid form of clubfoot deformity, results from retained tibialis posterior and tibialis anterior function in the child with a mid-lumbar neurological deficit (Fig. 54–3). The first line of treatment is casting to reduce the deformity, but surgery to produce a stable ankle joint is usually inevitable. A hindfoot valgus deformity with residual forefoot adduction is a common complication. Rigid fusions such as triple arthrodesis are associated with later development of neuropathic joints.[36] Children with paresis of the tibialis posterior are at risk for congenital convex pes valgus or rocker-bottom deformity. Surgical correction is designed to balance the hindfoot and forefoot musculature. Spasticity of foot muscles is more commonly associated with calcaneus deformities than with equinus deformities.[7]

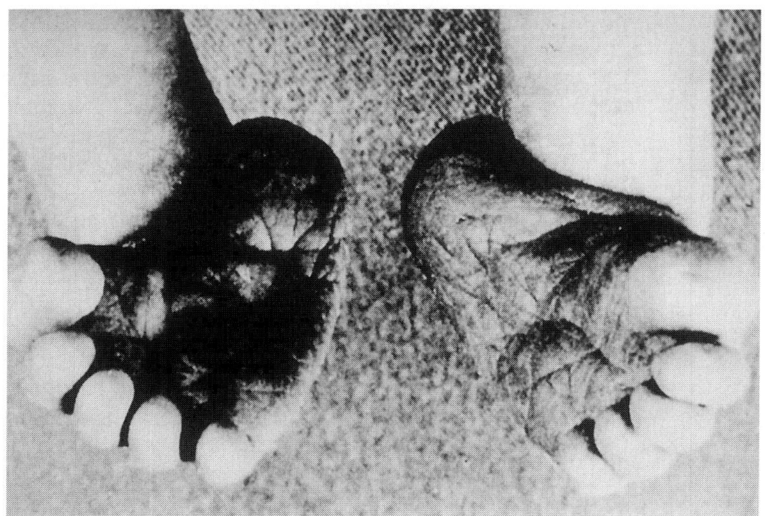

FIGURE 54–3. Equinovarus foot deformity is more commonly seen at birth and during early infancy.

Flexible, flail feet or S1-innervated ankles may drift into pure equinus deformity. This can be an indication for prescription of a neutrally positioned ankle-foot orthosis. Plantar flexion contracture of greater than 20 degrees is unlikely to improve with stretching and may require serial casting or soft tissue releases. Pes cavus requires little treatment until adolescence, when weight bearing may lead to skin ulceration. When necessary, metatarsal osteotomies and orthoses can successfully redistribute forces around the foot. Loss of foot intrinsic balance may produce a cock-up toe deformity at the great toe, best treated with tendon lengthening. Hindfoot valgus can be treated with orthoses until it exceeds 7 degrees (Fig. 54–4). Deformity beyond this amount requires tendon transfers for young children, epiphyseal interruption in older children, and supramalleolar osteotomy in adolescents.[36]

Spine. Spinal deformity in MMC usually occurs in one of three forms: (1) scoliosis with lordosis, (2) kyphosis, or (3) rigid congenital malformation.[36] There is a direct correlation between the level of spinal lesion and the incidence of scoliosis; 100% of patients with thoracic lesions develop a scoliosis of 45 degrees or more. The incidence is only 60% in patients with a lesion at the L4 level, and less than half of them will need surgical correction. When scoliosis accompanies high-level paraplegia, it occurs in early childhood or infancy, is usually C-shaped, and is always progressive. When scoliosis develops as a result of hydromyelia or syrinx formation it is often more S-shaped, occurs at any time, and may improve after treatment of the hydromyelia if the curve has not progressed beyond 50 degrees. Scoliosis that presents in later childhood may be the first sign of secondary CNS complications such as lipoma, dermoid tumors, or tethered cord.[8]

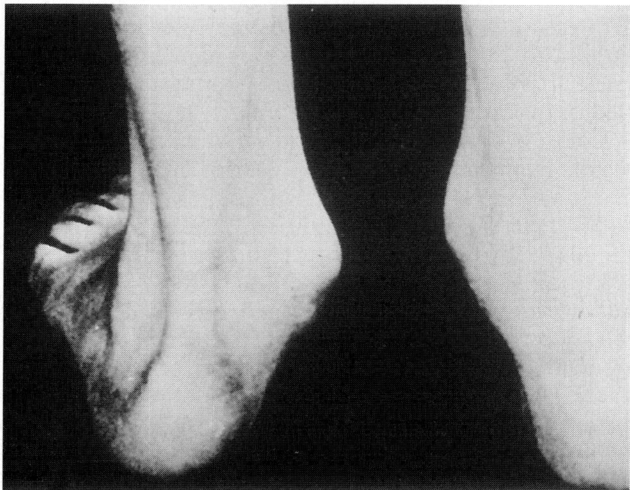

FIGURE 54–4. Calcaneovalgus deformity is commonly seen in later years.

Kyphosis in MMC is almost always progressive, and conservative management is rarely effective. Curves of 100 degrees or more are commonly seen by age 3. The most common form is the supple, collapsing C-shaped curve with kyphosis, which may have its apex at any point from the lower thoracic vertebrae to the lumbosacral joint. The kyphosis that presents at birth is associated with vertebral malformations. The rigid apex is commonly in the high- to mid-lumber region, and there is a compensatory lordosis above it. Rarely, children present with partial aplasia of the lumbar spine, which also results in kyphosis. The goals of treatment in kyphosis are to preserve or maintain abdominal height and allow room for abdominal contents, to relieve pressure on the diaphragm, and to prevent pressure sores. If kyphosis is allowed to approach 180 degrees, treatment becomes impossible.[36] Children with large congenital malformations of the vertebral column may require anterior and posterior fusion in infancy. Those who do not undergo early correction may develop additional, progressive curves with growth of the spine (Fig. 54–5).

In all three forms of scoliosis the timing of surgical correction is critical. Spinal fusion performed too early will further limit vertebral growth; waiting may lead to progressive curves that are more difficult or impossible to treat. The most appropriate approach is to individual-

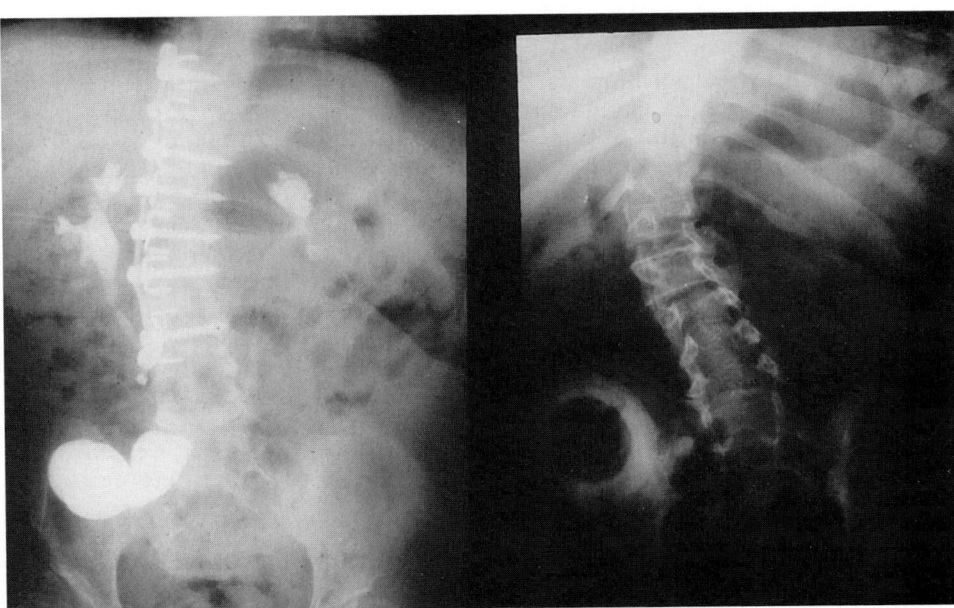

FIGURE 54–5. The risk for scoliosis is linearly correlated with age and inversely correlated with the level of the lesion.

ize treatment for each child and provide vigilant surveillance for spinal changes.

Fractures. Fractures occur in approximately 20% of children with MMC. The proximal and distal femur are the most frequently involved sites. In ambulatory patients, fractures often accompany falls. In nonambulatory children, fractures may occur with minor trauma to their osteopenic extremities.[68] In the insensate lower extremity, fractures may escape detection initially. They present with erythema, swelling, local warmth, fever, and malaise. Frequently the white blood cell (WBC) count and erythrocyte sedimentation rate (ESR) are elevated, and it is not uncommon for the unsuspected fracture to be mistaken for a soft tissue infection. Fractures heal quickly in children with MMC. The bone forms exuberant calluses and rarely needs rigid fixation. Those patients who have casts for fractures or surgery are relatively more osteopenic immediately after treatment and are at greatest risk for new fractures in the period immediately following cast removal.[68]

Mobility

Lesion Level. Mobility—efficient, effective moving through space—may or may not include independent walking. Most children with MMC use a variety of methods to maintain mobility, including walking, assistive devices, and wheelchairs. Traditionally, walking in MMC patients has been linked to the level of the neurological lesion and the pattern of motor strength in the lower extremities. The guidelines have never been completely consistent; some authors have emphasized the importance of quadriceps strength while others have stressed hip abductors and knee flexors.[42] Using motor level to predict ambulation is difficult because the classic neurosegmental levels and motor correlates are probably more variable than originally thought, and because there is a wide range of ambulation potential among patients with similar patterns of segmental innervation. The influence of motor innervation may be moderated by other factors, including cognitive ability, musculoskeletal complications, surgery, motivation, obesity, and age.[43]

The complicated relationship of motor innervation and independent ambulation resists reduction to a simple formula that could be used to predict ambulation potential. One recent study[42] attempted to clarify this issue by studying serial manual muscle tests in a large, stable population of children with MMC over a long period of time. In this study iliopsoas strength was a robust predictor of independent ambulation. Grade 4 to 5 iliopsoas strength was most often associated with community ambulation; grade 0 to 3 iliopsoas strength was always associated with wheelchair dependence. The ability to walk without assistive devices was strongly associated with grade 4 to 5 gluteal and tibialis anterior strength. Those patients with a combination of strong hip flexors and weak gluteus medius muscles were most likely to experience deterioration in muscle strength regardless of age.

Orthoses. Four principles govern the use of orthoses in children with MMC. (1) Orthotic devices may be used to prevent deformity. Splints and orthoses are most effective at maintaining correction of deformities that have been attained by casting or surgery. Their ability to prevent the development of or alter the progression of spontaneous deformity, for example, pes planus or scoliosis, is not well established in this population. (2) Orthotic devices can be used to support normal joint alignment and mechanics when they are carefully fabricated for that purpose. (3) Children with MMC have various patterns of muscular weakness that interfere with normal gait. In that setting orthoses may be used to control range of motion during gait. (4) Special orthotic devices, particularly those that provide support or augment mobility, may be used to facilitate function.[32]

In addition to the many variations of knee and ankle-foot orthoses, three unique and extensive bracing systems are used to facilitate function for children with MMC. The parapodium provides structural support from the midthorax to the floor. It is often jointed at the hip and knee to accommodate both standing and sitting positions. This allows the child to maintain an upright, weight-bearing position and to ambulate with a swing-through gait regardless of the level of paralysis. The swivel walker is a modification of the parapodium that was initially designed in Great Britain for children with limb deficiency resulting from the thalidomide crisis of the 1960s.[32] It has a dual footplate system that translates trunk rotation into forward movement. The reciprocating gait orthosis (RGO) joins two hip-knee-ankle-foot orthoses (HKAFOs) with an elaborate cable system to link hip flexion at each hip with hip extension on the contralateral side. All three of these systems have the advantage of simulating upright ambulation, but none approaches the energy efficiency of normal walking. Children using HKAFOs with a swing-through gait have greater gait velocity than children using the RGO and a reciprocating gait pattern, but they walk with higher energy consumption.[16]

Functional Mobility. There is a strong cultural imperative to encourage disabled children to maintain an upright weight-bearing position and if possible to ambulate with as little assistive equipment as possible. With appropriate support, surgery, extensive bracing, and therapy, many children with MMC with high-level lesions can become community ambulators.[13] This point of view has validity in a psychological sense. Standing and walking may have great value in the minds of individual children and their parents and should be supported for these reasons. Efficient, functional mobility, however, is often better achieved with these children by providing them with a wheelchair. Rarely is it necessary to make an exclusive choice of ambulation and bracing or wheeled mobility; judicious use of both modalities in different settings to achieve separate goals is often the best solution.

It is important to separate a cultural imperative from the clinical arguments that are frequently offered as justification for aggressive upright mobility regimens. An upright stance has been purported to improve urinary tract function by facilitating urine flow by gravity, but no scientific data exist to support this suggestion. Ambulation has been cited as a helpful adjunct in bowel function, but there is no evidence of its usefulness. Improved cardiopulmonary fitness is provided as an argument for aggressive ambulation with assistive devices, but abundant research suggests that energy expenditure for patients with disabilities is usually maintained at a constant level at the expense of decreased velocity and endurance. There are likely more opportunities for aerobic fitness available to wheelchair racers than to persons who must depend on braces and crutches for ambulation.[68]

The most commonly cited argument for weight bearing is the development of osteopenia and the increased risk of fractures in nonambulatory patients. It is true that these patients are more osteopenic than ambulatory children, but the risk of fracture is more closely associated with surgery and immobilization than with lack of weight bearing. Ambulatory children with MMC have a higher frequency of orthopedic procedures and therefore more risk of fractures.[68] Weight bearing is encouraged to counteract the risk of lower extremity contractures and deformity, but the association has never been clearly defined. It has been suggested that keeping children upright and weight bearing will prevent the development of obesity. One recent study comparing the users of standing frames and wheelchairs found the opposite to be true.[37] Maintaining an upright posture does not reduce the risk of decubitus formation; it only changes the pattern of skin breakdown. Wheelchair users have more gluteal lesions and ambulators have more foot involvement.[37, 68]

The purpose of this discussion is not to discourage ambulation and weight-bearing activities for patients with high-level lesions but to place the emphasis on walking in a functional context. The cultural and individual benefits of being upright should be considered in combination with the energy efficiency of wheelchair use so that appropriate choices can be made that will support each individual patient's needs and goals.

Skin Breakdown

Morbidity and Cost. In one clinic population the incidence of skin breakdown in children with MMC was reported to be 43%. The prevalence of skin breakdown noted at annual evaluations increased steadily from infancy to age 10 years, then leveled off to between 20% and 25% of patients.[52]

Frequent Sites. Skin breakdown occurs most commonly as a result of unrelieved pressure over anesthetic areas. Lacerations, burns, dermatitis, and even cold injury in anesthetic areas can also cause serious skin breakdown. In patients with MMC, higher rates of skin breakdown are seen in those who have mental retardation, large head size, kyphoscoliosis, or chronic soiling. Normal bony prominences or orthopedic deformities are common sites of skin ulceration from pressure or shear forces, and in children with MMC the most common sites of breakdown are over the perineum, over a gibbus deformity, and in the lower extremities. Nonambulatory patients have the highest frequency of ulceration of the perineum or gibbus, whereas the highest frequency of lower extremity breakdown occurs in ambulatory patients with lower lumbar motor levels.[53]

Prevention. Because of the high frequency and cost of skin breakdown, all patients with MMC should receive periodic examinations for and preventive guidance against skin breakdown. The child must learn that meticulous hygiene and daily inspection of insensate skin is important. Whenever a child receives a new spinal or lower extremity orthosis, a sequential wearing schedule should be used to monitor for sites of excessive pressure.[3] Ambulatory patients should be cautioned against walking barefoot, especially outdoors or on hot pavement. Patients who use wheelchairs need adjustment of seating to prevent pelvic obliquity or pressure over bony prominences. There is no preferred wheelchair cushion for patients with MMC, but gel cushions should not be left outdoors in cold climates because they may become cold enough to induce freeze burns.[51]

The fact that the incidence of skin breakdown increases as children with MMC grow larger speaks to the need to learn effective pressure relief whether from standing or sitting surfaces, but it will likely require many years of adult supervision before the child incorporates such habits into his or her daily routine.

Treatment. The medical management of skin breakdown in children with MMC is no different than for other diagnoses. Attention to relief of pressure or shear forces, hygiene, debridement, and nutrition is important. For wounds that extend beneath subcutaneous tissues, surgical closure may be necessary. Owing to the young age of the patient and the possibility of repeat surgery for skin breakdown, surgeons should plan the closure to allow for the greatest number of future options. Primary closure or skin rotation is preferable to myocutaneous flaps for first procedures.[35]

Obesity

Adults with spinal cord injury have a 10% to 30% reduction in basal metabolic rate and total daily energy expenditure as a result of decreased lean body mass from paralyzed muscle. Similar data are not available for children with MMC, but dieting studies document that on average, children with MMC ingest 25% fewer calories than their peers, and yet 27% to 90% are reported to be obese. The reduction in lean body mass and decreased activity that reduce the total daily energy expenditure are inversely related to the level of the lesion; higher-level lesions result in lower energy expenditure. Once a child with MMC becomes obese, the reduced energy expenditure makes further weight loss even more difficult. Dietary management should begin in infancy with anticipatory guidance and nutritional education. Weight reduction is extremely difficult, requiring professional assistance to maintain adequate protein and vitamin intake while severely restricting calories. Dietary intervention is most appropriately invested in preventing obesity because the outcome of weight reduction efforts is disappointingly poor.[67]

Psychological and Social Issues

Intellectual and Personal Development. Any individual's capacity to understand and cope with the world is much more complex than the single score on an intelligence test, but the imperfect representation of cognitive skill provided by IQ tests at least affords a crude measure for comparison of groups. When children with MMC as a large heterogeneous group are compared with nondisabled peers on the short-form Wechsler Intelligence Scale for Children, Revised (WISC-R), their scores are skewed toward the lower end. Only 6% of children with MMC score in the high-average to extremely high range, compared with 27% of controls. Seventy-five percent of children with MMC score in the low-average to extremely low range, compared with 25% of matched peers.[2] IQ scores have been correlated with level of lesion: higher-level lesions are associated with lower scores, lower lesions with better performance. IQ scores are adversely affected by the presence of CNS infection and shunt malformation.[71] The combination of cognitive impairment and significant physical disabilities makes training in self-care both challenging and difficult. It is not surprising that children with MMC develop activities of daily living (ADL) skills later and less efficiently than their peers and that families unwittingly reinforce dependence in their attempts to meet the normal requirements and constraints of daily life.

Perhaps most important is the effect MMC has on a child's self-concept and notion of competence. Recent investigation into this area suggests that when children with MMC are compared with matched nondisabled controls, they view themselves as less competent in academic, athletic, and social domains of self-concept even though they recognize these as areas of great importance in personal and social functioning. Peer social acceptance and social comparisons are highly valued by children with MMC, but they feel less supported by classmates than nondisabled children do. The discrepancy between social importance and self-competence for adolescents with MMC is greatest in the area of physical appearance.[2]

Clearly, interventions to foster independence in children with MMC must be distributed among several areas. The higher likelihood of cognitive impairment suggests the need for individualized education. Physical disability requires adaptive strategies for self-care. Interventions must be devised to develop greater levels of self-perception and self-competence so that these children can interact effectively with the remainder of society.

Family. MMC does not affect individuals so much as it affects families. The family is irreversibly changed by the presence of a disabled child, and the child is affected by the family's response. Most social science research now agrees that the family's response to the disabled child probably plays a greater role in emotional development than the disability itself.[22]

The family must be supported in its attempt to develop competence and coping with the stressors that accompany the care of a disabled child. There are at least nine different stressors, all of which may be operative at different times. They include modification of family goals and dreams, altered relationships, increased burden of care and reduction of free time, financial burdens, altered school performance and programming, modifications to the home, medical problems, social isolation, and grieving. Of these, medically related stress is predominant in infancy, but it eventually gives way to all the others in turn and in combination.[21]

Those who would attempt to support families in their care for the child with MMC have an armamentarium of at least six resources to offer. They are (1) attention to factors that promote the health and energy *of the caregivers,* (2) problem-solving strategies that allow families to adapt, (3) social skills so that family members can better communicate their needs to one another and the community, (4) social and emotional support from people outside the family, (5) material resources in the form of money, goods, or services, and (6) positive beliefs that maintain hope and sustain effective coping during difficult periods.[22]

One very practical source of help for families is the Spina Bifida Association of America. This organization provides education, advocacy, and support for patients and their families. Early referral can assist the family in developing relationships with other families who can provide practical advice and counseling that is based on their own personal experiences. The address of the association is listed at the end of this chapter.

MYELOMENINGOCELE IN ADULTS

Description of a New Disease

Before surgical closure of open neural tube defects in newborns became a common practice, most affected infants did not survive. Significant morbidity plagued those who did survive in the form of urinary tract infections, renal failure, hydrocephalus, and scoliosis. The combination of improved surgical practices, new antibiotics, changing patterns of medical ethics, and the willingness of health care professionals to manage patients with MMC using a team approach has made long-term survival possible.

Until recently, physicians had virtually no experience in caring for adults with MMC. Many relied on their understanding of spinal cord injury to guide their approach toward adults with MMC, only to find that functional and independent living skills were not commensurate with those expected based on level of physical impairment. Factors such as onset of impairment at birth, intellectual deficits, and difficulties in achieving bladder and bowel continence contribute to delayed social maturation throughout childhood and adolescence. Family expectations and opportunities for social interactions and vocational experiences probably contribute to dependency as well.

Only limited descriptive information is available on the types of medical complications and psychosocial difficulties of adults with MMC, but rehabilitation principles derived from other conditions can be applied to these problems. Periodic screening for change in neurological status, development of joint disease, deterioration of renal function, or development of pressure ulcers is essential.

Skin Breakdown. Pressure ulcers are a major cause of morbidity in adolescents and adults with MMC. In one series of young adults aged 19 to 27 years old, 85% had had skin breakdown requiring hospitalization, and 70% had continuing problems with skin ulcers. About half had only occasional breakdown, but one-fourth had nearly continuous problems.[20] Skin breakdown over the feet can be extremely difficult to heal and can cause loss of ambulation due to need for pressure relief or surgical amputation.

Musculoskeletal Complications and Joint Disease. Joint pain and degeneration can cause adults to become more dependent on a wheelchair for mobility. Those with sensory levels at L3 or L4 are particularly likely to lose the ability to be community ambulators in young adulthood.[28] Upper extremity joints such as the shoulder and elbow may become painful from overuse. Lower extremity joints may become Charcot joints in the second and third decade as a result of an orthopedic deformity, abnormal dynamic forces, and impaired sensation. Clinicians should give careful consideration to joint protection for young children with MMC.

Scoliosis does not appear to progress beyond adolescence, but its presence may cause ongoing problems with posture and seating, the development of pressure ulcers, loss of ambulation, impaired respiratory function, and pain.

Late Neurological Changes. Neurological deterioration in adults with MMC can occur as a result of shunt obstruction, syringomyelia, or tethering of the spinal cord. Most children with MMC and hydrocephalus do not seem to outgrow the need for a shunt as adults.[40] Hydromyelia causing upper extremity pain, paresthesias, and weakness has been reported as a late development in adults.[69] Tethering of the spinal cord and herniated disks have occurred in adults, often in association with pregnancy.[69] Symptoms from tethered cord can be exacerbated by forward bending, childbirth, and trauma.

Renal and Urological Problems. Renal failure is one of the most serious complications facing adults with MMC. In one study of 61 adults at age 25 years, 31% had renal damage and 15% were being treated for hypertension.[28] While the primary causes are most often reflux and recurrent infection, other contributing factors include hypertension, shunt nephritis, amyloidosis, and calculi. Patients with MMC appear to be good candidates for dialysis, with better survival rates than for diabetic patients with end-stage renal disease. Renal transplantation has also been used successfully.[50]

Late complications of previous urological surgery can also occur, including rupture of an enterocystoplasty and erosion or failure of an implanted artificial sphincter. Regular urological follow-up is important to monitor renal function, treat infections, and identify complications such as calculi formation or renal failure. Serum creatinine is not a good marker of glomerular filtration rate in patients with MMC because these children have widely varying body types and total muscle mass.[57] Radioisotope renal scan is a better measure of renal function.

Fertility. Studies have indicated that adolescents with MMC have similar expectations regarding marriage and reproduction as do adolescents without MMC, but they have considerably less experience with dating and knowledge of sexual functioning, family planning, and birth control.[23]

Girls, but not boys, with MMC have been observed to physically mature earlier than peers and same-sex family members without MMC. They also tend to reach menarche sooner than the national mean.[23]

Studies to date of the sexuality of adults with MMC have relied on self-report of function. Women report various degrees of genital sensation, while many men report the ability for erection and ejaculation, but none of these correlates with level of motor function. Most adults with MMC are reported to have satisfactory sexual function.[11] Men with MMC have been reported to father children, but some data suggest that primary testicular failure with low serum testosterone and elevated follicle-stimulating and luteinizing hormones may be common and that the prognosis for fertility may be poor.[60] Women with MMC have successfully conceived and carried to term without major complications, although urinary tract infections have been commonly reported.[11]

Affective Disorders

Adolescents with MMC often have low self-esteem and frequent doubts concerning their health, physical condition, and sexual functioning. Delayed social responsibility is also prominent, manifested by lack of chore assignments at home, social contacts with younger children as opposed to peers, and a paucity of friends.[19]

Adults with MMC are reported to have a range of adjustments from well adapted to poorly motivated, apathetic, and dependent personalities.[20] Intelligence and level of paralysis are associated with good adjustment. Social isolation is a frequent problem, with many adults reporting few friends and infrequent memberships in clubs or groups. Problems with physical access and attitudes of persons without disabilities compound social isolation.[66] While this is a high-risk group for psychosocial problems, suicide has not been reported in higher than expected frequency.

Vocational Issues

In large clinic series, most adults with MMC are reported to have completed high school and about half continued in postsecondary education.[20, 39, 74] About 25% of adults with MMC report employment.[20, 38] They mainly performed routine, non-manual work, had average working hours, but received below-average pay. Most enjoyed their jobs and were well accepted by peers at work, but job retention was poor.[38, 74] Adolescents with MMC appear to have unrealistic ideas about training and skill requirements compared with their peers, and are less often assigned chores at home, even chores well within their physical abilities.

Independent Living

Various rates of living away from parents have been reported in different cultures, ranging from over 60% in the United States to 15% in Great Britain.[20, 39] In one study, one-third of adults with MMC were fully independent—employed, financially independent, homeowners, and free of psychological problems. The other two-thirds required Social Security income and various levels of support from family and friends. Many have limited abilities to do cooking, shopping, or use public transportation.[39] Factors associated with independence include sensory level below L3, no ventriculoperitoneal shunt, IQ $\geq$ 80, no epilepsy, community ambulation skills, no pressure sores and freedom from incontinence pads.[28]

Planning for postsecondary education, vocation, and independent living should begin in early adolescence. Under the 1990 Amendments of the Education of the Handicapped Act, Public Law 101-476, schools must include transition services in the Individualized Education Program (I.E.P.) of a student receiving special education services by age 16 years. Such services are meant to be a coordinated plan for moving the child beyond school to such outcomes as vocational training, employment, adult services, independent living, and community participation. Clinicians can contribute to this process by reminding parents and schools to initiate such planning, and by providing information about physical and health conditions that may influence the process.[62]

For further information on spina bifida, the reader is referred to: The Spina Bifida Association of America, 1700 Rockville Pike, Suite 540, Rockville, MD 20852, telephone 301-770-SBAA.

REFERENCES

1. Agnarsson U, Warde C, McCarthy G, et al: Anorectal function of children with neurological problems: I. Spina bifida. Dev Med Child Neurol 1993; 35:893–902.
2. Appleton PE, Mincho P, Ellis N, et al: The self concept of young people with spina bifida: A population based study. Dev Med Child Neurol 1994; 36:198–215.
3. Banta JV, Lin J, Peterson M, et al: The team approach in the care of the child with myelomeningocele. J Prosthet Orthot 1989; 2:263–273.
4. Bishop DT: Multifactorial inheritance. In Emery AEH, Rimoin DL (eds): Principles and Practice of Medical Genetics. New York, Churchill Livingstone, 1990, pp 165–174.
5. Bosco PJ, Bauer SB, Colodny AH, et al: The long-term results of artificial sphincters in children. J Urol 1991; 146:396–399.
6. Brockelhurst G: The nature of spina bifida. In Brockelhurst G (ed): Spina Bifida for the Clinician. London, Spastics International, 1976, pp 1–7.
7. Broughton NS, Graham G, Menelaus MB: The high incidence of foot deformities in patients with high level spina bifida. J Bone Joint Surg Br 1994; 76:548–550.
8. Bunch WA, Scarff TB, Dronch V: Progressive loss in myelomeningocele patients. Orthop Trans 1983; 7:185.
9. Carmel P: The Arnold-Chiari malformation. In Section of Pediatric Neurosurgery of the American Association of Neurological Surgeons (eds): Pediatric Neurosurgery: Surgery of the Developing Nervous System, ed 2. Philadelphia, WB Saunders, 1989, pp 53–70.
10. Carter CO: Clues to aetiology of neural tube malformations. Dev Med Child Neurol 1974; 16(suppl 32):3–15.
11. Cass AS, Bloom BA, Luxenberg M: Sexual function in adults with myelomeningocele. J Urol 1986; 136:425–426.
12. Chan A, Robertson EF, Haan EA, et al: Prevalence of neural tube defects in South Australia, 1966–1991: Effectiveness and impact of prenatal diagnosis. Br Med J 1993; 307:703–706.
13. Charney EB, Melchionni JB, Smith DR: Community ambulation by children with myelomeningocele and high-level paralysis. J Pediatr Orthop 1991; 11:579–582.
14. Coniglio SJ, Anderson SM, Ferguson JE: Functional motor outcome in children with myelomeningocele: A correlation with anatomic level on prenatal ultrasound. Dev Med Child Neurol 1996; 38:675–680.
15. Cowchock S, Ainbender E, Prescott G, et al: The recurrence risk for neural tube defects in the United States: A collaborative study. Am J Med Genet 1980; 5:309–314.
16. Cuddeford TJ, Frelling RP, Thomas SS, et al: Energy consumption in children with myelomeningocele: A comparison between reciprocating gait orthoses and hip-knee-ankle-foot orthosis ambulators. Dev Med Child Neurol 1997; 34:239–242.
17. Czeizel AE, Dudas I: Prevention of the first occurrence of neural tube defects by periconceptional vitamin supplementation. N Engl J Med 1992; 327:1832–1835.

18. Dietrich S, Okamoto G: Bowel training for children with neurogenic dysfunction: A follow-up. Arch Phys Med Rehabil 1982; 63:166–170.
19. Dorner S: Adolescents with spina bifida: How they see their situation. Arch Dis Child 1976; 51:439–444.
20. Dunne KB, Shurtleff DB: The adult with meningomyelocele: A preliminary report. In McLaurin RL (ed): Spina Bifida: A Multidisciplinary Approach. New York, Praeger, 1986, pp 38–51.
21. Ferembac D: Frequency of spina bifida occulta in prehistoric human skeletons. Nature 1963; 197:100.
22. Friedman W, Schaffer J: Family adjustments and contributions. In Shurtleff DB (ed): Myelodysplasias and Extrophies: Significance, Prevention and Treatment. New York, Grune & Stratton, 1986, pp 399–409.
23. Furmen L, Mortimer JC: Menarche and menstrual function in patients with myelomeningocele. Dev Med Child Neurol 1994; 36:910–917.
24. Greenberg F, James LM, Oakley GP: Estimates of birth prevalence rates of spina bifida in the United States from computer-generated maps. Am J Obstet Gynecol 1983; 145:570–573.
25. Hamilton RA, Dorman JC: Neural tube defects–prenatal diagnosis and management. Ulster Med J 1992; 61:127–133.
26. Hays R, Jordan R, McLaughlin J, et al: Central ventilatory dysfunction in myelodysplasia: An independent determination of survival. Dev Med Child Neurol 1989; 31:366–370.
27. Hays RM, Erickson D, Astley S: Tethered cord syndrome in meningo-myelocele: Analysis of clinical features for early diagnosis. Arch Phys Med Rehabil 1989; 70:A–45.
28. Hunt GM, Powlton A: Open spina bifida: A complete cohort reviewed 25 years after closure. Dev Med Child Neurol 1995; 37:19–29.
29. Just M, Schwartz M, Ernest J: Magnetic resonance imaging of dysgraphic myelodysplasia. Childs Nerv Sys 1986; 4:149–153.
30. Kimura DK, Mayo M, Shurtleff D: Urinary tract management. In Shurtleff DB (ed): Myelodysplasias and Extrophies: Significance, Prevention and Treatment. New York, Grune & Stratton, 1986, pp 243–266.
31. King JC, Currie DM, Wright E: Bowel training in spina bifida: Importance of education, patient compliance, age, and anal reflexes. Arch Phys Med Rehabil 1993; 75:243–247.
32. Knutson LM, Clark DE: Orthotic devices for ambulation in children with cerebral palsy and myelomeningocele. Phys Ther 1991; 71:947–960.
33. Laurence KM, James N, Miller MH, et al: Double-blind randomized controlled trial of folate treatment before conception to prevent recurrence of neural-tube defects. Br Med J 1981; 282:1509–1511.
34. Lie HR, Lagergren J, Rasmussen F, et al: Bowel and bladder control of children with myelomeningocele: A Nordic study. Dev Med Child Neurol 1991; 33:1053–1061.
35. Linder RM, Morris D: The surgical management of pressure ulcers: A systematic approach based on staging. Decubitus 1990; 3:32–38.
36. Lindseth RE, Dias LS, Drennan JC: Myelomeningocele. Instruct Course Lect 1991; 40:271–291.
37. Liptak G, Shurtleff D, Bloss J, et al: Mobility aids for children with high level myelomeningocele: Parapodium vs wheelchair. Dev Med Child Neurol 1992; 34:787–796.
38. Lonton AP, Loughlin AM, O'Sullivan AM: The employment of adults with spina bifida. Z Kinderchir 1984; 39(suppl 2):132–134.
39. Lonton AP, O'Sullivan AM, Loughlin AM: Spina bifida adults. Z Kinderchir 1983; 38(suppl 2):110–112.
40. Lorber J, Pucholt V: When is a shunt no longer necessary? An investigation of 300 patients with hydrocephalus and myelomeningocele: 11–22 year follow-up. Z Kinderchir 1981; 34:327–329.
41. Luthy DA, Wardinsky T, Shurtleff DB, et al: Cesarean section before the onset of labor and subsequent motor function in infants with meningomyelocele diagnosed antenatally. N Engl J Med 1991; 324:662–666.
42. McDonald C, Jaffe K, Mosca V, et al: Ambulatory outcome of children with myelomeningocele: Effect of lower extremity muscle strength. Dev Med Child Neurol 1991; 33:482–490.
43. McDonald C, Jaffe K, Shurtleff D, et al: Modifications to the traditional description of neurosegmental intervention in myelomeningocele. Dev Med Child Neurol 1991; 33:473–481.
44. McEnory G, Borzyskowski M, Cox TCS: The spinal cord in neurologically stable spina bifida: An MRI study. Dev Med Child Neurol 1992; 34:342–347.
45. McGuire EJ: Neuroanatomy and neurophysiology. In McLaurin RL (ed): Spina Bifida: A Multidisciplinary Approach. New York, Praeger, 1986, pp 246–252.
46. McGuire EJ, Woodside JR, Borden TA, et al: Prognostic value of urodynamic testing in myelodysplastic patients. J Urol 1981; 126:205–209.
47. McLone DG, Czyzewsky D, Raimondi AJ, et al: Central nervous system infections as a limiting factor in intelligence of children born with myelomeningocele. Pediatrics 1982; 70:338–342.
48. Milunsky A, Ulcickas M, Rothman KJ, et al: Maternal heat exposure and neural tube defects. JAMA 1992; 268:882–885.
49. MRC Vitamin Study Research Group: Prevention of neural tube defects: Results of the Medical Research Counsel vitamin study. Lancet 1991; 338:131–137.
50. Muralikrishna GS, Rodger RSC, Macdougall AI, et al: Renal replacement treatment in patients with spina bifida or spinal cord injury. Br Med J 1989; 299:1506.
51. Odderson IR, Jaffe KM, Sleicher CA, et al: Gel wheelchair cushions: A potential cold weather hazard. Arch Phys Med Rehabil 1991; 72:1017–1020.
52. Okamoto GA, Lamers JV, Shurtleff DB: Skin breakdown in patients with myelomeningocele. Arch Phys Med Rehabil 1983; 64:20–23.
53. Okamoto GA, Sousa J, Telzrow RW, et al: Toileting skills in children with myelomeningocele: Rates of learning. Arch Phys Med Rehabil 1984; 65:182–185.
54. Ontzigt JGC, Los FJ, Grobee DE, et al: The risk of spina bifida aperts after first trimester exposure to valproate in a prenatal cohort. Neurology 1992; 42(suppl 15):119–125.
55. O'Rahilly R, Gardner E: The initial development of the human brain. Acta Anat 1979; 104:123–133.
56. Petersen M: Tethered cord syndrome in myelodysplasia: Correlation between level of lesion and height at time of presentation. Dev Med Child Neurol 1992; 34:604–610.
57. Quan A, Adams R, Ekmark E, et al: Serum creatinine is a poor marker of glomerular filtration rate in patients with spina bifida. Dev Med Child Neurol 1997; 39:808–810.
58. Raimondi AJ: Hydrocephalus. In Raimondi AJ (ed): Pediatric Neurosurgery: Theoretic Principles. Art of Surgical Techniques. New York, Springer-Verlag, 1987, pp 453–455.
59. Recommendations for the use of folic acid to reduce the number of cases of spina bifida and other neural tube defects. MMWR 1992; 41:1–7.
60. Reilly JM, Oates RD: Preliminary investigation of the potential fertility status of postpubertal males with myelodysplasia (abstract). J Urol 1992; 147:251A.
61. Roberts HE, Moore CA, Cragan JD, et al: Impact of prenatal diagnosis on the birth prevalence of neural tube defects, Atlanta 1990–1991. Pediatrics 1995; 96:830–833.
62. Ross B: Meeting the educational needs of children with disabilities: A collaborative management approach. Phys Med Rehabil Clin North Am 1991; 2:781–800.
63. Sandford MK, Kissling GE, Joubert PE: Neural tube defect etiology: New evidence concerning maternal hyperthermia, health, and diet. Dev Med Child Neurol 1992; 34:661–675.
64. Seller MJ: Risks in spina bifida. Dev Med Child Neurol 1994; 36:1021–1025.
65. Selzman AA, Elder JS, Mapstone TB: Urologic consequences of myelodysplasia and other congenital abnormalities of the spinal cord. Urol Clin North Am 1993; 20:485–504.
66. Shaffer J, Friedrich W: Young adult psychosocial adjustment. In Shurtleff DB (ed): Myelodysplasias and Extrophies: Significance, Prevention and Treatment. New York, Grune & Stratton, 1986, pp 421–430.
67. Shurtleff D: Dietary management. In Shurtleff DB (ed): Myelodysplasias and Extrophies: Significance, Prevention and Treatment. New York, Grune & Stratton, 1986, pp 285–295.
68. Shurtleff D: Mobility. In Shurtleff DB (ed): Myelodysplasias and Extrophies: Significance, Prevention and Treatment. New York, Grune & Stratton, 1986, pp 314–320.
69. Shurtleff D, Dunne K: Adults and adolescents with meningomyelocele. In Shurtleff DB (ed): Myelodysplasias and Extrophies:

Significance, Prevention and Treatment. New York, Grune & Stratton, 1986, pp 433–448.
70. Shurtleff D, Shurtleff H: Decision making for the treatment or nontreatment of congenitally malformed individuals. In Shurtleff DB (ed): Myelodysplasias and Extrophies: Significance, Prevention and Treatment. New York, Grune & Stratton, 1986, pp 3–24.
71. Shurtleff D, Stuntz JT: Back closure. In Shurtleff DB (ed): Myelodysplasias and Extrophies: Significance, Prevention and Treatment. New York, Grune & Statton, 1986, pp 117–138.
72. Shurtleff D, Stuntz JT, Hayden: Hydrocephalus. In Shurtleff DB (ed): Myelodysplasias and Extrophies: Significance, Prevention and Treatment. New York, Grune & Stratton, 1986, pp 139–180.
73. Slater JE: Rubber anaphylaxis. N Engl J Med 1989; 320:1126–1130.
74. Smith AD: Adult spina bifida survey in Scotland: Educational attainment and employment. Z Kinderchir 1983; 38(suppl): 107–109.
75. Sousa JC, Gordon LH, Shurtleff DB: Assessing the development of daily living skills in patients with spina bifida. Dev Med Child Neurol 1976; 18(suppl 37):134–142.
76. Spindel MR, Bauer SB, Dyro FM, et al: The changing neurologic lesion in myelodysplasia. JAMA 1987; 258:1630–1633.
77. Steinbok P, Irvine B, Cochrane DD, et al: Long-term outcome and complications of children born with meningomyelocele. Childs Nerv Syst 1992; 8:92–96.
78. Sussman GL, Tarlo S, Dolovich J: The spectrum of IgE mediated responses to latex. JAMA 1991; 265:2844–2847.
79. Tamaki N, Shirataki K, Kojima N, et al: Tethered cord syndrome of delayed onset following repair of myelomeningocele. J Neurosurg 1988; 69:393–398.
80. Task Force on Allergic Reaction to Latex: Committee Report. J Allergy Clin Immunol 1993; 92:16–18.
81. Uehling DT, Smith J, Meyer J, et al: Impact of an intermittent catheterization program in children with myelomeningocele. Pediatrics 1985; 76:892–895.
82. Van Hala S, Nelson VS, Hurvitz EA, et al: Bladder management in patients with pediatric onset neurogenic bladders. J Spinal Cord Med 1997; 20:410–415.
83. Warpinski JR, Folgert J, Cohen M, et al: Allergic reaction to latex: A risk factor for unsuspected anaphylaxis. Allergy Proc 1991; 12:95–102.
84. White JJ, Suzuki H, Shafie ME, et al: A physiologic rationale for the management of neurologic rectal incontinence in children. Pediatrics 1972; 49:888–893.
85. Wolraich ML, Hawtrey C, Mapel J, et al: Results of clean intermittent catheterization for children with neurogenic bladders. Urology 1983; 22:479–482.
86. Yen IH, Khoury MJ, Erickson JD, et al: The changing epidemiology of neural tube defects: United States. Am J Dis Child 1992; 146:857–861.

55

CHAPTER

Frederick S. Frost, M.D.

Spinal Cord Injury Medicine

Through thousands of years of human history, spinal cord injury (SCI) was considered a terminal medical condition. A number of factors, principally the discovery of modern antibiotics in an era of evolving societal attitudes toward persons with disability, have allowed countless individuals the opportunity not only to survive their injury, but to lead happy and productive lives (Table 55–1).

Organized efforts to deliver medical and rehabilitative care to this population began to take shape during the 1930s. The innovative work of British Army officer George Riddoch, Sir Ludwig Guttman at Stoke Mandeville Hospital in England, and Donald Munro at Boston City Hospital demonstrated that specialized treatment centers could successfully address the unique medical problems of these patients and promote successful community reintegration.[109] Subsequent attempts to establish regional referral networks for SCI care in Europe and the United States have met with a number of obstacles. Improved access to quality rehabilitation facilities close to home has made travel to regional centers less attractive to patients and families. Health care market forces also have played a role in limiting referrals to specialty centers. Competition for patients is often intense, and third-party payers may restrict the patients' choice of providers. These factors, while limiting the percentage of persons treated at specialized spinal cord centers, have not diminished the impact of such programs on the quality of care provided to this population worldwide. The United States Department of Education and the Veterans Administration have funded programs supporting hospital-based systems of comprehensive SCI care that have established and raised standards of patient care for nearly 30 years.

The benefits of SCI programs utilizing a system approach (i.e., coordination of emergency rescue, acute, rehabilitation, follow-up, and vocational services) have been documented. Patients admitted immediately after injury to such coordinated centers demonstrate better outcomes, including fewer medical complications,[145, 589] increased efficiency of rehabilitation gains,[264] higher percentages of discharges to private residences,[151] and reduced length of acute hospitalization and hospital charges. The most important contributions of such specialized programs, however, often go unnoticed. Clinicians and researchers at these centers have educated thousands of health care providers, founded and directed national and international academic and advocacy organizations, and contributed hundreds of research articles to the published literature in this field.

Recognizing the quality and scope of this research literature and the unique aspects of medical care in this setting, the Accreditation Council of Graduate Medical Education in the United States approved educational program training requirements in spinal cord injury medicine in 1996. By fulfilling these requirements, physicians who have completed an approved residency program in any American Board of Medical Specialties (ABMS) field relevant to SCI treatment become eligible for special qualifications examination and designation as a specialist in spinal cord injury medicine. The management of persons with spinal cord dysfunction requires a team and interspecialty approach, with contributions from relevant medical and surgical specialties as well as other health care professionals. The specialist in spinal cord injury medicine is trained to serve as the leader of this team.

Improvements in the acute treatment of SCI now allow even the most severely injured individuals to survive, placing a greater emphasis on the goal of improving quality of life. Persons with SCI no longer consider medical issues to be paramount in their existence; issues

TABLE 55–1 Life Expectancy for Persons with Spinal Cord Injuries Who Survive at Least 24 Hours Post Injury, by Age at Injury and Neurological Category (Frankel Grade)

	Life Expectancy (Years)				
Age at Injury	*Normal**	*C1–C4 Injury (Grade A, B, C)*	*C4–C8 Injury (Grade A, B, C)*	*T1–S5 Injury (Grade A, B, C)*	*Grade D*
5	70.8	37.3	47.7	55.7	61.4
10	65.9	32.9	43.1	51.0	56.6
15	61.0	28.5	38.4	46.3	51.8
20	56.3	25.3	34.3	42.1	47.5
25	51.6	22.4	30.5	38.1	43.3
30	46.9	19.3	26.5	34.0	39.0
35	42.2	16.5	22.9	30.0	34.6
40	37.6	14.2	19.5	26.2	30.3
45	33.0	12.2	16.4	22.6	26.0
50	28.6	9.7	13.1	18.7	21.9
55	24.4	7.3	10.2	15.0	18.1
60	20.5	5.0	7.8	11.6	14.8
65	16.9	3.5	5.8	8.9	11.8
70	13.6	2.2	4.0	6.7	9.0
75	10.7	1.3	2.7	4.8	6.7
80	8.1	0.3	1.6	3.2	4.6

* Normal values are from 1988 U.S. life tables for the general population.
Adapted from DeVivo MJ, Stover SL: Long term survival and causes of death. In Stover SL, DeLisa JA, Whiteneck GG (eds): Spinal Cord Injury: Clinical Outcomes from the Model Systems. Gaithersburg, MD, Aspen, 1995, p 297.

of community reintegration and socialization top the list of disability-related problems reported by this group.[193] As a person with a new injury regains health and confidence in his or her abilities, successful adjustment is promoted by a separation of the disabled person from the medical model of rehabilitation.[137, 449] Hospitals and physicians focus on illness, and chronic dependence on this system for emotional and social support forms a major barrier to reintegration. There is a common misperception that disabled persons need a lifetime of constant medical supervision. In reality, the rate of rehospitalization for medical complications actually declines as years pass after injury,[129] suggesting that adaptation to injury occurs on both a physiological and a psychological level. The ultimate goal of medical treatment is to allow these individuals the opportunity to live a satisfying personal and vocational life that is not dominated by medical problems.

EPIDEMIOLOGY

The differential diagnosis of spinal cord diseases resulting in paralysis is noted in Table 55–2. Persons with cancer metastatic to the spinal cord and those with degenerative spinal diseases outnumber patients with traumatic SCI.[404, 525] This heterogeneous group of patients is often overlooked in the provision of medical and rehabilitation services, usually because of advanced age or co-morbid medical conditions. Although a comprehensive discussion of all spinal cord diseases is beyond the scope of this chapter, most of the concepts of care related to traumatic SCI are pertinent and applicable to nontraumatic myelopathies.

Traumatic SCI is an uncommon condition. Not including persons who die at the scene of the accident, approximately 10,000 persons sustain SCI in the United States each year.[63, 177, 292, 312] Estimates of incidence in industrialized nations are similar, typically between 20 and 40 new cases per 1 million population each year. Prevalence studies estimate that 200,000 persons with SCI are living in the United States.[142, 211, 230, 255] The economic cost of SCI in the United States has been estimated at $7.2 billion per year.[149] The majority of injuries occur in young people, and the cumulative loss of years of potential employment, productivity, and good health creates a huge financial burden that, in many cases, must be absorbed by the social welfare and public health care systems. For many state Medicaid programs, SCI ranks among the most costly diagnoses.[317]

The United States Department of Education established the National Spinal Cord Injury Statistical Center (NSCISC) Database in 1973, based on the early data collection work of the Rehabilitation Services Administration (RSA) and Dr. John Young at the Barrow Neurologic Institute in Phoenix, Arizona. Since its inception, 24 Model Spinal Cord Injury Systems have submitted data on hundreds of variables related to their treatment of more than 18,000 injured persons. These data provide a detailed and reliable base of information regarding the scope and natural history of this condition.

SCI primarily affects young men. In the NSCISC database,[411] there has been no variation in the four-to-one male to female ratio of injury over the last two decades, although the average age at injury (currently 31.5 years) has slowly risen. The proportion of those older than 60 years at injury has nearly doubled (4.7% versus 9.7%) over the last 20 years. Both of these trends are consistent with the increase in median age of the general population. More than half (63.4%) of NSCISC patients were employed or in school at the time of their injury, and 53.7% were unmarried.

Significant changes in the racial distribution of persons included in this database have been observed. Al-

TABLE 55–2 Differential Diagnosis of Spinal Cord Injury

Traumatic (e.g., Fractures, Dislocations, Contusions)

Cervical (C1–C8)
Thoracic (T1–T12)
Lumbar (L1–L5)
Sacral
Multiple

Nontraumatic

Motor Neuron Diseases

Amyotrophic lateral sclerosis
Spinal muscular atrophy
Other motor neuron diseases

Spondylotic Myelopathies

Spondylolysis, spondylolisthesis
Spinal stenosis
Disk herniation, ruptures
Atlantoaxial instability

Infectious and Inflammatory Diseases

Multiple sclerosis
Epidural abscesses
Transverse myelitis
Poliomyelitis, post-poliomyelitis
Osteomyelitis
Arachnoiditis
Human immunodeficiency virus infection
Chronic inflammatory demyelinating polyradiculoneuropathy
Acute inflammatory demyelinating polyradiculoneuropathy

Neoplastic Diseases

1. Intradural intramedullary
   Primary: ependymoma, astrocytoma
   Metastatic: lung, breast, lymphoma, colorectal, head/neck, renal
2. Intradural extramedullary
   Primary: meningioma, neurofibroma, nerve sheath schwannoma, embryonal tumors
   Metastatic: leukemia/lymphoma, adenocarcinoma, untreated primary CNS tumors
3. Extradural
   Primary: myeloma, neuroblastoma, osteosarcoma, Ewing's sarcoma
   Metastatic: breast, lung, prostate, thyroid, kidney, lymphoma, gastrointestinal

Vascular Disorders

Ischemic myelopathy
Arteriovenous malformations

Toxic/Metabolic Conditions

Radiation-induced myelopathy
Subacute combined degeneration

Congenital/Developmental Disorders

Spina bifida
Developmental syringomyelia
Myelodysplasia

though the majority of persons injured are caucasian, large increases in the percentage of injuries sustained by African-American and Hispanic persons have been noted since the 1970s, especially in urban centers. Non-caucasian populations are disproportionately affected, when compared to racial frequencies in the general population.

The NASCIS database also shows a declining proportion of injuries due to motor vehicle crashes and sporting activities, while the proportion of injuries from acts of violence has nearly tripled since 1973.[507] Motor vehicle collisions (36.6%) have remained the most common cause of injury since 1991, followed by acts of violence (27.9%), falls (21.4%), and sports injuries (6.5%).[411] Injuries sustained by diving into water, both in the recreational and in the competitive setting, are arbitrarily classified as sporting injuries and constitute the most frequent cause of injury in this group. Several studies have confirmed that causes of injury differ by geographic region, race, age, and sex.[216] After age 45, falls supplant motor vehicle collisions as the most common cause of injury. As might be expected, women incur fewer injuries in sporting activities than men. In the African-American and Hispanic populations, acts of violence, not motor vehicle collisions, account for the majority of injuries.

Many of these injuries are preventable. Estimates of the rate of alcohol intoxication among those sustaining SCI range between 17% and 49%.[190, 263, 417] The majority of injuries occur on Saturday and Sunday, and the peak incidence occurs in the month of July.

ANATOMY, TERMINOLOGY, AND CLASSIFICATION OF INJURY

The International Standards for Neurological and Functional Classification of Spinal Cord Injury[11] provide a uniform language for description and analysis of traumatic spinal cord disorders. The classification of injuries is based on knowledge of the anatomy and function of the spinal cord and segmental nerves (Fig. 55–1).

The spinal cord extends from the foramen magnum to the lower border of the first lumbar vertebra, where it reaches a conical termination, the conus medullaris. Thirty-one functional segments (8 cervical, 12 thoracic, 5 lumbar, 5 sacral, and 1 coccygeal) receive and supply the paired dorsal and ventral root filaments that comprise the spinal nerves. The first cervical nerve, which usually lacks dorsal root fibers, has no corresponding dermatome. It exits the vertebral canal between the atlas and the occiput. The first seven cervical nerves exit the foramina above the vertebrae of their same number. The eighth cervical nerve emerges between C7 and T1. All the spinal nerves below this level exit the vertebral canal from the foramina beneath the vertebrae of the same number.

Knowledge of the blood supply of the spinal cord is helpful in understanding a number of injury syndromes.[486] The spinal cord is supplied by branches of the vertebral arteries and by anterior and posterior radicular arteries that arise from segmental vessels (i.e., ascending cervical, deep cervical, internal thoracic, intercostal, lumbar, and sacral arteries) and penetrate through the intervertebral foramina on the ventral surfaces of the nerve roots. A single radicular artery may become either an anterior or a posterior radicular artery, or it may divide to become both.[522]

Each vertebral artery gives rise to a posterior and an anterior spinal artery, but the anterior spinal arteries unite to form a single anterior midline vessel at the level of the medulla. The anterior spinal artery supplies the anterior two-thirds of the spinal cord, and is dependent on anastomotic branches from the anterior radicular arteries as it descends below the cervical spinal cord. In the thoracic region, the anterior spinal artery can be narrow and irregular, which places the spinal cord at risk should segmental vessels be occluded. The paired posterior spinal arteries supply the posterior third of the spinal cord, receiving blood from the posterior radicular arteries. They form a discontinuous plexus of vessels on the posterior surface of the spinal cord medial to the dorsal roots.

Radicular arteries vary considerably in number, and are most frequently located along the left side in the thoracic and lumbar regions. A large-caliber anterior radicular artery, the artery of Adamkiewicz, usually enters with a left lower thoracic or upper lumbar spinal root. This region of the spinal cord, along with the upper thoracic levels (which receive weak supply from the intercostal arteries), is particularly vulnerable to vascular compromise.

Accurate description and classification of an SCI depends on an appreciation of these anatomical arrangements and the performance of a detailed and systematic neurological examination of residual motor and sensory function. The injury is described both in terms of severity and in terms of the segmental level at which neurological impairment is noted. The examination is more than an exercise in neuroanatomy. The information obtained allows the clinician to counsel the patient about the potential for neurological improvement, as well as the future prognosis for function.

A useful SCI examination in the emergency setting requires the participation of an alert and cooperative patient but is often limited by concomitant brain injury, therapeutic sedation, or the influence of drug or alcohol intoxication.[358, 373] The initial examination is important in establishing an initial level of injury and for detecting secondary injuries to the cord during the first few days of hospitalization. For prognostic purposes, however, an examination at 72 hours is more reliable.[75] Evaluations of residual muscle and sensory function are the central elements of the examination. Examination of muscle stretch reflexes, including the bulbocavernosus reflex, is useful in assessing lesions of the lower motor neurons. In many instances, however, *spinal shock* can be encountered, in which upper motor neuron sensory and motor loss is associated with areflexia below the level of injury. Spinal shock is a poorly defined phenomenon. Reflex activity can often be detected by an electrophysiological study when it is not clinically apparent.[238] If lower motor neuron injury is not present, reflex activity typically returns over the course of weeks or months. The presence of spinal shock is of marginal prognostic significance, since a reliable examination and prognostic evaluation can be carried out when spinal shock is present.

The American Spinal Injury Association (ASIA) Impairment Scale (Fig. 55–1) is a modification of the Frankel classification,[181, 548] which has been used in almost every study of neurological outcomes in this population. It describes the degree of motor and sensory preservation below the level of injury and allows for description of the residual function of the injured spinal cord.[106] Injuries are rated along a spectrum ranging from functionally complete (grade A) to full motor and sensory preservation (grade E). Other clinical syndromes describe lesions that affect specific areas of the spinal cord. *Tetraplegia* results from an injury to the spinal cord within the cervical canal, with neurological deficits observed in the upper extremities, trunk, lower extremities, and visceral functions. In *paraplegia,* arm and hand function is normal, but deficits in neural control of the trunk, lower extremities, and visceral functions are brought about by SCI in the thoracic, lumbar, or sacral segments.

Central cord syndrome,[471] the most common of these clinical syndromes, is often associated with neck hyperextension injuries in older individuals with spondylosis.[252, 383, 462] This is an incomplete injury, characterized by weakness that is more severe in the arms than in the legs. Pathological findings of necrosis in the central spinal cord have been attributed to the sparse vascular supply in this area and to injury mechanics that place the greatest pressures on the center of the cord. The pattern of neurological deficit has traditionally been explained by the claim that the corticospinal tract is somatotopically organized, with fibers supplying upper extremity function lying medially, closer to the area of injury. There is limited evidence to support such organization, however, and other explanations for this syndrome have been suggested.[333] Traumatic central cord syndrome in the upper cervical spine is often referred to as *cruciate paralysis,*[43, 150] thought to result from midline damage to the rostral portion of the pyramidal decussation.

Brown-Séquard syndrome[463] is seen in association with a cord hemisection. Lesions of this type are characterized by ipsilateral muscle weakness and proprioception deficits. On the contralateral side, there is loss of sensation to pinprick caudal to one segment below the level of the lesion and loss of thermal sensation caudal to two segments below the lesion level. A clean hemisection injury is rare, and patients often exhibit lesions that mix characteristics of Brown-Séquard and central cord syndromes.

The *anterior cord syndrome* results from a lesion involving the anterior spinal artery or from direct trauma to the anterior two-thirds of the spinal cord. This can occur with retropulsion of disk or bone fragments and is sometimes associated with flexion injury of the cervical spine.[11] Anterior cord syndrome allows relative preservation of proprioception and light touch and deep-pressure sensation, but pain sensation and motor function are diminished below the level of injury.

The terms *conus medullaris syndrome* and *cauda equina syndrome* are often confused and misapplied in the description of lesions at the caudal region of the neuraxis.[424] Both syndromes are considered "paraplegic" injuries. A lesion of the conus medullaris is characterized by devastating deficits in bowel and bladder function, a symmetrical sensory deficit in the saddle distribution, and relatively minor deficits in lower extremity function. The deficits associated with cauda equina syndrome are asymmetrical and areflexic. The

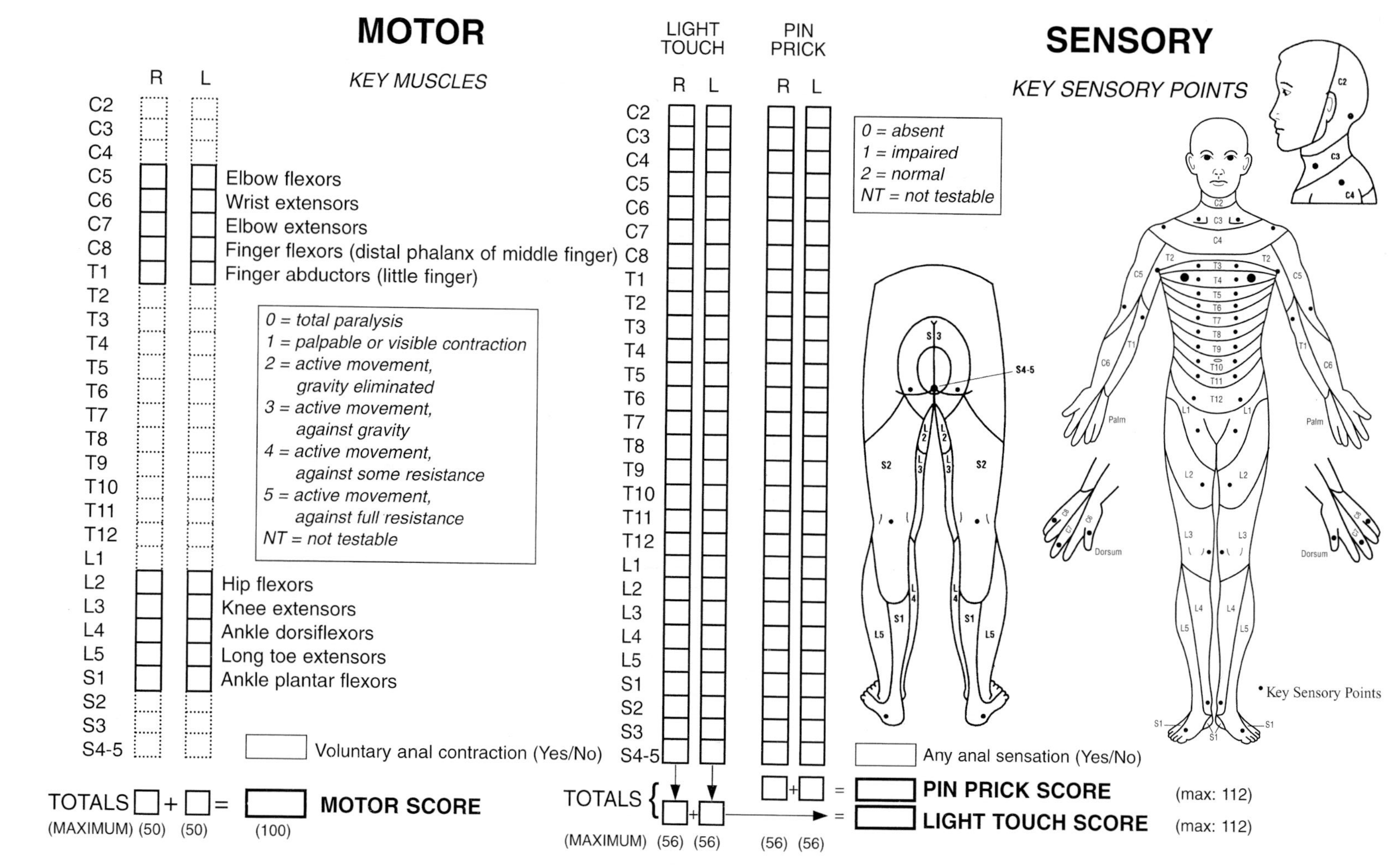

STANDARD NEUROLOGICAL CLASSIFICATION OF SPINAL CORD INJURY

MOTOR

KEY MUSCLES

	R	L	
C2			
C3			
C4			
C5			Elbow flexors
C6			Wrist extensors
C7			Elbow extensors
C8			Finger flexors (distal phalanx of middle finger)
T1			Finger abductors (little finger)
T2			
T3			
T4			
T5			
T6			
T7			
T8			
T9			
T10			
T11			
T12			
L1			
L2			Hip flexors
L3			Knee extensors
L4			Ankle dorsiflexors
L5			Long toe extensors
S1			Ankle plantar flexors
S2			
S3			
S4-5			

0 = total paralysis
1 = palpable or visible contraction
2 = active movement, gravity eliminated
3 = active movement, against gravity
4 = active movement, against some resistance
5 = active movement, against full resistance
NT = not testable

☐ Voluntary anal contraction (Yes/No)

TOTALS ☐ + ☐ = ☐ **MOTOR SCORE**
(MAXIMUM) (50) (50) (100)

SENSORY

KEY SENSORY POINTS

	LIGHT TOUCH R	LIGHT TOUCH L	PIN PRICK R	PIN PRICK L
C2				
C3				
C4				
C5				
C6				
C7				
C8				
T1				
T2				
T3				
T4				
T5				
T6				
T7				
T8				
T9				
T10				
T11				
T12				
L1				
L2				
L3				
L4				
L5				
S1				
S2				
S3				
S4-5				
TOTALS				
(MAXIMUM)	(56)	(56)	(56)	(56)

0 = absent
1 = impaired
2 = normal
NT = not testable

☐ Any anal sensation (Yes/No)

☐ **PIN PRICK SCORE** (max: 112)
☐ **LIGHT TOUCH SCORE** (max: 112)

NEUROLOGICAL LEVEL
The most caudal segment with normal function
SENSORY R ☐ L ☐
MOTOR R ☐ L ☐

COMPLETE OR INCOMPLETE? ☐
Incomplete = Any sensory or motor function in S4-S5

ASIA IMPAIRMENT SCALE ☐

ZONE OF PARTIAL PRESERVATION
Partially innervated segments
SENSORY R ☐ L ☐
MOTOR R ☐ L ☐

Version 4p
GHC 1996

FIGURE 55–1. *See legend on opposite page*

ASIA IMPAIRMENT SCALE

- ☐ **A = Complete:** No motor or sensory function is preserved in the sacral segments S4-S5.
- ☐ **B = Incomplete:** Sensory but not motor function is preserved below the neurological level and includes the sacral segments S4-S5.
- ☐ **C = Incomplete:** Motor function is preserved below the neurological level, and more than half of key muscles below the neurological level have a muscle grade less than 3.
- ☐ **D = Incomplete:** Motor function is preserved below the neurological level, and at least half of key muscles below the neurological level have a muscle grade of 3 or more.
- ☐ **E = Normal:** motor and sensory function is normal

CLINICAL SYNDROMES

- ☐ Central Cord
- ☐ Brown-Sequard
- ☐ Anterior Cord
- ☐ Conus Medullaris
- ☐ Cauda Equina

FIGURE 55–1. Standard neurological classification of spinal cord injury. (From American Spinal Association: International Standards for Neurological and Functional Classification of Spinal Cord Injury. Atlanta, American Spinal Injury Association, 1996.)

muscles affected exhibit atrophy and atonia. Patients with symmetrical weakness in lower extremity muscles across multiple myotomes are likely to have sustained a traumatic myelopathy above the level of the conus.

The *neurological level of injury* (Fig. 55–1) is defined as the most caudal neurological segment that retains normal sensory and motor function on both sides of the body. Often the neurological level of injury is different from the skeletal level of injury, and the segments where normal function is found often differ by side of body and in terms of sensory versus motor testing.[11] Up to four different segments can identify the neurological level (i.e., R-sensory, L-sensory, R-motor, and L-motor). In these instances, the assignment of a single neurological level might be misleading, and the injury is best described by detailing the four segments. Dermatomes and myotomes are assessed at 28 key sensory points and ten key muscles on each side. Muscles are graded from 0 (total paralysis) to 5 (provides full resistance).[123] The motor level (the lowest normal motor segment, which can differ by side of the body) is defined by the lowest key muscle that has a grade of 3 or better, provided that all the key muscles represented by segments above that level are judged to be normal (grade 5). Light touch and pinprick are used to determine the Sensory Index Score (SIS), with a maximum score of 224 for normal sensation. The Motor Index Score (MIS) is determined by adding the manual muscle test scores of the ten key muscles on each side, with a maximum of 100 points (20 key muscles with grade 5 strength).

A careful rectal examination is required to determine whether the injury is complete or incomplete. A complete lesion is defined as the absence of sensory or motor function in the lowest sacral segment. The use of this definition, proposed by Waters et al,[548] identifies a distinct subpopulation of injured persons who rarely change to incomplete status. If deep anal sensation or sensation at the anal mucocutaneous junction is reliably demonstrated or if there is voluntary control of the external anal sphincter, the lesion is incomplete.

NEUROLOGICAL PROGNOSIS AND FUNCTIONAL OUTCOMES

Virtually all patients who survive traumatic SCI experience some neurological recovery. For some patients this recovery results in an improved level of function. Recovery can be monitored by clinical examination and electrodiagnostic studies.[342] Recovery of neurological function in the segments near the zone of injury, or "root recovery," is distinguished from global improvements in spinal cord function that result in changes of injury grades within the ASIA Impairment Scale. In general, the best prognosis is in patients who initially exhibit some spared motor function and in those in whom neurological recovery is noted early after injury.[92, 180, 181, 367, 514, 614]

A number of studies[153, 549, 555, 565] have shown that in the interval between 1 month and 1 year post injury, the rate of motor recovery rapidly declines in the first 6 months, although gains in strength can be seen as late as 2 years after injury.[154] Patients with incomplete injuries recover faster in the zone of injury than those with complete injuries, but their degree of recovery is not necessarily greater.[355] Nearly all muscles with grade 1/5 or 2/5 strength 1 month after injury recover up to 3/5 (antigravity) strength by 1 year. Muscles with 0/5 strength that are located at the first neurological level below the most caudal segment having motor function typically recover antigravity strength in about one-third of cases. If the 0/5 muscle is two segments below the most caudal level exhibiting motor function, functional recovery is extremely rare.[549] The weakness of upper extremity muscles in tetraplegia likely reflects varying degrees of upper motor neuron and lower motor neuron damage. Electrodiagnostic analysis of compound muscle action potentials, as well as root mean square measurements of surface electromyographic (EMG) activity during voluntary muscle contractions, often helps distinguish upper from lower motor neuron weakness. Reha-

TABLE 55–3 Percentage Change in Frankel Grades from Admission to Discharge: 5658 Admissions Within 24 Hours of Injury, 1972–1992

Admission Grade	Discharge Grade				
	A	*B*	*C*	*D*	*E*
A	**88.8**	5.0	2.9	2.8	0
B	4.9	**48.9**	15.6	27.6	0.7
C	1.9	0.8	**41.4**	53.3	1.3
D	0.5	0.5	0.8	**90.3**	6.5
E	33.3	33.3	0	0	**33.3**

Data from Ditunno JF, et al. Functional Outcomes. In Stover SL, et al (eds): Spinal Cord Injury: Clinical Outcomes from the Model Systems. Gaithersburg, MD, Aspen, 1995, p 173.

bilitation efforts can be tailored on the basis of this information.[342]

Longitudinal studies utilizing the ASIA Impairment Scale and its predecessor, the Frankel classification,[181] have generated considerable data to describe the potential for recovery caudal to the zone of injury. Patients with complete injuries (grade A) have a poor prognosis for improvement, with estimates of changes in grade after such an injury ranging between 0% and 9%.[41, 42, 181, 358, 500, 605] Although late conversion of ASIA impairment grade A cases certainly can occur,[549, 559] retrospective analysis of these relatively rare cases has, in many instances, shown that concurrent conditions (e.g., concurrent brain injury, sedation) might have prevented an accurate initial examination.[367] The best information regarding conversion between grades comes from the NSCISC Model Systems database (Table 55–3). Analysis of Frankel grade changes within a group of over 5000 patients illustrates the more favorable outcome in those with incomplete injuries.[155]

Preservation of sensation alone carries an intermediate prognosis for neurological improvement. Preservation of pinprick sensation conveys a greater potential for ambulation recovery than preservation of light touch sensation, presumably due to the proximity of the spinothalamic and corticospinal tracts.[121, 180] The NSCISC data confirm the contention that persons with sparing of motor function below the zone of injury, including those with central cord syndrome and Brown-Séquard syndrome, have the best prognosis for recovery.[60, 180, 426, 463] The majority of persons with central cord syndrome ultimately attain functional use of their hands and control of bladder and bowel function. Recovery of ambulation in these patients correlates with a younger age at injury.[426] Patients with Brown-Séquard-type injuries have the best outlook; over 90% reach ambulatory status at 6 months post injury.[60, 341]

Functional Outcomes

The functional abilities of persons with SCI should be assessed in the areas of mobility, locomotion, feeding, dressing, grooming, bathing, and toileting (Table 55–4). Although these skills are generally described in reference to motor levels of injury,[48, 346, 597] many persons can master tasks that would not be predicted from the level of lesion alone.[592] Performance is influenced by

TABLE 55–4 Expectations for Function by Motor Level of Injury

Motor Level of Injury	Activities of Daily Living	Mobility and Locomotion
C1–C4	Feeding possible with balanced forearm orthoses Computer access by tongue, breath, voice controls Weight shifts with power tilt and recline chair Mouth stick use	Operate power chair with tongue, chin, or breath controller
C5	Drink from cup, feed with static splints and setup Oral/facial hygiene, writing, typing with equipment Dressing upper body possible Side-to-side weight shifts	Propel chair with hand rim projections short distances on smooth surfaces Power chair with hand controller
C6	Feed, dress upper body with setup Dressing lower body possible Forward weight shifts	Bed mobility with equipment Level surface transfers with assistance Propel chair indoors with coated hand rims
C7	Independent feeding, dressing, bathing with adaptive equipment, built-up utensils	Independent bed mobility Independent level surface transfers Wheelchair use outdoors (power chair for school or work)
C8	Independent in feeding, dressing, bathing Bowel and bladder care with setup	Propel chair, including curbs/wheelies Wheelchair-to-car transfers
T1	Independent in feeding, dressing, bathing Independent in bowel and bladder care	Transfer from floor to wheelchair
T2–L1	Independent in all self-care	Stand with braces for exercise Independent in transfers and wheelchair mobility
L2	Independent in all self-care	Potential for swing-to gait with long leg braces indoors Use of forearm crutches
L3	Independent in all self-care	Potential for community ambulation Potential for ambulation with short leg braces
L4–S1	Independent in all self-care	Potential for ambulation without assistive devices

such variables as age, body habitus, general health, concurrent injuries, spinal instrumentation, intelligence, and motivation.[599] In many instances complete independence in the performance of these tasks is not physically possible. In other situations, independent performance is possible but time constraints, energy costs, and environmental barriers are prohibitive.[564] A careful assessment of the patient's personal needs and social support is necessary to correctly identify the functional tasks that will be the most relevant after discharge from the rehabilitation setting. Insistence on independent functioning at all costs is often counterproductive. The most productive disabled individuals develop strategies to become successfully *interdependent*—making the most of help that is available from family, friends, hired assistants, and co-workers.

Several measurement and evaluation tools have been developed that allow clinicians to document and measure changes in functional status. Although these were developed chiefly in response to fiscal pressures, they have allowed clinicians to evaluate the efficacy and efficiency of the rehabilitation techniques employed in this setting in a scientific manner. The Functional Independence Measure (FIM)[248] has gained widespread use and has demonstrated validity and reliability. In the International Standards for Neurological and Functional Classification of Spinal Cord Injury, the FIM has been adopted as a means of systematic collection of outcome data for research and program evaluation purposes (see Chapter 8).

Although the general application of such uniform measurement tools as the FIM has facilitated many improvements in medical and rehabilitation care, their relevance to SCI treatment is often overestimated. Mobility and locomotion skills typically receive heavy emphasis in these scales, while gains in medical stability, patient and family knowledge, and community integration are not well represented. For persons with tetraplegia, what they learn about their bodies, their condition, and their potential represents much of the true benefit of their time in the hospital rehabilitation setting. They learn to engage caregivers and to direct the caregiver's assistance. In this situation, the patient with high tetraplegia might make remarkable progress toward a successful home discharge while showing virtually no improvement on functional outcome scales. The Quadriplegic Index of Function[229] and the Modified Barthel Index[597] have been developed in hopes of better describing functional gains in this population. The patient's level of disability might also not be the best predictor of handicap or of ultimate life quality. Studies employing measures such as the Craig Handicap Assessment and Reporting Technique[594] and the Life Situation Questionnaire[315] have demonstrated that the SCI patient's disability is just one of many determinants of outcomes in personal and vocational settings.[141]

THE REHABILITATION PROCESS

Through its staff and traditions, the successful hospital rehabilitation program imparts the understanding that it is possible to lead a happy and productive life despite the tragic losses associated with SCI. Despite a trend toward shorter hospitalizations for persons with SCI, the rehabilitation process in the broadest sense extends for years after the injury. It is impossible to measure the magnitude of personal loss experienced by a person with tetraplegia. Readjustment and adaptation can be a slow process, a critical point to consider when planning for the provision of rehabilitation services. While physical restrictions might be overcome fairly rapidly by environmental modifications and assistive equipment, the loss of freedom and change in body image cannot be reconciled so quickly. Adults with a new and severe disability must be allowed, if possible, to restart life at their own pace. A premature and unsuccessful return to the workplace, for example, only reinforces negative perceptions of the disabled held by the patient, the family, and the employer.

The rehabilitation process for persons with acute SCI begins in the intensive care setting. During this time, many medical and surgical problems occupy the attention of the doctors, nurses, patients, and families. Nevertheless, it is important to maintain a focus on the patient's projected functional potential and to anticipate problems that can have a long-term functional impact. Clinicians often debate difficult decisions regarding acute spinal surgery and cardiopulmonary management while the basic elements of nursing and rehabilitation care are ignored. The benefits of timely and proficient treatment in the intensive care setting can be negated by the development of a pressure ulcer that results in weeks of restricted activity.

The initial therapy process focuses on joint protection and maintenance of range of motion (ROM). Proper positioning in bed is critical, and ROM exercises are carried out one to three times a day, depending on the degree of muscle tone present in the extremities. Although most patients will experience arm, shoulder, and spinal pain in this setting, careful instruction of family members in these techniques can offer an excellent opportunity for their active involvement. In tetraplegic persons, particular care is taken to guard against shortening of shoulder adductor muscles, which would limit shoulder abduction. The wrists and ankles often need protective splints to preserve ROM (Fig. 55–2).

In the face of such a devastating medical condition, patients, family, and staff members often place an inappropriate urgency on starting strengthening exercise and aggressive conditioning programs. This can be particularly harmful in tetraplegic persons with borderline pulmonary reserve. Many of these patients are in a catabolic state, using all of their energy just to breathe and clear their lungs of secretions. There is nothing to be gained at this point by insisting that the patient sit in a chair for extended periods or engage in resistive exercises.

Patients and families benefit from meeting with members of the rehabilitation team early in the hospital course. Education regarding the rehabilitation process often helps reduce feelings of ignorance and helplessness. There is no single best way to counsel patients and families regarding prognosis. These discussions must take into account the patient's premorbid personality,

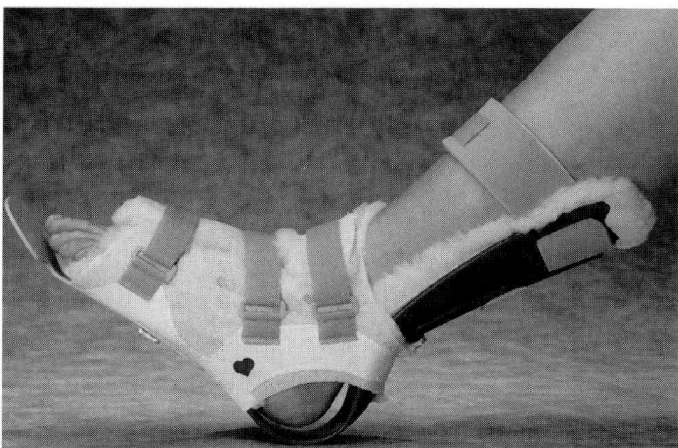

FIGURE 55–2. Heel suspension ankle-foot orthosis. (Courtesy of Mulitpodus boot/RCAI Inc.)

maturity, and status in life. Clinicians worried about creating false hope are as likely to create false pessimism. An overview of the rehabilitation process must not ignore the obvious; most persons with SCI are young, and 80% are male. Many were injured by violent acts or have a history of risk-taking behavior. Their disability occurs at a time when they are only beginning to develop an adult identity. In this setting, the need for counseling and support usually quickly outpaces the need for medical intervention.

As the patient achieves medical stability, effective use of resources requires that therapy be *goal oriented.* The program should be designed to achieve significant progress toward realistic functional goals. The patient, not the process, must be kept at the center of attention. In the optimal situation, the therapy disciplines work cooperatively with the nursing staff to promote the carryover of learned techniques into the daily routine. Integration of the family in this setting must be carried out with sensitivity, respecting that while the period of rehabilitation treatment is brief, many family members will be called on to serve as lifelong caregivers. The therapy team must be willing to work *within* the constraints of dysfunctional family relationships. Trying to drive a wedge between family members or to inappropriately change family dynamics in this setting is often counterproductive.

Scheduled meetings with the patient and family are an important part of the SCI rehabilitation process. These meetings should be carefully managed, productive, and occur at a minimum expense of staff treatment time. The meeting provides an opportunity for the team to show that a coordinated rehabilitation plan is being developed—a plan that is based on the input of the patient and family and on a genuine concern for the patient's individual needs. Patients and families bring considerable anxiety to these meetings. Team members best respond to this tension by presenting a positive, confident, and competent demeanor. Differences in opinion among staff members should be resolved prior to the meeting. Adequate preparation allows team members to give presentations that are succinct and well-coordinated. Inexperienced team members should be adequately supervised, and communication should include a careful avoidance of excessive medical jargon. Even when a large number of family members are present, team members must remember to address their comments directly to the patient.

This is a poor setting for resolving conflict between the team and the patient or family. Confronting a group of professionals in a hospital meeting room can be a threatening experience for the patient and family. Rehabilitation hospital language, rules, and culture are invariably unfamiliar. Team members should make every effort to interact on an individual basis with the patient and family before the meeting, to identify questions and remedy concerns. It is the job of the rehabilitation team member to bring solutions, rather than problems, to the table.

The central issue of prognosis must be addressed early on in the rehabilitation course. While the team typically sets goals based on the patient's current physical capabilities and the economic constraints of short hospital stays, patients usually set goals based on hopes for recovery. Team members must acknowledge this inherent conflict. Patients usually want a cure, not rehabilitation. It is important to give patients permission to hope for a full recovery, even as we know that the best medical opinion is not for full recovery.[398] Over the course of their stay, most patients gradually learn to view their disability from a different perspective, allowing them to make realistic plans for the immediate future.

Patients are required to assimilate a large amount of information in a short time period. The best rehabilitation programs offer a highly structured educational environment. Ideally, each patient should have a completely individualized treatment plan. This eclectic approach is usually not practical, however, as multiple therapists and three shifts of nurses cannot adequately master dozens of different treatment approaches. Poor communication among staff members and an inconsistent level of understanding of treatment plans become immediately apparent to the patient, with resulting loss of the team's credibility. There are many means by which the patient can achieve success with bladder, bowel, skin, and mobility management. However, it is best to develop a small number of treatment protocols and ensure that they are taught in a confident, consistent, and competent manner.

SPECIAL COMPONENTS OF THE REHABILITATION PROCESS

The treatment team can call on a wide variety of rehabilitation approaches to augment or restore function lost after paralysis. Traditional therapeutic exercise, functional training, and aerobic conditioning are augmented by the use of adaptive equipment and orthotic devices, tendon transfer surgery, and functional electrical stimulation. These modalities facilitate community reintegration by enhancing community reintegration and vocational rehabilitation.

Assistive Devices

The ability of the person with SCI to manipulate the environment might depend on the proper prescription of assistive devices and adaptive equipment (Table 55–5). Occupational therapists specialize in the instruction of patients in the use of devices (adapted utensils, long-handled reachers, sock and pant pullers, button hooks) that circumvent deficits in upper extremity function (see Chapter 25). Although some assistive devices may cost only a few dollars, items such as wheelchairs, adapted vehicles, and environmental control devices are expensive. These products should be prescribed by a person knowledgeable in the field. Those with limited experience often overprescribe, employing more technology than is necessary to solve a mobility problem or an environmental barrier. A higher level of technology does not guarantee a higher level of function. As devices become more complicated, breakdowns become more common, and the crucial fit at the user-device interface becomes more tenuous.

The best SCI rehabilitation programs make available a variety of sample assistive devices (wheelchairs, computers, adapted vehicles) that allow the patient to evaluate each item before a prescription is made (Fig. 55–3). Staff members should not feel compelled to order expensive equipment prior to the date of hospital discharge. In many instances, equipment vendors are willing to provide loaner equipment for a brief period until the definitive prescription is made. A wheelchair that is appropriate for a young SCI patient at 8 weeks post injury, for example, might be quite inappropriate at 12 weeks, as balance, strength, weight distribution, and even neurological status continue to change.

The goals of wheelchair prescription are to enhance mobility and locomotion, maximize pulmonary function, and prevent postural deformities, pain, and pressure sores (see Chapters 18 and 31).[306, 511, 579, 609] The newfound freedom afforded by a wheelchair can bring about a remarkable change in attitude and enhanced participation in newly injured patients who have spent weeks in bed. The treatment team helps the patient establish priorities for wheelchair use, anticipating the variety of situations and environments that the patient will encounter. The team must make clear the long-term importance of preventing pressure ulcers and protecting the shoulder joints. Compromises must be made with any prescription. The fastest and lightest wheelchair might be too unstable. The best cushion might restrict transfers to and from the chair, or it might require considerable maintenance.

The minimalist "use it or lose it" view emphasizes that patients should use the least amount of technology possible. Persons with lower level tetraplegia, however, are often appropriate for powered mobility. The energy saved from pushing the chair can be used for wheelchair transfers, weight shifts, and vocational activities, reducing the long-term wear and tear on joints and soft tissues. For those who need advanced technology and customized seating systems, rehabilitation engineers can help patients navigate through the enormous array of commercial components that are available. Despite aggressive marketing and advertising claims, the differences between many commercial components are negligible. An experienced local vendor can help guide choices. Whenever possible, these systems should be easily repairable in the patient's own community.

Computers play an ever-increasing role in SCI rehabilitation. Modifications of workstations in the rehabilitation hospital computer laboratory can allow the patient to improve arm strength and hand function while learning computer skills. Keyboards and peripheral devices can be adapted in a fashion that requires the patient to use specific muscle groups in isolation. In young patients, such activities take the place of traditional and less stimulating methods of strengthening (i.e., pegboards, finger ladders, arts and crafts, finger putty). Many disabled persons find unique opportunities to socialize, network, and gather information over the Internet. The computer can be even more important in the vocational rehabilitation setting. Breath-, voice-, and tongue-activated controllers now permit persons with no arm function to operate computers in an efficient fashion, and these controls can be integrated into a power wheelchair control system (Fig. 55–3). Computer access may be the best remedy for the consistently low rate of return to work in this population.[143]

Upper Extremity Functional Intervention

The techniques used to augment upper limb function range from simple splinting and positioning approaches to the most complex neuroprosthetic interventions. In the intensive care setting of acute SCI, attention to basic joint positioning and protection sets the stage for later work on strengthening and dexterity. For persons with tetraplegia through the C7 level, proper hand position is maintained by resting splints, which allow tightening of the flexor tendons. Many families and patients desire a cosmetic, "flat hand" position, and education regarding the use of tenodesis for hand function needs to be undertaken. Preventing of elbow flexor shortening can spell the difference between independent and assisted wheelchair transfers.[233] Maintenance of pronation range at the elbow is also critical, allowing patients to work with palms down in tabletop activities. As spinal and medical stability is achieved, work on strengthening innervated muscles can begin. For anxious patients with only a few functioning muscles, there is a high risk of muscle overwork and soft tissue strain. The treating occupational therapist should establish a monitored program of strengthening. Most patients with SCI report shoulder, neck, and arm pain early on, and these symptoms should be carefully monitored by the physician.

Patients can learn to compensate for impaired muscles by substitution movements, utilizing gravity and momentum and creating multiarticular closed kinetic chains (Table 55–6).[139, 351, 357, 612] These substitution movements can be used to improve respiratory function, to assist with weight shifting and transfer skills, and to facilitate proper hand positioning and dexterity. Compensatory patterns (use of two hands, mouth, or chin) are also used.

TABLE 55–5 Interventions and Supplies

International Classification System by Motor Level	C2	C3	C4	C5	C6	C7	C8	T1	T2–T5	T6–L1	L2	L3	L4	L5	S1	S2–S4
Self-Care/Orthoses																
Mouth stick	S	S	S													
Balanced forearm orthosis				U	S											
Drop-arm commode										S	S	S	S			
Bath bench				U	U	U	U	U	U	S	S	S	S	S	S	
Utensil cuffs/adaptation				U	U	U	S									
Skin mirror				S	U	U	U	U	U	U	S	S				
Reacher/long-handled sponge					U	U	U	U	U	S	S	S				
Resting hand splints	S	S	S	S	S	S	S									
Long opponens splint	U	U	U	U	S											
Short opponens splint					U	U	S	S								
Suppository inserter					S	S	S	S								
Rope ladder/leg lifter				U	U	U	S	S	S							
Rolling shower chair	S	S	S	S	S	S										
Electric leg bag opener	U	U	U	S	S	S										
Adapted leg bag clamp					U	U	U	S	S							
Mobility/Functional Restoration																
Tongue touch controller	S	S	S													
Sip-and-puff/chin switch	S	S	S													
Adapted personal computer	U	U	U	U	U	S	S									
Power recline wheelchair	U	U	U	U	S	S	S	S	S							
Power wheelchair	U	U	U	U	U	S	S	S	S							
Lightweight manual chair				U	U	U	U	U	U	U	S	S	S			
Wheelchair ramp	U	U	U	U	U	U	U	U	U	U	S	S	S			
Wheelchair cushion	U	U	U	U	U	U	U	U	U	U	U	U	U			
Transfer board	U	U	U	U	U	U	S	S	S							
Transfer lift device	U	U	U	U	S	S	S									
Auto hand controls						U	U	U	U	U	U	U	U			
Van with lift	U	U	U	U	S	S	S	S	S	S						
Adapted van driving system					U	U	S	S	S	S						
Leg braces									S	S	U	U	U	U	S	

Tendon Transfer and Neuroprostheses																
Phrenic nerve pacemaker	S	S	S													
Hand grasp neuroprosthesis				S	S											
Elbow extension transfer				S	S											
Tenodesis grip transfer					S	S										
One-stage pinch transfer					S	S										
Two-stage finger transfer					S	S										
Intrinsic transfers					S	S										
Bladder neuroprosthesis	S	S	S	S	S	S	S	S	S	S						
Medical Devices																
Primary and backup ventilator	U	U	S													
Aerosol nebulizer	U	U	S													
Portable suction machine	U	U	S													
Abdominal binder	U	U	U	U	U	U	U	U	S	S						
Elastic stockings	U	U	U	U	U	U	S	S	S	S	S	S	S			
Ankle-foot boots	U	U	U	U	U	S	S	S	S	S	S	S	S			
Blood pressure cuff and stethoscope	U	U	U	U	U	U	U	U	U							
Electric hospital bed	U	U	U	U	U	S	S	S	S	S						
Special mattress	S	S	S	S	S	S	S	S	S	S						
Urinary catheter supplies	U	U	U	U	U	U	U	U	U	U	U	S	S	S	S	
Suppositories/gloves	U	U	U	U	U	U	U	U	U	U	U	U	U	S	S	
Incontinence pads	U	U	U	U	U	U	U	U	U	S	S	S	S			
Grab bars				S	S	S	S	S	S	S	S	S	S	S		
Arm ergometer				S	S	S	S									

Key: U Usually required
S Sometimes required
Rarely required

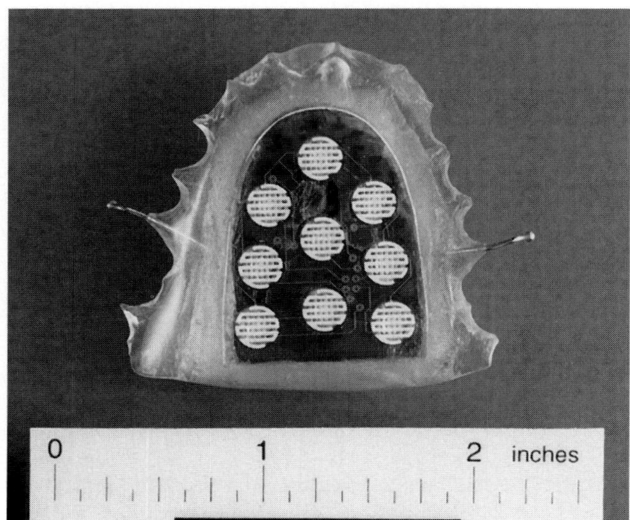

FIGURE 55–3. Tongue-touch keypad controller is fitted into a dental retainer, allowing persons with limited hand function to operate wheelchairs, computer keyboards, and environmental controls. (Courtesy of newAbilities Systems Inc., Palo Alto CA.)

Upper limb orthoses are commonly prescribed for persons with injury levels between C4 and C8. Balanced forearm orthoses and mobile arm supports augment weak deltoid and biceps muscles. These devices employ a counterweight/fulcrum mechanism to support the distal forearm, allowing the patient with a C4 or C5 injury to position the hand for tabletop activities (see Chapters 15 and 25). The devices can be used for strengthening, training, and as functional assist devices.

Persons with a C5 injury can position their hands but need long opponens orthoses to provide wrist stability. This static splint can be fabricated to include utensil slots and penholders. Functional neuromuscular stimulation devices have been studied in persons with this level of injury for nearly 40 years.[347] An implanted multichannel neuroprosthesis developed at Case–Western Reserve University is now commercially available.[300] This system provides persons injured at the C5 and C6 level with active hand grasp capabilities, controlled by sensors activated by contralateral shoulder muscles.

Functional abilities improve significantly with the addition of wrist extensor muscles at the C6 level of injury.[598] Active wrist extension results in tenodesis of the hand. This passive movement is characterized by the opposition of thumb and index finger, with flexion of the fingers occurring as the wrist extends against static finger flexor tendons. With wrist control at the C6 level, patients can use short opponens orthoses or utensil cuffs to feed themselves. The Rancho Wrist Driven Flexor Hinge Orthosis utilizes a mechanical ratchet lock to improve tenodesis pinch force. Although this device is expensive and patient acceptance is only fair, some patients can achieve sufficient pinch strength to perform urinary catheterization and bowel routine maneuvers. As an alternative, a simple tenodesis orthosis ("RIC orthosis") can be fabricated by the occupational therapist for the purposes of training and evaluation.

Patients with injury levels C7 and C8 need few orthotic interventions. The addition of finger extension and wrist flexion can augment grasp strength. Short opponens splints and utensil cuffs are often utilized. Pencil and utensil use can often be accomplished by weaving the device through the fingers, provided that sufficient tightness of the finger flexors is present. For those with C8 finger flexors, utensils with built-up handles can improve grip stability.

Upper Extremity Tendon Transfers

Tendon transfers and upper limb reconstructive surgery, long available only at select SCI centers, have recently gained more acceptance as a useful means of restoring elbow extension, wrist extension, and rudimentary hand function. Tendon transfers impart a significant improvement in function, both in adults and in children.[186, 277, 392, 393, 401, 610] These procedures are considered 1 year post injury, keeping in mind that upper limb muscle recovery (especially in wrist extensors) can occur over the course of 2 years or more.[153] This period allows patients to assess their upper extremity capabilities and compensatory strategies in their home and vocational environment, and to identify their goals for intervention. Patients with remote tetraplegia can also be considered, but outcomes are often less predictable.[270] In selecting appropriate candidates for these procedures, it is important to acknowledge that many patients can achieve a high level of upper limb function with the conservative means detailed above. Although the surgery itself is typically brief, splinting and prolonged immobilization of the arms might render the patient totally dependent for 3 to 6 weeks,[288, 392] and preoperative functional abilities can be temporarily lost. This can result in a major disruption in the patient's personal and vocational life,

TABLE 55–6 Common Muscle Substitutions After Spinal Cord Injury

Desired Action	Alternative Muscle
Triceps: extension of the elbow	1. External rotation of humerus at shoulder + gravity + eccentric contraction of biceps 2. Pectoralis major/anterior deltoid through closed kinetic chain
Flexor digitorum: finger flexion	Tenodesis with wrist extension
Wrist flexion	Gravity + eccentric contraction of wrist extensors
Finger intrinsic muscles: abduction	Lateral action of finger extensors
Pronator teres: forearm pronation	Adduction/internal rotation of humerus
Intercostal muscles: active lung expiration	Sternal pectoralis major action on thorax
Elevation of pelvis	Latissimus dorsi (shoulder depression) through closed kinetic chain

and requirements for caregiver assistance are commonly altered.

The International Classification of the Upper Limb in Quadriplegia (Table 55–7)[370] is used to describe the residual upper limb function where surgical management is considered. To achieve designation of a motor group, the tested muscles must achieve a grade of 4 or 5. This classification system also takes into account the importance of sensation. Patients who depend on visual feedback because of impaired finger sensation are less likely to have a positive functional outcome, and are not candidates for bilateral reconstruction.[186]

Restoring elbow extension in persons with C5 level injuries by posterior deltoid to triceps muscle transfer enables overhead and forward reaching and enhances performance of grooming, hygiene, and tabletop activities. Brachioradialis transfers to the wrist extensors produce a weak tenodesis grip and allow patients to manipulate light objects without an orthosis.[186, 401, 557] For those with C6 and C7 level injuries, there are many surgical options that can restore key-pinch and palmar grasp function (Table 55–7).

TABLE 55–7 Surgery to Enhance Upper Extremity Function in Tetraplegia: International Classification[370]

	Available Muscles Grade 4–5/5	Transfers and Reconstruction—Examples
Motor Groups		
0	None below elbow	Posterior deltoid to triceps (Moberg, 1975,[392] 1975) Biceps to triceps (Zancolli, 1979[610])
1	Brachioradialis (BR)	BR to ECRB (Freehafer, 1967) Flexor pollicus longus (FPL) tenodesis (McDowell, 1986[370])
2	ECRL	BR to ECRB/L BR to FPL (Waters, 1985)
3	ECRB	ECRL to flexor digitorum profundus (FDP) (Lamb, 1972)
4	Pronator Teres (PT)	BR to FDP + PT opponensplasty (Freehafer, 1984[186]) Two-stage House procedure (1985[277])
5	FCRB	As above
6	Finger extensors	As above, without finger extensor transfer
7	Thumb extensors	As above, without thumb extension transfer
8	Partial finger flexors	FDS lasso for intrinsic balance (House, 1985[277])
9	Lacks intrinsics only	Two-stage Zancolli procedure (1979[610])
Sensory Groups		
O	Ocular sensibility; two-point discrimination > 10 mm in the thumb	
Cu	Cutaneous sensibility; two-point discrimination < 10 mm in the thumb	

Abbreviations: ECRL, extensor carpi radialis longus; ECRB, extensor carpi radialis brevis; FCRB, flexor carpi radialis brevis; EDC, extensor digitorum communis; EPL, extensor pollicis longus; FDS, flexor digitorum sublimis.

Once healing has occurred, a successful outcome depends on closely supervised and coordinated postsurgical rehabilitation. Occupational therapy is essential to ensure proper positioning and gradual muscle reeducation and to diminish the formation of scar tissue. For hand transfers, night splints are used for 3 months to maintain transfer tightness.[272] All of this requires considerable commitment and motivation on the part of the patient.

Lower Extremity Functional Interventions

Walking is a goal of every person with newly acquired paralysis. Persons who ambulate at the community level after SCI usually have retained at least 4/5 strength in both hip flexors and in at least one quadriceps muscle.[280, 346] It is possible for almost every patient to achieve some type of vertical posture through the use of orthoses, standing frames or standing wheelchairs.[592] Although the psychological benefit of this activity might be high, there is little evidence that standing or limited ambulation is of physiological benefit in reducing osteoporosis or any of the other adverse medical sequelae of injury.[54] It is uncommon for patients with thoracic level paraplegia to use long leg braces for ambulation outside of the house. Rejection rates for long leg braces can be as high as 75%. Most of these patients don them only for exercise, or lose interest entirely once the high energy cost of their use becomes apparent. The energy expenditure of ambulation with long leg braces can be increased as much as 12 times per unit distance.[220, 377]

Ambulation outcomes are optimized when attention is given during the acute phase of injury to maintenance of hip extension and ankle dorsiflexion ROM through exercises and splinting (see Fig. 55–2). Factors that contribute to loss of joint ROM (heterotopic ossification, spasticity, pain) should receive aggressive treatment. Patients with leg weakness might need excessive lumbar lordosis to balance in the standing position, but this degree of spinal range of motion can be absent in those with lumbosacral spinal fusions. These persons also place unusual and excessive forces across sites of spinal fractures during standing activities, raising the risk of instrumentation and fusion failure in the first few months after injury.

Prediction of ambulation recovery is commonly based on examination of motor function shortly after injury. The presence of quadriceps function is a positive indicator of ambulation potential.[122] An ambitious prospective study carried out by researchers at Rancho Los Amigos Hospital detailed the neurological and functional recovery and function of 263 patients with paraplegia.[550, 554] There is a strong correlation between the physiological determinants of gait and the ASIA lower extremity motor score (five ASIA muscles each side graded 0 to 5, maximum score = 50).[556] Lower extremity motor score at 1 month is predictive of further motor recovery and the achievement of community ambulation status at 1 year. The majority of patients with lower extremity motor score greater than 10 at 1 month achieve community ambulation status at 1 year. Use of such a scoring system has disadvantages, however. The lower extremity motor score of incomplete tetraplegic patients might be the same as that for persons with incomplete paraplegia, but upper extremity deficits limit the use of assistive devices. In addition, the relationship between manual muscle test grade and contractile strength is nonlinear, and considerable variability in muscle performance among individuals can be attributed to body size and physical conditioning.

Lower extremity bracing (see Chapter 16) can help compensate for deficits in muscle strength, but energy costs associated with extensive bracing usually prohibit community-level ambulation.[551] Traditional knee-ankle-foot orthoses (KAFOs), or long leg braces, include a upper and lower thigh band, drop locks, and a double-action ankle joint. Custom-molded thermoplastic calf and shank sleeves are now commonly used in place of leather bands and extended metal uprights. Extension of the brace to include hip and trunk bands is possible for persons who lack hip control, but this does not enhance function.[545] The lighter Scott-Craig KAFO design allows easier donning and doffing and more efficient ambulation.[416] The lower calf and thigh bands of the standard KAFO are eliminated. In addition, this brace includes a hinged anterior tibial band, with snap locks, a bail knee lock, a proximal thigh band, and a reinforced footplate. The tibial band generates a force close to the knee for added stability, analogous to a patellar tendon-bearing prosthesis. It is not likely that patients will continue to use their braces after training unless they can ambulate nonstop more than 300 yards and use their braces all day.[105, 412]

Community ambulation is promoted through the use of a reciprocal gait pattern, a pattern that is virtually impossible using bilateral long leg braces.[559] Reciprocating orthoses have been developed that transform a passive rigid orthosis into an active, articulating orthosis by simulating hip flexion (see Chapter 16).[477] Examples of this design include the Louisiana State University Reciprocal Gait Orthosis,[160] the Hip Guidance Orthosis (HGO, or Parawalker),[423] and the Advanced Reciprocating Gait Orthosis (ARGO).

These devices allow the lower limb to advance when body weight is shifted from side to side. This is carried out by an isocentric mechanism or reciprocating cable incorporated into articulated hip joints. These orthoses are expensive to fabricate and require considerable formal therapy training for safe use. Adults with SCI can use them for therapeutic ambulation indoors on smooth surfaces. Patients often resort to swing-to gait patterns, abandoning the reciprocal motion. The ARGO has a modular design that allows the patient to test a temporary orthosis before committing to a definitive prescription. Prescription of these braces is best reserved for patients who have demonstrated consistent and regular use of their KAFOs.[285] There is no evidence that these braces offer a better long-term acceptance rate than standard KAFOs. Children with SCI might be better candidates for these interventions than adults, owing to differences in body habitus and energy levels.

Researchers in the field of functional neuromuscular stimulation have attempted to improve standing and gait performance by means of electrical stimulation of upper motor neuron paralyzed muscles, and by combining this stimulation with lower limb bracing.[310] Research on standing by persons with SCI began in 1960,[293] and the first commercial system (Parastep, Sigmedics) became available in 1990. This system requires the use of a walker and stimulation of the glutei and quadriceps for standing. The peroneal nerve is stimulated to produce a reflex flexion withdrawal response of the hip and forward stepping. Other systems (e.g., the Parawalker) combine orthoses and stimulation.[160, 273, 432, 489] Such hybrid designs can offer the potential for energy conservation, since reciprocating orthoses used in combination with functional neuromuscular stimulation devices have been shown to be more energy efficient than the latter alone or reciprocating orthosis systems alone.[273] A multichannel, fully implanted system has long been under study, but issues of practicality and reliability remain.[359] Simple surface electrical stimulation of the quadriceps muscle alone can be used for standing exercise[591] in many patients.

At the present time the clinical applications of lower extremity functional neuromuscular stimulation systems are limited, and decades of research have failed to achieve results that are superior to standard orthotic management. The cost of fitting such systems and their rehabilitation is high, and the distances that can be traveled are short. Electrical stimulation reverses the natural recruitment order of muscle fibers, resulting in severe and accelerated fatigue compared with that induced by normal muscle contraction. Fatigue of electrically stimulated muscles is an important limiting factor in lower extremity applications. Patients with intact or partial sensation can also find the stimulation painful or uncomfortable. It has been estimated that less than 11% of SCI persons are appropriate for these systems.[284] Patients who are most likely to benefit from participation in functional neuromuscular stimulation research are those who are coping well with their disabilities and have realistic expectations.[262, 595, 596]

Driver Rehabilitation

Driver rehabilitation is a critical component of successful community reintegration, even though funding support is often limited.[307, 435] The driver rehabilitation program evaluates driving ability and training needs, assists with state licensing issues, recommends passenger vehicles and modifications, and offers counseling regarding utilization of community transit services. Occupational and physical therapists, rehabilitation engineers, and vehicle technicians are important members of the team. Particular expertise is required for prescription of auto and van modifications. A prescription for van modifications should not be dispensed until the driver has been tested using the specific adapted driving equipment being considered.

Assessment of driving potential involves evaluation of vision, cognition, dynamic balance, and level of spasticity, as well as an assessment of the client's available muscle strength, proprioception, and ROM. Seating systems are assessed, with the focus on stability, field of vision, access to controls, and ease in transferring in and out of the vehicle. For persons with paraplegia, simple and effective vehicle hand controls have been available for over 50 years. For persons with tetraplegia, several commercially available vehicle guidance systems are available, employing joystick, computerized servo-control, and zero-effort technologies. Although these systems are in fairly common use, their safety and reliability have not been adequately studied.

Vocational Rehabilitation

Over 63% of persons in the NSCISC database reported being employed or in school at the time of their injury.[411] Return to work after injury is recognized as one of the indicators of recovery from injury, and some consider it a gauge of rehabilitation success.[151] Estimates of employment rates after injury range from 13% to 48%, with much of the variation attributed to inconsistent definition of the term "working."[518] In the NSCISC group, 37% of persons with paraplegia and 30% of persons with tetraplegia were employed by injury year 8. This information confirms other studies, from which a profile regarding post-injury re-employment can be drawn.[141, 143, 314, 353, 580] Those with paraplegia have higher re-employment rates than those with tetraplegia. Persons with incomplete injuries and those who incur SCI at a younger age are more likely to become employed. A lower employment rate occurs with low pre-injury education levels, minority race, and poor pre-injury vocational experience.[151] Several disincentives, chiefly the risk of losing disability income and public-funded medical insurance, make a return to work an unattractive proposition for many. In addition, despite the passage of the Americans With Disabilities Act in 1990, persons with disabilities are often subjected to discrimination and prejudice in the employment setting. The vocational counselor on the SCI treatment team helps age-appropriate clients negotiate these barriers by evaluating their background and re-employment potential, by developing a plan for job reentry, and by facilitating contact with supportive state and local agencies. There is good evidence that completion of such a program makes employment more likely.[143] There is more at stake than wages and productivity, since work provides a sense of purpose and the motivation to keep oneself healthy and active (see Chapter 35).[542]

MEDICAL CONDITIONS

With so many persons surviving for decades after their injuries, the myriad effects of paralysis on virtually every organ system have come into clearer focus. For each patient, the spectrum of medical issues changes over time, and they are confronted with unique medical challenges as they progress from intensive care treatment through hospital rehabilitation and into a phase of long-term medical homeostasis. Despite the wealth of information on these problems, most physicians do not appreciate the most basic elements of SCI care. Some physicians, overwhelmed by the patient's deficits, consider them fragile and impossibly complex, and parcel their problems out to a confusing array of specialists. Others push forward, utilizing treatment methods applicable to common medical conditions (pneumonia, urinary tract infection, fractures, skin lesions) with no special accommodations for this population. Of course, the best practice lies between these extremes. While there is no substitute for experience in this field, mastery of a small repertoire of basic treatment approaches can greatly enhance any physician's ability to handle these medical problems, especially in the chronic phase of care.

As is true in any life endeavor, youthful good health, physical attractiveness, an engaging personality, intelligence, adequate finances, and good family support are assets that support success. The medical profile of each patient, including injury-related as well as pre-injury medical conditions, constitutes only one of the factors that affect outcome. Most patients at the time of SCI also suffer associated trauma to other organ systems. The most common concurrent injuries documented in the NSCISC database are fractures (29%), loss of consciousness (28%), and pneumothorax and hemothorax (17%).[216] In the specialized centers that contribute to the NSCISC database, these conditions (and others) contribute to an average 15-day acute care hospital length of stay, followed by an average of 44 days in the rehabilitation hospital.[411] Persons with tetraplegia and those with complete injuries need longer hospitalizations. The costs of hospitalization account for over 80% of the total injury costs during the first year post injury.[606]

After initial hospital discharge, medical illnesses prompting readmission are common in the first years post injury, with a slight decline in frequency as years pass.[129, 313] It is likely that a bimodal distribution exists—studies have yet to detect the increase in rehospitalization expected at the end of life. Risk factors for readmission include younger age, nursing home residence, fewer trips outside the home, Frankel grade A and B status, and a lower educational level.[129, 313, 388] Urinary tract infections are the most frequent admitting diagnosis, although admissions for pressure ulcers account for more hospital days and generate greater human and financial costs.

Changes in survival and injury demographics have resulted in an increased interest in the problems faced by elderly persons with SCI and persons who have survived their injury for many decades.[147] Older persons with new-onset SCI have a different course than their younger counterparts, one that is characterized by a slower pace of rehabilitation and longer hospitalizations. Most elderly patients with adequate cognitive abilities benefit from rehabilitation services after injury, although goals are typically less ambitious. This is especially true for those with complete paraplegia, who are less likely to be independent in more complex skills such as dressing and transfers.[599]

The 1991 study of aging with SCI carried out by researchers at Craig Hospital in Denver analyzed the interaction between the aging process and preexisting paralysis.[572, 573] This study and others have helped to confirm the suggestion that such an interaction leads to a greater disability at an earlier age than expected.[144, 517, 586, 587] Over 25% of all individuals with SCI are now more than 20 years post injury.[49] Compared to persons recently injured, these individuals move into their later years with very different goals, perspectives, and priorities. The physician who treats persons with SCI must be especially skilled in moving between acute rehabilitation and chronic condition management.[376]

Renal diseases accounted for the majority of deaths after SCI in previous decades, and amyloidosis was also commonly seen, secondary to the presence of unresolved, recurrent infectious and inflammatory conditions.[318] The causes of death after SCI now approach those seen in the general population, although many cause-specific mortality rates remain above normal. Although pulmonary causes are now the most common cause of death, the ratio of actual to expected deaths is highest for septicemia. Clinicians should be aware of the high risk for suicide in SCI patients. A large epidemiological study of 5131 SCI patients showed that unintentional injuries and suicides are the leading cause of death in persons with paraplegia as well as in all SCI patients less than 55 years old.[146] Statistics regarding cause of death differ for injury subgroups, including age and level and grade of injury. For 435 persons with ventilator-dependent quadriplegia, DeVivo and Ivie[148] found the overall 1-year survival rate to be 25.4% and the 15-year survival rate to be 16.8%.

Psychological Issues

Traumatic SCI has been described as one of the most devastating calamities in life.[239] Almost every sphere of a person's life is affected, and adjustment to SCI is a challenge to all persons. Counseling services should be made available to all patients with SCI. It is unfortunate that some of the most pressing psychological and social needs of the patient are met by resources that are often diminished by financial cutbacks. The mental health model approach of Morris[398] allows the patient to receive these services in a way that does not imply that a specific psychiatric need or problem exists beyond the SCI itself. The psychologist should address such issues as the acceptance of impairment and the impact of the disability on the family and on sexual and vocational roles. The psychologist can be helpful to other team members as well, recommending approaches to the patient and helping to clarify patients' behavior in terms of adaptation to injury. All rehabilitation team members should be considered counselors. Even when ample psychological support is available, the time spent by patients in direct psychotherapy is much less than the hours spent with nurses, attendants, and therapy staff. The psychologist can often be most effective in the role of "counseling the counselors," ensuring that staff members serve each patient's emotional needs in a professional and therapeutic manner.

The assumption that most persons with SCI are clinically depressed is incorrect.[114] Even though it is difficult to apply the usual diagnostic criteria for depression to this population, several studies have shown that the overall incidence of depressive illness on the SCI rehabilitation unit is only moderate. When depression is diagnosed, the psychologist works with the injured person and the physician to develop a treatment plan. Many persons need several years to adapt psychologically to SCI.[519] Poor adaptation and depression often lead to medical complications, which can cause more adaptation and depression problems.

Alcohol and substance abuse can be involved as a cause of the injury itself and can continue after discharge from rehabilitation. Up to 50% of persons develop problems with substance abuse after SCI.[266] Substance abuse treatment should be initiated during the initial rehabilitation period and continued after discharge as needed.[265] Substance abuse typically results in poor compliance with pressure ulcer prevention activities, catheterization schedules, and medical therapies. Substance abuse often leads to covert self-destructive behavior and can be disruptive to the family as well.[588]

Cognitive deficits are common in persons with SCI and can interfere with the rehabilitation process.[399, 450, 460] Closed head injury occurs in up to 57% of SCI persons.[127] Closed head injury in SCI patients often went unrecognized in the past. Cognitive deficits are often multifactorial and can relate to substance abuse, learning disabilities, and other medical conditions. The team should be aware of these deficits and how they affect the person's ability to cooperate and participate in therapy. Strategies should be devised to determine the best descriptive techniques to illustrate a skill that must be learned. Neuropsychological evaluation gives insight into the person's behavior and allows the team to deal with the person on a more consistent and therapeutic basis (see Chapter 4).

The most pressing need for counseling support in this population arises over the long term, after hospital discharge. For disabled persons with suboptimal support systems, the cumulative effect of years of isolation, inactivity, or neglect can produce changes in psychological status that have a profound effect on health and quality of life. The aging or death of a patient's caregiver can bring about devastating life changes. Disability is often associated with poverty. Investigation of the patient's current social, financial, and family resources is the most important element of the health interview at a routine physician visit. Physical and sexual abuse of disabled persons is common. Physicians must be attuned to this fact and feel comfortable making inquiries if suspicions arise. Ongoing psychotherapy is rarely an option, due to difficulties with transportation, payor coverage, and limited psychology resources. Comprehensive care of persons with SCI requires that health care facilities maintain a referral relationship with organized, community-based peer support and independent living programs. For individuals with a recent SCI, exposure to a successful disabled role model is invaluable in many respects. Such exposure removes the person from an illness-based system of emotional support and helps redirect the focus back onto family, vocational, and social issues.

Respiratory System

The leading cause of death in persons with SCI is pneumonia, and diseases of the respiratory system are the underlying cause of death in over 20% of this population.[89, 140, 500] The clinical manifestations of pulmonary disease in this population are numerous and include ventilatory failure, pulmonary edema, pneumonia, atelectasis, restrictive lung disease, pneumothorax, hemothorax, lung contusion, and the need for tracheostomy. Persons with high cervical SCI or concomitant chest injuries and those injured later in life are at particular risk.[140, 571, 575] Although this risk extends through the chronic phase of SCI, the pulmonary complications seen during the acute phase of injury are the most debilitating and the most difficult and expensive to treat. Up to 50% of acutely injured persons develop pulmonary complications during the first month post injury, most commonly those with injuries from the C1 to C4 levels.[178, 283]

The muscles involved in normal pulmonary ventilation include the diaphragm, the intercostal muscles, the accessory neck muscles, and the abdominal muscles. The abdominal muscles are active primarily during forceful expiration and in producing cough.[590] Following SCI, the nature and magnitude of the changes in ventilatory function and cough depend on the level of neurological injury. Injuries between T7 and T12 impair abdominal muscle function, reducing forceful expiration and cough. In higher level thoracic and cervical injuries, intercostal muscle function is diminished or absent, affecting both inspiratory and expiratory function. In the first weeks after injury, flaccid intercostal muscle paralysis can result in paradoxical collapse of the rib cage during inspiration, further reducing ventilatory efficiency. As spasticity develops after a few weeks, this paradoxical movement is reduced and function improves.[356] Since the diaphragm is supplied by cervical roots C3, C4, and C5, it is common for persons injured above the C4 level to need ventilator support. For those with high-level injuries, accessory muscles of respiration in the neck can sustain acutely injured patients long enough to survive until emergency treatment arrives. These muscles (sternocleidomastoid, trapezius, platysma, mylohyoid, and sternohyoid) can generate tidal volumes of several hundred cubic centimeters. They are particularly effective during the chronic phase of injury, but are effective only during waking hours and are easily fatigued. Accessory muscles, including the clavicular portion of the pectoralis major, can also help produce the small active expiratory volumes seen in tetraplegic patients during the acute phase of injury.[138] Tetraplegic patients usually have a reduction in all measures of pulmonary function with the exception of residual volume. Residual volume is increased due to lack of active expiratory effort.[241, 469]

The chief pulmonary concerns during the acute phase of care are ventilation, oxygenation, secretion management, atelectasis, and segmental collapse. For acutely injured tetraplegic patients, initial energy requirements and tissue oxygen consumption are low. If no associated chest injuries are present, pulmonary status can remain stable for the first few days after injury. In a 5-year, multicenter collaborative prospective study published in 1994, Jackson and Groomes[283] detailed the scope of pulmonary morbidity in 261 persons with neurological injuries between C1 and T12, finding that 67% experienced significant pulmonary complications, most commonly atelectasis. Ventilatory failure and aspiration occurred earliest (mean 4.5 days), followed by atelectasis (mean 17.7 days) and pneumonia (mean 24.5 days). This late decline coincides with the onset of mucous hypersecretion and muscle fatigue. Biochemical sputum analysis in this setting reveals a secretory pattern similar to that seen in cystic fibrosis. Although the sputum quickly becomes colonized with bacteria in the intensive care setting, relatively few white cells are noted. This hypersecretory state is likely neurological in nature and has been attributed to unopposed vagal nerve stimulation of the airway submucosal glands.[53] A tracheostomy tube is frequently inserted to facilitate airway suctioning and secretion clearance. Cough assistance maneuvers can be carried out by nurses and respiratory therapists and produce a modest increase in expiratory flow. Insufflation-exsufflation machines can be used with or without tracheostomy tubes and have been shown to facilitate air stacking and achieve expiratory flow rates nearer to the 6 to 7 liters per second necessary for an effective cough (Figure 55–4).[25, 103] Nebulized acetylcysteine, anticholinergic antimuscarinic bronchodilators, human recombinant DNase, and atropine have been used for secretion management, but their efficacy is unproved.[533] Drying of secretions increases the risk of mucous plugging. Patients must be kept well hydrated, but overzealous hydration (i.e., in an attempt to normalize typical low blood pressures) can result in pulmonary edema. Secretion volume can be so high in some instances that suctioning every 15 minutes is required.

The problem of secretion management, combined with diminished ventilation of the lower lung segments, places these patients at high risk for pneumonia and segmental collapse. Over 36% of tetraplegic patients experience atelectasis with lung volume loss, and 31% develop pneumonia (most commonly in the left lower lobe).[178, 283] Curved-tip suction catheters can assist in suctioning the left mainstem bronchus, which is com-

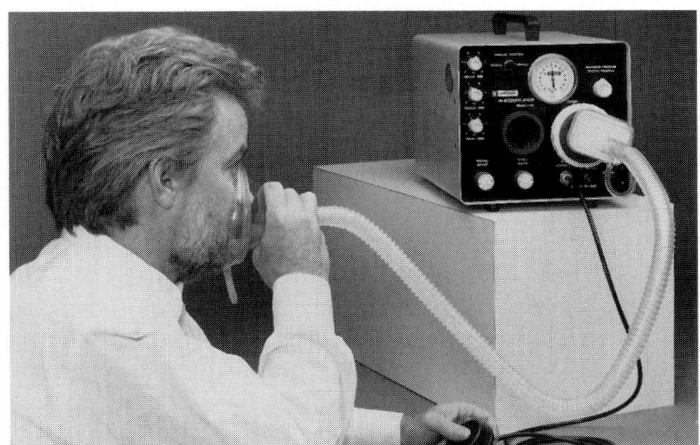

FIGURE 55–4. Mechanical insufflator-exsufflator for assistance with cough and clearance of pulmonary secretions. (Courtesy of J.H. Emerson Co., Cambridge, MA.)

monly missed with standard suctioning techniques.[185] Treatment with frequent bronchoscopic suctioning, combined with larger ventilator tidal volumes (15 mL/kg of ideal body weight) can be helpful.[431] In many cases segmental collapse follows a protracted and relapsing course. Prone Trendelenburg positioning promotes postural drainage of the left lower lobe, but unfortunately the hospital staff may resist this positioning because of difficulty in viewing the patient's face. The patient is typically placed in the supine Trendelenburg or semi-Fowler's position, with gravity drainage of secretions directed toward the lower left segments.

Body positioning is also important to facilitate ventilation. In contrast to other pulmonary conditions, patients with tetraplegia exhibit higher vital capacities when positioned flat in bed. The mechanisms underlying this phenomena are complex but likely relate to improved diaphragm function as the abdominal contents splint the lower rib cage. The reduction in vital capacity seen when these patients are seated upright can be counteracted to some extent by placement of an elastic abdominal binder. For obese persons and those already on positive pressure ventilation, these positioning effects are less significant, but their importance increases during periods of weaning.

Intubation and ventilation are usually undertaken based on objective measures of pulmonary function. Patients with new cervical injuries commonly experience a reduction in vital capacity of 24% to 31% of the predicted value.[195, 321, 325] Blood gases in these patients exhibit hypoxemia and normal $Paco_2$, and the ventilation-perfusion mismatch is usually attributed to microatelectasis. Signs of impending ventilatory failure include (1) a climbing respiratory rate and arterial CO_2 concentration in conjunction with a dropping tidal volume, (2) a drop in vital capacity to a level less than 15 mL/kg ideal body weight, (3) a drop in maximal inspiratory pressure to less than 20 cm H_2O, and (4) a neurological level of C3 or higher.[321, 397, 438] Pulmonary function can improve steadily over the acute course, even without concurrent neurological recovery. By 3 months, most tetraplegic patients can be expected to attain 60% of predicted vital capacity.[325] Ventilator weaning has been demonstrated in 80% of C4 SCI patients and in 57% of C3 SCI patients.[575] Considerable patience is required, as weaning protocols used for emphysema and heart failure patients are not applicable in this situation.[23, 289] Most authors argue for timed, progressive ventilator-free breathing, as opposed to synchronized intermittent mandatory ventilation (SIMV) weaning. The benefits of pressure support are yet to be clearly defined in this population, although intermittent positive pressure ventilation techniques have been shown to enhance noninvasive treatment of ventilatory failure via nasal or mouth masks.[26, 431] These promising noninvasive approaches decrease the need for tracheostomy ventilation but are not yet widely used. Most intensive care physicians remain unfamiliar with the equipment and techniques. Measurements of arterial CO_2 must accompany pulse oximetry measurements during the weaning process, since they provide an early and more sensitive indicator of respiratory muscle fatigue.

There are several special considerations in the management of tracheostomy care in this population. These considerations are based on the knowledge that pulmonary function improves quickly in most patients and that decannulation can usually be carried out in the weeks after injury as the need for suctioning and positive pressure treatments is reduced. Early on, a cuffed tracheostomy tube is usually needed that provides a good airway seal and anchors against heavy ventilation tubing. When pressure support is not needed, cuff deflation or a switch to cuffless cannulas can be considered. Cuffless tubes allow air to pass the vocal cords for phonation. For persons on ventilators, delivered volumes are increased to compensate for the air that bleeds cephalad through the vocal cords during the inflation phase. This step is taken gradually, since anxiety and fear interfere with the process.

A variety of special tracheostomy tubes are available that promote vocalization. Fenestrated tubes and one-way-valve devices work well, but they can become clogged by secretions and require frequent manipulation of the sensitive tracheotomy site. Their safe use requires that all staff understand the details of their function. Fenestrated tubes can irritate the posterior airway and promote formation of granulation tissue. Progression to a cuffless tube and progressive downsizing of the tube give the patient a sense of accomplishment during a time when functional gains are typically slow in coming. Tracheostomy tube changes should be carried out by an experienced individual. Patients who are not able to move air around a deflated cuff need special attention. The tracheal rings can be weakened by chronic inflammation, and excessive granulation tissue might be present. The tracheostomy tube might be serving as a splint for a damaged airway, and removal can result in airway collapse under the negative pressure of a deep breath.

The removal of the tracheostomy tube is warranted when the patient demonstrates an effective cough. Those who can cough secretions past a small-caliber cuffless tube into their mouth, and patients who can partially dislodge their tube with coughing, are certainly candidates for decannulation. With proper noninvasive support, decannulation can be carried out when peak cough flows are greater than 160 L/min.[26] Although frequent chest radiographs are not cost-effective in this population,[487] they should be obtained before decannulation to evaluate for an occult lung process such as pleural effusion and to document the overall lung status.

Patients with injuries above the segments innervating the phrenic nerve are candidates for phrenic nerve pacemaker implantation.[215] Although this technology is expensive and requires a lifelong tracheostomy, it has been shown to be a safe and reliable method for long-term ventilatory support. Benefits include reducing the need for heavy ventilator equipment, a reduction in sinus symptoms through better humidification of the upper airway, and improved taste sensation.[328] Persons with marginal ventilatory status and those with late, chronic decline in gas exchange are good candidates for noninvasive pulmonary support aids.[24, 27]

In the chronic phase of SCI, pulmonary issues remain at the forefront. Breathlessness and wheezing are common complaints, and bronchial hyperreactivity has been described.[173] Development of kyphoscoliosis can result in a reduction in lung compliance and vital capacity. Pregnancy and gastrointestinal dysmotility with gaseous distention of the viscera can interfere with diaphragmatic function. Nighttime oxygen desaturation is often noted in patients with chronic tetraplegia, presumably due to the reduced use of accessory muscles during sleep.[70] Resistive inspiratory muscle training can be useful in reducing respiratory complaints and complications.[466] Smoking cessation and vaccination programs (influenza and pneumococcal) are important components of long-term follow-up care.[124]

Changes in Body Composition and in Metabolic and Endocrine Function

The striking changes in body composition and physiological processes that occur with acute SCI often result in clinical problems that require active intervention and management. Soon after injury, body weight declines.[118, 322] There is a decrease in total body water, fat, and protein. Loss of protein results in increased urea nitrogen excretion. Both extracellular and intracellular water are decreased, but the preferential loss of intracellular water leads to the relative expansion of extracellular fluid stores. This is presumably due to failure of end organ responses to changes in electrolytes and atrial natriuretic factor (which is increased after injury).[83, 84, 480] Muscle tissue loss leads to decreased exchangeable potassium and increased exchangeable sodium, further exacerbating the expansion of extracellular fluid. Hyperkalemia and cardiac arrest can occur with administration of succinylcholine, a drug that must not be used in SCI patients.[74] Other electrolyte disturbances that have been described in the acute phase include hyperphosphatemia, hypermagnesuria, hyperuricosuria without hyperuricosemia, and decreased urine creatinine.[97, 99] Hyperosmolar hyponatremia (Na < 130 mmol/L) is also seen, especially in acute tetraplegia. Most patients are asymptomatic, but serious complications can result if the condition is ignored.[481] Disorders in sodium regulation can occur as a result of excessive fluid resuscitation or impaired cortisol response.[279] Anemia is common after acute SCI.[274, 278] This anemia is normochromic normocytic, with low levels of iron and transferrin. Total iron-binding capacity is reduced. Erythropoietin levels are usually normal.[96]

A number of abnormalities in endocrine function accompany acute injury. At rest, steady-state excretion of corticosteroids in the urine is normal, and serum measures of aldosterone, catecholamines, and methylhydroxymandelic acid are similar to those of resting, healthy subjects.[98] In the stimulated state, such as after surgery, the expected increases in these measurements are absent in persons with SCI, probably because of loss of integrated neuroendocrine function.[101, 279]

Changes in energy expenditure occur in the acute phase of paralysis. Acute SCI patients require up to 54% fewer calories than would be predicted by their weight.[118] The higher the level of injury, the greater the reduction in basal energy expenditure. The inability of tetraplegic and high paraplegic patients to control their body temperature is most striking in the period immediately after injury.[237, 395, 509] Close monitoring of ambient and body temperature is required in the acute phase after injury. These patients retain the ability to mount a febrile response to infectious conditions. In the phase of initial treatment after injury, multiple potential precipitants of fever are usually present. An awareness of the phenomenon of temperature instability in these patients must not be used as a rationalization for an incomplete search for another fever source. Patients without leukocytosis should be evaluated for venous thromboembolism and heterotopic ossification as a source of their fever. As a patient progresses into the rehabilitation hospital and into the chronic phase of injury, sensitivity to ambient temperature remains, although the striking dysregulation seen in the intensive care unit typically resolves.

Other body changes are most marked in the chronic phase of injury. Glucose intolerance is a common finding,[161] and hyperinsulinemia is noted. The insulin resistance is due in part to abnormal muscle utilization, decreased lean body mass, and increased fat body mass. Muscle fiber types can change during the chronic phase, with a gradual increase in the percentage of type II fibers, a factor that exacerbates insulin resistance.[231, 349] Anemia in chronic SCI persons is common, ranging in incidence from 30% to 56%,[274, 427, 527] with blood indices indicating an anemia of chronic disease. Chronic SCI patients continue to demonstrate lower rates of energy expenditure than predicted.[118, 394]

Calcium Metabolism and Osteoporosis

Any form of immobilization alters calcium metabolism, but the structural and physiological changes associated with SCI predispose these patients to a variety of complications. These include hypercalcemia, bone fractures, nephrolithiasis, and renal failure.[7, 33] As early as 10 days post injury, hypercalciuria develops, reaching a peak between 1 and 6 months post injury.[47, 100] This calcium is derived from bone resorption, as increased levels of urinary phosphate, hydroxyproline, and glycosaminoglycans are also observed. There is an initial suppression of parathyroid hormone (PTH) that reaches its nadir at 3 months and returns to the normal range at 6 months. Pathological studies demonstrate an increased number of osteoclasts in bone, reaching a peak at 16 weeks post injury, with diminished bone formation and mineralization.[391, 495] Hypercalcemia is seen in some patients. Risk factors for hypercalcemia include childhood or adolescent SCI, male sex, complete injuries, tetraplegia, dehydration, and prolonged immobilization.[365, 368, 515] Treatment of hypercalcemia in adults is similar to that used in children, including use of IV fluids, loop diuretics, pamidronate, and calcitonin.[86, 382, 389] Limitation of dietary calcium and vitamin D intake is not recommended.[495]

The degree of lower extremity bone loss after injury has been correlated with the occurrence of fractures.[200, 201, 250, 282, 442] Bone loss is most severe in regions having neurological deficits.[47, 201] Garland et al,[200] in a study of the bone density of persons with both acute and chronic (greater than 10 years) SCI, found that 50% of the acutely injured patients and 90% of those with chronic SCI had proximal tibial densities below the fracture threshold. The weight-bearing vertebral column is generally spared these severe effects, and spinal bone density can even improve as time passes after injury, especially in females.[36, 332] Patients with significant osteopenia of the spinal column should be investigated to determine whether secondary causes of osteoporosis are present.

A number of interventions have been studied in the hope of preventing and treating disorders of calcium metabolism in these subjects. Physical activity, including wheelchair use, frame-assisted standing, and tilt table, might improve calcium balance in the acute phase, but no effect on bone density has been demonstrated.[295] Functional electrical stimulation cycle ergometry can provide modest reductions in the rate of bone loss, sustained only during the period of application.[250, 329] Patients with chronic SCI can benefit from correction of nutritional deficiencies. Patients often restrict dietary calcium because of fear of renal lithiasis. Combined with several factors that result in vitamin D deprivation, the serum calcium can be further lowered in this group, resulting in stimulation of the parathyroid glands. Many individuals with chronic SCI are prone to secondary hyperparathyroidism and further bone loss, remediable by vitamin D and calcium supplementation.[33]

Antiresorptive therapies, including hormone treatment, calcitonin, and third-generation bisphosphonates, offer promising potential treatment alternatives.[164] The utility of these agents has been demonstrated in other diseases featuring rapid bone turnover. Estrogen therapy should be considered for women with SCI, just as it is used in the nondisabled population. The marginally increased risk of venous thrombosis associated with estrogen use in most patients is outweighed by the inevitable, tangible, and immediate problem of fractures and osteoporosis. The newer biphosphonates have been effective in preventing acute bone loss in rats exposed to weightless conditions. One of these drugs (tiludronate) has been shown to reduce bone resorption without impairing bone formation in persons with paraplegia.[91]

Cardiovascular Conditions

The alterations in cardiovascular physiology and risk factors for coronary heart disease after SCI merit special attention. Cardiac arrhythmias and orthostatic hypotension are common problems, especially during the acute phase of treatment. Over the long term, patients are predisposed to the development of accelerated and premature coronary artery disease.[34, 603] Cardiovascular diseases account for 46% of all deaths in SCI persons more than 30 years post injury, and the prevalence of asymptomatic coronary disease in persons with tetraplegia can be as high as 70%.[34, 35]

The vagus nerve exits the central nervous system (CNS) at the brainstem and is spared in SCI. Injuries to the spinal cord above the upper thoracic levels block the compensatory sympathetic impulses that exit toward the sympathetic cervical ganglia, resulting in impaired vasoconstrictor tone, reduced cardiac contractility and heart rate.[170, 182, 302, 330,434] Bradycardia is seen in all patients with complete tetraplegia, and in up to 71% of patients with Frankel class C or D tetraplegia.[330] Severe sinus slowing can necessitate treatment with temporary transvenous pacemakers, atropine, or sympathomimetic drugs.[212, 324, 330] The response to atropine can be blunted in this group. Bradycardia peaks around injury day 4 and resolves over the next 2 weeks in most instances. Bradycardia can be exacerbated by hypoxia and by activation of vagovagal reflexes during tracheal suctioning.[21, 182, 212] Hyperoxygenation before suctioning can help remedy this problem. Atrioventricular block, ventricular tachycardia, supraventricular tachyarrthymias, and cardiac arrest have also been described in cervical and high thoracic level injuries. Decreased heart rate and cardiac index can be treated with dopamine and dobutamine. However, pulmonary and systemic vascular resistance, as well as central venous pressures, are typically not as responsive to treatment.[334] A Swan-Ganz catheter is essential in gauging fluid replacement in these hypotensive patients.

As the SCI patient enters the rehabilitation phase of care, orthostatic hypotension can occur, resulting in lightheadedness, dizziness, nausea, loss of consciousness, and seizures.[236, 239] This condition is most prominent in persons with higher injury levels. Plasma adrenaline and noradrenaline levels respond to changes in body position significantly less than in noninjured control subjects.[209, 219, 403] Symptom relief can often be obtained through the use of recliner wheelchairs with elevating leg rests, elastic compression stockings, and abdominal binders. In some instances, short-term (1- to 2-month) treatment with salt, ephedrine, or fluorinated steroids is helpful.[232] Tilt table treatments are sometimes employed, but the patient's tolerance of such sessions has little bearing on the ability to achieve wheelchair sitting without symptomatic hypotension.

Although symptomatic orthostatic hypotension usually resolves soon after injury, persons with high injury levels can retain low blood pressure readings on a lifelong basis. Systolic readings in the 80 to 90 mm Hg range are not uncommon. Sometimes healthy, asymptomatic patients present with blood pressures that are virtually inaudible. This phenomenon makes the diagnosis of sepsis particularly difficult. Other long-term issues relate to the alteration in cardiovascular risk factors, including reduced cardiac output, glucose intolerance, an unfavorable lipid profile, a decrease in lean body mass, and reduced physical conditioning.[85, 496, 543] Tetraplegic patients with coronary artery disease often do not experience angina, due to interruption of cardiac nociceptive afferent fibers, necessitating a higher index of suspicion when the clinician is faced with intermittent or exercise-induced symptoms. Angina must remain in the differential diagnosis of left shoulder and arm pain. Reduced serum HDL cholesterol is seen in both tetraplegic and paraplegic patients, possibly related to hyperinsulinemia and increased hepatic triglyceride production.[34, 71, 268]

A complete fasting lipid profile is recommended for all SCI adults 20 years of age and older at least once every 5 years.[34] Indications for lipid-lowering drugs are the same as for the general population. Bile acid–binding resins are usually avoided in this group, however, due to the side effects of constipation, gas, and interference with absorption of nutrients. Exercise in persons with SCI, both with arm ergometry and electrically stimulated programs, can bring about increased HDL cholesterol levels, reversal of ventricular atrophy, and a reduction in the risk for developing cardiovascular disease.[71, 409, 491] For SCI persons at risk, exercise tolerance tests can be performed via arm ergometry, or thallium stress testing can be used (see Chapter 32).

Venous Thromboembolism

The potentially devastating consequences of venous thrombosis make prevention, diagnosis, and appropriate treatment very important in SCI patients. Pulmonary embolism (PE) and deep venous thrombosis (DVT) represent manifestations of a single condition, venous thromboembolism.[532] Autopsy studies of deaths in acute SCI patients report the incidence of death from PE to be as high as 37%.[516] PE is the third leading cause of death in all SCI patients in the first year post injury.[140] The risk of DVT during the months immediately following injury is also high. Studies of the incidence of DVT vary widely, depending on the type of diagnostic test that is used. Studies employing modern diagnostic techniques (Doppler ultrasound [US], fibrinogen scanning, venography) place the risk of DVT between 40% and 100%.[95, 202, 380, 381, 406] Risk prior to 72 hours post SCI appears to be low,[227] but over 80% of DVTs will occur within the first 2 weeks. The risk of DVT is maximal between days 7 and 10.[381, 457] PE is estimated to occur in approximately 5% of acute SCI patients.[140, 339, 544] For the paralyzed SCI patient, venous stasis in the flaccid lower extremities plays the principal role in clot development. Another factor could be the transient hypercoagulable state that has been described.[457] Reduced fibrinolytic activity and increased factor VII activity have also been reported.[405, 430] In immobilized patients without paralysis, thromboses are rare, suggesting that impaired autonomic input to the venous system might also play a role.[406]

The risk profiles for venous thrombosis differ when considering DVT and PE. Those with complete injuries are at higher risk for DVT than those with incomplete lesions. Patients with paraplegic injuries are at higher risk than tetraplegic patients for DVT, while an increased risk of PE is associated with tetraplegia, less spasticity, and greater body mass.[224] The incidence of DVT is similar for SCI persons in all age groups, while the incidence of PE peaks in years 61 to 75. Both DVT and PE occur with higher frequency in males with SCI.[443]

Physical examination is especially unreliable in the diagnosis of DVT in SCI patients.[406, 544, 561] Because of impaired of vasomotor tone in the legs, changes in volume and appearance are seen daily, and serial leg measurements are of little value.[510] The clinician is armed only with a strong index of suspicion and a willingness to employ more sensitive diagnostic tests, either as routine surveillance or as an adjunct to frequent leg examinations. Signs of DVT include unilateral edema, an increase in collateral vein markings, low-grade fever of unknown etiology, and changes in pain or leg sensation patterns in persons with incomplete SCI.

Duplex US with manual compression has become widely used as a convenient, sensitive, and specific noninvasive method of DVT diagnosis in symptomatic patients.[331, 570, 585] This technique is less sensitive as a case finding tool in asymptomatic patients, even in those at high risk for DVT.[131] Duplex US is limited, however, in that there is poor visualization of the venous system proximal to the femoral veins, poor sensitivity for calf vein thrombosis, and difficulties with imaging in the presence of heterotopic ossification.[594] If vena cava thrombosis is suspected, spiral computed tomography (CT) and magnetic resonance imaging (MRI) are particularly useful, with sensitivities and specificities in the 80% to 90% range.[281, 448]

Ventilation-perfusion lung scans are regarded as definitive only when normal or high probability readings are obtained. Scans read as low or intermediate probability are best followed by another study, such as US of the legs or pulmonary angiography. Contrast venography is still the gold standard for diagnosis of DVT, although it is underutilized because of inconvenience, patient discomfort, and the risks of allergic reactions and phlebitis.[247] Contrast venography should be considered when noninvasive testing is equivocal, or when noninvasive testing is negative in the setting of high clinical suspicion. Contrast venography should also be considered in the setting of recurrent DVT, when noninvasive testing is less reliable.[281] The search for serum laboratory markers that might assist in the diagnosis of acute thrombosis has focused mainly on the study of factor VIII and the breakdown products of cross-linked fibrin, especially d-dimer. A number of d-dimer assays are now commercially available.[326] A low d-dimer concentration has a high negative predictive value for thromboembolism,[3] but significant methodological problems with the test limit the usefulness of published estimates of d-dimer diagnostic accuracy.[40, 299, 429] D-dimer levels are elevated by a variety of co-morbid conditions (e.g., infections, surgery), and these elevations can persist for months after acute SCI.[62] In addition, the specificity of d-dimer in DVT diagnosis is low in asymptomatic patients, so its use as a surveillance test is limited.[120]

The Consortium for Spinal Cord Medicine[111] engaged in an exhaustive review of the medical literature relevant to thrombosis in SCI, and published clinical practice guidelines for the prevention of thromboembolism in 1997. Both mechanical and pharmacological methods of prevention were analyzed, and prophylaxis regimens were stratified based on estimates of relative patient risks (Table 55–8).

A number of mechanical treatments have proved effective in reducing the incidence of DVT, including ROM exercises, rotation beds, gradient elastic stockings, lower extremity electrical stimulation, external pneumatic leg compression, and the venous foot

TABLE 55–8 Guidelines for the Prevention of Thromboembolism in Spinal Cord Injury: Clinical Decision Table

Level of Risk	Motor Incomplete	Motor Complete	Motor Complete with Other Risk*
Intensity of prophylaxis			
Low	Compression hose Compression boots +	Compression hose Compression boots +	Compression hose Compression boots +
Intermediate	UH: 5000 U q 12 h	UH: Dose adjusted to high normal aPTT; or LMWH: 30 mg twice daily	UH: Dose adjusted to high normal aPTT; or LMWH: 30 mg twice daily ±
High	—	—	Inferior vena cava filter
Duration of prophylaxis			
	Compression boots: 2 wk Anticoagulants: while in hospital for ASIA class D and up to 8 wk for ASIA class C	Compression boots: 2 wk Anticoagulants: at least 8 wk	Compression boots: 2 wk Anticoagulants: 12 wk or until discharge from rehabilitation

Abbreviations: UH, unfractionated heparin; aPTT, activated partial thromboplastin time; LMWH, low molecular weight heparin.
* Other risk factors: lower limb fracture, previous thrombosis, cancer, heart failure, obesity, age over 70.
From The Consortium for Spinal Cord Medicine: Clinical practice guideline: Prevention of thromboembolism in spinal cord injury. Spinal Cord Med 1997; 20:259–284.

pump.[39, 111] External pneumatic compression devices are widely available and have been applied successfully in the SCI population.[228, 379] To ensure proper use, frequent examination of the underlying skin is necessary to detect evidence of pressure damage, abrasions, or bruising. If their use is instituted later than 72 hours post injury, testing to exclude the presence of leg thrombi should be undertaken.

Vena cava filter insertion is often considered in patients with complete motor paralysis due to lesions in the high cervical cord, patients with poor cardiac reserve, and in patients for whom bedside clinical assessment for DVT might be obscured by obesity or dark skin color. Vena cava filters are also employed in the setting of failed prophylaxis, in those with contraindications for pharmacological prophylaxis (bleeding risks in the CNS, lungs, or gastrointestinal [GI] tract), and for the treatment of thrombus in the vena cava. Filter use can be complicated by caval perforation or thrombosis and by filter migration or dislodgment during cough assistance maneuvers.[28] These potential risks should not prevent the insertion of filters or the use of cough assistance in appropriate patients.

Considerable progress has been made in the development of pharmacological strategies to prevent thrombosis. Evidence supporting the use of subcutaneous low-dose unfractionated heparin (5000 units, two or three times a day) comes chiefly from small, retrospective studies.[226] Higher doses of subcutaneous unfractionated heparin (10,000 to 15,000 units, twice daily) are more effective,[226] but bleeding complications are significant, and monitoring of aPTT levels is cumbersome. Prophylaxis with oral warfarin carries the same need for frequent blood tests, and its prophylactic effect is also inversely related to the risk of bleeding.[484] The presence of vitamin K deficiency in SCI patients and the potential for interactions with the multiplicity of drugs used in the acute setting make monitoring of warfarin prophylactic therapy even more problematic.[223]

New low molecular weight heparins have shown promise for use in propyhylaxis when used alone or in combination with mechanical modalities. Like standard heparin, low molecular weight heparins bind to antithrombin III, potentiating inhibitory actions against activated factor Xa and thrombin.[225, 378] The low molecular weight heparins, however, are unable to bind thrombin directly, do not reduce platelet activity, and do not change vascular permeability. These factors can allow for equivalent anticoagulant effects with reduced bleeding risks. These preparations also exhibit better subcutaneous absorption, longer half-life, and smoother anticoagulant response. They require only once or twice daily dosing. Initial experience with low molecular weight heparins in SCI patients has demonstrated both an improved safety profile and superior thrombosis prevention when compared to earlier modes of treatment.[224, 227, 254] There is little scientific data dealing with the duration of prophylaxis. For some patients, thrombosis development might only be delayed for the period during which preventive measures are employed.

When the diagnosis of proximal DVT or PE is confirmed, either low molecular weight heparin or unfractionated IV heparin should be administered. Therapies and mobilization are usually withheld for 4 to 7 days after diagnosis. Treatment of calf vein thrombosis has been more controversial. As an alternative to anticoagulation, some clinicians choose to follow calf thromboses with serial noninvasive tests to monitor for proximal extension. This approach is often impractical, however, and there is mounting evidence that the long-term complications of calf DVT can be as problematic as proximal DVT. In light of this, most of the patients with calf DVT in this high-risk group are best treated with full anticoagulation for at least 3 months.

The FDA recently approved one of the low molecular weight heparins (enoxaparin) for an indication in the treatment of DVT. Enoxaparin is administered subcutaneously, on a weight-based dose, once or twice a day.

When compared to IV unfractionated heparin, these drugs present a lower risk of thrombocytopenia and osteopenia.[281] Because of their favorable dose-response characteristics, monitoring is unnecessary in most patients. Warfarin remains the drug of choice for long-term treatment, and is begun on the first day of anticoagulant therapy in most settings. Careful monitoring of the International Normalized Ratio (INR) is essential in the SCI patient. Dietary changes, drug interactions, and co-morbidities interfere with dosing and response to the drug. The INR of 2.5 provides good protection against further thrombosis and is associated with no more bleeding complications than an INR of 2.0. The optimal duration of warfarin therapy in this patient population is also controversial, but treatment should be administered for a minimum of 3 to 6 months, in hopes of reducing the recurrence rate and the risk of chronic postthrombotic syndrome, with chronic lower extremity edema and skin ulceration.

There are few studies that examine the long-term risk of venous thromboembolism, but there is a much lower rate of occurrence than in the acute phase of SCI.[443] Persons with longstanding SCI who are readmitted to the hospital for medical or surgical illnesses are at similar risk for thrombosis development as other immobilized, hospitalized patients.[303] Reinstitution of prophylactic measures should be considered in this setting.

Autonomic Dysreflexia

Autonomic dysreflexia is an acute syndrome of massive sympathetic discharge that is triggered by a noxious stimulus. It occurs in persons with spinal cord lesions above the level of the sympathetic splanchnic outflow, which usually couples with the spinal cord at T6.[319] It is characterized by severe paroxysmal hypertension, pounding headache, sweating, nasal congestion, facial flushing, piloerection, and reflex bradycardia.[259] The incidence has been reported to range from 48% to 83% of tetraplegic and high paraplegic patients. Most persons do not experience signs and symptoms in the first 2 months post injury.[169, 340] Autonomic dysreflexia occurs most commonly in persons with injuries above T6, but occasionally it is seen in persons with injury levels as low as T10.[213] It can be seen in association with both incomplete and complete injuries. All patients with injuries above the mid-thoracic spinal cord levels will exhibit *autonomic dysregulation,* with very low baseline blood pressures and orthostatic hypotension.

Autonomic dysreflexia is a distinct entity. It is episodic in nature, and extremely high blood pressure is the sentinel sign. The most common cause by far is bladder distention. Other causes include bowel impaction, pressure sores, ingrown toenails, tight clothing, tight shoes and leg bag straps, urinary tract infections, and uterine contractions in pregnant women.[107, 372] Invasive procedures such as bladder catheterization, rectal stimulation, cystometrography,[340] and extracorporeal shock wave lithotripsy are known to precipitate this response.[77, 291]

This condition is generated by spinal cord and splanchnic reflex mechanisms that remain operative despite the SCI. The triggering events noted above produce afferent impulses that are transmitted to the dorsal column and spinothalamic tracts. As these tracts ascend, they synapse with sympathetic neurons in the intermediolateral columns and generate a generalized sympathetic reflex response. Normally, descending supraspinal inhibitory signals modulate these autonomic reflexes, but due to the spinal lesion above the sympathetic outflow, inhibitory impulses cannot effectively descend in the sympathetic chain to block the autonomic response. The result is peripheral and splanchnic vasoconstriction and the development of acute hypertension. Sweating and piloerection also occur as a result of the mass sympathetic discharge. Baseline serum catecholamine levels are low after SCI, raising the suspicion that a denervation hypersensitivity to adrenergic stimulation contributes to this condition.

With the increase in blood pressure, the aortic arch and carotid sinus receptors are stimulated, which can result in reflex bradycardia and vasodilation above the level of the lesion. The vasodilation is manifested as facial flushing, sweating, and nasal congestion (Fig. 55–5).[169] Signs and symptoms can vary slightly between patients (i.e., some patients exhibit tachycardia, not bradycardia), but the bedside diagnosis of this condition

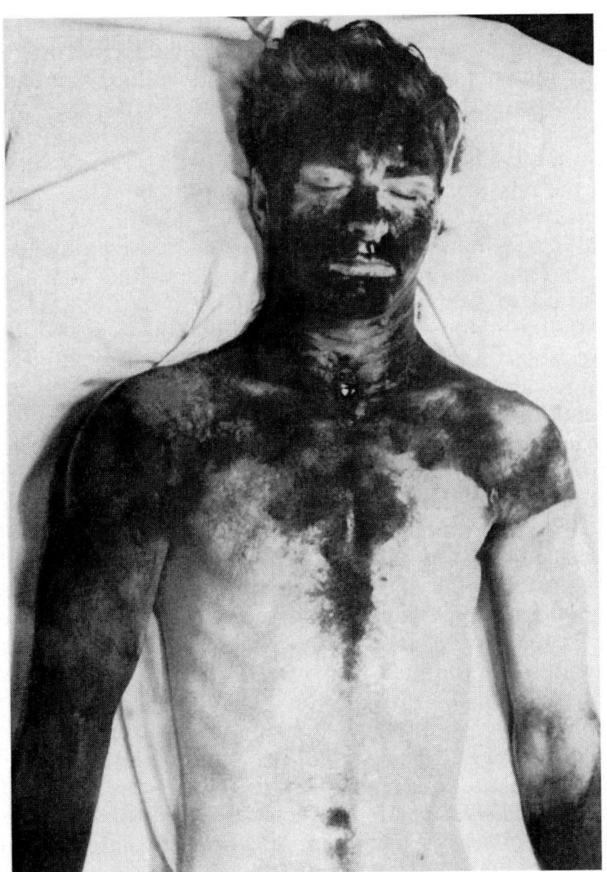

FIGURE 55–5. Illustration from Sir Ludwig Guttmann's text.[238, 239] Patient with acute autonomic dysreflexia, with Quinizarin skin dye applied to outline the neurological segments exhibiting reflex sweating. A blood pressure cuff was removed from the left arm. (Reproduced by permission of Blackwell Scientific Publications.)

is rarely ambiguous. A diagnostic challenge might exist in elderly patients or in pregnant women. Some elderly patients with recent motor incomplete injuries will exhibit the essential systolic hypertension that afflicted them prior to their injury. In pregnant women, hypertension can represent pre-eclampsia. In both of these situations, hypertension is asymptomatic and nonepisodic.

Complications that develop from autonomic dysreflexia are usually secondary to severe hypertension. The elevated blood pressure can result in life-threatening complications, including confusion, visual disturbance, loss of consciousness, encephalopathy, intracerebral hemorrhage, seizures, electrocardiographic changes, atrial fibrillation, acute myocardial failure, and pulmonary edema.[169, 415, 436, 593] In pregnant women with SCI, intracerebral hemorrhage and death during labor also have been reported.[2, 213]

Detailed reviews of the clinical treatment practices for autonomic dysreflexia have been done,[69] and based on the available scientific literature, the Consortium for Spinal Cord Medicine published a clinical practice guideline, Acute Management of Autonomic Dysreflexia, in 1997.[112] Treatment of an acute episode generally focuses on identifying and eliminating the cause. The first action taken is to place the patient in an upright sitting position with, if possible, the legs dangling over the bedside. This maneuver makes use of the natural orthostatic hypotensive response in SCI patients and can lower the blood pressure and reduce headache symptoms. Tight clothing and constrictive devices (catheter straps, belts) should be removed. The blood pressure and pulse are frequently monitored. A quick survey of the possible instigating causes should be done, beginning with the urinary system. This step might require bladder catheterization, irrigating an existing indwelling catheter, changing a catheter, or utilizing lidocaine anesthetic jelly, if available.

If these steps do not result in a reduction in blood pressure, rectal impaction should be suspected. Pharmacological management should be considered at this point, as stool removal digitally can exacerbate the episode. Opinion varies regarding the level of blood pressure that warrants pharmacological treatment. The treating physician should be aware that the baseline systolic blood pressure after a tetraplegic or high paraplegic injury falls in the 90 to 100 mm Hg range. Systolic pressures in the 150 mm Hg range typically represent significant hypertension. Rapid-onset, short-duration antihypertensive medications that can be used include nitrates, nifedipine, prazosin, hydralazine, mecamylamine, and IV diazoxide.[69, 77, 169] If 2% nitroglycerin ointment is used, 1 inch can be applied to the skin above the level of SCI and wiped off as the blood pressure is lowered. Nifedipine has been used safely in autonomic dysreflexia, but its use has declined as a result of multiple reports of hypotensive complications in patients with essential hypertension. Once the blood pressure is lowered, examination for fecal impaction (using lidocaine jelly lubricant) and for other inciting causes can be done. Headaches can persist for hours after the hypertension is treated; they usually respond to acetaminophen. Oral medications and regional, spinal, and epidural anesthesia have been used as pretreatment for episodes that are anticipated in association with surgical or diagnostic procedures. Epidural anesthesia is usually effective in the obstetrical setting.[498, 560]

Although most episodes of autonomic dysreflexia are easily remedied, the patient who experiences recurrent episodes presents one of the most difficult diagnostic and therapeutic challenges in SCI medicine. The triggering mechanism is often obscure, or the putative trigger is not easily remedied (pressure ulcer, bowel distention, fractures). In these situations, a suppressive therapeutic agent is usually needed. Over the years, ganglionic blocking agents (guanethidine, mecamylamine, and phenoxybenzamine) have been used in this setting.[69, 90, 169] Rarely prescribed, these drugs are difficult to obtain and questionable in efficacy. Newer alpha-adrenergic receptor blockers (e.g., terazosin) are reasonable options. The physician should be cautious in prescribing large doses of antihypertensive agents to a patient with a baseline systolic pressure of less than 100 mm Hg. In practice, however, these agents are usually well tolerated, suppressing hypertensive spikes while having little effect on baseline cardiovascular indices. If the medication successfully suppresses episodes, it can be discontinued after 3 to 4 weeks, assuming that the problem that triggered the events has been corrected. Pudendal nerve blocks, posterior rhizotomy, and cordectomy have been used in selected cases to obliterate the autonomic afferent input and reduce the response.

Prevention of recurrent episodes includes proper bladder and bowel management and skin care. Also vital is patient and family education regarding the prevention, causes, presentation, and treatment of autonomic dysreflexia. At discharge from rehabilitation, patients at risk for autonomic dysreflexia should be prescribed appropriate antihypertensive medications to use in an emergency setting, and the patient and family should be schooled in their use. Patients should also be aware that many physicians in emergency departments are unaware of autonomic dysreflexia and can confuse it with other causes of hypertension. Patients should learn how to explain this condition to treating medical personnel, and they should know how to refer others to telephone contact with clinicians knowledgeable in its treatment.

Pressure Ulcers

The importance of preventing pressure ulcers in the SCI patient cannot be overemphasized.[601] Their impact in terms of morbidity, diminished quality of life, and monetary expense can only be estimated; however, treatment of a severe single ulcer can produce more than $58,000 in hospital charges, a figure that does not take into account the cost in terms of lost days of work, social isolation, and contribution to chronic illness (see Chapter 31).[4]

Fuhrer et al,[194] in a community-based survey of SCI persons, noted that 33% had at least one pressure ulcer and 13.6% had a stage 3 or 4 ulcer. In the acute phase of injury, most pressure sores occur on the sacrum. By year 2 post injury, the ischium is the most common site of involvement, followed by the sacrum, trochanter, and heel.[602] Pressure ulcers are preventable.[421] For persons admitted to the Model Spinal Cord Injury Care Systems, the incidence of severe pressure sores is only 2%.[602]

Persons with myelopathy constitute a special group within the vast population of patients with pressure sores. In these individuals ulcers typically occur at a younger age and more frequently require surgical treatment.[338] The effect of SCI on skin and soft tissue pressure tolerance is poorly understood. It is well recognized, however, that persons with myelopathy have a much higher incidence of severe pressure sores than persons with other paralytic conditions (e.g., amyotrophic lateral sclerosis).[546] An autonomic or neurovascular deficit in soft tissue maintenance might underlie this phenomenon.[245, 506]

Pressure ulcers will not heal unless the pressure is removed. Negotiation around this point is rarely appropriate. An hour of sitting on an ischial ulcer can cause damage that might require weeks of bedrest to reverse. Special beds and cushions by themselves neither prevent nor heal pressure sores. The patient or caregiver must carry out regular weight-shifting and pressure relief maneuvers. Extensive counseling should be started early and continued in the years following injury. Most patients cannot appreciate the disastrous implications until a serious pressure ulcer develops.

Treatment of a pressure ulcer can require weeks or months of restricted activity, increased caregiver support, and time lost from work or school. Physicians involved with the treatment process should examine their attitudes about pressure sore development. It is tempting to blame these events on a patient's self-neglect and lack of adherence to medical advice. Patients who return with multiple recurrent sores are the most vividly remembered, but most patients who present with a serious ulcer have one-time occurrences.[19] The prevention of pressure ulcers usually involves many factors—genetic/physical predisposition, environmental and social resources, good health maintenance habits, and good luck. To say that pressure ulcers are preventable is not to say that they are easily prevented. Clinicians should keep in mind that the SCI, not the patient, is the problem. Experienced clinicians project a positive and therapeutic demeanor in this setting, looking forward to preventing further occurrences. Physicians must also contend with a dizzying and ever-changing array of dressings and potions used to treat ulcers, ranging from saline dressings to recombinant DNA platelet-derived growth factor. Few convincing studies have examined the cost-effectiveness of individual wound healing preparations.[113] Staff members are likely to gravitate toward expensive, new dressing products. As an illustration, the staff members involved in one study judged a sham, placebo dressing to be the most effective treatment after being told that it emitted electromagnetic waves.[176] Ulcers will heal if the basic elements of care are followed, medical status is optimized, pressure is removed, the ulcer is cleaned, and a moist environment for re-epithelialization is provided (see Chapter 31).

Surgical consultation is usually needed if the ulcer has eroded to underlying bone or bursa. It is possible to treat these ulcers without surgery, but draining sinuses and large scars are commonly encountered that can predispose to chronic tissue breakdown. Surgical treatment can provide the individual with well-padded, durable weight-bearing areas. On the other hand, each pressure ulcer operation "steals" tissue from an adjoining area of the body to fill the defect. For ulcers on the seated surface of the body, there are only a limited number of procedures that can be performed, short of lower limb amputation. Each surgical option that is used represents an option that is no longer available should a recurrence develop. For some body surfaces, the problems with surgical closure can be worse than the ulcer itself. For example, deep ulcers at the elbows and malleoli are often small but are especially frustrating to treat. Traction on these sores by joint motion guarantees undermining, and the soft tissue coverage might only be millimeters in thickness. Surgical treatment of elbow sores is fraught with difficulties, and requires immobilization of the joint and restriction of wheelchair mobility. In many instances, the physician must curb the desire to cure, and simply allow the patient to coexist with a clean, open ulcer over an extended period of time. If surgery is not planned for a chronic ulcer, antibiotic treatment should be reserved for instances where systemic illness or obvious spread of local infection is noted.

Surgery does not cure the problem of pressure ulcers.[311] Repair and healing of ulcers has to be accompanied by a graduated program of remobilization and rehabilitation, a thorough review of remediable environmental precipitants,[447] and education in the rehabilitation setting to teach methods to prevent recurrence. Re-instruction on pressure relief maneuvers should be carried out, including forward-leaning seated weight shifts and prone positioning in bed[269] Such educational efforts are an important element of lifelong follow-up care in the SCI clinic, as the effects of aging with a disability place patients at progressively higher risk for skin complications.

Urological Issues: Implementing a Bladder Management Program

Over the past 50 years, the urological treatment of persons with SCI has improved as physicians have gained a better understanding of bladder physiology and the management of urinary tract complications. The neurophysiology, natural history, and complications of neurogenic bladder dysfunction are discussed in detail in Chapter 27. There are many reasonable options for bladder management after SCI. There is no single method that meets the medical and social needs of all patients. Given the magnitude of choices, it is best when the SCI center staff selects a small number of applicable management options and teaches them well, rather than confuse patients and caregivers with an eclectic mix of techniques.

The medical priorities of urological management in this population are simple: regular voiding with low bladder residual urine, low baseline bladder pressures, and continence.[385] Intermittent catheterization comes to the mind of many clinicians when confronted with a person with SCI. A successful intermittent catheterization program involves much more than a timed catheterization schedule. It requires the active participation of the patient to monitor and adjust oral fluid intake, and constant adjustments of the intermittent catheterization schedule in response to a variety of variables. Intermittent catheterization is usually inappropriate in the acute, ICU setting,[344] when the patient is receiving IV fluids, and when dietary intake and urinary output are inconsistent. Intermittent catheterization, either as a long-term answer or as a means of promoting recovery of reflex voiding function, is best reserved for a time when the patient's urinary output and clinical status are stabilized. In the hospital setting, urinary bacterial colonization occurs in just 3 or 4 days. In the acute setting it is better to have a low-pressure colonized urine (with indwelling catheter) than a distended bladder with high-pressure colonized urine (as can occur when the nursing staff struggles to catch up with irregular and high urine output). Avoidance of mechanical detrusor damage from bladder overdistention in the ICU is extremely important.

Some patients, particularly those with incomplete injuries, regain normal voiding function. Those with more severe deficits who retain hand function can be expected to maintain a long-term catheter-free state with intermittent self-catheterization. Another group of SCI patients, mainly men who can use condom catheters, can potentially maintain a catheter-free state by triggering regular reflex bladder emptying. Intermittent catheterization can be used for these groups, either as a definitive program or as a means to achieve continent or reflex voiding.[240]

Education should begin in the hospital, with nurses teaching proper catheterization technique that is then carried out every 4 to 6 hours.[582] Catheterization volume in the 400 to 500 mL range is the goal. Care must be taken to avoid both overdistention and excessive voluntary fluid restriction and low urine output. Catheterization volumes are often large at night, as renal plasma flow increases in the supine position. Wide variability in catheterization volumes is expected early on. When large volumes occur, the patient is typically discouraged. The staff should offer reassurance rather than admonition.

Some patients begin to pass urine between catheterizations. If the long-term goal is to remain on intermittent catheterization, continence can be promoted by the use of anticholinergic medication.[513] This helps avoid the double inconvenience of an incontinence pad or condom catheter. After discharge, "clean technique" rather than sterile catheterization is tolerated in most situations.[304, 366] Specialized catheters with self-contained urinary collection bags are convenient, but funding for them is often limited.[583] If the goal is reflex or continent voiding, a neurourology evaluation is important. In these patients, intermittent catheterization is continued until adequate bladder emptying and low baseline bladder pressures are demonstrated by cystometrography. There is no magic number that designates a safe post-void residual urine. Volumes in the 100-mL range are reasonable, but higher residual volumes might be tolerated if the patient empties the bladder at shorter (2- to 3-hour) intervals. High pressure or overflow voiding secondary to high outflow resistance (detrusor-sphincter dyssynergia) must be avoided.[210] Management at this point should be directed by physicians with expertise in neurourology. A variety of methods are available to promote complete bladder emptying with reasonable bladder pressures.[456]

There is no external collecting device useful for women, and some men are unable to wear a condom catheter. A few highly motivated persons who lack hand function can reliably engage caregivers to perform intermittent catheterization, but such a practice creates an inconvenience for both parties. Other patients, despite a variety of sophisticated interventions, cannot maintain proper detrusor pressures. Indwelling catheters are a convenient and reasonable alternative for these individuals. Although there are many known complications associated with their use, they can be used successfully with proper self-care and regular medical follow-up. Suprapubic catheters can be used and have many advantages, although the risk of bladder stones is similar to that seen with urethral catheters.[352, 429] Suprapubic catheters do not restrict sexual function, are easily replaced, reduce the incidence of urethral erosions, and avoid catheter contact with other structures that are potentially infected (urethra, prostate, seminal vesicles). All SCI persons with indwelling catheters benefit from anticholinergic medication (to block the bladder reflexes from "fighting" the foreign object) and from regular follow-up with cystoscopy. Persons with indwelling catheters are at slightly higher risk for bladder neoplasms[345] and at high risk for stone development. Cystoscopy is the best means of surveillance for these conditions. Calcium bladder sludge, not free floating stones, is the most common cause of catheter blockage. Bladder sediment is rarely detected by US or plain radiography.

Asymptomatic bacteriuria is generally not treated in persons who use catheters. Even persons on intermittent catheterization commonly develop urinary colonization. Antibiotics are generally reserved for persons symptomatic with fever and leukocytosis and for those demonstrating catheter blockage, increased spasticity, or very foul urine. Overuse of antibiotics is common in SCI persons. Physicians should resist the urge to dispense antibiotics to treat vague symptoms, since this practice promotes bacterial resistance as well as vaginal and urethral candidiasis.[503]

Surgical manipulation of the genitourinary tract has evolved over the past 50 years, and several new surgical options are available. Continent diversion and bladder augmentation procedures have been studied in this population, and promising results have been seen, especially in the treatment of females with neurogenic bladder dysfunction.[218, 396] It is important that these operations be performed by a team of clinicians who have sufficient experience in their implementation in persons with SCI.[45]

Gastrointestinal Complications and Practical Management

Gastrointestinal disorders rank seventh as a cause of death in persons with SCI.[16] Dysfunction of this system has a profound impact on medical morbidity, maintenance of body image, need for caregiver support, and hospital discharge destination. More than one-third of surveyed persons with paraplegia ranked the loss of bowel and bladder control as the most significant functional loss associated with their respective injury—more important than the paralysis of their legs.[251] Difficulties in maintaining bowel continence can have an impact on virtually every aspect of life, interfering with fulfillment of interpersonal, sexual, and employment roles (see Chapter 28, and recent comprehensive review articles on this subject[192, 497]).

Studies of GI complaints have traditionally focused on the acute post-injury period, when ileus, fecal impaction, and upper GI bleeding are most prominent.[221] More recent investigations have assessed the importance of GI problems over the long term, finding that delayed bowel emptying, hemorrhoids, and lower GI tract bleeding are common problems.[115, 499] For persons with chronic SCI, the deleterious effects of decades of suppository use, digital evacuation, and chronic constipation are just now being determined as more SCI individuals present with declining satisfaction with their bowel function.

In the intensive care unit, swallowing and nutritional problems are common.[327] Dysphagia affects nearly 20% of tetraplegic patients,[581] brought about by excessive neck extension in halo devices, soft tissue swelling after anterior neck surgery, poor coordination with ventilator cycling, tracheostomy pain, and concomitant head or cranial nerve injuries. In most cases dysphagia is due to pharyngeal stage problems.[323, 528] Videofluoroscopy can be employed as a diagnostic aid in this setting.[490] In all persons with cervical spine injury, special attention must be given to ensure that esophageal perforation has not occurred at the time of initial trauma. Treatment includes careful supervision of feeding, use of compensatory positioning, and training in supraglottic swallowing and Mendelsohn maneuvers.[360] The prognosis for return of normal swallowing is good in this population.[528]

Even with supplemental tube feeding, nutritional support can be inadequate. Poor tolerance of tube feeding and ileus commonly limit replacement of the huge protein losses associated with injury. Appetite is often poor early on but improves with the establishment of a good bowel routine, correction of dehydration, and resumption of activity. Most patients are constipated at the time of discharge from the intensive care unit. In some instances, only liquid stool passes around a fecal impaction, giving the false impression of diarrhea. Diarrhea can occur in this setting, especially when *Clostridium difficile* and other pathogens colonize the bowel as a complication of liberal antibiotic use. A plain radiograph of the abdomen can be very helpful in patients with constipation. Typically, solid stool is seen in the cecum, which is an abnormal finding. Constipation is best relieved through digital and chemical rectal evacuation, avoiding the use of strong oral cathartics that invariably further distend a poorly motile GI tract.

Although upper GI problems[20, 461] are commonly seen in this population (slow stomach emptying, gallstones, superior mesenteric artery syndrome), bowel emptying is the major concern for most patients. In the acute setting, accurate records of stool output are critical to the development of a bowel routine. In persons with complete SCI, the primary deficits are the lack of sphincter control and reduced bowel motility associated with diminished physical activity. If sphincter control is absent, success depends on the development of "therapeutic constipation," balancing the factors of bowel motility and continence.

Persons with injuries in the lumbar cord or conus can lack the rectal reflex actions that normally expel stool. These patients are best managed with a program of digital stool removal, usually carried out daily. Often mobility and self-care skills are mastered long before the bowel routine is stabilized—a special problem with reduced length of acute hospital stay. Those with SCI in the cervical and thoracic regions who lack sphincter function can use rectal medications (suppositories or enemas), usually every second or third day. These chemical methods save time and provide an extended period of continence between bowel routines. Daily suppository use is usually not recommended. Many persons must be convinced to abandon their pre-injury bowel habits to use a less frequent schedule of every other day. Daily chemical use often results in overstimulation of the rectum and leads to mucous incontinence. Strong oral cathartic medications are avoided; their time of onset is unpredictable and their use precludes the development of a normal column of stool in the colon, increasing the risk of incontinence. Stool consistency is regulated by the use of medium-grade dietary fiber. Persons who are nonambulatory have difficulty hydrating and mobilizing coarse fiber breads and bran. Oral supplements (e.g., psyllium, docusate) are sometimes helpful if the patient has difficulty maintaining a healthy diet.

The most frustrating clinical problems occur when the patient has chronically damaged the colon with decades of infrequent bowel emptying or is bedridden. These persons commonly require oral motility agents (e.g., lactulose, magnesium cathartics) to prevent recurrent fecal impaction, making continence nearly impossible. Physical mobilization and a high level of daily activity are of critical importance in maintaining a successful bowel emptying program.

NEUROLOGICAL ISSUES AFTER INJURY

Pain Syndromes

Most SCI persons experience problems with pain. The pain associated with trauma to bone and soft tissue structures usually disappears within weeks of injury, but subsequent chronic pain problems are estimated to affect between 48% and 94% of this population.[159, 444, 454] For some of these patients, pain problems become a disabling preoccupation.[604] *Nociceptive pain,* generated by noxious stimuli in normally innervated body parts, can often be effectively managed by standard therapeutic modalities, injections, NSAIDs, and remediation of the pathological process that precipitates the pain stimulus.[414, 418, 521] *Neurogenic pain,* associated with injury to nerve roots, cauda equina, and the spinal cord, however, constitutes one of the most enigmatic clinical syndromes faced by patients, clinicians, and researchers. Ragnarsson et al[444] have provided a detailed and thoughtful review of the physiological basis and management strategies for this condition.

Some special causes of nociceptive pain after SCI warrant mention. Nociceptive pain sensation can vary in quality and localization can be inaccurate, but symptoms usually follow a reproducible pattern. Visceral pain (possibly transmitted through sensory fibers in the vagus nerve, pleura, peritoneum, and diaphragm) is often perceptible, even in higher level injuries, and can indicate pelvic or abdominal pathology.[20, 50, 87, 221, 461] Shoulder dysfunction, compression mononeuropathies,[128, 207] degenerative joint disease, trauma, and late spinal deformity and spasticity can precipitate pain complaints.[9, 465]

Neurogenic pain can be further described as radicular, segmental, or deafferentation central pain (DCP).[444] Pain near the level of the cord lesion can be nociceptive, radicular, or segmental. *Radicular pain,* caused by nerve root damage or arachnoiditis, can be unilateral or bilateral. It is confined to predictable areas near the root dermatomes. Electrodiagnostic studies often demonstrate root viability, although impaired nerve conduction and sensory potentials can be seen.[159] Nerve root blocks offer pain relief for many of these patients. *Segmental pain* is bilateral in many instances, and has also been described as "border zone pain," associated with hyperalgesia and hypersensitivity in two or three dermatomes adjacent to the level of SCI. Pain with cauda equina syndrome is a well-recognized variant of segmental pain, often described as a burning or tingling in the buttocks, anus, genitals, and feet. A constricting band can be felt around the trunk in persons with thoracic injuries. Another form of segmental pain, "burning hands syndrome" (or "stingers"), is experienced in many persons with incomplete tetraplegia or minor cord contusions. This is often difficult to distinguish from *reflex sympathetic dystrophy* (also known as complex regional pain syndrome).[207, 540] If the diagnostic criteria of Kozin et al[309] are fulfilled, standard treatment measures for complex regional pain syndrome are often helpful.

Deafferentation central pain is characterized by vague, nondermatomal symptoms originating caudal to the cord lesion that lacks reliable nociceptive precipitants.[541] This type of pain is common and extremely difficult to treat. Riddoch described this condition in 1917,[452] and in 1919 Holmes stated, "I have not, I think seen . . . any condition associated with such intense suffering."[276] Symptoms can be worsened by a variety of events (changes in body position, bladder infections, pressure ulcers) but are neither precipitated by them or relieved when these secondary conditions are remediated.[126, 128] The terms dysesthesias and phantom pain are often used in this setting, but are less specific than DCP.[374] This pain is variably described, but once it starts, it is continuous. It can begin weeks or months after SCI.[61, 76] It is likely that the pain impulses are generated in segments of the spinal cord just above the lesion, although a complex interaction involving supraspinal deafferentation changes in the thalamus and cortical sensory areas has also been postulated.[336, 375] Persons who develop neurogenic pain in the chronic phase of injury should be evaluated for syringomyelia.[459]

There is no single intervention, invasive or noninvasive, that is reliably effective in the treatment of segmental and deafferentation central pain. Judicious treatment of these conditions involves recognition of this fact and an appreciation of the complex physical and psychosocial factors that influence the impact that pain exerts on a patient's life. Despite the frustrating nature of the problem, patients must be reassured that, in the vast majority of instances, the usual pattern is for pain to become more tolerable or manageable.[133, 521] Commonly, this adaptation comes with an improvement in activity level and other psychosocial factors.[80]

The list of medications that have been used for DCP and segmental pain is long and continues to grow.[126, 261, 363] Medications are considered if symptoms restrict activity or sleep, beginning with aspirin, acetaminophen, and NSAIDs. Tricyclic antidepressants (e.g., amitriptyline, doxepin) have been used for decades in this setting. These drugs act by diminishing the presynaptic uptake of serotonin and norepinephrine. Trazadone has been studied in persons with SCI, with poor results. Newer antidepressants (fluoxetine, sertraline, venalafaxine) have not been well studied in this population. Anticonvulsants (carbamazepine, clonazepam, phenytoin, gabapentin) have also been prescribed, often in combination with antidepressant medication.[134] Their use is limited by the need for laboratory tests and by a number of side effects. Mexiletine is a local anesthetic and antiarrhythmic agent that has not been found to have a significant effect on DCP.[94] Narcotic analgesics are sometimes prescribed.

Although some pain specialists have advocated more liberal use of narcotic drugs in chronic pain conditions, these recommendations are difficult to put into daily practice. Patients with DCP typically experience their symptoms with or without narcotic medication. Many of these patients are taking several other medications for several other medical problems, and the risk of polypharmacy and toxicity is high. It is difficult to justify the use of opiates or opiate derivatives, especially in light of their side-effect profile. Constipation can become a significant side effect of these medications.

Over the years persons with spinal cord pain syndromes have been subjected to a large variety of ablative and invasive procedures. Spinal subarachnoid anesthesia has been used for diagnostic purposes[350] and has temporarily reduced pain symptoms in the majority of subjects. Intrathecal baclofen, morphine, and clonidine have also been studied. Transcutaneous nerve stimulation is best employed in the setting of nociceptive, radicular, or segmental pain.[134, 175, 242] Dorsal column electrical stimulation has also been attempted.[348, 410, 451] In addition, ablative surgical and injection procedures have been carried out at virtually every level of the neuraxis, with marginal benefit.[569] Of these, dorsal root entry zone microcoagulation has been well studied and is still used in selected centers.[189, 410] This procedure requires a multiple level laminectomy, with microthermal lesions created in the substantia gelatinosa just above the level of the cord lesion. This destructive procedure is reserved for a carefully selected group of patients in whom other interventions have failed.

Progressive Posttraumatic Cystic Myelopathy (Syringomyelia)

Syringomyelia is a recognized cause of progressive myelopathy. Syringomyelia is idiopathic in some cases, but usually it is associated with developmental anomalies of the foramen magnum, spinal cord tumors, or as a late complication of spinal cord trauma. Posttraumatic syringomyelia has been termed progressive posttraumatic cystic myelopathy (PPCM).[222] The classic clinical signs of PPCM include a dissociated loss of pain and temperature sensation, usually in the distal upper extremities. The most common initial symptom of PPCM is pain. PPCM has been noted as early as 2 months post injury and as late as 23 years.[600] Estimates of the incidence of PPCM range from 0.3% to 8%.[163, 523] Spinal cord cysts and myelomalacia are frequently seen on MRI after traumatic injury. The incidence figures vary according to the imaging modality employed and the criteria by which syringomyelia is defined. This condition is probably more frequent in persons with paraplegia. The pathological processes that generate cystic spinal cord changes are not well understood.[294, 578]

Symptoms of posttraumatic syringomyelia commonly consist of segmental or radicular pain, late motor and sensory loss, increased spasticity, and hyperhydrosis.[44, 364, 459, 492] Horner's syndrome and respiratory insufficiency can be seen with cysts that extend into the brainstem.[31, 530] Symptoms can also be positional. Radiological diagnosis is now much improved with the use of T1-weighted high-resolution MRI.[576] Gadolinium images are helpful in differentiating between syrinx and myelomalacia in posttraumatic cases.[222] Electrodiagnosis, including central motor conduction times and motor-evoked potentials, can also be a sensitive diagnostic modality.[343]

The treatment of PPCM has long been controversial. Asymptomatic cysts and those smaller than 1 cm are not considered for surgical treatment and are followed with serial clinical examinations and follow-up MRI. Surgery is considered if one or more signs or symptoms are encountered in the presence of larger cysts. Surgical treatment usually consists of a midline myelotomy, with placement of a shunt tube to continuously drain the cyst into the subarachnoid space. Desired surgical outcomes include resolution of clinical symptoms and persisting collapse of the cyst cavity. Treatment outcomes vary considerably among investigators.[163, 459, 531] Studies with long-term follow-up report less favorable postoperative results than those that present a shorter postoperative observation period.

Spasticity

A comprehensive review of the pathophysiology and treatment of spasticity is found in Chapter 29. The evaluation and treatment of spasticity in persons with SCI are comparable to that done in persons with other types of upper motor neuron neurological diseases.[298]

The evolution of uncontrolled muscle stretch reflexes is common during the period of initial inpatient rehabilitation and is a source of great interest to and misunderstanding among patients and families. The acknowledgment that this new movement is expected and is of little prognostic significance can be difficult. Spasticity is usually not painful. In some cases, however, spasticity can be so powerful as to make wheelchair use and transfers dangerous. Spasticity is not a problem that is separate from SCI; it is inseparable from the problem of muscle weakness and is part and parcel of upper motor neuron disease. Functional restrictions often arise, less from poorly functional spastic muscles than from the interference that spastic limbs present to positioning and the functional movements of normally innervated muscles.

Spastic hypertonia does not always require treatment. Many SCI patients use extensor muscle tone to assist with standing, transfers, and ambulation. Spasticity preserves muscle mass and might lessen the incidence of venous thrombosis. Treatment is indicated only if the spasticity interferes with the performance of self-care, gait, wheelchair positioning, and transfer activities, disrupts sleep, or causes excessive pain or joint deformity. Spasticity also contributes to the development of pressure ulcers. An unexplained worsening of spasticity can signal the development of a secondary condition, such as spinal instability or syringomyelia. Virtually any noxious stimulus, such as pressure ulcers, urinary tract infections, urolithiasis, or constipation, can worsen muscle spasms. Evaluation for such contributing factors is the first element in the comprehensive management of this condition.

A daily routine of prolonged muscle stretching is the foundation for management of spasticity.[56, 297] The reduction in hypertonia that follows can last for several hours. Spasticity is probably most severe in persons with motor incomplete spinal cord lesions. Early after injury, flexor tone usually predominates, but this can change to an extensor pattern as time passes.[384] In some instances, the problem is focal. Flexor spasticity at the elbow, for example, might respond to local treatment with muscle or nerve blocks, serial splinting, or orthopedic surgery intervention. A variety of nonpharmacological treatments have been tried, with variable effectiveness in this setting.[108] If the problem with abnormal tone is generalized, medications are considered. Four medications—baclofen, diazepam, dantrolene, and tizanidine—are indicated for use in SCI. Symptom relief can be modest with these drugs; clinicians must be familiar with their mechanisms of action and their significant side effects (see Chapter 29).

Baclofen, diazepam, and tizanidine act on the CNS. Baseline liver function tests are useful before initiating treatment with these antispasticity medications. Baclofen is often used as a first-line agent, with a starting dose of 5 mg three times a day in adults.[130] The maximum recommended dosage is 80 mg/day, but many clinicians use up to 120 mg/day. Abrupt discontinuation of the drug can result in seizures, and SCI persons with renal insufficiency require dose adjustment.[5, 512]

Diazepam is a safe and effective drug. Tolerance to its cognitive effects develops rapidly, and the antispasticity effects can persist indefinitely. Adult dosages of 10 to 40 mg/day are used.[297] Its use is contraindicated in persons with a history of alcohol, drug, or medication abuse. A paradoxical response is occasionally seen with diazepam, resulting in insomnia, hostility, or anxiety. Dosage increases in diazepam should be undertaken carefully.

Tizanidine treatment starts with 4 mg taken at bedtime. Its dose can be increased in very small increments to obtain the desired effects, an advantage over treatment with clonidine.[408] Most patients will require 12 to 36 mg/day in three or four divided doses. Problems with low blood pressure are expected with alpha-2 agonist drugs but are uncommon in the SCI population. The concurrent use of tizanidine and clonidine is not recommended.

Dantrolene acts peripherally at the neuromuscular junction. It is initiated at a dose of 25 mg, which can be increased slowly to a maximum of 400 mg/day in divided doses. This agent weakens innervated and noninnervated muscles in a nonselective fashion. Rarely, serious hepatotoxicity can occur. This risk is higher in females, persons older than 35 years, persons on estrogen therapy, and those taking high doses of the drug.[524, 577]

Clonidine, both in oral and in transdermal forms,[563, 584] has been studied as a spasticity agent in SCI patients.[584] Its use can be limited by the side effects of constipation, hypotension, and lethargy.[158] Gabapentin has also been studied. Doses above 400 mg three times a day are usually needed to produce a clinical response.[234, 439] A number of other drugs have been suggested, including cannabis.[354]

Intrathecal baclofen, delivered through an implanted programmable pump and catheter system, has been used for more than a decade for spasticity in persons with SCI (Fig. 55–6). The magnitude of spasticity relief is remarkable in comparison with that achieved with oral medication, but this invasive treatment is not appropriate for all patients.[1, 104, 425] Regular pump refills are needed on a lifelong basis and must be carried out by experienced nursing staff. In some instances, tachyphylaxis is encountered, and intrathecal morphine is temporarily substituted. Marketing of this device has focused on its benefits related to improved function, but it is also quite useful in persons who are chronically bedconfined. In these patients, severe spasticity often prevents proper positioning and hygiene of the perineal area. Other surgical options for the treatment of spasticity exist (see Chapter 29).[168, 271, 296, 440, 474]

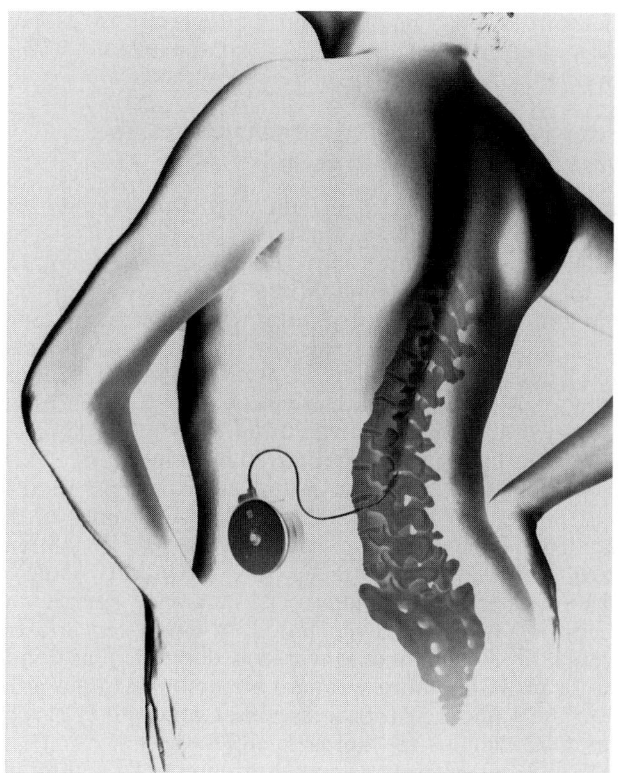

FIGURE 55–6. Programmable pump and catheter system for the intrathecal delivery of baclofen. (Courtesy of Medtronic Inc.)

ORTHOPEDIC AND MUSCULOSKELETAL ISSUES

Spinal Fractures

Although most persons with spinal fractures do not sustain SCI, most persons with SCI have spinal fractures. There are as many types of spine fractures as there are mechanisms of injury, and the study of spinal fractures occurring in conjunction with myelopathy has been limited by the lack of a widely accepted system to describe the bone trauma. Several textbooks and reviews cover decades of investigation on this expansive topic in appropriate detail.[8, 41, 42, 57, 82, 116, 275, 335, 362, 386, 493]

Initial orthopedic trauma care attempts to identify and immobilize fractures to lessen the risk of further neurological injury. The degree of spinal instability is then assessed, with consideration of the severity and stability of the neurological deficit. There is no single indicator of spinal stability, since stability is a relative term that takes into account both radiographic and clinical assessments. Even patients who have undergone spinal instrumentation and spinal immobilization with an orthosis can still have a high degree of spinal instability. As an example, many elderly patients who sustain fractures associated with ankylosing spondylitis remain at high risk for further neurological injury despite aggressive spine management. An understanding of the three-column concept of Holdsworth[275] and the components of cervical stability described by Allen et al[8] are helpful in quantifying the severity of ligamentous or bony injury. The fracture classification of Meyer[387] allows more detailed analysis of spinal stability by assessing vertebral displacement (in any plane), angulation and compression of vertebral bodies, canal compromise, and loss of vertebral height.

The goals of spinal treatment are to realign the spine, promote proper healing, prevent late deformity, and protect damaged neural tissue. Great controversy exists regarding the indications for spinal surgery and the timing of its application. It is of extreme importance that these patients be treated by an experienced spine traumatology team. There are dozens of compelling reasons to treat the spine surgically, but there is sparse evidence in human studies that surgery promotes neurological recovery over and above that expected on the basis of spontaneous improvement, either at the root or at the spinal cord level.[558] Surgery is sometimes advocated as a means of providing early patient mobilization, but for patients with severe neurological injuries at the cervical or high thoracic level, this benefit is questionable. With expert nursing and therapy care, little time is lost when the spinal immobilization period is used to enhance healing of associated injuries, nutrition, pulmonary status, and strength in preparation for the added stress imposed by sitting.[156, 611]

Spinal Orthoses

Proper management of spinal orthoses is an important part of the acute rehabilitation process (see Chapter 17). Several authors have detailed the application of these devices in the setting of spinal trauma, along with the degree of spinal immobilization that is provided.[22, 46, 179, 289, 552] The rehabilitation team works closely with the spinal surgeon and orthotist to ensure that braces are applied and maintained properly and that consistent directions for wear are given. No amount of orthotic adjustment can make a spinal brace comfortable, although return visits from the orthotist and encouragement from the rehabilitation team can reassure and comfort the patient. In some instances, the spinal brace temporarily restricts rehabilitation training (transfers, self-catheterization, bed mobility). Achievement of some therapy goals might have to be delayed until the spine has healed and the brace has been removed.

The halo orthosis is an effective means of reducing spinal motion, both for conservative and for postoperative management. This device provides superior restriction of cervical motion at most levels, although this restriction is not complete.[552] When properly applied it is remarkably well tolerated and needs little adjustment. Extra caution should be used when considering halo placement for persons with delirium, acute psychosis, or schizophrenia and for patients with severe skull osteoporosis (e.g., elderly rheumatoid patients). Swallowing difficulties and choking sensations can occur when the halo ring locks the neck in excessive extension. Most patients report occasional creaking and popping noises associated with the halo superstructure. Adjustment is usually not necessary unless there is obvious motion in the halo frame. Halo pin sites are cleaned daily. Inspection is facilitated by careful trimming of scalp hair around the posterior pins. Halo pins need not be disturbed unless cellulitis, drainage, or pain occurs at the pin site. Infected sites require pin replacement. Pain at the insertion site or tracking of the hole can indicate a loose or infected pin. When pin problems arise, pin tightness should be checked by an experienced examiner utilizing a torque wrench. A pin torque of 6 to 8 pounds per inch should be achieved within one complete wrench turn. A pin that spins with little resistance should be investigated and likely replaced.

Heterotopic Ossification

Heterotopic ossification is a poorly understood medical condition characterized by the development of para-articular ossification, usually on the flexor surfaces of larger joints. It occurs in persons with neurological diseases, usually within the region of their motor deficits. It also is seen in persons who have sustained burns and in persons who have undergone total hip arthroplasty. The factors that connect these three disparate groups of patients and predispose to the development of heterotopic bone are unknown. This process of true ossification (trabecular bone formation) is distinct from ectopic calcification, or mineralization of soft tissue structures, that is noted in a variety of medical and traumatic conditions. Its incidence in persons with SCI has been reported to range from 16% to 53%.[529] In the majority of SCI patients, ectopic bone is an incidental finding on plain radiographs and without clinical or functional significance.[505, 567] Of those developing heterotopic ossification, only 18% to 37% have disabling ROM limitations, and less than 5% develop ankylosis of the affected joint (Fig. 55–7).[197, 198, 568]

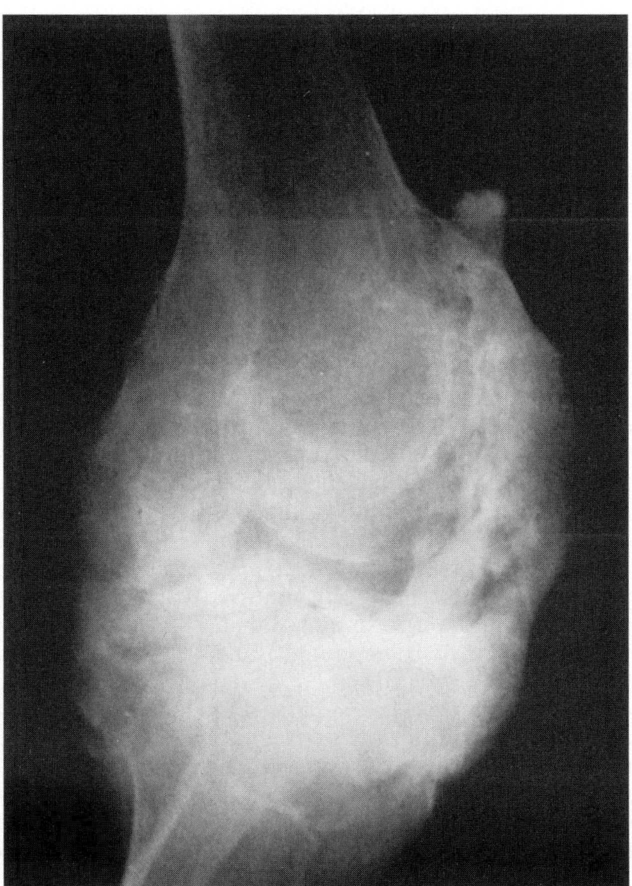

FIGURE 55–7. Plain radiograph of a knee, with ankylosis from heterotopic ossification.

The onset of heterotopic ossification is generally within 6 months after injury, with the most frequent occurrence between 1 and 4 months.[501, 567] It has been reported to occur as early as 20 days post injury. The initial presentation of heterotopic ossification rarely occurs more than 1 year after injury. The most commonly involved areas, in decreasing order, are the hips, knees, shoulders, and elbows.[502, 567] Involvement of the axial skeleton and smaller joints in the extremities is very rare. In comparison to heterotopic ossification found in traumatic brain injury and hip replacement patients, there appear to be specific patterns of formation in SCI patients. About the hip, heterotopic ossification is most commonly located anteriorly and generally forms between the anterior superior iliac spine and the lesser trochanter.[502] At the knee, involvement of the medial aspect is most commonly noted.

The pathogenesis of heterotopic ossification remains unclear. Its development is thought to be related to local metabolic, circulatory, or biochemical factors that stimulate a metaplastic response of mesenchymal cells.[286] Since it is also commonly found in patients who have sustained traumatic brain injury, the possibility of alteration in neural control over the differentiation of mesenchymal cells into osteoblasts has been suggested.[505] The presence or absence of spasticity has not been shown to be associated with the development of heterotopic ossification.[502] Although the presence of a pressure ulcer near a proximal joint increases the risk of developing heterotopic ossification,[257, 320] other conditions, including severe spasticity and aggressive ROM exercise, have not been demonstrated to be risk factors.[502]

Ectopic bone is extra-articular, often leaving the joint capsule intact. It forms in the connective tissue between the muscle planes and not within the muscle itself. The bone can be contiguous with the skeleton but generally does not involve the periosteum. Mature heterotopic ossification has histological features similar to those of a fracture callus. The bone is a lamellar corticospongiosal bone with a thin cortex, tightly latticed spongiosum, and occasional haversian systems.[458]

The initial clinical features of heterotopic ossification are nonspecific. The most common presentation is a warm, swollen, erythematous extremity. It can be confused with acute deep venous thrombosis. Swelling in the extremity is usually localized, and within several days a more circumscribed, firm mass can be noted within the area of edema.[501] Early symptoms can include pain and restriction of joint motion. During the initial presentation, the differential diagnosis includes cellulitis, septic arthritis, bone tumor, Baker's cyst, and venous thrombosis.[419, 567, 594]

Plain radiographs are of limited use in the early diagnosis of this condition. The first evidence of calcification might not appear for weeks after the clinical presentation.[501] An elevated serum alkaline phosphatase level can assist in differentiating early heterotopic ossification from other conditions,[199, 419] but serum levels are frequently abnormal secondary to other causes (spinal fracture, concomitant long bone injuries). Serial alkaline phosphatase levels are better used in following the progression of bone deposition rather than in the initial diagnosis. Increased 24-hour urinary prostaglandin E_2 levels can aid in early diagnosis.[473] The triple-phase bone scan, performed using radiolabeled diphosphates, is very helpful for early detection of heterotopic ossification. The first two phases, dynamic blood flow study and static scan for blood pool, are the most sensitive for early detection (Fig. 55–8).[184, 419] Ultrasonography is essential in differentiating this process from thrombosis and is also helpful in the diagnosis of heterotopic bone. Early in the course, an echolucent zone of muscle often encloses a broad reflective zone across the area of clinical suspicion.[437, 488]

When the diagnosis is confirmed, initial treatment involves passive ROM exercises to maintain joint mobility. There is no evidence in human studies that this approach increases the ultimate amount of bone formation. Misguided discontinuation of passive ROM exercise can result in decreased motion in the affected joint and possibly in ankylosis.[315, 502, 567] Disodium etidronate is effective in limiting the extent of heterotopic ossification when this treatment is started early in the course.[314, 501] It appears to be much less effective when used later in the disease course, regardless of dosage or duration of treatment.[29, 199] Larger doses of disodium etidronate have recently been employed in hopes of producing greater reduction in bone formation.[30] Other medications, most notably indomethacin and warfarin, have been studied in the treatment of this condition. In some instances these drugs are combined with radiation therapy to the affected joint.[78, 183, 197]

The complications of heterotopic ossification can include peripheral nerve entrapment,[73] the development of pressure ulcers,[257] an increased risk of DVT,[256] and extra-articular joint ankylosis. In these situations, surgical resection of the bone can be considered. Surgical resection of the bone would seem to be a simple solution to the problem, but complication rates approach 80%, even in experienced hands.[199] There is conflicting opinion regarding the timing of surgery and the modes of perioperative care. Conventional surgical approaches have included a delay of 12 to 18 months between diagnosis and surgery, ostensibly to allow the bone mass to mature before resection. Problems arise when conventional tests for bone maturity (bone scan, radiography, alkaline phosphatase levels) fail to correctly identify those with mature bone.[199, 505] Nuclear medicine scans can show activity for many months after the initial diagnosis, and the patient can have progressive loss of joint mobility during this waiting period. Recent reports of early resection of heterotopic bone in combination with drug and radiation treatment appear promising.[30, 369, 468] The surgical procedure is often more complicated than anticipated. The surgeon often encounters a "nest" of bone that is perforated by tortuous blood vessels and nerves, and no distinct tissue planes are apparent. Total resection is not undertaken. The goal of free ROM is obtained with a limited wedge resection, to reduce postoperative "dead space." A hematoma develops in the dead space soon after surgery. A fever can be present, and the operate limb is often warm and swollen. The question of perioperative DVT is always a consider-

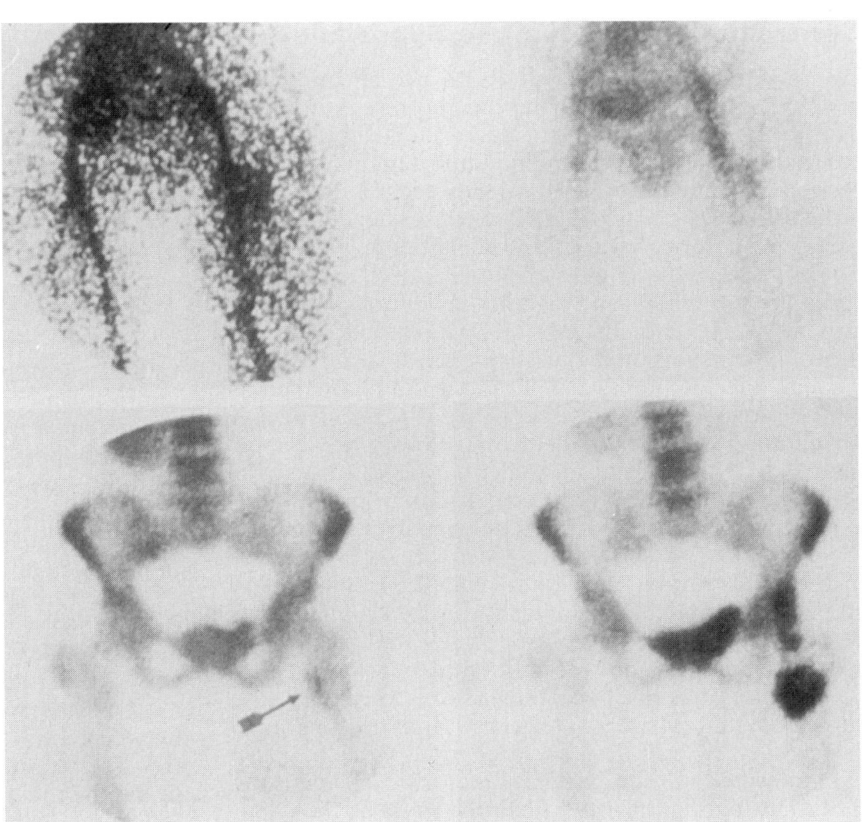

FIGURE 55–8. Triple-phase bone scan showing the formation of heterotopic ossification about the left hip. (From Orzel JA, Rudd TG: Heterotopic bone formation: Clinical laboratory and imaging correlation. J Nucl Med 1985; 26:125–132.)

ation in this setting, where anticoagulation can certainly aggravate the healing process. Wound infection can occur; experience and close clinical observation are necessary to determine whether a soft tissue or deep infection is present. The majority of patients exhibit recurrence of bone after surgery.[199, 505] With proper care, joint ROM can be preserved despite this recurrence. Many surgeons begin drug treatment with disodium etidronate and use radiation in the perioperative setting.[30, 197, 468, 470, 504] Careful positioning and turning in bed is necessary to protect the operated limb from excessive stretching and to prevent trauma to the swollen operative site.

Limb Fractures

In the acute setting, limb fractures are the most common traumatic condition associated with SCI.[216] Despite striking changes in bone metabolism during this phase, long bone and spinal fractures heal well with standard orthopedic care, including internal and external fixation.[197] The presence of longstanding myelopathy markedly raises the risk of leg fractures.[191] Fractures that occur in the chronic phase of injury present a number of unique treatment challenges. These fractures are often discovered after a minor or incidental trauma. In some instances the patient cannot identify the precipitating event. Most of these fractures occur just above or just below the knee.[187] The patient presents with malaise, clinical signs of fever, and swelling and redness of the affected limb. Venous thrombosis and cellulitis are always included in the differential diagnosis.

In the chronic phase of injury, upper extremity fractures, and leg fractures in ambulatory patients, are treated with the same techniques as are used in nondisabled populations. The treating physician confronts a unique set of circumstances when faced with leg fractures in persons who are nonambulatory. These fractures are radiographically striking, and osteopenia is severe. The temptation to instrument the fracture is great; however, severe muscle and soft tissue atrophy is present, the patients often lack sensation in the area, and they might not be able to properly splint the area due to spasticity. Patients often benefit from a short (2- to 3-day) period of bedrest when fever is present. After this, quick mobilization is undertaken with fracture stabilization provided by soft splint materials. In the nonambulatory patient, a limited degree of limb shortening and angulation of the fracture site is tolerated, but avoidance of rotational deformities is a priority. Hard cast materials can produce pressure ulcers. If the patient is careful with limb positioning and wheelchair transfers, hard cast immobilization is not necessary.

Persons with fractures of the leg are usually advised to elevate the limb while in the wheelchair. This practice is risky because elevation of the leg changes wheelchair positioning, shifting weight over the seated surface and placing the patient at high risk for seated pressure ulcers. If tissue edema is an issue, frequent recumbent rest periods out of the wheelchair are a better option. Although conservative care is used if possible in the chronic phase, subtrochanteric and proximal femur fractures rarely heal properly without internal fixation.[187]

Contractures and Overuse Syndromes

Pain and restrictions in joint ROM are an important problem in both the acute and the chronic setting. Preventing contractures and soft tissue shortening is time-consuming and inconvenient but important because correction of joint deformities once they occur is even more difficult. The intensity of ROM exercises needed to prevent joint deformity varies among patients, but education regarding the consequences of range restrictions (pressure sores, pain, and mobility restrictions) is important for every patient. Joint ROM restrictions result from muscle shortening, spasticity, capsular adhesions, trauma, and joint ankylosis. In the acute phase, splints at the wrists and ankles (see Fig. 55–2) and proper positioning of the shoulders and elbows are important.[233, 475] Nonambulatory patients who can lie in the prone position greatly reduce their risk of pressure ulcers and hip and knee flexion contractures. Achieving the prone position should be a goal for every SCI patient in the acute setting, as soon as spinal and pulmonary stability permit. Regional injection of neurolytic agents or botulinum toxin can be used in selected instances if spasticity restricts joint mobility and pharmacological management has not been satisfactory. Muscle release surgery requires special expertise and postoperative care.[166]

Patients with lower extremity motor deficits place an inordinate amount of weight-bearing stress on the upper extremities, either for wheelchair propulsion, transfers, or crutch walking. In the weight-bearing upper extremity, there is an increased prevalence of shoulder impingement, tears of the rotator cuff, carpal instability, and carpal tunnel syndrome. These conditions probably arise from muscle imbalance, repetitive loading, and postural abnormalities.[9, 37, 207, 208, 472, 520] Shoulder pain is reported in more than one-half of surveyed patients with SCI.[217, 414, 482, 783] Patients with upper extremity dysfunction can be treated with standard musculoskeletal modalities, including NSAIDs and injection, but a review of their mobility techniques by an experienced physical or occupational therapist is of utmost importance. The emphasis of treatment must be on joint conservation. This raises special concerns for many patients, from elite long-distance wheelchair athletes to overweight persons performing independent transfers.[59] A power wheelchair is sometimes the best means of preserving shoulder function into the later years for those with the potential to perform independent wheelchair transfers. Persons with progressive signs of nerve entrapment, shoulder impingement, and rotator cuff pathology are candidates for standard surgical decompression or repair.[81, 376]

PEDIATRIC SPINAL CORD INJURY

Across the United States, 5% of SCIs occur in children and adolescents under the age of 15.[110, 206, 244, 249, 301, 420] Just as in the adult population, motor vehicle collisions are the most common cause of injury (38% to 64%).[535] Young children (under the age of 8 years) are at special risk for sustaining automobile-inflicted injuries as pedestrians. Sporting activities, acts of violence, and falls are other common causes of traumatic paralysis. Sporting injuries, mostly from diving, account for 23% of injuries in this group and are seen more frequently in older children and adolescents.[216] Injuries from violence have increased over the past two decades. Even the youngest children are not spared; 15% of children under age 8 are injured by violent acts.[17, 535]

Other injury mechanisms are rare but unique to this group.[15, 79, 305] Neonatal SCIs are seen in approximately 1 in 60,000 births.[428] Rotational injuries from forceps trauma result in high cervical injuries. Cervicothoracic injuries can occur with breech deliveries, and thoracic lesions can arise as a result of perinatal umbilical artery trauma or paradoxical air embolism through transitional cardiovascular shunts.[535] In older children, injury can be associated with atlantoaxial instability (e.g., in Down's syndrome), juvenile rheumatoid arthritis, and in the setting of skeletal dysplasias, such as Morquio's syndrome or metatopic dwarfism.

In contrast to the population of persons injured as adults, girls and boys are equally represented in the youngest injury cohorts.[244, 301, 464, 535] In addition, the mechanisms and epidemiology of spinal injury differ between children and adults. Nearly 70% of spinal injuries in children result in paraplegia, probably because of the high incidence (64%) of motor vehicle trauma in this group.[535] Lap belt injuries, commonly seen in children weighing less than 40 lb, are brought about by flexion-distraction trauma over a restraint situated above the pelvic brim. These injuries are characterized by abdominal wall bruising and intra-abdominal injuries, with vertebral compression at any level in the lumbar spine.[508] Neurological lesions in this setting are variable. Deficits can be seen as high as the mid-thoracic spinal cord, implicating vascular trauma.[18] In the cervical spine, very high lesions (C1 to C3), which are rare in adults, are overrepresented in this group, accounting for 10% of injuries. This is most likely due to the proportionately large head and weak neck muscles in small children.[464] In the emergency setting, these anatomical differences necessitate the use of pediatric spine immobilization boards with cranial openings, to allow an anatomical alignment during transport and initial treatment.

In the immature spine, excessive elasticity, shallow, horizontal facet joints, and fragile vertebral end-plates contribute to the high incidence of SCI in the setting of normal spinal radiographs.[249, 316, 422] The incidence of SCI without radiographic abnormality is 63% in children under the age of 10.[93, 422] Despite the normal radiographic appearance, these children are more likely to develop a complete neurological injury and to have a poor neurological prognosis.[422] Adding even greater uncertainty to the emergency department evaluation of childhood trauma, in up to 25% of children with SCI there is a delay, lasting hours to days, between the traumatic episode and the appearance of neurological deficits.[243, 249] Newer MRI techniques are extremely helpful in this setting,[174] detailing soft tissue injury in 65% of children with SCI without radiographic abnormalities.

The resources needed to appropriately address the special needs of children with SCI are rarely available close to home. Even pediatricians can lack experience and training in this rare condition, and the treatment concepts applied to other disabling conditions of childhood (e.g., congenital scoliosis, myelomeningocele, cerebral palsy) are rarely relevant in this setting. The child with acquired paralysis must be treated in a milieu where clinicians understand the long-term implications of the condition and apply interventions that are developmentally appropriate. Even the youngest children should be given a role in decision making. There is a wide variability among patients in the capacity to communicate, understand, and cooperate. Children injured at birth present altogether different problems for the treatment team than those injured in adolescence. In addition, these injuries affect every aspect of family functioning.[12] Clinicians must be prepared to spend extra time with family members, providing anticipatory guidance and support. Centers that treat adults with SCI might not be able to meet the unique medical and psychological needs of this heterogeneous group.

In many respects, the medical management of children with SCI parallels that of adults. Although venous thromboembolism is diagnosed less frequently in children, the disastrous potential of clots that go undetected has led to the recommendation that all children should receive thromboprophylaxis,[111, 224, 441] with aggressive physical and pharmacological measures. The goals of acute pulmonary management are the same in children as in adults: to maintain appropriate oxygenation and reduce the effects of atelectasis and pneumonia. Alveolar ventilation requirements, however, are higher in children due to a higher metabolic rate. The compliance of the immature rib cage is also increased, necessitating bilateral pacing in infants by means of phrenic nerve electrostimulation.[562]

Methods of neurogenic bowel management in children are analogous to those used in adults. For children with intact sacral reflexes, a regular schedule of rectal emptying promoted by chemical or digital stimulation of the anorectum should be established. Children with lumbar and sacral injuries might lack sacral reflexes and need daily digital removal of stool. Considerable latitude should be given to younger children, who typically approach the problems of bowel continence at their own pace. The ultimate goal is to eliminate the use of diapers prior to kindergarten or first grade.[539] Older children and adolescents are prone to bowel emptying difficulties secondary to irregular dietary habits. Supplementation with moderate amounts of fiber supplements is often necessary.[192]

The presence of nonspecific GI complaints in an adolescent with SCI can indicate the presence of hypercalcemia. This usually appears within the first 3 months post injury and affects 10% to 23% of persons with SCI; it is most common in young males.[368, 407, 515] Clinical manifestations can include nausea, abdominal pain, vomiting, poor appetite, polydipsia, and mental status changes. The increase in bone turnover characteristic of growing children, combined with the increased bone resorption seen in acute SCI, might be responsible for the high incidence of hypercalcemia in this population.[539] In most instances, IV hydration, combined with administration of furosemide, facilitates renal excretion of calcium and symptom relief within 3 to 4 days. If this treatment is not successful, the use of calcitonin, given twice daily through the subcutaneous route, should be instituted. Etidronate disodium is not used in growing children because of the potential for development of a rachitic syndrome.[485] Close follow-up is needed after treatment, since prolonged hypercalcemia is associated with the development of urinary tract lithiasis and renal failure.

Proper urological management of the pediatric patient also minimizes the risk of renal complications by reducing risk factors such as cystitis, pyelonephritis, vesicoureteral reflux, and trauma from long-term catheter use.[526] Children should undergo routine urodynamic evaluations, renal US, and voiding cystourethrography to assess the function and coordination of the bladder and sphincter. The goals of treatment are the same as in adults—establishment of a plan that maintains low detrusor pressures and allows complete bladder emptying. For children under the age of 4, continence is not a primary concern, and diapers can be used if detrusor pressures are low and reflux is not present. Intermittent catheterization can be started at any age, even in infants,[136, 290] if recurrent infections or vesicoureteral reflux are noted. Bladder volumes range from 30 mL in neonates to over 350 mL in pre-adolescents.[566] An attempt to wean children from diapers should begin at an age-appropriate time, usually around 4 years. Parents are trained to perform clean intermittent catheterization, and continence is facilitated by pharmacological treatment with such agents as oxybutinin, imipramine, terazosin, propantheline, desmopressin, and pseudoephedrine.[165] Self-catheterization can be introduced as early as age 5, but many children, especially boys, might not be developmentally ready until age 8 or 9.

Intermittent catheterization programs are not successful in many children. Poor hand function, high-pressure, low-capacity bladders unresponsive to drug treatment, unacceptable drug side effects, inability to restrict fluid intake, and inconvenience are common reasons for abandoning intermittent catheterization. In older boys, condom catheters can be used, but they are only appropriate after a thoughtful and detailed analysis of baseline voiding function, as sphincterotomy is rarely performed in this setting. Indwelling urethral or suprapubic catheters allow the child considerable autonomy and convenience in the school setting, advantages that must be weighed against the increased risks of lower urinary tract trauma and calculus formation.

Families should be reminded that there is no perfect method of management of the neuropathic urinary tract. Even the best intermittent catheterization programs do not eliminate the risk of instrumentation trauma and infection.[157, 371] Counseling should emphasize the minimal use of antibiotics. The indications for prophylactic and acute antibiotic treatment are the same for children as they are for adults. Surgical reconstruction of the lower urinary tract, including construction of bowel loop diversions, continent catheterizable stomas, and bladder augmentation procedures, remains a reasonable option for children with recurrent symptomatic infections and evidence of upper urinary tract deterioration despite best efforts at conservative management. Consideration of a surgical reconstruction procedure must not be seen as an indication of failure on the part of parents or the patient.

Planning for any surgery should involve consideration of latex allergy and the risk of anaphylaxis when exposed to latex products in the operating suite. Up to 18% of children with SCI demonstrate positive skin testing for latex,[308, 537] precipitated by early and repeated contact with the allergenic proteins present in raw latex and extracts of finished rubber products in catheters and latex gloves. Life-threatening anaphylactic reactions can be the presenting sign of latex allergy in up to 30% of latex-sensitive children. Contact dermatitis and urticaria, wheezing, and angioedema are other presenting factors. If skin testing is not available, all children with SCI should be considered at risk. In many hospitals, these patients are automatically treated in latex-free medical environments, and perioperative prophylactic doses of glucocorticoids and antihistamines are given.

Notwithstanding the considerable attention given to medical concerns, the central focus of injured children and their parents relates to disability, and walking is their primary goal. The medical, orthopedic, and musculoskeletal benefits of achieving standing and walking are regularly misrepresented and overstated. Studies demonstrating that upright activities change the natural history of this condition are lacking.[285] Despite this fact, clinicians should understand that the desire to walk becomes an issue of profound psychological and social importance. Standing facilitates childhood recreational, educational, vocational, and leisure activities.[538]

Success in achieving ambulation depends on a number of factors, chiefly neurological level of injury, motivation, body size, and musculoskeletal integrity. For patients with residual arm function, castor carts can be used at 9 to 12 months to allow exploration of their environment. At 18 to 24 months, a wheelchair can be prescribed as a primary means of mobility for tetraplegic children, and as a concurrent mobility device for those who are learning to walk with assistive devices.[402] As in adults, children with lesions at L3 and below and those with International Classification D injuries have a favorable prognosis for long-term community ambulation.[280, 538] Younger children might benefit from high levels of energy and motivation, favorable trunk to leg proportions, and lean body build. They can sometimes achieve surprising levels of mobility despite higher neurological lesions. The use of standing frames and parapodia can be initiated at 10 to 12 months of age, even in individuals with quadriplegia. These devices allow children free use of their hands, and, given flat terrain, good head control, and joint flexibility, they can be used for rudimentary ambulation, using a swivel-rocking motion.[538] Cosmetic issues and reduced stability as the child grows taller usually restrict the use of these devices beyond the third grade. For children with thoracic and lumbar injuries, progression to orthoses that promote gait can begin at 12 to 18 months.

The muscle requirements for gait and orthosis prescription in this population are similar to those in adults. Children with good pelvis control and hip flexor strength are candidates for KAFO bracing. The hyperlordotic posture required for KAFO use places excessive stress on a recently fractured spine and can exacerbate the spinal deformities commonly seen in these patients. Because of this, children should begin standing only after sufficient spinal healing and stability are attained, and those with higher injuries are best served with KAFOs or reciprocating gait orthoses (RGOs).[119] RGOs are expensive, heavy, and require considerable maintenance. Although RGOs are designed to promote a reciprocal gait, many children use them with crutches and a swing-to pattern. Children fitted with RGOs are likely to use them only for household ambulation.[538] Newer RGOs with hydraulic assist components have been developed and might offer greater potential for community ambulation. Functional electrical stimulation to promote standing and gait has also been studied in children. These systems have demonstrated a good safety profile and show potential for providing a higher level of mobility for those with thoracic injuries.[58, 400]

Special attention should be given to orthosis prescription and fabrication in the pediatric setting. Particular vigilance for the development of pressure ulcers is required. Many braces allow for adjustment as the child grows, but repair, replacement, and training costs are not avoidable. Children who do not, for whatever reason, make use of their preliminary, simple orthoses will not use more complex and advanced systems. Counseling and discussion of parents' expectations and feelings of failure becomes even more important as the child reaches adolescence. Social goals, motivation, body habitus, and physical capabilities undergo major changes at this time. The patient should be given latitude in establishing his or her own priorities. In many instances, progressive musculoskeletal complications tip the balance toward use of a wheelchair for locomotion.

Acquired deformities at the hip are common after pediatric SCI. Hip instability is found in 78% of spastic hips and 89% of flaccid hips, and occurs with increased frequency in children injured before age 5.[51, 453, 536] Over the course of time, hip flexion contractures and subluxation occur as a result of muscle imbalance, poor socket development, and trauma. In those with paraplegia, it is unclear whether this represents the cause or the result of reduced ambulation as the child grows. As in adults, the hip is especially difficult to target with conservative treatment (stretching, nerve blocks, muscle injections). The muscles and nerves responsible are not easily isolated or stretched. It is best to place the emphasis of care on prevention. Once the joint demonstrates ankylosis or frank dislocation, attempts at surgical repair are complicated, and rarely successful.

Family members should be well versed in stretching techniques, and prone sleeping is encouraged. Spasticity management with baclofen and clonidine can be initiated. In children under the age of 6, diazepam might be the best choice, owing to difficulties with dosing of the other drugs and the constipation associated with clonidine.[539] Although the radiographic appearance and examination findings of hip dislocation are striking, this condition is often irrelevant from a functional standpoint. Children with hip dislocation can continue to use long leg braces, and the sitting position is rarely compromised. Advanced hip flexion deformities, however, might bring about more functional restrictions. For young people who are community ambulators, frequent examination allows the clinician to discover abnormalities in hip ROM at their earliest stage, when surgical soft tissue releases can best be utilized.

Frequent examination is even more critical in the management of late spinal deformity. As periods of rapid growth occur, spinal deformity can advance, sometimes over just a few months. Scoliosis is ubiquitous in children with spinal injuries that occur before skeletal maturity. Up to 67% will need surgery to prevent further loss of thoracoabdominal capacity, cardiopulmonary reserve, and musculoskeletal integrity.[135] The concepts applied to treatment of scoliosis in the able-bodied child have little pertinence for this population. Noting a prevalence of 91% to 100%, Betz has advocated the use of prophylactic spinal bracing in all children, before any curve develops,[52] along with prescription of an appropriate wheelchair and encouragement of ambulation. Lightweight plastic spinal orthoses are used, and refitted frequently as the child grows. The goal is to reduce or forestall the progression of spinal deformity until at least age 10, when the child has developed sufficient adult trunk height. At this time, corrective surgery for curves measuring more than 40 degrees are best considered.

The multiple surgical and medical issues that arise represent only part of the challenge that children with SCI and their families face. The life satisfaction of adults who had SCI as children is inversely associated with medical complications, but issues of education, socialization and recreation, and employment are also of extreme importance.[534] Rehabilitation services focus on family attitudes and resources, with the acknowledgment that the child's adaptation strategies will change as new challenges are faced.[253] Psychological assessment and ongoing support are important in helping the patient and family deal with the issues of independence, social development, and self-esteem. These are normal concerns for any child, but they are underscored when a disability is present. Education of parents regarding community recreation resources, peer support groups, camp opportunities, and financial resources is as important as education regarding medical issues.[12]

Most important in this setting is the social development of the injured child. After the acute treatment phase, school issues should be placed at the forefront of the rehabilitation plan (Table 55–9). The importance of school extends beyond academics.[402] Children depend on school to confirm and validate their individuality as they develop roles and relationships within a group setting. For the school-age child, the student role must be reintroduced in the hospital, as early as possible after injury. The process of returning to school after hospital discharge is a complicated one, and the school reentry plan should be developed immediately. As a group, students with SCI demonstrate good participation once they return to school, although performance expectations might be lower and strong vocational counseling support is necessary.[162, 361] Although career goals might have to be adjusted to be consistent with physical abilities, it is imperative that the child with SCI be given responsibilities equal to the level of their peers. In this population, educational and vocational success have a greater bearing on adult life satisfaction than injury severity or duration of disability.[534]

TABLE 55–9 Discharge School Planning Points for the Patient with Pediatric Spinal Cord Injury

- Initiate contact with school system personnel immediately to develop an individual educational plan.
- Continue schooling within the rehabilitation hospital as soon as the child is medically stable.
- Avoid placement into new schools and separation from peer groups.
- Avoid segregation into special education classes, but tap into special education programs to take advantage of related services (e.g., transportation, computer access, physical/occupational/respiratory therapies, personal assistance services).
- Educate school nurses, teachers, and classmates regarding spinal cord injury.
- Anticipate transportation problems. Adolescents and parents will not accept bus transportation with mentally retarded children.
- Recess and break periods are important. Do not use these for bladder management or nursing care.
- Ensure the student privacy for toileting.
- Discourage the GED route for high school students.
- In the United States, the law protects educational rights; children must be educated in the least restrictive environment possible.

Adapted from Massagli TL, Dudgeon BJ, Ross BW: Education, performance and vocational participation after spinal cord injury in childhood. Arch Phys Med Rehabil 1996; 77:995–999; and Mulcahey MJ: Unique management needs of pediatric spinal cord injury patients. J Spinal Cord Injury Med 1997; 20(1):25–29.

THERAPEUTIC AND REGENERATIVE THERAPIES

Because of the numerous mechanisms of trauma and the wide variety of neurological manifestations of SCI, the prospect for discovery of a single, effective drug treatment for paralysis remains remote. Nevertheless, enthusiasm for cure research has risen in the past three decades, based on the exciting possibility that a combination of pharmacological, bioengineering, genetic, surgical, and rehabilitative strategies can be used to reduce or reverse neurological deficits. As survival is no longer the primary issue for these patients, interest in the field of paralysis research is high, having long been fueled by compelling media images of young men suddenly paralyzed by injury or war. The publication of the second National Spinal Cord Injury Study (NASCIS II) in 1990[65] marked an era of new optimism in the field. Despite widespread skepticism and therapeutic nihilism, a new drug treatment was found to be effective in reducing the neurological sequelae of acute SCI and was put to clinical use throughout the world.

The experimental approach to the problem of acute SCI began nearly 100 years ago. Alfred Allen, a neurologist from Philadelphia, developed a reliable animal model for SCI utilizing a weight drop onto an exposed spinal cord. This produced a consistent, predictable neurological lesion. His histological analysis of these injuries formed the basis of our understanding of the progression in pathological tissue response after injury. He noted that the spinal cord appeared virtually undamaged in the first few minutes after injury, but shortly thereafter, petechial venous hemorrhages in the gray matter were seen, followed by formation of a central necrotic cavity. He postulated that the neurological deficits resulted from a cascade of damage that occurred in the hours after blunt trauma. He speculated that this secondary damage was brought about by factors released from damaged nervous system tissue and from interruption of normal vascular flow.

Remarkable refinements in laboratory sciences have allowed a new generation of researchers to broaden their scope of research. Sophisticated chemical analysis can be performed at the cellular level. These analyses have generated a detailed understanding of the secondary injury that occurs shortly after the initial cord trauma. Quantification of axonal loss is possible. In SCI cats,[55] significant motor improvement can be supported by remarkably few (5% to 10%) surviving axons. This fact alone fosters hope in a scientific community that once thought millions of axons would need to be restored in order to improve function.

Other investigations provide hope for persons with longstanding paralysis. Advancements in cell and tissue culture techniques have allowed scientists to investigate the possibility of transplantation of neural tissue that might bridge the gap left by chronic injury, and implantation of cells that are programmed to secrete beneficial substances into the damaged area. In addition, it has long been known that the white matter tracts surrounding the central necrosis of cord injury are often anatomically intact but have lost their conductive properties. Electrophysiological analysis at the cellular level now allows the evaluation of drugs that might improve local conduction to the point that functional transmission is established.

Of all the venues of research, the most exciting has been the study of treatments that might salvage or preserve residual function during the period of secondary injury to the spinal cord (Table 55–10). The cumulative effect of a variety of secondary injury processes determines how many axons will survive. Numerous pathological events have been described, events that might act independently or serve to amplify one another. Spinal cord cooling[6] and steroids[607] were the first agents that were studied extensively in the animal contusion model. Hypothermia treatments reached the level of human trials, but no significant effects on recovery were encountered.

The study of high-dose methylprednisolone in acute cord injury arose out of numerous encouraging animal studies. These reports noted that a single bolus of this drug given after injury significantly improved spinal cord blood flow, prevented decreases in extracellular calcium, and reduced total lesion volume.[13, 246, 607]

TABLE 55–10 Secondary Injury to the Spinal Cord

Pathophysiological Process	Potential Therapeutic Agents
Damage to membrane lipids • Occurs minutes after injury • Phospholipid hydrolysis by prostaglandins and leukotrienes • Free radical lipid peroxidation (enzymatic)	Methylprednisolone Tirilazad
Inflammation/autoimmune destruction • Invasion of macrophages, microglia • Release of pro-inflammatory cytokines and eicosanoids • Precursor to programmed cell death and demyelination	Methylprednisolone Interleukins (e.g., IL-10, IL-6) Interleukin-1 antagonist protein Anti-inflammatory cytokines Calcinurin inhibitors
Damage to membrane-bound enzymatic and receptor systems	Methylprednisolone/tirilazad
Tissues lose ability to regulate ionic concentrations • Calcium and sodium move into cells • Potassium and magnesium move out of cells	NMDA receptor antagonists (MK-801) 4-Aminopyridine Methylprednisolone/Tirilazad
Increases in levels of excitatory amino acids	NMDA receptor antagonists GM-1 Ganglioside
Ischemia/microvascular damage (Blood flow falls to 40% of normal after 2–3 hr)	Nimodipine Methylprednisolone/tirilazad Tissue cooling Naloxone
Edema	Methylprednisolone/tirilazad

Bringing these findings to the bedside, the multicenter NASCIS I study was completed in 1983. In that study, methylprednisolone, in dosages of 100 or 1000 mg/day, was started within 48 hours of injury and continued for 10 days.[64] Over 300 patients were randomized in this project, without placebo controls. No significant difference could be demonstrated in the neurological recovery of patients treated with the two doses of methylprednisolone. In retrospect, investigators suspected that the 48-hour window in which treatment could be started was too long; animal studies had shown efficacy of steroids only when used immediately after injury. In 1985 the NASCIS II study was initiated.[65] That study examined the use of the opiate receptor antagonist naloxone, which had shown promise in promoting locomotion recovery in animal SCI models.[171] The study also evaluated methylprednisolone, given in much larger doses than in NASCIS I (30 mg/kg bolus followed by 5.4 mg/kg/hr for 23 hours).[65] A placebo group was enrolled, and 80% of patients received treatment within 12 hours after injury. When changes in motor function at 6 weeks, 6 months, and 1 year were considered, there was a clear and statistically significant trend toward increasing recovery in those treated with methylprednisolone. When patients were evaluated by testing of 14 muscle groups, patients with complete injuries recovered 20% of motor function after methylprednisolone treatment, compared with an 8% improvement in placebo-treated patients.[66, 608] Among patients with incomplete injuries, those given methylprednisolone recovered 75% of what they had lost, compared to 59% recovery in patients given placebo.

As the average patient had received almost 10 grams of methylprednisolone in the study, concern over adverse drug effects from the use of such high doses of steroids prompted analysis of over 40 different potential medical complications. No statistically significant association between steroid use and medical complications could be demonstrated. In addition, no beneficial effect on neurological recovery could be demonstrated with naloxone. Subsequent analysis of this data showed that patients treated with steroids between 8 and 12 hours after injury actually fared worse than patients in the placebo group.

The complex dose-response relationship of methylprednisolone is not surprising. Animal studies have demonstrated a variable effect of the drug that depends on both the time of administration and the severity of injury.[67] The third National Acute Spinal Cord Injury Study (NASCIS III)[68] examined more closely the issue of treatment timing, examining two methylprednisolone treatment protocols as well as a treatment arm that utilized tirilazad, a novel 21-amino steroid. Tirilazad is 100 times more potent than methylprednisolone in blocking lipid peroxidation but has no corticosteroid receptor activity or immunosuppressive properties. The NASCIS III, whose results were published in 1997, concluded that a 48-hour course of methylprednisolone was more effective than a 24-hour course if patients were treated between 3 and 8 hours after injury. For those treated before 3 hours after injury, there was no difference between those treated with 24-hour versus 48-hour infusions. Neurological recovery in all groups, including the tirilazad group, was comparable to the best outcomes in the NASCIS II study, indicating that tirilazad could serve as a substitute for methylprednisolone.

The three NASCIS studies have drawn considerable attention, and controversy persists regarding the analysis of data and conclusions of the studies.[196, 413] Nevertheless, these studies reshaped both the clinical treatment and the future of experimental investigation of SCI. Many questions remain regarding the use of these drugs, and the exact mechanism of their action is unclear. Injuries from gunshot wounds, so common in many urban medical centers, were excluded from these studies.[260, 337] Other investigators have published results of follow-up studies, but these involved small numbers of patients and were neither blinded nor randomized nor placebo-controlled. With relatively small differences in clinical outcomes between patients, there is a high risk for false positive or false negative results. Full-scale clinical trials are necessary to prove the efficacy of new treatments. Placebo-controlled trials are no longer considered ethical, and future acute drug treatments must prove themselves in comparison to methylprednisolone and tirilazad.

In addition to the use of steroids in the acute setting, considerable attention has been drawn to the use of monosialic ganglioside (GM-1) as a subacute treatment for the first 3 to 4 weeks after injury. Gangliosides are acidic glycosphingolipids, which are thought to stimulate the repair of injured nerve cells. Geisler et al[204] studied patients who received 48 hours of methylprednisolone, followed by 4 to 6 weeks of GM-1 given as a daily intramuscular injection. In a randomized study of 37 patients, GM-1 significantly improved motor recovery. A multicenter randomized trial of GM-1 in over 800 patients was initiated in 1992, utilizing a 24-hour course of methylprednisolone followed by a 6- to 8-week course of GM-1. Results of this study are still undergoing analysis.[205]

The mechanisms of neurological improvement in the months after injury are not well understood. Initial recovery in the zone of injury, related to reversal of conduction block, occurs within 6 weeks of injury. Strength change after this time period is attributed to peripheral nerve sprouting and muscle hypertrophy, but there is limited evidence to support these concepts.[467] In animal models, nascent axons are seen traversing necrotic central spinal cord cavities,[38] raising the possibility that recovery in the months following injury is a result of CNS regeneration and plasticity. Strategies to promote and enhance such regenerative and restorative processes have now been described and have reached the level of human trials.

Noting that a layer of clinically silent, demyelinated, but anatomically intact white matter often rings the central necrotic cavity of contusion injuries,[608] scientists have hoped to manipulate the local chemical environment to improve conductivity in this tissue. The drug 4-aminopyridine (4-AP), a potassium channel blocker, improves axonal conduction and synaptic transmission in injured neurons in vitro and has been used, with marginal success, to promote neurological function in persons with multiple sclerosis.[258] 4-AP is a nonselective stimulant of the nervous system, leading to such side effects as seizures and hypertension. Tissue levels have been difficult to control, owing to the lipophilic nature of the drug. Even intrathecal administration has been limited by pooling near the port of the intrathecal catheter. New time-released oral preparations might prove to be an effective delivery vehicle.

Because this substance is easily formulated and available, much of its experimental use to date has been indiscriminate and poorly controlled. Initial studies in persons with SCI fail to present compelling evidence that this drug, in its current formulation, can produce consistent improvement in neurological function. It has shown promise as a symptomatic therapy for spasticity and neurogenic pain disorders in persons with incomplete SCI. Fortunately, a randomized, blinded, placebo-controlled multicenter study is currently underway to study the feasibility, safety, and efficacy of its use. The use of 4-AP in combination with the cell replacement and regeneration strategies described below has yet to be studied.

The seminal work of Ramon y Cajal, who in 1928 described the inability of spinal axons to regenerate,[445] defined the challenge for dozens of neuroscientists hoping to find the key to CNS repair. In 1981, David et al[125] demonstrated that peripheral nerve grafts into rat spinal cords allowed bridging of spinal cord lesions, through which brainstem-derived axons could be routed. This work was instrumental in demonstrating that, contrary to longstanding opinions, CNS neurons were capable of long-distance regeneration after injury, and researchers have recently made significant progress in understanding the cellular events that lead to such regrowth.

Working on the theory that the CNS environment inhibits recovery, Caroni and Schwab[88] isolated two proteins in myelin that inhibit axon growth. Using monoclonal antibodies directed against these neurite growth-inhibition proteins, they were able to promote axonal regeneration in the rat spinal cord transection model. Investigators have also implicated chondroitin-6-sulfate as an inhibitory factor.[167] In fetal development, neurite growth arrest is associated with increased levels of this proteoglycan.

Other proteins, called neurotrophins,[132] have recently been found to stimulate nerve growth. One of these growth factors, NT3, when used in combination with Schwab's antibody preparation (IN1), was found to enhance functional recovery in the mammalian spinal cord.[72] Several laboratories are also investigating the role of cellular adhesion molecules (CAM) in axonal growth. These molecules, present on membrane surfaces, are believed to guide growing axons and might be the natural antagonists to the growth-inhibiting proteins.[476] Furthermore, once the neurons are induced to grow, the chemical environment can be modified to attract them to appropriate synaptic connections and repel them from inappropriate ones. The netrin family of protein molecules has shown this capability in vitro.[478]

Over the past 10 years, a number of other substances have been reported to stimulate growth of CNS tissue, including fibroblast growth factor, brain-derived neurotrophic factor, epidermal growth factor, and insulin growth factor. Systematic investigation of these agents requires thousands of experiments and is well beyond the capabilities of any single laboratory. Collaborative projects, such as the Multicenter Animal Spinal Cord Injury Study (MASCIS), funded by the National Institutes of Health, help speed the process of bringing regenerative treatments to human trials.

Scientists now work with the knowledge that the local nervous system environment can be modified to be less hostile to tissue regrowth, and with sophisticated tissue processing techniques. Attempts to modify the local environment by surgical transposition of vascularized omentum to the damaged human spinal cord have not demonstrated encouraging results in humans.[102] In this setting, the possibility of cell replacement therapy and nervous system tissue transplantation becomes even more attractive. Cell replacement therapy research has focused on three major strategies: (1) the genetic modification of cells (e.g., fibroblasts), reprogrammed to secrete growth-supporting, rescue, and guidance-type molecules; (2) implantation of homotypic Schwann cells, which promote repair by establishing a path for regrowth or by remyelination of damaged areas; and (3) implantation of progenitor or stem cells, which can be driven to differentiate into neurons or glial cells. Years of preparatory study in the animal laboratory have demonstrated the feasibility of all three strategies. Most notably, embryonic tissue grafts to spinal cord lesions can be induced to survive, differentiate, and facilitate recovery of locomotion.[14] Researchers have now brought nervous system cell replacement and tissue transplantation strategies to the level of human investigation.[214, 613]

Animal studies have brought a wealth of knowledge regarding cell replacement therapy and its potential role in human SCI.[446] The milieu of injury plays a role in the survival of graft material. Transection lesions present a more hostile environment than the more common and clinically relevant contusion lesions. Adult homotypic solid tissue grafts usually do not serve as an efficient medium for host regrowth. Fetal brainstem and spinal cord tissue grafts delivered in suspension to a central injury cavity demonstrate good survival; novel neurons and dendrites develop over the course of months after grafting. Neocortical tissue grafts, however, can produce regrowth that is aggressive and malignant. In addition, there is a short window of opportunity for successful grafting, lasting only a few weeks after injury.

Many questions remain regarding this technique, not the least of which are the political and ethical issues raised related to human trials. Although animal grafts have been shown to survive and differentiate, it is not known whether the histologically evident new neurons and synapses represent functional circuitry or whether these fibers develop from the graft, the host, or both. The relative success of grafting in contusion injuries, as opposed to transection injuries, indicates that improvement in rat hind limb function might be attributable to the graft's effect on the demyelinated but viable host white matter that is often seen surrounding contusion injuries.[214] It is less likely that a novel circuitry has developed that results in improved function. Animal transplants can be carried out with minimal processing of graft material, but human transplants require immunosuppression of the host and special screening and testing of transplanted tissue, which reduces graft survivability. Promising results in human cerebral fetal tissue transplants for Parkinson's disease have led the way for trials in spinal cord disease.[188]

The Brazilian neurosurgeon Tarcisio Barros[32] has attempted human allograft transplantation of sural nerve to severed spinal cord in several patients with acute complete transection from gunshot injuries. Although no significant neurological recovery has been documented in these patients, transplantation in the setting of such devastating tissue destruction represents the most difficult paradigm for evaluation. Cell replacement therapy or grafting has not been carried out in patients with acute contusion injuries, chiefly out of ethical concern that myelotomy and manipulation of the injured spinal cord during the transplantation process might result in further damage. Investigators have now chosen another group of patients for pilot study: those with remote injuries who are experiencing progressive neurological worsening due to posttraumatic syringomyelia. Researchers at the University of Florida and at the Craig Hospital in Denver are currently utilizing progenitor cells from human embryonic tissue as a novel means of filling spinal cord cysts that have not responded to traditional surgical drainage procedures.[172] The purposes of these trials are to demonstrate the feasibility and safety of human allograft fetal tissue transplantation and to determine whether progressive syrinx enlargement can be arrested. If successful, efficacy studies in persons with chronic stable neurological deficits will follow.

Although the role of rehabilitation strategies in the treatment of humans with tissue replacement therapies has not been studied, studies of locomotor function in transplanted animals have, without exception, employed task-specific training, under the assumption that activity-dependent neural plasticity plays an important role in neurological improvement.[494] Sensory and proprioceptive feedback is a critical determinant of functional recovery in animals.[10, 152] By making major chemical and structural modifications in the area surrounding a spinal cord lesion, scientists have created a new neurological environment, one in which the traditional rules of regeneration and recovery may not apply. It is likely that repair and recovery will be organized by the rehabilitation experience of this new neurological environment.

REFERENCES

1. Abel NA, Smith RA: Intrathecal baclofen for treatment of intractable spinal spasticity. Arch Phys Med Rehabil 1994; 75:54–58.
2. Abouleish E: Hypertension in a paraplegic parturient. Anesthesiology 1980; 53:348.
3. Adema E, Gebert U: Pooled patient samples as a reference material for D-dimer. Thrombos Res 1995; 80:85–88.
4. Adkins RH, Waters RL, Kendall K: The cost of pressure sores in the treatment of acute spinal injury. Am Spinal Inj Assoc Digest, Atlanta 1988.
5. Aisen ML, Dieta M, McDowell F, et al: Baclofen toxicity in a patient with subclinical renal insufficiency. Arch Phys Med Rehabil 1994; 75:109–111.
6. Albin MS, White RJ, Yashom D, et al: Effects of localized cooling on spinal cord trauma. J Trauma 1969; 9(12):1000–1008.
7. Albright F, Reifenstein EC: The Parathyroid Glands and Metabolic Bone Disease. Baltimore, Williams & Wilkins, 1948.
8. Allen B, Ferguson R, Lehmann T, et al: A mechanistic classification of closed indirect fractures and dislocations of the lower cervical spine. Spine 1982; 7:1–27.
9. Aljure J, Eltorai I, Gradley WE, et al: Carpal tunnel syndrome in paraplegic patients. Paraplegia 1985; 23:182–186.
10. Alstermark B, Gorska T, Johannisson T, et al: Effects of dorsal column transection in the upper cervical segments on visually guided forelimb movements. Neurosci Res 1986; 3:462–466.
11. American Spinal Injury Association: International standards for neurological classification of spinal cord injury. Spinal Cord 1997; 35:266–274.
12. Anderson CJ: Psychosocial and sexuality issues in pediatric spinal cord injury. Top Spinal Cord Injury Rehabil 1997; 3(2):70–78.
13. Anderson DK, Means ED, et al: Microvascular perfustion and metabolism in injured spinal cord after methylprednisolone. J Neurosurg 1982; 56:106–113.
14. Anderson DK, Reier PJ, Wirth ED: Delayed grafting of fetal CNS grafts in chronic compression lesions of the adult cat spinal cord. Restor Neurol Neurosci 1991; 2:309–325.
15. Anderson JM, Schutt AH: Spinal injury in children. Mayo Clin Proc 1980; 55:499–504.
16. Apple DF Jr, Hudson LM (eds): Spinal cord injury: The model. In Proceedings of the National Consensus Conference on Catastrophic Illness and Injury. Atlanta, Georgia Regional Spinal Cord Injury Care System, Shephard Center for Treatment of Spinal Injuries, 1990.
17. Apple DF, Anson CA, Hunter JD, et al: Spinal cord injury in youth. Clin Pediatr 1995; 34(2):90–95.
18. Apple DF, Murray HH: Lap belt injuries in children. In Betz RR, Mulcahey MJ (eds): The Child with a Spinal Cord Injury. Rosemont, IL, American Academy of Orthopedic Surgeons, 1996.
19. Apple DF Jr: The new bicycle. Top Spinal Cord Injury Rehabil 1996; 2(1):v–vi.
20. Apstein MD, Dalecki-Chipperfield K: Spinal cord injury is a risk factor for gallstone disease. Gastroenterology 1987; 92:966–968.
21. Arrowood JA, Mohanty PK, Thames MD: Cardiovascular problems in the spinal cord-injured patient. Phys Med Rehabil 1987; 1:443–456.
22. Askins V, Eismont FJ: Efficacy of five cervical orthoses in restricting cervical motion. Spine 1997; 22:1193–1198.
23. Bach JR: Inappropriate weaning and late onset ventilatory failure of individuals with traumatic quadriplegia. Paraplegia 1993; 31:430–438.
24. Bach JR: New approaches in the rehabilitation of the traumatic high level quadriplegic. Am J Phys Med Rehabil 1991; 70:13–19.
25. Bach JR: Mechanical insufflation-exsufflation: Comparison of peak expiratory flows with manually assisted and unassisted coughing techniques. Chest 1993; 104:1553–1562.
26. Bach JR, Saporito LR: Criteria for extubation and tracheostomy tube removal for patients with ventilatory failure: A different approach to weaning. Chest 1996; 110:1566–1571.
27. Bach JR, O'Connor K: Electrophrenic ventilation: A different perspective. J Am Paraplegia Soc 1991; 14:9–17.
28. Balshi JD, Cantelmo NL, Menzoian JO: Complications of caval interruption by Greenfield filter in quadriplegics. J Vasc Surg 1989; 9:553–562.
29. Banovac K, Gonzalez F: Evaluation and management of heterotopic ossification in patients with spinal cord injury. Spinal Cord 1997; 35:158–162.
30. Banovac K, Gonzalez F, Renfree KJ: Treatment of heterotopic ossification after spinal cord injury. J Spinal Cord Med 1997; 20:60–65.
31. Barnett H, Botterell E, Jousse A, et al: Progressive myelopathy as a sequel to traumatic paraplegia. Brain 1966; 89:159–174.
32. Barros TEP, Azze RJ: Peripheral nerve bridges to spinal cord injury: Preliminary results. In Spinal Cord Injury Instructional Course. São Paulo, Brazil, University of São Paulo, 1998.
33. Bauman WA, Garland DE, Schwartz E: Calcium metabolism and osteoporosis in individuals with spinal cord injury. Top Spinal Cord Injury Rehabil 1997; 2(4):84–95.
34. Bauman WA: Carbohydrate and lipid metabolism in individuals after spinal cord injury. Top Spinal Cord Injury Rehabil 1997; 2(4):1–22.
35. Bauman WA, Adkins RH, Waters RL: Cardiovascular risk factors: Prevalence in 300 subjects with SCI (abstract). J Spinal Cord Med 1996; 19:56A.
36. Bauman WA, et al: A comparison of regional bone density in monozygotic twins with chronic paraplegia. J Spinal Cord Med 1996; 19:122–125.
37. Bayley JC, Cochran TP, Sledge CB: The weight bearing shoulder: The impingement syndrome in paraplegics. J Bone Joint Surg Am 1987; 69:676–678.
38. Beattie MS, Bresnahan JC, Kormon J, et al: Endogenous repair after spinal cord contusion injuries in the rat. Exp Neurol 1997; 148:453–463.
39. Becker D, Gonzalez M, Gentil A, Kormon J, et al: Prevention of deep vein thrombosis in patients with acute spinal cord injuries: Use of rotating treatment tables. Neurosurgery 1987; 20:675–677.
40. Becker DM, Philbrick JT, Bachhuber TL, et al: D-dimer testing and acute venous thromboembolism. Arch Intern Med 1996; 156:939–946.
41. Bedbrook GM: Spinal injuries with tetraplegia and paraplegia. J Bone Joint Surg Br 1979; 61:267–284.
42. Bedbrook GM, Sedgley GI: The management of spinal injuries: Past and present. Int Rehabil Med 1980; 2:45–61.

43. Bell HS: Paralysis of both arms from injury of the upper portion of the pyramidal decussation: "Cruciate paralysis." J Neurosurg 1997; 33:376–380.
44. Ben Zur PH: Intermittent Horner's syndrome: Recurrent, alternate Horner's syndrome in cervical cord injury. Ann Ophthalmol 1975; 7:955–962.
45. Bennett JK, Foote JE, Green BG, et al: Bladder augmentation: Indications and long term management. Top Spinal Cord Inj Rehabil 1996; 1(3):36–44.
46. Benzel EC, et al: Postoperative stabilization of the posttraumatic thoracic and lumbar spine: A review of concepts and orthotic techniques. J Spinal Disord 1989; 2(1):47–51.
47. Bergman P, Herlporn A, Schoutens A, et al: Longitudinal study of calcium and bone metabolism in paraplegic patients. Paraplegia 1977–78; 15:147–159.
48. Bergstrom EMK, Frankel HR, Galer IAR, et al: Physical ability in relation to anthropometric measurements in persons with complete spinal cord lesion below the sixth cervical segment. Int Rehabil Med 1985; 7:51–55.
49. Berkowitz M, Harvey C, Greene CG, et al: The Economic Consequences of Traumatic Spinal Cord Injury. New York, Demos, 1992.
50. Berlly MH, Wilmot CB: Acute abdominal emergencies during the first four weeks after spinal cord injury. Arch Phys Med Rehabil 1984; 65:687–690.
51. Betz RR, Beck T, Huss GK, et al: Hip instability in children with spinal cord injury. J Am Paraplegia Soc 1994; 17:119–122.
52. Betz RR: Orthopedic problems in the child with spinal cord injury. Top Spinal Cord Injury Rehabil 1997; 3(2):9–19.
53. Bhaskar KR, Brown R, O'Sullivan DD, et al: Bronchial mucus hypersecretion in acute quadriplegia. Am Rev Respir Dis 1991; 143:630–638.
54. Biering-Sorenson F, Bohr H, Schaadt O: Bone mineral content of the lumbar spine and lower extremities years after spinal cord lesion. Paraplegia 1988; 26:293–301.
55. Blight AR, DeCrescito V: Morphometric analysis of experimental spinal cord injury in the cat. Neuroscience 1986; 19:321–341.
56. Bohannon RW: Tilt table standing for reducing spasticity after spinal cord injury. Arch Phys Med Rehabil 1993; 74:1121–1122.
57. Bohlman H: Acute fractures and dislocations of the cervical spine. J Bone Joint Surg Am 1979; 61:1119–1142.
58. Bonaroti D, Betz RR, Mulcahey MJ, et al: The functional comparison of FES and KAFO's in an ambulatory child with a complete thoracic level spinal cord injury. J Spinal Cord Med 1997; 20(1):147.
59. Bonninger ML, Robertson RN, Wolff M, et al: Upper extremity nerve entrapments in elite wheelchair racers. Am J Phys Med 1996; 75:170–175.
60. Bosch A, Stauffer ES, Nickel VL: Incomplete traumatic quadriplegia: A ten year review. JAMA 1979; 216:473–480.
61. Botterell EH, Callaghan JC, Jousse AT: Pain in paraplegia: Clinical management and surgical treatment. Proc R Soc Med 1953; 47:281–288.
62. Boudaoud L, Roussi J, Lortat-Jacob S, et al: Endothelial fibrinolytic reactivity and the risk of deep venous thrombosis after spinal cord injury. Spinal Cord 1997; 35:151–157.
63. Bracken MB, Freeman DH Jr, Hellenbrand K: Incidence of acute traumatic hospitalized SCI in the United States, 1970–77. Am J Epidemiol 1981; 113:615–622.
64. Bracken MB, Collins WF, Freeman DF, et al: Efficacy of methylprednisolone in acute spinal cord injury. JAMA 1984; 251:45–52.
65. Bracken MB, Shepard MJ, Collins WF, et al: A randomized, controlled trial of methylprednisolone or naloxone in the treatment of acute spinal-cord injury. N Engl J Med 1990; 322:1405–1411.
66. Bracken MB, Shepard MJ, Collins WF Jr, et al: Methylprednisolone or naloxone treatment after acute spinal cord injury: 1-year follow-up data. J Neurosurg 1992; 76:23–31.
67. Bracken MB, Holford TR: Effects of timing of methylprednisolone or naloxone administration on recovery of segmental and long tract function. J Neurosurg 1993; 79:500–507.
68. Bracken MB, Shepard MJ, Holford TR, et al: Administration of methylprednisolone for 24 or 48 hours or tirilazad mesylate for 48 hours in the treatment of acute spinal cord injury. JAMA 1997; 277:1597–1604.
69. Braddom RL, Rocco JF: Autonomic dysreflexia: A survey of current treatment. Am J Phys Med Rehabil 1991; 70:234–241.
70. Braun SR, Giovannioni R, Levin AB: Oxygen saturation during sleep in patients with spinal cord injury. Am J Phys Med 1982; 61:302–309.
71. Brenes G, Dearwater S, Shapera R, et al: High density lipoprotein cholesterol concentrations in physically active and sedentary spinal cord–injured patients. Arch Phys Med Rehabil 1986; 67:445–450.
72. Bregman BS, Kunkel-Bagden E, Schell L, et al: Recovery from spinal cord injury mediated by antibodies to neurite growth inhibitors. Nature 1995; 378:498–501.
73. Brooke MM, Heard DL, deLateur BJ, et al: Heterotopic ossification and peripheral nerve entrapment: Early diagnosis and excision. Arch Phys Med Rehabil 1991; 72:425–429.
74. Brooke MM, Donovan WH, Stolov WC: Paraplegia: Succinylcholine induced hyperkalemia and cardiac arrest. Arch Phys Med Rehabil 1978; 59:306–309.
75. Brown PH, Marino RJ, Herbison GL, et al: The 72 hour examination as a predictor of recovery in motor complete quadriplegia. Arch Phys Med Rehabil 1991; 72:546–550.
76. Burke DC: Pain in paraplegia. Paraplegia 1973; 10:297–313.
77. Burnstein A, Richlin D, Sotolongo JR: Nifedipine pretreatment for prevention of autonomic hyperreflexia during anesthesia-free extracorporeal shock wave lithotripsy. J Urol 1992; 147:676–677.
78. Buschbacher R, McKinely W, Buschbacher L, et al: Warfarin in prevention of heterotopic ossification. Am J Phys Med Rehabil 1992; 71:86–91.
79. Byers RK: Spinal cord injuries during birth. Dev Med Child Neurol 1975; 17:103–110.
80. Cairns DM, Adkins RH, Scott MD: Pain and depression in acute traumatic spinal cord injury: Origins of chronic problematic pain? Arch Phys Med Rehabil 1996; 77:329–335.
81. Campbell CC, Koris MJ: Etiologies of shoulder pain in cervical spinal cord injury. Clin Orthop 1996; 322:140–145.
82. Capen DA, Zigler JE, Garland DE: Surgical stabilization in cervical spine trauma. Contemp Orthop 1987; 14(2):25–32.
83. Cardus D, McTaggart WG: Body composition in spinal cord injury. Arch Phys Med Rehabil 1985; 66:257–259.
84. Cardus D, McTaggart WG: Total body water and its distribution in men with spinal cord injury. Arch Phys Med Rehabil 1984; 65:509–512.
85. Cardus D, Ribas-Cardus F, McTaggart WG: Coronary risk in spinal cord injury: Assessment following a multivariate approach. Arch Phys Med Rehabil 1992; 73:930–933.
86. Carey DE, Raisz LG: Calcitonin therapy in prolonged immobilization hypercalcemia. Arch Phys Med Rehabil 1985; 66:640–644.
87. Carey ME, Nance FC, Kirgis HD, et al: Pancreatitis following spinal cord injury. J Neurosurg 1977; 47:917–922.
88. Caroni P, Schwab ME: Two membrane protein fractions from rat central myelin with inhibitory properties for neurite growth and fibroblast. Cell Biol 1988; 106:1281–1288.
89. Carter RE: Experiences with high tetraplegics. Paraplegia 1979; 17:140–146.
90. Chancellor MB, Erhard MJ, Hirsch IH, et al: Prospective evaluation of terazosin for the treatment of autonomic dysreflexia. J Urol 1994; 151:111–113.
91. Chappard D, Minaire P, Privat C, et al: Effects of tiludronate on bone loss in paraplegic patients. J Bone Miner Res 1995; 10:112–117.
92. Cheng L, Crozier KS, Zorn G, et al: Spinal cord injury: Prognosis for ambulation based on recovery of quadriceps function. J Am Paraplegia Soc 1991; 14:94–98.
93. Chesire DJE: The paediatric syndrome of traumatic myelopathy without demonstrable vertebral injury. Paraplegia 1977–78; 15:74–85.
94. Chiou-Tan FY, Tuel SM, Johnson JC, et al: Effect of mexiletine on spinal cord injury dysesthetic pain. Am J Phys Med Rehabil 1996; 75:84–87.
95. Clagett GP, Anderson FA, Heit J, et al: Prevention of venous thromboembolism. Chest 1995; 108(suppl 4):312S–334S.
96. Claus-Walker J, Dunn CD: Spinal cord injury and serum erythropoietin. Arch Phys Med Rehabil 1984; 65:370–374.
97. Claus-Walker J, Halstead LS: Metabolic and endocrine changes in spinal cord injury: I. The nervous system before and after

transection of the spinal cord. Arch Phys Med Rehabil 1981; 62:595–601.

98. Claus-Walker J, Halstead LS: Metabolic and endocrine changes in spinal cord injury: III. Less quanta of sensory input plus bedrest and illness. Arch Phys Med Rehabil 1982; 63:628–631.
99. Claus-Walker J, Halstead LS: Metabolic and endocrine changes in spinal cord injury: IV. Compounded neurologic dysfunctions. Arch Phys Med Rehabil 1982; 63:632–638.
100. Claus-Walker J, Spencer WA, Carter RE, et al: Bone metabolism in quadriplegia: Dissociation between calciuria and hydroxyprolinuria. Arch Phys Med Rehabil 1975; 56:327–332.
101. Claus-Walker J, Vallbona C, Caster RE, et al: Resting and stimulated endocrine function in human subjects with cervical spinal cord transection. J Chronic Dis 1971; 24:193–207.
102. Clifton GL, Donovan WH, Dimitrijevic MM, et al: Omental transposition in chronic spinal cord injury. Spinal Cord 1996; 34:193–203.
103. Clough P: Glossopharyngeal breathing: Its application with a traumatic quadriplegic patient. Arch Phys Med Rehabil 1983; 64:384–385.
104. Coffey RJ, Cahill D, Steers W, et al: Intrathecal baclofen for intractable spasticity of spinal origin: Results of a long-term multicenter study. J Neurosurg 1993; 78:226–232.
105. Coghlan JK, Robinson CE, Newmarch B: Lower extremity bracing in paraplegia: A follow-up study. Paraplegia 1980; 1:25–32.
106. Cohen ME, Sheehan TP, Herbison GJ: Content validity and reliability of the International Standards for Neurological Classification of Spinal Cord Injury. Top Spinal Cord Injury Rehabil 1996; 1(4):15–31.
107. Colachis SC: Autonomic hyperreflexia in spinal cord injury associated with pulmonary embolism. Arch Phys Med Rehabil 1991; 72:1014–1016.
108. Collins K, Oswald P, Burger G, et al: Customized adjustable orthoses: Their use in spasticity. Arch Phys Med Rehabil 1985; 66:397–398.
109. Collins WF: Historical introduction to spinal cord injury: The contributions of Allen, Riddoch and Guttmann. In Benzel E, Tator CH (eds): Contemporary Management of Spinal Cord Injury 1995. Park Ridge, IL, American Association of Neurological Surgeons, 1995.
110. Colorado Department of Public Health and Environment: 1995 Annual Report of the Spinal Cord Injury Early Notification System. Denver, Colorado Department of Transportation Printing Office, 1996.
111. The Consortium for Spinal Cord Medicine: Clinical practice guideline: Prevention of thromboembolism in spinal cord injury. Spinal Cord Med 1997; 20:259–284.
112. The Consortium for Spinal Cord Medicine: Clinical practice guideline: Acute management of autonomic dysreflexia. Spinal Cord Med 1997; 20:284–311.
113. The Consortium for Spinal Cord Medicine: Clinical practice guideline: Pressure ulcer prevention and treatment. Washington, DC, Paralyzed Veterans of America, September 1999.
114. The Consortium for Spinal Cord Medicine: Clinical practice guideline: Depression following spinal cord injury: A clinical practice guideline for primary care physicians. Washington, DC, Paralyzed Veterans of America, September 1998.
115. Cosman BC, Stone JM, Perkash I: The gastrointestinal system. In Whiteneck GG (ed): Aging With Spinal Cord Injury. New York, Demos, 1993, pp 117–127.
116. Cotler JM, Cotler HB (eds): Spinal Fusion: Science and Technique. New York, Springer-Verlag, 1990.
117. Coughlan JK, Robinson CE, Newmarch B, et al: Lower extremity bracing in paraplegia: A follow-up study. Paraplegia 1980; 18:25–32.
118. Cox SR, Weiss SM, Posuniak EA, et al: Energy expenditure after spinal cord injury: An evaluation of stable rehabilitation patients. J Trauma 1985; 25:419–423.
119. Creitz L, Nelson VS, Haubenstricker L, et al: Orthotic prescriptions. In Betz RR, Mulcahey MJ (eds): The Child with a Spinal Cord Injury. Rosemont, IL, American Academy of Orthopedic Surgeons, 1996.
120. Crippa L, D'Angelo SV, Tomassini L, et al: The utility and cost effectiveness of D-dimer measurements in the diagnosis of deep vein thrombosis. Haematologica 1997; 82:446–451.
121. Crozier K, Graziani V, Ditunno JF: Prognosis for ambulation based on sensory examination in patients who are initially motor complete. Arch Phys Med Rehabil 1991; 72:119–125.
122. Crozier KS, Cheng LL, Graziani V, et al: Spinal cord injury: Prognosis for ambulation based on quadriceps recovery. Paraplegia 1992; 30:762–767.
123. Daniels L, Worthingham C: Muscle Testing Techniques of Manual Examination, ed 5. Philadelphia, WB Saunders, 1996.
124. Darouiche RO, Groover J, Rowland J: Pneumococcal vaccination for patients with spinal cord injury. Arch Phys Med Rehabil 1993; 74:1354–1357.
125. David S, Aguayo AJ: Axonal elongation into peripheral nervous system bridges after central nervous system injury in adult rats. Science 1981; 214:931–933.
126. Davidoff G, Guarracini M, Roth E, et al: Trazodone hydrochloride in the treatment of dysesthetic pain in traumatic myelopathy: A randomized, double-blind placebo-controlled study. Pain 1987; 29:151–163.
127. Davidoff G, Morris J, Roth E, et al: Cognitive dysfunction and mild closed head injury in traumatic spinal cord injury. Arch Phys Med Rehabil 1985; 66:489–491.
128. Davidoff G, Roth E, Guarracini M, et al: Function-limiting dysesthetic pain syndrome among traumatic spinal cord injury patients: A cross-sectional study. Pain 1987; 29:39–48.
129. Davidoff G, Schultz JS, Lieb T, et al: Rehospitalization after initial rehabilitation for acute spinal cord injury: Incidence and risk factors. Arch Phys Med Rehabil 1990; 71:121–124.
130. Davidoff RA: Antispasticity drugs: Mechanisms of action. Neurology 1985; 17:107–116.
131. Davidson BL, Elliott CG, Lensing AWA, et al: Low accuracy of color Doppler ultrasound in the detection of proximal leg thrombosis in asymptomatic high-risk patients. Ann Intern Med 1992; 117:735–738.
132. Davies AM, Thoenen H, Barde YA: Different factors from the central nervous system and periphery regulate the survival of sensory neurons. Nature 1986; 319:497–499.
133. Davis R: Pain and suffering following spinal cord injury. Clin Orthop 1975; 112:76–80.
134. Davis R, Lentini R: Transcutaneous nerve stimulation for treatment of pain in patients with spinal cord injury. Surg Neurol 1975; 4:100–101.
135. Dearolf WW III, Betz RR, Vogel LC, et al: Scoliosis in pediatric spinal cord injured patients. J Pediatr Orthop 1990; 10:214–218.
136. Decter RM, Bauer SB: Urologic management of spinal cord injury in children. Urol Clin North Am 1993; 20:475–483.
137. DeJong G, Branch LG, Corcoran PJ: Independent living outcomes in spinal cord injury: Multivariate analyses. Arch Phys Med Rehabil 1984; 65:66–73.
138. DeTroyer A, Estenne M, Heilporn A: Mechanism of active expiration in tetraplegic subjects. N Engl J Med 1986; 314:740–744.
139. DeTroyer A, Estenne M: Review article: The expiratory muscles in tetraplegia. Paraplegia 1993; 29:359–363.
140. DeVivo M, Black K, Stover S: Causes of death during the first 12 years after spinal cord injury. Arch Phys Med Rehabil 1993; 74:248–254.
141. DeVivo MJ, Fine PR: Employment status of spinal cord-injured patients 3 years after injury. Arch Phys Med Rehabil 1982; 63:200–203.
142. DeVivo MJ, Fine PR, Maetz HM, et al: Prevalence of spinal cord injury: A re-estimation employing life table techniques. Arch Neurol 1980; 37:707–708.
143. DeVivo MJ, Rutt RD, Stover SL, et al: Employment after spinal cord injury. Arch Phys Med Rehabil 1987; 68:494–498.
144. DeVivo MJ, Kartus PL, Rutt RD: The influence of age at time of spinal cord injury on rehabilitation outcomes. Arch Neurol 1990; 47:687–691.
145. DeVivo, Kartus PL, Stover SL, et al: Benefits of early admission to an organized spinal cord injury care system. Paraplegia 1990; 28:545–555.
146. DeVivo MJ, Kartus PL, Stover SL: Cause of death for patients with spinal cord injuries. Arch Intern Med 1989; 149:1716–1734.
147. DeVivo MJ, Rutt RD, Black KJ, et al: Trends in spinal cord injury demographics and treatment outcomes between 1973 and 1986. Arch Phys Med Rehabil 1992; 73:424–430.

148. DeVivo MJ, Ivie CS: Life expectancy of ventilatory dependent persons with spinal cord injuries. Chest 1995; 108:226–232.
149. DeVivo MJ, Whiteneck GG, Charles ED: The economic impact of spinal cord injury. In Stover SL, DeLisa JA, Whiteneck GG (eds): Spinal Cord Injury: Clinical Outcomes from the Model Systems. Gaithersburg, MD, Aspen, 1995, pp 234–271.
150. Dickman CA, Hadley MN, Pappas CTE, et al: Cruciate paralysis: A clinical and radiographic analysis of injuries to the cervicomedullary junction. J Neurosurg 1990; 73:850–858.
151. Dijkers MP, Buda Abela M, Gans BM, et al: The aftermath of spinal cord injury. In Stover SL, DeLisa JA, Whiteneck GG (eds): Spinal Cord Injury: Clinical Outcomes from the Model Systems. Gaithersburg, MD, Aspen, 1995, pp 185–212.
152. Dimitrijevic MR, Faganel J, et al: Suprasegmentally induced motor unit activity in paralyzed muscles of patients with established spinal cord injury. Ann Neurol 1984; 16:216–221.
153. Ditunno JF, Sipski ML, Posuniak EA, et al: Wrist extensor recovery in traumatic quadriplegia. Arch Phys Med Rehabil 1987; 68:287–290.
154. Ditunno JF Jr, Stover SL, Freed MM, et al: Motor recovery of the upper extremities in traumatic quadriplegia: A multicenter study. Arch Phys Med Rehabil 1992; 73:431–436.
155. Ditunno JF, Cohen ME, Formal C, et al: Functional outcomes. In Stover SL, DeLisa JA, Whiteneck GG (eds): Spinal Cord Injury: Clinical Outcomes from the Model Systems. Gaithersburg, MD, Aspen, 1995, pp 170–184.
156. Donovan WH: Operative and nonoperative management of spinal cord injury: A review. Paraplegia 1994; 32:375–388.
157. Donovan WH, Stolov WC, et al: Bacteriuria during intermittent catheterization following spinal cord injury. Arch Phys Med Rehabil 1978; 59:351–357.
158. Donovan WH, Carter RE, Rossi D, et al: Clonidine effect on spasticity: A clinical trial. Arch Phys Med Rehabil 1988; 69: 193–194.
159. Donovan WH, Dimitrijevic MR, Dahm L, et al: Neurophysiological approaches to chronic pain following spinal cord injury. Paraplegia 1982; 20:135–146.
160. Douglas R, Larson PF, D'Ambrosia R, et al: The LSU reciprocation gait orthosis. Orthopedics 1983; 6:834–839.
161. Duckworth WC, Jallepalli P, Solomon SS: Glucose intolerance in spinal cord injury. Arch Phys Med Rehabil 1983; 64:107–110.
162. Dudgeon BJ, Massagli TL, Ross BW: Educational participation of children with spinal cord injury. Am J Occup Ther 1997; 51:553–561.
163. Dworkin G, Staas W: Posttraumatic syringomyelia. Arch Phys Med Rehabil 1985; 66:329–331.
164. Elias AN, Gwinup G: Immobilization osteoporosis in paraplegia. J Am Paraplegia Soc 1992; 15:163–170.
165. Eller DA, Austin PF, Tanguay S, et al: Daytime functional bladder capacity as a predictor of response to desmopressin in monosymptomatic nocturnal enuresis. Eur Urol 1998; Suppl 3:25–29.
166. Eltorai I, Montroy R: Muscle release in the management of spasticity in spinal cord injury. Paraplegia 1990; 28:433–440.
167. Emerling DE, Lander AD: Inhibitors and promotors of thalamic neuron adhesion and outgrowth. Neuron 1996; 17:1089–1100.
168. Erickson DL, Blacklock JB, Michaelson M, et al: Control of spasticity by implantable continuous flow morphine pump. Neurosurgery 1985; 16:215–217.
169. Erickson RP: Autonomic hyperreflexia: Pathophysiology and medical management. Arch Phys Med Rehabil 1980; 61:431–440.
170. Evans DE, Kobrine AI, Rizzoli HV: Cardiac arrhythmias accompanying acute compression of the spinal cord. J Neurosurg 1980; 52:52–59.
171. Faden AI, Jacobs TP, et al: Opiate antagonist improves neurologic recovery after spinal injury. Science 1980; 211:493–494.
172. Falci S, Holtz A, Akesson E, et al: Obliteration of a posttraumatic spinal cord cyst with solid human embryonic spinal cord grafts. J Neurotrauma 1997; 14:875–884.
173. Fein ED, Grimm DR Lesser M: The effects of ipratropium bromide on histamine-induced bronchoconstriction in subjects with cervical spinal cord injury. J Asthma 1998; 35:49–55.
174. Felsberg GJ, Tien RD, Osumi AK, et al: Utility of MR imaging in pediatric spinal cord injury. Pediatr Radiol 1995; 25:131–135.
175. Fenollosa P, Pallares J, Cervera J, et al: Chronic pain in the spinal cord injured: Statistical approach and pharmacological treatment. Paraplegia 1993; 6:48–56.
176. Fernie GR, Dornan J: The problems of clinical trials with new systems of preventing or healing decubiti. In Kenedi RM, Couden JM, Scales JT (eds): Bedsore Biomechanics. Baltimore, University Park Press, 1976, pp 315–320.
177. Fine PR, DeVivo MJ, McEachran AB: Incidence of acute traumatic hospitalized spinal cord injury in the United States: 1970–1977. Am J Epidemiol 1982; 15:475–477.
178. Fishburn MJ, Marino RS, Ditunno JF: Atelectasis and pneumonia in acute spinal cord injury. Arch Phys Med Rehabil 1990; 71:197–200.
179. Fisher SV, Bowar JF, Awad EA, et al: Cervical orthoses: Effect on cervical spine motion. Arch Phys Med Rehabil 1977; 58: 109–115.
180. Folman Y, Masri WE: Spinal cord injury: Prognostic indicators. Injury 1989; 20:92–95.
181. Frankel HL, Hancock DO, Hyslop G, et al: The value of postural reduction in the initial management of closed injuries of the spine with paraplegia and tetraplegia. Paraplegia 1969; 7: 179–192.
182. Frankel HL, Mathras CJ, Spalding JMK: Mechanisms of reflex cardiac arrest in tetraplegic patients. Lancet 1975; 2:1183–1185.
183. Freebourn TM, Barber DB, Able AC: The treatment of immature heterotopic ossification in spinal cord injury with combination surgery, radiation therapy and NSAID. Spinal Cord 1999; 37:50–53.
184. Freed JH, Hahn H, Menter MD, et al: The use of the three-phase bone scan in the early diagnosis of heterotopic ossification (HO) and in the evaluation of Didronel therapy. Paraplegia 1982; 20:208–216.
185. Freedman AP: Suctioning the left bronchial tree in the intubated adult. Crit Care Med 1982; 10:43–45.
186. Freehafer AA, Kelly CM, Peckham PH: Tendon transfer for the restoration of upper limb function after a cervical spinal cord injury. J Hand Surg Am 1984; 9:887–893.
187. Freehafer AA: Limb fractures in patients with spinal cord injury. Arch Phys Med Rehabil 1995; 76:823–827.
188. Freeman TB: From transplants to gene therapy for Parkinson's disease. Exp Neurol 1997: 144:47–50.
189. Friedman A, Nashold BS: Dorsal root entry zone lesions for relief of pain related to spinal cord injury. J Neurosurg 1986; 65:465–469.
190. Frisbie JH, Tun CG: Drinking and spinal cord injury. J Am Paraplegia Soc 1984; 7:71–73.
191. Frisbie JH: Fractures after myelopathy: The risk quantified. J Spinal Cord Med 1997; 20(1):66–69.
192. Frost F: Spinal cord injury: Gastrointestinal implications and management. Top Spinal Cord Injury Rehabil 1998; 4(2):56–80.
193. Fuhrer MJ, Rintala DH, Hart KA, et al: Relationship of life satisfaction to impairment, disability, and handicap among persons with spinal cord injury living in the community. Arch Phys Med Rehabil 1992; 73:552–558.
194. Fuhrer MF, Garber SL, Rintala DH, et al: Pressure ulcers in community resident persons with spinal cord injury: Prevalence and risk factors. Arch Phys Med Rehabil 1993; 74:1172–1177.
195. Fugl-Meyer AR: Effects of respiratory muscle paralysis in tetraplegic and paraplegic patients. Scand J Rehabil Med 1971; 3:141–150.
196. Galandiuk S, Raque G, Appel S, et al: The two-edged sword of large dose steroids for spinal cord trauma. Ann Surg 1993; 218:419–427.
197. Garland DE: Clinical observations on fractures and heterotopic ossification in the spinal cord and traumatic brain injured populations. Clin Orthop 1988; 233:86–101.
198. Garland DE: A clinical perspective on common forms of acquired heterotopic ossification. Clin Orthop 1991; 263:13–29.
199. Garland DE, Orwin JF: Resection of heterotopic ossification in patients with spinal cord injuries. Clin Orthop 1989; 242:169–176.
200. Garland DE, Maric Z, Adkins R, et al: Bone mineral density about the knee in spinal cord-injured patients with pathologic fractures. Contemp Orthop 1993; 26:375–379.
201. Garland DE, Foulkes G, Adkins RH, et al: Regional osteoporosis following incomplete spinal cord injury. Contemp Orthop 1994; 28:134–138.
202. Geerts WH, Code KI, Jay RM, et al: A prospective study of venous thromboembolism after major trauma. N Engl J Med 1994; 331:1601–1606.

203. Gerhart KA, Bergstrom E, Charlifue SW, et al: Long-term spinal cord injury: Functional changes over time. Arch Phys Med Rehabil 1993; 74:1030–1034.
204. Geisler FH, Dorsey FC, Coleman WP: Recovery of motor function after spinal-cord injury: A randomized, placebo-controlled trial with GM-1 ganglioside. N Engl J Med 1991; 324:1829–1838.
205. Geisler FH: Clinical trials of pharmacotherapy for spinal cord injury. Ann NY Acad Sci 1998; 845:374–381.
206. Geisler WO, Jousse AT, Wynne-Hones M, et al: Survival in traumatic spinal cord injury. Paraplegia 1983; 21:364–373.
207. Gellman H, Chandler DR, Petrasek J, et al: Carpal tunnel syndrome in paraplegic patients. J Bone Joint Surg Am 1988; 4: 517–519.
208. Gellman H, Sie I, Water RL: Late complications of the weight bearing upper extremity in the paraplegic patient. Clin Orthop 1988; 233:132–135.
209. Genard JM, Arias A, Berlan M, et al: Pharmacological evidence of alpha 1- and 2-adrenergic supersensitivity in orthostatic hypotension due to spinal cord injury: A case report. Eur J Clin Pharmacol 1991; 41:593–596.
210. Gerridzen RG, Thijssen AM, Dehoux E: Risk factors for upper urinary tract deterioration in chronic spinal cord-injured patients. J Urol 1992; 147:416–418.
211. Gibson CJ: Overview of spinal cord injury. Phys Med Rehabil Clin North Am 1992; 3:699–709.
212. Gilgoff IS, Ward SLD, Hohn AR: Cardiac pacemaker in high spinal cord injury. Arch Phys Med Rehabil 1991; 72:601–603.
213. Gimovsky ML, Ojeda A, Ozaki R, et al: Management of autonomic hyperreflexia associated with a low thoracic spinal cord lesion. Obstet Gynecol 1985; 153:223–224.
214. Giovanini MA, Reier PJ, Eskin TA, et al: Characteristics of human fetal spinal cord grafts in the adult rat spinal cord. Exp Neurol 1997; 148:523–543.
215. Glen WWL, Phelps MA: Diaphragm pacing by electrical stimulation of the phrenic nerve. Neurosurgery 1985; 17:974–984.
216. Go BK, DeVivo MJ, Richards JS: The epidemiology of spinal cord injury. In Stover SL, et al (eds): Spinal Cord Injury: Clinical Outcomes from the Model Systems. Gaithersburg, MD, Aspen, 1995, pp 21–55.
217. Goldstein B, Young J, Excobedo EM: Rotator cuff repairs in individuals with paraplegia. Am J Phys Med Rehabil 1997; 76:316–322.
218. Goldwasser B, Webster GD: Continent urinary diversion. J Urol 1985; 134:227–236.
219. Gonzalez F, Chang JY, Banovac K, et al: Autoregulation of cerebral blood flow in patients with orthostatic hypotension after spinal cord injury. Paraplegia 1991; 29:1–7.
220. Gordon EE , Vanderwalde H: Energy requirements in paraplegic ambulation. Arch Phys Med Rehabil 1956; 37:276–285.
221. Gore RM, Mintzer RA, Calenoff L: Gastrointestinal complications of spinal cord injury. Spine 1981; 6:538–544.
222. Green BA, Lee TT, Madsen PW, et al: Management of posttraumatic cystic myelopathy. Top Spinal Cord Injury Med 1997; 2(4):36–46.
223. Green D, Hull RD, Mammem EF, et al: Deep vein thrombosis in spinal cord injury. Chest 1992; 102:633S–635S.
224. Green D: Prophylaxis of thromboembolism in spinal cord injured patients. Chest 1994; 102:649S–651S.
225. Green D, Chen D, Chmiel JS, et al: Prevention of thromboembolism in spinal cord injury: Role of low molecular weight heparin. Arch Phys Med Rehabil 1994; 75:290–292.
226. Green D, Lee M, Ito V, et al: Fixed vs adjusted dose heparin in the prophylaxis of thromboembolism in spinal cord injury. JAMA 1988; 260:1255–1258.
227. Green D, Lee M, Lim A, et al: Prevention of thromboembolism after spinal cord injury using low-molecular weight heparin. Ann Intern Med 1990; 113:571–574.
228. Green D, Rossi E, Yao J, et al: Deep vein thrombosis in spinal cord injury: Effect of prophylaxis with calf compression, aspirin and dipyridamole. Paraplegia 1982; 20:227–234.
229. Gresham GE, Labi MLC, Dittmar SS, et al: The Quadriplegia Index of Function (QIF): Sensitivity and reliability demonstrated in a study of thirty quadriplegic patients. Paraplegia 1986; 24:38–42.
230. Griffin MR, O'Fallon WM, Opitz JL, et al: Mortality, survival, and prevalence: Traumatic spinal cord injury in Olmsted County, MN, 1935–1981. J Chronic Dis 1985; 38:643–653.
231. Grimby G, Broberg C, Krotkiewska I, et al: Muscle fiber composition in patients with traumatic cord lesion. Scand J Rehabil Med 1976; 8:37–42.
232. Groomes TE, Huang CT: Orthostatic hypotension after spinal cord injury: Treatment with fludrocortisone and ergotamine. Arch Phys Med Rehabil 1991; 72:56–58.
233. Grover J, Gellman H, Waters RL: The effect of a flexion contracture of the elbow on the ability to transfer in patients who have quadriplegia at the sixth cervical level. J Bone Joint Surg Am 1996; 78:1397–1400.
234. Gruenthal M, Mueller M, Olson WL, et al: Gabapentin for the treatment of spasticity in patients with spinal cord injury. Spinal Cord 1997; 35:686–689.
235. Guttmann L: Management of the Quinizarin-test. Postgrad Med J 1947; 23:353–366.
236. Guttmann L: Disorders of vasomotor control. In Spinal Cord Injuries: Comprehensive Management and Research. Oxford, Blackwell, 1973, pp 271–280.
237. Guttmann L, Silver J, Wyndham C: Thermoregulation in the spinal man. J Physiol 1958; 142:406–418.
238. Guttmann L, Silver J: Electromyographic studies on reflex activity of the intercostals and abdominals in cervical cord lesions. Paraplegia 1965; 3:1–6.
239. Guttmann L: Spinal Cord Injuries: Comprehensive Management and Research, ed 1. Boston, Blackwell, 1973, pp 183–184.
240. Guttmann L, Frankel H: The value of intermittent catheterization in the early management of traumatic paraplegia and tetraplegia. Paraplegia 1966; 4:63–82.
241. Haas F, Axen K, Pineda H, et al: Temporal pulmonary function changes in cervical cord injury. Arch Phys Med Rehabil 1985; 66:139–144.
242. Hachen HJ: Psychological, neurophysiological, and therapeutic aspects of chronic pain: Preliminary results with transcutaneous electrical stimulation. Paraplegia 1977; 15:353–367.
243. Hachen HJ: Spinal cord injury in children and adolescents: Diagnostic pitfalls and therapeutic considerations in the acute stage. Paraplegia 1977–78; 15:55–64.
244. Hadley MN, Zabramski JM, et al: Pediatric spinal trauma: Review of 122 cases of spinal cord and vertebral column injuries. J Neurosurg 1988; 68:18–24.
245. Hagisawa S, Ferguson-Pell M, Cardi M, et al: Assessment of skin blood content and oxygenation in spinal cord injured subjects during reactive hyperemia. J Rehabil Res Dev 1994; 31:1–14.
246. Hall ED, Braughler JM: Glucocorticoid mechanisms in acute spinal cord injury: A review. Surg Neurol 1982; 18:320–327.
247. Hall R, Hirsch J, Sackett DL, et al: Combined use of leg scanning and impedance plethysmography in suspected deep venous thrombosis: An alternative to venography. N Engl J Med 1977; 296:1497–1500.
248. Hamilton BB, Granger CV, Sherwin FS, et al: A uniform national data system for medical rehabilitation. In Fuhrer MJ (ed): Rehabilitation Outcomes: Analysis and Measurement. Baltimore, Paul H Brookes, 1987, p 137.
249. Hamilton MG, Mayles ST: Pediatric spinal injury: Review of 174 hospital admissions. J Neurosurg 1992; 77:700–704.
250. Hangartner TN, Rodgers MM, Glaser RM, et al: Tibial bone density loss in spinal cord-injured patients: Effects of FES exercise. J Rehabil Res Dev 1994; 31:50–61.
251. Hansen R, Franklin M: Sexual loss in relation to other functional losses for spinal cord injured males. Arch Phys Med Rehabil 1976; 57:291–293.
252. Hardy AG: Cervical spinal cord injury without bony injury. Paraplegia 1977; 14:296–305.
253. Harper DC: Paradigms for investigating rehabilitation and adaptation to childhood disability and chronic illness. J Pediatr Psychol 1991; 16:533–542.
254. Harris S, Chen D, Green D: Enoxaparin for thromboembolism prophylaxis in spinal cord injury. Am J Phys Med Rehabil 1996; 75:1–3.
255. Harvey C, Rothschild BB, Asmann AJ, et al: New estimates of traumatic SCI prevalence: A survey-based approach. Paraplegia 1990; 28:537–544.

256. Haselkorn J, Britell CW, Cardenas DD: Diagnostic imagery of heterotopic ossification with co-existent deep-venous thrombosis in flaccid paraplegia. Arch Phys Med Rehabil 1991; 72:227–229.
257. Hassard G: Heterotopic bone formation about the hip and unilateral decubitus ulcers in spinal cord injury. Arch Phys Med Rehabil 1975; 56:355–358.
258. Hayes KC: 4-Aminopyridine and spinal cord injury: A review. Restor Neurol Neurosci 1994; 6:259–270.
259. Head H, Riddoch G: The automatic bladder, excessive sweating and some other reflex conditions in gross injuries of the spinal cord. Brain 1917; 40:188–263.
260. Heary RF, Vaccaro AR, Mesa JJ, et al: Steroids and gunshot wounds to the spine. Neurosurgery 1997; 41:576–583.
261. Heilporn A: Two therapeutic experiments on stubborn pain in spinal cord lesions: Coupling melitracen-flupenthixen and the transcutaneous nerve stimulation. Paraplegia 1977; 15:368–372.
262. Heinemann AW, Magiera-Planey R: Evaluating the special needs of functional neuromuscular stimulation research candidates. J Med Eng Technol 1985; 9:167–173.
263. Heinemann AW, Doll M, Schnoll S: Treatment of alcohol abuse in persons with recent spinal cord injury. Alcohol Health World 1989; 13:111–117.
264. Heinemann AW, Yarkony GM, Roth EJ, et al: Functional outcome following spinal cord injury: A comparison of specialized spinal cord injury center vs general hospital short term care. Arch Neurol 1989; 46:1098–1102.
265. Heinemann AW, Doll MD, Armstrong KJ, et al: Substance abuse and receipt of treatment by persons with long-term spinal cord injuries. Arch Phys Med Rehabil 1991; 72:482–487.
266. Heinemann AW, Donohue R, Keen M, et al: Alcohol use by persons with recent spinal cord injury. Arch Phys Med Rehabil 1988; 69:619–624.
267. Heinemann AW, Magier-Planey R, Schiro-Geist C, et al: Mobility for persons with spinal cord injury: An evaluation of two systems. Arch Phys Med Rehabil 1987; 68:90–93.
268. Heldenberg D, Rubenstein A, Levtor O, et al: Serum lipids and lipoprotein concentrations in young quadriplegic patients. Atherosclerosis 1981; 39:163–167.
269. Henderson JL, Price SH, Brandstater ME, et al: Efficacy of three measures to relieve pressure in seated persons with spinal cord injury. Arch Phys Med Rehabil 1994; 75:535–539.
270. Hentz VR, Brown M, Keoshian LA: Upper-limb reconstruction in quadriplegia: Functional assessment and proposed treatment modifications. J Hand Surg Am 1983; 8:119–130.
271. Herz DA, Parsons KC, Pearl L: Percutaneous radiofrequency foraminal rhizotomies. Spine 1983; 8:729–732.
272. Hill JP: Surgical options after spinal cord injury. In Yarkony GM (ed): Spinal Cord Injury: Medical Management and Rehabilitation. Gaithersburg, MD, Aspen, 1994, pp 137–141.
273. Hirokawa S, Grimm M, Le T, et al: Energy consumption in paraplegic ambulation using the reciprocating gait orthosis and electric stimulation of the thigh muscles. Arch Phys Med Rehabil 1990; 71:687–694.
274. Hirsch GH, Menarch MR, Anton HA: Anemia after traumatic spinal cord injury. Arch Phys Med Rehabil 1991; 72:195–201.
275. Holdsworth F: Fractures, dislocation and fracture-dislocation of the spine. J Bone Joint Surg Am 1970; 52:1534–1551.
276. Holmes G: Pain of Central Origin: Contributions to Medical and Biological Research. New York, Hober, 1919, p 235.
277. House JH, Shannen MA: Restoration of strong grasp and lateral pinch in tetraplegia: A comparison of two methods of thumb control in each patient. J Hand Surg Am 1985; 10:22–29.
278. Huang CT, DeVivo MJ, Stover SL: Anemia in acute phase of spinal cord injury. Arch Phys Med Rehabil 1990; 71:3–7.
279. Huang TS, Wang YH, Lee SH, et al: Impaired hypothalamus-pituitary-adrenal axis in men with spinal cord injuries. Am J Phys Med Rehabil 1998; 77:108–112.
280. Hussey RW, Stauffer ES: Spinal cord injury: Requirements for ambulation. Arch Phys Med Rehabil 1973; 54:544–547.
281. Hyers TM: Venous thromboembolism. Am J Respir Crit Care Med 1999; 159:1–14.
282. Ingram RR, Suman RK, Freeman PA: Lower limb fractures in the chronic spinal cord-injured patients. Paraplegia 1989; 28:133–139.
283. Jackson AB, Groomes TE: Incidence of respiratory complications following spinal cord injury. Arch Phys Med Rehabil 1994; 75:270–275.
284. Jaeger RJ, Yarkony GM, Roth EJ, et al: Estimating the user population of a simple electrical stimulation system for standing. Paraplegia 1990; 28:505–511.
285. Jaeger RJ, Yarkony GM, Roth EJ: Rehabilitation technology for standing and walking after spinal cord injury. Am J Med Rehabil 1989; 198:128–133.
286. Jensen LL, Halar E, Little JW, et al: Neurogenic heterotopic ossification. Am J Phys Med 1988; 66:351–363.
287. Johnson K, Grant T, Peterson P: Ventilator weaning for the patient with high level tetraplegia. Top Spinal Cord Injury Rehabil 1997; 2(3):11–20.
288. Johnstone BR, Jordan CJ, Buntine JA: A review of surgical rehabilitation of the upper limb in quadriplegia. Paraplegia 1988; 26:317–339.
289. Jones RF, Snowdon E, Coan J, et al: Bracing of thoracic and lumbar spine fractures. Paraplegia 1987; 25:386–393.
290. Joseph DB, Bauer SB, Colodny AH, et al: Clean intermittent catheterization of infants with neurogenic bladder. Pediatrics 1989; 84:78–82.
291. Kabalin JN, Lennon S, Grill HS, et al: Incidence and management of autonomic dysreflexia and other intraoperative problems encountered in spinal cord injury patients undergoing extracorporeal shock wave lithotripsy without anesthesia on a second generation lithotriptor. J Urol 1993; 149:1064–1067.
292. Kalsbeek WD, McLaurin RL, Harris BSH, et al: The National Head and Spinal Cord Injury Survey: Major findings. J Neurosurg 1980; 53:S19–S43.
293. Kantrowitz A: Electronic Physiologic Aids: A Report of the Maimonides Hospital. Brooklyn, NY, Maimonides Hospital, 1960.
294. Kao CC, Chang LW: The mechanism of spinal cord cavitation following spinal cord transection. J Neurosurg 1977; 46:197–209.
295. Kaplan PE, Rodin W, Gilbert E, et al: Reduction of hypercalciuria in tetraplegia after weight-bearing and strengthening exercises. Paraplegia 1981; 19:289–293.
296. Kasdon DL, Lathi ES: A prospective study of radiofrequency rhizotomy in the treatment of posttraumatic spasticity. Neurosurgery 1984; 15:526–529.
297. Katz RT: Management of spasticity. Am J Phys Med Rehabil 1988; 67:108–116.
298. Katz RT, Rymer WZ: Spastic hypertonia: Mechanisms and measurement. Arch Phys Med Rehabil 1989; 70:144–155.
299. Kearon C, Julian JA, Newman TE, et al: Noninvasive diagnosis of deep venous thrombosis. McMaster Diagnostic Imaging Practice Guidelines Initiative. Ann Intern Med 1998; 128:663–677.
300. Keith MW, Peckham PH, Thrope GB, et al: Functional neuromuscular stimulation neuroprostheses for the tetraplegic hand. Clin Orthop 1988; 233:25–33.
301. Kewalramani LS, Kraus JF, Sterling HM: Acute spinal cord lesions in a pediatric population. Paraplegia 1980; 18:206–219.
302. Kessler KM, Pina I, Green BA, et al: Cardiovascular findings in quadriplegic and paraplegic patients and in normal subjects. Am J Cardiol 1986; 58:525–530.
303. Kim SW, Charallel JT, Park KW, et al: Prevalence of deep venous thrombosis in patients with chronic spinal cord injury. Arch Phys Med Rehabil 1994; 75:965–968.
304. King RB, Carlson CE, Mervine J, et al: Clean and sterile intermittent catheterization methods in hospitalized patients with spinal cord injury. Arch Phys Med Rehabil 1992; 73:798–802.
305. Koch BM, Eng GM: Neonatal spinal cord injury. Arch Phys Med Rehabil 1979; 60:378–380.
306. Kohlmeyer KM, Yarkony GM: Functional outcome after spinal cord injury rehabilitation. In Yarkony GM (ed): Spinal Cord Injury: Medical Management and Rehabilitation. Rockville, MD, Aspen, 1994.
307. Kohlmeyer KM, Rom C: Driver assessment. In Yarkony GM (ed): Spinal Cord Injury: Medical Management and Rehabilitation. Rockville, MD, Aspen, 1994.
308. Konz KR, Chia JK, Kurup VP, et al: Comparison of latex hypersensitivity among patients with neurologic defects. J Allergy Clin Immunol 1995; 95:950–954.

309. Kozin F, Ryan LM, Carerra GF, et al: The reflex sympathetic dystrophy syndrome: III. Am J Med 1981; 70:23–30.
310. Krajl A, Bajd T: Functional Electrical Stimulation: Standing and Walking after Spinal Cord Injury. Boca Raton, FL, CRC Press, 1989.
311. Kraft Fine C: Utilizating a day hospital program as part of a pressure ulcer management program continuum. Top Spinal Cord Injury Rehabil 1996; (2)1:42–50.
312. Kraus JF, Franti CE, Riggins RS, et al: Incidence of traumatic spinal cord lesions. J Chronic Dis 1975; 28:471–492.
313. Krause JS, Crewe NM: Chronologic age, time since injury and time of measurement: Effect on adjustment after spinal cord injury. Arch Phys Med Rehabil 1991; 72:91–100.
314. Krause JS: Employment after spinal cord injury. Arch Phys Med Rehabil 1992; 73:163–169.
315. Krause JS, Sternberg M: Aging and spinal cord injury: The role of chronologic age, time since injury and environmental change. Rehabil Psychol 1998; 42:287–302.
316. Kriss VM, Kriss TC: SCIWORA in infants and children. Clin Pediatr 1996; 35(3):119–124.
317. Kronick R, Zhou Z, Dreyfus T: Making risk adjustment work for everyone. Inquiry 1995; 32:41–55.
318. Kuhlemeier KV, Lloyd LK, Stover SL: Long-term followup of renal function after spinal cord injury. J Urol 1985; 134:510–513.
319. Kurnick NB: Autonomic hyperreflexia and its control in patients with spinal cord lesions. Ann Intern Med 1956; 44:678–686.
320. Lal S, Hamilton B, Heinemann A, et al: Risk factors for heterotopic ossification in spinal cord injury. Arch Phys Med Rehabil 1989; 70:387–390.
321. Lanig IS, Lammertse DP: The respiratory system in spinal cord injury. Phys Med Rehabil Clin North Am 1992; 3:725–740.
322. Lavin GT, Huang CT, DeVivo MJ, et al: Nutritional status during the acute stage of spinal cord injury. Am J Phys Med Rehabil 1989; 70:277–282.
323. Lazzara G, Lazarus C, Logemann SA: Swallowing disorders in spinal cord-injured patients. ASHA 1985; 28:123.
324. Leaf DA, Buhl RA, Adkins RH: Risk of cardiac dysrhythmias in chronic spinal cord injury patients. Paraplegia 1993; 31:571–575.
325. Ledsome JR Sharp JM: Pulmonary function in acute cervial cord injury. Am Rev Respir Dis 1981; 124:41–44.
326. Lee AY, Ginsberg JS: The role of D-dimer in the diagnosis of venous thromboembolism. Curr Opin Pulmon Med 1997; 3: 275–279.
327. Lee BY, Agarwal N, Corcoran L, et al: Assessment of nutritional and metabolic status of paraplegics. J Rehabil Res Dev 1985; 22:11–17.
328. Lee MY, Kirk PM, Yarkony GM: Rehabilitation of quadriplegic patients with phrenic nerve pacers. Arch Phys Med Rehabil 1989; 70:549–552.
329. Leeds EM, Klose SK, Ganz W, et al: Bone mineral density after bicycle ergometry training. Arch Phys Med Rehabil 1990; 71:207–279.
330. Lehmann KB, Lane JG, Piepmeier JM, et al: Cardiovascular abnormalities accompanying acute spinal cord injury in humans: Incidence, time course and severity. J Am Coll Cardiol 1987; 10:46–52.
331. Lensing A, Prandoni P, Brandjes D, et al: Detection of deep-vein thrombosis by real-time B-mode ultrasonography. N Engl J Med 1989; 320:342–345.
332. Leslie WD, Nance PW: Dissociated hip and spine demineralization: A specific finding in spinal cord injury. Arch Phys Med Rehabil 1993; 74:960–964.
333. Levi AD, Tator CH, Bunge RP: Clinical syndromes associated with disproportionate weakness of the upper versus the lower extremities after cervical spinal cord injury. Neurosurgery 1996; 38:179–185.
334. Levi L, Aizik W, Belzberg H: Hemodynamic parameters in patients with acute cervical cord trauma: Description, intervention and prediction of outcome. Neurosurgery 1993; 33:1007–1017.
335. Levine AM, Garfin SR, Eismont FJ, et al: Spine Trauma. Philadelphia, WB Saunders, 1993.
336. Levitt M, Levitt JH: The deafferentation syndrome in monkeys: Dysesthesias of spinal origin. Pain 1981; 10:129–147.
337. Levy ML, Gans W, Wijesinghe HS, et al: Use of methylprednisolone as an adjunct in the management of patients with penetrating spinal cord injury. Neurosurgery 1996; 39:1141–1148.
338. Lewis VL: Surgical management of pressure ulcers. In Yarkony GM (ed): Spinal Cord Injury: Medical Management and Rehabilitation. Gaithersburg, MD, Aspen, 1994, pp 85–95.
339. Lim AC, Roth EJ, Green D: Lower limb paralysis: Its effect on the recanalization of deep-vein thrombosis. Arch Phys Med Rehabil 1992; 73:331–333.
340. Lindan R, Joiner E, Freehafer AA, et al: Incidence and clinical features of autonomic dysreflexia in patients with spinal cord injuries. Paraplegia 1980; 18:285–292.
341. Little JW, Halar E: Temporal course of motor recovery after Brown-Séquard spinal cord injury. Paraplegia 1985; 23:39–45.
342. Little JW, Powers RK, Michelson P, et al: Electrodiagnosis of upper limb weakness in acute quadriplegia. Am J Phys Med Rehabil 1994; 73:15–22.
343. Little JW, Robinson LR, Goldstein B, et al: Electrophysiological findings in post-traumatic syringomyelia: Implications for clinical management. J Am Paraplegia Soc 1995; 15(2):44–52.
344. Lloyd LK, Kuhlemeier KV, Fine PR: Initial bladder management in spinal cord injury: Does it make a difference? J Urol 1986; 135:523.
345. Locke JR, Hill DE, Walzer Y: Incidence of squamous cell carcinoma in patients with long-term catheter drainage. J Urol 1985; 133:1034–1035.
346. Long C II, Lawton EB: Functional significance of spinal cord lesion level. Arch Phys Med Rehabil 1955; 36:249–255.
347. Long C II, Masciarelli VD: An electrophysiologic splint for the hand. Arch Phys Med Rehabil 1963; 44:499–503.
348. Long DM, Erickson DE: Stimulation of the posterior columns of the spinal cord for relief of intractable pain. Surg Neurol 1975; 4:134–141.
349. Lotta S, Scelsi R, Alfonsi E, et al: Morphometric and neurophysiological analysis of skeletal muscle in paraplegic patients with traumatic cord lesion. Paraplegia 1991; 29:247–252.
350. Loubser PG, Donovan WH: Diagnostic spinal anesthesia in chronic spinal cord injury pain. Paraplegia 1991; 29:29–36.
351. Loveridge B, Dubo H: Breathing pattern in chronic quadriplegia. Arch Phys Med Rehabil 1990; 71:495–499.
352. MacDiarmid SA, Arnold EP, Palmer NB, et al: Management of spinal cord injured patients by indwelling suprapubic catheterization. J Urol 1995; 154 (2 Pt 1):492–494.
353. MacKenzie EJ, Shapiro S, Smith RT, et al: Factors influencing return to work following hospitalization for traumatic injury. Am J Public Health 1987; 77:329–334.
354. Malec J, Harvey RF, Cayner JJ: Cannabis effect on spasticity in spinal cord injury. Arch Phys Med Rehabil 1982; 63:116–118.
355. Mange KC, Marino RJ, Gregory PC, et al: The course of motor recovery at the zone of injury in complete spinal cord injury. Arch Phys Med Rehabil 1992; 73:437–440.
356. Mansel JK, Norman JR: Respiratory complications and management of spinal cord injuries. Chest 1990; 97:1446–1452.
357. Marciello MA, Herbison GJ, Cohen ME, et al: Elbow extension using anterior deltoids and upper pectorals in spinal cord injured subjects. Arch Phys Med Rehabil 1995; 76:426–432.
358. Marino RJ, Crozier KS, et al: Neurologic examination and functional assessment after spinal cord injury. Phys Med Rehabil Clin North Am 1992; 3:829–852.
359. Marsolais EB, Kobetic R: Development of a practical electrical stimulation system for restoring gait in the paralyzed patient. Clin Orthop 1988; 233:64–74.
360. Martin B: Treatment of dysphagia in adults. In Cherney LR (ed): Clinical Management of Dysphagia in Adults and Children. Gaithersburg, MD, Aspen, 1994, pp 153–183.
361. Massagli TL, Dudgeon BJ, Ross BW: Educational performance and vocational participation after spinal cord injury in childhood. Arch Phys Med Rehabil 1996; 77:995–999.
362. Matthews PJ, Carlson CE: Spinal Cord Injury: A Guide to Rehabilitation Nursing. Rockville, MD, Aspen, 1987.
363. Maury M: About pain and its treatment in paraplegics. Paraplegia 1977; 15:349–352.
364. Maynard F: Posttraumatic cystic myelopathy in motor incomplete quadriplegia presenting as progressive orthostasis. Arch Phys Med Rehabil 1984; 65:30–32.
365. Maynard FM: Immobilization hypercalcemia following spinal cord injury. Arch Phys Med Rehabil 1986; 67:41–44.

366. Maynard FM, Glass J: Management of the neuropathic bladder by clean intermittent catheterization: 5 year outcomes. Paraplegia 1987; 25:106–110.
367. Maynard FM, Glenn GR, Fountain S, et al: Neurological prognosis after traumatic quadriplegia. J Neurosurg 1979; 50:611–616.
368. Maynard FM, Imai K: Immobilization hypercalcemia in spinal cord injury. Arch Phys Med Rehabil 1977; 58:16–24.
369. McAuliffe JA, Wolfson AH: Early excision of heterotopic ossification about the elbow followed by radiation therapy. J Bone Joint Surg Am 1997; 79:749–755.
370. McDowell CL, Moberg EA, House JH: The Second International Conference on Surgical Rehabilitation of the Upper Limb in Tetraplegia (Quadriplegia). J Hand Surg Am 1986; 11:604–608.
371. McGuire EJ, Savastano JA: Long term follow up of spinal cord injury patients managed by intermittent catheterization. J Urol 1983; 129:775–776.
372. McGregor JA, Meeuwsen J: Autonomic hyperreflexia: A mortal danger for spinal cord-damaged women in labor. Am J Obstet Gynecol 1985; 151:330–333.
373. Meinecke FW: Some thoughts about neurological recovery in spinal cord injury. Paraplegia 1985; 23:78.
374. Melzack R, Loeser JD: Phantom body pain in paraplegics: Evidence for a central nervous pattern generating mechanism for pain. Pain 1978; 4:195–210.
375. Melzack R: Phantom limbs and the concept of aneuromatrix. Trends Neurosci 1990; 13:88–92.
376. Menter RR: Aging with a spinal cord injury. Phys Med Rehabil Clin North Am 1992; 3:879–891.
377. Merkel KD, Miller NE, Westbrook PR, et al: Energy expenditure of paraplegic patients standing and walking with two knee-ankle-foot orthoses. Arch Phys Med Rehabil 1984; 65:121–124.
378. Merli G: Management of deep vein thrombosis in spinal cord injury. Chest 1992; 102:652S–657S.
379. Merli G, Crabbe S, Doyle L, et al: Mechanical plus pharmacological prophylaxis for deep vein thrombosis in acute spinal cord injury. Paraplegia 1992; 30:558–562.
380. Merli G, Crabbe S, Paluzzi R, et al: Etiology, incidence, and prevention of deep vein thrombosis in acute spinal cord injury. Arch Phys Med Rehabil 1993; 74:199–205.
381. Merli G, Herbison G, Ditunno J, et al: Deep vein thrombosis in acute spinal cord-injured patients. Arch Phys Med Rehabil 1988; 69:661–664.
382. Merli GJ, McElwain GE, Adler AG, et al: Immobilization hypercalcemia in acute spinal cord injury treated with etidronate. Arch Intern Med 1984; 144:1286–1288.
383. Merriam WF, Taylor TKF, Ruff SJ, et al: A reappraisal of acute traumatic central cord syndrome. J Bone Joint Surg Br 1986; 68:708–713.
384. Merritt JL: Management of spasticity in spinal cord injury. Mayo Clin Proc 1981; 56:614–622.
385. Merritt JL: Residual urine volume: Correlate of urinary tract infection in patients with spinal cord injury. Arch Phys Med Rehabil 1981; 62:558–561.
386. Meyer PR Jr: Surgery of Spine Trauma. New York, Churchill Livingstone, 1989.
387. Meyer PR Jr: A new spine fracture classification system. Presented at the American Academy of Physical Medicine and Rehabilitation 58th Assembly, Chicago, October 1996.
388. Meyers AR, Feltin M, Master RJ, et al: Rehospitalization and spinal cord injury: Cross sectional survey of adults living independently. Arch Phys Med Rehabil 1985; 66:704–708.
389. Meythaler JM, Tuel SM, Cross LL: Successful treatment of immobilization hypercalcemia using calcitonin and etidronate. Arch Phys Med Rehabil 1993; 74:316–319.
390. Mikelberg R, Reid S: Spinal cord lesions and lower extremity bracing: An overview and follow-up study. Paraplegia 1981; 19:379–385.
391. Minaire P, Meunier P, Edouard C, et al: Quantitative histological data on disuse osteoporosis: Comparison with biological data. Calcif Tissue Res 1974; 17:57–73.
392. Moberg EA: Surgical treatment for absent single-hand grip and elbow extension in quadriplegia. J Bone Joint Surg Am 1975; 57:196–206.
393. Mohammand K, Rothwell A, Sinclair S, et al: Upper limb surgery for tetraplegia. J Bone Joint Surg Br 1992; 74:873–879.
394. Mollinger LA, Sparr GB, El Ghatet AZ, et al: Daily energy expenditure and basal metabolic rates of patients with spinal cord injury. Arch Phys Med Rehabil 1985; 66:420–426.
395. Montgomerie JZ: Infections in patients with spinal cord injuries. Clin Infect Dis 1997; 25:1285–1292.
396. Moreno JG, Lofti MA, Rivas DA, et al: Continent urinary diversion using an umbilical stoma in quadriplegic patients (abstract). J Am Paraplegia Soc 1994; 17:125.
397. Morgan MDL, Silver JR, Williams SJ: The respiratory system of the spinal cord patient. In Bloch RF, Basbaum M (eds): Management of Spinal Cord Injuries. Baltimore, Williams & Wilkins, 1986, pp 78–116.
398. Morris J: Spinal injury and psychotheraphy: A treatment philosophy. In Yarkony GM (ed): Spinal Cord Injury: Medical Management and Rehabilitation. Rockville, MD, Aspen, 1994.
399. Morris J, Roth E, Davidoff G: Mild closed head injury and cognitive deficits in spinal cord-injured patients: Incidence and impact. J Head Trauma Rehabil 1986; 1:31–42.
400. Moynahan M, Mullin C, Cohn J, et al: FES program for standing and mobility in adolescents with spinal cord injury. Arch Phys Med Rehabil 1996; 77:1005–1013.
401. Mulcahey MJ: An overview of the upper extremity in pediatric spinal cord injury. Top Spinal Cord Injury Rehabil 1997; 3(2):48–55.
402. Mulcahey MJ: Unique management needs of pediatric spinal cord injury patients: Rehabilitation. J Spinal Cord Injury Med 1997; 20(1):25–29.
403. Munro AF, Robinson R: The catecholamine content of the peripheral plasma in human subjects with complete transverse lesions of the spinal cord. J Physiol 1960; 154:244–253.
404. Murray PK, Kusior MF: Epidemiology of nontraumatic and traumatic spinal cord injury. Arch Phys Med Rehabil 1984; 65:634.
405. Myllynen P, Kammonen M, Rokkanen P, et al: The blood F VIII:Ag/F VIII:C ratio as an early indicator of deep venous thrombosis during post-traumatic immobilization. J Trauma 1987; 27:287–290.
406. Myllynen P, Kammonen M, Rokkanen P, et al: DVT and pulmonary embolism in patients with acute spinal cord injury: A comparison with non-paralyzed patients immobilized due to spine fractures. J Trauma 1985; 25:541–543.
407. Nand S, Goldschmidt JW: Hypercalcemia and hyperuricemia in young patients with spinal cord injury. Arch Phys Med Rehabil 1976; 57:553–555.
408. Nance PW, Bugaresti J, et al: Efficacy and safety of tizanidine in the treatment of spasticity in patients with spinal cord injury. Neurology 1994; 44(suppl 9):44–53.
409. Nash MS, Bilsker S, Marcillo AE, et al: Reversal of adaptive left ventricular atrophy following electrically-stimulated exercise training in human tetraplegics. Paraplegia 1991; 29:590–599.
410. Nashold BS, Friedman H: Dorsal column stimulation for control of pain: Preliminary report on 30 patients. J Neurosurg 1972; 36:590–597.
411. National Spinal Cord Injury Statistical Center: Spinal Cord Injury: Facts and Figures at a Glance 1998. Birmingham, University of Alabama at Birmingham, 1998.
412. Natvig H, McAdam R: Ambulation without wheelchairs for paraplegics with complete lesions. Paraplegia 1978–79; 16:142–146.
413. Nesathurai S: Steroids and spinal cord injury: Revisiting the NASCIS2 and NASCIS3 trials. J Trauma Injury Infect Crit Care 1998; 45:1088–1093.
414. Nicholas PJR, Norman PA, Ennis JR: Wheelchair user's shoulder? Shoulder pain in patients with spinal cord lesions. Scand J Rehabil Med 1979; 11:29–32.
415. Nieder RM, O'Higgins JW, Aldrete JA: Autonomic hyperreflexia in urologic surgery. JAMA 1970; 213:867–869.
416. O'Daniel WE, Hahn HR: Follow-up usage of the Scott-Craig orthosis in paraplegia. Paraplegia 1981; 19:373–378.
417. O'Donnell J, Cooper J, Gessner J, et al: Alcohol, drugs, and spinal cord injury. Alcohol Health Res World 1981; 6:27–29.
418. Ohry A, Brooks ME, Steinbach TV, et al: Shoulder complications as a cause of delay in rehabilitation of spinal cord-injured patients. Paraplegia 1978; 16:310–316.
419. Orzel JA, Rudd TG: Heterotopic bone formation: Clinical, laboratory and imaging correlation. J Nucl Med 1985; 26:125–132

420. Osenbach RK, Menezes AH: Pediatric spinal cord and vertebral column injury. Neurosurgery 1992; 20:385–390.
421. Panel for the Prediction and Prevention of Pressure Ulcers in Adults: Pressure ulcers in adults: Prediction and prevention. AHCPR publication no 92-0047, Clinical Practice Guideline no 3. Rockville, MD, Agency for Health Care Policy and Research, Public Health Service, US Department of Health and Human Services, 1992.
422. Pang D: Spinal cord injury without radiographic abnormalities in children. J Neurosurg 1982; 57:114–129.
423. Patrick JH, McClelland MR: Low energy reciprocal walking for the adult paraplegic. Paraplegia 1985; 23:113–117.
424. Paulakis AJ, Siroky MB, Goldstein I, et al: Neurologic findings in conus medullaris and cauda equina injury. Arch Neurol 1983; 40:570–573.
425. Penn RD: Intrathecal baclofen for spasticity of spinal origin: Seven years of experience. J Neurosurg 1992; 77:236–240.
426. Penrod LE, Hegde SK, Ditunno JF: The effect of age on prognosis for ambulation in acute traumatic central cord syndrome. ASIA Abstracts Digest, ASIA 14th Annual Scientific Meeting, 1988, p 75.
427. Perkash A, Brown M: Anemia in patients with spinal cord injury. J Am Paraplegia Soc 1986; 9:10–15.
428. Perlman M: Neonatal spinal cord injury in the infant. In Betz RR, Mulcahey MJ (eds): The Child with a Spinal Cord Injury. Rosemont, IL, American Academy of Orthopedic Surgeons, 1996.
429. Perrier A: Non-invasive diagnosis of pulmonary embolism. Haematologica 1997; 82:328–331.
430. Petaja J, Myllynen P, Rokkanen P, et al: Fibrinolysis and spinal injury: relationships to posttraumatic deep vein thrombosis. Acta Chir Scand 1989; 155:241–246.
431. Peterson P: Pulmonary physiology and medical management. In Whiteneck G, Lammertse DP, Manley S, et al (eds): The Management of High Quadriplegia. New York, Demos, 1989, pp 35–50.
432. Petrofsky JS, Phillips CA, Douglas R, et al: A computer-controller walking system: The combination of an orthosis with functional electrical stimulation. J Clin Eng 1986; 11:121–133.
433. Philipi R, Kuhn W, Zach GA, et al: Survey of the neurological evaluation of 300 spinal cord injuries seen within 24 hours of injury. Paraplegia 1990; 18:337–346.
434. Piepmeier JM, Lehmann KB, Lane JG: Cardiovascular instability following acute cervical spinal cord trauma. Cent Nerv Syst Trauma 1985; 2:153–160.
435. Pierce S: Legal consideration for a driver rehabilitation program. Phys Disabil 1993; 16:1.
436. Pine ZM, Miller SD, Alonso JA: Atrial fibrillation associated with autonomic dysreflexia. Am J Phys Med Rehabil 1991; 70:271–273.
437. Pistarini C, Carlevati S, Contardi A, et al: Use of ultrasonography methods in the diagnosis of neurogenic paraosteoarthropathy in spinal cord injury. Recent Prog Med 1995; 86:483–488.
438. Polatty RC, McElaney MA, Marcelino V: Pulmonary complications in the spinal cord injury patient. In Ozer MN, Schmitt JK (eds): Medical Complications of Spinal Cord Injury. Phys Med Rehabil State Art Rev 1987; 1:353–373.
439. Priebe MM, Sherwood AM, Graves DE, et al: Effectiveness of gabapentin in controlling spasticity: A quantitative study. Spinal Cord 1997; 35:171–175.
440. Putty TK, Shapiro SA: Efficacy of dorsal longitudinal myelotomy in treating spinal spasticity: A review of 20 cases. J Neurosurg 1991; 75:397–401.
441. Radecki RT, Gaebler-Spira D: Deep vein thrombosis in the disabled pediatric population. Arch Phys Med Rehabil 1994; 75:248–250.
442. Ragnarsson KT, Seli H: Lower extremity fractures after spinal cord injury: A retrospective study. Arch Phys Med Rehabil 1981; 62:418–423.
443. Ragnarsson KT, Hall KM, Wilmot CB, et al: Management of pulmonary cardiovascular and metabolic conditions after spinal cord injury. In Stover SL, DeLisa JA, Whiteneck GG (eds): Spinal Cord Injury: Clinical Outcomes from the Model Systems. Gaithersburg, MD, Aspen, 1995, pp 79–99.
444. Ragnarsson KT: Management of pain in persons with spinal cord injury. J Spinal Cord Med 1997; 20:186–199.
445. Ramon y Cajal S: Degeneration and Regeneration of the Nervous System. London, Oxford University Press, 1928.
446. Reier PJ, Anderson DK, et al: Neural tissue transplantation and CNS trauma. J Neurotrauma 1992; 9(suppl 1):S223–S248.
447. Reger SI, Navarro RR, Neth DC: Computerized shape reproduction for custom contoured wheelchair seating systems. J Rehabil Res Dev 1991; 28:467–468.
448. Remy-Jardin MJ, Reiny J, Deschildre F, et al: Diagnosis of acute pulmonary embolism with spiral CT: Comparison with pulmonary angiography and scintigraphy. Radiology 1996; 200: 699–706.
449. Richards JS: Psychological adjustment to spinal cord injury during the first discharge year. Arch Phys Med Rehabil 1986; 67:362–365.
450. Richards JS, Brown L, Hagglund K, et al: Spinal cord injury and concomitant traumatic brain injury: Results of a longitudinal investigation. Am J Phys Med Rehabil 1988; 67:211–216.
451. Richardson RR, Meyer PR, Cerullo LJ: Neurostimulation in the modulation of the intractable paraplegic and traumatic neuroma pains. Pain 1980; 8:75–84.
452. Riddoch G: The reflex functions of the completely divided spinal cord in man compared with those associated with less severe lesions. Brain 1917–1918; 40:617 and 41:264–402.
453. Rink P, Miller F: Hip instability in SCI patients. J Pediatr Orthop 1990; 10:583–587.
454. Rintala DH, Loubser PG, Castro J, et al: Chronic pain in a community based sample of men with spinal cord injury. Arch Phys Med Rehabil 1998; 76:604–614.
455. Rosman N, Spira E: Paraplegic use of walking braces: Survey. Arch Phys Med Rehabil 1974; 55:310–314.
456. Ross JC, Gibbon NOK, Sunder GSO: Division of the external urethal sphincter in the neuropathic bladder: A twenty-year review. Br J Urol 1976; 48:649–656.
457. Rossi E, Green D, Rosen J, et al: Sequential changes in factor VIII and platelets preceding deep vein thrombosis in patients with spinal cord injury. Br J Haematol 1980; 45:143–151.
458. Rossier AB, Bussat P, Infante F, et al: Current facts on para-osteo-arthropathy (POA). Paraplegia 1973; 11:36–78.
459. Rossier AB, Foo D, Shillito J, et al: Posttraumatic cervical syringomyelia: Incidence, clinical presentation, electrophysiological studies, syrinx protein and results of conservative and operative treatment. Brain 1985; 108:439–461.
460. Roth E, Davidoff G, Thomas P: A controlled study of neuropsychological deficits in acute spinal cord injury. Paraplegia 1989; 27:480–489.
461. Roth EJ, Fenton LL, Gaebler-Spira DJ, et al: Superior mesenteric artery syndrome in acute traumatic quadriplegia: Case reports and literature review. Arch Phys Med Rehabil 1991; 72:417–420.
462. Roth EJ, Lawler MH, Yarkony GM: Traumatic central cord syndrome: Clinical features and functional outcomes. Arch Phys Med Rehabil 1990; 71:18–23.
463. Roth EJ, Park T, Pang T, et al: Traumatic cervical Brown-Séquard and Brown-Séquard-plus syndromes: The spectrum of presentations and outcomes. Paraplegia 1991; 29:582–589.
464. Ruge JR, Sinson GP, McLone DG, et al: Pediatric spinal injury: The very young. J Neurosurg 1988; 68:25–30.
465. Rush PJ: The rheumatic manifestations of traumatic spinal cord injury. Semin Arthritis Rheum 1989; 19:77–89, 290.
466. Rutchik A, Weissman AR, Almenoff PL: Resistive inspiratory muscle training in subjects with chronic cervical spinal cord injury. Arch Phys Med Rehabil 1998; 73:293–297.
467. Sahgal V, Sahgal S, Subramani V: Morphometric and histochemical correlation of recovery after spinal transection. Paraplegia 1980; 18:391–396.
468. Sauter-Bihl ML, Liebermeister E, Heinze HG, et al: The radiotherapy of heterotopic ossification in paraplegia. Strahlenther Onkol 1995; 171:454–459.
469. Scanlon PD, Loring SH, Pichurko BM, et al: Respiratory mechanics in acute quadriplegia: Lung and chest wall compliance and dimensional changes during respiratory maneuvers. Am Rev Respir Dis 1987; 135:367–371.

470. Schaeffer MA, Sosner J: Heterotopic ossification: Treatment of established bone with radiation therapy. Arch Phys Med Rehabil 1995; 76:284–286.
471. Schneider RC, Cherry G, Pantek H: Central cervical spinal cord injury with special reference to the mechanics involved in hyperextension injuries of cervical spine. J Neurosurg 1954; 11: 546–577.
472. Schroer W, Lacey S, Frost F, et al: Carpal instability in the weight bearing upper extremity. J Bone Joint Surg Am 1996; 78:1838–1843.
473. Schurch B, Capaul M, Vallotton MB, et al: Prostaglandin E2 measurements: Their value in the early diagnosis of heterotopic ossification in spinal cord injury patients. Arch Phys Med Rehabil 1997; 78:687–691.
474. Scott BA, Weinstein Z, Chiteman R, et al: Intrathecal phenol and glycerin in metrizamide for treatment of intractable spasms in paraplegia. J Neurosurg 1985; 63:125–127.
475. Scott JA, Donovan WH: The prevention of shoulder pain and contracture in the acute tetraplegic patient. Paraplegia 1981; 19:313–319.
476. Schachner M: Neural recognition molecules and synaptic plasticity. Curr Opin Cell Biol 1997; 9:627–634.
477. Seleski S: Orthotic prescription principles. J Spinal Cord Med 1996; 19:97–98.
478. Serafini T, Colamarino SA, et al: Netrin-1 is required for commissural axon guidance in the developing vertebrate nervous system. Cell 1996; 87:1001–1014.
479. Sheriff MK, Foley S, McFarlane J, et al: Long-term suprapubic catheterisation; clinical outcome and satisfaction survey. Spinal Cord 1 1998; 36:171–176.
480. Sica DA, Midha M, Aronoff G, et al: Atrial natriuretic factor in spinal cord injury. Arch Phys Med Rehabil 1993; 74:969–972.
481. Sica DA, Midha M, Zawada E, et al: Hyponatremia in spinal cord injury. J Am Paraplegia Soc 1990; 13:78–83.
482. Sie IH, Waters RL, Adkins RH, et al: Upper extremity pain the postrehabilitation spinal cord-injured patient. Arch Phys Med Rehabil 1992; 73:44–48.
483. Silfverskiold J, Waters RL: Shoulder pain and functional disability in spinal cord injury patients. Clin Orthop 1996; 322:140–145.
484. Silver JR: The prophylactic use of anticoagulant therapy in the prevention of pulmonary embolism in 100 consecutive spinal cord injury patients. Paraplegia 1974; 12:188–196.
485. Silverman SL, Hurvitz EA, Nelson VS, et al: Rachitic syndrome after disodium etidronate therapy in an adolescent. Arch Phys Med Rehabil 1994; 75:118–120.
486. Sliwa JA, Maclean IC: Ishemic myelopathy: A review of spinal vasculature and related clinical syndromes. Arch Phys Med Rehabil 1992; 73:365–372.
487. Sliwa JA, Mason K, Yarkony G, et al: The value of routine chest roentgenograms on admission for rehabilitation after traumatic spinal cord injury. Am J Phys Med Rehabil 1994; 73:84–88.
488. Snoecx M, DeMuynck M, Van Laere M: Association between muscle trauma and heterotopic ossification in spinal cord-injured patients: Reflections on their causal relationship and the diagnostic value of ultrasonography. Paraplegia 1995; 33:464–468.
489. Solomonow M, Baratta R, Hirokawa S, et al: The RGO generation II: Muscle stimulation powered orthosis as a practical walking system for thoracic paraplegics. Orthopedics 1989; 12:1309–1315.
490. Sonies BC: Dysphagia: A model for differential diagnosis for adults and children. In Cherney LR (ed): Clinical Management of Dysphagia in Adults and Children. Gaithersburg, MD, Aspen, 1994, pp 133–152.
491. Sorg RJ: HDL-cholesterol: Exercise formula. Results of long-term (six-year) strenuous swimming exercise in a middle-aged male with paraplegia. J Ortho Sports Phys Ther 1993; 17:1951–1959.
492. Stanworth PA: The significance of hyperhidrosis in patients with post-traumatic syringomyelia. Paraplegia 1982; 20:282–287.
493. Stauffer ES, Rhodes ME: Surgical stabilization of the cervical spine after trauma. Arch Surg 1976; 111:652–662.
494. Stelzner DJ, Cullen JM: Do propriospinal projections contribute to hindlimb recovery when all long tracts are cut in neonatal or weanling rats? Exp Neurol 1991; 114:193–205.
495. Stewart AF, Adler M, Byers CM, et al: Calcium homeostasis in immobilization: Example of resorptive hypercalciuria. N Engl J Med 1982; 306:1136–1140.
496. Stiens SA, Johnson MC II, Lyman PJ: Cardiac rehabilitation in patients with spinal cord injuries. Phys Med Rehabil Clin North Am 1995; 6:263–296.
497. Stiens SA, Bergman SB, Goetz LL: Neurogenic bowel dysfunction after spinal cord injury: Clinical evaluation and rehabilitative management. Arch Phys Med Rehabil 1997; 78(suppl 3):S86–S102.
498. Stirt JA, Marco A, Conklin KA: Obstetric anesthesia for a quadriplegic patient with autonomic hyperreflexia. Anesthesiology 1979; 51:560–562.
499. Stone JM, NinoMurcia M, Wolfe UA: Chronic gastrointestinal problems in spinal cord injury patients: A prospective analysis. Am J Gastroenterol 1990; 85:1114–1119.
500. Stover SL, Fine PR (eds): Spinal Cord Injury: The Facts and Figures. Birmingham, University of Alabama at Birmingham, 1986.
501. Stover SL, Hahn HR, Miller JM: Disodium etidronate in the prevention of heterotopic ossification following spinal cord injury (preliminary report). Paraplegia 1976; 14:146–156.
502. Stover SL, Hataway CJ, Zeiger HE: Heterotopic ossification in spinal cord-injured patients. Arch Phys Med Rehabil 1975; 56:199–204.
503. Stover SL, Lloyd LK, Waites KB, et al: Urinary tract infection in spinal cord injury. Arch Phys Med Rehabil 1989; 70:47–54.
504. Stover SL, Niemann KM, Miller JM: Disodium etidronate in the prevention of post-operative recurrence of heterotopic ossification in spinal cord injury patients. J Bone Joint Surg Am 1976; 58:683–688.
505. Stover SL, Niemann KM, Tulloss JR: Experience with surgical resection of heterotopic bone in spinal cord injury patients. Clin Orthop 1991; 263:71–77.
506. Stover SL, Omura EF, Buell AB: Clinical skin thickening following spinal cord injury studied by histopathology. J Am Paraplegia Soc 1994; 17(2):44–49.
507. Stover SL: Review of forty years of rehabilitation issues in spinal cord injury. J Spinal Cord Med 1995; 18:175–182.
508. Sturm PF, Glass RB, Sivit CJ, et al: Lumbar compression fractures secondary to lap belt use in children. J Pediatr Orthop 1995; 15:521–523.
509. Sugarman B: Fever in quadriplegic persons. Arch Phys Med Rehabil 1982; 63:639–640.
510. Swarczinski C, Dijkers M: The value of serial leg measurements for monitoring deep vein thrombosis in spinal cord injury. J Neurosci Nurs 1991; 23:306–314.
511. Taylor SJ: Powered mobility evaluation and technology. Top Spinal Cord Injury Rehabil 1995; 1(1):23–36.
512. Terrance CF, Fromm GH: Complications of baclofen withdrawal. Arch Neurol 1981; 38:588–589.
513. Thuroff JW, Bunke B, Ebner A, et al: Randomized, double-blind, multicenter trial on treatment of frequency, urgency and incontinence related to detrusor hyperactivity: Oxybutynin versus propantheline versus placebo. J Urol 1991; 145:813–817.
514. Tominaga L: Periodic, neurological-functional assessment for cervical cord injury. Paraplegia 1989; 27:227–232.
515. Tori JA, Hill LL: Hypercalcemia in children with spinal cord injury. Arch Phys Med Rehabil 1978; 59:443–447.
516. Tribe C: Cause of death in the early and late stages of paraplegia. Paraplegia 1963; 1:19–47.
517. Trieschmann RB: Aging with a Disability. New York, Demos, 1987.
518. Trieschmann RB: Spinal Cord Injuries: Psychological, Social and Vocational Rehabilitation, ed 2. New York, Demos, 1988.
519. Trieschmann RB (ed): Spinal Cord Injuries: Psychological, Social and Vocational Adjustment. Elmsford, NY, Pergamon Press, 1976.
520. Tun CG, Upton J: The paraplegic hand: Electrodiagnostic studies and clinical findings. J Hand Surg Am 1988; 13:716–719.
521. Tunks E, Bahry N, Rausbaum M: Pain in spinal cord-injured patients. In Bloch RF, Rausbaum M (eds): Management of Spinal Cord Injuries. Baltimore, Williams & Wilkins, 1986, pp 180–211.
522. Turnbull IM: Blood supply of the spinal cord: Normal and pathological considerations. Clin Neurosurg 1973; 20:56–84.

523. Umbach I, Heilport A: Post-spinal cord injury syringomyelia. Paraplegia 1991; 29:219–221.
524. Utili R, Boitnott JK, Zimmerman HJ: Dantrolene-associated hepatic injury: Incidence and character. Gastroenterology 1977; 72:610–616.
525. Van Dellen JR: Spinal cord trauma. In Bradley W, Daroff RB, et al (eds): Neurology in Clinical Practice, ed 2. Boston, Butterworth-Heinemann, 1995, pp 971–979.
526. Van Hala S, Nelson VS, Hurvitz EA: Bladder management in patients with pediatric onset neurogenic bladders. J Spinal Cord Med 1997; 20:410–415.
527. Vaziti ND, Eltorai IM, Segal S, et al: Erythropoietin profile in spinal cord-injured patients. Arch Phys Med Rehabil 1993; 74:65–67.
528. Veis SL, Logemann SA: Dysphagia after spinal cord injury (abstract). ASHA 1991; 33:112.
529. Venier LH, Ditunno JF: Heterotopic ossification in the paraplegic patient. Arch Phys Med Rehabil 1971; 52:475–479.
530. Vernon J, Silver J, Ohry A: Post-traumatic syringomyelia. Paraplegia 1982; 20:339–364.
531. Vernon J, Silver J, Symon L: Post-traumatic syringomyelia: The results of surgery. Paraplegia 1983; 21:37–46.
532. Virchow R: Neuer Fall von todlichen Embolie der Lungenarterie. Arch Pathol Anat 1856; 10:225–228.
533. Voelker KG, Chetty KG, Mahutte CK: Resolution of recurrent atelectasis in spinal cord injury patients with administration of recombinant human DNase. Intensive Care Med 1996; 22:582–584.
534. Vogel LC, Klaas SJ, Lubicky JP, et al: Long term outcomes and life satisfaction of adults who had pediatric spinal cord injuries. Arch Phys Med Rehabil 1998; 79:1496–1503.
535. Vogel LC, DeVivo MJ: Etiology and demographics. In Betz RR, Mulcahey MJ (eds): The Child with a Spinal Cord Injury. Rosemont, IL, American Academy of Orthopedic Surgeons, 1996.
536. Vogel LC, Gogia RS, Lubicky JP: Hip abnormalities in children with spinal cord injury. J Spinal Cord Med 1995; 18:172–175.
537. Vogel LC, Schrader T, Lubicky JP: Latex allergy in children and adolescents with spinal cord injury. J Pediatr Orthop 1995; 15:517–520.
538. Vogel LC, Lubicky JP: Ambulation with parapodia and reciprocating gait orthoses in pediatric spinal cord injury. Dev Med Child Neurol 1995; 37:957–964.
539. Vogel LC, Pontari MA: Pediatric Spinal Cord Injury Issues: Medical Issues. Top Spinal Cord Injury Rehabil 1997; 3(2):20–30.
540. Wainapel SF, Freed MM: Reflex sympathetic dystrophy in quadriplegia: Case report. Arch Phys Med Rehabil 1984; 65:35–36.
541. Waisbrod H, Hanse D, Gerbershagen HU: Chronic pain in paraplegics. Neurosurgery 1984; 15:933–934.
542. Walker BC, Holstein S: Vocational rehabilitation and spinal cord injury. In Yarkony GM (ed): Spinal Cord Injury: Medical Management and Rehabilitation. Rockville, MD, Aspen, 1994.
543. Walker J, Shepard RJ: Cardiac risk factors immediately following spinal injury. Arch Phys Med Rehabil 1993; 74:1129–1133.
544. Waring WP, Karunas RS: Acute spinal cord injuries and the incidence of clinically occurring thromboembolic disease. Paraplegia 1991; 29:8–16.
545. Warren CG, Lehmann JF, deLateur BJ: Pelvic band use in orthotics for adult paraplegic patients. Arch Phys Med Rehabil 1975; 56:221–223.
546. Watanabe S, Yamada K, Ono S, et al: Skin changes in patients with amyotrophic lateral sclerosis: Light and electron microscopic observations. J Am Acad Dermatol 1987; 17:1006–1012.
547. Waters R, Hislop H, Perry J: Walking and wheelchair energetics in persons with paraplegia. Phys Ther 1980; 60:1133–1139.
548. Waters RL, Adkins RH, Yakura JS: Definition of complete spinal cord injury. Paraplegia 1991; 9:573–581.
549. Waters RL, Adkins RH, Yakura JS, et al: Motor and sensory recovery following complete tetraplegia. Arch Phys Med Rehabil 1993; 74:242–247.
550. Waters RL, Adkins RH, Yakura JS, et al: Motor and sensory recovery following incomplete paraplegia. Arch Phys Med Rehabil 1994; 75:67–72.
551. Waters RL, Miller L: A physiological rationale for orthotic prescription in paraplegia. Clin Prosthet Orthot 1987; 2:66–73.
552. Waters RL, Adkins RH, Nelson R, et al: Cervical spinal cord trauma: Evaluation and nonoperative treatment with halo-vest immobilization. Contemp Orthop 1987; 14:35–45.
553. Waters RL, Yakura JS, Adkins R, et al: Determinants of gait performance following spinal cord injury. Arch Phys Med Rehabil 1989; 70:811–818.
554. Waters RL, Yakura JS, Adkins RH, et al: Recovery following complete paraplegia. Arch Phys Med Rehabil 1992; 73:784–789.
555. Waters RL, Adkins RH, Yakura JS, et al: Motor and sensory recovery following complete tetraplegia. Arch Phys Med Rehabil 1993; 74:242–247.
556. Waters RL, Adkins R, Yakura J: Prediction of ambulatory performance based on motor scores derived from standards of the American Spinal Injury Association. Arch Phys Med Rehabil 1994; 74:756–760.
557. Waters RL, Sie IH, Gellman H, et al: Functional hand surgery following tetraplegia. Arch Phys Med Rehabil 1996; 77: 86–93.
558. Waters RL, Adkins RH, Yakura JS, et al: Effect of surgery on motor recovery following traumatic spinal cord injury. Spinal Cord 1996; 34:188–192.
559. Waters RL: Functional prognosis of spinal cord injuries. J Spinal Cord Injury Med 1996; 19(2):89–105.
560. Watson DW, Downey GO: Epidural anesthesia for labor and delivery of twins of a paraplegic mother. Anesthesiology 1980; 52:257–261.
561. Watson N: Anticoagulant therapy in the prevention of venous thrombosis and pulmonary embolism in spinal cord injury. Paraplegia 1978–79; 16:265–269.
562. Weese-Mayer DE, Hunt CE, Brouillette RT, et al: Diaphragm pacing in infants and children. J Pediatr 1992; 120:1–8.
563. Weingarden SI, Belen JG: Clonidine transdermal system for treatment of spasticity in spinal cord injury. Arch Phys Med Rehabil 1992; 73:876–877.
564. Weingarden SI, Martin C: Independent dressing after spinal cord injury: A functional time evaluation. Arch Phys Med Rehabil 1989; 70:518–519.
565. Welch RD, Lobley SJ, O'Sullivan SB, et al: Functional independence in quadriplegia: Critical levels. Arch Phys Med Rehabil 1986; 676:235–240.
566. Wen JG, Tong EC: Cystometry in infants and children with no apparent voiding symptoms. Br J Urol 1998; 81:468–473.
567. Wharton GE, Morgan TH: Ankylosis in the paralyzed patient. J Bone Joint Surg Am 1970; 52:105–112.
568. Wharton GW: Heterotopic ossification. Clin Orthop 1975; 112:142–149.
569. White J, Kjellberg R: Posterior spinal rhizotomy: A substitute for cordotomy in the relief of localized pain in patients with normal life-expectancy. Neurochirurgia 1973; 16:141.
570. White RH, McGahan JP, Daschbuch MM, et al: Diagnosis of deep-vein thrombosis using duplex ultrasound. Ann Intern Med 1989; 11:1297–1304.
571. Whiteneck G (ed): The management of High Quadriplegia. New York, Demos, 1989.
572. Whiteneck GG, Charlifue SW, Frankel HL: Mortality, morbidity and psychosocial outcomes of persons spinal cord-injured more than 20 years. Paraplegia 1992; 30:617–630.
573. Whiteneck G, Menter R, Charlifue S: Impairment, disability handicap and medical expenses of persons aging with spinal cord injury. Paraplegia 1991; 26:613–619.
574. Whiteneck GG, Charlifue SW, Gerhart KA, et al: Quantifying handicap: A new measure of long-term rehabilitation outcomes. Arch Phys Med Rehabil 1992; 73:519–525.
575. Wicks AB, Menter RR: Long-term outlook in quadriplegic patients with initial ventilator dependency. Chest 1986; 90:406–410.
576. Wilberger JE, Maroon JC, Prostko ER, et al: Magnetic resonance imaging and intraoperative neurosonography in syringomyelia. Neurosurgery 1987; 20:599–605.
577. Wilkinson SP, Portmann B, Williams R: Hepatitis from dantrolene sodium. Gut 1979; 20:33–36.
578. Williams B: On the pathogenesis of syringomyelia: A review. J R Soc Med 1980; 73:798–806.
579. Wilson AB: The evolution of wheelchairs. Top Spinal Cord Injury Rehabil 1995; 1(1):42–53.
580. Wilson WC, Hensley BS, Owens JR: Vocational outcomes of spinal cord injured clients in Virgina: A ten-year study. Fishersville, VA, Woodrow Wilson Rehabilitation Center, 1984.

581. Wise MF, Milani JC: Dysphagia in spinal cord injury (abstract). Presented at the 13th annual meeting of the American Spinal Injury Association, Boston, March 1987, abstract 30.
582. Wu Y: Total bladder care for the spinal cord-injured patient. Ann Acad Med Singapore 1983; 12:387–399.
583. Wu Y, King RB, Hamilton BB, et al: RIC-Wu catheter kit: New device for an old problem. Arch Phys Med Rehabil 1980; 61:455–459.
584. Yablon SA, Sipski ML: Effect of transdermal clonidine on spinal spasticity: A case series. Am J Phys Med Rehabil 1993; 72:154–157.
585. Yao J: Deep vein thrombosis in spinal cord-injured patients: Evaluation and assessment. Chest 1992; 1026:645S–648S.
586. Yarkony GM: Aging after traumatic spinal cord injury. In Felsenthal G, Garrison SJ, Steinberg FU (eds): Rehabilitation of the Aging and Elderly Patient. Baltimore, Williams & Wilkins, 1993, pp 391–396.
587. Yarkony GM: Aging skin, pressure ulcerations and spinal cord injury. In Whiteneck GG (ed): Aging with Spinal Cord Injury. New York, Demos, 1993, pp 39–92.
588. Yarkony GM: Medical complications in rehabilitation. In Heinemann AW (ed): Substance Abuse and Physical Disability. Binghamton, NY, Haworth Press, 1993, pp 93–106.
589. Yarkony GM, Bass LM, Keenan V III, et al: Contractures complicating spinal cord injury: Incidence and comparison between spinal cord centre and general hospital acute care. Paraplegia 1985; 23:265.
590. Yarkony GM, Jaeger R, Turba R, et al: Cough in spinal cord-injured patients: Comparison of three methods to produce cough. Arch Phys Med Rehabil 1993; 74:1358–1361.
591. Yarkony GM, Jaeger RJ, Roth E, et al: Functional neuromuscular stimulation for standing after spinal cord injury. Arch Phys Med Rehabil 1990; 71:201–206.
592. Yarkony GM, Jones R, Hedman G, et al: Jones-Hedman walker modification for C7 quadriplegic patient: Case study in team cooperation. Arch Phys Med Rehabil 1986; 67:54–55.
593. Yarkony GM, Katz RT, Wu YC: Seizures secondary to autonomic dysreflexia. Arch Phys Med Rehabil 1986; 67:345–349.
594. Yarkony GM, Lee MY, Green D, et al: Heterotopic ossification pseudophlebitis. Am J Med 1989; 87:342–344.
595. Yarkony GM, Roth EJ, Cybulski GR, et al: Neuromuscular stimulation in spinal cord injury: I. Restoration of functional movement of the extremities. Arch Phys Med Rehabil 1992; 73:78–86.
596. Yarkony GM, Roth EJ, Cybulski GR, et al: Neuromuscular stimulation in spinal cord injury: II. Prevention of secondary complications. Arch Phys Med Rehabil 1992; 73:195–200.
597. Yarkony GM, Roth EJ, Heinemann AW, et al: Benefits of rehabilitation for traumatic spinal cord injury: Multivariate analysis in 711 patients. Arch Neurol 1987; 44:93.
598. Yarkony GM, Roth EJ, Heinemann AW, et al: Rehabilitation outcomes in C6 tetraplegia. Paraplegia 1988; 26:177–185.
599. Yarkony GM, Roth EJ, Heinemann AW, et al: Spinal cord injury rehabilitation outcome: The impact of age. J Clin Epidemiol 1988; 41:173–177.
600. Yarkony GM, Sheffler LR, Smith J, et al: Early onset posttraumatic cystic myelopathy complicating spinal cord injury. Arch Phys Med Rehabil 1994; 75:102–105.
601. Yarkony GM: Pressure ulcers: A review. Arch Phys Med Rehabil 1994; 75:908–917.
602. Yarkony GM, Heinemann AW: Pressure ulcers. In Stover SL, DeLisa JA, Whiteneck GG (eds): Spinal Cord Injury: Clinical Outcomes from the Model Systems. Gaithersburg, MD, Aspen, 1995, pp 104–111.
603. Yekutrel M, Brooks ME, Ohry A, et al: The prevalence of hypertension, ischemic heart disease and diabetes in traumatic spinal cord-injured patients and amputees. Paraplegia 1989; 27:58–62.
604. Yezierski RP: Pain following spinal cord injury: The clinical problem and experimental studies. Pain 1996; 68:185–194.
605. Young JS, Dexter WR: Neurological recovery distal to the zone of injury in 172 cases of closed traumatic spinal cord injury. Paraplegia 1978; 16:39–45.
606. Young JS, Burns PE, Bowen AM: Spinal Cord Injury Statistics: Experience of Regional Model Spinal Cord Injury Systems. Phoenix, AZ, Good Samaritan Medical Center, 1982.
607. Young W, Flamm ES: Effect of high dose corticosteroid therapy on blood flow, evoked potentials and extracellular calcium in experimental spinal cord injury. J Neurosurg 1982; 57:667–673.
608. Young W: Acute, restorative and regenerative therapy of spinal cord injury. In Piepmeier JM (ed): The Outcome Following Traumatic Spinal Cord Injury. Mount Kisco, NY, Futura, 1992.
609. Zacharkow D: Wheelchair Posture and Pressure Sores. Springfield, IL, Charles C Thomas, 1984, pp 12–53.
610. Zancolli E: Structural and Dynamic Bases of Hand Surgery, ed 2. Philadelphia, JB Lippincott, 1979, pp 229–262.
611. Zejdlik CM: Management of Spinal Cord Injury. Belmont, CA, Wadsworth, 1983.
612. Zerby SA, Herbison GJ, Marino RJ, et al: Elbow extension using anterior deltoid and upper pectorals. Muscle Nerve 1994; 17:1472–1474.
613. Zomba EA, Cain LD, Everhart AW: Transplant therapy: Recovery of function after spinal cord injury. J Neurotrauma 1997; 14:479–506.
614. Zorn GW, Crozier KS, Cheng LL, et al: Quadriceps recovery in Frankel C spinal cord injury. J Am Paraplegia Soc 1991; 14:90–94.

56

CHAPTER

Karen L. Andrews, M.D., Thom W. Rooke, M.D., and Phala A. Helm, M.D.

Vascular Disease: Evaluation and Management

Rehabilitation of the patient with vascular disease includes the evaluation and management of arterial, venous, and lymphatic diseases. The goals of optimal management are to decrease morbidity and to enhance function.

ARTERIAL DISEASE

Epidemiology

Peripheral arterial disease is a relatively common manifestation of systemic atherosclerosis; it affects 5% of persons 50 years of age and 20% of persons older than 70 years.[21, 43] The most frequent presentation of arterial occlusive disease is intermittent claudication. Epidemiologic studies have demonstrated that limb-threatening ischemia develops in as few as 2% to 5% of patients with intermittent claudication monitored for up to 10 years.[57] There is an overall reduction of 10 years in life expectancy among patients with peripheral vascular disease, with mortality primarily due to coronary artery disease and diabetes mellitus with its associated complications. The mortality rate in patients with peripheral vascular disease is 20% to 30% 5 years after diagnosis, 40% to 72% after 10 years, and 74% after 15 years. About 75% of the deaths are caused by cardiovascular events.[11]

Etiology

There are many causes of arterial occlusive disease, the most common of which is atherosclerosis obliterans (ASO). Other disease processes include thromboangiitis obliterans (Buerger's disease), vasospastic disorders (Raynaud's phenomenon, livedo reticularis, and acrocyanosis), thrombosis, embolism, dissection, vasculitis, and fibromuscular dysplasia.

Atherosclerosis

Atherosclerosis in its advanced form is a systemic disorder involving the coronary, cerebral, pulmonary, renal, and peripheral vessels. The earliest pathologic manifestation of atherosclerosis appears to be the intimal streak, although the eventual progression of streaks to fibrous or complicated plaques remains uncertain.[80] The plaques tend to develop at branch points, bifurcations, zones of rapid tapering, and areas where arteries follow a tortuous course.[79] These are all areas of low shear stress, where there is separation from unidirectional laminar blood flow, reversal of flow, and turbulence.[60] There is an inverse relation between shear stress and rate of lumen narrowing. Although low shear stress is associated with atherogenesis and disease progression, regions of moderate to high shear stress are relatively spared from intimal thickening as long as flow remains unidirectional and axially aligned.[60] Atherosclerosis typically involves multiple levels of the arterial tree; however, it tends to be a segmental disease in which intervening arterial segments can be remarkably free of involvement or minimally involved. Associated conditions can affect the location of disease. In diabetics, ASO occurs with equal frequency in both femoral and tibial arteries, whereas in nondiabetics the most common sites of severe disease are the abdominal aorta and iliac and femoral arteries.[49]

Potentially reversible factors that increase the risk of atherosclerosis include smoking, hyperlipidemia, hypertension, diabetes, and obesity. Most people younger than 65 years who have atherosclerosis have one or more identifiable risk factors. The presence of multiple risk factors further increases the risk of atherosclerosis. Cigarette smoking is by far the most common risk factor, competing with juvenile diabetes mellitus and certain rare congenital hyperlipidemias as the most serious.[26] Smoking acts synergistically with other risk factors such as hypertension or hypercholesterolemia to enhance progression of atherosclerotic lesions. The calculated risk of developing claudication is 15 times higher in male smokers than nonsmokers, 7 times higher in female smokers than nonsmokers, and directly related to the number of cigarettes smoked.[26]

Thromboangiitis Obliterans (Buerger's Disease)

Thromboangiitis obliterans (Buerger's disease) is a disease involving thrombosis and inflammation of small peripheral arteries and veins. The process tends to begin in the smaller peripheral arteries of the extremities. Lesions are usually located distal to the knee or elbow.[79] Most theories implicate some component of cigarette smoking that predisposes the arterial wall to inflammation, possibly through the formation of immune complexes.

Vasospasm

Raynaud's phenomenon most frequently involves the hands but can also affect the feet. With exposure to cold or emotional stress, spasm of the small arteries and arterioles results in ischemia (pallor or cyanosis), pain, and subsequent vasodilatation with hyperemia. Raynaud's phenomenon can be idiopathic or occur as a manifestation of a potentially serious underlying systemic disease.

Other Causes of Arterial Occlusive Disease

Thrombosis, embolism, and arterial dissection are discussed in the following sections on acute and chronic arterial occlusion.

Clinical Evaluation

Acute Arterial Occlusion

The clinical presentation in acute arterial occlusion includes sudden onset of toe, foot, and leg pain associated with absence of pulse and coolness and discoloration of the skin in a patchy irregular configuration (Fig. 56–1). The findings are frequently described as the "6 P's"—pulselessness, pain, polar (cold), pallor, paresthesia, and paralysis. The major causes of acute arterial occlusion are embolism, thrombosis, trauma, and dissection. If the patient has had a recent myocardial infarction, atrial fibrillation, or other source of possible embolus and has normal pulses in the contralateral extremity and no history of claudication, acute embolic disease is likely. The most common cause of acute arterial embolism is cardiac (atrial fibrillation, recent myocardial infarction, cardiomyopathy, native or prosthetic heart valve replacement, and, rarely, atrial myxoma). If previous symptoms of claudication are present in a patient with no cardiac dysfunction, the diagnosis of thrombosis is most likely. With acute arterial occlusion associated with aortic dissection, findings might also include excruciating precordial or intrascapular pain, moderate to severe hypertension, congestive heart failure, hemiplegia, anuria or hematuria, and acute intestinal ischemia.

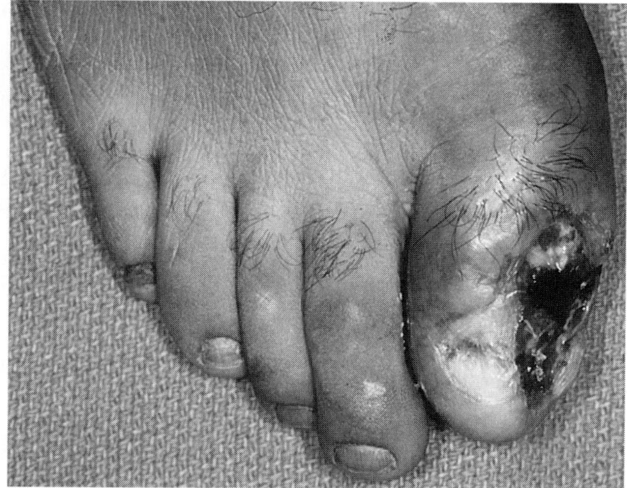

FIGURE 56–1. Ischemic changes in a great toe after arterial embolus.

Chronic Arterial Occlusion

Chronic arterial occlusive disease can usually be diagnosed from the history and physical examination. Unless complicated by thrombus or embolus, the symptoms and signs associated with atherosclerosis obliterans rarely have an abrupt onset. The most common symptom is intermittent claudication. Lower extremity claudication has two diagnostic clinical features. First, it is reproduced with a consistent level of exercise from one occasion to the next. Second, it completely resolves within minutes after the exercise has been discontinued.[41]

The site of claudication is a rough indicator for the level of occlusion.[50] Patients with occlusion at or above the ankle can present with claudication in the arch of the foot. Calf claudication suggests occlusion at or above the calf. Patients with isolated aortoiliac disease generally present with buttock pain or sexual dysfunction. To determine the severity of ischemia, the clinician should look for elevation pallor and dependent rubor and quantitate the venous filling time. Elevation pallor is determined by raising the leg to a 90-degree angle; if pallor develops within 60 seconds, the patient has mild occlusive disease; within 30 seconds, moderate disease; and within 15 seconds, severe disease.[49] When the legs are returned to a dependent position, the venous filling time (i.e., the time it takes for the small veins of the feet to distend with blood) can be determined. Normal venous filling time is classically described as 20 seconds, but this value is altered with associated congestive heart failure, venous insufficiency, pulmonary hypertension, or tricuspid regurgitation.

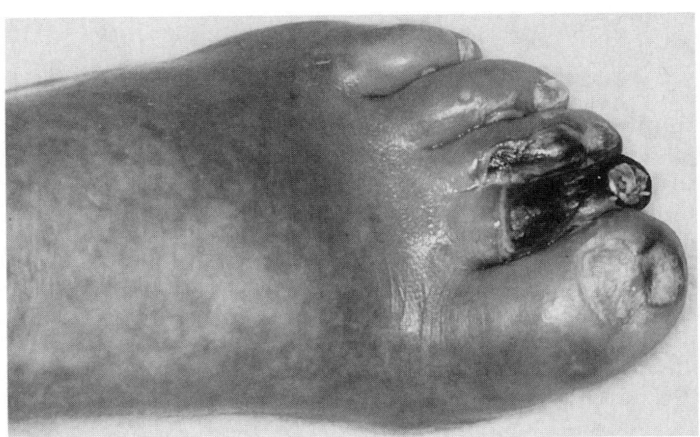

FIGURE 56–2. Chronic arterial occlusive disease with associated ischemia, trophic changes, rubor, edema, ulcerations, and gangrenous changes (second and third toes).

As the disease process advances, resting blood flow rates are affected, and ischemia at rest and impaired skin metabolism result. Clinical findings of ischemia can include trophic changes, dependent rubor, paresthesias (which may be partially or completely relieved with dependency), cutaneous ulceration, and gangrene. As the disease process advances, resting blood flow rates are affected, and ischemia at rest and impaired skin metabolism result (Fig. 56–2).

Vascular Testing

Noninvasive Studies

If ischemia is noted on clinical examination, noninvasive studies can delineate the degree and level of ischemia and the potential for healing. They can also provide a baseline for future comparison.[78] When patients present with symptoms that occur during exercise, some form of exercise evaluation should be performed. When patients present primarily with symptoms at rest, an evaluation can be performed without exercise testing (Table 56–1).

Segmental Pressure

Measurement of supine resting ankle pressure is the most common noninvasive study performed on patients with suspected vascular disease. The arterial systolic blood pressure in a given limb segment is determined by inflating a cuff around that segment and slowly deflating the cuff until pedal arterial blood flow (in the posterior tibial artery of the ankle or the dorsalis pedis artery of the foot) is detected with continuous-wave doppler or by feeling for the return of pulses. (A stethoscope is not sensitive enough to reliably assess the return of blood flow.) Variations in systemic pressure between individuals are corrected by expressing the absolute ankle pressure as a ratio relative to the brachial pressure (ankle/brachial index, ABI). The ABI is interpreted as follows: $\geq$0.9, normal; 0.8 to 0.9, mild; 0.5 to 0.8, moderate; and $\leq$0.5, severe.[61] In patients with mild symptoms of claudication, the ABI might be normal at rest but reduced after exercise. At rest, the vascular resistance of the leg is relatively high, and flow through a stenotic lesion can be sufficient to maintain normal distal pressure. After exercise, the vascular resistance is lower and blood flow through the stenosis might not be sufficient to keep the distal pressure from decreasing.[68]

Traditionally, post-exercise ABIs are determined by having the patient walk on a treadmill for 5 minutes at 2 miles per hour up a 10% to 12% grade. Under these conditions, not all patients achieve maximal exertion. Walking time in repeated tests may vary as much as 50% within the same subject.[42] In contrast, using a progressive increase in workload (a 3.5% increase in grade every 3 minutes until maximum symptoms of claudication are achieved), Hiatt found that the reproducibility of the variables measured at maximum exercise ranged from 7% to 13%.[42] In addition, the fall in ankle pressure after exercise was greater after walking at 3 mph than at 2 mph despite similar arm pressures at maximum exercise in both protocols. As a result, the 3-mph protocol is recommended when testing patients with mild or questionable arterial disease.[42]

Segmental limb pressure measurements extend the application of ankle pressure measurements and provide a more precise determination of the anatomy of the occlusive process.[26] Continuous-wave doppler is still used to assess posterior tibial or dorsalis pedis blood flow, but this time the occlusion cuffs are placed at "high"-thigh, above-knee, below-knee, and ankle locations. The measured limb pressures can exceed the measured brachial pressure in normal persons by up to 30 mm Hg. Limb pressure equal to or less than the brachial

TABLE 56–1 Noninvasive Vascular Studies Used to Diagnose Arterial Disease

Vascular Disease	Anatomic	Hemodynamic/Functional	Disadvantages
Arterial	Continuous wave doppler	Continuous wave doppler	Operator dependent Limited ability to quantify disease severity
	Pulse volume recording		Poor reproducibility
	Segmental pressure	Segmental pressure	
	Ankle/brachial index		Cannot be interpreted if vessels noncompressible
	$TcPO_2$ (amputation level)	$TcPO_2$	Limited availability
"Small vessel" (arteriolar)		$TcPO_2$	Limited availability

artery pressure indicates significant aortoiliac or proximal femoral arterial occlusive disease. A gradient of more than 20 mm Hg between any adjacent segment is an abnormal finding.[26] Falsely high readings can be obtained in patients with large thighs, when the cuff width is too narrow, or when the arteries are noncompressible because of medial calcification associated with diseases or other conditions. Falsely low readings can result when too wide a cuff is used on a thin thigh. Interpretation can also be difficult with multilevel arterial occlusive disease.

Continuous Wave Doppler

A normal flow waveform in peripheral arteries is characterized by a triphasic doppler signal during each cardiac cycle (Fig. 56–3A). The first component is a strong, high-frequency signal in the forward direction which corresponds to systole, and it is followed in early diastole by a short period of reverse flow. Later in diastole, the third component is forward prior to the subsequent heartbeat. Biphasic signals are observed in the absence of disease in distal arteries or when the peripheral resistance is low. Distal to a stenosis, the waveform becomes monophasic, characterized by a blunted peak velocity and the absence of a reverse component (Fig. 56–3B). If the probe is positioned directly over the stenotic segment, a very high-frequency signal occurs during systole and diastole as a result of increased velocity through the narrowed segment.[79]

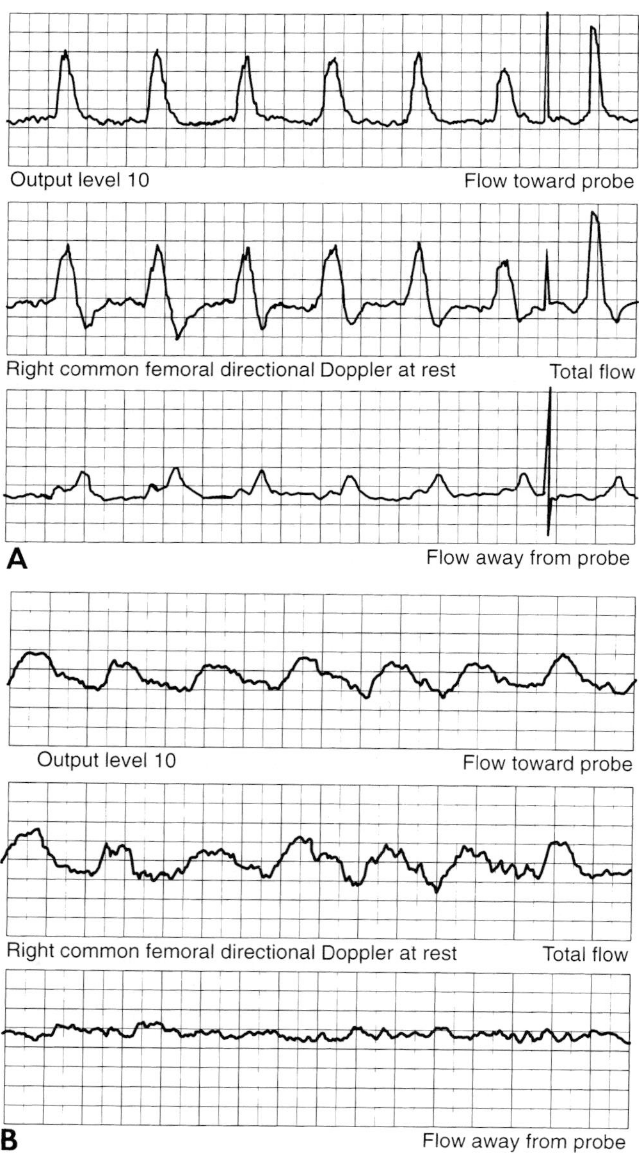

FIGURE 56–3. Doppler arterial wave forms. *A.* Normal triphasic signal. *B.* Blunted monophasic signal distal to stenosis.

Plethysmography

Plethysmography can be used to measure mean blood flow by recording the rate of increase in limb volume after sudden interruption of venous outflow. To perform a plethysmographic flow measurement, the limb is placed in a neutral, relaxed position, and the venous occlusion cuff is rapidly inflated. Blood that flows into the limb becomes trapped, and the limb expands. The rate at which expansion occurs is measured by the plethysmograph, from which arterial inflow can be estimated.[68]

Digital plethysmography can be performed with either strain-gauge or photoelectric instrumentation. Toe pressures evaluate obstructive disease in the digital vessels or pedal arch. This test is useful for the evaluation of patients with noncompressible ankle or leg arteries, because it is unusual for digital arteries to be affected by this process. The digital artery pressure is also used as a guide to the likelihood of spontaneous healing of superficial cutaneous lesions. A toe/brachial index greater than 0.60 is normal. If the absolute pressure is 30 mm Hg or less, healing is unlikely to occur.[61]

Transcutaneous Oxygen Tension

Transcutaneous oxygen tension ($TcPO_2$) is an objective indicator of ischemia of the skin in a patient with peripheral occlusive arterial disease.[2, 62, 69, 73] $TcPO_2$ measurements are relatively simple and reproducible. They also provide information regarding the physiologic importance of blood flow impairment. Oxygen-sensing electrodes with a surface temperature of 45°C are attached to the skin and allowed to equilibrate until stable. A reference electrode is placed on the chest, and other electrodes are placed over the area of interest. In a standard study of the lower extremities, two electrodes are placed on the dorsum of each foot. With the patient supine, $TcPO_2$ values are recorded and the regional perfusion indices ($TcPO_2$ foot/$TcPO_2$ chest) are calculated. The feet are then elevated to 30 degrees for 3 minutes, and the $TcPO_2$ measurements are repeated.[73] If the $TcPO_2$ value is 20 torr or less, healing is not likely to occur, whereas $TcPO_2$ values of more than 40 torr are associated with healing. If the $TcPO_2$ value decreases into the borderline zone of 20 to 40 torr, measuring the values after leg elevation improves the predictability of outcome.[2, 69] The regional perfusion index is important for patients who have cardiac or pulmonary dysfunction that produces variable degrees of systemic oxygen desaturation.[62]

Duplex Ultrasonography

Duplex ultrasonography combines a pulsed doppler with real-time B mode scanning. Duplex scanning combines exact anatomic localization of disease with physiologic blood flow studies to define the hemodynamic significance of the lesion.[26] The expense of this equipment limits its utilization as a general screening tool[68] (see the section on venous studies later in this chapter).

Magnetic Resonance Angiography

Magnetic resonance imaging can yield images of sufficient quality that peripheral vascular disease might also be diagnosed and visualized by noninvasive means.[54]

Invasive Studies

Arteriography

Although physiologic testing is excellent for screening and follow-up, arteriography remains the most accurate procedure for evaluation of arterial anatomy (Fig. 56–4). If surgery is anticipated, arteriography is usually needed to determine the length of arterial occlusion, level of distal reconstruction, and patency of the plantar arch. In the presence of inflow vessel disease, special arteriographic techniques such as digital subtraction angiography may be necessary for visualization of distal runoff vessels.[26, 79] Patients with arterial occlusive disease can also have renal disease, and consequently are at high risk for renal failure if contrast material is used. This risk must be considered whenever arteriography is contemplated.

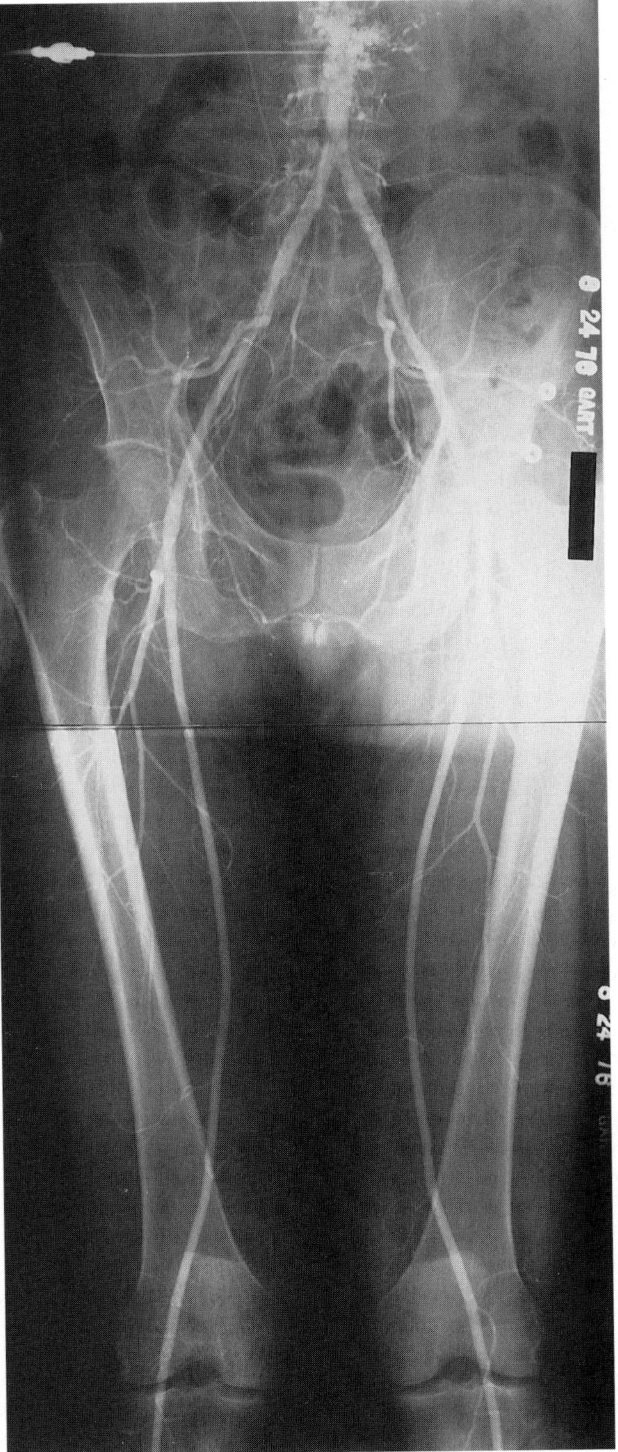

FIGURE 56–4. Angiogram showing mild atherosclerosis obliterans in a patient with pseudoclaudication.

Testing for Associated Diseases

When evaluating the patient with atherosclerotic occlusive disease, especially if surgical intervention is planned, it is important that the clinical evaluation define and quantify any associated cardiovascular, renal, and pulmonary problems. In patients with suspected coronary artery disease who must undergo peripheral vascular surgery, the perioperative mortality rate is approximately four times higher than for those without coronary artery disease, and the perioperative morbidity is also markedly increased.[32] Because many patients with vascular disease are sedentary and lack symptoms of coronary artery disease, it is easy to miss asymptomatic but hemodynamically significant coronary disease, despite obtaining a thorough history and physical examination.

The prevalence of serious coronary artery disease ranges from 37% to 78% in patients undergoing an operation for peripheral vascular disease.[32] Although operations involving aortic cross-clamping exert a greater acute systemic hemodynamic stress than femoral popliteal surgery, late cardiac morbidity and mortality are significant in all patients with atherosclerotic disease who undergo such procedures.[32] Through preoperative identification of high-risk patients, intensive medical therapy and monitoring can stabilize the patient preoperatively and potential intraoperative problems can be anticipated. During the postoperative period, careful hemodynamic monitoring and continued cardiac surveillance are mandatory.[32]

Rest and Exercise Electrocardiography

A 12-lead electrocardiogram (ECG) is almost universally recorded during the preoperative period. In patients requiring vascular surgery, up to 35% of those with a normal 12-lead ECG will have an abnormal exercise ECG.[32] ECG-monitored exercise testing has been shown to correlate with the risk of myocardial infarction. Patients who achieve less than 85% of their maximal predicted heart rate have a postoperative cardiac complication rate of 24%, whereas this rate is only 6% in patients whose heart rate exceeds 85% of the maximal predicted value.[26] Clearly, exercise testing is limited in patients who have severe claudication, rest ischemia, or prior amputation. The primary advantage of exercise testing is its wide availability and modest cost. Although ECG-monitored stress testing is being replaced by other tests that do not require exercise, it is still a useful means to obtain objective information regarding the relative degree of impairment imposed by claudication, pulmonary insufficiency, or coronary artery disease (see Chapter 32).

Exercise Thallium-201 Scintigraphy

Exercise thallium-201 scintigraphy (or related tests using provocative agents such as adenosine or dipyridamole and uptake agents such as sestamibi) are useful for screening patients with peripheral vascular disease for coronary artery disease because they are minimally invasive and can assess the extent of myocardium at risk. Exercise (or dobutamine, dipyridamole, or other agents) cause coronary vasodilation. During exercise (or drug administration in the case of patients who are unable to exercise), the difference in perfusion between myocardium supplied by normal coronary arteries and that supplied by stenotic, nondistensible vessels is accentuated. Thallium-201 is promptly absorbed by areas of normal perfusion and serves as a marker for viable myocardium. When the patient is rescanned 3 hours later, uptake of thallium-201 is delayed in areas of potentially ischemic myocardium. No uptake is noted in areas of infarcted tissue.[26] Although this test is highly sensitive, it has limited specificity. Nevertheless, it is well suited to the preoperative screening of patients with peripheral vascular disease. Only patients with significant thallium-201 redistribution require further cardiac evaluation. In general, patients with a history of chronic stable angina, those with a single uncomplicated myocardial infarction more than 6 months previously, or those in whom dobutamine thallium-201 scintigraphy shows no more than a small area of redistribution need no further cardiac evaluation.[26] Patients with a history of more severe cardiac disease and thallium-201 redistribution involving two or more vessels are at increased risk for postoperative cardiac complications, and further cardiac evaluation such as cardiac catheterization should be considered.

Treatment

Ideally, all ischemic limbs should be restored to a functional, pain-free state with appropriate management. Unfortunately, extensive vascular disease or underlying medical illness can preclude revascularization. Many patients with severe rest pain note a temporary decrease in their pain with dependency. This can be explained in part by an increase in hydrostatic pressure, which allows better perfusion to the ischemic tissue. Unless the pain is adequately controlled with narcotics, tricyclic antidepressants, anticonvulsants, or other measures, the patient will keep the involved extremity dependent. Continued dependency results in edema, decreased arterial flow, decreased perfusion, and further ischemia.

Acute Arterial Occlusion

Thrombosis

Acute thrombosis is generally best managed with an initial course of heparin therapy followed by arteriography to define the lesion and the status of the inflow and outflow vessels. Lytic therapy or urgent surgical revascularization might be required. Early intervention can prevent neuromuscular injury, enhance limb salvage, and avoid myonecrosis, myoglobinuria, and associated renal failure. In less severe cases where immediate revascularization is unnecessary, elective revascularization at a later date might be required to alleviate symptoms of chronic ischemia.

Embolic Ischemia

Heparin should be given as soon as the diagnosis of acute arterial embolus is suspected. Initial heparin requirements are frequently much higher than anticipated, and large doses of heparin can be required to inhibit coagulation and to prevent clot propagation. When results of sensory and motor examination are normal, the limb generally shows rapid improvement with anticoagulation. Early recognition and correction of an offending proximal lesion or cardiac abnormality are important.[26] The restoration of adequate perfusion is essential, but returning blood flow to the microcirculation might not be easy in the presence of swollen endothelial and perivascular cells.

Advanced ischemia is characterized by absent motor and sensory function, muscle tenderness and rigidity, limb pallor (without elevation), and prolongation of the venous filling time to more than 1 minute.[49] With marked motor deficit, muscle rigidity, or anesthesia on clinical examination, early amputation must be considered. Revascularization of such an ischemic limb can result in a mortality rate of 50% to 75% because of the effects of metabolic products on the renal and pulmonary systems (reperfusion syndrome).[26]

Dissection

Treatment of aortic dissection depends on location. If the dissection is located in the ascending aorta (Stanford type A), management includes control of arterial systolic blood pressure and emergency surgical repair. If the dissection occurs in the descending thoracic or abdominal aorta (Stanford type B), medical management of pain and arterial blood pressure is usually the treatment of choice. Surgical repair is generally reserved for patients who have significant vascular occlusion, persistent pain, progression of the dissection, or aneurysm formation.[26] Paraplegia is a possible surgical complication.

Chronic Arterial Occlusion

The ultimate goal is to develop effective therapy that prevents progression of the disease process and possibly promotes regression of existing lesions. It is important that the correct diagnosis and cause of the underlying disease process be identified before proceeding with treatment. Controllable risk factors such as smoking, diabetes, hyperlipidemia, hypertension, and gross obesity, as discussed previously, should be addressed with appropriate pharmacological approaches, dietary measures, or behavior modifications.

Patient and Family Education

Therapeutic success is most likely with an educated patient and family. It is important to discuss in detail the diffuse and progressive nature of atherosclerosis, the importance of controlling risk factors, and measures to protect the ischemic limb.

Protection from Trauma

Most amputations in persons with occlusive peripheral arterial disease result from some type of trauma (thermal, chemical, or mechanical) superimposed on a limb with chronic occlusive disease.[26, 76] Thermal injury is prevented by avoiding excess heat (heating pad, hot water). Warm outer footwear is recommended in the winter to protect against cold. Because a low skin temperature augments sympathetic tone, keeping an ischemic limb warm with vascular boots (Fig. 56–5) attenuates sympathetic tone, avoids vasoconstriction, and improves local cutaneous blood flow and $TcPO_2$.[71] Although vascular boots have a nonskid interface, they are not designed to protect ischemic or neuropathic feet during ambulation. Chemicals, corn remedies, and antiseptics should be avoided to prevent chemical trauma. Mechanical trauma can be caused by poorly fitting footwear.

Footwear

The use of rocker-sole shoes, to lessen the work of the gastrocnemius soleus muscle groups during ambulation, increases walking distance and can be a useful addition to the nonsurgical management of calf claudication.[67] Metal, double-upright, ankle-foot orthoses to eliminate ankle motion have also been studied. Despite the added weight, fixed ankle, appearance, and change of gait pattern, most patients noted an increase in their walking distance and were pleased with the results obtained with the use of this orthosis.[44]

Exercise

For many years, the main exercises for patients with occlusive arterial disease were the passive movements developed by Buerger, who theorized that blood vessels would accept a greater function in blood transfer if they were alternately emptied and distended.[8] The formation of collaterals was attempted by a series of exercises that consisted of the following sequence. The limbs were supported in an elevated position at an angle of 60 degrees to 90 degrees for 30 to 180 seconds or the minimum time required to produce blanching. Following the onset of blanching, the feet were permitted to hang down over the edge of the bed or table for 2 to 5 minutes or as long as necessary to produce reactive hyperemia or rubor, plus one additional minute (total time not to exceed 5 minutes). Next, the legs were placed in a horizontal position for 3 to 5 minutes. This cycle was repeated six or seven times at a sitting, and the entire sequence was repeated several times during a day.[8] Oscillating beds were also used to alternately fill the limb with blood and then drain it by positional changes.[19] The angle of depression of the oscillating bed was adjusted to suit the physiologic need. Readjustments were made as circulation improved. The aim on the upswing of the bed was to maintain sufficient elevation long enough for the veins to collapse but not to produce pallor in the capillary bed of the toes. With time, these passive interventions were prescribed less frequently as other therapeutic measures came into vogue. Wisham showed that passive postural movements did not enhance blood flow. Instead, increased flow occurred during and shortly after active exercise and appeared to increase in relation to the intensity of exercise.[84] Foley recommended exercise to stimulate collateral blood flow and improve the metabolic state of the ischemic tissues.[30]

The first randomized controlled trial of exercise training in persons with arterial occlusive disease demonstrated an improvement in treadmill walking distance with exercise.[53] Exercise increases the demand for blood to the lower extremities. In a normal arterial system, demand is primarily met by arterial vasodilatation. Although flow rates increase dramatically during exercise, arterial perfusion pressure remains essentially unchanged.[26] With atherosclerosis, the capability of the arterial system to supply peak blood flow is progressively reduced. At rest, maximal blood flow goes to the skin; during exercise, most of the increase in blood flow is shunted to the active muscle beds. Several studies have shown the beneficial effects of physical training in patients with intermittent claudication.[25, 48] Improved peripheral utilization of oxygen, walking technique, and glycolytic and oxidative metabolic capacity have been suggested as reasons for the improvement with training.[48] Although some believe that graded exercise stimulates the growth of collateral vessels,[1] Eckroth et al[25] found that maximal calf blood flow did not increase in parallel with increases in walking ability. This finding does not support the belief that physical training is directly associated with the development of collateral circulation. Another study found a dramatic increase in walking distances after a supervised, graduated-exercise program without an associated increase in resting ankle brachial indices, which suggests that the increased walking distance is due to an increase in the oxidative capacity of muscle. Such a metabolic change is supported by biochemical

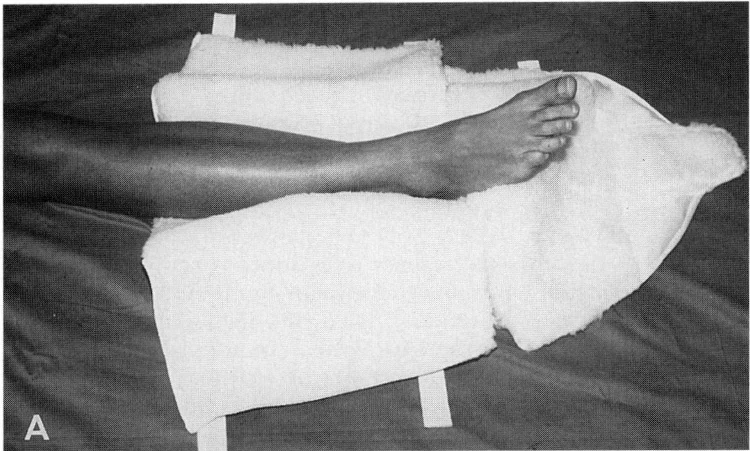
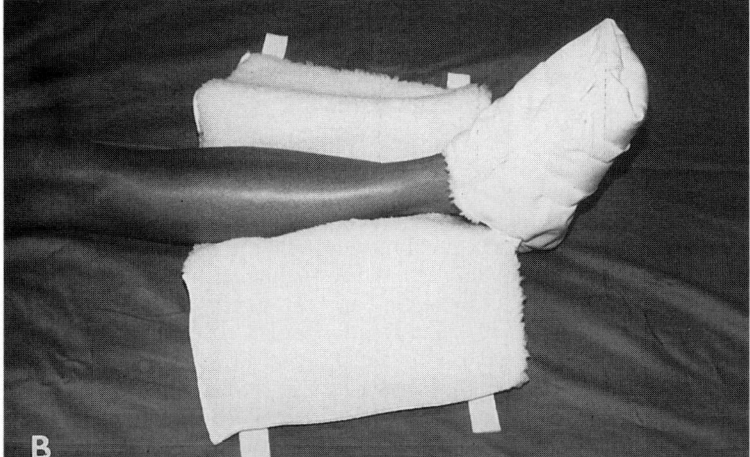
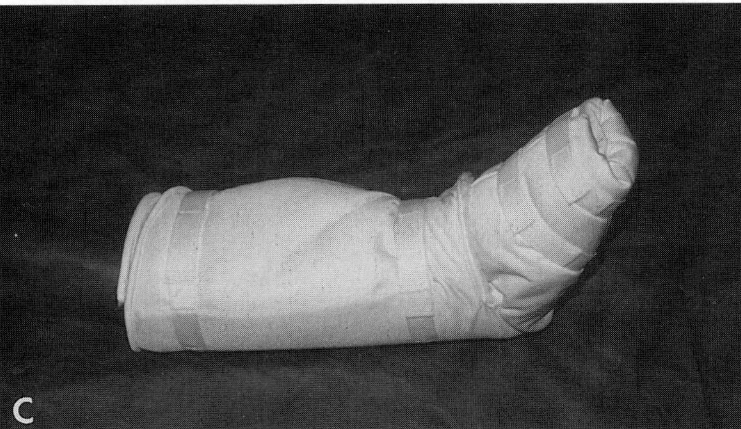

FIGURE 56–5. *A, B,* and *C.* Vascular boots are fabricated using cotton fleece with a nonskid sole. They lessen sympathetic tone, avoid vasoconstriction, and improve local cutaneous blood flow and transcutaneous oxygen tension.

evidence that the activity of glycolytic and mitochondrial enzymes in calf muscle tissue is positively correlated with walking distance in patients with claudication who receive physical training.[20] Walking programs must be individualized; however, the usual prescription has a goal of 30 to 60 minutes, 3 to 5 days per week at a pace of 2 miles per hour, as allowed by cardiac precautions.[20, 25] The patient should rest after symptoms of claudication develop.[1, 26] Improvement will be gradual over a period of 3 to 6 months.[20]

Risk Factor Modification

Peripheral artery disease and coronary artery disease are both manifestations of atherosclerotic disease and have similar risk factors: age, gender (estrogen status), family history, tobacco abuse, hypercholesterolemia, hypertension, diabetes mellitus, and physical inactivity. Patients should be counseled to modify these risk factors into a favorable profile to decrease their risk for further progression of atherosclerotic disease and its sequelae.

In addition, if premature atherosclerosis is detected, the patient's first-degree relatives should be screened for heritable risk factors such as homocysteine and possibly familial lipoproteinemia.

Medication

Vasodilators. The general aim of drug therapy for arterial occlusive disease is to increase oxygen delivery. Although vasodilator drugs have been shown to increase blood flow to the limbs and various organs in animal experiments and in humans with vasospastic disorders, their use in peripheral obstructive vascular disease remains questionable.[12] An ideal drug for treatment of peripheral vascular diseases would dilate blood vessels and increase blood flow only in areas of deficient blood supply. Such agents do not currently exist. In some circumstances, vasodilation in areas without diseased vessels can actually steal flow from the affected area.[12] Because β-adrenergic blockade can cause peripheral vasoconstriction, it has been recommended that β-adrenergic blockers be avoided in patients with arterial occlusive disease.

Anticoagulants and Antiplatelet Agents. Platelet aggregation can exacerbate arterial occlusive disease by causing mechanical occlusion of small arteries or by releasing serotonin and stimulating local vasospasm.[26] There is no evidence that fibrinolytic agents, anticoagulants, or antiplatelet agents are directly effective in the treatment of intermittent claudication. Cyclooxygenase inhibitors such as aspirin decrease both prostacycline production and thromboxane production. The former effect is proaggregatory and possibly vasoconstrictive, whereas the latter is antiaggregatory. Although aspirin is widely used for patients with arterial occlusive disease, its best-documented effects relate to prevention of coronary and vascular graft thrombosis rather than intermittent claudication.[26]

Hemorrhelogic Agents. Pentoxifylline (Trental) increases red cell deformability, decreases plasma viscosity, and diminishes platelet aggregation by decreasing fibrinogen concentration. It also increases resting and hyperemic extremity blood flow, presumably through its rheologic effects.[26, 65] Reports in the literature about the degree of clinical improvement in patients taking pentoxifylline for the treatment of intermittent claudication have been variable.[65, 75] In one pilot study, 10 subjects showed a significant increase in exercise tolerance, and 8 of 10 subjects demonstrated a significant increase in right dorsalis pedis arterial flow on noninvasive testing after pentoxifylline treatment.[75] Because pentoxifylline is a methylxanthine derivative, this drug should not be used in persons intolerant of this class of compounds (i.e., caffeine, theophylline).

Antioxidant Agents. Oxidation of low-density lipoprotein cholesterol tends to promote atherosclerotic disease development. Free radical injury of endothelial cells is prevented by antioxidant networks. Endogenous systems include glutathionine reductase and nonenzymatic antioxidant free radical scavengers (vitamins E, C, and β-carotene). Although the data are preliminary, several animal studies and epidemiologic data suggest that vitamins E, C, and β-carotene might retard atherosclerosis.[17] There might be a role for treatment of patients with peripheral arterial occlusive disease with antioxidant medications (vitamins E and C); however, final recommendations await a large-scale study of the effects of antioxidants in patients with peripheral arterial disease.

Revascularization

Angioplasty. Percutaneous transluminal angioplasty is an established treatment for claudication in patients with arterial occlusive disease. Angioplasty is indicated for focal stenosis or short segmental occlusions in which the adjacent vessels are relatively free of disease. Angioplasty is associated with a low incidence of morbidity, and 5-year patency rates of 80% to 90% have been reported for iliac lesions, as opposed to 60% to 70% for superficial femoral artery lesions.[20] A recent study suggested that supervised graduated exercise therapy produces better long-term improvement in mean distance walked before claudication and maximal walking distance in patients suitable for angioplasty than does angioplasty itself.[20] One advantage of angioplasty is that the inpatient stay is short, typically around 48 hours.

Surgery. Vascular reconstruction is indicated in patients with incapacitating claudication, rest pain, gangrene, and tissue loss, especially when the ankle/brachial index is less than 0.4 or the forefoot $TcPO_2$ is less than 30 mm Hg.[26]

Aortoiliac Occlusive Disease. The standard operation for aortoiliac disease is an aortobifemoral bypass. In selected patients with unilateral disease, limited operations such as femoral-femoral (fem-fem) bypass or iliofemoral bypass can be considered. Contralateral disease progression or atherosclerotic occlusive disease of the donor iliac artery in the fem-fem bypass can result in steal, from which ischemia develops in the previously asymptomatic donor leg. The advantages of these limited procedures are lack of manipulation of contralateral flow and a lower surgical risk (especially the fem-fem bypass, which is an extra-anatomic procedure).

Infrainguinal Occlusive Disease. Patients with superficial femoral or proximal popliteal occlusion in whom the arteries distal to the popliteal area are patent might be candidates for a femoral-popliteal bypass. When a femoral-popliteal bypass is not possible, a more distal bypass to the posterior tibial, anterior tibial, or peroneal arteries can be considered. The dorsalis pedis, posterior tibial, lateral tarsal, deep metatarsal arch, and medial and lateral plantar arteries have been used to provide successful bypass outflow even when the plantar arch is not patent or other major pedal arteries are occluded.[36, 38] The patency and limb salvage rates for inframalleolar revascularization are comparable to those obtained with femoral popliteal or femoral tibial bypasses.[36] The dorsalis pedis bypass has been especially beneficial for patients with diabetes whose occlusive disease frequently involves the tibial and peroneal vessels and spares the inframalleolar circulation.[33, 64] Femoral popliteal bypass grafting can prove technically successful but not relieve symptoms if extensive tibial disease is present. When this situation occurs, secondary bypass grafting to the dorsal pedal artery usually relieves symptoms.[64]

Other Measures

Sympathectomy. As reconstructive procedures have extended to distal vessels, sympathectomy has been performed less frequently. Limbs with inoperable arterial disease, ischemic cutaneous ulceration, pain at rest, or pregangrenous changes can be considered for sympathetic denervation. The primary effect of sympathectomy seems to be enhancing pain relief rather than augmenting blood flow to the ischemic limb. A diabetic neuropathy can frequently cause autosympathectomy. It is imperative to document the presence of sympathetic nerve function in such cases before proceeding with surgical sympathectomy.[9] Although specific neuroautonomic testing can be performed, a simpler approach is to assess the effects of a temporary sympathetic block.

Intermittent Venous Occlusion/Pneumatic End-Diastolic Leg Compression. Skin blood flow, as reflected by $TcPO_2$, can be augmented acutely in ischemic limbs by intermittent venous occlusion with an externally applied inflatable cuff[73, 74] (Fig. 56–6). The mechanism proposed to explain the increased flow is analogous to the pumping action of the calf muscle during walking.[50] A cuff is strapped to the leg and connected to a compressor that rapidly inflates the cuff with air, delivering a short pulse of 80 to 100 mm Hg every 20 seconds. The transient inflation imitates the effects of normal gait by generating vigorous hemodynamic impulses throughout the veins each time the lower extremity is compressed. In addition to these mechanical factors, the altered flow and shear forces generated by the inflation of the pneumatic cuff may mediate the release of endothelial and humoral factors having local and systemic effects.[50] Other devices, which apply intermittent circumferential pneumatic compression to the foot or lower limb during cardiac diastole, show promise as adjunct measures to augment limb perfusion.

Chelation Therapy. Intravenous administration of fluids containing chelating compounds such as ethylenediaminetetraacetate (EDTA) have been advocated for treatment of advanced arterial occlusive disease on the premise that calcium salts leached from the vascular lesions might potentiate regression of the disease. Because of the lack of objective documentation of the effectiveness and the nephrotoxic effects of this treatment, it is most commonly used only as an adjunctive measure of last resort.

Amputation

With advances in limb salvage procedures, it is important to review carefully the risk-to-benefit and cost-to-benefit ratios with the patient before each intervention. Although in the later stage of disease each patient has a choice between amputation or delay, the choices often are a relatively pain-free, comfortable prosthesis or salvage of a painful, ulcerated, or gangrenous foot. In the older person, the time required for medical care and hospitalization becomes more and more significant. Frequent hospitalizations and non-weight-bearing status of a year's duration can represent 20% of the remaining life of a 70-year-old patient. Most patients choose a shorter procedure enabling them to spend as much as possible of their remaining life in comfort.[31]

VENOUS DISEASE

Venous disease includes deep venous thrombosis (DVT), recurrent DVT, superficial thrombophlebitis, and chronic venous insufficiency. In all cases, it is important to make an accurate diagnosis before initiating therapy.

Epidemiology

More than 250,000 new cases of DVT occur each year, resulting in approximately 500,000 patients presenting

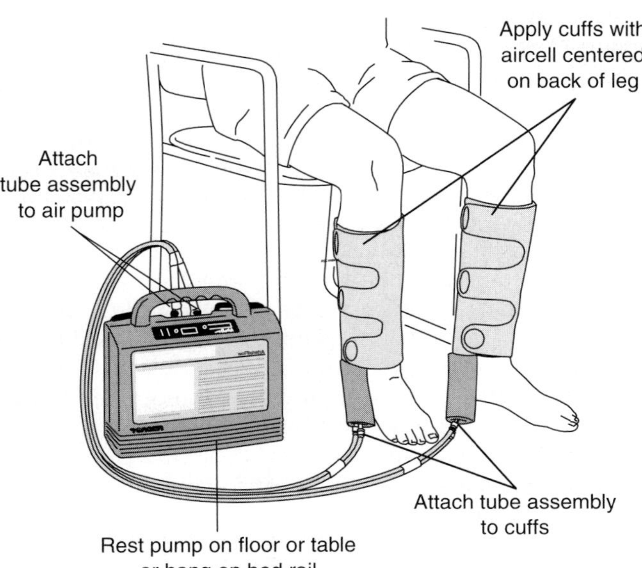

FIGURE 56–6. Intermittent venous occlusion can augment skin blood flow and decrease dependent edema. (Courtesy of Aircast, Inc.).

for the treatment of venous stasis ulcers.[18] Lindner found that 80% of patients followed for 5 to 10 years after venographically documented thrombosis had some symptoms of venous hypertension in association with valvular incompetence. Specifically, 49% had varicosities, 62% edema, 34% hyperpigmentation, and 4% ulceration. The location of the thrombosis influenced the probability of subsequent complications; 100% of iliac, 94% of femoral, and 40% of calf thrombosis were symptomatic.[55]

Etiology and Pathogenesis

Venous Thromboembolism

Thrombi frequently arise from clots that form in the cusps of venous valves and propagate into the major venous channel. Another site for thrombus development is at the entrance of a tributary vein; the thrombus can go on to occlude a major venous channel by prograde or retrograde propagation. Many small venous thrombi fortunately undergo rapid thrombolytic dissolution. For large thrombi, organization begins after 3 to 4 days. Recanalization can require a period of several months or more. Fibrous bands or strictures can form in the vein. Usually, but not always, venous valves are destroyed or lose their normal function as the fibrotic process thickens the venous wall and cusp.[26] Superficial venous thrombosis alone is not thought to have any serious morbidity unless a saphenous vein thrombus propagates and involves the common femoral vein.

The pathogenesis of DVT is outlined by Virchow's postulates: change in blood flow, alterations in the vessel wall, and variation in coagulability of the blood. Risk factors associated with the development of acute DVT include prior history of DVT, immobilization, postoperative state, age (older than 40 years), cardiac disease, limb trauma, post-thrombotic state or coagulation abnormalities, hormonal therapy, pregnancy and postpartum state, obesity, and advanced neoplasm.[26, 66] A complete medical workup should be done for any patient with an unexplained deep or superficial venous thrombosis to rule out cancer, inflammatory bowel disease, blood dyscrasias, or intrinsic clotting disease.

Chronic Venous Insufficiency

Many factors can result in the development of venous insufficiency, including heredity, local trauma, thrombosis, and intrinsic defects in the veins or valves themselves. To understand the pathogenesis of venous insufficiency, a basic review of the anatomy and function of leg veins is necessary. The venous system of the lower extremity is divided into three groups: (1) the superficial veins (great and small saphenous veins and their tributaries) (Fig. 56–7) which are subcutaneous and not well supported by the overlying tissues and skin; (2) the perforating (communicating) veins, which connect the superficial venous system with the deep venous system; and (3) the deep veins, which are supported externally by a strong fascial layer and the surrounding musculature.[56] The communicating pathways are variable from one person to another. They are most commonly located

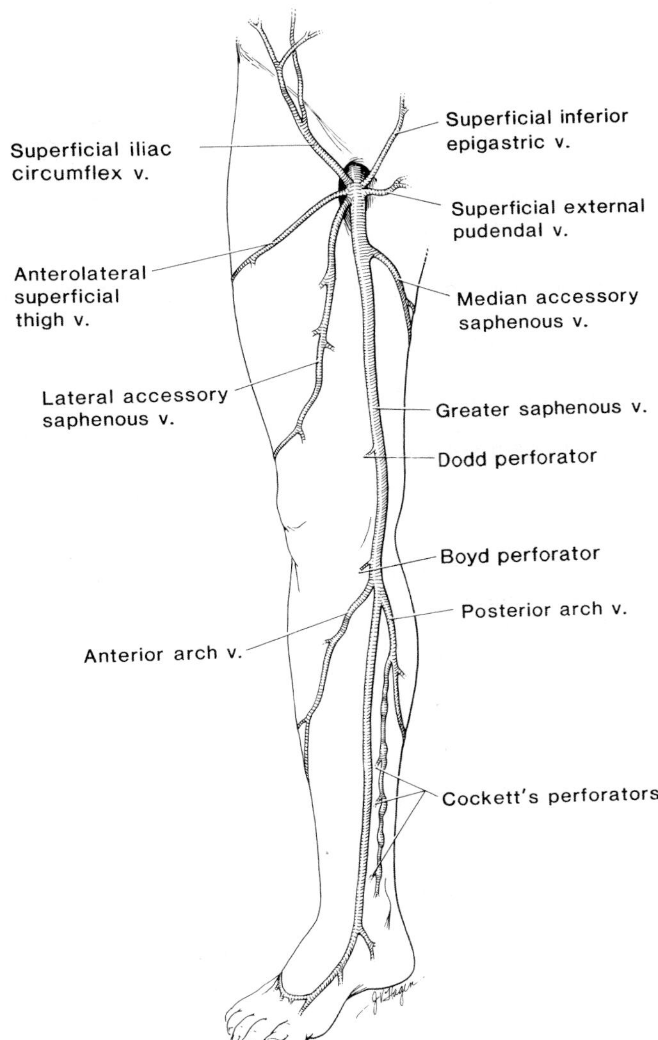

FIGURE 56–7. Normal anatomy of the greater saphenous vein and its tributaries. (Courtesy of Mayo Foundation.)

on the medial aspect of the calf but can be found at the thigh level.

Venous flow is based on a force that pushes the blood proximally (such as gravity or the calf muscle), an adequate outflow, and the presence of competent valves limiting reflux. Any disruption of these components results in chronic venous hypertension.[46] Normally the pressure in the leg vein is equal to the hydrostatic pressure from a vertical column of blood extending to the right atrium of the heart. At the ankle level, the hydrostatic pressure is about 90 mm Hg.[56] The pumping action of the calf muscles during exercise reduces this venous pressure by two-thirds. Even slight muscular movements during normal standing will lower the pressure.[56] Patients with venous insufficiency might fail to reduce ankle pressure, can show a rapid return of venous pressure to resting levels at the end of exercise, or experience a combination of both. The time required for the ankle vein pressure to return to resting levels after exercise is an indicator of the degree of reflux in the limb. Nicolaides found that elevated ambulatory venous pressure is associated with an increased incidence of ulceration.[59] When ambulatory venous pressure is below 30 mm Hg, the incidence of ulceration is zero. The incidence of ulceration increases linearly, reaching 100% when the ambulatory venous pressure is greater than 90 mm Hg.[59] The superficial leg veins carry 10% to 15% of the venous return. Incompetent valves in the superficial veins alone do not cause serious venous hypertension. Venous insufficiency develops only when the valves in the perforator or deep veins are incompetent. Ultimately, venous hypertension is the result of valve damage and retrograde venous blood flow to the superficial veins. Retrograde flow can occur with (1) faulty communication and superficial venous valves; (2) damage to the deep vein valves; (3) deep vein occlusion; and (4) muscle dysfunction and pump failure from fibrosis, neuropathies, and inflammatory disease.

Chronic venous insufficiency is usually the result of congenital or acquired valvular incompetence and less frequently obstruction of the veins.[35] Postthrombotic syndrome (venous occlusion and/or valve destruction after thrombosis) develops in 67% to 80% of patients after DVT.[22] A significant proportion of patients with chronic venous insufficiency have primary valvular incompetence with no history of phlebographic evidence of DVT.[35]

Several theories exist regarding the changes in the subcutaneous tissue of patients with chronic venous insufficiency. One hypothesis is that venous hypertension leads to venular dilatation and increased capillary permeability, with transudation of fibrinogen and hemosiderin from the capillaries into the subcutaneous tissue.[7] This theory proposes that the pericapillary fibrin acts as a diffusion barrier and the overlying dermis becomes hypoxic. There are no in vivo studies to document that pericapillary fibrin cuffs act as a diffusion barrier.[14, 27] A second hypothesis relates to the accumulation of white blood cells in the dermal capillaries of patients with venous disease. Trapped white cells release free radicals and inflammatory mediators, which are actively responsible for tissue injury.[15] Polymorphonuclear leukocytes, particularly those attached to capillary endothelium, may become activated, causing release of cytoplasmic granules containing proteolytic enzymes. In addition, a nonmitochondrial respiratory burst permits these cells to release free radicals (most notably the superoxide radical), which have destructive effects on lipid membranes, proteins, and many connective tissue compounds. Chemotactic leukotrienes are also released and attract more polymorphonuclear cells.[14] The true mechanism by which venous hypertension leads to induration and fibrosis of the skin (lipodermosclerosis) and ulceration remains unclear. It is apparent, however, that venous hypertension sets the stage for adverse conditions that eventually lead to skin damage and impaired healing.[45]

History and Clinical Findings

Venous Thromboembolism

Relevant history includes the patient's symptoms or presence of potential risk factors. Clinical findings associated with DVT include pain, tenderness, unilateral ankle or calf edema, palpable induration or cord, and pain produced by extreme dorsiflexion of the foot. Unfortunately, most clinical signs and symptoms attributed to DVT have been statistically analyzed and found to have a poor predictive value for determining the presence or absence of DVT.[22] It is therefore essential to perform objective testing (such as ultrasound duplex scanning) when DVT is suspected.

Chronic Venous Insufficiency

A complete history and clinical examination are ordinarily sufficient to diagnose venous insufficiency and to determine whether it involves the superficial, deep, or perforating veins individually or in combination. Symptoms of chronic venous insufficiency are highly variable and depend on the degree and duration of insufficiency. Patients generally note aching, edema, skin changes, decreased activity tolerance, and progressive leg pain with prolonged standing. If the patient states that the symptoms are unrelieved by leg elevation, especially overnight, the diagnosis of venous insufficiency should be questioned.[46] The earliest sign of chronic venous insufficiency is edema of the lower legs. At first, this is associated with an upright posture and is noticeable mainly in the evening. Early in the disease, intermittent soft pitting edema is present, but fibrosis eventually develops and the skin demonstrates firm induration. Pigmentation develops next, especially in the medial perimalleolar areas. Venous hypertension causes transudation of serous fluid and red blood cells into the subcutaneous tissue. Hemoglobin from the red blood cells breaks down to produce the pigment hemosiderin. A weepy pruritic dermatitis can develop, and recurrent secondary cellulitis is a fairly common complication. Chronic venous insufficiency results in chronic edema, scarring, obliteration of cutaneous lymphatics, decreased skin integrity, hemosiderin deposition (with brownish discoloration), dermatitis, and ulceration. Fortunately, not all patients with incompetent valves are symptomatic.

Vascular Testing

Although the evaluation of venous disease is accomplished principally with the history and physical examination, noninvasive testing modalities can complement these examinations (Table 56–2).

Impedance Plethysmography

Impedance plethysmography assesses volume changes at rest produced by a proximal, pneumatic, veno-occlusive cuff. The normal leg swells when a veno-occlusive tourniquet is placed and rapidly returns to its normal size when the tourniquet is released. Venous volume measured by electrical impedance normally shows a quick return to baseline levels, usually within 3 to 4 seconds. In the presence of a proximal lower-extremity DVT, the venous system will already be "maximally" filled. When the cuff is inflated, there is little additional increase in venous volume, and after tourniquet release the return to baseline is delayed.[68]

TABLE 56–2 Noninvasive Vascular Studies Used to Diagnose Venous Disease, Lymphedema, Arteriovenous Fistula, and Arteriovenous Malformation Fistula

Vascular Disease	Anatomic	Hemodynamic/Functional	Disadvantages
Venous			
Insufficiency	Continuous wave doppler		Operator dependent
		Exercise venous plethysmography	
	Duplex ultrasonography	Duplex ultrasonography	Expense
Obstruction	Continuous wave doppler		Operator dependent
		Strain gauge outflow plethysmography	Limited availability
		Impedence plethysmography	Variable accuracy
	Duplex ultrasonography	Duplex ultrasonography	Expense
Lymphedema		Lymphoscintigraphy	
Arteriovenous fistula		Continuous wave doppler	
		Pulse volume recording	Poor reproducibility
Arteriovenous malformation	Magnetic resonance imaging		Expense

Exercise Venous Plethysmography

Lower limb venous function is tested by performing a plethysmographic evaluation of limb volume before, during, and after exercise. In a normal individual, plethysmography shows a progressive decrease in leg volume during exercise followed by a period after exercise when the volume slowly returns to normal. In venous insufficiency, the exercise-induced decrease in venous volume is less than expected. In addition, when venous incompetence is present, the post-exercise return in volume will be more rapid than expected. Exercise venous plethysmography provides a quick and relatively inexpensive way to document or screen for venous incompetence. It also yields quantitative information about the severity of venous insufficiency that is not readily obtained with other noninvasive methods.[70]

Duplex Scanning

Duplex scanning is used to diagnose deep or superficial venous thrombosis, assess venous incompetence, and map the superficial veins before surgical harvest for bypass operations. The diagnosis of venous thrombosis can be established by demonstrating noncompressibility of the vein with use of real-time, two-dimensional, B-mode imaging (Fig. 56–8). If the veins do not collapse under a force sufficient to distort the arteries, intraluminal thrombus is assumed to be present. Older thrombi can appear echogenic or match the echogenicity of the vein wall and surrounding tissue. The pulsed-wave doppler confirms the lack of venous flow, and provides indirect evidence that spontaneous flow through the vein has disappeared (by the absence of phasic changes with respiration or the reduction or absence of augmentation). Duplex scanning can also document the presence of venous incompetence, identify the anatomic sites involved, and quantify the severity.[72]

Treatment

Superficial Thrombophlebitis

Superficial thrombophlebitis is treated with elevation and superficial heat. Appropriate compressive stockings, 30 to 40 mm Hg, should be worn when ambulating. Aspirin or nonsteroidal anti-inflammatory medications can be administered for pain relief. It is doubtful that these medications significantly diminish the potential

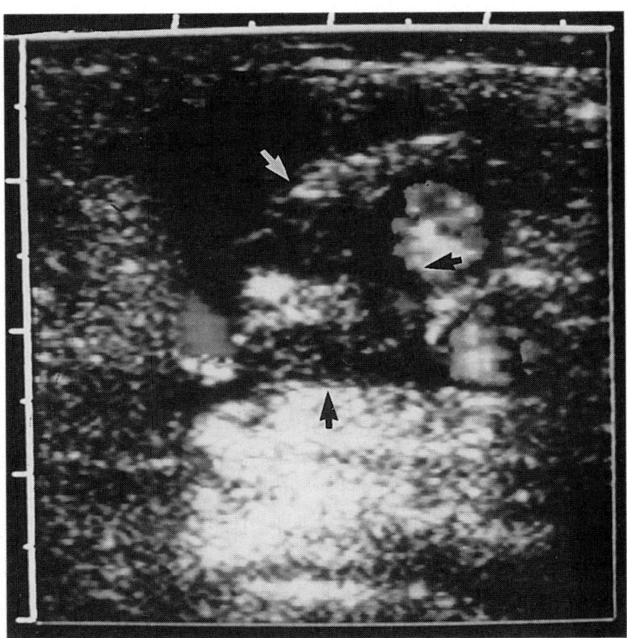

FIGURE 56–8. Duplex scan showing venous thrombus. In this cross-sectional view, the arrows outline a femoral vein that is filled with thrombus. A small channel around the clot continues to carry venous blood. The arteries are normal.

extension of the phlebitic process. If the process extends near the saphenofemoral junction, a duplex examination should clarify the status of the deep veins. If deep veins are also thrombosed, the patient should be treated for DVT.[26]

Deep Venous Thrombosis

Standard therapy for acute DVT consists of anticoagulation,[47] bed rest, elevation, and support of the extremity (Table 56–3).

Chronic Venous Insufficiency

Patient Education

Patient education is important in the management of chronic venous insufficiency. Patients must understand the disease process and the correct use of measures to decrease edema. Since venous hypertension is the physiologic cause of the damage in chronic venous insufficiency, the first step of treatment should be to reduce the venous pressure. When elevation is used for edema control, the extremity must be elevated above the level of the heart. Patients should lie on a sofa or sit in an orthopedic chair to elevate the legs appropriately above the heart. Periodic elevation of the legs, with the toes about 20 cm above heart level, relieves edema effectively by lowering the hydrostatic pressure to nearly zero.[56] The optimal duration and frequency of leg elevations are not known but should be tailored to the severity of disease.

Compression

Compressive dressings aid venous return by compressing the leg and increasing the interstitial tension. Compression of dilated, engorged superficial and intramuscular veins indirectly increases the efficiency of the calf pump mechanism.[56] With no history of congestive heart failure and no evidence of venous obstruction on noninvasive studies, lower extremity volume can be stabilized with an intermittent pneumatic compression pump. Compressive wraps should be used between pumping sessions. After the volume stabilizes, the patient can be measured for stockings. Elastic stockings should provide graduated compression, exerting most pressure at the ankle, less at the calf, and least pressure at the thigh. Greatest patient compliance is achieved by prescribing knee-length, graduated compression stockings with a pressure gradient of 30 to 40 mm Hg. In patients with concomitant arterial disease, lower compression might be required to avoid further compromise of arterial inflow by the extrinsic compression.

TABLE 56–3 Initial Treatment[1] of Acute DVT

Method	Agent	Duration of Rx
Conventional	IV Heparin	5+ days[2]
Outpatient	Subcutaneous low-molecular–weight heparin	5+ days[2]
Lytic	IV: Urokinase Streptokinase TPA	1–3 days

[1] All patients with DVT/PE need to have "Initial Treatment" followed by 3–6 months of coumadin.
[2] Heparin and coumadin must be overlapped a minimum of 5 days.

Exercise

The value of exercise in the management of chronic venous insufficiency has not been conclusively demonstrated. Exercises involving the leg musculature such as walking, bicycling, or swimming, promote muscle tone in the calf and enhance venous return. Exercise, however, produces variable reductions in venous hypertension. Patients with chronic venous stasis due to incompetent deep vein valves generally do not obtain as much reduction in venous pressure as do those in which the primary defect is due to incompetent perforator valves.[29]

Medication

Pentoxifylline has been evaluated in an attempt to alter the leukocyte trapping in tissues. This drug reduces leukocyte adhesiveness and the release of oxygen free radicals and has been shown to be effective in the treatment of venous leg ulcers in early trials.[3, 16]

Surgery

Surgical intervention for chronic venous insufficiency can include ligation of perforators, direct valve repair, vein segment transposition, or axillary valve autotransplantation.[36]

Sclerotherapy

Sclerotherapy (which uses the injection of an irritant substance into the vein) can also be used to obliterate incompetent veins in certain settings.[35, 46, 83] Sclerotherapy is used for the treatment of spider veins, small distal varicose veins, and venous insufficiency resulting from superficial and perforator incompetence.[48, 83] With sclerotherapy, a substance that irritates the endothelial lining is injected into a vein, followed by compression until the vein walls are permanently fused. Elastic compression is suggested for at least 6 weeks after treatment. Complications are rare and usually minor. The most frequent types of morbidity include skin discoloration, thrombophlebitis, and hematoma formation. Allergic or anaphylactic reactions to the sclerosing agent are very rare but have been observed. Skin or fat necrosis can occur if a large amount of concentrated solution is injected outside the vein.[36]

LYMPHATIC DISEASE

Etiology

Lymphedema is the abnormal accumulation of water and protein in the skin and subcutaneous tissues, and is classified as either primary or secondary. Primary lymphedema is due to aplastic or hypoplastic lymphatic trunks. Secondary lymphedema can occur after recurrent infection, tumor, lymphoproliferative disease, or injury to the lymphatic system stemming from surgical excision, trauma, or irradiation.[26] Lymphedema develops when the lymphatic load exceeds the transfer capacity of the lymphatic system. It becomes manifest if all the compensatory mechanisms (collateral lymphatic circulation, spontaneous lymphogenous anastomosis, and the proteolytic activity of tissue macrophages) are exhausted. This explains why lymphedema often develops several months—or even years—after interruption of the lymphatic pathways.[26] Without treatment, the protein-rich interstitial fluid is replaced by fibrinoid material. Inflammatory cells accumulate, and progressive fibrosis, sclerosis, and (in the final stage) elephantiasis develop. Lymphangiosarcoma, a severe late complication of secondary lymphedema, is rare.[26]

History and Clinical Findings

For evaluation of a swollen limb, it is important to determine the underlying diagnosis. Malignancy or metastatic disease must be excluded. Peripheral examination of the limb with lymphedema helps to differentiate it from other causes of peripheral edema. The edema usually involves the dorsal forefoot but spares the metatarsal phalangeal joint (Fig. 56–9). Dark pigmentary changes of the skin and prominent veins are unusual. Although ulceration is characteristic of more advanced cases of chronic venous insufficiency, it is rare in lymphedema.

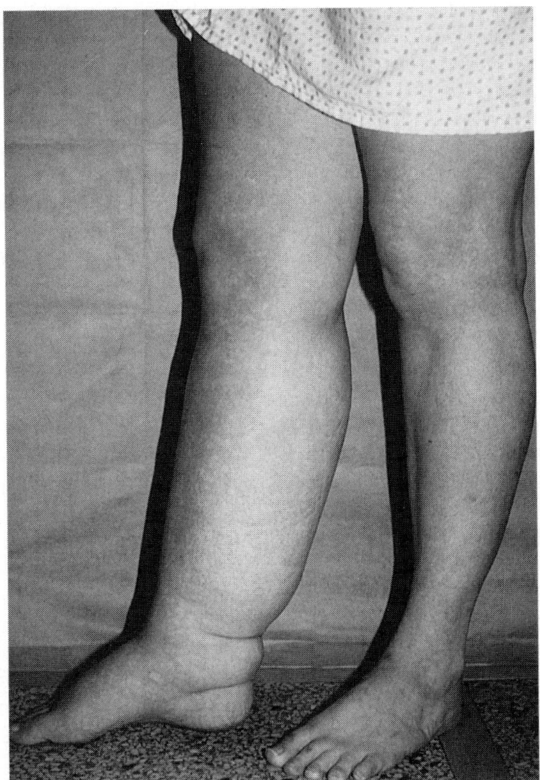

FIGURE 56–9. Lymphedema of right lower extremity. Note that the edema involves the dorsal forefoot but spares the metatarsal phalangeal joint.

Evaluation

Lymphoscintigraphy provides a functional assessment of lymph transport capacity and identifies major morphologic abnormalities of the lymphatic system. Lymphoscintigraphy also differentiates purely venous edema from mixed or lymphatic edema.[34] If venous disease is in question, noninvasive studies of the venous system should be obtained, including impedance plethysmography or duplex scanning. Magnetic resonance or computerized tomographic imaging may be needed to evaluate for malignancy or other problems.

Treatment

The goals of treatment for lymphedema are to preserve skin integrity, soften subcutaneous tissues, avoid lymphangiitis, reduce limb size,[26] and avoid contracture. In severe lymphedema, hospitalization can be required for 2 or 3 days to control limb volume with bedrest and a lymphedema sling (Fig. 56–10).

Compression

The use of compression in the management of lymphedema is based on the Starling hypothesis of counteracting forces driving water through the capillary wall.[77] Pneumatic single-chamber compression at 60 to 80 mm Hg, or sequential compression at 80 to 130 mm Hg as tolerated, is used twice daily for 3 or 4 days until the volume is stabilized. Volumetric or circumferential measurements are obtained after each treatment to monitor progress.

Manual decongestive massage and isometric exercises are used to increase venous and lymphatic flow and reduce edema. The massage and exercises are done with the extremity elevated to provide a gravity assist when mobilizing the fluid. The patient is instructed in a program of bandaging, elevation, and exercise to be done between treatments.[77]

After reduction of edema, new fluid will accumulate in the tissue space unless the volume is restricted by external support. This support is commonly supplied by compressive bandages or stockings. Elastic graded-compression stockings are prescribed at 30 to 40 or at 40 to 50 mm Hg. The patient should be supplied with two pairs to allow cleaning of one pair while wearing the other. Two pairs of stockings typically should last the patient about 4 to 6 months. Selective refractory patients can benefit from simultaneously using two compressive stockings, 40 to 50 mm Hg and 50 to 60 mm Hg. Donning is facilitated by applying the lower-compression garment first. Depending on the location of the edema, a knee-high garment over a thigh-high garment might be adequate.

The patient must be instructed in meticulous skin care to avoid fungal infection or injury. Long-sleeved shirts or pants should be worn to avoid insect bites, cuts, or abrasions. Needle sticks or intravenous lines should never be permitted in the lymphedematous extremity. Patients should avoid exposure to extreme temperatures, such as in a hot tub. A general conditioning program and weight loss are encouraged.

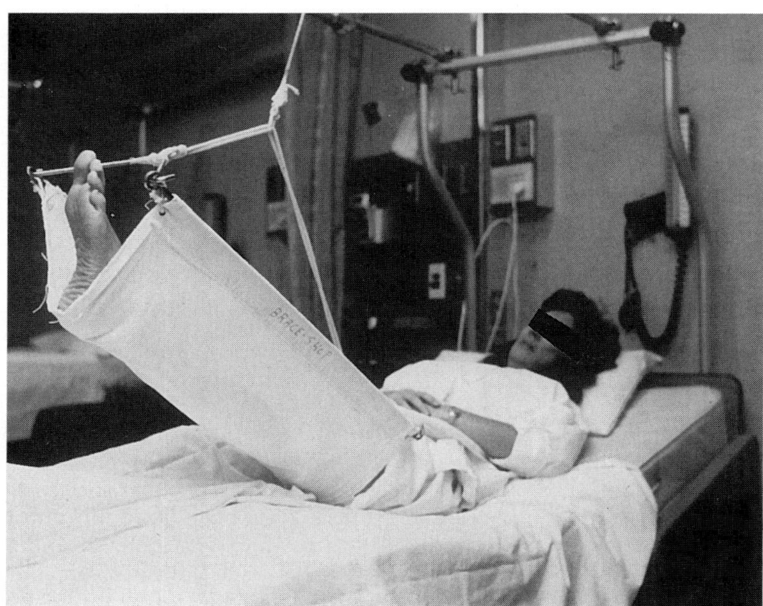

FIGURE 56–10. Bedrest with a lymphedema sling at 60° can be used for initial management of severe lymphedema.

Medications

Any evidence of infection needs immediate treatment. Patients can be given a supply of antibiotics with instructions to start treatment at the first sign of infection. The cause of cellulitis is almost always group A streptococci. If the patient has no allergies, penicillin is the drug of choice.

Benzopyrones can reduce the volume of high-protein edema by stimulating proteolysis, but are not available for use in North America. Flavonoids (benzo-[γ]-pyrone) are available and can be beneficial in the treatment of lymphedema, although gastric irritation can be a problem.[10]

The use of diuretics in the management of lymphedema is controversial. They decrease the water and sodium content of the interstitial space but have no effect on the protein content of the extravascular fluid.[26] With chronic use, these agents generally become ineffective. Diuretics can be used for temporary relief in severe lymphedema or to provide symptomatic relief for patients with a terminal malignancy.

Surgery

Surgery for lymphedema is indicated in only a small percentage of patients. Operations are either excisional or physiologic. The excisional operations (such as the Charles or Homan procedure) are aimed at removing excess tissue to decrease the volume of the extremity. The physiologic operations consist of lymphatic-to-lymphatic or lymphatic-to-venous anastomosis,[26, 63] which, it is hoped, will improve drainage. None of these operations is considered curative.

ARTERIOVENOUS FISTULAS AND ARTERIOVENOUS MALFORMATION

Etiology

Vascular malformations are classified as either congenital or acquired. The extent of the arterial component in a congenital arteriovenous malformation (AVM) is related to the stage of embryologic maturity at the time of developmental arrest. Acquired arteriovenous fistulae result from surgical construction of angioaccess for dialysis, penetrating injuries, infection, neoplasm, and aneurysmal erosion.

History and Clinical Findings

A history of penetrating trauma should promote a high index of suspicion of possible acquired arteriovenous fistula. In the acute phase, a pulsating hematoma, palpable thrill, and bruit are present.[79] When the peripheral pulse remains intact and the distal systolic pressures are normal, the fistula can be considered relatively small from a hemodynamic standpoint. If pulses are decreased or absent and the distal pressure is low, a large-volume shunt is indicated. In rare instances, the amount of blood siphoned by the fistula can produce heart failure, peripheral ischemia, or gangrene.[79]

Ischemia can develop early after fistula construction for dialysis in a patient with pre-existing arterial disease. It is more frequently a late manifestation, causing an increase in size of the arteriovenous fistula and reversal of flow in the distal radial artery. Clinical findings include pain, paresthesias, and muscular weakness in the affected extremity. These symptoms become more prominent during dialysis.[26]

Clinical presentation of a congenital AVM can be evident at birth. Most deep-seated AVMs are not evident until adolescence or early adulthood. An AVM causes symptoms with growth of the angiomatous mass, thrombosis of varicosities, or circulatory compromise.[26] Clinical presentations are variable. Swelling, discoloration, pain, an enlarged swollen limb, dermatitis, or ulceration may occur with all types of congenital vascular malformations[26] (Fig. 56–11).

Evaluation

The goals of evaluation are to establish the presence and type of lesion, to determine the hemodynamic ef-

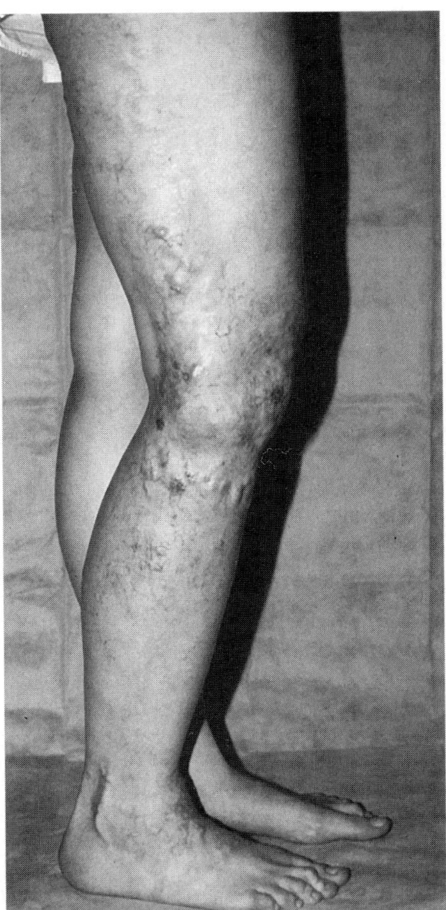

FIGURE 56–11. Arteriovenous malformation involving right lower extremity with associated varicosities and leg-length discrepancy.

fects, and to define the anatomic extent and involvement of adjacent structures.

To understand the hemodynamics of an arteriovenous fistula, it is imperative to understand the direction of flow in each of its component branches. Because a fistula markedly reduces the peripheral resistance, blood flow in the proximal artery loses its triphasic characteristic. Flow is always increased, particularly during diastole, and no reversed component is observed. Blood flow in the proximal vein increases and shows a pulsatile pattern. The direction of flow in the distal artery and vein can be either toward or away from the fistula. High resistance in the proximal artery and distal vascular bed, in combination with relatively low resistance at the site of the fistula and in the arterial collaterals, favors retrograde flow in the distal artery. Flow in the proximal artery and arterial collaterals is always directed toward the periphery, and the flow in the proximal vein and venous channels is always directed centrally.[79] The same diagnostic studies used to evaluate chronic arterial occlusive disease in the extremities, and to a lesser extent venous insufficiency, can provide useful information about the fistula. Continuous-wave doppler shows a high-flow, low-resistance pattern with loss of end-systolic reversal and considerable flow continuing throughout diastole.[26]

Magnetic resonance imaging is the best technique to evaluate patients with congenital vascular malformations. It defines hypertrophy of bone, muscle, or subcutaneous tissue and images varicose veins and hemangiomas in the subcutaneous space and muscles.[37]

Treatment

Early recognition and management of an acquired arteriovenous fistula are preferred. Management of large, chronic arteriovenous fistulae is complicated. Bleeding can be profuse from multiple arterial and venous collateral vessels in the area.[26] Elastic support is beneficial to treat symptoms of chronic venous insufficiency, protect the extremity from minor external trauma,[37] and preserve skin integrity by reducing the distal venous backup pressure. Appropriate footwear is important to accommodate limb hypertrophy and compensate for leg-length discrepancy. Physical therapy intervention should maintain mobility of joints and soft tissues and preserve a normal gait pattern. Orthopedic intervention can be beneficial to avoid or correct leg-length discrepancy.

VASCULAR WOUNDS

Etiology

Nonhealing vascular wounds result from (1) ischemia (arterial and small vessel disease), (2) venous insufficiency, and (3) neuropathy.

History and Clinical Findings

Ischemic

Ischemic ulcers typically result from a minor laceration, abrasion, or pressure in a limb with compromised blood flow. These lead to a chronic, painful ulcer that forms because the blood supply is insufficient to meet the increased demands of healing. Ischemic ulcers typically occur in the distal extremity.[23] Ulcers below the ankle with a pale or gray, nongranulating base are usually the result of major arterial insufficiency (Fig. 56–12). Simultaneous appearance of livedo reticularis and cutaneous toe infarcts (with subsequent ulceration) suggests atheromatous embolization, but these conditions can occur less commonly in periarteritis nodosa, systemic lupus erythematosus, or livedoid vasculitis. Small vessel ischemic ulcers are usually located on the leg and have areas of cutaneous infarction which coalesce and proceed to ulceration[49] (Fig. 56–13).

Venous

With a history of chronic venous insufficiency, clinical findings include edema, hyperpigmentation, and soft tissue fibrosis.[24] Ulcers are typically located on the medial perimalleolar area of the lower extremity (Fig. 56–14). Upper extremity ulcerations are not caused by chronic venous insufficiency unless an arteriovenous fistula is present.[28, 49]

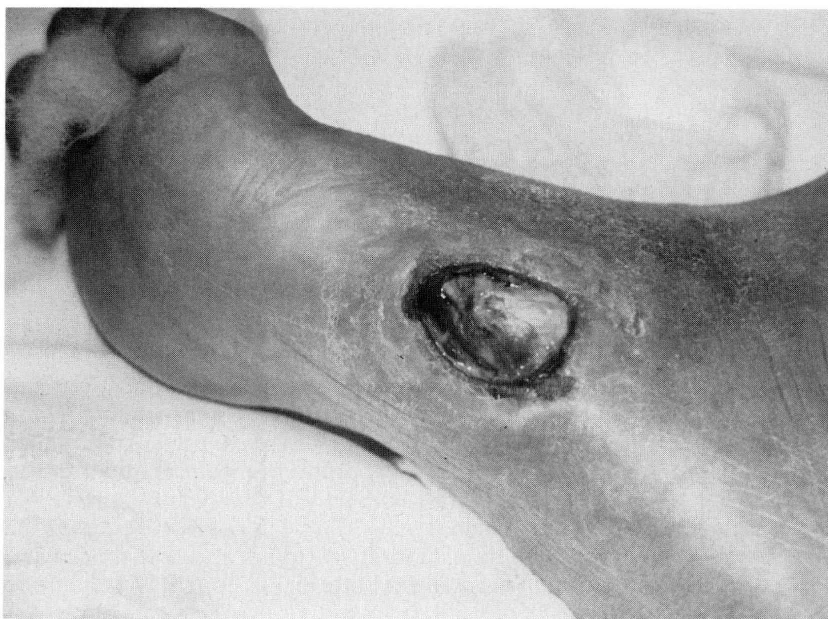

FIGURE 56–12. Arterial occlusive disease in a patient with history of mechanical trauma and subsequent ulcer formation.

Neuropathic

In patients with a history of autonomic and peripheral neuropathy, clinical findings can include decreased perspiration, dry skin, dependent rubor, impaired sensation, and denervation of foot intrinsic muscles with associated clawfoot deformity. Charcot changes can be present, including medial tarsal subluxation, pronation, forefoot valgus, increased width, and decreased length. Ulcers are typically located at the metatarsal heads, pulp or tip of a rigid great toe, lateral surface of the foot at the base of the metatarsal, heel, or midfoot (in the area of a collapsed navicula or cuboid). Neuropathic ulcers are characteristically painless and rimmed by callus; they can be present for years before the patient seeks medical consultation (Fig. 56–15).

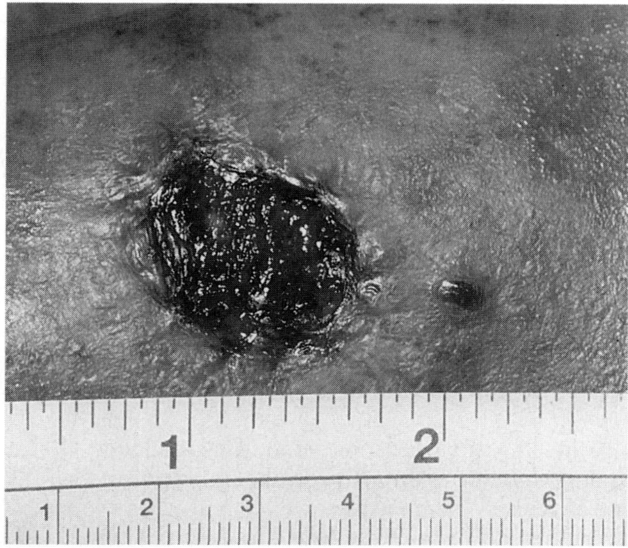

FIGURE 56–13. Hypertensive ischemic ulcers with areas of cutaneous infarction.

Controversy exists whether neuropathic ulcers can occur with an isolated neuropathic process or only in association with arterial or small vessel insufficiency. Studies by Brand[4, 5] suggest that neuropathic ulcers result from repetitive trauma. Brand studied the histology of rat paws after repetitive stress and determined that an increase in temperature always occurred with repetitive stress. If the increase was followed immediately by a gradual return to normal, this change was thought to be due to simple reactive hyperemia. If the temperature increase continued for 10 or more minutes, biopsies showed edema and collections of inflammatory cells.

When the repetitions continued at a force equal to walking 7 miles per day at a fast pace on hard ground, epithelial hypertrophy with marked inflammation and necrosis of deeper tissues was noted at day 3. Ulceration occurred at day 10. When the same experiment was performed with 20% fewer daily repetitions and breaks on weekends, hypertrophy occurred without significant breakdown.[4, 5] It can be inferred from this study that in patients with normal sensation, inflammation makes feet tender and the tender spot is spared further stress until inflammation subsides. With a neuropathic foot, pain is no longer present to provide this feedback.

A study of the recurrence of neuropathic ulcerations revealed that nearly half of the recurrences were solely attributable to failure to comply with the prescribed program.[40] Although a foot ulceration can be extensive, a lack of subjective pain often causes the patient to ignore a non-weightbearing recommendation. To the person who has lost sensation, the limb does not just feel incompetent, it feels "dead." The body image of such a person excludes the dead part. It is the medical team's responsibility to convey that pain sensation can be compensated by "intelligent anticipation."[5]

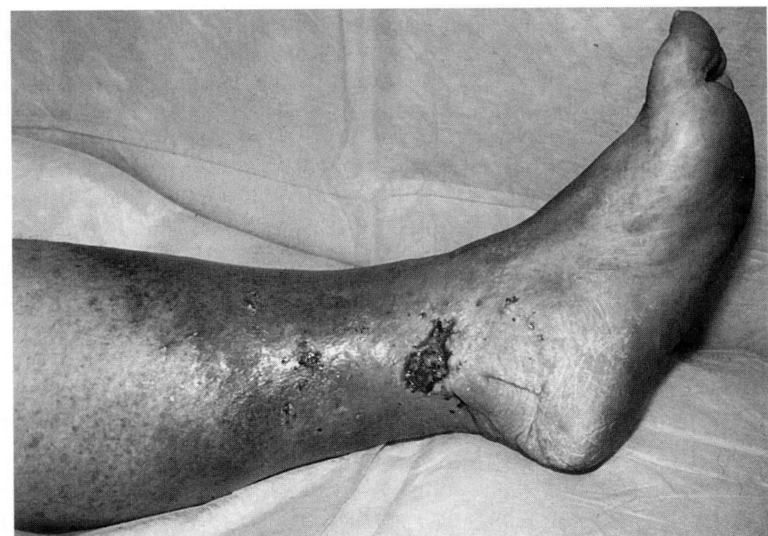

FIGURE 56–14. Chronic venous insufficiency with edema, hyperpigmentation, soft tissue fibrosis, and stasis ulcer.

Treatment

Wound care principles include (1) removal of devitalized tissue; (2) optimization of the wound environment to promote granulation and re-epithelialization; (3) avoidance of maceration, trauma, friction, or shearing forces; (4) relief of pressure; and (5) evaluation for reversible underlying conditions that may predispose to ulcer development or impede wound healing.

Debridement

Simple sharp debridement using topical lidocaine and occasionally surgical debridement might be necessary. Necrotic debris not only causes a foreign body reaction, but also provides an ideal environment for microorganisms. Dead tissue, whether black and dry or yellow and fibrinous, also prevents proper assessment of the wound depth. Wounds with a small amount of superficial necrotic tissue can be mechanically debrided gently using saline moistened coarse mesh gauze. Enzymatic agents cannot remove a hardened, black eschar or a large amount of necrotic tissue; however, they can loosen the eschar to facilitate sharp debridement. Whirlpool, shower cart, or pulsed-water (Waterpik) debridement can be useful adjuncts for ongoing debridement of large ulcers.

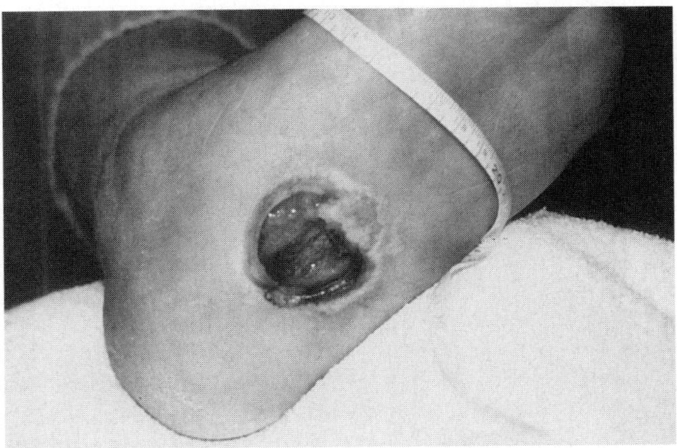

FIGURE 56–15. Large, painless, neuropathic ulcer with surrounding callus.

Indications for surgical debridement include the presence of a draining sinus, an infected nongranulating ulcer, an abscess, osteomyelitis, necrotic abscess formation, exposed nonviable tissue, and exposed nongranulating cartilage or bone surface.[6] In a patient with a chronic ulcer, the diagnosis of osteomyelitis can be extremely difficult. Although bone scans are generally used to diagnose osteomyelitis, in some cases magnetic resonance imaging may be more sensitive for detecting the early bone changes of osteomyelitis.[6] Once the presence of osteomyelitis is established, the area of infected bone should be debrided or excised.

Caution must be used to limit the debridement to devitalized tissue. It is important to evaluate the arterial supply carefully before sharp debridement. If the blood supply is inadequate, the margin of debridement is at risk for necrosis. With distal ischemia (dry gangrene) in a patient who is not a candidate for debridement or distal amputation, management can include protection of the extremity while awaiting demarcation and subsequent autoamputation in the affected region. Autoamputation is used to preserve as much of the residual limb as possible.

Wound Care Products

Many products are available for the treatment of wounds, but formal protocols are needed to evaluate the efficacy and cost of most. The faster rate of healing observed in wounds that are kept moist has been attributed to the avoidance of tissue injury during dressing removal and the fact that desiccation of the wound inhibits epithelialization.[51] It has been recently discovered that moisture-retentive dressings also facilitate dissolution of necrotic and fibrinous tissue (autolysis and fibrinolysis). Dressings that promote lysis of necrotic tissue and fibrin can facilitate the release of growth factors and reduce time to healing.[51]

A variety of new dressing materials are available. These dressings generally provide painless debridement, stimulate granulation tissue, encourage epithelialization, reduce wound pain, provide protection, and decrease frequency of dressing changes. With any wound care product, the skin surrounding the wound should be monitored for erythema, swelling, pain, or maceration. Erythema, swelling, and pain might be caused by unrelieved pressure or adverse reactions to wound care treatments. Skin maceration caused by prolonged contact of wound fluid with the skin is a sign that the topical wound care treatment selected is inappropriate for the patient.

Hyperbaric Oxygen Therapy

Although enhanced wound healing is a postulated benefit of adjunctive therapy with hyperbaric oxygen, the paucity of randomized controlled trials makes it difficult to assess the efficacy of hyperbaric oxygen. A trial of adjunctive therapy with hyperbaric oxygen at 2.0 to 2.5 atmospheres for 90 to 120 minutes can be considered for patients with ischemic wounds if the periulcer transcutaneous oxygen tension is shown to increase during treatment.[81]

Electrical Stimulation

Electrical stimulation has been demonstrated to enhance wound healing through effects on blood flow, edema reduction, anti-bacterial properties, cellular migration, fibroblast activity, and wound tensile strength.[52] The ideal parameters for clinical use have not yet been fully determined.

Vacuum

Polyvinyl foam under negative pressure using a vacuum has recently been shown to facilitate granulation tissue production while maintaining a relatively clean wound bed. As long as the vacuum is intact, the polyvinyl foam can remain in place for approximately one week.[58]

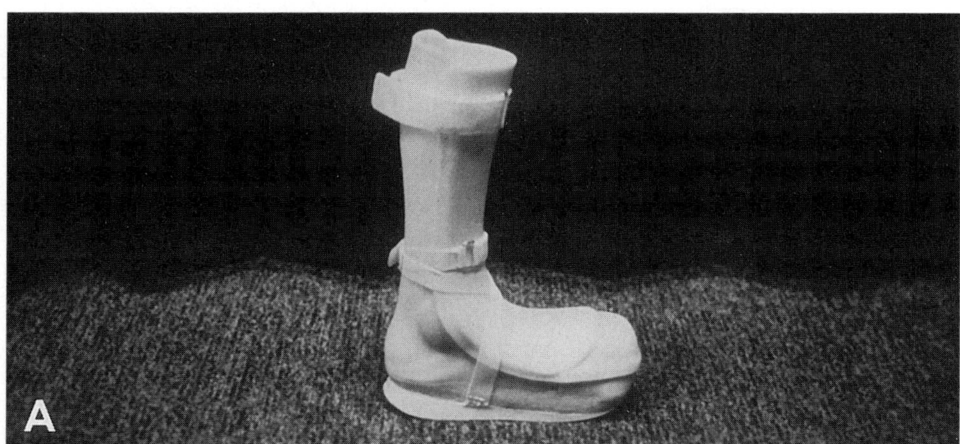

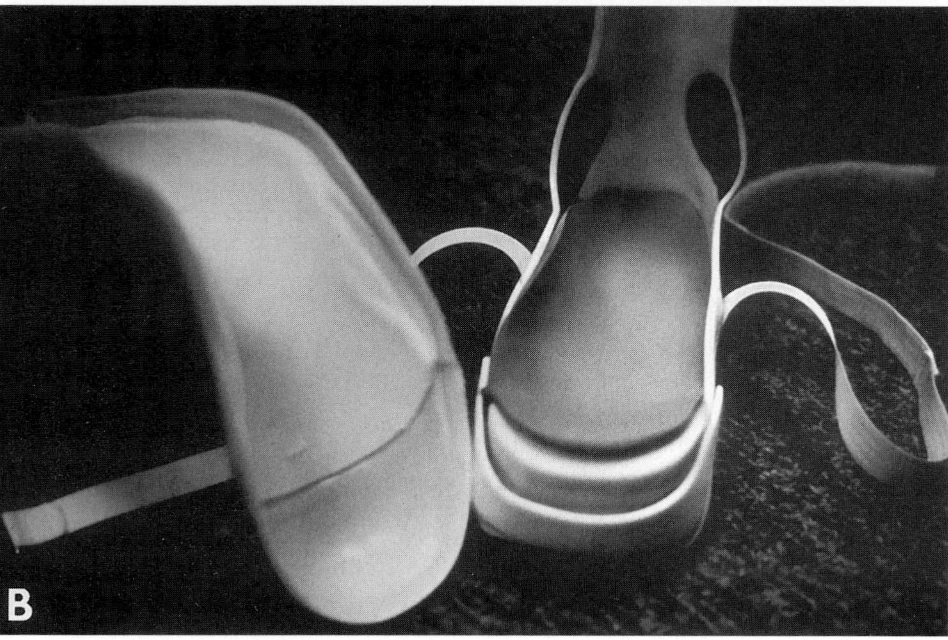

FIGURE 56–16. *A* and *B.* Custom total-contact, bivalved polypropylene ankle foot orthosis with custom foot bed. (Courtesy of Gretchen Hecht, CPO Sawtooth Orthotics, Boise.)

Protective Footwear

After the infection has been contained, edema controlled, and necessary revascularization performed, it is important to arrange for proper protective footwear. Total-contact casting has been shown to be beneficial for the treatment of neuropathic ulcers.[39, 82] The total-contact cast redistributes weightbearing forces, decreases edema, protects the wound and surrounding tissues, decreases sheer forces, localizes infection, protects the foot from outside contaminants, and provides immobilization of the wound and Charcot joint.[13, 39] In previous research, casting allowed healing of even the most chronic neuropathic ulceration in an average of 33 to 38 days.[39, 82] A custom total-contact, bivalved polypropylene ankle-foot orthosis (AFO) with custom foot bed (Fig. 56–16) has been tried recently. It is indicated if patients are unable to return for cast changes, or if the referring physician desires continued access to the wound.

Although the use of this AFO appears promising, it has not been formally studied. When either a total-contact cast or a custom bivalved AFO is used, footwear on the sound side must be adjusted to avoid a leg-length discrepancy. After initial healing, a total-contact sandal with a custom foot bed of moderate density, closed-cell, polyethylene foam and poron (PPT) interface can be fabricated. The patient wears this sandal for approximately 2 weeks until proceeding with definitive footwear. Definitive footwear includes an extra-depth shoe and a moderate-density inlay. Footwear for the insensitive foot should accommodate rather than attempt to correct skeletal deformities. A rocker-bottom sole can help to further dissipate the forces of ambulation.[4]

REFERENCES

1. Abramson DI: Physiologic basis for the use of physical agents in peripheral vascular disorders. Arch Phys Med Rehab 1965; 46:216.
2. Bacharach JM, Rooke TW, Osmundson PJ, et al: Predictive value of transcutaneous oxygen pressure and amputation success by use of supine and elevation measurements. J Vasc Surg 1992; 15:558.
3. Barbarino C: Pentoxifylline in the treatment of venous leg ulcers. Curr Med Res Opin 1992; 12:547.
4. Brand PW [Project Director]: The Cycle of Repetitive Stress on Insensitive Feet. Project Booklet. Supported in part by Social and Rehabilitation Service Grant No. RC 75 MPO. United States Public Health Service Hospital, Carville, Louisiana, 1975.
5. Brand PW: The Quest for Artificial Pain (Course Program). Presented at the American Association of Electrodiagnostic Medicine meeting, October 7, 1993, New Orleans, pp 7–18.
6. Brodsky JW, Schneidler C: Diabetic foot infections. Orthop Clin North Am 1991; 22:473.
7. Browse NL, Burnand KG: The cause of venous ulceration. Lancet 1982; 2:243.
8. Buerger L: The Circulatory Disturbances of the Extremities. Philadelphia, WB Saunders, 1924.
9. Carter SA: The relationship of distal systolic pressures to healing of skin lesions in limbs with arterial occlusive disease, with special reference to diabetes mellitus. Scand J Clin Lab Invest 1973; 31(suppl 128):239.
10. Casley-Smith JR, Morgan RG, Piller NB: Treatment of lymphedema of the arms and legs with 5,6-benzo-[α]-pyrone. N Engl J Med 1993; 329:1158.
11. Coffman JD: Intermittent claudication: Be conservative. N Engl J Med 1991; 325:577.
12. Coffman JD: Vasodilator drugs in peripheral vascular disease. N Engl J Med 1979; 300:713.
13. Coleman WC, Brand PW, Birke JA: The total contact cast: A therapy for plantar ulceration on insensitive feet. J Am Podiat Assoc 1984; 74:548.
14. Coleridge Smith PD: Pathogenesis of chronic venous insufficiency and possible effects of compression and pentoxifylline. Yale Biol Med 1993; 66:47.
15. Coleridge Smith PD, Thomas P, Schurr JH, Dormandy JA: Causes of venous ulceration: A new hypothesis. Br Med J 1988; 296:1726.
16. Colgan MP, Dormandy JA, Jones PW, et al: Oxpentifylline treatment of venous ulcers of the leg. Br Med J 1990; 300:972.
17. Cooke JP, Ma AO: Medical therapy of peripheral arterial occlusive disease. Surg Clin North Am 1995; 75:569.
18. Coon WW, Willis PW, Keller JB: Venous thromboembolism and other venous disease in the Tecumseh community health study. Circulation 1973; 48:839.
19. Council on Physiotherapy: Sanders vasocillator acceptable. JAMA 1938; 111:2016.
20. Creasy TS, McMillan PJ, Fletcher EW, et al: Is percutaneous transluminal angioplasty better than exercise for claudication? Preliminary results from a prospective randomized trial. Eur J Vasc Surg 1990; 4:135.
21. Criqui MH, Fronek A, Barrett-Connor E, et al: The prevalence of peripheral arterial disease in a defined population. Circulation 1985; 71:510.
22. Cronan JJ: Venous thromboembolic disease: The role of US. Radiology 1993; 186:619.
23. DeWeese JA, Leather R, Porter J: Practice guidelines: Lower extremity revascularization. J Vasc Surg 1993; 18:280.
24. Dodd HJ, Gaylarde PM, Sarkany I: Skin oxygen tension in venous insufficiency of the lower leg. J R Soc Med 1985; 78:373.
25. Ekroth R, Dahlof A-G, Gundevall B, et al: Physical training of patients with intermittent claudication: Indications, methods, and results. Surgery 1978; 84:640.
26. Ernst CB, Stanley JC (eds): Therapy in Vascular Surgery, ed 2. Philadelphia, BC Decker, 1991.
27. Falanga V: Venous ulceration. J Dermatol Surg Oncol 1993; 19:764.
28. Falanga V, Kirsner R, Katz MH, et al: Pericapillary fibrin cuffs in venous ulceration: Persistence with treatment and during ulcer healing. J Dermatol Surg Oncol 1992; 18:409.
29. Fitzpatrick JE: Stasis ulcers: Update on a common geriatric problem. Geriatrics 1989; 44:19–31.
30. Foley WT: Treatment of gangrene of the feet and legs by walking. Circulation 1957; 15:689.
31. Friedmann LW: Selecting the therapeutic alternative for rehabilitating patients with occlusive arterial disease. Vasc Surg 1977; 11:321.
32. Gersh BJ, Rihal CS, Rooke TW, et al: Evaluation and management of patients with both peripheral vascular and coronary artery disease. J Am Coll Cardiol 1991; 18:203.
33. Gibbons GW, Marcaccio EJ Jr, Burgess AM, et al: Improved quality of diabetic foot care, 1984 vs 1990. Arch Surg 1993; 128:576.
34. Gloviczki P, Calcagno D, Schirger A, et al: Noninvasive evaluation of the swollen extremity: Experiences with 190 lymphoscintigraphic examinations. J Vasc Surg 1989; 9:683.
35. Gloviczki P, Merrell SW: Surgical treatment of venous disease. Cardiovasc Clin 1992; 22:81.
36. Gloviczki P, Morris SM, Bower TC, et al: Microvascular pedal bypass for salvage of the severely ischemic limb. Mayo Clin Proc 1991; 66:243.
37. Gloviczki P, Stanson AW, Stickler GB, et al: Klippel-Trenaunay syndrome: The risks and benefits of vascular interventions. Surgery 1991; 110:469.
38. Gupta SK, Girishkumar H: Lower extremity revascularization. J Cardiovasc Surg 1993; 34:229.
39. Helm PA, Walker SC, Pullium G: Total contact casting in diabetic patients with neuropathic foot ulcerations. Arch Phys Med Rehabil 1984; 65:691.
40. Helm PA, Walker SC, Pullium GF: Recurrence of neuropathic ulceration following healing in a total contact cast. Arch Phys Med Rehabil 1991; 72:967.
41. Hertzer NR: The natural history of peripheral vascular disease: Implications for its management. Circulation 1991; 83(suppl 1): 112.

42. Hiatt WR, Nawaz D, Regensteiner JG, Hossack KF: Evaluation of exercise performance in patients with peripheral vascular disease. J Cardiopulm Rehabil 1988; 12:525.
43. Hiatt WR, Regensteiner JG, Wolfel EE: Special populations in cardiovascular rehabilitation. Cardiol Clin 1993; 11:309–321.
44. Honet JC, Strandness DE Jr, Stolov WC, et al: Short-leg bracing for intermittent claudication of the calf. Arch Phys Med Rehab 1968; 49:578.
45. Ibrahim S, MacPherson DR, Goldhaber SZ: Chronic venous insufficiency: Mechanisms and management. Am Heart J 1996; 132:856.
46. Jamieson WG: State of the art of venous investigation and treatment. Can J Surg 1993; 36:119.
47. Janssen MCH, Nováková IRO, Verbruggen H, et al: New developments in the treatment of deep venous thrombosis. Netherlands J Med 1997; 50:36.
48. Jonason T, Jonzon B, Ringqvist I, et al: Effect of physical training on different categories of patients with intermittent claudication. Acta Med Scand 1979; 206:253.
49. Juergens JL, Spittell JA Jr, Fairbairn JF II: Peripheral Vascular Disease, ed 5. Philadelphia, WB Saunders, 1980.
50. Koch CA: External leg compression in the treatment of vascular disease. Angiology 1997; 48:S3.
51. Kerstein MD: The scientific basis of healing. Adv Wound Care 1997; 10:30.
52. Kloth LC, McCulloch JM: Promotion of wound healing with electrical stimulation. Adv Wound Care 1996; 9:42.
53. Larsen OA, Lassen NA: Effect of daily muscular exercise in patients with intermittent claudication. Lancet 1966; 2:1093.
54. Lauffer RB, Parmelee DJ, Dunham SU, et al: MS-325: Albumin-targeted contrast agent for MR angiography. Radiology 1998; 207:529.
55. Lindner DJ, Edwards JM, Phinney ES, et al: Long-term hemodynamic and clinical sequelae of lower extremity deep venous thrombosis. Vasc Surg 1986; 4:436.
56. Lofgren KA: Surgical management of chronic venous insufficiency. Acta Chir Scand Suppl 1988; 544:62.
57. McDaniel MD, Cronenwett JL: Basic data related to the natural history of intermittent claudication. Ann Vasc Surg 1989; 3:273.
58. Müllner T, Mrkonjic L, Kwasny O, Vécsei V: The use of negative pressure to promote the healing of tissue defects: A clinical trial using the vacuum sealing technique. Br J Plast Surg 1997; 50:194.
59. Nicolaides AN, Hussein MK, Szendro G, et al: The relation of venous ulceration with ambulatory venous pressure measurements. J Vasc Surg 1993; 17:414.
60. Niebauer J, Cooke JP: Cardiovascular effects of exercise: Role of endothelial shear stress. J Am Coll Cardiol 1996; 28:1652.
61. Orchard TJ, Strandness DE Jr: Assessment of Peripheral Vascular Disease in Diabetes: Report and recommendations of an international workshop sponsored by the American Heart Association and the American Diabetes Association; 18–20 September 1992, New Orleans, Louisiana. Diabetes Care 1993; 16:1199.
62. Osmundson PJ, Rooke TW, Hallett JW: Effect of arterial revascularization on transcutaneous oxygen tension of the ischemic extremity. Mayo Clin Proc 1988; 63:897.
63. Pappas CJ, O'Donnell TF: Long-term results of compression treatment for lymphedema. J Vasc Surg 1992; 16:555.
64. Pomposelli FB Jr, Jepsen SJ, Gibbons GW, et al: Efficacy of the dorsal pedal bypass for limb salvage in diabetic patients: Short-term observations. J Vasc Surg 1990; 11:745.
65. Porter JM, Cutter BS, Lee BY, et al: Pentoxifylline efficacy in the treatment of intermittent claudication: Multicenter controlled double-blind trial with objective assessment of chronic occlusive arterial disease patients. Am Heart J 1982; 104:66.
66. Porter JM, Rutherford RB, Claggett JP, et al: Reporting standards in venous disease. J Vasc Surg 1988; 8:172.
67. Richardson JK: Rocker-soled shoes and walking distance in patients with calf claudication. Arch Phys Med Rehab 1991; 72:554.
68. Rooke TW: The noninvasive vascular laboratory. Cardiovasc Clin 1992; 22:27.
69. Rooke TW: The use of transcutaneous oximetry in the noninvasive vascular laboratory. Int Angiol 1992; 11:36.
70. Rooke TW, Heser JL, Osmundson PJ: Exercise strain-gauge venous plethysmography: Evaluation of "new" device for assessing lower limb venous incompetence. Angiology 1992; 43:219.
71. Rooke TW, Hollier LH, Osmundson PJ: The influence of sympathetic nerves on transcutaneous oxygen tension in normal and ischemic lower extremities. Angiology 1987; 38:400.
72. Rooke TW, Martin RP: Lower extremity venous imaging for the echocardiologist. J Am Soc Echo 1990; 3:158.
73. Rooke TW, Osmundson PJ: Effect of intermittent venous occlusion on transcutaneous oxygen tension in lower limbs with severe arterial occlusive disease. Int J Cardiol 1988; 21:76.
74. Rooke TW, Osmundson PJ: Variability and reproducibility of transcutaneous oxygen tension measurements in the assessment of peripheral vascular disease. Angiology 1989; 40:695.
75. Schwartz RW, Logan NM, Johnson PJ, et al: Pentoxifylline increases extremity blood flow in diabetic atherosclerotic patients. Arch Surg 1989; 124:434.
76. Spittell JA Jr: Conservative management of occlusive peripheral arterial disease. Cardiovasc Clin 1992; 22:209.
77. Stillwell GK, Redford JWB: Physical treatment of postmastectomy lymphedema. Proc Staff Meet Mayo Clin 1958; 33:1.
78. Strandness DE Jr, Langlois YE, Roederer GO: Noninvasive evaluation of vascular disease. In Haimovici H (ed): Vascular Surgery: Principles and Techniques, ed 2. New York, Appleton-Century-Crofts, 1984, pp 19–42.
79. Strandness DE Jr, Langlois YE, Roederer GO: Preoperative evaluation of vascular disease. In Haimovici H (ed): Vascular Surgery: Principles and Techniques, ed. 2 New York, Appleton-Century-Crofts, 1984, pp 43–64.
80. Strandness DE Jr, Sumner DS: Applications of ultrasound to the study of arteriosclerosis obliterans. Angiology 1975; 26:187.
81. Tibbles PM, Edelsberg JS: Hyperbaric-oxygen therapy. New Eng J Med 1996; 334:1642.
82. Walker SC, Helm PA, Pullium G: Total contact casting and chronic diabetic neuropathic foot ulcerations: Healing rates by wound location. Arch Phys Med Rehabil 1987; 68:217.
83. Weiss RA: Evaluation of the venous system by doppler ultrasound and photoplethysmography or light reflection rheography before sclerotherapy. Semin Dermatol 1993; 12:78.
84. Wisham L, Abramson A, Ebel A: The value of exercise in peripheral arterial disease. JAMA 1953; 153:10.

READING LIST

Berni GA, Bandyk DF, Zierler RE, et al: Streptokinase treatment of acute arterial occlusion. Ann Surg 1983; 198:185.

Cooke JP, Creager MA: Management of the patient with intermittent claudication. Vasc Med Rev 1991; 2:19–31.

Mills JL, Beckett WC, Taylor SM: The diabetic foot: Consequences of delayed treatment and referral. South Med J 1991; 84:970.

Rooke TW, Osmundson PJ: The influence of age, sex, smoking, and diabetes on lower limb transcutaneous oxygen tension in patients with arterial occlusive disease. Arch Intern Med 1990; 150:129.

Sørlie D, Myhre K, Mjøs OD: Exercise and post-exercise metabolism of the lower leg in patients with peripheral arterial insufficiency. Scand J Clin Lab Invest 1978; 38:635.

Strandness DE Jr, Priest RE, Gibbons GE: Combined clinical and pathological study of diabetic and nondiabetic peripheral arterial disease. Diabetes 1964; 13:366.

57

CHAPTER

Theresa A. Gillis, M.D., and Fae H. Garden, M.D.

Principles of Cancer Rehabilitation

The number of people who have survived 5 years or more with a history of cancer is now estimated to be 4 million.[48] As this number continues to grow, medical professionals will have to redefine what is meant by "cancer survivor" to take into consideration various quality-of-life issues that were not relevant a decade ago.

DEFINING THE NEED FOR CANCER REHABILITATION

That cancer patients develop functional deficits resulting from their disease and treatment has been discussed in the medical literature for years.[61] Although it has been stated that "almost all patients with cancer can benefit from a rehabilitation assessment and intervention,"[42] convincing oncologists and oncologic surgeons of these needs and of the potential role of rehabilitation services has been a challenge.

With the exception of stomach and cervical tumors, the incidence rates for all of the major cancers have been increasing over the past four decades.[29] Advances in early cancer detection, combined with aggressive multimodality treatments, are allowing more people with cancer to live longer. These cancer survivors frequently face significant physical and psychosocial problems that adversely influence their quality of life (Fig. 57–1). Ganz et al[40] surveyed 500 patients with colorectal, lung, and prostate cancer who had been living with cancer for over a year and found that more than 80% reported gait problems, with 50% indicating that these problems were severe. Significant problems in activities of daily living (ADL) and vocational pursuits were also reported (Fig. 57–2). It has been estimated that up to 50% of persons with cancer may meet the diagnostic criteria for clinical depression.[100] The severity of the depression often correlates with the degree of physical impairment. With early intervention by a rehabilitation team, long-term disability caused by cancer and cancer therapy can be prevented or minimized. The typical members of a cancer rehabilitation team include a physiatrist, nurse, physical therapist, occupational therapist, recreational therapist, social worker, psychologist or psychiatrist, pharmacist, dietitian, speech-language pathologist and chaplain. If the primary care physician is other than the physiatrist, he or she provides the management focusing on critical medical issues that affect discharge and hospital care.

TYPES OF CANCER REHABILITATION

The general rehabilitation goals of cancer patients are similar to those of patients with impairments caused by other diseases. They include obtaining independent mobility and independence in basic ADL, with or without assistive devices. Rehabilitation goals can be further defined according to when they are applied in the different stages of the disease.[96] The goal of *preventive rehabilitation therapy* is to achieve maximal function in patients considered to be cured or in remission. For patients whose cancer is progressing, the goals of *supportive rehabilitation therapy* include providing adaptive self-care equipment in an attempt to offset what can be a steady decline in the patient's functional skills. Range-of-motion (ROM) exercises and bed mobility techniques can be taught in order to prevent the adverse consequences of immobility (see also Chapter 34). *Palliative rehabilitation therapy* goals are to improve or maintain comfort and function during the terminal stages of the disease.[49] The application of orthoses, mo-

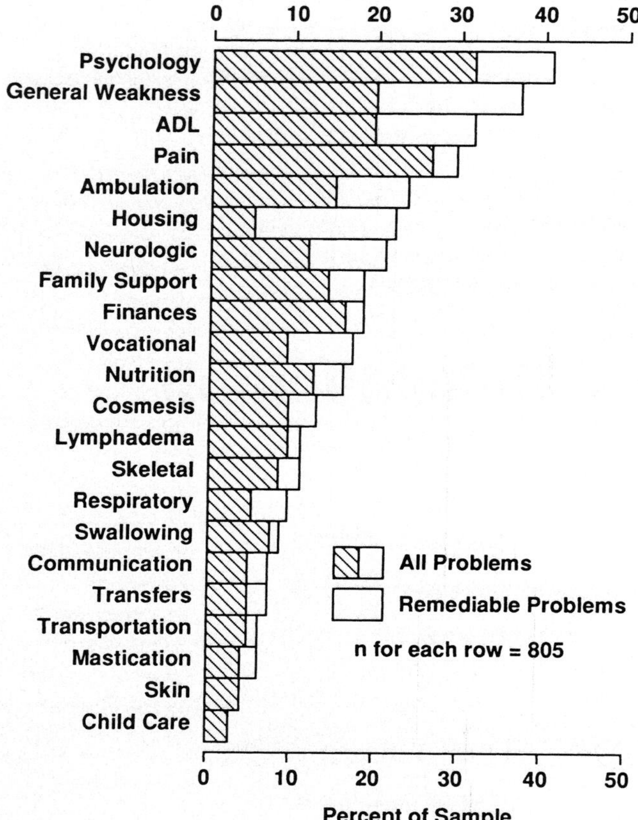

FIGURE 57–1. Percentage of people in sample with one or more rehabilitation problems. (From Lehmann JF, DeLisa JA, Warren CG, et al: Cancer rehabilitation: Assessment of need, development and evaluation of a model of care. Arch Phys Med Rehabil 1978; 59:412.)

dalities, and assistive equipment can be useful as an adjunct to pharmacological pain management.

CAUSES AND MANAGEMENT OF FUNCTIONAL IMPAIRMENT IN CANCER PATIENTS

Complications of Disuse and Bed Rest

The complications of immobility are described in detail in Chapter 34. These complications are pertinent in the cancer patient because of the typically prolonged period of illness, treatment, and recovery. Special issues in the cancer patient include the side effects of chemotherapy, especially from therapy with cardiotoxic drugs. When possible, a conditioning program started prior to cancer treatment is advisable.

Nutritional Concerns of Cancer Patients

Diet

Dietary factors have been in the research and medical spotlight recently as an important environmental influence on cancer prevention. The value and benefit of nutrition is generally recognized in the medical management and rehabilitation of cancer patients, and many cancer patients place appetite and ability to eat at the top of the list of items determining their sense of physical well-being.[16]

The comprehensive cancer treatment team should include a registered dietitian. The dietitian can initiate a screening process that takes into account the tumor type and treatment plan to determine whether a patient's nutritional status is at risk. From anthropometric data, an estimate of adult calorie and protein needs can be made. Caloric intake should generally be between 115% and 130% of resting energy expenditure. Protein needs range from 1.5 to 2.5 g/kg/day.[16, 67] Calorie and protein needs will vary depending on the type and extent of the tumor, as well as the type of treatment being used. The

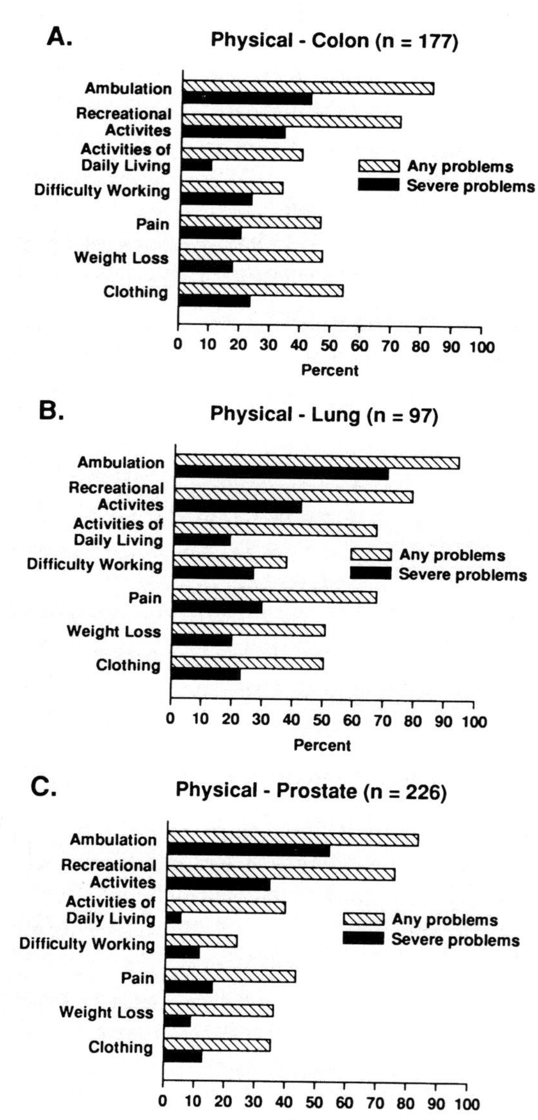

FIGURE 57–2. Constitutional and physical problems in colon (*A*), lung (*B*), and prostate (*C*) cancer patients living with cancer for more than a year since diagnosis. (From Haskell CM: Cancer Treatment, ed 3. Philadelphia, WB Saunders, 1990, p 885.)

impact of various surgical procedures on the nutritional status of cancer patients is summarized in Table 57–1.

Radiation Effects

Radiation therapy can also affect feeding and nutrition. Treatments to the head and neck area can produce alterations in taste and in saliva production. Distortion of food temperature and texture sensations can occur from radiation changes to the oral mucosa. Swallowing difficulties can result as well (see Chapter 26). Radiation treatments delivered to the stomach and intestines often lead acutely to nausea, vomiting, cramps, and diarrhea. Chronic complications include partial or complete intestinal obstruction, intestinal perforation, gastrointestinal bleeding, malabsorption, and enteral fistulas.[105] Attempts to feed patients who have sustained radiation damage to the intestines usually begin with lactose-free, low-residue oral diets and progress to enteral feedings or parenteral nutrition in more refractory cases.[70] Parenteral nutrition is recommended for patients who have lost 20% or more of their body weight.[30, 102]

Chemotherapy Effects

Cancer chemotherapeutic agents target the cell processes of malignant tumors. The rapidly reproducing cells of the bone marrow and gastrointestinal tract are vulnerable to the effects of chemotherapy as well. Nausea, vomiting, and anorexia are common initial gastrointestinal side effects. Severe and recurrent vomiting may cause vitamin B_1 deficiency, with resultant beriberi. The late effects of chemotherapy include stomatitis, mucosal ulceration, cheilosis, glossitis, and pharyngitis.

Numerous nutritional deficiencies can result from the use of antimetabolite drugs such as methotrexate. Folic acid metabolism, which is necessary for the synthesis of DNA, is inhibited by this drug. This inhibition causes a folic acid deficiency that results in macrocytic anemia, leukopenia, and an ulcerative stomatitis. The antimetabolites 5-fluorouracil and 6-mercaptopurine prevent nucleic acid synthesis by interfering with thiamine in DNA synthesis. Clinical signs of thiamine deficiency can be noted in the lips and oral cavity. Vitamin K deficiency results from long-term treatment with antibiotics such as moxalactam disodium, which can result in ecchymosis and a pronounced bleeding tendency.

TABLE 57–1 Potential Adverse Effects of Various Surgical Procedures on Nutrition in Cancer Patients

Procedure	Potential Adverse Effect
Neck dissection/glossectomy	Impaired mastication Impaired swallowing Impaired taste Impaired smell
Esophageal resection with vagotomy	Gastric stasis Diarrhea Steatorrhea
Pancreatomy	Diabetes mellitus Impaired digestion
Bowel resection	Malabsorption (short bowel syndrome) Vitamin deficiency (B_{12}, D, A)
Gastrectomy	Impaired digestion Malabsorption Megaloblastic anemia Hypoglycemia

Learned Food Aversion

During the course of cancer treatment, patients often reject specific foods or certain flavors. Although the exact mechanism for learned food aversion is unknown, it has been described as a variant of classical conditioning. The types of foods most susceptible to learned food aversion are meats, vegetables, and caffeinated beverages.[70] Various methods have been used to try to prevent learned food aversion. These include advising patients to eat very little before therapies.[6]

Proper nutritional support can be an important adjunct to cancer treatments.[67] Aggressive intervention to correct nutrient deficiencies and to maintain good nutritional status should be ongoing throughout the rehabilitation process. The use of appetite-stimulating drugs such as megestrol can improve quality of life in cancer patients with anorexia. When needed, enteral or parenteral feeding supplementation is useful in preventing weight loss, malnutrition, dehydration, and weakness.

Sexual Function in the Cancer Patient

The potential for sexual alteration or dysfunction is often ignored in cancer treatment plans. Yet both the cancer and the cancer treatment can affect this aspect of living (see Chapter 30). Inclusion of the possible impact of treatment on sexuality can be part of the informed consent procedure.[104]

Although most patients select treatments regardless of the potential for disfigurement, some refuse to risk the loss of a sex organ or body part. Sexual partners can contribute to sexual dysfunction by fostering dependent role changes or reacting in a negative way to the patient's physical disfigurement. Economic stress caused by the treatment can lead to marital problems that are expressed by avoidance of sexual contact. These issues must be sought out and addressed.

Concerns of Women

Although mastectomy has no direct physical effect on a woman's sexual response, the emotional effects of the procedure can have a profound negative impact. Fear of partner rejection can lead to avoidance of sexual intercourse. Encouraging partners to resume sexual activity as early as possible helps break this cycle.[56]

Women who have undergone pelvic surgery can feel a sense of guilt related to a false belief that sexual intercourse contributed to their disease.[12] Fear of disease recurrence can cause these women to avoid resumption of sexual activity. Women need to be counseled about the possible need for vaginal dilators to prevent stenosis as well as the possibility of bleeding with intercourse. The need for artificial lubrication and possibly a change from customary sexual positions should be discussed.

Regardless of a patient's age, the loss of fertility can precipitate a grief reaction. Presurgical preparation and counseling can reduce some of the psychodynamic causes of sexual dysfunction.

The side effects of chemotherapy and radiation therapy include nausea, fatigue, hair loss, and weight changes. These, along with hormonal depletion, can produce additional psychological and physical impediments to resuming sexual relationships.

Concerns of Men

Surgical treatment of prostate cancer can cause damage to the vascular or nerve pathways, resulting in impotence, retrograde ejaculation, or infertility. Orchiectomy has obvious hormonal and reproductive implications. Preoperative and pretreatment discussions of reproductive concerns should include consideration of sperm banking if permanent sterilization is anticipated.

Pelvic and abdominal radiation can produce fatigue, diarrhea, and erectile dysfunction. Irradiation of the urethra can cause painful ejaculation.[26] The effects of chemotherapy can adversely affect self-image, libido, and sexual performance. Sexual rehabilitation can include the use of erectile assistive devices and surgical reconstruction of the penis.

Neuropsychological Abnormalities

The neurobehavioral abnormalities found in tumor patients range from subtle problems with attention and motivation to frank delirium and clouding of consciousness. These deficits can be either primary, due to the tumor, or secondary, due to the treatment. They can also result from chronic illness, depression, or immobility.

Primary Tumor Effects

The majority of patients with primary or metastatic brain tumors have cognitive impairments that vary according to the location and size of the tumor. The pattern of neuropsychological deficits in patients with primary brain tumors can differ from those seen in cerebrovascular accidents or traumatic brain injury. Patients with brain tumors can have milder cognitive deficits and greater variability in the nature and extent of these deficits than patients with strokes in similar anatomical sites.[2] Even after extensive surgical resection of brain tissue, patients with slow-growing tumors often do not demonstrate neuropsychological deficits, perhaps because of a reorganization of cognitive functions to other brain regions.[75] Patients with rapidly growing tumors, such as glioblastoma multiforme, exhibit behavioral and cognitive deficits secondary to rapid destruction of white matter tracts, increased intracranial pressure, and metabolic deficits.[76] Improvements in cognitive and physical function have been noted in brain tumor patients receiving 10 mg of methylphenidate twice daily. Patients receiving this dosage showed increased stamina and motivation to perform activities in our center.

Radiation Effects

Additional effects on neuropsychological functioning can occur as a result of radiation therapy. The acute effects of radiation (during the time of treatment) are mostly symptomatic (headache and nausea). Subacute effects can occur 1 to 4 months after therapy is completed. At this time a reversible demyelination occurs in approximately 14% of brain tumor patients.[57] It is only by a gradual improvement in functional status during the ensuing 4 months that these symptoms can be distinguished from those caused by early tumor recurrence.[51] Delayed effects of radiation treatment can manifest 6 months to a year after therapy. The therapeutic dose of radiation for brain tumors can cause necrosis within 6 months of treatment.[79] Most of these lesions develop within the white matter of the forebrain.[110] In addition to focal necrosis, the delayed effects of brain irradiation can include atrophy, calcification, necrotizing leukoencephalopathy, aneurysms, and the formation of secondary cancers.[57]

Chemotherapy Effects

Chemotherapy, once believed to cause only early and reversible effects on cognition, is now recognized to be able to cause marked and prolonged neurobehavioral deficits. It is estimated that as many as 18% of neurologically normal cancer patients who have received chemotherapy have cognitive deficits 3 weeks after therapy is discontinued.[74] Deficits include impairments in visual-perceptive abilities, verbal memory, and judgment. Survivors of brain tumors who have received multimodality therapy (chemotherapy plus radiation) can have more profound impairments of intellectual function than those who receive single-modality treatment.[50] As cancer therapy becomes more effective, an increasing number of survivors will be in need of cognitive and vocational rehabilitation services.

Cancer Pain

Defining the Problem

The World Health Organization (WHO) estimates that 25% of all cancer patients die with unrelieved pain.[20] Up to 60% of patients at all stages of the disease process experience significant pain.[9] Most of this pain can be adequately relieved by oral analgesics.[109, 111] Unrelieved pain can be a risk factor for suicide in cancer patients.[14]

Etiology

Cancer pain can result from direct tumor invasion of pain-sensitive tissues or can be secondary to treatment or diagnostic procedures (Table 57–2). It can also be unrelated to any of these factors.

Treatment

An algorithm for medical decision making in the treatment of cancer pain has been devised by the WHO (Fig. 57–3). This three-step analgesic drug ladder outlines the use of nonopioid analgesics, opioid analgesics, and adjuvants for progressively more severe pain. Nonopioid analgesics, such as nonsteroidal anti-inflammatory drugs (NSAIDs), are associated with a ceiling effect for analgesia. Exceeding the maximum dosage range can result in organ toxicity that can mask similar toxici-

TABLE 57–2 Causes of Treatment-Related Pain in Cancer Patients

Chemotherapy-related pain
Oral mucositis
Peripheral neuropathy
Acute and chronic herpetic pain
Osteonecrosis secondary to steroids
Pseudorheumatism
Radiation-related pain
Osteoradionecrosis
Myelopathy
Brachial plexopathy
Lumbar plexopathy
Radiation-induced peripheral nerve tumors
Postsurgical pain
Post mastectomy
Post nephrectomy
Post thoracotomy
Post radical neck dissection
Residual limb and phantom limb
Procedure-related pain
Bone marrow biopsy
Bone biopsy
Lumbar puncture and spinal headache
Venipuncture

From Campa JA, Payne R: Pain syndromes due to cancer treatment. In Patt R (ed): Cancer Pain. Philadelphia, JB Lippincott, 1993, p 42.

ties from antineoplastic agents if the two are used concomitantly.

Opioid agonists do not exhibit ceiling effects. Dosing is guided by efficacy and is limited by side effects (Table 57–3). Long-acting oral preparations, particularly sustained-release morphine, are commonly used. Breakthrough pain can be treated with immediate-release "rescue doses" of morphine. Patients with moderate to severe pain requiring opioid therapy for more than a few days can be treated with a long-acting semisynthetic narcotic such as oxycodone hydrochloride. The recommended initial dose of oxycodone hydrochloride is 10 mg every 12 hours in patients not already taking opioid medications. A 5 mg immediate-release dosage is also available for breakthrough pain. Transdermal fentanyl provides an alternative method of analgesia with a longer duration for a given dose. It takes up to 24 hours for blood concentrations of fentanyl to stabilize after the application of a patch. Although oral administration is preferred, transdermal, rectal, and intravenous routes are indicated in some patients. Spinal routes, both epidural and intrathecal, can be employed with internal delivery systems that allow patients to be fully ambulatory. Children often need larger doses of opioids to achieve adequate pain relief.[72]

Tolerance to analgesia is an infrequent problem and is usually managed by changing doses or agents.[38] Physical dependence develops with chronic opioid use. *Addiction,* defined as a behavioral syndrome of compulsive, harmful use not requiring the existence of physical dependence or tolerance,[53] is not likely to occur in patients without a substance abuse history.[94] If necessary, the reduction of opiate dosing can be done slowly. The autonomic symptoms of withdrawal can be partly alleviated by the use of transdermal clonidine.[64]

Adjuvant drugs include antidepressants, anticonvulsants, benzodiazepines, neuroleptics, psychostimulants, antihistamines, corticosteroids, and calcitonin. These medications are chosen to supplement analgesics for their specific secondary effects or to treat side effects. Radiation therapy can also be highly effective in treating pain by shrinking the tumor mass.[52]

A significant number of patients whose pain does not respond to oral therapy might be helped by anesthetic procedures, such as nerve blocks. Surgical ablation of nervous structures by procedures such as rhizotomy or cordotomy can also play a role in pain relief for certain patients. There is, however, a risk of developing a delayed pain syndrome following such surgical deafferentation.

Deafferentation pain can be caused by a loss of normal sensory input when a peripheral nerve is severed or involved by tumor. Transcutaneous electrical nerve stimulation can provide some patients with relief. In addition, carefully selected patients might also benefit from surgical implantation of stimulation devices.[32]

LATE EFFECTS OF CANCER TREATMENT

Effects of Radiation Therapy

Myelopathy

The effects of radiation to the spinal cord and peripheral nervous systems are multifactorial and cannot be

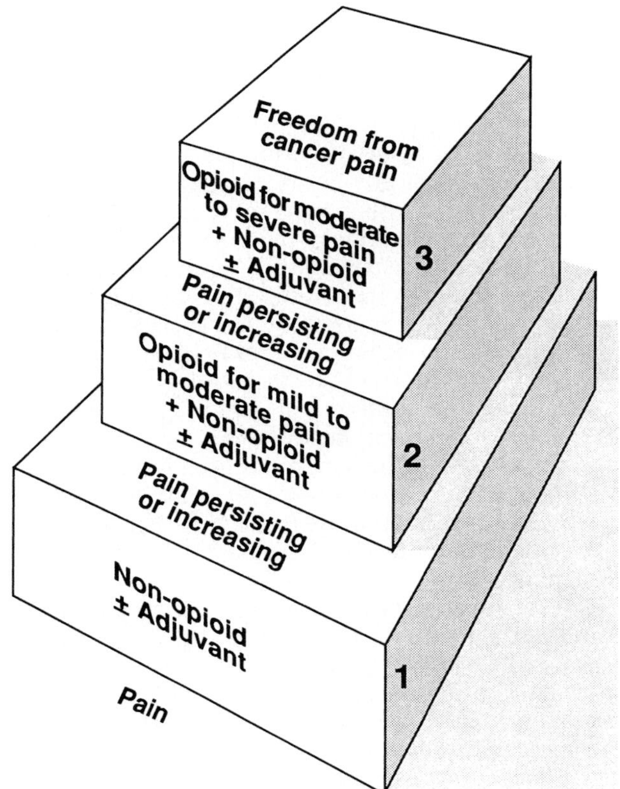

FIGURE 57–3. The WHO three-step analgesic ladder. (From Cancer Pain Relief and Palliative Care: Report of a WHO Expert Committee. Technical Report Series, no 804. Geneva, World Health Organization, 1990.)

TABLE 57–3 Oral and Parenteral Opioid Analgesic Equivalences and Relative Potency of Drugs as Compared with Morphine

	Parenteral (mg)	Oral (mg)	Conversion Factor (IV to PO)	Duration (Parenteral, Oral) (hr)
Narcotic Agonists				
Morphine	10	30	3.0[#]	3–4
Controlled-release morphine				
MS Contin	—	30	—	12
Roxanol SR	—	30	—	8
Methadone (Dolophine)*	10	20	2.0	4–8
Hydromorphone (Dilaudid)	1.5	7.5	5.0	2–3
Fentanyl†	100 μg	—	—	1
Meperidine (Demerol)‡	75	300	4.0	2–3
Levorphanol (Levo-Dromoran)	2	4	2.0	3–6
Codeine	130	200	1.5	3–4
Oxycodone (Roxicodone, component of Percodan, Tylox)§	—	30	—	3–5
Hydrocodone (Lortab, component of Vicodin)§	—	200‖	—	3–5
Propoxyphene (Darvon, component of Darvocet)*§	—	200	—	3–6
Mixed Agonist-Antagonists ¶				
Pentazocine (Talwin)	60	180	3.0	2–4
Nalbuphine (Nubain)	10	—	—	4–6
Butorphanol (Stadol)	2	—	—	4–6

* Long half-life; observe for drug accumulation and side effects.
† Available in transdermal system (Duragesic) supplying 25, 50, 75, or 100 μg.
‡ Not recommended for long-term or high-dose use because of CNS toxic metabolites (normeperidine, norpropoxyphene).
§ With the exception of Roxicodone and Darvon, these drugs are combined with acetylsalicylic acid (ASA) or acetaminophen in doses from 325 to 750 mg. Dosage must be monitored for safe limits of ASA or acetaminophen.
‖ Equivalence data not substantiated; thought to approximate codeine.
¶ Note. Drugs from this category should NOT be used in combination with narcotic agonist drugs. Converting a patient from an agonist to an agonist-antagonist could precipitate a withdrawal crisis in the narcotic-dependent patient.
\# Conversion factor listed is for chronic dosing: single doses may require 6:1 factor.
Courtesy of C. Stratton Hill, Jr., M.D., and the Texas Cancer Pain Initiative, Houston.

entirely attributed to dosage, site, or technique. The most common form of radiation-induced spinal cord injury is a transient myelopathy that occurs in patients being treated for head and neck tumors or lymphoma. The syndrome typically develops after a latent period of 1 to 30 months, with a peak onset at 4 to 6 months.[31] A transient demyelination of the ascending sensory neurons in the posterior column and lateral spinothalamic tract is postulated as the pathogenesis for this disorder. The clinical onset is marked by electrical shock sensations or paresthesias that radiate from the cervical spine to the extremities. The paresthesias are typically symmetrical and do not follow a dermatomal distribution.[66] Myelography and computed tomography (CT) are typically negative, and the syndrome usually resolves in 1 to 9 months.[31] The occurrence of transient radiation myelopathy does not put a person at a higher risk for the development of more severe delayed radiation-induced myelopathy.[31]

Delayed myelopathy is an irreversible condition with a reported incidence of 1% to 12%.[99] The onset of symptoms usually occurs 9 to 18 months after completion of treatment,[31] with most cases identified within 30 months. The latent period for delayed myelopathy decreases with increased radiation dose and is shortened in children.[65] The onset of symptoms usually begins with lower extremity paresthesias, followed by sphincter dysfunction and weakness. A partial Brown-Séquard syndrome consisting of sensory changes on one side and motor weakness or pyramidal tract signs on the opposite side can develop below the level of the injury. Functional deficits typically occur progressively and depend, for the most part, on the level of neurological injury. A central pain syndrome can be present in up to 20% of patients with radiation myelopathy. Patients typically note pain in their midback region and dysesthetic sensations in their lower extremities. Central pain syndrome may show some clinical response to treatment with tricyclic antidepressant, steroid, or anticonvulsant medications.

Plexopathy

Brachial plexopathy is a well-recognized complication of radiotherapy in patients with breast, lung, and mediastinal tumors, as well as lymphoma and other neoplasms. The latent period between the end of radiotherapy and the appearance of clinical symptoms ranges from 1 month to 15 years.[35] Chemotherapy can enhance the radiation-induced effects on nerve tissue and decrease the latency period for the development of plexopathy.[87] The predominant initial symptoms are paresthesias and pain (Table 57–4). Clinical signs include sensory loss, decreased or absent reflexes, and weakness.

Distinguishing between radiation-induced brachial plexopathy and that due to neoplastic infiltrations is often a clinical challenge. Horner's syndrome and pain are more common in neoplastic plexopathy, whereas extremity lymphedema is more common in radiation

TABLE 57–4 Differential Diagnosis Between Cancerous and Postradiation Brachial Plexopathies

Parameter	Cancerous	Postradiation
Incidence	10 times more common	Dose-related
Initial symptom	Pain 90%	Numbness, paresthesia, pain in less than 20%
Signs	Predominantly lower trunk	Predominantly upper trunk
Progression rate	Slow	Insidious, self-limiting
Latency	Months to over 20 yr; mean: several years	
Tumor progression	CT: focal lesions in over 90%	CT: loss of planes, no focal lesions
EMG		Myokymia

Abbreviations: EMG, electromyography; CT, computed tomography. From Hildebrand J: Lesions of the peripheral nervous system. In Hildebrand J (ed): Management in Neuro-Oncology. Berlin, Springer-Verlag, 1992, p 80.

plexopathy.[60] Electrodiagnosis has also been used to help differentiate between metastatic and radiation-induced plexopathy. Myokymic discharges and abnormal sensory conduction studies are more common in patients with radiation plexopathy than in those with neoplastic plexopathy.[46]

Rehabilitation management of radiation plexopathy includes providing adequate pain relief, maximizing the remaining function, and preventing the complications of immobility. After acute pain and inflammation have subsided, patients can be started on low-resistance weight exercises, which are gradually increased to a full shoulder and arm rehabilitation program. Neck rehabilitation exercises should be included, especially when the upper portion of the plexus has been injured. The shoulder often requires the support of a sling to prevent glenohumeral subluxation. Substitutes for lost hand and arm function include the use of flexor-hinge tenodesis and opponens splints. Wheelchair users with brachial plexopathy can benefit from using a balanced forearm orthosis for feeding and self-care. A functional arm orthosis attached to a hip cap can be constructed for the ambulatory patient.

Lumbosacral plexopathy is reported less frequently than brachial plexopathy but can occur in patients with colorectal and gynecological tumors who undergo radiation therapy. Symptoms often present bilaterally although seldom symmetrically (Table 57–5). Pain or paresthesias usually precede the development of motor symptoms, which include weakness and muscle atrophy.[82]

Effects of Chemotherapy

Neurotoxicity is a common complication for cancer chemotherapy. A progressive distal symmetrical sensory neuropathy occurs with cisplatin treatment.[39] Vincristine and cytarabine also have peripheral neuropathy as a principal toxic and dose-limiting side effect (see Chapter 47). Encephalopathies, cerebellar syndromes, myelopathy, and stroke-like syndromes can all occur after the administration of various chemotherapeutic agents.

Bleeding Problems

Both chemotherapeutic and radiotherapeutic procedures can cause thrombocytopenia. Exercise in the presence of thrombocytopenia can increase the risk of intra-articular bleeding. Bleeding from the lungs or oral and nasal mucosa can also occur. In general, platelet levels below 10,000/mL preclude exercise therapy, and the risk of intracerebral bleeding becomes significant below this level.[3, 55] Some centers allow aerobic but not resistive activities in patients with platelet counts between 10,000 and 20,000/mL.[3, 92]

REHABILITATION ISSUES IN SPECIFIC CANCERS

Breast Cancer

Eighteen percent of all cancer deaths in women are due to breast cancer, and it remains the leading cause of death for women 40 to 55 years of age.[80]

Surgical Options

Standard treatment has evolved from radical mastectomies to breast conservation strategies. Radical mastectomy requires resection of both the pectoralis major and minor muscles and the axillary lymph nodes. This leads to significant shoulder dysfunction, pain, lymphedema, and emotional trauma. Modified radical mastectomies, which spare the pectoralis major but include axillary dissection, are now more common. Other surgical options include lumpectomy and segmental (partial) or simple (total) mastectomy with or without axillary dissection. Varying combinations of radiotherapy, hormonal therapy, and adjuvant chemotherapy augment

TABLE 57–5 Differential Diagnosis Between Cancerous and Postradiation Lumbosacral Plexopathies

Parameter	Cancerous	Postradiation
Primaries	Colorectal, sarcomas, lymphomas, breast carcinoma	Cervical ovarian carcinoma; dose-related
Initial symptom	Pain in 70% to 80%	Weakness in about 50%
Signs	Bilateral in 10% to 25%	Bilateral in 80%
Latency	Variable	Median 5 yr; 1 to 31 yr
Tumor progression	Focal CT/MRI abnormalities	No focal abnormalities
EMG		Myokymia

Abbreviations: CT, computed tomography; MRI, magnetic resonance imaging; EMG, electromyography. From Hildebrand J: Lesions of the peripheral nervous system. In Hildebrand J (ed): Management in Neuro-Oncology. Berlin, Springer-Verlag, 1992, p 80.

the surgery and have reduced mortality. A common breast reconstruction procedure is the transverse rectus abdominis muscle (TRAM) flap (Fig. 57–4), which leads to a weakened abdominal musculature in some patients.[47, 62] Other reconstruction options include the use of tissue expanders followed by prosthetic implants, and latissimus dorsi transfers.

Rehabilitation Issues

The most common rehabilitation needs of women undergoing modified radical mastectomy or segmental mastectomy during the first month after primary treatment are identified in Figure 57–5.[41] The mobility limitations and weakness affect these patients' daily functional tasks, such as household chores, driving, lifting, and overall physical activity level. Early physical therapy has been shown to improve postoperative shoulder motion,[93] while delayed therapy is associated with poor range of motion.[37]

In postmastectomy patients who have not undergone reconstruction, shoulder abduction and flexion to 45 to 90 degrees is permitted immediately postoperatively. Some physicians prefer the use of abduction slings or pillows immediately postoperatively, with the goal of ensuring painless shoulder movement within this range.[4, 27] Immediate postoperative therapies can safely consist of hand pumping, wrist and elbow ROM exercise, elevation, scapular mobility, and postural exercises. Deep breathing and methods of relaxation are appropriate as well. A gentle, supine, passive shoulder ROM program to 90 degrees of flexion and abduction is begun, with external and internal rotation performed to tolerance. When surgical drains are removed, active and active-assisted range can be increased. At this time, wall climbing, wand, and overhead pulley exercises are also added. After all sutures have been removed, more aggressive ROM exercise is pursued. The use of physical modalities may be necessary at this point to reduce painful muscle splinting. Scar massage is generally begun 1 month postoperatively. Instructions for a home exercise program and a follow-up physical therapy assessment should ideally be included in every case. ROM exercise is particularly critical during and after radiation treatment to lessen the likelihood of fibrotic contracture formation.

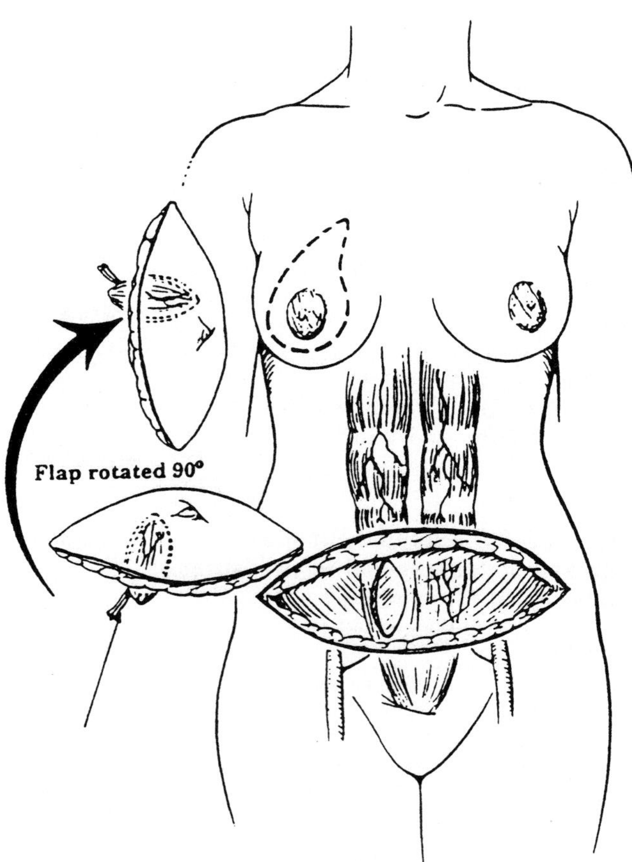

FIGURE 57–4. Transverse rectus abdominis muscle flap breast reconstruction in which the skin, subcutaneous tissue, and a portion of the rectus abdominis muscle and rectus sheath are removed from the lower abdomen and transferred to the chest for shaping into a breast mound. (From Miller MJ, Ross MR: Pregnancy following breast reconstruction with autogenous tissue. Cancer Bull 1993; 45:546–548.)

Lymphedema

Lymphedema is a frequent complication of breast cancer treatment. The overall incidence of this condition following mastectomy is 25.5%, climbing to 38.3% in patients undergoing axillary node clearance and radiation therapy.[58] Arm swelling can occur transiently in the immediate postoperative period, and this early form may resolve spontaneously. It can also occur as a result of cellulitis, requiring the use of antibiotics and analgesics and avoidance of compression until the infection resolves. The onset of lymphedema 2 years or more after treatment can be a sign of recurrent tumor occluding the lymphatic system. Occasionally, venous Doppler or radiolabeled venous flow studies may be necessary to diagnose thrombosis. Lymphedema is painless but is often accompanied by sensations of tightness or heaviness, and it is associated with neck or shoulder discomfort as the limb grows larger. A gradual progression occurs if left untreated, with an increased risk of cellulitis, further lymphatic damage, and extremity enlargement in a vicious cycle.

Education regarding lymphedema detection, prevention, and avoidance of infection is critical for all patients following lymphatic injury by surgery or irradiation. Early and aggressive treatment reduces the likelihood of chronic lymphatic overload, inflammation, and infection. Elevation, manual lymphatic drainage, compressive bandaging and garments, and pneumatic pumps may be employed in treatment.[7, 11, 21, 114, 116] Microsurgical techniques for lymphatic reconstruction are under investigation[83, 66] but have limited use at present. Benzopyrones, which stimulate macrophage breakdown of lymphatic proteins,[22] have not been approved for use in the United States. Patients must be taught a lifelong management plan for their lymphedema (see chapter 56).

Pain

A variety of pain symptoms have been reported in breast cancer patients. Chest wall tenderness is common

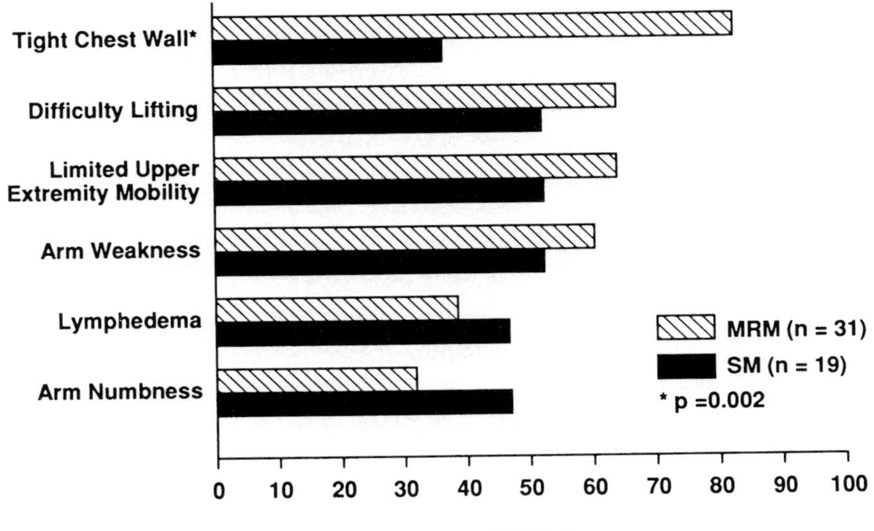

FIGURE 57–5. Most frequent physical problems directly related to breast cancer patients by type of primary treatment. MRM, modified radical mastectomy; SM, simple mastectomy. (From Ganz PA, Schag CC, Polinsky ML, et al: Rehabilitation needs and breast cancer: The first month after primary therapy. Breast Cancer Res Treat 1987; 10:243–253.)

after radiation treatment and can continue for years after treatment.[44] Allodynia or dysesthesia often occurs in the distribution of the intercostobrachial nerve. Adhesive capsulitis of the shoulder, transient brachial plexus neuritis, and acute and chronic radiation-related plexopathies can also occur. Phantom breast pain has also been described, affecting at least 10% of mastectomy patients.[59] It occurs more commonly in women with premastectomy pain.

Cosmetic Concerns

Cosmetic rehabilitation attempts to restore a woman's external physical appearance can be accomplished by the use of temporary breast forms made of fluffed cotton or lamb's wool. These can be given to the woman postoperatively, prior to discharge. A permanent prosthesis can usually be fitted 3 to 8 weeks after surgery, when the chest wall edema has resolved and the tissue is well healed. Both immediate and delayed reconstruction options exist, and irradiated skin in the axilla and chest are not contraindications. Some women choose to forgo reconstruction, often out of fear of recurrent tumor in the remaining breast tissue.[34]

Bone and Soft Tissue Tumors

Bone and soft tissue sarcomas are uncommon, accounting for just 0.5% to 1.0 % of adult malignancies in the United States,[19] but the rehabilitation concerns of these patients are particularly pertinent. The most common sarcoma in both adults and children is osteosarcoma of the knee or proximal humerus.[25] With advances in treatment, the 5-year survival rate for these tumors has advanced to nearly 80%.[103]

Amputation remains the preferred procedure for most high-grade malignancies of the distal lower extremity. Amputation at this level provides superior function and less morbidity than salvage or reconstruction surgery. Amputation might be unavoidable for very proximal tumors, especially when associated with intrapelvic extension.

Tumor amputees differ from dysvascular and traumatic amputees in several ways. Chemotherapy-induced fatigue, anemia, nausea, and cardiovascular toxic effects can sharply diminish functional capacity.[71, 113] Wound healing is often delayed over irradiated ports, and skin may be less tolerant of prosthesis wear. Anorexia with weight loss, muscle atrophy, and fluid shifts during chemotherapy can delay definitive prosthesis fabrication.[23] Many tumor amputees are children, with different cosmetic and functional concerns than those of adults. Amputee and prosthetic management is discussed in Chapters 13 and 14.

Criteria for limb salvage procedures include the ability to totally resect the tumor without sacrifice of major nerves and vessels, and the ability of a reconstruction to provide function equal or superior to that of an appropriate prosthesis. Pathological fractures and distant metastases are contraindications to such procedures. Limb salvage procedures are increasing in frequency and are associated with long-term survival and local recurrence rates equivalent to those of amputation.[18]

Metastatic Bone Lesions

The most frequently encountered bone tumors are metastatic in origin. Prostate carcinoma accounts for 60% of all bone metastases in men, and carcinomas of the breast account for 70% of all metastatic lesions in women.[1] The pathogenesis of bone metastasis is not well known. Skeletal metastases appear to arise primarily through hematogenous spread.[36] Batson[5] described a venous system connecting to and bypassing pulmonary, portal, and caval venous flow (Fig. 57–6). This network of veins has multidirectional flow determined by external pressure and related to biomechanical action and position. It is commonly believed to be a major hematogenous route for the spread of metastasis.

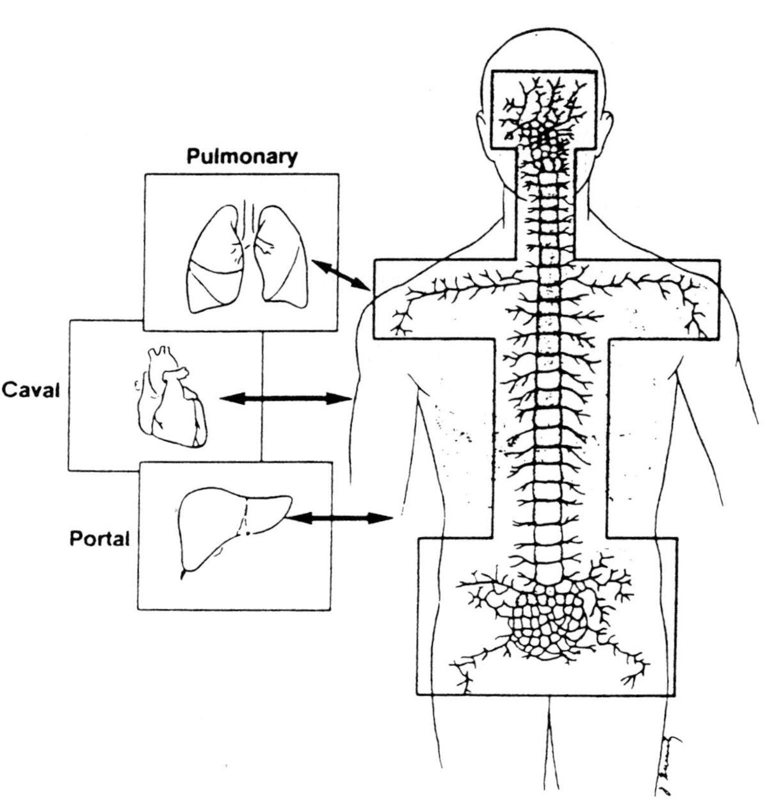

FIGURE 57–6. Batson's plexus of veins. (Modified from Batson OV: The function of the vertebral veins and their role in the spread of metastasis. Ann Surg 1940; 112:138–149.)

Patients with symptomatic bone lesions complain of localized pain that increases in severity and frequency, and is often worse at night than during the day. Pain was rated as moderate or severe in intensity in nearly 80% of patients presenting with symptomatic lesions.[54] Patients may develop reduced ROM at involved hips or shoulders, and increased pain with axial loading of involved long bones. Such symptoms in cancer patients should prompt a search for metastases, starting with radiographs for most sites and MRI for spinal complaints. Radionuclide bone scintigraphy is helpful when radiographs are inconclusive but metastasis is suspected.[13] However, in cases of lung tumor, melanoma, and multiple myeloma, bone scans frequently have false negative results.[13]

Long Bone Involvement

Pathological fractures occur in 10% to 30% of patients with metastatic bone lesions. These fractures are most common in the long bones, especially the femur and humerus.[68, 95] Bone strength is determined by both cortical and trabecular structure. Cortical destruction makes bone particularly susceptible to torsion and rotation fractures because such forces are no longer transmitted uniformly through the cortex (Fig. 57–7).

Efforts have been made to define the risk of pathological fracture at metastatic sites, in order to determine the need for preemptive surgical treatment. Most guidelines suggest increase fracture risk, and therefore appropriateness for surgical stabilization, when painful lesions are greater than 2.5 cm in diameter, occupy 50% or more of bony cortical diameter, or involve greater than 50% of medullary cross-sectional area or cortex.[68] Determining such involvement may be facilitated by CT coronal views. Surgical fixation usually involves removal of the tumor through curettage, with the use of methyl methacrylate, intramedullary rods, modular prostheses, or other hardware to repair the defect. Radiation treatments create transient softening of bone and theoretically increase the fracture risk for 6 to 8 weeks.[52] Reduced weight bearing may be recommended during this time for patients not treated with surgical fixation.

Vertebral Involvement

Metastases to the spine often involve the vertebral body, although they can settle in the paravertebral tissues, and they most frequently occur within the thoracic spine.[108] Pain can arise from epidural or root compression, intraosseous pressure from growing tumor cells, or mechanical instability. Severe neck or back pain or radicular or myelopathic findings require an immediate MRI evaluation and consideration of bolus dosing of methylprednisolone to prevent spinal cord compression. Goals of treatment should include pain control, avoidance of neurological compromise by tumor or spinal instability, local tumor control, and maximizing patient function. Pain can respond to external-beam radiation therapy, chemotherapy, bone-seeking radioisotopes, or surgical stabilization, individually or in combination.[73, 84] Management may also include the use of external orthoses and analgesic medications.

Head and Neck Tumors

Head and neck cancers constitute about 5% of all malignancies.[115] The larynx is the most commonly affected site, followed by the oral cavity, pharynx, and salivary gland. Malignant disease of the head and neck region can result in profound swallowing and nutritional prob-

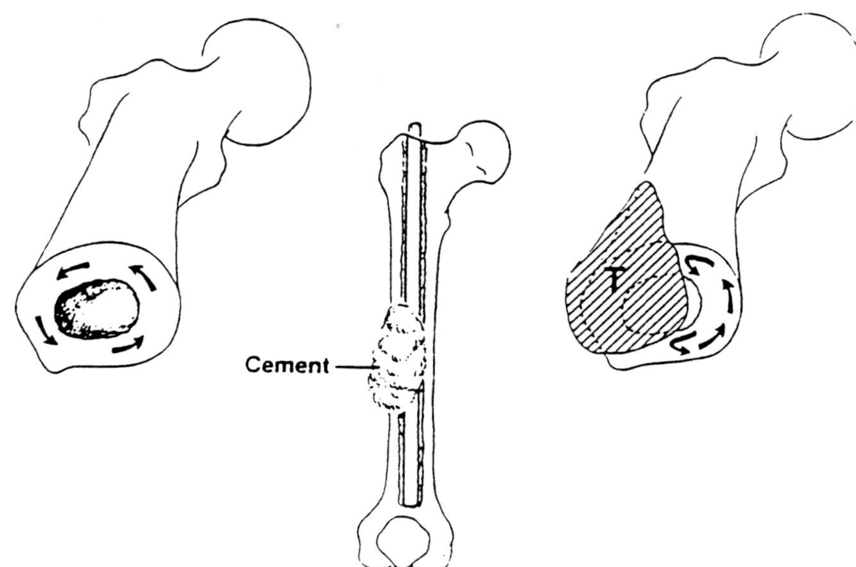

FIGURE 57–7. Schema demonstrating the biomechanical basis of intramedullary fixation of a bone with a large tumor defect. The normal rotational stress forces (*curved arrows*) are transmitted by the cortex in a uniform manner. A tumor defect (T) causes a stress riser that weakens the bone by 70% to 90% in torsion (rotation). The bone can be reconstructed by removing the tumor and reconstructing the defect with a combination of polymethylmethacrylate and intramedullary rod fixation. (From DeVita J, Hellman S, Rosenberg SA, et al (eds): Cancer: Principles and Practice of Oncology, ed 3. Philadelphia, JB Lippincott, 1989, p 2231.)

lems. The sensory functions of vision, hearing, balance, taste, and smell can be altered either by the disease or by its treatment. The goals of treatment, which include (1) eradication of cancer, (2) maintenance of adequate physiological function, and (3) achievement of socially acceptable cosmesis, can only be achieved through a multidisciplinary approach.

Surgery and radiotherapy can be, in some cases, curative.[115] Delayed surgical problems may arise and include deficits in swallowing (see Chapter 26) and speech (see Chapter 3).

Shoulder

Of special concern to the physiatrist are the shoulder impairment and chronic neck pain that can occur following radical neck dissection. The spinal accessory nerve is usually sacrificed during radical neck dissection. It can be incised in the lower neck where it enters the trapezius muscle and in the upper neck where it enters the sternocleidomastoid muscle. Postoperative shoulder problems occur with the loss of trapezius muscle function (Fig. 57–8). This causes the scapulae to move laterally, and deepens the axilla. Strengthening of the levator

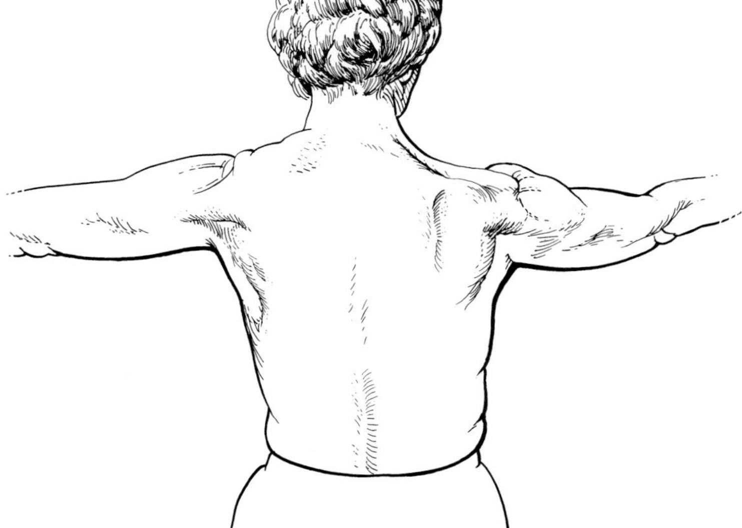

FIGURE 57–8. Scapular winging following radical neck dissection with trapezius muscle weakness.

scapulae, rhomboids, and serratus anterior, while not capable of completely substituting for trapezius function, can diminish pain and improve scapular stability and shoulder elevation.

The pectoralis muscle group is the main antagonist of the trapezius. Unopposed pull of the pectoralis muscles following radical neck dissection results in shoulder contracture with the scapulae in a protracted position.[28] Avoiding contracture of this muscle group is a major goal of postoperative rehabilitation. Table 57–6 outlines a sample postoperative exercise program for shoulder rehabilitation following radical neck dissection.

Neck

Unilateral disruption of the sternocleidomastoid, platysma, omohyoid, and diagnostic muscles can lead to asymmetrical neck motion.[28] These patients often need to support their neck and head with their hands when changing from a supine to sitting position. Following bilateral radical neck dissection, a patient is unable to flex the neck against gravity. In both cases, a passive ROM program can be initiated once sutures are removed. This can be advanced to active resistive strengthening by the 4th to 6th postoperative week. Scar massage and daily stretching following radiation therapy is essential to maintain mobility.

TABLE 57–6 Sample Postoperative Exercise Program for Head and Neck Cancer Patients

I. A. To be done lying on your back on a firm surface, with your hips and knees bent and your feet flat on the mat:
1. Keeping the back of your shoulders in contact with the mat, move your shoulders toward your ears and then relax.
2. With hands at your side and elbows straight, raise your arms forward and over your head. You may assist with your other hand, if necessary.
3. With hands at your side and elbows straight, move your arms away from your body toward your ear, keeping your arms in contact with the mat.
4. Clasp hands behind neck and push elbows back into the mat. Hold for a count of 5 and then relax without bringing your elbows forward.

B. To be done sitting on a straight-backed chair:
1. With your hands on your hips, try to touch your elbows together behind you.

II. A. To be done sitting on a straight-backed chair, maintaining good posture:
1. Slowly bring your head forward, touching chin to chest, then back as far as possible.
2. Tilt your head to the side, bringing your ear toward your shoulder without turning your head or raising your shoulder.
3. Rotate your head as far as possible to look over your shoulder without allowing the shoulder to come forward.

III. A. To be done standing in a corner:
1. Place one hand on each wall, holding elbows away from sides, and lean forward into the corner.

IV. A. To be done lying on your stomach with a pillow under your waist:
1. With your arms at a 90-degree angle to your body, raise your arms off the mat toward the ceiling.
2. a. With arms at sides, raise your head and then your shoulders. When you can perform this exercise with ease, substitute the following exercise in its place.
b. With your hands clasped behind your neck, raise your head and then your shoulders off the mat, keeping your elbows back.

V. A. To be done sitting on a straight-backed chair, maintaining good posture:
1. Slowly open and close your mouth. Do not force your mouth open or clench your teeth tightly.
2. With your jaws slightly apart, move your lower jaw from side to side.
3. With your jaws slightly apart, move your lower jaw forward and then back.

Spinal Cord Lesions

Tumor involvement of the spinal cord can result from primary or metastatic lesions. Primary tumors (meningiomas, neurofibromas, gliomas) are relatively rare. The majority of tumors affecting the spinal cord are metastatic in origin, and 95% are extradural.[89]

Most extradural metastases arise from the vertebral body and result in compression of the anterior aspect of the spinal cord (Fig. 57–9). The thoracic spine has a smaller ratio of canal to cord diameter than the lumbar or cervical segments; approximately 70% of diagnosed spinal metastasis occur in the thoracic spine.[45] The clinical presentation of spinal cord compression often involves complaints of pain that becomes worse in the recumbent position. Multiple spinal levels can be simultaneously involved. The development of bowel or bladder dysfunction can indicate spinal cord compromise, yet the onset of such symptoms may be obscured in patients taking opiates or adjuvant analgesics, which may cause constipation and urinary retention. Slowly evolving symptoms are indicative of gradual cord impingement and may respond to corticosteroids and radiotherapy. The rapid evolution of paraparesis over several hours usually signifies arterial compromise by tumor invasion or pressure, with a more guarded prognosis for recovery.

Treatment

The optimal surgical approach and stabilization procedures for metastatic spine lesions remain controversial.[86, 90, 106] Stability is of special concern if the tumor involves two or three vertebrae. Halo fixation, while providing the greatest stability to the cervical spine, is often poorly tolerated and unacceptable to many cancer patients. Sternal-occipital-mandibular immobilization is usually better tolerated and provides adequate flexion and extension stability to the lower cervical segments. The Philadelphia and similar hard collars can provide acceptable stability in flexion and extension for higher levels, but do not sufficiently restrict rotation and lateral bending in the lower cervical segments (see Chapter 17).

The "clamshell"-style thoracic-lumbar-sacral orthosis may be used to provide thoracic and lumbar support. However, its considerable support may not be an option for patients with painful rib or iliac crest metastases, friable or intolerant skin from steroid or radiation therapy, or dyspnea due to lung tumors or restrictive lung disease. Less restrictive devices serve only as proprioceptive cues but may still provide comfort and are more easily tolerated.

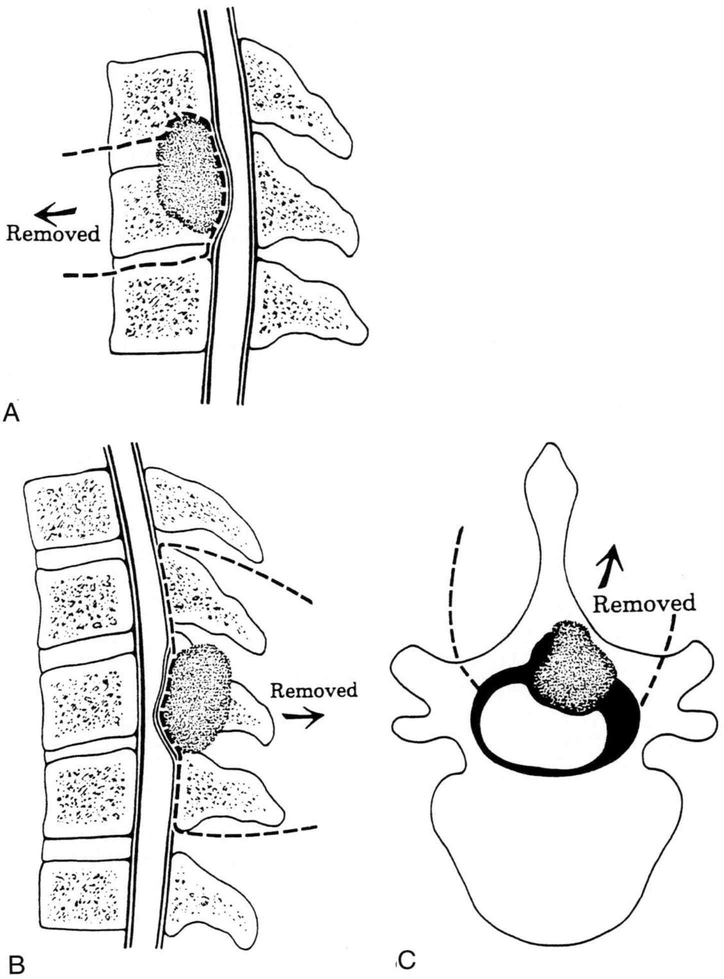

FIGURE 57–9. *A.* Most spinal metastases occur in the vertebral column anterior to the spinal canal. When surgery is indicated for tumors anterior to the spinal canal, surgical excision of the tumor and involved vertebral body with immediate stabilization of the spinal column effectively reverses compression of the spinal cord. *B* and *C.* Cord compression by tumors posterior to the spinal canal can be successfully relieved by laminectomy (removal of the laminae and spinous processes one level above and one level below the site of tumor) and tumor excision. (From DeVita JT, Hellman S, Rosenberg SA, et al (eds): Cancer: Principles and Practice of Oncology, ed 3. Philadelphia, JB Lippincott, 1989, p 1981.)

Brain Tumors

The rehabilitation of brain tumor patients differs from that for stroke or traumatic brain injury patients due to differences in the patterns of recovery. Normal brain tissue can be compressed or destroyed by tumor in discrete areas. The location of the lesion determines the resultant neurological deficits, which can be entirely reversed when focal pressure is relieved. Some patients experience dramatic improvement in function within hours after surgical resection. Most patients have a significant return of function when the tumor involvement is not extensive.[85]

The incidence of and mortality from primary brain tumors are increasing.[8] In 1993, 17,500 people in the United States were expected to be diagnosed with primary brain tumors.[10] More than 90% of the primary malignant tumors of the brain in adults are high-grade astrocytomas, and of these, the most common is glioblastoma multiforme.[97] Low-grade astrocytomas are the most common primary brain tumors in children. Medulloblastomas account for 20% of all intracranial tumors in children and are usually located near the cerebellar vermis.[63] Pediatric primary tumors tend to be infratentorial, while those in adults are more likely supratentorial. Metastatic lesions comprise roughly 25% to 30% of all intracranial tumors. Lung, gastrointestinal, and urinary tract tumors account for the majority of these metastases in men. In women, breast, lung, gastrointestinal, and melanoma primary tumors dominate.[107]

Symptoms and Signs

The presenting symptoms and signs of brain tumor involvement can include headache, weakness, seizures, and changes in cognition. Headache is the most common symptom. Weakness, the most common focal sign, is present on physical examination in 65% of patients.[112] Seizures occur in 20% of patients with supratentorial tumors. These are often focal motor or sensory seizures and localized to the area of tumor involvement, although they may be generalized. Nausea and vomiting are more common in patients with infratentorial lesions and in children.

Rehabilitation Issues

Despite improvements in the median survival rates of primary brain tumor patients and advances in the treatment of metastatic gliomas, survival for many of these patients is limited. Many patients with glioblastoma multiforme or high-grade astrocytoma die within 2 years.[112] Rehabilitation for brain tumor patients can dramatically improve the quality of their remaining life. Efforts directed toward preventing skin breakdown and contractures, progressive mobilization and transfer training, and relearning of activities of daily living are appropriate. Speech therapy is indicated for patients with aphasia, dysarthria, and dysphagia[81] and, together with neuropsychology, can provide compensatory strategies for patients with cognitive impairments.

PEDIATRIC CANCER REHABILITATION

The most common childhood cancer is leukemia (30% to 40%), especially acute lymphocytic leukemia (ALL), followed by central nervous system (CNS) tumors (20%), bone cancer (7%), and neuroblastoma (5%).[98]

Cancer deaths in children have decreased by approximately 50% in the past 25 years owing to improvement in detection and treatment.[33] Many survivors of childhood cancer have chronic neurological and musculoskeletal problems caused by the tumor or treatment. Brain irradiation done either as a primary treatment or as a prophylactic method is associated with cognitive decline, particularly when performed on children less than 7 years old.[24] Significant decreases in visuomotor and fine motor skills, along with attrition in arithmetic skills, spatial memory, and intelligence quotient (IQ) scores, have been reported following CNS irradiation in children.[78] Direct tumor effects and combined therapies also contribute to cognitive function decline.[89]

Children being treated for brain tumors can experience cerebellar disturbances and hemiparesis. Changes in visual acuity and oculomotor function can occur as well.[88] Hearing losses from chemotherapy, particularly vincristine, may also restrict normal childhood activities. Children treated for ALL are at increased risk of falling behind a grade level or needing special education classes.[17]

Musculoskeletal concerns of the pediatric cancer patient include the development of spinal deformities (kyphosis and scoliosis), especially when radiation is given during periods of rapid skeletal growth.[77] Bone sarcoma and the effects of limb salvage surgery or amputation are discussed above. Childhood growth patterns are frequently abnormal after completion of cancer treatment.

Most children with cancer experience pain, and in nearly two-thirds of cases the pain is treatment related.[77] Direct effects of tumors, including bone metastases and nerve compression, are also important causes of pain. The pharmacological treatment of cancer pain in children includes narcotics, NSAIDs, tricyclic antidepressants, amphetamines, and topical preparations. Oral meperidine use is avoided in children because its toxic metabolite, normeperidine, can cause seizures. Fentanyl is a short-half-life narcotic that is effective for use in acute pain from outpatient surgical procedures.

Children with cancer have a 17% incidence of developing a second malignancy by 20 years of age.[97] Radiation and chemotherapy are potential carcinogens. Chronic immunodeficiency following treatment and genetic predisposition also play a role in secondary tumor development.

SUMMARY

The number of people with a history of cancer who have survived 5 years or more continues to increase. Advances in early cancer detection, combined with aggressive multimodality treatments, are causing medical professionals to consider quality of life issues that were not relevant a decade ago. Outcome studies suggest that significant benefits may be derived from rehabilitation for various oncology diagnoses.[15, 43, 69, 85, 91, 101] Many communities and cancer centers now recognize that early intervention by a rehabilitation team can minimize long-term disability caused by cancer and cancer therapy.

REFERENCES

1. Abrams HL, Spiro R, Goldstein N: Metastases in carcinoma: Analysis of 1000 cases. Cancer 1950; 23:74–85.
2. Anderson SW, Damasio H, Tranel D: Neuropsychological impairments associated with lesions caused by tumor or stroke. Arch Neurol 1990; 47:397–405.
3. Andrykowsky MA, Henslee PJ, Farrall MG: Physical and psychosocial functioning of adult survivors of allogenic bone marrow transplantation. Bone Marrow Transplant 1989; 4:75–81.
4. Barbash S, Anathakrishnan N, Mohan CR: Postoperative positioning after mastectomy and other procedures in the pectoral region. Aust NZ J Surg 1982; 52:293.
5. Batson OV: The function of the vertebral veins and their role in the spread of metastases. Ann Surg 1940; 112–188.
6. Bernstein I, Webster MM, Bernstein ID: Food aversions in children receiving chemotherapy for cancer. Cancer 1982: 50:2961–2963.
7. Bertelli G, Venturini M, Forno G, et al: An analysis of prognostic factors in response to conservative treatment of postmastectomy lymphedema. Surg Gynecol Obstet 1992; 175:455–460.
8. Bondy ML, Wrensch M: Update on brain cancer epidemiology. Cancer Bull 1993; 45:365–369.
9. Bonica JJ: Treatment of cancer pain: Current status and future needs. In Fields HL, Dubner R, Cervero F, et al (eds): Advances in Pain Research and Therapy, vol 9. New York, Raven Press, 1985, pp 589–616.
10. Boring CC, Squires TS, Tong T: Cancer statistics, 1993. CA 1993; 43:7–26.
11. Boris M, Weindorf S, Lasinski B: Lymphedema reduction by noninvasive complex lymphedema therapy. Oncology 1994; 9:95–106.
12. Bos G: Sexuality of gynecologic cancer patients: Influence of traditional role patterns. In Aaronson NK, Beckmann JH (eds): The Quality of Life of Cancer Patients, New York, Raven Press, 1987, pp 207–213.
13. Brage ME, Simon MA: Evaluation, prognosis and medical treatment considerations of metastatic bone tumors. Orthopedics 1992; 15:589–594.
14. Breitbart W: Suicide. In Holland J, Rowland J (eds): Handbook of Psycho-Oncology. New York, Oxford University Press, 1990, pp 291–299.
15. Bunting RW, Boublik M, Blevins FT, et al: Functional outcome of pathologic fracture secondary to malignant disease in a rehabilitation hospital. Cancer 1992; 69:98–102.
16. Burgess J: Cancer therapy. In Skipper A: Dietitians' Handbook of Enteral and Parenteral Nutrition. Rockville, MD, Aspen, 1989, p 121.
17. Byrd R: Late effects of treatment of cancer in children. Pediatr Clin North Am 1985; 32:835–851.

18. Cammisa FP, Glasser DB, Otis JC, et al: The Van Nes tibial rotationplasty. J Bone Joint Surg Am 1990; 72:1541–1547.
19. Cancer Facts and Figures—1988. New York, American Cancer Society, 1988, p 8.
20. Cancer Pain Relief and Palliative Care. Geneva, World Health Organization, 1990.
21. Casley-Smith JR, Casley-Smith JR: Modern treatment of lymphoedema. Mod Med Austral 1992; 35:70–83.
22. Casley-Smith JR, Margan RG, Piller NB: Treatment of lymphedema of the arms and legs with 5,6, benzo-[a]-pyrone. N Engl J Med 1993; 329:1158–1163.
23. Cole WG, Klein RW, van Lith M, et al: Prosthetic programme after above-knee amputation in children with sarcomata. J Bone Joint Surg Br 1982; 64:586–589.
24. Copeland DR, Fletcher JM, Pfefferbaum-Levine B, et al: Neuropsychological sequelae of childhood cancer and long term survivors. Pediatrics 1985; 75:745–753.
25. Dahlin DC, Coventry MB: Osteogenic sarcoma: A study of six hundred cases. J Bone Joint Surg Am 1967; 49:101.
26. Davis M, Das S: Psychosexual support for genitourinary cancer patients. In Crawford ED, Das S (eds): Current Genitourinary Cancer Surgery. Philadelphia, Lea & Febiger, 1990, pp 669–674.
27. Degenshein GA: Mobility of the arm following radical mastectomy. Surg Gynecol Obstet 1977; 145:77.
28. DeLisa JA, Miller RM, Melnick RR, et al: Rehabilitation of the cancer patient. In DeVita VT, Hellman S, Rosenberg SA (eds): Cancer Principles and Practice of Oncology, ed 2. Philadelphia, JB Lippincott, 1989, pp 2155–2188.
29. Devesa SS, Silverman DT, Young JL, et al: Cancer incidence and mortality trends among whites in the United States 1947–1984. JNCI 1977; 79:701.
30. Douglass HO: Nutritional support of the cancer patient. Hosp Formulary 1984; 19:220–234.
31. Dropcho EJ: Central nervous system injury by therapeutic irradiation. Neurol Clin 1991; 9:969–988.
32. Duncan GH, Bushnell MC, Marchand S: Deep brain stimulation: A review of basic research and clinical studies. Pain 1991; 45:49–60.
33. Ellenberg L, McComb JG, Siegel SE, et al: Factors affecting intellectual outcome in pediatric brain tumor patients. Neurosurgery 1987; 21:638–644.
34. Fallowfield LJ, Baumm M, Maguire GP: Effects of breast conservation on psychological morbidity associated with diagnosis and treatment of early breast cancer. Br Med J 1986; 293:1331.
35. Fardin P, Lelli S, Negrin P, et al: Radiation-induced brachial plexopathy: Clinical and electromyographical considerations in 13 cases. Electromyogr Clin Neurophysiol 1990; 30:277–282.
36. Fidler IJ, Radinsky R: Genetic control of cancer metastasis. JNCI 1990; 82:160–168.
37. Flew TJ: Wound drainage following radical mastectomy: The effect of restriction of shoulder movement. Br J Surg 1979; 66:302.
38. Foley KM: Pharmacologic approaches to cancer pain management. In Fields HL, Dubner R, Cervero F, et al (eds): Advances in Pain Research and Therapy, vol 9. New York, Raven Press, 1985, pp 629–653.
39. Forman A: Peripheral neuropathy in cancer patients: Clinical types, etiology, and presentation. Oncology 1990; 4:85–89.
40. Ganz PA, Coscarelli Schag CA, Heinrich RL: Rehabilitation. In Haskell CM (ed): Cancer Treatment. Philadelphia, WB Saunders, 1990, pp 883–892.
41. Ganz PA, Schag CC, Polinsky ML, et al: Rehabilitation needs and breast cancer: The first month after primary therapy. Breast Cancer Res Treat 1987; 10:243.
42. Ganz PA: Current issues in cancer rehabilitation. Cancer 1990; 654:742–751.
43. Garstang SV, Gillis TA, Graves DE: Maintenance of functional gains following inpatient cancer rehabilitation. Arch Phys Med Rehabil (in press).
44. Gerber L, Lampert M, Wood C, et al: Comparison of pain, motion, and edema after modified radical mastectomy vs local excision with axillary dissection and radiation. Breast Cancer Res Treat 1992; 21:139.
45. Gilbert RW, Kim JH, Posner JB: Epidural spinal cord compression from metastatic tumor: Diagnosis and treatment. Ann Neurol 1978; 3:40–51.
46. Harper CM, Thomas JE: Distinction between neoplastic and radiation-induced brachial plexopathy, with emphasis on the role of EMG. Neurology 1989; 39:502–506.
47. Hartrampf CR: The transverse abdominal island flap for breast reconstruction: A 7-year experience. Clin Plast Surg 1988; 15:703.
48. Herold AH, Roetzheim HG: Cancer survivors. Primary Care 1992; 4:779–791.
49. Hinterbuchner C: Rehabilitation of the disability cancer. NY State J Med 1978; 78:1066–1069.
50. Hochberg FH, Slotnick B: Neuropsychologic impairment in astrocytoma survivors. Neurology 1980; 30:172–177.
51. Hoffman WF, Levia VA, Wilson CB: Evaluation of malignant glioma patients during the post irradiation period. J Neurosurg 1979; 50:624–628.
52. Hoskin PJ: Scientific and clinical aspects of radiotherapy in the relief of bone pain. Cancer Surv 1988; 7:69–86.
53. Jaffe JH: Drug addiction and drug abuse. In Gilman AG, Goodman LS, Rall TW, et al (eds): The Pharmacologic Basis of Therapeutics, ed 8. New York, Macmillan, 1985, pp 532–581.
54. Janjan NA, Payne R, Gillis T, et al: Presenting symptoms in patients referred to a multidisciplinary clinic for bone metastases. J Pain Symptom Manage 1998; 16:171–178.
55. Jones AL, Miller JL: Bone marrow morbidity of chemotherapy. In Plowman PN, McElwain TJ, Meadows AT, et al (eds): Complications of Cancer Management. Oxford, Butterworth-Heinemann, 1991, p 371.
56. Kaplan HS: A neglected issue: The sexual side effects of current treatments for breast cancer. J Sex Marital Ther 1992; 18:3–19.
57. Kingsley DPE, Kendll BE: CT of the adverse effects of therapeutic radiation of the central nervous system. AJNR 1981; 2:453–460.
58. Kissen MW: Risk of lymphedema following the treatment of breast cancer. Br J Surg 1986; 73:580.
59. Kroner K, Knudsen UB, Skov J, et al: Long-term phantom breast syndrome after mastectomy. Clin J Pain 1992; 8:346.
60. Lederman RJ, Wilbourn AJ: Brachial plexopathy: Recurrent cancer or radiation. Neurology 1984; 34:1331–1335.
61. Lehmann JF, DeLisa JA, Warren CG, et al: Cancer rehabilitation: Assessment of need, development and evaluation of a model of care. Arch Phys Med Rehabil 1978; 59:410–419.
62. Lejour M, Dome M: Abdominal wall function after rectus abdominis transfer. Plast Reconstr Surg 1991; 87:1054.
63. Levin VA, Gutin PH, Leibel S: Neoplasms of the central nervous system. In DeVita VT Jr, Hellman S, Rosenberg SA (eds): Cancer: Principles and Practice of Oncology, ed 4. Philadelphia, JB Lippincott, 1993, pp 1679–1737.
64. Levinson SF: Rehabilitation of the patient with cancer of human immunodeficiency virus. In DeLisa JA (ed): Rehabilitation Medicine: Principle and Practice, ed 2. Philadelphia, JB Lippincott, 1993, pp 916–933.
65. Liebel SA, Guten PH, Davis RL: Tolerance of the brain and spinal cord. In Guten PH (ed): Radiation Injury to the Nervous System. New York, Raven Press, 1991, pp 239–256.
66. Louton RB, Terranova WA: The use of suction curettage as an adjunct to the management of lymphedema. Ann Plast Surg 1989; 22:354–357.
67. Maillet JO: The cancer patient. In Lang CE: Nutritional Support in Critical Care. Rockville, MD, Aspen, 1987, p 250.
68. Mandi A, Szepesi K, Moroxz I: Surgical treatment of pathologic fractures from metastatic tumors of long bones. Orthopedics 1991; 14:43–50.
69. Marciniak CM, Sliwa JA, Spill G, et al: Functional outcome following rehabilitation of the cancer patient. Arch Phys Med Rehabil 1996; 77:54–57.
70. Mattes RD, Arnold C, Boraas M: Learned food aversions among cancer chemotherapy patients. Cancer 1987; 60:2576–2580.
71. McElwain TJ: Cardiac morbidity of chemotherapy. In Plowman PN, McElwain TJ, Meadows AT (eds): Complications of Cancer Management. Oxford, Butterworth-Heinemann, 1991, pp 182–192.
72. McGrath PA: Pain in Children: Nature, Assessment and Treatment. New York, Guilford Press, 1990.
73. Mercadanate S: Malignant bone pain: Pathophysiology and treatment. Pain 69; 1997:1–18.

74. Meyers CA, Abbruzzese JL: Cognitive functioning in cancer patients: Effect of previous treatment. Neurology 1992; 42: 434–436.
75. Meyers CA, Berman SA, Hayman A, et al: Pathological left-handedness and preserved function associated with a slowly evolving brain tumor. Dev Med Child Neurol 1992; 34:1102–1117.
76. Meyers CA, Scheibel RS: Early detection and diagnosis of neurobehavioral disorders in cancer patients. Oncology 1990; 4: 115–122.
77. Miser AW, Miser JS: The treatment of cancer pain in children. Pediatr Clin North Am 1989; 36:979–999.
78. Mulhern RK, Horowitz ME, Kovnar EH, et al: Neurodevelopmental status of infants and young children treated for brain tumors with pre-irradiation chemotherapy. J Clin Oncol 1989; 7:1660–1666.
79. Nakagaki H, Brunhart G, Kemper TL, et al: Monkey brain damage from radiation in the therapeutic range. J Neurosurg 1976; 44:3–11.
80. National Center for Health Statistics: Vital Statistics of the United States, vol 2. Mortality. Part A. US Department of Health and Human Services publication (PHS) no 90-110. Washington, DC, US Department of Health and Human Services, Public Health Service, 1990.
81. Newton HB, Newton C, Pearl D, et al: Swallowing assessment in primary brain tumor patients with dysphagia. Neurology 1994; 44:1927–1932.
82. Numata K, Ito M: A case of delayed radiation lumbosacral plexopathy. Brain Nerve 1990; 42:629–633.
83. O'Brien BM, Mellow CG, Khazanchi RK, et al: Long-term results after microlymphatico-venous anastomoses for the treatment of obstructive lymphedema. Plast Reconstr Surg 1990; 85:562–572.
84. O'Connor MI, Currier BL: Metastatic disease of the spine. Orthopedics 1992; 15:611–620.
85. O'Dell MW, Barr K, Spanier D, et al: Functional outcome of inpatient rehabilitation in persons with brain tumors. Arch Phys Med Rehabil 1998; 79:1530–1534.
86. O'Neil J, Gardner V, Armstrong G: Treatment of tumors of thoracic and lumbar spinal column. Clin Orthop 1988; 227: 103–112.
87. Olsen NK, Pfeiffer P, Mondrup K, et al: Radiation induced brachial plexus neuropathy in breast cancer patients. Acta Oncol 1990; 29:885–890.
88. Peckham VC: Learning disabilities in long term survivors of childhood cancer: Concern for parents and teachers. Int Disabil Stud 1991; 13:141–145.
89. Perrin RG, McBroom RJ, Perrin RG: Metastatic tumors of the cervical spine. Clin Neurosurg 1992; 37:740–755.
90. Perrin RG, McBroom RJ: Spinal fixation after anterior decompression for symptomatic spinal metastases. Neurosurgery 1988; 22:324–327.
91. Philip PA, Ayyangar R, Vanderbilt J, et al: Rehabilitation outcome in children after treatment of primary brain tumor. Arch Phys Med Rehabil 1994; 75:36–39.
92. Poliquin CM: Post-bone marrow transplant patient management. Yale J Biol Med 1990; 63:495–502.
93. Pollard R, Callum KG, Altman DG, et al: Shoulder movement following mastectomy. Clin Oncol 1976; 2:343.
94. Porter J, Jick H: Addiction rare in patients treated with narcotics. N Engl J Med 1980; 302:123.
95. Pugh J, Sherry H, Futterman B, et al: Biomechanics of pathologic fractures. Clin Orthop 1982; 169:109–114.
96. Ragnarsson KT: Principles of cancer rehabilitation medicine. In Holland JF (ed): Cancer Medicine. Philadelphia, Lea & Febiger, 1993, p 1054.
97. Ries LAG, Hankey BF, Miller BA, et al: Cancer Statistics Review 1973–1988. US Department of Health and Human Services publication (NIH) no 91-2789. Bethesda, MD, National Cancer Institute, 1991.
98. Ryan BR: Principles of pediatric oncology. In Lewis MM (ed): Musculoskeletal Oncology: A Multidisciplinary Approach. Philadelphia, WB Saunders, 1992, pp 73–86.
99. Schultheiss TE, El-Jahdi AM: Statistical analysis of two hundred radiation myelopathy cases. Presented at the Seventh International Congress of Radiation Research, 1983, D:3–41.
100. Shakin EJ, Heiligenstein E, Holland JC: Psychiatric complications of cancer. In Plowman PN, McElwain TJ, Meadows A (eds): Complications of Cancer Management, Oxford, Butterworth-Heinmann, 1991, p 423.
101. Sherer M, Meyers CA, Bergloff P: Efficacy of postacute brain injury rehabilitation for patients with primary malignant brain tumors. Cancer 1997; 80:250–257.
102. Silvain C, Besson I, Ingrand P, et al: Long-term outcome of severe radiation enteritis treated by total parenteral nutrition. Dig Dis Sci 1992; 37:1065–1071.
103. Sim FH: Primary bone malignancies: Current advances that improve survival. J Musculoskel Med 1987; 4:49.
104. Smith DB, Babaian RJ: The effects of treatment for cancer on male fertility and sexuality. Cancer Nurs 1992; 15:271–275.
105. Smith DH, Decosse JJ: Radiation damage to the small intestine. World J Surg 1986; 10:189–194.
106. Sundaresan N, Galicich JH, Lane JM, et al: Treatment of neoplastic epidural cord compression by vertebral body resection and stabilization. J Neurosurg 1985; 63:676–684.
107. Takakura K, Sano K, Hoho S, et al: Metastatic Tumors of the Central Nervous System. Tokyo, Igaku-Shoin, 1982.
108. Tubiana-Hulin M: Incidence, prevalence and distribution of bone metastases. Bone 1991; 12(suppl 1):S9–S10.
109. Ventafridda V, Tamburini M, Caraceni A, et al: A validation study of the WHO method for cancer pain relief. Cancer 1987; 59:850–856.
110. Wakisaka S, O'Neill RR, Kemper TL, et al: Delayed brain damage in adult monkeys from radiation in the therapeutic range. Radiat Res 1979; 80:277–291.
111. Walker VA, Hoskin PJ, Hanks GW, et al: Evaluation of WHO analgesic guidelines for cancer pain in a hospital-based palliative care unit. J Pain Symptom Manage 1988; 3:145–149.
112. Wallner KE, Galicich JH, Krol G, et al: Patterns of failure following treatment for glioblastoma multiforme and anaplastic astrocytoma. Int J Radiat Oncol Biol Phys 1989; 16:1405–1409.
113. Weesner KM, Bledsoe M, Chaurenet A, et al: Exercise echocardiography in the detection of anthracycline cardiotocicity. Cancer 1991; 66:435–438.
114. Yamazaki Z, Idezuki Y, Nemoto T, et al: Clinical experiences using pneumatic massage therapy for edematous limbs over the last 10 years. Angiology 1988; 39:154–163.
115. Zagars G, Norante JD: Head and Neck Tumors in Clinical Oncology, ed 6. New York, American Cancer Society, 1983, pp 230–261.
116. Zanolla R, Monzeglio C, Balzarini A, et al: Evaluation of the results of three different methods of postmastectoy lymphedema treatment. J Surg Oncol 1984; 26:210–213.

58 CHAPTER

M. Catherine Spires, M.D.

Rehabilitation of Patients with Burns

The human and economic cost of burn injuries is enormous. More than 70,000 persons are hospitalized each year for burn injury.[4] Men in the 18- to 25-year age group are most at risk for sustaining a significant thermal injury. Burn size and the patient's age are the cardinal determinants of survival. Mortality is highest in the very young and the elderly,[102] and is greater in females than in males with comparable injuries.[96] The average person believes that a serious burn injury is the most devastating trauma a person can survive.[92]

Burn injury is not a new problem. Mankind has struggled with burn injuries since the discovery of fire. Documents as early as the Ebers's Papyrus in 1600 B.C. specify burn treatment techniques.[42] Hippocrates stressed cleaning burn wounds with wine or water to avoid suppuration.[34] Cornelius Celsus, in first-century Rome, described one of the first surgical excisions of a contracted burn scar.[77]

With the advent of grafting techniques, early closure of burn wounds became possible, significantly improving survival rates. Pollack performed one of the earliest free skin autografts in 1871.[35] The development of the drum dermatome by Padgett and Hood in 1939 and the mesh dermatome by Tanner and Vandeput in 1963 made covering larger wounds possible through autografts.[35] These advances and the refinement of allograft and heterograft techniques resulted not only in early wound closure and increased survival, but also in reduced pain, fluid losses, and infection.

Evans devised a method of calculating fluid loss from burn injury based on the percentage of body surface area burned and the patient's weight.[29] More accurate fluid resuscitation improved survival rates. The commonly used fluid replacement formulas of Parkland and Baxter are based on the initial work of Evans.[8]

Modern burn treatment is the result of a long history of medical and technological advances. The survival rate of seriously burned patients has increased dramatically, especially in the past three decades. More patients are returning to active lives at home, at work, and in the community. The physiatrist is uniquely trained to manage the complex rehabilitation problems of burn injuries and to aid burn patients in returning to a full and productive life.

THE INTEGUMENT

The skin is the largest organ of the body and serves multiple functions. It is composed of a network of specialized epithelial and dermal cells, collagen, elastic fibers, small blood vessels, and nerve endings. Skin is a complex organ that acts as a mechanical barrier to protect internal organs from chemicals and foreign material. It is essential to fluid homeostasis, thermoregulation, and the body's immunological defense.

Skin Components

Skin consists of two major components, the epidermis and the dermis (Fig. 58–1). The epidermis has four layers—the stratum corneum, stratum granulosum, stratum spinosum, and stratum basale. A fifth layer, the stratum lucidum, is present on the palms of the hands and the soles of the feet. The stratum corneum is the resilient, semitransparent outermost layer that acts as a barrier to water transfer. The deepest layer, the stratum basale, is the major site of cell mitosis. Keratinocytes are the most numerous cells of the epidermis (Fig. 58–2). Originating in the stratum basale, keratinocytes migrate to the stratum corneum, undergoing keratinization. During this process, keratinocytes flatten and become anucleate, and leave a protective protein layer of keratin on the skin surface.[14]

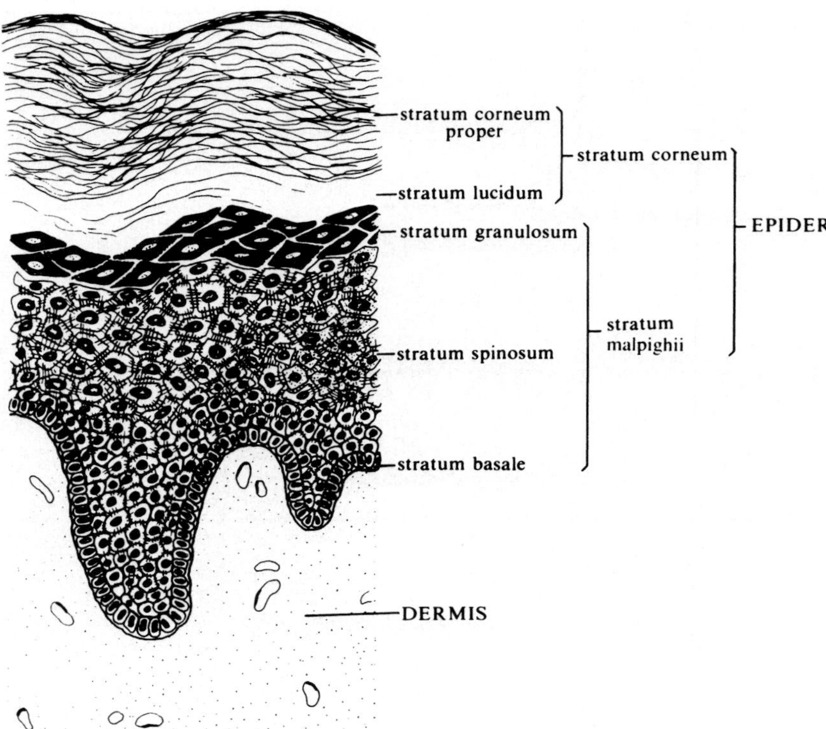

FIGURE 58–1. The histological characteristics of normal skin. Notice that the stratum lucidum is found only on the palms of hands and the soles of feet. (From Borysenko M, Beringer T: Functional Histology, ed 2. Boston, Little, Brown, 1984, p 228.)

The epidermis has a number of appendages. Hair follicles are lined by epidermal cells, which are in continuity with the epidermis and serve as a reservoir of epidermal cells in the event of injury. The sebaceous glands produce sebum, which moisturizes the skin. Eccrine glands dissipate heat through production of sweat and are essential in thermoregulation.

The epidermis is nourished by the underlying dermis. Undulating projections of the dermis, rete pegs, fit intimately with the stratum basale and reduce shear forces during mechanical manipulation. Rete pegs are underdeveloped in children and atrophied in the elderly. The dermis is composed of elastic fibers and loosely arranged collagen, which tend to be oriented in parallel with the epidermis (Fig. 58–3).

Mechanical Properties of Skin

Skin has properties that allow it to resist mechanical forces and yet allow for normal bodily motion. Stress is the force applied per unit area, whereas strain is the change in length created by an applied force. A typical stress-strain curve for skin is shown in Figure 58–4. Skin demonstrates complex responses to loading. Three phases are typically used to describe the mechanical response of skin. Skin compliance is greatest during

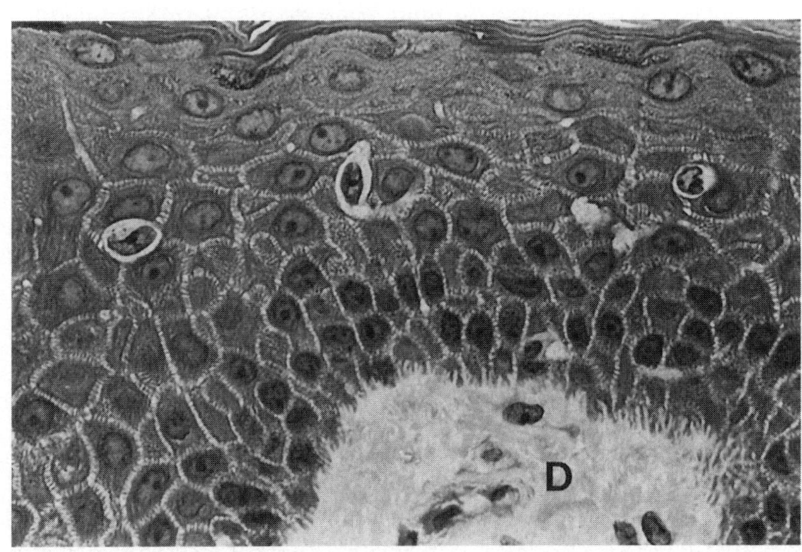

FIGURE 58–2. Light microscopy of epidermis, with the dermis (D) indicated. Note the abundance of keratinocytes joined by desmosomes. (From Borysenko M, Beringer T: Functional Histology, ed 2. Boston, Little, Brown, 1984, p 231.)

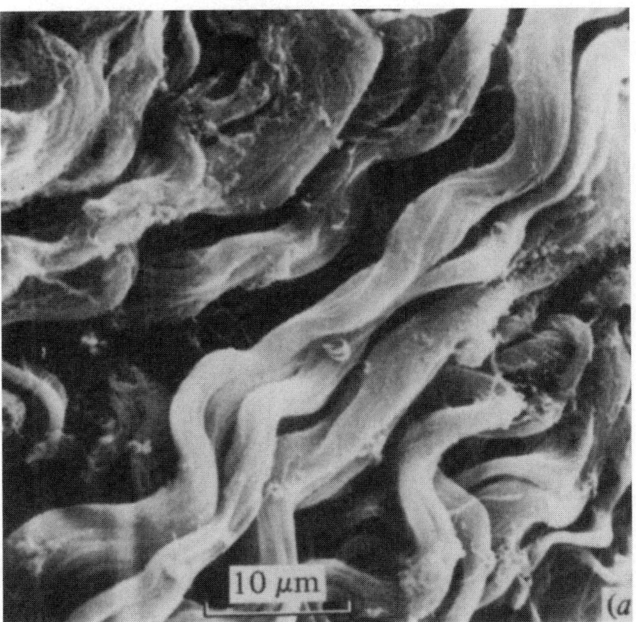

FIGURE 58–3. Electron micrograph of collagen bundles found in dermis. (From Millington PF, Wilkinson R: Skin. Cambridge, Cambridge University Press, 1983, p 85.)

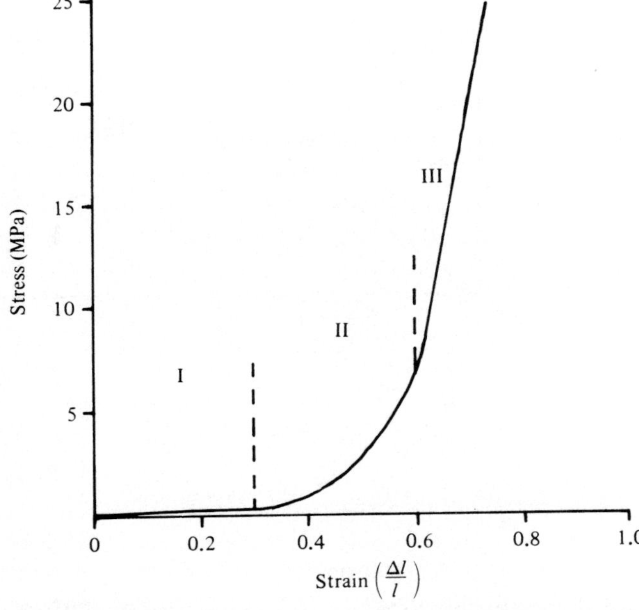

FIGURE 58–4. The stress-strain curve for skin. The various phases of skin response to elongation are indicated by roman numerals. (From Millington PF, Wilkinson R: Skin. Cambridge, Cambridge University Press, 1983, p 85.)

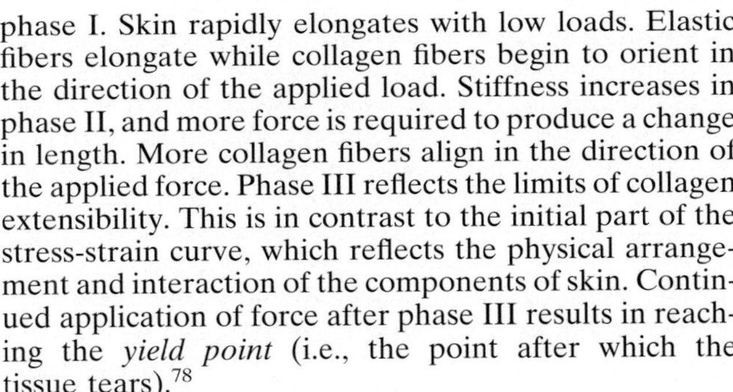

phase I. Skin rapidly elongates with low loads. Elastic fibers elongate while collagen fibers begin to orient in the direction of the applied load. Stiffness increases in phase II, and more force is required to produce a change in length. More collagen fibers align in the direction of the applied force. Phase III reflects the limits of collagen extensibility. This is in contrast to the initial part of the stress-strain curve, which reflects the physical arrangement and interaction of the components of skin. Continued application of force after phase III results in reaching the *yield point* (i.e., the point after which the tissue tears).[78]

Skin demonstrates a preconditioning effect. Consecutively applying and removing a load initially shows a noncoincident stress-strain curve. With repetition, the curves become very similar and nearly superimposable. The initial changes in the stress-strain curve with repetitious loading occur as a result of phase I elongation. However, after several force applications, phase I shows little change. Once this occurs, the skin is considered to be *preconditioned,* and the stress-strain characteristics of the skin are stabilized (Fig. 58–5).[78] The stress-strain curve also varies by tissue type, as demonstrated in Figure 58–6.[73] With injury and subsequent scarring, the

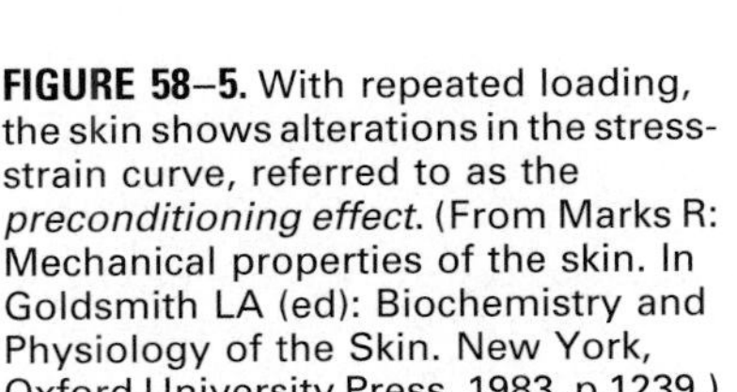

FIGURE 58–5. With repeated loading, the skin shows alterations in the stress-strain curve, referred to as the *preconditioning effect.* (From Marks R: Mechanical properties of the skin. In Goldsmith LA (ed): Biochemistry and Physiology of the Skin. New York, Oxford University Press, 1983, p 1239.)

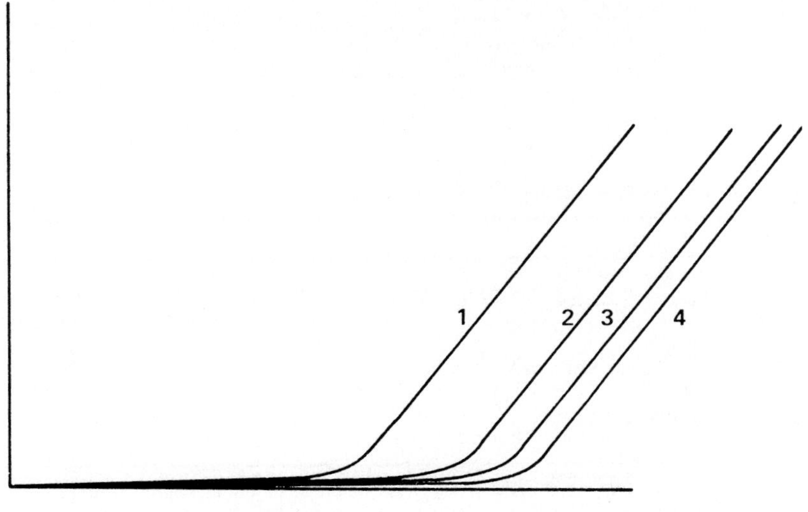

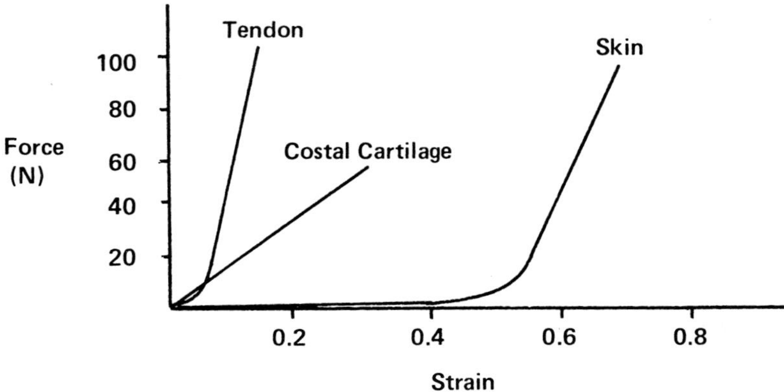

FIGURE 58–6. The stress-strain curves for tendon and cartilage compared with that of skin. (From Marks R: Mechanical properties of the skin. In Goldsmith LA (ed): Biochemistry and Physiology of the Skin. New York, Oxford University Press, 1983, p 1238.)

stress-strain relationship of skin is altered because higher collagen content decreases skin extensibility.[78] Awareness of these biomechanical principles becomes important for rehabilitation interventions of stretching and splint application.

MEDICAL AND SURGICAL MANAGEMENT OF BURN INJURY

The vast majority of burn injuries are thermal, resulting from flame or hot liquids. Chemical and electrical injuries are less frequent. The extent of tissue injury depends on the intensity and duration of heat exposure. A significant difference between chemical and thermal injury is the duration of tissue destruction. Heat injury ceases after the source is removed, whereas chemicals continue to destroy tissue until they are inactivated by neutralizing agents or until the chemical reaction with the tissue is complete.

Medical Management

The first priorities in medical management are interrupting the burning process and assessing the airways, breathing, and circulation. Further evaluation includes assessment of the total body surface area (TBSA) burned, burn depth, the presence or absence of inhalation injury, and involvement of specialized body regions (e.g., face, hands, perineum). The patient's age, the presence of other injuries, and the patient's premorbid medical condition are also considered. The amount of fluid needed to restore and maintain hemodynamic stability is calculated using the Brooke, Parkland, or other formulas for fluid resuscitation.[8, 29, 75] Clinical response determines further fluid needs. Close monitoring for infection and cardiopulmonary complications is required on an ongoing basis.

Classification of Burn Severity

The American Burn Association classifies a burn injury as minor, moderate, or severe based on patient age, extent and depth of injury, and associated injuries (Table 58–1). Patients with moderate and severe burns require hospitalization. Major injuries, which include inhalation burns and burns of the eyes, ears, face, feet, or perineum, should be treated in a specialized burn center.[4]

Burn injury extent is determined by the TBSA injured. The easiest method of calculating TBSA is the *rule of nines* (Fig. 58–7). Eleven areas of the body are assigned a surface area value of 9%, with a twelfth area, the perineum, assigned a value of 1%.[82] For children, this method is less accurate because the head, particularly during the first year of life, is larger in relation to the body size than is an adult's head. The Lund and Browder chart (Fig. 58–8) accounts for these developmental differences.[75]

TABLE 58–1 Burn Injury Classification

Type of Injury	Major Burn	Moderate Burn	Minor Burn
Partial-thickness burns			
Children	>20% TBSA	10% to 20% TBSA	<10% TBSA
Adults	>25% TBSA	15% to 25% TBSA	<15% TBSA
Full-thickness burns	>10% TBSA	2% to 10% TBSA	<2% TBSA
Injury to face, eyes, ears, feet, or perineum	+	—	—
Inhalation injury	+	—	—
Electrical injury	+	—	—
Comorbid factors of age, other trauma, or premorbid illness	+	—	—

Abbreviations: TBSA, total body surface area; +, presence of this injury or comorbidity indicates a major burn requiring care at a burn center.

From American Burn Association: Hospital and pre-hospital resources for optimal care of patients with burn injury: Guidelines for development and operation of burn center. J Burn Care Rehabil 1990; 11:98–104.

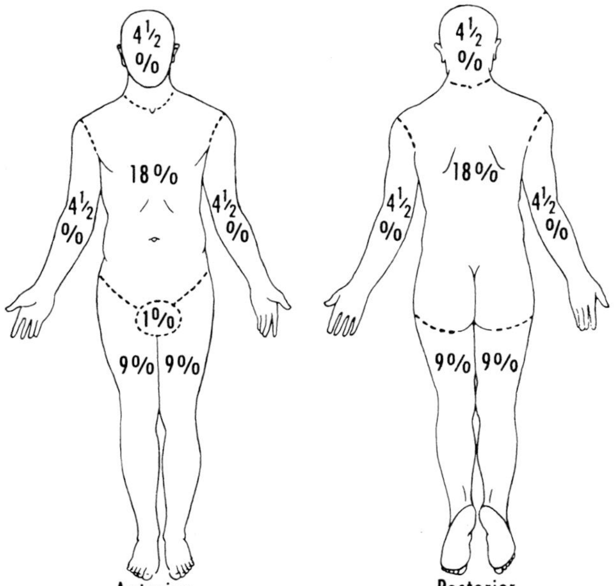

FIGURE 58–7. Rule of nines used to determine body surface area injured. (From Moylan JA: First aid and transportation of burned patients. In Artz CP, Moncrief JA, Pruitt BA (eds): Burns: A Team Approach. Philadelphia, WB Saunders, 1979, p 153.)

Burn injury depth refers to the extent to which the epidermis and dermis are injured (Fig. 58–9). Superficial burns, also called first-degree burns, cause local erythema and pain. Partial-thickness burns, or second-degree burns, are classified as superficial partial-thickness or deep partial-thickness burns. In superficial partial-thickness injuries, blistering occurs because of microvascular damage and an associated increase in capillary permeability. Sensory nerve endings are exposed, and the wound is painful.

In a deep partial-thickness wound, the dermis and the entire epidermis are injured. Only the skin appendages are spared. Spontaneous healing can occur, but it is associated with significant scarring. Poor cosmesis and function typically result.

In full-thickness burn injuries, or third-degree burns, the entire thickness of the dermis is devitalized. Because skin appendages are destroyed, the wound cannot heal by re-epithelization. Dermal blood vessels are destroyed, and the wound bed is avascular.

Even the most experienced clinicians can have difficulty distinguishing a deep partial-thickness injury from a full-thickness injury (Fig. 58–10). In fact, poor wound care, wound infection, or impaired perfusion can convert a deep partial-thickness injury to a full-thickness injury.

In the literature and in the clinical setting, a growing trend is to refer to burn depth in descriptive terms, that is, superficial partial-thickness, deep partial-thickness, and full-thickness burns, rather than first-, second-, and third-degree burns. The descriptive classification has the advantage of relaying a quick and accurate verbal description of the burn injury.

Principles of Wound Care

The goals of wound care are to facilitate wound healing, prevent infection, decrease pain, reduce scarring and contracture, and prepare the wound for any necessary grafting. Infection can cause sepsis or convert the wound

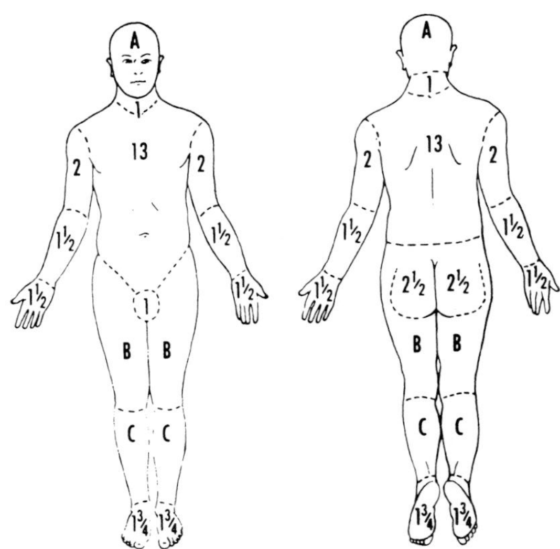

Relative Percentage of Areas Affected by Growth

	Age in Years					
	0	1	5	10	15	Adult
A—½ of head	9½	8½	6½	5½	4½	3½
B—½ of one thigh	2¾	3¼	4	4¼	4½	4¾
C—½ of one leg	2½	2½	2¾	3	3¼	3½

FIGURE 58–8. Lund and Browder method of determining skin surface area; method corrects for differences in percentage of body surface areas by age. (From McManus WF: Immediate emergency department care. In Artz CP, Moncrief JA, Pruitt BA (eds): Burns: A Team Approach. Philadelphia, WB Saunders, 1979, p 154.)

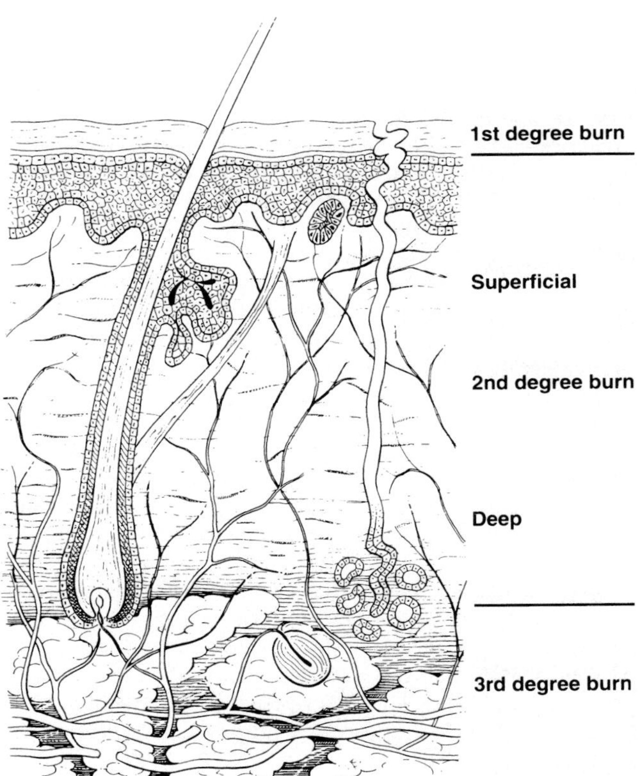

FIGURE 58–9. Normal skin histological characteristics, with depth of burn injury indicated. (From Kucan JO: Burn and trauma. In Ruberg RL, Smith DJ Jr (eds): Plastic Surgery: A Core Curriculum. St Louis, Mosby–Year Book, 1994, p 212.)

to a deeper-thickness injury. Burn wounds are covered by an eschar, which is necrotic tissue composed of denatured collagen, elastin, and protein. Because eschar favors wound infection and delays healing, debridement is initiated early. Debridement removes devitalized tissue and provides a viable base for wound healing and grafting.

Debridement is done by several techniques: mechanical, enzymatic, and surgical. Mechanical debridement includes techniques such as hydrotherapy and wet-to-dry dressing techniques. The wet-to-dry dressing technique involves placing saline-soaked gauze over the wound and allowing the dressing to nearly dry. Necrotic tissue adheres to the dressing as the gauze dries and is removed when the dressing is changed. This provides a simple and inexpensive debridement, but it can be painful and cause local bleeding. Its use is limited by the size of the wound to be debrided. To prevent desiccation of the wound, the dressing requires changing every 6 to 8 hours.

Hydrotherapy, via immersion or spraying a burn directly, is a reasonably comfortable way to remove dressings and loosen devitalized tissue. It is a time-consuming and labor-intensive procedure. Other disadvantages include hypothermia and bacterial cross-contamination between patients if meticulous care of hydrotherapy equipment is not maintained. Disposable liners are available to reduce cross-contamination. Hydrotherapy can be combined with other forms of mechanical debridement.

Several debriding enzymes, such as sutilains, are available for topical application to burn eschar. Enzymatic action includes proteolysis, fibrinolysis, and collagenolysis, with specificity varying from agent to agent. Enzymatic debridement can reduce the need for surgical debridement. Exercise and splinting programs are not contraindicated during enzymatic treatment. Disadvantages include increased pain and fluid loss. The amount of body surface area being enzymatically treated at one time should be limited to less than 20% TBSA. Localized irritation, cellulitis, and elevation in body temperature might also occur. Bleeding can occur at the interface between the eschar and the viable tissue.[103]

Surgical debridement excises the nonviable tissue by either sequential or fascial excision. The latter removes tissue down to the fascia, which ensures a viable wound bed but leaves a significant tissue defect. Sequential

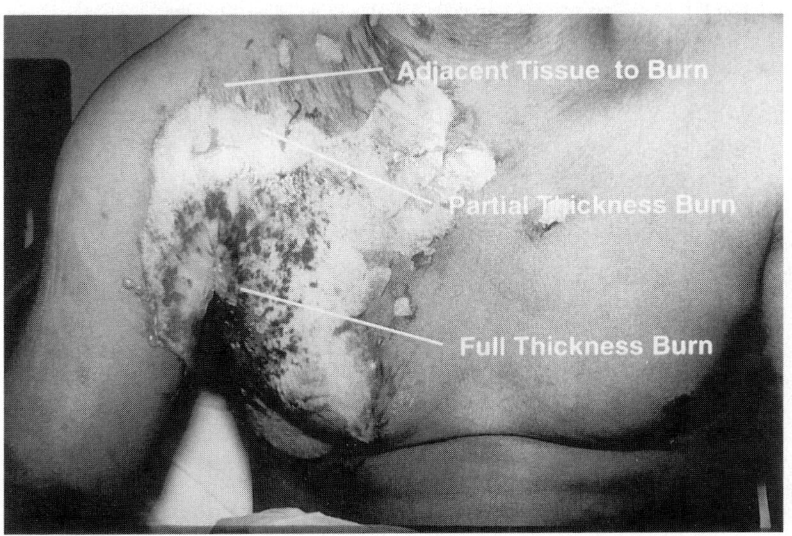

FIGURE 58–10. The clinical appearance of partial-thickness and full-thickness burns.

excision consists of sequential removal of thin slices of tissue until bleeding is observed. The bleeding indicates a viable wound bed. Although it is less likely to sacrifice viable tissue, sequential excision causes greater blood loss and requires extensive surgical experience.

Burn injury can cause massive edema. Compartment syndromes can develop, particularly with circumferential burns, that result in neurovascular compromise and potential limb loss. Escharotomies can be performed to relieve pressure by incising through the burned tissue at specified areas, which avoid flexor surfaces, of the upper and lower extremities (Fig. 58–11). Incision is also done over the chest wall if eschar interferes with respiration by preventing chest expansion. Circumferential upper or lower extremity burns require monitoring to ensure that compartment pressures do not exceed 40 mm Hg. If this pressure is reached, fasciotomies are indicated to prevent neurovascular compromise, which can also lead to amputation of the extremity.

Wound Dressings and Grafts

Biological dressings (i.e., biological tissue used for covering wounds) provide a means of early burn wound closure. Early closure reduces pain, promotes healing, and decreases bacterial proliferation. Early wound closure reduces evaporative fluid loss and metabolic rate. The primary types of biological dressings include heterografts (such as porcine grafts) and homografts (such as cadaver grafts). Homografts are considered the best biological dressing but are obtained primarily from cadaver donors and can be limited in supply. Biological dressings are often used to achieve early wound closure until an autograft (i.e., the surgical transfer of the patient's skin from one body site to another) is feasible. A biological dressing can also be used as a test graft to see if a wound is ready to accept an autograft.

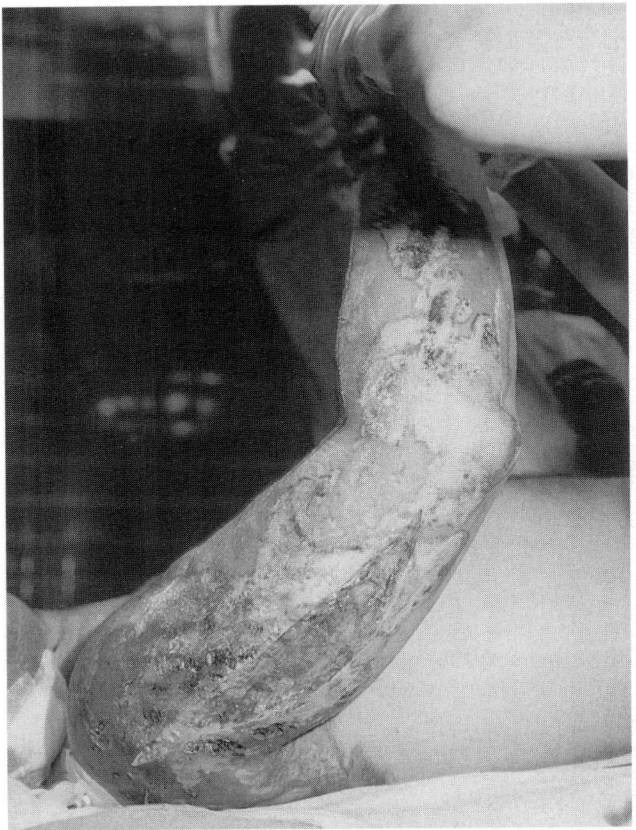

FIGURE 58–11. Escharotomy of the right upper arm to reduce pressure created by a circumferential burn.

Synthetic wound dressings include polyvinyl chlorides, polyurethanes, and other plastic membranes. The advantage of these temporary dressings includes water and gas permeability, but they fail to adhere to the wound bed, and fluids accumulate under the dressings.[83] Nylon mesh bonded to silicone (Biobrane) adheres to and successfully covers both partial- and full-thickness wounds. Like biological dressings, however, this type of dressing does not adhere to wounds having high bacterial counts.[39]

Topical antimicrobials are applied to burns and wounds after debridement and grafting to reduce bacterial proliferation. Sulfadiazine and mafenide acetate are two of the most commonly used topical agents. Mafenide acetate penetrates eschar, but it can cause pain as well as acidosis and leukopenia. Sulfadiazine is also a broad-spectrum topical antibiotic, but it does not penetrate eschar as mafenide acetate does. It has the advantage of causing less pain and is not associated with leukopenia or acidosis.

Autografting can be performed once the wound is free of devitalized tissue and infection. Split-thickness skin graft can be meshed or applied in sheets. Meshing is a process in which small, staggered, parallel slits are made in the graft to allow it to be expanded 1.5 times or more its original size. The interstices epithelialize, and the pattern of the mesh persists after wound healing (Figs. 58–12 and 58–13). The greater the degree to which the mesh is expanded, the poorer the cosmetic appearance. Mesh grafts are valuable when donor sites are limited and large areas need to be covered. Split-thickness grafts can be applied in sheets without meshing. These grafts are durable, limit contracture formation, and produce better cosmesis for covering the face, neck, and hands. Full-thickness grafts are useful for specialized areas, such as the palms of the hands, and are frequently used in reconstructive procedures.

Wound Healing

Wound healing involves three simultaneous processes: epithelization, scar formation (repair of the dermis), and wound contraction. Inflammation begins immediately after injury. This process spans a complex array of events, including initial vasoconstriction followed by vasodilation, marked changes in capillary permeability, and chemotaxis (which attracts neutrophils, macrophages, and lymphocytes). This period is marked by erythema, increased heat, edema, and pain. The inflammatory phase not only controls infection but also heralds the onset of the proliferative stage of healing by attracting fibroblasts.

Once inflammation is established, epithelium migrates from the edges of the wound or from epidermal

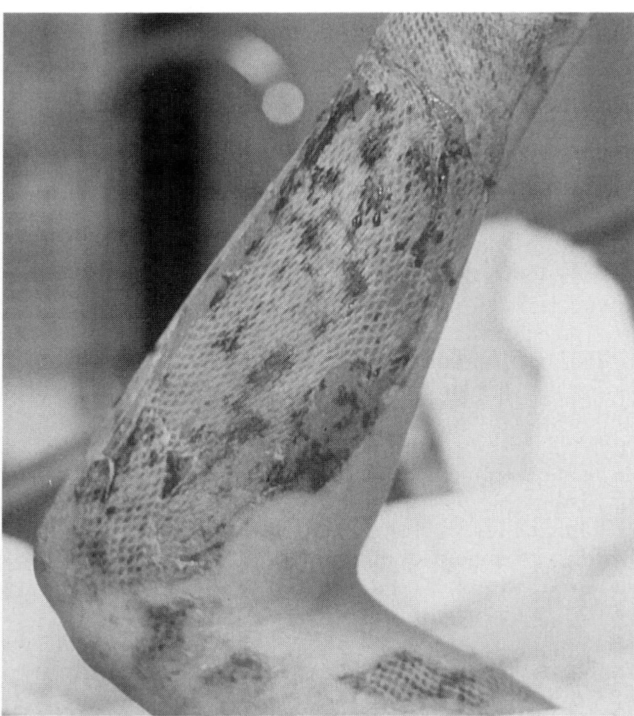

FIGURE 58–12. The appearance of a meshed split-thickness autograft during the acute postgrafting period.

appendages. If the burn involves the epidermis and superficial dermis, epithelialization is the primary process. However, with deep partial-thickness injuries and full-thickness injuries, both epithelialization and restoration of the dermis are crucial.

Fibroblastic activity is the hallmark of the proliferative wound healing phase. During this phase, fibroblasts synthesize collagen, which is the predominant protein found in scar tissue. Collagen gives tensile strength to the wound. Simultaneously, angiogenesis occurs to provide the vascular support needed for the reparative wound activities. Capillary proliferation produces the classic granular appearance of granulation tissue.

Wound contraction is the active movement of the wound edges toward the center of a wound, shrinking the defect size and aiding closure. The degree of contraction achieved depends on the looseness and redundancy of the surrounding skin. For instance, a wound involving the skin of the buttock results in greater wound contraction and reduction of the wound size than does one involving the the less mobile skin of the lateral malleolus. Fibroblasts appear to be the primary cells involved in wound contraction.[88]

Inflammation and angiogenesis resolve as the scar matures. The tissue becomes paler and flatter. Collagen synthesis is balanced by collagen degradation. The rete pegs do not reappear immediately and require months to form. This contributes to the scarred skin's reduced ability to tolerate applied forces.

ELECTRICAL BURN INJURIES

Electrical burn injuries account for approximately 3% of burn admissions and result in approximately 800 deaths per year.[44, 63] Injuries can be mild or can result in death from cardiac asystole. Electrical injuries are classified as low-tension-line or high-tension-line injuries. High-tension-line injuries result from exposure to greater than 1000 V. Amperage is also important. In general, the greater the amperage, the greater the injury. Electrical injuries occur predominantly in men younger than 30 years who work with high-voltage equipment or high-tension wires. Low-tension electrical injuries usually occur in residential settings.[63]

On superficial evaluation, electrical injuries can deceptively appear minor. The entrance site is typically small and charred, whereas the exit wound can be more explosive in appearance. Patients need careful evaluation to ensure that a serious underlying injury is not overlooked. The average TBSA injured in electrical burns is approximately 12%.[38] Electrical injuries can be further compounded if the clothing catches on fire, causing more extensive skin injury.

The damage of electrical exposure results from the heat produced as the current passes through various tissues. According to Joule's law, $J = I^2 RT$, the amount of heat produced (J) is related to the square of the amperage (I), the tissue resistance (R), and the duration

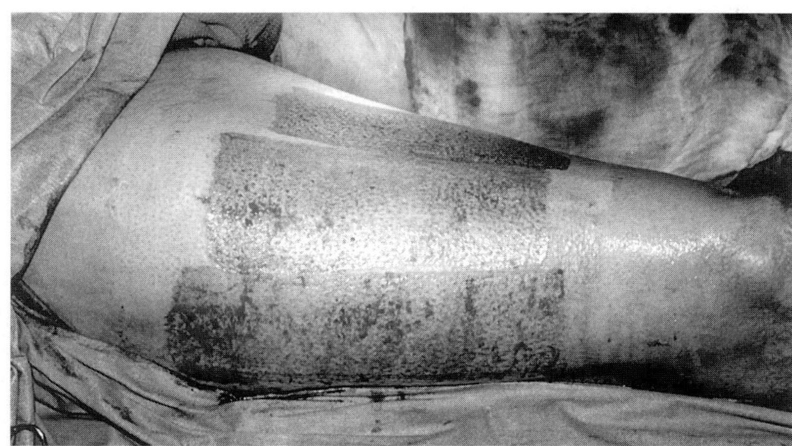

FIGURE 58–13. Donor site appearance after skin harvesting for autografting.

of exposure (T). Bone produces the most resistance, resulting in the greatest heat production. Although nerves and blood vessels provide the least resistance, they can sustain significant injury because they are more heat sensitive. As a consequence, the majority of the injuries sustained are in deep tissues.[81]

The cross-sectional area of the particular body part affects the density of current and the amount of heat generated. Body parts with a small cross-sectional area, such as fingers and toes, can sustain massive injury (Figs. 58–14A and B).[81] Extensive muscle and soft tissue necrosis often results in amputation. One-fourth to nearly one-half of patients hospitalized for electrical burns require limb amputation, and some require multiple limb amputations.[38, 52, 94] The upper extremity is the most common limb amputated.[37, 63] Haberal[37] reported that 27% of the 94 electrically injured patients he studied required major limb amputations. In the study, 80% of the major limb amputations involved the upper extremity. The right upper extremity accounted for two-thirds of these amputations. One-fourth of these patients required shoulder disarticulations; the remainder underwent above-elbow and below-elbow amputations.

Neurological Sequelae

Immediate neurological problems include loss of consciousness, anoxic encephalopathy, peripheral neuropathies, and spinal cord injury. Persistent coma correlates with a poor prognosis and often results in death.[36] Spinal cord injury, according to some sources the most common permanent neurological sequela of electrical injury,[81] typically occurs when the current travels from one extremity to another.[62] Peripheral neuropathies generally occur in the injured limb but can also be seen in the nonburned limb.[31] Although the pathophysiology of late-appearing neurological deficits is unknown, spinal cord injury and peripheral neuropathies can be observed as late as 2 years post injury. Late-appearing deficits generally have a poorer prognosis than those manifesting early in the course. With electrical injuries to the head and neck, serial eye examinations are required because cataracts can occur up to 3 years after the injury.[57, 81, 110]

REHABILITATION

Rehabilitation from a burn injury continues long after discharge, in some cases for life. The overall goal is to assist the individual in achieving the optimal level of functioning. During the acute period, more specific goals include promoting wound healing and preventing complications by preserving joint function, strength, endurance, and functional abilities. Goals are individualized according to the location, depth, and distribution of burn injuries and the individual's previous functional level, and should be continually assessed and modified as the patient improves. The extent of injury correlates with survival as well as with time required to return to independent functioning. Age, previous level of independence, premorbid medical conditions, and other injuries must be considered when assessing the burn patient.

Positioning

Proper positioning is fundamental to burn rehabilitation. Positioning prevents contracture formation, controls edema, and maintains tissues in an elongated state. Pain causes burn patients to assume a primarily flexed and adducted position that inadvertently favors contracture development. However, body parts should generally be positioned to maintain burned tissues in their elongated state. Typically, limbs should be positioned in extension and abduction (Fig. 58–15). The positioning program must be individualized in accordance with the injury sites. Proper positioning can be achieved using splints, strategically placed pillows, and foam wedges.

Splinting

Splinting should be considered in several circumstances. Contractures can develop quickly during burn healing.

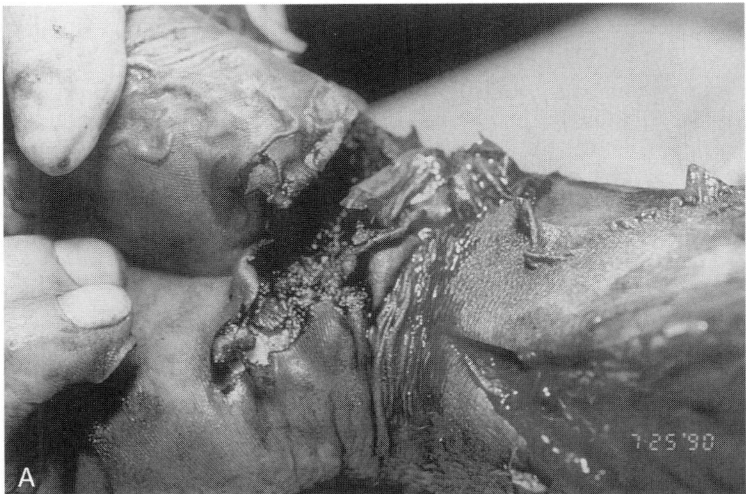

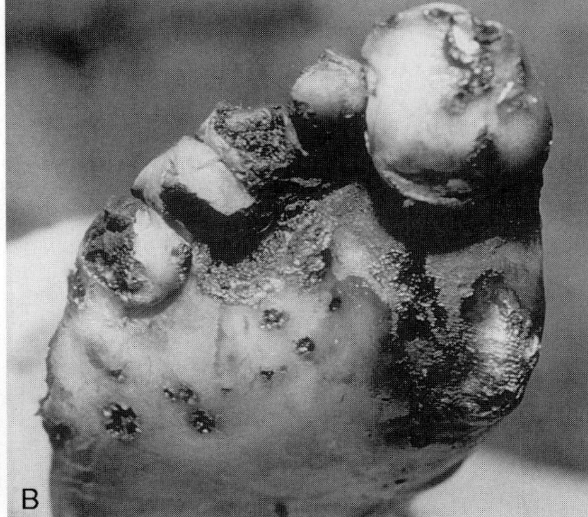

FIGURE 58–14. Electrical burn: entrance site (*A*); exit site (*B*).

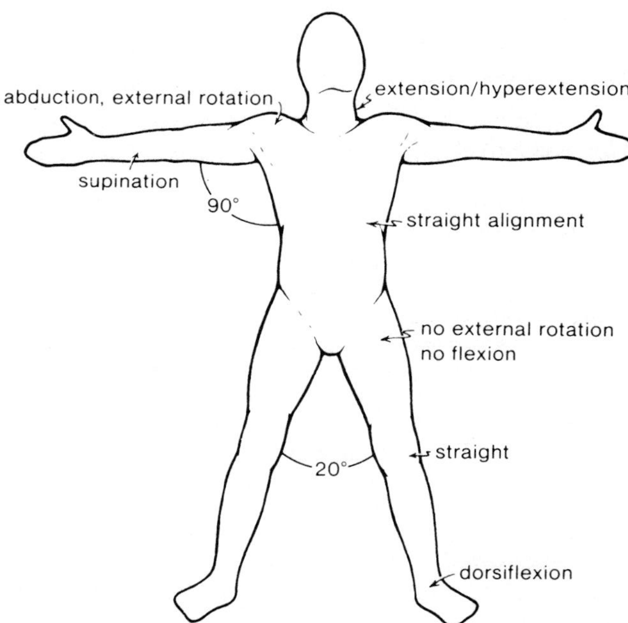

FIGURE 58–15. Suggested positioning guidelines for prevention of burn contractures. (From Helm PA, Kevorkian CG, Lushbaugh M, et al: Burn injury: Rehabilitation management in 1982. Arch Phys Med Rehabil 1982; 63:8.)

Contracture would interfere with joint function when a partial- or full-thickness burn overlies a joint surface or the skin near a joint. Splints are used to maintain proper anticontracture positions and range of motion (ROM) in joints at risk for development of contractures. Serial splinting and serial casting techniques are both nonoperative means of gaining ROM through sustained stretch and pressure.

Splints are also used to protect newly placed skin grafts and to shield injured anatomical structures, such as tendons, from further trauma. Splints can also be designed to prevent scarring in areas in which an important body contour would be lost, such as the anterior neck surface.

It is important to consider the benefits and risks of splinting. Splinting is labor-intensive and adds significant cost to patient care. Splinting is cost-effective, however, if it reduces the need for surgery or prevents loss of function.

Not all burned areas require splinting. Areas of superficial partial-thickness burns usually heal without scar contracture formation and do not require splinting. Unburned areas generally do not require splinting unless they are at risk for contracture development secondary to immobilization. For example, prolonged bed rest could cause joint motion to be lost in an unburned area such as the ankle. Splinting should be considered if full passive ROM is not present at a joint.

Splint materials must be compatible with topical medications and wound dressings. Prefabricated or custom splints can be used but require proper fitting. Care should be taken to ensure that the splints do not create pressure over bony prominences and delicate healing tissues. Splints should be easy to don and doff. "User-friendly" splints increase the likelihood that they will be used, and the complications of incorrect use will be avoided. Inexpensive and remoldable materials are best suited to accommodate changes as healing occurs.

The universal burn splint, unfortunately, does not exist. The type of splint used depends on the area burned, the depth of injury, the patient's functional status, and the patient's ability to participate in positioning and exercise programs. A wide variety of splints can be designed and fabricated. A splinting program should focus on motions at risk as well as ROM that is difficult to regain (e.g., shoulder flexion and abduction, elbow and knee extension). Splints can be fabricated for virtually any part of the body, including the mouth, face, neck, and axilla.

A resting hand splint maintains the hand in a functional position. The position of function is the hand splinted in full interphalangeal extension, 60 to 80 degrees of metacarpophalangeal flexion, thumb abduction, and wrist extension (Fig. 58–16).[44, 67] This position provides balance between the extensor and flexor tendons and places the ligaments and joint structures under maximum stretch to prevent shortening by inflammation and edema.[67]

Splints for the upper and lower extremities are among the most common. Lower extremity splints include such devices as the hip abduction splint to limit hip adduction, the knee extension splint to prevent knee flexion contractures, and the posterior footdrop splint to maintain the ankle in a neutral position. Individualized splints, unique to the patient's needs, can be fabricated. An example of such a customized foot splint is shown in Figure 58–17.

Plantar flexion deformity is a common problem. Prefabricated posterior footdrop splints are commercially available but still require modification to ensure proper fit. These splints can also be readily made by creating a gutter- or trough-shaped splint and attaching a footplate to hold the ankle in a neutral position. The trough can be lengthened to include positioning of the knee in extension.

Exercise in Burn Rehabilitation

Exercise is fundamental to maximizing patient function and overall outcome. Factors to consider in prescribing an exercise program include the extent, depth, and location of the injury. In general, the risk of contracture increases with increasing burn depth. The risk of exercise disrupting wound healing requires regular wound inspection, particularly in the case of deep partial-thickness and full-thickness burns over joint surfaces. Stretching can also disrupt already tenuous joint and tendon structures.

Preexisting medical conditions, such as cardiovascular or pulmonary disease, also affect the type of exercise prescribed. The stress of fluid resuscitation can complicate the recovery of patients with cardiovascular disease. Because deconditioning occurs rapidly in burn patients (see Chapter 34), principles of cardiac rehabilitation are often as important in these situations as burn exercise principles (see Chapter 32).

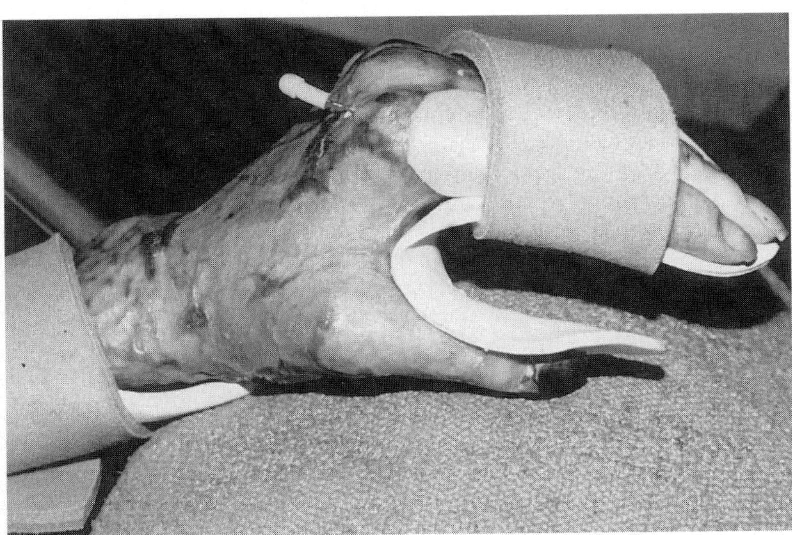

FIGURE 58–16. The left hand splinted in the position of function after skin grafting.

The initial exercise program should focus on preserving ROM and maintaining strength. Active forms of exercise are indicated for patients who are alert and able to participate. For obtunded or critically ill patients, the slow, controlled movement of passive ROM exercise is appropriate. While the patient is under anesthesia, passive ROM techniques can be applied to determine true joint ROM and factors limiting motion.

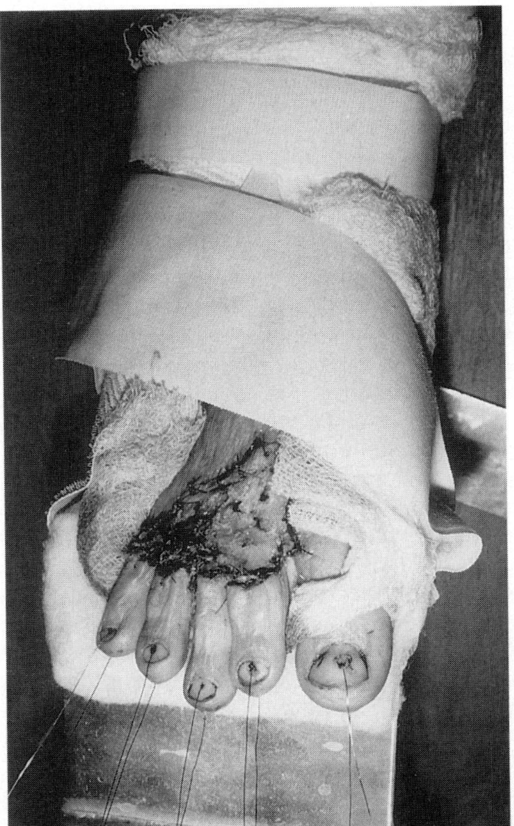

FIGURE 58–17. Customized splint designed to hold the foot in a neutral position while also preventing a hyperextension deformity at the metatarsophalangeal joints after dorsal foot autograft.

In the case of the patient who can actively move a joint but who is unable to achieve full ROM, active assistive ROM (AAROM) exercise is appropriate. The patient does as much of the ROM as possible, then a steady prolonged stretch or assistance is applied to complete the ROM. The stretch can be provided manually or by using devices such as pulleys and weights. Pain can limit stretching in some patients, so scheduling exercise shortly after pain medication administration is helpful.

Applying the principle of skin preconditioning (i.e., stretching the skin several times until phase I of the stress-strain curve stabilizes) can improve the success of a stretching program. Preconditioning can be done by moving a joint to its end ROM several times before applying a sustained stretch. Stretching can be sustained until the stretched tissue blanches. The blanching indicates that dermal capillary flow is impeded and correlates with early phase III of the skin stress-strain relationship (see Fig. 58–4). With overstretching beyond phase III, the yield point is reached and passed (i.e., the point in the stress-strain curve at which tissue integrity deteriorates).[78] Once normal joint ROM is achieved, active exercise is preferred.

Various types of strengthening protocols can be initiated, including progressive resistive exercises and circuit training (see Chapter 20). Endurance training should not be overlooked but requires careful monitoring in the patient with cardiac or pulmonary disease (see Chapters 32 and 33).

Ambulation and Mobility

Ambulation and mobility are important elements of a comprehensive rehabilitation program. Early ambulation maintains balance, lower extremity function, and a sense of well-being and decreases the risk of deep venous thrombosis. While ambulation should start as soon as possible after admission, it can be limited by medical status, the presence of new skin grafts, the depth and extent of lower extremity burns, and previous medical conditions, such as peripheral vascular disease. After lower extremity grafting, placing the legs in a dependent position is generally not permitted for up to 5 to 10 days. Although the protocol for the timing of ambulation varies among facilities, the underlying principle is to begin ambulation once competent circulation is established in the graft and the risk of venous pooling, which can cause graft loss, is reduced. Once ambulation is initiated, recent graft and deep tissue injuries of the lower extremities require elastic wraps or stockings. Elastic supports prevent venous stasis, control edema, reduce the risk of local trauma, and decrease pain induced by the dependent position. Before ambulation is begun, it is advisable to have the patient dangle the lower extremities (e.g., sit with the legs hanging over the edge of the bed) to evaluate the predisposition for edema formation. Wounds should be assessed before and after ambulation to note any ill effects.

Gait deviations are frequent and reflect the injured areas of the body (see Chapter 5). Reduced trunk and pelvic mobility, decreased weight shifting, and inadequate hip and knee extension are common. Some deviations spontaneously resolve with wound healing, but others require therapeutic intervention. Mirrors can provide feedback to patients for self-correction of posture and gait abnormalities. Assistive devices can optimize gait patterns (see Chapter 25).

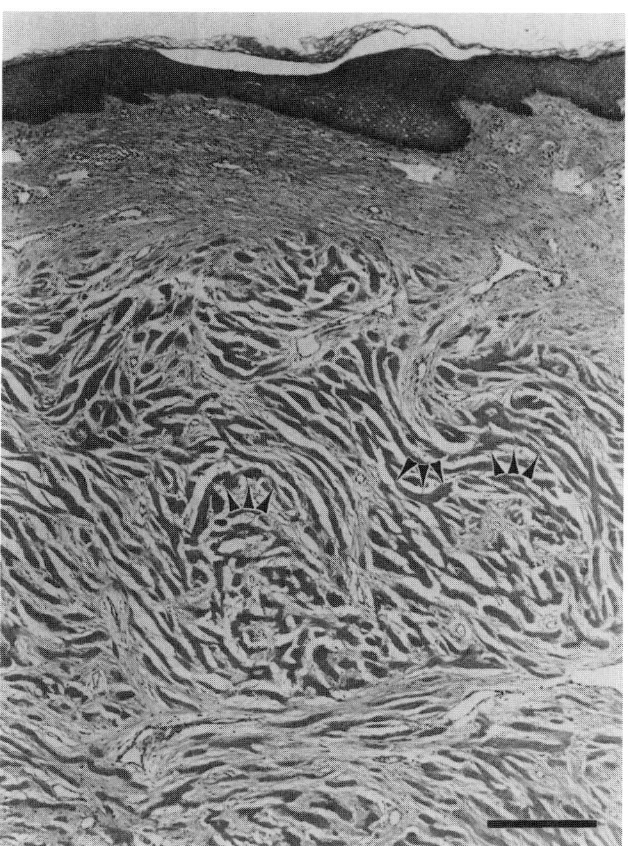

FIGURE 58–18. Whorled pattern of collagen in hypertrophic scar. Compare with the normal skin depicted in Figure 58–2. (From Staley MJ, Richard RL: Scar management. In Richard RL, Staley MJ (eds): Burn Care and Rehabilitation. Philadelphia, FA Davis, 1994, p 384.)

Scar Rehabilitation

The appearance of a wound is frequently satisfactory immediately after closure. However, over the next 1 to 3 months, hypertrophic scarring can occur with deep partial-thickness and full-thickness burn injuries. Hypertrophic scars are characteristically red, raised, and rigid.[1] The significance of these scars varies according to their location, with scarring over joints or on the face having a significant effect on function and appearance. Linares and Larson[68] describe three stages of burn scarring: immature, semimature, and mature. The immature nonhypertrophic scar is red and flat, whereas the immature hypertrophic scar is red but is also indurated and raised. In nonhypertrophic scars, the collagen fibers are aligned nearly parallel to the skin surface, an arrangement that resembles normal skin histologically. Hypertrophic scars demonstrate random collagen orientation, with fibers arranged in whorls and nodules (Fig. 58–18).

As normal and hypertrophic scars mature, the vascularity is reduced, the redness fades, and hypertrophic scars show a decrease in whorls and nodules on histological examination. With maturity, both types show a predominance of collagen in parallel arrays. Clinically, both scars are soft and pale. A hypertrophic scar requires up to 2 years to reach maturity, whereas a nonhypertrophic scar might mature in weeks to months.[1, 52]

Mechanical pressure alters the orientation of the collagen fibers found in hypertrophic scarring. Kischer and co-workers examined hypertrophic scars with electron microscopy and found that pressure-treated hypertrophic scars appeared to mature more rapidly.[60] Collagen fibers were more likely to be in parallel, and collagen nodules occurred less frequently.[53]

The risk of hypertrophic scarring increases with the depth of injury and length of time required for healing. Certain anatomical locations are associated with greater incidence of hypertrophic scarring (e.g., buttocks and chest) (Fig. 58–19). The risk of hypertrophic scarring is reported by some authors to be greater in more darkly pigmented skin types.[24, 95]

It is generally accepted that pressure-treated scars have a better functional and cosmetic outcome. The application of continuous pressure through garments, orthoses, and splints is the primary nonsurgical modality used to control hypertrophic scarring. The mechanism by which pressure suppresses hypertrophic scarring is unclear, but it has been hypothesized that pressure causes decreased capillary perfusion and decreased tissue oxygenation, resulting in reduced cellular activity and collagen synthesis.[87]

Treatment options for scar suppression include custom-fitted pressure garments (Fig. 58–20), elastic bandages, and custom-made elastic or rigid face masks. Pressure applied to the healing area should be at least 25 mm Hg, as it should exceed normal capillary pressure. Pressure is applied at least 23 hours per day. Uneven

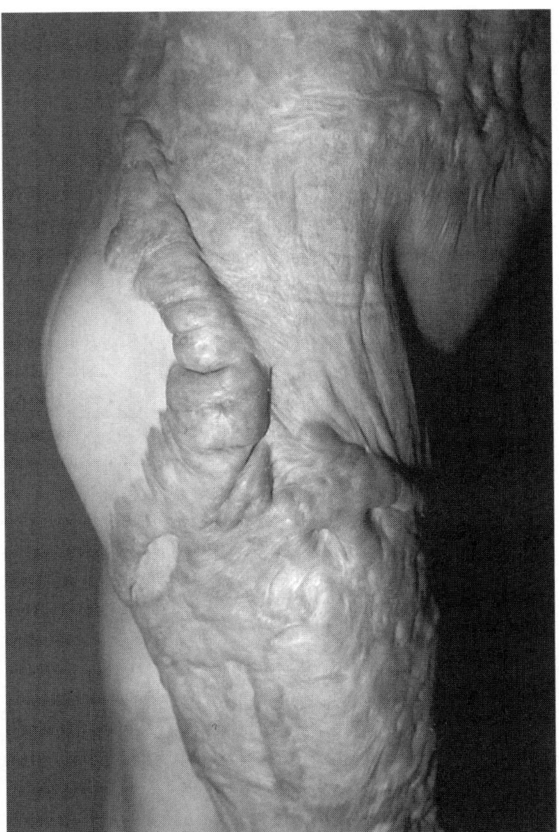

FIGURE 58–19. Lateral view of the lower trunk, buttock, and thigh showing extensive hypertrophic scarring that limits hip range of motion.

anatomical areas to which it is difficult to apply pressure, such as the web spaces of the hand, often require custom inserts. These pieces of silicone or moldable plastic are placed under pressure garments and orthoses to create a more intimate fit.

The application of pressure should continue until the scar is mature. Patient education is essential for pressure therapy compliance. The garments can be fabricated in varying colors, but patients often do not like the garment's appearance, regardless of color or type. In addition, pressure garments and devices are expensive and are often hot and difficult to don. Complications of pressure therapy garments include superficial abrasions from the shear forces produced by the garment and local dermatitis. In the young child, pressure effects on skeletal growth require monitoring. Frequent adjustments to accommodate growth spurts are necessary.[65]

Facial Burns

Facial burns have a significant impact on a person's appearance and state of well-being. Cosmesis and preservation of facial function are major priorities. Acutely, facial burns should alert the physician to possible inhalation injury. The risk of eye injury is also increased in facial burns. Facial wounds require an experienced wound care physician. Wounds expected to heal in less than 3 weeks often do not require early surgery and are less likely to develop significant scarring.[22, 93]

Custom-made elastic face masks and transparent orthoses are available for controlling facial scarring. The highly contoured features of the face, especially the central face, make scar control problematic. The goal is to preserve facial contours, especially the nasal profile and the shape of the mouth and eyes. Silicone and other materials can be added to face masks to achieve better pressure application in hard-to-control regions, such as the nasolabial fold.[22, 113]

Microstomia orthoses can be fabricated or purchased to maintain the normal mouth aperture (Fig. 58–21). Early splinting reduces the need for corrective surgery.[93, 113] Scarring can severely distort the nose, affecting cosmesis and respiratory function. Custom-fitted nasal trumpets (Fig. 58–22), which can be fabricated from low-temperature thermoplastic materials, can successfully maintain the nasal openings.[21, 55]

Unlike other body regions, pressure is contraindicated during the acute and recovery phase of ear burns. Ears require protection to avoid the development of pressure necrosis and chondritis. Specialized foam protectors and headgear can be designed.[41, 56]

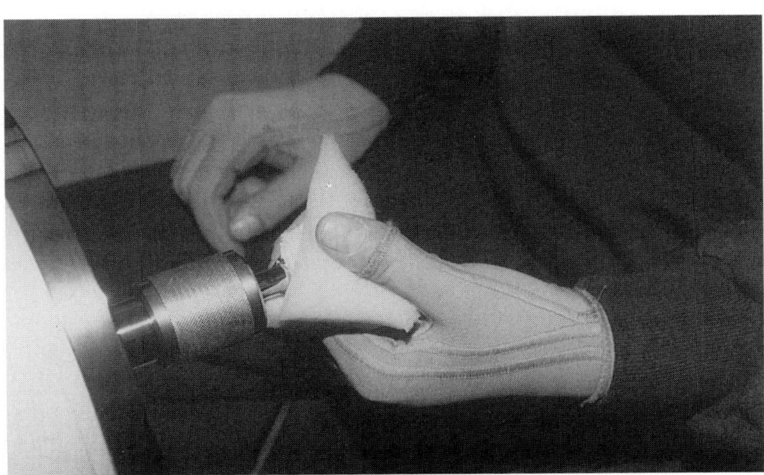

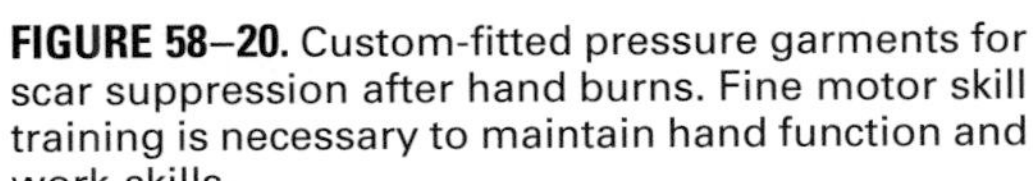

FIGURE 58–20. Custom-fitted pressure garments for scar suppression after hand burns. Fine motor skill training is necessary to maintain hand function and work skills.

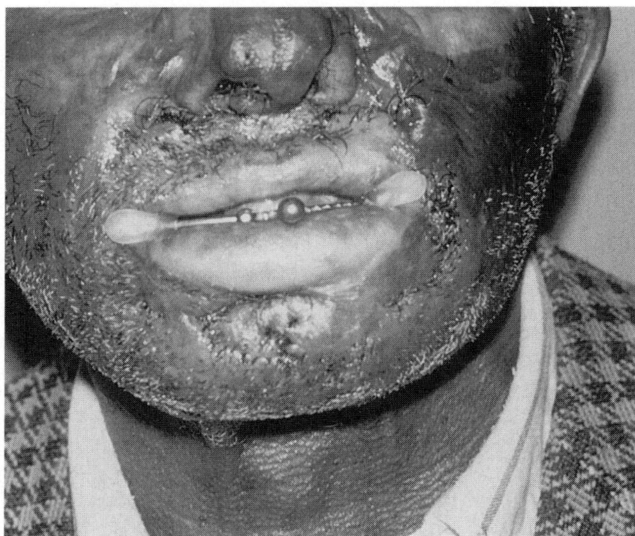

FIGURE 58–21. Microstomia splint to maintain oral commissure after facial burns.

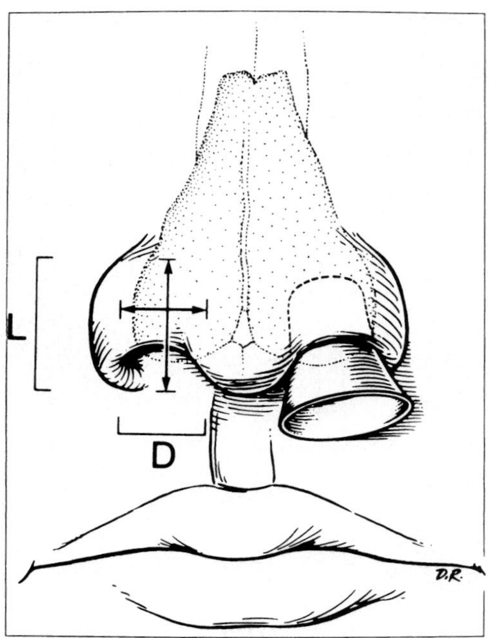

FIGURE 58–22. Nasal trumpet used to maintain patency and contour of nasal openings. The method of measuring for length (L) and depth (D) of the orthosis is indicated. (From Johnson J, Candia J, LaTrenta G, et al: A nasal trumpet orthosis to maintain nares openings and respiratory function for patients with facial burns: A case report. J Burn Care Rehabil 1992; 13:677.)

Hand Rehabilitation

Hands are the most common site of burn injury.[99] Because of the highly specialized functions of the hand, the burned hand requires the care of burn specialists experienced in hand management. Treatment goals include edema control, early wound closure, rapid return of hand function, and prevention of hand deformities (Fig. 58–23). Many types of hand deformities can result from deep partial-thickness and full-thickness injuries. The type of deformity relates to the location of the burn injury (e.g., burns of the thenar eminence and first web space cause thumb adduction contracture). Common deformities of the hand include wrist flexion contractures, metacarpophalangeal (MCP) hyperextension contractures, and interphalangeal (IP) flexion contractures. Bands of hypertrophic scarring can develop and limit hand function.

After the hand is assessed for potential hypertrophic scarring and contracture formation, a well-designed program of exercise, splinting, and hypertrophic scar suppression should be prescribed. Exercise coupled with splint use, when indicated, can prevent hand deformities and restore optimal hand function. When splints are used, they should maintain the hand in an anticontracture position, which prevents the anticipated deformity. The dorsum or the full circumference of the hand is frequently injured. These injuries require that the hand be splinted in the position of function—that is, IP joint

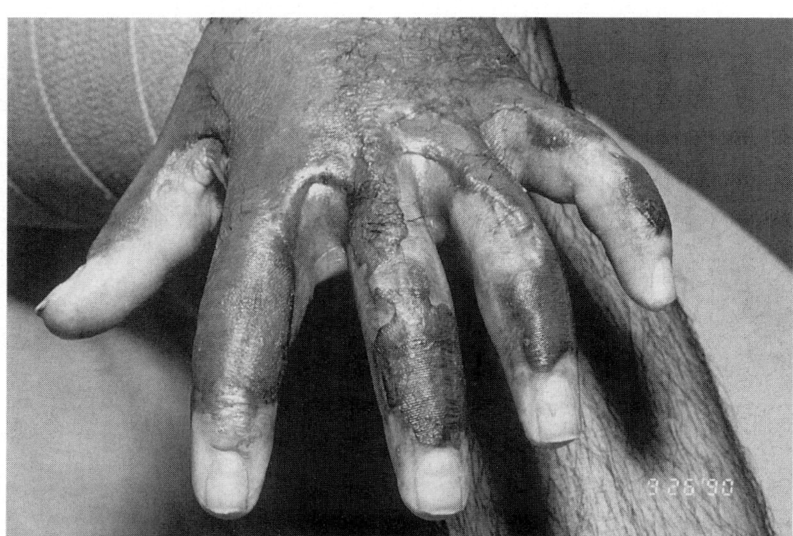

FIGURE 58–23. Hypertrophic scarring on dorsum of hand that limits flexion of metacarpophalangeal and interphalangeal joints.

extension, MCP joint flexion, thumb abduction, and wrist extension. This position preserves the maximal length and mobility of the extensor hood mechanism. Splint design should also preserve the transverse arch of the hand. In addition to static splints that hold the hand in a prescribed position, dynamic splints are available to facilitate ROM restoration or to substitute for a particular motion. Dynamic splints provide force in a specific plane, generally through elastic traction, while allowing motion in other planes.

Exposed tendons and joints of the hand demand specialized treatment. Any exposed tendons require dressings that will keep them moist, because dehydration can lead to tendon rupture. Exposed tendons are splinted in a slackened position. Once the wound is covered, passive ROM exercises can be performed judiciously. If the joint capsule is intact, gentle active exercise can be done. This exercise should be done under the supervision of an experienced therapist. The risk of septic arthritis is increased in open or exposed joints.

NEUROMUSCULAR COMPLICATIONS

Peripheral nerve injury after burns is common but not well recognized. Neurological involvement includes focal nerve compression, multiple mononeuropathies, and generalized peripheral neuropathies. Focal mononeuropathies commonly occur secondary to positioning, improperly applied splints, or bulky dressings.[45] Helm and associates[45] found that footdrop secondary to a peroneal neuropathy at the fibular head was the most common neuropathy, followed by median and ulnar mononeuropathies. The incidence of brachial plexopathies was also significant.

Multiple mononeuropathies can also occur. Marquez and co-workers[74] reported a prevalence of 2%, and noted that multiple mononeuropathies were more likely to develop in males than in females (4.3 : 1). Electrodiagnostic studies showed predominantly axonal involvement. The mononeuropathies were asymmetrical and were more likely to occur in the upper limbs (3 : 1); they were not always found in burned regions. Also, the neuropathies did not consistently correlate with compression from positioning, dressings, or splints.

Henderson and colleagues[49] first proposed that burn injuries are intrinsically associated with generalized peripheral neuropathy. Approximately 15% of the inpatients had peripheral neuropathy, which occurred primarily in patients who had injuries on more than 20% of TBSA. The type of peripheral neuropathy was not characterized.[49]

Helm and others[43] studied 88 patients with major burns who complained of persistent weakness or easy fatigability. A generalized peripheral neuropathy was found in 52%, but whether this was primarily an axonal or a demyelinating process was not reported.[43] Like the findings of Henderson and colleagues,[49] the incidence correlated with the amount of TBSA affected (i.e., neuropathy was more likely to occur in adults with more than 20% TBSA injury and in children with more than 30% TBSA injury). The study by Marquez and colleagues[47] showed electrodiagnostic evidence of a predominance of motor, rather than sensory, axonal peripheral neuropathy. Electrodiagnostically, these findings are consistent with critical care polyneuropathy seen in patients with multiple organ failure, as described by Bolton and others.[12] The generalized peripheral neuropathy of the burn patient might be a subset of critical care polyneuropathy. The etiology of the peripheral neuropathy of burns has not been established, but neurotoxicity from antibiotics and the possibility of a circulating neurotoxin from the burn injury itself have been hypothesized.[49, 80, 101]

HETEROTOPIC OSSIFICATION

Heterotopic ossification (HO) occurs after serious burns and represents abnormal calcification of soft tissues surrounding a joint. The risk of HO is increased in injuries that affect 20% or more of TBSA. Heterotopic ossification is more likely to occur the longer wounds remain open and the patient remains immobile. Evans documented an incidence of 2% in 1400 patients.[28] The most common site was the posterior elbow. The second most common site was the hip in children and the shoulder in adults. The site of ossification does not necessarily correlate with the location of burn injuries and can occur in single or multiple joints.

HO can cause progressive loss of joint ROM and nerve entrapment mononeuropathies. HO can spontaneously resolve in some cases. If HO significantly interferes with function and is unresponsive to nonsurgical treatment, surgery is indicated. Surgical excision is typically not performed until the bone has matured to reduce the risk of recurrence. Serial bone scans appear to be the most reliable method of determining when HO has matured.[27] Surgery has been performed earlier in the case of nerve entrapment associated with progressive neurological loss, despite the risk of HO recurrence.[111]

BURN-INDUCED AMPUTATION

Limb amputation can be necessary after severe burn injury, particularly after electrical burns. Electrical injury is the leading cause of amputation in the burn patient population.[76] The basic principles of amputee rehabilitation apply (see Chapters 13 and 14). The preprosthetic problems are similar to those with other amputations, but additional problems can occur, such as skin fragility, hypertrophic scarring, burn contractures, and altered skin sensation. The prosthesis might have to be fitted over scar tissue or previous graft sites, which can be less tolerant than normal of the shear forces created by the prosthesis. Blistering and open sores can develop more easily, forcing the patient to temporarily discontinue prosthesis use. These complications generally respond to local treatment. Newer prosthetic materials, such as silicone-impregnated sheaths and gel liners, can reduce shear stress and decrease the incidence of secondary skin disruption.

Painful bony spurs can occur at the distal end of the residual limb, especially with electrical injuries. Helm and Walker[46] noted that bony spurs occurred in 82% of patients who had electrical injuries and required amputation. The mean time from diagnosis to amputation was 38 weeks. Surgical revision was required in approximately 12% of cases. The pathophysiological process that causes the bone spur formation is not known.

Prosthesis fitting and training in burn patients is often complicated by the presence of wounds, multiple amputations, or ongoing medical problems. Successful prosthesis use can be achieved in patients with multiple amputations, but more intensive rehabilitation efforts are required.[54, 64, 108]

Malone and co-workers[71] demonstrated a high rate of successful upper extremity prosthesis use when patients were fitted within 30 days of amputation. Fletchall and Hickerson[33] have demonstrated that this principle is important in the burn population as well. Although their sample was small, a high rate of prosthesis use was reported in patients fitted within 30 days of the last definitive surgical procedure on the amputated upper limb. All patients were independent in self-care and used the prosthesis within 2 weeks of receipt. Self-care activities included eating, dressing, grooming, and using the toilet without assistance. Patients were able to return to driving, homemaking, and avocational interests in a mean of 2.5 months (range, 1.5 to 5 months).

PEDIATRIC BURNS

Mortality rates are higher for infants than adolescents or young adults. Children younger than 1 year are at greater risk for mortality than during subsequent preschool and school years.[96] More than half of the 26,000 children hospitalized each year for burns are younger than 5 years.[19] Children ages 6 months to 2 years account for more than half of pediatric burn admissions.[104] This correlates with the developmental stages during which children rapidly acquire motor skills that allow them to get into potentially dangerous situations. Burn treatment of pediatric patients is somewhat different from that of adults. The TBSA-to-body-weight ratio of children is greater than that of adults until adolesence. This predisposes children to even more significant fluid loss from evaporation and injury. Thermoregulation is more easily disturbed because of the relatively large body surface. Fluid resuscitation protocols should be adjusted to the child's weight and height.

The causes of burns in children are also different from those in adults. Scalding is the most common burn experienced by children. In children 4 years of age and under, 75% of all burns are due to scalding.[26] Burn injury is a common form of child abuse. Nonaccidental injuries account for approximately 10% to 28% of pediatric burns.[32, 104] Of all nonaccidental injuries experienced by children, 10% are due to burns.[90] The child who experiences a nonaccidental scald injury is typically younger than 2 years.[32] The hospital course for children who sustain nonaccidental scald burns is significantly longer, and their medical course tends to be more complicated.[50]

The clinician must recognize the characteristics of nonaccidental injuries, because 30% to 70% of abused children suffer a repeat injury.[90] Prompt medical and psychosocial care should be initiated. Characteristics that indicate a nonaccidental injury include the following: a history of injury that does not correlate with the type and location of injury observed on examination; uniform burn depth; sharp lines of demarcation between burned and nonburned areas; symmetrical wounds (i.e., in a stocking or glove pattern); an absence of splash marks in scald injuries; and the presence of other injuries in various stages of healing. All states require physicians to report any injuries caused by abuse or suspected abuse to the appropriate child protection agencies. Reporting procedures vary from state to state.[84]

The rehabilitation program is based on the child's injury and developmental stage. Children are often unable to cooperate with many aspects of therapy and do not understand long-term goals. Loss of function, such as hand dexterity and ROM, not only interferes with activities appropriate to the child's current developmental level, but also can limit future academic and vocational success (Fig. 58–24). Therapeutic success often depends on making therapy fun by incorporating age-appropriate recreation and play activities. Educating the child's family and establishing rapport with the child and family early in the course can improve participation, long-term compliance, and final outcome. Both the child and the family need emotional, social, and medical support to achieve the best rehabilitative outcome.

A child's size often makes positioning, splinting, and fitting of compression garments challenging. Children's growth makes more frequent modification of splints and custom-fitted pressure garments necessary. Skeletal and dental development can be compromised by compression therapy. For example, it is important to monitor jaw development and dental alignment during the use of face masks and orthoses to avoid malocclusion.[30, 65]

It is fairly common for children to regress emotionally, socially, and developmentally during the acute period of a burn injury. This should be temporary, and if it does not appear to be resolving, developmental screening is indicated. The Denver Developmental Screening Test is appropriate for children age 6 years and younger, and it is easy to administer. The type and location of injury have to be taken into account to avoid an inaccurate diagnosis of developmental delay. More in-depth assessments are also available to assess developmental delays if needed (see Chapter 2).

GERIATRIC BURNS

Skin atrophies with age, which results in deeper burn injuries in geriatric patients. Mortality rates are higher, since the risk of death increases with age from the middle years onward.[96] The likelihood of survival is markedly decreased by the presence of an inhalation injury in all age groups, but it is accentuated in elderly persons.[51]

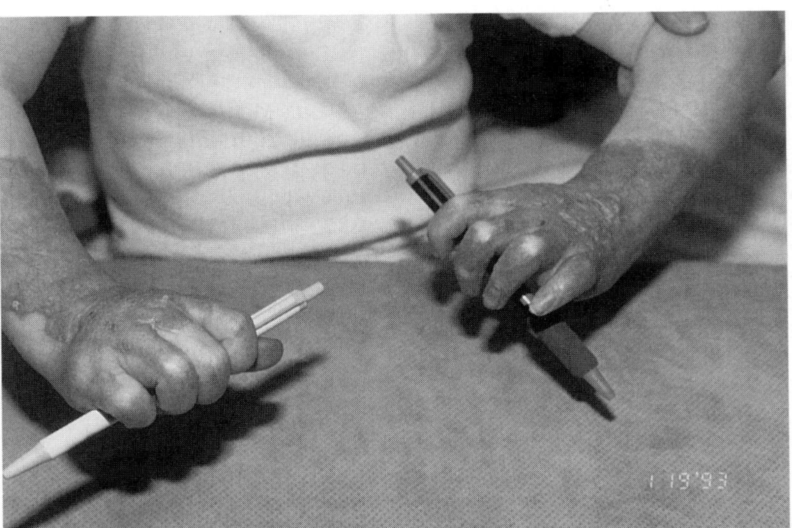

FIGURE 58–24. Notice blanching of interphalangeal joints with flexion. Significant loss of range of motion has occurred and limits fine motor skills, such as ability to write and manipulate small objects.

Cardiopulmonary disease, diabetes mellitus, peripheral vascular disease, and other preexisting medical conditions can complicate burn management in the elderly.

The geriatric patient can be at increased risk for burn injury because of premorbid mobility limitations, visual deficits, impaired sensation, and cognitive problems. Knowledge about the patient's functional level prior to the burn injury is important in planning the rehabilitation program. The patient who was previously marginally independent will likely be dependent in some aspects of mobility or performance of ADL at discharge. However, many geriatric patients are able to return to a home setting and avoid permanent placement in an extended care facility. Keys and associates[59] noted that only 5% of their patients required nursing home placement. Factors that predicted need for an extended care facility were both medical and social.

Geriatric patients often experience an initial drop in independence at discharge because of wound care, deconditioning, and outpatient therapy needs. Early involvement of social services can identify patients whose social and medical situation requires nursing home placement or a setting with additional support services. Early planning for home health care services can prevent or shorten stays in an extended care facility and enable a geriatric patient to return home.[59, 72, 105]

The elderly appear to have less hypertrophic scarring[58] and tend to experience slower healing than the young.[21, 66] Decreased scarring might be due to their reduced fibroblastic activity and collagen synthesis.[58] When the risk of hypertrophic scarring is evident, elderly persons can be less accepting of pressure garments because of difficulty in donning the garments and their high cost. The inclusion of zippers in pressure garments can make donning and doffing more feasible.

Splinting, positioning, and exercise principles in this population are similar to those of other adults. Splints require careful monitoring because of increased skin fragility and decreased sensation secondary to scarring and preexisting disease. Early mobilization is imperative because the effects of immobility occur more rapidly and are more pronounced in elderly persons.[13] Elderly persons typically have less cardiac reserve and decreased maximal oxygen consumption and cardiac work capacity.[89] Regardless of activity level, the number of motor units and overall muscle mass declines with age.[100] Although exercise programs should reflect these differences, well-designed exercise programs can assist geriatric patients in making significant gains in strength and endurance. Exercise protocols should emphasize functional activities of ambulation and mobility in addition to ROM and basic strengthening. Functional mobility is a first priority.

PSYCHOLOGICAL ADJUSTMENT

Pre-injury psychological status is a strong predictor of a patient's long-term emotional status after a serious burn. Patients who were previously well-adjusted emotionally are likely to continue to demonstrate appropriate emotional adjustment. Previous psychological dysfunction is likely to be accentuated by burn trauma.[91, 107] Burn patients with previous emotional dysfunction are also more likely to have medical complications and significantly longer hospital stays.[11, 17]

Premorbid psychiatric disorders tend to be more frequent in patients who sustain burns than in the general population. It appears that psychiatric disorder predisposes an individual to a burn injury.[94] The epidemiology of burns shows that alcohol, senility, and psychiatric disease all predispose individuals to burn injuries.[70] Approximately 45% to 69% of patients hospitalized for burns have a premorbid psychiatric history, including alcohol and substance abuse.[11, 85, 94] A history of depression increases the likelihood that patients sustained injury as a consequence of risk-enhancing behaviors.[94] An increase in stressful life events in the prior year is also associated with an increased risk of burns.[85]

A model describing the psychological adjustment of the seriously burned adult is outlined by Watkins and coworkers.[114] This model assumes no previous psychiatric illness. Rather than operating within a psychoanalytical paradigm, it describes the issues that patients face from the onset of injury to the completion of psychological recovery. It also assumes that psychological adaptation does not parallel physical recovery. The sequential stages proposed include survival anxiety, pain, search for meaning, investment in recuperation, acceptance of losses, investment in rehabilitation, and reintegration of identity. They suggest that if each stage is not successfully resolved, psychological complications are likely to occur. Therefore, interventions are proposed to facilitate resolution of each stage of recovery and ultimately a healthy emotional adjustment.

Delirium, adjustment disorders, major depression, and post-traumatic stress disorder are the most commonly seen psychiatric disorders during recovery from a burn injury.[115] Delirium, a transient disorder, is the most common, occurring in more than half of hospitalized burn patients.[94] The etiology is often multifactorial, resulting from sepsis, anoxia, anemia, liver and renal dysfunction, and other organic causes. Pediatric and geriatric patients are at greater risk for development of delirium. With correction of the underlying cause, the delirium resolves.[6]

Adjustment disorder is the second most frequently encountered disorder.[115] It occurs within 3 months of a stressful event and typically resolves within 6 months of termination of the stressor. It can persist longer in the presence of chronic conditions, such as a disabling medical condition or financial difficulties resulting from unemployment.[2] Depression and anxiety are frequently present. Anticipatory anxiety (e.g., an exaggerated expectation of pain with dressing changes or ROM exercise) is particularly common among patients with burn injuries. Individualized psychotherapeutic intervention and judiciously prescribed medications are indicated for these problems.[115]

Major depression and post-traumatic stress disorder are significant complications of burn injury. Serial evaluation and awareness of the potential for these complications can lead to early intervention, which can help prevent loss of function and improve rehabilitative outcome.

OUTPATIENT REHABILITATION

Planning for discharge should begin as early as possible. Education of the patient and family builds a foundation for all aspects of rehabilitation, including outpatient treatment. An outpatient rehabilitation program is influenced by a number of factors: the patient's social support system, functional status, ongoing need for physical and occupational therapy, wound care requirements, return to work/school criteria, availability of community services, and financial resources.

At discharge, the patient should be independent in all aspects of care in order to return home. If not, arrangements for appropriate outpatient services need to be in place prior to discharge. Home treatment programs usually involve a daily exercise regimen of stretching and strengthening, endurance training, use of pressure garments and splints, and wound care. Splints are often used and require that the patient learn the purpose and proper application of the devices. Visiting nurses can help reduce the risk of complications by assisting in wound care, monitoring wound healing and medication administration, and educating the patient about burn injury recovery.

The need for physical and occupational therapy does not end at discharge. The patient should ideally be referred to therapists with previous experience in treating burn injuries on an outpatient basis. Therapy programs need to continue the focus on ROM, strengthening, endurance, mobility, and gait.

It is common for patients to return to communities in which rehabilitation resources for the patient with burn injuries are limited. Regular follow-up, specific recommendations, and periodic communication with the community medical and allied health personnel can help to ensure quality rehabilitative care.

Skin that has been injured by burns has special needs. Moisturizers are required to control dryness, itching, and cracking. The skin must be protected from ultraviolet light because it is less tolerant and will burn more easily. Protection from sun and other sources of ultraviolet radiation is most critical during the period of scar maturation (i.e., the first 1 to 2 years).

During the months and years that follow discharge from the hospital, patients often require reconstructive surgery to correct or prevent deformity and loss of function (Fig. 58–25). Reconstructive surgery is typically delayed until scar maturation is achieved. An immature scar is more vascular, and local tissue response to the trauma of surgery is greater than in the mature scar. As a result, surgical outcomes are less favorable. However, if severe deformity is developing, surgery can be performed early to prevent irreversible loss of function (e.g., ectropion of the eyelid, which can lead to corneal damage and loss of vision). Serial procedures are often required to address cosmesis, function, or impaired physical maturation (e.g., female breast development). Because scar tissue does not expand with growth, children might need multiple operations during their growing years to correct and prevent loss of function and to improve cosmetic outcome.

Determining the timing of surgical releases and other reconstructive procedures requires consideration of the body region burned as well as the patient's age, lifestyle, occupation, and medical and psychological well-being. Though restoration of function is typically the first priority, cosmesis can be more important in cases of severe facial burns. The function and appearance of the hands and face generally are given the highest priority. After consideration of all factors, an overall surgical plan needs to be established that reflects the identified priorities and needs of the patient.

After discharge, the patient faces the task of family and community reintegration. Self-esteem can be significantly altered by changes in appearance and functional abilities. After a burn injury, women and girls have lower self-esteem than men and boys who experience comparable injuries.[86] Physical attractiveness is known to be more important for self-esteem in females

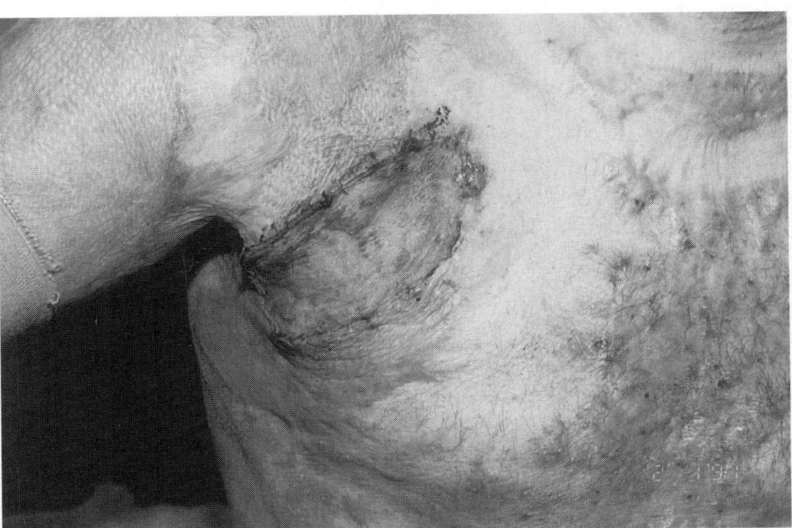

FIGURE 58–25. Right anterior axillary split-thickness skin graft performed to release an axillary contracture that limits shoulder range of motion. Note the healed mesh graft on the proximal arm. The interstices created by meshing the graft before it was applied persist.

than in males. This correlation is also seen in persons with burn injuries.[15] Persons with burn scars often do not experience the empathy from others that is typically seen with other disabilities. Burn patients can be seen as unattractive.[10] Children with facial, buttocks, or genital injuries are at increased risk of depression and poor self-esteem.[19]

Studies indicate that the greater the patient's perception of social support from family and friends, the more positive is the body image and the higher the sense of self-esteem. Symptoms of depression occur less frequently in this group of patients as well.[15, 86] Social support appears to be a key factor in a person's psychological adaptation to a burn injury.[61] The family should be educated about the key role that they and friends play in the patient's psychological recovery and continued sense of well-being.

WORK ISSUES

Returning to work is an issue of major importance to many burn patients. The TBSA injured, followed by the percentage of full-thickness and partial-thickness burns, correlates most strongly with the time needed to return to work.[47] The presence of hand burns,[48] the type of employment, and age are also significant factors.[16, 20] Overemphasis on ROM without adequate attention to the importance of endurance, strength, and power required in work settings can delay return to employment.[23]

Special problems affecting return to work include pruritus, skin fragility, heat and cold intolerance, altered sensation, and impaired coordination and dexterity. Burn injuries often occur at work, and affected individuals can have difficulty returning to the site of their injury. In the case of severe injury, approximately 20% to 50% of patients require a change in occupation.[20, 98] Vocational counselors can provide the patient and rehabilitation team with the expertise required to identify an appropriate occupation.

Work hardening is a highly structured work program that focuses on the tasks that a patient needs to be able to perform a given job (see Chapter 45). Individualized programs of training are developed after the individual's current level of function has been determined. Productivity, safety, work attitude, physical tolerance, and the specific demands of the job are weighed. The hallmark of work hardening is job simulation. The study by Zeller and associates[116] demonstrates that persons with major burn injuries can achieve a high level of vocational success; up to 90% of patients in the study returned to work.

Fewer than 1% of all disability claims approved by Social Security are due to burns.[98] Evaluation of back-to-work status and impairment ratings typically stress limitations of ROM.[5] Medical reports supporting impairment ratings should also address the unique long-term impairments in mobility, including standing and walking tolerance, hand function, skin fragility, sensitivity to ultraviolet light and chemicals, chronic pain and pruritus, heat and cold intolerance, impaired strength and sensation, and cardiopulmonary limitations.

Many patients are unfortunately lost to follow-up. A number of variables can hinder follow-up care. These variables are often interrelated and include the distance from the patient's home to the regional burn center, type of insurance, age, marital status, availability of social support, mental health, work status, educational background, and financial status.[61, 98] These issues need to be considered and potential problems addressed prior to discharge from the hospital, and they should be reevaluated at outpatient follow-up appointments. Ongoing care by specialists trained in burn care and rehabilitation optimizes the long-term outcome of the burn-injured individual.

SUMMARY

Rehabilitation should begin at the time of the acute admission. Serious burn injury results in multisystem trauma and has implications far beyond skin loss. Collaboration between the physiatrist and the burn surgeon managing the patient's acute medical and surgical care should begin immediately on the patient's admission to the burn unit. Integrating the expertise of the burn surgeon and the physiatrist helps ensure that all aspects of patient care are addressed and that the patient will receive the full complement of burn care services needed to achieve an optimal functional and cosmetic outcome. Because of the complexity and long-term effects of burns, patients need the expertise of a multidisciplinary burn care team that is composed of physicians, nurses, physical and occupational therapists, social workers, psychologists, speech pathologists, and other allied health personnel. The physiatrist is pivotal in directing the team in the planning and implementation of an individualized rehabilitation program for each patient. Many burns result in long-term functional impairments, and successful rehabilitation often requires years of effort. Success ultimately depends on the combined effort and commitment of the patient and the burn care rehabilitation team.

REFERENCES

1. Abston S: Scar reaction after thermal injury and prevention of scars and contractures. In Boswick JA (ed): The Art and Science of Burn Care. Rockville, MD, Aspen, 1987, pp 359–371.
2. Adler R: Burns are different: The child psychiatrist on the pediatric burn ward. J Burn Care Rehabil 1992; 13:28–32.
3. American Burn Association: Hospital and pre-hospital resources for optimal care of patients with burn injury: Guidelines for development and operation of burn center. J Burn Care Rehabil 1990; 11:98–104.
4. American Medical Association's Council on Scientific Affairs: Guide to Evaluation of Permanent Impairment, ed 4. Chicago, American Medical Association, 1993.
5. American Psychiatric Association: Adjustment disorder. In Diagnostic and Statistical Manual of Mental Disorders, ed 4. Washington, DC, American Psychiatric Association, 1994, pp 623–627.
6. Andreasen NJ, Noyes R, Hartford CR, et al: Management of emotional reactions in seriously burned adults. N Engl J Med 1972; 286:65–69.
7. Armstrong LE, Winent DM, Swasey PR, et al: Using isokinetic dynamometry to test ambulatory patients with multiple sclerosis. Phys Ther 1983; 63:74–79.
8. Baxter CR: Fluid volume and electrolyte changes in the early post burn period. Clin Plast Surg 1974: 1:693–709.
9. Bernstein N: Emotional Care of the Facially Burned and Disfigured. Boston, Little, Brown, 1976, p 288.
10. Bernstein N: Marital and sexual adjustment of severely burned patients: Medical aspects of human sexuality. Clin Plast Surg 1982; 9(3):337–346.
11. Berry CC, Wachtel TL, Frank HA: An analysis of factors which predict mortality in hospitalized burn patients. Burns 1982; 9:38.
12. Bolton CF, Young GB, Zochodne DW: The neurological complications of sepsis. Ann Neurol 1993; 33:94–100.
13. Bortz WM II: Disuse and aging. JAMA 1982; 248:1203–1208.
14. Borysenko M, Beringer T: Functional Histology. Boston, Little, Brown, 1984, pp 228–231.
15. Bowden ML, Feller I, Tholen D, et al: Self esteem in severely burned patients. Arch Phys Med Rehabil 1980; 61:449–452.
16. Bowden ML, Thomson PD, Prasad JK: Factors influencing return to employment after a burn injury. Arch Phys Med Rehabil 1989; 70:772–774.
17. Brezel BS, Kassenbrock JM, Stein JM: Burn in substance abusers and in neurologically and mentally impaired patients. J Burn Care Rehabil 1988; 9:169–171.
18. Campbell JL, La Clave LJ: Clinical depression in pediatric burn patients. Burns 1987; 13:213–217.
19. Centers for Disease Control and Prevention: Childhood injuries in the United States. Am J Dis Child 1990; 144:627–646.
20. Cheng S: Changes in occupational role performance after a severe burn: A retrospective study. Am J Occup Ther 1989; 43:17.
21. Chvapil M, Koopmann CF: Age and other factors regulating wound healing. Otolaryngol Clin North Am 1982; 15:259–270.
22. Covey MH: Occupational therapy. In Boswick JA (ed): The Art and Science of Burn Care. Rockville, MD, Aspen, 1987, pp 285–298.
23. Cronan R, Hammond J, Ward CG: The value of isokinetic exercise and testing in burn rehabilitation and determination of back to work status. J Burn Care Rehabil 1990; 11:224–227.
24. Deitch EA, Wheelahan TM, Rose MP, et al: Hypertrophic burn scars. J Trauma 1983; 23:895.
25. Dunphy JE, Van Winkle W: Repair and regeneration. New York, McGraw-Hill, 1969, pp 87–94.
26. East MK, Jones CA, Feller I, et al: Epidemiology of burns in children. In Carvajal HF, Parks DH (eds): Burns in Children. Chicago, Year Book Medical Publishers, 1988, p 20.
27. Edlich RF: Heterotopic calcification and ossification in the burn patient. J Burn Care Rehabil 1985; 6:363–368.
28. Evans EB: Orthopaedic measures in the treatment of severe burn. J Bone Joint Surg Am 1966; 48:643–669.
29. Evans ET, Purnell OJ, Robinett PW, et al: Fluid and electrolyte requirements in severe burns. Ann Surg 1952; 135:804.
30. Fader P: Preserving function and minimizing deformity. In Carvajal HF, Parks DH (eds): Burns in Children. Chicago, Year Book Medical Publishers, 1988, p 335.
31. Farrell DF, Starr A: Delayed neurologic sequelae of electrical injuries. Neurology 1968; 18:600–606.
32. Feldman KW, Schaller RT, Feldman JA, et al: Tap water scald burns in children. Pediatrics 1978; 62:1–7.
33. Fletchall S, Hickerson WL: Early upper extremity prosthetic fit in patients with burns. J Burn Care Rehabil 1991; 12:234.
34. Fraser PM: Ptolemaic Alexandria, vol 1. Oxford, Clarendon Press, 1937.
35. Freshwater MF, Krizek TJ: Skin grafting of burns: A centennial tribute to George David Pollack. J Trauma 1971; 11:862.
36. Grube BJ, Heimbach DM, Engrav LH, et al: Neurologic consequences of electrical burns. J Trauma 1990; 30:254–258.
37. Haberal J: Electrical burns: A five year experience: 1985 Evans Lecture. J Trauma 1986; 26:103–109.
38. Hammond JS, Ward CG: High voltage electrical injuries: Management and outcome of 60 cases. South Med J 1988; 81:1351–1352.
39. Hansbrough JF: Biologic dressings. In Boswick JA (ed): The Art and Science of Burn Care. Rockville, MD, Aspen, 1987, p 57.
40. Hansbrough JF, Zapata-Sirvent R, Carroll WJ, et al: Clinical experience with Biobrane biosynthetic dressing in the treatment of partial thickness burns. Burns 1984; 10:415–419.
41. Harries CA, Pegg SP: Foam ear protectors for burnt ears. J Burn Care Rehabil 1989; 10:183.
42. Haynes BW Jr: The history of burn care. In Boswick JA (ed): The Art and Science of Burn Care. Rockville, MD, Aspen, 1987, pp 3–9.
43. Helm PA, Johnson ER, Carlton AM: Peripheral neurological problems in the acute burn patient. Burns 1977; 3:123–125.
44. Helm PA, Kevorkian CG, Lushbaugh M, et al: Burn injury: Rehabilitation management in 1982. Arch Phys Med Rehabil 1982; 63:6–16.
45. Helm PA, Pandian G, Heck E: Neuromuscular problems in the burn patient: Causes and prevention. Arch Phys Med Rehabil 1985; 66:451–453.
46. Helm PA, Walker SC: New bone formation at amputation sites in electrically burn-injured patients. Arch Phys Med Rehabil 1987; 68:284–286.
47. Helm PA, Walker SC: Return to work after burn injury. J Burn Care Rehabil 1992; 13:53.
48. Helm PA, Walker SC, Peyton SA: Return to work following hand burns. Arch Phys Med Rehabil 1986; 67:297.
49. Henderson B, Koepke GH, Feller I: Peripheral polyneuropathy among patients with burns. Arch Phys Med Rehabil 1971; 52:149–152.
50. Hummel RP, Greenhalgh DG, Barthel PP, et al: Outcome and socioeconomic aspects of suspected child abuse scald burns. J Burn Care Rehabil 1993; 14:121.

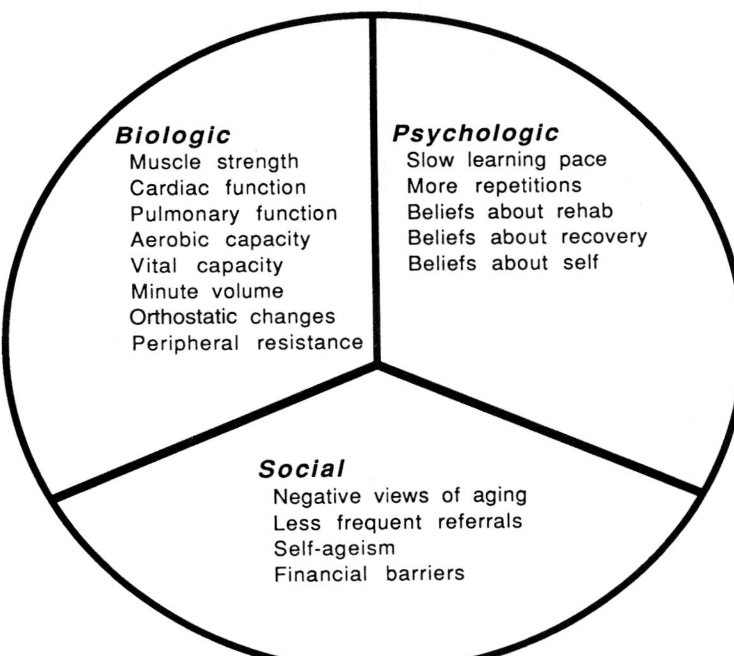

FIGURE 59–2. Age-related factors that may affect rehabilitation. (From Brummel-Smith K: Rehabilitation. In Ham RJ, Sloane PD (eds): Primary Care Geriatrics: A case-based approach. St. Louis, CV Mosby, 1992, p 141.)

the effects of disuse caused by inactivity or injury. An example is the patient with a humeral fracture who has lost extremity strength and mobility. A portion of this functional loss might be reversible and is secondary to the disuse subsequent to the immobilization that occurred during the treatment of the injury. Not uncommonly, such a patient might regain strength and partial motion but have a permanent partial loss of range of motion (ROM) of the shoulder. In this case, the rehabilitation program restored partial function to the shoulder. The same patient could also sustain loss of strength and motion in the rest of the involved extremity because of

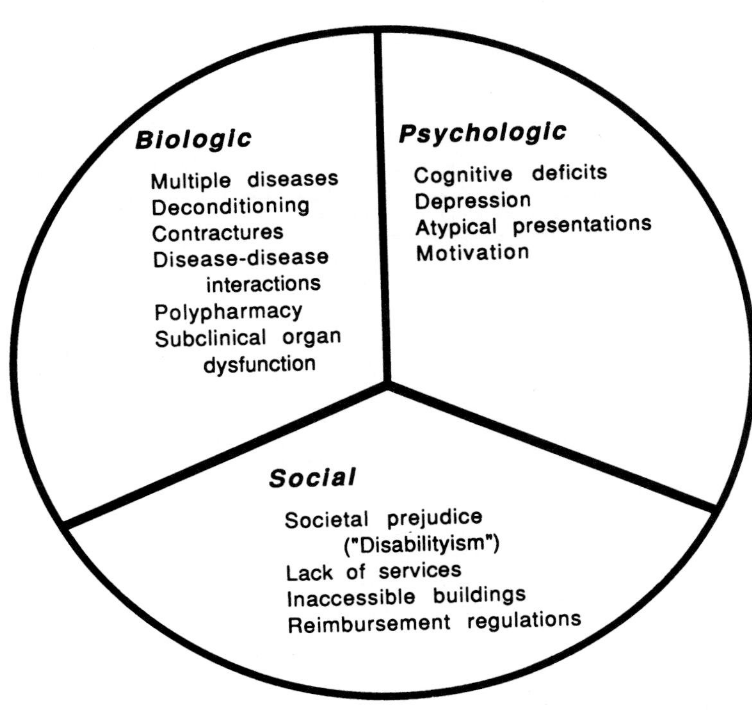

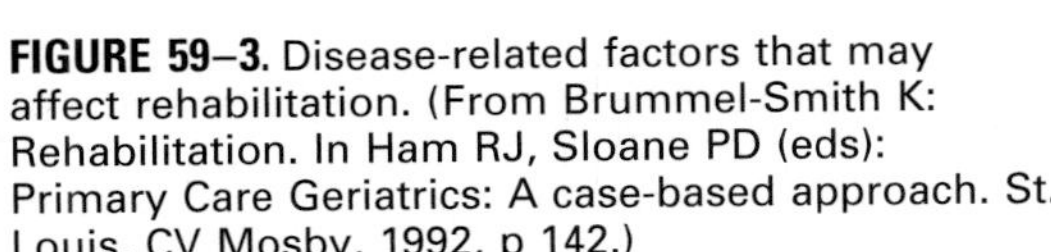
FIGURE 59–3. Disease-related factors that may affect rehabilitation. (From Brummel-Smith K: Rehabilitation. In Ham RJ, Sloane PD (eds): Primary Care Geriatrics: A case-based approach. St. Louis, CV Mosby, 1992, p 142.)

shoulder immobilization during treatment. This disuse can be avoided by preventive rehabilitation. This preventive concept should be broadened to include all geriatric patients by remembering the "use it or lose it" concept.[7]

Medical treatment of impairment is the third integral part of geriatric rehabilitation. Treatment is needed to cure when possible, or at least to stabilize the disease process when cure is not possible. Many of the impairments of the elderly are chronic and incurable but manageable, thus preventing or delaying progression and complications and associated disability.

BIOLOGY AND PHYSIOLOGY OF AGING

Body Composition

Body composition changes with aging (Table 59–2). There is a gradual loss of lean tissue and an increase in fat. The loss of lean tissue reflects loss of muscle mass: total body muscle mass, limb muscle volume, muscle cross-sectional area, and muscle fiber number and area.[27] Body fat increases to 30% of body weight at age 80 years as compared to 15% at age 30, which should be taken into account when prescribing fat-soluble drugs.[65] Bone mineral is lost; peak bone density occurs in the 30s and 40s and thereafter gradually declines.

Postural Changes of Aging

Figures 59–4 and 59–5 illustrate the postural changes that occur with aging.[38] Figure 59–4 shows the progressive anterior thrust of the head and extension of the cervical spine, accentuated thoracic kyphosis, and straightening of the lumbar spine. Increased extension of the arms and scapular protraction at the shoulders is associated with flexion of the elbows, ulnar deviation at the wrists, and finger flexion. In the lower extremity, there is an increase in hip and knee flexion and a decrease in ankle dorsiflexion. During ambulation, there is diminished arm swing and a shorter step length.[46]

Figure 59–5 illustrates the widening of the bony pelvis with aging. The angle of the femoral neck to the shaft increases, resulting in a valgus deformity of the hips.[65] Progressive widening of the standing base with aging is noted. In women, the knees can develop varus deformities with narrowing of the standing base.

The functional effect of these postural changes is to require a shift of the center of gravity of the body away from its previous location just anterior to the first or second sacral level and to shift the plumb line of the body so that it no longer favors extension of the lower extremity joints in relaxed standing. Consequently, patients must adjust their individual standing posture to maintain the erect position. Steinberg[64] points out that the center of gravity is shifted behind the hips by flexing the knees and that this may require the use of ambulatory aids such as a cane.

In addition to the described anatomical effects on posture, there are physiological effects noted. Increased postural sway occurs with aging.[17] The ability to balance on one leg with eyes either closed or open decreases.[6] Righting reflexes decrease and reaction time increases.

Normal Neurological Changes of Aging

In order to be able to recognize pathological changes in the elderly patient, it is necessary to know what is "normal" in aging. Table 59–3 lists frequently found neurological changes that are normal in elderly patients. As an example, absent ankle jerks and diminished vibratory sense in the distal legs of an elderly person do not necessarily indicate the presence of a peripheral neuropathy if they occur without the presence of other appropriate history or physical findings. Conversely, the absence of an expected finding in a disease state can occur in the elderly and can confuse the clinical picture.

TABLE 59–2 Changes in Biological Functions in Response to Aging, Inactivity, Weightlessness, and Exercise

Function	Aging	Inactivity	Weightlessness	Exercise
$\dot{V}o_2$max	Decreased	Decreased		Increased
Cardiac output	Decreased	Decreased		Increased not for older
Systolic BP	Increased		Increased	Decreased
Orthostatic tolerance	Decreased	Decreased	Decreased	Increased
Body water	Decreased	Decreased	Decreased	
RBC mass	Decreased	Decreased	Decreased	
Thrombosis	Increased	Increased		Decreased
Serum lipids	Increased	Increased		Decreased
HD lipoprotein	Increased over age 80 yr			Increased
Lean body mass	Decreased	Decreased	Decreased	
Muscle strength	Decreased	Decreased	Decreased	Increased
Calcium	Decreased	Decreased	Decreased	
Glucose tolerance	Decreased	Decreased		Increased
EEG dominant frequency	Decreased	Decreased		Increased

Abbreviations: $\dot{V}o_2$max, maximum oxygen consumption; BP, blood pressure; RBC, red blood cell; HD, high density; EEG, electroencephalogram.
From Stineman MG, Granger CV: Outcome studies and analysis: Principles of rehabilitation that influence outcome analysis. In Felsenthal G, Garrison SJ, Steinberg FU (eds): Rehabilitation of the Aging and Elderly Patient. Baltimore, Williams & Wilkins, 1994, p 512.

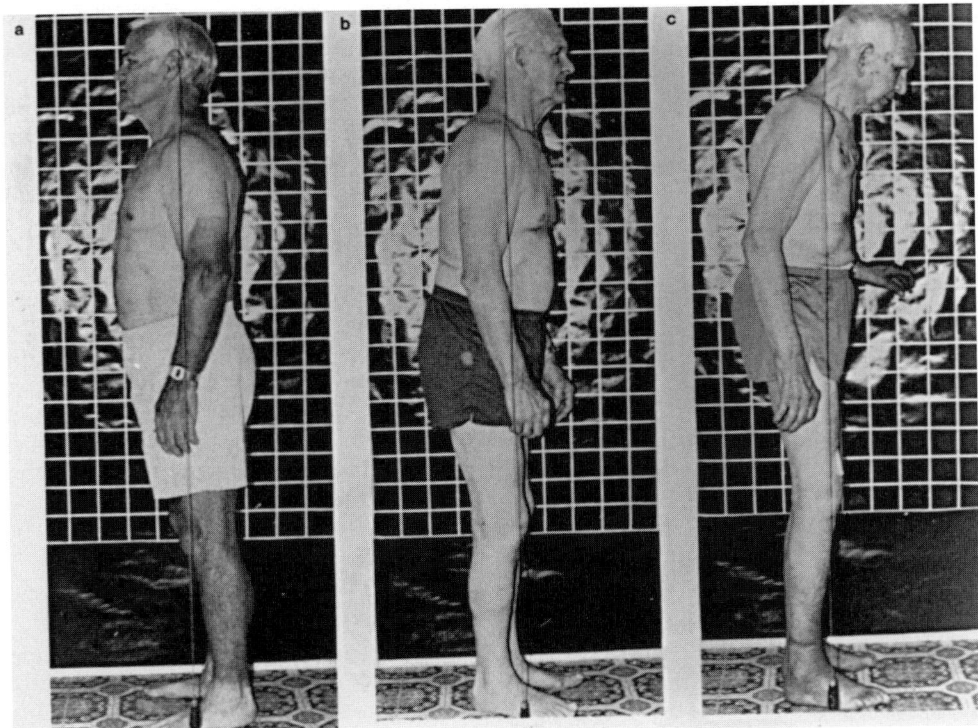

FIGURE 59–4. Lateral posture of a 60-year-old man (*a*), a 78-year-old man (*b*), and a 93-year-old man (*c*).

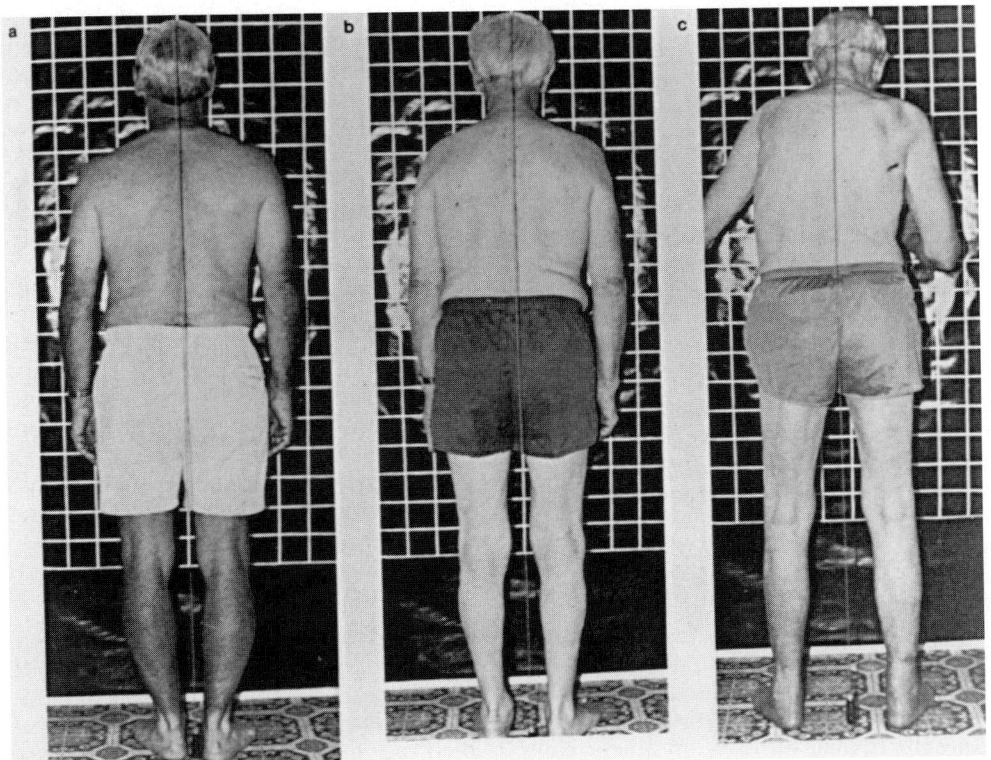

FIGURE 59–5. Posterior posture of a 60-year-old man (*a*), a 78-year-old man (*b*), and a 93-year-old man (*c*).

TABLE 59–3 Frequent Neurological Changes in Elderly Patients

Eye signs
- Small, irregular pupils
- Diminished reaction to light and near reflex
- Diminished range of movement on convergence and upward gaze
- Slowed pursuit movements with cogwheeling

Motor signs
- Tendency to tremor (>69 yr, 43% have hand tremor, 7% have head tremor [titubation])
- Gait: short-stepped or broad-based with diminished associated movements
- Dysmetria (in all >65 yr)
- Dysdiadochokinesia
- Atrophy of interossei (thenar wasting in 66%, anterior tibial wasting in 25%)
- Increased muscle tone: legs more than arms, proximal more than distal
- Diminished muscle strength: legs more than arms, proximal more than distal

Sensory signs
- Diminished vibratory sense distally, legs much more than arms
- Possible change in proprioception
- Mildly increased threshold for light touch, pain, and temperature
- Impaired double simultaneous stimulation

Reflex signs
- Diminished or absent ankle jerks
- Some reduction in knee, biceps, and triceps reflexes
- Abdominal reflex sometimes lost
- Babinski's sign may not occur (when it would in younger patients)
- Primitive reflexes occur in 20% to 25% (palmomental, snout, and nuchocephalic [doll's eyes])

From Ham RJ: Assessment. In Ham RJ, Sloane PD (eds): Primary Care Geriatrics: A Case-Based Approach. St Louis, Mosby–Year Book, 1992, p 87.

For example, Babinski's response does not always occur in upper motor neuron lesions in the elderly as it does in younger patients.

It should be emphasized that just because a physical finding is normal for an elderly patient, it still might have functional significance. For instance, loss of upward gaze is seen in elderly patients. The normal limit of upward gaze in the young adult is 40 to 45 degrees, but by the eighth decade it is reduced to an average of 16 degrees.[12] Mechanical neck problems are also common in the elderly, and this combination of restricted cervical motion and vertical gaze can make it difficult for a patient to see wall clocks, exit signs, room numbers, and other orienting information.[37] In an attempt to compensate for this, the patient might lean backward, contributing to imbalance and a possible fall.

Diminished muscle strength occurs in the elderly with the lower limbs more involved than the upper limbs and with greater weakness proximally than distally. One common functional complaint in the elderly is increasing difficulty arising from a chair or toilet seat. Physical examination frequently reveals little except functionally decreased strength in the limb girdle muscles, especially the hip extensors. These muscles no longer have the strength required to lift the patient's body weight against gravity from the sitting to the standing position. Exercise by itself does not always rectify this loss of functional strength, and accommodation and education are then necessary. Patients are typically more functional if seated in chairs with firm seats supporting their hips and knees at 90-degree angles, with their feet flat on the floor. The chairs should have armrests. The patients should be instructed to move their buttocks to the front of the chair and to flex their knees to bring their feet under the front edge of the chair and under their buttocks. Many patients will also need to use their arms to assist in coming to their feet.

The decline in cognitive function with normal aging, as demonstrated by the Baltimore Longitudinal Study of Aging,[58] tends to be of small magnitude. In fact some functional measures, such as vocabulary, digit span forward, and memory for text, actually improve with aging. Mentation changes in the elderly are more likely to be associated with pathological conditions such as dementia, depression, or delirium.

Skin

Aging changes that occur in the skin include decreases in moisture content, epidermal renewal, elasticity, blood supply, and sensitivity to touch, pain, and temperature. The effect of these changes is to make the patient, particularly if thin or malnourished, more susceptible to injury (pressure sores) or infection.

Cardiopulmonary Changes

Cardiac changes that occur with aging include decreased cardiac reserve, contractile function, heart rate, and response to exercise. Blood pressure tends to rise with aging. Pulmonary function mildly decreases with a decline in vital capacity. However, the main functional deficits secondary to the cardiopulmonary system are due to disease and not aging changes.[3, 4]

Urological Changes

Changes of the urinary system due to aging are functionally significant. Urinary frequency, hesitancy, retention, and nocturia are common complaints in both sexes and relate to anatomical and physiological aging changes of the kidney and bladder. Bladder capacity is reduced and reduced and residual volume increased. Prostatic hypertrophy is almost universal among elderly men. A reduction in creatinine clearance can predispose the elderly to toxic effects of renally excreted drugs unless dosage adjustments are made and renal function is monitored.

Hydration

The elderly have approximately a 25% decrease in thirst perception as compared to the young. In addition, they can be placed in situations with a limited access to water, leading to an increased risk of dehydration. Moreover, medications (diuretics or laxatives) might increase the elderly person's need for water to maintain adequate hydration.[45] Many diseases common in the elderly and many drugs commonly used by the elderly (antidepressents, analgesics, cancer chemotherapy agents) can cause the syndrome of inappropriate antidiuretic hormone secretion and lead to water retention and hyponatremia.

Temperature

Elderly people have impairment of their thermoregulatory mechanisms and are more susceptible to hyperthermia and hypothermia.[69] The febrile response to infection and other inflammatory diseases can fail to develop in the elderly and can lead to a missed diagnosis.[36]

EXERCISE

Bortz[7] emphasized that using one's physical capacities was necessary to prevent their loss. He stated it succinctly as the "use it or lose it" principle. This principle indicates that the decrease in physiological functioning in the elderly is not inevitably due to the aging process but is also due to inactivity. (The effects of deconditioning and inactivity are discussed in Chapter 34.) Figure 59–6 indicates that if inactive elderly persons initiate an appropriate exercise program, they can "lessen" their physiological age as measured by maximum oxygen consumption ($\dot{V}o_2max$).[34] Table 59–4 summarizes the adaptations to strength conditioning in older men, and Table 59–5 summarizes the adaptations to aerobic conditioning in older men and women. Flexibility and ROM have also been reported to improve in the elderly with exercise.[61]

In order to maintain function, critical ROM should be maintained in the major joints. In the upper extremity, ROM of the shoulder should allow abduction to at least 90 degrees, with sufficient internal rotation to touch the lower back and external rotation to touch the back of the head. ROM of the forearm should allow a minimum of 45 degrees of pronation and supination with wrist flexion of 45 degrees and extension of 30 degrees. Finger flexion should be to within 1 inch of the palm. In the lower extremity, hip extension should be to at least neutral and flexion to 90 degrees. Knee extension should be to neutral and flexion to 110 degrees. Ankle dorsiflexion should be to neutral.

Precautions and contraindications have to be considered before initiating an exercise program in the elderly.[27] Cardiac status has to be determined and any unstable or untreated cardiovascular impairment should be considered as a possible contraindication. Limited ROM and arthritic joint involvement might require modification of the exercise program. Any coexisting medical conditions—anemia, hyperthyroidism, etc.—should be under optimal management. The possible impact of any medications on the ability to safely exercise and the consequent need for modification of the exercise program must be considered, for example, symptomatic treatment of upper respiratory symptoms with decongestants. High temperature and humidity might necessitate modification of the exercise program.

PHARMACOLOGY AND SUBSTANCE ABUSE

Because of physiological changes affecting liver and kidney function, and the absorption and distribution of drugs, the elderly are more sensitive to medication effects than younger people.[52] Table 59–6 lists drugs causing functional impairments in mobility, bladder continence, and mental state. Elderly individuals take an

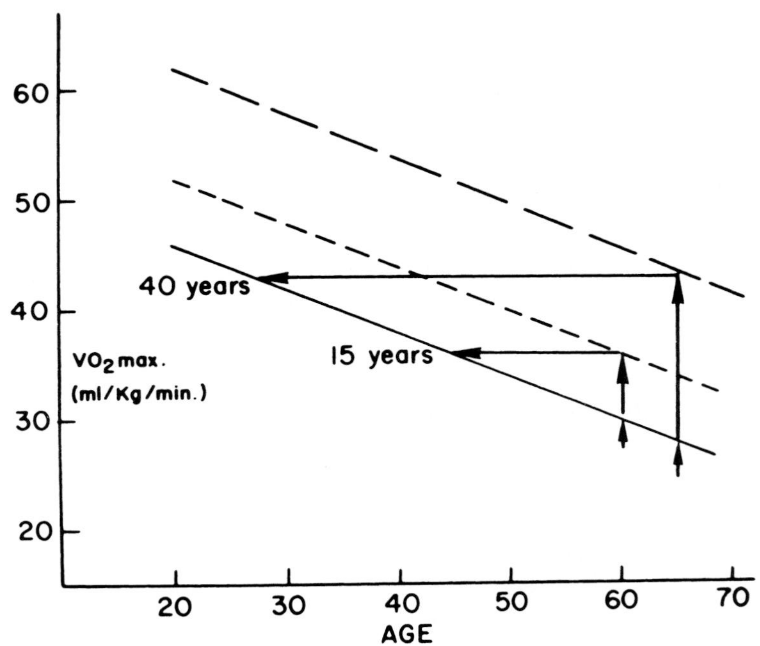

FIGURE 59–6. Potential improvement in $\dot{V}O_2max$ with age changes. *Top line:* athletes. *Middle line:* moderately active persons. *Bottom line:* sedentary persons. (From Hodgson J: Age and aerobic capacity of urban midwestern males. Thesis, University of Minnesota, Minneapolis, 1971.)

TABLE 59–4 Adaptations to Strength Conditioning in Older Men

Variable	Range of Reported Improvements
Strength	
Static	↑ 13%–72%
1 RM	↑ 9%–227%
Isokinetic	↑ 7%–29%
Strength gain/day	
Static	↑ 0.3%–4.0%
1 RM	↑ 3%–5%
Isokinetic	↑ 0.2%–0.5%
Isokinetic work	↑ 18%–21%
Torque-velocity curve	↑ Velocity at a given torque
Muscle size	
Cross-sectional area (on CT)	↑ 9%–12%
Type I fiber area	↑ 31%–38%
Type II fiber area	↑ 26%–52%
Mean fiber area	↑ 27%
Turnover of muscle protein (from urinary 3-methylhistidine)	↑ 41%
Muscle fiber type distribution	No change
Integrated electromyographic activity	↑ 23%
Muscle membrane Na^+-K^+ pumps	↑ 40%
Sarcoplasmic reticulum Ca^{2+}-ATPase	Decrease with age is prevented
Aerobic power ($\dot{V}O_2$max)	↑ 0%–6%
Maximum exercise heart rate	No change
Maximum exercise blood pressure	No change
Hemoglobin concentration	No change
Blood volume	No change
Capillary density per fiber	↑ 15%
Oxidative enzyme activity (citrate synthase)	↑ 30%

Abbreviations: RM, range of movement; CT, computed tomography; $\dot{V}O_2$max, maximum oxygen consumption.

From Frontera WR, Meredity CN: Exercise in the rehabilitation of the elderly. In Felsenthal G, Garrison SJ, Steinberg FU (eds): Rehabilitation of the Aging and Elderly Patient. Baltimore, Williams & Wilkins, 1994, p 40.

average of five medications, and the incidence of adverse reactions increases with the number of medications.[20] In addition, the elderly take many nonprescription medications and receive their prescribed medications from different sources. Interactions between these medications can be subtle and gradual in onset but ultimately can have a significantly detrimental effect on function. Elderly patients admitted to a rehabilitation service often show improvement in function only after their medication regimens have been modified or eliminated.

Substance abuse (e.g., alcohol) is common among the elderly, with a reported incidence of up to 20% in some studies.[59] A mnemonic useful for screening for alcoholism in elderly patients is CAGE: *C*ut down ("Have you tried to cut down on your drinking?"); *A*nnoyed or angry ("Have others annoyed or angered you by criticizing your drinking?"); *G*uilty ("Have you ever felt guilty about your drinking?"); *E*ye-opener ("Have you used alcohol to steady your nerves or to reduce the effects of a hangover?").[25]

With the need to be cognizant of polypharmacy and substance abuse, it is important to have guidelines for medication use in elderly rehabilitation patients (Table 59–7). A useful acronym for rational drug therapy in the elderly is MASTER: *m*inimize number of drugs used; *a*lternatives should be considered; *s*tart low and go slow; *t*itrate therapy; *e*ducate patient; *r*eview regularly.[66]

FUNCTIONAL ASSESSMENT

Various aspects of functional assessment are covered in Chapters 1, 2, 6, and 8. In the elderly, assessment tools measuring ADL and instrumental ADL have particular significance. If used to document the patient's status initially and serially, accurate comparison can lead to

TABLE 59–5 Adaptations to Aerobic Conditioning in Older Men and Women

Variable	Range of Reported Improvements
Ventilation	
During submaximal exercise	
Minute ventilation	↓ 9%–15%
During maximal exercise	
Minute ventilation	↑ 20%–30%
% Maximal voluntary ventilation	↑ 16%
Cardiac function	
During submaximal exercise	
Heart rate	↓ 9–20 beats/min
Stroke volume	↑ 8%
Cardiac output	No change
During maximal exercise	
Heart rate	No change
Stroke volume	↑ 6%–28%
Cardiac output	↑ 0%–34%
Circulation	
Total hemoglobin	↑ 7%
Blood volume	↑ 8%
Systemic vascular resistance during submaximal exercise	↓ 5%–18%
Leg blood flow during maximal exercise	↑ 42%
Muscle metabolism	
Fiber type distribution	No change or increased type IIA
Capillary density	No change
In vitro oxidative capacity	↑ 128%
Oxidative enzyme activity	↑ 0%–45%
Glycogen stores	↑ 10%–28%
Mitochondrial number, mean volume, and volume fraction	No change
During submaximal exercise	
Arteriovenous O_2 difference	No change
Blood lactate	↓ 21%–44%
During maximal exercise	
Arteriovenous O_2 difference	↑ 14%
Integrated response	
Submaximal $\dot{V}O_2$	No change
$\dot{V}O_2$max	↑ 11%–30%

Abbreviations: $\dot{V}O_2$, oxygen uptake; $\dot{V}O_2$max, maximum oxgen consumption.

From Frontera WR, Meredith CN: Exercise in the rehabilitation of the elderly. In Felsenthal G, Garrison SJ, Steinberg FU (eds): Rehabilitation of the Aging and Elderly Patient. Baltimore, Williams & Wilkins, 1994, p 42.

TABLE 59–6 Drug-Induced Impairment

Drug	Impairment
Antiepileptics	
Phenytoin	Osteoporosis, osteomalacia, neuropathy, sedation, cerebellar dysfunction, delirium, skin disorders
Barbiturates	Sedation, ataxia, skin disorders, behavior changes, respiratory depression, hypotension
Carbamazepine	Dizziness, sedation, ataxia, anemia, water retention, cardiac arrhythmias, vision disorders
Clonazepam	Sedation, respiratory depression, hypotension
Ethosuximide	Sedation, movement disorders, skin disorders
Valproate	Sedation, tremor, ataxia
Psychiatric	
Neuroleptics	Extrapyramidal symptoms, orthostatic hypotension, impaired balance, incontinence (central inhibition), dementia, constipation
Sedative hypnotics	Sedation, incontinence (oversedation), dementia
Lithium	Arthralgias, myopathies, polyuria, behavior changes, drowsiness, ataxia, impaired memory, skin disorders, confusion
Antidepressants	
Tricyclics	Sedation, delirium, constipation, urine retention, cardiac arrhythmias, orthostatic hypotension
Monoamine oxidase inhibitors	Irritability, agitation, tremor, urine retention, hypertension
Serotonin uptake inhibitors	Varies in sedative vs. stimulant effects
Other cyclics	Varies in sedative vs. stimulant effects
Parkinsonian Agents	
Dopamine Agonists	Postural hypotension, delirium
Anticholinergic	Delirium, constipation, urine retention
Amantadine	Orthostatic hypotension, delirium, depression, skin disorders
Analgesics	
Aspirin	Hypertension, impaired hearing, tinnitus, edema
Other nonsteroidal anti-inflammatory agents	Hypertension, edema
Narcotics (opioid)	Delirium, sedation, constipation, respiratory depression
Autonomic-Cardiovascular	
Cholinergics	Bronchoconstriction, bradycardia
Anticholinergics (antimuscarinics)	Blurred vision, urine retention, constipation, tachycardias, delirium
Alpha-2 agonists (central)	Sedation, bradycardia, depression
Adrenergic agonists	Restlessness, tremors, hypertension, tachycardia
Beta-receptor blockers	Bronchoconstriction, bradycardia, cardiac failure, orthostatic hypotension, depression, lethargy, sleep disorders, behavior changes
Calcium channel blockers	Hypotension, peripheral edema, muscle weakness, bradycardia
Diuretics	Hypotension, weakness, electrolyte imbalance, glucose abnormalities
Alpha antagonists (peripheral)	Hypotension, incontinence (stress)
Other	
Corticosteroids	Arthralgias, myopathies, osteoporosis, osteomalacia, glucose levels, behavior changes, depression, electrolyte abnormalities
Antihistamines	Sedation, urine retention, behavior changes

TABLE 59–7 Guidelines for Medication Use During Rehabilitation of Older Adults

Maintain a HIGH index of suspicion for medication toxicities.
Obtain accurate over-the-counter and prescription medication histories.
Review that each medication is still indicated.
Record a clear diagnosis for which each medication, especially psychotropic medication, is prescribed.
Gradually eliminate unnecessary medications.
Review that medication dosages are correct.
Simplify medication schedules as much as possible.
Clarify with patients that they are willing and able to take medications.
Educate patient and family about indications for medications and their side effects.

From Siebens H: Issues on medication use and substance abuse in older adults. In Felsenthal G, Garrison SJ, Steinberg FU (eds): Rehabilitation of the Aging and Elderly Patient. Baltimore, Williams & Wilkins, 1994, p 354.

early diagnosis and intervention at the first sign of functional deterioration.

Assessment tools can also be used to determine the cognitive status of the patient.[39] The Mini-Mental State Examination (MMSE)[26] (Table 59–8) is an example of a screening tool that can be used to help detect and assess dementia. It can be administered rapidly and accurately and can be used to follow cognitive improvement or deterioration over time. The MMSE can also be used to screen for delirium. The Geriatric Depression Scale[8] (Table 59–9) was developed to screen for the common symptoms of depression in the elderly.

Gait and balance instruments (Table 59–10) are also useful functional assessment instruments, allowing both diagnostic assessment and longitudinal evaluation of patient function. Tinetti and Ginter[67] have shown that an assessment that reproduces mobility maneuvers is a better method of assessing functional mobility than neuromuscular findings on a physical examination.

Impairment of driving significantly limits an older person's ability to function independently in the community. Factors identified as suggestive of the potential for adverse driving events include near vision acuity worse than 20/40, limited neck rotation, and poor performance on a test of visual attention such as the number cancellation task.[44]

Balance

Balance is a key component of mobility. It depends on the interaction of multiple systems—the peripheral nervous system, proprioception, vestibular and cerebellar function, and visual acuity. In addition, adequate muscle strength in the extensors of the hips and knees and normal ankle muscles are necessary for normal balance. When one component of the balance equation is impaired, the others can substitute, but when more than one component is affected, often balance is impaired. With normal aging, each component of the balance equation can be impaired (see Tables 59–3 and 59–10).

Gait

The basics of gait are covered in Chapter 5 and aging changes affecting gait are noted above under postural changes of aging and balance. Table 59–10 indicates that men develop a gait pattern of small steps with a wide base during walking and standing. Women typically develop a waddling style of gait with a narrow walking and standing base. During ambulation, the swing phase decreases and the period of double support increases.[46, 47] These changes and the postural changes that require muscular contraction to maintain joint extension increase the energy cost of ambulation. The aging person typically compensates for this increased energy demand by using a slower walking speed.

Pathological gait patterns in the elderly can be due to neurological or musculoskeletal causes and are often diagnostic of the underlying disease. Examples of abnormal gait patterns and their causes include circumduction (hemiparesis); scissoring (upper motor neuron disease); festinating (Parkinson's disease); ataxia (vitamin deficiency, cervical spondylosis, cerebellar dysfunction); apraxia (normal pressure hydrocephalus); senility (arterial degeneration); and waddling (muscle weakness).[35] Other musculoskeletal causes of pathological gait include problems of the feet, hip, knee, and lumbar spine. The importance of a hip extension deficit has been emphasized by Steinberg.[64]

FALLS

Falls and near falls occur in about one-third of the elderly.[11] While only 3% to 5% of falls result in fractures, 90% of fractures of the hip, pelvis, and forearm result from falls.[63] Normal aging changes that contribute to falls are listed in Tables 59–3, 59–11 to 59–13. Tables 59–13 and 59–14 list risk factors in the home. Additional environmental factors include inclement weather and unfamiliar surroundings (Table 59–13). Psychological factors include inattention, depression, and cognitive impairment. Living alone is a sociological risk factor. Iatrogenic causes are listed under medications in Table 59–13. Some illnesses associated with falls are listed in Table 59–13. Sometimes falls are a prodrome of a not as yet clinically apparent illness or infection. Strategies for reducing the risk of falls are listed in Table 59–12 and guidelines for home safety are listed in Table 59–14. One of the most significant consequences of falling is

TABLE 59–8 Mini-Mental State Examination

I. Orientation (Ask the following questions)

What is today's date?	Date (e.g., Jan. 21)	☐
What is the year?	Year	☐
What is the month?	Month	☐
What day is today?	Day (e.g., Monday)	☐
Can you also tell me what season it is?	Season	☐
Can you also tell me the name of this hospital (clinic)?	Hospital (clinic)	☐
What floor are we on?	Floor	☐
What town or city are we in?	Town or city	☐
What county are we in?	County	☐
What state are we in?	State	☐

II. Immediate Recall

Ask the subject if you may test his/her memory. Then say "ball, flag, tree" clearly and slowly, about 1 sec for each. After you have said all three, ask him/her to repeat them. This first repetition determines his/her score (0–3), but keep saying them until he/she can repeat all three, up to six tries. If he/she does not eventually learn all three, recall cannot be meaningfully tested.	"Ball" "Flag" "Tree" Number of trials: ______	☐ ☐ ☐

III. Attention and Calculation

Ask the subject to begin with 100 and count backward by 7. Stop after five subtracts (93, 86, 79, 72, 65). Score the total number of correct answers.	"93" "86" "79" "72" "65"	☐ ☐ ☐ ☐ ☐
If the subject cannot or will not perform "the count backward test"task, ask him/her to spell the word "world" backward. The score is the number of letters in correct order. For example, *dlrow* is 5, *dlorw* is 3.	D L R O W	☐ ☐ ☐ ☐ ☐

IV. Recall

Ask the subject to recall the 3 words you previously asked him/her to remember. Score 0–3.	"Ball" "Flag" "Tree"	☐ ☐ ☐

V. Language

NAMING Show the subject a wrist watch and ask him/her what it is. Repeat for pencil.	Watch Pencil	☐ ☐
REPETITION Ask the subject to repeat, "No ifs, ands, or buts."	Repetition	☐
3-STAGE COMMAND Give the subject a piece of plain blank paper and say, "Take the paper in your right hand, fold it in half and put it on the floor."	Takes paper in right hand Folds paper in half Puts paper on floor	☐ ☐ ☐
READING On a blank piece of paper print this sentence "Close your eyes," in letters large enough for the subject to see clearly. Ask him/her to read it and do what it says. Score correct only if he/she actually closes his/her eyes.	Closes eyes	☐
WRITING Give the subject a blank piece of paper and ask him/her to write a sentence. It is to be written spontaneously. It must contain a subject and a verb and be sensible. Correct grammar and punctuation are not necessary.	Writes sentence	☐
COPYING On a clean piece of paper, draw intersecting pentagons, each side about 1 inch, and ask subject to copy it exactly as it is. All 10 angles must be present and two must intersect to score one point. Tremor and rotation are ignored.	Draws pentagons	☐

e.g.

Deriving Total Score

Sum the number of correct replies to the test items. If item "world spelled backward" was used then add the number of correct letters given in proper sequence (one to five). The maximum score is 30 for this test.

TOTAL SCORE ☐

Reproduced with permission from Folstein MF, Folstein SE, McHugh PR: Mini-Mental State: A practical method for grading the cognitive state of patients for the clinician. J Psychiatr Res 1975; 12:189–198; and Kewas CH: Evaluation of cognition in the elderly rehabilitation patient. In Felsenthal G, Garrison SJ, Steinberg FU (eds): Rehabilitation of the Aging and Elderly Patient. Baltimore, Williams & Wilkins, 1994, pp 289–294.

TABLE 59–9 Geriatric Depression Scale*

1. Are you basically satisfied with your life?	Yes/No
2. Have you dropped many of your activities and interests?	Yes/No
3. Do you feel that your life is empty?	Yes/No
4. Do you often get bored?	Yes/No
5. Are you hopeful about the future?	Yes/No
6. Are you bothered by thoughts you can't get out of your head?	Yes/No
7. Are you in good spirits most of the time?	Yes/No
8. Are you afraid that something bad is going to happen to you?	Yes/No
9. Do you feel happy most of the time?	Yes/No
10. Do you often feel helpless?	Yes/No
11. Do you often get restless and fidgety?	Yes/No
12. Do you prefer to stay at home, rather than going out and doing new things?	Yes/No
13. Do you frequently worry about the future?	Yes/No
14. Do you feel you have more problems with memory than most?	Yes/No
15. Do you think its wonderful to be alive now?	Yes/No
16. Do you often feel downhearted and blue?	Yes/No
17. Do you feel pretty worthless the way you are now?	Yes/No
18. Do you worry a lot about the past?	Yes/No
19. Do you find life very exciting?	Yes/No
20. Is it hard for you to get started on new projects?	Yes/No
21. Do you feel full of energy?	Yes/No
22. Do you feel that your situation is hopeless?	Yes/No
23. Do you think that most people are better off than you are?	Yes/No
24. Do you frequently get upset over little things?	Yes/No
25. Do you frequently feel like crying?	Yes/No
26. Do you have trouble concentrating?	Yes/No
27. Do you enjoy getting up in the morning?	Yes/No
28. Do you prefer to avoid social gatherings?	Yes/No
29. Is it easy for you to make decisions?	Yes/No
30. Is your mind as clear as it used to be?	Yes/No

* A cutoff score of 9 has a sensitivity of 90% and a specificity of 80%; a cutoff score of 11 has a sensitivity of 84% and a specificity of 95%; a cutoff score of 14 has a sensitivity of 80% and a specificity of 100%.

From Brink TL, Yesavage JA, Lum O, et al: Screening tests for geriatric depression. Clin Gerontol 1982; 1:37–43.

TABLE 59–10 Position Changes, Balance Maneuvers, and Gait Components Included in Functional Mobility Assessment

Mobility Maneuvers	Conditions Defining Maneuver Done With Difficulty
Position Change or Balance Maneuver	
Getting up from chair*†	Does not get up with single movement, pushes up with arms or moves forward in chair first, unsteady on first standing
Sitting down in chair*†	Plops in chair, does not land in center
Withstanding nudge on sternum (examiner pushes lightly on sternum three times)	Moves feet, grabs object for support, feet not touching side by side
Eyes closed	Same as above (tests patient's reliance on visual input for balance)
Neck turning	Moves feet; grabs object for support; feet not touching side by side; complains of vertigo, dizziness, or unsteadiness
Reaching up	Unable to reach up to full shoulder flexion standing on tiptoes; unsteady; grabs object for support
Bending over	Unable to bend over to pick up small object (e.g., pen) from floor; grabs object to pull up on; requires multiple attempts to rise
Gait Component or Maneuver‡	
Initiation	Hesitates, stumbles, grabs object for support
Step height (raising feet while stepping)†§	Does not clear floor consistently (scrapes or shuffles), raises foot too high (>2 in.)
Step continuity§	After first few steps, does not consistently begin raising one foot as other foot touches floor
Step symmetry§	Step length not equal (pathological side usually has longer step length; problem may be in hip, knee, ankle, or surrounding muscles)
Path deviation‖	Does not walk in straight line; weaves from side to side
Turning†	Stops before initiating turn, staggers; sways; grabs object for support

* Hard, armless chair.

† Included in analysis.

‡ Patient walks down hallway at "usual pace," and comes back using usual walking aid. Examiner observes single component of gait at a time (analogous to heart examination).

§ Best observed from side of patient.

‖ Best observed from behind patient.

From Tinetti ME, Ginter SF: Indentifying mobility dysfunctions in elderly patients: Standard neuromuscular examination or direct assessment. JAMA 1988; 259:1189.

TABLE 59–11 Normal Aging Changes That Predispose to Falls and Injuries

Visual impairments
- Presbyopia and decreases in accommodative capacity, visual acuity, night vision, peripheral vision, glare tolerance, impaired blue-green discrimination, and contrast sensitivity

Nervous system impairments
- Reduced righting reflexes, proprioceptive input, and cerebral function; increased reaction time; lessened awareness of vibration, touch, and temperature; increased distractibility

Musculoskeletal impairments
- Osteopenia; musculoskeletal stiffness; reduced or uncoordinated muscle control

Cardiovascular impairments
- Postural hypotension

Gait changes
- Women: waddling gait, narrow walking and standing base
- Men: Small-stepped gait, wide walking and standing base

Auditory impairments
- Reduced speech discrimination
- Increased high-frequency threshold
- Wax accumulation

Adapted from Tideiksaar R: Falls in the elderly: An approach to management. Phys Assistant 1988; 10:114–132; and Barclay AM: Falls in the elderly: Is prevention possible? Postgrad Med 1988; 83:241–248.

TABLE 59–12 Strategies for Reducing Risk of Falls

Risk Factor	Interventions	
	Medical	*Rehabilitative or Environmental*
Reduced visual acuity, dark adaptation, and perception	Refraction; cataract extraction	Home safety assessment
Reduced hearing	Removal of cerumen; audiological evaluation	Hearing aid if appropriate (with training); reduction in background noise
Vestibular dysfunction	Avoidance of drugs affecting the vestibular system; neurological or ear, nose, and throat evaluation, if indicated	Habituation exercises
Proprioceptive dysfunction, cervical degenerative disorders, and peripheral neuropathy	Screening for vitamin B_{12} deficiency and cervical spondylosis	Balance exercises; appropriate walking aid; correctly sized footwear with firm soles; home safety assessment
Dementia	Detection of reversible causes; avoidance of sedative or centrally acting drugs	Supervised exercise and ambulation; home safety assessment
Musculoskeletal disorders	Appropriate diagnostic evaluation	Balance-and-gait training; muscle-strengthening exercises; appropriate walking aid; home safety assessment
Foot disorders (calluses, bunions, deformities)	Shaving of calluses; bunionectomy	Trimming of nails; appropriate footwear
Postural hypotension	Assessment of medications; rehydration; possible alteration in situational factors (e.g., meals, change of position)	Dorsiflexion exercises; pressure-graded stockings; elevation of head of bed; use of tilt table if condition is severe
Use of medications (sedatives: benzodiazepines, phenothiazines, antidepressants; antihypertensives; others: antiarrhythmics, anticonvulsants, diuretics, alcohol)	Steps to be taken: 1. Attempted reduction in the total number of medications taken 2. Assessment of risks and benefits of each medication 3. Selection of medication, if needed, that is least centrally acting, is least associated with postural hypotension, and has shortest action 4. Prescription of lowest effective dose 5. Frequent reassessment of risks and benefits	

Modified from Tinetti ME, Speechley M: Risk factors for falls among elderly persons living in the community. N Engl J Med 1989; 320:1056.

TABLE 59–13 Some Factors Implicated in Traumatic Fractures in the Elderly

- Aspects of aging
  - Primary osteoporosis
  - Impaired balance/vision
  - Alteration in gait
  - Loss in muscle/fat "padding" at hip
  - Falls forward (Colles' fracture/humerus) vs. falls down (hip/pelvic)
- Environment
  - Outdoor
    - Cracked walkway
    - Poor lighting
    - Poor weather
    - Uneven ground
    - Crime (assault and battery)
  - Indoor
    - Throw rugs
    - Wires across path
    - Slippery tub
    - Poor lighting
    - Stairs/railings
    - Pet causing a fall
- Genetic
  - Sex (females > males)
  - Race (white > black)
- Illnesses
  - Cerebrovascular accident
  - Syncopal episodes
  - Hypotensive illnesses
  - Secondary osteoporosis
    - Hyperthyroidism
    - Hypoparathyroidism, etc.
  - Osteomalacia
  - Parkinson's disease
  - Dementia
  - Arthritis
  - Paraparesis
  - Previous fracture
- Lifestyle
  - Exercise/nutrition
  - Alcoholism/other abused drugs
  - Bed rest/immobilization
  - Shoe style
- Medications
  - Benzodiazepines
  - Tricyclic antidepressants
  - Antipsychotic medications
  - Corticosteroids (secondary osteoporosis)
  - Barbiturates

From Stein BD, Felsenthal G: Rehabilitation of fractures in the geriatric population. In Felsenthal G, Garrison SJ, Steinberg FU (eds): Rehabilitation of the Aging and Elderly Patient. Baltimore, Williams & Wilkins, 1994, p 123.

the fear of another fall, with subsequent immobility, weakness, and isolation.

COMMON IMPAIRMENTS

Table 59–15 lists the common disorders that are typically seen by a geriatric rehabilitation team. The impairment groups for patients admitted to our geriatric rehabilitation unit, which is geared to the rehabilitation needs of the frail elderly (average patient age of 80), are listed in Table 59–16. Survey data from the National Center for Health Statistics (Fig. 59–7) indicate that of the 10 most common chronic conditions with morbidity in the age 65+ group, at least two—arthritis and orthopedic impairment—are commonly managed by the rehabilitation team. The other disorders listed in Table 59–17 are also seen in our patients[21] as comorbidities that require management to ensure that the patient's rehabilitation can proceed. Failure to manage these conditions can cause them to worsen and delay or complicate the rehabilitation process.

Our data indicate that these patients have multiple diagnoses, with a mean of six.[21] The disability caused by a specific impairment does not act in isolation from those associated with the other impairments. This interaction of impairments can have a cascade effect[20] in that the overall cumulative disability can greatly exceed the individual summated disabilities. As seen in Figure 59–8, each impairment has a limited associated disability, but that disability augments the limited disability caused by the patient's other impairments. This creates a greater total disability and a much more complicated management problem for the patient, the rehabilitation team, and the family.

Each of these common impairments is encountered not only in the elderly but also in patients of any age seen by the physiatrist and the rehabilitation team. These impairments are discussed in detail in other chapters. The following comments are specific to the impact of these impairments on elderly patients.

Pain

The majority of elderly people will, at some time, have a serious pain problem. Musculoskeletal pain is the most common type reported. Data show, for example, that approximately 75% of nursing home patients have pain problems. Taking a pain history requires special care regarding secondary gain or hidden agendas, which in the elderly can include loneliness, a planned family vacation, etc. In addition, hearing loss, dementia, pseudodementia (delirium or depression), and underreporting of symptoms by the patient all can influence the accuracy of information. Information from significant others can often be used to piece together a fuller picture of the problem. The physical examination for these patients has several potential unique findings (Table 59–18). Laboratory and radiographic studies to help sort out these problems are frequently more difficult because of severe contractures, kyphosis, confusion, agitation, or inaccessible veins. Since the elderly are more sensitive to medications and at greater risk of polypharmacy, physical measures should be the cornerstone of treatment of musculoskeletal pain in the elderly, with appropriate caution. A clinical practice guideline, the Management of Chronic Pain in Older Persons, gives specific recom-

TABLE 59–14 Guidelines for Home Safety

Problem Area	Risk Potential for Falls	Modifications to Recommend
Floors	High polish or wet surfaces may cause slipping	In bathrooms, use nonslip tiles, nonslip adhesive strips on floor next to tub, sink, and toilet, or indoor-outdoor carpeting; on linoleum floors, use slip-resistant floor wax with minimal buffing; use nonskid floor mat by kitchen sink to guard against wet floor
Carpets	Thick pile and carpet borders may cause tripping	Suggest carpets of low pile
Area rugs and mats	Rugs and mats may slide out from under person	Use rugs and mats with nonskid backing, or apply double-faced adhesive tape as backing
Lighting	Low or uneven lighting may obscure hazards	Increase lighting in high-risk areas, e.g., stairs, bathroom, bedroom
Glare	Visual impairment and distraction may be produced by glare from bright lights (especially sunlight) on polished floors and from unshielded light bulbs	Use polarized window glass, or apply tinted material to windows to eliminate glare without reducing light; reduce flood glare by repositioning light sources
Stairs	Poor lighting may contribute to tripping on stairway	Place light switches at top and bottom of stairway to avoid traveling up and down in the dark, or place night-lights by top and bottom step to provide visual cuing of steps; apply colored nonskid adhesive strips to stair edges; set maximum step rise at 6 in.
Handrails	Lack of support may result from missing or improper handrails	Place cylindrical rails 1–2 in. away from wall on both sides, with ends turned in and extending beyond top and bottom steps to provide easy grasping and signal top and bottom step
Sink edge and towel bar	Weak towel bar or wet, slippery sink edge may not provide adequate support	Replace towel bars with nonslip grab bars
Toilet seat	Transfer falls often occur because seat is too low	Advise use of elevated toilet with grab bars placed on wall next to toilet
Wet bathtub and shower floor surfaces	Slipping and falling are common on wet surfaces	Place nonslip adhesive rubber strips or suction-cup mat on tub floor; install nonslip grab bars in and around tub and shower; advise use of shower chair and flexible hand-held shower hose for patients with balance impairment
Bed height	Transfer falls are more common if height is not optimal	Adjust bed height distance from patella to floor (18 in. from top of mattress to floor allows for safest transfer by most persons)
Soft bed mattress	Poor sitting balance and support may lead to falls from bed	Bed mattress edges should be firm enough to support a seated person without sagging
Chair height	Transfer falls from low chairs are common	Replace low chairs with more suitable ones (chair height should be 14–16 in. from seat edge to floor; armrests should be present 7 in. above the seat and extend 1–2 in. beyond the seat edge for maximal leverage)
Shelf height	Reaching or bending to retrieve objects from high or low shelves leads to imbalance and falling	Rearrange frequently used kitchen and closet items to avoid excessive reacing and bending; encourage use of hand-held reach tools
Gas range	Difficult-to-see dial may not be turned off and may cause gas leak; fall may be first sign of gas asphyxiation with impaired smell	Mark on and off dial positions clearly
Temperature	Low room temperature may cause hypothermia; falls may be secondary to hypothemia	Maintain indoor temperature at 72°F in winter

Adapted from Tideiksaar R: Falls in the elderly: An approach to management: Phys Assistant 1988; 10:114–132; and Christiansen J, et al: The prevention of falls in later life: A report of the Kellogg International Work Group on the Prevention of Falls in the Elderly. Dan Med Bull 1987; 34:1–24.

TABLE 59–15 Common Disorders Seen in the Geriatric Rehabilitation Team Setting

Amputation	Joint replacement
Arthritis	Lymphedema
Burns	Neuropathy
Cancer	Osteoporosis
Cardiovascular disorders	Pain syndromes (acute)
Chronic pain	Parkinson's disease
Chronic pulmonary disease	Peripheral vascular disease
Contractures	Postural disorders/falls
Deconditioning	Pressure sores
Disk disorders	Spinal cord injury
Fracture	Spinal stenosis
Head injury	Stroke
Immobility	Trauma

Adapted from Reichel W: Clinical Aspects of Aging, ed 3. Baltimore, Williams & Wilkins, 1989, p 184.

TABLE 59–16 Geriatric Rehabilitation Unit Administration Impairment Groups—1997 to 1998

	Patients	
Impairment	*n*	%
Orthopedic	35	(33)
Stroke	27	(25)
Debility	11	(10)
Neurological	9	(8)
Pulmonary	9	(8)
Brain	4	(4)
Cardiac	4	(4)
Amputee	2	(2)
Arthritis	2	(2)
Spinal cord	1	(1)
Medically complex	1	(1)
Other	2	(2)
Total	107	100%

Data from Levondale Hebrew Geriatric Center and Hospital.

mendations for assessment and pharmacological treatment of chronic pain (Tables 59–19 to 59–21).[2]

Spinal problems are common causes of pain in the elderly. Spondylitic changes are present in up to 82% of persons in their sixth decade. Cervical disk degeneration presents most commonly at C5–6, followed by C6–7 and C4–5. Cervical spondylitic myelopathy is the most common reason for spinal cord dysfunction in patients over the age of 55. Lumbosacral spinal stenosis is commonly seen in the elderly. It typically produces bilateral symptoms that are worse with standing or walking. Sitting down or flexing the spine while standing usually relieves these symptoms.[19]

At least 25% of the elderly have shoulder pain, usually of soft tissue origin. Elbow, wrist, and hand pain occur commonly due to C7 radiculopathy, medial or lateral epicondylitis, median or ulnar nerve entrapment, de Quervain's tenosynovitis, or generalized arthritis. Hip pain is frequently due to arthritis, trochanteric bursitis, or radiculopathy at L5 or S1. Arthritis and trauma (sometimes even trivial trauma) can be major reasons for knee pain. Atrophic fat pads, bony deformities in the foot, and ill-fitting shoes can cause tendinitis, nerve

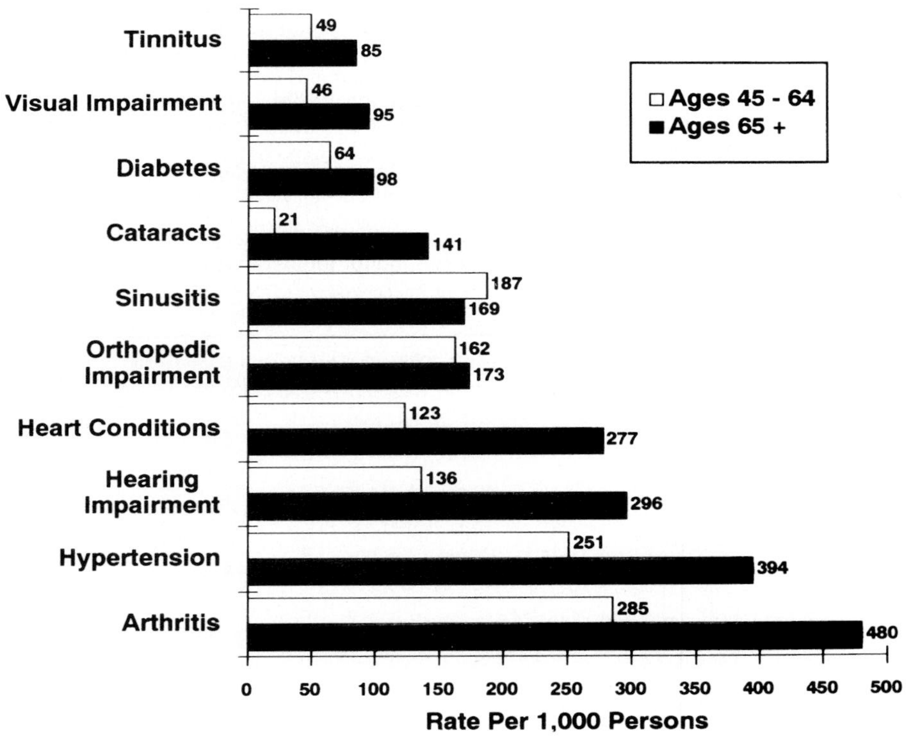

FIGURE 59–7. Morbidity from top ten chronic conditions, 1986. (From National Center for Health Statistics: Current estimates from the National Health Interview Survey, United States, 1986. Vital and Health Statistics Series 10, No. 164, October 1987.)

TABLE 59–17 Most Frequent Diagnoses—Primary or Secondary

Diagnoses	Patients	
	n	%
Hypertension	36	43.9
Arteriosclerotic heart disease	35	42.7
Cerebrovascular accidents	31	37.8
Peripheral vascular disease	25	30.5
Diabetes mellitus	24	29.3
Fractures	22	26.8
Osteoarthritis	17	20.7
Neuropsychiatric	13	15.9
Deconditioned	12	14.6
Decubitus ulcers	10	12.2

From Felsenthal G, Cohen BS, Hilton EB, et al: The physiatrist as primary physician for patients on an inpatient rehabilitation unit. Arch Phys Med Rehabil 1984; 65:375–378.

entrapments, and tenosynovitis. These pain problems can usually be eliminated or ameliorated by physical medicine management.[54]

Dysphagia

Motor function of the lips, tongue, and masticatory muscles slows with aging. Often multiple gestures of the tongue are made prior to swallowing. The latency from entry of the bolus into the pharynx until the elevation of the larynx increases with age. The amplitude of esophageal contractions decreases with age. The clinical significance of these changes is not known. However, the effects of other problems on swallowing in the aged are known, such as medication side effects, psychosocial factors (feeding dependency), neurological disorders, inflammatory muscle disease, scleroderma, cervical spine disorders, cancer, and tracheostomy.[51]

Arthritis

Arthritis is not only more common in the elderly, it may present differently in the elderly than in younger people. For example, the shoulder is typically more involved in the elderly with rheumatoid arthritis than in younger persons. A patient with osteoarthritis of the hip has a smaller chance of having hip osteoporosis and hip fractures. Older persons have smaller muscle fibers and fewer anterior horn cells than younger people. In addition, the tendons, ligaments, and capsules surrounding joints lose elasticity, as evidenced by a decrease in joint ROM and a sense of stiffness in older persons. ROM exercises for joints should start at a few degrees and should be done gently. The patient often resists needed assistive devices such as canes and walkers because of their stigma of aging and disability. If shown that the device can reduce pain, the patient may at least decide to use it privately, if not publicly. Joint replacement surgery can be of great help in medically intractable joint dysfunction, especially of the hip and knee.[49]

Osteoporosis and Paget's Disease

Acute symptomatic osteoporosis from vertebral fractures can be treated with bed rest and physical measures. Flank pain can be caused by severe kyphoscoliosis with the rib cage rubbing the pelvic rim. Back-strengthening exercises contribute to good posture and skeletal support, but flexion exercises of the spine are not recommended owing to the possibility of anterior wedge fractures (see Chapter 41). Paget's disease in the elderly can lead to fractures, rare cancerous changes, total joint replacement, and paraplegia.[60]

Fractures

Osteoporosis and falls are the reason for the great majority of fractures of the wrist, hip, and shoulder. Extensive rehabilitation is often needed for these patients, with an inpatient rehabilitation stay needed for some.

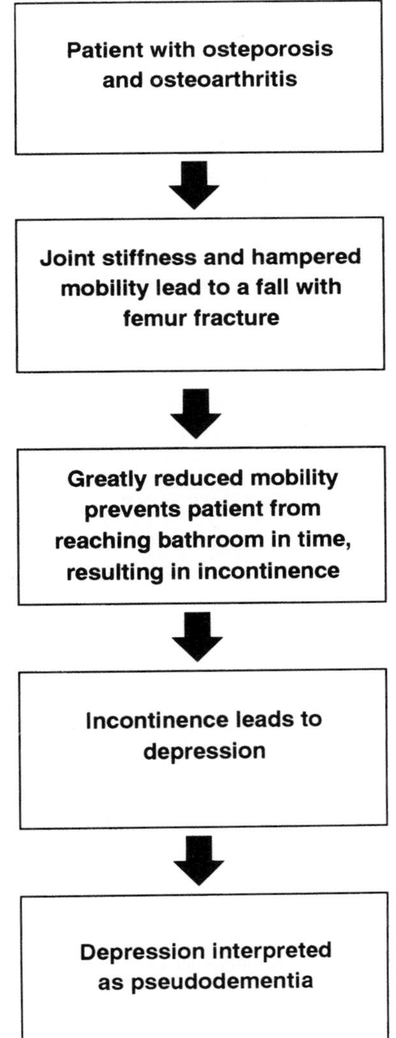

FIGURE 59–8. Cascade effect of a disability is greater than the sum of the individual disabilities.

TABLE 59–18 Examples of Geriatric Physical Examination Issues for the Pain Patient

Clinical Problem	Functional Consequence	Pain, Other Consequences
Hamstring and back extensor muscle contractures, decreased range of motion of heel cords (from high heels)	Excess knee and hip flexion and abnormal spinal postures to avoid falling from a heel cord contracture	Pain at multiple sites from fatigue and muscle overuse; give attention to heel cords
Restriction of upward gaze	Compensation by neck extension and lordosis, with foraminal narrowing, facet compression, and alterations in balance	Radicular compression at foramen with pain; increased risk of dizziness and falls
Orthostatic hypotension	Alterations in balance and gait	Differentiate from other neuromusculoskeletal reasons for altered gait

Weight bearing and ROM are important issues. After a subcapital hip fracture, repair by pinning will often require restricted weight bearing for 6 weeks or longer. Should a hemiarthroplasty have been performed, restrictions in hip motion to prevent dislocation (no flexion greater than 90 degrees, no adduction past the midline, and no internal rotation) are taught. The use of long-handled devices and "knee spreader" pillows are helpful tools for the approximately 3 months that the motion restrictions are in place. If the hemiarthroplasty is cemented, weight bearing is typically not restricted. However, the porous ingrowth type of prosthesis often requires reduced weight bearing for 6 weeks or more. Intertrochanteric fractures treated with sliding screw and plate fixation are variably followed by restricted weight bearing or weight bearing as tolerated, depending on the severity of the fracture and the orthopedic surgeon's approach to weight bearing after such procedures. Family support during rehabilitation is critical. Concomitant deep venous thrombosis, stroke, pain, and peripheral neuropathy may be present. Pelvic fractures, if severe, might need prolonged bed rest (with its risks) as part of the treatment. Colles' fractures can be severely disabling and also result in carpal tunnel syndrome.[63]

Stroke

Older persons are more at risk of being institutionalized after a stroke. Patients who typically have not been in a student situation for 50 or 60 years often have difficulty learning new ways to accomplish tasks. Multi-infarct dementia can be a confounding problem. The geriatric patient is also susceptible to osteoporosis, impaired au-

TABLE 59–19 Pharmacological Management of Chronic Pain in Older Persons: Acetaminophen and Nonsteroidal Anti-inflammatory Drugs*†

Drug	Maximum Dosage	Pharmacologic Changes	Precautions and Recommendations
Acetaminophen‡§ (Tylenol)	4000 mg/24 hr (q 4–6 hr dosing)	Hepatotoxic above maximum dose	Avoid exceeding maximum recommended dose
Aspirin‡§	4000 mg/24 hr (q 4–6 hr dosing)	Gastric bleeding; abnormal platelet function	Avoid high doses for prolonged periods of time
Ibuprofen‡ (Motrin, Advil, Nuprin, etc.)	2400 mg/24 hr (q 6–8 hr dosing)	Gastric, renal, and abnormal platelet function may be dose dependent; constipation, confusion, and headaches may be more common in older patients	Avoid high doses for prolonged periods of time
Naproxen‡§ (Naprosyn)	1000 mg/24 hr (q 8–12 hr dosing)	Similar toxicity to ibuprofen	Avoid high doses for prolonged periods of time
Choline magnesium trisalicylate‡‖ (Trilisate)	5500 mg/24 hr (q 8–12 hr dosing)	Prolonged half-life of 8-12 hr; similar toxicity to ibuprofen; classic salicylate toxicity may develop at high dose	Tests for salicylate levels may be necessary occasionally to avoid toxicity

* Limited number of representative examples only for demonstrative purposes. Comprehensive lists of other classes of NSAIDs and a multitude of brand names can be found elsewhere. There is no evidence of increased efficacy or decreased adverse effects (other than specific allergic sensitivities) to warrant the extremely high costs of most proprietary variations.

† Clinicians should monitor the literature closely for availability and cost-risk-benefit analyses of the cyclooxygenase-2-inhibitor class of NSAIDs, which should be commercially available soon.

‡ Available in liquid form.

§ Available in suppository form.

‖ Minimum platelet dysfunction.

From AGS Panel on Chronic Pain in Older Persons: The management of chronic pain in older persons. J Am Geriatr Soc 1998; 46:635–651.

TABLE 59–20 Pharmacological Management of Chronic Pain in Older Persons: Opioid Analgesic Drugs

Drug	Oral Equivalent	Starting Dosage	Aging Effects	Precautions and Recommendations
Short-acting drugs				
Morphine sulfate (Roxanol, MSIR)	30 mg	15–30 mg q 4 hr	Intermediate half-life; older people are more sensitive than younger people to side effects	Start low and titrate to comfort; continuous use for continuous pain; intermittent use for episodic pain; anticipate and prevent side effects
Codeine (plain codeine, Tylenol with codeine, other combinations)	120 mg	30–60 mg q 4–6 hr	Acetaminophen-NSAID* combinations limit dose; constipation is a major issue	Begin bowel program early; do not exceed recommended maximum dose
Hydrocodone (Vicoden, Lortab, others)	30 mg	5–10 mg q 3–4 hr	Acetaminophen-NSAID* combinations limit dose; toxicity similar to morphine	Anticipate and prevent side effects; begin bowel program early; do not exceed recommended maximum dose
Oxycodone (Roxicodone, Oxy IR, Percodan, Tylox, Percocet)	20–30 mg	5–10 mg q 3–4 hr	Acetaminophen-NSAID* combinations limit dose; toxicity similar to morphine; oxycodone is available as a single agent	Anticipate and prevent side effects; begin bowel program early; do not exceed recommended maximum dose
Hydromorphone (Dilaudid)	7.5 mg	1.5 mg q 3–4 hr	Half-life may be shorter than morphine (3 hr); toxicity similar	Similar to morphine; start low and titrate to comfort; give continuously (q 3–4 hr) for continuous chronic pain disorders
Long-acting drugs				
Sustained-release* morphine (MS Contin,† Kadian,‡§ Oramorph SR†)	30 mg	15–30 mg q 12 hr or 24-hr equivalent of total prior analgesics in divided doses q 12 hr	Rarely requires more frequent dosing than recommended on package insert	Escalate dose slowly because of possible drug accumulation; immediate-release opioid analgesic often necessary for breakthrough pain
Sustained-release* oxycodone (Oxycontin)	20–30 mg	10–20 mg q 12 hr or 24-hr equivalent of total prior analgesics in divided doses q 12 hr	Similar to sustained-released morphine	Immediate-release opioid often necessary for breakthrough pain
Transdermal fentanyl (Duragesic)	NA (see package insert)	>25 μg/hr; not recommended in opioid-naive patients	Effective activity may exceed 72 hr in older patient (transdermal patches designed for 3-day duration of action)	Titrate slowly using immediate-release analgesics for breakthrough pain; peak effects of first dose may take 18–24 hr

* These preparations are *not* to be broken, crushed, or dissolved. They must be used as formulated to provide continuous-release activity.
† Every 24 hour dosing.
‡ Every 8–12 hour dosing.
§ Capsules can be opened and contents sprinkled on applesauce for easier ingestion without altering activity of the drug.
From AGS Panel on Chronic Pain in Older Persons: The management of chronic pain in older persons. J Am Geriatr Soc 1998; 46:635–651.

ditory and visual abilities, polypharmacy, osteoarthritis, skin fragility, and the stresses of older families[30] (see Chapter 50).

Traumatic Brain Injury

Falling is the most common cause of traumatic brain injury (TBI) in those more than 65 years of age, and pedestrian accidents yield the most fatalities. Alcohol is involved commonly, especially with men. Advancing medical and neurological illnesses often increase the severity of the injury as well as its mortality. Reemployment is usually not a goal in the elderly. Protection from a second fall is a major goal to prevent further TBI and fractures. Selected elderly patients will benefit from an intensive comprehensive rehabilitation program that includes physical therapy, cognitive rehabilitation, behavioral management, dysphagia and communication treatment, and fall prevention.[24] (see Chapter 49).

Motor Neuron Disease and Parkinson's Disease

These well-known diseases occur in the elderly. Attention to dysphagia, respiratory problems, self-care, bal-

TABLE 59–21 Pharmacological Management of Chronic Pain in Older Persons: Nonopioid Analgesics and Adjuvant Drugs

Drug	Starting Dose (PO)	Specific Indications	Pharmacological Changes	Precautions and Recommendations
Corticosteroids (prednisone)	2.5–5.0 mg/day	Inflammatory disease	Increased risk of hyperglycemia, osteopenia, and Cushing phenomenon	Avoid high dose for long-term use
Antidepressants (amitriptyline, desipramine, doxepin, imipramine, nortriptyline)	10 mg HS	Neuropathic pain, sleep disturbance	Increased sensitivity to side effects, especially anticholinergic effects	Monitor carefully for anticholinergic adverse effects; desipramine may be as effective as amitriptyline with fewer side effects; start at lowest available dose, 10 mg, and titrate HS dose upward by 10 mg every 3–5 days
Anticonvulsants				
Clonazapam	0.25–0.5 mg	Neuropathic pain		
Carbamazepine (Tegratol)	100 mg	Only for lancinating pain (e.g., trigeminal neuralgia)	Can cause somnolence, ataxia, dizziness, leukopenia, thrombocytopenia, and rarely aplastic anemia	Start at 100 mg q.d., increase slowly bid, 200 mg q.d., then b.i.d.; check LFTs, CBC, RF at baseline; CBC at 2 then 8 wk
Gabapentin (Neurontin)	100 mg	Neuropathic pain	May prove to have less serious side effects than carbamazepine	Start with low dose (100 mg) and titrate up slowly to effect; neuropathic doses not yet established; titrate to t.i.d. dosing; monitor for idiosyncratic side effects (e.g., ankle swelling, ataxia); dose range for efficacy anecdotally reported as 100–800 mg t.i.d.
Anti-arrhythmics				
Mexiletine (Mexitil)	150 mg	Neuropathic pain	Side effects such as tremor, dizziness, unsteadiness, paresthesias are common; rarely hepatic damage and blood dyscrasias occur	Avoid use in patients with preexisting heart disease; start with low dose and titrate slowly; recommend initial and follow-up ECGs; titrate to t.i.d. to q.i.d. dosing
Local Anesthetics (intravenous) Lidocaine	3–5 mg/kg infused every 15–30 min	Diagnostic test	Delirium common	May be useful predictor of response to mexiletine or other oral local anesthetics for neuropathic pain; diagnostic test only in a monitored environment where seizure, delirium, airway control, and hemodynamic alterations can be managed
Other agents				
Baclofen	5 mg	Neuropathic pain, muscle spasms	Probable increased sensitivity and decreased clearance	Monitor for weakness, urinary dysfunction; avoid abrupt discontinuation due to CNS irritability

Abbreviations: CBC, complete blood cell count; CNS, central nervous system; ECG, electrocardiogram; HS, hour of sleep or at bedtime; LFT, liver function tests; RF, renal function.

From AGS Panel on Chronic Pain in Older Persons: The management of chronic pain in older persons. J Am Geriatr Soc 1998; 46:635–651.

ance and mobility, nutrition, and psychotherapy is important[41] (see Chapters 46 and 51).

Peripheral Nervous System Impairments

Elderly persons have decreased or lost vibratory sense (up to 82%) and ankle muscle stretch reflexes (up to 70%). Drug-related and toxic neuropathies, nutritional and alcoholic neuropathies, and postherpetic, diabetic, entrapment, rheumatic, carcinomatous, and paraproteinemic neuropathies are common in the elderly (see Chapter 47). Neuromuscular junction changes and muscle atrophy are commonly seen. Carefully timed exercises and energy conservation are important with myasthenia gravis. Appropriate exercise in the elderly has a proven successful record. Electrodiagnostic changes in the aged are well documented (see Chapter 11).[16]

Visual Impairments

Vision is a major factor contributing to balance and is an important factor in the risk of falling. Visual impairment is especially challenging when combined with a mobility impairment, as in an amputee or stroke patient. Poor vision often results in social isolation, impaired morale, and a decreased sense of well-being. Cataracts, age-related macular degeneration, glaucoma, and diabetic retinopathy are amenable in varying degrees to visual rehabilitative services.[68]

Hearing Loss

The incidence of significant hearing loss appears to be between 25% to 50% in those more than 65 years of age. The varying types of sensorineural hearing loss can be clarified by audiometric evaluation. Often patients refuse to wear hearing aids because of sound distortion, impaired dexterity in their use or adjustment, uncomfortable fit, or vanity (see Chapter 3).[31]

Peripheral Vascular Disease and Ischemic Skin Ulceration

Intermittent claudication should be distinguished from similar complaints of discomfort in the aged caused by arthritis, neural entrapment syndromes, diabetic neuropathy, and spinal stenosis. Proper foot care, including appropriate shoes, is part of the spectrum of care. Chronic venous insufficiency and lymphedema can be helped with compression garments in selected patients. Skin ulceration, especially in the malnourished older person, needs careful, aggressive treatment (see Chapters 31 and 56).[53]

Foot Disorders

The geriatric ankle and foot can be likened to a "fatigued trampoline" which has decreased shock absorption and spring abilities as a result of problems such as bony disfigurement, joint disorders, muscle imbalances, and skin and toenail disorders. Aging can result in insensitive feet with increased potential for ulceration and decreased ability to heal. Strengthening and other physical therapies, proper foot care, proper shoe selection with appropriate orthoses as needed, and appropriate podiatric treatment are important.[18]

Sexual Function

Sexual activity is affected by age-related changes in female and male hormonal levels; alterations in vision, hearing, and smell; negative social attitudes toward sexuality in the elderly; erectile and ejaculatory changes; vaginal dryness and dyspareunia; urinary stress incontinence; decreases in muscle strength and endurance; and limitations in movement from osteoarthritis. Additional problems in sexual functioning can arise from medical illnesses such as benign prostatic hypertrophy, hysterectomy, diabetes mellitus, primary hypothyroidism, cardiovascular disease, hypertension, degenerative joint disease, stroke, and mental illness. Drugs can also cause sexual dysfunction. After an accurate history and physical examination, one approach to treatment is staged levels of sexual counseling. This can range from "permission" to talk about sexual concerns, to increasing amounts of information, to therapy (see Chapter 30).[29] Another approach is medication.

AGING WITH A DISABILITY

Poliomyelitis

Of the more than 640,000 living people in the United States who have experienced paralytic poliomyelitis, more than 50% report having excessive fatigue, progressive weakness, pain, loss of function, and occasionally muscle atrophy 30 to 40 years after the acute episode. This is often referred to as the post-polio syndrome (see Chapter 46). The diagnosis requires evidence of a prior episode of poliomyelitis, a characteristic pattern of recovery from that episode, and exclusion of other conditions that could cause the new symptoms. An interdisciplinary evaluation is essential. Management includes careful strengthening, conservative pain treatment with heavy emphasis on physical medicine and rehabilitation techniques, appropriate orthoses, referral to a pulmonologist if needed, and attention to psychological issues.[32]

Spinal Cord Injury

Survivors of a spinal cord injury in the United States can expect a much longer survival than in decades past. Those more than 55 years old are more likely to have medical problems (see also Chapter 55).[55] Motor function, rather than age, is the predominant limiting factor in attainment of functional goals after a spinal cord injury. Age is associated with a lower statistical chance of achieving some of the functional goals, such as dressing, bathing, stair climbing, and complex transfers. The aging family also poses care issues for the newly injured geriatric patient as well as the aging patient with a chronic spinal cord injury. Psychological issues in aging are compounded by a spinal cord injury.[70]

Multiple Sclerosis

Weakness and fatigue in multiple sclerosis (MS) from upper motor neuron lesions is compounded by age-related peripheral nerve changes, muscle atrophy, and diminished cardiopulmonary reserve. Exercise is important to promote general fitness. Elderly MS patients often have to cope with problems such as hyperthermia, decreased skin sensation, diminished special senses, impairments of the genitourinary and gastrointestinal systems, cognitive dysfunctions, and affective disorders. Psychological, vocational, financial, and recreational issues in dealing with MS are compounded by the psychological issues of aging (see Chapter 52).[13]

Aging with Pediatric-Onset Disabilities

Chronic back pain (from poor posture), scoliosis, cervical spine pain (from heavy use of the neck owing to disability), the sequelae of hip dislocation, and spastic deformities of the feet and toes have been reported in adults with *cerebral palsy.* A high incidence of bowel, bladder, skin, cognitive, and dystonic problems is found. There is decreased access to medical care after the school years are completed.

Epilepsy in adulthood is more common in those with *Down sydrome* than in the general population. Pathological findings of neurofibrillary tangles and neuritic plaques suggest a link between Down syndrome and Alzheimer's disease and raise the question as to whether this is associated with an observed cognitive deterioration. Atlantoaxial instability, commonly with pain, is reported in 9% to 12% of Down syndrome patients.[48]

Persons with *spina bifida* can have late sequelae from hydromyelia, tethered cord, symptomatic Arnold-Chiari malformation, and inclusion dermoids, all of which can be surgically treated. Shunt failure, urinary and renal system dysfunction, arthritis, rotator cuff injury, and entrapment neuropathies can all occur in the aging person with spina bifida.[48]

REHABILITATION

In this era of fiscal constraint, we cannot deliver maximum quantity of medical services to all our patients but must utilize our medical resources to maximum benefit for the most patients. This requires matching our patients to the most appropriate site or level of care and to the optimal level or intensity of medical service needed to achieve significant functional goals in the most cost-effective manner. Figure 59–9 is a flow chart illustrating the concept of selecting the most appropriate setting for rehabilitation care.

The selection of patients who can significantly benefit from rehabilitation services is still an inexact science. It is difficult in all age groups, but especially among the elderly. The goals for each patient must be functionally significant and achievable within a reasonable period of time and with reasonable patient effort. Rules of thumb abound to aid selection of the appropriate patient, but they all have exceptions. They tend to work well when applied to large groups of patients but may be inappropriate when applied to the individual patient. Most have not been validated by research data. Clinical judgment and experience still form the best basis for patient selection.

One prevalent notion is that an incontinent patient cannot benefit from rehabilitation services. This judgment, however, precludes an assessment that might reveal a treatable cause such as infection or overflow or stress incontinence. In the case of bowel incontinence, treatable diarrhea or impaction might be present. Occasionally, gait abnormality, lack of privacy, or architectural barriers can be the cause of the incontinence. The most significant factor is the patient's concern about the incontinence. If the patient is unconcerned, the functional prognosis is worse.

Another prevalent notion that is used to determine patient selection is that a patient with dementia cannot benefit from a rehabilitation program.[57] Our experience indicates that the degree of dementia diminishes but does not preclude the patient's benefiting from rehabilitation services, depending on the goal(s) set by the patient, family, and rehabilitation team. If the goal is to discharge the patient to a noninstitutional setting, then there is evidence that patients with mild dementia succeed as often as those without dementia.[15] The presence of a significant other can be as important a determining factor as the presence of dementia.[21, 22] Three factors that interact to determine whether a patient can be discharged to a noninstitutional setting are ADL status; cognitive, judgment, and safety status; and the social support system.

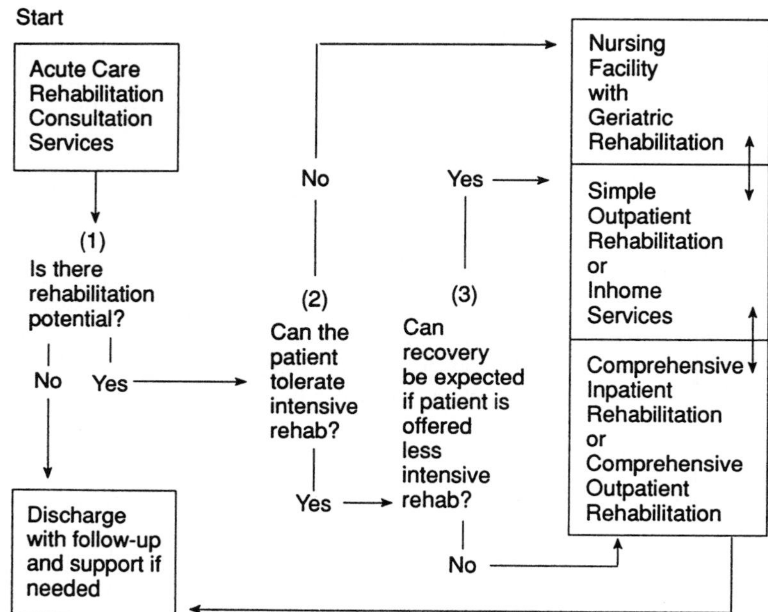

FIGURE 59–9. Flow chart for entry and movement through geriatric rehabilitation services. Clinical questions (nonboxed elements) are asked in sequence. Each care phase or intervention mode is boxed.

TREATMENT SITE

As indicated in Figure 59–9, the elderly rehabilitation patient can be treated appropriately in multiple sites, ranging from the acute hospital or rehabilitation unit of a hospital to the subacute unit or skilled nursing facility, to home care or outpatient rehabilitation. Each site must be modified for the special needs of the elderly in order to accomplish the rehabilitation goals. These modifications can be both architectural and programmatic.

Architectural and environmental factors that should be considered in designing living areas for the elderly are listed in Tables 59–12, 59–13, and 59–14. Increased intensity of lighting is needed to compensate for the decrease in light reaching the retina. Night lighting should be used to identify areas such as the toilet and bathroom. Acoustics should be designed to decrease background noise. Floor coverings should permit use of adaptive mobility equipment. Avoid deep pile carpeting and slippery floor surfaces. Energy-absorbing flooring materials can decrease the likelihood of injury secondary to a fall. Floor space in rooms and passageways should be sufficient to allow for wheelchairs and other adaptive equipment. Light switches, shelves, counters, and so forth should be accessible from a wheelchair. Colors should be used to identify different functional areas, and patient rooms should be painted different colors to allow easy identification. There should be space for personal belongings and to allow display of photographs and other mementos.

Reality orientation should be emphasized. In any institution or program, it is easy to lose track of the day of the week as well as the date. Clocks and calendars should be placed on units and in patient areas, including rooms. Daily schedules should be posted and patients given the responsibility of learning and following a schedule. Holidays, birthdays, and scheduled events should be part of the daily routine, and local and world news should be included.[14] Ideally, patients should be taken outside at least occasionally to reorient to the weather, day vs. night, the season, etc.

MOTIVATION

It is much easier to gain the cooperation of elderly patients for a rehabilitation program if they can see the benefits of what they are being asked to do. Abstract goals such as improving strength, balance, dexterity, ambulation distance, etc. are often insufficient to ensure cooperation. Concrete goals such as getting to the toilet or to a meal are more realistic and more likely to get patient cooperation. Learning what is important to the patient is the key to formulating goals that are significant both to the patient and the team. Brummel-Smith[9] has expressed this relationship as an equation, motivation $= (W \times E \times R)/C$, where W is what the patient wants, E is what the patient expects, R is the reinforcement or reward, and C is the cost, be it physical, economic, emotional, or social.

PRINCIPLES OF MANAGEMENT

Table 59–22 lists the principles of geriatric rehabilitation discussed in this chapter. Emphasis is placed on the multiple impairments found in the elderly patient and on the management rather than cure of these impairments. These impairments interact to cause disability that in many ways is unique to the individual patient. The varying goals and expectations of each patient and his or her family also contribute to this uniqueness. The planning and management by the rehabilitation team must take into consideration these differences between patients. No single plan fits all patients.

PRESCRIPTION MODIFICATION

Several factors unique to the elderly must be taken into consideration when writing a rehabilitation prescription for an elderly patient. Hunt[36] has emphasized homeostatic malfunctions in the elderly. Several of these must be considered as precautions when treating the elderly. As noted previously, temperature regulation can be problematic and the environment in which elderly patients exercise should be neither too hot nor too cold. The sense of thirst diminishes in the elderly, and monitoring for dehydration is a necessity. Transient circulatory insufficiency such as postural hypotension can occur and lead to falls and syncope. Postural instability can also lead to falls. Pain complaints can be diffuse and nonspecific, with both a higher threshold and decreased tolerance reported.[23] Cardiopulmonary impairments are common, and appropriate precautions should be exercised. Similarly, medications can affect the ability to participate in therapy and increase the risk of therapy (anticoagulants).

DISCHARGE PLANNING

Insightful discharge planning is critical if the patient is to avoid institutionalization. Discharge planning should begin simultaneously with the rehabilitation referral. The goals of the patient should be ascertained, as well

TABLE 59–22 Principles of Rehabilitation Management of the Elderly Patient

1. Ascertain level of function (functional assessment)
2. Ascertain available resources and options
3. Avoid immobilization
4. Be aware of altered physiological reactions
5. Determine patient's significant goals, motivation
6. Determine family expectations (psychosocial issues)
7. Differentiate between delirium, dementia, and depression
8. Emphasize function; management not diagnosis; cure
9. Emphasize task-specific exercise; simplify program
10. Encourage socialization and stimulation
11. Minimize medications
12. Realize that function may not be regained
13. Recognize that patients have multiple interacting impairments
14. Understand that improvement occurs in slow increments

as the ability of the family or other support system to help in meeting these goals. The bottom-line functional abilities required for the family to be able or willing to take a patient home should be determined. These functional abilities can include continence, taking meals, self-dressing, and the like. Unless there is adequate family or community support, even patients capable of self-care might not go home because of deficits in community reentry items, for example, shopping.[21] Not uncommonly, family support is lacking, since many aging patients have lost their spouses and live alone. Community services become increasingly important, as does the availability of companions or assisted living arrangements. These resources vary in availability throughout the country and can be determining factors in whether a patient can avoid institutionalization.

LEGAL AND ETHICAL ISSUES

Laws dealing with the elderly differ among different jurisdictions. Each state has its own rules governing informed consent, patients' competence, and the right to refuse treatment. Similarly, different states have different regulations governing the right to die, advance directives, living wills, and durable powers of attorney. All of these legal issues affect patient management[1] and should be known to the rehabilitation team functioning in a given jurisdiction.

Ethical issues in taking care of the elderly are becoming more complex. Physicians no longer have the fiscal ability to do everything for every patient. The ethical dilemma in determining how much to do and whether to do it involves the wishes of the patient and the family and the laws pertaining to each jurisdiction. Society is further complicating this discussion with a continuing reordering of the health care delivery system and possible rationing of health care resources available to the individual.[5]

OUTCOME

Rehabilitation of the elderly can be very successful and professionally rewarding. Although we must accept the irreversibility of aging and the concomitant physical and social changes and losses, we should also realize that with appropriate rehabilitation and social support (family and community), most elderly patients can be kept in the community or returned to their own homes or other community living arrangements. With the application of rehabilitation methodologies discussed in this chapter, their quality of life can be maintained or improved. Most elderly patients live in the community, and even among those aged 85 and above, only 15% of men and 25% of women live in a nursing home.[56] Discharge data from our geriatric rehabilitation unit indicate that we discharge over 70% of our patients to a noninstitutional setting. Our challenge as rehabilitation professionals is not to give in to the biases of ageism, but to employ our abilities in assisting our elderly patients to maintain the quality and dignity of their lives.

REFERENCES

1. Allen B, McCrary SV: Legal aspects of geriatric rehabilitative care. In Felsenthal G, Garrison SJ, Steinberg FU (eds): Rehabilitation of the Aging and Elderly Patient. Baltimore, Williams & Wilkins, 1994, pp 539–549.
2. AGS Panel on Chronic Pain in Older Persons: The management of chronic pain in older persons. J Am Geriatr Soc 1998; 46:635–651.
3. Anderson JM: Heart disease and cardiac rehabilitation in the elderly patient. In Felsenthal G, Garrison SJ, Steinberg FU (eds): Rehabilitation of the Aging and Elderly Patient. Baltimore, Williams & Wilkins, 1994, pp 253–262.
4. Bach JR: Pulmonary assessment and management of the aging and older patient. In Felsenthal G, Garrison SJ, Steinberg FU (eds): Rehabilitation of the Aging and Elderly Patient. Baltimore, Williams & Wilkins, 1994, pp 263–273.
5. Banja JD: Ethical issues in caring for the elderly. In Felsenthal G, Garrison SJ, Steinberg FU (eds): Rehabilitation of the Aging and Elderly Patient. Baltimore, Williams & Wilkins, 1994, pp 551–560.
6. Bohannon R, Larkin P, Cook A, et al: Decrease in timed balance test scores with aging. Phys Ther 1984; 64:1067–1070.
7. Bortz WM II: Effect of exercise on aging—effect of aging on exercise. J Am Geriatr Soc 1980; 28:49–51.
8. Brink TL, Yesavage JA, Lum O, et al: Screening tests for geriatric depression. Clin Gerontol 1982; 1:37–43.
9. Brummel-Smith K: Rehabilitation. In Cassel CK (ed): Geriatric Medicine. New York, Springer-Verlag, 1990, p 129.
10. Butler RN: A disease called ageism. J Am Geriatr Soc 1990; 38:178–180.
11. Campbell AJ, Reinkin J, Allan BC, et al: Falls in the old age: A study of frequency and related clinical factors. Age Ageing 1981; 10:264–270.
12. Chamberlin W: Restrictions in upward gaze with advancing age. Am J Ophthalmol 1971; 71:341–346.
13. Cobble ND, Miller JR, Grigsby J, et al: Aging with multiple sclerosis. In Felsenthal G, Garrison SJ, Steinberg FU (eds): Rehabilitation of the Aging and Elderly Patient. Baltimore, Williams & Wilkins, 1994, pp 427–436.
14. Diamond PT, Butler DH, Felsenthal G: Inpatient episodic care settings: I. Geriatric rehabilitation unit. In Felsenthal G, Garrison SJ, Steinberg FU (eds): Rehabilitation of the Aging and Elderly Patient. Baltimore, Williams & Wilkins, 1994, pp 467–471.
15. Diamond PT, Felsenthal G, Macciocchi SN, et al: Effect of cognitive impairment on rehabilitation outcome. Am J Phys Med Rehabil 1996; 75:40–43.
16. Dumitru D, Gershkoff A, Walsh NE: Peripheral nervous/muscular system. In Felsenthal G, Garrison SJ, Steinberg FU (eds): Rehabilitation of the Aging and Elderly Patient. Baltimore, Williams & Wilkins, 1994, pp 227–241.
17. Era P, Heikkinen E: Postural sway during standing and unexpected disturbance of balance in random samples of men of different ages. J Gerontol 1985; 40:287–295.
18. Esquenazi A, Thompson E: Management of foot disorders in the elderly. In Felsenthal G, Garrison SJ, Steinberg FU (eds): Rehabilitation of the Aging and Elderly Patient. Baltimore, Williams & Wilkins, 1994, pp 153–161.
19. Fast A: Disorders of the cervical and lumbosacral Spine. In Felsenthal G, Garrison SJ, Steinberg FU (eds): Rehabilitation of the Aging and Elderly Patient. Baltimore, Williams & Wilkins, 1994, pp 141–151.
20. Felsenthal G, Cohen BS, Hilton EB, et al: The physiatrist as primary physician for patients on an inpatient rehabilitation unit. Arch Phys Med Rehabil 1984; 65:375–378.
21. Felsenthal G, Glomski N, Jones D: Medication education in an inpatient geriatric rehabilitation unit. Arch Phys Med Rehabil 1986; 67:27–29.
22. Felsenthal G: Rehabilitating older patients: Primary care evaluation, treatment, and resources. Geriatrics 1989; 44:81–90.
23. Ferrell BA: Pain management in elderly people. J Am Geriatr Soc 1991; 39:64–73.
24. Fishman L: Rehabilitation of elderly patients after traumatic brain injury. In Felsenthal G, Garrison SJ, Steinberg FU (eds): Rehabilitation of the Aging and Elderly Patient. Baltimore, Williams & Wilkins, 1994, pp 187–214.

25. Fleming KC, Evans JM, Weber DC, et al: Practical functional assessment of elderly persons: A primary-care approach. Mayo Clin Proc 1995; 70:890–910.
26. Folstein MF, Folstein SE, McHugh PR: Mini-Mental State. A practical method for grading the cognitive state of patients for the clinician. J Psychiatr Res 1975; 12:189–198.
27. Frontera WR, Meredith CN: Exercise in the rehabilitation of the elderly. In Felsenthal G, Garrison SJ, Steinberg FU (eds): Rehabilitation of the Aging and Elderly Patient. Baltimore, Williams & Wilkins, 1994, pp 35–36.
28. Fulton JP, Katz S, Jack SS, et al: Physical functioning of the aged, United States, 1984. Vital and Health Statistics, series 10, no 167, 1989.
29. Garden F: Sexual function in the elderly. In Felsenthal G, Garrison SJ, Steinberg FU (eds): Rehabilitation of the Aging and Elderly Patient. Baltimore, Williams & Wilkins, 1994, pp 319–325.
30. Garrison SJ: Geriatric stroke rehabilitation. In Felsenthal G, Garrison SJ, Steinberg FU (eds): Rehabilitation of the Aging and Elderly Patient. Baltimore, Williams & Wilkins, 1994, pp 175–186.
31. Goins MA: Geriatric hearing loss. In Felsenthal G, Garrison SJ, Steinberg FU (eds): Rehabilitation of the Aging and Elderly Patient. Baltimore, Williams & Wilkins, 1994, pp 339–350.
32. Halstead LS: Poliomyelitis. In Felsenthal G, Garrison SJ, Steinberg FU (eds): Rehabilitation of the Aging and Elderly Patient. Baltimore, Williams & Wilkins, 1994, pp 415–425.
33. Hing E, Sekscenski E, Strahan G: The National Nursing Home Survey: 1985 summary for the United States. Vital and Health Statistics, series 13, no 97, 1989.
34. Hodgson J: Age and aerobic capacity of urban midwestern males. Thesis, University of Minnesota, Minneapolis, 1971.
35. Hough JC: Falls and falling. In Ham RJ, Sloane PD (eds): Primary Care Geriatrics: A Case-Based Approach. St Louis, Mosby–Year Book, 1992, pp 362–377.
36. Hunt TE: Homeostatic malfunctions in the aged. BC Med J 1980; 22:379–381.
37. Hutton JT, Shapiro I, Christians MA: Functional significance of restricted upgaze. Arch Phys Med Rehabil 1982; 63:617–619.
38. Kaufman T: Posture and age. Top Geriatr Rehabil 1987; 2(4):13–26.
39. Kawas CH: Evaluation of cognition in the elderly rehabilitation patient. In Felsenthal G, Garrison SJ, Steinberg FU (eds): Rehabilitation of the Aging and Elderly Patient. Baltimore, Williams & Wilkins, 1994, pp 289–294.
40. Kingston ER, Hirshorn BA, Cornman JM: Ties That Bind: The Interdependence of Generations. Washington, DC, Seven Locks Press; 1986.
41. Jain SS, DeLisa JA: Degenerative central nervous system diseases. In Felsenthal G, Garrison SJ, Steinberg FU (eds): Rehabilitation of the Aging and Elderly Patient. Baltimore, Williams & Wilkins, 1994, pp 215–226.
42. Magaziner J: Demographic and epidemiologic considerations for developing preventive strategies in the elderly. Md Med J 1989; 38:115–120.
43. Manton KG, Corder L, Stallard E: Chronic disability trends in elderly United States populations: 1982–1994. Proc Natl Acad Sci USA 1997; 94:2593–2598.
44. Marottoli RA, Richardson ED, Stowe MH, et al: Development of a test battery to identify older drivers at risk for self-reported adverse driving events. J Am Geriatr Soc 1998; 46:562–568.
45. Morley JE, Silver AJ: Nutrition needs and deficiencies in old age. In Felsenthal G, Garrison SJ, Steinberg FU (eds): Rehabilitation of the Aging and Elderly Patient. Baltimore, Williams & Wilkins, 1994, pp 61–62.
46. Murray MP, Kory RC, Clarkson BH: Walking patterns in healthy old men. J Gerontol 1969; 24:169–178.
47. Murray MP, Kory RC, Sepic SB: Walking patterns of normal women. Arch Phys Med Rehabil 1970; 51:637–650.
48. Nelson MR, Alexander MA: Pediatric-onset disabilities. In Felsenthal G, Garrison SJ, Steinberg FU (eds): Rehabilitation of the Aging and Elderly Patient. Baltimore, Williams & Wilkins, 1994, pp 407–413.
49. Nicholas JJ, Rosenberg AN: Arthritis and arthroplasties. In Felsenthal G, Garrison SJ, Steinberg FU (eds): Rehabilitation of the Aging and Elderly Patient. Baltimore, Williams & Wilkins, 1994, pp 97–106.
50. Owens NJ, et al: The relationship between comprehensive functional assessment and optimal pharmacotherapy in the older patient. DICP 1989; 23:847–854.
51. Palmer JB, DuChane AS: Rehabilitation of swallowing disorders in the elderly. In Felsenthal G, Garrison SJ, Steinberg FU (eds): Rehabilitation of the Aging and Elderly Patient. Baltimore, Williams & Wilkins, 1994, pp 275–287.
52. Parker B, Vestal RE: Pharmacology and aging. In Felsenthal G, Garrison SJ, Steinberg FU (eds): Rehabilitation of the Aging and Elderly Patient. Baltimore, Williams & Wilkins, 1994, pp 65–71.
53. Redford JB: Peripheral vascular disease and ischemic skin ulceration. In Felsenthal G, Garrison SJ, Steinberg FU (eds): Rehabilitation of the Aging and Elderly Patient. Baltimore, Williams & Wilkins, 1994, pp 163–173.
54. Reischer MA, Spindler HA: Rehabilitation management of pain in the elderly. In Felsenthal G, Garrison SJ, Steinberg FU (eds): Rehabilitation of the Aging and Elderly Patient. Baltimore, Williams & Wilkins, 1994, pp 303–317.
55. Roth EJ, Lovell L, Heinemann AW, et al: The older adult with a spinal cord injury. Paraplegia 1992; 30(7):520–526.
56. Schneider EL, Gurainik JM: The aging of America: Impact on health care costs. JAMA 1990; 263:2335–2340.
57. Schuman JE, Beattie EJ, Steed DA, et al: Geriatric patients with and without intellectual dysfunction: effectiveness of standard rehabilitation program. Arch Phys Med Rehabil 1981; 62:612–618.
58. Shock NW, Greulich RC, Costa PT, et al: Normal Human Aging: The Baltimore Longitudinal Study of Aging. US Department of Health and Human Services, Baltimore City Hospitals, 1984.
59. Siebens H: Issues on medication use and substance abuse in older adults. In Felsenthal G, Garrison SJ, Steinberg FU (eds): Rehabilitation of the Aging and Elderly Patient. Baltimore, Williams & Wilkins, 1994, pp 351–361.
60. Sinaki M, Nicholas JJ: Metabolic bone disease and aging. In Felsenthal G, Garrison SJ, Steinberg FU (eds): Rehabilitation of the Aging and Elderly Patient. Baltimore, Williams & Wilkins, 1994, pp 107–122.
61. Smith EL, Di Fabio RP, Gilligan K: Exercise intervention and physiologic function in the elderly. Top Geriatr Rehabil 1990; 6(1):57–68.
62. Sonn U, Grimby G: Assistive devices in an elderly population studied at 70 and 76 years of age. Disabil Rehabil 1994; 16(2):85–92.
63. Stein BD, Felsenthal G: Rehabilitation of fractures in the geriatric population. In Felsenthal G, Garrison SJ, Steinberg FU (eds): Rehabilitation of the Aging and Elderly Patient. Baltimore, Williams & Wilkins, 1994, pp 123–139.
64. Steinberg FU: Gait disorders in the aged. J Am Geriatr Soc 1972; 20:537–540.
65. Steinberg FU: Medical evaluation, assessment of function and potential, and rehabilitation plan. In Felsenthal G, Garrison SJ, Steinberg FU (eds): Rehabilitation of the Aging and Elderly Patient. Baltimore, Williams & Wilkins, 1994, pp 81–82.
66. Stratton MA: Geriatric pharmacotherapy. Pharmaguide to Hosp Med 1991; 4(3):1.
67. Tinetti ME, Ginter SF: Identifying mobility dysfunctions in elderly patients: Standard neuromuscular examination or direct assessment. JAMA 1988; 259:1190–1193.
68. Wainapel SF: Visual impairments. In Felsenthal G, Garrison SJ, Steinberg FU (eds): Rehabilitation of the Aging and Elderly Patient. Baltimore, Williams & Wilkins, 1994, pp 327–337.
69. Wongsurawat N: Temperature regulation in the aged. In Felsenthal G, Garrison SJ, Steinberg FU (eds): Rehabilitation of the Aging and Elderly Patient. Baltimore, Williams & Wilkins, 1994, pp 73–78.
70. Yarkony GM: Aging after a traumatic spinal cord injury. In Felsenthal G, Garrison SJ, Steinberg FU (eds): Rehabilitation of the Aging and Elderly Patient. Baltimore, Williams & Wilkins, 1994, pp 391–396.
71. Zimmerman SI, Fox K, Magaziner J: Demography and epidemiology of disabilities in the aged. In Felsenthal G, Garrison SJ, Steinberg FU (eds): Rehabilitation of the Aging and Elderly Patient. Baltimore, Williams & Wilkins, 1994, pp 11–20.

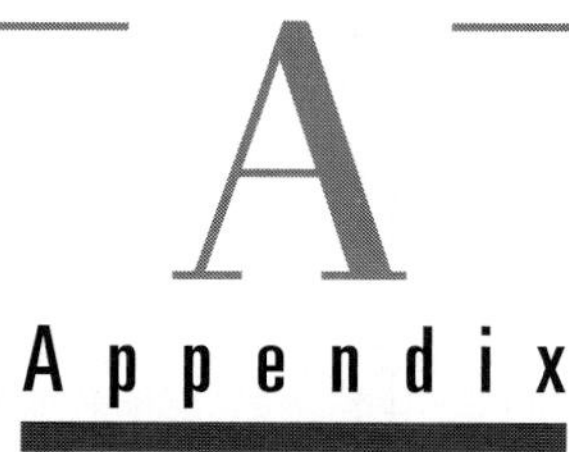

Appendix A

Organizations of Interest

American Geriatrics Society
770 Lexington Avenue, Suite 300
New York, NY 10021
Tel.: (212) 308-1414
Fax: (212) 832-8646
Website: http://www.americangeriatrics.org
E-mail: info.amger@americangeriatrics.org

National Institute on Aging Information Clearinghouse
P.O. Box 8057
Gaithersburg, MD 20857
Toll-free tel.: (800) 222-2225
Toll-free TTY: (800) 222-4225

National Institute on Disability and Rehabilitation Research
U.S. Department of Education

ABLEDATA
8455 Colesville Road, Suite 935
Silver Spring, MD 20910
Tel.: (301) 608-8998
TTY: (301) 608-8912
Fax: (301) 608-8958
Toll free: (800) 227-0216
Website: http://www.abledata.com/

National Rehabilitation Information Center
8455 Colesville Road, Suite 935
Silver Spring, MD 20910
Tel.: (301) 588-9284
Fax: (301) 587-1967
Toll-free information service: (800) 346-2742
Voice and TTY: (800) 227-0216
Website: http://www.naric.com/naric

60 CHAPTER

Michael W. O'Dell, M.D., Mary E. Dillon, M.D., and Anthony A. Oreste, M.D.

Rehabilitation Management in Persons with AIDS and HIV Infection

OVERVIEW OF AIDS AND HIV INFECTION

Epidemiology

In 1981, the U.S. Centers for Disease Control and Prevention (CDC) began receiving reports of *Pneumocystis carinii* pneumonia (PCP) in previously healthy, homosexual men.[64] A similar clinical presentation was soon evident in other groups, most notably intravenous (IV) drug users and persons with hemophilia. In 1983, the French scientist Luc Montagnier identified a human retrovirus, later renamed human immunodeficiency virus (HIV), as the cause of a profound cellular immune system dysfunction, which became known as acquired immunodeficiency syndrome (AIDS).[68]

As of June 1998, over 665,000 cases of AIDS had been reported to the CDC, of which over 401,000 had resulted in death.[27] After exponential increases in AIDS incidence through the 1980s, the epidemic plateaued, and actual decreases were reported in 1995. These decreases have continued through 1997, predominantly because of effective, new anti-HIV therapies that have altered the natural history of infection and slowed progression to the development of AIDS.[27] AIDS deaths declined 42% between 1996 and 1997, with a 15% drop in new diagnoses during the same time period.[27] However, the groups hardest hit by AIDS in recent years (those infected through heterosexual transmission, IV drug users, women) experienced less impressive declines. The least decreases were observed among African Americans (9%) and among those infected by heterosexual transmission (6% for women and 3% for men).[24] The AIDS epidemic continues to claim a disproportionate number of ethnic minorities. From July 1997 through June 1998, African Americans and Hispanics accounted for 60% of AIDS cases in men and 78% in women.[27]

Despite public impression to the contrary, HIV has rather restricted modes of transmission, limited to intimate sexual contact, exposure to infected blood or blood products, and perinatal transmission from mother to fetus.[55] There are actually no risk groups for HIV infection, only risk behaviors. There are no convincing data to support the notion that transmission occurs with any frequency through casual contact.[59] The high prevalence of unrecognized HIV infection in victims of trauma who may require rehabilitation services,[11, 99, 103] combined with the numerous opportunities for exposure to body fluids in the setting of rehabilitation, necessitates education in, and strict adherence to, universal precautions by all rehabilitation professionals in all patient encounters.[88]

Biology, Natural History, and Treatment

HIV is a member of the lentivirus subfamily of human retroviruses, recognized for their tendency to invade the nervous system, to have a long latency period, and to fail to elicit an effective neutralizing humoral immune response, which results in persistent viremia. HIV has a direct, primary destructive effect on various body tissues, including the intestines, glial cells, and bone marrow. The more important secondary pathological effect, however, is the invasion and eventual destruction of the CD4+ subpopulation of T lymphocytes, resulting in a collapse of cellular mediated immunity.[66]

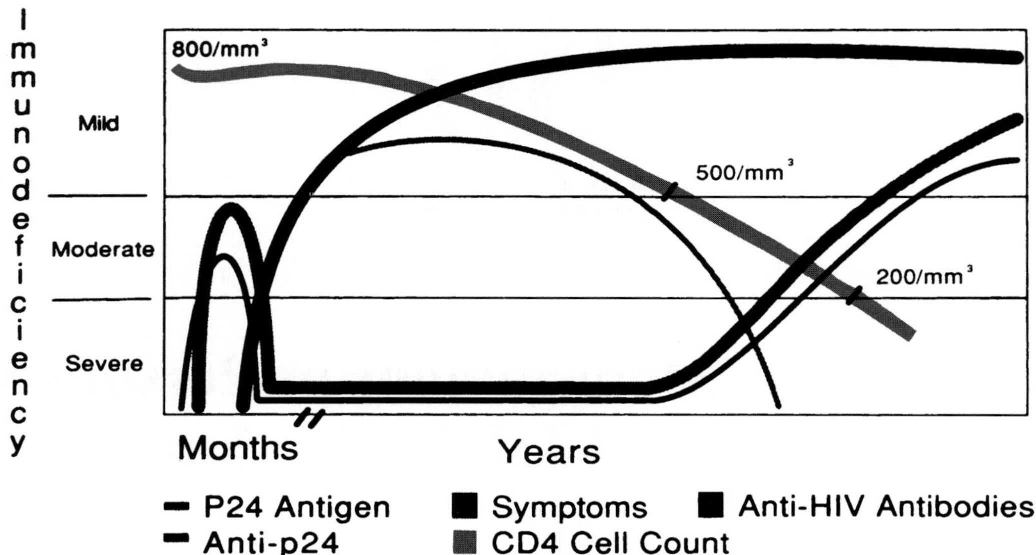

FIGURE 60–1. Natural history of immunological parameters and symptoms in persons with HIV infection. Symptoms are most prominent at the time of initial HIV infection (briefly) and after CD4+ T-lymphocyte counts drop below 500 cells/mL. It may take many years for symptoms to develop after HIV infection. A person is considered to have AIDS only with major symptoms or a CD4+ count below 200 cells/mL. (Courtesy of Dr. Jon Fuller, Boston City Hospital.)

AIDS is only the end-stage manifestation of chronic infection with HIV; that is, *AIDS* and *HIV infection* are not synonymous (Fig. 60–1).[138] Within a few weeks of initial HIV infection, symptoms occur that are typical of an acute viral syndrome, including fever, sweats, rash, nausea, diarrhea, and nonexudative pharyngitis. Antibodies to HIV can usually be detected within 1 to 3 months after infection.[55] The acute infection is followed by a period of relative clinical latency characterized by extensive viral replication and low but steadily increasing viral loads. The time from infection to development of symptoms varies, with a range of 2 to 15 years[55] and a median of 10 to 12 years.[33, 34] Hoover et al[79] found signs and symptoms even in those with asymptomatic HIV infection, but the functional significance of deficits prior to AIDS is debatable.[114] There is a steady decline of immune function during this "asymptomatic" phase. CD4+ T-lymphocyte counts, normally in the 500 to 1500/mL range, decline by approximately 50 to 80/mL/yr, with persons experiencing increasingly severe symptoms as counts drop below the 500/mL mark.[55, 76]

The more familiar clinical manifestations generally occur quite late in the course of HIV infection, after significant immunocompromise and the development of AIDS.[55] Although the manifestations of AIDS are legion, certain pathogens tend to be associated with particular organ systems. Examples are listed in Table 60–1. Cutaneous Kaposi's sarcoma is the most common presenting cancer, followed by lymphoma of the central nervous system (CNS).[128] Other late manifestations related to a direct effect of HIV include constitutional symptoms (particularly "HIV wasting syndrome"), cytopenias, and neurological disease such as AIDS-dementia complex and myelopathy.[12]

In 1993, the CDC[30] revised the system by which HIV infection is classified (Table 60–2). The 1993 classification consists of nine mutually exclusive categories based on both clinical parameters (group A—asymptomatic; group B—symptomatic but without an AIDS-defining illness; and group C—AIDS) and CD4+ counts (≥500/mL, 200–499/mL, and <200/mL, respectively), and is applicable only to persons over age 13 years. Under this new 1993 classification, persons with CD4+ counts under 200/mL meet the case surveillance definition of AIDS, regardless of clinical symptomatology.

The latter part of the 1990s has witnessed dramatic advances in the understanding of HIV pathogenesis, antiretroviral therapy, and measurement of viral load with plasma HIV RNA assays. The nature of the HIV

TABLE 60–1 Common Organ System Involvement for Selected Pathogens in AIDS

Pathogen and Class	Typical Site of Involvement
Parasites	
Toxoplasma gondii	Brain
Cryptosporidium	Gastrointestinal (GI) tract
Pneumocystis carinii	Lung
Fungi	
Candida albicans	Mouth, esophagus, vulva, and vagina
Cryptococcus neoformans	Meninges, lung
Viruses	
Cytomegalovirus	Retina, lungs, nervous system, GI tract
Herpes simplex, varicella-zoster	Cutaneous, esophagus, brain
JC virus	Brain—white matter
Mycobacteria	
Mycobacterium tuberculosis	Lungs, meninges, disseminated
Mycobacterium avium-intracellulare	GI tract, bone marrow, disseminated

TABLE 60–2 1993 Revised CDC Classification System for HIV Infection

	Clinical Categories*		
CD4+ Cell Count	*Group A: Asymptomatic, Acute HIV, or PGL*	*Group B: Symptomatic,† not Group A or C*	*Group C: AIDS Indicator Conditions*
≥500/mL	A1	B1	C1
200–499/mL	A2	B2	C2
<200/mL	A3	B3	C3

Abbreviation: PGL, persistent generalized lymphadenopathy.

* The categories italicized in the table represent the expanded AIDS surveillance case definition. All patients will be reported as having AIDS based on the AIDS indicator conditions or a CD4+ cell count <200/mL.

† Includes, but is not limited to, bacterial infections (pneumonia, meningitis, endocarditis, or sepsis); vulvovaginal candidiasis persistent >1 mo and poorly responsive to treatment; thrush and oral hairy leukoplakia; severe cervical dysplasia or carcinoma; shingles with two episodes or >1 dermatome; idiopathic thrombocytopenia purpura; listeriosis; nocardiosis; pelvic inflammatory disease; peripheral neuropathy; constitutional symptoms such as fever or diarrhea for >1 mo.

Data from 1993 Revised classification system for HIV infection and expanded case surveillance case definition for AIDS among adolescents and adults. MMWR 1992; 41:1–19.

viral replication process is proliferative, with rapid viral turnover (10^{10} virons produced and destroyed each day, with a virion half-life of 6 hours or less).[69] It is this rapid replication of HIV that causes progressive damage and deterioration of immune system function, resulting in patient susceptibility to opportunistic infections, malignancies, neurological disease, and ultimately death.[29] The error-prone nature of RNA virus replication also results in very high levels of genetic mutations.[34] The combination of rapid rates of virus replication with a high rate of mutation leads to rapid development of drug resistance, particularly in the presence of inadequate antiretroviral therapies or patient noncompliance.[45]

Plasma HIV RNA assay is the most sensitive and reliable measurement of plasma viral load, reflecting the magnitude of HIV viral replication and the associated rate of CD4+ T-cell destruction.[29] The extent of immune system damage that has already occurred in an HIV-infected person is indicated by the CD4+ T-cell count,[29] which, when combined with plasma HIV RNA levels, provides the most accurate assessment of the relative risk of disease progression and time to death.[98] Other measurements used to assess risk for disease progression, such as p_{24} antigen, neopterin, and β_2-microglobin, are less reliable than plasma HIV RNA assays.[29] More sensitive assays are being developed that demonstrate detection limits down to approximately 50 copies of RNA/mL.[69]

Since 1995, two or three new antiretroviral agents have been approved yearly (Table 60–3).[69] These agents are HIV reverse transcriptase inhibitors of the nucleoside, non-nucleoside, or nucleotide subclasses. Once HIV enters the cell, viral RNA undergoes reverse transcription to produce integrated double-stranded DNA. HIV protease inhibitors are the final class of drugs. HIV protease activity is essential during the final maturation process of an infectious viron. The main antiviral action of HIV protease inhibitors is to block the infectivity of nascent virons and to prevent subsequent waves of infection.[58] These agents have no effect on infected cells with integrated viral DNA.[58] Commonly used drugs and associated side effects are listed in Table 60–4.

Antiretroviral monotherapy is no longer recommended for treatment of HIV-infected persons, except in some cases to suppress perinatal transmission.[29] Combination therapy has proved to be the most effective approach to accomplish maximal suppression of viral replication, to minimize the risk of developing drug-resistant HIV variants, and to maximize protection from continuing immune system damage.[29] Choices for initiating therapy are expanding rapidly; however, the current recommended standard for initial therapy consists of a protease inhibitor combined with two nucleoside reverse transcriptase inhibitors.[29, 69] The decision to initiate therapy in the asymptomatic patient is complex, and careful counseling about the multiple risks and benefits of treatment is required. The principles relating to changing or modifying treatment, and considerations for primary HIV infection, pregnancy, and postexposure prophylaxis, have been extensively outlined.[24, 28, 29, 58]

Plasma HIV RNA levels are the best measure of the effectiveness of antiretroviral therapy. The goal of combination antiretroviral therapy is to suppress plasma HIV RNA levels below the limit of detection. Studies of the kinetics of HIV replication indicate that levels of plasma HIV RNA decline measurably within days of initial therapy, fall to approximately 1% of their initial levels within 2 weeks, and reach a steady state (hopefully below the level of detection) within approximately 8 weeks.[29] Suppression of plasma HIV levels below the limits of detection indicates profound inhibition of new cycles of virus replication, which will substantially prolong disease-free survival. It does not mean the infection has been eradicated or that the risk of transmission has been eliminated.

Most, if not all, infected patients have a small amount of virus in long-lived cellular reservoirs, and HIV replication may be continuing in various tissues such as lym-

TABLE 60–3 Antiretroviral Agents (Approved or in Advanced Development)

- Nucleoside analog reverse transcriptase inhibitors
  - Zidovudine (ZDV, AZT)
  - Didanosine (ddI)
  - Zalcitabine (ddC)
  - Stavudine (d4T)
  - Lamivudine (3TC)
  - Abacavir (1592U89)
- Non-nucleoside reverse transcriptase inhibitors
  - Nevirapine
  - Delavirdine
  - Efavirenz (DMP-266)
- Nucleotide analog reverse transcriptase inhibitors
  - Adefovir dipivoxil
- Protease inhibitors
  - Saquinavir
  - Ritonavir
  - Indinavir
  - Nelfinavir
  - Amprenavir (141W94, VX-478)

TABLE 60–4 Summary of Antiretroviral Medications

Medication Class	Generic Name	Trade Name	
NRTI	Zidovudine	Retrovir	Bone marrow suppression, anemia, neutropenia, GI intolerance, headache, insomnia, asthenia
NRTI	Didanosine (ddI)	Videx	Pancreatitis, peripheral neuropathy, nausea, diarrhea
NRTI	Zalcitabine (ddC)	Hivid	Peripheral neuropathy, stomatitis
NRTI	Stavudine (d4T)	Zerit	Peripheral neuropathy
NRTI	Lamivudine (3TC)	Epivir	Minimal toxicity
NNRTI	Nevirapine	Viramune	Rash, increased transaminase levels, hepatitis
NNRTI	Delavirdine	Rescriptor	Rash, headache
PI	Indinavir	Crixivan	Nephrolithiasis, GI intolerance, nausea, indirect bilirubinemia (inconsequential), headache, asthenia, blurred vision, dizziness, rash, metallic taste, thrombocytopenia, hyperglycemia
PI	Ritonavir	Norvir	GI intolerance, nausea, vomiting, diarrhea, paresthesias, hepatitis, asthenia, taste perversion, increased triglycerides (up to 200%), transaminase, uric acid, and CPK elevation, hypergylcemia
PI	Saquinavir	Invirase	GI intolerance, nausea, diarrhea, headache, increased transaminase enzymes, hyperglycemia
PI	Saquinavir	Fortovase	GI intolerance, nausea, diarrhea, abdominal pain, dyspepsia, headache, increased transaminase enzymes, hyperglycemia
PI	Nelfinavir	Viracept	Diarrhea, hyperglycemia

Abbreviations: NRTI, nucleoside reverse transcriptase inhibitor; NNRTI, non-nucleoside reverse transcriptase inhibitor; PI, protease inhibitor; GI, gastrointestinal.

Adapted from Centers for Disease Control: Guidelines for the use of antiretroviral agents in HIV-infected adults and adolescents. MMWR 1998; 47:43–82.

phatic tissue and the CNS, in which it is no longer detected by HIV RNA assays.[28, 58] The future challenges of HIV eradication in infected patients include activating these latently infected, resting CD4+ T-cell reservoirs, thereby allowing these cells to achieve active infection and death while released virons are unable to infect new cells via antiretroviral therapy.[3]

REHABILITATION MEDICINE AND HIV INFECTION

The AIDS epidemic has influenced virtually every medical specialty, including the field of physical medicine and rehabilitation. We have accumulated an initial base of knowledge in the epidemiology and management of HIV and AIDS-related disability. Although neither widely recognized nor widely reported, clinical experience in managing HIV-related disability among rehabilitation professionals is probably common, particularly in urban practices. Rehabilitation interventions will undoubtedly continue to focus on disability. However, given the remarkable changes in HIV treatments and their impact on the clinical manifestations of the disease, it would be futile to speculate on the specific impairments leading to those disabilities. As survival increases, secondary disability from the various treatment regimens may be of particular importance.[80]

The epidemiology of functional deficits throughout the spectrum of HIV infection has been delineated to some degree over the past few years. Using a self-report disability measure administered to persons with HIV living in the community, O'Dell and colleagues[114] found that less than 10% of persons with HIV infection prior to AIDS reported any type of functional limitation. Moreover, disability levels in this group were somewhat higher than in an age-, education-, and race-matched group without HIV infection. The authors estimated that between 30,000 and 150,000 persons with HIV infection prior to AIDS might be living with some degree of functional limitation. In persons with an AIDS diagnosis from the same study population, 20% to 30% reported at least some limitation in activities of daily living (ADL), and up to 50% reported some limitation in instrumental ADL.[113] In these cross-sectional and other longitudinal studies, the degree of HIV disability was strongly related to the number of reported symptoms,[113, 114] overall health status,[57, 113, 114] and fatigue,[57, 113, 114, 146] with little influence by demographic variables.[113, 114, 137] Recent longitudinal data suggest that HIV-related physical disability fluctuates considerably over time, with physical functional status improving in 15%, worsening in 42%, and remaining unchanged in 43% over a 1-year period.[57]

HIV disease remains a moving target in terms of planning for rehabilitation services. Recent plateaus in the number of new AIDS diagnoses and number of deaths might, on the surface, suggest a decreased demand for rehabilitation services.[139] There are, however, excellent and consistent data to support a strong association between symptoms or constellations of symptoms in HIV infection and functional deficits.[57, 113, 114, 146] Disabling symptoms can persist among persons living longer. New, more disabling symptoms could arise as a result of improved treatments, as well as secondary disability as a result of those treatments. On the other hand, better primary anti-HIV treatments might decrease the use of prophylactic medications and subsequent side effects.[80] Recent evidence suggests that rehabilitation physicians are providing more care to persons with HIV, although details are scarce.[7] Access to rehabilitation services might well be among the most important factors in the provision of rehabilitation services to persons with HIV infection. Managed care, including both private and public health insurances, could significantly limit the degree and types of services available. Stigma and fears on the part of rehabilitation professionals might also have an impact and are discussed later.[107]

Many kinds of rehabilitation interventions are appropriate in persons with HIV infection. O'Connell and Levinson[106] identified impaired mobility (76%), difficulty with self-care (57%), impaired cognition (29%), and uncontrolled pain (37%) in 51 outpatient rehabilitation consultations in persons with AIDS. Their prescribed interventions included therapeutic exercise (73%), gait aids (45%), bathroom and safety equipment (45%), orthoses (29%), vocational counseling (4%), pain management (29%), and whirlpool treatment (10%). In another study of 37 AIDS patients discharged from an acute care hospital, O'Dell et al[111] found that 22 (59%) needed human assistance in at least one of 18 areas on the Functional Independence Measure, and 12 (32%) needed assistance in more than five of 18 areas on the measure. Assistance was most often needed with stair climbing, ambulation, bowel management, and lower extremity dressing.[111] Interventions in the hospital setting appear to be quite similar to those used in a typical rehabilitation population.[109]

The course of the AIDS epidemic has changed in the last few years, but the future remains as unclear as ever. Rehabilitation physicians and professionals will continue to evaluate and treat persons with HIV-related disability, providing a variety of services, perhaps increasingly in the vocational realm (discussed later). The remainder of this chapter reviews the clinical manifestations of AIDS and HIV infection, outlines potential rehabilitation interventions, and discusses the psychosocial considerations for both patients and the rehabilitation team. For additional information, readers can refer to one of several available texts on the topic.[15, 48, 60, 110]

CLINICAL MANIFESTATIONS OF HIV INFECTION AND THE REHABILITATION APPROACH

For the sake of simplicity, the clinical manifestations of HIV infection are grouped as neurological (either central or peripheral) and non-neurological. Single impairments rarely lead to a specific disability. Fluctuating, multiple medical and neurological impairments are the rule, especially in late HIV disease. The approach to rehabilitation is discussed after the description of each complication.

Neurological Manifestations

Because multiple pathogens infecting multiple levels of the nervous system are common in persons with HIV infection, a few principles regarding the neurological manifestations of HIV infection bear review.[42] First, certain neurological processes tend to occur during certain clinical disease stages or CD4+ ranges (Fig. 60–2.) For example, demyelinating peripheral neuropathies tend to occur early in HIV infection. Most cerebral opportunistic infections occur quite late, after CD4+ counts fall well below 200 mL. Second, it is common for central and peripheral nervous system processes to

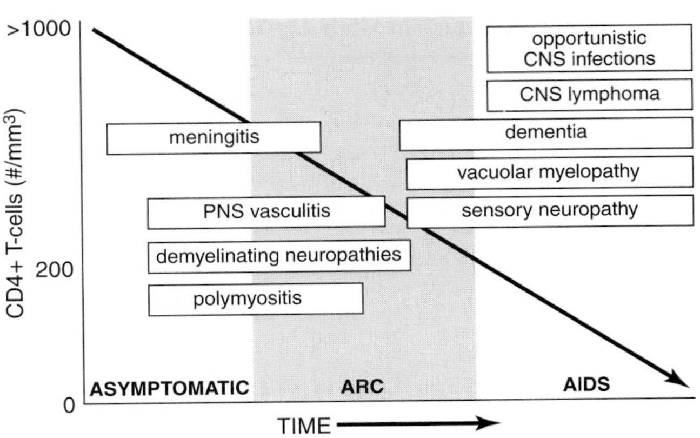

FIGURE 60–2. The major neurological complications of HIV infection plotted against their general time of occurrence after infection and blood CD4+ count. Most of the neurological morbidity and mortality occurs during AIDS (CD4+ <200/mm³). (ARC = AIDS-related complex.) (Modified with permission, from Glass JD, Johnson RT: Human immunodeficiency virus and the brain. Annu Rev Neurosci 1996;19:1–26, by Annual Reviews http://www.AnnualReviews.org)

occur simultaneously—for example, painful peripheral neuropathy in conjunction with AIDS-dementia complex. Multiple processes can also occur within one part of the neuraxis, as in the simultaneous occurrence of peripheral neuropathy and myopathy. Third, the potential effects of systemic disease and of medication side effects must be considered in the neurological differential diagnosis. For example, medical conditions can exacerbate the functional importance of a subclinical neurological process (e.g., hypoxemia from severe pulmonary disease can worsen mental status in mild AIDS-dementia complex). Exacerbation of subtle cognitive and motor deficits can also be related to new cerebral infections, mood disorders, or medication side effects.[42, 90] Finally, even though persons with AIDS are severely immunocompromised, the clinician should not fail to consider more common causes of nervous system dysfunction in appropriate circumstances. Examples include alcohol-induced peripheral neuropathy or myelopathy due to degenerative or discogenic disease in the appropriate clinical setting.

Central Nervous System Complications

Typical CNS diseases in HIV infection are outlined in Table 60–5 by cause, deficits, and prognosis.[87] Table 60–6 explores the presentation and differential diagnosis of CNS disease in HIV infection. Diffuse processes in HIV-related CNS disease can be broadly viewed within the traumatic brain injury model in terms of intervention, focal processes within the stroke model, and myelopathies, analogous to rehabilitation in spinal cord injury (SCI) (Table 60–7).[72, 86, 87] Although the intensity of treatment and the importance of maximizing quality of life over relatively short periods of time might differ, the general approach to managing functional deficits in AIDS is no different from that used for corresponding non-HIV processes.[72, 109, 112] In this sense, HIV rehabilitation directly parallels the philosophy of cancer rehabilitation (see Chapter 57).[87, 88, 112]

TABLE 60–5 Causes of CNS Dysfunction in HIV-Related Disease

Cause	Frequency	Cognitive Deficits	Focal CNS Deficits	Blindness	Myelopathy	Rehabilitation Prognosis
Viruses						
Primary HIV encephalitis	65%–90%	+++	−	−	++	Good early Poor late
CMV encephalitis	Up to 90%	++	±	−	+	Fair
CMV retinitis	20%–25%	−	−	+++	−	Good
PML (JC virus)	Up to 3.8%	++	+++	±	−	Very poor
Herpes simplex	Rare	+	++	±	+	Generally good
Varicella-zoster	Rare	+	±	−	+	Good
Epstein-Barr virus	Common	±	±	−	±	Generally good
Others	Rare	±	±	±	±	Variable
Bacteria						
Mycobacterium tuberculosis	Rare	+	+	−	±	Good except drug-resistant
Mycobacterium avium-intracellulare	Rare	+	−	−	−	Poor when disseminated
Others	Very rare	±	±	±	±	Variable
Fungi						
Cryptococcal meningitis	9%	+++	+	±	±	Variable (40% mortality)
Others	Very rare	±	±	±	±	Variable
Protozoa						
Toxoplasmosis	>2%	+	+++	±	−	Excellent with medical treatment
Malignancies						
Primary CNS lymphoma	1.5%	+	+++	±	−	Poor
Metastatic (Kaposi's sarcoma)	Rare	+	+++	±	±	Fair–poor
Cerebrovascular	Rare	++	+++	±	±	Poor
Multiple sclerosis	Unknown	+	+++	+	+++	

Abbreviations: CNS, central nervous system; CMV, cytomegalovirus; PML, progressive multifocal leukoencephalopathy; +++, usually present; ++, very common; +, common; ±, occasionally present; −, not found.

From Levinson SF, Merritt L: Disability due to CNS impairment. Phys Med Rehabil 1993; 7:s101–s118.

Diffuse Processes

Presentation

The most common diffuse CNS processes are AIDS-dementia complex (also termed HIV-1-associated cognitive/motor deficits) and cryptococcal meningitis.[87, 123] Less frequent processes include viral encephalopathies (e.g., cytomegalovirus infection), bacterial meningitis (e.g., tuberculous and syphilitic meningitis), lymphomatous meningitis, and secondary metabolic abnormalities.[123] It is also important to consider the relative contribution of mood disorders (i.e., anxiety and depression) and medication side effects to the appearance of cognitive deficits.[72] Mild cognitive dysfunction is common in patients with focal neurological presentations, particularly cerebral toxoplasmosis.

AIDS-dementia complex (ADC) is a relentlessly progressive encephalopathy characterized by cognitive, motor, and behavioral impairment.[123] As opposed to Alzheimer's disease, which is distinguished primarily by memory dysfunction, ADC is classified as a subcortical dementia and is characterized by slowness of thought, inattention, and forgetfulness. It resembles the cognitive and motor presentation of Parkinson's disease. Arousal and insight are well preserved until quite late. Motor deficits include lower extremity weakness and gait abnormalities, ataxia, cogwheel rigidity, and tremor.[96] Behavioral manifestations include apathy and even frank psychoses. ADC is almost always a late complication of AIDS, usually occurring when CD4+ counts fall below 250/mL. Although the incidence of cognitive deficits ranges from 25% to 80% (depending on

TABLE 60–6 Differential Diagnosis of Four Common Central Nervous System Complications of AIDS

Disorder	Temporal Evaluation	Alertness	Number of Lesions	Type of Lesions	Location of Lesions
Cerebral toxoplasmosis	Days	Reduced	Multiple	Spherical enhancement, mass effect	Cortex, basal ganglia
Primary CNS lymphoma	Days to weeks	Variable	1 or few	Diffuse enhancement, mass effect	Periventricular, white matter
Progressive multifocal leukoencephalitis	Weeks	Preserved	Multiple	Nonenhancing, no mass effect	White matter, adjacent to cortex
AIDS-dementia complex	Weeks to months	Preserved	None, multiple or diffuse	Increased T2 signal, no enhancement or mass effect	White matter, basal ganglia

From DeVita VT, Hellman S, Rosenberg SA (eds): AIDS: Etiology, Diagnosis, Treatment, and Prevention, ed 4. Philadelphia, Lippincott-Raven, 1997, p 340.

TABLE 60–7 Models of Neurorehabilitation in HIV Infection

Traditional Rehabilitation	HIV Considerations
Focal Presentation: Stroke Model	
Predominantly elderly patients	Predominantly young age
Vocational needs usually low	Vocational needs variable
Cause usually known	Cause often unknown
Survival: several years	Survival: months to a few years
Insurance coverage typical (Medicare)	Insurance coverage variable
Diffuse Presentation: TBI Model	
Static to improving impairment	Temporarily static impairment in treatable processes, ADC progressive
Extended survival	Shorter survival
Medically stable	Medical stability variable
Insight often impaired	Insight intact until late
Behavioral problems common	Behavioral problems potentially complicated by risk of HIV exposure to staff and patients
Disposition often difficult	Disposition may be further complicated by HIV discrimination
HIV Myelopathy: SCI Model	
Relatively static	Progressive
Extended survival	Short survival
Paraparesis or tetraparesis	Usually paraparesis
Functional level predictable	Functional level uncertain
Mild cognitive deficits	Possibly severe cognitive deficits (ADC)

Abbreviations: TBI, traumatic brain injury; ADC, AIDS-dementia complex; SCI, spinal cord injury.

the study and the criteria used), the incidence of severe dementia is only about 5% to 10%.[32, 96] The diagnosis is made by excluding other potential causes. Neuroimaging typically shows only brain atrophy.[123] Evidence is gradually accumulating showing that antiretroviral medications can prevent, slow, or reverse ADC, to some degree.[32, 54, 96, 123]

Cryptococcal meningitis is seen in about 5% to 10% of persons with AIDS, with extraneural presentation of the fungal infection being rather unusual.[123] Symptoms generally occur for less than 3 weeks prior to diagnosis and include headache, fever, and mental status changes. The diagnosis is confirmed by laboratory examination of CSF or blood for cryptococcal antigens. Neuroimaging studies are usually normal. Treatment consists of initiation and lifetime maintenance with fluconazole, possibly after induction with amphotericin B.[123] Other CNS fungal infections that have been reported in the setting of AIDS include aspergillosis, candidiasis, and histoplasmosis.

Rehabilitation Approach

Rehabilitation professionals can adapt a treatment approach similar to that used in traumatic brain injury, remembering that speed of processing is prominently impaired in ADC. The progressive nature of the late manifestations of AIDS necessitates an emphasis on relatively short-term, functionally based goals. Mild to moderate cognitive deficits can limit the rehabilitation potential of persons with the more focal neurological deficits.

Early in the course of cognitive attrition, performance can be enhanced with compensatory strategies such as memory notebooks, verbal monitoring of tasks, presenting limited amounts of material, reducing environmental distraction, and providing a structured daily routine.[9, 72] Although the patient should be the focus of intervention for as long as feasible, caretakers should be involved quite early when ADC is diagnosed, in light of the generally poor prognosis.[88] Some degree of neuropsychological testing may be indicated. This is especially true in mild or more slowly progressing cases, when specific delineation of cognitive deficits is needed for vocational adjustment and planning.[9, 72]

Psychosocial interventions are paramount. Counseling for patients, partners, family, and caretakers can facilitate adjustment to disability. Legal matters, such as preparation of living wills, power of attorney, and guardianship, should be addressed early, while the patient is mentally competent.[9, 72]

Focal Processes

Presentation

The approach to the diagnosis and treatment of focal (or multifocal) cerebral processes in persons with HIV infection has undergone substantial re-evaluation over the past 5 years.[8, 94] Prophylactic antibiotics have dramatically decreased the incidence of cerebral toxoplasmosis, and longer survival in an immunocompromised state may be contributing to the increased incidence of primary CNS lymphoma. Both events potentially change initial treatment and management decisions for focal brain lesions.[8] Progressive multifocal leukoencephalopathy (PML) may also be occurring with greater relative frequency and may respond to combination antiretroviral therapy.[8, 14, 80] Cranial magnetic resonance imaging (MRI) is more sensitive than computed tomography (CT) in demonstrating small lesions and in determining lesion age.[70] There also appears to be an important role of single-photon emission computed tomography (SPECT), particularly in differentiating toxoplasmosis from CNS lymphoma.[9]

Toxoplasma gondii is a single-cell protozoan, intracellular parasite. Although infection usually manifests with focal signs, it is common to see these deficits superimposed on an underlying encephalopathy.[94] The typical clinical presentation occurs over 1 to 2 weeks, with fatigue, fever, and progressive hemiparesis and/or aphasia, depending on the site of the lesion. CT of the brain usually shows multiple (sometimes single), ring-enhancing lesions with a propensity for the basal ganglia and frontoparietal lobes. MRI might show lesions in the absence of CT findings. Although empirical treatment with 2 weeks of pyrimethamine and sulfadiazine prior to brain biopsy has been the standard of care, the dramatic drop in the incidence of toxoplasmosis has called this practice into question.[9, 94] A clinical response with drug therapy requires lifetime maintenance to prevent recurrence. The prognosis is favorable for patients with CNS opportunistic infections, with survival of a year not infrequent.

Cerebrovascular disease (HIV-CVD) is seen clinically in persons with HIV infection; however, whether it is due to HIV infection remains unclear. Including all stages of HIV infection, a 1% to 2% incidence has been suggested.[120] In general, ischemic infarctions (associated with endocarditis or opportunistic infections) are more common than hemorrhagic strokes (associated with thrombocytopenia, CNS lymphoma, or Kaposi's sarcoma).[120] As in strokes in young persons in general, often no specific cause is found.[116] Engstrom et al[51] reported that survival following HIV-related stroke in the late 1980s ranged from a few days to 2 years.

Progressive multifocal leukoencephalopathy (PMI) is a CNS demyelinating disorder seen in about 4% to 5% of persons with AIDS and results from infection with papovavirus.[14] Cognitive and visual complaints and weakness in the absence of fever are the most common clinical presentations. The diagnosis is made by observing the typical nonenhancing, multiple low-density white matter lesions on brain CT and confirmed histopathologically after brain biopsy. Although the prognosis remains poor for the vast majority of patients, up to 7% will show some recovery and live longer than a year after diagnosis.[14] There is also very preliminary evidence that the clinical course of PML can be altered with the use of highly active antiretroviral therapies.[80] Treatment with cytosine and adenine arabinoside, as well as other experimental agents, has generally been disappointing, however.[14]

Primary CNS lymphoma is seen in 1% to 3% of persons with AIDS. With the decreasing incidence of cerebral toxoplasmosis, its importance in the differential diagnosis of cerebral mass lesion in AIDS may be increasing.[9] The presentation is variable, including solitary or multiple intracerebral masses, lymphomatous meningitis, and localized intradural spinal masses. Lymphoma appears on radiographs as single or multiple discrete lesions, with some degree of surrounding edema and contrast enhancement. SPECT can be helpful in differentiating lymphoma from toxoplasmosis. Treatment consists primarily of radiotherapy, with chemotherapy in selected patients.[1] Survival is usually measured in months, but can be longer in certain subgroups. Patients often succumb to other complications of AIDS.[1]

Uncommon neurological presentations in HIV infection include a fulminant variant of multiple sclerosis[65] and parkinsonian symptoms, particularly exacerbated by neuroleptic medications.[100]

Rehabilitation Approach

The approach to rehabilitation in focal CNS disease is similar to that used in stroke rehabilitation.[72, 86, 112, 116, 130] As is seen in non-HIV-related stroke, the impairment resolves somewhat with specific treatment and the resultant decrease in perilesion edema and diminution of the mass. O'Dell and Sasson[116] and Silwa and Smith[130] have reported on the rehabilitation approach to HIV-related hemiparesis. Interventions include providing appropriate orthoses (at both the wrist and ankle); treating spasticity using baclofen, assistive devices, and therapeutic exercise; and enhancing communication abilities. These interventions are best accomplished with an interdisciplinary rehabilitation team. Because of parallel tracking, clinicians should check carefully for concomitant peripheral neuropathy before prescribing orthoses. Basic rehabilitation concerns such as preventing skin compromise and contractures, maintaining bowel and bladder function, and ensuring safety of swallowing are no different from routine rehabilitation practice. Painful sequelae such as complex regional pain syndrome, musculoskeletal shoulder pain, and central pain syndrome are also seen with HIV-CVD and hemiparesis. The team should be aware of mild to moderate cognitive deficits that can affect new learning and the teaching of compensatory strategies. Education of family members or significant others should be initiated in nearly all cases.

Myelopathy

Presentation

Spinal cord involvement is found in 20% to 50% of persons with AIDS at autopsy.[41] HIV-associated myelopathy, termed *vacuolar myelopathy,* tends to affect the dorsolateral portion of the thoracic and cervical spinal cord, almost always in very advanced disease. The resulting clinical picture is one of ataxia and mild to moderate weakness with spasticty progressing over 1 to 4 months. Earlier associations between HIV myelopathy and both vitamin B_{12} deficiency pathologically and ADC clinically remain controversial. Other causes of spinal cord impairment include infection (HTLV-1, toxoplasmosis, syphilis, herpes, mycobacteria), lymphoma, and vitamin deficiency.[41] Neuroimaging of the spine is critical to rule out treatable causes.

Although high-dose antiretroviral medication has been suggested as treatment, no prospective data have been offered.[41] Recent reports of some improvement in impairment associated with HIV myelopathy[47] and cognitive function[49] with oral methionine are encouraging. The prognosis is variable, as symptoms can remain mild or the syndrome might rapidly progress.

Rehabilitation Approach

As in rehabilitation for non-HIV myelopathy, aggressive management of bladder dysfunction is a high priority. The exact type of bladder dysfunction depends on the level of spinal cord involvement and the presence of concomitant conditions such as peripheral or autonomic neuropathy. Trials of urological medications are warranted as well as initiation of intermittent catheterization, if indicated. Because of the multiple enteric pathogens seen in the setting of HIV infection, constipation is unusual.

Orthotic devices and adaptive equipment should be prescribed with clear functional goals in mind, such as facilitating ease of transfers, standing, and decreasing the burden of care for caretakers.[72] Evaluation for concomitant peripheral neuropathy should accompany any orthotic prescription. In many cases, fatigue and overall debilitation preclude all but household mobility.[86]

NEUROMUSCULAR COMPLICATIONS

Abnormalities at virtually every level of the peripheral neuromuscular system have been implicated in HIV infection. Although dysfunction of anterior horn cells, the autonomic nervous system, and the neuromuscular junction have been reported, peripheral neuropathy and myopathy are far more common.[85, 108, 131]

Peripheral Neuropathic Pain

There are several types of peripheral neuropathy associated with pain in HIV infection, each differing somewhat in clinical presentation (Table 60–8).[109] The most common is distal symmetrical polyneuropathy (DSP), caused by a dying-back type of axonopathy.[132] DSP presents with distal pain, paresthesia, and burning, with hyporeflexia and relatively normal strength. Symptoms tend to manifest late in the disease process, develop over weeks to months, and persist once present. There are several case reports of a painful axonal neuropathy resulting from a necrotizing vasculitis discovered on nerve biopsy.[20] This condition occurred relatively early in HIV infection, had a more rapid onset, and had asymmetrical clinical features, which helped differentiate it from DSP. DSP is treated with nonspecific interventions such as narcotics, tricyclic antidepressants, and antiepileptics. Inadequate control of symptoms is a common problem. In the patients with vasculitic neuropathy, corticosteroid treatment led to rapid relief of pain, followed by arrest of the neuropathic process.[20]

Medication-induced (iatrogenic) neuropathies present in a similar manner but over a shorter period of time (days to weeks). The most likely sources are the antiretroviral treatments ddI, d4T, and especially ddC.[37, 125] In the case of ddC treatment, peripheral neuropathy is the most frequent dose-limiting adverse effect and is generally reversible on discontinuation of treatment.[3] Other potential sources include the antituberculous drugs (rifampin, ethambutol, isoniazid); vincristine, sometimes used to treat Kaposi's sarcoma; and dapsone, which is used in PCP prophylaxis.[108] Studies of dapsone in HIV infection, however, fail to show peripheral neuropathy as a prominent side effect.[19, 83] Progressive polyradiculomyelopathy (PPR) is a severe, usually fatal infection of nerve roots and the cauda equina. This infection is commonly due to cytomegalovirus and less often *M. tuberculosis*.[39, 85, 132] Symptoms include extreme pain in a lumbosacral distribution, lower extremity weakness, and urine retention. Rapid diagnosis is important because treatment can arrest or partly reverse this otherwise fatal infection.[122] Empirical therapy with antituberculous drugs should be considered in some cases of PPR, together with ganciclovir or foscarnet.[39] Lastly, depending on the cranial, spinal, or peripheral nerve involved, mononeuropathies (either simplex or multiplex) may be a cause of neuromuscular pain. Although in some cases the symptoms progress, the prognosis in mononeuropathy is generally good.[133]

Neuromuscular Weakness

Causes of neuromuscular weakness include acute and chronic inflammatory demyelinating polyneuropathies (AIDP and CIDP, respectively) and myopathy, as well as PPR and mononeuropathy simplex or multiplex, discussed above (Table 60–9). True neuromuscular weakness should be distinguished from weakness associated with deconditioning and HIV-related fatigue, which are quite common.[91] AIDP (developing over days) and CIDP (developing over weeks) both present primarily with weakness. The acute form is similar in presentation to Guillain-Barré syndrome and is known to occur occasionally at the time of HIV seroconversion. Generally, AIDP and CIDP tend to occur earlier in the disease course.[85, 132] Cornblath et al[38] have suggested that the acute form is associated with more severe functional deficits. Plasmapheresis generally improves the symptons in AIDP and CIDP.[85, 132]

Sketetal muscle disorders in HIV-infected patients can be classified into (1) HIV-associated myopathies, (2) zidovudine (AZT) myopathy, (3) HIV wasting syndrome, and (4) opportunistic infections and tumoral infiltration of muscle.[31] Myopathy associated with HIV infection has no particular predilection for a given disease stage.[132] Although somewhat controversial,[85, 131, 132] AZT myopathy is usually seen after 9 months or more of drug use, with severe myalgias a more prominent symptom on presentation.[85] HIV wasting syndrome has been defined as the unintentional loss of more than 10%

TABLE 60–8 Etiologies of Neuromuscular Pain in HIV Infection

Diagnosis	Etiology	CDC Clinical Category*	Clinical Presentation
Distal symmetrical polyneuropathy	Dying-back axonopathy	B, C	Gradual onset of pain, paresthesia, decreased ankle jerk reflex and vibration sense, mild distal weakness
Progressive polyradiculopathy	Cauda equina infection with cytomegalovirus	C	Rapid onset of pain and lower extremity weakness, urine retention, loss of ankle jerk reflex and patellar reflexes
Mononeuropathy multiplex/simplex	Vasculitis and immune complex	C	Variable, depending on particular nerve affected

*See Table 60–2.
From O'Dell MW: Rehabilitation management of HIV neuromuscular disease. Phys Med Rehabil 1993; 7:S83–S99.

TABLE 60–9 Etiologies and Classification of Neuromuscular Weakness in HIV Infection

Diagnosis	Etiology	CDC Clinical Category*	Clinical Presentation
AIDP	Immune-mediated	A, B	Proximal and distal weakness, areflexia, mild sensory signs, onset over days, autonomic dysfunction
CIDP	Immune-mediated	A, B	Proximal and distal weakness, areflexia, mild sensory signs, onset over weeks, relative lack of autonomic dysfunction
Myopathy	Likely immune-mediated	A, B, C	Gradual onset, proximal weakness, myalgia in lower extremities, "wasting syndrome" a possible variant
Progressive polyradiculomyelopathy	Cytomegalovirus, TB	C	Rapid-onset paraparesis/paraplegia, decreased ankle jerk reflex and patellar reflex, urinary retention
Mononeuropathy multiplex/simplex	Immune-mediated, vasculitis	C	Variable, depending on the nerve affected

*See Table 60–2.
Abbreviations: AIDP, CIDP, acute and chronic inflammatory demyelinating polyneuropathies; TB, tuberculosis.
From O'Dell MW: Rehabilitation management of HIV neuromuscular disease. Phys Med Rehabil 1993; 7:S83–S99.

of body weight, plus either chronic diarrhea or chronic weakness and documented fever in the absence of a concurrent illness other than HIV infection.[31] This syndrome is likely due to metabolic and/or nutritional factors, and studies on the use of oral anabolic steroids (e.g., oxandrolone) have shown a positive impact on the weight and well-being of HIV-infected patients.[16]

Autonomic Neuropathy

Autonomic neuropathy is fairly common in AIDS and HIV infection,[127, 129] but its functional significance is unclear. There is a variable relationship between autonomic neuropathy and disease stage or presence of peripheral neuropathy. Several studies have demonstrated autonomic dysfunction even in patients not complaining of autonomic symptoms.[85, 131, 132] Rehabilitation implications can include exaggerated orthostasis when increasing mobility after a long period of bedrest, and the need to carefully monitor drugs known to cause orthostasis. An additional concern is the potential impact of autonomic neuropathy on bladder function.

NON-NEUROLOGICAL MANIFESTATIONS

As with neurological disease, single, isolated medical complications can be seen early in the course of HIV infection, but are unusual in AIDS. There is a multitude of medical manifestations of HIV infection.[55] Only the more common conditions, or those that substantially affect a rehabilitation effort, are addressed here.

Pulmonary Manifestations

Presentation

Pulmonary disease is one of the most common and most disabling manifestations of HIV infection.[55] Not only are primary functional limitations related to lung pathological changes, but poor endurance can substantially limit rehabilitation interventions for other neurological and non-neurological impairments.

The most common pulmonary process is bacterial pneumonia, although PCP is more often a cause of death.[97] Bacterial pneumonias seen frequently include *Streptococcus pneumoniae* and *S. viridans, Hemophilus influenzae,* and *Pseudomonas aeruginosa*. Tuberculosis (TB)[126] and CMV[97] are also common among persons with AIDS. Drug-resistant strains of TB and the possibility of transmission in both the hospital and community settings complicate management.[126] *Mycobacterium avium-intracellulare* (MAI) does not often cause pneumonia in isolation, but it is common at extrapulmonary sites and is difficult to treat. Fungal opportunistic pulmonary infections include *Cryptococcus neoformans, Histoplasma capsulatum,* and *Aspergillus fumigatus*. Fungal causes usually occur in the setting of fungicemia. Viral pneumonias and MAI infections usually occur in conjunction with other pathogens. Non-Hodgkin's lymphoma and Kaposi's sarcoma are the most common lung malignancies, with the latter having a particularly poor prognosis.[97] In addition, upper respiratory tract infections, sinusitis, and bronchitis are seen more frequently in persons with HIV infection.[126]

Rehabilitation Approach

Celli has suggested two primary goals for pulmonary rehabilitation in persons with HIV infection: (1) "to control, alleviate, and, as much as possible, reverse the symptoms and pathophysiologic processes leading to respiratory impairment," and (2) to "improve quality of life and prolong it."[26, 72] These goals are the same as for any pulmonary rehabilitation program.

Although any patient who experiences pulmonary symptoms is a candidate for rehabilitation, the best results are obtained in persons early in the course of pulmonary impairment *and* early in the overall course of HIV disease. In addition to the standard pulmonary rehabilitation interventions, Celli suggests smoking cessation, oxygen therapy, exercise conditioning, breathing techniques, chest physiotherapy, nutritional evaluation, and psychological support as appropriate. Use of bronchodilators is also helpful for some patients. A modified 6-minute walking test using a visual analog scale for induced dyspnea can be used as both an evaluatory and outcome measure tool. At a minimum, the ability to perform ADL should improve following intervention (see Chapter 33).

Cardiac Manifestations

Presentation

Cardiac disease can occur as a direct result of HIV infection, from infection or tumor, or iatrogenically as a side effect of treatment.[10] The most common cardiac manifestations in HIV infection are myocarditis, pericardial effusions, and cardiomyopathy leading to left ventricular dysfunction.[147] Less frequent are valvular abnormalities of both infectious and noninfectious causes.[147] It is unclear whether elevated triglycerides and cholesterol associated with newer antiretroviral therapies and longer survival times will result in more ischemic disease.[89]

Most HIV cardiac disease is asymptomatic, with morbidity occurring in only 6% to 7% of the population.[147] Abnormalities tend to be seen more with advanced disease and in IV drug abusers.[147] Although both cardiac and pulmonary disease can cause fatigue and shortness of breath, pulmonary abnormalities are far more common in HIV infection and are usually considered first by clinicians.[89] Cardiac disease should be considered in patients whose symptoms are out of proportion to the demonstrated pulmonary abnormalities.

Rehabilitation Approach

The approach to rehabilitation in HIV-related cardiac disease typically resembles that used with patients with congestive heart failure.[91] The use of medications such as digitalis, vasodilators, and diuretics is an important adjunct in maximizing function.[147] Vitamin and selenium supplementation may play a role.[147] As in most types of cardiac rehabilitation, the benefits are more likely due to peripheral adaptations rather than changes in actual cardiac function.[144] Exercise in persons with non-HIV left ventricular dysfunction has been found to be safe and effective.[36, 146] The end points of exercise training are fatigue and dyspnea, rather than the end points of pain, arrhythmias, or hypotension seen in ischemic disease. Programs should be designed around "long-duration, low-intensity" exercise, increasing the duration of effort before increasing the intensity when progressing.[144] Fatigue rather than dyspnea signals the need for rest breaks.[144] Although there is uncertainty about the long-term impact of exercise on either mortality or morbidity (in both HIV- and non-HIV-infected persons), short-term increases in quality of life and functional performance have been documented (see Chapter 32).

Rheumatological Manifestations

Presentation

There are multiple rheumatological manifestations of HIV, including myopathies, vasculitides, sicca syndrome, arthralgias, arthritis, and fibromyalgia.[82] Only the last three are discussed here. Rheumatological complications may occur more frequently in the homosexual than in the IV drug user risk behavior group.[91] Arthralgias are common, with data from early studies suggesting an incidence of about 35% to 40% in homosexuals[18, 22] versus 11% in IV drug users.[102] Knees, shoulders, and elbows are the joints most often affected. The treatment approach is symptomatic, using nonsteroidal anti-inflammatory drugs (NSAIDs) and other analgesics.[91]

HIV-related arthritis tends to affect the lower extremities, especially the ankles and knees,[82] resulting in difficulty in ambulation. The etiology of HIV-associated arthritis is probably multifactorial, related both to the virus itself and secondarily to immunological dysfunction or infections with other microorganisms.[82]

The myalgias and arthralgias seen in the setting of HIV infection can be either independent manifestations of the disease or components of fibromyalgia.[91] The prevalence of fibromyalgia[91] in HIV infection is 11% to 29% and probably exceeds that seen in either general medicine or rheumatology clinics. It can contribute significantly to both the pain and fatigue seen in persons with HIV infection in the outpatient setting.

Rehabilitation Approach

In the acute phase of rheumatic disease, rest, isometric exercise, and immobilization are the mainstays of treatment.[72] Orthotic devices help provide pain relief acutely and support unstable joints chronically. Progressive resistance exercise and further joint mobilization can begin as the acute synovitis revolves. NSAIDs and other analgesics, intra-articular steroids (if arthritis is limited to a few joints), low-dose cyclosporin, and possibly AZT are all pharmacological options.[82, 91] For fibromyalgia, treatment approaches include NSAIDs, trigger point injections, cyclobenzaprine and amitriptyline, and aerobic exercise if the patient can tolerate it (see Chapter 19).[72, 82, 91]

Fatigue

Fatigue is one of the most functionally limiting aspects of chronic HIV infection.[21, 72, 134] Fatigue might be the single most frequent symptom in persons with HIV infection,[91, 119] occurring in 6% to 9% of those even with "asymptomatic" HIV infection to 54% to 56% of ambulatory AIDS patients.[21, 79, 91] The cause of HIV-related fatigue is undoubtedly multifactorial, with contributions from both physical (peripheral) and psychological (central) sources.[43, 91, 134] Several studies have suggested that psychological causes (e.g., depression) might be relatively more important,[21, 91, 115, 134] perhaps as a result of preexisting physical disability.[67] Although fatigue can be seen as an isolated symptom, especially early in the disease course, it is more frequent later in the course and can be the primary limitation in the rehabilitation of other significant impairments.[72, 91]

Rehabilitation Approach

Identification and treatment of a correctable cause, for example, severe anemia, malnutrition, endocrine dysfunction, cardiomyopathy, fibromyalgia, or overt depression, should be the first step in evaluation.[91] Despite the number of medications required by many persons with HIV infection, fatigue as a medication side effect appears to be relatively unusual.[91] In most cases, no specific cause is found for fatigue (personal communication, Dennis McShane, M.D., 1993).

Behavioral modification in the form of education in energy conservation and work simplification techniques is the intervention with the least risk.[109] A recent randomized trial indicated that a seven-session educational program did not achieve statistically significant benefit in reducing fatigue.[62] There are no well-researched medications for specific use in HIV-associated fatigue. Wagner and colleagues,[143] however, found dextroamphetamine improved "low energy" in an open trial in 18 of 19 depressed patients with AIDS. Other potential choices might include amantadine and methylphenidate.[91] Dietary supplementation with fatty acids has been found useful in patients with chronic fatigue syndrome.[13]

PSYCHOSOCIAL AND REHABILITATION TEAM ISSUES

Like other predominantly young populations with newly acquired disabilities, persons with HIV infection must face the psychologically devastating reality of the need for physical care, financial assistance, and changing social worth. However, persons with HIV infection and AIDS face unequaled social stigma, discrimination, loss of mental acuity and personal relationships, and difficulty accessing health care,[46] while confronting existential and spiritual questions and their own mortality.[5] Addressing wide-ranging disabilities and handicaps is fundamental to rehabilitation medicine, making it a medical specialty uniquely qualified to address the need for physical, psychological, social, and financial interventions and support among persons with HIV infection. To adequately meet the needs of HIV-infected clients, rehabilitation professionals must maximize their knowledge of HIV and minimize their own anxiety.[4]

Emotional Sequelae

The emotional trauma that confronts persons with HIV infection and AIDS is rooted in a series of catastrophic events. Challenged by a progressive disease with a poor prognosis and no definitive cure, they face losses of bodily function, physical stamina, mental acuity, employability, career, financial autonomy, independence, and significant relationships.[78] An eroding sense of professional and social self-worth requires new coping skills to confront financial insecurity and the need for assistance.[46] Stressors are numerous, including fear of infecting others, prognosis, loss of confidentiality, the prejudices of society, and potential rejection by family and friends. In addition, there are major decisions to be made regarding putting one's affairs in order, sharing the diagnosis, and disclosure of sexual orientation. In one study, persons with AIDS rated the most salient stressors they experienced as worrying about their health or the future (49%), talking with others about their diagnosis (11%), and dealing with lifestyle changes (15%).[140]

Persons with asymptomatic HIV infection are at great risk for emotional distress, due to a persistent uncertainty about developing AIDS.[140] The caregivers of persons with AIDS, often infected themselves, must deal with bereavement stemming from the eerie sense of watching their own future unfold, while often mourning multiple deaths in their community. As the epidemic wears on, social support decreases and distress and depression increase.[75] Women with HIV disease face the additional stressors of parenting, pregnancy, and child custody. As Holland and Tross[78] have noted, "The ability of patients to tolerate the consequences of the disease depends on their psychological ability to cope based on emotional strength and the availability of social support."

Literature from other disease conditions supports the theory that psychosocial factors, including social support, can reduce morbidity and improve survival.[136] Those who successfully cope with the diagnosis frequently develop new psychological skills.[140] Factors such as an increased use of active coping strategies, relaxation exercises, use of more functional appraisals, and elicitation of social supports and the decreased use of denial or avoidance as coping strategies can be key to longer-term emotional well-being, social functioning, and physical functioning in persons with HIV.[92]

Discrimination

Persons with HIV infection and AIDS can face discrimination in the form of loss of confidentiality and employment, denial of insurance, limited access to health care, and denial of public services, including housing.[25, 46, 104] Confronted with homophobia, prejudice against IV drug users, and unfounded fear of contagion, patients face the adverse effects of legislation placing constraints on homosexual behavior, requiring mandatory HIV screening, and restricting jobs.[25, 140] Such misconceptions have served to misinform large segments of society, leading to fear and prejudices[2, 23] and causing barriers that prevent persons with HIV from receiving life-care services.[74] Studies have shown that misinformation about HIV transmission and negative attitudes toward homosexuals are strong predictors for support of stringent restrictions against persons with AIDS.[124] The widespread AIDS awareness movement and public education have helped lessen such attitudes.

Legislation and Access to Health Care

Access to health care and financial support is a significant problem for many persons with HIV infection and AIDS. As the disease progresses, many develop a work disability, with resulting loss of regular income and health insurance. The legislative response to AIDS has been limited. The Rehabilitation Act of 1973 prohibits discrimination against qualified disabled persons by organizations that receive federal grants or other forms of financial assistance.[101] In 1987, the U.S. Supreme Court found AIDS to be a communicable disease that is considered a handicap.[101] In 1990, the Americans with Disabilities Act was signed into effect, further extending protection from job discrimination into the public and private sector.[101] In 1993, the rules governing Social Security disability benefits as they apply to persons with AIDS were liberalized. Special attention was given to women and others with manifestations of HIV infection who did not previously qualify for disability benefits.[35]

Public health insurance plays a large role in financing the health care of people with HIV or AIDS.[56] Medicare coverage remains limited, however, because only a percentage of AIDS patients live long enough to qualify for benefits.[101] State-sponsored Medicaid-type programs frequently do not cover many of the expenses incurred, such as outpatient services, medications, durable equipment, in-home health care services, or care in skilled nursing facilities.[46] These gaps have been spanned by the tremendous array of volunteer services. Currently, thousands of organizations nationwide provide a host of these unmet services and needs.[46, 117, 124]

The Role of Rehabilitation

The demographics of HIV and AIDS are shifting toward minorities and the urban poor. Rehabilitation professionals have the skills to enhance quality of life and maximize functional status for these patients. Such interventions may eventually lower health care costs.[88]

The need for rehabilitation professionals to provide care for persons with HIV and AIDS is well established.[88, 109, 111, 112] The rehabilitation team can intervene to prevent further complications, enhance affected and unaffected systems, provide adaptive equipment, recommend environmental modifications, and provide psychological techniques for support and adjustment to disability.[72] To be successful, the rehabilitation team must place the individual at the center of the team and coordinate interventions with the services available from community-based HIV/AIDS service organizations.[72] The rehabilitation team should also reach out to the caregivers (both traditional family members and nontraditional caregivers) and offer emotional, physical, and social support for their roles.[121, 141]

Unique Rehabilitation Team Issues

Rehabilitation teams providing HIV rehabilitation are faced with several unique issues. The team must be comfortable with alternative lifestyles and nontraditional family dynamics. Often rehabilitation becomes an arena of confrontation between nontraditional significant others and biological family members. Learning to understand these emotionally charged dynamics and counseling all parties involved are essential to achieving the patient's wishes. Other important issues include establishing who will be the primary caregivers, assigning power of attorney, establishing a legal guardian for the patient, and addressing preparations for death.

Women and Children with HIV Infection or AIDS

The number of children orphaned by mothers with AIDS is growing rapidly. It is estimated that in the United States, 82,000 children under 17 years old will have been orphaned by AIDS by the year 2000.[105] Many low-income mothers and their children confront poverty, substandard housing, lack of access to health care, and inadequate child welfare systems, but mothers with HIV and their children also bear the burdens of discrimination, oppression, and the stigmatization of living with a deadly virus.[93] They want professionals to provide services in a respectful, nonjudgmental manner to help them have better lives,[93] access resources that can support their parenting skills,[84] and assist them in developing permanency plans for surviving children.[50, 95] Children with HIV and those orphaned by AIDS have unique needs for health, societal, and psychological support, to provide constant love, nurturing, and access to medical and social interventions.[6, 105, 118] In Cincinnati, Ohio, one mother whose child died of AIDS responded to this population's unique needs by founding FACE (For AIDS Children Everywhere). This agency provides a host of services, including counseling, meals, assistance with housing, transportation, and even holiday gifts for HIV-positive families.[40]

Vocational Rehabilitation

A 1986 survey of disabled Americans by Harris concluded, "not working is perhaps the truest definition of what it means to be disabled in this country."[142] The first nationwide survey of people with HIV and AIDS, by the National Association of People with AIDS, in 1992, indicated that their most important concern was having enough money. Approximately one-half of the respondents noted minor or major problems funding basic necessities, food, rent, and health care. Two-thirds reported incomes of less than $1000 a month. Other studies have shown that prior to the onset of symptoms, persons with HIV and AIDS are employed at the same rate as other Americans.[142] Following the development of symptoms, however, the rate of employment declines sharply and is associated with the loss of private health insurance and loss of income.[81] In San Francisco, a study from one AIDS clinic found 51% of clients developed a work disability within 3 years of onset of symptoms, with an estimated loss of 42% to 89% of the working life of the population.[101]

There are many barriers and disincentives to working for those with HIV infection or AIDS. In addition to a fluctuating physical condition, many persons lack education, job skills, transportation, and options for job accommodations. Women with HIV infection are more likely to be minority or uneducated.[44] A major disincentive is the need to declare inability to work to be eligible for federal disability benefits.[17, 142] Many end up preferring the guaranteed income and federal medical insurance to the option of inconsistent employment and limited medical coverage. Other daily activity options like volunteer work can provide the therapeutic benefits of being in the workforce without endangering private or public disability benefits.[72]

In 1990, the Rehabilitation Services Administration published its first policy statement on serving clients with HIV. The policy recognizes HIV infection as a physical disability qualifying clients for vocational rehabilitation services, to the extent that clients meet other eligibility criteria.

In 1993, Vachon[142] published a list of eight recommendations to improve employment among persons with HIV or AIDS and thereby improve their quality of life and minimize lost working life while extending their contribution to taxes and Social Security. Studies by Farnham and Gorsky[53] suggest that the illness-based costs incurred by a business employing an HIV-infected worker are less than costs measured from a societal perspective, and that businesses may benefit from keeping an HIV-infected employee on the job as long as possible, particularly because of the skills and productivity the employee brings to the job.[52, 53]

However, it is important to carefully approach vocational rehabilitation with this population. All factors—psychological, emotional, social, physical, and financial—that affect people living with HIV should be considered before considering return to work.[72]

REFERENCES

1. Aboulafia DM, Mitsuyasu RT: Lymphomas and other cancers associated with acquired immunodeficiency syndrome. In DeVito VT, Hellman S, Rosenberg SA (eds): AIDS: Biology, Diagnosis, Treatment, and Prevention, ed 4. Philadelphia, Lippincott-Raven, 1997, pp 319–330.
2. Abrams DI, Dilley JW, Maxey LM, et al: Routine care and psychosocial support of the patient with the acquired immunodeficiency syndrome. Med Clin North Am 1986; 70:707–720.
3. Adkins JC, Peters DH, Faulds D: Zalcitabine: An update of its pharmacodynamic and pharmacokinetic properties and clinical efficacy in the management of HIV infection. Drugs 1997; 53:1054–1080.
4. All AC, Fried JH: Factors influencing anxiety concerning HIV/AIDS in rehabilitation workers. J Rehabil 1996; 62:17–21.
5. All AC, Fried JH: Psychosocial issues surrounding HIV infection that affect rehabilitation. J Rehabil 1994; 64:8–12.
6. American Academy of Pediatrics, Committee on Pediatric AIDS: Planning for children whose parents are dying of HIV/AIDS. Pediatrics 1999; 103:509–511.
7. American Academy of Physical Medicine and Rehabilitation. Physiatrist 1997; 13:6.
8. Ammassari A, Scoppettuolo G, Murri R, et al: Changing disease patterns in focal brain lesion-causing disorders in AIDS. J AIDS Hum Retrovirol 1998; 18:365–371.
9. Auerbach V: Neuropsychological issues in HIV infection: Implications for rehabilitation management. Phys Med Rehabil 1993; 7:s119–s127.
10. Barbaro G, Lorenzo GD, Grisorio B, et al: Incidence of dilated cardiomyopathy and detection of HIV in myocardial cells of HIV-positive patients. N Engl J Med 1998; 339:1093–1099.
11. Baker JL, Kelen GD, Siverton KT, et al: Unsuspected human immunodeficiency virus in critically ill emergency room patients. JAMA 1987; 257:2609–2611.
12. Bartlett JG: The Johns Hopkins Hospital Guide to Medical Care of Patients with HIV Infection, ed 3. Baltimore, Williams & Wilkins, 1993.
13. Behan PO, Behan WMH, Horrobin D: Effect of high doses of essential fatty acids on the postviral fatigue syndrome. Acta Neurol Scand 1990; 82:209–216.
14. Berger JR, Gallo BV, Concha M: Progressive multifocal leukoencephalopathy. In Berger JR, Levy RM (eds): AIDS and the Nervous System. Philadelphia, Lippincott-Raven, 1997, pp 569–594.
15. Berger JR, Levy RM: AIDS and the Nervous System, ed 2. Philadelphia, Lippincott-Raven, 1997.
16. Berger JR, Pall L, Hall CD, et al: Oxandrolone in AIDS wasting myopathy. AIDS 1996; 10:1657–1662.
17. Berkowitz E: Disabled Policy: America's Program for the Handicapped. A Twentieth Century Fund Report. New York, Cambridge University Press, 1987.
18. Berman A, Espinoza LR, Diaz JD, et al: Rheumatic manifestations of human immunodeficiency virus infection. Am J Med 1988; 85:59–64.
19. Blum RN, Miller LA, Gaggini LC, et al: Comparative trial of dapsone versus trimethoprim/sulfamethoxazole for primary prophylaxis of *Pneumocystis carinii* pneumonia. J AIDS 1992; 5:341–347.
20. Bradley WG, Verma A: Painful vasculitic neuropathy in HIV-1 infection: Relief of pain with prednisone therapy. Neurology 1996; 47:1446–1451.
21. Brietbart W, McDonald MV, Rosebfield B, et al: Fatigue in ambulatory AIDS patients. J Pain Symptom Management 1998; 15:159–167.
22. Buskila D, Gladman DD, Langevita P, et al: Rheumatologic manifestations of infection with the human immunodeficiency virus (HIV). Clin Exp Rheumatol 1990; 8:567–573.
23. Capitanio JP, Lerche NW: Psychosocial factors and disease progression in simian AIDS: A preliminary report. AIDS 1991; 5:1103–1106.
24. Carpenter CC, Fischl MA, Hammer SM, et al: Antiretroviral therapy for HIV infection in 1998: Updated recommendations of the International AIDS Society-USA Panel. JAMA 1998; 280:78–86.
25. Cassens BJ: Social consequences of the acquired immunodeficiency syndrome. Ann Intern Med 1985; 103:768–771.
26. Celli BR: Pulmonary rehabilitation of the patient with AIDS. In Mukand J (ed): Rehabilitation for Patients with HIV Disease. New York, McGraw-Hill, 1991, pp 131–139.
27. Centers for Disease Control: HIV/AIDS Surveillance Report: U.S. HIV and AIDS cases reported through June 1998. Midyear edition, vol 10, no 1. Bethesda, MD, Centers for Disease Control, 1998.
28. Centers for Disease Control: Guidelines for the use of antiretroviral agents in HIV-infected adults and adolescents. MMWR 1998; 47:43–82.
29. Centers for Disease Control: Report of the NIH Panel to Define Principles of Therapy of HIV Infection. MMWR 1998; 47:1–39.
30. Centers for Disease Control: 1993 revised classification system for HIV infection and expanded case surveillance case definition for AIDS among adolescents and adults. MMWR 1992; 41:1–19.
31. Chariot P, Gherarde R: Myopathy and HIV Infection. Curr Opin Rheumatol 1995; 7:497–502.
32. Chiesi A, Vella S, Dally LG, et al: Epidemiology of AIDS dementia complex in Europe. LAUDS in Europe Study Group. J AIDS Hum Retrovirol 1996; 11:39–44.
33. Coffin JM: HIV Population dynamics in vivo: Implications for genetic variation, pathogenesis, and therapy. Science 1995; 267:483–489.
34. Coffin JM: HIV viral dynamics. AIDS 1996; 10 (suppl 3): S75–S84.
35. Collins H: New rules let more people get HIV disability benefits. Philadelphia Inquirer, June 30, 1993.
36. Conn EH, Williams RS, Wallace AG: Exercise response before and after physical conditioning in patients with severely depressed left ventricular function. Am J Cardiol 1982; 49:296–300.
37. Connolly KJ, Allan JD, Fitch H, et al: Phase I study of 2′-3′-dideoxyinosine administered orally twice daily to patients with AIDS or AIDS-related complex and hematologic intolerance to zidovudine. Am J Med 1991; 91:471–478.
38. Cornblath DR, McAuthor JC, Kennedy PGE, et al: Inflammatory demyelinating peripheral neuropathies associated with human T-cell lymphocytic virus type III infection. Ann Neurol 1987; 21:32–40.
39. Corral I, Quereda C, Casado JL, et al: Acute polyradiculopathies in HIV-infected Patients. J Neurol 1997; 244:499–504.
40. Curnutte M: One of the faces of AIDS. Cincinnati Enquirer, March 21, 1999.
41. Dal Pan GJ, Berger JR: Spinal cord disease in human immunodeficiency virus infection. In Berger JR, Levy RM (eds): AIDS

and the Nervous System. Philadelphia, Lippincott-Raven, 1997, pp 173–187.

42. Dal Pan GJ, McArthur JC, Harrison MJG: Neurological symptoms in human immunodeficiency virus syndrome. In Berger JR, Levy RM (eds): AIDS and the Nervous System. Philadelphia, Lippincott-Raven, 1997, pp 141–172.
43. Darko DF, Milter MM, Miller JC: Growth hormone, fatigue, poor sleep, and disability in HIV infection. Neuroendocrinology 1998; 67:317–324.
44. Davidson AJ, Bertram SL, Lezotte DC, et al: Comparison of health status, socioeconomic characteristics, and knowledge and use of HIV-related resources between HIV-infected women and men. Med Care 1998; 36:1676–1684.
45. Deeks SG, Smith M, Holodnly M, et al: HIV protease inhibitors: A review for clinicians. JAMA 1997; 277:145–153.
46. Dillon ME: Psychosocial aspects of AIDS: HIV and handicap. Phys Med Rehabil 1993; 7:s189–s201.
47. DiRocco A, Tagliati M, Danisi F, et al: A pilot study of L-methionine for the treatment of AIDS-associated myelopathy. Neurology 1998; 51:266–268.
48. DeVita VT, Hellman S, Rosenberg SA (eds): AIDS: Etiology, Diagnosis, Treatment, and Prevention, ed 4. Philadelphia, Lippincott-Raven, 1997.
49. Dorfman D, DiRocco A, Simpson DM, et al: Oral methionine may improve neuropsychological function in patients with AIDS myelopathy: Results of an open-label trial. AIDS 1997; 11:1066–1067.
50. Draimin BH, Gamble I, Shire A, et al: Improving permanency planning in families with HIV disease. Child Welfare 1998; 77:180–194.
51. Engstrom JW, Lowenstien DH, Bredesen DE: Cerebral infarction and transient neurologic deficits associated with acquired immunodeficiency syndrome. Am J Med 1989; 86:528–532.
52. Farnham PG: Defining and measuring the costs of the HIV epidemic to business firms. Public Health Rep 1994; 109:311–318.
53. Farnham PG, Gorsky RD: Costs to business for an HIV-infected worker. Inquiry 1994; 31:76–88.
54. Ferrando S, van Gorp W, McElhiney M, et al: Highly active antiretroviral treatment in HIV infection: Benefits for neuropsychological function. AIDS 1998; 12:F65–F70.
55. Fishman N, MacGregor RR: Basic biology and clinical manifestations of HIV infection. Phys Med Rehabil 1993; 7:s9–s28.
56. Fleishman JA: Transitions in insurance and employment among people with HIV infection. Inquiry 1998; 35:36–48.
57. Fleishman JA, Crystal S: Functional status transitions and survival in HIV disease: Evidence from the AIDS Cost and Service Utilization Survey. Med Care 1998; 36:533–543.
58. Flexner C: HIV-protease inhibitors. N Engl J Med 1998; 338:1281–1292.
59. Friedland G, Kahl P, Saltzman B, et al: Additional evidence for a lack of transmission of HIV infection by close interpersonal (causal) contact. AIDS 1990; 4:638–644.
60. Galantino ML (ed): Clinical Assessment and Treatment of HIV: Rehabilitation of a Chronic Illness. Thoroughfare, NJ, Slack, 1992.
61. Gardner W, Preator K: Children of seropositive mothers in the US AIDS epidemic. J Soc Issues 1996; 52:177–195.
62. Gifford AL, Laurent DD, Gonzales VM, et al. Pilot randomized trial of education to improve self-management skills of men with symptomatic HIV/AIDS. J AIDS Hum Retrovirol 1998; 18: 136–144.
63. Glass JD, Johnson RT: Human immunodeficiency virus and the brain. Annu Rev Neurosci 1996; 19:1–26.
64. Gottleib MS, Schroff R, Schanker HM, et al: *Pneumocystis carinii* pneumonia and mucosal candidiasis in previously healthy homosexual men. N Engl J Med 1981; 305:1425–1431.
65. Gray F, Chimelli L, Mohr M, et al: Fulminating multiple sclerosis-like leukoencephalopathy revealing human immunodeficiency virus infection. Neurology 1991; 41:105–109.
66. Greene WC: The molecular biology of human immunodeficiency virus type-1 infection. N Engl J Med 1991; 324:308–317.
67. Griffith KW, Rabkin JG, Remien RH, et al: Disease severity, physical limitations, and depression in HIV-infected men. J Psychosom Res 1998; 44:219–227.
68. Grmek MD: History of AIDS: The Emergence of a Modern Pandemic. Princeton, NJ, Princeton University Press, 1990.
69. Hammer SM, Yeni P: Antiretroviral therapy: Where are we? AIDS 1998; 12 (suppl A): s181–s188.
70. Hansman-Whiteman ML, Post JD, Sklar EML: Neuroimaging of acquired immunodeficiency syndrome. In Berger JR, Levy RM (eds): AIDS and the Nervous System. Philadelphia, Lippincott-Raven, 1997, pp 297–381.
71. Harris L: The ICD Survey of Disabled Americans: Bringing Disabled Americans into the Mainstream. New York, 1986.
72. Health Canada: Rehabilitation Services: Adult Intervention. In A Comprehensive Guide for the Care of Persons with HIV Disease. Module 7—Rehabilitation Services. Toronto, Health Canada, 1998, pp 35–62.
73. Heaton RK, Velin RA, McCutchan A, et al: Neuropsychological impairment in human immunodeficiency virus-infection: Implications for employment. Psychosom Med 1994; 56:8–17.
74. Heckman TG, Somlai AM, Peters J, et al: Barriers to care among persons living with HIV/AIDS in urban and rural areas. AIDS Care 1998; 10:365–375.
75. Hedge R: Psychosocial aspects of HIV infection. AIDS Care 1991; 3:409–412.
76. Hirsh MS, D'Aquila RT: Therapy for human immunodeficiency virus infection. N Engl J Med 1993; 328:1686–1695.
77. Hoffman MA: HIV disease and work: Effect on the individual, workplace, and interpersonal contexts. J Vocat Behav 1997; 51:163–201.
78. Holland JC, Tross S: The psychosocial and neuropsychological sequelae of the acquired immunodeficiency syndrome and related disorders. Ann Intern Med 1985; 103:760–764.
79. Hoover DR, Saah AJ, Bacellar H, et al: Signs and symptoms of "asymptomatic" HIV-1-infected homosexual men. J AIDS 1993; 6:66–71.
80. Jacobsen MA, French M: Altered natural history of AIDS-related opportunistic infections in the era of potent combination antiretroviral therapy. AIDS 1998; 12 (suppl A):S157–S163.
81. Kass NE, Munoz A, Chen B, et al: Changes in employment, insurance, and income in relation to HIV status and disease progression. J AIDS 1994; 7:86–91.
82. Kaye BR: Rheumatologic manifestations of HIV infection. Clin Rev Allergy Immunol 1996; 14:385–416.
83. Kemper CA, Tucker RM, Land OS, et al: Low-dose dapsone prophylaxis of *Pneumocystis carinii* pneumonia in AIDS and AIDS-related complex. AIDS 1990; 4:1145–1148.
84. Kotchick BA, Brody G, Armistead L, et al: The impact of maternal HIV infection on parenting in inner-city African American families. J Fam Psychol 1997; 11:447–461.
85. Lange DJ: Neuromuscular diseases associated with HIV-1 infection. Muscle Nerve 1994; 17:16–30.
86. Levinson SF, Fine SM: Rehabilitation of individuals with human immunodeficiency virus. In DeLisa JA, Gans BM (eds): Rehabilitation Medicine: Principles and Practice. Philadelphia, Lippincott-Raven, 1998, pp 1319–1335.
87. Levinson SF, Merritt L: Disability due to CNS impairment. Phys Med Rehabil 1993; 7:s101–s118.
88. Levinson SF, O'Connell PG: Rehabilitation dimensions of AIDS: A review. Arch Phys Med Rehabil 1991; 72:690–696.
89. Lipshultz SE: Dilated cardiomyopathy in HIV-infected patients (editorial). N Engl J Med 1998; 339:1153–1154.
90. Lopez OL, Becker JT, Banks G, et al: Development of subtle neurological signs after systemic illness in HIV-infected individuals. Eur Neurol 1996; 36:71–75.
91. Lubeck DP, Nobunaga AI, Williams C, et al: Rehabilitation of selected non-neurologic HIV disability. Phys Med Rehabil 1993; 7:s131–s153.
92. Lutgendorf S, Antoni MH, Schneiderman N, et al: Psychosocial counseling to improve quality of life in HIV infection. Patient Educ Counsel 1994; 24:217–235.
93. Marcenko MO, Samost L: Living with HIV/AIDS: The voices of HIV-positive mothers. Social Work 1999; 44:36–45.
94. Mariuz P, Bosler E, Luft BJ: Toxoplasmosis. In Berger JR, Levy RM (eds): AIDS and the Nervous System. Philadelphia, Lippincott-Raven, 1997, pp 641–659.
95. Mason S: Custody planning with HIV-affected families: Considerations for child welfare workers. Child Welfare 1998; 77: 161–177.

96. McArthur JC, Selnes OA: Human immunodeficiency virus-associated dementia. In Berger JR, Levy RM (eds): AIDS and the Nervous System. Philadelphia, Lippincott-Raven, 1997, pp 527–567.
97. McGuinness G: Changing trends in the pulmonary manifestations of AIDS. Radiol Clin North Am 1997; 35:1029.
98. Mellors JW, Munoz A, Giorgi JV, et al: Plasma viral load and CD4+ lymphocytes as prognostic markers of HIV-1 infection. Ann Intern Med 1997; 126:946–954.
99. Meythaler JM, Cross LL: Traumatic spinal cord injury complicated by AIDS-related complex. Arch Phys Med Rehabil 1988; 69:219–222.
100. Mirsattari SM, Power C, Nath A: Parkinsonism in HIV infection. Movement Disord 1998; 13:684–689.
101. Mukand J, Starkeson EC, Melvin JL: Public policy issues for the rehabilitation of patients with HIV-related disability. In Mukand J (ed): Rehabilitation for Patients with HIV Disease. New York, McGraw-Hill, 1991, pp 1–20.
102. Munoz-Fernandez S, Cardenal A, Balsa A, et al: Rheumatic manifestations in 556 patients with human immunodeficiency virus infection. Semin Arthritis Rheum 1991; 21:30–39.
103. Naugle RI: Catastrophic minor head injury. Arch Clin Neuropsychiatry 1987; 2:93–100.
104. Nichols SE: Psychosocial reactions of persons with the acquired immunodeficiency syndrome. Ann Intern Med 1985; 103: 765–767.
105. Nicholas SW, Abrams EJ: The "silent" legacy of AIDS children who survive their parents and siblings. JAMA 1992; 268:3478–3479.
106. O'Connell PG, Levinson SF: Experience with rehabilitation in the acquired immunodeficiency syndrome. Am J Phys Med Rehabil 1991; 70:195–200.
107. O'Dell MW: Rehabilitation in HIV infection: New applications for old knowledge. Phys Med Rehabil 1993; 7:s1–s8.
108. O'Dell MW: Rehabilitation management of HIV neuromuscular disease. Phys Med Rehabil 1993; 7:s83–s99.
109. O'Dell MW: Rehabilitation medicine consultation in persons hospitalized with AIDS. Am J Phys Med Rehabil 1993; 72:90–96.
110. O'Dell MW (ed): HIV-related disability: Assessment and management. Phys Med Rehabil 1993, no 7 (special issue).
111. O'Dell MW, Crawford A, Bohi E, et al: Disability in persons hospitalized with AIDS. Am J Phys Med Rehabil 1991; 70:91–95.
112. O'Dell MW, Dillon ME: Rehabilitation in adults with human immunodeficiency virus-related diseases. Am J Phys Med Rehabil 1992; 71:183–190.
113. O'Dell MW, Hubert H, Lubeck DP, et al: Physical disability in a cohort of persons with AIDS: Data from the AIDS Time Health-Oriented Study. AIDS 1996; 10:667–673.
114. O'Dell MW, Hubert H, Lubeck DP, et al: Pre-AIDS disability: Data from the AIDS Time Health-Oriented Study. Arch Phys Med Rehabil 1998; 79:1200–1205.
115. O'Dell MW, Riggs RV: Correlates of HIV-related fatigue: A pilot study. Disability and Rehabilitation 1996; 18:249–254.
116. O'Dell MW, Sasson NL: Hemiparesis in HIV infection: Rehabilitation approach. Am J Phys Med Rehabil 1992; 71:291–296.
117. O'Dowd MA: Psychosocial issues in HIV infection. AIDS 1988; 2:s201–s205.
118. Papola P, Alvarez M, Cohen HJ: Developmental and service needs of school-age children with human immunodeficiency virus infection: A descriptive study. Pediatrics 1994; 94:914–918.
119. Perdices M, Dunbar N, Grunseit A, et al: Anxiety, depression, and HIV-related symptomatology across the spectrum of HIV disease. Aust NZ J Psychiatry 1992; 26:560–566.
120. Pinto AN: AIDS and cerebrovascular disease. Stroke 1996; 27:538–543.
121. Poindexter CC, Linsk NL: Sources of support in a sample of HIV-affected older minority caregivers. Families Society. J Contemp Hum Serv 1998; 79:491–503.
122. Price RW: Neurological complications of HIV infection. Lancet 1996; 348:445–452.
123. Price RW, Brew BJ: Central and peripheral nervous system complications. In DeVito VT, Hellman S, Rosenberg SA (eds): AIDS: Biology, Diagnosis, Treatment, and Prevention, ed 4. Philadelphia, Lippincott-Raven, 1997, pp 331–353.
124. Price V, Hsu ML: Public opinion about AIDS policies: The role of misinformation and attitudes toward homosexuals. Public Opin Q 1992; 56:29–52.
125. Rana KZ, Dudley MN: Clinical pharmacokinetics of stavudine. Clin Pharmacokinet 1997; 33:276–284.
126. Rosen MJ: Overview of pulmonary complications. Clin Chest Med 1996; 17:621–631.
127. Ruttimann S, Hilti P, Spinas GA, et al: High frequency of human immunodeficiency virus-associated autonomic neuropathy. Arch Intern Med 1991; 152:485–501.
128. Safai B, Diaz B, Schwartz J: Malignant neoplasms associated with human immunodeficiency syndrome infection. CA Cancer J Clin 1992; 42:74–95.
129. Shahmanesh M, Bradbeer CS, Edwards A, et al: Autonomic dysfunction in patients with human immunodeficiency virus infection. Int J Stud AIDS 1990; 2:419–423.
130. Silwa JA, Smith JC: Rehabilitation of neurologic disability related to human immunodeficiency syndrome. Arch Phys Med Rehabil 1991; 72:759–762.
131. Simpson DM, Citak KA, Godfrey E, et al: Myopathies associated with human immunodeficiency virus and zidovudine. Neurology 1993; 43:971–976.
132. Simpson DM, Wolfe DE: Neuromuscular complication of HIV infection and its treatment. AIDS 1991; 5:917–926.
133. So YT, Olney RK: The natural history of mononeuropathy multiplex and simplex in patients with HIV infection (abstract). Neurology 1991; 41 (suppl 1): 375.
134. Soucy MD: Fatigue and depression: Assessment in human immunodeficiency virus disease. Nurse Pract Forum 1997; 8:121–125.
135. Souheaver HG, Benshoff JJ, Wright WR, et al: AIDS knowledge among rehabilitation professionals. J Rehabil 1996; 62:21–26.
136. Speigel D, Bloom JR, Kraemer HC, et al: Effect of psychosocial treatment on survival of patients with metastatic breast cancer. Lancet 1989; 334:888–891.
137. Stanton DL, Wu AW, Moore RD, et al: Functional status of persons with HIV infection in an ambulatory setting. J AIDS 1994; 7:1050–1056.
138. Steger KA: Epidemiology, natural history, and staging. In Libman H, Witzburg RA (eds): HIV Infection: A Clinical Manual. Boston, Little, Brown, 1993, pp 3–24.
139. Steinbrook R: Caring for people with human immunodeficiency virus infection. N Engl J Med 1998; 339:1926–1928.
140. Tross S, Hirsch DA: Psychological distress and neuropsychological complications of HIV infection and AIDS. Am Psychol 1988; 43:929–934.
141. Turner HA, Pearlin LI, Mullan JT: Sources and determinants of social support for caregivers of persons with AIDS. J Health Soc Behav 1998; 39:137–151.
142. Vachon RA: Employment assistance and vocational rehabilitation for persons with HIV or AIDS: Policy, practice and prospects. Phys Med Rehabil 1993; 7:s203–s224.
143. Wagner GJ, Rabkin JG, Rabkin R: Dextroamphetamine as a treatment for depression and low energy in AIDS patients: A pilot study. J Psychosom Res 1997; 42:407–411.
144. Wenger NK: Patients with left ventricular dysfunction and congestive heart failure. In Wenger NK (ed): Rehabilitation of the Coronary Patient. New York, Churchill Livingstone, 1992, pp 403–413.
145. Williams RS: Exercise testing of patients with ventricular dysfunction and heart failure. Cardiovasc Clin 1985; 15:219–231.
146. Wilson IB, Cleary PD: Clinical predictors of declines in physical functioning in persons with AIDS: Results of a longitudinal study. J AIDS Hum Retrovirol 1997; 16:343–349.
147. Yunis NA, Stone VE: Cardiac manifestations of HIV/AIDS: A review of disease spectrum and clinical management. J AIDS Hum Retrovirol 1998; 18:145–154.

61

CHAPTER

Mark A. Young, M.D., and Steven A. Stiens, M.D.

Rehabilitation Aspects of Organ Transplantation

The last decade has seen a rapid evolution of the art and science of organ transplantation. This has created a new group of patients needing rehabilitation services. But while the volume of patients undergoing organ transplantation continues to rise, the organ shortage remains acute, so that many appropriate patients must languish on the waiting list for transplantation (Fig. 61–1). For those facing incurable disease, transplantation offers a way to beat the physical challenges of living with end-stage disease. The hope is that transplantation will provide patients with a better quality of life, as well as added years in which to enjoy it.[8] The goal of rehabilitation of the transplantation patient is to improve functional outcome and speed the return to a lifestyle as near to normal as possible.

As new milestones in organ transplant science are steadily developed, the role of rehabilitation continues to expand into new domains. One new development has been the improvement of limb transplant techniques, recently resulting in a pioneering new "hand transplant" procedure. The vital role of rehabilitation in the functional restorative aftercare of this inaugural American limb transplant recipient has achieved international prominence (Fig. 61–2).[92]

The longevity of years post-organ transplant is increasing for several reasons—improved surgical techniques; advances in immunology and pharmacology that prevent rejection of the transplanted organ; and comprehensive, optimally timed, well coordinated rehabilitation.[26] Although the importance of comprehensive post-transplant care is self-evident, there is a dearth of literature outlining the fundamental principles of the transplantation rehabilitation process.[118] This chapter is designed to present an introduction to this new rehabilitation frontier, outlining the physiatric approach to solid organ transplantation. There are more than 19 transplantable organ systems (Fig. 61–3); however, we focus on the four most common solid organ transplant areas seen in rehabilitation—*cardiac, pulmonary, renal,* and *liver* transplantations. Rehabilitation also has a great impact on *bone marrow transplantation* (BMT), a non-solid organ transplant. Though not addressed in this chapter, management of the disabling musculoskeletal sequelae of BMT is discussed in detail in other sources.[38, 119]

ORGAN TRANSPLANTATION EPIDEMIOLOGY AND TRENDS

An estimated 64,000 Americans are currently waiting for a heart, lung, heart-lung, liver, or kidney transplant.[106] The United Network for Organ Sharing (UNOS), a private organization that runs the organ allocation system, estimates that 4000 people died in 1998 before they could get a donor organ (see Fig. 61–1). There is considerable competition for donor organs. New state and federal laws are, however, facilitating donation of organs, and the epidemiological trends are shifting[121]; hence, physiatrists are likely to see an increasing number of transplantation patients seeking rehabilitation in the future.

Until the early 1980s, few medical centers performed transplants and organ allocation was performed on a local or regional basis. With improvements in transplant survival, the federal government recognized the importance of having a national, centrally coordinated organ

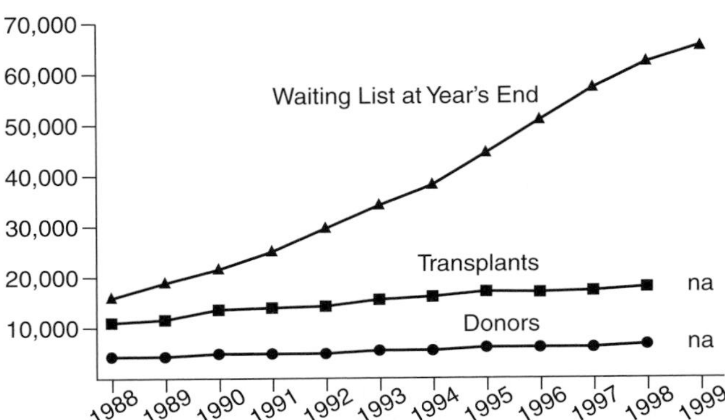

FIGURE 61–1. Cadaveric donors, cadaveric organ transplants, and waiting list at year's end.

distribution system that provides all patients with an equal chance of receiving donor organs. In 1999, the Institute of Medicine, a division of the National Academy of Sciences, reported its evaluation of the current organ procurement and allocation system. They found that the current system has generally worked reasonably well. However, they recommended significant improvements in both its fairness and effectiveness.[75] Consequently, it is likely that the current system of organ procurement and allocation, which has been in place since Congress passed the National Organ Transplant Act in 1984, will be revamped in the next few years.

One current federal policy change likely to result in an increasing number of transplant survivors requiring rehabilitation services is the effort to change organ allocation methodology. The new organ allocation system chooses recipients on the basis of medical criteria rather than geography. This will facilitate donation of organs to the "sickest" patients. Since these medically complex transplant survivors typically require prolonged hospitalization, they are more likely to need admission to a rehabilitation center/unit.[120]

Through its Scientific Registry, UNOS currently collects data on every solid organ transplant performed in the United States. These include kidney, kidney-pancreas, liver, pancreas, heart, heart-lung, lung, and intestinal transplant procedures. Data collected include treatment, clinical factors, and demographic variables as well as their relation to outcome in the form of graft and patient survivals. Survival data are stratified by such variables as first versus repeat transplants, degree of histocompatibility, recipient age, and medical status. Survival data are collected on all patients until the patient dies or the transplanted organ is lost. Data are also collected on all organ donors, both living and cadaveric.[72]

THE PHYSIATRIST'S ROLE IN ORGAN TRANSPLANT REHABILITATION

The need for rehabilitative aftercare for the transplant patient is growing. The transplantation rehabilitation process is a longitudinal, coordinated, interdisciplinary-team endeavor.[104] Because it is very helpful to determine the history and extent of functional deficits associated with end-stage organ damage, the physiatric baseline evaluation should be performed *prior* to surgery. The physiatrist should conduct a thorough musculoskeletal, neurologic, and functional assessment of the patient (Table 61–1). Emphasis should be placed on the maintenance of bodily systems that are likely to be adversely affected by immobilization. This includes contracture prevention, deep vein thrombosis and pulmonary embolism preventive measures, skin maintenance, and preservation of bowel and bladder function. The prevention of disuse atrophy of major muscle groups can be addressed through bedside isometric exercise protocols. A therapeutic plan emphasizing exercise and remobilization should be generated that takes into account the patient's presurgical functional status. As in all areas of rehabilitation, adequate consideration of the patient's psychosocial status and the impact of the impairment on handicap and disablement must be made.[102] During each step of the process, adequate communication with other members of the transplant team is essential.

After transplantation, close ongoing daily surveillance is needed to assure adequate immune system sup-

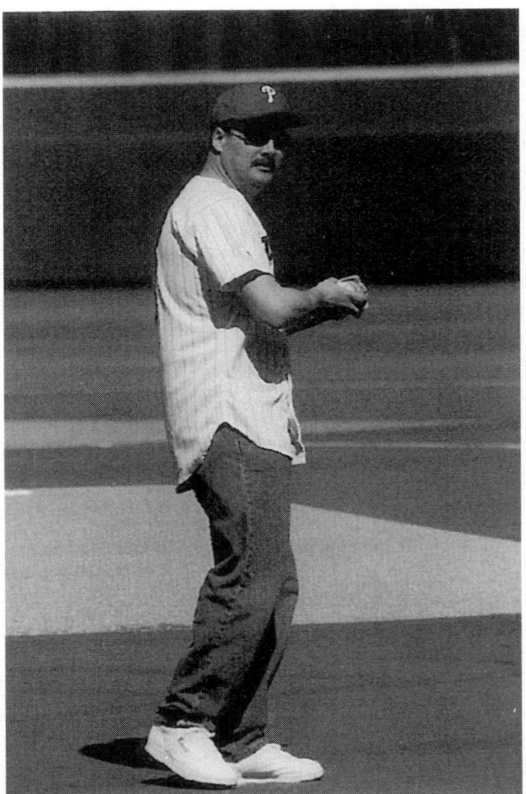

FIGURE 61–2. Matthew Scott—the first person in the United States to have a donor hand transplant—tries out his new left hand at the Phillies home opener. (Reprinted with permission from Sephton S: Mission possible. Adv Dir Rehabil 1999 (June): p 51.)

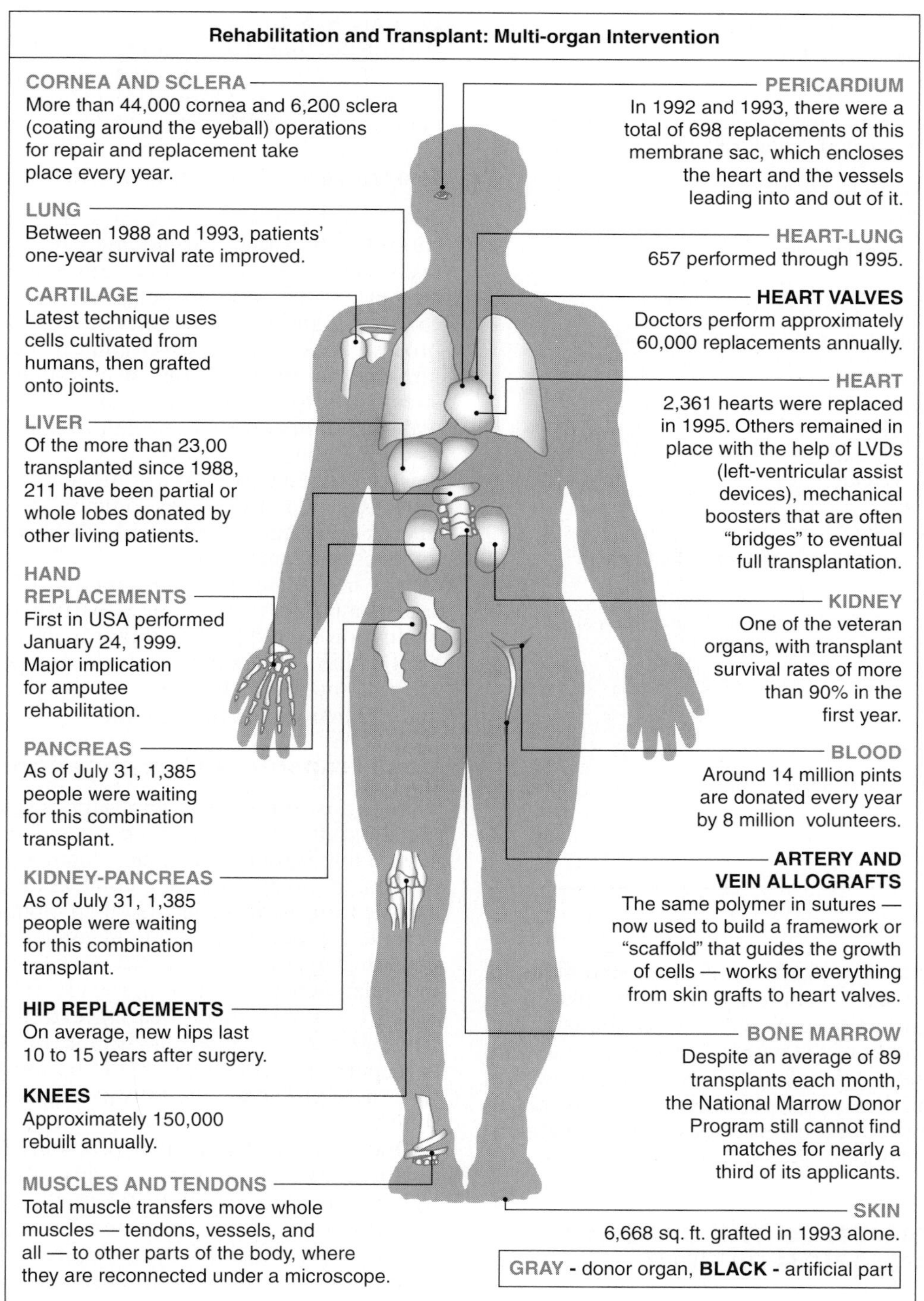

FIGURE 61–3. Transplantation rehabilitation: An organ system perspective (U.S. figures only, except where indicated). *Gray:* Donor organ; *black:* artificial part. *Sources:* United Network for Organ Sharing, Eye Bank Association of America, American Association of Tissue Banks, Baylor College of Medicine, National Marrow Donor Program, Columbia-Presbyterian Medical Center. (Redrawn from *Time,* Fall 1996.)

TABLE 61–1 Transplantation and Rehabilitation Assessment

Physiatric History

Diagnosis resulting in transplantation
Functional history (premorbid and post-transplant)
  Mobility status
  Use of assistive/adaptive devices
  Activities of daily living
  Community and household activities
  Cognition and communication
  Vocation
Past medical and surgical history (presurgical)
Review of systems
Evidence of end organ damage (neuropathy, retinopathy)
Prior rehabilitation interventions
Medications/allergies/diet

Psychosocial History

Living arrangements
Family and friendship support
Use of drugs and alcohol
Psychiatric history

Rehabilitation Examination

Musculoskeletal assessment of the transplant patient
Inspection
Palpation
Joint assessment (range of motion and contractures)
Manual muscle testing

Functional Examination

Mobility
ADLs

Neurologic Examination

Alertness and mental status
Cranial nerve
Motor and sensory
Reflexes
Communication

pression, prevent opportunistic infection, and maintain rehabilitation goals.[69] Emphasis should be placed on the underlying functional, medical, socioeconomic, and psychological needs of the patient.[98] Since patients who have undergone a transplant typically present with a multitude of medical co-morbidities, it is important to include any appropriate precautions in the rehabilitation plan prescription.

REHABILITATION OF THE CARDIAC TRANSPLANTATION PATIENT

Epidemiology of Cardiac Transplantation

The 90-day survival rate of patients undergoing heart transplant improved to 60% in the decade following inauguration of the procedure.[99] With continuing refinements in surgical technique, more than 2000 heart transplants were performed throughout the world by 1990. In 1998, 2340 heart transplants and 45 heart-lung transplants were performed in the United States alone. Currently more than 4000 patients are awaiting a heart transplant, and 227 are awaiting heart-lung transplantation.[106] Survival rates have consistently improved since the first heart transplant in 1967; the current survival rates are 81% for one year and 78% for five years.[96] It is estimated that survival rates after heart transplantation will continue to improve due to improved rejection prevention, better surgical techniques, and enhancement of anti-rejection methodology.

Pretransplant Considerations

Just as rehabilitative outcomes frequently hinge on choosing the "right" candidate, the success of heart transplantation depends on careful selection of suitable patients.[85] Appropriate selection also increases the chances of success in the rehabilitative and restorative process. Patients with proven clinical evidence of declining cardiac function and irreversible heart disease should be prioritized. Several cardinal criteria have been elaborated for cardiac transplant candidate selection,[103] as outlined in Table 61–2.

Congestive heart failure is the leading indication for heart transplantation. Less common indications for cardiac transplantation include idiopathic cardiomyopathy and post-partum cardiomyopathy.[59] Physiatric evaluation is helpful in the determination of whether heart transplantation is right for a particular patient. This evaluation should include a thorough review of the patient's physical health, expected changes in quality of life with the transplant, potential risk for complications, and a functional status baseline.

Post-Transplant Complications

Among post-transplant complications the most dreaded are allograft failure from rejection and immunosuppression complications including infection, neurological deficits, and physiological complications. One study of cardiac transplant recipients on an inpatient rehabilitation unit reported multiple secondary complications including hypertension, nutritional limitations, neuromuscular deficits, and compression fractures.[48] Stress fractures of the weight-bearing extremities have also been described,[64] most likely due to steroid-induced osteoporosis. Physiatrists should be intimately familiar with these problems, and fully prepared to evaluate and treat them.

One of the most immediate problems during the early postoperative period is the inability of the transplanted right ventricle to cope with pre-existing pulmonary hypertension. Pulmonary hypertension can be associated with chronic left-sided heart failure. Often the heart requires ionotrophic support during the period immedi-

TABLE 61–2 Indications for Cardiac Transplantation

Having life-threatening recurrent arrhythmia uncontrolled by medicine or electrophysiologic means
Reduced VO_2 max less than 14/mL/kg/min and severe limitations in life activity
Having severe angina without successful revascularization
Heart failure/CHF consistently uncontrollable by medical therapy

From Tayler A, Bergin J: Cardiac transplantation for the cardiologist not trained in transplantation. Am Heart J 1995; 129:578–592.

ately following transplant. The physiatrist is usually seeing the patient in an intensive care unit at this stage of the postoperative course, and typically prescribes low-intensity bedside exercises.

Many patients develop cyclosporine-related hypertension due to cyclosporine-induced renal vasoconstriction superimposed on chronic renal hypoperfusion, third spacing of fluids, and an abnormal distribution of blood flow.[19, 39, 67, 74, 109] Cyclosporine is believed to elicit afferent glomerular arteriolar vasoconstriction through an increase in transmembrane calcium flux in mesangial and vascular smooth muscle cells.[64, 74] Blood pressures should be closely monitored with morning blood pressure values used as a guide to antihypertensive therapy.[19, 74] This can be achieved in most cases without interruption of the exercise therapy regimen. Alternative cyclosporine dosing regimens, calcium channel antagonists, and angiotensin-converting enzyme inhibitors are preferred therapies to promote arteriolar dilation,[15, 61, 107] and can help facilitate full participation in the rehabilitative process.

Cardiac transplantation can lead to neurologic complications including metabolic encephalopathy, stroke, central nervous system infection, seizures, and psychosis. These potential complications are most likely to occur during the acute post-transplant period, although they can also surface during the rehabilitative/restorative phase.[96] The mechanism of stroke includes particulate embolism, air embolism, or inadequacy of perfusion during the transplantative process.

Once the post-transplant patient has achieved circulatory stability, another ongoing major challenge is preventing immunologic rejection. The cardiac transplant recipient is generally less immunologically depressed than the renal transplant patient. This is due to the prolonged uremia associated with kidney failure. Rehabilitation professionals must be mindful of the systemic and metabolic effects of transplant anti-rejection medications. A summary of the side effects of some of the most frequently used immunosuppressive agents is provided in Table 61–3. See Table 61–4 for the monitoring parameters for immunosuppresive medication.

Acute rejection in cardiac transplantation is a major complication that can be heralded by fulminant exacerbation of congestive heart failure (CHF), development of peripheral edema, premature atrial contractions, and/or by diastolic gallop and sudden marked reduction in exercise capacity. Chronic rejection can manifest itself as accelerated graft atherosclerosis.[42, 71, 111] At one year post-transplantation, 10% to 15% of patients have developed accelerated graft atherosclerosis, which rises to 35% to 50% by the fifth postoperative year.[2, 3, 29] Denervation produces an up-regulation of muscarinic receptors, which facilitates increased calcium influx in the coronary arteries of the transplanted heart. This leads to more diffuse, circumferential narrowing of the arterial lumenal diameters. Ultimately this type of coronary artery disease is a key barrier to the long-term survival of cardiac transplant patients; however, recent studies suggest that this condition can be improved with calcium channel blockers.[29, 91]

Beyond the postoperative complications just outlined, the leading cause of death in post-cardiac transplant patients is infection. The types of infections include mediastinitis, pneumonia, urinary tract infections, or intravenous catheter-induced sepsis.[45, 70, 108] Such problems tend to beset patients especially during the first two years following the cardiac transplant.[37, 71, 73] Bacterial and viral infections account for 47% and 41% of infections, respectively. Infections caused by fungus and protozoa account for 12% of post-transplant morbidity. Adequate washing of the hands for a full 10 seconds both before and after direct contact with the transplant patient is imperative.

Exercise Considerations in Cardiac Transplantation

Early in the history of cardiac transplantation, it was considered inadvisable to start an exercise protocol immediately following the surgery. However, new research suggests a vitally important role for the initiation of exercise therapy beginning within a month after transplant surgery. Benefits that accrue from this include improved strength, enhancement of aerobic capacity, and improved physical work capability. The number of heart transplantation recipients enrolled in rehabilitation and maintenance exercise programs continues to rise.[10]

Recent evidence suggests that supervised exercise programs should be a standard of care for heart transplant patients.[57] A 1999 article reported on a study in which 27 patients discharged within two weeks after receiving a heart transplant were randomly divided into two groups. One group of 14 patients was assigned to participate in a six-month structured aerobics exercise program involving sitting-to-standing exercises. Each patient in the structured exercise group worked with a physical therapist and had a customized program of muscular strength and aerobics training. The second group of 13 patients received only written instructions about exercises they should do at home, with no supervised sessions. All 27 patients were tested for muscle strength, aerobic capacity, and flexibility within one month of receiving a heart transplant, and tested again six months later. While all the patients showed an improvement in all areas, those in the structured exercise group showed significantly better results. Muscle strength, measured by the number of times a patient could stand from a sitting position repetitively for one minute, improved 125% for the exercise group (from a mean of 10.6 times per minute to a mean of 23.9 times). The control group of patients who had received only written instructions showed an 18% gain, increasing from 10.4 times per minute to 12.3. Aerobic capacity, tested by peak oxygen consumption, increased 49% in the group receiving formal exercise training, compared to just 18% in the control group.

Studies such as these offer compelling evidence for introducing exercise soon after organ transplantation. Patients tolerate exercise well after cardiac transplantation, and progressive endurance training is a beneficial component of treatment.[94] A controlled study designed

TABLE 61–3 Systemic and Metabolic Effects of Transplant Rejection Drugs

Adverse Effects	Clinical Manifestations
Azathioprine	
Bone marrow depression	Leukopenia, thrombocytopenia, anemia
Hepatotoxicity	Elevated bilirubin level Elevated alkaline phosphatase, AST, ALT Jaundice
Increased risk of malignancy when associated with high doses of multiple agents	Dependent on type and location of malignancy
Orthoclone (Okt3)	
Pyrexia, malaise	Fever, chills, flulike symptoms Headache, diarrhea
Respiratory distress associated with initial doses and fluid overload	Chest tightness, dyspnea, wheezing
Increased risk of malignancy when associated with high doses of multiple agents	Dependent on type and location of malignancy
Antithymocyte Preparations	
Anaphylactic reactions	Hypotension, dyspnea, wheezing, fever, chills
Serum sickness associated with antibody formation to foreign protein	Fever, joint pain
Bone marrow depression associated with prolonged use in conjunction with azathioprine	Leukopenia Thrombocytopenia Anemia
Local inflammatory reactions associated with IM administration	Pain, redness, extreme muscle soreness, swelling
Increased risk of malignancy when associated with high doses of multiple agents	Dependent on type and location of malignancy
FK506	
Nephrotoxicity associated with high doses	Elevated BUN and creatine levels Decreased urine output
Hyperkalemia	Elevated potassium levels
Insomnia	Sleep disturbances
Malaise	Headache, nausea, and vomiting associated with IV administration
Cyclosporine	
Nephrotoxicity	Elevated BUN and creatine Decreased urine output Weight gain, edema
Hypertension	Elevated blood pressure
Hepatotoxicity	Elevated bilirubin level Elevated alkaline phosphatase, aspartate aminotransferase (AST), and alanine aminotransferase (ALT) levels Jaundice
Hyperterichosis	Hirsutism
Tremors, seizures	Fine motor tremors, especially hands Associated paresthesias Seizure activity
Increased risk of malignancy when associated with high doses of multiple agents	Dependent on type and location of malignancy
Gingival hyperplasia	Growth of gums over teeth Bleeding gums
Corticosteroids	
Aseptic necrosis of bone, osteoporosis	Pain in weight-bearing joints Pathologic fractures
Hyperglycemia, steroid-induced diabetes mellitus	Elevated serum glucose Polydipsia, polyuria
Salt and water retention	Weight gain/fluctuations associated with edema
Hypertension	Elevated blood pressure
Skin alterations	
Acne	Rash or pimples on face and/or trunk
Sun sensitivity	Susceptibility to sunburn
Hirsutism	Excessive hair growth on face, trunk, extremities
Growth retardation in children	Failure to reach normal height for age
Gastritis/gastrointestinal ulcerations	Abdominal pain, dysphagia Hematermesis, guaiac-positive stools
Cataracts	Visual acuity problems

TABLE 61–4 Immunosuppressive Medication Monitoring for Physiatrists

Side Effects	Monitor
Prednisone	
GI irritability	Stool occult blood, Hct
Water, fluid retention	Daily weight
Diabetes mellitus	Fasting, urine glucose
Cyclosporine	
Nephrotoxicity	BUN, creat. (lavender tube)
Hepatotoxicity	LFTs
Drug toxicity	Cyclosporine level
Azathioprine	
Pancytopenia	CBC
Hepatotoxicity	LFTs

to determine the effect of resistance exercise training on bone metabolism in heart transplant recipients also produced positive results. Within two months after heart transplantation, about 3% of whole-body bone mineral density (BMD) is lost, due to decreases in trabecular bone. Six months of resistance exercise, consisting of low back exercise that isolates the lumbar spine and a regimen of variable resistance exercises, restored BMD toward pretransplantation levels. Research has suggested that resistance exercise is osteogenic, and should be initiated early after heart transplantation[12] (see also Chapter 41).

While almost every cardiac transplant patient will face episodes of graft rejection, it is rarely necessary to curtail the patient's exercise workout during episodes of moderate rejection. However, when the patient shows signs of new arrhythmias, hypotension, or fever, the physiatrist can adjust the exercise regimen to balance medical management with restorative rehabilitative services. The patient's long-term prognosis generally becomes poorer as rejection episodes increase in frequency and severity. Clinical and physiological monitoring of the patient is essential in maximizing the patient's prognosis and function.

Physiology of the Transplanted Heart

Customization of exercise programs for each transplant patient entering rehabilitation is essential, and requires an understanding of the physiology of the transplanted heart. The normal heart is innervated and hence affected by the sympathetic nervous system, which activates chronotropic and ionotrophic effects. The sympathetic nervous system enhances venous return, cardiac output, and stroke volume. A transplanted heart is denervated and consequently achieves a maximal heart rate more slowly then a normal heart solely through a response to circulating catecholamines. After an exercise session or ambulation activity, the heart transplant patient experiences a more gradual return to baseline. Despite the denervation, cardiac output in the transplanted heart is increased in response to dynamic activity.

When orthotopic heart transplant is performed, the complete denervation of the heart leads to a loss of the autonomic nervous system control mechanism. Reliance is then placed on circulating catecholamines for adjustment of heart rate during exercise activity. The denervated heart has a higher than normal resting heart rate, and is typically affected by carotid massage, valsalva maneuver, and body inclination.[60, 98, 113] The most widely accepted explanation for this higher than normal heart rate is the loss of vagal tone associated with denervation.[4, 35, 89, 90, 114]

When the patient begins to exercise, heart rate can increase slightly as a result of either the Bainbridge reflex[93] or the increased rate of ventricular work.[122] There is usually a delay of 3 to 5 minutes in the onset of cardiac acceleration. The gradual heart rate increase can continue into the recovery period, and the patient might also experience a slower than normal return to pre-exercise heart rate.[66, 110] The peak heart rate achieved during maximal exercise is considerably lower in cardiac transplant recipients than in age-matched control subjects.[21, 60, 66, 110] See Table 61–5 for a summary of cardiac transplant on various cardiovascular parameters.

Because heart transplant patients display this unusual cardioacceleratory response to exercise, exercise prescriptions based on target heart rates have limited utility, and are not recommended.[79] More beneficial measures of exercise intensity may be blood pressure reserve,[33, 77] perceived exertion,[9, 77] or the dyspnea index.[87] Blood pressure reserve is the difference between the maximal systolic (or diastolic) blood pressure and the resting systolic (or diastolic) blood pressure.

The resting stroke volume of patients with transplanted hearts is less than that of individuals without transplantation.[52] Despite this, cardiac output is virtually normal.[52, 68] Most patients experience a rapid increase in stroke volume of about 20% when they begin their exercise regimen.[23, 60, 68, 100] Subsequent increases in stroke volume or cardiac output during prolonged submaximal exercise are mediated by inotropic responses to circulating catecholamines.[50, 52, 55, 68]

The effect of transplantation on blood pressure is that both systolic and diastolic blood pressures are higher than expected; however, pulse pressure is essentially normal at rest.[18, 40, 52] Diastolic blood pressure can decline early in submaximal exercise because of reduced peripheral resistance.[40, 41, 49, 50] The peak systolic blood pressure is less than that of individuals without cardiac transplants, but diastolic blood pressure is not much different.

The transplanted heart has lower oxygen consumption during submaximal exercise than the nontransplanted heart.[14, 53–55, 78, 101] Oxygen consumption at the anaerobic threshold is also considerably lower than that of age-matched normal individuals.[53, 78, 101] According to Braith et al,[11] the decrement in peak oxygen consumption seen in transplant recipients is due in part to changes in skeletal muscle.

Aerobic cardiovascular conditioning programs and exercise regimens emphasizing endurance tasks have been shown to improve the ability of heart transplant patients to participate in higher levels of activities of daily living (ADL) in the community.[7] It is generally held that organ transplant survivors can perform exer-

TABLE 61–5 Effect of Cardiac Transplantation on Selected Cardiovascular Variables

Systolic Blood Pressure						
Heart Rate	**Stroke Volume**	**Systolic**	**Diastolic**	**PAP**	**VO_2**	**Serum (Lactate)**
Rest						
Greater than normal	Less than normal; little (Bainbridge reflex) or no positional change	Greater than normal	Greater than normal	Slightly greater than normal (although usually lower than pretransplantation)		Greater than normal
Submaximal Exercise						
Little or no immediate increase; delayed slow rise	Increase initially due to Frank-Starling mechanism; late increases due to circulating	Greater than normal	May fall initially due to reduced peripheral resistance	Greater than normal (rate of change is greater than normal)	Less than normal (absolute value)	Greater than normal
Maximal Exercise						
Blunted peak (less than predicted for age) Peak cardiac output, thus about 25% less than normal	Peak only 40–50% greater than most	Peak is less than normal	About the same		Less than normal (absolute value); relative anaerobic threshold is slightly higher than normal	Not markedly different

PAP, pulmonary arterial pressure; VO_2, oxygen consumption.

TABLE 61–6 Most Common Primary Diagnosis in Pulmonary Transplant Rehabilitation Patients

Pulmonary vascular disease
- Primary pulmonary hypertension
- Eisenmenger's syndrome
- Cardiomyopathy with pulmonary hypertension

Obstructive lung disease
- Emphysema—idiopathic
- Emphysema—alpha-antitrypsin deficiency
- Cystic fibrosis
- Bronchiectasis
- Post-transplant obliterative bronchiolitis

Rejection
- Acute, chronic

Side effects of immunosuppressive therapy

Psychosocial issues

cise and physical training routines and obtain effects comparable to those achieved by normal individuals of similar age.[56] Studies in the rehabilitation literature have focused on the hemodynamic responses to upright exercise after cardiac transplantation,[51] as well as the cardiovascular response to gait training and ambulation in hemiparetic heart recipients.[95]

PULMONARY TRANSPLANT REHABILITATION

The number of pulmonary transplantations is increasing steadily as a therapeutic option for patients having declining lung function for whom all other treatments have been exhausted. Surgeons typically perform lung transplants for patients with acquired end-stage pulmonary disease or congenital disease. Indications for lung transplant include chronic obstructive pulmonary disease (COPD), pulmonary hypertension, cystic fibrosis, alpha-1 antitrypsin deficiency, and sarcoidosis. Not all patients with decreased heart and lung function are candidates for transplantation and common contraindications are noted in Table 61–6. According to UNOS, more than 3000 patients were on the waiting list for a lung transplant in July of 1999 and more than 200 were awaiting a heart-lung transplant. In 1998, there were 849 lung transplantations and 45 heart-lung transplantations in the United States. The role of rehabilitation and its restorative aftercare is critical for these patients to achieve improved quality of life and longevity.

Rehabilitation, Exercise, and Complications in the Preoperative Period

In the preoperative period patients need rehabilitation for two reasons. The first reason is to physically prepare for the transplant operation itself. The second is to manage failing strength, decreased thoracic mobility, and altered posture. To optimize the patient's physical condition, physiatrists typically prescribe exercise that improves ventilation, mucociliary clearance, aerobic conditioning, strength, and flexibility. Supplemental oxygen should be administered as needed.[25]

Patients awaiting a lung transplant should be encouraged to remain as active as possible. Compared to education alone, pulmonary rehabilitation has been shown to increase exercise performance and to decrease muscle fatigue and shortness of breath.[82] Increased tolerance of exercise also reduces morbidity after thoracotomies.[97] Patients should enroll in a local pulmonary rehabilitation program[1] that provides a supervised exercise regimen tailored to personal needs. Both before and after transplantation, the exercise regimen should be prescribed using guidelines for the type of exercise to be performed, its frequency, intensity, and duration. The exercise prescription typically includes the use of either a cycle ergometer or treadmill. Some patients with higher exercise capacity can eventually use a stair climber apparatus.

Upper extremity exercise has been safely used in rehabilitation programs,[34, 81] although it can contribute to dyspnea. In patients with severe pulmonary disease, upper limb exercise can result in decreased exercise duration and dyssynchronous thoracoabdominal breathing. Upper limb exercise should be approached with caution prior to transplantation.[20]

Interval rather than continuous training is often more appropriate for patients with end-stage lung disease because it puts less stress on ventilatory demand.[1] Rest periods can be gradually decreased so that the patient advances toward periods of continuous exercise.[1] Diaphragmatic and segmental breathing exercises can increase lung volume and gas exchange.[62] Exercise training of inspiratory muscles can improve their function,[80] and might help improve overall function of the pulmonary system. Energy conservation exercises can help the patient adjust to the low functional capacity caused by advanced pulmonary disease.

Physiatrists can use a variety of methods to determine the level of exercise intensity suitable for each patient. Target heart rates have been applied to patients with lung disease.[44] Exercise regimens using 60% of peak heart rate as a target, as determined by an exercise test, have been demonstrated to increase exercise tolerance.[1, 44] In patients with severe lung disease, predicted maximal heart rates are usually not attained with exercise testing because exercise is limited by pulmonary rather than cardiac function.

To prescribe and monitor exercise intensity in patients with dyspnea, one helpful tool is the "dyspnea

TABLE 61–7 Contraindications to Heart-Lung Transplantation

Absolute Contraindications

- Significant systemic or multisystem disease
- Active extrapulmonary infection
- Cachexia or obesity
- Current cigarette smoking
- Psychiatric illness
- Drug or alcohol abuse

Relative Contraindications

- Corticosteroid therapy
- Previous cardiothoracic surgery

index," which evaluates the number of breaths a patient needs to take while counting out loud from one to fifteen.[87] An alternative measure is the dyspnea scale in which the patient rates the degree of dyspnea during exercise.[1] A third alternative is the Borg Rating Scale of Perceived Exertion (RPE),[9] which provides a rating of the overall effort needed during an activity or at rest. This scale asks the patient to evaluate all bodily sensations that indicate the effort of exercise. The RPE has been used effectively in combination with other measures.[5]

During the preoperative period acute changes in the patient's health status due to advancing disease can occur. The patient might, for example, have to cease exercising altogether until clinically stable,[63] and hospitalization might be required if the patient's lung function continues to decline. This deterioration should move the patient's name closer to the top of the transplant waiting list, and some lung transplant programs require the patient to move closer to the operating center so that they can be more closely monitored.[32, 104]

Acute Postoperative Rehabilitation

The transplanted lung is denervated, which leads to an impaired cough reflex. This can result in ineffective clearance of airway secretions, necessitating chest physical therapy (PT). Diaphragmatic dysfunction can also be present in lung transplant recipients, which can be evaluated with electrodiagnostic studies. The problems associated with the transplant procedure itself are frequently compounded by intubation and mechanical ventilation, prolonged static positioning during surgery, immunosuppression, pain, recumbency, and restricted mobility.[6, 17]

Bedrest in these patients can cause orthostatic intolerance, reduced ventilation, increased resting heart rate, and decreased oxygen uptake.[22, 27, 88] Altering the patient's position from supine to side-lying or upright can increase drainage from chest tubes, as well as promote drainage of pulmonary secretions.[58, 123, 124] The decreased mucociliary clearance associated with denervated lungs[28] can contribute to increased susceptibility to infection in the early postoperative period. The patient should be assisted with airway clearance, beginning on the first postoperative day if the patient is stable. Patients who are mechanically ventilated can benefit from a combination of shaking and hyperinflation with a manual ventilation bag.[112]

Following extubation, the patient can use the active-cycle-of-breathing technique or a Flutter valve device. Positive expiratory pressure therapy has been used in the post-transplant period.[47] Removing secretions requires an effective cough, but patients find it difficult to cough because of incisional pain and decreased sensation in the transplanted airway due to lung denervation.[30] Coughing technique can be improved using adequate pain control and optimal positioning. The patient should be encouraged to sit upright during coughing, since this produces the greatest expiratory flow rates.[117]

Huff coughing, performed without closing the glottis, has been demonstrated to produce a larger volume of expired air at a higher flow rate than conventional coughing.[43] For patients unable to generate substantial airflow, the technique of stacking breaths before the expulsion phase can increase the effectiveness of a cough. Splinted coughing, with a pillow against the incision, can help reduce the pain. Incisional pain can limit activity progression, deep breathing exercises, and coughing. Patients may complain of pain originating from the chest tube sites and from the abdomen (if an omental wrap is used). Epidural analgesia can help in pain management and allows the patient to participate more enthusiastically in rehabilitation.

Exercise Considerations

Progressive activity should be initiated on the first postoperative day, beginning with range of motion exercises. These can be advanced to transfers out of bed to a chair and then to ambulation. After the patient leaves the intensive care unit, rehabilitation should continue to focus on alveolar ventilation, mucociliary transport, and ventilation perfusion matching to optimize the efficiency of oxygen transport. Thoracic mobility might be improved by instructing the patient in chest and upper extremity mobilization exercises.[17] Breathing exercises should be included in the thoracic mobility and cardiovascular exercise programs, coughing and airway clearance, and general activities.

As the patient progresses, a treadmill and cycle ergometer can be introduced in the isolation exercise room, allowing the patient to improve cardiovascular endurance and strength without coming into contact with other patients. Pulmonary transplant recipients can often perform their exercise program well enough to obtain effects comparable with those achieved in healthy individuals of similar age. Denervation of the lungs does not impair the ability to increase ventilation during physical exertion, and most studies show that physical training results in an improved endurance and strength.[56] Before discharge from the hospital the patient should progress to stair climbing, which is the hallmark of recovery, since advanced pulmonary disease typically has made it impossible for most patients to do this for a period of weeks to years.

Cardiopulmonary exercise testing has demonstrated areas of limitation in exercise capacity after lung transplantation. Aerobic capacity, judged by maximal oxygen uptake, typically remains reduced at 32% to 60% of the predicted value.[85, 116] This reduction in aerobic capacity is thought to underlie the exercise limitations in lung transplant patients. Abnormalities of gas exchange and ventilation-perfusion are not thought to play a major role in the reduced exercise capacity of single lung transplant patients. Many other factors may contribute to reduced exercise reserve, including chronic deconditioning and muscle atrophy. Peripheral muscle work capacity is reduced following lung transplant and is predominantly responsible for exercise performance limitation.

Following lung transplantation, patients usually achieve considerable restoration of functional ability. Improvement in exercise tolerance has been demonstrated by an increase in six-minute walk distances after transplantation.[6,24,31,65,115] One center reported that no lung transplant recipients stopped a maximal symptom-limited exercise test because of dyspnea, as the main complaint was lower limb discomfort or pain.[46]

Medical Complications

To prevent acute and chronic rejection, patients are placed on triple drug immunosuppressant regimens consisting of cyclosporine, azathioprine, and prednisone. Recently a new generation of immunosuppressant medications has emerged including FK 506 (Tacrolimus), rapamycin (Sirolimus), and leflunomide. While these drugs are very helpful in averting acute and/or chronic rejection, they are fraught with significant side effects. A majority of acute rejection episodes occur during the initial three months following transplantation. Chronic rejection can also occur, and can manifest as a sudden decrease in the one-second forced expiratory ventilation (FEV-1). This is produced histologically as bronchiolitis obliterans.

Infection is the most common complication in lung transplantation and can lead to premature death if not properly recognized and treated. Physiatrists should be aware of common pathogens associated with infection. Cytomegalovirus is a common viral pathogen and generally appears 14 to 100 days postoperatively. The diagnosis of its infection can be made with a bronchoscopic lavage and biopsy. Fungal pathogens include Candida, Aspergillus, and Pneumocystis.

RENAL TRANSPLANT REHABILITATION

Kidney transplantation is being performed with increasing frequency as the number of people with end-stage renal failure continues to rise. In 1998, there were 11,990 kidney transplants, 4016 of whom received kidneys from living donors. There were also 965 kidney-pancreas transplants in the United States during that year. UNOS reported that, in mid-1999, more than 42,000 patients were on the kidney transplant waiting list, while another 1900 patients were awaiting a kidney-pancreas transplant.

Many renal failure patients seek a kidney transplant because they are unable to perform even the most basic tasks of everyday life. A majority of patients are unable to work because they are physically unable to sustain the energy required for work activity. However, the greatly enhanced survival rate of patients who have received a transplant, coupled with the net increase in procedures performed each year, has resulted in a growing number of patients now requiring rehabilitation and restorative services.

Post-surgical complications include bleeding, infection, and rejection. Kidney rejection is often heralded by malaise, anorexia, fever, hypertension, blood urea nitrogen (BUN) elevation, kidney enlargement with localized tenderness, and leucocytosis. Immunosuppressant medications typically include prednisone, azathioprine, and cyclosporine. Clinical signs of kidney rejection often arise during post-acute rehabilitation and include graft site tenderness, reduced urinary output, edema, and elevated temperature. See Table 61–8 for a complete list of the signs associated with kidney transplant rejection.

Rehabilitation Considerations in Renal Transplant

Many factors affect the renal transplant recipient's ability to exercise. It is well known that chronic renal failure imposes stress on the cardiovascular system. Electrolyte imbalances including sodium and water retention can increase preload at the right and left ventricles. With an increase in circulatory volume, hypertension is worsened, increasing afterload. This contributes to the development of hypertrophy, decreased compliance, and increased stiffness of the ventricles.

Patients with compromised renal function who engage in aerobic exercise may diminish renal perfusion and in so doing reduce the glomerular filtration rate. This can lead to a compromised ability to conserve water. Since patients with kidney disease often have anemia, they might not have the energy to tolerate much exercise. However, there are several ways to increase the patient's ability to exercise, including exercise training and treatment with recombinant human erythropoietin (epoetin). A successful kidney transplant can increase a patient's exercise capacity to near normal values for sedentary healthy individuals.

Exercise training after transplant further increases exercise capacity and counteracts some of the negative side effects of glucocorticoid therapy, such as muscle wasting and excessive weight gain. Studies have shown that before epoetin administration exercise training in patients on dialysis can increase exercise tolerance by 25%. Similar increases are observed after correction of anemia with epoetin, although the increase in exercise capacity is small. Because of the fatigue feeling, physiatrists frequently need to encourage renal patients to exercise and improve their physical functioning.[76]

Just as the ability to exercise is significantly impaired in chronic renal patients, patients who have received transplanted kidneys also demonstrate exercise intolerance.[36] Several factors contribute to this, including skeletal muscle atrophy, anemia, and cardiovascular deconditioning. Low levels of available red blood cells and hemoglobin can cause fatigue and decreased work capacity.

Often, kidney transplants are performed in conjunction with pancreas transplants for patients with severe end organ damage resulting from diabetes mellitus. An

TABLE 61–8 Clinical Signs of Kidney Transplant Rejection Arising in Post Acute Rehabilitation

Tenderness at graft site
Decrease in urine output
Sudden increase in weight: 3 to 5 pounds in a 24-hour period
Edema—usually begins in hands and feet
Elevated temperature
Elevated serum creatine above the individual baseline

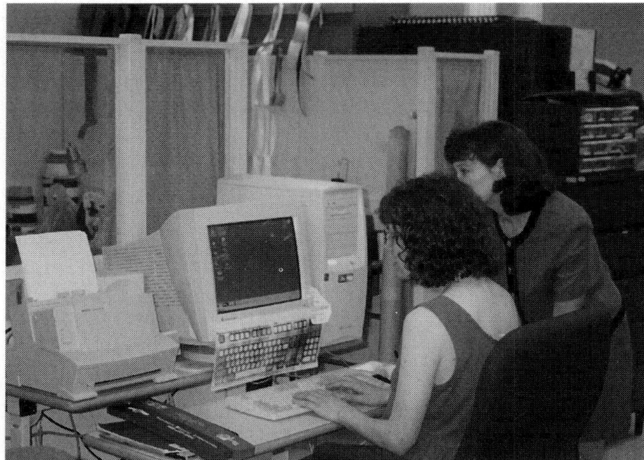

FIGURE 61–4. Patient receiving vocational rehabilitation services at the Maryland Rehabilitation Center after a successful kidney-pancreas transplant.

increasing number are surviving and moving on to rehabilitation and vocational rehabilitation services (Fig. 61–4).

LIVER TRANSPLANT REHABILITATION

The first liver transplantation was performed at the University of Colorado in 1963. Clinical outcomes of this complex surgical procedure improved dramatically in the 1980s when anti-rejection medications such as cyclosporine became widely available. Improved survival due to better surgical techniques and optimization of immunosuppression has led to improved survival and a larger number of referrals to rehabilitation centers. The current one-year survival rate post-liver transplant is approximately 80% to 90%, while the five-year patient survival rate is about 70%. The commitment of the transplant team (Fig. 61–5) to rehabilitative care is a key factor in enhancing the patient's longevity and quality of life.

There are many patients awaiting liver transplantation, representing an extreme shortage of human livers. This shortage was, in fact, central to the debate on revamping the way human organs are distributed.[75] According to UNOS, more than 13,000 patients were on the waiting list for a liver transplant in mid-1999. In 1998, 4450 liver transplants were performed in the United States.

Quality of life issues following liver transplantation are heightening in importance as survival rates continue to improve. A survey conducted by Robinson et al[83] tracked the progress of 31 patients after liver transplantation. Forty-seven percent of the patients surveyed reported abnormal function in at least one limb and 13% reported developing gout. Sixty-one percent reported severe impairment in endurance before the transplant, with 48% unable to ambulate outside the house. After the transplant, only 6% reported severely impaired endurance. Three years after the transplant, 39% of patients reported that they were employed full-time while 26% were homemakers.

Often, kidney transplants are performed in conjunction with pancreas transplants for patients with severe end organ damage resulting from diabetes mellitus. An increasing number are surviving and moving on to rehabilitation and vocational rehabilitation services.

Indications for Liver Transplant and Presurgical Considerations

One of the most common reasons for liver transplantation is the development of hepatic failure. Occasionally, physiatrists see these patients during the "wait and see" pretransplant phase. Depending on chronicity, this population varies widely in degree of deconditioning and debility. In general, patients with liver failure fall into two major categories:

1. *Fulminant hepatic failure.* These patients develop liver failure after a toxic episode or secondary to viral hepatitis. This type of liver failure characteristically occurs acutely and without warning in otherwise healthy patients. Although fulminant liver failure patients are markedly deconditioned and fatigued, they seldom require immediate urgent transplantation after presentation of their disease. By virtue of their prior good health, fulminant hepatic failure patients tend to be well-nourished and have limited functional deficits.
2. *Chronic liver failure.* This group includes patients with autoimmune disease, chronic hepatitis C, alcoholic cirrhosis, sclerosing cholangitis, inborn errors of metabolism such as alpha I antitrypsinase deficiency, and primary biliary cirrhosis.

A common denominator seen in the liver failure population is the presence of hepatocellular dysfunction. Laboratory abnormalities commonly associated with hepatocellular dysfunction include thrombocytopenia, prothrombin time elevations, leukopenia secondary to splenomegaly, and anemia. Other major medical issues associated with hepatocellular damage and liver failure include portal hypertension and ascites. Patients with portal hypertension can require frequent endoscopic procedures and blood transfusions.

Other features associated with the disease include neurologic dysfunction, fatigue, and forgetfulness. Bronster et al[13] report that neurologic complications are

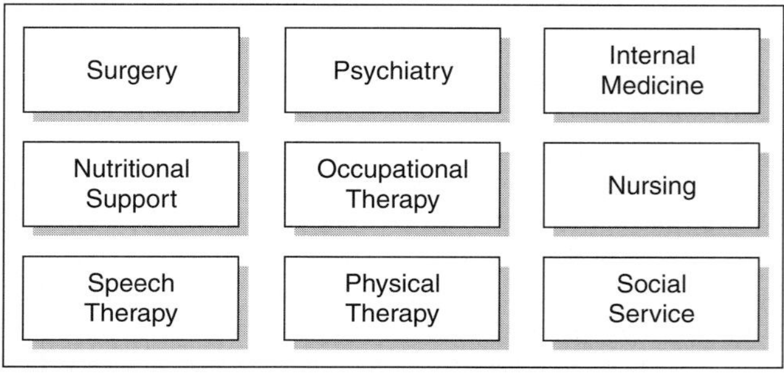

FIGURE 61–5. Members of the transplant rehabilitation team.

TABLE 61–9 Complications of Liver Transplant Arising on Rehabilitation Unit

Primary graft nonfunction
Hemorrhage
Biliary leak, obstruction, or stricture
Hepatic artery or portal vein thrombosis
Infection
  Viral, bacterial, opportunistic
Rejection
  Acute, chronic
Side effects of immunosuppressive therapy
Psychosocial issues

common after liver transplantation, causing considerable morbidity and mortality. Neurologic complications are frequently the result of the therapeutic interventions required to maintain function of the transplanted liver. Recognizing the early signs of drug-related neurotoxicity is the first step in preventing the development of more severe problems. (See Table 61–9.) Careful perioperative management of fluids, particularly sodium and glucose levels, can help reduce the risk of CPM.[120]

A generalized decline in functional ability often occurs in chronic liver disease, making rehabilitation an important intervention. Functional ability deterioration is attributable to the generalized decrement in cognitive and mental function, as well as the physical loss of muscle mass and malnutrition. Malnutrition in pre-liver transplant patients is due to a number of factors. Metabolic abnormalities, such as hyperbilirubinemia, can induce nausea and anorexia. The presence of ascites can promote excessive protein loss and worsen the nitrogen balance. Protein losses through ascites can exacerbate negative nitrogen balance, which can lead to muscle atrophy and skin fragility. Chronic fatigue in this population is also a concern. The enzymes typically used to track graft function following liver transplant are specified in Table 61–10.

Rehabilitation Concerns in the Liver Transplant Patient

A number of critical priorities exist in the promotion of functional well-being in the transplant patient. A customized rehabilitation plan should begin with a comprehensive presurgical evaluation. Physical therapy should be initiated immediately after the transplant recipient has achieved surgical stabilization. A special emphasis must be placed on sustaining the patient's nutritional status. Priorities should include restoration of muscle mass and strength through graded isometric exercises, as well as enhancement of aerobic endurance. Early mobilization postoperatively should be achieved. The liver transplant patient receiving rehabilitative services should be monitored carefully for signs of rejection and for liver failure.

TABLE 61–10 Enzymes Used to Monitor Graft Function Following Liver Transplantation

Enzyme	Normal Range
Transaminases	
AST	7–40 U/L
ALT	7–35 U/L
Phosphatases	
Alkaline phosphatase	30–115 IU/L
Gamma GT (GGT)	5–55 U/L

AST, Aspartate aminotransferase—previously known as SGOT; ALT, alanine aminotransferase—previously known as SGPT.

Normal reported enzyme values will vary from laboratory to laboratory, depending on the specific methods to measure enzymes in each setting.

SUMMARY

Our society has been dramatically influenced by the development of organ transplantation science. Recent

TABLE 61–11 Transplantation Rehabilitation: Patient Family Education

Basic immune system
Purpose of immunosuppression
Activities related to immunosuppression:
  Avoiding crowds during high immunosuppression
  Wearing mask in hospital and clinic
  Care of cuts and wounds
  Mouth care/dental visits
  Notifying transplant team of exposure to diseases (influenza, chicken pox, measles, etc.)
Other activities:
  Exercise (walking, bicycling, swimming if no T-tube or open wounds)
  Restrictions on lifting and driving after major abdominal surgery (3–6 months)
  Sexual activity/birth control
  Care of T-tube (usually removed after 3 months)
Medications—proper administration, side effects, and purpose:
  Immunosuppressants
  Prophylactics (antivirals, antibiotics, antifungals, antacids)
  Others (antihypertensives, multivitamins, etc.)
Home monitoring responsibilities (how, why, and what to do if abnormal):
  Blood pressure readings
  Temperature
  Stool for occult blood
  Urine for glucose or blood
  Daily weight
  Quality of urine (cloudy, dark, normal)
  Quality of stools (tan/clay colored, black, maroon, normal)
Dietary:
  Restrictions (fat, sugar, salt)
  Balanced diet, low-calorie snacks
  Expected increase in appetite and fat deposition due to steroids
Signs and symptoms of infection and rejection—what to do and whom to call:
  Symptoms are so similar for these two that notifying the transplant team is paramount
Medical follow-up:
  Biopsies (usually 3 and 6 months, then yearly; and with dysfunction)
  Frequent transplant clinic visits (blood tests, radiographic tests)
  Routine check-ups with referring and transplant physicians
  Cancer monitoring (annual PAP smear, self breast exam, testicular exam, mammogram, stool for occult blood)
  Routine dental visits (prophylactic antibiotics prior to visit)

technological discoveries and breakthroughs have created a new type of physiatric practice, that of transplant rehabilitation. Life-saving treatment of disease by organ transplantation is becoming standard practice. Transplant patients are enjoying more active and meaningful lives due to early rehabilitation intervention.[119] A cautious and progressive rehabilitation program typically results in organ recipients' returning to a more active lifestyle—one that includes exercise, work, recreation, and travel. Another role of the rehabilitation team has been the education of patients and families regarding the transplant process and how to better cope with it (Table 61–11). As transplant science progresses, it is predicted that the need for transplant rehabilitation services will continue to grow.

ACKNOWLEDGMENTS

The authors acknowledge with gratitude the assistance of Dr. Leon Reinstein in facilitating this chapter. Thanks to Joseph Powers and Annie Mihalyo for rendering editorial assistance and to Soma Gupta of the Novartis Transplantation Learning Center. Very special thanks are due to Norma and Jeff Beaver for sharing their graphic and editorial skills.

REFERENCES

1. ACSM Guidelines for Exercise Testing and Prescription, ed 4. Philadelphia, Lea & Febiger; 1991, pp 60–62, 86–109, 134–165.
2. Ardehali A: Heart transplantation, accelerated graft atherosclerosis. Adv Card Surg 1995; 6:195–205.
3. Barry WH: Mechanisms of immune-mediated myocyte injury. Circulation 1994; 89:2421–2432.
4. Beck W, Barnard CN, Schrire V: Heart rate after cardiac transplantation. Circulation 1969; 40:437–445
5. Belman MJ: Exercise in chronic obstructive pulmonary disease. Clin Chest Med 1986; 7:585–597.
6. Biggar DG, Malen JF, Trulock EP, et al: Pulmonary rehabilitation before and after lung transplantation. In Kasaburi R, Petty TL (eds): Principles and Practice of Pulmonary Rehabilitation. Philadelphia, WB Saunders, 1993, pp 459–467.
7. Block E, Montmayor J, Adler JC, Alba A: Influence of exercise on a heart transplant patient. Arch Phys Med Rehabil 1990; 71(2):153–155.
8. Bonsel GJ, Essink-Bot ML, Klompmaker IJ, Sloof MJH: Assessment of the quality of life before and following liver transplantation. Transplantation 1992; 53(4):796–800.
9. Borg G: Psychophysical basis of perceived exertion. Med Sci Sports Exer 1982; 14:377–381.
10. Braith RW: Exercise training in patients with CHF and heart transplant recipients. Med Sci Sports Exer 1998; 30(suppl 10): S367–S378.
11. Braith RW, Limacher MC, Leggett SH, Pollock ML: Skeletal muscle strength in heart transplant recipients. J Heart Lung Transplant 1993; 12:1018–1023.
12. Braith RW, Mills RM, Welsch MA, et al: Resistance exercise training restores bone mineral density in heart transplant recipients. J Am Coll Cardiol 1996; 28(6):1471–1477.
13. Bronster DJ, Emre S, Mor E, et al: Neurologic complications of orthotopic liver transplantation. Mount Sinai J Med 1994; 61(1):63–69.
14. Brubaker PH, Berry MJ, et al: Relationship of lactate and ventilatory thresholds in cardiac transplant patients. Med Sci Sports Exer 1993; 25:191–196.
15. Bunke M, Ganzel B: Effects of calcium antagonists on renal function in hypertensive heart transplant recipients. J Heart Lung Transplant 1992; 2:1194–1199.
16. Bunke M, Sloan R, Brier M, Ganzel B: An improved glomerular filtration rate in cardiac transplant recipients with once a day cyclosporine dosing. Transplantation 1995; 59:537–540.
17. Butler BB: Physical therapy in heart and lung transplantation. In Hillegas E, Sadowski S (eds): Cardiopulmonary Physical Therapy, ed 3. St Louis, Mosby–Year Book, 1995, pp 404–422.
18. Campeau L, Pospisil L, et al: Cardiac catheterization findings at rest and after exercise in patients following cardiac transplantation. Am J Cardiol 1970; 25:523–528.
19. Cavero PG, Sudhir K, Galli F, et al: Effect of orthotopic cardiac transplantation on peripheral vascular function in congestive heart failure: Influence of cyclosporine therapy. Am Heart J 1994; 127:1581–1587.
20. Celli BR, Rassulu J, Make BJ: Dyssynchronous breathing during arm but not leg exercise patients with chronic air flow obstruction. N Engl J Med 1986; 314:1485–1490.
21. Cerretelli P, Marconi C, et al: Gas exchange kinetics in heart transplant recipients. Chest 1992; 101:199S–205S.
22. Chase GA, Grave C, Rowell LB: Independence of changes in functional and performance capacities attending prolonged bed rest. Aerospace Med 1966; 37:1232–1237.
23. Christos SC, Katch V, Crowley DC, et al: Hemodynamic responses to upright exercise of adolescent cardiac transplant recipients. J Pediatr 1992; 121:312–316.
24. Cooper JD, Patterson GA, Grossman R, et al: Double-lung transplant for advanced chronic obstructive lung disease. Am Rev Respir Dis 1989; 139:303–307.
25. Connors G, Hilling L (eds): AACVPR Guidelines for Pulmonary Rehabilitation Programs. Champaign, IL, Human Kinetics Inc, 1993, pp 1–10.
26. Daly RC: Lung transplantation: Where are we today? Mayo Clin Proc 1997; 72:77–78.
27. Dean E: Effect of body position on pulmonary function. Phys Ther 1985; 65:613–618.
28. Dolovich M, Rossman C, Chambers C, et al: Mucociliary function in patients following single lung or lung/heart transplantation. Am Rev Respir Dis 1987; 135:363 [Abstract].
29. Drexler H, Schroeder JS: Unusual forms of ischemic heart disease. Curr Opin Cardiol 1994; 9:457–464.
30. Egan TM, Kaiser LR, Cooper JD: Lung transplantation. Curr Prob Surg 1989; 26:673–752.
31. Egan TM, Westerman JH, Lambert CJ Jr, et al: Isolated lung transplantation for end-stage lung disease: A viable therapy. Ann Thorac Surg 1992; 53:590–596.
32. Egan TM, Westerman JH, Mill MR, et al: Lung transplantation at UNC: The first year. N C Med J 1991; 52:325–329.
33. Ehrmann J, et al: Cardiovascular responses of heart transplant recipients to graded exercise testing. J Appl Physiol 1992; 73: 260–264.
34. Ellis BE, Ries AL: Upper extremity exercise training in pulmonary rehabilitation. J Cardiopulm Rehabil 1991; 11:227–231.
35. Folino AF, Baja G, Miorelli M, et al: Heart rate variability in patients with orthotopic heart transplantation: Long-term follow-up. Clin Cardiol 1993; 16:539–542.
36. Gallagher-Lepak S: Functional capacity and activity level before and after renal transplantation. Anna J 1991; 18(4):378–382, 406.
37. Gentry LO: Cardiac transplantation and related infections. Semin Respir Infect 1993; 8:199–206.
38. Grant J, Young MA, Pidcock FS, Christenson JR: Physical medicine and rehabilitation management of chronic graft vs. host disease in bone marrow transplantation. Rehabil Oncol 1997; 15(3):13–15.
39. Greenberg A, Egel JW, Thompson ME, et al: Early and late forms of cyclosporine nephrotoxicity: Studies in cardiac transplant recipients. Am J Kidney Dis 1987; 9:12–22.
40. Greenberg ML, Uretsky BF, et al: Long-term hemodynamic follow-up of cardiac transplant patients treated with cyclosporine and prednisone. Circulation 1985; 71:487–494.
41. Griepp RB, Stinson ED, Dong E Jr, et al: Hemodynamic performance of the transplanted human heart. Surgery 1971; 70:88–96.
42. Hanto DW, Mohanakumar T: Transplant immunology. *In* Greenfield U, Mulholland MW, Oldham KT, Zelenock GB (eds): Surgery Scientific Principles and Practice. Philadelphia, JB Lippincott, 1993, pp 461–590.

43. Hietpas B, Roth R, Jensen W: Huff coughing and airway patency. Resp Care 1979; 24:710–714.
44. Hodgkin JE, Litzau KL: Exercise training target heart rates in chronic obstructive pulmonary disease. Chest 1988; 94:S30.
45. Hosenpud JD, Novick RJ, Breen TJ, Daily OP: Registry of the International Society for Heart and Lung Transplantation: Eleventh official report—1994. J Heart Lung Transplant 1994; 13:561–570.
46. Howard DK, Iademarco EJ, Trulock EP: The role of cardiopulmonary exercise testing in lung and heart-lung transplantation. Clin Chest Med 1994; 15:405–420.
47. Ishii K, Devins J: Lung transplantation: A case study. Cardiopulm Phys Ther 1992; 3(1):17–19.
48. Joshi A, Kevorkian CG: Rehabilitation after cardiac transplantation. Am J Phys Med Rehabil 1997; 76(3):249–254.
49. Kao AC, Van Trigt PR, et al: Central and peripheral limitations to upright exercise in untrained cardiac transplant recipients. Circulation 1994; 89:2605–2615.
50. Kao AC, Van Trigt PR, Shaeffer-McCall GS, et al: Allograft diastolic dysfunction and chronotropic incompetence limit cardiac output response to exercise two to six years after heart transplantation. J Heart Lung Transplant 1995; 14:11–22.
51. Kappagoda CT, et al: The hemodynamic responses to upright exercise after orthotopic cardiac transplant. Arch Phys Med Rehabil 1993; 74(5):484–489.
52. Kavanagh T, Yacoub MH, et al: Cardiorespiratory responses to exercise training after orthotopic cardiac transplantation. Circulation 1988; 77:162–171.
53. Kavanagh T, Yacoub MH: Exercise training in patients after heart transplantation. Ann Acad Med Singapore 1992; 21: 372–378.
54. Keteyian S, Marks CR, Levine AB, et al: Cardiovascular responses of cardiac transplant patients to arm and leg exercise. Eur J Appl Physiol 1994; 68:441–444.
55. Keteyian SJ, Marks CR, Levine AB, et al: Cardiovascular responses to submaximal arm and leg exercise in cardiac transplant patients. Med Sci Sports Exer 1994; 26:420–424.
56. Kjaer M, Beyer N, Secher NH: Exercise and organ transplantation. Scand J Med Sci Sports 1999; 9(1):1–14.
57. Kobashigawa JA, Leaf DA, Lee N, et al: A controlled trial of exercise rehabilitation after heart transplantation. N Engl J Med 1999; 340(4):272–277.
58. Lannefors L, Wollmer P: Mucus clearance with three chest physiotherapy regimens in cystic fibrosis: A comparison between postural drainage, PEP, and physical exercise. Eur Respir J 1992; 5:748–753.
59. Latlief G, Young MA: Cardiac transplantation in a post-partum female. Arch Phys Med Rehabil 1994; September [Abstract].
60. Leenen FH, Davies RA, Fourney A: Role of cardiac beta 2-receptors in cardiac responses to exercise in cardiac transplant patients. Circulation 1995; 91:685–690.
61. Legault L, Olgilvie RI, Cardella CJ, Leenen PH: Calcium antagonists in heart transplant recipients: Effects on cardiac and renal function and cyclosporine pharmacokinetics. Can J Cardiol 1993; 9:398–404.
62. Levenson CR: Breathing exercises. In Zadai CC (ed): Pulmonary Management in Physical Therapy. New York, Churchill Livingstone, 1992, pp 136–140.
63. Limberg TM: Case study 1. In Connors G, Hilling L (eds): AACVPR Guidelines for Pulmonary Rehabilitation Programs. Champaign, IL, Human Kinetics Inc, 1993, pp 111–115.
64. Lucas TS, Einhorn TA: Stress fracture of the femoral neck during rehabilitation after heart transplantation. Arch Phys Med Rehabil 1993; 74(9):1004–1006.
65. Mal H, Sleiman C, Jebrak G, et al: Functional results of single-lung transplantation for chronic obstructive lung disease. Am J Respir Crit Care Med 1994; 149:1476–1481.
66. Martin TW, Gaucher J, et al: Response to upright exercise after cardiac transplantation. Clin Cardiol 1994; 17:292–300.
67. McGiffin D, Kirklin JK, Nafiel DC: Acute renal failure after heart transplantation and cyclosporine therapy. J Heart Transplant 1985; 4:396–399.
68. Meyer M, Rahmel A, Marconi C, et al: Adjustment of cardiac output to step exercise in heart transplant recipients. Z Kardiol 1994; 83(suppl 3):103–109.
69. Midthun DE, McDougall JC, Peters SG, Scott JP: Medical management and complications in the lung transplant recipient. Mayo Clin Proc 1997; 72:175–184.
70. Miller LW, Naftel DC, Bourge RC, et al: Infection after heart transplantation: A multi-institutional study—Cardiac Transplant Research Database Group. J Heart Lung Transplant 1994; 13: 381–393.
71. Mills RM Jr: Transplantation and the problems afterward including coronary vasculopathy. Clin Cardiol 1994; 17:287–290.
72. Noman DJ: UNOS: The development, objectives and future of the National Organ Transplant Network. New Dev Transplant 1994; 1(1).
73. Norberg D, de Marchena E, Mitrani A, Bolooki H: Cardiac transplantation: University of Miami/Jackson Memorial Hospital experience. J Florida Med Assoc 1994; 81:414–417.
74. O'Connell JB, Bourge RC, Costanzo-Nordin MR, et al: Cardiac transplantation: Recipient selection, donor procurement, and medical follow-up—a statement for health professionals from the Committee on Cardiac Transplantation of the Council on Clinical Cardiology, American Heart Association. Circulation 1992; 86:1061–1079.
75. Organ Procurement and Transplantation: Assessing Current Policies and the Potential Impact of the DHHS Final Rule. Institute of Medicine: Committee on Organ Procurement and Transplantation Policy, Division of Health Sciences Policy. National Academy Press, Washington, DC, 1999.
76. Painter P: The importance of exercise training in rehabilitation of patients with end stage renal disease. Am J Kidney Dis 1994; 24(suppl 1):S2–S9, S31–S32.
77. Pate RR, Blair SN, et al: Guidelines for Exercise Testing and Prescription, ed 4. Philadelphia, Lea & Febiger, 1991, p 314.
78. Paterson DH, Cunningham DA, et al: Oxygen uptake kinetics in cardiac transplant recipients. J Appl Physiol 1994; 77:1935–1940.
79. Pope SE, Stinson EB, Daughters GTD, et al: Exercise response of the denervated heart in long-term cardiac transplant recipients. Am J Cardiol 1980; 46:213–218.
80. Reid WD, Dechman G: Considerations when testing and training the respiratory muscles. Phys Ther 1995; 75:971–982.
81. Ries AL: Position paper of the American Association on Cardiovascular and Pulmonary Rehabilitation: Scientific basis of pulmonary rehabilitation. J Cardiopulm Rehabil 1990; 10:418–441.
82. Ries AL, Kaplan RM, Limberg TM, et al: Effects of pulmonary rehabilitation on physiologic and psychosocial outcomes in patients with chronic obstructive pulmonary disease. Ann Intern Med 1995; 122:823–832.
83. Robinson LR, Switala J, Tarter RE, Nicholas JJ: Functional outcome after liver transplantation: A preliminary report. Arch Phys Med Rehabil 1990; 71(6):426–427.
84. Rosenblum DS, Rosen ML, Pine ZM, Rosen SH, Borg-Stein J: Health status and quality of life following cardiac transplantation. Arch Phys Med Rehabil 1993; 74(5):490–493.
85. Ross DJ, Waters PF, Mohsenifar Z, et al: Hemodynamic responses to exercise after lung transplantation. Chest 1993; 103:46–53.
86. Sadowsky HS: Interventions in cardiac and cardiopulmonary transplants. In Scully R, Barnes MR (eds): Physical Therapy. Philadelphia, JB Lippincott 1989, pp 787–795.
87. Sadowsky HS, Rohrkemper KF, Quon SYM: Activity end-point guidelines. In Rehabilitation of Cardiac and Cardiopulmonary Recipients. Stanford University Hospital, 1986, appendix 1.
88. Saltin B, Blomquist G, Mitchell JH: Response to exercise after bed rest and after turning: A longitudinal study of adaptive changes in oxygen transport and body composition. Circulation 1968; 38(suppl 7):1–78.
89. Savin WM, Haskell WL, Schroeder JS, Stinson EB: Cardiorespiratory responses of cardiac transplant patients to graded symptom limited exercise. Circulation 1980; 62:55–60.
90. Schrire V, Barnard CN, Beck W: Some electrocardiographic changes in human heart transplants. Isr J Med Sci 1969; 5:931–937.
91. Schroeder JS, Gao SZ, Alderman EL, et al: A preliminary study of diltiazem in the prevention of coronary artery disease in heart transplant recipients. N Engl J Med 1993; 328:164–170.
92. Sephton S: Mission possible. Adv Dir Rehabil June 1999; pp 51–54.

93. Shaver JA, Leon DF, Gray SD, et al: Hemodynamic observations after cardiac transplantation. N Engl J Med 1969; 281:822–827.
94. Shephard RJ: Responses to acute exercise and training after cardiac transplantation: A review. Can J Sport Sci 1991; 16(1):9–22.
95. Sliwa JA, Andersen S, Griffin J: Cardiovascular responses to gait training and ambulation in a hemiparetic heart recipient. Arch Phys Med Rehabil 1990; 71(6):424–425.
96. Sliwa JA, Blendonohy PM: Stroke rehabilitation in a patient with a history of heart transplantation. Arch Phys Med Rehabil 1988; 69(11):973–975.
97. Smith TP, Kinasewitz GT, Tucker WY, et al: Exercise capacity as a predictor of post-thoracotomy morbidity. Am Rev Respir Dis 1984; 129:730–734.
98. Sokal EM: Quality of life after orthotopic transplantation in children. An overview of physical, psychological and social outcome. Eur J Pediatr 1995; 154:171–175.
99. Solis E, Kaye MP: The registry of the International Society For Heart Transplantation. J Heart Transplant 1986; 5:2–5.
100. Spes CH, Schnaack SD, et al: Cardiac function during graded bicycle exercise: Doppler echocardiographic findings in normal subjects and heart transplant recipients. Z Kardiol 1993; 82: 324–331.
101. Squires RW: Exercise training after cardiac transplantation. Med Sci Sports Exerc 1991; 23:686–694.
102. Stiens S, O'Young B, Young MA: The person, disablement and the process of rehabilitation. In Physical Medicine and Rehabilitation Secrets. Philadelphia, Hanley & Belfus, 1997, pp 1–4.
103. Tayler A, Bergin J: Cardiac transplantation for the cardiologist not trained in transplantation. Am Heart J 1995; 129:578–592.
104. Toronto Lung Transplant Group: Experience with single-lung transplantation for pulmonary fibrosis. JAMA 1988; 259:2258–2262.
105. Tuel SM, Meythaler JM, Cross LL: Inpatient Comprehensive Rehabilitation after Liver Transplantation. Am J Phys Med Rehabil 1991; 70(5):242–245.
106. United Network Organ System Report 1999.
107. Valentine H, Keogh A, McIntosh N, et al: Cost containment: Co-administration of diltiazem with cyclosporine, after heart transplantation. J Heart Lung Transplant 1992; 2(part 1):1–7.
108. Vaska PL: Common infections in heart transplant patients. Am J Crit Care 1993; 2:145–156.
109. Ventura HO, Lavie CJ, Messerli FH, et al: Cardiovascular adaptation to cyclosporine-induced hypertension. J Hum Hypertens 1994; 8:233–237.
110. Verani MS, Nishimura S, et al: Cardiac function after orthotopic heart transplantation: Response to postural changes exercise, and beta adrenergic blockade. J Heart Lung Transplant 1994; 13:181–193.
111. Von Scheidt W, Kembes BM, Reichart B, et al: Percutaneous transluminal coronary angioplasty of focal coronary lesions after cardiac transplantation. Clin Invest 1993; 71:524–530.
112. Webber BA, Pryor JA: Physiotherapy skills: Techniques and adjuncts. In Webber BA, Pryor JA (eds): Physiotherapy for Respiratory and Cardiac Problems. Edinburgh, Scotland: Churchill Livingstone, 1993, pp 116–127.
113. Wechsler ME, Giardina EG, Sciacca RR, et al: Increased early mortality in women undergoing cardiac transplantation. Circulation 1995; 91:1029–1035.
114. Wenting GJ, vd Meiracker AH, Simoons MI, et al: Circadian variation of heart rate but not of blood pressure after heart transplantation. Transplant Proc 1987; 19:2554–2555.
115. Williams TJ, Grossman RF, Maurer JR: Long-term functional follow-up of lung transplant recipients. Clin Chest Med 1990; 11:347–358.
116. Williams TJ, Patterson GA, McClean NZ, et al: Maximal exercise testing in single and double lung transplant recipients. Am Rev Respir Dis 1992; 145:101–105.
117. Yamazaki S, Owaga J, Shohzu A, et al: Intrapleural cough pressure in patients after thoracotomy. J Thorac Cardiovasc Surg 1980; 80:600–605.
118. Young M: (Book review) "Physical Medicine & Rehabilitation." JAMA September 24, 1997.
119. Young MA, Steins SA, McGill D, et al: Rehabilitation of the patient requiring transplantation. In Grabois M (ed): Physical Medicine & Rehabilitation: The Complete Approach. Cambridge, MA, Blackwell Science, 1999, pp 622–650.
120. Young MA, Young MM: Organ Transplant Rehabilitation Perspectives. Abstract Proceedings of the 11th European Congress of PM&R, Gothenburg, Sweden, May 27, 1999.
121. Young MA, Young MM: Rehabilitation of the Transplant Patient: An International Perspective. Abstract Proceedings of the Second Mediterranean Congress of PM&R, Valencia, Spain, May 23, 1999; p 446.
122. Yusuf S, Mitchell A, Yacoub MH: Interrelation between donor and recipient heart rates during exercise after heterotopic cardiac transplantation. Br Heart J 1985; 54:173–178.
123. Zadai CC: Physical therapy for the acutely ill medical patient. Phys Ther 1981; 61:1746–1753.
124. Zausmer E: Bronchial drainage: Evidence supporting the procedures. Phys Ther 1968; 48:586–591.

INDEX

Note: Page numbers in *italics* refer to illustrations; page numbers followed by t refer to tables.

B

C

D

I

N

T

U

V

ISBN 0-7216-8076-3